D1572754

Remington and Klein's Infectious Diseases of the Fetus and Newborn Infant

Remington and Klein's Infectious Diseases of the Fetus and Newborn Infant

EIGHTH EDITION

Christopher B. Wilson, MD
Director, Discovery & Translational Sciences
Global Health Program
Bill & Melinda Gates Foundation
Seattle, Washington

Victor Nizet, MD
Professor of Pediatrics and Pharmacy
University of California San Diego School of Medicine and Skaggs School of Pharmacy and Pharmaceutical Sciences
La Jolla, California;
Physician, Rady Children's Hospital
San Diego, California

Yvonne A. Maldonado, MD
Professor of Pediatrics and of Health Research and Policy
Chief, Division of Pediatric Infectious Diseases
Department of Pediatrics
Stanford University School of Medicine
Stanford, California;
Berger-Raynolds Packard Distinguished Fellow
Lucile Salter Packard Children's Hospital at Stanford
Palo Alto, California

Jack S. Remington, MD
Professor Emeritus, Department of Medicine
Division of Infectious Diseases and Geographical Medicine
Stanford University School of Medicine
Stanford, California;
Marcus Krupp Research Chair Emeritus
Research Institute
Palo Alto Medical Foundation
Palo Alto, California

Jerome O. Klein, MD
Professor, Department of Pediatrics
Boston University School of Medicine;
Maxwell Finland Laboratory for Infectious Diseases
Boston Medical Center
Boston, Massachusetts

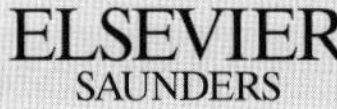

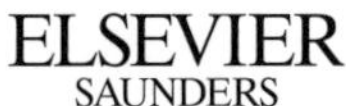

ELSEVIER
SAUNDERS

1600 John F. Kennedy Blvd.
Ste. 1800
Philadelphia, PA 19103-2899

Remington and Klein's Infectious Diseases of the Fetus and Newborn Infant, Eighth Edition

ISBN: 978-0-323-24147-2

Notices

Knowledge and best practice in this field are constantly changing. As new research and experience broaden our understanding, changes in research methods, professional practices, or medical treatment may become necessary.

Practitioners and researchers must always rely on their own experience and knowledge in evaluating and using any information, methods, compounds, or experiments described herein. In using such information or methods they should be mindful of their own safety and the safety of others, including parties for whom they have a professional responsibility.

With respect to any drug or pharmaceutical products identified, readers are advised to check the most current information provided (i) on procedures featured or (ii) by the manufacturer of each product to be administered, to verify the recommended dose or formula, the method and duration of administration, and contraindications. It is the responsibility of practitioners, relying on their own experience and knowledge of their patients, to make diagnoses, to determine dosages and the best treatment for each individual patient, and to take all appropriate safety precautions.

To the fullest extent of the law, neither the Publisher nor the authors, contributors, or editors assume any liability for any injury and/or damage to persons or property as a matter of products liability, negligence or otherwise, or from any use or operation of any methods, products, instructions, or ideas contained in the material herein.

Library of Congress Cataloging-in-Publication Data

Infectious diseases of the fetus and newborn infant.
Remington and Klein's infectious diseases of the fetus and newborn infant / [edited by] Christopher B. Wilson, Victor Nizet, Yvonne A. Maldonado, Jack S. Remington, Jerome O. Klein. -- Eighth edition.
p. ; cm.
Preceded by Infectious diseases of the fetus and newborn infant / [edited by] Jack S. Remington ... [et al.]. 7th ed. c2011.
Includes bibliographical references and index.
ISBN 978-0-323-24147-2 (hardcover : alk. paper)
I. Wilson, Christopher B. (Christopher Bruce), 1946- , editor. II. Nizet, Victor, editor. III. Maldonado, Yvonne A., editor. IV. Remington, Jack S., 1931- , editor. V. Klein, Jerome O., 1931- , editor. VI. Title.
[DNLM: 1. Communicable Diseases. 2. Fetal Diseases. 3. Infant, Newborn, Diseases. 4. Infant, Newborn. WC 100]
RJ275
618.92'01--dc23

2014043452

Executive Content Strategist: Kate Dimock
Content Development Specialist: Margaret Nelson
Publishing Services Manager: Anne Altepeter
Project Manager: Louise King
Design Direction: Ashley Miner

Printed in China

Last digit is the print number: 9 8 7 6 5 4 3 2 1

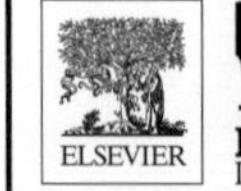

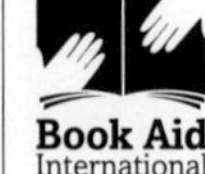

To those most dear to us
Sherryl, Alyssa and Bryan, Amelia and Floyd
C.B.W.

Christine, Oliver, Pierre, Maria, Alex, Aliza, and Hannah
V.N.

Lauren, Stephen, Lindsey, Alfonso and Aida, Ann, and Ramiro
Y.A.M

Francoise, Lynne, David, Amanda, Aaron, and Nathan
J.S.R.

Linda, Andrea, Bennett, Adam, Zachary, Alex, Evan, and Dana
J.O.K.

And to the mentors, colleagues, fellows, and students who have enriched our academic and personal lives, and to the physicians and the women and infants with infectious diseases for whom they care

Contributors

Kristina M. Adams Waldorf, MD
Associate Professor, Department of Obstetrics and Gynecology, University of Washington, Seattle, Washington
Obstetric Factors Associated with Infections of the Fetus and Newborn Infant

Stuart P. Adler, MD
Professor, Department of Microbiology and Immunology, Medical College of Virginia, Virginia Commonwealth University, Richmond, Virginia
Human Parvovirus

Carol J. Baker, MD
Professor, Department of Pediatrics and Molecular Virology and Microbiology, Baylor College of Medicine; Attending Physician, Department of Pediatrics, Section of Infectious Diseases, Texas Children's Hospital, Houston, Texas
Group B Streptococcal Infections

Elizabeth D. Barnett, MD
Professor of Pediatrics, Boston University School of Medicine; Director, International Clinic, Boston Medical Center, Boston, Massachusetts
Bacterial Infections of the Respiratory Tract

Catherine M. Bendel, MD
Associate Professor, Department of Pediatrics, University of Minnesota Medical School, Minneapolis, Minnesota
Candidiasis

Daniel K. Benjamin, Jr., MD, PhD, MPH
Professor of Pediatrics, Duke University Medical Center; Faculty Associate Director, Duke Clinical Research Institute, Durham, North Carolina
Clinical Pharmacology of Antiinfective Drugs

Lars Bode, PhD
Associate Professor, Divisions of Neonatology and Pediatric Gastroenterology, Hepatology, and Nutrition, Department of Pediatrics, University of California San Diego, La Jolla, California
Human Milk

Robert Bortolussi, MD, FRCPC
Professor, Departments of Pediatrics and Microbiology and Immunology, Dalhousie University, Halifax, Nova Scotia, Canada
Listeriosis

John S. Bradley, MD
Professor of Pediatrics, Division of Infectious Diseases, Department of Pediatrics, University of California San Diego School of Medicine; Division of Infectious Diseases, Rady Children's Hospital San Diego, La Jolla, California
Staphylococcal Infections

William Britt, MD
Charles A. Alford Professor of Pediatric Infectious Diseases, Pediatrics, Microbiology, and Neurobiology, The University of Alabama at Birmingham, Birmingham, Alabama
Cytomegalovirus

James D. Cherry, MD, MSc
Distinguished Research Professor of Pediatrics, David Geffen School of Medicine at University of California Los Angeles; Attending Physician, Pediatric Infectious Diseases, Mattel Children's Hospital UCLA, Los Angeles, California
Bordetella pertussis *and Other* Bordetella *spp. Infections; Enterovirus, Parechovirus, and Saffold Virus Infections*

Susan E. Coffin, MD, MPH
Professor of Pediatrics, Division of Infectious Diseases, Department of Infection Prevention and Control, The Children's Hospital of Philadelphia, Philadelphia, Pennsylvania
Health Care–Associated Infections in the Nursery

James E. Crowe, Jr., MD, PhD
Director, Vanderbilt Vaccine Center, Professor and Ann Scott Carell Chair, Departments of Pediatrics and Pathology, Microbiology, and Immunology, Vanderbilt University, Nashville, Tennessee
Prevention of Fetal and Early Life Infections Through Maternal–Neonatal Immunization

Carl T. D'Angio, MD
Professor, Departments of Pediatrics and Medical Humanities and Bioethics, University of Rochester School of Medicine and Dentistry; Golisano Children's Hospital, University of Rochester Medical Center, Rochester, New York
Laboratory Aids for Diagnosis of Neonatal Sepsis

Gary L. Darmstadt, MD, MS
Senior Fellow, Global Development Division, Bill & Melinda Gates Foundation, Seattle, Washington
Neonatal Infections: A Global Perspective

Toni Darville, MD
Chief of Infectious Diseases, Department of Pediatrics, Children's Hospital of North Carolina at Chapel Hill; Professor of Pediatrics and Microbiology/Immunology, Department of Pediatrics, University of North Carolina at Chapel Hill, Chapel Hill, North Carolina
Chlamydia *Infections*

Simon R.M. Dobson, MD, FRCPC
Director and Clinical Associate Professor, Pediatric Infectious Diseases, British Columbia Children's Hospital, Vancouver, British Columbia, Canada
Syphilis

Morven S. Edwards, MD
Professor of Pediatrics, Baylor College of Medicine; Attending Physician, Department of Pediatrics, Section of Infectious Diseases, Texas Children's Hospital, Houston, Texas
Group B Streptococcal Infections

Joanne E. Embree, MD, FRCPC
Professor, Department of Pediatrics and Child Health, Department of Medical Microbiology and Infectious Diseases, University of Manitoba, Winnipeg, Manitoba, Canada
Gonococcal Infections

Henry M. Feder, Jr., MD
Professor of Pediatrics, Connecticut Children's Medical Center, Hartford, Connecticut; Professor of Pediatrics and Family Medicine, University of Connecticut Health Center, Farmington, Connecticut
Borrelia *Infections: Lyme Disease and Relapsing Fever*

Justus Garweg, MD
Associate Professor of Ophthalmology, University of Bern; Berner Augenklinik am Lindenhofspital, Bern, Switzerland; Swiss Eye Institute, Rotkreuz, Switzerland
Toxoplasmosis

Anne A. Gershon, MD
Professor, Pediatrics, Columbia University College of Physicians and Surgeons, New York, New York
Varicella, Measles, and Mumps

Ronald S. Gibbs, MD
Professor, Department of Obstetrics and Gynecology, Associate Dean for Continuing Medical Education, University of Colorado, Aurora, Colorado
Obstetric Factors Associated with Infections of the Fetus and Newborn Infant

Francis Gigliotti, MD
Professor and Chief of Infectious Diseases, Vice Chair of Academic Affairs, Department of Pediatrics, University of Rochester School of Medicine and Dentistry, Rochester, New York
Pneumocystis *and Other Less Common Fungal Infections*

Michael G. Gravett, MD
Professor and Vice-Chairperson, Department of Obstetrics and Gynecology, University of Washington; Scientific Director, Global Alliance for the Prevention of Prematurity and Stillbirth, Seattle, Washington
Obstetric Factors Associated with Infections of the Fetus and Newborn Infant

Kathleen M. Gutierrez, MD
Associate Professor, Department of Pediatrics, Division of Pediatric Infectious Disease, Stanford University School of Medicine, Stanford, California
Herpes Simplex Virus Infections

Willem A. Hanekom, MB, ChB
Deputy Director, Tuberculosis, Global Health Program, Bill & Melinda Gates Foundation, Seattle, Washington
Tuberculosis

R. Doug Hardy, MD
Pediatric Infectious Diseases, Medical City Children's Hospital, Dallas, Texas
Mycoplasmal Infections

Thomas R. Hawn, MD, PhD
Professor, Division of Allergy and Infectious Diseases, Department of Medicine, University of Washington, Seattle, Washington
Tuberculosis

Ulrich Heininger, MD
Professor and Chairperson, Pediatric Infectious Diseases, University Children's Hospital; Member, Medical Faculty, University of Basel, Basel, Switzerland
Bordetella pertussis *and Other* Bordetella *spp. Infections*

David K. Hong, MD
Clinical Assistant Professor, Department of Pediatrics/Infectious Diseases, Stanford University, Stanford, California; Chief, Pediatric Infectious Diseases, Department of Pediatrics, Santa Clara Valley Medical Center, San Jose, California
Developmental Immunology and Role of Host Defenses in Fetal and Neonatal Susceptibility to Infection

Wikrom Karnsakul, MD
Assistant Professor, Johns Hopkins Pediatric Liver Center, Johns Hopkins University School of Medicine, Baltimore, Maryland
Hepatitis

François Kieffer, MD
Staff Physician, Neonatal Intensive Care Unit, Armand Trousseau Hospital–APHP, Paris, France
Toxoplasmosis

Jae H. Kim, MD, PhD
Clinical Professor of Pediatrics, Divisions of Neonatology and Pediatric Gastroenterology, Hepatology, and Nutrition, Department of Pediatrics, University of California San Diego, La Jolla, California
Human Milk

David W. Kimberlin, MD
Professor of Pediatrics, Sergio Stagno Endowed Chair in Pediatric Infectious Diseases, Co-Director, Division of Pediatric Infectious Diseases, The University of Alabama at Birmingham, Birmingham, Alabama
Herpes Simplex Virus Infections

Jerome O. Klein, MD
Professor, Department of Pediatrics, Boston University School of Medicine; Maxwell Finland Laboratory for Infectious Diseases, Boston Medical Center, Boston, Massachusetts
Current Concepts of Infections of the Fetus and Newborn Infant; Bacterial Sepsis and Meningitis; Bacterial Infections of the Respiratory Tract; Bacterial Infections of the Urinary Tract

William C. Koch, MD, FAAP, FIDSA
Associate Professor of Pediatrics, Division of Infectious Diseases, Virginia Commonwealth University School of Medicine; Attending Physician, Children's Hospital of Richmond, Virginia Commonwealth University, Richmond, Virginia
Human Parvovirus

Tobias R. Kollmann, MD, PhD
Associate Professor, Department of Pediatrics, Division of Infectious Diseases, University of British Columbia, Vancouver, British Columbia, Canada
Listeriosis; Syphilis

Paul Krogstad, MD
Professor, Department of Pediatrics and Molecular and Medical Pharmacology, David Geffen School of Medicine at University of California Los Angeles; Attending Physician, Mattel Children's Hospital UCLA, Los Angeles, California
Enterovirus, Parechovirus, and Saffold Virus Infections

Damian J. Krysan, MD, PhD
Associate Professor, Vice Chair for Research, Departments of Pediatrics and Microbiology & Immunology, University of Rochester School of Medicine and Dentistry, Rochester, New York
Pneumocystis *and Other Less Common Fungal Infections*

David B. Lewis, MD
Professor of Pediatrics, Chief, Division of Immunology, Allergy, and Rheumatology, Department of Pediatrics, Stanford University School of Medicine, Stanford, California; Attending Physician, Lucile Salter Packard Children's Hospital, Palo Alto, California
Developmental Immunology and Role of Host Defenses in Fetal and Neonatal Susceptibility to Infection

Lucy L. Linley, MB, ChB
Department of Pediatrics and Child Health, Health Sciences Faculty, University of Cape Town, Cape Town, South Africa
Tuberculosis

Sarah S. Long, MD
Professor of Pediatrics, Drexel University College of Medicine; Chief, Section of Infectious Diseases, St. Christopher's Hospital for Children, Philadelphia, Pennsylvania
Bacterial Infections of the Urinary Tract

Yalda C. Lucero, MD, PhD
Pediatric Gastroenterologist, Assistant Professor of Pediatrics, Faculty of Medicine, University of Chile; Hospital Luis Calvo Mackenna, Santiago, Chile
Microorganisms Responsible for Neonatal Diarrhea

Timothy L. Mailman, MD
Associate Professor, Department of Pediatrics and Microbiology and Immunology, Dalhousie University, IWK Health Centre, Halifax, Nova Scotia, Canada
Listeriosis

Yvonne A. Maldonado, MD
Professor of Pediatrics and of Health Research and Policy, Chief, Division of Pediatric Infectious Diseases, Department of Pediatrics, Stanford University School of Medicine, Stanford, California; Berger-Raynolds Packard Distinguished Fellow, Lucile Salter Packard Children's Hospital at Stanford, Palo Alto, California
Current Concepts of Infections of the Fetus and Newborn Infant; Human Immunodeficiency Virus/Acquired Immunodeficiency Syndrome in the Infant; Less Common Viral Infections; Malaria and Less Common Protozoan and Helminth Infections

Mona Marin, MD
Medical Epidemiologist, Centers for Disease Control and Prevention, Atlanta, Georgia
Varicella, Measles, and Mumps

Julia A. McMillan, MD
Professor of Pediatrics, Department of Pediatrics, Johns Hopkins School of Medicine, Baltimore, Maryland
Less Common Viral Infections

Martha Muller, MD
Associate Professor, Department of Pediatrics, University of New Mexico, Albuquerque, New Mexico
Bacterial Infections of the Bones and Joints; Focal Bacterial Infections

Delma J. Nieves, MD
Clinical Instructor, Pediatric Infectious Diseases, University of California Irvine School of Medicine/Children's Hospital of Orange County, Orange, California
Bordetella pertussis *and Other* Bordetella *spp. Infections*

Victor Nizet, MD
Professor of Pediatrics and Pharmacy, University of California San Diego School of Medicine and Skaggs School of Pharmacy and Pharmaceutical Sciences, La Jolla, California; Physician, Rady Children's Hospital, San Diego, California
Current Concepts of Infections of the Fetus and Newborn Infant; Bacterial Sepsis and Meningitis; Focal Bacterial Infections; Group B Streptococcal Infections; Staphylococcal Infections

James Nuttall, MB, ChB
Department of Pediatrics and Child Health, Health Sciences Faculty, University of Cape Town, Cape Town, South Africa
Tuberculosis

Miguel L. O'Ryan, MD
Professor and Director, Microbiology and Mycology Program, Institute of Biomedical Sciences, Faculty of Medicine, University of Chile, Santiago, Chile
Microorganisms Responsible for Neonatal Diarrhea

Pearay L. Ogra, MD
Professor Emeritus, School of Medicine and Biomedical Sciences, State University of New York at Buffalo, Buffalo, New York; Former John Sealy Distinguished Chair, Professor and Chair of Pediatrics, University of Texas Medical Branch at Galveston, Galveston, Texas
Human Milk

Gary D. Overturf, MD
Professor Emeritus, Pediatrics and Pathology, Department of Pediatrics, University of New Mexico School of Medicine; Medical Director, Infectious Diseases, Department of Pathology, TriCore Reference Laboratories, Albuquerque, New Mexico
Bacterial Infections of the Bones and Joints; Focal Bacterial Infections

François Peyron, MD, PhD
Professor, Institute for Parasitology and Medical Mycology, Hospices Civils de Lyon, Lyon, France
Toxoplasmosis

Stanley A. Plotkin, MD
Professor Emeritus of Pediatrics, University of Pennsylvania, Philadelphia, Pennsylvania; Executive Advisor to the Chief Executive Officer, Sanofi Pasteur Inc., Doylestown, Pennsylvania
Rubella

Octavio Ramilo
Henry G. Cramblett Chair in Pediatric Infectious Diseases, Professor, Department of Pediatrics, Ohio State University; Chief, Division of Infectious Diseases, Department of Pediatrics, Nationwide Children's Hospital, Columbus, Ohio
Mycoplasmal Infections

Susan E. Reef, MD
Medical Epidemiologist, Global Immunization Division, Centers for Disease Control and Prevention, Atlanta, Georgia
Rubella

Jack S. Remington, MD
Professor Emeritus, Department of Medicine, Division of Infectious Diseases and Geographical Medicine, Stanford University School of Medicine, Stanford, California; Marcus Krupp Research Chair Emeritus, Research Institute, Palo Alto Medical Foundation, Palo Alto, California
Current Concepts of Infections of the Fetus and Newborn Infant

Julia S. Sammons, MD, MSCE
Assistant Professor of Clinical Pediatrics, The University of Pennsylvania Perelman School of Medicine; Medical Director and Hospital Epidemiologist, Department of Infection Prevention and Control, The Children's Hospital of Philadelphia, Philadelphia, Pennsylvania
Health Care–Associated Infections in the Nursery

Kathleen B. Schwarz, BA, MAT, MD
Professor of Pediatrics, Department of Pediatrics, Johns Hopkins University School of Medicine, Baltimore, Maryland
Hepatitis

Jane F. Seward, MBBS, MPH
Deputy Director, Division of Viral Diseases, National Center for Immunization and Respiratory Diseases, Centers for Disease Control and Prevention, Atlanta, Georgia
Varicella, Measles, and Mumps

Avinash K. Shetty, MD, FAAP, FIDSA
Professor of Pediatrics, Chief, Pediatric Infectious Diseases, Wake Forest School of Medicine; Brenner Children's Hospital, Winston-Salem, North Carolina
Human Immunodeficiency Virus/Acquired Immunodeficiency Syndrome in the Infant

Barbara J. Stoll, MD
George W. Brumley, Jr., Professor and Chair, Department of Pediatrics, Emory University School of Medicine and Children's Healthcare of Atlanta, Atlanta, Georgia
Neonatal Infections: A Global Perspective

Jorge J. Velarde, MD, PhD
Assistant in Medicine, Division of Infectious Diseases, Boston Children's Hospital, Boston, Massachusetts
Microorganisms Responsible for Neonatal Diarrhea

Kelly C. Wade, MD, PhD, MSCE
Associate Professor, Clinical Pediatrics, Perelman School of Medicine, University of Pennsylvania; Attending Neonatologist, The Children's Hospital of Philadelphia, Philadelphia, Pennsylvania
Clinical Pharmacology of Antiinfective Drugs

Martine Wallon, MD, MPH, PhD
Adjunct Professor, Institute for Parasitology and Medical Mycology, Hospices Civils de Lyon, Lyon, France
Toxoplasmosis

Geoffrey A. Weinberg, MD
Professor of Pediatrics, Department of Pediatrics, University of Rochester School of Medicine and Dentistry; Director, Pediatric HIV Program, Golisano Children's Hospital, University of Rochester Medical Center, Rochester, New York
Laboratory Aids for Diagnosis of Neonatal Sepsis

Christopher B. Wilson
Director, Discovery & Translational Sciences, Global Health Program, Bill & Melinda Gates Foundation, Seattle, Washington
Current Concepts of Infections of the Fetus and Newborn Infant

Terry W. Wright, PhD
Associate Professor, Departments of Pediatrics and Microbiology & Immunology, University of Rochester Medical Center, Rochester, New York
Pneumocystis *and Other Less Common Fungal Infections*

Anita K.M. Zaidi, MBBS, SM
Director, Enteric and Diarrheal Diseases, Global Health Program, Bill & Melinda Gates Foundation, Seattle, Washington
Neonatal Infections: A Global Perspective

Preface

Major advances in biology and medicine made during the past several decades have contributed greatly to our understanding of infections that affect the fetus and newborn. As the medical, social, and economic impact of these infections becomes more fully appreciated, the time is again appropriate for an intensive summation of existing information on this subject. Our goal for the eighth edition of this text is to provide a complete, critical, and contemporary review of this information. We have directed the book to all students of medicine interested in the care and well-being of infants, and hope to include among our readers medical students, residents and fellows, practicing physicians, microbiologists, and health care workers. We believe the text to be of particular importance for infectious disease specialists; obstetricians and physicians who are responsible for the pregnant woman and her developing fetus; pediatricians and family physicians who care for newborn infants; and primary care physicians, neurologists, audiologists, ophthalmologists, psychologists, and other specialists who are responsible for children who suffer the sequelae of infections acquired in utero or during the first month of life.

The scope of this book encompasses infections of the fetus and newborn, including infections acquired in utero, during the delivery process, and in early infancy. When appropriate, sequelae of these infections that affect older children and adults also are included. Infection in the adult is described when pertinent to recognition of infection in the pregnant woman and her developing fetus and newborn infant. The first chapter provides an introductory overview of the subsequent chapters, general information, and a report on new developments and new challenges in this area. Each subsequent chapter covers a distinct topic in depth and when appropriate touches on issues that overlap with the theme of other chapters or refers the reader to those chapters for relevant information. Chapters in Sections II, III, and IV cover specific types of infection, and each includes a review of the history, microbiology, epidemiology, pathogenesis and pathology, clinical signs and symptoms, diagnosis, prognosis, treatment, and prevention of the infection. Chapters in Sections I and V address issues of a more general nature.

For two of us (Jack S. Remington and Jerome O. Klein), it has been an extraordinary experience and privilege over the past 45 years to be participants in reporting the advances in understanding and management of the infectious diseases of the fetus and newborn infant. Consider the virtual elimination in the developed world of some infectious diseases (e.g., rubella, early-onset group B streptococcal diseases); the recognition of new diseases (e.g., Borrelia, HIV); the increased survival and vulnerability to infection of the very low-birth-weight infant; the introduction of new antimicrobial agents, in particular antiviral and antifungal drugs; and increased emphasis on immunization of women in the childbearing years to prevent transmission of disease to the fetus and neonate. Of importance now and in the future is the recognition of the universality of infectious diseases. Of particular concern are the continued high mortality rates of infectious diseases for infants in the first weeks of life, particularly in low- and middle-income countries. Increased efforts are important to extrapolate advances in care of the pregnant woman and her newborn infant from developed countries to regions with limited resources.

The seventh edition of this text was published in 2011. In the ensuing 4 years, there have been several notable changes. The current edition includes a new chapter on pertussis, whose re-emergence warranted a more in-depth discussion than possible within another chapter. Conversely, the editors elected not to continue with a dedicated chapter on smallpox, incorporating relevant information into the chapter on less common viral infections. In many cases, authors have updated chapters they wrote for earlier editions, incorporating new knowledge, describing current practice, and bringing in new co-authors where appropriate. As has been our practice with each new edition, we have sought to completely refresh some chapters by collaborating with new authors, while thanking the previous authors for their important contributions to past editions. Major revisions of most chapters suggest the importance of new information about infections of the fetus and newborn infant.

Each author is a recognized authority in the field and has made significant contributions to our understanding of infections in the fetus and newborn infant. Almost all were supported, in part or totally, during their training period, and subsequently, by funds obtained from the National Institutes of Health, national health research funding agencies in other countries, or private agencies such as the March of Dimes and the Bill & Melinda Gates Foundation. The major advances in medicine during this period would not have been possible without these funding mechanisms and the freedom given to the investigators to pursue programs of their own choosing. The medical advances represented in this text are also a testimony to the trustees of agencies and the legislators and other federal officials who provided research funds from the 1960s to the present day.

Two of us (Remington and Klein) were fellows at the Thorndike Memorial Laboratory, Harvard Medical Unit, Boston City Hospital in the early 1960s under the supervision of Maxwell Finland. Although subsequently we worked in separate areas of investigation on the two coasts, one of us as an internist and the other as a pediatrician, we maintained close contact, and because of a mutual interest in infections of the fetus and newborn infant and their long-term effects, we joined forces to develop this text.

Christopher B. Wilson joined us in editing the sixth, seventh, and now eighth editions. Chris trained in immunology and infectious diseases in Palo Alto, then joined the University of Washington for 30 years before moving to the

Bill & Melinda Gates Foundation. Because Drs. Remington and Klein consider themselves sons of Maxwell Finland, Chris is representative of the many "grandsons and granddaughters" of Dr. Finland. Yvonne A. Maldonado is an expert in pediatric HIV infection and is chief of the Division of Pediatric Infectious Diseases at Stanford University School of Medicine. Victor Nizet is a pediatric physician-scientist and expert in bacterial pathogenesis and innate immunity; he is a division chief and program director at the University of California, San Diego Schools of Medicine and Pharmacy.

We are indebted to our teachers and associates, and especially to individuals such as Dr. Maxwell Finland, who guided our training and helped to promote our development as physician-scientists through the early stages of our careers. We also wish to express our appreciation to Margaret Nelson, Stefanie Jewell-Thomas, Kate Dimock, and Louise King of Elsevier, for guiding this project to a successful conclusion, and to Ms. Valerie Berland for her editorial assistance.

Jack S. Remington

Jerome O. Klein

Christopher B. Wilson

Yvonne A. Maldonado

Victor Nizet

Contents

SECTION IV PROTOZOAN, HELMINTH, AND FUNGAL INFECTIONS

SECTION V DIAGNOSIS AND MANAGEMENT

SECTION I

GENERAL INFORMATION

SECTION OUTLINE

1 Current Concepts of Infections of the Fetus and Newborn Infant

YVONNE A. MALDONADO, VICTOR NIZET, JEROME O. KLEIN, JACK S. REMINGTON, and CHRISTOPHER B. WILSON

CHAPTER OUTLINE

Overview

Current concepts of pathogenesis, microbiology, diagnosis, and management of infections of the fetus and newborn are reviewed in this chapter with the goal of providing a brief synthesis and overview. Information within this chapter regarding specific infections or syndromes is illustrative only. Detailed discussions are provided in the subsequent sections, to which the reader should refer to gain the more comprehensive knowledge needed to properly evaluate and manage these conditions.

The first section of the book contains chapters providing the global perspective on fetal and neonatal infections as well as chapters addressing obstetric factors, immunity, host defenses, and the role of human breast milk in fetal and neonatal infections. Chapters containing detailed information about specific bacterial, viral, protozoan, helminthic, and fungal infections follow in subsequent sections. The final section contains chapters addressing nosocomial infections, the diagnosis and therapy of infections in the fetus and neonate, and prevention of fetal and neonatal infections through immunization of the mother or neonate.

Important changes continue to occur in the epidemiology, diagnosis, prevention, and management of infectious diseases of the fetus and newborn infant since publication of the last edition of this book. Some of these changes are noted in Table 1-1 and are discussed in this and the relevant chapters.

To keep pace with these changes, with the eighth edition, the editors have sought to streamline the references while maintaining full citation formats both in the print and online editions. All chapters have been updated through extensive revisions, and in some cases, new chapters have been prepared by different authors to provide a fresh viewpoint on certain key topics. There is no longer a separate chapter devoted to smallpox, information about which is now incorporated into Chapter 30 (Less Common Viral Infections). Conversely, with the resurgence of pertussis cases in the United States and elsewhere, a new Chapter 21 on pertussis has been prepared by James Cherry.

Substantial progress has been made toward reducing the burden of infectious diseases in the fetus and newborn infant. The incidence of early-onset group B streptococcal (GBS) disease has been reduced by aggressive use of intrapartum chemoprophylaxis, in particular, as guided by the culture-based screening strategy now recommended for universal use in the United States and several other countries. Vertical transmission of human immunodeficiency virus (HIV) has been reduced by identification of the infected mother and subsequent treatment, including broader recommendations for the use of antiretroviral regimens among pregnant and postpartum women that are practical in countries with high prevalence but limited resources.

There has been a substantial commitment of resources by government agencies and philanthropies, such as the Bill and Melinda Gates Foundation, the Clinton Health Access

Table 1-1 Changes in Epidemiology and Management of Infectious Diseases of the Fetus and Newborn Infant

Epidemiology	Increased viability of very-low-birth-weight infants at risk for invasive infectious diseases Increased number of multiple births (often of very low birth weight) because of successful techniques for management of infertility Global perspective of vertically transmitted infectious diseases Global decline in infant mortality but lesser decline of neonatal mortality
Diagnosis	Polymerase chain reaction assay for diagnosis of infection in mother, fetus, and neonate Relative decrease in use of fetal blood and chorionic villus sampling and increase in use of amniotic fluid sampling for diagnosis of fetal infectious diseases
Prevention	Intrapartum antibiotic prophylaxis widely implemented to prevent early-onset group B streptococcal infection Antiretroviral therapy in pregnancy and postpartum to prevent transmission of HIV to fetus
Treatment	Spread within nurseries of multiple antibiotic-resistant bacterial pathogens Increased use of vancomycin for β-lactam–resistant gram-positive infections Increased use of acyclovir for infants with suspected herpes simplex infection Use of ganciclovir or valganciclovir for overtly symptomatic congenital CMV

CMV, Cytomegalovirus; *HIV*, human immunodeficiency virus.

Table 1-2 Useful Internet Sites for Physicians Interested in Infectious Diseases of the Fetus and Newborn Infant

Agency for Healthcare Research and Quality	http://www.ahrq.gov
American Academy of Pediatrics	http://www.aap.org
American College of Obstetricians and Gynecologists	http://www.acog.org
Centers for Disease Control and Prevention	http://www.cdc.gov
Food and Drug Administration	http://www.fda.gov
Immunization Action Coalition	http://www.immunize.org
Information on AIDS Trials	http://www.aidsinfo.nih.gov
March of Dimes	http://www.marchofdimes.com
Morbidity and Mortality Weekly Report	http://www.cdc.gov/mmwr
National Center for Health Statistics	http://www.cdc.gov/nchs
Pediatric Infectious Diseases Society	http://www.pids.org
General academic information	http://www.googlescholar.com; http://www.ncbi.nlm.nih.gov/pubmed

Initiative, and Save the Children, among others, to combat global infectious diseases in mothers and children. Global mortality for children younger than 5 years fell by 41% between 1990 and 2011 from a rate of 87 to 51 deaths per 1000 live births, but still totals 6.9 million deaths per year globally. Neonatal mortality has not declined as quickly and now constitutes 40% of total under-5-years mortality, and great disparities remain; the global neonatal mortality rates in 2011 in the United States and European regions are 6.1 and 13 per 1000 live births, respectively, but in the African region the rate is 106 per 1000 live births[1] (www.who.int/gho/child_health/mortality/mortality_under_five_text/en/index.html). Stillbirths, defined as late fetal deaths at greater than 1000 g or greater than 28 weeks of gestation, are estimated at 3 million cases annually, with 99% occurring in low- and middle-income countries.[2] Whereas infection accounts for approximately one third of neonatal deaths globally, it accounts for a considerably smaller fraction in the United States.

Setbacks facing initiatives to reduce the global burden of infectious disease in the fetus and newborn infant include the continuing epidemic of HIV infection in sub-Saharan Africa, particularly among women, and the lack of finances to provide effective treatment for these women and their newborn infants. In the United States, infectious disease challenges include the increase in antimicrobial resistance among nosocomial pathogens and in the incidence of invasive fungal infections among infants of extremely low birth weight. Moreover, the rate of pertussis is rising, notably so in older children and adolescents in the United States and other countries, with disproportional impact on morbidity and mortality of the newborn. This rising prevalence is likely due, in part, to accelerated waning of immunity associated with the use of acellular vaccines, which have supplanted the killed whole-cell vaccine primarily in high-resource settings.[3,4]

Use of the Internet continues to expand rapidly, allowing access to information hitherto unavailable to physicians or parents. Physicians may obtain current information about diseases and management as well as various guidelines for diagnosis and treatment. Interested parents who have access to the Internet can explore various websites that present a vast array of information but, unfortunately, also misinformation. As an example of the latter, a case of neonatal tetanus was associated with the use of cosmetic facial clay (Indian Healing Clay) as a dressing on an umbilical cord stump. The product had been publicized as a healing salve by midwives on an Internet site dedicated to "cord-care."[5] The antivaccination movement is active on the Internet, deploying a variety of tactics and rhetoric to effectively spread their messages.[6] Because much of the information on the Internet is from commercial sources and parties with varying interests and expertise, physicians should be prepared to assist interested parents and patients in finding Internet sites of genuine value. Several Internet sites pertinent to infectious diseases of the fetus and newborn infant are listed in Table 1-2.

Vital statistics relevant to infectious disease risk in neonates in the United States for 2010 to 2011 are listed in Table 1-3.[1] The disparities in birth weight, prenatal care, and neonatal mortality among different racial and ethnic groups in the United States are important to note and to consider in the context of the global disparities noted above.

The number of infectious diseases in fetuses and newborn infants must be extrapolated from selected studies (see chapters on specific diseases). Approximately 1% of newborn infants shed cytomegalovirus (CMV), greater than 4% of infants are born to mothers infected with *Chlamydia*

Table 1-3 Percentage of Births with Selected Characteristics by Race and Hispanic Origin of Mother in the United States*

	RACIAL/ETHNIC ORIGIN OF MOTHER							
	ALL RACES		NON-HISPANIC WHITE		NON-HISPANIC BLACK		HISPANIC	
	2010	**1990**	**2010**	**1990**	**2010**	**1990**	**2010**	**1990**
MOTHER								
<20 years old	9.3	12.8	6.7	9.6	15.2	23.2	13.1	16.8
≥40 years old	2.9	1.2	3.0	1.2	2.3	0.8	2.4	1.2
Diabetes during pregnancy	5.1	2.1	4.7	2.2	4.5	1.8	5.2	2.0
Cesarean delivery	32.8	22.7	32.6	23.4	35.5	22.1	31.8	21.2
INFANT								
Birth weight†								
LBW	8.2	7.0	7.1	5.6	13.5	13.3	7.0	6.1
VLBW	1.5	1.3	1.2	0.9	3.0	2.9	1.2	1.0
Gestational age‡								
Preterm	12.0	10.6	10.8	8.5	17.1	18.9	11.8	11.0
Preterm early	3.5	3.3	2.9	2.4	6.1	7.4	3.3	3.2
Preterm late	8.5	7.3	7.8	6.1	11.0	11.5	8.5	7.8

Modified from Hamilton BE, Hoyert DL, Martin JA, et al: Annual summary of vital statistics—2010-2011. *Pediatrics* 131:548-558, 2013.
*All values are in percent births.
†*LBW*, low birth weight (<2500 g); *VLBW*, very low birth weight (<1500 g).
‡Preterm early: <34 weeks of gestation; late preterm: 34-36 weeks of gestation.

trachomatis, and bacterial sepsis develops in 1 to 4 infants per 1000 live births. Since the institution of intrapartum chemoprophylaxis in the United States, the number of infants with early-onset GBS disease has declined, with reduction in incidence from approximately 1.5 cases to 0.29 case per 1000 live births.[7] In the United States, the use of maternal highly active antiretroviral treatment and peripartum chemoprophylaxis reduced the rate of mother-to-child transmission of HIV from approximately 25% of infants born to mothers who received no treatment to less than 2%; less complex but practical regimens of intrapartum prophylaxis have helped to reduce the rate of perinatal HIV transmission in the developing world.[8-10] Recently revised World Health Organization (WHO) guidelines (www.who.int/hiv/pub/guidelines/arv2013/intro/rag/en/index2.html) now also recommend that all HIV-infected pregnant and breastfeeding women and HIV-infected partners of monogamous HIV-uninfected pregnant women receive highly active antiretroviral treatment regardless of their CD4 T-cell numbers, which should help to further lower the rates of HIV transmission in resource-limited settings. Among sexually transmitted diseases, the rate of congenital syphilis had declined substantially in the United States to 13.4 per 100,000 live births in 2000[11]; however, after 14 years of decline, the rate of congenital syphilis increased in 2006 and 2007 from 9.3 to 10.5 cases per 100,000 live births, in parallel with the increase in the syphilis rates among the general population.[12] Immunization has virtually eliminated congenital rubella syndrome in newborn infants of U.S.-born mothers, but cases continue to occur in infants of foreign-born mothers; the mothers of 24 of 26 infants with congenital rubella born between 1997 and 1999 were foreign born, 21 of them Hispanic.[13] Efforts led by the Pan American Health Organization to eliminate congenital rubella syndrome in the Americas by 2010 appears to have been successful, with the last case reported in 2009, providing impetus for a global attack on the problem through universal immunization.[7]

Consequences of perinatal infections vary depending on whether the infection occurs in utero or during the intrapartum or postpartum periods. Infection acquired in utero can result in resorption of the embryo, abortion, stillbirth, malformation, intrauterine growth restriction, prematurity, or the untoward sequelae of chronic postnatal infection. Infection acquired during the intrapartum or early postpartum period may result in severe systemic disease that leads to death or the establishment of persistent postnatal infection. In utero infection and intrapartum infections may lead to late-onset disease. Such infections may not be apparent at birth but may manifest with signs or symptoms weeks, months, or years later, as exemplified by chorioretinitis of *Toxoplasma gondii* infection, hearing loss of rubella, and immunologic defects that result from HIV infection. The immediate and the long-term effects of these infections constitute a major problem throughout the world.

Infections of the Fetus

PATHOGENESIS

Pregnant women are not only exposed to infections prevalent in the community but are also likely to reside with young children or to associate with groups of young children, which represents a significant additional factor in exposure to infectious agents. Most infections in pregnant women affect the upper respiratory and gastrointestinal tracts, and either resolve spontaneously without therapy or are readily treated with antimicrobial agents. Such infections usually remain localized and have no effect on the developing fetus. The infecting organism may invade the bloodstream, however, and subsequently infect the placenta and fetus.

Successful pregnancy is a unique example of immunologic tolerance—the mother must be tolerant of her allogeneic fetus (and vice versa). The basis for maternal-fetal tolerance is not completely understood but is known to reflect local modifications of host defenses at the maternal-fetal interface and more global changes in immunologic competence in the mother. Specific factors acting locally in the placenta include indoleamine 2,3-dioxygenase, which suppresses cell-mediated immunity by catabolizing the essential amino acid tryptophan, and regulatory proteins that prevent complement activation.[14,15] Based on data from murine models, there is an accumulating body of evidence that pregnancy is associated with maternal-fetal tolerance that depends in part on the development of maternal regulatory T-cell–mediated tolerance to fetal antigens inherited from the father.[16] Regulatory T cells are also relatively more abundant and active in the human fetus, whose T-cell populations are also otherwise naïve in phenotype and function (see Chapter 4). Further, as pregnancy progresses, a general shift from T-helper type 1 (Th1) cell-mediated immunity to T-helper type 2 (Th2) responses also occurs in the mother.[17, 18] Nonetheless, because Th1 cell-mediated immunity is important in host defense against intracellular pathogens, the reduced Th1 bias established during normal gestation may compromise successful immunity against organisms such as *T. gondii*. In addition, it has been proposed that a strong curative Th1 response against an organism may overcome protective T-regulatory and Th2 activity at the maternal-fetal interface, resulting in fetal loss.

Transplacental spread and invasion of the bloodstream after maternal infection is the usual route by which the fetus becomes infected. Uncommonly, the fetus may be infected by extension of infection in adjacent maternal tissues and organs, including the peritoneum and the genitalia, during parturition, or as a result of invasive methods for the diagnosis and therapy of fetal disorders, such as the use of monitors, chorionic villus biopsy, sampling of fetal blood, and intrauterine transfusion.

Microorganisms of concern are listed in Table 1-4 and include those identified in the acronym *TORCH*: *T. gondii*, rubella virus, CMV, and herpes simplex virus (HSV). As a point of historical interest, the *O* in TORCH originally stood for "other infections/pathogens," reflecting an early appreciation of this possibility. A new acronym is needed to include other, well-described causes of in utero infection: syphilis, enteroviruses, varicella-zoster virus (VZV), HIV, Lyme disease *(Borrelia burgdorferi)*, and parvovirus. In certain geographic areas, *Plasmodium* and *Trypanosoma cruzi* are responsible for in utero infections. *TORCHES CLAP* (see Table 1-4) is an inclusive acronym. Case reports indicate other organisms that are unusual causes of infections transmitted by a pregnant woman to her fetus, including *Brucella melitensis*,[19] *Coxiella burnetii* (Q fever),[20] *Babesia microti* (babesiosis),[21] human T-cell lymphotropic virus (HTLV) types 1 and 2 (although the main route of transmission of these viruses is through breastfeeding),[22,23] hepatitis G and TT viruses,[24,25] human herpesvirus 6,[26,27] and dengue.[28]

Table 1-4 Suggested Acronym for Microorganisms Responsible for Infection of the Fetus: TORCHES CLAP

TO	*Toxoplasma gondii*
R	Rubella virus
C	Cytomegalovirus
H	Herpes simplex virus
E	Enteroviruses
S	Syphilis (*Treponema pallidum*)
C	Chickenpox (varicella-zoster virus)
L	Lyme disease (*Borrelia burgdorferi*)
A	AIDS (HIV)
P	Parvovirus B19

AIDS, Acquired immunodeficiency syndrome; *HIV*, human immunodeficiency virus.

Among these other organisms, investigators from France reported that *Coxiella burnetti* (the causative agent of the zoonotic disease Q fever) infection of the pregnant woman is associated with untoward pregnancy outcomes, including spontaneous abortion, intrauterine fetal demise, preterm delivery, and intrauterine growth retardation in a large majority (81%) of untreated women.[20] Restricting their analysis to women in whom such complications were not evident at presentation, complications were observed in 14 of 21 women who were not treated and 7 of 16 who received long-term (>5 weeks) daily cotrimoxazole therapy (P = .047). They acknowledge the noncontrolled nature of their data and the possible selection bias but nonetheless propose that such therapy be given to all pregnant women with proven *Coxiella burnetti* infection. However, other, though smaller, reports have not observed a high rate of complications and would restrict such therapy to women with symptomatic acute infection or chronic Q fever.[29]

Before rupture of fetal membranes, organisms in the genital tract may invade the amniotic fluid and infect the fetus. These organisms can invade the placenta through microscopic defects in the membranes, particularly in devitalized areas overlying the cervical os. It also is possible that microorganisms gain access to the fetus from descending infection through the fallopian tubes in women with salpingitis or peritonitis, or from direct extension of an infection in the uterus, such as myometrial abscess or cellulitis. Available evidence does not suggest, however, that transtubal or transmyometrial passage of microbial agents is a significant route of fetal infection.

Invasive techniques developed for in utero diagnosis and therapy are potential sources of infection for the fetus. Abscesses have been observed in infants who had scalp punctures for fetal blood sampling or electrocardiographic electrodes attached to their scalps. Cases of osteomyelitis of the skull and streptococcal sepsis have followed local infection at the site of a fetal monitoring electrode[30]; HSV infections at the fetal scalp electrode site also have been reported. Intrauterine transfusion for severe erythroblastosis diagnosed in utero also has resulted in infection of the fetus. In one case, CMV infection reportedly resulted from intrauterine transfusion[31]; in another instance, contamination of donor blood with a gram-negative coccobacillus, *Acinetobacter calcoaceticus*, led to an acute placentitis and subsequent fetal bacteremia.[32]

Fetal infection in the absence of rupture of internal membranes usually occurs transplacentally after invasion of the maternal bloodstream. Microorganisms in the blood may be carried within white blood cells or attached to erythrocytes, or they may be present in serum independent of cellular elements.

Microbial Invasion of the Maternal Bloodstream

The potential consequences of invasion of the mother's bloodstream by microorganisms or their products (Fig. 1-1) include placental infection without infection of the fetus, fetal infection without infection of the placenta, absence of fetal and placental infection, and infection of placenta and fetus (see Chapter 3 for additional discussion of this topic).

Placental Infection Without Infection of the Fetus. After reaching the intervillous spaces on the maternal side of the placenta, organisms can remain localized in the placenta without affecting the fetus. Evidence that placentitis can occur independently of fetal involvement has been shown for maternal tuberculosis, syphilis, malaria, coccidioidomycosis, CMV, rubella virus, and mumps vaccine virus infection. The reasons for the lack of spread to the fetus after placental infection are unknown. Defenses of the fetus that may operate after placental infection include the villous trophoblast, placental macrophages, and locally produced immune factors, such as antibodies and cytokines.

Fetal Infection Without Overt Infection of the Placenta. Microorganisms may traverse the chorionic villi directly through pinocytosis, placental leaks, or diapedesis of infected maternal leukocytes and erythrocytes. Careful histologic studies usually reveal areas of placentitis sufficient to serve as a source of fetal infection, however.

Absence of Fetal and Placental Infection. Invasion of the bloodstream by microorganisms is common in pregnant women, yet in most cases, neither fetal nor placental infection results. Bacteremia may accompany abscesses, cellulitis, bacterial pneumonia, pyelonephritis, appendicitis, endocarditis, or other pyogenic infections; nevertheless, placental or fetal infection as a consequence is rare. In most cases, the fetus is likely protected through efficient clearance of microbes by maternal innate or preexisting adaptive immunity.

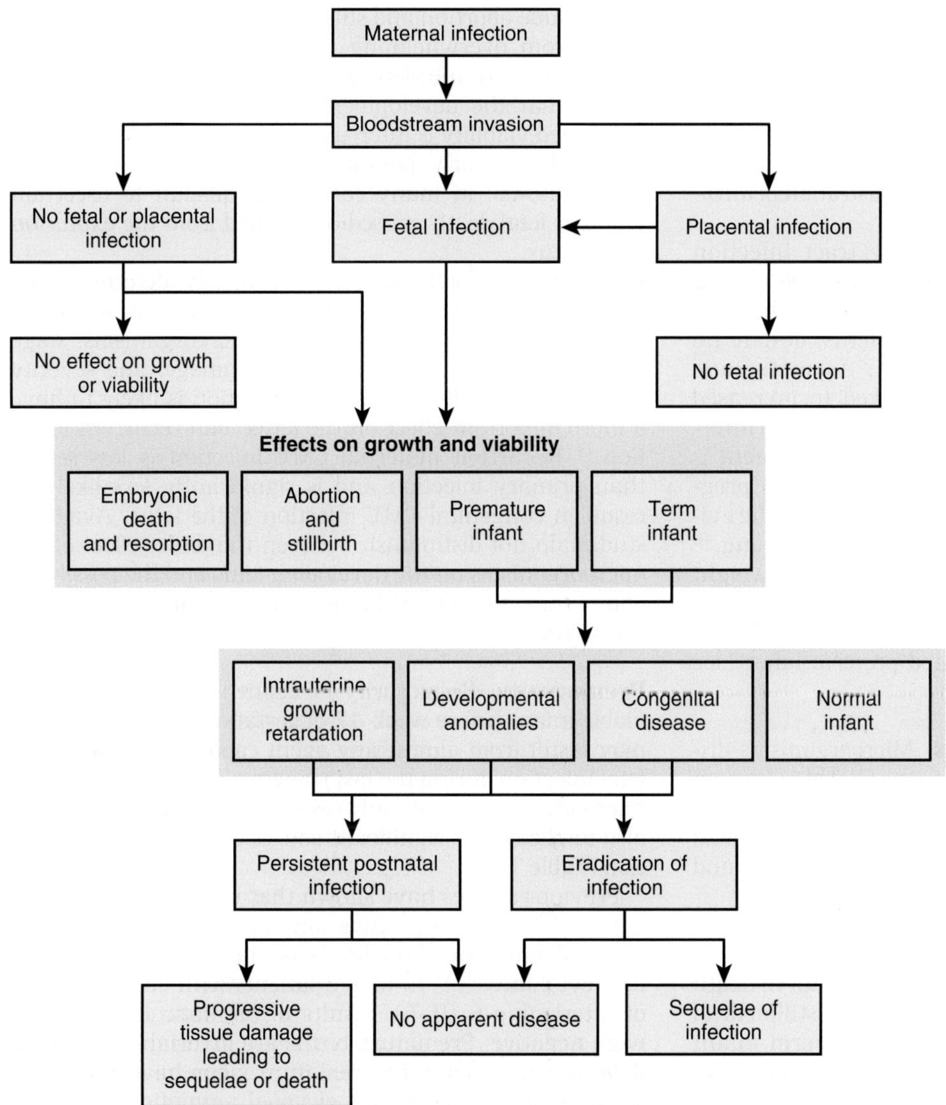

Figure 1-1 Pathogenesis of hematogenous transplacental infections.

Many bacterial diseases of the pregnant woman, including typhoid fever, pneumonia, gram-negative bacterial sepsis, and urinary tract infections, may affect the developing fetus without direct microbial invasion of the placenta or fetal tissues. Similarly, protozoan infection in the mother, such as malaria, and systemic viral infections, including varicella, variola, and measles, also may affect the fetus indirectly. Fever, anoxia, circulating toxins, or metabolic and hematologic derangements in the mother concomitant with these infections can affect the pregnancy, possibly resulting in abortion, stillbirth, or premature delivery.

The effects of microbial toxins on the developing fetus are uncertain. The fetus may be adversely affected by toxic shock in the mother secondary to *Staphylococcus aureus* or *Streptococcus pyogenes* infection.[33] Botulism in pregnant women has not been associated with disease in infants.[34,35] A unique case of Guillain-Barré syndrome in mother and child shows that infection-induced, antibody-mediated autoimmune disease in the mother may be transmitted to her infant. In this case, the disease was diagnosed in the mother during week 29 of pregnancy. A healthy infant was delivered vaginally at 38 weeks of gestation, while the mother was quadriplegic and on respiratory support. On day 12 of life, the infant developed flaccid paralysis of all limbs with absence of deep tendon reflexes, and cerebrospinal fluid (CSF) examination revealed increased protein concentration without white blood cells.[36] The delay in onset of paralysis in the infant seemed to reflect transplacentally transferred blocking antibodies specifically directed at epitopes of the mature, but not the fetal, neuromuscular junction. The infant improved after administration of intravenous immunoglobulin.[37]

The association of maternal urinary tract infection with premature delivery and low birth weight is a well-studied example of a maternal infection that adversely affects growth and development of the fetus, despite no evidence of fetal or placental infection. Asymptomatic bacteriuria in pregnancy has been linked to increased low-birth-weight deliveries.[38,39] A meta-analysis of interventional studies concluded that antibiotic treatment is effective in reducing the risk of pyelonephritis in pregnancy and the risk for preterm delivery, although the evidence supporting this latter conclusion is not as strong.[40] The basis for the premature delivery and low birth weight of infants of mothers with bacteriuria remains obscure[41] and may, in part, reflect an altered maternal genital tract microbiome and dysbiosis-associated preterm labor (see Chapter 3).

Infection of Placenta and Fetus. Microorganisms disseminate from the infected placenta to the fetal bloodstream through infected emboli of necrotic chorionic tissues or through direct extension of placental infection to the fetal membranes, with secondary amniotic fluid infection and aspiration by the fetus.

Infection of the Embryo and Fetus

Hematogenous transplacental spread may result in death and resorption of the embryo, abortion and stillbirth of the fetus, and live birth of a premature or term infant who may or may not be healthy. The effects of fetal infection may appear in a live-born infant as low birth weight (resulting from intrauterine growth restriction), developmental anomalies, congenital disease, or none of these. Infection acquired in utero may persist after birth and cause significant abnormalities in growth and development that may be apparent soon after birth or may not be recognized for months or years. The variability of the effects of fetal infection is emphasized by reports of biovular twin pregnancies that produced one severely damaged infant and one infant with minimal or no detectable abnormalities.[42-47]

Embryonic Death and Resorption. Various organisms may infect the pregnant woman in the first few weeks of gestation and cause death and resorption of the embryo. Because loss of the embryo usually occurs before the woman realizes she is pregnant or seeks medical attention, it is difficult to estimate the incidence of this outcome for any single infectious agent. The incidence of early pregnancy loss after implantation from all causes has been estimated to be 31%. The proportion of cases of loss because of infection is unknown.[48]

Abortion and Stillbirth. The earliest recognizable effects of fetal infection are seen after 6 to 8 weeks of pregnancy and include abortion and stillbirth. Intrauterine death may result from overwhelming fetal infection, or the microorganisms may interfere with organogenesis to such an extent that the development of functions necessary for continued viability is interrupted. The precise mechanisms responsible for early spontaneous termination of pregnancy are unknown; in many cases, it is difficult to ascertain whether fetal death caused or resulted from the expulsion of the fetus.

Numerous modifying factors probably determine the ultimate consequence of intrauterine infection, including virulence or tissue tropism of the microorganisms, stage of pregnancy, associated placental damage, and severity of the maternal illness. Primary infection is likely to have a more important effect on the fetus than recurrent infection.[49] Recurrent maternal CMV infection is less severe than primary infection and is significantly less likely to result in congenital CMV infection of the fetus. Available studies do not distinguish between the direct effect of the microorganisms on the developing fetus and the possibility of an indirect effect attributable to illness or poor health of the mother.

Prematurity. Prematurity is defined as the birth of a viable infant before week 37 of gestation. Premature birth may result from almost any agent capable of establishing fetal infection during the last trimester of pregnancy. Many microorganisms commonly responsible for prematurity are also implicated as significant causes of stillbirth and abortion (Table 1-5).

Previous studies have shown that women in premature labor with bacteria-positive amniotic fluid cultures have elevated amniotic fluid levels of multiple proinflammatory cytokines.[50-55] In many patients with elevated levels of interleukin-6 (IL-6), results of amniotic fluid culture were negative. Premature births are invariably observed, however, in women in premature labor having positive amniotic fluid culture and elevated amniotic fluid levels

Table 1-5 Effects of Transplacental Fetal Infection on the Fetus and Newborn Infant

	DISEASE				
Organism	**Prematurity**	**Intrauterine Growth Restriction/Low Birth Weight**	**Developmental Anomalies**	**Congenital Disease**	**Persistent Postnatal Infection**
Viruses	CMV HSV Rubeola Smallpox HBV HIV*	CMV Rubella VZV* HIV*	CMV Rubella VZV Coxsackievirus B* HIV*	CMV Rubella VZV HSV Mumps* Rubeola Vaccinia Smallpox Coxsackievirus B Poliovirus HBV HIV LCV Parvovirus	CMV Rubella VZV HSV HBV HIV
Bacteria	*Treponema pallidum* *Mycobacterium tuberculosis* *Listeria monocytogenes* *Campylobacter fetus* *Salmonella typhi*			*T. pallidum* *M. tuberculosis* *L. monocytogenes* *C. fetus* *S. typhi* *Borrelia burgdorferi*	*T. pallidum* *M. tuberculosis*
Protozoa	*Toxoplasma gondii* *Plasmodium** *Trypanosoma cruzi*	*T. gondii* *Plasmodium* *T. cruzi*		*T. gondii* *Plasmodium* *T. cruzi*	*T. gondii* *Plasmodium*

CMV, Cytomegalovirus; *HBV*, hepatitis B virus; *HIV*, human immunodeficiency virus; *HSV*, herpes simplex virus; *LCV*, lymphocytic choriomeningitis virus; *VZV*, varicella-zoster virus.

*Association of effect with infection has been suggested and is under consideration.

of IL-6. To clarify further the role of elevated levels of IL-6 in amniotic fluid, Hitti and colleagues[51] amplified bacterial DNA encoding 16S ribosomal RNA (rRNA) by using a polymerase chain reaction (PCR) assay to detect infection in amniotic fluid of women in premature labor whose membranes were intact. In patients who were culture-negative, PCR assay detected bacterial infection in a significant percentage of those with elevated IL-6 levels. These data suggest that 33% of women in premature labor with culture-negative amniotic fluid but with elevated IL-6 levels may have infected amniotic fluid. The investigators concluded that the association between infected amniotic fluid and premature labor may be underestimated on the basis of amniotic fluid cultures and that a broad-spectrum bacterial 16S rDNA PCR assay may be useful for detecting prenatal infection. The utility of amniotic fluid testing for IL-6 and other biomarkers in predicting risk for preterm birth is discussed further in Chapter 3.

In recent years, many studies have explored how abnormal composition of the vaginal flora, maternal vaginal colonization with *Ureaplasma* or *Mycoplasma* spp., or development of bacterial vaginosis (BV) during pregnancy can influence the risk of preterm birth.[56,57] Meta-analyses of recent interventional studies of antibiotic administration to correct such dysbiosis during the first trimester are, to date, inconclusive with respect to reducing preterm birth.[58,59] Further advances in the detection of microbes and the assessment of microbial diversity through high-throughput, next-generation sequencing–based assessment offer the promise to better understand the role of microbes in preterm labor and its untoward consequences (see Chapter 3).

Intrauterine Growth Restriction and Low Birth Weight. Infection of the fetus may result in birth of an infant who is small for gestational age. Although many maternal infections are associated with low-birth-weight infants and infants who are small for gestational age, causal evidence is sufficient only for congenital rubella, VZV infection, toxoplasmosis, and CMV infection, although it is likely that congenital syphilis can, in some cases, also result in intrauterine growth restriction (see Chapter 16).

The organs of infants dying with congenital rubella syndrome or congenital CMV infection contain reduced numbers of morphologically normal cells.[60,61] By contrast, in infants who are small for gestational age with growth deficit from noninfectious causes, such as maternal toxemia or placental abnormalities, the parenchymal cells are normal in number but have a reduced amount of cytoplasm, presumably because of fetal malnutrition.[62,63]

Developmental Anomalies and Teratogenesis. CMV, rubella virus, and VZV cause developmental anomalies in the human fetus. Coxsackieviruses B3 and B4 have been associated with congenital heart disease. Although the pathogenetic mechanisms responsible for fetal abnormalities produced by most infectious agents remain obscure, histologic studies of abortuses and congenitally infected infants have suggested that some viruses render these effects through mediating cell death, alterations in cell growth, or chromosomal damage. Inflammation and tissue destruction, rather than teratogenic activity, seem to be responsible for the widespread structural abnormalities characteristic of congenital syphilis, transplacental HSV and VZV infection, and toxoplasmosis. Infants with

Table 1-6 Clinical Manifestations of Neonatal Infection Acquired In Utero or at Delivery

Rubella Virus	Cytomegalovirus	*Toxoplasma gondii*	Herpes Simplex Virus	*Treponema pallidum*	Enteroviruses
Hepatosplenomegaly	Hepatosplenomegaly	Hepatosplenomegaly	Hepatosplenomegaly	Hepatosplenomegaly	Hepatosplenomegaly
Jaundice	Jaundice	Jaundice	Jaundice	Jaundice	Jaundice
Pneumonitis	Pneumonitis	Pneumonitis	Pneumonitis	Pneumonitis	Pneumonitis
Petechiae *or* purpura	Petechiae *or* purpura	Petechiae *or* purpura	Petechiae *or* purpura	Petechiae *or* purpura	Petechiae *or* purpura
Meningoencephalitis	Meningoencephalitis	Meningoencephalitis	Meningoencephalitis	Meningoencephalitis	Meningoencephalitis
Hydrocephalus	Hydrocephalus	Hydrocephalus*	Hydrocephalus	Adenopathy	Adenopathy
Adenopathy	Microcephaly*	Microcephaly	Microcephaly	Maculopapular exanthems*	Maculopapular exanthems
Hearing deficits	Intracranial calcifications*	Maculopapular exanthems	Maculopapular exanthems	Bone lesions*	Paralysis*
Myocarditis	Hearing deficits	Intracranial calcifications*	Vesicles*	Glaucoma	Myocarditis*
Congenital defects*	Chorioretinitis *or* retinopathy	Myocarditis	Myocarditis	Chorioretinitis *or* retinopathy	Conjunctivitis *or* keratoconjunctivitis
Bone lesions*	Optic atrophy	Bone lesions	Chorioretinitis *or* retinopathy	Uveitis	
Glaucoma*		Chorioretinitis *or* retinopathy*	Cataracts		
Chorioretinitis *or* retinopathy*		Cataracts	Conjunctivitis *or* keratoconjunctivitis*		
Cataracts*		Optic atrophy			
Microphthalmia		Microphthalmia			
		Uveitis			

*Has special diagnostic significance for this infection.

congenital toxoplasmosis may have microcephaly, hydrocephalus, or microphthalmia, but these manifestations usually result from an intense necrotizing process involving numerous organisms and are more appropriately defined as lesions of congenital infection, rather than as effects of teratogenic activity of the organism.

Some mycoplasmas[64] and viruses[65,66] produce chromosomal damage in circulating human lymphocytes or in human cells in tissue culture. The relationship of these genetic aberrations to the production of congenital abnormalities in the fetus is unknown.

Congenital Disease. Clinical evidence of intrauterine infections, resulting from tissue damage or secondary physiologic changes caused by the invading organisms, may be present at birth or may manifest soon thereafter or years later. The clinical manifestations of infection acquired in utero or at delivery in the newborn infant are summarized in Table 1-6. Signs of widely disseminated infection may be evident during the neonatal period in infants with congenital rubella; toxoplasmosis; syphilis; or congenital CMV, HSV, or enterovirus infection. These signs include jaundice, hepatosplenomegaly, and pneumonia, each of which reflects lesions caused by microbial invasion and proliferation, rather than by defects in organogenesis. Although these signs of congenital infection are not detected until the neonatal period, the pathologic processes responsible for their occurrence have been progressing for weeks or months before delivery. In some infants, the constellation of signs is sufficient to suggest the likely congenital infection (Table 1-7). In other infants, the signs are transient and self-limited and resolve as neonatal defense mechanisms control the spread of the microbial agent and tissue destruction. If damage is severe and widespread at the time of delivery, survival of the infant is unlikely.

It is frequently difficult to determine whether an infection in the newborn infant was acquired in utero, intrapartum, or postpartum. If the onset of clinical signs after birth occurs within the minimal incubation period for the disease (e.g., 3 days for enteroviruses, 10 days for VZV and rubella viruses), it is likely that the infection was acquired before delivery. The interval between malaria exposure in the mother and congenital malaria in the infant can be prolonged; one case of congenital malaria resulting from *Plasmodium malariae* occurred in an infant born in the United States 25 years after the mother had emigrated from China.[67] Children with perinatal HIV infection can be diagnosed by 6 months of age using a DNA (or RNA) PCR method, which has largely replaced other approaches for viral detection.[68] A variable fraction (less than half) of

Table 1-7 Syndromes in the Neonate Caused by Congenital Infections

Microorganism	Signs
Toxoplasma gondii	Hydrocephalus, diffuse intracranial calcification, chorioretinitis
Rubella virus	Cardiac defects, sensorineural hearing loss, cataracts, microcephaly, "blueberry muffin" skin lesions, hepatomegaly, interstitial pneumonitis, myocarditis, disturbances in bone growth, intrauterine growth restriction
CMV	Microcephaly, periventricular calcifications, jaundice, petechiae or purpura, hepatosplenomegaly, intrauterine growth restriction
HSV	Skin vesicles or scarring, eye scarring, microcephaly or hydranencephaly, vesicular skin rash, keratoconjunctivitis, meningoencephalitis, sepsis with hepatic failure
Treponema pallidum	Bullous, macular, or eczematous skin lesions involving palms and soles; rhinorrhea; dactylitis and other signs of osteochondritis and periostitis; hepatosplenomegaly; lymphadenopathy
VZV	Limb hypoplasia, cicatricial skin lesions, ocular abnormalities, cortical atrophy
Parvovirus B19	Nonimmune hydrops fetalis
HIV	Severe thrush, failure to thrive, recurrent bacterial infections, calcification of basal ganglia

CMV, Cytomegalovirus; *HIV*, human immunodeficiency virus; *HSV*, herpes simplex virus; *VZV*, varicella-zoster virus.

children with perinatal HIV contract the infection in utero, depending on the setting and maternal treatment.[69] Virus-negative infants who later become virus-positive may have been infected in the intrapartum or early postpartum period, including via breastfeeding, especially when neither the infant nor the mother is receiving antiretroviral prophylaxis while breastfeeding. In this situation, up to a 54% increase in postpartum HIV transmission associated with breastfeeding has been documented.[69,70]

Healthy Infants. Most newborn infants infected in utero by rubella virus, *T. gondii*, CMV, HIV, or *Treponema pallidum* have no signs of congenital disease. Fetal infection by a limited inoculum of organisms or with a strain of low virulence or pathologic potential may underlie this low incidence of clinical disease in infected infants. Alternatively, gestational age may be the most important factor in determining the ultimate consequences of prenatal infection. When congenital rubella and toxoplasmosis are acquired during the last trimester of pregnancy, the incidence of clinical disease in the infected infants is lower than when microbial invasion occurs during the first or second trimester. Congenital syphilis most commonly results from exposure during the second or third trimesters but can be transmitted to the fetus in the first trimester.

Absence of clinically apparent disease in the newborn may be misleading. Careful observation of infected but healthy-appearing children over months or years often reveals defects that were not apparent at birth. The failure to recognize such defects early in life may be due to the inability to test young infants for the sensory and developmental functions involved. Hearing defects identified years after birth may be the only manifestation of congenital rubella. Significant sensorineural deafness and other central nervous system deficiencies have affected children with congenital CMV infection who were considered to be normal during the neonatal period. In utero infection with *Toxoplasma*, rubella, and CMV may have manifestations that are difficult to recognize, including failure to thrive, visual defects, and minimal-to-severe brain dysfunction, including motor, learning, language, and behavioral disorders. Infants infected with HIV are usually asymptomatic at birth and for the first few months of life. The median age of onset for signs of congenital HIV infection is approximately 3 years, but many children remain asymptomatic for more than 5 years. Signs of perinatal infection related to HIV include failure to thrive, persistent diarrhea, recurrent suppurative infections, and diseases associated with opportunistic infections that occur weeks to months or years after birth. Of particular concern is a report by Wilson and colleagues[71] showing stigmata of congenital *T. gondii* infection, including chorioretinitis and blindness, in almost all of 24 children at follow-up evaluations; the children had serologic evidence of infection but were without apparent signs of disease at birth and either did not receive treatment or received inadequate treatment.

Because abnormalities may become obvious only as the child develops and fails to reach appropriate physiologic or developmental milestones, it is crucial to perform careful and thorough follow-up examinations in infants born to women with known or suspected infections during pregnancy.

Persistent Postnatal Infection. Microbial agents may continue to survive and replicate in tissues for months or years after in utero infection. Rubella virus and CMV have been isolated from various body fluid and tissue compartments over long periods from healthy-appearing children and children with abnormalities at birth. Progressive tissue destruction has been shown in some congenital infections, including rubella; toxoplasmosis; syphilis; tuberculosis; malaria; and CMV, HSV, and HIV infection. Recurrent skin and eye infections can occur as a result of HSV infection acquired in utero or at the time of delivery. A progressive encephalitis occurred in children with congenital rubella infection; stable clinical manifestations of congenital infection over many years were followed by deterioration of motor and mental functions at ages 11 to 14 years.[72,73] Rubella virus was subsequently isolated from the brain biopsy specimen of a 12-year-old child. Finally, fetal parvovirus B19 infection can persist for months after birth with persistent anemia because of suppressed hematopoiesis.[74]

The mechanisms responsible for maintaining or terminating chronic fetal and postnatal infections are only partially understood. Humoral immune responses, as determined by measurement of either fetal immunoglobulin M (IgM) or IgA antibodies or specific IgG antibodies that develop in the neonatal period, seem to be intact in almost all infants (see Chapter 4). The importance of cell-mediated immunity, cytokines, complement, antimicrobial peptides, and other host defense mechanisms remains to be adequately defined; at present, there is insufficient evidence to support a causal relationship between deficiencies in any one of these factors and persistent postnatal infection. All of the diseases associated with persistent postnatal infection—with the exception of rubella, but including syphilis; tuberculosis; malaria; toxoplasmosis; hepatitis; and CMV, HSV, VZV, and HIV infections—can also produce prolonged and, in certain instances, lifelong infection when acquired later in life.

EFFICIENCY OF TRANSMISSION OF MICROORGANISMS FROM MOTHER TO FETUS

The efficiency of transmission from the infected, immunocompetent mother to the fetus varies among microbial agents and can vary with the trimester of pregnancy. In utero transmission of rubella virus and *T. gondii* occurs mainly during primary infection, whereas in utero transmission of CMV, HIV, and *T. pallidum* can occur in consecutive pregnancies. The risk of congenital rubella infection in fetuses of mothers with symptomatic rubella was high in the first trimester (90% before 11 weeks of gestation), declined to a nadir of 25% at 23 to 26 weeks, and then increased to 67% after 31 weeks. Infection in the first 11 weeks of gestation was uniformly teratogenic, whereas no birth defects occurred in infants infected after 16 weeks of gestation.[75] By contrast, the frequency of stillbirth and clinical and subclinical congenital *T. gondii* infections among offspring of women who acquired the infection during pregnancy was lowest in the first trimester (14%), increased in the second trimester (29%), and was highest in the third trimester (59%).[76]

Congenital CMV infection can result both from primary and recurrent infections. On the basis of studies in Birmingham, Alabama, and other centers, Whitley and Stagno and their colleagues[77,78] estimate that 1% to 4% of women have primary infection during pregnancy, 40% of these women transmit the infection to their fetuses, and 5% to 15% of the infants have signs of CMV disease. Congenital infection as a result of recurrent CMV infection occurs in 0.5% to 1% of live births, but less than 1% of the infected infants have clinically apparent disease.

The transmission rate of HIV infection from an untreated mother to the fetus is estimated to be about 25%, but the data are insufficient to identify efficiency of transmission in each trimester. Risk of transmission does not seem to be greater in mothers who acquire primary infection during pregnancy than in mothers who were infected before they became pregnant.[79]

DIAGNOSIS OF INFECTION IN THE PREGNANT WOMAN

Clinical Diagnosis

Symptomatic or Clinical Infection. In many instances, infection in the pregnant woman and congenital infection in the newborn infant can be suspected on the basis of clinical signs or symptoms. Careful examination can be sufficient to suggest a specific diagnosis, particularly when typical clinical findings are accompanied by a well-documented history of exposure (see Tables 1-6 and 1-7).

Asymptomatic or Subclinical Infection. Many infectious diseases with serious consequences for the fetus are difficult or impossible to diagnose in the mother solely on clinical grounds. Asymptomatic or subclinical infections may be caused by rubella virus, CMV, *T. gondii*, *T. pallidum*, HSV, and HIV. Most women infected with these organisms during pregnancy have no apparent signs of disease; only 50% of women infected with rubella virus have a rash, and although occasional cases of CMV mononucleosis are recognized, these constitute a very small proportion of women who acquire primary CMV infection during pregnancy. Similarly, the number of women with clinical manifestations of toxoplasmosis is less than 10%, and few women have systemic illness associated with primary HSV infection. The genital lesions associated with HSV infection and syphilis are often not recognized.

Recurrent and Chronic Infection. Some microorganisms can infect a susceptible person more than once, and when such reinfections occur in a pregnant woman, the organism can affect the fetus. These reinfections are generally associated with waning host immunity, but low levels of circulating antibodies may be detectable. Such specific antibodies would be expected to provide some protection against hematogenous spread and transplacental infection; however, fetal disease has followed reexposure of immune mothers to vaccinia,[80] variola,[81] and rubella[82] viruses.

In addition, an agent capable of persisting in the mother as a chronic asymptomatic infection could infect the fetus long after the initial infection. Such delayed infection is common for congenital CMV and HIV infections, which have been observed in infants from consecutive pregnancies in the same mother. Reports of infection of the fetus as a result of chronic maternal infection have been cited in cases of malaria,[83] syphilis,[84] hepatitis,[85] herpes zoster[47] and herpes simplex,[86] and *T. gondii* infection.[87] In the case of *T. gondii*, congenital transmission from a chronically infected woman occurs almost solely when the woman is immunocompromised during pregnancy.

Preconceptional Infection. The occurrence of acute infection immediately before conception may result in infection of the fetus, and the association may go unrecognized. Congenital rubella has occurred in the fetus in cases in which the mother was infected 3 weeks to 3 months before conception. A prolonged viremia or persistence of virus in the maternal tissues may be responsible for infection of the embryo or fetus. The same phenomenon has occurred rarely in cases of maternal infection with *T. gondii*.[88]

Isolation and Identification of Infectious Agents

General Approach. Diagnostic tests for microorganisms or infectious diseases are part of routine obstetric care; special care is warranted for selected patients with known or suspected exposure to the infectious agent or clinical signs of infection. Table 1-8 lists general categories of diagnostic tests and interventions that may be required in the event of a diagnosis. The specific interventions for each disease are discussed in subsequent chapters.

The most direct mode of diagnosis is isolation of the microbial agent from tissues and body fluids such as blood, CSF, or urine. Isolation of the agent must be considered in context with its epidemiology and natural history in the host. Isolation of an enterovirus from stool during the summer months may represent colonization, rather than significant infection, with risk of hematogenous spread to the fetus. Isolation of an enterovirus from an atypical body fluid or identification of a significant increase in antibody titer would be necessary to define an acute infectious process.

Tests for the presence of hepatitis B virus (HBV) surface antigen (HBsAg) should be performed in all pregnant women. The Centers for Disease Control and Prevention (CDC) has estimated that 16,500 births occur each year in the United States to women who are positive for HBsAg. Infants born to HBsAg-positive mothers may have a 90% chance of acquiring perinatal HBV infection. If maternal infection is identified soon after birth, use of hepatitis B immunoglobulin combined with hepatitis B vaccine is an effective mode of prevention of infection. For these reasons, the Advisory Committee on Immunization Practices of the U.S. Public Health Service[89] and the American Academy of Pediatrics (AAP)[7] recommend universal screening of all pregnant women for HBsAg.

The seminal publication by Daffos and colleagues[90] in 1983, in which fetal blood sampling for prenatal diagnosis was first described, provided a method for diagnosing various infections in the fetus that previously could be diagnosed only after birth. Their methods were widely adopted and have contributed significantly to our understanding of the immune response of the fetus to various pathogens, including rubella virus, VZV, CMV, and *T. gondii*,[91-94] and to a more objective approach to treating infection in the fetus before birth.

Fetal blood sampling and amniocentesis are performed with ultrasound guidance. The method is not free of risk; amniocentesis alone carries a risk of fetal injury or death of 1%,[54,95] and fetal blood sampling carries a risk of approximately 1.4%.[96] Because the amniotic fluid contains viruses

Table 1-8 Management of Infections in the Pregnant Woman

Microorganism	Diagnostic Test	First Visit	Third Trimester	At Delivery	Intervention*
ROUTINE CARE					
Mycobacterium tuberculosis	Tuberculin skin test	+			Chest radiograph, culture, antituberculous therapy
Gonorrhea	Culture		+		Antibiotic therapy
Hepatitis B	Serology	+			HBIG and hepatitis B vaccine to the infant within 12 hr of birth†
Chlamydia		+	+		Antibiotic therapy
Syphilis	Serology	+	+	+	Antibiotic therapy
Rubella	Serology	+			Postpartum vaccine
Group B *Streptococcus*	Culture		+		Intrapartum antibiotic prophylaxis
Herpes simplex virus	Examination, PCR, culture	+	+	+	Cesarean section‡ Antiviral therapy
Influenza	None needed				Vaccination
Neonatal pertussis	None needed				Vaccination for each pregnancy
SPECIAL CARE IF EXPOSED OR WITH CLINICAL SIGNS					
CMV	Serology	+			Education regarding hygiene to prevent infection
HIV	ELISA + Western blot, RNA testing	+			Antiretroviral therapy
Malaria	Rapid diagnostic testing, blood smear	+			IPTp and bed nets, antimalarial treatment
Parvovirus	Ultrasonography, serology				Intrauterine transfusion
Toxoplasmosis	Serology, PCR assay (amniotic fluid)				Anti-*Toxoplasma* therapy
VZV	Examination, PCR, ultrasonography				Antiviral therapy

Modified from table prepared by Riley L, Fetter S, Geller D: Boston City Hospital and Boston University School of Medicine.
ELISA, Enzyme-linked immunosorbent assay; *HBIG*, hepatitis B immune globulin; *HIV*, human immunodeficiency virus; *IPTp*, intermittent preventive therapy in pregnancy; *PCR*, polymerase chain reaction; *VZV*, varicella-zoster virus.
*See appropriate chapters.
†Hepatitis B immunoglobulin only in neonates born to women with high-risk factors, and in addition, hepatitis B vaccine for neonate.
‡When signs or symptoms of active genital herpes simplex virus are present at the onset of labor.

or bacteria shed from the placenta, skin, urine, or tracheal fluid of the infected fetus, this fluid may also be used to detect the infecting organism by culture, antigen detection test, or the presence of its nucleic acids by PCR. Amniotic fluid analysis is generally preferred over fetal blood sampling for this purpose and because the procedure, in experienced hands, appears to have a lower risk of complications than fetal blood sampling. Fetal blood can be examined for the same factors and antibodies formed by the fetus against the pathogen (e.g., IgA or IgM antibodies). These procedures are usually performed during or after week 18 of gestation. In any case, the decision to perform either procedure should be predicated on expectation that the information obtained will affect management. A fetus at high risk for infection (e.g., the fetus of a nonimmune woman who acquired infection with *T. gondii*, cytomegalovirus, or rubella virus during pregnancy) may be evaluated and followed by ultrasound examination to detect abnormalities such as dilation of the cerebral ventricles that suggest the presence of fetal infection.

Isolation, Culture, and Polymerase Chain Reaction. Isolation of CMV and rubella virus[97] and demonstration of HBsAg[98] from amniotic fluid obtained by amniocentesis have been reported. As PCR techniques have proved to be sensitive and specific for diagnosing many infections in the pregnant woman, fetus, and newborn, in many instances, isolating the infectious agent to make a definitive diagnosis is no longer necessary if PCR techniques are used. PCR techniques decrease the time to diagnosis and increase the sensitivity for diagnosis of many infectious agents, as exemplified by the prenatal diagnosis of infections caused by parvovirus,[99,100] CMV,[101-103] *T. gondii*,[104,105] and rubella virus.[106,107]

As with all diagnostic testing, caution is required in interpreting the results of prenatal PCR testing, however, because the sensitivity of PCR results on amniotic fluid is uncertain. One third of cases of congenital toxoplasmosis yield a negative result on amniotic fluid PCR assay,[105,107] and infants with congenital rubella may have negative amniotic fluid PCR assay results but positive fetal blood tests. Also, false-positive rates of 5% for viral DNA detection in fluids obtained for genetic testing have been observed when congenital fetal infection was not suspected or documented. Combined diagnostic approaches in which PCR is used in concert with fetal serology and other diagnostic modalities (e.g., serial fetal ultrasonography) to test amniotic fluid and fetal blood may offer the greatest sensitivity and predictive power in cases in which congenital infection is suspected, and this information is important in management decisions.[105,108]

Cytologic and Histologic Diagnosis. Histologic review of cytologic preparations and tissue sections is no longer used as the primary method of diagnosing maternal infections; however, it may provide a preliminary diagnosis of certain infections. Cervicovaginal smears or cell scrapings from the base of vesicles are valuable in diagnosing VZV and HSV infections. Typical histologic changes include multinucleated giant cells and intranuclear inclusions. The diagnosis of acute toxoplasmosis can be made from characteristic histologic changes in lymph nodes or by demonstration of the tachyzoite in biopsy or autopsy specimens of infected tissues. These morphologic approaches have been replaced, however, by more specific methods, such as PCR and serologic testing, to detect VZV, HSV, CMV, and toxoplasmosis. Detailed descriptions of the changes associated with infections of the placenta are presented in a monograph by Fox.[109] Examination of the placental parenchyma, the membranes, and the cord may provide valuable information for diagnosis of the infection and identification of the mode of transmission to the fetus (in utero or ascending infection).

Serologic Diagnosis. The serologic diagnosis of infection in the pregnant woman most often requires demonstration of elevated antibody titer against the suspected agent. Ideally, the physician should have available information about the patient's serologic status at the onset of pregnancy to identify women who are unprotected against *T. pallidum*, *T. gondii*, and rubella virus or who are infected with HBV or HIV. Many obstetricians have adopted this valuable practice.

Difficulties in interpreting serologic test results seldom arise when patients are seen shortly after exposure or at the onset of symptoms. In certain infections, including rubella and toxoplasmosis, however, a relatively rapid increase in antibody levels may preclude demonstration of a significant titer increase, especially in patients who are tested more than 7 days after the onset of the suspected illness. In these circumstances, a diagnosis may be obtained through the measurement of antibodies that increase more slowly over several weeks. Demonstration of IgA and IgE antibodies (in addition to the more conventional use of tests for IgG and IgM antibodies) is useful in the early diagnosis of infection in the pregnant woman, fetus, and newborn, and this should serve as an impetus for commercial firms to make these methods more widely available for health care providers. The same pertains to IgG avidity tests, which have proved accurate in ruling out recently acquired infection with *T. gondii*,[110] CMV,[111,112] and rubella virus.[113,114] At present, these tests require special techniques and are not performed routinely by most laboratories, so local or state health departments should be consulted for further information regarding their availability.

Use of Skin Tests. Routine skin tests for diagnosis of tuberculosis should be considered a part of prenatal care. Tuberculin skin tests can be administered to the mother without risk to the fetus.

Universal Screening

Prenatal care in the United States includes routine screening for serologic evidence of syphilis and rubella infection; culture or antigen evidence of *Chlamydia trachomatis*, group B streptococcus, or HBV infection; screening for urinary tract infection; and skin testing for tuberculosis. Evidence that treatment of the HIV-infected mother significantly reduces virus transmission to the fetus has led to recommendations by the U.S. Public Health Service for universal HIV screening of all pregnant women in the United States. Current CDC guidelines support voluntary HIV testing under conditions that simplify consent procedures, while preserving a woman's right to refuse testing, that is, an opt-out approach.[8,115,116]

Pregnant women with known HIV infection should be monitored and given appropriate treatment to enhance maternal and fetal health and to prevent maternal-to-fetal transmission. Pregnant women should be examined carefully for the presence of HIV-related infections, including gonorrhea, syphilis, and *C. trachomatis*. Baseline antibody titers should be obtained for opportunistic infections, such as *T. gondii*, which are observed commonly in HIV-infected women and which may be transmitted to their fetuses. More detailed information on management of the HIV-infected pregnant woman and her infant is given in Chapter 22.

DIAGNOSIS OF INFECTION IN THE NEWBORN INFANT

Infants with congenital infection as a result of rubella virus, CMV, HSV, *T. gondii*, or *T. pallidum* may present similarly with one or more of the following abnormalities: purpura, jaundice, hepatosplenomegaly, pneumonitis, and meningoencephalitis. Some findings have specific diagnostic significance (see Tables 1-5 and 1-6). Diagnostic tests for specific agents are described in detail in the relevant chapters, and general features are briefly reviewed here; a discussion of laboratory tests that may aid in the diagnosis of neonatal sepsis is given in Chapter 36.

In certain congenital infections, the organism may be isolated or its nucleic acids detected from tissues and body fluids. Infants may excrete CMV and rubella virus in the urine for weeks to months after birth. *T. pallidum* may be found in the CSF, in nasal secretions, and in syphilitic skin lesions. In infants with congenital HIV infection, approximately 30% are PCR positive at birth, but nearly 100% are positive by 4 to 6 months of life.

Serologic tests are available through state or commercial laboratories for the TORCH group of microorganisms

(*T. gondii*, rubella virus, CMV, and HSV) and for certain other congenitally acquired infections. To distinguish passively transferred maternal IgG antibody from antibody produced by the neonate in response to infection in utero, it is necessary to obtain two blood specimens from the infant. Because the half-life of IgG is approximately 3 weeks, the first sample is obtained soon after birth, and the second sample should be obtained at least two half-lives, or approximately 6 weeks, after the first specimen.

IgA, IgE, and IgM antibodies do not cross the placenta. Antigen-specific IgA, IgE, and IgM antibodies in the infant's blood provide evidence of current infection, but few commercial laboratories use reliable assays for these antibodies for the purpose of identifying congenital infections (as described in a Public Health Advisory from the U.S. Food and Drug Administration outlining the limitations of *Toxoplasma* IgM commercial test kits).

Although most congenital infections occur as a single entity, many HIV-infected mothers are coinfected with other infectious agents that may be transmitted to the newborn. A neonate born to a mother with HIV infection should be considered at risk for other sexually transmitted diseases, such as syphilis, gonorrhea, and *C. trachomatis* infection. Coinfection also has been documented for CMV.[117,118]

PREVENTION AND MANAGEMENT OF INFECTION IN THE PREGNANT WOMAN

Prevention of Infection

The pregnant woman should avoid contact with individuals with communicable diseases, particularly if she is known to be naïve to those infections. In some cases, specific measures can be taken. The pregnant woman should use barrier methods during intercourse with her sexual partner if he has a vesicular lesion on the penis that may be associated with HSV or if he is known or suspected to be infected with HIV. The WHO also recommends that HIV-infected partners of HIV-uninfected women in monogamous long-term relationships should be treated with highly active antiretroviral therapy regardless of their CD4 T-cell count, to prevent transmission to the uninfected partner.

Pregnant women should avoid eating raw or undercooked lamb, pork, and beef because of risk of *T. gondii* contamination. They also should avoid contact with cat feces or objects or materials contaminated with cat feces because these are highly infectious if they harbor oocysts of *T. gondii* (see Chapter 31). Pregnant women should not eat unpasteurized dairy products (including all soft cheeses), prepared meats (hot dogs, deli meat, and pâté), and undercooked poultry because these foods often contain *Listeria monocytogenes*, which is associated with maternal infection, miscarriage, fetal infection, and stillbirth (see Chapter 13), as well as other pathogens such as enterohemorrhagic *E. coli* 0157 and *Staphylococcus aureus*.

Prevention of infection in the mother and of transmission of maternal infection to the fetus and neonate through antimicrobial therapy is discussed in Chapter 3 and in chapters on the relevant infections. Prevention through active or passive immunization of the mother or neonate is discussed in Chapter 38.

Infections Acquired by the Newborn Infant During Birth

PATHOGENESIS

The developing fetus is protected from the microbial flora (microbiota) of the maternal genital tract. Initial colonization of the newborn and of the placenta usually occurs after rupture of maternal membranes. If delivery is delayed after membranes rupture, components of the vaginal microbiota can ascend and, in some cases, produce inflammation of fetal membranes, umbilical cord, and placenta (see Chapter 3). Fetal infection also can result from aspiration of infected amniotic fluid. Some viruses are present in the genital secretions (HSV, CMV, HBV, or HIV) or blood (HBV, hepatitis C virus, or HIV). If delivery occurs shortly after rupture of the membranes, the infant can be colonized during passage through the birth canal, where various, potentially pathogenic microorganisms may be present. These include gram-positive cocci (staphylococci and streptococci); gram-negative cocci and coccobacilli *(Neisseria gonorrhoeae* and *Haemophilus influenzae);* gram-negative enteric bacilli *(Escherichia coli, Proteus* spp., *Klebsiella* spp., *Pseudomonas* spp., *Salmonella*, and *Shigella);* anaerobic bacteria; viruses (CMV, HSV, rubella virus, and HIV); fungi (predominantly *Candida albicans*); *C. trachomatis*; mycoplasmas and ureaplasmas; and protozoa *(Trichomonas vaginalis* and *T. gondii).* The newborn is initially colonized on the skin; mucosal surfaces, including the nasopharynx, oropharynx, conjunctivae, umbilical cord, and external genitalia; and the gastrointestinal tract (from swallowing infected amniotic fluid or vaginal secretions). In most infants, the organisms proliferate at these sites without causing illness. A few infants become infected by direct extension from the sites of colonization (e.g., otitis media from nasopharyngeal colonization). Alternatively, invasion of the bloodstream can ensue, with subsequent dissemination of infection. The umbilical cord was a particularly common portal of entry for systemic infection before local disinfection methods became routine because the devitalized tissues are an excellent medium for bacterial growth and because thrombosed umbilical vessels provide direct access to the bloodstream. Microorganisms also can infect abrasions or skin wounds. At present, the most frequent routes for bloodstream invasion are the lung from aspirated infected amniotic fluid or vaginal contents and the gastrointestinal tract from transmigration of microbial flora across the gut wall.

Infants who develop bacterial sepsis often have specific risk factors absent in infants who do not develop significant infections. Among these factors are preterm delivery at gestational age less than 37 weeks, low birth weight, prolonged rupture of maternal membranes, maternal intra-amniotic infection, traumatic delivery, and fetal anoxia. Relative immaturity of the immune system is considered to be one factor increasing risk of infection during the neonatal period. The role of host defenses in neonatal infection is discussed in detail in Chapter 4.

Preterm birth is the most significant risk factor for acquisition of infections in infants immediately before or during delivery or in the nursery. Because of the increasing number of infants with extremely or very low birth weight, infection remains an important cause of morbidity and mortality. Expansion of treatments for infertility has continued to increase the number of pregnancies with multiple births (see Table 1-3), and a gestational age of less than 28 weeks is common in multiparity. A summary of 6215 very-low-birth-weight neonates (birth weight, 401 to 1500 g) from the National Institute of Child Health and Human Development Neonatal Research Network reported a 2% incidence of early-onset sepsis, 3% incidence of meningitis, and remarkable 36% incidence of blood culture–positive late-onset sepsis.[119] Infection rate was inversely correlated with birth weight and gestational age; rates of early-onset sepsis were 6% at 22 weeks and 1% at 28 weeks, and rates of late-onset sepsis were 58% at 22 weeks and 20% at 28 weeks. Mortality and morbidity were inversely related to gestational age regardless of whether the infant also experienced late-onset sepsis.

The effectiveness of certain innate host defense mechanisms of the neonate remains controversial. Vernix caseosa contains antimicrobial proteins (see Chapter 4), and retention of vernix probably provides a protective barrier to the skin. Breast milk influences the composition of the fecal flora by suppression of *E. coli* and other gram-negative enteric bacilli and encouragement of *Lactobacillus* growth. In addition, breast milk contains secretory IgA, lysozymes, white blood cells, and lactoferrin (an iron-binding protein that significantly inhibits the growth of *E. coli* and other microorganisms); however, the role of these constituents in mitigating colonization and systemic infection in the neonate acquired at or shortly after birth is uncertain (see Chapter 5).

The virulence of the invading microorganism is also a factor in the pathogenesis of neonatal sepsis. Certain phage types of *S. aureus* (types 80 and 81) were responsible for most cases of disease in the staphylococcal pandemic of the 1950s. Phage group 2 *S. aureus* strains have been responsible for staphylococcal scalded skin syndrome sometimes seen in neonates (toxic epidermal necrolysis). Other evidence suggests that the K1 capsular antigens of *E. coli* and type III strains of group B streptococcus possess virulence properties that enhance their propensity for invasion of the blood-brain barrier during bacteremia, compared with non-K1 and non–type III strains of the same species, respectively.

MICROBIOLOGY

The agents responsible for early-onset (before 7 days) neonatal sepsis are found in the maternal birth canal.[120,121] Most of these organisms are considered to be saprophytic but occasionally can be responsible for maternal infection and its sequelae, including endometritis and puerperal fever. Before the introduction of the sulfonamides and penicillin in the 1940s, gram-positive cocci, particularly group A streptococci, were responsible for most cases of neonatal sepsis. After the introduction of antimicrobial agents, gram-negative enterics, in particular *E. coli*, were the predominant causes of serious bacterial infections of the newborn. An increase in serious neonatal infection caused by group B streptococci was noted in the early 1970s, and group B streptococci and *E. coli* continue to be the most frequent causative agents for early-onset neonatal sepsis and late-onset sepsis in term infants. By contrast, late-onset (after 7 days) sepsis in preterm neonates, remaining in the neonatal intensive care unit for weeks or months, is typically caused by commensal organisms (e.g., coagulase-negative staphylococci and *Candida* spp.) and organisms acquired from the mother and from the nursery environment.

The bacteria responsible for neonatal sepsis are discussed in Chapter 6. Mycoplasmas, anaerobic bacteria, and viruses (including HSV, HBV, CMV, and HIV) that colonize the maternal genital tract are also acquired during birth.

DIAGNOSIS

Review of the maternal record provides important clues for diagnosis of infection in the neonate. Signs of illness during pregnancy; exposure to sexual partners with transmissible infections; and results of cultures (e.g., for *C. trachomatis*, *N. gonorrhoeae*, or group B streptococci), serologic tests (e.g., for HIV infection, rubella, HBV, hepatitis C virus, or syphilis), and tuberculin skin tests or chest radiographs should be identified in the pregnancy record. The delivery chart should be checked for peripartum events that indicate risk of sepsis in the neonate, including premature rupture of membranes; prolonged duration (>18 hours) of rupture of membranes; evidence of fetal distress and fever; or other signs of maternal infection, such as bloody diarrhea, respiratory or gastrointestinal signs (i.e., enterovirus), indications of large concentrations of pathogens in the genitourinary tract (as reflected in bacteriuria caused by group B streptococci), and evidence of invasive bacterial infections in prior pregnancies.

The clinical diagnosis of systemic infection in the newborn can be difficult because the initial signs of infection may be subtle and nonspecific. Not only are the signs of infectious and noninfectious processes similar, but also the signs of in utero infection are indistinguishable from signs of infections acquired during the birth process or during the first few days of life. Respiratory distress, lethargy, irritability, poor feeding, jaundice, emesis, and diarrhea are associated with various infectious and noninfectious causes.

Some clinical manifestations of neonatal sepsis, such as hepatomegaly, jaundice, pneumonitis, purpura, and meningitis, are common to many infections acquired in utero or during delivery. Certain signs are related to specific infections (see Tables 1-6 and 1-7). Many signs of congenital infection are not evident at birth. HBV infection should be considered in an infant with onset of jaundice and hepatosplenomegaly between 1 and 6 months of age; CMV infection acquired at or soon after delivery may be associated with an afebrile protracted pneumonitis; enterovirus infection should be considered in an infant with CSF pleocytosis in the first months of life. Most infants with congenital HIV infection do not have signs of disease during the first months of life. Uncommonly, signs may be present at birth. Srugo and colleagues[122] described an infant with signs of meningoencephalitis at 6 hours of life; HIV was subsequently isolated from CSF. Clinical manifestations associated with infection by specific agents are discussed in greater detail in the relevant chapters.

Most early-onset bacterial infections are nonfocal except in the circumstance of respiratory distress at or shortly after birth, in which the chest radiograph reveals pneumonia.

Focal infections are frequent with late-onset neonatal sepsis and include otitis media, pneumonia, soft tissue infections, urinary tract infections, septic arthritis, osteomyelitis, and peritonitis. Bacterial meningitis is of particular concern because of the substantial mortality rate and the significant morbidity in survivors. Few infants have overt meningeal signs, and a high index of suspicion and examination of the CSF are required for early diagnosis.

Available routine laboratory methods can provide limited assistance in the diagnosis of systemic infections in the newborn infant, as described in Chapter 36. Immunoglobulin is produced by the fetus and newborn infant in response to infection, and increased levels of IgM have been measured in the serum of newborns with infections acquired transplacentally (i.e., syphilis, rubella, cytomegalic inclusion disease, toxoplasmosis, and malaria). Increased levels of IgM may also result from postnatally acquired bacterial infections. Not all infected infants have increased levels of serum IgM, however, and some infants who do have elevated concentrations of total IgM are apparently uninfected; thus increased levels of total IgM are neither sufficiently specific nor sensitive for clinical decision making.

Because inflammation of the placenta and umbilical cord may accompany peripartum sepsis, pathologic examination of sections of these tissues may assist in the diagnosis of infection in the newborn. Histologic evidence of inflammation may also be noted in the absence of evidence of neonatal sepsis, however. In the immediate postnatal period, gastric aspirate, pharyngeal mucus, or fluid from the external ear canal has been used to delineate exposure to potential pathogens, but are not useful in the diagnosis of neonatal sepsis.

Isolation of microorganisms from a usually sterile site, such as blood, CSF, or skin vesicle fluid, or from a suppurative lesion or a sterilely obtained sample of urine remains the only valid method of diagnosing systemic infection. Aspiration of any focus of infection in a critically ill infant (e.g., needle aspiration of middle ear fluid in an infant with otitis media or from the joint or metaphysis of an infant with osteoarthritis) should be performed to determine the etiologic agent. In infants with very low birth weight, commensal microorganisms, such as coagulase-negative staphylococci, *Enterococcus*, or *Candida*, isolated from a usually sterile body site should be considered pathogens until proven otherwise. Culture of infectious agents from the nose, throat, skin, umbilicus, or stool indicates colonization; these agents may include the pathogens that are responsible for the disease but, in themselves, do not establish the presence of active systemic infection.

PCR assays are useful to detect the nucleic acid of various important pathogens, including viruses and *Pneumocystis jirovecii*. When appropriate, serologic studies should be performed to ascertain the presence of in utero or postnatal infection for pathogens, such as HIV, rubella, parvovirus B19, *T. gondii*, and *T. pallidum*. For some of these infections (e.g., rubella), the diagnostic serologic assay measures IgG. To distinguish passively transferred maternal antibody from antibody derived from infection in the neonate, it is necessary to obtain two blood specimens from the infant. Because the half-life of IgG is estimated to be 23 days, the first sample is obtained soon after birth, and the second sample should be obtained at least two half-lives, or approximately 6 weeks, after the first specimen. Measurement of IgM antibody provides evidence of current infection in the neonate, but none of these assays has proven reliability at present.

MANAGEMENT

Successful management of neonatal bacterial sepsis depends on a high index of suspicion based on maternal history and infant signs, prompt initiation of appropriate antimicrobial therapy while diagnostic tests are performed, and meticulous supportive measures. If the physician suspects bacterial infection in a newborn, culture specimens should be obtained, and treatment with appropriate antimicrobial agents should be initiated immediately. In general, initial therapy must provide coverage against gram-positive cocci, particularly group B and other streptococci, *Listeria monocytogenes*, and gram-negative enteric bacilli. Ampicillin is the preferred agent with effectiveness against gram-positive cocci and *L. monocytogenes*. Most experts prefer ampicillin and gentamicin therapy for early-onset presumptive sepsis and for initial therapy for *E. coli*, GBS, and *L. monocytogenes* infections, with the addition of cefotaxime for presumptive bacterial meningitis.[7] The choice of therapy for gram-negative infections depends on the current pattern of antimicrobial susceptibility in the local community. Intrapartum antimicrobial therapy can yield drug concentrations in the blood of the newborn infant sufficient to suppress growth of group B streptococci and possibly other susceptible organisms in blood obtained for culture. An algorithm has been devised to guide empirical management of neonates born to mothers who received intrapartum antimicrobial prophylaxis for prevention of early-onset GBS infection or in whom prophylaxis was indicated but not given at least 4 hours before delivery,[7] and the algorithm is discussed in Chapter 12.

The choice of antibacterial drugs should be reviewed when results of cultures and susceptibility tests become available. The clinician should take care to select drugs that have been studied for appropriate dose, interval of dosing, and safety in neonates, especially for very-low-birth-weight infants, and that have the narrowest antimicrobial spectrum that would be effective (see Chapter 37). The duration of therapy depends on the initial response to the appropriate antibiotics—typically 10 days in most infants with sepsis, pneumonia, or minimal or absent focal infection; a minimum of 14 days for uncomplicated meningitis caused by group B streptococci or *L. monocytogenes*; and 21 days for gram-negative enteric bacilli.[123] The clinical pharmacology of antibiotics administered to the newborn infant is unique and cannot be extrapolated from adult data on absorption, excretion, and toxicity. The safety of new antimicrobial agents is a particular concern because toxic effects may not be detected until several years later (see Chapter 37).

Development of antimicrobial drug resistance in microbial pathogens is a constant concern. Group B streptococci remain uniformly susceptible to penicillins and cephalosporins, but many isolates now are resistant to erythromycin and clindamycin.[124] Administration of one or two doses of a penicillin or cephalosporin as part of a peripartum prophylactic regimen for prevention of GBS infection in the neonate should not significantly affect the genital flora, but monitoring should be continued to detect alterations in flora and antibiotic susceptibility. Because the nursery is a small, closed community, development of resistance is a greater concern with nosocomial infections than with infections acquired in utero or at delivery.

Antiviral therapies are available for newborns infected with HSV (acyclovir), VZV (acyclovir), HIV (combination antiretroviral therapy), and overtly symptomatic CMV (ganciclovir or valganciclovir). Because early use of acyclovir for herpes simplex infections in neonates has been associated with improved outcome, physicians may choose to begin therapy for presumptive HSV disease and reevaluate when information on clinical course and results of cultures and PCR assay become available. A phase II trial examining safety, pharmacodynamics, and efficacy of ganciclovir treatment for symptomatic congenital CMV infection established the safe dose in infants and showed an antiviral effect with suppression of viruria.[125, 126] Neutropenia (63%), thrombocytopenia, and altered hepatic enzymes were noted in most of the infants, with nearly half of the infants requiring dosage adjustments because of severe neutropenia. A phase III randomized, controlled trial of intravenous ganciclovir for 6 weeks in 100 CMV-infected infants with central nervous system involvement at birth showed that ganciclovir treatment maintained hearing or allowed hearing improvement in 84% of infants, compared with 41% of control infants[126]; neurodevelopmental delays were also significantly reduced at 6 and 12 months of age in the treated compared to the control infants.[127] Twice daily oral valganciclovir administered for 6 weeks or 6 months twice daily in amounts expected to achieve blood concentrations of valganciclovir (VGCV) comparable to those achieved with intravenous ganciclovir in the phase III trial is currently being evaluated by the National Institute of Allergy and Infectious Diseases Collaborative Antiviral Study Group. Preliminary results suggest that 6 months of oral VGCV with symptomatic congenital CMV improves audiologic and neurodevelopmental outcomes through at least 2 years of age.[128] The use of hyperimmune gamma globulin preparations to prevent or modify perinatal infections have been used with some success after newborn exposure to some pathogens, such as varicella, but with equivocal results for others, such as cytomegalovirus.[129-131] Further information regarding treatment of these infections is provided in the relevant chapters.

PREVENTION

Immunoprophylaxis

Passive immunoprophylaxis with specific hyperimmune immunoglobulin or monoclonal antibody preparations is indicated for the prevention of hepatitis B, varicella, and respiratory syncytial virus infection in infants at risk for these infections. Details are provided in Chapter 38.

Universal immunization of infants with hepatitis B vaccine has been recommended by the AAP since 1992.[132] Prior strategies of selective vaccination in high-risk populations and serologic screening of all pregnant women for HBsAg had little impact on control of HBV infections or their sequelae, and public health authorities believe that infant immunization offers the most feasible approach to universal protection and eventual eradication of the disease. Infants born to HBsAg-positive women should be immunized at birth and receive hepatitis B immunoglobulin at or shortly after birth. This prevention strategy may be improved if a birth dose of hepatitis B vaccine is universally recommended, providing additional coverage for infants whose maternal records are incorrect or unavailable before hospital discharge.

Chemoprophylaxis

After administration to the mother, antimicrobial agents capable of crossing biologic membranes can achieve pharmacologic concentrations in the fetus comparable with concentrations in well-vascularized maternal tissues. Prevention of newborn GBS infection by administration of ampicillin to the mother was first shown by Boyer and colleagues[133] and other investigators in 1983 (see Chapter 12). A prevention strategy initially recommended by the AAP in 1992[134] was revised in 1997, and current recommendations from the CDC are endorsed by the AAP, the American College of Obstetricians and Gynecologists, and the American Academy of Family Physicians. These organizations recommend universal culture screening of all pregnant women at 35 to 37 weeks of gestation and administration of intravenous penicillin during labor to those who are culture positive, the only exception being women with GBS bacteriuria during pregnancy or women who have had a previous neonate with invasive GBS infection; these groups should always receive intravenous penicillin during labor.[7]

Fetal drug concentrations can exceed 30% of the maternal blood concentrations,[135] and concentrations bactericidal against group B streptococci can be achieved in amniotic fluid 3 hours after a maternal dose (see Chapters 12 and 37). Parenteral antimicrobial therapy administered to the mother in labor essentially treats the fetus earlier in the course of the intrapartum infection. If the fetus has been infected, the regimen is treatment, not prophylaxis, and for some infected fetuses, the treatment administered in utero is insufficient to prevent early-onset GBS disease.[136]

Other modes of chemoprophylaxis administered to the neonate include ophthalmic drops or ointments for prevention of gonococcal ophthalmia and antiretroviral therapy for infants born to HIV-infected mothers. Empirical administration of antibacterial agents to infants with minimal or ambiguous clinical signs is considered therapy for presumed sepsis and should not be considered prophylaxis.

Infections of the Newborn Infant in the First Month of Life

When fever or other signs of systemic infection occur in the first weeks or months of life, various sources of infection should be considered: (1) congenital infections with onset in utero; (2) infections acquired during the birth process from the maternal genital tract; (3) infections acquired in the nursery; (4) infections acquired in the household after discharge from the nursery; and (5) infection that suggests an anatomic defect, underlying immunologic disease, or metabolic abnormality.

PATHOGENESIS AND MICROBIOLOGY

Congenital Infections

Signs of congenital infection may not appear for weeks, months, or years after birth. Diagnosis and management are discussed in the disease chapters.

Infections Acquired During Delivery

Although maternal intrapartum prophylaxis has reduced the incidence of early-onset GBS disease (by >80% in a Pittsburgh survey),[137] the regimen has had no impact on the incidence of late-onset disease,[138] with signs occurring from 6 to 89 days of life and up to 6 months of age in infants with very low birth weight. The pathogenesis of late-onset GBS disease remains obscure, but it is likely that even when vertical transmission from the mother at birth is prevented, exposure to either the mother (in whom colonization resumes after delivery) or other colonized family members and caregivers can serve as a source for colonization through direct contact. It is unknown why sepsis develops without warning in an infant who has no risk factors for sepsis and was well for days to weeks; this concern also is relevant in infants who acquire late-onset disease as a result of *E. coli* and *L. monocytogenes*.

Nursery-Acquired Infections

After arrival in the nursery, the newborn may become infected by various mechanisms involving either human carriers or contaminated materials and equipment. Human sources in the hospital include personnel, mothers, and other infants. The methods of transmission may include the following:

- Respiratory droplet spread from adults or other newborn infants. Outbreaks of respiratory virus infections, including influenza, respiratory syncytial, and parainfluenza viruses, in prolonged-stay nurseries are frequent.[136] Methods for identification and control are provided in Chapter 35.
- Carriage of the microorganism on the hands of hospital personnel. A study has suggested that the hands may be not only a means of transmission, but also a significant reservoir of bacteria.[139]
- Suppurative lesions. Although spread of staphylococcal and streptococcal infections to infants or mothers may be associated with asymptomatic carriers, the most serious outbreaks have been caused by a member of the medical or nursing staff with a significant lesion.
- Human milk. CMV, HIV, HSV, hepatitis C virus, HTLV-1,[140] HTLV-2,[141] and HBsAg have been identified in mother's milk and may be transmitted to the neonate by this route. CMV-infected milk from banks can be dangerous for infants lacking passively transferred maternal antibody, especially among premature infants. The risk of breast-milk transmission of hepatitis C appears to be low and avoidance of breastfeeding by a hepatitis C infected mother is not recommended.

Breast-milk transmission of HIV is of concern because of the importance of breastfeeding in providing nutrition and immunologic protection in the first year of life. Breast milk has been documented as the likely source of HIV infection in neonates whose mothers were transfused with HIV-infected blood after delivery or in whom disease developed postpartum through sexual contact.[142] Because of the importance of breastfeeding for infant nutrition and survival, WHO guidelines for infant feeding of HIV-exposed infants living in resource-poor settings recommend exclusive breastfeeding through 6 months, with extended breastfeeding through 12 months, and several antiretroviral options for prevention of mother to child transmission.[143-145] By contrast, in the United States and Western Europe, HIV-infected mothers are discouraged from breastfeeding because other forms of nutrition are available.[146] The recommendation also notes that in some regions and cultures, women are stigmatized for not breastfeeding, and alternatives such as formula are unaffordable or unsafe. The number of antenatal women in developing countries that lack resources for prevention in pregnancy has reached alarming proportions: 70% of women at a prenatal clinic in Zimbabwe and 30% of women in urban areas in six African countries were infected. The United Nations survey indicated that by 2000, breastfeeding would be responsible for more than one third (>200,000) of children newly infected with HIV, unless some attempts were made to limit this route of transmission.[147] Current efforts to prevent breastfeeding transmission include improved universal testing of pregnant women for HIV infection as well as dissemination of prophylactic regimens for pregnant women and their newborns.[148] However, availability of such regimens appears to be limited to approximately 45% of HIV-infected pregnant women in low- and middle-income countries.[149]

Infection of breast milk by bacterial pathogens, such as *S. aureus*, group B streptococci, *L. monocytogenes*,[150] and *Salmonella* spp., can result in neonatal disease. Bacteria that are components of skin flora, including *Staphylococcus epidermidis* and α-hemolytic streptococci, are frequently cultured from freshly expressed human milk and are unlikely to be associated with disease in the breastfed infant. Other possible sources of infection in the nursery include the following:

- Blood used for replacement or exchange transfusion in neonates should be screened for safety using validated, efficacious methods, including tests for hepatitis B antigen and anti–hepatitis B core antibody, hepatitis C antibody and nucleic acids, HIV antibody and nucleic acids, West Nile Virus nucleic acids, HTLV-1 and HTLV-2 antibodies, CMV antibody, *Trypanosoma cruzi*, and *Plasmodium* spp. in malaria-endemic areas.
- Equipment has been implicated in common-source nursery outbreaks, usually including contaminated solutions used in nebulization equipment, room humidifiers, and bathing solutions. Several gram-negative bacteria, including *Pseudomonas aeruginosa*, *Serratia marcescens*, and *Flavobacterium*, are able to multiply in aqueous environments at room temperature. In recent years, few solution-related or equipment-related outbreaks caused by these organisms have been reported because of the scrupulous infection control practices enforced in most intensive care nurseries.
- Catheterization of the umbilical vein and artery has been associated with sepsis, umbilical cellulitis, and abscess formation, but careful hygienic practices with insertion

of these devices make these complications rare. Intravenous alimentation using central venous catheters has been lifesaving for some infants, but also is associated with increased risk for catheter-related bacteremia or fungemia.

- Parenteral feeding with lipid emulsions has been associated with neonatal sepsis caused by coagulase-negative staphylococci and *Candida* and *Malassezia* spp. Strains of staphylococci isolated from infected ventricular shunts or intravascular catheters produce a biofilm that promotes adherence and growth of colonies on the surfaces and in the walls of catheters manufactured with synthetic polymers. The biofilm also protects the bacteria against antibiotics and phagocytosis. The introduction of lipid emulsion through the venous catheter provides nutrients for growth of the bacteria and fungi.[151]

Hand hygiene remains the most important element in controlling the spread of infectious diseases in the nursery (see Chapter 35). Hand hygiene measures should be implemented before and after every patient contact. Surveys of hospital employees indicate that rigorous adherence to hand hygiene, although the most simple of infection control techniques, is still lacking in most institutions. A study by Brown and colleagues[152] in a Denver neonatal intensive care unit indicated that compliance with appropriate hand-washing techniques was low for medical and nursing personnel. Compliance was monitored using a direct observation technique; of 252 observed encounters of nurses, physicians, and respiratory therapists with infants, 25% of the personnel broke contact with the infant by touching self (69%) or touching another infant (4%), and 25% did not wash before patient contact.

Waterless, alcohol-based hand hygiene products are routinely used in nurseries, with surveys indicating their rapid acceptance by nursery personnel, including physicians. Their ease of application and time saved through reduction in the need for hand washing should increase adherence with hand hygiene recommendations.

Community-Acquired Infections

The newborn infant is susceptible to many of the infectious agents that colonize other members of the household and caregivers. The physician should consider illnesses in these contacts before discharging an infant from the hospital. If signs of an infectious disease develop after 15 to 30 days of life in an infant who was healthy at discharge and had no significant risk factors during gestation or delivery, the infection was probably acquired from a household or community contact. Suppurative lesions related to *S. aureus* in a household member can expose an infant to a virulent strain capable of disseminated infection. A careful history of illness in family members can suggest the source of the infant's disease (e.g., respiratory viruses, skin infections, prolonged illness with coughing).

Conversely, an infant can be a source of infection for household contacts. An infant with congenital rubella syndrome can shed virus for many months and is a significant source of infection for susceptible close contacts. The same is true for an infant with vesicular lesions of herpes simplex or a syphilitic infant with rhinitis or skin rash.

Infections That Indicate Underlying Abnormalities

Infection may serve as a first clue indicating an underlying anatomic, metabolic, or immune system abnormality. Infants with galactosemia, iron overload, chronic granulomatous disease, and leukocyte adhesion defects are susceptible to certain invasive bacterial infections. Genitourinary infection in the first months of life can suggest an anatomic or a physiologic defect of the urinary tract. Similarly, otitis media in the first month of life may be an indication of a midline defect of the palate or a eustachian tube dysfunction. Meningitis caused by agents that are less invasive (e.g., coagulase-negative staphylococci) can be a clue to the presence of a dermoid sinus tract to the intradural space. In infants with underlying humoral immune defects, systemic infections may not develop until passively acquired maternal antibody has dissipated. Because the half-life of IgG is about 3 weeks, such infections are likely to occur after 3 months of age.

References

1. Hamilton BE, Hoyert DL, Martin JA, et al: Annual summary of vital statistics: 2010-2011, *Pediatrics* 131:548-558, 2013.
2. Lawn JE, Kerber K, Enweronu-Laryea C, Cousens S: 3.6 million neonatal deaths— what is progressing and what is not? *Semin Perinatol* 34:371-386, 2010.
3. Tartof SY, Lewis M, Kenyon C, et al: Waning immunity to pertussis following 5 doses of DTaP, *Pediatrics* 131:e1047-e1052, 2013.
4. Witt MA, Arias L, Katz PH, et al: Reduced risk of pertussis among persons ever vaccinated with whole cell pertussis vaccine compared to recipients of acellular pertussis vaccines in a large US cohort, *Clin Infect Dis* 56:1248-1254, 2013.
5. U.S. Food and Drug Administration: Med Bull 8, Summer 1998.
6. Kata A: Anti-vaccine activists, Web 2.0, and the postmodern paradigm—an overview of tactics and tropes used online by the anti-vaccination movement. *Vaccine* 30:3778-3789, 2012.
7. Pickering LK, editor: *Red book: report of the Committee on Infectious Diseases*, ed 29, Elk Grove Village, Ill, 2012, American Academy of Pediatrics.
8. American Academy of Pediatrics Committee on Pediatric AIDS: HIV testing and prophylaxis to prevent mother-to-child transmission in the United States, *Pediatrics* 122:1127-1134, 2008.
9. Sullivan JL: Prevention of mother-to-child transmission of HIV—what next? *J Acquir Immune Defic Syndr* 34((Suppl 1):S67-S72, 2003.
10. World Health Organization: Expert consultation on new and emerging evidence on the use of antiretroviral drugs for the prevention of mother-to-child transmission of HIV, November 17-19, 2008. Available at http://www.who.int/hiv/topics/mtct/mtct_conclusions_consult.pdf. Accessed April 21, 2014.
11. Centers for Disease Control and Prevention: Congenital syphilis—United States, 2000, *MMWR Morb Mortal Wkly Rep* 50:573-577, 2001.
12. Centers for Disease Control and Prevention: Sexually transmitted disease surveillance, 2007—syphilis, 2008. Available at http://cdc.gov/std/stats07/syphilis.htm.
13. Centers for Disease Control and Prevention: Control and prevention of rubella: evaluation and management of suspected outbreaks, rubella in pregnant women, and surveillance for congenital rubella syndrome, *MMWR Recomm. Rep* 50(RR-12):1-23, 2001.
14. Mellor AL, Chandler P, Lee GK, et al: Indoleamine 2,3-dioxygenase, immunosuppression and pregnancy, *J Reprod Immunol* 57:143-150, 2002.
15. Xu C, Mao D, Holers VM, et al: A critical role for murine complement regulator crry in fetomaternal tolerance, *Science* 287:498-501, 2000.
16. Rowe JH, Ertelt JM, Xin L, Way SS: Pregnancy imprints regulatory memory that sustains anergy to fetal antigen, *Nature* 490:102-106, 2012.
17. Gaunt G, Ramin K: Immunological tolerance of the human fetus, *Am J Perinatol* 18:299-312, 2001.

18. Chaouat G, Zourbas S, Ostojic S, et al: A brief review of recent data on some cytokine expressions at the materno-foetal interface which might challenge the classical TH1/TH2 dichotomy, *J Reprod Immunol* 53:241-256, 2002.
19. Chheda S, Lopez SM, Sanderson EP: Congenital brucellosis in a premature infant, *Pediatr Infect Dis J* 16:81-83, 1997.
20. Carcopino A, Raoult D, Bretelle F, Boubli L, Stein A: Managing Q fever during pregnancy: the benefits of long-term cotrimoxazole therapy, *Clin Infect Dis* 45:548-555, 2007.
21. New DL, Quinn JB, Qureshi MZ, Sigler SJ: Vertically transmitted babesiosis, *J Pediatr* 131:163-164, 1997.
22. Fujino T, Nagata Y: HTLV-I transmission from mother to child, *J Reprod Immunol* 47:197-206, 2000.
23. Van Dyke RB, Heneine W, Perrin ME, et al: Mother-to-child transmission of human T-lymphotropic virus type II, *J Pediatr* 127:924-928, 1995.
24. Schroter M, Polywka S, Zöllner B, et al: Detection of TT virus DNA and GB virus type C/hepatitis G virus RNA in serum and breast milk: determination of mother-to-child transmission, *J Clin Microbiol* 38:745-747, 2000.
25. Feucht HH, Zollner B, Polywka S, Laufs R: Vertical transmission of hepatitis G, *Lancet* 347:615-616, 1996.
26. Adams O, Krempe C, Kögler G, et al: Congenital infections with human herpesvirus 6, *J Infect Dis* 178:544-546, 1998.
27. Lanari M, Papa I, Venturi V, et al: Congenital infection with human herpesvirus 6 variant B associated with neonatal seizures and poor neurological outcome, *J Med Virol* 70:628-632, 2003.
28. Chye JK, Lim CT, Ng KB, et al: Vertical transmission of dengue, *Clin Infect Dis* 25:1374-1377, 1997.
29. Boden K, Brueckman A, Wagner-Wiening C, et al: Maternofetal consequences of *Coxiella burnetii* infection in pregnancy: a case series of two outbreaks, *BMC Infect Dis* 12:359, 2012.
30. Overturf GD, Balfour G: Osteomyelitis and sepsis: severe complications of fetal monitoring, *Pediatrics* 55:244-247, 1975.
31. King-Lewis PA, Gardner SD: Congenital cytomegalic inclusion disease following intrauterine transfusion, *BMJ* 2:603-605, 1969.
32. Scott JM, Henderson A: Acute villous inflammation in the placenta following intrauterine transfusion, *J Clin Pathol* 25:872-875, 1972.
33. Centers for Disease Control and Prevention: Congenital syphilis—United States, 2003-2008, *MMWR Morb Mortal Wkly Rep* 59:413-417, 2010.
34. St Clair EH, DiLiberti JH, O'Brien ML: Letter: observations of an infant born to a mother with botulism, *J Pediatr* 87:658, 1975.
35. Robin L, Herman D, Redett R: Botulism in pregnant women, *N Engl J Med* 335:823-824, 1996.
36. Luijckx GJ, Vles J, de Baets M, et al: Guillain-Barré syndrome in mother and newborn child, *Lancet* 349:27, 1997.
37. Buchwald B, de Baets M, Luijckx GJ, Toyka KV: Neonatal Guillain-Barré syndrome: blocking antibodies transmitted from mother to child, *Neurology* 53:1246-1253, 1999.
38. Naeye RL: Causes of the excessive rates of perinatal mortality and prematurity in pregnancies complicated by maternal urinary-tract infections, *N Engl J Med* 300:819-823, 1979.
39. Savage WE, Hajj SN, Kass EH: Demographic and prognostic characteristics of bacteriuria in pregnancy, *Medicine (Baltimore)* 46:385-407, 1967.
40. Smaill F: Antibiotics for asymptomatic bacteriuria in pregnancy, *Cochrane Database Syst*, 2001. Rev. (2):CD000490.
41. Millar LK, Cox SM: Urinary tract infections complicating pregnancy, *Infect Dis Clin North Am* 11:13-26, 1997.
42. Shearer WT, Schreiner RL, Marshall RE, Barton LL: Cytomegalovirus infection in a newborn dizygous twin, *J Pediatr* 81:1161-1165, 1972.
43. Stokes JH, Beerman H: *Modern clinical syphilology, diagnosis, treatment: case study*, Philadelphia, 1968, WB Saunders.
44. Ray CG, Wedgwood RJ: Neonatal listeriosis: six case reports and a review of the literature, *Pediatrics* 34:378-392, 1964.
45. Marsden JP, Greenfield CRM: Inherited smallpox, *Arch Dis Child* 9:309, 1934.
46. Forrester RM, Lees VT, Watson GH: Rubella syndrome: escape of a twin, *BMJ* 1:1403, 1966.
47. Feldman GV: Herpes zoster neonatorum, *Arch Dis Child* 27:126-127, 1952.
48. Wilcox AJ, Weinberg CR, O'Connor JF, et al: Incidence of early loss of pregnancy, *N Engl J Med* 319:189-194, 1988.
49. Brabin BJ: Epidemiology of infection in pregnancy, *Rev Infect Dis* 7:579-603, 1985.
50. Hillier SL, Witkin SS, Krohn MA, et al: The relationship of amniotic fluid cytokines and preterm delivery, amniotic fluid infection, histologic chorioamnionitis, and chorioamnion infection, *Obstet Gynecol* 81:941-948, 1993.
51. Hitti J, Riley DE, Krohn MA, et al: Broad-spectrum bacterial rDNA polymerase chain reaction assay for detecting amniotic fluid infection among women in premature labor, *Clin Infect Dis* 24:1228-1232, 1997.
52. Romero R, Yoon BH, Mazor M, et al: The diagnostic and prognostic value of amniotic fluid white blood cell count, glucose, interleukin-6, and Gram stain in patients with preterm labor and intact membranes, *Am J Obstet Gynecol* 169:805-816, 1993.
53. Romero R, Yoon BH, Mazor M, et al: A comparative study of the diagnostic performance of amniotic fluid glucose, white blood cell count, interleukin-6, and Gram stain in the detection of microbial invasion in patients with preterm premature rupture of membranes, *Am J Obstet Gynecol* 169:839-851, 1993.
54. Roper EC, Konje JC, De Chazal RC, et al: Genetic amniocentesis: gestation-specific pregnancy outcome and comparison of outcome following early and traditional amniocentesis, *Prenat Diagn* 19:803-807, 1999.
55. Jacobsson B, Mattsby-Baltzer I, Andersch B, et al: Microbial invasion and cytokine response in amniotic fluid in a Swedish population of women in preterm labor, *Acta Obstet Gynecol Scand* 82:120-128, 2003.
56. Donders GG, Guashcino S, Peters K, Tacchi R, Lauro V; for the VARIANT1 Study Group: A multicenter, double-blind, randomized, placebo-controlled study of rifaximin for the treatment of bacterial vaginosis. *Int J Gynaecol Obstet* 120:131-136, 2013.
57. Capoccia R, Greub G, Baud D: Ureaplasma urealyticum, mycoplasma hominis and adverse pregnancy outcomes, *Curr Opin Infect Dis* 26:231-240, 2013.
58. Brocklehurst P, Gordon A, Heatley E, Milan SJ: Antibiotics for treating bacterial vaginosis in pregnancy, *Cochrane Database Syst* Rev 1:CD000262, 2013
59. Lamont RF, Nhan-Chang CL, Sobel JD, et al: Treatment of abnormal vaginal flora in early pregnancy with clindamycin for the prevention of spontaneous preterm birth: a systematic review and metaanalysis, *Am J Obstet Gynecol* 205:177-190, 2011.
60. Naeye RL, Blanc W: Pathogenesis of congenital rubella, *JAMA* 194:1277-1283, 1965.
61. Naeye RL: Cytomegalic inclusion disease: the fetal disorder, *Am J Clin Pathol* 47:738-744, 1967.
62. Naeye RL, Kelly JA: Judgment of fetal age. 3. The pathologist's evaluation, *Pediatr Clin North Am* 13:849-862, 1966.
63. Naeye RL: Infants of prolonged gestation: a necropsy study, *Arch Pathol* 84:37-41, 1967.
64. Allison AC, Paton GR: Chromosomal abnormalities in human diploid cells infected with mycoplasma and their possible relevance to the aetiology of Down's syndrome (mongolism), *Lancet* 2:1229-1230, 1966.
65. Nichols WW: The role of viruses in the etiology of chromosomal abnormalities, *Am J Hum Genet* 18:81-92, 1966.
66. Nusbacher J, Hirschhorn K, Cooper LZ: Chromosomal abnormalities in congenital rubella, *N Engl J Med* 276:1409-1413, 1967.
67. Centers for Disease Control and Prevention: Congenital malaria in children of refugees—Washington, Massachusetts, Kentucky, *MMWR Morb Mortal Wkly Rep* 30:53-55, 1981.
68. Nesheim S, Palumbo P, Sullivan K, et al: Quantitative RNA testing for diagnosis of HIV-infected infants, *J Acquir Immune Defic Syndr* 32:192-195, 2003.
69. Shetty AK, Maldonado Y: Antiretroviral drugs to prevent mother-to-child transmission of HIV during breastfeeding, *Curr HIV Res* 11:102-125, 2013.
70. Coovadia HM, Brown ER, Fowler MG, et al: for the HPTN 046 protocol team: Efficacy and safety of an extended nevirapine regimen in infant children of breastfeeding mothers with HIV-1 infection for prevention of postnatal HIV-1 transmission (HPTN 046): a randomized, double-blind, placebo-controlled trial. *Lancet* 379:221-228, 2012.
71. Wilson CB, Remington JS, Stagno S, Reynolds DW: Development of adverse sequelae in children with subclinical congenital *Toxoplasma* infection, *Pediatrics* 66:767-774, 1980.

72. Townsend JJ, Baringer JR, Wolinsky JS, et al: Progressive rubella panencephalitis: late onset after congenital rubella, *N Engl J Med* 292:990-993, 1975.
73. Weil ML, Itabashi H, Cremer NE, et al: Chronic progressive panencephalitis due to rubella virus simulating subacute sclerosing panencephalitis, *N Engl J Med* 292:994-998, 1975.
74. Donders GG, Van Lierde S, Van Elsacker-Niele AM, et al: Survival after intrauterine parvovirus B19 infection with persistence in early infancy: a two-year follow-up, *Pediatr Infect Dis J* 13:234-236, 1994.
75. Miller E, Cradock-Watson JE, Pollock TM: Consequences of confirmed maternal rubella at successive stages of pregnancy, *Lancet* 2:781-784, 1982.
76. Desmonts G, Couvreur J: 1979 Congenital toxoplasmosis: a prospective study of the offspring of 542 women who acquired toxoplasmosis during pregnancy. In Thalhammer O, Baumgarten K, Pollack A, editors: *Pathophysiology of congenital disease*, Stuttgart, 1979, Georg Thieme, pp 51-60.
77. Fowler KB, Stagno S, Pass RF, et al: The outcome of congenital cytomegalovirus infection in relation to maternal antibody status, *N Engl J Med* 326:663-667, 1992.
78. Stagno S, Whitley RJ: Herpesvirus infections of pregnancy. Part I. Cytomegalovirus and Epstein-Barr virus infections, *N Engl J Med* 313:1270-1274, 1985.
79. Roongpisuthipong A, Siriwasin W, Simonds RJ, et al: HIV seroconversion during pregnancy and risk for mother-to-infant transmission, *J Acquir Immune Defic Syndr* 26:348-351, 2001.
80. Green DM, Reid SM, Rhaney K: Generalised vaccinia in the human foetus, *Lancet* 1:1296-1298, 1966.
81. Sharma R, Jagdev DK: Congenital smallpox, *Scand J Infect Dis* 3:245-247, 1971.
82. Eilard T, Strannegard O: Rubella reinfection in pregnancy followed by transmission to the fetus, *J Infect Dis* 129:594-596, 1974.
83. Harvey B, Remington JS, Sulzer AJ: IgM malaria antibodies in a case of congenital malaria in the United States, *Lancet* 1:333-335, 1969.
84. Nelson NA, Struve VR: Prevention of congenital syphilis by treatment of syphilis in pregnancy, *JAMA* 161:869-872, 1956.
85. Zuckerman AJ, Taylor PE: Persistence of the serum hepatitis (SH-Australia) antigen for many years, *Nature* 223:81-82, 1969.
86. Nahmias AJ, Alford CA, Korones SB: Infection of the newborn with herpesvirus hominis, *Adv Pediatr* 17:185-226, 1970.
87. Desmonts G, Couvreur J, Thulliez P: Congenital toxoplasmosis: 5 cases of mother-to-child transmission of pre-pregnancy infection, *Presse Med* 19:1445-1449, 1990.
88. Vogel N, Kirisits M, Michael E, et al: Congenital toxoplasmosis transmitted from an immunologically competent mother infected before conception, *Clin Infect Dis* 23:1055-1060, 1996.
89. Centers for Disease Control and Prevention: Hepatitis B virus: a comprehensive strategy for eliminating transmission in the United States through universal childhood vaccination. Recommendations of the Immunization Practices Advisory Committee (ACIP), *MMWR Recomm Rep* 40(RR-13):1-25, 1991.
90. Daffos F, Capella-Pavlovsky M, Forestier F: Fetal blood sampling via the umbilical cord using a needle guided by ultrasound: report of 66 cases, *Prenat Diagn* 3:271-277, 1983.
91. Daffos F, Forestier F, Grangeot-Keros L, et al: Prenatal diagnosis of congenital rubella, *Lancet* 2:1-3, 1984.
92. Daffos F, Forestier F, Capella-Pavlovsky M, et al: Prenatal management of 746 pregnancies at risk for congenital toxoplasmosis, *N Engl J Med* 318:271-275, 1988.
93. Hohlfeld P, Vial Y, Maillard-Brignon C, et al: Cytomegalovirus fetal infection: prenatal diagnosis, *Obstet Gynecol* 78:615-618, 1991.
94. Grangeot-Keros L, Pillot J, Daffos F, Forestier F: Prenatal and postnatal production of IgM and IgA antibodies to rubella virus studied by antibody capture immunoassay, *J Infect Dis* 158:138-143, 1988.
95. Hanson FW, Happ RL, Tennant FR, et al: Ultrasonography-guided early amniocentesis in singleton pregnancies, *Am J Obstet Gynecol* 162:1376-1381, 1990.
96. Ghidini A, Sepulveda W, Lockwood CJ, Romero R: Complications of fetal blood sampling, *Am J Obstet Gynecol* 168:1339-1344, 1993.
97. Skvorc-Ranko R, Lavoie H, St-Denis P, et al: Intrauterine diagnosis of cytomegalovirus and rubella infections by amniocentesis, *Can Med Assoc J* 145:649-654, 1991.
98. Papaevangelou G, Kremastinou T, Prevedourakis C, Kaskarelis D: Hepatitis B antigen and antibody in maternal blood, cord blood, and amniotic fluid, *Arch Dis Child* 49:936-939, 1974.
99. Torok TJ, Wang QY, Gary GW Jr, et al: Prenatal diagnosis of intrauterine infection with parvovirus B19 by the polymerase chain reaction technique, *Clin Infect Dis* 14:149-155, 1992.
100. Wattre P, Dewilde A, Subtil D, et al: A clinical and epidemiological study of human parvovirus B19 infection in fetal hydrops using PCR Southern blot hybridization and chemiluminescence detection, *J Med Virol* 54:140-144, 1998.
101. Lazzarotto T, Varani S, Guerra B, et al: Prenatal indicators of congenital cytomegalovirus infection, *J Pediatr* 137:90-95, 2000.
102. Lazzarotto T, Gabrielli L, Foschini MP, et al: Congenital cytomegalovirus infection in twin pregnancies: viral load in the amniotic fluid and pregnancy outcome, *Pediatrics* 112:153-157, 2003.
103. Revello MG, Sarasini A, Zavattoni M, et al: Improved prenatal diagnosis of congenital human cytomegalovirus infection by a modified nested polymerase chain reaction, *J Med Virol* 56:99-103, 1998.
104. Hohlfeld P, Daffos F, Costa JM, et al: Prenatal diagnosis of congenital toxoplasmosis with a polymerase-chain-reaction test on amniotic fluid, *N Engl J Med* 331:695-699, 1994.
105. Romand S, Wallon M, Franck J, et al: Prenatal diagnosis using polymerase chain reaction on amniotic fluid for congenital toxoplasmosis, *Obstet Gynecol* 97:296-300, 2001.
106. Bosma TJ, Corbett KM, Eckstein MB, et al: Use of PCR for prenatal and postnatal diagnosis of congenital rubella, *J Clin Microbiol* 33: 2881-2887, 1995.
107. Gay-Andrieu F, Marty P, Pialat J, et al: Fetal toxoplasmosis and negative amniocentesis: necessity of an ultrasound follow-up, *Prenat Diagn* 23:558-560, 2003.
108. Enders G, Bäder U, Lindemann L, et al: Prenatal diagnosis of congenital cytomegalovirus infection in 189 pregnancies with known outcome, *Prenat Diagn* 21:362-377, 2001.
109. Fox H: *Pathology of the placenta*, Philadelphia, 1978, WB Saunders.
110. Liesenfeld O, Montoya JG, Kinney S, et al: Effect of testing for IgG avidity in the diagnosis of Toxoplasma gondii infection in pregnant women: experience in a U.S. reference laboratory, *J Infect Dis* 183:1248-1253, 2001.
111. Nigro G, Anceschi MM, Cosmi EV: Clinical manifestations and abnormal laboratory findings in pregnant women with primary cytomegalovirus infection, *Br J Obstet Gynaecol* 110:572-577, 2003.
112. Revello MG, Gerna G: Diagnosis and management of human cytomegalovirus infection in the mother, fetus, and newborn infant, *Clin Microbiol Rev* 15:680-715, 2002.
113. Tang JW, Aarons E, Hesketh LM, et al: Prenatal diagnosis of congenital rubella infection in the second trimester of pregnancy, *Prenat Diagn* 23:509-512, 2003.
114. Gutierrez J, Rodríguez MJ, De Ory F, et al: Reliability of low-avidity IgG and of IgA in the diagnosis of primary infection by rubella virus with adaptation of a commercial test, *J Clin Lab Anal* 13:1-4, 1999.
115. Centers for Disease Control and Prevention: Revised recommendations for HIV screening of pregnant women, *MMWR Recomm Rep* 50(RR-19):63-85, 2001.
116. American College of Obstetrics and Gynecology Committee on Obstetric Practice: ACOG Committee Opinion No. 418: prenatal and perinatal human immunodeficiency virus testing: expanded recommendations, *Obstet Gynecol* 112:739-742, 2008.
117. Mussi-Pinhata MM, Yamamoto AY, Figueiredo LT, et al: Congenital and perinatal cytomegalovirus infection in infants born to mothers infected with human immunodeficiency virus, *J Pediatr* 132: 285-290, 1998.
118. Thomas DL, Villano SA, Riester KA, et al: Perinatal transmission of hepatitis C virus from human immunodeficiency virus type 1-infected mothers. Women and Infants Transmission Study, *J Infect Dis* 177:1480-1488, 1998.
119. Stoll BJ, Hansen NI, Bell EF, et al: Neonatal outcomes of extremely preterm infants from the NICHD Neonatal Research Network, *Pediatrics* 126:443-456, 2010.
120. Rosebury T: *Microorganisms indigenous to man*, New York, 1962, McGraw-Hill.
121. Gorbach SL, Menda KB, Thadepalli H, Keith L: Anaerobic microflora of the cervix in healthy women, *Am J Obstet Gynecol* 117: 1053-1055, 1973.
122. Srugo I, Wittek AE, Israele V, et al: Meningoencephalitis in a neonate congenitally infected with human immunodeficiency virus type 1, *J Pediatr* 120:93-95, 1992.

123. Fernandez M, Hickman ME, Baker CJ: Antimicrobial susceptibilities of group B streptococci isolated between 1992 and 1996 from patients with bacteremia or meningitis, *Antimicrob Agents Chemother* 42:1517-1519, 1998.
124. Biedenbach DJ, Stephen JM, Jones RN: 2003 Antimicrobial susceptibility profile among β-haemolytic *Streptococcus* spp. Collected in SENTRY antimicrobial surveillance program—North America, *Diagn Microbiol Infect Dis* 46:291-294, 2001.
125. Whitley RJ, Cloud G, Gruber W, et al: Ganciclovir treatment of symptomatic congenital cytomegalovirus infection: results of a phase II study. National Institute of Allergy and Infectious Diseases Collaborative Antiviral Study Group, *J Infect Dis* 175:1080-1086, 1997.
126. Kimberlin DW, Lin CY, Sánchez PJ, et al: Effect of ganciclovir therapy on hearing in symptomatic congenital cytomegalovirus disease involving the central nervous system: a randomized, controlled trial, *J Pediatr* 98:16-25, 2003.
127. Oliver SE, Cloud GA, Sánchez PJ, et al: Neurodevelopmental outcomes following ganciclovir therapy in symptomatic congenital cytomegalovirus infections involving the central nervous system, *J Clin Virol* 46(Suppl 4):S22-S26, 2009.
128. Kimberlin DW, Jester P, Sanchez PJ, et al: Six months versus six weeks of oral valganciclovir for infants with symptomatic congenital cytomegalovirus (CMV) disease with and without central nervous system (CNS) involvement: results of a phase III, randomized, double-blind, placebo-controlled, multinational study. Oral presentation, ID Week, October 5, 2013, San Francisco.
129. Nigro G, Adler SP, La Torre R, Best AM: Passive immunization during pregnancy for congenital cytomegalovirus infection, *N Engl J Med* 353:1350-1362, 2005.
130. Revello MG: Role of antibodies and CMI in preventing congenital CMV. Presented at The Development and Evaluation of Human Cytomegalovirus Vaccines, Public Workshop, January 10, 2012. The Food and Drug Administration (FDA) Center for Biologics Evaluation and Research (CBER), the National Institutes of Health, the National Institute of Allergy and Infectious Diseases (NIAID), the Centers for Disease Control and Prevention and the National Vaccine Program Office. Available at http://videocast.nih.gov/launch.asp?17050. Accessed April 21, 2014.
131. Adler SP: Primary maternal cytomegalovirus infection during pregnancy: do we have a treatment option? *Clin Infect Dis* 55:504-506, 2012.
132. American Academy of Pediatrics Committee on Infectious Diseases: Universal hepatitis B immunization, *Pediatrics* 89:795-800, 1992.
133. Boyer KM, Gadzala CA, Burd LI, et al: Selective intrapartum chemoprophylaxis of neonatal group B streptococcal early-onset disease. I. Epidemiologic rationale, *J Infect Dis* 148:795-801, 1983.
134. American Academy of Pediatrics Committee on Infectious Diseases and Committee on Fetus and Newborn: Guidelines for prevention of group B streptococcal (GBS) infection by chemoprophylaxis, *Pediatrics* 90:775-778, 1992.
135. MacAulay MA, Abou-Sabe M, Charles D: Placental transfer of ampicillin, *Am J Obstet Gynecol* 96:943-950, 1966.
136. Moisiuk SE, Robson D, Klass L, et al: Outbreak of parainfluenza virus type 3 in an intermediate care neonatal nursery, *Pediatr Infect Dis J* 17:49-53, 1998.
137. Brozanski BS, Jones JG, Krohn MA, Sweet RL: Effect of a screening-based prevention policy on prevalence of early-onset group B streptococcal sepsis, *Obstet Gynecol* 95:496-501, 2000.
138. Schrag S, Gorwitz R, Fultz-Butts K, Schuchat A: Prevention of perinatal group B streptococcal disease. Revised guidelines from CDC, *MMWR Recomm Rep* 51(RR-11):1-22, 2002.
139. Knittle MA, Eitzman DV, Baer H: Role of hand contamination of personnel in the epidemiology of gram-negative nosocomial infections, *J Pediatr* 86:433-437, 1975.
140. Nagamine M, Nakashima Y, Uemura S, et al: DNA amplification of human T lymphotropic virus type I (HTLV-I) proviral DNA in breast milk of HTLV-I carriers, *J Infect Dis* 164:1024-1025, 1991.
141. Heneine W, Woods T, Green D, et al: Detection of HTLV-II in breastmilk of HTLV-II infected mothers, *Lancet* 340:1157-1158, 1992.
142. Dunn DT, Newell ML, Ades AE, Peckham CS: Risk of human immunodeficiency virus type 1 transmission through breastfeeding [see comments], *Lancet* 340:585-588, 1992.
143. World Health Organization: Breast feeding/breast milk and human immunodeficiency virus (HIV), *Wkly Epidemiol Rec* 33:245, 1987.
144. World Health Organization: Guidelines on HIV and infant feeding 2010: principles and recommendations for infant feeding in the context of HIV and a summary of evidence. Available at http://www.who.int/maternal_child_adolescent/documents/9789241599535/en/. Accessed April 21, 2014.
145. World Health Organization: Antiretroviral drugs for treating pregnant women and preventing HIV infection in infants: recommendations for a public health approach, 2010 version. Available at http://whqlibdoc.who.int/publications/2010/9789241599818_eng.pdf. Accessed April 21, 2014.
146. American Academy of Pediatrics Work Group on Breastfeeding: Breastfeeding and the use of human milk, *Pediatrics* 100: 1035-1039, 1997.
147. Altman LK: AIDS brings a shift on breast-feeding, New York Times, 1998. July 26, 1998. Available at http://www.nytimes.com/1998/07/26/world/aids-brings-a-shift-on-breast-feeding.html? Accessed July 1, 2014.
148. World Health Organization: Rapid advice: use of antiretroviral drugs for treating pregnant women and preventing HIV infection in infants. Available at http://www.who.int/hiv/pub/mtct/rapid_advice_mtct.pdf. Accessed April 21, 2014.
149. World Health Organization: Mother-to-child transmission of HIV. Available at http://www.who.int/hiv/topics/mtct/en/index.html. Accessed April 21, 2014.
150. Svabic-Vlahovic M, Pantić D, Pavićić M, Bryner JH: Transmission of *Listeria monocytogenes* from mother's milk to her baby and to puppies, *Lancet* 2:1201, 1988.
151. Klein JO: From harmless commensal to invasive pathogen—coagulase-negative staphylococci, *N Engl J Med* 323:339-340, 1990.
152. Brown J, Froese-Fretz A, Luckey D, et al: High rate of hand contamination and low rate of hand washing before infant contact in a neonatal intensive care unit, *Pediatr Infect Dis J* 15:908-910, 1996.

2 Neonatal Infections: A Global Perspective

ANITA K.M. ZAIDI, GARY L. DARMSTADT, and BARBARA J. STOLL

CHAPTER OUTLINE

Among the greatest challenges in global public health are to eliminate the gaps between high- and low-income countries in health care resources, provide access to preventive and curative services, and improve health outcomes. Although child and infant mortality burden has declined substantially in recent decades,[1] neonatal mortality, especially deaths in the first week of life, has changed relatively little.[2] Worldwide, an estimated 2.9 million neonatal deaths occur annually, accounting for 44% of deaths in children younger than 5 years.[3] The vast majority (99%) of these deaths occur in low- and middle-income countries (LMICs),[4] in the context of poverty, high-risk maternal and newborn care practices, poor care seeking and access to quality care, and poorly functioning health systems. Causes of neonatal mortality, especially in low-income countries, are difficult to ascertain, partly because many of these deaths occur at home, unattended by medical personnel, in settings without vital registration systems, and partly because critically ill neonates often present with nondiagnostic signs and symptoms of disease.

Serious infections, intrapartum-related neonatal deaths (i.e., "birth asphyxia"),[5] and complications of prematurity are the major direct causes of neonatal death worldwide.[1,4] Malnutrition and low birth weight (LBW) underlie the majority of these deaths.[6] Globally, serious neonatal infections cause an estimated 27.5% of neonatal deaths.[1] In very high mortality settings (neonatal mortality rate [NMR] > 45 per 1000 live births), neonatal infections are estimated to cause 40% to 50% of all neonatal deaths.[4,7] Neonatal mortality related to infection could be substantially reduced by simple, known preventive interventions before and during pregnancy, labor, and delivery, and preventive and curative interventions immediately after birth and in the early days of life.[8-12]

In this chapter, we review the global burden of infectious diseases in the newborn, direct and indirect causes of neonatal mortality attributed to infection, specific infections of relevance in LMICs, and strategies to reduce both the incidence of neonatal infection and morbidity and mortality in infants who do become infected.

Global Burden of Neonatal Infections

INFECTION AS A CAUSE OF NEONATAL DEATH

The majority of infection-related neonatal deaths are thought to be caused by bacterial sepsis and meningitis, respiratory infection, neonatal tetanus, diarrhea, and omphalitis. Very little is known about viral infections in the newborn period in LMICs. Neonatal deaths caused by infection may occur early in the neonatal period, in the first 7 days of life, and are usually attributable to infection acquired during the peripartum process. Late neonatal deaths, those occurring from 8 to 28 days of life, are most commonly caused by acquisition of pathogens from the environment in which the vulnerable newborn is placed.

In LMICs, because about half of births and most neonatal deaths occur at home and are not attended by medical personnel, deaths are underreported, and information on cause of death is often incomplete. Remarkably few published studies worldwide present detailed surveillance data on numbers of births and neonatal deaths and on probable causes of death. Although hospital-based studies are important for accurately determining causes of morbidity and mortality, they may not reflect what is happening in the community and, because of selection bias, may not be representative of the population. A recent review summarized 32 community-based studies that were published from 1990 to 2007.[13] Infection-specific mortality was found to range from 2.7 per 1000 live births in South Africa to 38.6 per 1000 live births in Somalia. Overall, 8% to 80% (median, 36.5%; interquartile range, 26%-49%) of all neonatal deaths in developing countries were found to be attributable to infections.[13] However, significant data gaps exist, especially from low-resource countries. There is a need for carefully conducted population-based studies that assess the number and causes of neonatal deaths resulting from bacterial and viral infections in LMICs.

In the absence of better data, global estimates for causes of neonatal deaths have been derived through statistical modeling, extrapolating from evidence available from several countries at different levels of development and neonatal mortality rates.[1] According to these estimates, infections are the second largest cause of neonatal mortality, accounting for 27.5% of all neonatal deaths; sepsis, pneumonia, and meningitis together account for 22.5% of neonatal deaths, whereas tetanus and diarrhea account for 2.5% each.[1] This translates to 0.8 million neonatal deaths caused by infections, most of which can be averted with appropriate prevention and management.[8,14] Using available data, it is estimated that between 252,000 to 552,000 neonatal deaths resulting from sepsis, pneumonia, or meningitis occur in developing countries each year[1] (Table 2-1). The range is large because of the imprecision of available data.

INCIDENCE OF NEONATAL SEPSIS, BACTEREMIA, AND MENINGITIS AND ASSOCIATED MORTALITY

Hospital and community-based studies from LMICs have been reviewed recently to determine the incidence of neonatal sepsis, bacteremia, and meningitis; the case-fatality rates (CFRs) associated with these infections; and the spectrum of bacterial pathogens in different regions of the world.[13,15-17] The vast majority of studies did not distinguish among maternally acquired, community-acquired, and nosocomial infections. Population-based studies from developing countries have reported clinical sepsis rates ranging from 49 to 170 per 1000 live births.[13] The majority of studies reported sepsis-associated case fatality rates greater than 30%. A carefully conducted recent population-based surveillance study from Mirzapur, a rural part of Bangladesh, attempted to capture all births and all cases of sepsis in a well-defined population through active, household-level surveillance.[18] The incidence of clinically suspected neonatal infection was approximately 50 per 1000 live births.[18] However, improvements continue to be made in the clinical algorithm used in Integrated Management of Newborn and Childhood Illness (IMNCI) to identify newborns with clinically suspected serious infections. Further refinements will likely lead to lower estimates when clinical signs of lower specificity, such as fast breathing, are removed.

Information on incidence rates of neonatal bacteremia (sepsis confirmed by isolation of bacteria from the blood) from developing countries is extremely limited. The median incidence of blood culture confirmed sepsis was 16 per 1000 live births in developing countries, among 18 studies reviewed recently.[13] Berkley and colleagues[19] reported a bacteremia rate of 5.5 per 1000 live births in rural Kenya, most likely an underestimate because only infants presenting to their referral hospital from the surrounding catchment area were included, and no active case finding through community surveillance was conducted. In Mirzapur, Bangladesh, active population-based, household-level newborn illness surveillance detected an incidence rate of bacteremia of 3.0 per 1000 person-neonatal periods.[18] Comparative figures for early-onset neonatal bacteremia reported in the United States range from 0.8 to 1 per 1000 live births.[20,21] Population-based surveillance studies with a focus on early birth detection in home-delivered babies and both bacterial and viral etiology of serious infections in young infants are currently underway in Bangladesh, India, and Pakistan

Table 2-1 Incidence* of Neonatal Causes of Death in Different Regions in 2010

	World	Africa	Americas	Eastern Mediterranean	Europe	Southeast Asia	Western Pacific
Pneumonia	325 (209-470)	109 (80-154)	5 (4-6)	43 (31-67)	7 (4-9)	153 (78-227)	11 (5-17)
Sepsis/meningitis	393 (252-552)	156 (127-227)	16 (8-18)	57 (43-90)	10 (8-13)	145 (74-245)	12 (8-18)
Tetanus	58 (20-276)	27 (9-190)	1 (1-7)	14 (4-59)	1 (0-5)	15 (4-38)	1 (0-5)
Diarrhea	50 (17-151)	19 (9-55)	0 (0-1)	6 (2-19)	0 (0-1)	20 (4-68)	4 (1-8)
Others	2246 (1848-2851)	753 (634-886)	115 (110-120)	324 (278-373)	91 (81-103)	762 (460-1093)	224 (166-271)
Total	3072	1064	137	444	108	1096	252

Modified from Liu L, Johnson HL, Cousens S, et al: Global, regional, and national causes of child mortality: an updated systematic analysis for 2010 with time trends since 2000, *Lancet* 379:2151-2161, 2012; [table 2].

*In thousands (uncertainty range).

and will provide more reliable estimates of incidence of sepsis and bacteremia in South Asian newborns.

Very few studies on neonatal meningitis were available to evaluate incidence and CFRs by region. The incidence of neonatal meningitis ranged from 0.33 to 7.3 per 1000 live births (average, 1 per 1000 live births), with CFRs ranging from 13% to 59%.[22]

BACTERIAL PATHOGENS ASSOCIATED WITH INFECTIONS IN DIFFERENT GEOGRAPHIC REGIONS

Historical reviews from developed countries have demonstrated that the predominant organisms responsible for neonatal infections change over time.[23,24] Prospective microbiologic surveillance is therefore important to guide empirical therapy and identify potential targets for vaccine development, identify new agents of importance for neonates, recognize epidemics, and monitor changes over time. Moreover, the organisms associated with neonatal infection are different in different geographic areas, reinforcing the need for local microbiologic surveillance. In areas where blood cultures in sick neonates cannot be performed, knowledge of the bacterial flora of the maternal genital tract may serve as a surrogate marker for organisms causing early-onset neonatal sepsis, meningitis, and pneumonia. The vast majority of studies on the causes of neonatal sepsis and meningitis are hospital reviews that include data on infants born in hospitals as well as those transferred from home or other facilities.

A recent review highlighted the scarcity of data on pathogens associated with neonatal sepsis and meningitis in LMICs.[17] This review found 63 studies published between 1980 and 2007 that reported etiologic data from LMICs.[17] The review also included findings from the Young Infant Clinical Signs Studies and community-based data from Karachi. Only 12 of these studies focused on community-acquired infections. In most of the remaining studies, it was difficult to determine whether infections were of maternal origin or were hospital- or community-acquired. Because of insufficient information provided, assumptions of community acquired infections were made if this was implied by the study setting. Therefore the possible inclusion of some nosocomial infections cannot be ruled out. Also, the infants' ages at the time of infection were not always specified. The studies varied in the detail with which culture methods were presented.

Table 2-2 gives further details about the distribution of organisms by geographic region. The review found 19 studies that reported etiologic data for the entire neonatal period. In the aggregated data of these studies, the ratio of gram-negative to gram-positive organisms was 1.6:1, and *Staphylococcus aureus*, *Escherichia coli*, and *Klebsiella* spp. collectively caused

Table 2-2 Etiology of Community-Acquired Neonatal Sepsis in Low- and Middle-Income Countries by Region

	AFRICA		EAST ASIA AND PACIFIC		MIDDLE EAST AND CENTRAL ASIA		SOUTH ASIA		ALL REGIONS	
Organism Isolated	***N***	**%**	***N***	**%**	***N***	**%**	***N***	**%**	***N***	**%**
Total	1058	100	915	100	256	100	365	100	2594	100
Staphylococcus aureus	112	10.59	146	15.96	51	19.92	36	9.86	345	13.30
Streptococcus pyogenes	71	6.71	8	0.87	2	0.78	3	0.82	84	3.24
Group B streptococci	161	15.22	2	0.22	20	7.81	26	7.12	209	8.06
Group D streptococci/*Enterococcus*	4	0.38			13	5.08	22	6.03	39	1.50
Group G streptococci	1	0.09	1	0.11					2	0.08
Streptococcus pneumoniae	129	12.19	4	0.44	7	2.73	7	1.92	147	5.67
Other *Streptococcus* species/unspecified	3	0.28	40	4.37	1	0.39	43	11.78	87	3.35
Other gram positives	72	6.81					2	0.55	74	2.85
All gram positives	553	52.27	201	21.97	94	36.72	139	38.08	987	38.05
Klebsiella species	82	7.75	134	14.64	49	19.14	85	23.29	350	13.49
Escherichia coli	94	8.88	237	25.9	68	26.56	44	12.05	443	17.08
Pseudomonas species	7	0.66	134	14.64	8	3.13	37	10.14	186	7.17
Enterobacter species	3	0.28	52	5.68	8	3.13	15	4.11	78	3.01
Serratia species			39	4.26	2	0.78			41	1.58
Proteus species	5	0.47			7	2.73	1	0.27	13	0.50
Salmonella species	118	11.15	4	0.44			2	0.55	124	4.78
Citrobacter species							4	1.10	4	0.15
Haemophilus influenzae	12	1.13	1	0.11	2	0.78	1	0.27	16	0.62
Neisseria meningitidis	11	1.04			3	1.17			14	0.54
Acinetobacter species			94	10.27	2	0.78	13	3.56	109	4.20
Other gram negatives	132	12.48	19	2.08	1	0.39	20	5.48	172	6.63
All gram negatives	464	43.86	714	78.03	150	58.59	222	60.82	1550	59.75
Other	41	3.88			12	4.69	4	1.10	57	2.20

Modified from Zaidi AK, Thaver D, Ali SA, Khan TA: Pathogens associated with sepsis in newborns and young infants in developing countries, *Pediatr Infect Dis J* 28(Suppl 1):S10-S18, 2009; with permission.

almost half of all infections. This pattern was consistent across all regions except Africa, where gram-positive organisms were predominant because of higher frequency of *S. aureus, Streptococcus pneumoniae,* and *Streptococcus pyogenes.*

Forty-four studies presented the etiology of early-onset neonatal sepsis in LMICs; all were facility-based studies. One fourth of all episodes of early-onset neonatal sepsis were caused by *Klebsiella* spp., 18% by *S. aureus,* 15% by *E. coli,* 7% by group B streptococci (GBS), and 12% were caused collectively by *Acinetobacter* spp. and *Pseudomonas* spp. The overall ratio of gram-negative to gram-positive organisms was 2:1. However, in African countries, the ratio of gram-positive to gram-negative organisms was 1:1, with a larger proportion of infections caused by *S. aureus* and GBS. *Pseudomonas* spp. and *Acinetobacter* spp. were found to be more common in East Asian, Pacific, and South Asian countries. *S. aureus* was relatively uncommon in East Asia and Latin America compared with other regions.

The review also found 11 studies that reported etiologic data on community-acquired infections occurring between 7 and 59 days of life. Almost half of the isolates in this age group were from the large World Health Organization (WHO)-sponsored multicenter Young Infant Study conducted in the early 1990s in four developing countries: Ethiopia, The Gambia, Papua New Guinea, and the Philippines.[25-32] The ratio of gram-negative to gram-positive organisms in this group was 0.8:1, with higher proportions of *Salmonella* spp., *Haemophilus influenzae, S. pneumoniae,* and *S. pyogenes,* compared with the first week of life.[17] Additional data on etiology of serious infections in the first 2 months of life is forthcoming from the second Young Infant Clinical Sign Study.[33]

Although data are limited, studies involving home-delivered babies or babies from maternity hospitals and rural referral hospitals found gram-negative organisms to be more than three times as common as gram-positive organisms (ratio of 3:1 among home births, 3.5:1 among rural referral hospitals).[17] Three gram-negative bacteria (*E. coli, Klebsiella* spp., and *Pseudomonas* spp.) accounted for 43% to 64% of all infections, and the gram-positive *S. aureus* accounted for 8% to 21% of all infections. Among babies born at home, gram-negative organisms were responsible for 77% of all neonatal infections. In Mirzapur, Bangladesh, among home-born newborns identified through population-based household surveillance, half of all culture-proven episodes of suspected sepsis were due to gram-negative organisms, including *Klebsiella* spp., *Pseudomonas* spp., *Acinetobacter* spp., and *Enterobacter* spp. Among gram-positive cultures, *S. aureus* was the most common isolate, responsible for one third of all positive cultures.[18]

The ongoing study evaluating pathogens of neonatal infections in South Asia (ANISA study) will provide valuable information on etiology of infections in low resource community settings.

Incidence of Group B Streptococcal Colonization and Infection

Although GBS remains the most important bacterial pathogen associated with early-onset neonatal sepsis and meningitis in many developed countries (especially among term infants),[34] studies from developing countries present a different picture. The most striking finding is the significantly lower rate of GBS sepsis reported in South Asia, Central Asia, East Asia, the Middle East, and the Pacific, and the high rate reported from Africa (see Table 2-2). Another recent review showed GBS incidence of 0.67 and 1.21 per 1000 live births in the Americas and Africa, respectively, compared with only 0.02 per 1000 live births in Southeast Asia.[35]

It is unclear why neonates in many LMICs are rarely infected with GBS. The most important risk factor for invasive GBS disease in the neonate is exposure to the organism via the mother's genital tract. Other known risk factors include young maternal age, preterm birth, prolonged rupture of the membranes, maternal chorioamnionitis, exposure to a high inoculum of a virulent GBS strain, and a low maternal serum concentration of antibody to the capsular polysaccharide of the colonizing GBS strain.[36] In the United States, differences in GBS colonization rates have been identified among women of different ethnic groups that appear to correlate with infection in newborns. In an attempt to understand the low rates of invasive GBS disease reported among neonates in many LMICs, Stoll and Schuchat[37] reviewed 34 studies published between 1980 and 1998 that evaluated GBS colonization rates in women. These studies reported culture results from 7730 women, with an overall colonization rate of 12.7%. Studies using culture methods judged to be appropriate found significantly higher colonization rates than those that used inadequate methods (675 of 3801 women [17.8%] vs. 308 of 3929 [7.8%]). When analyses were restricted to studies with adequate methods, the prevalence of colonization by region was Middle East/North Africa, 22%; Asia/Pacific, 19%; sub-Saharan Africa, 19%; India/Pakistan, 12%; and the Americas, 14%. Further data is needed from studies using state-of-the-art methodologies for detection of GBS in low- and middle-income countries.

The distribution of GBS serotypes varied among studies. GBS serotype III, the most frequently identified invasive serotype in the West, was identified in all studies reviewed and was the most frequently identified serotype in one half of the studies. Serotype V, which has only recently been recognized as a cause of invasive disease in developed countries,[38] was identified in studies from Peru[39] and The Gambia.[40] Monitoring serotype distribution is important because candidate GBS vaccines are considered for areas with high rates of disease.

With estimated GBS colonization rates among women in many LMICs estimated at about 15% to 20%, higher rates of invasive neonatal disease than have been reported would be expected. Low rates of invasive GBS disease in some LMICs may be due to lower virulence of strains, genetic differences in susceptibility to disease, as-yet unidentified beneficial cultural practices, or high concentrations of transplacentally acquired protective antibody in serum (i.e., a mother may be colonized yet have protective concentrations of type-specific GBS antibody).

In LMICs where most deliveries occur at home, infants with early-onset sepsis often become sick and die at home or are taken to local health care facilities, where a diagnosis of possible sepsis may be missed, or where blood cultures cannot be performed. In these settings, there may be underdiagnosis of infection by early-onset pathogens, including GBS. In the WHO Young Infants Study,[25] 1673 infants were evaluated in the first month of life; only 2 had cultures positive for GBS. The absence of GBS in this study cannot be explained by the evaluation of insufficient numbers of sick neonates (360 of the1673 infants were younger than 1 week).

Data suggest that heavy colonization with GBS may increase the risk of delivering a preterm LBW infant.[41] Population differences in the prevalence of heavy GBS colonization have been reported in the United States, where African Americans have a significantly higher risk of heavy colonization. If heavy colonization is more prevalent among women in LMICs and results in an increase in numbers of preterm LBW infants, GBS-related morbidity may appear as illness and death related to prematurity. By contrast, heavy colonization could increase maternal type-specific GBS antibody concentrations, resulting in lower risk of neonatal disease. Further studies in LMICs are needed to explore these important issues.

ANTIMICROBIAL RESISTANCE IN NEONATAL PATHOGENS

Rising rates of antimicrobial resistance among common pathogens involved in neonatal infections are being observed in LMICs.[42] However, limited published information is available on antimicrobial resistance patterns among neonatal pathogens from community settings where a large proportion of births take place at home. A recent review identified only 10 studies during 1990 to 2007, including two unpublished works, that contributed resistance data from community settings in low- and middle-income countries, primarily regarding *Klebsiella* spp., *E. coli, and S. aureus*.[42] Compared with data from hospital settings, resistance rates were lower in community-acquired infections. Among *E. coli*, greater than 70% of isolates were resistant to ampicillin, and 13% were resistant to gentamicin. Among *Klebsiella* spp., all were resistant to ampicillin and 60% to gentamicin.[42] However, resistance to third-generation cephalosporins was uncommon, and methicillin-resistant *S. aureus* (MRSA) occurred rarely.[42] Another recent review identified 19 studies from 13 different countries on resistance patterns from community settings. The study showed high rates of resistance of gram-negative bacteria and *S. aureus*.[43] However, it is unclear how many of these infections were truly maternally or community acquired. Additional data on antimicrobial resistance patterns of neonatal pathogens encountered in home-delivered babies are needed to develop evidence-based guidelines for management. The ANISA study mentioned earlier will provide much-needed information from South Asia on antimicrobial resistance among neonatal pathogens among home-born infants.

By contrast, several studies from hospitalized infants in hospitals from LMICs show alarming antimicrobial resistance rates among neonatal pathogens in hospital nurseries. A large recent review showed that greater than 70% of neonatal isolates from hospitals of LMICs were resistant to ampicillin and gentamicin—the recommended regimen for the management of neonatal sepsis.[44,45] Resistance was also documented against expensive second- and third-line agents; 46% of *E. coli* and 51% of *Klebsiella* spp. were resistant to the third-generation cephalosporin cefotaxime.[45] Equally disturbing was the high prevalence of MRSA isolates, especially in South Asia, where they comprised 56% of all isolates.[45] Pan-resistant *Acinetobacter* spp. infections are also now widely reported.[46,47] In these resource-constrained settings, many multidrug-resistant pathogens are now unfortunately untreatable, and high mortality rates are observed.[48]

NOSOCOMIAL INFECTIONS

Hospitals in LMICs are ill-equipped to provide hygienic care to the vulnerable newborn infant.[45,49] A recent review of the rates of neonatal infections among hospital-born babies in LMICs found rates to be 3 to 20 times higher than those observed in industrialized countries.[45,49] Moreover, a high proportion of infections in the early neonatal period were due to *Klebsiella* spp., *Pseudomonas* spp., and *S. aureus*, rather than organisms typically associated with the maternal birth canal, suggesting acquisition from the hospital environment, rather than the mother.[45] Overall, gram-negative rods were found to be predominant, comprising 60% of all positive cultures from newborns. *Klebsiella* spp. were found to be the major pathogens, present in 23% of cases, followed by *S. aureus* (16.3%) and *E. coli* (12.2%).[45]

High nosocomial infection rates observed among hospital-born babies in LMICs are attributable to lack of aseptic delivery and hand hygiene; lack of essential supplies, such as running water, soap, and gloves; equipment shortages; lack of sterilization facilities; lack of knowledge and training regarding adequate sterilization; overcrowded and understaffed health facilities; and inappropriate and prolonged use of antibiotics.[45]

Hospital Infection Control

Lack of attention to infection control increases the newborn's risk of acquiring a nosocomial pathogen from the hospital environment.[45] Urgent attention to improving infection control practices in hospitals that care for mothers and newborns is required if survival gains from promoting institutional delivery are to be fully realized. Several cost-effective strategies to reduce infection transmission in hospitals of LMICs have been discussed in recent reviews of hospital-acquired neonatal infections.[45,50,51]

Hand hygiene remains the most important infection control practice. However, in many LMICs, hospital delivery wards and nurseries lack sinks and running water. For such settings, alcohol-based hand rubs are an attractive option. Several studies have shown the efficacy of use of hand rubs by hospital staff in reducing rates of colonization and infection among neonates.[52,53] Although commercially available alcohol-based hand gels are expensive, costs may be offset by significant reduction in nosocomial infections. Also, low-cost solutions can be prepared by hospital pharmacies by combining 20 mL of glycerin, sorbitol, glycol, or propylene with 980 mL of greater than 70% isopropanol.[45] Addition of 0.5% chlorhexidine prolongs the bactericidal effect but increases expense.[45]

Attention to aseptic technique during intrapartum care for the mother and cutting the umbilical cord is particularly important. Reducing the number of vaginal examinations reduces the risk of chorioamnionitis. A systematic review of the use of vaginal chlorhexidine treatment included two large, nonrandomized, nonblinded hospital-based trials from Malawi and Egypt that reported neonatal outcomes.[54-56] Both found that the use of 0.25% chlorhexidine wipes during vaginal examinations and application of another wipe for the neonate soon after birth significantly reduced early neonatal deaths (Egypt: 2.8 vs. 4.2% in intervention vs. control groups, respectively, P = .01) and neonatal mortality caused by infections (Malawi: odds ratio [OR], 0.5; 95% confidence interval [CI], 0.29 to 0.88; Egypt: 0.22% vs. 0.84% in intervention vs. control groups, respectively, P = .004).[57,58] However, a hospital-based trial from South Africa found no impact of maternal vaginal and newborn skin cleansing with chlorhexidine on rates of neonatal sepsis or the vertical acquisition of potentially pathogenic bacteria among neonates.[59] Rates of infection in the South African trial, however, were exceedingly low, and the study lacked power to reach a definitive conclusion.

Topical application of emollients that serve to augment the barrier for invasion of pathogenic microbes through immature skin of premature infants has also shown promise. Daily applications of sunflower seed oil in very premature infants hospitalized in Bangladesh and Egypt have been shown to substantially reduce nosocomial infections by about 40% to 50% and mortality by 26% in Bangladesh.[60-62] Another trial in Pakistan has shown similar results (Z. Bhutta, unpublished data). A randomized, controlled, community-based trial of the impact of improved skin care practices, including modifications of oil (sunflower seed oil instead of mustard oil) and oil application techniques (gentle instead of the usual cultural practice of vigorous massage) is underway in India; another study of the impact of a substitution of sunflower seed oil for mustard oil is underway in Nepal.

Appropriate measures are also needed to address infection transmission that may occur through reuse of critical items that come into contact with sterile body sites, mucous membranes, or broken skin. Improper sterilization and defective reprocessing of these items has been associated with higher rates of *Pseudomonas* infections in a study from Indonesia.[63] A study from Mexico identified several faults in the reprocessing chain, such as inadequate monitoring of sterilization standards and use of inappropriate sterilization agents.[64]

Fluid reservoirs, such as those used in suctioning and respiratory care, can also be a source of infection in critical care areas. Targeted respiratory tract care with focused education campaigns has been found to be effective in reducing infection rates in developing countries.[65] In the face of outbreaks, point sources of contamination, such as intravenous fluids and medications, must be investigated and eliminated. Systematic reviews have found no evidence of the benefit of routine gowning by health personnel or infant attendants in hospital nurseries.[66]

Several studies have also examined the impact of "bundled" or packaged interventions in controlling hospital-acquired infections among children in developing countries. These packages include several infection control interventions, such as use of alcohol-based hand rubs, bedside checklists to monitor adequate infection control practices, appropriate antibiotic use policies, simple algorithms for effective treatment of neonatal sepsis, decreasing the degree of crowding in wards, increasing the number of infection control nurses, and establishing guidelines for appropriate handling of intravenous catheters and solutions. Although the results from these studies have varied in the degree of success, they have all reported decreases in nosocomial infections through implementation of such interventions.[67]

Selected Neonatal Infections

ACUTE RESPIRATORY INFECTIONS/PNEUMONIA

The onset of pneumonia in neonates may occur early (acquired during birth from organisms that colonize or infect the maternal genital tract) or late (acquired later from organisms in the hospital, home, or community). Although only a few studies of the bacteriology of neonatal pneumonia have been performed, the findings suggest that organisms causing pneumonia are similar to those that cause neonatal sepsis.[68,69] The role of viruses and agents such as *Bordetella pertussis* in neonatal pneumonia, especially in LMICs, remains unclear. Recent studies from developed countries suggest that viruses, including respiratory syncytial virus, parainfluenza viruses, adenoviruses, and influenza viruses, contribute to respiratory morbidity and mortality, especially during epidemic periods (G.L. Darmstadt, unpublished data).[70,71] Maternal influenza vaccination during pregnancy in Bangladesh reduced febrile respiratory illnesses in their young infants by one third, compared with infants of mothers not receiving influenza vaccine, suggesting an important role for influenza viruses in neonatal acute respiratory infections (ARI).[72]

Because of similarities in presentation, pneumonia in neonates is very difficult to differentiate from neonatal sepsis or meningitis, and all three diseases are often grouped under one category and treated similarly. Therefore assessing the true burden of neonatal respiratory infections is very difficult. A respiratory rate greater than 60 per minute in an infant younger than 2 months has been proposed as a sensitive sign of serious illness and possible pneumonia by the WHO, but concerns about low specificity resulting from conditions such as transient tachypnea of the newborn and upper respiratory infections remain to be addressed.[33] In a review of the causes of neonatal mortality, Liu and colleagues[1] estimated that 325,000 neonatal deaths caused by pneumonia occur annually in LMICs. In a carefully conducted community-based study in rural India, published in 1993, Bang and associates[73] determined that 66% of pneumonia deaths in the first year of life occurred in the neonatal period.

It is difficult to determine the incidence of neonatal ARI/pneumonia in LMICs because many sick neonates are never referred for medical care. In a large community-based study of ARI in Bangladeshi children, the highest incidence of ARI was in children younger than 5 months.[72] In the study by Bang and associates,[73] there were 64 cases of pneumonia among 3100 children (incidence of 21/1000), but this finding underestimates the true incidence because it was known that many neonates were never brought for care. A community-based study conducted by English and colleagues[74] in Kenya found the incidence of pneumonia to be as high as 81 per 1000 for children younger than 2 months. The risk of pneumonia and of ARI-related death increases in infants who are LBW and/or malnourished and in those who are not breastfed.[75,76] In a study of LBW infants in India[77] in which infants were visited weekly and mothers queried about disease, there were 61 episodes of moderate-to-severe ARI among 211 LBW infants and 125 episodes among 448 normal-weight infants. Although 33% of episodes occurred in LBW infants, 79% of the deaths occurred in this weight group.

Management of pneumonia in neonates follows the same principles as neonatal sepsis because the syndrome is difficult to distinguish clinically from sepsis. Trials are underway in Nigeria, Kenya, Democratic Republic of Congo, and Pakistan evaluating the efficacy of therapy in young infants who present with fast breathing as their sole clinical sign of illness.

DIARRHEA

Although diarrheal diseases are important killers of children younger than 1 year, most deaths resulting from diarrhea during infancy occur in the second 6 months of life.[78,79] Worldwide, only 1% of deaths in the neonatal period are attributed to diarrhea.[1] The high prevalence of breastfeeding in the first month of life in LMICs most likely protects breast-fed newborns from diarrhea.[80,81]

Kotloff and colleagues[79] studied the etiology and burden of moderate-to-severe diarrhea in Kenya, Mali, Mozambique, The Gambia, Bangladesh, India, and Pakistan. The investigators enrolled 4029 infants over a period of 3 years and compared them with 4878 matched control subjects. Four pathogens were significantly associated with moderate-to-severe diarrhea: rotavirus, *Cryptosporidium*, *Shigella*, and enterotoxigenic *E. coli*. Rotavirus was the most common agent, with an incidence of 7 episodes per 100 child-years during infancy. Black and colleagues[82] performed community studies of diarrheal epidemiology and etiology in a periurban community in Peru. The incidence of diarrhea was 9.8 episodes per child in the first year of life and did not differ significantly by month of age (0.64-1.0 episode per child-month). Mahmud and colleagues[83] prospectively followed a cohort of 1476 Pakistani newborns from four different communities. Eighteen percent of infants evaluated in the first month of life (180/1028) had diarrhea.

Although home births still account for many of the births in LMICs, those born in hospitals are at risk for nosocomial diarrheal infections. Aye and associates[84] studied diarrheal morbidity in neonates born at the largest maternity hospital in Rangoon, Myanmar. Diarrhea was a significant problem, with rates of 7 cases per 1000 live births for infants born vaginally and 50 per 1000 for infants delivered by cesarean section. These differences were attributed to the following: infants born by cesarean section remained hospitalized longer, were handled more by staff and less by their own mothers, and were less likely to be exclusively breastfed.

Rotavirus is one of the most important causes of diarrhea among infants and children worldwide, occurring most commonly in infants aged 3 months to 2 years. In LMICs, most rotavirus infections occur early in infancy.[79] There are few reports of rotavirus diarrhea in newborns.[85] It appears that in most cases, neonatal infection is asymptomatic, and that neonatal infection may protect against severe diarrhea in subsequent infections.[86-88] Neonates are generally infected with unusual rotavirus strains that may be less virulent and may serve as natural immunogens.[89] Exposure to the asymptomatic rotavirus I321 strain, in particular, has been shown to confer protection against symptomatic diarrheal episodes caused by rotavirus among neonates.[90]

The rate of infection among neonates, however, may be more common than was previously thought. Cicirello and associates[89] screened 169 newborns at six hospitals in Delhi, India and found a rotavirus prevalence of 26%. Prevalence increased directly with length of hospital stay. More recently, Ramani and associates[91] found the prevalence of rotavirus among neonates with gastrointestinal symptoms to be as high as 55% in a tertiary hospital in southern India. Gladstone and colleagues[92] studied a cohort of 373 children in India and found 56% were infected with rotavirus by 6 months of age. Rotavirus was identified in 15.2% of all diarrheal episodes. The high prevalence of neonatal infections in India (and perhaps in other low-resource country settings) could lead to priming of the immune system and have implications for vaccine efficacy. Several of the community-based studies reviewed earlier present data on diarrhea as a cause of neonatal death.[93-102] In these studies, diarrhea was responsible for 1% to 12% of all neonatal deaths. In 9 of the 10 studies, 70 of 2673 neonatal deaths (3%) were attributed to diarrhea. Whereas diarrhea is more common in infants after 6 months of age, it is also associated with morbidity and, in some cases, mortality, for neonates in LMICs.

OMPHALITIS

In LMICs, aseptic delivery techniques and hygienic cord care have markedly decreased the occurrence of umbilical infection or omphalitis. Furthermore, prompt diagnosis and antimicrobial therapy have decreased morbidity and mortality if omphalitis develops. Omphalitis continues to be an important problem, however, where clean delivery and hygienic cord care practices remain a challenge, particularly among the world's 60 million home births, which account for nearly half of all births, as well as for many facility-based births in low-resource settings.[103,104] The necrotic tissue of the umbilical cord is an excellent medium for bacterial growth. The umbilical stump is rapidly colonized by bacteria from the maternal genital tract and from the environment. This colonized necrotic tissue, in close proximity to umbilical vessels, provides microbial pathogens with direct access to the bloodstream. Thus invasion of pathogens via the umbilicus may occur with or without the presence of signs of omphalitis, such as redness, pus discharge, swelling, or foul odor.[105,106]

Omphalitis is associated with increased risk of mortality.[107] Omphalitis may remain a localized infection or may spread to the abdominal wall, the peritoneum, the umbilical or portal vessels, or the liver. Infants who present with abdominal wall cellulitis or necrotizing fasciitis have a high incidence of associated bacteremia (often polymicrobial) and a high mortality rate.[104,108,109]

Limited data are available on risk factors and incidence of umbilical infections from LMICs, especially from community settings. Overall, incidence of omphalitis in hospital-based studies has ranged from 2 to 77 per 1000 hospital-born infants, with the CFR ranging from 0% to 15%.[103-116] Mullany and colleagues[106] defined clinical algorithms for identification of umbilical infections and reported a 15% incidence of mild omphalitis, defined as the presence of moderate redness (<2 cm extension of redness onto the abdominal skin at the base of the cord stump) and a 1% incidence of severe omphalitis, defined as severe redness with pus, among 15,123 newborn babies identified in rural Nepal through community-based household surveillance.[105,110] In Pemba, Tanzania, 9550 cord assessments in 1653 infants identified an omphalitis rate ranging from 1%, based on a definition of moderate to severe redness with pus discharge, to 12.0%, based on the presence of pus and foul odor.[103] Mir and colleagues[116] recently studied the burden and etiology of omphalitis from a community setting in Karachi, Pakistan, with a high proportion of unskilled home deliveries, and found the incidence of omphalitis to be 21%, with 2% of cases associated with sepsis.

A key risk factor for development of omphalitis in the community included topical applications of potentially unclean substances (e.g., mustard oil). Hand washing by the birth attendant with soap provided in the clean delivery kit, consistent hand washing by the mother, and the practice of skin-to-skin care reduced the risk of omphalitis.[103]

Some information on microbiologic etiology of omphalitis from LMICs is available. Over a 2-year period, Güvenç and associates[114] identified 88 newborns with omphalitis at a university hospital in eastern Turkey. Gram-positive organisms were isolated from 68% of umbilical cultures; gram-negative organisms were isolated from 60%, and multiple organisms were cultured in 28% of patients. Airede[111] studied 33 Nigerian neonates with omphalitis. Aerobic bacteria were isolated from 70%, and anaerobic bacteria were isolated from 30%. Sixty percent of the aerobic isolates were gram-positive organisms, and polymicrobial isolates were common. Faridi and colleagues[113] in India identified gram-negative organisms more frequently than gram-positive organisms (57% vs. 43%), but *S. aureus* was the single most frequent isolate (28%). In a study from Papua New Guinea, umbilical cultures were performed in 116 young infants with signs suggestive of omphalitis. The most frequently isolated organisms were group A β-hemolytic streptococci (44%), *S. aureus* (39%), *Klebsiella* spp. (17%), *E. coli* (17%), and *Proteus mirabilis* (16%).[29] In infants with both omphalitis and bacteremia, *S. aureus*, *S. pyogenes*, and *Klebsiella pneumoniae* were isolated from both sites. In Thailand, postdischarge follow-up cultures from 180 newborns yielded a positive culture in all cases, mostly commonly for *Klebsiella* spp. (60%), *E. coli* (37%), *Enterobacter* spp. (32%), and *S. aureus*.[117] In Oman, cultures from 207 newborns with signs of omphalitis yielded a positive culture in 191 cases; 57% were positive for *S. aureus*, 14% for *E. coli*, and 10% for *Klebsiella* spp.[118]

Community-based data on the etiology of omphalitis in LMICs are scarce, particularly from African settings. Two recent studies in South Asia reported the etiology of omphalitis in community settings. Mir and colleagues[116] in Pakistan identified *S. aureus* as the most common pathogen (52%), followed by *S. pyogenes* (18%), GBS (10%), *Pseudomonas* spp. (8.9%), *Aeromonas* spp. (3.2%), and *Klebsiella* spp. (2%). However, Mullany and colleagues[119] identified gram-negative organisms as more commonly causing colonization of the umbilical stump among newborns who received dry cord care in Bangladesh. Gram-negative organisms were isolated in 76.3% of all swabs, compared with 55.2% of swabs that yielded gram-positive organisms (mainly *S. aureus*). Among gram-negative organisms, *E. coli* was the most common organism (43%), followed by *K. pneumoniae* (34%) and *Pseudomonas* spp. (25%).

The method of caring for the umbilical cord after birth affects both bacterial colonization, time to cord separation, and risk for infection and mortality.[120-122] Hygienic delivery and postnatal care practices, including hand washing and clean cord care, are important interventions to reduce risk of omphalitis and death.[10,122] Clean birth kits, which package together items such as a sterile blade, sterile cord tie, and soap, are promoted in many settings, especially for home births, although evidence for impact of birth kits on reducing rates of omphalitis and neonatal mortality is limited.[123-128]

During a study of pregnancy in a rural area of Papua New Guinea, Garner and colleagues[129] detected a high prevalence of neonatal fever and umbilical infection, which were associated with the subsequent development of neonatal sepsis. They designed an intervention program for umbilical cord care that included maternal health education and umbilical care packs containing acriflavine spirit and new razor blades. Neonatal sepsis was significantly less frequent in the intervention group. Mullany and colleagues[105] demonstrated a 75% reduction (95% CI, 47% to 88%) in severe umbilical cord infections and a 24% reduction (95% CI, −4% to 55%) in all-cause neonatal mortality in a large (n = 15,123) community-based trial of 4% chlorhexidine cord cleansing, applied once daily for 8 of the first 10 days of life, compared with dry cord care. In infants enrolled within the first 24 hours of life, mortality was significantly reduced by 34% (95% CI, 5% to 54%) in the chlorhexidine cord cleansing group. In a third study arm, soap and water did not reduce infection or mortality risk, compared with dry cord care. Chlorhexidine treatment delayed cord separation by about 1 day. However, this was not associated with increased risk of omphalitis.[130] Soofi and colleagues[131] in Pakistan and Arifeen and colleagues[132] in Bangladesh also found that use of 4% chlorhexidine application resulted in significant reduction of omphalitis and neonatal deaths.

A WHO expert review panel convened in September 2012 reviewed the evidence for use of chlorhexidine for cord care in low-income countries. The panel recommended chlorhexidine for routine cord care in home-delivered infants. However, formal guidance on this from WHO is awaited. Because of lack of sufficient evidence from hospital settings, clean cord care is still recommended for hospital-born infants, although it is acknowledged that antiseptics might benefit infants in settings where harmful substances are traditionally applied.[133]

TETANUS

Neonatal tetanus, caused by *Clostridium tetani*, is an under-reported "silent" illness. The disease may go unrecognized because it attacks newborns in the poorest countries of the world in the first few days of life, often while they are still confined to home, because of a high and rapid CFR

(85% untreated)[134] and because of poor access to medical care.[135-137] The surveillance case definition of neonatal tetanus is relatively straightforward, that is, the ability of a newborn to suck at birth and for the first few days of life, followed by inability to suck starting between 3 and 10 days of age, spasms, stiffness, convulsions, and death.[138]

Neonatal tetanus is a completely preventable disease. It can be prevented by immunizing the mother before or during pregnancy and/or by ensuring a clean delivery, clean cutting of the umbilical cord, and proper care of the cord in the days after birth.[10] Clean delivery practices have additional benefits: prevention of other maternal and neonatal infections, in addition to tetanus. Tetanus threatens mothers as well as babies, and tetanus-related mortality is a complication of both induced abortion and childbirth in unimmunized women.[139] Immunization of women with at least three doses of tetanus toxoid vaccine provides complete prevention against both maternal and neonatal tetanus.

The Maternal and Neonatal Tetanus Elimination Initiative of the United Nations Children's Fund (UNICEF), the WHO, the United Nations Population Fund (UNFPA), and other partners, established in 1999, has led to the vaccination of hundreds of millions of women of childbearing age against tetanus, either through vaccination campaigns or during routine antenatal care (ANC) visits. Between 2000 and 2013, 31 countries, 19 of 35 states in India, and 29 of 33 provinces in Indonesia eliminated tetanus.[140,141] An estimated 74% of women of childbearing age in developing countries are now adequately protected from tetanus, associated with marked and rapid declines in global deaths attributed to tetanus, from an estimated 146,000 in 2000 to 58,000 in 2010.[1] Only an estimated 1% of global neonatal deaths are now attributed to tetanus. Progress continues, and the elimination of maternal and neonatal tetanus remains a global goal.[1]

OPHTHALMIA NEONATORUM

Ophthalmia neonatorum, defined as purulent conjunctivitis in the first 28 days of life, remains a common problem in many LMICs. The risk of infection in the neonate is directly related to the prevalence of maternal infection and the frequency of ocular prophylaxis. Infants born in areas of the world with high rates of sexually transmitted diseases (STDs) are at greatest risk.

Data on incidence and bacteriologic spectrum from specific countries are limited. Although a wide array of agents are cultured from infants with ophthalmia neonatorum,[142-144] *Neisseria gonorrhoeae* (the gonococcus) and *Chlamydia trachomatis* are the most important etiologic agents from a global perspective[143,145-150] and share similar mechanisms of pathogenesis. Infection is acquired from an infected mother during passage through the birth canal or through an ascending route. Clinical examination alone cannot distinguish infection caused by one etiologic agent from infection caused by another; each produces a purulent conjunctivitis. However, gonococcal ophthalmia may appear earlier and is typically more severe than chlamydial conjunctivitis. Untreated gonococcal conjunctivitis may lead to corneal scarring and blindness, whereas the risk of severe ocular damage is low with chlamydial infection. Without ocular prophylaxis, ophthalmia neonatorum will develop in 30% to 42% of infants born to mothers with untreated *N. gonorrhoeae* infection[146,148,149] and in approximately 30% of infants exposed to *Chlamydia*.[148]

A 5-year study from Iran showed *S. aureus* to be the major organism responsible for ophthalmia neonatorum.[151] Similar predominance of *S. aureus* has been reported from Argentina and Pakistan.[152,153] The reasons for these differences in etiology are not well understood, and data from the lowest-resource countries are not available.

Strategies to prevent or ameliorate ocular morbidity related to ophthalmia neonatorum include (1) primary prevention of STDs; (2) antenatal screening for and treatment of STDs, particularly gonorrhea and *Chlamydia* infection; (3) eye prophylaxis at birth; and (4) early diagnosis and treatment of ophthalmia neonatorum.[149] For developing countries, eye prophylaxis soon after birth is the most cost-effective and feasible strategy in settings where STD rates are high. Eye prophylaxis is used primarily to prevent gonococcal ophthalmia. Primary prevention of STDs in LMICs is limited, although promotion of condom use has been successful in reducing STDs in some countries.[154,155] Screening women at prenatal and STD clinics and treatment based on a syndromic approach (i.e., treat for possible infections in all women with vaginal discharge without laboratory confirmation) is cost-effective but may lead to overtreatment of uninfected women and missed cases.

Eye prophylaxis consists of cleaning the eyelids and instilling an antimicrobial agent into the eyes as soon after birth as possible. The agent should be placed directly into the conjunctival sac (using clean hands), and the eyes should not be flushed after instillation. Infants born both vaginally and by cesarean section should receive prophylaxis. Although no agent is 100% effective at preventing disease, the use of 1% silver nitrate solution (introduced by Credé in 1881)[156] dramatically reduced the incidence of ophthalmia neonatorum. This inexpensive agent is still widely used in many parts of the world. The major problems with silver nitrate are that it may cause chemical conjunctivitis in up to 50% of infants, and it has limited antimicrobial activity against *Chlamydia*.[149,157,158] In LMICs where heat and improper storage may be a problem, evaporation and concentration are particular concerns. Although 1% tetracycline and 0.5% erythromycin ointments are commonly used and are as effective as silver nitrate for the prevention of gonococcal conjunctivitis, these agents are more expensive and unavailable in many parts of the world. Moreover, silver nitrate appears to be a better prophylactic agent in areas where penicillinase-producing *N. gonorrhoeae* (PPNG) is a problem.[159]

The ideal prophylactic agent for low-resource settings would have a broad antimicrobial spectrum and also be available and affordable. Povidone-iodine is an inexpensive, nontoxic topical agent that is potentially widely available. Recent studies suggest that it may be useful in preventing ophthalmia neonatorum. A prospective masked, controlled trial of ocular prophylaxis using 2.5% povidone-iodine solution, 1% silver nitrate solution, or 0.5% erythromycin ointment was conducted in Kenya.[160] Of 3117 neonates randomized to receive a study drug, 13.1% in the povidone-iodine group versus 15.2% of those who received erythromycin and 17.5% in the silver nitrate group developed infectious conjunctivitis ($P < .01$). The high rates of infection in this study despite ocular prophylaxis are striking. Although there was no significant difference among agents in prevention of gonococcal ophthalmia (1% or less for each agent), povidone-iodine was most effective in preventing chlamydial conjunctivitis. A 2003 study by the same group compared prophylaxis with one drop and with two drops of the povidone-iodine solution instilled in both eyes at birth in 719 Kenyan neonates. No cases of *N. gonorrhoeae* infection were identified. Double application did not change the rates of infection with *C. trachomatis* (4.2% and 3.9%).[161] Although the antimicrobial spectrum of povidone-iodine is wider than that of the other topical agents[162] and antibacterial resistance has not been demonstrated,[87] published data on the efficacy of povidone-iodine against PPNG are not yet available. Of note, 2.5% povidone-iodine might also be useful as an antimicrobial agent for cord care, which is of relevance in the prevention of omphalitis (see earlier discussion). Another trial in Iran compared the efficacy of topical povidone-iodine versus erythromycin as prophylactic agents for ophthalmia neonatorum, compared with no prophylaxis.[163] Among 330 infants studied, ophthalmia neonatorum developed in 9% of neonates receiving povidone-iodine, 18% of neonates receiving erythromycin, and 22% of the neonates receiving no prophylaxis. Further studies are needed on the safety and efficacy of povidone-iodine in LMICs.

The frequency of practice of ocular prophylaxis in LMICs is unknown. In consideration of the high rates of STDs among pregnant women in many low-resource settings, eye prophylaxis is an important blindness prevention strategy. For infants born at home, a single dose of antimicrobial agent for ocular prophylaxis could be added to birth kits and potentially distributed to trained birth attendants during ANC, although more information about the feasibility and acceptability of this approach is needed. The strategy of ocular prophylaxis is more cost-effective than early diagnosis and appropriate treatment. Furthermore, in areas of the world in which access to medical care is limited and effective drugs are scarce or unavailable, it may be the only viable strategy.

No prevention strategy is 100% effective. Even with prophylaxis, 5% to 10% of infants will develop ophthalmia. All infants with ophthalmia must be given appropriate treatment, even if they received prophylaxis at birth. A single dose of either ceftriaxone (2–50mg/kg intravenously [IV] or intramuscularly [IM], not to exceed 125mg) or cefotaxime (100mg/kg, IV or IM) is effective therapy for gonococcal ophthalmia caused by both PPNG and non PPNG strains.[159] Gentamicin and kanamycin also have been shown to be effective therapeutic agents and may be more readily available in some settings. Rarely, gonococcal infection acquired at birth may become disseminated, resulting in arthritis, septicemia, and even meningitis. Neonates with disseminated gonococcal disease require systemic therapy with ceftriaxone (25-50mg/kg once daily) or cefotaxime (25mg/kg IM or IV twice daily) for 7 days for arthritis or sepsis or 10 to 14 days for meningitis. If a lumbar puncture cannot be performed and meningitis cannot be ruled out in an infant with evidence of dissemination, the longer period of therapy should be chosen.[159] Infants with chlamydial conjunctivitis should receive a 2-week course of oral erythromycin (50 mg/kg/day in four divided doses). After the immediate neonatal period, oral sulfonamides may be used.[159]

Table 2-3 Statistics on the world epidemic of HIV and AIDS

	Estimate	Range
People living with HIV/AIDS in 2011	34.0 million	30.3-36.1 million
Adults living with HIV/AIDS in 2011	30.7 million	28.2-34.0 million
Women living with HIV/AIDS in 2011	16.7 million	14.2-16.9 million
Children living with HIV/AIDS in 2011	3.3 million	1.9-2.3 million
People newly infected with HIV in 2011	2.5 million	2.2-3.2 million
Children newly infected with HIV in 2011	0.33 million	0.33-0.41 million
AIDS deaths in 2011	1.7 million	1.8-2.3 million
Child AIDS deaths in 2011	0.23 million	0.25-0.29 million

Modified from Joint United Nations Programme on HIV/AIDS: *UNAIDS report on the global AIDS epidemic, 2012.* Available at http://www.unaids.org/en/media/unaids/contentassets/documents/epidemiology/2012/gr2012/20121120_unaids_global_report_2012_with_annexes_en.pdf.
AIDS, Acquired immunodeficiency syndrome; *HIV*, human immunodeficiency virus.

HUMAN IMMUNODEFICIENCY VIRUS (HIV) INFECTION

The Joint United Nations Programme on HIV/AIDS (UNAIDS) and the WHO estimate that in 2011 approximately 34 million people worldwide were infected with HIV and new infections were occurring at a rate of approximately 2.5 million per year.[164] Most HIV infections occur in LMICs; greater than 90% of those infected live in sub-Saharan Africa, Asia, Latin America, or the Caribbean. Women are particularly vulnerable to HIV infection; worldwide, approximately 50% of cases occur in women. The proportion of women infected with HIV has increased in many regions, with women representing approximately 58% of HIV infections in sub-Saharan Africa. An estimated 330,000 children were infected with HIV in 2011, mostly by maternal-to-child transmission, either in utero, at the time of delivery, or through breastfeeding.[164]

Because HIV increases deaths among young adults, the acquired immunodeficiency syndrome (AIDS) epidemic has resulted in a generation of AIDS orphans. As of 2011, about 17.3 million children younger than 18 years have lost one or both parents to AIDS, with the vast majority in sub-Saharan Africa.[165] It is well known that maternal mortality increases neonatal and infant deaths, independent of HIV infection. Global estimates for 2011, including the number of people living with HIV infection/AIDS, the number newly infected, and total AIDS deaths, are presented in Table 2-3.

Transmission: Reducing the Disparity Between Low- and High-Income Countries

Risk factors for mother-to-child transmission of HIV include maternal health and severity of disease, obstetric factors, maternal coinfection with other STDs, prematurity/LBW, and infant feeding practices (Table 2-4). In most developed

Table 2-4 Risk Factors Associated With Mother-to-Child Transmission of HIV

Risk Factor	Possible Mechanism of Mother-to-Child Transmission of Infection
MATERNAL HEALTH	
Advanced HIV disease	High viral load and low CD4 T cells
Primary HIV infection	High viral load; lack of immune response
No maternal anti-retroviral treatment	High viral load
OBSTETRIC FACTORS	
Vaginal delivery	Exposure to HIV-infected genital secretions
Episiotomies and vaginal tears	Exposure to HIV-infected blood
Instrumental deliveries	Exposure of breached infant skin to secretions containing HIV
Chorionic villus biopsy or amniocentesis	Increased risk of placental microtransfusion
Fetal electrode monitoring	Breach in infant skin and exposure to infected secretions
Prolonged rupture of fetal membranes	Prolonged exposure to HIV-infected secretions
Chorioamnionitis	Ascending infection
Low birth weight	Impaired fetal or placental membranes
Prematurity	Impaired fetal or placental membranes
MATERNAL COINFECTION	
Malaria (placental malaria)	Increased viral load, disruption in placental architecture
HSV-2	Increased plasma viral load, increased shedding of HIV in genital secretions, genital ulcers
Other STDs	Genital ulcerations and exposure to HIV-infected blood or genital secretions
INFANT FEEDING	
Breastfeeding	Mastitis, cell-free and cell-associated virus
Mixed feeding	Contaminated formula or water used in preparing formula may cause gastroenteritis leading to microtrauma to infant's bowel and provides entry to HIV virus
Miscellaneous factors	
Infant-mother HLA concordance	HLA molecules on the surface of HIV-infected maternal cells are recognized as 'self' by cytotoxic T-lymphocytes or NK cells of the infant and are therefore less likely to be destroyed
Maternal HLA homozygosity	Increased viral load
Presence of CCR5 Δ32 mutation in T cells of exposed infants	Decreased susceptibility to HIV infection

Modified from Paintsil E, Andiman A: Update on successes and challenges regarding mother-to-child transmission of HIV, *Curr Opin Pediatr* 21:94-101, 2009.
HIV, Human immunodeficiency virus; *HLA*, human leukocyte antigen; *HSV-2*, herpes simplex virus type 2; *NK*, natural killer; *STDs*, sexually transmitted diseases.

countries, a package of evidence-based interventions, including use of antiretroviral (ARV) drugs, elective cesarean section before the onset of labor and before rupture of membranes, and avoidance of breastfeeding has reduced vertical transmission of HIV to 1% to 2%, with virtual elimination of transmission in some settings.[166-169] Without interventions, it is estimated that 20% to 45% of infants may become infected.[170] Some progress has been made in reducing mother-to-infant transmission of HIV in areas where services in the public sector have been scaled up.[171] In 2010 UNICEF committed to the goal of virtual elimination of mother-to-child transmission of HIV by 2015.[172] Although this target is achievable, more resources need to be focused on implementation strategies to prevent vertical transmission.[171]

Breastfeeding and Human Immunodeficiency Virus

Although breastfeeding by HIV-positive mothers is discouraged in Europe and North America, where safe and affordable alternatives to breast milk are available, the issue of breastfeeding and HIV is much more complicated in developing countries, where breastfeeding has proven benefits and where artificial feeding has known risks. Benefits of breastfeeding include decreased risk of diarrhea and other infectious diseases, improved nutritional status, and decreased infant mortality.[173,174] Research conducted over the past 20 years has increased understanding of mother-to-child transmission of HIV through breast milk.[175-179] Risk factors for transmission of HIV via breast milk include maternal factors (e.g., recent infection or advanced maternal disease, low CD4 counts, viral load in breast milk and plasma, mastitis/breast abscess, and duration of breastfeeding), infant factors (e.g., prematurity, oral thrush, being fed breast milk as well as non–breast-milk alternatives, resulting in "mixed" infant feeding), and viral factors (viral load, clade C).[177] Three interventions have been shown to reduce late mother-to-child transmission via breastfeeding: complete avoidance of breastfeeding, exclusive breastfeeding rather than mixed feeding, and ARV prophylaxis for the lactating mother and for the infant who is breastfeeding.[177-180]

In 2006 UNAIDS, the WHO, and UNICEF issued a joint policy statement on HIV and infant feeding to help decision makers in different countries develop their own policies regarding feeding practices in the context of HIV infection.[180] The policy statement was further updated in 2010, with significant changes made to encourage wider use of ARVs.[181] The policy encourages national health authorities to recommend one infant feeding practice for all HIV-positive mothers to be promoted and supported by maternal, newborn, and child health services, as opposed to individualized counseling approaches recommended in the past. National health authorities should endorse either breastfeeding while receiving ARVs (to the mother or infant) or avoidance of all breastfeeding, depending on a careful assessment taking into account major factors, including HIV prevalence, background infant and child mortality rates, current infant and young child feeding practices and nutritional status of infants, availability of clean water and sanitation, socioeconomic status of the population, and quality of health services, including provision of interventions for prevention of mother-to-child transmission (PMTCT) of HIV. Mothers need ongoing counseling and support to optimally feed their infants. The policy also recommends that women who breastfeed and receive ARVs (or whose infants are receiving ARVs) should exclusively breastfeed their infants for 6 months and continue breastfeeding until 12 months of age.

Prevention of Human Immunodeficiency Virus Infection in Low- and Middle-Income Countries

Primary prevention of HIV infection among women of childbearing age is the most successful but most difficult way to prevent the infection of infants. Improving the social status of women, education of both men and women, ensuring access to information about HIV infection and its prevention, promotion of safer sex through condom use, social marketing of condoms, and treatment of other STDs that increase the risk of HIV transmission are potential strategies that have been successful at reducing HIV infection. A goal for health services in LMICs is to provide interventions to reduce sexual transmission of HIV, with special focus on reducing infections during pregnancy and among women who are breastfeeding, and to prevent unintended pregnancies among women infected with HIV.

Prevention of Transmission From an Infected Mother to Her Infant

Antiretroviral Strategies. The era of antiretroviral therapy (ART) to reduce vertical transmission of HIV started in 1994 with publication of the Pediatric AIDS Clinical Trials Groups (ACTG) Protocol 076.[182] This trial, performed in the United States and France, demonstrated that 3′-azido-3′-deoxythymidine (AZT; zidovudine) administered orally to HIV-infected pregnant women with no prior treatment with ARV drugs during pregnancy, beginning at 14 to 34 weeks of gestation and continuing throughout pregnancy and then intravenously during labor to the mother, and orally to the newborn for the first 6 weeks of life, reduced perinatal transmission by 67.5%, from 25.5% (95% CI, 18.4% to 32.5%) to 8.3% (95% CI, 3.9% to 12.8%). The regimen was recommended as standard care in the United States and quickly became common practice. Studies over the past 15 years have shown that a variety of ARV regimens among pregnant women can reduce mother-to child transmission of HIV. Moreover, these studies have shown that it is feasible to provide ART and prophylaxis to women in LMICs and thus substantially reduce mother-to-child transmission throughout the world.[183-186] A trial from Kenya showed success and feasiblity of a maternal triple-ARV regimen from late pregnancy through 6 months of breastfeeding for PMTCT, with HIV transmission rates at birth, 6 weeks, 6 months, 12 months, and 24 months of 2.5%, 4.2%, 5.0%, 5.7%, and 7.0%, respectively.[175] Another trial in Malawi showed decreased risk of HIV-1 transmission with the continued use of maternal ARVs for 28 weeks postpartum (in addition to intrapartum nevirapine), compared with the control group given ARVs for 1 week only (4% vs. 7%).[176] ART requires the identification of HIV-infected women early enough in pregnancy to allow them access to therapy; therefore a system for voluntary, confidential HIV counseling and testing must be in place. In 2011 only 57% of pregnant women in LMICs had access to effective ARV regimens for PMTCT. In sub-Saharan Africa, home to 92% of pregnant women living with HIV, the percentage of pregnant women living with HIV who receive antiretroviral therapy or prophylaxis is now 59% (53%-66%). Reported coverage is believed to be substantially lower in South and Southeast Asia (18% [13%-23%]) and in the Middle East and North Africa (7% [6%-9%]).[163]

Cesarean Section to ReduceTransmission of Human Immunodeficiency Virus. Meta-analyses of North American and European studies performed in the late 1990s found that elective cesarean section reduced the risk of mother-to-child transmission of HIV by greater than 50%.[187,188] For mothers on highly active ART and with low viral loads, the benefits of delivery by cesarean section for reducing perinatal transmission of HIV are uncertain, especially in low-resource settings where risks of operative complications are high.[189]

Integrated Health Care Programs

Successful programs to reduce mother-to-child transmission of HIV require integration with health care services for women and children. These programs provide early access to adequate ANC; voluntary and confidential counseling and HIV testing for women and their partners; ARV drugs during pregnancy and delivery for HIV-positive women; improved care during labor and delivery; counseling for HIV-positive women regarding choices for infant feeding; support for HIV-positive women with ongoing health care and ARVs for life and follow-up for their infants; and access to voluntary family planning information, services, and supplies (Box 2-1).

Human Immunodeficiency Virus and Child Survival

Although there have been tremendous gains in child survival over the past 3 decades, with reductions worldwide in deaths caused by diarrhea, pneumonia, malaria, vaccine-preventable diseases, and neonatal conditions, especially neonatal infections,[190,191] the AIDS epidemic threatens to undermine this dramatic trend in some countries in sub-Saharan Africa.[192] In sub-Saharan Africa, AIDS has become a leading cause of death among infants and children, although globally it causes just 3% of under-5 mortality.[190,191] Moreover, there is a complex link between increasing mortality of children younger than 5 years

Box 2-1 Package of Essential Services for High-Quality Maternal Care

Package of Routine Quality Antenatal and Postpartum Care for All Women Regardless of HIV Status

1. Health education, information on prevention and care for HIV and sexually transmitted infections, including safer sex practices, pregnancy including antenatal care, birth planning and delivery assistance, malaria prevention, optimal infant feeding, and family planning counseling and related services
2. Provider-initiated HIV testing and counseling, including HIV testing and counseling for women of unknown status at labor and delivery or postpartum
3. Couple and partner HIV testing and counseling, including support for disclosure
4. Promotion and provision of male and female condoms
5. HIV-related gender-based violence screening
6. Obstetric care, including history taking and physical examination
7. Maternal nutritional support
8. Counseling on infant feeding
9. Psychosocial support
10. Birth planning, birth preparedness (including pregnancy and postpartum danger signs), including skilled birth attendants
11. Tetanus vaccination
12. Iron and folic acid supplementation
13. Syphilis screening and management of sexually transmitted diseases
14. Risk reduction interventions for injecting drug users

Additional Package of Services for Women Living With HIV

1. Additional counseling and support to encourage partner testing, adoption of risk reduction and disclosure
2. Clinical evaluation, including clinical staging of HIV disease
3. Immunologic assessment (CD4 cell count) where available
4. ARV therapy when indicated
5. Counseling and support on infant feeding based on knowledge of HIV status
6. ARV prophylaxis for prevention of mother-to-child transmission of HIV provided during the antepartum, intrapartum, and postpartum periods
7. Cotrimoxazole prophylaxis where indicated
8. Additional counseling and provision of services as appropriate to prevent unintended pregnancies
9. Supportive care, including adherence support
10. Additional counseling and provision of services as appropriate to prevent unintended pregnancies
11. Tuberculosis screening and treatment when indicated; preventive therapy (isoniazid prophylaxis) when appropriate
12. Advice and support on other prevention interventions, such as safe drinking water
13. Supportive care, including adherence support and palliative care and symptom management

Additional Package of Services for All Women Regardless of HIV Status in Specific Settings

1. Malaria prevention and treatment
2. Counseling, psychosocial support and referral for women who are at risk of or have experienced violence
3. Counseling and referral for women with a history of harmful alcohol or drug use
4. De-worming
5. Consider retesting late in pregnancy where feasible in generalized epidemics

Essential Postnatal Care for HIV-Exposed Infants and Young Children

1. Completion of ARV prophylaxis regimen as necessary
2. Routine newborn and infant care, including routine immunization and growth monitoring
3. Cotrimoxazole prophylaxis
4. Early HIV diagnostic testing and diagnosis of HIV-related conditions
5. Continued infant feeding counseling and support, especially after HIV testing and at 6 months
6. Nutritional support throughout the first year of life, including support for optimal infant feeding practices and provision of nutritional supplements and replacement foods if indicated
7. ARV therapy for children living with HIV when indicated
8. Treatment monitoring for all children receiving ARV therapy
9. Isoniazid prophylaxis when indicated
10. Counseling on adherence support for caregivers
11. Malaria prevention and treatment where indicated
12. Diagnosis and management of common childhood infections and conditions and Integrated Management of Childhood Illness (IMCI) strategy
13. Diagnosis and management of tuberculosis and other opportunistic infections

ARV Regimens Recommended by the WHO for Treating Pregnant Women and Preventing HIV Infection in Infants: Promoting More Efficacious ARV Regimens

1. The WHO recommends ART for all pregnant women who are eligible for treatment. Initiation of ART in pregnant women will address not only their health needs but will also significantly reduce HIV transmission to their infants. In addition, by securing the health of women, it also improves child well-being and survival.
2. For pregnant women with HIV who do not yet require ART, ARV prophylactic regimens are recommended for mother-to-child transmission prevention. The recommended regimens by the WHO are based on AZT (from 28 weeks of pregnancy or as soon as possible thereafter) plus single-dose nevirapine plus a maternal 7-day tail of AZT and 3TC and 1 week of AZT for the infant.
3. Updated WHO guidelines recommend lifelong ART (one simplified triple regimen) for all pregnant and breastfeeding women with HIV, regardless of their clinical stage or CD4 cell count. This is referred to as Option B+.

Modified from the World Health Organization (WHO), United Nations Children's Fund, Interaction Task Team: Guidance on global scale-up of the prevention of mother-to-child transmission of HIV. © WHO 2007. Available at http://www.who.int/hiv/mtct/PMTCT_enWEBNov26.pdf. Accessed January 6, 2014.

ART, Antiretroviral therapy; *ARV*, antiretroviral; *AZT*, 3′-azido-3′-deoxythymidine (zidovudine); *HIV*, human immunodeficiency virus; *3TC*, lamivudine; *WHO*, World Health Organization.

and high rates of HIV prevalence in adults, related to both mother-to-child transmission of HIV and the compromised ability of parents who are ill themselves to care for young children.[193] With success of PMTCT programs, increasing numbers of HIV-exposed but uninfected infants are being born.[194] A challenge for health care systems is to ensure that these infants have access to health care and remain healthy. Programs for HIV/AIDS prevention and treatment have been developed largely as vertical programs that now need to be linked to broader efforts to improve maternal, neonatal, and child health care, including family planning services in LMICs.

TUBERCULOSIS

In 2010 tuberculosis (TB) caused 1.2 million deaths worldwide and caused 4.6% of all deaths in women aged 15 to 49 years.[195] After HIV/AIDS, TB is the second leading cause of death from infectious causes among women of childbearing age (15-44 years), with an estimated 228,000 deaths occurring annually in this population.[196] The vast majority of the world's disability-adjusted life years, or DALYs (99.4%), and deaths (99.6%) caused by TB occur in LMICs.[196,197] TB during pregnancy may have adverse consequences for mother and baby, including increased risk of miscarriage, prematurity, LBW, and neonatal death.[198-202] Without adequate treatment, half of all neonates born with congenital TB may eventually die.[198] Adverse perinatal outcomes are increased in mothers who have late diagnosis or incomplete or irregular therapy.[199] Ideally diagnosis and treatment of TB in women should occur before pregnancy.

The lung remains the most common site of infection; however, the prevalence of extrapulmonary TB is increasing. Although congenital TB is rare, the fetus may become infected by hematogenous spread in a woman with placentitis by swallowing or aspirating infected amniotic fluid or by direct contact with an infected cervix at the time of delivery.[198,202] The most common route of infection of the neonate, however, is through airborne transmission of *Mycobacterium tuberculosis* from an infected, untreated mother to her infant. Infected newborns are at particularly high risk of developing severe disease, including fulminant septic shock with disseminated intravascular coagulation and respiratory failure.[202,203] The diagnosis of neonatal TB may be facilitated by using a set of diagnostic criteria developed by Cantwell and colleagues.[204] These include demonstration of primary hepatic complex/caseating granulomas in the liver, tuberculous infection of the placenta or maternal genital tract, and demonstration of lesions during the first week of life.

The resurgence of TB and the increased risk of TB among those who are infected with HIV are well known. In areas where HIV is endemic, TB rates have been increasing.[205,206] Pregnant women who are coinfected with HIV may be at increased risk for placental or genital TB, resulting in an increased risk of transmission to the fetus.[207] In addition, neonates born with TB/HIV coinfection have been shown to be at higher risk of severe, rapidly progressive HIV disease.[208] In areas of the world where both TB and HIV are endemic, the key to preventing neonatal TB is early identification of maternal TB and HIV serostatus, based primarily on maternal history and relevant investigations of the mother and newborn and initiation of effective treatment.[198,209]

MALARIA

From a global perspective, malaria is one of the most important infectious diseases. Half of the world's population lives in areas with malaria risk. The disease is mainly confined to poorer tropical areas of Africa, Asia, and Latin America. In 2010 an estimated 660,000 deaths occurred resulting from malaria, with 86% of these occurring in children younger than 5 years.[210] Countries in sub-Saharan Africa account for greater than 90% of malaria cases and 88% of malaria cases among children younger than 5 years.[211]

The true burden of congenital malaria remains unknown. Studies in Africa have shown that 7% to 10% of newborns may have malaria parasites in their cord blood,[212] whereas other studies have shown a very low prevalence of parasitemia.[213] Four species of the malaria parasite infect humans: *Plasmodium falciparum*, *Plasmodium vivax*, *Plasmodium ovale*, and *Plasmodium malariae*. *P. falciparum* is responsible for the most severe form of disease and is the predominant parasite in tropical Africa, Southeast Asia, the Amazon area, and the Pacific. Groups at greatest risk for severe disease and death are young nonimmune children, pregnant women (especially primigravidas), and nonimmune adults.[214]

Malaria in Pregnancy

Preexisting levels of immunity determine susceptibility to infection and severity of disease.[214-218] In areas of high endemicity or high stable transmission, where there are high levels of protective immunity, the effects of malaria on the mother and fetus are less severe than in areas where malaria transmission is low or unstable (i.e., sporadic, periodic). It is unclear why pregnant women (even with preexisting immunity) are at increased risk for malaria. The most severe maternal complications (cerebral malaria, pulmonary edema, renal failure) occur in women who have lived previously in nonendemic areas and who have little or no immunity to *P. falciparum*. Severe malaria may result in pregnancy-related maternal death.

Malaria parasitemia is more common, and the parasite burden tends to be higher in pregnant than in nonpregnant women.[215,217] This increase in both prevalence and density of parasitemia is highest in primiparous women and decreases with increasing parity.[217] The greater severity in primiparous women from endemic areas appears to be attributable in part to a pregnancy-restricted *P. falciparum* variable surface protein present on parasitized erythrocytes; because primiparous women have not been previously exposed to this antigen, they lack immunity to it, allowing this protein to bind to placental chondroitin sulfate and parasitized erythrocytes to become sequestered in the placenta.[219] The parasite burden is highest in the second trimester and decreases with increasing gestation.[218,220,221] The most important effects of malaria on pregnant women are severe anemia[215,222] and placental infection.[214-218,223,224] The prevalence of anemia can be as high as 78%, and anemia is more common and more severe in primigravidas.[223]

Perinatal Outcome

Perinatal outcome is directly related to placental malaria. Malaria is associated with an increase in spontaneous abortions, stillbirths, preterm delivery, and intrauterine growth restriction, particularly in areas where malaria is acquired by nonimmune women.[218,225-227] Reported rates of fetal loss range from 9% to 50%.[217] The uteroplacental vascular space is thought to be a relatively protected site for parasite sequestration and replication.[224,228] Placental malaria is characterized by the presence of parasites and leukocytes in the intervillous space, pigment within macrophages, proliferation of cytotrophoblasts, and thickening of the trophoblastic basement membrane.[223] Placental infection may alter the function of the placenta, reducing oxygen and nutrient transport and resulting in intrauterine growth restriction, and may allow the passage of infected red blood cells to the fetus, resulting in congenital infection. In primigravidas living in endemic areas, placental malaria occurs in 16% to 63% of women, whereas in multigravidas, the prevalence is much lower at 12% to 33%.[215,217]

The most profound effect of placental malaria is the reduction of birth weight.[218,225,229,230] Both *P. falciparum* and *P. vivax* infection during pregnancy are associated with a reduction in birth weight.[225,231] Steketee and associates[229] have estimated that in highly endemic settings, placental malaria may account for approximately 13% of cases of LBW secondary to intrauterine growth restriction. Of importance, malaria is one of the few preventable causes of LBW. Because LBW is a major determinant of neonatal and infant mortality in developing countries, malaria may indirectly increase mortality by increasing LBW.[232]

Congenital Malaria

Transplacental infection of the fetus also may occur. It is relatively rare in populations with prior immunity (0.1%-1.5%),[215] but more common in nonimmune mothers. It is thought that the low rate of fetal infection concomitant with a high incidence of placental infection is due in part to protection from transplacental maternal antibodies.[233,234]

The clinical characteristics of neonates with congenital malaria (i.e., malaria parasitemia on peripheral blood smear) include fever, respiratory distress, pallor, anemia, hepatomegaly, jaundice, and diarrhea. There is a high mortality rate with congenital infection.[235] The global burden of disease related to congenital malaria is unknown.

Prevention and Treatment of Malaria in Pregnancy

Pregnant women living in malaria-endemic areas need access to services that can provide prompt, safe, and effective treatment for malaria. Among at-risk pregnant populations in stable-/high-transmission areas, the WHO recommends that malaria control strategies include ANC, a dose of intermittent preventive treatment (IPT) (e.g., with sulfadoxine-pyrimethamine) at each ANC visit during the second and third trimester, the early and consistent use of insecticide-treated bed nets during pregnancy through the postpartum period, effective case management of malaria, and screening and treatment of anemia frequently resulting from malaria infection.[236,237] In low-transmission areas, case management is emphasized.[237] Malaria prevention guidelines have been recently updated, and since October 2012, the WHO has recommended IPT at each scheduled ANC visit after the first trimester.[210]

Prophylaxis and Treatment Using Antimalarial Drugs

There are a limited number of safe and effective antimalarials available for use in pregnancy. For a drug to be considered safe, it must be safe for the mother, for the fetus, and ideally for the breastfeeding infant.[238,239] Historically, chloroquine, the safest, cheapest, most widely available antimalarial drug, was the agent of choice for the prevention and treatment of malaria in pregnancy.[238] However, in all areas where *P. falciparum* is prevalent, the parasite is at least partially resistant to chloroquine, and resistance to sulfadoxine-pyrimethamine, the first-line drug for IPT in pregnancy, is increasing.[240,241] New drug development has been impeded by the fact that pregnant women have been excluded for ethical reasons from drug development programs because of the justified fear of risks to the fetus.[242,243]

A 2006 systematic review on drugs for preventing malaria in pregnant women examined studies on antimalarial prophylaxis and IPT.[244] Chemoprophylaxis or IPT is associated with reduced maternal disease, including anemia and placental infection. One study found that the incidence of placental malaria is reduced by prophylaxis, even when chloroquine is used in areas with chloroquine-resistant malaria.[245] In addition, antimalarial prophylaxis was seen to have a positive effect on birth weight, risk of preterm delivery, and neonatal mortality (risk ratio [RR], 0.73; 95% CI, 0.53 to 0.99).[244]

A major problem with both chemoprophylaxis and prompt therapy for known or suspected infection is that it is often difficult to deliver services to pregnant women, especially those who live in areas remote from health centers. IPT involves single-dose treatment of a safe and effective antimalarial given to women in malaria-endemic areas at each ANC visit, with the presumption that they are at high risk of malaria infection. Recent studies from Africa have demonstrated that IPT can reduce the incidence of malaria and its adverse consequences substantially.[246,247] A recent study in Mozambique showed that IPT reduced neonatal mortality by 61% in the population under study.[248] In 2000 the WHO recommended IPT with sulfadoxine-pyrimethamine in malaria-endemic areas where *P. falciparum* is resistant to chloroquine and sensitive to sulfadoxine-pyrimethamine.[249] This drug is not bitter and is relatively well tolerated. In areas where malaria transmission is lower and *P. vivax* as well as *P. falciparum* are a problem, finding an appropriate drug regimen is more difficult.[250] In these areas and where *P. falciparum* is resistant to sulfadoxine-pyrimethamine, further research on the safety and efficacy of alternative antimalarial drugs for both prevention and treatment of malaria in pregnancy, including artemisinin-based combination therapies (ACTs), is urgently needed.[243]

Current WHO recommendations for treatment of malaria in pregnancy include quinine plus clindamycin during the first trimester. If this treatment fails or is unavailable, or there is uncertainty regarding patient compliance, ACT is indicated. For the second and third trimesters, ACT known to be effective in the region should be used.[251]

Prevention Using Insecticide-Treated Nets

Although the benefits of antimalarial chemoprophylaxis have been established, poor compliance and increasing drug resistance have led to trials of alternative prevention strategies.[252] The use of insecticide-treated nets (ITNs) has been successful in reducing childhood morbidity and mortality in malaria-endemic areas.[253-255] A systematic review of ITN use during pregnancy in Africa associated their use with a reduced risk of placental malaria in all pregnancies (RR, 0.79; 95% CI, 0.63 to 0.98), reduced risk of LBW (RR, 0.77; 95% CI, 0.61 to 0.98) and reduced risk of fetal loss in the first to fourth pregnancy (RR, 0.67; 95% CI, 0.47 to 0.97).[256] The use of social marketing and incentives, such as voucher and discounted net programs, has increased bed-net coverage and use.[257,258] An additional benefit of bed-net use is protection of the neonate, who almost always sleeps with the mother in these settings.[257] A pooled analysis of studies of ITN use in early childhood found a reduction in all-cause child mortality associated with the use of ITNs (RR, 0.82; 95% CI, 0.76 to 0.89).[14] Although there is clear evidence of the impact of ITNs in Africa, further data are needed from trials of ITNs in Latin America and Asia, and areas of high *P. vivax* transmission.[256]

Malaria Control Strategies and Challenges

Comprehensive malaria prevention and treatment strategies implementing the interventions recommended by the WHO can have dramatic effects on child health outcomes. A program that achieved high coverage of multiple malaria control measures in Equatorial Guinea was associated with reduced prevalence of malaria infection (OR, 0.31; 95% CI, 0.2 to 0.46), and led to an overall reduction in under-5 mortality from 152 per 1000 to 55 per 1000 live births (hazard ratio [HR], 0.34; 95% CI, 0.23 to 0.49).[259] Results from other African settings of high malaria transmission have also been promising.[260]

Effective vaccination against malaria could be a powerful strategy for control. Several vaccine candidates are undergoing field evaluation for potential use in public health programs.[261,262] Of these, clinical development of the RTS,S/AS01 vaccine is the most advanced and expected to gain licensure in 2015.[261] The RTS,S/AS01 vaccine targets the pre-erythrocytic stages in the life cycle of the parasite and has shown modest efficacy of 31.3% (95% CI, 23.6 to 38.3) against prevention of malaria in African infants in the per-protocol population.[263] Vaccine efficacy against severe malaria was 36.6% (95% CI, 4.6 to 57.7).[263]

Studies have shown an association between malaria and HIV in pregnancy, with an increase in the risk of maternal malaria and of placental malaria in HIV-positive mothers, although the influence of malaria on the clinical course of HIV infection remains unclear.[264-266] There is some suggestion that coinfection with malaria and HIV infection in pregnancy may be linked with increased mother-to-child transmission of HIV and both perinatal and early infant mortality, as well as postneonatal morbidity.[267,268] IPT with sulfadoxine-pyrimethamine is less effective in preventing malaria in HIV-infected than uninfected women, underscoring the need for research to expand the arsenal of safe and effective antimalarials. Furthermore, interactions between antimalarial and ARV drugs are poorly understood.[267] There remains a need for effective, practical, and well-tolerated strategies to prevent and treat malaria in women with HIV.

Indirect Causes of Neonatal Death Related to Infection

In addition to direct infectious causes of neonatal deaths, there are many indirect causes that contribute to infectious deaths in developing countries. These contributory factors have socioeconomic as well as medical roots. Sociocultural factors include poverty, illiteracy, low social status of women, lack of political power (for women and children) and lack of will in those who have power, gender discrimination (for both mother and neonate), harmful traditional or cultural practices, poor hygiene, lack of clean water and sanitation, the cultural belief that a sick newborn is doomed to die and that the family is powerless to alter fate, the family's inability to recognize danger signs in the newborn, inadequate access to high-quality medical care (either because it is unavailable, unaffordable, or because of the lack of transport for emergency care) or the lack of supplies or appropriate drugs, and maternal death.[269-274] Medical factors that may also contribute to an infectious neonatal death include poor maternal physical and mental health, untreated maternal infections (including STDs, urinary tract infection, and chorioamnionitis), failure to fully immunize the mother against tetanus, unhygienic and inappropriate management of labor and delivery, unsanitary cutting and care of the umbilical cord, failure to promote early and exclusive breastfeeding, and prematurity and/or LBW.[269,270,275-278] To promote change, families must be empowered and mobilized to identify illness and to seek care. Health care workers (of all levels) must know what to do and must have the resources, including commodities, to support needed therapy. Moreover, better maternal care, both preventive and curative, is preventive medicine for the newborn.

Coordinated activities are needed to bring about change that is sustainable by countries on their own, over the long haul. This will involve a multidisciplinary approach—bringing together people with different interests, from different backgrounds, different agencies, different government ministries—to seek solutions to problems and to implement change at the local level. Finally, it will involve the global acknowledgment that this is the right thing to do (i.e., a moral imperative) and therefore the long-term commitment of substantial funding to help provide needed services to low-resource, high maternal and neonatal–mortality countries in a coordinated way that is responsive to the needs of countries. A major remaining challenge is to link science and medicine with social solutions through a global commitment to long-term, long-lasting change so that improvements in both maternal and newborn health can be achieved and sustained.

Strategies to Prevent and Treat Infection in the Neonate

Strategies to prevent or reduce neonatal infections and to reduce morbidity and mortality in those newborns in whom infection develops involve putting into practice what is

Box 2-2 Interventions to Reduce Neonatal Infections or to Reduce Infection-Associated Mortality in Low- and Middle-Income Countries[10,12,14]

Periconceptual Care

Folic acid supplementation to prevent neural tube defects (and associated risk of infectious morbidity and mortality)

Antenatal Care

Tetanus immunization
- Maternal influenza immunization
- Primary prevention of sexually transmitted disease, including human immunodeficiency virus infection, through maternal education and safer sex using condoms
- Diagnosis and treatment of sexually transmitted diseases (e.g., syphilis), urinary tract infection (including detection and treatment of asymptomatic bacteriuria), malaria, tuberculosis
- Intermittent presumptive treatment for malaria
- Sleeping under an insecticide-treated bed net
- Balanced protein-energy supplements in food-insecure populations

Intrapartum/Delivery Care

Skilled maternal and immediate newborn care
- Antibiotics for preterm premature rupture of membranes
- Corticosteroids for preterm labor (to prevent respiratory distress syndrome/hyaline membrane disease)
- Optimal management of complications, including fever, premature rupture of membranes, puerperal sepsis
- Clean delivery
- Clean cutting of the umbilical cord and clean cord care
- Immediate breastfeeding

Postnatal Care

Immediate, exclusive breastfeeding
- Hand washing
- Thermal care to prevent and manage hypothermia
- Skin-to-skin care
- Emollient therapy (e.g., sunflower seed oil for very preterm infants)
- Case management for pneumonia

known and creating innovative ways to make these interventions feasible in a developing country context. In addition to facility-based care, use of simple, cost-effective technologies that are potentially available and feasible for use in the community and at first-level health facilities could have a major impact in reducing morbidity and mortality related to neonatal infection. Moreover, public health, medical, and social interventions all have a role to play in reducing the global burden of neonatal infection. Several potential interventions are reviewed here (Box 2-2).

MATERNAL IMMUNIZATION TO PREVENT NEONATAL DISEASE

There is growing interest in the use of maternal immunization to protect neonates and very young infants from infection through passively acquired transplacental or breast-milk antibodies, or both (see Chapter 38).[279-281] Immunization of pregnant women with tetanus toxoid has dramatically reduced cases of neonatal tetanus and is the classic example of maternal immunization and subsequent passive immunization to protect the newborn as well as the mother.[141,282] Because most immunoglobulin G (IgG) antibody is transported across the placenta in the last 4 to 6 weeks of pregnancy, maternal immunization to prevent neonatal disease through transplacental antibodies is most promising for term rather than preterm newborns, as the former will have adequate antibody levels at birth. Boosting breast-milk antibodies by immunizing the mother is a potential strategy for reducing infection in both term and preterm infants.

Vaccination of mothers against influenza has been shown to reduce maternal and neonatal morbidity and holds promise as an effective strategy for improving maternal and perinatal outcomes.[283] Despite the fact that no study to date has demonstrated an increased risk of either maternal complications or adverse fetal outcomes associated with inactivated influenza vaccination,[281,284] compliance remains poor. A recent study in Bangladesh[285] revealed a greater burden of influenza in infants than had been predicted and, moreover, showed that maternal influenza vaccination provided significant protection to infants as well as their mothers. Vaccinating mothers against influenza reduced laboratory-proven influenza in their infants by 68% from birth to 6 months of age and also reduced episodes of maternal influenza-like illnesses by 35%. Other ongoing and recently completed studies in Mali, South Africa, and Nepal will increase our understanding of the benefits of maternal immunization with influenza vaccine. To achieve protection, influenza vaccines need to be administered during each pregnancy. This would require strengthening of current antenatal immunization programs, which have limited reach, and education on the benefits of the vaccine to overcome the general reluctance to intervene in healthy pregnant women.

Other vaccines currently being developed or field tested to reduce or prevent neonatal infection by maternal immunization include vaccines against GBS, *S. pneumoniae*, and *H. influenzae*.[286-295] Because most neonatal GBS disease, especially the most severe, occurs in the first hours of life, maternal immunization to provide passive protection to the neonate is a potentially important strategy.[35,296] A problem with GBS vaccines has been poor immunogenicity, resulting in more recent interest in the potential of conjugate vaccines.[297] GBS polysaccharide–tetanus toxoid conjugates are safe in adults and elicit antibody levels above what is likely to be passively protective for neonates.[289,290] Multivalent vaccines, which could provide protection against multiple GBS serotypes, are particularly promising.[288]

Pneumococcal polysaccharide vaccines have been administered safely to pregnant women.[292,294] A study from Bangladesh reported that pneumococcal vaccination during pregnancy increased type-specific IgG serum antibody in both mother and infant.[293] Cord blood levels of antibody were about half those of the mother, with IgG1 subclass antibodies preferentially transferred to the infant. The estimated antibody half-life in the infant was 35 days. Immunization increased breast-milk antibody as well. However, in a study of the 23-valent pneumococcal vaccine given to women before pregnancy, neither mothers nor infants had significantly elevated pneumococcus-specific antibody at delivery.[293] If passive immunization does not interfere with active immunization of young infants, vaccination of pregnant women could potentially be used to prevent pneumococcal disease in early infancy, followed by active immunization of the older infant; however, this requires further research.

Maternal pertussis vaccination has been an area of recent debate. There has been a substantial increase in reported cases of pertussis in the United States. In 2012 there were 41,880 reported cases and 14 deaths in infants younger than 1 year,[298] causing the Centers for Disease Control and Prevention (CDC) to recommend the use of tetanus toxoid, reduced diphtheria toxoid, and acellular pertussis vaccine (Tdap) during every pregnancy. However, the resurgence of pertussis has not been uniform worldwide.[299] With varying incidence trends and lack of data from developing countries, surveillance to understand disease burden in early infancy and effectiveness of maternal pertussis vaccination to prevent neonatal disease are needed.[300]

Additional studies of the safety, efficacy, and effectiveness of immunizing pregnant women with specific vaccines are needed. Studies must address issues of safety to the mother, fetus, and young infant. Vaccines are not routinely tested for safety in pregnant women, so most safety data come from animal studies or postlicensure pregnancy registries and adverse event reporting systems. However, based on accumulated evidence, vaccines against diphtheria, tetanus, and influenza have been recommended for use in pregnancy. Studies must assess protection against specific diseases (e.g., sepsis, pneumonia, meningitis) as well as protection against all-cause neonatal and infant mortality. Local epidemiology must also be considered because HIV and malaria can reduce the amount of antibody transferred to the fetus, lowering the benefits of maternal immunization programs in highly endemic areas. The subsequent response of the infant to active immunization also must be evaluated, to ensure that passive immunization does not interfere with the infant's ability to mount an immune response. Therefore in LMICs, studies must be carried out in settings in which it is possible to maintain surveillance throughout infancy.

NEONATAL IMMUNIZATION

Protection of young infants against vaccine-preventable diseases requires vaccines that are immunogenic in early life (see Chapter 38).[301] Bacillus Calmette-Guérin (BCG), hepatitis B, and oral poliovirus vaccines are currently given to neonates within the first days of life in many LMICs. The BCG vaccine, developed early in this century, is a live-attenuated strain of *Mycobacterium bovis*. The WHO promotes the use of BCG in newborns to prevent TB, and this vaccine is widely used in developing countries in which TB is a common and potentially lethal disease. Although approximately 3 billion doses have been given, the efficacy of this vaccine is still debated. Vaccine efficacy in many prospective trials and case-control studies of vaccine use at all ages ranges from possibly harmful to 90% protective.[302] One meta-analysis of BCG studies in newborns and infants concluded that the vaccine was effective and reduced infection in children by greater than 50%.[303] It was estimated that the 100 million BCG vaccinations given to infants in 2002 prevented nearly 30,000 cases of tuberculous meningitis (5th to 95th centiles; range, 24,063-36,192) in children during their first 5 years of life, or one case for every 3435 vaccinations (range, 27,710-4177), and 11,486 cases of miliary tuberculosis (range, 7304-16,280), or one case for every 9314 vaccinations (range, 6172-13,729).[304] At a cost of U.S. $2 to $3 per dose, BCG vaccination costs U.S. $206 ($150-$272) per year of healthy life gained, considered highly cost-effective. BCG reduced the risk of pulmonary TB, TB meningitis, disseminated TB, and death from TB. Factors that may explain the variability of responses to BCG vaccination in different studies and populations include use of a wide variety of vaccine preparations, regional differences in environmental flora that may alter vaccine response, and population differences.[279] The safety of BCG in immunocompromised patients (e.g., those with HIV infection) is of significant concern, and the WHO has made HIV infection in infants a full contraindication to BCG vaccination.[305]

Hepatitis B vaccination of newborns was the first demonstration of newborn vaccination to prevent neonatal infections and subsequent adult sequelae.[306] Studies from both developed and developing countries have shown that hepatitis B vaccine administered in the immediate newborn period can significantly reduce the rate of neonatal infection and the development of a chronic hepatitis B surface antigen carrier state.[307] The efficacy of vaccine alone (without hepatitis B immune globulin [HBIG]) has allowed developing countries that cannot screen pregnant women and do not have HBIG to make a major impact in reducing the infection of newborns. The WHO recommends that all countries include hepatitis B vaccine in their routine childhood immunization programs.[308]

With the global problem of increasing antibiotic resistance, maternal and neonatal immunizations have become even more important strategies to pursue. In LMICs, issues of vaccine cost, availability, and efficacy in the field are particularly pressing and are major barriers to the use of vaccines that are known to be safe and effective. The Global Alliance for Vaccines and Immunizations (GAVI), established in 1999 with funding from the Bill & Melinda Gates Foundation and others, is working to address these issues. Since 2000, 370 million additional children were immunized with vaccines funded by GAVI, and more than 5.5 million premature deaths were averted.[309]

ANTENATAL CARE AND PREVENTION OF NEONATAL INFECTION

The care and general well-being of the mother are inextricably linked to the health of her newborn. ANC can play an important role in the prevention or reduction of neonatal infections.[310] Both preventive and curative interventions directed toward the mother can have beneficial effects on the fetus or newborn or both. Tetanus immunization of the pregnant woman is an essential component of any developing country's ANC program and, as discussed earlier, will prevent neonatal tetanus.[311,312] The diagnosis and treatment of STDs—especially syphilis, gonorrhea, and chlamydial infection—can have a significant impact on neonatal morbidity and mortality.[313,314] In areas of the world in which syphilis is endemic, congenital syphilis may be an important cause of neonatal morbidity and mortality.[315] Antenatal treatment of gonorrhea and chlamydial infection can prevent neonatal infection with these agents: ophthalmia neonatorum (for gonorrhea and chlamydial infection), disseminated gonorrhea, and neonatal respiratory disease (for chlamydial infection).[313,314] Moreover, STDs and maternal urinary tract infection increase the mother's risk of puerperal sepsis, with its associated increased risk of neonatal sepsis. In malaria-endemic areas, treatment of maternal malaria can have an impact on newborn health, particularly through a reduction in the incidence of LBW.[316]

ANC also is an important setting for maternal education regarding danger signs during pregnancy, labor, delivery, and the early postpartum period—especially maternal fever, prolonged or premature rupture of the membranes, and prolonged labor—and danger signs to watch for in the newborn. Moreover, it is the time and place for the mother to plan where and by whom she will be delivered and for the health care worker to stress the importance of a clean delivery, preferably with a skilled birth attendant. Antenatal visits, including home visits by a community health worker, also provide an opportunity to educate the mother on birth and newborn care preparedness, including anticipation of breastfeeding and keeping the infant warm, which are important for prevention of neonatal infections.

INTRAPARTUM AND DELIVERY CARE AND PREVENTION OF NEONATAL INFECTION

It is universally recognized that poor aseptic techniques during labor and delivery, including performing procedures with unclean hands and unclean instruments and unhygienic cutting of the umbilical cord, are major risk factors for both maternal and neonatal infections.[317,318] It is essential to promote safe and hygienic practices at every level of the health care system where women deliver (i.e., home, first-level health clinic, district or referral hospital). Proper management of labor and delivery can have a significant impact on the prevention of neonatal infection. It is important to emphasize the need for clean hands, clean perineum, clean delivery surface, clean instruments, clean cord care, avoidance of harmful traditional practices, prevention of unnecessary vaginal examinations, prevention of prolonged labor, and optimal management of pregnancy complications, including prolonged rupture of the membranes, maternal fever, and chorioamnionitis/puerperal sepsis.[22,319,320]

Prophylactic antibiotic use in women with preterm rupture of membranes (PROM) has been shown to reduce the risk of neonatal infections (RR, 0.67; 95% CI, 0.52 to 0.85) and chorioamnionitis (RR, 0.66; 95% CI, 0.46 to 0.96) in a recent Cochrane review.[321] However, it is unclear whether there is any effect on neonatal mortality reduction or long-term benefit to the newborn.[321] Evidence regarding choice of antibiotic regimen to use is lacking. The combination of amoxicillin-clavulanate in women with PROM is associated with a substantially increased risk of necrotizing enterocolitis in newborns (RR, 4.72; 95% CI, 1.57 to 14.23).[321] For mothers delivering in LMIC hospitals, the benefit of prophylactic antibiotics in women with PROM is not known.

POSTNATAL CARE AND PREVENTION OF NEONATAL INFECTION

The birth attendant is responsible for observation of the newborn at and after birth and deciding that the newborn is healthy and ready to be "discharged" to the care of the mother. It is important to link postpartum care of the mother with surveillance and care of the newborn. The postnatal visit(s) should be used for health education and negotiation of improved household practices, as well as to detect and treat the sick newborn and to evaluate the mother. Birth attendants need to be trained to identify problems in the newborn, to treat simple problems (e.g., skin infections), and to refer newborns with conditions that are potentially life-threatening (e.g., suspected sepsis). Moreover, they should provide all new mothers with breastfeeding support and give advice regarding personal hygiene/cleanliness and other prevention strategies, such as clean cord care, thermal care, and immunization. Survival of medically stable preterm infants weighing less than 2000 g has been shown to be substantially improved (51% reduction in neonatal mortality) through Kangaroo Mother Care, which provides warmth; promotes breastfeeding, maternal-infant bonding, and growth; and reduces infections.[322] Improvement in domestic hygiene should be encouraged, including sanitary disposal of wastes, use of clean water, and hand washing, so that the newborn enters a clean home and is less likely to encounter pathogenic organisms. Community interventions need to be designed and modified to meet the needs of mothers and newborns in different settings in different countries with varying policies on the role of frontline workers in the recognition and management of infections.

Despite its importance, postnatal care is one of the most neglected aspects of maternal and newborn care in LMICs. Although a number of simple, low-cost preventive interventions are available that can avert a substantial proportion of deaths attributed to infections, including immediate and exclusive breastfeeding, thermal care, hand washing, chlorhexidine cleansing of the cord, and skin-to-skin care,[8,10,12,14] few data are available on coverage with postnatal care (i.e., a postnatal visit with a health care provider within 2 days of delivery). In 12 African countries, recent Demographic and Health Survey data indicated that less than 10% of newborns, on average, received an early postnatal care visit.[323]

The importance of early postnatal care was highlighted in a study in Sylhet, Bangladesh, where, overall, a 34% reduction (95% CI, 7% to 53%) in neonatal mortality was achieved through implementation of a package of maternal and neonatal interventions, aimed primarily at prevention and treatment of infections, delivered by community health workers through antenatal and postnatal home visits.[324] However, further analysis revealed that a 64% reduction (95% CI, 45% to 77%) in mortality was seen among the newborns who had an early postnatal home visit within the first 2 days of life, whereas no mortality impact was found among those who were visited only after the first 2 days.[325] Another study of promotion of healthy, preventive household newborn care practices (e.g., birth preparedness, clean delivery, skin-to-skin care, breastfeeding, clean cord and skin care, thermal care) through home visitation and community meetings by trained community health workers in a very high mortality setting in Uttar Pradesh, India, resulted in a 54% reduction (95% CI, 40% to 65%) in all-cause neonatal mortality.[326] Serious infections appeared to be the most important cause of death that was averted, and establishment of skin-to-skin care was fundamental to empowering women and promoting breastfeeding. Similar findings were also reported from a large study in rural Sindh, Pakistan, which showed decreased neonatal mortality through community-based intervention packages.[327] A review of studies from South Asia showed a reduced risk of neonatal death (RR, 0.62; 95% CI, 0.44 to 0.87) and stillbirth (RR, 0.76; 95% CI, 0.65 to 0.89), and a significant improvement in antenatal and neonatal practice indicators with home visits for neonatal care by community health workers.[328] There is also emerging evidence regarding the importance of early postnatal care in community settings from Africa. A cluster, randomized trial on the effect of home visitation in Ghana showed increased uptake of key maternal and newborn care behaviors and higher rates of facility births, resulting in an 8% reduction of neonatal mortality in the intervention areas (RR, 0.92; 95% CI, 0.75 to 1.12) compared with control areas.[329]

Breastfeeding

The promotion of early and exclusive breastfeeding is one of the most important interventions for the maintenance of newborn health and the promotion of optimal growth and development.[22] Breastfeeding is especially important in developing countries, where safe alternatives to breast milk are often unavailable or too expensive. Moreover, poor hygiene and a lack of clean water and clean feeding utensils make artificial formula an important vehicle for the transmission of infection. Breast milk has many unique antiinfective factors, including secretory immunoglobulin A (IgA) antibodies, lysozyme, and lactoferrin (see Chapter 5). In addition, breast milk is rich in receptor analogues for certain epithelial structures that microorganisms need for attachment to host tissues, an initial step in infection.[330] Many studies have shown that breastfeeding reduces the risk of infectious diseases, including neonatal sepsis, diarrhea, and possibly respiratory tract infection,[331-336] and that breastfeeding protects against infection-related neonatal and infant mortality.[8,10,337-340] A recent review showed that infants exclusively breastfed for 6 months had a significant reduction in risk of gastrointestinal and respiratory infections and showed no deficits in growth compared with infants breastfed for only 3 to 4 months.[341]

The HIV epidemic has raised questions about the safety of breastfeeding in areas in which there is a high prevalence of HIV infection among lactating women.[342-352] HIV can be transmitted through breastfeeding. A major question for any setting is whether the benefits of breastfeeding outweigh the risk of postnatal transmission of HIV through breast milk.[344] For many areas of the world where infectious diseases, especially diarrheal diseases, are a primary cause of infant death, breastfeeding, even when the mother is HIV infected, remains the safest mode of infant feeding. However, as noted above and outlined in new guidelines issued by WHO, national health authorities in each country need to develop guidance for feeding options for all HIV-infected mothers in their country, based on consideration of locally relevant factors that maximize chance of infant survival.[353]

MANAGEMENT OF NEONATAL INFECTION

If the mother develops a puerperal infection, the newborn requires special attention and should be treated for presumed sepsis.[310] Prolonged rupture of the membranes, maternal fever during labor, and chorioamnionitis are particular risk factors for early-onset neonatal sepsis and pneumonia.[354-356] Ideally high-risk infants who are born at home should be referred to the nearest health care facility for observation and antibiotic therapy. In practice, this may be either impossible or unacceptable to the family, as evidenced by high rates of noncompliance with referral in many settings,[273,274,324,326,357] and ways to deliver care to the mother and the newborn in the home must be developed and evaluated.

Identification of Neonates with Infection

If untreated, infections in newborns can rapidly become severe and life-threatening. Therefore early identification and appropriate treatment of newborns with infection are critical to survival. In LMICs, where access to care may be limited, diagnosis and treatment are particularly difficult. It is important to recognize maternal and neonatal factors that increase risk of infection in the newborn. These include maternal infections during pregnancy (STDs, urinary tract infection, others), premature or prolonged rupture of membranes, prolonged labor, fever during labor, unhygienic obstetric practices or cord care, poor hand washing practices, prematurity/LBW, artificial feeding, and generally unhygienic living conditions.[269,275,276]

In areas without sophisticated technology and the diagnostic help of laboratory tests and radiographic studies, treatment decisions must be made on the basis of the history and findings on physical examination. The WHO Young Infants Study was designed to identify clinical predictors of serious neonatal infections and enrolled more than 3000 sick infants younger than 2 months who presented to health facilities in Ethiopia, The Gambia, Papua New Guinea, and the Philippines.[358] In multivariable analysis, 14 signs were independent predictors of severe disease: reduced feeding ability, absence of spontaneous movement, temperature greater than 38° C, drowsiness or unconsciousness, a history of a feeding problem or change in activity, state of agitation, the presence of lower chest indrawing (retractions), respiratory rate greater than 60 per minute, grunting, cyanosis, a history of convulsions, a bulging fontanel, and slow digital capillary refill. The presence of any one of these signs had a sensitivity for severe disease (sepsis, meningitis, hypoxemia, or radiologically proven pneumonia) of 87% and a specificity of 54%; reducing the list to 9 signs only slightly reduced sensitivity (83%) but significantly improved specificity (62%).[358] More recently, 8899 young infants who presented to health facilities in six countries (India, Bangladesh, Pakistan, Ghana, South Africa, Bolivia) with a complaint of illness were enrolled in a second Young Infant Clinical Signs Study.[33] Seven signs were found to be associated with severe illness requiring referral level care in the first week of life: history of difficulty feeding, history of convulsions, movement only when stimulated, respiratory rate of 60 breaths per minute or greater, severe chest indrawing, and temperature of 37.5° C or greater or less than 35.5° C. These signs had a sensitivity and specificity of 85% and 75%, respectively, in infants younger than 1 week.[33] Studies in Bangladesh have recently sought to validate the ability of community health workers to use the clinical signs recommended by the WHO Young Infant Studies during routine household surveillance to identify neonates needing referral level care. In Sylhet, 288 newborns were assessed independently for the presence of clinical signs suggestive of very severe disease by community health workers and by study physicians. Compared with the physician's gold standard assessment, community health workers correctly classified very severe disease in newborns with a sensitivity of 91%, specificity of 95%, and kappa value of 0.85 ($P < .001$).[359] In Mirzapur, Bangladesh, community health workers' classification of very severe disease showed a sensitivity of 73%, a specificity of 98%, a positive predictive value of 57%, and a negative predictive value of 99%.[360] In addition to clinical signs, community health workers gathered historical information on neonatal illness. A history of a feeding problem, as reported by the mother to a physician, was significantly associated with the presence of a severe feeding problem, particularly a lack of ability to suck, as assessed by community health workers. Because assessing breastfeeding is complex, time-consuming, and difficult for male physicians because of cultural sensitivity, a reported history may substitute for an observed feeding problem in the algorithm, substantially simplifying the assessment. Thus it appears that trained and supervised community health workers can use a diagnostic algorithm to identify severely ill newborns with high validity.

Antibiotic Treatment of Neonates with Infection

Currently, the drugs most frequently used to treat suspected severe neonatal infections are a combination of penicillin or ampicillin and an aminoglycoside (usually gentamicin).[361] The WHO continues to recommend that young infants (from birth up to 2 months of age) with signs of severe infection should be referred for inpatient care and treated with intravenous broad-spectrum antibiotics—a combination of a benzyl penicillin and an aminoglycoside, such as gentamicin, for 10 to 14 days.

If 90% of neonates with infections received timely and appropriate antibiotic therapy, it is estimated that 30% to 70% of global neonatal deaths attributed to infections could be averted.[10,362] However, most infants with suspected serious infections in developing countries do not currently receive adequate treatment; inpatient care is not feasible for most families, either because treatment is available only in tertiary care facilities that are not accessible or because hospitalization is not affordable or acceptable to families.[324,357] In a study in Sylhet, Bangladesh, for example, two thirds of families with a newborn infant identified by a community health worker as having suspected serious infection refused referral to the hospital, despite the offer of transportation and free care.[363] Moreover, in many settings, placement and management of an intravenous line is not possible, and thus parenteral antibiotic therapy must be delivered by intramuscular injections. In this context, extended-interval gentamicin regimens have been recommended as the preferred mode of aminoglycoside dosing,[124,364,365] and evidence is accumulating that procaine penicillin may be a feasible alternative to multiple daily dosing regimens with ampicillin.[363]

Eliminating the need for multiple daily contacts with the patient to deliver antibiotics makes it more feasible for frontline workers in low-resource settings to potentially treat neonates with suspected infections, either at peripheral health facilities or possibly even in the home in situations where compliance with referral to a hospital is not possible.[363,366] A series of studies have been completed in Bangladesh, Pakistan, Nigeria, Kenya, and the Democratic Republic of Congo in newborns whose families refused referral to hospital, testing the equivalence of simplified regimens of antibiotic treatment that require fewer injections over the course of treatment (e.g., combinations of injectable gentamicin and oral amoxicillin) for infants with fast breathing or with clinical signs of suspected serious infections; results are forthcoming.[367-370] Currently available antibiotics for treatment of serious neonatal infections in developing countries have been reviewed recently.[371,372]

Ideally antibiotic therapy should be tailored to the specific microbiologic needs of a particular patient or, if patient-level data is not available, for the geographic region based on local surveillance data, especially if blood cultures are not performed and cannot be used to guide therapy, as is the case in most low- and middle-income settings. In reality, however, surveillance data also is generally not available. In addition, issues related to drug supply, availability, quality, and cost must be addressed. The problem of antibiotic resistance is now recognized to be a global problem, and the emergence of antibiotic-resistant pathogens is particularly alarming in hospitals in low-resource settings. The widespread availability of antibiotics in many LMICs, even directly to families outside contact with the formal health system, and indiscriminate and inappropriate antibiotic use in both the health and agriculture sectors contribute to this problem.[373]

Appropriate treatment of neonatal infections is one of the most important child survival interventions.[10,362] However, where it is not possible to deliver parenteral antibiotic therapy in a health facility, community-based case management is emerging as a viable alternative to facility-based care.* Recent data suggest that well-trained and supervised primary health care workers, including community health workers conducting routine household surveillance, are capable of identifying and treating sick newborns.[359,360,379] In a pooled analysis of five controlled trials of community-based management of neonatal pneumonia (four using cotrimoxazole, one ampicillin or penicillin), all-cause neonatal mortality was reduced by 27% (95% CI, 18% to 35%), and pneumonia-specific mortality was reduced by 42% (95% CI, 22% to 57%).[380] Another recent review using Grading of Recommendations, Assessment, Development, and Evaluation (GRADE)[381] criteria to assess the evidence showed reductions in all-cause neonatal mortality (RR, 0.75; 95% CI, 0.64 to 0.89) and neonatal pneumonia-specific mortality (RR, 0.58; 95% CI, 0.41 to 0.82) with timely case management.[362] A 62% reduction in neonatal mortality was also demonstrated in

*References 10-12, 324, 357, 359, 360, 362, 367, 374-378.

a nonrandomized controlled study in rural Maharashtra, India, in which village health workers conducted home visits and identified and treated neonates with suspected serious infections with a combination of oral cotrimoxazole and injectable gentamicin. The CFR declined from 16.6% before the intervention to 2.8% after the intervention ($P < .05$). Similarly, in a cluster, randomized controlled trial in rural Sylhet, Bangladesh, community health workers identified sick newborns and referred them to a health facility for treatment. If the family refused referral, the community health workers provided treatment in the home with injectable procaine penicillin and gentamicin, resulting in a 34% reduction (95% CI, 7% to 53%) in neonatal mortality compared with the control arm, where the usual services of the government of Bangladesh and a variety of private providers were available. In Sylhet, although there was only 32% compliance of referrals of sick newborns to hospital by community health workers, another 42% accepted injectable antibiotic treatment at home, indicating that with the addition of home-based treatment, approximately three fourths of sick neonates received curative antibiotic treatment from qualified providers and/or community health workers. CFR for treatment of neonates with suspected serious infections was 14.2% at health facilities and 4.4% in the hands of the community health workers. After controlling for differences in background characteristics and illness signs among treatment groups, newborns treated by community health workers had a HR of 0.22 (95% CI, 0.07 to 0.71) for death during the neonatal period, and those treated by qualified providers had a HR of 0.61 (95% CI, 0.37 to 0.99), compared with newborns who received no treatment or were treated by untrained providers.[363] An individually randomized controlled trial in young infants with possible serious bacterial infection, whose families refused hospital referral in low-income communities of Karachi, Pakistan, showed that injectable procaine penicillin and gentamicin given as once-daily injections in primary care clinics had a cure rate of 91%. Ceftriaxone gave similar results, but higher failure rates were noted with trimethoprim-sulfamethoxazole and gentamicin combination therapy.

Integrated Management of Neonatal Illness

An integrated approach to the sick child, including the young infant, has been developed by the WHO and UNICEF.[382] This strategy promotes prompt recognition of disease, appropriate therapy using standardized case management, referral of serious cases, and prevention through improved nutrition (breastfeeding of the neonate) and immunization. This approach stresses diagnosis using simple clinical signs, defined through the Young Infant Clinical Signs Studies, that can be taught to health care workers at all levels. The health care worker assesses the child by questioning the mother and examining the child, classifies the illness as serious or not, and determines if the infant needs urgent treatment and referral, specific treatment and advice, or only simple advice and home management. Importance of breastfeeding is stressed, and follow-up instructions are given. All young infants are checked for specific danger signs that equate with need for emergency care and urgent referral. Because the signs of serious bacterial infection in the newborn are not easily recognized, every young infant with danger signs is given treatment for a possible bacterial infection.[383]

MATERNAL EDUCATION AND SOCIOECONOMIC STATUS

Maternal education, literacy, and overall socioeconomic status are powerful influences on the health of both mother and newborn.[384-387] Education of girls must be promoted and expanded so that women of reproductive age know enough to seek preventive services, understand the implications of danger signs during labor and delivery and in their newborns, recognize that they must obtain referral care for obstetric or newborn complications, and are able to navigate the health system and receive timely, quality care. Improvements in education and socioeconomic status are obviously linked. They may affect child health by allowing the mother a greater voice in the family with greater decision-making power, making her better informed about domestic hygiene, disease prevention, or disease recognition, or enhancing her ability to seek medical attention outside the home and to comply with medical advice.

Conclusion

Neonatal infections cause a massive burden of mortality and morbidity, with the vast majority occurring in LMICs in settings characterized by high-risk household practices, poor care seeking and access to quality care, and weak health systems. Attention to the triad of mother, fetus, and newborn is particularly important in addressing neonatal infections. Surveillance for infections is limited, but available data indicate that antibiotic resistance is increasing. A number of preventative and curative interventions are available, which, if implemented effectively at large scale, could avert the majority of neonatal infection-related deaths around the world. Moreover, development of new and adapted tools and technologies holds promise for expanding the availability and impact of interventions to prevent deaths caused by infections. Implementation challenges, however, continue to limit coverage with interventions. Renewed commitment is needed to deliver evidence-based interventions at the community level and to improve care at health facilities. For long-term success, newborn services must be integrated with reproductive, maternal, and child health and nutrition programs.

Acknowledgment

The authors are grateful to Dr. Danyal Thaver for excellent assistance with article references and editing of this chapter.

References

1. Liu L, Johnson HL, Cousens S, et al: Global, regional, and national causes of child mortality: an updated systematic analysis for 2010 with time trends since 2000, *Lancet* 379:2151-2161, 2012.
2. Lawn JE, Kinney MV, Black RE, et al: Newborn survival: a multi-country analysis of a decade of change, *Health Policy Plan* 27(Suppl 3): iii6-iii28, 2012.
3. United Nations Children's Fund. Levels and trends in child mortality, 2013. Available at http://www.unicef.org/media/files/2013_IGME_child_mortality_Report.pdf. Accessed October 16, 2013.

4. Lawn JE, Cousens S, Zupan J: 4 million neonatal deaths: when? Where? Why? *Lancet* 365:891-900, 2005.
5. Lawn JE, Lee AC, Kinney M, et al: Two million intrapartum-related stillbirths and neonatal deaths: where, why, and what can be done? *Int J Gynaecol Obstet* 107(Suppl 1):S5-S19, 2009.
6. Bhutta ZA, Ahmed T, Black RE, et al: What works? Interventions for maternal and child undernutrition and survival, *Lancet* 371: 417-440, 2008.
7. Baqui AH, Darmstadt GL, Williams EK, et al: Rates, timing and causes of neonatal deaths in rural India: implications for neonatal health programmes, *Bull World Health Organ* 84:706-713, 2006.
8. Adam T, Lim SS, Mehta S, et al: Cost effectiveness analysis of strategies for maternal and neonatal health in developing countries, *BMJ* 331:1107, 2005.
9. Bhutta ZA, Zaidi AK, Thaver D, et al: Management of newborn infections in primary care settings: a review of the evidence and implications for policy? *Pediatr Infect Dis J* 28(Suppl 1):S22-S30, 2009.
10. Darmstadt GL, Bhutta ZA, Cousens S, et al: Evidence-based, cost-effective interventions: how many newborn babies can we save? *Lancet* 365:977-988, 2005.
11. Darmstadt GL, Black RE, Santosham M: Research priorities and postpartum care strategies for the prevention and optimal management of neonatal infections in less developed countries, *Pediatr Infect Dis J* 19:739-750, 2000.
12. Darmstadt GL, Walker N, Lawn JE, et al: Saving newborn lives in Asia and Africa: cost and impact of phased scale-up of interventions within the continuum of care, *Health Policy Plan* 23:101-117, 2008.
13. Thaver D, Zaidi AK: Burden of neonatal infections in developing countries: a review of evidence from community-based studies, *Pediatr Infect Dis J* 28(Suppl 1):S3-S9, 2009.
14. Bhutta ZA, Ali S, Cousens S, et al: Alma-Ata: Rebirth and Revision 6 Interventions to address maternal, newborn, and child survival: what difference can integrated primary health care strategies make? *Lancet* 372:972-989, 2008.
15. Ganatra HA, Zaidi AK: Neonatal infections in the developing world, *Semin Perinatol* 34:416-425, 2010.
16. Waters D, Jawad I, Ahmad A, et al: Aetiology of community-acquired neonatal sepsis in low and middle income countries, *J Glob Health* 1:154-170, 2011.
17. Zaidi AK, Thaver D, Ali SA, et al: Pathogens associated with sepsis in newborns and young infants in developing countries, *Pediatr Infect Dis J* 28(Suppl 1):S10-S18, 2009.
18. Darmstadt GL, Saha SK, Choi Y, et al: Population-based incidence and etiology of community-acquired neonatal bacteremia in Mirzapur, Bangladesh: an observational study, *J Infect Dis* 200:906-915, 2009.
19. Berkley JA, Lowe BS, Mwangi I, et al: Bacteremia among children admitted to a rural hospital in Kenya, *N Engl J Med* 352:39-47, 2005.
20. Stoll BJ, Hansen NI, Sánchez PJ, et al: Early onset neonatal sepsis: the burden of group B streptococcal and E. coli disease continues, *Pediatrics* 127:817-826, 2011.
21. Weston EJ, Pondo T, Lewis MM, et al: The burden of invasive early-onset neonatal sepsis in the United States, 2005-2008, *Pediatr Infect Dis J* 30:937-941, 2011.
22. Stoll BJ: The global impact of neonatal infection, *Clin Perinatol* 24: 1-21, 1997.
23. Bennett R, Eriksson M, Melen B, et al: Changes in the incidence and spectrum of neonatal septicemia during a fifteen-year period, *Acta Paediatr Scand* 74:687-690, 1985.
24. Gladstone IM, Ehrenkranz RA, Edberg SC, et al: A ten-year review of neonatal sepsis and comparison with the previous fifty-year experience, *Pediatr Infect Dis J* 9:819-825, 1990.
25. World Health Organization Young Infants Study Group: The bacterial etiology of serious infections in young infants in developing countries: results of a multicenter study, *Pediatr Infect Dis J* 18(Suppl 10): S17-S22, 1999.
26. World Health Organization Young Infants Study Group: Clinical prediction of serious bacterial infections in young infants in developing countries, *Pediatr Infect Dis J* 18(Suppl 10):S23-S31, 1999.
27. World Health Organization Young Infants Study Group: Conclusions from the WHO multicenter study of serious infections in young infants, *Pediatr Infect Dis J* 18(Suppl 10):S32-S34, 1999.
28. Gatchalian SR, Quiambao BP, Morelos AM, et al: Bacterial and viral etiology of serious infections in very young Filipino infants, *Pediatr Infect Dis J* 18(Suppl 10):S50-S55, 1999.
29. Lehmann D, Michael A, Omena M, et al: The bacterial and viral etiology of severe infection in children aged less than three months in the highlands of Papua New Guinea, *Pediatr Infect Dis J* 18(Suppl 10): S42-S49, 1999.
30. Lehmann D, Sanders RC, Marjen B, et al: High rates of *Chlamydia trachomatis* infections in young Papua New Guinean infants, *Pediatr Infect Dis J* 18(Suppl 10):S62-S69, 1999.
31. Muhe L, Tilahun M, Lulseged S, et al: Etiology of pneumonia, sepsis and meningitis in infants younger than three months of age in Ethiopia, *Pediatr Infect Dis J* 18(Suppl 10):S56-S61, 1999.
32. Mulholland EK, Ogunlesi OO, Adegbola RA, et al: Etiology of serious infections in young Gambian infants, *Pediatr Infect Dis J Suppl* 18:S35-S41, 1999.
33. Young Infants Clinical Signs Study Group: Clinical signs that predict severe illness in children under age 2 months: a multicentre study, *Lancet* 371:135-142, 2008.
34. Moore MR, Schrag SJ, Schuchat A: Effects of intrapartum antimicrobial prophylaxis for prevention of group-B-streptococcal disease on the incidence and ecology of early-onset neonatal sepsis, *Lancet Infect Dis* 3:201-213, 2003.
35. Edmond KM, Kortsalioudaki C, Scott S, et al: Group B streptococcal disease in infants aged younger than 3 months: systematic review and meta-analysis, *Lancet* 379:547-556, 2012.
36. Centers for Disease Control and Prevention: Prevention of perinatal group B streptococcal disease. Revised Guidelines from CDC, *MMWR Morb Mortal Wkly Rep* 51(RR-11):1-22, 2002.
37. Stoll BJ, Schuchat A: Maternal carriage of group B streptococci in developing countries, *Pediatr Infect Dis J* 17:499-503, 1998.
38. Blumberg HM, Stephens DS, Modansky M, et al: Invasive group B streptococcal disease: the emergence of serotype V, *J Infect Dis* 173:365-373, 1996.
39. Collins TS, Calderon M, Gilman RH, et al: Group B streptococcal colonization in a developing country: its association with sexually transmitted disease and socioeconomic factors, *Am J Trop Med* 59:633-636, 1998.
40. Suara RO, Adegbola RA, Baker CJ, et al: Carriage of group B streptococci in pregnant Gambian mothers and their infants, *J Infect Dis* 70:1316-1319, 1994.
41. Regan JA, Klebanoff MA, Nugent RP, et al: Colonization with group B streptococci in pregnancy and adverse outcome. VIP Study Group, *Am J Obstet Gynecol* 174:1354-1360, 1996.
42. Thaver D, Ali SA, Zaidi AK: Antimicrobial resistance among neonatal pathogens in developing countries, *Pediatr Infect Dis J* 28(Suppl 1): S19-S21, 2009.
43. Downie L, Armiento R, Subhi R, et al: Community-acquired neonatal and infant sepsis in developing countries: efficacy of WHO's currently recommended antibiotics—systematic review and meta-analysis, *Arch Dis Child* 98:146-154, 2013.
44. World Health Organization: Management of the child with a serious infection or severe malnutrition: guidelines for care at the first-referral level in developing countries, Geneva, 2000, World Health Organization.
45. Zaidi AK, Huskins WC, Thaver D, et al: Hospital-acquired neonatal infections in developing countries, *Lancet* 365:1175-1188, 2005.
46. Chan PC, Huang LM, Lin HC, et al: Control of an outbreak of pan-drug-resistant *Acinetobacter baumannii* colonization and infection in a neonatal intensive care unit, *Infect Control Hosp Epidemiol* 28: 423-429, 2007.
47. Zingg W, Posfay-Barbe KM, Pittet D: Healthcare-associated infections in neonates, *Curr Opin Infect Dis* 21:228-234, 2008.
48. Saleem AF, Ahmed I, Mir F, Ali SR, Zaidi AK: Pan-resistant Acinetobacter infection in neonates in Karachi, Pakistan, *J Infect Dev Ctries* 4:30-37, 2009.
49. Srivastava S, Shetty N: Healthcare-associated infections in neonatal units: lessons from contrasting worlds, *J Hosp Infect* 65:292-306, 2007.
50. Schulman J, Wirtschafter DD, Kurtin P: Neonatal intensive care unit collaboration to decrease hospital-acquired bloodstream infections: from comparative performance reports to improvement networks, *Pediatr Clin North Am* 56:865-892, 2009.
51. Sandora TJ: Prevention of healthcare-associated infections in children: new strategies and success stories, *Curr Opin Infect Dis* 23: 300-305, 2010.
52. Brown SM, Lubimova AV, Khrustalyeva NM, et al: Use of an alcohol-based hand rub and quality improvement interventions to improve hand hygiene in a Russian neonatal intensive care unit, *Infect Control Hosp Epidemiol* 24:172-179, 2003.

53. Ng PC, Wong HL, Lyon DJ, et al: Combined use of alcohol hand rub and gloves reduces the incidence of late onset infection in very low birthweight infants, *Arch Dis Child Fetal Neonatal Ed* 89:F336-F340, 2004.
54. Goldenberg RL, McClure EM, Saleem S, et al: Use of vaginally administered chlorhexidine during labor to improve pregnancy outcomes, *Obstet Gynecol* 107:1139-1146, 2006.
55. McClure EM, Goldenberg RL, Brandes N, et al: The use of chlorhexidine to reduce maternal and neonatal mortality and morbidity in low-resource settings, *Int J Gynaecol Obstet* 97:89-94, 2007.
56. Mullany LC, Darmstadt GL, Tielsch JM: Safety and impact of chlorhexidine antisepsis interventions for improving neonatal health in developing countries, *Pediatr Infect Dis J* 25:665-675, 2006.
57. Taha TE, Biggar RJ, Broadhead RL, et al: Effect of cleansing the birth canal with antiseptic solution on maternal and newborn morbidity and mortality in Malawi: clinical trial, *BMJ* 315:216-219, 1997. discussion 220.
58. Bakr AF, Karkour T: Effect of predelivery vaginal antisepsis on maternal and neonatal morbidity and mortality in Egypt, *J Womens Health (Larchmt)* 14:496-501, 2005.
59. Cutland CL, Madhi SA, Zell ER, et al: Chlorhexidine maternal-vaginal and neonate body wipes in sepsis and vertical transmission of pathogenic bacteria in South Africa: a randomised, controlled trial, *Lancet* 19:19, 2009.
60. Darmstadt GL, Badrawi N, Law PA, et al: Topically applied sunflower seed oil prevents invasive bacterial infections in preterm infants in Egypt: a randomized, controlled clinical trial, *Pediatr Infect Dis J* 23:719-725, 2004.
61. Darmstadt GL, Saha SK, Ahmed AS, et al: Effect of topical treatment with skin barrier-enhancing emollients on nosocomial infections in preterm infants in Bangladesh: a randomised controlled trial, *Lancet* 365:1039-1045, 2005.
62. Darmstadt GL, Saha SK, Ahmed AS, et al: Effect of skin barrier therapy on neonatal mortality rates in preterm infants in Bangladesh: a randomized, controlled, clinical trial, *Pediatrics* 121:522-529, 2008.
63. Rhinehart E, Goldmann DA, O'Rourke EJ: Adaptation of the Centers for Disease Control guidelines for the prevention of nosocomial infection in a pediatric intensive care unit in Jakarta, Indonesia, *Am J Med* 91:213S-220S, 1991.
64. Zaidi M, Angulo M, Sifuentes-Osornio J: Disinfection and sterilization practices in Mexico, *J Hosp Infect* 31:25-32, 1995.
65. Berg DE, Hershow RC, Ramirez CA, et al: Control of nosocomial infections in an intensive care unit in Guatemala City, *Clin Infect Dis* 21:588-593, 1995.
66. Webster J, Pritchard MA: Gowning by attendants and visitors in newborn nurseries for prevention of neonatal morbidity and mortality, *Cochrane Database Syst Rev* (3) CD003670, 2003.
67. Darmstadt GL, Nawshad Uddin Ahmed AS, Saha SK, et al: Infection control practices reduce nosocomial infections and mortality in preterm infants in Bangladesh, *J Perinatol* 25:331-335, 2005.
68. Misra S, Bhakoo ON, Ayyagiri A, et al: Clinical and bacteriological profile of neonatal pneumonia, *Indian J Med Res* 93:366-370, 1991.
69. Patwari AK, Bisht S, Srinivasan A, et al: Aetiology of pneumonia in hospitalized children, *J Trop Pediatr* 42:15-19, 1996.
70. Monto AS: Lehmann, Acute respiratory infections (ARI) in children: prospects for prevention, *Vaccine* 16:1582-1588, 1998.
71. Ploin D, Liberas S, Thouvenot D, et al: Influenza burden in children newborn to eleven months of age in a pediatric emergency department during the peak of an influenza epidemic, *Pediatr Infect Dis J* 22:S218-S222, 2003.
72. Zaman K, Baqui AH, Yunus M, et al: Acute respiratory infections in children: a community-based longitudinal study in rural Bangladesh, *J Trop Pediatr* 43:133-137, 1997.
73. Bang AT, Bang RA, Morankar VP, et al: Pneumonia in neonates: can it be managed in the community? *Arch Dis Child* 68:550-556, 1993.
74. English M, Ngama M, Mwalekwa L, et al: Signs of illness in Kenyan infants aged less than 60 days, *Bull World Health Organ* 82:323-329, 2004.
75. Victora CG, Kirkwood BR, Ashworth A, et al: Potential interventions for the prevention of childhood pneumonia in developing countries: improving nutrition, *Am J Clin Nutr* 70:309-320, 1999.
76. Arifeen S, Black RE, Antelman G, et al: Exclusive breastfeeding reduces acute respiratory infection and diarrhea deaths among infants in Dhaka slums, *Pediatrics* 108:e67, 2001.
77. Datta N, Kumar V, Kumar L, et al: Application of case management to the control of acute respiratory infections in low-birth-weight infants: a feasibility study, *Bull World Health Organ* 65:77-82, 1987.
78. Walker CL, Rudan I, Liu L, et al: Global burden of childhood pneumonia and diarrhoea, *Lancet* 381:1405-1416, 2013.
79. Kotloff KL, Nataro JP, Blackwelder WC, et al: Burden and aetiology of diarrhoeal disease in infants and young children in developing countries (the Global Enteric Multicenter Study, GEMS): a prospective, case-control study, *Lancet* 382:209-222, 2013.
80. Golding J, Emmett PM, Rogers IS: Gastroenteritis, diarrhoea and breast feeding, *Early Hum Dev* 49(Suppl):S83-103, 1997.
81. Huttly SR, Morris SS, Pisani V: Prevention of diarrhoea in young children in developing countries, *Bull World Health Organ* 75: 163-174, 1997.
82. Black RE, Lopez de Romaña G, Brown KH, et al: Incidence and etiology of infantile diarrhea and major routes of transmission in Huascar, Peru, *Am J Epidemiol* 129:785-799, 1989.
83. Mahmud A, Jalil F, Karlberg J, et al: Early child health in Lahore, Pakistan: VII. Diarrhoea, *Acta Paediatr Suppl* 390:79-85, 1993.
84. Aye DT, Bact D, Sack DA, et al: Neonatal diarrhea at a maternity hospital in Rangoon, *Am J Public Health* 81:480-481, 1991.
85. Haffejee IE: The epidemiology of rotavirus infections: a global perspective, *J Pediatr Gastroenterol Nutr* 20:275-286, 1995.
86. Bhan MK, Lew JF, Sazawal S, et al: Protection conferred by neonatal rotavirus infection against subsequent diarrhea, *J Infect Dis* 168:282-287, 1993.
87. Bishop RF, Barnes GL, Cipriani E, et al: Clinical immunity after neonatal rotavirus infection: a prospective longitudinal study in young children, *N Engl J Med* 309:72-76, 1983.
88. Fischer TK, Valentiner-Branth P, Steinsland H, et al: Protective immunity after natural rotavirus infection: a community cohort study of newborn children in Guinea-Bissau, West Africa, *J Infect Dis* 186:593-597, 2002.
89. Cicirello HG, Das BK, Gupta A, et al: High prevalence of rotavirus infection among neonates born at hospitals in Delhi, India: predisposition of newborns for infection with unusual rotavirus, *Pediatr Infect Dis J* 13:720-724, 1994.
90. Vethanayagam RR, Ananda Babu M, Nagalaxmi KS, et al: Possible role of neonatal infection with the asymptomatic reassortant rotavirus (RV) strain I321 in the decrease in hospital admissions for RV diarrhea, Bangalore, India, 1988-1999, *J Infect Dis* 189: 2282-2289, 2004.
91. Ramani S, Sowmyanarayanan TV, Gladstone BP, et al: Rotavirus infection in the neonatal nurseries of a tertiary care hospital in India, *Pediatr Infect Dis J* 27:719-723, 2008.
92. Gladstone BP, Ramani S, Mukhopadhya I, et al: Protective effect of natural rotavirus infection in an Indian birth cohort, *N Engl J Med* 365:337-346, 2011.
93. Bhatia S: Patterns and causes of neonatal and postneonatal mortality in rural Bangladesh, *Stud Fam Plann* 20:136-146, 1989.
94. De Francisco A, Hall AJ, Schellenberg JR, et al: The pattern of infant and childhood mortality in Upper River Division, The Gambia, *Ann Trop Paediatr* 13:345-352, 1993.
95. Garg SK, Mishra VN, Singh JV, et al: Neonatal mortality in Meerut district, *Indian J Med Sci* 47:222-225, 1993.
96. Islam MS, Rahaman MM, Aziz KM, et al: Infant mortality in rural Bangladesh: an analysis of causes during neonatal and postneonatal periods, *J Trop Pediatr* 28:294-298, 1982.
97. Kandeh BS: Causes of infant and early childhood deaths in Sierra Leone, *Soc Sci Med* 23:297-303, 1986.
98. Khan SR, Jalil F, Zaman S, et al: Early child health in Lahore, Pakistan: X. Mortality, *Acta Paediatr* 390(Suppl):109-177, 1993.
99. Knobel RH, Yang WS, Ho MS: Urban-rural and regional differences in infant mortality in Taiwan, *Soc Sci Med* 39:815-822, 1994.
100. Kumar V, Datta N, Saini SS: Infant mortality in a rural community development block in Haryana, *Indian J Pediatr* 49:795-802, 1982.
101. Singhal PK, Mathur GP, Mathur S, et al: Neonatal morbidity and mortality in ICDS urban slums, *Indian Pediatr* 27:485-488, 1990.
102. Sivagnanasundram C, Sivarajah N, Wijayaratnam A: Infant deaths in a health unit area of Northern Sri Lanka, *J Trop Med Hyg* 88: 401-406, 1985.
103. Mullany LC, Faillace S, Tielsch JM, et al: Incidence and risk factors for newborn umbilical cord infections on Pemba Island, Zanzibar, Tanzania, *Pediatr Infect Dis J* 28:503-509, 2009.

104. Cushing AH: Omphalitis: a review, *Pediatr Infect Dis* 4:282-285, 1985.
105. Mullany LC, Darmstadt GL, Khatry SK, et al: Topical applications of chlorhexidine to the umbilical cord for prevention of omphalitis and neonatal mortality in southern Nepal: a community-based, cluster-randomised trial, *Lancet* 367:910-918, 2006.
106. Mullany LC, Darmstadt GL, Katz J, et al: Development of clinical sign based algorithms for community based assessment of omphalitis, *Arch Dis Child Fetal Neonatal Ed* 91:F99-104, 2006.
107. Mullany LC, Darmstadt GL, Katz J, et al: Risk of mortality subsequent to umbilical cord infection among newborns of southern Nepal: cord infection and mortality, *Pediatr Infect Dis J* 28:17-20, 2009.
108. Sawin RS, Schaller RT, Tapper D, et al: Early recognition of neonatal abdominal wall necrotizing fasciitis, *Am J Surg* 167:481-484, 1994.
109. Samuel M, Freeman NV, Vaishnav A, et al: Necrotizing fasciitis: a serious complication of omphalitis in neonates, *J Pediatr Surg* 29:1414-1416, 1994.
110. Mullany LC, Darmstadt GL, Katz J, et al: Risk factors for umbilical cord infection among newborns of southern Nepal, *Am J Epidemiol* 165:203-211, 2007.
111. Airede AI: Pathogens in neonatal omphalitis, *J Trop Pediatr* 38: 129-131, 1992.
112. Bhardwaj N, Hasan SB: High perinatal and neonatal mortality in rural India, *J R Soc Health* 60-63, 1993.
113. Faridi MM, Rattan A, Ahmad SH: Omphalitis neonatorum, *J Indian Med Assoc* 91:283-285, 1993.
114. Güvenç H, Güvenç M, Yenioğlu H, et al: Neonatal omphalitis is still common in eastern Turkey, *Scand J Infect Dis* 23:613-616, 1991.
115. Güvenç H, Aygün AD, Yaşar F, Soylu F, et al: Omphalitis in term and preterm appropriate for gestational age and small for gestational age infants, *J Trop Pediatr* 43:368-372, 1997.
116. Mir F, Tikmani SS, Shakoor S, et al: Incidence and etiology of omphalitis in Pakistan: a community-based cohort study, *J Infect Dev Ctries* 5:828-833, 2011.
117. Chamnanvanakij S, Decharachakul K, Rasamimaree P, et al: A randomized study of 3 umbilical cord care regimens at home in Thai neonates: comparison of time to umbilical cord separation, parental satisfaction and bacterial colonization, *J Med Assoc Thai* 88: 967-972, 2005.
118. Sawardekar KP: Changing spectrum of neonatal omphalitis, *Pediatr Infect Dis J* 23(1):22-26, 2004.
119. Mullany LC, Saha SK, Shah R, et al: Impact of 4.0% chlorhexidine cord cleansing on the bacteriologic profile of the newborn umbilical stump in rural Sylhet District, Bangladesh: a community-based, cluster-randomized trial, *Pediatr Infect Dis J* 31:444-450, 2012.
120. Rush J, Chalmers I, Enkin M: Care of the new mother and baby. In Chalmers I, Enkin M, Keirse MJ, editors: *Effective care in pregnancy and childbirth*, New York, 1989, Oxford University Press, pp 1333-1346.
121. Baley JE, Fanaroff AA: Neonatal infections: I. Infection related to nursery care practices. In Sinclair JC, Bracken MB, editors: *Effective care of the newborn infant*, New York, 1992, Oxford University Press, pp 454-476.
122. Mullany LC, Darmstadt GL, Tielsch JM: Role of antimicrobial applications to the umbilical cord in neonates to prevent bacterial colonization and infection: a review of the evidence, *Pediatr Infect Dis J* 22:996-1002, 2003.
123. Balsara ZP, Hussein MH, Winch PJ, et al: Impact of clean delivery kit use on clean delivery practices in Beni Suef Governorate, *Egypt. J Perinatol* 29:673-679, 2009.
124. Hossain M, Chowdhury NA, Shirin M, et al: Simplified gentamicin dosing for treatment of sepsis in Bangladeshi neonates, *J Health Pop Nutr* 27:640-645, 2009.
125. Jokhio AH, Winter HR, Cheng KK: An intervention involving traditional birth attendants and perinatal and maternal mortality in Pakistan, *N Engl J Med* 352:2091-2099, 2005.
126. Mosha F, Winani S, Wood S, et al: Evaluation of the effectiveness of a clean delivery kit intervention in preventing cord infection and puerperal sepsis among neonates and their mothers in rural Mwanza Region, Tanzania, *Tanzan Health Res Bull* 7:185-188, 2005.
127. Tsu V: Nepal Clean Home Delivery Kit: evaluation of the health impact, Seattle, 2000, PATH.
128. Winani S, Wood S, Coffey P, et al: Use of a clean delivery kit and factors associated with cord infection and puerperal sepsis in Mwanza, Tanzania, *J Midwifery Womens Health* 52:37-43, 2007.
129. Garner P, Lai D, Baea M, et al: Avoiding neonatal death: an intervention study of umbilical cord care, *J Trop Pediatr* 40:24-28, 1994.
130. Mullany LC, Darmstadt GL, Khatry SK, et al: Impact of umbilical cord cleansing with 4.0% chlorhexidine on time to cord separation among newborns in southern Nepal: a cluster-randomized, community-based trial, *Pediatrics* 118:1864-1871, 2006.
131. Soofi S, Cousens S, Imdad A, et al: Topical application of chlorhexidine to neonatal umbilical cords for prevention of omphalitis and neonatal mortality in a rural district of Pakistan: a community-based, cluster-randomised trial, *Lancet* 379:1029-1036, 2012.
132. Arifeen SE, Mullany LC, Shah R, et al: The effect of cord cleansing with chlorhexidine on neonatal mortality in rural Bangladesh: a community-based, cluster-randomised trial, *Lancet* 379:1022-1028, 2012.
133. World Health Organization: Pocket book of hospital care for children: guidelines for the management of common childhood illnesses, ed 2, Geneva, 2013, World Health Organization.
134. Stroh G, Kyu UA, Thaung U, et al: Measurement of mortality from neonatal tetanus in Burma, *Bull World Health Organ* 65:309-316, 1987.
135. World Health Organization, United Nations Children's Fund, World Bank: State of the world's vaccines and immunization, Geneva, 2002, World Health Organization.
136. United Nations Children's Fund: The progress of nations 2000, New York, 2000, UNICEF.
137. World Health Organization: Maternal and neonatal tetanus elimination by 2005. Strategies for achieving and maintaining elimination, Geneva, 2000, World Health Organization.
138. Lawn JE, Wilczynska-Ketende K, Cousens SN: Estimating the causes of 4 million neonatal deaths in the year 2000, *Int J Epidemiol* 35: 706-718, 2006.
139. Rochat R, Akhter HH: Tetanus and pregnancy-related mortality in Bangladesh, *Lancet* 354:565, 1999.
140. World Health Organization: Maternal and neonatal tetanus elimination, 2013. Available at http://www.who.int/immunization_monitoring/diseases/MNTE_initiative/en/index4.html. Accessed October 16, 2013.
141. Blencowe H, Lawn J, Vandelaer J, et al: Tetanus toxoid immunization to reduce mortality from neonatal tetanus, *Int J Epidemiol* 39(suppl 1): i102-109, 2010.
142. Nsanze H, Dawodu A, Usmani A, et al: Ophthalmia neonatorum in the United Arab Emirates, *Ann Trop Paediatr* 16:27-32, 1996.
143. Pandey KK, Bhat BV, Kanungo R, et al: Clinico-bacteriological study of neonatal conjunctivitis, *Indian J Pediatr* 57:527-531, 1990.
144. Verma M, Chhatwal J, Varughese PV: Neonatal conjunctivitis: a profile, *Indian Pediatr* 31:1357-1361, 1994.
145. Fransen L, Nsanze H, Klauss V, et al: Ophthalmia neonatorum in Nairobi, Kenya: the roles of *Neisseria gonorrhoeae* and *Chlamydia trachomatis*, *J Infect Dis* 153:862-869, 1986.
146. Galega F, Heymann D, Nasah B: Gonococcal ophthalmia neonatorum: the case for prophylaxis in tropical Africa, *Bull World Health Organ* 62:95-98, 1984.
147. Laga M, Meheus A, Piot P: Epidemiology and control of gonococcal ophthalmia neonatorum, *Bull World Health Organ* 67:471-477, 1989.
148. Laga M, Plummer FA, Nzanze H, et al: Epidemiology of ophthalmia neonatorum in Kenya, *Lancet* 2:1145-1148, 1986.
149. Laga M, Plummer FA, Piot P, et al: Prophylaxis of gonococcal and chlamydial ophthalmia neonatorum: a comparison of silver nitrate and tetracycline, *N Engl J Med* 318:653-657, 1988.
150. Sergiwa A, Pratt BC, Eren E, et al: Ophthalmia neonatorum in Bangkok: the significance of *Chlamydia trachomatis*, *Ann Trop Paediatr* 13:233-236, 1993.
151. Amini E, Ghasemi M, Daneshjou K: A five-year study in Iran of ophthalmia neonatorum: prevalence and etiology, *Med Sci Monit* 14:CR90-CR96, 2008.
152. Di Bartolomeo S, Higa M, Janer M, et al: [Neonatal conjunctivitis in a hospital at Gran Buenos Aires. Last 5 years update], *Rev Argent Microbiol* 37:139-141, 2005.
153. Gul SS, Jamal M, Khan N: Ophthalmia neonatorum, *J Coll Physicians Surg Pak* 20:595-598, 2010.
154. Hanenberg R, Rojanapithayakorn W, Kunasol P, et al: Impact of Thailand's HIV-control programme as indicated by the decline of sexually transmitted diseases, *Lancet* 344:243-246, 1994.
155. Nelson K, Celentano DD, Eiumtrakol S, et al: Changes in sexual behavior and decline in HIV infection among young men in Thailand, *N Engl J Med* 335:297-303, 1996.
156. Credé KSF: Die Verhütung der Augenentzündung der Neugeborenen, *Arch Gynekol* 17:50-53, 1881.

157. Hammerschlag MR, Cummings C, Roblin PM, et al: Efficacy of neonatal ocular prophylaxis for the prevention of chlamydial and gonococcal conjunctivitis, *N Engl J Med* 320:768-772, 1989.
158. Zanoni D, Isenberg S, Apt L: A comparison of silver nitrate with erythromycin for prophylaxis against ophthalmia neonatorum, *Clin Pediatr* 31:295-298, 1992.
159. Pickering LK, editor: 2000 Red book: report of the Committee on Infectious Diseases, ed 25, Elk Grove Village, Ill.
160. Isenberg SJ, Apt L, Wood M: A controlled trial of povidone-iodine as prophylaxis against ophthalmia neonatorum, *N Engl J Med* 332:562-566, 1995.
161. Isenberg S, Apt L, Del Signore M, et al: A double application approach to ophthalmia neonatorum prophylaxis, *Br J Ophthalmol* 87: 1449-1452, 2003.
162. Benevento W, Murray P, Reed CA, et al: The sensitivity of *Neisseria gonorrhoeae, Chlamydia trachomatis*, and herpes simplex type II to disinfection with povidone-iodine, *Am J Ophthalmol* 109:329-333, 1990.
163. Ali Z, Khadije D, Elahe A, et al: Prophylaxis of ophthalmia neonatorum comparison of betadine, erythromycin and no prophylaxis, *J Trop Pediatr* 53:388-392, 2007.
164. World Health Organization (WHO)/Joint United Nations Programme on HIV/AIDS (UNAIDS): Global report: UNAIDS report on the global AIDS epidemic, Geneva, 2012, WHO/UNAIDS.
165. Luo C: Innovation for elimination of new HIV infections in children by 2015 and keeping mother alive, 2012. Available at http://www.unicef.org/supply/files/4-EMTCT_innovation.pdf. Accessed May 20, 2013.
166. Panel on Treatment of HIV-Infected Pregnant Women and Prevention of Perinatal Transmission: Recommendations for use of antiretroviral drugs in pregnant HIV-1-infected women for maternal health and interventions to reduce perinatal HIV transmission in the United States. Available at http://aidsinfo.nih.gov/contentfiles/lvguidelines/PerinatalGL.pdf. Accessed May 20, 2013.
167. Taylor GP, Clayden P, Dhar J, et al: British HIV Association guidelines for the management of HIV infection in pregnant women 2012, *HIV Med* 13(Suppl 2):87-157, 2012.
168. Townsend CL, Cortina-Borja M, Peckham CS, et al: Low rates of mother-to-child transmission of HIV following effective pregnancy interventions in the United Kingdom and Ireland, 2000-2006, *AIDS* 22:973-981, 2008.
169. Committee on Pediatric AIDS: Infant feeding and transmission of human immunodeficiency virus in the United States, *Pediatrics* 131:391-396, 2013.
170. De Cock KM, Fowler MG, Mercier E, et al: Prevention of mother-to-child HIV transmission in resource-poor countries: translating research into policy and practice, *JAMA* 283:1175-1182, 2000.
171. Tudor Car L, Brusamento S, Elmoniry H, et al: The uptake of integrated perinatal prevention of mother-to-child HIV transmission programs in low- and middle-income countries: a systematic review, *PLoS One* 8:e56550, 2012.
172. United Nations Children's Fund: Children and AIDS: fifth stocktaking report, New York, 2010, United Nations Children's Fund.
173. Effect of breastfeeding on infant and child mortality due to infectious diseases in less developed countries: a pooled analysis. WHO Collaborative Study Team on the Role of Breastfeeding on the Prevention of Infant Mortality, *Lancet* 355:451-455, 2000.
174. Jones G, Steketee RW, Black RE, et al: How many child deaths can we prevent this year? *Lancet* 362:65-71, 2003.
175. Thomas TK, Masaba R, Borkowf CB, et al: Triple-antiretroviral prophylaxis to prevent mother-to-child HIV transmission through breastfeeding—the Kisumu Breastfeeding Study, Kenya: a clinical trial, *PLoS Med* 8:e1001015, 2011.
176. Jamieson DJ, Chasela CS, Hudgens MG, et al: Maternal and infant antiretroviral regimens to prevent postnatal HIV-1 transmission: 48-week follow-up of the BAN randomised controlled trial, *Lancet* 379:2449-2458, 2012.
177. Coovadia H: Current issues in prevention of mother-to-child transmission of HIV-1, *Curr Opin HIV AIDS* 4:319-324, 2009.
178. Horvath T, Madi BC, Iuppa IM, et al: Interventions for preventing late postnatal mother-to-child transmission of HIV, *Cochrane Database Syst Rev* CD006734, 2009.
179. Kuhn L, Reitz C, Abrams EJ: Breastfeeding and AIDS in the developing world, *Curr Opin Pediatr* 21:83-93, 2009.
180. World Health Organization (WHO)/Joint United Nations Programme on HIV/AIDS (UNAIDS): HIV and infant feeding update 2006, Geneva, 2006, WHO/UNAIDS.
181. World Health Organization: HIV and infant feeding 2010: an updated framework for priority action (2012), Geneva, 2012, World Health Organization.
182. Connor EM, Sperling RS, Gelber R, et al: Reduction of maternal-infant transmission of human immunodeficiency virus type 1 with zidovudine treatment. Pediatric AIDS Clinical Trials Group Protocol 076 Study Group, *N Engl J Med* 331:1173-1180, 1994.
183. World Health Organization/United Nations Children's Fund: The Interaction Task Team (IATT) on Prevention of HIV Infection in Pregnant Women, Mothers and Their Children: Guidance on global scale-up of the prevention of mother-to-child transmission of HIV: towards universal access for women, infants and young children and eliminating HIV and AIDS among children, Geneva, 2007, World Health Organization.
184. Paintsil E, Andiman WA: Update on successes and challenges regarding mother-to-child transmission of HIV, *Curr Opin Pediatr* 21:94-101, 2009.
185. Spensley A, Sripipatana T, Turner AN, et al: Preventing mother-to-child transmission of HIV in resource-limited settings: the Elizabeth Glaser Pediatric AIDS Foundation experience, *Am J Public Health* 99:631-637, 2009.
186. World Health Organization: Joint United Nations Programme on HIV/AIDS: Antiretroviral drugs for treating pregnant women and preventing HIV infection in infants: towards universal access, Geneva, 2006, World Health Organization.
187. The mode of delivery and the risk of vertical transmission of human immunodeficiency virus type 1: a meta-analysis of 15 prospective cohort studies. The International Perinatal HIV Group, *N Engl J Med* 340:977-987, 1999.
188. Read JS, Newell MK: Efficacy and safety of cesarean delivery for prevention of mother-to-child transmission of HIV-1, *Cochrane Database Syst Rev* CD005479, 2005.
189. Read JS: Cesarean section delivery to prevent vertical transmission of human immunodeficiency virus type 1. Associated risks and other considerations, *Ann N Y Acad Sci* 918:115-121, 2000.
190. Black RE, Morris SS, Bryce J: Where and why are 10 million children dying every year? *Lancet* 361:2226-2234, 2003.
191. Bryce J, Boschi-Pinto C, Shibuya K, et al: WHO estimates of the causes of death in children, *Lancet* 365:1147-1152, 2005.
192. Menu E, Scarlatti G, Barré-Sinoussi F, et al: Mother-to-child transmission of HIV: developing integration of healthcare programmes with clinical, social and basic research studies. Report of the International Workshop held at Chobe Marina Lodge, Kasane, Botswana, 21-25 January 2003, *Acta Paediatr* 92:1343-1348, 2003.
193. Bennett JV, Rogers MF: Child survival and perinatal infections with human immunodeficiency virus, *Am J Dis Child* 145:1242-1247, 1991.
194. Filteau S: The HIV-exposed, uninfected African child, *Trop Med Int Health* 14:276-287, 2009.
195. Lozano R, Naghavi M, Foreman K, et al: Global and regional mortality from 235 causes of death for 20 age groups in 1990 and 2010: a systematic analysis for the Global Burden of Disease Study, *Lancet* 380:2095-2128, 2010.
196. World Health Organization: Women and health: today's evidence, tomorrow's agenda, Geneva, 2009, World Health Organization.
197. Murray CJ, Vos T, Lozano R, et al: Disability-adjusted life years (DALYs) for 291 diseases and injuries in 21 regions, 1990-2010: a systematic analysis for the Global Burden of Disease Study, *Lancet* 380:2197-2223, 2010.
198. Loto OM, Awowole I: Tuberculosis in pregnancy: a review, *J Pregnancy* 379271, 2012.
199. Figueroa-Damián R, Arredondo-García JL: Neonatal outcome of children born to women with tuberculosis, *Arch Med Res* 32:66-69, 2001.
200. Jana N, Vasishta K, Jindal SK, et al: Perinatal outcome in pregnancies complicated by pulmonary tuberculosis, *Int J Gynecol Obstet* 44:119-124, 1994.
201. Smith KC: Congenital tuberculosis: a rare manifestation of a common infection, *Curr Opin Infect Dis* 15:269-274, 2002.
202. Starke JR: Tuberculosis: an old disease but a new threat to the mother, fetus, and neonate, *Clin Perinatol* 24:107-127, 1997.
203. Mazade MA, Evans EM, Starke JR, et al: Congenital tuberculosis presenting as sepsis syndrome: case report and review of the literature, *Pediatr Infect Dis J* 20:439-442, 2001.
204. Cantwell MF, Shehab ZM, Costello AM, et al: Brief report: congenital tuberculosis, *N Engl J Med* 330:1051-1054, 1994.
205. Lawn SD, Churchyard G: Epidemiology of HIV-associated tuberculosis, *Curr Opin HIV AIDS* 4:325-333, 2009.

206. Abdool Karim SS, Churchyard GJ, Karim QA, et al: HIV infection and tuberculosis in South Africa: an urgent need to escalate the public health response, *Lancet* 374:921-933, 2009.
207. Adhikari M, Pillay T, Pillay D: Tuberculosis in the newborn: an emerging disease, *Pediatr Infect Dis J* 16:1108-1112, 1997.
208. Pillay T, Adhikari M, Mokili J, et al: Severe, rapidly progressive human immunodeficiency virus type 1 disease in newborns with coinfections, *Pediatr Infect Dis J* 20:404-410, 2001.
209. Adhikari M: Tuberculosis and tuberculosis/HIV co-infection in pregnancy, Semin Fetal Neonatal Med 14:234-240, 2009.
210. World Health Organization: World malaria report 2012, Geneva, 2012, World Health Organization.
211. World Health Organization: WHO Global Malaria Programme: World malaria report 2008, Geneva, 2008, World Health Organization.
212. Fischer PR: Malaria and newborns, *J Trop Pediatr* 49:132-134, 2003.
213. Mwaniki MK, Talbert AW, Mturi FN, et al: Congenital and neonatal malaria in a rural Kenyan district hospital: an eight-year analysis, *Malar J* 9:313, 2010.
214. Shulman CE, Dorman EK: Importance and prevention of malaria in pregnancy, *Trans R Soc Trop Med Hyg* 97:30-35, 2003.
215. Brabin BJ: An analysis of malaria in pregnancy in Africa, *Bull World Health Organ* 61:1005-1016, 1983.
216. Steketee RW, Wirima JJ, Slutsker L, et al: The problem of malaria and malaria control in pregnancy in sub-Saharan Africa, *Am J Trop Med Hyg* 55:2-7, 1996.
217. McGregor IA: Epidemiology, malaria, and pregnancy, *Am J Trop Med Hyg* 33:517-525, 1984.
218. Nosten F, ter Kuile F, Maelankirri L, et al: Malaria during pregnancy in an area of unstable endemicity, *Trans R Soc Trop Med Hyg* 85: 424-429, 1991.
219. Duffy PE: *Plasmodium* in the placenta: parasites, parity, protection, prevention and possibly preeclampsia, *Parasitology* 134(Pt 13):1877-1881, 2007.
220. Gilles HM, Lawson JB, Sibelas M, et al: Malaria, anaemia and pregnancy, *Ann Trop Med Parasitol* 63:245-263, 1969.
221. Egwunyenga OA, Ajayi JA, Duhlinska-Popova DD: Malaria in pregnancy in Nigerians: seasonality and relationship to splenomegaly and anaemia, *Indian J Malariol* 34:17-24, 1997.
222. Seal SL, Mukhopadhay S, Ganguly RP: Malaria in pregnancy, *J Indian Med Assoc* 108:487-490, 2010.
223. Matteelli A, Caligaris S, Castelli F, et al: The placenta and malaria, *Ann Trop Med Parasitol* 91:803-810, 1997.
224. McGregor IA, Wilson ME, Billewicz WZ: Malaria infection of the placenta in The Gambia, West Africa; its incidence and relationship to stillbirth, birthweight and placental weight, *Trans R Soc Trop Med Hyg* 77:232-244, 1983.
225. Albiti AH, Adam I, Ghouth AS: Placental malaria, anaemia and low birthweight in Yemen, *Trans R Soc Trop Med Hyg* 104:191-194, 2010.
226. Okoko BJ, Enwere G, Ota MO: The epidemiology and consequences of maternal malaria: a review of immunological basis, *Acta Trop* 87:193-205, 2003.
227. Okoko BJ, Ota MO, Yamuah LK, et al: Influence of placental malaria infection on fetal outcome in the Gambia: twenty years after Ian Mcgregor, *J Health Popul Nutr* 20:4-11, 2002.
228. Galbraith RM, Fox H, Hsi B, et al: The human maternal-foetal relationship in malaria: II. Histological, ultrastructural and immunopathological studies of the placenta, *Trans R Soc Trop Med Hyg* 74:61-72, 1980.
229. Steketee RW, Wirima JJ, Hightower AW, et al: The effect of malaria and malaria prevention in pregnancy on offspring birthweight, prematurity, and intrauterine growth retardation in rural Malawi, *Am J Trop Med Hyg* 55:33-41, 1996.
230. Bouvier P, Breslow N, Doumbo O, et al: Seasonality, malaria, and impact of prophylaxis in a West African village: II. Effect on birthweight, *Am J Trop Med Hyg* 56:384-389, 1997.
231. Nosten F, McGready R, Simpson JA, et al: Effects of *Plasmodium vivax* malaria in pregnancy, *Lancet* 354:546-549, 1999.
232. Luxemburger C, McGready R, Kham A, et al: Effects of malaria during pregnancy on infant mortality in an area of low malaria transmission, *Am J Epidemiol* 154:459-465, 2001.
233. Chizzolini C, Trottein F, Bernard FX, et al: Isotypic analysis, antigen specificity, and inhibitory function of maternally transmitted *Plasmodium falciparum*-specific antibodies in Gabonese newborns, *Am J Trop Med Hyg* 45:57-64, 1991.
234. Nguyen-Dinh P, Steketee RW, Greenberg AE, et al: Rapid spontaneous postpartum clearance of *Plasmodium falciparum* parasitemia in African women, *Lancet* 2:751-752, 1988.
235. Ibhanesebhor SE: Clinical characteristics of neonatal malaria, *J Trop Pediatr* 41:330-333, 1995.
236. Brabin BJ, Warsame M, Uddenfeldt-Wort U, et al: Monitoring and evaluation of malaria in pregnancy—developing a rational basis for control, *Malar J* 7(Suppl 1):S6, 2008.
237. World Health Organization Regional Office for Africa (WHO/AFRO): A strategic framework for malaria prevention and control during pregnancy in the African region, Brazzaville, Republic of the Congo, 2004, WHO/AFRO.
238. Wolfe MS, Cordero JF: Safety of chloroquine in chemosuppression of malaria during pregnancy, *BMJ* 290:1466-1467, 1985.
239. Newman RD, Parise ME, Slutsker L, et al: Safety, efficacy and determinants of effectiveness of antimalarial drugs during pregnancy: implications for prevention programmes in *Plasmodium falciparum*-endemic sub-Saharan Africa, *Trop Med Int Health* 8:488-506, 2003.
240. United Nations Children's Fund: The progress of the nations 1997, New York, 1997, United Nations Children's Fund.
241. ter Kuile FO, van Eijk AM, Filler SJ: Effect of sulfadoxine-pyrimethamine resistance on the efficacy of intermittent preventive therapy for malaria control during pregnancy: a systematic review, *JAMA* 297:2603-2616, 2007.
242. Nosten F, McGready R, Looareesuwan S, et al: Editorial: maternal malaria: time for action, *Trop Med Int Health* 8:485-487, 2003.
243. Nosten F, McGready R, d'Alessandro U, et al: Antimalarial drugs in pregnancy: a review, *Curr Drug Saf* 1:1-15, 2006.
244. Garner P, Gulmezoglu AM: Drugs for preventing malaria in pregnant women, *Cochrane Database Syst Rev* 4:CD000169, 2006.
245. Cot M, Roisin A, Barro D, et al: Effect of chloroquine chemoprophylaxis during pregnancy on birth weight: results of a randomized trial, *Am J Trop Med Hyg* 46:21-27, 1992.
246. Shulman CE, Dorman EK, Cutts F, et al: Intermittent sulphadoxine-pyrimethamine to prevent severe anaemia secondary to malaria in pregnancy: a randomised placebo-controlled trial, *Lancet* 353: 632-636, 1999.
247. Schultz LJ, Steketee RW, Chitsulo L, et al: Evaluation of maternal practices, efficacy, and cost-effectiveness of alternative antimalarial regimens for use in pregnancy: chloroquine and sulfadoxine-pyrimethamine, *Am J Trop Med Hyg* 55(Suppl 1):87-94, 1996.
248. Menendez C, Bardají A, Sigauque B, et al: Malaria prevention with IPTp during pregnancy reduces neonatal mortality, *PLoS One* 5:e9438, 2010.
249. World Health Organization Expert Committee on Malaria: WHO Technical Report Series Number 892, Geneva, 2000, World Health Organization, pp 1-74.
250. Steketee RW: Malaria prevention in pregnancy: when will the prevention programme respond to the science, *J Health Popul Nutr* 20: 1-3, 2002.
251. World Health Organization: Guidelines for the treatment of malaria, ed 2, Geneva, 2010, World Health Organization.
252. Heymann DL, Steketee RW, Wirima JJ, et al: Antenatal chloroquine chemoprophylaxis in Malawi: chloroquine resistance, compliance, protective efficacy and cost, *Trans R Soc Trop Med Hyg* 84:496-498, 1990.
253. Alonso PL, Lindsay SW, Armstrong JR, et al: The effect of insecticide-treated bed nets on mortality of Gambian children, *Lancet* 337: 1499-1502, 1991.
254. Nevill CG, Some ES, Mung'ala VO, et al: Insecticide-treated bednets reduce mortality and severe morbidity from malaria among children on the Kenyan coast, *Trop Med Int Health* 1:139-146, 1996.
255. Binka FN, Kubaje A, Adjuik M, et al: Impact of permethrin impregnated bednets on child mortality in Kassena-Nankana district, Ghana: a randomized controlled trial, *Trop Med Int Health* 1: 147-154, 1996.
256. Gamble C, Ekwaru JP, ter Kuile FO, Insecticide-treated nets for preventing malaria in pregnancy, *Cochrane Database Syst Rev* CD003755, 2006.
257. Marchant T, Schellenberg JA, Edgar T, et al: Socially marketed insecticide-treated nets improve malaria and anaemia in pregnancy in southern Tanzania, *Trop Med Int Health* 7:149-158, 2002.
258. Hanson K, Marchant T, Nathan R, et al: Household ownership and use of insecticide treated nets among target groups after implementation of a national voucher programme in the United Republic of Tanzania: plausibility study using three annual cross sectional household surveys, *BMJ* 339:b2434, 2009.

259. Kleinschmidt I, Schwabe C, Benavente L, et al: Marked increase in child survival after four years of intensive malaria control, *Am J Trop Med Hyg* 80:882-888, 2009.
260. Eriksen J, Schwabe C, Benavente L, et al: Effectiveness of a community intervention on malaria in rural Tanzania: a randomised controlled trial, *Afr Health Sci* 10:332-340, 2010.
261. von Seidlein L, Bejon P: Malaria vaccines: past, present and future, *Arch Dis Child* 98:981-985, 2013.
262. Schwartz L, Brown GV, Genton B, et al: A review of malaria vaccine clinical projects based on the WHO rainbow table, *Malar J* 11:11, 2012.
263. Agnandji ST, Lell B, Fernandes JF, et al: A phase 3 trial of RTS,S/AS01 malaria vaccine in African infants, *N Engl J Med* 367:2284-2295, 2012.
264. Brahmbhatt H, Kigozi G, Wabwire-Mangen F, et al: The effects of placental malaria on mother-to-child HIV transmission in Rakai, Uganda, *Aids* 17:2539-2541, 2003.
265. Ladner J, Leroy V, Karita E, et al: Malaria, HIV and pregnancy, *Aids* 17:275-276, 2003.
266. van Eijk AM, Ayisi JG, ter Kuile FO, et al: HIV increases the risk of malaria in women of all gravidities in Kisumu, Kenya, *Aids* 17:595-603, 2003.
267. Briand V, Badaut C, Cot M: Placental malaria, maternal HIV infection and infant morbidity, *Ann Trop Paediatr* 29:71-83, 2009.
268. Ticconi C, Mapfumo M, Dorrucci M, et al: Effect of maternal HIV and malaria infection on pregnancy and perinatal outcome in Zimbabwe, *J Acquir Immune Defic Syndr* 34:289-294, 2003.
269. Bale JR, Stoll BJ, Lucas AO, editors: Improving birth outcomes: meeting the challenge in the developing world, Washington, DC, 2003, Institute of Medicine, National Academies Press.
270. Save the Children: State of the world's mothers, Washington, DC, 2012.
271. United Nations Statistics Division: The world's women 1995: trends and statistics. Social statistics and indicators, New York, 1995, United Nations.
272. Tomasevski K: Women and human rights, Atlantic Highlands, NJ, 1993, Zed Books.
273. Herbert HK, Lee AC, Chandran A, et al: Care seeking for neonatal illness in low- and middle-income countries: a systematic review, *PLoS Med* 9:e1001183, 2014.
274. Owais A, Sultana S, Stein AD, et al: Why do families of sick newborns accept hospital care? A community-based cohort study in Karachi, Pakistan, *J Perinatol* 31:586-592, 2011.
275. Save the Children: The state of the world's newborns: a report from saving newborn lives, Washington, DC, 2001, Save the Children.
276. World Health Organization: Mother-baby package: implementing safe motherhood in countries, Geneva, 1994, World Health Organization, Division of Family Health, Maternal Health and Safe Motherhood Programme.
277. World Health Organization: Maternal and perinatal infections: a practical guide: report of a WHO consultation, Geneva, 1991, World Health Organization. WHO/MCH/91.10.
278. World Health Organization: Maternal care for the reduction of perinatal and neonatal mortality, Geneva, 1986, World Health Organization.
279. Fischer GW, Ottolini MG, Mond JJ: Prospects for vaccines during pregnancy and in the newborn period, *Clin Perinatol* 24:231-249, 1997.
280. Vicari M, Dodet B, Englund J: Protection of newborns through maternal immunization, *Vaccine* 21:3351, 2003.
281. Lindsey B, Kampmann B, Jones C: Maternal immunization as a strategy to decrease susceptibility to infection in newborn infants, *Curr Opin Infect Dis* 26:248-253, 2013.
282. Roper MH, Vandelaer JH, Gasse FL: Maternal and neonatal tetanus, *Lancet* 370:1947-1959, 2007.
283. Ortiz JR, Neuzil KM, Ahonkhai VI, et al: Translating vaccine policy into action: a report from the Bill & Melinda Gates Foundation Consultation on the prevention of maternal and early infant influenza in resource-limited settings, *Vaccine* 30:7134-7140, 2012.
284. Tamma PD, Ault KA, del Rio C, et al: Safety of influenza vaccination during pregnancy, *Am J Obstet Gynecol* 20:20, 2009.
285. Zaman K, Roy E, Arifeen SE, et al: Effectiveness of maternal influenza immunization in mothers and infants, *N Engl J Med* 359:1555-1564, 2008.
286. Baker CJ, Rench MA, Edwards MS, et al: Immunization of pregnant women with a polysaccharide vaccine of group B streptococcus, *N Engl J Med* 319:1180-1185, 1988.
287. Baker CJ, Edwards MS: Group B streptococcal conjugate vaccines, *Arch Dis Child* 88:375-378, 2003.
288. Baker CJ, Rench MA, Fernandez M, et al: Safety and immunogenicity of a bivalent group B streptococcal conjugate vaccine for serotypes II and III, *J Infect Dis* 188:66-73, 2003.
289. Baker CJ, Rench MA, McInnes P: Immunization of pregnant women with group B streptococcal type III capsular polysaccharide-tetanus toxoid conjugate vaccine, *Vaccine* 21:3468-3472, 2003.
290. Lin FY, Philips 3rd JB, Azimi PH, et al: Level of maternal antibody required to protect neonates against early-onset disease caused by group B *Streptococcus* type Ia: a multicenter, seroepidemiology study, *J Infect Dis* 184:1022-1028, 2001.
291. Mulholland K, Suara RO, Siber G, et al: Maternal immunization with *Haemophilus influenzae* type b polysaccharide-tetanus protein conjugate vaccine in The Gambia, *JAMA* 275:1182-1188, 1996.
292. O'Dempsey TJ, McArdle T, Ceesay SJ, et al: Immunization with a pneumococcal capsular polysaccharide vaccine during pregnancy, *Vaccine* 14:963-970, 1996.
293. Santosham M, Englund JA, McInnes P, et al: Safety and antibody persistence following *Haemophilus influenzae* type b conjugate or pneumococcal polysaccharide vaccines given before pregnancy in women of childbearing age and their infants, *Pediatr Infect Dis J* 20:931-940, 2001.
294. Shahid NS, Steinhoff MC, Hoque SS, et al: Serum, breast milk, and infant antibody after maternal immunisation with pneumococcal vaccine, *Lancet* 346:1252-1257, 1995.
295. Englund JA, Glezen WP, Thompson C, et al: *Haemophilus influenzae* type b-specific antibody in infants after maternal immunization, *Pediatr Infect Dis J* 16:1122-1130, 1997.
296. Schrag SJ: Group B streptococcal vaccine for resource-poor countries, *Lancet* 378:11-12, 2011.
297. Michon F, Uitz C, Sarkar A, et al: Group B streptococcal type II and III conjugate vaccines: physicochemical properties that influence immunogenicity, *Clin Vaccine Immunol* 13:936-943, 2006.
298. Centers for Disease Control and Prevention: Updated recommendations for use of tetanus toxoid, reduced diphtheria toxoid, and acellular pertussis vaccine (Tdap) in pregnant women–Advisory Committee on Immunization Practices (ACIP), 2012, *MMWR Morb Mortal Wkly Rep* 62:131-135, 2013.
299. Jackson DW, Rohani P: Perplexities of pertussis: recent global epidemiological trends and their potential causes, *Epidemiol Infect* 142:1-13, 2014.
300. Forsyth K, Thisyakorn U, von König CH, et al: Pertussis control in the Asia-Pacific region: a report from the Global Pertussis Initiative, *Southeast Asian J Trop Med Public Health* 43:699-711, 2012.
301. Marchant A, Newport M: Prevention of infectious diseases by neonatal and early infantile immunization: prospects for the new millennium, *Curr Opin Infect Dis* 13:241-246, 2000.
302. Smith PG: Case-control studies of the efficacy of BCG against tuberculosis. International Union Against Tuberculosis. In XXVIth IUAT World Conference on Tuberculosis and Respiratory Diseases, Singapore, 1987, Professional Postgraduate Services International.
303. Colditz GA, Berkey CS, Mosteller F, et al: The efficacy of bacillus Calmette-Guérin vaccination of newborns and infants in the prevention of tuberculosis: meta-analyses of the published literature, *Pediatrics* 96:29-35, 1995.
304. Trunz BB, Fine P, Dye C: Effect of BCG vaccination on childhood tuberculous meningitis and miliary tuberculosis worldwide: a meta-analysis and assessment of cost-effectiveness, *Lancet* 367:1173-1180, 2006.
305. Hesseling AC, Cotton MF, Fordham von Reyn C, et al: Consensus statement on the revised World Health Organization recommendations for BCG vaccination in HIV-infected infants, *Int J Tuberc Lung Dis* 12:1376-1379, 2008.
306. Delage G, Remy-Prince S, Montplaisir S: Combined active-passive immunization against the hepatitis B virus: five-year follow-up of children born to hepatitis B surface antigen-positive mothers, *Pediatr Infect Dis J* 12:126-130, 1993.
307. Andre FE, Zuckerman AJ: Review: protective efficacy of hepatitis B vaccines in neonates, *J Med Virol* 44:144-151, 1994.
308. World Health Organization: Expanded programme on immunization: global advisory group, *Wkly Epidemiol Rec* 3:11-16, 1992.
309. Global Alliance for Vaccines and Immunizations: GAVI's impact, 2013. Available at http://www.gavialliance.org/about/mission/impact/. Accessed May 20, 2013.
310. World Health Organization: The prevention and management of puerperal infections: report of a technical working group, Geneva, 1992, World Health Organization.

311. World Health Organization: The global elimination of neonatal tetanus: progress to date, *Bull World Health Organ* 72:155-164, 1994.
312. World Health Organization/United Nations Children's Fund: Maternal care for the reduction of perinatal and neonatal mortality. A joint WHO/UNICEF statement, Geneva, 1986, World Health Organization.
313. Gerbase AC, Rowley JT, Mertens TE: Global epidemiology of sexually transmitted diseases, *Lancet* 351(Suppl 3):2-4, 1998.
314. Moodley P, Sturm AW: Sexually transmitted infections, adverse pregnancy outcome and neonatal infection, *Semin Neonatol* 5: 255-269, 2000.
315. Walker DG, Walker GJ: Forgotten but not gone: the continuing scourge of congenital syphilis, *Lancet Infect Dis* 2:432-436, 2002.
316. Kuate Defo B: Epidemiology and control of infant and early childhood malaria: a competing risks analysis, *Int J Epidemiol* 24: 204-217, 1995.
317. Seale AC, Mwaniki M, Newton CR, et al: Maternal and early onset neonatal bacterial sepsis: burden and strategies for prevention in sub-Saharan Africa, *Lancet Infect Dis* 9:428-438, 2009.
318. van Dillen J, Zwart J, Schutte J, et al: Maternal sepsis: epidemiology, etiology and outcome, *Curr Opin Infect Dis* 23:249-254, 2010.
319. Edmond K, Zaidi A: New approaches to preventing, diagnosing, and treating neonatal sepsis, *PLoS Med* 7:e1000213, 2010.
320. Blencowe H, Cousens S, Mullany LC, et al: Clean birth and postnatal care practices to reduce neonatal deaths from sepsis and tetanus: a systematic review and Delphi estimation of mortality effect, *BMC Public Health* 11(suppl 3):S11, 2011.
321. Kenyon S, Boulvain M, Neilson JP: Antibiotics for preterm rupture of membranes, *Cochrane Database Syst Rev* (8):CD001058, 2010.
322. Lawn JE, Mwansa-Kambafwile J, Horta BL, et al: 'Kangaroo mother care' to prevent neonatal deaths due to preterm birth complications, *Int J Epidemiol* 39(suppl 1):i144-i154, 2010.
323. Partnership for Maternal, Newborn, and Child Health: In Lawn JE, Kerber KJ, editors: *Opportunities for Africa's newborns: practical data, policy and programmatic support for newborn care in Africa*, Cape Town, 2006, South Africa. Partnership for Maternal, Newborn and Child Health.
324. Baqui AH, El-Arifeen S, Darmstadt GL, et al: Effect of community-based newborn-care intervention package implemented through two service-delivery strategies in Sylhet district, Bangladesh: a cluster-randomised controlled trial, *Lancet* 371:1936-1944, 2008.
325. Baqui AH, Ahmed S, El Arifeen S, et al: Effect of timing of first postnatal care home visit on neonatal mortality in Bangladesh: a observational cohort study, *BMJ* 339:b2826, 2009.
326. Kumar V, Mohanty S, Kumar A, et al: Effect of community-based behaviour change management on neonatal mortality in Shivgarh, Uttar Pradesh, India: a cluster-randomised controlled trial, *Lancet* 372:1151-1162, 2008.
327. Bhutta ZA, Soofi S, Cousens S, et al: Improvement of perinatal and newborn care in rural Pakistan through community-based strategies: a cluster-randomised effectiveness trial, *Lancet* 377:403-412, 2011.
328. Gogia S, Sachdev HS: Home visits by community health workers to prevent neonatal deaths in developing countries: a systematic review, *Bull World Health Organ* 88:658-666B, 2010.
329. Kirkwood BR, Manu A, ten Asbroek AH, et al: Effect of the Newhints home-visits intervention on neonatal mortality rate and care practices in Ghana: a cluster randomised controlled trial, *Lancet* 381:2184-2192, 2013.
330. Hanson LA, Hahn-Zoric M, Berndes M, et al: Breast feeding: overview and breast milk immunology, *Acta Paediatr Jpn* 36:557-561, 1994.
331. Ashraf RN, Jalil F, Zaman S, et al: Breast feeding and protection against neonatal sepsis in a high risk population, *Arch Dis Child* 66:488-490, 1991.
332. Brown KH, Black RE, Lopez de Romaña G, et al: Infant-feeding practices and their relationship with diarrheal and other diseases in Huascar (Lima), *Peru. Pediatrics* 83:31-40, 1989.
333. De Zoysa I, Rea M, Martines J: Why promote breastfeeding in diarrhoeal disease control programmes? *Health Policy Plan* 6:371-379, 1991.
334. Feachem RG, Koblinsky MA: Interventions for the control of diarrhoeal diseases among young children: promotion of breast-feeding, *Bull World Health Organ* 62:271-291, 1984.
335. Glezen WP: Epidemiological perspective of breastfeeding and acute respiratory illnesses in infants, *Adv Exp Med Biol* 310:235-240, 1991.
336. Narayanan I, Black RE, Lopez de Romaña G, et al: Randomised controlled trial of effect of raw and holder pasteurised human milk and of formula supplements on incidence of neonatal infection, *Lancet* 2:1111-1113, 1984.
337. Habicht JP, DaVanzo J, Butz WP: Does breastfeeding really save lives, or are apparent benefits due to biases? *Am J Epidemiol* 123:279-290, 1986.
338. Srivastava SP, Sharma VK, Jha SP: Mortality patterns in breast versus artificially fed term babies in early infancy: a longitudinal study, *Indian Pediatr* 31:1393-1396, 1994.
339. Victora CG, Smith PG, Vaughan JP, et al: Infant feeding and deaths due to diarrhea. A case-control study, *Am J Epidemiol* 129: 1032-1041, 1989.
340. Victora CG, Smith PG, Vaughan JP, et al: Evidence for protection by breast-feeding against infant deaths from infectious diseases in Brazil, *Lancet* 2:319-322, 1987.
341. Kramer MS, Kakuma R: Optimal duration of exclusive breastfeeding, *Cochrane Database Syst Rev* (8):CD003517, 2012.
342. Bertolli J, St Louis ME, Simonds RJ, et al: Estimating the timing of mother-to-child transmission of human immunodeficiency virus in a breast-feeding population in Kinshasa, Zaire, *J Infect Dis* 174: 722-726, 1996.
343. Bobat R, Moodley D, Coutsoudis A, et al: Breastfeeding by HIV-1-infected women and outcome in their infants: a cohort study from Durban, South Africa, *AIDS* 11:1627-1633, 1997.
344. Brahmbhatt H, Gray RH: Child mortality associated with reasons for non-breastfeeding and weaning: is breastfeeding best for HIV-positive mothers? *Aids* 17:879-885, 2003.
345. Dunn DT, Newell ML, Ades AE, et al: Risk of human immunodeficiency virus type 1 transmission through breastfeeding, *Lancet* 340:585-588, 1992.
346. Ekpini ER, Wiktor SZ, Satten GA, et al: Late postnatal mother-to-child transmission of HIV-1 in Abidjan, Côte d'Ivoire, *Lancet* 349:1054-1059, 1997.
347. Fowler MG, Newell ML: Breast-feeding and HIV-1 transmission in resource-limited settings, *J Acquir Immune Defic Syndr* 30:230-239, 2002.
348. Kourtis AP, Butera S, Ibegbu C, et al: Breast milk and HIV-1: vector of transmission or vehicle of protection? *Lancet Infect Dis* 3:786-793, 2003.
349. Kreiss J: Breastfeeding and vertical transmission of HIV-1, *Acta Paediatr Suppl* 421:113-117, 1997.
350. Tess BH, Rodrigues LC, Newell ML, et al: Breastfeeding, genetic, obstetric and other risk factors associated with mother-to-child transmission of HIV-1 in São Paulo State, Brazil. São Paulo Collaborative Study for Vertical Transmission of HIV-1, *Aids* 12:513-520, 1998.
351. Van de Perre P: Postnatal transmission of human immunodeficiency virus type 1: the breast-feeding dilemma, *Am J Obstet Gynecol* 173:483-487, 1995.
352. World Health Organization (WHO)/Joint United Nations Programme on HIV/AIDS (UNAIDS): HIV and infant feeding: a policy statement developed collaboratively by UNAIDS, WHO, and UNICEF, Geneva, 1998, WHO/UNAIDS. pp 20-21.
353. World Health Organization: HIV and infant feeding: an updated framework for priority action, 2010. Available at http://apps.who.int/iris/bitstream/10665/75152/1/FWC_MCA_12.1_eng.pdf. Accessed October 16, 2013.
354. Raghavan M, Mondal GP, Bhat BV, et al: Perinatal risk factors in neonatal infections, *Indian J Pediatr* 59:335-340, 1992.
355. Airede AI: Prolonged rupture of membranes and neonatal outcome in a developing country, *Ann Trop Paediatr* 12:283-288, 1992.
356. Asindi AA, Omene JA: Prolonged rupture of membrane and neonatal morbidity, *East Afr Med J* 57:707-711, 1980.
357. Bang AT, Bang RA, Baitule SB, et al: Effect of home-based neonatal care and management of sepsis on neonatal mortality: field trial in rural India, *Lancet* 354:1955-1961, 1999.
358. Weber MW, Carlin JB, Gatchalian S, et al: Predictors of neonatal sepsis in developing countries, *Pediatr Infect Dis J* 22:711-717, 2003.
359. Baqui AH, Arifeen SE, Rosen HE, et al: Community-based validation of assessment of newborn illnesses by trained community health workers in Sylhet district of Bangladesh, *Trop Med Int Health* 5:5, 2009.
360. Darmstadt GL, Baqui AH, Choi Y, et al: Validation of community health workers' assessment of neonatal illness in rural Bangladesh, *Bull World Health Organ* 87:12-19, 2009.
361. Klein JO: Bacterial sepsis and meningitis. In Remington JS, Klein JO, editors: *Infectious diseases of the fetus and newborn infant*, Philadelphia, 2000, WB Saunders, pp 943-998.

362. Zaidi AK, Ganatra HA, Syed S, et al: Effect of case management on neonatal mortality due to sepsis and pneumonia, *BMC Public Health* 11(suppl 3):S13, 2011.
363. Baqui AH, Arifeen SE, Williams EK, et al: Effectiveness of home-based management of newborn infections by community health workers in rural Bangladesh, *Pediatr Infect Dis J* 28:304-310, 2009.
364. Darmstadt GL, Hossain MM, Jana AK, et al: Determination of extended-interval gentamicin dosing for neonatal patients in developing countries, *Pediatr Infect Dis J* 26:501-507, 2007.
365. Darmstadt GL, Miller-Bell M, Batra M, et al: Extended-interval dosing of gentamicin for treatment of neonatal sepsis in developed and developing countries, *J Health Popul Nutr* 26:163-182, 2008.
366. Zaidi AK, Tikmani SS, Warraich HJ, et al: Community-based treatment of serious bacterial infections in newborns and young infants: a randomized controlled trial assessing three antibiotic regimens, *Pediatr Infect Dis J* 31:667-672, 2012.
367. Zaidi AK, Tikmani SS, Sultana S, et al: Simplified antibiotic regimens for the management of clinically diagnosed severe infections in newborns and young infants in first-level facilities in Karachi, Pakistan: study design for an outpatient randomized controlled equivalence trial, *Pediatr Infect Dis J* 32(9 suppl 1):S19-25, 2013.
368. AFRIcan NEonatal Sepsis Trial Group: Simplified regimens for management of neonates and young infants with severe infection when hospital admission is not possible: study protocol for a randomized, open-label equivalence trial, *Pediatr Infect Dis J* 32(9 Suppl 1): S26-S32, 2013.
369. AFRIcan NEonatal Sepsis Trial Group: Treatment of fast breathing in neonates and young infants with oral amoxicillin compared with penicillin-gentamicin combination: study protocol for a randomized, open-label equivalence trial, *Pediatr Infect Dis J* 32(9 suppl 1):S33-S38, 2013.
370. Qazi SA, Wall S, Brandes N, et al: An innovative multipartner research program to address detection, assessment and treatment of neonatal infections in low-resource settings, *Pediatr Infect Dis J* 32(9 suppl 1):S3-6, 2013.
371. Darmstadt GL, Batra M, Zaidi AK: Oral antibiotics in the management of serious neonatal bacterial infections in developing country communities, *Pediatr Infect Dis J* 28(Suppl 1):S31-S36, 2009.
372. Darmstadt GL, Batra M, Zaidi AK: Parenteral antibiotics for the treatment of serious neonatal bacterial infections in developing country settings, *Pediatr Infect Dis J* 28(Suppl 1):S37-S42, 2009.
373. Roess AA, Winch PJ, Ali NA, et al: Animal husbandry practices in rural Bangladesh: potential risk factors for antimicrobial drug resistance and emerging diseases, *Am J Trop Med Hyg* 89:965-970, 2013.
374. Baqui AH, Rahman M, Zaman K, et al: A population-based study of hospital admission incidence rate and bacterial aetiology of acute lower respiratory infections in children aged less than five years in Bangladesh, *J Health Popul Nutr* 25:179-188, 2007.
375. Bhutta ZA, Darmstadt GL, Hasan BS, et al: Community-based interventions for improving perinatal and neonatal health outcomes in developing countries: a review of the evidence. Pediatrics 115(Suppl 2): 519-617, 2005.
376. Haws RA, Thomas AL, Bhutta ZA, et al: Impact of packaged interventions on neonatal health: a review of the evidence, *Health Policy Plan* 22:193-215, 2007.
377. Bang AT, Reddy HM, Deshmukh MD, et al: Neonatal and infant mortality in the ten years (1993 to 2003) of the Gadchiroli field trial: effect of home-based neonatal care, *J Perinatol* 25(Suppl 1):S92-107, 2005.
378. Winch PJ, Gilroy KE, Wolfheim C, et al: Intervention models for the management of children with signs of pneumonia or malaria by community health workers, *Health Policy Plan* 20:199-212, 2005.
379. Darmstadt G, El Arifeen S, Choi Y, et al: Household surveillance of severe neonatal illness by community health workers in Mirzapur, Bangladesh: coverage and compliance with referral, *Health Policy Plan* 25:112-124, 2010.
380. Sazawal S, Black RE: Effect of pneumonia case management on mortality in neonates, infants, and preschool children: a meta-analysis of community-based trials, *Lancet Infect Dis* 3:547-556, 2003.
381. Guyatt GH, Oxman AD, Schünemann HJ, et al: GRADE guidelines: a new series of articles in the Journal of Clinical Epidemiology, *J Clin Epidemiol* 64:380-382, 2011.
382. World Health Organization: Integrated management of the sick child, *Bull World Health Organ* 73:735-740, 1995.
383. World Health Organization, United Nations Children's Fund: Integrated management of childhood illness chart booklet, 2008. Available at http://whqlibdoc.who.int/publications/2008/9789241597289_eng.pdf. Accessed October 16, 2013.
384. Bank TW: World development report 1993: investing in health, New York, 1993, Oxford University Press.
385. Bicego GT, Boerma JT: Maternal education and child survival: a comparative study of survey data from 17 countries, *Soc Sci Med* 36:1207-1227, 1993.
386. van Ginneken JK, Lob-Levyt J, Gove S: Potential interventions for preventing pneumonia among young children in developing countries: promoting maternal education, *Trop Med Int Health* 1: 283-294, 1996.
387. Victora CG, Johnson HL, Cousens S, et al: Maternal education in relation to early and late child health outcomes: findings from a Brazilian cohort study, *Soc Sci Med* 34:899-905, 1992.

3 Obstetric Factors Associated with Infections of the Fetus and Newborn Infant

KRISTINA M. ADAMS WALDORF, RONALD S. GIBBS, and MICHAEL G. GRAVETT

CHAPTER OUTLINE

Overview

Obstetric infections remain an important and potentially preventable contributor to maternal and neonatal morbidity and mortality. Intraamniotic infection (IAI) is associated with 20% of all preterm births (PTBs) and 50% of extreme PTBs at 28 weeks of gestation or less.[1,2] PTB, defined as birth at less than 37 completed weeks of gestation, is one of the leading causes of adverse outcomes of pregnancy. In the United States, in 2011, nearly one in every eight neonates was born prematurely.[3] Prematurity accounts for 70% of all perinatal deaths and half of long-term neurologic morbidity in the United States, and globally prematurity is now the second leading underlying cause of under-5 childhood mortality.[4] In most cases, the underlying cause of preterm labor is not apparent, but evidence from many sources points to a relationship between PTB and genitourinary tract infections.[5,6] In addition to the genitourinary tract, infection leading to PTB may arise in the placenta or from a more remote site, such as the periodontal tissues.[7-10] Newer information has suggested that subclinical infection is responsible not only for PTB but also for many serious neonatal sequelae, including periventricular leukomalacia, cerebral palsy, bronchopulmonary dysplasia, and necrotizing enterocolitis.[11-18] In addition, one quarter to one third of PTBs are preceded by preterm premature rupture of the membranes (PPROM),[19] which is associated with an increased risk of maternal endometritis and neonatal sepsis. Maternal endometritis can develop into puerperal sepsis, which is an infection of the genital tract that begins any time between rupture of membranes or onset of labor and the 42nd postpartum day. Puerperal sepsis is the third leading cause of maternal mortality globally, accounting for 10% to 12% of all maternal deaths.[20,21] This chapter will focus on these entities and their consequences.

Infections not related specifically to pregnancy (e.g., human immunodeficiency virus [HIV], curable sexually transmitted infections, tuberculosis, and malaria) are also important contributors to maternal and neonatal mortality and morbidity. HIV is the leading non-obstetric infectious cause of maternal death in sub-Saharan Africa and also increases the risk for puerperal sepsis compared with HIV-negative women.[22,23] Tuberculosis is an important comorbidity among HIV-infected women in Africa. For example, an autopsy study from Mozambique found that 8.5% of maternal deaths were due to tuberculosis in the context of a 53% HIV prevalence rate.[24] Similarly, malaria is an important contributor to maternal mortality in endemic regions; placental malaria is associated with stillbirth, preterm delivery, and low birth weight.[25] Finally, the World Health Organization estimates that 340 million treatable sexually transmitted infections occur each year (e.g., syphilis, gonorrhea, chlamydial infections, trichomoniasis) and are associated with a wide range of adverse pregnancy outcomes. These and other non-obstetric infections are covered in detail elsewhere in this book. In this chapter, we focus on infection as a cause of PTB and neonatal morbidity and mortality.

Infection as a Cause of Preterm Birth

Intraamniotic infection (IAI), prematurity, and PPROM are important risk factors for neonatal infectious morbidity and mortality. IAI occurs in 1% to 4% of all pregnant women and is the main cause of the earliest PTBs that impart the greatest risk of neonatal mortality and morbidity.[26,27] Synonymous terms applied to IAI include clinical chorioamnionitis, amnionitis, and amniotic fluid infection. We use the term IAI to encompass a clinical syndrome, distinct from bacterial colonization of amniotic fluid (also referred to as microbial invasion of the amniotic cavity) and from histologic inflammation of the placenta (i.e., histologic chorioamnionitis). Histologic chorioamnionitis is characterized by a polymorphonuclear leukocyte infiltration of the chorioamnion and occurs more frequently than clinical IAI, especially at term.

IAI is an important contributor to PTB, occurring in approximately 20% (range, 9%-39%) of all women in preterm labor when assessed by standard laboratory culture of the amniotic fluid (Table 3-1).[2,28-34] Amplification of bacterial DNA encoding 16S ribosomal RNA (rDNA) is a more sensitive test and detects IAI in a greater number of women with preterm labor (range, 11%-56%).[29,34] The rate of IAI also appears to increase in pregnancies with a lower gestational age. In a study of 105 women in preterm labor, IAI was diagnosed by culture in 67% (4/6) at 23 to 24 weeks, 36% (5/14) at 25 to 26 weeks, 17% (2/12) at 27 to 28 weeks, and 11% (4/36) at 33 to 34 weeks of gestation.[2]

PATHOGENESIS

Before labor and membrane rupture, amniotic fluid is usually sterile. The physical and chemical barriers formed by intact fetal membranes (chorioamnion) and the cervical mucus are usually effective in preventing entry of bacteria. With the onset of labor or with membrane rupture, bacteria from the lower genital tract may enter the amniotic cavity. The origin of IAI was originally postulated to occur in four discrete stages of an ascending IAI (Fig. 3-1A). The first stage represents a shift in vaginal or cervical microbial flora with trafficking of bacteria into the cervix. An example of stage I is bacterial vaginosis (BV), a heterogeneous vaginal condition associated with perturbed vaginal flora and loss of healthy *Lactobacillus* organisms. In stage II, bacteria ascend from the vagina or cervix into the choriodecidua, the specialized

Table 3-1 Prevalence of a Positive Culture and/or PCR Test for Bacteria in the Amniotic Fluid of Women in Preterm Labor with Intact Membranes

Author (year)	*N*	Culture	PCR	Culture and PCR Combined	Reference
Watts (1992)	105	19%	—	—	2
Romero (1989)	264	9%			28
Hitti (1997)	69	23%	30%	32%	29
Markenson (1997)	54	9%	56%	56%	30
Oyarzun (1998)	50	12%	46%	46%	31
DiGiulio (2008)	166	10%	11%	15%	32
Han (2009)	26	39%	50%	50%	33
Marconi (2011)	20	—	40%	—	34

Modified from Table 1 in DiGuilio DB: Diversity of microbes in amniotic fluid. *Semin Fetal Neonatal Med* 17:2-11, 2012.
PCR, Polymerase chain reaction.

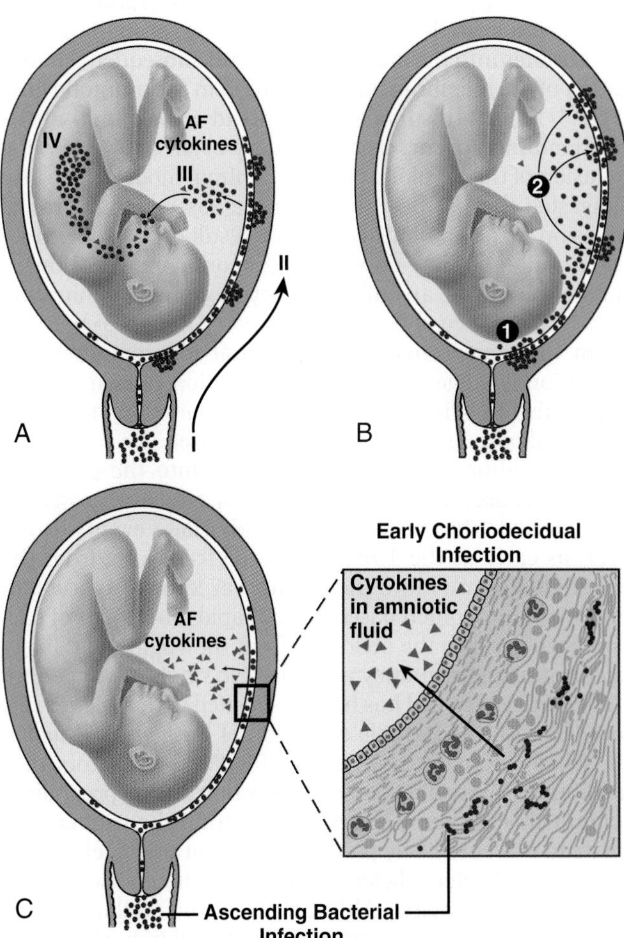

Figure 3-1 Conceptual models of how intraamniotic infection or inflammation may occur during pregnancy. **A,** A choriodecidual infection begins with overgrowth of pathogenic organisms in the vagina and cervix (stage I). Next, the infection ascends to the choriodecidua (stage II), where the microbes invade the amniotic cavity (stage III). Then the fetus becomes infected through aspiration of the amniotic fluid or via the umbilical cord, leading to fetal injury (stage IV). **B,** In this model, bacteria traffic into the amniotic fluid (step 1), propagate within the amniotic fluid (step 2), and subsequently colonize the chorioamnion. **C,** A transient or limited choriodecidual infection is also possible that does not result in bacterial colonization of the amniotic fluid. Bacteria that penetrate the choriodecidua trigger local cytokine production. Cytokines may then pass into the amniotic fluid and induce preterm birth or fetal lung injury. Chorioamnionitis may not be apparent at the time of birth either because of limited placental sampling or complete resolution of the infection. *AF,* Amniotic fluid. (Modified from Romero R, Mazor M: Infection and preterm labor, *Clin Obstet Gynecol* 31:553-584, 1988.)

endometrium of pregnancy. The inflammatory response here facilitates trafficking of organisms into the chorioamnion, leading to chorioamnionitis. In stage III, bacteria invade chorionic vessels (choriovasculitis) and migrate through the amnion into the amniotic cavity to cause IAI. Bacteria recovered from the amniotic fluid and fetal membranes generally consist of organisms that colonize the vagina, including gram-positive (group B streptococci [GBS]), gram-negative (e.g. *Escherichia coli, Gardnerella vaginalis*), and anaerobic (*Mycoplasma hominis*) bacteria (Table 3-2).[28,35,37] Once bacteria invade the amniotic cavity, bacteria may then gain access to the fetus through several potential mechanisms, culminating in stage IV; fetal bacteremia, sepsis, and pneumonia.[38]

Alternatively, an ascending IAI has been hypothesized to occur, which emphasized rapid trafficking through the fetal membranes into the amniotic fluid with subsequent colonization of the membranes from bacteria in the amniotic fluid (Fig. 3-1B). In this model, widespread colonization of the chorioamnion occurs as a secondary event after microbial invasion of the amniotic cavity.[39] Animal models have also suggested that PTB can occur in the absence of microbial invasion of the amniotic cavity as a result of choriodecidual colonization of a low-dose of bacteria or lipopolysaccharide (LPS), leading to an inflammatory response culminating in both clearance of the bacteria and PTB (Fig. 3-1C).[40,41] From this perspective, choriodecidual inflammation is a transitional stage of ascending infection. Regardless of mechanism, IAI is likely dependent on bacterial inoculum, microbial pathogenicity and host response.

Investigation of bacterial trafficking into the pregnant uterus has been limited in humans for ethical reasons; no animal model has been used to study these events. However, as early as the 1960s, bacterial trafficking from the lower genital tract into the uterus was known to occur in nonpregnant women based on the rapid movement of carbon particles into the abdomen from the vagina and likely occurs during pregnancy as well.[42] No single lower genital tract bacteria studied has been associated with a higher risk for PTB with the possible exception of *Trichomonas vaginalis*, which increases the risk of PPROM.[43-46] Factors that facilitate an ascending bacterial infection during pregnancy remain elusive. Immune responses within the vagina, cervix, and placenta likely play an important role to eliminate pathogenic bacteria before invasion of the chorioamnion and amniotic cavity. Although a robust inflammatory response may trigger preterm labor, not all individuals will deliver preterm, underscoring the role of host-pathogen interactions in the process.[47]

The inflammatory response triggered by bacteria is a central mechanism of PTB and fetal injury. Perinatal research has focused on small immunologic proteins called cytokines and chemokines, which are frequently detected in the amniotic fluid and cord blood of preterm neonates with an IAI. Frequently studied cytokines associated with PTB include interleukin-1β (IL-1β), IL-6, IL-8, tumor necrosis factor-α (TNF-α), and C-X-C motif chemokine ligand (CXCL) 10. Many different placental tissues produce cytokines in response to bacterial stimulation, including amniotic epithelium, chorion, decidua and trophoblast cells.[48-51] IL-1β and TNF-α are considered key inflammatory cytokines because amniotic fluid infusion of either is capable of

Table 3-2 Microbial Diversity Within the Amniotic Fluid From Women in Preterm Labor with Intact Membranes as Detected by Culture and PCR

	CULTURE		PCR	
Bacterial Species	**% Positive (No. Positive / Total *N**)**	**Reference**	**% Positive (No. Positive/ Total *N**)**	**Reference**
GENITAL MYCOPLASMAS				
Ureaplasma spp.	25% (6/24)	28	10% (2/21)	33
	35% (7/20)	2		
	13% (4/30)	36		
	61% (14/23)	37		
	19% (3/16)	32	16% (3/19)	32
	24% (5/21)	33		
Mycoplasma spp.	17% (4/24)	28	5% (1/19)	32
	5% (1/20)	2		
	7% (2/30)	36		
	6% (1/16)	32	10% (2/21)	33
ANAEROBES				
Bacteroides spp.	13% (3/24)	28	14% (3/21)	33
	40% (8/20)	2		
Fusobacterium spp.	21% (5/24)	28	33% (7/21)	33
	35% (7/20)	2		
	31% (5/16)	32	4% (2/50)	31
	25% (4/16)	33	26% (5/19)	32
AEROBES				
Group B streptococci	4% (1/24)	28	5% (1/19)	32
	0% (0/20)	2		
	7% (2/30)	36		
	6% (1/16)	32	10% (2/21)	33
	13% (2/16)	33		
Escherichia coli	0% (0/24)	28	26% (13/50)	31
	0% (0/20)	2		
	13% (2/16)	33		
Gardnerella vaginalis	13% (3/24)	28	—	
	15% (3/20)	2		
	13% (2/16)	32	—	
FASTIDIOUS, NONCULTIVATABLE BACTERIA				
Leptotrichia amnionii	—		11% (2/19)	32
			5% (1/21)	33
Sneathia sanguinegens	—		21% (4/19)	32
			14% (3/21)†	33
FUNGI				
Candida albicans	10% (2/20)	2	11% (2/19)	32
	7% (2/30)	36		
	6% (1/16)	32		

PCR, Polymerase chain reaction.
*Total *N* represents all the positive cultures or PCR tests reported in the study.
†A positive PCR test for *L. sanguinegens* (*N* = 1) and *S. sanguinegens* (*N* = 2) in the original study were combined into *S. sanguinegens* because of a recent change in nomenclature.

inducing PTB in a nonhuman primate model.[47] Although infusion of IL-6 does not induce PTB, murine IL-6 knockouts deliver 1 day later than expected and are refractory to LPS stimulated PTB.[52] This suggests that IL-6 may play an important role in controlling the progression of labor and facilitating PTB. IL-6 and other cytokines can also stimulate prostaglandin production by amniotic epithelium and the decidua, which further drive labor.[53]

Another model of placental infection may be specific to *Listeria monocytogenes*, an aerobic gram-positive rod associated with PTB and stillbirth.[54-56] In this case, hematogenous spread of the bacteria occurs after ingestion of colonized food (e.g., unpasteurized cheese). Next, bacteria invade the extravillous trophoblast cells, which are specialized invasive placental cells that form the placenta vascular bed. Within the extravillous trophoblast cells, *L. monocytogenes* is efficiently confined for a period of time within vacuolar compartments destined for lysosome degradation. Over time, the placenta becomes a dangerous nidus of infection and continuously reseeds maternal organs until the placenta is expulsed with delivery.[57,58] Maternal deaths may occur as a result, which is also the case for other virulent organisms with hematogenous spread such as group A streptococci.[59] The mechanism of stillbirth may result from an impaired response of the normally immunosuppressive maternal T-regulatory ($Foxp3^+$) cells to fetal antigens.[60]

IAI may also develop as a consequence of obstetric procedures such as cervical cerclage, diagnostic amniocentesis, cordocentesis (percutaneous umbilical cord blood sampling), or intrauterine transfusion. After cervical cerclage, data regarding infectious complications are reported to range from 1% to 18%, but this may also be a consequence of cervical shortening and dilation.[59,61,62] After diagnostic amniocentesis, rates of IAI range from 0% to 1%.[63] Chorioamnionitis is a rare complication of chorionic villus sampling. Although IAI is very rare after percutaneous umbilical blood sampling, and the fetal loss rate accompanying this procedure is only 1% to 2%, infection is responsible for a high percentage of losses and may lead to life-threatening maternal complications.[64]

Clinical risk factors for IAI have implicated low parity, a greater number of vaginal examinations in labor, longer labor, greater duration of membrane rupture, and internal fetal monitoring.[65] The most significant clinical risk factor is membrane rupture longer than 12 hours.[66] Meconium staining of the amniotic fluid has also been associated with an increased risk of chorioamnionitis (4.3% vs. 2.1%).[67] Prior spontaneous and elective abortion (at <20 weeks) in the immediately preceding pregnancy has also been associated with development of IAI in the subsequent pregnancy.[68]

HISTOLOGIC CHORIOAMNIONITIS

A consistent observation is that placentas in PTBs are more likely to show evidence of inflammation (i.e., histologic chorioamnionitis). In a series of 3500 consecutive placentas, Driscoll found infiltrates of polymorphonuclear cells in 11%.[69] Clinically evident infection developed in only a few of the women in the study, but the likelihood of neonatal sepsis and death was increased. An association has also been established between histologic chorioamnionitis and chorioamnion infection (defined as the recovery of microorganisms from the chorioamnion).[70] Overall, the organisms found in the chorioamnion are similar to organisms found in the amniotic fluid in cases of clinical IAI. This array of organisms supports an ascending route for chorioamnion infection in most cases. The rate of histologic chorioamnionitis increases with decreasing gestational age at delivery. In one study, when birth weight was greater than 3000 g, the percentage of placentas showing histologic chorioamnionitis was less than 20%; when birth weight was less than 1500 g, the percentage was 60% to 70%.[71]

ANIMAL MODELS

Pregnant mice, rabbits and sheep have been used to identify inflammatory mediators in the PTB pathway and potential therapeutic targets that might improve neonatal outcome. Together, data from multiple animal models have been critical for understanding the inflammatory cascade occurring in the placenta, amniotic fluid, fetus and mother, which is necessary to prevent development of IAI, PTB, and early-onset neonatal infections. However, many animal models are sufficiently different from humans in terms of hormonal events associated with parturition and placental structure to limit their translational potential.

The model that most closely resembles human pregnancy in both placentation and hormonal events of pregnancy is the chronically instrumented nonhuman primate (NHP) model, using either pregnant rhesus or pigtail macaques. A major strength of the NHP model lies in the ability to longitudinally correlate data from maternal, fetal, and amniotic fluid samples with uterine contractility over time in individual animals. Experiments in the NHP model have elucidated the primary role for maternal and fetal inflammation in mediating infection-associated PTB. For example, experiments in the NHP model demonstrated that immunomodulators (dexamethasone, indomethacin) that can suppress the inflammatory response in combination with antibiotics could prolong pregnancy in women with IAI from GBS.[72] Further study is required to demonstrate fetal safety of this approach, as well as efficacy, in animal models.

Animal models have also delineated the role of specific inflammatory mediators in PTB and therapeutic potential of their antagonists.

- *IL-1β and TNF-α:* IL-1β and TNF-α are cytokines elevated in the amniotic fluid of women with IAI and appear to play a critical role in infection-induced PTB in animal models.[73,74] Infusion of IL-1β into the amniotic fluid of NHP leads uniformly to PTB, whereas high-dose TNF-α caused PTB in about half the animals.[47] However, the overexpression of the natural IL-1 receptor antagonist in transgenic mice could not inhibit IL-1β induction of PTB.[75] Pretreatment with an antibody to TNF-α was shown to reduce PTB and fetal death.[76]
- *IL-6 and IL-8:* In human studies, amniotic fluid IL-6 and IL-8 has been implicated in the cytokine cascade, culminating in PTB.[77,78] In NHP, intraamniotic infection or inflammation induced by GBS, LPS, and other pathogens elevates IL-6 and IL-8 in amniotic fluid. However, isolated infusions of IL-6 or IL-8 into the amniotic fluid do not cause PTB.[47] This suggests a hierarchy of cytokine

effects on preterm labor, with IL-1β and TNF-α playing a more important role than either IL-6 or IL-8. Recently, IL-6 has been postulated to facilitate labor progression, because there is a slight delay in normal parturition and LPS-induced PTB in IL-6 knockout mice.[52]

- N-*acetylcysteine (NAC):* Oxidative stress is implicated in PPROM by promoting apoptosis and collagen weakening through production of reactive oxygen species (ROS).[79,80] ROS are unstable molecules released by immune cells during bacterial killing and from mitochondria that are capable of widespread membrane damage. NAC counteracts oxidative stress and has shown promise in delaying PTB in mice and rats. Administration of NAC in a murine model of LPS-induced PTB was associated with a significant delay in delivery, reduction in oxidative stress, and greater fetal survival.[81] In rats, NAC was shown to significantly attenuate an LPS-induced cytokine response in maternal serum and amniotic fluid.[82]
- *Toll-like receptors (TLRs):* TLRs are a family of pattern recognition receptors that activate the innate and adaptive immune systems after recognition of bacterial pathogens. PTB has been shown to occur in mice after activation of either TLR2, TLR3, TLR4, or TLR9 by their respective ligands: lipotechoic acid or peptidoglycan, polyinosinic:polycytidylic acid (poly[I:C]), LPS, and cytosine-phosphate-guanosine (CpG) dinucleotide, respectively.[83-85] Research has focused on TLR4 because gram-negative bacteria are commonly associated with PTB, and TLR4 recognizes LPS from the outer cell membrane of gram-negative microbes.[35,86] LPS-induced PTB does not occur in TLR4 knockout mice.[84] Furthermore, pretreatment with a TLR4 antagonist in the NHP model completely suppressed LPS-induced uterine activity and amniotic fluid cytokines and prostaglandins.[87]
- *Matrix metalloproteinases (MMPs):* Elevated amniotic fluid MMP-8 is a powerful predictor of spontaneous PTB in humans.[88] MMP-1 is also elevated in the placenta during labor.[89] A nonspecific MMP inhibitor (GM6001; EMD Biosciences, San Diego, CA) significantly inhibited LPS-induced PTB in a murine model, suggesting that at least one (or more) MMP is critical for inducing labor in the setting of inflammation or infection.[90] Endothelin-1 (ET-1) has recently been shown in the mouse to act in the same molecular pathway as MMP-1 for infection-associated PTB.[91] Inhibition of ET-1 through endothelin receptor antagonists or RNA interference also inhibits PTB.[92]

MICROBIOLOGY

The cause of IAI is often polymicrobial, involving aerobic and anaerobic organisms (see Table 3-2). In a microbiologic controlled study, amniotic fluid cultures from women with and without IAI were compared.[93] Patients with IAI were more likely to have 10^2 colony-forming units (CFU)/mL of any isolate, any number of high virulence isolates, and more than 10^2 CFU/mL of a high-virulence isolate (e.g., GBS, *Escherichia coli,* and enterococci). Although GBS and *E. coli* were isolated with only modest frequency (15% and 8%, respectively), if detected in the amniotic fluid, they are strongly associated with maternal or neonatal bacteremia (25% and 33%, respectively). The isolation of low-virulence organisms, such as lactobacilli, diphtheroids, and

Table 3-3 Association of Lower Genitourinary Tract Infections with Preterm Birth

Infection	Odds or Hazard Ratio for Preterm Birth (95% Confidence Interval)	Reference
Ureaplasma urealyticum	1.0 (0.18-1.2)	45
Chlamydia trachomatis	2.42* (1.37-4.27)	94
Neisseria gonorrhea	1.77* (1.05-3.00)	94
Trichomonas vaginalis	1.59* (1.18-2.14)	94
Bacterial vaginosis	1.3 (1.1-1.4)	107
Bacteriuria	1.64 (1.35-1.78)	324

*These hazard ratios were calculated for a "very preterm birth" defined as delivery before 33 weeks. *Chlamydia, Trichomonas,* and gonorrhea were also significantly associated with later preterm births.

Staphylococcus epidermidis, was similar in the IAI and control groups. Common amniotic fluid isolates and odds ratios (ORs) for the association of specific bacterial species with PTB are shown in Table 3-3. Several sexually transmitted infections also appear to be risk factors for PTB, including *Neisseria gonorrhea, Chlamydia trachomatis,* and *Trichomonas vaginalis.*[43,94]

Mycoplasma hominis and *Ureaplasma* species have been consistently recovered from amniotic fluid at a higher frequency than other bacteria but usually in association with other bacteria of known virulence. Some have questioned whether these bacteria cause PTB or may secondarily invade the amniotic cavity in the setting of another primary infection. Amniotic fluid inoculation of either *M. hominis* or *Ureaplasma* species induced PTB, chorioamnionitis, and fetal pneumonia in NHP. PTB occurred between 2.5 to 15 days after *Ureaplasma parvum* inoculation (10^7 CFU) and 17 to 30 days after *M. hominis* inoculation (10^5-10^7 CFU).[95] Genital mycoplasmas (*Ureaplasma urealyticum* and *M. hominis*) have also been associated with fetal and neonatal morbidity in human studies. In one study of neonates born between 23 and 32 weeks' gestation, positive umbilical cord blood cultures for genital mycoplasmas were detected in 23%.[96] Patients with spontaneous preterm delivery had a significantly higher rate of blood cultures positive for *U. urealyticum* or *M. hominis* or both than patients with indicated preterm delivery (34.7% vs. 3.2%; $P < .0001$) The earlier the gestational age at delivery, the more likely the culture was positive. In addition, newborns with a positive blood culture had a higher frequency of a neonatal systemic inflammatory response syndrome, higher serum concentrations of IL-6, and more frequent histologic evidence of placental inflammation than neonates with negative cultures. Bacteria within the amniotic fluid have also been identified by broad-range polymerase chain reaction (PCR) targeting the bacterial ribosomal unit 16S.[29,32,97] This technique allows the identification of fastidious or unculti-vatable microbes and has confirmed the heterogeneous and polymicrobial nature of amniotic fluid infection.

Maternal genital tract colonization with GBS may lead to neonatal sepsis, especially when birth occurs prematurely, or when the membranes have been ruptured for prolonged intervals. Several studies have found an association between GBS colonization of the lower genital tract and PTB or an earlier term birth.[44,98] In many other studies, no association between GBS genital colonization and preterm labor or delivery was found.[99] In contrast with the conflicting data regarding genital colonization with GBS, GBS bacteriuria has been consistently associated with preterm delivery, and treatment of this bacteriuria resulted in a marked reduction in prematurity (37.5% in the placebo group vs. 5.4% in the treatment group).[100-102] In a randomized treatment trial of erythromycin versus placebo in women colonized with GBS, erythromycin use was not shown to be effective in prolonging gestation or increasing birth weight.[103]

BV is a vaginal infection characterized by perturbations of the vaginal flora, high concentrations of certain bacterial species (e.g., *G. vaginalis*), and reductions in vaginal lactobacilli that has also been associated with IAI and PTB. The prevalence of BV varies by population, with rates of 8% in pregnant U.S. white women[104], 23% in pregnant U.S. black women,[104] and 44% in nonpregnant Kenyan women.[105] BV is associated with an increased PTB risk (1.4- to 3-fold or greater) thought to occur from an ascending vaginal infection resulting from loss of normal, healthy *Lactobacillus* flora and acquisition of a particularly pathogenic bacterial species.[27,106-109] Another possibility is that BV acts locally in the lower genital tract to facilitate ascending infection by other organisms.

Bacteria associated with BV have been detected in amniotic fluid and placenta, suggesting that trafficking of vaginal microbes into the uterus occurs during pregnancy.[32,71,110] Molecular techniques now enable identification of recognized bacterial species that are highly specific for BV but had not previously been detected using standard cultivation methods.[111] These bacteria are fastidious or uncultivable and include species such as *Leptotrichia amnionii* that are detected using PCR for bacterial DNA encoding 16S rRNA. There is striking heterogeneity in the microbial communities within BV, which has led to the hypothesis that one or more specific bacterial species may be responsible for the increased PTB risk. In contrast, the vaginal microbiota from women with normal, healthy vaginal flora is typically fairly homogeneous with between one and six bacterial species in the vagina dominated by *Lactobacillus*.[111]

BV may interact with genetic susceptibility and environmental factors to increase the risk of spontaneous PTB. Maternal carriers of a single nucleotide polymorphism in the TNF-α gene 2 *(TNF2)* were at significantly increased risk of spontaneous PTB (OR, 2.7; 95% confidence interval [CI], 1.7 to 4.5) in a case-control study. However, the association between *TNF2* and PTB was modified by the presence of BV; mothers with a "susceptible" genotype and BV had an increased odds of PTB compared with mothers who did not.[112] This association has not been confirmed at present but represents an interesting hypothesis for the interaction between a genetic predisposition and vaginal microbes in the susceptibility to PTB.

Viruses have also been detected in the amniotic fluid of asymptomatic women in the second trimester, suggesting that the hematogenous spread of viruses to the placenta occurs with a low frequency. Several studies have determined that between 2.2% and 8.4% of low-risk women with normal fetuses on ultrasonography in the second trimester have detectable genome sequences from at least one of eight viruses: human herpesvirus 6 (HHV6), adenoviruses, Epstein-Barr virus, varicella zoster virus, herpes simplex virus, parvovirus B19, human cytomegalovirus (HCMV), and enteroviruses.[113] The most commonly detected virus in amniotic fluid in these studies was HHV6, recovered from 1.0% of patients. No significant changes in amniotic fluid white blood cell count, glucose, or IL-6 level were associated with viral invasion of the amniotic cavity. Of the inflammatory mediators tested, only CXCL 10 was associated with HCMV viral load. In general, however, viruses have not been linked to IAI, and fetal morbidity or mortality appears rare.

DIAGNOSIS OF INTRAAMNIOTIC INFECTION

The diagnosis of IAI requires a high index of suspicion because the clinical signs and symptoms may be subtle and occur late in the course of the infection. Clinical features of IAI include maternal fever greater than or equal to 37.8° C, maternal leukocytosis greater than 15,000/mm^3, maternal tachycardia greater than 100 beats per minute, fetal tachycardia greater than 160 beats per minute, uterine tenderness, and foul-smelling amniotic fluid.[26] Maternal leukocytosis supports the diagnosis of clinical IAI, although recent administration of antenatal corticosteroids may cause a mild leukocytosis.[114] The presence of a left shift (i.e., an increase in the proportion of neutrophils, especially immature forms), however, is particularly suggestive of clinical IAI. Malodorous amniotic fluid and uterine tenderness, although more specific for IAI, occur in a minority of cases. Other causes of fever in the parturient, such as epidural analgesia and concurrent infection of the urinary tract or other organ systems, must be considered.

Amniotic Fluid Testing

Direct examination of the amniotic fluid is desirable to confirm the diagnosis of IAI because clinical signs are inconsistent. Samples can be collected transabdominally by amniocentesis or transvaginally by aspiration of amniotic fluid through an intrauterine pressure catheter. Although amniotic fluid microbial cultures are important in ascertaining the etiology of the infection, they require 48 to 72 hours to provide results and thus cannot be used immediately to guide therapy. Adjunctive, rapid diagnostic tests, including Gram stain, amniotic fluid white cell count, and amniotic fluid glucose concentration, are therefore frequently used.[115,116] In one study directly comparing these tests with amniotic fluid culture, amniotic fluid glucose level and Gram stain were the most specific for predicting a positive amniotic fluid culture (Table 3-4).[117,118] The combination of Gram stain with amniotic fluid glucose concentration is superior to any individual rapid adjunctive test currently widely available. The combination of Gram stain and an amniotic fluid glucose of less than or equal to 14 mg/dL had a sensitivity of 91% and a specificity of 81% when compared with amniotic fluid culture and those are the two most widely used adjunctive tests to diagnose IAI. Other diagnostic tools reported include measurement of amniotic fluid IL-6,[119] MMP-8,[120] or the detection of inflammatory mediators by proteomic analysis of amniotic fluid[121,122] or cervicovaginal secretions.[123] These tests, although sensitive and specific for the diagnosis of IAI, are not widely available or used at this time. Finally, detection of microorganisms by

Table 3-4 Diagnostic Value of Amniotic Fluid Testing in Detection of Positive Amniotic Fluid Culture in Patients with Preterm Labor and Intact Membranes

Diagnostic Test	Sensitivity	Specificity	Positive Predictive Value	Negative Predictive Value
Gram stain	7/11 (64%)	108/109 (99%)	7/8 (88%)	108/112 (96%)
IL-6	11/11 (100%)	90/109 (83%)	11/30 (37%)	90/90 (100%)
WBC count	7/11 (64%)	103/109 (95%)	7/13 (54%)	103/107 (96%)
Glucose	9/11 (82%)	80/109 (82%)	9/29 (31%)	89/91 (98%)
Gram stain plus WBC count	10/11 (91%)	102/109 (94%)	10/17 (59%)	102/103 (99%)
Gram stain plus glucose	10/11 (91%)	88/109 (81%)	10/31 (33%)	88/89 (99%)
Gram stain plus glucose plus WBC count	10/11 (91%)	85/109 (78%)	10/34 (29%)	85/86 (99%)

Modified from Romero R, Yoon BH, Mazor M, et al: The diagnostic and prognostic value of amniotic fluid white blood cell count, glucose, interleukin-6, and Gram stain in patients with preterm labor and intact membranes. *Am J Obstet Gynecol* 169:805-816, 1993.
IL-6, Interleukin-6; *WBC,* white blood cell.
WBC ≥ 50 cells/mm^3 on Gram stain.
Glucose threshold ≤ 14 mg/dL.

PCR, to detect DNA encoding 16S rRNA, may be useful for the rapid diagnosis of IAI in the future. The PCR assay has a higher sensitivity than culture for detection of microorganisms in the amniotic fluid, particularly in patients whose amniotic fluid is culture negative, but other markers indicate evidence of an inflammatory response.[29-31]

Recently, the detection of amniotic fluid "sludge," hyperechogenic material within the amniotic fluid identified by ultrasonography, has also been described as a diagnostic marker for microbial colonization of amniotic fluid and IAI.[124] In a retrospective case-control study, patients with "sludge" had a significantly higher rate of spontaneous preterm delivery; a higher frequency of clinical chorioamnionitis, histologic chorioamnionitis, and funisitis; a higher frequency of PPROM; and a shorter median ultrasound-to-delivery interval.[125] In addition, the combination of a cervical length less than 25 mm and "sludge" conferred a 15-fold increased odds for spontaneous preterm delivery at less than 28 weeks when compared with women with a normal cervical length and no amniotic fluid sludge (OR, 14.8; 95% CI, 3.9 to 56.5). By comparison, the increased risk of preterm delivery at less than 28 weeks was 6.8 (95% CI, 1.2 to 39.5) for those with a short cervix alone and 9.1 (95% CI, 2.9 to 28.6) for those with amniotic fluid sludge alone, respectively.

In the setting of premature rupture of the membranes (PROM), diagnosis of IAI is usually based on clinical criteria because oligohydramnios may preclude successful sampling of amniotic fluid. The incidence of microbial colonization and IAI are therefore likely underestimated. Risks of colonization and of IAI vary with gestational age and with labor. The rate of positive amniotic fluid cultures for microorganisms is higher with PPROM (32.4%) than with preterm labor with intact membranes (12.8%).[126] In addition, among women with PROM the risk of microbial invasion of the amniotic after the onset of labor is as high as 75%.[127]

Proteomics

Timely interventions to prevent neonatal sepsis in the setting of IAI would require early diagnosis, which is challenging because the clinical signs and symptoms tend to occur as late manifestations, and adjunctive laboratory tests have limited predictive value or require an invasive amniocentesis. Proteomics has been applied to investigate differentially expressed proteins in the amniotic fluid, cervicovaginal fluid, and maternal serum predictive of IAI (Fig. 3-2). Multiple proteins in the amniotic fluid were differentially expressed in NHF as early as 12 hours after experimental IAI and before clinical signs or symptoms of infection, including azurocidin, calgranulin B, and a proteolytic fragment of insulin-like growth factor binding protein-1 (IGFBP-1).[121] Validation of these biomarkers among a cohort of women in preterm labor with intact fetal membranes yielded a sensitivity of 100% and a specificity of 91%.[121] A limitation of this approach is the requirement for an amniocentesis, which many providers are reluctant to perform in women with preterm labor. In the nonhuman primate, 27 proteins were differentially expressed in the cervicovaginal fluid after experimental *U. parvum* infection.[128] In a cohort of 170 women in preterm labor with intact fetal membranes, 15 differentially expressed proteins in vaginal fluid were associated with subclinical IAI.[123] A four-analyte immunoassay panel developed from these differentially expressed proteins was able to correctly classify 89% of patients as infected or not infected and included α1-acid glycoprotein, IGFBP-1, calgranulin C, and cystatin A. In maternal serum, proteomics identified a reduction in three peptides associated with the inter-α-trypsin inhibitor heavy chain–4 protein in women destined to have a PTB.[129]

TREATMENT OF INTRAAMNIOTIC INFECTION

Management guidelines for the treatment of women in preterm labor and the use of antibiotics in preterm labor and PPROM are presented in Box 3-1 and Table 3-5. Antibiotics have not been shown to improve neonatal outcomes or prolong pregnancy in women in preterm labor with intact membranes. However, antibiotic therapy is important to prevent postpartum endometritis and has been studied in the prevention of IAI. Progesterone therapy has been discovered to prevent PTB in a small subset of women, but it is unknown whether it prevents IAI and is, therefore, not discussed.[130,131]

Antenatal Antibiotics to Prevent Intraamniotic Infection

Antibiotics given during prenatal care to patients at increased risk of preterm delivery have not shown benefit

Maternal Serum

Proteomic biomarkers predictive of subsequent spontaneous PTB after sampling of maternal serum at 24-28 weeks

- Corticotrophin-releasing factor
- Tumor necrosis factor-α receptor type 1
- Thrombin antithrombin complex
- Defensin
- Ferritin
- Lactoferrin

Amniotic Fluid

Predictive of intraamniotic infection and imminent preterm birth

- Azurocidin
- Calgranulin A
- Calgranulin B
- Calgranulin C
- Insulin-like growth factor binding protein-1, proteolytic fragment (11 kDa)
- Neutrophil defensin-1
- Neutrophil defensin-2

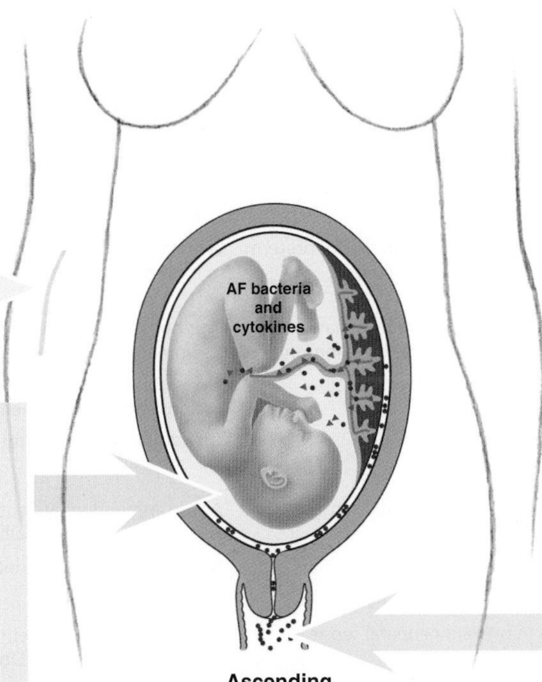

Vaginal Fluid

Predictive of intraamniotic infection

- α1-acid glycoprotein
- α1-antitrypsin
- Complement component 3
- Calgranulin C
- Lysozyme
- Matrix metalloproteinase-9
- Insulin-like growth factor binding protein-1
- Vitamin D binding protein
- Haptoglobin
- Fatty acid binding protein
- Involucrin
- Fibronectin

Figure 3-2 Proteomic markers identified in the amniotic fluid, cervicovaginal fluid, and maternal serum—identified as linked to preterm birth or intraamniotic infection. *AF*, Amniotic fluid; *PTB*, preterm birth. (From Gravett MG, Novy MJ, Rosenfeld RG, et al: Diagnosis of intra-amniotic infection by proteomic profiling and identification of novel biomarkers, *JAMA* 292:462-469, 2004; Buhimschi IA, Christner R, Buhimschi CS: Proteomic biomarker analysis of amniotic fluid for identification of intra-amniotic inflammation, *BJOG* 112:173-181, 2005; Hitti J, Lapidus JA, Lu X, et al: Noninvasive diagnosis of intraamniotic infection: proteomic biomarkers in vaginal fluid, *Am J Obstet Gynecol* 203:32 e31-e38, 2010; and Esplin MS, Merrell K, Goldenberg R, et al: Proteomic identification of serum peptides predicting subsequent spontaneous preterm birth, *Am J Obstet Gynecol* 204:391.e1-e8, 2011.

Box 3-1 Management Principles of Preterm Labor

The following recommendations and conclusions are based on good and consistent scientific evidence (Level A):

- A single course of corticosteroids to promote fetal lung maturation is recommended for pregnant women between 24 weeks of gestation and 34 weeks of gestation who are at risk of preterm delivery within 7 days.
- Accumulated available evidence suggests that magnesium sulfate reduces the severity and risk of cerebral palsy in surviving infants if administered when birth is anticipated before 32 weeks of gestation. Hospitals that elect to use magnesium sulfate for fetal neuroprotection should develop uniform and specific guidelines for their departments regarding inclusion criteria, treatment regimens, concurrent tocolysis, and monitoring in accordance with one of the larger trials.
- Evidence supports the use of first-line tocolytic treatment with β-adrenergic agonist therapy, calcium channel blockers, or nonsteroidal antiinflammatory drugs for short-term prolongation of pregnancy (up to 48 hours) to allow the administration of antenatal steroids.
- Maintenance therapy with tocolytics is ineffective for preventing preterm birth and improving neonatal outcomes and is not recommended for this purpose.
- Antibiotics should not be used to prolong gestation or improve neonatal outcomes in women with preterm labor and intact membranes.

The following recommendations and conclusions are based on limited and inconsistent scientific evidence (Level B):

- A single course of repeat antenatal corticosteroids should be considered in women whose prior course of antenatal corticosteroids was administered at least 7 days previously and who remain at risk of preterm birth before 34 weeks of gestation.
- Bed rest and hydration have not been shown to be effective for the prevention of preterm birth and should not be routinely recommended.
- The positive predictive value of a positive fetal fibronectin test result or a short cervix alone is poor and should not be used exclusively to direct management in the setting of acute symptoms.

Reproduced from American College of Obstetrics and Gynecology; Committee on Practice Bulletins—Obstetrics: ACOG practice bulletin no. 127: management of preterm labor, Obstet Gynecol *119:1308-1317, 2012.*

Table 3-5 Suggested Guidelines on the Use of Antibiotics to Prevent Preterm Birth or for Treatment of Preterm Labor with Intact Membranes or Preterm Premature Rupture of Membranes

Opinion	Comment
DURING PRENATAL CARE	
Treat *Neisseria gonorrhoeae* and *Chlamydia trachomatis* infection.	Screening and treatment of these two sexually transmitted organisms should follow standard recommendations to prevent spread to sexual partner(s) and the newborn. Published nonrandomized trials show improved pregnancy outcome with treatment.
Treat bacteriuria, including group B streptococcal bacteriuria.	Screening and treatment for bacteriuria is a standard practice to prevent pyelonephritis. A meta-analysis concluded that bacteriuria is directly associated with preterm birth.
Screen for and treat bacterial vaginosis in patients at high risk for preterm birth. In these high-risk women, treat with oral metronidazole for ≥1 week.	A meta-analysis has shown benefit with this treatment in women with high-risk pregnancies.
Treat symptomatic *Trichomonas vaginalis* infection to relieve maternal symptoms, but do not screen for or treat asymptomatic trichomoniasis.	This opinion is based on randomized trials in asymptomatic infected women.
Do not treat *Ureaplasma urealyticum* genital colonization.	One double-blind treatment trial that corrected for confounding infections showed no benefit.
Do not treat group B streptococcal genital colonization.	One double-blind treatment trial showed no benefit.
WITH PRETERM LABOR AND INTACT MEMBRANES	
Give group B streptococcal prophylaxis to prevent neonatal sepsis.	As recommended by Centers for Disease Control and Prevention and American College of Obstetricians and Gynecologists.
Do not give antibiotics routinely to prolong pregnancy.	A meta-analysis concluded that antibiotics gave no neonatal benefit.
WITH PRETERM PREMATURE RUPTURE OF THE MEMBRANES	
Give group B streptococcal prophylaxis to prevent neonatal sepsis.	As recommended by Centers for Disease Control and Prevention and American College of Obstetricians and Gynecologists.
Give additional antibiotics (ampicillin or amoxicillin plus erythromycin) in pregnancies at 24 to 34 weeks.	Meta-analyses concluded that there was substantial benefit to the neonate. Controversy exists as to whether there is benefit between 32 to 34 weeks.

in preventing IAI. Early studies found a decrease in low-birth-weight infants delivered of women who received oral erythromycin for 6 weeks in the third trimester compared with placebo.[132,133] A larger multicenter study of more than 1100 women with genital *U. urealyticum* found no change in any measured outcomes (gestational age at birth, low birth weight) when women were randomly assigned to receive placebo or erythromycin beginning at 26 to 30 weeks of gestation and continuing until 35 weeks.[134] Treatment of *U. urealyticum* in pregnancy to prevent prematurity remains experimental.

Two retrospective, nonrandomized studies have reported reductions in preterm labor, PROM, and low birth weight through antenatal treatment of *C. trachomatis* infection.[135,136] In the first study, patients successfully treated for *C. trachomatis* had significantly lower rates of PROM and premature labor than patients who failed to have *C. trachomatis* eradicated. In the second study, adverse outcome was assessed among three large groups: *C. trachomatis*–positive but untreated (*N* = 1110), *C. trachomatis*–positive and treated (*N* = 1327), and *C. trachomatis*–negative (*N* = 9111). The *C. trachomatis*–positive but untreated group had higher rates of PROM, low birth weight, and perinatal mortality than the other two groups. The only randomized treatment trial for *C. trachomatis* in pregnancy led to conflicting results, however.[137] In this latter study, the rate of pregnancies resulting in low-birth-weight infants was reduced in three of the five centers but not significantly reduced in the remaining two. A more recent large study found that treatment of *C. trachomatis* in midpregnancy was not associated with a decreased frequency of PTB.[138] At the present time, it is the standard of care to treat women with *C. trachomatis* infection, not so much to prevent preterm labor but to prevent spread of the sexually transmitted disease.

Treatment with metronidazole should be offered to women who have symptomatic *T. vaginalis* infection in pregnancy, to relieve maternal symptoms and prevent spread of a sexually transmitted disease. Metronidazole is safe for use in the first trimester of pregnancy.[139] However, in one study when pregnant women with asymptomatic *T. vaginalis* infection at 24 to 29 weeks of gestation were randomly assigned to receive either metronidazole or placebo, rates of PTB were increased in the group given metronidazole.[140] Caution is therefore advised if treating asymptomatic trichomoniasis in the late second or third trimester.

To date, antibiotic treatment trials of BV have generally not reduced PTB despite overwhelming evidence that BV is consistently related to PTB, amniotic fluid infection, and chorioamnionitis.[71,108-110,141-145] Several methodologic problems with prior trials include (1) BV treatment too late in pregnancy to prevent significant microbial trafficking into the uterus, (2) antibiotics tested were ineffective against many uncultivable pathogens,[146,147] (3) failure to establish a *Lactobacillus*-dominant flora to prevent recurrence, and (4) lack of follow-up to document resolution. In Tanzanian women, a single course of metronidazole resulted in a shift from one BV-associated microbiota profile to another but rarely resulted in return of a *Lactobacillus*-dominant flora.[148] The route of antibiotic administration may also be

Table 3-6 Antibiotic Regimens to Prevent Endometritis in Women with IAI

Antibiotic	Dose	Comment	Reference
Ampicillin + Gentamicin	*Ampicillin:* 2 g IV every 6 hours, plus *gentamicin:* 5.0 mg/kg IV once daily (normal renal function)	Fetal levels are threefold higher with once-daily versus standard (1.5 mg/kg) dosing of gentamicin ▪ If penicillin allergic, may substitute ampicillin with vancomycin 1 g IV every 12 hours. ▪ Clindamycin 900 mg IV every 8 hours should be added to this regimen for women undergoing cesarean section or used as a substitute for ampicillin to achieve better anaerobic bacterial coverage.	325-327
Ampicillin-sulbactam	3 g IV every 6 hours		328
Ticarcillin-clavulanate	3.1 g (3 g ticarcillin + 100 mg clavulanate) IV every 4 hours		329
Cefoxitin	2 g IV every 6 hours		330
Cefotetan	2 g IV every 12 hours		330
Piperacillin-tazobactam	3.375 g IV every 6 hours		331

From Hopkins L, Smaill F: Antibiotic regimens for management of intraamniotic infection, *Cochrane Database Syst Rev* (3):CD003254, 2002.
IAI, Intraamniotic infection; *IV*, intravenous.
Data does not support an ideal antimicrobial regimen for the treatment of IAI to prevent postpartum endometritis. Ampicillin and gentamicin are inexpensive and highly effective.

a key factor in resolution; a recent report suggests that oral metronidazole is effective at clearing BV-associated species, such as *Leptotrichia* and *Sneathia*, but intravaginal metronidazole is not.[147] Vaginal microbial communities are also dynamic during pregnancy and may derive from an intestinal reservoir.[149,150] With advancing gestation, there is an increasing representation of proteobacteria (gram-negative bacteria) in the third trimester, an overall reduction in species richness (number of taxa), and a reduction in within-subject (alpha) diversity.[149] There may also be a unique window of PTB susceptibility in early pregnancy during which vaginal bacteria can colonize the endometrial cavity, which would favor earlier therapy of BV to prevent preterm labor.

An American College of Obstetricians and Gynecologists practice bulletin on assessment of risk factors for PTB has advocated that BV screening and treatment of high-risk or low-risk women would not be expected to reduce the overall rate of PTB.[151] In certain populations of high-risk women, such as women with prior PTB and BV early in pregnancy, many experts still recommend treatment of BV diagnosed early in pregnancy.[152]

Lack of consistent findings in antibiotic trials for BV to prevent PTB raises the question of why antibiotics have been effective in so few clinical situations. One explanation is that bacterial vaginosis is microbially very heterogenous, and only a subset of the women with bacterial vaginosis may harbor particularly pathogenic microbes for preterm labor. Second, treatment trials may have targeted therapy too late in pregnancy to be effective in preventing ascending infection that leads to PTB. Finally, antibiotics administered may not have been completely effective in eradicating fastidious bacteria.

For reasons other than prevention of PTB, detection and treatment of *N. gonorrhoeae, C. trachomatis*, and bacteriuria are appropriate. Future research is urgently needed, however, to identify markers in women who are in preterm labor as a result of infection, in whom intervention with antibiotics or other novel therapies is most likely to be beneficial. In addition, detection of women genetically predisposed to infection-induced PTB is important. Some investigators have identified associations between polymorphisms (single nucleotide polymorphisms [SNPs]) in the cytokine gene complexes, including TNF-α and PPROM or spontaneous PTB.[153-155] Further research is needed, however, to determine if screening for these SNPs can inform or impact clinical management.

PREVENTION OF POSTPARTUM ENDOMETRITIS AFTER INTRAAMNIOTIC INFECTION DIAGNOSIS

Several principles guide the treatment of IAI. First, IAI is frequently a polymicrobial infection, involving both facultative and anaerobic microorganisms; broad-spectrum parenteral antibiotics are indicated mainly to eradicate the infection and prevent postpartum endometritis. Antibiotic therapy should be begun in the intrapartum period, as soon as the diagnosis is confirmed. Delivery, except under very unusual circumstances (e.g., listeriosis), is warranted by usual obstetric indications.

Antibiotic Choice

Several broad-spectrum antibiotics are appropriate for the treatment of IAI to prevent postpartum endometritis (Table 3-6). A combination of parenteral ampicillin and an aminoglycoside, such as gentamicin, has traditionally been used because of excellent activity against common neonatal pathogens, including GBS and *E. coli*. However, these agents provide little anaerobic coverage. Therefore, clindamycin may be added to this regimen for patients with IAI who undergo cesarean delivery to prevent postpartum endometritis. Because dysfunctional labor leads to cesarean delivery in many patients with IAI, the consequence of this treatment protocol is that a high proportion of patients with IAI will ultimately require triple therapy, with its associated expense and potential toxicity. For most infections, single-agent therapy with a broad-spectrum antibiotic is equally efficacious and cost effective. Recommended intravenous regimens include cefotetan, cefoxitin, or penicillins combined with β-lactamase inhibitors, such as timentin/clavulanate or piperacillin/tazobactam. Because of the greater risk of postpartum endometritis after cesarean delivery, the chosen antibiotic regimen should be continued until the patient has been afebrile and symptoms resolved for at least 24 hours in those patients delivered by cesarean. For patients delivering vaginally, the duration of antibiotic therapy is arbitrary. Most patients defervesce promptly and more than one dose of antibiotics postpartum may be unnecessary.[156]

Among women in preterm labor with intact membranes, there have been several studies and meta-analyses studying the effect of various antibiotic regimens. The ORACLE II study showed no delay in delivery and no improvement in a composite outcome that included neonatal death, chronic lung disease, or cerebral anomaly.[157] In the Cochrane meta-analysis, 7428 women in 11 trials were assessed.[158] The relative risk (RR) for neonatal death in the antibiotic treatment group was 1.52 (95% CI, 0.99 to 2.34). There was a significant reduction in postpartum intrauterine infection with use of antibiotics, but this reduction was not seen as sufficient justification for widespread use of antibiotics in preterm labor. In a subanalysis, the reviewers looked at trials using antibiotics that were active against anaerobes (i.e., metronidazole or clindamycin). There were significant benefits in delivery within 7 days and in neonatal intensive care unit admissions. These benefits were not accompanied, however, by significant reductions in major end points, such as PTB, perinatal mortality, or neonatal sepsis.

In two studies with varying durations of antibiotic therapy after delivery complicated by IAI, there was no significant difference in rate of endometritis or postpartum fever.[156,159] In one study, however, there was a 2.5-fold increase in wound infection rate in patients who did not receive scheduled postpartum antibiotics (5% vs. 1.8%). Based on these studies, it seems that when antibiotic treatment is initiated early, a short course of therapy in the puerperium is sufficient therapy in most patients.

More recent studies have addressed the issue of duration of antibiotic therapy postpartum in cases of IAI. One randomized trial compared single-dose versus multidose postpartum treatment of mothers and reported that single-dose treatment was accompanied by a shorter time to discharge (33 vs. 57 hours; $P = .001$).[156] The single-dose group had a nearly threefold increase in failure of therapy, but this did not achieve statistical significance (11% vs. 3.7%; $P = .27$). Although not statistically significant, this threefold increase in "failed therapy" elicits concern regarding single-dose postpartum therapy for IAI.

Timing of Antibiotic Therapy

In the past, there was debate regarding timing of antibiotic administration, but it has now become standard to begin treatment during labor, as soon as possible after the maternal diagnosis of IAI is made. Three studies, including a randomized clinical trial, have shown benefits from intrapartum antibiotic therapy compared with immediate postpartum treatment.[93,160,161] In a large, nonrandomized allocation of intrapartum versus immediate postpartum treatment, intrapartum antibiotic therapy was associated with a significant decrease in neonatal bacteremia (2.8% vs. 19.6%; $P < .001$) and a reduction in neonatal death from sepsis (0.9% versus 4.3%; $P = .07$).[93] Another large study showed an overall reduction in neonatal sepsis ($P = .06$), especially bacteremia caused by GBS (0% vs. 4.7%; $P = .004$), with use of intrapartum treatment.[160]

After maternal intravenous administration, these antibiotics rapidly penetrate into the fetal compartment and achieve therapeutic concentrations in cord blood.[162] Studies comparing intrapartum with postpartum treatment have consistently reported a lower incidence of neonatal sepsis with intrapartum therapy.[93,160,161] In the only randomized, prospective trial of intrapartum versus postpartum treatment, there were significant reductions in neonatal sepsis or pneumonia in those receiving intrapartum treatment (0% vs. 32% among those with postpartum treatment; $P < .05$) and a 2-day reduction in the average neonatal hospital length of stay.[161] Maternal postpartum febrile morbidity was also reduced by intrapartum treatment.

Delivery as Therapy

Delivery is essential for adequate treatment, and prompt action should begin at the time of diagnosis; unless the expected time to delivery is remote, cesarean section should be reserved for usual obstetric indications. There is no advantage to cesarean delivery, per se, and it increases maternal risk of postpartum febrile morbidity. There are few data regarding the effect of the duration of the time interval from the diagnosis of infection until delivery on neonatal infectious morbidity. A critical time period beyond which maternal and neonatal complications increase has not been identified. Most patients with IAI deliver within 5 to 7 hours. Several studies, however, found no increase in neonatal infections for an interval of at least 12 hours among patients receiving intrapartum antibiotic treatment.[163-165] Whether or not intervals longer than 12 hours increase the risk of neonatal infections has not been determined. The combination of villous edema, hyperthermia, and fetal infection may contribute to fetal acidosis. Fetal tachycardia may be associated with maternal pyrexia but is also an independent predictor of fetal sepsis and pneumonia. Persistent fetal tachycardia may therefore portend an ill neonate that will require resuscitation and support. Personnel skilled in neonatal resuscitation should therefore be present for the delivery.

NEONATAL OUTCOMES

Chorioamnionitis was previously considered a maternal infection, but evidence implicates the fetus in an inflammatory response that culminates in PTB. Challenges in diagnosing IAI confound the interpretation of studies of resulting fetal injury. Most studies use a histologic or clinical diagnosis of chorioamnionitis as a proxy for IAI. Not only is the clinical diagnosis of IAI often missed, but histologic chorioamnionitis may involve only segments of the fetal chorioamnion and be missed by the routine and limited placental sampling for histopathology. Despite these limitations, several studies associated chorioamnionitis with injury to the fetal lung (bronchopulmonary dysplasia [BPD]), brain[166,167] (periventricular leukomalacia [PVL], intraventricular hemorrhage [IVH], cerebral palsy [CP]), bowel[18] (necrotizing enterocolitis [NEC]), and eye[168] (retinopathy of prematurity [ROP]). The pathogenesis of fetal lung and brain injury in utero is strongly linked to the inflammatory response to infection (Fig. 3-3). A systemic proinflammatory cytokine response may also occur in the fetus ("fetal inflammatory response syndrome"), which

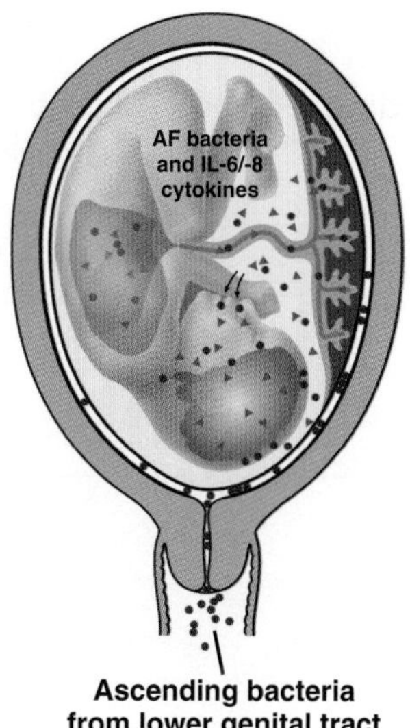

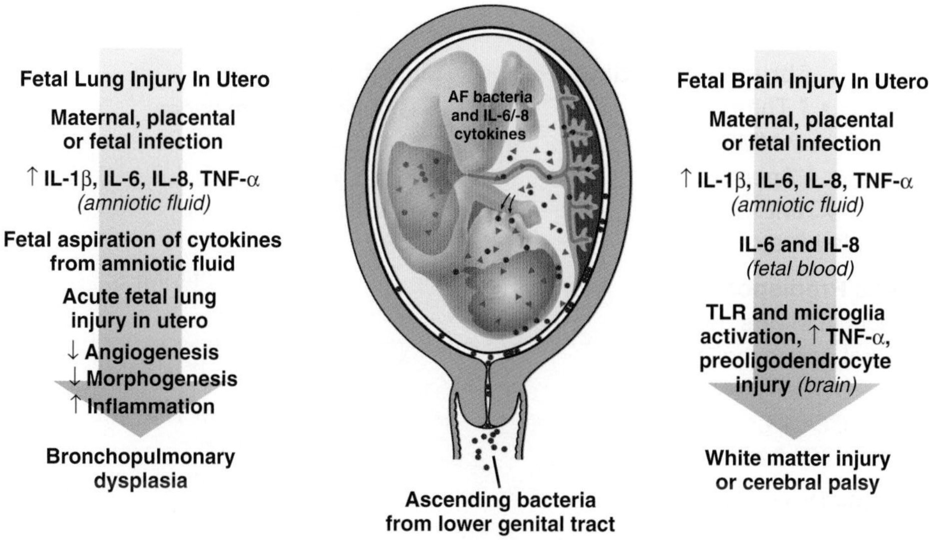

Figure 3-3 Biologic events link intraamniotic and choriodecidual infection with cytokine production in the amniotic fluid or fetus and subsequent fetal lung and brain injury in utero. *AF*, Amniotic fluid; *IL*, interleukin; *TLR*, Toll-like receptor; *TNF*, tumor necrosis factor.

is associated with significant neonatal morbidity.[169-171] When the fetal systemic inflammatory response persists after birth, the risk of injury to multiple organs becomes greater.

Fetal Lung Injury

Intraamniotic inflammation and infection are important risk factors for BPD, a chronic lung disease affecting one third of preterm infants weighing less than 1500 g.[17,172,173] BPD is characterized by arrested alveolar development, impaired pulmonary angiogenesis, inflammation, and interstitial fibrosis.[174,175] Other insults to the fetal lung also play a role in pathogenesis of BPD, including mechanical ventilation (barotrauma, hyperoxia, oxidative stress) and sepsis.[17,176] The link between chorioamnionitis and BPD was only modest in a recent large meta-analysis with more than 15,000 subjects from 59 studies (OR, 1.58; 95% CI, 1.11 to 2.24).[177] A stronger link has been established between elevated cytokines in the amniotic fluid, cord blood, and neonatal serum and BPD, neonatal morbidity, and mortality (increased IL-8, IL-10; decreased RANTES [regulated on activation, normal T-cell expressed and secreted]).[172,178-180] Fetal lung inflammation in the sheep and nonhuman primates has also been associated with intrauterine infection and elevated amniotic fluid cytokines.[181-184] The mechanisms responsible for fetal lung injury have not been well characterized but likely involve proinflammatory cytokines or exposure to bacterial products. The fetal lung becomes exposed to amniotic fluid cytokines and possibly to bacterial products through swallowing movements that occur normally in utero. In the nonhuman primate, elevations of amniotic fluid cytokines were associated with shifts in fetal lung gene expression characteristic of decreased angiogenesis and morphogenesis, which is critical for normal lung growth.

Fetal Brain Injury

Fetal brain injury is also associated with intrauterine infection and inflammation, but discrepancies in study results illustrate the complexity of studying how perinatal events influence long-term neurodevelopmental outcomes. Studies are conflicting as to whether periventricular leukomalacia (PVL) is associated with chorioamnionitis.[185,186] However, levels of inflammatory cytokines are increased in the amniotic fluid of infants with white matter lesions (i.e., PVL), and there is overexpression of these cytokines in neonatal brain with PVL.[13] Experimental intrauterine infection or inflammation in animal models also leads to brain white matter lesions.[14,187,188] Several lines of evidence have also linked intrauterine inflammation with CP, which is a neurodevelopmental disorder that is now the most common cause of severe physical disability in childhood.[12,185,189,190] In contrast, a secondary data analysis from the Alabama Preterm Birth Study did not find an increased risk of severe neurodevelopmental outcomes among children born between 23 and 32 weeks of gestation with in utero exposure to inflammation.[191]

Mechanisms of fetal brain injury induced by intrauterine infection and inflammation may occur through a direct cytokine or pathogen injury or in combination with other insults such as hypoxia and oxidative stress. Cytokines and inflammatory cells are common to many pathways associated with fetal brain injury, including infection, hypoxia-ischemia, reperfusion, and toxin-mediated injury.[167] Elevations of IL-1β and IL-6 in the amniotic fluid have been associated with PVL.[192] Cytokines in the fetal blood may change the permeability of the blood-brain barrier, allowing microbial invasion of the cerebrospinal fluid. The cells vulnerable to injury in the fetal brain are white matter oligodendrocyte progenitor cells (preoligodendrocytes), which can be injured by activated microglia (brain macrophages), and free radical attack.[193,194] TNF-α has been specifically linked with brain injury induced by microglia.[195] When preoligodendrocytes are injured, normal differentiation into myelin-forming oligodendrocytes may not occur, which increases the risk for neurodevelopmental abnormalities such as CP.[196] The combination of placental inflammation and white matter injury in extremely premature infants was associated with CP.[197] In studies of neonatal brain pathology, noncystic PVL is also a risk factor for CP and was associated with reactive microglial accumulations.[198] Animal models further support the association between placental inflammation, activation of fetal microglia, and subsequent motor deficits.[194,199]

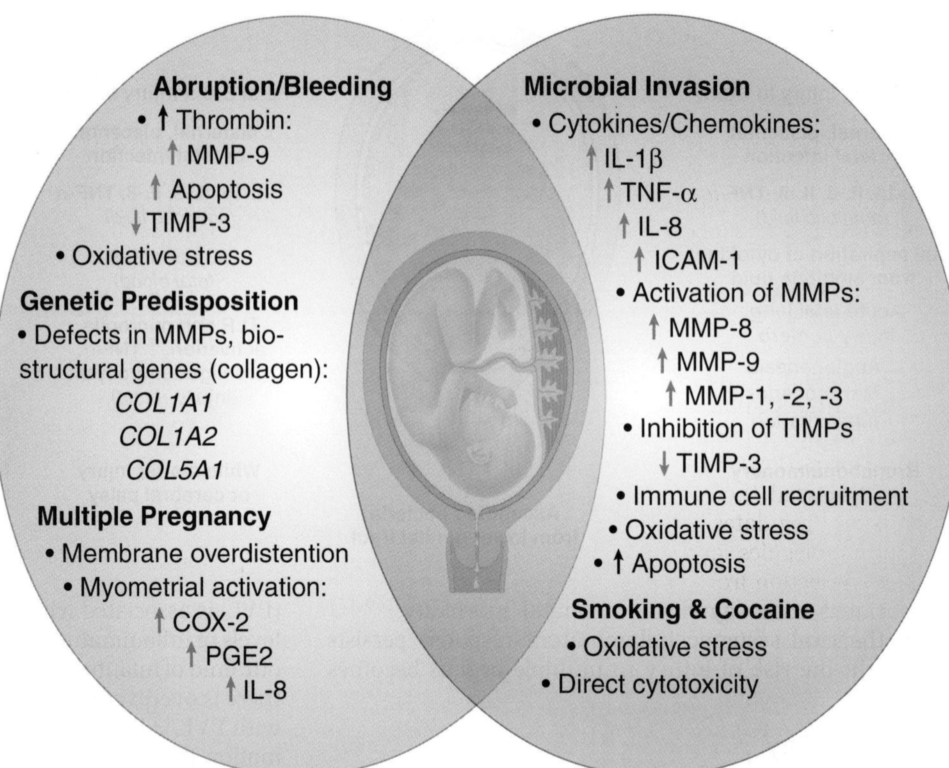

Figure 3-4 Several biologic pathways have been linked to preterm premature rupture of the membranes, which may act synergistically to weaken the membranes. *COX,* Cyclooxygenase; *ICAM,* intercellular adhesion molecule; *IL,* interleukin; *MMP,* matrix metalloproteinase; *TIMP,* tissue inhibitors of metalloproteinases; *TNF-α,* tumor necrosis factor-α.

Magnesium Sulfate for Neuroprotection

The use of magnesium sulfate in women in preterm labor was significantly associated with a reduced risk of cerebral palsy in a randomized controlled trial of 2241 women.[200] Whether magnesium sulfate confers neuroprotection in the setting of IAI is unknown, but several of the hypothesized mechanisms target cellular injury induced by infection and inflammation.[201] For example, magnesium decreases production of proinflammatory cytokines and oxygen free radicals produced during hypoxic-ischemic reperfusion.[202] Magnesium may also increase blood flow to the fetal brain by reducing constriction of the cerebral arteries.[203] Use of magnesium sulfate in women in preterm labor is now the standard of care, depending on gestational age, and likely to also confer neuroprotection in the setting of IAI.

Premature Rupture of Membranes

Before the onset of labor, PROM is common and occurs in 8% of deliveries.[204] When fetal membranes rupture preterm (PPROM), the etiology is often related to an underlying infection, which can result in morbidity for the mother and fetus. PPROM occurs in approximately 1% to 2% of all pregnancies and is implicated in 30% of all PTBs.[205] Despite some progress in prolonging the latent period after membrane rupture, PPROM remains a leading contributor to the overall problem of premature birth. The impact of PTBs from PPROM is greatest in low- and middle-income countries, where most childhood deaths associated with prematurity occur.[206]

Several clinical risk factors have been associated with PPROM, including low body mass index, bacterial vaginosis or infection, placental bleeding (abruption), heavy smoking, cocaine use, genetic predisposition, short cervix (<25 mm) or cervical incompetence, cervical operations and lacerations, multiple pregnancies, and polyhydramnios.[207-210] Multiparous women with a prior history of PTB, short cervix, and a positive fetal fibronectin had a 31-fold higher risk of PROM and delivery before 35 weeks, compared with women without these risk factors (25% vs. 0.8%; $P = .001$).[211] Sexual intercourse may also increase the risk of PROM, which has been hypothesized to result from microbial attachment to sperm.[212] Progesterone therapy seems to be effective in reducing the risk of recurrent PTB secondary to spontaneous preterm labor.[213-217] Whether or not progesterone specifically decreases the incidence of recurrent preterm birth after PPROM is unknown as prior studies have either not reported PPROM incidence or excluded women with PPROM in the index birth.[130,218] Once PPROM has occurred, progesterone therapy does not delay preterm birth.[219]

Common biologic pathways, discussed below, that lead to chorioamnion weakening are activated by many of the conditions associated with PPROM and likely act synergistically (Fig. 3-4). Understanding factors contributing to membrane biomechanical strength and pathways that lead to membrane weakening is the first step to developing new therapies.

NATURAL HISTORY OF PREMATURE RUPTURE OF THE MEMBRANES AND PRETERM PREMATURE RUPTURE OF THE MEMBRANES

When women are managed expectantly after PROM at term, approximately half will give birth within 5 hours, and 95% will give birth within 28 hours of membrane rupture.[220] After PPROM, the latency period between membrane rupture and delivery is much longer than at term. More than half of women with PPROM will have a latency period of at least 24 hours (57%-83%),[221,222] and up to 40% may have a latency period as long as 1 week (19%-41%).[221,223] Latency periods are also longer the earlier in gestation that PPROM occurs. Between 25 and 32 weeks of gestation, at least one third of women with PPROM had a latent period of 3 days, but only 5% to 16% had a similar latency if rupture occurred between 35 and 37 weeks. With expectant management, 3% to 13% may anticipate the cessation of leakage of amniotic fluid and continuation of pregnancy.[224,225]

BIOMECHANICAL STRENGTH OF THE CHORIOAMNION

The composition of the fetal membranes is an important element to understanding its mechanical strength and why rupture may occur prematurely. The fetal membranes are composed of two layers, the amnion and chorion, which are collectively called the chorioamnion. The chorioamnion contains and regulates amniotic fluid volume, selectively transports molecules, and helps protect the fetus from an ascending infection from vaginal bacteria.[226] The amnion is a thin avascular layer adjacent to the amniotic fluid, which has greater biomechanical strength than the thicker chorion layer.[227-229] Intracellular cytoskeletal proteins and intermediate filaments within amniotic epithelium likely provide the amnion with some of its shear strength. Descending filaments, which include types I and III collagen, are anchored to the basement membrane of the amniotic epithelium. Additional resistance to shear stress may be provided by elastin molecules within the compact layer of the amnion, but this is controversial.[230,231] The chorion provides the bulk of the chorioamnion membrane and undergoes active remodeling throughout pregnancy. The chorion appears to rupture before the amnion in a video analysis of puncture testing of the fetal membranes.[229] The earliest biologic events contributing to PPROM may involve weakening and thinning of the chorion.

Calculations of the mechanical load on the fetal membranes suggests that the chorioamnion is under significant stress and is closer to a failure threshold (rupture) than other tissues in the body (aorta).[232] A weak region of the chorioamnion has been identified over the cervix in both term and preterm membranes; the membrane rupture site is generally in this location.[231,233,234] Histologically, the chorioamnion at the rupture site has disrupted collagen fibrils, chorion thinning, and sometimes absent decidua, which has been referred to as the "zone of altered morphology."[231]

PATHOGENESIS

Infection and Inflammation, Matrix Metalloproteinase Activation, and Oxidative Stress

Perhaps the most common and well-studied pathway of PPROM is infection, which may occur as a limited infection of the chorioamnion without bacterial trafficking into the amniotic fluid (Fig. 3-5A) or with frank amniotic fluid invasion (Fig. 3-5B).[235] Evidence of chorioamnion infection can be detected in nearly half of all women with PPROM.[227] The earlier in gestation that PPROM occurs, the more likely that infection plays a role. A positive amniotic fluid bacterial culture occurs in approximately 18% to 38% of all PPROM cases.[120,127,236-239] The odds of eventual PPROM in women in spontaneous preterm labor with intact membranes is very high if bacteria are detected within the amniotic fluid (OR, 27).[240] An inflammatory cascade begins after microbial invasion of the placenta, leading to production of inflammatory cytokines and chemokines that are also typical in preterm labor with intact membranes (i.e., IL-1β, TNF-α, IL-6).[241] TNF-α and IL-1β are both associated with biomechanical membrane weakening in vitro when applied to full-thickness membranes.[242] Cytokines, particularly TNF-α, also initiate other pathways to membrane weakening, including recruitment of other immune cells (neutrophils, macrophages), activation of MMP, oxidative stress, and induction of apoptosis within the chorioamnion.[233,234,243-248]

Collagen fibrils within the chorioamnion are susceptible to degradation by MMP, which is a family of zinc enzymes that become elevated near term and also in IAI and PPROM.[227,249] MMPs not only degrade extracellular matrix proteins such as collagens but can also activate cytokines and chemokines, release ligands to induce apoptosis, and cleave cell surface receptors. The best-characterized MMP in PPROM is MMP-9, but MMP-8 activity also correlates with chorioamnionitis, funisitis, and poor neonatal outcomes.[250,251] The activity of many other MMPs is increased in chorioamnion or amniotic fluid in preterm labor (intact membranes) or PPROM: MMP-1, MMP-2, MMP-3, MMP-10, MMP-11, MMP-13, and MMP-14.[252] Tissue inhibitors of metalloproteinases (TIMPs) act to prevent MMP enzymatic degradation of the chorioamnion and are also elevated in PPROM.

Infection also induces oxidative stress within the chorioamnion, which leads to apoptosis, collagen weakening, and widespread membrane damage.[79,253] Oxidative stress occurs during bacterial killing when immune cells release ROS, which inflict damage through several mechanisms: collagen cleavage, MMP-9 activation, DNA damage, catalytic enzyme release, and lipid peroxidation. There is also histologic evidence of oxidative stress in membranes after PPROM.[80] The link between cigarette smoking and PPROM is also likely through oxidative stress.[254] The antioxidant properties of amniotic fluid may help to prevent membrane damage from oxidative stress resulting from infection or cigarette smoking. Antioxidant activity of amniotic fluid increases from the second to the third trimester, which means that there is a lesser capacity of the amniotic fluid to buffer oxidative stress within the membranes during the late second trimester, when cases of infection-associated PPROM are more likely to occur.[255] Unfortunately, clinical trials of the antioxidants vitamin C and E had mixed results, but these vitamins unexpectedly were associated with an increase in PPROM rates over placebo in a single large clinical trial (4.6% vs. 1.7%; RR, 2.68; $P = .025$).[256-258] Further studies are needed to investigate the therapeutic potential of inhibition of oxidative stress for the prevention of PPROM.

Abruption (Placental Bleeding) and Thrombin

Abruption is a clinical risk factor for PPROM, which is thought to be mediated by the production of thrombin after activation of the coagulation cascade.[235] In a small case-control study of women with a prior history of PPROM, complexes of thrombin-antithrombin in maternal plasma were predictive of eventual PPROM.[259] After blood vessel injury, blood becomes exposed to tissue factor and prothrombin is cleaved to make thrombin. Thrombin production results

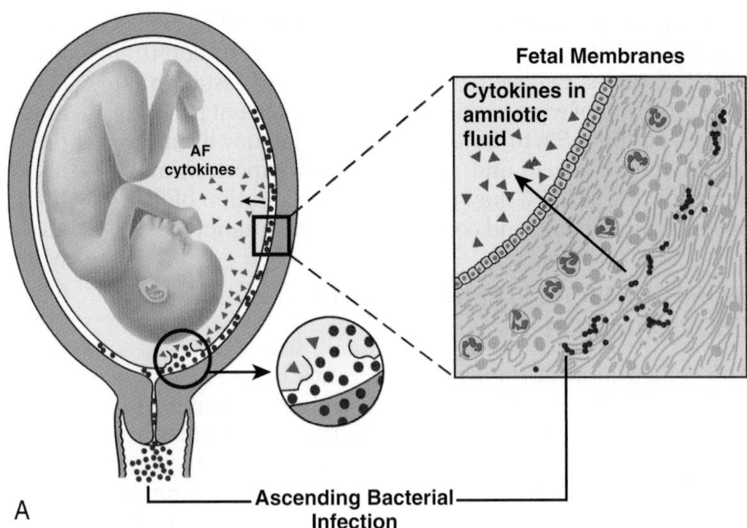

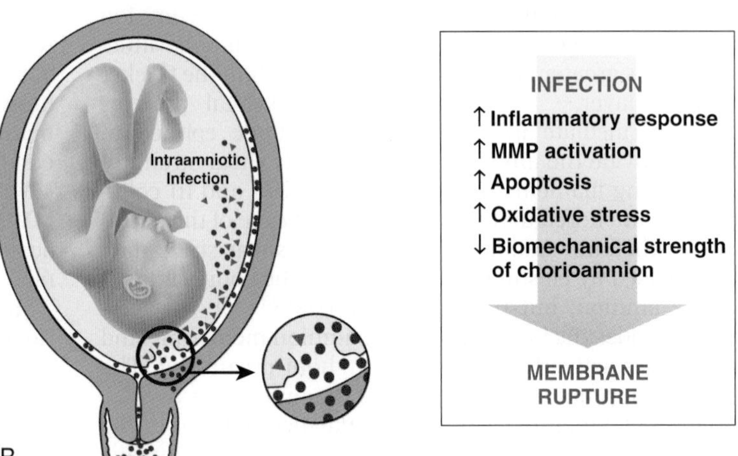

Figure 3-5 Conceptual models of how preterm premature rupture of the membranes may occur after intraamniotic infection or inflammation. **A,** A limited choriodecidual infection in the lower uterine segment induces cytokine production, apoptosis, matrix metalloproteinase activation, and recruitment of immune cells, leading to loss of cytostructural integrity and membrane rupture. **B,** Another possibility is that microbes first invade the amniotic cavity near the lower uterine segment and then secondarily colonize the chorioamnion at other sites. Trafficking of organisms into the amniotic fluid further amplifies the inflammatory response and weakening of the chorioamnion. Histologically, infection of the chorioamnion leads to chorion thinning, apoptotic loss of amniotic epithelial cells, and an overall loss of architecture. Membrane rupture occurs as a result of the inflammatory response, microbial byproducts (proteases), or as a direct pathogenic effect of the organism. *AF,* Amniotic fluid; *MMP,* matrix metalloproteinase. (A and B modified from Romero R, Mazor M: Infection and preterm labor, *Clin Obstet Gynecol* 31:553-584, 1988.)

in activation of many biologic pathways associated with PPROM: inflammation (e.g., IL-8), MMP activation (MMP-1, MMP-9), apoptosis and oxidative stress.[260-266] Thrombin has also been shown to weaken the fetal membranes in a dose-dependent manner, possibly through MMP-9 activity and poly–ADP ribose polymerase (PARP) cleavage.[242] PARP is involved in DNA repair, and cleavage is associated with apoptosis. Although exposure of chorioamnion explants to TNF-α and IL-1β also results in weakening, only thrombin weakens isolated amnion.[242,267] Weakening of amnion explants can be inhibited by pretreatment with α-lipoic acid (antioxidant), which suggests that membrane weakening induced by thrombin also acts through oxidative stress.[268]

Genetic Predisposition

A genetic predisposition to PPROM was recognized in the 1960s for women with Ehlers-Danlos syndrome, which is characterized by defects in collagen genes or collagen processing.[269,270] In the first report of 18 women with Ehlers-Danlos, PPROM occurred in 13 of the 14 PTBs.[270] If the fetus was affected with Ehlers-Danlos, the risk of PPROM in the pregnancy was nearly double that of women with an unaffected fetus (50% vs. 20%). Women with other connective tissue disorders, such as restrictive dermopathy and osteogenesis imperfecta type II, also have a higher risk of PPROM.[269] PPROM has been specifically linked to fetal carriage of variants or defects in collagen genes *(COL1A1, COL1A2, COL5A1)* or related proteins involved in collagen processing (cartilage associated protein *[CRTAP]*, leucine proline–enriched proteoglycan 1 *[LEPRE1]*, and zinc metallopeptidase STE24 *[ZMPSTE24]*).[269]

Genetic variants within genes related to inflammatory potential, collagen processing, and MMP activation have also been investigated in PPROM. A functional SNP within the *SERPINH1* gene (-656 C/T) has been associated with an increased risk of PPROM; of interest, this gene variant is enriched in women of West African ancestry, and African-American ethnicity is associated with an increased risk of PTB.[271] Other gene variants affecting the function of MMP and immune and apoptosis pathways are also implicated in PPROM.[153,272-276]

DIAGNOSIS

In most cases, PROM is readily diagnosed by history, physical findings, and simple laboratory tests, such as determination of pH or detection of ferning. Several tests have been evaluated in the diagnosis of PROM, with most having a

Table 3-7 Diagnostic Value of Tests to Diagnose Membrane Rupture

Test/Reference	Cutoff	Sensitivity (%)	Specificity (%)	PPV (%)	NPV (%)	Comments	Reference
Nitrazine (pH)	Positive/negative	90-97	16-70	63-75	80-93	Gold standard, but not as sensitive and specific as newer tests	333, 334
Ferning and/or pooling	Positive/negative	51-98	70-88	84-93	87-97		335
Placental alpha-1 microglobulin (PAMG-1, AmniSure ROM Test)	>5.0 ng/mL	98-99	88-100	98-100	91-99	Highly accurate, easy to perform bedside test. Reliable across a wide gestational age range (11-42 weeks)	336-339
AmnioSense (absorbent pad)	pH > 5.2	98.3	70	65-70	98		
Fetal fibronectin	>50 ng/mL	97-98	70-97	74-93	98-100		340
AFP (ROM Check)	>30 µg/1	90-94	95-100	94-100	91-94		341-343
Urea and creatinine	Urea > 0.12 mg/dL and creatinine >0.6 mg/dL	90-100	87-100	94-100	91-100		344
Diamine oxidase	>25 µIU/test	83	90-100	100	89		
Lactate (Lac test)	≥4.5 mmol/L	79-86	88-92	88-92	78-87		345
IGFBP-1 (PROM-TEST and AMNI Check)	>3 µg/L	74-97	74-98	73-97	56-95		333, 334, 346, 347
Prolactin	>30-50 µIU/mL	70-95	76-78	72-84	75-93		343, 348, 349
β-hCG	>40-65 µIU/mL	68-95	70-95	73-91	78-97		350, 351
Tampon test (vaginal tampon + AF inoculation of indigo blue)	Positive/negative	Unknown					204

Modified from Di Renzo, Roura LC, Facchinetti F, et al: Guidelines for the management of spontaneous preterm labor: identification of spontaneous preterm labor, diagnosis of preterm premature rupture of membranes, and preventive tools for preterm birth, *J Matern Fetal Neonatal Med* 24:659-667, 2011.
AF, Amniotic fluid; *AFP,* α-fetoprotein; *β-hCG,* beta subunit of human chorionic gonadotropin; *IGFBP-1,* insulin-like growth factor binding protein-1; *NPV,* negative predictive value; *PAMG-1,* placental α-microglobulin 1; *PPV,* positive predictive value; *ROM,* rupture of membranes.

sensitivity and specificity greater than 85% (Table 3-7). Although these tests are fairly accurate, they can yield false-positive and false-negative results, especially in women with small amounts of amniotic fluid in the vagina. Another test involves inserting a vaginal tampon and then injecting a dilute solution of indigo carmine blue into the amniotic fluid. The tampon is inspected 30 minutes later for blue dye. Methylene blue should not be used because of reported methemoglobinemia in the fetus. This test requires an amniocentesis, which may not be feasible after rupture of membranes, and the accuracy of diagnosis is unknown. An immunoassay for placenta α1-microglobulin (abundant in amniotic fluid but barely detectable in normal cervicovaginal secretions) has a high diagnostic accuracy but is not widely available.[277] Ultrasound examination has also been used as a diagnostic technique because oligohydramnios supports a diagnosis of PROM.

Because of the frequency and potential severity of maternal and fetal infections after PROM, various tests have been studied as predictors of infection, but none are ideal. All women with PPROM should receive a thorough physical examination, focusing on possible evidence of chorioamnionitis. Abnormal physical examination findings that could support a diagnosis of chorioamnionitis include maternal or fetal tachycardia; uterine tenderness; and detection of a purulent, foul-smelling discharge. Maternal fever is often a late sign of chorioamnionitis, especially in PPROM.

Several authors have evaluated the use of amniocentesis and microscopic examination of amniotic fluid for the diagnosis of IAI in the setting of PPROM. An elevated amniotic fluid MMP-8 is a sensitive test for IAI after PPROM (90% sensitivity, 80% specificity, 77% positive predictive value) and predicts shorter latency, chorioamnionitis, and neonatal morbidity.[120] However, MMP-8 assays are not widely available clinical tests at this time. The use of amniocentesis may also result in complications such as trauma, placental bleeding, initiation of labor, or introduction of infection, although these are rare.[278]

Most practitioners do not routinely perform amniocentesis in women with PPROM because the procedure has uncertain value. Most patients with PROM and positive amniotic fluid culture results are in labor within 48 hours; amniotic fluid culture results are often delayed and available only after delivery. Some patients have a positive culture result but no clinical evidence of infection, which could lead to the unnecessary delivery of a preterm infant. Overall, it has not been shown that clinical decisions based on data from amniocentesis lead to an improved perinatal outcome.[279]

MANAGEMENT OF PREMATURE RUPTURE OF THE MEMBRANES AND PRETERM PREMATURE RUPTURE OF THE MEMBRANES

Management guidelines for PROM and PPROM are driven by the gestational age of the fetus and potential for viability if delivered (Fig. 3-6, see Table 3-5). If the patient will not be delivered immediately, a digital examination should be deferred because examination may introduce bacteria into

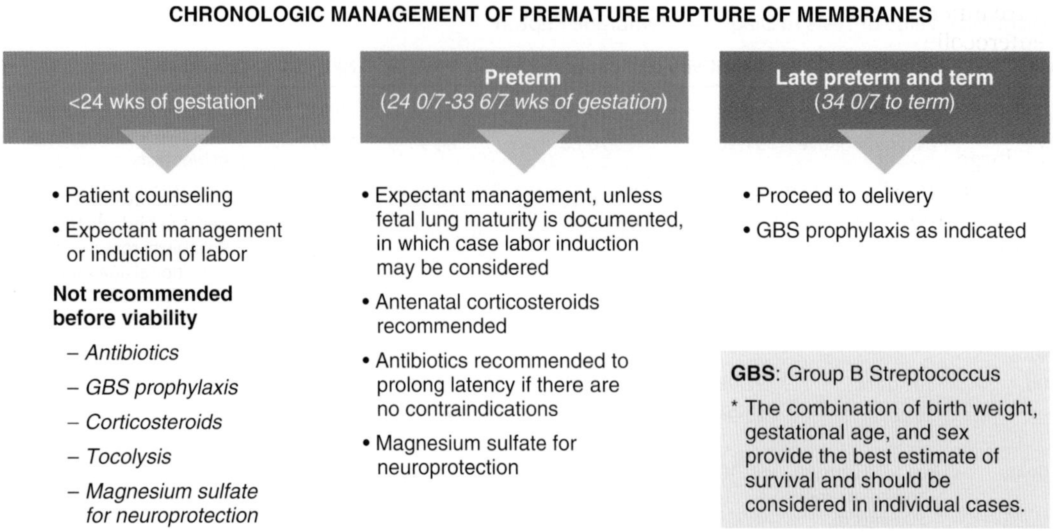

CHRONOLOGIC MANAGEMENT OF PREMATURE RUPTURE OF MEMBRANES

<24 wks of gestation*	Preterm (24 0/7-33 6/7 wks of gestation)	Late preterm and term (34 0/7 to term)
• Patient counseling • Expectant management or induction of labor **Not recommended before viability** – *Antibiotics* – *GBS prophylaxis* – *Corticosteroids* – *Tocolysis* – *Magnesium sulfate for neuroprotection*	• Expectant management, unless fetal lung maturity is documented, in which case labor induction may be considered • Antenatal corticosteroids recommended • Antibiotics recommended to prolong latency if there are no contraindications • Magnesium sulfate for neuroprotection	• Proceed to delivery • GBS prophylaxis as indicated **GBS**: Group B Streptococcus * The combination of birth weight, gestational age, and sex provide the best estimate of survival and should be considered in individual cases.

Figure 3-6 Management guidelines for preterm premature rupture of the membranes by the gestational age at membrane rupture. *MMP,* Matrix metalloproteinase. (Modified from American College of Obstetrics and Gynecology; Committee on Practice Bulletins—Obstetrics: ACOG practice bulletin no. 127: management of preterm labor, *Obstet Gynecol* 119:1308-1317, 2012.)

the uterus and shorten the latent phase. In a comparison of outcomes, women with digital examination after PROM had a significantly shorter latency period, more maternal infections, and more positive amniotic fluid cultures.[280]

Preterm Premature Rupture of the Membranes Before Fetal Viability

The recommended approaches to PPROM before 23 to 24 weeks of gestation include labor induction or expectant management because the fetus is not yet viable. With expectant management for PROM before fetal viability, the latency period is relatively long (mean, 12-19 days; median, 6-7 days), [281-285] although this may not achieve a gestational age consistent with neonatal survival. Neonatal survival depends on the gestational age at membrane rupture and duration of the latent period. In cases with PPROM at less than 23 weeks, the perinatal survival rate was 13% to 47%; with PPROM at 24 to 26 weeks, it was 50%. The incidence of stillbirth is greater (15%) with midtrimester PPROM than with later PPROM (1%). The incidence of lethal pulmonary hypoplasia is 50% to 60% when membrane rupture occurs before 19 weeks.[286] Although maternal clinically evident infections are common (chorioamnionitis: 35%-59% and endometritis: 13%-17%) few of these infections are serious; however, maternal death from sepsis has been reported.[283,285] If labor induction is chosen, after appropriate counseling, it can be facilitated by usual obstetric methods such as oxytocin or misoprostol administration.

Preterm Premature Rupture of the Membranes Between 24 and 34 Weeks

Some studies of preterm pregnancies have found an increased rate of chorioamnionitis with an increasing length of the latency period,[287,288] whereas others have not.[289] In patients with PPROM, digital vaginal examination should be avoided until labor develops, although transperineal ultrasonography can be used safely to assess cervical length without increasing the risk of infection.[290] Some studies noted that prolonged rupture of membranes decreased the incidence of respiratory distress syndrome (RDS),[208,291] but others noted no significant effect.[223,288,289,292] These discrepancies may be explained by differences in experimental design (e.g., grouping of various gestational ages) or in definitions of clinical complications.

Administration of antibiotics during latency has been found to increase the latency period from rupture of membranes to delivery, prolong pregnancy, and reduce maternal and neonatal morbidity in the setting of PPROM between 24 and 34 weeks of gestation.[293] In a meta-analysis, the benefits of latency antibiotics included a significant reduction in chorioamnionitis, IVH, and confirmed neonatal sepsis.[294] There was a significant decrease in the number of women delivering within 1 week of membrane rupture (OR, 0.56), but no significant differences were seen in necrotizing enterocolitis, RDS, or perinatal mortality. The evidence currently supports use of antibiotics in PPROM to prolong latency and to decrease maternal and neonatal infectious complications. Administration of latency antibiotics for PPROM before 24 weeks has not been well studied, and is not recommended.

Two large trials are of particular note. In the first, the National Institute of Child Health and Human Development (NICHD) Maternal-Fetal Medicine Units Network conducted a large, multicenter trial of antibiotics after PPROM but did not use tocolytics or corticosteroids.[295] Patients with PPROM between 24 and 32 weeks were included. Patients were randomly assigned to receive intravenous antibiotic therapy consisting of ampicillin (2 g intravenously every 6 hours) and erythromycin (250 mg intravenously every 6 hours) for the first 48 hours, followed by 5 days of oral therapy of amoxicillin (250 mg every 8 hours) and enteric-coated erythromycin base (333 mg orally every 8 hours) or placebo. Twice as many patients in the antibiotic treatment group remained pregnant after 7 days, and 21-day composite neonatal morbidity was significantly reduced in the antibiotic treatment group (53% vs. 44%; $P < .05$). Individual neonatal complications occurred significantly less often in the antibiotic treatment group, including RDS, stage 3/4 necrotizing enterocolitis, patent ductus arteriosus, and BPD. Infections occurred significantly less frequently with antibiotic therapy, including neonatal GBS-associated sepsis, neonatal sepsis, and pneumonia.

The second large trial was the multicenter ORACLE trial of oral antibiotics in women with PPROM at less than 37 weeks.[296] More than 4800 patients were randomly assigned to receive oral erythromycin, amoxicillin/clavulanic acid, erythromycin and amoxicillin/clavulanic acid, or placebo for up to 10 days. All of the antibiotic regimens prolonged pregnancy compared with placebo. However, amoxicillin/clavulanic acid increased the risk for neonatal necrotizing enterocolitis (1.9% vs. 0.5%; P = .001), and these regimens containing amoxicillin/clavulanic acid are not recommended.

The Cochrane Library has reviewed antibiotic use in PPROM in more than 6000 women in 19 trials.[297] This meta-analysis also found that antibiotic use in PPROM was associated with an increased latent period at 48 hours and 7 days and reduction in major neonatal comorbid conditions or indicators, such as neonatal infection, surfactant use, oxygen therapy, and abnormalities on head ultrasound examination before hospital discharge. There was an increased risk of necrotizing enterocolitis in two trials involving 2492 infants, in which amoxicillin/clavulanic acid was administered to the mother (RR, 4.6; 95% CI, 1.98 to 10.72).

Because of concerns for development of resistant organisms, another question involves duration of antibiotic therapy in PPROM. Two small trials have evaluated this question. Segel and associates[298] compared 3 days and 7 days of ampicillin (given as 2 g intravenously every 6 hours for 48 hours, followed by either 1 or 5 days of oral ampicillin 500 mg every 6 hours) in patients at 24 to 33 weeks with PPROM. In 48 patients, there was no difference in 7-day latency and no difference in rates of chorioamnionitis, postpartum endometritis, and neonatal morbidity and mortality. Lewis and colleagues[299] studied 3 versus 7 days of ampicillin/sulbactam (3 g intravenously every 6 hours) and similarly found no difference in outcomes between groups. Current recommendations call for 7 days of antibiotics, usually ampicillin/amoxicillin and erythromycin, following the dosing from the NICHD trial, although azithromycin (1 g intravenously, followed by 250 mg orally for 5 days) may be substituted for erythromycin.[295]

Antenatal Corticosteroids and Tocolytics

Administration of a single course of antenatal corticosteroids has been demonstrated to reduce respiratory distress and other adverse neonatal outcomes and should be offered after PPROM. A National Institutes of Health Consensus Development Panel in 1995 recommended that corticosteroids be given in the absence of IAI to women with PPROM at less than 30 to 32 weeks of gestation because the benefits of corticosteroids may outweigh the risk at this gestational age, particularly of IVH. As the number of patients receiving corticosteroids with PPROM greater than 32 weeks of gestation was small, the consensus panel chose to restrict its recommendation to less than 32 weeks of gestation. The American College of Obstetrics & Gynecology recommended a single course of corticosteroids before 34 0/7 weeks in women with PPROM (see Table 3-5).[204]

Tocolytics have been shown to prolong pregnancy by approximately 48 hours in women in preterm labor with intact membranes, but their efficacy with PPROM is unclear. Two small randomized controlled trials assessed use of tocolytics in the presence of PROM.[300,301] Both trials found no significant increase in time to delivery or in birth weight and no decrease in RDS or neonatal hospital stay. These studies did not use antibiotics or corticosteroids, however. In a patient with PPROM and contractions, a diagnosis of IAI must be excluded before consideration of tocolytics. Tocolytics may be considered in the early third trimester in order to administer antenatal corticosteroids. However, regardless of type (e.g., β-adrenergic agonists, calcium channel blockers, nonsteroidal antiinflammatory drugs, or oxytocin antagonists), tocolytics do not improve neonatal outcome beyond 48 hours of administration and increase the risk of chorioamnionitis and endometritis.[302,303,304]

Determination of Fetal Lung Maturity

Some clinicians determine the status of fetal pulmonary maturity and proceed with delivery if the lungs are mature. Amniotic fluid may be collected by amniocentesis or from the posterior vagina. Either the presence of phosphatidylglycerol or a lecithin/sphingomyelin ratio greater than 2 in amniotic fluid has been reported to be a good predictor of pulmonary maturity. In a case series with PPROM before 36 weeks, patients were delivered if phosphatidylglycerol was present in the vaginal pool or there was evidence of spontaneous labor or sepsis.[305] Of 214 patients, 47 had phosphatidylglycerol present initially and were delivered. Of the remaining 167, 36 (21%) were subsequently found to have phosphatidylglycerol; these 36 patients were induced or delivered by cesarean, and none had RDS. Evidence of maternal infection developed in 8 (5%) and spontaneous labor developed in 123 (74%) of the 167 patients. Although phosphatidylglycerol in amniotic fluid from the vagina reliably predicted fetal lung maturity, its absence did not mean that RDS would develop. Of 131 patients who did not show phosphatidylglycerol in the vaginal pool in any sample, 82 (62%) were delivered of infants who did not develop RDS. A separate study of 201 patients, using a rapid immunoassay (Amniostat-FLM test; Hana Biologics, Irvine, CA) to detect phosphatidylglycerol from vaginal pool samples from women with PPROM, confirmed the reliability of vaginal phosphotidylglycerol to detect fetal lung maturity.[306]

Antenatal Surveillance

Hospitalization is recommended for PPROM occurring at 24 to 34 weeks of gestation until delivery because infection can develop during the latency period, and few studies have evaluated outpatient management. We recommend daily fetal heart rate monitoring (non–stress testing) and weekly assessment of amniotic fluid volume by ultrasonography. Nonreassuring fetal status, clinical chorioamnionitis, and significant vaginal bleeding are indications for delivery regardless of gestational age.

Preterm Premature Rupture of the Membranes Between 34 to 37 Weeks

Management of PPROM between 34 and 37 weeks of gestation remains controversial, but most evidence would favor labor induction. Mercer and colleagues[307] compared expectant management and immediate induction in 93 pregnancies complicated by PROM between 32 and 36 weeks and 6 days, when mature fetal lung profiles were documented. They found significant prolongation of latent period and of maternal hospitalization, increased neonatal length of stay, and increased antimicrobial use in the expectant management group despite no increase in documented neonatal sepsis. These investigators concluded that in women with PPROM at 32 through 36 weeks with a mature fetal lung profile, immediate induction of labor reduces the duration of hospitalization in the mother and neonate. When pregnancies complicated by PPROM at 30 to 34 weeks of gestation were studied and randomized to expectant management versus immediate induction, there was no significant difference in fetal complications (i.e., necrotizing enterocolitis, neonatal sepsis, RDS, or perinatal death) between the groups.[308] There was an increased incidence of chorioamnionitis and a longer antepartum hospitalization with expectant management.

Two recent randomized controlled trials (PPROM Expectant Management versus Induction of Labor [PPROMEXIL] Study) evaluated delivery versus expectant management between 34 weeks and 37 weeks of gestation and included a total of 736 women.[309,310] Induction of labor significantly reduced the risk of chorioamnionitis (1.6% at 34 weeks vs. 5.3% at 37 weeks of gestation; RR, 0.31; 95% CI, 0.1 to 0.8). However, induction of labor did not produce a statistically significant reduction in the rate of neonatal sepsis, RDS, or cesarean delivery. Taken together with other studies, these data suggest benefit to induction of labor for PPROM at 34 to 37 weeks without evidence of increased maternal or neonatal risk.

Premature Rupture of the Membranes After 37 Weeks

Approximately 8% of pregnant women at term experience PROM, although contractions begin spontaneously within 24 hours of membrane rupture in 80% to 90% of patients.[311] When more than 24 hours elapses after membrane rupture at term, the incidence of neonatal infection is approximately 1%, but this risk increases to 3% to 5% when clinical chorioamnionitis is diagnosed.[312]

After confirmation of PROM, gestational age and fetal position should be confirmed and antenatal testing used to assess fetal status. GBS prophylaxis should be given based on prior culture results or intrapartum risk factors if cultures have not been previously performed. A recent meta-analysis of 12 randomized controlled trials (6814 women) found that induction of labor after PROM at term reduced the time to delivery and the rates of chorioamnionitis, endometritis, and admission to the neonatal intensive care unit without increasing the rates of cesarean delivery or operative vaginal delivery.[313]

In one of the largest prospective studies, four management schemes in women with PROM at term were evaluated: (1) immediate induction with oxytocin; (2) immediate induction with vaginal prostaglandin E2; (3) expectant management for up to 4 days, followed by oxytocin induction; and (4) expectant management, followed by prostaglandin E2 induction.[220] Although no differences in cesarean section rates or frequency of neonatal sepsis were found, an increase in chorioamnionitis was noted in the expectant management groups, and all deaths not caused by congenital anomalies occurred in the expectant management group. Patient satisfaction was higher among those women assigned to the immediate induction. A secondary analysis showed five variables as independent predictors of neonatal sepsis: clinical chorioamnionitis (OR, 5.89), presence of GBS (OR, 3.08), seven to eight vaginal examinations (OR, 2.37), duration of ruptured membranes 24 to 48 hours (OR, 1.97), greater than 48 hours from membrane rupture to active labor (OR, 2.25), and maternal antibiotics before delivery (OR, 1.63).

Confirming the association between length of PROM and neonatal sepsis, another study investigated how the interval of membrane rupture and delivery affects the risk of neonatal sepsis and whether duration of labor (defined as the interval between onset of regular contractions and delivery) influences the risk.[314] The investigators showed that the risk of neonatal sepsis increased independently and nearly linearly with duration of membrane rupture up to 36 hours, with an OR of 1.29 for each 6-hour increase in membrane rupture duration. The risk also increased with increasing birth weight, increasing gestational age, primiparity, and male infant gender. Duration of labor was not an independent risk factor for neonatal sepsis.

If the cervix is favorable, labor induction with oxytocin is recommended for women with PROM at term. If the condition of the cervix is unfavorable, induction with appropriate doses of prostaglandins may be used before use of oxytocin. Intrapartum antibiotic prophylaxis against GBS should be used according to the Centers for Disease Control and Prevention guidelines[315] (described more fully in Chapter 12). There is insufficient evidence to justify the routine use of prophylactic antibiotics with PROM at term in the absence of an indication for GBS prophylaxis.[204]

MATERNAL AND NEONATAL OUTCOMES

Maternal Outcomes

Maternal infectious complications are common after PPROM or PROM. IAI occurs in approximately 15% to 25% and is related to earlier gestational age at membrane rupture.[164,282,316] Postpartum endometritis occurs in approximately 15% to 20% of women. Although maternal infectious morbidity is common, maternal mortality is rare. Sepsis occurs in approximately 1% of mothers with PPROM but usually does not result in death. Placental abruption after PROM is reported in 4% to 6% of cases, severalfold higher than the rate of 0.5% to 1% in the general population.[317]

Neonatal Outcomes

The most significant risks to the fetus after PPROM are complications of prematurity. The most common complication among neonates with PPROM is RDS, which is found in 10% to 40% of neonates. Neonatal sepsis, IVH, and necrotizing enterocolitis are also associated with prematurity, but these are less common and occur infrequently after term PROM. Neonatal sepsis is documented in less than 10% of neonates, even in the setting of maternal IAI.[318] Other complications of PROM, especially in preterm pregnancies, include malpresentation and umbilical cord prolapse. Differences in study design have led to a wide variation of reported complications for the neonate after PPROM attributable to major differences in populations studied, gestational age, definitions, and management.

When latent periods in preterm pregnancies are prolonged, pulmonary hypoplasia is an additional neonatal complication. Although the rate of pulmonary hypoplasia seems to depend on the gestational age of PROM and the remaining amount of amniotic fluid surrounding the fetus, reported rates vary.[286,319,320] One study reported that if severe oligohydramnios is present, there is nearly a 100% probability of lethal pulmonary hypoplasia when PROM occurs before 23 weeks.[320] Others reported that the incidence of pulmonary hypoplasia is approximately 50% when rupture occurs before 19 weeks.[321,322] When PPROM occurred before 26 weeks, but there was a long interval until delivery (e.g., >5 weeks), one study found a 27% incidence of pulmonary hypoplasia.[319] Pulmonary hypoplasia is rare if PPROM occurs after 26 weeks of gestation and is poorly predicted by ultrasonography.[286,320] Ultrasound estimates of interval fetal lung growth include lung length, chest circumference, chest circumference–abdominal circumference ratio, or chest circumference–femur length ratio.

In addition to the risk of pulmonary hypoplasia, neonates may have skeletal deformities because of in utero compression. Nonskeletal restriction deformities of prolonged intrauterine crowding similar to features of Potter syndrome include abnormal facies with low-set ears and epicanthal folds. Limbs may be malpositioned and flattened.[323]

Conclusion

Approximately four million babies die in the first week of life each year globally. PTB remains the largest contributor to neonatal deaths after exclusion of congenital anomalies. Obstetric infections are an important cause of not only PTB but also neonatal and maternal sequelae (e.g., BPD, cerebral palsy, endometritis). Although our understanding of the pathogenesis of preterm labor and PPROM has advanced over the last 3 decades, we still lack an effective preventive therapy for IAI. Although magnesium sulfate has emerged as a therapy to ameliorate fetal neurologic injury, we lack a similar strategy to prevent fetal lung injury. Several therapies that downregulate inflammation have shown promise in animal models to delay preterm birth, but future studies need to comprehensively assess fetal outcomes with these treatments to determine if prolonging pregnancy in the setting of IAI treatment is safe.

References

1. Romero R, Espinoza J, Kusanovic JP, et al: The preterm parturition syndrome, *BJOG* 113(Suppl 3):17-42, 2006.
2. Watts DH, Krohn MA, Hillier SL, Eschenbach DA: The association of occult amniotic fluid infection with gestational age and neonatal outcome among women in preterm labor, *Obstet Gynecol* 79: 351-357, 1992.
3. Martin JA, Hamilton BE, Ventura SJ, Osterman MJK, Mathews TJ: Births: final data for 2011, *Natl Vital Stat Rep* 62:1-90, 2013.
4. Lawn JE, Kinney MV, Black RE, et al: Newborn survival: a multi-country analysis of a decade of change, *Health Policy Plan* 27(Suppl 3): iii6-iii28, 2012.
5. Gibbs R, Romero R, Hillier S, Eschenbach D, Sweet R: A review of premature birth and subclinical infection, *Am J Obstet Gynecol* 166:1515-1528, 1992.
6. Minkoff H: Prematurity: infection as an etiologic factor, *Obstet Gynecol* 62:137-144, 1983.
7. Jarjoura K, Devine PC, Perez-Delboy A, et al: Markers of periodontal infection and preterm birth, *Am J Obstet Gynecol* 192:513-519, 2005.
8. Boggess KA, Madianos PN, Preisser JS, Moise KJ Jr, Offenbacher S: Chronic maternal and fetal *Porphyromonas gingivalis* exposure during pregnancy in rabbits, *Am J Obstet Gynecol* 192:554-557, 2005.
9. Lopez R: Periodontal disease and adverse pregnancy outcomes, *Evid Based Dent* 9:48, 2008.
10. Kjersti Aagaard, Jun Ma, Kathleen M. Antony, et al: The placenta harbors a unique microbiome, *Sci Transl Med* 6:237, 2014.
11. Gibson CS, MacLennan AH, Goldwater PN, Dekker GA: Antenatal causes of cerebral palsy: associations between inherited thrombophilias, viral and bacterial infection, and inherited susceptibility to infection, *Obstet Gynecol Surv* 58:209-220, 2003.
12. Murphy DJ, Sellers S, MacKenzie IZ, Yudkin PL, Johnson AM: Case-control study of antenatal and intrapartum risk factors for cerebral palsy in very preterm singleton babies, *Lancet* 346:1449-1454, 1995.
13. Yoon BH, Romero R, Kim CJ, et al: High expression of tumor necrosis factor-alpha and interleukin-6 in periventricular leukomalacia, *Am J Obstet Gynecol* 177:406-411, 1997.
14. Yoon BH, Kim CJ, Romero R, et al: Experimentally induced intrauterine infection causes fetal brain white matter lesions in rabbits, *Am J Obstet Gynecol* 177:797-802, 1997.
15. Hartling L, Liang Y, Lacaze-Masmonteil T: Chorioamnionitis as a risk factor for bronchopulmonary dysplasia: a systematic review and meta-analysis, *Arch Dis Child Fetal Neonatal Ed* 97:F8-F17, 2012.
16. Jobe AH: Blood cytokines and BPD, *J Pediatr* 154:A2, 2009.
17. Kramer BW, Kallapur S, Newnham J, Jobe AH: Prenatal inflammation and lung development, *Semin Fetal Neonatal Med* 14:2-7, 2009.
18. Been JV, Lievense S, Zimmermann LJ, Kramer BW, Wolfs TG: Chorioamnionitis as a risk factor for necrotizing enterocolitis: a systematic review and meta-analysis, *J Pediatr* 162:236-242, 2013. e232.
19. Goldenberg RL, Culhane JF, Iams JD, Romero R: Epidemiology and causes of preterm birth, *Lancet* 371:75-84, 2008.
20. Khan KS, Wojdyla D, Say L, Gulmezoglu AM, Van Look PF: WHO analysis of causes of maternal death: a systematic review, *Lancet* 367:1066-1074, 2006.
21. Hogan MC, Foreman KJ, Naghavi M, et al: Maternal mortality for 181 countries, 1980-2008: a systematic analysis of progress towards Millennium Development Goal 5, *Lancet* 375:1609-1623, 2010.
22. Sebitloane HM, Mhlanga RE: Changing patterns of maternal mortality (HIV/AIDS related) in poor countries, *Best Pract Res Clin Obstet Gynaecol* 22:489-499, 2008.
23. Zvandasara P, Hargrove JW, Ntozini R, et al: Mortality and morbidity among postpartum HIV-positive and HIV-negative women in Zimbabwe: risk factors, causes, and impact of single-dose postpartum vitamin A supplementation, *J Acquir Immune Defic Syndr* 43:107-116, 2006.
24. Menendez C, Romagosa C, Ismail MR, et al: An autopsy study of maternal mortality in Mozambique: the contribution of infectious diseases, *PLoS Med* 5:e44, 2008.
25. Schantz-Dunn J, Nour NM: Malaria and pregnancy: a global health perspective, *Rev Obstet Gynecol* 2:186-192, 2009.
26. Gibbs RS, Duff P: Progress in pathogenesis and management of clinical intraamniotic infection, *Am J Obstet Gynecol* 164(5 Pt 1):1317-1326, 1991.
27. Goldenberg RL, Hauth JC, Andrews WW: Intrauterine infection and preterm delivery, *N Engl J Med* 342:1500-1507, 2000.
28. Romero R, Sirtori M, Oyarzun E, et al: Infection and labor. V. Prevalence, microbiology, and clinical significance of intraamniotic infection in women with preterm labor and intact membranes, *Am J Obstet Gynecol* 161:817-824, 1989.
29. Hitti J, Riley DE, Krohn MA, et al: Broad-spectrum bacterial rDNA polymerase chain reaction assay for detecting amniotic fluid infection among women in premature labor, *Clin Infect Dis* 24:1228-1232, 1997.
30. Markenson GR, Martin RK, Tillotson-Criss M, et al: The use of the polymerase chain reaction to detect bacteria in amniotic fluid in pregnancies complicated by preterm labor, *Am J Obstet Gynecol* 177:1471-1477, 1997.
31. Oyarzun E, Yamamoto M, Kato S, et al: Specific detection of 16 micro-organisms in amniotic fluid by polymerase chain reaction and its correlation with preterm delivery occurrence, *Am J Obstet Gynecol* 179:1115-1119, 1998.

32. DiGiulio DB, Romero R, Amogan HP, et al: Microbial prevalence, diversity and abundance in amniotic fluid during preterm labor: a molecular and culture-based investigation, *PLoS One* 3:e3056, 2008.
33. Han YW, Shen T, Chung P, Buhimschi IA, Buhimschi CS: Uncultivated bacteria as etiologic agents of intra-amniotic inflammation leading to preterm birth, *J Clin Microbiol* 47:38-47, 2009.
34. Marconi C, de Andrade Ramos BR, Peracoli JC, Donders GG, da Silva MG: Amniotic fluid interleukin-1 beta and interleukin-6, but not interleukin-8 correlate with microbial invasion of the amniotic cavity in preterm labor, *Am J Reprod Immunol* 65:549-556, 2011.
35. Hillier SL, Krohn MA, Kiviat NB, Watts DH, Eschenbach DA: Microbiologic causes and neonatal outcomes associated with chorioamnion infection, *Am J Obstet Gynecol* 165(4 Pt 1):955-961, 1991.
36. Hitti J, Tarczy-Hornoch P, Murphy J, et al: Amniotic fluid infection, cytokines, and adverse outcome among infants at 34 weeks' gestation or less, *Obstet Gynecol* 98:1080-1088, 2001.
37. Yoon BH, Romero R, Lim JH, et al: The clinical significance of detecting *Ureaplasma urealyticum* by the polymerase chain reaction in the amniotic fluid of patients with preterm labor, *Am J Obstet Gynecol* 189:919-924, 2003.
38. Romero R, Mazor M: Infection and preterm labor, *Clin Obstet Gynecol* 31:553-584, 1988.
39. Kim MJ, Romero R, Gervasi MT, et al: Widespread microbial invasion of the chorioamniotic membranes is a consequence and not a cause of intra-amniotic infection, *Lab Invest* 89:924-936, 2009.
40. Adams Waldorf KM, Gravett MG, McAdams RM, et al: Choriodecidual group B streptococcal inoculation induces fetal lung injury without intra-amniotic infection and preterm labor in Macaca nemestrina, *PloS One* 6:e28972, 2011.
41. Grigsby PL, Novy MJ, Waldorf KM, Sadowsky DW, Gravett MG: Choriodecidual inflammation: a harbinger of the preterm labor syndrome, *Reprod Sci* 17:85-94, 2010.
42. Egli GE, Newton M: The transport of carbon particles in the human female reproductive tract, *Fertil Steril* 12:151-155, 1961.
43. Cotch MF, Pastorek JG 2nd, Nugent RP, et al: *Trichomonas vaginalis* associated with low birth weight and preterm delivery. The Vaginal Infections and Prematurity Study Group, *Sex Transm Dis* 24:353-360, 1997.
44. Regan JA, Klebanoff MA, Nugent RP, et al: Colonization with group B streptococci in pregnancy and adverse outcome. VIP Study Group, *Am J Obstet Gynecol* 174:1354-1360, 1996.
45. Carey JC, Blackwelder WC, Nugent RP, et al: Antepartum cultures for *Ureaplasma urealyticum* are not useful in predicting pregnancy outcome. The Vaginal Infections and Prematurity Study Group, *Am J Obstet Gynecol* 164:728-733, 1991.
46. Cotch MF, Hillier SL, Gibbs RS, Eschenbach DA: Epidemiology and outcomes associated with moderate to heavy *Candida* colonization during pregnancy. Vaginal Infections and Prematurity Study Group, *Am J Obstet Gynecol* 178:374-380, 1998.
47. Sadowsky DW, Adams KM, Gravett MG, Witkin SS, Novy MJ: Preterm labor is induced by intraamniotic infusions of interleukin-1beta and tumor necrosis factor-alpha but not by interleukin-6 or interleukin-8 in a nonhuman primate model, *Am J Obstet Gynecol* 195:1578-1589, 2006.
48. Keelan JA, Sato T, Mitchell MD: Interleukin (IL)-6 and IL-8 production by human amnion: regulation by cytokines, growth factors, glucocorticoids, phorbol esters, and bacterial lipopolysaccharide, *Biol Reprod* 57:1438-1444, 1997.
49. Fortunato SJ, Menon RP, Swan KF, Menon R: Inflammatory cytokine (interleukins 1, 6 and 8 and tumor necrosis factor-alpha) release from cultured human fetal membranes in response to endotoxic lipopolysaccharide mirrors amniotic fluid concentrations, *Am J Obstet Gynecol* 174:1855-1861, 1996; discussion 1861-1852.
50. Denison FC, Kelly RW, Calder AA, Riley SC: Cytokine secretion by human fetal membranes, decidua and placenta at term, *Hum Reprod* 13:3560-3565, 1998.
51. Griesinger G, Saleh L, Bauer S, Husslein P, Knofler M: Production of pro- and anti-inflammatory cytokines of human placental trophoblasts in response to pathogenic bacteria, *J Soc Gynecol Invest* 8:334-340, 2001.
52. Robertson SA, Christiaens I, Dorian CL, et al: Interleukin-6 is an essential determinant of on-time parturition in the mouse, *Endocrinology* 151:3996-4006, 2010.
53. Furuta I, Yamada H, Sagawa T, Fujimoto S: Effects of inflammatory cytokines on prostaglandin E(2) production from human amnion cells cultured in serum-free condition, *Gynecol Obstet Invest* 49: 93-97, 2000.
54. Boucher M, Yonekura ML: Perinatal listeriosis (early-onset): correlation of antenatal manifestations and neonatal outcome, *Obstet Gynecol* 68:593-597, 1986.
55. Petrilli ES, D'Ablaing G, Ledger WJ: *Listeria monocytogenes* chorioamnionitis: diagnosis by transabdominal amniocentesis, *Obstet Gynecol* 55(3 Suppl):5S-8S, 1980.
56. Fleming AD, Ehrlich DW, Miller NA, Monif GR: Successful treatment of maternal septicemia due to *Listeria monocytogenes* at 26 weeks' gestation, *Obstet Gynecol* 66(3 Suppl):52S-53S, 1985.
57. Bakardjiev AI, Theriot JA, Portnoy DA: *Listeria monocytogenes* traffics from maternal organs to the placenta and back, *PLoS Pathog* 2:e66, 2006.
58. Zeldovich VB, Robbins JR, Kapidzic M, Lauer P, Bakardjiev AI: Invasive extravillous trophoblasts restrict intracellular growth and spread of Listeria monocytogenes, *PLoS Pathog* 7:e1002005, 2011.
59. van Dillen J, Zwart J, Schutte J, van Roosmalen J. Maternal sepsis: epidemiology, etiology and outcome, *Curr Opin Infect Dis* 23:249, 2010.
60. Rowe JH, Ertelt JM, Xin L, Way SS: *Listeria monocytogenes* cytoplasmic entry induces fetal wastage by disrupting maternal Foxp3+ regulatory T cell-sustained fetal tolerance, *PLoS Pathog* 8:e1002873, 2012.
61. Mitra AG, Katz VL, Bowes WA Jr, Carmichael S: Emergency cerclages: a review of 40 consecutive procedures, *Am J Perinatol* 9: 142-145, 1992.
62. Harger JH: Comparison of success and morbidity in cervical cerclage procedures, *Obstet Gynecol* 56:543-548, 1980.
63. Eddleman KA, Malone FD, Sullivan L, et al: Pregnancy loss rates after midtrimester amniocentesis, *Obstet Gynecol* 108:1067-1072, 2006.
64. Wilkins I, Mezrow G, Lynch L, Bottone EJ, Berkowitz RL: Amnionitis and life-threatening respiratory distress after percutaneous umbilical blood sampling, *Am J Obstet Gynecol* 160:427-428, 1989.
65. Soper DE, Mayhall CG, Dalton HP: Risk factors for intraamniotic infection: a prospective epidemiologic study, *Am J Obstet Gynecol* 161:562-566, 1989; discussion 566-568.
66. Soper DE, Mayhall CG, Froggatt JW: Characterization and control of intraamniotic infection in an urban teaching hospital, *Am J Obstet Gynecol* 175:304-309, 1996; discussion 309-310.
67. Tran SH, Caughey AB, Musci TJ: Meconium-stained amniotic fluid is associated with puerperal infections, *Am J Obstet Gynecol* 189: 746-750, 2003.
68. Krohn MA, Germain M, Muhlemann K, Hickok D: Prior pregnancy outcome and the risk of intraamniotic infection in the following pregnancy, *Am J Obstet Gynecol* 178:381-385, 1998.
69. Driscoll SG: The placenta and membranes. In Charles D, Finlands M, editors: *Obstetrical and perinatal infections*, Philadelphia, 1973, Lea & Febiger.
70. Russell P: Inflammatory lesions of the human placenta: I. Clinical significance of acute chorioamnionitis, *Am J Diagn Gynecol Obstet* 1:127, 1979.
71. Hillier SL, Martius J, Krohn M, et al: A case-control study of chorioamnionic infection and histologic chorioamnionitis in prematurity, *N Engl J Med* 319:972-978, 1988.
72. Gravett MG, Adams KM, Sadowsky DW, et al: Immunomodulators plus antibiotics delay preterm delivery after experimental intraamniotic infection in a nonhuman primate model, *Am J Obstet Gynecol* 197:518 e511-e518, 2007.
73. Romero R, Brody DT, Oyarzun E, et al: Infection and labor. III. Interleukin-1: a signal for the onset of parturition, *Am J Obstet Gynecol* 160(5 Pt 1):1117-1123, 1989.
74. Romero R, Manogue KR, Mitchell MD, et al: Infection and labor. IV. Cachectin-tumor necrosis factor in the amniotic fluid of women with intraamniotic infection and preterm labor, *Am J Obstet Gynecol* 161:336-341, 1989.
75. Yoshimura K, Hirsch E: Effect of stimulation and antagonism of interleukin-1 signaling on preterm delivery in mice, *J Soc Gynecol Investig* 12:533-538, 2005.
76. Holmgren C, Esplin MS, Hamblin S, et al: Evaluation of the use of anti-TNF-alpha in an LPS-induced murine model, *J Reprod Immunol* 78:134-139, 2008.
77. Romero R, Avila C, Santhanam U, Sehgal PB: Amniotic fluid interleukin 6 in preterm labor. Association with infection, *J Clin Invest* 85:1392-1400, 1990.

78. Romero R, Ceska M, Avila C, et al: Neutrophil attractant/activating peptide-1/interleukin-8 in term and preterm parturition, *Am J Obstet Gynecol* 165(4 Pt 1):813-820, 1991.
79. Longini M, Perrone S, Vezzosi P, et al: Association between oxidative stress in pregnancy and preterm premature rupture of membranes, *Clin Biochem* 40:793-797, 2007.
80. Menon R, Boldogh I, Hawkins HK, et al: Evidence of oxidative stress and premature senescence in preterm premature rupture of the human fetal membranes recapitulated in vitro, *Am J Pathol* 184:1740, 2014.
81. Buhimschi IA, Buhimschi CS, Weiner CP: Protective effect of N-acetylcysteine against fetal death and preterm labor induced by maternal inflammation, *Am J Obstet Gynecol* 188:203-208, 2003.
82. Beloosesky R, Gayle DA, Amidi F, et al: N-acetyl-cysteine suppresses amniotic fluid and placenta inflammatory cytokine responses to lipopolysaccharide in rats, *Am J Obstet Gynecol* 194:268-273, 2006.
83. Ilievski V, Lu SJ, Hirsch E: Activation of toll-like receptors 2 or 3 and preterm delivery in the mouse, *Reprod Sci* 14:315-320, 2007.
84. Elovitz MA, Wang Z, Chien EK, Rychlik DF, Phillippe M: A new model for inflammation-induced preterm birth: the role of platelet-activating factor and Toll-like receptor-4, *Am J Pathol* 163:2103-2111, 2003.
85. Sun Y, Qin X, Shan B, et al: Differential effects of the CpG-Toll-like receptor 9 axis on pregnancy outcome in nonobese diabetic mice and wild-type controls, *Fertil Steril* 99:1759-1767, 2013.
86. Poltorak A, He X, Smirnova I, et al: Defective LPS signaling in C3H/HeJ and C57BL/10ScCr mice: mutations in Tlr4 gene, *Science* 282:2085-2088, 1998.
87. Adams Waldorf KM, Persing D, Novy MJ, Sadowsky DW, Gravett MG: Pretreatment with toll-like receptor 4 antagonist inhibits lipopolysaccharide-induced preterm uterine contractility, cytokines, and prostaglandins in rhesus monkeys, *Reprod Sci* 15:121-127, 2008.
88. Yoon BH, Oh SY, Romero R, et al: An elevated amniotic fluid matrix metalloproteinase-8 level at the time of mid-trimester genetic amniocentesis is a risk factor for spontaneous preterm delivery, *Am J Obstet Gynecol* 185:1162-1167, 2001.
89. Vu TD, Yun F, Placido J, Reznik SE: Placental matrix metalloproteinase-1 expression is increased in labor, *Reprod Sci* 15:420-424, 2008.
90. Koscica KL, Ananth CV, Placido J, Reznik SE: The effect of a matrix metalloproteinase inhibitor on inflammation-mediated preterm delivery, *Am J Obstet Gynecol* 196:551 e1-e3, 2007.
91. Olgun NS, Patel HJ, Stephani R, Lengyel I, Reznik SE: Blockade of endothelin-1 with a novel series of 1,3,6-trisubstituted-2-carboxy-quinol-4-ones controls infection-associated preterm birth, *Am J Pathol* 177:1929-1935, 2010.
92. Wang W, Yen H, Chen CH, et al: Prevention of inflammation-associated preterm birth by knockdown of the endothelin-1-matrix metalloproteinase-1 pathway, *Mol Med* 16:505-512, 2010.
93. Gibbs RS, Blanco JD, St Clair PJ, Castaneda YS: Quantitative bacteriology of amniotic fluid from women with clinical intraamniotic infection at term, *J Infect Dis* 145:1, 1982.
94. Mann JR, McDermott S, Gill T: Sexually transmitted infection is associated with increased risk of preterm birth in South Carolina women insured by Medicaid, *J Matern Fetal Neonatal* 23:563-568, 2010.
95. Novy MJ, Duffy L, Axthelm MK, et al: *Ureaplasma parvum* or *Mycoplasma hominis* as sole pathogens cause chorioamnionitis, preterm delivery, and fetal pneumonia in rhesus macaques, *Reprod Sci* 16: 56-70, 2009.
96. Goldenberg RL, Andrews WW, Goepfert AR, et al: The Alabama Preterm Birth Study: umbilical cord blood *Ureaplasma urealyticum* and *Mycoplasma hominis* cultures in very preterm newborn infants, *Am J Obstet Gynecol* 198:43 e41-e45, 2008.
97. DiGuilio DB: Diversity of microbes in amniotic fluid, *Semin Fetal Neonatal Med* 17:2-11, 2012.
98. Mitchell K, Brou L, Bhat G, et al: Group B *Streptococcus* colonization and higher maternal IL-1beta concentrations are associated with early term births, *J Matern Fetal Neonatal* 26:56-61, 2013.
99. Gibbs RS, Romero R, Hillier SL, Eschenbach DA, Sweet RL: A review of premature birth and subclinical infection, *Am J Obstet Gynecol* 166:1515-1528, 1992.
100. Moller M, Thomsen AC, Borch K, Dinesen K, Zdravkovic M: Rupture of fetal membranes and premature delivery associated with group B streptococci in urine of pregnant women, *Lancet* 2:69-70, 1984.
101. White CP, Wilkins EG, Roberts C, Davidson DC: Premature delivery and group B streptococcal bacteriuria, *Lancet* 2:586, 1984.
102. Thomsen AC, Morup L, Hansen KB: Antibiotic elimination of group-B streptococci in urine in prevention of preterm labour, *Lancet* 1:591-593, 1987.
103. Klebanoff MA, Regan JA, Rao AV, et al: Outcome of the Vaginal Infections and Prematurity Study: results of a clinical trial of erythromycin among pregnant women colonized with group B streptococci, *Am J Obstet Gynecol* 172:1540-1545, 1995.
104. Goldenberg RL, Klebanoff MA, Nugent R, et al: Bacterial colonization of the vagina during pregnancy in four ethnic groups. Vaginal Infections and Prematurity Study Group, *Am J Obstet Gynecol* 174:1618-1621, 1996.
105. Bukusi EA, Cohen CR, Meier AS, et al: Bacterial vaginosis: risk factors among Kenyan women and their male partners, *Sex Transm Dis* 33:361-367, 2006.
106. Klebanoff MA, Hillier SL, Nugent RP, et al: Is bacterial vaginosis a stronger risk factor for preterm birth when it is diagnosed earlier in gestation? *Am J Obstet Gynecol* 192:470-477, 2005.
107. Leitich H, Bodner-Adler B, Brunbauer M, et al: Bacterial vaginosis as a risk factor for preterm delivery: a meta-analysis, *Am J Obstet Gynecol* 189:139-147, 2003.
108. Hillier SL, Nugent RP, Eschenbach DA, et al: Association between bacterial vaginosis and preterm delivery of a low-birth-weight infant. The Vaginal Infections and Prematurity Study Group, *N Engl J Med* 333:1737-1742, 1995.
109. Meis PJ, Goldenberg RL, Mercer B, et al: The preterm prediction study: significance of vaginal infections. National Institute of Child Health and Human Development Maternal-Fetal Medicine Units Network, *Am J Obstet Gynecol* 173:1231-1235, 1995.
110. Hillier SL, Krohn MA, Cassen E, et al: The role of bacterial vaginosis and vaginal bacteria in amniotic fluid infection in women in preterm labor with intact fetal membranes, *Clin Infect Dis* 20(Suppl 2):S276-S278, 1995.
111. Fredricks DN, Fiedler TL, Marrazzo JM: Molecular identification of bacteria associated with bacterial vaginosis, *N Engl J Med* 353: 1899-1911, 2005.
112. Macones GA, Parry S, Elkousy M, et al: A polymorphism in the promoter region of TNF and bacterial vaginosis: preliminary evidence of gene-environment interaction in the etiology of spontaneous preterm birth, *Am J Obstet Gynecol* 190:1504-1508, 2004; discussion 1503A.
113. Gervasi MT, Romero R, Bracalente G, et al: Viral invasion of the amniotic cavity (VIAC) in the midtrimester of pregnancy, *J Matern Fetal Neonatal Med* 25:2002-2013, 2012.
114. Edwards RK: Chorioamnionitis and labor, *Obstet Gynecol Clin North Am* 32:287-296, 2005.
115. Kiltz RJ, Burke MS, Porreco RP: Amniotic fluid glucose concentration as a marker for intra-amniotic infection, *Obstet Gynecol* 78: 619-622, 1991.
116. Hussey MJ, Levy ES, Pombar X, Meyer P, Strassner HT: Evaluating rapid diagnostic tests of intra-amniotic infection: Gram stain, amniotic fluid glucose level, and amniotic fluid to serum glucose level ratio, *Am J Obstet Gynecol* 179(3 Pt 1):650-656, 1998.
117. Greig PC, Ernest JM, Teot L: Low amniotic fluid glucose levels are a specific but not a sensitive marker for subclinical intrauterine infections in patients in preterm labor with intact membranes, *Am J Obstet Gynecol* 171:365-370, 1994; discussion 370-371.
118. Romero R, Yoon BH, Mazor M, et al: The diagnostic and prognostic value of amniotic fluid white blood cell count, glucose, interleukin-6, and gram stain in patients with preterm labor and intact membranes, *Am J Obstet Gynecol* 169:805-816, 1993.
119. Romero R, Yoon BH, Kenney JS, et al: Amniotic fluid interleukin-6 determinations are of diagnostic and prognostic value in preterm labor, *Am J Reprod Immunol* 30:167-183, 1993.
120. Kim KW, Romero R, Park HS, et al: A rapid matrix metalloproteinase-8 bedside test for the detection of intraamniotic inflammation in women with preterm premature rupture of membranes, *Am J Obstet Gynecol* 197:292, e1-e5, 2007.
121. Gravett MG, Novy MJ, Rosenfeld RG, et al: Diagnosis of intra-amniotic infection by proteomic profiling and identification of novel biomarkers, *JAMA* 292:462-469, 2004.
122. Buhimschi IA, Christner R, Buhimschi CS: Proteomic biomarker analysis of amniotic fluid for identification of intra-amniotic inflammation, *BJOG* 112:173-181, 2005.
123. Hitti J, Lapidus JA, Lu X, et al: Noninvasive diagnosis of intraamniotic infection: proteomic biomarkers in vaginal fluid, *Am J Obstet Gynecol* 203:32.e1-e8, 2010.

124. Romero R, Kusanovic JP, Espinoza J, et al: What is amniotic fluid 'sludge'? *Ultrasound Obstet Gynecol* 30:793-798, 2007.
125. Kusanovic JP, Espinoza J, Romero R, et al: Clinical significance of the presence of amniotic fluid 'sludge' in asymptomatic patients at high risk for spontaneous preterm delivery, *Ultrasound Obstet Gynecol* 30:706-714, 2007.
126. Goncalves LF, Chaiworapongsa T, Romero R: Intrauterine infection and prematurity, *Ment Retard Dev Disabil Res Rev* 8:3-13, 2002.
127. Romero R, Quintero R, Oyarzun E, et al: Intraamniotic infection and the onset of labor in preterm premature rupture of the membranes, *Am J Obstet Gynecol* 159:661-666, 1988.
128. Gravett MG, Thomas A, Schneider KA, et al: Proteomic analysis of cervical-vaginal fluid: identification of novel biomarkers for detection of intra-amniotic infection, *J Proteome Res* 6:89-96, 2007.
129. Esplin MS, Merrell K, Goldenberg R, et al: Proteomic identification of serum peptides predicting subsequent spontaneous preterm birth, *Am J Obstet Gynecol* 204:391. e1-e8, 2011.
130. Meis PJ, Klebanoff M, Thom E, et al: Prevention of recurrent preterm delivery by 17 alpha-hydroxyprogesterone caproate, *N Engl J Med* 348:2379-2385, 2003.
131. da Fonseca EB, Bittar RE, Carvalho MH, Zugaib M: Prophylactic administration of progesterone by vaginal suppository to reduce the incidence of spontaneous preterm birth in women at increased risk: a randomized placebo-controlled double-blind study, *Am J Obstet Gynecol* 188:419-424, 2003.
132. Kass EH, McCormack WM, Lin JS, Rosner B, Munoz A: Genital mycoplasmas as a cause of excess premature delivery, *Trans Assoc Am Physicians* 94:261-266, 1981.
133. McCormack WM, Rosner B, Lee YH, et al: Effect on birth weight of erythromycin treatment of pregnant women, *Obstet Gynecol* 69:202-207, 1987.
134. Eschenbach DA, Nugent RP, Rao AV, et al: A randomized placebo-controlled trial of erythromycin for the treatment of *Ureaplasma urealyticum* to prevent premature delivery. The Vaginal Infections and Prematurity Study Group, *Am J Obstet Gynecol* 164:734-742, 1991.
135. Cohen I, Veille JC, Calkins BM: Improved pregnancy outcome following successful treatment of chlamydial infection, *JAMA* 263: 3160-3163, 1990.
136. Ryan GM Jr, Abdella TN, McNeeley SG, Baselski VS, Drummond DE: *Chlamydia trachomatis* infection in pregnancy and effect of treatment on outcome, *Am J Obstet Gynecol* 162:34-39, 1990.
137. Martin DH, Eschenbach DA, Cotch MF, et al: Double-blind placebo-controlled treatment trial of *Chlamydia trachomatis* endocervical infections in pregnant women, *Infect Dis Obstet Gynecol* 5:10-17, 1997.
138. Andrews WW, Klebanoff MA, Thom EA, et al: Midpregnancy genitourinary tract infection with *Chlamydia trachomatis*: association with subsequent preterm delivery in women with bacterial vaginosis and *Trichomonas vaginalis*, *Am J Obstet Gynecol* 194:493-500, 2006.
139. Burtin P, Taddio A, Ariburnu O, Einarson TR, Koren G: Safety of metronidazole in pregnancy: a meta-analysis, *Am J Obstet Gynecol* 172(2 Pt 1):525-529, 1995.
140. Klebanoff MA, Carey JC, Hauth JC, et al: Failure of metronidazole to prevent preterm delivery among pregnant women with asymptomatic *Trichomonas vaginalis* infection, *N Engl J Med* 345:487-493, 2001.
141. Martius J, Krohn MA, Hillier SL, et al: Relationships of vaginal *Lactobacillus* species, cervical *Chlamydia trachomatis*, and bacterial vaginosis to preterm birth, *Obstet Gynecol* 71:89-95, 1988.
142. Hitti J, Hillier SL, Agnew KJ, et al: Vaginal indicators of amniotic fluid infection in preterm labor, *Obstet Gynecol* 97:211-219, 2001.
143. Carey JC, Klebanoff MA, Hauth JC, et al: Metronidazole to prevent preterm delivery in pregnant women with asymptomatic bacterial vaginosis. National Institute of Child Health and Human Development Network of Maternal-Fetal Medicine Units, *N Engl J Med* 342:534-540, 2000.
144. Joesoef MR, Hillier SL, Wiknjosastro G, et al: Intravaginal clindamycin treatment for bacterial vaginosis: effects on preterm delivery and low birth weight, *Am J Obstet Gynecol* 173:1527-1531, 1995.
145. McGregor JA, French JI, Jones W, et al: Bacterial vaginosis is associated with prematurity and vaginal fluid mucinase and sialidase: results of a controlled trial of topical clindamycin cream, *Am J Obstet Gynecol* 170:1048-1059, 1994; discussion 1059-1060.
146. Mitchell C, Balkus J, Agnew K, Lawler R, Hitti J: Changes in the vaginal microenvironment with metronidazole treatment for bacterial vaginosis in early pregnancy, *J Womens Health (Larchmt)* 18:1817-1824, 2009.
147. Mitchell CM, Hitti JE, Agnew KJ, Fredricks DN: Comparison of oral and vaginal metronidazole for treatment of bacterial vaginosis in pregnancy: impact on fastidious bacteria, *BMC Infect Dis* 9:89, 2009.
148. Hummelen R, Fernandes AD, Macklaim JM, et al: Deep sequencing of the vaginal microbiota of women with HIV, *PLoS One* 5:e12078, 2010.
149. Koren O, Goodrich JK, Cullender TC, et al: Host remodeling of the gut microbiome and metabolic changes during pregnancy, *Cell* 150:470-480, 2012.
150 Marrazzo JM, Fiedler TL, Srinivasan S, et al: Extravaginal reservoirs of vaginal bacteria as risk factors for incident bacterial vaginosis, *J Infect Dis* 205:1580-1588, 2012.
151. American College of Obstetricians and Gynecologists: ACOG Practice Bulletin. Assessment of risk factors for preterm birth. Clinical management guidelines for obstetrician-gynecologists. Number 31, October 2001. (Replaces Technical Bulletin number 206, June 1995; Committee Opinion number 172, May 1996; Committee Opinion number 187, September 1997; Committee Opinion number 198, February 1998; and Committee Opinion number 251, January 2001), *Obstet Gynecol* 98:709-716, 2001.
152. Iams JD, Romero R, Culhane JF, Goldenberg RL: Primary, secondary, and tertiary interventions to reduce the morbidity and mortality of preterm birth, *Lancet* 371:164-175, 2008.
153. Roberts AK, Monzon-Bordonaba F, Van Deerlin PG, et al: Association of polymorphism within the promoter of the tumor necrosis factor alpha gene with increased risk of preterm premature rupture of the fetal membranes, *Am J Obstet Gynecol* 180:1297-1302, 1999.
154. Genc MR, Gerber S, Nesin M, Witkin SS: Polymorphism in the interleukin-1 gene complex and spontaneous preterm delivery, *Am J Obstet Gynecol* 187:157-163, 2002.
155. Ferrand PE, Parry S, Sammel M, et al: A polymorphism in the matrix metalloproteinase-9 promoter is associated with increased risk of preterm premature rupture of membranes in African Americans, *Mol Hum Reprod* 8:494-501, 2002.
156. Chapman SJ, Owen J: Randomized trial of single-dose versus multiple-dose cefotetan for the postpartum treatment of intrapartum chorioamnionitis, *Am J Obstet Gynecol* 177:831-834, 1997.
157. Kenyon SL, Taylor DJ, Tarnow-Mordi W: Broad-spectrum antibiotics for spontaneous preterm labour: the ORACLE II randomised trial. ORACLE Collaborative Group, *Lancet* 357:989-994, 2001.
158. King J, Flenady V: Prophylactic antibiotics for inhibiting preterm labour with intact membranes, *Cochrane Database Syst Rev* (4):CD00024657, 2002.
159. Edwards RK, Duff P: Single additional dose postpartum therapy for women with chorioamnionitis, *Obstet Gynecol* 102(5 Pt 1):957-961, 2003.
160. Gilstrap LC 3rd, Leveno KJ, Cox SM, et al: Intrapartum treatment of acute chorioamnionitis: impact on neonatal sepsis, *Am J Obstet Gynecol* 159:579-583, 1988.
161. Gibbs RS, Dinsmoor MJ, Newton ER, Ramamurthy RS: A randomized trial of intrapartum versus immediate postpartum treatment of women with intra-amniotic infection, *Obstet Gynecol* 72:823-828, 1988.
162. Gilstrap LC 3rd, Bawdon RE, Burris J: Antibiotic concentration in maternal blood, cord blood, and placental membranes in chorioamnionitis, *Obstet Gynecol* 72:124-125, 1988.
163. Gibbs RS, Castillo MS, Rodgers PJ: Management of acute chorioamnionitis, *Am J Obstet Gynecol* 136:709-713, 1980.
164. Garite TJ, Freeman RK: Chorioamnionitis in the preterm gestation, *Obstet Gynecol* 59:539-545, 1982.
165. Silver RK, Gibbs RS, Castillo M: Effect of amniotic fluid bacteria on the course of labor in nulliparous women at term, *Obstet Gynecol* 68:587-592, 1986.
166. Ahn HM, Park EA, Cho SJ, Kim YJ, Park HS: The association of histological chorioamnionitis and antenatal steroids on neonatal outcome in preterm infants born at less than thirty-four weeks' gestation, *Neonatology* 102:259-264, 2012.
167. McAdams RM, Juul SE: The role of cytokines and inflammatory cells in perinatal brain injury, *Neurol Res Int* 2012:561494, 2012.

168. Chen ML, Allred EN, Hecht JL, et al: Placenta microbiology and histology and the risk for severe retinopathy of prematurity, *Invest Ophthalmol Vis Sci* 52:7052-7058, 2011.
169. Yoon BH, Romero R, Kim KS, et al: A systemic fetal inflammatory response and the development of bronchopulmonary dysplasia, *Am J Obstet Gynecol* 181:773-779, 1999.
170. Yoon BH, Romero R, Park JS, et al: The relationship among inflammatory lesions of the umbilical cord (funisitis), umbilical cord plasma interleukin 6 concentration, amniotic fluid infection, and neonatal sepsis, *Am J Obstet Gynecol* 183:1124-1129, 2000.
171. Yoon BH, Romero R, Yang SH, et al: Interleukin-6 concentrations in umbilical cord plasma are elevated in neonates with white matter lesions associated with periventricular leukomalacia, *Am J Obstet Gynecol* 174:1433-1440, 1996.
172. Lee J, Oh KJ, Yang HJ, et al: The importance of intra-amniotic inflammation in the subsequent development of atypical chronic lung disease, *J Matern Fetal Neonatal Med* 22:917-923, 2009.
173. Stroustrup A, Trasande L: Epidemiological characteristics and resource use in neonates with bronchopulmonary dysplasia: 1993-2006, *Pediatrics* 126:291-297, 2010.
174. Speer CP: Inflammation and bronchopulmonary dysplasia, *Semin Neonatol* 8:29-38, 2003.
175. Jobe AH: The new bronchopulmonary dysplasia, *Curr Opin Pediatr* 23:167-172, 2011.
176. Van Marter LJ, Dammann O, Allred EN, et al: Chorioamnionitis, mechanical ventilation, and postnatal sepsis as modulators of chronic lung disease in preterm infants, *J Pediatr* 140:171-176, 2002.
177. Hartling L, Liang Y, Lacaze-Masmonteil T: Chorioamnionitis as a risk factor for bronchopulmonary dysplasia: a systematic review and meta-analysis, *Arch Dis Child Fetal Neonatal Ed* 97:F8-F17, 2012.
178. Yoon BH, Romero R, Jun JK, et al: Amniotic fluid cytokines (interleukin-6, tumor necrosis factor-alpha, interleukin-1 beta, and interleukin-8) and the risk for the development of bronchopulmonary dysplasia, *Am J Obstet Gynecol* 177:825-830, 1997.
179. Ghezzi F, Gomez R, Romero R, et al: Elevated interleukin-8 concentrations in amniotic fluid of mothers whose neonates subsequently develop bronchopulmonary dysplasia, *Eur J Obstet Gynecol Reprod Biol* 78:5-10, 1998.
180. Ambalavanan N, Carlo WA, McDonald SA, et al: Identification of extremely premature infants at high risk of rehospitalization, *Pediatrics* 128:e1216-e1225, 2011.
181. Kallapur SG, Willet KE, Jobe AH, Ikegami M, Bachurski CJ: Intra-amniotic endotoxin: chorioamnionitis precedes lung maturation in preterm lambs, *Am J Physiol Lung Cell Mol Physiol* 280:L527-L536, 2001.
182. Kramer BW, Moss TJ, Willet KE, et al: Dose and time response after intraamniotic endotoxin in preterm lambs, *Am J Respir Crit Care Med* 164:982-988, 2001.
183. Kramer BW, Kramer S, Ikegami M, Jobe AH: Injury, inflammation, and remodeling in fetal sheep lung after intra-amniotic endotoxin, *Am J Physiol Lung Cell Mol Physiol* 283:L452-L459, 2002.
184. McAdams RM, Vanderhoeven J, Beyer RP, et al: Choriodecidual infection downregulates angiogenesis and morphogenesis pathways in fetal lungs from *Macaca nemestrina*, *PloS One* 7:e46863, 2012.
185. Wu YW, Colford JM Jr: Chorioamnionitis as a risk factor for cerebral palsy: a meta-analysis, *JAMA* 284:1417-1424, 2000.
186. Maleki Z, Bailis AJ, Argani CH, Askin FB, Graham EM: Periventricular leukomalacia and placental histopathologic abnormalities, *Obstet Gynecol* 114:1115-1120, 2009.
187. Elovitz MA, Brown AG, Breen K, et al: Intrauterine inflammation, insufficient to induce parturition, still evokes fetal and neonatal brain injury, *Int J Dev Neurosci* 29:663-671, 2011.
188. Patrick LA, Gaudet LM, Farley AE, et al: Development of a guinea pig model of chorioamnionitis and fetal brain injury, *Am J Obstet Gynecol* 191:1205-1211, 2004.
189. Grether JK, Nelson KB: Maternal infection and cerebral palsy in infants of normal birth weight, *JAMA* 278:207-211, 1997.
190. Wu YW, Escobar GJ, Grether JK, et al: Chorioamnionitis and cerebral palsy in term and near-term infants, *JAMA* 290:2677-2684, 2003.
191. Andrews WW, Cliver SP, Biasini F, et al: Early preterm birth: association between in utero exposure to acute inflammation and severe neurodevelopmental disability at 6 years of age, *Am J Obstet Gynecol* 198:466.e1-466.e11, 2008.
192. Yoon BH, Jun JK, Romero R, et al: Amniotic fluid inflammatory cytokines (interleukin-6, interleukin-1beta, and tumor necrosis factor-alpha), neonatal brain white matter lesions, and cerebral palsy, *Am J Obstet Gynecol* 177:19-26, 1997.
193. Back SA, Han BH, Luo NL, et al: Selective vulnerability of late oligodendrocyte progenitors to hypoxia-ischemia, *J Neurosci* 22:455-463, 2002.
194. McAdams RM, Juul SE: The role of cytokines and inflammatory cells in perinatal brain injury, *Neurol Res Int* 2012:561494, 2012.
195. Li J, Ramenaden ER, Peng J, et al: Tumor necrosis factor alpha mediates lipopolysaccharide-induced microglial toxicity to developing oligodendrocytes when astrocytes are present, *J Neurosci* 28:5321-5330, 2008.
196. Volpe JJ, Kinney HC, Jensen FE, Rosenberg PA: The developing oligodendrocyte: key cellular target in brain injury in the premature infant, *Int J Dev Neurosci* 29:423-440, 2011.
197. Leviton A, Allred EN, Kuban KC, et al: Microbiologic and histologic characteristics of the extremely preterm infant's placenta predict white matter damage and later cerebral palsy, the ELGAN study, *Pediatr Res* 67:95-101, 2010.
198. Verney C, Pogledic I, Biran V, et al: Microglial reaction in axonal crossroads is a hallmark of noncystic periventricular white matter injury in very preterm infants, *J Neuropathol Exp Neurol* 71:251-264, 2012.
199. Burd I, Balakrishnan B, Kannan S: Models of fetal brain injury, intrauterine inflammation, and preterm birth, *Am J Reprod Immunol* 67:287-294, 2012.
200. Rouse DJ, Hirtz DG, Thom E, et al: A randomized, controlled trial of magnesium sulfate for the prevention of cerebral palsy, *N Engl J Med* 359:895-905, 2008.
201. Marret S, Doyle LW, Crowther CA, Middleton P: Antenatal magnesium sulphate neuroprotection in the preterm infant, *Semin Fetal Neonatal Med* 12:311-317, 2007.
202. Hoffman DJ, Marro PJ, McGowan JE, Mishra OP, Delivoria-Papadopoulos M: Protective effect of MgSO4 infusion on nmda receptor binding characteristics during cerebral cortical hypoxia in the newborn piglet, *Brain Res* 644:144-149, 1994.
203. Macdonald RL, Curry DJ, Aihara Y, et al: Magnesium and experimental vasospasm, *J Neurosurg* 100:106-110, 2004.
204. Practice bulletins no: 139: premature rupture of membranes, *Obstet Gynecol* 122:918-930, 2013.
205. Parry S, Strauss JF 3rd: Premature rupture of the fetal membranes, *N Engl J Med* 338:663-670, 1998.
206. Liu L, Johnson HL, Cousens S, et al: Global, regional, and national causes of child mortality: an updated systematic analysis for 2010 with time trends since 2000, *Lancet* 379:2151-2161, 2012.
207. Evaldson G, Lagrelius A, Winiarski J: Premature rupture of the membranes, *Acta Obstet Gynecol Scand* 59:385-393, 1980.
208. Eggers TR, Doyle LW, Pepperell RJ: Premature rupture of the membranes, *Med J Aust* 1:209-213, 1979.
209. Harger JH, Hsing AW, Tuomala RE, et al: Risk factors for preterm premature rupture of fetal membranes: a multicenter case-control study, *Am J Obstet Gynecol* 163(1 Pt 1):130-137, 1990.
210. Mercer BM, Goldenberg RL, Moawad AH, et al: The preterm prediction study: effect of gestational age and cause of preterm birth on subsequent obstetric outcome. National Institute of Child Health and Human Development Maternal-Fetal Medicine Units Network, *Am J Obstet Gynecol* 181(5 Pt 1):1216-1221, 1999.
211. Mercer BM, Goldenberg RL, Meis PJ, et al: The Preterm Prediction Study: prediction of preterm premature rupture of membranes through clinical findings and ancillary testing. The National Institute of Child Health and Human Development Maternal-Fetal Medicine Units Network, *Am J Obstet Gynecol* 183:738-745, 2000.
212. Naeye RL: Factors that predispose to premature rupture of the fetal membranes, *Obstet Gynecol* 60:93-98, 1982.
213. da Fonseca EB, Bittar RE, Carvalho MH, Zugaib M: Prophylactic administration of progesterone by vaginal suppository to reduce the incidence of spontaneous preterm birth in women at increased risk: a randomized placebo-controlled double-blind study, *Am J Obstet Gynecol* 188:419-424, 2003.
214. Petrini JR, Callaghan WM, Klebanoff M, et al: Estimated effect of 17 alpha-hydroxyprogesterone caproate on preterm birth in the United States, *Obstet Gynecol* 105:267-272, 2005.
215. Romero R, Nicolaides K, Conde-Agudelo A, et al: Vaginal progesterone in women with an asymptomatic sonographic short cervix in the midtrimester decreases preterm delivery and neonatal morbidity: a systematic review and metaanalysis of individual patient data, *Am J Obstet Gynecol* 206:124.e1-19, 2012.

216. Hassan SS, Romero R, Vidyadhari D, et al: Vaginal progesterone reduces the rate of preterm birth in women with a sonographic short cervix: a multicenter, randomized, double-blind, placebo-controlled trial, *Ultrasound Obstet Gynecol* 38:18-31, 2011.
217. da Fonseca EB, Bittar RE, Carvalho MH, Zugaib M: Prophylactic administration of progesterone by vaginal suppository to reduce the incidence of spontaneous preterm birth in women at increased risk: a randomized placebo-controlled double-blind study, *Am J Obstet Gynecol* 188:419, 2003.
218. Briery CM, Veillon EW, Klauser CK, et al: Women with preterm premature rupture of the membranes do not benefit from weekly progesterone, *Am J Obstet Gynecol* 204:54, 2011.
219. Hannah ME, Ohlsson A, Farine D, et al: Induction of labor compared with expectant management for prelabor rupture of the membranes at term. TERMPROM Study Group, *N Engl J Med* 334:1005-1010, 1996.
220. Kappy KA, Cetrulo CL, Knuppel RA, et al: Premature rupture of the membranes at term. A comparison of induced and spontaneous labors, *J Reprod Med* 27:29-33, 1982.
221. Kappy KA, Cetrulo CL, Knuppel RA, et al: Premature rupture of the membranes: a conservative approach, *Am J Obstet Gynecol* 134:655-661, 1979.
222. Christensen KK, Christensen P, Ingemarsson I, et al: A study of complications in preterm deliveries after prolonged premature rupture of the membranes, *Obstet Gynecol* 48:670-677, 1976.
223. Cox SM, Williams ML, Leveno KJ: The natural history of preterm ruptured membranes: what to expect of expectant management, *Obstet Gynecol* 71:558-562, 1988.
224. Johnson JW, Egerman RS, Moorhead J: Cases with ruptured membranes that "reseal", *Am J Obstet Gynecol* 163:1024-1030, 1990; discussion 1030-1022.
225. Brace RA: Physiology of amniotic fluid volume regulation, *Clin Obstet Gynecol* 40:280-289, 1997.
226. Parry S, Strauss JF 3rd: Premature rupture of the fetal membranes, *N Engl J Med* 338:663-670, 1998.
227. Oxlund H, Helmig R, Halaburt JT, Uldbjerg N: Biomechanical analysis of human chorioamniotic membranes, *Eur J Obstet Gynecol Reprod Biol* 34:247-255, 1990.
228. Arikat S, Novince RW, Mercer BM, et al: Separation of amnion from choriodecidua is an integral event to the rupture of normal term fetal membranes and constitutes a significant component of the work required, *Am J Obstet Gynecol* 194:211-217, 2006.
229. Bryant-Greenwood GD: The extracellular matrix of the human fetal membranes: structure and function, *Placenta* 19:1-11, 1998.
230. Malak TM, Bell SC: Structural characteristics of term human fetal membranes: a novel zone of extreme morphological alteration within the rupture site, *Br J Obstet Gynaecol* 101:375-386, 1994.
231. Joyce EM, Moore JJ, Sacks MS: Biomechanics of the fetal membrane prior to mechanical failure: review and implications, *Eur J Obstet Gynecol Reprod Biol* 144(Suppl 1):S121-S127, 2009.
232. El Khwad M, Stetzer B, Moore RM, et al: Term human fetal membranes have a weak zone overlying the lower uterine pole and cervix before onset of labor, *Biol Reprod* 72:720-726, 2005.
233. El Khwad M, Pandey V, Stetzer B, et al: Fetal membranes from term vaginal deliveries have a zone of weakness exhibiting characteristics of apoptosis and remodeling, *J Soc Gynecol Investig* 13:191-195, 2006.
234. Lannon SM, Vanderhoeven JP, Eschenbach DA, Gravett MG, Waldorf KM: Synergy and interactions among biological pathways leading to preterm premature rupture of membranes, *Reprod Sci* 21:1215-1227, 2014.
235. Santolaya-Forgas J, Romero R, Espinoza J, et al: Prelabor rupture of membranes. In Reece EA, Hobbins JC, editors: *Clinical obstetrics: the fetus and the mother*, 3rd ed, Malden, Mass, 2007, Blackwell Publishing, pp 1130-1188.
236. Garite TJ, Freeman RK, Linzey EM, Braly P: The use of amniocentesis in patients with premature rupture of membranes, *Obstet Gynecol* 54:226-230, 1979.
237. Shim SS, Romero R, Hong JS, et al: Clinical significance of intra-amniotic inflammation in patients with preterm premature rupture of membranes, *Am J Obstet Gynecol* 191:1339-1345, 2004.
238. Romero R, Baumann P, Gomez R, et al: The relationship between spontaneous rupture of membranes, labor, and microbial invasion of the amniotic cavity and amniotic fluid concentrations of prostaglandins and thromboxane B2 in term pregnancy, *Am J Obstet Gynecol* 168(6 Pt 1):1654-1664; 1993; discussion 1664-1658.
239. Guinn DA, Goldenberg RL, Hauth JC, et al: Risk factors for the development of preterm premature rupture of the membranes after arrest of preterm labor, *Am J Obstet Gynecol* 173:1310-1315, 1995.
240. Cobo T, Kacerovsky M, Palacio M, et al: Intra-amniotic inflammatory response in subgroups of women with preterm prelabor rupture of the membranes, *PLoS One* 7:e43677, 2012.
241. Kumar D, Schatz F, Moore RM, et al: The effects of thrombin and cytokines upon the biomechanics and remodeling of isolated amnion membrane, in vitro, *Placenta* 32:206-213, 2011.
242. Fortunato SJ, Menon R, Lombardi SJ: Role of tumor necrosis factor-alpha in the premature rupture of membranes and preterm labor pathways, *Am J Obstet Gynecol* 187:1159-1162, 2002.
243. Jacobsson B, Aaltonen R, Rantakokko-Jalava K, Morken NH, Alanen A: Quantification of *Ureaplasma urealyticum* DNA in the amniotic fluid from patients in PTL and pPROM and its relation to inflammatory cytokine levels, *Acta Obstet Gynecol Scand* 88:63-70, 2009.
244. Romero R, Mazor M, Sepulveda W, et al: Tumor necrosis factor in preterm and term labor, *Am J Obstet Gynecol* 166:1576-1587, 1992.
245. Yui J, Garcia-Lloret M, Wegmann TG, Guilbert LJ: Cytotoxicity of tumour necrosis factor-alpha and gamma-interferon against primary human placental trophoblasts, *Placenta* 15:819-835, 1994.
246. Paavola LG, Furth EE, Delgado V, et al: Striking changes in the structure and organization of rat fetal membranes precede parturition, *Biol Reprod* 53:321-338, 1995.
247. Canzoneri BJ, Feng L, Grotegut CA, et al: The chorion layer of fetal membranes is prematurely destroyed in women with preterm premature rupture of the membranes, *Reprod Sci* 20:1246-1254, 2013.
248. Strauss JF 3rd: Extracellular matrix dynamics and fetal membrane rupture, *Reprod Sci* 20:140-153, 2013.
249. Biggio JR Jr, Ramsey PS, Cliver SP, et al: Midtrimester amniotic fluid matrix metalloproteinase-8 (MMP-8) levels above the 90th percentile are a marker for subsequent preterm premature rupture of membranes, *Am J Obstet Gynecol* 192:109-113, 2005.
250. Athayde N, Edwin SS, Romero R, et al: A role for matrix metalloproteinase-9 in spontaneous rupture of the fetal membranes, *Am J Obstet Gynecol* 179:1248-1253, 1998.
251. Menon R, Fortunato SJ: The role of matrix degrading enzymes and apoptosis in rupture of membranes, *J Soc Gynecol Investig* 11:427-437, 2004.
252. Woods JR Jr: Reactive oxygen species and preterm premature rupture of membranes-a review, *Placenta* 22(Suppl A):S38-S44, 2001.
253. Menon R, Fortunato SJ, Yu J, et al: Cigarette smoke induces oxidative stress and apoptosis in normal term fetal membranes, *Placenta* 32:317-322, 2011.
254. Burlingame JM, Esfandiari N, Sharma RK, Mascha E, Falcone T: Total antioxidant capacity and reactive oxygen species in amniotic fluid, *Obstet Gynecol* 101:756-761, 2003.
255. Plessinger MA, Woods JR Jr, Miller RK: Pretreatment of human amnion-chorion with vitamins C and E prevents hypochlorous acid-induced damage, *Am J Obstet Gynecol* 183:979-985, 2000.
256. Mercer BM, Abdelrahim A, Moore RM, et al: The impact of vitamin C supplementation in pregnancy and in vitro upon fetal membrane strength and remodeling, *Reprod Sci* 17:685-695, 2010.
257. Spinnato JA 2nd, Freire S, Pinto e Silva JL, et al: Antioxidant supplementation and premature rupture of the membranes: a planned secondary analysis, *Am J Obstet Gynecol* 199(433):e431-e438, 2008.
258. Rosen T, Kuczynski E, O'Neill LM, Funai EF, Lockwood CJ: Plasma levels of thrombin-antithrombin complexes predict preterm premature rupture of the fetal membranes, *J Matern Fetal Med* 10:297-300, 2001.
259. Stephenson CD, Lockwood CJ, Ma Y, Guller S: Thrombin-dependent regulation of matrix metalloproteinase (MMP)-9 levels in human fetal membranes, *J Matern Fetal Neonatal Med* 18:17-22, 2005.
260. Chen D, Dorling A: Critical roles for thrombin in acute and chronic inflammation, *J Thromb Haemost* 7(Suppl 1):122-126, 2009.
261. Park KW, Jin BK: Thrombin-induced oxidative stress contributes to the death of hippocampal neurons: role of neuronal NADPH oxidase, *J Neurosci Res* 86:1053-1063, 2008.
262. Lopez JJ, Salido GM, Gomez-Arteta E, Rosado JA, Pariente JA: Thrombin induces apoptotic events through the generation of reactive oxygen species in human platelets, *J Thromb Haemost* 5:1283-1291, 2007.
263. Harger JH, Hsing AW, Tuomala RE, et al: Risk factors for preterm premature rupture of fetal membranes: a multicenter case-control study, *Am J Obstet Gynecol* 163(1 Pt 1):130-137, 1990.
264. Rosen T, Schatz F, Kuczynski E, et al: Thrombin-enhanced matrix metalloproteinase-1 expression: a mechanism linking placental abruption with premature rupture of the membranes, *J Matern Fetal Neonatal Med* 11:11-17, 2002.

265. Matta P, Lockwood CJ, Schatz F, et al: Thrombin regulates monocyte chemoattractant protein-1 expression in human first trimester and term decidual cells, *Am J Obstet Gynecol* 196(268):e261-e268, 2007.
266. Puthiyachirakkal M, Lemerand K, Kumar D, et al: Thrombin weakens the amnion extracellular matrix (ECM) directly rather than through protease activated receptors, *Placenta* 34:924-931, 2013.
267. Moore RM, Schatz F, Kumar D, et al: Alpha-lipoic acid inhibits thrombin-induced fetal membrane weakening in vitro, *Placenta* 31:886-892, 2010.
268. Anum EA, Hill LD, Pandya A, Strauss JF 3rd: Connective tissue and related disorders and preterm birth: clues to genes contributing to prematurity, *Placenta* 30:207-215, 2009.
269. Barabas AP: Ehlers-Danlos syndrome: associated with prematurity and premature rupture of foetal membranes; possible increase in incidence, *Br Med J* 2:682-684, 1966.
270. Wang H, Parry S, Macones G, et al: A functional SNP in the promoter of the SERPINH1 gene increases risk of preterm premature rupture of membranes in African Americans, *Proc Natl Acad Sci U S A* 103:13463-13467, 2006.
271. Fujimoto T, Parry S, Urbanek M, et al: A single nucleotide polymorphism in the matrix metalloproteinase-1 (MMP-1) promoter influences amnion cell MMP-1 expression and risk for preterm premature rupture of the fetal membranes, *J Biol Chem* 277:6296-6302, 2002.
272. Kalish RB, Nguyen DP, Vardhana S, et al: A single nucleotide A>G polymorphism at position -670 in the Fas gene promoter: relationship to preterm premature rupture of fetal membranes in multifetal pregnancies, *Am J Obstet Gynecol* 192:208-212, 2005.
273. Kalish RB, Vardhana S, Normand NJ, Gupta M, Witkin SS: Association of a maternal CD14 -159 gene polymorphism with preterm premature rupture of membranes and spontaneous preterm birth in multi-fetal pregnancies, *J Reprod Immunol* 70:109-117, 2006.
274. Annells MF, Hart PH, Mullighan CG, et al: Interleukins-1, -4, -6, -10, tumor necrosis factor, transforming growth factor-beta, FAS, and mannose-binding protein C gene polymorphisms in Australian women: risk of preterm birth, *Am J Obstet Gynecol* 191:2056-2067, 2004.
275. Fuks A, Parton LA, Polavarapu S, et al: Polymorphism of Fas and Fas ligand in preterm premature rupture of membranes in singleton pregnancies, *Am J Obstet Gynecol* 193(3 Pt 2):1132-1136, 2005.
276. Lee SE, Park JS, Norwitz ER, et al: Measurement of placental alpha-microglobulin-1 in cervicovaginal discharge to diagnose rupture of membranes, *Obstet Gynecol* 109:634-640, 2007.
277. Yeast JD, Garite TJ, Dorchester W: The risks of amniocentesis in the management of premature rupture of the membranes, *Am J Obstet Gynecol* 149:505-508, 1984.
278. Feinstein SJ, Vintzileos AM, Lodeiro JG, et al: Amniocentesis with premature rupture of membranes, *Obstet Gynecol* 68:147-152, 1986.
279. Lewis DF, Major CA, Towers CV, et al: Effects of digital vaginal examinations on latency period in preterm premature rupture of membranes, *Obstet Gynecol* 80:630-634, 1992.
280. Taylor J, Garite TJ: Premature rupture of membranes before fetal viability, *Obstet Gynecol* 64:615-620, 1984.
281. Beydoun SN, Yasin SY: Premature rupture of the membranes before 28 weeks: conservative management, *Am J Obstet Gynecol* 155:471-479, 1986.
282. Moretti M, Sibai BM: Maternal and perinatal outcome of expectant management of premature rupture of membranes in the midtrimester, *Am J Obstet Gynecol* 159:390-396, 1988.
283. Major CA, Kitzmiller JL: Perinatal survival with expectant management of midtrimester rupture of membranes, *Am J Obstet Gynecol* 163:838-844, 1990.
284. Dinsmoor MJ, Bachman R, Haney EI, Goldstein M, Mackendrick W: Outcomes after expectant management of extremely preterm premature rupture of the membranes, *Am J Obstet Gynecol* 190:183-187, 2004.
285. Rotschild A, Ling EW, Puterman ML, Farquharson D: Neonatal outcome after prolonged preterm rupture of the membranes, *Am J Obstet Gynecol* 162:46-52, 1990.
286. Fayez JA, Hasan AA, Jonas HS, Miller GL: Management of premature rupture of the membranes, *Obstet Gynecol* 52:17-21, 1978.
287. Schreiber J, Benedetti T: Conservative management of preterm premature rupture of the fetal membranes in a low socioeconomic population, *Am J Obstet Gynecol* 136:92-96, 1980.
288. Perkins RP: The neonatal significance of selected perinatal events among infants of low birth weight. II. The influence of ruptured membranes, *Am J Obstet Gynecol* 142:7-16, 1982.
289. Schutte MF, Treffers PE, Kloosterman GJ, Soepatmi S: Management of premature rupture of membranes: the risk of vaginal examination to the infant, *Am J Obstet Gynecol* 146:395-400, 1983.
290. Berkowitz RL, Kantor RD, Beck GJ, Warshaw JB: The relationship between premature rupture of the membranes and the respiratory distress syndrome. An update and plan of management, *Am J Obstet Gynecol* 131:503-508, 1978.
291. Jones MD Jr, Burd LI, Bowes WA Jr, Battaglia FC, Lubchenco LO: Failure of association of premature rupture of membranes with respiratory-distress syndrome, *N Engl J Med* 292:1253-1257, 1975.
292. Kenyon S, Boulvain M, Neilson J: Antibiotics for preterm rupture of the membranes: a systematic review, *Obstet Gynecol* 104(5 Pt 1):1051-1057, 2004.
293. Mercer BM, Arheart KL: Antimicrobial therapy in expectant management of preterm premature rupture of the membranes, *Lancet* 346:1271-1279, 1995.
294. Mercer BM, Miodovnik M, Thurnau GR, et al: Antibiotic therapy for reduction of infant morbidity after preterm premature rupture of the membranes. A randomized controlled trial. National Institute of Child Health and Human Development Maternal-Fetal Medicine Units Network, *JAMA* 278:989-995, 1997.
295. Kenyon SL, Taylor DJ, Tarnow-Mordi W: Broad-spectrum antibiotics for preterm, prelabour rupture of fetal membranes: the ORACLE I randomised trial. ORACLE Collaborative Group, *Lancet* 357:979-988, 2001.
296. Kenyon S, Boulvain M: Antibiotics for preterm premature rupture of membranes, *The Cochrane Database System Rev*(2)CD001058, 2000.
297. Segel SY, Miles AM, Clothier B, Parry S, Macones GA: Duration of antibiotic therapy after preterm premature rupture of fetal membranes, *Am J Obstet Gynecol* 189:799-802, 2003.
298. Lewis DF, Adair CD, Robichaux AG, et al: Antibiotic therapy in preterm premature rupture of membranes: are seven days necessary? A preliminary, randomized clinical trial, *Am J Obstet Gynecol* 188:1413-1416, 2003; discussion 1416-1417.
299. Garite TJ, Keegan KA, Freeman RK, Nageotte MP: A randomized trial of ritodrine tocolysis versus expectant management in patients with premature rupture of membranes at 25 to 30 weeks of gestation, *Am J Obstet Gynecol* 157:388-393, 1987.
300. Weiner CP, Renk K, Klugman M: The therapeutic efficacy and cost-effectiveness of aggressive tocolysis for premature labor associated with premature rupture of the membranes, *Am J Obstet Gynecol* 159:216-222, 1988.
301. Decavalas G, Mastrogiannis D, Papadopoulos V, Tzingounis V: Short-term verus long-term prophylactic tocolysis in patients with preterm premature rupture of membranes, *Eur J Obstet Gynecol Reprod Biol* 59:143-147, 1995.
302. Fontenot T, Lewis DF: Tocolytic therapy with preterm premature rupture of membranes, *Clin Perinatol* 28:787-796, vi, 2001.
303. Mackeen AD, Seibel-Seamon J, Grimes-Dennis J, Baxter JK, Berghella V: Tocolytics for preterm premature rupture of membranes, *Cochrane Database Syst Rev*(10)CD007062, 2011.
304. Brame RG, MacKenna J: Vaginal pool phospholipids in the management of premature rupture of membranes, *Am J Obstet Gynecol* 145:992-1000, 1983.
305. Lewis DF, Towers CV, Major CA, et al: Use of Amniostat-FLM in detecting the presence of phosphatidylglycerol in vaginal pool samples in preterm premature rupture of membranes, *Am J Obstet Gynecol* 169:573-576, 1993.
306. Mercer BM, Crocker LG, Boe NM, Sibai BM: Induction versus expectant management in premature rupture of the membranes with mature amniotic fluid at 32 to 36 weeks: a randomized trial, *Am J Obstet Gynecol* 169:775-782, 1993.
307. Cox SM, Leveno KJ: Intentional delivery versus expectant management with preterm ruptured membranes at 30-34 weeks' gestation, *Obstet Gynecol* 86:875-879, 1995.
308. van der Ham DP, van der Heyden JL, Opmeer BC, et al: Management of late-preterm premature rupture of membranes: the PPROMEXIL-2 trial, *Am J Obstet Gynecol* 207:276.e1-e10, 2012.
309. van der Ham DP, Vijgen SM, Nijhuis JG, et al: Induction of labor versus expectant management in women with preterm prelabor rupture of membranes between 34 and 37 weeks: a randomized controlled trial, *PLoS Med* 9:e1001208, 2012.

310. Caughey AB, Robinson JN, Norwitz ER: Contemporary diagnosis and management of preterm premature rupture of membranes, *Rev Obstet Gynecol* 1:11-22, 2008.
311. Gerdes JS: Clinicopathologic approach to the diagnosis of neonatal sepsis, *Clin Perinatol* 18:361-381, 1991.
312. Dare MR, Middleton P, Crowther CA, Flenady VJ, Varatharaju B: Planned early birth versus expectant management (waiting) for prelabour rupture of membranes at term (37 weeks or more), *Cochrane Database Syst Rev*(1)CD005302, 2006.
313. Herbst A, Kallen K: Time between membrane rupture and delivery and septicemia in term neonates, *Obstet Gynecol* 110:612-618, 2007.
314. Verani JR, McGee L, Schrag SJ: Prevention of perinatal group B streptococcal disease–revised guidelines from CDC, 2010, *MMWR Recomm Rep* 59(RR-10):1-36, 2010.
315. Kenyon S, Boulvain M, Neilson JP: Antibiotics for preterm rupture of membranes, *Cochrane Database Syst Rev*(8)CD001058, 2010.
316. Gonen R, Hannah ME, Milligan JE: Does prolonged preterm premature rupture of the membranes predispose to abruptio placentae? *Obstet Gynecol* 74(3 Pt 1):347-350, 1989.
317. Mercer BM: Management of premature rupture of membranes before 26 weeks' gestation, *Obstet Gynecol Clin North Am* 19:339-351, 1992.
318. Nimrod C, Varela-Gittings F, Machin G, Campbell D, Wesenberg R: The effect of very prolonged membrane rupture on fetal development, *Am J Obstet Gynecol* 148:540-543, 1984.
319. Vergani P, Ghidini A, Locatelli A, et al: Risk factors for pulmonary hypoplasia in second-trimester premature rupture of membranes, *Am J Obstet Gynecol* 170(5 Pt 1):1359-1364, 1994.
320. Lauria MR, Gonik B, Romero R: Pulmonary hypoplasia: pathogenesis, diagnosis, and antenatal prediction, *Obstet Gynecol* 86:466-475, 1995.
321. Rizzo G, Capponi A, Angelini E, Mazzoleni A, Romanini C: Blood flow velocity waveforms from fetal peripheral pulmonary arteries in pregnancies with preterm premature rupture of the membranes: relationship with pulmonary hypoplasia, *Ultrasound Obstet Gynecol* 15:98-103, 2000.
322. Lauria MR, Gonik B, Romero R: Pulmonary hypoplasia: pathogenesis, diagnosis, and antenatal prediction, *Obstet Gynecol* 86:466-475, 1995.
323. Romero R, Oyarzun E, Mazor M, et al: Meta-analysis of the relationship between asymptomatic bacteriuria and preterm delivery/low birth weight, *Obstet Gynecol* 73:576-582, 1989.
324. French LM, Smaill FM: Antibiotic regimens for endometritis after delivery, *The Cochrane Database Syst Rev*(4)CD001067, 2004.
325. Lyell DJ, Pullen K, Fuh K, et al: Daily compared with 8-hour gentamicin for the treatment of intrapartum chorioamnionitis: a randomized controlled trial, *Obstet Gynecol* 115(2 Pt 1):344-349, 2010.
326. Locksmith GJ, Chin A, Vu T, Shattuck KE, Hankins GD: High compared with standard gentamicin dosing for chorioamnionitis: a comparison of maternal and fetal serum drug levels, *Obstet Gynecol* 105:473-479, 2005.
327. Gall S, Koukol DH: Ampicillin/sulbactam vs. clindamycin/gentamicin in the treatment of postpartum endometritis, *J Reprod Med* 41:575-580, 1996.
328. Faro S, Martens M, Phillips LE, et al: Ticarcillin disodium/clavulanate potassium versus clindamycin/gentamicin in the treatment of postpartum endometritis, *J Reprod Med* 33(6 Suppl):603-606, 1988.
329. MacGregor RR, Graziani AL, Samuels P: Randomized, double-blind study of cefotetan and cefoxitin in post-cesarean section endometritis, *Am J Obstet Gynecol* 167:139-143, 1992.
330. Rosene K, Eschenbach DA, Tompkins LS, Kenny GE, Watkins H: Polymicrobial early postpartum endometritis with facultative and anaerobic bacteria, genital mycoplasmas, and *Chlamydia trachomatis*: treatment with piperacillin or cefoxitin, *J Infect Dis* 153:1028-1037, 1986.
331. Hopkins L, Smaill F: Antibiotic regimens for management of intraamniotic infection, *Cochrane Database Syst Rev*(3)CD003254, 2002.
332. Gaucherand P, Salle B, Sergeant P, et al: Comparative study of three vaginal markers of the premature rupture of membranes. Insulin like growth factor binding protein 1 diamine-oxidase pH, *Acta Obstet Gynecol Scand* 76:536-540, 1997.
333. Erdemoglu E, Mungan T: Significance of detecting insulin-like growth factor binding protein-1 in cervicovaginal secretions: comparison with nitrazine test and amniotic fluid volume assessment, *Acta Obstet Gynecol Scand* 83:622-626, 2004.
334. Smith RP: A technic for the detection of rupture of the membranes. A review and preliminary report, *Obstet Gynecol* 48:172-176, 1976.
335. Petrunin DD, Griaznova IM: Petrunina IuA, Tatarinov IuS. [Immunochemical identification of organ specific human placental alphalglobulin and its concentration in amniotic fluid], *Akush Ginekol (Mosk)*62-64, 1977.
336. Cousins LM, Smok DP, Lovett SM, Poeltler DM: AmniSure placental alpha microglobulin-1 rapid immunoassay versus standard diagnostic methods for detection of rupture of membranes, *Am J Perinatol* 22:317-320, 2005.
337. Boltovskaia MN, Zaraiskii EI, Fuks BB, et al: [Histochemical and clinical-diagnostic study of placental alpha 1-microglobulin using monoclonal antibodies], *Biull Eksp Biol Med* 112:397-400, 1991.
338. Lee SE, Park JS, Norwitz ER, et al: Measurement of placental alpha-microglobulin-1 in cervicovaginal discharge to diagnose rupture of membranes, *Obstet Gynecol* 109:634-640, 2007.
339. Lockwood CJ, Senyei AE, Dische MR, et al: Fetal fibronectin in cervical and vaginal secretions as a predictor of preterm delivery, *N Engl J Med* 325:669-674, 1991.
340. Kishida T, Yamada H, Negishi H, et al: Diagnosis of premature rupture of the membranes in preterm patients, using an improved AFP kit: comparison with ROM-check and/or nitrazine test, *Eur J Obstet Gynecol Reprod Biol* 69:77-82, 1996.
341. Li HY, Chang TS: Vaginal fluid creatinine, human chorionic gonadotropin and alpha-fetoprotein levels for detecting premature rupture of membranes, *Zhonghua Yi Xue Za Zhi (Taipei)* 63:686-690, 2000.
342. Shahin M, Raslan H: Comparative study of three amniotic fluid markers in premature rupture of membranes: prolactin, beta subunit of human chorionic gonadotropin, and alpha-fetoprotein, *Gynecol Obstet Invest* 63:195-199, 2007.
343. Kafali H, Oksuzler C: Vaginal fluid urea and creatinine in diagnosis of premature rupture of membranes, *Arch Gynecol Obstet* 275:157-160, 2007.
344. Wiberg-Itzel E, Cnattingius S, Nordstrom L: Lactate determination in vaginal fluids: a new method in the diagnosis of prelabour rupture of membranes, *BJOG* 112:754-758, 2005.
345. Jeurgens-Borst AJ, Bekkers RL, Sporken JM, van den Berg PP: Use of insulin like growth factor binding protein-1 in the diagnosis of ruptured fetal membranes, *Eur J Obstet Gynecol Reprod Biol* 102:11-14, 2002.
346. Lockwood CJ, Wein R, Chien D, et al: Fetal membrane rupture is associated with the presence of insulin-like growth factor-binding protein-1 in vaginal secretions, *Am J Obstet Gynecol* 171:146-150, 1994.
347. Buyukbayrak EE, Turan C, Unal O, Dansuk R, Cengizoglu B: Diagnostic power of the vaginal washing-fluid prolactin assay as an alternative method for the diagnosis of premature rupture of membranes, *J Matern Fetal Neonatal Med* 15:120-125, 2004.
348. Koninckx PR, Trappeniers H, Van Assche FA: Prolactin concentration in vaginal fluid: a new method for diagnosing ruptured membranes, *Br J Obstet Gynaecol* 88:607-610, 1981.
349. Esim E, Turan C, Unal O, Dansuk R, Cengizglu B: Diagnosis of premature rupture of membranes by identification of beta-HCG in vaginal washing fluid, *Eur J Obstet Gynecol Reprod Biol* 107:37-40, 2003.
350. Kim YH, Park YW, Kwon HS, Kwon JY, Kim BJ: Vaginal fluid beta-human chorionic gonadotropin level in the diagnosis of premature rupture of membranes, *Acta Obstet Gynecol Scand* 84:802-805, 2005.
351. Di Renzo GC, Roura LC, Facchinetti F, et al: Guidelines for the management of spontaneous preterm labor: identification of spontaneous preterm labor, diagnosis of preterm premature rupture of membranes, and preventive tools for preterm birth, *J Matern Fetal Neonatal Med* 24:659-667, 2011.
352. American College of Obstetrics and Gynecology; Committee on Practice Bulletins—Obstetrics: ACOG practice bulletin no. 127: management of preterm labor, *Obstet Gynecol* 119:1308-1317, 2012.

4 Developmental Immunology and Role of Host Defenses in Fetal and Neonatal Susceptibility to Infection

DAVID K. HONG and DAVID B. LEWIS

CHAPTER OUTLINE

CHAPTER OUTLINE

The human fetus and neonate are unduly susceptible to infection with a wide variety of microbes, many of which are not pathogenic in more mature individuals. This susceptibility results from limitations of both innate and adaptive (antigen-specific) immunity and their interactions. This chapter focuses on the ontogeny of the immune system in the fetus, neonate, and young infant and the relationship between limitations in immune function and susceptibility to specific types of infection.

The immune system includes innate protective mechanisms against pathogens provided by the skin, respiratory and gastrointestinal epithelia, and other mucosa; humoral factors, such as cytokines (Tables 4-1 and 4-2) and complement components (Fig. 4-1); and innate and adaptive immune mechanisms mediated by hematopoietic cells, including mononuclear phagocytes (circulating monocytes and tissue macrophages), granulocytes, dendritic cells (DCs), and lymphocytes. Certain nonhematopoietic cells, such as follicular dendritic cells and thymic epithelial cells, also play important roles in adaptive immunity.

Innate immunity, unlike adaptive immunity to be discussed later, does not require prior exposure to be immediately effective and is equally efficient on primary and subsequent encounter with a microbe but does not provide long-lasting protection against reinfection. Innate defenses consist of fixed epithelial barriers and resident tissue macrophages, which act immediately or within the first minutes to hours of encounter with a microbe. These "frontline" defenses are sufficient for protection from the vast majority of microbes in the environment, which do not produce disease in healthy individuals. If the microbial insult is too great or the organism is able to evade these initial defenses, these cells release mediators that incite an inflammatory response, through which soluble and cellular defenses are recruited and help to limit or eradicate the infection over the next hours to days and to initiate the antigen-specific immune response that follows.

Epithelial Barriers

Epithelia form a crucial physical and chemical barrier against infection. Tight junctions between epithelial cells prevent direct entry of microbes into deeper tissues, and physical injury that disrupts epithelial integrity can greatly increase the risk for infection. In addition to providing a physical barrier, mechanical and chemical factors and colonization by commensal microbes contribute to the protective functions of the skin and of the mucosal epithelia of the gastrointestinal and respiratory tracts.

ANTIMICROBIAL PEPTIDES AND PROTEINS

A general feature of epithelial defenses is the production of one or more antimicrobial peptides, which include the α-defensins and β-defensins and the cathelicidin LL-37. Defensins and cathelicidin have direct antimicrobial activity against gram-positive and gram-negative bacteria and some fungi; viruses, such as, influenza and respiratory syncytial virus (RSV); and protozoa.[1-4] Some of these antimicrobial peptides also exhibit proinflammatory and immunomodulatory activities.

There are six known human α-defensins: human neutrophil proteins (HNP) 1 to 4 and human defensins (HD) 5 and 6. HNPs 1 to 4 are expressed in leukocytes (white blood cells). HD-5 and HD-6 are produced and secreted by Paneth cells, located at the base of crypts in the small intestine. There are at least six human β-defensins, but only four (hBD-1 to -4) have been well characterized. hBD-1 is constitutively expressed by skin keratinocytes, whereas exposure to bacteria or proinflammatory cytokines, including tumor necrosis factor-α (TNF-α) and interleukin-1β (IL-1β) (see Tables 4-1 and 4-2), induces expression of hBD-2 and hBD-3 in keratinocytes and hBD-4 in lung epithelial cells, respectively. hBD-2 appears to be a normal component of human amniotic fluid, with levels increasing in the setting of chorioamnionitis and preterm labor.[5] hBD-1 and hBD-2 are active against gram-negative bacteria and streptococci but are less active against *Staphylococcus aureus*, whereas hBD-3 is broadly active against gram-positive and gram-negative bacteria and *Candida* species. The cathelicidin LL-37 is expressed in leukocytes, for instance, neutrophils, mononuclear phagocytes, and mast cells,[4,6] and its expression is induced by microbes and proinflammatory cytokines in epithelial cells of the skin, gut, and respiratory tract; LL-37 is active against gram-positive and

Table 4-1 Major Human Cytokines and Tumor Necrosis Factor Family Ligands: Structure, Cognate Receptors, and Receptor-Mediated Signal Transduction Pathways

Cytokine Family	Members	Structure	Cognate Receptor Family	Proximal Signal Transduction Pathways
IL-1		β-Trefoil, monomers; processed and secreted	IL-1 receptor (IL-1R) superfamily (three immunoglobulin-like ectodomains)	MyD88, IRAKs, NF-κB, MAPK, JNK
IL-1 subfamily	IL-1α, IL-1β, IL-33, IL-1 receptor antagonist (RA)			
IL-18 subfamily	IL-18, IL-37			
IL-36 subfamily	IL-36α, IL-36β, IL-36γ, IL-36RA, IL-38			
Hematopoietin	IL-2–IL-7, IL-9–IL-13, IL-15, IL-17, IL-19 to IL-32, IL-34, IL-35, CSFs, oncostatin-M, IFNs (α, β, γ, and others); class II subfamily consists of IL-10, IL-19, IL-20, IL-22, IL-24, IL-26, IFNs (including IFN-αs, IFN-β, IL-27/28)	Four α-helical; monomers except for IL-5 and IFNs (homodimers) and IL-12, IL-23, IL-27, IL-30, IL-35 (heterodimers); secreted	Hematopoietin receptors	JAK tyrosine kinases/STAT, SRC kinases, PI3K, PKB
TNF ligand	TNF-α, lymphotoxin-α, lymphotoxin-β, CD27L, CD30L, CD40L, OX40L, TRAIL, others	β-Jellyroll, homotrimers; type II membrane proteins and secreted	TNF receptor family	TRAFs and proteins mediating apoptosis
TGF-β	TGF-β1, TGF-β2, TGF-β3, bone morphogenetic proteins	Cysteine knot; processed and secreted	TGF-β receptors type 1 and type 2 heterodimers (intrinsic serine threonine kinases)	SMAD proteins
Chemokines		Three-stranded β-sheet; all but fractalkine are secreted	Seven membrane-spanning domains	G protein–mediated
CXC ligand subfamily	CXCL1-14, CXCL16		CXCR1 to CXCR6	
CC ligand subfamily	CCL1-5, CCL7, CCL8, CCL11, CCL13 to CCL28		CCR1 to CCR10	
C ligand subfamily	XCL1 (lymphotactin), XCL2 (SCM-1β)		XCR1	
CX3C ligand subfamily	CX3CL (fractalkine)		CX3CR1	

CSF, Colony-stimulating factor; *IFN,* interferon; *IL,* interleukin; *IRAK,* IL-1 receptor–associated serine/threonine kinase; *JAK,* Janus tyrosine kinase; *JNK,* c-Jun N-terminal kinase; *MAPK,* mitogen-activated protein kinase; *NF-κB,* nuclear factor-kappa B; *PI3K,* phosphoinositide-3-kinase; *PKB,* protein kinase B; *RA,* receptor antagonist; *SMAD,* SMA- and MAD-related; *SRC,* sarcoma (family); *STAT,* signal transducer and activator of transcription; *TGF,* transforming growth factor; *TNF,* tumor necrosis factor; *TRAFs,* TNF-α receptor–associated factors; *TRAIL,* TNF-related apoptosis–inducing ligand.

gram-negative bacteria but less active against *S. aureus* than hBD-3[7]; it also has activity in vitro against RSV[3] and in vivo against influenza A virus.[2]

In addition to the defensins, other antimicrobial proteins also contribute to epithelial defenses. These include the C-type lectin hepatocarcinoma-intestine-pancreas/pancreatic-associated protein (HIP/PAP), which is expressed by Paneth cells and enterocytes and which binds to gram-positive bacterial peptidoglycan[8]; phospholipase A2 (PLA2), which hydrolyses bacterial membrane phospholipids and is produced by Paneth cells and mononuclear phagocytes[4]; psoriasin (S100A7), which is produced by keratinocytes[9] and inhibits gram-negative bacteria; and RNase7, which is expressed by the skin and the gastrointestinal and genitourinary epithelia,[10] and inhibits gram-positive bacteria, including *S. aureus* skin colonization.[11,12]

SKIN

The barrier function of the skin is mediated primarily by its outermost layer, the *stratum corneum,* which consists of keratinocytes and the lipid rich matrix that surrounds them. These lipids, particularly ceramides, inhibit microbial growth, as does the low pH environment they help to create. The lipid content and acidic pH of the skin are established postnatally, reaching maturity by 2 to 4 weeks in term neonates but at a later age in premature neonates. Epithelial integrity and the antimicrobial barrier this provides are easily disrupted at this age. The skin of neonates is also coated by a water, protein, and lipid-rich material, the vernix caseosa. The skin is rapidly colonized by environmental bacteria after birth, creating a normal flora of commensal bacteria that help to prevent colonization by pathogens. This flora normally consists of coagulase-negative staphylococci (e.g., *Staphylococcus epidermidis*), micrococci, and other species.[13] Commensal bacteria, such as *S. epidermidis,* may play a protective role in the skin by secreting lipopeptides that bind to Toll-like receptor 2 (TLR2) on neonatal keratinocytes and stimulating them to produce hBD-2 and hBD-3[14]; the role of TLRs in innate immunity is discussed in detail later. The organisms that make up the initial microbiota of the skin in newborns are heavily influenced by the mode of delivery,

Table 4-2 Immunoregulatory Effects of Select Cytokines, Chemokines, and Tumor Necrosis Factor (TNF) Ligand Family Proteins

Cytokine	Principal Cell Source	Major Biologic Effects
IFN-γ	T cells and NK cells	Pleiotropic, including enhancement of MΦ activation and antigen processing and MHC expression; promotes Th1 differentiation of activated CD4 T cells; regulates B-cell isotype switching
IL-1α, IL-1β	Many cell types; MΦ are a major source	Fever, inflammatory response, cofactor in T- and B-cell growth
IL-2	T cells	T-cell > B-cell growth, increased cytotoxicity by T and NK cells, increased cytokine production and sensitivity to apoptosis by T cells, growth and survival of regulatory T cells
IL-3	T cells	Growth of early hematopoietic precursors (also known as multi-CSF)
IL-4	T cells, mast cells, basophils, eosinophils	Required for IgE synthesis; enhances B-cell growth and MHC class II expression; promotes T-cell growth and Th2 differentiation, mast-cell growth factor; enhances endothelial VCAM-1 expression
IL-5	T cells, NK cells, mast cells, basophils, eosinophils	Eosinophil growth, differentiation, and survival
IL-6	MΦ, fibroblasts, T cells	Hepatic acute-phase protein synthesis, fever, T-cell and B-cell growth and differentiation
IL-7	Stromal cells of bone marrow and thymus	Essential thymocyte growth factor, promotes survival and homeostatic proliferation of peripheral T cells
IL-8 (CXCL8)	MΦ, endothelial cells, fibroblasts, epithelial cells, T cells	Chemotaxis and activation of neutrophils
IL-10	MΦ, T, cells, B cells, NK cells, keratinocytes, eosinophils	Inhibits cytokine production by T cells and mononuclear cell inflammatory function and MHC expression; promotes B-cell growth and isotype switching; inhibits NK-cell cytotoxicity
IL-12	DCs, MΦ	Induces Th1 and TFH differentiation of CD4 T cells
IL-13	T cells (Th2) and mast cells	Promotes B-cell isotype switching to IgE, mucous production by epithelial cells
IL-15	DCs, MΦ	Pleiotropic, including enhancement of NK-cell differentiation and survival and function of CD8 T cells
IL-21	T cells	Pleiotropic, including promotion of B-cell growth, plasma-cell differentiation, NK-cell cytotoxicity
IL-23	DCs, MΦ	Promotes Th17 differentiation of activated CD4 T cells
TNF-α	MΦ, T cells, NK cells	Fever and inflammatory response effects similar to IL-1, shock, hemorrhagic necrosis of tumors, and increased VCAM-1 expression on endothelium; induces catabolic state
CD40 ligand (CD154)	T cells, lower amounts by B cells and DCs	B-cell growth factor; promotes isotype switching, promotes IL-12 production by DCs; activates MΦ
Fas ligand	Activated T cells, NK cells retina, testicular epithelium	Induces apoptosis of cells expressing Fas, including effector B and T cells
Flt-3 ligand	Bone marrow stromal cells	Potent DC growth factor; promotes growth of myeloid and lymphoid progenitor cells in conjunction with other cytokines
G-CSF	MΦ, fibroblasts, epithelial cells	Growth of granulocyte precursors
GM-CSF	MΦ, endothelial cells, T cells	Growth of granulocyte-MΦ precursors and DCs; enhances granulocyte-MΦ function and B-cell antibody production
CCL3 (MIP-1α)	MΦ, T cells	MΦ chemoattractant; T-cell activator
CCL5 (RANTES)	MΦ, T cells, fibroblasts, epithelial cells	MΦ and memory T-cell chemoattractant; enhances T-cell activation; blocks HIV coreceptor
TGF-β	MΦ, T cells, fibroblasts, epithelial cells, others	Inhibits MΦ activation; inhibits Th1 T-cell responses

CSF, Colony-stimulating factor; *DC*, dendritic cell; *G-CSF*, granulocyte colony-stimulating factor; *GM-CSF*, granulocyte-macrophage colony-stimulating factor; *HIV*, human immunodeficiency virus; *IL*, interleukin; *MΦ*, mononuclear phagocytes; *MHC*, major histocompatibility complex; *MIP*, macrophage inhibitory protein; *NK*, natural killer; *RANTES*, regulated on activation, normal T-cell expressed and secreted; *TFH*, T-follicular helper; *TGF*, transforming growth factor; *Th1*, T helper 1; *Th17*, T helper 17; *VCAM-1*, vascular cell adhesion molecule-1.

with vaginally delivered infants acquiring bacterial communities similar to the vaginal microbiome.[15]

Antimicrobial peptides are expressed by neonatal keratinocytes and are present in the *vernix caseosa*. As in adults, the *stratum corneum* of skin from normal term neonates contains hBD-1.[16] By the end of the second trimester of gestation, fetal skin constitutively expresses hBD-3, psoriasin, and RNase7,[17] and neonatal skin expresses hBD-2 and LL-37,[16,18] which are absent or present only in very low amounts in the skin of normal adults. The mechanisms underlying the apparent constitutive production of hBD-2 and LL-37 by neonatal keratinocytes are not known, but their presence may help to provide an immediate barrier against bacterial invasion during the initial exposure of the neonate to environmental microbes. *Vernix caseosa* may augment skin defenses and contains HNPs 1 to 3 and additional antibacterial proteins, including lysozyme and psoriasin (S100A7).[19,20]

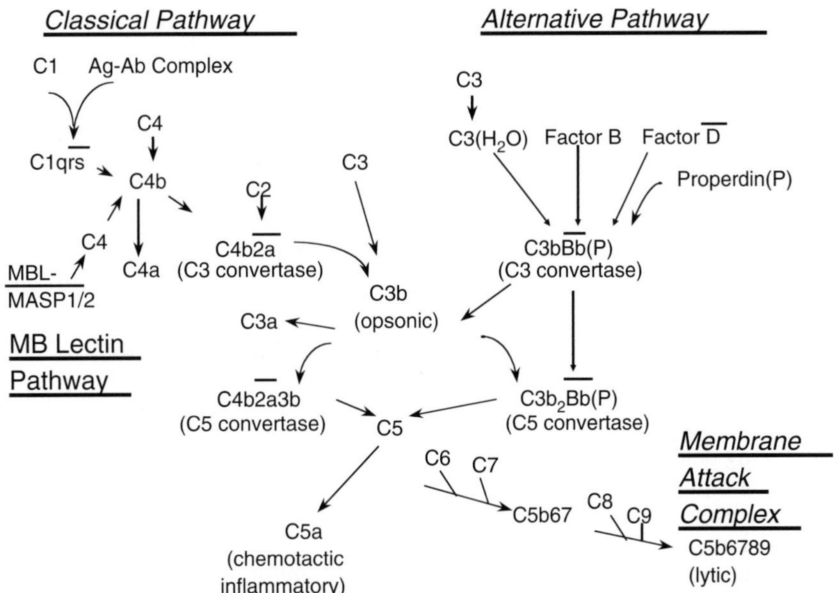

Figure 4-1 Complement activation. Classical and mannose-binding lectin (MBL) pathways of activation intersect with the alternative pathway at C3. The MBL pathway of activation is identical to the classical pathway, starting with the cleavage of C4. When C3 is activated, this is followed by activation of the terminal components, which generate the membrane attack complex (C5b6789). Enzymatically active proteases, which serve to cleave and activate subsequent components, are shown with an overbar.

THE GASTROINTESTINAL TRACT

The proximal gastrointestinal epithelium of the mouth and esophagus consists of a squamous epithelium, whereas the stomach, small intestine, and colon have a columnar epithelium with microvilli, which, along with intestinal peristalsis, help to maintain the longitudinal movement of fluid. The acidic pH of the stomach acts as a chemical barrier in adults. Gastric acidification is not yet fully developed in neonates, but digestion of milk lipids by gastric lipases may compensate in part by generating free fatty acids.[21] The gastrointestinal tract is coated with a mucin-rich glycocalyx, which forms a viscous coating that helps to protect the epithelium and to which commensal intestinal bacteria bind.[22] The composition of the intestinal glycocalyx in neonates differs from adults and may contribute to differences in commensal flora.

The application of high-throughput, comprehensive, culture-independent molecular approaches to assess microbial diversity has shown that the commensal intestinal flora of humans is a highly diverse ecologic system consisting of approximately 10^{14} microorganisms, representing the most abundant and diverse microbial community in our body and exceeding the numbers (by a factor of 10) and genetic content of human cells in an individual. In adults, colonic and stool flora are dominated by gram-negative anaerobic bacteria *(Bacteroides)* and one phylum of gram-positive bacteria (Firmicutes), whereas Actinobacteria, Proteobacteria, and Verrucomicrobia, although found in many people, are typically minor constituents, and aerobic gram-negative bacteria (e.g., *Escherichia coli*) are present in much lower abundance.[23] The composition of stool flora in the first year of life is highly dynamic. Based on a longitudinal study of 14 term infants from whom serial samples were collected from birth to 1 year of age, the flora of individual infants differs substantially from one infant to another in the first months of life, initially most closely resembling the maternal fecal, vaginal, or breast-milk flora.[24] In addition, the bacterial composition in infants is highly influenced by environmental factors, such as mode of delivery, geographic location, and life events, such as illness, antibiotic use, and changes in diet.[15,25,26] This interindividual variability typically diminishes over time and by 1 year of age converges on a pattern similar to that found in adults. As more data become available linking microbiota composition to disease states, there will be a better understanding of how such factors affect the intestinal flora and, perhaps modulate the risk for necrotizing enterocolitis (NEC) and other inflammatory, infectious or allergic diseases in neonates and infants.

The dynamic interaction between host and microbe in the gut has an important impact on nutrition, intestinal homeostasis and development of innate and adaptive immunity.[22] Such immunity, in turn, restricts these microbes to the gut and primes the immune system to respond properly to dangerous microbes. For example, recent murine studies have shown that commensal bacteria are important for systemically maintaining a relatively low threshold for activation in mononuclear phagocytes, which allows these cells to efficiently respond to systemic viral infection.[27] Commensal bacteria appear to act by helping to maintain the appropriate epigenetic structure of promoters of genes involved in the antiviral inflammatory response so that these genes can be efficiently expressed in response to innate immune receptor engagement.[28] Other murine studies have found a similar requirement of commensal bacteria for maintaining an appropriate threshold for DC function—in this case, the response to necrotic cells.[29] If this priming of innate immune function by commensals occurs in humans, which appears likely, then limitations in neonatal innate immune cellular function would be expected to be most prominent immediately after birth, with increases in function as the commensal flora is established postnatally.

At the same time, commensal bacteria dampen the response to the normal flora, harmless environmental antigens, and self-antigens to prevent self-injury. Certain intestinal epithelial cells play special roles in intestinal immunity: goblet cells produce mucus, Paneth cells (located at the base of small intestinal crypts) secrete antimicrobial factors, and M cells deliver, by transcytosis, a sample of the distal small intestinal microbiota to antigen-presenting DCs located beneath the epithelium; some DCs also directly sample the intestinal lumen of the distal small intestine.

The intestinal epithelium can directly recognize and respond to microbes using a limited set of invariant cell surface, endosomal, and cytosolic innate immune pattern recognition receptors, including TLRs and others described later. How commensals prime innate and adaptive immunity in the gut without inducing deleterious inflammation and how potentially dangerous pathogens are discriminated from harmless commensals is an area of active investigation. This is achieved in part by innate immune receptor location. For example, intestinal epithelial cells normally express few or no TLRs on their luminal surface, where they are in contact with commensals. Conversely, pathogens that invade through or between epithelial cells can be recognized by endosomal TLRs, cytosolic innate immune recognition receptors, and TLRs located on the basolateral surface of epithelial cells. Moreover, certain commensal bacteria inhibit signaling and inflammatory mediator production downstream of these receptors[22,30] or induce antiinflammatory cytokine production,[31] thereby actively suppressing gut inflammation. The importance of one of these antiinflammatory cytokines, IL-10, in maintaining intestinal immune homeostasis after birth has been dramatically demonstrated by patients with genetic immunodeficiencies of IL-10 or its receptor components, all of whom present with severe inflammatory bowel disease in early infancy.[32]

Adaptation of the intestinal epithelium to avoid unwarranted inflammatory responses to the normal flora is developmentally and/or environmentally regulated. Human 20- to 24-week fetal small intestinal organ cultures produced much more of the proinflammatory cytokine IL-8 (see Tables 4-1 and 4-2) when exposed to bacterial lipopolysaccharide (LPS) or IL-1 than similar cultures from infants or adults.[33] Developmental differences in inflammatory signaling may also contribute to aberrant intestinal inflammation in preterm neonates with NEC.[34] Recently, neonatal CD71^{+} erythroid cells in the mouse have been shown to have immunosuppressive properties to dampen immune activation in response to rapid colonization of microorganisms in the gut,[35] and it will be of interest to determine if these cells play a similar role in the human intestine.

Intestinal epithelial cells produce and secrete defensins and other antimicrobial factors. Epithelial cells of the esophagus, stomach, and colon constitutively produce hBD-1 and LL-37, and produce hBD-2, hBD-3, and hBD-4 in response to infection and inflammatory stimuli.[36] Intrinsic host defense of the small intestine is provided by Paneth cells, which constitutively produce HD-5 and lysozyme.[37] The abundance of HD-5 in the neonatal small intestine correlates with the abundance of Paneth cells, which are present but much less abundant in the midgestation fetus than at term and which, in turn, are much less abundant than in adults. These data suggest that intrinsic small intestinal defenses may be compromised in human neonates, particularly when preterm. However, a study in the mouse suggests another possibility. The intestinal epithelium of neonatal mice expresses abundant amounts of cathelicidin, which is lost by 14 days of postnatal age, by which time Paneth cells expressing murine defensins reach adult numbers.[38] Whether a similar "switch" in intestinal antimicrobial defenses occurs in humans is not known.

THE RESPIRATORY TRACT

The respiratory tract is second only to the gut in epithelial surface area. The upper airways and larger airways of the lung are lined by pseudostratified ciliated epithelial cells, with smaller numbers of mucin-producing goblet cells, whereas the alveoli are lined by nonciliated type I pneumocytes and by smaller numbers of surfactant-producing type II pneumocytes. Airway surface liquid and mucociliary clearance mechanisms provide an important first line of defense. Airway surface liquid contains a number of antimicrobial factors, including lysozyme, secretory leukoprotease inhibitor (SLPI), defensins and LL-37, and surfactant apoproteins A and D (SP-A, SP-D).[39] Collectively, these factors likely account for the lack of microbes in the lower respiratory tract of normal individuals.

Lung parenchymal cells express a diverse set of TLRs and other innate immune receptors. Lower airway epithelial cells express and respond to ligands for TLR2, TLR4, and TLR5,[40] whereas airway epithelial cells express TLR3, TLR7, and TLR9 primarily on the apical surface in the human trachea.[41] However, to our knowledge, there are no data carefully comparing TLR function in the airways of the human fetus and neonate versus human adults; data from neonatal sheep (and rodents) indicate developmental differences. TLR2 and TLR4 are expressed in the lungs of fetal sheep in the latter part of gestation: messenger RNA (mRNA) abundance increases from 20% of adult values at the beginning of the third trimester to 50% at term.[42] TLR4 mRNA was present in the airway epithelium and parenchyma, whereas TLR2 expression was found primarily in inflammatory cells after intraamniotic administration of LPS, which resulted in increased expression of TLR2 and TLR4. TLR3 expression was approximately 50% of adult values and unchanged in response to LPS. Similar developmental differences have been observed in mice.[43] In the human fetal lung, transcripts for TLR2, TLR3, TLR5, TLR6, TLR7, TLR8, and TLR10 increase between 3 months and 4 to 5 months of gestation, whereas TLR4 expression remains unchanged.[44] However, the relationship of these TLR mRNA levels to protein expression, the cellular sources of these transcripts, and the biologic activity of these TLRs during fetal development, which requires the presence of intracellular signaling adapters, for instance, MyD88 (myeloid differentiation primary response protein 88), and in some cases, accessory surface molecules, for instance, CD14 and MD2 for TLR4 signaling, remains unclear.

Airway epithelial cells express hBD-1 constitutively and hBD-2, hBD-3, hBD-4 ,and LL-37 in response to a variety of microbial stimuli and inflammatory cytokines, including IL-1.[6,39] Lung explants from term but not preterm fetuses expressed hBD-2 and smaller amounts of hBD-1 (although the amount even at term appeared to be less than at older ages) but did not contain hBD-3 mRNA.[45] By contrast, LL-37 mRNA was present and appeared not to vary at these ages. Consistent with these findings, tracheal aspirates from mechanically ventilated term, but not preterm neonates, contained hBD-2, whereas lower amounts of LL-37 were found, but these amounts were similar in aspirates from term and preterm neonates. However, another study found no difference in the abundance of hBD-1, hBD-2, and LL-37 in aspirates from ventilated neonates, ranging in ages from 22 to 40 weeks.[46]

Surfactant proteins SP-A and SP-D are produced by type II pneumocytes and by Clara cells, which are progenitors of ciliated epithelial cells located at the bronchoalveolar junction. SP-A and SP-D are members of the collectin family. Collectins are involved in both antimicrobial host defense as well as the clearance of apoptotic cells by human alveolar macrophages and other mononuclear phagocytes. Collectins bind to carbohydrates, including mannose, glucose, and fucose, found on the surface of gram-positive and gram-negative bacteria, yeasts, and some viruses, including RSV.[47] Once bound, collectins can result in aggregation of microbes, which may inhibit their growth or facilitate their mechanical removal, or they can opsonize microbes, that is, facilitate their ingestion by phagocytic cells. Mice lacking SP-A or SP-D have impaired lung clearance of group B streptococci (GBS), *Haemophilus influenzae, Pseudomonas aeruginosa,* and RSV.[48,49] SP-A and SP-D are detectable in human fetal lungs by 20 weeks of gestation,[50] and amounts appear to increase with increasing fetal maturity and in response to antenatal steroid administration.[51,52] Low levels of SP-A or SP-D are correlated with a higher risk of infection and the development of chronic lung disease in premature infants.[53]

SUMMARY

The skin of neonates, particularly preterm neonates, is more readily disrupted and lacks the protection provided by an acidic pH until approximately 1 month of postnatal age. Counterbalancing these factors is the constitutive production in neonates of a broader array of antimicrobial peptides by the skin epithelium and the presence of such peptides in the *vernix caseosa*. The lack of an acidic pH in the stomach may facilitate the establishment of the protective commensal flora, which at birth varies substantially from infant to infant, converging by 1 year of age to resemble adult flora. The lack of gastric acidity and diminished numbers of antimicrobial peptide-producing Paneth cells in the small intestine of preterm and, to a lesser degree, term neonates may increase their risk for enterocolitis and invasion by pathogens; these deficits may be counterbalanced by more robust production of antimicrobial peptides by other intestinal epithelial cells, but as yet, this has only been demonstrated in animal models. Innate defenses of the respiratory epithelium—TLRs, antimicrobial peptides, SP-A, and SP-D—mature in the last trimester. Consequently, these defenses may be compromised in preterm infants. Reduced numbers of resident alveolar macrophages may further impair lung innate defenses in preterm infants (see "Mononuclear Phagocytes").

Complement and Other Humoral Mediators of Innate Immunity

COLLECTINS, PENTRAXINS, AND FICOLINS

C-reactive protein (CRP) and mannose-binding lectin (MBL) are soluble proteins that can bind to structures found on the surface of microbes and infected or damaged host cells and facilitate their clearance by phagocytes. Both are produced by the liver. Their concentrations in the blood increase in response to infection and tissue injury as part of the acute-phase response, allowing them to contribute to early host defense to infection and the clearance of damaged cells.

CRP is a member of the pentraxin family of proteins,[54] which binds to phosphocholine and other lipids and carbohydrates on the surface of certain gram-positive bacteria, particularly *Streptococcus pneumoniae,* fungi, and apoptotic host cells. It does not cross the placenta. Term and preterm neonates can produce CRP as well as adults.[55] Values of CRP in cord blood from term infants are low, rising to concentrations found in adult blood in the first days of life, paralleling a postnatal increase in serum IL-6 and microbial colonization.[56]

MBL (like SP-A and SP-D described earlier) is a member of the collectin family and binds to carbohydrates, including mannose, glucose, and fucose, on the surface of bacteria, yeasts, and some viruses.[57] When bound, MBL activates complement and enhances phagocytosis by neutrophils and macrophages. Engagement of MBL is impeded by capsular polysaccharides of most virulent bacterial pathogens. MBL abundance in neonates is affected by three interacting variables: MBL genotype, gestational age, and postnatal age. In neonates with a MBL genotype lacking mutations, MBL concentrations are 50% to 75% of those in adults and reach adult values by 7 to 10 days and 20 weeks of age in term and preterm neonates, respectively.[58,59] Concentrations are more than fivefold lower, and these increases are less evident in those with variant MBL genotypes. Preterm neonates with low concentrations of MBL found in those with variant genotypes appear to be at greater risk for sepsis or pneumonia.[59-61]

Ficolins are multimeric lectins and come in three forms: L-ficolin (ficolin-2), which is made by the liver; H-ficolin (ficolin-3), which is produced by the liver and lung; and M-ficolin (ficolin-1), which is produced by mononuclear phagocytes. All three ficolins are detectable in serum and can activate the lectin-dependent complement pathway, which is described later. Ficolins recognize acetylated compounds, including *N*-acetyl-glucosamine, *N*-acetyl-galactosamine, *N*-acetylneuraminic acid, and sialic acid and bind bacteria, such as *S. aureus,* GBS, *Salmonella,* and *E. coli.*[62,63] Although serum levels of ficolins are highly variable, in one study,[64] all three ficolins were in lower concentration in prematurely born infants compared with term neonates and older children and adults; only M-ficolin in children older than 1 year and H-ficolin in term neonates and children were comparable to the values found in adults. However, despite these differences, there were still substantial levels of all three ficolins in premature infants, and it is unclear to what extent these modest decreases limit lectin-dependent complement activation and predispose to neonatal bacteremia and sepsis.[65]

COMPLEMENT

The complement system is composed of serum proteins that can be activated sequentially through one of three pathways—the classical, MBL, and alternative pathways, each of which leads to the generation of activated C3, C3, and C5 convertases and the membrane attack complex (see Fig. 4-1).[66]

Classical and Mannose-Binding Lectin Pathways

Activation of the classical pathway is initiated when antibodies capable of engaging C1q to their Fc portion (immunoglobulin M [IgM], IgG1, IgG2, and IgG3 in humans) complex with microbial (or other) antigens. After C1q binds to the immune complex, there is sequential binding of C1r and C1s to C1q. C1s can then cleave C4, followed by C2, and the larger fragments of these bind covalently to the surface of the microbe or particle, forming the classical pathway C3 convertase (C2aC4b). C3 convertase cleaves C3, thereby liberating C3b, which binds to the microbe or particle, and C3a, which is released into the fluid phase. This pathway can also be activated directly by CRP. When CRP binds to the surface of a microbe, its conformation is altered such that it can bind C1q and activate the classical pathway.[67] Similarly, when MBL or ficolins engage the surface of a microbe, their confirmation is altered, creating a binding site for mannose-binding lectin–associated serine protease (MASP)1 and MASP2.[68] MASP2, in turn, cleaves C4 and C2, leading to the formation of the C3 convertase.[63] Independently of their activation of downstream complement components, Clq and MBL can also bind apoptotic cells and initiate their uptake into mononuclear phagocytes by macropinocytosis.[69]

Alternative Pathway

The alternative pathway is activated constitutively by the continuous low-level hydrolysis of C3 in solution, creating a binding site for factor B. This complex is in turn cleaved by factor D, generating C3b and Bb. If C3b and Bb bind to a microorganism, they form a more efficient system, which binds and activates additional C3 molecules, depositing C3b on the microbe and liberating C3a into the fluid phase. This interaction is facilitated by factor P (properdin) and inhibited by alternative pathway factors H and I. The classical pathway, by creating particle-bound C3b, also can activate the alternative pathway, thereby amplifying complement activation. This amplification step may be particularly important in the presence of small amounts of antibody. Bacteria vary in their capacity to activate the alternative pathway, which is determined by their ability to bind C3b and to protect the complex of C3b and Bb from the inhibitory effects of factors H and I. Sialic acid, a component of many bacterial polysaccharide capsules, including those of GBS and *E. coli* K1, favors factor H binding. Thus many bacterial pathogens are protected from the alternative pathway by their capsules and/or by proteins that bind to factor H. Antibody is needed for efficient opsonization of such organisms.

Terminal Components, Membrane Attack Complex, and Biologic Consequences of Complement Activation

Binding of C3b on the microbial surface facilitates microbial killing or removal through the interaction of C3b with CR1 receptors on phagocytes. C3b also is cleaved to C3bi, which binds to the CR3 receptor (Mac-1, Cd11b-CD18) and CR4 receptor (CD11c-CD18). C3bi receptors are β_2 integrins, which are present on neutrophils, mononuclear phagocytes, and certain other cell types and also play a role in leukocyte adhesion. Along with IgG antibody, which binds to Fcγ receptors on phagocytes, C3b and C3bi promote phagocytosis and killing of bacteria and fungi. Bound C3b, together with C4b and C2a or together with Bb, form C5 convertases, which cleave C5. The smaller fragment, C5a, is released into solution. The larger fragment, C5b, triggers the recruitment of the terminal components, C6 to C9, which together form the membrane attack complex. This complex is assembled in lipid-containing cell membranes, which include the outer membrane of gram-negative bacteria and the plasma membrane of infected host cells. Once assembled in the membrane, this complex can lyse the cell. Such lysis appears to be a central defense mechanism against meningococcal and systemic gonococcal infection. Certain gram-negative organisms have mechanisms to impede complement-mediated lysis, and gram-positive bacteria are intrinsically resistant to complement-mediated lysis because they do not have an outer membrane.

The soluble fragment of C5, C5a, and, to a more limited degree, C3a and C4a cause vasodilatation and increase vascular permeability. C5a also is a potent chemotactic factor for phagocytes. In addition to these roles for complement in innate immunity, complement facilitates B-cell responses to T-cell–dependent antigens as discussed in the section B-Cell Activation and Immune Selection.

Complement in the Fetus and Neonate

Complement components are synthesized by hepatocytes and, for some components, also by macrophages. Little, if any, maternal complement is transferred to the fetus. Fetal synthesis of complement components can be detected in tissues as early as 6 to 14 weeks of gestation, depending on the specific complement component and tissue examined.[70]

Table 4-3 summarizes published reports on classical pathway complement activity (CH_{50}) and alternative pathway complement activity (AP_{50}) and individual complement components in neonates. Substantial individual variability is seen, and in many term neonates, values of individual complement components or of CH_{50} or AP_{50} are within the adult range. Alternative pathway activity and components are more consistently decreased than are classical pathway activity and components. The most marked deficiency is in the terminal complement component C9, which correlates with poor killing of gram-negative bacteria by serum from neonates. The C9 deficiency in neonatal serum appears to be a more important factor in the inefficient killing of *E. coli* K1 than the deficiency in antigen-specific IgG antibodies.[71] Preterm infants demonstrate a greater and more consistent decrease in both classical and alternative pathway complement activity and components.[72] Mature but small-for-gestational-age infants have values similar to those for healthy term infants.[73] The concentration of most complement proteins increases postnatally and reaches adult values by 6 to 18 months of age.[74]

Opsonization is the process whereby soluble factors present in serum or other body fluids bind to the surface

Table 4-3 Summary of Published Complement Levels in Neonates

	MEAN % OF ADULT LEVELS	
Complement Component	**Term Neonate**	**Preterm Neonate**
CH_{50}	56-90 (5)*	45-71 (4)
AP_{50}	49-65 (4)	40-55 (3)
Clq	61-90 (4)	27-58 (3)
C4	60-100 (5)	42-91 (4)
C2	76-100 (3)	67-96 (2)
C3	60-100 (5)	39-78 (4)
C5	73-75 (2)	67 (1)
C6	47-56 (2)	36 (1)
C7	67-92 (2)	72 (1)
C8	20-36 (2)	29 (1)
C9	<20-52 (3)	<20-41 (2)
B	35-64 (4)	36-50 (4)
P	33-71 (6)	16-65 (3)
H	61 (1)	—
C3bi	55 (1)	—

Data from Johnston RB, Stroud RM: Complement and host defense against infection, *J Pediatr* 90:169-179, 1977; Notarangelo LD, Chirico G, Chiara A, et al: Activity of classical and alternative pathways of complement in preterm and small for gestational age infants, *Pediatr Res* 18:281-285, 1984; Davis CA, Vallota EH, Forristal J: Serum complement levels in infancy: age related changes, *Pediatr Res* 13:1043-1046, 1979; Lassiter HA, Watson SW, Seifring ML, et al: Complement factor 9 deficiency in serum of human neonates, *J Infect Dis* 166:53-57, 1992; Wolach B, Dolfin T, Regev R, et al: The development of the complement system after 28 weeks' gestation, *Acta Paediatr* 86:523-527, 1997; and Zilow G, Brussau J, Hauck W, et al: Quantitation of complement component C9 deficiency in term and preterm neonates, *Clin Exp Immunol* 97:52-59, 1994.
*Number of studies.

of microbes (or other particles) and thereby enhance their phagocytosis and killing. Some organisms are effective activators of the alternative pathway, whereas others require antibody to activate complement. Thus, depending on the organism, opsonic activity reflects antibody, MBL, ficolin, CRP, classical or alternative complement pathway activity, or combinations of these. Accordingly, it is not surprising that the efficiency with which neonatal sera opsonize organisms is quite variable. For example, although opsonization of *S. aureus* was normal in neonatal sera in all studies, opsonization of GBS, *S. pneumoniae, E. coli,* and other gram-negative rods was decreased against some strains and in some studies but not in others.[75]

Neonatal sera generally are less able to opsonize organisms in the absence of antibody.[75] This difference is compatible with deficits in the function of the alternative and MBL pathways and with the moderate reduction in alternative pathway components. This difference is not due to a reduced ability of neonatal sera to initiate complement activation through the alternative pathway. Neonatal sera also are less able to opsonize some strains of GBS in a classical pathway–dependent but antibody-independent manner. The deficit in antibody-independent opsonization is accentuated in sera from premature neonates, in whom there is significantly reduced levels of circulating MBL, MASP, and all three ficolins[64] and may be further impaired by the depletion of complement components in septic neonates.

Sera from term neonates generate less chemotactic activity than adult sera. This diminished activity reflects a defect in complement activation rather than lack of antibody.[76,77] These observations notwithstanding, preterm and term neonates do generate substantial amounts of activated complement products in response to infection in vivo.[78]

SUMMARY

Compared with adults, neonates have moderately diminished alternative complement pathway activity, slightly diminished classical complement pathway activity, and decreased abundance of some terminal complement components. Neonates with much reduced concentrations of MBL resulting from genetic variation and prematurity appear to be at greater risk for sepsis or pneumonia. Consistent with these findings, neonatal sera are less effective than adult sera in opsonization when concentrations of specific antibody are limiting and in the generation of complement-derived chemotactic activity; these differences are greater in preterm than in term neonates. These deficiencies, in concert with phagocyte deficits described later, may contribute to delayed inflammatory responses and impaired bacterial clearance in neonates.

Phagocytes

HEMATOPOIESIS

Phagocytes as well as all leukocytes of the immune system are derived from self-renewing, pluripotent hematopoietic stem cells (HSCs), which have the capacity for indefinite self-renewal (Fig. 4-2). Most circulating HSCs in cord blood and adult bone marrow are identified by their $CD34^+CD45^+CD133^+CD143^+$ surface phenotype, combined with a lack of expression of CD38 and markers found on specific lineages of mature leukocytes; for instance, they lack CD3, a T-cell marker, and are thus CD34 positive and lineage-marker negative ($CD34^+Lin^-$).[79] HSCs are generated during ontogeny from embryonic para-aortic tissue, fetal liver, and bone marrow.[80] The yolk sac, which is extraembryonic, is a major site of production of primitive erythrocytes and some primitive mononuclear phagocytes, starting at about the third week of embryonic development. HSCs that give rise to both erythrocyte and all nonerythroid hematopoietic cell lineages appear in the fetal liver after 4 weeks of gestation and in the bone marrow by 11 weeks of gestation. Liver-mediated hematopoiesis ceases by 20 weeks of gestation, with the bone marrow becoming the sole site of hematopoiesis thereafter. All major lineages of hematopoietic cells that are part of the immune system are present in the human by the beginning of the second trimester.

HSCs can subsequently differentiate into common lymphoid progenitors or common myeloid-erythroid progenitors (see Fig. 4-2). Common lymphoid progenitors give rise to T, B, and natural killer (NK) lymphocytes, which will be discussed in later sections of this chapter. Common myeloid-erythroid progenitors give rise to the megakaryocyte, erythroid, and myeloid lineages. Myeloid and lymphoid cells represent the two largely distinct but functionally

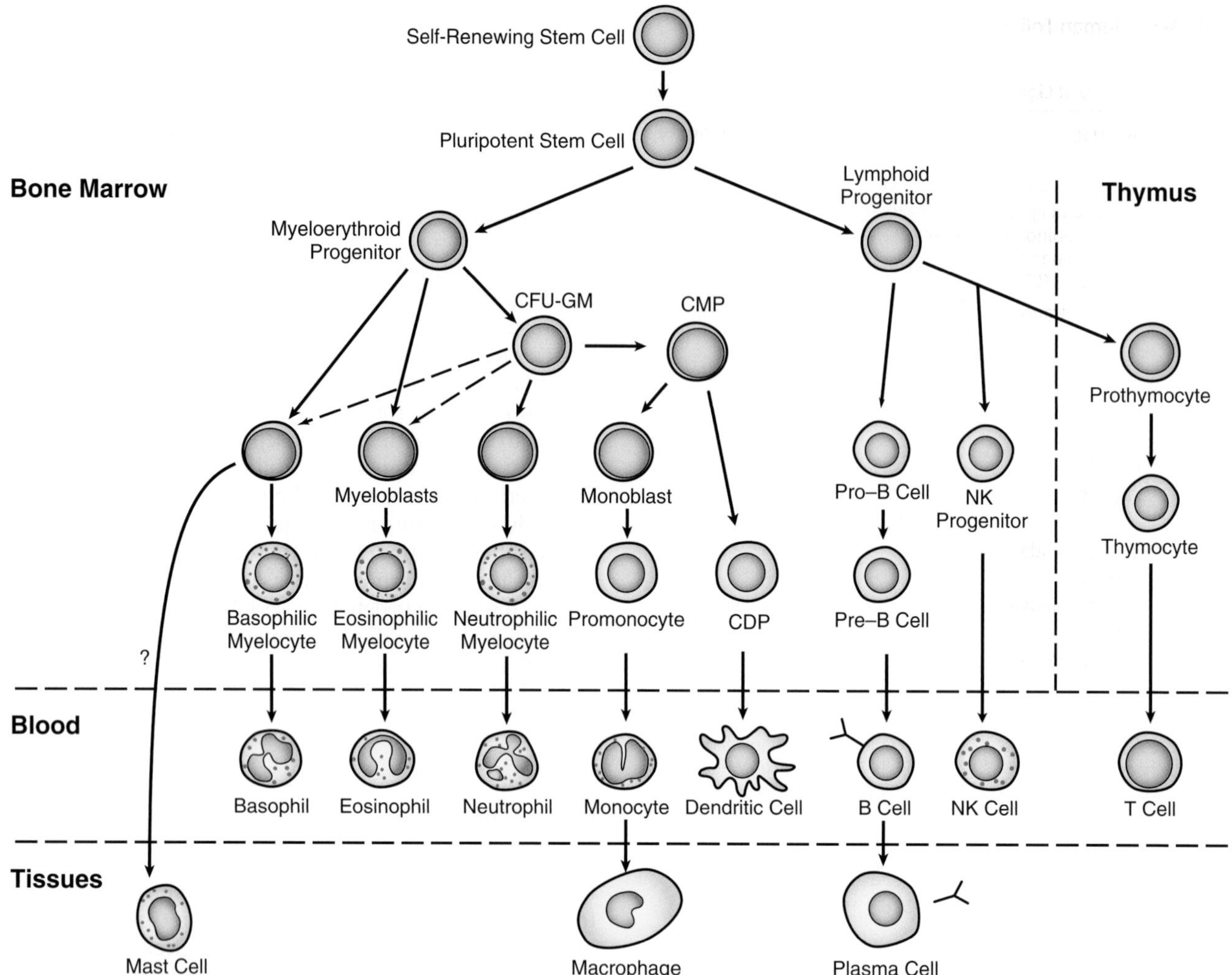

Figure 4-2 Myeloid and lymphoid differentiation and the tissue compartments in which they occur. *CDP*, Committed dendritic cell progenitor; *CFU-GM*, colony-forming unit–granulocyte-macrophage; *CMP*, common myeloid progenitor; *NK*, natural killer.

interrelated immune cell lineages, with DCs, which are myeloid derived, providing a key functional bridge between these lineages (see "Dendritic Cells" later).

As was first described in mice and birds, fetal HSCs and adult HSCs in humans appear to give rise to T-cell populations that have distinct properties. For example, HSCs of the second trimester of pregnancy give rise to naïve CD4 T cells that have many features of regulatory T cells (see "Regulatory T Cells" in the "T Cells and Antigen Presentation" section), whereas those of the adult give rise to naïve CD4 T cells that tend to become effector cells rather than regulatory cells.[81] This appears to be a cell-intrinsic property of fetal versus adult HSCs,[81] and it is possible that other HSC derivatives, such as monocytes[82] and NK cells,[83] may also differ between the fetus and adult because of these developmentally related cell-intrinsic properties.

PHAGOCYTE PRODUCTION BY THE BONE MARROW

Phagocytes are derived from a common precursor myeloid stem cell, which often is referred to as the colony-forming unit–granulocyte-monocyte (CFU-GM) (see Fig. 4-2). The formation of myeloid stem cells from pluripotent HSCs and further differentiation of the myeloid precursor into mature granulocytes and monocytes are governed by bone marrow stromal cells and soluble colony-stimulating factors (CSFs) and other cytokines (see Table 4-2).[80] In response to an infectious or inflammatory stimulus, the production of granulocyte-specific colony-stimulating factor (G-CSF), granulocyte-macrophage–specific colony-stimulating factor (GM-CSF), and certain other cytokines is increased, resulting in increased production and release of granulocytes and monocytes. Similarly, when given exogenously, these factors enhance production and function of the indicated cell lineages.

INNATE IMMUNE PATTERN RECOGNITION RECEPTORS USED BY LEUKOCYTES

Monocytes, macrophages, DCs, neutrophils, and other cells of the innate immune system use invariant innate immune pattern receptors to discriminate between microbes and self, or things that are "dangerous" or are not. These receptors recognize microbial structures (commonly referred to as pathogen-associated molecular patterns [PAMPs] and

Table 4-4 Human Toll-like Receptors (TLRs)

TLR	Microbial Ligands	Site of Interaction with Ligand	Signal Transduction/Effector Molecules	Expression by Antigen-Presenting Cells
TLR1	See TLR2	Cell surface	MyD88-dependent induction of cytokines	Monocytes and B cells > cDCs
TLR2	Bacterial peptidoglycan, lipoteichoic acid and lipopeptides; mycobacterial lipoarabinomannan, recognition of some ligands is mediated by TLR2/TLR1 or TLR2/TLR6 heterodimers	Cell surface	MyD88-dependent induction of cytokines	Monocytes and cDCs > B cells
TLR3	Double-stranded RNA	Endosome	TRIF-dependent induction of type I IFNs and cytokines	cDCs
TLR4	LPS, RSV	Cell surface	MyD88-dependent and TRIF-dependent induction of cytokines; TRIF-dependent induction of type I IFNs	Monocytes > cDCs
TLR5	Flagellin	Cell surface	MyD88-induction of cytokines	Monocytes > cDCs
TLR6	See TLR2	Cell surface	MyD88-dependent induction of cytokines	Monocytes and cDCs, B cells > pDCs
TLR7	Single-stranded RNA, imidazoquinoline drugs	Endosome	MyD88-dependent induction of type I IFNs and cytokines	pDCs and B cells >> cDCs > monocytes
TLR8	Single-stranded RNA, imidazoquinoline drugs	Endosome	MyD88-dependent induction of type I IFNs and cytokines	Monocytes and cDCs >> B cells
TLR9	Unmethylated CpG DNA	Endosome	MyD88-dependent induction of cytokines and type I IFNs	pDCs and B cells
TLR10	Viral RNA-protein complexes	Unknown	Unknown	Monocytes (postviral infection), B cells > cDCs and pDCs

cDCs, Conventional dendritic cells; *CpG*, cytosine-guanine dinucleotide; *IFN*, interferon; *LPS*, lipopolysaccharide; *MyD88*, myeloid differentiation primary response protein 88; *pDCs*, plasmacytoid dendritic cells; *RSV*, respiratory syncytial virus; *TLR*, Toll-like receptor; *TRIF*, TIR-domain-containing adaptor-inducing interferon-β.

danger-associated molecular patterns [DAMPS]), produced by infected or injured host cells—molecules such as uric acid, adenosine triphosphate (ATP), heat shock proteins (HSPs), and high-mobility group box 1 (HMGB1) protein. Recognition is followed by signals that activate the innate immune response.

Toll-like Receptors

Toll-like receptors are a family of structurally related proteins and are the most extensively characterized set of innate immune pattern recognition receptors. Ten different TLRs have been defined in humans.[84] Their distinct ligand specificities, subcellular localization, and patterns of expression by specific cell types are shown in Table 4-4.

TLR4 forms a functional LPS receptor with myeloid differentiation (MD-2) protein, a soluble protein required for surface expression of the TLR4/MD-2 receptor complex. CD14, which is expressed abundantly on the surface of monocytes and also exists in a soluble form in the plasma, facilitates recognition by the TLR4/MD-2 complex and is essential for recognition of smooth LPS present on pathogenic gram-negative bacteria. TLR2, which forms a heterodimer with TLR1 or TLR6, recognizes bacterial lipopeptides, lipoteichoic acid, and peptidoglycan, and this recognition is facilitated by CD14. TLR2 has a central role in the recognition of gram-positive bacteria and also contributes to recognition of fungi, including *Candida* species.[84] TLR5 recognizes bacterial flagellin. Consistent with their role in recognition of microbial cell surface structures, these TLRs are displayed on the cell surface.

By contrast, TLRs 3, 7, 8, and 9 recognize nucleic acids: TLR3 binds double-stranded RNA, TLR7 and TLR8 bind single-stranded RNA, and TLR9 binds nonmethylated cytosine-guanine dinucleotide (CpG)-containing DNA. These TLRs appear primarily to function in antiviral recognition and defense,[85] and TLR9 also contributes to defense against bacteria and fungi.[86,87] These TLRs preferentially recognize features of nucleic acids that are more common in microbes than mammals, but their specificity may be as much based on location as nucleic sequence: TLRs 3, 7, 8, and 9 detect nucleic acids in a location where they should not be found—acidified late endolysosomes.[85] Individuals lacking TLR3; TRIF (TIR-domain–containing adaptor-inducing interferon-β), which is required for intracellular signaling by TLR3; or a protein UNC93B, required for proper localization of TLRs 3, 7, 8, and 9 to endosomes, are unduly susceptible to infection with herpesviruses, particularly primary herpes simplex encephalitis.[88]

A conserved cytoplasmic Toll/IL-1 receptor (TIR) domain links TLRs to downstream signaling pathways by interacting with adaptor proteins, including myeloid differentiation primary response protein 88 (MyD88) and TRIF. MyD88 is involved in signaling downstream of all TLRs with the exception of TLR3, which signals solely through TRIF. TLR signaling via MyD88 leads to the activation and translocation of the transcription factor nuclear factor kappa B (NF-κB) to the nucleus and to the induction or activation by extracellular signal-regulated kinase (ERK)/p38/c-Jun *N*-terminal kinase (JNK)/mitogen-activated protein kinases (MAPK) of other transcription factors, resulting in the production of the proinflammatory cytokines, including TNF-α, IL-1, and IL-6. Production of the antiinflammatory and immunomodulatory cytokine IL-10 is dependent on signal transducer and activator of transcription 3 (STAT3) activation in addition to NF-κB and MAPK activation.[89]

In addition to these transcription factors, activation of interferon regulatory factor 3 (IRF3) and/or IRF7 is required for the induction of type I interferons (IFNs), which are key mediators of antiviral innate immunity.[90] Activation of IRF3 and the production of type I IFNs downstream of TLR4 are dependent on TRIF. TRIF is also essential for the activation of IRF3 and for the production of type I IFNs and other cytokines via TLR3. Conversely, TLRs 7, 8, and 9 use the adaptor MyD88 to activate IRF7 and to induce the production of type I IFNs and other cytokines. Consistent with their role in detection of bacterial but not viral structures, TLR2 and TLR5 do not induce type I IFNs.

The production of IL-12 and IL-27 (but not of the structurally related cytokine IL-23) is, like the production of type I IFNs, dependent on IRF3 and IRF7.[90,91] Consequently, signals via TLR3, TLR4, and TLR7/8, but not via TLR2 and TLR5, can induce the production of these two cytokines; by contrast, each of these TLRs, except TLR3, which signals exclusively via TRIF, can induce the production of IL-23. IL-23 promotes the production of IL-17 and IL-22, which contribute to host defenses to extracellular bacterial and fungal pathogens, whereas IL-12 and IL-27 stimulate interferon-gamma (IFN-γ) production by NK cells and thereby facilitate defense against viruses and other intracellular pathogens. Thus, through the concerted regulation of IL-12, IL-27, and type I IFNs, IRF3 and IRF7 link TLR recognition to host defenses against intracellular pathogens.

Recent studies have also found that engagement of TLR7 and/or TLR8 can induce the production of high levels of IL-1β in a caspase-1–dependent manner in monocytes and DCs.[92-94] As discussed immediately below, IL-1β secretion in response to many non-TLR stimuli involves the activation of caspase-1 by the inflammasome and the caspase-1–dependent cleavage of pro–IL-1β,[95] but it is unclear if caspase-1 activation by the TLR7/8 pathway involves the inflammasome or a novel mechanism.

Nucleotide-Binding Domain– and Leucine-Rich Repeat–Containing Receptors (NLRs)

NLRs are a family of 22 proteins in humans, most of which play a role in innate immunity activation in response to microbial products or endogenously derived danger signals.[95] These include nucleotide oligomerization domain 1 (NOD1), NOD2, and NLRP3 (also known as NALP3), which recognize components of bacterial peptidoglycan; NLRP3 is also involved in responses to components of gram-positive bacteria, including bacterial RNA and DNA, products of injured host cells such as uric acid, and noninfectious foreign substances, including asbestos and aluminum salts, which are widely used as the adjuvant alum[96]; NOD-like receptor C4 (NLRC4) (also known as IL-1-converting enzyme protease activating factor, or IPAF) is involved in responses to *Salmonella* and, like TLR5, the PAMP recognized is flagellin.[96] NOD1 and NOD2 can activate MAP kinase and NF-κB pathways and proinflammatory cytokines in synergy with TLRs. By contrast, NLRP3 interacts with the mitochondrial antiviral signaling (MAVS) adaptor protein to activate the inflammasome, a protein platform that activates caspase-1, which, in turn, cleaves pro–IL-1 and pro–IL-18, allowing the secretion of the mature forms of these inflammatory cytokines.[97] NLRC4 directly binds to caspase-1 and induces its activation.[97] In addition to leading to IL-1 and IL-18 secretion, caspase-1 activation results in pores in the cell membrane and, as a consequence, a form of cell death known as pyroptosis.

Three NLR members that are not associated with inflammasomes—CTIIA, NLRC5, and NLRP10—have distinct roles in augmenting antigen presentation rather than in regulating innate immunity responses: CTIIA (class II activator) is a transcriptional coactivator that is essential for the upregulation of major histocompatibility complex (MHC) class II expression by IFN-γ[98]; NLRC5, also known as CITA, plays an analogous role for the IFN-γ–dependent enhancement of the MHC class I antigen presentation pathway by augmenting transcription of the MHC class I heavy and light chain genes and transporter associated with antigen processing (TAP)-1;[99] NLRP10 appears to play an essential role in the migration of DCs from inflamed tissues via afferent lymphatics to the TD areas of draining lymph nodes.[100]

Retinoic Acid–Inducible Gene-I–Like Receptors

There are three members of the retinoic acid–inducible gene-I (RIG)-I–like receptor (RLR) family: RIG-I, melanoma-differentiation–associated protein (MDA-5), and Laboratory of Genetics and Physiology 2 (LGP2).[101] RLRs are present in the cytoplasm of nearly all mammalian cells, where they provide rapid, cell-intrinsic, antiviral surveillance. RIG-I is important for host resistance to a wide variety of RNA viruses, including influenza, parainfluenza, and hepatitis C virus, whereas MDA-5 is important for resistance to picornaviruses. RIG-I and MDA-5 interact with a common signaling adaptor (MAVS or IFN-β–promoter stimulator 1 [IPS-1]), which, like TRIF in the TLR3/4 pathway, induces the phosphorylation of IRF3 to stimulate type I IFN production.

C-Type Lectin Receptors

C-type lectin receptors (CLRs) are a family of surface proteins, which include DC-SIGN (dendritic cell–specific ICAM-3–grabbing nonintegrin), a receptor on DCs that is involved in their interaction with human immunodeficiency virus (HIV); the macrophage mannose receptor; dectin-1 and dectin-2, which are expressed by DCs and macrophages; and CLEC9A, which facilitates the uptake of necrotic material by DCs.[102,103] Dectin-1 and dectin-2 bind to fungi, such as *Candida*, and activate cytokine production by a signaling pathway that involves the spleen tyrosine kinase (Syk) and caspase activation and recruitment domain 9 (CARD9),[104] an adaptor protein that links Syk activity to the induction of NF-κB and activator protein-1 (AP-1), resulting in the production of cytokines. The recognition by dectins of the hyphal forms of fungi, which is indicative of invasion rather than colonization of a tissue,[105] results in the preferential induction of cytokines, for instance, IL-1β, IL-6, and IL-23, that favor naïve CD4 T cells recognizing fungal antigens differentiating into Th17 cells. The secretion of IL-1β after dectin-1 engagement involves the processing of pro–IL-1β via a novel caspase-8 inflammasome rather than a canonical caspase-1–containing inflammasome.[106] The importance of this pathway for fungal host defense is illustrated by the patients prone to opportunistic fungal infection who have genetic deficiencies of dectin, CARD9, or IL-17.[107]

Cytoplasmic DNA Receptors

Cytoplasmic receptors for double-stranded DNA are found in leukocytes and other cell types that, upon binding of DNA, lead to the production of type I IFNs. The best characterized of these receptors involves cyclic guanosine monophosphate–adenosine monophosphate (GMP-AMP) synthase (cGAS) coupled with the STING (stimulator of interferon genes) adaptor protein.[108] Upon DNA binding, cGAS synthesizes a novel cyclic dinucleotide, cyclic guanosine monophosphate–adenosine monophosphate (cGAMP), that binds to STING, which, in turn, activates kinase pathways that result in IRF3 phosphorylation and its translocation to the nucleus where type I IFN transcription is induced. The source of the DNA can be viral or bacterial and, unlike TLR9 DNA recognition, there is no preference for a particular nucleotide sequence, and the cytosine methylation status of CpGs also does not influence receptor activity. STING may also be coupled with other mammalian cytoplasmic DNA receptors, such as DDX41, but their role in host defense versus that of cGAS remains unclear.[109] STING and innate immune responses can also be directly triggered by cyclic dinucleotides that are generated by bacteria, for instance, during intracellular infection with *Listeria monocytogenes*, but are biochemically distinct from the cyclic dinucleotides generated by cGAS.

Decoding the Nature of the Threat Through Combinatorial Receptor Engagement

The differing molecular components of specific microbes result in the engagement of different combinations of innate immune recognition receptors. The innate immune system uses combinatorial receptor recognition patterns to decode the nature of the microbe and then tailors the ensuing early innate response and the subsequent antigen-specific response to combat that specific type of infection. Extracellular bacteria engage TLRs 2, 4, and/or 5 on the cell surface and also activate NLRs, providing a molecular signature of this type of pathogen. This leads to the production of proinflammatory cytokines and IL-23 to recruit neutrophils and support the development of a T-helper (Th)17-type T-cell response (see "Differentiation of Activated Naïve T Cells into Effector and Memory Cells"). Fungal products engage TLR2 and dectins, leading to a similar response.[104,110] Conversely, virus recognition via TLRs 3, 7, 8, 9, and RLRs (for RNA viruses) and cGAS/STING (for DNA viruses) stimulates the production of type I IFNs and IFN-induced chemokines (e.g., CXCL10), which, in turn, induce and recruit CD8 and Th1 CD4 T cells. Nonviral intracellular bacterial pathogens also induce type I IFNs, such as via the TLR9 and cGAS/STING pathways, which collaborate with signals from cell surface TLRs and NLRs to induce the production of IL-12, resulting in Th1-type responses. The importance of these innate sensing mechanisms is underscored by strategies that pathogenic microbes have evolved to evade them and the mediators they induce.

NEUTROPHILS

Production

Polymorphonuclear leukocytes or granulocytes, including neutrophils, eosinophils, and basophils, are derived from CFU-GM. Neutrophils are the principal cells of interest in relation to defense against pyogenic pathogens. The first identifiable committed neutrophil precursor is the myeloblast, which sequentially matures into myelocytes, metamyelocytes, bands, and mature neutrophils. Myelocytes and more mature neutrophilic granulocytes cannot replicate and constitute the postmitotic neutrophil storage pool. The postmitotic neutrophil storage pool is an important reserve because these cells can be rapidly released into the circulation in response to inflammation. Mature neutrophils enter the circulation, where they remain for approximately 8 to 10 hours and are distributed equally and dynamically between circulating cells and those cells adherent to the vascular endothelium. After leaving the circulation, neutrophils do not recirculate and die after approximately 24 hours. Release of neutrophils from the marrow may be enhanced in part by cytokines, including IL-1, IL-17, and TNF-α, in response to infection or inflammation.

Neutrophil precursors are detected at the end of the first trimester, appearing somewhat later than macrophage precursors.[111] Mature neutrophils are first detected by 14 to 16 weeks of gestation, but at midgestation, the numbers of postmitotic neutrophils in the fetal liver and bone marrow remain markedly lower than in term newborns and adults.[112] By term, the numbers of circulating neutrophil precursors are 10- to 20-fold higher in the fetus and neonate than in the adult, and neonatal bone marrow also contains an abundance of neutrophil precursors.[113] However, the rate of proliferation of neutrophil precursors in the human neonate appears to be near maximal,[114] suggesting that the capacity to increase numbers in response to infection may be limited.

At birth, neutrophil counts are lower in preterm than term neonates and in neonates born by cesarean section without labor. Within hours of birth, the numbers of circulating neutrophils increase sharply.[115,116] The number of neutrophils normally peaks shortly thereafter, whereas the fraction of neutrophils that are immature (bands and less mature forms) remains constant at about 15%. Peak counts occur at approximately 8 hours in infants born at greater than 28 weeks gestation and at approximately 24 hours in those born at less than 28 weeks gestation, then decline to a stable level by approximately 72 hours in those born without complications. Thereafter, the lower limit of normal for term and preterm neonates is approximately 2500 and 1000 per μL, respectively, and the upper limit of normal is approximately 7000 per μL for both term and preterm neonates.

Values may be influenced by a number of additional factors. Most important is the response to sepsis. Septic infants may have normal or increased neutrophil counts. Sepsis and other perinatal complications, including maternal hypertension, periventricular hemorrhage, and severe asphyxia, can cause neutropenia, however, and severe or fatal sepsis often is associated with persistent neutropenia, particularly in preterm neonates.[117] Neutropenia may be associated with increased margination of circulating neutrophils, which occurs early in response to infection. However, neutropenia that is sustained often reflects depletion of the neonate's limited postmitotic neutrophil storage pool. Septic neutropenic neonates in whom the neutrophil storage pool is depleted are more likely to die than are those with normal neutrophil storage pools.[117] Leukemoid reactions also are observed at a frequency of approximately 1% in term neonates in the absence of an identifiable cause. Such reactions appear to reflect increased neutrophil production.

Circulating G-CSF levels in healthy infants are highest in the first hours after birth, and levels in premature neonates are generally higher than in term neonates.[118] Levels decline rapidly in the neonatal period and more slowly thereafter. Plasma G-CSF levels tend to be elevated in infected neonates.[118] Mononuclear cells and monocytes from midgestation fetuses and premature neonates generally produce less G-CSF and GM-CSF after stimulation in vitro than comparable adult cell types, whereas cells from term neonates produce amounts that are similar to or modestly less than those of adults.[119,120]

Migration to Sites of Infection or Injury

After release from the bone marrow into the blood, neutrophils circulate until they are called upon to enter infected or injured tissues. Neutrophils adhere selectively to endothelium in such tissues but not in normal tissues. The adhesion and subsequent migration of neutrophils through blood vessels into tissues and to the site of infection result from a multistep process, which is governed by the pattern of expression on their surface of adhesion molecules and receptors for chemotactic factors and by the local patterns and gradients of adhesion molecule and chemotactic factors in the tissues.

The adhesion molecules involved in neutrophil migration from the blood into tissues include selectins, integrins, and the molecules to which they adhere.[121] The selectins are named by the cell types in which they are primarily expressed: L-selectin by leukocytes, E-selectin by endothelial cells, and P-selectin by platelets and endothelial cells. L-selectin is constitutively expressed on leukocytes and appears to bind to tissue- or inflammation-specific carbohydrate-containing ligands on endothelial cells. E-selectin and P-selectin are expressed on activated not resting endothelial cells or platelets. E- and P-selectin bind to sialylated glycoproteins on the surface of leukocytes, including P-selectin glycoprotein ligand-1. L-selectin binds to glycoproteins and glycolipids, which are expressed on vascular endothelial cells in specific tissues. The integrins are a large family of heterodimeric proteins composed of an α and a β chain. The β_2 integrins LFA-1 (CD11a-CD18) and Mac-1 (CD11b-CD18) play a critical role in neutrophil function because neutrophils do not express other integrins in substantial amounts. The β_2 integrins are constitutively expressed on neutrophils, but their abundance and avidity for their endothelial ligands are increased after activation of neutrophils in response to chemotactic factors. Their endothelial ligands include intercellular adhesion molecule 1 (ICAM-1) and ICAM-2. Both are constitutively expressed on endothelium, but ICAM-1 expression is increased markedly by exposure to inflammatory mediators, including IL-1, TNF-α, and LPS.

Chemotactic factors may be derived directly from bacterial components, such as *n*-formylated-Met-Leu-Phe (fMLP) peptide; from activated complement, including C5a; and from host cell lipids, including leukotriene B_4 (LTB_4). In addition, a large family of chemotactic cytokines (chemokines) is synthesized by macrophages and many other cell types (see Tables 4-1 and 4-2). Chemokines constitute a cytokine superfamily, with more than 50 members known at present, most of which are secreted and of relatively low molecular weight.[122] Chemokines attract various leukocyte populations, which bear the appropriate G protein–linked chemokine receptors. They can be divided into four families according to their pattern of amino-terminal cysteine residues: CC, CXC, C, and CX3C (X represents a noncysteine amino acid between the cysteines). A nomenclature for the chemokines and their receptors has been adopted, in which the family is first denoted (e.g., CC), followed by L for ligand (the chemokine itself) and a number, or followed by R (for receptor) and a number. Functionally, chemokines also can be defined by their principal function—homeostatic or inflammatory cell migration—and by the subsets of cells on which they act. Neutrophils are attracted by the subset of CXC chemokines that contain a glutamine-leucine-arginine motif, including the prototypical neutrophil chemokine CXLC8, also known as IL-8.

These adhesion molecules and chemotactic factors act in a coordinated fashion to allow neutrophil recruitment. In response to injury or inflammatory cytokines, E-selectin and P-selectin are expressed on the endothelium of capillaries or postcapillary venules. Neutrophils in the blood adhere to these selectins in a low-avidity fashion, allowing them to roll along the vessel walls. This step is transient and reversible unless a second, high-avidity interaction is triggered. If, at the time of the low-avidity binding, neutrophils also encounter chemotactic factors released from the tissues or from the endothelium itself, they rapidly upregulate the avidity and abundance of LFA-1 and Mac-1 on the neutrophil cell surface. This process results in high-avidity binding of neutrophils to endothelial cells, which, in the presence of a gradient of chemotactic factors from the tissue to the blood vessel, induces neutrophils to migrate across the endothelium and into the tissues by diapedesis.

The profound importance of integrin- and selectin-mediated leukocyte adhesion is illustrated by the genetic leukocyte adhesion deficiency (LAD) syndromes.[123] In LAD 1, deficiency of the common β_2 integrin chain (CD18) results in inability of leukocytes to exit the bloodstream and reach sites of infection and injury in the tissues. Affected patients are profoundly susceptible to infections with pathogenic and nonpathogenic bacteria and may present in early infancy with delayed separation of the umbilical cord, omphalitis, and severe bacterial infection without pus formation. Two related syndromes, LAD 2 and LAD 3, are due, respectively, to a defect in synthesis (fucosylation) of the carbohydrate selectin ligands and mutations in the gene encoding kindlin-3, a protein required for integrin activation.[123]

Migration of Neonatal Neutrophils

The ability of neonatal neutrophils to migrate from the blood into sites of infection and inflammation is reduced or delayed, and the transition from a neutrophilic to mononuclear cell inflammatory response is delayed.[111] This diminished delivery of neutrophils may result in part from defects in adhesion and chemotaxis.

Adhesion of neonatal neutrophils under resting conditions is normal or at most modestly impaired, whereas adhesion of activated cells is deficient.[124] Adhesion and rolling of neonatal neutrophils to activated endothelium under conditions of flow similar to those found in capillaries or postcapillary venules is variable but on average approximately 50% of that observed with adult neutrophils.[110,125] This decreased adhesion appears to reflect, at least in part, decreased abundance and shedding of L-selectin and decreased binding of neonatal neutrophils to P-selectin.[125] Resting neonatal and adult neutrophils have similar amounts of Mac-1 and LFA-1 on their plasma membrane, but neonatal neutrophils have a reduced ability to upregulate expression of these integrins after exposure to chemotactic agents.[125,126] Reduced integrin upregulation is associated with a parallel decrease in adhesion to activated endothelium or ICAM-1 suggesting that a deficit in adhesion underlies the diminished ability of neonatal neutrophils to migrate through endothelium into tissues, particularly in preterm neonates.[125,127]

In nearly all studies in which neutrophil migration has been examined in vitro, chemotaxis of neonatal neutrophils was less than that of adult neutrophils.[75] The response of neonatal neutrophils to a variety of chemotactic factors, including fMLP, LTB_4, and neutrophil-specific chemokines, including IL-8, is reduced.[128-130] Chemotactic factor binding and dose response patterns of neonatal neutrophils appear similar to adult neutrophils, whereas downstream processes, including expression of Ras-related C3 botulinum toxin substrate 2 (Rac2), the increases in the free (nonprotein bound) intracellular calcium concentration $[Ca^{2+}]_i$ and inositol phospholipid generation and the change in cell membrane potential are impaired. An additional factor may be the reduced deformability of neonatal neutrophils, which may limit their ability to enter the tissues after binding to the vascular endothelium. Decreased generation of chemotactic factors in neonatal serum may compound the intrinsic chemotactic deficits of neonatal neutrophils. However, the generation of other chemotactic agents, such as LTB_4, by neonatal neutrophils appears to be normal.[131]

Phagocytosis

Having reached the site of infection, neutrophils must bind, phagocytose, and kill the pathogen.[132] Opsonization greatly facilitates this process. Neutrophils express on their surface receptors for multiple opsonins, including receptors for the Fc portion of the IgG molecule (Fcγ receptors): FcγRI (CD64), FcγRIIA (CD32), and FcγRIIIB (CD16).[133] Neutrophils also express receptors for activated complement components C3b and C3bi, which are bound by CR1, CR3 (CD11b-CD18), and CR4 (CD11c-CD18), respectively. Opsonized bacteria bind and cross link Fcγ and C3b-C3bi receptors. This cross linkage transmits a signal for ingestion and for the activation of the cell's microbicidal mechanisms.

Under optimal in vitro conditions, neutrophils from healthy neonates bind and ingest gram-positive and gram-negative bacteria as well as or only slightly less efficiently than an adult's neutrophils.[75] However, the concentrations of opsonins are reduced in serum from neonates, in particular, preterm neonates, and when concentrations of opsonins are limited,[134] neutrophils from neonates ingest bacteria less efficiently than those from adults. Consistent with this finding, phagocytosis of bacteria by neutrophils from preterm, but not term, neonates is reduced compared with adult neutrophils when assayed in whole blood.[135-137] Why neonatal neutrophils have impaired phagocytosis when concentrations of opsonins are limiting is incompletely understood. Basal expression of receptors for opsonized bacteria is not greatly different. Neutrophils from neonates, particularly preterm neonates, express greater amounts of the high-affinity FcγRI, lesser amounts of FcγRIII, and similar or slightly reduced amounts of FcγRIIA at birth, compared with adults; values in preterm neonates approach those of term neonates by 1 month of age.[138] Expression of complement receptors on neutrophils from term neonates and adults is similar, but reduced expression of CR3 on neutrophils from preterm neonates has been reported in some studies.[138,139] Neutrophils from preterm neonates also are less able to upregulate CR3 in response to LPS and chemotactic factors.[140-142] Lower expression of proteins involved in the engulfment process, including Rac2 as noted above, may also contribute to impaired phagocytosis when concentrations of opsonins are limited.

Killing

After ingestion, neutrophils kill ingested microbes through oxygen-dependent and oxygen-independent mechanisms. Oxygen-dependent microbicidal mechanisms are of central importance, as illustrated by the severe compromise in defenses against a wide range of pyogenic pathogens (with the exception of catalase-negative bacteria) observed in individuals with a genetic defect in this system.[143] Children with this disorder have a defect in one of several proteins that constitute the phagocyte oxidase, which is activated during receptor-mediated phagocytosis. The assembly of the oxidase in the plasma membrane results in the generation and delivery of reactive oxygen metabolites, including superoxide anion, hydrogen peroxide, and hydroxyl radicals. These oxygen radicals, along with the granule protein myeloperoxidase, are discharged into the phagocytic vacuole, where they collaborate in killing ingested microbes. In addition to this oxygen-dependent pathway, neutrophils contain other granule proteins with potent microbicidal activity, including the defensins HNPs 1 to 4, LL-37, elastase, cathepsin G, and a protein that binds selectively to and helps to kill gram-negative bacteria, bactericidal permeability-increasing (BPI) protein.[144]

Oxygen-dependent and oxygen-independent microbicidal mechanisms of neutrophils from neonates and adults do not differ greatly.[145,146] Generation of superoxide anion and hydrogen peroxide by neutrophils from term neonates is generally similar to or greater than by cells from adults in response to soluble stimuli.[147,148] Although a modest reduction in the generation of reactive oxygen metabolites by neutrophils from preterm compared with term neonates was seen in response to some strains of coagulase-negative staphylococci, this was not observed with other strains nor with a strain of GBS and is of uncertain significance.[149] By contrast, LPS primes adult neutrophils for increased production of reactive oxygen metabolites, but priming is much reduced with neonatal neutrophils, which could limit their efficacy in response to infection in vivo.[142,150] The few studies of oxygen-independent microbicidal mechanisms suggest that neonatal neutrophils contain and release reduced amounts of BPI (approximately two to threefold) and lactoferrin (approximately twofold) compared with adult neutrophils but contain or release comparable amounts of myeloperoxidase, defensins, and lysozyme.[145,146,151,152]

Consistent with these findings, killing of ingested gram-positive and gram-negative bacteria and *Candida* organisms by neutrophils from neonates and adults is generally similar.[145,146] However, variable and usually mildly decreased bactericidal activity has been noted against *Pseudomonas aeruginosa*,[153] *S. aureus*,[154] and certain strains of GBS.[75] Deficits in killing of engulfed microbes by neonatal neutrophils are more apparent at high ratios of bacteria to neutrophils, as is killing by neutrophils from sick or stressed neonates (i.e., those born prematurely or who have sepsis, respiratory impairment, hyperbilirubinemia, premature rupture of membranes, or hypoglycemia).

Neutrophils also function in trapping and killing extracellular bacteria in neutrophil extracellular traps (NETs), which consist of a complex of DNA, histones, granule enzymes, and antimicrobial proteins that are extruded from the cell.[155] Neonatal neutrophils from both term and preterm infants are unable to form NETs and therefore have impaired extracellular bacterial killing in vitro.[156]

Activation by Innate Immune Receptors

Although neutrophils were formally viewed by many as cells highly specialized for the uptake and killing of bacteria and fungi, human neutrophils also express a variety of innate immune receptors that are functional, including all TLRs except TLR3 and TLR7, NLRs (NOD2 and NLRP3), and RLRs (RIG-I and MDA-5).[157-159] Moreover, neutrophils respond to TLR agonists or NOD2 ligands with production of IL-8 and other chemokines, superoxide generation, and shedding of L-selectin,[157] and they also produce IL-1β after NLRP3 activation.[158] In mice, neutrophil-derived IL-1β is sufficient for the formation of abscesses in *S. aureus* infection, with cytokine production involving both TLRs and NLRs.[160] This suggests that neutrophils may be an important in vivo source of proinflammatory cytokines, at least in certain contexts. There is little information on neonatal neutrophil activation by innate immune receptors. One study of infants with severe RSV found that neutrophils of the blood and lung had reduced expression of TLR4.[161] As TLR4 is a receptor for RSV G protein, it is plausible that this decreased expression could contribute to the disease severity.

Neutrophil Clearance and Resolution of Neutrophilic Inflammation

One to 2 days after egress from the bone marrow, neutrophils undergo apoptosis and are efficiently cleared by tissue macrophages without producing inflammation or injury. In the context of infection or sterile inflammation, their survival is prolonged by CSFs and other inflammatory mediators, allowing them to aid in microbial clearance, while at the same time augmenting or perpetuating tissue injury. Studies from several groups have shown that spontaneous and anti-Fas–induced apoptosis of isolated neonatal neutrophils is reduced when these cells are cultured in vitro.[111,162-164] The greater survival of neonatal than adult neutrophils was associated with reduced expression of the apoptosis-inducing Fas receptor and pro-apoptotic members of the Bcl-2 family.[162] The increased survival of neonatal neutrophils has led some to speculate that this may help to compensate for the neonate's limited neutrophil storage pool in protection against infection, but this might also contribute to persistent untoward inflammation and tissue injury.[111]

Effects of Immunomodulators

After systemic treatment with G-CSF and GM-CSF, the numbers of neutrophils increase in neonates, as does expression of CR3 on these cells.[114] The increased numbers likely reflect increased production and survival.[162,164] GM-CSF and IFN-γ enhance the chemotactic response of neonatal neutrophils,[114,165] although, at high concentrations, GM-CSF inhibits chemotaxis while augmenting oxygen radical production.[166] Of potential concern, indomethacin, which is used clinically to facilitate ductal closure in premature neonates, impairs chemotaxis of cells from term and preterm neonates.[167]

EOSINOPHILS

In adults and older children, eosinophils represent a small percentage of the circulating granulocytes. In the healthy fetus and neonate, eosinophils commonly represent a larger fraction (10%-20%) of total granulocytes than in adults.[168] Numbers of eosinophils increase postnatally, peaking at the third to fourth week of postnatal life. A relative increase in the abundance of eosinophils in inflammatory exudates of various causes is also seen in neonates, paralleling their greater numbers in the circulation.[169] Thus eosinophil-rich inflammatory exudates do not so strongly suggest the presence of allergic disease or helminthic infection, as they do in older individuals, and are not associated with increased amounts of circulating IgE. The degree of eosinophilia is greater yet in preterm neonates and in those with Rh disease, total parenteral nutrition, and transfusions.[170] The basis for the eosinophilic tendency of the neonate is not known. By contrast to the diminished migration of neonatal neutrophils, neonatal eosinophils exhibit greater spontaneous and chemotactic factor–induced migration than adult eosinophils.[168] Their greater numbers and ability to migrate may contribute to the relatively greater abundance of eosinophils in neonatal inflammatory infiltrates, including those seen in physiologic conditions such as erythema toxicum.

MONONUCLEAR PHAGOCYTES

Production and Differentiation of Monocytes and Resident Tissue Macrophages

Together, monocytes and tissue macrophages are referred to as mononuclear phagocytes. Under steady-state conditions, monocytes are released from the bone marrow within 24 hours and circulate in the blood for 1 to 3 days before moving to the tissues,[171] where they differentiate into tissue macrophages. All monocytes express CD14, which serves as a co-receptor for recognition of LPS by TLR4/MD-2. CD14 is commonly used as a lineage marker for these cells because it is the only cell type that expresses it in high amounts. Additional commonly used mononuclear phagocyte markers include CD68, a glycoprotein that binds to low density lipoprotein, and CD163, a scavenger receptor for hemoglobin-haptoglobin complexes. Monocytes also express histocompatibility leukocyte antigen (HLA)-DR (MHC class II) and can present antigens to CD4 T cells, which is discussed in detail in the section "Antigen Presentation by Classical Major Histocompatibility Complex Molecules," although the amounts expressed and efficiency of antigen presentation are less than by DCs. Monocytes are heterogeneous. In the healthy adult circulation, CD14$^+$ monocytes can be divided into three subsets based on their levels of expression of CD14 and CD16 (a Fc receptor for IgG)—CD14^{++}CD16$^-$, CD14$^+$CD16$^+$, and CD14^{dim}CD16^{++}, which comprise approximately 85%, 6%, and 9% of total blood monocytes, respectively.[172,173] CD14^{++}CD16$^-$ monocytes have relatively low levels of surface expression of CD11c, CD80/86, CD163, and HLA-DR compared with CD14$^+$CD16$^+$ monocytes.[172,174] Both CD11c, a β_2 integrin molecule, and L-selectin (CD62-L), are involved in leukocyte adhesion, and CD80 and CD86 are important for co-stimulation to T cells. The CD14^{dim}CD16^{++} cell subset, which was only recently described,[172] is highly responsive to viral nucleic acids but not bacterial products, such as LPS, although this point is controversial. Studies in humanized mice suggest that CD14^{dim}CD16^{++} monocytes "patrol" the endothelium in an L-selectin–dependent manner.[172]

Macrophages are resident in tissues throughout the body and include distinct populations of alveolar macrophages (lung), histiocytes (interstitial connective tissue), Kupffer cells (liver), microglia (brain), and osteoclasts (bone).[175] Macrophages have multiple functions, including the clearance of dead host cells (efferocytosis),[176] phagocytosis and killing of microbes, secretion of inflammatory mediators, and presentation of antigen to T cells. They can also act to limit or suppress inflammation in certain contexts and promote tissue repair. With the exception of inflammatory macrophages, which are similar to neutrophils in being short-lived, most macrophage populations are relatively long-lived cells, but their life span may vary from days to possibly years, depending on the particular macrophage population.

Macrophages are detectable as early as 4 weeks of fetal life in the yolk sac and are found shortly thereafter in the liver and then in the bone marrow.[177] Recent studies in mice indicate that the major tissue subsets, including liver Kupffer cells and lung alveolar, splenic, and peritoneal macrophages, are established before birth (21 days of gestation) and are subsequently maintained by proliferation in situ rather than by replenishment from circulating monocytes.[178] These findings, along with others documenting tissue macrophage proliferation in the mouse in diverse inflammatory responses, for instance, tissue nematode infection[179] and atherosclerosis,[180] suggest that tissue macrophage proliferation could be an important part of human mononuclear cell homeostasis and regulation by inflammation.

The capacity of the fetus and the neonate to produce monocytes is at least as great as that of adults.[181] The numbers of monocytes per volume of blood in neonates are equal to or greater than those in adults.[182] Cord blood has a similar fraction of monocytes that are CD14^{++}CD16$^-$ and CD14$^+$CD16$^+$ as adult peripheral blood.[174] Cord blood monocytes express approximately 50% as much HLA-DR as adult monocytes, and a larger fraction of neonatal monocytes lack detectable HLA-DR[183]; this reduced expression in cord blood applies to both the CD14^{++}CD16$^-$ and CD14$^+$CD16$^+$ subsets.[174] In contrast, other surface markers are expressed similarly, with the CD14$^+$CD16$^+$ subset of both cord blood and adult peripheral blood having significantly higher levels of CD11c, CD80/86, and CD163 than CD14^{++}CD16$^-$ monocytes.[174] To the best of our knowledge, there have been no studies reporting the frequency and phenotype of the recently described CD14^{dim}CD16^{++} monocyte subset in human neonates.[172]

The numbers of tissue macrophages in human neonates are not well characterized. Limited data in humans, which are consistent with data in nonhuman primates and other mammals, suggest that the lung contains few macrophages until shortly before term.[184] Postnatally, the numbers of lung macrophages increase to adult levels by 24 to 48 hours in healthy monkeys.[185] A similar increase occurs in humans, although the data are less complete and by necessity derived from individuals with clinical problems necessitating tracheobronchial lavage.[186] The blood of premature neonates contains increased numbers of pitted erythrocytes or erythrocytes containing Howell-Jolly bodies,[187] suggesting that the ability of splenic and liver macrophages to clear these effete cells, and perhaps microbial cells, may be reduced in the fetus and premature infant.

Migration to Sites of Infection and Delayed Hypersensitivity Responses

Like neutrophils, mononuclear phagocytes express the adhesion molecules L-selectin and β_2 integrins. These cells also express substantial amounts of the $\alpha_4\beta_1$ integrin very late antigen-4 (VLA-4) , allowing them, unlike neutrophils, to adhere efficiently to endothelium expressing vascular cell adhesion molecule 1 (VCAM-1), the ligand for VLA-4.[121] Interaction of VLA-4 with VCAM-1 allows monocytes to enter tissues in states in which there is little or no neutrophilic inflammation.[188] Chemokines that are chemotactic for neutrophils are not generally chemotactic for monocytes, and vice versa. Monocytes respond to a range of CC chemokines, such as CCL2 (monocyte chemotactic protein-1 [MCP-1]).[189]

The acute inflammatory response is characterized by an initial infiltration of neutrophils that is followed within 6 to 12 hours by influx of mononuclear phagocytes.[171] Some inflammatory responses, including delayed-type hypersensitivity (DTH) reactions induced by the injection of antigens, for instance, purified protein derivative (PPD), to which the individual is immune (i.e., has developed an antigen-specific T-cell response) are characterized by the influx of mononuclear phagocytes and lymphocytes with very minimal or no initial neutrophilic phase.[190]

The influx of monocytes into sites of inflammation, including DTH responses, is delayed and attenuated in neonates compared with adults.[191,192] This is true even when antigen-specific T-cell responses are evident in vitro, suggesting that decreased migration of monocytes and lymphocytes into the tissues is predominantly responsible for the poor response in neonates. Whether this delay results from impaired chemotaxis of neonatal monocytes or impaired generation of chemotactic factors or both is unresolved

Antimicrobial Properties of Monocytes and Macrophages

Although neutrophils ingest and kill pyogenic bacteria more efficiently, resident macrophages are the initial line of phagocyte defense against microbial invasion in the tissues. When the microbial insult is modest, these cells are sufficient. If not, they produce cytokines and other inflammatory mediators to direct the recruitment of circulating neutrophils and monocytes from the blood. Monocytes and macrophages express receptors that allow them to bind to microbes. These receptors include FcγRI, II, and III, which bind IgG-coated microbes[193]; FcαR, which binds IgA-coated microbes[194]; and the CR1 and CR3 receptors, which bind microbes coated with C3b and C3bi, respectively.[195] Microbes bound through these receptors are efficiently engulfed by macrophages and once ingested can be killed by microbicidal mechanisms using many methods similar to those used by neutrophils. Mononuclear phagocytes generate reactive oxygen metabolites but in lesser amounts than neutrophils. Circulating monocytes, but not tissue macrophages, contain myeloperoxidase, which facilitates the microbicidal activity of hydrogen peroxide. The expression of microbicidal granule proteins differs somewhat in mononuclear phagocytes and neutrophils; for instance, human mononuclear phagocytes express β-defensins but not α-defensins, whereas neutrophils express both.[196]

The microbicidal activity of resident tissue macrophages is relatively modest, especially compared with the robust activity of neutrophils. This limited activity may be important in allowing macrophages to remove dead or damaged host cells and small numbers of microbes without excessively damaging host tissues. However, in response to infection, macrophage microbicidal and proinflammatory functions are enhanced in a process referred to as classical (M1) macrophage activation.[197,198] Macrophage activation results from the integration of signals from TLRs and other innate immune pattern recognition receptors and receptors for activated complement components, immune complexes, cytokines, and ligands produced by other immune cells, including IFN-γ, CD40 ligand, TNF-α, and GM-CSF.[198,199]

The increased antimicrobial activity of M1-activated macrophages results in part from increased expression of FcγRI, enhanced phagocytic activity, and increased production of reactive oxygen metabolites. Other antimicrobial mechanisms induced by activation of these cells include the catabolism of tryptophan by indoleamine 2,3-dioxygenase, scavenging of iron, and production of nitric oxide and its metabolites by the inducible nitric oxide synthase (iNOS). The last is a major mechanism by which activated murine macrophages inhibit or kill a variety of intracellular pathogens. However, the role of nitric oxide in the antimicrobial activity of human macrophages is controversial, although polymorphisms of the iNOS gene locus in humans have been associated with the host susceptibility to *Mycobacteria tuberculosis.*[200] Activated mononuclear phagocytes also secrete a number of noncytokine products that are potentially important in host defense mechanisms. These include complement components, fibronectin, and lysozyme.

Classical (M1) activation of macrophages plays a critical role in defense against infection with intracellular bacterial and protozoan pathogens that replicate within phagocytic vacuoles. Support for this notion comes from studies in humans and mice with genetic deficiencies that impair the activation of macrophages by IFN-γ. Humans with genetic defects involving IL-12, which induces IFN-γ production by NK and T cells, the IL-12 receptor, the IFN-γ receptor or the transcription factor STAT1, which is activated via this receptor, suffer unduly from infections with mycobacteria and *Salmonella.*[201] Treatment of humans with antagonists of TNF-α also impair antimycobacterial defenses.[202] Patients with the hyper-IgM syndrome, which is due to a defect in CD40 ligand, or with autosomal recessive hyper-IgM due to a mutation in CD40, the receptor for CD40 ligand, are predisposed to disease caused by *Pneumocystis jirovecii* and *Cryptosporidium parvum,* in addition to the problems they experience from defects in antibody production (see section CD4 T-Cell Help for Antibody Production).[203] These findings are consistent with the notion that IFN-γ, TNF-α, and CD40 ligand–mediated M1 macrophage activation is important in host defense against these pathogens and that these molecules activate macrophages, at least in part, in a nonredundant manner.

By contrast to this canonical pathway of macrophage activation, macrophages exposed to cytokines produced by Th2 cells, such as IL-4, which are induced by infection with parasitic helminths and as part of allergic responses, are activated in an alternative manner.[198,204,205] These alternatively activated macrophages, also termed M2 cells, dampen acute inflammation, impede the generation of reactive nitrogen products, limit proinflammatory T-cell responses, and foster fibrosis through the production of arginase and other mediators. Although best characterized in mice, this alternative pathway appears to be relevant in humans as well, and a recent study suggests that there is substantial additional diversity in the function of human macrophage subsets beyond the M1 and M2 paradigms.[206]

Antimicrobial Activity and Activation of Neonatal Monocytes and Macrophages. Monocytes from human neonates and adults ingest and kill *S. aureus, E. coli,* and GBS with similar efficiency.[207-211] Consistent with these findings, the production of microbicidal oxygen metabolites by neonatal and adult monocytes is similar.[210,212-215] Neonatal and adult monocytes, monocyte-derived macrophages, and fetal macrophages are comparable in their ability to prevent herpes simplex virus (HSV) from replicating within them.[216,217] And although neonatal monocytes may be slightly less capable of killing HSV-infected cells than adult monocytes in the absence of antibody, they are equivalent in the presence of antibody.[218,219]

The ability of neonatal and adult monocyte-derived macrophages (monocytes cultured in vitro) to phagocytose GBS, other bacteria, and *Candida* through receptors for mannose-fucose, IgG, and complement components is similar. Despite comparable phagocytosis, neonatal monocyte-derived macrophages kill *Candida* and GBS less efficiently. Moreover, GM-CSF, but not IFN-γ, activates neonatal monocyte-derived macrophages to produce superoxide anion and to kill these organisms, whereas both of these cytokines activate adult macrophages.[220-222] The lack of response to IFN-γ by neonatal macrophages was associated with normal binding to its receptor but decreased activation of STAT1.[220] Studies with alveolar macrophages from newborn and, particularly, premature newborn monkeys[223] and other mammals also have shown reduced phagocytic and/or microbicidal activity, suggesting this might apply to humans. By contrast to these reports of decreased antimicrobial activity and failure of macrophage activation by IFN-γ, blood monocytes and IFN-γ–treated monocyte-derived and placental macrophages from neonates kill and restrict the growth of *Toxoplasma* as effectively as cells from adults.[224,225]

Mononuclear Phagocytes Produce Cytokines and Other Mediators That Regulate Inflammation and Immunity

Monocytes and macrophages produce cytokines, chemokines, colony-stimulating factors and other mediators in response to ligand binding by TLRs and other pattern recognition receptors expressed by these cells (described in the next section), cytokines produced by other cell types, activated complement components and other mediators, and engagement of CD40 on their surface by CD40 ligand expressed on activated CD4 T cells. These include the cytokines IL-1α, IL-1β, TNF-α, and IL-6, which induce the production of prostaglandin E2, which, in turn, induces fever, accounting for the antipyretic effect of drugs that inhibit prostaglandin synthesis. Fever may have a beneficial role in host resistance to infection by inhibiting the growth of certain microorganisms and by enhancing host immune responses. TNF-α, IL-1, and IL-6 also act on the liver to induce the acute-phase response, which is associated with decreased albumin synthesis and increased synthesis of certain complement components, fibrinogen, CRP, and MBL. G-CSF, GM-CSF, and macrophage-specific colony-stimulating factor (M-CSF) enhance the production of their respective target cell populations, increasing the numbers of phagocytes available. At the sites of infection or injury, TNF-α and IL-1 increase endothelial cell expression of adhesion molecules, including E-selectin and P-selectin, ICAM-1, and VCAM-1, increase endothelial cell procoagulant activity and enhance neutrophil adhesiveness by upregulating β_2 integrin expression. IL-6 may help to terminate neutrophil recruitment into tissues and to facilitate a switch from an inflammatory infiltrate rich in neutrophils to one dominated by monocytes and lymphocytes.[226] IL-8 and other Glu-Leu-Arg (ELR)-containing CXC chemokines enhance the avidity of neutrophil β_2 integrins for ICAM-1 and attract neutrophils into the inflammatory-infectious focus; CC chemokines play a similar role in attracting mononuclear phagocytes and lymphocytes. These and additional factors contribute to edema, redness, and leukocyte infiltration, which characterize inflammation.

In addition to secreting cytokines that regulate the acute inflammatory response and play a crucial role in host defense to extracellular bacterial and fungal pathogens, monocytes and macrophages (and DCs, see later) produce cytokines that mediate and regulate defense against intracellular viral, bacterial, and protozoan pathogens. Type I IFNs directly inhibit viral replication in host cells,[227] as do IFN-γ and TNF-α.[228] IL-12, IL-23, and IL-27 are members of a family of heterodimeric cytokines that help to regulate T-cell and NK-cell differentiation and function.[229] IL-12 is composed of IL-12/23 p40 and p35; IL-23 is composed of IL-12/23 p40 and p19; and IL-27 is composed of Epstein-Barr virus–induced gene 3 protein (EBI-3) and p28.[229] IL-12, in concert with IL-15 and IL-18, enhance NK-cell lytic function and production of IFN-γ and facilitate the development of type 1 CD4 T helper (Th1) and CD8 effector T cells, which are discussed more fully in the section "Differentiation of Activated Naïve T Cells into Effector and Memory Cells" and which play a critical role in control of infection with intracellular bacterial, protozoal, and viral pathogens. IFN-γ activates macrophages, allowing them to control infection with intracellular pathogens, and enhances their capacity to produce IL-12 and TNF-α, which, in turn, amplifies IFN-γ production by NK cells and causes T cells to differentiate into IFN-γ–producing Th1 T cells.[230] IL-27 also facilitates IFN-γ production, while at the same time inducing the expression of IL-10, which dampens inflammatory and Th1 T-cell responses to limit tissue injury. By contrast, IL-23 favors IL-17–producing Th17 T-cell responses, in which IL-17 promotes neutrophil production, acute inflammation, and defense to extracellular pathogens.

The production of cytokines by mononuclear phagocytes normally is restricted temporally and anatomically to cells in contact with microbial products, antigen-stimulated T cells, or other agonists. When excess production of proinflammatory cytokines occurs systemically, septic shock and disseminated intravascular coagulation may ensue,[231] underscoring the importance of closely regulated and anatomically restricted production of proinflammatory mediators. Tight control of inflammation normally is achieved by a combination of positive and negative feedback regulation. For example, TNF-α, IL-1, and microbial products that induce their production also cause macrophages to produce cytokines that attenuate inflammation and dampen immunity, including IL-10[231] and the IL-1 receptor antagonist.[232] Inflammation is also attenuated by the production of antiinflammatory lipid mediators (resolvins), including the lipoxins, protectins, and maresins.[233]

Cytokine Production, Toll-like Receptors, and Regulation of Innate Immunity and Inflammation by Neonatal Monocytes and Macrophages

Much of the older literature suggested that blood mononuclear cells (BMCs) obtained from cord blood or neonatal peripheral blood were less efficient in general than adult BMC in the production of cytokines in response to LPS, other TLR ligands, or whole bacteria. BMCs consist of monocytes, DCs, and B, T, and NK lymphocytes. Because of the greater than 10-fold abundance of monocytes compared with DCs in blood and BMCs, and the relatively limited production by lymphocytes of cytokines in response to TLR agonists, monocytes were likely to be the predominant source for most of these cytokines. The recent development of routine flow cytometric analysis of 6- to 12-color monoclonal antibody staining for intracellular cytokines and surface markers applied to BMC now permits an assessment of the levels of production of multiple cytokines per cell for each cell type. Also, because of simplicity and a desire to minimize manipulations that might activate or alter blood leukocyte function, many recent studies have been done with whole blood to which TLR ligands are added directly ex vivo, with cytokine production evaluated by enzyme-linked immunosorbent assay (ELISA) or bead-based fluorescent assays or, in some cases, by multiparameter flow cytometry. The findings for recent flow cytometric studies using whole blood or BMC will be emphasized here, although secreted cytokine levels will also be included where the likely cell source can be inferred. As TLR3 and TLR9 are expressed by certain DC population but not monocytes, and monocytes, in general, produce type I IFN poorly, the results for type I IFN production and other cytokines in response to TLR3 or TLR9 ligands in whole-blood assays will be discussed separately in the section "Dendritic Cells: The Link Between Innate and Adaptive Immunity."

The preponderance of the currently available data does not support the notion of a general inability of neonatal monocytes (and, as discussed later, DCs) to produce cytokines, but rather suggests a difference in the nature of their response.

There is a clear, substantial, and with rare exception, consistent deficit in the production of IL-12p70 and IFN-γ in response to TLR agonists that act on monocytes (TLR2, TLR4, TLR7/8).[234,235] In assays using whole blood or BMC, the IFN-γ produced is probably mainly derived from NK cells responding to IL-12p70 rather than from T cells. These deficits of cord blood leukocytes are likely cell intrinsic because they are consistently observed with either whole-blood assays or assays of BMC cultured with heterologous adult serum or with fetal calf serum. As discussed in the section "Dendritic Cells: The Link Between Innate and Adaptive Immunity," there are also marked reductions in type I IFN production by DCs in cord blood. Because type I IFNs synergize with IL-12p70 and IFN-γ in promoting Th1 development from naïve CD4 T cells,[236] this cytokine profile combined with T-cell intrinsic mechanisms, which are discussed later, would be expected to limit the generation of Th1 effectors in neonates, as has been observed in neonatal HSV infection. As LPS-induced IL-12p70 production by monocytes is itself markedly increased by IFN-γ, it is noteworthy that IL-12p70 secretion and IL-12p35 mRNA expression in cord blood after combined LPS and IFN-γ stimulation is decreased, and this decrease persisted until at least 1 month of age.[237] Whole-blood assays indicate that adult levels of production of IL-12p70 in response to LPS are achieved by 6 months of age.[238] A large body of evidence, including from human genetic immunodeficiencies, has clearly demonstrated that IL-12p70 and IFN-γ are essential for Th1-type immune control of pathogens, especially mycobacteria. Thus it is plausible that these antigen-presenting cell (APC) limitations in Th1 cytokine production are an important mechanism contributing to the well-described vulnerability of the neonate and young infant to *Mycobacterium* tuberculosis infection.[239]

A similar deficit in TNF-α production is evident in response to stimulation with TLR2, TLR3, TLR4, and TLR5 agonists,[183,234,237,240,241] particularly when whole blood is used or BMC or monocytes are cultured in high (≥50%) concentrations of neonatal serum. In contrast, TNF-α production in response to TLR8 agonists or whole gram-positive or gram-negative bacteria is similar.[242] Further, in flow cytometric analysis of BMC cultured in adult serum, production of TNF-α by cord blood and adult peripheral blood monocytes was similar.[235] As discussed later, these findings are explained at least in part by the presence of an inhibitory factor in cord blood plasma and suggest that any cell-intrinsic limitations in TNF-α production by cord blood monocytes may be relatively subtle.

In any case, with the exception of TNF-α, production by neonatal cells of cytokines central to host defense against extracellular bacterial and fungal pathogens, acute inflammation, and Th17-type responses appear not to be greatly decreased and, in some cases, is more robust. IL-1 production by cells from term neonates and adults is similar or, at most, marginally reduced. In response to TLR agonists, neonatal monocytes produced equal or greater amounts of IL-6, IL-23, and IL-10, compared with adult cells, but were less able to produce multiple cytokines simultaneously.[243] In one recent longitudinal study of the ontogeny of TLR-mediated cytokine responses in South African infants, this high level of production of IL-6 and IL-23, which was particularly robust in response to TLR2 agonists, gradually declined in the first year of life to adult peripheral blood levels.[244] As IL-1, IL-6, and IL-23 production by APCs instructs the differentiation of naïve CD4 T cells into Th17-type effector cells, these findings are in agreement with apparently intact Th17 immunity in the neonate.[245] Although some early studies suggested that the production of the immunoregulatory and antiinflammatory cytokine IL-10 by neonatal cells was reduced,[246,247] most studies have found greater production of IL-10 by whole blood and equal or greater production by BMCs.[234,241,242,248,249] These high levels of IL-10 in whole-blood assays, which are particularly prominent after TLR2 stimulation, gradually decline to adult levels in the first year of life, indicating that they are not merely a feature of cord blood leukocytes.

The basis for lower production of certain cytokines by neonatal monocytes and macrophages in response to microbial products that signal through TLRs is incompletely understood. Cell surface expression of TLR2, TLR4, and TLR8 by adult and neonatal monocytes is similar in most studies,[183,250,251] and expression of CD14, which facilitates responses to LPS and TLR2 agonists, is similar or, at most, slightly reduced on neonatal monocytes.[183,240,251-255] Monocytes from premature infants express less TLR2 and TLR4 at birth but increase their expression to amounts comparable to term infants by 2 weeks of age.[256] By reverse-transcriptase polymerase chain reaction (RT-PCR) analysis, neonatal and adult monocytes contain similar amounts of TLRs 1 to 9, MD-2, CD14, MyD88, TIR domain-containing adaptor protein (TIRAP), and interleukin-1 receptor-associated kinase 4 (IRAK4) mRNA.[240] One group reported that neonatal monocytes have reduced amounts of MyD88 protein[253] but found no difference between adult and neonatal monocytes in LPS-induced activation of ERK1/2 and p38 kinases and phosphorylation and degradation of inhibitor of kappa B (IκB), events that are downstream of MyD88.[253] Moreover, decreased expression of MyD88 is not sufficient to explain the diminished induction of HLA-DR and CD40 on neonatal monocytes in response to LPS,[183] or of CD40 and CD80 on neonatal dendritic cells in response to LPS and polyinosinic:polycytidylic (poly [I:C]) acid,[241] because these TLR ligands induce co-stimulatory molecules by TRIF- and type I IFN–dependent but MyD88-independent pathways.[257-260]

Humoral Influences on Mononuclear Phagocyte Cytokine Production. Levy and colleagues[240,261] identified adenosine as a factor in cord blood plasma that inhibited TNF-α production but preserved IL-6 production by monocytes in response to TLR2, TLR4, and TLR7 ligands. Compared with adult monocytes, cord blood monocytes also had a greater sensitivity to adenosine-induced (most likely A3 receptor–mediated) accumulation of cyclic adenosine monophosphate (cAMP). Adenosine was modestly elevated in cord blood compared with adult peripheral blood plasma, and the elevated cAMP had an inhibitory effect on TLR2- or TLR4-induced TNF-α but not on IL-6 production, and it was associated with decreased p38 kinase activation. In contrast, with TLR8 stimulation, cord blood plasma did not reduce the levels of p38 activation by monocytes or diminish the amounts of TNF-α, IL-1β, and multiple other cytokines produced.[94,240,262] The increased amounts of adenosine may be related, in part, to hypoxia occurring during the birth process, to the relatively low amounts of adenosine deaminase (which converts adenosine to inosine) in cord blood, and to increased adenosine generation by ectoenzymes that convert ATP/adenosine diphosphate (ADP) to adenosine.[263] In addition to adenosine, estrogen and progesterone are also at high levels in the fetus during pregnancy and in cord blood. These hormones may contribute to the suppressive effect of cord blood on TLR-induced monocyte proinflammatory cytokine production by inhibiting TLR-dependent activation of NF-κB activity, and, as in the case of adenosine, cord blood monocytes may have greater sensitivity to the inhibitory effects of these hormones than adult cells.[264]

It is plausible that immunosuppressive effect of humoral factors, such as adenosine, may be a transient phenomenon alleviated shortly after birth. This possibility is supported by studies that found that cord blood plasma, but not plasma from 1-month-old infants, suppressed IL-12p70 production and increased IL-10 production by adult peripheral BMCs treated with LPS and IFN-γ.[237,265] Moreover, a study of rhesus macaques evaluating TLR-induced cytokine production using whole-blood assays found that, similar to humans, TNF-α and IL-1β production by cord blood cells in response to TLR2/6 agonist stimulation was markedly reduced compared with the amounts produced by adult peripheral blood cells, but cytokine production from blood at 1 week of age was similar to (TNF-α) or exceeded that of adult blood (IL-1β);[94] whether this normalization by 1 week after birth reflects decreases in adenosine levels or monocyte sensitivity to adenosine or some other mechanism remains unclear.

Compared with blood from healthy adults, neonatal cord blood contains lower amounts of soluble CD14 and similar or modestly reduced amounts of soluble LPS-binding protein (LBP); concentrations of CD14 and LBP rise to adult levels in the first week of life and rise further in response to infection, as they do in adults.[266] The reduced amounts of these two proteins may account for the earlier observation that neonatal cord blood contains lower amounts of a soluble protein(s) that facilitates the response of monocytes to LPS.[252] However, the addition of soluble CD14 to neonatal plasma did not restore TNF-α production by neonatal monocytes.

Resolution of Mononuclear Phagocytic Inflammation

The resolution of mononuclear phagocytic inflammation involves the secretion of antiinflammatory cytokines, such as IL-10, IL-1 receptor antagonist,[232] and resolvin lipid mediators.[233] Phagocytosis-induced cell death (PICD) after ingestion of bacteria may also potentially be beneficial or harmful to the host, depending on whether cell death results in the death of the ingested microbe or its release into the extracellular space.[267] As was observed for neonatal neutrophils, cord blood monocytes had reduced PICD compared with adult peripheral blood monocytes,[268] which could contribute to persistent inflammation and sequelae, such as bronchopulmonary dysplasia and periventricular leukomalacia, in septic neonates.

SUMMARY

The most critical deficiency in phagocyte defenses in the term neonate and particularly in the preterm neonate is the limited ability to accelerate neutrophil production in response to infection. This age-specific limitation appears to result in large part from a limited neutrophil storage pool and perhaps a more limited ability to increase neutrophil production in response to infection. Impaired migration of neutrophils into tissues is likely to also be a factor, whereas phagocytosis and intracellular killing do not appear to be greatly impaired. However, the inability of neonatal neutrophils to form extracellular traps and the subsequent defect in extracellular bacterial killing may contribute to the increased susceptibility of neonates to bacterial infection. Persistent inflammation and tissue injury may result from impaired clearance of infection and protracted neutrophilic inflammation once the infection is cleared.

Monocytes and macrophages are detected in early fetal life and are present in blood and tissues by late gestation in numbers similar to adults. An exception is lung alveolar macrophages, which are few in number before birth, increase rapidly after birth in term neonates, but may be delayed in preterm neonates. Recruitment of monocytes to sites of infection and inflammation is slower than in adults. Ingestion and killing of pathogens by neonatal monocytes is as competent as in adults, but neonatal macrophages may be less efficient and be activated less efficiently by IFN-γ. Whereas expression by neonatal and adult monocytes of TLRs and other innate immune receptors appears not to differ greatly, their responses to stimulation via these receptors differ. In response to most but not all microbial stimuli, neonatal blood mononuclear cells produce (1) substantially lower amounts of IL-12 and type I IFNs, which are cytokines produced primarily by DCs and important for defense against intracellular pathogens; (2) moderately less TNF-α; (3) similar or somewhat greater amounts of other proinflammatory cytokines and IL-23, which are cytokines that are important in defense against extracellular bacterial and fungal pathogens; and (4) similar or greater amounts of the antiinflammatory and immunoregulatory cytokine IL-10.

Dendritic Cells: the Link between Innate and Adaptive Immunity

OVERVIEW

Dendritic cells, which have aptly been referred to as sentinels of the immune system, derive their name from the characteristic cytoplasmic protrusions or "dendrites" found on their mature form. DCs are bone marrow–derived myeloid cells that are found in all tissues and also circulate in the blood, where they represent approximately 0.5% to 1% of circulating leukocytes. Some DCs that are newly produced by the bone marrow enter into the blood and exit directly into lymphoid tissues, where they permanently reside as lymphoid tissue (LT) DCs. Other newly produced circulating DCs exit into the nonlymphoid tissues and are known as migratory DCs, which later migrate via afferent lymphatics into lymph nodes, particularly after exposure to inflammatory stimuli.

Human DCs can be divided into two major groups of cells that express high levels of the CD11c/CD18 β_2 integrin protein, hereafter referred to as conventional DCs (cDCs) and plasmacytoid cells (pDCs), which are $CD11c^-$ and express other distinct markers, such as CD123 (a component of the IL-3 receptor). Langerhans cells, which are also $CD11c^+$, are a migratory DC of squamous epithelium that has a distinct developmental origin from other DCs and will be discussed separately, as will inflammatory DCs, which are derived from mature monocytes rather than immature bone marrow precursors.

The DC cell surface lacks molecules characteristic of other bone marrow–derived cell lineages (a feature that is termed Lin^-), including molecules that are typically expressed on T cells (e.g., CD3-ε), monocytes or neutrophils (e.g., CD14), B cells (e.g., CD19 or CD20), and natural killer (NK) cells (e.g., CD16 or CD56). Resting DCs express MHC class II, and, upon activation/maturation, express greater amounts than any other cell type in the body. Relatively high amounts of MHC class I are also expressed. The role of MHC molecules in the presentation of antigenic peptide to T cells is discussed later in the section "Antigen Presentation by Classic Major Histocompatibility Complex Molecules."

cDC and pDC development in the bone marrow requires the expression by DC precursors of Flt3, a cytokine receptor, and its binding to the Flt3 ligand, which is mainly produced by nonhematopoietic stromal cells. Murine studies suggest that the DC and monocyte lineages are derived from a common bone marrow cell precursor, the monocyte and DC progenitor (MDP), which can differentiate into either monocytes or committed DC progenitors (CDPs).[269,270] The CDP gives rise to pre-cDCs, which enter the blood and then are presumed to rapidly enter into lymphoid or nonlymphoid organs, where, respectively, they differentiate in situ into immature lymphoid tissue cDCs or migratory cDCs. In the mouse, this final differentiation step includes the acquisition of their final DC subset surface phenotype, the characteristic cytoplasmic protrusions, and probing behavior.[271] pDCs leaving the bone marrow appear to be immature functionally but otherwise fully differentiated. Unlike cDCs, pDCs only acquire cytoplasmic protrusions and high levels of MHC class II after they undergo terminal maturation by exposure to pathogen-derived products or viral infection.

CONVENTIONAL DENDRITIC CELLS

Conventional dendritic cells (cDCs) play a unique and essential role in the initiation and modulation of the adaptive immune response as well as the maintenance of tolerance to self-proteins. They integrate signals from receptors that recognize microbial-derived PAMPs or DAMPs; the latter are of host origin and include molecules that are induced by inflammation, danger, or cellular stress, which are frequently induced in the setting of infection.[272] In the absence of these warning signs of infection, there is a constant low-level turnover of both migratory and lymphoid tissue cDCs.[273] By mechanisms that are poorly understood, some migratory cDCs in uninflamed tissues undergo a maturation process and travel via the afferent lymphatics to lymph nodes, where they interact with T cells in the T-cell–rich extrafollicular areas. These migratory cDCs play a central role in maintaining a state of T-cell tolerance to self-peptides derived from tissue proteins by presenting them to T cells in the absence of co-stimulatory signals required for T-cell activation.[274] This results in self-antigen–specific T cells that either die by apoptosis or that become anergic or regulatory cells, which are suppressive rather than immunostimulatory.[275] Resident lymphoid tissue DCs may also participate in tolerance induction for self-peptides of proteins expressed within lymphoid tissues in steady-state conditions.

Alternatively, in cases of infection within the tissues, immature migratory cDCs take up microbes and microbial antigens by micropinocytosis and macropinocytosis of extracellular fluid and particulate debris from perturbed tissues and process proteins into peptides, which are loaded onto MHC class I and class II molecules. At the same time, cDCs start to express on their surface the CCR7 chemokine receptor and to lose expression of receptors for chemokines that target them to nonlymphoid tissues. This change in chemokine receptor expression enhances cDC migration via lymphatics to T-cell–rich areas of the draining lymph nodes, which constitutively express chemokines that bind to CCR7 (CCL19 and CCL21). Concomitant with their migration to the draining lymph nodes, cDCs mature and cease their pinocytotic uptake and display on their cell surface high amounts of MHC molecules enriched for antigenic peptides derived from previously internalized microbes and antigens. These peptide-MHC complexes are present on the surface of mature DCs in great abundance, as are the co-stimulatory molecules CD40, CD80 (B7-1), and CD86 (B7-2), which together allow these cells to present antigens to T cells in a highly effective manner (see Antigen Presentation by Classic Major Histocompatibility Complex Molecules). A similar maturation process most likely occurs in situ with lymphoid tissue cDCs in response to lymphoid tissue inflammation. Because activated DCs display very high levels of peptide/MHC complexes and co-stimulatory ligands, they are the most efficient APCs for initiating the T-cell immune response to neoantigens, that is, antigens that have not been previously encountered by the host. However, cDCs are also important for maximizing the memory T-cell response to bacterial and viral pathogens.[276]

cDCs not only play a critical role in T-cell activation, they influence the quality of the T-cell response that ensues through the production of cytokines. Naïve CD4 T cells may become Th1, Th2, Th9, Th17, Th22, or T-follicular helper (TFH) effector cells,[230] each with a distinct cytokine-secretion profile and role in host defense. The secretion by DCs of particular cytokines instructs CD4 T-cell effector differentiation. For example, IL-12, IL-27, and type I IFNs instruct naïve CD4 T cells to produce IFN-γ and to differentiate into Th1 cells, which help to protect against intracellular bacteria, by multiple effects on mononuclear phagocytes, as well as certain viruses. IL-1, IL-6, TGF-β, and IL-23 induce differentiation to Th17 cells, which secrete IL-17A and IL-17F and help to protect against extracellular bacteria and fungi by increasing neutrophil production and activity and the expression in mucosal tissues of antimicrobial peptides and proteins. Th2 cell development is instructed by IL-33, thymic stromal lymphopoietin (TSLP), and IL-4 (from a non–T-cell source, such as basophils or innate lymphoid cells), and Th2 cells produce IL-4, IL-5, and IL-13 to protect against infections with multicellular pathogens, such as worms, but also are important in the pathogenesis of allergic disorders.

cDC migration and maturation can be triggered by a variety of stimuli, including pathogen-derived products that are recognized directly by innate immune receptors, by cytokines, including IL-1, TNF-α, and type I IFNs (see Tables 4-1 and 4-2), and by engagement of CD40 on the DC surface by CD40 ligand (CD154) on the surface of activated CD4 T cells (Table 4-5). Given their role as early detectors of infection or perturbations that are often associated with infection, it is not surprising that cDCs express a great diversity of receptors for PAMPs, including TLRs, NLRs, CLRs, and RLRs.[277-280] Human cDCs express multiple TLRs but do not express TLR9 (see Table 4-4) and consequently are not activated by unmethylated CpG DNA, a potent inducer of IFN-α production by pDCs, which do express TLR9. Unlike pDCs (and monocytes), cDCs express TLR3 (see Table 4-4), which, along with RIG-I, allows them to produce type I IFNs and other cytokines in response to double-stranded RNAs, including poly I:C. cDCs also express receptors for DAMPs, such as extracellular ATP and heat shock proteins, as well as receptors that facilitate the uptake of necrotic cell debris.

Given that the role of cDCs in regulating T-cell immunity is highly nuanced and potentially involves the recognition of diverse types of pathogens in different tissues, it is perhaps not surprising that cDCs are heterogeneous in their ontogeny, location, migration, phenotype, and function. In the human, there is specialization of cDC function that is carried out by two major subsets of human cDCs: CD1c$^+$ and CD141$^+$ cDCs.

CD1c$^+$ cDCs, which outnumber CD141$^+$ cDCs by about 10-fold, are the major population of cDCs in the blood, tissues, and lymphoid organs and appear to be the human equivalent of the murine CD11b$^+$ cDC subset.[281] CD1c$^+$ cDCs are equipped with a wide range of pattern recognition receptors and respond well to ligands for TLRs 1 to 8 and express high levels of the dectin-1 and dectin-3 CLRs, which are involved in fungal recognition. They produce TNF-α, IL-8, IL-10, IL-12, and IL-23. Like murine CD11b cDCs, they are particularly good stimulators of CD4 T cells, and, based on their cytokine profile, are likely important for the induction of both Th1 and Th17 immunity. They have a relatively limited ability to cross present antigens to and stimulate CD8 T cells. The importance of CD1c$^+$ cDCs in mycobacterial immunity is supported by the report of an infant with disseminated bacillus Calmette-Guérin (BCG) infection with an IRF8 missense mutation that results in selective depletion of CD1c$^+$ cDCs and, as a consequence, impaired TLR7/8 ligand–induced IL-12p70 production by peripheral blood mononuclear cells (PBMCs).[282] Because CD1c is involved in nonclassical antigen presentation of

Table 4-5 Selected Pairs of Surface Molecules Involved in T-Cell–Antigen-Presenting–Cell (APC) Interactions

T Cell Surface Molecule	T Cell Distribution	Corresponding Ligands on APCs	APC Distribution
CD2	Most T cells; higher on memory cells, lower on adult naïve and neonatal T cells	LFA-3 (CD58), CD59	Leukocytes
CD4	Subset of αβ T cells with predominantly helper activity	MHC class II β chain	DCs MΦ, B cells, others (see text)
CD5	All T cells	CD72	B cells, MΦ
CD8	Subset of αβ T cells with predominantly cytotoxic activity	MHC class I heavy chain	Ubiquitous
LFA-1 (CD11a/CD18)	All T cells; higher on memory cells, lower on adult naïve and neonatal T cells	ICAM-1 (CD54)	Leukocytes (ICAM-3 > ICAM-1, ICAM-2) and endothelium (ICAM-1, ICAM-2); most ICAM-1 expression requires activation
		ICAM-2 (CD102)	
		ICAM-3 (CD50)	
CD28	Most CD4 T cells, subset of CD8 T cells	CD80 (B7-1)	DCs, MΦ, activated B cells
		CD86 (B7-2)	
ICOS	Effector and memory T cells, particularly CD4$^+$ T follicular helper cells, not on resting naïve cells	B7RP-1 (ICOS-L, B7h)	B cells, MΦ, DCs, endothelial cells
VLA-4 (CD49d/CD29)	All T cells; higher on memory cells, lower on adult naïve and neonatal T cells	VCAM-1 (CD106)	Activated or inflamed endothelium (increased by TNF, IL-1, IL-4)
ICAM-1 (CD54)	All T cells; higher on memory cells, lower on adult virgin and neonatal T cells	LFA-1 (CD11a/CD18)	Leukocytes
CTLA-4 (CD152)	Activated T cells	CD80	DCs, MΦ, activated B cells, activated T cells
		CD86	
CD40 ligand (CD154)	Activated CD4 T cells; lower on neonatal CD4 T cells	CD40	DCs, MΦ, B cells, thymic epithelial cells
PD-1	Activated CD4 and CD8 T cells	PD-L1, PD-L2	DCs, MΦ, B cells, regulatory T cells

CTLA-4, Cytotoxic T-lymphocyte antigen-4; *DCs*, dendritic cells; *ICAM*, intercellular adhesion molecule; *ICOS*, inducible co-stimulator; *IL*, interleukin; *LFA*, leukocyte function antigen; *MΦ*, mononuclear phagocytes; *MHC*, major histocompatibility complex; *PD-1*, programmed death molecule-1; *TNF*, tumor necrosis factor; *VCAM*, vascular cell adhesion molecule; *VLA-4*, very late antigen-4.

mycobacterial products (mycoketides and lipopeptides) to T cells, limitations in mycobacterial antigen presentation might also have played a role in this patient.

CD141$^+$ cDCs, which appear to be the human equivalent of the murine CD8α$^+$CD103$^+$ cDC subset, comprise about 10% of human blood cDCs (i.e., only about 0.1% of PBMCs). CD141$^+$ cDCs are also found among resident cDCs of lymphoid tissue, including lymph node, tonsil, and spleen, and nonlymphoid tissues, including the skin, liver, and lung. Like murine CD8α$^+$CD103$^+$ cDCs, human CD141$^+$ cDCs express the CLEC9A CLR, which facilitates the uptake of necrotic cellular material for antigen processing, and are highly efficient at cross-presentation, in which externally derived proteins that are taken up by endocytosis, pinocytosis, or by CLEC9A are diverted from loading onto MHC class II molecules and, instead, are loaded onto MHC class I molecules for presentation to CD8 T cells (see Antigen Presentation by Classic Major Histocompatibility Complex Molecules). These DCs are capable of efficiently phagocytosing dead cells by using CLEC9. In contrast to mice, in which CD8α$^+$ DCs are highly specialized for cross-presentation, most other human DC populations also have some capacity to cross present antigens to CD8 T cells. CD141$^+$ cDCs produce high levels of IFN-λ (IL-28/29), TNF-α, and the chemokine CXCL10 after engagement of TLR3 by poly I:C, a mimic of viral double-stranded RNA.

Neonatal Conventional Dendritic Cells

Conventional dendritic cells overall constitute a similar fraction (0.5%-1.0%) of blood mononuclear cells in neonates, children, and adults, but cDCs only constitute about 25% of the total of circulating DCs in neonates, whereas cDCs constitute about 75% of the total in adults.[183,283-286] The absolute numbers of cDCs remain constant from the neonatal period into adulthood, whereas the fraction and absolute numbers of pDCs decline with increasing postnatal age, reaching numbers similar to adults at greater than or equal to 5 years of age.[285] To the best of our knowledge, the relative proportion of circulating cDCs in the newborn that are CD1c$^+$ and CD141$^+$ has not yet been reported. It is likely that the CD1c$^+$ cDC subset predominates in the neonatal circulation as in the adult circulation (10:1 ratio with respect to CD141$^+$ cells), so that the results of cDC (Lin$^-$CD11c$^+$) studies using cord blood or infant peripheral blood mainly reflect the properties of the CD1c$^+$ subset.

Older flow cytometric studies[183,241,283] reported that expression of MHC class II (HLA-DR), CD40, CD80, and CD86 on cord blood and adult peripheral blood cDCs were similar, although a more recent study found that the basal surface expression of HLA-DR and CD80 on cord blood cDCs was substantially decreased compared with circulating adult cDCs.[238] Although cord blood cDCs can stimulate allogeneic cord blood T cells in vitro,[284,287,288] it is unclear whether neonatal cDCs are as proficient as adult cDCs in processing and presenting foreign antigens to T cells. Limitations in cord blood cDC antigen presentation are plausible because cord blood cDCs do not upregulate CD40 and CD80 to the same degree as adult cDCs in response to agonists for TLR2/6 (macrophage-activated lipopeptide [MALP]), TLR3 (poly I:C), TLR4 (LPS), or TLR7, whereas TLR8 agonists induce equivalent increases in expression.[241,262] Decreased maturation of cord blood cDCs was also observed in response to pertussis toxin.[289]

Flow cytometric studies of cytokine expression by cord blood cDCs indicate that they were approximately 50% as efficient as adult cDCs at producing TNF-α in response to LPS,[183] whereas TNF-α production in response to TLR8 agonists was similar.[262] In contrast to TNF-α, IL-1α and IL-6 production by adult cDCs and cDCs from cord blood of term infants in response to LPS was similar,[183] as was production of IL-12/IL-23p40 in response to most TLR agonists.[234] However, cDCs in the cord blood of premature infants have markedly lower responses to these stimuli,[290] which is paralleled by reduced secretion of IL-23 by cord blood mononuclear cell cultures. Given the importance of IL-23 production by cDCs in instructing naïve CD4 T cells for differentiation into Th17 effector cells, it is plausible that premature infants may have compromised Th17 immunity, which may increase their risk of extracellular bacterial and fungal infection.

However, these limitations in cDC function present at birth may be quite transient. A recent longitudinal study of a cohort of South African infants that evaluated cDC cytokine accumulation of TNF-α, IL-6 and IL-12/23p40 by flow cytometry after whole-blood stimulation with TLR agonists found that the cytokine level per cell was higher at 2 weeks of age compared with adults.[244] This enhanced cytokine accumulation was consistent in that it was observed for multiple cytokines (TNF-α, IL-6, and IL-12/23p40) and after stimulation with TLR2/1, TLR4, or TLR7/8 agonists. Of interest, in most cases, the cytokine level per cell gradually declined to adult levels by 1 year of age. This apparently rapid postnatal maturation cDC function may not be limited to cytokine production capacity because there are also marked increases in the cDC expression of HLA-DR and CD80 by 3 months of age compared with at birth.[238]

Earlier studies using stimulation of whole blood or unfractionated blood mononuclear cells also indicated that cord blood cDC responses to TLR3 stimulation were substantially reduced compared with those of adults. TLR3-induced cDC function can be inferred after poly I:C stimulation of whole blood or blood mononuclear cells because poly I:C activates blood cells primarily via TLR3, and cDCs are the only cell type in blood that expresses substantial amounts of TLR3. Therefore the observation that poly I:C–stimulated cord blood and cord blood mononuclear cells had modestly diminished production of type I IFNs and markedly decreased production of IL-12p70 suggested that cord blood cDCs had decreased TLR3-dependent function.[241,291] The production of IFN-γ by poly I:C–stimulated cord blood and cord blood mononuclear cells also likely reflected diminished TLR3-mediated IL-12p70 and type I IFN production by cDCs, which, in turn, resulted in diminished production of IFN-γ by cord blood NK cells (see Fetal and Neonatal Natural Killer Cell-Mediated Cytotoxicity and Cytokine Production).

Several studies suggest that the reduced TLR3-mediated cDC function increases during the first month of life. For example, a study in The Gambia found that poly I:C stimulation of whole blood induced significantly higher levels of TNF-α and IFN-γ at 1 month of age compared with at birth (cord blood).[292] Similarly, a study of Belgian infants showed a significant increase in IL-12p70 secretion after poly

I:C whole blood stimulation at 1 month of age compared with at birth.[237] In a longitudinal study of South African infants peripheral blood samples from 2-week-old infants had substantially higher levels of IL-12p70, IL-23, IFN-γ, and chemokines that are upregulated by IFN-γ (MCP-1 and IFN-γ–induced protein-10[IP-10]) than did adult blood samples,[244] and these high levels declined to those of adults by approximately 1 year of age. In contrast to these studies, which indicated rapid postnatal acquisition of adult levels of competency for TLR3-induced cDC function, one study of Canadian infants found that poly I:C treatment of cord blood mononuclear cells induced levels of IL-12/23p40, IL-12p70, IFN-γ, and type I IFN that were substantially lower than those of adult peripheral blood mononuclear cells, and they remained so at 1 and 2 years of age.[235] These different results, at least those in the first month of life, could reflect humoral factors, such as adenosine or maternally derived hormones, acting to reduce the cDC-derived production of cytokines in whole blood. However, the precise basis for these findings is unclear, and there is precedent for substantially different levels of TLR-induced cytokine production by cDCs when they are assayed as purified cells versus in whole-blood assays.[293]

A recent study used transcriptional profiling to compare the response of DCs (a mixture of cDCs and pDCs) from cord blood and adult peripheral blood to incubation with RSV.[294] Of interest, cord blood DCs had a transcriptional profile indicating increased transforming growth factor (TGF)-β– and TGF-β–dependent gene expression, and secreted increased levels of TGF-β compared with adult DCs. When RSV-infected DCs were co-cultured with autologous circulating T cells, the adult co-cultured cells secreted relatively high levels of IL-12p70, TNF-α, IL-2, IL-10, IL-13, and IFN-γ, whereas the cord blood co-cultured cells secreted low levels of these cytokines and, compared to the adult cell co-cultures, high levels of IL-1β, IL-4, IL-6, and IL-17. Blockade of TGF-β signaling using a chemical inhibitor in the cord blood co-cultures markedly increased IL-12p70 secretion and more modestly enhanced the levels of other cytokines, such as IL-1β and IL-6. This approach did not address to what extent the results are due to differences between adult and neonatal T-cell populations, that is, a substantial fraction of effector memory T-cells were already committed to the Th1 lineage in adult preparations, whereas the cord blood T-cells were predominantly uncommitted antigenically-naïve T-cells. The importance of cDCs versus pDCs for TGF-β production is also unclear. Despite these limitations, the findings suggest that cord blood cDCs in response to RSV secrete a cytokine milieu (high levels of IL-1β, IL-6, and TGF-β and low levels IL-12p70) that favor Th17 differentiation rather than Th1 differentiation, which could contribute to the immunopathogenesis of RSV infection in young infants.

PLASMACYTOID DENDRITIC CELLS

Plasmacytoid dendritic cell have a Lin− $CD11c^-$ $HLA\text{-}DR^+$ CD123(IL-3 receptor)$^+$ CD303(BDCA-2)$^+$ CD304(BDCA4; neuropilin)$^+$ surface phenotype.[295] They also express CD4 and CD45RA.[296] Immature pDCs are found in the blood and secondary lymphoid organs. In contrast to migratory cDCs, pDCs appear to migrate to secondary lymphoid organs from the blood via entry into high endothelial venules. They also accumulate at particularly high levels in inflamed lymph nodes. Their characteristic function is the capacity to produce high levels of type I IFNs and certain other cytokines, which achieve systemic levels and directly help to protect the host from viral infection in particular. Although pDCs in the blood and uninflamed tissues have a very limited capacity for antigen uptake and presentation, stimulation of these cells via TLR7 or TLR9 results in their upregulation of CCR7 and migration to T-cell–rich areas of lymph nodes, upregulation of HLA-DR and co-stimulatory molecules, and increased capacity to present antigen to T cells, including cross-presentation of antigen to the CD8 T-cell subset. Consistent with their specialized function, pDCs express only high levels of two TLRs—TLR7, which allows them to respond to single-stranded RNA from RNA viruses such as influenza, parainfluenza, RSV, and HIV-1, and TLR9, which allows them to respond to unmethylated CpG DNA from bacteria, such as *S. aureus*, and DNA viruses, such as HSV.[295] Because pDCs are the only circulating leukocyte that expresses TLR9, the production of type I IFN by CpG stimulation of whole blood or BMC is often used to infer pDC function. pDCs also express CLRs that are mainly involved in antigen uptake, for instance, BDCA-2 (CLEC4C), DEC-205, dectin-1, DCIR (dendritic cell immunoreceptor), and Fc receptor CD32, rather than innate immune receptors that are directly linked to proinflammatory intracellular signaling pathways.

Neonatal Plasmacytoid Dendritic Cells

Cells with the histologic features of immature pDCs are found in fetal lymph nodes between 19 to 21 weeks of gestation.[297] Using flow cytometry, pDC-lineage cells ($Lin^-CD11c^-CD4^+CD45RA^+CD123^+$) have been identified in fetal liver and bone marrow as early as 16 weeks of gestation; these can be further divided into $CD34^+$ and $CD34^-$ subsets that are likely to be pro-pDCs and immature pDCs, respectively. Of interest, both fetal liver pro-pDCs and immature pDCs were capable of high levels of type I IFN production in response to stimulation with irradiated HSV-1, indicating this function of pDCs is established early in ontogeny.

The absolute concentration of pDCs in the term neonate is approximately twofold higher than in the adult and gradually declines after birth, reaching numbers similar to adults at greater than or equal to 5 years of age.[285] The biologic significance of the predominance of pDCs in the neonatal circulation is uncertain. In the prematurely born neonate, there is a trend for a greater proportion of cord blood pDCs with a pro-pDC ($CD34^+$) surface phenotype than is observed in adult blood.

Compared with adult pDCs, multiple studies have found that cord blood pDCs produce less type I IFNs in response to unmethylated CpG oligonucleotide, a potent TLR9 ligand.[283,298,299] or to TLR7 agonists.[298] Because pDCs appear to be the main sources of type I IFN in response to CpG oligonucleotide stimulation of whole blood or blood mononuclear cells, type I IFN production from these cells can be attributed to pDCs. Thus diminished type I IFN expression in 4-day-old neonates suggests that decreased pDC function persists until at least this age,[283] These reductions in type I IFN production in response to TLR7 and TLR9 agonists are more pronounced in the cord blood of prematurely born infants[290,300] and are associated with greater immaturity of premature infant pDCs, based on their decreased expression of CD304 (BDCA-4) and "immature" morphology by electron microscopy. The defect in neonatal pDC type I IFN production in response to CpG stimulation appears to result in part from impaired activation and translocation of IRF7 to the nucleus.[298] Consistent with these findings, TNF-α is more modestly reduced, and production of IL-6 is comparable to adult pDCs.[298]

In addition to diminished type I IFN responses, cord blood pDCs also express lower amounts of HLA-DR, CD40, CD80, CD86, and CCR7 after stimulation with TLR7 or TLR9 agonists than adult pDCs.[283,298,301] Cord blood pDCs may also have a tendency for reduced survival during culture with CpG oligonucleotides, which could contribute to their reduced responses to these stimuli.[299]

In older studies, type I IFN production by blood cells from neonates in response to direct viral stimulation was significantly diminished, for instance, to HSV,[302] cytomegalovirus (CMV),[298] and parainfluenza virus.[241,303] As for stimulation by TLR7 or TLR9 ligands, this reduced type I IFN response to herpesviruses was associated with decreased IRF7 cytoplasmic to nuclear translocation.[298] However, a recent report[299] found that type I IFN production in response to influenza A virus (live or heat-inactivated), HIV, or HSV was similar for cord blood and adult peripheral blood pDCs, regardless of whether whole blood, blood mononuclear cells, or purified pDCs were used. The production of TNF-α and the chemokines CCL3 and CCL4 in this study were also similar for cord blood and adult peripheral blood pDCs by using these assay conditions.[299] The reasons for these different findings remain unclear, but they raise the possibility that production of such cytokines by neonatal pDCs may be as competent as those of adults in response to strong viral stimulation. Therefore additional studies to determine pDC function ex vivo in the setting of neonatal viral infection will be of interest.

In limited studies, the age at which responses to TLR ligands become comparable to adult cells has been assessed. CpG-induced upregulation of HLA-DR and CD80 on pDCs did not reach adult levels until 6 to 9 months of age. pDC-derived chemokine production (interferon gamma induced protein 10 [IP-10] and monokine induced by gamma interferon [MIG]) in whole blood was lower during the first year of life compared with adult pDCs. Of interest, pDC-derived IL-6, IL-8, IL-10, and IL-1β were significantly higher than in adult cells from 3 months of age onward, suggesting that neonatal pDCs have a unique cytokine profile that may inhibit Th1 responses (i.e., IL-10) and promote Th17 responses (IL-6 and IL-1β). Consistent with this finding, which suggested a maturation of pDC function by 9 months of age, one study[235] found that pDC production of TNF-α and IL-6 in response to either TLR7/8 or TLR9 agonists at 1 year of age was similar to those of adult pDCs.

LANGERHANS CELLS

Langerhans cells are a unique type of DC found only in the epidermis, in the interstices of keratinocytes, where they can be differentiated from dermal cDCs by their expression of CD1a and Birbeck granules and lack of expression of the factor XIIIa coagulation factor. Langerhans cells also express high levels of Langerin (CD207), although this is not specific for this cell type because subsets of cDCs also express Langerin but do so at lower levels.[269] Langerhans cells are distinct from other DC populations in their ability to undergo local self-renewal in the epidermis (for up to 10 years after limb transplant) and their dependence on M-CSF for their development rather than the Flt3 ligand or GM-CSF.[304] Langerhans cells do not express TLRs 2, 4, and 5, which may account for their limited responsiveness to bacterial stimulation. In uninflamed human skin Langerhans cells seem to mainly be involved in the maintenance of tolerance by selectively promoting the activation of skin-resident regulatory T cells, but in response to infection, for instance, the injection into skin of *Candida albicans*, can present antigen to skin-resident pathogen-specific memory T cells.[305] However, cell lineage tracing studies suggest that Langerhans cells may play a relatively minor role compared with migratory dermal cDCs in the activation of T cells in the draining lymph nodes, even though they may cross present protein antigens as efficiently as cDCs.

In the embryonic mouse, Langerhans cells appear to arise largely from fetal liver monocytes that seed the skin before bone marrow hematopoiesis initiates. This may also apply to humans because Langerhans cells can be detected in human embryonic skin as early as 6 to 7 weeks of gestation.[306,307] However, there is little information as to the function of Langerhans cells in the human fetus and neonate.

INFLAMMATORY AND MONOCYTE-DERIVED DENDRITIC CELLS

Murine inflammatory DCs, in contrast to cDCs, are derived from mature monocytes that are exposed to strong inflammatory stimuli, such as LPS or gram-negative bacteria. Murine inflammatory DCs, like cDCs, have cytoplasmic protrusions, upregulate CCR7, home to T-cell areas of peripheral lymphoid tissue, and can efficiently present antigen to and activate CD4 and CD8 T cells; however, inflammatory DCs are distinct in expressing DC-SIGN (CD209a).[308] Human inflammatory DCs with many of these features, and that are likely to have been derived from monocytes, have been described in psoriatic skin,[309,310] inflammatory tumor ascites fluid, and synovial fluid of patients with rheumatoid arthritis.[311] Cells similar, although not identical to, inflammatory DCs can be generated by culturing monocytes in GM-CSF plus IL-4 to produce monocyte-derived DCs (moDCs), which can then be matured by treatment with TNF-α.

Whether inflammatory DCs occur in the neonate in settings of strong inflammatory stimuli, such as bacterial sepsis, is not known. Studies comparing neonatal and adult moDCs suggest that the capacity of neonatal monocytes to differentiate into inflammatory DCs that can instruct Th1 immunity is limited. Most studies have found that neonatal moDCs produce much less IL-12p70 in response to LPS, poly I:C, and TLR8 ligands or engagement of CD40 than adult moDCs.[312-314] Reduced production of IL-12p70 is due to reduced amounts of the IL-12p35 component, whereas the p40 component that is common to IL-12p70 and IL-23 (IL-12/23p40) is produced in similar amounts by neonatal and adult cells. Diminished IL-12p35 production appears to result from a defect in IRF3 binding to and remodeling of the IL-12p35 promoter, whereas more proximal aspects of signaling resulting in IRF3 translocation from the cytoplasm to the nucleus appear to be intact.[315,316] Although neonatal moDCs stimulated with live *Mycobacterium bovis* BCG[317] or with a TLR8 agonist plus LPS or poly I:C secreted much less IL-12 than adult moDCs, when moDCs were stimulated with these combinations of TLR ligands in cultures also containing autologous naïve CD4 T cells, comparable IL-12–dependent IFN-γ production was observed.[314] Together, these observations suggest that defective production of IFN-γ–inducing cytokines, including IL-12, by neonatal DCs can be overcome by combined signaling from TLRs, NLRs, and direct physical interactions between T cells and DCs.

SUMMARY

DCs are detectable by 16 weeks of gestation. At birth, the concentration of cDCs is similar and the concentration of pDCs greater than in adult blood. Although adult and neonatal blood cDCs and moDCs express on their surface the MHC class II molecule HLA-DR and co-stimulatory molecules in similar abundance, expression by neonatal DCs increases less in response to stimulation via TLRs. TLR-stimulated neonatal cDCs and moDCs generally produce substantially less IL-12 and type I IFNs, cytokines that contribute to early innate defenses and subsequent T-cell–mediated defenses against intracellular pathogens. By contrast, these neonatal DCs produce proinflammatory cytokines and IL-23, which are important in defense against extracellular bacterial and fungal pathogens, more efficiently than their adult counterparts. These differences may limit the ability of neonatal DCs to activate naïve pathogen-specific T cells and, in particular, to induce IFN-γ–producing Th1 T-cell responses rather than Th17 or Th2 T-cell responses. However, neonatal DCs may be able to produce IL-12 and support IFN-γ production by neonatal T cells in response to combinatorial activation of innate immune receptors and when in contact with T cells. Whether neonatal pDCs are deficient in the production of type I IFNs, IFN-dependent chemokines, and other functions during in vivo viral infections remains unclear; these cells are markedly less responsive to stimulation with chemical TLR7 and TLR9 agonists.

Natural Killer Cells and Innate Lymphoid Cells

NATURAL KILLER CELLS

Overview and Development

NK cells are large granular lymphocytes with cytotoxic function, which, unlike T and B lymphocytes, lack antigen-specific T-cell receptor (TCR) or B-cell receptor (BCR) receptors characteristic of the adaptive immune system and instead express a diverse array of activating and inhibitory receptors. Although NK cells are generally considered to be a component of the innate rather than adaptive immune system, in mouse models they can be primed by infection, such as with herpesviruses, and retain certain features of memory/effector T cells, such as enhanced cytotoxicity and cytokine secretion for at least several months postinfection. In clinical practice, NK cells are usually defined as lymphoid cells that express CD16 and CD56 but not CD3, that is, have a $CD16^+CD56^+CD3^-$ surface phenotype. Virtually all circulating NK cells from adults also express the NK-cell–specific NKp30 and NKp46 receptors, along with CD2 and CD161, and approximately 50% express CD57, but these molecules are found on other lymphocyte types as well.

The fetal liver produces NK cells as early as 6 weeks of gestation, but the bone marrow is the major site for NK-cell production from late gestation onward. NK cells are derived from bone marrow cells that lack surface molecules specific for other cell lineages (i.e., $CD34^+Lin^-$ cells) but express CD7 or CD38. NK-cell development is dependent on the IL-15/IL-15 receptor (which consists of the IL-15 receptor α chain, the IL-2 receptor β chain, and the common γ chain)/Janus tyrosine kinase 3 (JAK3) pathway. Based on the lack of NK-cell development in genetic immunodeficiencies, human NK-cell development also requires adenylate kinase 2 and the GATA binding protein 2 transcription factor.[318] In vitro studies suggest a NK lineage cell developmental sequence in which CD161 is acquired early in NK development. At the next developmental stage, NKp30, NKp46, 2B4, and NKG2D are expressed on the cell surface, followed by members of the killer cell inhibitor receptor (KIR) family, CD94-NKG2A, CD2, and CD56; the function of these molecules is discussed in the sections that follow.

NK cells are functionally defined by their natural ability to lyse virally infected or tumor target cells in a non–HLA-restricted manner that does not require prior sensitization. NK cells preferentially recognize and kill cells expressing ligands for activating receptors that are not antigen-specific in conjunction with reduced or absent expression of self-HLA class I molecules, a property referred to as natural cytotoxicity.[319] These ligands for activating receptors are characteristically increased in response to stresses, such as infection or malignant transformation. This is in contrast with cytotoxic CD8 T cells, which are triggered to lyse targets after the recognition of foreign antigenic peptides bound to self-HLA class I molecules or self-peptides bound to foreign HLA class I molecules. NK cells also have the ability to kill target cells that are coated with IgG antibodies, a process known as antibody-dependent cellular cytotoxicity (ADCC). ADCC requires the recognition of IgG bound to the target cell by the NK-cell FcγRIIIB receptor (CD16).

Mature NK cells can be subdivided into $CD56^{hi}CD16^{lo}$ and $CD56^{lo}CD16^{hi}$ populations.[320] $CD56^{hi}CD16^{lo}$ cells usually are only a minority of mature NK cells in the circulation but express CCR7 and L-selectin and predominate in lymph node tissue. $CD56^{hi}CD16^{lo}$ cells have limited cytotoxic capacity but produce cytokines and chemokines efficiently, whereas the inverse is true for $CD56^{lo}CD16^{hi}$ NK cells.[321] These features suggest that the $CD56^{hi}CD16^{lo}$ subset could regulate lymph node T cells and DCs through cytokine secretion. Developmental studies suggest that $CD56^{hi}CD16^{lo}$ NK cells are less mature than $CD56^{lo}CD16^{hi}$ NK cells, but the precise precursor-product relationship of these subsets under various conditions in vivo has not been firmly established.

NK cells are particularly important in the early containment of viral infections, especially with pathogens that may initially avoid control by adaptive immune mechanisms.

Infection of host cells by the herpesvirus group, including HSV, CMV, and varicella-zoster virus (VZV), and some adenoviruses leads to decreased surface expression of HLA class I molecules. Viral protein–mediated decreases in expression of HLA class I may limit the ability of CD8 T cells to lyse virally infected cells and to clonally expand from naïve precursors. These virus-mediated effects may be particularly important during early infection, when CD8 T cells with appropriate antigen specificity are present at a low frequency. By contrast, decreased HLA class I expression in conjunction with the expression of ligands for activating receptors facilitates recognition and lysis by NK cells. The importance of NK cells in the initial control of human herpesvirus infections is suggested by the observation that persons with selective deficiency of NK-cell numbers or function are prone to severe infection with HSV, CMV, and VZV.

Natural Killer Cell Receptors

NK-cell cytotoxicity is regulated by a complex array of inhibitory and activating receptor–ligand interactions with target cells (Fig. 4-3). The expression of multiple combinations of inhibitory and activating receptors leads to a large amount of NK-cell diversity. By some estimates, there are 6000 to 30,000 different NK-cell populations within an individual.[322] Individual NK cells in the bone marrow appear to undergo a tuning process so that the threshold for their activation is appropriate for their particular repertoire of receptors. NK-cell activation is inhibited by recognition of HLA class I molecules expressed on nontransformed, uninfected cells; this recognition is presumed to provide a net inhibitory signal that predominates over activating signals. Infection or other perturbations of the host target cell, such as malignant transformation, can reduce the amount of HLA class I on the cell surface, thereby reducing inhibitory signaling, and upregulate other molecules that promote NK-cell activation, such as MHC class I–related chains A and B (MICA and MICB).

There are two major families of inhibitory NK-cell receptors that recognize HLA class I molecules in humans: KIR and the CD94-containing C-type lectin families.[323,324] KIRs with a long cytoplasmic domain transmit signals that inhibit NK-cell activation; most, although not all, NK cells express one or more inhibitory KIRs on their surface. Most NK cells, including all those not expressing any inhibitory KIRs, also express inhibitory CD94-NKG2A receptors.[325] KIRs bind to polymorphic HLA-B, HLA-C, or HLA-A molecules,[324] whereas CD94-NKG2A binds to HLA-E, which is monomorphic (HLA molecules are discussed later in the sections "Antigen Presentation by Classic Major Histocompatibility Complex Molecules" and "Nonclassic Antigen-Presentation Molecules"). Because HLA-E reaches the cell surface only when its peptide binding groove is occupied by hydrophobic peptides derived from the leader sequences of HLA-A, HLA-B, and HLA-C molecules,[326] the amount of HLA-E on the cell surface reflects the overall levels of HLA-A, HLA-B, and HLA-C molecules on that cell.[327]

In addition to CD94-NKG2A, a third group of inhibitory receptors that broadly recognize HLA class I molecules are the leukocyte immunoglobulin-like receptors B1 and B2 (LILRB1 and LILRB2). LILRB1 and LILRB2, also referred to as LIR1/CD85J and LIR2/CD85d, bind to HLA-A, HLA-B, and HLA-C molecules, as well as the nonconventional class

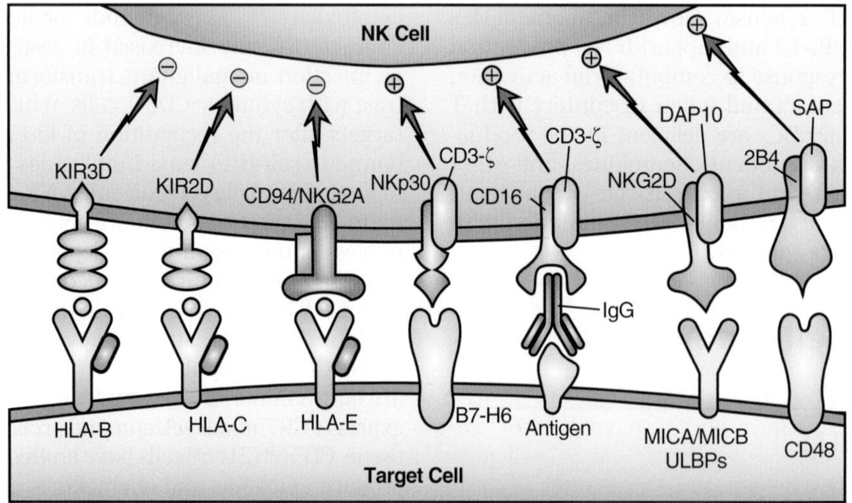

Figure 4-3 Positive and negative regulation of NK-cell cytotoxicity by receptor–ligand interactions. NK-cell cytotoxicity is inhibited by engagement of KIR by MHC class I molecules, such as HLA-B and HLA-C. In addition, NK cells are inhibited when CD94-NKG2A complex, a member of the C-type lectin family, on the NK cell is engaged by HLA-E. HLA-E binds hydrophobic leader peptides derived from HLA-A, HLA-B, and HLA-C molecules and requires these for its surface expression. Thus HLA-E surface expression on a potential target cell indicates the overall production of conventional MHC class I molecules. These inhibitory influences on NK-cell cytotoxicity are overcome if viral infection of the target cell results in decreased MHC class I and HLA-E levels. NK-cell cytotoxicity is positively regulated by the engagement of NKG2D, which interacts with MICA, MICB, and ULBPs; 2B4, which interacts with CD48; and natural cytotoxicity receptors, such as NKp30 and, not shown, NKp46, for which the ligands on the target cell induced by infection are unknown. CD16 is an Fc receptor for IgG and mediates antibody-dependent cellular cytotoxicity against cells coated with antibody, for instance, against viral proteins found on the cell surface. Positive receptors mediate their intracellular signals via associated CD3-ζ, DAP10 or DAP12 proteins. *DAP,* DNAX-activating protein; *HLA,* human leukocyte antigen; *IgG,* immunoglobulin G; *KIR,* killer inhibitory receptors; *MHC,* major histocompatibility complex; *MICA* and *MICB,* MHC class I–related chains A and B; *NK,* natural killer; *SAP,* SLAM-associated protein; *ULBPs,* UL16-binding proteins (UL16 is a cytomegalovirus protein).

I molecules HLA-E, HLA-F, and HLA-G. HLA-G is the only HLA class I molecule constitutively expressed on the surface of fetal trophoblasts. Thus the interaction of LILRB1 and LILRB2 with HLA-G is thought to protect the placenta from injury by maternal NK cells.[328]

Countering the effects of these inhibitory receptors are multiple types of activating receptors. NKG2D is found on NK cells as well as in certain T-cell populations. NKG2D recognizes MICA, MICB, and UL16-binding proteins (ULBPs 1-4).[329] MICA and MICB are nonclassical HLA class I molecules that are expressed on stressed or infected cells. ULBPs are a group of HLA class I–like molecules expressed on many cell types that were first identified and named based on their ability to bind to the human CMV UL16 viral protein. In human CMV infection, UL16 probably limits NK-cell– and T-cell–mediated activation by binding to ULBPs internally and preventing their surface expression on the infected cell.[329]

NK cells also express NKp30, NKp44, and NKp46. NKp44 and NKp46 can trigger NK-cell cytotoxicity through their recognition of influenza virus hemagglutinin and Sendai (parainfluenza family) virus hemagglutinin-neuraminidase.[330] These receptors also recognize ligands on tumor cells and cells infected with herpesviruses, but with the exception of NKp30, which recognizes the tumor ligand B7-H6,[319] the definitive nature of the ligands is not known.

The proteins 2B4 (CD244) and NTBA are members of the signaling lymphocytic-activation molecule (SLAM) protein family and are expressed on most NK cells.[331] 2B4 binds to CD48, whereas the ligand for NTBA remains unclear. Both 2B4 and NTBA engagement triggers NK-cell activation through SLAM-associated protein (SAP), an intracellular adapter protein that is mutated in the X-linked lymphoproliferative syndrome.

Finally, NK cells may express KIRs with short cytoplasmic tails, which unlike their counterparts with long cytoplasmic tails, activate NK cells by a DNAX-activating protein 12 (DAP12) signaling mechanism.[319] Also, unlike CD94-NKG2A, CD94-NKG2C is an activating receptor complex that also activates via DAP12 signaling. These activating KIRs and CD94-NKG2C and their respective inhibitory forms have identical or very similar ligand specificities. How NK cells integrate the effects on natural cytotoxicity of these multiple inhibitory and activating receptors, particularly those that recognize the same or similar ligands, remains unclear.

Natural Killer Cell Cytotoxicity

After binding via adhesion molecule interactions and activation, NK cells release perforin and granzymes from preformed cytotoxic granules into a synapse formed between the NK cell and its target, leading to death by apoptosis of the target cell. NK cell–mediated cytotoxicity also may be mediated by Fas ligand or TRAIL (TNF-related apoptosis-inducing ligand) expressed on the activated NK cell surface. Fas–Fas ligand interactions appear not to be essential for human NK cell control of viral infections because persons with dominant-negative mutations of the Fas or Fas ligand genes develop autoimmunity but do not experience an increased severity of virus infections.[332] In contrast with natural cytotoxicity, in which perforin/granzyme-dependent mechanisms appear to be predominant, ADCC appears to use both perforin/granzyme- and Fas ligand–dependent cytotoxic mechanisms.[333]

Natural Killer Cell Cytokine Responsiveness and Dependence

NK cell proliferation and cytotoxicity are enhanced in vitro by cytokines produced by T cells (IL-2, IFN-γ), APCs (IL-1β, IL-12p70, IL-18, and type I IFNs), and nonhematopoietic cells (IL-15, stem cell factor, Flt3 ligand, IFN-β). IL-15, which appears critical for the development of NK cells, also promotes the survival of mature NK cells and, like IL-12, increases the expression of perforin and granzymes. A subset of NK cells found in mucosal-associated lymphoid tissues responds to IL-23 by producing cytokines, including IL-22, that help to protect the gut from bacterial pathogens.[320]

Natural Killer Cell Cytokine and Chemokine Production

NK cells are also important producers of IFN-γ and TNF-α in the early phase of the immune response to viruses, and IFN-γ may promote the development of CD4 T cells into Th1 effector cells (see "Differentiation of Activated Naïve T Cells into Effector and Memory Cells"). NK-cell–mediated IFN-γ production may be induced by the ligation of surface β1 integrins on the NK-cell surface,[334] as well as by the cytokines IL-1, IL-12, IL-15, and IL-18,[335] which are produced by DCs and mononuclear phagocytes. The combination of IL-12 and IL-15 also potently induces NK cells to produce the CC chemokine macrophage inhibitory protein-1α (MIP-1α; CCL-3),[336] which may help to attract other types of mononuclear cells to sites of infection, where NK-cell–mediated lysis takes place.[337] NK cells from HIV-infected persons also are able to produce a variety of CC chemokines, including MIP-1α, MIP-1β (CCL-4), and RANTES (regulated on activation, normal T-cell expressed and secreted; CCL-5) in response to treatment with IL-2 alone; these chemokines may help prevent HIV infection of T cells and mononuclear phagocytes by acting as antagonists of the HIV co-receptor CCR5.[338] NK cells also can be triggered to produce a similar array of cytokines during ADCC in vitro, but the role of such ADCC-derived cytokines in regulating immune responses in vivo is poorly defined. Some of the cytokine-dependent mechanisms by which NK cells, T cells, and APCs may influence each other's function, such as in response to infection with viruses and other intracellular pathogens, are summarized in Figure 4-4.

Natural Killer Cells of the Maternal Decidua and Human Leukocyte Antigen G

The maternal decidua contains a prominent population of NK cells, which may help contribute to the maintenance of pregnancy. NK cells belonging to the $CD56^{hi}CD16^{lo}$ subset, which have a high capacity for cytokine production but low capacity for cytotoxicity, predominate. Murine studies suggest that maternal NK-cell–derived cytokines, such as IFN-γ, may help to remodel the spiral arteries of the placenta. Although the NK-cell populations of the decidua have a low capacity for cytotoxicity, their presence in a tissue lacking expression of HLA-A, HLA-B, and HLA-C molecules could potentially contribute to placental damage and fetal rejection. As noted earlier, the expression by human fetal trophoblast of HLA-G is thought to protect this tissue

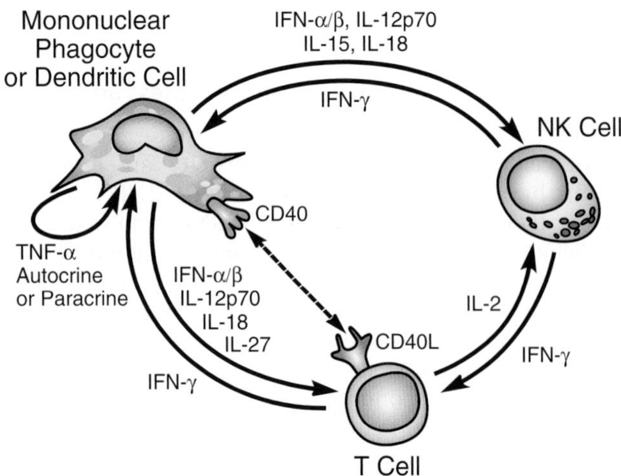

Figure 4-4 Cytokines link innate and antigen-specific Th1 immune mechanisms against intracellular pathogens. Activation of T cells by antigen-presenting cells, such as dendritic cells and mononuclear phagocytes, results in the expression of CD40 ligand (CD40L) and the secretion of cytokines, such as interleukin-2 (IL-2) and interferon-γ (IFN-γ). Mononuclear phagocytes are activated by IFN-γ and the engagement of CD40 with increased microbicidal activity. Mononuclear phagocytes produce tumor necrosis factor-α (TNF-α), which enhances their microbicidal activity in a paracrine or autocrine manner. Mononuclear phagocytes and dendritic cells also secrete cytokines IFN-α/β, IL-12p70, IL-18, and IL-27. These cytokines promote Th1 effector cell differentiation, and most also promote activation of natural killer (NK) cells. Mononuclear phagocytes and dendritic cells, as well as nonhematopoietic cells, also secrete IL-15, which is particularly important for NK-cell maturation and the generation and homeostasis of effector and memory CD8 T cells. NK-cell activation is augmented further by other cytokines, such as IL-2 and IL-21, which are produced by CD4 T cells and other cell types. Activated NK cells secrete IFN-γ, which enhances mononuclear phagocyte activation and Th1 effector-cell differentiation futher.

from attack by maternal NK cells through binding to the inhibitory receptors LILRB1 and LILRB2.[328]

Natural Killer–Cell Numbers and Surface Phenotype in the Fetus and Neonate

Circulating NK cells become increasingly abundant during the second trimester,[339,340] and at term, their numbers in the neonatal circulation (approximately 15% of total lymphocytes) are typically the same as or greater than in adults.[339] Relatively high frequencies of NK cells are found in the fetal liver, lung, and spleen, whereas frequencies in the bone marrow and mesenteric lymph nodes are relatively low.[83] The fraction of blood neonatal and adult NK cells that are $CD56^{hi}CD16^{-/lo}$ (approximately 10%) and $CD56^{lo}CD16^{+}$ NK cells (approximately 90%) is similar.[341,342] Earlier studies of cell surface molecule expression on neonatal NK cells varied in their conclusions regarding the expression of molecules involved with adhesion, activation, inhibition, and cytotoxicity by neonatal NK cells. More recent studies using newer and more reliable methods suggest that neonatal NK cells have decreased expression of ICAM-1 but similar expression of other adhesion molecules, similar or greater expression of the inhibitory CD94-NKG2A complex but reduced expression of the inhibitory LILRB1 (LIR1) receptor, similar or greater expression of the activating NKp30 and NKp46 receptors, similar or slightly reduced expression of the activating NKG2D receptor, and similar to reduced surface expression of CD57.[341,342] The abundance of the cytotoxic molecules perforin, granzyme B, Fas ligand, and TRAIL is as great or greater in neonatal NK cells as in adult NK cells.[342] Thus these findings suggest that neonatal NK cells differ phenotypically from but are not simply immature versions of adult NK cells.

Congenital viral or *Toxoplasma* infection during the second trimester can increase the number of circulating NK cells,[340] which have phenotypic features of activated cells.[343]

Fetal and Neonatal Natural Killer Cell–Mediated Cytotoxicity and Cytokine Production

Recent studies of NK cells of the fetal lung and other tissues have found that KIR-expressing cells are hyporesponsive in terms of cytotoxicity compared with those of adult peripheral blood or lung tissue. Fetal tissue NK-cell function also appears to be substantially more sensitive to the suppressive effects of TGF-β than adult NK cells.[83] The cytotoxic function of circulating NK cells increases progressively during fetal life to reach values approximately 50% (a range of 15%-60% in various studies) of those in adult cells at term, as determined in assays using tumor cell targets and either unpurified or NK cell–enriched preparations.[75] Reduced cytotoxic activity by neonatal NK cells has been observed in studies using cord blood from vaginal or cesarean section deliveries or peripheral blood obtained 2 to 4 days after birth[344]; full function is not achieved until at least 9 to 12 months of age. Decreased cytotoxic activity by neonatal NK cells compared with adult cells also is consistently observed with HSV- and CMV-infected target cells.[345,346] By contrast, both neonatal and adult NK cells had equivalent cytotoxic activity against HIV-1–infected cells.[347] These results suggest that ligands on the target cell or the target cell's intrinsic sensitivity to induction of apoptosis may influence fetal and neonatal NK-cell function. The mechanisms of these pathogen-related differences remain unclear but may contribute to the severity of neonatal HSV infection. Paralleling the reduction in natural cytotoxic activity of neonatal cells, ADCC of neonatal mononuclear cells is approximately 50% of that of adult mononuclear cells, including against HSV-infected targets.

The reduced cytotoxic activity of neonatal NK cells appears not to reflect decreased expression of cytotoxic molecules but, instead, may result from diminished adhesion to target cells, perhaps as a result of decreased expression of ICAM-1 or diminished recycling of cells to kill multiple targets.[342,348,349] However, the mechanisms responsible for diminished neonatal NK-cell cytotoxicity have not been conclusively defined. Cytokines, including IL-2, IL-12, IL-15, IFN-α, IFN-β, and IFN-γ, can augment the cytotoxic activity of neonatal NK cells, as they do for adult NK cells,[75] and with fetal tissue NK cells, the augmentation of cytotoxicity may exceed that for adult NK cells.[83] Consistent with the ability of IL-2 and IFN-γ to augment their cytolytic activity, neonatal NK cells express on their surface receptors for IL-2/IL-15 and IFN-γ in numbers that are equal to or greater than those of adult NK cells.[350] Treatment of neonatal NK cells with ionomycin and phorbol myristate acetate (PMA) also enhances natural cytotoxicity to levels present in adult NK cells.[351] This increase is blocked by inhibitors of granule exocytosis, indicating that decreased release of granules containing perforin and granzyme may contribute to reduced neonatal NK cytotoxicity. Finally, decreased neonatal NK cytotoxicity is not determined at the level of the precursor cells of the NK-cell lineage: Donor-derived NK cells appear early after cord blood transplantation, with good cytotoxicity effected through the perforin/granzyme and Fas–Fas ligand cytotoxic pathways.[352]

Neonatal NK cells produce IFN-γ as effectively as adult NK cells in response to exogenous IL-2, IL-12, IL-18, HSV,[353] and polyclonal stimulation with ionomycin and PMA, but fewer neonatal NK cells express TNF-α than do adult NK cells after ionomycin and PMA stimulation.[354] Neonatal NK cells produce chemokines that suppress the growth of HIV strains that use CCR5 as a co-receptor to infect CD4 T cells but not those strains that use CXCR4 as a receptor.[338]

INNATE LYMPHOID CELLS

Innate lymphoid cells (ILCs) are a family of lymphocytes derived from a common developmental pathway that is closely related to NK cells. ILCs are involved in tissue development and immunity. Like NK cells, they are distinguished from other cell types by their absence of antigen-specific T-cell receptors or B-cell receptors, a lack of DC or myeloid cell markers, and a lymphoid morphology. ILCs lack most markers and receptors that are characteristic of NK cells and typically have a relatively limited ability to mediate cell-mediated cytotoxicity. Their distinct functional feature is their ability to secrete cytokines in patterns that in many cases follow the patterns of CD4 T-cell helper (Th) effector subsets (see "Regulation of CD4 Effector T-Cell Subset Differentiation"). Subsets of ILCs have now been described that have the cytokine production profiles of several of the T-helper effector cell subsets, that is, they secrete cytokines in a mutually exclusive pattern that is characteristic of the major Th effector subsets, including IFN-γ (Th1), IL-4 and/or IL-13 (Th2), and IL-17 and/or IL-22 (Th17). Human ILCs were first described in the lymph nodes and spleen of the second trimester fetus and have a $Lin^{-}CD45^{mid}CD127^{hi}$ surface phenotype.[355] These cells can be found in the mesentery of the human fetal intestine as early 8 to 9 weeks of gestation before the appearance of distinct lymph nodes in the second trimester of pregnancy. They appear to be analogous to murine lymphoid tissue inducer (LTi) cells in playing a role in lymph node organogenesis by expressing lymphotoxin-α, lymphotoxin-β, and IL-17 and inducing mesenchymal cells to increase expression of adhesion molecules important in lymphoid tissue organogenesis.[356]

More recent studies reveal that IL-17/IL-22– and IL-4/IL-13–producing ILCs are found in mucosal tissues, including within the epithelium and in lymphoid-associated tissues such as Peyer patches and the lamina propria.[357] They are intimately involved in interactions between epithelial cells, immune cells, and commensal microbes and help to maintain mucosal homeostasis. Based on murine studies, ILCs of the intestines appear to present antigens on MHC class II molecules to CD4 T cells, but rather than inducing activation, they limit CD4 T-cell responses to intestinal commensal bacteria.[358] Also, based on murine studies, their IL-22 production likely helps maintain high levels of defensins and other antimicrobial proteins and mucosal integrity, and their IL-17 and IL-22 production is likely an important firs-tline defense against bacterial and fungal pathogens. However, like Th17 cells, dysregulated expression of these cytokines by ILCs has been associated with inflammatory bowel disease.[357] Human IFN-γ–secreting ILCs have also been implicated in the pathogenesis of inflammatory bowel disease.[359] IL-4/IL-13–secreting ILCs are potentially first responders to mucosal infection with multicellular parasites, such as worms, but, like Th2 cells, may also play an important role in the pathogenesis of allergic diseases.[360] Little is known of ILCs in the intestines of the neonate and young infant, but given the importance of these cells in mucosal homeostasis and regulation of commensal bacteria, such knowledge may be important in understanding normal mucosal immune development after birth as well as the pathogenesis of certain diseases such as NEC.

SUMMARY

NK cells appear early during gestation and are present in normal numbers by mid to late gestation. However, certain phenotypic features of NK cells differ from those of adult NK cells. Neonatal NK cells appear to be as capable as adult cells of producing IFN-γ and chemokines that inhibit the ability of CCR5-trophic HIV strains to infect CD4 T cells but may produce less TNF-α and chemokines that inhibit infection by CXCR4-trophic strains of HIV. Compared with adult NK cells, neonatal NK cells have decreased cytotoxicity to many types of target cells, including HSV- and CMV-infected but not HIV-infected cells. This decreased cytotoxicity is particularly evident in the tissues. Neonatal NK cell cytotoxicity can be augmented by incubation with cytokines, such as IL-15 in vitro, suggesting a potential immunotherapeutic strategy, and can also be expanded into large numbers for cellular immunotherapy.

T Cells and Antigen Presentation

OVERVIEW

T cells are so named because the vast majority of these cells originate in the thymus. They, along with B cells, which in mammals develop in the bone marrow, comprise the adaptive or antigen-specific immune system. T cells play a central role in antigen-specific immunity because they directly mediate and regulate cellular immune responses and play a critical role in facilitating antigen-specific humoral immune responses by B cells. Most T cells recognize antigen in the form of peptides bound to MHC molecules on APCs. Antigen-specific TCRs are heterodimeric molecules composed of either α and β chains (αβ-TCRs) (Fig. 4-5) or γ and δ chains (γδ-TCRs), with the amino-terminal portion of each of these chains variable and involved in antigen recognition. This variability is generated, in large part, as a result of TCR gene rearrangement of variable (V), diversity (D), and joining (J) segments. The TCR on the cell surface is invariably associated with the nonpolymorphic complex of CD3 proteins, which include CD3-γ, -δ, -ε, and -ζ (see Fig. 4-5). The cytoplasmic domains of proteins of the CD3 complex include 10 immunoreceptor tyrosine-based activation motifs (ITAMs), which serve as docking sites for the lck and ZAP-70 (CD3 zeta-associated protein of 70 kilodaltons) intracellular tyrosine kinases that transduce proximal activation signals to the interior of the cell after the TCR has been engaged by antigen.

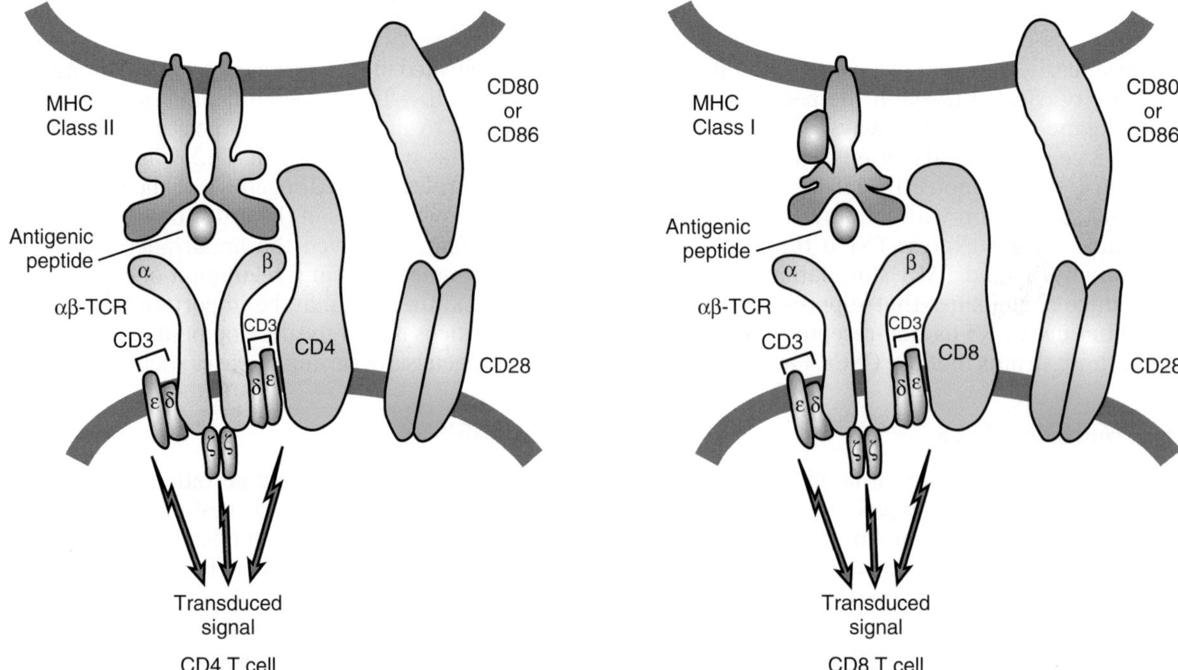

Figure 4-5 T-cell recognition of antigen and activation. αβ T-cell receptor (αβ-TCR) recognizes antigen presented by the antigen-presenting cell (APC) in the form of antigenic peptides bound to major histocompatibility complex (MHC) molecules on the APC surface. Most CD4 T cells recognize peptides bound to MHC class II, whereas most CD8 T cells recognize peptides bound to MHC class I. This MHC restriction is the result of a thymic selection process and is due in part to an intrinsic affinity of the CD4 and CD8 molecules for the MHC class II and class I molecules, respectively. Once antigen is recognized, the CD3 protein complex, which is invariably associated with the TCR, acts as docking site for tyrosine kinases that transmit activating intracellular signals. Interaction of the T-cell CD28 molecule with either CD80 (B7-1) or CD86 (B7-2) provides an important co-stimulatory signal to the T cell, leading to complete activation, rather than partial activation or functional inactivation (anergy).

Most T cells that bear an αβ-TCR (or αβ T cells), also express on their surface the CD4 or CD8 co-receptors in a mutually exclusive manner and are commonly referred to as CD4 or CD8 T cells, respectively. Nearly all CD8 T cells recognize protein antigens in the form of 7- to 9-mer peptide fragments bound to MHC class I molecules of the classic type (HLA-A, HLA-B, and HLA-C in humans). CD4 T cells recognize antigen presented by MHC class II molecules (HLA-DR, HLA-DP, and HLA-DQ in humans); most of these antigens are in the form of peptide fragments typically ranging between 12 to 22 amino acids in length. MHC class II presentation of certain zwitterionic bacterial polysaccharides, such as those derived from *Bacteroides fragilis*, can also occur.[31]

APCs, which include DCs, mononuclear phagocytes, and B cells, constitutively express both MHC class I and class II molecules, which allows them to present antigenic peptides to CD8 and CD4 T cells, respectively. DCs are particularly important for presentation to T cells that are antigenically naïve and that have not been previously activated by foreign antigen. γδ T cells, which mainly recognize stress-induced molecules rather than peptide/MHC complexes, have distinct immune functions from αβ T cells and are discussed later in a separate section.

ANTIGEN PRESENTATION BY CLASSIC MAJOR HISTOCOMPATIBILITY COMPLEX MOLECULES

Major Histocompatibility Complex Class Ia

MHC class Ia proteins are heterodimers of a heavy chain that is polymorphic and a monomorphic light chain, β_2-microglobulin. Antigenic peptides 8 to 10 amino acids in length bind to a cleft formed by two domains of the heavy chain (Fig. 4-6; see Fig. 4-5). There are three different types of MHC class Ia molecules—HLA-A, HLA-B, and HLA-C—which are all highly polymorphic and for which there are 1833, 2459, and 1507 different protein allotypes, respectively, that are encoded by molecularly defined alleles.[361] The greatest degree of polymorphism is found in the region encoding the antigenic cleft, which results in considerable differences among individuals in their ability to present antigenic peptides to T cells. The CD8 molecule has an affinity for a nonvariable domain of the heavy chain that is not involved in binding peptide and that contributes to T-cell activation. Most peptides bound to MHC class Ia molecules are derived from proteins synthesized de novo within host cells (see Fig. 4-6), with the majority derived from recently translated proteins rather than as a result of turnover of stable proteins.[362] This helps minimize any delay in detecting pathogen-derived peptides that may result from recent infection. In uninfected cells, these peptides are derived from host proteins; that is, they are self-peptides. Recently synthesized host proteins that are targeted for degradation, for example, because of misfolding or defective posttranslational modification, are a major source of self-peptides that bind to MHC class Ia. After intracellular infection, such as with a virus, peptides derived from viral proteins endogenously synthesized within the cell bind to and are presented by MHC class Ia. Antigenic peptides are derived predominantly by enzymatic cleavage of proteins in the cytoplasm by the proteasome. A specific peptide transporter or pump, the transporter associated with antigen processing (TAP), then shuttles peptides formed in

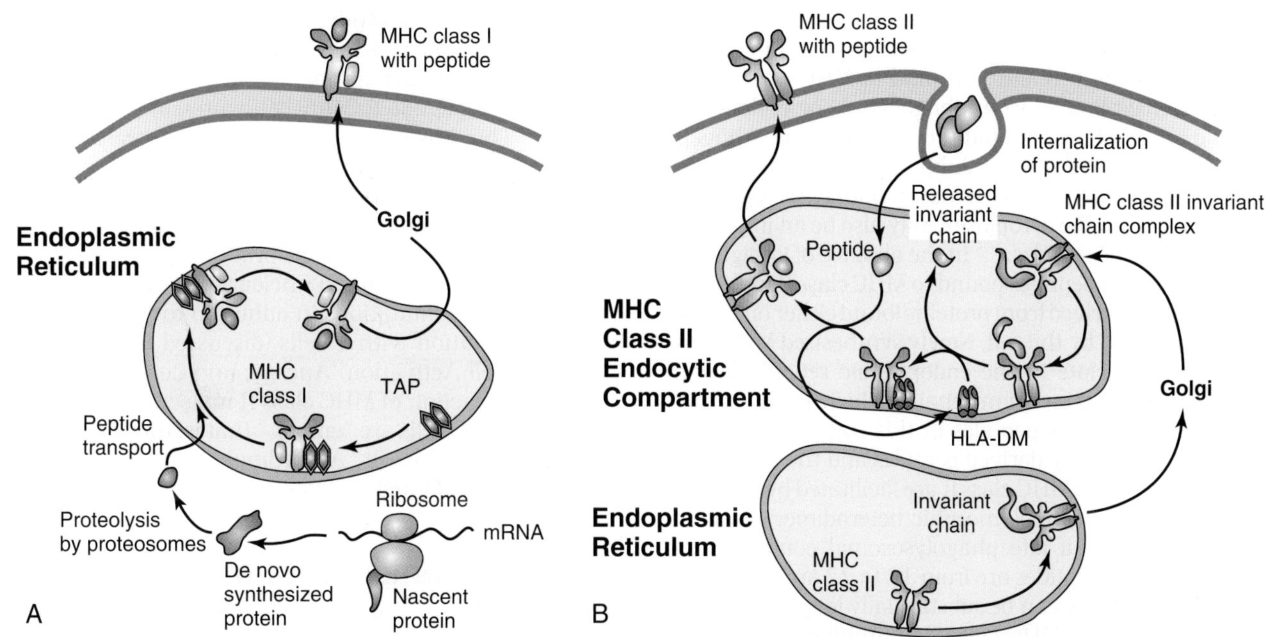

Figure 4-6 Intracellular pathways of antigen presentation. **A,** Foreign peptides that bind to MHC class I are predominantly derived from cytoplasmic proteins synthesized de novo within the cell. Viral proteins entering cells after fusion of an enveloped virus with the cell membrane may also enter this pathway. Dendritic cells are particularly efficient at taking up proteins for the MHC class I pathway by micropinocytosis or macropinocytosis. These cells can also transfer proteins taken up as part of necrotic or apoptotic debris into the MHC class I pathway, a process known as cross-presentation. Cytoplasmic proteins are degraded by proteasomes into peptides, which then enter into the endoplasmic reticulum via the TAP (transporter associated with antigen processing) system. Peptide binding by de novo synthesized MHC class I takes place within the endoplasmic reticulum. **B,** Foreign peptides that bind to MHC class II are mainly derived from either internalization proteins found in the extracellular space or that are components of cell membrane or endosomal compartments in which pathogens, such as Mycobacteria, are sequestered. The invariant chain binds to recently synthesized MHC class II and prevents peptide binding until a specialized cellular compartment for MHC class II peptide loading is reached. In this compartment, the invariant chain is proteolytically cleaved and released, and peptides derived from internalized proteins may now bind to MHC class II. The HLA-DM molecule facilitates the loading of peptide within this compartment. In dendritic cells, proteins that enter into the MHC class II antigen presentation pathway can be transferred to the MHC class I pathway by cross-presentation. *HLA,* Human leukocyte antigen; *MHC,* major histocompatibility complex; *mRNA,* messenger RNA.

the cytoplasm to the endoplasmic reticulum, where peptides are able to bind to recently synthesized MHC class Ia molecules.[362] Peptide binding stabilizes the association of the heavy chain with β_2-microglobulin in this compartment and allows the complex to transit to the cell surface.

MHC class Ia molecules and the cell components required for peptide generation, transport, and MHC class Ia binding are virtually ubiquitous in the cells of vertebrates. The advantage to the host is that cytotoxic CD8 T cells can then recognize and lyse cells infected with intracellular pathogens in most tissues. The abundance of MHC class I molecules is increased by exposure to type I IFNs and IFN-γ, which also can induce the expression of modest amounts of MHC class Ia molecules on cell types that normally lack expression, including neuronal cells.

DCs are unique in their ability to present antigenic peptides on MHC class Ia molecules by an additional pathway, known as cross-presentation, in which extracellular proteins that are taken up as large particles (phagocytosis), as small particles (macropinocytosis), or in soluble form (micropinocytosis) are transferred from endocytic vesicles to the cytoplasm. Once these proteins are in the cytoplasm, they undergo proteasome-mediated degradation and loading onto MHC class Ia molecules through TAP. Cross-presentation is essential for the induction of primary CD8 T-cell responses directed toward antigens of pathogens that do not directly infect APCs (e.g., most viruses) and therefore cannot be directly loaded into the MHC class Ia pathway. Cross-presentation is enhanced by exposure of DCs to type I IFNs.[363] Cross-presentation may also be facilitated by the reduced nicotinamide adenine dinucleotide phosphate oxidase complex,[364] which helps limit acidification that can destroy protein-derived epitopes.

Major Histocompatibility Complex Class II

In MHC class II molecules, an α and a β chain each contribute to the formation of the antigenic peptide-binding groove (see Fig. 4-6). The three major types of human MHC class II molecules—HLA-DR, HLA-DP, and HLA-DQ—are highly polymorphic, particularly in the region encoding the peptide-binding cleft. In humans and primates, HLA-DR allelic diversity is mediated solely by the HLA-DR β chain because the HLA-DR α chain is essentially monomorphic (only two highly similar proteins). HLA-DRβ protein is encoded mainly at the DRB1 locus, for which there are 1047 distinct amino acid sequences encoded by 1411 molecularly defined alleles.[361] Some HLA-DRβ proteins may be encoded by less polymorphic loci, such DRB3, DRB4, and DRB5, which are closely linked to DRB1. The HLA-DPα, HLA-DPβ, HLA-DQα, and HLA-DQβ gene loci are highly polymorphic and encode 19, 205, 32, and 337 distinct proteins, respectively.[361] HLA-DR is expressed at substantially higher levels than HLA-DP or HLA-DQ, which probably accounts for its predominance as the restricting MHC class II type for many CD4 T-cell immune responses. Analogous to the CD8 molecule and MHC class I, the CD4 molecule has affinity for a domain of the MHC class II β chain distinct from the region that forms part of the peptide-binding groove. In contrast with MHC class Ia, peptides that bind to MHC class II proteins are derived mostly from phagocytosis or endocytosis of soluble or membrane-bound proteins or from pathogens that are sequestered in intracellular compartments (see Fig. 4-6).[362] Autophagy, which removes damaged organelles and microbes from the cytoplasm, may also be an important cytosolic source of peptides.[365] In the absence of foreign proteins, a majority of peptides bound to MHC class II molecules are self-peptides derived from proteins found either on the cell surface or secreted by the cell. Newly synthesized MHC class II molecules associate in the endoplasmic reticulum with a protein called the invariant chain, which impedes their binding of endogenous peptides in this compartment. The loading of exogenously derived peptides and the removal of invariant chain from MHC class II are facilitated by HLA-DM (see Fig. 4-6),[362] a nonpolymorphic heterodimeric protein, and likely occur in a late phagolysosomal compartment. Most MHC class II peptides are from 12 to 22 amino acids in length, although they can be substantially longer.

The distribution of MHC class II in uninflamed tissues is much more restricted than MHC class Ia, with constitutive MHC class II mainly limited to APCs, such as DCs, mononuclear phagocytes, and B cells. Limiting MHC class II expression in most situations to these cell types makes teleologic sense because the major function of these professional APCs is to process foreign antigen for recognition by CD4 T cells. Many other cell types can be induced to express MHC class II and, in some cases, present antigen to CD4 T cells, as a consequence of tissue inflammation or exposure to cytokines, particularly IFN-γ but also TNF-α or GM-CSF (see Tables 4-1 and 4-2).

Major Histocompatibility Complex Molecule Expression and Antigen Presentation in the Fetus and Neonate

The expression of MHC class I and class II molecules by fetal tissues is evident by 12 weeks of gestation, and all of the major APCs, including mononuclear phagocytes, B cells, and DCs,[366] are present by this time. Fetal tissues are vigorously rejected after transplantation into non–MHC-matched hosts, indicating that surface MHC expression is sufficient to initiate an allogeneic response, probably by host cytotoxic CD8 T cells. However, this vigorous allogeneic response does not exclude more subtle deficiencies in antigen presentation in the fetus and neonate, particularly under more physiologic conditions that more stringently test APC function. The amount of MHC class Ia expression on neonatal lymphocytes is lower than on adult cells[367] and this could limit the ability of lymphocytes infected by pathogens to be lysed by cytotoxic CD8 T cells.

For technical reasons, most studies of human neonatal DC antigen presentation have involved using autologous or allogeneic monocyte-derived dendritic cells (moDCs) to activate T cells. Neonatal and adult moDCs are similarly efficient in processing exogenous protein and presenting antigenic peptides, leading to the activation of autologous naïve T cells. A similar ability to cross present soluble protein to CD8 T cells has also been reported,[301] although neonatal moDC function may not be indicative of that by human primary neonatal cDCs.

By contrast, in one study, neonatal monocytes were inferior to adult monocytes in presentation of either whole protein antigen, in which antigen processing was required, or of exogenous peptide to HLA-DR expressing T-cell hybridomas.[368] This was not accounted for by decreased expression of either MHC class II or co-stimulatory molecules, such as CD80 or CD86, by neonatal monocytes, and because this applied to both whole protein and exogenously added peptides, a defect only in antigen processing is unlikely. The precise mechanisms remain unclear but could involve neonatal monocyte limitations in adhesion to or immunologic synapse formation with T cells (discussed later in the section on T-Cell Activation, Anergy, and Co-Stimulation). A substantial fraction of MHC class II molecules on neonatal, but not adult, B cells are "empty," that is, they lack peptides in the binding groove.[369] Accordingly, neonatal B cells may be functionally limited as APCs.

NONCLASSIC ANTIGEN-PRESENTATION MOLECULES

Human Leukocyte Antigen E

Human leukocyte antigen E (HLA-E) is a nonclassic and essentially monomorphic class Ib MHC molecule similar to conventional MHC class Ia in its dependency on the proteasome for the generation of peptides and its obligate association with β_2-microglobulin. In contrast with conventional MHC class Ia molecules, HLA-E preferentially binds hydrophobic peptides, including those derived from the amino-terminal leader sequences of most alleles of HLA-A, HLA-B, and HLA-C.[370] Low levels of HLA-E surface expression can be detected on most cell types, consistent with the nearly ubiquitous distribution of HLA-A, HLA-B, HLA-C, and the TAP system. An important role for HLA-E is to interact with the CD94-containing receptors on NK lymphocytes and to regulate their function (see earlier section on Natural Killer Cell Receptors). HLA-E is also expressed on fetal-derived extravillous trophoblasts of the human placenta. Because trophoblast cells lack expression of most conventional MHC class Ia molecules, the surface expression of HLA-E may limit the lysis of these cells by maternal or fetal NK cells.[371]

Human Leukocyte Antigen G

Human leukocyte antigen G (HLA-G), which, like HLA-E, is also expressed at high levels by human cytotrophoblasts within the maternal uterine wall, has limited polymorphism but otherwise is quite similar to MHC class Ia in its association with β_2-microglobulin and structure. HLA-G occurs as either an integral membrane protein or a secreted isoform.[372] As for HLA-E, HLA-G is capable of engaging regulatory receptors on NK cells and may serve to limit NK-cell–mediated cytotoxicity against trophoblasts (see "Natural Killer Cells of the Maternal Decidua and Human Leukocyte Antigen G"). In this context, the hydrophobic leader sequence of HLA-G may provide a peptide that is particularly effective for HLA-E–mediated regulation of NK-cell cytotoxicity.[371] Soluble HLA-G is present at relatively high levels in the serum of pregnant women[372] and in lower amounts in cord blood and in the peripheral blood of nonparous women and men. The in vivo function of soluble HLA-G remains unclear, but it may inhibit immune responses. Consistent with this proposed function, soluble HLA-G (and class Ia molecules) can induce Fas (CD95)-dependent apoptosis of activated CD8 T cells, by engaging CD8 and increasing surface expression of Fas ligand (CD95L).[373,374]

Major Histocompatibility Class I–Related Chains A and B

MHC class I–related chains A and B (MICA and MICB, respectively) have limited but clear homology with conventional MHC class I molecules. In contrast with conventional MHC class I, however, they lack a binding site for CD8, are not associated with β_2-microglobulin, and do not appear to be involved with the presentation of peptide antigens. Instead, these molecules are expressed on stressed intestinal epithelial cells, such as those experiencing heat shock, and on other cell types in response to infection with viruses, such as those of the herpesvirus group. The expression of MICA and MICB transcripts in the unstressed cell is under negative control by cellular microRNAs, which themselves are downregulated by stress.[375] MICA and MICB are ligands for NKG2D found on most NK cells, some CD8 T cells, and certain populations of γδ T cells (e.g., those expressing Vγ9Vδ2 TCRs).[376] NKG2D can either directly activate or act in concert with TCR-mediated signals to activate the cells that express it.[377]

CD1

The human CD1 locus includes five nonpolymorphic genes, CD1a to CD1e. CD1 molecules associate with β_2-microglobulin but have limited structural homology with either MHC class I or MHC class II proteins. In humans, they are expressed mainly on APCs, including DCs and B cells. CD1a and CD1c are involved in the presentation of lipids unique to microorganisms, such as lipopeptides, phosphomycoketides, and sulfoglycolipids, to clonally diverse T cells,[378-380] as well as endogenously derived lipids, for instance, CD1a presentation of squalene and wax esters of the skin.[381] In contrast, the T-cell response to CD1b bound to mycolic acid lipid from *Mycobacterium tuberculosis* includes both T cells with a restricted αβ-TCR (GEM [germline-encoded mycolyl-lipid reactive] T cells) as well as more clonally diverse T cells.[382] CD1d presents microbial and self-lipid antigens to natural killer T (NKT) cells, a specialized T-cell population with a highly restricted αβ-TCR repertoire (discussed in more detail later).[378] CD1e, which is only expressed intracellularly, influences antigen presentation to T cells by transferring lipid antigens to other CD1 molecules.[383] Antigen processing and loading of CD1 molecules involves endocytic pathways,[378,384] at least some of which intersect with those involved in peptide loading of MHC class II molecules. Little is known of the adequacy of antigen presentation by CD1 molecules in the human fetus or neonate.

PROTHYMOCYTES AND EARLY THYMOCYTE DIFFERENTIATION

Thymic Ontogeny

With the exception of a subset of the T cells found in the gut and perhaps the liver, most αβ T cells develop from immature progenitor cells within the unique microenvironment of the thymus. The thymus does not have a population of self-replenishing stem cells and requires a continual input of thymocyte progenitor cells (prothymocytes) to maintain thymocytopoiesis. The entry of prothymocytes from the circulation into the thymus appears to occur cyclically rather than continuously, resulting in waves of thymocyte development.

The thymic rudiment (lacking hematopoietic cells) arises from the endoderm of the third pharyngeal pouch[385] at weeks 4 to 5 of gestation. An interstitial deletion of a 1.5 to 3 megabase (Mb) region of the human chromosome 22q11.2 region is the most frequent genetic cause of the DiGeorge/velocardial facial syndrome, and results in hypoplasia of tissues deriving from the third pharyngeal pouches, including the thymus.[386] A murine model suggests that haploinsufficiency for two genes located within the human 22q11.2 deleted segment, *Tbx1* and *Crkl*, is responsible for this hypoplasia.[387]

The prothymocyte is an early derivative of, but not identical with, a fully totipotent HSC. The human prothymocyte of the fetal bone marrow has a $CD7^+CD34^{hi}CD45RA^{hi}Lin^-$ (lacking markers for the mature T-cell, B-cell, NK-cell, erythroid, and myeloid cell lineages) surface phenotype.[388] This cell population is replaced in the postnatal bone marrow by a $CD7^-CD10^+CD24^-CD34^+$ cell population as the likely major prothymocyte population.[389] Human fetal prothymocytes not only have T-cell differentiation potential but retain the capacity to differentiate along B-cell, NK-cell, and myeloid, but not erythroid, lineages.[388] Whether postnatal human prothymocytes retain a capacity for myeloid and erythroid lineage differentiation is controversial.[389,390]

The first waves of human fetal $CD7^+$ prothymocytes derived from the liver probably enter into the thymic rudiment when it lacks a vasculature at about 8 weeks of gestation,[388] with later ones entering through postcapillary venules at the cortical medullary junction. Newly entering prothymocytes rapidly encounter perivascular thymic epithelial cells[388] that express the delta-like ligands. These ligands engage the Notch 1 protein on the prothymocyte cell to rapidly promote its T-lineage commitment, as evidenced by the expression of T-cell specific genes, and the suppression of B-cell development. The rapid induction of the expression of these T-cell–specific genes may be facilitated by their having an open chromatin structure, starting at the HSC stage[391]; this chromatin configuration likely continues through the prothymocyte stage.

Intrathymic cellular progeny of the entering prothymocyte gives rise to the three major subsets of thymocytes characteristic of the second and third trimester fetal and postnatal human thymus (Fig. 4-7). These subsets are named according to their pattern of surface expression of CD4 and CD8 and are further characterized by their surface expression of αβ-TCR complexes. Thymocytes can be classified as double negative ($CD4^-CD8^-$), expressing little or no CD4 or CD8 (hence, double negative) or $CD3^-CD4^-CD8^-$ (and therefore sometimes referred to as triple negative) and are direct products of the entering prothymocyte; double positive ($CD4^+CD8^+$), expressing medium levels of αβ-TCR–CD3 and are derived from the most mature double-negative cells; and single positive ($CD4^+CD8^-$ and $CD4^-CD8^+$), expressing high levels of αβ-TCR–CD3 and are derived from

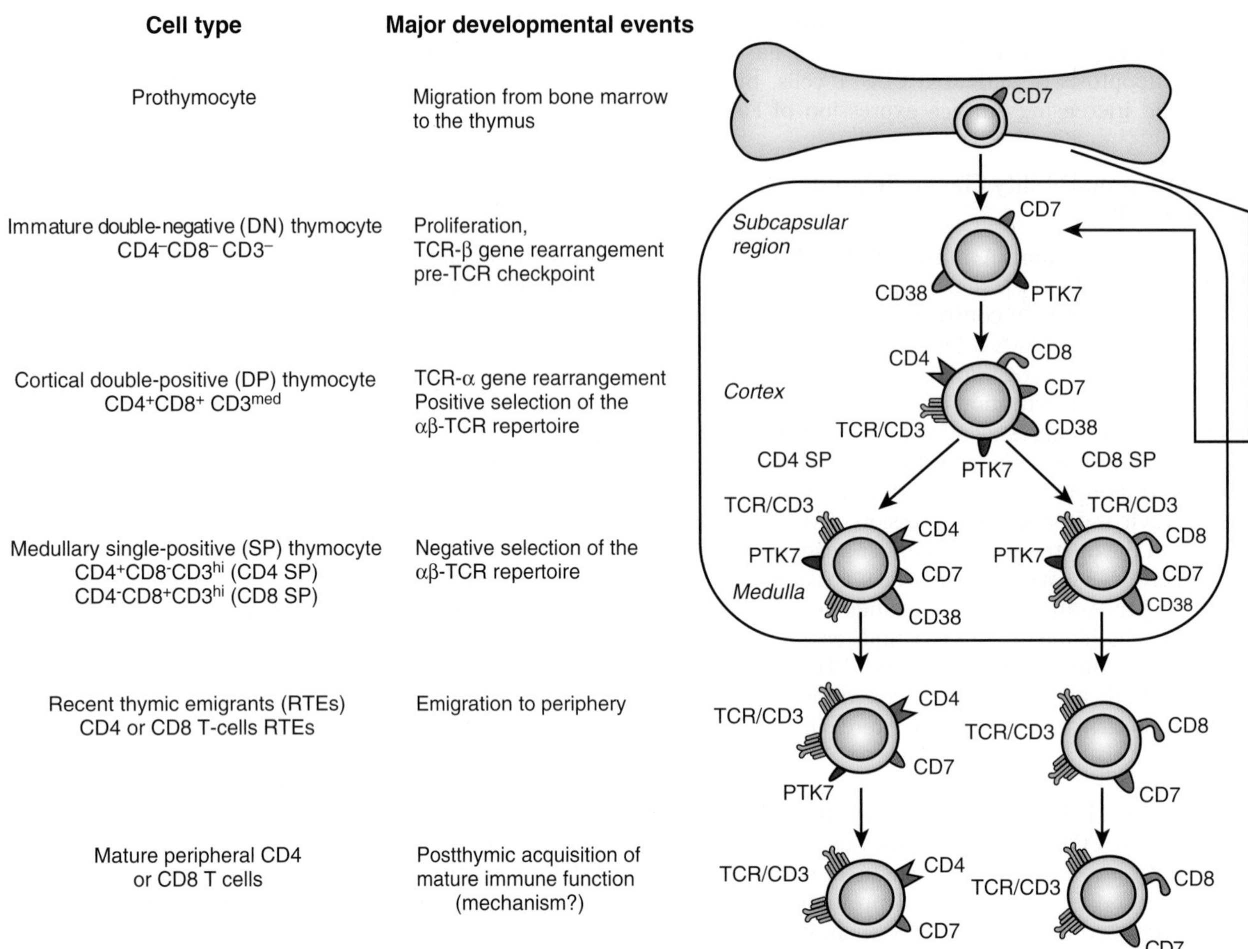

Figure 4-7 Putative stages of human αβ T-cell receptor-positive (TCR⁺) thymocyte development. Prothymocytes from the bone marrow or fetal liver, which express CD7, enter the thymus via vessels at the junction between the thymic cortex and medulla. They differentiate to progressively more mature αβ-TCR⁺ thymocytes, defined by their pattern of expression of the αβ-TCR/CD3 complex, CD4, CD8, CD38, and protein tyrosine kinase 7 (PTK7). TCR-β and TCR-α chain genes are sequentially rearranged in the outer cortex. Positive selection occurs mainly in the central thymic cortex by interaction with thymic epithelial cells, and negative selection occurs mainly in the medulla by interaction with thymic dendritic cells and medullary cells. After these selection processes, medullary thymocytes emigrate into the circulation and colonize the peripheral lymphoid organs as CD4 and CD8 T cells with high levels of the αβ-TCR/CD3 complex. These recent thymic emigrants (RTEs) also contain high levels of signal joint T-cell receptor excision circles (sjTRECs), which are a circular product of TCR gene rearrangement. Most RTEs in adults probably lack CD38 surface expression. In contrast, in neonates, most peripheral T cells retain surface expression of CD38 and have high amounts of sjTRECs compared with adult peripheral T cells. PTK7 is expressed at high levels during all stages of human intrathymic development. PTK7⁺ naïve CD4 T cells in the adult circulation are an RTE population. As in the case of CD38, neonatal CD4 and CD8 T cells have uniformly high levels of PTK7 surface expression.

double-positive cells. In humans, there is also an intermediate stage between double-negative and double-positive thymocytes, which is characterized by a $CD4^{lo}CD8^-CD3^-$ (immature single positive) surface phenotype.[392]

A fetal triple-negative ($CD3^-CD4^-CD8^-$) thymocyte population that is also $CD1a^-CD7^+CD34^{hi}CD45RA^{hi}$ likely includes prothymocytes that have recently immigrated into the thymus.[388] In the postnatal thymus, this most recent thymic immigrant population is replaced by a triple-negative population that is $CD1a^-CD7^-CD10^+CD34^{hi}CD45RA^{hi}$. Triple-negative thymocytes undergo progressive differentiation, which involves alterations in expression of CD34, CD38, and CD1a and in which the progeny of recent thymic immigrants progressively differentiate into $CD1a^+CD34^-CD38^-$, $CD1a^+CD34^-CD38^+$, and $CD1a^+CD34^+CD38^+$ thymocytes to become $CD4^{lo}CD8^-CD3^-$ (immature single-positive) cells.[390] During this differentiation, thymocytes move outward in the cortex toward the subcapsular region, a process that is accompanied by proliferation driven by the binding of Wnt, IL-7, and Flt3 ligand to their specific receptors on the thymocyte cell surface.[393] Once thymocytes reach the outer cortex, they then reverse course and move from the outer to the inner cortex as double-positive thymocytes.[394] Finally, double-positive cells become single-positive thymocytes in the medulla, which exit the thymus as mature but naïve (i.e., they have not yet encountered and are thus naïve to the antigen they are capable of recognizing) T cells probably through blood vessels located in the medulla (see Fig. 4-7).

Thymocytes expressing proteins that are characteristic of T-lineage cells, including CD4, CD8, and the αβ-TCR–CD3 complex, are found shortly after initial thymus colonization at 8.5 weeks of gestation.[395] By 12 weeks of gestation, the pattern of expression of a number of other proteins expressed by thymocytes, such as CD2, CD5, CD38, and the CD45 isoforms, matches that in the postnatal thymus.

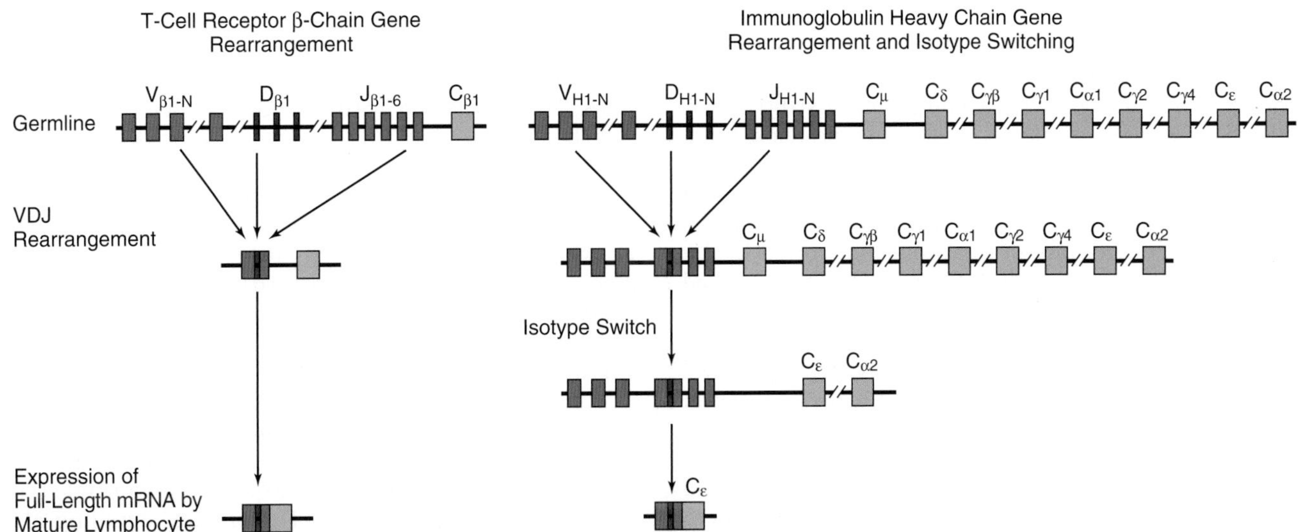

Figure 4-8 The T-cell receptor (TCR) and immunoglobulin genes are formed by rearrangement in immature lymphocytes. The TCR-β chain gene and the immunoglobulin heavy chain genes are shown as examples. A similar process is involved with rearrangement of the TCR-α, -δ, and -γ chain genes, and with the immunoglobulin light chain genes. Rearrangement involves the joining of dispersed segments of V (variable), D (diversity), and J (joining) gene segments with the deletion of intervening DNA. This allows expression of a full-length messenger RNA (mRNA) transcript that can be translated into a functional protein, provided that there are no premature translational stop codons. Immunoglobulin heavy chain genes undergo an additional rearrangement called isotype switching, in which the C (constant) region segment is changed without alteration of the antigen- combining site formed by the V, D, and J segments. The isotype switch from immunoglobulin M (IgM) to IgE is shown.

Concurrently, a clear architectural separation between the thymic cortex and medulla is evident,[396] with Hassall corpuscles observable in the thymic medulla shortly thereafter.[397] By 14 weeks of gestation, the three major human thymocyte subsets (double negative [$CD4^-CD8^-$], double positive [$CD4^+CD8^+$], and mature single positive [$CD4^+CD8^-$ and $CD4^-CD8^+$]) characteristic of the postnatal thymus are found (see Fig. 4-7). Fetal thymocyte expression of the chemokine receptors CXCR4 and CCR5, which also are major co-receptors for entry of HIV-1, has been found by 18 to 23 weeks of gestation[398] and is likely to be present earlier.

Thymic cellularity increases dramatically during the second and third trimesters of fetal gestation. Transient thymic involution, mainly the loss of cortical double-positive ($CD4^+CD8^+$) thymocytes, which is evident within 1 day after birth, probably begins at the end of the third trimester.[399] This involution may be a consequence of the elevation in circulating levels of glucocorticoids that occurs during the third trimester before delivery. Thymic recovery is evident by 1 month after delivery and is paralleled by a sharp decline in glucocorticoid levels within hours after birth.[399] This transient involution is followed by a resumption of increased thymic cellularity, with peak cellularity and thymus size probably attained at about 1 year of age.[400] When complete thymectomy is performed during the first year of life, subsequent circulating numbers of CD4 and CD8 T cells are decreased, indicating the importance of postnatal thymocyte production for the maintenance of the peripheral T-cell compartment.[401]

There is gradual replacement of thymic cellularity of the cortex and medulla by fat after early childhood, with single-positive thymocytes within the medulla being relatively spared compared with cortical double-positive thymocytes.[402] Nevertheless, the thymus remains active in T-cell production through the fourth decade of life[403-406] and is also capable of increasing its output of antigenically naïve T cells in response to severe T-cell lymphopenia (e.g., after intense cytoablative chemotherapy, treatment with highly active combination antiretroviral therapy for HIV infection).[407] The mechanisms by which increased thymocytopoiesis is triggered by severe lymphopenia are unclear but may include the increased production of IL-7, which is plausible because IL-7 administration increases recent thymic emigrant output in healthy adults.[408]

INTRATHYMIC GENERATION OF T-CELL RECEPTOR DIVERSITY

Overview

T (and B) lymphocytes undergo a unique developmental event, the generation of a highly diverse repertoire of antigen receptors through DNA recombination, a process referred to as V(D)J recombination. This diversity is generated through the random rearrangement and juxtaposition into a single exon of variable (V), diversity (D), and joining (J) segments to form in each cell a unique TCR-α and TCR-β gene sequence (Fig. 4-8). V(D)J recombination is a highly ordered process that is controlled at multiple levels and is restricted to T- and B-lineage cells that express the two recombination-activating genes, *RAG1* and *RAG2*. Recombination of the TCR genes is further restricted to cells of the T lymphocyte rather than B lymphocyte lineage by mechanisms (e.g., histone acetylation) that allow RAG proteins access to the TCR genes only in T-cell progenitors. The RAG proteins are critically involved in the initiation of the recombination process; they recognize and cleave conserved sequences flanking each V, D, and J segment. Other proteins, including a high-molecular-weight DNA-dependent protein kinase catalytic subunit (DNA-PKcs) and its associated Ku70 and Ku80 proteins, DNA ligase IV and its associated XRCC4 protein, Artemis, and Cernunnos-XLF, then perform nonhomologous DNA end-joining (NHEJ) repair of the cleaved V(D)J segments. Unlike RAG proteins, these other proteins involved in NHEJ DNA repair are expressed in most cells and are involved in repair of double-stranded DNA breaks induced by cell damage, such as radiation. Genetic deficiency of any of the proteins involved in the rearrangement process results in a form of severe combined immunodeficiency (SCID) because both T-cell and B-cell development depend on the surface expression of rearranged TCR and immunoglobulin genes, respectively.[409]

The complementarity-determining regions (CDRs) of the TCR and immunoglobulin molecules are those that are involved in forming the three-dimensional structure that binds with antigen. The V segments encode the CDR1 and CDR2 regions for both TCR chains. The CDR3 region, where the distal portion of the V segment joins the (D)J segment, is a particularly important source of αβ-TCR diversity for peptide-MHC recognition, and is the center of the antigen-binding site for peptide-MHC complexes. CDR3 (also known as junctional) diversity is achieved by multiple mechanisms. These mechanisms include the following:

1. The addition of one or two nucleotides that are palindromic to the end of the cut gene segment (termed P-nucleotides); these nucleotides are added as part of the process of asymmetrical repairing of "hairpin" ends (the two strands of DNA are joined at the ends) that are generated by RAG endonuclease activity;
2. The activity of terminal deoxytransferase (TdT; also referred to as "deoxynucleotidyltransferase, terminal" or DNTT), which randomly adds nucleotides (called N-nucleotides) to the ends of segments undergoing rearrangement; TdT addition is a particularly important mechanism for diversity generation because every three additional nucleotides encodes a potential codon, potentially increasing repertoire diversity by a factor of 20.
3. Exonuclease activity that results in a variable loss of nucleotide residues, as part of the DNA repair process.

Together, the mechanisms for generating diversity can theoretically result in as many as 10^{15} types of αβ-TCR. In reality, the final repertoire of naïve T cells in the adult human circulation is on average a total of approximately 10^6 different TCR-β chains, each pairing on average with at least 25 different TCR-α chains.[410] This results in a maximum of about 10^8 different combinations of TCR-α and TCR-β chains for the naïve T-cell αβ-TCR repertoire. Because in young adults, the body has approximately 2×10^{11} CD4 T cells and 1×10^{11} CD8 T cells,[411,412] of which about 50% belong to the naïve subset, the average clonal size (all clones express an identical αβ-TCR) for a naïve T cell is approximately 500 to 1000.[410,413]

RAG expression is present by the double-negative thymocyte stage, with the TCR-γ chain and TCR-δ chain genes typically undergoing rearrangement first.[414] The TCR-β gene becomes accessible to RAG proteins before the TCR-α gene, and it is the first to undergo rearrangement (a small fraction of double-negative cells may undergo productive rearrangements of the TCR-γ and TCR-δ genes, and this is discussed in more detail in the section on γδ T cells). The TCR-β chain D segment first rearranges to a downstream J segment, with the deletion of intervening DNA. This is followed by rearrangement of a V segment to the DJ segment, resulting in a contiguous (VDJ) β-chain gene segment, which is joined to the constant (C) region segment by mRNA splicing. If a VDJ segment lacks premature translation stop codons, the TCR-β chain protein may be expressed on the thymocyte surface in association with a pre–TCR-α chain protein (pre-Tα) and the CD3 complex proteins. This pre-Tα complex signals intracellularly and thereby instructs the thymocyte to increase its surface expression of CD4 and CD8, to start rearrangement of the TCR-α chain gene, and to stop rearrangement of the other TCR-β chain allele.[415] This inhibition of TCR-β chain gene rearrangement results in allelic exclusion so that greater than 99% of αβ T cells express only a single type of TCR-β chain gene.[416] Pre-Tα complex signaling also results in multiple rounds of cell division of the thymocyte, which improves the chances that some of the progeny will have both a productive TCR-β and TCR-α gene rearrangement.

Rearrangement of the TCR-α chain gene then occurs at the double-positive stage and involves the joining of V segments directly to J segments, without intervening D segments. If successful, this leads to the expression of an αβ-TCR heterodimer on the cell surface in association with CD3 proteins to form the TCR-CD3 complex. Allelic exclusion is ineffective for the TCR-α chain gene, and it is estimated that as many as one third of peripheral human αβ T cells may express two types of TCR-α chains.[417] RAG protein expression normally ceases in cortical thymocytes, limiting TCR gene rearrangement to progenitor thymocytes.

Fetal and Neonatal T-Cell Receptor Repertoire

The generation of the αβ-TCR repertoire by the process of V(D)J recombination of the TCR-β and then TCR-α genes probably occurs within a few days after colonization of the thymus by prothymocytes. The use of D and J segments in rearrangement of the TCR-β chain gene in the thymus at approximately 8 weeks of gestation is less diverse than at 11 to 13 weeks of gestation or subsequently.[75] This restriction is not explained by an effect of positive or negative selection in the thymus because it applies to D-to-J rearrangements, which are not expressed on the immature thymocyte cell surface. The CDR3 region of the TCR-β chain transcripts is reduced in length and sequence diversity in the human fetal thymus between 8 and 15 weeks of gestation. This is probably due to decreased amounts of the TdT enzyme, which performs N-nucleotide addition during V(D)J recombination. TdT is detectable by 13 weeks of gestation, and fetal TdT activity and CDR3 length both increase during the second trimester. Exonuclease activity ("nucleotide nibbling"), in which there is variable trimming of the length of V(D)J segments before their joining by Artemis and, possibly, a long isoform of TdT, remains relatively constant from the second trimester onward. Vα and Vβ segment use in the thymus and peripheral lymphoid organs is diverse. The αβ-TCR repertoire of cord blood T cells that is expressed on the cell surface is characterized by a diversity of TCR-β use and CDR3 length that is similar to that of antigenically naïve T cells in adults and infants, indicating that the functional preimmune repertoire is fully formed by birth.

Because the CDR3 region of the TCR chains is a major determinant of antigen specificity,[418] decreased CDR3 diversity, in conjunction with restricted use of DJ segments, theoretically could limit recognition of foreign antigens by the fetal αβ-TCR repertoire, particularly during the first trimester. The effects of any potential "holes" in the αβ-TCR repertoire of the human fetus from limitations in CDR3 are likely to be subtle, however, particularly after the second trimester, when V segment use is diverse. This is suggested by the fact that the T-cell response to immunization and viral challenge generally is normal in mice that are completely deficient in TdT as a result of selective gene targeting.[419]

Repertoire analysis using CDR3 spectratyping suggests that there is greater oligoclonal expansion of αβ T cells during the third trimester, particularly after 28 weeks of gestation, than in adults, and that these oligoclonal expansions involve a variety of different Vβ segment families.[420] Whether this oligoclonal expansion is antigen driven, such as by a response to maternally derived immunoglobulins (e.g., immunoglobulin idiotypes),[421] or, more likely, is a form of homeostatic proliferation, is unknown.

T-CELL RECEPTOR EXCISION CIRCLES

The V(D)J recombination process that joins the TCR gene segments also generates double-stranded circular DNA byproducts of the intervening sequences, termed T-cell receptor excision circles or TRECs. TRECs appear to be stable throughout the life of a T-lineage lymphocyte. Because they lack a DNA origin of replication, TRECs are diluted at the population level by cell proliferation.[422] For example, the level of DβJβ TRECs, which are formed during Dβ to Jβ rearrangement of the TCR-β gene locus during the double-negative stage of thymocyte development, are at the highest concentration in this cell population.[423] The marked thymocyte proliferation after surface expression of a TCR-β/pre-Tα complex is indicated by the observation that double-positive thymocytes lacking αβ-TCR/CD3 surface complexes, which have not yet achieved a productive TCR-α gene rearrangement, have only 4% of the concentration of DβJβ TRECs per cell as do double-negative cells[423]; this suggests that about 4 to 5 mitoses occur between these two stages of thymocyte development. At the double-positive αβ-TCR/CD3^{neg} stage of thymocyte development, most TCR-α gene loci first undergo a rearrangement that deletes much of the TCR-δ gene locus, which is located between clusters of Vα and Jα segments. This rearrangement forms a signal joint (sj) between the δRec segment and the downstream ψJα segment and a sjTREC that contains the deleted Dδ, Jδ, and Cδ segments (Fig. 4-9); this irreversibly commits the TCR-α/δ gene locus undergoing this rearrangement to the αβ-TCR differentiation pathway.[424] This rearrangement is followed by a second V(D)J recombination event, discussed in the previous section, in which Vα is joined to Jα to form a recombined Vα-Jα-Cα gene segment and a coding joint (cj)TREC.

sjTRECs, which are the result of a signal joint (sj) forming between a δRec segment and a downstream ψJα segment in the TCR-α gene (see Fig. 4-9), have been the predominant type of TREC assayed in human studies. In most αβ T cells, both TCR-α/δ gene loci have undergone δRec/ψJα joining, with the maximal theoretical level of sjTREC content per T-lineage cell being two. The highest levels of

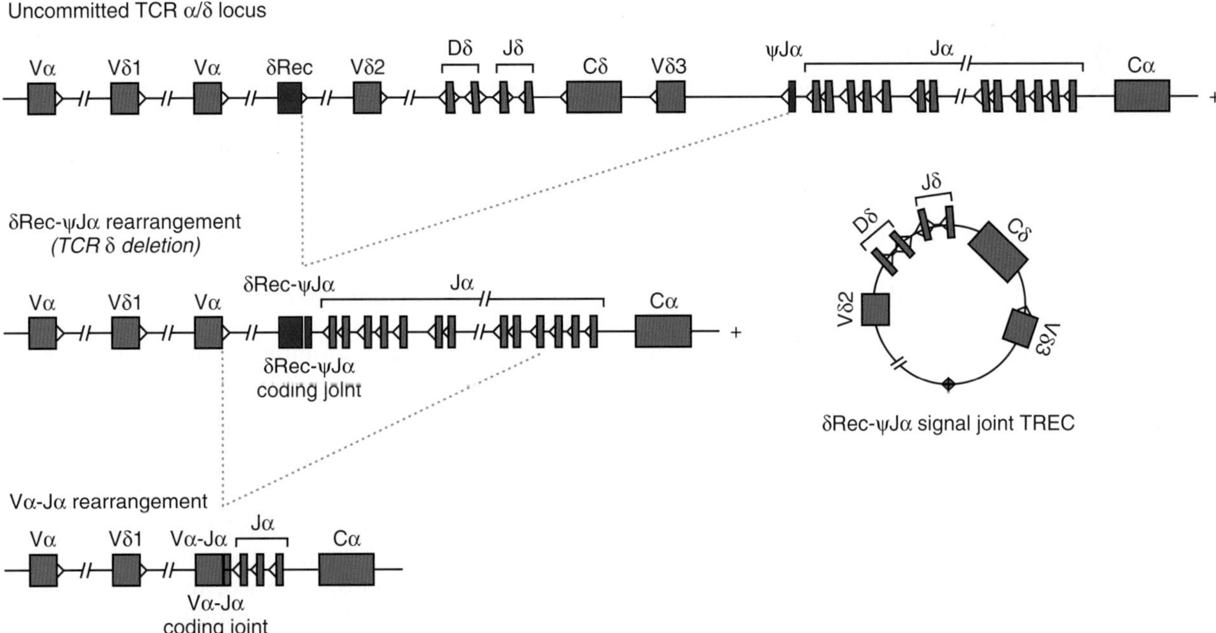

Figure 4-9 Sequential rearrangements in the T-cell receptor (TCR)-α/δ locus generate signal joint T-cell receptor excision circles (sjTRECs) and Vα-Jα rearrangements. Rearrangement of the δRec to the Jα segment results in a commitment to the αβ-TCR lineage because this deletes the C and J segments that are necessary to encode a productive TCR-δ chain. The δRec-ψJα rearrangement also generates an sjTREC, which is commonly used for monitoring peripheral T-cell populations for their recent thymic origin. The δRec-ψJα rearrangement is followed by TCR-α (Vα-Jα) rearrangements, which if productive result in expression of an αβ-TCR on the thymocyte cell surface. Most thymocytes that express αβ-TCRs have molecular evidence of nonproductive rearrangements of portions of the TCR-δ gene locus (not shown).

sjTRECs that have been measured are 1.5 copies per cell for $CD4^+CD8^+\alpha\beta^-$TCR/$CD3^-$ human fetal thymocytes.[425,426] As fetal thymocytes progress to the $CD4^+CD8^+CD3^{mid}$ and the mature single-positive stage ($CD4^+CD8^-CD3^{hi}$ or $CD4^-CD8^+CD3^{hi}$) stages, the sjTREC content declines to 0.7 and 0.6 copies per cell, respectively.[425,426] This indicates that the maturation of double-positive into single-positive thymocytes, which occurs by the process of positive selection described later, is accompanied by approximately one cell division. The sjTREC content of neonatal CD4 T cells is significantly higher than adult antigenically naïve CD4 T cells, indicating that a greater fraction of the adult naïve CD4 T-cell subset has undergone cell division, most likely in the form of homeostatic proliferation, than in the neonate. Such homeostatic proliferation, in which the naïve CD4 T cells retain their characteristic surface phenotype, that is, $CD45RA^{hi}$L-$selectin^{hi}$, appears to occur as protein tyrosine kinase 7 $(PTK7)^+$ CD4 recent thymic emigrants (RTEs) mature into $PTK7^-$ naïve CD4 T cells because the sjTREC content of $PTK7^+$ CD4 RTEs is significantly higher than that of $PTK7^-$ naïve CD4 T cells.[406] The ratio of sjTRECs and DβJβ TRECs (generated during Dβ-to-Jβ gene segment rearrangement) in peripheral naïve T cells has also been used to infer the relative amount of intrathymic proliferation occurring between the double-negative and double-positive stages of thymic development, with higher values indicating greater amounts of proliferation.[423] In certain states, such as HIV infection, this ratio is reduced in peripheral T cells indicating that the infection has a deleterious impact on the intrathymic production of T cells.[423]

THYMOCYTE SELECTION AND LATE MATURATION

Positive and Negative Selection

Thymocytes that have successfully rearranged and express αβ-TCRs and have a $CD4^+CD8^+$ surface phenotype (see Fig. 4-7) undergo a selective process that tests the appropriateness of their TCR specificity, known as positive selection.[415] Positive selection requires that the αβ-TCR recognize self-peptides bound to MHC molecules displayed on epithelial cells of the thymic cortex. If the TCR has sufficient but not too high affinity for self-peptide–MHC complexes, the thymocyte receives a signal allowing its survival. If this signal is absent or weak, the thymocyte dies by apoptosis as a result of activation of caspases, a family of intracellular cysteine proteases. Too strong a signal in the thymic cortex may also not result in effective positive selection. Recent studies indicate that the default pathway of maturation of a positively selected double-positive thymocyte is to become a mature $CD4^-CD8^+$ single-positive cell. If however, the double-positive thymocyte receives a relatively strong signal via the αβ-TCR/CD3 complex, this increases the expression of the GATA-binding protein-3 (GATA-3), a transcription factor, that induces the T-helper inducing POZ/Kruppel-like (ThROK) transcription factor. ThPOK then acts to help upregulate its own expression as well as prevent the loss of CD4 expression by binding to and inhibiting silencer elements in both of these genes.[427] This directs the double-positive thymocyte to become a $CD4^+CD8^-$ single-positive cell and ultimately a naïve CD4 T cell. Positive selection also extinguishes *RAG* gene expression, terminating further TCR-α rearrangement. Effective positive selection by MHC class I and MHC class II molecules requires that cortical thymic epithelial cells express a novel β5t catalytic subunit of the proteasome and the proteolytic enzyme cathepsin L, respectively. This requirement most likely reflects the importance of generating a specialized set of peptides for positive selection, although the identities of these peptides remain to be defined.

Positively selected $CD4^{hi}CD8^-$ and $CD4^-CD8^{hi}$ thymocytes enter the medulla, where they undergo a second selection process called negative selection, in which they are eliminated by apoptosis if their TCR has too high an affinity for self-peptide–MHC complexes expressed on medullary DCs. Negative selection helps eliminate αβ T cells with TCRs that could pose a risk of autoimmune reactions and is an important influence on the final TCR repertoire. Thymic epithelial cells found in the medulla express a diverse array of tissue-specific self-antigens (e.g., insulin, myelin basic protein) that help in this elimination. Individual thymic medullary epithelial cells only express some of these self-antigen proteins, and this expression is acquired in an apparently stochastic manner. The protein encoded by the autoimmune regulator *(AIRE)* gene plays a key role in enhancing the ectopic expression of these tissue-specific or developmentally regulated proteins by thymic epithelial cells. *AIRE* appears to help release stalled RNA polymerase II molecules on the promoters of these ectopically expressed genes.[428] The importance of *AIRE* is indicated by the high frequency of autoimmune endocrine disease in patients with *AIRE* gene defects, particularly hypoadrenalism, hypoparathyroidism, and type 1 diabetes mellitus. *AIRE* defects also frequently result in severe mucocutaneous candidiasis because of the development of autoantibodies to IL-17A, IL-17F, and IL-22.[429] *AIRE* may also play a similar role in inducing peripheral T-cell tolerance in the lymph nodes by increasing ectopic antigen expression by extrathymic AIRE-expressing cells (eTACs), which comprise a bone marrow–derived APC population that is distinct from DCs.[430] As a net result of either the failure to productively rearrange the TCR-α or TCR-β chain gene, the lack of positive selection, or the occurrence of negative selection, only about 2% to 3% of the progeny of hematopoietic lymphoid precursors that enter the thymus emerge as mature single-positive thymocytes.

Because the region forming the peptide-binding groove of MHC molecules is highly polymorphic in the human population (see section on Antigen Presentation by Classic Major Histocompatibility Complex Molecules), a result of positive selection is that T cells have a strong preference for recognizing a particular foreign peptide bound to self-MHC, rather than to the MHC of an unrelated person. On the other hand, the fact that a TCR has intrinsic affinity for MHC molecules[431] accounts for the ability of an APC bearing foreign MHC molecules to activate a substantial proportion (up to several percent) of T cells—the allogeneic response. In the allogeneic response, T cells are activated by novel antigen specificities that are thought to result from the combination of a foreign MHC with multiple self-peptides.[432] Because these self-peptide–foreign MHC specificities are not expressed in the thymus of that individual, T cells capable of recognizing them have not been eliminated by the negative selection process in the medulla.

THYMOCYTE GROWTH AND DIFFERENTIATION FACTORS

The factors within the thymic microenvironment that are essential for thymocyte development include key cytokines produced by thymic epithelial cells, such as IL-7. Persons lacking a functional IL-7 receptor, because of a genetic deficiency of either the IL-7 receptor α chain or the common γ chain (γc) cytokine receptor (CD132) with which the α chain associates, have abortive thymocyte development and lack mature αβ T cells.[409] A similar phenotype is observed with genetic deficiency of the JAK-3 tyrosine kinase, which is associated with the cytoplasmic domain of the γc cytokine receptor and delivers activation signals to the interior of the cell. Human fetal B-cell development is spared in these human genetic immunodeficiencies, although a lack of γc-dependent cytokine receptors, such as that for IL-21, results in these B cells having intrinsic functional defects.

Thymocyte Postselection Maturation

$CD4^+CD8^-$ and $CD4^-CD8^+$ thymocytes are the most mature αβ T-lineage cell population in the thymus and predominate in the thymic medulla. Many of the functional differences between peripheral CD4 and CD8 T cells appear to be established during the later stages of thymic maturation, presumably as a result of differentiation induced by positive selection: Mature $CD4^+CD8^-$ thymocytes, like peripheral CD4 T cells, are enriched in cells that can secrete certain cytokines, such as IL-2, and in providing help for B cells in producing immunoglobulin.[433,434] $CD4^-CD8^+$ thymocytes, like peripheral CD8 T cells, are relatively limited in their ability to produce IL-2 but, once primed by antigen, are effective in mediating cytotoxic activity.[433] In preparation for thymic emigration, the last stages of single-positive thymocyte maturation include increased levels of the Kruppel-like factor 2 (KLF-2) transcription factor, which in turn, appears to increase the thymocyte expression of the sphingosine-1-phosphate receptor.[435] Thymocytes are then directed to emigrate into the blood and/or lymph, both of which have high concentrations of sphingosine-1-phosphate compared with the medulla.

NAÏVE T CELLS

CD4 and CD8 Recent Thymic Emigrants

Mature $CD4^{hi}CD8^-$ and $CD4^-CD8^{hi}$ single-positive thymocytes enter into the circulation as RTEs, joining the antigenically naïve CD4 and CD8 αβ T-cell compartments, respectively (see Fig. 4-7). In humans, RTEs of the CD4 T-cell lineage are identified by their expression of PTK7, a member of the receptor tyrosine kinase family.[406] The function of PTK7 appears to promote cell survival and protection from apoptosis (Swati Acharya and D.B. Lewis, unpublished observations, 2014). This protein has no known ligands and appears to be a catalytically inactive kinase because it lacks a functional ATP-binding cassette in its cytoplasmic domain.[436] Approximately 5% of circulating naïve CD4 T cells from healthy young adults are $PTK7^+$, and these cells are highly enriched in their sjTREC content compared with $PTK7^-$ naïve CD4 T cells but otherwise have a similar surface phenotype.[406] As expected for an RTE cell population, $PTK7^+$ naïve CD4 T cells have a highly diverse αβ-TCR repertoire, similar to that of the overall naïve CD4 T-cell population, and rapidly decline in the circulation after complete thymectomy (performed for the treatment of myasthenia gravis).[406] As described below, $PTK7^+$ naïve CD4 T cells (hereafter referred to as $PTK7^+$ CD4 RTEs) from healthy adults have reduced activation-dependent function compared with $PTK7^-$ naïve CD4 T cells.

Virtually all CD4 T cells and most CD8 T cells of the neonate express high levels of surface protein and mRNA transcripts for PTK7, which is a marker for CD4 RTEs in older children and adults[406] (Christopher Haines and D.B. Lewis, unpublished observations, 2014). Although this high level of PTK7 expression by the neonatal naïve CD4 T cells may be explained, in part, by their being highly enriched in RTEs, it is likely that PTK7 expression is regulated differently in neonatal CD4 T cells compared with adult naïve CD4 T cells based on two observations: First, there is a higher level of expression of PTK7 per neonatal naïve CD4 T cell compared with adult PTK7 CD4 RTEs.[406] Second, there are a few, if any, $PTK7^-$ cells among circulating neonatal naïve CD4 T cells even though studies of older children undergoing complete thymectomy suggest that most $PTK7^+$ CD4 RTEs are converted to $PTK7^-$ naïve CD4 T cells over a 3-month period,[406] and at least some neonatal T cells are likely to have emigrated from the thymus more than 6 months previously.

The expression of CD103 ($\alpha_E\beta_7$ integrin) appears to be a marker for CD8, but not CD4, T-lineage RTEs.[426] As for $PTK7^+$ CD4 RTEs, the thymic dependence of this circulating CD8 RTE population has been demonstrated by the impact of complete thymectomy,[426] and these cells are relatively enriched in sjTRECs compared with $CD103^-$ naïve CD8 T cells. It remains unclear whether $CD103^+$ naïve CD8 T cells in the adult circulation differ in function from those of the $CD103^-$ naïve CD8 T-cell subset.

Naïve T-Cell Entry into Lymphoid Tissue, Recirculation, and Survival

Human naïve CD4 T cells have a $CD45RA^{hi}CD45RO^{lo}CD27^{hi}$ $L\text{-}selectin^{hi}\alpha_4\beta_1{}^-CD11a^{lo}$ surface phenotype.[437] Naïve T cells, including RTEs, preferentially home to the secondary lymphoid tissue, which includes the lymph nodes, spleen, Peyer patches, and mucosa-associated lymphoid tissue (MALT), and then recirculate through these compartments along with the rest of the antigenically naïve CD4 and CD8 T-cell populations. Egress of RTEs from the thymus as well as of naïve T cells and B cells from secondary lymphoid tissue requires that these cell types express sphingosine-1-phosphate (S1P) receptors. S1P, the receptor ligand, is at higher concentrations in the blood and lymph than in the thymus and secondary lymphoid tissue, which directs these cells to exit the tissues and enter into these fluids.[438] Bronchus-associated lymphoid tissue (BALT), a type of MALT, typically appears only after birth, and is another potential site for naïve T-cell homing and recirculation.[439]

Development of secondary lymph node tissues is dependent on signaling by lymphotoxin (LT) α and β members of the TNF cytokine gene family (see Table 4-1). Peripheral lymphoid organogenesis involves lymphoid tissue inducer cells, which are $CD45^+CD4^+CD3^-$ innate lymphoid cells that express surface $LT\alpha\beta_2$ trimers that engagei the LTβ receptor on stromal cells. This induces stromal cells to become stromal organizers by increasing their expression of adhesion molecules (VCAM-1, ICAM-1, and mucosal vascular addressin cell adhesion molecule-1 [MADCAM-1]) and of chemokines (CXCL13, CCL19, and CCL21) which attracts naïve B cells and T cells as well as more lymphoid tissue inducer cells, ultimately resulting in fully formed peripheral lymph nodes.[440]

As described for DCs, migration of fully mature naïve T cells and RTEs, which both express high levels of the CCR7 chemokine receptor and L-selectin,[406] into the peripheral lymphoid organs is determined in part by the local patterns and gradients of chemokine receptor ligands in tissues (see Tables 4-1 and 4-2) and ligands for adhesion molecules. L-selectin, which is constitutively expressed on many types of leukocytes, including naïve and certain subsets of memory T cells, binds to multivalent carbohydrate ligands displayed on specific protein or lipid backbones on the cell surface. T-cell surface expression of L-selectin allows their binding to the peripheral lymph node addressin, which is expressed on the surface of the specialized high endothelium of the postcapillary venules (HEV) in the peripheral lymph nodes, Peyer patches, and tonsils.[441] Tethered to the surface of the HEV is the chemokine, CCL21, which binds to CCR7 on the surface of RTEs and naïve T cells. CCL21 and another CCR7 ligand, CCL19, are produced by stromal cells and perhaps some APCs in the lymph node. The engagement of CCR7 on naïve T cells by CCL21 triggers signals leading to an increase in the affinity of LFA-1, allowing the naïve T cells to bind avidly to the LFA-1 ligands ICAM-1 and ICAM-2 on the vascular endothelium. This stops T-cell rolling, allowing the T cell to undergo diapedesis across the endothelium and to enter the T-cell zones of the lymph node. There, CCL19 is produced by DCs, resulting in the juxtaposition of naïve T cells and DCs.[441]

Based on elegant studies in mice, the survival of naïve T cells in the periphery has been shown to be dependent on two major exogenous factors. The first is continuous interaction with self-peptide–MHC complexes, which appears to be particularly important for the survival of the antigenically naïve T-cell populations.[442] Whether this survival signal is analogous to positive selection in the thymus in its requirements for a diverse self-peptide repertoire remains unclear. The second major factor appears to be signals provided by IL-7 binding to IL-7 receptors on naïve CD4 and CD8 T cells.[443] It is unclear if human naïve T cells have similar requirements for their survival in the periphery, and, if so, whether RTEs and more mature naïve T cells differ in their dependence on these αβ-TCR/CD3 and cytokine receptor signals.

ONTOGENY OF NAÏVE T-CELL SURFACE PHENOTYPE

Circulating T cells are detectable as early as 12.5 weeks of gestation, demonstrating the emigration of mature T-lineage cells from the thymus.[444] By 14 weeks of gestation, CD4 and CD8 T cells are found in the fetal liver and spleen, and CD4 T cells are detectable in lymph nodes.[445] The percentage of T cells in the fetal (or in the case of very preterm birth, premature infant) circulation gradually increases during the second and third trimesters of pregnancy through approximately 6 months of age,[445] followed by a gradual decline to adult levels during childhood.[446] The ratio of CD4 to CD8 T cells in the circulation is relatively high during fetal life (about 3.5) and gradually declines with age.[446] The levels of expression of the αβ-TCR, CD3, CD4, CD5, CD8, and CD28 proteins on fetal and neonatal αβ T cells are similar to those in adult T cells (D.B. Lewis, unpublished data, 2008).[447]

CD31

CD31, also known as platelet endothelial cell adhesion molecule-1 (PECAM-1), is expressed in large amounts on most adult peripheral CD4 T cells that have a naïve ($CD45RA^{hi}$) surface phenotype but is absent or decreased on most memory CD4 T cells. A small fraction of $CD45RA^{hi}$ CD4 T cells that are $CD31^{lo}$ appears and gradually increases with ageing, especially after adulthood, and these cells have very low sjTREC content and an oligoclonal rather than polyclonal αβ-TCR repertoire compared with either $PTK7^+$ CD4 RTEs (which are uniformly $CD31^{hi}$) or $PTK7^-$ $CD31^{hi}$ naïve CD4 T cells.[448,449] The $CD31^{lo}$ naïve CD4 T-cell populations appears to be the result of homeostatic proliferation of $CD31^{hi}$ naïve CD4 T cells rather than reversion of memory/effector cells to a CD45RA surface phenotype because these cells lack a capacity to express cytokines characteristic of memory/effector cells, such as IFN-γ.

Most neonatal $CD45RA^{hi}$ T cells are $CD31^{hi}$, but approximately 10% to 20% have been reported to be $CD31^{lo}$.[450] It is unclear if the neonatal $CD31^{lo}$ subset of naïve CD4 T cells has low levels of sjTRECs, similar to that found in adult $CD31^{lo}$ naïve CD4 T-cell subset, which would suggest that these cells have undergone extensive proliferation compared with most neonatal CD4 T cells. Alternatively, a finding of high sjTREC content in $CD31^{lo}$ naïve CD4 T cells of the neonate would suggest that this population may be an immature population that gives rise to $CD31^{hi}$ naïve CD4 T cells. As neonatal CD4 T cells are uniformly $PTK7^{hi}$, and PTK7 expression by adult CD4 RTEs is lost in an in vitro model of homeostatic proliferation using a cytokine cocktail,[406] the latter possibility appears to be more likely.

CD38

CD38 is an ectoenzyme that generates cyclic adenosine diphosphate ribose (cADPR), a metabolite that induces intracellular calcium mobilization. It is expressed on most thymocytes, some activated peripheral blood T cells and B cells, plasma cells, and DCs. Unlike adult naïve T cells, virtually all peripheral fetal and neonatal T cells express very high levels of the CD38 molecule,[451-453] suggesting that peripheral T cells in the fetus and neonate may represent a thymocyte-like immature transitional population. One study found that CD38 expression on circulating T cells persisted through 1 month of age,[454] but it is unclear at what age expression is lost thereafter. There is no substantial difference in CD38 expression by adult circulating $PTK7^+$ CD4 RTEs and $PTK7^-$ naïve CD4 T cells,[406] indicating that this persistence of high levels of CD38 expression is unique to the naïve T-cell compartment of the fetus and neonate. In contrast with circulating fetal and neonatal T cells, a significant fraction of T cells in the fetal spleen between 14 and 20 weeks of gestation lack CD38 expression,[455] which suggests that CD38 may be downregulated on entry into secondary lymphoid tissue. As discussed later, a significant fraction of splenic CD4 T cells in the fetus appear to belong to the regulatory T-cell subset, and it is plausible that this subset may have only relatively low levels of CD38 expression, based on analysis of adult regulatory T cells.[456] Neonatal CD4 T cells lose expression of CD38 after in vitro culture with IL-7 for 10 days,[457] which implies that this cytokine promotes further maturation independently of engagement of the αβ-TCR–CD3 complex. The precursor-product relationship between CD38$^+$ and CD38$^-$ peripheral naïve T cells in humans is unclear.

The role of CD38 in the function of human T cells and other cell types also is unknown. In mice, CD38 is required for chemokine-mediated migration of mature DCs into secondary lymphoid tissue, and as a consequence, CD38 deficiency impairs humoral immunity to TD antigens. Of interest, mice, in contrast with humans, have relatively low levels of thymocyte expression of CD38, and CD38 deficiency in these animals does not have a clear impact on thymocyte development or intrinsic T-cell function. One recent report also suggests that CD38 might, in conjunction with two other cell surface ectoenzymes (CD203a and CD73), be involved in the generation of adenosine from cADPR.[458] This observation, which needs confirmation, is of interest given the overall immunosuppressive effects of adenosine.

CD45 Isoforms

Circulating T cells in the term and preterm (22 to 30 weeks of gestation) neonate and in the second- and third-trimester fetus predominantly express a CD45RA^{hi}CD45RO^{lo} surface phenotype,[453,459,460] which also is found on antigenically naïve T cells of adults. About 30% of circulating T cells of the term neonate are CD45RA^{lo}CD45RO^{lo},[461] a surface phenotype that is rare in circulating adult T cells. Because these CD45RA^{lo}CD45RO^{lo} T cells are functionally similar to neonatal CD45RA^{hi}CD45RO^{lo} T cells and become CD45RA^{mid}CD45RO^{lo} T cells when incubated in vitro with fibroblasts,[461] they appear to be immature thymocyte-like cells rather than mature naïve cells that have been activated in vivo to express the CD45RO isoform.

Most studies have found that the healthy neonate and the late-gestation fetus lack circulating CD45RO^{hi} T cells, consistent with their limited exposure to foreign antigens. A lack of surface expression of other memory/effector markers, such as β_1 integrins (e.g., VLA-4), and, in the case of CD8 T cells, KIRs[462] and CD11b,[463,464] also is consistent with an antigenically naïve population predominating in the healthy neonate.

A postnatal precursor-product relationship between CD45RA^{hi}CD45RO^{lo} and CD45RA^{lo}CD45RO^{hi} T cells is suggested by the fact that the proportion of αβ T cells with a memory/effector phenotype and the capacity of circulating T cells to produce cytokines, such as IFN-γ, both gradually increase, whereas the proportion of antigenically naïve T cells decreases, with increasing postnatal age.[446,465] These increases in the ability to produce cytokines and expression of the CD45RO^{hi} phenotype presumably are due to cumulative antigenic exposure and T-cell activation, leading to the generation of memory T cells from antigenically naïve T cells.

In premature or term neonates who are stressed, a portion of circulating T-lineage cells are CD3^{lo} and co-express CD1, CD4, and CD8,[452] a phenotype characteristic of immature thymocytes of the cortex.[466] It is likely that stress results in the premature release of cortical thymocytes into the circulation, but the immunologic consequences of this release are unclear.

A minority but substantial proportion of T cells in the second trimester fetal spleen are CD45RA^{lo}CD45RO^{hi}, a T-cell population that is absent from the spleen of young infants.[460] These fetal CD45RO^{hi} T cells have a diverse αβ-TCR repertoire and express high levels of CD25 (IL-2 receptor α chain) and proliferate with IL-2.[461] In contrast with adult CD45RO^{hi} T cells, however, these fetal spleen CD45RO^{hi} T cells express low surface levels of CD2 and LFA-1 and proliferate poorly after activation with either anti-CD2 or anti-CD3 monoclonal antibody (mAb), suggesting that they are not fully functional.[460] As discussed in the section Fetal and Neonatal Tregs, many features of this cell population are consistent with their being regulatory T cells (Tregs), which have recently been shown to be prominent in both the spleen and lymph nodes of the fetus.[467,468] The extent to which these fetal spleen CD45RO^{hi} T cells contribute to the postnatal (Treg or non-Treg) peripheral T-cell compartment, however, is unknown.

HOMEOSTATIC PROLIFERATION

Spontaneous Naïve Peripheral T-Cell Proliferation

Naïve T cells may undergo proliferation by processes that are distinct from those of full activation by cognate antigen and appropriate co-stimulation, and such proliferative processes may make a significant contribution to expansion of the peripheral T-cell pool during development. Based on flow cytometric analysis of expression of the Ki67 antigen, a significantly higher fraction of naïve (CD45RO^{lo}) CD4 and CD8 T cells in the third-trimester fetus and the term neonate are spontaneous in cell cycle than the fraction of adult naïve T cells.[413] The highest levels are observed at 26 weeks of gestation, and these gradually decline with gestational age. Even at term, however, the reported frequencies of Ki67$^+$ naïve CD4 and CD8 T cells—approximately 1.4% and 3.2%, respectively—are sevenfold higher than those of adult naïve T cells and are substantially higher than those observed for adult CD45RO^{hi} T cells.[413] These results are supported by other in vitro assays of mitosis, such as the incorporation of tritiated (^{3}H)-thymidine or the loss of fluorescence after labeling cell membranes with carboxyfluorescein succinimidyl ester (CFSE)[469] (D.B. Lewis, unpublished results, 2014).

A substantial proportion of both CD4 and CD8 T cells of the neonate express the killer cell lectin-like receptor G1 (KLRG1),[470] an inhibitory receptor that is also expressed by NK cells and that interacts with cadherins. These KLRG1$^+$ neonatal T cells have naïve surface phenotype, a normal proliferative response to anti-CD3 and CD28 mAb, and a diverse αβ-TCR repertoire but reduced sjTREC content compared with their KLRG1$^-$ counterparts.[470] Based on these findings, it is plausible that the KLRG1$^+$ subset of naïve T cells of the neonate may be enriched for cells that have undergone homeostatic proliferation.

Although the mechanism underlying this proliferation of human fetal and neonatal naïve T cells is unclear, it differs from that in rodent models of homeostatic proliferation, including in the neonatal mouse,[471] in that the proliferation occurs in the absence of peripheral lymphopenia. As discussed next, one potential explanation for this increased spontaneous proliferation is an increased sensitivity of fetal and neonatal T cells to cytokines, such as IL-7, which is also a feature of circulating PTK7$^+$ CD4 RTEs of adults.[406] Future studies are needed to determine if spontaneously proliferating naïve T cells in fetus and neonate (and proliferating PTK7$^+$ CD4 RTEs in adults) have a diverse TCR repertoire (as would be predicted by a model of generalized increased sensitivity to cytokines) and whether they can be distinguished from noncycling cells by other markers, such as those that are induced during naïve T-cell proliferation in the setting of peripheral lymphopenia, and by reduced sjTREC content.

Antigen-Independent Naïve T-Cell Proliferation in Response to IL-7 and IL-15

Murine studies show that homeostatic proliferation in the lymphopenic host and survival of naïve CD4 and CD8 T cells depends on IL-7.[407] Human neonatal naïve CD4 T cells are capable of higher levels of polyclonal cell proliferation than adult naïve CD4 T cells in response to IL-7,[413,472-474] so it is plausible that IL-7–dependent proliferation could account for the high rate of spontaneous CD4 T-cell proliferation in the human fetus and neonate, and contribute to the normal and rapid expansion of the peripheral CD4 T-cell compartment at this age. The increased IL-7 proliferative response is associated with increased expression of the CD127 (IL-7 receptor α-chain component) by neonatal naïve CD4 T cells compared with adult naïve CD4 T cells,[472,474,475] although surface expression of the other component of the IL-7 receptor, the γc cytokine receptor chain (CD132), was actually decreased on neonatal naïve CD4 T cells compared with that on adult naïve T cells in one study.[474] This increased expression of the IL-7 receptor α chain by neonatal naïve CD4 T cells is not observed for PTK7$^+$ CD4 RTEs in adults,[406] indicating that the increased responsiveness of RTEs to IL-7 may be mediated by a different mechanism (see directly below).

Murine studies also indicate that positive selection results in a dramatic upregulation of both the IL-7 receptor α chain and the γc cytokine receptor on CD3^{hi} (mature) CD4$^+$CD8$^-$ and CD8$^+$CD4$^-$ single-positive thymocytes.[475] In vitro thymic organ culture experiments suggest that IL-7 plays a key role in the postselection expansion of these single-positive thymocyte populations by a mechanism that does not involve αβ-TCR engagement.[475] Human CD4-single positive thymocytes have also been shown to have an increased proliferative response to IL-7,[476] suggesting that this increased IL-7 sensitivity also applies to late thymocyte maturation in humans. These observations, taken with the finding that human PTK7$^+$ CD4 RTEs also have an increased proliferative response to IL-7 compared with PTK7$^-$ naïve CD4 T cells, even though there are no differences in surface expression of either component of the IL-7 receptor[406] (C. Haines and D.B. Lewis, unpublished observations, 2014), suggests that the mechanism for this increased IL-7 sensitivity by neonatal CD4 T cells is (1) likely to be downstream of cytokine receptor binding and (2) shared with mature CD4$^+$CD8$^-$ thymocytes and PTK7$^+$ CD4 RTEs.

Whether IL-7 not only contributes to extrathymic expansion of naïve CD4 T cells but also influences their maturation remains unclear. IL-7 treatment of neonatal naïve CD4 T cells for relatively long periods (7 or 14 days) does not decrease expression of CD45RA or L-selectin and does not increase the expression of CD45RO.[457,472,477,478] The extent to which IL-7 treatment, alone, of neonatal naïve CD4 T cells results in acquisition of a phenotype with selective features of both naïve and memory/effector cells remains contentious: Results are conflicting regarding whether IL-7 treatment increases surface expression of CD11a, a memory/effector cell marker; the activation-dependent proteins CD25 and CD40 ligand; or the capacity of neonatal CD4 T cells to produce Th1 and Th2 cytokines.[457,472] IL-7 in combination with a cocktail of other cytokines (IL-6, IL-10, IL-15, and TNF-α) has been shown to result in the loss of PTK7 surface expression by adult PTK7$^+$ CD4 RTEs,[406] but it is unknown if PTK7 downregulation is accompanied by an increased capacity for Th1 effector function by adult RTEs and if this downregulation occurs with such treatment of neonatal T cells.

Naïve CD4 and CD8 T-cell survival in adults requires interactions between the αβ-TCR and self-peptide/MHC molecules on immature DCs as well as engagement of the T-cell IL-7 receptor by IL-7 on fibroblastic reticular cells found in the T-cell zone of secondary lymphoid organs; IL-15 may also play a role in CD8 T-cell survival.[442] Human neonatal naïve CD8 T cells are more responsive to treatment with a combination of IL-7 and IL-15 than is the analogous adult cell population, as indicated by loss of CFSE staining with culture after in vitro labeling.[413] Whether this enhanced effect is related to increased levels of IL-15 receptors on neonatal T cells is unknown. Also unclear are the effects of treatment with this combination of cytokines on neonatal naïve CD8 T-cell phenotype and function.

NAÏVE T-CELL ACTIVATION, ANERGY, AND CO-STIMULATION

If naïve T cells of the lymph nodes encounter DCs presenting cognate peptide-MHC complexes, they stop migrating and remain there. If they do not encounter such DCs, they migrate through the lymph node to the efferent lymph and thereby return to the bloodstream. Thus naïve T cells continually circulate between the blood and secondary lymphoid tissues, allowing them the opportunity to continuously sample APCs for their cognate antigen. Because they regulate this homeostatic recirculation of naïve T cells, CCL19 and CCL21 are referred to as homeostatic chemokines.

When naïve CD4 T cells first encounter foreign peptide–MHC complexes during a primary immune response, they extinguish expression of lung Kruppel-like factor (LKLF), a transcription factor that maintains naïve T cells in a resting state,[479] allowing them to become activated. The TCR-CD3 complex is linked to an intricate and highly interconnected complex of kinases, phosphatases, and adapter molecules that together transduce signals in response to engagement of the TCR and, in αβ T cells, the appropriate CD4 or CD8 co-receptor by cognate peptide-MHC complexes (Fig. 4-10; see Fig. 4-5).[480] Lipid rafts play a critical role in facilitating the assembly of signaling complexes at specific regions of the plasma membrane at high local concentrations; these complexes contained in lipid microdomains, in turn, recruit adapters and signal-transducing proteins.[481] Proximal activation events include the activation of the Lck and ZAP-70 tyrosine kinases and phospholipase C, followed by elevation of inositol triphosphate, which leads to the release of calcium into the cytoplasm from the endoplasmic reticulum. This increase in free intracellular ($[Ca^{2+}]_i$) is sensed by the stromal interaction molecule 1 (STIM1) and STIM2 proteins of the endoplasmic reticulum, which interact with and open calcium-release activated calcium (CRAC) channels of the cell membrane, resulting in a 10-fold increase in $[Ca^{2+}]_i$ and full T-cell activation.[482]

An increased calcium concentration activates calcineurin, allowing the translocation of nuclear factor of activated T cells (NFAT) transcription factors from the cytosol to the nucleus. Concurrent activation of the ERK/MAPK pathway enhances activation of other transcription factors, including AP-1/activating transcription factor (ATF). T-cell activation also activates the NF-κB transcription factor by a pathway that involves protein kinase C-θ and the caspase recruitment domain-containing membrane-associated guanylate kinase protein-1 (CARMA1)/Bcl10/Malt1 trimolecular complex.[480] Collectively, these transcription factors induce the transcription of genes encoding key proteins for activation, such as cytokines, for instance, IL-2, cell-cycle regulators, and, in cytotoxic T cells, proteins involved in killing other cells, such as perforins.

Full naïve T-cell activation that leads to cytokine production and cell proliferation requires that signaling through the trimolecular αβ-TCR–peptide–MHC complex exceeds a specific threshold as well as co-stimulatory signaling pathways. Low-affinity interactions that do not trigger full T-cell activation, particularly in the absence of co-stimulation, may lead to a state of long-term unresponsiveness to subsequent stimulation, which is referred to as anergy. Anergy may help maintain tolerance by mature T cells to certain self-antigens, in particular, those that are not expressed in the thymus in sufficient abundance to induce negative selection. At least in certain contexts, anergy may be the result of activation of caspase-3 and the cleavage by that enzyme of intracellular signaling molecules required for T-cell activation, for instance, Vav1 and adapter molecules,[483] rendering the T cell unresponsive to subsequent encounters with optimal amounts of peptide–MHC antigen complexes and co-stimulatory molecules. The induction of E3 ubiquitin ligases, such as Cbl-b, also appear to play an important role in anergy.[484]

The best-characterized co-stimulatory signal is provided by the engagement of CD28 on the T cell with CD80 (B7-1) or CD86 (B7-2) on APCs (see Table 4-5).[485] CD80 and CD86 are related proteins that are expressed at low levels on immature DCs, mononuclear phagocytes, and B cells and at increased levels after LPS exposure, B-cell receptor cross-linking, and CD40 signaling (see Fig. 4-10). Thus APCs primed by these factors, and, in particular, mature DCs, express high levels of CD80 and CD86. CD80 and CD86 both bind to CD28, which is constitutively expressed on T cells, thereby lowering the strength or duration of TCR signaling needed for full activation.[486] Another B7 family member, inducible co-stimulator (ICOS) ligand and its receptor on T cells, ICOS, which is homologous to CD28, are important for driving the differentiation of activated T cells into specialized effector lineages, such as Th17 cells and TFH cells, which are discussed more later. Other members of the family, such as PD-1 (programmed death-1) and PD-2, when engaged on the T cell by PD ligands act to dampen the T-cell response by inducing T-cell apoptosis.[485] The expression of high levels of these PD-1 or PD-2 may result in T cells being "exhausted," that is, having a

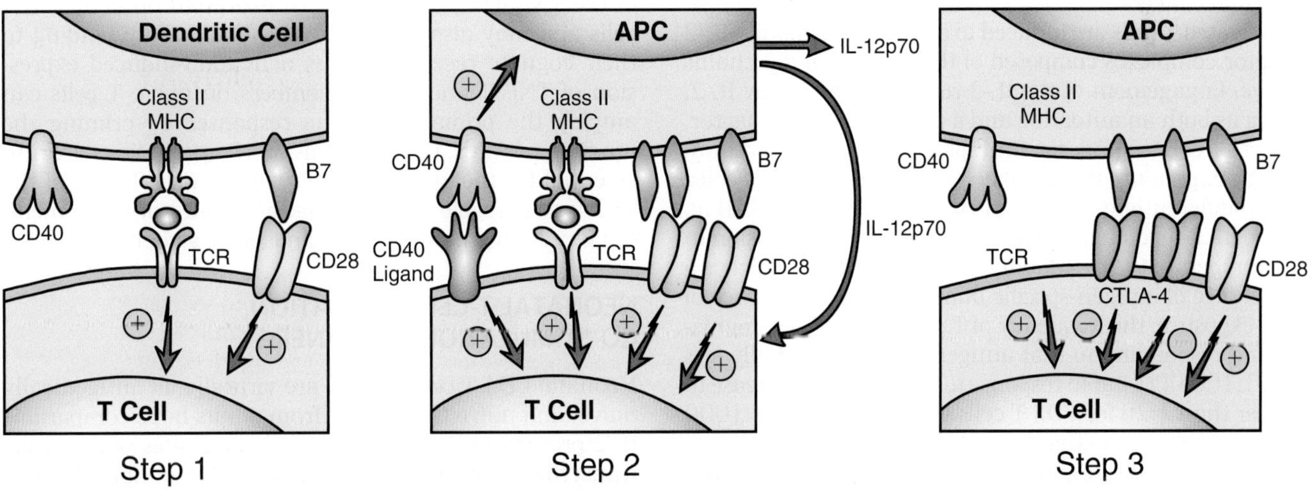

Figure 4-10 T-cell–antigen-presenting cell (APC) interactions early during the immune response to peptide antigens. A Th1 type major histocompatibility complex (MHC) class II–restricted response by CD4 T cells is shown as an example. Dendritic cells are probably the most important APC for antigenically naïve T cells and constitutively express CD80 or CD86 (B7 molecules), CD40 and MHC class II molecules on their cell surface. Engagement of αβ T-cell receptor (αβ-TCR) on the CD4 T cell by antigenic peptides bound to MHC molecules on the dendritic cell, in conjunction with co-stimulation provided by interactions of B7 (CD80/86) with CD28, leads to full T-cell activation (step 1). The activated T cell expresses CD40 ligand (CD154) on its surface, which engages CD40 on the dendritic cell; this increases B7 expression on the dendritic cell enhancing T-cell co-stimulation (step 2). CD40 engagement also activates the dendritic cell to produce cytokines, such as IL-12p70. IL-12p70, in turn, promotes the proliferation and differentiation of T cells into Th1-type effector cells that produce high levels of interferon-γ. Cytotoxic T-lymphocyte antigen-4 (CTLA-4 [CD152]) is expressed on the T cells during the later stages of T-cell activation. Engagement of CTLA-4 by B7 molecules on the APC delivers negative signals that help terminate T-cell activation (step 3).

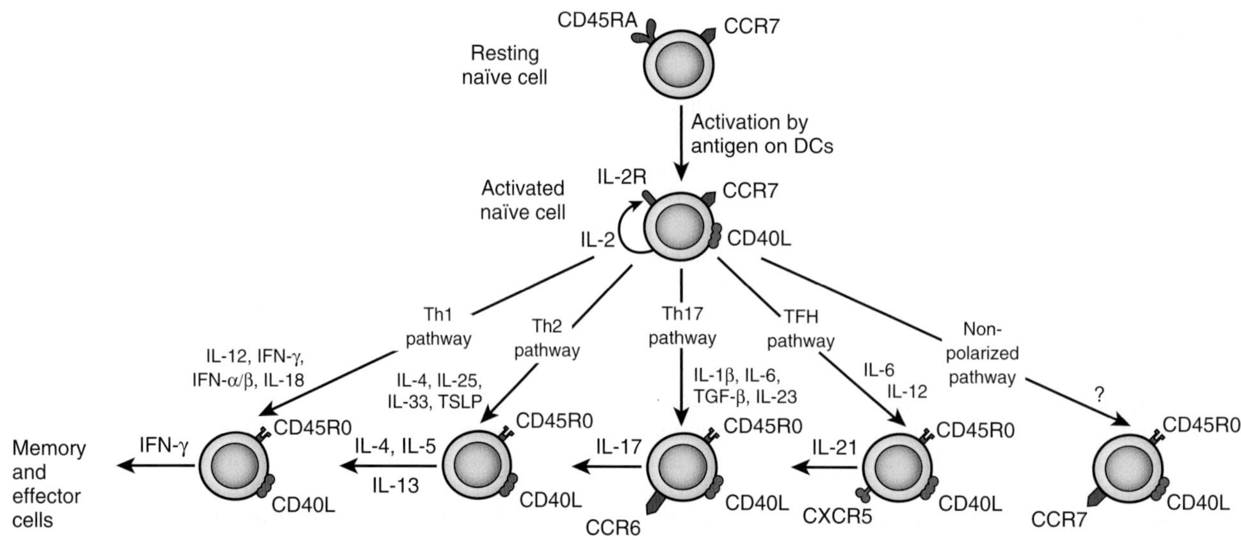

Figure 4-11 Differentiation of antigenically naïve CD4 T cells into Th1, Th2, unpolarized, and T-follicular helper memory and effector T cells. Antigenically naïve CD4 T cells express high levels of the CD45RA isoform of the CD45 surface protein tyrosine phosphatase. They are activated by antigen presented by antigen-presenting cells (APCs) to express CD40 ligand and interleukin-2 (IL-2) and to undergo clonal expansion and differentiation, which is accompanied by expression of the CD45R0 isoform and loss of the CD45RA isoform. Exposure of differentiating memory stem CD4 T cells to IL-12p70, IFN-γ, and type I interferon (IFN-α/β) favors their differentiation into Th1 memory and effector cells that secrete IFN-γ, whereas exposure to IL-4 from non–T-cell sources, such as basophils, and dendritic cells (DCs) that have been exposed to thymic stromal lymphopoietin , IL-25, and IL-33 favors their differentiation into Th2 cells that secrete IL-4, IL-5, and IL-13. Th17 cell differentiation is favored by exposure of differentiating CD4 T cells to IL-1β, IL-6, IL-23 and transforming growth factor-β (TGF-β), whereas T-follicular helper (TFH) cell differentiation is favored by exposure of activated CD4 T cells to IL-12 and IL-6. TFH cells, which express high levels of CXCR5, move into B-cell follicle areas, where they express CD40 ligand (CD40L) and IL-21 and provide help for B-cell responses. Many memory and effector cells are nonpolarized and do not express Th1, Th2, or Th17 cytokines. They may be enriched for cells that continue to express the CCR7 chemokine receptor, which favors their recirculation between the blood and the lymph nodes and spleen. Additional subsets with distinct cytokine secretion patterns include Th9 cells, which express IL-9, and Th22 cells, which express IL-22 (not shown). In a currently favored model (not shown), memory cells are maintained by a self-renewing stem cell memory CD4 T-cell population that gives rise to more differentiated central memory-cell populations that are $CCR7^+$ and L-selectin$^+$. Central memory cells, in turn, give rise to effector memory cells that are $CCR7^-$ and L-selectin$^-$ and express other chemokine receptors that target these cells to nonlymphoid tissues. Memory cells rechallenged with antigen undergo rapid clonal expansion into secondary effector cells that mediate the same functions as the initial memory population. Most effector cells eventually die by apoptosis.

limited capacity for effector function, and such populations are frequently seen in chronic infections, such as HIV, and in certain cancers.[487]

Activated T cells are induced to express high-affinity IL-2 receptor complexes composed of the IL-2R α and β chains and γc. Engagement of the IL-2 receptor complex by IL-2, acting as both an autocrine and a paracrine growth factor, triggers T cells to undergo multiple rounds of proliferation, thereby expanding the numbers of antigen-specific T cells, and to differentiate into memory and effector T cells (Fig. 4-11). IL-2–mediated proliferation leads to an expansion in the numbers of the responding T-cell population, which is a key feature of antigen-specific immunity. In the absence of prior exposure, the frequency of T cells capable of recognizing and responding to that antigen is small, generally less than 1:100,000, but in response to infection can increase to greater than 1:20 for CD8 T cells and greater than 1:1000 for CD4 T cells in less than a week.[488]

Activated T cells, especially those of the CD4 T-cell subset, also express on their surface CD40 ligand (CD154 or TNFSF5), a member of the TNF ligand family (see Tables 4-1 and 4-5), which engages the CD40 molecule on B cells, DCs, and mononuclear phagocytes.[489,490] As mentioned previously, CD40 engagement induces the expression of CD80 and CD86 on these APCs and induces DCs to produce IL-12 family heterodimeric cytokines, such as IL-12p70 (see Fig. 4-10). Interactions between CD40 and CD40 ligand appear to play an important role in vivo in the expansion of CD4 T cells during a primary immune response but may be less critical for expansion of CD8 T cells. Several other members of the TNF ligand family can be expressed on activated T cells and may also stimulate APC function by binding to their cognate receptors. Thus activation-induced expression of TNF ligand family members on naïve T cells can amplify the primary immune responses by priming the function of APCs. CD40 ligand–CD40 interactions are also essential for the generation of memory CD4 T cells of the Th1 type (capable of producing IFN-γ but not IL-4), memory B cells, and immunoglobulin isotype switching.[489,490]

NEONATAL T-CELL ACTIVATION, CO-STIMULATION, AND ANERGY

Neonatal CD4 T cells, which are virtually all antigenically naïve, and naïve CD4 T cells from adults have comparable IL-2 protein and mRNA expression and rates of IL-2 gene transcription if strong (and potentially nonphysiologic) activators of T cells are used, such as calcium ionophores or mitogenic lectins combined with phorbol esters.[75] These findings suggest that neonatal T cells have a normal capacity to produce IL-2 under optimal conditions of activation. Neonatal T cells also produce IL-2 and proliferate as well as do adult T cells in response to anti-CD3 mAb if optimal CD28 co-stimulation is provided,[491] indicating that CD28-mediated signaling is intact. However, decreased IL-2 production by neonatal T cells has been observed using more physiologic activation conditions. For example, compared with adult naïve CD4 T cells, neonatal naïve CD4 T cells produced less IL-2 mRNA and expressed fewer high-affinity IL-2 receptors in response to stimulation with anti-CD2 mAb.[492-494] These differences were abrogated when phorbol ester, which bypasses proximal signaling pathways and directly activates the Ras signaling pathway, was included,[492] suggesting that the capacity to express IL-2 and high-affinity receptors is not absolutely limited for neonatal cells, but signals leading to their induction may not be transmitted efficiently. Similarly, the production of IL-2 by neonatal naïve CD4 T cells was reduced compared with that by adult CD45RA^{hi} CD4 T cells after allogeneic stimulation with adult monocyte-derived DCs, a system that closely mimics physiologic T-cell activation by foreign peptide–self-MHC complexes.[495] Together, these observations argue that neonatal T cells may be intrinsically limited in their ability to produce IL-2 in response to physiologic activation.

The ability of activated T cells to efficiently divide in response to IL-2 depends on the expression of the high-affinity IL-2 receptor, which consists of CD25 (IL-2 receptor α chain), β chain (shared with the IL-15 receptor), and the γc cytokine receptor chain (shared with the specific receptors for IL-4, IL-7, IL-9, IL-15, and IL-21). In contrast with IL-2 production, neonatal T cells appear to express similar or higher amounts of CD25 after stimulation with anti-CD3 mAb. This finding is consistent with the signal transduction pathways leading to the induction of CD25 being in part distinct from those involved in IL-2 production, and with neonatal T cells having a relatively selective limitation in signals required for cytokine production rather than a generalized limitation at an early step of the activation cascade. Thus activated neonatal T cells proliferate in response to exogenous IL-2 as well as or better than adult T cells, as indicated by ^{3}H-thymidine incorporation.[496] Older studies[75] have found that neonatal T cells may also be less able to differentiate into effector cells in response to neoantigens, and this limitation is associated with diminished proliferation and the production of IL-2.

Superantigens activate T cells by binding to a portion of the TCR-β chain outside of the peptide antigen recognition site but otherwise mimic activation by peptide-MHC complexes in most respects. Neonatal T cells differ from adult naïve CD45RA^{hi} T cells in their tendency to become anergic rather than competent for increased cytokine secretion after priming with bacterial superantigen bound to MHC class II–transfected murine fibroblasts.[497] This anergic tendency is developmentally regulated because CD4$^+$CD8$^-$ thymocytes, the immediate precursors of antigenically naïve CD4 T cells, also are prone to anergy when treated under these conditions.[498] Consistent with this anergic tendency, newborns with toxic shock syndrome–like exanthematous disease, in which the Vβ2-bearing T-cell population is markedly expanded in vivo by the superantigen TSST-1, have a greater fraction of anergic Vβ2-bearing T cells than is found in adults with TSST-1–mediated toxic shock syndrome.[499]

Earlier studies[75] also found that neonatal, but not adult, CD4 T cells primed by alloantigen, in the form of Epstein-Barr virus (EBV)-transformed human B cells, become nonresponsive to restimulation by alloantigen or by a combination of anti-CD3 and anti-CD28 mAbs, possibly because of a lack of Rat sarcoma (Ras) signaling. A large body of murine studies suggest that T-cell signaling in which a calcium signal is not accompanied by robust activation of the transcription factor activator protein-1 (AP-1), which is downstream of Ras activation, results in anergy.[500] The induction of anergy results in the expression of E3 ubiquitin ligases, such Cbl-b, that help maintain the anergic state.[501] A recent study supports that idea that neonatal CD4 T cells may be prone to anergy because anti-CD3 mAb treatment of these cells resulted in high levels of calcium flux (significantly higher than adult naïve CD4 T cells), decreased induction of transcription mediated by AP-1, and increased induction of Cbl-b.[502] Of interest, this enhanced calcium signaling, which was due at least in part to increased expression of microRNA-181a, was also seen in PTK7$^+$ CD4 RTEs of adult peripheral blood.[502] Because enhanced calcium signaling resulting from increased microRNA-181a has also been observed in murine thymocyte development,[503] the anergic tendency of neonatal CD4 T cells may also apply to RTEs and may represent the retention of thymocyte-like phenotype. Together, these results suggest that neonatal and, presumably, fetal T cells have a greater tendency to become anergic, particularly under conditions in which production of inflammatory mediators or co-stimulation (e.g., by CD40, CD80, or CD86 on the APC) may be limited.

ICOS expression by circulating neonatal and adult CD4 T cells has been reported to be similar,[504] but it is unclear if neonatal CD4 T cells are as responsive to signals after ICOS ligand engagement as adult CD4 T cells, that is, for the differentiation into Th17 and TFH cells, which are discussed immediately below. There is also limited information on the expression of PD and PD ligand proteins on neonatal T cells.

DIFFERENTIATION OF ACTIVATED NAÏVE T CELLS INTO EFFECTOR AND MEMORY CELLS

Effector CD4 T-Cell Subsets Are Defined by Their Patterns of Cytokine Production

Fully activated naïve CD4 T cells differentiate into effector cells that have a CD45RA^{lo}CD45RO^{hi} surface phenotype as well as increased expression of adhesion molecules, such as CD11a.[505] The functions of effector T cells, particularly those of the CD4 subset, are mediated in large part by the multiple additional cytokines they produce that are not produced by naïve T cells. Most of these cytokines are secreted, although some (e.g., some members of the TNF ligand family) may be predominantly expressed on the T-cell surface. These cytokines include IL-3, IL-4, IL-5, IL-9, IL-10, IL-13, IL-17A, IL-17F, IL-21, IL-22, IFN-γ, GM-CSF, CD40 ligand, TNF-α, Fas ligand, OX40 ligand, and 41BB ligand.[506-508] Table 4-2 summarizes the major immunomodulatory effects of T-cell–derived cytokines and of cytokines produced by other cell types that act on T cells.

IFN-γ is the signature cytokine produced by Th1 effector cells, which also produce substantial amounts of IL-2, lymphotoxin-α, and TNF-α but little or no IL-4, IL-5, IL-13, IL-17, or IL-21. By contrast, IL-4 is the signature cytokine of Th2 cells, which also produce IL-5 and IL-13 but little or no IFN-γ, IL-2, IL-17, or IL-21. Human Th17 cells secrete IL-17A and IL-17F, two members of the IL-17 family. A minor subset of human Th17 cells expresses IL-22 and IFN-γ (also referred to as Th22 cells) and, in contrast to murine Th17 cells, most express TNF-α but not IL-6.[509] TFH cells are particularly efficient producers of IL-21, a cytokine that may also be involved in their generation from naïve CD4 T cells,[510] and may also express cytokines characteristic of either Th1, Th2, or Th17 cells. CD4 effector T cells producing effector cytokines of both Th1 and Th2 types are commonly referred to as Th0 cells, which often are seen after vaccination with protein antigens.[511] The generation of Th0 cells in vitro seems to be favored by the presence of large amounts of IL-2 in the absence of cytokines that polarize differentiation toward particular effector cell subsets. The majority of circulating adult memory CD4 T cells appear to be nonpolarized, that is, not belonging to the Th1, Th2, Th17, or TFH subsets based on their capacity for cytokine expression and their expression of chemokine receptors.[512] These nonpolarized memory cells can likely give rise to more polarized cell subsets after activation and proliferation in the context of appropriate instructional signals that are described later.

In addition to their differing cytokine profiles, these four Th effector subsets differ in their repertoire of chemokine receptors, which influence their localization and function in vivo. Human Th1 cells preferentially express CCR5 and CXCR3. In contrast, most Th2 cells express CCR4, but only a minority of Th1 cells do.[512] The expression of CCR5 by most Th1 cells and monocytes allows these two cell types to be concurrently recruited to sites of inflammation,[513] which may enhance the activation of mononuclear phagocytes by Th1-derived IFN-γ. The ligands for CCR4, CCL17, and CCL22 are commonly expressed by leukocytes at sites of allergic disease, which attracts Th2 cells that contribute to allergic pathogenesis. Most human Th17 cells express CCR6,[509] which helps target these cells to tissues, such as inflamed gastrointestinal epithelium, that produce high levels of CCL20, the sole ligand for CCR6.[514] TFH cells express high amounts of CXCR5, whose sole ligand is CXCL13, a chemokine produced by stromal cells of the B-cell follicle. This CXCR5–CXCL13 interaction helps retain TFH in the B-cell follicles, where they can provide help for antibody production.[515]

REGULATION OF CD4 EFFECTOR T-CELL SUBSET DIFFERENTIATION

The cytokine milieu[230] as well as the strength of TCR signaling (determined by antigen dose and the strength of peptide binding)[516] encountered by activated naïve CD4 T cells appear to be the major determinants affecting expression of key master transcriptional regulatory factors that direct Th subset differentiation.[517] Th1 effector development is favored by exposure to high levels of IL-12p70 and IL-18 produced by APCs and to IFN-γ produced by NK cells and other T cells (see Figs. 4-4 and 4-11), which support induction of the Th1 master regulatory transcription factor T-bet. In humans, but less so in mice, type I IFNs also promote Th1 differentiation, although they cannot replace IL-12p70 in this process.[518] The importance of IL-12 in the development of robust Th1 responses is demonstrated by the limited Th1 responses observed in patients with defects of IL-12 or IL-12 receptor signaling.[519,520] Th2 development is favored when CD4 T cells initially are activated in the relative absence of Th1 promoting cytokines and in the presence of TSLP, IL-4, IL-25, and IL-33 (an IL-1 family member); the latter are mainly derived from epithelial sources[521] (see Fig. 4-11), whereas the usual non–T-cell source of IL-4 may be basophils or innate lymphoid cells, depending on the particular immunologic context.[522,523] GATA-3 is the master regulator transcription factor for Th2 T-cell development.[524] Th17 cell development is favored by exposure to IL-1β, IL-6, and TGF-β, as well as IL-21, IL-23, and TNF-α,[525] and requires RORγt and RORα as master regulator transcription factors. TFH cell development in humans appears to be promoted by a variety of cytokines, including IL-6, IL-12, IL-21, and IL-23.[515,526,527] Based on murine studies, ICOS–ICOS ligand interactions between CD4 T cells and B cells in the lymphoid follicle are also likely important.[515] The master transcriptional regulation of TFH differentiation appears to be Bcl6.[528]

CD4 T-Cell Help for Antibody Production

CD4 T cells play a crucial role in the regulation of B-cell proliferation, immunoglobulin class switching, affinity maturation, and memory B-cell generation in response to proteins or protein conjugates. The enhancement of B-cell responses is commonly referred to as T-cell help. This process is critically dependent on the recognition through the αβ-TCR of cognate peptide-MHC complexes on B cells and on multiple contact-dependent interactions between members of the TNF ligand–TNF receptor families (see Table 4-1) and the CD28-B7 families (see Table 4-5). Recently activated CD4 T cells that express CXCR5 migrate to B-cell follicles and provide key help for antibody production as TFH cells that secrete IL-21 and express surface CD40 ligand[515] (see Fig. 4-11). CXCR5 is the receptor for CXCL13 (BCA-1), a chemokine produced by stromal cells of the B-cell follicle. The function of these TFH cells in providing B-cell help is discussed in more detail in the section CD4 T-Cell Help for Naive B-Cell Activation.

The importance of cognate T-cell help is clearly illustrated by the phenotype of patients with X-linked hyper–immunoglobulin M (hyper-IgM) syndrome, who have genetic defects in the expression of CD40 ligand.[490] In affected individuals, the marked paucity of immunoglobulin isotypes other than IgM and inability to generate memory B-cell responses indicate that these responses critically depend on the engagement of CD40 on B cells by CD40 ligand on T cells. Engagement of CD40 on B cells in conjunction with other signals provided by cytokines, such as IL-4 and IL-21, markedly enhances immunoglobulin production and class switching and B-cell survival.[529]

Activated and memory CD4 T cells also express ICOS, a receptor for the ICOS ligand, which is constitutively expressed on B cells and a variety of other cell types. ICOS co-stimulates the T-cell response and promotes the development of Th2 and TFH responses. ICOS ligand engagement on the B cell by ICOS also is important for enhancing B-cell differentiation and IgG production. The identification of ICOS deficiency as one cause of common variable immunodeficiency, in which there is profound hypogammaglobulinemia and poor antibody responses to vaccination[530] demonstrates the importance of ICOS–ICOS ligand interactions in humans.

Soluble cytokines produced by activated T cells influence the amount and type of immunoglobulin produced by B cells. Experiments in mice in which the IL-2, IL-4, IL-5, or IFN-γ gene or, in some cases, their specific receptors and associated STAT signaling molecules have been disrupted by gene targeting suggest that these cytokines are important for the proper regulation of B-cell immunoglobulin isotype expression. For example, inactivation of the IL-4 gene, components of the high-affinity IL-4 receptor, or the STAT6 protein involved in IL-4 receptor signal transduction results in a greater than 90% decrease in IgE production, whereas the production of other antibody isotypes is largely unperturbed.[531] IL-21 secretion by T cells may be important for immunoglobulin production by B cells not only because of direct effects on B-cell antibody secretion and differentiation into plasma cells but also because of IL-21 promoting TFH development in an autocrine or paracrine manner.[515]

Overview of Memory T Cells

Although greater than 90% of antigen-specific effector T cells generated during a robust primary immune response die, a fraction of effector cells persist as memory T cells. Memory T cells account for the enhanced secondary T-cell response to subsequent challenge: This reflects both the substantially greater frequency of antigen-specific memory T cells (approximately 1:100 to 1:10,000) than that of antigen-specific T cells in a naïve host (approximately 1:100,000 for most antigens) and the enhanced functions of memory compared with those of naïve T cells.[532] Memory T cells retain many of the functions of the effector T cells that characterized the immune response from which the memory T cells arose. These functions include a lowered threshold for activation and the ability to produce more rapidly the effector cytokines that characterized the effector T-cell subset from which they arose, that is, Th1, Th2, Th17, or TFH cells. Turnover of human memory T cells occurs slowly but more rapidly than that of naïve T cells.[532] Antigen-specific memory T-cell populations appear to persist (in humans most likely for decades) in the absence of further contact with foreign antigenic peptide–MHC complexes.[533]

Recent studies indicate that long-term human T-cell memory resides within a T-cell subset with stem cell–like properties of self-renewal.[534] Based on analysis of non–human primates,[535] these T stem cell–like memory (TSCM) cells, which are mainly localized in lymph nodes and not on mucosal surfaces, are the least differentiated memory subset (in terms of acquisition of memory-cell markers), and are likely precursors to central memory T cells. Humans genetically deficient in CD40 ligand have reduced CD4 T-cell recall responses to previously administered protein vaccines,[536,537] indicating that CD40–CD40 ligand–mediated signals are important for memory CD4 T-cell generation and/or maintenance.

Like effector cells, most human memory CD4 T cells can be distinguished from naïve cells by their surface expression of the CD45RO rather than the CD45RA isoform of CD45 (see Fig. 4-11).[532] In addition, memory and effector T cells typically express higher levels of adhesion molecules, such as the $\alpha_4\beta_1$ and CD11a/CD18 integrins, than levels observed on naïve T cells (see Table 4-5).[505,538] About 40% of circulating adult CD4 T cells have this CD45RA^{lo} CD45RO^{hi} ($\alpha_4\beta_1{}^{hi}$) memory/effector surface phenotype, and a fraction of these cells are L-selectin^{hi}, belonging to the central memory cell subset,[539] which is discussed later. In persistent viral infection, a subset of memory CD4 T cells express PD-1, and this expression is associated with impaired T-cell function in cases of HIV-1 infection.

Activation and propagation of CD45RA^{hi}CD45RO^{lo} CD4 T cells in vitro results in their acquisition of memory/effector cell–like features, including a lower threshold for activation, a CD45RA^{lo}CD45RO^{hi} phenotype in most cases, an enhanced ability to produce effector cytokines, (e.g., IFN-γ, IL-4, IL-17, and IL-21), and an increased ability to provide help for B-cell antibody production. These findings support the notion that CD45RA^{hi} T cells are precursors of CD45RO^{hi} T cells and that this differentiation occurs after T-cell activation; these findings also are consistent with the observation that the CD45RA^{lo}CD45RO^{hi} cell subset consists mainly of memory T cells that respond to recall antigens.[532]

Memory CD8 T cells are similar to those of the CD4 subset in expressing a CD45RA^{lo}CD45RO^{hi} surface phenotype and, by comparison to their naïve precursors, in possessing an enhanced capacity to produce multiple cytokines as well as molecules involved in cell-mediated cytotoxicity, such as perforins and granzymes.[540] In addition, unlike memory CD4 T cells, a substantial subset of these CD45RO^{hi} CD8 T cells express CD11b, CD57, killer inhibitory receptors (KIRs), and NKG2D.[541,542] As described earlier for NK cells, binding of KIRs on memory CD8 T cells to self-HLA-A, HLA-B, or HLA-C molecules might be expected to raise the threshold for activation of KIR$^+$ CD8 T cells by antigenic peptide–MHC complexes; however, human KIR$^+$ CD8 T cells appear to be functionally equivalent to the KIR$^-$ subset.[543] NKG2D expression on the other hand may serve as a means to enhance CD8 T-cell effector function.[542]

Human effector CD8 T cells also can be distinguished from circulating naïve CD8 T cells by surface phenotype: Most human CD8 effector cells have a CD45RA^{hi}CD27$^-$CD28$^-$ surface phenotype and a high capacity to directly mediate cytotoxicity (high levels of intracellular perforin and granzyme staining) and to produce Th1-type effector cytokines, including TNF-α and IFN-γ.[505,540] By contrast, naïve CD8 T cells have a CD45RA^{hi}CD27$^+$CD28$^+$ surface phenotype and a limited ability to mediate cytotoxicity and to secrete these cytokines.

The tissue localization of memory T cells is determined by differential expression of adhesion molecules and chemokine receptors. Distinct central (lymphoid homing) and effector (non–lymphoid tissue homing) memory T-cell populations in humans have been identified.[544] Recent studies suggest that TSCMs of the lymph nodes give rise in situ to central memory T cells.[535] Central memory T cells express CCR7 receptor and high levels of L-selectin, whereas most effector memory T cells lack CCR7 and express low levels of L-selectin. Most effector memory T cells express adhesion molecules other than L-selectin that help target them to specific tissues. Central memory CD4 T cells typically demonstrate reduced antigen-specific expression of certain cytokines, such as IFN-γ, compared with the effector memory subset, whereas IL-2 production is similar or higher by the central memory subset compared with effector memory CD4 T cells.[545,546]

The central memory pool may be a larger fraction of the memory pool for CD4 than for CD8 T cells. Human central memory CD4 T cells also have a lower turnover[547] and are more responsive to maintenance signals provided by cytokines, such as IL-2 and IL-7, compared with effector memory CD4 T cells.[548] Although the precursor-product relationship between central and effector memory T cells is as yet uncertain, there is strong evidence that central memory CD4 T cells are the precursors of effector memory cells at least in primates. For example, in chronic simian immunodeficiency virus infection, a progressive decline in central memory CD4 T cells ultimately results in effector memory CD4 T-cell insufficiency and increased viral-induced disease.[549]

Turnover of memory CD4 and CD8 T cells appears to be much more frequent than that of their naïve counterparts, suggesting that the process is a dynamic one.[532] Unlike with naïve T cells, the maintenance of memory T cells appears not to require continued contact with self-peptide–MHC complexes but does require IL-7 and IL-15.[533] Most CD4 T-cell memory cells require both cytokines for survival, whereas most memory CD8 T cells require IL-15 but not IL-7 for survival.[533]

Memory T-Cell Activation

When memory T cells reencounter antigenic peptide–MHC complexes ("recall antigen") as part of the secondary response, they are activated and undergo expansion and differentiation into a secondary effector population. The secondary immune response to recall antigen is typically more rapid and robust than the primary response to an antigen that has never been encountered previously. This difference is due both to the greater frequency of antigen-specific memory T cells than of naïve T cells with TCRs that recognize the same antigens and to the enhanced function of these memory T cells and their secondary effector progeny. Compared with naïve T cells, memory T cells in general have a lower activation threshold, are less dependent on these co-stimulatory signals, and can commit to proliferate after engagement of their αβ-TCR more quickly than naïve T cells. This increased responsiveness of memory T cells is the result of reprogramming of gene expression by epigenetic changes, such as DNA methylation, histone modifications, and chromatin remodeling of genes involved in effector functions, such as the IFN-γ genetic locus, as well as alterations in transcription factors.[517,550,551] There are also differences between memory T cells and naïve T cells in certain features of proximal and distal signal transduction pathways after αβ-TCR engagement, which likely enhance signal strength in memory cells.[552] The quality of the effector immune response may also be enhanced at the individual T-cell level. For example, individual secondary effectors generated from memory CD8 T cells may express both perforin and effector cytokines, whereas primary effectors generated from naïve CD8 T cells may express either perforin or cytokines, but not both.[553]

Postnatal Ontogeny of Memory CD4 T-Cell Subsets

The memory CD4 T-cell subset in infants and young children has a significantly higher ratio of central memory to effector memory CD4 T cells than in adults.[545] The frequency of effector memory CD4 T cells that can produce IFN-γ and the amount of IFN-γ produced per cell in response to bacterial superantigen, however, are similar in the blood of infants and young children and adults.[545] This finding indicates that effector memory cells generated during infancy are functionally similar to those of adults. It is likely that the greater proportion of central memory cells also applies to memory CD4 T-cell responses that occur in the first few months of life, but this remains to be shown. The mechanism responsible for the greater fraction of central memory cells in infants and children is unclear. One possibility is that the decreased proportion of effector memory CD4 T cells may reflect reduced activity of IL-12–dependent Th1 pathways because effector memory CD4 T cells are markedly reduced in IL-12Rβ1 deficiency, which ablates IL-12p70.[519]

PRODUCTION OF CYTOKINES, CHEMOKINES, AND TUMOR NECROSIS FACTOR–LIGAND PROTEINS BY NEONATAL T CELLS

CD4 T-Cell Cytokine Production

In contrast with IL-2, the production of most other cytokines or their cognate mRNAs by unfractionated neonatal T cells or the CD4 T-cell subset appears to be reduced after short-term stimulation, including with anti-CD3 mAb, mitogen, or pharmacologic agents (e.g., the combination of calcium ionophore and phorbol ester) compared with that in adult T cells.[75] For most cytokines (IL-3, IL-4, IL-5, IL-6, IL-10, IL-13, IFN-γ, and GM-CSF), this is a marked reduction; for a few, such as TNF-α, the reduction is modest. As with neonatal T cells, naïve T cells from adults have a reduced capacity to produce most of these cytokines compared with that of adult memory/effector T cells, although adult naïve T cells may produce substantial amounts of IL-13.[554] The low capacity of neonatal T cells to produce IFN-γ and IL-4 is due to an almost complete absence of IFN-γ and IL-4 mRNA–expressing cells,[555] which is paralleled by a lack of cells expressing detectable levels of these cytokines after polyclonal activation and analysis by flow cytometry after intracellular staining.[354,556,557] Together, these results suggest that much of the apparent deficiency in cytokine production by neonatal T cells is accounted for in part by the fact that almost all neonatal T cells are naïve and the lack of antigenic experience.

As discussed in the section "Dendritic Cells: The Link Between Innate and Adaptive Immunity," the limited capacity of neonatal cDCs to produce IL-12p70 in response to TLR stimulation suggests that this is likely an important contributor to limitations in the development of Th1 responses in the neonate and infant. However, when purified neonatal or adult naïve CD4 T cells are stimulated in parallel by using a potent allogeneic stimulus in the form of a pool of moDCs from multiple unrelated donors, there is markedly lower IFN-γ production by neonatal T cells.[495] This finding strongly suggests that the capacity of neonatal naïve CD4 T cells to produce IFN-γ is due, at least in part, to a cell-autonomous mechanism.

IL-10 production by anti-CD3 mAb and IL-2–stimulated neonatal CD4 T cells, although reduced after short-term stimulation, may be substantially higher than by adult naïve CD4 T cells after more prolonged incubation.[558] Whether these IL-10–producing neonatal CD4 T cells are derived from non-Treg versus natural Treg cell populations is uncertain, but regardless, increased production of IL-10 by T cells in vivo would be expected to inhibit both antigen-presenting cell and effector T-cell function.[559]

CD8 T-Cell Cytokine and Chemokine Production

Cytokine production by neonatal CD8 T cells has not been as well characterized as for the CD4 T-cell subset. The lack of a memory (CD45RO^{hi}) CD8 T-cell subset in the neonate appears to account for reduced production of the chemokine CCL-5 (RANTES) by neonatal T cells compared with that by adult cells.[560] A striking result, which needs to be confirmed, is that neonatal naïve CD8 T cells produce substantially more IL-13, which is characteristic of Th2 immune responses, than that produced by analogous adult cells after stimulation with anti-CD3 and anti-CD28 mAbs and exogenous IL-2.[561] It will be of interest to determine if this unusual cytokine profile also applies to antigen-specific immune responses, for instance, to viral pathogens, by neonatal CD8 T cells.

Postnatal Ontogeny of Cytokine Production

Neonatal T cells have been intensively studied for their cytokine secretion phenotype, but relatively little is known regarding the postnatal ontogeny of T-cell cytokine production during the first year of life. A study using phytohemagglutinin as a stimulus found that the capacity of peripheral blood lymphocytes obtained from newborns was similar to cord blood in having a low capacity to produce IFN-γ, IL-4, and IL-10.[562] The capacity of peripheral blood lymphocytes to produce all three of these cytokines gradually increased during the first year of life,[562] consistent with the acquisition of increased cytokine production because of the progressive acquisition of memory T cells resulting from exposure to foreign antigens. A more recent longitudinal study using fluorescent barcoding to allow pooling of multiple stimulation conditions for flow cytometric analysis found that tetanus toxoid–specific and PPD-specific CD4 T cells (as assessed by simultaneous expression of IFN-γ and CD69) significantly increased between 6 months and 12 months of age.[563]

CD40 Ligand

Durandy and colleagues[564] reported that a substantial proportion of circulating fetal T cells present between 19 and 31 weeks of gestation expressed CD40 ligand in vitro in response to polyclonal activation. Whether fetal T cells that can express CD40 ligand have a distinct surface phenotype from those lacking this capacity is unclear. By contrast, T cells from later-gestational-age fetuses and from neonates have a much more limited capacity to produce CD40 ligand after activation with calcium ionophore and phorbol ester.[75]

Expression of CD40 ligand by activated neonatal CD4 T cells remains reduced for at least 10 days postnatally but is almost equal to adult cells by 3 to 4 weeks after birth[564] (D.B. Lewis, unpublished data, 2010). In most of these studies, activated neonatal CD4 T cells derived from cord blood expressed markedly lower amounts of CD40 ligand surface protein and mRNA than did either adult CD45RA^{hi} or CD45RO^{hi} CD4 T cells. Thus decreased CD40 ligand expression may not be due to the lack of a memory/effector population in the neonatal T-cell compartment but may represent a true developmental limitation in cytokine production.

Decreased CD40 ligand production by neonatal T cells also has been documented in the mouse,[565] suggesting that it may be a feature of RTEs. Consistent with this idea, human CD4$^+$CD8$^-$ thymocytes, the immediate precursors of RTEs, also have a low capacity to express CD40 ligand.[566,567] However, adult PTK7$^+$ CD4 RTEs have similar levels of CD40 ligand expression as PTK7$^-$ naïve CD4 T cells,[406] indicating that the capacity for activation-induced CD40 ligand expression is upregulated before thymic emigration or shortly thereafter, at least in adults. As with most T-cell–derived cytokines characteristic of effector cells, when neonatal T cells are strongly activated in vitro into an effector-like T-cell population, they acquire a markedly increased capacity to produce CD40 ligand on restimulation, demonstrating that this reduction is not a fixed phenotypic feature.[564,566]

In view of the importance of CD40 ligand in multiple aspects of the immune response,[490] limitations in CD40 ligand production could contribute to decreased antigen-specific immunity mediated by Th1 effector cells and B cells in the neonate. However, the initial studies showing a relative deficiency of CD40 ligand expression by neonatal T cells were done by stimulating blood mononuclear cells with calcium ionophore and phorbol ester, a combination that maximizes the production of CD40 ligand but that may not accurately mimic physiologic T-cell activation. However, similarly reduced CD40 ligand surface expression by purified unfractionated or CD4 naïve neonatal T cells also has been observed after stimulation with stimuli that engage the αβ-TCR–CD3 complex either alone or in combination with anti-CD28 mAb,[568,569] suggesting that this reduction is likely to be applicable to physiologic T-cell activation. Others, however, have found equivalent levels of CD40 ligand expression by neonatal and adult T cells using anti-CD3 mAb stimulation,[570,571] suggesting that the particular in vitro conditions used (e.g., the particular anti-CD3 mAb and cell culture conditions) may influence the outcome of the assay.

The ability of neonatal and adult T cells to produce CD40 ligand in response to allogeneic stimulation, a condition that should closely mimic T-cell activation through the recognition of foreign peptide–MHC complexes, has also been evaluated. One study found that CD40 ligand expression by neonatal T cells was similar to that by adult T cells after 5 days of allogeneic stimulation with irradiated adult monocyte-derived DCs.[572] By contrast, another study[495] found that CD40 ligand expression by purified neonatal naïve CD4 T cells was substantially less than in adult naïve CD4 T cells after 24 to 48 hours of stimulation. This reduced CD40 ligand production was accompanied by reduced IL-12p70 production (by moDCs) and IL-2 and IFN-γ production (by naïve CD4 T cells). Together, these studies suggest that CD40 ligand surface expression initially may be more limited for neonatal naïve CD4 T cells, but that with longer term stimulation, at least in vitro, this limitation can be overcome.

Other Tumor Necrosis Factor Family Ligands

Fas ligand, another member of the TNF ligand family, plays a key role in inducing apoptotic cell death on target cells that express Fas on the surface. Human Fas or Fas ligand deficiency is associated with antibody-mediated autoimmunity and lymphoid hyperplasia but not with defects in viral clearance.[573] Neonatal T cells have decreased Fas ligand expression after anti-CD3 and anti-CD28 mAb stimulation compared with that in adult cells.[569] Neonatal and adult CD4 T cells express similar surface levels of Fas.[504] Iwama and colleagues[574] reported that circulating levels of Fas ligand are elevated in newborns, but the cellular source of this protein and its functional significance are unclear. The role of Fas–Fas ligand interactions in regulating apoptosis of neonatal T cells is discussed in the section Regulation of T-cell Expansion by Apoptosis.

Mechanisms for Decreased Cytokine, Chemokine, and TNF Ligand Production by Neonatal T Cells

For many cytokine and TNF ligand genes, a key event leading to de novo gene transcription is an activation-induced increase in the concentration of free intracellular calcium ($[Ca^{2+}]_i$), which is required for NFAT nuclear location and transcriptional activity.[575] Certain studies comparing adult and neonatal unfractionated or CD4 T cells have suggested that neonatal T cells have substantial limitations in proximal signal transduction events that are required for the cytokine and TNF ligand expression. These limitations include a generalized decrease in the overall level of activation-induced tyrosine phosphorylation of intracellular proteins compared with that in unfractionated adult T cells,[576] decreased activation-induced phosphorylation of CD3-ε, decreased phosphorylation and enzyme activity of the Lck and ZAP-70 tyrosine kinases and the ERK2, JNK, and p38 kinases,[569] reduced basal expression of protein kinase C β1, ε, θ, and ζ,[577] and reduced basal and activation-induced levels of phospholipase C isoenzymes.[578]

It remains unclear if these reported deficiencies in proximal signal transduction events described above apply specifically to neonatal naïve T cells but not to adult naïve T cells because these studies used unfractionated adult T cells. In a recent study in which such a direct comparison was made, neonatal naïve CD4 T cells actually had higher $[Ca^{2+}]_i$ flux after anti-CD3 mAb stimulation than adult naïve CD4 T cells, but the induction of AP-1–dependent transcription was reduced, resulting in an anergy-like phenotype with increased expression of Cbl-b expression in the neonatal cells.[502] Another study[579] found that activation by anti-CD3 plus anti-CD26 mAb was markedly less effective for inducing proximal signaling events, such as phosphorylation of Lck, and proliferation for neonatal T cells compared with adult naïve T cells. This poor activation by anti-CD26 mAb was associated with CD26 being located outside lipid raft microdomains in neonatal T cells, whereas in activated adult naïve T cells CD26 was a lipid raft component. Although the importance of CD26 in physiologic T-cell activation remains uncertain, these observations are of interest because they suggest that further analysis of the composition of the lipid raft microdomains of neonatal versus adult naïve T cells may provide additional insights into limitations of neonatal T-cell activation.

Reduced IL-4 and IFN-γ mRNA expression by polyclonally activated neonatal CD4 and CD8 T cells, compared with that observed in adult T cells after stimulation through an αβ-TCR–CD3 complex or pharmacologic activation with calcium ionophore and phorbol ester, is due primarily to reduced transcription of these cytokine genes.[75] IFN-γ and IL-4 are expressed mainly by memory/effector T-cell populations, rather than by the naïve T-cell populations. Thus the reduced expression of these cytokines by neonatal T cells can be accounted for by the lack of memory/effector cells in the circulating neonatal T-cell population. For many genes, including the IFN-γ gene, DNA methylation of the locus represses transcription by decreasing the ability of transcriptional activator proteins to bind to regulatory elements, such as promoters and enhancers. Thus it is of interest that reduced expression of IFN-γ by neonatal T cells may also result in part from greater methylation of DNA in the IFN-γ gene locus in neonatal naïve CD4 T cells than adult naïve T cells.[580] With a detailed understanding of epigenetic alterations of the IFN-γ gene locus during T-cell development and by naïve versus memory T cells now available,[550,551] a higher resolution comparison of naïve T cells from neonates and adults for these epigenetic modifications may provide new insights as to mechanisms for decreased IFN-γ expression by neonatal T cells.

In addition to decreased cytokine gene transcription, decreased cytokine mRNA stability also may contribute to reduced cytokine production by neonatal T cells. For example, decreased IL-3 production by neonatal T cells appears to be due mainly to reduced IL-3 mRNA stability, rather than to decreased gene transcription.[581] The mechanism for this reduced mRNA stability remains unclear. Decreased mRNA stability also has been observed for other cytokines after stimulation of cord blood mononuclear cells,[247] but whether this also holds for purified neonatal T cells has not been addressed.

Cytokine Production by Neonatal T Cells after Short-Term In Vitro Differentiation

The generation of effector T cells from naïve precursors in response to antigen in vivo can be mimicked by in vitro stimulation, such as by engagement of the αβ-TCR–CD3 complex in conjunction with accessory cells (non–T cells contained in BMCs) and exogenous cytokines. Neonatal T cells, if polyclonally activated under conditions that favor repeated cell division (strong activation stimuli in common with the provision of exogenous IL-2), resemble antigenically naïve adult T cells in efficiently acquiring the characteristics of effector cells. These characteristics include a $CD45RA^{lo}CD45RO^{hi}$ surface phenotype, an enhanced ability to be activated by anti-CD2 or anti-CD3 mAb, and an increased capacity to produce cytokines (e.g., IL-4, IFN-γ).[75]

Although neonatal CD4 T cells can be effectively primed for expression of effector cytokines by strong mitogenic stimuli and provision of cytokines, such as IL-2, as already noted, their capacity to differentiate into Th1 effector cells under more physiologic conditions may be more limited: Neonatal naïve CD4 T cells stimulated with allogeneic DCs were found to have decreased frequency of $IFN\text{-}\gamma^+$ cells, based on intracellular cytokine staining, compared with that observed in adult naïve CD4 T cells in response to short-term (i.e., 24 to 48 hours of duration) stimulation by allogeneic DCs.[495]

This decreased expression of IFN-γ by neonatal CD4 T cells activated under these more physiologic conditions of DC-mediated allogeneic stimulation probably is due to several factors. First, neonatal CD4 T cells are less effective than adult naïve cells at inducing the co-cultured DCs to produce

IL-12p70,[495] a key cytokine for promoting Th1 differentiation and IFN-γ production.[520] This reduced IL-12 production is attributable, at least in part, to reduced expression of CD40 ligand by neonatal CD4 T cells in response to allogeneic stimulation using DCs[495] because engagement of CD40 on DCs by CD40 ligand is an important mechanism for inducing IL-12 production.[582] Second, CD40 ligand is also important for the activation and differentiation of antigen-specific CD4 T cells, including those with Th1 immune function.[536,537] Third, neonatal CD4 T cells may have decreased expression of certain transcription factors, such as the NFATc2 protein,[583,584] although this finding is controversial[585]; such a reduction could limit the induction of IFN-γ gene transcription as well as IL-2 and CD40 ligand expression in response to T-cell activation.[586] Fourth, as already noted, the greater methylation of DNA of the IFN-γ genetic locus in neonatal T cells than in adult naïve T cells may also contribute to a reduced and delayed acquisition of IFN-γ production after activation in vitro.[580] Together, these mechanisms intrinsic to the T cell, as well as immaturity of cDC function (see earlier), may account for the delayed acquisition of IFN-γ production by antigen-specific CD4 T cells after infection in the neonatal period (see "Antigen-Specific T-Cell Function in the Fetus and Neonate").

In contrast to impaired Th1 generation by neonatal CD4 T cells, it has been argued that there is skewing toward Th2 development in the human fetus and neonate, similar to what has been observed in neonatal mice.[587] There is also considerable interest in using the production of Th2 cytokines by cord blood mononuclear cells or T cells as a predictor of the later development of atopic disease. Although some early studies suggested that, under certain in vitro conditions, neonatal T cells might proliferate more in response to IL-4 and have a greater tendency to become Th2 effectors than adult T cells,[75] it should be noted that a skewing for increased production of IL-4 by neonatal CD4 T cells was not observed after stimulation with allogeneic DCs.[495] However, a recent study did find markedly higher levels of IL-4 production by cord blood CD4 T cells from premature infants, but not term infants, after priming in "neutral" conditions, that is, anti-CD3 and anti-CD28 mAb and IL-2,[245] raising the possibility of Th2 skewing in the fetus.

Cytokine Production After Long-Term In Vitro Generation of Effector CD4 T Cells

Activated neonatal CD4 T cells can be differentiated in vitro into either Th1- or Th2-like effector cells by incubation for several days to weeks with IL-12 and anti–IL-4 antibody or with IL-4 and anti-IL-12 antibody, respectively.[75] Consistent with this ability to differentiate into Th1 cells, activated neonatal and adult naïve CD4 T cells upregulate expression of the IL-12Rβ1 and IL-12Rβ2 chains similarly.[588,589] In many cases, IL-2 is added after the initial activation phase to promote survival and expansion of the effector cells. Treatment of neonatal T cells with IL-4 and anti–IL-12 upregulates GATA-3, the master regulator transcription factor promoting Th2 effector generation.[230] Treatment of neonatal CD4 T cells with the combination of IL-12 is effective at inducing T-bet, the master regulator transcription factor promoting Th1 effector generation.[230] Mature single-positive ($CD4^+CD8^-$ or $CD4^-CD8^+$) fetal thymocytes obtained as early as 16 weeks of gestation can be also differentiated into either Th1 or Th2 effector cells by such cytokine treatment,[590] indicating that the capacity to acquire a polarized cytokine profile is established relatively early in fetal life. However, this ability to acquire high levels of cytokine production may not necessarily apply to more physiologic conditions of stimulation.

Higher levels of IL-17, indicative of Th17 generation, are produced by purified naïve CD4 T cells from cord blood, compared with adult peripheral blood, after anti-CD3 and anti-CD28 mAb stimulation and an optimal Th17 cytokine cocktail (IL-1, IL-6, IL-23, and low doses of TGF-β).[245] Of interest, even higher levels of IL-17 are obtained from premature infant naïve CD4 T cells under these conditions. This suggests that the capacity for Th17 immunity may be greater than in adults. In support of a cell-autonomous mechanism for this enhanced Th17 generation, neonatal naïve CD4 T cells express substantially higher levels of transcripts for proteins that promote Th17 differentiation, including IL-23R, RORγt, STAT3, and TGF-β receptor, than do adult naïve CD4 T cells.[245] This greater capacity for IL-17 production by neonatal naïve CD4 T has been attributed to a small $CD161^+$ subset that is absent from the circulating adult naïve CD4 T-cell compartment. Despite its expression of CD161 (also known as NK1.1 in mice), which is broadly expressed on NK and NKT cells, this $CD161^+$ T-cell population is distinct from NKT cells, based on its diverse αβ-TCR repertoire and in being MHC class II rather than CD1d restricted.[591] One possibility to explain these age-related differences is that the $CD161^+$ population may preferentially home after birth to sites known to be rich for the generation of Th17 cells, such as gastrointestinal mucosa, and does not subsequently recirculate.

To the best of our knowledge, neonatal and adult naïve CD4 T cells have not been directly compared for their ability to differentiate in vitro into TFH-like cells. Cord blood naïve CD4 T cells incubated with anti-CD3 and anti-CD28 mAbs and cytokines that activate via STAT3 (IL-6, IL-21, or IL-27) acquire certain TFH-like features, such as ICOS and IL-21 expression and increased help for B-cell antibody production.[527] It is unclear whether these or other conditions, for instance, IL-12p70, also increase expression of Bcl-6 and surface proteins characteristic of human TFH cells, such as CXCR5 and PD-1.[515]

T CELL–MEDIATED CYTOTOXICITY

T cell–mediated cytotoxicity involves two major pathways: through the secretion of the perforin and granzyme cytotoxins or through the engagement of Fas by Fas ligand (Fig. 4-12). The growing use of cord blood for hematopoietic cell transplantation and the finding that its use is associated with reduced graft-versus-host disease compared with that seen with adult bone marrow have led to great interest in the capacity of neonatal T cells to mediate cytotoxicity and to potentiate graft rejection.

Early studies[75] mostly used unfractionated mononuclear cells as a source of killer cells in a variety of non–antigen-specific assays. Reduced cytotoxicity was observed with lectin-activated cord blood lymphocytes, particularly if purified T cells were used. Most studies also found that neonatal T cells were moderately less effective than adult T cells as cytotoxic effector cells after priming by allogeneic

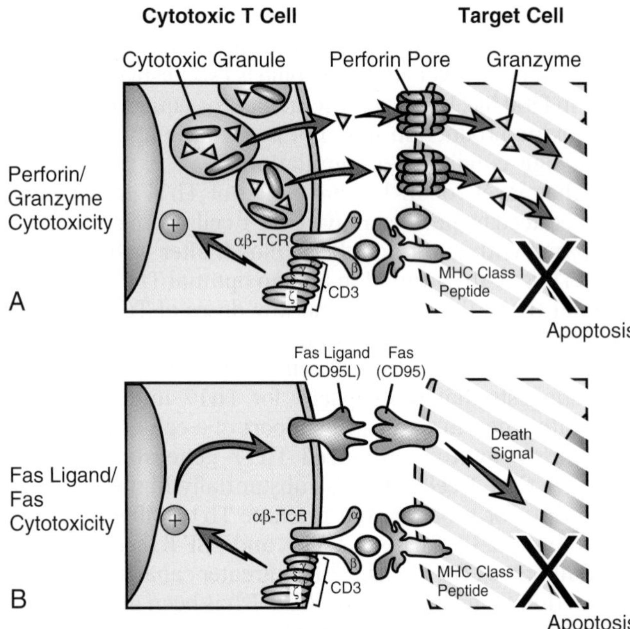

Figure 4-12 Two major mechanisms of antigen-specific major histocompatibility complex (MHC) class I–restricted T-cell–mediated cytotoxicity. Engagement of the αβ T-cell receptor (αβ-TCR) of CD8 T cells by antigenic peptides bound to MHC class I molecules on the target cell leads to T-cell activation and target cell death. **A,** Cytotoxicity may occur by the extracellular release of the contents of cytotoxic granules from the T cell, including perforins, granzymes, and other cytotoxins, such as granulysin. Perforins introduce pores by which granzymes can enter into the target cell, leading to the triggering of apoptosis and cell death. **B,** Activation of T cells results in their surface expression of Fas ligand, which engages Fas on the target cell, resulting in the delivery of a death signal culminating in apoptosis. Other related molecules, such as TRAIL (TNF-related apoptosis-inducing ligand), may also play a role in cytotoxicity (not shown).

stimulation. As with the acquisition of Th1 effector function by neonatal CD4 T cells, more substantial defects in T cell–mediated cytotoxicity by neonatal T cells after allogeneic priming were observed when no exogenous cytokines, such as IL-2, were added, suggesting that this decreased cytolytic activity might be physiologically significant in vivo. The mechanism for reduced neonatal T-cell–mediated cytotoxicity remains poorly understood.

The capacity of fetal T cells to mediate cytotoxicity has until recently not received as much scrutiny, despite its relevance to the development of fetal therapy using HSCs. CD8 T cells bearing αβ-TCRs can be cloned as polyclonal lines from human fetal liver by 16 weeks of gestation.[592,593] These CD8 T-cell lines have proliferative activity in response to allogeneic stimulation, but their reactivity toward HLA antigens and their cytolytic activity are not known. More compelling are studies documenting robust fetal effector CD8 T-cell responses, including clonal expansion and perforin expression, in response to congenital CMV infection[594]; however, other studies have observed limitations in IFN-γ secretion as well as recognition of specific viral antigens[595,596] (see "T-Cell Response to Congenital Infection"). Nevertheless, these findings demonstrate that the capacity to generate a functional CD8 T-cell effector population in vivo is established in utero, at least under conditions of chronic stimulation.

EFFECTOR T-CELL MIGRATION

As already noted, the differential expression of chemokine receptors by T cells is important in their selective trafficking either to sites where naïve T cells may potentially encounter antigen for the first time, such as the spleen and lymph nodes, or to inflamed tissues for effector functions.[189] CCR7 expression by naïve T cells allows these cells to recirculate between the blood and uninflamed lymphoid organs, which constitutively express the two major ligands for CCR7: CCL19 and CCL21. Naïve T cells in the adult express CCR1, CCR7, and CXCR4 on their surface and have low to undetectable levels of CCR5. The role served by CCR1 and CXCR4 expression on naïve T cells is unclear, and CCR1 may be nonfunctional in this cell type.[597] Neonatal naïve T cells have a phenotype similar to those of adult naïve cells, except that they lack CCR1 surface expression, and unlike adult naïve T cells, they do not increase CXCR3 expression, nor do they decrease CCR7 expression, after activation by means of anti-CD3 and anti-CD28 mAbs.[447,598] The CCR7 expressed on neonatal T cells is functional and mediates chemotaxis of these cells in response to CCL19 and CCL21.[599] These results suggest that activated neonatal T cells may be limited in their capacity to traffic to nonlymphoid tissue sites of inflammation and, instead, may continue to recirculate between the blood and peripheral lymphoid organs.

CCR5 recognizes a number of chemokines that are produced at high levels by leukocytes at sites of inflammation, including CCL2 (MIP-1α), CCL4 (MIP-1β), and CCL5 (RANTES), and is an important chemokine receptor for the entry of T cells into inflamed or infected tissues. Neonatal T cells can increase their surface expression of CCR5 in response to stimulation by mitogen or IL-2.[600] The observation that CCR5 is expressed by fetal mesenteric lymph node T cells during the second trimester of pregnancy[397] suggests that CCR5 can be upregulated in vivo by a mechanism that does not involve foreign antigenic stimulation. CCR5 expression on CD4 T cells gradually increases after birth, in parallel with the appearance of memory cells, suggesting that this process occurs in vivo as part of memory cell generation.[601]

Neonatal naïve CD4 T cells also have the capacity after long-term in vitro differentiation in the presence of polarizing cytokines (IL-12 and anti-IL-4 for Th1, and IL-4 and anti-IL-12 for Th2) to acquire the ability to produce chemokines characteristic of Th1 or Th2 effectors The Th1 effectors generated in vitro from either neonatal or adult naïve CD4 T-cell precursors tend to express CXCR3, CCR5, and CX3CR1, whereas Th2 effectors tend to express CCR4 and, to a lesser extent, CCR3.[602-604] Studies of freshly isolated memory CD4 T cells suggest that expression of CXCR3 and CCR4 may be more accurate predictors of cells with Th1 and Th2 cytokine profiles, respectively.[512,605] In many cases, a combination of chemokine receptors, for example, CXCR3 and CCR5 for the Th1 cytokine producers, may be the most predictive of highly polarized patterns of cytokine production by memory T cells.[512]

TERMINATION OF THE T-CELL EFFECTOR RESPONSE

To prevent excessive immune responses, mechanisms for terminating the T-cell response operate on multiple levels.

CD45 is a protein tyrosine phosphatase that promotes T-cell activation by counteracting the phosphorylation of tyrosine residues that inhibit the function of tyrosine kinases involved in T-cell activation, such as Lck. Because dimerization of CD45 impedes its phosphatase activity, it is possible that the preferential expression of the low-molecular-weight CD45RO isoform on effector CD4 T cells may facilitate CD45 dimerization and thereby attenuate the immune response.[606] T-cell activation is also limited by the engagement of cytotoxic T-lymphocyte antigen-4 (CTLA-4) (i.e., CD152) on the T cell by CD80 and CD86 on the APC. CTLA-4 is expressed mainly on the T-cell surface during the later stages of activation. How CTLA-4 acts to terminate T-cell activation is controversial. The engagement of the B7 family member PD-1 on activated T cells by its B7 family ligands PDL1 (B7-H1) and PDL2, expressed on APCs (see Table 4-5) and in certain tissues, also dampens the effector T-cell response, particularly within parenchymal tissues. As mentioned previously, increased PD-1 expression on memory CD4 T cells, as in HIV infection or certain cancers, is associated with "exhaustion" and poor effector function. The importance of CTLA-4 and PD-1 in limiting endogenous T-cell responses in cancer has been dramatically demonstrated by the ability of neutralizing antibody to CTLA-4 or to PD-1/PD-1 ligand to enhance T-cell responses to tumors in cancer patients and decrease tumor burden.[607]

Regulation of T-Cell Expansion by Apoptosis

The elimination of effector T cells by apoptosis is important for lymphocyte homeostasis, with a failure of this process resulting in autoimmunity and severe immunopathology, such as hemophagocytosis.[608] Activated T cells express surface Fas molecules[609] and downregulate expression of the intracellular Bcl-2 and Bcl-xL proteins that protect against apoptosis.[610] Effector T cells may also have increased expression of other Bcl-2 family members that either antagonize Bcl-2 and Bcl-xL, such as Bad and Bim, or that directly promote apoptosis downstream, such as Bax and Bcl-xS.[608] The balance between the activity of prosurvival and proapoptotic Bcl-2 family members determines whether the integrity of mitochondria is maintained, which when lost causes the release of proteins that trigger apoptosis, such as cytochrome c. This net apoptotic tendency is countered by signals through the IL-2 receptor complex, which maintains/increases expression of Bcl-X_L, making effector T cells highly dependent on IL-2 (or other cytokines that signal through the γc cytokine receptor) for their survival.[608]

Apoptosis can be studied using effector T cells that are generated in vitro from naïve precursors either by acutely withdrawing exogenous cytokines, such as IL-2, used in effector generation, and/or by reactivating the effector cells (e.g., using anti-CD3 mAb). This Bcl-2–regulated pathway of apoptosis can also be induced by cytotoxic drugs, such as glucocorticoids. In addition, activated T cells upregulate their expression of Fas and other receptors, such as the p55 (type I) and p75 (type II) TNF-α receptors (TNFRs), which contain cytoplasmic death domains. The ligation of Fas by Fas ligand on another cell results in the activation of a death-receptor–regulated pathway of apoptosis, and a similar process occurs with the engagement of surface TNFRs.[608,611] An early event in the death-receptor–regulated pathway is the activation of caspase-8, a member of a group of proteases that are primarily involved in the regulation of apoptosis and that are associated with the cytoplasmic domains of death receptors. The Bcl-2–regulated and death-receptor–regulated pathways of apoptosis have a final common pathway in which downstream effector caspases (caspases-3, -6, and -7) proteolytically cleave a group of proteins that irrevocably commit the cell to undergo apoptosis. These include activation of caspase-activated DNase, which is involved in the internucleosomal cleavage of genomic DNA into 200 to 300 bp fragments characteristic of apoptosis.[608]

Circulating mononuclear cells from cord blood, including naïve CD4 T cells, are more prone than those from the adult circulation to undergo spontaneous apoptosis in vitro.[473,477,612,613] The mechanism is most likely mediated by the Bcl-2–regulated pathway of apoptosis and probably does not involve Fas engagement because Fas levels are low to undetectable on freshly isolated neonatal lymphocytes, including CD4 and CD8 T cells[613-616]; high levels of Fas expression are limited mainly to memory/effector cells, which are largely absent in the neonatal circulation.[615] The increased tendency of neonatal naïve CD4 and unfractionated T cells to undergo apoptosis may be related to their expression of a lower ratio of Bcl-2 (anti-apoptotic) to Bax (pro-apoptotic) proteins compared with adult T cells.[473,617] Neonatal naïve T cells also have a more marked decrease than adult T cells in expression of Bcl-2 and Bcl-X_L, which like Bcl-2 is anti-apoptotic, after 7 days in culture without exogenous cytokines.[477] Treatment of neonatal naïve CD4 T cells with IL-7 can block spontaneous apoptosis[457,477,478]; this effect is accompanied by increased expression of Bcl-2 and Bcl-X_L.[457,477] The tendency for neonatal T cells to spontaneously undergo apoptosis in mononuclear cell culture can also be blocked by incubation with insulin-like growth factor-1 (IGF-1),[613] but the mechanism involved remains unclear. The circulating levels of non–cell-associated Fas, TNF-α, and p55 TNFR increase in the first several days after birth,[618] and it has been proposed that the apoptotic tendency of neonatal lymphocytes may be downregulated in the immediate postnatal period by the ability of these soluble factors to inhibit engagement by their respective cell-associated ligand pairs.

Although neonatal T cells have an increased tendency to undergo spontaneous apoptosis, their activation in vitro (priming) may render them less prone than adult T cells to undergo apoptosis by Fas ligand or TNF-α engagement, probably because they express less Fas, p55 TNFR, TNFR-associated death domain (TRADD) (which associates in the cytoplasm with procaspase-8), and effector caspases, such as caspase-3.[617,619] By contrast, restimulation of primed neonatal T cells using anti-CD3 mAb induces greater apoptosis than occurs with use of similarly treated adult T cells; this anti-CD3 mAb–induced pathway in neonatal cells appears to be Fas independent.[619] These results suggest a mechanism by which the clonal expansion of neonatal T cells might be limited after activation through the αβ-TCR–CD3 complex and the means to counteract this apoptotic tendency, such as administration of IL-2, other exogenous γc cytokine receptor–using cytokines, or IGF-1 or IL-6 (which is induced by IGF-1 in cultures of neonatal mononuclear cell culture).[620] It remains unclear, however, whether adult naïve T cells primed under the same conditions as for neonatal T cells retain the tendency of unfractionated adult T cells for greater Fas-mediated and p55 TNFR–mediated apoptosis and reduced anti-CD3 mAb–mediated apoptosis. A tendency for greater apoptosis after anti-CD3 stimulation of neonatal CD4 T cells does not appear to be due to their consisting mainly of RTEs because we have found no significant differences between the frequency of apoptotic cells after CD3 and CD28 mAb stimulation of adult PTK7$^+$ CD4 RTEs and PTK7$^-$ naïve CD4 T cells (D.B. Lewis, unpublished observations, 2008).

Neonatal circulating mononuclear cells, probably including T cells, also are more prone than adult mononuclear cells to undergo apoptosis after engagement of surface MHC class I by mAb treatment,[612] apparently through a mechanism independent of Fas–Fas ligand interactions. The physiologic importance of the spontaneous and MHC class I–induced apoptotic pathways for fetal lymphocytes is unclear. It is plausible that an increased tendency of fetal T lymphocytes to undergo apoptosis after engagement of MHC class I might be a mechanism to maintain tolerance against noninherited maternal alloantigens.

An important caveat of most of the studies of T-cell apoptosis described above is that they have mainly used cord blood from term deliveries as a T-cell source. Thus it is unclear if this pro-apoptotic tendency of neonatal naïve T cells applies to the fetus or early postnatal period, and, if so, is influenced by prematurity and circulating levels of glucocorticoids. In most studies, there also has not been a direct comparison of neonatal T cells, which are predominantly antigenically-naïve, with antigenically-naïve adult T cells. Furthermore, non-Treg populations have not been assessed separately from neonatal Tregs, which appear to be intrinsically resistant to apoptosis (see later).

UNIQUE PHENOTYPE AND FUNCTION OF THE FETAL T-CELL COMPARTMENT

As discussed in the sections on CD45 Isoforms and Fetal and Neonatal Tregs, a substantial proportion of splenic T cells of the second trimester fetus, but not the young infant, are CD45RA^{lo}CD45RO^{hi}.[460] Most likely these fetal T cells, which have a diverse αβ-TCR repertoire, are mainly regulatory T cells (see Regulatory T Cells, later) because they have both phenotypic features, for instance, high levels of surface CD25 and functional features, for instance, high proliferative responses to IL-2 but limited activation by anti-CD3 mAb,[460] that are suggestive of this T-cell subset.[467,468] It is unclear if the CD45RA^{lo}CD45RO^{hi} subset of the second trimester fetus has substantial differences from circulating or splenic T cells of the neonate in terms of function after mAb stimulation.

Mucosal T cells are present in the fetal intestine by 15 to 16 weeks of gestation, and these cells have the capacity to secrete substantial amounts of IFN-γ after treatment with anti-CD3 mAb in combination with exogenous IFN-α.[621] IFN-α in vitro helps direct differentiation of circulating naïve CD4 T cells, including those of the neonate, toward a Th1 effector cytokine profile dominated by production of IFN-γ and not IL-4, IL-5, or IL-13, although it does not replace a requirement for IL-12p70 in this context. Because type I IFN–mediated secretion of IL-12p70 by DCs has been identified,[622] endogenously produced IL-12p70 could play a role in IFN-γ production by human fetal intestine in response to anti-CD3 mAb and exogenous IFN-α. Although it is not clear what T-cell type is the major source of IFN-γ in this tissue, these observations also suggest the possibility that a similar Th1 skewing of T-cell responses might occur in cases of fetal viral infection involving the intestine in which type I IFNs are induced.

Fetal Extrathymic T-Cell Differentiation

The human fetal liver contains rearranged VDJ transcripts of the TCR-β chain as early as 7.5 weeks of gestation, and pre-Tα transcripts can be found as early 6 weeks of gestation.[592,593] This raises the possibility that extrathymic differentiation of αβ-TCR–bearing T cells could occur in the fetal liver before such differentiation in the thymus. In the adult liver, CD4$^+$CD8$^-$ and CD4$^-$CD8$^-$ T cells with characteristics distinct from those of natural killer T cells (which also may have, in part, an extrathymic origin) have been described in conjunction with detection of transcripts for pre-Tα and the *RAG* genes. Thus it is possible that some liver T cells may be generated in situ even in adults.

Extrathymic differentiation of αβ T cells may occur in the fetal intestine because the lamina propria of the fetal intestine contains CD3$^-$CD7$^+$ lymphocytes expressing pre-Tα transcripts as early as 12 to 14 weeks of gestation, and these cells have the capacity to differentiate into αβ T cells.[623] Although it is unclear if these CD3$^-$CD7$^+$ precursor cells have a thymic or other origin, the Vβ repertoire of αβ T-lineage cells in the fetal intestine differs substantially from that of contemporaneous fetal αβ T-lineage cells found in the circulation, suggesting their independent origin.[623] A thymus-independent origin for these cells is supported by a recent study of intestine tissue at 16 weeks of gestation from an athymic fetus because of a homozygous null mutation for FOXN1.[624] Intestinal tissue from this fetus, as well as that from a normal fetus, expressed pre-Tα, RAG1, and RAG2 transcripts, and contained small numbers of CD8 T cells with a CD45RA naïve phenotype. These intestinal-derived CD8 T cells apparently circulated because their Vβ repertoire was oligoclonal and very similar to that of T cells in the cord blood.[624] The lamina propria and epithelium of the jejunum are potential sites of extrathymic T-cell development in adults in that immature lymphocytes with markers indicative of T-lineage commitment (CD2$^+$CD7$^+$CD3$^-$) are found at these sites, and these cells co-localize with transcripts for pre-Tα and the *RAG1* gene.[625] A recent report suggests that the tonsils of children could also potentially serve as an extrathymic site of T-cell production because this tissue contains TdT$^+$ lymphocyte populations that indicate increasing levels of differentiation along the T-lineage pathway up to a double-positive stage (CD4$^+$CD8$^+$αβ-TCR$^+$).[626] These tonsillar lymphocyte subsets also express transcripts for RAG1, pre-Tα, and ThPOK in amounts similar to their phenotypic counterparts in the thymus.

REGULATORY T CELLS

Overview

Regulatory T cells (hereafter referred to as Tregs) are αβ T cells that are critical for inhibiting immune responses to autoantigens,[627] transplantation antigens, and antigens derived from normal endogenous bacterial flora of the gut[628]; Tregs may also be important in maintenance of maternal-fetal tolerance.[629] Tregs are highly enriched within the small fraction of circulating human CD4 T cells that are CD25^{hi}, express the Foxp3 transcription factor, and have low or undetectable surface levels of CD127 (IL-7 receptor α chain).[630] CD25 is the IL-2 receptor α chain, which in conjunction with the IL-2 receptor β chain and the γc cytokine receptor chain, comprises the high-affinity IL-2 receptor. CD25^{hi} CD4 Tregs depend on IL-2 and high-affinity IL-2 receptors for their generation and maintenance,[631] as well as signaling via the STAT5b pathway.[632] In addition to CD25^{hi} CD4 Tregs, other cell types with regulatory activity include certain subsets of CD8$^+$ or CD4$^-$CD8$^-$ T cells and of B cells. CD25^{hi} CD4 Tregs can be generated in the thymus (referred to as natural Tregs) or from peripheral CD4 T cells (referred to as adaptive or peripherally derived Tregs). Human natural Tregs may be generated from CD4$^+$CD8$^-$ medullary thymocytes by a process of "secondary positive selection," in which these cells interact with thymic DCs displaying high levels of self-antigen and co-stimulatory molecules. These DCs are proposed to display high levels of co-stimulatory molecules as a result of their exposure to TSLP, an IL-7–like cytokine, produced by thymic epithelial cells of the Hassall's corpuscle.[633] TSLP production by placental trophoblasts has also been implicated in inducing maternal decidual T cells to differentiate into Tregs.[634]

Natural Tregs predominate in the healthy fetus and neonate, require the FoxP3 transcription factor for their intrathymic development, and have a circulating surface phenotype similar to that of most non-Treg naïve CD4 T cells, that is, CD45RA^{hi}CD45RO^{lo}Fas$^-$.[635] The expression of the Helios transcription factor has been proposed to distinguish natural Tregs from adaptive Tregs,[636] although this distinction is controversial and not absolute.[637,638] Genetic deficiency of Foxp3 (IPEX [immune dysregulation, polyendocrinopathy, enteropathy, X-linked] syndrome) results in an absence of circulating Tregs and the early postnatal or congenital onset of a severe T-cell–mediated autoimmune disease (enteritis, type 1 diabetes mellitus, and other autoimmune endocrinopathies).

Adult peripheral blood CD25^{hi} CD4 Tregs that have a Fox P3$^+$CD45RA^{lo}CD45RO^{hi}Fas$^+$ phenotype are presumed to be mainly adaptive Tregs, an idea supported by the observation that most of these cells appear to have a memory CD4 T-cell origin based on their in vivo labeling properties.[639] Adult adaptive Tregs are heterogeneous and can be divided into distinct Th1-like (CXCR3$^+$), Th2-like (CXCR3$^-$CCR4$^+$CCR6$^-$), Th17-like (CXCR3$^-$CCR4$^+$CCR6$^+$CCR10$^-$ and CD161$^+$), and Th22-like (CXCR3$^-$CCR4$^+$CCR6$^+$CCR10$^+$) cell subsets, based on their chemokine receptor/CD161 surface phenotype similarity to Th effector-cell populations. Although these FoxP3$^+$ Treg subsets retain their capacity to suppress immune responses similar to natural Tregs,[640,641] in some cases, they can also secrete cytokines that are typically considered proinflammatory, for instance, Th1-like Tregs produce IFN-γ and Th17-like Tregs produce IL-17. Proinflammatory cytokine production by Tregs may promote immune tolerance rather than effector function, possibly because of concurrent production of IL-10 and other concurrent immunosuppressive mechanisms, which are discussed below. The specialization in chemokine receptors presumably allows targeting of Tregs to adaptive immune responses occurring in the tissues.

Treg-mediated suppression requires activation through the αβ-TCR (e.g., antigenic peptide–MHC), but thereafter, regulatory T-cell–mediated suppression is not antigen specific. Mechanisms of inhibition may include the production of cytokines, such as IL-10, TGF-β, or IL-35 (a novel heterodimeric cytokine consisting of IL-12/IL-23p40 and EBI-3); expression of surface molecules, such as CTLA-4; and by competing for cytokines, for instance, IL-2, on which effector T-cell responses are dependent.[642] Tregs may also "regulate" effector T-cell responses by killing other T cells and/or APCs.[630] Adaptive Tregs may also mediate suppression by the production of adenosine and prostaglandin E2, both of which elevate intracellular cyclic adenosine monophosphate (cAMP) and inhibit proinflammatory signaling pathways in T cells and other cell types.

Fetal and Neonatal Tregs

CD25^{hi} CD4 Tregs, as assessed by their lack of CD127 expression and enrichment for Foxp3 mRNA or protein expression, are about 5% to 10% of circulating CD4 T cells in neonates,[75] including those who are prematurely born.[504] These neonatal Tregs are enriched in demethylation of the FoxP3 promoter at the TSDR (Treg-specific demethylated region) that is associated with robust and stable suppressor activity.[643] These circulating Tregs are most likely predominantly produced intrathymically based on their naïve surface phenotype, that is, CD45RA^{hi}CD45RO^{lo}Fas$^-$,[635,644] and high levels of intracellular Helios expression,[645,646] whereas most circulating adult Tregs have a phenotype indicating prior activation, suggesting that they are induced rather than natural Tregs.[647] These neonatal CD25^{hi} CD4 Tregs are resistant to Fas ligand–mediated apoptosis, as would be expected because of their limited Fas expression.[635] Neonatal Tregs include approximately 10% of cells that may be precommitted to IL-17 production based on their expression of CD161 or CCR6. Such IL-17–precommited cells constitute a substantially larger portion of circulating adult Tregs.[641]

CD4$^+$CD8$^-$ intrathymic precursors of CD25^{hi} CD4 Tregs are identifiable in the fetal thymus between 13 to 17 weeks of gestation and display an antigenically naïve surface phenotype (CD45RA^{hi}CD45RO^{lo}CD69$^-$Fas$^-$).[467] After leaving the thymus, these FoxP3$^+$ CD25^{hi} CD4 Tregs enter into the fetal lymph nodes and spleen, where they acquire a phenotype indicative of activation (CD45RA^{lo}CD45RO^{hi} CD69$^+$Fas$^+$cytoplasmicCTLA-4$^+$). Despite their strikingly different surface phenotypes, both the mature intrathymic CD25^{hi} CD4 Treg precursors and the Tregs found in peripheral lymphoid tissue have a similar ability to suppress the activation of autologous CD25$^-$ CD4 T cells in vitro.[467] A relatively large fraction of these CD25$^-$ CD4 and CD8 T cells in fetal lymphoid tissue express CD69 and secrete IFN-γ in the absence of CD25^{hi} CD4 Tregs, indicating that they are previously activated effector cells and suggesting that active inhibition by Tregs is an important mechanism constraining potentially untoward effector T-cell responses in utero.[468]

Taken together, the above results suggest that natural Tregs in the human fetus acquire the capacity for suppression in the thymus before their emigration to the periphery. After entering into the peripheral lymphoid tissues, they appear to encounter potentially autoreactive CD25$^-$ CD4 T cells, and thereby gain Treg activity. This implies that peripheral non-Treg T cells in the fetus have an αβ-TCR repertoire that is highly enriched for autoreactive specificities, an idea supported by studies of the murine neonatal peripheral T-cell compartment.[648]

In normal human pregnancy, maternal hematopoietic cells, the phenotype of which is still unclear, are routinely detectable in the fetal lymph nodes, where they appear to be responsible for the induction of fetal Tregs that are specific for maternal alloantigens.[649] Whether these fetal Tregs are first generated intrathymically or are adaptive Tregs that are induced from naïve CD4 T-cell precursors remains unclear, but fetal lymph node naïve non-Treg CD4 T cells clearly have an enhanced capacity to become Tregs compared with adult naïve CD4 T cells.[649] This greater propensity for Treg differentiation by fetal lymph node naïve CD4 T cells appears to be a property conferred by their origin from fetal HSCs.[81] It is unclear at what age this HSC-autonomous propensity for Treg generation is replaced by a capacity for effector T-cell generation similar to that of adult peripheral naïve CD4 T cells. The observation that specific tolerance by T cells to noninherited maternal alloantigens persists in most individuals until at least late childhood[650] suggests that Treg function that begins during fetal life can be quite durable, and could, at least in some cases, impact regulation of postnatal immune responses.[649]

In contrast to the fetus, FoxP3$^+$ CD25^{hi} CD4 Tregs are rare in mesenteric lymph node tissue of healthy adults.[468] This suggests that there is a dramatic postnatal decline in Tregs of the peripheral lymphoid organs, which might reflect a reduced requirement postnatally for Treg-mediated peripheral tolerance of the naïve T cells. These findings, which suggest a high level of CD25^{hi} CD4 Treg activity in the fetus, may also account for the presence at birth of autoimmune disease, such as type 1 diabetes, in some cases of genetic deficiency of Foxp3, a disorder in which natural Treg development is ablated.[651]

Most studies, but not all, have found that cord blood CD25^{hi} CD4 Tregs have an ability similar to adult peripheral Tregs to inhibit CD25$^-$ T-cell activation.[75] Intact neonatal Treg function is also indicated by the observation that in cases of newborns who were HIV-1 exposed but uninfected at birth, the removal of CD25^{hi} CD4 Tregs from cord blood strongly augments HIV-1–specific CD4 and CD8 T-cell responses.[652] Studies have also found that reduced Treg activity in the cord blood, either in absolute terms[653] or as decreased ratio of Tregs to Th2-type CD4 T cells at birth, may be a risk factor for children to subsequently develop allergic disease. A reduced frequency of Tregs relative to non-Treg T-cell populations has also been reported in the lamina propria of the ileum affected with NEC from premature infants compared with age-matched tissue from controls.[654] Although it is plausible that impaired Treg function could contribute to NEC pathogenesis, the selective increases in non-Tregs compared with Tregs could also reflect a differential effect of inflammation on the accumulation, proliferation, and/or survival of these two T-cell populations.

NATURAL KILLER AND MUCOSAL-ASSOCIATED INVARIANT T CELLS

Overview of Natural Killer T Cells

Natural killer T (NKT) cells are so named because they express αβ-TCRs in conjunction with CD161 (NKR-P1A), the human orthologue of the mouse NK1.1 protein, and other NK-cell markers, including CD56, CD57, CD94/NKG2A, and NKG2D. Like murine NKT cells, human NKT cells have a highly restricted repertoire of αβ-TCR (TCR-α chains containing the Vα24Jα18 segments in association with TCR-β chains containing Vβ11 segments) and recognize antigens presented by the nonclassic MHC molecule, CD1d, rather than by MHC class I or class II molecules. Bacterially derived CD1d-restricted antigens that can be recognized by the invariant αβ-TCR of NKT cells include α-galactosylceramides derived from *Borrelia burgdorferi*, *Sphingomonas*, and *Bacteroides*,[655,656] and diacylglycerol-containing glycolipids from gram-positive bacteria, including GBS and *Streptococcus pneumoniae*.[657] NKT cells can also recognize endogenously produced β-linked glycolipids, such as β-galactosylceramide, bound to CD1d, and this recognition may serve as microbial-induced danger signal.[658] Based on studies in adults, the presentation of self-lipids by CD1d$^+$ B cells may be essential for the maintenance of NKT cells.[659] In addition to their invariant TCR, many NKT cells also express high levels of cytokine receptors, particularly for IL-12. Based on mouse models of bacterial infection, the direct activation of NKT cells by IL-12 may be a more important protective mechanism than their activation by microbial antigens engaging their αβ-TCR,[660] although this point is controversial. NKG2D-dependent but TCR-independent activation of NKT cells, for instance, for cytotoxic activity, can also occur.[661]

Based on murine studies, the intrathymic commitment to the NKT lineage occurs when immature thymocytes expressing the invariant αβ-TCR are able to interact with CD1d$^+$ CD4$^+$CD8$^+$ double-positive thymocytes; β-galactosylceramide, which is normally expressed in the thymus, may serve as a positive selecting ligand bound to CD1d.[658] NKT-cell development in both humans and mice also depends on signaling via the SLAM family, which uses SAP for intracellular signaling. Thus NKT cells are absent in genetic SAP deficiency (X-linked lymphoproliferative syndrome).[662] The intrathymic development of NKT cells is also distinct from that for conventional αβ T cells in that NKT-lineage cells do not acquire a CD45RA^{hi} naïve surface phenotype before their thymic emigration and instead retain a uniformly CD45RO^{hi} phenotype in the periphery.[663] In addition, unlike conventional αβ T cells, NKT thymocytes acquire a high capacity to produce effector T-cell cytokines, such as IFN-γ and IL-4, before their thymic emigration.[664]

NKT cells have the ability to secrete high levels of inflammatory cytokines, including IFN-γ, IL-4, IL-17, IL-21, and GM-CSF and to express Fas ligand and TRAIL on their cell surface on primary stimulation, a capacity not observed with most antigenically naïve αβ T cells. This rapid ability to secrete cytokines, such as IFN-γ, occurs because these cells constitutively express IL-4 and IFN-γ mRNA, with cell activation resulting in the rapid translation of cytokine mRNA into protein that is secreted.[550,664] Thus NKT cells can potentially be an early source of cytokines that are characteristically secreted by Th1, Th2, Th17, or TFH cells. Some NKT cells also secrete IL-10 after activation,[665] which may in part mediate their regulatory activity on other effector cell populations. NKT cells are also enriched for preformed cytoplasmic stores of perforin and granzymes[665] that allows them to rapidly carry out cell-mediated cytotoxicity in contrast to naïve CD8 T cells, which initially lack such cytotoxic capacity and only acquire it after their differentiation into effector cells.

In adults, NKT cells that express the $V\alpha24^+$ $\alpha\beta$-TCR can be divided into $CD4^+CD8^-$ and $CD4^-CD8^-$ cell subsets. The $CD4^+V\alpha24^+$ subset has higher levels of L-selectin (CD62L) and lower surface expression of CD11a and secretion of IFN-γ and cytotoxins (perforin and granzyme A) than does the $CD4^-CD8^-V\alpha24^+$ subset,[665,666] which has high levels of expression of CCR5.[663] This suggests that the $CD4^+V\alpha24^+$ NKT cells may preferentially recirculate in secondary lymphoid tissue and act as regulatory cells, whereas $CD4^-CD8^-$ $V\alpha24^+$ NKT cells may mainly serve as effector cells at sites of extra–lymphoid tissue inflammation. Adult NKT-cell activation and maintenance appear to require antigen presenting by $CD1d^+$ B cells, a function that is impaired with patients with systemic lupus erythematosus.[659]

Although the physiologic role of NKT cells in host defense remains poorly understood, they may provide an important source of early cytokines that influence the later phases of innate immunity and the nature of the subsequent adaptive immune response. The ability of NKT cells to produce large amounts of cytokines in response to IL-12 or NKG2D engagement, alone, raises the possibility that antigen recognition by the invariant $\alpha\beta$-TCR may not play a role in this early innate response but rather be only required for the intrathymic development of these NKT cells. NKT cells have also been implicated as negative regulators of certain T-cell–mediated immunopathologic responses because relative deficiency of their numbers has been associated with certain autoimmune diseases, graft-versus-host disease after hematopoietic cell transplantation, and asthma.

NKT Cells of the Fetus and Neonate

NKT-lineage cells are present in the human fetal thymus by the beginning of the second trimester of gestation, and their relative frequencies, compared with the other thymocyte subsets, declines with increasing gestational age[663] because of rapid expansion of thymocytes differentiating along the conventional $\alpha\beta$ T-cell pathway. Fetal and postnatal thymic NKT cells are largely $CD4^+CD45RO^+$, with only a small percentage expressing CD161[663,664]; NKT cells in cord blood have a similar phenotype, except for greater expression of CD161.[663] Human fetal thymic NKT cells express high levels of IL-7 receptors, and their development appears to be largely IL-7-dependent. IL-7 treatment of both fetal thymic NKT cells and NKT cells in peripheral cord blood results in marked proliferation, the induction of effector cytokine production, that is, IFN-γ and IL-4, and increased expression of CD161, indicating increased differentiation.[663,664] Extrathymic fetal NKT-cell populations are found in the small intestine, where they may comprise up to 5% of all T cells in this tissue, as well as the T cells of the lung, spleen, and mesenteric lymph nodes.[667] Those NKT cells found in the fetal small intestine are distinct from those of fetal peripheral lymphoid tissue because they share many features of adult peripheral blood NKT cells, including higher CD161 expression, a greater capacity to produce IFN-γ, and lower levels of expression of L-selectin, CCR7, and CD4.[667] Murine studies suggest that commensal bacteria may be important for NKT-cell expansion and maturation, but the finding of a human NKT-cell population with mature features in the fetal intestine before bacterial colonization of the gut suggests a different mechanism is responsible. One possibility is that this maturation is due to the presentation of endogenous glycolipids by CD1d, which is abundantly expressed in the fetal intestine.[667]

Using a rigorous assay for NKT-cell detection by flow cytometry—that is, the binding of tetramers of CD1d loaded with α-galactosylceramide—neonates, infants, and older children have a similar mean frequency of circulating NKT cells (approximately 0.06% of circulating lymphocytes); this frequency is modestly but significantly lower than the mean frequency of 0.2% for adult peripheral blood.[668] At all ages, there is striking individual variation in values, with frequencies ranging from less than 0.001% to greater than 0.5 % of circulating lymphocytes.[668] The basis for this great variability and its immunologic impact are unknown. Cord blood NKT cells differ from those of adult peripheral blood in lacking the $CD4^-CD8^-$ subset and expressing lower levels of CD161 and higher levels of proteins involved in lymphoid tissue homing, for instance, L-selectin and CCR7.[663,664,669] Cord blood NKT cells also express higher levels of CD25 than those of adult blood and can be activated by lower doses of CD1d-restricted antigens.[669] Compared with their adult peripheral blood counterparts, cord blood NKT cells also produce a substantially higher ratio of IL-4 to IFN-γ in response to most stimuli, such as anti-CD3 and anti-CD28 mAb or phorbol ester and calcium ionophore.[664,670] This Th2 bias is largely accounted for by skewing of the relatively small $CD4^-CD8^-$ subset of cord blood NKT cells toward high levels of IL-4 production and limited IFN-γ production.[671] Consistent with their relatively high capacity to simultaneously produce IFN-γ and IL-4, both cord blood and adult peripheral blood NKT cells constitutively express high levels of T-bet and GATA3, the respective master transcription factors for Th1 and Th2 cytokine gene expression, and have IL-4 and IFN-γ genetic loci that are relatively hypomethylated and poised for transcription compared with conventional naïve CD4 $\alpha\beta$ T cells.[664]

Mucosal-Associated Invariant T Cells

Mucosal-associated invariant T (MAIT) cells are a population of $CD8^+$ or $CD8^-CD4^-$ $\alpha\beta$ T cells that predominantly express an invariant $V\alpha7.2$ and $J\alpha33$ TCR-α chain and that are activated by antigen presentation by MR1, a MHC class I–like protein that is widely expressed on hematopoietic and epithelial cells. Antigen for the MAIT-cell $\alpha\beta$-TCR consists of bacterial- or fungal-derived metabolites of the riboflavin biosynthetic pathway, which bind to MRI at a site analogous to the peptide-binding groove used by conventional MHC class I heavy chains.[672] MAIT cells that express high levels of CD161 and the IL-18 receptor α chain (IL-18Rα) have the ability to produce both Th17 and Th1 cytokines in response to stimulation with calcium ionophore and phorbol ester, anti-CD3 and anti-CD28 mAb, or IL-12 and IL-18 treatment.[673] MAIT cells also express a variety of cytokines and can kill bacterially infected epithelial cells.[674] MAIT cells of healthy adults constitute up to 10% of circulating $\alpha\beta$ T cells, are predominantly $CD8^+$, and uniformly have a memory ($CD45RA^{lo}CD45RO^{hi}$) cell surface phenotype.[675-677] MAIT cells are a predominant $\alpha\beta$ T-cell type in the liver and the lamina propria of the healthy intestine[678] and are also found in lung tissue.[679] MAIT cells express high levels of CCR6 and CXCR6 chemokine receptors, which is consistent with their tissue-homing properties to the liver and intestines.[678] Murine studies have shown that MAIT cells can mediate protection against mycobacterial and gram-negative bacterial infection,[676] including pulmonary infection with *Francisella.*[680]

MAIT cells develop in the thymus and, based on murine studies, this development appears to be mediated by MR1-expressing double-positive thymocytes.[681] Unlike developing NKT cells, the mature precursors of MAIT cells of the human thymus have an antigenically naïve ($CD45RA^{hi}$ $CD45RO^{lo}$) surface phenotype.[675] Intrathymic MAIT-cell precursors, which are $CD161^{hi}V\alpha7.2^{+}$ but IL-$18R^{lo}$, are detectable at 18 weeks of gestation. In the periphery, MAIT cells that have an activated and proliferative phenotype, that is, IL-$18R\alpha^{hi}CD45RO^{+}Ki67^{+}$, are easily detected in the small intestine, liver, and lung between 18 and 23 weeks of gestation.[682] It is plausible that fetal tissue MAIT cells, which express high levels of IL-7 receptors, may undergo homeostatic proliferation driven by locally derived IL-7. Fetal extra–lymphoid tissue MAIT cells appear to have substantial function; for instance, those of the fetal intestine can secrete IFN-γ and IL-22 in response to paraformaldehyde-fixed *Escherichia coli* and anti-CD28 mAb.[682] Collectively, these findings suggest that MAIT cells of the fetus constitute a functional cell population that develops in the absence of exposure to commensal microbes, and that could mediate host defense against intrauterine bacterial and fungal infection.

MAIT cells in the cord blood of neonates, which constitute approximately 0.7% of circulating αβ T cells, express similar high levels of CD161 and IL-18Rα as their adult counterpart.[678] In contrast to adult peripheral blood MAIT cells, those of cord blood have a predominant antigenically naïve ($CD45RA^{hi}CD45RO^{lo}$) surface phenotype, and are predominantly $CD4^{-}CD8^{-}$ rather than $CD8^{+}$.[675,678] It is possible that circulating MAIT cells in the neonate are mainly recent thymic emigrant precursor cells that are in transit to extra–lymphoid tissues, where they may mature and acquire a memory phenotype, as apparently occurs in the fetus,[682] whereas MAIT cells in adult peripheral blood may be mature cells that have reentered the blood from the liver, intestine, and gut. The frequency of circulating MAIT cells gradually increases after birth, reaching the frequency of adult cells by approximately 1 to 2 years of age, and a predominance of a memory-cell surface phenotype is evident by 3 months of age.[678]

GAMMA-DELTA T CELLS

Phenotype and Function

Gamma-delta T cells, which express a TCR heterodimer consisting of a gamma (γ) and a delta (δ) chain in association with the CD3 complex proteins, are rarer than αβ T cells in most tissues, including the blood, where they constitute approximately 1% to 10% of circulating T cells in adults. A major exception is certain epithelial tissues, such as those of the intestine, where γδ T cells predominate among intraepithelial lymphocytes (IELs). Although some γδ-TCRs can recognize peptide antigens presented by classic MHCs, most directly recognize the three-dimensional structures of protein or nonprotein molecules in a MHC-independent manner, akin to antibody recognition of antigen. The specificity of γδ-TCRs for activating ligands has been best characterized for human γδ T cells expressing TCRs that use Vγ9 (using an older but still commonly used nomenclature) and Vδ2 variable segments, which are hereafter referred to as Vγ9Vδ2 T cells. The recognition by the Vγ9Vδ2 TCR of phosphoantigens, that is, nonpeptidic pyrophosphomonoester compounds, results in cell proliferation and the secretion of cytokines, chemokines, and preformed cytotoxins (perforins, granzymes, granulysin).[683] These phosphoantigens can be derived from mycobacteria and other bacterial species, plasmodia, or from host cellular isopentenyl phosphates (IPPs) that are involved in cholesterol biosynthesis from mevalonate. The cellular levels of IPPs can be increased by metabolic stress from intracellular infection after treatment with certain drugs, for instance, aminobisphosphonates, or after oncogenic transformation. The precise mechanism by which the Vγ9Vδ2 TCR recognizes exogenous or endogenous phosphoantigens remains unclear but requires all three CDR regions of both the TCR-γ and TCR-δ chains[684] and does not involve MHC class I or class II or CD1 recognition. Although there is limited information on activating ligands for other human γδ T-cell populations,[683] some examples include the γδ-TCRs of $V\delta1^{+}$ IELs binding to the MICA protein[685] and those of circulating $V\delta1^{+}$ T cells binding to endogenous sulphatides bound to CD1d.[686] Because γδ T cells frequently express multiple types of activating receptors that are also found on NK cells, for instance, NKG2D, NKp30, and NKp44, the relative role of the γδ-TCR versus these other receptors remains unclear in many immunologic contexts, for instance, the lysis of tumor cells.[687]

In addition to resident sites of γδ T-cell accumulation, increased numbers of these cells are found in the intestine involved with inflammatory bowel disease, the skin lesions of patients with leprosy, psoriasis, and erythema nodosum, and in the blood in cases of malaria and acute and chronic herpesvirus infections. Subpopulations of γδ T cells express adhesion molecules that allow them to enter these tissues, such as cutaneous leukocyte antigen for the skin, but compared with conventional αβ T cells, their expression of chemokine receptors is much more limited.[688,689]

Most activated γδ T cells express high levels of perforin, serine esterases, Fas ligand, and granulysin and are capable of cytotoxicity against tumor cells and other cell targets, such as infected cells. γδ T cells also can secrete a variety of cytokines in vitro, including TNF-α, IFN-γ, IL-4, IL-17, and IL-22,[690] as well as chemokines that may help recruit inflammatory cells to the tissues. Cytokine production can be potently activated by products from live bacteria, such as isobutylamine, and by type I IFN or by agents that potently induce it, such as oligonucleotides containing unmethylated CpG motifs. Human Vγ2Vδ2 T cells, after adoptive transfer into genetically immunodeficient mice, can mediate rapid and potent protection against gram-positive and gram-negative bacteria[691] and influenza virus.[692] The protective effect of Vγ2Vδ2 T cells for influenza A virus may be due to perforin/granzyme-mediated cellular cytotoxicity as well as the secretion of cytokines with antiviral activity, for instance, TNF-α and IFN-γ.

Ontogeny of Gamma-Delta T-Cell Production and T-Cell Receptor Gene Rearrangements

Only about 2% to 5% of T-lineage cells of the thymus and peripheral blood express γδ-TCR in most persons.[693] Unlike in most αβ T cells, whose development requires an intact thymus, a significant proportion of γδ T cells can develop by a thymic-independent pathway, and normal numbers of γδ T cells are found in cases of complete thymic aplasia[693] and in the human fetus before the first waves of thymically derived T cells.[694] This may be explained, at least in part, by the differentiation of γδ T cells directly from primitive lymphohematopoietic precursor cells found in the small intestine, as has been demonstrated in the mouse.[695]

The human TCR-γ and TCR-δ chain genes undergo a programmed rearrangement of dispersed segments analogous to that of the TCR-β and TCR-α chain genes. Most circulating adult human γδ T cells lack evidence of TCR-β chain gene rearrangement,[696] indicating that commitment to this lineage mainly is the result of a double-negative thymocyte expressing both a productive TCR-γ and TCR-δ chain gene rearrangement. High levels of signaling through Notch receptors, particularly Notch3, on immature thymocytes may favor TCR-γ and TCR-δ rearrangement over TCR-β rearrangement.[697] The expression of a functional γδ-TCR results in strong cell signaling that suppresses TCR-β rearrangement. Alternatively, if the TCR-β chain gene is productively rearranged (but not both the TCR-γ and TCR-δ genes), signals from the pre-TCR complex favor progression to the $CD4^{pos}CD8^{pos}$ stage where positive selection of αβ-TCR^+ cells can take place. Most γδ T cells lack surface expression of either CD4 or CD8α/CD8β heterodimers, consistent with their not undergoing a process of positive selection that is obligatory for αβ T cells. Whether human γδ T cells undergo negative selection is unclear.

Rearranged TCR-δ genes are first expressed extrathymically in the liver and primitive gut between 6 and 9 weeks of gestation.[698,699] Rearrangement of the human TCR-γ and TCR-δ genes in the fetal thymus begins shortly after its colonization with lymphoid cells, with TCR-δ protein detectable by 9.5 weeks of gestation.[700] γδ T cells comprise about 10% of the circulating T-cell compartment at 16 weeks, a percentage that gradually declines to less than 3% by term.[459,701]

Although there is potential for the formation of a highly diverse γδ-TCR repertoire, peripheral γδ T cells use only a small number of V segments, which vary with age and with tissue location. These can be divided into two major groups, Vγ9Vδ2 cells and Vδ1 cells, in which a Vδ1-bearing TCR-δ chain predominantly pairs with a TCR-γ chain by using a Vγ segment other than Vγ9. Most γδ-TCR^+ thymocytes in the first trimester of fetal life express Vδ2 segments. This is followed by γδ-TCR^+ thymocytes that express Vδ1, which predominate at least through infancy in the thymus. Most circulating fetal and neonatal γδ T cells also are Vδ1 bearing, with only about 10% bearing Vδ2,[702] and these Vδ1 cells constitute the predominant γδ T-cell population of the small intestinal epithelium after birth. In contrast with the early-gestation fetal thymus and the fetal and neonatal circulation, Vδ2 T cells predominate in the fetal liver and spleen early during the second trimester,[703,704] and appear before αβ-TCR^+ thymocytes,[700,705] suggesting that they are produced extrathymically by the fetal liver.

As indicated by TCR spectratyping, the TCR-δ chains using either Vδ1 or Vδ2 segments usually are oligoclonal at birth.[706,707] Because this oligoclonality also is characteristic of the adult γδ T-cell repertoire, this is not due to postnatal clonal expansion but reflects an intrinsic feature of this cell lineage. By age 6 months, γδ T cells bearing Vγ9 Vδ2 segments become predominant and remain so during adulthood,[708] probably because of their preferential expansion in response to ubiquitous antigen(s), such as endogenous bacterial flora.

Ontogeny of Gamma-Delta T-Cell Function

Antigenically naïve and experienced subsets of γδ T cells can be distinguished using markers commonly applied to αβ T cells; for instance, naïve γδ T cells can be identified by their $CD45RA^{hi}CD45RO^{lo}CD27^{hi}CD1a^{lo}$ surface phenotype.[709] By these criteria, circulating γδ T cells of the neonate are predominantly antigenically naïve, whereas those of the adult are almost uniformly memory cells.[709] Neonatal γδ T cells proliferate in vitro in response to mycobacterial lipid antigens,[710] and Vγ2Vδ2 T cells of the neonate also proliferate in response to isoprenyl phosphate and IL-2 or to high doses of HMB-PP ([E]-4-hydroxy-3-methyl-2-butenyl pyrophosphate), a potent bacterially derived phosphoantigen, although less effectively than their adult cell counterparts.[711,712] However, neonatal Vγ2Vδ2 T cells are not intrinsically limited in their ability to proliferate under all circumstances because bisphosphonates induce levels of proliferation that are similar to their adult peripheral blood counterparts.[712]

Circulating neonatal γδ T cells express lower levels of serine esterases and perforin than do adult γδ T cells, suggesting they are less effective cytotoxic cells.[711,713] γδ T-cell clones derived from cord blood also have a markedly reduced capacity to mediate cytotoxicity against tumor cell extracts.[701] Because these neonatal clones also have lower CD45RO surface expression than that observed in the adult clones, their reduced activity may reflect their antigenic naïveté. In contrast with freshly isolated neonatal αβ T cells, activation and propagation of these fetal and neonatal γδ T cells in culture (e.g., with exogenous IL-2) do not enhance their function. However, the combination of bisphosphonate and IL-23 substantially enhanced the expression of cytotoxic mediators (perforin, granzyme A, granzyme B, and granulysin) by cord blood Vγ2Vδ2 T cells,[712] although it is unclear whether this also enhanced cell-mediated cellular cytotoxicity. The function of fetal liver γδ T cells remains unclear, although one older report suggests that they have cytotoxic reactivity against maternal MHC class I[705] and thereby may prevent engraftment of maternal T cells.

The capacity of neonatal γδ T cells for cytokine production is also markedly reduced under some conditions, but not all. For example, virtually no cord blood Vγ2Vδ2 T cells produce IFN-γ in response to isoprenyl phosphate,[709,714] whereas IFN-γ production by these circulating cells in 1- to 2-year-old infants is only slightly reduced compared with that of adults.[709] Compared with those of adult peripheral blood, cord blood Vγ2Vδ2 T cells, particularly those from preterm or small-for-gestational pregnancies, also have reduced IFN-γ and TNF-α production in response to influenza A virus.[715] The impaired IFN-γ production by cord blood Vγ2Vδ2 T cells can be markedly enhanced by the addition of TNF-α but not IL-12, reflecting their having similar levels of receptors for TNF-α but not for IL-12 compared with adult Vγ2Vδ2 T cells.[714] Moreover, certain stimuli, such as bisphosphonate compounds, are relatively effective at inducing IFN-γ production, by neonatal Vγ2Vδ2 T cells. The combination of bisphosphonate with IL-23 not only increases IFN-γ secretion but also generates a subset of neonatal Vγ2Vδ2 T cells that produce IL-17 but not IFN-γ; of interest, the production of IFN-γ was enhanced, but no IL-17 was expressed when adult peripheral blood Vγ2Vδ2 T cells were stimulated under these conditions.[712] This tendency of activated neonatal γδ T cells to mediate Th17-like responses is reminiscent of that observed for activated neonatal naïve CD4 T cells, suggesting that there may be common mechanisms among T-lineage cells of the fetus and neonate that favor the production of IL-17.

As discussed in more detail in the section "T-Cell Response to Congenital Infection," congenital infection with CMV results in the expansion of a distinct Vγ8Vδ1 T-cell population in the fetus.[716] Thus, as is true for conventional CD8 T-cell responses, the γδ T-cell response to congenital viral infection can be relatively robust.

ANTIGEN-SPECIFIC T-CELL FUNCTION IN THE FETUS AND NEONATE

Delayed Cutaneous Hypersensitivity, Graft Rejection, and Graft-versus-Host Disease

Skin test reactivity to cell-free antigens assesses a form of delayed cutaneous hypersensitivity (DTH) that requires the function of antigen-specific CD4 T cells. Skin test reactivity to common antigens, such as *Candida*, streptokinase-streptodornase, and tetanus toxoid, usually is not detectable in neonates.[717-719] Absence of such reactivity reflects a lack of antigen-specific sensitization because in vitro T-cell reactivity to these antigens also is absent. When leukocytes, and presumably antigen-specific CD4 T cells, from sensitized adults were adoptively transferred to neonates, children, or adults; however, only neonates failed to respond to antigen-specific skin tests.[720] This finding indicates that the neonate may be deficient in other components of the immune system required for DTH, such as APCs and production of inflammatory chemokines or cytokines. Such deficiencies may account, at least in part, for diminished skin reactivity in the neonate after specific sensitization or after intradermal injection with T-cell mitogens.[192,721] Diminished skin reactivity to intradermally administered antigens persists postnatally up to 1 year of age.[721]

Neonates, including those born prematurely, are capable of rejecting foreign tissues, such as skin grafts, although rejection may be delayed compared with adults.[722] Experiments using human–SCID mouse chimeras also suggest that second-trimester human fetal T cells are capable of becoming cytotoxic effector T cells in response to foreign antigens and in rejecting solid tissue allografts.[723] Clinical transplantation of fetal blood from one unaffected fraternal twin to another did not result in marrow engraftment, despite a sharing of similar MHC haplotypes; instead, there was a postnatal recipient cytotoxic T-cell response against donor leukocytes.[724] A T-cell response to alloantigens can also be detected in newborns after in utero irradiated red blood cell transfusions from unrelated donors.[725,726] Thus fetal T cells appear similar to neonatal T cells in being able to mediate allogeneic responses in vivo, including graft rejection.

Another indication that neonatal T cells can mediate allogeneic responses is the fact that blood transfusions rarely induce graft-versus-host disease in the neonate. Rare cases of persistence of donor lymphocytes and of graft-versus-host disease have developed after intrauterine transfusion in the last trimester as well as in transfused premature neonates, however.[727-730] Because the infusion of fresh leukocytes induces partial tolerance to skin grafts,[722] tolerance for transfused lymphocytes might occur by a similar mechanism, predisposing the fetus or neonate to graft-versus-host disease. Together, these observations suggest a partial immaturity in T-cell and inflammatory mechanisms required for DTH and for graft rejection.

T-Cell Reactivity to Environmental Antigens

Specific antigen reactivity theoretically can develop in the fetus by exposure to antigens transferred from the mother, by transfer of antigen-specific maternal lymphocytes, or by infection of the fetus itself. Several studies suggest that fetal T cells have become primed to environmental or dietary protein allergens as a result of maternal exposure and transfer to the fetus.[75,731] A criticism of these studies is that the antigen-specific proliferation is low compared with the basal proliferation of cord blood mononuclear cells, and direct detection of cytokine-producing T cells by flow cytometry has not been reported. In addition, many of these studies used antigen extracts rather than defined recombinant proteins or peptides, and these may have nonspecific stimulatory effects.

Fetal T-Cell Sensitization to Maternally Administered Vaccines and Maternally Derived Antigens

In contrast with protein allergens, there is only one report in which antigen-specific fetal T-cell priming to influenza vaccination has been detected using a flow cytometric assay after staining T cells with fluorochrome-labeled influenza hemagglutinin peptide/HLA-DR (MHC class II) tetramers.[732] This study, which needs to be confirmed, contrasts with one in which maternal vaccination during the last trimester of pregnancy with tetanus toxoid or inactivated influenza virus A or B did not result in detectable neonatal T-cell responses using lymphocyte blastogenesis assays.[733] The use of corroborating assays that are reliable for the detection of very low frequencies of T cells, such as enzyme-linked immunosorbent spot-forming cell (ELISPOT) assays, might allow a better definition of the extent of fetal T-cell sensitization by maternal vaccination. In any case, the neonatal CD4 T-cell responses induced by maternal immunization are of a much lower frequency than those after postnatal vaccination responses in children,[734] and their durability is unknown. Together, this suggests that fetal sensitization to foreign proteins may be relatively inefficient, particularly when exposure is temporally limited. Whether this reflects relatively inefficient maternal-fetal transfer of protein antigens or intrinsic limitations of the fetus for antigen presentation and T-cell priming, or both, is unclear. Even if it is assumed that the capacity for fetal T cells to be primed by foreign antigens is similar to that of antigenically naïve adult T cells, the immune response to maternally derived foreign vaccine proteins by fetal T cells would be expected to be poor compared with the maternal response because antigen probably enters into the fetal circulation with little if any accompanying activation of the innate response required for efficient T-cell activation.

Growing evidence, however, suggests that fetal T-cell sensitization can occur in cases of antigen exposure resulting from chronic infection of the mother with parasites or viruses: Parasite (schistosomal, filarial, and plasmodial) antigen-specific cytokine production by peripheral blood lymphocytes, probably of T-cell origin, was detectable at birth in infants without congenital infection who were born to infected mothers.[735,736] Of interest, this apparent T-cell immunity persisted for at least 1 year after birth in the absence of postnatal infection with parasites and was associated with downregulation of *M. bovis* BCG–specific IFN-γ production after neonatal administration of BCG vaccine.[735] These results suggest that fetal exposure to parasitic antigens without infection can downregulate subsequent postnatal Th1 responses to unrelated antigens. HIV peptide–specific IL-2 production by cord blood CD4 T cells also has been reported in uninfected infants born to HIV-infected mothers, suggesting that fetal T-cell sensitization can occur in cases of chronic viral infection of the mother without congenital infection.[737]

Maternal Transfer of T-Cell Immunity to the Fetus

The older literature contains many reports of cord blood lymphocyte proliferation or cytokine production in response to antigens that the fetus is presumed not to have encountered. These antigen responses, for instance, for PPD, *Mycobacterium leprae*, measles, or rubella, have been attributed to passive transfer of T-cell immunity from the mother. The responses usually are weak and may represent laboratory artifacts rather than true sensitization because complex antigen mixtures were used that likely may activate T cells in a non–MHC-restricted manner. Although maternal-to-fetal transfer of leukocytes, particularly T cells, occurs, their number in the fetus is very low (usually < 0.1%)[738] unless the neonate or infant has a severe defect of T cells that normally prevents maternal T-cell engraftment, such as SCID.[739] Accordingly, detectable antigen-specific cellular immunity by conventional assays is unlikely for immunocompetent neonates. Thus, reports of T-cell responses in healthy neonates as a result of transfer of maternal immunity should remain suspect unless the T-cell population is identified, for instance, by flow cytometry, and its antigen specificity and MHC restriction are demonstrated.

T-CELL RESPONSE TO CONGENITAL INFECTION

CD4 T Cells

Pathogen-specific T-cell proliferative responses and cytokine responses (IL-2 and IFN-γ) in infants and children with congenital infection (e.g., with *Treponema pallidum*, CMV, VZV, or *Toxoplasma*) are often much lower than such responses in infants and children with postnatal infection, or are absent entirely.[75] These studies used blood mononuclear cells and mainly detected CD4 T-cell responses because antigen preparations (e.g., whole-cell lysates of virally infected cells) and the APC populations (e.g., peripheral blood monocytes and B cells as the predominant APCs, with few cDCs) favor activation of MHC class II–restricted rather than class I–restricted responses. These reduced CD4 T-cell responses are particularly true with first- or second-trimester infections. Similarly, a recent study of neonates with congenital exposure to hepatitis C virus failed to find hepatitis C–specific CD4 T-cell responses in cord blood,[740] although there were some relatively subtle perturbations of Treg surface phenotype and T-cell cytokine production to polyclonal stimulation. With severe infections in the first trimester, a direct deleterious effect on T-cell development is possible. T cells from infants and children with congenital toxoplasmosis, however, retain the ability to respond to alloantigen, mitogen, and, in one case, tetanus toxoid.[741]

Whereas markedly diminished responses in congenitally, compared with postnatally, acquired infection in infancy are common, this may not be observed in all cases. For example, one study found that nearly all neonates with congenital *Toxoplasma* infection, similar to older *Toxoplasma*-immune individuals, had T-cell responses to soluble *Toxoplasma* antigens, measured as antigen-stimulated induction of CD25 (IL-2 receptor α chain).[742] In another study from the same group, among infants younger than 1 year who received antenatal treatment for in utero *Toxoplasma* infection, antigen-specific IFN-γ production was detected in 94%.[743] Marchant and colleagues[744] found that CMV-specific CD4 T-cell responses, measured as antigen-stimulated cytokine and CD154 expression, were weaker in the blood of infants than in adults in The Gambia; there was no difference in the responses of infants with congenital CMV infection versus infection acquired in the first 3 months of life.[7]

Congenital infections may also have a positive impact on heterologous postnatal immune responses. For example, infants congenitally infected with *Trypanosoma cruzi*, the agent of Chagas disease, had substantially higher peripheral blood mononuclear cell IFN-γ responses, likely mainly derived from Th1 cells, to hepatitis B surface antigen (HBsAg) and diphtheria and tetanus toxoids, compared with uninfected infants, including those were exposed to *T. cruzi*.[745]

Several groups have evaluated the impact on the adaptive immunity of African neonates who have had high levels of fetal exposure to maternally derived *Plasmodium falciparum* antigens as a result of the accumulation of infected maternal red blood cells in the placenta but who were not congenitally infected with malaria. In this situation, malaria antigen–induced CD4 T-cell cytokine production (IFN-γ, IL-2, IL-5, and/or IL-13) was detectable in these neonates,[746,747] indicating that dual Th1- and Th2-type immune responses may develop after fetal exposure to pathogenic antigens from the mother. A subgroup of neonates exposed as fetuses to *Plasmodium* antigens may develop tolerance, as assessed by the production of IL-10 but not proinflammatory cytokines produced by cord blood mononuclear cells, and be at a greater risk for the postnatal acquisition of malaria.[746]

This in utero priming by plasmodial antigens was not associated with altered frequencies of Tregs or of naïve or central or effector memory CD4 T cells in cord blood compared with unexposed neonates.[644,748,749] and did not alter the capacity of cord blood mononuclear cells to produce cytokines (IL-2, IL-4, IL-6, IL-10, TNF-α, and IFN-γ) in response to polyclonal stimulation with anti-CD3 and anti-CD28 mAbs.[748] However, there was increased expression of HLA-DR and CD25 by the small populations of central and effector memory CD4 T cells of neonates who were *Plasmodium* antigen exposed,[749] which may account for their cord blood mononuclear cells supporting higher levels of HIV production, at least in vitro.[750] There may also be a longer-term impact on other adaptive immune responses; for instance, in utero plasmodial antigen exposure was associated with decreased PPD-specific Th1 responses at one year of age in children who received routine neonatal BCG vaccination.[751]

The reduced CD4 T-cell responses seen in many types of congenital infection may be the result of antigen-specific unresponsiveness (e.g., anergy, deletion, or ignorance–the failure of the CD4 T cell to be initially activated by antigen). As discussed earlier, it is unlikely that a decreased TCR repertoire limits these immune responses, particularly after the second trimester onward.

CD8 T Cells

By comparison with responses of CD4 T cells, CD8 T-cell responses to congenital infections appear to be relatively robust. In congenital CMV infection, high frequencies of CMV-specific CD8 T cells were detectable by staining with CMV peptide–MHC class I tetramers, and these cells demonstrated IFN-γ and perforin expression, cytolytic activity, and oligoclonal αβ-TCR expansion, similar to those of chronically infected adults.[594] Other studies found that although the CMV-infected fetuses and their transmitter mothers had similar levels of activated, effector/memory, and memory CMV-specific CD8 T cells, there was impaired secretion by fetal CD8 T cells of IFN-γ in response to CMV antigen or CD3 and CD28 mAb stimulation,[595,596] and this impairment was associated with decreased viral clearance. Similarly, most newborns with congenital HIV-1 infection had detectable HIV-specific cytotoxic T-cell responses within the first week of life, indicating that fetal T cells were activated by viral antigens.[752] Congenital infection with *T. cruzi* also results in a marked expansion of CD8 T cells over CD4 T cells, with evidence of oligoclonality of the TCR repertoire, indicating that this is antigen driven.[753] These CD8 T cells are enriched in markers for activation (HLA-DR^{hi}), memory (CD45RO^{hi}), and end-stage effector cells (CD28^{-}), and for cytotoxicity (perforin^{+}), and have markedly greater capacity to produce IFN-γ and TNF-α than is seen in CD8 T cells from uninfected newborns; in comparison with CD8 T cells, CD4 T cells in these congenitally infected newborns appear to have undergone much less clonal expansion and acquisition of effector function.[753] Congenital infection with viruses or *Toxoplasma* during the second and third trimesters may result in the appearance of CD45RO^{hi} memory T cells and an inverse ratio of CD4 to CD8 T cells,[75] findings that also suggest that fetal CD8^{+} T cells are activated and expanded in response to serious infection. These alterations in CD45RO expression by T cells in congenital infection may persist at least through early infancy.

Gamma-Delta T Cells

The cord blood of most neonates with congenital CMV infection contains an expanded Vγ8Vδ1 T-cell population that has effector features, including a CD27^{-}CD28^{-} surface phenotype, and high levels of expression of transcripts for IFN-γ, multiple activating receptors that are also found on NK cells, and cytotoxins.[716] Clones from this Vγ8Vδ1 T-cell population killed CMV-infected target cells, suggesting that this γδ T-cell population may help limit CMV infection in vivo. Of interest, these Vγ8Vδ1 T cells for the most part lack N-terminal nucleotide addition in the CDR3 regions of the rearranged TCR-γ and TCR-δ chain genes, which are essentially germline encoded.[716] This contrasts with the prominence of N-nucleotide additions in the CDR3 regions of most αβ T cells and suggests that a highly conserved interaction occurs between the CMV-induced antigen and the antigen-binding site of the Vγ8Vδ1 TCR occurs in most individuals with congenital CMV. γδ T cells with these features were found as early as 21 weeks of gestation, indicating that, as for CD8 αβ T-cell responses, vigorous CMV-specific γδ T-cell responses can be mounted in the fetus and may play an important role in prenatal host defense.[716] Future studies defining the CMV-induced antigen that Vγ8Vδ1 T cells recognize, and whether an expanded population of these cells occurs in postnatal CMV infection, and can be induced by vaccination, will be of interest.

T-CELL RESPONSE TO POSTNATAL INFECTIONS AND VACCINATION IN EARLY INFANCY

CD4 T-Cell Responses to Postnatal Infection

Postnatal infection with HSV in the neonatal period results in antigen-specific proliferation and cytokine (IL-2 and IFN-γ) production by CD4 T cells. These responses are substantially delayed, however, compared with those in adults with primary HSV infection.[754,755] It is unclear at what postnatal age the kinetics of this response become similar to those in adults. Studies of CMV-specific CD4 T-cell immunity (expression of IL-2, IFN-γ, and CD40 ligand) in older infants and young children with primary infection found substantially reduced responses compared with those in adults with infection of similar duration.[545] This reduced CD4 T-cell response was associated with persistent shedding of the virus into secretions.[545] As noted above, the magnitude of CMV-specific CD4 T-cell responses in infants infected in utero or in the first 3 months of life was similar, and the CD4 T-cell responses of both groups of infants remained less than those of adults for at least the first 2 years of life.[744] Of interest, as in congenital CMV infection,[594-596] older infants and young children with primary CMV infection had robust CMV-specific CD8 T-cell responses similar to those in adults.[545,756,757]

CD4 T-Cell Responses to Postnatal Immunization with Inactivated Vaccines

One older study of vaccinated infants between 6 and 12 months of age also demonstrated lower IL-2 production in response to tetanus toxoid than that observed in older children and adults.[758] This finding suggests that either antigen-specific memory CD4 T-cell generation or function is decreased during early infancy. Whether this reflects limitations in antigen processing, T-cell activation and co-stimulation, or proliferation and differentiation remains unclear. Postvaccination tetanus toxoid–specific CD4 T cells that accumulate at 4 months are mainly TH0-like cells (high levels of expression of IL-2 and TNF-α but little or no IFN-γ or Th2 cytokines) with a CCR7^{hi}CD45RA^{lo} surface phenotype indicative of central memory cells.[759] A similar cytokine profile and surface phenotype has been reported for pertussis-specific CD4 T cells in 9-month-old infants after multiple DTaP (diphtheria-tetanus–acellular pertussis) vaccinations, whereas pertussis-specific CD4 T cells in adults post-TdaP (tetanus toxoid–reduced diphtheria toxoid–acellular pertussis) vaccination have greater numbers of cells that are polyfunctional, that is, simultaneously express IFN-γ, IL-2, and TNF-α, and that have a CCR7$^-$CD45RA$^-$ effector memory-cell phenotype.[760] It should be noted that, in this study, TdaP was likely stimulating a recall response in the adults, who, unlike the infants, would have been previously primed by immunization with whole-cell pertussis-containing vaccines or pertussis infection, which may have contributed to the differences observed. In any case, these results suggest that infants tend to develop less robust Th1 responses and polyfunctional cytokine responses to inactivated vaccines during their primary immunization series than adults receiving booster vaccines, but, compared with adults, infants may preferentially accumulate central memory T cells, which are associated with relatively durable immune responses (see "Overview of Memory T Cells").

Based largely on murine studies, human neonates and young infants have been suggested to have skewing of CD4 T-cell responses toward a Th2 cytokine profile, although this may be an oversimplification. For example, an older study in which total cytokine production by PBMCs stimulated with tetanus toxoid was evaluated, both Th1 (IFN-γ) and Th2 (IL-5 and IL-13) memory responses occur, particularly after the third vaccine dose at 6 months of age.[511] The tetanus toxoid–specific Th1 response, in some cases, transiently decreased by 12 months of age, whereas Th2 responses did not.[511,761] Using a similar assay, greater cross-reacting material (CRM)197-specific Th2 responses were observed in infants who received a series of CRM197-conjugated pneumococcal polysaccharide, starting at birth rather than beginning at 1 month of age[762]; this Th2 skewing of the infants vaccinated at birth resolved by 9 months of age.[763] However, no such age-related Th2 skewing was recently observed in a flow cytometric analysis comparing pertussis-specific CD4 T cells responses of infants versus adults after immunization with pertussis vaccine.[760] It remains to be shown that vaccine antigen-specific CD4 T cells are the source of the Th2 cytokines in infant blood samples. It is possible that other cellular sources in peripheral blood mononuclear may mediate Th2 cytokine production, for instance, CD8 T cells, which, in the neonate, have the ability as antigenically naïve cells to produce high amounts of IL-13 in response to activation.[561]

CD4 T-Cell Responses to Postnatal Immunization with Live-Attenuated Vaccines

In contrast with postnatally acquired herpesvirus infections or inactivated vaccine antigens, BCG vaccination at birth versus 2 months or 4 months of age appeared equally effective in inducing peripheral blood mononuclear cell CD4 T-cell proliferative and IFN-γ responses to PPD, extracellular *M. tuberculosis* antigens, and an *M. tuberculosis* intracellular extract in infants in The Gambia.[764,765] In this cross-sectional analysis, the responses were robust not only at 2 months after immunization but were also measurable at 1 year of age, and no skewing toward Th2 cytokine production was noted.[764,765] A recent longitudinal analysis using flow cytometry extended these findings, revealing that BCG-specific CD4 T cells are detectable as early as 3 weeks after vaccination at birth in South African infants, with peak responses achieved at approximately 10 weeks of age, followed by a gradual decline until 1 year of age.[759] These BCG-specific CD4 T cells have a Th1-like cytokine profile (IFN-γ predominant with less expression of TNF-α and IL-2) with little or no detection of IL-17,[759] and predominantly central memory-cell (CCR7^{hi}CD45RA^{lo}bcl-2^{hi}) phenotype, particularly those that accumulate from the peak response onward. Together, this suggests that the BCG-specific CD4 T-cell response of infants is a blend between an effector memory-like one, in terms of Th1 cytokine profile, but central memory-like in terms of chemokine receptor expression.

Although the early cross-sectional studies in The Gambia suggested that there was little impact of delaying BCG vaccination on the subsequent immune response, this group later reported that neonatally vaccinated infants may have a delay in the appearance of BCG-specific CD4 T cells expressing CD40 ligand until after 1 year of age.[766] Moreover, a more recent flow cytometric study using direct ex vivo stimulation in whole blood rather than stimulation of isolated blood mononuclear cells compared neonatal BCG vaccination with vaccination delayed until 10 weeks of age in South African infants and found that the frequencies of BCG-specific CD4 T cells (particularly polyfunctional cells coexpressing IFN-γ, IL-2, and TNF-α) were greater with delayed vaccination; this augmented immunity was particularly evident at 1 year of age.[767] By contrast to the results of these studies from South Africa and The Gambia, in Uganda, vaccination with BCG shortly after birth compared with 6 weeks of age-induced greater numbers of IFN-γ– and/or perforin-expressing CD4 and CD8 T cells and of proliferating T cells that had greater capacity to produce IFN-γ, TNF-α, and IL-2 at the individual cell level[768]; the same approach was used, and some of the same investigators conducted the Ugandan and South African studies, suggesting that the differences are likely to reflect local biologic rather than technical differences. Consistent with this notion, using a similar whole-blood assay, infants vaccinated in the United Kingdom had more robust production of Th1-related cytokines than infants in Malawi, who had a cytokine profile skewed toward Th17 cytokine production.[769] In addition, the season of birth (wet season vs. dry season) in tropical areas may influence the CD4 T-cell response to neonatal BCG vaccination,[766] as may the strain of BCG used.[770] Thus the magnitude and quality of CD4 T-cell immunity may be influenced by the timing of administration and by particular geographic and environmental contexts, as is the case for the apparent protective benefits of BCG immunization.[771] It should also be pointed out that one study has found that Th1 responses induced by BCG vaccination at birth do not correlate with protection against tuberculosis[772] and that readily assayed and robust immune correlates of protection against tuberculosis have not yet been identified.

Flow cytometry analysis of BCG-stimulated whole-blood samples obtained from vaccinated infants also indicates an important contribution of lymphocyte populations other than CD4 T cells, for instance, CD8 T cells, γδ T cells, and NK cells to IFN-γ production.[773,774] Thus future studies in which multiparameter cytometry is used to evaluate the cellular sources of cytokine production in whole-blood assays may help clarify mechanisms that influence the outcome of BCG vaccination under these various conditions.

Early BCG immunization can also have an impact on the adaptive immune responses to heterologous antigens. BCG given at birth increased Th1- and Th2-specific responses and antibody titers to HBsAg given simultaneously.[765] BCG given at birth did not enhance the Th1 response to tetanus toxoid given at 2 months of age but did increase the Th2 response (IL-13 production). It is likely that BCG vaccination may accelerate DC maturation so that these cells can augment either Th1 or Th2 responses. This BCG-induced maturation may also differ among BCG strains because Th1 responses to tetanus toxoid at 1 year of age were higher in infants who were vaccinated at birth with BCG-Denmark compared with other strains.[770] It has also been suggested that BCG immunization in the neonatal period and in early infancy reduces overall mortality unrelated to any effect on tuberculosis[775]; however, these provocative findings and the potential underlying mechanisms have yet to be assessed in randomized controlled trials.

The T-cell–specific response to oral poliovirus vaccine (OPV), another live vaccine, suggests a decreased Th1 response. Neonates given OPV at birth and at 1, 2, and 3 months of age demonstrate lower OPV-specific CD4 T-cell proliferation and IFN-γ production and have fewer IFN-γ–positive cells compared with adults who were immunized as children but not recently reimmunized.[776] By contrast, their antibody titers were higher than those in adults, suggesting that CD4 T-cell help for B cells is not impaired. It is plausible that OPV may be less effective at inducing a Th1 response than BCG in neonates and young infants because of its limited replication, site of inoculation, or ability to stimulate APCs in a manner conducive to Th1 immunity, relative to BCG, which induces persistent infection in the recipient.

CD8 T Cells

As discussed, CD8 T-cell responses to CMV infection acquired in utero[594] or during infancy and early childhood[545,756,777] are robust, and it is likely that this also applies for infection acquired perinatally or during early infancy. CD8 T-cell responses to HIV can be detected by 6 weeks of age in all perinatally infected infants,[778] and the frequency and cell surface phenotype of HIV-specific CD8 T cells between 3 to 6 months after perinatal infection are similar to that observed in adults after acute infection.[779] However, there may be qualitative differences in the infant and adult immune response in that HIV-specific T cells of infants are often less polyfunctional, that is, defined as the ability of single cells to express multiple cytokines (IL-2, IFN-γ, and TNF-α) and to secrete cytotoxic granules, than those of adults. HIV-Gag–specific T cells are absent in young infants with perinatal infection and often remain low during the first 2 years of life,[780] whereas this is less frequent after acute adult infection. HIV Gag–specific T-cell responses are a good prognostic factor for viral containment in both infants and adults, including elite controllers,[780-782] but the mechanism for this remains to be established. HIV-1 infection may inhibit antigen-specific immunity by depleting circulating DCs, impairing antigen presentation, decreasing thymic T-cell output, and promoting T-cell apoptosis. In addition, maintenance of HIV-specific CD8 T cells with effector function depends on HIV-specific CD4 T cells and may be selectively and severely impaired by the virus. Surprisingly, some of the inhibitory effects of HIV-1 infection also may occur in HIV-exposed but uninfected infants born to HIV-infected mothers,[783,784] with suppression of HIV-specific T-cell responses by Tregs appearing to be an important contributor.

In one older study, RSV-specific cytotoxicity was more pronounced and frequent in infants 6 to 24 months of age than in younger infants.[785] These results, which need to be repeated using more current assays, suggest that the CD8 T-cell response to RSV gradually increases with postnatal age. Murine studies indicate that RSV infection suppresses CD8 T-cell–mediated effector activity (IFN-γ production and cytolytic activity) and that only transient memory CD8 T-cell responses occur after infection. Longitudinal studies of CD8 T-cell immunity to RSV in children and adults after primary and secondary infection will be of interest to determine if this immunoevasive mechanism applies to humans.

SUMMARY

T-cell function in the fetus and neonate is impaired compared with that in adults. Diminished functions include T-cell participation in cutaneous DTH and, as also discussed in the next section, T-cell help for B-cell differentiation. Selectively decreased cytokine production by fetal and neonatal T cells, such as decreased IFN-γ secretion and expression of CD40 ligand, may contribute to these deficits. In the case of IFN-γ, the predominance in the fetus and neonate of recent thymic emigrants may contribute to this immaturity in cytokine secretion. The repertoire of αβ-TCR probably is adequate, except in early gestation. After fetal or neonatal infection, the acquisition of CD4 T-cell antigen-specific responses typically is delayed. In vitro studies suggest that deficiencies of DC function and activation and differentiation of antigenically naïve CD4 T cells into memory/effector T cells may be contributory. In contrast with diminished CD4 T-cell function, conventional CD8 T cell–mediated cytotoxicity and cytokine production in response to strong chronic stimuli, such as congenital CMV infection or allogeneic cells, appear to be intact in the fetus and neonate. Responses by innate-like T-cell populations, such as γδ T cells, may also be relatively robust in the setting of congenital infection. The mother does not transfer T-cell–specific immunity to the fetus. T-cell sensitization of the fetus may occur with maternal vaccination, but it is unclear if in utero sensitization occurs to allergens.

B Cells and Immunoglobulin

OVERVIEW

Mature B cells are lymphocytes that are identifiable by their surface expression of immunoglobulin. Immunoglobulin, which is synonymous with antibody, is a heterotetrameric protein consisting of two identical heavy chains and two identical light chains linked by disulfide bonds (Fig. 4-13).

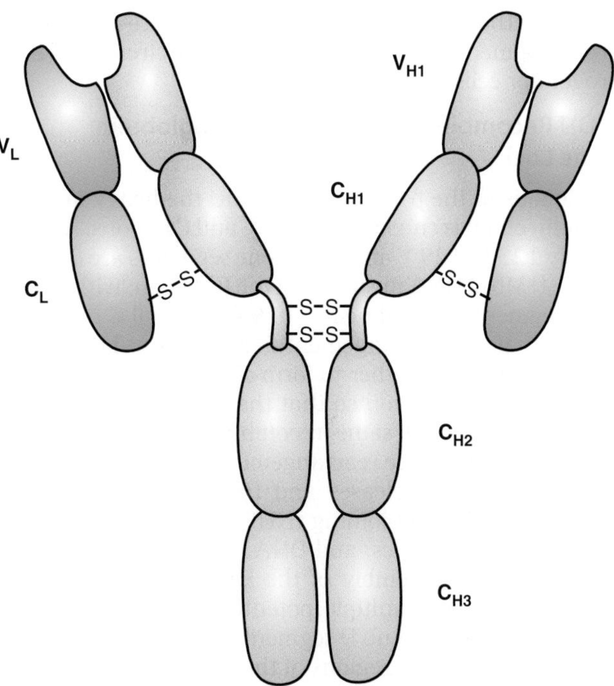

Figure 4-13 Structure of an immunoglobulin molecule. The immunoglobulin molecule consists of two heavy chains *(brown shading)* and two light chains *(blue shading)* linked together by disulfide bonds. The antigen-combining site is formed by amino-terminal region of the heavy and light chains contained in the V_H and V_L domains of the heavy and light chains, respectively. For immunoglobulin G (IgG), IgD, and IgA, the constant region C_{H3} domain of the heavy chain encodes isotype or subclass specificity, which determines the ability of the immunoglobulin to fix complement, bind to Fc receptors, and be actively transported from the mother to the fetus during gestation. IgM and IgE (not shown) are structurally similar, except that they contain an additional C_{H4} domain conferring these properties, and they lack a hinge region.

As with the TCR, the amino-terminal portion of the antibody chains is highly variable as a consequence of the assembly of V, D, and J gene segments (heavy chain) or V and J segments (light chain) to a monomorphic constant (C) region. These amino-terminal regions of a pair of heavy and light chains form the antigen-binding fragment (Fab) portion of immunoglobulin, which contains the antigen-binding site (see Fig. 4-13).

As with the TCR, the variable region of each chain can be subdivided into three hypervariable CDR1, CDR2, and CDR3 regions, and four intervening, less variable framework regions. The three-dimensional folding of the antibody molecules results in the approximation of the three CDR regions into a contiguous antigen recognition site, with CDR3 located at the center and the CDR1 and CDR2 regions forming the outer border of the site. Antibody molecules are distinct from the αβ-TCR, however, because they typically recognize antigens found on intact proteins or other molecules, such as complex carbohydrates. Thus the B-cell recognition of antigen is typically highly sensitive to its three-dimensional structure.

The constant regions of the heavy and light chains consist of three constant heavy (C_H) domains and one constant light (C_L) domain, respectively (see Fig. 4-13). The heavy chains also have a hinge region at which the two halves are joined by disulfide bonds. The heavy chain C region is the Fc portion of immunoglobulin and contains sites that determine complement fixation, placental transport, and binding to leukocyte Fc receptors. The portion of the heavy chain C region encoded by the last exon of the heavy chain gene defines antibody isotype or isotype subclass, of which there are nine in humans: IgM, IgD, IgG1, IgG2, IgG3, IgG4, IgA1, IgA2, and IgE. Light chains comprise two types, kappa and lambda, each containing a distinct type of C region. In isotype switching, the C region at the carboxy terminus of the immunoglobulin heavy chain gene is replaced with another isotype-specific segment, but the antigen-combining site at the amino terminus is preserved.

In addition to their secretion of antibodies, mature B cells express MHC class II and also may participate in antigen processing and presentation to CD4 T cells. They may also serve as a source of effector cytokines, for instance, IFN-γ, and as regulators (suppressors) of immune responses (regulatory B cells or Bregs), by secretion of immunosuppressive cytokines, such as IL-10.

In cases in which the antigen has multiple and identical surface determinants (e.g., complex polysaccharides, certain viral proteins with repetitive motifs) and multiple surface immunoglobulins (sIgs) are cross-linked, antigen binding alone may be sufficient to induce B-cell activation without cognate (direct cell-cell interaction) help from T cells. In this case, other signals derived from non–T cells, such as cytokines, or from microorganisms, such as bacterial lipoproteins or pathogen-derived DNA, may enhance antibody responses.

EARLY B-CELL DEVELOPMENT AND IMMUNOGLOBULIN REPERTOIRE FORMATION

Pro–B-Cell and Pre–B-Cell Maturation

The pro–B cell is the most immature cell type that is known to have differentiated along the B-lineage. Human pro–B cells of the adult bone marrow and of cord blood have a $CD10^{hi}CD19^{-}CD34^{hi}$ surface phenotype[786] and are probably derived from a $CD10^{-}$L-selectin^{hi} precursor that can give rise to all lymphoid lineages.[787] Human pro–B cells also express key transcription factors that promote and maintain B-cell lineage differentiation, including early B-cell factor (EBF) and Pax5. Pro-B cells also express RAG, TdT, and CD79 proteins and undergo D-to-J and then V-to-DJ immunoglobulin heavy chain gene rearrangements.[788] D-to-J heavy-chain gene rearrangements also may occur in immature lymphocytes that are not committed to the B lineage, such as thymocytes, but V-to-DJ rearrangement is a characteristic feature of committed B-lineage cells. In cases in which the immunoglobulin heavy chain is productively rearranged, it is expressed cytoplasmically and on the B-lineage cell surface as part of the pre-BCR complex, which consists of a surrogate light chain (a VpreB and a λ5/14.1 segment) in association with Ig-α (CD79a) and Ig-β (CD79b) heterodimers. Expression of the pre-BCR complex defines the pre–B-cell stage, and pre–B cells have a $CD10^{hi}CD19^{hi}$ surface phenotype. CD34 expression decreases during the pro–B-cell to pre–B-cell transition.

The heavy chain gene usually rearranges first, initially with a joining of a D segment to a J segment. D-to-J heavy chain gene rearrangement and protein expression are followed by the joining of a V segment to the D-to-J segment.

Productive V(D)J rearrangement results in the expression of full-length heavy chain protein in the cytoplasm. In humans, the first easily recognized pre–B cells are those that contain cytoplasmic IgM heavy chains but no light chains or sIg. The expression of the pre-BCR by the pre–B cell blocks rearrangement of the other heavy chain gene allele (allelic exclusion) and results in proliferation of the pre–B cell, with concurrent downregulation of RAG and TdT activity.[789]

The human pro–B-cell to pre–B-cell transition is dependent on the ability to form a functional pre-BCR complex. This transition is blocked by mutations in either the Cμ segment of the heavy chain gene, Ig-α, Ig-β, the cytoplasmic Btk tyrosine kinase, or B-cell linker (BLNK) cytoplasmic adapter protein, all of which compromise pre-BCR signal transduction. No known ligand for the human pre-BCR has been defined, and much of its extracellular domain of heavy chain is dispensable for its function. This suggests that the pre-BCR may have ligand-independent basal signaling function. Such ligand-independent function is supported by a structural study that found that the human pre-BCR receptor can dimerize in the absence of any ligand and probably cannot recognize antigens because of steric blockade of the heavy chain binding site by the surrogate light chain.[790] After a burst of cell proliferation, the pre–B cell exits from cycling, upregulates RAG and TdT activity, and proceeds with immunoglobulin light chain rearrangement.

After the expression of the pre-BCR, a similar process of gene rearrangement subsequently occurs to assemble light chain genes from V and J segments. Allelic exclusion also usually acts at the light chain level so that only a single type of light chain is produced. Kappa light chain gene rearrangement usually occurs first, and if neither kappa chain gene rearrangement is productive, this apparently permits lambda chain gene rearrangement to proceed. In approximately 35% of B cells a kappa receptor excision circle (KREC) is generated from the kappa light chain locus and the content of KRECs can be used similar to TRECs in T-lineage cells to monitor de novo production of naïve cells, for instance, after hematopoietic stem cell transplantation.[791] Approximately 60% of human immunoglobulin molecules use kappa light chains, and the remainder use lambda light chains. If rearrangement and expression of a complete kappa or lambda light chain subsequently occur, a functional immunoglobulin molecule is assembled and expressed as sIg. The end result of allelic exclusion is that a B cell usually synthesizes only a single immunoglobulin protein. Compared with that of the heavy chain, allelic exclusion of immunoglobulin light chains is relatively "leaky" such that 0.2% to 0.5% of circulating B cells express both a kappa and a lambda light chain in their surface IgM.

Pre–B cells are first detected in the human fetal liver and omentum by 8 weeks of gestation and in the fetal bone marrow by 13 weeks of gestation.[792] By midgestation, the bone marrow is the predominant site of pre–B-cell development.[793] B-cell lymphopoiesis occurs solely in the bone marrow after 30 weeks of gestation and for the remainder of life.[794] The neonatal circulation contains higher levels of $CD34^+CD38^-$ progenitor cells that are capable of differentiating into B cells than are found in the bone marrow compartment of children or adults.[795] Cord blood has circulating $IgM^-CD34^+CD19^+Pax\text{-}5^+$ B-cell progenitor cells that span the early–B-cell, pro–B-cell, and pre–B-cell stages of development; CD10 expression by these circulating B-cell progenitor cells is variable.[796]

V(D)J Recombination of the Immunoglobulin Gene Loci

Analogous to the β chain of the TCR, the heavy immunoglobulin chain is encoded by V, D, J, and C regions. Approximately 123 to 129 V and 27 D gene segments are dispersed over 1.0 Mb of DNA upstream of the JC region, with 9 different J segments located near 5 to 9 functional C regions.[797] Antibody gene rearrangement is required to bring the V, D, and J regions together to form a single exon that is juxtaposed to the C region so that the gene can be expressed (see Fig. 4-8). The same recombinase enzyme complex required for TCR gene rearrangement, including the RAG1 and RAG2 endonucleases and the proteins involved in nonhomologous end-joining (NHEJ) DNA repair (Artemis, Cernunnos, DNA-PKcs, and DNA ligase IV), mediates this process.[798] The assembly of the kappa and lambda light chain genes from multiple potential segments is similar, except that there are no D segments. As in the TCR chains, the CDR1 and CDR2 regions of the antigen-combining site are encoded entirely by the V segments, and the CDR3 is encoded at the junction of the V, D, and J segments. Antibody diversity, like TCR diversity, is generated by the juxtaposition of various combinations of V, D, and J segments and by imprecision in the joining process itself resulting from exonucleolytic activity, random nucleotide addition by the TdT enzyme, and resolution of hairpin ends as P nucleotides. In the case of the heavy chain gene, D-to-D joining can also occur, and D segments also can rearrange by inversion or deletion. Together, these mechanisms permit a theoretical immunoglobulin repertoire of more than 10^{12} specificities to be generated from fewer than 10^3 somatic gene segments. For reasons that are not clear, however, immunoglobulin heavy chain V segment usage by immature pre–B cells and antigenically naïve B cells appears to be dominated by relatively few segments.[799,800] Thus actual immunoglobulin diversity is less than would be predicted if segment usage were completely random. As in the case of the TCR genes, the CDR3 region appears to be the most important source of diversity. Further diversification is possible later in B-cell differentiation by processes known as receptor editing and somatic mutation, which are described later.

V(D)J Segment Usage in the Fetus and Neonate

The primary or preimmune immunoglobulin repertoire, which consists of all antibodies that can be expressed before encounter with antigen, is determined by the number of different B-cell clones with distinct antigen specificity and is limited during the initial stages of B-cell development in the fetus, compared with that in the adult. In the early to midgestation human fetus, the set of V segments used to generate the heavy chain gene is smaller than in the adult.[801] The V segments are scattered throughout the heavy chain gene locus.[802] Differences in the usage of particular heavy chain D and J segments between the first and second trimesters and term also have been identified.[801] These developmental differences are intrinsic rather than the result of environmental influences because they occur in immature B-cell precursors lacking a pre-BCR complex.

By the third trimester, the V and D segment heavy chain gene repertoire of peripheral B cells appears to be similar to that of the adult, although there may be overrepresentation of certain segments[803,804] and underuse of certain J_H segments.[804] Certain heavy chain V segments expressed in adult B cells are not found in neonatal B cells,[805,806] but it is unlikely that this severely limits the neonatal humoral immune response. Other V segments, such as V_H3, are present at a greater frequency in the preimmune Ig repertoire.[806,807] This increased representation may confer on antibody molecules the ability to bind protein A of *S. aureus*, thus providing some intrinsic protection during the perinatal period.

CDR3 Length and Terminal Deoxytransferase

The length of the CDR3 region of the immunoglobulin heavy chain, which is formed at the junction of the V segment with the D and J segments, is shorter in the midgestation fetus than at birth[808] or in adulthood.[809] This is due, in part, to decreased TdT, which is responsible for N-nucleotide additions. This decreased TdT expression is an intrinsic property of neonatal $CD34^+$ precursor cells not yet committed to the B lineage because in vitro differentiation of B-lineage cells from neonatal $CD34^+$ cells results in lower amounts of TdT than are present in similar cells from adults.[810]

Up to 25% of heavy chain CDR3 regions in fetal B cells lack N additions, and in the remaining, the size of the N-nucleotide additions is smaller than for neonatal or adult CDR3 regions. The CDR3 region is the most hypervariable portion of immunoglobulins, and a short CDR3 region significantly reduces the diversity of the fetal immunoglobulin repertoire.[805] The CDR3 region of the heavy chain gene remains relatively short at the beginning of the third trimester and gradually increases in length until birth.[803,811,812] Because the CDR3 region is at the center of the antigen-binding pocket of the antibody, reduced CDR3 diversity could limit the efficiency of the fetal antibody response. The importance of shortened CDR3 regions by themselves in limiting antibody responses might be subtle, however, because gene knockout mice lacking TdT produce apparently normal antibody responses after immunization or infection.[419] Nevertheless, a combination of lack of TdT and limitations in V and D usage could limit the ability of the fetal B cells to recognize a full spectrum of antibody responses to foreign antigens, particularly before midgestation.

In mice, premature expression of TdT during fetal development achieved by transgenesis was detrimental in adulthood by preventing the appearance of certain natural (preimmune) antibody specificities, for instance, reactive with phosphorylcholine, which increased the susceptibility of the animals to bacterial infection.[813] It is interesting that the combination of decreased TdT activity and the preferential use of D7-27, which is the shortest of the D segments, results in particularly short CDR3 regions in the human fetus and neonate.[804] It has been proposed that these limitations in CDR3 length, combined with preferential use of V_H6-1, may be important in generating natural IgM antibody specificities, such as for single-stranded DNA, that may be protective in the fetus and neonate, for instance, by helping eliminate fetal apoptotic cells.[804]

B-CELL MATURATION, PREIMMUNE SELECTION, AND ACTIVATION

Receptor Editing, Clonal Deletion, and Clonal Anergy

Immature B cells of the bone marrow that have successfully produced a productive heavy and light chain express these as IgM on the cell surface. A large proportion of these sIgs are autoreactive, that is, they bind with relatively high affinity to molecules on other cell types within the bone marrow microenvironment and peripheral lymphoid organs.[814] Such self-reactivity and BCR signaling at this stage of development maintains RAG activity, with the result that the B cell frequently undergoes a secondary V-to-J light chain rearrangement. This involves V segments located 5′ and J segments that are located 3′ to the current VJ rearrangement. If this eliminates sIg autoreactivity, the lack of BCR-mediated cell signaling turns off RAG activity, and the B cell enters into the circulation as a new emigrant (transitional) B cell to complete its maturation. If not, additional light chain rearrangement can occur. Analysis of patients with genetic immunodeficiencies of signaling pathways involved in TLR recognition unexpectedly found an accumulation of autoreactive B cells, indicating that IRAK-4– and MyD88-dependent signaling is involved in the receptor editing process.[815] Most immature autoreactive B cells can be converted to nonautoreactivity by receptor editing, thereby allowing most B cells with productive Ig heavy chain rearrangements to contribute to the final repertoire.

Those persistently autoreactive B cells are probably eliminated by a process of clonal deletion, which involves apoptosis induced by strong BCR signaling,[814] or anergy, in which the B cells are functionally inactivated.[816] In healthy human adults, circulating anergic B cells have been identified as having an $IgD^+IgM^-CD27^-$ surface phenotype,[816] many of which also lack CD21 surface expression.[817] These anergic B cells have a predominantly autoreactive BCR antigen specificity and a reduced capacity to increase intracellular calcium and increase tyrosine phosphorylation after BCR engagement.[816,817] IgD^+IgM^- anergic B cells constitute about 3% of all circulating B cells in healthy adults,[816] but their frequency in the neonate and infant is unclear.

New Emigrant (Transitional) versus Fully-Mature Naïve B Cells

The initial expression of sIg by B-lineage cells is in the form of both the IgM and IgD isotypes. This is the result of alternative mRNA splicing of the exons of the heavy chain gene. In human adults, these $IgM^{hi}IgD^{hi}$ transitional B cells can be identified in the bone marrow and circulation by their high levels of expression of CD5, CD10, CD24, CD38, and low levels of Bcl-2 and of the ABCB1 transporter.[818-822] These cells also are enriched for Ki67 staining, indicating they have recently undergone proliferation. Analogous to T-lineage cells, these circulating transitional B cells can be considered as recent bone marrow emigrants (or new emigrants for short) that undergo a post–bone marrow phase of peripheral maturation into fully mature naïve B cells. These transitional B cells can be further divided into a less mature $CD21^-$ subset that has higher levels of IgD and Ki67 staining than the more mature $CD21^+$ subset.[823] The immature $CD21^-$ subset of transitional B cells is distinct from a

CD21⁻ B-cell population found in adult peripheral blood, which identifies anergic cells and which has a fully mature naïve B-cell surface phenotype, that is, CD38⁻.[817] As new emigrant B cells mature into naïve B cells, their expression of CD5, CD10, CD24, CD38, and Ki67 decline and ABCB1 is upregulated.[819]

The maturation of new emigrant B cells into fully mature antigenically-naïve B cells includes negative selection of B cells with autoreactive BCRs that have entered into the periphery and that have somehow escaped central tolerance mechanisms in the bone marrow.[824] Although the mechanisms involved in this secondary checkpoint for B-cell tolerance remain poorly understood, it may involve, at least in part, the death of autoreactive B cells because of their greater dependence for survival on BAFF (B-cell activating factor), a member of the TNF ligand superfamily, than nonautoreactive B cells.[815] This peripheral tolerance checkpoint also appears to require CD4 T-cell–derived signals, as the proportion of B cells that have autoreactive BCRs is significantly increased in antigenically-naïve B cells of patients with genetic defects affecting CD40 ligand or MHC class II.[825] It is plausible that the increased frequency of autoreactive naïve B cells in patients with MHC class II deficiency may reflect decreased numbers of MHC class II–restricted CD25$^+$ CD4 Tregs in these individuals.[826]

New emigrant B cells may also be subject to the influence of positive selection, which in mice can influence whether a B cell differentiates into particular B-cell subsets, such as follicular B cells versus marginal zone B cells, which are discussed later. Positive selection requires an intact BCR complex and presumably involves either some interaction of the antigen-combining site of the BCR with self-molecules or tonic signaling by the BCR complex,[827] or both. In contrast with positive selection of thymocytes, which involves mainly cortical epithelial cells that present self-peptides, the nature and cellular sources of the ligands involved remain obscure. Evidence for positive selection of B cells in the human as early as fetal life comes from comparisons of the immunoglobulin repertoire of pre–B cells and transitional B cells versus that of mature naïve B cells.[828]

The new emigrant B-cell subset of adults is also enriched in B cells that have the capacity to express IL-10 after in vitro treatment with strong stimuli.[829] Such IL-10–producing B cells are prominent in certain autoimmune diseases and have been proposed to serve as negative regulators of adaptive immune responses. The fraction of new emigrant B cells in the adult that can express IL-10 and potentially mediate regulatory function is unknown. It is also unclear whether IL-10–producing B cells with a new emigrant surface phenotype are a phenotypically and functionally stable population or can further mature into fully mature naïve B cells, a process that is discussed later.

Follicular B-Cell Maturation

New emigrant B cells that escape negative selection and have undergone positive selection become fully mature naïve IgM^{hi}IgD^{hi}CD27$^{lo/-}$ABCB1$^+$ follicular B cells.[819,830] Follicular B cells include most of those that are involved in adaptive immune responses to T-cell–dependent antigens, such as proteins and protein-carbohydrate conjugates, and are the predominant naïve B-cell subset of cells in the circulation or secondary lymphoid tissue. Marginal zone and B-1 B cells, which have distinct roles from follicular B cells in immunity, are discussed separately. Like naïve T cells, the naïve B cells have a very slow rate of turnover in vivo[819,831] and express CXCR4, CXCR5, and CCR7, which promotes their recirculation between the follicles of the peripheral lymphoid organs, including the spleen, lymph nodes, and Peyer patches, and the blood and lymph.[832] The CXCR5 chemokine receptor recognizes CXCL13, which is produced within the follicles and promotes entry into and retention by the follicle. Other B-cell functions that concurrently mature include a decreased tendency to undergo apoptosis after BCR engagement, an increased responsiveness to T-cell help (e.g., CD40 ligand and soluble cytokines, such as IL-21), increased expression of CD86, and maturation of intracellular signaling in response to BCR engagement. In addition to secondary lymphoid tissue, follicular B cells may also home to the perisinusoidal areas of bone marrow, which are also enriched in DCs that may provide important signals for B-cell survival.

Fetal and Neonatal B-Cell Frequency and Surface Phenotype

B cells expressing surface IgM are present by 10 weeks of gestation.[792] The frequency of B cells in tissues rapidly increases so that by 22 weeks of gestation, the proportion of B cells in the spleen, blood, and bone marrow is similar to that in the adult. The concentration of B cells in the circulation is higher during the second and third trimesters than at birth.[833] After birth, the concentration of B cells increases to peak levels between 6 to 12 months of age, followed by a gradual decrease throughout childhood and adolescence, until adult values are reached.[834]

Circulating neonatal B cells are highly enriched in the new emigrant cell subset[819] based on their IgM$^+$IgD$^+$ CD24$^+$CD38$^+$ABCB1$^-$ surface phenotype and high levels of CD5, CD10, and Ki67. Approximately 70% to 75% of cord blood B cells are new emigrants, the majority of which express CD21, which identifies a subset of these cells that are the least mature[835]; about 25% to 30% are fully naïve B cells.[819,836] CD27$^+$ B cells, which include most memory B cells in adults, are low to undetectable in cord blood,[834] consistent with the antigenic naiveté of the healthy newborn. Together, these findings account for earlier reports of higher levels of IgM, CD5, CD10, and CD38 surface expression and lower levels of CD11a, CD21, CD44, CD54 (ICAM-1), and L-selectin[75] by cord blood B cells than those of the adult circulation. Most fetal spleen B cells express CD5 and CD10,[837,838] indicating that new emigrant B cells predominate in the spleen. As for RTEs, the predominance of new emigrant B cells in the fetus and neonate is consistent with the likely high level of production of B cells at this age.

Unfractionated neonatal B cells and CD27$^-$/IgM$^+$ adult B cells of the circulation have similar levels of surface IgD, CD19, CD22, CD23, CD40, CD44, CD80, CD81, CD86, CCR6, and CXCR5,[75] but neonatal B cells may have modestly lower levels of CCR7.[839] Neonatal naïve B cells differ from their adult counterparts in having significantly lower expression of the IL-4 receptor α chain and responsiveness to IL-4 as assessed by tyrosine phosphorylation of STAT6.[840] However, the importance of this decreased expression is uncertain because IL-4 treated neonatal B cells that receive CD40 ligand stimulation are able to effectively undergo isotype switching to

IgE[841] (see "Isotype Switching and Immunoglobulin Production by Fetal and Neonatal B Cells").

Absolute B-cell numbers in the circulation double in the first 6 months of life from those at birth, and this is mainly due to expansion of fully mature naïve B cells and, to a lesser extent, transitional B cells.[842] After 6 months, there is a gradual decline to adult values, which is complete by adolescence. The frequency of new emigrant B cells in the circulation gradually declines with age.[834,842]

B-CELL ACTIVATION AND IMMUNE SELECTION

As with T cells, B cells receive additional regulatory signals from the engagement of surface molecules other than the BCR that act as either co-stimulatory or inhibitory molecules. Of the co-stimulatory molecules, a complex consisting of CD19, CD21, and CD81 is best defined. CD21, also known as complement receptor 2, binds the CD3d fragment of the C3 complement component. CD19 transmits intracellular activation signals after complement binding to CD21. Effective signaling after engagement of the BCR requires that key proximal signaling molecules are appropriately compartmentalized by means of lipid rafts, which are specialized cholesterol and glycosphingolipid microdomains of the plasma cell membrane.[843] In this context, CD81 may be particularly important for partitioning CD19/CD21/BCR complexes into lipid rafts so that antigen engagement will be effective for B-cell activation. Antigen-BCR interactions that are not accompanied by co-stimulation may result in B-cell death by autophagy rather than cell activation.[844]

The encounter of naïve B cells with antigen recognized by the sIg triggers their activation and proliferation under appropriate conditions. In contrast to αβ T cells, which recognize antigen in the form of processed fragments bound to the antigen-presenting grooves of MHC molecules, most B-cell sIgs recognize antigen in a nondenatured form so that antigen recognition is highly sensitive to any alterations in the three-dimensional shape, such as posttranslational modifications. Naïve B cells may encounter such nondenatured antigens presented by conventional DCs shortly after the B cell enters the lymph node or spleen via high endothelial venules before it enters the follicle. Alternatively, naïve B cells entering the follicle may have soluble antigens shuttled to them by other B cells or presented by follicular dendritic cells, a resident nonhematopoietic cell of the follicle. A specialized macrophage population of the subcapsular sinus of the lymph node may also present larger antigens, such as viruses, particulates, or immune complexes to B cells. The relative importance of these different mechanisms for antigen presentation to naïve B cells likely varies depending on the nature of the antigen and the sites at which it is acquired by APCs.[845]

B cells are activated to proliferate and differentiate into antibody-secreting cells after surface immunoglobulin (sIg) binds antigen. The sIg molecule is invariably associated with the nonpolymorphic membrane proteins, Ig-α (CD79a) and Ig-β (CD79b), which, in conjunction with sIg, constitute the BCR. Ig-α and Ig-β, which are structural and functional homologues of the CD3 complex proteins, are expressed as disulfide-linked heterodimers and contain immunoreceptor tyrosine-based activation motifs (ITAMs) in their cytoplasmic tails. ITAMs act as docking sites for signaling molecules, such as the Lyn and Syk tyrosine kinases, which comprise signaling pathways that ultimately alter gene transcription and initiate an activation program.[846] As with naïve T cells, activation of naïve B cells by BCR engagement has a relatively high signal threshold compared with that of memory cells, a feature that may prevent inappropriate activation by low-affinity self-antigens. This is followed by activation of the phospholipase C/protein kinase C, Ras, and alternative NF-κB/Rel pathways that ultimately alter gene transcription. The CD19 molecule also has a cytoplasmic domain that serves as a docking site for several tyrosine kinases that provide co-stimulation when the CD19/CD21 complex is engaged by complement fragments, such as C3d. Engagement of CD40 on the B cell by CD40 ligand on the CD4 T cell also contributes to activation by inducing the alternative NF-κB/Rel transcription factor pathway. In the case of protein antigens, BCR engagement is followed by antigen internalization and entry into the MHC class II antigen presentation pathway. Activation also increases B-cell expression of CCR7, which promotes B-cell movement toward the outer border of the T-cell zone, and of OX40 ligand (TNFSF4) and CD30 ligand (TNFSF8), each of which can provide T-cell co-stimulation.

Negative Regulation of B-Cell Signaling

As for T cells, the activation of B cells is tightly regulated, and several surface molecules provide inhibitory signals that ensure that full activation requires overcoming a high signaling threshold, thereby limiting the risk of activation by low affinity autoantigens. These include CD22 and CD72, both of which contain intracellular immunoreceptor tyrosine-based inhibition motifs (ITIMs) that, when phosphorylated, recruit tyrosine phosphatases, such as SHP-1 and SHP-2, and inositol phosphatases, such as SHIP-1, that limit B-cell activation signals via the BCR and co-stimulatory molecules, such as CD21. In addition, B cells express FcRγIIb, an ITIM-containing Fc receptor that mediates negative signaling when antibody simultaneously engages this receptor via its Fc moiety and binds to antigen on the BCR surface.[847] Surface expression of FcγRIIb is reduced on neonatal B cells,[848] possibly rendering them less subject to the inhibitory effect of antigen-antibody complexes.

CD4 T-Cell Help for Naïve B-Cell Activation

For B cells to be activated effectively and to produce antibody against protein and protein-carbohydrate conjugate antigens requires help from CD4 T cells in most cases. This help is in the form of soluble cytokines, such as IL-21, and of cell surface–associated signals, such as CD40 ligand, which is transiently expressed on the surface of activated CD4 T cells.[849] In T-cell–dependent activation, antigenically naïve CD4 T cells probably are first activated by DCs independently of B cells. CD4 T cells that are activated by DCs bearing antigenic peptide–MHC class II complexes and CD80-CD86 co-stimulatory molecules express CD40 ligand, OX40, ICOS, and CXCR5. These activated CD4 T cells may either leave the lymphoid organ to become effector or memory T cells of the various subsets, for instance, Th1, Th2, or Th17, or Tregs, or become TFH cells that are specialized to provide help to B cells in the follicle. In humans, the generation of TFH cells from naïve CD4 T cells is favored by exposure to DC-derived cytokines, such as IL-12p70, which induces the expression of CXCR5, ICOS, IL-21, and Bcl6.[526,850] This CXCR5 expression promotes movement of these CD4 T cells to the outer border of the T-cell zone, to contact antigen-activated B cells at the edge of the follicular zone. Here, CD4 T-cell activation is reinforced by recognition of antigenic peptides displayed on MHC class II molecules of the B cell, and the interaction between ICOS on the T cell with ICOS ligand on the B cells maintains TFH-cell differentiation. These CXCR5^{hi} CD4 T cells then enter into the follicle, where they provide help to B cells as TFH cells by expressing CD40 ligand, secreting IL-21 and other cytokines, and providing ICOS-dependent B-cell co-stimulation. As discussed earlier in the T-cell section CD40 Ligand, surface levels of CD40 ligand by circulating neonatal CD4 T cells are reduced compared with that by naïve adult CD4 T cells. Although this reduction could limit B-cell help for antibody responses, it is unclear if such reductions apply to TFH cells of the neonate and infant in vivo.

B-Cell Selection in Germinal Centers of the Follicle

During the initial immune response, most antigenically naïve follicular B cells are derived from clones expressing antibody variable regions with relatively low affinity for antigen. As in the case of the TCR, activation through the BCR is also not necessarily an all-or-none phenomenon. For example, high-affinity binding to IgM of the BCR may allow B-cell proliferation to occur in the absence of any T-cell help, whereas lower-affinity binding may result in proliferation only in the presence of additional T-cell–derived signals. Antigen-specific B cells that proliferate strongly within the B-cell follicle lead to the formation of germinal centers. The more avidly the B cell binds antigen, the stronger is the stimulus to proliferate. One major source of antigen for triggering the extensive B-cell proliferation of the germinal center may be provided by antigen complexed with antibody bound to Fc receptors on follicular DCs, The follicular DC is a nonhematopoietic cell type that appears to have the unusual capacity to bind antigen-antibody complexes for long periods on their cell surface. As already noted, follicular B cells may also receive antigen from other B cells that enter into the follicle or by their interactions with DCs upon entry into the lymph node from the circulation or with macrophages of the subcapsular sinus.[845] True germinal centers in the spleen and lymph nodes are absent during fetal life but appear during the first months after postnatal antigenic stimulation.[851]

Somatic Hypermutation

Immunoglobulin variants are generated among germinal center B cells by the process of somatic hypermutation, in which immunoglobulin genes accumulate apparently random point mutations within productively rearranged V, D, and J segments.[852] These variants undergo a selection process favoring B cells that bear sIg with high affinity for antigen. Such high-affinity immunoglobulin provides high levels of BCR signaling, favoring germinal center B-cell survival rather than a default pathway of apoptosis. Somatic hypermutation requires activation-induced cytidine deaminase (AID), which appears to be expressed only by germinal center B cells,[853] and error-prone DNA polymerases.[854] AID deaminates deoxycytidine residues in single-stranded DNA to deoxyuridines, which are processed by DNA replication, base excision, or mismatch repair to restore normal base pairing between the two DNA strands, resulting in somatic hypermutation. The effects of the mutator are focused on the variable region of immunoglobulin and its immediate flanking sequences. The peak of somatic mutation is approximately 10 to 12 days after immunization with a protein antigen. Somatic mutation is an important means for increasing antibody affinity, but it may also result in the acquisition of autoimmunity. Thus human B cells with newly acquired autoreactivity as a result of somatic mutation are not subject to receptor editing or other tolerance mechanisms.

Most neonatal and fetal immunoglobulin heavy chain gene variable regions appear not to have undergone somatic mutation,[806,808] consistent with the predominance of antigenically-naïve new emigrant B cells in the fetus and neonate. By contrast, somatic mutations are detectable in some neonatal B cells expressing IgG or IgA transcripts,[812] and the mutational frequency per length of DNA is similar to that of adult B cells. In contrast to follicular B cells, in which somatic hypermutation appears to occur only in germinal centers, a subset of IgM$^+$IgD$^+$CD27$^+$ B cells found in cord blood and in the fetal spleen demonstrate somatic hypermutation before the general appearance of germinal centers.[855] In this context, extrafollicular somatic hypermutation appears to serve as a means to broaden the preimmune immunoglobulin repertoire of this B-cell subset. This early competency for somatic hypermutation by fetal B cells is supported by the similar ability of cord blood and adult peripheral blood B cells to increase expression of AID and error-prone polymerases in response to BCR engagement.[854]

MEMORY B CELLS

Most memory B cells are CD27$^+$ and express surface immunoglobulins other than IgM, for instance, IgG or IgA, as a result of having undergone immunoglobulin isotype switching,[856] a process that is described below. However, a recent study examining memory B-cell populations in adult peripheral blood for their surface phenotype, replication history (based on KREC content), and immunoglobulin somatic hypermutation has concluded that there are five distinct subsets, which originate from three different pathways[857]: Three subsets that are generated in germinal center responses include (1) CD27$^+$ cells that IgM$^-$ and are either IgG$^+$ or IgA$^+$, which are the predominant phenotype of circulating memory B cells in the adult and are derived from consecutive germinal center reactions; (2) CD27$^+$ cells that are IgM$^+$(IgD$^-$), which are derived from primary germinal center reactions; and (3) CD27$^-$IgG$^+$ cells, which are about 25% of the circulating IgG$^+$ B cells in adults[858] and which demonstrate that CD27 is not an invariant marker for memory B cells in humans. The two memory cell subsets that are not germinal center–dependent, as indicated by their presence in CD40 or CD40 ligand–deficient patients, are (1) CD27$^+$IgM$^+$IgD$^+$ cells, which are prominent in systemic immune responses involving the marginal zone of the spleen (see "The Marginal Zone and Marginal Zone B Cells") and (2) CD27$^-$IgA$^+$ cells, which may be derived from local responses, particularly in the gut. These germinal center–independent responses are discussed later.

Germinal center B cells that receive appropriate survival signals leave the germinal center to persist as memory B cells. Most follicular memory B cells are $CD27^{hi}$ and have undergone isotype switching so that they are IgM^-IgD^-. They also lack the ABCB1 naïve B-cell marker.[819] The turnover of memory B cells is approximately fivefold higher than naïve B cells, based on their high levels of labeling in vivo and expression of the Ki67 antigen. Germinal center–derived memory B cells of the $CD27^-IgG^+$ subset are $ABCB1^-$ cells and express BCRs that have mainly undergone isotype switching to IgG1 or IgG3 but not to IgG2.[819] Human memory B cells are also heterogeneous in their expression of CD19, CD21, CD24, CD25, CD38, and FcRH4 (an inhibitory receptor), and these markers can be used to define additional memory B-cell subsets,[859] which are not considered here.

The engagement of CD40 on germinal center B cells by CD40 ligand on T cells is absolutely required for germinal center–dependent memory B-cell generation. Efficient memory B-cell generation requires the binding by CD21 on B cells of C3 complement components, such as C3d. Memory B cells enter the recirculating lymphocyte pool, where they preferentially colonize the skin and mucosa, sites that are likely to have direct contact with antigen. Once memory B cells are generated, they appear to persist indefinitely even in the absence of any subsequent exposure to the inciting antigen.[860] $CD27^+$ memory B cells that are dependent on germinal centers for their formation, that is, the $CD27^+IgG^+$, $CD27^+IgA^+$, and $CD27^+IgM^+IgD^-$ B-cell subsets, are typically not detectable in the circulation of the healthy fetus or neonate,[834] consistent with limited B-cell exposure to foreign antigens in utero. About 1% of cord blood B cells have a $CD27^-IgG^+$ memory cell phenotype, and the frequency of this phenotype increases with postnatal age, although there is wide individual variation.[834] Whether the neonatal $CD27^-IgG^+$ memory B-cell subset is similar to that of adults[857] in its germinal center dependence and in having somatic hypermutation of its immunoglobulin genes is unclear.

B CELLS AS ANTIGEN-PRESENTING CELLS

B cells express all of the proteins of the MHC class II antigen presentation pathway and can serve as APCs to CD4 T cells. Memory B cells are probably more effective than antigenically naïve B cells in simulating CD4 T cells because they constitutively express higher surface levels of CD80 or CD86 molecules that provide T cell co-stimulation. Interactions between ICOS on the T cell and ICOS ligand on the B cell may also be essential for inducing and maintaining TFH differentiation.[515] The preferential source of protein for antigenic peptides presented to T cells by B cells probably is sIg-protein complexes internalized from the cell surface. The internalized proteins are degraded to peptides that can then be presented back on the B-cell surface bound to MHC class II molecules. Because the sIg-antigen interaction is of high affinity, B-cell antigen presentation theoretically permits CD4 T cells to be activated at relatively low concentrations of antigen.

Circulating neonatal B cells have lower levels of MHC class II than those observed for adult splenic B cells but proliferate at least as well as adult splenic B cells after MHC class II engagement.[861] Moreover, circulating third-trimester fetal and adult B cells were recently reported to express similar amounts of MHC class II.[862] However, there is limited information as to the capacity of fetal and neonatal B cells to serve as APCs for CD4 T cells.

SWITCHING OF IMMUNOGLOBULIN ISOTYPE AND CLASS AND ANTIBODY PRODUCTION

Isotype Switching

Human B cells produce five isotypes of antibody: IgM, IgD, IgG, IgA, and IgE. The IgG and IgA isotypes can be, respectively, divided into the IgA1 and IgA2 and the IgG1, IgG2, IgG3, and IgG4 subclasses. During their process of differentiation into plasma cells, B cells are able to change from IgM to other antibody isotypes without changing antigen specificity (see Fig. 4-8). With the exception of IgD expression, this switching usually involves isotype recombination, the genetic replacement of the IgM-specific portion of the constant region ($C\mu$) of the heavy chain with a new isotype-specific gene segment. As in V(D)J recombination, the intervening DNA is excised as a large circle. Isotype recombination is mediated by switch regions that are positioned immediately upstream of each of the isotype-specific C regions, with the exception of IgD. Successive multiple isotype switching by a single B cell also can occur, for example, IgM to IgA to IgG to IgE.

Genetic studies of the hyper-IgM syndrome, in which there is a generalized block in isotype switching from IgM to other isotypes, have revealed that the process requires interactions between CD40 ligand on the T cell and CD40 on the B cell, the AID gene product (which also is required for somatic hypermutation), and the uracil *N*-glycolyase (UNG) enzyme.[853] There are also CD40-independent signals for such switching, such as provided by TLR9 found in the B-cell endosomal compartment binding to unmethylated CpG DNA, for instance, derived from bacteria or viruses. The molecular biology of switch recombination, like V(D)J recombination, involves double-stranded DNA breaks, in this case, induced by the sequential action of AID, UNG, and an apurinic/apryimidinic endonuclease rather than the RAG proteins. These breaks are repaired by the NHEJ proteins involved in V(D)J recombination[798] as well as additional proteins.[853] Secreted cytokines derived from T cells or other cell types play an important role in promoting or inhibiting switching to a specific isotype. For example, IL-4 or IL-13 is absolutely required for isotype switching to IgE, a process that can be inhibited by the presence of IFN-γ. In some instances, hormones also may play a role in isotype switching. For example, vasoactive intestinal peptide in conjunction with CD40 engagement can induce human B cells to produce high levels of IgA1 and IgA2.[863] Also, murine studies indicate that vitamin A metabolites, such as all-trans–retinoic acid secreted by DCs, may promote B-cell isotype switching to IgA.[864]

CD4 T-cell and CD40-ligand–independent isotype switching to IgA mediated by two other members of the TNF ligand superfamily—APRIL (a proliferation-inducing ligand) and BAFF (B-cell activator factor) —has also been described in mice and likely also applies to humans.[865] These cell surface proteins, which are expressed by a variety of cell types, including intestinal epithelium, may play an important role in the development of IgA plasma cells in the gut in response to commensal bacteria.[866]

During a primary immune response, isotype switching by B cells appears to occur shortly after these cells enter into the follicle.[867] These B cells may have received the requisite T-cell–derived signals (i.e., cytokines and CD40 ligand) during their interaction with T cells at the border between the follicle and T-cell zones. Switch recombination after primary immunization is evident in peripheral lymphoid tissue 4 days after immunization with protein antigen and peaks between 10 and 18 days.[868] Switch recombination also is triggered during memory B-cell responses, is detectable within 24 hours of secondary immunization, and peaks between 3 and 4 days.[869]

Generation of Plasma Cells and the Molecular Basis for Immunoglobulin Secretion

Some activated B cells become plasmablasts and migrate to extrafollicular regions of the lymph node or spleen, where they become short-lived plasma cells that mainly produce IgM. Differentiation of these plasma cells does not require and may be inhibited by the CD40 ligand–CD40 interaction. In the absence of CD40 engagement, germinal center B cells that have survived the selection process probably differentiate to memory B cell populations. Memory B cells appear to have a low threshold to become relatively long-lived plasma cells in an antigen-dependent manner, and this antigen-dependent conversion, as well as antigen-independent division within the memory B-cell pool, appears to account for the typically lifelong maintenance of serologic (antibody) memory in humans after natural infection.[860] In this case, the level of memory B cells attained after infection or vaccination would be the main determinant of antibody levels. Human memory B cells can differentiate into plasma cells in response to antigen-independent mechanisms, such as exposure to oligonucleotides containing unmethylated CpG DNA or activated T cells. Such polyclonal activation of memory B cells has been proposed to maintain levels of specific antibody for a lifetime once a memory B-cell response has been generated.[860]

Plasma-cell differentiation in humans is potently induced by IL-21 derived from TFH cells and potentially other cellular sources.[870] Plasma-cell generation from B cells involves the downregulation of the Bcl6 protein and the upregulation of the BLIMP-1 (B-lymphocyte–induced maturation protein-1) and X box–binding protein 1 (XBP1) transcription factors. XBP1 drives B cell differentiation into a fully mature plasma cell that is capable of extremely high levels of antibody production. The membrane-bound form of immunoglobulin is slightly longer than the secreted form and contains a carboxy-terminal region that anchors the molecule in the cell membrane. Plasma-cell differentiation results in switch to a secretory form of immunoglobulin that lacks this membrane-anchoring segment and the loss of sIg expression as a result of a change in splicing of the heavy chain mRNA. Plasma cells, rather than mature B cells, account for most of the secreted antibody during both primary and secondary immune responses.

B-cell differentiation into plasma cells is also likely accompanied by increases in CXCR4 expression, which helps target these cells to niches in the bone marrow containing stromal cells that secrete the CXCR4 ligand CXCL12 (SDF-1). Plasma cells are concentrated in peripheral lymphoid tissue, liver, and bone marrow, as well as in lymphoid tissue of the gastrointestinal and respiratory tracts.

Isotype Switching and Immunoglobulin Production by Fetal and Neonatal B Cells

Early in vitro studies of neonatal immunoglobulin production used pokeweed mitogen (PWM), a polyclonal activator of both T and B cells. In this system, immunoglobulin production was low compared with that in adults, and mixing experiments suggested that neonatal T cells acted as suppressors of immunoglobulin production by either adult or neonatal B cells. Further fractionation of the T-cell populations in this assay suggested that in the absence of memory/effector T cells, antigenically naïve ($CD45RA^{hi}CD45RO^{lo}$) $CD4^+$ T cells of either the neonate or the adult acted as suppressors of antibody production.[871] The relevance of the suppression to neonatal B-cell responses in vivo remains unclear, however. In any case, priming of neonatal or adult antigenically naïve CD4 T cells in vitro resulted in their acquisition of a $CD45RA^{lo}CD45RO^{hi}$ phenotype and, concurrently, an ability to enhance rather than suppress PWM-induced immunoglobulin production.[871] This increased capacity for B-cell help probably reflects the fact that priming of naïve T cells enhances expression of CD40 ligand and cytokines needed for T-cell–dependent help for B-cell responses.

When B cells are activated by exogenous cytokines (e.g., IL-4, IL-10, or cytokine-containing supernatants from activated T cells) and a cellular source of CD40 ligand (e.g., CD40 ligand–expressing fibroblasts) or EBV infection, neonatal B-cell production of IgM, IgG1, IgG2, IgG3, IgG4, and IgE is similar to that in adult antigenically naïve B cells.[75] This is not unexpected because neonatal B cells are highly enriched in new emigrant B cells,[819,821,822,836] and this B-cell subset in adults and fully mature naïve B cells are similarly efficient in undergoing isotype switching and secreting switched antibody[836]; neonatal B cells treated under these conditions also have robust signaling based on tyrosine phosphorylation of STAT6 by IL-4 and of STAT3 by IL-21 and secrete high levels of IgE.[841]

Isotype switching is associated with cell division, and neonatal and adult B cells demonstrate a similar acquisition of switching beginning after the third cell division.[872] Pre–B cells have the capacity for isotype switching even during fetal ontogeny: For example, isotype switching to IgE and IgG4 by fetal B and pre–B cells at 12 weeks of gestation can be induced in vitro.[873] IgA1 and IgA2 are produced in similar amounts by antigenically naïve fetal and adult B cells on stimulation with anti-CD40 antibody and vasoactive intestinal peptide hormone. Fetal pre–B cells also can synthesize IgA under these conditions.[874] When human fetal or neonatal B cells develop in, or are adoptively transferred into, SCID mice, they are capable of isotype switching and immunoglobulin production if appropriate T-cell–derived signals are present.[723,875,876]

Other studies, however, suggest that isotype switching and antibody production by fetal and neonatal B cells is limited compared with these processes in antigenically naïve (IgM^+IgD^+) adult B cells. Durandy and colleagues[564] found that IgM, IgG, and IgE production by fetal B cells at midgestation was substantially lower than that of neonatal or adult B cells, suggesting an intrinsic hyporesponsiveness to CD40 or cytokine receptor engagement, or both. Neonatal B cells produce substantially less IgA than do adult naïve B cells in the presence of adult T cells stimulated by anti-CD3 mAb (as a source of CD40 ligand) and exogenous cytokines, such as IL-10.[877] These limitations of fetal and neonatal isotype switching and antibody production probably reflect intrinsic limitations of B-cell function, particularly when T-cell help may be limited. Such limited production is not due to decreased activation or proliferation because neonatal B cells proliferate normally in response to engagement of CD40 or surface IgM, or both.[878]

Neonatal T cells activated for a few hours provide less help for neonatal B-cell immunoglobulin production and isotype switching than do similarly treated adult T cells.[566] Because this help probably is through CD40 ligand, reduced expression of CD40 ligand (or similar activation-induced molecules) by naïve neonatal T cells in the first few hours after activation may limit fetal and neonatal B-cell immune responses. More prolonged activation of neonatal CD4 T cells results in a cell population that is able to provide help for neonatal B cells,[871] and it is likely that this increase in helper function is due to increased CD40 ligand. Whether decreased neonatal DC function also contributes to diminished B-cell responses has not been determined.

Between 8 and 11 weeks of gestation, transcripts for IgA and IgG can be detected in the liver,[879] and IgM and IgG synthesis have been detected as early as 12 weeks of gestation in fetal organ cultures.[880] By 16 weeks of gestation, fetal bone marrow B cells expressing sIg of all heavy chain isotypes are detectable.[881] Immunoglobulin-secreting plasma cells are detectable by week 15 of gestation, and those secreting IgG and IgA by 20 and 30 weeks of gestation, respectively.[882] The stimulus for isotype switching during fetal development remains unclear because in the adult, isotype switching typically occurs in response to B-cell activation by foreign protein antigens. These findings in bone marrow contrast with a flow cytometric study in which nonspecific binding was carefully excluded, and neonatal B cells expressing surface IgG or IgA were below the limit of detectability (i.e., <1% of circulating B cells).[883]

In general, neonatal B cells can differentiate into IgM-secreting plasma cells as efficiently as adult cells. However, TD immunoglobulin production by neonatal B cells is more readily inhibited by agents that raise intracellular cyclic adenosine monophosphate (cAMP), such as prostaglandin E2.[884]

IgA plasma cells are largely absent from the infant intestine until after 1 month of age, and their subsequent appearance coincides with increased expression of APRIL and its receptors within isolated lymphoid follicles of the gut.[865] In contrast, CD40 ligand and CD40 expression were expressed within isolated lymphoid follicles before 1 month. Collectively, this suggests that isotype switching to IgA in the infant intestine occurs postnatally and may be driven by an APRIL-dependent process rather than by CD4 T-cell–derived CD40 ligand. In mice, this APRIL-dependent CD40 ligand–independent pathway for the development of IgA plasma cells in the gut is induced by commensal bacteria,[866] and it is likely that the postnatal acquisition of commensal bacteria plays a similar role in humans.

THE MARGINAL ZONE AND MARGINAL ZONE B CELLS

The human spleen has distinct anatomic sites that may play specialized roles in the production of antibody against blood-derived particulate antigens and purified repetitive carbohydrate antigens. Important examples of such carbohydrate antigens are the capsular polysaccharides of pathogenic bacteria, such as *Streptococcus pneumoniae, Neisseria meningitidis,* and *Haemophilus influenzae.* Antigens and leukocytes enter the spleen through vascular sinusoids located in the red pulp that are in proximity to the marginal zone (MZ) area. The white pulp area contains periarteriolar sheaths of lymphocytes, mainly T cells, as well as periarteriolar follicles, which are mainly B cells. These, in turn, are surrounded by the MZ, which contains loose clusters of B cells, DCs, macrophages, and some CD4 T cells, and that are in close contact with the blood; neutrophils may also be a normal cellular component of the human MZ,[885] although this remains controversial.

B cells of the human MZ of the adult spleen are predominantly CD27$^+$IgM$^+$IgD$^+$ and, in contrast to murine B cells found in the MZ, have BCRs encoded by somatically mutated immunoglobulin genes.[885] These CD27$^+$IgM$^+$IgD$^+$ B cells, which also express CD1c and CD21 but not CD23, are hereafter referred to as MZ B cells. Although it is possible that in adults a fraction of this cell population may be germinal center–derived,[886] most of these germinal cell–dependent cells are probably contained within the CD27$^+$IgM$^+$IgD$^-$ subset (see "Memory B Cells"). MZ B cells are of interest because they appear to mediate most of the IgM antibody response to unconjugated polysaccharides,[887] which are T-cell–independent type II antigens. In contrast to the murine MZ B cells, which appear not to recirculate once they arise in the spleen from new emigrant B cells, human B cells with this marginal zone phenotype are found in substantial numbers in the human adult circulation, the inner wall of the subcapsular sinus of lymph nodes, the epithelium of tonsillar crypts, and the subepithelial dome of intestinal Peyer patches.[885] Also based on murine studies, somatic hypermutation was formally thought to be limited to B cells undergoing activation in germinal centers. However, human MZ B cells retain their somatic hypermutated immunoglobulin receptors in genetic disorders that prevent germinal center formation, such as deficiency of CD40, CD40 ligand, ICOS, and SH2D1A (SAP),[490] strongly arguing for the existence of a germinal center–independent pathway. The tissue microenvironment in which such germinal center–independent somatic hypermutation by MZ B cells occurs remains unclear.

MZ B cells have unique phenotypic and functional properties that may be important in their rapidly producing IgM in response to bloodborne particulate antigens, such as bacteria, in addition to their having direct access to the blood and to circulating DCs that may bear these antigens. Compared with naïve follicular B cells, MZ zone B cells express higher levels of CD21, which may facilitate the binding of C3d-coated bloodborne antigens, such as encapsulated bacteria.[888] MZ B cells are also more readily activated by non-BCR signals, such as through TLRs, and more rapidly become effector cells than naïve follicular B cells after activation. This enhanced reactivity may be important in their being able to respond to purified polysaccharide antigens in the absence of T-cell–derived signals.[889] MZ B cells also appear "poised" to rapidly differentiate into IgM$^+$ plasmablasts because of their constitutive expression of B-lymphocyte–induced maturation protein-1 (BLIMP-1), which promotes plasma-cell differentiation.[890]

The hyposplenic or asplenic state invariably compromises the human antibody response to purified polysaccharides, such as capsular polysaccharide components of the 23-valent pneumococcal vaccine. Splenic MZ B cells may be required for the generation of antibody responses to purified polysaccharide antigens, accounting for the loss of these responses with splenectomy. However, this could also be due to the removal of other cell types and/or a specialized splenic microenvironment required for the response to purified polysaccharide antigens. This immune response does not absolutely require T-cell help (see section Response to T-Cell–Independent Antigens). Immunization with T-cell–independent antigens before human splenectomy maintains the capacity of the immune system to respond to these antigens subsequently.[891] This finding suggests that the activation of splenic B cells recognizing polysaccharide antigens may result in their migration and persistence in other lymphoid organs. The pathways by which capsular polysaccharide antigens reach the MZ are unknown, and the role that human MZ DCs, macrophages, or neutrophils play in activating MZ B cells to produce antibody to purified polysaccharides remains poorly understood. How human splenic MZ B cells involved in the response to purified polysaccharide antigens differentiate from naïve precursors, presumably transitional B cells,[885] also remains unclear.

Recent work suggests that MZ B cells can also undergo substantial amounts of switch recombination in response to either T-cell–independent or T-cell–dependent antigens that engage their BCR. In the case of TI switching, macrophages, DCs, sinus lining cells, and, possibly, neutrophils, that inhabit the MZ secrete BAFF and APRIL, which bind to TACI (transmembrane activator and CAML interactor), a specific receptor that is expressed at high levels by MZ B cells. This binding results in the induction of isotype switching by a TLR-like pathway that involves MyD88 and other components of TLR signaling. This BAFF/APRIL-mediated switching pathway works cooperatively with the engagement of TLR ligands and, in the case of T-cell–dependent pathways, with CD40 signals.[885]

Marginal Zone B Cells of the Fetus and Neonate

Circulating MZ B cells are detectable at birth in relatively low numbers and gradually increase to adult levels by approximately 2 to 3 years of age.[834] Of interest, these MZ B cells have a diverse immunoglobulin repertoire similar to that of conventional naïve B cells rather than a more skewed repertoire typical for memory B cells that have undergone isotype switching. Together, these observations argue that IgM$^+$IgD$^+$CD27$^+$ B cells are distinct from conventional follicular B cells in that somatic hypermutation occurs outside of germinal centers and generates mutated immunoglobulin sequence as part of preimmune mechanism. Consistent with this idea, CD27$^+$IgM$^+$IgD$^+$ B cells with somatically mutated immunoglobulin genes are detectable in the circulation, liver, mesenteric lymph nodes, spleen, and bone marrow as early as 14 weeks of gestation,[855] even though germinal centers and presumably antigen exposure are absent until after birth. Somatic hypermutation of this fetal B-cell population may occur in the mesenteric lymph nodes and liver because cells in these tissues express the AID enzyme required for this process, whereas fetal spleen tissue does not. The somatic hypermutation does not appear to require T-cell help because it occurs normally in human CD27$^+$IgM$^+$IgD$^+$ B cells developing from human hematopoietic stem cells in RAG2/common gamma-chain knockout nude mice, which lack T cells.[855]

Although the marginal zone of the spleen does not achieve its mature configuration until about 2 years of age, CD27$^+$IgM$^+$IgD$^+$ B cells have been identified in the marginal zone as early as 8 months of age.[892] Thus, if the CD27$^+$IgM$^+$IgD$^+$ MZ B-cell population is required for the responses to unconjugated polysaccharides, the inability of infants less than 2 years of age to respond to such vaccines is not accounted for by an absence of this splenic B-cell subset. Rather, the deficiency is likely to be due at least in part to a qualitative defect in this CD27$^+$IgM$^+$IgD$^+$ B-cell subset or in the other cells involved in its activation, such as the macrophages, DCs, lining cells, or, possibly, neutrophils, of the MZ. One such factor may be the reduced expression on B cells from preterm and, to a lesser degree, term neonates of receptors for the BAFF and APRIL, such as TACI.[893] However, it is unclear whether this observation also applies to MZ B-cell subset of neonates.

B-1 CELLS AND NATURAL IMMUNOGLOBULIN M

In mice, a B-cell subset that has been termed B-1 has a distinct tissue distribution restricted largely to the peritoneal and pleural cavities and special functional features, such as a tendency for polyreactive antibody specificities, particularly of the IgM isotype, compared with the bulk of B cells, which are termed B-2. Murine naïve B-1 cells and MZ B cells both are important contributors to the early and rapid production of IgM in response to bloodborne particulate antigens and to other T-cell–independent antigens.[894] Murine B-1 cells are commonly reactive with both self-antigens, such as DNA, and foreign antigens, such as viral proteins or bacteria-derived products, such as phosphorylcholine, and they also appear to be essential for the production of natural antibodies that provide protection against encapsulated bacteria and for the antibody response to unconjugated polysaccharides. In mice, B-1 cells constitute the major source of the low amounts of circulating "natural" IgM present at birth and produced in the absence of antigenic stimulation, and animals lacking the ability to secrete natural IgM have an increased susceptibility to acute peritonitis from endogenous bacteria. Although natural IgM antibodies are of low affinity, they can activate complement, which may allow antigenically naïve B cells to become activated as a result of receiving co-stimulation via CD21 (complement receptor 2). In addition to their role in host defense, natural IgM antibodies may also play a role in removing apoptotic cells.[804]

One group has recently identified human B-1 cells as having a CD20$^+$CD27$^+$CD43$^+$CD70$^-$ surface phenotype,[895] which constitutes 3% to 11% of cord blood B cells. These cells, which are hereafter referred to as putative human B-1 cells, were similar to murine B-1 cells in their greater tendency to spontaneously express IgM, efficiently stimulate allogeneic T cells in culture, and to be activated in response to a tyrosine phosphatase inhibitor (vanadate), compared with either naïve B cells or memory B cells.[895] In this study, CD43 expression was used to distinguish putative B-1 cells in cord blood and adult peripheral blood from $CD27^+$ B-cell populations, including MZ B cells.[895] Unlike MZ B cells of cord blood, putative B-1 cells had very low levels of somatic hypermutation, suggesting that they constitute two distinct $CD27^+$ B-cell populations in cord blood. However, to the best of our knowledge, a direct comparison of MZ B cells and B-1 cells in the functional assays described above has not been performed. Putative B-1 cells have been reported to constitute 90% of $CD27^+$ B cells in cord blood, with their frequency gradually declining to approximately 40% in the adult circulation.[895] About 10% of putative B-1 cells in cord blood and adult peripheral blood are $CD11b^+$, and this subset, which is more effective than the $CD11b^-$ subset in allogeneic stimulation of T cells, is markedly increased in the circulation of patients with systemic lupus erythematosus.[896]

A recent study of the B-cell responses of nonhuman primates (NHPs) to immunization with a T-cell–independent type II antigen suggests that B-1 cells in primates and mice share a number of phenotypic and functional features.[897] Similar to murine peritoneal B-1 cells, a substantial fraction of B cells of the NHP peritoneum and omentum were $CD11b^+IgM^+CD27^{lo}$ and demonstrated constitutive activation of STAT3 and enrichment of BCR reactivity with phosphorylcholine.[897] After intravenous immunization with a T-cell–independent type II antigen, antigen-specific IgM^+ B cells with a $CD11b^+CD27^{hi}$ surface phenotype were detectable in the circulation for up to 3 weeks postvaccination. By 6 weeks after immunization, antigen-specific $CD11b^+$ B-1 cells with a $CD27^+IgM^+IgD^+$ surface phenotype were found in the spleen but not lymph nodes.[897] These findings suggest that in NHPs, and likely humans, B-1 cells found in peritoneum, omentum, and possibly other serosal sites may be activated by circulating T-cell–independent type II antigens, acquire CD27 expression, and enter the spleen, where they may persist as $CD27^+IgM^+IgD^+$ cells enriched for CD11b expression. Thus it is plausible that the $CD27^+IgM^+IgD^+$ B-cell population of the human spleen MZ is heterogeneous and may include previously activated B-1 cells. The relationship of these $CD11b^+$ B cell populations in NHPs with the previously discussed $CD11b^+$ subset of $CD20^+CD27^+CD43^+CD70^-$ putative B-1 cells in cord blood and adult peripheral blood[896] remains unclear.

It may be of interest in future studies to determine if CD11b expression by human splenic $CD27^+IgM^+IgD^+$ B cells enriches for B-1 cells, and if antigenically naïve ($CD27^-$) B-1 cells analogous to those found in NHPs can be identified in the human peritoneum and omentum. Because the study of NHPs also found that the numbers of $CD11b^+CD27^-$ peritoneal and omental tissue B-1 cells increased substantially between birth and 18 months of age,[897] it is plausible that a delayed appearance after birth of serosal human B-1 cells could contribute, at least in part, to limitations in the ability of the neonate and young infant to respond to T-cell–independent type II antigens (see "Response to T-Cell–Independent Antigens").

As discussed in the section "Immunoglobulin Synthesis by the Fetus and Neonate," total circulating IgM concentrations are very low in the fetus and healthy newborn. Nevertheless, antigen microarrays have revealed that most cord blood sera have IgM antibodies that react with multiple self-antigens, such as single-stranded DNA, whereas such reactivity is lacking in maternal IgM.[898,899] Some autoreactivity was observed with cord blood IgA, although to a much lesser degree than for IgM. The importance of natural IgM in human host defense in the fetus and neonate and its B-cell source are unclear.

REGULATORY B CELLS

Murine regulatory B cells, like Tregs, limit inflammation and autoimmunity, with those producing IL-10 (B10 cells) being the best characterized. Murine B10 cells produce IL-10 after strong stimulation, for instance, the combination of LPS, phorbol ester, and calcium ionophore, constitute about 1% to 3% of splenic B cells, and are enriched for a $CD1d^{hi}CD5^+CD19^{hi}$ surface phenotype.[900] However, this combination of markers is shared with multiple distinct B-cell subsets so that the precursor product relationship of B10 cells with other B-cell subsets remains unclear. Human B10 cells that can inhibit the in vitro activation of autologous T cells by an IL-10–dependent mechanism have been reported to be enriched in a subset of adult peripheral blood $CD19^+CD38^{hi}CD24^{hi}$ B cells.[901] This surface phenotype is shared with immature transitional B cells (see above section, "New Emigrant (Transitional) versus Fully Mature Naïve B Cells"), and it is unclear if B10 function is an intrinsic property of most transitional B cells or, alternatively, may be mediated by a distinct subset of $CD19^+CD38^{hi}CD24^{hi}$ cells that may or may not be a bona fide transitional population.[901] If B10 function is an intrinsic property of transitional B cells, then it is plausible that the high levels of transitional B cells in the fetus and young infant could limit B-cell–dependent activation of CD4 T cells in early life. Such an intrinsic property would account for the relatively high frequency (up to 7%) of cord blood B cells that can produce IL-10 after prolonged and strong stimulation, for instance, LPS and CD40 agonist, followed by phorbol ester and calcium ionophore, compared with adult peripheral blood B cells.[829] It would also account for the observation that IL-10 production by adult B cells stimulated under these conditions is contained mainly within cells having a transitional $CD19^+CD38^{hi}CD24^{hi}$ phenotype.[829] To the best of our knowledge, IL-10 production by human B cells directly ex vivo has not been demonstrated, except in one report where this was observed after hematopoietic stem cell transplantation using cord blood.[902] Thus the importance of B10 cells in regulating immunity in vivo in health remains unclear.

T-CELL–DEPENDENT AND T-CELL–INDEPENDENT RESPONSES BY B CELLS

Overview

The chronology of the response to different antigens differs, depending on the need for cognate T-cell help (Table 4-6). Largely on the basis of findings on murine studies, antigens can be divided into those dependent on a functional thymus and cognate help (direct cell-cell interactions) provided by mature αβ T cells (T-cell–dependent antigens [TD]) and those partially or completely independent of T-cell help

Table 4-6 Hierarchy of Antibody Responsiveness

Species	Type of Antigen	Examples of Antigen	Age at Onset of Antibody Response
Mouse	T-cell dependent	TNP-KLH	Birth
	T-cell independent type I	TNP–*Brucella abortus*	Birth
	T-cell independent type II	TNP-Ficoll	Delayed (2-3 wk of age)
Human	T-cell dependent	Tetanus toxoid, HBsAg, *Haemophilus influenzae* conjugate vaccine, bacteriophage ΦX174	Birth
	T-cell independent type I	TNP–*B. abortus*	Birth
	T-cell independent type II	Bacterial capsular polysaccharides (*H. influenzae* type b, *Neisseria meningitidis, Streptococcus pneumoniae,* GBS)	Delayed (6-24 mo of age)

GBS, Group B streptococci; *HBsAg,* hepatitis B surface antigen; *KLH,* keyhole limpet hemocyanin; *TNP,* trinitrophenol.

(T-cell–independent antigens [TI]). The TI antigens can be further divided into TI type I and TI type II, in accordance with their dependence on cytokines produced by T cells (or other cells).

Most proteins are TD antigens requiring cognate T-cell–B-cell interaction for production of antibodies (other than small amounts of IgM). The antibody response to TD antigens is characterized by the generation of memory B cells and long-lived plasma cells with somatically mutated, high-affinity immunoglobulin and the potential for isotype switching.

TI type I antigens are those that bind to B cells and directly activate them in vitro to produce antibody without T cells or exogenous cytokines. In the human, one such TI type I antigen is fixed *Brucella abortus*. TI type II antigens are mostly polysaccharides with multiple identical subunits and certain proteins that contain multiple determinants of identical or similar antigenic specificity. Responses to these antigens are enhanced in vitro and in vivo by cytokines, including IL-6, IL-12, IFN-γ, GM-CSF,[75] as well as BAFF and APRIL.[885] NK cells, T cells, NKT cells, macrophages, DCs, and, possibly, neutrophils may provide these cytokines. TI type II responses also are enhanced by bacterially derived TLR ligands, including lipopolysaccharide, lipoproteins, and unmethylated CpG DNA.[75,885] The response to TI type II antigens is characterized by the lack of B-cell memory and is restricted largely to the IgM and IgG2 isotypes.[903] The IgM response to TI type II antigens appears to be mediated mainly by MZ B cells, which have a high degree of somatic hypermutation of their immunoglobulin genes that appears to be generated before their encountering antigen. Immunization with TI type II antigens may result in the appearance of additional somatic hypermutation of the antibody produced by MZ B cells,[904] although whether this represents the expansion of previously mutated clones that were undetectable before immunization versus additional somatic hypermutation remains unclear. Such additional antigen-induced somatic hypermutation is a controversial mechanism because most studies have found that MZ B cells of the spleen and circulation have undetectable levels of the AID enzyme, which is absolutely required for somatic hypermutation.

Response to T-Cell Dependent Antigens

The capacity of the neonate to respond to TD antigens is well established at birth (see Table 4-6) and is only modestly reduced in comparison with the response in the adult. Any of several mechanisms, alone or in combination, may be responsible for this modest reduction: decreased DC interactions or interactions with CD4 T cells or B cells, limitations in CD4 T-cell activation and expansion into a T-helper/effector-cell population, impaired cognate interactions between CD4 T cells and B cells, or an intrinsic B-cell defect. Another possibility is that TD antigens preferentially upregulate CD22, which raises the threshold for B-cell activation, on neonatal compared with adult B cells.[905] Because neonatal B cells are highly enriched for the new emigrant subset, it is plausible that this subset may be less effective at responding to TD antigens than fully mature naïve B cells, which predominate in the nonmemory B-cell compartment of adults.

A study comparing the RSV F protein–specific heavy chain antibody responses in RSV-infected neonates and adults revealed a distinct use of variable heavy chain segments in the neonates, suggesting that there are major age-related differences in the selection of antibody specificities. Of importance, there was also significantly less somatic hypermutation of the immunoglobulin heavy chain gene and decreased N-nucleotide addition in the antibody response of neonates compared with adults. These differences would be expected to result in a relatively poor RSV-specific antibody response in the neonate and young infant. Whether isotype switching is limited in TD responses in the neonate in response to infection is less clear. Although this is plausible, given that CD40 ligand expression by activated neonatal CD4 T cells may be decreased,[564,566,568,906] studies are needed to determine if reductions in CD40 ligand expression by antigen-specific T cells also occurs in response to neonatal vaccination, and, if so, whether such reduced expression correlates with reduced memory B-cell development, decreased isotype switching, and somatic hypermutation. An additional factor that may contribute to the modest reduction in TD antibody production, is the reduced expression on B cells (nearly all of which are naïve $IgM^+IgD^+CD27^-$ follicular B cells) from preterm and, to a lesser degree, term neonates of the receptors for BAFF and APRIL; these receptors help promote TD differentiation into plasma cells, plasma cell survival,[893] and TI isotype switching.[885]

Response to T-Cell–Independent Antigens

Antibody production by human neonatal B cells to a TI type I antigen in vitro *(Brucella abortus)* is only modestly reduced[907] (see Table 4-6). This reduction may reflect a decreased ability of antigen-activated B cells to proliferate rather than a decreased precursor frequency of antigen-specific clones.[907]

In humans and mice, the response to TI type II antigens is the last to appear chronologically (see Table 4-6). This helps to account for the neonate's susceptibility to infection with encapsulated bacteria, such as GBS, and the poor response to polysaccharide antigens from other capsulated bacterial pathogens until approximately 2 to 3 years of age. The poor response in neonates is associated with their relatively low levels of circulating MZ ($IgM^+IgD^+CD27^+$) B cells, that are characteristically found in the MZ of the spleen and other extrafollicular sites, such as in the tonsil. However, recent studies have documented these cells in the MZ region of the spleen and blood in substantial numbers during the first 2 years of life, arguing that the poor response to TI type II antigens is not simply a quantitative defect of this B-cell subset. Rather, the decreased responses to TI type II antigens during early childhood probably reflect an intrinsic immaturity of $IgM^+IgD^+CD27^+$ B cells, perhaps including decreased expression of BAFF and APRIL receptors,[893] or decreased function of other cell types that support their differentiation and function.

Decreased expression of CD21 on neonatal B cells has been proposed as a possible mechanism for limitations in TI type II response in the neonate.[908,909] CD19 is expressed in association with CD21, the type 2 complement receptor, and serves to transduce B-cell–activating signals when CD21 is engaged by C3 complement components,[910] thereby inducing polysaccharide-reactive B cells to proliferate in vivo. Genetic disruption experiments in mice support the idea that the type 2 complement receptor, which includes CD21 and CD35 in mice, is important for TI type II antibody responses to pathogens, such as *Streptococcus pneumoniae*.[888] In vitro studies of human splenic tissue suggest that TI type II antigens activate complement and bind C3 and then localize to MZ splenic B cells expressing complement receptors.[903] However, whether $IgM^+IgD^+CD27^+$ B cells of the neonate and young infant have reduced CD21 expression compared with those of older children and adults remains unclear. Similarly, the degree to which reduced expression of receptors for BAFF and APRIL on neonatal B cells, particularly of those born prematurely, contributes to impaired TI type II antibody responses in human neonates is uncertain.

Dextran-conjugated antiimmunoglobulin mAbs have been used to mimic the events in TI type II antibody responses in vitro.[911] Human neonatal B cells proliferated to this stimulus as well as adult B cells, suggesting that the lack of the neonatal TI type II response is not due to an intrinsic limitation in their activation via sIg cross-linking.[912] B cells that respond to dextran-conjugated antiimmunoglobulin mAbs, however, may be enriched for B-cell types, such as new emigrant B cells and fully mature naïve B cells, that are functionally distinct from $IgM^+IgD^+CD27^+$ B cells that respond to polysaccharides or other TI type II antigens.

The response of human cord blood and adult peripheral blood B cells to CpG oligonucleotides is similar in terms of cell proliferation, the production of chemokines (CCL3 [MIP-1α] and CCL4 [MIP-1β]), and upregulation of CD86 and MHC class II expression.[839] This indicates that neonatal B-cell expression of TLR9 is similar to that of the adult and the TLR9 signaling pathway, which involves MyD88, is intact. These findings are consistent with a recent study[904] showing that new emigrant B cells of the adult and neonate express high levels of TLR9 and are capable of secreting IgM and IgG after stimulation with CpG oligonucleotides in the absence of added exogenous cytokines, including detectable levels of serotype-specific antipneumococcal polysaccharide IgM antibody. This stimulus also increases new emigrant B-cell expression of AID and BLIMP-1, consistent with the acquisition of the ability to secrete isotype-switched IgG, and the acquisition of a plasmablast surface phenotype by a substantial cell fraction.[904]

Of interest, some of these CpG oligonucleotides-stimulated new emigrant B cells of the neonate acquire a $CD27^+IgM^+$ surface phenotype reminiscent of the $IgM^+IgD^+CD27^+$ MZ B-cell subset of the spleen and circulation[904] (see above section on The Marginal Zone and Marginal Zone B Cells) These observations raise the possibility that new emigrant B cells in the neonate and young infant may give rise to the $IgM^+IgD^+CD27^+$ B-cell subset implicated in the IgM response to TI type II antigens, and that this maturation may be enhanced by exposure to bacterial-derived products, such as CpG-containing DNA, in an antigen-independent manner. Because a striking feature of the $IgM^+IgD^+CD27^+$ B-cell subset is its high degree of preimmune somatic hypermutation of the immunoglobulin genes, an analysis of the immunoglobulin repertoire of IgM^+CD27^+ B cells generated from adult or cord blood new emigrant B cells will be of interest in future studies. It is important to note that this hypothesized postnatal pathway for $IgM^+IgD^+CD27^+$ B-cell maturation is distinct from a pathway that is operative in the fetus in which these somatically hypermutated preimmune IgM^+ B cells are generated in a sterile environment.[855] The signals within the fetal microenvironment that drive this somatic hypermutation remain unclear. Finally, the TLR9 pathway also is capable of inducing naïve adult B cells to produce IL-12p70, a key cytokine for promoting Th1 differentiation and which also promotes TFH differentiation in humans, as discussed earlier, but it is unknown whether neonatal B cells are also capable of IL-12p70 production under these conditions.

SPECIFIC ANTIBODY RESPONSE BY THE FETUS TO MATERNAL IMMUNIZATION AND CONGENITAL INFECTION

Response to Fetal Immunization in Animal Models

Early studies by Silverstein and colleagues[913] of the antibody response of fetal sheep and rhesus monkeys to immunization with foreign proteins were conceptually important in establishing two major features of the ontogeny of B-cell immune competence for TD antigens in larger mammals. First, immune competence for TD antigens is established early during fetal ontogeny: Primary immunization of fetal rhesus monkeys between 103 and 127 days of gestation (out of a total of 160 days) with sheep red blood cells (SRBCs), a TD antigen, results in the formation of SRBC-reactive B cells in the spleen; reimmunization 3 weeks later results in a rapid antibody response using IgG. In fetal sheep, the antibody response to bacteriophage ΦX174 occurs as early as 40 days after conception,[914] and again, isotype switching is evident during the fetal response. Together, these findings suggest that the B-cell response to protein antigens, including isotype switching and, probably, memory-cell generation, are functional during fetal life. Second, these responses occur in a predictable, stepwise fashion for particular antigens. For example, in fetal sheep, the antibody response to keyhole limpet hemocyanin and lymphocytic choriomeningitis virus are first detectable at about 80 and 120 days, respectively, after conception.[914] These differences in the responsiveness to particular antigens are not explained by limitations in the repertoires of surface Ig or αβ-TCRs.

No correlation exists between the physical or chemical characteristics of particular antigens and their immunogenicity during ontogeny. For example, bacteriophage ΦX174 and bacteriophage T4 both are particulate antigens that should interact in a similar manner. In fetal sheep, however, bacteriophage T4 becomes immunogenic 60 days after ΦX174 does so. Baboon fetuses immunized with HBsAg vaccine have a robust IgG antibody response, and this response is boosted by postnatal immunization.[915]

Response to Maternal Immunization

In studies by one group of investigators, antibody responses by the human fetus may occur after maternal immunization with tetanus toxoid during the third trimester but not earlier, as shown by the presence of IgM tetanus antibodies at birth.[916,917] Whether tetanus-specific IgG responses at birth are reduced, as suggested by reports of reduced CD4 T-cell responses to tetanus vaccine in young infants,[758] remains unclear. Infants with tetanus-specific antibodies at birth had enhanced secondary antibody responses after tetanus immunization, indicating that fetal antigen exposure was a priming event rather than a tolerizing one.[916] By contrast, Englund and associates[733] were unable to demonstrate neonatal tetanus toxoid–specific IgM antibody or T-cell proliferation after maternal tetanus toxoid vaccination in the third trimester. Similarly, no fetal response to maternal immunization with inactivated trivalent influenza vaccine was noted.[733] However, one study found that maternal immunization with a split influenza vaccine during the second and third trimesters of pregnancy resulted in detectable IgM-specific responses to influenza proteins in cord blood.[732] If adequate fetal antibody responses to maternal vaccination with polysaccharide-protein conjugate vaccines occurred, such vaccines could be used during pregnancy to ensure that protective antibody levels were present at birth.

Response to Intrauterine Infection

Specific antibody may be present at birth to agents of intrauterine infection, including rubella virus, CMV, HSV, VZV, and *Toxoplasma gondii* and often can be used to diagnose congenital infection. Not all fetuses have an antibody response to intrauterine infection, however; specific IgM antibody was undetectable in 34% of infants with congenital rubella,[918] 19% to 33% of infants with congenital *Toxoplasma* infection,[919,920] and 11% of infants with congenital CMV infection.[921] When congenital infection is severe during the first or second trimester, antibody production may be delayed until late childhood.[922] This delay may reflect a lack of T-cell help, because antigen-specific T-cell responses often are reduced in parallel with B-cell responses.

Congenital *Toxoplasma* infection may lead to detectable IgE and IgA anti-*Toxoplasma* antibodies at birth or during early infancy.[923] Similarly, filaria- or schistosome-specific IgE is present in the sera of most newborns after maternal filiariasis or schistosomiasis.[924] Thus TD isotype switching and immunoglobulin production occurs during fetal life, at least for certain pathogens. In fact, with some infectious agents, such as *Toxoplasma*, IgA or IgE antibodies may be more sensitive than IgM antibodies for diagnosis of congenital infection. The titers of IgA and IgE anti-*Toxoplasma* antibodies may be lower at 20 to 30 weeks of gestation than after birth,[925-927] however, indicating that their production may be delayed in the context of congenital infection.

POSTNATAL SPECIFIC ANTIBODY RESPONSES

Specific Antibody Responses by the Neonate and Young Infant to Protein Antigens

Immunization of neonates usually elicits or at least primes for a protective response to protein antigens, including tetanus and diphtheria toxoids,[928] OPV,[929] *Salmonella* flagellar antigen,[930,931] bacteriophage ΦX174,[932] and HBsAg (with hepatitis B vaccine).[933] The response to some vaccines, however, may be less vigorous in the neonate than in older children or adults. A diminished primary response to recombinant hepatitis B vaccine has been noted in term neonates lacking maternally derived HBsAg antibody, compared with that in unimmunized children and adults.[933,934] The ultimate anti-HBsAg titers achieved in neonates after secondary and tertiary immunizations are similar to those in older children, indicating that neonatal immunization does not result in tolerance.[933] If initial immunization is delayed until 1 month of age, the antibody response to primary hepatitis B vaccination is increased and nearly equivalent to that in older children, suggesting that the developmental limitations responsible for reduced antibody responses are transient.[933,935] Similarly, 2-week-old infants immunized with a single dose of diphtheria or tetanus toxoid demonstrated delayed production of specific antibody compared with that in older infants, but by 2 months of age, their responses were similar to that of 6-month-old infants.[936] The switch from IgM to IgG also may be delayed after neonatal vaccination for some (e.g., *Salmonella* H vaccine[931] but not all (e.g., bacteriophage ΦX174[932]) antigens. Immunization of infants born to HIV-infected mothers with recombinant HIV-1 gp120 vaccine in MF59 adjuvant, beginning at birth, also resulted in high antibody titers, indicating that early postnatal vaccination is not tolerogenic.[937]

Unlike with other vaccines, in newborns given whole-cell pertussis vaccination, not only may they demonstrate a poor initial antibody response, but their subsequent antibody response to certain antigenic components, such as pertussis toxin, may be less than in infants initially immunized at 1 month of age or older,[938-940] suggesting low-level tolerance. Whole-cell pertussis vaccine immunization of premature infants (born at 28-36 weeks of gestation) at 2 months of age elicited responses similar to those in 2-month-old term infants,[929] indicating that this putative tolerigenic period wanes rapidly and is relatively independent of gestational age. This low-level tolerance was restricted to the pertussis component of the whole-cell pertussis vaccine because an inhibitory effect has not been observed after administration of diphtheria or tetanus toxoid[928] or hepatitis B vaccine given within 48 hours of birth.[933] A more recent study[941] also found that neonatal immunization with acellular pertussis vaccine combined with diphtheria and tetanus toxoids also resulted in lower subsequent pertussis-specific antibody responses than when vaccination was delayed. In contrast, and for unclear reasons, no such inhibition of pertussis-specific antibody responses was observed when the acellular pertussis vaccine was administered alone shortly after birth.[942,943] Administration of OPV at birth enhanced, rather than inhibited, the response to subsequent immunization, also indicating that immunization through the mucosal route does not produce tolerance.[944]

The antibody response to measles vaccine given at 6 months of age is significantly less than when the vaccine is given at 9 or 12 months of age, even when there is control for the inhibitory effect of maternal antibody.[945] This decreased response is not due to a lack of measles-specific T cells, because measles antigen–specific T-cell proliferation and IL-12 and IFN-γ proliferation were similar in the three age groups.[945-947] Although the basis for this reduced response is not known, early vaccination as young as 6 months does not impair the antibody and T-cell response after a second dose of vaccine at 12 months.[948] Thus there is no evidence for tolerigenic effects from early measles vaccination.

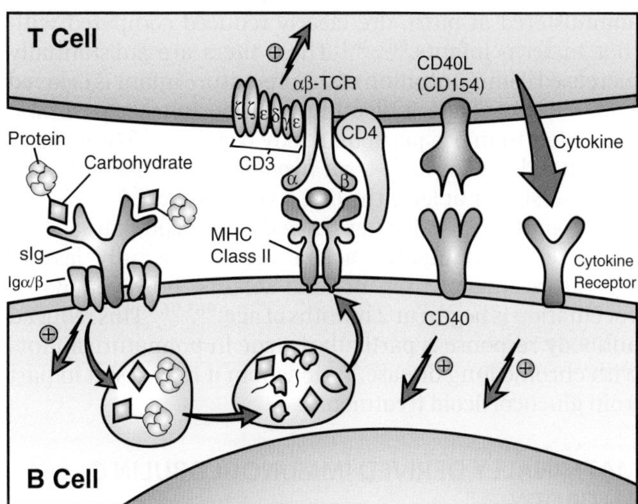

Figure 4-14 Interactions between B cells and T cells in the response to vaccines consisting of purified carbohydrate (e.g., bacterial capsular polysaccharide) covalently linked to protein carrier. The carbohydrate moiety of the conjugate is bound by surface immunoglobulin (sIg) on B cells, resulting in the internalization of the conjugate. Peptides derived from the protein moiety of the conjugate are presented by major histocompatibility complex (MHC) class II on the B cell, resulting in the activation of the T cell and expression of CD40 ligand (CD40L). Engagement of CD40 on the B cell by CD40L, in conjunction with cytokines secreted by the T cell, such as IL-21, results in carbohydrate-specific B-cell proliferation, immunoglobulin isotype switching, secretion of antibody, and memory B-cell generation. *TCR*, T-cell receptor.

Specific Antibody Responses by the Term Neonate to Polysaccharide and Polysaccharide-Protein Conjugates

In contrast with the response to protein antigens, the newborn's response to polysaccharide antigens is absent or severely blunted, as demonstrated by an inability to mount an antibody response to unconjugated *Haemophilus influenzae* type b (Hib) polysaccharide vaccine or to GBS capsular antigens after infection. The response to some polysaccharide antigens can be demonstrated by 6 months of age, but the response to vaccination with Hib, most pneumococcal serotype polysaccharides, and *Neisseria meningitidis* type C is poor until 18 to 24 months of age.[949] The delayed postnatal appearance of MZ B cells in the spleen has been proposed to account for this delayed response (see section Response to T-Cell–Independent Antigens), although this suggestion remains controversial and functional differences in the response of such cells is likely also to be a factor, as noted in the preceding sections.

Coupling of the Hib polysaccharide to a protein carrier converts a TI type II antigen to a TD antigen.[950] This is accompanied by an enhanced magnitude and higher-avidity antibody response on subsequent boosting, presumably resulting from TD memory B-cell generation and somatic hypermutation. The early interactions between T cells and B cells in response to such carbohydrate-protein conjugate vaccines are summarized in Figure 4-14. Conjugation of Hib polysaccharide to tetanus or diphtheria toxoid does not change the repertoire of the antibodies produced from that of the free polysaccharide.[951,952]

The neonatal response to Hib conjugate vaccines mimics, in most respects, the response to other T-dependent antigens in that covalent conjugation of Hib capsular polysaccharide to a protein carrier renders it immunogenic in infants as young as 2 months of age and primes for an enhanced antibody response to unconjugated vaccine given at 12 months of age. Because the response to the unconjugated vaccine usually is poor at this age, the conjugate vaccine acts by inducing Hib polysaccharide-specific B-cell memory.[952] Similarly, the administration of a single dose of Hib polysaccharide–tetanus toxoid conjugate to term neonates as early as a few days of age may enhance the antibody response to unconjugated Hib polysaccharide vaccine at 4 months of age.[953] This enhanced response is weak, however, and did not occur when neonates were primed with tetanus toxoid, followed by immunization with conjugate vaccine at 2 months of age.[954]

Vaccination with protein–capsular polysaccharide conjugate vaccines containing polysaccharides of *S. pneumoniae* (types 4, 6B, 9V, 14, 18C, 19F, and 23F in the Danish nomenclature)[955] and *N. meningitidis* (types A and C)[956] is immunogenic in 2-month-old infants and primes them for subsequent memory responses. Immunization of neonates within 3 days of birth with a 7-valent *S. pneumoniae*–CRM197 protein conjugate vaccine in a New Guinean population resulted in similar levels of serotype-specific *S. pneumoniae* antibody after completion of a three-dose series, as when the first dose was delayed until 1 month of age,[763] indicating there was no tolerogenic effect of early vaccination.

Antibody Responses by the Premature Infant to Immunization

Preterm neonates of 24 weeks of gestation or greater produce antibody to protein antigens such as diphtheria toxoid, diphtheria-pertussis-tetanus vaccine, and oral and inactivated poliovirus vaccines as well as do term neonates, when the vaccines are administered at 2, 4, and 6 months of age.[929,957-960] The antibody response in premature infants to multiple doses of hepatitis B vaccine, initially administered at birth, are clearly reduced compared with that in term infants.[961,962] These titers are substantially increased if immunization of the premature infant is delayed until 5 weeks of age, indicating the importance of postnatal age rather than of a particular body weight.[963] The benefits of such a delay for long-term hepatitis B–specific antibody levels persist for at least the first 3 years of life.[964]

The antibody levels after three doses of Hib polysaccharide–tetanus conjugate vaccine are significantly less in premature infants than in term infants, however, when vaccination is begun at 2 months of age.[965,966] This reduced antibody response is particularly true in premature infants with chronic lung disease,[967] in whom it may result in part from glucocorticoid treatment.

MATERNALLY DERIVED IMMUNOGLOBULIN G ANTIBODY

The transfer of IgG to the fetus depends on the recognition of maternal IgG through its Fc domain. IgG is internalized by the syncytiotrophoblast, possibly by pinocytosis, and binds to FcRn (also known as the Brambell receptor, FcRB) in the early endosome.[968] FcRn is a unique β_2-microglobulin–associated nonpolymorphic member of the MHC class I family, which lacks a functional peptide-binding groove and, instead, uses a different region of the molecule to bind the Fc domain of IgG.[969] IgG bound to FcRn undergoes transcytosis across the syncytiotrophoblast and is released into the fetal circulation. In addition to the syncytiotrophoblast, FcRn is widely expressed by nonplacental tissues, where it binds to pinocytosed IgG and recycles it to the circulation.[970] This recycling system accounts for the very long half-life of IgG. FcRn may also play a role in the targeting of antibody-antigen complexes taken up by DCs for cross-presentation to CD8 T cells.

Maternal IgG and FcRn expression can be detected in placental syncytiotrophoblasts during the first trimester,[971] but transport does not occur until about 17 weeks of gestation. The maternally derived placental cytotrophoblast, which is found between the syncytiotrophoblast and the fetal endothelium during the first trimester, may act as a barrier to IgG transport. This cytotrophoblast layer becomes discontinuous as the villous surface area expands during the second trimester.[971]

IgG is detectable in the fetus by 17 weeks of gestation, after which circulating concentrations rise steadily, reaching half of the term concentration by about 30 weeks, and equaling that of the mother by about 38 weeks.[972,973] In some instances, fetal IgG concentrations may exceed those of the mother.[974,975]

The fetus synthesizes little IgG; the concentration in utero is almost solely maternally derived (Fig. 4-15).[976] Accordingly, the degree of prematurity is reflected in proportionately lower neonatal IgG concentrations. The IgG2 concentration in cord blood relative to that in maternal blood is low at birth, particularly in preterm infants, whereas

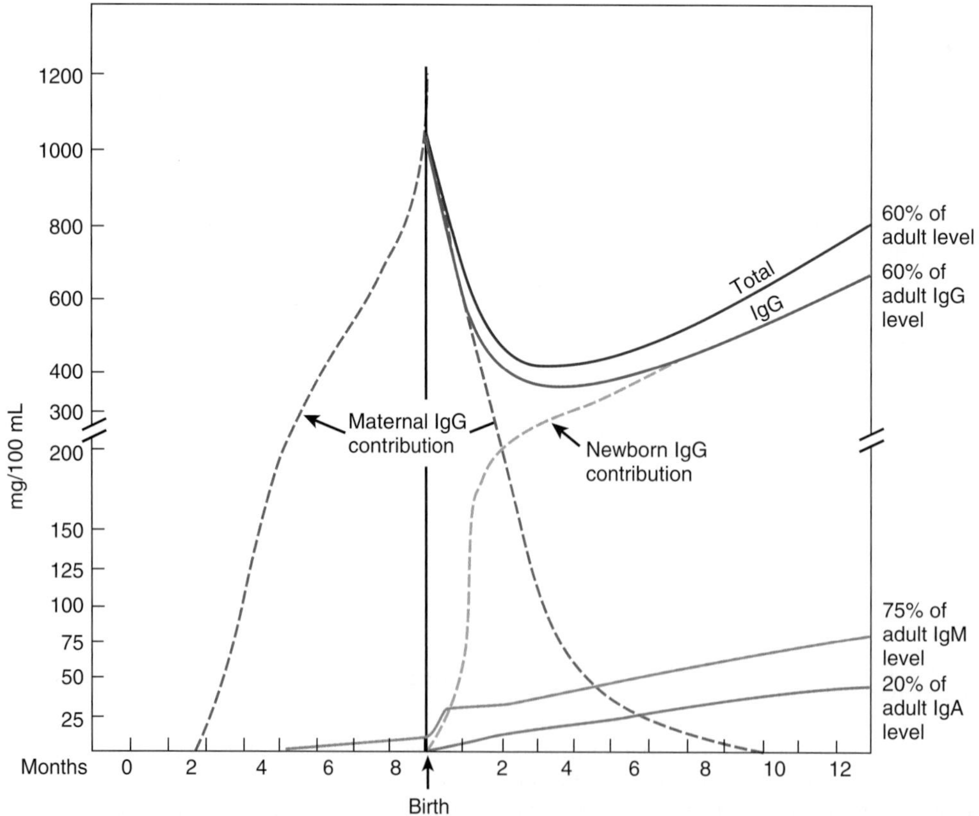

Figure 4-15 Immunoglobulin (IgG, IgM, and IgA) levels in the fetus and in the infant in the first year of life. IgG of the fetus and newborn infant is predominantly of maternal origin. Maternal IgG disappears by age 9 months, by which time endogenous synthesis of IgG by the infant is well established. IgM and IgA of the neonate are entirely endogenously synthesized because maternal IgM and IgA do not cross the placenta. (Data from Saxon A, Stiehm ER: The B-lymphocyte system. In Stiehm ER, editor: *Immunologic disorders in infants and children*, ed 3, Philadelphia, 1989, WB Saunders, pp 40-67.)

the overall fetal-to-maternal ratio is usually near 1.0 for the other IgG subclasses.[977-979] The low IgG2 concentration appears to reflect a relatively low affinity of FcRn for IgG2. IgM, IgA, and IgD do not cross the placenta, although there is some evidence for IgE crossing in some pregnancies by an unknown mechanism.[980,981] Evidence for transamniotic transfer of IgG to the fetus also is lacking.[975]

Placental Transfer of Specific Antibodies

The fetus receives IgG antibodies against antigens to which the mother has been exposed by infection or vaccination. For example, in mothers immunized with Hib capsular polysaccharide antigen at 34 to 36 weeks of gestation, concentrations of anticapsular antibody are high, resulting in protective antibody levels in their infants for approximately the first 4 months of life. In the absence of recent immunization or natural exposure, the maternal antibody IgG antibody titer may be too low to protect the neonate. Protection of the infant may be absent even if the mother is protected because she has memory B cells and can mount a rapid recall antibody response on infectious challenge. In addition, if maternal antibodies are primarily IgM, such as antibodies to E. *coli* and *Salmonella*,[930,931] the fetus will not be protected because IgM does not traverse the placenta. Finally, premature infants may not receive sufficient amounts of IgG for protection because the bulk of maternal IgG is transferred to the fetus after 34 weeks of gestation,[982] thereby accounting for the greater susceptibility of premature compared with term neonates to certain infections, such as with VZV.[983]

Inhibition of Neonatal Antibody Responses by Maternal Antibodies. Maternal antibody also may inhibit the production by the fetus or newborn of antibodies of the same specificity. This inhibition varies with the maternal antibody titer and with the type and amount of antigen. Maternal antibody markedly inhibits the response to measles and rubella vaccine but not mumps vaccine[984]; this is the reason for delaying measles-mumps-rubella (MMR) vaccine until at least 12 months of age in the developed world. Inhibition of the response to these live-attenuated viral vaccines may result in part from the binding of maternal antibody to immunogenic epitopes, thereby inhibition antigen binding to surface Ig on the antigen-specific B cells of the infant (i.e., masking), and from reduced replication of vaccine virus.

Maternal antibodies also may inhibit the neonatal and young infant response to certain nonreplicating vaccines, such as whole-cell pertussis vaccine,[940] diphtheria toxoid,[985] *Salmonella* flagellar antigen,[931] and inactivated poliovirus vaccine,[986] but not others, such as Hib conjugate vaccine.[987] Maternal antibody may mask the immunogenic epitope, and formation of maternal IgG antibody-antigen complexes may inhibit activation of B cells via surface Ig by simultaneous engagement of the inhibitory FcγRII receptor by the IgG component of the complex.[847] Alternatively, maternal antibody may lead to the rapid clearance of vaccine antigen and decreased immunogenicity. Of interest, maternal antibodies may actually enhance rather than inhibit the T-cell response to postnatal vaccination, as in the case of tetanus toxoid.[988] Finally, for certain antibodies, such as anti-HbsAg, neither maternal antibodies nor hepatitis B immune globulin administration has a substantial inhibitory effect on the newborn's immune response to hepatitis B vaccination.

IMMUNOGLOBULIN SYNTHESIS BY THE FETUS AND NEONATE

Immunoglobulin G

IgG is the predominant immunoglobulin isotype at all ages (Table 4-7).[989] In adults, IgG1 is the predominant subclass, accounting for approximately 70% of total IgG; IgG2, IgG3, and IgG4 account for approximately 20%, 7%, and 3% of the total, respectively.[990] Passively derived maternal IgG is the source of virtually all of the IgG subclasses detected in the fetus and neonate. Because the IgG plasma half-life is

Table 4-7 Levels of Immunoglobulins in Sera of Normal Subjects by Age*

	IgG		IgM		IgA		TOTAL IMMUNOGLOBULINS	
Age	**mg/dL**	**% Adult Level**	**mg/dL**	**% Adult Level**	**mg/dL**	**% Adult Level**	**mg/dL**	**% Adult Level**
Newborn	1031 ± 200†	89 ± 17	11 ± 5	11 ± 5	2 ± 3	1 ± 2	1044 ± 201	67 ± 13
1-3 mo	430 ± 119	37 ± 10	30 ± 11	30 ± 11	21 ± 13	11 ± 7	418 ± 127	31 ± 9
4-6 mo	427 ± 186	37 ± 16	43 ± 17	43 ± 17	28 ± 18	14 ± 9	498 ± 204	32 ± 13
7-12 mo	661 ± 219	58 ± 19	54 ± 23	55 ± 23	37 ± 18	19 ± 9	752 ± 242	48 ± 15
13-24 mo	762 ± 209	66 ± 18	58 ± 23	59 ± 23	50 ± 24	25 ± 12	870 ± 258	56 ± 16
25-36 mo	892 ± 183	77 ± 16	61 ± 19	62 ± 19	71 ± 37	36 ± 19	1024 ± 205	65 ± 14
3-5 yr	929 ± 228	80 ± 20	56 ± 18	57 ± 18	93 ± 27	47 ± 14	1078 ± 245	69 ± 17
6-8 yr	923 ± 256	80 ± 22	65 ± 25	66 ± 25	124 ± 45	62 ± 23	1112 ± 293	71 ± 20
9-11 yr	1124 ± 235	92 ± 20	79 ± 33	80 ± 33	131 ± 60	66 ± 30	1334 ± 254	85 ± 17
12-16 yr	946 ± 124	82 ± 11	59 ± 20	60 ± 20	148 ± 63	74 ± 32	1153 ± 169	74 ± 12
Adult	1158 ± 305	100 ± 26	99 ± 27	100 ± 27	200 ± 61	100 ± 31	1457 ± 353	100 ± 24

Modified from Stiehm ER, Fudenberg HH: Serum levels of immune globulins in health and disease: a survey, *Pediatrics* 37:715, 1966.

*The values were derived from measurements made for 296 normal children and 30 adults. Levels were determined by the radial diffusion technique, using specific rabbit antisera to human immunoglobulins.

†1 SD.

about 21 days, these maternally derived levels fall rapidly after birth. IgG synthesized by the neonate and that derived from the mother are approximately equal at 2 months of age, and by 10 to 12 months of age, the IgG is nearly all derived from synthesis by the infant. As a consequence of the fall in passively derived IgG and increased synthesis of IgG, values reach a nadir of approximately 400mg/dL in term infants at 3 to 4 months of age and rise thereafter (see Table 4-7 and Fig. 4-15). The premature infant has lower IgG concentrations at birth, which reach a nadir at 3 months of age; mean IgG values of 82 and 104mg/dL are observed in infants born at 25 to 28 and 29 to 32 weeks of gestation, respectively.

By 1 year of age, the total IgG concentration is approximately 60% of that in adults. IgG1 and IgG3 subclasses reach adult concentrations by 8 years of age, whereas IgG2 and IgG4 do so by 10 and 12 years of age, respectively.[991] As discussed earlier, maternal IgG may inhibit certain postnatal antibody responses by binding to FcγRIIb receptors and by rapidly clearing or masking potential antigens. The slow onset of IgG synthesis in the neonate, however, is predominantly an intrinsic limitation of the neonate, rather than an effect of maternal antibody; indeed, a similar pattern of IgG development was observed in a neonate born to a mother with untreated agammaglobulinemia.[992]

The slow rise in IgG2 concentrations parallels the poor antibody response to bacterial polysaccharide antigens, which are predominantly IgG2.[993] Of interest, the postpartum order in which adult levels of isotype expression are achieved closely parallels the chromosomal order of the heavy chain gene segments that encode these isotypes. Thus postnatal regulation of isotype switching is mediated in part at the heavy chain gene locus.

Although passive maternal antibody plays an important role in protection, it limits the value of antigen-specific IgG levels in the diagnosis of immunodeficiency or infection in the young infant.

Immunoglobulin M

IgM is the only isotype besides IgG that binds and activates complement. IgM has a half-life in the blood of 5 days. The concentration of IgM in the blood increases from a mean of 6 mg/dL in infants born at less than 28 weeks of gestation to 11 mg/dL at term,[994,995] which is approximately 8% of the maternal IgM level. This IgM, which is likely to be preimmune (i.e., not the result of a B-cell response to foreign antigens), is enriched for polyreactive antibodies. Murine studies suggest that such natural IgM plays an important role in innate defense against infection, allowing time for the initiation of antigen-specific B-cell response; it also enhances antigen-specific B-cell responses through its ability to fix complement and thereby co-stimulate B-cell activation through CD21.[910] Some of the human neonatal IgM is monomeric and therefore nonfunctional, however, as opposed to its usual pentameric functional form.[996,997]

Postnatal IgM concentrations rise rapidly for the first month and then more gradually thereafter, presumably in response to antigenic stimulation (see Fig. 4-15 and Table 4-7). By 1 year of age, values are approximately 60% of those in adults. The postnatal rise is similar in premature and in term infants.[996] Elevated (greater than 20 mg/dL) IgM concentrations in cord blood suggest possible intrauterine infections,[998] but many infants with congenital infections have normal cord blood IgM levels.[921]

Immunoglobulin A

IgA does not cross the placenta, and its concentration in cord blood usually is 0.1 to 5.0 mg/dL, approximately 0.5% of the levels in maternal sera.[995] Concentrations are similar in term and in premature neonates,[994] and both IgA1 and IgA2 are present. IgA has a half-life in the blood of 6 days. Secretory IgA can be detected in the saliva of neonates as early as 3 days after birth.[999]

At birth, the frequency of IgA1- and IgA2-bearing B cells in the blood is equivalent. Subsequently, a preferential expansion of the IgA1-bearing cell population occurs.[1000] Concentrations of IgA in serum increase to 20% of those in adults by 1 year of age and rise progressively through adolescence (see Table 4-7). Increased cord blood IgA concentrations are observed in some infants with congenital infection[998] and is common in those infected with HIV by vertical transmission. IgA has a relatively short half-life in plasma of approximately 5 days. Secretory IgA is present in substantial amounts in the saliva by 10 days after birth.[1001]

Immunoglobulin D

IgD is detectable by sensitive techniques in serum from cord blood in term and premature infants.[994,1002] Mean serum levels at birth are approximately 0.05 mg/dL[995] and increase during the first year of life.[1003] IgD is also detectable in the saliva of newborn infants.[1001] Circulating or salivary IgD has no clear functional role in normal humoral immunity because mice in which IgD expression has been eliminated by gene targeting have normal immune responses by other antibody isotypes. Elevated levels of IgD are associated in some cases with proinflammatory states, such as in mevalonate kinase deficiency,

Immunoglobulin E

Although IgE synthesis by the fetus is detectable as early as 11 weeks, concentrations of IgE in cord blood are typically low, with a mean of approximately 0.5% of that of maternal levels.[995] IgE concentrations are higher in infants born at 40 to 42 weeks of gestation than in those born at 37 to 39 weeks.[995] The rate of postnatal increase varies and is greater in infants predisposed to allergic disease or who have greater environmental exposure to allergens.[1004,1005] The concentration of IgE at birth appears to have limited predictive value for later development of atopic disease for most individuals.[1005,1006] Maternofetal transfer of IgE appears to be a common cause of elevated IgE at birth.[980,981] Based on murine experiments, one potential mechanism for such transfer may be IgG anti-IgE complexes being transported via FcRn.[1007]

SUMMARY

The neonate is partially protected from infection by passive maternal IgG antibody, predominantly transferred during the latter third of pregnancy. Fetal IgG concentrations are equal to or higher than maternal concentrations after 34 weeks of gestation. The inability of the neonate to produce antibodies in response to polysaccharides, particularly bacterial capsular polysaccharides, limits resistance to bacterial pathogens to which the mother has little or no IgG antibody. The basis for this defect remains unclear, but it may reflect an intrinsic limitation of B-cell function or a deficiency in the anatomic microenvironment required for B cells to develop in extra–lymphoid tissue or to become activated and differentiate into plasma cells. By contrast, the neonatal IgM response to most protein antigens is intact and only slightly limited for IgG responses to certain vaccines. Nevertheless, a clear difference between neonates and older infants has been observed in the magnitude of the antibody response to most protein neoantigens, but this difference rapidly resolves after birth. The antibody response of the neonate to viral infection may also be more limited. The predominance of transitional B cells in fetus and neonate may account, in part, for limitations in function. A limited antibody response of premature infants to immunization with protein antigens occurs during the first month of life but not subsequently. Thus chronologic (i.e., postnatal) age is a more important determinant of antibody responses to T-cell-dependent antigens than gestational age. Isotype expression by B cells after immunization with T-cell-dependent antigens is limited by altered T-cell function, such as reduced CD40 ligand production, intrinsic limitations of B cell maturation and function, and, likely, other cell types that augment B-cell activation in vivo. These limitations are exaggerated in the fetus.

Immunologic Approaches to Prevent or Treat Fetal and Neonatal Infections

OVERVIEW

Vaccination (i.e., active immunization) is a key approach by which to prevent infectious diseases beyond the neonatal period, but only a few vaccines whose safety and benefit have been demonstrated are indicated for use in newborns. In the United States, only hepatitis B vaccine is routinely administered in the newborn period, whereas, in other parts of the world, BCG and oral poliovirus vaccine may also be given to neonates. Immunization of the mother before or during pregnancy is another mechanism by which to protect the neonate and young infant. This protection is achieved either through transfer of maternal antibodies to the fetus, as noted above, that is, the fetus and newborn are passively immunized, or by preventing the mother from acquiring an infection that she may transmit to her fetus or infant. This topic is discussed in Chapter 38. The remainder of this chapter briefly reviews other immunologic approaches to protect or treat the fetus and neonate, through administration of immunoglobulin or antibody preparations or other immunomodulatory agents.

U.S. FOOD AND DRUG ADMINISTRATION–APPROVED USES OF PASSIVE IMMUNIZATION IN THE MOTHER AND NEWBORN INFANT

Polyclonal antibody preparations for use in humans are prepared from plasma collected from large numbers of human donors. Donors are screened to identify and exclude individuals whose blood is at higher risk to contain transmissible agents, and additional measures are taken during the purification and formulation steps to remove or inactivate such agents. Immunoglobulins, usually the IgG fraction, are purified and formulated into a preparation suitable for administration; if formulated for intravenous use, these preparations are referred to as intravenous immunoglobulin (IVIG). In some cases, donors are selected based on their having high titers of antibodies to specific agents, which preparations are referred to as hyperimmune globulins. Administration of conventional or hyperimmune immunoglobulin preparations can provide temporary antibody-based immunity against those agents for which antibodies are given in sufficient amounts to have functional activity against that organism in the recipient; this approach is referred to as passive immunization.

Monoclonal antibodies that are fully human or which were originally generated in another species, usually mouse, and then humanized, that is, by replacement of murine constant regions of the immunoglobulin chains with those of human, are now in common use, in particular to treat human autoimmune diseases and cancer. One mAb is licensed for the prevention of infection in the United States—palivizumab, which is a mAb against RSV. Palivizumab is recommended for infants at high risk for severe RSV disease, which includes infants born at less than 32 weeks' gestation or with chronic lung disease of prematurity or hemodynamically significant congenital heart disease. Such infants should receive up to five monthly doses during seasons of the year when RSV is prevalent. More detailed information regarding approved uses of passive immunization is provided in the 29th edition of the *American Academy of Pediatrics Red Book*.[1008]

Two hyperimmune globulins are recommended for use in the neonatal period in the United States. Hepatitis B immune globulin should be given to newborns of mothers who are HBsAg positive concurrently with the birth dose of hepatitis B vaccine but at a different site, both given preferably within 12 hours of birth. If the mother's hepatitis B status is unknown, vaccine should be given but hepatitis B immune globulin withheld until the mother's status is known, and, if found to be positive, given as soon as possible thereafter. Varicella-zoster immune globulin is indicated (1) for newborn infants whose mothers have signs and symptoms of varicella from 5 days before to 2 days after delivery; (2) for hospitalized premature infants born at greater or equal to 28 weeks of gestation who have been exposed to varicella or herpes zoster and whose mothers do not have evidence of immunity to varicella; and (3) regardless of their mother's varicella status, for exposed, hospitalized premature infants born before 28 weeks of gestation or who weigh less than or equal to 1000 g at birth.

EXPLORATORY EVALUATION OF PASSIVE IMMUNIZATION FOR OTHER INDICATIONS

Prevention or Treatment of Neonatal Sepsis with Intravenous Immunoglobulin

Numerous studies have evaluated the use of IVIG for the prevention of nosocomial or late-onset pyogenic infections in premature neonates. The most recent 2013 Cochrane analysis identified 19 randomized controlled trials in which IVIG was used for the prevention of sepsis in the setting of neonatal intensive care units; these trials included a total of approximately 5000 infants born at less than 37 weeks or at a birth weight of less than 2500 g.[1009] When combined, these studies showed a significant reduction in sepsis (relative risk [RR], 0.85; 95% confidence interval [CI], 0.74 to 0.98) and a significant reduction of one or more episodes of any serious infection (RR, 0.82; 95% CI, 0.74 to 0.92). However, overall mortality was not significantly decreased (RR, 0.89; 95% CI, 0.75 to 1.05), nor was there any significant difference in the incidence of necrotizing enterocolitis, bronchopulmonary dysplasia, or intraventricular hemorrhage, or in the length of hospital stay. The authors of these reports and others[1010] concluded that IVIG is not indicated for prophylaxis in preterm neonates and neonates with low birth weight because there is no effect on long-term outcome and little or no effect on short-term outcomes. Moreover, they concluded that the evidence base is sufficiently rich that future studies of this nature are not indicated.

Similarly, various studies have been performed to determine whether IVIG would improve the outcome in neonates with suspected or proven sepsis. These studies have differed in design and have been performed in countries with differing rates of neonatal sepsis, management approaches, and preparations of IVIG. To address this heterogeneity and to provide a more definitive result, a more comprehensive randomized and controlled International Immunotherapy Study (INIS) trial was conducted to investigate the use of IVIG as adjunctive therapy for suspected or proven serious neonatal infections, the results of which were published in 2011.[1011] This INIS study involved 3493 infants enrolled in 113 hospitals in nine countries. The primary outcome variable—death or major disability at the age of 2 years—was observed in 686 of 1759 IVIG-treated infants (39.0%) and in 677 of 1734 infants (39.0%) who received placebo (RR, 1.00; 95% CI, 0.92 to 1.08). There were also no significant differences in the incidence of subsequent sepsis episodes or rates of major or minor disability at 2 years of age.

After this report, a Cochrane analysis was published in 2013.[1012] This analysis included the results of the INIS study and seven additional randomized or quasi-randomized studies evaluating a total of 3871 infants less than 28 days of postnatal age who received adjunct therapy with IVIG for suspected or proven bacterial/fungal infection, compared with placebo or no intervention.[1012] There was no significant difference in mortality regardless of whether the analyses included infants with clinically suspected infection at trial entry (RR, 0.94; 95% CI, 0.80 to 1.12), proven infection at trial entry (RR, 0.95; 95% CI, 0.74 to 1.21), or either clinically suspected or proven infection at trial entry (RR, 1.00; 95% CI, 0.86 to 1.16). There was also no significant difference in death or major disability at 2 years corrected age or in length of hospital stay. Similarly, the aggregate results in studies in which IgM-enriched IVIG rather than conventional IVIG was used as adjunctive treatment for suspected infection (three studies [$n = 164$]) did not show a statistically significant benefit (RR, 0.57; 95% CI, 0.31 to 1.04; $P = .06$). Based on the cumulative data, adjunctive therapy with IVIG is not recommended in the management of neonatal sepsis.

Cytomegalovirus Hyperimmune Intravenous Immunoglobulin

Cytomegalovirus hyperimmune IVIG is prepared from pooled adult human plasma selected for high titers of antibody to CMV. It is licensed for use in the United States for the prophylaxis of CMV disease associated with transplantation of kidney, lung, liver, pancreas, and heart in older subjects. Results of an uncontrolled study in pregnant women with documented primary CMV infection during pregnancy and with CMV-positive amniotic fluid suggested that administration soon after seroconversion may decrease the risk of symptomatic congenital CMV disease in their infants.[1013] In a subsequent trial, 123 women in whom primary infection occurred at 5 to 26 weeks' gestation were randomized to receive CMV IVIG or placebo every 4 weeks until 36 weeks of gestation.[1014] Congenital infection was documented in 18 of 61 (30%) of the treated women and 27 of 62 (44%) of the control subjects. This 14% reduction in the infection rate (95% CI, −35% to 31%) was not statistically significant ($P = .13$), nor were there any significant differences in secondary outcome variables), although the number of adverse obstetric events was greater in the treatment group (13% vs. 2%, $P = .06$). Two additional randomized controlled trials addressing this question are underway. However, at present, the use of CMV IVIG to prevent congenital CMV infection is not recommended.

NEUTROPHIL TRANSFUSIONS

Neutrophil transfusions enhance survival rate in certain animal models of neonatal sepsis, but the clinical efficacy of neutrophil transfusion in human neonates with sepsis is uncertain. Three of five controlled studies showed statistically significant improvement in the survival rate for neonates receiving granulocyte transfusions compared with infants not receiving this therapy.[1015] Nonetheless, small sample sizes and differences in entry criteria for treatment and control groups, in methods of neutrophil preparation, in numbers of neutrophils per transfusion, in numbers of transfusions, and in bacterial pathogens causing disease preclude a meaningful meta-analysis of these studies. Although neutrophil storage pool depletion has been used as a selection criterion for neonates for whom transfusion may be beneficial, the difficulty in ascertainment of neutrophil storage pool size in clinical practice and the failure of this parameter to predict outcome in some studies make this measure an imperfect criterion in clinical practice. The utility of neutrophil transfusions is compromised further by the difficulty in obtaining these cells in a timely fashion and the potential complications of transfusions, including the risk of infection. For these reasons, neutrophil transfusions cannot be recommended as routine therapy for neonates with suspected or proven sepsis.

COLONY-STIMULATING FACTORS

Recombinant G-CSF and GM-CSF augment granulocyte production and function in neonatal animals and provide some protection against challenge with pyogenic bacteria, including GBS, in neonatal animal models. These findings prompted clinical trials to determine if administration of recombinant G-CSF or GM-CSF to human neonates would result in increased levels of circulating neutrophils and protect at-risk neonates from sepsis. Four randomized trials of prophylaxis with recombinant GM-CSF and one comparative observational study of prophylaxis with recombinant G-CSF were conducted.[1015-1017] These studies showed that G-CSF and GM-CSF increase circulating neutrophil counts and seem to be well tolerated.

The most recent and largest randomized trial of 280 neonates[1018] and a meta-analysis of the results from the four GM-CSF trials showed no reduction in the rate of sepsis or mortality.[1016] A small, nonrandomized observational study found that prophylactic administration of G-CSF to neutropenic infants with low birth weight born to mothers with preeclampsia led to a reduction in proven bacterial infections in these patients.[1019] No randomized controlled trials with G-CSF have been conducted, however; thus its utility as a prophylactic agent is essentially untested. The evidence does not support the prophylactic use of G-CSF or GM-CSF in neonates.

Whereas the evidence that prophylaxis is not beneficial is clear, results of treatment studies are more favorable. Administration of G-CSF to human neonates 26 to 40 weeks of gestational age with presumed early-onset sepsis was shown to increase significantly the numbers of circulating neutrophils, bone marrow neutrophil storage pool size, and neutrophil expression of CR3 receptors (CD11b/CD18) without adverse effects.[1020-1022] The 2003 Cochrane meta-analysis of all causes of mortality in 257 infants with suspected sepsis from seven randomized clinical trials showed, however, that survival was not improved by adjunctive treatment with G-CSF or GM-CSF; G-CSF was used in most of these studies.[1016] A subset analysis from three of these studies that included 97 infants with neutropenia (absolute neutrophil count less than 1700 per μL) showed an apparent reduction in mortality (RR, 0.34; 95% CI, 0.12 to 0.92). In an earlier meta-analysis of five studies involving 73 neonates who received G-CSF and 82 controls by Bernstein and colleagues,[1023] the mortality rate was significantly reduced ($P < .05$), but if data from two nonrandomized trials were excluded, there was no significant difference (observed risk, 0.43; 95% CI, 0.14 to 1.23; $P = .13$). More recently, a randomized, blinded controlled trial conducted in Kolkata, India, showed clear benefit.[1024] In this study, premature infants born at less than 34 weeks gestation and weighing less than 2500 g with at least one positive blood culture and an absolute neutrophil count of less than 1500/mm^3 for more than 24 hours were randomized to receive three daily injections of G-CSF or a placebo, along with conventional therapy. Similar to other studies of neonatal sepsis in South Asia, gram-negative bacterial pathogens, particularly *Klebsiella pneumoniae* and *Pseudomonas aeruginosa*, were isolated in the majority. Deaths in the group receiving G-CSF (4/39 = 10%) were significantly reduced compared with the control group (14/39 = 35%; $P < .05$), and the duration of hospitalization was also significantly shortened. No significant adverse effects of G-CSF adjunctive therapy were noted in these studies; also, one long-term follow-up study found no adverse effects. Thus the data regarding the use of G-CSF for adjunctive therapy of neonatal sepsis indicate that it is safe and may be useful in some contexts but are currently insufficient to support routine use.

References

1. Selsted ME, Ouellette AJ: Mammalian defensins in the antimicrobial immune response, *Nat Immunol* 6:551-557, 2005.
2. Barlow PG, Svoboda P, Mackellar A, et al: Antiviral activity and increased host defense against influenza infection elicited by the human cathelicidin LL-37, *PloS One* 6:e25333, 2011.
3. Currie SM, Findlay EG, McHugh BJ, et al: The human cathelicidin LL-37 has antiviral activity against respiratory syncytial virus, *PloS One* 8:e73659, 2013.
4. Gallo RL, Hooper LV: Epithelial antimicrobial defence of the skin and intestine, *Nat Rev Immunol* 12:503-516, 2012.
5. Soto E, Espinoza J, Nien JK, et al: Human beta-defensin-2: a natural antimicrobial peptide present in amniotic fluid participates in the host response to microbial invasion of the amniotic cavity, *J Matern Fetal Neonatal Med* 20:15-22, 2007.
6. Parker D, Prince A: Innate immunity in the respiratory epithelium, *Am J Respir Cell Mol Biol* 45:189-201, 2011.
7. Kisich KO, Howell MD, Boguniewicz M, et al: The constitutive capacity of human keratinocytes to kill *Staphylococcus aureus* is dependent on beta-defensin 3, *J Invest Dermatol* 127:2368-2380, 2007.
8. Cash HL, Whitham CV, Behrendt CL, et al: Symbiotic bacteria direct expression of an intestinal bactericidal lectin, *Science* 313: 1126-1130, 2006.
9. Glaser R, Harder J, Lange H, et al: Antimicrobial psoriasin (s100a7) protects human skin from *Escherichia coli* infection, *Nat Immunol* 6:57-64, 2005.
10. Harder J, Schroder JM: RNase 7, a novel innate immune defense antimicrobial protein of healthy human skin, *J Biol Chem* 277:46779-46784, 2002.
11. Zanger P, Holzer J, Schleucher R, et al: Constitutive expression of the antimicrobial peptide RNase 7 is associated with *Staphylococcus aureus* infection of the skin, *J Infect Dis* 200:1907-1915, 2009.
12. Simanski M, Dressel S, Gläser R, et al: RNase 7 protects healthy skin from *Staphylococcus aureus* colonization, *J Invest Dermatol* 130:2836-2838, 2010.
13. Carr DL, Kloos WE: Temporal study of the staphylococci and micrococci of normal infant skin, *Appl Environ Microbiol* 34:673-680, 1977.
14. Li D, Lei H, Li Z, et al: A novel lipopeptide from skin commensal activates TLR2/CD36-p38 MAPK signaling to increase antibacterial defense against bacterial infection, *PloS One* 8:e58288, 2013.
15. Dominguez-Bello MG, Costello EK, Contreras M, et al: Delivery mode shapes the acquisition and structure of the initial microbiota across multiple body habitats in newborns, *Proc Natl Acad Sci U.S.A* 107:11971-11975, 2010.
16. Marchini G, Lindow S, Brismar H, et al: The newborn infant is protected by an innate antimicrobial barrier: peptide antibiotics are present in the skin and vernix caseosa, *Br J Dermatol* 147: 1127-1134, 2002.
17. Schuster C, Gläser R, Fiala C, et al: Prenatal human skin expresses the antimicrobial peptide RNase 7, *Arch Dermatol Res* 305:545-549, 2013.
18. Dorschner RA, Lin KH, Murakami M, et al: Neonatal skin in mice and humans expresses increased levels of antimicrobial peptides: innate immunity during development of the adaptive response, *Pediatr Res* 53:566-572, 2003.
19. Akinbi HT, Narendran V, Pass AK, et al: Host defense proteins in vernix caseosa and amniotic fluid, *Am J Obstet Gynecol* 191: 2090-2096, 2004.
20. Tollin M, Bergsson G, Kai-Larsen Y, et al: Vernix caseosa as a multicomponent defence system based on polypeptides, lipids and their interactions, *Cell Mol Life Sci* 62:2390-2399, 2005.
21. Newburg DS: Innate immunity and human milk, *J Nutr* 135: 1308-1312, 2005.
22. Artis D: Epithelial-cell recognition of commensal bacteria and maintenance of immune homeostasis in the gut, *Nat Rev Immunol* 8:411-420, 2008.
23. Lozupone CA, Stombaugh JI, Gordon JI, et al: Diversity, stability and resilience of the human gut microbiota, *Nature* 489:220-230, 2012.
24. Palmer C, Bik EM, DiGiulio DB, et al: Development of the human infant intestinal microbiota, *PLoS Biol* 5:e177, 2007.
25. Yatsunenko T, Rey FE, Manary MJ, et al: Human gut microbiome viewed across age and geography, *Nature* 486:222-227, 2012.

26. Koenig JE, Spor A, Scalfone N, et al: Succession of microbial consortia in the developing infant gut microbiome, *Proc Natl Acad Sci U.S.A* 108(Suppl 1):4578-4585, 2011.
27. Abt MC, Osborne LC, Monticelli LA, et al: Commensal bacteria calibrate the activation threshold of innate antiviral immunity, *Immunity* 37:158-170, 2012.
28. Ganal SC, Sanos SL, Kallfass C, et al: Priming of natural killer cells by nonmucosal mononuclear phagocytes requires instructive signals from commensal microbiota, *Immunity* 37:171-186, 2012.
29. Young JA, He TH, Reizis B, et al: Commensal microbiota are required for systemic inflammation triggered by necrotic dendritic cells, *Cell Rep* 3:1932-1944, 2013.
30. Tien MT, Girardin SE, Regnault B, et al: Anti-inflammatory effect of *Lactobacillus casei* on *Shigella*-infected human intestinal epithelial cells, *J Immunol* 176:1228-1237, 2006.
31. Mazmanian SK, Kasper DL: The love-hate relationship between bacterial polysaccharides and the host immune system, *Nat Rev Immunol* 6:849-858, 2006.
32. Shah N, Kammermeier J, Elawad M, et al: Interleukin-10 and interleukin-10-receptor defects in inflammatory bowel disease, *Curr Allergy Asthma Rep* 12:373-379, 2012.
33. Nanthakumar NN, Fusunyan RD, Sanderson I, et al: Inflammation in the developing human intestine: a possible pathophysiologic contribution to necrotizing enterocolitis, *Proc Natl Acad Sci U.S.A* 97:6043-6048, 2000.
34. Gribar SC, Richardson WM, Sodhi CP, et al: No longer an innocent bystander: epithelial Toll-like receptor signaling in the development of mucosal inflammation, *Mol Med* 14:645-659, 2008.
35. Elahi S, Ertelt JM, Kinder JM, et al: Immunosuppressive CD71+ erythroid cells compromise neonatal host defence against infection, *Nature* 504:158-162, 2013.
36. Wehkamp J, Schauber J, Stange EF: Defensins and cathelicidins in gastrointestinal infections, *Curr Opin Gastroenterol* 23:32-38, 2007.
37. Salzman NH, Underwood MA, Bevins CL: Paneth cells, defensins, and the commensal microbiota: a hypothesis on intimate interplay at the intestinal mucosa, *Semin Immunol* 19:70-83, 2007.
38. Menard S, Förster V, Lotz M, et al: Developmental switch of intestinal antimicrobial peptide expression, *J Exp Med* 205:183-193, 2008.
39. Grubor B, Meyerholz DK, Ackermann MR: Collectins and cationic antimicrobial peptides of the respiratory epithelia, *Vet Pathol* 43:595-612, 2006.
40. Mayer AK, Muehmer M, Mages J, et al: Differential recognition of TLR-dependent microbial ligands in human bronchial epithelial cells, *J Immunol* 178:3134-3142, 2007.
41. Ioannidis I, Ye F, McNally B, et al: Toll-like receptor expression and induction of type I and type II interferons in primary airway epithelial cells, *J Virol* 87:3261-3270, 2013.
42. Hillman NH, Moss TJ, Nitsos I, et al: Toll-like receptors and agonist responses in the developing fetal sheep lung, *Pediatr Res* 63: 388-393, 2008.
43. Harju K, Glumoff V, Hallman M: Ontogeny of Toll-like receptors TLR2 and TLR4 in mice, *Pediatr Res* 49:81-83, 2001.
44. Petrikin JE, Gaedigk R, Leeder JS, et al: Selective Toll-like receptor expression in human fetal lung, *Pediatr Res* 68:335-338, 2010.
45. Starner TD, Agerberth B, Gudmundsson GH, et al: Expression and activity of beta-defensins and LL-37 in the developing human lung, *J Immunol* 174:1608-1615, 2005.
46. Schaller-Bals S, Schulze A, Bals R: Increased levels of antimicrobial peptides in tracheal aspirates of newborn infants during infection, *Am J Respir Crit Care Med* 165:992-995, 2002.
47. Haagsman HP, Hogenkamp A, van Eijk M, et al: Surfactant collectins and innate immunity, *Neonatology* 93:288-294, 2008.
48. Giannoni E, Sawa T, Allen L, et al: Surfactant proteins A and D enhance pulmonary clearance of *Pseudomonas aeruginosa*, *Am J Respir Cell Mol Biol* 34:704-710, 2006.
49. LeVine AM, Elliott J, Whitsett JA, et al: Surfactant protein-D enhances phagocytosis and pulmonary clearance of respiratory syncytial virus, *Am J Respir Cell Mol Biol* 31:193-199, 2004.
50. Stahlman MT, Gray ME, Hull WM, et al: Immunolocalization of surfactant protein-D (SP-D) in human fetal, newborn, and adult tissues, *J Histochem Cytochem* 50:651-660, 2002.
51. Stray-Pedersen A, Vege A, Stray-Pedersen A, et al: Post-neonatal drop in alveolar SP-A expression: biological significance for increased vulnerability to SIDS? *Pediatr Pulmonol* 43:160-168, 2008.
52. Hilgendorff A, Schmidt R, Bohnert A, et al: Host defence lectins in preterm neonates, *Acta Paediatr* 94:794-799, 2005.
53. Bersani I, Speer CP, Kunzmann S: Surfactant proteins A and D in pulmonary diseases of preterm infants, *Expert Rev Anti Infect Ther* 10:573-584, 2012.
54. Mantovani A, Garlanda C, Doni A, et al: Pentraxins in innate immunity: from C-reactive protein to the long pentraxin PTX3, *J Clin Immunol* 28:1-13, 2008.
55. Ainbender E, Cabatu EE, Guzman DM, et al: Serum C-reactive protein and problems of newborn infants, *J Pediatr* 101:438-440, 1982.
56. Angelone DF, Wessels MR, Coughlin M, et al: Innate immunity of the human newborn is polarized toward a high ratio of IL-6/TNF-alpha production in vitro and in vivo, *Pediatr Res* 60:205-209, 2006.
57. Eisen DP, Minchinton RM: Impact of mannose-binding lectin on susceptibility to infectious diseases, *Clin Infect Dis* 37:1496-1505, 2003.
58. Lau YL, Chan SY, Turner MW, et al: Mannose-binding protein in preterm infants: developmental profile and clinical significance, *Clin Exp Immunol* 102:649-654, 1995.
59. Dzwonek AB, Neth OW, Thiébaut R, et al: The role of mannose-binding lectin in susceptibility to infection in preterm neonates, *Pediatr Res* 63:680-685, 2008.
60. de Benedetti F, Auriti C, D'Urbano LE, et al: Low serum levels of mannose binding lectin are a risk factor for neonatal sepsis, *Pediatr Res* 61:325-328, 2007.
61. Frakking FN, Brouwer N, van Eijkelenburg NK, et al: Low mannose-binding lectin (MBL) levels in neonates with pneumonia and sepsis, *Clin Exp Immunol* 150:255-262, 2007.
62. Aoyagi Y, Adderson EE, Rubens CE, et al: L-ficolin/mannose-binding lectin-associated serine protease complexes bind to group B streptococci primarily through N-acetylneuraminic acid of capsular polysaccharide and activate the complement pathway, *Infect Immun* 76:179-188, 2008.
63. Matsushita M: Ficolins in complement activation, *Mol Immunol* 55:22-26, 2013.
64. Sallenbach S, Thiel S, Aebi C, et al: Serum concentrations of lectin-pathway components in healthy neonates, children and adults: mannan-binding lectin (MBL), M-, L-, and H-ficolin, and MBL-associated serine protease-2 (MASP-2), *Pediatr Allergy Immunol* 22:424-430, 2011.
65. Cedzynski M, Swierzko AS, Kilpatrick DC: Factors of the lectin pathway of complement activation and their clinical associations in neonates, *J Biomed Biotechnol* 2012:363246, 2012.
66. Lambris JD, Ricklin D, Geisbrecht BV: Complement evasion by human pathogens, *Nat Rev Microbiol* 6:132-142, 2008.
67. Manfredi AA, Rovere-Querini P, Bottazzi B, et al: Pentraxins, humoral innate immunity and tissue injury, *Curr Opin Immunol* 20:538-544, 2008.
68. Degn SE, Thiel S: Humoral pattern recognition and the complement system, *Scand J Immunol* 78:181-193, 2013.
69. Ogden CA, deCathelineau A, Hoffmann PR, et al: C1q and mannose binding lectin engagement of cell surface calreticulin and CD91 initiates macropinocytosis and uptake of apoptotic cells, *J Exp Med* 194:781-795, 2001.
70. Kohler PF: Maturation of the human complement system. I. Onset time and sites of fetal C1q, C4, C3, and C5 synthesis, *J Clin Invest* 52:671-677, 1973.
71. Lassiter HA, Watson SW, Seifring ML, et al: Complement factor 9 deficiency in serum of human neonates, *J Infect Dis* 166:53-57, 1992.
72. Johnston RB Jr, Altenburger KM, Atkinson AW Jr, et al: Complement in the newborn infant, *Pediatrics* 64:781-786, 1979.
73. Notarangelo LD, Chirico G, Chiara A, et al: Activity of classical and alternative pathways of complement in preterm and small for gestational age infants, *Pediatr Res* 18:281-285, 1984.
74. Davis CA, Vallota EH, Forristal J: Serum complement levels in infancy: Age related changes, *Pediatr Res* 13:1043-1046, 1979.
75. Lewis DB, Wilson CB: Developmental immunology and role host defenses in fetal and neonatal susceptibility to infection. In Remington JS, Klein JO, Wilson CB, et al, editors: *Infectious Diseases of the fetus and newborn infant*, ed 7, Philadelphia, 2011, Elsevier, pp 80-191.
76. Raghunathan R, Miller ME, Everett S, et al: Phagocyte chemotaxis in the perinatal period, *J Clin Immunol* 2:242-245, 1982.
77. Anderson DC, Hughes BJ, Edwards MS, et al: Impaired chemotaxigenesis by type III group B streptococci in neonatal sera: relationship to diminished concentration of specific anticapsular antibody and abnormalities of serum complement, *Pediatr Res* 17:496-502, 1983.

78. Zilow EP, Hauck W, Linderkamp O, et al: Alternative pathway activation of the complement system in preterm infants with early onset infection, *Pediatr Res* 41:334-339, 1997.
79. Jokubaitis VJ, Sinka L, Driessen R, et al: Angiotensin-converting enzyme (CD143) marks hematopoietic stem cells in human embryonic, fetal, and adult hematopoietic tissues, *Blood* 111:4055-4063, 2008.
80. Fernandez KS, de Alarcon PA: Development of the hematopoietic system and disorders of hematopoiesis that present during infancy and early childhood, *Pediatr Clin North Am* 60:1273-1289, 2013.
81. Mold JE, Venkatasubrahmanyam S, Burt TD, et al: Fetal and adult hematopoietic stem cells give rise to distinct T cell lineages in humans, *Science* 330:1695-1699, 2010.
82. Krow-Lucal ER, Kim CC, Burt TD, et al: Distinct functional programming of human fetal and adult monocytes, *Blood* 123:1897-1904, 2014.
83. Ivarsson MA, Loh L, Marquardt N, et al: Differentiation and functional regulation of human fetal NK cells, *J Clin Invest* 123:3889-3901, 2013.
84. Kawai T, Akira S: The role of pattern-recognition receptors in innate immunity: Update on Toll-like receptors, *Nat Immunol* 11:373-384, 2010.
85. Blasius AL, Beutler B: Intracellular Toll-like receptors, *Immunity* 32:305-315, 2010.
86. Bhan U, Lukacs NW, Osterholzer JJ, et al: TLR9 is required for protective innate immunity in gram-negative bacterial pneumonia: role of dendritic cells, *J Immunol* 179:3937-3946, 2007.
87. Zhang Y, Wang F, Bhan U, et al: TLR9 signaling is required for generation of the adaptive immune protection in Cryptococcus neoformans-infected lungs, *Am J Pathol* 177:754-765, 2010.
88. Sancho-Shimizu V, Pérez de Diego R, Lorenzo L, et al: Herpes simplex encephalitis in children with autosomal recessive and dominant TRIF deficiency, *J Clin Invest* 121:4889-4902, 2011.
89. Huang Y, Li T, Sane DC, et al: IRAK1 serves as a novel regulator essential for lipopolysaccharide-induced interleukin-10 gene expression, *J Biol Chem* 279:51697-51703, 2004.
90. Ikushima H, Negishi H, Taniguchi T: The IRF family transcription factors at the interface of innate and adaptive immune responses, *Cold Spring Harb Symp Quant Biol* 78:105-116, 2013.
91. Molle C, Goldman M, Goriely S: Critical role of the IFN-stimulated gene factor 3 complex in TLR-mediated IL-27p28 gene expression revealing a two-step activation process, *J Immunol* 184:1784-1792, 2010.
92. Hurst J, Prinz N, Lorenz M, et al: TLR7 and TLR8 ligands and antiphospholipid antibodies show synergistic effects on the induction of IL-1beta and caspase-1 in monocytes and dendritic cells, *Immunobiology* 214:683-691, 2009.
93. Ward JR, West PW, Ariaans MP, et al: Temporal interleukin-1beta secretion from primary human peripheral blood monocytes by P2X7-independent and P2X7-dependent mechanisms, *J Biol Chem* 285:23147-23158, 2010.
94. Philbin VJ, West PW, Ariaans MP, et al: Imidazoquinoline Toll-like receptor 8 agonists activate human newborn monocytes and dendritic cells through adenosine-refractory and caspase-1-dependent pathways, *J Allergy Clin Immunol* 130:195-204, 2012. e9.
95. Zhong Y, Kinio A, Saleh M: Functions of Nod-like receptors in human diseases, *Front Immunol* 4:333, 2013.
96. Khare S, Luc N, Dorfleutner A, et al: Inflammasomes and their activation, *Crit Rev Immunol* 30:463-487, 2010.
97. Wen H, Miao EA, Ting JP: Mechanisms of Nod-like receptor-associated inflammasome activation, *Immunity* 39:432-441, 2013.
98. Devaiah BN, Singer DS: CIITA and its dual roles in MHC gene transcription, *Front Immunol* 4:476, 2013.
99. Meissner TB, Li A, Kobayashi KS: NLRC5: a newly discovered MHC class I transactivator (CITA), *Microbes Infect* 14:477-484, 2012.
100. Eisenbarth SC, Luc N, Dorfleutner A, et al: NLRP10 is a Nod-like receptor essential to initiate adaptive immunity by dendritic cells, *Nature* 484:510-513, 2012.
101. Ramos HJ, Gale M Jr: RIG-I like receptors and their signaling crosstalk in the regulation of antiviral immunity, *Curr Opin Virol* 1:167-176, 2011.
102. Kerrigan AM, Brown GD: Syk-coupled C-type lectin receptors that mediate cellular activation via single tyrosine based activation motifs, *Immunol Rev* 234:335-352, 2010.
103. Drummond RA, Brown GD: Signalling C-type lectins in antimicrobial immunity, *PLoS Pathog* 9:e1003417, 2013.
104. LeibundGut-Landmann S, Gross O, Robinson MJ, et al: Syk- and CARD9-dependent coupling of innate immunity to the induction of T helper cells that produce interleukin 17, *Nat Immunol* 8:630-638, 2007.
105. Gow NA, van de Veerdonk FL, Brown AJ, et al: *Candida albicans* morphogenesis and host defence: discriminating invasion from colonization, *Nat Rev Microbiol* 10:112-122, 2012.
106. Gringhuis SI, Kaptein TM, Wevers BA, et al: Dectin-1 is an extracellular pathogen sensor for the induction and processing of IL-1beta via a noncanonical caspase-8 inflammasome, *Nat Immunol* 13:246-254, 2012.
107. Puel A, Cypowyj S, Maródi L, et al: Inborn errors of human IL-17 immunity underlie chronic mucocutaneous candidiasis, *Curr Opin Allergy Clin Immunol* 12:616-622, 2012.
108. Xiao TS, Fitzgerald KA: The cGAS-STING pathway for DNA sensing, *Mol Cell* 51:135-139, 2013.
109. Burdette DL, Vance RE: STING and the innate immune response to nucleic acids in the cytosol, *Nat Immunol* 14:19-26, 2013.
110. Acosta-Rodriguez EV, Rivino L, Geginat J, et al: Surface phenotype and antigenic specificity of human interleukin 17-producing T helper memory cells, *Nat Immunol* 8:639-646, 2007.
111. Koenig JM, Yoder MC: Neonatal neutrophils: the good, the bad, and the ugly, *Clin Perinatol* 31:39-51, 2004.
112. Laver J, Duncan E, Abboud M, et al: High levels of granulocyte and granulocyte-macrophage colony-stimulating factors in cord blood of normal full-term neonates, *J Pediatr* 116:627-632, 1990.
113. Ohls RK, Li Y, Abdel-Mageed A, et al: Neutrophil pool sizes and granulocyte colony-stimulating factor production in human midtrimester fetuses, *Pediatr Res* 37:806-811, 1995.
114. Banerjea MC, Speer CP: The current role of colony-stimulating factors in prevention and treatment of neonatal sepsis, *Semin Neonatol* 7:335-349, 2002.
115. Mouzinho A, Rosenfeld CR, Sánchez PJ, et al: Revised reference ranges for circulating neutrophils in very-low-birth-weight neonates, *Pediatrics* 94:76-82, 1994.
116. Manroe BL, Weinberg AG, Rosenfeld CR, et al: The neonatal blood count in health and disease. I. Reference values for neutrophilic cells, *J Pediatr* 95:89-98, 1979.
117. Christensen RD, Calhoun DA, Rimsza LM: A practical approach to evaluating and treating neutropenia in the neonatal intensive care unit, *Clin Perinatol* 27:577-601, 2000.
118. Gessler P, Kirchmann N, Kientsch-Engel R, et al: Serum concentrations of granulocyte colony-stimulating factor in healthy term and preterm neonates and in those with various diseases including bacterial infections, *Blood* 82:3177-3182, 1993.
119. English BK, Hammond WP, Lewis DB, et al: Decreased granulocyte-macrophage colony-stimulating factor production by human neonatal blood mononuclear cells and T cells, *Pediatr Res* 31:211-216, 1992.
120. Schibler KR, Liechty KW, White WL, et al: Production of granulocyte colony-stimulating factor in vitro by monocytes from preterm and term neonates, *Blood* 82:2478-2484, 1993.
121. Herter J, Zarbock A: Integrin regulation during leukocyte recruitment, *J Immunol* 190:4451-4457, 2013.
122. Charo IF, Ransohoff RM: The many roles of chemokines and chemokine receptors in inflammation, *N Engl J Med* 354:610-621, 2006.
123. Badolato R: Defects of leukocyte migration in primary immunodeficiencies, *Eur J Immunol* 43:1436-1440, 2013.
124. Anderson DC, Hughes BJ, Wible LJ, et al: Impaired motility of neonatal PMN leukocytes: relationship to abnormalities of cell orientation and assembly of microtubules in chemotactic gradients, *J Leuk Biol* 36:1-15, 1984.
125. Anderson DC, Abbassi O, Kishimoto TK, et al: Diminished lectin-, epidermal growth factor-, complement binding domain-cell adhesion molecule-1 on neonatal neutrophils underlies their impaired CD18-independent adhesion to endothelial cells in vitro, *J Immunol* 146:3372-3379, 1991.
126. McEvoy LT, Zakem-Cloud H, Tosi MF: Total cell content of CR3 (CD11b/CD18) and LFA-1 (CD11a/CD18) in neonatal neutrophils: relationship to gestational age, *Blood* 87:3929-3933, 1996.
127. Anderson DC, Rothlein R, Marlin SD, et al: Impaired transendothelial migration by neonatal neutrophils: abnormalities of Mac-1 CD11b/CD18-dependent adherence reactions, *Blood* 76:2613-2621, 1990.

128. Dos Santos C, Davidson D: Neutrophil chemotaxis to leukotriene B4 in vitro is decreased for the human neonate, *Pediatr Res* 33: 242-246, 1993.
129. Tan ND, Davidson D: Comparative differences and combined effects of interleukin-8, leukotriene B4, and platelet-activating factor on neutrophil chemotaxis of the newborn, *Pediatr Res* 38:11-16, 1995.
130. Fox SE, Lu W, Maheshwari A, et al: The effects and comparative differences of neutrophil specific chemokines on neutrophil chemotaxis of the neonate, *Cytokine* 29:135-140, 2005.
131. Kikawa Y, Shigematsu Y, Sudo M: Leukotriene B4 biosynthesis in polymorphonuclear leukocytes from blood of umbilical cord, infants, children, and adults, *Pediatr Res* 20:402-406, 1986.
132. Underhill DM, Goodridge HS: Information processing during phagocytosis, *Nat Rev Immunol* 12:492-502, 2012.
133. Bruhns P: Properties of mouse and human IgG receptors and their contribution to disease models, *Blood* 119:5640-5649, 2012.
134. Miller ME: Phagocyte function in the neonate: selected aspects, *Pediatrics* 64:709-712, 1979.
135. Fujiwara T, Kobayashi T, Takaya J, et al: Plasma effects on phagocytic activity and hydrogen peroxide production by polymorphonuclear leukocytes in neonates, *Clin Immunol Immunopathol* 85:67-72, 1997.
136. Falconer AE, Carr R, Edwards SW: Impaired neutrophil phagocytosis in preterm neonates: lack of correlation with expression of immunoglobulin or complement receptors, *Biol Neonate* 68: 264-269, 1995.
137. Falconer AE, Carr R, Edwards SW: Neutrophils from preterm neonates and adults show similar cell surface receptor expression: analysis using a whole blood assay, *Biol Neonate* 67:26-33, 1995.
138. Fjaertoft G, Håkansson L, Foucard T, et al: CD64 (Fcgamma receptor I) cell surface expression on maturing neutrophils from preterm and term newborn infants, *Acta Paediatr* 94:295-302, 2005.
139. Adinolfi M, Cheetham M, Lee T, et al: Ontogeny of human complement receptors CR1 and CR3: expression of these molecules on monocytes and neutrophils from maternal, newborn and fetal samples, *Eur J Immunol* 18:565-569, 1988.
140. Henneke P, Osmers I, Bauer K, et al: Impaired CD14-dependent and independent response of polymorphonuclear leukocytes in preterm infants, *J Perinat Med* 31:176-183, 2003.
141. Jones DH, Schmalstieg FC, Dempsey K, et al: Subcellular distribution and mobilization of Mac-1 CD11b/CD18 in neonatal neutrophils, *Blood* 75:488-498, 1990.
142. Qing G, Rajaraman K, Bortolussi R: Diminished priming of neonatal polymorphonuclear leukocytes by lipopolysaccharide is associated with reduced CD14 expression, *Infect Immun* 63:248-252, 1995.
143. Segal BH, Leto TL, Gallin JI, et al: Genetic, biochemical, and clinical features of chronic granulomatous disease, *Medicine (Baltimore)* 79:170-200, 2000.
144. Rigby KM, DeLeo FR: Neutrophils in innate host defense against Staphylococcus aureus infections, *Semin Immunopathol* 34:237-259, 2012.
145. Hill HR: Biochemical, structural, and functional abnormalities of polymorphonuclear leukocytes in the neonate, *Pediatr Res* 22:375-382, 1987.
146. Johnston RB Jr: Function and cell biology of neutrophils and mononuclear phagocytes in the newborn infant, *Vaccine* 16:1363-1368, 1998.
147. Strunk T, Temming P, Gembruch U, et al: Differential maturation of the innate immune response in human fetuses, *Pediatr Res* 56: 219-226, 2004.
148. Chudgar UH, Thurman GW, Ambruso DR: Oxidase activity in cord blood neutrophils: a balance between increased membrane associated cytochrome b558 and deficient cytosolic components, *Pediatr Blood Cancer* 45:311-317, 2005.
149. Bjorkqvist M, Jurstrand M, Bodin L, et al: Defective neutrophil oxidative burst in preterm newborns on exposure to coagulase-negative staphylococci, *Pediatr Res* 55:966-971, 2004.
150. Al-Hertani W, Yan SR, Byers DM, et al: Human newborn polymorphonuclear neutrophils exhibit decreased levels of MYD88 and attenuated p38 phosphorylation in response to lipopolysaccharide, *Clin Invest Med* 30:E44-E53, 2007.
151. Nupponen I, Turunen R, Nevalainen T, et al: Extracellular release of bactericidal/permeability-increasing protein in newborn infants, *Pediatr Res* 51:670-674, 2002.
152. Levy O, Martin S, Eichenwald E, et al: Impaired innate immunity in the newborn: newborn neutrophils are deficient in bactericidal/permeability-increasing protein, *Pediatrics* 104:1327-1333, 1999.
153. Cocchi P, Marianelli L: Phagocytosis and intracellular killing of *Pseudomonas aeruginosa* in premature infants, *Helv Paediatr Acta* 22:110-118, 1967.
154. Coen R, Grush O, Kauder E: Studies of bactericidal activity and metabolism of the leukocyte in full-term neonates, *J Pediatr* 75: 400-406, 1969.
155. Brinkmann V, Reichard U, Goosmann C, et al: Neutrophil extracellular traps kill bacteria, *Science* 303:1532-1535, 2004.
156. Yost CC, Cody MJ, Harris ES, et al: Impaired neutrophil extracellular trap (NET) formation: a novel innate immune deficiency of human neonates, *Blood* 113:6419-6427, 2009.
157. Hayashi F, Means TK, Luster AD: Toll-like receptors stimulate human neutrophil function, *Blood* 102:2660-2669, 2003.
158. Ekman AK, Cardell LO: The expression and function of Nod-like receptors in neutrophils, *Immunology* 130:55-63, 2010.
159. Berger M, Hsieh CY, Bakele M, et al: Neutrophils express distinct RNA receptors in a non-canonical way, *J Biol Chem* 287: 19409-19417, 2012.
160. Cho JS, Guo Y, Ramos RI, et al: Neutrophil-derived IL-1beta is sufficient for abscess formation in immunity against *Staphylococcus aureus* in mice, *PLoS Pathog* 8:e1003047, 2012.
161. Halfhide CP, Brearey SP, Flanagan BF, et al: Neutrophil TLR4 expression is reduced in the airways of infants with severe bronchiolitis, *Thorax* 64:798-805, 2009.
162. Hanna N, Graboski S, Laskin DL, et al: Effects of ibuprofen and hypoxia on neutrophil apoptosis in neonates, *Biol Neonate* 86: 235-239, 2004.
163. Molloy EJ, O'Neill AJ, Grantham JJ, et al: Labor promotes neonatal neutrophil survival and lipopolysaccharide responsiveness, *Pediatr Res* 56:99-103, 2004.
164. Molloy EJ, O'Neill AJ, Grantham JJ, et al: Granulocyte colony-stimulating factor and granulocyte-macrophage colony-stimulating factor have differential effects on neonatal and adult neutrophil survival and function, *Pediatr Res* 57:806-812, 2005.
165. Hill HR, Augustine NH, Jaffe HS: Human recombinant interferon gamma enhances neonatal polymorphonuclear leukocyte activation and movement, and increases free intracellular calcium, *J Exp Med* 173:767-770, 1991.
166. Cairo MS, van de Ven C, Toy C, et al: Recombinant human granulocyte-macrophage colony-stimulating factor primes neonatal granulocytes for enhanced oxidative metabolism and chemotaxis, *Pediatr Res* 26:395-399, 1989.
167. Kamran S, Usmani SS, Wapnir RA, et al: In vitro effect of indomethacin on polymorphonuclear leukocyte function in preterm infants, *Pediatr Res* 33:32-35, 1993.
168. Moshfegh A, Lothian C, Halldén G, et al: Neonatal eosinophils possess efficient eotaxin/IL-5- and N-formyl-methionyl-leucyl-phenylalanine-induced transmigration in vitro, *Pediatr Res* 58:138-142, 2005.
169. Smith JB, Kunjummen RD, Kishimoto TK, et al: Expression and regulation of L-selectin on eosinophils from human adults and neonates, *Pediatr Res* 32:465-471, 1992.
170. Bhat AM, Scanlon JW: The pattern of eosinophilia in premature infants. A prospective study in premature infants using the absolute eosinophil count, *J Pediatr* 98:612, 1981.
171. van Furth R, Raeburn JA, van Zwet TL: Characteristics of human mononuclear phagocytes, *Blood* 54:485-500, 1979.
172. Cros J, Cagnard N, Woollard K, et al: Human CD14dim monocytes patrol and sense nucleic acids and viruses via TLR7 and TLR8 receptors, *Immunity* 33:375-386, 2010.
173. Wong KL, Tai JJ, Wong WC, et al: Gene expression profiling reveals the defining features of the classical, intermediate, and nonclassical human monocyte subsets, *Blood* 118:e16-e31, 2011.
174. Sohlberg E, Saghafian-Hedengren S, Bremme K, et al: Cord blood monocyte subsets are similar to adult and show potent peptidoglycan-stimulated cytokine responses, *Immunology* 133:41-50, 2011.
175. Galli SJ, Borregaard N, Wynn TA: Phenotypic and functional plasticity of cells of innate immunity: macrophages, mast cells and neutrophils, *Nat Immunol* 12:1035-1044, 2011.

176. Korns D, Frasch SC, Fernandez-Boyanapalli R, et al: Modulation of macrophage efferocytosis in inflammation, *Front Immunol* 2:57, 2011.
177. Kelemen E, Jaanossa M: Macrophages are the first differentiated blood cells formed in human embryonic liver, *Exp Hematol* 8: 996-1000, 1980.
178. Hashimoto D, Chow A, Noizat C, et al: Tissue-resident macrophages self-maintain locally throughout adult life with minimal contribution from circulating monocytes, *Immunity* 38:792-804, 2013.
179. Jenkins SJ, Ruckerl D, Thomas GD, et al: IL-4 directly signals tissue-resident macrophages to proliferate beyond homeostatic levels controlled by CSF-1, *J Exp Med* 210:2477-2491, 2013.
180. Robbins CS, Hilgendorf I, Weber GF, et al: Local proliferation dominates lesional macrophage accumulation in atherosclerosis, *Nat Med* 19:1166-1172, 2013.
181. Ueno Y, Koizumi S, Yamagami M, et al: Characterization of hemopoietic stem cells (CFUc) in cord blood, *Exp Hematol* 9:716-722, 1981.
182. Weinberg AG, Rosenfeld CR, Manroe BL, et al: Neonatal blood cell count in health and disease. II. Values for lymphocytes, monocytes, and eosinophils, *J Pediatr* 106:462-466, 1985.
183. Drohan L, Harding JJ, Holm B, et al: Selective developmental defects of cord blood antigen-presenting cell subsets, *Hum Immunol* 65:1356-1369, 2004.
184. Alenghat E, Esterly JR: Alveolar macrophages in perinatal infants, *Pediatrics* 74:221-223, 1984.
185. Jacobs RF, Wilson CB, Smith AL, et al: Age-dependent effects of aminobutyryl muramyl dipeptide on alveolar macrophage function in infant and adult macaca monkeys, *Am Rev Resp Dis* 128:862-867, 1983.
186. Blahnik MJ, Ramanathan R, Riley CR, et al: Lipopolysaccharide-induced tumor necrosis factor-alpha and IL-10 production by lung macrophages from preterm and term neonates, *Pediatr Res* 50:726-731, 2001.
187. Freedman R, Johnston D, Mahoney MJ, et al: Development of splenic reticuloendothelial function in neonates, *J Pediatr* 96:466-468, 1980.
188. Hyduk SJ, Cybulsky MI: Role of alpha4beta1 integrins in chemokine-induced monocyte arrest under conditions of shear stress, *Microcirculation* 16:17-30, 2009.
189. Bachelerie F, Ben-Baruch A, Burkhardt AM, et al: International union of pharmacology. Update on the extended family of chemokine receptors and introducing a new nomenclature for atypical chemokine receptors, *Pharmacol Rev* 66:1-79, 2014.
190. Luster AD: The role of chemokines in linking innate and adaptive immunity, *Curr Opin Immunol* 14:129-135, 2002.
191. Bullock JD, Robertson AF, Bodenbender JG, et al: Inflammatory response in the neonate re-examined, *Pediatrics* 44:58-61, 1969.
192. Uhr JW, Dancis J, Neumann CG: Delayed-type hypersensitivity in premature neonatal humans, *Nature* 187:1130-1131, 1960.
193. Baerenwaldt A, Lux A, Danzer H, et al: Fcgamma receptor IIb (FcgammaRIIb) maintains humoral tolerance in the human immune system in vivo, *Proc Natl Acad Sci U S A* 108:18772-18777, 2011.
194. Monteiro RC, Van De Winkel JG: IgA Fc receptors, *Annu Rev Immunol* 21:177-204, 2003.
195. Sengelov H: Complement receptors in neutrophils, *Crit Rev Immunol* 15:107-131, 1995.
196. Duits LA, Ravensbergen B, Rademaker M, et al: Expression of beta-defensin 1 and 2 mRNA by human monocytes, macrophages and dendritic cells, *Immunology* 106:517-525, 2002.
197. Ehrt S, Schnappinger D, Bekiranov S, et al: Reprogramming of the macrophage transcriptome in response to interferon-gamma and *Mycobacterium tuberculosis*: signaling roles of nitric oxide synthase-2 and phagocyte oxidase, *J Exp Med* 194:1123-1140, 2001.
198. Gordon S, Martinez FO: Alternative activation of macrophages: mechanism and functions, *Immunity* 32:593-604, 2010.
199. McCoy CE, O'Neill LA: The role of Toll-like receptors in macrophages, *Front Biosci* 13:62-70, 2008.
200. Azad AK, Sadee W, Schlesinger LS: Innate immune gene polymorphisms in tuberculosis, *Infect Immun* 80:3343-3359, 2012.
201. Bustamante J, Boisson-Dupuis S, Jouanguy E, et al: Novel primary immunodeficiencies revealed by the investigation of paediatric infectious diseases, *Curr Opin Immunol* 20:39-48, 2008.
202. Harris J, Keane J: How tumour necrosis factor blockers interfere with tuberculosis immunity, *Clin Exp Immunol* 161:1-9, 2010.
203. Lougaris V, Badolato R, Ferrari S, et al: Hyper immunoglobulin M syndrome due to CD40 deficiency: clinical, molecular, and immunological features, *Immunol Rev* 203:48-66, 2005.
204. Martinez FO, Gordon S, Locati M, et al: Transcriptional profiling of the human monocyte-to-macrophage differentiation and polarization: new molecules and patterns of gene expression, *J Immunol* 77:7303-7311, 2006.
205. Van Dyken SJ, Locksley RM: Interleukin-4- and interleukin-13-mediated alternatively activated macrophages: roles in homeostasis and disease, *Annu Rev Immunol* 31:317-343, 2013.
206. Xue J, Schmidt SV1 Sander J, et al: Transcriptome-based network analysis reveals a spectrum model of human macrophage activation, *Immunity* 40:274-288, 2014.
207. Becker ID, Robinson OM, Bazán TS, et al: Bactericidal capacity of newborn phagocytes against group B beta-hemolytic streptococci, *Infect Immun* 34:535-539, 1981.
208. Weston WL, Carson BS, Barkin RM, et al: Monocyte-macrophage function in the newborn, *Am J Dis Child* 131:1241-1242, 1977.
209. Dretschmer RR, Stewardson RB, Papierniak CK, et al: Chemotactic and bactericidal capacities of human newborn monocytes, *J Immunol* 117:1303-1307, 1976.
210. Hawes CS, Kemp AS, Jones WR: In vitro parameters of cell-mediated immunity in the human neonate, *Clin Immunol Immunopathol* 17: 530-536, 1980.
211. Orlowski JP, Sieger L, Anthony BF: Bactericidal capacity of monocytes of newborn infants, *J Pediatr* 89:797-801, 1976.
212. Speer CP, Ambruso DR, Grimsley J, et al: Oxidative metabolism in cord blood monocytes and monocyte-derived macrophages, *Infect Immun* 50:919-921, 1985.
213. Speer CP, Wieland M, Ulbrich R, et al: Phagocytic activities in neonatal monocytes, *Eur J Pediatr* 145:418-421, 1986.
214. Speer CP, Gahr M, Wieland M, et al: Phagocytosis-associated functions in neonatal monocyte-derived macrophages, *Pediatr Res.* 24:213-216, 1988.
215. Conly ME, Speert DP: Human neonatal monocyte-derived macrophages and neutrophils exhibit normal nonopsonic and opsonic receptor-mediated phagocytosis and superoxide anion production, *Biol Neonate* 60:361-366, 1991.
216. Plaeger-Marshall S, Ank BJ, Altenburger KM, et al: Replication of herpes simplex virus in blood monocytes and placental macrophages from human neonates, *Pediatr Res* 26:135-139, 1989.
217. Mintz L, Drew WL, Hoo R, et al: Age-dependent resistance of human alveolar macrophages to herpes simplex virus, *Infect Immun* 28:417-420, 1980.
218. Kohl S: Herpes simplex virus immunology: problems, progress, and promises, *J Infect Dis* 152:435-440, 1985.
219. Milgrom H, Shore SL: Assessment of monocyte function in the normal newborn infant by antibody-dependent cellular cytotoxicity, *J Pediatr* 91:612-614, 1977.
220. Marodi L: Deficient interferon-gamma receptor-mediated signaling in neonatal macrophages, *Acta Paediat* 91:117-119, 2002.
221. Marodi L, Kaposzta R, Nemes E: Survival of group B streptococcus type III in mononuclear phagocytes: differential regulation of bacterial killing in cord macrophages by human recombinant gamma interferon and granulocyte-macrophage colony-stimulating factor, *Infect Immun* 68:2167-2170, 2000.
222. Marodi L, Káposzta R, Campbell DE, et al: Candidacidal mechanisms in the human neonate. Impaired IFN-gamma activation of macrophages in newborn infants, *J Immunol* 153:5643-5649, 1994.
223. Kurland G, Cheung AT, Miller ME, et al: The ontogeny of pulmonary defenses: alveolar macrophage function in neonatal and juvenile rhesus monkeys, *Pediatr Res* 23:293-297, 1988.
224. Wilson CB, Haas JE: Cellular defenses against toxoplasma gondii in newborns, *J Clin Invest* 73:1606-1616, 1984.
225. Berman JD, Johnson WD Jr: Monocyte function in human neonates, *Infect Immun* 19:898-902, 1978.
226. Jones SA: Directing transition from innate to acquired immunity: defining a role for IL-6, *J Immunol* 175:3463-3468, 2005.
227. Taniguchi T, Takaoka A: The interferon-alpha/beta system in antiviral responses: a multimodal machinery of gene regulation by the IRF family of transcription factors, *Curr Opin Immunol* 14:111-116, 2002.
228. Boehm U, Klamp T, Groot M, et al: Cellular responses to interferon-gamma, *Annu Rev Immunol* 15:749-795, 1997.

229. Goriely S, Goldman M: The interleukin-12 family: new players in transplantation immunity? *Am J Transplant* 7:278-284, 2007.
230. Yamane H, Paul WE: Early signaling events that underlie fate decisions of naive CD4(+) T cells toward distinct T-helper cell subsets, *Immunol Rev.* 252:12-23, 2013.
231. Schulte W, Bernhagen J, Bucala R: Cytokine in sepsis: potent immunoregulators and potential therapeutic targets—an updated view, *Mediators Inflamm* 2013:165974, 2013.
232. van de Veerdonk FL, Netea MG: New insights in the immunobiology of IL-1 family members, *Front Immunol* 4:167, 2013.
233. Spite M, Claria J, Serhan CN: Resolvins, specialized proresolving lipid mediators, and their potential roles in metabolic diseases, *Cell Metab* 19:21-36, 2014.
234. Kollmann TR, Crabtree J, Rein-Weston A, et al: Neonatal innate TLR-mediated responses are distinct from those of adults, *J Immunol* 183:7150-7160, 2009.
235. Corbett NP, Blimkie D, Ho KC, et al: Ontogeny of Toll-like receptor mediated cytokine responses of human blood mononuclear cells, *PloS One* 5:e15041, 2010.
236. de Jong EC, Smits HH, Kapsenberg ML: Dendritic cell-mediated T cell polarization, *Springer Semin Immunopathol* 26:289-307, 2005.
237. Belderbos ME, van Bleek GM, Levy O, et al: Skewed pattern of Toll-like receptor 4-mediated cytokine production in human neonatal blood: low LPS-induced IL-12p70 and high IL-10 persist throughout the first month of life, *Clin Immunol* 133:228-237, 2009.
238. Nguyen CN, Schnulle PM, Chegini N, et al: Neonatal neutrophils with prolonged survival secrete mediators associated with chronic inflammation, *Neonatology* 98:341-347, 2010.
239. Vanden Driessche K, Persson A, Marais BJ, et al: Immune vulnerability of infants to tuberculosis, *Clin Dev Immunol* 2013:781320, 2013.
240. Levy O, Zarember KA, Roy RM, et al: Selective impairment of TLR-mediated innate immunity in human newborns: neonatal blood plasma reduces monocyte TNF-alpha induction by bacterial lipopeptides, lipopolysaccharide, and imiquimod, but preserves the response to R-848, *J Immunol* 173:4627-4634, 2004.
241. De Wit D, Tonon S, Olislagers V, et al: Impaired responses to Toll-like receptor 4 and Toll-like receptor 3 ligands in human cord blood, *J Autoimmun* 21:277-281, 2003.
242. Karlsson H, Hessle C, Rudin A: Innate immune responses of human neonatal cells to bacteria from the normal gastrointestinal flora, *Infect Immun* 70:6688-6696, 2002.
243. Kollmann TR, Crabtree J, Rein-Weston A, et al: Neonatal innate TLR-mediated responses are distinct from those of adults, *J Immunol* 183:7150-7160, 2009.
244. Reikie BA, Adams RC, Ruck CE, et al: Ontogeny of Toll-like receptor mediated cytokine responses of South African infants throughout the first year of life, *PloS One* 7:e44763, 2012.
245. Black A, Bhaumik S, Kirkman RL, et al: Developmental regulation of TH17-cell capacity in human neonates, *Eur J Immunol* 42:311-319, 2012.
246. Chang M, Suen Y, Lee SM, et al: Transforming growth factor-beta 1, macrophage inflammatory protein-1 alpha, and interleukin-8 gene expression is lower in stimulated human neonatal compared with adult mononuclear cells, *Blood* 84:118-124, 1994.
247. Chheda S, Palkowetz KH, Garofalo R, et al: Decreased interleukin-10 production by neonatal monocytes and T cells: relationship to decreased production and expression of tumor necrosis factor-alpha and its receptors, *Pediatr Res* 40:475-483, 1996.
248. Seghaye MC, Heyl W, Grabitz RG, et al: The production of pro- and anti-inflammatory cytokines in neonates assessed by stimulated whole cord blood culture and by plasma levels at birth, *Biol Neonate* 73:220-227, 1998.
249. Yerkovich ST, Wikström ME, Suriyaarachchi D, et al: Postnatal development of monocyte cytokine responses to bacterial lipopolysaccharide, *Pediatr Res* 62:547-552, 2007.
250. Dasari P, Zola H, Nicholson IC: Expression of Toll-like receptors by neonatal leukocytes, *Pediatr Allergy Immunol* 22:221-228, 2011.
251. Sadeghi K, Berger A, Langgartner M, et al: Immaturity of infection control in preterm and term newborns is associated with impaired Toll-like receptor signaling, *J Infect Dis* 195:296-302, 2007.
252. Cohen L, Haziot A, Shen DR, et al: CD14-independent responses to LPS require a serum factor that is absent from neonates, *J Immunol* 155:5337-5342, 1995.
253. Yan SR, Qing G, Byers DM, et al: Role of MYD88 in diminished tumor necrosis factor alpha production by newborn mononuclear cells in response to lipopolysaccharide, *Infect Immun* 72:1223-1229, 2004.
254. Liu E, Tu W, Law HK, et al: Changes of CD14 and CD1a expression in response to IL-4 and granulocyte-macrophage colony-stimulating factor are different in cord blood and adult blood monocytes, *Pediatr Res* 50:184-189, 2001.
255. Kampalath B, Cleveland RP, Kass L: Reduced CD4 and HLA-DR expression in neonatal monocytes, *Clin Immunol Immunopathol* 87:93-100, 1998.
256. Shen CM, Lin SC, Niu DM, et al: Development of monocyte Toll-like receptor 2 and Toll-like receptor 4 in preterm newborns during the first few months of life, *Pediatr Res* 73:685-691, 2013.
257. Hoebe K, Beutler B: LPS, dsRNA and the interferon bridge to adaptive immune responses: TRIF, TRAM, and other TIR adaptor proteins, *J Endotoxin Res* 10:130-136, 2004.
258. Hoebe K, Janssen EM, Kim SO, et al: Upregulation of costimulatory molecules induced by lipopolysaccharide and double-stranded RNA occurs by TRIF-dependent and TRIF-independent pathways, *Nat Immunol* 4:1223-1229, 2003.
259. Iwasaki A, Medzhitov R: Toll-like receptor control of the adaptive immune responses, *Nat Immunol* 5:987-995, 2004.
260. Akira S, Takeda K: Functions of Toll-like receptors: lessons from KO mice, *Curr Rev Biol* 327:581-589, 2004.
261. Levy O, Coughlin M, Cronstein BN, et al: The adenosine system selectively inhibits TLR-mediated TNF-alpha production in the human newborn, *J Immunol* 177:1956-1966, 2006.
262. Levy O, Suter EE, Miller RL, et al: Unique efficacy of Toll-like receptor 8 agonists in activating human neonatal antigen-presenting cells, *Blood* 108:1284-1290, 2006.
263. Pettengill M, Robson S, Tresenriter M, et al: Soluble ecto-5′-nucleotidase (5′-NT), alkaline phosphatase, and adenosine deaminase (ADA1) activities in neonatal blood favor elevated extracellular adenosine, *J Biol Chem* 288:27315-27326, 2013.
264. Giannoni E, Guignard L, Knaup Reymond M, et al: Estradiol and progesterone strongly inhibit the innate immune response of mononuclear cells in newborns, *Infect Immun* 79:2690-2698, 2011.
265. Belderbos ME, Levy O, Stalpers F, et al: Neonatal plasma polarizes TLR4-mediated cytokine responses towards low IL-12p70 and high IL-10 production via distinct factors, *PloS One* 7:e33419, 2012.
266. Berner R, Fürll B, Stelter F, et al: Elevated levels of lipopolysaccharide-binding protein and soluble CD14 in plasma in neonatal early-onset sepsis, *Clin Diagn Lab Immunol* 9:440-445, 2002.
267. Lammas DA, Stober C, Harvey CJ, et al: ATP-induced killing of mycobacteria by human macrophages is mediated by purinergic P2X7 receptors, *Immunity* 7:433-444, 1997.
268. Gille C, Dreschers S, Leiber A, et al: The CD95/CD95L pathway is involved in phagocytosis-induced cell death of monocytes and may account for sustained inflammation in neonates, *Pediatr Res* 73:402-408, 2013.
269. Merad M, Sathe P, Helft J, et al: The dendritic cell lineage: ontogeny and function of dendritic cells and their subsets in the steady state and the inflamed setting, *Annu Rev Immunol* 31:563-604, 2013.
270. Haniffa M, Collin M, Ginhoux F: Ontogeny and functional specialization of dendritic cells in human and mouse, *Adv Immunol* 120: 1-49, 2013.
271. Cahalan MD, Parker I: Choreography of cell motility and interaction dynamics imaged by two-photon microscopy in lymphoid organs, *Annu Rev Immunol* 26:585-626, 2008.
272. Nace G, Evankovich J, Eid R, et al: Dendritic cells and damage-associated molecular patterns: endogenous danger signals linking innate and adaptive immunity, *J Innate Immun* 4:6-15, 2012.
273. Villadangos JA, Schnorrer P: Intrinsic and cooperative antigen-presenting functions of dendritic-cell subsets in vivo, *Nat Rev Immunol* 7:543-555, 2007.
274. Idoyaga J, Fiorese C, Zbytnuik L, et al: Specialized role of migratory dendritic cells in peripheral tolerance induction, *J Clin Invest* 123:844-854, 2013.
275. Manicassamy S, Pulendran B: Dendritic cell control of tolerogenic responses, *Immunol Rev* 241:206-227, 2011.
276. Zammit DJ, Cauley LS, Pham QM, et al: Dendritic cells maximize the memory CD8 T cell response to infection, *Immunity* 22:561-570, 2005.
277. Liu D, Rhebergen AM, Eisenbarth SC: Licensing adaptive immunity by NOD-like receptors, *Front Immunol* 4:486, 2013.
278. Szabo A, Rajnavolgyi E: Collaboration of Toll-like and RIG-I-like receptors in human dendritic cells: triggering antiviral innate immune responses, *Am J Clin Exp Immunol* 2:195-207, 2013.

279. Cerboni S, Gentili M, Manel N: Diversity of pathogen sensors in dendritic cells, *Adv Immunol* 120:211-237, 2013.
280. van Kooyk Y: C-type lectins on dendritic cells: key modulators for the induction of immune responses, *Biochem Soc Trans* 36: 1478-1481, 2008.
281. Collin M, McGovern N, Haniffa M: Human dendritic cell subsets, *Immunology* 140:22-30, 2013.
282. Hambleton S, Salem S, Bustamante J, et al: IRF8 mutations and human dendritic-cell immunodeficiency, *N Engl J Med* 365:127-138, 2011.
283. De Wit D, Olislagers V, Goriely S, et al: Blood plasmacytoid dendritic cell responses to CpG oligodeoxynucleotides are impaired in human newborns, *Blood* 103:1030-1032, 2004.
284. Borras FE, Matthews NC, Lowdell MW, et al: Identification of both myeloid CD11c+ and lymphoid CD11c- dendritic cell subsets in cord blood, *Br J Haematol* 113:925-931, 2001.
285. Teig N, Moses D, Gieseler S, et al: Age-related changes in human blood dendritic cell subpopulations, *Scand J Immunol* 55:453-457, 2002.
286. Hagendorens MM, Ebo DG, Schuerwegh AJ, et al: Differences in circulating dendritic cell subtypes in cord blood and peripheral blood of healthy and allergic children, *Clin Exp Allergy* 33:633-639, 2003.
287. Sorg RV, Kogler G, Wernet P: Functional competence of dendritic cells in human umbilical cord blood, *Bone Marrow Transplant* 22(Suppl 1):S52-S54, 1998.
288. Sorg RV, Kogler G, Wernet P: Identification of cord blood dendritic cells as an immature CD11c− population, *Blood* 93:2302-2307, 1999.
289. Tonon S, Goriely S, Aksoy E, et al: *Bordetella pertussis* toxin induces the release of inflammatory cytokines and dendritic cell activation in whole blood: impaired responses in human newborns, *Eur J Immunol* 32:3118-3125, 2002.
290. Lavoie PM, Huang Q, Jolette E, et al: Profound lack of interleukin (IL)-12/IL-23p40 in neonates born early in gestation is associated with an increased risk of sepsis, *J Infect Dis* 202:1754-1763, 2010.
291. Wilson CB, Kollmann TR: Induction of antigen-specific immunity in human neonates and infants, *Nestle Nutr Workshop Ser Pediatr Program* 61:183-195, 2008.
292. Burl S, Townend J, Njie-Jobe J, et al: Age-dependent maturation of Toll-like receptor-mediated cytokine responses in gambian infants, *PloS One* 6:e18185, 2011.
293. Hemont C, Neel A, Heslan M, et al: Human blood mDC subsets exhibit distinct TLR repertoire and responsiveness, *J Leukoc Biol* 93:599-609, 2013.
294. Thornburg NJ, Shepherd B, Crowe JE Jr: Transforming growth factor beta is a major regulator of human neonatal immune responses following respiratory syncytial virus infection, *J Virol* 84: 12895-12902, 2010.
295. Mathan TS, Figdor CG, Buschow SI: Human plasmacytoid dendritic cells: From molecules to intercellular communication network, *Front Immunol* 4:372, 2013.
296. Blom B, Ho S, Antonenko S, et al: Generation of interferon alpha-producing predendritic cell (pre-DC)2 from human CD34(+) hematopoietic stem cells, *J Exp Med* 192:1785-1796, 2000.
297. Olweus J, BitMansour A, Warnke R, et al: Dendritic cell ontogeny: a human dendritic cell lineage of myeloid origin, *Proc Natl Acad Sci U S A* 94:12551-12556, 1997.
298. Danis B, George TC, Goriely S, et al: Interferon regulatory factor 7-mediated responses are defective in cord blood plasmacytoid dendritic cells, *Eur J Immunol* 38:507-517, 2008.
299. Zhang X, Lepelley A, Azria E, et al: Neonatal plasmacytoid dendritic cells (pDCs) display subset variation but can elicit potent anti-viral innate responses, *PloS One* 8:e52003, 2013.
300. Schuller SS, Sadeghi K, Wisgrill L, et al: Preterm neonates display altered plasmacytoid dendritic cell function and morphology, *J Leukoc Biol* 93:781-788, 2013.
301. Gold MC, Robinson TL, Cook MS, et al: Human neonatal dendritic cells are competent in MHC class I antigen processing and presentation, *PloS One* 2:e957, 2007.
302. Cederblad B, Riesenfeld T, Alm GV: Deficient herpes simplex virus-induced interferon-alpha production by blood leukocytes of preterm and term newborn infants, *Pediatr Res* 27:7-10, 1990.
303. Neustock P, Kruse A, Bein G, et al: Failure to detect type 1 interferon production in human umbilical cord vein endothelial cells after viral exposure, *J Interfer Cytokine Res* 15:129-135, 1995.
304. Hoeffel G, Wang Y, Greter M, et al: Adult langerhans cells derive predominantly from embryonic fetal liver monocytes with a minor contribution of yolk sac-derived macrophages, *J Exp Med* 209:1167-1181, 2012.
305. Seneschal J, Wang Y, Greter M, et al: Human epidermal langerhans cells maintain immune homeostasis in skin by activating skin resident regulatory T cells, *Immunity* 36:873-884, 2012.
306. Foster CA, Holbrook KA: Ontogeny of Langerhans cells in human embryonic and fetal skin: cell densities and phenotypic expression relative to epidermal growth, *Am J Anat* 184:157-164, 1989.
307. Schuster C, Vaculik C, Fiala C, et al: HLA-DR+ leukocytes acquire CD1 antigens in embryonic and fetal human skin and contain functional antigen-presenting cells, *J Exp Med* 206:169-181, 2009.
308. Cheong C, Matos I, Choi JH, et al: Microbial stimulation fully differentiates monocytes to DC-SIGN/CD209(+) dendritic cells for immune T cell areas, *Cell* 143:416-429, 2010.
309. Lowes MA, Chamian F, Abello MV, et al: Increase in TNF-alpha and inducible nitric oxide synthase-expressing dendritic cells in psoriasis and reduction with efalizumab (anti-CD11a), *Proc Natl Acad Sci U. S.A* 102:19057-19062, 2005.
310. Hansel A, Günther C, Ingwersen J, et al: Human SLAN (6-sulfo Lanac) dendritic cells are inflammatory dermal dendritic cells in psoriasis and drive strong TH17/TH1 T-cell responses, *J Allergy Clin Immunol* 127:787-794, 2011. e1-e9.
311. Segura E, Amigorena S: Identification of human inflammatory dendritic cells, *Oncoimmunol* 2:e23851, 2013.
312. Goriely S, Vincart B, Stordeur P, et al: Deficient IL-12(p35) gene expression by dendritic cells derived from neonatal monocytes, *J Immunol* 166:2141-2146, 2001.
313. Langrish CL, Buddle JC, Thrasher AJ, et al: Neonatal dendritic cells are intrinsically biased against Th-1 immune responses, *Clin Exp Immunol* 128:118-123, 2002.
314. Krumbiegel D, Zepp F, Meyer CU: Combined Toll-like receptor agonists synergistically increase production of inflammatory cytokines in human neonatal dendritic cells, *Hum Immunol* 68:813-822, 2007.
315. Aksoy E, Albarani V, Nguyen M, et al: Interferon regulatory factor 3-dependent responses to lipopolysaccharide are selectively blunted in cord blood cells, *Blood* 109:2887-2893, 2007.
316. Goriely S, Van Lint C, Dadkhah R, et al: A defect in nucleosome remodeling prevents IL-12(p35) gene transcription in neonatal dendritic cells, *J Exp Med* 199:1011-1016, 2004.
317. Liu E, Law HK, Lau YL: BCG promotes cord blood monocyte-derived dendritic cell maturation with nuclear Rel-b up-regulation and cytosolic I kappa B alpha and beta degradation, *Pediatr Res.* 54:105-112, 2003.
318. Jouanguy E, Gineau L, Cottineau J, et al: Inborn errors of the development of human natural killer cells, *Curr Opin Allergy Clin Immunol* 13:589-595, 2013.
319. Finton KA, Strong RK: Structural insights into activation of antiviral NK cell responses, *Immunol Rev* 250:239-257, 2012.
320. Cella M, Fuchs A, Vermi W, et al: A human natural killer cell subset provides an innate source of IL-22 for mucosal immunity, *Nature* 457:722-725, 2009.
321. Loza MJ, Perussia B: The IL-12 signature: NK cell terminal CD56+high stage and effector functions, *J Immunol* 172:88-96, 2004.
322. Horowitz A, Strauss-Albee DM, Leipold M, et al: Genetic and environmental determinants of human NK cell diversity revealed by mass cytometry, *Sci Transl Med* 5, 2013. 208ra145.
323. Natarajan K, Dimasi N, Wang J, et al: Structure and function of natural killer cell receptors: multiple molecular solutions to self, nonself discrimination, *Annu Rev Immunol* 20:853-885, 2002.
324. Parham P: Taking license with natural killer cell maturation and repertoire development, *Immunol Rev* 214:155-160, 2006.
325. Lanier LL: NK cell receptors, *Annu Rev Immunol* 16:359-393, 1998.
326. O'Callaghan CA: Natural killer cell surveillance of intracellular antigen processing pathways mediated by recognition of HLA-E and Qa-1b by CD94/NKG2 receptors, *Microbes Infect* 2:371-380, 2000.
327. Croy BA, Esadeg S, Chantakru S, et al: Update on pathways regulating the activation of uterine natural killer cells, their interactions with decidual spiral arteries and homing of their precursors to the uterus, *J Reprod Immunol* 59:175-191, 2003.
328. Morel E, Bellon T: Hla class I molecules regulate IFN-gamma production induced in NK cells by target cells, viral products, or immature dendritic cells through the inhibitory receptor ILT2/CD85j, *J Immunol* 181:2368-2381, 2008.

329. Odom CI, Gaston DC, Markert JM, Cassady KA: Human herpesviridae methods of natural killer cell evasion, *Adv Virol* 359869:2012, 2012.
330. Wu J, Chalupny NJ, Manley TJ, et al: Intracellular retention of the MHC class I-related chain B ligand of NKG2D by the human cytomegalovirus UL16 glycoprotein, *J Immunol* 170:4196-4200, 2003.
331. Snyder MR, Weyand CM, Goronzy JJ: The double life of NK receptors: stimulation or co-stimulation? *Trends Immunol* 25:25-32, 2004.
332. Arkwright PD, Rieux-Laucat F, Le Deist F, et al: Cytomegalovirus infection in infants with autoimmune lymphoproliferative syndrome (ALPS), *Clin Exp Immunol* 121:353-357, 2000.
333. Eischen CM, Schilling JD, Lynch DH, et al: Fc receptor-induced expression of fas ligand on activated NK cells facilitates cell-mediated cytotoxicity and subsequent autocrine NK cell apoptosis, *J Immunol* 156:2693-2699, 1996.
334. Mainiero F, Gismondi A, Soriani A, et al: Integrin-mediated Ras-extracellular regulated kinase (Erk) signaling regulates interferon gamma production in human natural killer cells, *J Exp Med* 188:1267-1275, 1998.
335. Hunter CA, Chizzonite R, Remington JS: IL-1 beta is required for IL-12 to induce production of IFN-gamma by NK cells. A role for IL-1 beta in the T cell-independent mechanism of resistance against intracellular pathogens, *J Immunol* 155:4347-4354, 1995.
336. Bluman EM, Bartynski KJ, Avalos BR, et al: Human natural killer cells produce abundant macrophage inflammatory protein-1 alpha in response to monocyte-derived cytokines, *J Clin Invest* 97: 2722-2727, 1996.
337. Tay CH, Szomolanyi-Tsuda E, Welsh RM: Control of infections by NK cells, *Curr Top Microbiol Immunol* 230:193-220, 1998.
338. Bernstein HB, Kinter AL, Jackson R, et al: Neonatal natural killer cells produce chemokines and suppress HIV replication in vitro, *AIDS Res Hum Retroviruses* 20:1189-1195, 2004.
339. Nakazawa T, Agematsu K, Yabuhara A: Later development of fas ligand-mediated cytotoxicity as compared with granule-mediated cytotoxicity during the maturation of natural killer cells, *Immunology* 92:180-187, 1997.
340. Bradstock KF, Luxford C, Grimsley PG: Functional and phenotypic assessment of neonatal human leucocytes expressing natural killer cell-associated antigens, *Immunol Cell Biol* 71:535-542, 1993.
341. Sundstrom Y, Nilsson C, Lilja G, et al: The expression of human natural killer cell receptors in early life, *Scand J Immunol* 66: 335-344, 2007.
342. Dalle JH, Menezes J, Wagner E, et al: Characterization of cord blood natural killer cells: implications for transplantation and neonatal infections, *Pediatr Res* 57:649-655, 2005.
343. Braakman E, Sturm E, Vijverberg K, et al: Expression of CD45 isoforms by fresh and activated human gamma delta T lymphocytes and natural killer cells, *Int Immunol* 3:691-697, 1991.
344. Merrill JD, Sigaroudinia M, Kohl S: Characterization of natural killer and antibody-dependent cellular cytotoxicity of preterm infants against human immunodeficiency virus-infected cells, *Pediatr Res* 40:498-503, 1996.
345. Webb BJ, Bochan MR, Montel A, et al: The lack of NK cytotoxicity associated with fresh HUCB may be due to the presence of soluble HLA in the serum, *Cell Immunol* 159:246-261, 1994.
346. Harrison CJ, Waner JL: Natural killer cell activity in infants and children excreting cytomegalovirus, *J Infect Dis* 151:301-307, 1985.
347. Jenkins M, Mills J, Kohl S: Natural killer cytotoxicity and antibody-dependent cellular cytotoxicity of human immunodeficiency virus-infected cells by leukocytes from human neonates and adults, *Pediatr Res* 33:469-474, 1993.
348. McDonald T, Sneed J, Valenski WR, et al: Natural killer cell activity in very low birth weight infants, *Pediatr Res* 31:376-380, 1992.
349. Georgeson GD, Szony BJ, Streitman K, et al: Natural killer cell cytotoxicity is deficient in newborns with sepsis and recurrent infections, *Eur J Pediatr* 160:478-482, 2001.
350. Lin SJ, Yang MH, Chao HC, et al: Effect of interleukin-15 and Flt3-ligand on natural killer cell expansion and activation: umbilical cord vs. adult peripheral blood mononuclear cells, *Pediatr Allergy Immunol* 11:168-174, 2000.
351. Condiotti R, Nagler A: Effect of interleukin-12 on antitumor activity of human umbilical cord blood and bone marrow cytotoxic cells, *Exp Hematol* 26:571-579, 1998.
352. Brahmi Z, Hommel-Berrey G, Smith F, et al: NK cells recover early and mediate cytotoxicity via perforin/granzyme and fas/fasL pathways in umbilical cord blood recipients, *Hum Immunol* 62: 782-790, 2001.
353. Nomura A, Takada H, Jin CH, et al: Functional analysis of cord blood natural killer cells and T cells: a distinctive interleukin-18 response, *Exp Hematol* 29:1169-1176, 2001.
354. Schatt S, Holzgreve W, Hahn S: Stimulated cord blood lymphocytes have a low percentage of Th1 and Th2 cytokine secreting T cells although their activation is similar to adult controls, *Immunol Lett* 77:1-2, 2001.
355. Cupedo T, Crellin NK, Papazian N, et al: Human fetal lymphoid tissue-inducer cells are interleukin 17-producing precursors to RORc+ CD127+ natural killer-like cells, *Nat Immunol* 10:66-74, 2009.
356. Cupedo T: Human lymph node development: an inflammatory interaction, *Immunol Lett* 138:4-6, 2011.
357. Spits H, Cupedo T: Innate lymphoid cells: emerging insights in development, lineage relationships, and function, *Annu Rev Immunol* 30:647-675, 2012.
358. Hepworth MR, Monticelli LA, Fung TC, et al: Innate lymphoid cells regulate CD4+ T-cell responses to intestinal commensal bacteria, *Nature* 498:113-117, 2013.
359. Bernink J, Mjosberg J, Spits H: Th1- and Th2-like subsets of innate lymphoid cells, *Immunol Rev* 252:133-138, 2013.
360. Mjosberg J, Bernink J, Golebski K, et al: The transcription factor GATA3 is essential for the function of human type 2 innate lymphoid cells, *Immunity* 37:649-659, 2012.
361. Robinson J, Halliwell JA, McWilliam H, et al: The IMGT/HLA database, *Nucl Acids Res* 41:D1222-D1227, 2013.
362. Blum JS, Wearsch PA, Cresswell P: Pathways of antigen processing, *Annu Rev Immunol* 31:443-473, 2013.
363. Le Bon A, Tough DF: Type I interferon as a stimulus for cross-priming, *Cytokine Growth Factor Rev* 19:33-40, 2008.
364. Mantegazza AR, Savina A, Vermeulen M, et al: NADPH oxidase controls phagosomal pH and antigen cross-presentation in human dendritic cells, *Blood* 112:4712-4722, 2008.
365. Deretic V, Saitoh T, Akira S: Autophagy in infection, inflammation and immunity, *Nat Rev Immunol* 13:722-737, 2013.
366. Fossum S: The life history of dendritic leukocytes, *Curr Top Pathol* 79:101-124, 1989.
367. Keever CA, Abu-Hajir M, Graf W, et al: Characterization of the alloreactivity and anti-leukemia reactivity of cord blood mononuclear cells, *Bone Marrow Transplant* 15:407-419, 1995.
368. Canaday DH, Chakravarti S, Srivastava T, et al: Class II MHC antigen presentation defect in neonatal monocytes is not correlated with decreased MHC-II expression, *Cell Immunol* 243:96-106, 2006.
369. Garban F, Ericson M, Roucard C, et al: Detection of empty HLA class II molecules on cord blood B cells, *Blood* 87:3970-3976, 1996.
370. Miller JD, Weber DA, Ibegbu C, et al: Analysis of HLA-E peptide-binding specificity and contact residues in bound peptide required for recognition by CD94/NKG2, *J Immunol* 171:1369-1375, 2003.
371. Ishitani A, Sageshima N, Hatake K: The involvement of HLA-E and -F in pregnancy, *J Reprod Immunol* 69:101-113, 2006.
372. Hunt JS: Stranger in a strange land, *Immunol Rev* 213:36-47, 2006.
373. Fournel S, Aguerre-Girr M, Huc X, et al: Cutting edge: Soluble HLA-G1 triggers CD95/CD95 ligand-mediated apoptosis in activated CD8+ cells by interacting with CD8, *J Immunol* 164:6100-6104, 2000.
374. Contini P, Ghio M, Poggi A, et al: Soluble HLA-A, -B, -C, and -G molecules induce apoptosis in T and NK CD8+ cells and inhibit cytotoxic T cell activity through CD8 ligation, *Eur J Immunol* 33:125-134, 2003.
375. Stern-Ginossar N, Gur C, Biton M, et al: Human microRNAs regulate stress-induced immune responses mediated by the receptor NKG2D, *Nat Immunol* 9:1065-1073, 2008.
376. Das H, Groh V, Kuijl C, et al: MICA engagement by human Vgamma2Vdelta2 T cells enhances their antigen-dependent effector function, *Immunity* 15:83-93, 2001.
377. Gonzalez S, Groh V, Spies T: Immunobiology of human NKG2D and its ligands, *Curr Top Microbiol Immunol* 298:121-138, 2006.
378. Cohen NR, Garg S, Brenner MB: Antigen presentation by CD1 lipids, T cells, and NKT cells in microbial immunity, *Adv Immunol* 102:1-94, 2009.

379. Kasmar AG, Van Rhijn I, Magalhaes KG, et al: Cutting edge: CD1a tetramers and dextramers identify human lipopeptide-specific T cells ex vivo, *J Immunol* 191:4499-4503, 2013.
380. Ly D, Kasmar AG, Cheng TY, et al: CD1c tetramers detect ex vivo T cell responses to processed phosphomycoketide antigens, *J Exp Med* 210:729-741, 2013.
381. de Jong A, Cheng TY2, Huang S3, et al: CD1a-autoreactive T cells recognize natural skin oils that function as headless antigens, *Nat Immunol* 15:177-185, 2014.
382. Van Rhijn I, Kasmar A, de Jong A, et al: A conserved human T cell population targets mycobacterial antigens presented by CD1b, *Nat Immunol* 14:706-713, 2013.
383. Facciotti F, Cavallari M, Angénieux C, et al: Fine tuning by human CD1e of lipid-specific immune responses, *Proc Natl Acad Sci U.S.A* 108:14228-14233, 2011.
384. Van Rhijn I, Ly D, Moody DB: CD1a, CD1b, and CD1c in immunity against mycobacteria, *Adv Exp Med Biol* 783:181-197, 2013.
385. Gordon J, Wilson VA, Blair NF, et al: Functional evidence for a single endodermal origin for the thymic epithelium, *Nat Immunol* 5:546-553, 2004.
386. Hollander G, Gill J, Zuklys S, et al: Cellular and molecular events during early thymus development, *Immunol Rev* 209:28-46, 2006.
387. Guris DL, Duester G, Papaioannou VE, et al: Dose-dependent interaction of Tbx1 and Crkl and locally aberrant ra signaling in a model of del22q11 syndrome, *Dev Cell* 10:81-92, 2006.
388. Haddad R, Guimiot F, Six E, et al: Dynamics of thymus-colonizing cells during human development, *Immunity* 24:217-230, 2006.
389. Six EM, Bonhomme D, Monteiro M, et al: A human postnatal lymphoid progenitor capable of circulating and seeding the thymus, *J Exp Med* 204:3085-3093, 2007.
390. Weerkamp F, Baert MR, Brugman MH, et al: Human thymus contains multipotent progenitors with T/B lymphoid, myeloid, and erythroid lineage potential, *Blood* 107:3131-3137, 2006.
391. Maes J, Maleszewska M, Guillemin C, et al: Lymphoid-affiliated genes are associated with active histone modifications in human hematopoietic stem cells, *Blood* 112:2722-2729, 2008.
392. Kraft DL, Weissman IL, Waller EK: Differentiation of CD3-4-8- human fetal thymocytes in vivo: characterization of a CD3-4+8- intermediate, *J Exp Med* 178:265-277, 1993.
393. Staal FJ, Luis TC, Tiemessen MM: Wnt signalling in the immune system: Wnt is spreading its wings, *Nat Rev Immunol* 8:581-593, 2008.
394. Misslitz A, Bernhardt G, Forster R: Trafficking on serpentines: molecular insight on how maturating T cells find their winding paths in the thymus, *Immunol Rev* 209:115-128, 2006.
395. Horst E, Meijer CJ, Duijvestijn AM, et al: The ontogeny of human lymphocyte recirculation: high endothelial cell antigen (HECA-452) and CD44 homing receptor expression in the development of the immune system, *Eur J Immunol* 20:1483-1489, 1990.
396. Gilhus NE, Matre R, Tonder O: Hassall's corpuscles in the thymus of fetuses, infants and children: immunological and histochemical aspects, *Thymus* 7:123-135, 1985.
397. Kitchen SG, Zack JA: Distribution of the human immunodeficiency virus coreceptors CXCR4 and CCR5 in fetal lymphoid organs: implications for pathogenesis in utero, *AIDS Res Hum Retroviruses* 15:143-148, 1999.
398. Vandenberghe P, Delabie J, de Boer M, et al: In situ expression of B7/BB1 on antigen-presenting cells and activated B cells: an immunohistochemical study, *Int Immunol* 5:317-321, 1993.
399. Ramos SB, Garcia AB, Viana SR, et al: Phenotypic and functional evaluation of natural killer cells in thymectomized children, *Clin Immunol Immunopathol* 81:277-281, 1996.
400. Weerkamp F, de Haas EF, Naber BA, et al: Age-related changes in the cellular composition of the thymus in children, *J Allergy Clin Immunol* 115:834-840, 2005.
401. Baroni CD, Valtieri M, Stoppacciaro A, et al: The human thymus in ageing: histologic involution paralleled by increased mitogen response and by enrichment of OKT3+ lymphocytes, *Immunology* 50:519-528, 1983.
402. Poulin JF, Viswanathan MN, Harris JM, et al: Direct evidence for thymic function in adult humans, *J Exp Med* 190:479-486, 1999.
403. Mackall CL, Fleisher TA, Brown MR, et al: Age, thymopoiesis, and CD4+ T-lymphocyte regeneration after intensive chemotherapy, *N Engl J Med* 332:143-149, 1995.
404. Hakim FT, Memon SA, Cepeda R, et al: Age-dependent incidence, time course, and consequences of thymic renewal in adults, *J Clin Invest* 115:930-939, 2005.
405. Vrisekoop N, den Braber I, de Boer AB, et al: Sparse production but preferential incorporation of recently produced naive T cells in the human peripheral pool, *Proc Natl Acad Sci U.S.A* 105:6115-6120, 2008.
406. Haines CJ, Giffon TD, Lu LS, et al: Human CD4+ T cell recent thymic emigrants are identified by protein tyrosine kinase 7 and have reduced immune function, *J Exp Med* 206:275-285, 2009.
407. Guimond M, Fry TJ, Mackall CL: Cytokine signals in T-cell homeostasis, *J Immunother* 28:289-294, 2005.
408. Sportes C, Hakim FT, Memon SA, et al: Administration of rhIL-7 in humans increases in vivo TCR repertoire diversity by preferential expansion of naive T cell subsets, *J Exp Med* 205:1701-1714, 2008.
409. Buckley RH: Molecular defects in human severe combined immunodeficiency and approaches to immune reconstitution, *Annu Rev Immunol* 22:625-655, 2004.
410. Arstila TP, Casrouge A, Baron V, et al: A direct estimate of the human alphabeta T cell receptor diversity, *Science* 286:958-961, 1999.
411. Westermann J, Pabst R: Distribution of lymphocyte subsets and natural killer cells in the human body, *Clin Invest* 70:539-544, 1992.
412. Haase AT: Population biology of HIV-1 infection: viral and CD4+ T cell demographics and dynamics in lymphatic tissues, *Annu Rev Immunol* 17:625-656, 1999.
413. Schonland SO, Zimmer JK, Lopez-Benitez CM, et al: Homeostatic control of T-cell generation in neonates, *Blood* 102:1428-1434, 2003.
414. Dik WA, Pike-Overzet K, Weerkamp F, et al: New insights on human T cell development by quantitative T cell receptor gene rearrangement studies and gene expression profiling, *J Exp Med* 201:1715-1723, 2005.
415. von Boehmer H: Selection of the T-cell repertoire: receptor-controlled checkpoints in T-cell development, *Adv Immunol* 84: 201-238, 2004.
416. Padovan E, Giachino C, Cella M, et al: Normal T lymphocytes can express two different T cell receptor beta chains: implications for the mechanism of allelic exclusion, *J Exp Med* 181:1587-1591, 1995.
417. Padovan E, Casorati G, Dellabona P, et al: Expression of two T cell receptor alpha chains: dual receptor T cells, *Science* 262:422-424, 1993.
418. Davis MM: The evolutionary and structural 'logic' of antigen receptor diversity, *Semin Immunol* 16:239-243, 2004.
419. Gilfillan S, Bachmann M, Trembleau S, et al: Efficient immune responses in mice lacking N-region diversity, *Eur J Immunol* 25:3115-3122, 1995.
420. Schelonka RL, Raaphorst FM, Infante D, et al: T cell receptor repertoire diversity and clonal expansion in human neonates, *Pediatr Res* 43:396-402, 1998.
421. Grunewald J, Janson CH, Wigzell H: Biased expression of individual T cell receptor V gene segments in CD4+ and CD8+ human peripheral blood T lymphocytes, *Eur J Immunol* 21:819-822, 1991.
422. Dion ML, Sekaly RP, Cheynier R: Estimating thymic function through quantification of T-cell receptor excision circles, *Methods Mol Biol* 380:197-213, 2007.
423. Dion ML, Poulin JF, Bordi R, et al: HIV infection rapidly induces and maintains a substantial suppression of thymocyte proliferation, *Immunity* 21:757-768, 2004.
424. Hazenberg MD, Verschuren MC, Hamann D, et al: T cell receptor excision circles as markers for recent thymic emigrants: basic aspects, technical approach, and guidelines for interpretation, *J Mol Med* 79:631-640, 2001.
425. Okamoto Y, Douek DC, McFarland RD, et al: Effects of exogenous interleukin-7 on human thymus function, *Blood* 99:2851-2858, 2002.
426. McFarland RD, Douek DC, Koup RA, et al: Identification of a human recent thymic emigrant phenotype, *Proc Natl Acad Sci U.S.A* 97:4215-4220, 2000.
427. Bell JJ, Bhandoola A: Putting ThPOK in place, *Nat Immunol* 9:1095-1097, 2008.
428. Giraud M, Yoshida H, Abramson J, et al: Aire unleashes stalled RNA polymerase to induce ectopic gene expression in thymic epithelial cells, *Proc Natl Acad Sci U.S.A* 109:535-540, 2012.
429. Wolff AS, Sarkadi AK, Maródi L, et al: Anti-cytokine autoantibodies preceding onset of autoimmune polyendocrine syndrome type I features in early childhood, *J Clin Immunol* 33:1341-1348, 2013.

430. Gardner JM, Metzger TC, McMahon EJ, et al: Extrathymic Aire-expressing cells are a distinct bone marrow-derived population that induce functional inactivation of CD4(+) T cells, *Immunity* 39: 560-572, 2013.
431. Zerrahn J, Held W, Raulet DH: The MHC reactivity of the T cell repertoire prior to positive and negative selection, *Cell* 88:627-636, 1997.
432. Housset D, Malissen B: What do TCR-pMHC crystal structures teach us about MHC restriction and alloreactivity? *Trends Immunol* 24:429-437, 2003.
433. Ceredig R, Glasebrook AL, MacDonald HR: Phenotypic and functional properties of murine thymocytes. I. Precursors of cytolytic T lymphocytes and interleukin 2-producing cells are all contained within a subpopulation of "mature" thymocytes as analyzed by monoclonal antibodies and flow microfluorometry, *J Exp Med* 155:358-379, 1982.
434. Ceredig R, Dialynas DP, Fitch FW, et al: Precursors of T cell growth factor producing cells in the thymus: ontogeny, frequency, and quantitative recovery in a subpopulation of phenotypically mature thymocytes defined by monoclonal antibody GK-1.5, *J Exp Med* 158:1654-1671, 1983.
435. Weinreich MA, Hogquist KA: Thymic emigration: when and how T cells leave home, *J Immunol* 181:2265-2270, 2008.
436. Blume-Jensen P, Hunter T: Oncogenic kinase signalling, *Nature* 411:355-365, 2001.
437. De Rosa SC, Herzenberg LA, Roederer M: 11-color, 13-parameter flow cytometry: Identification of human naive T cells by phenotype, function, and T-cell receptor diversity, *Nat Med* 7:245-248, 2001.
438. Schwab SR, Cyster JG: Finding a way out: lymphocyte egress from lymphoid organs, *Nat Immunol* 8:1295-1301, 2007.
439. Xu B, Wagner N, Pham LN, et al: Lymphocyte homing to bronchus-associated lymphoid tissue (BALT) is mediated by L-selectin/PNAD, alpha4beta1 integrin/VCAM-1, and LFA-1 adhesion pathways, *J Exp Med* 197:1255-1267, 2003.
440. Vondenhoff MF, Kraal G, Mebius RE: Lymphoid organogenesis in brief, *Eur J Immunol* 37(Suppl 1):S46-S52, 2007.
441. Forster R, Davalos-Misslitz AC, Rot A: CCR7 and its ligands: balancing immunity and tolerance, *Nat Rev Immunol* 8:362-371, 2008.
442. Sprent J, Surh CD: Normal T cell homeostasis: the conversion of naive cells into memory-phenotype cells, *Nat Immunol* 12:478-484, 2011.
443. Carrette F, Surh CD: IL-7 signaling and CD127 receptor regulation in the control of T cell homeostasis, *Semin Immunol* 24:209-217, 2012.
444. Pahal GS, Jauniaux E, Kinnon C, et al: Normal development of human fetal hematopoiesis between eight and seventeen weeks' gestation, *Am J Obstet Gynecol* 183:1029-1034, 2000.
445. Settmacher U, Volk HD, Jahn S, et al: Characterization of human lymphocytes separated from fetal liver and spleen at different stages of ontogeny, *Immunobiology* 182:256-265, 1991.
446. Hannet I, Erkeller-Yuksel F, Lydyard P, et al: Developmental and maturational changes in human blood lymphocyte subpopulations, *Immunol Today* 13:215-218, 1992.
447. Sato K, Kawasaki H, Nagayama H, et al: Chemokine receptor expressions and responsiveness of cord blood T cells, *J Immunol* 166:1659-1666, 2001.
448. Kimmig S, Przybylski GK, Schmidt CA, et al: Two subsets of naïve T helper cells with distinct T cell receptor excision circle content in human adult peripheral blood, *J Exp Med* 195:789-794, 2002.
449. Kohler S, Wagner U, Pierer M, et al: Post-thymic in vivo proliferation of naive CD4+ T cells constrains the TCR repertoire in healthy human adults, *Eur J Immunol* 35:1987-1994, 2005.
450. Delespesse G, Yang LP, Ohshima Y, et al: Maturation of human neonatal CD4+ and CD8+ T lymphocytes into Th1/Th2 effectors, *Vaccine* 16:1415-1419, 1998.
451. Gerli R, Rambotti P, Cernetti C, et al: A mature thymocyte-like phenotypic pattern on human cord circulating T-lymphoid cells, *J Clin Immunol* 4:461-468, 1984.
452. Wilson M, Rosen FS, Schlossman SF, et al: Ontogeny of human T and B lymphocytes during stressed and normal gestation: phenotypic analysis of umbilical cord lymphocytes from term and preterm infants, *Clin Immunol Immunopathol* 37:1-12, 1985.
453. Tsegaye A, Wolday D, Otto S, et al: Immunophenotyping of blood lymphocytes at birth, during childhood, and during adulthood in HIV-1-uninfected Ethiopians, *Clin Immunol* 109:338-346, 2003.
454. Gerli R, Cernetti C, Spinozzi F, et al: Lymphocyte surface antigens: a longitudinal study during the first month of human life, *Int J Tissue React* 6:537-540, 1984.
455. Asma GE, Van den Bergh RL, Vossen JM: Use of monoclonal antibodies in a study of the development of T lymphocytes in the human fetus, *Clin Exp Immunol* 53:429-436, 1983.
456. Rallon NI, Cernetti C, Spinozzi F, et al: Level, phenotype and activation status of CD4+Foxp3+ regulatory T cells in patients chronically infected with human immunodeficiency virus and/or hepatitis C virus, *Clin Exp Immunol* 155:35-43, 2009.
457. Hassan J, Reen DJ: IL-7 promotes the survival and maturation but not differentiation of human post-thymic CD4+ T cells, *Eur J Immunol* 28:3057-3065, 1998.
458. Horenstein AL, Cernetti C, Spinozzi F, et al: A CD38/CD203a/CD73 ectoenzymatic pathway independent of CD39 drives a novel adenosinergic loop in human T lymphocytes, *Oncoimmunology* 2:e26246, 2013.
459. Peakman M, Buggins AG, Nicolaides KH, et al: Analysis of lymphocyte phenotypes in cord blood from early gestation fetuses, *Clin Exp Immunol* 90:345-350, 1992.
460. Byrne JA, Stankovic AK, Cooper MD: A novel subpopulation of primed T cells in the human fetus, *J Immunol* 152:3098-3106, 1994.
461. Bofill M, Akbar AN, Salmon M, et al: Immature CD45RA(low) RO(low) T cells in the human cord blood. I. Antecedents of CD45RA+ unprimed T cells, *J Immunol* 152:5613-5623, 1994.
462. D'Andrea A, Lanier LL: Killer cell inhibitory receptor expression by T cells, *Curr Top Microbiol Immunol* 230:25-39, 1998.
463. Azuma M, Cayabyab M, Phillips JH, et al: Requirements for CD28-dependent T cell-mediated cytotoxicity, *J Immunol* 150:2091-2101, 1993.
464. Azuma M, Phillips JH, Lanier LL: CD28- T lymphocytes. Antigenic and functional properties, *J Immunol* 150:1147-1159, 1993.
465. Frenkel L, Bryson YJ: Ontogeny of phytohemagglutinin-induced gamma interferon by leukocytes of healthy infants and children: evidence for decreased production in infants younger than 2 months of age, *J Pediatr* 111:97-100, 1987.
466. Spits H: Development of alphabeta T cells in the human thymus, *Nat Rev Immunol* 2:760-772, 2002.
467. Cupedo T, Nagasawa M, Weijer K, et al: Development and activation of regulatory T cells in the human fetus, *Eur J Immunol* 35: 383-390, 2005.
468. Michaelsson J, Mold JE, McCune JM, et al: Regulation of T cell responses in the developing human fetus, *J Immunol* 176:5741-5748, 2006.
469. Lyons AB: Analysing cell division in vivo and in vitro using flow cytometric measurement of CFSE dye dilution, *J Immunol Methods* 243:147-154, 2000.
470. Marcolino I, Przybylski GK, Koschella M, et al: Frequent expression of the natural killer cell receptor KLRG1 in human cord blood T cells: correlation with replicative history, *Eur J Immunol* 34: 2672-2680, 2004.
471. Min B, McHugh R, Sempowski GD, et al: Neonates support lymphopenia-induced proliferation, *Immunity* 18:131-140, 2003.
472. Fukui T, Katamura K, Abe N, et al: IL-7 induces proliferation, variable cytokine-producing ability and IL-2 responsiveness in naïve CD4+ T-cells from human cord blood, *Immunol Lett.* 59:21-28, 1997.
473. Hassan J, Reen DJ: Human recent thymic emigrants—identification, expansion, and survival characteristics, *J Immunol* 167:1970-1976, 2001.
474. Dardalhon V, Jaleco S, Kinet S, et al: IL-7 differentially regulates cell cycle progression and HIV-1-based vector infection in neonatal and adult CD4+ T cells, *Proc Natl Acad Sci U.S.A* 98:9277-9282, 2001.
475. Hare KJ, Jenkinson EJ, Anderson G: An essential role for the IL-7 receptor during intrathymic expansion of the positively selected neonatal T cell repertoire, *J Immunol* 165:2410-2414, 2000.
476. Okazaki H, Ito M, Sudo T, et al: Il-7 promotes thymocyte proliferation and maintains immunocompetent thymocytes bearing alpha beta or gamma delta T-cell receptors in vitro: synergism with IL-2, *J Immunol* 143:2917-2922, 1989.

477. Soares MV, Borthwick NJ, Maini MK, et al: IL-7-dependent extrathymic expansion of CD45RA+ T cells enables preservation of a naïve repertoire, *J Immunol* 161:5909-5917, 1998.
478. Webb LM, Foxwell BM, Feldmann M: Putative role for interleukin-7 in the maintenance of the recirculating naïve CD4+ T-cell pool, *Immunology* 98:400-405, 1999.
479. Buckley AF, Kuo CT, Leiden JM: Transcription factor LKLF is sufficient to program t cell quiescence via a c-myc-dependent pathway, *Nat Immunol* 2:698-704, 2001.
480. Smith-Garvin JE, Koretzky GA, Jordan MS: T cell activation, *Annu Rev Immunol* 27:591-619, 2009.
481. Dustin ML, Depoil D: New insights into the T cell synapse from single molecule techniques, *Nat Rev Immunol* 11:672-684, 2011.
482. Shaw PJ, Qu B, Hoth M, et al: Molecular regulation of CRAC channels and their role in lymphocyte function, *Cell Mol Life Sci* 70:2637-2656, 2013.
483. Puga I, Rao A, Macian F: Targeted cleavage of signaling proteins by caspase 3 inhibits T cell receptor signaling in anergic T cells, *Immunity* 29:193-204, 2008.
484. Paolino M, Penninger JM: Cbl-b in T-cell activation, *Semin Immunopathol* 32:137-148, 2010.
485. Bour-Jordan H, Esensten JH, Martinez-Llordella M, et al: Intrinsic and extrinsic control of peripheral T-cell tolerance by costimulatory molecules of the CD28/ B7 family, *Immunol Rev* 241:180-205, 2011.
486. Keir ME, Butte MJ, Freeman GJ, et al: PD-1 and its ligands in tolerance and immunity, *Annu Rev Immunol* 26:677-704, 2008.
487. Araki K, Youngblood B, Ahmed R: Programmed cell death 1-directed immunotherapy for enhancing T-cell function, *Cold Spring Harb Symp Quant Biol* 78: 239-247, 2013.
488. Spellberg B, Edwards JE Jr: Type 1/type 2 immunity in infectious diseases, *Clin Infect Dis* 32:76-102, 2001.
489. Quezada SA, Jarvinen LZ, Lind EF, et al: CD40/CD154 interactions at the interface of tolerance and immunity, *Annu Rev Immunol* 22:307-328, 2004.
490. Notarangelo LD, Lanzi G, Peron S, et al: Defects of class-switch recombination, *J Allergy Clin Immunol* 117:855-864, 2006.
491. Cayabyab M, Phillips JH, Lanier LL: CD40 preferentially costimulates activation of CD4+ T lymphocytes, *J Immunol* 152:1523-1531, 1994.
492. Hassan J, O'Neill S, O'Neill LA, et al: Signalling via CD28 of human naïve neonatal T lymphocytes, *Clin Exp Immunol* 102:192-198, 1995.
493. Hassan J, Rainsford E, Reen DJ: Linkage of protein kinase C-beta activation and intracellular interleukin-2 accumulation in human naïve CD4 T cells, *Immunology* 92:465-471, 1997.
494. Hassan J, Reen DJ: Cord blood CD4+CD45RA+ T cells achieve a lower magnitude of activation when compared with their adult counterparts, *Immunology* 90:397-401, 1997.
495. Chen L, Cohen AC, Lewis DB: Impaired allogeneic activation and T-helper 1 differentiation of human cord blood naive CD4 T cells, *Biol Blood Marrow Transplant* 12:160-171, 2006.
496. Wilson CB, Westall J, Johnston L, et al: Decreased production of interferon-gamma by human neonatal cells. Intrinsic and regulatory deficiencies, *J Clin Invest* 77:860-867, 1986.
497. Takahashi N, Imanishi K, Nishida H, et al: Evidence for immunologic immaturity of cord blood T cells. Cord blood T cells are susceptible to tolerance induction to in vitro stimulation with a superantigen, *J Immunol* 155:5213-5219, 1995.
498. Imanishi K, Seo K, Kato H, et al: Post-thymic maturation of migrating human thymic single-positive T cells: thymic CD1a-CD4+ T cells are more susceptible to anergy induction by toxic shock syndrome toxin-1 than cord blood CD4+ T cells, *J Immunol* 160: 112-119, 1998.
499. Takahashi N, Kato H, Imanishi K, et al: Immunopathophysiological aspects of an emerging neonatal infectious disease induced by a bacterial superantigen, *J Clin Invest* 106:1409-1415, 2000.
500. Chappert P, Schwartz RH: Induction of T cell anergy: integration of environmental cues and infectious tolerance, *Curr Opin Immunol* 22:552-559, 2010.
501. Paolino M, Thien CB, Gruber T, et al: Essential role of E3 ubiquitin ligase activity in Cbl-b-regulated T cell functions, *J Immunol* 186:2138-2147, 2011.
502. Palin AC, Ramachandran V, Acharya S, et al: Human neonatal naive CD4+ T cells have enhanced activation-dependent signaling regulated by the microRNA miR-181a, *J Immunol* 190:2682-2691, 2013.
503. Li QJ, Chau J, Ebert PJ, et al: Mir-181a is an intrinsic modulator of T cell sensitivity and selection, *Cell* 129:147-161, 2007.
504. Takahata Y, Nomura A, Takada H, et al: CD25+CD4+ T cells in human cord blood: an immunoregulatory subset with naive phenotype and specific expression of forkhead box P3 (foxP3) gene, *Exp Hematol* 32:622-629, 2004.
505. Appay V, van Lier RA, Sallusto F, et al: Phenotype and function of human T lymphocyte subsets: consensus and issues, *Cytometry A* 73:975-983, 2008.
506. Borish LC, Steinke JW: 2. Cytokines and chemokines, *J Allergy Clin Immunol* 111:S460-S475, 2003.
507. Locksley RM: The roaring twenties, *Immunity* 28:437-439, 2008.
508. Croft M: The role of TNF superfamily members in T-cell function and diseases, *Nat Rev Immunol* 9:271-285, 2009.
509. Liu H, Rohowsky-Kochan C: Regulation of IL-17 in human CCR6+ effector memory T cells, *J Immunol* 180:7948-7957, 2008.
510. Silver JS, Hunter CA: With a little help from their friends: Interleukin-21, T cells, and B cells, *Immunity* 29:7-9, 2008.
511. Rowe J, Macaubas C, Monger T, et al: Heterogeneity in diphtheria-tetanus-acellular pertussis vaccine-specific cellular immunity during infancy: relationship to variations in the kinetics of postnatal maturation of systemic Th1 function, *J Infect Dis* 184:80-88, 2001.
512. Kim CH, Rott L, Kunkel EJ, et al: Rules of chemokine receptor association with T cell polarization in vivo, *J Clin Invest* 108:1331-1339, 2001.
513. Viola A, Molon B, Contento RL: Chemokines: coded messages for T-cell missions, *Front Biosci* 13:6341-6353, 2008.
514. Williams IR: CCR6 and CCL20: Partners in intestinal immunity and lymphorganogenesis, *Ann N.Y Acad Sci* 1072:52-61, 2006.
515. Tangye SG, Ma CS, Brink R, et al: The good, the bad and the ugly—TFH cells in human health and disease, *Nat Rev Immunol* 13: 412-426, 2013.
516. Tubo NJ, Pagán AJ, Taylor JJ, et al: Single naive CD4+ T cells from a diverse repertoire produce different effector cell types during infection, *Cell* 153:785-796, 2013.
517. Josefowicz SZ: Regulators of chromatin state and transcription in CD4 T-cell polarization, *Immunology* 139:299-308, 2013.
518. Ramos HJ, Davis AM, George TC, et al: IFN-alpha is not sufficient to drive Th1 development due to lack of stable T-bet expression, *J Immunol* 179:3792-3803, 2007.
519. Cleary AM, Tu W, Enright A, et al: Impaired accumulation and function of memory CD4 T cells in human IL-12 receptor beta 1 deficiency, *J Immunol* 170:597-603, 2003.
520. Filipe-Santos O, Bustamante J, Chapgier A, et al: Inborn errors of IL-12/23- and IFN-gamma-mediated immunity: molecular, cellular, and clinical features, *Semin Immunol* 18:347-361, 2006.
521. Saenz SA, Taylor BC, Artis D: Welcome to the neighborhood: epithelial cell-derived cytokines license innate and adaptive immune responses at mucosal sites, *Immunol Rev* 226:172-190, 2008.
522. Min B, Brown MA, Legros G: Understanding the roles of basophils: breaking dawn, *Immunology* 135:192-197, 2012.
523. Mirchandani AS, Besnard AG, Yip E, et al: Type 2 innate lymphoid cells drive CD4+ Th2 cell responses, *J Immunol* 192:2442-2448, 2014.
524. Zhu J, Paul WE: CD4 T cells: fates, functions, and faults, *Blood* 112:1557-1569, 2008.
525. Korn T, Bettelli E, Oukka M, et al: IL-17 and Th17 cells, *Annu Rev Immunol* 27:485-517, 2009.
526. Schmitt N, Bustamante J, Bourdery L, et al: IL-12 receptor beta1 deficiency alters in vivo T follicular helper cell response in humans, *Blood* 121:3375-3385, 2013.
527. Ysebrant de Lendonck L, Eddahri F, Delmarcelle Y, et al: Stat3 signaling induces the differentiation of human ICOS(+) CD4 T cells helping B lymphocytes, *PloS One* 8:e71029, 2013.
528. Choi YS, Yang JA, Crotty S: Dynamic regulation of Bcl6 in follicular helper CD4 T (Tfh) cells, *Curr Opin Immunol* 25:366-372, 2013.
529. Ettinger R, Kuchen S, Lipsky PE: The role of IL-21 in regulating B-cell function in health and disease, *Immunol Rev* 223:60-86, 2008.
530. Schaffer AA, Salzer U, Hammarström L, et al: Deconstructing common variable immunodeficiency by genetic analysis, *Curr Opin Genet Dev* 17:201-212, 2007.
531. Geha RS, Jabara HH, Brodeur SR: The regulation of immunoglobulin E class-switch recombination, *Nat Rev Immunol* 3:721-732, 2003.

532. Beverley PC: Kinetics and clonality of immunological memory in humans, *Semin Immunol* 16:315-321, 2004.
533. Surh CD, Sprent J: Homeostasis of naive and memory T cells, *Immunity* 29:848-862, 2008.
534. Gattinoni L, Salzer U, Hammarström L, et al: A human memory T cell subset with stem cell-like properties, *Nat Med* 17:1290-1297, 2011.
535. Lugli E, Dominguez MH, Gattinoni L, et al: Superior T memory stem cell persistence supports long-lived T cell memory, *J Clin Invest* 123:594-599, 2013.
536. Ameratunga R, Lederman HM, Sullivan KE, et al: Defective antigen-induced lymphocyte proliferation in the X-linked hyper-IgM syndrome, *J Pediatr* 131:147-150, 1997.
537. Levy J, Espanol-Boren T, Thomas C, et al: Clinical spectrum of X-linked hyper-IgM syndrome, *J Pediatr* 131:47-54, 1997.
538. Hamann D, Baars PA, Rep MH, et al: Phenotypic and functional separation of memory and effector human CD8+ T cells, *J Exp Med* 186:1407-1418, 1997.
539. Lanzavecchia A, Sallusto F: Understanding the generation and function of memory T cell subsets, *Curr Opin Immunol* 17:326-332, 2005.
540. Appay V, Rowland-Jones SL: Lessons from the study of T-cell differentiation in persistent human virus infection, *Semin Immunol* 16:205-212, 2004.
541. McMahon CW, Raulet DH: Expression and function of NK cell receptors in CD8+ T cells, *Curr Opin Immunol* 13:465-470, 2001.
542. Ogasawara K, Lanier LL: NKG2D in NK and T cell-mediated immunity, *J Clin Immunol* 25:534-540, 2005.
543. van der Veken LT, Campelo MD, van der Hoorn MA, et al: Functional analysis of killer Ig-like receptor-expressing cytomegalovirus-specific CD8+ T cells, *J Immunol* 182:92-101, 2009.
544. Sallusto F, Lanzavecchia A: Heterogeneity of CD4+ memory T cells: functional modules for tailored immunity, *Eur J Immunol* 39: 2076-2082, 2009.
545. Tu W, Chen S, Sharp M, et al: Persistent and selective deficiency of CD4+ T cell immunity to cytomegalovirus in immunocompetent young children, *J Immunol* 172:3260-3267, 2004.
546. Stubbe M, Vanderheyde N, Pircher H, et al: Characterization of a subset of antigen-specific human central memory CD4+ T lymphocytes producing effector cytokines, *Eur J Immunol* 38:273-282, 2008.
547. Macallan DC, Wallace D, Zhang Y, et al: Rapid turnover of effector-memory CD4(+) T cells in healthy humans, *J Exp Med* 200: 255-260, 2004.
548. Riou C, Yassine-Diab B, Van grevenynghe J, et al: Convergence of TCR and cytokine signaling leads to Foxo3a phosphorylation and drives the survival of CD4+ central memory T cells, *J Exp Med* 204:79-91, 2007.
549. Okoye A, Meier-Schellersheim M, Brenchley JM, et al: Progressive CD4+ central memory T cell decline results in CD4+ effector memory insufficiency and overt disease in chronic SIV infection, *J Exp Med* 204:2171-2185, 2007.
550. Schoenborn JR, Wilson CB: Regulation of interferon-gamma during innate and adaptive immune responses, *Adv Immunol* 96: 41-101, 2007.
551. Thurman RE, Rynes E, Humbert R, et al: The accessible chromatin landscape of the human genome, *Nature* 489:75-82, 2012.
552. Kannan A, Huang W, Huang F, et al: Signal transduction via the T cell antigen receptor in naive and effector/memory T cells, *Int J Biochem Cell Biol* 44:2129-2134, 2012.
553. Veiga-Fernandes H, Walter U, Bourgeois C, et al: Response of naive and memory CD8+ T cells to antigen stimulation in vivo, *Nat Immunol* 1:47-53, 2000.
554. Jung T, Wijdenes J, Neumann C, et al: Interleukin-13 is produced by activated human CD45RA+ and CD45RO+ T cells: modulation by interleukin-4 and interleukin-12, *Eur J Immunol* 26:571-577, 1996.
555. Lewis DB, Yu CC, Meyer J, et al: Cellular and molecular mechanisms for reduced interleukin 4 and interferon-gamma production by neonatal T cells, *J Clin Invest* 87:194-202, 1991.
556. Krampera M, Vinante F, Tavecchia L, et al: Progressive polarization towards a T helper/cytotoxic type-1 cytokine pattern during age-dependent maturation of the immune response inversely correlates with CD30 cell expression and serum concentration, *Clin Exp Immunol* 117:291-297, 1999.
557. Krampera M, Tavecchia L, Benedetti F, et al: Intracellular cytokine profile of cord blood T- and NK cells and monocytes, *Haematologica* 85:675-679, 2000.
558. Rainsford E, Reen DJ: Interleukin 10, produced in abundance by human newborn T cells, may be the regulator of increased tolerance associated with cord blood stem cell transplantation, *Br J Haematol* 116:702-709, 2002.
559. Mosser DM, Zhang X: Interleukin-10: new perspectives on an old cytokine, *Immunol Rev* 226:205-218, 2008.
560. Hariharan D, Ho W, Cutilli J, et al: C-C chemokine profile of cord blood mononuclear cells: RANTES production, *Blood* 95:715-718, 2000.
561. Ribeiro-do-Couto LM, Boeije LC, Kroon JS, et al: High IL-13 production by human neonatal T cells: neonate immune system regulator? *Eur J Immunol* 31:3394-3402, 2001.
562. Vigano A, Esposito S, Arienti D, et al: Differential development of type 1 and type 2 cytokines and beta-chemokines in the ontogeny of healthy newborns, *Biol Neonate* 75:1-8, 1999.
563. Stam J, Abdulahad W, Huitema MG, et al: Fluorescent cell barcoding as a tool to assess the age-related development of intracellular cytokine production in small amounts of blood from infants, *PloS One* 6:e25690, 2011.
564. Durandy A, De Saint Basile G, Lisowska-Grospierre B, et al: Undetectable CD40 ligand expression on T cells and low B cell responses to CD40 binding agonists in human newborns, *J Immunol* 154:1560-1568, 1995.
565. Flamand V, Donckier V, Demoor FX, et al: CD40 ligation prevents neonatal induction of transplantation tolerance, *J Immunol* 160:4666-4669, 1998.
566. Nonoyama S, Penix LA, Edwards CP, et al: Diminished expression of CD40 ligand by activated neonatal T cells, *J Clin Invest* 95:66-75, 1995.
567. Fuleihan R, Ahern D, Geha RS: CD40 ligand expression is developmentally regulated in human thymocytes, *Clin Immunol Immunopathol* 76:52-58, 1995.
568. Jullien P, Cron RQ, Dabbagh K, et al: Decreased CD154 expression by neonatal CD4+ T cells is due to limitations in both proximal and distal events of T cell activation, *Int Immunol* 15:1461-1472, 2003.
569. Sato K, Nagayama H, Takahashi TA: Aberrant CD3- and CD28-mediated signaling events in cord blood T cells are associated with dysfunctional regulation of Fas ligand-mediated cytotoxicity, *J Immunol* 162:4464-4471, 1999.
570. Splawski JB, Nishioka J, Nishioka Y, et al: CD40 ligand is expressed and functional on activated neonatal T cells, *J Immunol* 156:119-127, 1996.
571. Reen DJ: Activation and functional capacity of human neonatal CD4 T cells, *Vaccine* 16:1401-1408, 1998.
572. Matthews NC, Wadhwa M, Bird C, et al: Sustained expression of CD154 (CD40L) and proinflammatory cytokine production by alloantigen-stimulated umbilical cord blood T cells, *J Immunol* 164:6206-6212, 2000.
573. Oliveira JB, Gupta S: Disorders of apoptosis: mechanisms for autoimmunity in primary immunodeficiency diseases, *J Clin Immunol* 28(Suppl 1):S20-S28, 2008.
574. Iwama H, Akutsu H, Kuretake S, et al: Serum concentrations of soluble Fas antigen and soluble Fas ligand in mother and newborn, *Arch Gynecol Obstet* 263:108-110, 2000.
575. Oh-hora M, Rao A: Calcium signaling in lymphocytes, *Curr Opin Immunol* 20:250-258, 2008.
576. Ansart-Pirenne H, Soulimani N, Tartour E, et al: Defective IL-2 gene expression in newborn is accompanied with impaired tyrosine-phosphorylation in T cells, *Pediatr Res* 45:409-413, 1999.
577. Hii CS, Costabile M, Mayne GC, et al: Selective deficiency in protein kinase c isoenzyme expression and inadequacy in mitogen-activated protein kinase activation in cord blood T cells, *Biochem J* 370:497-503, 2003.
578. Miscia S, Di Baldassarre A, Sabatino G, et al: Inefficient phospholipase C activation and reduced Lck expression characterize the signaling defect of umbilical cord T lymphocytes, *J Immunol* 163:2416-2424, 1999.
579. Kobayashi S, Ohnuma K, Uchiyama M, et al: Association of CD26 with CD45RA outside lipid rafts attenuates cord blood T-cell activation, *Blood* 103:1002-1010, 2004.
580. White GP, Watt PM, Holt BJ, et al: Differential patterns of methylation of the IFN-gamma promoter at CpG and non-CpG sites underlie differences in IFN-gamma gene expression between human neonatal and adult CD45RO- T cells, *J Immunol* 168:2820-2827, 2002.

581. Suen Y, Lee SM, Qian J, et al: Dysregulation of lymphokine production in the neonate and its impact on neonatal cell mediated immunity, *Vaccine* 16:1369-1377, 1998.
582. Cella M, Scheidegger D, Palmer-Lehmann K, et al: Ligation of CD40 on dendritic cells triggers production of high levels of interleukin-12 and enhances T cell stimulatory capacity: T-T help via APC activation, *J Exp Med* 184:747-752, 1996.
583. Kadereit S, Mohammad SF, Miller RE, et al: Reduced NFAT1 protein expression in human umbilical cord blood T lymphocytes, *Blood* 94:3101-3107, 1999.
584. Kiani A, García-Cózar FJ, Habermann I, et al: Regulation of interferon-gamma gene expression by nuclear factor of activated T cells, *Blood* 98:1480-1488, 2001.
585. O'Neill RM, Reen DJ: Equivalent functional nuclear factor of activated T cell 1 mRNA and protein expression in cord blood and adult T cells, *Transplantation* 76:1526-1528, 2003.
586. Macian F, Lopez-Rodriguez C, Rao A: Partners in transcription: NFAT and AP-1, *Oncogene* 20:2476-2489, 2001.
587. Adkins B: Heterogeneity in the CD4 T cell compartment and the variability of neonatal immune responsiveness, *Curr Immunol Rev* 3:151-159, 2007.
588. Rogge L, Barberis-Maino L, Biffi M, et al: Selective expression of an interleukin-12 receptor component by human T helper 1 cells, *J Exp Med* 185:825-831, 1997.
589. Bofill M, Almirall E, McQuaid A, et al: Differential expression of the cytokine receptors for human interleukin (IL)-12 and IL-18 on lymphocytes of both CD45RA and CD45RO phenotype from tonsils, cord and adult peripheral blood, *Clin Exp Immunol* 138: 460-465, 2004.
590. Yamaguchi E, de Vries J, Yssel H: Differentiation of human single-positive fetal thymocytes in vitro into IL-4- and/or IFN-gamma-producing CD4+ and CD8+ T cells, *Int Immunol* 11:593-603, 1999.
591. Cosmi L, De Palma R, Santarlasci V, et al: Human interleukin 17-producing cells originate from a CD161+CD4+ T cell precursor, *J Exp Med* 205:1903-1916, 2008.
592. Renda MC, Fecarotta E, Dieli F, et al: Evidence of alloreactive T lymphocytes in fetal liver: Implications for fetal hematopoietic stem cell transplantation, *Bone Marrow Transplant* 25:135-141, 2000.
593. Renda MC, Fecarotta E, Maggio A, et al: In utero fetal liver hematopoietic stem cell transplantation: is there a role for alloreactive T lymphocytes? *Blood* 96:1608-1609, 2000.
594. Marchant A, Appay V, Van Der Sande M, et al: Mature CD8(+) T lymphocyte response to viral infection during fetal life, *J Clin Invest* 111:1747-1755, 2003.
595. Elbou Ould MA, Luton D, Yadini M, et al: Cellular immune response of fetuses to cytomegalovirus, *Pediatr Res.* 55:280-286, 2004.
596. Pedron B, Guerin V, Jacquemard F, et al: Comparison of CD8+ T cell responses to cytomegalovirus between human fetuses and their transmitter mothers, *J Infect Dis* 196:1033-1043, 2007.
597. Sato K, Kawasaki H, Morimoto C, et al: An abortive ligand-induced activation of CCR1-mediated downstream signaling event and a deficiency of CCR5 expression are associated with the hyporesponsiveness of human naïve CD4+ T cells to CCL3 and CCL5, *J Immunol* 168:6263-6272, 2002.
598. Berkowitz RD, Beckerman KP, Schall TJ, et al: CXCR4 and CCR5 expression delineates targets for HIV-1 disruption of T cell differentiation, *J Immunol* 161:3702-3710, 1998.
599. Christopherson K, Brahmi Z, Hromas R: Regulation of naïve fetal T-cell migration by the chemokines Exodus-2 and Exodus 3, *Immunol Lett* 69:269-273, 1999.
600. Mo H, Monard S, Pollack H, et al: Expression patterns of the HIV type 1 coreceptors CCR5 and CXCR4 on CD4+ T cells and monocytes from cord and adult blood, *AIDS Res Hum Retroviruses* 14:607-617, 1998.
601. Auewarakul P, Sangsiriwut K, Pattanapanyasat K, et al: Age-dependent expression of the HIV-1 coreceptor CCR5 on CD4+ lymphocytes in children, *J Acquir Immune Defic Syndr* 24:285-287, 2000.
602. Langenkamp A, Messi M, Lanzavecchia A, et al: Kinetics of dendritic cell activation: impact on priming of Th1, Th2 and nonpolarized T cells, *Nat Immunol* 1:311-316, 2000.
603. Bonecchi R, Bianchi G, Bordignon PP, et al: Differential expression of chemokine receptors and chemotactic responsiveness of type 1 T helper cells (Th1s) and Th2s, *J Exp Med* 187:129-134, 1998.
604. Fraticelli P, Sironi M, Bianchi G, et al: Fractalkine (CX3CL1) as an amplification circuit of polarized Th1 responses, *J Clin Invest* 107:1173-1181, 2001.
605. Chipeta J, Komada Y, Zhang XL, et al: Neonatal (cord blood) T cells can competently raise type 1 and 2 immune responses upon polyclonal activation, *Cell Immunol* 205:110-119, 2000.
606. Hermiston ML, Xu Z, Weiss A: CD45: a critical regulator of signaling thresholds in immune cells, *Annu Rev Immunol* 21:107-137, 2003.
607. Ceeraz S, Nowak EC, Noelle RJ: B7 family checkpoint regulators in immune regulation and disease, *Trends Immunol* 34:556-563, 2013.
608. Strasser A: The role of Bh3-only proteins in the immune system, *Nat Rev Immunol* 5:189-200, 2005.
609. Akbar AN, Borthwick N, Salmon M, et al: The significance of low bcl-2 expression by CD45RO T cells in normal individuals and patients with acute viral infections. The role of apoptosis in T cell memory, *J Exp Med* 178:427-438, 1993.
610. Nelson BH, Willerford DM: Biology of the interleukin-2 receptor, *Adv Immunol* 70:1-81, 1998.
611. Tibbetts MD, Zheng L, Lenardo MJ: The death effector domain protein family: regulators of cellular homeostasis, *Nat Immunol* 4: 404-409, 2003.
612. El Ghalbzouri A, Drénou B, Blancheteau V, et al: An in vitro model of allogeneic stimulation of cord blood: induction of fas independent apoptosis, *Hum Immunol* 60:598-607, 1999.
613. Tu W, Cheung PT, Lau YL: Insulin-like growth factor 1 promotes cord blood T cell maturation and inhibits its spontaneous and phytohemagglutinin-induced apoptosis through different mechanisms, *J Immunol* 165:1331-1336, 2000.
614. Drenou B, Choqueux C, El Ghalbzouri A, et al: Characterisation of the roles of CD95 and CD95 ligand in cord blood, *Bone Marrow Transplant* 22:S44-S47, 1998.
615. Potestio M, Pawelec G, Di Lorenzo G, et al: Age-related changes in the expression of CD95 (Apo1/Fas) on blood lymphocytes, *Exp Gerontol* 34:659-673, 1999.
616. Kuntz TB, Christensen RD, Stegner J, et al: Fas and fas ligand expression in maternal blood and in umbilical cord blood in preeclampsia, *Pediatr Res* 50:743-749, 2001.
617. Aggarwal S, Gollapudi S, Yel L, et al: TNF-alpha-induced apoptosis in neonatal lymphocytes: TNFRp55 expression and downstream pathways of apoptosis, *Genes Immun* 1:271-279, 2000.
618. Malamitsi-Puchner A, Sarandakou A, Tziotis J, et al: Evidence for a suppression of apoptosis in early postnatal life, *Acta Obstet Gynecol Scand* 80:994-997, 2001.
619. Aggarwal S, Gupta A, Nagata S, et al: Programmed cell death (apoptosis) in cord blood lymphocytes, *J Clin Immunol* 17:63-73, 1997.
620. Law HK, Tu W, Liu E, et al: Insulin-like growth factor I promotes cord blood T cell maturation through monocytes and inhibits their apoptosis in part through interleukin-6, *BMC Immunol* 9:74, 2008.
621. Monteleone G, Pender SL, Wathen NC, et al: Interferon-alpha drives T cell-mediated immunopathology in the intestine, *Eur J Immunol* 31:2247-2255, 2001.
622. Gautier G, Humbert M, Deauvieau F, et al: A type I interferon autocrine-paracrine loop is involved in Toll-like receptor-induced interleukin-12p70 secretion by dendritic cells, *J Exp Med* 201:1435-1446, 2005.
623. Howie D, Spencer J, DeLord D, et al: Extrathymic T cell differentiation in the human intestine early in life, *J Immunol* 161:5862-5872, 1998.
624. Fusco A, Panico L, Gorrese M, et al: Molecular evidence for a thymus-independent partial T cell development in a Foxn1(-/-) athymic human fetus, *PloS One* 8:e81786, 2013.
625. Bas A, Hammarstrom SG, Hammarstrom ML: Extrathymic TCR gene rearrangement in human small intestine: identification of new splice forms of recombination activating gene-1 mRNA with selective tissue expression, *J Immunol* 171:3359-3371, 2003.
626. McClory S, Hughes T, Freud AG, et al: Evidence for a stepwise program of extrathymic T cell development within the human tonsil, *J Clin Invest* 122:1403-1415, 2012.
627. d'Hennezel E, Piccirillo CA: Functional plasticity in human FoxP3(+) regulatory T cells: implications for cell-based immunotherapy, *Hum Vaccin Immunother* 8:1001-1005, 2012.
628. Bollrath J, Powrie FM: Controlling the frontier: regulatory T-cells and intestinal homeostasis, *Semin Immunol* 25:352-357, 2013.
629. Burt TD: Fetal regulatory T cells and peripheral immune tolerance in utero: implications for development and disease, *Am J Reprod Immunol* 69:346-358, 2013.

630. Roncarolo MG, Battaglia M: Regulatory T-cell immunotherapy for tolerance to self antigens and alloantigens in humans, *Nat Rev Immunol* 7:585-598, 2007.
631. Sakaguchi S, Yamaguchi T, Nomura T, et al: Regulatory T cells and immune tolerance, *Cell* 133:775-787, 2008.
632. Cohen AC, Nadeau KC, Tu W, et al: Cutting edge: decreased accumulation and regulatory function of CD4+ CD25(high) T cells in human STAT5b deficiency, *J Immunol* 177:2770-2774, 2006.
633. Liu YJ: A unified theory of central tolerance in the thymus, *Trends Immunol* 27:215-221, 2006.
634. Li DJ, Guo PF: The regulatory role of thymic stromal lymphopoietin (TSLP) in maternal-fetal immune tolerance during early human pregnancy, *J Reprod Immunol* 83:106-108, 2009.
635. Fritzsching B, Oberle N, Pauly E, et al: Naive regulatory T cells: a novel subpopulation defined by resistance toward CD95L-mediated cell death, *Blood* 108:3371-3378, 2006.
636. Thornton AM, Korty PE, Tran DQ, et al: Expression of Helios, an Ikaros transcription factor family member, differentiates thymic-derived from peripherally induced FoxP3+ T regulatory cells, *J Immunol* 184:3433-3441, 2010.
637. Yadav M, Stephan S, Bluestone JA: Peripherally induced Tregs—role in immune homeostasis and autoimmunity, *Front Immunol* 4:232, 2013.
638. Himmel ME, MacDonald KG, Garcia RV, et al: Helios+ and Helios− cells coexist within the natural FoxP3+ T regulatory cell subset in humans, *J Immunol* 190:2001-2008, 2013.
639. Vukmanovic-Stejic M, Zhang Y, Cook JE, et al: Human CD4+ CD25hi FoxP3+ regulatory T cells are derived by rapid turnover of memory populations in vivo, *J Clin Invest* 116:2423-2433, 2006.
640. Duhen T, Duhen R, Lanzavecchia A, et al: Functionally distinct subsets of human FoxP3+ Treg cells that phenotypically mirror effector Th cells, *Blood* 119:4430-4440, 2012.
641. Pesenacker AM, Bending D, Ursu S, et al: CD161 defines the subset of FoxP3+ T cells capable of producing proinflammatory cytokines, *Blood* 121:2647-2658, 2013.
642. Pandiyan P, Zheng L, Ishihara S, et al: CD4+CD25+FoxP3+ regulatory T cells induce cytokine deprivation-mediated apoptosis of effector CD4+ T cells, *Nat Immunol* 8:1353-1362, 2007.
643. Nettenstrom L, Alderson K, Raschke EE, et al: An optimized multi-parameter flow cytometry protocol for human T regulatory cell analysis on fresh and viably frozen cells, correlation with epigenetic analysis, and comparison of cord and adult blood, *J Immunol Methods* 387:81-88, 2013.
644. Flanagan KL, Halliday A, Burl S, et al: The effect of placental malaria infection on cord blood and maternal immunoregulatory responses at birth, *Eur J Immunol* 40:1062-1072, 2010.
645. Ayyoub M, Raffin C, Valmori D: Comment on Helios+ and Helios− cells coexist within the natural FoxP3+ T regulatory cell subset in humans, *J Immunol* 190:4439-4440, 2013.
646. MacDonald KG, Han JM, Himmel ME, et al: Response to comment on Helios+ and Helios− cells coexist within the natural FoxP3+ T regulatory cell subset in humans, *J Immunol* 190:4440-4441, 2013.
647. Akbar AN, Vukmanovic-Stejic M, Taams LS, et al: The dynamic co-evolution of memory and regulatory CD4+ T cells in the periphery, *Nat Rev Immunol* 7:231-237, 2007.
648. Smith H, Chen IM, Kubo R, et al: Neonatal thymectomy results in a repertoire enriched in T cells deleted in adult thymus, *Science* 245:749-752, 1989.
649. Mold JE, Michaëlsson J, Burt TD, et al: Maternal alloantigens promote the development of tolerogenic fetal regulatory T cells in utero, *Science* 322:1562-1565, 2008.
650. Hirayama M, Azuma E, Komada Y: Tolerogenic effect of non-inherited maternal antigens in hematopoietic stem cell transplantation, *Front Immunol* 3:135, 2012.
651. Ochs HD, Gambineri E, Torgerson TR: IPEX, FoxP3 and regulatory T-cells: a model for autoimmunity, *Immunol Res* 38:112-121, 2007.
652. Legrand FA, Nixon DF, Loo CP, et al: Strong HIV-1-specific T cell responses in HIV-1-exposed uninfected infants and neonates revealed after regulatory T cell removal, *PloS One* 1:e102, 2006.
653. Smith M, Tourigny MR, Noakes P, et al: Children with egg allergy have evidence of reduced neonatal CD4(+)CD25(+)CD127(lo/−) regulatory T cell function, *J Allergy Clin Immunol* 121:1460-1466, 2008. 1466.e1-e7.
654. Weitkamp JH, Koyama T, Rock MT, et al: Necrotising enterocolitis is characterised by disrupted immune regulation and diminished mucosal regulatory (FoxP3)/effector (CD4, CD8) T cell ratios, *Gut* 62:73-82, 2013.
655. Kinjo Y, Wu D, Kim G, et al: Recognition of bacterial glycosphingolipids by natural killer T cells, *Nature* 434:520-525, 2005.
656. Wieland Brown LC, Penaranda C, Kashyap PC, et al: Production of alpha-galactosylceramide by a prominent member of the human gut microbiota, *PLoS Biol* 11:e1001610, 2013.
657. Kinjo Y, Illarionov P, Vela JL, et al: Invariant natural killer T cells recognize glycolipids from pathogenic gram-positive bacteria, *Nat Immunol* 12:966-974, 2011.
658. Brennan PJ, Tatituri RV, Brigl M, et al: Invariant natural killer T cells recognize lipid self antigen induced by microbial danger signals, *Nat Immunol* 12:1202-1211, 2011.
659. Bosma A, Abdel-Gadir A, Isenberg DA, et al: Lipid-antigen presentation by CD1d(+) B cells is essential for the maintenance of invariant natural killer T cells, *Immunity* 36:477-490, 2012.
660. Brigl M, Tatituri RV, Watts GF, et al: Innate and cytokine-driven signals, rather than microbial antigens, dominate in natural killer T cell activation during microbial infection, *J Exp Med* 208: 1163-1177, 2011.
661. Kuylenstierna C, Björkström NK, Andersson SK, et al: NKG2D performs two functions in invariant NKT cells: direct TCR-independent activation of NK-like cytolysis and co-stimulation of activation by CD1d, *Eur J Immunol* 41:1913-1923, 2011.
662. Veillette A, Perez-Quintero LA, Latour S: X-linked lymphoproliferative syndromes and related autosomal recessive disorders, *Curr Opin Allergy Clin Immunol* 13:614-622, 2013.
663. Sandberg JK, Stoddart CA, Brilot F, et al: Development of innate CD4+ alpha-chain variable gene segment 24 (valpha24) natural killer T cells in the early human fetal thymus is regulated by IL-7, *Proc Natl Acad Sci U.S.A* 101:7058-7063, 2004.
664. de Lalla C, Festuccia N, Albrecht I, et al: Innate-like effector differentiation of human invariant NKT cells driven by IL-7, *J Immunol* 180:4415-4424, 2008.
665. Sandberg JK, Bhardwaj N, Nixon DF: Dominant effector memory characteristics, capacity for dynamic adaptive expansion, and sex bias in the innate valpha24 NKT cell compartment, *Eur J Immunol* 33:588-596, 2003.
666. Sandberg JK, Fast NM, Palacios EH, et al: Selective loss of innate CD4(+) V alpha 24 natural killer T cells in human immunodeficiency virus infection, *J Virol* 76:7528-7534, 2002.
667. Loh L, Ivarsson MA, Michaëlsson J, et al: Invariant natural killer T cells developing in the human fetus accumulate and mature in the small intestine, *Mucosal Immunol* 7:1233-1243, 2004.
668. Berzins SP, Cochrane AD, Pellicci DG, et al: Limited correlation between human thymus and blood nkt cell content revealed by an ontogeny study of paired tissue samples, *Eur J Immunol* 35: 1399-1407, 2005.
669. Ladd M, Sharma A, Huang Q, et al: Natural killer T cells constitutively expressing the interleukin-2 receptor alpha chain early in life are primed to respond to lower antigenic stimulation, *Immunology* 131:289-299, 2010.
670. Kadowaki N, Antonenko S, Ho S, et al: Distinct cytokine profiles of neonatal natural killer T cells after expansion with subsets of dendritic cells, *J Exp Med* 193:1221-1226, 2001.
671. Harner S, Noessner E, Nadas K, et al: Cord blood Valpha24-Vbeta11 natural killer T cells display a Th2-chemokine receptor profile and cytokine responses, *PloS One* 6:e15714, 2011.
672. Birkinshaw RW, Kjer-Nielsen L, Eckle SB, et al: MAITs, MR1 and vitamin B metabolites, *Curr Opin Immunol* 26:7-13, 2014.
673. Ussher JE, Bilton M, Attwod E, et al: CD161++ CD8+ T cells, including the MAIT cell subset, are specifically activated by IL-12+IL-18 in a TCR-independent manner, *Eur J Immunol* 44:195-203, 2014.
674. Le Bourhis L, Dusseaux M, Bohineust A, et al: MAIT cells detect and efficiently lyse bacterially-infected epithelial cells, *PLoS Pathogens* 9:e1003681, 2013.
675. Martin E, Treiner E, Duban L, et al: Stepwise development of MAIT cells in mouse and human, *PLoS Biol* 7:e54, 2009.
676. Le Bourhis L, Martin E, Péguillet I, et al: Antimicrobial activity of mucosal-associated invariant T cells, *Nat Immunol* 11:701-708, 2010.
677. Reantragoon R, Corbett AJ, Sakala IG, et al: Antigen-loaded MR1 tetramers define T cell receptor heterogeneity in mucosal-associated invariant T cells, *J Exp Med* 210:2305-2320, 2013.

678. Dusseaux M, Martin E, Serriari N, et al: Human MAIT cells are xenobiotic-resistant, tissue-targeted, CD161hi IL-17-secreting T cells, *Blood* 117:1250-1259, 2011.
679. Gold MC, Cerri S, Smyk-Pearson S, et al: Human mucosal associated invariant T cells detect bacterially infected cells, *PLoS Biol.* 8:e1000407, 2010.
680. Meierovics A, Yankelevich WJ, Cowley SC: MAIT cells are critical for optimal mucosal immune responses during in vivo pulmonary bacterial infection, *Proc Natl Acad Sci U.S.A* 110:3119-3128, 2013.
681. Seach N, Cerri S, Smyk-Pearson S, et al: Double-positive thymocytes select mucosal-associated invariant T cells, *J Immunol* 191: 6002-6009, 2013.
682. Leeansyah E, Loh L, Nixon DF, et al: Acquisition of innate-like microbial reactivity in mucosal tissues during human fetal MAIT-cell development, *Nat Commun* 5:3143, 2014.
683. Vantourout P, Hayday A: Six-of-the-best: unique contributions of γδ T cells to immunology, *Nat Rev Immunol* 13:88-100, 2013.
684. Wang H, Fang Z, Morita CT: Vgamma2Vdelta2 T cell receptor recognition of prenyl pyrophosphates is dependent on all CDRs, *J Immunol* 184:6209-6222, 2010.
685. Xu B, Pizarro JC, Holmes MA, et al: Crystal structure of a γδ T-cell receptor specific for the human MHC class I homolog MICA, *Proc Natl Acad Sci U.S.A* 108:2414-2419, 2011.
686. Bai L, Picard D, Anderson B, et al: The majority of CD1d-sulfatide-specific T cells in human blood use a semiinvariant Vdelta1 TCR, *Eur J Immunol* 42:2505-2510, 2012.
687. Correia DV, Lopes A, Silva-Santos B: Tumor cell recognition by γδ T lymphocytes: T-cell receptor vs. NK-cell receptors, *Oncoimmunology* 2:e22892, 2013.
688. Laggner U, Di Meglio P, Perera GK, et al: Identification of a novel proinflammatory human skin-homing Vgamma9Vdelta2 T cell subset with a potential role in psoriasis, *J Immunol* 187:2783-2793, 2011.
689. Mann ER, McCarthy NE, Peake ST, et al: Skin- and gut-homing molecules on human circulating γδ T cells and their dysregulation in inflammatory bowel disease, *Clin Exp Immunol* 170:122-130, 2012.
690. Ness-Schwickerath KJ, Jin C, Morita CT: Cytokine requirements for the differentiation and expansion of IL-17A- and IL-22-producing human Vgamma2Vdelta2 T cells, *J Immunol* 184:7268-7280, 2010.
691. Wang L, Kamath A, Das H, et al: Antibacterial effect of human Vgamma2Vdelta2 T cells in vivo, *J Clin Invest* 108:1349-1357, 2001.
692. Tu W, Zheng J, Liu Y, et al: The aminobisphosphonate pamidronate controls influenza pathogenesis by expanding a gamma delta T cell population in humanized mice, *J Exp Med* 208:1511-1522, 2011.
693. Borst J, Vroom TM, Bos JD, et al: Tissue distribution and repertoire selection of human gamma delta T cells: comparison with the murine system, *Curr Top Microbiol Immunol* 173:41-46, 1991.
694. McVay LD, Carding SR: Extrathymic origin of human gamma delta T cells during fetal development, *J Immunol* 157:2873-2882, 1996.
695. Saito H, Kanamori Y, Takemori T, et al: Generation of intestinal T cells from progenitors residing in gut cryptopatches, *Science* 280:275-278, 1998.
696. Joachims ML, Chain JL, Hooker SW, et al: Human alpha beta and gamma delta thymocyte development: TCR gene rearrangements, intracellular TCR beta expression, and gamma delta developmental potential—differences between men and mice, *J Immunol* 176:1543-1552, 2006.
697. Van de Walle I, Waegemans E, De Medts J, et al: Specific Notch receptor-ligand interactions control human TCR-αβ/γδ development by inducing differential Notch signal strength, *J Exp Med* 210:683-697, 2013.
698. McVay LD, Jaswal SS, Kennedy C, et al: The generation of human gamma delta T cell repertoires during fetal development, *J Immunol* 160:5851-5860, 1998.
699. McVay LD, Carding SR: Generation of human gamma delta T-cell repertoires, *Crit Rev Immunol* 19:431-460, 1999.
700. Haynes BF, Heinly CS: Early human T cell development: analysis of the human thymus at the time of initial entry of hematopoietic stem cells into the fetal thymic microenvironment, *J Exp Med* 181:1445-1458, 1995.
701. Bukowski JF, Morita CT, Brenner MB: Recognition and destruction of virus-infected cells by human gamma delta CTL, *J Immunol* 153:5133-5140, 1994.
702. Musha N, Yoshida Y, Sugahara S, et al: Expansion of CD56+ NK T and gamma delta T cells from cord blood of human neonates, *Clin Exp Immunol* 113:220-228, 1998.
703. Erbach GT, Semple JP, Osathanondh R, et al: Phenotypic characteristics of lymphoid populations of middle gestation human fetal liver, spleen and thymus, *J Reprod Immunol* 25:81-88, 1993.
704. Wucherpfennig KW, Liao YJ, Prendergast M, et al: Human fetal liver gamma/delta T cells predominantly use unusual rearrangements of the T cell receptor delta and gamma loci expressed on both CD4+CD8- and CD4-CD8- gamma/delta T cells, *J Exp Med* 177:425-432, 1993.
705. Miyagawa Y, Matsuoka T, Baba A, et al: Fetal liver T cell receptor gamma/delta+ T cells as cytotoxic T lymphocytes specific for maternal alloantigens, *J Exp Med* 176:1-7, 1992.
706. Beldjord K, Beldjord C, Macintyre E, et al: Peripheral selection of V delta 1+ cells with restricted T cell receptor delta gene junctional repertoire in the peripheral blood of healthy donors, *J Exp Med* 178:121-127, 1993.
707. Shen J, Andrews DM, Pandolfi F, et al: Oligoclonality of Vdelta1 and Vdelta2 cells in human peripheral blood mononuclear cells: TCR selection is not altered by stimulation with gram-negative bacteria, *J Immunol* 160:3048-3055, 1998.
708. Parker CM, Groh V, Band H, et al: Evidence for extrathymic changes in the T cell receptor gamma/delta repertoire, *J Exp Med* 171:1597-1612, 1990.
709. De Rosa SC, Andrus JP, Perfetto SP, et al: Ontogeny of gamma delta T cells in humans, *J Immunol* 172:1637-1645, 2004.
710. Tsuyuguchi I, Kawasumi H, Ueta C, et al: Increase of T-cell receptor gamma/delta-bearing T cells in cord blood of newborn babies obtained by in vitro stimulation with mycobacterial cord factor, *Infect Immun* 59:3053-3059, 1991.
711. Li J, Li H, Mao H, et al: Vgamma9Vdelta2-T lymphocytes have impaired antiviral function in small-for-gestational-age and preterm neonates, *Cell Mol Immunol* 10:253-260, 2013.
712. Moens E, Brouwer M, Dimova T, et al: IL-23R and TCR signaling drives the generation of neonatal Vgamma9Vdelta2 T cells expressing high levels of cytotoxic mediators and producing IFN-gamma and IL-17, *J Leukoc Biol* 89:743-752, 2011.
713. Smith MD, Worman C, Yüksel F, et al: T gamma delta-cell subsets in cord and adult blood, *Scand J Immunol* 32:491-495, 1990.
714. Campos Alberto EJ, Shimojo N, Aoyagi M, et al: Differential effects of tumour necrosis factor-alpha and interleukin-12 on isopentenyl pyrophosphate-stimulated interferon-gamma production by cord blood Vgamma9 T cells, *Immunology* 127:171-177, 2009.
715. Li J, Li H, Mao H, et al: Vγ9Vδ2-T lymphocytes have impaired antiviral function in small-for-gestational-age and preterm neonates, *Cell Mol Immunol* 10:253-260, 2013.
716. Vermijlen D, Brouwer M, Donner C, et al: Human cytomegalovirus elicits fetal gamma delta T cell responses in utero, *J Exp Med* 207:807-821, 2010.
717. Steele RW, Suttle DE, LeMaster PC, et al: Screening for cell-mediated immunity in children, *Am J Dis Child* 130:1218-1221, 1976.
718. Munoz AI, Limbert D: Skin reactivity to *Candida* and streptokinase-streptodornase antigens in normal pediatric subjects: Influence of age and acute illness, *J Pediatr* 91:565-568, 1977.
719. Franz ML, Carella JA, Galant SP: Cutaneous delayed hypersensitivity in a healthy pediatric population: diagnostic value of diptheria-tetanus toxoids, *J Pediatr* 88:975-977, 1976.
720. Warwick W, Good RA, Smith RT: Failure of passive transfer of delayed hypersensitivity in the newborn human infant, *J Lab Clin Med* 56:139-147, 1960.
721. Bonforte RJ, Topilsky M, Siltzbach LE, et al: Phytohemagglutinin skin test: A possible in vivo measure of cell-mediated immunity, *J Pediatr* 81:775-780, 1972.
722. Fowler R Jr, Schubert WK, West CD: Acquired partial tolerance to homologous skin grafts in the human infant at birth, *Ann N.Y. Acad Sci* 87:403-428, 1960.
723. Rouleau M, Namikawa R, Antonenko S, et al: Antigen-specific cytotoxic T cells mediate human fetal pancreas allograft rejection in SCID-hu mice, *J Immunol* 157:5710-5720, 1996.

724. Orlandi F, Giambona A, Messana F, et al: Evidence of induced non-tolerance in HLA-identical twins with hemoglobinopathy after in utero fetal transplantation, *Bone Marrow Transplant* 18:637-639, 1996.
725. Vietor HE, Bolk J, Vreugdenhil GR, et al: Alterations in cord blood leukocyte subsets of patients with severe hemolytic disease after intrauterine transfusion therapy, *J Pediatr* 130:718-724, 1997.
726. Vietor HE, Hawes GE, van den Oever C, et al: Intrauterine transfusions affect fetal T-cell immunity, *Blood* 90:2492-2501, 1997.
727. Naiman JL, Punnett HH, Lischner HW, et al: Possible graft-versus-host reaction after intrauterine transfusion for Rh erythroblastosis fetalis, *N Engl J Med* 281:697-701, 1969.
728. Parkman R, Mosier D, Umansky I, et al: Graft-versus-host disease after intrauterine and exchange transfusions for hemolytic disease of the newborn, *N Engl J Med* 290:359-363, 1974.
729. Berger RS, Dixon SL: Fulminant transfusion-associated graft-versus-host disease in a premature infant, *J Am Acad Dermatol* 20:945-950, 1989.
730. Flidel O, Barak Y, Lifschitz-Mercer B, et al: Graft versus host disease in extremely low birth weight neonates, *Pediatrics* 89:689-690, 1992.
731. Prescott S, Macaubas C, Holt BJ, et al: Transplacental priming of the human immune system to environmental allergens: universal skewing of initial T cell responses toward the Th2 cytokine profile, *J Immunol* 160:4730-4737, 1998.
732. Rastogi D, Wang C, Mao X, et al: Antigen-specific immune responses to influenza vaccine in utero, *J Clin Invest* 117: 1637-1646, 2007.
733. Englund JA, Mbawuike IN, Hammill H, et al: Maternal immunization with influenza or tetanus toxoid vaccine for passive antibody protection in young infants, *J Infect Dis* 168:647-656, 1993.
734. Zeman AM, Holmes TH, Stamatis S, et al: Humoral and cellular immune responses in children given annual immunization with trivalent inactivated influenza vaccine, *Pediatr Infect Dis J* 26: 107-115, 2007.
735. Malhotra I, Mungai P, Wamachi A, et al: Helminth- and bacillus Calmette-Guérin-induced immunity in children sensitized in utero to filariasis and schistosomiasis, *J Immunol* 162:6843-6848, 1999.
736. King CL, Malhotra I, Wamachi A, et al: Acquired immune responses to *Plasmodium falciparum* merozoite surface protein-1 in the human fetus, *J Immunol* 168:356-364, 2002.
737. Kuhn L, Coutsoudis A, Moodley D, et al: T-helper cell responses to HIV envelope peptides in cord blood: against intrapartum and breast-feeding transmission, *AIDS* 15:1-9, 2001.
738. Lo Y, Lo ES, Watson N, et al: Two-way traffic between mother and fetus: biologic and clinical implications, *Blood* 88:4390-4395, 1996.
739. Muller SM, Ege M, Pottharst A, et al: Transplacentally acquired maternal T lymphocytes in severe combined immunodeficiency: A study of 121 patients, *Blood* 98:1847-1851, 2001.
740. Babik JM, Cohan D, Monto A, et al: The human fetal immune response to hepatitis C virus exposure in utero, *J Infect Dis* 203: 196-206, 2011.
741. McLeod R, Mack DG, Boyer K, et al: Phenotypes and functions of lymphocytes in congenital toxoplasmosis, *J Lab Clin Med* 116: 623-635, 1990.
742. Fatoohi AF, Cozon GJ, Wallon M, et al: Cellular immunity to *Toxoplasma gondii* in congenitally infected newborns and immunocompetent infected hosts, *Eur J Clin Microbiol Infect Dis* 22:181-184, 2003.
743. Chapey E, Wallon M, Debize G, et al: Diagnosis of congenital toxoplasmosis by using a whole-blood gamma interferon release assay, *J Clin Microbiol* 48:41-45, 2010.
744. Miles DJ, Sande MV, Kaye S, et al: CD4(+) T cell responses to cytomegalovirus in early life: a prospective birth cohort study, *J Infect Dis* 197:658-662, 2008.
745. Dauby N, Alonso-Vega C, Suarez E, et al: Maternal infection with *Trypanosoma cruzi* and congenital Chagas disease induce a trend to a type 1 polarization of infant immune responses to vaccines, *PLoS Negl Trop Dis* 3:e571, 2009.
746. Malhotra I, Dent A, Mungai P, et al: Can prenatal malaria exposure produce an immune tolerant phenotype? A prospective birth cohort study in Kenya, *PLoS Med* 6:e1000116, 2009.
747. Metenou S, Suguitan AL Jr, Long C, et al: Fetal immune responses to *Plasmodium falciparum* antigens in a malaria-endemic region of Cameroon, *J Immunol* 178:2770-2777, 2007.
748. Soulard V, Amadoudji Zin M, Fitting C, et al: Placental malaria-associated suppression of parasite-specific immune response in neonates has no major impact on systemic CD4 T cell homeostasis, *Infect Immun* 79:2801-2809, 2011.
749. Steiner KL, Amadoudji Zin M, Fitting C, et al: In utero activation of fetal memory T cells alters host regulatory gene expression and affects HIV susceptibility, *Virology* 425:23-30, 2012.
750. Steiner K, Myrie L, Malhotra I, et al: Fetal immune activation to malaria antigens enhances susceptibility to in vitro HIV infection in cord blood mononuclear cells, *J Infect Dis* 202:899-907, 2010.
751. Walther B, Miles DJ, Waight P, et al: Placental malaria is associated with attenuated CD4 T-cell responses to tuberculin PPD 12 months after BCG vaccination, *BMC Infect Dis* 12:6, 2012.
752. Thobakgale CF, Ramduth D, Reddy S, et al: Human immunodeficiency virus-specific CD8+ T-cell activity is detectable from birth in the majority of in utero-infected infants, *J Virol* 81:12775-12784, 2007.
753. Hermann E, Truyens C, Alonso-Vega C, et al: Human fetuses are able to mount an adult-like CD8 T-cell response, *Blood* 100: 2153-2158, 2002.
754. Sullender WM, Miller JL, Yasukawa LL, et al: Humoral and cell-mediated immunity in neonates with herpes simplex virus infection, *J Infect Dis* 155:28-37, 1987.
755. Burchett SK, Corey L, Mohan KM, et al: Diminished interferon-gamma and lymphocyte proliferation in neonatal and postpartum primary herpes simplex virus infection, *J Infect Dis* 165:813-818, 1992.
756. Chen SF, Tu WW, Sharp MA, et al: Antiviral CD8 T cells in the control of primary human cytomegalovirus infection in early childhood, *J Infect Dis* 189:1619-1627, 2004.
757. Gibson L, Piccinini G, Lilleri D, et al: Human cytomegalovirus proteins pp65 and immediate early protein 1 are common targets for CD8(+) T cell responses in children with congenital or postnatal human cytomegalovirus infection, *J Immunol* 172:2256-2264, 2004.
758. Clerici M, DePalma L, Roilides E, et al: Analysis of T helper and antigen-presenting cell functions in cord blood and peripheral blood leukocytes from healthy children of different ages, *J Clin Invest* 91:2829-2836, 1993.
759. Soares AP, Kwong Chung CK, Choice T, et al: Longitudinal changes in CD4(+) T-cell memory responses induced by BCG vaccination of newborns, *J Infect Dis* 207:1084-1094, 2013.
760. Sharma SK, Pichichero ME: Functional deficits of pertussis-specific CD4+ T cells in infants compared to adults following DTaP vaccination, *Clin Exp Immunol* 169:281-291, 2012.
761. Rowe J, Macaubas C, Monger TM, et al: Antigen-specific responses to diphtheria-tetanus-acellular pertussis vaccine in human infants are initially Th2 polarized, *Infect Immun* 68:3873-3877, 2000.
762. van den Biggelaar AH, Richmond PC, Pomat WS, et al: Neonatal pneumococcal conjugate vaccine immunization primes T cells for preferential Th2 cytokine expression: a randomized controlled trial in Papua New Guinea, *Vaccine* 27:1340-1347, 2009.
763. van den Biggelaar AH, Pomat W, Bosco A, et al: Pneumococcal conjugate vaccination at birth in a high-risk setting: no evidence for neonatal T-cell tolerance, *Vaccine* 29:5414-5420, 2011.
764. Marchant A, Goetghebuer T, Ota MO, et al: Newborns develop a Th1-type immune response to *Mycobacterium bovis* bacillus Calmette-Guérin vaccination, *J Immunol* 163:2249-2255, 1999.
765. Ota MO, Vekemans J, Schlegel-Haueter SE, et al: Influence of *Mycobacterium bovis* bacillus Calmette-Guérin on antibody and cytokine responses to human neonatal vaccination, *J Immunol* 168:919-925, 2002.
766. Miles DJ, van der Sande M, Crozier S, et al: Effects of antenatal and postnatal environments on CD4 T-cell responses to *Mycobacterium bovis* BCG in healthy infants in the Gambia, *Clin Immunol* 15: 995-1002, 2008.
767. Kagina BM, Abel B, Bowmaker M, et al: Delaying BCG vaccination from birth to 10 weeks of age may result in an enhanced memory CD4 T cell response, *Vaccine* 27:5488-5495, 2009.
768. Lutwama F, Kagina BM, Wajja A, et al: Distinct T-cell responses when BCG vaccination is delayed from birth to 6 weeks of age in Ugandan infants, *J Infect Dis* 209:887-897, 2014.

769. Lalor MK, Floyd S, Gorak-Stolinska P, et al: BCG vaccination induces different cytokine profiles following infant BCG vaccination in the UK and Malawi, *J Infect Dis* 204:1075-1085, 2011.
770. Anderson EJ, Webb EL, Mawa PA, et al: The influence of BCG vaccine strain on mycobacteria-specific and non-specific immune responses in a prospective cohort of infants in Uganda, *Vaccine* 30:2083-2089, 2012.
771. Mangtani P, Abubakar I, Ariti C, et al: Protection by BCG vaccine against tuberculosis: a systematic review of randomized controlled trials, *Clin Infect Dis* 58:470-480, 2014.
772. Kagina BM, Abel B, Scriba TJ, et al: Specific T cell frequency and cytokine expression profile do not correlate with protection against tuberculosis after bacillus Calmette-Guérin vaccination of newborns, *Am J Respir Crit Care Med* 182:1073-1079, 2010.
773. Murray RA, Mansoor N, Harbacheuski R, et al: Bacillus Calmette Guérin vaccination of human newborns induces a specific, functional CD8+ T cell response, *J Immunol* 177:5647-5651, 2006.
774. Zufferey C, Germano S, Dutta B, et al: The contribution of non-conventional T cells and NK cells in the mycobacterial-specific IFNgamma response in bacille Calmette-Guérin (BCG)-immunized infants, *PloS One* 8:e77334, 2013.
775. Aaby P, Whittle H, Benn CS: Vaccine programmes must consider their effect on general resistance, *B.M.J* 344:e3769, 2012.
776. Vekemans J, Ota MO, Wang EC, et al: T cell responses to vaccines in infants: defective IFNgamma production after oral polio vaccination, *Clin Exp Immunol* 127:495-498, 2002.
777. Luzuriaga K, Holmes D, Hereema A, et al: HIV-1-specific cytotoxic T lymphocyte responses in the first year of life, *J Immunol* 154: 433-443, 1995.
778. Shalekoff S, Meddows-Taylor S, Gray GE, et al: Identification of human immunodeficiency virus-1 specific CD8+ and CD4+ T cell responses in perinatally-infected infants and their mothers, *AIDS* 23:789-798, 2009.
779. Slyker JA, John-Stewart GC, Dong T, et al: Phenotypic characterization of HIV-specific CD8+ T cells during early and chronic infant HIV-1 infection, *PloS One* 6:e20375, 2011.
780. Huang S, Dunkley-Thompson J, Tang Y, et al: Deficiency of HIV-Gag-specific T cells in early childhood correlates with poor viral containment, *J Immunol* 181:8103-8111, 2008.
781. Nqoko B, Day CL, Mansoor N, et al: HIV-specific Gag responses in early infancy correlate with clinical outcome and inversely with viral load, *AIDS Res Hum Retroviruses* 27:1311-1316, 2011.
782. Turk G, Ghiglione Y, Falivene J, et al: Early Gag immunodominance of the HIV-specific T-cell response during acute/early infection is associated with higher CD8+ T-cell antiviral activity and correlates with preservation of the CD4+ T-cell compartment, *J Virol* 87:7445-7462, 2013.
783. Nielsen SD, Jeppesen DL, Kolte L, et al: Impaired progenitor cell function in HIV-negative infants of HIV-positive mothers results in decreased thymic output and low CD4 counts, *Blood* 98:398-404, 2001.
784. Chougnet C, Kovacs A, Baker R, et al: Influence of human immunodeficiency virus–infected maternal environment on development of infant interleukin-12 production, *J Infect Dis* 181:1590-1597, 2000.
785. Chiba Y, Higashidate Y, Suga K, et al: Development of cell-mediated cytotoxic immunity to respiratory syncytial virus in human infants following naturally acquired infection, *J Med Virol* 28:133-139, 1989.
786. Ichii M, Oritani K, Yokota T, et al: The density of CD10 corresponds to commitment and progression in the human B lymphoid lineage, *PloS One* 5:e12954, 2010.
787. Kohn LA, Hao QL, Sasidharan R, et al: Lymphoid priming in human bone marrow begins before expression of CD10 with upregulation of L-selectin, *Nat Immunol* 13:963-971, 2012.
788. Pieper K, Grimbacher B, Eibel H: B-cell biology and development, *J Allergy Clin Immunol* 131:959-971, 2013.
789. Martensson IL, Keenan RA, Licence S: The pre-B-cell receptor, *Curr Opin Immunol* 19:137-142, 2007.
790. Bankovich AJ, Raunser S, Juo ZS, et al: Structural insight into pre-B cell receptor function, *Science* 316:291-294, 2007.
791. Mensen A, Ochs C, Stroux A, et al: Utilization of TREC and KREC quantification for the monitoring of early T- and B-cell neogenesis in adult patients after allogeneic hematopoietic stem cell transplantation, *J Transl Med* 11:188, 2013.
792. Solvason N, Chen X, Shu F, et al: The fetal omentum in mice and humans. A site enriched for precursors of CD5 B cells early in development, *Ann N.Y. Acad Sci* 65:10-20, 1992.
793. Nishimoto N, Kubagawa H, Ohno T, et al: Normal pre-B cells express a receptor complex of Mu heavy chains and surrogate light-chain proteins, *Proc Natl Acad Sci U.S.A* 88:6284-6288, 1991.
794. Nunez C, Nishimoto N, Gartland GL, et al: B cells are generated throughout life in humans, *J Immunol* 156:866-872, 1996.
795. Arakawa-Hoyt J, Dao MA, Thiemann F, et al: The number and generative capacity of human B lymphocyte progenitors, measured in vitro and in vivo, is higher in umbilical cord blood than in adult or pediatric bone marrow, *Bone Marrow Transplant* 24:1167-1176, 1999.
796. Sanz E, Alvarez-Mon M, Martínez- AC, et al: Human cord blood CD34+Pax-5+ B-cell progenitors: single-cell analyses of their gene expression profiles, *Blood* 101:3424-3430, 2003.
797. Watson CT, Steinberg KM, Huddleston J, et al: Complete haplotype sequence of the human immunoglobulin heavy-chain variable, diversity, and joining genes and characterization of allelic and copy-number variation, *Am J Hum Genet* 92:530-546, 2013.
798. Lieber MR: The mechanism of double-strand DNA break repair by the nonhomologous DNA end-joining pathway, *Annu Rev Biochem* 79:181-211, 2010.
799. Stewart AK, Huang C, Stollar BD, et al: High-frequency representation of a single VH gene in the expressed human B cell repertoire, *J Exp Med* 177:409-418, 1993.
800. Kraj P, Rao SP, Glas AM, et al: The human heavy chain Ig V region gene repertoire is biased at all stages of B cell ontogeny, including early pre-B cells, *J Immunol* 158:5824-5832, 1997.
801. Schroeder HW Jr, Ippolito GC, Shiokawa S: Regulation of the antibody repertoire through control of HCDR3 diversity, *Vaccine* 16:1383-1390, 1998.
802. Schutte ME, Ebeling SB, Akkermans-Koolhaas KE, et al: Deletion mapping of Ig VH gene segments expressed in human CD5 B cell lines. JH proximity is not the sole determinant of the restricted fetal VH gene repertoire, *J Immunol* 149:3953-3960, 1992.
803. Zemlin M, Schelonka RL, Bauer K, et al: Regulation and chance in the ontogeny of B and T cell antigen receptor repertoires, *Immunol Res* 26:265-278, 2002.
804. Meffre E, Salmon JE: Autoantibody selection and production in early human life, *J Clin Invest* 117:598-601, 2007.
805. Sanz I: Multiple mechanisms participate in the generation of diversity of human H chain CDR3 regions, *J Immunol* 147:1720-1729, 1991.
806. Mortari F, Newton JA, Wang JY, et al: The human cord blood antibody repertoire. Frequent usage of the VH7 gene family, *Eur J Immunol* 22:241-245, 1992.
807. Silverman GJ, Sasano M, Wormsley SB: Age-associated changes in binding of human B lymphocytes to a VH3-restricted unconventional bacterial antigen, *J Immunol* 151:5840-5855, 1993.
808. Raaphorst FM, Timmers E, Kenter MJ, et al: Restricted utilization of germ-line VH3 genes and short diverse third complementarity-determining regions CDR3 in human fetal B lymphocyte immunoglobulin heavy chain rearrangements, *Eur J Immunol* 22:247-251, 1992.
809. Raaphorst FM, Raman CS, Tami J, et al: Human Ig heavy chain CDR3 regions in adult bone marrow pre-B cells display an adult phenotype of diversity: evidence for structural selection of DH amino acid sequences, *Int Immunol* 9:1503-1515, 1997.
810. Hirose Y, Kiyoi H, Itoh K, et al: B-cell precursors differentiated from cord blood CD34+ cells are more immature than those derived from granulocyte colony-stimulating factor-mobilized peripheral blood CD34+ cells, *Immunology* 104:410-417, 2001.
811. Cuisinier AM, Fumoux F, Moinier D, et al: Rapid expansion of human immunoglobulin repertoire VH, V kappa, V lambda expressed in early fetal bone marrow, *New Biol* 2:689-699, 1990.
812. Mortari F, Wang JY, Schroeder HJ: Human cord blood antibody repertoire. Mixed population of VH gene segments and CDR3 distribution in the expressed C alpha and C gamma repertoires, *J Immunol* 150:1348-1357, 1993.
813. Benedict CL, Kearney JF: Increased junctional diversity in fetal B cells results in a loss of protective anti-phosphorylcholine antibodies in adult mice, *Immunity* 10:607-617, 1999.
814. Wardemann H, Nussenzweig MC: B-cell self-tolerance in humans, *Adv Immunol* 95:83-110, 2007.

815. Meffre E: The establishment of early B cell tolerance in humans: lessons from primary immunodeficiency diseases, *Ann N.Y. Acad Sci* 1246:1-10, 2011.
816. Duty JA, Szodoray P, Zheng NY, et al: Functional anergy in a subpopulation of naive B cells from healthy humans that express autoreactive immunoglobulin receptors, *J Exp Med* 206:139-151, 2009.
817. Isnardi I, Ng YS, Menard L, et al: Complement receptor 2/CD21- human naive B cells contain mostly autoreactive unresponsive clones, *Blood* 115:5026-5036, 2010.
818. Sims GP, Ettinger R, Shirota Y, et al: Identification and characterization of circulating human transitional B cells, *Blood* 105: 4390-4398, 2005.
819. Wirths S, Lanzavecchia A: ABCB1 transporter discriminates human resting naive B cells from cycling transitional and memory B cells, *Eur J Immunol* 35:3433-3441, 2005.
820. Ettinger R, Sims GP, Fairhurst AM, et al: IL-21 induces differentiation of human naive and memory B cells into antibody-secreting plasma cells, *J Immunol* 175:7867-7879, 2005.
821. Cuss AK, Avery DT, Cannons JL, et al: Expansion of functionally immature transitional B cells is associated with human-immunodeficient states characterized by impaired humoral immunity, *J Immunol* 176:1506-1516, 2006.
822. Marie-Cardine A, Divay F, Dutot I, et al: Transitional B cells in humans: characterization and insight from B lymphocyte reconstitution after hematopoietic stem cell transplantation, *Clin Immunol* 127:14-25, 2008.
823. Suryani S, Fulcher DA, Santner-Nanan B, et al: Differential expression of CD21 identifies developmentally and functionally distinct subsets of human transitional B cells, *Blood* 115:519-529, 2010.
824. Suryani S, Tangye SG: Therapeutic implications of advances in our understanding of transitional B-cell development in humans, *Expert Rev Clin Immunol* 6:765-775, 2010.
825. Herve M, Isnardi I, Ng YS, et al: CD40 ligand and MHC class II expression are essential for human peripheral B cell tolerance, *J Exp Med* 204:1583-1593, 2007.
826. Isnardi I, Ng YS, Srdanovic I, et al: IRAK-4- and MYD88-dependent pathways are essential for the removal of developing autoreactive B cells in humans, *Immunity* 29:746-757, 2008.
827. Monroe JG: ITAM-mediated tonic signalling through pre-BCR and BCR complexes, *Nat Rev Immunol* 6:283-294, 2006.
828. Brezinschek HP, Brezinschek RI, Lipsky PE: Analysis of the heavy chain repertoire of human peripheral B cells using single-cell polymerase chain reaction, *J Immunol* 155:190-202, 1995.
829. Iwata Y, Matsushita T, Horikawa M, et al: Characterization of a rare IL-10-competent B-cell subset in humans that parallels mouse regulatory B10 cells, *Blood* 117:530-541, 2011.
830. Klein U, Rajewsky K, Kuppers R: Human immunoglobulin (Ig) M+IgD+ peripheral blood B cells expressing the CD27 cell surface antigen carry somatically mutated variable region genes: Cd27 as a general marker for somatically mutated (memory) B cells, *J Exp Med* 188:1679-1689, 1998.
831. Macallan DC, Wallace DL, Zhang Y, et al: B-cell kinetics in humans: rapid turnover of peripheral blood memory cells, *Blood* 105: 3633-3640, 2005.
832. Allen CD, Okada T, Cyster JG: Germinal-center organization and cellular dynamics, *Immunity* 27:190-202, 2007.
833. Schultz C, Reiss I, Bucsky P, et al: Maturational changes of lymphocyte surface antigens in human blood: comparison between fetuses, neonates and adults, *Biol Neonate* 78:77-82, 2000.
834. van Gent R, van Tilburg CM, Nibbelke EE, et al: Refined characterization and reference values of the pediatric T- and B-cell compartments, *Clin Immunol* 133:95-107, 2009.
835. Smet J, Mascart F, Schandene L: Are the reference values of B cell subpopulations used in adults for classification of common variable immunodeficiencies appropriate for children? *Clin Immunol* 138:266-273, 2011.
836. Avery DT, Bryant VL, Ma CS, et al: IL-21-induced isotype switching to IgG and IgA by human naive B cells is differentially regulated by IL-4, *J Immunol* 181:1767-1779, 2008.
837. Punnonen J, Aversa GG, Vandekerckhove B, et al: Induction of isotype switching and IgG production by CD5+ and CD10+ human fetal B cells, *J Immunol* 148:3398-3404, 1992.
838. LeBien TW, Wörmann B, Villablanca JG, et al: Multiparameter flow cytometric analysis of human fetal bone marrow B cells, *Leukemia* 4:354-358, 1990.
839. Tasker L, Marshall-Clarke S: Functional responses of human neonatal B lymphocytes to antigen receptor cross-linking and CpG DNA, *Clin Exp Immunol* 134:409-419, 2003.
840. Tian C, Kron GK, Dischert KM, et al: Low expression of the interleukin (IL)-4 receptor alpha chain and reduced signalling via the IL-4 receptor complex in human neonatal B cells, *Immunology* 119: 54-62, 2006.
841. Avery DT, Ma CS, Bryant VL, et al: STAT3 is required for IL-21-induced secretion of IgE from human naive B cells, *Blood* 112:1784-1793, 2008.
842. Schatorje EJ, Gemen EF, Driessen GJ, et al: Age-matched reference values for B-lymphocyte subpopulations and CVID classifications in children, *Scand J Immunol* 74:502-510, 2011.
843. Gupta N, DeFranco AL: Lipid rafts and B cell signaling, *Semin Cell Dev Biol* 18:616-626, 2007.
844. McLeod IX, He Y: Roles of autophagy in lymphocytes: reflections and directions, *Cell Mol Immunol* 7:104-107, 2010.
845. Harwood NE, Batista FD: Antigen presentation to B cells, *F1000 Biol Rep* 2:87, 2010.
846. Cambier JC, Getahun A: B cell activation versus anergy; the antigen receptor as a molecular switch, *Immunol Lett* 128:6-7, 2010.
847. Nimmerjahn F, Ravetch JV: FcGammaRs in health and disease, *Curr Top Microbiol Immunol* 350:105-125, 2011.
848. Jessup CF, Ridings J, Ho A, et al: The Fc receptor for IgG (Fc Gamma RII; CD32) on human neonatal B lymphocytes, *Hum Immunol* 62:679-685, 2001.
849. Tangye SG, Deenick EK, Palendira U, et al: T cell-B cell interactions in primary immunodeficiencies, *Ann N.Y. Acad Sci* 1250:1-13, 2012.
850. Ma CS, Suryani S, Avery DT, et al: Early commitment of naive human CD4(+) T cells to the T follicular helper (TFH) cell lineage is induced by IL-12, *Immunol Cell Biol* 87:590-600, 2009.
851. Zheng B, Kelsoe G, Han S: Somatic diversification of antibody responses, *J Clin Immunol* 16:1-11, 1996.
852. Kuppers R, Zhao M, Hansmann ML, et al: Tracing B cell development in human germinal centres by molecular analysis of single cells picked from histological sections, *EMBO J* 12:4955-4967, 1993.
853. Kracker S, Gardes P, Durandy A: Inherited defects of immunoglobulin class switch recombination, *Adv Exp Med Biol* 685:166-174, 2010.
854. Bowen AL, Tian C, LaFleur BJ, et al: Transcriptional control of activation-induced cytidine deaminase and error-prone DNA polymerases is functionally mature in the B cells of infants at birth, *Hum Immunol* 67:43-46, 2006.
855. Scheeren FA, Nagasawa M, Weijer K, et al: T cell-independent development and induction of somatic hypermutation in human IgM+ IgD+ CD27+ B cells, *J Exp Med* 205:2033-2042, 2008.
856. Kaminski DA, Wei C, Qian Y, et al: Advances in human B cell phenotypic profiling, *Front Immunol* 3:302, 2012.
857. Berkowska MA, Driessen GJ, Bikos V, et al: Human memory B cells originate from three distinct germinal center-dependent and -independent maturation pathways, *Blood* 118:2150-2158, 2011.
858. Fecteau JF, Cote G, Neron S: A new memory CD27-IgG+ B cell population in peripheral blood expressing VH genes with low frequency of somatic mutation, *J Immunol* 177:3728-3736, 2006.
859. Sanz I, Wei C, Lee FE, et al: Phenotypic and functional heterogeneity of human memory B cells, *Semin Immunol* 20:67-82, 2008.
860. Lanzavecchia A, Sallusto F: Human B cell memory, *Curr Opin Immunol* 21:298-304, 2009.
861. Garban F, Truman JP, Lord J, et al: Signal transduction via human leucocyte antigen class II molecules distinguishes between cord blood, normal, and malignant adult B lymphocytes, *Exp Hematol* 26:874-884, 1998.
862. Jones CA, Holloway JA, Warner JO: Phenotype of fetal monocytes and B lymphocytes during the third trimester of pregnancy, *J Reprod Immunol* 56:45-60, 2002.
863. Cerutti A: The regulation of IgA class switching, *Nat Rev Immunol* 8:421-434, 2008.
864. Duriancik DM, Lackey DE, Hoag KA: Vitamin A as a regulator of antigen presenting cells, *J Nutr* 140:1395-1399, 2010.
865. Gustafson CE, Higbee D, Yeckes AR, et al: Limited expression of APRIL and its receptors prior to intestinal IgA plasma cell development during human infancy, *Mucosal Immunol* 7:467-477, 2014.
866. Macpherson AJ, Gatto D, Sainsbury E, et al: A primitive T cell-independent mechanism of intestinal mucosal IgA responses to commensal bacteria, *Science* 288:2222-2226, 2000.

867. Pape KA, Kouskoff V, Nemazee D, et al: Visualization of the genesis and fate of isotype-switched B cells during a primary immune response, *J Exp Med* 197:1677-1687, 2003.
868. Ochs HD, Winkelstein J: *Disorders of the B-cell system*, Philadelphia, 1996, WB Saunders.
869. Ochs HD, Hollenbaugh D, Aruffo A: The role of CD40L (gp39)/CD40 in T/B cell interaction and primary immunodeficiency, *Semin Immunol* 6:337-341, 1994.
870. Moens L, Tangye SG: Cytokine-mediated regulation of plasma cell generation: IL-21 takes center stage, *Front Immunol* 5:65, 2014.
871. Clement LT: Isoforms of the CD45 common leukocyte antigen family: markers for human T-cell differentiation, *J Clin Immunol* 12:1-10, 1992.
872. Tangye SG, Ferguson A, Avery DT, et al: Isotype switching by human B cells is division-associated and regulated by cytokines, *J Immunol* 169:4298-4306, 2002.
873. Punnonen J, Cocks BG, de Vries JE: IL-4 induces germ-line IgE heavy chain gene transcription in human fetal pre-B cells. Evidence for differential expression of functional IL-4 and IL-13 receptors during B cell ontogeny, *J Immunol* 155:4248-4254, 1995.
874. Kimata H, Fujimoto M: Induction of IgA1 and IgA2 production in immature human fetal B cells and pre-B cells by vasoactive intestinal peptide, *Blood* 85:2098-2104, 1995.
875. Ueno Y, Ichihara T, Hasui M, et al: T-cell-dependent production of IgG by human cord blood b cells in reconstituted SCID mice, *Scand J Immunol* 35:415-419, 1992.
876. Vandekerckhove BA, Jones D, Punnonen J, et al: Human IgG production and isotype switching in severe combined immunodeficient-human mice, *J Immunol* 151:128-137, 1993.
877. Splawski J, Yamamoto K, Lipsky P: Deficient interleukin-10 production by neonatal T cells does not expalin their ineffectiveness at promoting neonatal B cell differentiation, *Eur J Immunol* 28: 4248-4256, 1998.
878. Gagro A, McCloskey N, Challa A, et al: CD5-positive and CD5-negative human B cells converge to an indistinguishable population on signalling through B-cell receptors and CD40, *Immunology* 101:201-209, 2000.
879. Baskin B, Islam KB, Smith CI: Characterization of the CDR3 region of rearranged alpha heavy chain genes in human fetal liver, *Clin Exp Immunol* 112:44-47, 1998.
880. Gitlin D, Biasucci A: Development of gamma G, gamma A, gamma M, beta IC-beta IA, C 1 esterase inhibitor, ceruloplasmin, transferrin, hemopexin, haptoglobin, fibrinogen, plasminogen, alpha 1-antitrypsin, orosomucoid, beta-lipoprotein, alpha 2-macroglobulin, and prealbumin in the human conceptus, *J Clin Invest* 48:1433-1446, 1969.
881. Dosch HM, Lam P, Hui MF, et al: Concerted generation of Ig isotype diversity in human fetal bone marrow, *J Immunol* 143:2464-2469, 1989.
882. Gathings WE, Kubagawa H, Cooper MD: A distinctive pattern of B cell immaturity in perinatal humans, *Immunol Rev* 57:107-126, 1981.
883. Wedgwood JF, Weinberger BI, Hatam L, et al: Umbilical cord blood lacks circulating B lymphocytes expressing surface IgG or IgA, *Clin Immunol Immunopathol* 84:276-282, 1997.
884. Splawski JB, Lipsky PE: Prostaglandin E2 inhibits T cell-dependent Ig secretion by neonatal but not adult lymphocytes, *J Immunol* 152:5259-5267, 1994.
885. Cerutti A, Cols M, Puga I. Marginal zone B cells: Virtues of innate-like antibody-producing lymphocytes, *Nat Rev Immunol* 13:118-132, 2013.
886. Seifert M, Kuppers R: Molecular footprints of a germinal center derivation of human IgM+(IgD+)CD27+ B cells and the dynamics of memory B cell generation, *J Exp Med* 206:2659-2669, 2009.
887. Kruetzmann S, Rosado MM, Weber H, et al: Human immunoglobulin M memory B cells controlling Streptococcus pneumoniae infections are generated in the spleen, *J Exp Med* 197:939-945, 2003.
888. Haas KM, Hasegawa M, Steeber DA, et al: Complement receptors CD21/35 link innate and protective immunity during *Streptococcus pneumoniae* infection by regulating IgG3 antibody responses, *Immunity* 17:713-723, 2002.
889. Zandvoort A, Timens W: The dual function of the splenic marginal zone: essential for initiation of anti-TI-2 responses but also vital in the general first-line defense against blood-borne antigens, *Clin Exp Immunol* 130:4-11, 2002.
890. Martins G, Calame K: Regulation and functions of BLIMP-1 in T and B lymphocytes, *Annu Rev Immunol* 26:133-169, 2008.
891. Amlot PL, Hayes AE: Impaired human antibody response to the thymus-independent antigen, DNP-ficoll, after splenectomy, Implications for post-splenectomy infections, *Lancet* 1:1008-1011, 1985.
892. Weller S, Mamani-Matsuda M, Picard C, et al: Somatic diversification in the absence of antigen-driven responses is the hallmark of the IgM+ IgD+ CD27+ B cell repertoire in infants, *J Exp Med* 205:1331-1342, 2008.
893. Kaur K, Chowdhury S, Greenspan NS, et al: Decreased expression of tumor necrosis factor family receptors involved in humoral immune responses in preterm neonates, *Blood* 110:2948-2954, 2007.
894. Martin F, Kearney JF: B1 cells: Similarities and differences with other B cell subsets, *Curr Opin Immunol* 13:195-201, 2001.
895. Griffin DO, Holodick NE, Rothstein TL: Human B1 cells in umbilical cord and adult peripheral blood express the novel phenotype CD20+ CD27+ CD43+ CD70+, *J Exp Med* 208:67-80, 2011.
896. Griffin DO, Rothstein TL: A small CD11b(+) human B1 cell subpopulation stimulates T cells and is expanded in lupus, *J Exp Med* 208:2591-2598, 2011.
897. Yammani RD, Haas KM: Primate B-1 cells generate antigen-specific B cell responses to T cell-independent type 2 antigens, *J Immunol* 190:3100-3108, 2013.
898. Mouthon L, Nobrega A, Nicolas N, et al: Invariance and restriction toward a limited set of self-antigens characterize neonatal IgM antibody repertoires and prevail in autoreactive repertoires of healthy adults, *Proc Natl Acad Sci U.S.A* 92:3839-3843, 1995.
899. Merbl Y, Zucker-Toledano M, Quintana FJ, et al: Newborn humans manifest autoantibodies to defined self molecules detected by antigen microarray informatics, *J Clin Invest* 117:712-718, 2007.
900. Kalampokis I, Yoshizaki A, Tedder TF: IL-10-producing regulatory B cells (B10 cells) in autoimmune disease, *Arthritis Res Ther* 15(Suppl 1):S1, 2013.
901. Blair PA, Noreña LY, Flores-Borja F, et al: CD19(+)CD24(hi)-CD38(hi) B cells exhibit regulatory capacity in healthy individuals but are functionally impaired in systemic lupus erythematosus patients, *Immunity* 32:129-140, 2010.
902. Beaudette-Zlatanova BC, Le PT, Knight KL, et al: A potential role for B cells in suppressed immune responses in cord blood transplant recipients, *Bone Marrow Transplant* 48:85-93, 2013.
903. Rijkers GT, Sanders EA, Breukels MA, et al: Infant B cell responses to polysaccharide determinants, *Vaccine* 16:1396-1400, 1998.
904. Capolunghi F, Cascioli S, Giorda E, et al: CpG drives human transitional B cells to terminal differentiation and production of natural antibodies, *J Immunol* 180:800-808, 2008.
905. Viemann D, Schlenke P, Hammers HJ, et al: Differential expression of the B cell-restricted molecule CD22 B lymphocytes depending upon antigen stimulation, *Eur J Immunol* 30:550-559, 2000.
906. Fuleihan R, Ahern D, Geha RS: Decreased expression of the ligand for CD40 in newborn lymphocytes, *Eur J Immunol* 24:1925-1928, 1994.
907. Golding B, Muchmore AV, Blaese RM: Newborn and Wiskott-Aldrich patient B cells can be activated by TNP-*Brucella abortus*: evidence that TNP-*Brucella abortus* behaves as a T-independent type 1 antigen in humans, *J Immunol* 133:2966-2971, 1984.
908. Griffioen AW, Toebes EA, Zegers BJ, et al: Role of CR2 in the human adult and neonatal in vitro antibody response to type 4 pneumococcal polysaccharide, *Cell Immunol* 143:11-22, 1992.
909. Timens W, Rozeboom T, Poppema S: Fetal and neonatal development of human spleen: an immunohistological study, *Immunology* 60:603-609, 1987.
910. Rickert RC: Regulation of B lymphocyte activation by complement C3 and the B cell coreceptor complex, *Curr Opin Immunol* 17: 237-243, 2005.
911. Snapper CM, Mond JJ: A model for induction of T cell-independent humoral immunity in response to polysaccharide antigens, *J Immunol* 157:2229-2233, 1996.
912. Halista SM, Johnson-Robbins LA, El-Mohandes AE, et al: Characterization of early activation events in cord blood B cells after stimulation with t cell-independent activators, *Pediatr Res.* 43:496-503, 1998.
913. Silverstein AM, Prendergast RA, Parshall CJ Jr: Cellular kinetics of the antibody response by the fetal rhesus monkey, *J Immunol* 104:269-271, 1970.
914. Silverstein A: *Ontogeny of the immune response: a perspective*, New York, 1977, Raven Press.

915. Watts AM, Stanley JR, Shearer MH, et al: Fetal immunization of baboons induces a fetal-specific antibody response, *Nat Med* 5: 427-430, 1999.
916. Gill TJ, Repetti CF, Metlay LA, et al: Transplacental immunization of the human fetus to tetanus by immunization of the mother, *J Clin Invest* 72:987-996, 1983.
917. Vanderbeeken Y, Sarfati M, Bose R, Delespesse G: In utero immunization of the fetus to tetanus by maternal vaccination during pregnancy, *Am J Reprod Immunol Microbiol* 8:39-42, 1985.
918. Enders G: Serologic test combinations for safe detection of rubella infections, *Rev Infect Dis* 7:S113-S122, 1985.
919. Naot Y, Desmonts G, Remington JS: IgM enzyme-linked immunosorbent assay test for the diagnosis of congenital *Toxoplasma* infection, *J Pediatr* 98:32-36, 1981.
920. Chumpitazi BF, Boussaid A, Pelloux H, et al: Diagnosis of congenital toxoplasmosis by immunoblotting and relationship with other methods, *J Clin Microbiol* 33:1479-1485, 1995.
921. Griffiths PD, Stagno S, Pass RF, et al: Congenital cytomegalovirus infection: diagnostic and prognostic significance of the detection of specific immunoglobulin M antibodies in cord serum, *Pediatrics* 69:544-549, 1982.
922. Aase JM, Noren GR, Reddy DV, et al: Mumps-virus infection in pregnant women and the immunologic response of their offspring, *N Engl J Med* 286:1379-1382, 1972.
923. Pinon JM, Toubas D, Marx C, et al: Detection of specific immunoglobulin E in patients with toxoplasmosis, *J Clin Microbiol* 28: 1739-1743, 1990.
924. King CL, Malhotra I, Mungai P, et al: B cell sensitization to helminthic infection develops in utero in humans, *J Immunol* 160: 3578-3584, 1998.
925. Desmonts G, Daffos F, Forestier F, et al: Prenatal diagnosis of congenital toxoplasmosis, *Lancet* 1:500-504, 1985.
926. Stepick-Biek P, Thulliez P, Araujo FG, et al: IgA antibodies for diagnosis of acute congenital and acquired toxoplasmosis, *J Infect Dis* 162:270-273, 1990.
927. Decoster A, Darcy F, Caron A, et al: Anti-p30 IgA antibodies as prenatal markers of congenital *Toxoplasma* infection, *Clin Exp Immunol* 87:310-315, 1992.
928. Dengrove J, Lee EJ, Heiner DC, et al: IgG and IgG subclass specific antibody responses to diphtheria and tetanus toxoids in newborns and infants given DTP immunization, *Pediatr Res* 20:735-739, 1986.
929. Smolen P, Bland R, Heiligenstein E, et al: Antibody response to oral polio vaccine in premature infants, *J Pediatr* 103:917-919, 1983.
930. Fink C, Miller WE Jr, Dorward B, et al: The formation of macroglobulin antibodies II. Studies on neonatal infants and older children, *J Clin Invest* 41:1422-1428, 1962.
931. Smith R, Eitzman DV: The development of the immune response, *Pediatrics* 33:163-183, 1964.
932. Uhr J, Dancis J, Franklin EC, et al: The antibody response to bacteriophage phi-X 174 in newborn premature infants, *J Clin Invest* 41:1509-1513, 1962.
933. West DJ: Clinical experience with hepatitis B vaccines, *Am J Infect Control* 17:172-180, 1989.
934. Lee SS, Lo YC, Young BW, et al: A reduced dose approach to hepatitis B vaccination for low-risk newborns and preschool children, *Vaccine* 13:373-376, 1995.
935. Greenberg DP: Pediatric experience with recombinant hepatitis B vaccines and relevant safety and immunogenicity studies, *Pediatr Infect Dis J* 12:438-445, 1993.
936. Dancis J, Osborn JJ, Kunz HW: Studies of the immunology of the newborn infant. IV. Antibody formation in the premature infant, *Pediatrics* 12:151-157, 1953.
937. McFarland EJ, Borkowsky W, Fenton T, et al: Human immunodeficiency virus type 1 (HIV-1) gp120-specific antibodies in neonates receiving an HIV-1 recombinant gp120 vaccine, *J Infect Dis* 184:1331-1335, 2001.
938. Peterson J: Immunization in the young infant. Response to combined vaccines, *Am J Dis Child* 81:484-491, 1951.
939. Provenzano R, Wetterow LH, Sullivan CL: Immunization and antibody response in the newborn infant. I. Pertussis inoculation within twenty-four hours of birth, *N Engl J Med* 273:959-965, 1965.
940. Baraff LJ, Leake RD, Burstyn DG, et al: Immunologic response to early and routine DTP immunization in infants, *Pediatrics* 73: 37-42, 1984.
941. Halasa NB, O'Shea A, Shi JR, et al: Poor immune responses to a birth dose of diphtheria, tetanus, and acellular pertussis vaccine, *J Pediatr* 153:327-332, 2008.
942. Belloni C, De Silvestri A, Tinelli C, et al: Immunogenicity of a three-component acellular pertussis vaccine administered at birth, *Pediatrics* 111:1042-1045, 2003.
943. Knuf M, Schmitt HJ, Wolter J, et al: Neonatal vaccination with an acellular pertussis vaccine accelerates the acquisition of pertussis antibodies in infants, *J Pediatr* 152:655-660, 2008. 660.e1.
944. Schoub BD, Johnson S, McAnerney J, et al: Monovalent neonatal polio immunization—a strategy for the developing world, *J Infect Dis* 157:836-839, 1988.
945. Gans HA, Arvin AM, Galinus J, et al: Deficiency of the humoral immune response to measles vaccine in infants immunized at age 6 months, *JAMA* 280:527-532, 1998.
946. Gans HA, Maldonado Y, Yasukawa LL, et al: IL-12, IFN-gamma, and T cell proliferation to measles in immunized infants, *J Immunol* 162:5569-5575, 1999.
947. Gans H, Yasukawa L, Rinki M, et al: Immune responses to measles and mumps vaccination of infants at 6, 9, and 12 months, *J Infect Dis* 184:817-826, 2001.
948. Gans HA, Yasukawa LL, Alderson A, et al: Humoral and cell-mediated immune responses to an early 2-dose measles vaccination regimen in the United States, *J Infect Dis* 190:83-90, 2004.
949. Smith DH, Peter G, Ingram DL, et al: Responses of children immunized with the capsular polysaccharide of *Haemophilus influenzae*, type b, *Pediatrics* 52:637-644, 1973.
950. Schlesinger Y, Granoff DM: Avidity and bactericidal activity of antibody elicited by different *Haemophilus influenzae* type b conjugate vaccines. The Vaccine Study Group, *JAMA* 267:1489-1494, 1992.
951. Adderson EE, Shackelford PG, Quinn A, et al: Restricted Ig H chain V gene usage in the human antibody response to *Haemophilus influenzae* type b capsular polysaccharide, *J Immunol* 147:1667-1674, 1991.
952. Granoff DM, Holmes SJ, Osterholm MT, et al: Induction of immunologic memory in infants primed with *Haemophilus influenzae* type b conjugate vaccines, *J Infect Dis* 168:663-671, 1993.
953. Eskola J, Kayhty H: Early immunization with conjugate vaccines, *Vaccine* 16:1433-1438, 1998.
954. Lieberman JM, Greenberg DP, Wong VK, et al: Effect of neonatal immunization with diphtheria and tetanus toxoids on antibody responses to *Haemophilus influenzae* type b conjugate vaccines, *J Pediatr* 126:198-205, 1995.
955. Hsu KK, Pelton SI: Heptavalent pneumococcal conjugate vaccine: current and future impact, *Expert Rev Vaccines* 2:619-631, 2003.
956. Conterno LO, Silva Filho CR, Rüggeberg JU: Conjugate vaccines for preventing meningococcal C meningitis and septicaemia, *Cochrane Database Syst Rev* (3):CD001834, 2006.
957. Bernbaum JC, Daft A, Anolik R, et al: Response of preterm infants to diphtheria-tetanus-pertussis immunizations, *J Pediatr* 107: 184-188, 1985.
958. Koblin BA, Townsend TR, Muñoz A, et al: Response of preterm infants to diphtheria-tetanus-pertussis vaccine, *Pediatr Infect Dis J* 7:704-711, 1988.
959. Adenyi-Jones SC, Faden H, Ferdon MB, et al: Systemic and local immune responses to enhanced-potency inactivated poliovirus vaccine in premature and term infants, *J Pediatr* 120:686-689, 1992.
960. Shinefield H, Black S, Ray P, et al: Efficacy, immunogenicity and safety of heptavalent pneumococcal conjugate vaccine in low birth weight and preterm infants, *Pediatr Infect Dis J* 21:182-186, 2002.
961. Lau YL, Tam AY, Ng KW, et al: Response of preterm infants to hepatitis B vaccine, *J Pediatr* 121:962-965, 1992.
962. Freitas da Motta MS, Mussi-Pinhata MM, Jorge SM, et al: Immunogenicity of hepatitis B vaccine in preterm and full term infants vaccinated within the first week of life, *Vaccine* 20:1557-1562, 2002.
963. Kim SC, Chung EK, Hodinka RL, et al: Immunogenicity of hepatitis B vaccine in preterm infants, *Pediatrics* 99:534-536, 1997.
964. Linder N, Vishne TH, Levin E, et al: Hepatitis B vaccination: long-term follow-up of the immune response of preterm infants and comparison of two vaccination protocols, *Infection* 30:136-139, 2002.
965. Greenberg DP, Vadheim CM, Partridge S, et al: Immunogenicity of *Haemophilus influenzae* type b tetanus toxoid conjugate vaccine in young infants. The Kaiser-UCLA Vaccine Study Group, *J Infect Dis* 170:76-81, 1994.

966. Heath PT, Booy R, McVernon J, et al: Hib vaccination in infants born prematurely, *Arch Dis Child* 88:206-210, 2003.
967. Washburn LK, O'Shea TM, Gillis DC, et al: Response to *Haemophilus influenzae* type b conjugate vaccine in chronically ill premature infants, *J Pediatr* 123:791-794, 1993.
968. Rath T, Kuo TT, Baker K, et al: The immunologic functions of the neonatal Fc receptor for IgG, *J Clin Immunol* 33(Suppl 1):S9-S17, 2013.
969. Firan M, Bawdon R, Radu C, et al: The MHC class I-related receptor, FcRn, plays an essential role in the maternofetal transfer of gamma-globulin in humans, *Int Immunol* 13:993-1002, 2001.
970. Roopenian DC, Akilesh S: FcRn: the neonatal Fc receptor comes of age, *Nat Rev Immunol* 7:715-725, 2007.
971. Simister NE: Human placental Fc receptors and the trapping of immune complexes, *Vaccine* 16:1451-1455, 1998.
972. Kohler PF, Farr RS: Elevation of cord over maternal IgG immunoglobulin: evidence for an active placental IgG transport, *Nature* 210:1070-1071, 1966.
973. Gusdon JP Jr: Fetal and maternal immunoglobulin levels during pregnancy, *Am J Obstet Gynecol* 103:895-900, 1969.
974. Pitcher-Wilmott RW, Hindocha P, Wood CB: The placental transfer of IgG subclasses in human pregnancy, *Clin Exp Immunol* 41:303-308, 1980.
975. Landor M: Maternal-fetal transfer of immunoglobulins, *Ann Allergy Asthma Immunol* 74:279-283, 1995.
976. Martensson L, Fudenberg HH: Gm genes and gamma G-globulin synthesis in the human fetus, *J Immunol* 94:514-520, 1965.
977. Hay FC, Hull MG, Torrigiani G: The transfer of human IgG subclasses from mother to foetus, *Clin Exp Immunol* 9:355-358, 1971.
978. Oxelius VA, Svenningsen NW: IgG subclass concentrations in preterm neonates, *Acta Paediatr Scand* 73:626-630, 1984.
979. Malek A, Sager R, Schneider H: Maternal-fetal transport of immunoglobulin G and its subclasses during the third trimester of human pregnancy, *Am J Reprod Immunol* 32:8-14, 1994.
980. Bonnelykke K, Pipper CB, Bisgaard H: Sensitization does not develop in utero, *J Allergy Clin Immunol* 121:646-651, 2008.
981. Bonnelykke K, Pipper CB, Bisgaard H: Transfer of maternal IgE can be a common cause of increased IgE levels in cord blood, *J Allergy Clin Immunol* 126:657-663, 2010.
982. Morell A, Sidiropoulos D, Herrmann U, et al: IgG subclasses and antibodies to group B streptococci, pneumococci, and tetanus toxoid in preterm neonates after intravenous infusion of immunoglobulin to the mothers, *Pediatr Res* 20:933-936, 1986.
983. Linder N, Waintraub I, Smetana Z, et al: Placental transfer and decay of varicella-zoster virus antibodies in preterm infants, *J Pediatr* 137:85-89, 2000.
984. Sato H, Albrecht P, Reynolds DW, et al: Transfer of measles, mumps, and rubella antibodies from mother to infant. Its effect on measles, mumps, and rubella immunization, *Am J Dis Child* 133:1240-1243, 1979.
985. Vahlquist B: Response of infants to diphtheria immunization, *Lancet* 1:16-18, 1949.
986. Perkins F, Yetts R, Gaisford W: Response of infants to a third dose of poliomyelitis vaccine given 10 to 12 months after primary immunization, *BMJ* 1:680-682, 1959.
987. Panpitpat C, Thisyakorn U, Chotpitayasunondh T, et al: Elevated levels of maternal anti-tetanus toxin antibodies do not suppress the immune response to a *Haemophilus influenzae* type b polyribosylphosphate-tetanus toxoid conjugate vaccine, *Bull World Health Org* 78:364-371, 2000.
988. Rowe J, Poolman JT, Macaubas C, et al: Enhancement of vaccine-specific cellular immunity in infants by passively acquired maternal antibody, *Vaccine* 22:3986-3992, 2004.
989. Stiehm ER, Fudenberg HH: Serum levels of immune globulins in health and disease: a survey, *Pediatrics* 37:715-727, 1966.
990. Lee SI, Heiner DC, Wara D: Development of serum IgG subclass levels in children, *Monogr Allergy* 19:108-121, 1986.
991. Ochs HD, Wedgwood RJ: IgG subclass deficiencies, *Annu Rev Med* 38:325-340, 1987.
992. Kobayashi RH, Hyman CJ, Stiehm ER: Immunologic maturation in an infant born to a mother with agammaglobulinemia, *Am J Dis Child* 134:942-944, 1980.
993. Granoff DM, Shackelford PG, Pandey JP, et al: Antibody responses to *Haemophilus influenzae* type b polysaccharide vaccine in relation to Km 1 and G2m 23 immunoglobulin allotypes, *J Infect Dis* 154:257-264, 1986.
994. Cederqvist LL, Ewool LC, Litwin SD: The effect of fetal age, birth weight, and sex on cord blood immunoglobulin values, *Am J Obstet Gyn* 131:520-525, 1978.
995. Avrech OM, Samra Z, Lazarovich Z, et al: Efficacy of the placental barrier for immunoglobulins: correlations between maternal, paternal and fetal immunoglobulin levels, *Int Arch Allergy Immunol* 103:160-165, 1994.
996. Allansmith M, McClellan BH, Butterworth M, et al: The development of immunoglobulin levels in man, *J Pediatr* 72:276-290, 1968.
997. Perchalski JE, Clem LW, Small PJ: 7S gamma-M immunoglobulins in normal human cord serum, *Am J Med Sci* 256:107-111, 1968.
998. Alford CJ, Stagno S, Reynolds DW: Diagnosis of chronic perinatal infections, *Am J Dis Child* 129:455-463, 1975.
999. Fitzsimmons SP, Evans MK, Pearce CL, et al: Immunoglobulin A subclasses in infants' saliva and in saliva and milk from their mothers, *J Pediatr* 124:566-573, 1994.
1000. Conley ME, Kearney JF, Lawton AR 3rd, et al: Differentiation of human B cells expressing the IgA subclasses as demonstrated by monoclonal hybridoma antibodies, *J Immunol* 125:2311-2316, 1980.
1001. Seidel BM, Schulze B, Kiess W, et al: Determination of secretory IgA and albumin in saliva of newborn infants, *Biol Neonate* 78: 186-190, 2000.
1002. Josephs SH, Buckley RH: Serum IgD concentrations in normal infants, children, and adults and in patients with elevated IgE, *J Pediatr* 96:417-420, 1980.
1003. Haraldsson A, Weemaes CM, Jónasdóttir S, et al: Serum immunoglobulin D in infants and children, *Scand J Immunol* 51:415-418, 2000.
1004. Bazaral M, Orgel HA, Hamburger RN: IgE levels in normal infants and mothers and an inheritance hypothesis, *J Immunol* 107: 794-801, 1971.
1005. Edenharter G, Bergmann RL, Bergmann KE, et al: Cord blood-IgE as risk factor and predictor for atopic diseases, *Clin Exp Allergy* 28:671-678, 1998.
1006. Chang WT, Sun HL, Lue KH, et al: Predictability of early onset atopic dermatitis by cord blood IgE and parental history, *Acta Paediatr Taiwan* 46:272-277, 2005.
1007. Hogan SP: Neonatal Fc receptor (FcRn) and maternal-to-newborn IgE absorption, *Clin Exp Allergy* 42:1656-1659, 2012.
1008. American Academy of Pediatrics: In Pickering LK, editor: *Red book: 2012 report of the Committee on Infectious Diseases*, ed 29, Elk Grove Village, Ill, 2012, American Academy of Pediatrics.
1009. Ohlsson A, Lacy JB: Intravenous immunoglobulin for preventing infection in preterm and/or low birth weight infants, *Cochrane Database Syst Rev* (7):CD000361, 2013.
1010. The INIS Study: International Neonatal Immunotherapy Study: non-specific intravenous immunoglobulin therapy for suspected or proven neonatal sepsis: an international, placebo controlled, multicentre randomised trial, *BMC Pregnancy Childbirth* 8:52, 2008.
1011. Group IC, Brocklehurst P, Farrell B, et al: Treatment of neonatal sepsis with intravenous immune globulin, *N Engl J Med* 365: 1201-1211, 2011.
1012. Ohlsson A, Lacy JB: Intravenous immunoglobulin for suspected or proven infection in neonates, *Cochrane Database Syst Rev* (7):CD001239, 2013.
1013. Nigro G, Adler SP, La Torre R, et al: Passive immunization during pregnancy for congenital cytomegalovirus infection, *N Engl J Med* 353:1350-1362, 2005.
1014. Revello MG, Lazzarotto T, Guerra B, et al: A randomized trial of hyperimmune globulin to prevent congenital cytomegalovirus, *N Engl J Med* 370:1316-1326, 2014.
1015. Suri M, Harrison L, Van de Ven C, et al: Immunotherapy in the prophylaxis and treatment of neonatal sepsis, *Curr Opin Pediatr* 15:155-160, 2003.
1016. Carr R, Modi N, Doré C: G-CSF and GM-CSF for treating or preventing neonatal infections, *Cochrane Database Syst Rev* (3):CD003066, 2013.
1017. Carr R, Brocklehurst P, Doré CJ, et al: Granulocyte-macrophage colony stimulating factor administered as prophylaxis for reduction of sepsis in extremely preterm, small for gestational age neonates (the programs trial): a single-blind, multicentre, randomised controlled trial, *Lancet* 373:226-233, 2009.
1018. Marlow N, Morris T, Brocklehurst P, et al: A randomised trial of granulocyte-macrophage colony-stimulating factor for neonatal sepsis: outcomes at 2 years, *Arch Dis Child Fetal Neonatal Ed* 98:F46-F53, 2013.

1019. Kocherlakota P, La Gamma EF: Preliminary report: rhG-CSF may reduce the incidence of neonatal sepsis in prolonged preeclampsia-associated neutropenia, *Pediatrics* 102:1107-1111, 1998.
1020. Rosenthal J, Healey T, Ellis R, et al: A two-year follow-up of neonates with presumed sepsis treated with recombinant human granulocyte colony-stimulating factor during the first week of life, *J Pediatr* 128:135-137, 1996.
1021. Gillan ER, Christensen RD, Suen Y, et al: A randomized, placebo-controlled trial of recombinant human granulocytes colony stimulatoring factor administration in newborn infants with presumed sepsis: significant induction of peripheral and bone marrow neutrophilia, *Blood* 84:1427-1433, 1994.
1022. Drossou-Agakidou V, Kanakoudi-Tsakalidou F, Sarafidis K, et al: Administration of recombinant human granulocyte-colony stimulating factor to septic neonates induces neutrophilia and enhances the neutrophil respiratory burst and beta2 integrin expression. Results of a randomized controlled trial, *Eur J Pediatr* 157: 583-588, 1998.
1023. Bernstein HM, Pollock BH, Calhoun DA, et al: Administration of recombinant granulocyte colony-stimulating factor to neonates with septicemia: a meta-analysis, *J Pediatr* 138:917-920, 2001.
1024. Chaudhuri J, Mitra S, Mukhopadhyay D, et al: Granulocyte colony-stimulating factor for preterms with sepsis and neutropenia: a randomized controlled trial, *J Clin Neonatol* 1:202-206, 2012.

5 Human Milk

JAE H. KIM, LARS BODE, and PEARAY L. OGRA

CHAPTER OUTLINE

Mother's milk delivered naturally through breastfeeding has been the sole source of infant nutrition in mammalian species for millions of years. Since human beings learned to domesticate cattle about 10,000 years ago, nonhuman mammalian milk also has been used to supplement or replace maternal milk in the human infant. The development and widespread use of commercially prepared infant formula products have been phenomena of the 20th century and notably of the past 6 decades. Such products provide an alternative to breastfeeding that is useful in certain situations. Nonetheless, compelling evidence demonstrates that breastfeeding is an ideal source of infant nutrition whose use is associated with lower rates of postnatal infant mortality in the United States and in other parts of the world.[1-3] Human milk helps to protect the infant against a wide variety of infections and to reduce the risk for allergic and autoimmune diseases, the risk of obesity and its complications, and the risk for certain types of neoplasms later in life, and it has been associated with slightly better performances on tests of cognitive development in some studies.[3] For these reasons, the American Academy of Pediatrics (AAP) and the World Health Organization (WHO) recommend that in the absence of specific contraindications (see "Benefits and Risks of Human Milk") healthy term infants should be exclusively breastfed or fed expressed breast milk beginning within the first hour after birth through 6 months of age and supported with breastfeeding until at least 1 year of age.[1-3] This chapter reviews existing information on major aspects of the physiologic, nutritional, and bioactive components of human milk.

Developmental Anatomy of the Mammary Gland

ANATOMY AND DEVELOPMENT

The mammary gland is an apocrine, milk-secreting gland with a compound tubuloalveolar architecture made up of cells from the ectoderm and mesoderm of the early embryo.[4,5] Mesoderm and epidermal cells are intimately positioned with each other to form an assemblage of collecting ducts that end in terminal duct lobular units with hollow alveolar ductules that can differentiate to produce and expel milk. Similar to other organ structures, organogenesis occurs very early in gestation. The rudimentary mammary tissue undergoes several developmental changes during morphogenesis and lactogenesis: In the 4-mm human embryo, the breast tissue appears as a tiny mammary band on the chest wall[6,7]; by the 7-mm embryonic stage, the mammary band develops into the mammary line, along which eventually develops the true mammary anlage; by the 12-mm stage, a primitive epithelial nodule develops; and by the 30-mm stage, the primitive mammary bud appears. These initial phases of development take place in both genders (Table 5-1). Further development in the male, however, appears to be limited by androgenic or other male-associated substances.[8,9] Castration in male rat embryos early in gestation leads to female breast development, whereas ovariectomy in the female does not alter the course of development of the mammary anlage. Toward the end of pregnancy, initial phases of fetal mammary differentiation seem to occur under the influence

Table 5-1 Possible Endocrine Factors in Growth of Human Female Mammary Glands

Clinical State	Growth Characteristics	Maturational Hormones
Prenatal	Rudimentary	None
Infancy	Rudimentary	None
Puberty	Growth and budding of milk ducts	Growth hormone, prolactin-estrogen, corticosteroids, prolactin (high doses)
Pregnancy	Growth of acinar lobules and alveoli	Estrogen, progesterone, prolactin, growth hormone, corticosteroids
Parturition	Alveolar growth	Prolactin, corticosteroids
Lactational growth of tissue	None	None
Secretory products	Casein, α-lactalbumin	Prolactin, insulin, corticosteroids

of placental and transplacentally acquired maternal hormones, with transient development of the excretory and lactiferous ductular systems. Such growth, differentiation, and secretory activities are transient and regress soon after birth.[9,10]

POSTNATAL DEVELOPMENT

Postnatal development occurs in five distinct stages: puberty, pregnancy, lactation, involution, and menopause. Each stage requires a specific set of morphogenetic changes in glandular structure and function. Cycles of cell proliferation, differentiation, and involution may recur until menopause.[4] At thelarche, and later on at menarche, true mammary growth and development begin in association with rapidly increasing levels of estrogens, progesterone, growth hormone, insulin, adrenocorticosteroids, and prolactin.[10,11] Estrogens appear to be important for the growth and development of the ductular system, and progestins for lobuloalveolar development. Final differentiation of the breast associated with growth and proliferation of the acinar lobes and alveoli continues to be influenced by the levels of estrogen and progesterone. Other peptide hormones, such as prolactin, insulin, and placental chorionic somatomammotropin, appear to be far more important for the subsequent induction and maintenance of lactation.

Prolactin secretion from the pituitary gland is under neural control and the increasing innervation of the breast throughout pregnancy is regulated by estrogens.[11] Intense neural input in virgin and parturient but not in currently pregnant mammals has been shown to result in lactation. For example, lactation in goats can be induced by milking maneuvers. Adoptive breastfeeding also is well documented in primitive human societies. Sudden and permanent cessation of suckling can result in the termination of milk secretion and involution of the breast to the pre-pregnant state as the concentrations of prolactin decline. Estrogen and progesterone also may amplify the direct effects of prolactin or may induce additional receptors for this peptide hormone on appropriate target tissues in the breast.

Physiology of Lactation

ENDOCRINE CONTROL OF MAMMARY GLAND FUNCTION

Breast tissue is responsive to hormones, even as a rudimentary structure, as illustrated by the secretion of "witch's milk" by both male and female newborns in response to exposure to maternal secretion of placental lactogen, estrogens, and progesterone.[7] The secretion of this early milk ceases after exposure to maternal hormones has waned. Sexual differentiation, marked by puberty, is the next major stage in mammary development. As pointed out earlier, androgens inhibit the development of mammary tissue in the male, whereas the development of mammary tissue in the female is dependent on estrogen, progesterone, and pituitary hormones.[12] The postpubertal mammary gland undergoes cyclic changes in response to the release of hormones that takes place during the menstrual cycle. The last stage of development occurs during menopause, when the decline in estrogen secretion results in some atrophy of mammary tissue.

During the menstrual cycle, the mammary gland responds to the sequential release of estrogen and progesterone with a hyperplasia of the ductal system that continues through the secretory phase and declines with the onset of menstruation. The concentration of prolactin modestly increases during the follicular stage of the menstrual cycle but remains constant during the secretory phase.[13] Prolactin secretion appears to be held in readiness for the induction and maintenance of lactation.

INITIATION AND MAINTENANCE OF LACTATION

Pregnancy is marked by profound hormonal changes reflecting major secretory contributions from the placenta, the hypothalamus, and the pituitary gland, with contributions from a number of other endocrine glands (e.g., the pancreas, thyroid, and parathyroid). Increased estrogen and progesterone levels during pregnancy stimulate secretion of prolactin from the pituitary, whereas placental lactogen appears to inhibit the release of a prolactin-inhibiting factor from the hypothalamus. Prolactin, lactogen, estrogen, and progesterone all aid in preparing the mammary gland for lactation. Initially in gestation, an increased growth of ductule and lobuloalveolar tissue occurs in response to estrogen and progesterone. In the beginning of the second trimester, secretory material begins to appear in the luminal cells. By the middle of the second trimester, mammary development has advanced sufficiently to permit lactation to occur should parturition take place.

Once the infant is delivered, a major regulatory factor, the placenta, is lost and new regulatory factors, including the maternal-infant interaction and neuroendocrine regulation, are gained for control of lactation. Loss of placental hormone secretion results in an endocrine hypothalamic stimulation of prolactin release from the anterior pituitary gland, as well as neural stimulation of oxytocin from the posterior pituitary. The stimulation of the nipple by suckling activates a neural pathway that results in release of both prolactin and oxytocin. Prolactin is responsible for stimulating milk production, whereas oxytocin stimulates milk ejection (the combination is known as the let-down reflex). Oxytocin also stimulates uterine contractions, which the mother may feel while she is breastfeeding; this response helps to restore the uterus to pre-pregnancy tone.

Milk production and ejection are thus dependent on the complex interaction of stimulation by the infant's suckling, neural reflex of the hypothalamus to such stimulation, release of hormones from the anterior and posterior pituitary, and response of the mammary gland to these hormones to complete the cycle.

MILK SECRETION

Milk is produced as the result of synthetic mechanisms within the mammary gland, as well as the transport of components from blood. Milk-specific proteins are synthesized in the mammary secretory cells, packaged in secretory vesicles, and exocytosed into the alveolar lumen. Lactose is secreted into the milk in a similar manner, whereas many monovalent ions, such as sodium, potassium, and chloride, are dependent on active transport systems based on sodium-potassium adenosine triphosphatases (Na^+/K^+-ATPases). In some situations, the mammary epithelium, which may behave as a "mammary barrier" between the interstitial fluid derived from blood and the milk because of the lack of space between these cells, may "leak," permitting direct diffusion of components into the milk. This barrier results in the formation of different pools or compartments of milk components within the mammary gland and is responsible for maintaining gradients of these components from the blood to the milk.

Lipid droplets can be observed within the secretory cells of the mammary gland and are surrounded by a milk fat globule membrane. These fat droplets appear to fuse with the apical membrane of the secretory cells and then to be either exocytosed or "pinched off" into the milk,[12] growing as they fuse with one another.[14] Some whole cells also are found in milk, including leukocytes, macrophages, lymphocytes, and mammary epithelial cells. The mechanisms by which these cells enter the milk are complex and include, among others, specific cellular receptor-mediated homing of antigen-specific lymphocytes.

As the structure of the mammary gland is compartmentalized, so is that of the milk. The gross composition of milk consists of cytoplasm encased by cellular membranes in milk fat globule membranes (fat compartments made up of fat droplets), a soluble compartment containing water-soluble constituents, a casein micelle compartment containing acid-precipitable proteins with calcium and lactose, and a cellular compartment. The relative amounts of these components change during the course of lactation, generally with less fat and more protein in early lactation than in late lactation.

Colostrum is the first postpartum milk that is produced and is generally very dense in protein and fat content and has an enriched amount of immunologic factors compared with mature milk. Colostrum gives way to a transitional milk during the first week of life, where water content increases. Mature milk is relatively constant during the next ensuing months until weaning. Mode of delivery appears to also influence macronutrient composition of colostrum, with vaginal delivery versus cesarean section being associated with higher protein content.[15] In addition, there are strong influences of maternal diet on fatty acid profiles in colostrum and later milk.[16,17] Maternal age may also positively influence fat content in colostrum and may be related to increased fat synthesis or reduced water production.[18] Thus the infant consumes a dynamic complex solution that has physical properties permitting unique separation of different functional constituents from one another, presumably in forms that best support growth and development.

LACTATION PERFORMANCE

Successful lactation performance depends on continued effective contributions from the neural, endocrine, and maternal-infant interactions that were initiated at the time of delivery. The part of this complex behavior most liable to inhibition is the mother-child interaction. Early and frequent attachment of the infant to the breast is mandatory to stimulate the neural pathways essential to maintaining prolactin and oxytocin release.

A healthy newborn infant placed between the mother's breasts will locate a nipple and begin to suck spontaneously within the first hour of birth.[19] This rapid attachment to the mother may reflect olfactory stimuli from the breast received by the infant at birth.[20] Frequent feedings are necessary for the mother to maintain an appropriate level of milk production for the infant's proper growth and development. Programs to support lactation performance must emphasize proper maternal-infant bonding, relaxation of the mother, support for the mother, technical assistance to initiate breastfeeding properly and to cope with problems, and reduction of environmental hindrances. Such hindrances may include lack of rooming-in in the hospital, use of supplemental formula feeds, and lack of convenient daycare for working mothers.

Lactation ceases when suckling stops; therefore any behavior that reduces the amount of suckling by the infant initiates weaning or the end of lactation. Introduction of water in bottles or of one or two bottles of formula a day may begin the weaning process, regardless of the time after parturition, but can be most damaging to the process when the mother-infant dyad is first establishing lactation. In some cases where breast milk has not come in and newborns have dropped greater than 5% weight, discrete amounts of supplemental formula may improve breastfeeding success.[21]

There are physiologic consequences to women who never lactate. Parous women aged 50 years or younger who had never lactated had higher prevalence of hypertension, obesity, and diabetes. Long-term cancer risk for breast and ovarian cancer are also reduced in women who have lactated.[22,23]

Components of Human Milk and Their Potential Benefits for the Breastfed Infant

Human milk contains a rich diversity of nutrients, including proteins and peptides, lipids, carbohydrates, vitamins, minerals, electrolytes, and trace metals. The distribution and relative content of various nutritional substances found in human milk are presented in Box 5-1. The chemical composition often exhibits considerable variation among lactating women and in the same woman at different times of lactation,[24] as well as between samples obtained from mothers of preterm infants and from mothers of full-term infants.[25,26] The appropriate amounts of each nutrient must be considered within these constraints.

Box 5-1 Distribution of Secretory Products in Human Milk*

Water: 86%-87.5%;
Total solids: 11.5 g

Nutritional Components

Lactose: 6.9-7.2 g
Fat: 3.0-4.4 g
Oligosaccharides: 0.5-2 g
Protein: 0.9-1.03 g
α-Lactalbumin: 150-170 mg
β-Lactoglobulin: trace
Serum albumin: 50 mg

Nitrogen-Containing Components

Total protein: 0.9-1.2 g
Whey protein nitrogen: 75-78 mg
Casein protein nitrogen: 38-41 mg
Nonprotein nitrogen: 25% of total nitrogen
Urea: 0.027 g
Creatinine: 0.021 g
Glucosamine: 0.112 g

Vitamins

C: 4.5-5.5 mg
Thiamine: (B1): 12-15 μg
Niacin: 183.7 μg
B6: 11-14 μg
B12: <0.05 μg
Biotin: 0.6-0.9 μg
Folic acid: 4.1-5.2 μg
Choline: 8-9 mg
Inositol: 40-46 mg
Pantothenic acid: 200-240 μg
A (retinol): 54-56 μg
D: <0.42 IU
E: 0.56 μg
K: 1.5 μg

Electrolytes, Minerals, and Trace Metals

Sodium: 15-17.5 mg
Potassium: 51-55 mg
Calcium: 32-43 mg
Phosphorus: 14-15 mg
Chloride: 38-40 mg
Magnesium: 3 mg
Iron: 0.03 mg
Zinc: 0.17 mg
Copper: 15-105 μg
Iodine: 4.5 μg
Manganese: 1.5-2.4 μg
Fluoride: 5-25 μg
Selenium: 1.8-3.2 μg
Boron: 8-10 μg

*Estimates based on amount per deciliter.

PROTEINS, PEPTIDES, AND NONPROTEIN NITROGEN

The total protein concentration in mature, term human milk is approximately 0.9 to 1.2 g/dL. Protein concentrations are significantly higher in the milk of women with preterm deliveries.[27] Protein concentrations are highest in colostrum and decrease over the first 4 to 6 weeks of life regardless of gestational age at delivery.[27,28] Milk protein concentrations are generally not affected by maternal diet but increase with maternal body weight for height and decrease in women who produce higher milk volumes.[29]

Human milk proteins can largely be classified into three groups: caseins, whey proteins, and mucins (milk fat globule membrane proteins). Caseins and whey proteins contribute the largest part, and their ratio and composition vary over the course of lactation.[30] The whey-to-casein protein ratio in humans may change during lactation, with the whey component ranging from 90% (early milk) to 60% (mature milk) to 50% (late milk).[31] In contrast, mucins constitute a smaller percentage of total milk protein, and their concentration changes little during lactation.[32] Human milk proteins provide the thriving infant with a source of essential amino acids (nutritional proteins) but also exert physiologic activities to further benefit infant health (bioactive proteins). Most milk proteins are both nutritional and bioactive. Recent technical advances in proteomics have dramatically expanded our knowledge about human milk proteins. In 2010, 285 unique proteins were identified from human milk; in 2012, the inventory was updated to 761 entries. In addition, human milk contains peptides that are either originally present in the milk or released from milk proteins after proteolytic cleavage in the infant's gastrointestinal system (protein-derived peptides). Furthermore, approximately 25% of the human milk nitrogen comes in the form of nonprotein nitrogen and includes compounds such as urea, uric acid, creatine, creatinine, amino acids, and nucleotides. Milk proteins, peptides, and nonprotein nitrogen compounds will be reviewed in the following sections.

Nutritional Proteins

Caseins are a family of phosphoproteins that make up 20% to 45% of the protein in human milk. In contrast, caseins constitute greater than 80% of the total protein in bovine milk. β-Casein is the major protein found in human milk. The protein binds to calcium at its phosphorylated regions, which enables the caseins to form micelles that improve casein digestibility for the infant. The soluble κ-casein is believed to stabilize the casein micelles.

The major whey protein in human milk is α-lactalbumin, comprising about 25% to 35% of the total protein. It has a well-balanced amino acid composition with a high content of essential amino acids. α-Lactalbumin fragments have not been found in the stool of term or preterm infants, suggesting that it is well used. However, in vitro proteolysis generates α-lactalbumin fragments with bifidogenic or bactericidal properties as described in the section "Protein-Derived Peptides." Although α-lactalbumin is the major whey protein in human milk, β-lactoglobulin is the major whey protein in bovine milk (and is not found in human milk).[33] A consistent fraction of human milk whey protein is made up of serum albumin. Its source remains unclear; some evidence indicates that it may be synthesized in the mammary gland.[34] Most of the serum albumin, however, probably is synthesized outside the mammary gland. In addition to α-lactalbumin, the whey protein fraction contains all of the proposed functional proteins in human milk (immunoglobulins, lysozyme, lactoferrin, enzymes, cytokines, peptide hormones) that are described in the sections that follow.

Bioactive Proteins and Peptides

Whereas a major proportion of human milk protein is composed of the nutritional proteins just described, a significant number of the remaining proteins serve a variety of functions, either other than or in addition to the nutritional support of the neonate. These proteins include carrier proteins, enzymes, hormones, growth factors, immunoglobulins, and cytokines. Whether these proteins are still functional once they have been ingested by the neonate has not always been established, but it is clear that human milk supplies a mixture that is potentially far more complex than just nutritional substrate.

Carrier Proteins. A number of nutrients are supplied to the neonate bound to proteins found in human milk. This binding may play an important role in making these nutrients bioavailable. Lactoferrin is an iron-binding protein that is apparently absorbed intact by the infant.[35] Lactoferrin may be important in the improved absorption of iron by the infant from human milk compared with that from cow's milk preparations, which contain little lactoferrin.[36] Lactoferrin also may bind other minerals, including zinc and manganese, although the preferred mineral form appears to be the ferric ion. However, greater than 90% of the lactoferrin in human milk is in the iron-unsaturated form (apo-lactoferrin). The apo-form has very high affinity for iron, thereby withholding iron from iron-dependent pathogens. For example, the iron-sequestering, bacteriostatic activity of lactoferrin has been shown to inhibit the growth of *Cronobacter* (previously *Enterobacter*) *sakazakii*, a foodborne pathogen known to cause diarrhea in infants.[37] Lactoferrin also has bactericidal activity, killing a variety of infant disease-relevant pathogens such as *Vibrio cholerae*.[38] Oral lactoferrin prophylaxis has been recently shown to reduce the incidence of late-onset sepsis in infants weighing less than 1500 g and most effectively in infants weighing less than 1000 g. A statistically significant reduction in late-onset sepsis was observed in infants weighing less than 1500 g who received lactoferrin (relative ratio [RR], 0.34; 95% confidence interval [CI], 0.17 to 0.70); more research is currently underway to determine the utility of lactoferrin in clinical use.[39,40]

A number of other proteins appear to be important as carriers of vitamins and hormones. Folate-binding, vitamin B_{12}–binding, and vitamin D–binding proteins all have been identified in human milk. These proteins appear to have some resistance to proteolysis, especially when they are saturated with the appropriate vitamin ligand.[41] Serum albumin acts as a carrier of a number of ligands, whereas α-lactalbumin acts as a carrier for calcium. Finally, proteins that bind thyroid hormone and corticosteroids have been reported to be present in human milk, although serum albumin may in part fulfill this function.[42,43]

Enzymes. The activity of several dozen enzymes has been detected in human milk.[44] Most of these enzymes appear to originate from the blood, with a few originating from secretory epithelial cells of the mammary gland. Little is known about the role of these enzymes, other than lysozyme and the lipases, in human milk. The enzymes found in human milk range from ATPases to antioxidant enzymes, such as catalase, to phosphatases and glycolytic enzymes. Although these enzymes have important roles in normal body metabolism, it is not clear how many of them either function in the milk itself or survive ingestion by the infant to function in the neonate.

Lysozyme appears to have a part in the antibacterial function of human milk, whereas the lipases have a more nutrient-related role in modulating fat metabolism for the neonate. Lysozyme is present in human milk at relatively high concentrations and is known to degrade the cell walls of gram-positive bacteria. Lactoferrin may in some contexts promote bacterial killing by lysozyme. A key feature of this defense is structural antimicrobial peptide motifs on the *N*-terminus of the protein.[45]

Two main lipases have been identified in human milk, a pancreatic lipase–related protein 2 (PLRP2) and a bile salt–stimulated lipase (BSSL).[46] PLRP2 appears to be involved in determining the pattern of lipids found in human milk by regulating uptake into milk at the level of the mammary gland. Human milk BSSL is an acid-stable protein that compensates for the low activity of lipases secreted into the digestive tract during early development. Thus these two enzymes regulate both the amount and the pattern of lipid that appears in milk as well as the extremely efficient absorption of lipid by the infant. Pasteurization of human milk inactivates these enzymes and decreases lipid use.[47]

Hormones and Growth Factors. Human milk contains several growth factors with potential effects on the intestine, vasculature, nervous system, and endocrine system.[48] Epidermal growth factor (EGF) is critical to maturation and repair of the intestinal mucosa. EGF is resistant to low stomach pH and digestive enzymes and reaches the intestine. There, it may stimulate intestinal cells and alter DNA and protein synthesis, cell division, and absorbance of water and glucose. EGF concentrations are highest in colostrum and decrease over the course of lactation.[49,50] Even in mature milk, average EGF concentrations are 100-fold higher than in maternal serum. Preterm milk contains higher EGF concentrations than term milk.[49,50] Human milk also contains insulin-like growth factor (IGF)-1 and -2 as well as IGF-binding proteins and IGF-specific proteases.[51-53] Concentrations are highest in colostrum and decrease over the course of lactation. Breastfed infants have higher serum IGF-1 concentrations than formula-fed infants, but the exact physiologic role and function of human milk IGF and IGF-related proteins remains unclear.[54] In addition, human milk contains transforming growth factor-β (TGF-β), vascular endothelial growth factor (VEGF), erythropoietin

(Epo), calcitonin, and somatostatin, as well as brain-derived neurotropic factor (BDNF) and glial cell line–derived neurotropic factor (GDNF).[3,55-59] However, data on how these hormones affect infant health are limited and often extrapolated from in vitro systems or animal models.

Human milk also contains several metabolism-regulating hormones, such as adiponectin, leptin, resistin, and ghrelin.[60-63] Adiponectin concentrations in the mother's milk correlate inversely with infant weight and body mass index, but whether or not there is a causal relationship whereby adiponectin contributes to a reduced incidence of overweight and obesity later in life remains unclear.[61,62]

In addition, a variety of gastrointestinal peptides have been identified in human milk. Presumably, the supply of these various factors to the infant through the milk compensates for their possible deficiency in the infant during early development.

Immunoglobulins. As observed in other peripheral mucosal sites, the major class of immunoglobulin in human colostrum and milk is the 11S secretory immunoglobulin A (sIgA). Other isotypes, namely, 7S IgA, IgG, IgM, IgD, and IgE, also are present. The 11S IgA exists as a dimer of two 7S IgA molecules linked together by a polypeptide chain, the J-chain, and is associated with a nonimmunoglobulin protein referred to as the secretory component. The sIgA protein constitutes about 75% of the total nitrogen content of human milk. The IgA dimers produced by plasma cells at the basal surface of the mammary epithelium are bound by the polymeric immunoglobulin receptor on the basolateral surface of mammary epithelial cells, which transports them through these cells, where they are released into the alveolar spaces as an 11S IgA dimer associated with a portion of the polymeric immunoglobulin receptor referred to as the secretory component.[64]

Sequential quantitation of class-specific immunoglobulin in human colostrum and mature milk has demonstrated that the highest levels of sIgA and IgM are present during the first few days of lactation (Fig. 5-1). Levels of IgA are 4 to 5 times greater than those of IgM, 20 to 30 times greater than those of IgG, and 5 to 6 times greater than those of serum IgA.[65] As lactation progresses, IgA declines to levels that range from 20 to 27 mg/g of protein, and IgM levels decline to 3.5 to 4.1 mg/g of protein. IgG levels do not show any significant change during early and late lactation and usually are maintained in the range of 1.4 to 4.9 mg/g of protein (see Fig. 5-1). Although a dramatic and rapid decline in milk IgA and IgM occurs during the first week of life, this decrease is more than balanced by an increase in the volume of milk produced as the process of lactation becomes established (Table 5-2; see Fig. 5-1).

It has been estimated that the breastfed infant may consistently receive an amount of about 1 g of IgA each day and approximately 1% of this amount for IgM and IgG.[66,67] Most ingested IgA is eliminated in the feces, although up to 10% may be absorbed from the intestine into the circulation within the first 18 to 24 hours after birth.[68] Feces of breastfed infants contain functional antibodies present in the ingested milk.[69] Other studies also support the finding of prolonged survival of milk IgA in the gastrointestinal tract. Infants fed human milk have demonstrated the presence of all immunoglobulin classes in the feces. Fecal IgA content was three to four times greater than that of IgM after human milk feeding. Comparative studies on survival of human milk IgA and bovine IgG in the neonatal intestinal tract have suggested that the fecal content of IgA may be 14 to 20 times greater after human milk feeding than that of bovine IgG after feeding of bovine immune globulin.[70]

Endogenous production of secretory IgA by the infant's mucosal immune system increases progressively in the postnatal period.[71] Nonetheless, breastfed infants have

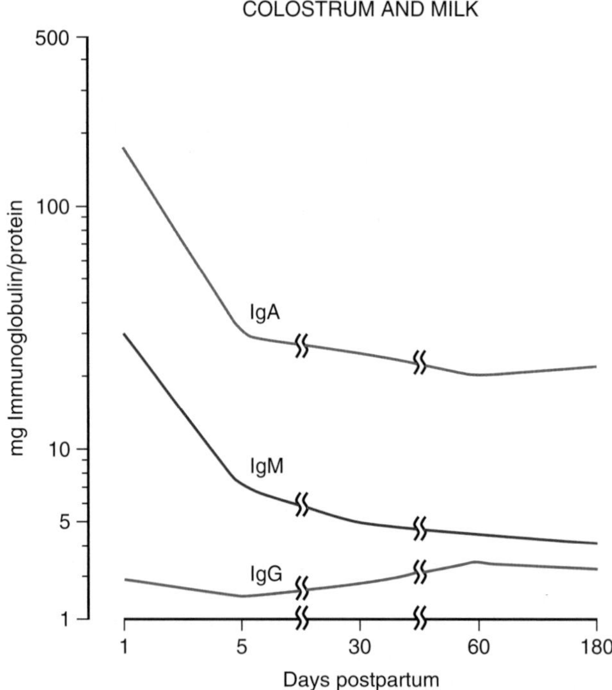

Figure 5-1 Comparison of the mean levels of IgG, IgA, and IgM in colostrum and milk at different intervals after the onset of lactation in mothers who were breastfeeding. (Data from Ogra SS, Ogra PL: Immunologic aspects of human colostrum and milk. II. Characteristics of lymphocyte reactivity and distribution of E-rosette forming cells at different times after the onset of lactation, *J Pediatr* 92:550-555, 1978.)

Table 5-2 Level of Immunoglobulins in Human Milk and Estimates of Delivery of Lactational Immunoglobulins to the Breastfeeding Neonate Over the Course of Lactation*

	PERCENTAGE OF TOTAL PROTEINS REPRESENTED BY IMMUNOGLOBULIN			OUTPUT OF IMMUNOGLOBULIN (mg/24 hr)		
Day Postpartum	**IgG**	**IgM**	**IgA**	**IgG**	**IgM**	**IgA**
1	7	3	80	80	120	11,000
3	10	45	45	50	40	2,000
7	1-2	4	20	25	10	1,000
7-28	1-2	2	10-15	10	10	1,000
<50	1-2	0.5-1	10-15	10	10	1,000

From Ogra SS, Ogra PL: *Components of immunologic reactivity in human colostrum and milk*, New York, 1979, Raven Press; and Losonsky GA, Ogra PL: *Mucosal immune system*, Orlando, Fla, 1984, Grune & Stratton.
*Estimates based on the available data for total immunoglobulin and daily protein synthesis.

substantially greater concentrations of fecal sIgA than formula-fed infants. Prentice and colleagues[72] found approximately 10-fold and approximately 4-fold higher concentrations of sIgA in the stools of breastfed than formula-fed infants at 6 and 12 weeks of postnatal age, respectively, even though only approximately 15% to 20% of ingested sIgA appeared in the feces.

IgA antibodies found in milk possess specificity for infectious agents endemic to or pathogenic for the intestinal and respiratory tracts. These antibodies may be present in the milk in the absence of specific circulating IgA. In a study in which pregnant women were given oral feedings of *Escherichia coli* 083, development of IgA antibody in human milk was evident in the absence of detectable serum antibody-specific responses.[73] In another study, investigators have observed similar responses in animal models by using intrabronchial immunization with *Streptococcus pneumoniae*. These and other studies[74-77] have strongly supported the concept of a bronchomammary as well as an enteromammary axis of immunologic reactivity in the breast.

Maternal immunity can be transferred to the infant via antigen-specific sIgA and other immunoglobulins in the mother's milk and thereby prevent adherence and penetration of both bacterial and dietary antigens that would otherwise provoke inflammation in the intestinal mucosa.[78-80] Colostrum and milk can inhibit the activity of *E. coli* and *V. cholerae* enterotoxins in experimental settings.[81] The antitoxic activity of human milk appears to correlate well with its IgA content but not with its IgM and IgG content. Precoating of *V. cholerae* with specific sIgA protects infant mice from disease.[82] Similar results have been obtained by using specific purified milk sIgA in preventing *E. coli*– and *Shigella dysenteriae*–induced disease in rabbits.[83]

Cytokines. In the 1990s, several cytokines, chemokines, and growth factors that mediate the effector phases of natural and specific immunity were discovered in human milk, and many more have been identified subsequently. Moreover, human milk displays a number of biologic activities characteristic of cytokines, including the stimulation of growth, differentiation of immunoglobulin production by B cells,[84-86] enhancement of thymocyte proliferation,[87] inhibition of interleukin-2 (IL-2) production by T cells,[88] and suppression of IgE production.[89] IL-1β[90] and tumor necrosis factor-α (TNF-α)[91] were the first two cytokines quantified in human milk. In colostrum, TNF-α is present mainly in fractions of molecular weight 80 to 195 kDa, probably bound to its soluble receptors.[92] Milk TNF-α is secreted both by milk macrophages[91,93] and by the mammary epithelium.[94]

IL-6 was first demonstrated in human milk by a specific bioassay[95] and also has been demonstrated by immunoassays.[91,94,96,97] In like manner, IL-6 is localized in high-molecular-weight fractions of human milk.[96] The association of IL-6 with its own receptor has not been studied in milk, although the expression of IL-6 receptor by the mammary epithelium[94] and in secreted form in the milk[92] may explain the high molecular weight of this cytokine in human milk. The expression of IL-6 messenger ribonucleic acid and protein in milk cells and in the mammary gland epithelium suggests that both milk mononuclear cells and the mammary gland are likely major sources of this cytokine.[93,94,98]

The presence of interferon-γ (IFN-γ) in human milk also has been reported,[94,97,99] although some investigators have found significant levels of IFN-γ only in milk samples obtained from mothers whose infants had been delivered by cesarean section. The significance of this observation is not clear. Whether this IFN-γ is bioactive, as well as its source, also remains to be determined.[99]

Chemokines are a novel class of small cytokines with discrete target cell selectivity that are able to recruit and activate different populations of leukocytes, and they are grouped into families defined by the spacing between cysteine residues (see Chapter 4). In CXC, cysteine pairs are separated by one amino acid, whereas in CC chemokines, paired cysteines are adjacent to each other. Certain CXC chemokines that contain an ELR (glutamic acid–leucine-arginine) motif, including CXCL8 (also known as IL-8) and CXCL1 (GRO-α), predominantly attract neutrophils, whereas basophils, eosinophils, dendritic cells, monocytes, and specific subsets of T and B lymphocytes are attracted by specific CC chemokines and non-ELR CXC chemokines. The presence of a number of CXC and CC chemokines has been described in human milk.[98,100-102]

Although it is tempting to speculate that cytokines present in milk may be able to interact with mucosal tissues in the respiratory and alimentary tracts of the recipient infant, the functional expression of specific receptors for cytokines on epithelial or lymphoid cells in the airway and gastrointestinal mucosa has not been fully explored.[103] A receptor-independent mechanism of cytokine uptake by the gastrointestinal mucosa during the neonatal period has not been demonstrated to date.

Whether and to what extent cytokines in human milk contribute to the beneficial effects of human milk in the gut and elsewhere is largely unknown. Indirect evidence suggests that IL-7, which is a growth factor for T-cell progenitors (and for memory T cells), in human milk may support thymic growth. Thymus size was found to be larger in breastfed than formula-fed 4-month-old infants in Denmark,[104] and thymus size and IL-7 content of breast milk were directly correlated with each other in exclusively breastfed infants in The Gambia.[105] In the latter study, reduced human milk content of IL-7 was observed in the "hungry season" in association with reduced thymus size and thymic production of T cells; however, whether IL-7 in breast milk was absorbed intact and causally related to greater thymus size or was merely a surrogate for other factors cannot be determined from this study.

Protein-Derived Peptides

In addition to the proteins and peptides already present in human milk, a number of bioactive peptides have been identified that are derived from milk proteins. These protein-derived peptides are encrypted within the sequence of parental milk proteins and are released after enzymatic digestion in the infant's stomach and intestine. The size of these bioactive protein-derived peptides are in the range of 2 to 20 amino acids, and some of them are known to have multiple functions.[106,107] Some of them exert their bioactive function directly in the gastrointestinal tract (preabsorptive bioactive peptides); others are absorbed in the intestine and function at peripheral sites (postabsorptive bioactive peptides). These bioactive peptides can be derived from both caseins and whey proteins.

The open and flexible structure of caseins allows for easy access of digestive enzymes to release bioactive peptides. For example, caseinophosphopeptides (CPPs) are casein-derived phosphopeptides that are thought to facilitate calcium ion absorption through vitamin D–independent mechanisms.[108,109] Glycomacropeptide (GMP) is derived from the highly glycosylated *C*-terminus of κ-casein. GMP has bifidogenic effects and promotes the growth of *Bifidobacterium bifidum* and *Bifidobacterium infantis*[110]; bifidobacteria are more prevalent in exclusively breastfed infants [79] and have other effects that are thought to be beneficial, suggesting that GMP may help to promote a beneficial gut microbiota.[111] GMP was also shown to have antiadhesive properties against certain pathogens, including *Helicobacter pylori*, enteropathogenic *E. coli*, *Salmonella typhimurium*, and *Shigella flexneri*.[112-114] Although α-lactalbumin is one of the major nutritive whey proteins in human milk that provides the neonate with essential amino acids, it is also a considerable source of bioactive peptides. Lactoferrin has a variety of bioactive functions; some are only exerted after enzymatic digestion in the intestine and the release of lactoferrin-derived bioactive peptides.[115] For example, the antimicrobial potency of some of the lactoferrin-derived peptides is higher than that of the intact, undigested lactoferrin itself. Most of the studies on protein-derived peptides stem from bovine milk, but a growing body of work suggests that human milk proteins also deliver bioactive peptides. Future research is needed to fully describe the role of these human milk protein–derived bioactive peptides in the context of infant health and disease.[106,107]

Nonprotein Nitrogen

Nonprotein nitrogen contributes up to 15% to 30% of the total nitrogen in human milk and consists of free amino acids, peptides, urea, ammonia, carnitine, polyamines, nucleic acids, and nucleotides.[48] The significance of the presence of these components is not always clear, but when they are not fed, as in the case of infant formulas that contain little taurine[116] or of soy formulas that contain little carnitine,[117] apparent deficiencies that may influence the development of the infant occur. Taurine is important for bile salt conjugation as well as for support of appropriate development of the brain and retina,[118,119] whereas carnitine appears to be important for appropriate fatty acid metabolism.[120]

Nucleotides constitute 2% to 5% of nonprotein nitrogen and serve as structural backbones of DNA and RNA and play important roles in cell replication and metabolism, store cellular energy, mediate intracellular metabolic processes, and support protein synthesis.[121,122] Levels of nucleotides in human milk are much higher than those found in previously made infant formulas. Some infant formulas now are supplemented with nucleotides to levels closer to those in breast milk.[123] The level of nucleotides in human milk varies greatly between individuals and may be related to maternal diet and ethnicity.[124] Requirements for nucleotides are higher during periods of stress, and it has been proposed that nucleotides are conditionally essential to infants.[125] Infants fed formula with nucleotide supplementation had lower risk of diarrhea, higher natural killer–cell activities, and produced higher antibody responses to *Haemophilus influenzae* type b, diphtheria toxoid, and oral polio vaccines when compared with infants who did not receive supplementation.[123] There is still controversy as to the presence of any growth advantage with nucleotide supplementation in infant formulas. However, a recent randomized controlled study demonstrated a significant advantage in nucleotide-supplemented infants regarding growth in head circumference, with a mean difference in Z scores at 8 weeks of 0.4 (95% CI, 0.1 to 0.7; $P = .006$), which remained significant after adjustment for potential confounding factors ($P = .002$), and weight at 8 weeks of age was also greater.[126] Nucleotide supplementation was associated with a relative increase in abundance of *Bifidobacterium* spp. compared with *Bacteroides* spp., *Porphyromonas* spp., or *Prevotella* spp. in infants' fecal microbiota, but whether these changes in the microbiota are causally related to the improved growth is not known.[127] An older study reported improved rates of growth in rapidly growing infants born small for gestational age,[128] but additional work is required to validate the beneficial effects of dietary nucleotides in infants with specific clinical conditions.

LIPIDS

Lipids (fats) provide about half of the calories in human milk and are supplied in the form of fat globules enclosed in plasma membranes derived from the mammary epithelial cells.[129] The lipid content is highest in colostrum and decreases from transitional to mature milk. There is a diurnal variation in lipid content but an even larger variation between milk collected at the beginning (foremilk) and the end (hindmilk) of the feeding.[130] During the feeding, the lipid content increases so that hindmilk has a higher fat content than foremilk.

Most of the lipids are provided as triglycerides and with a minor part as phospholipids, cholesterol, and glycolipids. The fatty acid pattern differs in breast milk from mothers delivering very preterm, preterm, or term and further—from colostrum to transitional to mature milk.[131] Most of the fatty acids are saturated, with a predominance of palmitic acid (16:0). Besides saturated and monounsaturated fatty acids, breast milk supplies the neonate with essential fatty acids (EFA) and long-chain polyunsaturated fatty acids (LCPUFA). Humans cannot synthesize EFA because the desaturases for introducing a double bond at carbons 3 and 6 (counted from the methyl end) are missing. The essential fatty acid linoleic acid (18:2ω6) supplies about 10% of the calories derived from the lipid fraction. Several different elongases and desaturases transform EFAs to LCPUFAs, such as arachidonic acid (AA), docosahexaenoic acid (DHA), and eicosapentaenoic acid (EPA), which serve as substrates for a wide range of bioactive metabolites, including eicosanoids, lipoxins, resolvins, and protectins. Different fatty acids compete as substrates for the different elongases and desaturases, and different substrates lead to different bioactive metabolites with sometimes opposing effects. The EFA and LCPUFA contents in human milk mainly depend on the mother's diet. The mother's long-term diet affects the mother's lipid profile stored in her adipose tissue, which then feeds into the lipid composition of her milk. The mother's short-term diet affects milk lipid composition directly. For instance, there is a high correlation between the mother's fish intake and the DHA concentrations in her plasma and her breast milk.[132] Therefore the maternal diet should receive special attention during both pregnancy and lactation.

DHA is important for neurologic development, including visual acuity. The brain is mainly built of lipids, and DHA constitutes 40% of the fatty acids in the gray matter,[133,134] concentrated in the synaptic membranes. The retina is the organ with the highest DHA content, especially in the rod outer segment. Sensibility of the retina is very susceptible to low DHA concentrations.[135,136] Fatty acids also influence gene expression, which might affect long-term neurodevelopment and metabolism. The most vulnerable to inadequate specific fatty acid intake are preterm infants, who have limited capacity to generate enough LCPUFAs on their own despite having the synthetic enzymes present. As a result, infant formulas for both term and preterm formulas are now supplemented with LCPUFAs because, originally, designed formulas were based on plant lipids and therefore did not contain appreciable amounts of LCPUFAs, although systematic reviews have concluded that insufficient evidence is present to recommend LCPUFA supplementation for term and preterm formulas.[137,138] However, in preterm infants, levels of DHA two to three times the levels found in current preterm formulas or average breast milk have resulted in improved neurodevelopmental outcomes.[139] Therefore the exact dosing for preterm infants still needs to be determined. For the term infant, there is some recent long-term evidence that LCPUFA supplementation may be beneficial. This includes improved visual acuity by 12 months of age in those infants who received LCPUFA supplementation in their infant formula.[140] Early infant formula fatty acid supplementation also led to faster information processing in children followed up to age 6 years compared with those who only received unsupplemented formula.[141]

Cholesterol is an important lipid constituent of human milk (12 mg/dL) even if it is a small fraction of total fat content (0.5%).[142] Breastfed infants consume very high amounts of cholesterol per kg of body weight compared with adults (more than 10-fold). Cholesterol is found in only trace amounts in commercial formulas. It has been suggested that early breastfeeding associated with high measured total blood serum cholesterol may actually prevent some of the risks of developing cardiovascular diseases later in life.[143,144] Additional research is required to determine the potential role that early cholesterol consumption may play in later cardiovascular health.

CARBOHYDRATES

Lactose

Lactose is the primary sugar found in human milk and usually is the carbohydrate chosen for the preparation of commercial formulas. Lactose supplies approximately one third the energy (of a total 67 kcal/dL) taken in by the infant from human milk. Lactose (a disaccharide of glucose and galactose) also may be important to the neonate as a carrier of galactose, which may be more readily incorporated into gangliosides in the central nervous system than galactose derived from glucose in the neonate.[145] Also, glycogen may be synthesized more efficiently from galactose than from glucose in the neonate because of the relatively low activity of glucokinase in early development.[146] Human milk also contains a significant amount of other sugars, including glucose and galactose and more than 150 different oligosaccharides.

Oligosaccharides

Human milk oligosaccharides (HMOs) represent the third most abundant component of human milk after lactose and lipids, with concentrations often exceeding that of total protein.[147-150] One liter of mature milk contains between 10 and 20 g HMOs. The concentrations in colostrum are even higher. In contrast, today's infant formulas contain only trace amounts of HMOs but are often supplemented with structurally different nonhuman oligosaccharides, namely galactooligosaccharides (GOSs) and fructooligosaccharides (FOSs).[150]

HMOs are resistant to the low pH in the infant stomach and to digestion by brush border and pancreatic enzymes and reach the infant colon intact and at high concentrations.[151-155] HMOs are prebiotics because they are selectively metabolized by certain bacteria that may be beneficial to infant health and well-being. The resulting metabolites may benefit the infant but also contribute to shaping an environment in the intestinal lumen that further selects for beneficial bacteria and against potential pathogens.[156-161]

In addition, HMOs are antiadhesive agents because they serve as soluble decoy receptors for pathogen attachment. Many viruses, bacteria, as well as protozoan parasites, need to attach to the intestinal surface to reside in and colonize the intestinal lumen or invade the host. The initial attachment is often via complex sugars on either the host's intestinal surface or the microorganisms themselves. HMOs often resemble some of these sugar epitopes, compete for binding, and thus reduce the chance for a microorganism to attach to the host's intestinal surface. Microorganisms that cannot bind are often washed out of the feces. Thus HMOs may contribute to a lower risk of enteric infections observed in breastfed infants compared with formula-fed infants. For example, tissue culture studies revealed that *Campylobacter jejuni*, one of the most common causes of bacterial diarrhea, binds to $\alpha(1,2)$-fucosylated sugars on epithelial cells. The same sugar epitopes are part of HMOs and are able to inhibit *C. jejuni* binding to epithelial cells.[162] A cohort study later revealed that these observations made in tissue culture translate to human infants. Infants who receive mother's milk with high concentrations of $\alpha(1,2)$-fucosylated HMOs had a significantly lower ($P = .001$) incidence of moderate- to severe diarrhea of all causes than infants who received milk with low levels of these specific HMOs.[163] HMOs also interfere with the attachment of *H. influenzae*, *Streptococcus pneumoniae*, enteropathogenic *E. coli*, or the protozoan parasite *Entamoeba histolytica*.[164-166] Moreover, human milk can interfere with the binding of human immunodeficiency virus (HIV) envelope antigen gp120 to CD4 molecules on T cells or to the DC-SIGN receptor on dendritic cells.[167,168] Although these data stem from in vitro models, a recent report from a cohort study conducted in Zambia suggests that mothers whose milk HMO concentrations were above the median were less likely to transmit HIV to their infants (odds ratio [OR], 0.45; 95% CI, 0.21 to 0.97; $P = .04$ after adjustment for CD4 count and breast-milk HIV RNA concentrations), whereas the proportion of 3′-sialyllactose

(3′-SL) per total HMOs was higher among transmitting than among nontransmitting women ($P = .003$) and correlated with higher plasma and breast-milk HIV RNA and lower CD4 counts.[150]

In addition to their prebiotic and antiadhesive effects, HMOs have been shown to alter immune responses locally in the infant's intestine, but also systemically. Although most of the HMOs are either metabolized by intestinal bacteria or are excreted with the infant's feces, approximately 1% of the HMOs is absorbed, reaches the systemic circulation, and is excreted intact with the infant's urine.[153-155] Given the high concentrations of HMOs in milk, a 1% absorption rate is still able to yield systemic HMO concentrations in the low-to-middle μg/mL range, which could lead to additional effects throughout the body. HMOs in the urine might contribute to a reduced incidence of urinary tract infections in breastfed infants compared with formula-fed infants.[169] Most data on the benefits of HMOs are currently limited to studies in tissue culture or animal models. Recent advances in high-throughput screening of HMO profiles from hundreds or even thousands of milk samples will enable clinical cohort studies to link individual HMOs with infant health and disease. Moreover, individual HMOs are becoming available in quantities and qualities for the use in clinical studies to test their efficacy in human infants.

VITAMINS

Vitamin D

Human milk typically contains a vitamin D concentration of 25 IU (international units) per liter or less, which alone does not provide infants with an adequate intake. Although most breastfed infants are able to synthesize additional vitamin D through routine sunlight exposure, avoidance of direct sunlight has limited this source of vitamin D. The low content of vitamin D in human milk has been related to the development of rickets in a few breastfed infants.[170] Therefore the AAP and Institute of Medicine (IOM) currently recommend that all breastfed infants, including preterm infants, receive 400 IU of oral vitamin D drops daily, beginning during the first 2 months of life and continuing until adequate amounts of vitamin D are provided through daily consumption by the infant of fortified formula or milk.[3,171,172]

Vitamin E

The vitamin E content (mainly α-tocopherol) is higher in human milk than in bovine milk. α-Tocopherol concentrations in colostrum are higher than that of transitional and mature milk. In well-nourished populations, supplementing the mother's diet with vitamin E has only limited effects on vitamin E concentration in human milk. α-Tocopherol functions mostly as a chain-breaking antioxidant that prevents propagation of lipid peroxidation, modulates immune function, affects cell signaling, regulates gene expression, and contributes to several metabolic processes in the human body.

Vitamin K

Human milk contains 1 to 4 μg/L of vitamin K1. Bleeding in infants caused by vitamin K deficiency is rare (0.25%-1.7% incidence), but can be severe. Thus the AAP recommends 0.5 to 1.0 mg vitamin K1 administered to all infants shortly after birth.

Vitamin B

Poor maternal status of vitamins such as thiamine (B_1), riboflavin (B_2), vitamin B_6, and vitamin B_{12} causes concentrations of these nutrients to be low in breast milk and the infant to become deficient. In contrast, in maternal folate depletion, breast-milk folate concentrations are maintained. The prevalence of maternal deficiency of these vitamins is uncertain but certainly higher in developing countries with limited availability of high-quality food sources.

MINERALS

The mineral content of human milk is low relative to that of infant formulas and very low compared with that of cow's milk, from which most formulas are prepared, so that although human milk is sufficient to support growth and development, it also presents a fairly low solute load to the developing kidney. The levels of major minerals tend to decline during lactation, with the exception of magnesium, but with considerable variability among women tested.[27,173] Sodium, potassium, chloride, calcium, zinc, and phosphorus all appear to be more bioavailable in human milk than in infant formulas, reflecting their lower concentrations in human milk. Iron is readily bioavailable to the infant from human milk but may have to be supplemented later in lactation.[36,174] Dietary influences may affect levels of calcium and copper but not other minerals.[175] Preterm infants fed human milk require supplements of calcium, phosphorus, sodium, and iron.[176]

CELLS

In addition to its nutritive and bioactive biochemical components, milk contains maternal cells that are live in fresh milk and that might have specific functions for the breastfed infant.[177] There are strong interpersonal and intrapersonal variations in the amount and composition of cells in human milk. Human milk can contain between 10,000 and 13,000,000 cells/mL.[178,179] Colostrum often contains more cells than transitional and mature milk. At least three different cell types have been reported in human milk: leukocytes, epithelial cells, and stem cells. These three categories are reviewed in more detail as follows.

Leukocytes

In addition to the many biochemical immune modulators already described, human milk contains blood-derived leukocytes that are believed to be transported into the milk via the paracellular pathway.[177] Depending on the stage of lactation and the health of the mother or the infant, leukocytes may constitute the majority of the cells in human milk. Leukocyte content in colostrum varies within a wide range (13.2%-70.4%). Infection of the mother or the infant is associated with an increase in milk leukocytes, which decreases when the infection resolves. The predominant leukocyte types in colostrum are macrophages (40%-50%), followed by polymorphonuclear neutrophils (40%-50%), and lymphocytes (5%-10%). Greater than 80% of the lymphocytes are T cells, and only 5% to 6% are B cells.[180,181] In fresh milk, many of these cells are live, activated, and motile.[182,183] Data from animal models suggest that they cross the infant's intestinal epithelial barrier and are engrafted in different organs and tissues, including mesenteric lymph nodes, liver, and spleen.[184-187] Milk leukocytes are thought to protect the mother's lactating mammary gland from infections and may provide a benefit to the infant, although this remains to be demonstrated.[188] In contrast to colostrum, leukocyte content in mature milk is rather low but also increases in response to infections in the breastfeeding mother or the breastfed infant.

Epithelial Cells

Human milk contains both ductal and alveolar, luminal-epithelial, and myoepithelial cells. Over the years and based on newly acquired data, three different hypotheses developed about why epithelial cells occur in milk. At first, it was thought that epithelial cells are the product of apoptosis. Later, evidence showed that the majority of epithelial cells in freshly expressed milk are viable and can be propagated in primary culture to form functioning mammospheres.[189,190] This led to the second hypothesis, that milk epithelial cells passively detached from ducts and alveoli in the process of milk synthesis and secretion, for instance, because of the vacuum applied to the ducts during suction.[191] The most recent data supports a third hypothesis, that epithelial cells are detached in an active process that is driven by differential gene expression. As a result, the cells become more motile, leading to an active detachment. Milk epithelial cells often occur as clusters that can be isolated and cultured for further analysis.[192,193] Whether the presence of these cells is biologically useful or merely reflects physiologic turnover is not known.

Stem Cells

Cell preparations from fresh human milk are able to expand in culture and form different colony types that can be maintained through multiple passages.[192-195] This observation led to the hypothesis that human milk contains breast-milk stem cells (hBSCs). The hypothesis was confirmed when researchers discovered that some human milk cells express the stem cell markers CK5 and nestin, as well as the stem/progenitor cell markers p63 and CD49f.[190,191,196] These cells were able to self-renew and differentiate into luminal and myoepithelial cells. Most recently, it was discovered that some of these hBSCs express pluripotency markers, such as the transcription factors OCT4, SOX2, and NANOG.[189] As with most milk components, there is wide interpersonal and intrapersonal variation in hBSC content and expression levels of stem/progenitor cell and pluripotency markers. What factors influence this variation has not yet been determined. hBSCs are able to differentiate into cells of the mammary gland lineage that synthesize and secrete milk-specific proteins and other components. Most intriguing, however, are results that demonstrated the ability of hBSCs to also differentiate into cells of other lineages, including cells with properties of adipocytes, cardiomyocytes, chondrocytes, osteoblasts, neurons, hepatocytes, and pancreatic beta cells.[189] The discovery of pluripotent hBSCs that are capable of differentiating into cells from all three germ layers opened an entirely new area of human milk research. Future studies will have to show how hBSCs impact the breastfed infant and whether they have the potential to be used in the context of regenerative medicine.[177]

Overall, the presence of viable cells in human milk, whether they are leukocytes, epithelial cells, or stem cells, raises the question of how they affect the breastfed infant. Considering the concentration of cells in human milk and the milk volume consumed, it can be estimated that thousands or even millions of viable cells are ingested by the breastfed infant with each and every feed. Research in animals has shown that some of these cells are able to cross infant epithelial barriers and are engrafted in infant tissues and organs.[184-187] This has mainly been shown for leukocytes but may also be possible for epithelial cells and stem cells, causing a microchimerism with maternal cells (i.e., detected as cells containing only maternal DNA) engrafted in infant tissues (i.e., infant DNA with maternal and paternal contribution). Potential lifelong consequences are unknown and need further investigation.[197]

BACTERIA

Traditionally, bacteria in human milk had been associated with infections and perceived as harmful for the breastfeeding mother and the breastfed infant. Several studies, however, reported the presence of bacteria even in the milk of healthy women without any clinical or subclinical signs of infection. Newer culture-independent techniques based on 16S ribosomal RNA sequencing led to a more comprehensive description of the human milk microbiome.[198-200] The human milk microbiome tends to be stable over time and is highly personalized.[199] Although the bacterial composition varies between mothers, most milk samples contain a set of core bacteria that include *Streptococcus, Staphylococcus, Pseudomonas, Corynebacteria, Propionibacterium, Sphingomonas,* and Bradyrhizobiaceae. Although it is now generally accepted that milk from healthy women is not sterile, the origin of the human milk microbiome remains uncertain.[198,201,202] One hypothesis is that human milk microbes are derived from the mother's skin and/or the infant's oral flora. The second hypothesis is that the microbes stem from the mother's gastrointestinal tract. It suggests that permeability in the mother's intestine is increased, which allows bacteria to enter the bloodstream and reach the mammary gland. The third hypothesis is that microbes in the mother's intestine are sampled by specialized dendritic cells that transport selected bacteria to the mammary gland. If the second or third hypothesis proves to be correct, it will be intriguing to study how a manipulation of the mother's intestinal microbiome with prebiotics, probiotics, or antibiotics might impact the human milk microbiome and affect not only maternal but also infant health. Bacteria in human milk could protect the infant against infections and contribute to the maturation of the immune system.[202] On the other hand, dysbiosis may lead to mammary gland infections (mastitis), which remains one of the main reasons for women to stop breastfeeding.

Benefits and Risks of Human Milk

BENEFITS

Gastrointestinal Homeostasis

The development of mucosal integrity in the gut appears to depend on maturation of the mucosal tissue itself and the establishment of a normal gut flora. The former represents anatomic and enzymatic blockades to invasion of microorganisms and antigens, and the latter, an inhibition of colonization by pathogenic bacteria. Although permeability of the neonatal gut to immunoglobulin is rather short-lived, damaged neonatal gut is permeable to a host of other proteins and macromolecules for several weeks or longer. Peptides derived from proteins and bovine serum albumin can enter the circulation and induce a circulating antibody response.[203] The inflamed or ischemic gut is even more porous to both antigens and pathogens. A variety of proven and presumed mechanisms for the role of both sIgA and the normal flora have been proposed to compensate for these temporary inadequacies.[204]

Prevention of Diarrhea

Extensive epidemiologic evidence supports a "prophylactic value" of exclusive breastfeeding in the first 6 months of life, with the addition of complementary feeding thereafter, in the prevention or amelioration of diarrheal disease in infants and young children in developed and developing nations and is summarized in several reviews.[1,205-208] These earlier findings are supported by a recent Cochrane analysis that concluded that infants who continue exclusive breastfeeding for 6 months or more appear to have a significantly reduced risk of gastrointestinal and respiratory infection, at least in the Iranian and Nigerian studies, compared with those who breastfeed for less than 4 months. Historically, a preventive and therapeutic role for breastfeeding has been suggested in nursery outbreaks of diarrheal disease caused by enteropathogenic strains of *E. coli*[209] and rotavirus.[210] Earlier observations have shown a reduced rate of diarrhea in breastfed infants, even in the face of milk contamination with *E. coli* and *Shigella* spp.[211]

Cholera is rare in infancy, especially in endemic areas where the prevalence of breastfeeding is high. The experience with an outbreak of cholera in Guinea-Bissau lends support to the possibility that breastfeeding is an important variable in protecting against cholera in infancy. In this study, the risk of diarrheal disease caused by cholera was reduced from 29% to 7% in breastfed children (RR for breastfed children, 0.19; 95% CI, 0.04 to 0.91, adjusted for age) and in those breastfed children who developed disease, maternal milk contained lower concentrations of anti–cholera toxin IgA/total IgA (median, 2.0 units/mL) than in the breastfed children who did not develop diarrheal disease (median, 17.4 units/mL).[212]

Ample experimental animal data on the value of specific colostral antibody in preventing diarrheal illness are available from studies of colostral deprivation. These include colibacteriosis associated with *E. coli* K88 in swine; rotaviral gastroenteritis in cattle, swine, and sheep; and diarrheal illness associated with transmissible gastroenteritis of swine.[213] In addition, the diverse serotypes of aerobic, gram-negative bacilli present in the oropharynx and the gastrointestinal tract of the neonate may serve as a source of antigen to boost the presensitized mammary glands, leading to a further modulation of specific bacterial growth in the mucosa.[214]

Case-control studies of enteric viral infections in breastfed infants suggest that breastfeeding may more often protect infants from severe disease and hospitalization rather than from infection itself.[215,216] This is also the case for the protection provided by rotavirus vaccines.[217] Notable in this regard are conflicting data regarding the impact of breastfeeding on risk for human rotaviral infection and disease. A community-based study in Germany, Switzerland, and Austria showed a protective effect of breastfeeding on the incidence of acute rotavirus gastroenteritis.[218] However, in developed countries, most rotavirus infections in neonates are asymptomatic, regardless of breastfeeding or bottle feeding,[219-221] and on the basis of careful clinical observations, Bishop and co-workers[222] in Australia questioned the positive effects of breastfeeding in rotavirus infection. Consistent with this point, the risk of rotavirus-associated diarrheal disease in hospitalized infants in Uganda was not lower in those who were breastfeeding (OR, 1.08; 95% CI, 0.52 to 2.25; $P = 0.8$).[223] Thus, although breastfeeding protects against many causes of diarrheal disease, the magnitude of the benefit can vary, and the mechanisms of such protection remain to be more fully defined.[215,216]

Necrotizing Enterocolitis

Necrotizing enterocolitis (NEC) is a complex gastrointestinal inflammatory condition that occurs principally in very premature infants and is often associated with hypoxia, gut mucosal ischemia, and necrolysis.[224,225] Evidence supports the notion that NEC is associated with an exaggerated immunologic or inflammatory response in the host.[226,227] A role for a gestational age window of susceptibility to dysregulated inflammation in the timing of NEC may be present as NEC occurs after several weeks in the smallest preterm infants compared with the first week for older preterm infants.[228] Outbreaks of NEC related to *Klebsiella* and *Salmonella* spp. secondary to banked human milk feedings have been documented.[229-231] However, although NEC has been associated in some cases with a specific pathogen, most cases are not caused by a single organism.

Clinical manifestations include abdominal distention, gastric retention, and bloody diarrhea. Classic radiographic findings include air in the bowel wall (pneumatosis intestinalis), air in the portal system, and free infradiaphragmatic air (signifying perforation). A breakdown in the mucosal defense leads to dysregulated inflammation from unchecked invasion of pathogenic bacteria. Treatment involves decompression, systemic antibiotics, and, often, surgery.[67,232-236]

The prevention of NEC is the primary management for this condition. A number of studies have demonstrated a beneficial role of human milk in preventing or modifying the severity of NEC in high-risk preterm infants, in particular the potential for an exclusively human milk diet with human milk versus bovine-based fortifiers to lead to a 50% reduction of all NEC and 90% reduction of surgical NEC.[237-243] And although some other pediatric centers have claimed a virtual absence of NEC in human milk–fed infants with slowly advancing feeding protocols, others have not.[244,245]

In an asphyxiated neonatal rat model of NEC, the condition could be prevented with feeding of maternal milk. Although cellular components in human milk are obvious candidates, most preterm diets have limited mammalian cells because of storage, freezing, or use of donor human milk. It also is possible that antibody and nonspecific factors play a role, including establishment of a physiologic gut microbiota with associated beneficial effects on intestinal integrity and homeostasis and gut intrinsic immune processes (see Chapter 4).[111,246,247]

Use of broad-spectrum antibiotics is standard therapy when NEC has developed, and this is based on the assumption that reducing pathogenic bacterial burden is supportive of gut restitution. The most effective combination of antibiotics has not been determined clearly for the treatment of NEC.[248] Past strategies of enteral antibiotic regimens have been associated with reduced NEC incidence, but concerns for antibiotic resistance limited this approach.[249] Conversely, however, retrospective data from the National Institute of Child Health and Human Development Neonatal Research Network and others have associated longer initial empirical antibiotic use after birth with NEC incidence.[250-252] Presumably, initial antibiotics may significantly alter gut microflora and increase the chances for NEC to occur.[253] Antenatal antibiotic use has also been a risk factor for the development of NEC.[254]

Thus NEC continues to present a medical challenge whose etiopathogenesis remains to be more fully defined. Although breastfeeding may be protective, a number of other factors are clearly related to the mechanism of mucosal injury and the pathogenesis of this condition.

Neonatal Sepsis

There is a body of evidence suggesting that the incidence of bacteremia among preterm infants fed breast milk is significantly lower than that among those receiving formula feedings or no feeding.[255-260] Other studies have, however, failed to demonstrate protection against systemic infection in breastfed infants.[261-263] These controversies notwithstanding, there is substantial support for the notion that the use of human milk for very-low-birth weight (VLBW) neonates reduces the risk of late-onset sepsis.[239,264-266, 267]

Prevention of Atopy and Allergy

Since the first report in 1936, numerous publications have addressed the effect of infant feeding on the development of atopic disease and asthma.[268] Breastfeeding has been reported to have a prophylactic benefit on the development of atopic disease and asthma. The first prospective long-term study, with extended follow-up from infancy until the age of 17 years, found that the prevalence of atopy was significantly higher in those infants with short-duration (<1 month) or no breastfeeding than in infants with intermediate-duration (1-6 months) or prolonged (>6 months) breastfeeding. The differences in the prevalence of atopy persisted when the groups were divided according to positive or negative atopic heredity.[269] Furthermore, the atopy manifestations in the different infant feeding groups did not remain constant with age. In particular, respiratory allergy, including asthma, increased greatly in prevalence up to the age of 17 years, with a prevalence at this age as high as 64% in the group with short-duration or no breastfeeding.[269] In another prospective, longitudinal study of the prevalence and risk factors for acute and chronic respiratory illness in childhood, investigators examined the relationship of infant feeding to recurrent wheezing at age 6 years and the association of wheezing early in life with lower respiratory tract illnesses.[270] Children who were never breastfed had significantly higher rates of recurrent wheezing at 6 years of age, but in this study, increasing the duration of breastfeeding beyond 1 month was not associated with significantly lower rates of recurrent wheezing. The beneficial effect of breastfeeding was apparent for children both with and without wheezing lower respiratory tract illnesses in the first 6 months of life. In contrast with the findings of the first study, however, the beneficial effect of breastfeeding was significant only among nonatopic children.[270]

How might breastfeeding confer long-lasting protection against allergic sensitization? Multiple synergistic mechanisms may contribute (1) maturation of the recipient gastrointestinal and airway mucosa, promoted by growth factors present in human milk[271-273]; (2) inhibition of antigen absorption by milk sIgA[274]; (3) reduced incidence of mucosal infections and consequent sensitization to bystander antigens[275]; (4) impact of breast milk on the infant's microbiota[224,276]; and (5) direct immunomodulatory activity of human milk components on the recipient infant[103] and differences in exposure to potential allergens.

Secretory IgA, along with the intestinal glycocalyx and intestinal enzymes, might impede the development of allergic sensitization, in part via a process of immune exclusion, whereby immune processes help to impede foreign macromolecular transport across the immature gut and its consequences in terms of the generation of circulating antibody or immune complexes. Beginning with the observations of IgA-deficient patients, it has become clear that the absence of the IgA barrier in the gut is associated with both an increased incidence of circulating antibodies directed against many food antigens and an increased occurrence of atopic-allergic diseases.[274] The neonate is similar in some respects to the IgA-deficient patient,[277] and increased transintestinal uptake of food antigen with consequent circulating antibody formation in the premature infant has been reported.[278] Immune exclusion is not an absolute rule, however, because uptake of some antigens across the gut may be enhanced rather than blocked by interaction with antibody at the mucosal surface.

In addition to immune exclusion, prolonged breastfeeding could also protect against atopy by direct exclusion—if the mother's milk is the infant's sole food, ingestion by the infant is precluded unless the mother consumes the food and food antigens are transported into her milk.[279] In this regard, intact bovine milk proteins and other food antigens and antibodies have been observed in samples of colostrum and milk.[10] In any case, such direct exclusion is not required because other studies have suggested that early breastfeeding, even of short duration, is associated with a decreased serum antibody response to cow's milk proteins.[280]

These potential biologic mechanisms and the studies noted above notwithstanding, there is considerable debate regarding the protective immune effects of early breastfeeding on the development of atopy and allergy, the duration and exclusivity of breastfeeding that results in benefit, the duration of that benefit after the termination of breastfeeding, and the importance of the act of breastfeeding in addition to the constituents of breast milk.[269,281-284] For example, one retrospective Korean study showed an increased risk for asthma in infants who were breastfed beyond 1 year.[285] Another reported that the protective effect of breastfeeding was not found for infants fed breast milk by bottle.[286]

Differences in conclusions may be related, at least in part, to methodologic issues. Kramer[287] conducted an extensive meta-analysis of 50 studies published before

1986 that focused on infant feeding and atopic disease. Seven of the 13 studies on asthma included in this analysis claimed a protective effect of breastfeeding, whereas 6 claimed no protection. In a number of the studies analyzed, early infant feeding history was obtained months or years after the feeding period, ascertainment of the infant feeding history was obtained by interviewers who were aware of the disease outcome, or insufficient duration and exclusivity of breastfeeding were documented; all were confounding variables. Failure to control for confounding variables was a common violation identified in several studies. For example, the effect of infant feeding on subsequent asthma may be confounded by other variables, including family history of atopic disease, socioeconomic status, and parental cigarette smoking. Only 1 of the 13 studies on asthma included in the meta-analysis adequately controlled for these confounding factors. Moreover, 3 of the studies that did not demonstrate a protective effect of breastfeeding on asthma had inadequate statistical power. The effect of infant feeding on the severity of outcome and on the age at onset of the disease was virtually ignored in most of the studies. This Cochrane analysis was updated in 2012, with the conclusion that in the 3 high-quality studies from Finland, Australia, and Belarus, no significant reduction in risk of atopic eczema, asthma, or other atopic outcomes was demonstrated.[288]

Special Considerations for the Premature Neonate

Many of the benefits of human milk evident in term neonates are also evident in very-low-birth weight (<1500 g) preterm neonates fed unfortified human milk, and the incidence of necrotizing enterocolitis also appears to be reduced. Nonetheless, the content of calcium, phosphorus, protein, sodium, vitamins, and energy in unfortified human milk is inadequate to meet the needs of the very-low-birth weight preterm neonate, and, if used as an exclusive source of nutrients, may be associated with impaired growth and nutrient deficiencies. Meta-analysis of studies comparing premature infants fed unfortified or fortified human milk found that fortified milk was associated with greater increases in weight, length, head circumference, and better nitrogen balance and bone mineral content, without an increase in feeding intolerance or complications.[238,289] Fortification with bovine milk–based fortifiers provides a rich source of multinutrient fortification for most preterm infants but may carry some added risk for the development of NEC compared with an exclusively human diet.

Other Benefits

As noted in the section on diarrheal disease, a 2012 Cochrane analysis concluded that infants who continue exclusive breastfeeding for 6 months or more appear to have not only a significantly reduced risk of gastrointestinal, but at least in the Iranian and Nigerian studies, a reduced risk of respiratory infections compared with those who breastfeed for less than 4 months.[288] Data are lacking in humans regarding passive protection on other mucosal surfaces, such as the eye, ear, or genitourinary tract. Some epidemiologic evidence suggests that recurrence of otitis media with effusion is strongly associated with early bottle feeding and that breastfeeding may confer protection against otitis media with effusion for the first 3 years of life.[290]

A number of other benefits have been associated with breastfeeding, including natural contraception during active nursing,[288,291] protection against sudden infant death syndrome,[292] diabetes,[293] obesity,[294] high cholesterol level, and ischemic heart disease later in life.[295] A reduced risk of breast cancer has also been shown in several studies, and a recent meta-analysis reported a pooled odds ratio of 0.72 (95% CI, 0.58 to 0.89),[296] for women who ever breastfed, although reduced risk was not found in another recent cohort study.[297] Several studies have demonstrated enhanced cognitive outcome in breastfed children, although controversy exists regarding the mechanisms by which such improved performance may occur.[298-301] The 2012 Cochrane analysis, based on the only study (from Belarus) that met their review criteria, concluded that 6 months of exclusive breastfeeding conferred no benefit (vs. 3 months of exclusive breastfeeding, followed by continued partial breastfeeding through 6 months) on cognitive ability or behavior at 6.5 years of age.[288]

NONINFECTIOUS RISKS

Human milk is the optimal form of nutrition for healthy term infants in almost all situations. The failure to initiate lactation properly during early breastfeeding may present a risk of dehydration to the infant because insufficient fluids may be ingested. Inappropriate introduction of bottles and pacifiers also may interfere with proper induction of lactation. Later in lactation, introduction of bottles may induce premature weaning as the result of a reduction in the milk supply. The Baby Friendly Hospital Initiative (BFHI) is a worldwide effort by the WHO and United Nations Children's Fund to promote best breastfeeding practices in delivery hospitals by following 10 important steps (www.unicef.org/programme/breastfeeding/baby.htm).

There are very few absolute contraindications to breastfeeding.[302] The most important reasons for cessation of breastfeeding include certain maternal medications and infection. Some circumstances have been identified in which continued breastfeeding should be conducted with caution to protect the infant. Infants with inherited metabolic diseases may also require alternative forms of nutrition instead of breast milk: neonates with galactosemia caused by deficiency of galactose-1-phosphate uridyltransferase should receive lactose-free milk (lactose is a glucose-galactose disaccharide); infants with phenylketonuria may receive some human milk to support their requirement for phenylalanine, and this may be best with concurrent blood levels of phenylalanine with alternative support of specially prepared commercial milks.[303,304] Mothers who have received radionuclides for diagnostic or therapeutic purposes should use alternative forms of nutrition for the days to weeks required for these compounds to be eliminated, as should mothers receiving certain chemotherapeutic and immunosuppressive agents and actively using drugs of abuse, including amphetamines, cocaine, heroin, and phencyclidine.[305] Breastfeeding and the use of cannabis substances is concerning, given reports of neurodevelopmental impairment, but it is not clear when the critical windows of exposure are.[306] Low-level maternal exposure to environmental chemicals and tobacco smoking should be avoided as much as possible but is not a contraindication to breastfeeding.

Antimicrobial agents taken by mothers only rarely represent a contraindication to breastfeeding. As first principles, antimicrobials that may be safely given to infants may be safely given to their lactating mothers, and blood concentrations that may be achieved through breast-milk ingestion are lower than therapeutic doses used in infants.[307] Breastfeeding by mothers receiving chloramphenicol is contraindicated because its use may be associated with fatal complications in newborn infants. The effects of metronidazole are uncertain, but to minimize exposure to this drug, which is mutagenic in bacteria, mothers receiving single-dose therapy should discontinue breastfeeding for 12 to 24 hours.[305] Excretion of antibiotics in human milk is also discussed in Chapter 37. The reader is also referred to the leading source of up-to-date information on maternal medications and breastfeeding, called LactMed (see LactMed tab at http://toxnet.nlm.nih.gov/).

Several instances of specific nutrient deficiencies in breastfed infants have been described, specifically related to lack of vitamin K, vitamin D, vitamin B_{12}, folic acid, vitamin C, and carnitine. In each of these instances, several case reports have appeared warning against deficiencies that have resulted in clinical consequences to the neonate. For example, hemorrhagic disease is almost exclusively reported in breastfed infants who did not receive vitamin K or received only one dose at birth. This can be successfully treated with vitamin K.[308] Endogenous vitamin D production versus dietary vitamin D is the primary means by which humans naturally obtain vitamin D. Breastfed infants are dependent on their maternal vitamin D stores. Cases of rickets in breastfed infants have been reported, particularly during winter among infants not exposed to the sun.[170,309] Vitamin D requirements can be best met with infant supplementation with oral vitamin D, although maternal high-dose vitamin D supplementation has also been suggested.[310] Mothers who practice unusual dietary habits, such as strict vegetarianism, may have reduced levels of vitamin B_{12} and folic acid in their milk, and deficiencies in breastfed infants of such mothers have been reported.[311-313] Deficiency of carnitine, a key amino acid responsible for fat metabolism, also has been reported to result in clinical symptoms in breastfed infants in mothers ingesting unusual diets.[120,314] However, these concerns can best be addressed in almost all cases by counseling mothers regarding nutritional practices and by the provision of supplemental vitamins and other micronutrients when appropriate; this is the case in the developed world and even more so in the developing world, where the untoward consequences of not breastfeeding are particularly great.[206]

Management of hyperbilirubinemia associated with breastfeeding has been an area of some controversy in the past. Two primary mechanisms occur in the development of jaundice with breastfeeding. Not enough breast-milk jaundice occurs early in lactation when milk supply does not meet fluid requirements of the infant. This can be accompanied by slower gastrointestinal transit that exacerbates the uptake of bilirubin through the enterohepatic circulation. Breast-milk jaundice occurs later in the first week of lactation and is suggested to be due to the several components in human milk, including progesterone metabolites, free fatty acids, inflammatory cytokines, and growth factors. Some recent evidence suggests a role for commensal bacteria, such as bifidobacteria, in protecting against the development of breast-milk jaundice.[315] Present recommendations are for continued breastfeeding with efforts to increase the volume of milk ingested, with the provision that with severe hyperbilirubinemia, a brief interruption of breastfeeding might be appropriate.[316]

INFECTIOUS RISKS

Human milk may contain infectious agents that are secreted into the milk, enter milk during lactation, or are acquired when milk is improperly collected, stored, and later fed to her infant. Formal training and evaluation of breastfeeding practices by trained caregivers is the best way to reduce these risks; routine culture or heat treatment of a mother's milk even when it is stored and later used to feed her infant is not cost-effective.[316]

Stored milk is now routinely used to feed infants when their mothers are not able to breastfeed directly because of work or travel constraints or when an infant is premature or otherwise unable to breastfeed effectively. Inadvertent feeding of stored milk from other than the birth mother has occurred in nurseries. If this occurs, the AAP recommends that this be handled in the same manner as if accidental exposure to blood or other body fluids has occurred[307] (see Chapter 35 for additional information).

In the United States, the Human Milk Banking Association of North America (www.hmbana.org/) collects human donor milk for the purpose of administration to infants whose mother's milk is not available or adequate. Members of this association follow guidelines formulated in consultation with the U.S. Food and Drug Administration (FDA) and Centers for Disease Control and Prevention (CDC). These guidelines help to assure that donors are screened for transmissable infectious agents and that the milk is carefully collected, processed, and stored. Using these practices, donor milk is collected and pooled, subjected to Holder pasteurization (62.5° C) for 30 minutes, which reliably kills bacteria and inactivates HIV and cytomegalovirus (CMV), and eliminates or substantially reduces the amounts of other viruses. The pooled milk is then tested to assure that it meets standards and frozen for later distribution and use.

Bacterial Infections

Transmission of bacterial pathogens, including *Staphylococcus aureus*, group B streptococci, mycobacteria, and other species may occur through breastfeeding (Table 5-3) Mastitis and breast abscesses may be associated with substantial concentrations of bacteria in the mother's milk. In general, feeding an infant from a breast affected by an abscess is not recommended.[307] Infant feeding on the affected breast may be resumed, however, 24 to 48 hours after drainage and the initiation of appropriate antibiotic therapy. Mastitis usually resolves with appropriate antimicrobial therapy and with continued lactation, even if feeding from the affected breast is temporarily interrupted. In both of these conditions, feeding from the unaffected breast need not be interrupted.

Mothers with active tuberculosis should refrain from breastfeeding for at least 2 weeks or longer after institution of appropriate treatment if they are considered contagious.

This recommendation also applies to the uncommon situation where mastitis or breast abscess is caused by *Mycobacterium tuberculosis*.[307]

Viral Infections

Viruses that have been detected in human milk include CMV, hepatitis B (HBV) and hepatitis C (HCV) viruses, herpes simplex virus (HSV), HIV-1, human T-lymphotropic virus type 1 (HTLV-1) and type 2 (HTLV-2), rubella virus, and West Nile virus (see Table 5-3).[3] Whether varicella virus is secreted into human milk is unknown. Although some of these viruses present a risk to infant, for most but not all, the benefits of breastfeeding to the infant are greater than the risk.

Cytomegalovirus Infection. Cytomegalovirus infection is a common perinatal infection. The virus is shed in the milk in about 25% of infected mothers. Although breastfeeding from infected mothers may result in seroconversion in up to 70% of breastfeeding neonates, the infection often is not associated with clinical symptoms of disease. Very-low-birth weight infants (born at <1500 g), however, may exhibit evidence of clinical disease, with thrombocytopenia, neutropenia, or hepatosplenomegaly seen in 50% of those infected through breastfeeding. The decision to breastfeed a premature baby by an infected mother should be based on weighing the potential benefits of human milk versus the risk of CMV transmission.[3]

Table 5-3 Infectious Agents Transmitted Through Breastfeeding

Organism	Transmission	Disease	Intervention
Cytomegalovirus	+	VLBW infants	Consider risk/benefit
Hepatitis B virus	+	+	HBIg/HB vaccine
Hepatitis C virus	HIV-positive mothers only	?	See text
Herpes simplex virus	+	+	See text
Human immunodeficiency virus	+	+	United States: Do not breastfeed*
HTLV-1	+	±	United States: Do not breastfeed*
HTLV-2	+	±	United States: Do not breastfeed
Rubella virus	+	0	None
West Nile virus	±	±	None
Group B streptococci	+	±	See text
Staphylococcus aureus	+	±	See text
Mycobacterium tuberculosis	+	+	See text

HB, Hepatitis B; *HBIg*, hepatitis B immunoglobulin; *HTLV*, human T-lymphotropic virus; *VLBW*, very low birth weight.
*In many other parts of the world, the benefits of breastfeeding often outweigh the risks of alternative methods of infant feeding. See text for discussion of risk versus benefit in other parts of the world.

Hepatitis B Virus Infection. Hepatitis B surface antigen (HBsAg) has been detected in milk of HBV-infected mothers. Nevertheless, breastfeeding does not increase the risk of HBV infection among these infants. Infants born to HBV-positive mothers should receive hepatitis B immune globulin (HBIg) and the initial dose of hepatitis B vaccine within 12 hours of birth, followed by the recommended series of hepatitis B vaccine without any delay in the institution of breastfeeding.[3]

Hepatitis C Virus Infection. The RNA of HCV and antibody to HCV have been detected in the milk from infected mothers. Transmission by means of breastfeeding, however, has not been documented in anti-HCV–positive, anti-HIV–negative mothers but is a theoretical possibility about which these mothers should be informed before deciding whether they will breastfeed. According to current guidelines, HCV infection is not a contraindication to breastfeeding, although mothers with cracked or bleeding nipples should consider refraining from breastfeeding until they have healed.[307]

Herpes Simplex Virus. Herpes simplex virus transmission directly from maternal breast lesions to their infants has been demonstrated. Women with lesions on one breast may feed from the other unaffected breast, making sure that lesions on the other breast or on other parts of the body are covered and using careful hand hygiene.[307]

Human Immunodeficiency Virus 1. A number of studies have demonstrated HIV in milk.[317-321] The findings include isolation of HIV from milk supernatants collected from symptom-free women and from cellular fractions of maternal milk, recovery of HIV virions in the histiocytes and cell-free extracts of milk by electron microscopy, and detection of viral DNA by polymerase chain reaction in greater than 70% of samples from HIV-seropositive lactating women.

Transmission of HIV through breastfeeding may account for up to one third of all HIV infections in infants globally, with risk of transmission being approximately 15% when breastfeeding continues beyond the first year of life.[322,323] The risk of postnatal HIV transmission appears to be constant throughout the first 18 months of life; thus risk is cumulative as duration of breastfeeding increases.[324] Risk of transmission via breast milk is greater when maternal HIV infection is acquired during lactation; when viral load is greater or maternal disease is more advanced; when babies are both breastfed and formula fed; when the mother has bleeding or cracked nipples, mastitis, or a breast abscess; and when the infant has thrush or certain other coinfections (see Chapter 21).

Current recommendations from the AAP[316-325] and other authorities[326] state that in populations such as that of the United States, in which the risk of death from infectious diseases and malnutrition is low and in which safe and effective alternative sources of feeding are readily available, HIV-infected women should be counseled not to breastfeed their infants nor to donate milk. A recent report found that highly active antiretroviral therapy (HAART) administered during pregnancy or postpartum suppresses HIV RNA, but not DNA, in breast milk.[327] At present, the AAP recommends that infants of HIV-infected mothers in the United States receiving HAART should not be breastfed.

Despite the potential risk of HIV infection in infants of HIV-infected breastfeeding mothers, consideration of cessation of breastfeeding must be balanced against the other beneficial effects described in this chapter. Thus, in areas of the world where infectious diseases and malnutrition are important causes of death early in life, the beneficial effects of breastfeeding often outweigh the potential risk of HIV transmission through breastfeeding. Studies in such settings have shown that HIV-free survival at 7 months of age is similar in exposed infants who were breastfed or formula fed from birth.[328-330] Studies in Africa demonstrate that exclusive breastfeeding in the first 6 months of life reduces the risk of HIV transmission compared with mothers who supplement breastfeeding with other foods and milk sources.[328,329,331] Thus, in areas of the world where the burden of infectious diseases and malnutrition is high and where alternatives to breast milk that provide adequate nutrition are not acceptable, affordable, feasible, and safe, the WHO recommends exclusive breastfeeding for the first 6 months of life, followed by complementary foods and breastfeeding through 12 months of age, for women whose HIV status is unknown and for women known to have HIV, accompanied in the latter group by postnatal infant or maternal antiretroviral prophylaxis to reduce HIV transmission during breastfeeding.[205,316,325,326,332] The WHO policy also stresses the need for continued support for breastfeeding by mothers who are HIV-negative, improved access to HIV counseling and testing, and government efforts to ensure uninterrupted access to nutritionally adequate human milk substitutes.[317]

Human T-Lymphotropic Viruses Types 1 and 2. Human T-lymphotropic virus type 1 is endemic in Japan, the Caribbean, and parts of South America. This infection can be transmitted from mother to infant, and this transmission occurs primarily through breastfeeding. HTLV-2 infection has been identified in some Native Americans and Native Alaskans and in some injection drug abusers in the United States and Europe. Mother-to-infant transmission of HTLV-2 has been demonstrated, although the frequency with which this occurs and the route of transmission are uncertain. Women in the United States who are known to be seropositive for HTLV-1 or HTLV-2 should not breastfeed. However, routine screening for HTLV-1 and HTLV-2 is not recommended.[317]

Rubella. Rubella virus has been recovered from milk after natural as well as vaccine-associated infection. It has not been associated with significant disease in infants, however, although transient seroconversion has been frequently demonstrated. No contraindication to breastfeeding exists in women recently immunized with currently licensed rubella vaccines.

West Nile Virus Infection. The RNA of West Nile virus has been detected in human milk, and seroconversion in breastfeeding infants also has been observed. Although West Nile virus can be transmitted in milk, the extent of transmission in humans remains rare.[333] Most infants and children infected with the virus to date have been asymptomatic or have had minimal disease.[317] Because the risk is uncertain, the AAP recommends that women in endemic areas may continue to breastfeed.

Current Trends in Breastfeeding

Both international and national organizations have endorsed breastfeeding as the optimal means of feeding for the healthy term infant.[317] In general, the percentage of mothers initiating breastfeeding in developing countries is 90% or greater, which both reflects the lack of other options and the severe health and economic consequences for bottle feeding their infants. In the United States, at one point in the early 1970s, the rate of breastfeeding initiation was as low as 25%. The rate of initiation has improved dramatically since that time. In the Infant Feeding Practices Survey (IFPS) II survey conducted by the FDA from 2005 to 2007, 83% of respondents initiated breastfeeding.[334] More recent establishment of benchmarks on a new Perinatal Care Core Measure Set by the Joint Commission on Accreditation of Health Care Organizations (JCAHO) has led to their mandatory reporting. In 2012, California reported that any breastfeeding during hospitalization occurred at an average of 92.2% of healthy term infants. The CDC 2013 Breastfeeding Report Card found that 77% of new mothers breastfed their babies, up from 71% about a decade ago. In 2010, 49% of mothers were still breastfeeding when their child was 6 months of age, and 27% were still doing so when their child was 1 year of age. In 2000, rates were 35% and 16%, respectively. From 2007 to 2011, the percentage of facilities with at least 90% of infants receiving skin-to-skin contact after vaginal birth increased from 40.8% to 54.4%, and the percentage of facilities with at least 90% of mothers and babies staying together in the same room throughout the stay increased from 30.8% to 37.1%.

The growth of the BFHI worldwide has expanded to include more than 16,000 institutions (www.who.int/nutrition/topics/bfhi/en/), and this initiative has been shown to improve the establishment of exclusive breastfeeding. In the United States as of 2014, there are 175 hospitals in 41 states that have the BFHI designation. This represents an increase from 2.9% to 6.9% of births occurring in a Baby Friendly status.

Healthy People 2020 is a national program introduced by the U.S. Department of Health and Human Services that provides science-based, 10-year national objectives for improving the health of all Americans (www.healthypeople.gov). It has set a reachable target of 8.1% of births taking place in a Baby Friendly hospital by 2020.

Within the United States, a variety of demographic patterns appear to be associated with breastfeeding behavior. Older mothers, mothers with a college education, and higher-income mothers all are more likely to breastfeed. By contrast, black and Hispanic mothers, mothers of lower socioeconomic status who are participants in the Women, Infants, and Children (WIC) program of the U.S. Department of Health and Human Services and mothers who live in the southern regions of the United States are much less likely to breastfeed. The low rate of breastfeeding for mothers enrolled in WIC is of particular concern because that agency has a specific policy to encourage breastfeeding. Approximately half of all mothers of infants born in the United States receive services through the WIC. In 2009, a new program called Special Supplemental Nutrition Program was introduced by WIC to encourage more breastfeeding by including greater food packages for those mothers who continue to breastfeed. Some data would suggest that these programs are associated with improved breastfeeding success.[335] Many states continue to depend on formula manufacturer rebates to fund part of their WIC programs, creating an apparent conflict of interest. The disturbing part of the demographic pattern of breastfeeding in the United States is that the infants of lower socioeconomic status mothers, who would accrue the greatest health and economic benefits from breastfeeding, are those least likely to be breastfed.[336,337]

Although demographic studies indicate who is breastfeeding, they do not explain the behavioral differences among groups of mothers. One of the more complete models designed to explain breastfeeding behavior includes components that address maternal attitudes and family, societal, cultural, and environmental variables.[338] Individual studies have shown that the maternal decision-making process is closely related to the social support and influence that come from the family members surrounding the mother.[339] The husband, in particular, appears to have a strong positive influence, whereas the mother's mother may have a negative influence on the breastfeeding decision. Social support appears to be different among ethnic groups, as are maternal attitudes; such differences may provide one explanation for differences in breastfeeding behavior among ethnic groups.[340,341]

Summary and Conclusions

Human milk contains a wide variety of soluble and cellular components with a diverse spectrum of biologic functions. The major milk components identified to date exhibit antimicrobial, antiinflammatory, proinflammatory, and/or immunoregulatory functions; cytotoxicity for tumor cells; ability to mature and repair tissue damage; and receptor analogue functions, as well as other metabolic effects. The biologic activities of different milk components are summarized in Table 5-4.

The major antimicrobial effects of human milk are associated with milk immunoglobulin, especially the sIgA isotype, which makes up to 80% of all immunoglobulins in the human body (see Figure 5-1 and Table 5-2). Milk antibodies appear to provide protection against many intestinal pathogens, such as *Campylobacter, Shigella, E. coli, V. cholerae, Giardia,* and rotavirus, and against respiratory pathogens such as respiratory syncytial virus. Milk antibodies also effectively neutralize toxins and a variety of human viruses. The role of small amounts of IgG and IgM in milk is uncertain. Lactoferrin, lysozyme, α-lactalbumin, and other milk proteins,

Table 5-4 Possible Role of Soluble and Cellular Factors Identified in Human Milk

Factor	Antimicrobial	Antiinflammatory	Proinflammatory	Immunoregulatory	Other
Immunoglobulin (sIgA)	+++	++		++	++
Other immunoglobulins	+++	+	++	+	
PMNs, macrophages	++		+	++	
Lactoferrin	+++	+++			
α-Lactalbumin		++			
CARBOHYDRATES					
Oligosaccharides	++	++			++
Glycoconjugates	++	++			++
Glycolipids					
Lipid and fat globules	++				
NUCLEOTIDES	+			++	++
Defensins	+			+	
Lysozymes	±				
CYTOKINES, CHEMOKINES					
TGF-β		++	++	++	++
IL-10		++	++	++	
IL-1			++	++	
TNF-α			++		
IL-6			++		
IL-7					++
Prostaglandins		++	++		
Leptin				++	++
Antiproteases		++			
Other growth factors		++		++	
sTLR2, sCD14		+++		++	

+ to +++, Minimal-to-moderate effect; *–*, no effect; *IL*, interleukin; *PMNs*, polymorphonuclear neutrophils (leukocytes); *sCD14*, soluble CD14 (protein marker); *sIgA*, secretory immunoglobulin A; *TGF-β*, transforming growth factor-β; *sTLR2*, soluble Toll-like receptor 2; *TNF-α*, tumor necrosis factor-α.

along with lipids, also contribute to the antimicrobial and immunomodulatory properties of human milk. Milk carbohydrates, particularly milk oligosaccharides, assist in modulating the microbial milieu of the infant's gut, acting largely as complex and diverse prebiotics. Milk also contains large numbers of cytokines, chemokines, growth factors, soluble Toll-like receptors, and CD14, which may modulate inflammatory and immunologic responses in the gut, although this remains to be clearly established. Polymorphonuclear neutrophils, macrophages, lymphocytes, and epithelial cells are observed in human milk, but their functions in milk are unknown; it is possible that their primary task is the antimicrobial defense of the mammary gland itself.

The passive transfer of the diversity of maternal biologic experiences to the neonate through the process of breastfeeding represents an essential component of the survival mechanism in the mammalian neonate. For millions of years, maternal products of lactation delivered through breastfeeding have been the sole source of nutrition and immunity during the neonatal and early infancy period for all mammals, including the human infant. During the past few centuries, however, human societies have undergone remarkable changes that have had a major impact on basic maternal-infant interaction, breastfeeding, and on our environment. Such changes include introduction of sanitation and nonhuman milk and formula feeds for neonatal nutrition, use of antimicrobial agents, introduction of processed foods, and exposure to newer environmental macromolecules and dietary antigens. These changes have had a profound impact on human homeostatic mechanisms that, at the same time, are opening up new insights into the importance of breastfeeding in the developing human neonate.

Comparative analysis of natural (traditional) forms of breastfeeding and artificial feeding modalities has demonstrated clearly that natural breastfeeding is associated with significant reduction in infant mortality and morbidity, protection against acute infectious diseases, and possible protection against allergic disorders and autoimmune disease; acute and chronic inflammatory disorders; obesity, diabetes mellitus, and other metabolic disorders; and development of certain malignancies later in life. This information has been reviewed by Hanson[342] in an elegant monograph and by others.[207] Despite the overwhelmingly protective role attributed to natural breastfeeding and the evolutionary advantages related to the development of lactation, several infectious agents have acquired, during the course of evolution, the ability to evade immunologic factors in milk and to use milk as the vehicle for maternal-to-infant transmission. The potential for the acquisition of infections such as those due to HIV, HTLV-1, HTLV-2, CMV, and possibly other pathogens highlights potential hazards of breastfeeding in some clinical situations. Nevertheless, we conclude that the development of lactation, a hallmark of mammalian evolution, is designed to enhance the survival of the neonate of the species through a remarkable spectrum of immediate and long-term protective functions.

References

1. Black RE, Allen LH, Bhutta ZA, et al: Maternal and child undernutrition: global and regional exposures and health consequences, *Lancet* 371:243-260, 2008.
2. Chen A, Rogan WJ: Breastfeeding and the risk of postneonatal death in the United States, *Pediatrics* 113:e435-e439, 2004.
3. Breastfeeding and the use of human milk, *Pediatrics* 129:e827-e841, 2012.
4. Sakakura T, Suzuki Y, Shiurba R: Mammary stroma in development and carcinogenesis, *J Mammary Gland Biol Neoplasia* 18: 189-197, 2013.
5. Macias H, Hinck L: Mammary gland development, *Wiley Interdiscip Rev Dev Biol* 1:533-557, 2012.
6. Kratochwil K: *Experimental analysis of the prenatal development of the mammary gland*, vol. 15. Basel, 1975, S. Karger.
7. Vorherr H: *The breast: morphology, physiology and lactation*, New York, 1974, Academic Press.
8. Goldman AS, Shapiro B, Neumann F: Role of testosterone and its metabolites in the differentiation of the mammary gland in rats, *Endocrinology* 99:1490-1495, 1976.
9. Kleinberg DL, Niemann W, Flamm E: Primate mammary development: effects of hypophysectomy, prolactin inhibition, and growth hormone administration, *J Clin Invest* 75:1943-1950, 1985.
10. Ogra SS, Ogra PL: *Components of immunologic reactivity in human colostrum and milk*, New York, 1979, Raven Press.
11. Pasteels JL: Control of mammary growth and lactation by the anterior pituitary: an attempt to correlate classic experiments on animals with recent clinical findings. In Kretchmern N, Rossi E, Sereni F, editors: *Milk and lactation, modern problems in paediatrics*, vol. 15, Basel, 1975, S. Karger.
12. Mepham TB: *Physiology of lactation*, Milton Keynes, England, 1987, Open University Press.
13. Frantz AG: Prolactin, *N Engl J Med* 298:201-207, 1978.
14. Cavaletto M, Giuffrida MG, Conti A: Milk fat globule membrane components–a proteomic approach, *Adv Exp Med Biol* 606:129-141, 2008.
15. Dizdar EA, Sari FN, Degirmencioglu H, et al: Effect of mode of delivery on macronutrient content of breast milk, *J Matern Fetal Neonatal Med* 27:1099-1102, 2014.
16. Gao YX, Zhang J, Wang C, et al: The fatty acid composition of colostrum in three geographic regions of China, *Asia Pac J Clin Nutr* 22:276-282, 2013.
17. Fidler N, Koletzko B: The fatty acid composition of human colostrum, *Eur J Nutr* 39:31-37, 2000.
18. Hausman Kedem M, Mandel D, Domani KA, et al: The effect of dvanced maternal age upon human milk fat content, *Breastfeed Med* 8:116-119, 2013.
19. Widström AM, Ransjo-Arvisson AB, Christensson K, et al: Gastric suction in healthy newborn infants, *Acta Paediatr Scand* 76: 566-572, 1987.
20. Varendi H, Porter RH, Winberg J: Does the newborn baby find the nipple by smell? *Lancet* 344:989-990, 1994.
21. Flaherman VJ, Aby J, Burgos AE, et al: Effect of early limited formula on duration and exclusivity of breastfeeding in at-risk infants: an RCT, *Pediatrics* 131:1059-1065, 2013.
22. do Carmo Franca-Botelho A, Ferreira MC, Franca JL, et al: Breastfeeding and its relationship with reduction of breast cancer: a review, *Asian Pac J Cancer Prev* 13:5327-5332, 2012.
23. Stuebe A: The risks of not breastfeeding for mothers and infants, *Rev Obstet Gynecol* 2:222-231, 2009.
24. Lönnerdal B, Forsum E, Hambraeus L: The protein content of human milk. I. A transversal study of Swedish normal mothers, *Nutr Rep Int* 13:125-134, 1976.
25. Schanler RJ, Oh W: Composition of breast milk obtained from mothers of premature infants as compared to breast milk obtained from donors, *J Pediatr* 96:679-681, 1980.
26. Sann L, Bienvenu F, Lahet C: Comparison of the composition of breast milk from mothers of term and preterm infants, *Acta Paediatr Scand* 70:115-116, 1981.
27. Bauer J, Gerss J: Longitudinal analysis of macronutrients and minerals in human milk produced by mothers of preterm infants, *Clin Nutr* 30:215-220, 2011.
28. Saarela T, Kokkonen J, Koivisto M: Macronutrient and energy contents of human milk fractions during the first six months of lactation, *Acta Paediatrica* 94:1176-1181, 2005.
29. Nommsen LA, Lovelady CA, Heinig MJ, Lonnerdal B, Dewey KG: Determinants of energy, protein, lipid, and lactose concentrations in human milk during the first 12 mo of lactation: the DARLING Study, *Am J Clin Nutr* 53:457-465, 1991.
30. Lönnerdal B: Nutritional and physiologic significance of human milk proteins, *Am J Clin Nutr* 77:1537S-1543S, 2003.

31. Kunz C, Lönnerdal B: Re-evaluation of the whey protein/casein ratio of human milk, *Acta Paediatr* 81:107-112, 1992.
32. Patton S, Huston GE: A method for isolation of milk fat globules, *Lipids* 21:170-174, 1986.
33. Hambraeus L: Proprietary milk versus human breast milk in infant feeding. A critical appraisal from the nutritional point of view, *Pediatr Clin North Am* 24:17-36, 1977.
34. Phillippy BO, McCarthy RD: Multi-origins of milk serum albumin in the lactating goat, *Biochim Biophys Acta* 584:298-303, 1979.
35. Spik G, Brunet B, Mazunier-Dehaine C, et al: Characterization and properties of the human and bovine lactoferrins extracted from the faeces of newborn infants, *Acta Paediatr Scand* 71:979-985, 1982.
36. Saarinen UM, Siimes MA, Dallman PR: Iron absorption in infants: high bioavailability of breast milk iron as indicated by extrinsic tag method of iron absorption and by the concentration of serum ferritin, *J Pediatr* 91:36-39, 1977.
37. Wakabayashi H, Yamauchi K, Takase M: Inhibitory effects of bovine lactoferrin and lactoferricin B on Enterobacter sakazakii, *Biocontrol Sci* 13:29-32, 2008.
38. Arnold RR, Brewer M, Gauthier JJ: Bactericidal activity of human lactoferrin: sensitivity of a variety of microorganisms, *Infect Immun* 28:893-898, 1980.
39. Pammi M, Abrams SA: Oral lactoferrin for the treatment of sepsis and necrotizing enterocolitis in neonates, *Cochrane Database Syst Rev* (10):CD007138, 2011.
40. Sherman MP, Miller MM, Sherman J, Niklas V: Lactoferrin and necrotizing enterocolitis, *Curr Opin Pediatr* 26:146-150, 2014.
41. Trugo NM, Newport MJ: Vitamin B12 absorption in the neonatal piglet. 2. Resistance of the vitamin B12-binding protein in sows' milk to proteolysis in vivo, *Br J Nutr* 54:257-267, 1985.
42. Oberkotter LV, Tenore A, Pasquariello PS, Zavod W: A thyroxine-binding protein in human breast milk similar to serum thyroxine-binding globulin, *J Clin Endocrinol Metab* 57:1133-1139, 1983.
43. Payne DW, Peng LH, Pearlman WH: Corticosteroid-binding proteins in human colostrum and milk and rat milk, *J Biol Chem* 251:5272-5279, 1976.
44. Blanc B: Biochemical aspects of human milk—comparison with bovine milk, *World Rev Nutr Diet* 36:1-89, 1981.
45. Ibrahim HR, Imazato K, Ono H: Human lysozyme possesses novel antimicrobial peptides within its N-terminal domain that target bacterial respiration, *J Agric Food Chem* 59:10336-10345, 2011.
46. Lindquist S, Hernell O: Lipid digestion and absorption in early life: an update, *Curr Opin Clin Nutr Metab Care* 13:314-320, 2010.
47. Andersson Y, Savman K, Blackberg L, Hernell O: Pasteurization of mother's own milk reduces fat absorption and growth in preterm infants, *Acta Paediatr* 96:1445-1449, 2007.
48. Lönnerdal B: Bioactive proteins in breast milk, *J Paediatr Child Health* 49(Suppl 1):1-7, 2013.
49. Dvorak B, Fituch CC, Williams CS, Hurst NM, Schanler RJ: Increased epidermal growth factor levels in human milk of mothers with extremely premature infants, *Pediatr Res* 54:15-19, 2003.
50. Dvorak B, Fituch CC, Williams CS, Hurst NM, Schanler RJ: Concentrations of epidermal growth factor and transforming growth factor-alpha in preterm milk, *Adv Exp Med Biol* 554:407-409, 2004.
51. Blum JW, Baumrucker CR: Colostral and milk insulin-like growth factors and related substances: mammary gland and neonatal (intestinal and systemic) targets, *Domest Anim Endocrinol* 23(1-2): 101-110, 2002.
52. Burrin DG: Is milk-borne insulin-like growth factor-I essential for neonatal development? *J Nutr* 127(Suppl 5):975S-979S, 1997.
53. Philipps AF, Kling PJ, Grille JG, Dvorak B: Intestinal transport of insulin-like growth factor-I (igf-I) in the suckling rat, *J Pediatr Gastroenterol Nutr* 35:539-544, 2002.
54. Buyukkayhan D, Tanzer F, Erselcan T, Cinar Z, Yonem O: Umbilical serum insulin-like growth factor 1 (IGF-1) in newborns: effects of gestational age, postnatal age, and nutrition, *Int J Vitam Nutr Res* 73:343-346, 2003.
55. Loui A, Eilers E, Strauss E, et al: Vascular endothelial growth factor (VEGF) and soluble VEGF receptor 1 (sFlt-1) levels in early and mature human milk from mothers of preterm versus term infants, *J Hum Lact* 28:522-528, 2012.
56. Penttila I: Effects of transforming growth factor-beta and formula feeding on systemic immune responses to dietary beta-lactoglobulin in allergy-prone rats, *Pediatr Res* 59:650-655, 2006.
57. Penttila IA: Milk-derived transforming growth factor-beta and the infant immune response, *J Pediatr* 156(Suppl 2):S21-S25, 2010.
58. Struck J, de Almeida P, Bergmann A, Morgenthaler NG: High concentrations of procalcitonin but not mature calcitonin in normal human milk, *Horm Metab Res* 34:460-465, 2002.
59. Fichter M, Klotz M, Hirschberg DL, et al: Breast milk contains relevant neurotrophic factors and cytokines for enteric nervous system development, *Mol Nutr Food Res* 55:1592-1596, 2011.
60. Martin LJ, Woo JG, Geraghty SR, et al: Adiponectin is present in human milk and is associated with maternal factors, *Am J Clin Nutr* 83:1106-1111, 2006.
61. Woo JG, Guerrero ML, Altaye M, et al: Human milk adiponectin is associated with infant growth in two independent cohorts, *Breastfeed Med* 4:101-109, 2009.
62. Woo JG, Guerrero ML, Guo F, et al: Human milk adiponectin affects infant weight trajectory during the second year of life, *J Pediatr Gastroenterol Nutr* 54:532-539, 2012.
63. Savino F, Sorrenti M, Benetti S, et al: Resistin and leptin in breast milk and infants in early life, *Early Hum Dev* 88:779-782, 2012.
64. Johansen FE, Braathen R, Brandtzaeg P: The J chain is essential for polymeric Ig receptor-mediated epithelial transport of IgA, *J Immunol* 167:5185-5192, 2001.
65. Ogra SS, Ogra PL: Immunologic aspects of human colostrum and milk. I. Distribution characteristics and concentrations of immunoglobulins at different times after the onset of lactation, *J Pediatr* 92:546-549, 1978.
66. McClelland DBL, McGrath J, Samson RR: Antimicrobial factors in human milk: studies of concentration and transfer to the infant during the early stages of lactation, *Acta Paediatr Scand Suppl* 271:1-20, 1978.
67. Kliegman RM, Pittard WB, Fanaroff AA: Necrotizing enterocolitis in neonates fed human milk, *J Pediatr* 95:450-453, 1979.
68. Ogra SS, Weintraub D, Ogra PL: Immunologic aspects of human colostrum and milk. III. Fate and absorption of cellular and soluble components in the gastrointestinal tract of the newborn, *J Immunol* 119:245-248, 1977.
69. Kenny JF, Boesman MI, Michaels RH: Bacterial and viral coproantibodies in breast-fed infants, *Pediatrics* 39:201-213, 1967.
70. Haneberg B: Immunoglobulins in feces from infants fed human or bovine milk, *Scand J Immunol* 3:191-197, 1974.
71. Weemaes C, Klasen I, Goertz J, et al: Development of immunoglobulin A in infancy and childhood, *Scand J Immunol* 58:642-648, 2003.
72. Prentice A, Ewing G, Roberts SB, et al: The nutritional role of breast-milk IgA and lactoferrin, *Acta Paediatr Scand* 76:592-598, 1987.
73. Goldblum RM, Ahlatedt S, Carlson B, et al: Antibody forming cells in human colostrum after oral immunization, *Nature* 257:797-799, 1975.
74. Fishaut JM, Murphy D, Neifert M, et al: The broncho-mammary axis in the immune response to respiratory syncytial virus, *J Pediatr* 99:186-191, 1981.
75. Orskov F, Sorenson KB: *Escherichia coli* serogroups in breast-fed and bottle-fed infants, *Acta Pathol Microbiol Scand B* 83:25-30, 1975.
76. van Genderen J: Diphtheria-antitoxin in Kolostrum und Muttermilch bei Menschen, *Z Immunutaetsforsch Allerg Klin Immunol* 83: 54-59, 1934.
77. Montgomery PC, Rosner BR, Cohn J, et al: The secretory antibody response: anti-DNP antibodies induced by dinitrophenylated type III pneumococcus, *Immunol Commun* 3:143-156, 1974.
78. Duerkop BA, Vaishnava S, Hooper LV: Immune responses to the microbiota at the intestinal mucosal surface, *Immunity* 31: 368-376, 2009.
79. Renz H, Brandtzaeg P, Hornef M: The impact of perinatal immune development on mucosal homeostasis and chronic inflammation, *Nat Rev Immunol* 12:9-23, 2012.
80. McClelland DBL, Samson RR, Parkin DM, et al: Bacterial agglutination studies with secretory IgA prepared from human gastrointestinal secretions and colostrum, *Gut* 13:450-458, 1972.
81. Stoliar OA, Pelley RP, Kaniecki-Green E, et al: Secretory IgA against enterotoxins in breast milk, *Lancet* 1:1258-1261, 1976.
82. Steele EJ, Chicumpa W, Rowley D: Isolation and biological properties of three classes of rabbit antibody in *Vibrio cholerae*, *J Infect Dis* 130:93-103, 1974.
83. Cantey JR: Prevention of bacterial infections of mucosal surfaces of immune secretory IgA, *Adv Exp Med Biol* 107:461-470, 1978.
84. Pittard III BK: Differentiation of cord blood lymphocytes into IgA-producing cells in response to breast milk stimulatory factor, *Clin Immunol Immunopathol* 13:430-434, 1979.
85. Juto P: Human milk stimulates B cell function, *Arch Dis Child* 60: 610-613, 1985.

86. Julius MH, Janusz M, Lisowski J: A colostral protein that induces the growth and differentiation of resting B lymphocytes, *J Immunol* 140:1366-1371, 1988.
87. Soder O: Isolation of interleukin-1 from human milk, *Int Arch Allergy Appl Immunol* 83:19-23, 1987.
88. Hooton JW, Pabst HF, Spady DW, et al: Human colostrum contains an activity that inhibits the production of IL-2, *Clin Exp Immunol* 86:520-524, 1991.
89. Sarfati M, Vanderbeeken Y, Rubio-Trujillo M, et al: Presence of IgE suppressor factors in human colostrum, *Eur J Immunol* 16: 1005-1008, 1986.
90. Munoz C, Endres S, van der Meer J, et al: Interleukin-1 beta in human colostrum, *Res Immunol* 141:501-513, 1990.
91. Rudloff HE, Schmalstieg FC, Mushtaha AA, et al: Tumor necrosis factor-α in human milk, *Pediatr Res* 31:29-33, 1992.
92. Buescher ES, Malinowska I: Soluble receptors and cytokine antagonists in human milk, *Pediatr Res* 40:839-844, 1996.
93. Skansen-Saphir U, Linfors A, Andersson U: Cytokine production in mononuclear cells of human milk studied at the single-cell level, *Pediatr Res* 34:213-216, 1993.
94. Basolo F, Conaldi PG, Fiore L, et al: Normal breast epithelial cells produce interleukins-6 and 8 together with tumor-necrosis factor: defective IL-6 expression in mammary carcinoma, *Int J Cancer* 55:926-930, 1993.
95. Saito S, Manuyama M, Kato Y, et al: Detection of IL-6 in human milk and its involvement in IgA production, *J Reprod Immunol* 20: 267-276, 1991.
96. Rudloff HE, Schmalstieg FC, Palkowetz KH, et al: Interleukin-6 in human milk, *J Reprod Immunol* 23:13-20, 1993.
97. Bocci V, von Bremen K, Corradeschi F, et al: Presence of interferon-α and interleukin-6 in colostrum of normal women, *Lymphokine Cytok Res* 12:21-24, 1993.
98. Srivastava MD, Srivastava A, Brouhard B, et al: Cytokines in human milk, *Res Commun Mol Pathol Pharmacol* 93:263-287, 1996.
99. Eglinton BA, Roberton DM, Cummins AG: Phenotype of T cells, their soluble receptor levels, and cytokine profile of human breast milk, *Immunol Cell Biol* 72:306-313, 1994.
100. Bottcher MF, Jenmalm MC, Bjorksten B: Cytokine, chemokine and secretory IgA levels in human milk in relation to atopic disease and IgA production in infants, *Pediatr Allergy Immunol* 14:35-41, 2003.
101. Groer MW, Shelton MM: Exercise is associated with elevated proinflammatory cytokines in human milk, *J Obstet Gynecol Neonatal Nurs* 38:35-41, 2009.
102. Takahata Y, Takada H, Nomura A, et al: Detection of interferon-gamma-inducible chemokines in human milk, *Acta Paediatr* 92:659-665, 2003.
103. Garofalo RP, Goldman AS: Expression of functional immunomodulatory and anti-inflammatory factors in human milk, *Clin Perinatol* 26:361-377, 1999.
104. Hasselbalch H, Jeppesen DL, Engelmann MD, Michaelsen KF, Nielsen MB: Decreased thymus size in formula-fed infants compared with breastfed infants, *Acta Paediatr* 85:1029-1032, 1996.
105. Ngom PT, Collinson AC, Pido-Lopez J, et al: Improved thymic function in exclusively breastfed infants is associated with higher interleukin 7 concentrations in their mothers' breast milk, *Am J Clin Nutr* 80:722-728, 2004.
106. Korhonen H, Pihlanto A: Food-derived bioactive peptides—opportunities for designing future foods, *Curr Pharm Des* 9:1297-1308, 2003.
107. Pihlanto A, Korhonen H: Bioactive peptides and proteins, *Adv Food Nutr Res* 47:175-276, 2003.
108. Mellander O: The physiological importance of the casein phosphopeptide calcium salts. II. Peroral calcium dosage of infants, *Acta Soc Med Ups* 55(5-6):247-255, 1950.
109. Ferranti P, Traisci MV, Picariello G, et al: Casein proteolysis in human milk: tracing the pattern of casein breakdown and the formation of potential bioactive peptides, *J Dairy Res* 71:74-87, 2004.
110. Bezkorovainy A, Topouzian N: *Bifidobacterium bifidus* var. Pennsylvanicus growth promoting activity of human milk casein and its derivatives, *Int J Biochem* 13:585-590, 1981.
111. Smith MI, Yatsunenko T, Manary MJ, et al: Gut microbiomes of Malawian twin pairs discordant for kwashiorkor, *Science* 339: 548-554, 2013.
112. Boren T, Falk P, Roth KA, Larson G, Normark S: Attachment of *Helicobacter pylori* to human gastric epithelium mediated by blood group antigens, *Science* 262:1892-1895, 1993.
113. Falk P, Roth KA, Boren T, et al: An in vitro adherence assay reveals that *Helicobacter pylori* exhibits cell lineage-specific tropism in the human gastric epithelium, *Proc Natl Acad Sci U S A* 90:2035-2039, 1993.
114. Bruck WM, Kelleher SL, Gibson GR, et al: The effects of alpha-lactalbumin and glycomacropeptide on the association of CaCo-2 cells by enteropathogenic *Escherichia coli, Salmonella typhimurium* and *Shigella flexneri, FEMS Microbiol Lett* 259:158-162, 2006.
115. Tomita M, Bellamy W, Takase M, et al: Potent antibacterial peptides generated by pepsin digestion of bovine lactoferrin, *J Dairy Sci* 74:4137-4142, 1991.
116. Järvenpää AL, Räihä NCR, Rassin DK, et al: Milk protein quantity and quality in the term infant. II. Effects on acidic and neutral amino acids, *Pediatrics* 70:221-230, 1982.
117. Novak M, Wieser PB, Buch M, et al: Acetyl-carnitine and free carnitine in body fluids before and after birth, *Pediatr Res* 13:10-15, 1979.
118. Gross SJ, Geller J, Tomarelli RM: Composition of breast milk from mothers of preterm infants, *Pediatrics* 68:490-493, 1981.
119. Rassin DK, Räihä NCR, Gaull GE: *Protein and taurine nutrition in infants*, New York, 1981, Raven Press.
120. Schmidt-Sommerfeld E, Novak M, Penn D, et al: Carnitine and development of newborn adipose tissue, *Pediatr Res* 12:660-664, 1978.
121. Maldonado J, Navarro J, Narbona E, Gil A: The influence of dietary nucleotides on humoral and cell immunity in the neonate and lactating infant, *Early Hum Dev* 65(Suppl):S69-S74, 2001.
122. Newburg DS, Walker WA: Protection of the neonate by the innate immune system of developing gut and of human milk, *Pediatr Res* 61:2-8, 2007.
123. Carver JD: Dietary nucleotides: effects on the immune and gastrointestinal systems, *Acta Paediatr Suppl* 88:83-88, 1999.
124. Liao KY, Wu TC, Huang CF, et al: Profile of nucleotides and nucleosides in Taiwanese human milk, *Pediatr Neonatol* 52:93-97, 2011.
125. Uauy R, Quan R, Gil A: Role of nucleotides in intestinal development and repair: implications for infant nutrition, *J Nutr* 124(Suppl 8):1436S-1441S, 1994.
126. Singhal A, Kennedy K, Lanigan J, et al: Dietary nucleotides and early growth in formula-fed infants: a randomized controlled trial, *Pediatrics* 126:e946-e953, 2010.
127. Singhal A, Macfarlane G, Macfarlane S, et al: Dietary nucleotides and fecal microbiota in formula-fed infants: a randomized controlled trial, *Am J Clin Nutr* 87:1785-1792, 2008.
128. Cosgrove M, Davies DP, Jenkins HR: Nucleotide supplementation and the growth of term small for gestational age infants, *Arch Dis Child Fetal Neonatal Ed* 74:F122-F125, 1996.
129. Jensen RG, Ferris AM, Lammi-Keefe CJ: Lipids in human milk and infant formulas, *Annu Rev Nutr* 12:417-441, 1992.
130. Mitoulas LR, Kent JC, Cox DB, et al: Variation in fat, lactose and protein in human milk over 24 h and throughout the first year of lactation, *Br J Nutr* 88:29-37, 2002.
131. Molto-Puigmarti C, Castellote AI, Carbonell-Estrany X, Lopez-Sabater MC: Differences in fat content and fatty acid proportions among colostrum, transitional, and mature milk from women delivering very preterm, preterm, and term infants, *Clin Nutr* 30:116-123, 2011.
132. Sabel KG, Strandvik B, Petzold M, Lundqvist-Persson C: Motor, mental and behavioral developments in infancy are associated with fatty acid pattern in breast milk and plasma of premature infants, *Prostaglandins Leukot Essent Fatty Acids* 86(4-5):183-188, 2012.
133. Clandinin MT, Chappell JE, Leong S, et al: Intrauterine fatty acid accretion rates in human brain: implications for fatty acid requirements, *Early Hum Dev* 4:121-129, 1980.
134. Kuipers RS, Luxwolda MF, Offringa PJ, et al: Fetal intrauterine whole body linoleic, arachidonic and docosahexaenoic acid contents and accretion rates, *Prostaglandins Leukot Essent Fatty Acids* 86(1-2):13-20, 2012.
135. Lauritzen L, Hansen HS, Jorgensen MH, Michaelsen KF: The essentiality of long chain n-3 fatty acids in relation to development and function of the brain and retina, *Prog Lipid Res* 40(1-2):1-94, 2001.
136. Simmer K, Patole S: Long-chain polyunsaturated fatty acid supplementation in preterm infants, *Cochrane Database Syst Rev* (1): CD000375, 2004.
137. Simmer K, Patole SK, Rao SC: Long-chain polyunsaturated fatty acid supplementation in infants born at term, *Cochrane Database Syst Rev* (12):CD000376, 2011.
138. Schulzke SM, Patole SK, Simmer K: Long-chain polyunsaturated fatty acid supplementation in preterm infants, *Cochrane Database Syst Rev* (2):CD000375, 2011.

139. Lapillonne A, Groh-Wargo S, Gonzalez CH, Uauy R: Lipid needs of preterm infants: updated recommendations, *J Pediatr* 162(Suppl 3):S37-S47, 2013.
140. Qawasmi A, Landeros-Weisenberger A, Bloch MH: Meta-analysis of LCPUFA supplementation of infant formula and visual acuity, *Pediatrics* 131:e262-e272, 2013.
141. Willatts P, Forsyth S, Agostoni C, et al: Effects of long-chain PUFA supplementation in infant formula on cognitive function in later childhood, *Am J Clin Nutr* 98:536S-542S, 2013.
142. Ontsouka EC, Albrecht C: Cholesterol transport and regulation in the mammary gland, *J Mammary Gland Biol Neoplasia* 19:43-58, 2014.
143. Rudnicka AR, Owen CG, Strachan DP: The effect of breastfeeding on cardiorespiratory risk factors in adult life, *Pediatrics* 119: e1107-e1115, 2007.
144. Owen CG, Whincup PH, Kaye SJ, et al: Does initial breastfeeding lead to lower blood cholesterol in adult life? A quantitative review of the evidence, *Am J Clin Nutr* 88:305-314, 2008.
145. Moser HW, Karnovsky ML: Studies on the biosynthesis of glycolipids and other lipids of the brain, *J Biol Chem* 234:1990-1997, 1959.
146. Kliegman RM, Miettinen EL, Morton S: Potential role of galactokinase in neonatal carbohydrate assimilation, *Science* 220:302-304, 1983.
147. Kunz C, Rudloff S, Baier W, Klein N, Strobel S: Oligosaccharides in human milk: structural, functional, and metabolic aspects, *Annu Rev Nutr* 20:699-722, 2000.
148. Newburg DS, Ruiz-Palacios GM, Morrow AL: Human milk glycans protect infants against enteric pathogens, *Annu Rev Nutr* 25:37-58, 2005.
149. German JB, Freeman SL, Lebrilla CB, Mills DA: Human milk oligosaccharides: evolution, structures and bioselectivity as substrates for intestinal bacteria, *Nestle Nutr Workshop Ser Paediatr Program* 62:205-218, 2008; discussion 218–222.
150. Bode L: Human milk oligosaccharides: every baby needs a sugar mama, *Glycobiology* 22:1147-1162, 2012.
151. Gnoth MJ, Rudloff S, Kunz C, Kinne RK: Investigations of the in vitro transport of human milk oligosaccharides by a Caco-2 monolayer using a novel high performance liquid chromatography-mass spectrometry technique, *J Biol Chem* 276:34363-34370, 2001.
152. Engfer MB, Stahl B, Finke B, Sawatzki G, Daniel H: Human milk oligosaccharides are resistant to enzymatic hydrolysis in the upper gastrointestinal tract, *Am J Clin Nutr* 71:1589-1596, 2000.
153. Rudloff S, Obermeier S, Borsch C, et al: Incorporation of orally applied (13)C-galactose into milk lactose and oligosaccharides, *Glycobiology* 16:477-487, 2006.
154. Rudloff S, Pohlentz G, Borsch C, Lentze MJ, Kunz C: Urinary excretion of in vivo ^{13}C-labelled milk oligosaccharides in breastfed infants, *Br J Nutr* 107:957-963, 2012.
155. Rudloff S, Pohlentz G, Diekmann L, Egge H, Kunz C: Urinary excretion of lactose and oligosaccharides in preterm infants fed human milk or infant formula, *Acta Paediatr* 85:598-603, 1996.
156. Chichlowski M, German JB, Lebrilla CB, Mills DA: The influence of milk oligosaccharides on microbiota of infants: opportunities for formulas, *Annu Rev Food Sci Technol* 2:331-351, 2011.
157. LoCascio RG, Ninonuevo MR, Freeman SL, et al: Glycoprofiling of bifidobacterial consumption of human milk oligosaccharides demonstrates strain specific, preferential consumption of small chain glycans secreted in early human lactation, *J Agric Food Chem* 55:8914-8919, 2007.
158. Sela DA, Chapman J, Adeuya A, et al: The genome sequence of *Bifidobacterium longum* subsp. *infantis* reveals adaptations for milk utilization within the infant microbiome, *Proc Natl Acad Sci U S A* 105:18964-18969, 2008.
159. Marcobal A, Barboza M, Froehlich JW, et al: Consumption of human milk oligosaccharides by gut-related microbes, *J Agric Food Chem* 58:5334-5340, 2010.
160. Marcobal A, Barboza M, Sonnenburg ED, et al: *Bacteroides* in the infant gut consume milk oligosaccharides via mucus-utilization pathways, *Cell Host Microbe* 10:507-514, 2011.
161. Asakuma S, Hatakeyama E, Urashima T, et al: Physiology of consumption of human milk oligosaccharides by infant gut-associated bifidobacteria, *J Biol Chem* 286:34583-34592, 2011.
162. Ruiz-Palacios GM, Cervantes LE, Ramos P, Chavez-Munguia B, Newburg DS: *Campylobacter jejuni* binds intestinal H(O) antigen (Fuc alpha 1, 2Gal beta 1, 4GlcNAc), and fucosyloligosaccharides of human milk inhibit its binding and infection, *J Biol Chem* 278:14112-14120, 2003.
163. Morrow AL, Ruiz-Palacios GM, Altaye M, et al: Human milk oligosaccharides are associated with protection against diarrhea in breast-fed infants, *J Pediatr* 145:297-303, 2004.
164. Jantscher-Krenn E, Lauwaet T, Bliss LA, et al: Human milk oligosaccharides reduce *Entamoeba histolytica* attachment and cytotoxicity in vitro, *Br J Nutr* 28:1839-1846, 2012.
165. Manthey CF, Autran CA, Eckmann L, Bode L: Human milk oligosaccharides protect against enteropathogenic *E. coli* (EPEC) attachment in vitro and EPEC colonization in suckling mice, *J Pediatr Gastroenterol Nutr* 58:167-170, 2014.
166. Andersson B, Porras O, Hanson LA, et al: Inhibition of attachment of *Streptococcus pneumoniae* and *Haemophilus influenzae* by human milk and receptor oligosaccharides, *J Infect Dis* 153:232-237, 1986.
167. Hong P, Ninonuevo MR, Lee B, Lebrilla C, Bode L: Human milk oligosaccharides reduce HIV-1-gp120 binding to dendritic cell-specific ICAM3-grabbing non-integrin (DC-SIGN), *Br J Nutr* 101: 482-486, 2009.
168. Newburg DS, Viscidi RP, Ruff A, et al: A human milk factor inhibits binding of human immunodeficiency virus to the CD4 receptor, *Pediatr Res* 31:22-28, 1992.
169. Lin AE, Autran CA, Espanola SD, Bode L, Nizet V: Human milk oligosaccharides protect bladder epithelial cells against uropathogenic *Escherichia coli* invasion and cytotoxicity, *J Infect Dis* 209: 389-398, 2014.
170. O'Connor P: Vitamin D-deficiency rickets in two breast-fed infants who were not receiving vitamin D supplementation, *Clin Pediatr* 16:361-363, 1977.
171. Institute of Medicine: Dietary reference intakes for calcium and vitamin D. Washington, DC, 2011, The National Academies Press.
172. Abrams SA: Committee on Nutrition. Calcium and vitamin D requirements of enterally fed preterm infants, *Pediatrics* 131: e1676-e1683, 2013.
173. Anderson RR: Variations in major minerals of human milk during the first 5 months of lactation, *Nutr Res* 12:701-711, 1992.
174. McMillan JA, Oski FA, Louire G, et al: Iron absorption from human milk, simulated human milk, and proprietary formulas, *Pediatrics* 60:896-900, 1977.
175. Maru M, Birhanu T, Tessema DA: Calcium, magnesium, iron, zinc and copper, compositions of human milk from populations with cereal and 'enset' based diets, *Ethiop J Health Sci* 23:90-97, 2013.
176. Bode L, Kuhn L, Kim HY, et al: Human milk oligosaccharide concentration and risk of postnatal transmission of HIV through breastfeeding, *Am J Clin Nutr* 96:831-839, 2012.
177. Hassiotou F, Geddes DT, Hartmann PE: Cells in human milk: state of the science, *J Hum Lact* 29:171-182, 2013.
178. Hassiotou F, Geddes D: Anatomy of the human mammary gland: current status of knowledge, *Clin Anat* 26:29-48, 2013.
179. Brooker BE: The epithelial cells and cell fragments in human milk, *Cell Tissue Res* 210:321-332, 1980.
180. Goldman AS, Goldblum RM: Transfer of maternal leukocytes to the infant by human milk, *Curr Top Microbiol Immunol* 222:205-213, 1997.
181. Xanthou M: Immune protection of human milk, *Biol Neonate* 74:121-133, 1998.
182. Smith CW, Goldman AS: The cells of human colostrum. I. In vitro studies of morphology and functions, *Pediatr Res* 2:103-109, 1968.
183. Smith CW, Goldman AS: Interactions of lymphocytes and macrophages from human colostrum: characteristics of the interacting lymphocyte, *J Reticuloendothel Soc* 8:91-104, 1970.
184. Weiler IJ, Hickler W, Sprenger R: Demonstration that milk cells invade the suckling neonatal mouse, *Am J Reprod Immunol* 4:95-98, 1983.
185. Zhou L, Yoshimura Y, Huang Y, et al: Two independent pathways of maternal cell transmission to offspring: through placenta during pregnancy and by breast-feeding after birth, *Immunology* 101: 570-580, 2000.
186. Jain L, Vidyasagar D, Xanthou M, et al: In vivo distribution of human milk leucocytes after ingestion by newborn baboons, *Arch Dis Child* 64(Spec No 7):930-933, 1989.
187. Schnorr KL, Pearson LD: Intestinal absorption of maternal leucocytes by newborn lambs, *J Reprod Immunol* 6:329-337, 1984.
188. Fetherston CM, Lee CS, Hartmann PE: Mammary gland defense: the role of colostrum, milk and involution secretion, *Adv Nutr Res* 10:167-198, 2001.
189. Hassiotou F, Beltran A, Chetwynd E, et al: Breastmilk is a novel source of stem cells with multilineage differentiation potential, *Stem Cells* 30:2164-2174, 2012.

190. Thomas E, Zeps N, Rigby P, Hartmann P: Reactive oxygen species initiate luminal but not basal cell death in cultured human mammary alveolar structures: a potential regulator of involution, *Cell Death Dis* 2:e189, 2011.
191. Cregan MD, Fan Y, Appelbee A, et al: Identification of nestin-positive putative mammary stem cells in human breastmilk, *Cell Tissue Res* 329:129-136, 2007.
192. Taylor-Papadimitriou J, Shearer M, Stoker MG: Growth requirements of human mammary epithelial cells in culture, *Int J Cancer* 20:903-908, 1977.
193. Buehring GC: Culture of human mammary epithelial cells: keeping abreast with a new method, *J Natl Cancer Inst* 49:1433-1434, 1972.
194. Gaffney EV, Polanowski FP, Blackburn SE, Lambiase JP: Origin, concentration and structural features of human mammary gland cells cultured from breast secretions, *Cell Tissue Res* 172:269-279, 1976.
195. Stoker M, Perryman M, Eeles R: Clonal analysis of morphological phenotype in cultured mammary epithelial cells from human milk, *Proc R Soc Lond B Biol Sci* 215:231-240, 1982.
196. Thomas E, Lee-Pullen T, Rigby P, et al: Receptor activator of NF-kappaB ligand promotes proliferation of a putative mammary stem cell unique to the lactating epithelium, *Stem Cells* 30:1255-1264, 2012.
197. Twigger AJ, Hodgetts S, Filgueira L, Hartmann PE, Hassiotou F: From breast milk to brains: the potential of stem cells in human milk, *J Hum Lact* 29:136-139, 2013.
198. Jeurink PV, van Bergenhenegouwen J, Jimenez E, et al: Human milk: a source of more life than we imagine, *Benef Microbes* 4: 17-30, 2013.
199. Hunt KM, Foster JA, Forney LJ, et al: Characterization of the diversity and temporal stability of bacterial communities in human milk, *PLoS One* 6:e21313, 2011.
200. Cabrera-Rubio R, Collado MC, Laitinen K, et al: The human milk microbiome changes over lactation and is shaped by maternal weight and mode of delivery, *Am J Clin Nutr* 96:544-551, 2012.
201. Fernandez L, Langa S, Martin V, et al: The microbiota of human milk in healthy women, *Cell Mol Biol (Noisy-le-Grand)* 59:31-42, 2013.
202. Fernandez L, Langa S, Martin V, et al: The human milk microbiota: origin and potential roles in health and disease, *Pharmacol Res* 69: 1-10, 2013.
203. Price D, Ackland L, Suphioglu C: Nuts 'n' guts: transport of food allergens across the intestinal epithelium, *Asia Pac Allergy* 3: 257-265, 2013.
204. Scaldaferri F, Pizzoferrato M, Gerardi V, Lopetuso L, Gasbarrini A: The gut barrier: new acquisitions and therapeutic approaches, *J Clin Gastroenterol* 46(Suppl):S12-S17, 2012.
205. Losonsky GA, Ogra PL: *Mucosal immune system*, Orlando, FL, 1984, Grune & Stratton.
206. Bhutta ZA, Ahmed T, Black RE, et al: What works? Interventions for maternal and child undernutrition and survival, *Lancet* 371: 417-440, 2008.
207. Labbok MH, Clark D, Goldman AS: Breastfeeding: maintaining an irreplaceable immunological resource, *Nat Rev Immunol* 4: 565-572, 2004.
208. Glass RI, Stoll BJ: The protective effect of human milk against diarrhea. A review of studies from Bangladesh, *Acta Paediatr Scand Suppl* 351:131-136, 1989.
209. Svirsky-Gross S: Pathogenic strains of coli (O;111) among prematures and the cause of human milk in controlling the outbreak of diarrhea, *Ann Pediatr (Paris)* 190:109-115, 1958.
210. Yolken RH, Wyatt RG, Mata L, et al: Secretory antibody directed against rotavirus in human milk-measurement by means of an ELISA, *J Pediatr* 93:916-921, 1978.
211. Mata LJ, Wyatt RG: The uniqueness of human milk: host resistance to infection, *Am J Clin Nutr* 24:976-986, 1971.
212. Qureshi K, Molbak K, Sandstrom A, et al: Breast milk reduces the risk of illness in children of mothers with cholera: observations from an epidemic of cholera in Guinea-Bissau, *Pediatr Infect Dis J* 25:1163-1166, 2006.
213. Sandine W, Muralidh KS, Elliker PR, et al: Lactic acid bacteria in food and health: a review with special references to enteropathogenic *Escherichia coli* as well as certain enteric diseases and their treatment with antibiotics and lactobacilli, *J Milk Food Technol* 35:691-702, 1972.
214. Lodinova R, Jouya V: Antibody production by the mammary gland in mothers after oral colonization of their infants with a nonpathogenic strain *E. coli* 083, *Acta Paediatr Scand* 66:705-708, 1977.
215. Duffy LC, Byers TE, Riepenhoff-Taltz M, et al: The effects of infant feeding on rotavirus-induced gastroenteritis: a prospective study, *Am J Public Health* 76:259-263, 1986.
216. Duffy LC, Riepenhoff-Talty M, Byers TE, et al: Modulation of rotavirus enteritis during breast-feeding, *Am J Dis Child* 140:1164-1168, 1986.
217. Heaton PM, Ciarlet M: Vaccines: the pentavalent rotavirus vaccine: discovery to licensure and beyond, *Clin Infect Dis* 45:1618-1624, 2007.
218. Plenge-Bonig A, Soto-Ramirez N, Karmaus W, et al: Breastfeeding protects against acute gastroenteritis due to rotavirus in infants, *Eur J Pediatr* 169:1471-1476, 2010.
219. Bishop RF, Cameron DJ, Barnes GL, et al: The aetiology of diarrhea in newborn infants, *Ciba Found Symp* 42:223-236, 1976.
220. Cameron DJ, Bishop RF, Veenstra AA, et al: Noncultivable viruses and neonatal diarrhea: fifteen-month survey in a newborn special care nursery, *J Clin Microbiol* 8:93-98, 1978.
221. Murphy AM, Albrey MB, Crewe EB: Rotavirus infections of neonates, *Lancet* 2:1149-1150, 1977.
222. Bishop RF, Cameron DJ, Veenstra AA, et al: Diarrhea and rotavirus infection associated with differing regimens for postnatal care of newborn babies, *J Clin Microbiol* 9:525-529, 1979.
223. Nakawesi JS, Wobudeya E, Ndeezi G, Mworozi EA, Tumwine JK: Prevalence and factors associated with rotavirus infection among children admitted with acute diarrhea in Uganda, *BMC Pediatr* 10:69, 2010.
224. Frantz ID 3rd, L'Heureux P, Engel RR, et al: Necrotizing enterocolitis, *J Pediatr* 86:259-263, 1975.
225. Bell MJ, Feigen RD, Ternberg JL: Changes in the incidence of necrotizing enterocolitis associated with variation of the gastrointestinal microflora in neonates, *Am J Surg* 138:629-631, 1979.
226. Grave GD, Nelson SA, Walker WA, et al: New therapies and preventive approaches for necrotizing enterocolitis: report of a research planning workshop, *Pediatr Res* 62:510-514, 2007.
227. Nanthakumar N, Meng D, Goldstein AM, et al: The mechanism of excessive intestinal inflammation in necrotizing enterocolitis: an immature innate immune response, *PLoS One* 6:e17776, 2011.
228. Sharma R, Hudak ML, Tepas JJ 3rd, et al: Impact of gestational age on the clinical presentation and surgical outcome of necrotizing enterocolitis, *J Perinatol* 26:342-347, 2006.
229. Pitt J, Barlow B, Heird WC: Protection against experimental necrotizing enterocolitis by maternal milk. I. Role of milk leucocytes, *Pediatr Res* 11:906-909, 1977.
230. Moriartey RR, Finer NN, Cox SF, et al: Necrotizing enterocolitis and human milk, *J Pediatr* 94:295-296, 1979.
231. Eibl MM, Wolf HM, Furnkranz H, et al: Prophylaxis of necrotizing enterocolitis by oral IgA-IgG: review of a clinical study in low birth weight infants and discussion of the pathogenic role of infection, *J Clin Immunol* 10:72S-77S, 1990.
232. Book LS, Overall JC, Herbst JJ, et al: Clustering of necrotizing enterocolitis: interruption by infection-control measures, *N Engl J Med* 297:984-986, 1977.
233. Bunton GL, Durbin GM, McIntosh M, et al: Necrotizing enterocolitis, *Arch Dis Child* 52:772-777, 1977.
234. Raval MV, Moss RL: Current concepts in the surgical approach to necrotizing enterocolitis, *Pathophysiology* 21:105-110, 2014.
235. Torrazza RM, Li N, Neu J: Decoding the enigma of necrotizing enterocolitis in premature infants, *Pathophysiology* 21:21-27, 2014.
236. Gordon PV, Swanson JR: Necrotizing enterocolitis is one disease with many origins and potential means of prevention, *Pathophysiology* 2014:13-19, 2013.
237. Boyd CA, Quigley MA, Brocklehurst P: Donor breast milk versus infant formula for preterm infants: systematic review and meta-analysis, *Arch Dis Child Fetal Neonatal Ed* 92:F169-F175, 2007.
238. Quigley MA, Henderson G, Anthony MY, McGuire W: Formula milk versus donor breast milk for feeding preterm or low birth weight infants, *Cochrane Database Syst Rev* (4):CD002971, 2007.
239. Schanler RJ: The use of human milk for premature infants, *Pediatr Clin North Am* 48:207-219, 2001.
240. Cristofalo EA, Schanler RJ, Blanco CL, et al: Randomized trial of exclusive human milk versus preterm formula diets in extremely premature infants, *J Pediatr* 163:1592-1595.e1, 2013.
241. Meinzen-Derr J, Poindexter B, Wrage L, et al: Role of human milk in extremely low birth weight infants' risk of necrotizing enterocolitis or death, *J Perinatol* 29:57-62, 2009.
242. Sullivan S, Schanler RJ, Kim JH, et al: An exclusively human milk-based diet is associated with a lower rate of necrotizing enterocolitis than a diet of human milk and bovine milk-based products, *J Pediatr* 156:562-567, 2010.

243. Lucas A, Cole TJ: Breast milk and neonatal necrotising enterocolitis, *Lancet* 336:1519-1523, 1990.
244. Stout G, Lambert DK, Baer VL, et al: Necrotizing enterocolitis during the first week of life: a multicentered case-control and cohort comparison study, *J Perinatol* 28:556-560, 2008.
245. Pietz J, Achanti B, Lilien L, Stepka EC, Mehta SK: Prevention of necrotizing enterocolitis in preterm infants: a 20-year experience, *Pediatrics* 119:e164-e170, 2007.
246. Pitt J: *Necrotizing enterocolitis: a model for infection-immunity interaction*, Orlando, FL, 1984, Grune & Stratton.
247. Koropatkin NM, Cameron EA, Martens EC: How glycan metabolism shapes the human gut microbiota, *Nat Rev Microbiol* 10:323-335, 2012.
248. Shah D, Sinn JK: Antibiotic regimens for the empirical treatment of newborn infants with necrotising enterocolitis, *Cochrane Database Syst Rev* (8):CD007448, 2012.
249. Bury RG, Tudehope D: Enteral antibiotics for preventing necrotizing enterocolitis in low birthweight or preterm infants, *Cochrane Database Syst Rev* (1):CD000405, 2001.
250. Abdel Ghany EA, Ali AA: Empirical antibiotic treatment and the risk of necrotizing enterocolitis and death in very low birth weight neonates, *Ann Saudi Med* 32:521-526, 2012.
251. Kuppala VS, Meinzen-Derr J, Morrow AL, Schibler KR: Prolonged initial empirical antibiotic treatment is associated with adverse outcomes in premature infants, *J Pediatr* 159:720-725, 2011.
252. Shah P, Nathan E, Doherty D, Patole S: Prolonged exposure to antibiotics and its associations in extremely preterm neonates—the Western Australian experience, *J Matern Fetal Neonatal Med* 26:1710-1714, 2013.
253. Zeissig S, Blumberg RS: Life at the beginning: perturbation of the microbiota by antibiotics in early life and its role in health and disease, *Nat Immunol* 15:307-310, 2014.
254. Weintraub AS, Ferrara L, Deluca L, et al: Antenatal antibiotic exposure in preterm infants with necrotizing enterocolitis, *J Perinatol* 32:705-709, 2012.
255. Weinberg RJ, Tipton G, Klish WJ, et al: Effect of breast-feeding on morbidity in rotavirus gastroenteritis, *Pediatrics* 74:250-253, 1984.
256. The influence of breast-feeding on the incidence of infectious illness during the first year of life. A report of the Research Sub-committee of the South-East England Faculty of the Royal College of General Practitioners, *Practitioner* 209:356-362, 1972.
257. Fallot ME, Boyd JL, Oski FA: Breast-feeding reduces incidence of hospital admissions for infection in infants, *Pediatrics* 65:1121-1124, 1980.
258. Hylander MA, Strobino DM, Dhanireddy R: Human milk feedings and infection among very low birth weight infants, *Pediatrics* 102:E38, 1998.
259. Glode MP, Sutton A, Robbins JB, et al: Neonatal meningitis due to *Escherichia coli* K1, *J Infect Dis* 136(Suppl):S93-S97, 1977.
260. Ellestad-Sayed J, Coodin FJ, Dilling LA, et al: Breast-feeding protects against infection in Indian infants, *Can Med Assoc J* 120:295-298, 1979.
261. Elger MS, Rausen AR, Silverio J: Breast vs. bottle feeding, *Clin Pediatr* 23:492-495, 1984.
262. Habicht JP, DaVanzo J, Butz WP: Does breast-feeding really save lives, or are apparent benefits due to biases? *Am J Epidemiol* 123:279-290, 1986.
263. Bauchner H, Leventhal JM, Shapiro ED: Studies of breast-feeding and infections. How good is the evidence? *JAMA* 256:887-892, 1986.
264. de Silva A, Jones PW, Spencer SA: Does human milk reduce infection rates in preterm infants? A systematic review, *Arch Dis Child Fetal Neonatal Ed* 89:F509-F513, 2004.
265. Furman L: Yes, human milk does reduce infection rates in very low birthweight infants, *Arch Dis Child Fetal Neonatal Ed* 91:F78, 2006.
266. Patel AL, Johnson TJ, Engstrom JL, et al: Impact of early human milk on sepsis and health-care costs in very low birth weight infants, *J Perinatol* 33:514-519, 2013.
267. Kramer MS: Breastfeeding and allergy: the evidence, *Ann Nutr Metab* 59(Suppl 1):20-26, 2011.
268. Grulee CG, Sanford HN: The influence of breast and artificial feeding on infantile eczema, *J Pediatr* 9:223-225, 1936.
269. Saarinen UM, Kajosaari M: Breast-feeding as prophylaxis against atopic disease: prospective follow-up study until 17 years old, *Lancet* 346:1065-1069, 1995.
270. Wright AL, Holberg CJ, Taussig LM, et al: Relationship of infant feeding to recurrent wheezing at age 6 years, *Arch Pediatr Adolesc Med* 149:758-763, 1995.
271. Klagsbrun M: Human milk stimulates DNA synthesis and cellular proliferation in cultured fibroblasts, *Proc Natl Acad Sci U S A* 75:5057-5061, 1978.
272. Okada M, Ohmura E, Kamiya Y, et al: Transforming growth factor (TGF)-α in human milk, *Life Sci* 48:1151-1156, 1991.
273. Saito S, Yoshida M, Ichijo M, et al: Transforming growth factor-beta (TGF-β) in human milk, *Clin Exp Immunol* 94:220-224, 1993.
274. Hanson LA, Ahlstedt S, Carlsson B, et al: Secretory IgA antibodies against cow's milk proteins in human milk and their possible effect in mixed feeding, *Int Arch Allergy Appl Immunol* 54:457-462, 1977.
275. Uhnoo IS, Freihort J, Riepenhoff-Talty M, et al: Effect of rotavirus infection and malnutrition on uptake of dietary antigen in the intestine, *Pediatr Res* 27:153-160, 1990.
276. Koenig JE, Spor A, Scalfone N, et al: Succession of microbial consortia in the developing infant gut microbiome, *Proc Natl Acad Sci U S A* 108(Suppl 1):4578-4585, 2011.
277. Brandtzaeg P: The secretory immune system of lactating human mammary glands compared with other exocrine organs, *Ann N Y Acad Sci* 409:353-382, 1983.
278. Rieger CHL, Rothberg RM: Development of the capacity to produce specific antibody to an ingested food antigen in the premature infant, *J Pediatr* 87:515-518, 1975.
279. Businco L, Marchetti F, Pellegrini G, et al: Prevention of atopic disease in "at risk newborns" by prolonged breast-feeding, *Ann Allergy* 51:296-299, 1983.
280. Eastham EJ, Lichauco T, Grady ML, et al: Antigenicity of infant formulas: role of immature intestine on protein permeability, *J Pediatr* 93:561-564, 1978.
281. Koletzko S, Sherman P, Corey M, et al: Role of infant feeding practices in development of Crohn's disease in childhood, *BMJ* 298:1617-1618, 1989.
282. Koletzko S, Griffiths A, Corey M, et al: Infant feeding practices and ulcerative colitis in childhood, *BMJ* 302:1580-1581, 1991.
283. Mayer EJ, Hamman RF, Gay EC, et al: Reduced risk of IDDM among breast-fed children, *Diabetes* 37:1625-1632, 1988.
284. Davis MK, Savitz DA, Grauford B: Infant feeding in childhood cancer, *Lancet* 2:365-368, 1988.
285. Hong S, Choi WJ, Kwon HJ, et al: Effect of prolonged breast-feeding on risk of atopic dermatitis in early childhood, *Allergy Asthma Proc* 35:66-70, 2014.
286. Soto-Ramirez N, Karmaus W, Zhang H, et al: Modes of infant feeding and the occurrence of coughing/wheezing in the first year of life, *J Hum Lact* 29:71-80, 2013.
287. Kramer MS: Does breast-feeding help protect against atopic disease? Biology, methodology, and a golden jubilee of controversy, *J Pediatr* 112:181-190, 1988.
288. Kramer MS, Kakuma R: Optimal duration of exclusive breastfeeding, *Cochrane Database Syst Rev* (8):CD003517, 2012.
289. Kuschel CA, Harding JE: Multicomponent fortified human milk for promoting growth in preterm infants, *Cochrane Database Syst Rev* (1):CD000343, 2004.
290. Saarinen UM: Prolonged breast-feeding as prophylaxis for recurrent otitis media, *Acta Paediatr Scand* 71:567-571, 1982.
291. Short RV: Breast-feeding, *Sci Am* 250:35-41, 1984.
292. Gunther M: The neonate's immunity gap, breast-feeding and cot death, *Lancet* 1:441-442, 1975.
293. Pettitt DJ, Forman MR, Hanson RL, et al: Breast-feeding and incidence of non-insulin-dependent diabetes mellitus in Pima Indians, *Lancet* 350:166-168, 1997.
294. Kramer MS: Do breast-feeding and delayed introduction of solid foods protect against subsequent obesity? *J Pediatr* 98:883-887, 1981.
295. Fall CHD, Barker DJP, Osmond C, et al: Relation of infant feeding to adult serum cholesterol concentration and death from ischaemic heart disease, *BMJ* 304:801-805, 1992.
296. Anothaisintawee T, Wiratkapun C, Lerdsitthichai P, et al: Risk factors of breast cancer: a systematic review and meta-analysis, *Asia Pac J Public Health* 25:368-387, 2013.
297. Butt S, Borgquist S, Anagnostaki L, Landberg G, Manjer J: Breastfeeding in relation to risk of different breast cancer characteristics, *BMC Res Notes* 7:216, 2014.

298. Rodgers B: Feeding in infancy and later ability and attainment: a longitudinal study, *Dev Med Child Neurol* 20:421-426, 1978.
299. Rogan WJ, Gladen BC: Breast-feeding and cognitive development, *Early Hum Dev* 31:181-193, 1993.
300. Horwood LJ, Fergusson DM: Breast-feeding and later cognitive and academic outcomes, *Pediatrics* 101:99, 1998.
301. Kramer MS, Aboud F, Mironova E, et al: Breastfeeding and child cognitive development: new evidence from a large randomized trial, *Arch Gen Psychiatry* 65:578-584, 2008.
302. Lawrence RM: Circumstances when breastfeeding is contraindicated, *Pediatr Clin North Am* 60:295-318, 2013.
303. Lamonica DA, Stump MV, Pedro KP, et al: Breastfeeding follow-up in the treatment of children with phenylketonuria, *J Soc Bras Fonoaudiol* 24:386-389, 2012.
304. Feillet F, Agostoni C: Nutritional issues in treating phenylketonuria, *J Inherit Metab Dis* 33:659-664, 2010.
305. Transfer of drugs and other chemicals into human milk, *Pediatrics* 108:776-789, 2001.
306. Jaques SC, Kingsbury A, Henshcke P, et al: Cannabis, the pregnant woman and her child: weeding out the myths, *J Perinatol* 34: 117-121, 2014.
307. Human milk. In Pickering LK, editor: *American Academy of Pediatrics. Red book: report of the Committee on Infectious Diseases*, Elk Grove Village, Ill, 2012, American Academy of Pediatrics.
308. McNinch A, Busfield A, Tripp J: Vitamin K deficiency bleeding in Great Britain and Ireland: British Paediatric Surveillance Unit Surveys, 1993-94 and 2001-02, *Arch Dis Child* 92:759-766, 2007.
309. Higinbotham MC, Sweetman L, Nyhan WL: A syndrome of methylmalonic aciduria, homocystinuria, megaloblastic anemia and neurologic abnormalities in a vitamin B12-deficient breast-fed infant of a strict vegetarian, *N Engl J Med* 299:317-323, 1978.
310. Basile LA, Taylor SN, Wagner CL, Horst RL, Hollis BW: The effect of high-dose vitamin D supplementation on serum vitamin D levels and milk calcium concentration in lactating women and their infants, *Breastfeeding Med* 1:27-35, 2006.
311. Zmora E, Gorodescher R, Bar-Ziv J: Multiple nutritional deficiencies in infants from a strict vegetarian commune, *Am J Dis Child* 133:141-144, 1979.
312. Nau SB, Stickler GB, Hawort JC: Serum 25-hydroxyvitamin D in infantile rickets, *Pediatrics* 57:221-225, 1976.
313. Citak FE, Citak EC: Severe vitamin B12 deficiency in a breast fed infant with pancytopenia, *J Trop Pediatr* 57:69-70, 2011.
314. Kanaka C, Schütz B, Zuppinger KA: Risks of alternative nutrition in infancy: a case report of severe iodine and carnitine deficiency, *Eur J Pediatr* 151:786-788, 1992.
315. Tuzun F, Kumral A, Duman N, Ozkan H: Breast milk jaundice: effect of bacteria present in breast milk and infant feces, *J Pediatr Gastroenterol Nutr* 56:328-332, 2013.
316. Section on Breastfeeding: Breastfeeding and the use of human milk, *Pediatrics* 129:e827-e841, 2012.
317. Thiry L, Sprecher-Goldberger S, Joncksheer T, et al: Isolation of AIDS virus from cell-free breast milk of three healthy virus carriers, *Lancet* 2:891-892, 1985.
318. Vogt MW, Witt DJ, Craven DE, et al: Isolation of HTLV-III/LAV from cervical secretions of women at risk of AIDS, *Lancet* 1:525-527, 1986.
319. Bucens M, Armstrong J, Stuckey M: Virologic and electron microscopic evidence for postnatal HIV transmission via breast milk. In *Fourth International Conference on AIDS*, Frederick, MD, 1988, University Publishing Group.
320. Vonesch N, Sturchio E, Humani AC, et al: Detection of HIV-1 genome in leukocytes of human colostrum from anti-HIV-1 seropositive mothers, *AIDS Res Hum Retroviruses* 8:1283-1287, 1992.
321. Ruff AJ, Coberly J, Halsey NA, et al: Prevalence of HIV-1 DNA and p24 antigen in breast milk and correlation with maternal factors, *J Acquir Immune Defic Syndr* 7:68-73, 1994.
322. Fowler MG, Lampe MA, Jamieson DJ, Kourtis AP, Rogers MF: Reducing the risk of mother-to-child human immunodeficiency virus transmission: past successes, current progress and challenges, and future directions, *Am J Obstet Gynecol* 197(Suppl 3):S3-S9, 2007.
323. Kourtis AP, Jamieson DJ, de Vincenzi I, et al: Prevention of human immunodeficiency virus-1 transmission to the infant through breastfeeding: new developments, *Am J Obstet Gynecol* 197(Suppl 3):S113-S122, 2007.
324. Breastfeeding, HIV International Transmission Study Group, Coutsoudis A, et al: Late postnatal transmission of HIV-1 in breast-fed children: an individual patient data meta-analysis, *J Infect Dis* 189:2154-2166, 2004.
325. Committee on Pediatric AIDS: Infant feeding and transmission of human immunodeficiency virus in the United States, *Pediatrics* 131:391-396, 2013.
326. Shearer WT: Breastfeeding and HIV infection, *Pediatrics* 121: 1046-1047, 2008.
327. Shapiro RL, Ndung'u T, Lockman S, et al: Highly active antiretroviral therapy started during pregnancy or postpartum suppresses HIV-1 RNA, but not DNA, in breast milk, *J Infect Dis* 192: 713-719, 2005.
328. Coovadia HM, Bland RM: Preserving breastfeeding practice through the HIV pandemic, *Trop Med Int Health* 12:1116-1133, 2007.
329. Coovadia HM, Rollins NC, Bland RM, et al: Mother-to-child transmission of HIV-1 infection during exclusive breastfeeding in the first 6 months of life: an intervention cohort study, *Lancet* 369:1107-1116, 2007.
330. Thior I, Lockman S, Smeaton LM, et al: Breastfeeding plus infant zidovudine prophylaxis for 6 months vs formula feeding plus infant zidovudine for 1 month to reduce mother-to-child HIV transmission in Botswana: a randomized trial: the Mashi Study, *JAMA* 296: 794-805, 2006.
331. Iliff PJ, Piwoz EG, Tavengwa NV, et al: Early exclusive breastfeeding reduces the risk of postnatal HIV-1 transmission and increases HIV-free survival, *AIDS* 19:699-708, 2005.
332. Wilfert CM, Fowler MG: Balancing maternal and infant benefits and the consequences of breast-feeding in the developing world during the era of HIV infection, *J Infect Dis* 195:165-167, 2007.
333. Hinckley AF, O'Leary DR, Hayes EB: Transmission of West Nile virus through human breast milk seems to be rare, *Pediatrics* 119: e666-e671, 2007.
334. Grummer-Strawn LM, Scanlon KS, Fein SB: Infant feeding and feeding transitions during the first year of life, *Pediatrics* 122(Suppl 2):S36-S42, 2008.
335. Langellier BA, Chaparro MP, Wang MC, Koleilat M, Whaley SE: The new food package and breastfeeding outcomes among women, infants, and children participants in Los Angeles County, *Am J Public Health* 104(Suppl 1):S112-S118, 2014.
336. Jensen E, Labbok M: Unintended consequences of the WIC formula rebate program on infant feeding outcomes: will the new food packages be enough? *Breastfeeding Med* 6:145-149, 2011.
337. Baumgartel KL, Spatz DL: American Academy of Nursing Expert Breastfeeding Panel: WIC (the Special Supplemental Nutrition Program for Women, Infants, and Children): policy versus practice regarding breastfeeding, *Nursing Outlook* 61:466-470, 2013.
338. Bentovim A: Shame and other anxieties associated with breastfeeding: a systems theory and psychodynamic approach, *Ciba Found Symp* 45:159-178, 1976.
339. Baranowski T, Bee DE, Rassin DK, et al: Social support, social influence, ethnicity and the breast-feeding decision, *Soc Sci Med* 17: 1599-1611, 1983.
340. Baranowski T, Rassin DK, Richardson CJ, et al: Attitudes toward breast-feeding, *J Dev Behav Pediatr* 7:367-372, 1986.
341. Baranowski T, Rassin DK, Richardson CJ, et al: Expectancies of infant-feeding methods among mothers in three ethnic groups, *Psychol Health* 5:59-75, 1990.
342. Hanson LA: *Immunobiology of human milk: how breastfeeding protects babies*, Amarillo, Tex, 2004, Pharmasoft Publishing.

SECTION II

BACTERIAL INFECTIONS

SECTION OUTLINE

6 Bacterial Sepsis and Meningitis

VICTOR NIZET and JEROME O. KLEIN

CHAPTER OUTLINE

Bacterial sepsis in the neonate is a clinical syndrome characterized by systemic signs of infection and accompanied by bacteremia in the first month of life. Meningitis in the neonate usually is a sequela of bacteremia and is discussed in this chapter because meningitis and sepsis typically share a common cause and pathogenesis. Infections of the bones, joints, and soft tissues and of the respiratory, genitourinary, and gastrointestinal tracts can be accompanied by bacteremia, but the cause, clinical features, diagnosis, and management of these infections are sufficiently different to warrant separate discussions. Bloodstream and central nervous system (CNS) infections caused by group B streptococci (GBS), *Staphylococcus aureus*, and coagulase-negative staphylococci (CoNS), *Neisseria gonorrhoeae*, *Listeria monocytogenes*, *Salmonella* spp., and *Mycobacterium tuberculosis* are described in detail in other individual chapters. Chapter 2 describes the features of neonatal sepsis and meningitis in developing regions.

The two patterns of disease, early-onset and late-onset, have been associated with systemic bacterial infections during the first month of life (Table 6-1). Early-onset disease typically presents as a fulminant, systemic illness during the first 24 hours of life (median age of onset approximately 6 hours), with the large majority of other cases presenting on the second day of life. Infants with early-onset disease can have a history of one or more obstetric complications, including premature or prolonged rupture of maternal membranes, preterm onset of labor, chorioamnionitis, and peripartum maternal fever, and many of the infants are premature or of low birth weight (LBW). Bacteria responsible for early-onset disease are acquired hours before delivery from the birth canal during delivery after overt or occult rupture of membranes. The mortality rate varies from 3% to as high as 50% in some series, especially with gram-negative pathogens. Late-onset disease has been variably defined for epidemiologic purposes as occurring after 72 hours to 6 days (e.g., GBS) of life. Very-late-onset infection caused by GBS (disease in infants older than 3 months) is discussed in Chapter 12. Term infants with late-onset infections can have a history of obstetric complications, but these are less characteristic than in early-onset sepsis or meningitis. Bacteria responsible for late-onset sepsis (LOS) and meningitis include those acquired from the maternal genital tract and organisms acquired after birth from human contacts or, infrequently, from contaminated hospital equipment or materials, where prolonged intensive care is needed for a neonate. The mortality rate usually is lower than that for early-onset sepsis but can vary between 2% and 40%, with the latter figure typically for very-low-birth-weight (VLBW) infants with gram-negative sepsis. Because different microorganisms are responsible for disease according to age at onset, the choice of antimicrobial agents also differs. Some organisms, such as *Escherichia coli*, groups A and B streptococci, and *L. monocytogenes*, can be responsible for early- and late-onset infections, whereas others, such as *S. aureus*, CoNS, and *Pseudomonas aeruginosa*, rarely cause early-onset and typically are associated with late-onset disease. The survival of VLBW infants with prolonged stays in the neonatal intensive care unit (NICU) has been accompanied by increased risk for nosocomial or hospital-associated infections and for very-late-onset disease[1] (see Chapter 35).

Table 6-1 Characteristics of Early-Onset and Late-Onset Neonatal Sepsis

Characteristic	Early Onset*	Late Onset†
Time of onset (days)	0-6	7-90
Complications of pregnancy or delivery	+	±
Source of organism	Mother's genital tract	Mother's genital tract; postnatal environment
Usual clinical presentation	Fulminant	Slowly progressive or fulminant
	Multisystem	Focal
	Pneumonia frequent	Meningitis frequent
Mortality rate (%)	3-50‡	2-40‡

*Many studies define early-onset sepsis as that which occurs in the first 72 hours of life; others in the first 5 or 6 days of life.
†Very small premature infants may have late-onset sepsis beyond 90 days of life.
‡Higher mortality rates in earlier studies.

Bacteriology

The changing pattern of organisms responsible for neonatal sepsis is well illustrated in a series of reports by pediatricians at the Yale–New Haven Hospital covering the period 1928 to 2003[2-8] (Table 6-2). Before development of the sulfonamides, gram-positive cocci, including *S. aureus* and β-hemolytic streptococci, caused most cases of neonatal sepsis. With the introduction of antimicrobial agents, gram-negative enteric bacilli, particularly *E. coli*, became the predominant cause of serious infection in the newborn. Reports for the periods of 1966 to 1978 and 1979 to 1988 document the rise to importance of GBS and *E. coli* as agents of neonatal sepsis. In the most recent analysis from 1989 to 2003, CoNS species, predominantly *Staphylococcus epidermidis*, emerged as the single most commonly identified agent of neonatal sepsis, with GBS, *E. coli*, *Enterococcus faecalis*, *S. aureus*, and *Klebsiella* spp. also occurring at substantial frequency. The latest reports also document the problem of sepsis in very premature and LBW infants who have survived with the aid of sophisticated life-support equipment and advances in neonatal intensive care; it is these infants for whom CoNS are particularly threatening. Emerging data from the same center indicate that intrapartum antibiotic prophylaxis protocols, although reducing the overall incidence of early-onset sepsis, may be influencing a higher proportion of septicemia attributable to ampicillin-resistant *E. coli*.[9]

The etiologic pattern of microbial infection observed at Yale Medical Center also has been reported in studies of neonatal sepsis carried out at other centers during the same intervals. Studies indicate that GBS and gram-negative enteric bacilli, predominantly *E. coli*, were the most frequent pathogens for sepsis, but other organisms were prominent

Table 6-2 Bacteria Causing Neonatal Sepsis at Yale–New Haven Hospital, 1928-2003

	NO. OF CASES						
Organism	**1928-1932***	**1933-1943†**	**1944-1957†**	**1958-1965‡**	**1966-1978§**	**1979-1988‖**	**1999-2003¶**
β-Hemolytic streptococci	15	18	11	8	86	83	155
Group A		16	5	0	0	0	0
Group B		2	4	1	76	64	86
Group D *(Enterococcus)*		0	1	7	9	19	65
Viridans streptococci						11	10
Staphylococcus aureus	11	4	8	2	12	14	70
Staphylococcus epidermidis						36	248
Streptococcus pneumoniae	2	5	3	2	2	2	0
Haemophilus spp.				1	9	9	5
Escherichia coli	10	11	23	33	76	46	106
Pseudomonas aeruginosa	1	0	13	11	5	6	33
Klebsiella and *Enterobacter* spp.	0	0	0	8	28	25	97
Others	0	6	4	9	21	38	54
Total no. of cases	39	44	62	73	239	270	784
Mortality rate for years	87%	90%	67%	45%	26%	16%	3%

*Data from Dunham EC: Septicemia in the newborn, *Am J Dis Child* 45:229, 1933.
†Data from Nyhan WL, Fousek MD: Septicemia of the newborn, *Pediatrics* 22:268, 1958.
‡Data from Gluck L, Wood HF, Fousek MD: Septicemia of the newborn, *Pediatr Clin North Am* 13:1131, 1966.
§Data from Freedman RM, Ingram DL, Cross I, et al: A half century of neonatal sepsis at Yale, *Am J Dis Child* 35:140, 1981.
‖Data from Gladstone IM, Ehrenkranz RA, Edberg SC, Baltimore RS: A ten-year review of neonatal sepsis and comparison with the previous fifty-year experience, *Pediatr Infect Dis J* 9:819, 1990.
¶Data from Bizzarro MJ, Raskind C, Baltimore RS, Gallagher PG: Seventy-five years of neonatal sepsis at Yale: 1928-2003, *Pediatrics* 116:595, 2005.

in some centers. *S. aureus* was an important cause of sepsis in the mid-1980s in Finland[10] and East Africa[11] and a more recently significant pathogen in Connecticut[7] and southern Israel.[12] *S. epidermidis* was responsible for 53% of cases in Liverpool,[13] CoNS account for 35% to 48% of all LOS in VLBW infants across the United States[14,15] and in Israel,[16] and *Klebsiella* and *Enterobacter* spp. were the most common bacterial pathogens in Tel Aviv.[17] Sepsis and focal infections in neonates in developing countries are further discussed in Chapter 2.

The Yale data also provide information about the microorganisms responsible for early- and late-onset bacterial sepsis (Table 6-3). GBS were responsible for most early-onset disease. CoNS, *S. aureus*, *E. coli*, *Enterococcus* spp., and *Klebsiella* spp. were the major pathogens of late-onset disease; a wide variety of gram-positive cocci and gram-negative bacilli are documented as causes of bacterial sepsis in the infant after age 30 days.

The mortality rates for neonatal sepsis over time are documented in the Yale Medical Center reports. In the pre-antibiotic era, neonatal sepsis usually was fatal. Even with the introduction of penicillins and aminoglycosides in the reports from 1944 to 1965, death resulted from sepsis in most infants. Concurrent with the introduction of NICUs and technologic support for cardiorespiratory and metabolic functions beginning in the early 1970s, the mortality rate was reduced to 16%. By 1989 to 2003, mortality from neonatal sepsis in this academic medical center was a rare event, occurring in only 3% of cases. A decline in the incidence of early-onset sepsis, commonly associated with more virulent pathogens, coupled with an increase in late and "late-late"–onset sepsis from CoNS and other commensal species (which together now account for nearly half of all cases), has contributed to the improved survival figures, along with continued advances in care and monitoring of the critically ill infant.

From 2005 to 2008, 658 cases of neonatal early-onset sepsis were reported to the Centers for Disease Control and Prevention (CDC) Active Bacterial Core surveillance (ABCs) sites in four states (California, Connecticut, Georgia, Minnesota), for an incidence of approximately 77 cases per 1000 live births (95% confidence interval [CI], 0.72 to 0.84) associated with a 10.9% mortality rate (Table 6-4).[18] The five most commonly reported pathogens were GBS (37.8%), *E. coli* (24.2%), viridans streptococci (17.9%), *S. aureus* (4.0%), and *Haemophilus influenzae* (4.0%). *E. coli* infections had the highest case fatality rate at 24.5%. Black preterm infants had the highest disease incidence (5.14 cases/1000 live births) and case fatality ratio (24.4%), whereas nonblack term infants had the lowest incidence (0.40 cases/1000 live births) and case fatality ratio (1.6%).[18] *E. coli* was the most common infection (1.18 cases/1000 live births) with the highest case fatality ratio (32.1%) among preterm infants, whereas GBS were the leading pathogens among term infants (0.22 cases/1000 live births), with no reported deaths.[18]

The incidence of neonatal sepsis showed a strong inverse correlation to birth weight in the latest Yale cohort: greater than 2000 g (0.2%), 1500 to 1999 g (2.5%), 1000 to 1499 g (9.4%), 750 to 999 g (14.8%), and less than 750 g (34.8%). Survival of VLBW infants (<1500 g) has been accompanied by an increased risk for invasive, nosocomial, or health care–associated bacterial infection as a cause of morbidity and mortality. The danger of sepsis is documented in a multicenter trial that enrolled 2416 VLBW infants in a study of the efficacy of intravenous immunoglobulin in

Table 6-3 Microbiology of Neonatal Sepsis at Yale–New Haven Hospital, 1989-2003

	NO. OF ISOLATES				
	AGE WHEN CULTURED (DAYS)				
Microorganism	**0-4**	**5-30**	**>30**	**Trans-ported Infants**	**Total**
Staphylococcus aureus	8	18	20	24	70
Coagulase-negative staphylococci	6	119	42	81	248
Group B streptococci	53	12	7	14	86
Enterococcus spp.	5	21	23	33	82
Viridans streptococci	0	3	3	4	10
Stomatococcus spp.	0	0	0	1	1
Bacillus spp.	1	0	1	0	2
Listeria monocytogenes	1	0	0	0	1
Escherichia coli	25	27	12	41	106
Klebsiella pneumoniae	0	20	9	18	47
Klebsiella oxytoca	0	7	8	4	19
Enterobacter aerogenes	0	1	3	4	8
Enterobacter agglomerans	0	3	1	0	4
Enterobacter cloacae	0	7	5	7	19
Serratia marcescens	0	6	10	7	23
Pseudomonas aeruginosa	2	14	4	13	33
Acinetobacter spp.	1	0	2	1	4
Proteus mirabilis	0	1	1	1	3
Citrobacter freundii	1	0	0	1	2
Haemophilus influenzae	5	0	0	0	5
Bacteriodes spp.	0	0	1	2	3
Yersinia enterocolitica	0	1	0	2	3
Other gram-negative rods	0	3	0	1	4
Candida and other fungi/ yeast	3	41	16	18	78
Total	112	304	169	277	862

Data from Bizzaro MJ, Raskind C, Baltimore RS, Gallagher PG: Seventy-five years of neonatal sepsis at Yale: 1928-2003, *Pediatrics* 116:595, 2005.

preventing nosocomial infections.[19] Sixteen percent of the VLBW infants developed septicemia at a median age of 17 days, with an overall mortality rate of 21% and a hospital stay that averaged 98 days; infants without sepsis had an overall mortality rate of 9% and 58-day average length of stay. Stoll and colleagues[20] reported recent patterns of pathogens causing early-onset sepsis in VLBW infants (400-1500 g) in the centers participating in the National Institute of Child Health and Human Development (NICHD) Neonatal Research Network (Table 6-5). Compared with earlier cohorts, a marked reduction in GBS infections (from 5.9-2.08/1000 live births) and an increase in *E. coli* infections (3.2-5.09/1000 live births) were noted, although the overall incidence of neonatal sepsis in this population did not change.

Organisms responsible for bacterial meningitis in the newborn are listed in Table 6-6, which summarizes data collected from 1932 to 1997 at neonatal centers in the United States,[21-24] The Netherlands,[25] Great Britain,[26,27] and Israel.[12] Gram-negative enteric bacilli and GBS currently are responsible for most cases. Organisms that cause acute bacterial meningitis in older children and adults—*Streptococcus pneumoniae, Neisseria meningitidis,* and type b and nontypeable *Haemophilus influenzae*—are relatively infrequent causes of meningitis in the neonate.[28] A nationwide survey of causative agents of neonatal meningitis in Sweden between 1976 and 1983 indicated a shift from bacterial to viral or unidentified microorganisms, with lower attributable mortality rates.[29]

GROUP B STREPTOCOCCI

Group B β-hemolytic streptococci were implicated in human disease shortly after the precipitin-grouping technique was described.[30] For the past 3 decades, GBS has been the most common pathogen causing invasive disease in neonates throughout the United States and western Europe (see Chapter 12).

Streptococcus agalactiae, the species designation of GBS, has a characteristic colonial morphology on suitable solid media. The organism produces a mucoid colony with a narrow zone of β-hemolysis on sheep blood–agar media. The GBS can be differentiated immunochemically on the basis of their type-specific polysaccharides. Ten capsular types—Ia, Ib, II, III, IV, V, VI, VII, VIII, and IX—have been characterized, and most invasive human isolates can be classified as one of these types, with serotypes Ia, III, and V the most prevalent in many recent epidemiologic surveys.

GBS have been isolated from various sites and body fluids, including throat, skin, wounds, exudates, stool, urine, cervix, vagina, blood, joint, pleural or peritoneal fluids, and cerebrospinal fluid (CSF). The organisms frequently are found in the lower gastrointestinal and genital tracts of adult women and men and in the lower gastrointestinal and upper respiratory tracts of newborns. Patterns of early-, late-, and very-late-onset disease have been associated with GBS (see Table 6-1). Early-onset disease presents as a multisystem illness, with rapid onset typically during the first day or two of life and is frequently characterized by severe respiratory distress. The pathogenesis is presumed to be similar to that of other forms of early-onset sepsis of neonates. The mortality rate is estimated at 8% but was previously as high as 50% in the 1970s.[31]

Clinical manifestations of late-onset neonatal sepsis are more insidious than those of early-onset disease, and meningitis is frequently a part of the clinical picture. However, some infants with meningitis have a fulminant onset with rapid progression to centrally mediated apnea. Many of the infants are products of a normal pregnancy and delivery and have no problems in the nursery. It is uncertain whether GBS infection was acquired at the time of birth and carried until disease developed, was acquired after delivery from the mother or other household contacts, or was acquired from other infants or personnel in the nursery. In late-onset infection, a majority of strains belong to serotype III. The mortality rate, estimated at 3%, is lower than that for early-onset disease. With increasing survival of extremely-low-birth-weight (ELBW) (<1000 g) infants, very-late-onset disease (>89 days) has been described in the past decade.[16]

In addition to sepsis and meningitis, other manifestations of neonatal disease caused by GBS include pneumonia,

Table 6-4 Invasive Early-Onset* Neonatal Sepsis Cases and Deaths, Centers for Disease Control Active Bacterial Core Surveillance, 2005-2008

	TOTAL		BLACK PRETERM		BLACK TERM		NONBLACK PRETERM		NONBLACK TERM	
	Cases (Rate)	**Deaths (CFR)**	**Cases (Rate)**	**Deaths (CFR)**	**Cases (Rate)**	**Deaths (CFR)**	**Cases (Rate)**	**Deaths (CFR)**	**Cases (Rate)**	**Deaths (CFR)**
Total	658 (0.77)	72 (10.9)	131 (5.14)	32 (24.4)	120 (0.89)	2 (1.7)	158 (2.27)	34 (21.5)	249 (0.040)	4 (1.6)
GBS	249 (0.29)	17 (6.8)	40 (1.57)	9 (22.5)	75 (0.55)	0 (0)	38 (0.55)	8 (21.1)	96 (0.15)	0 (0)
Escherichia coli	159 (0.19)	39 (24.5)	46 (1.81)	17 (37.0)	16 (0.12)	1 (6.3)	66 (0.95)	19 (28.8)	31 (0.05)	2 (6.5)
E. coli (Amp-R)	81 (0.09)	16 (19.8)	31 (1.22)	9 (29.0)	3 (0.02)	0 (0)	31 (0.45)	6 (19.4)	16 (0.03)	1 (6.3)
Viridans streptococci	118 (0.14)	3 (2.5)	16 (0.63)	2 (12.5)	16 (0.12)	0 (0)	18 (0.26)	0 (0)	68 (0.11)	1 (1.5)
Staphylococcus aureus	26 (0.03)	2 (7.7)	2 (0.08)	1 (50.0)	5 (0.04)	1 (20.0)	1 (0.01)	0 (0)	18 (0.03)	0 (0)
Haemophilus influenzae	26 (0.03)	4 (15.4)	10 (0.39)	1 (10.0)	0 (0)	0 (0)	12 (0.17)	3 (25.0)	4 (0.006)	0 (0)
Other pathogens	80 (0.09)	7 (8.9)	17 (0.67)	2 (11.8)	8 (0.06)	0 (0)	23 (0.33)	4 (17.4)	32 (0.05)	1 (3.1)

Data from Weston EJ, Pondo T, Lewis MM, et al: The burden of invasive early-onset neonatal sepsis in the United States, 2005–2008, *Pediatr Infect Dis J* 30:937, 2011.
Amp-R, Ampicillin-resistant; *CFR*, case-fatality ratio; *GBS*, group B streptococci.
Preterm, <37 weeks of gestation; term, ≥37 weeks of gestation
Rate is per 1000 live births.
Other pathogen categories include: *Enterococcus* spp. (*n* = 21), *Listeria monocytogenes* (*n* = 9), *Streptococcus pneumoniae* (*n* = 8), *Citrobacter koseri* (*n* = 7), *Klebsiella pneumoniae* (*n* = 6), group A *Streptococcus* (*n* = 3), *Streptococcus bovis* (*n* = 3), *Bacteroides fragilis* (*n* = 2), group G *Streptococcus* (*n* = 2).
*Occurring in infants the first 72 hours of life:

empyema, facial cellulitis, ethmoiditis, orbital cellulitis, conjunctivitis, necrotizing fasciitis, osteomyelitis, suppurative arthritis, and impetigo. Bacteremia without systemic or focal signs of sepsis can occur. GBS infection in pregnant women can result in peripartum infections, including septic abortion, chorioamnionitis, peripartum bacteremia, septic pelvic thrombophlebitis, meningitis, and toxic shock syndrome.[32]

GROUP A STREPTOCOCCI

Streptococcal puerperal sepsis has been recognized as a cause of morbidity and mortality among parturient women since the 16th century.[33-35] Neonatal group A streptococcal (GAS) infection now is reported infrequently[36-39] but can occur rarely in epidemic form in nurseries.[40-44] The reemergence of virulent GAS infections during the last 4 decades, including invasive disease and toxic shock syndrome, has been reflected in more case reports of severe disease in the pregnant woman and the newborn.[33-35]

GAS disease in the mother can affect the fetus or newborn in two clinical patterns. Maternal streptococcal bacteremia during pregnancy can lead to in utero infection resulting in fetal loss or stillbirth, or alternatively, acquisition of GAS from the maternal genital tract can cause early-onset neonatal sepsis similar to early-onset GBS disease. In the first form of disease, previously healthy pregnant women with influenza-like signs and symptoms have been reported. This presentation rapidly progressed to disseminated intravascular coagulopathy and shock, with high mortality and risk to the fetus or newborn.[45-47]

The features of 38 cases of neonatal invasive GAS infection from the literature were recently catalogued.[48] Overall mortality rate in neonatal invasive GAS infection was significantly high, at 31%. Most of these infants presented with early-onset infection (62%), with many occurring in the first 48 hours of life. A specific focus of GAS infection was documented in three quarters of cases; 42% of neonates had pneumonia, sometimes complicated by empyema, and 17% had a toxic-shock–like syndrome presentation. Among the cases of early-onset GAS infection, puerperal sepsis or toxic shock–like syndrome in the mother during the peripartum period was an associated factor in 62% of cases. In late-onset cases of neonatal GAS infection reviewed in this series, soft tissue infections, meningitis, and pneumonia were among the reported clinical manifestations. An earlier review by Greenberg and colleagues[49] on 15 cases of GAS neonatal infection yielded similar statistics on clinical presentations and mortality.

In addition to sepsis, meningitis, and toxin-mediated disease in the neonate, focal infections, including cellulitis,[38] omphalitis, pneumonia, empyema,[39] osteomyelitis, and parotitis,[37] have been reported. Because all GAS are susceptible to β-lactam antibiotics, the current strategy for prevention or treatment of infections caused by GBS also could apply to infections caused by GAS.

STREPTOCOCCUS PNEUMONIAE

Although pneumococcal infections in the neonate are unusual occurrences, they are associated with substantial morbidity and mortality.[50-53] Malhotra and colleagues[54] recently reported four infants with invasive neonatal pneumococcal infections that developed within the first 24 hours of life, with all four having clinical and radiologic features of pneumonia and a pattern of disease rather indistinguishable from typical severe early-onset GBS sepsis. One of the infants was a 33-week premature infant, and one of the mothers had chorioamnionitis before delivery. All four infants survived, with varying levels of supportive care,

Table 6-5 Characteristics and Mortality Rate of 389 U.S. Infants With Early-Onset Sepsis

	All Patients (N = 389)	Preterm (22-36 wk) with GBS or *E. coli*		Term (37+ wk) with GBS or *E. coli*		Overall with GBS or *E. coli*	
Infant Characteristics, *n* (%)		GBS (*n* = 43)	*E. coli* (*n* = 87)	GBS (*n* = 117)	*E. coli* (*n* = 20)	GBS (*n* = 160)	*E. coli* (*n* = 107)
BIRTH WEIGHT (G)							
401-1500	142 (37%)	27 (63)	66 (76)	0 (0)	0 (0)	27 (17)	66 (62)
1501-2500	51 (13%)	11 (26%)	20 (23%)	3 (3)	0 (0)	14 (9)	20 (19)
2501+	196 (50%)	5 (12)	1 (1)	114 (97)	20 (100)	119 (74)	21 (20)
INFANT GENDER							
Male	205 (53)	22 (51)	47 (54)	57 (49)	15 (75)	79 (49)	62 (58)
Female	184 (47)	21 (49)	40 (46)	60 (51)	5 (25)	81 (51)	45 (42)
DELIVERY							
Vaginal	181 (47)	18 (43)	29 (33)	63 (54)	9 (47)	81 (51)	37 (35)
Cesarean section	204 (53)	25 (57)	58 (67)	54 (46)	10 (53)	76 (49)	68 (65)
ROM > 18 hr PTD	127 (33)	19 (44)	54 (62)	17 (15)	4 (21)	36 (23)	58 (55)
SROM < 37 wk of gestation	157 (40)	30 (70)	75 (86)	NA	NA	NA	NA
SYMPTOMS < 72 HR PTD							
Maternal temperature > 38.0° C	102 (26)	3 (7)	27 (32)	42 (36)	6 (30)	45 (28)	33 (31)
Uterine or abdominal tenderness	56 (15)	6 (14)	26 (31)	4 (3)	0 (0)	10 (6)	26 (25)
Maternal tachycardia (>100 bpm)	115 (30)	14 (33)	36 (42)	30 (26)	7 (35)	44 (28)	43 (41)
Fetal tachycardia (>160 bpm)	120 (31)	11 (26)	34 (40)	40 (34)	7 (35)	51 (32)	41 (39)
PLACENTAL PATHOLOGY PERFORMED	248 (65)	33 (77)	72 (85)	49 (43)	13 (65)	82 (52)	85 (81)
HISTOLOGIC CHORIOAMNIONITIS	190 (77)	30 (91)	63 (88)	32 (65)	8 (62)	62 (76)	71 (84)
INFANT MORTALITY *n* (%)							
All Deaths	61 (16)	13 (30)	33 (38)	2 (2)	2 (10)	15 (9)	35 (33)
TIME OF DEATH							
0-3 days	35 (57)	7 (54)	21 (64)	1 (50)	1 (50)	8 (53)	22 (63)
4-7 days	12 (20)	1 (8)	7 (21)	1 (50)	1 (50)	2 (13)	8 (23)
8-14 days	3 (5)	0 (0)	2 (6)	0 (0)	0 (0)	0 (0)	2 (6)
>14 days	11 (18)	5 (38)	3 (9)	0 (0)	0 (0)	5 (33)	3 (9)

Data from Stoll BJ, Hansen NI, Sánchez PJ, et al: Early onset neonatal sepsis: the burden of group B streptococcal and *E. coli* disease continues, *Pediatrics* 127:817, 2011.

bpm, Beats per minute; *E. coli*, *Escherichia coli*; *GBS*, group B streptococci; *NA*, not available; *PTD*, prior to delivery; *ROM*, rupture of membranes; *SROM*, spontaneous rupture of membranes.

including extracorporeal membrane oxygenation in a child who also developed meningitis. Two infants were expected to suffer significant long-term sequelae. In another report, fatal pneumococcal bacteremia in a mother 4-weeks postpartum and the same disease and outcome in her healthy term infant who died at 6 weeks of age suggested an absence of protective antibody in mother and child.[55]

Hoffman and colleagues,[51] from the United States Multicenter Pneumococcal Surveillance Group, identified 20 cases of neonatal *S. pneumoniae* sepsis or meningitis in a review of 4428 episodes of pneumococcal infection at eight children's hospitals from 1993 to 2001. Ninety percent of the infants were born at term, with a mean age at the onset of infection of 18.1 days. Only two of the mothers had clinically apparent infections at the time of delivery. Eight neonates had meningitis and 12 had bacteremia; 4 of the bacteremic neonates also had pneumonia. The most common infecting pneumococcal serotypes were 19 (32%), 9 (18%), and 18 (11%). Penicillin and ceftriaxone nonsusceptibility were observed in 21.4% and 3.6% of isolates, respectively. Three deaths (15%) occurred, all within 36 hours of presentation. A case report of peripartum transmission of penicillin-resistant *S. pneumoniae* underlines concern that the increasing use of peripartum ampicillin to prevent GBS disease in the neonate may result in an increase in neonatal infections caused by β-lactam–resistant organisms.[52] A case of purulent pneumococcal pericarditis in a neonate has recently been reported.[56]

OTHER STREPTOCOCCI

Human isolates of group C and G streptococci form large β-hemolytic colonies that closely resemble those of GAS and share many virulence genes, including those encoding surface M proteins and the cytotoxin streptolysin S. Group C streptococci have been associated with puerperal sepsis, but neonatal sepsis or meningitis related to these organism is rare.[57-60] Likewise, group G streptococci are an infrequent cause of neonatal sepsis and pneumonia.[61-63] Maternal intrapartum transmission was the likely source for most

Table 6-6 Bacteria Associated With Neonatal Meningitis in Selected Studies

	NO. OF CASES OF ASSOCIATION								
Organism	**Boston, 1932-1957, 77 Cases[21]**	**Los Angeles, 1963-1968, 125 Cases[22]**	**Houston, 1967-1972, 51 Cases[24]**	**Multihospital Survey,* 1971-1973, 131 Cases[742]**	**The Netherlands, 1976-1982, 280 Cases[25]**	**Great Britain, 1985-1987, 329 Cases[26]**	**Dallas, 1969-1989, 257 Cases[24]**	**Israel, 1986-1994, 32 Cases[31†]**	**Great Britain, 1996-1997, 144 Cases[45]**
β-Hemolytic streptococci (group not stated)	9	12	—	—	—	—	—	—	—
β-Hemolytic streptococci									
Group A	—	—	1	2	—	—	—	—	—
Group B	—	—	18	41	68	113	134	6	69
Group D	—	—	—	2	4	—	—	—	1
Staphylococcus epidermidis or coagulase-negative *Staphylococcus*	—	5	—	3	—	9	—	2	2
Staphylococcus aureus	12	1	3	1	7	4	—	—	—
Streptococcus pneumoniae	7	4	3	2	6	21	18	—	8
Listeria monocytogenes	—	6	5	7	12	21	—	—	7
Escherichia coli	25	44	16‡	50	132	2	42	4	26
Pseudomonas aeruginosa	4	1	2	2	4	3	—	1	—
Klebsiella and *Enterobacter* spp.	3	13	‡	3	19	8	10	4	—
Proteus spp.	2	5	‡	4	5	8	3	2	—
Haemophilus spp.	—	2	2	3	2	12	—	—	1
Neisseria meningitidis	1	—	—	1	3	14	—	—	6
Salmonella spp.	2	4	—	3	3	2	4	—	1
Miscellaneous	12	28	1	7	15	32	46	—	23

*Survey of 16 newborn nurseries participating in neonatal meningitis study of intrathecal gentamicin under the direction of Dr. George McCracken, Jr.
†Authors report an additional nine cases of gram-positive and six cases of gram-negative meningitis with organisms not otherwise specified.
‡Authors report 16 cases related to enteric bacteria, including *Escherichia coli*, *Proteus* spp., and *Klebsiella-Enterobacter* group.

cases,[61] and concurrent endometritis and bacteremia in the mother and sepsis in the neonate have been reported.[62] Recently, a case of neonatal toxic streptococcal shock syndrome attributed to maternal transmission of a group C streptococcus was reported.[64]

Viridans streptococci are a heterogeneous group of α-hemolytic and nonhemolytic streptococci that are constituents of the normal flora of the respiratory and gastrointestinal tracts of infants, children, and adults. There are several classification schemes for these streptococci, and they may bear different designations in the literature. *Streptococcus bovis* is capable of causing neonatal sepsis and meningitis that is clinically similar to sepsis caused by GBS.[65,66] Rare cases of fulminant neonatal sepsis or meningitis caused by *Streptococcus mitis*,[67] *Streptococcus gallolyticus*,[68,69] and *Streptococcus alactolyticus*[70] have been reported.

Viridans streptococci accounted for 23% of isolates from cultures of blood and CSF obtained from neonates at the Jefferson Davis Hospital, Houston; only GBS were more common (28%) as a cause of neonatal sepsis.[71] In this series, most infants had early-onset infection with clinical features similar to those of sepsis caused by other pathogens, but 22.6% had no signs of infection. One infant had meningitis. The case-fatality rate was 8.8%. Sepsis related to viridans streptococci also has been reported from Finland,[10] Liverpool,[13] Indianapolis,[72] and Montreal.[73] Among ventilated neonates in a NICU in Ankara, Turkey, the most prominent bacteria in bronchioalveolar lavage cultures were multidrug-resistant viridans streptococci (66%), and these were also one of the most common bloodstream isolates (29%) in the same population.[74] It is clear from these studies that isolation of viridans streptococci from the blood culture of a neonate suspected to have sepsis cannot be considered a contaminant, as is the case in many other patient populations.

ENTEROCOCCUS SPECIES

Members of the genus *Enterococcus* (*E. faecalis* and *E. faecium*) were formerly classified as group D streptococci; but in the mid-1980s, genomic DNA sequence analysis revealed that taxonomic distinction was appropriate, and a unique genus was established.[75] Enterococci are differentiated from nonenterococci by their ability to grow in 6.5% sodium chloride broth and to withstand heating at 60° C for 30 minutes.

Most cases of enterococcal sepsis in the neonate are caused by *E. faecalis*, with a smaller number caused by *E. faecium*[65,76-80]; In the 4 years beginning in 1974, 30 neonates with enterococcal sepsis occurred among 30,059 deliveries at Parkland Memorial Hospital in Dallas.[76] During this period, enterococci were second only to GBS (99 cases) and were more common than *E. coli* (27 cases) as a cause of neonatal sepsis. The clinical presentation in most cases was similar to that of early-onset sepsis of any cause.[78] Among infants with respiratory distress as a prominent sign of infection, the chest radiographs were similar to those demonstrating the hyaline membrane–appearing pattern of GBS infection. Enterococcal bacteremia during the 10 years beginning January 1977 was reported in 56 neonates from the Jefferson Davis Hospital in Houston, Texas.[81] Patients were segregated among three clinical syndromes: early-onset disease was a mild illness with respiratory distress or diarrhea; late-onset infection often was severe with apnea, bradycardia, shock, and increased requirement for oxygen and mechanical ventilation; and many cases were nosocomial.[81] A large series of 100 cases of enterococcal bacteremia in neonates over a 20-year period at New York Hospital–Cornell Medical Center was evaluated by McNeeley and colleagues.[77] Common characteristics were the presence of a central venous catheter (77%) or a diagnosis of necrotizing enterocolitis (NEC; 33%).

In general, *Enterococcus* spp. are resistant to cephalosporins, are only moderately susceptible to penicillin G and ampicillin, and require the synergistic activity of penicillin, at high dosage, and an aminoglycoside for maximal bactericidal action; nonenterococcal strains are susceptible to penicillin G, ampicillin, and most cephalosporins. Vancomycin-resistant (VRE) *Enterococcus* has been reported from NICUs, causing illnesses clinically indistinguishable from vancomycin-sensitive strains,[77] yet raises concerns about the efficacy of antimicrobial agents currently approved for use in neonates.[82] Use of high doses of ampicillin is one option, but other drugs, including daptomycin[83] and the oxazolidinone linezolid,[84] may be required depending on the susceptibility pattern (see Chapter 37).

STAPHYLOCOCCUS AUREUS AND COAGULASE-NEGATIVE STAPHYLOCOCCI

S. aureus and CoNS, especially *S. epidermidis*, colonize skin and mucosa. Isolation of *S. aureus* from tissue, blood, or other body fluids usually is clearly associated with disease. Most episodes of sepsis caused by *S. aureus* are hospital acquired, and mortality can be high (23% among 216 Swedish neonates with *S. aureus* bacteremia during 1967 to 1984), with LBW as the most important risk factor.[85] Recently, reports of pneumonia and other severe nosocomial infection in neonates caused by community-acquired methicillin-resistant *S. aureus* (CA-MRSA) strains, including the epidemic USA300 clone, have been documented.[86-88] Molecular epidemiologic techniques have established direct transmission of CA-MRSA between postpartum women[89] and among NICU patients.[90]

CoNS include more than 30 different species. *S. epidermidis* is the dominant species of CoNS responsible for neonatal sepsis, but other species, including *Streptococcus capitis*, *Streptococcus hemolyticus* and *Streptococcus hominis*, have been identified as causes of sepsis in the newborn.[91] A well-documented increased incidence of CoNS sepsis[8,15,16,92] has accompanied the increased survival of VLBW and ELBW infants with developmentally immature immune systems and prolonged stay in NICUs. The CoNS infections have been associated with the introduction of invasive procedures for maintenance and monitoring of the infants, in particular long-term vascular access devices. Levels of serum complement and transplacental anti-CoNS immunoglobulin G (IgG) are inversely correlated with gestational age, and this relative deficiency in preterm infants contributes to their suboptimal opsonization and impaired bacterial killing of CoNS.[93,94] Because CoNS are present on the skin, isolation of these organisms from a single culture of blood can represent skin contamination but also can indicate bloodstream invasion. Collection of two cultures of blood at separate sites can assist in differentiating skin or blood-culture–bottle contamination from bloodstream invasion in the infant with suspected late-onset sepsis,[95] and adoption of a standard two blood-culture practice can reduce the number of neonates diagnosed with CoNS and exposed to intravenous antibiotic therapy.[96,97] The significance of a positive blood culture yielding CoNS is discussed in "Microbiologic Techniques."

Many episodes of sepsis caused by CoNS are associated with the use of vascular catheters. *S. epidermidis* and other CoNS species can adhere to and grow on surfaces of synthetic polymers used in the manufacture of catheters. Strains obtained from infected ventricular shunts or intravenous catheters produce a mucoid substance (i.e., slime or glycocalyx) that stimulates adherence of microcolonies to various surfaces in the environment and on epithelial surfaces, ultimately leading to establishment of a biofilm.[98,99] In addition to this adhesin function, the slime may protect staphylococci against antibiotics and host defense mechanisms, such as macrophage phagocytosis,[100] predisposing to persistent infection.[101] Parenteral nutrition with a lipid emulsion administered through a venous catheter having organisms adherent to the polymer provides nutrients for growth of the bacteria, leading to invasion of the bloodstream when the organisms reach an inoculum of sufficient size.[102]

Disease in newborn infants caused by *S. aureus* and CoNS is discussed in detail in Chapter 14.

LISTERIA MONOCYTOGENES

The potential of *L. monocytogenes* to contaminate food products and the resultant danger to immunocompromised patients and pregnant women was reconfirmed in a 2002 outbreak involving 46 patients in eight states. This outbreak resulted in seven deaths of adults and miscarriages or stillbirths in three pregnant women.[103] *Listeria* can be found in unprocessed animal products, including milk, meat, poultry, cheese, ice cream, and processed meats, and on fresh fruits and vegetables. The organism possesses several virulence factors that allow it to infect the fetal placental unit, survive and replicate within human cells, and achieve cell-to-cell spread.[104] Although most people exposed to *L. monocytogenes* do not develop illness, pregnant women can suffer fetal loss, and the neonate can develop early- or late-onset sepsis and meningitis. Neonatal disease caused by *Listeria* is discussed in detail in Chapter 13.

ESCHERICHIA COLI

Escherichia coli is second only to GBS as the most common cause of both early- and late-onset neonatal sepsis and meningitis.[9,105-107] Coliform organisms are prevalent in the maternal birth canal, and most infants are colonized in their lower gastrointestinal or respiratory tracts during or just before delivery. The antigenic structure of *E. coli* is complex; members of this species account for more than 145 different somatic (O) antigens, approximately 50 flagellar (H) antigens, and 80 different capsular (K) antigens. Although there is a wide genetic diversity of human commensal isolates of *E. coli*, strains causing neonatal pathology are derived from a limited number of clones.[108] One of these, the O18:K1:H7 clone, is distributed globally; meanwhile, others such as O83:K1 and O45:K1 are restricted to a smaller subset of countries.[109] The presence of a 134-kDa plasmid encoding iron aquisition systems and other putative virulence genes is characteristic of several of these clones, and loss of the plasmid reduces the virulence more than 100-fold in a neonatal rat model of *E. coli* meningitis.[110] In a recent analysis comparing *E. coli* with other agents of early-onset neonatal sepsis, infants with *E. coli* sepsis (n = 19) were more likely to be premature, of VLBW (<1500 g), and to have been associated with the intrapartum characteristics of fever, premature or prolonged rupture of membranes, antibiotic use, and presentation in the first 24 hours of life.[111] Fifteen of the 19 *E. coli* isolates in this study (79%) were ampicillin resistant, and three (16%) were gentamicin resistant; antepartum or intrapartum antibiotic exposure was associated with ampicillin-resistant *E. coli* sepsis.[111]

The K1 capsular antigen present in certain strains of *E. coli* is uniquely associated with neonatal meningitis.[112,113] The K1 antigen is polysialic acid that is immunochemically identical to the capsular antigen of group B *N. meningitidis*. McCracken and coworkers[114] found K1 strains in the blood or CSF of most (65/77) neonates with meningitis related to *E. coli*. These strains also were cultured from the blood of some infants (14/36) and adults (43/301) with sepsis but without meningitis. The K1 capsular antigen was present in 88% of 132 strains from neonates with *E. coli* meningitis reported from The Netherlands.[25] Infants with meningitis caused by K1 strains had significantly higher mortality and morbidity rates than did infants with meningitis caused by non-K1 *E. coli* strains.[112] The K1 strains have been present in the birth canal of mothers and subsequently in cultures from their newborns, indicating that these newborn infants acquired the organisms vertically from their mothers.[115,116] However, high rates of carriage of K1 strains by nursery personnel indicate that postnatal acquisition of the K1 strains in the nursery also may occur.[112,115]

The pathogenesis of *E. coli* K1 infection is hypothesized to begin with bacterial penetration of the gastrointestinal epithelium to enter the circulation, and efficient transcytosis of gastrointestinal epithelial cell monolayers by the pathogen has been demonstrated in tissue culture.[117] Next, the organisms can establish high-grade bacteremia in the immune-susceptible neonate through the complement resistance properties of its O lipopolysaccharide and K1 capsule–mediated impairment of opsonophagocytic killing.[118] Finally, the pathogen possesses a series of surface protein determinants (OmpA, IbeA-C, CNF1, etc.) that mediate binding to and invasion of brain endothelial cells, as demonstrated in human tissue culture experiments and the neonatal rat model of meningitis.[113]

KLEBSIELLA SPECIES

Klebsiella is a genus of Enterobacteriaceae that has emerged as a significant nosocomial pathogen in neonates.[119,120] The four recognized species include *Klebsiella pneumoniae, Klebsiella oxytoca, Klebsiella terrigena,* and *Klebsiella planticola. K. pneumoniae,* the most common human pathogen, and *K. oxytoca* cause neonatal infections of the bloodstream, urinary tract, CNS, lung, skin, and soft tissues.[121-123] Previously thought to be a nonpathogenic organism inhabiting soil and water, *K. planticola* has been implicated as a cause of neonatal sepsis.[124,125]

In a 4-year retrospective study from Israel,[126] *Klebsiella* spp. caused 31% of late-onset neonatal sepsis. Greenberg and colleagues[12] performed an 8-year prospective study of neonatal sepsis and meningitis at Soroka University Medical Center in Israel during 1986 to 1994; 49 (20%) of 250 cases were caused by *K. pneumoniae*, with a mortality rate of 29%. *Klebsiella* was also the most common single agent in recent reviews of sepsis in Jamaican[127] and Indian[128] neonates. Risk factors for infection included preterm, VLBW, prolonged rupture of membranes (>24 hours), and cesarean section or instrument delivery. *Klebsiella* spp. appear to be among the more common causes of liver abscess complicating bacteremia in the neonate.[129]

The reservoirs for transmission of *Klebsiella* infections include the hands of health care workers and the gastrointestinal tracts of hospitalized infants. Multidrug resistance, in the form of extended-spectrum β-lactamase production, of *Klebsiella* strains causing neonatal infections and nursery outbreaks has become a substantial problem in some nurseries and is associated with increased morbidity and mortality.[130-132] Enhanced infection-control measures and changes in use of routine broad-spectrum antibiotics can reduce the frequency of these serious infections.

ENTEROBACTER AND *CRONOBACTER* SPECIES

Among the *Enterobacter* spp., *Enterobacter cloacae, Enterobacter sakazakii,* and *Enterobacter hormaechei* have caused sepsis and a severe form of necrotizing meningitis in neonates.[133-135] In 2008, the taxonomy of *E. sakazakii* was revised, resulting in identification of five species belonging to a new genus, *Cronobacter*.[136]

Enterobacter septicemia was the most common nosocomial infection in neonates at the Ondokuz Mayis University Hospital in Samsun, Turkey, from 1988 to 1992.[137] Willis and Robinson[138] reviewed 17 cases of neonatal meningitis caused by *E. sakazakii;* cerebral abscess or cyst formation developed in 77% of the infants, and 50% of the infants died. Bonadio and colleagues[139] reviewed 30 cases of *E. cloacae* bacteremia in children, including 10 infants younger than 2 months. Of importance was the high frequency of multidrug resistance among isolates from patients in the

NICUs that was attributed to routine extended-spectrum cephalosporin use.[140] In a recent review of *Enterobacter* sepsis in 28 neonates from Taiwan, thrombocytopenia (66%) and increased band-form neutrophils (41%) were common laboratory features, with a reported clinical outcome of 11% mortality, 14% meningitis, and 7% brain abscess.[141]

In addition to the gastrointestinal tracts of hospitalized infants and hands of health care personnel, sources and modes of transmission of *Enterobacter* infections in the neonate include contaminated infant formula,[142,143] contaminated total parenteral nutrition fluid,[144,145] bladder catheterization devices,[144] and contaminated saline.[146] Effective infection-control measures require reinforcement of procedures, including proper hand hygiene, aseptic technique, isolation protocols, and disinfection of environmental surfaces.

Cronobacter spp. are an emerging group of opportunistic gram-negative pathogens that typically affect LBW neonates, causing life-threatening meningitis, sepsis, and NEC.[147] An outbreak of *C. sakazakii* in a French NICU in 1994 involved 17 cases, including 7 neonates with NEC, 1 case of sepsis, and 1 case of meningitis; 8 infants were colonized but asymptomatic; there were three deaths. Four separable pulse types of *C. sakazakii* were identified, but the deaths were attributable to only one.[148] *C. sakazakii* infection in vulnerable infants has often been linked to the consumption of contaminated powdered infant formula.[149]

CITROBACTER SPECIES

Organisms of the genus *Citrobacter* are gram-negative bacilli that are occasional inhabitants of the gastrointestinal tract and are responsible for disease in neonates and debilitated or immunocompromised patients. The genus has undergone frequent changes in nomenclature, making it difficult to relate the types identified in reports of newborn disease over the years. For example, in 1990, *Citrobacter koseri* replaced *Citrobacter diversus*.[150]

Citrobacter spp. are responsible for sporadic and epidemic clusters of neonatal sepsis and meningitis, and *C. koseri* is uniquely associated with brain abscesses.[150-155] Neonatal disease can occur as early- or late-onset presentations. Brain abscesses caused by *C. koseri* have been reported in a pair of twins.[156] Outbreaks of *C. koseri* in NICUs resulting in sepsis and meningitis, septic arthritis, and skin and soft tissue infections were reviewed by Doran.[150] Other focal infections in neonates caused by *Citrobacter* spp. include bone, pulmonary, and urinary tract infections.[150]

From 1960 to 1980, 74 cases of meningitis caused by *Citrobacter* spp. were reported to the CDC of the U.S. Public Health Service.[157] In 1999, Doran reviewed an additional 56 cases of neonatal meningitis caused by *Citrobacter* spp.[150] Combining results from the two studies, brain abscess developed in 73 (76%) of 96 patients for whom information was available. The pathogenesis of brain abscess caused by *C. koseri* is uncertain; cerebral vasculitis with infarction and bacterial invasion of necrotic tissues is one possible explanation.[153] Studies in the neonatal rat model suggest that the ability of *C. koseri* to survive phagolysosome fusion and persist intracellularly within macrophages could contribute to the establishment of chronic CNS infection and brain abscess.[158] Such persistence of *C. koseri* in the CNS is well illustrated by a case report of recovery of the organism from the CSF during a surgical procedure 4 years after treatment of neonatal meningitis.[152] The mortality rate for meningitis caused by *Citrobacter* spp. was about 30%; most of the infants who survived had some degree of mental retardation. A review of 110 survivors of *Citrobacter* meningitis revealed only 20 infants who were believed to have structurally intact brains and development that was age appropriate.[150]

Citrobacter spp. usually are resistant to ampicillin and variably susceptible to aminoglycosides. Serial neuroimaging is critical for the diagnosis of cerebral abscess in infants with *Citrobacter* meningitis.[159] Surgical drainage has been used in some cases with variable success. Choosing antimicrobial agents with the most advantageous susceptibility pattern and selected surgical drainage appears to be the most promising approach to therapy. High neutrophil and CNS penetration and favorable toxicity profiles suggest ciprofloxacin and meropenem as potential antibiotic treatment options for systemic infection or meningitis caused by *C. koseri*.[160] Plasmid profiles, biotypes, serotypes, and chromosomal restriction endonuclease digests are useful as epidemiologic markers for the study of isolates of *C. koseri*. Morris and colleagues[154] used these markers to investigate an outbreak of six cases of neonatal meningitis caused by *C. koseri* in three Baltimore hospitals between 1983 and 1985. Identification of a specific outer membrane protein associated with strains isolated from CSF but uncommon elsewhere can provide a marker for virulent strains of *C. koseri* according to some investigators.[155]

SERRATIA MARCESCENS

Like other members of Enterobacteriaceae, *Serratia marcescens* increasingly is associated with hospital-acquired infections among infants in the NICU.[161-163] Late-onset sepsis has occurred in infants infected from health care equipment,[162,164-166] the hands of heath care workers,[167] milk bottles,[161] aqueous solutions such as theophylline,[161] hand hygiene washes,[162] and lipid parenteral feeds.[165] The gastrointestinal tracts of hospitalized infants provide a reservoir for transmission and infection.[164] Investigation of an outbreak of multidrug-resistant *S. marcescens* in NICU identified exposure to inhalational therapy as an independent risk factor for acquisition.[168] Recently, three consecutive outbreaks caused by genetically unrelated *S. marcescens* clones occurred in a NICU over a 3-year period, with administration of total parenteral nutrition the only statistically significant risk factor identified by logistic regression.[169]

In a review of neonatal bacteremia and meningitis caused by *S. marcescens* by Campbell and colleagues,[170] 11 (29%) of 38 infants had meningitis as a complication of their bacteremia. Mean gestational age and birth weight were 28 weeks and 1099 g, respectively. All patients required mechanical ventilation, 90% had central venous catheters in situ, 90% had received prior antibiotics, 50% had a prior intraventricular hemorrhage, 40% had a hemodynamically significant patent ductus arteriosis treated medically or surgically, and 20% had NEC with perforation. All patients were treated for a minimum of 21 days with combination antimicrobial therapy that included a third-generation cephalosporin or an ureidopenicillin and an aminoglycoside, typically gentamicin. Three of 10 patients died. Four of the 7 survivors developed severe hydrocephalus requiring ventriculoperitoneal shunt placement and had poor neurologic outcome. Poor neurologic outcome also was documented in a report of *S. marcescens* brain abscess, resulting in multicystic encephalomalacia and severe developmental retardation.[171] Combination therapy with high-dose amikacin and meropenem was associated with clinical improvement in a case of *S. marcescens* brain abscess in a 34-week premature neonate.[172]

PSEUDOMONAS AERUGINOSA

Pseudomonas aeruginosa usually is a cause of late-onset disease in infants who are presumably infected from their endogenous flora or from equipment, from aqueous solutions, or occasionally from the hands of health care workers. An outbreak of *P. aeruginosa* sepsis in a French NICU was associated with contamination of a milk bank pasteurizer.[173] Stevens and colleagues[174] reported nine infants with *Pseudomonas* sepsis, four of whom presented in the first 72 hours of life. In three of these infants, the initial signs were those of respiratory distress, and chest radiographs were consistent with hyaline membrane disease. Noma (i.e., gangrenous lesions of the nose, lips, and mouth) in a neonate has been associated with bacteremia caused by *P. aeruginosa.*[175]

A retrospective review of sepsis in infants admitted over the 10-year period from 1988 through 1997 to the NICU at Children's Hospital of the King's Daughters in Norfolk, Virginia, identified 825 cases of LOS.[14] Infants with *Pseudomonas* sepsis had the highest frequency of clinically fulminant onset (56%), and 20 (56%) of the 36 (56%) infants with *Pseudomonas* sepsis died within 48 hours of blood-culture collection.

P. aeruginosa conjunctivitis in the neonate is a danger because it is rapidly destructive to the tissues of the eye and because it may lead to sepsis and meningitis. Shah and Gallagher[176] reviewed the course of 18 infants at Yale–New Haven Hospital NICU who had *P. aeruginosa* isolated from cultures of the conjunctiva during the 10 years beginning in 1986. Five infants developed bacteremia, including 3 with meningitis, and 2 infants died. A cluster of four fatal cases of *P. aeruginosa* pneumonia and bacteremia among neonates was traced by genotypic fingerprinting to their shared exposure to a health care worker experiencing intermittent otitis externa.[177] A case of fatal multidrug-resistant pseudomonal sepsis with ecthyma gangrenosum was recently reported in a premature neonate, shortly after the infant was discharged after a prolonged course of empirical antibiotic therapy secondary to maternal chorioamnionitis.[178]

SALMONELLA SPECIES

Non-Typhi *Salmonella* infection is an uncommon cause of sepsis and meningitis in neonates, but a significant proportion of cases of *Salmonella* meningitis occur in young infants. The CDC observed that approximately one third of 290 *Salmonella* isolates from CSF reported during 1968 to 1979 were from patients younger than 3 months, and more than one half were from infants younger than 1 year.[179] A 21-year review of gram-negative enteric meningitis in Dallas, beginning in 1969, identified *Salmonella* as the cause in 4 of 72 cases.[24] Investigators from Turkey reported 7 cases of neonatal meningitis caused by *Salmonella* during 1995 to 2001.[180] Two of the five survivors developed communicating hydrocephalus, and one had a subdural empyema. Cases of neonatal meningitis caused by *Salmonella enterica* ser. *Ancona,* in which the pathogen was isolated simultaneously from the newborn's CSF, parental fecal samples, and the mother's breast milk[181]; *S. enterica* ser. *Arizona* meningitis in a 13-day-old girl[182]; and septicemia caused by *S. Paratyphi* B[183] were recently reported.

Reed and Klugman[184] reviewed 10 cases of neonatal typhoid that occurred in a rural African hospital. Six of the infants had early-onset sepsis with acquisition of the organism from the maternal genital tract, and 4 had late-onset infection with acquisition from a carrier or an environmental source. Two neonates developed meningitis, and 3 died. Recurrent *S. entertidis* meningitis in a neonate after a 3-week course of ceftriaxone and ciprofloxacin was recently described.[185]

NEISSERIA MENINGITIDIS

Although *Neisseria meningitidis* is a leading cause of bacterial sepsis and meningitis among children and adolescents, it rarely is associated with invasive infection in neonates.[12,27,186] *N. meningitidis* may colonize the female genital tract[187] and has been associated with pelvic inflammatory disease.[188] The infant can be infected at delivery by organisms present in the maternal genital tract, or intrauterine infection can result during maternal meningococcemia.[189] Meningococcal sepsis is rare in the neonate, but more than 50 cases (including 13 from the preantibiotic era) have been described.[190,191] Early- and late-onset forms[191,192] of meningococcal sepsis in neonates have been reported. Purpura similar to that of meningococcemia in older children has been observed in a 15-day-old[193] and a 25-day-old infant.[194]

Shepard and colleagues[191] from the CDC reported 22 neonates with invasive meningococcal disease from a 10-year active, population-based surveillance of 10 states with diverse populations and more than 31 million persons. The average annual incidence was 9 cases per 100,000 people (vs. 973.8/100,000 for GBS). Sixteen patients had meningitis, and 6 of these also had meningococcemia. Six patients had early-onset disease. The overall mortality rate was 14%. Ten isolates were serogroup B, 4 were serogroup C, 3 were serogroup Y, 1 was nongroupable, and 4 were unavailable for analysis. Cases of meningococcal meningitis in infants successfully treated with no evidence of neurologic sequelae have been described.[195,196]

HAEMOPHILUS INFLUENZAE

Because of the introduction of *H. influenzae* type b conjugate vaccines in 1988, there has been a substantial decrease in the incidence in *H. influenzae* type b disease in infants and children in the United States and many other countries.[197,198] Given the estimated proportion of individuals that are completely immunized, the decrease in *H. influenzae* type b invasive disease has exceeded expectations. The reduction in *H. influenzae* carriage associated with vaccination and the consequent decreased transmission from immunized children to unimmunized infants and children likely explains this effect.[199,200]

Despite increased reporting of invasive infections caused by nontypeable *H. influenzae* in adults and older children,[201] such infections in neonates remain uncommon.[202-205] Five clinical syndromes have been associated with neonatal disease caused by *H. influenzae*: sepsis or respiratory distress syndrome, pneumonia, meningitis, soft tissue or joint infection, and otitis media or mastoiditis. The overall mortality rate was 5.5% for 45 cases reviewed by Friesen and Cho[206]; the mortality rate was 90% for 20 infants with a gestation lasting less than 30 weeks. Clinical and epidemiologic characteristics were similar to those of neonatal disease caused by GBS, including early- (within 24 hours of birth) and late-onset presentations, signs simulating respiratory distress syndrome, and a high mortality rate. Autopsy of infants with bacteremia related to nontypeable *H. influenzae* and signs of respiratory distress syndrome revealed hyaline membranes with gram-negative coccobacilli within the membranes, similar to findings of hyaline membranes caused by GBS.[207] Examination of placentas from mothers of infants with sepsis caused by nontypeable *H. influenzae* revealed acute chorioamnionitis and acute villitis in some.[203] *H. influenzae* also has been responsible for maternal disease, including bacteremia, chorioamnionitis,[208] acute or chronic salpingitis, and tubo-ovarian abscess.[204] Recently, a cluster of 8 cases of early-onset infections over 53 months caused by β-lactamase negative, nontypeable *H. influenzae* was reported from a NICU in Israel.[209] In this series, a presentation resembling pneumonia, rather than classic respiratory distress syndrome, characterized the infants' respiratory problems.

Neonatal sepsis caused by *Haemophilus parainfluenzae*[210] and *Haemophilus aphrophilus*[211] have also been reported.

ANAEROBIC BACTERIA

Improvements in techniques for isolation and identification of the various genera and species of anaerobic bacteria have provided a better understanding of the anaerobic flora of humans and their role in disease.[212] With the exception of *Clostridium tetani* and *Clostridium botulinum*, all of the anaerobic bacteria belong to the normal flora of humans. Anaerobes are present on the skin, in the mouth, in the intestines, and in the genital tract. They account for the greatest proportion of the bacteria of the stool. All are present in the intestines and have been isolated from the external genitalia or vagina of pregnant and nonpregnant women.[213] Newborns are colonized with these organisms during or just before delivery. A literature review by Brook[214] in 1990, on neonatal bacteremia caused by anaerobic bacteria, included 179 cases, with a mortality rate of 26%. *Bacteroides* and *Clostridium* spp. were the most common isolates. Predisposing factors for infection included premature rupture of membranes, preterm delivery, and NEC.

Anaerobic bacteria have been isolated from the blood of newborns with sepsis,[215-217] from various organs at autopsy,[218] from an infant with an adrenal abscess,[219] from an infant with an infected cephalhematoma,[220] and from infants with necrotizing fasciitis of the scalp associated with placement of a scalp electrode.[221] Feder[222] reviewed meningitis caused by *Bacteroides fragilis;* seven of nine reported cases occurred in neonates.

The incidence of neonatal sepsis caused by anaerobic bacteria remains uncertain, but recent data are available from some surveys that suggest the incidence is low (<5%).[12,14,214] Noel and colleagues[216] identified 29 episodes of anaerobic bacteremia in neonates in the intensive care unit (ICU) at New York Hospital during 18 years. Chow and coworkers[218] analyzed 59 cases of neonatal sepsis associated with anaerobic pathogens and classified them into four groups: transient bacteremia after premature rupture of membranes and maternal amnionitis, sepsis after postoperative complications, fulminant septicemia (in the case of clostridial infections), and intrauterine death associated with septic abortion. The mortality rate associated with neonatal anaerobic sepsis reported in the literature ranges from 4% to 38%.[218,223,224]

Serious infections of the bloodstream or CNS of neonates caused by *Bacillus cereus* have been reported,[225-227] and in certain cases have proven intractable and refractory to antibiotic therapy.[228,229] Magnetic resonance imaging of *B. cereus* meningoencephalitis reveals a pattern of hemorrhage and early cavitation accompanied by selective white matter destruction.[230] An outbreak of *B. cereus* infections in a NICU was traced to contamination of balloons used in mechanical ventilation.[231] *Bacteroides fragilis* has been identified as a cause of pneumonia, sepsis, or meningitis in the immediate newborn period.[232-234]

Infections caused by *Clostridium* spp. can be localized, as in the case of omphalitis,[235] cellulitis, and necrotizing fasciitis,[236] or can manifest as sepsis or meningitis.[237] Disease in neonates has been related to *Clostridium perfringens, Clostridium septicum, Clostridium sordellii, Clostridium butyricum, Clostridium tertium,* and *Clostridium paraputrificum.*[238] The presenting signs usually are similar to those of other forms of bacterial sepsis. Chaney[237] reported a case of bacteremia caused by *C. perfringens* in mother and child in which the neonate had classic features of adult clostridial sepsis, including active hemolysis, hyperbilirubinemia, and hemoglobinuria. Motz and colleagues[239] reviewed five cases of clostridial meningitis caused by *C. butyricum* and *C. perfringens*. Clostridial sepsis is accompanied by a high mortality rate.[237]

NEONATAL TETANUS

Neonatal tetanus is caused by the gram-positive anaerobic spore-forming bacillus, *C. tetani.* The organism is present in soil and can be present in human and animal feces. Infection usually occurs after contamination of the umbilical stump. Maternal and neonatal tetanus are important causes of mortality in developing countries, claiming an estimated 180,000 lives annually.[240] In the United States, tetanus in the newborn is exceedingly rare.[241] Since 1984, only three cases of neonatal tetanus have been reported.[241-243] The most recent case, reported from Montana in 1998, was an infant born to an unimmunized mother; the parents used a *C. tetani*–contaminated clay powder to accelerate drying of the umbilical cord. The use of this product had been promoted on an Internet site on "cord care" for use by midwives.[244]

In many developing countries, both the incidence and mortality of neonatal tetanus remain startlingly high.[245-248] Mustafa and colleagues[249] conducted a retrospective neonatal tetanus survey among rural and displaced communities in the East Nile province in the Sudan and observed an incidence of neonatal tetanus of 7.1 cases per 1000 live births, more than double that reported from the stable rural community (3.2/1000). In both communities, coverage with two doses of tetanus toxoid was about 58%. Mortality attributable to neonatal tetanus in Djakarta in 1982 was 6.9 deaths per 1000 live births, and in the island provinces of Indonesia, it was 10.7 deaths per 1000 live births.[250] Among 62 cases of neonatal tetanus in Ethiopia, 90% were born at home and 70% lacked antenatal care.[248] Three quarters of infants in this series died in hospital, and risk factors for fatal outcome included an incubation period of less than 1 week, onset of symptoms at less than 48 hours, tachycardia, and fever.[248] The mortality rate for neonates with tetanus in Lima, Peru was 45% and was not improved with use of intrathecal tetanus antitoxin.[251] However, a meta-analysis of intrathecal therapy in tetanus suggested benefit in adults but not in neonates.[252] A recent systematic review of prognostic factors in neonatal tetanus indicated that LBW and age of onset less than or equal to 5 to 7 days were crucial factors increasing the odds of death.[253]

Application of contaminated materials to the umbilical cord is associated with deep-rooted customs and rituals in developing countries. A case-control study to identify risk factors for neonatal tetanus in rural Pakistan identified application of ghee (i.e., clarified butter from the milk of water buffaloes or cows) to the umbilical wound as the single most important risk factor.[254] Although commercial ghee is available in Pakistan, the ghee used in rural areas is made at home from unpasteurized milk. Oudesluys-Murphy[255] observed that application of some materials, including ghee and a stone wrapped in wet cloth, increased the risk of neonatal tetanus among Yoruba women but that other practices of cord care decreased the incidence, including searing of the cord with heat in China during the Ming dynasty and use of a candle flame to scar the cord in Guatemala.

Neonatal tetanus is a preventable disease; use of hygienic techniques at delivery and a program of tetanus toxoid immunization of children and young adults, particularly of pregnant women, are effective in eliminating this lethal disease.[255,256] A systematic review of interventions to reduce neonatal tetanus mortality found vaccination of pregnant women with tetanus toxoid to be the key factor; in resource-poor countries such as Pakistan, this single intervention coupled with regular effective antenatal checkups and clean delivery practices effectively reduces neonatal tetanus.[257]

MIXED INFECTIONS

Multiple organisms frequently are present in brain, liver, or lung abscesses; lung aspirate after pneumonia; or pleural empyema, but multiple organisms are found infrequently in cultures of blood or CSF. When several species are found, the significance of each is uncertain because it is possible that one or more of the organisms in a mixed culture is a contaminant.

Bacteremia with more than one organism occurs in patients with immunodeficiency, major congenital abnormalities, or contamination of a body fluid with multiple organisms, as is present in peritonitis, typically as a sequela of severe NEC in the VLBW infant. Neonatal meningitis caused by *S. pneumoniae* and *Acinetobacter calcoaceticus*[258] and sepsis caused by *P. aeruginosa* and *Yersinia enterocolitica*[259] have been reported. Although included in a series of cases of neonatal sepsis by some investigators, mixed cultures are not identified by most. Mixed infections were reported by Tessin and coworkers[260] in 5% of 231 Swedish neonates, by Vesikari and associates[261] in 4% of 377 Finnish infants, and by Bruun and Paerregaard[262] in 7% of 81 Danish neonates. Faix and Kovarik[263] reviewed the records of 385 specimens of blood or CSF submitted to the microbiology laboratories at the University of Michigan Medical Center from September 1971 to June 1986. More than one organism was present in 38 specimens from 385 infants in the NICU; 15 (3.9%) infants had multiple pathogens associated with clinical signs of sepsis or meningitis. The mortality was high (60%). Factors predisposing to mixed infection included prolonged rupture of membranes (>24 hours), total parenteral nutrition, NEC, presence of an intravascular catheter or ventriculostomy, and entities associated with multiple pathogens, including peritonitis, pseudomembranous colitis, and hepatic necrosis. Chow and colleagues[218] reported polymicrobial bacteremia in eight newborns with anaerobic co-isolates or aerobic and anaerobic organisms in combination. An outbreak of polymicrobial bacteremia caused by *K. pneumoniae* and *E. cloacae* associated with use of a contaminated lipid emulsion was reported by Jarvis and colleagues.[264]

Mixed infections also can include bacteria and viruses or bacteria and fungi, typically *Candida*, in the situation of intravascular central catheter or peritoneal infections associated with bowel perforation. Sferra and Pacini[265] reported mixed viral-bacterial meningitis in five patients, including neonates with CSF isolates of enterovirus and GBS in a 10-day-old child and enterovirus and *Salmonella* in a 12-day-old child.

UNCOMMON BACTERIAL PATHOGENS

A large number of additional bacterial pathogens have been identified as rare or uncommon causes for neonatal sepsis and meningitis. These are listed in Table 6-7 with references, and were reviewed by Giacoia.[266]

Epidemiology

INCIDENCE OF SEPSIS AND MENINGITIS

The reported incidence of neonatal sepsis varies from less than 1 to 8.1 cases per 1000 live births.* The increased use of intrapartum antibiotic prophylaxis for women with GBS colonization, with or without other risk factors associated with neonatal GBS disease, has been associated with a 70% reduction in the incidence of early-onset GBS sepsis to 0.44 per 1000 live births in 1999, a rate comparable to that of LOS[7] (see Chapter 12).

*References 12, 18, 20, 119, 126, 260, 267-270.

Table 6-7 Unusual Pathogens Responsible for Neonatal Sepsis and Meningitis

Organism	Reference
Achromobacter spp.	743-745
Acinetobacter spp.	746-750
Bacillus anthracis	751
Bacillus cereus	226, 228, 231, 752
Borrelia (relapsing fever)	753, 754
Brucella spp.	755, 756
Burkholderia cepacia	757-759
Burkholderia pseudomallei	760
Campylobacter spp.	725, 761
Capnocytophaga spp.	762-764
Corynebacterium spp.	765, 766
Edwardsiella tarda	767-769
Escherichia hermanii	770, 771
Chryseobacterium (Flavobacterium) spp.	772, 773
Gardnerella vaginalis	774, 775
Helicobacter cinaedi	776
Lactobacillus spp.	777, 778
Leptospira spp.	779, 780
Leuconostoc spp.	781, 782
Morganella morganii	783-785
Mycoplasma hominis	786
Ochrobactrum anthropi	787
Pantoea agglomerans	788
Pasteurella spp.	722, 789, 790
Plesiomonas spp.	791-793
Proteus mirabilis	794-796
Pseudomonas pseudomallei	797
Psychrobacter immobilis	798
Ralstonia pickettii	799
Rothia dentocariosa	800
Shigella sonnei	801-803
Staphylococcus capitis	804
Stomatococcus mucilaginosus	805
Vibrio cholerae	806, 807
Yersinia enterocolitica	808, 809
Yersinia pestis	810

The incidence of meningitis usually is a fraction of the number of neonates with early-onset sepsis. During the 8-year period from 1986 to 1994 at the Soroka University Medical Center in southern Israel, Greenberg and colleagues[12] found incidences of neonatal bacterial sepsis and meningitis of 3.2 and 0.5 cases per 1000 live births, respectively. Certain pathogens that cause bloodstream invasion, such as GBS, *E. coli*, and *L. monocytogenes*, are more likely to be accompanied by meningeal invasion than others (e.g., *S. aureus*). Meningitis is more frequent during the first month of life than in any subsequent period.

CHARACTERISTICS OF INFANTS WHO DEVELOP SEPSIS

Host susceptibility, socioeconomic factors, obstetric and nursery practices, and the health and nutrition of mothers are important in the pathogenesis of neonatal sepsis and meningitis. Infants who develop sepsis, particularly early-onset disease, usually have a history of one or more risk factors associated with the pregnancy and delivery that significantly increase the risk for neonatal infection. These factors include preterm delivery or LBW, premature rupture of membranes (i.e., rupture before the onset of labor), prolonged time of rupture of membranes, maternal peripartum infection, septic or traumatic delivery, and fetal hypoxia.

Birth Weight

The factor associated most significantly with enhanced risk for bacterial sepsis and meningitis in neonates is LBW[12,18-20,271] (see Table 6-5). Infection is the most common cause of death in VLBW infants[271,272]; the diagnosis of early-onset sepsis in this population is associated with a threefold increase in mortality.[273] However, with the exception of infection caused by GBS, it is unusual for a term infant to develop early-onset sepsis after an uneventful pregnancy and delivery. In a U.K. study, neonates born weighing less than 2000 g acquired meningitis six times more frequently than did infants weighing greater than 2000 g.[27] The lower the infant's birth weight, the higher is the incidence of sepsis (see Table 6-5). An Israeli study of 5555 VLBW infants documented the increased risk of LOS with decreasing birth weight; LOS occurred in 16.8% of neonates with a birth weight of 1250 to 1500 g, 30.6% of neonates weighing 1000 to 1249 g, 46.4% of those weighing 750 to 999 g, and 53% of those weighing less than 750 g at birth.[16] In NICHD prospective disease surveillance from 2006 to 2009, the incidence of infection per 1000 live births was 0.57 for infants with birth weight greater than 2500 g, 1.38 for infants with birth weight 1500 to 2500 g, and 10.96 for infants of birth weight 400 to 1500 g.[20]

Risk Factors of Infant and Mother

The relative importance of other factors associated with systemic infection in the newborn is more difficult to define. Greenberg and coworkers[12] found that certain conditions were common in their prospective study of 229 infants with sepsis and meningitis: 130 (57%) were premature (<37 weeks of gestation), 64 (28%) were delivered by cesarean section or instrumental delivery, 43 (19%) had an Apgar score of less than 7 at 5 minutes, and 27 (2%) had a prolonged (>24 hours) interval after rupture of maternal membranes. Investigators in Pakistan[274] found that maternal urinary tract infection and maternal fever, vaginal discharge, and vaginal examinations during labor were maternal factors significantly associated with neonatal early-onset sepsis, whereas low Apgar scores at birth and the need for endotracheal intubation were significant neonatal risk factors.[20] Attack rates for early-onset sepsis are affected by birth weight, duration of rupture of membranes, and occurrence of maternal peripartum fever. Uterine or abdominal tenderness and/or maternal or fetal tachycardia are other suggestive signs (see Table 6-5).

Maternal fever during labor or after delivery suggests a concurrent infectious event in mother and infant, but noninfectious events may be responsible for maternal fever. Use of epidural analgesia for pain relief during labor is associated with increases in maternal temperature. Intrapartum fever of greater than 38° C (100.4° F) occurred an average of 6 hours after initiation of the epidural anesthesia in 14.5% of women receiving an epidural anesthetic, compared with 1.0% of women not receiving an epidural agent; the rate of fever increased from 7% in women with labors of less than 6 hours to 36% for labors lasting longer than 18 hours. There was no difference in the incidence of neonatal sepsis in the infants born to 1045 women who received epidural analgesia (0.3%), compared with infants born to women who did not have epidural analgesia (0.2%).[275] Fetal core temperature may be elevated during maternal temperature

Table 6-8 Selected Characteristics of Women,* Their Pregnancies, and Newborns

	PERCENT WITH CHARACTERISTICS	
Characteristic	**White Women**	**Black Women**
PREMATURE RUPTURE OF MEMBRANES: TIME FROM RUPTURE TO ONSET OF LABOR (HR)		
<8	70.9	56.7
8-23	18.3	21.9
24-48	5.4	11.7
≥49	5.4	9.7
PUERPERAL INFECTION	3.6	4.1
TYPE OF DELIVERY		
Vaginal vertex	91.7	92.4
Vaginal breech	3.3	2.6
Cesarean section	4.9	5.0
BIRTH WEIGHT < 2500 G	7.1	13.4
NEUTROPHILIC INFILTRATION OF		
Amnion	9.0	7.9
Chorion	13.1	15.6
Umbilical vein	14.6	7.5

Data from Niswander KR, Gordon M: *The women and their pregnancies. The Collaborative Perinatal Study of the National Institute of Neurological Diseases and Stroke. U.S. Department of Health, Education and Welfare Publication No. (NIH) 73-379,* Washington, DC, 1972, U.S. Government Printing Office.

*Approximately 18,700 white women and 19,800 black women were evaluated.

Table 6-9 Incidence of Fetal and Neonatal Infections by Sex

	NO. OF INFANTS		
Infection	**Male**	**Female**	**Ratio of Male to Female**
INTRAUTERINE INFECTIONS			
Syphilis	118	134	0.89
Tuberculosis	15	14	1.07
Toxoplasmosis	118	103	1.14
Listeriosis	26	37	0.70
PERINATAL SEPSIS			
Gram-negative organisms	82	34	2.41
Gram-positive organisms	58	31	1.87
PERINATAL MENINGITIS			
Gram-negative organisms	126	44	2.87
Gram-positive organisms	45	39	1.15

Data based on a review of the literature and study of Johns Hopkins Hospital case records, 1930-1963. Washburn TC, Medearis DN J, Childs B: Sex differences in susceptibility to infections, *Pediatrics* 35:57, 1965.

elevation, and increased temperature may be present transiently in the neonate after delivery.

Ethnicity

The Collaborative Perinatal Research Study provides historical information on 38,500 pregnancies[276]; selected data for white and black women are presented in Tables 6-4 and 6-8. Black women had a higher rate of premature rupture of membranes lasting more than 24 hours (21.4%), compared with white women (10.8%); black women had a higher rate of puerperal infection (4.1%), compared with white women (3.6%); and more black infants weighed less than 2500 g at birth (13.4%), compared with white infants (7.1%). Recent published data concurs with that observed 30 years ago. The National Center for Health Statistics reports continued disparities between blacks and whites in maternal and infant health indicators.[277] In 2010, significant differences were found between non-Hispanic blacks and the general population in terms of neonatal mortality (11.46 vs. 6.14 deaths/1000 live births), LBW (13.6% vs. 7.7%), and preterm delivery less than 37 weeks' gestation (17.1% vs. 12.0%). An earlier review of the literature from 1966 to 1994 reported significantly increased rates of severe histologic chorioamnionitis, maternal fever during labor, prolonged rupture of membranes, and early neonatal mortality from sepsis in blacks compared with whites.[278]

In a study of GBS disease in infants from the Atlanta metropolitan area,[268] black infants had a higher incidence than nonblack infants of early-onset disease; the risk of late-onset disease was 35 times greater in black than in white infants. Thirty percent of early-onset disease and 92% of late-onset disease could be attributed to black race, after controlling for other significant risk factors, such as LBW and maternal age younger than 20 years. The increased incidence of GBS disease in blacks of all ages was observed in a survey by the CDC in selected counties in California, Georgia, and Tennessee and the entire state of Oklahoma. The rate of disease of 13.5 cases per 100,000 blacks was significantly higher than the 4.5 cases per 100,000 whites. In neonates with early-onset infection, 2.7 cases per 1000 live births occurred in blacks and 1.3 cases per 1000 live births occurred in whites.[279] Maternal factors, such as socioeconomic status, nutrition, recently acquired sexually transmitted diseases, or racial differences in maternally acquired protective antibodies, may result in the increased risk of GBS disease among blacks.

Gender

Historical data have suggested that there is a predominance of male neonates affected by sepsis and meningitis but not by in utero infections[280,281] (Table 6-9). This difference partially may reflect the fact that female infants had lower rates of respiratory distress syndrome (i.e., hyaline membrane disease) than did male infants. Torday and colleagues[282] studied fetal pulmonary maturity by determining lecithin-to-sphingomyelin ratios and concentrations of saturated phosphatidylcholine and cortisol in amniotic fluid of fetuses between 28 and 40 weeks of gestation. Female infants had higher indices of pulmonary maturity than did male infants. These data provide a biochemical basis for the increased risk of respiratory distress syndrome in male infants and the possible role of these factors of pulmonary maturation in the development of pulmonary infection. Later studies failed to confirm a significant increased risk for bacterial sepsis and meningitis among male infants.[12,283-285]

Geographic Factors

The cause of neonatal sepsis varies from hospital to hospital and from one community to another. These differences probably reflect characteristics of the population served, including unique cultural features and sexual practices, local obstetric and nursery practices, and patterns of antimicrobial agent use. The bacteriology of neonatal sepsis and meningitis in western Europe† and Jamaica[288] is generally similar to that in the United States. In tropical areas, a somewhat different pattern can be observed.[289-291] In Riyadh, Saudi Arabia, from 1980 through 1984, *E. coli, Klebsiella,* and *Serratia* spp. were the dominant causes of neonatal sepsis; group B streptococci were an infrequent cause.[291] However, later data from this geographic location revealed *E. coli* and CoNS, respectively, were the most common pathogens causing early-onset and LOS.[292]

Every year four million neonatal deaths occur. About one third of the deaths are due to sepsis.[293,294] The highest numbers of neonatal deaths are in South Central Asian countries and sub-Saharan Africa. The global perspective of neonatal sepsis is discussed in Chapter 2. The most common isolates responsible for neonatal sepsis vary by country but include a wide spectrum of gram-negative and gram-positive species, the most common of which are *E. coli, S. aureus, Pseudomonas,* and *Klebsiella.*[295] Multidrug-resistant strains are an increasing threat to intervention programs.[296,297] In a recent meta-analysis of 19 neonatal sepsis studies identified from 13 developing countries, *Staphylococcus aureus, Klebsiella* spp., and *Escherichia coli* accounted for 55% (39%-70%) of culture-positive sepsis on weighted prevalence.[298]

GBS is the most frequent cause of early- and late-onset sepsis in the United States, but the rates and risk factors for maternal and neonatal GBS colonization and disease vary in different communities.[299-301] Amin and colleagues[299] in the United Arab Emirates evaluated 563 pregnant women from similar socioeconomic and ethnic backgrounds and reported a GBS colonization rate of 10.1%. In Athens, Greece, maternal and neonatal colonization rates were 6.6% and 2.4%, respectively, with a vertical transmission rate of 22.5%.[300] Middle-class women followed in the private setting were more frequently colonized with GBS than those followed in a public hospital. No association was found between colonization with GBS and maternal age, nationality, marital status, previous obstetric history, cesarean section, infant birth weight, or preterm birth.

Stoll and Schuchat[301] reviewed data on female genital colonization with GBS from 34 reports in the literature and emphasized the importance of appropriate specimen collection and inoculation into selective (antibiotic containing) broth media in the ascertainment of accurate colonization rates. Analysis of data from studies using adequate methods revealed regional GBS colonization rates of 12% in India and Pakistan, 19% in Asian and Pacific countries, 19% in sub-Saharan Africa, 22% in the Middle East and North Africa, and 14% in the Americas. A comparison of studies that did and did not use selective broth media revealed significantly higher GBS colonization rates in the populations where selective broth media was used to assess colonization. Other reasons for varying rates of GBS colonization and disease may include socioeconomic factors or differences in sexual practices, hygiene, or nutrition.

Socioeconomic Factors

The lifestyle pattern of mothers, including cultural practices, housing, nutrition, and level of income, appears to be important in determining infants at risk for infection. The most significant factors enhancing risk for neonatal sepsis are LBW and prematurity, and the incidence of these is inversely related to socioeconomic status. Various criteria for determining socioeconomic status have been used, but no completely satisfactory and reproducible standard is available. Maternal education, resources, and access to health care can affect the risk of neonatal sepsis. A CDC report[302] evaluating the awareness of perinatal GBS infection among women of childbearing age in the United States revealed that women with a high school education or less; women with a household income of less than $25,000; and women reporting black, Asian/Pacific Islander, or other ethnicity had lower awareness of perinatal GBS infections than other women.

Procedures

Most VLBW infants have one or more procedures that place them at risk for infection. Any disruption of the protective capability of the intact skin or mucosa can be associated with infection. In a multicenter study of NICU patients, increased risk of bacteremia was associated with parenteral nutrition, mechanical ventilation, peripherally inserted central catheters, peripheral venous catheters, and umbilical artery catheters.[303]

NURSERY OUTBREAKS OR EPIDEMICS

The nursery is a small community of highly susceptible infants where patients have contact with many adults, including parents, physicians, nurses, respiratory therapists, and diagnostic imaging technicians (see Chapter 14). Siblings may enter the nursery or mothers' hospital suites and represent an additional source of infection. In these circumstances, outbreaks or epidemics of respiratory and gastrointestinal illness, most of which is caused by nonbacterial agents, can occur. Spread of microorganisms to the infant occurs by droplets from the respiratory tracts of parents, nursery personnel, or other infants. Organisms can be transferred from infant to infant by the hands of health care workers. Individuals with open or draining lesions are especially hazardous agents of transmission.

Staphylococcal infection and disease are a concern in many nurseries in the United States (see Chapter 14). Epidemics or outbreaks associated with contamination of nursery equipment and solutions caused by *Proteus* spp., *Klebsiella* spp., *S. marcescens, Pseudomonas* spp., and *Flavobacterium* also have been reported. An unusual and unexplained outbreak of early-onset GBS sepsis with an attack rate of 14 per 1000 live births occurred in Kansas City during January through August of 1990.[304]

The availability of molecular techniques to distinguish bacterial strains provides an important epidemiologic tool in the investigation of nursery outbreaks. Previously, methods to determine strain relatedness relied on antibiotic susceptibility patterns, biochemical profiles, and plasmid or phage analysis.[154,305] More recent techniques permit the discrimination of strains based on bacterial chromosomal polymorphisms. Pulse-field gel electrophoresis, ribotyping, multilocus sequence typing, and polymerase chain reaction (PCR)-based methods are widely used tools to assign strain identity or relatedness.[306-308]

†References 10, 13, 26, 260-262, 267, 286, 287.

Antimicrobial agents play a major role in the ecology of the microbial flora in the nursery. Extensive and prolonged use of these drugs eliminates susceptible strains and allows proliferation of resistant subpopulations of neonatal flora. There is selective pressure toward colonization by microorganisms that are resistant to the antimicrobial agents used in the nurseries and, because of cross-resistance patterns, to similar drugs within an antimicrobial class.

A historical example of the selective pressure of a systemic antimicrobial agent is provided by Gezon and coworkers[41] in their use of benzathine penicillin G to control an outbreak of GAS disease. All infants entering the nursery during a 3-week period were treated with a single intramuscular dose of penicillin. Before institution of this policy, most strains of *S. aureus* in the nursery were susceptible to penicillin G. One week after initiation of the prophylactic regimen and for the next 2 years, almost all strains of *S. aureus* isolated from newborns in this nursery were resistant to penicillin G.

During a 4-month period in 1997, van der Zwet and colleagues[309] investigated a nosocomial nursery outbreak of gentamicin-resistant *K. pneumoniae* in which 13 neonates became colonized and 3 became infected. Molecular typing of strains revealed clonal similarity of isolates from 8 neonates. The nursery outbreak was terminated by the substitution of amikacin for gentamicin in neonates when treatment with an aminoglycoside was believed to be warranted. Development of resistance in gram-negative enteric bacilli also has been documented in an Israeli study after widespread use of aminoglycosides.[310]

Extensive or routine use of third-generation cephalosporins in the nursery, especially for all neonates with suspected sepsis, can lead to more rapid emergence of drug-resistant gram-negative enteric bacilli than occurs with the standard regimen of ampicillin and an aminoglycoside. Investigators in Brazil[130] performed a prospective investigation of extended-spectrum β-lactamase (ESBL)-producing *K. pneumoniae* colonization and infection during the 2-year period from 1997 to 1999 in the NICU. A significant independent risk factor for colonization was receipt of a cephalosporin and an aminoglycoside. Previous colonization was an independent risk factor for infection. In India, Jain and coworkers[140] concluded that indiscriminate use of third-generation cephalosporins was responsible for the selection of ESBL-producing, multiresistant strains in their NICU, where ESBL production was detected in 86.6% of *Klebsiella* spp., 73.4% of *Enterobacter* spp., and 63.6% of *E. coli* strains. Nosocomial infections in the nursery and their epidemiology and management are further discussed in Chapter 35.

Pathogenesis

The developing fetus is relatively protected from the microbial flora of the mother. However, procedures disturbing the integrity of the uterine contents, such as amniocentesis,[311] cervical cerclage,[312,313] transcervical chorionic villus sampling,[314] or percutaneous umbilical blood sampling,[311,315] can permit entry of skin or vaginal organisms into the amniotic sac, causing amnionitis and secondary fetal infection.

Initial colonization of the neonate usually takes place after rupture of the maternal membranes.[280,316] In most cases, the infant is colonized with the microflora of the birth canal during delivery. However, if delivery is delayed, vaginal bacteria may ascend the birth canal and, in some cases, produce inflammation of the fetal membranes, umbilical cord, and placenta.[317] Fetal infection can then result from aspiration of infected amniotic fluid,[318] leading to stillbirth, premature delivery, or neonatal sepsis.[311,317,319,320] The organisms most commonly isolated from infected amniotic fluid are GBS, *E. coli* and other enteric bacilli, anaerobic bacteria, and genital mycoplasmas.[311,319]

There are studies reporting that amniotic fluid inhibits the growth of *E. coli* and other bacteria because of the presence of lysozyme, transferrin, immune globulins (IgA and IgG but not IgM), zinc and phosphate, and lipid-rich substances.[320-326] The addition of meconium to amniotic fluid in vitro has resulted in increased growth of *E. coli* and GBS in some studies.[327,328] However, in other in vitro studies of the bacteriostatic activity of amniotic fluid, there is not inhibition of the growth of GBS.[329-331] Further discussion of bacterial inhibition by amniotic fluid is available in Chapter 3.

Infection of the mother at the time of birth, particularly genital infection, can play a significant role in the development of infection in the neonate. Transplacental hematogenous infection during or shortly before delivery (including the period of separation of the placenta) is possible, although it is more likely that the infant is infected just before or during passage through the birth canal. Among reports of concurrent bacteremia in mother and neonate are cases caused by *H. influenzae* type b,[332] *H. parainfluenzae*,[333] *S. pneumoniae*,[334,335] GAS,[336] *N. meningitidis*,[189] *Citrobacter* spp.,[337] and *Morganella morganii*,[338] and concurrent cases of meningitis have been reported as caused by *S. pneumoniae*,[339] *N. meningitidis*,[189] and GBS.[340] Many neonates are bacteremic at the time of delivery, which indicates that invasive infection occurred antepartum.[341] Infants with signs of sepsis during the first 24 hours of life also have the highest mortality rate.[10] These data suggest the importance of initiating chemoprophylaxis for women with GBS colonization or other risk factors for invasive disease in the neonate at the time of onset of labor (see Chapter 12).[342]

Microorganisms acquired by the newborn infant just before or during birth colonize the skin and mucosal surfaces, including the conjunctivae, nasopharynx, oropharynx, gastrointestinal tract, umbilical cord, and in the female infant, the external genitalia. Normal skin flora of the newborn includes CoNS, diphtheroids, and *E. coli*.[343] In most cases, the microorganisms proliferate at the initial site of attachment without resulting in illness. On occasion, contiguous areas may be infected by direct extension (e.g., sinusitis and otitis can occasionally occur from upper respiratory tract colonization).

Bacteria can be inoculated into the skin and soft tissue by obstetric forceps, and organisms may infect these tissues if abrasions or congenital defects are present. Scalp abscesses can occur in infants who have electrodes placed during labor for monitoring of heart rate.[81,344,345] The incidence of this type of infection in the hands of experienced clinicians, however, is generally quite low (0.1% to 5.2%).[346] A 10-year survey of neonatal enterococcal bacteremia detected 6 of 44 infants with scalp abscesses as the probable source of their bacteremia.[81] The investigators were unable from the data available to deduce whether these abscesses were associated with fetal scalp monitoring, intravenous infusion, or other procedures that resulted in loss of the skin barrier.

Transient bacteremia can accompany procedures that traumatize mucosal membranes, such as endotracheal suctioning.[347] Invasion of the bloodstream also can follow multiplication of organisms in the upper respiratory tract or other foci. Although the source of bacteremia frequently is inapparent, careful inspection can reveal a focus, such as an infected circumcision site or infection of the umbilical stump, in some neonates. Metastatic foci of infection can follow bacteremia and can involve the lungs, kidney, spleen, bones, or CNS.

Most cases of neonatal meningitis result from bacteremia. Fetal meningitis followed by stillbirth[348] or hydrocephalus, presumably because of maternal bacteremia and transplacentally acquired infection, has been described but is exceedingly rare. Although CSF leaks caused by spiral fetal scalp electrodes do occur, no cases of meningitis have been traced to this source.[349,350] After delivery, the meninges can be invaded directly from an infected skin lesion, with spread through the soft tissues and skull sutures and along thrombosed bridging veins,[316] but in most circumstances, bacteria gain access to the brain through the bloodstream to the choroid plexus during the course of sepsis.[348] Infants with developmental defects, such as a midline dermal sinus or myelomeningocele, are particularly susceptible to invasion of underlying nervous tissue.[24]

Brain abscesses can result from hematogenous spread of microorganisms (i.e., septic emboli) and proliferation in tissue that is devitalized because of anoxia or vasculitis with hemorrhage or infarction. Certain organisms are more likely than others to invade nervous tissue and cause local or widespread necrosis.[24] Most cases of meningitis related to *C. koseri* (formerly *C. diversus*) and *E. sakazakii* are associated with cyst and abscess formation. Other gram-negative bacilli with potential to cause brain abscesses include *Proteus, Citrobacter, Pseudomonas, S. marcescens,* and occasionally GBS.[155,170,351-353] Volpe[354] comments that bacteria associated with brain abscesses are those that cause meningitis with severe vasculitis.

HOST FACTORS PREDISPOSING TO NEONATAL BACTERIAL SEPSIS

Infants with one or more predisposing factors (e.g., LBW, premature rupture of membranes, septic or traumatic delivery, fetal hypoxia, maternal peripartum infection) are at increased risk for sepsis. Microbial factors such as inoculum size[355] and virulence properties of the organism[311] undoubtedly are significant. Immature function of phagocytes and decreased inflammatory and immune effector responses are characteristic of very small infants and can contribute to the unique susceptibility of the fetus and newborn (see Chapter 4).

Metabolic factors are likely to be important in increasing risk for sepsis and severity of the disease. Fetal hypoxia and acidosis can impede certain host defense mechanisms or allow localization of organisms in necrotic tissues. Infants with hyperbilirubinemia can suffer impairment of various immune functions, including neutrophil bactericidal activity, antibody response, lymphocyte proliferation, and complement functions (see Chapter 4). The indirect hyperbilirubinemia that commonly occurs with breastfeeding jaundice rarely is associated with neonatal sepsis.[356] Late-onset jaundice and direct hyperbilirubinemia can be the result of an infectious process. In one study from Turkey, more than one third of infants with late-onset direct hyperbilirubinemia had culture-proven sepsis, with gram-negative enteric bacteria, including *E. coli,* the most common etiologic agents.[357] Evidence of diffuse hepatocellular damage and bile stasis have been described in such infected and jaundiced infants.[358,359]

Hypothermia in newborns, generally defined as a rectal temperature equal to or less than 35° C (95° F), is associated with a significant increase in the incidence of sepsis, meningitis, pneumonia, and other serious bacterial infections.[360-363] In developing countries, hypothermia is a leading cause of death during the winter. Hypothermia frequently is accompanied by abnormal leukocyte counts, acidosis, and uremia, each of which can interfere with resistance to infection. However, the exact cause of increased morbidity in infants presenting with hypothermia remains poorly understood. In many infants, it is unclear whether hypothermia predisposes to or results from bacterial infection. For example, in a large outbreak of *S. marcescens* neonatal infections affecting 159 cases in Gaza City, Palestine, hypothermia was the single most common presenting symptom, recorded in 38% of cases.[364]

Infants with galactosemia have increased susceptibility to sepsis caused by gram-negative enteric bacilli, in particular *E. coli.*[365-367] Among 8 infants identified with galactosemia by routine newborn screening in Massachusetts, 4 had systemic infection caused by *E. coli.*[366] Three of these 4 infants died of sepsis and meningitis; the fourth infant, who had a urinary tract infection, survived. A survey of state programs in which newborns are screened for galactosemia revealed that among 32 infants detected, 10 had systemic infection, and 9 died of bacteremia. *E. coli* was the infecting organism in 9 of the infants. It appears that galactosemic neonates have an unusual predisposition to severe infection with *E. coli,* and bacterial sepsis is a significant cause of death among these infants. Depressed neutrophil function resulting from elevated serum galactose levels is postulated to be a possible cause of their predisposition to sepsis.[368,369] The gold standard for diagnosis of classic galactosemia is measurement of galactose-1-phosphate uridyltransferase (GALT) activity in erythrocytes, and the sole therapy is galactose restriction in the diet.[370] Shurin[368] observed that infants became ill when serum galactose levels were high and when glucose levels were likely to be low, and that susceptibility to infection diminished when dietary control was initiated.

Other inherited metabolic diseases have not been associated with a higher incidence of neonatal bacterial infection. A poorly documented increase in the relative frequency of sepsis has been observed among infants with hereditary fructose intolerance.[371] Infants with methylmalonic acidemia and other inborn errors of branched-chain amino acid metabolism manifest neutropenia as a result of bone marrow suppression by accumulated metabolites; however, no increased incidence of infection has been described in this group of infants.[372,373]

Iron may have an important role in the susceptibility of neonates to infection, but this continues to be controversial. Iron added to serum in vitro enhances the growth of many organisms, including *E. coli, Klebsiella* spp., *Pseudomonas* spp., *Salmonella* spp., *L. monocytogenes,* and *S. aureus.* The siderophore IroN is a proven virulence factor for the bacteremic phase of *E. coli* K1 sepsis and meningitis in the neonatal rat infection model.[374] Iron-binding proteins, lactoferrin and transferrin, are present in serum, saliva, and breast milk. However, the newborn has low levels of these proteins.[375] The iron sequestering capacity of oral bovine lactoferrin supplementation may be one contributing factor to its reported efficacy in prophylaxis of bacterial sepsis in VLBW infants.[376]

Barry and Reeve[377] demonstrated an increased incidence of sepsis in Polynesian infants who were treated with intramuscular iron as prophylaxis for iron-deficiency anemia. The regimen was shown to be effective in preventing anemia of infancy, but an extraordinary increase in bacterial sepsis occurred. The incidence of sepsis in newborns receiving iron was 17 cases per 1000 live births, whereas the incidence of sepsis in infants who did not receive iron was 3 cases per 1000 live births; during a comparable period, the rate of sepsis for European infants was 0.6 cases per 1000 live births. Special features of sepsis in the infants who received iron soon after birth were late onset, paucity of adverse perinatal factors, and predominance of *E. coli* as the cause of sepsis. During the period studied, *E. coli* was responsible for 26 of 27 cases of sepsis in iron-treated Polynesian infants and for none of three cases of sepsis in the infants who did not receive iron. Results of this study were similar to the experience reported by Farmer[378] for New Zealand infants given intramuscular iron. The incidence of meningitis caused by *E. coli* increased fivefold in infants who received iron and decreased when the use of iron was terminated. Conventional iron-supplemented human milk fortifiers, however, appear safe and do not contribute to a higher rate of sepsis in preterm infants.[379]

INFECTION IN TWINS

Studies have suggested a higher risk for contracting ascending intrauterine infection in the first than the second born of twins.[380,381] Comparing delivery methods, no difference was observed in the incidence of neonatal sepsis in twins delivered in the vertex/vertex position when compared with cases requiring uterine manipulation (vertex/breech extraction).[382] However, vaginal delivery of twin A, followed by cesarean delivery of twin B, may be associated with a higher rate of endometritis and neonatal sepsis when compared with cases where both twins are delivered by cesarean section.[383]

A recent large study from the NICHD Neonatal Research Network conducted from 2002 to 2008 identified LOS occurring in 25.0% (3797/15,178) of singleton and 22.6% (1196/5294) of multiple-birth infants with VLBW (401-1500 g).[384] CoNS accounted for 53.2% of episodes in singletons and 49.2% in multiples. A similar concordance of LOS in same-sex and unlike-sex twin pairs suggested that susceptibility to LOS among VLBW infants is not genetically determined.[384] No difference in complications or sepsis risk exists among twin pregnancies conceived spontaneously or through in vitro fertilization.[385]

Edwards and colleagues[386] studied GBS infection in 12 index cases of multiple gestations. Early-onset disease occurred in both twins in one pair and in one twin in five other pairs; late-onset infection occurred in both infants in two pairs and in one twin in four other pairs. Cases of late-onset GBS disease in twin pairs occurred closely in time to one another: 19 and 20 days in one set and at 28 and 32 days of age in the other set. In another case report of late-onset GBS infection in identical twins, twin A suffered fulminant fatal meningitis whereas twin B recovered completely. The GBS isolates proved to be genetically identical; clinical variables associated with the adverse outcome in twin A were longer duration of fever before antibiotics and the development of neutropenia.[387] In twins, the presence of virulent organisms in the environment, especially the maternal genital tract; their absence of specific maternal antibodies; and their similar genetic heritage probably contribute to the risk for invasive infection. It seems logical that twins, particularly if monochorionic, should have high rates of simultaneous early-onset infection, but it is particularly intriguing that some cases of late-onset disease occur in twins almost simultaneously. However, the incidence of infection in preterm twins co-bedding in the nursery did not differ from those cared for in separate beds.[388]

Infections in twins, including disease related to *Toxoplasma pallidum,* echoviruses 18 and 19, and *Toxoplasma gondii,* are discussed in Chapters 16, 25, and 31, respectively. Examples of neonatal infections in twins include those caused by GAS[389] (case report of streptococcal sepsis in a mother and infant twins), *Salmonella* spp.,[390] *C. koseri* (brain abscesses in twins,[156] malaria,[391,392] coccidioidomycosis,[393] cytomegalovirus infection,[394-396] and rubella[397]).

THE UMBILICAL CORD AS A FOCUS OF INFECTION

Historically, the umbilical cord was a particularly common portal of entry for systemic infection in the newborn, and infection by this route can still occur. The devitalized tissue is an excellent medium for bacterial growth, the recently thrombosed umbilical vessels provide access to the bloodstream, the umbilical vein is a direct route to the liver, and the umbilical artery and urachus are pathways to the pelvis.[398] Epidemics of erysipelas, staphylococcal disease, tetanus, and gas gangrene of the umbilicus were common in the 19th century. The introduction of simple hygienic measures in cord care resulted in a marked reduction of omphalitis.[399] In 1930, Cruickshank wrote, "in Prague, before antiseptic and aseptic dressing of the cord was introduced, sepsis neonatorum was as common as puerperal sepsis… after the introduction of cord dressing in the hospital the number of newborn children developing fever sank from 45% to 11.3%."[400,401]

Closure of the umbilical vessels and the subsequent aseptic necrosis of the cord begin soon after the infant takes the first breath; the umbilical arteries contract, the blood flow is interrupted, and the cord tissues, deprived of a blood supply, undergo aseptic necrosis. The umbilical stump acquires a rich flora of microorganisms. Within hours, the umbilical stump is colonized with large numbers of gram-positive cocci, particularly *Staphylococcus* spp., and shortly thereafter with fecal organisms.[401,402] These bacteria can invade the open umbilical wound, causing a localized infection with purulent discharge and, as a result of delayed obliteration of the umbilical vessels, bleeding from the umbilical stump. From this site, infection can proceed into the umbilical vessels, along the fascial planes of the abdominal wall, or into the peritoneum[401,403,404] (Fig. 6-1).

Although umbilical discharge or an "oozing" cord is the most common manifestation of omphalitis, periumbilical cellulitis and fasciitis are the conditions most often associated with hospitalization.[403] Infants presenting with fasciitis have a high incidence of bacteremia, intravascular coagulopathy, shock, and death.[403] Edema of the umbilicus and peau d'orange appearance of the surrounding abdominal skin, signaling obstruction of the underlying lymphatics, can be an early warning sign, whereas the pathognomonic purplish-blue discoloration implies advanced necrotizing fasciitis.[398] Septic embolization arising from the infected umbilical vessels is uncommon but can produce metastatic spread to various organs, including the lungs, pancreas, kidneys, and skin.[399] Such emboli can arise from the umbilical arteries and from the umbilical vein because final closure of the ductus venosus and separation of the portal circulation from the inferior vena cava and the systemic circulation are generally delayed until day 15 to day 30 of life.[405]

Complications of omphalitis, now a rare infection in developed countries because of modern umbilical cord care, include a variety of infections such as septic umbilical arteritis,[399,406] suppurative thrombophlebitis of the umbilical or portal veins or the ductus venosus,[406-408]

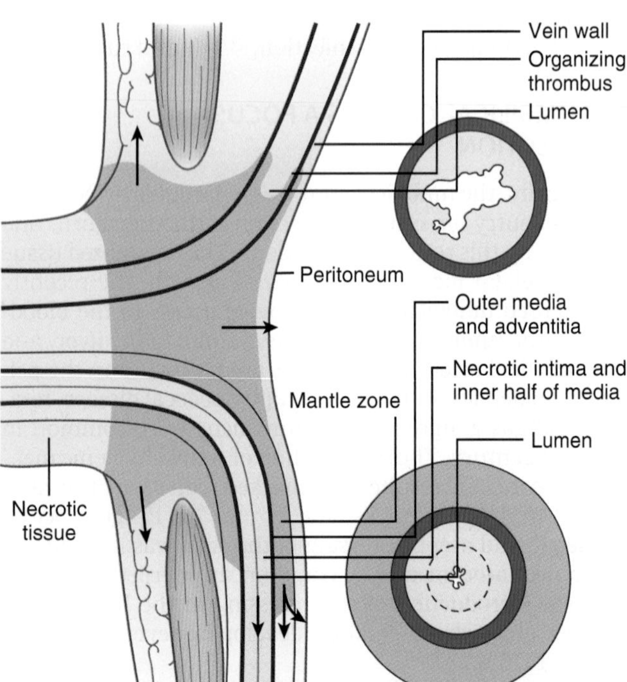

Figure 6-1 After birth, the necrotic tissue of the umbilical stump separates. This provokes some inflammation, which is limited by a fibroblastic reaction extending to the inner margin of the coarsely stippled area. The inner half of the media and the intima of the umbilical arteries become necrotic, but this does not stimulate an inflammatory reaction. *Arrows* indicate routes by which infection may spread beyond the granulation tissue barriers. Organisms invading the thrombus in the vein may disseminate by emboli. (Modified from Morison JE: *Foetal and neonatal pathology*, ed 3, Washington, DC, 1970, Butterworth.)

peritonitis,[404,406,407,409] intestinal gangrene,[404] pyourachus (infection of the urachal remnant),[410] liver abscess, endocarditis, pylephlebitis,[404,411] and subacute necrotizing funisitis.[412] Some of these infections can occur in the absence of signs of omphalitis.[399,406]

ADMINISTRATION OF DRUGS TO THE MOTHER BEFORE DELIVERY

Almost all antimicrobial agents cross the placenta. Antimicrobial drugs administered to the mother at term can alter the initial microflora of the neonate and can complicate the diagnosis of infection in the neonate. Chapter 37 reviews the clinical pharmacology of antimicrobial agents administered to the mother.

It is well established that studies have shown that corticosteroid administration to mothers in preterm labor to enhance pulmonary maturation in the fetus resulted in a significant decrease in the incidence and severity of neonatal respiratory distress syndrome but an increase in maternal infection, particularly endometritis, when compared with placebo[413]; however, the impacts of this practice on the risk of neonatal infection differed among early studies.[413,414] However, Roberts and Dalziel[415] recently performed large meta-analysis of 21 randomized controlled studies from the Cochrane Pregnancy and Childbirth Group Trials register, comprising in sum 3885 pregnant women and 4269 infants, and concluded that antenatal corticosteroid administration (betamethasone, dexamethasone, or hydrocortisone) given to women expected to deliver singleton or multiple pregnancies, whether labor was spontaneous, induced by membrane rupture, or electively induced, was associated with multiple favorable outcomes, including reduced neonatal death (risk ratio [RR], 0.69), intensive care admissions (RR, 0.80), and systemic infections in the first 48 hours of life (RR, 0.56).

Substance abuse during pregnancy can affect immune function in the neonate. Significant abnormalities in T-cell function and an apparent increased incidence of infections have been found during the first year of life among infants born to alcohol-addicted[416-418] and heroin-addicted[419,420] mothers. The adverse effects of cocaine and opiates on placental function, fetal growth and development, and prematurity also may predispose to a greater likelihood of neonatal infection.[420,421] Unfortunately, drug abuse is a multifactorial problem; it is virtually impossible to separate the consequences of direct pharmacologic effects on the fetus from those resulting from inadequate nutrition, lack of prenatal care, and infectious medical complications encountered in addicted pregnant women.[420,421]

ADMINISTRATION OF DRUGS OTHER THAN ANTIBIOTICS TO THE NEONATE

Administration of indomethacin to neonates for the closure of a patent ductus arteriosus (PDA) has been associated with a higher incidence of sepsis and NEC in the indomethacin-treated groups compared with infants treated with surgery or other medications.[422-424] The mechanism by which indomethacin predisposes LBW infants to sepsis is unknown. A recent meta-analysis of studies comparing ibuprofen with indomethacin for PDA closure did not identify differences in the incidence of sepsis, mortality, or duration of hospitalization.[425]

O'Shea and colleagues[426] described the outcomes of VLBW (500-1250 g) infants given dexamethasone at 15 to 25 days of age for the prevention of chronic lung disease. Among 61 infants treated with tapering doses of dexamethasone for 42 days, there was no increase in the incidence of sepsis or the number of sepsis evaluations in the treatment group when compared with a control population. Further trials of dexamethasone administration for chronic lung disease prophylaxis in VLBW infants confirmed a lack of increased risk for sepsis.[427]

A strong association between intravenous lipid administration to newborns and CoNS bacteremia has been established.[102,428] The role of lipid as a nutritional source for the bacteria, mechanical blockage of the catheter by deposition of lipid in the lumen, and the effect of lipid emulsions on the function of neutrophils and macrophages each might contribute to the observed increased risk for bacteremia. Avila-Figueroa and colleagues[428] identified exposure to intravenous lipids at any time during hospitalization as the single most important risk factor (odds ratio [OR], 9.4) for development of CoNS bacteremia in VLBW infants, calculating that 85% of these bacteremias were attributable to lipid therapy. A randomized trial found that changing intravenous tubing for lipid infusion in neonates every 24 hours instead of 72 hours may reduce bloodstream infections and mortality by approximately 50%.[429]

Recently, a surprisingly strong association between ranitidine therapy in neonates admitted to one NICU and the risk of late-onset bacterial sepsis was reported.[430] The mechanism for such an association remains unclear but certainly merits further analysis.

Pathology

Infants with severe and rapidly fatal sepsis generally have minimal or no histologic indication of an infectious process.[316,431] Findings typical of bacteremia, such as multiple disseminated abscesses of similar size, purulent vasculitis, and intravascular identification of bacteria, are evident in a minority of infants.[431] Shock accompanying sepsis sometimes causes findings such as periventricular leukomalacia and intraventricular hemorrhage, scattered areas of nonzonal hepatic necrosis, renal medullary hemorrhage, renal cortical or acute tubular necrosis, and adrenal hemorrhage and necrosis. Evidence of disseminated intravascular coagulopathy, manifested by strands of interlacing fibrin in the vessels or by a well-demarcated subarachnoid fibrinous hematoma, also can be present.[348,431] The pathology of infections of the respiratory, genitourinary, and gastrointestinal tracts and focal suppurative diseases is discussed in subsequent chapters.

The pathology of neonatal meningitis[348,432,433] and brain abscess[434,435] is similar to that in the older child and adult. The major features are ventriculitis (including inflammation of the choroid plexus), vasculitis, cerebral edema, infarction, cortical neuronal necrosis, and periventricular leukomalacia; chronic pathologic features include hydrocephalus, multicystic encephalomalacia and porencephaly, and cerebral cortical and white matter atrophy.[436] Significant collections of purulent material can be present in the sulci and subarachnoid space, particularly around the basal cisterns, of infants with meningitis. Because the fontanelles are open, exudative material can collect around the base of the brain without a significant increase in intracranial pressure. Hydrocephalus may result from closure of the aqueduct or the foramina of the fourth ventricle by purulent exudate or by means of inflammatory impairment of CSF resorption through the arachnoid channels.[348,437] Ventriculitis has been described in 20% to 90% of cases[24,348,437] and often is the reason for persistence of bacteria in CSF when obstruction ensues and for a slow clinical recovery.[438] Acute inflammatory cells infiltrate the ependymal and subependymal tissues, causing destruction of the epithelial lining of the ventricles. Hemorrhage, venous thrombosis, and subdural effusions often are present.

Brain abscesses and cysts in the neonate are distinguished by the relatively large size of the lesions and relatively poor capsule formation. They occur most frequently in association with meningitis caused by *C. koseri, E. sakazakii, S. marcescens,* and *Proteus mirabilis* and usually are located in the cerebrum, involving several lobes.[155,170,351,434] These organisms characteristically give rise to a hemorrhagic meningoencephalitis caused by intense bacterial infiltration of cerebral vessels and surrounding tissues. The resulting vascular occlusion is followed by infarction and widespread necrosis of cerebral tissue with liquefaction and formation of multiple loculated abscesses and cysts.[351,354]

CLINICAL MANIFESTATIONS

Signs of fetal distress can be the earliest indication of infection in neonates with sepsis, beginning at or soon after delivery. Fetal tachycardia in the second stage of labor was evaluated by Schiano and colleagues[439] as a sign of infection. Pneumonia or sepsis occurred in 3 of 8 infants with marked fetal tachycardia (>180 beats/min), in 7 of 32 infants with mild tachycardia (160-179 beats/min), and in 1 of 167 infants with lower heart rates. Maternal risk factors, such as premature rupture of membranes, foul-smelling amniotic fluid, and evidence of acute placental inflammation, are associated with increased risk of neonatal sepsis and should prompt detailed evaluation of the newborn.[440,441]

A low Apgar score, suggesting distress at or before delivery, also has been correlated with sepsis and associated adverse outcomes in the newborn period.[440,442] Infants delivered vaginally had a 56-fold higher risk of sepsis when the Apgar score was less than 7 at 5 minutes, compared with infants with higher Apgar scores.[443] Among infants with rupture of the amniotic membranes for 24 hours or more, St. Geme and colleagues[317] found a significant increase in the risk for perinatal bacterial infection among those with an Apgar score of less than 6 at 5 minutes but found no association with fetal tachycardia (>160 beats/min).

The Apgar score is well characterized in term infants but less so in premature infants who have the higher attack rates for sepsis. Because low Apgar scores (<3 at 1 minute, <6 at 5 minutes) were significantly associated with LBW and shorter gestation, the use of the score is less valuable as an indicator of sepsis in premature than in term infants.[444]

The earliest signs of sepsis often are subtle and nonspecific. Poor feeding, diminished activity, or just "not looking well" can be the only early evidence that infection is present. More prominent findings are respiratory distress, apnea, lethargy, fever or hypothermia, jaundice, vomiting, diarrhea, and skin manifestations, including petechiae, abscesses, and sclerema.[445]

The nonspecific and subtle nature of the signs of sepsis in newborns is even more problematic in identifying sepsis in the VLBW infant. In a study by Fanaroff and colleagues,[19] the clinical signs of LOS in 325 infants weighing 501 to 1500 g at birth included increasing apnea and bradycardia episodes (55%), increasing oxygen requirement (48%), feeding intolerance, abdominal distention or guaiac-positive stools (46%), lethargy and hypotonia (37%), and temperature instability (10%). Unexplained metabolic acidosis (11%) and hypoglycemia (10%) were the most common laboratory indicators of the metabolic derangement accompanying sepsis.

Bonadio and coworkers[446] attempted to determine the most reliable clinical signs of sepsis in more than 200 febrile infants from birth to 8 weeks of age. They found that changes in affect, peripheral perfusion, and respiratory status best identified those infants with serious bacterial infection. Alterations in feeding pattern, level of alertness, level of activity, and muscle tone also were present; however, these signs were less sensitive indicators. Recently, Kudawla and colleagues[447] developed a scoring system for late-onset neonatal sepsis in infants weighing between 1000 and 2500 g. Clinical parameters included lethargy, tachycardia, grunting, abdominal distension, increased prefeed residual gastric aspirates, fever, and chest retractions. However, these data needed to be combined with laboratory parameters such as elevated C-reactive protein (CRP) or absolute neutrophil or band count to achieve high sensitivity and specificity.[447]

Focal infection involving any organ can occur in infants with sepsis, but most often (excluding pneumonia or meningitis) this occurs in neonates with late-onset rather than early-onset disease. Evaluation of infants with suspected bacteremia must include a careful search for primary or secondary foci, such as meningitis, pneumonia, urinary tract infection, septic arthritis, osteomyelitis, peritonitis, or soft tissue infection.

Serious bacterial infections are uncommon in neonates without any clinical evidence of illness,[446] even among those with maternal risk factors for infection.[448] On occasion, bacteremia occurs without clinical signs.[449-451] Albers and associates[449] described the case histories of 3 infants without signs of illness for whom blood cultures were performed as part of a nursery study involving 131 infants. Blood was obtained from peripheral veins at different times during the first 10 days of life. The same pathogen was isolated repeatedly (i.e., three, three, and two times) from the blood of the 3 infants even though they remained well. The infants subsequently were treated with appropriate antimicrobial agents. Bacteremia caused by GBS can occur with minimal or no systemic or focal signs,[451-453] and it may be sustained over several days.[454] Most healthy appearing infants with GBS bacteremia were born at term and had early-onset (<7 days of age) infection. Similarly, among 44 neonates with enterococcal bacteremia, 3 (76%) of 18 with early-onset infection but none with late-onset infection appeared well.[81] The true incidence of bacteremia without clinical signs is uncertain because few cultures of blood are performed for infants who show no signs of sepsis.

Table 6-10 lists the common clinical signs of neonatal bacterial sepsis. Clinical signs of neonatal bacterial meningitis are given in Table 6-11. Noninfectious conditions that can present with clinical manifestations similar to those of sepsis are shown in Box 6-1.

FEVER AND HYPOTHERMIA

The temperature of the infant with sepsis may be elevated, depressed, or normal.[452-458] In a multicenter survey of nearly 250 infants with early-onset GBS bacteremia, approximately 85% had a normal temperature (36° C to 37.2° C [96.8° F to 99° F]) at the time of their admission to the NICU.[452] When comparing temperatures by gestational age, it was observed that term infants were more likely to have

Table 6-10 Clinical Signs of Bacterial Sepsis

Clinical Sign	Percent of Infants with Sign
Hyperthermia	51
Hypothermia	15
Respiratory distress	33
Apnea	22
Cyanosis	24
Jaundice	35
Hepatomegaly	33
Lethargy	25
Irritability	16
Anorexia	28
Vomiting	25
Abdominal distention	17
Diarrhea	11

Data from Nyhan WL, Fousek MD: Septicemia of the newborn, *Pediatrics* 22:268, 1958; Gluck L, Wood HF, Fousek MD: Septicemia of the newborn, *Pediatr Clin North Am* 13:1131, 1966; Moorman RS, Sell SH: Neonatal septicemia, *South Med J* 54:137, 1962; and Buetow KC, Klein SW, Lane RB: Septicemia in premature infants, *Am J Dis Child* 110:29, 1965.

Table 6-11 Clinical Signs of Bacterial Meningitis

Clinical Sign	Percent of Infants with Sign
Hypothermia or fever	62
Lethargy or irritability	52
Anorexia or vomiting	48
Respiratory distress	41
Bulging or full fontanelle	35
Seizures	31
Jaundice	28
Nuchal rigidity	16
Diarrhea	14

Data from Ziai M, Haggerty RJ: Neonatal meningitis, *N Engl J Med* 259:314, 1958; Holt DE, Halket S, de Louvois J, Harvey D: Neonatal meningitis in England and Wales: 10 years on, *Br Med J* 84:F85, 2001; Watson DG: Purulent neonatal meningitis: a study of forty-five cases, *J Pediatr* 50:352, 1957; and Yu JS, Grauang A: Purulent meningitis in the neonatal period, *Arch Dis Child* 38:391, 1963.

Box 6-1 Differential Diagnosis: Clinical Signs Associated With Neonatal Sepsis and Some Noninfectious Conditions

Respiratory Distress (Apnea, Cyanosis, Costal and Sternal Retraction, Rales, Grunting, Diminished Breath Sounds, Tachypnea)

Transient tachypnea of the newborn
Respiratory distress syndrome
Atelectasis
Aspiration pneumonia, including meconium aspiration
Pneumothorax
Pneumomediastinum
Central nervous system disease: hypoxia, hemorrhage
Congenital abnormalities, including tracheoesophageal fistula, choanal atresia, diaphragmatic hernia, hypoplastic lungs
Congenital heart disease
Cardiac arrhythmia
Hypothermia (neonatal cold injury)
Hypoglycemia
Neonatal drug withdrawal syndrome
Medication error with inhaled epinephrine

Temperature Abnormality (Hyperthermia or Hypothermia)

Altered environmental temperature
Disturbance of central nervous system thermoregulatory mechanism, including anoxia, hemorrhage, kernicterus
Hyperthyroidism or hypothyroidism
Neonatal drug withdrawal syndrome
Dehydration
Congenital adrenal hyperplasia
Vaccine reaction

Jaundice

Breast milk jaundice
Blood group incompatibility
Red cell hemolysis, including blood group incompatibility, glucose-6-phosphate dehydrogenase (G6PD) deficiency
Resorption of blood from closed space hemorrhage
Gastrointestinal obstruction, including pyloric stenosis
Extrahepatic or intrahepatic biliary tract obstruction
Inborn errors of metabolism, including galactosemia, glycogen storage disease type IV, tyrosinemia, disorders of lipid metabolism, peroxisomal disorders, defective bile acid synthesis (trihydroxycoprostanic acidemia)
Hereditary diseases, including cystic fibrosis, α1-antitrypsin deficiency, bile excretory defects (Dubin-Johnson, Rotor, Byler, Aagenaes syndrome)
Hypothyroidism
Prolonged parenteral hyperalimentation

Hepatomegaly

Red cell hemolysis, including blood group incompatibility, G6PD deficiency
Infant of a diabetic mother
Inborn errors of metabolism, including galactosemia, glycogen storage disease, organic acidemias, urea cycle disorders, hereditary fructose intolerance, peroxisomal disorders
Biliary atresia
Congestive heart failure
Benign liver tumors, including hemangioma, hamartoma
Malignant liver tumors, including hepatoblastoma, metastatic neuroblastoma, congenital leukemia

Gastrointestinal Abnormalities (Anorexia, Regurgitation, Vomiting, Diarrhea, Abdominal Distention)

Gastrointestinal allergy
Overfeeding, aerophagia
Intestinal obstruction (intraluminal or extrinsic)
Necrotizing enterocolitis
Hypokalemia
Hypercalcemia or hypocalcemia
Hypoglycemia
Inborn errors of metabolism, including galactosemia, urea cycle disorders, organic acidemias
Ileus secondary to pneumonia
Congenital adrenal hyperplasia
Gastric perforation
Neonatal drug withdrawal syndrome

Lethargy

Central nervous system disease, including hemorrhage, hypoxia, or subdural effusion
Congenital heart disease
Neonatal drug withdrawal syndrome
Hypoglycemia
Hypercalcemia
Familial dysautonomia

Seizure Activity (Tremors, Hyperactivity, Muscular Twitching)

Hypoxia
Intracranial hemorrhage or kernicterus
Congenital central nervous system malformations
Neonatal drug withdrawal syndrome
Hypoglycemia
Hypocalcemia
Hyponatremia, hypernatremia
Hypomagnesemia
Inborn errors of metabolism, including urea cycle disorders, organic acidemias, galactosemia, glycogen storage disease, peroxisomal disorders
Pyridoxine deficiency

Petechiae, Purpura, and Vesiculopustular Lesions

Birth trauma
Blood group incompatibility
Neonatal isoimmune thrombocytopenia
Maternal idiopathic thrombocytopenic purpura
Maternal lupus erythematosus
Drugs administered to mother
Giant hemangioma (Kasabach-Merritt syndrome)
Thrombocytopenia with absent radii (TAR) syndrome
Disseminated intravascular coagulopathy
Coagulation factor deficiencies
Congenital leukemia
Child abuse
Cutaneous histiocytosis

fever than preterm infants (12% vs. 1%), whereas preterm infants more frequently had hypothermia (13% vs. 3%). Phagocytes of the infant born after an uncomplicated labor can produce adult concentrations of interleukin-1 (IL-1), a potent pyrogen. The phagocytes of infants born after cesarean section have a markedly suppressed ability to produce this pyrogen.[459] In the studies reviewed in Table 6-10, approximately one half of the infants had fever. Hypothermia, which was mentioned in one study, occurred in 15% of the infants.

Fever is variably defined for newborns. A temperature of 38.0° C (100.4° F) measured rectally generally is accepted as the lower limit of the definition of fever. Although some clinical studies indicate that axillary,[460] skin-mattress,[461] and infrared tympanic membrane thermometry[462] are accurate and less dangerous than rectal measurements for obtaining core temperature, the reliability of these methods, particularly in febrile infants, has been questioned.[463-465] A recent study established that statistically significant differences are present between the rectal and axillary temperatures obtained in newborns during the first 4 days of life even with the same electronic temperature device.[466] Thus the current method of choice for determining the presence of fever in neonates is a rectal temperature taken at a depth of 2 to 3 cm past the anal margin. In infants with suspected sepsis without fever, it has been shown that a difference between core (rectal) and skin (sole of the foot) temperature of more than 3.5° C can be a more useful indicator of infection than measurement of core temperature alone.[458]

There is no study of temperatures in neonates that is prospective, assesses all infants (febrile and afebrile), includes rectal and axillary temperatures, includes preterm and term infants, and requires positive cultures of blood or other body fluids to define invasive bacterial infection. However, Voora and colleagues[467] observed 100 term infants in Chicago with an axillary or rectal temperature of 37.8° C (100.1° F) or higher during the first 4 days of life, and Osborn and Bolus[468] conducted a retrospective review of 2656 term infants in Los Angeles. Both groups of investigators reported that temperature elevation in healthy term infants was uncommon. Approximately 1% of neonates born at term had at least one episode of fever, measured as 37.8° C (100.1° F) or higher per axilla.[467] Temperature elevation infrequently was associated with systemic infection when a single evaluation occurred. None of 64 infants in these two studies who had a single episode of fever developed clinical evidence of systemic infection (cultures of blood or other body fluids were not obtained). By contrast, temperature elevation that was sustained for more than 1 hour frequently was associated with infection. Of 7 infants with sustained fever in the Osborn and Bolus study,[468] 5 had proven bacterial or viral infections. Of 65 infants reported by Voora and colleagues,[467] 10 had documented systemic bacterial disease. Temperature elevation without other signs of infection was infrequent. Only 1 infant (with cytomegalovirus infection) of the 5 Los Angeles infants had fever without other signs. Only 2 infants (with bacteremia caused by *E. coli* or GBS, respectively) of the 10 Chicago infants with fever and proven bacterial disease had no other signs of infection.

In addition to infection, fever may be caused by an elevation in ambient temperature, dehydration, retained blood or extensive hematoma, and damage to the temperature-regulating mechanisms of the CNS. Less common noninfectious causes of fever are hyperthyroidism, cystic fibrosis, familial dysautonomia, and ectodermal dysplasia. When thermoregulatory devices that monitor and modify infant temperature are introduced, the use of fever or hypothermia as a diagnostic sign of sepsis sometimes is impeded.

RESPIRATORY DISTRESS

Signs of respiratory distress, including tachypnea, grunting, flaring of the alae nasi, intercostal retractions, rales, and decreased breath sounds, are common and important findings in the infant suspected of having sepsis. Respiratory distress syndrome and aspiration pneumonia must be considered in the differential diagnosis. Apnea is one of the most specific signs of sepsis but usually occurs in the setting of a fulminant onset or after other nonspecific signs have been present for hours or days. Clinical signs of cardiovascular dysfunction, including tachycardia, arrhythmia, and poor peripheral perfusion, that occur in the absence of congenital heart disease are sensitive and specific signs of sepsis.

JAUNDICE

Jaundice is present in approximately one third of infants with sepsis and is a common finding in infants with urinary tract infection.[357,469-471] It can develop suddenly or subacutely and occasionally is the only sign of sepsis. Jaundice usually decreases after institution of appropriate antimicrobial therapy. It occurs in septic infants irrespective of the type of bacterial pathogen. A fatal case of acute kernicterus secondary to glucose-6-phosphate deficiency was misdiagnosed as neonatal sepsis.[472]

ORGANOMEGALY

The liver edge is palpable in premature infants and can extend to 2 cm below the costal margin in healthy term infants. Ashkenazi and colleagues[473] evaluated liver size in healthy term infants examined within 24 hours of birth and again between 72 and 96 hours. Measurements ranged between 1.6 and 4.0 cm below the costal margin, and there was no significant difference between early and late examinations. Reiff and Osborn[474] suggested that determination of liver span by palpation and percussion is a more reliable technique than identifying the liver projection below the costal margin. Hepatomegaly is a common sign of in utero infections and of some noninfectious conditions such as cardiac failure and metabolic diseases, including galactosemia and glycogen storage disease. Tender hepatomegaly can be a sign of bacterial liver abscess in neonates, a potential complication of misplaced central umbilical catheters.[129] Splenomegaly is less common than hepatomegaly and infrequently is mentioned in reports of bacterial sepsis of the newborn.[475]

Lymph nodes infrequently are palpable in newborns unless they are infected with viruses, spirochetes, or protozoa. Bamji and colleagues[476] examined 214 healthy neonates in New York and identified palpable nodes at one or more sites in one third of the infants. Embree and Muriithi[477] examined 66 healthy, term Kenyan neonates during the first 24 hours of life and found palpable axillary nodes (27.7%) but no palpable inguinal nodes. Adenopathy is a sign of congenital infection caused by rubella virus, *T. gondii, T. pallidum,* and enteroviruses. Adenitis can occur in drainage areas involved with bacterial soft tissue infection. Although adenopathy is not an important sign of systemic bacterial infection in neonates, cellulitis-adenitis syndrome, a rare clinical manifestation of late-onset GBS infection in infants, is a condition in which local inflammation can be the only initial sign of sepsis that can include concurrent meningitis.[478,479] Recently, cellulitis-adenitis syndrome was reported in a neonate with GAS sepsis.[480]

GASTROINTESTINAL SIGNS

Gastrointestinal disturbances, including poor feeding, regurgitation or vomiting, large gastric residuals in infants fed by tube, diarrhea, and abdominal distention, are common and significant early signs of sepsis. The first indications of illness can be a change in feeding pattern or lethargy during feedings.

SKIN LESIONS

A variety of skin lesions can accompany bacteremia, including cellulitis, abscess, petechiae, purpuric lesions, sclerema, erythema multiforme, and ecthyma.

NEUROLOGIC SIGNS

The onset of meningitis in the neonate is accompanied by identical signs of illness, as observed in infants with sepsis. Meningitis can be heralded by increasing irritability, alteration in consciousness, poor tone, tremors, lip smacking, or twitching of facial muscles or an extremity. Seizures were present in 31% of the infants reviewed in Table 6-11, but Volpe[354] identified seizures, in many cases subtle, in 75% of infants with bacterial meningitis. Approximately one half of the seizures were focal, and at their onset, they usually were subtle. Focal signs, including hemiparesis, horizontal deviation of the eyes, and cranial nerve deficits involving the seventh, third, and sixth cranial nerves, in that order of frequency, can be identified.[354] Because cranial sutures in the neonate are open and allow for expansion of the intracranial contents and for increasing head size, a full or bulging fontanelle can be absent.[453,481] The presence of a bulging fontanelle is not related to gestational age. Among 72 newborns with gram-negative enteric bacillary meningitis, a bulging fontanelle was seen in 18% and 17% of term and preterm infants, respectively.[24] Nuchal rigidity, an important sign in older children and adults, is uncommon in neonates.[24]

In addition to the physical findings observed in infants with meningitis, several investigators have reported the occurrence of fluid and electrolyte abnormalities associated with inappropriate antidiuretic hormone secretion, including hyponatremia, decreased urine output, and increased weight gain.[437,443] On occasion, the onset of meningitis has been followed by a transient or persistent diabetes insipidus.[481]

Early clinical signs of brain abscess in the newborn are subtle and frequently unnoticed by the physician or parent. Presenting signs include those of increased intracranial pressure (e.g., emesis, bulging fontanelle, enlarging head size, separated sutures), focal cerebral signs (e.g., hemiparesis, focal seizures), and acute signs of meningitis. Of six infants with brain abscesses described by Hoffman and colleagues,[434] two were febrile, two had seizures, and five had increased head size.

Other focal infections in the nervous system include pneumococcal endophthalmitis in a neonate with meningitis,[482] pseudomonal endophthalmitis in a premature neonate with LOS,[483] and epidural abscess caused by *S. aureus*.[484,485]

Diagnosis

The diagnosis of systemic infection in the newborn is difficult to establish on the basis of clinical findings alone. A history of one or more risk factors for neonatal sepsis associated with the pregnancy and delivery often is associated with early-onset infection, but there can be no clues before the onset of subtle signs in the term infant who develops LOS. The extensive list of conditions that must be considered in the differential diagnosis for the various signs that are associated with sepsis or meningitis and noninfectious conditions is given in Box 6-1. Laboratory tests to assist in the diagnosis of sepsis are discussed in Chapter 36, with recent explorations into the utility of various novel tools, such as acute phase reactants (e.g. CRP and procalcitonin), cytokines, and cell surface markers.[486]

MATERNAL HISTORY

Many infants, particularly those born prematurely, who develop systemic infection just before or shortly after delivery, are born to women who have one or more risk features for early-onset sepsis in their infants. These features include preterm labor, premature rupture of the membranes at any time during gestation, prolonged rupture of membranes, chorioamnionitis, prolonged labor, intrauterine scalp electrodes, and traumatic delivery. In 2010, the CDC revised its guidelines for the prevention of perinatal GBS disease,[487] a policy endorsed by the American Academy of Pediatrics (AAP)[488] and the American College of Obstetrics and Gynecology (ACOG).[489]

Per these recommendations, intrapartum antibiotic prophylaxis is recommended for pregnancies with

1. Previous infant with invasive GBS disease
2. GBS bacteriuria during any trimester of the current pregnancy
3. Positive GBS vaginal-rectal screening culture in late gestation (35-37 weeks) during current pregnancy
4. Unknown GBS status at the onset of labor (culture not done, incomplete, or results unknown) and any of the following:
    a. Delivery at less than 37 weeks of gestation
    b. Amniotic membrane rupture greater than or equal to 18 hours
    c. Intrapartum temperature greater than or equal to 100.4° F (≥38.0° C)

Conversely, intrapartum GBS prophylaxis is NOT indicated for pregnancies with

1. GBS colonization or GBS bacteriuria during a previous pregnancy, unless an indication for GBS prophylaxis is present for current pregnancy
2. Negative vaginal and rectal GBS screening culture in late gestation during the current pregnancy, regardless of intrapartum risk factors
3. Cesarean delivery performed before onset of labor on a woman with intact amniotic membranes, regardless of GBS colonization status or gestational age

MICROBIOLOGIC TECHNIQUES

Isolation of microorganisms from a usually sterile site, such as the blood, CSF, urine, other body fluids (e.g., peritoneal, pleural, joint, middle ear), or tissues (e.g., bone marrow, liver, spleen) remains the most valid method of diagnosing bacterial sepsis. Infectious agents cultured from the nose, throat, external auditory canal, skin, umbilicus, or stool indicate colonization and can include organisms that cause sepsis, but isolation of a microorganism from these sites does not establish invasive systemic infection. The limited sensitivity, specificity, and predictive value of body surface cultures in a NICU was documented by Evans and colleagues[490] using a database of 24,584 cultures from 3371 infants. These investigators strongly discouraged the use of cultures from these sites in diagnosing neonatal sepsis because of their poor correlation with the pathogen in the blood and their expense.

Culture of Blood

Isolation of a pathogenic microorganism from the blood or other body fluid is the only method to definitively establish the diagnosis of neonatal bacteremia/sepsis.

Methods. Technology has evolved from manually read, broth-based methods to continuously monitored, automated blood-culture systems that use enriched media for processing of blood-culture specimens. Automated and semiautomated systems for continuous blood-culture monitoring are standard in laboratories in the United States.[491-493] Before the widespread use of automated blood-culturing systems, lysis direct plating was the most often used method of isolating bacteria. Positive cultures were recognized by growth of colonies on agar and provided a rapid means to obtaining quantitative blood-culture results from pediatric patients. St. Geme and colleagues[494] used this technique to investigate the distinction of sepsis from contamination in cultures of blood growing CoNS; true CoNS infection is unlikely in infants with birth weight greater than 2000 g and gestation greater than 34 weeks.[97]

Time to Detection of a Positive Blood Culture. Bacterial growth is evident in most cultures of blood from neonates within 48 hours.[495-497] With use of conventional culture techniques and subculture at 4 and 14 hours, only 4 of 105 cultures that had positive results (1 GBS and 3 *S. aureus*) required more than 48 hours of incubation.[496] By use of a radiometric technique (BACTEC 460, Becton Dickinson, Sparks, MD), 40 of 41 cultures that grew GBS and 15 of 16 cultures with *E. coli* were identified within 24 hours.[497] Controlled experiments suggest that delayed entry of the collected blood-culture bottle into the automated blood-culture machine can significantly prolong the time to positivity for common newborn pathogens.[498]

Optimal Number of Cultures. The optimal number of cultures to obtain for the diagnosis of bacteremia in the newborn remains uncertain. A single blood culture from an infant with sepsis can be negative, but most studies suggest a sensitivity of 90% or slightly more. Sprunt[499] suggested the use of two blood cultures "not primarily to increase the yield of organisms…" but to "minimize the insecurity and debates over the meaning of the findings." In a study by Struthers and colleagues,[96] it was estimated that in 5% of neonates a second blood culture failed to substantiate the presence of CoNS, leading to an 8% reduction in antibiotic use. In the high-risk neonate, there is no doubt the need to initiate therapy promptly can make this practice difficult.

Optimal Volume of Blood. The optimal volume of blood needed to detect bacteremia in neonates has not been determined. Neal and colleagues[500] evaluated the volume of neonatal blood submitted for culture by physicians who were unaware of the study and found that the mean blood volume per patient was 1.05 mL. Dietzman and coworkers[501] suggested that 0.2 mL of blood was sufficient to detect bacteremia caused by *E. coli*. The relationship between colony counts of *E. coli* from blood cultures from infants with sepsis and meningitis and mortality was evaluated. Meningitis occurred only in neonates with more than 1000 colonies of *E. coli*/mL of blood. These data of Dietzman and associates[501] are supported by experimental results indicating that common pediatric pathogens can be reliably recovered from 0.5 mL of blood even when cultured at blood-to-broth ratios of 1:100.[502,503] More recent studies have found that in the circumstance of low-inoculum bacteremia (<10 colony-forming units/mL of blood), the collection of only 0.5 mL of blood proved inadequate for the reliable detection of common pathogens.[504-507] It appears that if one blood culture is to be collected before antimicrobial therapy is initiated, a volume of 1 mL or more will ensure the greatest sensitivity.

Cultures of Blood From Umbilical Vessels and Intravascular Catheters. Umbilical vessel and intravascular catheters are essential in the care of neonates in the ICU and are preferred blood-culture sampling sites.[508-510] Results of cultures of blood obtained from indwelling umbilical or central venous catheters can present ambiguities in interpretation (e.g., contamination versus catheter colonization vs. systemic infection). Obtaining blood cultures from a peripheral vessel and catheters in the ill-appearing neonate is useful in the interpretation of results. A recent prospective study of semiquantitive catheter tip cultures in a Brazilian NICU found that a cutoff point of approximately 100 colony forming units was predictive of clinically significant catheter-related infections, of which CoNS accounted for 75% of cases.[511]

Distinguishing Clinically Important Bacteremia From Blood-Culture Contamination. The increased use of intravascular catheters in neonates has resulted in an increase in the incidence of bacteremia, particularly that caused by CoNS, and uncertainty regarding the significance of some results. Investigators have considered criteria based on clinical signs and microbiologic factors.

Yale investigators[6] used the following criteria to define the role of commensal organisms in neonatal sepsis: one major clinical sign, such as apnea, bradycardia, core temperature greater than 38.0° C or less than 36.5° C documented at the time the blood culture was obtained, plus another blood culture positive for the same organism obtained within 24 hours of the first or an intravascular access device in place before major clinical signs occurred. Some microbiologic features can be useful in differentiating sepsis from contamination:

1. Time to growth in conventional media: The longer the time needed to detect growth (>2-3 days), the more likely that skin or intravascular line contamination was present.
2. Number of cultures positive: If peripheral and intravascular catheter specimens are positive, the presence of the organism in the blood is likely; if the catheter specimen alone is positive, intravascular line colonization may have occurred; if multiple cultures from an indwelling vascular catheter are positive or if a single culture is positive and the patient has had a clinical deterioration, a bloodstream infection must be presumed.
3. Organism type: Organisms that are part of skin flora (e.g., diphtheroids, nonhemolytic streptococci, CoNS) suggest contamination in certain cases as described previously, whereas known bacterial pathogens must be considered to be associated with sepsis. Contamination is more likely when multiple species grow in one blood-culture bottle, different species grow in two bottles, or only one of several cultures before or during antimicrobial therapy is positive.
4. Clinical signs: If the infant is well without use of antibiotics, growth of a commensal organism from a blood culture is more likely to be a contaminant.

In an attempt to resolve the question of sepsis versus contamination, investigators have used multiple-site blood cultures,[512] comparisons of results of cultures of blood and cultures of skin at the venipuncture site,[513] and quantitative blood cultures.[496] These techniques are of investigational interest, but the results do not suggest that any one is of sufficient value to be adopted for clinical practice. Healy and colleagues[514] suggest that isolation of CoNS of the same species or antimicrobial susceptibility from more than one blood culture or from one blood culture obtained from an indwelling catheter or a peripheral vessel and a normally sterile body site represents true infection if the patient is a premature infant with signs of clinical sepsis. In a recent study of premature neonates with birth weight less than 2000 g and gestation less than 34 weeks, total central lines placed, but not central line duration or presence in situ, predicted proved (OR, 3.5) and probable CoNS infection (OR, 2.7) by multivariate analysis, as did lethargy and gastric residuals.[97] At present, management of the sick premature infant, especially the VLBW patient, with a positive blood culture for CoNS requires that the organism be considered a pathogen and managed with appropriate antimicrobial agents. If the infant is well, the microbiologic results given earlier should be considered in the decision to continue or discontinue use of an antimicrobial agent. Another culture of blood should be obtained when the initial culture result is ambiguous.

Buffy-Coat Examination

The rapid diagnosis of bacteremia by identification of microorganisms in the buffy leukocyte layer of centrifuged blood is a method used for many years and has been evaluated for use in newborn infants.[515-521] By using Gram and methylene blue stains of the buffy-coat preparation, immediate and accurate information was obtained for 37 (77%) of 48 bacteremic, clinically septic infants in the four studies.[516-518,520] Positive results were found for gram-positive and gram-negative organisms. In contrast to findings reported for adult populations,[522] there were no false-positive results among almost 200 infants with negative blood cultures. Failure to identify organisms was attributed to extreme neutropenia in several patients.

The large inoculum of microorganisms in the blood of neonates with sepsis most probably explains the excellent sensitivity of leukocyte smears. Smears can be positive with as few as 50 colonies/mL of *S. aureus* in the peripheral blood; approximately 50% of neonates with *E. coli* bacteremia have higher concentrations.[501] *Candida* and *S. epidermidis* septicemia in young infants also has been diagnosed by this method.[523-525] Strom[526] reported reported that bacteria were identified in peripheral blood smears in 17 of 19 infants with septicemia. However, Rodwell and associates[527] were able to identify bacteria in direct blood smears for only 4 of 24 bacteremic neonates. It is likely that the disparity in these results reflects differences in patient populations, or distribution of etiologic agents or both. The buffy-coat examination of blood smears has become infrequently used in laboratories since the introduction of automated systems for continuous blood-culture monitoring.

Culture of Urine

Infants with sepsis can have a urinary tract origin or a concomitant urinary tract infection. The yield from culture of urine is low in early-onset sepsis and most often reflects metastatic spread to the bladder from the bacteremia, but in late-onset infection, the yield is substantially higher. Visser and Hall[528] found positive cultures of urine in only 1.6% of infants with early-onset sepsis compared with 7.4% of infants with LOS. DiGeronimo[529] performed a chart review of 146 clinically septic infants who had cultures of blood and urine. Of 11 infants with positive blood cultures, only 1 infant with GBS bacteremia had a positive urine culture. These data suggest that cultures of urine yield very limited information about the source of infection in infants with signs of sepsis before age 7 days. In contrast, it is apparent that urine should be collected for culture from infants with suspected LOS before initiation of antimicrobial therapy. Of interest, the presence of elevated leukocyte counts (≥10/high-power field) in urine of infants younger than 90 days is an accurate predictor of urinary tract infections complicated by bacteremia.[530]

Because of the difficulty in collecting satisfactory clean-voided specimens of urine from the newborn, bladder catheterization or suprapubic needle aspiration of bladder urine frequently is performed. These methods are simple and safe, and suprapubic bladder aspiration avoids the ambiguities inherent in urine obtained by other methods.[531-533] If a suprapubic aspirate cannot be performed for technical or medical reasons, catheterization is a satisfactory method of obtaining urine, although ambiguous results can occur because of contamination from the urethra, especially in VLBW neonates. Of note, application of a clinical pain scoring system using a blinded observer and video recording found suprapubic aspiration to produce more discomfort than transurethral catheterization in female and circumcized male infants younger than 2 months.[534]

Cultures of Tracheal Aspirates and Pharynx

Because of the association of pneumonia and bacteremia, investigators have sought to determine the risk of sepsis on the basis of colonization of the upper respiratory tract. Lau and Hey[535] found that among ventilated infants who became septic, the same organism usually was present in cultures of tracheal aspirate and blood. However, growth of a bacterial pathogen from a tracheal aspirate culture does not predict which infants will develop sepsis. Similarly, cultures of the pharynx or trachea do not necessarily predict the causative organism in the blood of a neonate with clinical sepsis.[536] A review of the literature by Srinivasan and Vidyasagar[537] suggest endotracheal aspirates are of poor sensitivity (≈50%), modest specificity (≈80%) and poor positive predictive value. Unless the patient has a change in respiratory status documented clinically and radiographically, routine use of cultures from the pharynx or trachea provide low diagnostic yield and seem unjustified given their expense.

Diagnostic Needle Aspiration and Tissue Biopsy

Direct aspiration of tissues or body fluids through a needle or catheter is used for the diagnosis of a wide variety of infectious and noninfectious diseases.[538] Aspiration of an infectious focus in lung, pleural space, middle ear, pericardium, bones, joints, abscess, and other sites provides immediate and specific information to guide therapy. Biopsy of the liver or bone marrow can assist in diagnosing occult infections, but this rarely is necessary.

Autopsy Microbiology

Two factors must be considered in interpreting bacterial cultures obtained at autopsy: The frequent isolation of organisms usually considered to be nonpathogenic and the difficulty of isolating fastidious organisms such as anaerobic bacteria. To minimize these problems, it is important that specimens be collected with proper aseptic technique and as early as possible after death.

It is a common belief that organisms in the intestinal and respiratory tracts gain access to tissues after death, but it also is possible that bacteremia occurs shortly before death and is not a postmortem phenomenon. Eisenfeld and colleagues[539] identified the same organisms in specimens obtained before and within 2 hours after death. Confusion in the interpretation of results of bacteriologic cultures often is obviated by the review of slides prepared directly from tissues and fluids. If antimicrobial treatment was administered before death, organisms can be observed on a smear even though they are not viable. Pathogens would be expected to be present in significant numbers and accompanied by inflammatory cells, whereas contaminants or organisms that invade tissues after death, if they are seen, would be present in small numbers with no evidence of an inflammatory process.[540,541]

Rapid Techniques for Detection of Bacterial Antigens in Body Fluid Specimens

In the 1970s, the limulus lysate assay for detection of endotoxin produced by gram-negative bacteria based on a gelation reaction between lysates of *Limulus* (horseshoe crab) amebocytes and bacterial endotoxin was investigated for diagnosis of neonatal meningitis with equivocal results.[542-546] Counterimmunoelectrophoresis also was used successfully for detecting the capsular polysaccharide antigens of various pathogenic bacteria, including *S. pneumoniae, N. meningitidis, H. influenzae,* and GBS (see Chapter 12) in CSF, serum, and urine. Less complex and more rapid detection methods have replaced these two assays.

Latex agglutination detection now is preferred because of its speed, simplicity, and greater sensitivity for selected organisms. Kits designed to detect cell wall or capsular or cell wall antigen released into body fluids are commercially available. Latex agglutination assays have been shown to be of potential benefit in early detection of bacterial antigens in the CSF of patients with acute meningitis, which may be of increased importance in the era of intrapartum antibiotic prophylaxis and its potential interference with culture yield. Among the prevalent bacterial pathogens in neonatal infections, only GBS is routinely analyzed by latex agglutination. However, *N. meningitidis* group B shares a common capsular antigen with the neonatal meningitis pathogen *E. coli* serotype K1, which should allow cross-identification of the latter by using a meningococcal latex reagent.[547] The sensitivity of latex agglutination methods for identifying infants with GBS meningitis varies between 73% and 100% for CSF and 75% and 84% for urine.[548] Possible cross-reactions have occurred when concentrated urine was tested. The GBS cell wall antigen can occasionally cross react with those from *S. pneumoniae,* CoNS, enterococci, and gram-negative enteric bacteria, including *P. mirabilis* and *E. cloacae.* False-positive results in urine for a positive latex agglutination test for GBS often were caused by contamination of bag specimens of urine with the streptococci from rectal or vaginal colonization.[549] The poor specificity of GBS antigen detection methods used with urine led to the U.S. Food and Drug Administration (FDA) recommendation in 1996 that these methods not be used except for testing of CSF and serum.

Lumbar Puncture and Examination of Cerebrospinal Fluid

Because meningitis can accompany sepsis with no clinical signs to differentiate between bacteremia alone and bacteremia with meningitis, a lumbar puncture (LP) should be considered for examination of the CSF in any neonate before initiation of therapy. Up to 15% of infants with sepsis have accompanying meningitis. The overall incidence of bacterial meningitis is less than 1 case per 1000 infants, but the incidence for LBW (<2500 g) infants or premature infants is severalfold higher than that for term infants. Data from the NICHD Neonatal Research Network surveyed 9641 VLBW infants who survived 3 days or more: 30% had one or more LPs and 5% of those who had a LP had late-onset meningitis.[550] For the diagnosis of some noninfectious CNS diseases in neonates (e.g., intracranial hemorrhage), cranial ultrasonography, and, occasionally, computed tomography or magnetic resonance imaging are the techniques of choice. For infants with hypoxic-ischemic encephalopathy, LP should be considered only for those infants in whom meningitis is a possible diagnosis.

Some investigators suggest that too many healthy term infants have a diagnostic evaluation for sepsis, including LP, based solely on maternal risk features and that the LP rarely provides clinically useful information. Other investigators have questioned the role of an admission LP in the premature infant with respiratory distress and found that the yield of the procedure is very low.[551-553] Of more than 1700 infants with respiratory distress syndrome evaluated for meningitis, bacterial pathogens were identified in the CSF of only 4. Three of the 4 infants with meningitis were bacteremic with the same pathogen.[553] A large, retrospective study assessed the value of LP in the evaluation of suspected sepsis during the first week of life and found that bacteria were isolated from 9 of 728 CSF specimens, but only 1 infant was believed to have bacterial meningitis.[554] Fielkow and colleagues[555] found no cases of meningitis among 284 healthy appearing infants who had a LP performed because of maternal risk factors, whereas 2.5% of 799 neonates with clinical signs of sepsis had meningitis regardless of maternal risk factors. In summary, the value of a LP has been established for infants with clinical signs of sepsis, but LP performed because of maternal risk features in a healthy appearing neonate is less likely to be useful.

The considerations are quite different for the VLBW neonate (400-1500 g), as documented in a recent study by Stoll and colleagues[550] performed through the NICHD Neonatal Research Network. A full one third (45/134) of these high-risk neonates with meningitis have negative blood cultures. Lower gestational age and prior sepsis were important risk factors for development meningitis, which carried a significant risk of mortality compared with uninfected infants (23% vs. 2%). These results indicate the critical importance of LP and suggest that meningitis may be significantly underdiagnosed in the VLBW population.[550]

Method of Lumbar Puncture. Lumbar puncture is more difficult to perform in the neonate than in the older child or adult; traumatic LPs resulting in blood in the CSF are more frequent, and care must be taken in the infant who is in respiratory distress. Gleason and colleagues[556] suggest that the procedure be performed with the infant in the upright position or, if performed in the flexed position, be modified with neck extension. Pinheiro and associates[557] evaluated the role of locally administered lidocaine before LP and found that the local anesthesia decreased the degree of struggling of the infant. However, other investigators have concluded that local anesthesia failed to influence physiologic changes in the neonate undergoing LP.[558] Fiser and colleagues[559] suggest that the administration of oxygen before LP prevents most hypoxemia resulting from this procedure in infants.

The physician can choose to withhold or delay LP in some infants who would be placed at risk for cardiac or respiratory compromise by the procedure. Weisman and colleagues[560] observed that transient hypoxemia occurred during LP performed in the lateral position (i.e., left side with hips flexed to place knees to chest) but occurred less frequently when the infant was in a sitting position or modified lateral position (i.e., left side with hips flexed to 90 degrees). Reasons for withholding LP in older children, such as signs of increased intracranial pressure, signs of a bleeding disorder, and infection in the area that the needle will traverse to obtain CSF, are less likely to be concerns in the neonate.

Ventricular puncture should be considered in the infant with meningitis who does not respond clinically or microbiologically to antimicrobial therapy because of ventriculitis, especially with obstruction between the ventricles and lumbar CSF. Ventriculitis is diagnosed on the basis of elevated white blood cell count (>100 cells/mm^3) or identification of bacteria by culture, Gram stain, or antigen detection. Ventricular puncture is a potentially hazardous procedure and should be performed only by a physician who is an expert in the technique.

If a Lumbar Puncture is Not Performed. Is it sufficient to culture only blood and urine for the diagnosis of neonatal bacterial meningitis? Visser and Hall[561] demonstrated that the blood culture was sterile when the CSF yielded a pathogen in 6 (15%) of 39 infants with bacterial meningitis. Franco and colleagues[562] reported that in 26 neonates with bacterial meningitis, only 13 had a positive blood culture. In surveys from two large data bases, NICUs managed by the Pediatrix Medical Group (Sunrise, FL)[563] and the NICHD Neonatal Research Network[550] results were similar: One third of infants at 34 or more weeks' estimated gestation with meningitis and one third of VLBW neonates with meningitis had negative blood cultures. A significant number of infants with meningitis will not have this diagnosis established unless a LP is performed.

Ideally the LP should be performed before the initiation of antimicrobial therapy, but there are alternative strategies for infants who may not tolerate the procedure. If the physician believes that LP would endanger the infant with presumed sepsis and meningitis, therapy should be initiated after blood (and urine for late-onset illness) is obtained for culture. After the infant is stabilized, LP should be performed. Even several days after the start of antibiotic therapy, CSF pleocytosis and abnormal CSF chemistry assays usually should identify the presence or absence of an inflammatory reaction, although CSF culture may be sterile.

Examination of Cerebrospinal Fluid. The cell content and chemistry of the CSF of healthy newborn infants differ from those of older infants, children, and adults (Table 6-12). The values vary widely during the first weeks of life, and the normal range must be considered in evaluation of CSF in infants suspected to have meningitis.[564-568] The cell content in the CSF of a neonate is higher than that in older infants. A recent analysis calculated the median CSF leukocyte count was significantly higher in infants who were aged less than or equal to 28 days (3/μL, 95th percentile: 19/μL) than in infants who were aged 29 to 56 days (2/μL, 95th percentile: 9/μL; $P < .001$).[569] Neutrophils often are present in the CSF of normal newborns, whereas more than a single neutrophil in the CSF of older infants or children should be

Table 6-12 Hematologic and Chemical Characteristics of Cerebrospinal Fluid in Healthy Newborns: Results of Selected Studies

Study (year)	No. of Patients	Age (days)	White Blood Cells* (mm³)	Neutrophils* (mm³)	Glucose* (mg/dL)	Protein* (mg/dL)
Naidoo[813] (1968)	135	1	12 (0-42)	7 (0-26)	48 (38-64)	73 (40-148)
	20	7	3 (0-9)	2 (0-5)	55 (48-62)	47 (27-65)
Sarff[488] (1976)	87	Most < 7	8.2 ± 7.1, median 5 (0-32)	61	52 (34-119)	90 (20-170)
Bonadio[565] (1992)	35	0-4 wk	11.0 ± 10.4, median 8.5	0.4 ± 1.4, median 0.15	46 ± 10.3	84 ± 45.1
	40	4-8 wk	7.1 ± 9.2, median 4.5	0.2 ± 0.4, median 0	46 ± 10.0	59 ± 25.3
Ahmed[566] (1996)	108	0-30	7.3 ± 13.9, median 4	0.8 ± 6.2, median 0	51.2 ± 12.9	64.2 ± 24.2

Data from Ahmed A, Hickey S, Ehrett S, et al: Cerebrospinal fluid values in the term neonate, *Pediatr Infect Dis J* 15:298, 1996.
*Expressed as mean with range (number in parentheses) or ± standard deviation unless otherwise specified.

Table 6-13 Hematologic and Chemical Characteristics of Cerebrospinal Fluid in Healthy Very-Low-Birth-Weight Infants

Birth Weight (g)	Age (days)	No. of Samples	Red Blood Cells (mm³) Mean (range)	White Blood Cells (mm³) Mean (range)	Polymorphonuclear Leukocytes (%) Mean (range)	Glucose (mg/dL) Mean (range)	Protein (mg/dL) Mean (range)
<1000	0-7	6	335 (0-1780)	3 (1-8)	11 (0-50)	70 (41-89)	162 (115-222)
	8-28	17	1465 (0-19,050)	4 (0-14)	8 (0-66)	68 (33-217)	159 (95-370)
	29-84	15	808 (0-6850)	4 (0-11)	2 (0-36)	49 (29-90)	137 (76-260)
1000-1500	0-7	8	407 (0-2450)	4 (1-10)	4 (0-28)	74 (50-96)	136 (85-176)
	8-28	14	1101 (0-9750)	7 (0-44)	10 (0-60)	59 (39-109)	137 (54-227)
	29-84	11	661 (0-3800)	8 (0-23)	11 (0-48)	47 (31-76)	122 (45-187)

Data from Rodriguez AF, Kaplan SL, Mason EO Jr: Cerebrospinal fluid values in the very low birth weight infant, *J Pediatr* 116:971, 1990.

considered abnormal. Similarly, protein concentration is higher in preterm than in term infants and highest in VLBW infants[568] (Table 6-13). In term infants, the total protein concentration decreases with age, reaching values of healthy older infants (<40 mg/dL) before the third month of life. In LBW or preterm infants, CSF leukocyte and protein concentrations decline with postnatal age and may not fall within normal values for older infants for several months after birth.[570] CSF glucose levels are lower in neonates than in older infants and can be related to the lower concentrations of glucose observed in blood. Healthy term infants can have blood glucose levels as low as 30mg/dL, and preterm infants may have levels as low as 20mg/dL.[568] The physiologic basis for the higher concentration of protein and the increased numbers of white blood cells in the CSF of healthy, uninfected preterm and term infants is unknown; explanations offered include possible mechanical irritation of the meninges during delivery and an increased permeability of the blood-brain barrier.

In nearly all of the studies of the CSF in newborns, normal or healthy refers to the absence of clinical manifestations at the time of examination of the CSF. Only the study by Ahmed and colleagues[566] included in the definition of normal the absence of viral infection defined by lack of evidence of cytopathic effect in five cell lines and negative PCR for enteroviruses. None of the studies included information about the health of the infant after the newborn period. It now is recognized that infants with congenital infections, such as rubella, cytomegalovirus infection, toxoplasmosis, acquired immunodeficiency syndrome, and syphilis, can have no signs of illness during the newborn period. Observations of these infants over the course of months or years can reveal abnormalities that are inapparent at birth. Until more data are available, it would appear prudent to observe carefully infants with white blood cells in excess of 20/mm³ or a protein level in excess of 100 mg/dL in the CSF and, if clinical signs indicate, to obtain paired serum samples for serologic assays and viral cultures from body fluids or tissues for congenital CNS infections (i.e., *T. gondii*, rubella virus, cytomegalovirus, herpes simplex virus, human immunodeficiency virus, and *T. pallidum*).

In newborns with bacterial meningitis, there can be thousands of white blood cells in the CSF, and neutrophils predominate early in the course of the disease.[21,564] The number of CSF leukocytes can vary greatly in infants with both gram-negative and gram-positive meningitis. The median number of cells/mm³ in the CSF of 98 infants with gram-negative meningitis was more than 2000 (range, 6-40,000), whereas the median number of cells/mm³ in 21 infants with GBS meningitis was less than 100 (range, 8 to >10,000).[564] The concentration of glucose in CSF usually is less than two thirds of the concentration in blood. The concentration of protein can be low (<30 mg/dL) or very high (>1000 mg/dL). CSF parameters observed in the healthy term neonate can overlap with those observed in the infant with meningitis.

A Gram-stain smear of CSF should be examined for bacteria, and appropriate media should be inoculated with the CSF specimen. Sarff and colleagues[564] detected organisms in Gram-stain smears of CSF in 83% of infants with GBS meningitis and in 78% of those with gram-negative meningitis. After initiation of appropriate antimicrobial therapy, gram-positive bacteria usually clear from the CSF within 36 hours, whereas in some patients with meningitis caused by gram-negative enteric bacilli cultures can remain positive for many days.[567]

Microorganisms can be isolated from CSF that has normal white blood cell and chemistry test values. Visser and Hall[561] reported normal CSF parameters (cell count <25; protein level <200 mg/dL) in 6 (15%) of 39 infants with culture-proven meningitis. Subsequent examination of the CSF identified an increase in the number of cells and protein level. Presumably, the initial LP was performed early in the course of meningitis before an inflammatory response occurred. Other investigators reported isolation of enterovirus[571] and *S. pneumoniae*[572] from the CSF of neonates in the absence of pleocytosis.

Identification of bacteremia without meningitis, defined by the absence of pleocytosis or isolation of a pathogen from culture of CSF, can be followed by meningeal inflammation on subsequent examinations. Sarman and colleagues[573] identified six infants with gram-negative bacteremia and initial normal CSF who developed evidence of meningeal inflammation 18 to 59 hours after the first examination. Although the investigators suggest that a diagnosis of gram-negative bacteremia in the neonate warrants repeat LP to identify the optimal duration of therapy, this recommendation could be broadened to include all infants with bacteremia and initial negative studies of CSF. Dissemination of the organisms from the blood to the meninges can occur after the first LP before sterilization of the blood by appropriate antimicrobial therapy occurs. This is especially likely to occur in neonates with intense bacteremia where sterilization by β-lactam agents (i.e., third-generation cephalosporins) is inoculum dependent.

Smith and colleagues[574] recently performed a large cohort study of CSF parameters in preterm neonates with meningitis. Analysis of first LPs of 4632 neonates of less than 34 weeks of gestation found significant differences in culture-proven meningitis cases versus controls in their CSF leukocyte count (110 cells/mm^3 vs. 6 cells/mm^3), total protein (217 mg/dL vs. 130 mg/dL), and glucose (43 mg/dL vs. 49 mg/dL). However the sensitivity for predicting meningitis was only 71% for CSF leukocyte count greater than 25 cells/mm^3, 61% for CSF protein greater than 170 mg/dL, and 32% for CSF glucose less than 24 mg/dL. The positive predictive value for each of these parameters was low (4%-10%), emphasizing the critical need for CSF culture to establish the diagnosis of meningitis. In terms of excluding meningitis, a normal CSF protein was the most useful parameter because 96% of premature neonates with meningitis had a CSF protein greater than 90 mg/dL.[574]

Investigators have sought a sensitive and specific CSF metabolic determinant of bacterial meningitis with little success. Among products that have been evaluated and found to be inadequate to distinguish bacterial meningitis from other neurologic disease (including cerebroventricular hemorrhage and asphyxia) are γ-aminobutyric acid,[575] lactate dehydrogenase,[576] and creatine kinase brain isoenzyme.[577] Cyclic-3′,5′-adenosine monophosphate was elevated in the CSF of neonates with bacterial meningitis, compared with the CSF of infants who had nonbacterial meningitis or a control group.[578] Elevated CSF concentrations of CRP have been reported for infants with bacterial meningitis who were older than 4 weeks[579,580]; however, the test was found to be of no value in neonates.[581] Current investigations of the proinflammatory cytokines IL-6 and IL-8 indicate that there is a cytokine response in the CSF after birth asphyxia and that these assays are not useful in detecting the infant with meningitis.[582,583]

The Traumatic Lumbar Puncture. A traumatic LP can result in blood in the CSF and can complicate the interpretation of the results for CSF white blood cell count and chemistries.[584] Schwersenski and colleagues[554] found that 13.8% of 712 CSF specimens obtained during the first week of life were bloody and that an additional 14.5% were considered inadequate for testing.

If the total number of white blood cells compared with the number of red blood cells exceeds the value for whole blood, the presence of CSF pleocytosis is suggested. Some investigators have found that the observed white blood cell counts in bloody CSF were lower than would be predicted based on the ratio of white-to-red blood cells in peripheral blood; the white blood cells lyse more rapidly than red blood cells, or the number of white blood cells is decreased for other reasons.[585-588] Several formulas have been used in an attempt to interpret cytologic findings in CSF contaminated by blood.[589-591] However, none of the corrections applied to bloody CSF can be used with confidence for excluding meningitis in the neonate.[592-594] In a cohort study of LPs performed at 150 neonatal units between 1997 and 2004, 39.5% (2519/6374) were traumatic, and 50 of these infants turned out to have meningitis by culture. The authors found correction of the leukocyte count to account for blood contamination resulted in loss of sensitivity and only marginal gain in specificity and therefore would not aid in the diagnosis of bacterial (or fungal) meningitis.[595]

Protein in CSF usually is elevated after a traumatic LP because of the presence of red blood cells. It has been estimated that an increase of approximately 2.0 mg/dL in CSF protein occurs for every 1000 red blood cells/μL in neonates and infants,[596] whereas a value of 1.1 mg/dL per 1000 red blood cells/mL applies in older children.[597] The concentration of glucose does not appear to be altered by blood from a traumatic LP; a low CSF glucose concentration should be considered an important finding even when associated with a traumatic LP.

Because a "bloody tap" is difficult to interpret, it can be valuable to repeat the LP 24 to 48 hours later. If the results of the second LP reveal a normal white blood cell count, bacterial meningitis can be excluded. Even if performed without trauma or apparent bleeding, CSF occasionally can be ambiguous because white blood cells can be elicited by the irritant effect of blood in the CSF.

Brain Abscess. Brain abscess is a rare entity in the neonate, usually complicating meningitis caused by certain gram-negative bacilli. The CSF in the infant with a brain abscess can demonstrate a pleocytosis of a few hundred cells with a mononuclear predominance and an elevated protein level. Bacteria may not be seen by Gram stain of the CSF if meningitis is not present. Sudden clinical deterioration and the appearance of many cells (>1000/mm^3), with a majority of polymorphonuclear cells, suggest rupture of the abscess into the CSF.

LABORATORY AIDS

Historically, aids in the diagnosis of systemic and focal infection in the neonate include peripheral white blood cell and differential counts, platelet counts, acute-phase reactants, blood chemistries, histopathology of the placenta and umbilical cord, smears of gastric or tracheal aspirates, and diagnostic imaging studies. New assays for diagnosis of early-onset sepsis, including serum concentrations of neutrophil CD11b,[598] granulocyte colony-stimulating factor (G-CSF),[599] IL receptor antagonist,[600] IL-6,[601-603] and procalcitonin,[604-606] serum amyloid A,[607] and prohepcidin[608] show promise for increased sensitivity and specificity compared with other laboratory assessments, such as white blood cell count, absolute neutrophil count, and acute-phase reactants. However, proinflammatory cytokines, including IL-1, IL-6, and tumor necrosis factor-α (TNF-α), have been identified in serum and CSF in infants after perinatal asphyxia, raising doubts about the specificity of some of these markers.[582,583,609,610] Mehr and Doyle[611] have reviewed the recent literature on cytokines as aids in the diagnosis of neonatal bacterial sepsis. These assays and procedures are discussed in detail in Chapter 36.

Recently, attention has focused to the use of real-time PCR technologies, often based on the 16S ribosomal RNA sequence of leading pathogens, as a tool for the accelerated culture-independent diagnosis of neonatal sepsis. Compared with the gold standard of blood culture, the evaluation of sensitivity and specificity of these PCR technologies and their consequent clinical utility has ranged from equivocal[612,613] to highly promising.[614,615] A recent study of multiplexed PCR, using 100 μL neonatal blood volume, demonstrated a higher sensitivity (90.5%) compared with blood culture (71.4%), including clinical sepsis cases, even though it had a lower specificity (80.0% vs. 100.0%).[616] Continued rapid advances in nucleic acid–based diagnostics are certain to be explored in this important clinical arena.

Management

If the maternal history or infant clinical signs suggest the possibility of neonatal sepsis, blood, CSF (all infants), and cultures of urine and other clinically evident focal sites should be collected (all infants with suspected late-onset infection). If respiratory abnormalities are apparent or respiratory status has changed, a radiograph of the chest should be performed. Because the clinical manifestations of sepsis can be subtle, the progression of the disease can be rapid, and the mortality rate remains high when compared with that for older infants with serious bacterial infection; thus empirical treatment should be initiated promptly. Many infants who have a clinical course typical of bacterial sepsis are treated empirically because of the imperfect sensitivity of a single blood culture in the diagnosis of sepsis.

CHOICE OF ANTIMICROBIAL AGENTS

Initial Therapy for Presumed Sepsis

The choice of antimicrobial agents for the treatment of suspected sepsis is based on knowledge of the prevalent organisms responsible for neonatal sepsis by age of onset and hospital setting as well as on their patterns of antimicrobial susceptibility. Initial therapy for the infant who develops clinical signs of sepsis during the first few days of life (early-onset disease) must include agents active against gram-positive cocci, particularly GBS, other streptococci, *L. monocytogenes*, and gram-negative enteric bacilli. Treatment of the infant who becomes septic while in the nursery after age 6 days (late-onset disease) must include therapy for hospital-acquired organisms, such as *S. aureus*, gram-negative enteric bacilli, CoNS (in the VLBW infant), and occasionally *P. aeruginosa*, as well as for maternally acquired etiologic agents.

GBS continue to demonstrate significant in vitro susceptibility to penicillins and cephalosporins. Of 3813 case isolates in active population-based surveillance conducted by the CDC between 1996 and 2003, all were sensitive to penicillin, ampicillin, cefazolin, and vancomycin.[617] However, new reports in the United States and Japan have identified GBS strains with reduced β-lactam susceptibility and first-step mutations in the PBPx2 protein reminiscent of the emergence of β-lactam resistance in pneumococci decades ago.[618,619] In the recent CDC surveillance, GBS resistance to clindamycin (15%) and erythromycin (30%) are also noted to be on the rise.[617]

In vitro studies[620-622] and experimental animal models of bacteremia,[623,624] however, indicate that the bactericidal activity of ampicillin and penicillin against GBS and *L. monocytogenes* is enhanced by the addition of gentamicin (synergy). Some physicians prefer to continue the combination of ampicillin and gentamicin for 48 to 72 hours, but once GBS is identified as the etiologic agent, the drug of choice for therapy is penicillin administered intravenously for the remainder of the treatment regimen. There are no clinical data to indicate that continuing an aminoglycoside in combination with a penicillin results in more rapid recovery or improved outcome for infected neonates (see Chapter 12).

Most strains of *S. aureus* that cause disease in neonates produce β-lactamase and are resistant to penicillin G and ampicillin. Many of these organisms are susceptible to the penicillinase-resistant penicillins, such as nafcillin, and to first-generation cephalosporins. Methicillin-resistant staphylococci that are resistant to other penicillinase-resistant penicillins and cephalosporins have been encountered in many nurseries in the United States. Antimicrobial susceptibility patterns must be monitored by surveillance of staphylococcal strains causing infection and disease in each NICU. Bacterial resistance must be considered whenever staphylococcal disease is suspected or confirmed in a patient, and empirical vancomycin therapy should be initiated until the susceptibility pattern of the organism is known. Virtually all staphylococcal strains isolated from neonates have been susceptible to vancomycin. Synergistic activity is provided by the combination of an aminoglycoside (see Chapter 14). Vancomycin- or glycopeptide-resistant *S. aureus* has been reported from Japan and the United States, but none of these strains has been isolated from neonates.

CoNS can cause systemic infection in VLBW infants and in neonates with or without devices such as an intravascular catheter or a ventriculoperitoneal shunt. Vancomycin is the drug of choice for treatment of serious CoNS infections.

If daily cultures from an indwelling device continue to grow CoNS, removal of the foreign material probably will be necessary to cure the infection.

Enterococcus species are only moderately susceptible to penicillin and highly resistant to cephalosporins. Optimal antimicrobial therapy for neonatal infections caused by *Enterococcus* includes ampicillin or vancomycin in addition to an aminoglycoside, typically gentamicin or tobramycin.

L. monocytogenes is susceptible to penicillin and ampicillin and resistant to cephalosporins. Ampicillin is the preferred agent for treating *L. monocytogenes*, although an aminoglycoside can be continued in combination with ampicillin if the patient has meningitis. Specific management of *L. monocytogenes* infection is discussed in Chapter 13.

The choice of antibiotic therapy for infections caused by gram-negative bacilli depends on the pattern of susceptibility for these isolates in the nursery that cares for the neonate. These patterns vary by hospital or community and by time within the same institution or community. Although isolates from neonates should be monitored to determine the emergence of new strains with unique antimicrobial susceptibility patterns, the general pattern of antibiotic susceptibility in the hospital is a good guide to initial therapy for neonates. The aminoglycosides, including gentamicin, tobramycin, netilmicin, and amikacin, are highly active in vitro against virtually all isolates of *E. coli, P. aeruginosa, Enterobacter, Klebsiella,* and *Proteus* spp.

Role of Third-Generation Cephalosporins and Carbapenems

The third-generation cephalosporins, cefotaxime, ceftriaxone, and ceftazidime, possess attractive features for therapy for bacterial sepsis and meningitis in newborns. These features include excellent in vitro activity against GBS and *E. coli* and other gram-negative enteric bacilli. Ceftazidime is highly active in vitro against *P. aeruginosa*. None of the cephalosporins is active against *L. monocytogenes* or *Enterococcus*, and activity against *S. aureus* is variable. These cephalosporins provide concentrations of drug at most sites of infection that greatly exceed the minimum inhibitory concentrations of susceptible pathogens, and there is no dose-related toxicity. Clinical and microbiologic results of studies of sepsis and meningitis in neonates suggest that the third-generation cephalosporins are comparable to the traditional regimens of penicillin and an aminoglycoside (see Chapter 37).[625-628] Because ceftriaxone can displace bilirubin from serum albumin, it is not recommended for use in neonates unless it is the only agent effective against the bacterial pathogen. Meropenem is a broad-spectrum carbapenem antibiotic with extended-spectrum antimicrobial activity, including against *P. aeruginosa*, and excellent CSF penetration that appears safe and efficacious in the neonate for treatment of most nosocomial gram-negative pathogens.[629]

The rapid development of resistance of gram-negative enteric bacilli when cefotaxime is used extensively for presumptive therapy for neonatal sepsis suggests that extensive use of third- or fourth-generation cephalosporins can lead to rapid emergence of drug-resistant bacteria in nurseries.[630] Also of concern, recent studies have identified a principal risk factor for development of invasive infection with *Candida* and other fungi in preterm neonates to be extended therapy with third-generation cephalosporins.[631,632] Empirical use of cefotaxime in neonates should be restricted to those with evidence of meningitis or with gram-negative sepsis. Continued cefotaxime therapy should be limited to those infants with gram-negative meningitis caused by susceptible organisms or those with ampicillin-resistant enteric infections.[633]

CURRENT PRACTICE

The combination of ampicillin and an aminoglycoside, usually gentamicin or tobramycin, is suitable for initial treatment of presumed early-onset neonatal sepsis.[634] If there is a concern for endemic or epidemic staphylococcal infection, typically occurring beyond 6 days of age, the initial treatment of late-onset neonatal sepsis should include vancomycin.

The increasing use of antibiotics, particularly in NICUs, can result in alterations in antimicrobial susceptibility patterns of bacteria and can necessitate changes in initial empirical therapy. This alteration of the microbial flora in nurseries where the use of broad-spectrum antimicrobial agents is routine supports recommendations from the CDC for the judicious use of antibiotics. The hospital laboratory must regularly monitor isolates of pathogenic bacteria to assist the physician in choosing the most appropriate therapy. The clinical pharmacology and dosage schedules of the various antimicrobial agents considered for neonatal sepsis are provided in Chapter 37.

CONTINUATION OF THERAPY WHEN RESULTS OF CULTURES ARE AVAILABLE

The choice of antimicrobial therapy should be reevaluated when results of cultures and susceptibility tests become available. The duration of therapy depends on the initial response to the appropriate antibiotics but should be 10 days, with sepsis documented by positive culture of blood and minimal or absent focal infection. The usual duration of therapy for infants with meningitis caused by gram-negative enteric bacilli is 21 days. However, in complicated cases of meningitis caused by gram-negative enteric bacilli, GBS, or other pathogens, the duration of therapy is variable and is best determined in consultation with an infectious diseases specialist.

The third-generation cephalosporins cefotaxime, ceftriaxone, and ceftazidime have important theoretical advantages for treatment of sepsis or meningitis compared with therapeutic regimens that include an aminoglycoside. Unlike the aminoglycosides, third-generation cephalosporins are not associated with ototoxicity and nephrotoxicity. However, little toxicity from aminoglycosides occurs when use is brief or when continued for the duration of therapy, if serum trough levels are maintained at less than 2 μg/mL. Because cephalosporins have no dose-related toxicity, measurements of serum concentrations, obligatory with the use of aminoglycosides beyond 72 hours or in infants with renal insufficiency, are unnecessary. However, routine use of the cephalosporins for presumptive sepsis therapy in neonates often leads to problems with drug-resistant enteric organisms. Extensive use of the third-generation cephalosporins in the nursery could result in the emergence of resistance caused by derepression of chromosomally mediated β-lactamases.[635] Cefotaxime is preferred to other third-generation cephalosporins for use in neonates because it has been used more extensively[626-628] and because it does not affect the binding of bilirubin.[635,636] Ceftazidime or meropenem in combination with an aminoglycoside should be used in therapy for *P. aeruginosa* meningitis because of their excellent in vitro activity and its good penetration into the CSF. Use of ceftriaxone in the neonate should be determined on a case-by-case basis because of its ability to displace bilirubin from serum albumin and result in biliary sludging.

MANAGEMENT OF THE INFANT WHOSE MOTHER RECEIVED INTRAPARTUM ANTIMICROBIAL AGENTS

Antimicrobial agents commonly are administered to women in labor who have risk factors associated with sepsis in the fetus, including premature delivery, prolonged rupture of membranes, fever, or other signs of chorioamnionitis or GBS colonization. Antimicrobial agents cross the placenta and achieve concentrations in fetal tissues that are parallel to concentrations achieved in other well-vascularized organs. Placental transport of antibiotics is discussed in more detail in Chapter 37.

Protocols for prevention of GBS infection in the newborn by administration of a penicillin to the mother were published in 1992 by ACOG[637] and the AAP.[638] These guidelines were revised in 1996 by the CDC,[639] in 1997 by the AAP,[640] and in 2002 by the CDC,[641] AAP, and ACOG.[642] Recent data suggest that nearly 50% of women receive intrapartum chemoprophylaxis because of the presence of one or more risk factors for neonatal sepsis or because of a positive antenatal screening culture for GBS.[643]

When ampicillin or penicillin is administered to the mother, drug concentrations in the fetus are achieved that are more than 30% of the concentrations in the blood of the mother.[644] Concentrations of penicillin, ampicillin, and cefazolin that are bactericidal for GBS are achieved in the amniotic fluid approximately 3 hours after completion of a maternal intravenous dose. Parenteral antibiotic therapy administered to a mother with signs of chorioamnionitis in labor essentially is treating the fetus early in the course of the intrapartum infection.[645,646] However, for some infected fetuses, the treatment administered in utero is insufficient to prevent signs of early-onset GBS disease. Although maternal intrapartum prophylaxis has been associated with a 75% decrease in the incidence of early-onset GBS disease since 1993,[647,648] the regimen has had no impact on the incidence of late-onset disease.[649]

The various algorithms prepared to guide empirical management of the neonate born to a mother with risk factors for GBS disease who received intrapartum antimicrobial prophylaxis for prevention of early-onset GBS disease focus on three clinical scenarios[647-650]:

1. Infants who have signs of sepsis should receive a full diagnostic evaluation and should be treated, typically with ampicillin and gentamicin, until laboratory studies are available.
2. Infants born at 35 or more weeks of gestation who appear healthy and whose mothers received intrapartum prophylaxis with penicillin, ampicillin, or cefazolin for 4 or more hours before delivery do not have to be evaluated or treated but should be observed in the hospital for 48 hours.
3. Infants who are less than 35 weeks of gestation, who appear healthy, and whose mothers received penicillin, ampicillin, or cefazolin for less than 4 hours before delivery should receive a limited evaluation, including a blood culture and a complete blood cell count with a differential count, and be observed for 48 hours in the hospital. The same management probably is necessary for infants of any gestation whose mothers received vancomycin for prophylaxis because nothing is known about the amniotic fluid penetration of this drug or its efficacy in preventing early-onset GBS disease.

The first two clinical scenarios are readily identified, but the third category often leads to controversy regarding optimal management. Recent recommendations for prevention and treatment of early-onset GBS infection are discussed in detail in Chapter 12.

Management of the infant born to a mother who received an antimicrobial agent within hours of delivery must include consideration of the effect of the drug on cultures obtained from the infant after birth. Intrapartum therapy provides some treatment of the infant in utero, and variable concentrations of drug will be present in the infant's body fluids. If the infant is infected and the bacterial pathogen is susceptible to the drug administered to the mother, cultures of the infant can be sterile despite a clinical course suggesting sepsis.

TREATMENT OF THE INFANT WHOSE BACTERIAL CULTURE RESULTS ARE NEGATIVE

Whether or not the mother received antibiotics before delivery, the physician must decide on the subsequent course of therapy for the infant who was treated for presumed sepsis and whose bacterial culture results are negative. If the neonate appears to be well and there is reason to believe that infection was unlikely, treatment can be discontinued at 48 hours. If the clinical condition of the infant remains uncertain and suspicion of an infectious process remains, therapy should be continued as outlined for documented bacterial sepsis unless another diagnosis becomes apparent. Significant bacterial infection can occur without bacteremia. Squire and colleagues[651] found that results of premortem blood cultures were negative in 7 (18%) of 39 infants with unequivocal infection at autopsy. Some infants with significant systemic bacterial infection may not be identified by the usual single blood-culture technique. The physician must consider this limitation when determining length of empirical therapy. However, if treatment for infection is deemed necessary, parenteral administration for 10 days is recommended.

MANAGEMENT OF THE INFANT WITH CATHETER-ASSOCIATED INFECTION

Investigators in Connecticut found that multiple catheters, LBW, low gestational age at birth, and low Apgar scores were significant risk factors for LOS.[509] Benjamin and colleagues[510] reported a retrospective study at Duke University conducted from 1995 to 1999 of all neonates who had central venous access. The goal of the Duke study was to evaluate the relationship between central venous catheter removal and outcome in bacteremic neonates. Infants bacteremic with *S. aureus* or a gram-negative rod who had their catheter retained beyond 24 hours had a 10-fold higher rate of infection-related complications than those in whom the central catheter was removed promptly. Compared with neonates who had three or fewer positive intravascular catheter blood cultures for coagulase-negative staphylococci, neonates who had four consecutive positive blood cultures were at significantly increased risk for end-organ damage and death. In neonates with central venous catheter–associated infection, prompt removal of the device is advised unless there is rapid clinical improvement and sterilization of blood cultures after initiation of therapy.

TREATMENT OF NEONATAL MENINGITIS

Because the pathogens responsible for neonatal meningitis are largely the same as those that cause neonatal sepsis, initial therapy and subsequent therapy are similar. Meningitis caused by gram-negative enteric bacilli can pose special management problems. Eradication of the pathogen often is delayed, and serious complications can occur.[24,122,352,637] The persistence of gram-negative bacilli in CSF despite bactericidal levels of the antimicrobial agent led to the evaluation of lumbar intrathecal[652] and intraventricular[653] gentamicin. Mortality and morbidity were not significantly different in infants who received parenteral drug alone or parenteral plus intrathecal therapy.[652] The study of the intraventricular gentamicin was stopped early because of the high mortality in the parenteral plus intraventricular therapy group.[653]

Feigin and colleagues[634] provide a review of the management of meningitis in children, including neonates. Ampicillin or penicillin G, initially with an aminoglycoside, are appropriate antimicrobial agents for treating infection caused by GBS. Cefotaxime has superior in vitro and in vivo bactericidal activity against many microorganisms.[626] Treatment of enteric gram-negative bacillary meningitis should include cefotaxime and an aminoglycoside until results of susceptibility testing are known.

If meningitis develops in a LBW infant who has been in the nursery for a prolonged period or in a neonate who has received previous courses of antimicrobial therapy for presumed sepsis, alternative empirical antibiotic regimens should be considered. Enterococci and antibiotic-resistant, gram-negative enteric bacilli are potential pathogens in these settings. A combination of vancomycin, an aminoglycoside, and cefotaxime may be appropriate. Ceftazidime or meropenem in addition to an aminoglycoside should be considered for *P. aeruginosa* meningitis.

Other antibiotics may be necessary for the treatment of highly resistant organisms. Meropenem,[654] ciprofloxacin,[655-657] or trimethoprim-sulfamethoxazole[658,659] can be the only antimicrobial agents active in vitro against bacteria that are highly resistant to broad-spectrum β-lactam antibiotics or aminoglycosides. Some of these drugs require careful monitoring because of toxicity to the newborn (see Chapter 37), and ciprofloxacin has not been approved for use in the United States in infants younger than 3 months. Definitive treatment of meningitis caused by gram-negative enteric bacilli should be determined by in vitro susceptibility tests, and assistance from an infectious diseases specialist can be helpful.

Use of dexamethasone as adjunctive treatment in childhood bacterial meningitis has been recommended based on reduction of neurologic sequelae in infants and children, in particular hearing loss, and especially in cases of *H. influenzae* type b meningitis. Only one randomized controlled study exists for neonates, conducted in 52 full-term neonates, and the mortality (22% dexamethasone vs. 28% controls) and morbidity at 24 months (30% vs. 39%) did not significantly differ between groups.[660]

If cultures of blood and CSF for bacterial pathogens by usual laboratory techniques are negative in the neonate with meningitis, the differential diagnosis of aseptic meningitis must be reviewed, particularly in view of diagnosing treatable infections (Table 6-14).

MANAGEMENT OF THE INFANT WITH A BRAIN ABSCESS

If purulent foci or abscesses are present, they should be drained. However, some brain abscesses resolve with medical therapy alone.[352,661] Brain abscesses can be polymicrobial or result from organisms that uncommonly cause meningitis, such as *Citrobacter*,[157,662] *Enterobacter*,[138] *Proteus*,[352] and *Salmonella* spp.[657] Aspiration of the abscess provides identification of the pathogens to guide rational antimicrobial therapy.

Table 6-14 Infectious and Noninfectious Causes of Aseptic Meningitis* in the Neonate

Cause	Disease
INFECTIOUS AGENT	
Bacteria	Partially treated meningitis Parameningeal focus (brain or epidural abscess) Tuberculosis
Viruses	Herpes simplex meningoencephalitis Cytomegalovirus Enteroviruses Rubella Acquired immunodeficiency syndrome Lymphocytic choriomeningitis Varicella
Spirochetes	Syphilis Lyme disease
Parasites	Toxoplasmosis Chagas disease
Mycoplasma	*Mycoplasma hominis* infection *Ureaplasma urealyticum* infection
Fungi	Candidiasis Coccidioidomycosis Cryptococcosis
NONINFECTIOUS CAUSES	
Trauma	Subarachnoid hemorrhage Traumatic lumbar puncture
Malignancy	Teratoma Medulloblastoma Choroid plexus papilloma and carcinoma

*Aseptic meningitis is defined as meningitis in the absence of evidence of bacterial pathogen detectable in cerebrospinal fluid by usual laboratory techniques.

TREATMENT OF THE INFANT WITH MENINGITIS WHOSE BACTERIAL CULTURE RESULTS ARE NEGATIVE

In the absence of a detectable bacterial pathogen, an aggressive diagnostic approach is necessary for the infant with meningitis, defined by CSF pleocytosis and variable changes in the concentration of CSF protein and glucose. The most frequent cause of aseptic or nontuberculous bacterial meningitis in the neonate is prior antimicrobial therapy resulting in negative blood and CSF cultures. Congenital infections need to be excluded. Treatable diseases, such as partially treated bacterial disease, meningoencephalitis caused by herpes simplex virus, syphilis, cytomegalovirus, toxoplasmosis, Lyme disease in regions where *Borrelia* is prevalent, tuberculosis, and malignancy, need to be considered in the differential diagnosis. The history of illness and contacts in the mother and family and epidemiologic features, such as animal exposures and recent travel, should be explored. Reexamination of the infant for focal signs of disease, including special techniques such as ophthalmologic examination, and consideration of appropriate diagnostic imaging studies of the long bones, skull, and brain can provide further information in determining the source of infection. Treatment of possible bacterial or nonbacterial causes of aseptic meningitis may be necessary before the results of culture, PCR, or serology tests are available to indicate the diagnosis.

TREATMENT OF ANAEROBIC INFECTIONS

The importance of anaerobic bacteria as a cause of serious neonatal infection is uncertain. *Clostridium, Peptococcus,* and *Peptostreptococcus* are highly sensitive to penicillin G, but *B. fragilis* spp. usually are resistant. If anaerobic organisms are known or suspected to be responsible for infection (as in peritonitis), initiating therapy with a clinically appropriate agent, such as clindamycin, metronidazole, meropenem, ticarcillin, or piperacillin/tazobactam, is warranted.

ADJUNCTIVE THERAPIES FOR TREATMENT OF NEONATAL SEPSIS

Despite appropriate antimicrobial and optimal supportive therapy, mortality rates resulting from neonatal sepsis remain high, especially for the VLBW infant. With the hope of improving survival and decreasing the severity of sequelae in survivors, investigators have considered adjunctive modes of treatment, including granulocyte transfusion, exchange transfusion, and the use of standard intravenous immune globulin (IVIG) or pathogen-specific polyclonal or monoclonal antibody reagents for deficits in neonatal host defenses. These therapies are discussed in further detail in Chapter 4. Pentoxifylline has been documented to reduce plasma TNF-α concentrations in premature infants with sepsis and to improve survival, but the number of infants treated (five of five survived) and number of controls (one of four survived) was too small to provide more than a suggestion of efficacy.[663] In neutropenic infants with sepsis, the administration of G-CSF and human granulocyte-macrophage colony-stimulating factor (GM-CSF) have had variable effects on outcome.[664-667] Although the results of selected studies indicate that some of these techniques improved survival, the potential adverse effects (e.g., graft-versus-host reaction, pulmonary leukocyte sequestration) are sufficiently concerning to warrant further study in experimental protocols.

IVIG preparations have been assessed for adjunctive therapy for neonatal sepsis based on the hypothesis that infected infants lack circulating antibodies against bacterial pathogens and that IVIG can provide some antibody for protection. Ohlsson and Lacy[668] performed a meta-analysis of eight randomized studies evaluating 3871 infants of IVIG for treatment of suspected or proven bacterial/fungal infection compared with placebo or no invention. No differences in mortality during hospital stay, length of hospital stay, or death or major disability at 2 years were identified, leading the authors to conclude that routine administration of IVIG to prevent mortality in infants with suspected or proven infection is not recommended. A critical and definitive study in this analysis was the, placebo-controlled multicenter trial in LBW or ventilated neonates (INIS [International Neonatal Immunotherapy Study]) comparing the adjunctive use of 10 mg/kg IVIG versus placebo at the time of suspected infection and 48 hours later; no difference in the primary outcome variables of mortality or major disability at 2 years were identified, nor were differences seen in secondary outcomes including the incidence of subsequent sepsis.[669]

Prognosis

Before the advent of antibiotics, almost all infants with neonatal sepsis died.[5] Dunham[2] reported that physicians used various treatments, including "erysipelas serum" and transfusions, without altering the course of the disease. The introduction of sulfonamides and penicillin and later introduction of broad-spectrum antibiotics, such as chloramphenicol and streptomycin, decreased the mortality rate to about 60%.[3,5] During this period, some infants undoubtedly died because of treatment with high dosages of chloramphenicol, which can cause cardiovascular collapse (i.e., gray baby syndrome).

The introduction of the aminoglycosides, first with kanamycin in the early 1960s and gentamicin late in that decade, vastly improved therapy for bacteremia caused by gram-negative organisms, the leading cause of sepsis at that time.[6] These therapies, together with an improved understanding of neonatal physiology and advances in life-support systems, combined to result in a steady decrease in neonatal mortality in the United States[6] and in Europe[260,261,286,670] during the period 1960 to 1985. Mortality rates for sepsis, including infants of all weights and gestational ages, decreased from 40% to 50% in the 1960s[4,6,286,670] to 10% to 20% in the 1970s and 1980s.[6,10,261,452,670] Population-based surveillance of selected counties in the United States conducted by the CDC from 1993 to 1998 reported 2196 cases of neonatal sepsis caused by GBS, of which 92 (4%) were fatal.[649]

The postnatal age at which infection occurs, once thought to be of prognostic significance, has become less important within the past 2 decades. Fulminant sepsis, with signs of illness present at birth or during the first day of life, has a high mortality rate, varying from 14% to 20%[6,12,261,288] to as high as 70%.[671] However, when infections occurring during the first 24 hours of life, most of which are caused by GBS, are excluded from the analysis, the percentage of deaths caused by early-onset sepsis does not differ significantly from that associated with late-onset infection.‡ Mortality from sepsis is higher for preterm than for term infants in virtually all published studies§ but is approximately the same for all major bacterial pathogens[10,260] (see Tables 6-4 and 6-5).

In recent surveys, the mortality rate for neonatal meningitis has declined from 25%[10,25,672,673] to 10% to 15%.[12,24,27,674,675] This decrease represents a significant improvement from prior years, when studies reported a case-fatality rate of more than 30%.[22,436,654,655,676] Mortality is greater among preterm than term infants.[12,24,27,677]

Significant sequelae develop in 17% to 60% of infants who survive neonatal meningitis caused by gram-negative enteric bacilli or GBS.[24,672-675] These sequelae include mental and motor disabilities, convulsive disorders, hydrocephalus, hearing loss, and abnormal speech patterns. The most extensive experience with the long-term observation of infants who had GBS meningitis as neonates was reported by Edwards and colleagues.[677] Sixty-one patients were treated between 1974 and 1979, and 21% died. Of the 38 survivors who were available for evaluation at 3 years of age or older, 29% had severe neurologic sequelae, 21% had minor deficits, and 50% were functioning normally. Presenting factors that were associated with death or severe disability included comatose or semicomatose state, decreased perfusion, total peripheral white blood cell count less than $5000/mm^3$, absolute neutrophil count less than $1000/mm^3$, and CSF protein level greater than 300mg/dL. A comparable study evaluating 35 newborns over a period of 3 to 18 years demonstrated more favorable outcomes, with 60% of survivors considered normal at the time of follow-up compared with sibling controls, 15% with mild-to-moderate neurologic residua, and 25% with major sequelae.[676] Franco and coworkers[675] reported the results of frequent and extensive neurologic, developmental, and psychometric assessments on a cohort of 10 GBS meningitis survivors followed for 1 to 14 years and found that 1 child had severe CNS damage; 5 children, including 1 with hydrocephalus, had mild academic or behavioral problems; and 4 children were normal.

The neurodevelopmental outcomes described for infants with gram-negative bacillary meningitis are similar to those reported for GBS meningitis. Unhanand and colleagues[24] reported findings from their 21-year experience with gram-negative meningitis at two hospitals in Dallas, Texas. Among 72 patients less than 28 days of age at the onset of symptoms, there were 60 survivors, 43 of whom were followed and evaluated for a period of at least 6 months. Neurologic sequelae, occurring alone or in combination, were described in 56% and included hydrocephalus (≈30%), seizure disorder (≈30%), developmental delay (≈30%), cerebral palsy (25%), and hearing loss (15%). Forty-four percent of the survivors were developmentally normal at follow-up. Among infants with gram-negative bacillary meningitis, thrombocytopenia, CSF white blood cell count greater than $2000/mm^3$, CSF protein greater than 200 mg/dL, CSF glucose–to–blood glucose ratio of less than 0.5, prolonged (>48 hours) positive CSF cultures, and elevated endotoxin and IL-1 concentrations in CSF were indicators of a poor outcome.[24,438,546,678] Investigators in England and Wales[675] found that independent predictors of adverse outcome 12 hours after admission were the presence of seizures, coma, ventilatory support, and leukopenia.

Computed tomography reveals a high incidence of CNS residua among newborns with meningitis. McCracken and colleagues[679] report that, among 44 infants with gram-negative bacillary meningitis, only 30% of computed tomographic scans were considered normal. Hydrocephalus was found in 20% of cases; areas of infarct, cerebritis, diffuse encephalomalacia, or cortical atrophy in 30%; brain abscess in about 20%; and subdural effusions in 7%. Two or more abnormalities were detected in about one third of infants.

The prognosis of brain abscess in the neonate is guarded because about one half of these children die, and sequelae such as hydrocephalus are common among survivors. Of 17 children who had brain abscess during the neonatal period and were followed for at least 2 years, only 4 had normal intellect and were free of seizures.[352] In neonates with brain abscess, the poor outcome probably is caused by destruction of brain parenchyma as a result of hemorrhagic infarcts and necrosis.

Prevention

OBSTETRIC FACTORS

Improvement in the health of pregnant women with increased use of prenatal care facilities has led to lower rates of prematurity. Increased use of antenatal steroids in pregnant women with preterm labor and of surfactant in their infants has resulted in significantly fewer cases of respiratory distress syndrome. More appropriate management of prolonged interval after rupture of maternal membranes, maternal peripartum infections, and fetal distress has improved infant outcome. Because these factors are associated with sepsis in the newborn, improved care of the mother should decrease the incidence of neonatal infection. The development of neonatal intensive care expertise and units with appropriate equipment has resulted in the survival of VLBW infants. Increasingly, obstetric problems are anticipated, and mothers are transferred to medical centers with NICUs before delivery.

CHEMOPROPHYLAXIS

The use of antibiotics to prevent infection can be valuable when they are directed against specific microorganisms for a limited time. In the neonate, the use of silver nitrate eye drops or intramuscular ceftriaxone to prevent gonococcal ophthalmia, vaccination with bacillus Calmette-Guérin (BCG) or prophylactic use of isoniazid to reduce morbidity from tuberculosis in infants who must return to endemic areas, and use of hexachlorophene baths to prevent staphylococcal disease have been recognized as effective modes of chemoprophylaxis. The value of using antimicrobial agents against unknown pathogens in infants believed to be at high risk of infection or undergoing invasive procedures is

‡References 6, 10, 81, 260, 261, 286, 452.

§References 7, 10, 12, 19, 260, 261, 451, 452.

uncertain. Studies of penicillin administered to the mother during labor for prevention of neonatal disease caused by GBS are reviewed earlier and in Chapter 12.

Prophylaxis using low-dose vancomycin as a strategy to prevent LOS in high-risk neonates has been the subject of several recent clinical investigations.[680-683] A meta-analysis incorporating these studies found that low-dose prophylactic vancomycin reduced the incidence of total neonatal nosocomial sepsis, and specifically CoNS sepsis in the preterm infants, but that mortality and length of NICU stay did not differ between the treatment and placebo groups.[684] A potential confounding factor in these studies is that low-dose vancomycin in the intravenous infusion may itself have prevented recovery of pathogens from blood cultures drawn from the central lines. Because clear clinical benefits have not been demonstrated, the rationale for routine prophylaxis with intravenous vancomycin cannot presently outweigh the theoretical concern of selection for antibiotic-resistant pathogens (e.g., vancomycin-resistant enterococci). An intriguing alternative approach was studied in a randomized prospective trial by Garland and colleagues[685]—the use of a vancomycin-heparin lock solution in peripherally inserted central catheters in VLBW and other critically ill neonates. The study found the antibiotic lock solution to be associated with a marked reduction in the incidence of catheter-associated bloodstream infections (5% vs. 30% in controls), providing proof-of-principle for wider investigation of this method that reduces systemic antibiotic exposure.[685]

MATERNAL FACTORS

The antiviral and antibacterial activity of human milk has been recognized for many years[686-689] and is discussed extensively in Chapter 5. Evidence that breastfeeding defends against neonatal sepsis and gram-negative meningitis was first reported more than 30 years ago from Sweden.[690] Studies carried out in Pakistan have shown that even partial breastfeeding appears to be protective among neonates in a resource-limited nation with a high neonatal mortality rate from clinical sepsis.[691] In a study from Georgetown University, human milk–fed VLBW infants had a significant reduction in sepsis or meningitis compared with exclusively formula-fed VLBW infants (OR, 0.47; 95% CI, 0.23 to .95).[692] Breastfed infants have a lower incidence of gastroenteritis, respiratory illness, and otitis media than those who are formula fed. A protective effect of breastfeeding against infections of the urinary tract also has been suggested.[693] Breastfeeding is also associated with general immune stimulatory effects, as evidenced by larger thymus size[694] and improved antibody responses to immunization.[695,696]

Lactoferrin is the major whey protein in human milk and has immunomodulatory activities. A study of bovine lactoferrin supplementation in VLBW neonates identified efficacy in decreasing the incidence of LOS. The decrease occurred for gram-positive bacteremia and fungemia.[376]

IMMUNOPROPHYLAXIS

The immaturity of the neonatal immune system is characterized by decreased levels of antibody against common pathogens; decreased complement activity, especially alternative pathway components; diminished polymorphonuclear leukocyte production, mobilization, and function; diminished T-lymphocyte cytokine production to many antigens; and reduced levels of lactoferrin and transferrin.[693] Recognition of these factors has resulted in attempts at therapeutic intervention aimed specifically at each component of the deficient immune response.[697]

Infants are protected from infection by passively transferred maternal IgG. To enhance the infant's ability to ward off severe infections, immunization of pregnant women and women in the childbearing years has been selectively adopted.[695,698-700] Programs to immunize pregnant women in resource-limited countries with tetanus toxoid have markedly decreased the incidence of neonatal tetanus. Investigational programs for immunization of pregnant women with polysaccharide pneumococcal, *H. influenzae* type b and GBS vaccines aim to provide infants with protection in the first months of life. Studies of safety and immunogenicity of polysaccharide conjugate vaccines for GBS show promise of a reduction in incidence of late- and early-onset disease in newborns.[700] Use of vaccines in pregnant women is discussed in Chapter 38.

Several clinical trials have explored the use of IVIG to correct the antibody deficiency of neonates, particularly very preterm newborns, and thereby reduce the incidence of sepsis. In 1994, the NICHD Neonatal Research Network reported a randomized clinical trial of 2416 subjects to determine the effects of prophylactic IVIG on the risk of sepsis in premature neonates.[701] No reduction in mortality, morbidity, nor incidence of nosocomial infections was achieved by IVIG administration. The use of hyperimmune IVIG preparations and human monoclonal antibodies to prevent specific infections (e.g., CoNS, *S. aureus*) in high-risk neonates is also an area of active exploration; however, although these products appear safe and well tolerated, no reduction in staphylococcal infection was documented in two recent large, randomized multicenter studies.[702,703] A systematic meta-analysis of 19 studies published through 2013, including approximately 5000 infants, calculated IVIG prophylaxis and provided a 3% to 4% reduction in nosocomial infections but did not reduce mortality nor other important clinical outcomes (e.g., NEC, length of hospital stay).[704] The cost of IVIG and the value assigned to these clinical outcomes will dictate use; the authors suggest there is no need for further randomized clinical trials, and that basic scientists and clinicians will need to explore new avenues for prophylaxis against bacterial infection in this special patient population.[704]

An interesting older study by Sidiropoulos and coworkers[705] explored the potential benefit of low-dose (12 g in 12 hours) or high-dose (24g daily for 5 days) IVIG given to pregnant women at risk for preterm delivery because of chorioamnionitis. Cord blood IgG levels were doubled in infants older than 32 weeks of gestational age whose mothers received the higher dosage schedule but were unaffected in infants born earlier, suggesting little or no placental transfer of IVIG before the 32nd week of gestation. Among the infants delivered after 32 weeks, 6 (37%) of 16 born to untreated mothers developed clinical, laboratory, or radiologic evidence of infection and required antimicrobial therapy, whereas none of 7 infants born to treated mothers became infected. Although this study suggests that intrauterine fetal prophylaxis can be beneficial in selected cases, widespread use of IVIG for all women having premature onset of labor is not feasible because of uncertain timing before delivery, widespread shortages of IVIG, and cost.

The decreased number of circulating polymorphonuclear leukocytes and reduced myeloid reserves in the bone marrow of newborns have been ascribed to impaired production of cytokines, IL-3, G-CSF, GM-CSF, TNF-α, and interferon-γ.[706,707] Considerable experience with in vitro myeloid cell cultures and animal models[708,709] suggested that cytokine or growth factor therapy to stimulate myelopoiesis could be an effective aid in preventing sepsis among newborns with hereditary or acquired congenital neutropenia. Individual studies of prophylactic GM-CSF in neonates were inconsistent in demonstrating that absolute neutrophil counts are increased or that the incidence of sepsis is reduced.[666,667,710] Very recently, a single-blind, multicenter randomly controlled trial of GM-CSF in 280 infants at or less than 31 weeks of gestation demonstrated that although neutrophil counts rose more rapidly in the treatment group in the first 11 days after study initiation, there was no difference in the incidence of sepsis nor improved survival associated with these changes.[711] It is important to note that although G-CSF therapy of severe congenital neutropenia reverses neutropenia, demonstrable functional deficiency of the neutrophils persists, and this probably explains why these neonates remain at significantly elevated risk of infection.[712]

The amino acid glutamine has been recognized as important for gut and immune function in critically ill adults, and recent attention has focused on its potential benefit to the neonate, especially because it is not included in standard intravenous amino acid solutions. A large, multicenter, double-blind clinical trial of glutamine supplementation was found not to decrease the incidence of sepsis nor the mortality in ELBW infants,[713] and this failure to provide a statistically significant benefit was borne out in a recent meta-analysis of seven randomized trials, including more than 2300 infants in total.[714]

A few recent studies have examined the effect of probiotic administration of *Lactobacillus* or *Bifidobacterium* spp., generally intended as prophylaxis against NEC in neonates, on the secondary outcome of systemic bacterial infection, yielding conflicting results.[715-717] A recent meta-analysis of nine trials randomizing 1425 infants suggests that enteral supplementation of probiotic bacteria reduced the risk of severe NEC, but there was no evidence of a comparable beneficial effect on the incidence of nosocomial sepsis.[718]

The iron-binding glycoprotein lactoferrin is a component of the innate immune system produced at mucosal sites and activated in response to infection or inflammation. By restricting microbial iron access and through the direct cell wall lytic activity of its component peptides, lactoferrin exhibits broad-spectrum antimicrobial activity.[719] Bovine lactoferrin, sharing 77% homology with the human protein, has been granted "generally recognized as safe" (GRAS) status by the FDA. A recent randomized study of bovine lactoferrin supplementation in VLBW neonates demonstrated a reduced rate of a first episode of LOS in the treatment group (RR, 0.34; 95% CI, 0.17 to 0.70).[376] Certainly, this simple and promising intervention deserves further exploration as a tool to reduce the incidence of nosocomial infection in this extremely high-risk population.

DECONTAMINATION OF FOMITES

Because contamination of equipment poses a significant infectious challenge for the newborn, disinfection of all materials that are involved in the care of the newborn is an important responsibility of nursery personnel. The basic mechanisms of large pieces of equipment must be cleaned appropriately or replaced because they have been implicated in nursery epidemics. The use of disposable equipment and materials packaged in individual units, such as containers of sterile water for a nebulization apparatus, are important advances in the prevention of infection. The frequency of catheter-associated CoNS sepsis has led to attempts to prevent bacterial colonization of intravascular catheters through use of attachment-resistant polymeric materials, antibiotic impregnation, and immunotherapy directed against adherence factors.[720] These procedures are reviewed in Chapter 35.

EPIDEMIOLOGIC SURVEILLANCE

Endemic Infection

Nursery-acquired infections can become apparent days to several months after discharge of the infant. A surveillance system that provides information about infections within the nursery and involves follow-up of infants after discharge should be established. Various techniques can be used for surveillance and are reviewed in Chapter 35.

Epidemic Infection

The medical and nursing staff must be aware of the possibility of outbreaks or epidemics in the nursery. Prevention of disease is based on the level of awareness of personnel. Infection in previously well infants who lack high-risk factors associated with sepsis must be viewed with suspicion. Several cases of infection occurring within a brief period, caused by the same or an unusual pathogen, and occurring in close physical proximity should raise concern about the possibility of a nursery outbreak. Techniques for management of infection outbreaks in nurseries are discussed in Chapter 35.

Sepsis in the Newborn Recently Discharged From the Hospital

When fever or other signs of systemic infection occur in the first weeks after the newborn is discharged from the nursery, appropriate management requires consideration of the possible sources of infection. Infection acquired at birth or from a household contact is the most likely cause. Congenital infection can be present with signs of disease that are detected after discharge. Late-onset infection from microorganisms acquired in the nursery can occur weeks or occasionally months after birth. Infection can occur after discharge because of underlying anatomic, physiologic, or metabolic abnormalities.

The newborn is susceptible to infectious agents that colonize or cause disease in other household members. If an infant whose gestation and delivery were uneventful is discharged from the nursery and develops signs of an infectious disease in the first weeks of life, the infection was probably acquired from someone in the infant's environment. Respiratory and gastrointestinal infections are common and can be accompanied by focal disease such as otitis media. A careful history of illnesses in household members can suggest the source of the infant's infection.

CONGENITAL INFECTION

Signs of congenital infection can appear or be identified after discharge from the nursery. Hearing impairment caused by congenital rubella or cytomegalovirus infection can be noticed by a parent at home. Hydrocephalus with gradually increasing head circumference caused by congenital toxoplasmosis can be apparent only after serial physical examinations. Chorioretinitis, jaundice, or pneumonia can occur as late manifestations of congenital infection. A LP may be performed in the course of a sepsis evaluation. CSF pleocytosis and increased protein concentration can be caused by congenital infection and warrant appropriate follow-up diagnostic studies.

LATE-ONSET DISEASE

Late-onset disease can present after the first week to months after birth as sepsis and meningitis or other focal infections. GBS (see Chapter 12) is the most frequent cause of LOS in the neonate, followed by *E. coli*. Organisms acquired in the nursery also can cause late-onset disease. Skin and soft tissue lesions or other focal infections, including osteomyelitis and pneumonia from *S. aureus*, can occur weeks after birth. The pathogenesis of LOS is obscure in many cases. The reason why an organism becomes invasive and causes sepsis or meningitis after colonizing the mucous membranes, skin, or upper respiratory, genitourinary, or gastrointestinal tracts remains obscure. Nosocomially acquired or health care–associated organisms are discussed in further detail in Chapter 35.

INFECTIONS IN THE HOUSEHOLD

Infection can be associated with an underlying anatomic defect, physiologic abnormality, or metabolic disease. The infant who fails to thrive or presents with fever can have a urinary tract infection as the first indication of an anatomic abnormality. Infants with lacrimal duct stenosis or choanal atresia can develop focal infection. Sepsis caused by gram-negative enteric bacilli occurs frequently in infants with galactosemia (see "Pathogenesis").

The infected infant can be an important source of infection to family members. In one study in New York,[721] 12.6% of household contacts developed suppurative lesions during the 10-month period after introduction into the home of an infant with a staphylococcal lesion. The incidence of suppurative infections in household contacts of infants without lesions was less than 2%. Damato and coworkers[720] demonstrated colonization of neonates with enteric organisms possessing R factor–mediated resistance to kanamycin and persistence of these strains for more than 12 months after birth. During the period of observation, one third of the household contacts of the infants became colonized with the same strain.

Infections in infants have been associated with bites or licks from household pets. *Pasteurella multocida* is part of the oral flora of dogs, cats, and rodents. A recent review of 25 cases of *P. multocida* infection in the neonatal period found animal exposure to cats and/or dogs in 52% of cases, the majority of which did not involve bites or trauma; the balance were felt to represent vertical transmission from an infected mother.[722] In one case report, a 5-week-old infant with *P. multocida* meningitis frequently was licked by the family dog, and the organism was identified in cultures of the dog's mouth but not of the parents' throats.[723] *P. multocida* sepsis and meningitis was reported in 2-month-old twin infants after household exposure to a slaughtered sheep.[724] A neonatal case of *Campylobacter jejuni* sepsis was proven genetically to result from transmission from the family dog.[725] The epidemiologic link between cats and dogs and infection in young infants suggests that parents should limit contact between pets and infants.

FEVER IN THE FIRST MONTH OF LIFE

Reviews of fever in the first weeks of life indicate that elevation of temperature (>38.8° C [101.8° F])[726-731] is relatively uncommon. However, when fever occurs in the young infant, the incidence of severe disease, including bacterial sepsis, meningitis, and pneumonia, is sufficiently high to warrant careful evaluation and conservative management.[726,732] Approximately 12% of all febrile (>38.0° C [100.4° F]) neonates presenting to emergency departments are found to have a serious bacterial infection.[733,734] Important pathogens in the age group include GBS and *E. coli*, and occult bacteremia and urinary tract infections are the most common foci of disease.[733,734]

A careful history of the pregnancy, delivery, nursery experience, interval since discharge from the nursery, and infections in the household should be obtained. Physical examination should establish the presence or absence of signs associated with congenital infection and late-onset diseases. Culture of blood and urine should be performed if no other focus is apparent, and culture of the CSF and a chest radiograph should be considered if the infant is believed to have systemic infection. Risk stratification algorithms have been evaluated to incorporate ancillary clinical testing in hopes of supplementing the often incomplete picture that emerges from history and physical examination.[732] For example, the "Rochester criteria" for analysis of febrile infants, originally proposed by Dagan and colleagues,[729] used criteria such as normal peripheral leukocyte count (5000-15,000/mm^3), normal absolute band neutrophil count (<1500/mm^3) and absence of pyuria to identify low-risk patients. However, when Ferrera and coworkers[728] retrospectively applied these criteria to the subset of patients in their first 4 weeks of life, 6% of the neonates fulfilling low-risk criteria actually had serious bacterial infections. Similarly, when groups of febrile newborns were retrospectively stratified as low risk by the "Philadelphia criteria"[735] or "Boston criteria,"[736] developed for older infants, it became apparent that 3.5% to 4.6% of the neonates with a serious bacterial infection would have been missed.[733,734]

Consequently, because of the inability to accurately predict serious bacterial infections in this age group, a complete sepsis evaluation should be performed and include a culture of blood, urine, and CSF; a complete blood cell and differential count; examination of CSF for cells, glucose, and protein; and a urinalysis. Although a peripheral blood cell count is routinely ordered, it is not sufficiently discriminatory to preclude the mandatory collection of blood for culture.[737,738] Unlike older infants,[739] the presence of signs consistent with a viral upper respiratory tract infection in the neonate does not obviate the need for a full diagnostic evaluation. Indeed, neonates infected with respiratory syncytial virus had equivalent rates of serious bacterial infection as those testing negative for the virus.[740] However, recent data suggests that febrile infants younger than 60 days and positive for influenza virus infection may indeed have lower rates of bacteremia and urinary tract infection than similar infants without influenza infection.[741]

Because of the high rates of serious bacterial infections, guidelines prepared by Baraff and colleagues[726] for the management of infants and children with fever without source state that all febrile infants younger than 28 days should be hospitalized for parenteral antibiotic therapy, regardless of the results of laboratory studies.

Acknowledgment

Drs. S. Michael Marcy, Carol Baker and Debra L. Palazzi contributed to this chapter in earlier editions. The authors are indebted to these scholars for their roles in the preparation of this chapter.

References

1. Gaynes RP, Edwards JR, Jarvis WR, et al: Nosocomial infections among neonates in high-risk nurseries in the United States, *Pediatrics* 93:357, 1996.
2. Dunham EC: Septicemia in the newborn, *Am J Dis Child* 45:229, 1933.
3. Nyhan WL, Fousek MD: Septicemia of the newborn, *Pediatrics* 22:268, 1958.
4. Gluck L, Wood HF, Fousek MD: Septicemia of the newborn, *Pediatr Clin North Am* 13:1131, 1966.
5. Freedman RM, Ingram DL, Cross I, et al: A half century of neonatal sepsis at Yale, *Am J Dis Child* 35:140, 1981.
6. Gladstone IM, Ehrenkranz RA, Edberg SC, et al: A ten-year review of neonatal sepsis and comparison with the previous fifty-year experience, *Pediatr Infect Dis J* 9:819, 1990.
7. Baltimore RS, Huie SM, Meek JI, et al: Early-onset neonatal sepsis in the era of group B streptococcal prevention, *Pediatrics* 108:1094, 2001.
8. Bizzarro MJ, Raskind C, Baltimore RS, et al: Seventy-five years of neonatal sepsis at Yale: 1928-2003, *Pediatrics* 116:595, 2005.
9. Bizzarro MJ, Dembry LM, Baltimore RS, et al: Changing patterns in neonatal *Escherichia coli* sepsis and ampicillin resistance in the era of intrapartum antibiotic prophylaxis, *Pediatrics* 121:689, 2008.
10. Vesikari R, Janas M, Gronroos P, et al: Neonatal septicemia, *Arch Dis Child* 60:542, 1985.
11. Winfred I: The incidence of neonatal infections in the nursery unit at the Ahmadu Bello University Teaching Hospital, Zaria, Nigeria, *East Afr Med J* 61:197, 1984.
12. Greenberg D, Shinwell ES, Yagupsky P, et al: A prospective study of neonatal sepsis and meningitis in Southern Israel, *Pediatr Infect Dis J* 16:768, 1997.
13. Hensey OJ, Hart CA, Cooke RWI: Serious infection in a neonatal intensive care unit: a two-year survey, *J Hyg (Camb)* 95:289, 1985.
14. Karlowicz MG, Buescher ES, Surka AE: Fulminant late-onset sepsis in a neonatal intensive care unit, 1988-1997, and the impact of avoiding empiric vancomycin therapy, *Pediatrics* 106:1387, 2000.
15. Stoll BJ, Hansen N, Fanaroff AA, et al: Late-onset sepsis in very low birth weight neonates: the experience of the NICHD Neonatal Research Network, *Pediatrics* 110:285, 2002.
16. Makhoul IR, Sujov P, Smolkin T, et al: Epidemiology, clinical, and microbiological characteristics of late-onset sepsis among very low birth weight infants in Israel: a national survey, *Pediatrics* 109:34, 2002.
17. Karpuch J, Goldberg M, Kohelet D: Neonatal bacteremia: a 4-year prospective study, *Isr J Med Sci* 19:963, 1983.
18. Weston EJ, Pondo T, Lewis MM, et al: The burden of invasive early-onset neonatal sepsis in the United States, 2005-2008, *Pediatr Infect Dis J* 30:937-941, 2011.
19. Fanaroff AA, Korones SB, Wright LL, et al: Incidence, presenting features, risk factors and significance of late onset septicemia in very low birth weight infants, *Pediatr Infect Dis* 17:593, 1998.
20. Stoll BJ, Hansen NI, Sánchez PJ, et al: Early onset neonatal sepsis: the burden of group B streptococcal and *E. coli* disease continues, *Pediatrics* 127:817-826, 2011.
21. Ziai M, Haggerty RJ: Neonatal meningitis, *N Engl J Med* 259:314, 1958.
22. Mathies AW Jr, Wehrle PF: *Management of bacterial meningitis*, Philadelphia, 1974, WB Saunders.
23. Yow MD, Baker CJ, Barrett FF, et al: Initial antibiotic management of bacterial meningitis, *Medicine (Baltimore)* 52:305, 1973.
24. Unhanand M, Mustafa MM, McCracken GH Jr, et al: Gram-negative enteric bacillary meningitis: a twenty-one-year experience, *J Pediatr* 122:15, 1993.
25. Mulder CJJ, van Alphen L, Zanen HC: Neonatal meningitis caused by *Escherichia coli* in the Netherlands, *J Infect Dis* 150:935, 1984.
26. de Louvois J, Blackbourn J, Hurley R, et al: Infantile meningitis in England and Wales: a two year study, *Arch Dis Child* 66:603, 1991.
27. Holt DE, Halket S, de Louvois J, et al: Neonatal meningitis in England and Wales: 10 years on, *Br Med J* 84:F85, 2001.
28. Moreno MT, Vargas S, Poveda R, et al: Neonatal sepsis and meningitis in a developing Latin American country, *Pediatr Infect Dis J* 13:516, 1994.
29. Bennhagen R, Svenningsen NW, Bekassy AN: Changing pattern of neonatal meningitis in Sweden: a comparative study 1976 vs. 1983, *Scand J Infect Dis* 19:587, 1987.
30. Lancefield RC: Serologic differentiation of human and other groups of hemolytic streptococci, *J Exp Med* 57:571, 1933.
31. Baker CJ, Barrett FF, Gordon RC, et al: Suppurative meningitis due to streptococci of Lancefield group B: a study of 33 infants, *J Pediatr* 82:724, 1973.
32. Schlievert PM, Gocke JE, Deringer JR: Group B streptococcal toxic shock-like syndrome: report of a case and purification of an associated pyrogenic toxin, *Clin Infect Dis* 17:26, 1993.
33. Mason KL, Aronoff DM: Postpartum group A streptococcus sepsis and maternal immunology, *Am J Reprod Immunol* 67:91, 2012.
34. Sriskandan S: Severe peripartum sepsis, *J R Coll Physicians Edinb* 41:339, 2011.
35. Hamilton SM, Stevens DL, Bryant AE: Pregnancy-related group a streptococcal infections: temporal relationships between bacterial acquisition, infection onset, clinical findings, and outcome, *Clin Infect Dis* 57:870, 2013.
36. Miyairi I, Berlingieri D, Protic J, et al: Neonatal invasive group A streptococcal disease: case report and review of the literature, *Pediatr Infect Dis J* 23:161, 2004.
37. Herrera Guerra AA, Osguthorpe RJ: Acute neonatal parotitis caused by *Streptococcus pyogenes*: a case report, *Clin Pediatr (Phila)* 49:499, 2010.
38. Martic J, Mijac V, Jankovic B, et al: Neonatal cellulitis and sepsis caused by group A *Streptococcus*, *Pediatr Dermatol* 27:528, 2010.
39. Erol S, Dilli D, Aydin B, et al: Pleural empyema due to group A beta-hemolytic streptococci in a newborn: case report, *Tuberk Toraks* 61:152, 2013.
40. Geil CC, Castle WK, Mortimer EA: Group A streptococcal infections in newborn nurseries, *Pediatrics* 46:849, 1970.
41. Gezon HM, Schaberg MJ, Klein JO: Concurrent epidemics of *Staphylococcus aureus* and group A *Streptococcus* disease in a newborn nursery-control with penicillin G and hexachlorophene bathing, *Pediatrics* 51:383, 1973.
42. Peter G, Hazard J: Neonatal group A streptococcal disease, *J Pediatr* 87:454, 1975.
43. Nelson JD, Dillon HC Jr, Howard JB: A prolonged nursery epidemic associated with a newly recognized type of group A streptococcus, *J Pediatr* 89:792, 1976.
44. Campbell JR, Arango CA, Garcia-Prats JA, et al: An outbreak of m serotype 1 group A *Streptococcus* in neonatal intensive care unit, *J Pediatr* 129:396, 1996.
45. Acharya U, Lamont CAR, Cooper K: Group A beta-hemolytic streptococcus causing disseminated intravascular coagulation and maternal death, *Lancet* 1:595, 1988.

46. Kavi J, Wise R: Group A beta-hemolytic streptococcus causing disseminated intravascular coagulation and maternal death, *Lancet* 1:993, 1988.
47. Swingler GR, Bigrigg MA, Hewitt BG, et al: Disseminated intravascular coagulation associated with group A streptococcal infection in pregnancy, *Lancet* 1:1456, 1988.
48. Miyairi I, Berlingieri D, Protic J, et al: Neonatal invasive group A streptococcal disease: case report and review of the literature, *Pediatr Infect Dis J* 23:161, 2004.
49. Greenberg D, Leibovitz E, Shinnwell ES, et al: Neonatal sepsis caused by *Streptococcus pyogenes*–resurgence of an old etiology? *Pediatr Infect Dis J* 18:479, 1999.
50. Westh H, Skibsted L, Korner B: *Streptococcus pneumoniae* infections of the female genital tract and in the newborn child, *Rev Infect Dis* 12:416, 1990.
51. Hoffman JA, Mason EO, Schutze G, et al: *Streptococcus pneumoniae* infections in the neonate, *Pediatrics* 112:1095, 2003.
52. McDonald LC, Bryant K, Snyder J: Peripartum transmission of penicillin-resistant *Streptococcus pneumoniae*, *J Clin Microbiol* 41:2258, 2003.
53. Prommalikit O, Mekmullica J, Pancharoen C, et al: Invasive pneumococcal infection in neonates: 3 case reports, *J Med Assoc Thai* 93(Suppl 5):S46, 2010.
54. Malhotra A, Hunt RW, Doherty RR: *Streptococcus pneumoniae* sepsis in the newborn, *J Paediatr Child Health* 48:E79, 2012.
55. Shaw PJ, Robinson DL, Watson JG: Pneumococcal infection in a mother and infant, *Lancet* 2:47, 1984.
56. Morris L, Groner A, Geiger M, et al: *Streptococcus pneumoniae* purulent pericarditis in a neonate, *Cardiol Young* 23:146, 2013.
57. Stewardson-Krieger P, Gotoff SP: Neonatal meningitis due to group C beta hemolytic *Streptococcus*, *J Pediatr* 90:103, 1977.
58. Quinn RJ, Hallett AF, Appelbaum PC, et al: Meningitis caused by *Streptococcus dysgalactiae* in a preterm infant, *Am J Clin Pathol* 70:948, 1978.
59. Hervas JA, Labay MV, Rullan G, et al: Neonatal sepsis and meningitis due to *Streptococcus equisimilis*, *Pediatr Infect Dis J* 4:694, 1985.
60. Arditi M, Shulman ST, Davis AT, et al: Group C β-hemolytic streptococcal infections in children: nine pediatric cases and review, *Rev Infect Dis* 11:34, 1989.
61. Dyson AE, Read SE: Group G streptococcal colonization and sepsis in neonates, *J Pediatr* 99:944, 1981.
62. Carstensen H, Pers C, Pryds O: Group G streptococcal neonatal septicemia: two case reports and a brief review of the literature, *Scand J Infect Dis* 20:407, 1988.
63. Auckenthaler R, Hermans PE, Washington JA II: Group G streptococcal bacteremia: clinical study and review of the literature, *Rev Infect Dis* 5:196, 1983.
64. Yamaoka S, Ogihara T, Yasui M, et al: Neonatal streptococcal toxic shock syndrome caused by *Streptococcus dysgalactiae* subsp, *Equisimilis Pediatr Infect Dis J* 29:979, 2010.
65. Fikar CR, Levy J: *Streptococcus bovis* meningitis in a neonate, *Am J Dis Child* 133:1149, 1979.
66. Gavin PJ, Thomson RB Jr, Horng SJ, et al: Neonatal sepsis caused by *Streptococcus bovis* variant (biotype ii/2): report of a case and review, *J Clin Microbiol* 41:3433, 2003.
67. Bignardi GE, Isaacs D: Neonatal meningitis due to *Streptococcus mitis*, *Rev Infect Dis* 11:86, 1989.
68. Thatrimontrichai A, Chanvitan P, Janjindamai W, et al: Early onset neonatal bacterial meningitis caused by *Streptococcus gallolyticus* subsp. *Pasteurianus*, *Southeast Asian J Trop Med Public Health* 43:145, 2012.
69. Onoyama S, Ogata R, Wada A, et al: Neonatal bacterial meningitis caused by *Streptococcus gallolyticus* subsp. *Pasteurianus*, *J Med Microbiol* 58:1252, 2009.
70. Toepfner N, Shetty S, Kunze M, et al: Fulminant neonatal sepsis due to *Streptococcus alactolyticus*: a case report and review, *APMIS* 122:654-656, 2014.
71. Broughton RA, Krafka R, Baker CJ: Non-group D alpha-hemolytic streptococci: new neonatal pathogens, *J Pediatr* 99:450, 1981.
72. Kumar SP, Delivoria-Papadopoulos M: Infections in newborn infants in a special care unit, *Ann Clin Lab Sci* 15:351, 1985.
73. Spigelblatt L, Saintonge J, Chicoine R, et al: Changing pattern of neonatal streptococcal septicemia, *Pediatr Infect Dis J* 4:56, 1985.
74. Gunlemez A, Atasay B, Guriz H, et al: Multi-resistant viridans streptococcal pneumonia and sepsis in the ventilated newborn, *Ann Trop Paediatr* 24:253, 2004.
75. Ludwig W, Seewaldt E, Kilpper-Balz R, et al: The phylogenetic position of *Streptococcus* and *Enterococcus*, *J Gen Microbiol* 131:543, 1985.
76. Siegel JD, McCracken GH Jr: Group D streptococcal infections, *J Pediatr* 93:542, 1978.
77. McNeeley DF, Saint-Louis F, Noel GJ: Neonatal enterococcal bacteremia: an increasingly frequent event with potentially untreatable pathogens, *Pediatr Infect Dis J* 15:800, 1996.
78. Alexander JB, Giacoia GP: Early onset nonenterococcal group D streptococcal infection in the newborn infant, *J Pediatr* 93:489, 1978.
79. Headings DL, Herrera A, Mazzi E, et al: Fulminant neonatal septicemia caused by *Streptococcus bovis*, *J Pediatr* 92:282, 1978.
80. Bavikatte K, Schreiner RL, Lemons JA, et al: Group D streptococcal septicemia in the neonate, *Am J Dis Child* 133:493, 1979.
81. Dobson SRM, Baker CJ: Enterococcal sepsis in neonates: features by age at onset and occurrence of focal infection, *Pediatrics* 85:165, 1990.
82. McNeeley DF, Brown AE, Noel GJ, et al: An investigation of vancomycin-resistant *Enterococcus faecium* within the pediatric service of a large urban medical center, *Pediatr Infect Dis J* 17:184, 1998.
83. Beneri CA, Nicolau DP, Seiden HS, et al: Successful treatment of a neonate with persistent vancomycin-resistant enterococcal bacteremia with a daptomycin-containing regimen, *Infect Drug Resist* 1:9-11, 2008.
84. Ergaz Z, Arad I, Bar-Oz B, et al: Elimination of vancomycin-resistant enterococci from a neonatal intensive care unit following an outbreak, *J Hosp Infect* 74:370, 2010.
85. Espersen F, Frimodt-Màller N, Rosdahl VT, et al: *Staphylococcus aureus* bacteremia in children below the age of one year, *Acta Paediatr Scand* 78:56, 1989.
86. Shane AL, Hansen NI, Stoll BJ, et al: Methicillin-resistant and susceptible *Staphylococcus aureus* bacteremia and meningitis in preterm infants, *Pediatrics* 129:e914, 2012.
87. Heinrich N, Mueller A, Bartmann P, et al: Successful management of an mrsa outbreak in a neonatal intensive care unit, *Eur J Clin Microbiol Infect Dis* 30:909, 2011.
88. Nubel U, Nachtnebel M, Falkenhorst G, et al: MRSA transmission on a neonatal intensive care unit: epidemiological and genome-based phylogenetic analyses, *PLoS One* 8:e54898, 2013.
89. Saiman L, O'Keefe M, Graham PL 3rd, et al: Hospital transmission of community-acquired methicillin-resistant *Staphylococcus aureus* among postpartum women, *Clin Infect Dis* 37:1313, 2003.
90. David MD, Kearns AM, Gossain S, et al: Community-associated methicillin-resistant *Staphylococcus aureus*: nosocomial transmission in a neonatal unit, *J Hosp Infect* 64:244, 2006.
91. Wang SM, Liu CC, Tseng HW, et al: *Staphylococcus capitis* bacteremia of very low birth weight premature infants at neonatal intensive care units: clinical significance and antimicrobial susceptibility, *J Microbiol Immunol Infect* 32:26, 1999.
92. Marchant EA, Boyce GK, Sadarangani M, et al: Neonatal sepsis due to coagulase-negative staphylococci, *Clin Dev Immunol* 2013:586076, 2013.
93. Strunk T, Richmond P, Simmer K, et al: Neonatal immune responses to coagulase-negative staphylococci, *Curr Opin Infect Dis* 20:370, 2007.
94. Power Coombs MR, Kronforst K, Levy O: Neonatal host defense against staphylococcal infections, *Clin Dev Immunol* 2013:826303, 2013.
95. Baumgart S, Hall SE, Campos JM, et al: Sepsis with coagulase-negative staphylococci in critically ill newborns, *Am J Dis Child* 137:461, 1983.
96. Struthers S, Underhill H, Albersheim S, et al: A comparison of two versus one blood culture in the diagnosis and treatment of coagulase-negative staphylococcus in the neonatal intensive care unit, *J Perinatol* 22:547, 2002.
97. Healy CM, Baker CJ, Palazzi DL, et al: Distinguishing true coagulase-negative staphylococcus infections from contaminants in the neonatal intensive care unit, *J Perinatol* 33:52, 2013.
98. Hall RT, Hall SL, Barnes WG, et al: Characteristics of coagulase negative staphylococci from infants with bacteremia, *Pediatr Infect Dis J* 6:377, 1987.
99. Otto M: Virulence factors of the coagulase-negative staphylococci, *Front Biosci* 9:841, 2004.
100. Shiau AL, Wu CL: The inhibitory effect of staphylococcus epidermidis slime on the phagocytosis of murine peritoneal macrophages is interferon-independent, *Microbiol Immunol* 42:33, 1998.

101. Dimitriou G, Fouzas S, Giormezis N, et al: Clinical and microbiological profile of persistent coagulase-negative staphylococcal bacteraemia in neonates, *Clin Microbiol Infect* 17:1684, 2011.
102. Freeman J, Goldmann DA, Smith NE, et al: Association of intravenous lipid emulsion and coagulase-negative staphylococcal bacteremia in neonatal intensive care units, *N Engl J Med* 323:301, 1990.
103. Centers for Disease Control and Prevention: Public health dispatch: outbreak of listeriosis—northeastern United States 2002, *MMWR Morb Mortal Wkly Rep* 51:950, 2002.
104. Posfay-Barbe KM, Wald ER: Listeriosis, *Semin Fetal Neonatal Med* 14:228, 2009.
105. Schrag SJ, Hadler JL, Arnold KE, et al: Risk factors for invasive, early-onset escherichia coli infections in the era of widespread intrapartum antibiotic use, *Pediatrics* 118:570, 2006.
106. Raymond J, Lopez E, Bonacorsi S, et al: Evidence for transmission of *Escherichia coli* from mother to child in late-onset neonatal infection, *Pediatr Infect Dis J* 27:186, 2008.
107. Soto SM, Bosch J, Jimenez de Anta MT, et al: Comparative study of virulence traits of *Escherichia coli* clinical isolates causing early and late neonatal sepsis, *J Clin Microbiol* 46:1123, 2008.
108. Bingen E, Picard B, Brahimi N, et al: Phylogenetic analysis of *Escherichia coli* strains causing neonatal meningitis suggests horizontal gene transfer from a predominant pool of highly virulent B2 group strains, *J Infect Dis* 177:642, 1998.
109. Bonacorsi S, Bingen E: Molecular epidemiology of *Escherichia coli* causing neonatal meningitis, *Int J Med Microbiol* 295:373, 2005.
110. Peigne C, Bidet P, Mahjoub-Messai F, et al: The plasmid of *Escherichia coli* strain S88 (o45:K1:H7) that causes neonatal meningitis is closely related to avian pathogenic *E. coli* plasmids and is associated with high-level bacteremia in a neonatal rat meningitis model, *Infect Immun* 77:2272, 2009.
111. Tsai CH, Chen YY, Wang KG, et al: Characteristics of early-onset neonatal sepsis caused by *Escherichia coli*, *Taiwan J Obstet Gynecol* 51:26, 2012.
112. McCracken GH Jr, Sarff LD: Current status and therapy of neonatal *E. coli* meningitis, *Hosp Pract* 9:57, 1974.
113. Kim KS: Current concepts on the pathogenesis of *Escherichia coli* meningitis: implications for therapy and prevention, *Curr Opin Infect Dis* 25:273, 2012.
114. Robbins JB, McCracken GH Jr, Gotschuch EC, et al: *Escherichia coli* K1 capsular polysaccharide associated with neonatal meningitis, *N Engl J Med* 290:1216, 1974.
115. Sarff LD, McCracken GH Jr, Schiffer MS, et al: Epidemiology of *Escherichia coli* K1 in healthy and diseased newborns, *Lancet* 1:1099, 1975.
116. Peter G, Nelson JS: Factors affecting neonatal *E. coli* K1 rectal colonization, *J Pediatr* 93:866, 1978.
117. Burns JL, Griffith A, Barry JJ, et al: Transcytosis of gastrointestinal epithelial cells by *Escherichia coli* K1, *Pediatr Res* 49:30, 2001.
118. Xie Y, Kim KJ, Kim KS: Current concepts on *Escherichia coli* K1 translocation of the blood-brain barrier, *FEMS Immunol Med Microbiol* 42:271, 2004.
119. Hervás JA, Ballesteros F, Alomar A, et al: Increase of *Enterobacter* in neonatal sepsis: a twenty-two-year study, *Pediatr Infect Dis J* 20:1134, 2001.
120. Gupta A: Hospital-acquired infections in the neonatal intensive care unit—*Klebsiella pneumoniae*, *Semin Perinatol* 26:340, 2002.
121. Sood SK, Mulvihill D, Daum RS: Intrarenal abscess caused by *Klebsiella pneumoniae* in a neonate: modern management and diagnosis, *Am J Perinatol* 6:367, 1989.
122. Basu S, Mukherjee KK, Poddar B, et al: An unusual case of neonatal brain abscess following *Klebsiella pneumoniae* septicemia, *Infection* 29:283, 2001.
123. Ozkan H, Kumtepe S, Turan A, et al: Perianal necrotizing fasciitis in a neonate, *Indian J Pediatr* 64:116, 1997.
124. Podschun R, Acktun H, Okpara J: Isolation of *Klebsiella planticola* from newborns in a neonatal ward, *J Clin Microbiol* 36:2331, 1998.
125. Westbrook GL, O'Hara CM, Roman SB, et al: Incidence and identification of *Klebsiella planticola* in clinical isolates with emphasis on newborns, *J Clin Microbiol* 38:1495, 2000.
126. Leibovitz E, Flidel-Rimon O, Juster-Reicher A, et al: Sepsis at a neonatal intensive care unit: a four-year retrospective study (1989-1992), *Israel J Med Sci* 33:734, 1997.
127. Bell Y, Barton M, Thame M, et al: Neonatal sepsis in Jamaican neonates, *Ann Trop Paediatr* 25:293, 2005.
128. Viswanathan R, Singh AK, Mukherjee S, et al: Aetiology and antimicrobial resistance of neonatal sepsis at a tertiary care centre in Eastern Iindia: a 3 year study, *Indian J Pediatr* 78:409, 2011.
129. Simeunovic E, Arnold M, Sidler D, et al: Liver abscess in neonates, *Pediatr Surg Int* 25:153, 2009.
130. Pessoa-Silva CL, Meurer Moreira B, Camara Almeida V, et al: Extended-spectrum beta-lactamase-producing *Klebsiella pneumoniae* in a neonatal intensive care unit: risk factors for infection and colonization, *J Hosp Infect* 53:198, 2003.
131. Roilides E, Kyriakides G, Kadiltsoglou I, et al: Septicemia due to multiresistant *Klebsiella pneumoniae* in a neonatal unit: a case-control study, *Am J Perinatol* 17:35, 2000.
132. Stone PW, Gupta A, Loughrey M, et al: Attributable costs and length of stay of an extended-spectrum beta-lactamase-producing *Klebsiella pneumoniae* outbreak in a neonatal intensive care unit, *Infect Control Hosp Epidemiol* 24:601, 2003.
133. Harbarth S, Sudre P, Dharan S, et al: Outbreak of *Enterobacter cloacae* related to understaffing, overcrowding, and poor hygiene practices, *Infect Control Hosp Epidemiol* 20:598, 1999.
134. Wenger PJ, Tokars JI, Brennan P, et al: An outbreak of *Enterobacter hormaechei* infection and colonization in an intensive care nursery, *Clin Infect Dis* 24:1243, 1997.
135. da Silva CL, Miranda LE, Moreira BM, et al: *Enterobacter hormaechei* bloodstream infection at three neonatal intensive care units in Brazil, *Pediatr Infect Dis J* 21:175, 2002.
136. Iversen C, Mullane N, McCardell B, et al: *Cronobacter* gen. nov., a new genus to accommodate the biogroups of *Enterobacter sakazakii*, and proposal of *Cronobacter sakazakii* gen. nov., comb. nov., *Cronobacter malonaticus* sp. nov., *Cronobacter turicensis* sp. nov., *Cronobacter muytjensii* sp. nov., *Cronobacter dublinensis* sp. nov., *Cronobacter* genomospecies 1, and of three subspecies and *Cronobacter dublinensis* subsp. *Lactaridi* subsp nov, *Int J Syst Evol Microbiol* 58:1442, 2008.
137. Gurses N: Enterobacter septicemia in neonates, *Pediatr Infect Dis J* 14:638, 1995.
138. Willis J, Robinson JE: *Enterobacter sakazakii* meningitis in neonates, *Pediatr Infect Dis J* 7:196, 1988.
139. Bonadio WA, Margolis D, Tovar M: *Enterobacter cloacae* bacteremia in children: a review of 30 cases in 12 years, *Clin Pediatr* 30:310, 1991.
140. Jain A, Roy I, Gupta MK, et al: Prevalence of extended-spectrum beta-lactamase-producing gram-negative bacteria in septicaemic neonates in a tertiary care hospital, *J Med Microbiol* 52:421, 2003.
141. Chen HN, Lee ML, Yu WK, et al: Late-onset *Enterobacter cloacae* sepsis in very-low-birth-weight neonates: experience in a medical center, *Pediatr Neonatol* 50:3, 2009.
142. Drudy D, Mullane NR, Quinn T, et al: *Enterobacter sakazakii*: an emerging pathogen in powdered infant formula, *Clin Infect Dis* 42:996, 2006.
143. Cronobacter species isolation in two infants—New Mexico, 2008, *MMWR Morb Mortal Wkly Rep* 58:1179, 2009.
144. Fok TF, Lee CH, Wong EMC, et al: Risk factors for *Enterobacter* septicemia in a neonatal unit: case-control study, *Clin Infect Dis* 27:1204, 1998.
145. Tresoldi AT, Padoveze MC, Trabasso P, et al: *Enterobacter cloacae* sepsis outbreak in a newborn unit caused by contaminated total parenteral nutrition solution, *Am J Infect Control* 28:258, 2000.
146. Cheng HS, Lin HC, Peng CT, et al: Outbreak investigation of nosocomial *Enterobacter cloacae* bacteraemia in a neonatal intensive care unit, *Scand J Infect Dis* 32:293, 2000.
147. Hunter CJ, Bean JF: *Cronobacter*: an emerging opportunistic pathogen associated with neonatal meningitis, sepsis and necrotizing enterocolitis, *J Perinatol* 33:581, 2013.
148. Townsend S, Hurrell E, Forsythe S: Virulence studies of *Enterobacter sakazakii* isolates associated with a neonatal intensive care unit outbreak, *BMC Microbiol* 8:64, 2008.
149. Yan QQ, Condell O, Power K, et al: *Cronobacter* species (formerly known as *Enterobacter sakazakii*) in powdered infant formula: a review of our current understanding of the biology of this bacterium, *J Appl Microbiol* 113:1, 2012.
150. Doran TI: The role of *Citrobacter* in clinical disease of children: review, *Clin Infect Dis* 28:384, 1999.
151. Lin FYC, Devol WF, Morrison C, et al: Outbreak of neonatal *Citrobacter diversus* meningitis in a suburban hospital, *Pediatr Infect Dis J* 6:50, 1987.

152. Eppes SC, Woods CR, Mayer AS, et al: Recurring ventriculitis due to *Citrobacter diversus*: clinical and bacteriologic analysis, *Clin Infect Dis* 17:437, 1993.
153. Foreman SD, Smith EE, Ryan NJ, et al: Neonatal *Citrobacter* meningitis; pathogenesis of cerebral abscess formation, *Ann Neurol* 16:655, 1984.
154. Morris JG, Lin FY, Morrison CB, et al: Molecular epidemiology of neonatal meningitis due to *Citrobacter diversus*: a study of isolates from hospitals in Maryland, *J Infect Dis* 154:409, 1986.
155. Kline MW, Mason EO Jr, Kaplan SL: Characterization of *Citrobacter diversus* strains causing neonatal meningitis, *J Infect Dis* 157:101, 1988.
156. Etuwewe O, Kulshrestha R, Sangra M, et al: Brain abscesses due to *Citrobacter koseri* in a pair of twins, *Pediatr Infect Dis J* 28:1035, 2009.
157. Graham DR, Band JD: *Citrobacter* brain abscess and meningitis in neonates, *JAMA* 1981:245, 1923.
158. Townsend SM, Pollack HA, Gonzalez-Gomez I, et al: *Citrobacter koseri* brain abscess in the neonatal rat: survival and replication within human and rat macrophages, *Infect Immun* 71:5871, 2003.
159. Plakkal N, Soraisham AS, Amin H: *Citrobacter freundii* brain abscess in a preterm infant: a case report and literature review, *Pediatr Neonatol* 54:137, 2013.
160. McPherson C, Gal P, Ransom JL: Treatment of *Citrobacter koseri* infection with ciprofloxacin and cefotaxime in a preterm infant, *Ann Pharmacother* 42:1134, 2008.
161. Fleisch F, Zimmermann-Baer U, Zbinden R, et al: Three consecutive outbreaks of *Serratia marcescens* in a neonatal intensive care unit, *Clin Infect Dis* 34:767, 2002.
162. Jang TN, Fung CP, Yang TL, et al: Use of pulsed-field gel electrophoresis to investigate an outbreak of *Serratia marcescens* infection in a neonatal intensive care unit, *J Hosp Infect* 48:13, 2001.
163. Dessi A, Puddu M, Testa M, et al: *Serratia marcescens* infections and outbreaks in neonatal intensive care units, *J Chemother* 21:493, 2009.
164. Newport MT, John JF, Michel YM, et al: Endemic *Serratia marcescens* infection in a neonatal intensive care nursery associated with gastrointestinal colonization, *Pediatr Infect Dis* 4:160, 1985.
165. Berthelot P, Grattard F, Amerger C, et al: Investigation of a nosocomial outbreak due to *Serratia marcescens* in a maternity hospital, *Infect Control Hosp Epidemiol* 20:233, 1999.
166. Cullen MM, Trail A, Robinson M, et al: *Serratia marcescens* outbreak in a neonatal intensive care unit prompting review of decontamination of laryngoscopes, *J Hosp Infect* 59:68, 2005.
167. Zaidi M, Sifuentes J, Bobadilla M, et al: Epidemic of *Serratia marcescens* bacteremia and meningitis in a neonatal unit in Mexico City, *Infect Control Hosp Epidemiol* 10:14, 1989.
168. Maragakis LL, Winkler A, Tucker MG, et al: Outbreak of multidrug-resistant *Serratia marcescens* infection in a neonatal intensive care unit, *Infect Control Hosp Epidemiol* 29:418, 2008.
169. Maltezou HC, Tryfinopoulou K, Katerelos P, et al: Consecutive *Serratia marcescens* multiclone outbreaks in a neonatal intensive care unit, *Am J Infect Control* 40:637, 2012.
170. Campbell JR, Diacovo T, Baker CJ: *Serratia marcescens* meningitis in neonates, *Pediatr Infect Dis J* 11:881, 1992.
171. Ries M, Deeg KH, Heininger U, et al: Brain abscesses in neonates—report of three cases, *Eur J Pediatr* 152:745, 1993.
172. Hirooka TM, Fontes RB, Diniz EM, et al: Cerebral abscess caused by *Serratia marcescens* in a premature neonate, *Arq Neuropsiquiatr* 65:1018, 2007.
173. Gras-Le Guen C, Lepelletier D, Debillon T, et al: Contamination of a milk bank pasteuriser causing a *Pseudomonas aeruginosa* outbreak in a neonatal intensive care unit, *Arch Dis Child Fetal Neonatal Ed* 88, 2003. F434.
174. Stevens DC, Kleiman MB, Schreiner RL: Early-onset *Pseudomonas* sepsis of the neonate, *Perinatol Neonatol* 6:75, 1982.
175. Ghosal SP, SenGupta PC, Mukherjee AK: Noma neonatorum: its aetiopathogenesis, *Lancet* 2:289, 1978.
176. Shah SS, Gallagher PG: Complications of conjunctivitis caused by *Pseudomonas aeruginosa* in a newborn intensive care unit, *Pediatr Infect Dis J* 17:97, 1998.
177. Zawacki A, O'Rourke E, Potter-Bynoe G, et al: An outbreak of *Pseudomonas aeruginosa* pneumonia and bloodstream infection associated with intermittent otitis externa in a healthcare worker, *Infect Control Hosp Epidemiol* 25:1083, 2004.
178. Basu S, Kumar A: Ecthyma gangrenosum in a premature low-birth-weight newborn, *J Wound Care* 20:587, 2011.
179. Centers for Disease Control and Prevention: Reported isolates of *Salmonella* from CSF in the United States, 1968-1979, *J Infect Dis* 143:504, 1981.
180. Totan M, Kucukoduk S, Dagdemir A, et al: Meningitis due to *Salmonella* in preterm neonates, *Turkish J Pediatr* 44:45, 2002.
181. Cooke FJ, Ginwalla S, Hampton MD, et al: Report of neonatal meningitis due to *Salmonella enterica* serotype *Agona* and review of breast milk-associated neonatal *Salmonella* infections, *J Clin Microbiol* 47:3045, 2009.
182. Lakew W, Girma A, Triche E: *Salmonella enterica* serotype arizonae meningitis in a neonate, *Case Rep Pediatr* 2013:813495, 2013.
183. Bhat P, Dias M, Hegde R, et al: *Salmonella paratyphi* B septicemia in a neonate, *J Clin Neonatol* 2:93-94, 2013.
184. Reed RP, Klugman KP: Neonatal typhoid fever, *Pediatr Infect Dis J* 13:774, 1994.
185. Fomda BA, Charoo BA, Bhat JA, et al: Recurrent meningitis due to *Salmonella enteritidis*: a case report from Kashmir India, *Indian J Med Microbiol* 30:474, 2012.
186. Schuchat A, Robinson K, Wenger JD, et al: Bacterial meningitis in the United States in 1995, *N Engl J Med* 337:970, 1997.
187. Fiorito SM, Galarza PG, Sparo M, et al: An unusual transmission of *Neisseria meningitidis*: neonatal conjunctivitis acquired at delivery from the mother's endocervical infection, *Sex Transm Dis* 28:29, 2001.
188. Cher DJ, Maxwell WJ, Frusztajer N, et al: A case of pelvic inflammatory disease associated with *Neisseria meningitidis* bacteremia, *Clin Infect Dis* 17:134, 1993.
189. Bhutta ZA, Khan IA, Agha Z: Fatal intrauterine meningococcal infection, *Pediatr Infect Dis J* 10:868, 1991.
190. Arango CA, Rathore MH: Neonatal meningococcal meningitis: case reports and review of literature, *Pediatr Infect Dis J* 15:1134, 1996.
191. Shepard CW, Rosenstein NE, Fischer M: Active bacterial core surveillance team. Neonatal meningococcal disease in the United States, 1990 to 1999, *Pediatr Infect Dis J* 22:418, 2003.
192. Jones RN, Stepack J, Eades A: Fatal neonatal meningococcal meningitis: association with maternal cervical-vaginal colonization, *JAMA* 236:2652, 1976.
193. Manginello FP, Pascale JA, Wolfsdorf J, et al: Neonatal meningococcal meningitis and meningococcemia, *Am J Dis Child* 133:651, 1979.
194. Clegg HW, Todres ID, Moylan FM, et al: Fulminant neonatal meningococcemia, *Am J Dis Child* 134:354, 1980.
195. Falcao MC, Andrade SB, Ceccon ME, et al: Neonatal sepsis and meningitis caused by *Neisseria meningitidis*: a case report, *Rev Inst Med Trop Sao Paulo* 49:191, 2007.
196. Tinsa F, Jallouli M, Ben Lassouad M, et al: Neonatal meningitis by *Neisseria meningitidis* B, *Tunis Med* 86:1014, 2008.
197. Adams WG, Deaver KA, Cochi SL, et al: Decline of childhood *Haemophilus influenzae* type b (Hib) disease in the hib vaccine era, *JAMA* 269:221, 1993.
198. Bisgard KM, Kao A, Leake J, et al: *Haemophilus influenzae* invasive disease in the United States, 1994-1995: near disappearance of a vaccine-preventable childhood disease, *Emerg Infect Dis* 4:229, 1998.
199. Murphy TV, Pastor P, Medley R, et al: Decreased *Haemophilus* colonization in children vaccinated with *Haemophilus influenzae* type b conjugate vaccine, *J Pediatr* 122:517, 1993.
200. Mohle-Boetani JC, Ajello G, Breneman E, et al: Carriage of *Haemophilus influenzae* type b in children after widespread vaccination with *Haemophilus influenzae* type b vaccines, *Pediatr Infect Dis J* 12:589, 1993.
201. Perdue DG, Bulkow LR, Gellin GB: Invasive *Haemophilus influenzae* disease in Alaskan residents aged 10 years and older before and after infant vaccination programs, *JAMA* 283:3089, 2000.
202. Barton LL, Cruz RD, Walentik C: Neonatal *Haemophilus influenzae* type C sepsis, *Am J Dis Child* 136:463, 1982.
203. Campognone P, Singer DB: Neonatal sepsis due to nontypeable *Haemophilus influenzae*, *Am J Dis Child* 140:117, 1986.
204. Wallace RJ Jr, Baker CJ, Quinones FJ, et al: Nontypable *Haemophilus influenzae* (biotype 4) as a neonatal, maternal and genital pathogen, *Rev Infect Dis* 5:123, 1983.
205. Falia TJ, Dobson SRM, Crook DWM, et al: Population-based study of non-typeable *Haemophilus influenzae* invasive disease in children and neonates, *Lancet* 341:851, 1993.

206. Friesen CA, Cho CT: Characteristic features of neonatal sepsis due to *Haemophilus influenzae*, *Rev Infect Dis* 8:777, 1986.
207. Lilien LD, Yeh TF, Novak GM, et al: Early-onset *Haemophilus* sepsis in newborn infants: clinical, roentgenographic, and pathologic features, *Pediatrics* 62:299, 1978.
208. Silverberg K, Boehm FH: *Haemophilus influenzae* amnionitis with intact membranes: a case report, *Am J Perinatol* 7:270, 1990.
209. Hershckowitz S, Elisha MB, Fleisher-Sheffer V, et al: A cluster of early neonatal sepsis and pneumonia caused by nontypable *Haemophilus influenzae*, *Pediatr Infect Dis J* 23:1061, 2004.
210. Bradley JS: *Haemophilus parainfluenzae* sepsis in a very low birth weight premature infant: a case report and review of the literature, *J Perinatol* 19:315, 1999.
211. Miano A, Cipolloni AP, Casadei GP, et al: Neonatal *Haemophilus aphrophilus* meningitis, *Helv Paediatr Acta* 31:499, 1977.
212. Gorbach SL, Bartlett JG: Anaerobic infections, *N Engl J Med* 290:1177, 1974.
213. Finegold SM: Anaerobic infections, *Surg Clin North Am* 60:49, 1980.
214. Brook I: Bacteremia due to anaerobic bacteria in newborns, *J Perinatol* 10:351, 1990.
215. Chow AW, Guze LB: Bacteroidaceae bacteremia: clinical experience with 112 patients, *Medicine (Baltimore)* 53:93, 1974.
216. Noel GJ, Laufer DA, Edelson PJ: Anaerobic bacteremia in a neonatal intensive care unit: an eighteen year experience, *Pediatr Infect Dis J* 7:858, 1988.
217. Mitra S, Panigrahi D, Narang A: Anaerobes in neonatal septicaemia: a cause for concern, *J Trop Pediatr* 43:153, 1997.
218. Chow AW, Leake RD, Yamauchi T, et al: The significance of anaerobes in neonatal bacteremia: analysis of 23 cases and review of the literature, *Pediatrics* 54:736, 1974.
219. Ohta S, Shimizu S, Fujisawa S, et al: Neonatal adrenal abscess due to *Bacteroides*, *J Pediatr* 93:1063, 1978.
220. Lee YH, Berg RB: Cephalhematoma infected with *Bacteroides*, *Am J Dis Child* 121:72, 1971.
221. Siddiqi SF, Taylor PM: Necrotizing fasciitis of the scalp: a complication of fetal monitoring, *Am J Dis Child* 136:226, 1982.
222. Feder HM Jr: *Bacteroides fragilis* meningitis, *Rev Infect Dis* 9:783, 1987.
223. Harrod JR, Stevens DA: Anaerobic infections in the newborn infant, *J Pediatr* 85:399, 1974.
224. Dunkle LM, Brotherton TJ, Feigin RD: Anaerobic infections in children: a prospective survey, *Pediatrics* 57:311, 1976.
225. Feder HM Jr, Garibaldi RA, Nurse BA, et al: *Bacillus* species isolates from cerebrospinal fluid in patients without shunts, *Pediatrics* 82:909, 1988.
226. Hilliard NJ, Schelonka RL, Waites KB: *Bacillus cereus* bacteremia in a preterm neonate, *J Clin Microbiol* 41:3441, 2003.
227. Manickam N, Knorr A, Muldrew KL: Neonatal meningoencephalitis caused by *Bacillus cereus*, *Pediatr Infect Dis J* 27:843, 2008.
228. John AB, Razak EA, Razak EE, et al: Intractable *Bacillus cereus* bacteremia in a preterm neonate, *J Trop Pediatr* 53:131, 2007.
229. Tuladhar R, Patole SK, Koh TH, et al: Refractory *Bacillus cereus* infection in a neonate, *Int J Clin Pract* 54:345, 2000.
230. Lequin MH, Vermeulen JR, van Elburg RM, et al: *Bacillus cereus* meningoencephalitis in preterm infants: neuroimaging characteristics, *AJNR Am J Neuroradiol* 26:2137, 2005.
231. Van Der Zwet WC, Parlevliet GA, Savelkoul PH, et al: Outbreak of *Bacillus cereus* infections in a neonatal intensive care unit traced to balloons used in manual ventilation, *J Clin Microbiol* 38:4131, 2000.
232. Yohannan MD, Vijayakumaran E, Remo C, et al: Congenital pneumonia and early neonatal septicemia due to *Bacteroides fragilis*, *Eur J Clin Microbiol Infect Dis* 11:472, 1992.
233. Keffer GL, Monif GR: Perinatal septicemia due to the Bacteroidaceae, *Obstet Gynecol* 71:463, 1988.
234. Feder HM Jr: *Bacteroides fragilis* meningitis, *Rev Infect Dis* 9:783, 1987.
235. Airede AI: Pathogens in neonatal omphalitis, *J Trop Pediatr* 38:129, 1992.
236. Kosloske A, Cushing AH, Borden TA, et al: Cellulitis and necrotizing fasciitis of the abdominal wall in pediatric patients, *J Pediatr Surg* 16:246, 1981.
237. Chaney NE: *Clostridium* infection in mother and infant, *Am J Dis Child* 134:1175, 1980.
238. Spark RP, Wike DA: Nontetanus clostridial neonatal fatality after home delivery, *Arizona Med* 40:697, 1983.
239. Motz RA, James AG, Dove B: *Clostridium perfringens* meningitis in a newborn infant, *Pediatr Infect Dis J* 15:708, 1996.
240. Roper MH, Vandelaer JH, Gasse FL: Maternal and neonatal tetanus, *Lancet* 370:1947, 2007.
241. Pascual FB, McGinley EL, Zanardi LR, et al: Tetanus surveillance—United States, 1998-2000, *MMWR Surveill Summ* 52:1, 2003.
242. Craig AS, Reed GW, Mohon RT, et al: Neonatal tetanus in the United States: a sentinel event in the foreign-born, *Pediatr Infect Dis J* 16:955, 1997.
243. Kumar S, Malecki LM: A case of neonatal tetanus, *South Med J* 84:396, 1991.
244. Centers for Disease Control and Prevention: Neonatal tetanus—Montana, 1998, *MMWR Morb Mortal Wkly Rep* 47:928, 1998.
245. Vandelaer J, Birmingham M, Gasse F, et al: Tetanus in developing countries: an update on the maternal and neonatal tetanus elimination initiative, *Vaccine* 21:3442, 2003.
246. Quddus A, Luby S, Rahbar M, et al: Neonatal tetanus: mortality rate and risk factors in Loralai District, Pakistan, *Int J Epidemiol* 31:648, 2002.
247. Idema CD, Harris BN, Ogunbanjo GA, et al: Neonatal tetanus elimination in Mpumalanga Province, South Africa, *Trop Med Int Health* 7:622, 2002.
248. Amsalu S, Lulseged S: Tetanus in a children's hospital in Addis Ababa: review of 113 cases, *Ethiop Med J* 43:233, 2005.
249. Mustafa BE, Omer MI, Aziz MI, et al: Neonatal tetanus in rural and displaced communities in the East Nile province, *J Trop Pediatr* 42:110, 1996.
250. Arnold RB, Soewarso TI, Karyadi A: Mortality from neonatal tetanus in Indonesia: results of two surveys, *Bull World Health Organ* 64:259, 1986.
251. Herrero JIH, Beltran RR, Sanchanz AMM: Failure of intrathecal tetanus antitoxin in the treatment of tetanus neonatorum, *J Infect Dis* 164:619, 1991.
252. Abrutyn E, Berlin JA: Intrathecal therapy in tetanus, *JAMA* 266:2262, 1991.
253. Lambo JA, Anokye EA: Prognostic factors for mortality in neonatal tetanus: a systematic review and meta-analysis, *Int J Infect Dis* 17:e1100, 2013.
254. Traverso HP, Kahn AJ, Rahim H, et al: Ghee application to the umbilical cord: a risk factor for neonatal tetanus, *Lancet* 1:486, 1989.
255. Oudesluys-Murphy AM: Umbilical cord care and neonatal tetanus, *Lancet* 1:843, 1989.
256. Schofield F: Selective primary health care: strategies for control of disease in the developing world. XXII. Tetanus: a preventable problem, *Rev Infect Dis* 8:144, 1986.
257. Khan AA, Zahidie A, Rabbani F: Interventions to reduce neonatal mortality from neonatal tetanus in low and middle income countries—a systematic review, *BMC Public Health* 13:322, 2013.
258. Gromisch DS, Gordon SG, Bedrosian L, et al: Simultaneous mixed bacterial meningitis in an infant, *Am J Dis Child* 119:284, 1970.
259. Pacifico L, Chiesa C, Mirabella S, et al: Early-onset *Pseudomonas aeruginosa* sepsis and *Yersinia enterocolitica* neonatal infection: a unique combination in a preterm infant, *Eur J Pediatr* 146:192, 1987.
260. Tessin I, Trollfors B, Thiringer K: Incidence and etiology of neonatal septicaemia and meningitis in western Sweden 1975-1986, *Acta Paediatr Scand* 79:1023, 1990.
261. Vesikari T, Isolauri E, Tuppurainen N, et al: Neonatal septicaemia in Finland 1981-85, *Acta Paediatr Scand* 78:44, 1989.
262. Bruun B, Paerregaard A: Septicemia in a Danish neonatal intensive care unit, 1984 to 1988, *Pediatr Infect Dis J* 10:159, 1991.
263. Faix RG, Kovarik SM: Polymicrobial sepsis among intensive care nursery infants, *J Perinatol* 9:131, 1989.
264. Jarvis WR, Hybsmith AK, Allen JR, et al: Polymicrobial bacteremia associated with lipid emulsion in a neonatal intensive care unit, *Pediatr Infect Dis J* 2:203, 1983.
265. Sferra TJ, Pacini DL: Simultaneous recovery of bacterial and viral pathogens from CSF, *Pediatr Infect Dis J* 7:552, 1988.
266. Giacoia GP: Uncommon pathogens in newborn infants, *J Perinatol* 14:134, 1994.
267. Hervás JA, Alomar A, Salva F, et al: Neonatal sepsis and meningitis in Mallorca, Spain, 1977-1991, *Clin Infect Dis* 16:719, 1993.
268. Schuchat A, Oxtoby M, Cochi S, et al: Population-based risk factors for neonatal group B streptococcal disease: results of a cohort study in metropolitan Atlanta, *J Infect Dis* 162:672, 1990.

269. Cordero L, Sananes M, Ayers LW: Bloodstream infections in a neonatal intensive-care unit: 12 years' experience with an antibiotic control program, *Infect Control Hosp Epidemiol* 20:242, 1999.
270. Persson E, Trollfors B, Brandberg LL, et al: Septicaemia and meningitis in neonates and during early infancy in the Göteborg area of Sweden, *Acta Paediatr* 91:1087, 2002.
271. Barton L, Hodgman JE, Pavlova Z: Causes of death in the extremely low birth weight infant, *Pediatrics* 103:446, 1999.
272. Stoll BJ, Hansen N: Infections in VLBW infants: studies from the nichd neonatal research network, *Semin Perinatol* 27:293, 2003.
273. Pisani V, Bizzarri B, Cardi V, et al: Early onset sepsis in very low birth weight newborn infants, *J Matern Fetal Neonatal Med* 25(Suppl 3):21, 2012.
274. Bhutta ZA, Yusuf K: Early-onset neonatal sepsis in pakistan: a case control study of risk factors in a birth cohort, *Am J Perinatol* 14:577, 1997.
275. Lieberman E, Lang JM, Frigoletto F Jr, et al: Epidural analgesia, intrapartum fever, and neonatal sepsis evaluation, *Pediatrics* 99:415, 1997.
276. Niswander KR, Gordon M: The women and their pregnancies. The collaborative perinatal study of the national institute of neurological diseases and stroke. U.S. Department of Health, Education and Welfare publication No. (NIH) 73-379, Washington, DC, 1972, U.S. Government Printing Office.
277. National Vital Statistics System, National Center for Health Statistics, U.S. Centers for Disease Control and Prevention. http://www.cdc.gov/nchs/nvss.htm.
278. Fiscella K: Race, perinatal outcome, and amniotic infection, *Obstet Gynecol Surv* 51:60, 1996.
279. Centers for Disease Control and Prevention: Group B streptococcal disease in the United States, 1990: report from a multistate active surveillance system, *MMWR Morb Mortal Wkly Rep* 41:25, 1992.
280. Benirschke K, Driscoll S: *The pathology of the human placenta*, New York, 1967, Springer-Verlag.
281. Washburn TC, Medearis DN Jr, Childs B: Sex differences in susceptibility to infections, *Pediatrics* 35:57, 1965.
282. Torday JS, Nielsen HC, Fencl MD, et al: Sex differences in fetal lung maturation, *Am Rev Respir Dis* 123:205, 1981.
283. Sinha A, Yokoe D, Platt R: Epidemiology of neonatal infections: experience during and after hospitalization, *Pediatr Infect Dis J* 22:244, 2003.
284. Schuchat A, Zywicki SS, Dinsmoor MJ, et al: Risk factors and opportunities for prevention of early-onset neonatal sepsis: a multicenter case-control study, *Pediatrics* 105:21, 2000.
285. Sohn AH, Garret DO, Sinkowitz-Cochran RL, et al: Prevalence of nosocomial infections in neonatal intensive care unit patients: results from the first national point-prevalence study, *J Pediatr* 139:821, 2001.
286. Speer C, Hauptmann D, Stubbe P, et al: Neonatal septicemia and meningitis in Göttingen, West Germany, *Pediatr Infect Dis J* 4:36, 1985.
287. Battisi O, Mitchison R, Davies PA: Changing blood culture isolates in a referral neonatal intensive care unit, *Arch Dis Child* 56:775, 1981.
288. MacFarlane DE: Neonatal group B streptococcal septicaemia in a developing country, *Acta Paediatr Scand* 76:470, 1987.
289. Ako-Nai AK, Adejuyigbe EA, Ajayi FM, et al: The bacteriology of neonatal septicaemiae in Ile-Ife, Nigeria, *J Trop Pediatr* 45:146, 1999.
290. Kuruvilla KA, Pillai S, Jesudason M, et al: Bacterial profile of sepsis in a neonatal unit in South India, *Indian Pediatr* 35:851, 1998.
291. Ohlsson A, Bailey T, Takieddine F: Changing etiology and outcome of neonatal septicemia in Riyadh, Saudi Arabia, *Acta Paediatr Scand* 75:540, 1986.
292. Kilani RA, Basamad M: Pattern of proven bacterial sepsis in a neonatal intensive care unit in Riyadh-Saudi Arabia: a 2-year analysis, *J Med Liban* 48:77, 2000.
293. Knippenberg R, Lawn JE, Darmstadt GL, et al: Systematic scaling up of neonatal care in countries, *Lancet* 365:1087, 2005.
294. Lawn JE, Cousens S, Zupan J: 4 million neonatal deaths: when? where? why? *Lancet* 365:891, 2005.
295. Vergnano S, Sharland M, Kazembe P, et al: Neonatal sepsis: an international perspective, *Arch Dis Child Fetal Neonatal Ed* 90:F220, 2005.
296. Rahman S, Hameed A, Roghani MT, et al: Multidrug resistant neonatal sepsis in Peshawar, Pakistan, *Arch Dis Child Fetal Neonatal Ed* 87:F52, 2002.
297. Blomberg B, Jureen R, Manji KP, et al: High rate of fatal cases of pediatric septicemia caused by gram-negative bacteria with extended-spectrum beta-lactamases in Dar es Salaam, Tanzania, *J Clin Microbiol* 43:745, 2005.
298 Downie L, Armiento R, Subhi R, et al: Community-acquired neonatal and infant sepsis in developing countries: efficacy of who's currently recommended antibiotics—systematic review and meta-analysis, *Arch Dis Child* 98:146, 2013.
299. Amin A, Abdulrazzaq YM, Uduman S: Group B streptococcal serotype distribution of isolates from colonized pregnant women at the time of delivery in United Arab Emirates, *J Infect* 45:42, 2002.
300. Tsolia M, Psoma M, Gavrili S, et al: Group B streptococcus colonization of Greek pregnant women and neonates: prevalence, risk factors and serotypes, *Clin Microbiol Infect* 9:832, 2003.
301. Stoll BJ, Schuchat A: Maternal carriage of group B streptococci in developing countries, *Pediatr Infect Dis J* 17:499, 1998.
302. Cogwill K, Taylor TH Jr, Schuchat A, et al: Report from the CDC. Awareness of perinatal group B streptococcal infection among women of childbearing age in the United States, 1999 and 2002, *J Womens Health* 12:527, 2003.
303. Beck-Sague CM, Azimi P, Fonseca SN, et al: Blood stream infections in neonatal intensive care unit patients: results of a multicenter study, *Pediatr Infect Dis J* 13:1110, 1994.
304. Adams WG, Kinney JS, Schuchat A, et al: Outbreak of early onset group B streptococcal sepsis, *Pediatr Infect Dis J* 12:565, 1993.
305. Cheasty T, Robertson R, Chart H, et al: The use of serodiagnosis in the retrospective investigation of a nursery outbreak associated with *Escherichia coli* O157:H7, *J Clin Pathol* 51:498, 1998.
306. Hoyen C, Rice L, Conte S, et al: Use of real time pulsed field gel electrophoresis to guide interventions during a nursery outbreak of *Serratia marcescens* infection, *Pediatr Infect Dis J* 18:357, 1999.
307. Olive DM, Bean P: Principles and applications of methods for DNA-based typing of microbial organisms, *J Clin Microbiol* 37:1661, 1999.
308. Dent A, Toltzis P: Descriptive and molecular epidemiology of gram-negative bacilli infections in the neonatal intensive care unit, *Curr Opin Infect Dis* 16:279, 2003.
309. van der Zwet WC, Parlevliet GA, Savelkoul PH, et al: Nosocomial outbreak of gentamicin-resistant *Klebsiella pneumoniae* in a neonatal intensive care unit controlled by a change in antibiotic policy, *J Hosp Infect* 42:295, 1999.
310. Raz R, Sharir R, Shmilowitz L, et al: The elimination of gentamicin-resistant gram-negative bacteria in newborn intensive care unit, *Infection* 15:32, 1987.
311. Gibbs RS, Duff P: Progress in pathogenesis and management of clinical intraamniotic infection, *Am J Obstet Gynecol* 164:1317, 1991.
312. Charles D, Edwards WR: Infectious complications of cervical cerclage, *Am J Obstet Gynecol* 141:1065, 1981.
313. Aarts JM, Brons JT, Bruinse HW: Emergency cerclage: a review, *Obstet Gynecol Surv* 50:459, 1995.
314. Fejgin M, Amiel A, Kaneti H, et al: Fulminant sepsis due to group B beta-hemolytic streptococci following transcervical chorionic villi sampling, *Clin Infect Dis* 17:142, 1993.
315. Wilkins I, Mezrow G, Lynch L, et al: Amnionitis and life-threatening respiratory distress after percutaneous umbilical blood sampling, *Am J Obstet Gynecol* 160:427, 1989.
316. Morison JE: *Foetal and neonatal pathology*, ed 3, Washington, DC, 1970, Butterworth.
317. St. Geme JW Jr, Murray DL, Carter J, et al: Perinatal bacterial infection after prolonged rupture of amniotic membranes: an analysis of risk and management, *J Pediatr* 104:608, 1984.
318. Blanc WA: Pathways of fetal and early neonatal infection: viral placentitis, bacterial and fungal chorioamnionitis, *J Pediatr* 59:473, 1961.
319. Hillier SL, Krohn MA, Kiviat NB, et al: Microbiologic causes and neonatal outcomes associated with chorioamnion infection, *Am J Obstet Gynecol* 165:955, 1991.
320. Yoder PR, Gibbs RS, Blanco JD, et al: A prospective, controlled study of maternal and perinatal outcome after intra-amniotic infection at term, *Am J Obstet Gynecol* 145:695, 1983.
321. Larsen B, Snyder IS, Galask RP: Bacterial growth inhibition by amniotic fluid. I. In vitro evidence for bacterial growth-inhibiting activity, *Am J Obstet Gynecol* 119:492, 1974.
322. Kitzmiller JL, Highby S, Lucas WE: Retarded growth of *E. coli* in amniotic fluid, *Obstet Gynecol* 41:38, 1973.
323. Axemo P, Rwamushaija E, Pettersson M, et al: Amniotic fluid antibacterial activity and nutritional parameters in term Mozambican and Swedish pregnant women, *Gynecol Obstet Invest* 42:24, 1996.
324. Scane TM, Hawkins DF: Antibacterial activity in human amniotic fluid: relationship to zinc and phosphate, *Br J Obstet Gynaecol* 91:342, 1984.

325. Nazir MA, Pankuch GA, Botti JJ, et al: Antibacterial activity of amniotic fluid in the early third trimester: its association with preterm labor and delivery, *Am J Perinatol* 4:59, 1987.
326. Baker SM, Balo NN, Abdel Aziz FT: Is vernix a protective material to the newborn? A biochemical approach, *Indian J Pediatr* 62:237, 1995.
327. Florman AL, Teubner D: Enhancement of bacterial growth in amniotic fluid by meconium, *J Pediatr* 74:111, 1969.
328. Hoskins IA, Hemming VG, Johnson TRB, et al: Effects of alterations of zinc-to-phosphate ratios and meconium content on group B *Streptococcus* growth in human amniotic fluid in vitro, *Am J Obstet Gynecol* 157:770, 1988.
329. Altieri C, Maruotti G, Natale C, et al: In vitro survival of *Listeria monocytogenes* in human amniotic fluid, *Zentralbl Hyg Umweltmed* 202:377, 1999.
330. Evaldson G, Nord CE: Amniotic fluid activity against *Bacteroides fragilis* and group B streptococci, *Med Microbiol Immunol* 170:11, 1981.
331. Eidelman AI, Nevet A, Rudensky B, et al: The effect of meconium staining of amniotic fluid on the growth of *Escherichia coli* and group B *Streptococcus*, *J Perinatol* 22:467, 2002.
332. Marston G, Wald ER: *Haemophilus influenzae* type B sepsis in infant and mother, *Pediatrics* 58:863, 1976.
333. Zinner SH, McCormack WM, Lee YH, et al: Puerperal bacteremia and neonatal sepsis due to *Haemophilus parainfluenzae*: report of a case with antibody titers, *Pediatrics* 49:612, 1972.
334. Tarpay MM, Turbeville DV, Krous HF: Fatal *Streptococcus pneumoniae* type III sepsis in mother and infant, *Am J Obstet Gynecol* 136:257, 1980.
335. Hughes BR, Mercer JL, Gosbel LB: Neonatal pneumococcal sepsis in association with fatal maternal pneumococcal sepsis, *Aust N Z J Obstet Gynaecol* 41:457, 2001.
336. Panaro NR, Lutwick LI, Chapnick EK: Intrapartum transmission of group A *Streptococcus*, *Clin Infect Dis* 17:79, 1993.
337. Mastrobattista JM, Parisi VM: Vertical transmission of a *Citrobacter* infection, *Am J Perinatol* 14:465, 1997.
338. Boussemart T, Piet-Duroux S, Manouana M, et al: *Morganella morganii* and early-onset neonatal infection, *Arch Pediatr* 11:37, 2004.
339. Tempest B: Pneumococcal meningitis in mother and neonate, *Pediatrics* 53:759, 1974.
340. Grossman J, Tompkins RL: Group B beta-hemolytic streptococcal meningitis in mother and infant, *N Engl J Med* 290:387, 1974.
341. Pyati SP, Pildes RS, Jacobs NM, et al: Penicillin in infants weighing two kilograms or less with early-onset group B streptococcal disease, *N Engl J Med* 308:1383, 1983.
342. Maberry MC, Gilstrap LC: Intrapartum antibiotic therapy for suspected intraamniotic infection: impact on the fetus and neonate, *Clin Obstet Gynecol* 34:345, 1991.
343. Sacks LM, McKitrick JC, MacGregor RR: Surface cultures and isolation procedures in infants born under unsterile conditions, *Am J Dis Child* 137:351, 1983.
344. Brook I, Frazier EH: Microbiology of scalp abscess in newborn, *Pediatr Infect Dis J* 11:766, 1992.
345. Freedman RM, Baltimore R: Fatal *Streptococcus viridans* septicemia and meningitis: a relationship to fetal scalp electrode monitoring, *J Perinatol* 10:272, 1990.
346. Cordero L, Anderson CW, Zuspan FP: Scalp abscess: a benign and infrequent complication of fetal monitoring, *Am J Obstet Gynecol* 146:126, 1983.
347. Storm W: Transient bacteremia following endotracheal suctioning in ventilated newborns, *Pediatrics* 65:487, 1980.
348. Singer DB: *Infections of fetuses and neonates*, Boston, 1991, Blackwell Scientific Publications.
349. Sorokin Y, Weintraub Z, Rothschild A, et al: Cerebrospinal fluid leak in the neonate—complication of fetal scalp electrode monitoring. Case report and review of the literature, *Isr J Med Sci* 26:633, 1990.
350. Nieburg P, Gross SJ: Cerebrospinal fluid leak in a neonate with fetal scalp electrode monitoring, *Am J Obstet Gynecol* 147:839, 1983.
351. Nagle RC, Taekman MS, Shallat RF, et al: Brain abscess aspiration in nursery with ultrasound guidance, *J Neurosurg* 65:557, 1986.
352. Renier D, Flandin C, Hirsch E, et al: Brain abscesses in neonates: a study of 30 cases, *J Neurosurg* 69:877, 1988.
353. Jadavji T, Humphreys RP, Prober CG: Brain abscesses in infants and children, *Pediatr Infect Dis* 4:394, 1985.
354. Volpe JJ: *Neurology of the newborn*, ed 2, Philadelphia, 1987, WB Saunders.
355. Dillon HC, Khare S, Gray BM: Group B streptococcal carriage and disease: a 6-year prospective study, *J Pediatr* 110:31, 1987.
356. Maisels MJ, Kring E: Risk of sepsis in newborns with severe hyperbilirubinemia, *Pediatrics* 90:741, 1992.
357. Tiker F, Tarcan A, Kilicdag H, et al: Early onset conjugated hyperbilirubinemia in newborn infants, *Indian J Pediatr* 73:409-412, 2006.
358. Haber BA, Lake AM: Cholestatic jaundice in the newborn, *Clin Perinatol* 17:483, 1990.
359. Rooney JC, Hills DJ, Danks DM: Jaundice associated with bacterial infection in the newborn, *Am J Dis Child* 122:39, 1971.
360. Dagan R, Gorodischer R: Infections in hypothermic infants younger than 3 months old, *Am J Dis Child* 138:483, 1984.
361. Johanson RB, Spencer SA, Rolfe P, et al: Effect of post-delivery care on neonatal body temperature, *Acta Paediatr* 81:859, 1992.
362. Michael M, Barrett DJ, Mehta P: Infants with meningitis without CSF pleocytosis, *Am J Dis Child* 140:851, 1986.
363. El-Radhy AS, Jawad M, Mansor N, et al: Sepsis and hypothermia in the newborn infant: value of gastric aspirate examination, *J Pediatr* 104:300, 1983.
364. Al Jarousha AM, El Qouqa IA, El Jadba AH, et al: An outbreak of *Serratia marcescens* septicaemia in neonatal intensive care unit in Gaza City, Palestine, *J Hosp Infect* 70:119, 2008.
365. Barr PH: Association of *Escherichia coli* sepsis and galactosemia in neonates, *J Am Board Fam Pract* 5:89, 1992.
366. Levy HL, Sepe SJ, Shih VE, et al: Sepsis due to *Escherichia coli* in neonates with galactosemia, *N Engl J Med* 297:823, 1977.
367. Kelly S: Septicemia in galactosemia, *JAMA* 216:330, 1971.
368. Shurin SB: *Escherichia coli* septicemia in neonates with galactosemia, *N Engl J Med* 297:1403, 1977.
369. Kobayashi RH, Kettelhut BV, Kobayashi A: Galactose inhibition of neonatal neutrophil function, *Pediatr Infect Dis J* 2:442, 1983.
370. Bosch AM: Classical galactosaemia revisited, *J Inherit Metab Dis* 29:516, 2006.
371. Odievre M, Gentil C, Gautier M, et al: Hereditary fructose intolerance. Diagnosis, management, and course in 55 patients, *Am J Dis Child* 132:605, 1978.
372. Guerra-Moreno J, Barrios N, Santiago-Borrero PJ: Severe neutropenia in an infant with methylmalonic acidemia, *Bol Assoc Med P R* 95:17, 2003.
373. Hutchinson RJ, Bunnell K, Thoene JG: Suppression of granulopoietic progenitor cell proliferation by metabolites of the branched-chain amino acids, *J Pediatr* 106:62, 1985.
374. Negre VL, Bonacorsi S, Schubert S, et al: The siderophore receptor iron, but not the high-pathogenicity island or the hemin receptor ChuA, contributes to the bacteremic step of *Escherichia coli* neonatal meningitis, *Infect Immun* 72:1216, 2004.
375. Weinberg ED: Iron and susceptibility to infectious disease, *Science* 184:952, 1974.
376. Manzoni P, Rinaldi M, Cattani S, et al: Bovine lactoferrin supplementation for prevention of late-onset sepsis in very low-birth-weight neonates: a randomized trial, *JAMA* 302:1421, 2009.
377. Barry DMJ, Reeve AW: Increased incidence of gram-negative neonatal sepsis with intramuscular iron administration, *Pediatrics* 60:908, 1977.
378. Farmer K: The disadvantages of routine administration of intramuscular iron to neonates, *N Z Med J* 84:286, 1976.
379. Berseth CL, Van Aerde JE, Gross S, et al: Growth, efficacy, and safety of feeding an iron-fortified human milk fortifier, *Pediatrics* 114:e699, 2004.
380. Usta IM, Nassar AH, Awwad JT, et al: Comparison of the perinatal morbidity and mortality of the presenting twin and its co-twin, *J Perinatol* 22:391, 2002.
381. Benirschke K: Routes and types of infection in the fetus and newborn, *Am J Dis Child* 99:714, 1960.
382. Alexander JM, Gilstrap LC 3rd, Cox SM, et al: The relationship of infection to method of delivery in twin pregnancy, *Am J Obstet Gynecol* 177:1063, 1997.
383. Alexander JM, Leveno KJ, Rouse D, et al: Cesarean delivery for the second twin, *Obstet Gynecol* 112:748, 2008.
384. Boghossian NS, Page GP, Bell EF, et al: Late-onset sepsis in very low birth weight infants from singleton and multiple-gestation births, *J Pediatr* 162:1120-1124.e1121, 2013.
385. Szymusik I, Kosinska-Kaczynska K, Bomba-Opon D, et al: IVF versus spontaneous twin pregnancies—which are at higher risk of complications? *J Matern Fetal Neonatal Med*, 25:2725, 2012.
386. Edwards MS, Jackson CV, Baker CJ: Increased risk of group B streptococcal disease in twins, *JAMA* 245:2044, 1981.

387. Doran KS, Benoit VM, Gertz RE, et al: Late-onset group B streptococcal infection in identical twins: insight to disease pathogenesis, *J Perinatol* 22:326, 2002.
388. LaMar K, Dowling DA: Incidence of infection for preterm twins cared for in cobedding in the neonatal intensive-care unit, *J Obstet Gynecol Neonatal Nurs* 35:193, 2006.
389. Nieburg PI, William ML: Group A beta-hemolytic streptococcal sepsis in a mother and infant twins, *J Pediatr* 87:453, 1975.
390. Larsen JG, Harra BA, Bottone EJ, et al: Multiple antibiotic resistant *Salmonella agora* infection in malnourished neonatal twins, *Mt Sinai J Med* 46:542, 1979.
391. Devlin HR, Bannatyne RM: Neonatal malaria, *Can Med Assoc J* 116:20, 1977.
392. Romand S, Bouree P, Gelez J, et al: Congenital malaria. A case observed in twins born to an asymptomatic mother, *Presse Med* 23:797, 1994.
393. Shafai T: Neonatal coccidioidomycosis in premature twins, *Am J Dis Child* 132:634, 1978.
394. Saigal S, Eisele WA, Chernesky MA: Congenital cytomegalovirus infection in a pair of dizygotic twins, *Am J Dis Child* 136:1094, 1982.
395. Duvekot JJ, Theewes BA, Wesdorp JM, et al: Congenital cytomegalovirus infection in a twin pregnancy: a case report, *Eur J Pediatr* 149:261, 1990.
396. Lazzarotto T, Gabrielli L, Foschini MP, et al: Congenital cytomegalovirus infection in twin pregnancies: viral load in the amniotic fluid and pregnancy outcome, *Pediatrics* 112:e153, 2003.
397. Montgomery RC, Stockdell K: Congenital rubella in twins, *J Pediatr* 76:772, 1970.
398. Fraser N, Davies BW, Cusack J: Neonatal omphalitis: a review of its serious complications, *Acta Paediatr* 95:519, 2006.
399. Forshall I: Septic umbilical arteritis, *Arch Dis Child* 32:25, 1957.
400. Cruickshank JN: Child life investigations: the causes of neo-natal death. Medical Research Council special report series no. 145, London, 1930, His Majesty's Stationery Office. 26.
401. Cushing AH: Omphalitis: a review, *Pediatr Infect Dis J* 4:282, 1985.
402. Rotimi VO, Duerden BI: The development of the bacterial flora in normal neonates, *J Med Microbiol* 14:51, 1981.
403. Mason WH, Andrews R, Ross LA, et al: Omphalitis in the newborn infant, *Pediatr Infect Dis J* 8:521, 1989.
404. Ameh EA, Nmadu PT: Major complications of omphalitis in neonates and infants, *Pediatr Surg Int* 18:413, 2002.
405. Meyer WW, Lind J: The ductus venosus and the mechanism of its closure, *Arch Dis Child* 41:597, 1966.
406. Morison JE: Umbilical sepsis and acute interstitial hepatitis, *J Pathol Bacteriol* 56:531, 1944.
407. Elliott RIK: The ductus venosus in neonatal infection, *Proc R Soc Med* 62:321, 1969.
408. Bedtke K, Richarz H: Nabelsepsis mit pylephlebitis, multiplen leberabscessen, lungenabscessen und osteomyelitis. Ausgang in heilung, *Monatsschr Kinderheilkd* 105:70, 1957.
409. Thompson EN, Sherlock S: The aetiology of portal vein thrombosis with particular reference to the role of infection and exchange transfusion, *Q J Med* 33:465, 1964.
410. MacMillan RW, Schullinger JN, Santulli TV: Pyourachus: an unusual surgical problem, *J Pediatr Surg* 8:387, 1973.
411. Navarro C, Blanc WA: Subacute necrotizing funisitis: a variant of cord inflammation with a high rate of perinatal infection, *J Pediatr* 85:689, 1974.
412. Ohlsson A: Treatment of preterm premature rupture of the membranes: a meta-analysis, *Am J Obstet Gynecol* 160:890, 1989.
413. Crowley P, Chalmers I, Keirse MJ: The effects of corticosteroid administration before preterm delivery: an overview of the evidence from controlled trials, *Br J Obstet Gynaecol* 97:11, 1990.
414. Vermillion ST, Soper DE, Bland ML, et al: Effectiveness of antenatal corticosteroid administration after preterm premature rupture of the membranes, *Am J Obstet Gynecol* 183:925, 2000.
415. Roberts D, Dalziel S: Antenatal corticosteroids for accelerating fetal lung maturation for women at risk of preterm birth, *Cochrane Database Syst Rev* (3); CD004454 2006.
416. Gottesfeld Z, Ullrich SE: Prenatal alcohol exposure selectively suppresses cell-mediated but not humoral immune responsiveness, *Int J Immunopharmacol* 17:247, 1995.
417. Johnson S, Knight R, Marmer DJ, et al: Immune deficiency in fetal alcohol syndrome, *Pediatr Res* 15:908, 1981.
418. Culver KW, Ammann AJ, Partridge JC, et al: Lymphocyte abnormalities in infants born to drug-abusing mothers, *J Pediatr* 111:230, 1987.
419. Morena V, Omeñaca Teres F, Moyano I, et al: Newborn infants of mothers addicted to heroin: study of 45 cases. *An Esp Pediatr* 28:9, 1988.
420. Woods JR Jr: Drug abuse in pregnancy, *Clin Obstet Gynecol* 36:221, 1993.
421. Chasnoff IJ, editor: *Drug use in pregnancy: mother and child*, Boston, 1986, MTP Press.
422. Ojala R, Ikonen S, Tammela O: Perinatal indomethacin treatment and neonatal complications in preterm infants, *Eur J Pediatr* 159:153, 2000.
423. Major CA, Lewis DF, Harding JA, et al: Tocolysis with indomethacin increases the incidence of necrotizing enterocolitis in the low-birth-weight neonate, *Am J Obstet Gynecol* 170:102, 1994.
424. Herson VC, Krause PJ, Einsenfeld LI, et al: Indomethacin-associated sepsis in very-low-birth-weight infants, *Am J Dis Child* 142:555, 1988.
425. Ohlsson A, Walia R, Shah S: Ibuprofen for the treatment of patent ductus arteriosus in preterm and/or low birth weight infants, *Cochrane Database Syst Rev* 4:CD003481, 2010. doi: 10.1002/14651858.CD003481.pub4. Review. Update in: Cochrane Database Syst Rev. 2013;4:CD003481. PubMed PMID: 20393936.
426. O'Shea TM, Kothadia JM, Klinepeter KL, et al: Follow-up of preterm infants treated with dexamethasone for chronic lung disease, *Am J Dis Child* 147:658, 1993.
427. Tapia JL, Ramirez R, Cifuentes J, et al: The effect of early dexamethasone administration on bronchopulmonary dysplasia in preterm infants with respiratory distress syndrome, *J Pediatr* 132:48, 1998.
428. Avila-Figueroa C, Goldmann DA, Richardson DK, et al: Intravenous lipid emulsions are the major determinant of coagulase-negative staphylococcal bacteremia in very low birth weight newborns, *Pediatr Infect Dis J* 17:10, 1998.
429. Matlow AG, Kitai I, Kirpalani H, et al: A randomized trial of 72- versus 24-hour intravenous tubing set changes in newborns receiving lipid therapy, *Infect Control Hosp Epidemiol* 20:487, 1999.
430. Bianconi S, Gudavalli M, Sutija VG, et al: Ranitidine and late-onset sepsis in the neonatal intensive care unit, *J Perinat Med* 35:147, 2007.
431. Barson AJ: *A postmortem study of infection in the newborn from 1976 to 1988*, New York, 1990, John Wiley & Sons.
432. Berman PH, Banker BQ: Neonatal meningitis: a clinical and pathological study of 29 cases, *Pediatrics* 38:6, 1966.
433. Stocker JT, Dehner LP: *Pediatric pathology*, Philadelphia, 1992, JB Lippincott.
434. Hoffman HJ, Hendrick EB, Hiscox JL: Cerebral abscesses in early infancy, *J Neurosurg* 33:172, 1970.
435. Watson DG: Purulent neonatal meningitis: a study of forty-five cases, *J Pediatr* 50:352, 1957.
436. Volpe JJ: *Neurology of the newborn*, ed 3, Philadelphia, 1995, WB Saunders.
437. Perlman JM, Rollins N, Sanchez PJ: Late-onset meningitis in sick, very-low-birth-weight infants: clinical and sonographic observations, *Am J Dis Child* 146:1297, 1992.
438. Gilles FH, Jammes JL, Berenberg W: Neonatal meningitis: the ventricle as a bacterial reservoir, *Arch Neurol* 34:560, 1977.
439. Schiano MA, Hauth JC, Gilstrap LC: Second-stage fetal tachycardia and neonatal infection, *Am J Obstet Gynecol* 148:779, 1984.
440. Shah GS, Budhathoki S, Das BK, et al: Risk factors in early neonatal sepsis, *Kathmandu Univ Med J (KUMJ)* 4:187, 2006.
441. Mwanyumba F, Inion I, Gaillard P, et al: Placental inflammation and perinatal outcome, *Eur J Obstet Gynecol Reprod Biol* 108:164, 2003.
442. Kermorvant-Duchemin E, Laborie S, Rabilloud M, et al: Outcome and prognostic factors in neonates with septic shock, *Pediatr Crit Care Med* 9:186, 2008.
443. Soman M, Green B, Daling J: Risk factors for early neonatal sepsis, *Am J Epidemiol* 121:712, 1985.
444. Hegyi T, Carbone T, Anwar M, et al: The Apgar score and its components in the preterm infant, *Pediatrics* 101:77, 1998.
445. Powell KR: Evaluation and management of febrile infants younger than 60 days of age, *Pediatr Infect Dis J* 9:153, 1990.
446. Bonadio WA, Hennes H, Smith D, et al: Reliability of observation variables in distinguishing infectious outcome of febrile young infants, *Pediatr Infect Dis J* 12:111, 1993.

447. Kudawla M, Dutta S, Narang A: Validation of a clinical score for the diagnosis of late onset neonatal septicemia in babies weighing 1000-2500 g, *J Trop Pediatr* 54:66, 2008.
448. Fielkow S, Reuter S, Gotoff SP: Cerebrospinal fluid examination in symptom-free infants with risk factors for infection, *J Pediatr* 119:971, 1991.
449. Albers WH, Tyler CW, Boxerbaum B: Asymptomatic bacteremia in the newborn infant, *J Pediatr* 69:193, 1966.
450. Petanovic M, Zagar Z: The significance of asymptomatic bacteremia for the newborn, *Acta Obstet Gynecol Scand* 80:813, 2001.
451. Howard JB, McCracken GH: The spectrum of group B streptococcal infections in infancy, *Am J Dis Child* 128:815, 1974.
452. Weisman LE, Stoll BJ, Cruess DF, et al: Early-onset group B streptococcal sepsis: a current assessment, *J Pediatr* 121:428, 1992.
453. Yagupsky P, Menegus MA, Powell KR: The changing spectrum of group B streptococcal disease in infants: an eleven-year experience in a tertiary care hospital, *Pediatr Infect Dis J* 10:801, 1991.
454. Ramsey PG, Zwerdling R: Asymptomatic neonatal bacteremia, *N Engl J Med* 295:225, 1976.
455. Yu JS, Grauang A: Purulent meningitis in the neonatal period, *Arch Dis Child* 38:391, 1963.
456. Solomon SL, Wallace EM, Ford-Jones EL, et al: Medication errors with inhalant epinephrine mimicking an epidemic of neonatal sepsis, *N Engl J Med* 310:166, 1984.
457. Bonadio WA, Hegenbarth M, Zachariason M: Correlating reported fever in young infants with subsequent temperature patterns and rate of serious bacterial infections, *Pediatr Infect Dis J* 9:158, 1990.
458. Messaritakis J, Anagnostakis D, Laskari H, et al: Rectal-skin temperature difference in septicaemic newborn infants, *Arch Dis Child* 65:380, 1990.
459. Dinarello CA, Shparber M, Kent EF Jr, et al: Production of leukocytic pyrogen from phagocytes of neonates, *J Infect Dis* 144:337, 1981.
460. Mayfield SR, Bhatia J, Nakamura K, et al: Temperature measurement in term and preterm neonates, *J Pediatr* 104:271, 1984.
461. Johnson KJ, Bhatia P, Bell EF: Infrared themometry of newborn infants, *Pediatrics* 87:34, 1991.
462. Schuman AJ: The accuracy of infrared auditory canal thermometry in infants and children, *Clin Pediatr* 32:347, 1993.
463. Anagnostakis D, Matsaniotis N, Grafakos S, et al: Rectal-axillary difference in febrile and afebrile infants and children, *Clin Pediatr* 32:268, 1993.
464. Weisse ME, Reagen MS, Boule L, et al: Axillary vs. rectal temperatures in ambulatory and hospitalized children, *Pediatr Infect Dis J* 10:541, 1991.
465. Freed GL, Fraley JK: Lack of agreement of tympanic membrane temperature assessments with conventional methods in a private practice setting, *Pediatrics* 89:384, 1992.
466. Hutton S, Probst E, Kenyon C, et al: Accuracy of different temperature devices in the postpartum population, *J Obstet Gynecol Neonatal Nurs* 38:42, 2009.
467. Voora S, Srinivasan G, Lilien LD, et al: Fever in full-term newborns in the first four days of life, *Pediatrics* 69:40, 1982.
468. Osborn LM, Bolus R: Temperature and fever in the full-term newborn, *J Fam Pract* 20:261, 1985.
469. Garcia FJ, Nager A: Jaundice as an early diagnostic sign of urinary tract infection in infancy, *Pediatrics* 109:846, 2002.
470. Bilgen H, Ozek E, Unver T, et al: Urinary tract infection and hyperbilirubinemia, *Turk J Pediatr* 48:51, 2006.
471. Shahian M, Rashtian P, Kalani M: Unexplained neonatal jaundice as an early diagnostic sign of urinary tract infection, *Int J Infect Dis* 16:e487, 2012.
472. Christensen RD, Yaish HM, Wiedmeier SE, et al: Neonatal death suspected to be from sepsis was found to be kernicterus with G6PD deficiency, *Pediatrics* 132:e1694, 2013.
473. Ashkenazi S, Mimouni F, Merlob P, et al: Size of liver edge in full-term, healthy infants, *Am J Dis Child* 138:377, 1984.
474. Reiff MI, Osborn LM: Clinical estimation of liver size in newborn infants, *Pediatrics* 71:46, 1983.
475. Sfeir J, Bloomfield J, Aspillaga C, et al: Early onset neonatal septicemia caused by *Listeria monocytogenes*, *Rev Chil Pediatr* 61:330, 1990.
476. Bamji M, Stone RK, Kaul A, et al: Palpable lymph nodes in healthy newborns and infants, *Pediatrics* 78:573, 1986.
477. Embree J, Muriithi J: Palpable lymph nodes, *Pediatrics* 81:598, 1988.
478. Monfort Gil R, Castells Vilella L, Pagone Tangorra F, et al: Group B streptococcus late-onset disease presenting as cellulitis-adenitis syndrome, *Ann Pediatr* 60:75, 2004.
479. Artigas Rodriguez S, Diaz Gonzalez P, et al: Group B streptococcus cellulitis-adenitis syndrome in neonates. Is it a marker of bacteremia? *An Esp Pediatr* 56:251, 2002.
480. Huber BM: Cellulitis-adenitis in a neonate with group A streptococcal sepsis, *Klin Padiatr* 226:82-83, 2014.
481. Bell AH, Brown D, Halliday HL, et al: Meningitis in the newborn: a 14 year review, *Arch Dis Child* 64:873, 1989.
482. Weintraub MI, Otto RN: Pneumococcal meningitis and endophthalmitis in a newborn, *JAMA* 219:1763, 1972.
483. Matasova K, Hudecova J, Zibolen M: Bilateral endogenous endophthalmitis as a complication of late-onset sepsis in a premature infant, *Eur J Pediatr* 162:346, 2003.
484. Nejat F, Ardakani SB, Khotaei GT, et al: Spinal epidural abscess in a neonate, *Pediatr Infect Dis J* 21:797, 2002.
485. Tang K, Xenos C, Sgouros S: Spontaneous spinal epidural abscess in a neonate. With a review of the literature, *Childs Nerv Syst* 17:629, 2001.
486. Shah BA, Padbury JF: Neonatal sepsis: an old problem with new insights, *Virulence* 5:170, 2014.
487. Verani JR, McGee L, Schrag SJ: Prevention of perinatal group B streptococcal disease—revised guidelines from CDC, 2010, *MMWR Recomm Rep* 59:1, 2010.
488. Baker CJ, Byington CL, Polin RA: Policy statement-recommendations for the prevention of perinatal group B streptococcal (GBS) disease, *Pediatrics* 128:611, 2011.
489. American College of Obstetricians and Gynecologists Committee on Obstetric Practice: ACOG Committee Opinion No. 485: prevention of early-onset group B streptococcal disease in newborns, *Obstet Gynecol* 117:1019, 2011.
490. Evans ME, Schaffner W, Federspiel CF, et al: Sensitivity, specificity, and predictive value of body surface cultures in a neonatal intensive care unit, *JAMA* 259:248, 1988.
491. Hertz D, Fuller D, Davis T, et al: Comparison of DNA probe technology and automated continuous-monitoring blood culture systems in the detection of neonatal bacteremia, *J Perinatol* 19:290, 1999.
492. Anderson JD, Trombley C, Cimolai N: Assessment of the Bactec NR660 blood culture system for the detection of bacteremia in young children, *J Clin Microbiol* 27:721, 1989.
493. Campos JM, Spainhour JR: Rapid detection of bacteremia in children with modified lysis direct plating method, *J Clin Microbiol* 22:674, 1985.
494. St. Geme JW 3rd, Bell LM, Baumgart S, et al: Distinguishing sepsis from blood culture contamination in young infants with blood cultures growing coagulase-negative staphylococci, *Pediatrics* 86:157, 1990.
495. Kurlat I, Stoll BJ, McGowan JE Jr: Time to positivity for detection of bacteremia in neonates, *J Clin Microbiol* 27:1068, 1989.
496. Pichichero MD, Todd JK: Detection of neonatal bacteremia, *J Pediatr* 94:958, 1979.
497. Rowley AH, Wald ER: Incubation period necessary to detect bacteremia in neonates, *Pediatr Infect Dis J* 5:590, 1986.
498. Jardine LA, Sturgess BR, Inglis GD, et al: Neonatal blood cultures: effect of delayed entry into the blood culture machine and bacterial concentration on the time to positive growth in a simulated model, *J Paediatr Child Health* 45:210, 2009.
499. Sprunt K, Commentary: In Gellis SS, editor: *1973 yearbook of pediatrics*, Chicago, 1973, Year Book Medical Publishers.
500. Neal PR, Kleiman MB, Reynolds JK, et al: Volume of blood submitted for culture from neonates, *J Clin Microbiol* 24:353, 1986.
501. Dietzman DE, Fischer GW, Schoenknecht FD: Neonatal *Escherichia coli* septicemia—bacterial counts in blood, *J Pediatr* 85:128, 1974.
502. Kennaugh JK, Gregory WW, Powell KR, et al: The effect of dilution during culture on detection of low concentrations of bacteria in blood, *Pediatr Infect Dis J* 3:317, 1984.
503. Jawaheer G, Neal TJ, Shaw NJ: Blood culture volume and detection of coagulase negative staphylococcal septicaemia in neonates, *Arch Dis Child* 76:57F, 1997.
504. Kellogg JA, Manzella JP, Bankert DA: Frequency of low-level bacteremia in children from birth to fifteen years of age, *J Clin Microbiol* 28:2181, 2000.
505. Kellogg JA, Ferrentino FL, Goodstein MH, et al: Frequency of low-level bacteremia in infants from birth to two months of age, *Pediatr Infect Dis J* 16:381, 1997.

506. Schelonka RL, Chai MK, Yoder BA, et al: Volume of blood required to detect common neonatal pathogens, *J Pediatr* 129:275, 1996.
507. Connell TG, Rele M, Cowley D, et al: How reliable is a negative blood culture result? Volume of blood submitted for culture in routine practice in a children's hospital, *Pediatrics* 119:891, 2007.
508. Pourcyrous M, Korones SB, Bada HS, et al: Indwelling umbilical arterial catheter: a preferred sampling site for blood cultures, *Pediatrics* 81:621, 1988.
509. Bhandari V, Eisenfeld L, Lerer T, et al: Nosocomial sepsis in neonates with single lumen vascular catheters, *Indian J Pediatr* 64:529, 1997.
510. Benjamin DK Jr, Miller W, Garges H, et al: Bacteremia, central catheters, and neonates: when to pull the line, *Pediatrics* 107:1272, 2001.
511. Marconi C, Cunha Mde L, Lyra JC, et al: Usefulness of catheter tip culture in the diagnosis of neonatal infections, *J Pediatr (Rio J)* 85:80, 2009.
512. Wiswell TE, Hachey WE: Multiple site blood cultures in the initial evaluation for neonatal sepsis during the first week of life, *Pediatr Infect Dis J* 10:365, 1991.
513. Hammerberg O, Bialkowska-Hobrzanska H, Gregson D, et al: Comparison of blood cultures with corresponding venipuncture site cultures of specimens from hospitalized premature neonates, *J Pediatr* 120:120, 1992.
514 Healy CM, Palazzi DL, Edwards MS, et al: Distinctive features of neonatal invasive staphylococcal disease, *Pediatrics* 114:953, 2004.
515. Humphrey AA: Use of the buffy layer in the rapid diagnosis of septicemia, *Am J Clin Pathol* 14:358, 1944.
516. Boyle RJ, Chandler BD, Stonestreet BS, et al: Early identification of sepsis in infants with respiratory distress, *Pediatrics* 62:744, 1978.
517. Faden HS: Early diagnosis of neonatal bacteremia by buffy-coat examination, *J Pediatr* 88:1032, 1976.
518. Storm W: Early detection of bacteremia by peripheral smears in critically ill newborns, *Acta Paediatr Scand* 70:415, 1981.
519. Kleiman MB, Reynolds JK, Schreiner RL, et al: Rapid diagnosis of neonatal bacteremia with acridine orange-stained buffy coat smears, *J Pediatr* 105:419, 1984.
520. Kite P, Millar MR, Gorham P, et al: Comparison of five tests used in diagnosis of neonatal bacteremia, *Arch Dis Child* 63:639, 1988.
521. Tak SK, Bhandari PC, Bhandari B: Value of buffy coat examination in early diagnosis of neonatal septicemia, *Indian Pediatr* 17:339, 1980.
522. Powers DL, Mandell GL: Intraleukocytic bacteria in endocarditis patients, *JAMA* 227:312, 1974.
523. Cattermole HEJ, Rivers RPA: Neonatal *Candida* septicaemia: diagnosis on buffy smear, *Arch Dis Child* 62:302, 1987.
524. Ascuitto RJ, Gerber MA, Cates KL, et al: Buffy coat smears of blood drawn through central venous catheters as an aid to rapid diagnosis of systemic fungal infections, *J Pediatr* 106:445, 1985.
525. Selby DM, Gautier G, Luban NLC, et al: Overwhelming neonatal septicemia diagnosed upon examination of peripheral blood smears, *Clin Pediatr* 29:706, 1990.
526. Strom W: Early detection of bacteremia by peripheral blood smears in critically ill newborns, *Acta Paediatr Scand* 70:415, 1981.
527. Rodwell RL, Leslie AL, Tudehope DI: Evaluation of direct and buffy coat films of peripheral blood for the early detection of bacteraemia, *Aust Paediatr J* 25:83, 1989.
528. Visser VE, Hall RT: Urine culture in the evaluation of suspected neonatal sepsis, *J Pediatr* 94:635, 1979.
529. DiGeronimo RJ: Lack of efficacy of the urine culture as part of the initial workup of suspected neonatal sepsis, *Pediatr Infect Dis J* 9:764, 1992.
530. Bonsu BK, Harper MB: Leukocyte counts in urine reflect the risk of concomitant sepsis in bacteriuric infants: a retrospective cohort study, *BMC Pediatr* 7:24, 2007.
531. Tobiansky R, Evans N: A randomized controlled trial of two methods for collection of sterile urine in neonates, *J Paediatr Child Health* 34:460, 1998.
532. Garcia Munoz MT, Cerezo Pancorbo JM, et al: Suprapubic bladder aspiration. Utility and complication, *An Esp Pediatr* 45:377, 1996.
533. Nelson JD, Peters PC: Suprapubic aspiration of urine in premature and term infants, *Pediatrics* 36:132, 1965.
534. Kozer E, Rosenbloom E, Goldman D, et al: Pain in infants who are younger than 2 months during suprapubic aspiration and transurethral bladder catheterization: a randomized, controlled study, *Pediatrics* 118:e51, 2006.
535. Lau YL, Hey E: Sensitivity and specificity of daily tracheal aspirate cultures in predicting organisms causing bacteremia in ventilated neonates, *Pediatr Infect Dis J* 10:290, 1991.
536. Finelli L, Livengood JR, Saiman L: Surveillance of pharyngeal colonization: detection and control of serious bacterial illness in low birth weight infants, *Pediatr Infect Dis J* 13:854, 1994.
537. Srinivasan HB, Vidyasagar D: Endotracheal aspirate cultures in predicting sepsis in ventilated neonates, *Indian J Pediatr* 65:79, 1998.
538. Klein JO, Gellis SS: Diagnostic needle aspiration in pediatric practice: with special reference to lungs, middle ear, urinary bladder, and amniotic cavity, *Pediatr Clin North Am* 18:219, 1971.
539. Eisenfeld L, Ermocilla R, Wirtschaffer D, et al: Systemic bacterial infections in neonatal deaths, *Am J Dis Child* 137:645, 1983.
540. Minckler TM, Newell GR, O'Toole WF, et al: Microbiology experience in human tissue collection, *Am J Clin Pathol* 45:85, 1966.
541. Pierce JR, Merenstein GB, Stocker JT: Immediate postmortem cultures in an intensive care nursery, *Pediatr Infect Dis J* 3:510, 1984.
542. Levin J, Poore TE, Zauber NP, et al: Detection of endotoxin in the blood of patients with sepsis due to gram-negative bacteria, *N Engl J Med* 283:1313, 1970.
543. Levin J, Poore TE, Young NS: Gram-negative sepsis. Detection of endotoxemia with the limulus test. With studies of associated changes in blood coagulation, serum lipids, and complement, *Ann Intern Med* 76:1, 1972.
544. Stumacher RJ, Kovnat MJ, McCabe WR: Limitations of the usefulness of the limulus assay for endotoxin, *N Engl J Med* 288:1261, 1973.
545. Elin RJ, Robinson RA, Levine AS, et al: Lack of clinical usefulness of the limulus test in the diagnosis of endotoxemia, *N Engl J Med* 293:521, 1975.
546. McCracken GH Jr, Sarff LD: Endotoxin in csf detection in neonates with bacterial meningitis, *JAMA* 235:617, 1976.
547. Sobanski MA, Gray SJ, Cafferkey M, et al: Meningitis antigen detection: interpretation of agglutination by ultrasound-enhanced latex immunoassay, *Br J Biomed Sci* 56:239, 1999.
548. McGowan KL: Diagnostic value of latex agglutination tests for bacterial infections, *Rep Pediatr Infect Dis* 8:31, 1992.
549. Sanchez PJ, Siegel JD, Cushion NB, et al: Significance of a positive urine group B streptococcal latex agglutination test in neonates, *J Pediatr* 116:601, 1990.
550. Stoll BJ, Hansen N, Fanaroff AA, et al: To tap or not to tap: high likelihood of meningitis without sepsis among very low birth weight infants, *Pediatrics* 113:1181, 2004.
551. Weiss MG, Ionides SP, Anderson CL: Meningitis in premature infants with respiratory distress: role of admission lumbar puncture, *J Pediatr* 119:973, 1991.
552. Hendricks-Munoz KD, Shapiro DL: The role of the lumbar puncture in the admission sepsis evaluation of the premature infant, *J Perinatol* 10:60, 1990.
553. Eldadah M, Frenkel LD, Hiatt IM, et al: Evaluation of routine lumbar punctures in newborn infants with respiratory distress syndrome, *Pediatr Infect Dis J* 6:243, 1987.
554. Schwersenski J, McIntyre L, Bauer CR: Lumbar puncture frequency and CSF analysis in the neonate, *Am J Dis Child* 145:54, 1991.
555. Fielkow S, Reuter S, Gotoff SP: Clinical and laboratory observations: cerebrospinal fluid examination in symptom-free infants with risk factors for infection, *J Pediatr* 119:971, 1991.
556. Gleason CA, Martin FJ, Anderson JV, et al: Optimal position for a spinal tap in preterm infants, *Pediatrics* 71:31, 1983.
557. Pinheiro JMB, Furdon S, Ochoa LF: Role of local anesthesia during lumbar puncture in neonates, *Pediatrics* 91:379, 1993.
558. Porter FL, Miller JP, Cole S, et al: A controlled clinical trial of local anesthesia for lumbar punctures in newborns, *Pediatrics* 88:663, 1991.
559. Fiser DH, Gober GA, Smith CE, et al: Prevention of hypoxemia during lumbar puncture in infancy with preoxygenation, *Pediatr Emerg Care* 9:81, 1993.
560. Weisman LE, Merenstein GB, Steenbarger JR: The effect of lumbar puncture position in sick neonates, *Am J Dis Child* 137:1077, 1983.
561. Visser VE, Hall RT: Lumbar puncture in the evaluation of suspected neonatal sepsis, *J Pediatr* 96:1063, 1980.
562. Franco SM, Cornelius VE, Andrews BF: Should we perform lumbar punctures on the first day of life? *Am J Dis Child* 147:133, 1993.
563. Garges HP, Moody MA, Cotten CM, et al: Neonatal meningitis: what is the correlation among cerebrospinal fluid cultures, blood cultures, and cerebrospinal fluid parameters? *Pediatrics* 117:1094, 2006.

564. Sarff LD, Platt LH, McCracken GH Jr: Cerebrospinal fluid evaluation in neonates: comparison of high-risk infants with and without meningitis, *J Pediatr* 88:473, 1976.
565. Bonadio WA, Stanco L, Bruce R, et al: Reference values of normal CSF composition in infants ages 0 to 8 weeks, *Pediatr Infect Dis J* 11:589, 1992.
566. Ahmed A, Hickey SM, Ehrett S, et al: Cerebrospinal fluid values in the term neonate, *Pediatr Infect Dis J* 15:298, 1996.
567. McCracken GH Jr: The rate of bacteriologic response to antimicrobial therapy in neonatal meningitis, *Am J Dis Child* 123:547, 1972.
568. Rodriguez AF, Kaplan SL, Mason EO Jr: Cerebrospinal fluid values in the very low birth weight infant, *J Pediatr* 116:971, 1990.
569. Kestenbaum LA, Ebberson J, Zorc JJ, et al: Defining cerebrospinal fluid white blood cell count reference values in neonates and young infants, *Pediatrics* 125:257, 2010.
570. Mhanna MJ, Alesseh H, Gori A, et al: Cerebrospinal fluid values in very low birth weight infants with suspected sepsis at different ages, *Pediatr Crit Care Med* 9:294, 2008.
571. Yeager AS, Bruhn FW, Clark J: Cerebrospinal fluid: presence of virus unaccompanied by pleocytosis, *J Pediatr* 85:578, 1974.
572. Moore CM, Ross M: Acute bacterial meningitis with absent or minimal CSF abnormalities: a report of three cases, *Clin Pediatr (Phila)* 12:117, 1973.
573. Sarman G, Moise AA, Edwards MS: Meningeal inflammation in neonatal gram-negative bacteremia, *Pediatr Infect Dis J* 14:701, 1995.
574. Smith PB, Garges HP, Cotton CM, et al: Meningitis in preterm neonates: importance of cerebrospinal fluid parameters, *Am J Perinatol* 25:421, 2008.
575. Hedner T, Iversen K, Lundborg P: Aminobutyric acid concentrations in the CSF of newborn infants, *Early Hum Dev* 7:53, 1982.
576. Engelke S, Bridgers S, Saldanha RL, et al: Cerebrospinal fluid lactate dehydrogenase in neonatal intracranial hemorrhage, *Am J Med Sci* 29:391, 1986.
577. Worley G, Lipman B, Gewolb IH, et al: Creatine kinase brain isoenzyme: relationship of CSF concentration to the neurologic condition of newborns and cellular localization in the human brain, *Pediatrics* 76:15, 1985.
578. Lin CY, Ishida M: Elevation of cAMP levels in CSF of patients with neonatal meningitis, *Pediatrics* 71:932, 1983.
579. Corrall CJ, Pepple JM, Moxon ER, et al: C-reactive protein in spinal fluid of children with meningitis, *J Pediatr* 99:365, 1981.
580. BenGershom E, Briggeman-Mol GJJ, de Zegher F: Cerebrospinal fluid C-reactive protein in meningitis: diagnostic value and pathophysiology, *Eur J Pediatr* 145:246, 1986.
581. Philip AGS, Baker CJ: Cerebrospinal fluid C-reactive protein in neonatal meningitis, *J Pediatr* 102:715, 1983.
582. Martin-Ancel A, Garcia-Alix A, Pascual-Salcedo D, et al: Interleukin-6 in the cerebrospinal fluid after perinatal asphyxia is related to early and late neurological manifestations, *Pediatrics* 100:789, 1997.
583. Sayman K, Blennow M, Gustafson K, et al: Cytokine response in cerebrospinal fluid after birth asphyxia, *Pediatr Res* 43:746, 1998.
584. Srinivasan L, Harris MC, Shah SS: Lumbar puncture in the neonate: challenges in decision making and interpretation, *Semin Perinatol* 36:445, 2012.
585. Chow G, Schmidley JW: Lysis of erythrocytes and leukocytes in traumatic lumbar punctures, *Arch Neurol* 41:1084, 1984.
586. Steele RW, Marmer DJ, O'Brien MD, et al: Leukocyte survival in CSF, *J Clin Microbiol* 23:965, 1986.
587. Osborne JP, Pizer B: Effect on the white cell count of contaminating CSF with blood, *Arch Dis Child* 56:400, 1981.
588. Novak RW: Lack of validity of standard corrections for white blood cell counts of blood-contaminated CSF in infants, *Am J Clin Pathol* 82:95, 1984.
589. Mayefsky JH, Roghmann KJ: Determination of leukocytosis in traumatic spinal tap specimens, *Am J Med* 82:1175, 1987.
590. Mehl A: Interpretation of traumatic lumbar puncture: a prospective experimental model, *Clin Pediatr* 25:523, 1986.
591. Mehl A: Interpretation of traumatic lumbar puncture: predictive value in the presence of meningitis, *Clin Pediatr* 25:575, 1986.
592. Bonadio WA, Smith DS, Goddard S, et al: Distinguishing CSF abnormalities in children with bacterial meningitis and traumatic lumbar puncture, *J Infect Dis* 162:251, 1990.
593. Naqvi SH, Dunkle LM, Naseer S, et al: Significance of neutrophils in CSF samples processed by cytocentrifugation, *Clin Pediatr* 22:608, 1983.
594. Bonadio WA: Bacterial meningitis in children whose CSF contains polymorphonuclear leukocytes without pleocytosis, *Clin Pediatr* 27:198, 1988.
595. Greenberg RG, Smith PB, Cotten CM, et al: Traumatic lumbar punctures in neonates: test performance of the cerebrospinal fluid white blood cell count, *Pediatr Infect Dis J* 27:1047, 2008.
596. Hines EM, Nigrovic LE, Neuman MI, et al: Adjustment of cerebrospinal fluid protein for red blood cells in neonates and young infants, *J Hosp Med* 7:325, 2012.
597. Nigrovic LE, Shah SS, Neuman MI: Correction of cerebrospinal fluid protein for the presence of red blood cells in children with a traumatic lumbar puncture, *J Pediatr* 159:158, 2011.
598. Weirich E, Rabin RL, Maldonado Y, et al: Neutrophil CD11b expression as a diagnostic marker for early-onset neonatal infection, *J Pediatr* 132:445, 1998.
599. Kennon C, Overturf G, Bessman S, et al: Granulocyte colony-stimulating factor as a marker for bacterial infection in neonates, *J Pediatr* 128:765, 1996.
600. Kuster H, Weiss M, Willeitner AE, et al: Interleukin-1 receptor antagonist and interleukin-6 for early diagnosis of neonatal sepsis 2 days before clinical manifestation, *Lancet* 352:1271, 1998.
601. Doellner H, Arntzen KJ, Haereid PE, et al: Interleukin-6 concentrations in neonates evaluated for sepsis, *J Pediatr* 132:295, 1998.
602. Panero A, Pacifico L, Rossi N, et al: Interleukin 6 in neonates with early and late onset infection, *Pediatr Infect Dis J* 16:370, 1997.
603. Harding D, Dhamrait S, Millar, et al: Is interleukin-6-174 genotype associated with the development of septicemia in preterm infants? *Pediatr* 112:800, 2003.
604. Resch B, Gusenleitner W, Muller WD: Procalcitonin and interleukin-6 in the diagnosis of early-onset sepsis of the neonate, *Acta Paediatr* 92:243, 2003.
605. Kordek A, Giedrys-Kalemba S, Pawlus B, et al: Umbilical cord blood serum procalcitonin concentration in the diagnosis of early neonatal infection, *J Perinatol* 23:148, 2003.
606. Chiesa C, Panero A, Rossi N, et al: Reliability of procalcitonin concentrations for the diagnosis of sepsis in critically ill neonates, *Clin Infect Dis* 26:664, 1998.
607. Cetinkaya M, Ozkan H, Koksal N, et al: Comparison of serum amyloid a concentrations with those of C-reactive protein and procalcitonin in diagnosis and follow-up of neonatal sepsis in premature infants, *J Perinatol* 29:225, 2009.
608. Yapakci E, Tarcan A, Celik B, et al: Serum pro-hepcidin levels in term and preterm newborns with sepsis, *Pediatr Int* 51:289, 2009.
609. Yoon BH, Romero R, Yang SH, et al: Interleukin-6 concentrations in umbilical cord plasma are elevated in neonates with white matter lesions associated with periventricular leukomalacia, *Am J Obstet Gynecol* 174:1433, 1996.
610. Dammann O, Leviton A: Maternal intrauterine infection, cytokines, and brain damage in the preterm newborn, *Pediatr Res* 42:1, 1997.
611. Mehr S, Doyle LW: Cytokines as markers of bacterial sepsis in newborn infants: a review, *Pediatr Infect Dis J* 19:879, 2000.
612. Reier-Nilsen T, Farstad T, Nakstad B, et al: Comparison of broad range 16S rDNA PCR and conventional blood culture for diagnosis of sepsis in the newborn: a case control study, *BMC Pediatr* 9:5, 2009.
613. Ohlin A, Backman A, Bjorkqvist M, et al: Real-time PCR of the 16S-rRNA gene in the diagnosis of neonatal bacteraemia, *Acta Paediatr* 97:1376, 2008.
614. Chan KY, Lam HS, Cheung HM, et al: Rapid identification and differentiation of gram-negative and gram-positive bacterial bloodstream infections by quantitative polymerase chain reaction in preterm infants, *Crit Care Med* 37:2441, 2009.
615. Chen LH, Duan QJ, Cai MT, et al: Rapid diagnosis of sepsis and bacterial meningitis in children with real-time fluorescent quantitative polymerase chain reaction amplification in the bacterial 16s rRNA gene, *Clin Pediatr (Phila)* 48:641, 2009.
616. Kasper DC, Altiok I, Mechtler TP, et al: Molecular detection of late-onset neonatal sepsis in premature infants using small blood volumes: proof-of-concept, *Neonatology* 103:268, 2013.
617. Castor ML, Whitney CG, Como-Sabetti K, et al: Antibiotic resistance patterns in invasive group B streptococcal isolates, *Infect Dis Obstet Gynecol* 2008:727505, 2008.
618. Dahesh S, Hensler ME, Van Sorge NM, et al: Point mutation in the group B streptococcal PBP2x gene conferring decreased susceptibility to beta-lactam antibiotics, *Antimicrob Agents Chemother* 52:2915, 2008.

619. Kimura K, Suzuki S, Wachino J, et al: First molecular characterization of group B streptococci with reduced penicillin susceptibility, *Antimicrob Agents Chemother* 52:2890, 2008.
620. Swingle HM, Bucciarelli RL, Ayoub EM: Synergy between penicillins and low concentrations of gentamicin in the killing of group b streptococci, *J Infect Dis* 152:515, 1985.
621. Baker CN, Thornsberry C, Facklam RR: Synergism, killing kinetics, and antimicrobial susceptibility of group A and B streptococci, *Antimicrob Agents Chemother* 19:716, 1981.
622. Schauf V, Deveikis A, Riff L, et al: Antibiotic-killing kinetics of group B streptococci, *J Pediatr* 89:194, 1976.
623. Deveikis A, Schauf V, Mizen M, et al: Antimicrobial therapy of experimental group B streptococcal infection in mice, *Antimicrob Agents Chemother* 11:817, 1977.
624. Backes RJ, Rouse MS, Henry NK, et al: Activity of penicillin combined with an aminoglycoside against group B streptococci in vitro and in experimental endocarditis, *J Antimicrob Chemother* 18:491, 1986.
625. Odio CM, Umana MA, Saenz A, et al: Comparative efficacy of ceftazidime vs. carbenicillin and amikacin for treatment of neonatal septicemia, *Pediatr Infect Dis J* 6:371, 1987.
626. Begue P, Floret D, Mallet E, et al: Pharmacokinetics and clinical evaluation of cefotaxime in children suffering from purulent meningitis, *J Antimicrob Chemother* 14:161, 1984.
627. Odio CM, Faingezicht I, Salas JL, et al: Cefotaxime vs. conventional therapy for treatment of bacterial meningitis of infants and children, *Pediatr Infect Dis J* 5:402, 1986.
628. Odio CM: Cefotaxime for treatment of neonatal sepsis and meningitis, *Diagn Microbiol Infect Dis* 22:111, 1995.
629. Bradley JS, Sauberan JB, Ambrose PG, et al: Meropenem pharmacokinetics, pharmacodynamics, and Monte Carlo simulation in the neonate, *Pediatr Infect Dis J* 27:794-799, 2008.
630. Bryan CS, John JF Jr, Pai MS, et al: Gentamicin vs. cefotaxime for therapy of neonatal sepsis, *Am J Dis Child* 139:1086, 1985.
631. Manzoni P, Farina D, Leonessa M, et al: Risk factors for progression to invasive fungal infection in preterm neonates with fungal colonization, *Pediatrics* 118:2359, 2006.
632. Benjamin DK Jr, Stoll BJ, Fanaroff AA, et al: Neonatal candidiasis among extremely low birth weight infants: risk factors, mortality rates, and neurodevelopmental outcomes at 18 to 22 months, *Pediatrics* 117:84-92, 2006.
633. Man P, Verhoeven BA, Verbrugh HA, et al: An antibiotic policy to prevent emergence of resistant bacilli, *Lancet* 355:973, 2000.
634. Feigin RD, McCracken GH, Klein JO: Diagnosis and management of meningitis, *Pediatr Infect Dis J* 11:785, 1992.
635. Bradley JS, Ching DLK, Wilson TA, et al: Once-daily ceftriaxone to complete therapy of uncomplicated group B streptococcal infection in neonates: a preliminary report, *Clin Pediatr* 31:274, 1992.
636. Kaplan SL, Patrick CC: Cefotaxime and aminoglycoside treatment of meningitis caused by gram-negative enteric organisms, *Pediatr Infect Dis J* 9:810, 1990.
637. American College of Obstetricians and Gynecologists: Group B streptococcal infections in pregnancy, Washington, DC, 1996, American College of Obstetricians and Gynecologists.
638. American Academy of Pediatrics Committee on Infectious Diseases and Committee on Fetus and Newborn: Guidelines for prevention of group B streptococcal (GBS) infection by chemoprophylaxis, *Pediatrics* 90:775, 1992.
639. Centers for Disease Control and Prevention: Prevention of perinatal group B streptococcal infection: a public health perspective, *MMWR Morb Mortal Wkly Rep* 45:1, 1996.
640. American Academy of Pediatrics, Committee on Infectious Diseases/ Committee on Fetus and Newborn: Revised guidelines for prevention of early-onset group B streptococcal infection, *Pediatrics* 99:489, 1997.
641. Schrag S, Gorwitz R, Fultz-Butts K, et al: Prevention of perinatal group B streptococcal disease. Revised guidelines from CDC, *MMWR Morb Mortal Wkly Rep* 51:1, 2002.
642. American College of Obstetricians and Gynecologists: ACOG Committee Opinion: number 279, December 2002. Prevention of early-onset group B streptococcal disease in newborns, *Obstet Gynecol* 100:1405, 2002.
643. Uy IP, D'Angio CT, Menegus M, et al: Changes in early-onset group B beta hemolytic streptococcus disease with changing recommendations for prophylaxis, *J Perinatol* 22:516, 2002.
644. MacAulay MA, Abou-Sabe M, Charles D: Placental transfer of ampicillin, *Am J Obstet Gynecol* 96:943, 1966.
645. Nau H: Clinical pharmacokinetics in pregnancy and perinatology. II. Penicillins, *Dev Pharmacol Ther* 10:174, 1987.
646. Adamkin DH, Marshall E, Weiner LB: The placental transfer of ampicillin, *Am J Perinatol* 1:310, 1984.
647. Brozanski BS, Jones JG, Krohn MA, et al: Effect of a screening-based prevention policy on prevalence of early-onset group B streptococcal sepsis, *Obstet Gynecol* 95:496, 2000.
648. Moore MR, Schrag SJ, Schuchat A: Effects of intrapartum antimicrobial prophylaxis for prevention of group-B-streptococcal disease on the incidence and ecology of early-onset neonatal sepsis, *Lancet Infect Dis* 3:201, 2003.
649. Schrag SJ, Zywicki S, Farley MM, et al: Group B streptococcal disease in the era of intrapartum antibiotic prophylaxis, *N Engl J Med* 342:15, 2000.
650. Gotoff SP, Boyer KM: Prevention of early-onset neonatal group B streptococcal disease, *Pediatr* 99:866, 1997.
651. Squire E, Favara B, Todd J: Diagnosis of neonatal bacterial infection: hematologic and pathologic findings in fatal and nonfatal cases, *Pediatrics* 64:60, 1979.
652 McCracken GH Jr, Mize SG: A controlled study of intrathecal antibiotic therapy in gram-negative enteric meningitis of infancy. Report of the neonatal meningitis cooperative study group, *J Pediatr* 89:66, 1976.
653. McCracken GH Jr, Mize SG, Threlkeld N: Intraventricular gentamicin therapy in gram-negative bacillary meningitis of infancy, *Lancet* 1:787, 1980.
654. Koksal N, Hacimustafaoglu M, Bagci S, et al: Meropenem in neonatal severe infections due to multiresistant gram-negative bacteria, *Ind J Pediatr* 68:15, 2001.
655. Khaneja M, Naprawa J, Kumar A, et al: Successful treatment of late-onset infection due to resistant *Klebsiella pneumoniae* in an extremely low birth weight infant using ciprofloxacin, *J Perinatol* 19:311, 1999.
656. van den Oever HL, Versteegh FG, Thewessen EA, et al: Ciprofloxacin in preterm neonates: case report and review of the literature, *Eur J Pediatr* 157:843, 1998.
657. Wessalowski R, Thomas L, Kivit J, et al: Multiple brain abscesses caused by *Salmonella enteritidis* in a neonate: successful treatment with ciprofloxacin, *Pediatr Infect Dis J* 12:683, 1993.
658. Levitz RE, Quintiliani R: Trimethoprim-sulfamethoxazole for bacterial meningitis, *Ann Intern Med* 100:881, 1984.
659. Spirer Z, Jurgenson U, Lazewnick R, et al: Complete recovery from an apparent brain abscess treated without neurosurgery: the importance of early CT scanning, *Clin Pediatr (Phila)* 21:106, 1982.
660. Daoud AS, Batieha A, Al-Sheyyab M, et al: Lack of effectiveness of dexamethasone in neonatal bacterial meningitis, *Eur J Pediatr* 158:230-233, 1999.
661. Tekerekoglu MS, Durmaz R, Ayan M, et al: Analysis of an outbreak due to *Chryseobacterium meningosepticum* in a neonatal intensive care unit, *New Microbiol* 26:57, 2003.
662. Kaplan AM, Itabashi HH, Yoshimori R, et al: Cerebral abscesses complicating neonatal *Citrobacter freundii* meningitis, *West J Med* 127:418, 1977.
663. Lauterbach R, Zembala M: Pentoxifylline reduces plasma tumour necrosis factor-alpha concentration in premature infants with sepsis, *Eur J Pediatr* 155:404, 1996.
664. Schibler KR, Osborn RA, Leung LY, et al: A randomized, placebo-controlled trial of granulocyte colony-stimulating factor administration to newborn infants with neutropenia and clinical signs of early-onset sepsis, *Pediatrics* 102:6, 1998.
665. Kocherlakota P, LaGamma EF: Preliminary report: rhG-CSF may reduce the incidence of neonatal sepsis in prolonged preeclampsia-associated neutropenia, *Pediatrics* 102:1107, 1998.
666. Bilgin K, Yaramis A, Haspolat K, et al: A randomized trial of granulocyte-macrophage colony-stimulating factor in neonates with sepsis and neutropenia, *Pediatrics* 107:36, 2001.
667. Ahmad A, Laborada G, Bussel J, et al: Comparison of recombinant granulocyte colony-stimulating factor, recombinant human granulocyte-macrophage colony-stimulating factor and placebo for treatment of septic preterm infants, *Pediatr Infect Dis J* 21:1061, 2002.
668 Ohlsson A, Lacy JB: Intravenous immunoglobulin for suspected or proven infection in neonates, *Cochrane Database Syst Rev* 7:CD001239, 2013. doi: 10.1002/14651858.CD001239.pub4.

669. Brocklehurst P, Farrell B, King A, et al: for the INIS Collaborative Group: Treatment of neonatal sepsis with intravenous immune globulin. *N Engl J Med* 365:1201, 2011. doi: 10.1056/NEJMoa1100441. PubMed PMID: 21962214.
670. Bennet R, Bergdahl S, Eriksson M, et al: The outcome of neonatal septicemia during fifteen years, *Acta Paediatr Scand* 78:40, 1989.
671. Placzek MM, Whitelaw A: Early and late neonatal septicaemia, *Arch Dis Child* 58:728, 1983.
672. de Louvois J: *Septicaemia and meningitis in the newborn*, New York, 1990, John Wiley & Sons.
673. Klinger G, Chin CN, Beyene J, et al: Predicting the outcome of neonatal bacterial meningitis, *Pediatr* 106:477, 2000.
674. Wald E, Bergman I, Chiponis D, et al: Long-term outcome of group B streptococcal meningitis, *Pediatrics* 77:217, 1986.
675. Franco SM, Cornelius VE, Andrews BF: Long-term outcome of neonatal meningitis, *Am J Dis Child* 146:567, 1992.
676. Horn KA, Zimmerman RA, Knostman JD, et al: Neurological sequelae of group B streptococcal neonatal infection, *Pediatrics* 53:501, 1974.
677. Edwards MS, Rench MA, Haffar AAM, et al: Long-term sequelae of group B streptococcal meningitis in infants, *J Pediatr* 106:717, 1985.
678. McCracken GH Jr, Mustafa M, Ramilo O, et al: Cerebrospinal fluid interleukin-1β and tumor necrosis factor concentrations and outcome from neonatal gram-negative enteric bacillary meningitis, *Pediatr Infect Dis J* 8:155, 1989.
679. McCracken GH Jr, Threlkeld N, Mize S, et al: Moxalactam therapy for neonatal meningitis due to gram-negative enteric bacilli: a prospective controlled evaluation, *JAMA* 252:1427, 1984.
680. Baier J, Bocchini JA Jr, Brown EG: Selective use of vancomycin to prevent coagulase-negative staphylococcal nosocomial bacteremia in high risk very low birth weight infants, *Pediatr Infect Dis J* 17:179, 1998.
681. Cooke RW, Nycyk JA, Okuonghuae H, et al: Low-dose vancomycin prophylaxis reduces coagulase-negative staphylococcal bacteraemia in very low birthweight infants, *J Hosp Infect* 37:297, 1997.
682. Kacica MA, Horgan MJ, Ochoa L, et al: Prevention of gram-positive sepsis in neonates weighing less than 1500 grams, *J Pediatr* 125:253, 1994.
683. Spafford PS, Sinkin RA, Cox C, et al: Prevention of central venous catheter-related coagulase-negative staphylococcal sepsis in neonates, *J Pediatr* 125:259, 1994.
684. Craft AP, Finer NN, Barrington KJ: Vancomycin for prophylaxis against sepsis in preterm neonates, *Cochrane Database Syst Rev* (2) CD001971, 2000.
685. Garland JS, Alex CP, Henrickson KJ, et al: A vancomycin-heparin lock solution for prevention of nosocomial bloodstream infection in critically ill neonates with peripherally inserted central venous catheters: a prospective, randomized trial, *Pediatrics* 116:e198, 2005.
686. Van de Perre P: Transfer of antibody via mother's milk, *Vaccine* 21:3374, 2003.
687. Hanson LA, Karlsson B, Jalil F, et al: *Antiviral and antibacterial factors in human milk*, New York, 1988, Raven Press.
688. Mathus NB, Dwarkadas AM, Sharma VK, et al: Anti-infective factors in preterm human colostrum, *Acta Paediatr Scand* 79:1039, 1990.
689. Isaacs CF, Kashyap S, Heird WC, et al: Antiviral and antibacterial lipids in human milk and infant formula feeds, *Arch Dis Child* 65:861, 1990.
690. Winberg J, Wessner G: Does breast milk protect against septicaemia in the newborn? *Lancet* 1:1091, 1971.
691. Ashraf RN, Jalil F, Zaman S, et al: Breast feeding and protection against neonatal sepsis in a high risk population, *Arch Dis Child* 66:488, 1991.
692. Hylander MA, Strobino DM, Dhanireddy R: Human milk feedings and infection among very low birth weight infants, *Pediatrics* 102:E38, 1998.
693. Coppa GV, Gabrielli OR, Giorgi P, et al: Preliminary study of breast-feeding and bacterial adhesion to uroepithelial cells, *Lancet* 1:569, 1990.
694. Hasselbalch H, Jeppesen DL, Engelmann MD, et al: Decreased thymus size in formula-fed infants compared with breastfed infants, *Acta Paediatr* 85:1029-1032, 1996.
695. Pabst HF, Godel J, Grace M, et al: Effect of breast-feeding on immune response to BCG vaccination, *Lancet* 1:295, 1989.
696. Silfverdal SA, Bodin L, Ulanova M, et al: Long term enhancement of the IgG2 antibody response to *Haemophilus influenzae* type b by breast-feeding, *Pediatr Infect Dis J* 21:816-821, 2002.
697. Cohen-Wolkowiez M, Benjamin DK Jr, Capparelli E: Immunotherapy in neonatal sepsis: advances in treatment and prophylaxis, *Curr Opin Pediatr* 21:177, 2009.
698. Englund JA, Glezen WP: Maternal immunization for the prevention of infection in early infancy, *Semin Pediatr Infect Dis* 2:225, 1991.
699. Vicari M, Dodet B, Englund J: Protection of newborns through maternal immunization, *Vaccine* 21:3351, 2003.
700. Baker CJ, Rench MA, McInnes P: Immunization of pregnant women with group B streptococcal type III capsular polysaccharide-tetanus toxoid conjugate vaccine, *Vaccine* 21:3468, 2003.
701. Fanaroff AA, Korones SB, Wright LL, et al: A controlled trial of intravenous immune globulin to reduce nosocomial infections in very-low-birth-weight infants. National Institute of Child Health and Human Development Neonatal Research Network, *N Engl J Med* 330:1107, 1994.
702. DeJonge M, Burchfield D, Bloom B, et al: Clinical trial of safety and efficacy of inh-a21 for the prevention of nosocomial staphylococcal bloodstream infection in premature infants, *J Pediatr* 151:260-265. e261, 2007.
703. Benjamin DK, Schelonka R, White R, et al: A blinded, randomized, multicenter study of an intravenous *Staphylococcus aureus* immune globulin, *J Perinatol* 26:290-295, 2006.
704. Ohlsson A, Lacy JB: Intravenous immunoglobulin for preventing infection in preterm and/or low birth weight infants, *Cochrane Database Syst Rev* 7:CD000361, 2013. doi: 10.1002/14651858. CD000361.pub3. Review. PubMed PMID: 23821390.
705. Sidiropoulos D, Herrman U Jr, Morell A, et al: Transplacental passage of intravenous immunoglobulin in the last trimester of pregnancy, *J Pediatr* 109:505, 1986.
706. Roilides E, Pizzo PA: Modulation of host defenses by cytokines: evolving adjuncts in prevention and treatment of serious infections in immunocompromised patients, *Clin Infect Dis* 15:508, 1992.
707. Roberts RL, Szelc CM, Scates SM, et al: Neutropenia in an extremely premature infant treated with recombinant human granulocyte colony-stimulating factor, *Am J Dis Child* 145:808, 1991.
708. Cairo MS, Agosti J, Ellis R, et al: A randomized, double-blind, placebo-controlled trial of prophylactic recombinant human granulocyte-macrophage colony-stimulating factor to reduce nosocomial infections in very low birth weight neonates, *J Pediatr* 134:64, 1999.
709. Yang KD, Bohnsack FJ, Hill HR: Fibronectin in host defense: implications in the diagnosis, prophylaxis and therapy of infectious diseases, *Pediatr Infect Dis J* 12:234, 1993.
710. Yoder MC: Therapeutic administration of fibronectin: current uses and potential applications, *Clin Perinatol* 18:325, 1991.
711. Carr R, Brocklehurst P, Dore CJ, et al: Granulocyte-macrophage colony stimulating factor administered as prophylaxis for reduction of sepsis in extremely preterm, small for gestational age neonates (the programs trial): a single-blind, multicentre, randomised controlled trial, *Lancet* 373:226, 2009.
712. Donini M, Fontana S, Savoldi G, et al: G-CSF treatment of severe congenital neutropenia reverses neutropenia but does not correct the underlying functional deficiency of the neutrophil in defending against microorganisms, *Blood* 109:4716, 2007.
713. Poindexter BB, Ehrenkranz RA, Stoll BJ, et al: Parenteral glutamine supplementation does not reduce the risk of mortality or late-onset sepsis in extremely low birth weight infants, *Pediatrics* 113:1209, 2004.
714. Tubman TR, Thompson SW, McGuire W: Glutamine supplementation to prevent morbidity and mortality in preterm infants, *Cochrane Database Syst Rev* (1):CD001457, 2008.
715. Lin HC, Su BH, Oh W: Oral probiotics prevent necrotizing enterocolitis, *J Pediatr* 148:849, 2006. author reply 850.
716. Lin HC, Su BH, Chen AC, et al: Oral probiotics reduce the incidence and severity of necrotizing enterocolitis in very low birth weight infants, *Pediatrics* 115:1, 2005.
717. Manzoni P, Mostert M, Leonessa ML, et al: Oral supplementation with *Lactobacillus casei* subspecies *rhamnosus* prevents enteric colonization by *Candida* species in preterm neonates: a randomized study, *Clin Infect Dis* 42:1735, 2006.
718. Alfaleh K, Anabrees J, Bassler D: Probiotics reduce the risk of necrotizing enterocolitis in preterm infants: a meta-analysis, *Neonatology* 97:93, 2009.
719. Orsi N: The antimicrobial activity of lactoferrin: current status and perspectives, *Biometals* 17:189, 2004.

720. Damato JJ, Eitzman DV, Baer H: Persistence and dissemination in the community of R-factors of nosocomial origin, *J Infect Dis* 129:205, 1974.
721. Klein JO: Family spread of staphylococcal disease following a nursery outbreak, *N Y State J Med* 60:861, 1960.
722. Nakwan N, Atta T, Chokephaibulkit K: Neonatal pasteurellosis: a review of reported cases, *Arch Dis Child Fetal Neonatal Ed* 94:F373, 2009.
723. Bhave SA, Guy LM: *Pasteurella multocida* meningitis in an infant with recovery, *BMJ* 2:741, 1977.
724. Guillet C, Join-Lambert O, Carbonnelle E, et al: *Pasteurella multocida* sepsis and meningitis in 2-month-old twin infants after household exposure to a slaughtered sheep, *Clin Infect Dis* 45:e80, 2007.
725. Wolfs TF, Duim B, Geelen SP, et al: Neonatal sepsis by *Campylobacter jejuni*: genetically proven transmission from a household puppy, *Clin Infect Dis* 32:E97, 2001.
726. Baraff LJ, Bass JW, Fleisher GR, et al: Practice guideline for the management of infants and children 0 to 36 months of age with fever without source. Agency for Health Care Policy and Research, *Ann Emerg Med* 22:1198, 1993.
727. Baker MD: Evaluation and management of infants with fever, *Pediatr Clin North Am* 46:1061, 1999.
728. Ferrera PC, Bartfield JM, Snyder HS: Neonatal fever: utility of the Rochester Criteria in determining low risk for serious bacterial infections, *Am J Emerg Med* 15:299, 1997.
729. Dagan R, Sofer S, Phillip M, et al: Ambulatory care of febrile infants younger than 2 months of age classified as being at low risk for having serious bacterial infections, *J Pediatr* 112:355, 1988.
730. King JC Jr, Berman ED, Wright PF: Evaluation of fever in infants less than 8 weeks old, *South Med J* 80:948, 1987.
731. Klein JO, Schlessinger PC, Karasic RB: Management of the febrile infant under three months of age, *Pediatr Infect Dis J* 3:75, 1984.
732. Ishimine P: Fever without source in children 0 to 36 months of age, *Pediatr Clin North Am* 53:167-194, 2006.
733. Baker MD, Bell LM: Unpredictability of serious bacterial illness in febrile infants from birth to 1 month of age, *Arch Pediatr Adolesc Med* 153:508, 1999.
734. Kadish HA, Loveridge B, Tobey J, et al: Applying outpatient protocols in febrile infants 1-28 days of age: can the threshold be lowered? *Clin Pediatr (Phila)* 39:81, 2000.
735. Baker MD, Bell LM, Avner JR: Outpatient management without antibiotics of fever in selected infants, *N Engl J Med* 329:1437, 1993.
736. Baskin MN, O'Rourke EJ, Fleisher GR: Outpatient treatment of febrile infants 28 to 89 days of age with intramuscular administration of ceftriaxone, *J Pediatr* 120:22, 1992.
737. Bonsu BK, Chb M, Harper MB: Identifying febrile young infants with bacteremia: is the peripheral white blood cell count an accurate screen? *Ann Emerg Med* 42:216, 2003.
738. Brown L, Shaw T, Wittlake WA: Does leucocytosis identify bacterial infections in febrile neonates presenting to the emergency department? *Emerg Med J* 22:256, 2005.
739. Greenes DS, Harper MB: Low risk of bacteremia in febrile children with recognizable viral syndromes, *Pediatr Infect Dis J* 18:258, 1999.
740. Levine DA, Platt SL, Dayan PS, et al: Risk of serious bacterial infection in young febrile infants with respiratory syncytial virus infections, *Pediatrics* 113:1728, 2004.
741. Krief WI, Levine DA, Platt SL, et al: Influenza virus infection and the risk of serious bacterial infections in young febrile infants, *Pediatrics* 124:30, 2009.
742. McCracken GH Jr: Personal communication, 1976.
743. Namnyak SS, Holmes B, Fathalla SE: Neonatal meningitis caused by *Achromobacter xylosoxidans*, *J Clin Microbiol* 22:470, 1985.
744. Hearn YR, Gander RM: *Achromobacter xylosoxidans*. An unusual neonatal pathogen, *Am J Clin Pathol* 96:211, 1991.
745. Molina-Cabrillana J, Santana-Reyes C, Gonzalez-Garcia A, et al: Outbreak of *Achromobacter xylosoxidans* pseudobacteremia in a neonatal care unit related to contaminated chlorhexidine solution, *Eur J Clin Microbiol Infect Dis* 26:435, 2007.
746. Christo GG, Shenoy V, Matthai J, et al: *Acinetobacter* sepsis in neonates, *Indian Pediatr* 30:1413, 1993.
747. Mishra A, Mishra S, Jaganath G, et al: *Acinetobacter* sepsis in newborns, *Indian Pediatr* 35:27, 1998.
748. Mittal N, Nair D, Gupta N, et al: Outbreak of *Acinetobacter* spp septicemia in a neonatal icu, *Southeast Asian J Trop Med Public Health* 34:365, 2003.
749. Kilic A, Li H, Mellmann A, et al: *Acinetobacter septicus* sp. Nov. Association with a nosocomial outbreak of bacteremia in a neonatal intensive care unit, *J Clin Microbiol* 46:902, 2008.
750. Simmonds A, Munoz J, Aguero-Rosenfeld M, et al: Outbreak of acinetobacter infection in extremely low birth weight neonates, *Pediatr Infect Dis J* 28:210, 2009.
751. Kadanali A, Tasyaran MA, Kadanali S: Anthrax during pregnancy: case reports and review, *Clin Infect Dis* 36:1343, 2003.
752. Manickam N, Knorr A, Muldrew KL: Neonatal meningoencephalitis caused by *Bacillus cereus*, *Pediatr Infect Dis J* 27:843, 2008.
753. Larsson C, Andersson M, Guo BP, et al: Complications of pregnancy and transplacental transmission of relapsing-fever borreliosis, *J Infect Dis* 194:1367, 2006.
754. Melkert PW, Stel HV: Neonatal *Borrelia* infections (relapsing fever): report of 5 cases and review of the literature, *East Afr Med J* 68:999, 1991.
755. Chheda S, Lopez SM, Sanderson EP: Congenital brucellosis in a premature infant, *Pediatr Infect Dis J* 16:81, 1997.
756. Giannacopoulos I, Eliopoulou MI, Ziambaras T, et al: Transplacentally transmitted congenital brucellosis due to *Brucella abortus*, *J Infect* 45:209, 2002.
757. Lee JK: Two outbreaks of *Burkholderia cepacia* nosocomial infection in a neonatal intensive care unit, *J Paediatr Child Health* 44:62, 2008.
758. Kahyaoglu O, Nolan B, Kumar A: *Burkholderia cepacia* sepsis in neonates, *Pediatr Infect Dis J* 14:815, 1995.
759. Doit C, Loukil C, Simon AM, et al: Outbreak of *Burkholderia cepacia* bacteremia in a pediatric hospital due to contamination of lipid emulsion stoppers, *J Clin Microbiol* 42:2227, 2004.
760. Abbink FC, Orendi JM, de Beaufort AJ: Mother-to-child transmission of *Burkholderia pseudomallei*, *N Engl J Med* 344:1171, 2001.
761. Krishnaswamy R, Sasidharan P, Rejjal A, et al: Early onset neonatal sepsis with *Campylobacter jejuni*: a case report, *Eur J Pediatr* 150:277, 1991.
762. Feldman JD, Kontaxis EN, Sherman MP: Congenital bacteremia due to *Capnocytophaga*, *Pediatr Infect Dis* 4:415, 1985.
763. Rosenman JR, Reynolds JK, Kleiman MB: *Capnocytophaga canimorsus* meningitis in a newborn: an avoidable infection, *Pediatr Infect Dis J* 22:204, 2003.
764. Edwards C, Yi CH, Currie JL: Chorioamnionitis caused by *Capnocytophaga*: case report, *Am J Obstet Gynecol* 173:244, 1995.
765 Berner R, Pelz K, Wilhelm C, et al: Fatal sepsis caused by *Corynebacterium amycolatum* in a premature infant, *J Clin Microbiol* 35:1011, 1997.
766. Platt MS: Neonatal *Haemophilus vaginalis (Corynebacterium vaginalis)* infection, *Clin Pediatr (Phila)* 10:513, 1971.
767 Vohra K, Torrijos E, Jhaveri R, et al: Neonatal sepsis and meningitis caused by *Edwardsiella tarda*, *Pediatr Infect Dis J* 7:814, 1988.
768. Okubadejo OA, Alausa KO: Neonatal meningitis caused by *Edwardsiella tarda*, *Br Med J* 3:357, 1968.
769. Mowbray EE, Buck G, Humbaugh KE, et al: Maternal colonization and neonatal sepsis caused by *Edwardsiella tarda*, *Pediatrics* 111:e296, 2003.
770. Dahl KM, Barry J, DeBiasi RL: *Escherichia hermannii* infection of a cephalohematoma: case report, review of the literature, and description of a novel invasive pathogen, *Clin Infect Dis* 35:e96, 2002.
771. Ginsberg HG, Daum RS: *Escherichia hermannii* sepsis with duodenal perforation in a neonate, *Pediatr Infect Dis J* 6:300, 1987.
772. Tekerekoglu MS, Durmaz R, Ayan M, et al: Analysis of an outbreak due to *Chryseobacterium meningosepticum* in a neonatal intensive care unit, *New Microbiol* 26:57, 2003.
773. Abrahamsen TG, Finne PH, Lingaas E: *Flavobacterium meningosepticum* infections in a neonatal intensive care unit, *Acta Paediatr Scand* 78:51, 1989.
774. Amaya RA, Al-Dossary F, Demmler GJ: *Gardnerella vaginalis* bacteremia in a premature neonate, *J Perinatol* 22:585, 2002.
775. Venkataramani TK, Rathbun HK: *Corynebacterium vaginale* (*Haemophilus vaginalis*) bacteremia: clinical study of 29 cases, *Johns Hopkins Med J* 139:93, 1976.
776. Orlicek SL, Welch DF, Kuhls TL: Septicemia and meningitis caused by *Helicobacter cinaedi* in a neonate, *J Clin Microbiol* 31:569, 1993.
777. Thompson C, McCarter YS, Krause PJ, et al: *Lactobacillus acidophilus* sepsis in a neonate, *J Perinatol* 21:258, 2001.
778. Cox SM, Phillips LE, Mercer LJ, et al: Lactobacillemia of amniotic fluid origin, *Obstet Gynecol* 68:134, 1986.

779. Gsell HO Jr, Olafsson A, Sonnabend W, et al: Intrauterine *Leptospirosis pomona*. 1st reported case of an intrauterine transmitted and cured leptospirosis, *Dtsch Med Wochenschr* 96:1263, 1971.
780. Shaked Y, Shpilberg O, Samra D, et al: Leptospirosis in pregnancy and its effect on the fetus: case report and review, *Clin Infect Dis* 17:241, 1993.
781. Yossuck P, Miller-Canfield P, Moffett K, et al: *Leuconostoc* spp sepsis in an extremely low birth weight infant: a case report and review of the literature, *W V Med J* 105:24, 2009.
782. Janow G, Lambert B, Scheiner M, et al: *Leuconostoc* septicemia in a preterm neonate on vancomycin therapy: case report and literature review, *Am J Perinatol* 26:89, 2009.
783. Sinha AK, Kempley ST, Price E, et al: Early onset *Morganella morganii* sepsis in a newborn infant with emergence of cephalosporin resistance caused by depression of AmpC beta-lactamase production, *Pediatr Infect Dis J* 25:376, 2006.
784. Dutta S, Narang A: Early onset neonatal sepsis due to *Morganella morganii*, *Indian Pediatr* 41:1155, 2004.
785. Casanova-Roman M, Sanchez-Porto A, Casanova-Bellido M: Early-onset neonatal sepsis caused by vertical transmission of *Morganella morganii*, *Scand J Infect Dis* 34:534, 2002.
786. Hata A, Honda Y, Asada K, et al: *Mycoplasma hominis* meningitis in a neonate: case report and review, *J Infect* 57:338, 2008.
787. Duran R, Vatansever U, Acunas B, et al: *Ochrobactrum anthropi* bacteremia in a preterm infant with meconium peritonitis, *Int J Infect Dis* 13:e61, 2009.
788. Aly NY, Salmeen HN, Lila RA, et al: *Pantoea agglomerans* bloodstream infection in preterm neonates, *Med Princ Pract* 17:500, 2008.
789. Thompson CM, Pappu L, Leukoff AH, et al: Neonatal septicemia and meningitis due to *Pasteurella multocida*, *Pediatr Infect Dis J* 3:559, 1984.
790. Cohen-Adam D, Marcus N, Scheuerman O, et al: *Pasteurella multocida* septicemia in a newborn without scratches, licks or bites, *Isr Med Assoc J* 8:657, 2006.
791. Fujita K, Shirai M, Ishioka T, et al: Neonatal *Plesiomonas shigelloides* septicemia and meningitis: a case and review, *Acta Paediatr Jpn* 36:450, 1994.
792. Terpeluk C, Goldmann A, Bartmann P, et al: *Plesiomonas shigelloides* sepsis and meningoencephalitis in a neonate, *Eur J Pediatr* 151:499, 1992.
793. Billiet J, Kuypers S, Van Lierde S, et al: *Plesiomonas shigelloides* meningitis and septicaemia in a neonate: report of a case and review of the literature, *J Infect* 19:267, 1989.
794. Kassim Z, Aziz AA, Haque QM, et al: Isolation of *Proteus mirabilis* from severe neonatal sepsis and central nervous system infection with extensive pneumocephalus, *Eur J Pediatr* 162:644, 2003.
795. Darby CP, Conner E, Kyong CU: *Proteus mirabilis* brain abscess in a neonate, *Dev Med Child Neurol* 20:366, 1978.
796. Velvis H, Carrasco N, Hetherington S: Trimethoprim-sulfamethoxazole therapy of neonatal *Proteus mirabilis* meningitis unresponsive to cefotaxime, *Pediatr Infect Dis* 5:591, 1986.
797. Lumbiganon P, Pengsaa K, Puapermpoonsiri S, et al: Neonatal melioidosis: a report of 5 cases, *Pediatr Infect Dis J* 7:634, 1988.
798. Lloyd-Puryear M, Wallace D, Baldwin T, et al: Meningitis caused by *Psychrobacter immobilis* in an infant, *J Clin Microbiol* 29:2041, 1991.
799. Kimura AC, Calvet H, Higa JI, et al: Outbreak of *Ralstonia pickettii* bacteremia in a neonatal intensive care unit, *Pediatr Infect Dis J* 24:1099, 2005.
800. Shin JH, Shim JD, Kim HR, et al: *Rothia dentocariosa* septicemia without endocarditis in a neonatal infant with meconium aspiration syndrome, *J Clin Microbiol* 42:4891, 2004.
801. Ruderman JW, Stoller KP, Pomerance JJ: Bloodstream invasion with *Shigella sonnei* in an asymptomatic newborn infant, *Pediatr Infect Dis* 5:379, 1986.
802. Aldrich JA, Flowers RP 3rd, Hall FK: *Shigella sonnei* septicemia in a neonate: a case report, *J Am Osteopath Assoc* 79:93, 1979.
803. Moore EE: *Shigella sonnei* septicaemia in a neonate, *Br Med J* 1:22, 1974.
804. Gras-Le Guen C, Fournier S, Andre-Richet B, et al: Almond oil implicated in a *Staphylococcus capitis* outbreak in a neonatal intensive care unit, *J Perinatol* 27:713, 2007.
805. Langbaum M, Eyal FG: *Stomatococcus mucilaginosus* septicemia and meningitis in a premature infant, *Pediatr Infect Dis J* 11:334, 1992.
806. Bose A, Philip JK, Jesudason M: Neonatal septicemia caused by *Vibrio cholerae* O:139, *Pediatr Infect Dis J* 19:166, 2000.
807. Kerketta JA, Paul AC, Kirubakaran VB, et al: Non-01 vibrio cholerae septicemia and meningitis in a neonate, *Indian J Pediatr* 69:909, 2002.
808. Thompson EC: *Yersinia enterocolitica* sepsis in a 3-week-old child, *J Natl Med Assoc* 86:783, 1994.
809. Challapalli M, Cunningham DG: *Yersinia enterocolitica* septicemia in infants younger than three months of age, *Pediatr Infect Dis J* 12:168, 1993.
810. White ME, Rosenbaum RJ, Canfield TM, et al: Plague in a neonate, *Am J Dis Child* 135:418, 1981.
811. Naidoo BT: The CSF in the healthy newborn infant, *S Afr Med J* 42:933, 1968.

7 Bacterial Infections of the Respiratory Tract

ELIZABETH D. BARNETT and JEROME O. KLEIN

CHAPTER OUTLINE

Infections of the Oral Cavity and Nasopharynx

PHARYNGITIS, RETROPHARYNGEAL CELLULITIS, AND RETROPHARYNGEAL ABSCESS

Neonates with bacterial infection of the oropharynx may present with pharyngeal inflammation with or without exudate or with retropharyngeal cellulitis or abscess. Clinical signs and symptoms include respiratory distress, poor feeding, and irritability. Infants can have submandibular swelling, and some may have a weak or hoarse cry. Infection may extend to the surrounding structures, leading to formation of deep neck abscess. Microorganisms identified as the etiologic agents of these infections and their manifestations of disease include the following:

Staphylococcus aureus: Although many children are colonized in the throat and nasopharynx with *S. aureus*, this organism is rarely a primary agent in the etiology of pharyngitis in infants (or adults). There have been reports, however, of localized abscesses in the oral cavity related to *S. aureus*. In 1936, Clark and Barysh[1] reported a case of retropharyngeal abscess in a 6-week-old infant. The infant was critically ill but recovered after incision and drainage of the abscess. A 6-day-old infant described in a report from India presented with stridor, dysphagia, and lateral cervical swelling. The infant was found to have a retropharyngeal abscess caused by *S. aureus*.[2] Steinhauer[3] reported a case of cellulitis of the floor of the mouth (Ludwig angina) in a 12-day-old infant. The infant was febrile and toxic; examination of the mouth revealed swelling under the tongue. Purulent material was subsequently drained from this lesion, and *S. aureus* was isolated from the pus. A laceration was noted in the floor of the mouth, and the author considered this wound to be the portal of entry of the infection. Increased incidence of methicillin-resistant *S. aureus* (MRSA) has been reflected in three reports of retropharyngeal abscesses caused by MRSA in infants 3 weeks to 3 months of age. The first case involved a 2-month-old infant in Japan (who also had evidence of penicillin-resistant *Pneumococcus*)[4]; the second was of a 3-week-old infant from Romania[5]; and the third report involved 3- and 4-month-old infants in the United States, one of whom had extension of the abscess into the mediastinum accompanied by venous thrombosis.[6]

Group A *Streptococcus:* Fever and pharyngeal inflammation may result from infection with group A *Streptococcus* (GAS) in the neonate.[7]

Streptococcus agalactiae: Retropharyngeal cellulitis has been associated with bacteremia caused by group B streptococci (GBS).[8-10] Affected neonates presented with poor feeding, noisy breathing, persistent crying, irritability, and widening of the retropharyngeal space on radiographs of the lateral neck. Stridor also may be associated with retropharyngeal abscess, as reported in a 13-day-old infant in Hong Kong.[11] A retropharyngeal abscess caused by GBS occurred in one of three neonates reported in a series of 31 cases of retropharyngeal abscess in Australian children during 1954 to 1990.[12,13] This infant was found to have a third branchial arch pouch that was subject to recurrent infection until age 5 years.

Listeria monocytogenes: Small focal granulomas on the mucous membrane of the posterior pharynx have been observed in neonates with *L. monocytogenes* infection. Necrosis of the granulomas can result in ulcers on the pharynx and tonsils.

Treponema pallidum: Mucous patches occur on the lips, tongue, and palate of infants with congenital *T. pallidum* infection. Rhinitis may appear after the first week of life.

Neisseria gonorrhoeae: A yellow mucoid exudate of the pharynx may be present simultaneously with ophthalmia with *N. gonorrhoeae* infection (A. Yu, personal communication, 1981). A case report of in utero gonococcal infection with involvement of multiple tissues included pharyngeal abscess.[14]

Enterococcus faecalis: In a case of retropharyngeal abscess, *E. faecalis* was isolated from a culture of aspirated pus, and two strains of coagulase-negative staphylococci occurred in a 2-week-old full-term infant from Australia.[13] The infant was severely ill and had atlantoaxial dislocation resulting in paraplegia. At autopsy, the findings included bacterial endocarditis, diffuse bilateral pneumonia, and renal infarcts.

Escherichia coli: E. coli can be a rare cause of infection of the pharyngeal cavity. Two strains of *E. coli* were isolated from pus from a retropharyngeal abscess in a 1-week-old infant.[13] The infant was afebrile on presentation and had significant midline pharyngeal swelling.

Infants may have coryza and other signs of upper respiratory tract disease secondary to infection with respiratory viruses. Infections with respiratory viruses may damage the respiratory mucosa, increasing susceptibility to bacterial infection of the respiratory tract. Eichenwald[15] described an apparent synergy of respiratory viruses and staphylococci that produced an upper respiratory tract infection called the "stuffy nose syndrome." The syndrome occurred only when both organisms were present. Eichenwald and coworkers[16] also documented increased dissemination of bacteria by newborns carrying staphylococci and echovirus 20 or adenovirus type 2 in the nasopharynx and coined the term "cloud babies" for these infants. Because these studies have not been repeated by other investigators, the significance of synergy of two or more microorganisms in neonatal respiratory infections remains uncertain.

NOMA

Noma (cancrum oris) is a destructive gangrenous process that may affect the nose, lips, and mouth. It occurs almost exclusively in malnourished children in developing countries; nutrient deficiencies have been postulated to play a role in its pathogenesis.[17] Although it is usually a chronic, destructive process in older children, in neonates it may be rapidly fatal. Affected neonates are usually premature and of low birth weight. In older children and adults, noma is caused by fusospirochetes such as *Fusobacterium necrophorum*.[18] The disease in neonates is usually due to *Pseudomonas aeruginosa*. Ghosal and coworkers[19] reported bacteriologic and histologic findings in 35 cases of noma in neonates in Calcutta. *P. aeruginosa* was isolated from blood or the gangrenous area in greater than 90% of the cases. In Israel, a full-term infant with bilateral choanal atresia who required an airway developed gangrenous lesions of the cheek on day 11 and palatal lesions that progressed to ulceration and development of an oronasal fistula. Cultures of material from the lesions grew *P. aeruginosa*.[20] Freeman and associates[21] reported the development of noma neonatorum in the third week of life in a 26-week-gestation premature infant; they suggested that this entity represents a neonatal form of ecthyma gangrenosum. Human immunodeficiency virus (HIV) testing has been recommended for infants in whom noma is diagnosed because of the difficulty distinguishing between early signs of noma and necrotizing diseases of the oral cavity associated with HIV infection.[22]

EPIGLOTTITIS

Epiglottitis caused by *S. aureus* in an 8-day-old infant was reported by Baxter[23] in a survey of experience with the disease at Montreal Children's Hospital from 1951 to 1965. Rosenfeld and associates[24] reported a case of epiglottitis caused by *S. aureus* in a 5-day-old infant. The infant presented with bradycardia, hoarseness, and inspiratory stridor and had diffuse inflammation of the arytenoids and epiglottis. *S. aureus* was cultured from pus on the epiglottic surface; blood culture was negative. Epiglottitis secondary to *Streptococcus sanguinis* in a newborn infant and secondary to GBS in an 11-week-old infant have also been reported.[25,26]

LARYNGITIS

Laryngitis in the newborn is rare. A newborn infant with congenital syphilis may have laryngitis and an aphonic cry. Hazard and coworkers[27] described a case of laryngitis caused by *Streptococcus pneumoniae*. A term infant was noted at 12 hours to have a hoarse cry, which progressed to aphonia during the next 3 days. Direct examination of the larynx revealed swelling and redness of the vocal cords. The infant was febrile (38.5° C), but the physical examination was unremarkable. *S. pneumoniae* was isolated from the amniotic fluid, the maternal cervix, and the larynx of the infant. The infant responded rapidly to treatment with parenteral penicillin G. Laryngitis may also be a sign of respiratory papillomatosis, usually associated with human papillomavirus. It has also been linked with acid reflux.[28]

INFECTION OF THE PARANASAL SINUSES

The paranasal sinuses of the fetus begin to differentiate at about the fourth month of gestation. The sinuses develop by local evagination of nasal mucosa and concurrent resorption of overlying bone. The maxillary and ethmoid sinuses are developed at birth and may be sites for suppurative infection. The sphenoid and frontal sinuses are rudimentary at birth and are not well defined until about 6 years of age.[29,30]

Inflammation may occur simultaneously in the paranasal sinuses, the middle ears, and the lungs. Autopsy may reveal that purulent exudate and leukocytic infiltration of the mucosa are present at one or more of these sites. Infection of the ethmoid and maxillary sinuses may be severe and life threatening in the newborn. Clinical manifestations include general signs of infection, such as fever, lethargy, irritability, and poor feeding, and focal signs indicative of sinus involvement (i.e., nasal congestion, purulent drainage from the nostrils, and periorbital redness and swelling). Proptosis may occur in severely affected children. Although any of the organisms responsible for neonatal sepsis may cause sinusitis, *S. aureus*, GAS, and GBS are responsible for most infections.[31-33] Suppurative infection of the maxillary sinus may progress to osteomyelitis of the superior maxilla (see Chapter 8).[32]

Blood specimens, nasopharyngeal secretions, and purulent drainage material (if present) should be obtained for culture before treatment. Antibacterial therapy must include a penicillinase-resistant penicillin or cephalosporin for activity against *S. aureus*, GAS, and GBS. If no material is available for examination of Gram-stained pus or if results of the preparation are ambiguous, initial therapy should include an aminoglycoside or a third-generation cephalosporin to ensure activity against gram-negative enteric bacilli (see discussion of management in Chapter 37). Surgical drainage of the infected site should be considered. Drainage of the suppurative maxillary sinus should be performed through the nose to avoid scars on the face and damage to the developing teeth.[32]

DIPHTHERIA

Neonatal diphtheria, although now extremely rare in the United States, was common before widespread immunization with diphtheria toxoid. Outbreaks occurred in hospital nurseries. One of the most striking reports described three separate epidemics in a "foundling hospital" in Tipperary, Ireland, during 1937 to 1941; 36 infants younger than 1 month were affected, and 26 died.[34] Goebel and Stroder[35] described 109 infants younger than 1 year with diphtheria in Germany during the period from the fall of 1945 to the summer of 1947: 59 infants were younger than 1 month, and 26 died. In a report from the Communicable Disease Unit of the Los Angeles County Hospital covering a 10-year period ending June 1950, 1433 patients were admitted to the hospital with diphtheria; 19 patients were younger than 1 year, but only 2 patients were younger than 1 month.[36] Diphtheria incidence continues to decline globally[37]; Mathur and associates[38] identified only three cases of neonatal diphtheria in India from 1974 to 1984.

Respiratory diphtheria has been well controlled in the United States since the introduction of diphtheria toxoid in the 1920s, although it remained endemic in some states through the 1970s.[39] The results of a survey of cases of diphtheria reported to the Centers for Disease Control and Prevention (CDC) of the U.S. Public Health Service, Atlanta, Georgia, for the period 1971 to October 1975 showed that no cases involved children younger than 1 month and that only six cases occurred in children younger than 1 year (the youngest was 5 months old) (G. Filice, personal communication, 1981). During the period 1980 to 1995, 41 cases of respiratory diphtheria were reported to the CDC; 4 (10%) were fatal, all of which occurred in unvaccinated children.[40] A single case of diphtheria has been reported in the United States since 2003.[41] Most cases of diphtheria in high-income countries are imported from countries where diphtheria remains endemic or where there is a resurgence of disease.[42] Reemergence of diphtheria in the newly independent states of the former Soviet Union underscored the need to maintain control measures in the United States, including universal childhood immunization, adult boosters, and maintenance of surveillance activities.[43] Maternal immunization may provide some protection to infants in the neonatal period before diphtheria vaccine is given.[44]

A newborn receives antibodies to *Corynebacterium diphtheriae* from the mother if she is immune, and the titers of mother and infant at birth are approximately equivalent.[45] Some degree of protection results in the neonate from this passively transferred antibody. Serologic surveys performed in the United States in the 1970s and 1980s suggested that 20% to 60% of adults older than 20 years may be susceptible to diphtheria.[46,47] Additional data from Europe confirmed that many adults remain susceptible to diphtheria.[48,49] As is the case in general with passively transferred immunity, protection depends on the level of maternal antibody at the time of the infant's birth, and protection decreases during the months after birth unless the infant is immunized.[50,51] Recommendations for one dose of tetanus toxoid-reduced diphtheria toxoid-acellular pertussis (Tdap) vaccine for all adults in the United States and for one dose of Tdap during every pregnancy should provide added protection to neonates against diphtheria.[52]

Neonatal diphtheria usually is localized to the nares. Diphtheria of the fauces is less common. The skin and mucous membranes may be affected; diphtheritic conjunctivitis was reported in an 8-day-old neonate.[36] Because isolation of *C. diphtheriae* requires inoculation of special culture media, notification of the laboratory about the possibility of diphtheria is important. Specimens of nasal and pharyngeal secretions may improve yield of positive cultures.[53] Infants suspected to have diphtheria should be isolated and receive penicillin or erythromycin to eradicate the organism from the respiratory tract or other foci of infection to terminate toxin production and decrease likelihood of transmission. The mainstay of therapy is diphtheria antitoxin, which should be administered as soon as the diagnosis of diphtheria is considered. This product is available in the United States from the CDC.[54]

PERTUSSIS

The pathophysiology, clinical features, treatment, and prevention of *Bordetella pertussis* infection are provided in detail in Chapter 21. Infants and young children in the United States are at the highest risk for pertussis and its complications.[55] Although the incidence of pertussis has declined markedly since 1934, when more than 250,000 cases were recorded, resurgence of disease since the early 1980s underscores the need for continued awareness of this disease.[56] Hospitalization rates for pertussis for infants were fairly constant from 1993 to 2004 in the United States, with rates highest for infants 1 to 2 months of age (293 hospitalizations per 100,000 live births).[57] Substantial numbers of cases of pertussis continued into the 2010s, with 14 deaths of infants younger than 1 year in 2012.[52]

Newborns may be exposed to pertussis through household or hospital contacts.[58] From 1959 to 1977, pertussis was diagnosed in 400 children in Dallas hospitals; 69 patients (17%) were younger than 12 weeks. An adult in the household with undiagnosed mild disease was the usual source of infection for these neonates and young infants.[59] Another risk factor for pertussis may be low birth weight. A study of cases of pertussis in Wisconsin infants and young children concluded that children of low birth weight were more likely than their normal birth weight counterparts to contract pertussis and to be hospitalized with the disease.[60] Fatal pertussis was identified through a pediatric hospital–based active surveillance system in 16 infants in Canada from 1991 to 2001; 15 of 16 infants were 2 months of age or younger. When fatal cases were matched with 32 nonfatal cases by age, date, and geography, pneumonia and leukocytosis were identified as independent predictors of a fatal outcome in hospitalized infants.[61] A more recent report described the histopathologic findings in the respiratory tracts of 15 infants younger than 4 months who died of pertussis. The findings suggested that the organism triggers a cascade of events, including pulmonary vasoconstriction and release of pertussis toxins leading to increased leukocyte mass and refractory pulmonary hypertension.[62]

Clinical presentation of pertussis in newborns is similar to the presentation in older children, but may lack some features typical of disease in older children. The incubation period ranges from 5 to 10 days. The initial sign usually is mild coughing, which may progress over several days to severe paroxysms with regurgitation and vomiting of food. The characteristic "whoop" may be absent in infants. The clinical picture of the most severely affected infants may be dominated by marked respiratory distress, cyanosis, and apnea, rather than significant cough. Fever is usually absent. Lymphocyte counts are frequently greater than 30,000/mm^3. Clinical signs of respiratory infection caused by *Chlamydia trachomatis* are similar to signs of pertussis (see Chapter 19).

Complications of pertussis in young infants include convulsions, bronchopneumonia, and hemorrhage. Bacterial and viral superinfection may occur. *B. pertussis* pneumonia may progress rapidly; pulmonary hypertension resulting from difficulty perfusing the congested lung may cause right-sided heart failure or fatal cardiac arrhythmias.[63] Long-term sequelae of whooping cough in infancy and early childhood were studied by Johnston and coworkers[64]; there was a significant reduction in forced vital capacity in adulthood in individuals who had pertussis before age 7 years compared with individuals who did not have pertussis. Diagnostic methods for pertussis depend on the immunization status of the patient and the duration of cough. Culture of a nasopharyngeal specimen, collected with a Dacron or calcium alginate swab and inoculated onto specialized agar (Regan-Lowe or Bordet-Gengou) is the most specific technique, but the organism is fastidious and may be difficult to isolate in individuals who have been immunized and in those with cough duration of more than 3 weeks. Direct fluorescent antibody testing of nasopharyngeal secretions has low sensitivity and variable specificity and is no longer recommended. Polymerase chain reaction (PCR) assay shows promise as a diagnostic tool[65,66]; although it may lack sensitivity in immunized individuals, it may still be more sensitive than culture. A Dacron swab must be used to collect the nasopharyngeal specimen because calcium alginate swabs are inhibitory to PCR. Although no U.S. Food and Drug Administration (FDA)-licensed test is available, the CDC has released a "best practices" document to guide PCR assays.[67] Serologic testing is available, but no commercial kit is licensed by the FDA, and diagnostic cutoff points have not been established. These tests also would be limited in the event of recent immunization with pertussis-containing vaccines.

Antimicrobial therapy may lessen severity of disease if it is given in the catarrhal stage, but it has no clinical effect after paroxysms occur. Antibiotic therapy eliminates carriage of organisms from the upper respiratory tract and is valuable in limiting communicability of infection, even if given late in the clinical course. Azithromycin, 10 mg/kg/day orally in one dose for 5 days, with a maximum daily dose of 600 mg, is the drug of choice for treatment or prevention of pertussis in infants younger than 1 month.[68] An alternative is erythromycin estolate, 40 mg/kg/day orally in four divided doses for 14 days.[68,69] Chemoprophylaxis is recommended for household and other close contacts, such as individuals in the hospital, including medical and surgical personnel.[68,70,71]

Two Tdap vaccines were licensed in 2005 to enhance protection against pertussis in adolescents and adults. Currently, immunization with Tdap vaccine is recommended during every pregnancy.[52,72,73] These vaccines have also been recommended for health care workers who have direct patient contact.[73]

Otitis Media

Otitis media in the newborn may be an isolated infection, or it may be associated with sepsis, pneumonia, or meningitis. Acute otitis media is defined as the presence of fluid in the middle ear (middle ear effusion) accompanied by an acute sign of illness. Middle ear effusion may be present without other signs of acute illness. Diagnostic criteria for otitis media in newborns are the same as in older children, but the vulnerability of the newborn and potential differences in the microbiology of otitis media in newborns, especially in the first 2 weeks of life, make it necessary to exercise special considerations in choosing antimicrobial therapy.

PATHOGENESIS AND PATHOLOGY

During fetal life, amniotic fluid bathes the entire respiratory tree, including the lungs, paranasal sinuses, and middle ear cleft. Amniotic fluid and cellular debris usually are cleared from the middle ear in most infants within a few days after birth.[74] In term infants, the middle ear usually is well aerated, with normal middle ear pressure and normal tympanic membrane compliance, within the first 24 hours.[75] A study of 68 full-term infants examined by otoscopy, tympanometry, and acoustic reflectometry within the first 3 hours of life revealed the presence of middle ear effusion in all neonates; fluid was absent at 72 hours of life in almost all infants.[76]

Studies of the middle ear at autopsy provide important information about the development of otitis media in the neonate. Inflammation in the lungs or paranasal sinuses usually was accompanied by inflammation in the middle ear.[31,74-78] deSa[74] examined 130 infants, including 36 stillborn infants, 74 neonates who died within 7 days of life, and 20 infants who died between 8 and 28 days. In 56 cases, the middle ear was aerated or contained a small amount of clear fluid. In 55 cases, amniotic debris was present; in 2 additional cases, cellular material was mixed with mucus. A purulent exudate was present in the middle ear of 17 infants; these exudates were cultured, and a bacterial pathogen was isolated from 13. Amniotic material was present in specimens obtained from most of the stillborn infants. Purulent exudate was not seen in the stillborn infants; the frequency of its presence increased with postnatal age at time of death. Of the 20 infants who lived for 7 or more days, 11 had purulent exudate in the middle ear. Each of the 17 infants with otitis media had one or more significant infections elsewhere; 12 had pneumonia, and 6 had meningitis. deSa[79] subsequently identified mucosal metaplasia and chronic inflammation in the middle ears of newborns receiving ventilatory support.

Factors that may affect the development of otitis media in the neonate include the nature of the amniotic fluid, the presence of other infectious processes, the need for resuscitative efforts (especially positive-pressure ventilation), the presence of anatomic defects such as cleft palate, the immunologic status of the infant, and the general state of health of the infant. Aspiration of infected amniotic fluid through the eustachian tube may be one factor in the development of otitis media in the neonate; dysfunction of the eustachian tube, which is shorter, wider, and more horizontal than in the older child, and failure to clear aspirated material from the middle ear probably have etiologic roles as well.[80,81] Piza and associates[82] speculated that infants born through thick meconium fluid may be at greater risk for otitis media because of the inflammatory nature of this fluid. deSa[74] noted that many infants in whom otitis media developed had required assistance in respiration and speculated that the pressure of ventilation efforts was responsible for propelling infected material into the middle ear. In infants, as in older children, middle ear effusion seems to be frequent in patients with nasotracheal tubes, and the effusion occurs first on the side of intubation.[83] Berman and colleagues[84] described an association between nasotracheal intubation for more than 7 days and the presence of middle ear effusion.

Infants with cleft palate are at high risk for recurrent otitis media and conductive hearing loss because of persistence of middle ear effusion. Attempts to reduce the incidence of permanent hearing impairment have included intensive monitoring of children with cleft palate for middle ear effusion and repair of these defects earlier in infancy. One study found, however, that early cleft palate repair did not reduce significantly the subsequent need for ventilating tubes in these children.[85]

Breastfed infants are at lower risk than bottle-fed infants for acute otitis media. Results of studies of Canadian Eskimo infants[86] and of infants in India,[87] Finland,[88] Denmark,[89] and the United States[90] indicate a significant decrease in the incidence of infection of the middle ear in breastfed infants compared with bottle-fed infants. A study from Cooperstown, New York, identified a significantly lower incidence of acute lower respiratory tract infection in infants who were breastfed, compared with infants who were bottle-fed; the incidence of otitis media was lower in the breastfed infants, but this difference was not statistically significant.[91] Infants in Boston who were breastfed had a lower risk for either having had one or more episodes of acute otitis media or having had recurrent acute otitis media (three or more episodes) during the first year of life. The protective association of breastfeeding did not increase with increased duration of breastfeeding; infants who were breastfed for 3 months had an incidence of otitis media in the first year of life that was as low as infants who were breastfed for 12 months.[92]

The beneficial effects of breastfeeding may be due to immunologic factors in breast milk or to development of musculature in the breastfed infant that may affect eustachian tube function and assist in promoting drainage of middle ear fluid. Alternatively, the findings could indicate harmful effects of bottle feeding, including the reclining or horizontal position of the bottle-fed infant that allows fluid to move readily into the middle ear,[93,94] allergy to one or more components in cow's milk or formula, or aspiration of fluids into the middle ear during feeding. The hypothesis that breast milk is protective is substantiated by results of studies of a special feeding bottle for infants with cleft palate. Among infants who were fed by this bottle containing breast milk, the number of days with middle ear effusion was less than in infants fed by this device containing formula, which suggests that protection was more likely to be due to a quality of the milk, rather than the mode of feeding.[95] Adherence of *S. pneumoniae* and *Haemophilus influenzae* to buccal epithelial cells was inhibited by human breast milk.[96]

Early onset of pneumococcal otitis media has been associated with low levels of cord blood pneumococcal immunoglobulin G (IgG) antibodies. Among a group of infants who had siblings with middle ear disease, low concentrations of cord blood antibody to pneumococcal serotype 14 or 19F were associated with earlier onset of otitis media.[97] Low cord blood antibody concentrations to serotype 19F predicted more episodes of otitis media over the first year of life in a cohort of 415 infants whose mothers enrolled in the study during pregnancy.[98] In these infants, early otitis media was associated significantly with type 14 IgG1 in the lowest quartile but not with type 19F IgG1 antibody or with either IgG2 antibody.[99] These findings prompted study of maternal immunization to prevent pneumococcal disease in neonates. Immunization of pregnant chinchillas with heptavalent pneumococcal vaccine resulted in reduced incidence and severity of experimental otitis in their infants.[100] Immunization of pregnant women in Bangladesh, The Gambia, the Philippines, and the United States with pneumococcal polysaccharide vaccine resulted in pneumococcal antibody concentrations that were higher at birth in infants of immunized mothers than in controls.[101-104] In addition, pneumococcal IgG antibody acquired by infants of immunized mothers had greater opsonophagocytic activity than that in control infants.[103]

Antibody to pneumococci in breast milk has been proposed to have a role in prevention of early otitis media. Early colonization with pneumococci or other bacteria is associated with early otitis media.[105] The role of antibodies to pneumococci in human milk in prevention of nasopharyngeal colonization of infants with pneumococci is controversial. A study in Sweden involving 448 mother-infant pairs failed to show reduction in carriage of pneumococci in neonates fed milk with anticapsular and antiphosphorylcholine activity and showed an increase in colonization when infants were fed milk with anti–cell wall polysaccharide antibody activity.[106] Maternal immunization with pneumococcal polysaccharide vaccine resulted in higher breast milk IgA antibodies to serotype 19F, but not type 6B.[101]

EPIDEMIOLOGY

The incidence of acute otitis media or middle ear effusion in the newborn is uncertain because of the paucity of definitive studies. Warren and Stool[107] examined 127 consecutive infants with birth weight less than 2300 g and found 3 with middle ear effusions (at 2, 7, and 26 days of life). Jaffe and coworkers[108] examined 101 Navajo infants within 48 hours of birth and identified 18 with impaired mobility of the tympanic membrane. Berman and colleagues[84] identified effusion in the middle ear of 30% of 125 consecutively examined infants who were admitted to a neonatal intensive care unit. The clinical diagnosis was corroborated by aspiration of middle ear fluid. The basis for the differences in incidence in the various studies is uncertain, but there may be an association with procedures used in the nurseries.

Acute otitis media is common in early infancy. In the prospective study of Boston children, 9% of children had an episode of middle ear infection by 3 months of age.[92] Age at the time of first episode of acute otitis media seems to be an important predictor for recurrent otitis media.[92,108,109] Children who experience a first episode during the first months of life are more likely to experience repeated infection than children whose first episode occurs after the first birthday. Additional risk factors include parental smoking and low socioeconomic status.[110,111]

Some host factors that also are present in infants with neonatal sepsis have been identified in infants with middle ear infection. The incidence of infection is higher in premature infants than in infants delivered at term in some studies[112,113] but not in the prospective study of Boston children.[92] Male infants are more frequently infected than female infants.[112] Otitis media also is associated with a prolonged interval after rupture of maternal membranes and with other obstetric difficulties.[74,114] Middle ear infection is more severe in Native Americans and Canadian Eskimos than in the general population, and it is likely that this is true in neonates and older infants as well.[86,108] Children with cleft palate have a high incidence of otitis media, which may begin soon after birth.[115] Prenatal, innate, and early environmental exposures were assessed in relation to early otitis media in a cohort of 596 infants followed prospectively from birth. In multivariable analysis, prenatal factors were not associated with early onset of otitis media, but environmental (day care, upper respiratory infection, birth in the fall) and innate factors (parental and sibling history of otitis media) were associated with early or recurrent otitis media, or both.[116]

MICROBIOLOGY

The bacteriology of otitis media in infants has been studied by investigators in Honolulu,[112] Dallas,[113] Huntsville,[117] Boston,[117] Denver,[81,84] Milwaukee,[118] Tampere Hospital in Finland,[119] and Beer-Sheva, Israel[120] (Table 7-1). *S. pneumoniae* and *H. influenzae* are isolated frequently from fluid aspirated from the middle ear in very young infants, as is the case in older infants and children. Although it has been suggested that otitis media in the youngest neonates

Table 7-1 Microbiology of Otitis Media in Newborn Infants

	PATIENTS			CAUSATIVE ORGANISM: NO. OF CASES (%)					
Author(s)	**Site (Years)**	**Age Range**	**No. in Series**	***Streptococcus pneumoniae***	***Haemophilus influenzae***	**Staphylococcal Species**	**Enteric Gram-negative Species**	**Other**	**Comment**
Bland[112]	Honolulu (1970-1971)	10-14 days 15-42 days	2 19*	1 (50) 0 (0)	0 (0) 3 (12)	0 (0) 5 (20)	1 (50) 13 (52)	0 (0) 1 (4)	Outpatients
Tetzlaff et al[113]	Dallas (1974-1976)	0-5 weeks	42*	13 (30)	11 (26)	NA†	8 (19)	12 (28)‡	Outpatients
Balkany et al[81]	Denver (1975-1976)	0-4 months	21	9 (43)	5 (24)	5 (24)	1 (4)	1 (4)	Outpatients
Berman et al[84]	Denver (1975-1976)	0-4 months	13*	0 (0)	0 (0)	6 (60)	4 (40)	0 (0)	NICU patients
Shurin et al[117]	Huntsville, Boston (1976)	0-6 weeks	17	4 (24)	2 (12)	0 (0)	1 (6)	3 (18)	Three nurseries
Karma et al[119]	Finland (1980-1985)	0-1 month 1-2 months	14 93	1 (7) 19 (20)	2 (14) 8 (9)	5 (35) 55 (60)	0 (0) 5 (5)	2 (14) 11 (11)	
Nozicka et al[118]	Milwaukee (1994-1995)	0-2 weeks 2-8 weeks	Unknown* Unknown*	1 (14) 5 (19)	1 (14) 0 (0)	0 (0) 9 (35)	2 (28) 3 (12)	3 (43) 9 (35)	"Nontoxic outpatients"
Turner et al[120]	Israel (1995-1999)	0-2 weeks 2-8 weeks	5 109*	2 (40) 54 (44)	0 (0) 41 (34)	0 (0) 0 (0)	3 (60) 7 (6)	0 (0) 15 (12)	Outpatients

NICU, Neonatal intensive care unit.
*In some infants, more than one organism was identified, or cultures of middle ear fluid yielded no growth.
†Nonpathogen in this study (NA, not applicable).
‡Includes group A and B streptococci, *Staphylococcus* species, *Neisseria* species, diphtheroids, and other hemolytic streptococci.

(<2 weeks of age) is caused more frequently by organisms associated with neonatal sepsis, such as GBS, *S. aureus*, and gram-negative enteric bacilli, this pattern does not emerge consistently when multiple studies are examined. Pneumococci were isolated from middle ear fluid in the first 2 weeks of life, and otitis associated with gram-negative enteric organisms and GBS occurred in older infants. Microbiology of middle ear disease in infants who are in neonatal intensive care nurseries may be an exception to the pattern associated with otitis media in previously healthy infants and may reflect pathogens present in the neonatal intensive care unit. In a small series of 13 such infants, only gram-negative enteric organisms and staphylococcal species were identified in the 10 samples of middle ear fluid from which bacteria were identified.[94] Table 7-1 shows the microbiology of middle ear isolates from eight studies of otitis media in infants; when possible, data from the youngest neonates have been separated from data from older infants.

Susceptibility patterns of organisms causing otitis media in newborns reflect local patterns. In general, trends toward increasing resistance of pneumococci to antibacterial agents and colonization and disease resulting from pneumococcal serotypes not present in the pneumococcal conjugate vaccine used routinely in the United States and other countries have been observed.

Gram-negative enteric bacilli have been the predominant organisms isolated at autopsy from purulent effusions of the middle ear. Of 17 infants studied by deSa,[74] 7 were found to have *E. coli*, and 6 had *P. aeruginosa*. β-Hemolytic streptococci (not further identified) were isolated from one infant, and no organism was recovered from the remaining 3 infants. Because pneumonia and meningitis accompanied otitis in all of these cases, the predominance of gram-negative pathogens in this series is not unexpected.

Congenital tuberculosis of the ear[121] and of the ear and parotid gland[122] has been reported in preterm infants from Hong Kong and Turkey. Both cases were notable for significant regional lymphadenopathy, lack of response to antibacterial therapy, and presence of active pulmonary tuberculosis in the mother. Authors of both reports suggest that there is continued need for a high index of suspicion for this disease in appropriate circumstances. Otitis media and bacteremia resulting from *P. aeruginosa* occurring at 19 days of life was thought to occur after inoculation of the organism during a water birth.[123] *B. pertussis* was isolated from middle ear fluid in a 1-month-old infant hospitalized with pertussis; intubation of the infant's airway may have facilitated spread of the organism from the nasopharynx to the middle ear.[124]

DIAGNOSIS

During the first few weeks of life, examination of the ear requires patience and careful appraisal of all of the structures of the external canal and the middle ear.[125] The diagnostic criteria for acute otitis media in the neonate are the same as in the older child: presence of fluid in the middle ear accompanied by signs of acute illness. Middle ear effusion and its effect on tympanic membrane mobility are best measured with a pneumatic otoscope. The normal tympanic membrane moves inward with positive pressure and outward with negative pressure. The presence of fluid in the middle ear dampens tympanic membrane mobility.

In the first few days of life, the ear canal is filled with vernix caseosa; this material is readily removed with a small curette or suction tube. The canal walls of the young infant are pliable and tend to expand and collapse with insufflation during pneumatic otoscopy. Continuing pneumatic insufflation as the speculum is advanced is helpful because the positive pressure expands the pliable canal walls. The tympanic membrane often appears thickened and opaque, and mobility may be limited during the first few days of life.[126] In many infants, the membrane is in an extreme oblique position, with the superior aspect proximal to the observer (Fig. 7-1). The tympanic membrane and the superior canal wall may appear to lie almost in the same plane, so it is often difficult to distinguish the point where the canal ends and the pars flaccida of the membrane begins. The inferior canal wall may bulge loosely over the inferior position of the tympanic membrane and move with positive pressure, simulating movement of the tympanic membrane. The examiner must distinguish between the movement of the canal walls and the movement of the membrane.

The following considerations are helpful in recognition of these structures: Vessels are seen within the tympanic membrane but are less apparent in the skin of the ear canal; the tympanic membrane moves during crying or respiration when the middle ear is aerated. The ear canals of most neonates permit entry of only a 2-mm-diameter speculum. Because the entire eardrum cannot be examined at one time owing to the small diameter of the speculum, quadrants must be examined sequentially. By 1 month of age, the infant's tympanic membrane has assumed an oblique position that is less marked than in the first few weeks of life and is similar to the position in the older child.

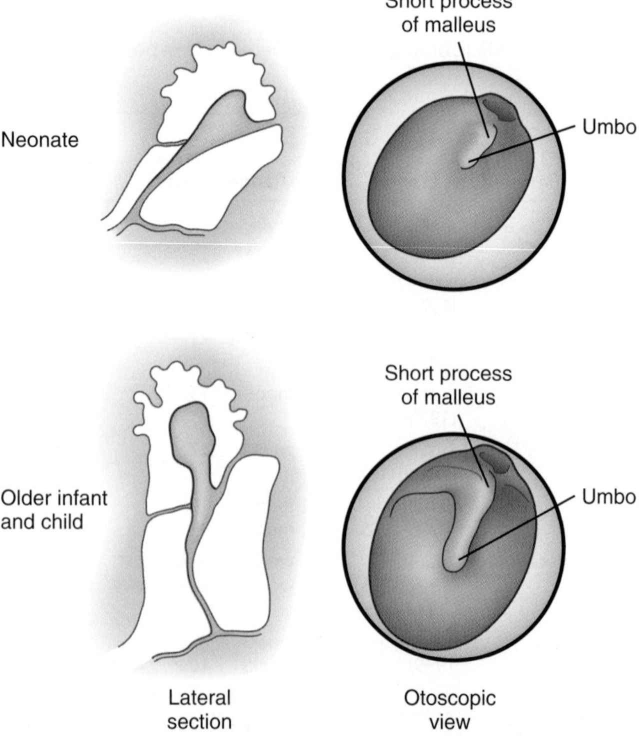

Figure 7-1 Lateral section of middle ear and otoscopic view of tympanic membrane in the neonate and older infant and child.

Tympanometry is of limited value in diagnosis of middle ear effusion in the neonate. The flat tympanogram indicative of effusion in children 6 months of age or older often is not present in younger infants, even when fluid is documented by aspiration.[127] Acoustic reflectometry may be advantageous compared with tympanometry in the neonate because it does not require insertion into the ear canal or the achievement of a seal within the canal, but there are insufficient data to identify sensitivity and specificity.[128]

Culture of the throat or nasopharynx is an imperfect method of identifying the bacterial pathogens responsible for otitis media. Many studies have shown the diagnostic value of needle aspiration of middle ear effusions (tympanocentesis) in acute otitis media. The specific microbiologic diagnosis defines the appropriate antimicrobial therapy and is sufficiently important in the sick neonate to warrant consideration of aspiration of the middle ear fluid. Aspiration of middle ear fluid is more difficult in the neonate than in the older child, and usually the assistance of an otolaryngologist (using an otoscope with a surgical head or an otomicroscope) is required.

When spontaneous perforation has occurred, the fluid exuding into the external canal from the middle ear is contaminated by the microflora from the canal. Appropriate cultures may be obtained by cleaning the canal carefully with 70% alcohol and obtaining cultures from the area of perforation as the fluid emerges or by needle aspiration through the intact membrane.

TREATMENT

Initial therapy for febrile or ill-appearing infants with otitis media during the first 2 weeks of life is similar to therapy for infants with neonatal sepsis. A penicillin and an aminoglycoside or third-generation cephalosporin should be used. Specific therapy can be provided if needle aspiration is performed and the pathogen is identified. Infants who remain in the nursery because of prematurity, low birth weight, or illness require similar management during the first 4 to 6 weeks of life. If the infant was born at term, had a normal delivery and course in the nursery, has been in good health since discharge from the nursery, is not ill appearing, and is 2 weeks of age or older, the middle ear infection probably is due to *S. pneumoniae* or *H. influenzae* and may be treated with an appropriate oral antimicrobial agent such as amoxicillin or amoxicillin-clavulanate.[129] The infant may be managed outside the hospital if he or she does not seem to have a toxic condition. For infants born at term who have acute otitis media and are in a toxic condition, the physician must consider hospitalization, cultures of blood and cerebrospinal fluid, and use of parenterally administered antimicrobial agents because of possible systemic infection, a focus of infection elsewhere, or presence of a resistant organism.

PROGNOSIS

Infants who have infections of the middle ear in the neonatal period seem to be susceptible to recurrent episodes of otitis media.[92,108,109] The earlier in life an infant has an episode of otitis media, the more likely he or she is to have recurrent infections. It is uncertain whether this means that an early episode of otitis media damages the mucosa of the middle ear and makes the child more prone to subsequent infection, or whether early infection identifies children with dysfunction of the eustachian tube or subtle or undefined immune system abnormalities who have a propensity to infection of the middle ear because of these abnormalities.

MASTOIDITIS

The mastoid air cells are not developed at birth and usually consist of only a single space each. Mastoiditis rarely occurs in neonates. One report cited a case of meningitis and mastoiditis caused by *H. influenzae* in a newborn.[130] Radiographs of the mastoid area showed a cloudy right antrum. At operation, the middle ear was normal, but the antrum was filled with infected mesenchymal tissue.

Pneumonia

Pneumonia, inflammation of the lungs, in the fetus and newborn can be classified into four categories according to the time and mode of acquisition of inflammation:

1. *Congenital pneumonia acquired by the transplacental route*: Pneumonia is one component of generalized congenital disease.
2. *Intrauterine pneumonia*: This is an inflammatory disease of the lungs found at autopsy in stillborn or live-born infants who die within the first few days of life, usually associated with fetal asphyxia or intrauterine infection, and includes infectious and noninfectious causes.
3. *Pneumonia acquired during birth*: Signs of pneumonia occur within the first few days of life, and infection is due to microorganisms that colonize the maternal birth canal.
4. *Pneumonia acquired after birth*: The illness manifests during the first month of life, either in the nursery or at home; sources of infection include human contacts and contaminated equipment.

Although helpful as a general framework for understanding neonatal pneumonia, these four categories have clinical features and pathologic characteristics that overlap. Management of pneumonia is essentially the same for all four categories, requiring aggressive supportive measures for the respiratory and circulatory systems along with treatment for the specific underlying infectious disorder.

Pneumonia in the neonate may be caused by viruses, bacteria, or parasitic organisms. Detailed information about causative organisms mentioned in this chapter other than bacteria is found in the appropriate chapters in this book; bacterial disease is covered in detail here.

Pneumonia acquired by the transplacental route may be caused by rubella, cytomegalovirus, herpes simplex virus, adenoviruses,[131] mumps virus,[132] *Toxoplasma gondii*, *L. monocytogenes*, or *T. pallidum*. Some of these organisms and enteroviruses, genital mycoplasmas, *Mycobacterium pneumoniae*,[133] *C. trachomatis*, and *M. tuberculosis* are also responsible for intrauterine pneumonia resulting from aspiration of infected amniotic fluid. Fatal pneumonitis caused by echovirus has also been reported in newborns (see Chapter 25).[134] Isolation of *Trichomonas vaginalis* from the tracheal aspirates of infants with pneumonia suggests a possible association of this organism with respiratory tract disease in the neonate.[135,136]

GBS is the most frequent cause of bacterial pneumonia acquired at delivery. Pneumonia caused by GBS and other bacteria, such as *E. coli* or *L. monocytogenes*, may resemble respiratory distress syndrome.

Pneumonias acquired after birth, either in the nursery or at home, include those caused by respiratory viruses, such as respiratory syncytial virus, influenza virus, or adenoviruses; gram-positive bacteria, such as pneumococci and *S. aureus*; gram-negative enteric bacilli; *Legionella pneumophila*[137]; *C. trachomatis*; *Mycoplasma*; and *Pneumocystis carinii*.[138] A fatal case of adenovirus serotype 14 with pathologic features consistent with bronchiolitis and acute respiratory distress syndrome occurred in a 12-day-old infant in 2006.[139] Pneumonia caused by nonbacterial microorganisms is discussed in the appropriate chapters. Bacterial pneumonia and neonatal sepsis acquired during or soon after birth share many features of pathogenesis, epidemiology, and management, and these aspects are discussed in Chapter 6. Discussion of pneumonia in the fetus and newborn not presented elsewhere in the text follows.

PATHOGENESIS AND PATHOLOGY

Congenital or Intrauterine Pneumonia

Histologic features of congenital or intrauterine pneumonia have been described from autopsy findings in infants who are stillborn or who die shortly after birth (usually within 24 hours). An inflammatory reaction is found in histologic sections of lung. Polymorphonuclear leukocytes are present in the alveoli and often are mixed with vernix and squamous cells. Infiltrates of round cells may be present in interstitial tissue of small bronchioles and interalveolar septa.[140-145] Alveolar macrophages may be present and have been associated with duration of postnatal life and inflammatory pulmonary lesions.[146] The inflammation is diffuse and usually is uniform throughout the lung. Bacteria are seen infrequently, and cultures for bacteria are often negative. Davies and Aherne[143] noted that the usual characteristics of bacterial pneumonia are missing in congenital pneumonia; among these characteristics are pleural reactions, infiltration or destruction of bronchopulmonary tissue, and fibrinous exudate in the alveoli.

The pathogenesis of congenital pneumonia is not well understood.[147] Asphyxia and intrauterine infection, acting alone or together, seem to be the most important factors.[143] It is thought that microorganisms of the birth canal contaminate the amniotic fluid by ascending infection after early rupture of maternal membranes or through minimal and often unrecognized defects in the membranes. Evidence of aspiration of amniotic fluid is frequent.[143] Naeye and colleagues[148-150] proposed that microbial invasion of the fetal membranes and aspiration of infected amniotic fluid constitute frequent causes of chorioamnionitis and congenital pneumonia. Bacteriologic studies have produced equivocal results, however. Many infants with congenital pneumonia do not have bacteria in their lungs, yet cultures of the lung of some infants without pneumonia do yield bacteria.[151] Fetal asphyxia or hypoxia seems to be a factor in most cases of congenital pneumonia. The asphyxia may cause death directly or by eliciting a pulmonary response consisting of hemorrhage, edema, and inflammatory cells. From his studies of congenital pneumonia, Barter[152] concluded that hypoxia or infection may produce similar inflammation in the lungs. In addition, Bernstein and Wang[153] found that evidence of fetal asphyxia was frequently present at autopsy in infants with congenital pneumonia who also had generalized petechial hemorrhage, subarachnoid and intracerebral hemorrhage, liver cell necrosis, or ulceration of the gastrointestinal mucosa.

Although it is likely that asphyxia and infection can produce similar inflammatory patterns in lungs of the fetus, available information is insufficient to determine which is more important or more frequent. In a review of fetal and perinatal pneumonia, Finland[154] concluded that "pulmonary lesions certainly play a major role in the deaths of the stillborn and of infants in the early neonatal period. Infection, on the other hand, appears to play only a minor role in what has been called 'congenital pneumonia,' that is, the inflammatory lesion seen in the stillborn or in those dying within the first few hours, or possibly the first day or two; it assumes greater importance in pneumonias that cause death later in the neonatal period." Davies[155] noted that the histologic presentation of congenital pneumonia seems to represent aspiration of materials in amniotic fluid, including maternal leukocytes and amniotic debris, rather than infection originating in the pulmonary air spaces. Evidence of infiltration of alveoli or destruction of bronchopulmonary tissue is rarely present.

Pneumonia Acquired During the Birth Process and in the First Month of Life

The pathology of pneumonia acquired during or after birth is similar to the pathology found in older children or adults. The lung contains areas of densely cellular exudate with vascular congestion, hemorrhage, and pulmonary necrosis.[143,153,156] Bacteria often are seen in sections of the lung. *S. aureus* (see Chapter 14) and *Klebsiella pneumoniae*[157,158] may produce extensive tissue damage, microabscesses, and empyema. Pneumatoceles are a common manifestation of staphylococcal pneumonia but also may occur in infections with *K. pneumoniae*[157,158] and *E. coli*.[159] Hyaline membranes similar to those seen in respiratory distress syndrome have been observed in the lungs of infants who died with pneumonia caused by GBS. Cocci were present within the membranes, and in some cases, exuberant growth that included masses of organisms was apparent. Although most thoroughly documented in cases of pneumonia caused by GBS, similar membranes have been seen in histologic sections of lungs of infants who died with pneumonia caused by *H. influenzae* and gram-negative enteric bacilli.[160]

The pathogenesis of pneumonia acquired at or immediately after birth is similar to the pathogenesis of neonatal sepsis and is discussed in Chapter 6. Presumably, aspiration of infected amniotic fluid or secretions of the birth canal are responsible for most cases of pneumonia acquired during delivery. After birth, the infant may become infected through human contact or contaminated equipment. Infants who receive assisted ventilation are at risk owing to the disruption of the normal barriers to infection because of the presence of the endotracheal tube and possible irritation of tissues near the tube. Bacteria or other organisms may invade the damaged tissue, which may result in tracheitis or tracheobronchitis.[161] Biofilm formation has been identified on endotracheal tubes from infants and a relationship between biofilm formation and lower respiratory tract infection in intubated neonates has been hypothesized.[162]

Ventilator-associated pneumonia may be prevented by reducing bacterial colonization of the aerodigestive tract and decreasing the incidence of aspiration. A review highlighted strategies for prevention of pneumonia in patients receiving mechanical ventilation, including nonpharmacologic strategies, such as attention to hand washing and standard precautions, positioning of patients, avoiding abdominal distention, avoiding nasal intubation, and maintaining ventilator circuits and suction catheters and tubing, and pharmacologic strategies, such as appropriate use of antimicrobial agents.[163] Newborns with congenital anomalies, such as tracheoesophageal fistula, choanal atresia, and diaphragmatic hernia, have an increased risk of developing pneumonia.

Lung abscess and empyema are uncommon in neonates and usually occur as complications of severe pneumonia. Abscesses also may occur as a result of infection of congenital cysts of the lung.

MICROBIOLOGY

Most information about the bacteriology of fetal and neonatal pneumonia has been derived from studies done at autopsy of stillborn infants and of infants who die during the first month of life. A study reviewing causes of death of infants with very low birth weight concluded, on the basis of histologic studies done at autopsy, that pneumonia was an underrecognized cause of death in these infants.[164] Barter and Hudson[151] reported bacteriologic studies at autopsy of infants with and without pneumonia. The incidence of bacteria in the lungs increased with age in infants dying with and without pneumonia. Among the infants with pneumonia, bacteria were cultured from the lungs of 55% of stillborn infants and infants who died during the first day of life, 70% of infants who died between 24 hours and 7 days of age, and 100% of infants who died between 7 and 28 days of age. Among the infants without pneumonia, bacteria were cultured from the lungs of 36% of stillborn infants and infants who died within the first 24 hours, 53% of infants who died between 24 hours and 7 days of age, and 75% of infants who died between 7 and 28 days of age. The bacterial species were similar in the infants with and without pneumonia, with the exception of GBS, which was found only in infants with pneumonia.

These results were corroborated by Penner and McInnis.[145] Bacteria were cultured from 92% of the lungs of fetuses and neonates with pneumonia and from 40% of the lungs of fetuses and neonates without pneumonia. Maden and associates[165] identified congenital pneumonia (defined by the presence of neutrophils in the alveolar spaces) in 45% of neonatal autopsy cases; isolated organisms included S. epidermidis, GBS, E. coli and Ureaplasma urealyticum. Barson[166] identified bacteria in lung cultures at autopsy of 252 infants dying with bronchopneumonia; positive cultures were obtained in 60% of infants dying on the first day of life and in 78% of infants dying between 8 and 28 days of age. Bacteria were cultured at autopsy from the lungs of many infants with and without pneumonia. Information about bacterial etiology of pneumonia also can be obtained by culturing blood, tracheal aspirates, and pleural fluid and by needle aspiration of the lungs of living children with pneumonia.

The bacterial species responsible for fetal and neonatal pneumonia are those present in the maternal birth canal; included in this flora are gram-positive cocci such as group A, group B, and group F[167] streptococci and gram-negative enteric bacilli, predominantly *E. coli* and, to a lesser extent, *Proteus, Klebsiella,* and *Enterobacter* species. For infants who remain hospitalized, microorganisms acquired postnatally may reflect the microbial environment of the inpatient setting. For infants who develop pneumonia in the community, typical organisms causing community-acquired pneumonia predominate. In the 1950s and 1960s, *S. aureus* was a common cause of neonatal pneumonia.

Few data exist about relative frequency of specific etiologic agents of neonatal pneumonia or incidence of pneumonia caused by specific organisms. One review of invasive pneumococcal disease monitored prospectively by the U.S. Pediatric Multicenter Pneumococcal Surveillance Group identified 29 cases of pneumococcal infection in infants younger than 30 days among 4428 cases in children; 4 of these were bacteremic pneumonia.[168] In addition to *S. pneumoniae,*[169-171] *H. influenzae*[160,172] and *Moraxella catarrhalis*[173] also are infrequent causes of pneumonia in newborns. Pneumonia caused by these organisms is frequently associated with bacteremia and sometimes with meningitis.[143,169,171,172] Many other organisms have been reported in association with pneumonia in neonates, including a fatal case of congenital pneumonia caused by *Pasteurella multocida* in a full-term neonate associated with maternal infection and colonization of the family cat with the same organism.[174] A case of pneumonia and sepsis caused by ampicillin-resistant *Morganella morganii* was reported from Texas[175]; the authors speculate about the role of increased use of intrapartum antibiotics in predisposing to colonization and infection with ampicillin-resistant organisms. A case of pneumonia caused by *Legionella pneumophila* occurred in a newborn after water birth.[176]

Certain bacteria are associated with a predilection for developing lung abscess or empyema. During the 1950s and 1960s, outbreaks of staphylococcal pneumonia occurred; many times these infections were accompanied by empyemas and pneumatoceles. Although rare in newborns, *H. influenzae* was associated with pneumonia and empyema[177] until its virtual disappearance after initiation of universal immunization in the early 1990s. Single or multiple abscesses may also be caused by GBS, *E. coli,* and *K. pneumoniae.*[178,179] Cavitary lesions may develop in pneumonia caused by *Legionella pneumophila.*[180] Lung abscess and meningitis caused by *Citrobacter koseri* was reported in a previously healthy 1-month-old infant.[181] Nosocomial infection secondary to *L. pneumophila* has been reported, including cases of fatal necrotizing pneumonia and cavitary pneumonia.[182] Reports have identified *Citrobacter diversus* as a cause of lung abscess[183] and *Bacillus cereus* as a cause of a necrotizing pneumonia in premature infants.[184]

Empyema can also be associated with extensive pneumonia. Empyema secondary to *E. coli* and *Klebsiella* has been reported in 6- and 8-day-old infants,[185] and *Serratia marcescens* was isolated from blood, tracheal aspirate, and empyema fluid in a premature neonate.[186] Cases of pleural empyema secondary to group A streptococci have been reported from the United Kingdom and Sweden.[187,188]

EPIDEMIOLOGY

Incidence

Table 7-2 presents the incidence of pneumonia at autopsy of stillborn and live-born infants. Pneumonia is a significant cause of death in the neonatal period,[189] and infection of amniotic fluid leading to pneumonia is an important cause of death in extremely premature infants.[190] The definition of pneumonia in the autopsy studies usually was based on the presence of polymorphonuclear leukocytes in the pulmonary alveoli or interstitium or both. The presence or absence of bacteria was not important in the definition of pneumonia. The incidence rates for congenital and neonatal pneumonia at autopsy are similar despite the different periods of study (1922-1999) and different locations[140-142,144,153,164,188-192] (with the single exception of a report from Helsinki[170]): 15% to 38% of stillborn infants and 20% to 32% of live-born infants had evidence of pneumonia. The incidence rates for pneumonia were similar in premature and in term infants. Rates of pneumonia derived from epidemiologic studies are scarce. Sinha and colleagues[193] reported an attack rate of 0.4 per 100 infants diagnosed during a nursery stay and 0.03 and 0.01 per 100 infants diagnosed at pediatric office visits and in hospital or emergency department visits. They acknowledged a paucity of data with which to compare their rates, which they derived from retrospective review of data from a large health maintenance organization.

Race and Socioeconomic Status

In two studies, black infants had pneumonia at autopsy significantly more often than white infants. The Collaborative Study of the National Institutes of Health[192] considered the incidence of pneumonia in live-born infants who died within the first 48 hours of life: 27.7% of black infants had evidence of pneumonia, whereas only 11.3% of white infants showed signs of this disease, and this difference was present in every weight group. In New York City, Naeye and coworkers[148] studied 1044 consecutive autopsies of newborn and stillborn infants; black infants had significantly more pneumonia (38%) than Puerto Rican infants (22%) or white infants (20%). The same study showed that the incidence of pneumonia in infants was inversely related to the level of household income. Infants from the families with the lowest income had significantly more pneumonia than infants from the families with the highest income. At comparable levels of household income, black infants had a higher incidence of neonatal pneumonia than Puerto Rican or white infants. These racial and economic differences were not readily explained by the authors or by other investigators.

Epidemic Disease

Pneumonia may be epidemic in a nursery because of a single source of infection, such as a suppurative lesion caused by *S. aureus* in a nursery employee or contamination of a common solution or piece of equipment, usually caused by *Pseudomonas*, *Flavobacterium*, or *Serratia marcescens*. Infection may also spread by droplet nuclei among infants or between personnel and infants. Epidemics of respiratory infection related to viruses also have been reported (see Chapters 30 and 35).

Developing Countries

Pneumonia is the leading cause of death in children worldwide. Although discussion of global efforts to address reduction of pneumonia morbidity and mortality are beyond the scope of this chapter, a few details are noted here. A survey of a rural area in central India revealed that the mortality rate for pneumonia in the first 29 days of life was 29 per 1000 live-born children (the rate during the first year was 49.6 per 1000 live-born children).[194] The aerobic bacteria grown from the vaginas of rural women were used

Table 7-2 Incidence of Congenital and Neonatal Pneumonia Based on Findings at Autopsy

	NO. WITH PNEUMONIA / TOTAL NO. OF INFANTS (%)						
	STILLBIRTHS			LIVE-BORN INFANTS			
Site (Years)	Premature	Term	Total	Premature	Term	Total	Age or Weight of Infants at Death
Helsinki (1951)[140]	5/13 (38)	9/32 (28)	14/45 (31)				
Helsinki (1946-1952)[156]				13 (30)	11 (26)	NA	<29 days
Newcastle (1955-1956)[141]			13/70 (90)			10/31 (32)	<7 days
Adelaide (1950-1951)[142]	5/44 (11)	10/53 (19)	15/97 (13)	9/32 (28)	3/8 (38)	12/40 (30)	Lived >6 hr after birth
Detroit (1956-1959)[151]						55/231 (24)	<7 days
Winnipeg (1954-1960)[189]	15/46 (33)						<750 g
Winnipeg (1954-1957)[190]						27/110 (25)	<7 days
Edinburgh (1922)[191]						22/80 (26)	8 hr-5 wk
NIH Collaborative (1959-1964)[192]				67/387 (17)	33/125 (26)	100/512 (20)	<48 hr
Manchester (1950-1954)[144]			28/273 (10)			59/219 (27)	<7 days
Los Angeles (1990-1993)[164]				25/111 (23)			<1000 g, <48 hr

NA, Not applicable; *NIH*, National Institutes of Health.

as a surrogate for likely pathogens of pneumonia in neonates.[195] Vaginal flora included *E. coli* and other gram-negative enteric bacilli and staphylococcal species in expected proportions but a relatively low rate of β-hemolytic streptococci (3.2%). Because of the lack of microbiologic information, syndrome-based management of infectious diseases is encouraged in the developing world. A meta-analysis of this approach found a reduction of pneumonia mortality of 42% in neonates managed in this fashion.[196]

Singhi and Singhi[197] studied the clinical signs of illness in Chandigarh infants younger than 1 month with radiologically confirmed pneumonia to determine how to increase accuracy of diagnosis of pneumonia by health care workers. Rural health care workers (most were illiterate) used revised World Health Organization criteria for pneumonia in infants, including respiratory rate greater than 60 breaths per minute, presence of severe chest indrawing (retraction), or both.[198] Cough and respiratory rate greater than 50 breaths per minute missed 25% of cases; decreasing the threshold respiratory rate to 40 breaths per minute increased the sensitivity. In the absence of cough, chest retraction or respiratory rate greater than 50 breaths per minute or both had maximal accuracy. Another study in Pakistan demonstrated the ability of rural health care workers to diagnose and treat severe pneumonia in the home setting.[199]

CLINICAL MANIFESTATIONS

Onset of respiratory distress at or soon after birth is characteristic of intrauterine or congenital pneumonia. Before delivery, fetal distress may be evident: The infant may be tachycardic, and the fetal tracing may show poor beat-to-beat variability or evidence of deep decelerations. Meconium aspiration may have occurred before delivery, suggesting fetal asphyxia and gasping. The infant may have episodes of apnea or may have difficulty establishing regular respiration. In some cases, severe respiratory distress is delayed, but it may be preceded by increasing tachypnea, apneic episodes, and requirement for increasing amounts of oxygen. The infant may have difficulty feeding, temperature instability, and other signs of generalized sepsis, including poor peripheral perfusion, disseminated intravascular coagulation, and lethargy.

Infants who acquire pneumonia during the birth process or postnatally may have signs of systemic illness, such as lethargy, anorexia, and fever. Signs of respiratory distress, including tachypnea, dyspnea, grunting, coughing, flaring of the alae nasi, irregular respirations, cyanosis, intercostal and supraclavicular retractions, rales, and decreased breath sounds, may be present at the onset of the illness or may develop later. Severe disease may progress to apnea, shock, and respiratory failure. Signs of pleural effusion or empyema may be present in suppurative pneumonias associated with staphylococcal infections, group A[200] and group B streptococcal infections, and *E. coli* infections.[201]

In a study of 103 neonates in New Delhi, Mathur and colleagues documented the sensitivity and specificity, respectively, of signs of neonatal pneumonia: cough (n = 13; 14%; 100%); difficulty in feeding (n = 91; 88%; 6%); chest retractions (n = 96; 93%; 36%); flaring of alae nasi (n = 50; 49%; 70%).[202]

DIAGNOSIS

Clinical Diagnosis

A history of premature delivery, prolonged interval between rupture of maternal membranes and delivery, prolonged labor, excessive obstetric manipulation, and presence of foul-smelling amniotic fluid frequently are associated with neonatal infection, including sepsis and pneumonia. The clinical manifestations of pneumonia may be subtle and nonspecific at the onset, and specific signs of respiratory infection may not be evident until late in the course of illness. Most commonly, pneumonia is associated with evidence of respiratory distress, including tachypnea, retractions, flaring of nasal alae, and increasing requirement for oxygen.

Radiologic Diagnosis

A chest radiograph is the most helpful tool for making the diagnosis of pneumonia. The radiograph of an infant with intrauterine pneumonia may contribute no information, however, or show only the coarse mottling of aspiration. If the radiologic examination is done early in the course of meconium or other aspiration pneumonias, typical radiologic features may not yet have developed. The radiograph of an infant with pneumonia acquired during or after birth may show streaky densities or confluent opacities. Peribronchial thickening, indicating bronchopneumonia, may be present. Pleural effusion, abscess cavities, and pneumatoceles are frequent in infants with staphylococcal infections but also may occur in pneumonia caused by group A streptococci, *E. coli*,[159] or *K. pneumoniae*.[158] Diffuse pulmonary granularity or air bronchograms similar to that seen in respiratory distress syndrome have been observed in infants with pneumonia related to GBS.[203] Computed tomography (CT) with contrast medium enhancement is beneficial in localizing pulmonary lesions such as lung abscess and distinguishing abscess from empyema, pneumatoceles, or bronchopleural fistulas.[179] Ultrasound examination was used to diagnose hydrothorax in utero at 32 weeks of gestation.[204]

Although it is impossible to distinguish bacterial from viral pneumonia on the basis of a chest radiograph alone, several features may help distinguish between the two. Findings that are more characteristic of viral pneumonias include hyperexpansion, atelectasis, parahilar peribronchial infiltrates, and hilar adenopathy, which is associated almost exclusively with adenovirus infection. Alveolar disease, consolidation, air bronchograms, pleural effusions, pneumatoceles, and necrotizing pneumonias are more characteristic of bacterial processes.[205]

Microbiologic Diagnosis

Because of the difficulty in accessing material from a suppurative focus in the lower respiratory tree, microbiologic diagnosis of pneumonia is problematic. Although cultures of material obtained from lung aspiration have been shown to yield bacterial pathogens in about one third of a group of seriously ill infants with lung lesions accessible to needle aspiration,[206] this rate of positive results is unlikely to be obtained in an unselected group of infants with pneumonia. Diagnosis may be based on isolating pathogens from other sites. When generalized systemic infection is present, cultures of blood, urine, or cerebrospinal fluid may yield a pathogen. Bacteremia may be identified in about 10% of febrile children with pneumonia.[207] If a pleural effusion is present and the bacterial diagnosis is not yet evident, pleural fluid biopsy or culture or both may be helpful. Bacterial cultures of the throat and nasopharynx are unrevealing or misleading because of the high numbers of respiratory pathogens present.

Tracheal aspiration through a catheter is frequently valuable when performed by direct laryngoscopy, but the aspirate may be contaminated when the catheter is passed through the nose or mouth. Sherman and colleagues[208] performed a careful study of the use of tracheal aspiration in diagnosis of pneumonia in the first 8 hours of life. Tracheal aspirates were obtained from 320 infants with signs of cardiorespiratory disease and abnormalities on the chest radiograph; 25 infants had bacteria present in the smear of the aspirate, and the same organisms were isolated from cultures of 14 of 25 aspirates. Thureen and colleagues[209] found that tracheal aspirate cultures failed to define an infectious cause of deterioration in ventilated infants. Positive tracheal aspirates were found with equal frequency among infants with clinically suspected lower respiratory tract infection and in "well" control subjects. Tracheal aspirate cultures may provide useful information about potential pathogens in pneumonia or bacteremia but rarely indicate the risk or timing of such complications.[210] Often, surveillance cultures of tracheal aspirate material are used to guide empirical therapy when a new illness develops in an infant with a prolonged course on a ventilator.

Bronchoscopy can provide visual, cytologic, and microbiologic evidence of bacterial pneumonia.[211] Aspiration of pulmonary exudate (lung puncture or "lung tap") can be used to provide direct, immediate, and unequivocal information about the causative agent of pneumonia.[206] This procedure is now performed rarely; most reports of its use in infants and young children precede the introduction of antimicrobial agents.[212,213]

Open lung biopsy has been used to identify the etiology of lung disease in critically ill infants and seems to have been most helpful at a time when corticosteroids for bronchopulmonary dysplasia were withheld if there was concern about pulmonary infection. Cheu and colleagues[214] identified three infections in 17 infants who had open lung biopsies: respiratory syncytial virus in 1 infant and *Ureaplasma urealyticum* in 2 infants. Although the optimal indications for use of corticosteroids in bronchopulmonary dysplasia are controversial,[215,216] in general corticosteroids are not withheld if indicated because of low likelihood of an infectious process.[217]

Histologic and Cytologic Diagnosis

The data of Naeye and coworkers[148] indicated that congenital pneumonia or pneumonia acquired during birth is almost always accompanied by chorioamnionitis, although chorioamnionitis may be present in the absence of pneumonia or other neonatal infections. These and other data[218] suggested that the presence of leukocytes in sections of placental membranes and of umbilical vessels or in Wharton jelly is valuable in diagnosing fetal and neonatal infections, including pneumonia and sepsis. Other investigators were less certain and believed that the presence of inflammation in the placenta or umbilical cord does not distinguish changes caused by hypoxia from those caused by infection.[152,153]

Culture of material obtained by aspiration of stomach contents usually is not helpful in diagnosing pneumonia because this material is contaminated by the flora of the upper respiratory tract. In addition, infants with pneumonia may have no evidence of the organism in the gastric aspirate.[219] There is some evidence, however, that microscopic examination of gastric contents may be useful in defining the presence of an inflammatory process in the lung after the first day of life. Because affected infants are unable to expectorate, they swallow bronchial secretions. During the first few hours of life, inflammatory cells present in the gastric aspirate are of maternal origin; however, after the first day, any polymorphonuclear leukocytes present are those of the infant. Tam and Yeung[219] showed that if greater than 75% of the cells in the gastric aspirate obtained from infants after the first day of life were polymorphonuclear leukocytes, pneumonia was usually present. A study by Pole and McAllister[220] did not confirm the value of gastric aspirate cytology in the diagnosis of pneumonia, however.

Primary ciliary dyskinesia is congenital and may manifest in the newborn period as respiratory distress. Infants with situs inversus are at risk for this condition. Consultation with a geneticist may be warranted; a biopsy specimen of nasal epithelium may be needed to identify the characteristic abnormal morphology of cilia of the immotile cilia syndrome.[221-223]

Immunologic Diagnosis

Immunologic response to various microorganisms responsible for pneumonia is used extensively as an aid to diagnosis with infections caused by GBS, *S. aureus* (see Chapters 12 and 14) and organisms that cause congenital infection (rubella virus, *T. gondii*, herpes simplex virus, cytomegalovirus, and *T. pallidum*). Giacoia and colleagues[224] prepared antigens from microorganisms isolated from bronchial aspirates and correlated specific antibodies and nonspecific IgM antibody with clinical and radiologic evidence of pneumonia. A significant immune response was identified in approximately one fourth of the patients studied. These data are of uncertain significance because of the difficulty of distinguishing immune response to organisms responsible for lower respiratory tract disease from the response to organisms colonizing the respiratory tree.[225]

Although controversial, testing of blood, urine, and cerebrospinal fluid for antigens to GBS, pneumococci, *H. influenzae*, and *Neisseria meningitidis* may provide helpful information for selected infants with generalized sepsis and pneumonia.[226] Interpretation of results must take into account possible contamination by organisms colonizing the area around the urethra (in the case of a bag specimen of urine) and possible interference with the test result caused by recent immunization against *H. influenzae* type b or pneumococci or recent infection owing to these organisms. Bedside cold agglutination testing may be helpful in the case of *Mycoplasma* infection, but the test has low sensitivity, so a negative result is not diagnostic.

Availability of rapid diagnostic tests for respiratory illness is becoming more widespread, and clinicians will need to determine what is available to them locally. In many settings, laboratory capability includes simultaneous testing for multiple viral and bacterial pathogens during the appropriate season.

DIFFERENTIAL DIAGNOSIS

Various noninfectious diseases and conditions may simulate infectious pneumonia. Respiratory distress syndrome (hyaline membrane disease), atelectasis, aspiration pneumonia, pneumothorax or pneumomediastinum, pulmonary edema and hemorrhage, pleural effusions of the lung (e.g., chylothorax), cystic lung disease, hypoplasia or agenesis, pulmonary infarct, and cystic fibrosis all have some signs and symptoms similar to pneumonia. Meconium aspirated into the distal air passages may produce chemical pneumonitis or segmental atelectasis.[227] Multifocal pulmonary infiltrates have been associated with feeding supplements containing medium-chain triglycerides.[228] Infants with immotile cilia syndrome may present within the first 24 hours of life with tachypnea, chest retraction, and rales. Results of prospective epidemiologic studies of neonatal respiratory diseases from Sweden[229] for the period 1976 to 1977 and from Lebanon[230] for the period 1976 to 1984 indicate that infection was second in frequency to hyaline membrane disease in both surveys. Avery and coworkers[231] presented clues to the diagnosis of diseases and conditions producing respiratory distress based on information from the maternal history and signs in the infant (Table 7-3).

Pneumonia may be superimposed on hyaline membrane disease. One survey showed that histologic evidence of pneumonia was present at autopsy in 16% of 1535 infants with hyaline membrane disease.[232] Foote and Stewart[233] showed, by chest radiography, that pneumonia modifies the reticulogranular pattern of hyaline membrane disease by replacing the air in the alveoli with inflammatory exudate. Any modification of the radiographic pattern typical of hyaline membrane disease should lead the physician to consider superinfection.

Ablow and colleagues[234] reported that infants with pneumonia caused by GBS who also showed clinical and radiologic signs of respiratory distress syndrome were easier to ventilate than infants who had hyaline membrane disease with a clinical picture suggestive of respiratory distress syndrome unassociated with infection. These findings are of limited value in identifying infection in individual infants and were not confirmed in a subsequent study by Menke and colleagues.[235]

Pleural fluid, usually limited to the lung fissures, occurs in many infants and may be related to slow resorption of fetal lung fluid, to transient tachypnea of the newborn, or to respiratory distress syndrome of noninfectious etiology. Large collections of fluid in the pleural space may represent bacterial empyema; noninfectious causes include chylothorax, hydrothorax (associated with hydrops fetalis, congestive heart failure, or transient tachypnea), meconium aspiration pneumonitis, or hemothorax related to hemorrhagic disease of the newborn.

The symptoms of cystic fibrosis may begin in early infancy. Of patients with newly diagnosed cases seen in a 5-year period at Children's Hospital Medical Center in Boston, 30% were younger than 1 year.[236] The authors described the histories of four children whose respiratory symptoms began before the infants were 1 month of age.

Table 7-3 Clues to Diagnosis of Types of Respiratory Distress

Information from Maternal History	Most Probable Condition in Infant
Peripartum fever	Pneumonia
Foul-smelling amniotic fluid	Pneumonia
Excessive obstetric manipulation at delivery	Pneumonia
Infection	Pneumonia
Premature rupture of membranes	Pneumonia
Prolonged labor	Pneumonia
Prematurity	Hyaline membrane disease
Diabetes	Hyaline membrane disease
Hemorrhage in days before premature delivery	Hyaline membrane disease
Meconium-stained amniotic fluid	Meconium aspiration
Hydramnios	Tracheoesophageal fistula
Pain medications	CNS depression
Use of reserpine	Stuffy nose
Traumatic or breech delivery	CNS hemorrhage, phrenic nerve paralysis
Fetal tachycardia or bradycardia	Asphyxia
Prolapsed cord or cord entanglements	Asphyxia
Postmaturity	Aspiration
Amniotic fluid loss	Hypoplastic lungs
Signs in the Infant	**Most Probable Associated Condition**
Single umbilical artery	Congenital anomalies
Other congenital anomalies	Associated cardiopulmonary anomalies
Situs inversus	Kartagener syndrome
Scaphoid abdomen	Diaphragmatic hernia
Erb palsy	Phrenic nerve palsy
Inability to breathe with mouth closed	Choanal atresia, stuffy nose
Gasping with little air exchange	Upper airway obstruction
Overdistention of lungs	Aspiration, lobar emphysema, pneumothorax
Shift of apical pulse	Pneumothorax, chylothorax, hypoplastic lung
Fever or increase in body temperature	Pneumonia
Shrill cry, hypertonia or flaccidity	CNS disorder
Atonia	Trauma, myasthenia, poliomyelitis, amyotonia
Frothy blood from larynx	Pulmonary hemorrhage
Head extended without neurologic findings	Laryngeal obstruction or vascular rings
Choking after feedings	Tracheoesophageal fistula or pharyngeal incoordination
Plethora	Transient tachypnea

From Avery ME, Fletcher BD, Williams RG: *The lung and its disorders in the newborn infant*, Philadelphia, 1981, WB Saunders.
CNS, Central nervous system.

The clinical course of the disease in young infants is characterized by a bronchiolitis-like syndrome with secondary chronic obstructive pulmonary disease and respiratory distress, coughing, wheezing, poor exchange of gases, cyanosis, hypoxia, and failure to thrive.

MANAGEMENT

Infants with bacterial pneumonia must receive prompt treatment with appropriate antimicrobial agents. Culture of blood and urine may identify a bacterial pathogen, especially in patients with generalized sepsis. Cerebrospinal fluid culture may be helpful if the infant is not too unstable for lumbar puncture. In intubated infants, tracheal aspirate smears may indicate the presence of inflammatory cells, and cultures may provide information about organisms colonizing the trachea.

Because the microbiology of pneumonia in the newborn is the same as that of sepsis, the guidelines for management discussed in Chapter 6 are applicable. Initial antimicrobial therapy should include a penicillin (usually ampicillin) or a penicillinase-resistant penicillin (if staphylococcal infection is a possibility) and an aminoglycoside or a third-generation cephalosporin. In situations in which resistant pneumococci or MRSA may be the cause of the pneumonia, vancomycin may be used for initial therapy until microbiologic data are available. The oxazolidinone antibiotic linezolid, an agent with a unique mechanism of action with activity against gram-positive organisms, has been studied in neonates. Sixty-three neonates with known or suspected resistant gram-positive infections were randomly assigned to receive linezolid or vancomycin. No difference in efficacy of the two agents was noted, and the authors concluded that linezolid is a safe and effective alternative to vancomycin in treatment of resistant gram-positive infections.[237]

Duration of therapy depends on the causative agent: Pneumonia caused by gram-negative enteric bacilli or GBS is treated for 10 days; disease caused by *S. aureus* may require 3 to 6 weeks of antimicrobial therapy, according to the severity of the pneumonia and the initial response to therapy. Empyema or lung abscesses may also require longer courses of therapy.

When clinical and radiologic signs of respiratory distress syndrome are present, infection caused by GBS or gram-negative organisms, including *H. influenzae*, is not readily distinguished from respiratory distress syndrome of noninfectious etiology. Until techniques are developed that can distinguish infectious from noninfectious causes of respiratory distress syndrome, it is reasonable to treat all infants who present with clinical and radiologic signs of the syndrome. Therapy is instituted for sepsis, as outlined earlier, after appropriate cultures have been taken. If the results of cultures are negative and the clinical course subsequently indicates that the illness was not infectious, the antimicrobial regimen is stopped. Because of concern over respiratory signs as a part of the initial presentation of sepsis and the rapid progression of bacterial pneumonia in neonates with associated high mortality rate, particularly pneumonia caused by GBS, early and aggressive therapy is warranted in infants with respiratory distress syndrome.

Antibiotics are only part of the management of the newborn with pneumonia; supportive measures, such as maintaining fluid and electrolyte balance, providing oxygen or support of respiration with continuous positive airway pressure, or instituting intubation and ventilation, are equally important. Drainage of pleural effusions may be necessary when accumulation of fluid results in respiratory embarrassment. Single or multiple thoracocenteses may be adequate when the volumes of fluid are small. If larger amounts are present, a closed drainage system with a chest tube may be needed. The tube should be removed as soon as its drainage function is completed because delay may result in injury to local tissues, secondary infection, and sinus formation. Empyema and abscess formation are uncommon but serious complications of pneumonia. They may occur in association with pneumonia caused by *S. aureus* and are discussed in detail in Chapter 14.

PROGNOSIS

Available data on the significance of pneumonia during early life have been obtained in large measure from autopsy studies. There is information about the natural course of pneumonia caused by *S. aureus* in infants (see Chapter 14), but few studies of the sequelae of pneumonia caused by other agents exist. Even autopsy studies are equivocal in determining the importance of pneumonia because respiratory disease may have been the cause of death, a contributing factor in death, or incidental to and apart from the main cause of death.[238,239] Pneumonia was said to be the sole cause of death in about 15% of neonatal deaths studied by Ahvenainen.[156] In the British Perinatal Mortality Study,[240] pulmonary infections were considered to be the cause of death in 5.5% of stillborn infants and infants dying in the neonatal period.

Ahvenainen[156] noted that pneumonia often is a fatal complicating factor in infants with certain underlying conditions, such as central nervous system malformations or disease, congenital heart disease, and anomalies of the gastrointestinal tract such as intestinal atresia. A prospective study of premature newborns found ventilator-associated pneumonia to occur frequently and to be significantly associated with death in extremely premature infants who remained in a neonatal intensive care unit for more than 30 days.[241]

The presence of pneumonia in the neonatal period has been implicated as a cause of chronic pulmonary disease in infancy and childhood. Pacifico and associates[242] found that isolation of *U. urealyticum* from the respiratory tract of premature low-birth-weight infants in the first 7 days of life was associated with early development of bronchopulmonary dysplasia and severe pulmonary outcome. Brasfield and colleagues[243] studied a group of 205 infants hospitalized with pneumonitis during the first 3 months of life and identified radiographic and pulmonary function abnormalities that persisted for more than 1 year.

References

1. Clark H, Barysh N: Retropharyngeal abscess in an infant of six weeks, complicated by pneumonia and osteomyelitis, with recovery: report of case, *Arch Pediatr* 53:417, 1936.
2. Ravindra C, Merchant R, Dalal S, et al: Retropharyngeal abscesses in infants, *Indian J Pediatr* 50:449, 1983.
3. Steinhauer PF: Ludwig's angina: report of a case in a 12-day-old boy, *J Oral Surg* 25:251, 1967.
4. Masaaki H, Hisashi I, Kyoko T: Retropharyngeal abscess in a 2-month-old infant—a case report, *Otolaryngol Head Neck Surg (Tokyo)* 75:651, 2003.

5. Falup-Pecurariu O, Leibovitz E, Pascu C, Falup-Pecurariu C: 2009 Bacteremic methicillin-resistant *Staphylococcus aureus* deep neck abscess in a newborn—case report and review of literature, *Int J Pediatr Otorhinolaryngol* 73, 1824.
6. Fleisch AF, Nolan S, Gerber J, et al: Methicillin-resistant *Staphylococcus aureus* as a cause of extensive retropharyngeal abscess in two infants, *Pediatr Infect Dis J* 26:1161, 2007.
7. Langewisch WH: An epidemic of group A, type 1 streptococcal infections in newborn infants, *Pediatrics* 18:438, 1956.
8. Asmar BI: Neonatal retropharyngeal cellulitis due to group B streptococcus, *Clin Pediatr (Phila)* 26:183, 1987.
9. Smith WL, Yousefzadeh DK, Yiu-Chiu VS, et al: Percutaneous aspiration of retropharyngeal space in neonates, *AJR Am J Roentgenol* 139:1005, 1982.
10. Bourgeois FT, Shannon MW: Retropharyngeal cellulitis in a 5-week-old infant, *Pediatrics* 109:e51, 2002.
11. Abdullah V, Ng SK, Chow SN, et al: A case of neonatal stridor, *Arch Dis Child Fetal Neonatal Ed* 87:224, 2002.
12. Coulthard M, Isaacs D: Retropharyngeal abscess, *Arch Dis Child* 66:1227, 1991.
13. Coulthard M, Isaacs D: Neonatal retropharyngeal abscess, *Pediatr Infect Dis J* 10:547, 1991.
14. Oppenheimer EH, Winn KJ: Fetal gonorrhea with deep tissue infection occurring in utero, *Pediatrics* 69:74, 1982.
15. Eichenwald HF: "Stuffy nose syndrome" of premature infants: an example of bacterial-viral synergism, *Am J Dis Child* 96:438, 1958.
16. Eichenwald HF, Kotsevalov O, Fasso LA: The "cloud baby": an example of bacterial-viral interaction, *Am J Dis Child* 100:161, 1960.
17. Enwonwu CO, Falkler Jr WA, Idigbe EO, et al: Pathogenesis of cancrum oris (noma): confounding interactions of malnutrition with infection, *Am J Trop Med Hyg* 60:223, 1999.
18. Falkler WA, Enwonwu JCO, Idigbe EO: Isolation of *Fusobacterium necrophorum* from cancrum oris (noma), *Am J Trop Med Hyg* 60:150, 1999.
19. Ghosal SP, Sen Gupta PC, Mukherjee AK, et al: Noma neonatorum: its aetiopathogenesis, *Lancet* 2:289, 1978.
20. Alkalay A, Mogilner BM, Nissim F, et al: Noma in a full-term neonate, *Clin Pediatr (Phila)* 24:528, 1985.
21. Freeman AF, Mancini AJ, Yogev R: Is noma neonatorum a presentation of ecthyma gangrenosum in the newborn? *Pediatr Infect Dis J* 21:83, 2002.
22. Enwonwu CO: Noma—the ulcer of extreme poverty, *N Engl J Med* 354:221, 2006.
23. Baxter JD: Acute epiglottitis in children, *Laryngoscope* 77:1358, 1967.
24. Rosenfeld RM, Fletcher MA, Marban SL: Acute epiglottitis in a newborn infant, *Pediatr Infect Dis J* 11:594, 1992.
25. Young N, Finn A, Powell C: Group B streptococcal epiglottitis, *Pediatr Infect Dis J* 15:95, 1996.
26. Bos AP, Fetter WP, Baerts W, et al: Streptococcal pharyngitis and epiglottitis in a newborn infant, *Eur J Pediatr* 151:874, 1992.
27. Hazard GW, Porter PJ, Ingall D: Pneumococcal laryngitis in the newborn infant: report of a case, *N Engl J Med* 271:361, 1964.
28. Ulualp SO, Rodriguez S, Cunningham S, et al: Pharyngeal pH monitoring in infants with laryngitis, *Otolaryngol Head Neck Surg* 137:776, 2007.
29. Davis WB: Anatomy of the nasal accessory sinuses in infancy and childhood, *Ann Otol Rhinol Laryngol* 27:940, 1918.
30. Wasson WW: Changes in the nasal accessory sinuses after birth, *Arch Otolaryngol* 17:197, 1933.
31. Benner MC: Congenital infection of the lungs, middle ears and nasal accessory sinuses, *Arch Pathol* 29:455, 1940.
32. Cavanagh F: Osteomyelitis of the superior maxilla in infants: a report on 24 personally treated cases, *BMJ* 1:468, 1960.
33. Howard JB, McCracken Jr GH: The spectrum of group B streptococcal infections in infancy, *Am J Dis Child* 128:815, 1974.
34. O'Regan JB, Heenan M, Murray J: Diphtheria in infants, *Ir J Med Sci* 6:116, 1943.
35. Goebel F, Stroder J: Diphtheria in infants, *Dtsch Med Wochenschr* 73:389, 1948.
36. Naiditch MJ, Bower AG: Diphtheria: a study of 1433 cases observed during a ten-year period at the Los Angeles County Hospital, *Am J Med* 17:229, 1954.
37. Galazka AM, Robertson SE: Diphtheria: patterns in the developing world and the industrialized world, *Eur J Epidemiol* 11:107, 1995.
38. Mathur NB, Narang P, Bhatia BD: Neonatal diphtheria, *Indian J Pediatr* 21:174, 1984.
39. Centers for Disease Control and Prevention: Toxigenic *Corynebacterium diphtheriae*—Northern Plains Indian Community, August-October 1996, *MMWR Morb Mortal Wkly Rep* 46:506, 1997.
40. Bisgard KM, Hardy IRB, Popovic T, et al: Virtual elimination of respiratory diphtheria in the United States [Abstract no. G12]. In *Abstracts of the 36th Interscience Conference on Antimicrobial Agents and Chemotherapy*, Washington, DC, 1995, American Society for Microbiology, p 160.
41. World Health Organization: Diphtheria reported cases. Available at http://apps.who.int/immunization_monitoring/globalsummary/timeseries/tsincidencediphtheria.html. Accessed December 16, 2013.
42. Centers for Disease Control and Prevention: 1995 Diphtheria acquired by US citizens in the Russian Federation and Ukraine—1994, *MMWR Morb Mortal Wkly Rep* 44:237, 1995.
43. Golaz A, Hardy IR, Strebel P, et al: Epidemic diphtheria in the newly independent states of the former Soviet Union: implications for diphtheria control in the United States, *J Infect Dis* 18(Suppl 1):S237, 2000.
44. Durbaca S: Antitetanus and antidiphtheria immunity in newborns, *Rom Arch Microbiol Immunol* 58:267, 1999.
45. Vahlquist B: The transfer of antibodies from mother to offspring, *Adv Pediatr* 10:305, 1958.
46. Crossley K, Irvine P, Warren JB, et al: Tetanus and diphtheria immunity in urban Minnesota adults, *JAMA* 242:2298, 1979.
47. Koblin BA, Townsend TR: Immunity to diphtheria and tetanus in inner-city women of child-bearing age, *Am J Public Health* 79:1297, 1989.
48. Maple PA, Efstratiou A, George RC, et al: Diphtheria immunity in UK blood donors, *Lancet* 345:963, 1995.
49. Galazka A: The changing epidemiology of diphtheria in the vaccine era, *J Infect Dis* 181(Suppl 1):S2, 2000.
50. Barr M, Glenny AT, Randall KJ: Concentration of diphtheria antitoxin in cord blood and rate of loss in babies, *Lancet* 2:324, 1949.
51. Cohen P, Scadron SJ: The effects of active immunization of the mother upon the offspring, *J Pediatr* 29:609, 1946.
52. Advisory Committee on Immunization Practices, Centers for Disease Control and Prevention: Updated recommendations for use of tetanus toxoid, reduced diphtheria toxoid, and acellular pertussis vaccine (Tdap) in pregnant women and persons who have or anticipate having close contact with an infant aged <12 months, 2012, *MMWR Morb Mortal Wkly Rep* 62:131, 2013. Available at http://www.cdc.gov/mmwr/preview/mmwrhtml/mm6207a4.htm. Accessed December 16, 2013.
53. Farizo KM, Strebel PM, Chen RT, et al: Fatal respiratory disease due to *Corynebacterium diphtheriae*: case report and review of guidelines for management, investigation, and control, *Clin Infect Dis* 16:59, 1993.
54. Centers for Disease Control and Prevention: Diphtheria, 2013. Available at http://www.cdc.gov/diphtheria/dat.html. Accessed December 16, 2013.
55. Centers for Disease Control and Prevention: Pertussis vaccination: use of acellular pertussis vaccines among infants and young children—recommendations of the Advisory Committee on Immunization Practices (ACIP), *MMWR Recomm Rep* 46(RR-7):2, 1997.
56. Centers for Disease Control and Prevention: Pertussis—United States, January 1992-June 1995, *MMWR Morb. Mortal Wkly Rep* 44:525, 1995.
57. Cortese MM, Baughman AL, Zhang R, et al: Pertussis hospitalizations among infants in the United States, 1993 to 2004, *Pediatrics* 121:484, 2008.
58. Sutter RW, Cochi SL: Pertussis hospitalizations and mortality in the United States, *JAMA* 267:386, 1992.
59. Nelson JD: The changing epidemiology of pertussis in young infants, *Am J Dis Child* 132:371, 1978.
60. Langkamp DL, Davis JP: Increased risk of reported pertussis and hospitalization associated with pertussis in low birth weight children, *J Pediatr* 128:654, 1996.
61. Mikelova LK, Halperin SA, Scheifele D, et al: Predictors of death in infants hospitalized with pertussis: a case-control study of 16 pertussis deaths in Canada, *J Pediatr* 143:576, 2003.
62. Paddock CD, Sanden GN, Cherry JD, et al: Pathology and pathogenesis of fatal *Bordetella pertussis* infection in infants, *Clin Infect Dis* 47:328, 2008.

63. Lovell MA, Miller AM, Hendley O: Pathologic case of the month: pertussis pneumonia, *Arch Pediatr Adolesc Med* 152:925, 1998.
64. Johnston IDA, Strachan DP, Anderson HR: Effect of pneumonia and whooping cough in childhood on adult lung function, *N Engl J Med* 338:581, 1998.
65. Edelman K, Nikkari S, Ruuskanen O, et al: Detection of *Bordetella pertussis* by polymerase chain reaction and culture in the nasopharynx of erythromycin-treated infants with pertussis, *Pediatr Infect Dis J* 15:54, 1996.
66. Dragsted DM, Dohn B, Madsen J, et al: Comparison of culture and PCR for detection of *Bordetella pertussis* and *Bordetella parapertussis* under routine laboratory conditions, *J Med Microbiol* 53:749, 2004.
67 Centers for Disease Control and Prevention: Pertussis (whooping cough): best practices for health care professionals on the use of polymerase chain reaction (PCR) for diagnosing pertussis. Available at http://www.cdc.gov/pertussis/clinical/diagnostic-testing/diagnosis-pcr-bestpractices.html. Accessed December 17, 2013.
68. Pickering LK, Baker CJ, Kimberlin DW, Long SS: Pertussis (whooping cough). In Pickering LK, editor: *Red book: 2009 report of the Committee on Infectious Diseases,* ed 28, Elk Grove Village, Ill, 2009, American Academy of Pediatrics, p 504.
69. Pichichero ME, Hoeger WJ, Casey JR: Azithromycin for the treatment of pertussis, *Pediatr Infect Dis J* 22:847-849, 2003.
70. Granstrom G, Sterner G, Nord CE, et al: Use of erythromycin to prevent pertussis in newborns of mothers with pertussis, *J Infect Dis* 155:1210, 1987.
71. Friedman DS, Curtis CR, Schauer SL, et al: Surveillance for transmission and antibiotic adverse events among neonates and adults exposed to a healthcare worker with pertussis, *Infect Control Hosp Epidemiol* 25:967, 2004.
72. Centers for Disease Control and Prevention: Prevention of pertussis, tetanus, and diphtheria among pregnant and post-partum women and their infants, *MMWR Morb Mortal Wkly Rep* 57:1, 2008.
73. Centers for Disease Control and Prevention: Prevention of tetanus, diphtheria and pertussis among adults: use of tetanus toxoid, reduced diphtheria toxoid, and acellular pertussis vaccine, *MMWR Morb Mortal Wkly Rep* 55:1, 2006.
74. deSa DJ: Infection and amniotic aspiration of middle ear in stillbirth and neonatal deaths, *Arch Dis Child* 48:872, 1973.
75. Keith RW: Middle ear function in neonates, *Arch Otolaryngol* 101:376, 1975.
76. Roberts DG, Johnson CE, Carlin SA, et al: Resolution of middle ear effusion in newborns, *Arch Pediatr Adolesc Med* 149:873, 1995.
77. McLellan MS, Strong JP, Johnson QR, Dent JH: Otitis media in premature infants: a histopathologic study, *J Pediatr* 61:53, 1962.
78. Johnson WW: A survey of middle ears: 101 autopsies of infants, *Ann Otol Rhinol Laryngol* 70:377, 1961.
79. deSa DJ: Mucosal metaplasia and chronic inflammation in the middle ear of infants receiving intensive care in the neonatal period, *Arch Dis Child* 158:24, 1983.
80. Bluestone CD: Pathogenesis of otitis media: role of eustachian tube, *Pediatr Infect Dis J* 15:281, 1996.
81. Balkany TJ, Berman SA, Simmons MA, et al: Middle ear effusions in neonates, *Laryngoscope* 88:398, 1978.
82. Piza J, Gonzalez M, Northrop CC, et al: Meconium contamination of the neonatal middle ear, *J Pediatr* 115:910, 1989.
83. Persico M, Barker GA, Mitchell DP: Purulent otitis media—a "silent" source of sepsis in the pediatric intensive care unit, *Otolaryngol Head Neck Surg* 93:330, 1985.
84. Berman SA, Balkany TJ, Simmons MA: Otitis media in neonatal intensive care unit, *Pediatrics* 62:198, 1978.
85. Nunn DR, Derkay CS, Darrow DH, et al: The effect of very early cleft palate closure on the need for ventilation tubes in the first years of life, *Laryngoscope* 105:905, 1995.
86. Schaefer O: Otitis media and bottle feeding: an epidemiological study of infant feeding habits and incidence of recurrent and chronic middle ear disease in Canadian Eskimos, *Can J Public Health* 62:478, 1971.
87. Chandra RK: Prospective studies of the effect of breast feeding on incidence of infection and allergy, *Acta Paediatr Scand* 68:691, 1979.
88. Pukander J: Acute otitis media among rural children in Finland, *Int. J Pediatr Otorhinolaryngol* 4:325, 1982.
89. Saarinen UM: Prolonged breast feeding as prophylaxis for recurrent otitis media, *Acta Paediatr Scand* 71:567, 1982.
90. Dewey KG, Heinig J, Nommsen-Rivers LA: Differences in morbidity between breast-fed and formula-fed infants, *J Pediatr* 126:696, 1995.
91. Cunningham AS: Morbidity in breast fed and artificially fed infants, *J Pediatr* 90:726, 1977.
92. Teele DW, Klein JO, Rosner B: Epidemiology of otitis media during the first seven years of life in children in Greater Boston: a prospective cohort study, *J Infect Dis* 160:83, 1989.
93. Duncan RB: Positional otitis media, *Arch Otolaryngol* 72:454, 1960.
94. Beauregard WG: Positional otitis media, *J Pediatr* 79:294, 1971.
95. Paradise JL, Elster BA: Breast milk protects against otitis media with effusion, *Pediatr Res* 18:283, 1984.
96. Andersson B, Porras O, Hanson LA, et al: Inhibition of attachment of *Streptococcus pneumoniae* and *Haemophilus influenzae* by human milk and receptor oligosaccharides, *J Infect Dis* 153:232, 1986.
97. Salazar JC, Daly KA, Giebink GS, et al: Low cord blood pneumococcal immunoglobulin G (IgG antibodies predict early onset acute otitis media in infancy), *Am J Epidemiol* 145:1048, 1997.
98. Becken ET, Daly KA, Lindgren BR, et al: Low cord blood pneumococcal antibody concentrations predict more episodes of otitis media, *Arch Otolaryngol Head Neck Surg* 127:517, 2001.
99. Lockhart NJ, Daly KA, Lindgren BR, et al: 2000 Low cord blood type 14 pneumococcal IgG1 but not IgG2 antibody predicts early infant otitis media, *J Infect Dis* 181:1979, 2000.
100. Hajek DM, Quartey M, Giebink GS: Maternal pneumococcal conjugate immunization protects infant chinchillas in the pneumococcal otitis media model, *Acta Otolaryngol* 122:262, 2002.
101. Shahid NS, Steinhoff MC, Hoque SS, et al: Serum, breast milk, and infant antibody after maternal immunization with pneumococcal vaccine, *Lancet* 346:1252, 1995.
102. O'Dempsey TJD, McArdle T, Ceesay SJ, et al: Immunization with a pneumococcal capsular polysaccharide vaccine during pregnancy, *Vaccine* 14:963, 1996.
103. Munoz FM, Englund JA, Cheesman CC, et al: Maternal immunization with pneumococcal polysaccharide vaccine in the third trimester of gestation, *Vaccine* 20:826, 2001.
104. Quimbao BP, Nohynek HM, Käyhty H, et al: Immunogenicity and reactogenicity of 23-valent pneumococcal polysaccharide vaccine among pregnant Filipino women and placental transfer of antibodies, *Vaccine* 25:4470, 2007.
105. Faden H, Duffy L, Wasielewski R, et al: Relationship between nasopharyngeal colonization and the development of otitis media in children, *J Infect Dis* 175:1440, 1997.
106. Rosen IAV, Håkansson A, Aniansson G, et al: Antibodies to pneumococcal polysaccharides in human milk: lack of relationship to colonization and acute otitis media, *Pediatr Infect Dis J* 15:498, 1996.
107. Warren WS, Stool SJE: Otitis media in low-birth-weight infants, *J Pediatr* 79:740, 1971.
108. Jaffe BF, Hurtado F, Hurtado E: Tympanic membrane mobility in the newborn (with seven months' followup), *Laryngoscope* 80:36, 1970.
109. Howie VM, Ploussard JH, Sloyer J: The "otitis-prone" condition, *Am. J Dis Child* 129:676, 1975.
110. Ey JL, Holberg CJ, Aldous MB, et al: Passive smoke exposure and otitis media in the first year of life, *Pediatrics* 95:670, 1995.
111. Stahlberg MR, Ruuskanen O, Virolainen E: Risk factors for recurrent otitis media, *Pediatr Infect Dis J* 5:30, 1986.
112. Bland RD: Otitis media in the first six weeks of life: diagnosis, bacteriology and management, *Pediatrics* 49:187, 1972.
113. Tetzlaff TR, Ashworth C, Nelson JD: Otitis media in children less than 12 weeks of age, *Pediatrics* 59:827, 1977.
114. McLellan MS, Strong JP, Vautier T, et al: Otitis media in the newborn: relationship to duration of rupture of amniotic membrane, *Arch Otolaryngol* 85:380, 1967.
115. Paradise JL, Bluestone CD: Early treatment of universal otitis media of infants with cleft palate, *Pediatrics* 53:48, 1974.
116. Daly KA, Brown JE, Lindgren BR, et al: Epidemiology of otitis media onset by six months of age, *Pediatrics* 103:1158, 1999.
117. Shurin PA, Howie VM, Pelton SI, et al: Bacterial etiology of otitis media during the first six weeks of life, *J Pediatr* 92:893, 1978.
118. Nozicka CA, Hanly JG, Beste DJ, et al: Otitis media in infants aged 0-8 weeks: frequency of associated serious bacterial disease, *Pediatr Emerg Care* 15:252, 1999.
119. Karma PH, Pukander JS, Sipilä MM, et al: Middle ear fluid bacteriology of acute otitis media in neonates and very young infants, *Int J Pediatr Otorhinolaryngol* 14:141, 1987.

120. Turner D, Leibovitz E, Aran A, Piglansky L, et al: Acute otitis media in infants younger than two months of age: microbiology, clinical presentation and therapeutic approach, *Pediatr Infect Dis J* 21:669, 2002.
121. Ng PC, Hiu J, Fok TF, et al: Isolated congenital tuberculosis otitis in a pre-term infant, *Acta Paediatr* 84:955, 1995.
122. Senbil N, Sahin F, Cağlar MK, et al: Congenital tuberculosis of the ear and parotid gland, *Pediatr Infect Dis J* 16:1090, 1997.
123. Parker PC, Boles RG: *Pseudomonas* otitis media and bacteremia following a water birth, *Pediatrics* 99:653, 1997.
124. Decherd ME, Deskin RW, Rowen JL, et al: *Bordetella pertussis* causing otitis media: a case report, *Laryngoscope* 113:226, 2003.
125. Eavey RD, Stool SE, Peckham GJ, et al: How to examine the ear of the neonate, *Clin Pediatr* 15:338, 1976.
126. Cavanaugh RM: Pneumatic otoscopy in healthy full-term infants, *Pediatrics* 79:520, 1987.
127. Pestalozza G, Cusmano G: Evaluation of tympanometry in diagnosis and treatment of otitis media of the newborn and of the infant, *Int J Pediatr Otorhinolaryngol* 2:73, 1980.
128. Barnett ED, Klein JO, Hawkins KA, et al: Comparison of spectral gradient acoustic reflectometry and other diagnostic techniques for detection of middle ear effusion in children with middle ear disease, *Pediatr Infect Dis J* 17:556, 1998.
129. Dowell SF, Butler JC, Giebink GS, et al: Acute otitis media: management and surveillance in an era of pneumococcal resistance—a report from the Drug-Resistant *Streptococcus pneumoniae* Therapeutic Working Group, *Pediatr Infect Dis J* 18:1, 1999.
130. Lee BT, Stingle WH, Ombres P, et al: Neonatal meningitis and mastoiditis caused by Haemophilus influenzae, *JAMA* 235:407, 1976.
131. Meyer K, Girgis N, McGravey V: Adenovirus associated with congenital pleural effusion, *J Pediatr* 107:433, 1985.
132. Reman O, Freymuth F, Laloum D, et al: Neonatal respiratory distress due to mumps, *Arch Dis Child* 61:80, 1986.
133. Srinivasjois RM, Kohan R, Keil AD, Smith NM: Congenital *Mycoplasma pneumoniae* pneumonia in a neonate, *Pediatr Infect Dis J* 27:474, 2008.
134. Boyd MT, Jordan SW, Davis LE: Fatal pneumonitis from congenital echovirus type 6 infection, *Pediatr Infect Dis J* 6:1138, 1987.
135. McLaren LC, Davis LE, Healy GR, James CG: Isolation of *Trichomonas vaginalis* from the respiratory tract of infants with respiratory disease, *Pediatrics* 71:888, 1983.
136. Hiemstra I, Van Bel F, Berger HM: Can *Trichomonas vaginalis* cause pneumonia in newborn babies? *BMJ* 289:355, 1984.
137. Shachor-Meyouhas Y, Kassis I, Bamberger E, et al: Fatal hospital-acquired *Legionella* pneumonia in a neonate, *Pediatr Infect Dis J* 29:280, 2010.
138. Hostoffer RW, Litman A, Smith PG, et al: *Pneumocystis carinii* pneumonia in a term newborn infant with a transiently depressed T lymphocyte count, primarily of cells carrying the CD4 antigen, *J Pediatr* 122:792, 1993.
139. Centers for Disease Control and Prevention: Acute respiratory disease associated with adenovirus serotype 14—four states, 2006-2007, *MMWR Morb Mortal Wkly Rep* 56:1181, 2007.
140. Ahvenainen EK: On congenital pneumonia, *Acta Paediatr* 40:1, 1951.
141. Anderson GS, Green CA, Neligan GA, Newell DJ, Russell JK: Congenital bacterial pneumonia, *Lancet* 2:585, 1962.
142. Barter R: The histopathology of congenital pneumonia: a clinical and experimental study, *J Pathol Bacteriol* 66:407, 1953.
143. Davies PA, Aherne W: Congenital pneumonia, *Arch Dis Child* 37:598, 1962.
144. Langley FA, McCredie Smith JA: Perinatal pneumonia: a retrospective study, *J Obstet Gynaecol Br Commonw* 66:12, 1959.
145. Penner DW, McInnis AC: Intrauterine and neonatal pneumonia, *Am J Obstet Gynecol* 69:147, 1955.
146. Alenghat E, Esterly JR: Alveolar macrophages in perinatal infants, *Pediatrics* 74:221, 1984.
147. Schaffer AJ: The pathogenesis of intrauterine pneumonia, I: a critical review of the evidence concerning intrauterine respiratory-like movements, *Pediatrics* 17:747, 1956.
148. Naeye RL, Dellinger WS, Blanc WA: Fetal and maternal features of antenatal bacterial infection, *J Pediatr* 79:733, 1971.
149. Naeye RL, Tafari N, Judge D, et al: Amniotic fluid infections in an African city, *J Pediatr* 90:965, 1977.
150. Naeye RL, Peters EC: Amniotic fluid infections with intact membranes leading to perinatal death: a prospective study, *Pediatrics* 61:171, 1978.
151. Barter RA, Hudson JA: Bacteriological findings in perinatal pneumonia, *Pathology* 6:223, 1974.
152. Barter RA: Congenital pneumonia, *Lancet* 1:165, 1962.
153. Bernstein J, Wang J: The pathology of neonatal pneumonia, *Am J Dis Child* 101:350, 1961.
154. Finland M: Fetal and perinatal pneumonia. In Charles D, Finland M, editors: *Obstetric and perinatal infections*, Philadelphia, 1973, Lea & Febiger, p 122.
155. Davies PA: Pathogen or commensal? *Arch Dis Child* 55:169, 1980.
156. Ahvenainen EK: Neonatal pneumonia, I: incidence of pneumonia during first month of life, *Ann Med Intern Fenn* 42(Suppl 17):1, 1953.
157. Thaler MM: *Klebsiella-Aerobacter* pneumonia in infants: a review of the literature and report of a case, *Pediatrics* 30:206, 1962.
158. Papageorgiou A, Bauer CR, Fletcher BD, Stern L: *Klebsiella* pneumonia with pneumatocele formation in a newborn infant, *Can Med Assoc J* 109:1217, 1973.
159. Kunh JP, Lee SB: Pneumatoceles associated with *Escherichia coli* pneumonias in the newborn, *Pediatrics* 51:1008, 1973.
160. Jeffery H, Mitchison R, Wigglesworth JS, et al: Early neonatal bacteraemia: comparison of group B streptococcal, other gram-positive and gram-negative infections, *Arch Dis Child* 52:683, 1977.
161. Rojas J, Flanigan TH: Postintubation tracheitis in the newborn, *Pediatr Infect Dis J* 5:714, 1986.
162. Jialin Y, Boman C, Guanxin L, Linyan H, Luquan L: Electron microscopic analysis of bacterial biofilm on tracheal tubes removed from intubated neonates and the relationship between bacterial biofilm and lower respiratory infections, *Pediatrics* 121:S121, 2008.
163. Kollef MH: The prevention of ventilator-associated pneumonia, *N Engl J Med* 340:627, 1999.
164. Barton L, Hodgman JE, Pavlova Z: Causes of death in the extremely low birth weight infant, *Pediatrics* 103:446, 1999.
165. Madan E, Meyer MP, Amortequi A: Chorioamnionitis: a study of organisms isolated in perinatal autopsies. *Ann Clin Lab Sci* 18:39, 1988.
166. Barson AF: A postmortem study of infection in the newborn from 1976 to 1988. In de Louvois J, Harvey D, editors: *Infection in the newborn*, New York, 1990, John Wiley, p 13.
167. Wells DW, Keeney GT: Group F *Streptococcus* associated with intrauterine pneumonia. Letter to the editor, *Pediatrics* 66:820, 1980.
168. Hoffman JA, Mason EO, Schutze GE, et al: *Streptococcus pneumoniae* infections in the neonate, *Pediatrics* 112:1095, 2003.
169. Rhodes PG, Burry VF, Hall RT, et al: Pneumococcal septicemia and meningitis in the neonate, *J Pediatr* 86:593, 1975.
170. Moriartey RR, Finer NN: Pneumococcal sepsis and pneumonia in the neonate, *Am J Dis Child* 133:601, 1979.
171. Naylor JC, Wagner KR: Neonatal sepsis due to Streptococcus pneumoniae, *Can Med Assoc J* 133:1019, 1985.
172. Collier AM, Connor JD, Nyhan WL: Systemic infection with *Haemophilus influenzae* in very young infants, *J Pediatr* 70:539, 1967.
173. Ohlsson A, Bailey T: Neonatal pneumonia caused by *Branhamella catarrhalis*, *Scand J Infect Dis* 17:225, 1985.
174. Andersson S, Larinkari U, Vartia T: Fatal congenital pneumonia caused by cat-derived *Pasteurella multocida*, *Pediatr Infect Dis J* 13:74, 1994.
175. Rowen JL, Lopez SM: *Morganella morganii* early onset sepsis, *Pediatr Infect Dis J* 17:1176, 1998.
176. Franzin L, Scolfaro C, Cabodi D, Valera M, Tovo PA: *Legionella pneumophila* pneumonia in a newborn after water birth: a new mode of transmission, *Clin Infect Dis J* 33:e103, 2001.
177. Brook I: Microbiology of empyema in children and adolescents, *Pediatrics* 85:722, 1990.
178. Siegel JD, McCracken GH: Neonatal lung abscess, *Am J Dis Child* 133:947, 1979.
179. Mayer T, Matlak ME, Condon V, Shasha I, Glasgow L: Computed tomographic findings of neonatal lung abscess, *Am J Dis Child* 139:39, 1982.
180. Famiglietti RF, Bakerman PR, Saubolle MA, et al: Cavitary legionellosis in two immunocompetent infants, *Pediatrics* 99:899, 1997.
181. Adler SC, Chusid MJ: *Citrobacter koseri* pneumonia and meningitis in an infant, *J Infect* 45:65, 2002.
182. Holmberg RE, Pavia AT, Montgomery D, et al: Nosocomial *Legionella* pneumonia in the neonate, *Pediatrics* 92:450, 1993.
183. Shamir R, Horev G, Merlob P, et al: *Citrobacter diversus* lung abscess in a preterm infant, *Pediatr Infect Dis. J* 9:221, 1990.
184. Vevon GP, Dunne Jr WM, Hicks MJ, et al: *Bacillus cereus* pneumonia in premature neonates: a report of two cases, *Pediatr Infect Dis J* 12:251, 1993.
185. Gupta R, Faridi MM, Gupta P: Neonatal empyema thoracis, *Indian J Pediatr* 63:704, 1996.

186. Khan EA, Wafelman LS, Garcia-Prats JA, et al: *Serratia marcescens* pneumonia, empyema and pneumatocele in a preterm neonate, *Pediatr Infect Dis J* 16:1003, 1997.
187. Thaarup J, Ellermann-Eriksen S, Sternholm J: Neonatal pleural empyema with group A *Streptococcus, Acta Paediatr* 86:769, 1997.
188. Nathavitharana KA, Watkinson M: Neonatal pleural empyema caused by group A *Streptococcus, Pediatr Infect Dis J* 13:671, 1994.
189. Briggs EJN, Hogg G: Pneumonia found at autopsy in infants weighing less than 750 grams, *Can Med Assoc J* 85:6, 1961.
190. Briggs EJN, Hogg G: Perinatal pulmonary pathology, *Pediatrics* 22:41, 1958.
191. Browne FJ: Pneumonia neonatorum, *BMJ* 1:469, 1922.
192. Fujikura T, Froehlich LA: Intrauterine pneumonia in relation to birth weight and race, *Am J Obstet Gynecol* 97:81, 1967.
193. Sinha A, Yokoe D, Platt R: Epidemiology of neonatal infections: experience during and after hospitalization, *Pediatr Infect Dis J* 22:244, 2003.
194. Bang AT, Bang RA, Morankar VP, et al: Pneumonia in neonates. Can it be managed in the community? *Arch Dis Child* 68:550, 1993.
195. Kishore K, Deorari AK, Singh M, et al: Early onset neonatal sepsis—vertical transmission from maternal genital tract, *Indian Pediatr J* 24:45, 1987.
196. Sazawal S, Black RE: Effect of pneumonia case management on mortality in neonates, infants, and preschool children: a meta-analysis of community-based trials, *Lancet Infect Dis* 3:547, 2003.
197. Singhi S, Singhi PD: Clinical signs in neonatal pneumonia, *Lancet* 336:1072, 1990.
198. World Health Organization: *Acute respiratory infections in children: case management in small hospitals in developing countries*, Geneva, 1990, World Health Organization.
199. Soofi S, Ahmed S: 2012 Effectiveness of community based management of severe pneumonia with oral amoxicillin in children aged 2-59 months in Matiari District, rural Pakistan: a cluster- randomized controlled trial, *Lancet* 379:729, 2012.
200. Petersen S, Astvad K: Pleural empyema in a newborn infant, *Acta Paediatr Scand* 65:527, 1976.
201. Gustavson EE: *Escherichia coli* empyema in the newborn, *Am J Dis Child* 140:408, 1986.
202. Mathur NB, Garg K, Kumar S: Respiratory distress in neonates with special reference to pneumonia, *Indian Pediatr* 39:529, 2002.
203. Ablow RC, Gross I, Effmann EL, et al: The radiographic features of early onset group B streptococcal neonatal sepsis, *Radiology* 124:771, 1977.
204. Thomas DB, Anderson JC: Antenatal detection of fetal pleural effusion and neonatal management, *Med J Aust* 2:435, 1979.
205. Steele RW, Thomas MP, Kolls JK: Current management of community-acquired pneumonia in children: an algorithmic guideline recommendation, *Infect Med* 16:46, 1999.
206. Klein JO: Diagnostic lung puncture in the pneumonias of infants and children, *Pediatrics* 44:486, 1969.
207. Teele DW, Pelton SI, Grant MJ, et al: Bacteremia in febrile children under 2 years of age: results of cultures of blood of 600 consecutive febrile children seen in a "walk-in" clinic, *J Pediatr* 87:227, 1975.
208. Sherman MP, Goetzman BW, Ahlfors CE, et al: Tracheal aspiration and its clinical correlates in the diagnosis of congenital pneumonia, *Pediatrics* 65:258, 1980.
209. Thureen PJ, Moreland S, Rodden DJ, et al: Failure of tracheal aspirate cultures to define the cause of respiratory deteriorations in neonates, *Pediatr Infect Dis J* 12:560, 1993.
210. Lau YL, Hey E: Sensitivity and specificity of daily tracheal aspirate cultures in predicting organisms causing bacteremia in ventilated neonates, *Pediatr Infect Dis J* 10:290, 1991.
211. Fan LL, Sparks LM, Dulinski JP: Applications of an ultrathin flexible bronchoscope for neonatal and pediatric airway problems, *Chest* 89:673, 1986.
212. Alexander HE, Craig HR, Shirley RG, Ellis C: Validity of etiology diagnosis of pneumonia in children by rapid typing from nasopharyngeal mucus, *J Pediatr* 18:31, 1941.
213. Bollowa JGM: Primary pneumonias of infants and children, *Public Health Rep* 51:1076, 1903.
214. Cheu MHW, Lally KP, Clark R, et al: Open lung biopsy in the critically ill newborn, *Pediatrics* 86:561, 1990.
215. Greenough A: Gains and losses from dexamethasone for neonatal chronic lung disease, *Lancet* 352:835, 1998.
216. Yeh TF, Lin YJ, Lin HC, et al: Outcomes at school age after postnatal dexamethasone therapy for lung disease of prematurity, *N Engl J Med* 350:1304, 2004.
217. Onland W, Offringa M, van Kaam A: Late (≥ 7 days) inhalation corticosteroids to reduce bronchopulmonary dysplasia in preterm infants. *Cochrane Database Syst Rev* 4:CD002311, 2012.
218. Aherne W, Davies PA: Congenital pneumonia, *Lancet* 1:234, 1962.
219. Tam ASY, Yeung CY: Gastric aspirate findings in neonatal pneumonia, *Arch Dis Child* 47:735, 1972.
220. Pole VRG, McAllister TA: Gastric aspirate analysis in the newborn, *Acta Paediatr Scand* 64:109, 1975.
221. Whitelaw A, Evans A, Corrin B: Immotile cilia syndrome: a new cause of neonatal respiratory distress, *Arch Dis Child* 56:432, 1981.
222. Ramet J, Byloos J, Delree M, et al: Neonatal diagnosis of the immotile cilia syndrome, *Chest* 89:138, 1986.
223. Ciliary dyskinesia and ultrastructural abnormalities in respiratory disease: *Lancet* 1:1370, 1988.
224. Giacoia GP, Neter E, Ogra P: Respiratory infections in infants on mechanical ventilation: the immune response as a diagnostic aid, *J Pediatr* 98:691, 1981.
225. Marks MI, Law B: Respiratory infections vs. colonization, *J Pediatr* 100:508, 1982.
226. Nigrovic LE, Kuppermann N, McAdam AJ, et al: Cerebrospinal latex agglutination fails to contribute to the microbiologic diagnosis of pretreated children with meningitis, *Pediatr Infect Dis J* 23:786, 2004.
227. Lung function in children after neonatal meconium aspiration, *Lancet* 2:317, 1988.
228. Smith RM, Brumley GW, Stannard MW: Neonatal pneumonia associated with medium-chain triglyceride feeding supplement, *J Pediatr* 92:801, 1978.
229. Hjalmarson O: Epidemiology of classification of acute, neonatal respiratory disorders: a prospective study, *Acta Paediatr Scand* 70:773, 1981.
230. Mounla NA: Neonatal respiratory disorders, *Acta Paediatr Scand* 76:159, 1987.
231. Avery ME, Fletcher BD, Williams RE: *The lung and its disorders in the newborn infant*, Philadelphia, 1981, WB Saunders.
232. Butler NR, Alberman ED: Clinicopathological associations of hyaline membranes, intraventricular haemorrhage, massive pulmonary haemorrhage and pulmonary infection. In *British Perinatal Mortality Survey, second report: perinatal problems*, Edinburgh, 1969, Livingstone, p 184.
233. Foote GA, Stewart JH: The coexistence of pneumonia and the idiopathic respiratory distress syndrome in neonates, *Br J Radiol* 46:504, 1973.
234. Ablow RC, Driscoll SG, Effmann EL, et al: A comparison of early-onset group B streptococcal infection and the respiratory distress syndrome of the newborn, *N Engl J Med* 294:65, 1976.
235. Menke JA, Giacoia GP, Jockin H: Group B beta hemolytic streptococcal sepsis and the idiopathic respiratory distress syndrome: a comparison, *J Pediatr* 94:467, 1979.
236. Lloyd-Still JD, Khaw KT, Schwachman H: Severe respiratory disease in infants with cystic fibrosis, *Pediatrics* 53:678, 1974.
237. Delville JG, Adler S, Azimi PH, et al: Linezolid versus vancomycin in the treatment of known or suspected resistant gram-positive infections in neonates, *Pediatr Infect Dis J* 22:S158, 2003.
238. Ahvenainen EK: A study of causes of neonatal deaths, *J Pediatr* 55:691, 1959.
239. Osborn GT: Discussion on neonatal deaths, *Proc R Soc Med* 51:840, 1958.
240. Butler NR, Bonham DG: *Perinatal mortality*, London, 1963, Livingstone.
241. Apisarnthanarak A, Holzmann-Pazgal G, Hamvas A, et al: Ventilator-associated pneumonia in extremely preterm neonates in a neonatal intensive care unit: characteristics, risk factors, and outcomes, *Pediatrics* 12:1283, 2003.
242. Pacifico L, Panero A, Roggini M, et al: *Ureaplasma urealyticum* and pulmonary outcome in a neonatal intensive care population, *Pediatr Infect Dis J* 16:579, 1997.
243. Brasfield DM, Stagno S, Whitley RJ, et al: Infant pneumonitis associated with cytomegalovirus, *Chlamydia, Pneumocystis* and *Ureaplasma*: follow-up, *Pediatrics* 79:76, 1987.

8

Bacterial Infections of the Bones and Joints

MARTHA MULLER and GARY D. OVERTURF

CHAPTER OUTLINE

Osteomyelitis

Osteomyelitis occurring in the first 2 months of life is uncommon. During the worldwide pandemic of staphylococcal disease from the early 1950s to the early 1960s, pediatric centers in Europe,[1-5] Australia,[6] and North America[6-11] reported the infrequent occurrence of neonatal osteomyelitis, accounting for only one or two admissions per year at each institution.[12-16] An overall incidence of neonatal osteomyelitis has been reported as 1 in 5000 to 15,000 live births.[17] With the introduction of invasive neonatal supportive care and the increased use of diagnostic and therapeutic procedures, there was concern that osteomyelitis and septic arthritis secondary to bacteremia might occur more frequently in the newborn.[18] Yet subsequent experience in Europe,[19-21] Canada,[22,23] and the United States[11,24,25] (J.D. Nelson, personal communication, 1987) during the decade 1970 to 1979 indicated little or no change in the incidence of this condition. Even in intensive care nurseries, despite an increasing problem with fungal (*Candida*) osteoarthritis,[26-30] the overall rate of occurrence of nosocomial bone and joint infections remained low at equal to or less than 2.6 per 1000 admissions.[28,31,32] Infections associated with invasive procedures, such as placement of intravascular catheters, may not appear (or be recognized) until days or weeks after the perinatal period, however.[18,28] Although the incidence has not changed, causative organisms have become increasingly resistant to antibiotics, as exemplified by the increased incidence of *Staphylococcus aureus* infections resistant to oxacillin (methicillin-resistant *S. aureus* [MRSA]).

Little had been published on the relative incidence of neonatal osteomyelitis during the 1980s and 1990s. An ongoing review of nursery infections at a Kaiser Permanente hospital in southern California revealed only 3 cases of osteomyelitis among 67,000 consecutive live births from 1963 to 1993, and none occurred in the final years (A. Miller, personal communication, 1993). A similar survey performed at two pediatric referral centers in Texas showed no significant variation in the number of annual admissions for this condition from 1964 to 1986[33] (J.D. Nelson, personal communication, 1987). One to 3 cases of bone or joint infection per 1000 admissions remains a reported incidence, almost identical to that noted in years past.[12-14,28,31,32]

In a review of more than 300 cases of neonatal osteomyelitis, male infants predominated over female infants (1.6:1). Premature infants acquire osteomyelitis with relatively greater frequency than term infants.[11,19,22,34-43] In a series of osteomyelitis, 17 of 30 proven cases were in premature infants, 4 occurred in term infants receiving intensive care, and *S. aureus* was responsible for 23 of the proven cases of osteomyelitis (methicillin-sensitive strains in 16 cases and MRSA in 7 cases).[44] *Escherichia coli* and group B streptococci (GBS) caused 3 and 2 cases, respectively. Risk factors for osteomyelitis and septic arthritis in premature infants have been mostly iatrogenic, including use of intravenous or intraarterial catheters, ventilatory support, and bacteremia with nosocomial pathogens.

Risk factors for osteomyelitis have been reviewed in detail in other publications.[45] Osteomyelitis and septic arthritis today are largely associated with nosocomial bacteria acquired with systemic infection during neonatal intensive care. Narang and colleagues[46] noted an incidence of 1 per 1500 in cases of bone and joint infections, with a mean gestational age of 34 weeks (range, 27-40) and mean birth weight of 2269 (range, 990-4750), emphasizing the high risk among premature infants. In addition to sepsis, both septic arthritis and osteomyelitis are risks for infection of the adjacent site, either the synovium or the bone. Box 8-1 reviews the known risk factors presented in most series. The neonate, and particularly the premature infant, is at much higher risk of multifocal osteomyelitis. For instance, Howan-Giles and Uren[47] found that two peaks of multifocal osteomyelitis occurred with the first peak of less than 6 weeks, accounting for 38% of the cases of multifocal osteomyelitis. The association of sepsis and/or urinary tract infections or urinary tract anomalies has frequently been observed.[48,49] The presence of certain focal or predisposing conditions has long been recognized, such as cephalohematomas and/or

Box 8-1 Risk Factors for Septic Arthritis and Osteomyelitis in Neonates

Prematurity

Sepsis

Urinary Tract Infection

Respiratory distress syndrome

Umbilical Artery Catheterization

Intravenous line infection
Breech delivery

Birth Trauma

Associated nerve palsies of the upper extremity

Cephalohematoma

Fetal scalp monitoring

Surgical Wounds

infection after fetal monitors with direct osteomyelitis of the skull. In addition, the associations of hip septic arthritis associated with breech delivery,[50] and of brachial palsy with septic arthritis of the hip and shoulder, respectively, have been recognized for the complication of joint infection. Cieslak and Rajnik[50-52] calculated a high incidence of septic arthritis or pelvic osteomyelitis among breech infants with an incidence of approximately 1 per 8000 or a relative risk of 4.1 compared with nonbreech infants. Abnormal uterine posture of the upper limb or associated radial nerve palsy has frequently been associated with septic arthritis.

Although osteomyelitis was rare in the past, more recent series have suggested that the frequency may be increasing in neonates. The spectrum of bacterial and fungal infections in Finland from 1985 to 1989 was studied with 2836 infections in children.[53] The incidence of osteomyelitis and septic arthritis in children 28 days of age or younger was 67.7 per 100,000 person-years, compared with rates of 262.2 and 2013.1 per 100,000 for meningitis and bacteremia, respectively; pneumonia (80.4 per 100,000) and pyelonephritis (143.8 per 100,000) also were more frequent than bone or joint infections. Studies from other countries have also suggested an increase in osteomyelitis; among 241 bone infections in Panamanian children, 9 occurred in neonates (3 cases were due to gram-negative bacilli; 3 cases, to *S. aureus*; 1 case, to GBS; and 2 cases, to other organisms).[54]

MICROBIOLOGY

Because most cases of neonatal osteomyelitis arise as a consequence of bacteremia, the organisms responsible for causing osteomyelitis reflect the changing trends in the etiology of neonatal sepsis. Before 1940, hemolytic streptococci were the predominant organisms responsible for sepsis in newborns[55] and frequently caused osteomyelitis.[56,57] Streptococci were implicated in most cases of osteomyelitis in neonates and infants younger than 6 months.[58]

After 1950, the incidence of *S. aureus* osteomyelitis increased. A review of reports from 1952 to 1972 showed that 85% of the infections were caused by *S. aureus*, 6% were caused by hemolytic streptococci (no groups specified), and 2% were due to *Streptococcus pneumoniae*; either no organisms or miscellaneous organisms (particularly gram-negative bacilli) were isolated in 7% of the cases.[2-6,11,37,40,59-65] MRSA has infected many nurseries and has been associated with disseminated infections of neonates, including endocarditis, skin and soft tissue infections, organ abscesses, and osteomyelitis and septic arthritis. Community-acquired strains of MRSA have become increasingly more common in neonatal units; at the present time, 50% or more of infections are caused by MRSA strains acquired outside of the hospital. Osteomyelitis and septic arthritis have been observed in these outbreaks as part of a general septic dissemination of MRSA to multiple organs and multiple sites (reviewed in Chapter 14).

Recognition of group B streptococcal sepsis in the late 1960s to the 1970s was associated with a concomitant increase in reported frequency of bone and joint infections caused by this organism.[12,26,66] This change in spectrum was reflected in U.S. reviews of osteomyelitis in infants hospitalized from 1965 to 1978, showing that GBS had become the most frequent agent.[11,25,67] This experience was not universal, however; newborn centers in Canada,[22] Sweden,[19] Spain,[68] Switzerland,[20] Nigeria,[69] and sections of the United States[33] continued to find *S. aureus* as the predominant cause of osteomyelitis, with GBS accounting for only a few cases. Although their relative importance may vary by region or institution, these two organisms have remained the most common cause of neonatal osteomyelitis.[34,35,42,70] A review of cases of occult bacteremia caused by GBS identified 147 children.[71] Eleven of these children had nonmeningeal foci, including 2 with septic arthritis and 2 with osteomyelitis. More recent cases of unusual sites of group B streptococcal osteomyelitis in the iliac wing[72] and the vertebrae[73] emphasize the renewed importance and frequency of this infection.

Osteomyelitis caused by gram-negative enteric bacilli is uncommon despite the frequency of neonatal bacteremia.[34,55,74,75] In Stockholm during 1969 to 1979, *E. coli* and *Klebsiella*/*Enterobacter* were responsible for about 30% of cases of neonatal septicemia[21] but only 5% of bone infections.[19] *S. aureus*, although also causing about 30% of neonatal bacteremia cases, was responsible for 75% of cases of osteomyelitis. Several other surveys performed within the past 2 decades show about 10% of cases of neonatal osteomyelitis to be due to gram-negative enteric bacilli,* although rates of 19%[69] and 45%[41,42,68] have been observed. A review of the literature has revealed isolated instances of hematogenous osteomyelitis in newborns caused by *E. coli*,† *Proteus* spp.,[19,25,62,76-80] *Klebsiella pneumoniae*,‡ *Enterobacter*,[68,77,85,86] *Serratia marcescens*,[25,68] *Pseudomonas* spp.,§ and *Salmonella* spp.[22,33,41,88-92]

Although bacteremia resulting from infected invasive devices is a common cause of enteric osteomyelitis, infection may occur directly by translocation from the gut or from urinary tract infection. Studies of neonatal rats have suggested that formula feeding enhances translocation of

*References 11, 20, 22, 33, 40, 70
†References 2, 8, 11, 19, 20, 25, 36, 40-42, 57, 62, 68, 76-81.
§References 25, 37, 40, 42, 57, 68, 87, 88.
‡References 19, 42, 43, 68, 81, 82-84.

enteric organisms, with subsequent infection of the bone,[93] although other organs were infected as well. Although translocation of bacteria occurred in 23% of breastfed rats, compared with 100% of formula-fed rats, positive bone cultures developed in 77% of the formula-fed rats, whereas none of the breastfed rats had positive cultures. A single case of a 4-week-old boy with urinary tract infection with *K. pneumoniae* and vesicoureteral reflux suggests that this site also may be a source of gram-negative enteric bone and joint infections.[94]

Whereas suppurative arthritis is the most common manifestation of gonococcal sepsis involving the skeletal system,[95] osteomyelitis is associated with sepsis as well and probably represents the site of primary infection in many cases.[40,96,97] Syphilitic osteitis and osteochondritis, although frequent in former years,[98] have been largely eliminated through serologic detection of disease during routine antenatal testing and institution of appropriate therapy for infected mothers. An increase in the incidence of syphilis among women of childbearing age has been reflected in a parallel increase in the frequency of neonatal syphilis and attendant problems of treponemal bone infection.[99,100]

Mycoplasma and *Ureaplasma* have been reported as rare causes of osteomyelitis in infants. In one infant, bone infection caused by *Mycoplasma hominis* developed in a sternotomy wound after cardiac surgery[101]; in another infant weighing 900 g with osteomyelitis of the hip and femur, the infection was caused by *Ureaplasma urealyticum*.[102] Tuberculous osteomyelitis is extremely rare in neonates, even in the presence of disseminated congenital tuberculosis.[103,104] Among a group of infants with widespread disease acquired in the perinatal or neonatal period, the youngest with skeletal involvement was 3 months of age.[97]

Candida species are also rare causes of neonatal osteomyelitis.[105,106] Pan and colleagues[107] reported a total of 22 cases of *Candida albicans* osteomyelitis in infants and children. All of the 19 neonates and infants presented in the review were thought to have sustained infection as a complication of candidemia during their neonatal intensive care unit hospitalization.[107] Of special note is the observation that the presentation of osteoarticular infections with *Candida* species may be delayed for several months, inclusive of treatment for previous systemic disease,[105-107] prompting the need for diligent monitoring after infection. Although *Candida albicans* has been the most common cause of bone and joint infections, Oleinik and colleagues[108] reported a case of osteomyelitis caused by antifungal resistant *Candida lusitaniae* successfully treated with a combination of 5-flucytosine and fluconazole, and Weisse and colleagues[109] have reported a case of arthritis caused by *Candida tropicalis* necessitating treatment with 5-flucytosine and amphotericin B.

PATHOGENESIS

Acute osteomyelitis is generally the rule for neonates with the infection.[110] Complications of pregnancy, labor, or delivery may precede the occurrence of neonatal osteomyelitis in one half of patients.[‖] Most bone and joint infections occur in a small or premature infant as a result of prolonged nosocomial exposures and multiple invasive procedures. Although anoxia (as from placenta previa, breech extraction, or fetal distress) or exposure to microorganisms (from premature rupture of membranes) can explain this association in some cases, the means whereby maternal or obstetric problems influence the likelihood of acquiring bone infection is generally unknown.

Microorganisms may reach the skeletal tissues of the fetus and newborn in one of four ways: (1) by direct inoculation, (2) by extension from infection in surrounding soft tissues, (3) as a consequence of maternal bacteremia with transplacental infection and fetal sepsis, and (4) by bloodborne dissemination in the course of neonatal septicemia. Although hematogenous dissemination is responsible for most cases, examples of other routes of infection have appeared occasionally in the literature. As noted previously (see "Microbiology"), other factors, such as preceding urinary tract infection or direct translocation of bacteria across the bowel wall, may explain bone or joint infection in some neonates.

Direct inoculation of bacteria resulting in osteomyelitis has followed femoral venipuncture,[38,79,80,111-113] radial artery puncture,[68] use of a fetal scalp monitor,[20,114-117] capillary blood sampling from the great toe[95,118] or heel,[20,68,70,119-123] and serial lumbar punctures.[124] Infection after surgical invasion of bony structures (e.g., median sternotomy for cardiac surgery) is uncommon.[125] Nevertheless, trauma has been associated with osteomyelitis of the neonate (an association that has been noted for osteomyelitis in older children); *S. aureus* osteomyelitis has occurred in a neonate at 3 weeks of age at the site of a perinatal fracture of the clavicle.[126]

Osteomyelitis caused by extension of infection from surrounding soft tissues usually is associated with organisms from an infected cephalohematoma involving the adjacent parietal bone.[115,127-131] A series of patients with *S. aureus* osteomyelitis of the skull associated with overlying scalp abscesses was reported in 1952.[132] Predisposing factors in these patients were thought to be prolonged, excessive pressure on the fetal head when it lay against the sacral promontory or symphysis pubis, secondary ischemic necrosis, and localization of infection. *E. coli* has also been associated with this phenomenon, including one report of infection in 2011 with an extended-spectrum β-lactamase–producing isolate.[131] Paronychia during the newborn period, although most frequently a source of sepsis and hematogenous dissemination of organisms, may extend into bony structures and cause phalangeal infection.[57]

Transplacental bacterial bone infection is most characteristic of syphilis (see Chapter 16). A rare exception, published as a case report in 1933, described a premature infant who died at 19 hours of age with evidence of subacute parietal bone osteomyelitis, meningitis, and cerebritis. Rupture of the amniotic sac immediately before delivery, histopathologic evidence of the prolonged course (at least 2 weeks) of the infection, and the lack of involvement of the overlying scalp epidermis indicate that despite apparent absence of maternal illness, this infant was infected transplacentally. The authors postulated that a primary infection occurred in the parietal bone, with secondary extension to the meninges and brain. Although organisms were not isolated, gram-positive diplococci were identified in infected tissues.[133]

Bloodborne dissemination of organisms, with metastatic seeding of the skeletal system through nutrient

‖References 11, 19, 22, 25, 40-42, 68.

arteries, is the major cause of neonatal osteomyelitis.[56,134] Before the advent of antibiotics, the long bones reportedly became infected in 10% of infants with bacteremia.[57,135] Since that time, early recognition and effective empirical therapy for bacterial sepsis led to a marked decrease in the incidence of this complication. Candidal invasion of the bloodstream has become a more frequent cause of bone and joint infections in small infants[¶] (also see Chapter 33).

The use of intravascular catheters has frequently been associated with bacterial and fungal osteomyelitis in neonates.[#] Septic embolization occurs from infected catheter-tip thrombi, producing relatively high-grade bacteremias; local hypoxia from partial occlusion of vessels by the catheter may also contribute to bone infections.[18,147] The most common etiologic agent has been *S. aureus*, but other microorganisms, such as *Klebsiella*,[84] *Proteus*,[75] *Enterobacter*,[85,86] and *Candida*,[26,28,77,136] have also been implicated. Because the iliac arteries are the most likely pathway for an arterial embolus originating in an aortic catheter tip, the hips or knees or both are involved in more than three fourths of patients.[*a] There is a very close correlation between the site of the catheter and localization of osteomyelitis in the ipsilateral leg.[18] The distribution of infection originating in umbilical vein catheters is less predictable[†a] The incidence of osteoarthritis varies greatly, ranging from 1 in 30[148] to less than 1 in 600[18] infants with umbilical artery catheters; it can be reduced significantly by proper attention to aseptic technique and careful monitoring of catheter placement combined with prompt catheter removal whenever possible.[18]

The disseminating focus of a bacteremia-producing metastatic abscess in bones is often unknown. Common primary sources include omphalitis[‡a] pustular dermatitis[§a] purulent rhinitis,[5,64,141] paronychia,[‖a] and mastitis.[4,59] In a few infants, sepsis with subsequent osteomyelitis has arisen from infected circumcisions,[8,38] operative sites,[8,70,80] intramuscular injections,[59,80] or varicella lesions.[11] Although gonococcal osteoarthritis originates most commonly from a purulent conjunctivitis, virtually any orifice may provide a portal of entry.[95]

Hematogenous infection of long bones is initiated in dilated capillary loops of the metaphysis, adjacent to the cartilaginous growth plate (physis), where blood flow slows, providing pathogenic bacteria with an ideal environment to multiply, resulting in abscess formation (Fig. 8-1).[17,134,142,143] When the infectious process localizes at this site, the following sequence may occur: (1) direct invasion and lysis of the cartilaginous growth plate; (2) spread from metaphyseal vessel loops into transphyseal vessels coursing through the growth plate and into epiphyseal vessels; or (3) rupture occurring laterally through the cortex into the joint, subperiosteal space, or surrounding soft tissues.[142,143] The large vascular spaces and thin spongy structure of metaphyseal cortex in infants permit early decompression of this primary abscess into the

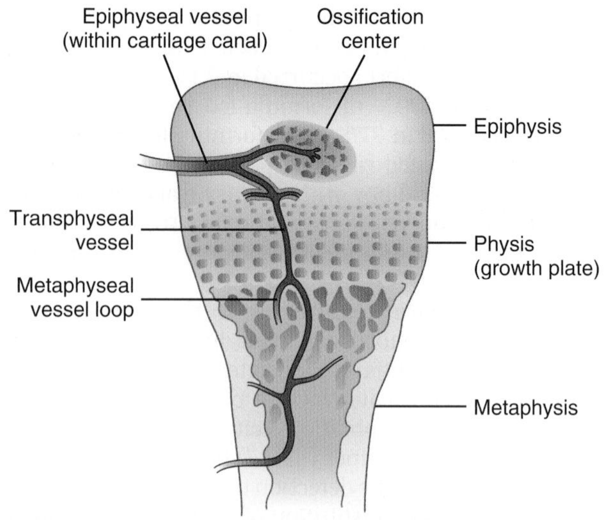

Figure 8-1 Schematic depiction of blood supply in the neonatal epiphysis. In children, normally there are two separate circulatory systems: (1) the metaphyseal loops, derived from the diaphyseal nutrient artery, and (2) the epiphyseal vessels, which course through the epiphyseal cartilage within structures termed cartilage canals. In the neonatal period, sinusoidal vessels, termed transphyseal vessels, connect these two systems. With ensuing skeletal maturation, these vessels disappear, and the epiphyseal and metaphyseal systems become totally separated.

subperiosteal space.[58,65] For this reason, the bone marrow compartment is seldom involved in neonates, and the term osteitis is probably more accurate than osteomyelitis.

After rupture into the subperiosteal space, the abscess dissects rapidly beneath loosely attached periosteum, often involving the entire length and circumference of the bone. As pressure increases from accumulating pus, there may be decompression through the thin, periosteal tissue into surrounding soft tissues, and a subcutaneous abscess may form. In the absence of surgical intervention, collected pus "points" and drains spontaneously through the skin, forming a sinus tract. When adequate decompression and drainage have been established, general supportive care often is sufficient to permit complete healing and resolution of osseous and soft tissue foci of infection.[56,58,144,145] Free communication between the original site of osteomyelitis and the subperiosteal space prevents the necrosis and extensive spread of infection through the bone shaft, which occurs frequently in older children and adults. Cortical sequestra are less common in infants, and because of the extreme richness of the newborn bone blood supply, sequestra often are completely absorbed, if they do form.[58] In addition, the efficient vasculature and fertility of the inner layer of the periosteum encourage early development of profuse new bone formation (involucrum), permitting remodeling of bone within a very short time after the infectious process has been controlled.[58,134]

The same characteristics of neonatal bone that serve to prevent many of the features of chronic osteomyelitis seen in older children are also responsible for complications occurring in neonates and young infants, such as epiphysitis and pyarthrosis. A consequence of the excellent bone blood supply in newborns is persistent fetal vessels that penetrate the cartilaginous epiphyseal plate and end in large venous lakes within the epiphysis.[134,142,143] Localization of

¶References 26, 28, 29, 35, 136, 137.
#References 11, 19, 22, 26, 28, 29, 42, 89-91, 138-146.
*aReferences 11, 18, 84, 86, 138, 147.
†aReferences 28, 85, 136, 139, 140, 147.
‡aReferences 4, 5, 11, 34, 41, 42, 59, 82, 86, 148, 149-151.
§aReferences 4, 11, 25, 35, 41, 59, 62, 68, 80.
‖aReferences 4, 5, 39, 61, 64, 80, 141.

organisms at these sites early in the course of osteomyelitis leads to an epiphysitis, with resultant severe damage of the cartilage cells on the epiphyseal side of the growth plate. When such damage occurs, it is generally irreparable[81,134] and ultimately results in arrest or disorganization of growth at the ends of the bone. By age 8 to 18 months, the vascular connections between metaphysis and epiphysis are obliterated, and the cartilaginous growth plate provides a barrier against the spread of infection that persists throughout childhood and adult life.[134,142,143]

Rapid decompression of the primary metaphyseal abscess through the adjacent cortex also permits ready entrance of pus into the articular space of the bones whose metaphyses lie within the articular capsule of the joint. Given the unique vascularity of the infant, suppurative arthritis of the hips, shoulders, elbows, and knees is frequently associated with osteomyelitis of the humerus or femur in infants.[¶a] This common extension of infection into the contiguous joint space is reported in 50% to 76% of infections.[13,15,107] When the infection originates in the epiphysis, pyarthrosis also may occur by direct extension of the primary abscess through the articular cartilage and into the joint space. Laxity of the surrounding musculature and increasing pressure secondary to purulence lend to distention of the joint capsule, and the increasing pressure may eventually produce a pathologic dislocation, particularly of the shoulder or hip joint.[107] The lytic action of pyogenic exudate within the joint[146,149] and ischemia produced by the high intraarticular tension often are sufficient to cause dissolution or separation of the entire head of the femur or humerus, both of which are composed almost completely of cartilage during the neonatal period.[#a] Although serious growth disturbances and deformities may result from septic arthritis at other sites, complete destruction of the joint is rare.

CLINICAL MANIFESTATIONS

Two distinct clinical syndromes that may be associated with suppurative bone involvement in the newborn period are (1) a benign form, with little or no evidence of infection (other than local swelling) or disability, related to an osteomyelitis involving one or more skeletal sites, and (2) a severe form, with systemic manifestations of sepsis predominating until multiple sites of bone and visceral involvement are noted as manifestations of the infant's underlying condition.[3,39,46,152] Reported to be influenced more by the offending organism than the host response,[13] the most likely cause of the benign form of neonatal osteomyelitis is a mild, transient bacteremia that arises peripherally and causes only minimal inflammation and suppuration. The experience of most investigators indicates that this form of illness represents most cases.[*b] Because fever is notably an unreliable sign in neonates with osteomyelitis,[23] the few series in which high fever and evidence of sepsis were noted as common presenting signs probably represent instances in which diagnosis was delayed, resulting in more advanced disease at presentation.[2,3,41,59] Infants with mild illness generally feed well, gain weight, and develop normally. Systemic manifestations are minimal, and the temperature is usually normal or only slightly elevated.[†b]

Neonates have an immature immune system that is thought to contribute to infections with organisms of low virulence, as well as a delay in the development of clinical signs.[16,106] As a result, the diagnosis may be missed until 2 to 4 weeks have elapsed, by which time bone destruction may be severe and widespread.[57,63,65,142] Even in intensive care nurseries, where infants are under continuous professional observation, osteomyelitis may be missed for days or weeks. Bone involvement may be discovered during a skeletal survey or computed tomography (CT) or magnetic resonance imaging (MRI) as an unsuspected site or sites of infection in an infant without known bone involvement; osteomyelitis also has been diagnosed as an incidental finding on chest or abdominal radiographs.[22,28,153]

The first signs that may be noted by parents or physicians are diffuse edema and swelling of an extremity or joint, usually without discoloration, accompanied by excessive irritability of the infant. Handling the infant causes increased discomfort, and prolonged episodes of crying may be noted during or after a diaper change or other physical manipulations of routine care. Examination reveals diminished spontaneous and reflex movement of the affected extremity, either because of pain (pseudoparalysis)[‡b] or because of weakness caused by an associated neuropathy.[154-157] Many authors endorse swelling and pseudoparalysis as the most diagnostic signs.[155] Pyarthrosis of the hip joint is characterized by maintenance of the hip in a flexed, abducted, and externally rotated (frog-leg) position.[154] Because the slightest degree of passive motion of an extremity may cause severe pain and prolonged crying, attempts to elicit a point of maximal bone tenderness are often unsuccessful.

As the suppurative process extends through the metaphyseal cortex into the surrounding subperiosteal and subcutaneous tissues, external signs of inflammation become more intense, and points of maximal swelling, redness, and heat are more readily discernible. In most cases, an inflammatory mass is directly adjacent to the involved metaphysis or joint, although when deeper skeletal structures (e.g., vertebrae or pelvis) are involved, the abscess may point in distant sites. Three infants have been described in whom vertebral osteomyelitis was not discovered, or even suspected, until after a large retroperitoneal abscess had developed.[6] An abscess arising from the proximal femur, ilium, or hip joint appears usually in the upper thigh, on the buttocks, or in the groin but occasionally also in the iliac fossa, where it can be palpated through the abdominal wall or rectum.[159] Even when infection is localized in the distal extremities, it is difficult to determine solely on clinical grounds whether the bone or adjacent joint or both are involved. Radiologic examinations and diagnostic aspiration of suspected joints are generally necessary to establish a diagnosis.

The striking feature of the benign form of neonatal osteomyelitis is the satisfactory general condition of the infant, despite the intensity of the local process; feeding and weight gain are undisturbed, and there is no evidence of involvement of visceral structures. Although deformity

[¶a] References 3, 4, 6, 11, 19, 22, 25, 26, 37, 67, 152, 153-157.
[#a] References 3, 36, 37, 149, 151, 158.
[*b] References 4, 6, 11, 19, 20, 22, 25, 34, 40, 42, 65, 70, 159-161.
[†b] References 4, 20, 34, 65, 70, 150, 160.
[‡b] References 25, 34, 42, 69, 70, 83, 143.

and disability may follow such infections, the fatality rate is exceedingly low, and healing is prompt.

By contrast, signs and symptoms of the severe form of neonatal osteomyelitis are predominantly those of a septic process with prolonged and intense bacteremia. Infants with this condition usually exhibit failure to thrive, with associated lethargy, refusal or vomiting of feedings, abdominal distention, jaundice, and other signs characteristic of sepsis in the newborn. Infection of the bones and joints may be noted almost simultaneously with onset of septicemia, or it may appear later, despite administration of antibiotics. The clinical evolution of the osteomyelitic process is identical to that in patients with the benign form of the disease. Early localizing signs and symptoms are frequently overshadowed by the systemic manifestations occurring in the infant. Evidence of a suppurative process in the bone may be discovered accidentally in the course of routine radiographic examinations, or it may not be apparent until formation of a local subcutaneous abscess directs attention to the underlying bone. The prognosis for these infants is guarded; death is generally caused by sepsis, with widespread and multiple foci of infection in the nervous system or viscera. The prognosis for the skeletal lesions among survivors is not different, however, from the prognosis for the benign form.

As group B streptococcal infections have become increasingly prevalent, a distinctive clinical picture associated with osteomyelitis has emerged for GBS.[25,67,70,162-166] Most cases are caused by the type III serotype of streptococci and manifest as a late-onset illness during the third and fourth weeks of life (mean age at diagnosis, 25 days). Predisposing factors commonly seen with osteomyelitis caused by other agents, such as maternal obstetric complications, difficulties in the early neonatal period, use of vascular catheters, or other manipulative procedures, are unusual with group B streptococcal disease. The male preponderance usually identified with neonatal osteomyelitis is reversed, with females more affected in a ratio of 1.5:1. Previously, in almost 90% of the infants described with this condition, only a single bone has been involved, most commonly the humerus (50%) or femur (33%), affecting the shoulder or knee. However, multifocal bone involvement in neonatal osteomyelitis has received increased recognition in the last decade.[17,103,164,165] In most cases, infants manifest the benign form of osteomyelitis without signs of systemic toxicity or involvement of other organ systems. Nevertheless, most are ill no more than 3 or 4 days before the diagnosis is established. Although affected joints are typically neither warm nor erythematous, local swelling, tenderness, and diminished movement of the affected extremity are usually severe enough for parents to seek early medical attention.

The distribution of bone involvement reported in the literature is shown in Table 8-1, with 741 infected sites among 485 patients. A single bone was involved in 324 patients, and multiple foci were involved in 161 patients (33%).[167,168] Because radiographic or radionuclide skeletal surveys, which often identify unsuspected foci of osteomyelitis,[§b] were generally not performed, the number of infants reported to have infection in multiple sites is probably falsely low. The high incidence of infections of the femur, humerus, and tibia in neonates has also been noted in adults[170] and older infants and children.[8,10,160,171] The relatively large number of cases of maxillary osteomyelitis is unique, however, to the newborn period; this entity is discussed separately later on.

[§b]References 19, 22, 28, 34, 153, 169.

Table 8-1 Distribution of Bone Involvement in 485 Newborns With Osteomyelitis

Bone	No. Sites*	% of Sites
Femur	287	39
62 Proximal		
91 Distal		
81 Unspecified		
Humerus	134	18
66 Proximal		
16 Distal		
51 Unspecified		
Tibia	102	14
47 Proximal		
11 Distal		
44 Unspecified		
Radius	34	5
5 Proximal		
17 Distal		
12 Unspecified		
Maxilla	30	4
Ulna	22	3
Clavicle	18	2
Tarsal bones	15	2
10 Calcaneous		
3 Talus		
2 Unspecified		
Metacarpals	14	2
Phalanges	12	2
Ribs	12	2
Skull	9	1
Fibula	9	1
Ilium	8	1
Metatarsals	7	1
Mandible	7	1
Scapula	7	1
Sternum	6	1
Vertebrae	5	1
Ischium	3	0.4
Patella	1	0.1

*Among infants, 33% had disease in more than one bone.

The exuberant new bone formation associated with osteomyelitis in the newborn period makes it difficult to determine the original foci of infection when radiographs are obtained late in the clinical course. For this reason, either the site of primary metaphyseal abscess was unspecified, or the infection was referred to as a "panosteitis" in many instances. In the femur, proximal, distal, and uncertain sites of early infection are equally distributed, whereas localization in the tibia and humerus occurs most often at proximal ends of bones; in the radius, distal osteomyelitis predominates. The major consequence of these patterns of infection is the high incidence of secondary purulent arthritis of the hips, shoulders, knees, and wrists; this secondary arthritis has been noted in virtually every large series of newborns with bone infection.

PROGNOSIS

From 1920 to 1940, reports of neonatal osteomyelitis cited mortality rates of 40% in neonates and young infants[58] but stressed an overall benign nature of the disease and the good prognosis for life and function if sepsis was not present.[56,58,144,145] The introduction of antimicrobial agents effective against the common infecting organisms was associated with a considerable reduction in mortality rates. Only 24 deaths (mortality rate 4.2%) were reported among approximately 575 newborns with osteomyelitis acquired from 1945 to 1990.[‖b]

The improved survival rate directed greater attention to a high incidence of residual joint deformities after neonatal osteomyelitis, particularly with hip and knee involvement or delayed diagnosis for more than 3 or 4 days.[¶b] With affected infants often sustaining permanent skeletal deformaties,[172] cited incidence rates for sequelae range from 6% to 50%.[173] The overall extent of growth disturbance is thought to be multifactorial, related to the area and location of physeal destruction, degree of associated hyaline cartilage damage and vascularity of chondroepiphysis.[174] Destruction or separation of the capital femoral epiphysis may result in serious disturbances of growth, usually combined with a marked coxa vara, valga, or magna; an unstable hip joint; flexion contractures; and abnormalities of gait.[#b] Damage to the cartilaginous growth plate in the knees also is often followed by disturbances in longitudinal growth and angulation at the site of infection, leading to genu varum or valgum, restricted motion, and instability of the joint.[*c] Although the consequences of shortening of bone and angular deformities are more serious in lower extremities, analogous growth disturbances may follow osteomyelitis of the humerus, radius, or ulna.[†c] Most of these data have been collected from infants with staphylococcal bone or joint infection; in contrast, the prognosis for full recovery is excellent after group B streptococcal infection.[25,67]

Although vertebral osteomyelitis in the newborn is unusual, the consequences can be grave. Collapse or complete destruction of one or more vertebral bodies may occur,[19,28,178-182] with severe kyphosis or paralysis caused by spinal cord compression appearing as late complications.[19,178,179] In most cases, vertebral involvement is not recognized until after paraspinal abscesses appear.[6,183-185]

The full clinical consequences of osteomyelitis in the newborn period may not be apparent for months to years. Despite a seemingly favorable outcome, even infants with minor bone or joint involvement should be followed to skeletal maturity to observe for the appearance of late deformity, dysfunction, or growth arrest.[80,81] Early evidence of skeletal destruction frequently requires multiple orthopedic procedures to stabilize a joint or to straighten a limb or equalize its length with that of the contralateral arm or leg. Descriptions of late regeneration of femoral epiphyses despite severe injury emphasize the remarkable healing potential and unpredictability of this illness.[175,176,186-190]

‖b References 2, 4-6, 11, 19, 20, 22, 25, 40-42, 63, 65, 68, 70, 85, 146, 151.

¶b References 36-38, 40, 41, 65, 80, 81, 172-174.

#b References 37, 65, 86, 101, 114, 151, 163, 164, 175, 176.

*c References 11, 35, 65, 81, 141, 177.

†c References 3, 20, 39, 65, 81, 178.

Chronic osteomyelitis and sequestration of necrotic bone had been thought to be uncommon complications before and after the availability of antibiotic therapy.[‡c] However, the apparent rarity of these complications in former years should be questioned, because in approximately 10% of infants with osteomyelitis who were studied by several groups of investigators, formation of sequestra occurred, and in many cases, sequestrectomy was required for complete cure.[§c]

Rare complications of neonatal osteomyelitis include epiphyseal[193] and osteochondroma (or exostosis) at the distal ulna after *S. aureus* osteomyelitis.[190] Early diagnosis of neonatal osteoarticular infections remains one of the most effective means of improving overall prognosis.[188]

DIAGNOSIS

Diagnosis of osteomyelitis in neonates is frequently difficult because their presentation differs from that seen in older children.[17,34] Plain film radiographs remain a mainstay in the establishment of the diagnosis of neonatal osteomyelitis. Experience with CT and MRI in the evaluation of neonatal bone infection is increasing, and use of these modalities is limited only by the ability to transport small neonates to facilities for imaging and the need for monitoring of anesthetized infants. CT and MRI may be used if plain radiographs, ultrasonography (of joints), and bone scans have not yielded a diagnosis.[194]

The earliest radiographic sign is swelling of soft tissue around the site of primary infection. Although this finding reflects spreading edema and inflammation that occur as pus breaks through metaphyseal cortex, it is nonspecific and serves only to define an area of inflammation. In addition, deeper soft tissue swelling may be challenging to discern in this population, given poorly characterized fascial planes and decreased subcutaneous fat.[110] The first distinct evidence of bone involvement appears as small foci of necrosis and rarefaction, most commonly located in the metaphysis adjoining the epiphyseal growth plate; this may be accompanied by capsular distention or widening of the joint space if inflammatory exudate or pus has entered the articular capsule. Lateral subluxation of the hip is a significant diagnostic tool for detection of septic arthritis.[160] In contrast to older children, in whom radiographic changes are commonly delayed for 3 weeks,[10,171] neonates almost always show definite signs of bone destruction after only 7 to 10 days.[‖c]

Extension of the suppurative process often produces widespread areas of cortical rarefaction, which, despite their appearance, infrequently result in significant bone sequestration. The presence of pus in the hip and shoulder joints may cause progressive lateral and upward displacement of the head of the femur[34,151,158,195] or humerus through stages of subluxation to pathologic dislocation. The absence in the newborn period of ossification centers, with the exception of those at the distal femur and proximal tibia, makes it very difficult to diagnose neonatal epiphysitis in any area but the knees.[177] For similar reasons,

‡c References 6, 39, 41, 58, 65, 144, 145.

§c References 2, 5, 22, 60, 85, 135, 155, 159, 191, 192.

‖c References 5, 11, 18, 25, 40, 62, 64, 169, 189.

epiphyseal separation or destruction of the head of the femur or humerus is difficult to distinguish radiologically from simple dislocation.[151,158]

In most infants, the reparative phase begins within 2 weeks after onset of infection. The first sign of healing is the formation of a thin layer of subperiosteal bone, which rapidly enlarges to form a thick involucrum between the raised periosteum and the cortex. Although bone destruction may continue at the same time, necrotic foci are rapidly absorbed and filled in as new bone is deposited. The entire process from the first signs of rarefaction to restoration of the cortical structure may last no longer than 2 months; however, several months usually elapse before minimal deformities disappear and remodeling of the shaft is complete. In some cases, well-circumscribed defects involving the metaphysis and epiphysis may persist for years.[177]

The benefit of using radiologic skeletal surveys in newborns with osteomyelitis should be emphasized, particularly because the occurrence of multiple sites of osteomyelitis is much more common in the neonatal period. Clinically unsuspected sites of infection can be discovered in a significant proportion of infants.[¶c]

Demonstration of such lesions may provide therapeutic benefits. In one series,[22] 4 of 7 areas of occult infection required aspiration or drainage, whereas in another study,[19] 3 of 17 hip joint infections were discovered on routine radiographs taken because the infant had osteomyelitis elsewhere. Plain film skeletal surveys for occult bone and joint infection are recommended in any infant with osteomyelitis.

As mentioned, experience with CT and MRI in the diagnosis of neonatal musculoskeletal infection is limited.[197,198] Although both procedures can be helpful adjuncts to clinical diagnosis and conventional radiography, they are slow and require heavy sedation—usually undesirable in a febrile septic infant—to prevent movement artifact and loss of resolution. CT provides good definition of cortical bone and is sensitive for early detection of bone destruction, periosteal reaction, and formation of sequestra. It has been used to particular advantage in diagnosis of osteomyelitis of the skull associated with infected cephalhematoma.[127,128] Plain radiographs of uninfected cephalohematomas can show soft tissue swelling, periosteal elevation, calcification, and even underlying radiolucency caused by bone resorption[191]—findings also consistent with bone infection. In such cases, CT has been able to define foci of bone destruction more accurately, helping to confirm the presence of osteomyelitis.

MRI is of limited value in defining structural changes in cortical bone, but it provides excellent anatomic detail of muscle and soft tissue, superior to that of any other imaging technique.[198] It is particularly useful in showing the early soft tissue edema seen adjacent to areas of bone involvement before the appearance of any osseous changes. MRI is also helpful in determining the presence of a periosteal abscess and assessing the need for surgical drainage. The major advantage of MRI over CT is the ability to detect inflammatory or destructive intramedullary disease. It is of greater advantage in older children and adults than in neonates, however, because involvement of the marrow compartment is uncommon in neonates. Both modalities provide excellent spatial resolution and anatomic detail; however, CT is best suited to cross-sectional views, whereas MRI can display anatomy with equal clarity in coronal and sagittal planes, permitting visualization in the plane most advantageous for accurate diagnosis. Absence of ionizing radiation is another distinct advantage of MRI over CT.

There has been increasing interest in the use of ultrasonography to detect bone infection and joint effusions.[191-202] Diagnosis of osteomyelitis is based on periosteal thickening or the presence of abscess formation, as indicated by periosteal elevation and separation from bone. The exact role of ultrasonography in diagnosis of neonatal osteoarthritis has continued to be defined. It currently seems most useful as a tool for defining the presence of fluid collections in joints or adjacent to bone and as a guide for needle aspiration or surgical drainage of these collections. The occurrence of false-positive or false-negative examinations, although infrequent, requires that infants with conflicting clinical findings be evaluated further by other techniques. Reports of successful diagnosis of osteomyelitis in neonates with ultrasonography include the diagnosis of rib infection in a 650-g infant with staphylococcal osteomyelitis.[203] Other series have included 2- to 6-week-old infants with osteomyelitis of the costochondral junction and ribs.[193,204]

Despite reports emphasizing the reliability of technetium-99m bone imaging in older infants and children,[205] experience with the use of this technique in neonates has been far less favorable.[22,35,42,169,206-210] In one study, among 10 newborns subsequently proved to have osteomyelitis involving 20 sites in all, only 8 of these sites were found to be abnormal or equivocal by technetium-99m scan.[206] Of the 12 sites that were normal by technetium-99m scan at 1 to 33 days (mean, 8 days) after onset of symptoms, 9 showed destructive changes in the corresponding radiograph. The increased radioactivity in areas of inflammatory hyperemia surrounding an osteomyelitic lesion, usually present in the early "blood-pool" images in children,[207] also was not seen, even in infants with ultimately positive delayed bone scans. Although false-negative bone scans also have been described in older infants,[211,212] the reason for the excessively high incidence among neonates is unknown. It has been suggested that the discrepancy is due either to differences in the pathophysiology of neonatal disease or to the inability of earlier gamma cameras to separate the increased activity of the growth plate in the first weeks of life from that of infection.[153,205]

As indicated by clinical studies, use of newer high-resolution cameras combined with electronic magnification may provide greater diagnostic accuracy.[153] However, in these studies, the investigators also used significantly (fourfold to sixfold) larger doses of technetium 99m, and almost all sites of involvement had radiographically detectable lesions at the time of diagnosis. It seems reasonable at the present time to limit the use of technetium-99m radionuclide scans to evaluation of infants with normal or equivocal radiographs in whom there is a strong clinical suspicion of osteomyelitis.

Among older patients, gallium-67 bone imaging has been shown to be valuable when results of the technetium-99m scan and appearance on plain films are normal

[¶c]References 19, 22, 28, 35, 169, 196.

and osteomyelitis is strongly suspected.[212] Studies performed in small infants and neonates have shown similar results.[211,213] The radiation burden of this isotope is high, however, and the probability that the results of a scan by themselves would influence therapy is low. The role of gallium-67 bone imaging in the diagnosis of neonatal bone and joint infections is very limited.

Needle aspiration of an inflammatory area may provide a rapid diagnosis.[25,40,42,70] Differentiation of subcutaneous from subperiosteal infection often is difficult; however, significant accumulations of pus aspirated from a periarticular abscess almost invariably are found to originate in bone rather than in the soft tissues.[2,143] Clinical or radiologic evidence of joint space infection, particularly in the hip and shoulder, requires immediate confirmation by needle aspiration. If no effusion is found and clinical signs persist, aspiration should be repeated within 8 to 12 hours. If there is doubt about whether the joint was actually entered, limited arthrography with small amounts of dye can readily be performed with an aspirating needle.[151,158] Most iodinated contrast materials do not interfere with bacterial growth from aspirated specimens.[214] Inserting a needle into the metaphyseal region or joint 24 hours before scanning does not interfere with the scintigraphic detection of osteomyelitis.[207-209]

The total peripheral white blood cell count is of little value in diagnosing neonatal osteomyelitis.[110] In more than 150 cases in which these values were recorded, the median peripheral leukocyte count was approximately 17,000 cells/mm^3 (mean, 20,000 cells/mm^3; range, 4000 to 75,100 cells/mm^3). Polymorphonuclear leukocytes usually represented about 60% of the white blood cells counted; frequently, the number of immature forms was higher than normal. Neonates with osteomyelitis usually have an erythrocyte sedimentation rate higher than 20 mm/hr.[#c]

Similar to leukocyte count, erythrocyte sedimentation rate is helpful for diagnosis and follow-up evaluation when elevated but cannot be used to rule out osteomyelitis when normal.[11,19,20,110,215] Alternatively, C-reactive protein is more useful than erythrocyte sedimentation rate as an acute-phase reactant in neonates, and most methods for C-reactive protein determination require only 0.1 mL of blood, as opposed to erythrocyte sedimentation rate, which may require 1 to 2 mL of blood.

DIFFERENTIAL DIAGNOSIS

The early descriptions of pyogenic neonatal osteomyelitis emphasized difficulties in distinguishing the pseudoparalysis and irritability that are characteristic of this condition from the symptoms of congenital syphilis and from true paralysis of congenital poliomyelitis.[216-218] The clinical course and radiologic examinations are generally sufficient to rule out polio and other neuroparalytic illnesses; however, the periosteitis and metaphyseal bone destruction that accompany congenital syphilis are frequently indistinguishable from bone alterations observed in infants with multicentric pyogenic osteomyelitis (see Chapter 16).[174,177] Similar osseous changes have been noted at birth in infants with congenital tumors or leukemia.[216-219]

Serial radiologic examinations may be necessary to distinguish a superficial cellulitis, subcutaneous abscess, or bursitis[220,221] from a primary bone infection, particularly when these conditions arise in a periarticular location. Similarly, a suppurative arthritis arising in the joint space, rather than in the adjacent metaphysis, can be defined as such only by determining that no destruction has occurred in bones contiguous to that joint.

The relative lack of any inflammatory sign other than edema is the only clinical feature that helps to differentiate between candidal and bacterial osteomyelitis.[26,28] *Candida* infections have been observed more frequently in recent years, particularly in premature infants, in whom antibiotic therapy, placement of umbilical catheters, and use of parenteral hyperalimentation, together with immature host defense mechanisms, predispose to candidal infection and dissemination.[*d]

The lesions of *Candida albicans* infection typically are seen as well defined ("punched-out") metaphyseal lucencies on radiographs but are less aggressive in appearance than the lesions of staphylococcal osteitis and often are surrounded by a slightly sclerotic margin.[†d]

Even when characteristic clinical circumstances and radiographic features are present, the diagnosis in almost all cases rests on identification of the organism by Gram stain or culture, although *Candida* organisms are frequently present concomitantly in blood cultures obtained during febrile episodes.

Several congenital viral lesions have also been associated with bone changes. Lesions caused by congenital rubella, although generally seen in the metaphyseal ends of the long bones, are distinct from the lesions of bacterial osteomyelitis during the early stages of pathogenesis and show no evidence of periosteal reaction during the reparative phase.[225] There is little likelihood of confusion of the radiographic features of bone pathology resulting from congenital cytomegalic inclusion disease[226,227] or from herpes simplex virus type 2 infections[228] with those of hematogenous osteomyelitis, particularly when radiographic findings are considered in context with the characteristic clinical signs and symptoms of these infections.

Numerous noninfectious conditions causing bone destruction or periosteal reaction may be confused with osteomyelitis on clinical and radiographic grounds and on the basis of radionuclide scan findings. These conditions include skeletal trauma caused by the birth process or caregiver abuse[153,229-231] or associated with osteogenesis imperfecta; congenital infantile cortical hyperostosis (Caffey disease)[153,230,232]; congenital bone tumors, metastases, and leukemia[152,217]; extravasation of calcium gluconate at an infusion site[233]; and prostaglandin E1 infusion.[234] The periosteal bone growth sometimes seen in normal infants, particularly premature infants, may produce a "double-contour" effect in long bones that appears to be similar to the early involucrum of healing osteomyelitis but is unassociated with evidence of bone destruction and metaphyseal changes and is never progressive.[235]

[#c]References 11, 19, 34, 67, 148, 164.

[*d]References 26, 28-30, 36-39, 86, 136, 222, 223.

[†d]References 26, 28, 36, 39, 40, 86, 223, 224.

THERAPY

Successful treatment of osteomyelitis or septic arthritis depends on prompt clinical diagnosis and identification of the infectious agent. Every effort should be made to isolate responsible organisms before therapy is initiated. Pus localized in skin, soft tissues, joint, or bone should be aspirated under strict aseptic conditions and sent to the laboratory for Gram stain, culture, and antibiotic susceptibility testing. Blood specimens for culture should be obtained; such cultures may be the only source of the pathogen.[‡d]

Because osteomyelitis generally is the consequence of a systemic bacteremia, a lumbar puncture should be considered. Any potential source of infection should be examined, including intravascular catheter tips.[237] Cerebrospinal fluid can occasionally be helpful when direct examination of suppurative material fails to provide an etiologic diagnosis. Choice of therapy should be guided by results of Gram stain, culture, and antibiotic susceptibilities.

When the cause of infection cannot be immediately determined, the initial choice of antimicrobial agents must be based on the presumptive bacteriologic diagnosis. Penicillinase-resistant penicillins (e.g., nafcillin, oxacillin) and vancomycin are active against *S. aureus*, group A streptococci and GBS, and *S. pneumoniae*, which together account for more than 90% of cases of osteoarthritis in neonates. Osteomyelitis caused by enteric organisms is sufficiently common to justify additional therapy with an aminoglycoside such as gentamicin, tobramycin, or amikacin or an extended-spectrum cephalosporin agent (cefotaxime) or the use of an extended-spectrum, *Pseudomonas*-active agent such as cefepime.

MRSA and most strains of coagulase-negative staphylococci are increasingly frequent causes of sepsis and other focal infections in neonates. Numerous outbreaks of nosocomial and community-acquired MRSA infections have been reported. Infants who acquire infection in nurseries where MRSA is prevalent or where community-acquired MRSA infections have occurred should be started on vancomycin, rather than a penicillin antibiotic.[169] Alternative antibiotics approved and licensed for treatment of MRSA infections in older children and adults, including daptomycin, linezolid, and quinupristin-dalfopristin, have not been fully evaluated or approved for use in neonates in the first 2 months of life and should be used on an individual basis only when the neonate cannot tolerate vancomycin because of acquired toxicity.

When bacterial culture and sensitivity data are available, treatment should be changed to the single safest and most effective drug. If group B streptococcal infection is confirmed, combination therapy with penicillin G (or ampicillin) and gentamicin should be given for 2 to 5 days, after which time penicillin G (or ampicillin) alone is adequate.[238] Standard disk susceptibility tests may falsely indicate sensitivity of MRSA to cephalosporins.[217] Use of β-lactam antibiotics is inappropriate for MRSA infections, and vancomycin should be continued for the full course of therapy. It is controversial whether the synergistic addition of an active aminoglycoside (e.g., gentamicin) to a penicillin antibiotic or vancomycin for a limited period (e.g., 5 days) enhances the clinical outcomes of infants with neonatal osteomyelitis caused by *S. aureus*.

All antibiotics should be given by the parenteral route, usually intravenously. There is no significant clinical advantage to intravenous over intramuscular administration, but the limited number of injection sites available in the newborn makes the intramuscular route impractical for use during prolonged periods. Intraarticular administration of antibiotics is unnecessary in the treatment of suppurative arthritis because adequate levels of activity have been shown in joint fluid after parenteral doses of most drugs that would be used for therapy.[236]Although there continues to be insufficient data detailing appropriate length of therapy in this population,[239] antibiotic therapy for either osteomyelitis or suppurative arthritis should be continued for at least 4 or 6 weeks after defervescence. Monitoring serum acute-phase proteins (particularly C-reactive protein) has been proposed as a useful way to determine resolution of infection and duration of therapy.[127,239-241]

There are insufficient data on the absorption and efficacy of orally administered antibiotics in the neonate to recommend their use routinely in this age group for treatment of osteoarthritis. Nevertheless, after an initial course of intravenous therapy, newborns have been treated successfully with oral dicloxacillin,[215,242,243] flucloxacillin,[34] fusidic acid,[34,35] and penicillin V[34,196] for additional periods ranging from 14 to 42 days. If sequential parenteral-oral therapy is used, adequacy of antibiotic absorption and efficacy must be closely monitored with regular clinical evaluation and, possibly, serum bactericidal titers or, preferably, direct measurement of antibiotic agents in blood.[196,243,244] It is likely, but unproved in the neonate, that the traditional antibiotics used for hematogenous osteomyelitis in older children (e.g., amoxicillin or cephalexin, in divided doses totaling 100 to 150 mg/kg/day) would be tolerated and effective, but these agents should be used only after successful parenteral therapy has been established and only under the supervision of physicians with adequate training.

To overcome the uncertainties of oral absorption while still allowing discharge of the patient from the hospital, home intravenous antibiotic therapy has been advocated as an alternative form of treatment.[27] Although home management for older children and adults is now widely accepted, experience with newborns is still limited; however, with proper family and medical support, it can be a successful alternative to inpatient treatment. Either carefully monitored oral therapy or, more frequently, the use of intravenous antibiotics given by peripheral intravenous central catheters or surgically implanted central catheters may be used.

Surgical drainage is indicated whenever there is a significant collection of pus in soft tissues. The need for drilling or "windowing" the cortex to drain intramedullary collections of pus is controversial.[11,19,20,34] There is no evidence, based on controlled studies, that these procedures are of any value in either limiting systemic manifestations or decreasing the extent of bone destruction. Open surgical drainage for relief of intraarticular pressure is a critical measure, however, for preserving the viability of the head of the femur or humerus in infants with suppurative arthritis of hip or shoulder joints.[6,37,172] Intermittent needle aspiration with saline irrigation usually is adequate for drainage of other, more readily accessible joints. Lack of improvement after 3 days, rapid reaccumulation of fluid, or loculation of pus and necrotic

[‡d] References 22, 33, 37, 40, 61, 64, 236.

debris in the joint may indicate the need for open drainage of these joints as well.[245]

Surgical drainage (arthrotomy) or needle aspiration is used for treatment of septic arthritis. There is increasing evidence that both septic hip and septic shoulders respond and heal better with the use of either surgical drainage or needle aspirations, and it is the consensus that both of these infections should be treated with antibiotics and drainage.[246-250] However, it is not clear that one modality is superior to the other, and there have been very few head-to-head trials of these methods of drainage. In addition, most studies have included children younger than 12 months, but not necessarily only newborn infants. Nunn and colleagues[251] conducted a prospective study of arthrotomy; 34% had a full and uncomplicated clinical and radiologic recovery and 66% had complications, but all patients treated within 5 days by arthrotomy and appropriate antibiotics had an uncomplicated recovery. However, Givon and colleagues[252] used ultrasound-guided needle aspiration and irrigation of the hip in 28 children; the mean number of aspirations was 3.6 (range, 3-5), and 75% of these children resumed walking after 24 hours. Four of these children did not improve and subsequently underwent arthrotomy. Last, Bos and colleagues[253] reviewed the late sequelae of shoulder septic arthritis in 8 neonates with 10 shoulder infections; all 10 shoulders were treated with repeated needle aspirations, followed by arthrotomy in 2. At follow-up (average, 14 years), 5 of the 10 shoulders had a full range of motion, and others had only minimal restriction. Shortening of the humerus was the most common sequelae and occurred in 3 of the 10 shoulders. The delay in diagnosis between the onset of symptoms and diagnosis was 1 day in 5 patients, 2 days in 3, and 7 days in 1; early diagnosis and treatment favored a better outcome.

The affected extremity should be immobilized until inflammation has subsided and there is radiologic evidence of healing. Prolonged splinting in a brace or cast is necessary when pathologic dislocation of the head of the femur accompanies pyarthrosis of the hip joint. Maintenance of adequate nutrition and fluid requirements is crucial in determining the ultimate course of the illness. Before the advent of antibiotics, attention to these factors alone often was adequate to ensure prompt healing of osseous lesions in infants who survived the initial septic process.[58]

Primary Septic Arthritis

Although septic arthritis often is a complication of neonatal osteomyelitis, it also can occur in the absence of demonstrable radiologic changes in adjacent bone. Once known as "Tom Smith's arthritis,"[254] infection usually is the result of synovial implantation of organisms in the course of a septicemia. Infrequently, traumatic inoculation of organisms into the articular capsule may occur as a consequence of femoral venipuncture.[38,69,111-113] As in osteomyelitis, there is a strong association between septic arthritis and placement of an umbilical catheter.[27] Whatever the source of infection, the presence of a concurrent osteomyelitis can never be ruled out completely because of the possibility that the original suppurative focus lay in the radiolucent cartilaginous portion of the bone, permitting entry of organisms to the joint by direct extension. The spectrum of agents responsible for primary septic arthritis is similar to that of organisms causing arthritis secondary to a contiguous osteomyelitis. Bacteria that have been isolated from blood or joints of newborns in two series are listed in Table 8-2. Exceedingly rare in neonates, unlike its anticipated presence in older children, group A *Streptococcus* was isolated from the elbow joint of a neonate in India.[255]

Table 8-2 Reported Spectrum and Organisms Isolated From Blood or Joints of Neonates With Primary Bacterial Arthritis (1972-1986)

Bacteria	No. Infants
Staphylococcus aureus	9
Group B streptococci	4
Streptococci, unspecified	2
Staphylococcus epidermidis	1
Haemophilus influenzae type b	0
Escherichia coli	0
Klebsiella pneumoniae	1
Pseudomonas aeruginosa	1
Neisseria gonorrhoeae	1

Data from J.D. Nelson, personal communication, 1987; Pittard WB 3rd, Thullen JD, Fanaroff AA: Neonatal septic arthritis, *J Pediatr* 88:621, 1976; and Jackson MA, Nelson JD: Etiology and medical management of acute suppurative bone and joint infections in pediatric patients, *J Pediatr Orthop* 2:313, 1982.

Signs and symptoms of purulent arthritis are virtually identical to the signs and symptoms seen in newborns with osteomyelitis.[246,256] Limitation in use of an extremity progressing to pseudoparalysis is characteristic of both conditions, and although external signs of inflammation tend to be more localized to the periarticular area, recognition of this feature is of little diagnostic value in individual cases. Data are insufficient to provide any meaningful comparison between the skeletal distribution of septic arthritis and that of osteomyelitis. Multiple joint involvement is common to both conditions, however. Involvement of the hip has been cited in up to 80% of cases.[15] In one series of 16 consecutive newborns with pyarthrosis, 22 joints were involved; 4 (25%) infants had multifocal infections.[33] A migratory polyarthritis, which may precede localization in a single joint by several days, is particularly characteristic of gonococcal arthritis, as is an extremely high frequency of knee and ankle involvement.[95] In a Malaysian series, the knee, hip, and ankle were involved in 10 cases of septic arthritis, and 9 of the 10 cases were caused by MRSA, exhibiting the frequent occurrence of septic arthritis caused by nosocomial pathogens in premature infants in neonatal intensive care units.[247]

The radiologic features, differential diagnosis, and therapy for septic arthritis are discussed under "Osteomyelitis." Long-term evaluations regarding prognosis after septic arthritis incurred during infancy are few and involve small volume patient cases.[248,249] However, recognition for this need to improve treatment options is increasing.[250]

Osteomyelitis of the Maxilla

Neonatal osteomyelitis of the maxilla is a distinct clinical entity, and early reports of neonatal osteomyelitis frequently focused exclusively on this entity. In terms of total numbers, maxillary osteomyelitis is a rare condition (there are <200 reported cases); yet in earlier surveys of neonatal bone infections, maxillary involvement was noted in approximately 25% of infants.[§d] The far lower incidence in children[8,10] and adults[170] is probably explained by earlier recognition and treatment of sinusitis in these age groups and by the lack of predisposing factors unique to the newborn.

The causative organism is most frequently *S. aureus*,[258-260] although hemolytic streptococci have been isolated on rare occasions from drainage sites.[260] Greater than 85% of all maxillary infections in infants occur in the first 3 months of life; the incidence is highest during the second to fourth weeks.[259-262] In most cases, the predisposing cause remains obscure.

Infants with sources of infection, such as skin abscesses or omphalitis, constitute a small minority.[260,262] It has been postulated that there is a relationship between breast abscess in the nursing mother and maxillary osteomyelitis[260,262,263]; however, it is unclear whether the maternal infection is a source or a result of the infant's condition.[264] The pathogenesis of bone infection after colonization of the infant by staphylococci is equally uncertain. In some cases, osteomyelitis is believed to result from extension from a contiguous focus of infection in the maxillary antrum. Alternatively, organisms may be bloodborne, establishing infection in the rich vascular plexus surrounding tooth buds.[262] Although the hematogenous route may be important in certain cases, particularly cases involving the premaxilla,[258] this explanation is incompatible with the fact that mandibular osteomyelitis or associated metastatic involvement of other structures is uncommon.[260] Another theory is that trauma or abrasion of the gum overlying the first molar is the primary route of introduction of organisms.[262]

The clinical course of maxillary osteomyelitis begins with acute onset of fever and nonspecific systemic symptoms. Shortly thereafter, redness and swelling of the eyelid appear and are frequently accompanied by conjunctivitis with a purulent discharge. Thrombosis of nutrient vessels and increasing edema may cause a proptosis or chemosis of the affected eye. In most infants, an early and diffuse swelling and inflammation of the cheek may localize to form an abscess or draining fistula below the inner or outer canthus of the eye; this is nearly always followed or accompanied by a purulent unilateral nasal discharge that is increased by pressure on the abscess. The alveolar border of the superior maxilla on the affected side is swollen and soft, as is the adjacent hard palate. Within a few days, abscesses and draining fistulas may form in these areas.[265] Sepsis and death are frequent in untreated cases. In most infants, the illness pursues a relatively chronic course characterized by discharge of premature teeth or numerous small sequestra of necrotic bone through multiple palatal and alveolar sinuses that have formed. The entire course may evolve over several days in severe cases, or it may extend for several weeks in mild or partially treated cases.

Neonatal maxillary osteomyelitis is frequently confused with either orbital cellulitis or dacryocystitis.[19,262,266] The early edema and redness of the cheeks that accompany acute osteomyelitis constitute an important differentiating feature, which is not observed in orbital cellulitis and occurs only as a late sign in infection of the lacrimal sac. Neither orbital cellulitis nor lacrimal sac infection is associated with a unilateral purulent nasal discharge. The early onset, limited area of involvement, and Gram stain characteristic of ophthalmia neonatorum should be sufficient, in most cases, to permit diagnosis of this condition. CT can be helpful in assessing the extent of infection and evaluating for possible complications, such as cerebral abscess.[265]

Therapy for maxillary osteomyelitis should be directed toward early adequate drainage of the maxillary empyema and contiguous abscess and should include appropriate parenterally administered antibiotics. Because most infections are due to *S. aureus* and group A streptococci, systemic use of a penicillinase-resistant penicillin (or vancomycin) alone should be sufficient as initial therapy, pending the results of bacterial cultures and sensitivity tests. The need for or desirability of instillation of antibiotics into the maxillary antrum is uncertain.

Before the advent of antibiotic therapy, the mortality rate for maxillary osteomyelitis was high, ranging from 15% to 75% in various series.[260,262,263,267] Children who survived often had severe facial and dental deformities. Later studies[260,262,267] showed a mortality rate of closer to 5%, although sequelae such as stenosis of the lacrimal duct, ectropion, permanent loss of teeth, malocclusion, and facial hemiatrophy are still seen.[11,259-261] In many instances, these complications could have been prevented through early recognition of the nature of the illness and prompt institution of appropriate therapy.

[§d]References 3, 6, 11, 58, 64, 257.

References

1. Craig WS: *Care of the newly born infant*, Baltimore, 1962, Williams & Wilkins.
2. Boyes J, Bremner AD, Neligan GA: Haematogenous osteitis in the newborn, *Lancet* 1:544, 1957.
3. Dennison WM: Haematogenous osteitis in the newborn, *Lancet* 2:474, 1955.
4. Masse P: L'ostéomyelité du nouveau-né, *Semaine Hôp Paris* 34:2812, 1958.
5. Contzen H: Die sogennante Osteomyelitis des Neugeborenen, *Dtsch Med Wochenschr* 86:1221, 1961.
6. Clarke AM: Neonatal osteomyelitis: a disease different from osteomyelitis of older children, *Med J Aust* 1:237, 1958.
7. Hall JE, Silverstein EA: Acute hematogenous osteomyelitis, *Pediatrics* 31:1033, 1963.
8. Green M, Nyhan WL Jr, Fousek MD: Acute hematogenous osteomyelitis, *Pediatrics* 17:368, 1956.
9. Hung W, McGavisk DF: Acute hematogenous osteomyelitis: a report of 36 cases seen at Children's Hospital 1950 to 1958, *Clin Proc Child Hosp* 16:163, 1960.
10. Morse TS, Pryles CV: Infections of the bones and joints in children, *N Engl J Med* 262:846, 1960.
11. Fox L, Sprunt K: Neonatal osteomyelitis, *Pediatrics* 62:535, 1978.
12. Baevsky RH: Neonatal group B beta-hemolytic *Streptococcus* osteomyelitis, *Am J Emerg Med* 17:619, 1999.
13. Barton LL, Villar RG, Rice SA: Neonatal group B streptococcal vertebral osteomyelitis, *Pediatrics* 98:459, 1996.
14. Korakaki E, Aligizakis A, Manoura A, et al: Methicillin-resistant *Staphylococcus aureus* osteomyelitis and septic arthritis in neonates: diagnosis and management, *Jpn J Infect Dis* 60:129, 2007.
15. Matic A, Gajdobranski D, Petković L, et al: Acute osteomyelitis and septic arthritis of the shoulder in premature neonates: report of two cases, *Med Pregl* 65:59, 2012.
16. Sandal G, Uras N, Akar M, et al: Iliac osteomyelitis in the newborn: a case report, *J Pediatr Orthop* 21:404, 2012.
17. Zhang J, Lee BH, Chen C: Gram-negative osteomyelitis: two case reports, *Neonatal Netw* 30:81, 2011.
18. Lim MO, Gresham EL, Franken EA Jr, et al: Osteomyelitis as a complication of umbilical artery catheterization, *Am J Dis Child* 131:142, 1977.

19. Bergdahl S, Ekengren K, Eriksson M: Neonatal hematogenous osteomyelitis: risk factors for long-term sequelae, *J Pediatr Orthop* 5:564, 1985.
20. Bamberger T, Gugler E: Die akute Osteomyelitis im Kindesalter, *Schweiz Med Wochenschr* 113:1219, 1983.
21. Bennet R, Eriksson M, Zetterström R: Increasing incidence of neonatal septicemia: causative organism and predisposing risk factors, *Acta Paediatr Scand* 70:207, 1981.
22. Mok PM, Reilly BJ, Ash JM: Osteomyelitis in the neonate with cerebral abscess, *Radiology* 145:677, 1982.
23. Dan M: Septic arthritis in young infants: clinical and microbiologic correlations and therapeutic implications, *Rev Infect Dis* 6:147, 1984.
24. Barton LL, Dunkle LM, Habib FH: Septic arthritis in childhood: a 13-year review, *Am J Dis Child* 141:898, 1987.
25. Edwards MS, Baker CJ, Wagner ML, et al: An etiologic shift in infantile osteomyelitis: the emergence of the group B streptococcus, *J Pediatr* 93:578, 1978.
26. Yousefzadeh DK, Jackson JH: Neonatal and infantile candidal arthritis with or without osteomyelitis: a clinical and radiographical review of 21 cases, *Skeletal Radiol* 5:77, 1980.
27. Pittard WB 3rd, Thullen JD, Fanaroff AA: Neonatal septic arthritis, *J Pediatr* 88:621, 1976.
28. Brill PW, Winchester P, Krauss AN, et al: Osteomyelitis in a neonatal intensive care unit, *Radiology* 13:83, 1979.
29. Johnson DE, Thompson TR, Green TP, et al: Systemic candidiasis in very low-birth-weight infants (≤1,500 grams), *Pediatrics* 73:138, 1984.
30. Turner RB, Donowitz LG, Hendley JO: Consequences of candidemia for pediatric patients, *Am J Dis Child* 139:178, 1985.
31. Goldmann DA, Durbin WA Jr, Freeman J: Nosocomial infections in a neonatal intensive care unit, *J Infect Dis* 144:449, 1981.
32. Townsend TR, Wenzel RP: Nosocomial bloodstream infections in a newborn intensive care unit, *Am J Epidemiol* 114:73, 1981.
33. Jackson MA, Nelson JD: Etiology and medical management of acute suppurative bone and joint infections in pediatric patients, *J Pediatr Orthop* 2:313, 1982.
34. Knudsen CJ, Hoffman EB: Neonatal osteomyelitis, *J Bone Joint Surg Br* 72:846, 1990.
35. Williamson JB, Galasko CSB, Robinson MJ: Outcome after acute osteomyelitis in preterm infants, *Arch Dis Child* 65:1060, 1990.
36. Baitch A: Recent observations of acute suppurative arthritis, *Clin Orthop* 22:157, 1962.
37. Obletz BE: Suppurative arthritis of the hip joint in premature infants, *Clin Orthop* 22:27, 1962.
38. Ross DW: Acute suppurative arthritis of the hip in premature infants, *JAMA* 156:303, 1954.
39. Thomson J, Lewis IC: Osteomyelitis in the newborn, *Arch Dis Child* 25:273, 1950.
40. Weissberg ED, Smith AL, Smith DH: Clinical features of neonatal osteomyelitis, *Pediatrics* 53:505, 1974.
41. Kumari S, Bhargava SK, Baijal VN, et al: Neonatal osteomyelitis: a clinical and follow-up study, *Indian J Pediatr* 15:393, 1978.
42. Deshpande PG, Wagle SU, Mehta SD, et al: Neonatal osteomyelitis and septic arthritis, *Indian J Pediatr* 27:453, 1990.
43. Wong M, Isaacs D, Howman-Giles R, et al: Clinical and diagnostic features of osteomyelitis in the first three months of life, *Pediatr Infect Dis* 14:1047, 1995.
44. Frederiksen B, Christiansen P, Knudsen FU: Acute osteomyelitis and septic arthritis in the neonate, risk factors and outcome, *Eur J Pediatr* 152:577, 1993.
45. Narang A, Mukhopadhyay K, Kumar P, et al: Bone and joint infection in neonates, *Indian J Pediatr* 65:461, 1998.
46. Howman-Giles R, Uren R: Multifocal osteomyelitis in childhood. Review by radionuclide bone scan, *Clin Nucl Med* 17:274, 1992.
47. Egan SC, LaSalle MD, Stock JA, et al: Septic arthritis secondary to vesicourethral reflux into a single ectopic ureter, *Pediatr Nephrol* 13:932, 1999.
48. deJesus LE, Fernandes A, Sias SM, et al: Neonatal osteomyelitis and complex nephro-ureteral duplication, *Surg Infect (Larchmt)* 12:73, 2011.
49. Cieslak TJ, Rajnik M: Fetal breech presentation predisposes to subsequent development of septic arthritis of the hip, *Pediatr Infect Dis J* 24:650, 2005.
50. Estienne M, Scaioli V, Zibordi F, et al: Enigmatic osteomyelitis and bilateral upper limb palsy in a neonate, *Pediatr Neurology* 32:56, 2005.
51. Lejman T, Strong M, Michno P: Radial nerve palsy associated with septic shoulder in neonates, *J Pediatr Orthop* 15:169, 1995.
52. Saarinen M, Takala AK, Koskenniemi E, et al: Spectrum of 2,836 cases of invasive bacterial or fungal infections in children: results of prospective nationwide five-year surveillance in Finland, *Clin Infect Dis* 21:1134, 1995.
53. Saez-Llorens X, Velarde J, Canton C: Pediatric osteomyelitis in Panama, *Clin Infect Dis* 19:323, 1994.
54. Freedman RM, Ingram DL, Gross I, et al: A half century of neonatal sepsis at Yale: 1928 to 1978, *Am J Dis Child* 135:140, 1981.
55. Dillehunt RB: Osteomyelitis in infants, *Surg Gynecol Obstet* 61:96, 1935.
56. Dunham EC: Septicemia in the newborn, *Am J Dis Child* 45:230, 1933.
57. Green WT, Shannon JG: Osteomyelitis of infants: a disease different from osteomyelitis of older children, *Arch Surg* 32:462, 1936.
58. Aractingi TR: Étude de 32 cas d'ostéomyélité du nouveauné, *Rev Chir Orthop* 47:50, 1961.
59. Dennison WM, MacPherson DA: Haematogenous osteitis of infancy, *Arch Dis Child* 27:375, 1952.
60. Hutter CG: New concepts of osteomyelitis in the newborn infant, *J Pediatr* 32:522, 1948.
61. Lindell L, Parkkulainen KV: Osteitis in infancy and early childhood: with special reference to neonatal osteitis, *Ann Paediatr Fenn* 6:34, 1960.
62. Kienitz M, Schulte M: Problematik bakterieller Infectionen des Früh- und Neuegeborenen, *Munch Med Wochenschr* 109:70, 1967.
63. Wolman G: Acute osteomyelitis in infancy, *Acta Paediatr Scand* 45:595, 1956.
64. Blanche DW: Osteomyelitis in infants, *J Bone Joint Surg Am* 34:71, 1952.
65. Howard JB, McCracken GH Jr: The spectrum of group B streptococcal infections in infancy, *Am J Dis Child* 128:815, 1974.
66. Memon IA, Jacobs NM, Yeh TF, et al: Group B streptococcal osteomyelitis and septic arthritis: its occurrence in infants less than 2 months old, *Am J Dis Child* 133:921, 1979.
67. Coto-Cotallo GD, Solís Sánchez G, Crespo Hernández M, et al: Osteomielitis neonatal: estudio de una serie de 35 casos, *Ann Esp Pediatr* 33:429, 1990.
68. Omene JA, Odita JC: Clinical and radiological features of neonatal septic arthritis, *Trop Geogr Med* 31:207, 1979.
69. Asmar BI: Osteomyelitis in the neonate, *Infect Dis Clin North Am* 6:117, 1992.
70. Garcia Pena BM, Harper MB, Fleisher GR: Occult bacteremia with group B streptococci in an outpatient setting, *Pediatrics* 102:67, 1998.
71. Choma TJ, Davlin LB, Wagner JS: Iliac osteomyelitis in the newborn presenting as nonspecific musculoskeletal sepsis, *Orthopedics* 17:632, 1994.
72. Barton LL, Villar RG, Rice SA: Neonatal group B streptococcal vertebral osteomyelitis, *Pediatrics* 98:459, 1996.
73. Speer CP, Hauptmann D, Stubbe P, et al: Neonatal septicemia and meningitis in Göttingen, West Germany, *Pediatr Infect Dis* 4:36, 1985.
74. Karpuch J, Goldberg M, Kohelet D: Neonatal bacteremia: a 4-year prospective study, *Isr J Med Sci* 19:963, 1983.
75. Levy HL, O'Connor JF, Ingall D: Neonatal osteomyelitis due to Proteus mirabilis, *JAMA* 202:582, 1967.
76. Müller WD, Urban C, Haidvogel M, et al: Septische Arthritis und Osteomyelitis als Komplikation neonataler Intensivpflege, *Paediatr Paedol* 14:469, 1979.
77. Bogdanovich A: Neonatal arthritis due to Proteus vulgaris, *Arch Dis Child* 23:65, 1948.
78. Omene JA, Odita JC, Okolo AA: Neonatal osteomyelitis in Nigerian infants, *Pediatr Radiol* 14:318, 1984.
79. Choi IH, Pizzutillo PD, Bowen JR, et al: Sequelae and reconstruction after septic arthritis of the hip in infants, *J Bone Joint Surg Am* 72:1150, 1990.
80. Peters W, Irving J, Letts M: Long-term effects of neonatal bone and joint infection on adjacent growth plates, *J Pediatr Orthop* 12:806, 1992.
81. Hensey JO, Hart CA, Cooke RWI: Serious infections in a neonatal intensive care unit: a two year survey, *J Hyg* 95:289, 1985.
82. Berant M, Kahana D: *Klebsiella* osteomyelitis in a newborn, *Am J Dis Child* 118:634, 1969.

83. White AA, Crelin ES, McIntosh S: Septic arthritis of the hip joint secondary to umbilical artery catheterization associated with transient femoral and sciatic neuropathy, *Clin Orthop* 100:190, 1974.
84. Nathanson I, Giacoia GP: *Klebsiella* osteoarthritis in prematurity: complication of umbilical artery catheterization, *N Y State J Med* 79:2077, 1979.
85. Voss HV, Göbel U, Kemperdick H, et al: *Enterobacter*-Osteomyelitis bei zwei Säuglingen, *Klin Paediatr* 187:465, 1975.
86. Gordon SL, Maisels MJ, Robbins WJ: Multiple joint infections with Enterobacter cloacae, *Clin Orthop* 125:136, 1977.
87. Bayer AS, Chow AW, Louie JS, et al: Gram-negative bacillary septic arthritis: clinical, radiographic, therapeutic, and prognostic features, *Semin Arthritis Rheum* 7:123, 1977.
88. Gajzago D, Gottche O: *Salmonella suipestifer* infections in childhood, *Am J Dis Child* 63:15, 1942.
89. Levinsky RJ: Two children with *Pseudomonas* osteomyelitis: the paucity of systemic symptoms may lead to delay in diagnosis, *Clin Pediatr* 14:288, 1975.
90. Konzert W: Über ein *Salmonella*-Osteomyelitis im Rahmen einer *Salmonella typhimurium* Epidemia auf einer Neugeborenen Station, *Wien Klin Wochenschr* 81:713, 1969.
91. Tur AJ, Gartoch OO: Ein Fall von Erkrankung eines frühgeborenen Kindes im ersten Lebensmonate an multiplier Arthritis durch den, *Bacillus suipestifer*, *Z Kinderheilkd* 56:696, 1934.
92. Adeyokunnu AA, Hendrickse RG: *Salmonella* osteomyelitis in childhood: a report of 63 cases seen in Nigerian children of whom 57 had sickle cell anemia, *Arch Dis Child* 55:175, 1980.
93. Steinwender G, Schimpl G, Sixl B, et al: Gut-derived bone infection in the neonatal rat, *Pediatr Res* 50:767, 2001.
94. Nair S, Schoeneman MJ: Septic arthritis in an infant with vesicoureteral reflux and urinary tract infection, *Pediatrics* 111:e195, 2003.
95. Kohen DP: Neonatal gonococcal arthritis: three cases and review of the literature, *Pediatrics* 53:436, 1974.
96. Gregory JE, Chison JL, Meadows AT: Short case report: gonococcal arthritis in an infant, *Br J Vener Dis* 48:306, 1972.
97. Cooperman MB: End results of gonorrheal arthritis: a review of seventy cases, *Am J Surg* 5:241, 1928.
98. Nabarro D: *Congenital syphilis*, London, 1954, Edward Arnold.
99. Zenker PN, Berman SM: Congenital syphilis: trends and recommendations for evaluation and management, *Pediatr Infect Dis J* 10:516, 1991.
100. Brion LP, Manuli M, Rai B, et al: Long-bone radiographic abnormalities as a sign of active congenital syphilis in asymptomatic newborns, *Pediatrics* 88:1037, 1991.
101. Lequier L, Robinson J, Vaudry W: Sternotomy infection with *Mycoplasma hominis* in a neonate, *Pediatr Infect Dis J* 14:1010, 1995.
102. Gjuric G, Prislin-Muskić M, Nikolić E, et al: *Ureaplasma urealyticum* osteomyelitis in a very low birth weight infant, *Perinat Med* 22:79, 1994.
103. Hughesdon MR: Congenital tuberculosis, *Arch Dis Child* 21:121, 1946.
104. Mallet R, Ribierre M, Labrune B, Breteaue C: Diffuse bony tuberculosis in the newborn (spina ventosa generalisata), *Semaine Hôp Paris* 44:36, 1968.
105. Harris MC, Pereira GR, Myers MD, et al: Candidal arthritis in infants previously treated for systemic candidiasis during the newborn period: report of three cases, *Pediatr Emerg Care* 16:249, 2000.
106. Merchant RH, Sanghvi KP, Sridhar N, et al: Nursery outbreak of neonatal fungal arthritis treated with fluconazole, *J Trop Pediatr* 43:106, 1997.
107. Pan N, Herzog R, Blanco JS, et al: *Candida albicans* osteomyelitis in an infant: a case report and literature review, *J Pediatr Orthop* 22:491, 2013.
108. Oleinik EM, Della-Latta P, Rinaldi MG, et al: *Candida lusitaniae* in premature infant, *Am J Perinatol* 10:313, 1993.
109. Weisse ME, Person DA, Berkenbaugh JT Jr: Treatment of *Candida* arthritis with flucytosine and amphotericin B, *J Perinatol* 13:402, 1993.
110. Offiah AC: Acute osteomyelitis and discitis: difference between neonates and older children, *Eur J Radiol* 60:221, 2006.
111. Nelson DL, Hable KA, Matsen JM: *Proteus mirabilis* osteomyelitis in two neonates following needle puncture, *Am J Dis Child* 125:109, 1973.
112. Asnes RS, Arendar GM: Septic arthritis of the hip: a complication of femoral venipuncture, *Pediatrics* 38:837, 1966.
113. Chacha PB: Suppurative arthritis of the hip joint in infancy: a persistent diagnostic problem and possible complication of femoral venipuncture, *J Bone Joint Surg Am* 53:538, 1971.
114. Overturf GD, Balfour G: Osteomyelitis and sepsis: severe complications of fetal monitoring, *Pediatrics* 55:244, 1975.
115. Plavidal FJ, Werch A: Fetal scalp abscess secondary to intrauterine monitoring, *Am J Obstet Gynecol* 125:65, 1976.
116. Brook I: Osteomyelitis and bacteremia caused by *Bacteroides fragilis*: a complication of fetal monitoring, *Clin Pediatr* 19:639, 1980.
117. McGregor JA, McFarren T: Neonatal cranial osteomyelitis: a complication of fetal monitoring, *Obstet Gynecol* 73:490, 1989.
118. Puczynski MS, Dvonch VM, Menendez CE, et al: Osteomyelitis of the great toe secondary to phlebotomy, *Clin Orthop* 190:239, 1984.
119. Lilien LD, Harris VJ, Ramamurthy RS, et al: Neonatal osteomyelitis of the calcaneus: complication of heel puncture, *J Pediatr* 88:478, 1976.
120. Myers MG, McMahon BJ, Koontz FP: Neonatal calcaneus osteomyelitis related to contaminated mineral oil, *Clin Microbiol* 6:543, 1977.
121. Blumenfeld TA, Turi GK, Blanc WA: Recommended site and depth of newborn heel skin punctures based on anatomical measurements and histopathology, *Lancet* 1:230, 1979.
122. Borris LC, Helleland H: Growth disturbance of the hind part of the foot following osteomyelitis of the calcaneus in the newborn: a report of two cases, *J Bone Joint Surg Am* 68:302, 1986.
123. Fernandez-Fanjul JL, Lopez-Sastre J, Coto-Cotallo D, et al: Osteomyelitis des Calcaneus beim Neugeborenen als Folge diagnostischer Fersenpunktionen, *Monatsschr Kinderheilkd* 127:515, 1979.
124. Bergman I, Wald ER, Meyer JD, et al: Epidural abscess and vertebral osteomyelitis following serial lumbar punctures, *Pediatrics* 72:476, 1983.
125. Edwards MS, Baker CJ: Median sternotomy wound infections in children, *Pediatr Infect Dis* 2:105, 1983.
126. Valerio PH: Osteomyelitis as a complication of perinatal fracture of the clavicle, *Eur J Pediatr* 154:497, 1995.
127. Mohon RT, Mehalic TF, Grimes CK, et al: Infected cephalohematoma and neonatal osteomyelitis of the skull, *Pediatr Infect Dis* 5:253, 1986.
128. Nightingale LM, Eaton CB, Fruehan AE, et al: 1986 Cephalohematoma complicated by osteomyelitis presumed due to *Gardnerella vaginalis*, *JAMA* 256, 1936.
129. Lee PYC: Case report: infected cephalohematoma and neonatal osteomyelitis, *J Infect* 21:191, 1990.
130. Chan MS, Wong YC, Lau SP, et al: MRI and CT findings of infected cephalohematoma complicated by skull vault osteomyelitis, venous sinus thrombosis and left cerebral hemorrhage, *Pediatr Radiol* 32:376, 2002.
131. Nakwan N, Nakwan N, Wannaro J, et al: Septicemia, meningitis and skull osteomyelitis complicating infected cephalohematoma caused by ESBL-producing *Esherichia coli*, *Southeast Asian J Trop Med Public Health* 42:148, 2011.
132. McCarthy D, Walker AHC, Matthews S: Scalp abscesses in the newborn: a discussion of their causation, *J Obstet Gynaecol Br Emp* 59:37, 1952.
133. Ladewig W: Über eine intrauterin entstandene umschriebene Osteomyelitis des Schädeldaches, *Virchows Arch Pathol Anat* 289:395, 1933.
134. Trueta J: Three types of acute haematogenous osteomyelitis, *J Bone Joint Surg Br* 41:671, 1959.
135. Todd RM: Septicaemia of the newborn: a clinical study of fifteen cases, *Arch Dis Child* 23:102, 1948.
136. Svirsky-Fein S, Langer L, Milbauer B, et al: Neonatal osteomyelitis caused by *Candida tropicalis*: report of two cases and review of the literature, *J Bone Joint Surg Am* 61:455, 1979.
137. Baley JE, Kliegman RM, Fanaroff AA: Disseminated fungal infections in very low-birth-weight infants: clinical manifestations and epidemiology, *Pediatrics* 73:144, 1984.
138. Rhodes PG, Hall RT, Burry VE, et al: Sepsis and osteomyelitis due to *Staphylococcus aureus* phage type 94 in a neonatal intensive care unit, *J Pediatr* 88:1063, 1976.
139. Qureshi ME: Osteomyelitis after exchange transfusion, *BMJ* 1:28, 1971.
140. Simmons PB, Harris LE, Bianco AJ: Complications of exchange transfusion: report of two cases of septic arthritis and osteomyelitis, *Mayo Clin Proc* 48:190, 1973.

141. Lindblad B, Ekingren K, Aurelius G: The prognosis of acute hematogenous osteomyelitis and its complications during early infancy after the advent of antibiotics, *Acta Paediatr Scand* 54:24, 1965.
142. Chung SMK: The arterial supply of the developing proximal end of the human femur, *J Bone Joint Surg Am* 58:961, 1976.
143. Ogden JA: Pediatric osteomyelitis and septic arthritis: the pathology of neonatal disease, *Yale J Biol Med* 52:423, 1979.
144. Cass JM: *Staphylococcus aureus* infection of the long bones in the newly born, *Arch Dis Child* 15:55, 1940.
145. Stone S: Osteomyelitis of the long bones in the newborn, *Am J Dis Child* 64:680, 1942.
146. Curtis PH, Klein L: Destruction of articular cartilage in septic arthritis, I: in vitro studies, *J Bone Joint Surg Am* 45:797, 1963.
147. deLorimier AA, Haskin D, Massie FS: Mediastinal mass caused by vertebral osteomyelitis, *Am J Dis Child* 111:639, 1966.
148. Knudsen FU, Petersen S: Neonatal septic osteoarthritis due to umbilical artery catheterisation, *Acta Paediatr Scand* 66:225, 1977.
149. Curtis PH, Klein L: Destruction of articular cartilage in septic arthritis, II: in vivo studies, *J Bone Joint Surg Am* 47:1595, 1965.
150. Obletz BE: Acute suppurative arthritis of the hip in the neonatal period, *J Bone Joint Surg Am* 42:23, 1960.
151. Glassberg GB, Ozonoff MB: Arthrographic findings in septic arthritis of the hip in infants, *Radiology* 128:151, 1978.
152. Greengard J: Acute hematogenous osteomyelitis in infancy, *Med Clin North Am* 30:135, 1946.
153. Bressler EL, Conway JJ, Weiss SC: Neonatal osteomyelitis examined by bone scintigraphy, *Radiology* 152:685, 1984.
154. Clay SA: Osteomyelitis as a cause of brachial plexus neuropathy, *Am J Dis Child* 136:1054, 1982.
155. Young RSK, Hawkes DL: Pseudopseudoparalysis. Letter to the editor, *Am J Dis Child* 137:504, 1983.
156. Isaacs D, Bower BD, Moxon ER: Neonatal osteomyelitis presenting as nerve palsy, *BMJ* 1:1071, 1986.
157. Obando I, Martin E, Alvarez-Aldean J, et al: Group B streptococcus pelvic osteomyelitis presenting as footdrop in a newborn infant, *Pediatr Infect Dis J* 10:703, 1991.
158. Kaye JJ, Winchester PH, Freiberger RH: Neonatal septic "dislocation" of the hip: true dislocation or pathological epiphyseal separation? *Radiology* 114:671, 1975.
159. DeWet IS: Acute osteomyelitis and suppurative arthritis of infants, *S Afr Med J* 28:81, 1954.
160. Ingelrans P, Fontaine G, Lacheretz M, et al: Les ostéoarthrites du nouveau-né et du nourrison: particulariteés étiologiques, diagnostiques et thérapeutiques: à propos de 35 observations, *Lille Med* 13:390, 1968.
161. Chung SMK, Pollis RE: Diagnostic pitfalls in septic arthritis of the hip in infants and children, *Clin Pediatr* 14:758, 1975.
162. Lai TK, Hingston J, Scheifele D: Streptococcal neonatal osteomyelitis, *Am J Dis Child* 134:711, 1980.
163. Ancona RJ, McAuliffe J, Thompson TR, et al: Group B streptococcal sepsis with osteomyelitis and arthritis: its occurrence with acute heart failure, *Am J Dis Child* 133:919, 1979.
164. McCook TA, Felman AH, Ayoub E: Streptococcal skeletal infections: observations in four infants, *AJR Am J Roentgenol* 130:465, 1978.
165. Chilton SJ, Aftimos SF, White PW: Diffuse skeletal involvement of streptococcal osteomyelitis in a neonate, *Radiology* 134:390, 1980.
166. Broughton RA, Edwards MS, Haffar A, et al: Unusual manifestations of neonatal group B streptococcal osteomyelitis, *Pediatr Infect Dis* 1:410, 1982.
167. Einstein RAJ, Thomas CG Jr: Osteomyelitis in infants, *AJR Am J Roentgenol* 55:299, 1946.
168. Stack JK, Newman W: Neonatal osteomyelitis, *Q Bull Northwest Univ Med Sch* 27:69, 1953.
169. Ish-Horowicz MR, McIntyre P, Nade S: Bone and joint infections caused by multiply resistant *Staphylococcus aureus* in a neonatal intensive care unit, *Pediatr Infect Dis J* 11:82, 1992.
170. Waldvogel FA, Medoff G, Swartz MN: *Osteomyelitis: clinical features, therapeutic considerations, and unusual aspects*, Springfield, Ill, 1971, Charles C Thomas.
171. Dich VQ, Nelson JD, Haltalin KC: Osteomyelitis in infants and children: a review of 163 cases, *Am J Dis Child* 129:1273, 1975.
172. Samilson RL, Bersani FA, Watkins MB: Acute suppurative arthritis in infants and children, *Pediatrics* 21:798, 1958.
173. Hallel T, Salvati EA: Septic arthritis of the hip in infancy: end result study, *Clin Orthop* 132:115, 1978.
174. Bennett OM, Namyak SS: Acute septic arthritis of the hip joint in infancy and childhood, *Clin Orthop* 281:123, 1992.
175. Halbstein BM: Bone regeneration in infantile osteomyelitis: report of a case with 14-year follow-up, *J Bone Joint Surg Am* 49:149, 1967.
176. Miller B: Regeneration of the lateral femoral condyle after osteomyelitis in infancy, *Clin Orthop* 65:163, 1969.
177. Roberts PH: Disturbed epiphyseal growth at the knee after osteomyelitis in infancy, *J Bone Joint Surg Br* 52:692, 1970.
178. Ekengren K, Bergdahl S, Eriksson M: Neonatal osteomyelitis: radiographic findings and prognosis in relation to site of involvement, *Acta Radiol Diagn* 23:305, 1982.
179. Mallet JF, Rigault P, Padovani JP, et al: Les cyphoses par spondylodiscite grave du nourrisson et du jeune enfant, *Rev Chir Orthop* 70:63, 1984.
180. Ammari LK, Offit PA, Campbell AB: Unusual presentation of group B streptococcus osteomyelitis, *Pediatr Infect Dis J* 11:1066, 1992.
181. Altman N, Harwood-Nash DC, Fitz CR, et al: Evaluation of the infant spine by direct sagittal computed tomography, *AJNR Am J Neuroradiol* 6:65, 1985.
182. Bolivar R, Kohl S, Pickering LK: Vertebral osteomyelitis in children: report of 4 cases, *Pediatrics* 62:549, 1978.
183. Bode H, Kunzer W: Dornfortsatzosteomyelitis der Brustwirbel 10 und 11 bei einem Neugeborenen, *Klin Paediatr* 197:65, 1985.
184. McCook TA, Felman AH, Ayoub E: Streptococcal skeletal infections: observations in four infections, *AJR Am J Roentgenol* 130:465, 1978.
185. Ein SH, Shandling B, Humphreys R, et al: Osteomyelitis of the cervical spine presenting as a neurenteric cyst, *J Pediatr Surg* 23:779, 1988.
186. Lloyd-Roberts GC: Suppurative arthritis of infancy: some observations upon prognosis and management, *J Bone Joint Surg Br* 42:706, 1960.
187. Singson RD, Berdon WE, Feldman F, et al: "Missing" femoral condyle: an unusual sequela to neonatal osteomyelitis and septic arthritis, *Radiology* 161:359, 1986.
188. Potter CMC: Osteomyelitis in the newborn, *J Bone Joint Surg Br* 36:578, 1954.
189. Troger J, Eissner D, Otte G, et al: Diagnose und Differentialdiagnose der akuten hämatogenen Osteomyelitis des Säuglings, *Radiologe* 19:99, 1979.
190. Vallcanera A, Moreno-Flores A, Gomez J, et al: Osteochondroma post osteomyelitis, *Pediatr Radiol* 26:680, 1996.
191. Harris VJ, Meeks W: The frequency of radiolucencies underlying cephalohematomas, *Pediatr Radiol* 129:391, 1978.
192. Einhorn M, Howard DB, Dagan R: The use of ultrasound in the diagnosis and management of childhood acute hematogenous osteomyelitis (abstract Publ 77) Thirty-First Interscience Conference on Antimicrobial Agents and Chemotherapy: Anaheim, Calif, October 1992.
193. Riebel TW, Nasir R, Nazarenko O: The value of sonography in the detection of osteomyelitis, *Pediatr Radiol* 26:291, 1996.
194. Jaramillo D, Treves ST, Kasser JR, et al: Osteomyelitis and septic arthritis in children: appropriate use of imaging to guide treatment, *Am J Radiol* 165:399, 1995.
195. Volberg FM, Sumner TE, Abramson JS, et al: Unreliability of radiographic diagnosis of septic hip in children, *Pediatrics* 74:118, 1984.
196. Perkins MD, Edwards KM, Heller RM, et al: Neonatal group B streptococcal osteomyelitis and suppurative arthritis: outpatient therapy, *Clin Pediatr* 28:229, 1989.
197. Schauwecker DS, Braunstein EM, Wheat LJ: Diagnostic imaging of osteomyelitis, *Infect Dis Clin North Am* 4:441, 1990.
198. Moore SG, Bisset GS 3rd, Siegel MJ, et al: Pediatric musculoskeletal MR imaging, *Radiology* 179:345, 1991.
199. Williamson SL, Seibert JJ, Glasier CM, et al: Ultrasound in advanced pediatric osteomyelitis: a report of 5 cases, *Pediatr Radiol* 21:288, 1991.
200. Abiri MM, Kirpekar M, Ablow RC: Osteomyelitis: detection with US, *Radiology* 172:509, 1989.
201. Zeiger MM, Dorr U, Schulz RD: Ultrasonography of hip joint effusions, *Skeletal Radiol* 16:607, 1987.
202. Velkes S, Ganel A, Chechick A: Important modality available in the diagnostic armamentarium of septic arthritis of the hip is ultrasonography, *Clin Orthop* 260:309, 1990.
203. Rubin LP, Wallach MT, Wood BP: Radiological case of the month, *Arch Pediatr Adolesc Med* 150:217, 1996.
204. Wright NB, Abbott GT, Carty HML: Ultrasound in children with osteomyelitis, *Clin Radiol* 50:623, 1995.
205. Harcke HT Jr: Bone imaging in infants and children: a review, *J Nucl Med* 19:324, 1978.

206. Ash JM, Gilday DL: The futility of bone scanning neonatal osteomyelitis: concise communication, *J Nucl Med* 21:417, 1980.
207. Gilday DL, Paul DJ: Diagnosis of osteomyelitis in children by combined blood pool and bone imaging, *Radiology* 117:331, 1975.
208. Canale ST, Harkness RM, Thomas PA, et al: Does aspiration of bones and joints affect results of later bone scanning? *J Pediatr Orthop* 5:23, 1985.
209. Traughber PD, Manaster BJ, Murphy K, et al: Negative bone scans of joints after aspiration or arthrography: experimental studies, *AJR Am J Roentgenol* 146:87, 1986.
210. Herndon WA, Alexieva BT, Schwindt ML, et al: Nuclear imaging for musculoskeletal infections in children, *J Pediatr Orthop* 5:343, 1985.
211. Lewin JS, Rosenfield NS, Hoffer PB, et al: Acute osteomyelitis in children: combined Tc-99m and Ga-67 imaging, *Radiology* 158:795, 1986.
212. Berkowitz ID, Wenzel W: "Normal" technetium bone scans in patients with acute osteomyelitis, *Am J Dis Child* 134:828, 1980.
213. Handmaker H, Giammona ST: Improved early diagnosis of acute inflammatory skeletal-articular diseases in children: a two-radiopharmaceutical approach, *Pediatrics* 73:661, 1984.
214. Melson GL, McDaniel RC, Southern PM, et al: In vitro effects of iodinated arthrographic contrast media on bacterial growth, *Radiology* 112:593, 1974.
215. Cole WG, Dalziel RE, Leitl S: Treatment of acute osteomyelitis in childhood, *J Bone Joint Surg Br* 64:218, 1982.
216. Rasool MN, Govender S: The skeletal manifestations of congenital syphilis: a review of 197 cases, *J Bone Joint Surg Br* 71:752, 1989.
217. Hiva SK, Ganapati JB, Patel JB: Early congenital syphilis: clinico-radiologic features in 202 patients, *Sex Transm Dis* 12:177, 1985.
218. McLean S: The roentgenographic and pathologic aspects of congenital osseous syphilis, *Am J Dis Child* 41:130, 1931.
219. Ewerbeck V, Bolkenius M, Braun A, et al: Knochentumoren und tumorähnliche Veränderungen im Neugeborenen-und Säuglingsalter, *Z Orthop* 123:918, 1985.
220. Meyers S, Lonon W, Shannon K: Suppurative bursitis in early childhood, *Pediatr Infect Dis* 3:156, 1984.
221. Brian MJ, O'Ryan M, Waagner D: Prepatellar bursitis in an infant caused by group B streptococcus, *Pediatr Infect Dis J* 11:502, 1992.
222. Keller MA, Sellers BB Jr, Melish ME, et al: Systemic candidiasis in infants: a case presentation and literature review, *Am J Dis Child* 131:1260, 1977.
223. Reiser VM, Rupp N, Färber D: Röntgenologische Befunde bei der septischen *Candida*-Arthritis, *Rofo* 129:335, 1978.
224. Businco L, Iannaccone G, Del Principe D, et al: Disseminated arthritis and osteitis by *Candida albicans* in a two month old infant receiving parenteral nutrition, *Acta Paediatr Scand* 66:393, 1977.
225. Rudolph AJ, Singleton EB, Rosenberg HS, et al: Osseous manifestations of the congenital rubella syndrome, *Am J Dis Child* 110:428, 1965.
226. Merten DF, Gooding CA: Skeletal manifestations of congenital cytomegalic inclusion disease, *Radiology* 95:333, 1970.
227. Jenson HB, Robert MF: Congenital cytomegalovirus infection with osteolytic lesions: use of DNA hybridization in diagnosis, *Clin Pediatr* 26:448, 1987.
228. Chalhub EG, Baenziger J, Feigen RD, et al: Congenital herpes simplex type II infection with extensive hepatic calcification, bone lesions and cataracts: complete postmortem examination, *Dev Med Child Neurol* 19:527, 1977.
229. Madsen ET: Fractures of the extremities in the newborn, *Acta Obstet Gynecol Scand* 34:41, 1955.
230. Caffey J: *Pediatric x-ray diagnosis*, 6th ed, Chicago, 1972, Year Book Medical Publishers.
231. Park HM, Kernek CB, Robb JA: Early scintigraphic findings of occult femoral and tibial fractures in infants, *Clin Nucl Med* 13:271, 1988.
232. Marshall GS, Edwards KM, Wadlington WB: Sporadic congenital Caffey's disease, *Clin Pediatr* 26:177, 1987.
233. Ravenel D: Cellulitis from extravasation of calcium gluconate simulating osteomyelitis, *Am J Dis Child* 137:402, 1983.
234. Ringel RE, Haney PJ, Brenner JI, et al: Periosteal changes secondary to prostaglandin administration, *J Pediatr* 103:251, 1983.
235. Ditkowsky SP, Goldman A, Barnett H, et al: Normal periosteal reactions and associated soft-tissue findings, *Clin Pediatr* 9:515, 1970.
236. Nelson JD: Follow up: the bacterial etiology and antibiotic management of septic arthritis in infants and children, *Pediatrics* 50:437, 1972.
237. Cooper GI, Hopkins CC: Rapid diagnosis of intravascular catheter-associated infection by direct Gram staining of catheter segments, *N Engl J Med* 312:1142, 1985.
238. Schauf V, Deveikis A, Riff L, et al: Antibiotic-killing kinetics of group B streptococci, *J Pediatr* 89:194, 1976.
239. Paakkonen M, Petola H: Management of a child with suspected septic arthritis, *Arch Dis Child* 97:287, 2012.
240. Sann L, Bienvenu F, Bienvenu J, et al: Evolution of serum prealbumin, C-reactive protein, and orosomucoid in neonates with bacterial infection, *J Pediatr* 105:977, 1984.
241. Philip AGS: Acute-phase proteins in neonatal infection, *J Pediatr* 105:940, 1984.
242. Fajardo JE, Bass JW, Lugo EJ, et al: Oral dicloxacillin for the treatment of neonatal osteomyelitis, *Am J Dis Child* 138:991, 1984.
243. Schwartz GJ, Hegyi T, Spitzer A: Subtherapeutic dicloxacillin levels in a neonate: possible mechanisms, *J Pediatr* 89:310, 1976.
244. Nelson JD: Options for outpatient management of serious infections, *Pediatr Infect Dis J* 11:175, 1992.
245. Dunkle LM: Towards optimum management of serious focal infections: the model of suppurative arthritis, *Pediatr Infect Dis J* 8:195, 1989.
246. Borella L, Goobar JE, Summitt RL, et al: Septic arthritis in childhood, *J Pediatr* 62:742, 1963.
247. Halder D, Seng QB, Malik AS, et al: Neonatal septic arthritis, *Southeast Asian J Trop Med Public Health* 27:600, 1996.
248. Dobbs MB, Sheridan JJ, Gordon JE, et al: Septic arthritis of the hip in infancy: long term follow-up, *J Pediatr Orthop* 23:162, 2003.
249. Jagodzinski NA, Kanwar R, Graham K, et al: Prospective evaluation of a shortened regimen of treatment for osteomyelitis and septic arthritis in children, *J Pediatr Orthop* 29:518, 2009.
250. Mortia M, Nakamura H, Kitano T: Comparison of clinical outcomes after treatment of hip arthritis caused by MRSA with that caused by non-MRSA in infants, *J Pediatr Orthop* 18:1, 2009.
251. Nunn TR, Cheung WY, Rollinson PD: A prospective study of pyogenic sepsis of the hip in childhood, *J Bone Joint Surg Br* 89:100, 2007.
252. Givon U, Liberman B, Schindler A, et al: Treatment of septic arthritis of the hip by repeated ultrasound-guided aspirations, *J Pediatr Orthop* 24:266, 2004.
253. Bos CF, Mol LJ, Obermann WR, et al: Late sequelae of neonatal septic arthritis of the shoulder, *J Bone Joint Surg Br* 80:645, 1998.
254. Nade S: Septic arthritis, *Best Pract Res Clin Rheumatol* 17:183, 2003.
255. Umadevi S, Kali A, Sreenivasan S, et al: Septic arthritis caused by group b Streptoccus in newborns. An unusual presentation, *J Clin Diagn Res* 7:1143, 2013.
256. Howard PJ: Sepsis in normal and premature infants with localization in the hip joint, *Pediatrics* 20:279, 1957.
257. Gilmour WN: Acute hematogenous osteomyelitis, *J Bone Joint Surg Br* 44:841, 1962.
258. Allibone EC, Mills CP: Osteomyelitis of the premaxilla, *Arch Dis Child* 36:562, 1961.
259. Boete G: Zur Frage der Spätschäden nach Kieferosteomyelitis von Säuglingen und Kleinkindern, *Arch Klin Exp Ohren Nasen Kehlkopfheilkd* 187:674, 1966.
260. Cavanagh F: Osteomyelitis of the superior maxilla in infants: a report on 24 personally treated cases, *BMJ* 1:468, 1960.
261. McCash CR, Rowe NL: Acute osteomyelitis of the maxilla in infancy, *J Bone Joint Surg Br* 35:22, 1953.
262. Wilensky AO: The pathogenesis and treatment of acute osteomyelitis of the jaws in nurslings and infants, *Am J Dis Child* 43:431, 1932.
263. Bass MH: Acute osteomyelitis of the superior maxilla in young infants. *Am J Dis Child* 70:382, 1954.
264. Webb JF: Newborn infants and breast abscesses of staphylococcal origin, *Can Med Assoc J* 70:382, 1954.
265. Wong SK, Wilhelmus KR: Infantile maxillary osteomyelitis, *J Pediatr Ophthalmol Strabismus* 23:153, 1986.
266. Burnard ED: Proptosis as the first sign of orbital sepsis in the newborn, *Br J Ophthalmol* 43:9, 1959.
267. Hahlbrock KH: Über die Oberkieferosteomyelitis des Säuglings, *Klin Monatsbl Augenheilkd* 145:744, 1964.

9 Bacterial Infections of the Urinary Tract

SARAH S. LONG and JEROME O. KLEIN

CHAPTER OUTLINE

In 1918, Helmholz[1] recognized the cryptogenic nature and underdiagnosis of urinary tract infection (UTI) in the newborn. His observations still hold true today. There are no specific signs of UTI in a newborn; the clinical presentation can vary, ranging from fever with or without other signs of septicemia to minimal changes such as alteration in feeding habits or poor weight gain. The diagnosis of UTI in a neonate is made only by the examination and culture of a properly obtained specimen of urine.

The reported incidence, clinical manifestations, and prognosis of UTI in neonates have varied significantly. There are at least two reasons for discrepant results obtained in studies of UTI: (1) different criteria have been used to define UTI, and (2) infants with different characteristics have been studied. Before 1960 clean-voided specimens were used almost exclusively for examination and culture of urine. It is now clear that contamination is frequent when this method is used; Schlager and coworkers[2] observed that 16 cultures of urine obtained by bag collection from 98 healthy newborns yielded greater than 10^4 colonies/mL of urine, with organisms that were found also on periurethral skin. The only reliable methods for obtaining urine for bacteriologic study are percutaneous aspiration and urethral catheterization of bladder urine.

Bacterial infections of the kidney and urinary tract in neonates are usually acquired at or after delivery. Fungal infections develop as nosocomial infections in infants with risk factors such as prematurity and use of intravascular catheters, parenteral alimentation, and broad-spectrum antibiotics, or after prolonged or intermittent catheterization of the urinary tract.[3,4] Viral infections, including rubella, herpes simplex, and cytomegalovirus infections, are responsible for in utero infection, although the organisms can be excreted in the urine for months after birth. Common bacterial infections of the urinary tract are reviewed here. For information about infection and disease of the kidney and urinary tract caused by other microorganisms, the reader is referred to the chapters on toxoplasmosis, rubella, cytomegalovirus, herpes simplex, syphilis, mycoplasmas, *Candida*, group B streptococci, gonorrhea, staphylococcal infection, and neonatal diarrhea *(Salmonella)*.

Epidemiology

The incidence of UTI in infants in the first month of life varies, ranging from 0.1% to 1% in older studies.[5-11] Using a national database for 2003, the rate of hospitalization for UTI was 53.6 per 100,000 population younger than 1 month.[12] The frequency may be 10% in infants of low birth weight[13] and 12% to 25% in infants of very low birth weight evaluated for sepsis (Table 9-1).[14,15] In contrast to the increased incidence of bacteriuria among females in other age groups, infection of the urinary tract in the first 3 months of life is more frequent in males.[2,5-10,15-17]

Infection of the urinary tract is usually sporadic, but clusters of cases, closely related in time, have been reported from nurseries in Cleveland[18] and Baltimore.[19] A nursery epidemic caused by *Serratia marcescens* was responsible for UTI and balanitis; the outbreak was caused by contamination of a solution applied to the umbilical cord.[20]

Surveys of infants born in U.S. Army medical centers and subsequently hospitalized for UTI indicate that uncircumcised boys have substantially more UTIs than circumcised boys in the first month and in months 2 to 12 of life.[11,21,22] In 1982, Ginsburg and McCracken[23] observed that 95% of 62 infant boys with UTI were uncircumcised. A case-control study performed in 112 infant boys in whom suprapubic aspiration or bladder catheterization had been performed for investigation of acute illness showed that all infants with UTI were uncircumcised, compared with 32% of control subjects.[24] Infection was associated with anatomic abnormalities in 26% of cases. In a meta-analysis of infants younger than 3 months who were evaluated for fever, rates of UTI were 7.5% for girls, 2.4% for circumcised boys, and 20.1% for uncircumcised boys.[25] The records of

Table 9-1 Incidence of Urinary Tract Infection in Newborn Infants: Results of Eight Studies

			SEX				BIRTH WEIGHT			
			MALE		FEMALE		MALE		FEMALE	
Study	**Methods Used to Obtain Urine**	**No. Infected/ No. Studied (%)**	**No. Surveyed**	**No. Infected**	**No. Surveyed**	**No. Infected**	**No. Surveyed**	**No. Infected**	**No. Surveyed**	**No. Infected**
Christchurch, NZ, 1968-1969[5]	CVS, SPA	14/1460 (0.95)	757	11	703	3	NS	—	NS	—
Göteborg, 1960-1966[6]	CVS	75*/57,000 (0.14)	NS	54	NS	21	NS	11	NS	64
New York, 1973[7†]	CVS, SPA	12/1042 (1.2)	493	7	549	5	206	6	836	6
Leeds, 1967[8]	CVS, SPA	8/600 (1.3)	309	7	291	1	NS	0	NS	8
Oklahoma City, 1974[13]	SPA	10/102 (10)	NS	NS	NS	NS	102	10	—	—
Lausanne, 1978[9†]	CVS, SPA	43/1762‡ (2.4)	1006	26	756	7	634§	10	1028‖	33
Göteborg, 1977-1980[10¶]	CVS, SPA	26/198 (0.81)	1502	23	1696	3	—	—	—	—
U.S. Army, 1975-1984[11#]	SPA, Ca	320/422,328 (0.08)	217, 116	162	205, 212	158	—	—	—	—

Ca, Catheter; *CVS*, clean-voided specimen; *NS*, not stated; *SPA*, suprapubic aspiration (of bladder urine).
*Five male infants with infection and suspected or proven obstruction malformation of urinary tract not included.
†Date of published report; years of study not provided.
‡Includes only infants <28 days of age who were admitted to neonatal intensive care unit.
§Results reported for premature infants (<259 days of gestation)
‖Results reported for term infants (≥259 days of gestation).
¶Results reported for infants 1 week to 2 months of age.
#Results reported for infants 1 week to 2 months of age who were hospitalized.

more than 136,000 boys born in U.S. Army hospitals from 1980 to 1985 were reviewed through the first month of life to compare clinical courses in uncircumcised and circumcised boys.[26] Of 35,929 uncircumcised boys, 88 (0.24%) had UTI, 33 had concomitant bacteremia, 3 had meningitis, 2 had renal failure, and 2 died. Complications followed 0.19% of 100,157 circumcisions (including 20 UTIs), and all were minor except for three episodes of hemorrhage leading to transfusion. Meta-analysis of nine published studies through 1992 yielded an overall 12-fold increased risk of infection in uncircumcised boys.[27]

Studies published in 1996 and 1998 using case-control and cohort design support the earlier observational studies,[11] with newer studies showing a three- to sevenfold increased risk for uncircumcised boys.[28,29] An investigation by the Cochrane Neonatal Group found no randomized or quasi-randomized controlled trial of circumcision to prevent UTI.[30] The American Academy of Pediatrics (AAP) has made a variety of statements regarding male circumcision after convening multidisciplinary workgroups and stakeholders to evaluate existing evidence. In 2012, the AAP concluded that the health benefits of newborn male circumcision outweigh the risks. Specific benefits considered were the prevention of UTI, penile cancer, and transmission of some sexually transmitted infections.[31]

Ritual Jewish circumcision performed on the eighth day of life (when periurethral bacterial colonization has been established) seems to have attendant risk for UTI. An epidemiologic study in Israel revealed excessive UTIs in boys only in the postcircumcision period, from days 9 to 20 of life.[32] A case-control study identified performance by a nonphysician (mohel) versus a physician as a risk factor for UTI (odds ratio, 4.34); the authors postulate the technique of hemostasis and duration of the shaft wrapping as responsible factors.[33]

Microbiology

Escherichia coli continues to be responsible for most community-acquired UTI in infants younger than 3 months, accounting for 90% or more cases reported through the 1990s,[34-36] with lower prevalence since, possibly related to widespread use of intrapartum chemoprophylaxis.[4,37] Many different O serotypes of *E. coli* have been associated with UTI in the general population; however, UTI in neonates was associated with a limited number of O:K:H serotypes with P fimbriae, adhesive capacity, hemolysin production, and serum resistance.[38] Serotypes of *E. coli* associated with diarrhea rarely cause UTI. Cultures of urine can be positive in infants with septicemia caused by group B streptococci, but primary infection of the urinary tract without septicemia is uncommon.[17,39] Community-associated UTI in neonates caused by *Staphylococcus aureus* with or without bloodstream infection has been reported.[37,40]

The incidence of neonatal UTI as a complication of intensive care has increased sharply in recent years; intensive care–associated UTI occurs in patients with and without urinary catheters.[3] Mean age at occurrence was 42 days in one large study.[41] Microbiology of neonatal nosocomial UTI is dramatically different from that observed in neonatal intensive care units in the 1970s (Table 9-2), with *E. coli* supplanted by other genera of Enterobacteriaceae, *Pseudomonas, Enterococcus, Candida,* and coagulase-negative staphylococci.[3,4,14,15,42-45] Multiple pathogens occasionally can be present as documented by bladder aspiration and bladder catheterization. *S. aureus* and *E. coli* have been responsible for localized suppurative disease of the urinary tract in neonates, including prostatitis, orchitis, and epididymitis.[46-49] Other examples of focal disease in the urinary tract include orchitis caused by *Pseudomonas aeruginosa*[50] and testicular abscess caused by *Salmonella enteritidis*.[51] Blood cultures frequently are positive in affected infants. In

Table 9-2 Pathogens Responsible for Urinary Tract Infections in Neonatal Intensive Care Units

	FREQUENCY (%) OF ISOLATIONS OF EACH PATHOGEN			
Organism	**1969-1978***	**1989-1992†**	**1991-2007‡**	**1997-2010§**
Escherichia coli	75.3	10.5	24.8	18
Klebsiella species	13.4	10.5	25.5	NR
Enterobacter species	1.4	12.3	14.3	NR
Other gram-negative species‖	NR	NR	NR	32
Enterococcus species	2.1	14	4.9	13
CoNS	1.4	31.6	4.3	14
Other gram-positive species	NR	NR	NR	5
Candida species	—	12.3	15.5	15
Other	6.4	8.8	8.7	NR

CoNS, Coagulase-negative *Staphylococcus; NR*, not recorded.
*Data from 139 patients in nurseries and intensive care nurseries.[5,6,8,9]
†Data from 50 patients in neonatal intensive care units.[41,43]
‡Data from 161 patients in neonatal intensive care units.[4,14,15,44]
§Data from 984 patients in 322 neonatal intensive care units; 97% were older than 3 days.[42]
‖Included *Enterobacter, Klebsiella, Serratia, Pseudomonas,* and *Proteus* species.

one large study of neonatal intensive care unit (NICU)-associated UTIs, 13% of infants had concordant urinary and blood pathogens; in multivariate analysis, only organism type (i.e., gram-positive cocci, such as *Staphylococcus* species, group B streptococcus, and *Candida* species) predicted concordant positive blood culture.[42]

Pathogenesis

In older children and adults, most UTIs are thought to occur by the ascending route after introduction of bacteria through the urethral meatus. Less frequently, bloodborne infection of the kidney occurs. In neonates, it is frequently difficult to know whether UTI was the cause or the result of bacteremia. The predominance of males with UTI among infants younger than 3 months contrasts with the predominance of females in all other age groups. This difference may reflect increased risk of UTI in young uncircumcised boys; increased prevalence of urinary and renal anomalies in boys; transient urodynamic dysfunction; vesicoureteral reflux (VUR), which predominantly affects male infants; and the occasional UTI that complicates circumcision. In addition, bacteremia is more frequent in male infants, and hematogenous invasion of the kidney can cause UTI.

ANATOMIC AND PHYSIOLOGIC ABNORMALITIES

Anatomic or physiologic abnormalities of the urinary tract play a role in the development and consequences of UTI in some infants. Of these, obstructive uropathy is the most important. Infection often is the first indication of an abnormality. UTI was the presenting sign in half of 40 infants younger than 2 months with anomalies of the kidneys or ureters reported in 1980.[52] Congenital obstruction of the urinary tract was diagnosed in 5 of 80 children with UTI studied in Göteborg[6] and in 2 of 60 children studied in Leeds[53]; important radiologic abnormalities of the urinary tract were identified in 10 of 46 infant boys and 3 of 13 infant girls younger than 3 months from 1972 to 1982 in Christchurch, New Zealand.[54]

VUR is identified in many infants with UTI who are examined by radiologic techniques. VUR is frequently the result of infection but also can be a primary defect. VUR is not a prerequisite for upper tract infection (i.e., pyelonephritis); in two studies, less than half of children with pyelonephritis diagnosed by scintigraphy had VUR.[55,56] Majd and coworkers[57] found that 23 of 29 (79%) children hospitalized for UTI and found to have VUR had pyelonephritis diagnosed by scintigraphy; 39 of 65 (60%) children without VUR were also found to have pyelonephritis. VUR can be a congenital abnormality. Fetal ultrasonography showed that 30 of 107 infants with prenatally diagnosed urinary tract abnormalities had VUR, which was the only abnormality found postnatally in 10 infants.[58] Gordon and colleagues[59] observed that 16 of 25 infants with dilation of the fetal urinary tract had VUR, which was of grade 3 to 5 severity in 79%. In Austrian infants, 39 urinary tract abnormalities detected prenatally were compared with 46 urinary tract abnormalities found after first UTI.[60] Obstructive lesions and multicystic dysplastic malformations of the kidneys accounted for 90% of all prenatally diagnosed malformations; VUR accounted for only 10%. By contrast, VUR accounted for 59% of abnormalities detected after the first UTI.

VUR detected prenatally has a male-to-female distribution of 6:1 (in contrast to VUR detected after UTI, when females predominate,[61]) may be determined developmentally by the site of the origin of the ureteral bud from the wolffian (mesonephric) duct, and in severe cases can be associated with congenital renal damage consisting of global parenchymal loss (so-called reflux nephropathy).[62] Gunn and colleagues[63] performed ultrasound examinations of 3228 fetuses; no renal tract abnormalities were detected before 28 weeks of gestation. Subsequently, 3856 fetuses were examined by ultrasonography after 28 weeks of gestation. Urinary tract anomalies were identified in 313 fetuses; 15 had major structural abnormalities, all of which were confirmed postnatally. In 298 (7.7%) of the fetuses, dilated renal pelvis with normal bladder was found; most of the cases resolved spontaneously, but 40 of the cases were confirmed postnatally to be due to serious abnormalities (usually obstruction or VUR).[64] In one study, preterm infants with nosocomial UTI had a lower incidence of VUR than that noted in term infants with nosocomial UTI[15]; however, in another study comparing 250 neonates (mean gestation age, 39 weeks) with community-associated UTI with 51 neonates (mean gestation age, 36 weeks) with nosocomial UTI, the neonates with nosocomial infection were more likely to have VUR and abnormal renal ultrasound examination.[4]

Isolated mild renal pyelectasis (i.e., <10 mm diameter of the collecting duct and without VUR) in fetuses is likely to be transient, unassociated with pathology or risk for UTI.[65,66] In one study, 54% of such cases had resolved in the first postnatal month, and 85% of the cases of moderate or severe pelviectasis had resolved or improved over the first

2 years of life.[67] Results of a long-term outcome study of 125 infants in the Netherlands with antenatal hydronephrosis suggested that a cutoff of less than 15 mm anterior-posterior diameter of the renal pelvis identified infants at low risk for UTI or surgical conditions and low incidence and benign course of VUR.[68] In a 2012 Argentinean study of 196 hydronephrotic kidneys in 236 infants with mild (5-15–mm anterior-posterior pelvic diameter), isolated antenatal hydronephrosis was followed for a mean of 15 months postnatally without antibiotic prophylaxis or neonatal voiding cystourethrography (VCUG) study; 38% of patients had intrauterine total resolution, 42% had postnatal total resolution, and only 1% (3 patients) had progression. Of 98 infants with bilateral hydronephrosis, 9% had a UTI during follow-up none had VUR. Of 38 infants with unilateral hydronephrosis, 10% had a UTI; 2 had low-grade reflux.[69] In a long-term study performed in the United Kingdom, of 425 infants with antenatally detected hydronephrosis, 284 had normal findings on neonatal ultrasound examination; the negative predictive value of normal ultrasound findings for subsequent UTI in the first year of life was 99%.[70]

In a 5-year retrospective statewide, cohort analysis of 522 Washington state infants with birth-hospital discharge diagnosis of antenatal hydronephrosis (not quantified further) and 2610 control infants, hospitalization for UTI in the first year of life was 5% versus 1% (relative risk [RR] 11.8; 95% confidence interval [CI] 6.8 to 20.5). RR for UTI was higher, especially among girls with antenatal hydronephrosis (RR, 36.3; 95% CI, 10.6 to 124.0).[71] In a 17-year study from a single institution in Seoul of 480 infants with antenatal and postnatal hydronephrosis without VUR, UTI developed in the first year of life in 39% of infants with obstructive uropathy, compared with 11% without obstructive uropathy ($P < .001$). Higher grade of hydronephrosis and presence of hydroureteronephrosis were associated with higher incidence of UTI.[72] Investigators from Montreal compared occurrence of UTIs and VUR in 148 children with low-grade (grade 1 and 2) and high-grade (grade 3 and 4) hydronephrosis detected prenatally. Children with anatomic abnormalities were excluded. UTIs were 3.6 times higher among the high-grade nephrosis group (11.1 infections/100 patient-years) compared with the low-grade hydronephrosis group (3.52 infections/100 patient-years); VUR was not an independent risk factor for UTI.[73]

In a long-term study in Toronto of 260 infants with a prenatal diagnosis of hydronephrosis, 25 also had VUR (grade 3 or higher in 73%), received antibiotic prophylaxis, and did not have surgical correction during 4 years of follow-up. Breakthrough infection occurred in only four patients. Improvement was seen in most of the children with VUR, and there was no difference in renal growth in children who had resolved versus unresolved VUR or high-grade versus low-grade VUR.[74] In a 2013 systematic review to evaluate the value of continuous antibiotic prophylaxis in reducing UTIs in this population, only 21 citations were included, of which 76% were of moderate or low quality. Pooled UTI rates in children younger than 2 years with low-grade hydronephrosis were similar regardless of receiving antibiotic prophylaxis (2.2%) or not (2.8%). In children with high-grade hydronephrosis, patients receiving prophylaxis had a significantly lower UTI rate (14.6%) compared with those not receiving prophylaxis (28.9%) ($P < .01$).[75] Postnatal management of prenatal hydronephrosis is controversial. Although experts favor evaluation of even mild cases by postnatal ultrasonography, and some favor VCUG,[76] recent evidence supports a broad trend to use VCUG and antibiotic prophylaxis judiciously.[69,73,75]

The outcome of interest for strategies to identify obstructive uropathy, hydronephrosis, VUR, and UTI is lessening renal damage. Except for obstructive uropathies, the relative impacts and benefits of special management of hydronephrosis and VUR are increasingly controversial. A National Institutes of Health multicenter, randomized, placebo-controlled, double-blind study has been designed to determine preventive effect of antimicrobial prophylaxis on recurrent UTI and renal scarring in children with primary VUR (i.e., not due to increased bladder pressure, as from a neurogenic bladder, outlet obstruction, or other vesicular anomalies).[77] Chesney and colleagues[78] commented on background knowledge and rationale for the study design. A few relevant points are as follows: (1) The percentage of patients with recurrent UTIs and VUR who develop renal scarring is small. (2) Many children, even those with high-grade VUR, do not develop scars. (3) Patients without VUR who have recurrent UTI can develop scars. (4) Older studies (with poorer outcomes) included patients with secondary VUR (i.e., high-pressure VUR) and genetic renal syndromes. (5) Trials of antimicrobial prophylaxis or surgery or both for VUR generally are underpowered and do not include a nonintervention arm. (6) In a Cochrane analysis using 10 trials involving 964 children, the authors could not conclude that identification and treatment of children with VUR conferred a long-term benefit.

BACTERIAL VIRULENCE

Bacterial virulence factors are likely to play an important role in the pathogenesis of UTIs. Strains of *E. coli* causing UTI are a selected sample of the fecal flora. Pyelonephritic isolates belong to a restricted number of serotypes, are resistant to the bactericidal effect of serum, attach to and invade uroepithelial cells, and produce hemolysins.[79] Pili on the bacterial cell surface that adhere to specific receptors on epithelial cells may play a role in development of UTI. Some of these features of pyelonephritic strains of *E. coli* have been shown in UTIs in newborns.[38]

The increased rate of UTIs in uncircumcised boys is likely to be associated with periurethral bacterial flora. During the first 6 months of life, uncircumcised boys have significantly higher total urethral bacterial colony counts and more frequent isolation and higher colony counts of uropathogenic organisms, such as *E. coli*, *Klebsiella/Enterobacter* species, *Proteus*, and *Pseudomonas*.[80] With increasing age, the foreskin is more easily retracted, and penile hygiene improves; by 12 months of age, the excessive periurethral flora and UTIs in uncircumcised boys almost disappear.[22,80]

Natural defenses in the urinary tract include antibacterial properties of urine, antiadherence mechanisms, mechanical effects of urinary flow and micturition, presence of phagocytic cells, antibacterial properties of the urinary tract mucosa, and immune mechanisms.[81] There is scant knowledge about these mechanisms in the newborn.

Pathology

The histologic appearance of acute pyelonephritis in newborns is similar to that in the adult. Neutrophils are present in the glomeruli, the tubules, and the interstitial tissues. The renal pelvis can show signs of acute inflammation, with loss of the lining epithelium and necrosis. Focal suppuration can be present in the kidney, prostate, or testis. In disease of longer duration, the interstitial tissue is infiltrated with lymphocytes, plasma cells, and eosinophils. The number of glomeruli may be decreased, and some may be hyalinized. The epithelium of tubules is atrophic, and the lumen is filled with colloid casts. Pericapsular fibrosis is present in some infants. If the infant dies within 6 months, there is little scarring or contraction of the kidney. Reversible hydronephrosis and hydroureter are observed manifestations of acute pyelonephritis in the neonate who has no anatomic abnormality or VUR. It is postulated that bacteria and endotoxins inhibit ureteral peristalsis.

Pathologic processes indicative of additional suppurative infections, such as otitis media, pneumonia, and meningitis, also can be seen in infants dying of acute infection of the urinary tract. Hepatocellular damage and bile stasis may be noted in liver sections from jaundiced infants.

Clinical Manifestations

The signs of UTI in neonates are varied and nonspecific. Five patterns generally are observed: (1) septicemia associated with early-onset (within the first 5 days of life) or late-onset (after 5 days of age) disease (see Chapter 6); (2) acute onset of fever without apparent source; (3) insidious illness marked by low-grade fever or failure to gain weight; (4) no apparent signs; and (5) localized signs of infection, including balanitis, prostatitis, urethritis, and orchitis.

The most frequent signs of acute UTI are associated with fever or septicemia or both (see Chapter 6) (Table 9-3).[4-6,8,9] Less acute and nonspecific manifestations also are common, and the presenting signs include poor weight gain, vomiting, and poor feeding. Fever was a less common feature of nosocomial UTI in one study, compared with community-associated cases.[4] Temperature instability was not significantly associated with UTI in a NICU case-control study; no clinical feature except increased age (75 vs. 29 days) was significantly associated with UTI.[45] Enlargement of the liver and spleen, distention of the abdomen, and palpable enlargement of a kidney can occur. Signs associated with renal anomalies (e.g., a single umbilical artery, supernumerary nipples, spina bifida, low-set ears, and anorectal abnormalities) are seen in some infants.

Table 9-3 Clinical Manifestations of Urinary Tract Infections in Newborn Infants

Clinical Manifestations	% of Infants with Manifestations*
Fever	55
Vomiting	27
Failure to thrive	26
Poor feeding	24
Irritability or lethargy	17
Jaundice	10
Diarrhea	8

Data from References 4-6, 8, 9.

*When sign was not mentioned in report, the number of infants in the report was removed from the denominator used to determine the percentage of infants with manifestations.

Jaundice is an important feature of UTI and can be the presenting sign[81]; it is frequently sudden in onset and clears rapidly after adequate antimicrobial therapy. Many infants with UTI and jaundice have positive blood cultures.[19] In one study of 306 infants admitted to the hospital within 21 days of birth solely because of indirect hyperbilirubinemia (mean peak serum bilirubin level, 18.5 mg/dL), 90% were breastfed, and none had a positive culture of urine or blood.[82] In other studies, however, 12 of 160 (7.5%) infants younger than 8 weeks[83] and 14 of 113 (12.2%) infants younger than 2 weeks[84] evaluated solely for jaundice had UTI confirmed by bladder catheterization. Infection was associated with elevated unconjugated bilirubin in very young infants and with elevated conjugated bilirubin in infants older than 8 days.[83] In 122 matched, healthy, control infants who were not jaundiced,[84] 8 had positive culture of bag urine specimens, none of which was confirmed by catheterized urine culture. In a study of 100 infants, whose sole abnormality was jaundice lasting beyond 2 weeks of age, all were breastfed, and 6 had UTI.[85]

A reported case of severe methemoglobinemia in a 3-week-old infant with *E. coli* UTI was postulated to result from nitrite-forming bacteria, but concurrent diarrhea, dehydration, and acidosis may have been precipitating factors.[86] Hyperammonemic encephalopathy caused by *Proteus* infection in children with urinary tract obstruction or atony also has been described.[87] Bacteriuria without apparent signs of illness also was documented occasionally in screening studies performed in the 1970s and 1980s.[5,7,10,13]

Abscesses of the prostate, testis, or epididymis usually manifest with additional signs of septicemia, including fever, vomiting, and diarrhea.[45-51] Local signs of inflammation, including tenderness and swelling over the surface of the infected organ, may be present. Urinary retention occurs in infants with prostatitis.[47] Renal abscess is rare in neonates; at least one case report in a neonate with congenital nephrotic syndrome has been published.[88]

UTI should be considered in the differential diagnosis for unexplained fever in early infancy. UTI with or without bacteremia is the most common cause of serious bacterial infection in infants younger than 3 months and evaluated because of fever; it was responsible for 79% of cases in a Utah study.[37] Presence of UTI has been studied in thousands of infants younger than 3 months who have been evaluated because of fever by practitioners in emergency department and office settings. Rates range from 5% to 13%, depending predominantly on prevalence of circumcision in the population.[89-94] Increase in UTIs is more evident in infants 1 to 3 months of age rather than in neonates.[89] In a New York study, prevalence of UTI in febrile infant boys (82% of whom were not circumcised) was 12.4%. In a Pittsburgh study, prevalence of UTI in febrile infant boys (2% of whom were not circumcised) was only 2.9%. In a multicenter prospective study of febrile infants younger than 2 months, 9% had UTI (21% of uncircumcised boys, 5% of girls, and 2% of circumcised boys).[95] In a study of 162 febrile Japanese infants younger than 8 weeks, 22 (13.8%) had UTI; 18 were boys, none of whom was circumcised.[96]

In a study of 2411 febrile children younger than 24 months and evaluated in an emergency department in Philadelphia, history of malodorous urine, prior history of UTI, and presence of abdominal tenderness were significantly associated with the diagnosis of UTI; these findings were present in less than 10% of infected infants, however, and only 8% to 13% of infants with findings had UTI confirmed.[36] In a retrospective study of 354 Boston infants younger than 24 months with confirmed UTI, irritability and decreased appetite were each reported in 50% of children; diarrhea, vomiting, lethargy, and respiratory congestion were reported in 25%; and malodorous urine, apparent dysuria, increased frequency of urination, and abdominal pain were reported in less than 10%.[17]

Diagnosis

Infection of the urinary tract is defined as the presence of bacteria in urine that was obtained without contamination from the urethra or external genitalia. UTI should be considered in all infants older than 3 days who have fever or other signs of septicemia or who have subtle and nonspecific signs of failure to thrive during the first months of life. At present, no clinical finding or simple laboratory test adequately defines the location of infection in the urinary tract of the infant. It is assumed that bacteriuria in the neonate indicates infection throughout the urinary tract (including the kidney). Studies of neonates with early-onset septicemia indicate that the yield for culture of urine is low.[14,15,97] Culture can be eliminated in evaluation of infants younger than 3 days for presumed sepsis.

CULTURE OF URINE

Although a negative result from culture of bag-collected urine indicates that the urine is sterile, 12% to 21% of bag-collected specimens yield results that are indeterminate or positive (colony count ≥ 10^4/mL),[2,34] and positive results must be verified by aspiration of bladder urine or by catheterization. There is frequently insufficient time for this stepwise approach before institution of therapy. The technique of needle aspiration of the bladder has been used extensively, is technically simple and safe, and causes minimal discomfort to the infant.[98] After most infected infants have urine specimens with bacterial colony counts of 10^5/mL or greater, any bacterial growth in urine obtained by suprapubic aspiration is significant.

Morbidity associated with suprapubic aspiration is minimal. Transient gross hematuria has been reported in 0.6% of 654 infants.[98] Gross bleeding that ceased only after cauterization was reported in one case.[99] Perforation of the bowel occurred in two cases, but this complication can be avoided if the infant's bladder is carefully defined through palpation or percussion.[99] A hematoma of the anterior wall of the bladder,[100] peritonitis,[101] and anaerobic bacteremia[102] have also been reported after suprapubic aspiration. These reports warranted publication because the cases are very uncommon. Suprapubic aspiration should not be performed, however, if the infant has recently voided, has abdominal distention, has poorly defined anomalies of the urinary tract, or has a hematologic abnormality that might result in hemorrhage.

Suprapubic aspiration of bladder urine should be performed at least 1 hour after the patient has voided. The infant should lie supine, with the lower extremities held in a frog-leg position. The suprapubic area is cleaned with iodine and alcohol. A 20-gauge, 1½-inch needle attached to a syringe is used to pierce the abdominal wall and bladder approximately 1 inch above the symphysis pubis. The needle is directed caudally toward the fundus of the bladder, and urine is aspirated gently. Vigorous aspiration should be avoided because the mucosa can be drawn in to block the needle opening. The aspirated urine is sent to the laboratory immediately in a sterile tube. Ultrasound examination may be useful in detecting the presence of urine in the bladder before suprapubic aspiration; with ultrasound-guided aspiration, the success rate for acquisition of an adequate sample of urine improved from 60% to 96%.[103]

Catheterization of the bladder using sterile technique also is an appropriate sampling method. The incidence of infection related to catheterization in infants is unknown. Urine for culture should be transported to the laboratory as soon as possible, but if a delay is unavoidable, the specimen must be refrigerated. Isolation of 10^3 colonies/mL or greater of urine obtained by catheter may represent significant bacteriuria in this age group.[104] In multiple studies of young children evaluated because of fever (relatively few of whom were neonates), approximately 80% of the children with bacteriuria had colony counts of 10^5/mL or greater. Significant pyuria, elevated serum level of C-reactive protein (CRP), isolation of a single enteric organism, and abnormality on renal scintigraphy were each decreasingly associated with lower colony counts, with only rare positive tests in children with colony counts of less than 10^4/mL.[16,17,35,105]

CULTURE OF BLOOD AND CEREBROSPINAL FLUID

Because bacteremia and meningitis can accompany UTI, cultures of the blood and cerebrospinal fluid should be obtained before therapy for UTI is begun if the neonate has fever or any signs of illness. Blood (but not cerebrospinal fluid) for culture also should be obtained from a neonate with UTI who has no specific or nonspecific signs of infection. In a study from Sweden in the 1970s,[6] lumbar puncture was performed before therapy in 31 neonates with UTI; 6 infants had purulent meningitis, and in 9 infants the cerebrospinal fluid was sterile but pleocytosis (22-200 white blood cells [WBCs]/mm^3) also was present. Blood was obtained for culture in 32 infants and was positive in 12 infants. Meningitis accompanied UTI in less than 2% of young Australian infants reported in 2007[106] and 1.2% of infants younger than 28 days in 2011,[107] and in 3% of infants in a multi-NICU study in the United States reported in 2013.[42] Although sterile cerebrospinal fluid pleocytosis has been reported in association with UTI in young infants, a 2008 report of a multicenter prospective study of 1025 febrile infants younger than 2 months, in which 91 had confirmed UTI, sterile cerebrospinal fluid pleocytosis was uncommon (was found in 0% to 8%, depending on the definition of pleocytosis). Overinterpretation of pleocytosis resulting from traumatic lumbar puncture may be the explanation for the previously reported association.[108]

Bacteremia was present in 11 of 35 (31%) infants in Dallas who were younger than 30 days and had UTI. The infants had been considered healthy when discharged from the nursery and were evaluated because of fever. Older infants with UTI were less likely to be bacteremic; positive cultures of blood occurred in 5 of 24 infants (21%) 1 to 2 months of age having UTI, 2 of 14 infants (14%) 2 to 3 months of age, and 1 of 18 infants (5.5%) 3 months of age or older.[23] Similarly, in Boston, bacteremia was present in 17 of 80 (21%) febrile infants with UTI and younger than 1 month, 8 of 59 (13%) 1 to 2 months of age, and 8 of 116 (7%) 2 to 6 months of age; 4 neonates had meningitis.[17] In Pittsburgh, incidence of bacteremia in community-associated UTI was higher in infants younger than 2 months (22%) than in older infants (3%).[109] No clinical finding or laboratory test discriminated between bacteremic and nonbacteremic infants.[17] In surveillance for UTI among 203,399 infants born in U.S. Army hospitals from 1985 to 1990, 23% of noncircumcised infant boys with UTI and younger than 3 months had concomitant bacteremia; incidence of bacteremia associated with UTI was not different from the incidence in circumcised boys or girls with UTI.[27] Incidence of bacteremia in neonatal nosocomial UTI is higher than in community-associated infection and is more associated with gram-positive organisms[42]; bacteremia occurred in 38% of cases of nosocomial UTI in one study.[14]

EXAMINATION OF URINE SEDIMENT

Many studies and a meta-analysis assessing presence of WBCs in the urine of newborn infants have been performed.[5,22,70,110-112] Healthy infants can have 10 WBCs/mm^3 of clean-voided urine.[111]

Neither presence nor absence of pyuria is completely reliable evidence for or against UTI. Many studies have assessed urine specimens for predictive values for UTI of WBCs or organisms or detection by dipstick of leukocyte esterase or reduction of nitrate. The following results are limited to studies of acutely ill, usually febrile infants whose urine was obtained by catheterization (or suprapubic aspiration where stated). Methods of assessing pyuria and definitions of UTI vary. Less than 10 WBCs per high-power field were present in 27% of unspun urine samples collected by suprapubic aspiration from Dallas infants with UTI (bacterial colony counts ≥ 10^5/mL).[23] Landau and coworkers[16] reported that among infants younger than 4 months and with positive urine cultures (colony counts ≥ 10^4/mL), 4 of 49 (8.2%) with acute pyelonephritis diagnosed by renal scintigraphy had less than 5 WBCs per high-power field (400×) in fresh, centrifuged urine, compared with 27 of 79 (34.2%) infants with UTI and negative results of scintigraphy.

Quantifying WBCs in uncentrifuged urine using a counting chamber is the most reproducible test for pyuria. Hoberman and colleagues[113] found pyuria (at least 10 WBCs/mm^3 of unspun urine) absent in 20% of 190 febrile infants younger than 24 months and with positive urine cultures (colony counts ≥ 5 × 10^4/mL) and present in 6.7% with negative cultures; a single patient, among 15 cases without pyuria, in whom renal scintigraphy was performed under protocol, had a positive result. In a study by Hansson and coworkers[114] of 366 infants younger than 1 year and with symptomatic UTI (colony counts ≥ 10^3/mL from suprapubic aspirate of urine), 80% had colony counts of 10^5/mL or greater, 13% had counts of 1 to 9 × 10^4/mL, and 7% had counts of 1 to 9 × 10^3/mL. Pyuria was significantly associated with increased colony count. In children with UTI with colony counts of less than 10^5/mL, sensitivity of pyuria (>10 WBCs/mm^3) was 69% compared with 88% for children with at least 10^5 colonies/mL. Nitrate reduction test was highly insensitive; 44% of the patients had a positive result when the colony count was at least 10^5/mL, and 11% had a positive result with lower counts.[35] Nitrate reduction would be expected to be negative in all cases in which non-Enterobacteriaceae, gram-positive cocci or *Candida*, are causative. Renal scintigraphy was not performed in the study of Hansson and coworkers[114] to estimate significance of UTI, but VUR was present equally in infants with high (30%) and low (38%) colony counts.

Dipstick test for leukocyte esterase and nitrite performs poorly in the diagnosis of UTI in infants. In the study by Hoberman and colleagues,[105] the test had a sensitivity of 53% and positive predictive value of 82% for detecting 10 or more WBCs/mm^3; nitrite determination had a sensitivity of 31% in identifying urine cultures with growth of at least 50,000 colonies/mL. Shaw and coworkers[115] reported dipstick results in 3873 febrile children younger than 2 years evaluated for UTI; sensitivity of a positive result (trace or greater for leukocyte esterase or positive nitrite) was 79%, and positive predictive value was 46% for isolation of at least 10,000 colonies/mL from urine culture.

Microscopic hematuria is present in some infants with UTI.[3,44] Gross hematuria usually is associated with other conditions (e.g., renal vein thrombosis, polycystic disease of the kidney, obstructive uropathy, Wilms tumor).[116]

Usefulness of Gram stain of urine specimens in predicting bacteriuria has been studied prospectively in febrile infants younger than 24 months. Smears were prepared using 2 drops of uncentrifuged urine on a slide within a standardized marked area 1.5 cm in diameter, which was then air dried, fixed, and stained. The presence of at least 1 organism per 10 high-power fields examined using oil immersion lens was considered a positive result. Sensitivity and positive predictive value were 81% and 43%, respectively, for isolation of at least 1 × 10^4 colonies/mL of urine in the study by Shaw and colleagues[115] and 93% and 57% for isolation of at least 5 × 10^4 colonies/mL in the study by Hoberman and coworkers.[105] The presence of pyuria and bacteriuria increased the positive predictive value for positive cultures in these studies to 85% and 88%, respectively.

EXAMINATION OF BLOOD

Elevated peripheral blood neutrophil count, band count, band-to-neutrophil ratio, and CRP level are documented in infants with UTI. These abnormalities, however, do not reliably discriminate presence, absence, or level of infection in the urinary tract or presence of bacteremia.[16,17,113] Hemolytic anemia frequently accompanies jaundice when the latter is present in infants with UTI. Results of the direct Coombs test usually are negative. The reticulocyte count can be normal or elevated.

Although signs of inflammatory response, such as elevated erythrocyte sedimentation rate (ESR), serum CRP, or procalcitonin, correlate generally with abnormal renal scintigraphy—findings that are suggestive of acute pyelonephritis in children with UTI—standardized cutoff values for stand-alone positive or negative predictive tests have not been possible. In 64 children studied, Majd and colleagues[57] found abnormal scans in 78% of children with ESR of at least 25 mm/hr, compared with 33% of children with lower ESR. Benador and coworkers[56] found that ESR greater than 20 mm/hr or CRP level greater than 10 mg/L had a sensitivity of 89% and specificity of 25% for identifying renal lesions among 73 children with UTI. Stokland and colleagues[117] correlated CRP level greater than 2 mg/dL at the time of acute infection with resultant renal scar in 157 children reevaluated 1 year later; sensitivity of elevated CRP was 92%, and positive and negative predictive values were 41% and 80%, respectively. In 153 children with fever and positive urine culture (colony count $\geq 5 \times 10^4$/mL), Hoberman and coworkers[113] reported significant correlations between evidence of pyelonephritis versus cystitis versus asymptomatic bacteriuria with mean peripheral WBC count (22,400/mm^3 vs. 14,600/mm^3 vs. 11,700/mm^3), ESR (44 mm/hr vs. 26.8 mm/hr vs. 15.3 mm/hr), and CRP (1 mg/dL vs. 0.27/dL vs. 0.3 mg/dL). In a study using cutoff values of 1 ng/mL for procalcitonin and 2 mg/dL for CRP, rates of sensitivity for detection of pyelonephritis in infants with UTI were similar (92%), but specificity of procalcitonin (62%) exceeded that of CRP (34%).[118]

CHEMICAL DETERMINATIONS

Hyperbilirubinemia is present in many infants with UTI; the percentage of conjugated bilirubin often is determined by the age of the infant at the onset of jaundice. During the first week of life, almost all of the bilirubin is unconjugated, but in the second week and thereafter, the fractionation is approximately equivalent. In 80 Boston infants younger than 1 month and with UTI, 11 (14%) had jaundice and hyperbilirubinemia; only 4 had bacteremia.[17] With the exception of changes in serum bilirubin, the results of serum hepatic enzyme tests generally are normal or only slightly abnormal. Azotemia and hyperchloremic acidosis are not unusual; serum bicarbonate concentrations were less than 20 mEq/L in 34.1% of 354 young children with UTI in one study.[17]

IMAGING OF THE URINARY TRACT

The major goal of imaging of the urinary tract in infants with UTI (and infants with abnormalities noted prenatally) is to identify important and correctable lesions, including urethral strictures, renal anomalies, obstructive uropathy, urethral valves in boys, and some cases of severe VUR, and to provide the opportunity to begin antibiotic prophylaxis against recurring UTIs in certain infants with reflux or hydronephrosis in whom surgery is not indicated. (See previous discussion of uncertainty of benefit of antibiotic prophylaxis and surgery for primary VUR or hydronephrosis.) Multiple imaging modalities are available, and each modality provides unique evaluations.[55,61,117,119-121] Ultrasonography can delineate the size, shape, and location of kidneys and contributes to the diagnosis of hydronephrosis, hydroureter, ureterocele, bladder distention, and stones but less so to VUR. Ultrasonography is the most noninvasive study, and its accuracy is dependent on the experience of the interpreter. It is an insensitive test for pyelonephritis but sometimes shows kidney enlargement with abnormal echogenicity. Renal ultrasonography performed to follow up on fetal studies should be postponed for at least 48 hours after birth to avoid a false-negative result from dehydration or low glomerular filtration rate characteristic of newborns.[119]

Renal cortical scintigraphy using technetium-99m–labeled dimercaptosuccinic acid or gluceptate is the most sensitive test for identifying acute pyelonephritis (i.e., focally or diffusely decreased cortical uptake of tracer without evidence of cortical loss, sometimes in an enlarged kidney) or chronic scarring (i.e., decreased uptake with corresponding cortical volume loss); scintigraphy also provides an estimate of renal function. Scintigraphy is the gold standard for diagnosis of acute pyelonephritis; 66% to 75% of children younger than 2 years with febrile UTI in multiple studies have a positive result.[56,57] Renal scintigraphy at the time of UTI was performed in a multicenter study in Spain. In a subset of infants younger than 30 days and with community-associated UTI (106 cases) and nosocomial UTI (15 cases), cortical defects were present in 31% and 73%, respectively. Although abnormal scintigraphy was significantly associated with abnormal ultrasonography and VCUG, 21% of study infants had abnormality by scintigraphy alone.[4]

VCUG using radiographic or radionuclide methodology is the best study to visualize the bladder and urethra and to detect VUR; radionuclide scanning is superior to a dye study for detection of intermittent reflux but is inferior for detection of urethral and bladder wall abnormalities and cannot be used to grade VUR. Both are invasive and associated with discomfort attendant with catheterization. A 24-day-old male infant with ureterovesical junction obstruction was found to have *E. coli* septicemia and UTI 6 days after elective VCUG, which did not show VUR.[122] A toxic reaction to the VCUG dye can occur in infants but is rare.

Ultrasonography and VCUG have been recommended for all neonates with UTI judged to be other than that secondary to septicemia. Male infants with community-associated first UTI diagnosed before 8 weeks of age have a higher incidence of VUR or anatomic abnormalities (22% of 45 male infants in one Israeli study) than that noted in older children.[123] Ultrasonography is performed at the time of infection to identify major renal and ureteral abnormalities. VCUG traditionally was delayed to permit resolution of inflammatory VUR; however, in clinical studies, acute pyelonephritis-associated VUR was present in only a minority of patients and was of low grade.[38,57,120] Recently published guidelines for management of UTI in children do not include performance of VCUG after the first UTI when good-quality ultrasonography shows normal kidneys and bladder; infants younger than 1 month are excluded from these guidelines.[124]

For infants who have undergone prenatal ultrasonography in an experienced center after 30 to 32 weeks of gestation and whose study findings were normal, or in infants who have had a normal postnatal ultrasonography, repeat ultrasonography at the time of first UTI is not necessary.[112,113,125,126] Renal scintigraphy is useful in diagnosis and management of selective cases of UTI.[127,128] Computed tomography is performed infrequently, such as when a mass lesion or abscess is suspected.

Management and Prevention

Management of UTI is aimed at halting infection rapidly, reconstituting normal fluid and acid-base status, and assessing medical or surgical interventions required to prevent subsequent episodes of UTI and kidney damage. Antimicrobial agents should be administered as soon as culture specimens of the blood, cerebrospinal fluid (if indicated), and urine have been obtained. The choice of antimicrobial agents for initial therapy and the dosage schedule are the same as outlined in Chapter 6 for septicemia (a penicillin and an aminoglycoside). A penicillinase-resistant penicillin (methicillin or oxacillin) should be used if an abscess of the kidney, prostate, or testis is present, which suggests infection with *S. aureus*; vancomycin may be appropriate when methicillin-resistant *S. aureus* organisms are prevalent in the community or nursery. Patients who have suspected hospital-acquired infection are frequently given vancomycin and an aminoglycoside as initial therapy because of the significant role of coagulase-negative staphylococci and *Enterococcus* species. The decision to use a third-generation cephalosporin is based on the patient's prior receipt of antibiotics, the patient's clinical state, and the knowledge of bacterial species indigenous in each neonatal intensive care unit.

Extended-spectrum β-lactamase–producing organisms of the family Enterobacteriaceae are increasingly problematic in neonatal nosocomial infections, including UTI. Gram stain of urine sediment is helpful in initiating empirical therapy for UTI, especially when fungal infection is considered. Therapeutic regimens should be reconsidered when the results of cultures and antimicrobial susceptibility tests are available, with the aim to narrow therapy and to avoid use of unnecessary or potentially toxic agents.

Effective antimicrobial agents sterilize the urine within 24 to 48 hours. A second specimen of urine often is obtained for examination and culture at about 48 hours. Persistence of bacteriuria or funguria implies that treatment is ineffective or that a foreign body, fungus ball, or obstruction is present.

The duration of antimicrobial therapy for UTI in neonates usually is 14 days. Longer therapy (up to 3 weeks) is necessary if there is a poor response or if an anatomic or physiologic abnormality suggests that relapse may occur if administration of the drug is not continued. Timing of change from parenterally to orally administered agents depends on rapidity of clinical and microbiologic response and the presence of bacteremia or anatomic, functional, or physiologic abnormalities and availability of a highly active oral agent. Parenteral therapy usually is given for at least 3 to 4 days in uncomplicated cases.[129,130] Clinical vigilance for nonspecific symptoms and signs of illness after conclusion of therapy is important so that recurrent infection can be detected and treated appropriately. Children with certain urinary tract anomalies, functional abnormalities, and high-grade VUR often are given prophylactic antibiotics continuously for extended periods until the condition improves or surgery is performed.[63,119] (See previous discussion of uncertainty of benefit of standard prophylaxis in primary VUR alone.) A systematic review of randomized controlled trials of prophylaxis revealed limited evidence for its efficacy.[131] A randomized trial in 576 older infants and children in Australia showed statistically significant but modest effect of trimethoprim-sulfamethoxazole over placebo in preventing UTIs (13% vs. 19%).[132] In a multicenter, randomized, controlled, follow-up trial of antimicrobial prophylaxis compared with no prophylaxis in 100 Italian infants with grades 2 through 4 VUR, prophylaxis had no effect on recurrences of UTI, renal scarring, or persistence of VUR. Recurrences in the prophylaxis group were caused by multidrug-resistant bacteria, whereas recurrences in the group not receiving prophylaxis all were due to antibiotic-susceptible *E. coli*.[133] A U.S. multicenter study to test this question in children with VUR is ongoing.[77,78] In 84 Turkish infants diagnosed prenatally with ureteropelvic junction obstruction and varying degrees of hydronephrosis, followed for 1 year with disodium carbon-14–methanearsonate scintigraphy without prophylaxis, no UTI or scarring occurred.[134] This study suggests that risk of UTI and benefit of prophylaxis in these patients also may be uncertain. If prophylaxis of UTI is given, amoxicillin, 20 mg/kg/day divided in doses administered every 12 hours, is the agent most frequently used in the neonate.

Measures that have been shown to reduce nosocomial UTIs in older children and adults should be applied to newborns. Evidence-based interventions include avoidance of unnecessary urinary catheterization, vigilance in hand hygiene, insertion and maintenance of a catheter in a sterile manner, and discontinuation of catheterization as soon as possible (i.e., daily evaluation of need to continue).[135]

Prognosis

The natural history of UTI in the newborn without underlying abnormality is incompletely described. Some infants with asymptomatic bacteriuria have infection that clears without use of antimicrobial agents.[5,6,136] Some infants with symptomatic infection respond readily to therapy and have no subsequent infections, although the likelihood of recurrences seems to be lower than that for older children. In the series from Göteborg[6] and Leeds,[8] recurrences occurred in 26% and 19% of infants, respectively; the second episode usually occurred during the first few months after the initial infection.

It is possible that inflammatory changes in the kidney early in life may lead to subsequent impairment of growth and development of the kidney and to epithelial damage, fibrosis, and vascular changes, but it is uncertain how frequently these events occur. In a study of 25 children with UTI in whom renal scintigraphy showed evidence of acute pyelonephritis and who underwent repeat scanning an average of 10.5 months later, 16 (64%) had corresponding scars.[56] In another study, 38% of 157 children (median age; 0.4 year at the time of asymptomatic UTI) had renal scars documented 1 year later.[117] Infants do not seem to be at increased risk for scarring compared with older children; in 50 infants younger than 1 year and with UTI and having abnormal scintigraphy acutely, repeat scintigraphy after an average of 3 months showed scars in 40%.[137]

Obstructive lesions associated with reflux during the neonatal period may be associated with progressive renal damage, whereas children with unobstructive reflux, regardless of severity, infrequently have progressive renal damage. The hypothesis that outcome depends on prevention of infection has been challenged.[77,78] For patients with UTI and underlying genitourinary abnormalities, long-term control of infection may be important. After that, prognosis depends on severity of the lesion and associated congenital renal syndromes.

References

1. Helmholz HF: Pyelitis in the newborn, *Med Clin North Am* 1:1451, 1918.
2. Schlager TA, Hendley JO, Dudley SM, et al: Explanation for false-positive urine cultures obtained by bay technique, *Arch Pediatr Adolesc Med* 149:170, 1995.
3. Lohr JA, Downs SM, Dudley S, et al: Hospital-acquired urinary tract infections in the pediatric patient: a prospective study, *Pediatr Infect Dis J* 13:8, 1994.
4. Sastre JB, Aparicio AR, Cotallo GD, et al: Urinary tract infection in the newborn: clinical and radioimaging studies, *Pediatr Nephrol* 22:1735, 2007.
5. Abbott GD: Neonatal bacteriuria: a prospective study of 1460 infants, *BMJ* 1:267, 1972.
6. Bergström T, Larson H, Lincoln K, et al: Studies of urinary tract infections in infancy and childhood. XII. Eighty consecutive patients with neonatal infection, *J Pediatr* 80:858, 1972.
7. Edelman CM Jr, Ogwo JE, Fine BP, et al: The prevalence of bacteriuria in full-term and premature newborn infants, *J Pediatr* 82:125, 1973.
8. Littlewood JM, Kite P, Kite BA: Incidence of neonatal urinary tract infection, *Arch Dis Child* 44:617, 1969.
9. Maherzi M, Guignard JP, Torrado A: Urinary tract infection in high-risk newborn infants, *Pediatrics* 62:521, 1978.
10. Wettergren B, Jodal U, Jonasson G: Epidemiology of bacteriuria during the first year of life, *Acta Paediatr Scand* 74:925, 1985.
11. Wiswell TE, Roscelli JD: Corroborative evidence for the decreased incidence of urinary tract infections in circumcised male infants, *Pediatrics* 78:96, 1986.
12. Yorita KL, Holman RC, Sejvar JJ, et al: Infectious disease hospitalizations among infants in the United States, *Pediatrics* 121:244, 2008.
13. Pendarvis BC, Chitwood LA, Wenzl JE: *Bacteriuria in the premature infant*, Washington, DC, 1969, American Society for Microbiology.
14. Tamim MM, Alesseh H, Aziz H: Analysis of the efficacy of urine culture as part of sepsis evaluation in the premature infant, *Pediatr Infect Dis J* 22:805, 2003.
15. Bauer S, Eliakim A, Pomeranz A, et al: Urinary tract infection in very low birth weight preterm infants, *Pediatr Infect Dis J* 22:426, 2003.
16. Landau D, Turner ME, Brennan J, et al: The value of urinalysis in differentiating acute pyelonephritis from lower urinary tract infection in febrile infants, *Pediatr Infect Dis J* 13:777, 1994.
17. Bachur R, Caputo GL: Bacteremia and meningitis among infants with urinary tract infections, *Pediatr Emerg Care* 11:280, 1995.
18. Sweet AY, Wolinsky E: An outbreak of urinary tract and other infections due to *E coli Pediatrics* 33:865, 1964.
19. Kenny JF, Medearis DN Jr, Klein WS, et al: An outbreak of urinary tract infections and septicemia due to *Escherichia coli* in male infants, *J Pediatr* 68:53, 1966.
20. McCormack RC, Kunin CM: Control of a single source nursery epidemic due to *Serratia marcescens*, *Pediatrics* 37:750, 1966.
21. Wiswell TE, Smith FR, Bass JW: Decreased incidence of urinary tract infections in circumcised male infants, *Pediatrics* 75:901, 1985.
22. Wiswell TE, Enzenauer RW, Holton ME, et al: Declining frequency of circumcision: implications for changes in the absolute incidence and male to female sex ratio of urinary tract infections in early infancy, *Pediatrics* 79:338, 1987.
23. Ginsburg CM, McCracken GH Jr: Urinary tract infections in young infants, *Pediatrics* 69:409, 1982.
24. Herzog LW: Urinary tract infections and circumcision: a case-control study, *Am J Dis Child* 143:348, 1989.
25. Shaikh N, Morone NE, Bost JE, et al: Prevalence of urinary tract infection in childhood: a meta-analysis, *Pediatr Infect Dis J* 27:302, 2008.
26. Wiswell TE, Geschke DW: Risks from circumcision during the first month of life compared with those for uncircumcised boys, *Pediatrics* 83:1011, 1989.
27. Wiswell TE, Hachey WE: Urinary tract infections and the uncircumcised state: an update, *Clin Pediatr* 32:130, 1993.
28. To T, Agha M, Dick PT, et al: Cohort study on circumcision of newborn boys and subsequent risk of urinary-tract infection, *Lancet* 352:1813, 1998.
29. Craig JC, Knight JF, Sureshkumar P, et al: Effect of circumcision on incidence of urinary tract infection in preschool boys, *J Pediatr* 128:23, 1996.
30. Jagannath VA, Fedorowicz Z, Sud V, et al: Routine neonatal circumcision for the prevention of urinary tract infection in infancy, *Cochrane Database System Rev*(11)CD009129, 2012.
31. American Academy of Pediatrics Task Force on Circumcision: *Pediatrics* 130:e756, 2012. Available at http://www.pediatrics.org/cgi/doi/10.1542/peds.2012-1990. Accessed June 5, 2014.
32. Cohen HA, Drucker MM, Vainer S, et al: Post-circumcision urinary tract infection, *Clin Pediatr* 31:322, 1992.
33. Harel L, Straussbergr R, Jackson S, et al: Influence of circumcision technique on frequency of urinary tract infections in neonates, *Pediatr Infect Dis J* 21:879, 2002.
34. Crain EF, Gershel JC: Urinary tract infections in febrile infants younger than 8 weeks of age, *Pediatrics* 86:363, 1990.
35. Hoberman A, Wald ER, Hickey RW, et al: Oral versus initial intravenous therapy for urinary tract infections in young febrile children, *Pediatrics* 104:79, 1999.
36. Shaw KN, Gorelick M, McGowan KL, et al: Prevalence of urinary tract infection in febrile young children in the emergency department, *Pediatrics* 102:390, 1998.
37. Glasgow TS, Young PC, Wallin J, et al: Association of intrapartum antibiotic exposure and late-onset serious bacterial infections in infants, *Pediatrics* 116:696, 2005.
38. Israele V, Darabi A, McCracken GH Jr: The role of bacterial virulence factors and Tamm-Horsfall protein in the pathogenesis of *Escherichia coli* urinary tract infection in infants, *Am J Dis Child* 141:1230, 1987.
39. Pena BM, Harper MB, Fleisher GR: Occult bacteremia with group B streptococci in an outpatient setting, *Pediatrics* 102:67, 1998.
40. Fortunov RM, Hulten KG, Hammerman WA, et al: Evaluation and treatment of community-acquired *Staphylococcus aureus* infections in term and late-preterm previously healthy neonates, *Pediatrics* 120:93, 2007.
41. Lohr JA, Donowitz LG, Sadler JE 3rd: Hospital-acquired urinary tract infection, *Pediatrics* 83:193, 1989.
42. Downey LC, Benjamin DK Jr, Clark RH, et al: Urinary tract infection concordance with positive blood and cerebrospinal fluid cultures in the neonatal intensive unit, *J Perinatol* 33:302, 2013.
43. Davies HD, Jones EL, Sheng RY, et al: Nosocomial urinary tract infections at a pediatric hospital, *Pediatr Infect Dis J* 11:349, 1992.
44. Sohn AH, Garrett DO, Sinkowitz-Cochran RL, et al: Prevalence of nosocomial infections in neonatal intensive care unit patients: results from the first national point-prevalence survey, *J Pediatr* 139:821, 2001.
45. Foglia EE, Lorch SA: Clinical predictors of urinary tract infection in the neonatal intensive care unit, *J Neonatal Perinatal Med* 5:327, 2012.
46. Williams DI, Martins AG: Periprostatic haematoma and prostatic abscess in the neonatal period, *Arch Dis Child* 35:177, 1960.
47. Mann S: Prostatic abscess in the newborn, *Arch Dis Child* 35:396, 1960.
48. Hendricks WM, Kellett GN: Scrotal mass in a neonate: testicular abscess, *Am J Dis Child* 129:1361, 1975.
49. Hemming VG: Bilateral neonatal group A streptococcal hydrocele infection associated with maternal puerperal sepsis, *Pediatr Infect Dis* 5:107, 1986.
50. McCartney ET, Stewart I: Suppurative orchitis due to *Pseudomonas aeruginosa J Pediatr* 52:451, 1958.
51. Foster R, Weber TR, Kleiman M, et al: *Salmonella enteritidis*: testicular abscess in a newborn, *J Urol* 130:790, 1983.

52. Bensman A, Baudon JJ, Jablonski JP, et al: Uropathies diagnosed in the neonatal period: symptomatology and course, *Acta Paediatr Scand* 69:499, 1980.
53. Littlewood JM: 66 infants with urinary tract infection in first month of life, *Arch Dis Child* 57:218, 1972.
54. Bourcher D, Abbott ED, Maling TMJ: Radiological abnormalities in infants with urinary tract infection, *Arch Dis Child* 59:620, 1984.
55. Andrich MP, Majd M: Diagnostic imaging in the evaluation of the first urinary tract infection in infants and young children, *Pediatrics* 90:436, 1992.
56. Benador D, Benador N, Slosman DO, et al: Cortical scintigraphy in the evaluation of renal parenchymal changes in children with pyelonephritis, *J Pediatr* 124:17, 1994.
57. Majd M, Rushton HG, Jantausch B, et al: Relationships among vesicoureteral reflux, P-fimbriated *Escherichia coli*, and acute pyelonephritis in children with febrile urinary tract infection, *J Pediatr* 119:578, 1991.
58. Najmaldin A, Burge DM, Atwell JD: Pediatric urology: fetal vesicoureteric reflux, *Br J Urol* 65:403, 1990.
59. Gordon AC, Thomas DF, Arthur RJ, et al: Prenatally diagnosed reflux: a follow-up study, *Br J Urol* 65:407, 1990.
60. Ring E, Zobel G: Urinary infection and malformations of urinary tract in infancy, *Arch Dis Child* 63:818, 1988.
61. Steele BT, De Maria J: A new perspective on the natural history of vesicoureteric reflux, *Pediatrics* 90:30, 1992.
62. Assael BM, Guez S, Marra G, et al: Congenital reflux nephropathy: a follow-up of 108 cases diagnosed perinatally, *Br J Urol* 82:252, 1998.
63. Gunn TR, Mora JD, Pease P: Outcome after antenatal diagnosis of upper urinary tract dilatation by ultrasonography, *Arch Dis Child* 63:1240, 1988.
64. Gunn TR, Mora JD, Pease P: Antenatal diagnosis of urinary tract abnormalities by ultrasonography after 28 weeks' gestation: incidence and outcome, *Am J Obstet Gynecol* 172:479, 1995.
65. Dremsek PA, Gindl K, Voitl P, et al: Renal pyelectasis in fetuses and neonates: diagnostic value of renal pelvis diameter in pre- and postnatal sonographic screening, *AJR Am J Roentgenol* 168:1017, 1997.
66. Thomas DFM, Madden NP, Irving HC, et al: Mild dilatation of the fetal kidney: a follow-up study, *Br J Urol* 74:236, 1993.
67. Cheng AM, Phan V, Geary DF, et al: Outcome of isolated antenatal hydronephrosis, *Arch Pediatr Adolesc Med* 158:38, 2004.
68. de Kort EH, Oetomo S, Zegers SH: The long-term outcome of antenatal hydronephrosis up to 15 millimetres justifies a noninvasive postnatal follow-up, *Acta Paediatr* 97:708, 2008.
69. Alconcher LF, Tombesi MM: Natural history of bilateral mild isolated antenatal hydronephrosis conservatively managed, *Pediatr Nephrol* 27:1119, 2012.
70. Moorthy I, Joshi N, Cook JV, et al: Antenatal hydronephrosis: negative predictive value of normal postnatal ultrasound—a 5 year study, *Clin Radiol* 58:964, 2003.
71. Walsh TJ, Hsieh S, Grady R, et al: Antenatal hydronephrosis and the risk of pyelonephritis hospitalization during the first year of life, *Pediatr Urol* 69:970, 2007.
72. Lee JH, Choi HS, Kim JK, et al: Nonrefluxing neonatal hydronephrosis and the risk of urinary tract infection, *J Urol* 179:1524, 2008.
73. Szymanski KM, Al-Said AN, Pippi Salle JL, et al: Do infants with prenatal hydronephrosis benefit from screening for vesicoureteral reflux? *J Urol* 188:576, 2012.
74. Upadhyay J, McLorie GA, Bolduc S, et al: 2003 Natural history of neonatal reflux associated with prenatal hydronephrosis: long-term results of a prospective study, *J Urol 169*, 1837.
75. Braga LH, Mijovoc H, Farrokhyar F, et al: Antibiotic prophylaxis for urinary tract infections in antenatal hydronephrosis, *Pediatrics* 131:e251, 2013. Available at http://www.pediatrics.org/cgi/doi/10.1542/peds.2012-1870. Accessed June 5, 2014.
76. Estrada CR Jr: Prenatal hydronephrosis: early evaluation, *Curr Opin Urol* 18:401, 2008.
77. Keren R, Carpenter MA, Hoberman A, et al: Rationale and design issues of the randomized intervention for children with vesicoureteral reflux (RIVUR) study, *Pediatrics* 122:S241, 2008.
78. Chesney RW, Carpenter MA, Moxey-Mims M, et al: Randomized intervention for children with vesicoureteral reflux (RIVUR): background commentary of RIVUR investigators, *Pediatrics* 122:S233, 2008.
79. Svanborg C, Hausson S, Jodal U, et al: Host-parasite interaction in the urinary tract, *J Infect Dis* 157:421, 1988.
80. Wiswell TE, Miller GM, Gelston HM Jr, et al: Effect of circumcision status on periurethral bacterial flora during the first year of life, *J Pediatr* 113:442, 1988.
81. Sobel JD: Pathogenesis of urinary tract infections, *Infect Dis Clin North Am* 1:751, 1987.
82. Maisels MJ, Kring E: Risk of sepsis in newborns with severe hyperbilirubinemia, *Pediatrics* 90:741, 1992.
83. Garcia FJ, Nager A: Jaundice as an early diagnostic sign of urinary tract infection in infancy, *Pediatrics* 112:1213, 2003.
84. Shahian M, Rashtian P, Kalani M: Unexplained neonatal jaundice as an early diagnostic sign of urinary tract infection, *Int J Inf Dis* 16:e487, 2012. Available at http://dx.doi.org/10.1016/j.ijid.2012.02.011. Accessed June 5, 2014.
85. Pashapour N, Nikibanhksh AA, Golmohammadlou S: Urinary tract infection in term neonates with prolonged jaundice, *Urol J* 4:91, 2007.
86. Luk G, Riggs D, Luque M: Severe methemoglobinemia in a 3-week-old infant with a urinary tract infection, *Crit Care Med* 19:1325, 1992.
87. Das A, Henderson D: Your diagnosis please, *Pediatr Infect Dis J* 15:922, 1996.
88. Crawford DB, Rasoulpour M, Dhawan VM, et al: Renal carbuncle in a neonate with congenital nephrotic syndrome, *J Pediatr* 93:78, 1978.
89. Watt K, Waddle E, Jhaveri R: Changing epidemiology of serious bacterial infections in febrile infants without localizing signs, *PLoS One* 5:e12448, 2010.
90. Krober MS, Bass JW, Powell JM, et al: Bacterial and viral pathogens causing fever in infants less than 3 months old, *Am J Dis Child* 139:889, 1985.
91. Amir J, Alpert G, Reisner SH, et al: Fever in the first months of life, *Isr J Med Sci* 20:447, 1984.
92. Hoberman A, Chao HP, Keller DM, et al: Prevalence of urinary tract infection in febrile infants, *J Pediatr* 123:17, 1993.
93. Byington CL, Rittichier KK, Bassett KE, et al: Serious bacterial infections in febrile infants younger than 90 days of age: the importance of ampicillin-resistant pathogens, *Pediatrics* 111:964, 2003.
94. Pantell RH, Newman TB, Bernzweig J, et al: Management and outcomes of care of fever in early infancy, *JAMA* 10:1261, 2004.
95. Zorc JJ, Levine DA, Platt SL, et al: Clinical and demographic factors associated with urinary tract infection in young febrile infants, *Pediatrics* 116:644, 2005.
96. Lin DS, Huang SH, Lin CC, et al: Urinary tract infection in febrile infants younger than eight weeks of age, *Pediatrics* 105:414, 2000.
97. DiGeronimo RJ: Lack of efficacy of the urine culture as part of the initial work up of suspected neonatal sepsis, *Pediatr Infect Dis J* 11:764, 1992.
98. Pryles CV, Saccharow L: Further experience with the use of percutaneous suprapubic aspiration of the urinary bladder: bacteriologic studies in 654 infants and children, *Pediatrics* 43:1018, 1969.
99. Weathers WT, Wenzl JE: Suprapubic aspiration: perforation of a viscus other than the bladder, *Am J Dis Child* 117:590, 1969.
100. Morell RE, Duritz G, Oltorf C: Suprapubic aspiration associated with hematoma, *Pediatrics* 69:455, 1982.
101. Schreiver RL, Skafish P: Complications of suprapubic bladder aspiration, *Am J Dis Child* 132:98, 1978.
102. Pass RF, Waldo FB: Anaerobic bacteremia following suprapubic bladder aspiration, *J Pediatr* 94:748, 1979.
103. Kiernan SC, Pinckert TL, Kesler M: Ultrasound guidance of suprapubic bladder aspiration in neonates, *J Pediatr* 123:789, 1993.
104. Pryles CV, Lüders D, Alkan MK: A comparative study of bacterial cultures and colony counts in paired specimens of urine obtained by catheter versus voiding from normal infants and infants with urinary tract infection, *Pediatrics* 27:17, 1961.
105. Hoberman A, Wald ER, Reynolds EA, et al: Pyuria and bacteriuria in urine specimens obtained by catheter from young children with fever, *J Pediatr* 124:513, 1994.
106. Vuillermin PJ, Starr M: Investigation of the rate of meningitis in association with urinary tract infection in infants 90 days of age or younger, *Emerg Med Australas* 19:464, 2007.
107. Tebruegge M, Pantazidou A, Clifford V, et al: The age-related risk of co-existing meningitis in children with urinary tract infection, *PLoS One* 6:e26576, 2011.

108. Shah SS, Zorc JJ, Levine DA, et al: Sterile cerebrospinal fluid pleocytosis in young infants with urinary tract infections, *J Pediatr* 153:290, 2008.
109. Pitetti RD, Choi S: Utility of blood cultures in febrile children with UTI, *Am J Emer Med* 20:271, 2002.
110. Littlewood JM: White cells and bacteria in voided urine of healthy newborns, *Arch Dis Child* 46:167, 1971.
111. Lincoln K, Winberg J: Studies of urinary tract infection in infancy and childhood, III: quantitative estimation of cellular excretion in unselected neonates, *Acta Paediatr Scand* 53:447, 1964.
112. Huicho L, Campos-Sanchez M, Alamo C: Metaanalysis of urine screening tests for determining the risk of urinary tract infection in children, *Pediatr Infect Dis J* 21:1, 2002.
113. Hoberman A, Wald ER, Reynolds EA, et al: Is urine culture necessary to rule out urinary tract infection in young febrile children? *Pediatr Infect Dis J* 15:304, 1996.
114. Hansson S, Brandstrom P, Larsson P: Low bacterial counts in infants with urinary tract infection, *J Pediatr* 132:180, 1998.
115. Shaw KN, McGowan KL, Gorelick MH, et al: Screening for urinary tract infection in infants in the emergency department: which test is best? *Pediatrics* 101:1, 1998.
116. Emanuel B, Aronson N: Neonatal hematuria, *Am J Dis Child* 128:204, 1974.
117. Stokland E, Hellström M, Jacobsson B, et al: Renal damage one year after first urinary tract infection: role of dimercaptosuccinic acid scintigraphy, *J Pediatr* 129:815, 1996.
118. Prat C, Domínguez J, Rodrigo C, et al: Elevated serum procalcitonin values correlate with renal scarring in children with urinary tract infection, *Pediatr Infect Dis J* 22:438, 2003.
119. Fine RN: Diagnosis and treatment of fetal urinary tract abnormalities, *J Pediatr* 121:333, 1992.
120. Strife CF, Gelfand MJ: Renal cortical scintigraphy: effect on medical decision making in childhood urinary tract infection, *J Pediatr* 129:785, 1996.
121. Dick PT, Feldman W: Routine diagnostic imaging for childhood urinary tract infections: a systematic overview, *J Pediatr* 128:15, 1996.
122. Slyper AH, Olson JC, Nair RB: Overwhelming *Escherichia coli* sepsis in ureterovesical junction obstruction without reflux, *Arch Pediatr Adolesc Med* 148:1102, 1994.
123. Goldman M, Lahat E, Strauss S, et al: Imaging after urinary tract infection in male neonates, *Pediatrics* 105:1232, 2000.
124. K. Roberts (chair) American Academy of Pediatrics Subcommittee on Urinary Tract Infection, Steering Committee on Quality Improvement and Management: Urinary tract infection: clinical practice guideline for the diagnosis and management of the initial UTI in febrile infants and children 2 to 24 months. *Pediatrics* 128:595, 2011.
125. Sasaki J, Parajuli N, Sharma P, et al: Utility of post-urinary tract infection (UTI) imaging in patients with normal prenatal renal ultrasound, *Clin Pediatr* 51:243, 2011.
126. Lowe LH, Patel MN, Gatti JM, et al: Utility of follow-up renal sonography in children with vesicoureteral reflux and normal initial sonogram, *Pediatrics* 113:548, 2004.
127. Hoberman A, Charron M, Hickey RW, et al: Imaging studies after a first febrile urinary tract infection in young children, *N Engl J Med* 348:195, 2003.
128. Stapleton FB: Imaging studies for childhood urinary infections, *N Engl J Med* 348:251, 2003.
129. Hellerstein S: Antibiotic treatment for urinary tract infections in pediatric patients, *Pediatrics* 112:1213, 2003.
130. Magin EC, García-García JJ, Sert SZ, et al: Efficacy of short-term intravenous antibiotic in neonates with urinary tract infection, *Pediatr Emerg Care* 23:83, 2007.
131. Williams G, Lee A, Craig J: Antibiotic for the prevention of urinary tract infection in children: a systematic review of randomized controlled trials, *J Pediatr* 138:868, 2001.
132. Craig JC, Simpson JM, Williams GJ, et al: Antibiotic prophylaxis and recurrent urinary tract infection in children, *N Engl J Med* 361:1748, 2009.
133. Pennesi M: Is antibiotic prophylaxis in children with vesicoureteral reflux effective in preventing pyelonephritis and renal scars? A randomized, controlled trial, *Pediatrics* 121:e1489, 2008.
134. Islek A, Guven AG, Koyun M, et al: Probability of urinary tract infection in infants with ureteropelvic junction obstruction: Is antibacterial prophylaxis really needed? *Pediatr Nephrol* 10:1837, 2011.
135. Lo E, Nicolle L, Classen D, et al: Strategies to prevent catheter-associated urinary tract infections in acute care hospitals, *Infect Control Hosp Epidemiol* 29:S41, 2008.
136. Hoffpauir CW, Guidry DJ: Asymptomatic urinary tract infection in premature infants, *Pediatrics* 45:128, 1970.
137. Benador D, Benador N, Slosman D, et al: Are younger children at highest risk of renal sequelae after pyelonephritis? *Lancet* 349:17, 1997.

10 Focal Bacterial Infections

GARY D. OVERTURF, MARTHA MULLER, and VICTOR NIZET

CHAPTER OUTLINE

Infections of the Liver

Bacterial infection of the hepatic parenchyma frequently is recognized as multiple, small inflammatory foci (hepatic microabscesses) observed as an incidental finding in infants dying with sepsis. Diffuse hepatocellular damage, often in conjunction with infection of several organ systems, may be present after transplacental passage of microorganisms to the fetal circulation. Liver involvement rarely may take the form of a solitary purulent abscess. Metastatic focal infections of the liver associated with bacteremia resolve with antimicrobial therapy, are not recognized, or are found only at postmortem examination. Rarely, they are clinically apparent as solitary[1] or multiple[2] large abscesses diagnosed during life.

Although metastatic infections are rare, it is difficult to ascertain their true incidence. In a survey of more than 7500 autopsies of children performed from 1917 to 1967, Dehner and Kissane[3] found only 3 neonates with multiple, small, pyogenic hepatic abscesses, whereas a review of approximately 4900 autopsies performed at Los Angeles Children's Hospital from 1958 to 1978 revealed 9 infants with pyogenic hepatic abscesses.[4] Among 175,000 neonates admitted from 1957 to 1977 to Milwaukee Children's Hospital, 2 died with hepatic microabscesses[5]; 3 patients with hepatic microabscesses were seen among 83,000 pediatric patients admitted to New York Hospital from 1945 to 1983.[6]

Solitary hepatic abscesses in newborns have also been reported rarely.[1,2,4] These infections frequently are associated with prematurity and umbilical vein catheterization,[4,5] or because of bacteremia, for instance, after sepsis caused by *Staphylococcus aureus*.[1]

MICROBIOLOGY

Etiologic agents in the infants described by Dehner and Kissane,[3] Moss and Pysher,[4] Chusid,[5] and Simeunovic and colleagues[7] have included *Escherichia coli*, *S. aureus*, *Pseudomonas aeruginosa*, *Klebsiella* spp., *Enterobacter* spp., *Neisseria gonorrhoeae*, and *Listeria monocytogenes*. The causative bacteria of solitary abscesses are generally the bacteria colonizing the umbilical stump,[8] including *S. aureus* (most common), *E. coli*, *Enterobacter* spp., *Klebsiella pneumoniae*, *P. aeruginosa*, and *Streptococcus pyogenes*. The observation of gas in abscesses[9,10] may indicate infection with anaerobes, a frequent cause of liver abscess in adults.[11]

The most common cause of intrauterine bacterial hepatitis, congenital listeriosis, characteristically involves the liver and adrenals (see Chapter 13). Typical lesions are histologically sharply demarcated areas of necrosis (miliary granulomatosis) or microabscesses containing numerous pleomorphic gram-positive bacilli.[12] Intrauterine tuberculosis results from maternal bacillemia with transplacental dissemination to the fetal bloodstream (see Chapter 18). Because the liver is perfused by blood and well oxygenated[13] and is the first organ that encounters tubercle bacilli, it is often severely involved.[12,14] The presence of primary liver foci is considered evidence for congenital tuberculous infection as a result of hematogenous spread through the umbilical vein.[15] Closed-needle biopsy may be less accurate in the diagnosis of hepatic granulomas, and open biopsy may be required to confirm liver and regional node involvement.[16] In addition to hepatomegaly, a clinical picture of fever with elevated serum immunoglobulin M (IgM) and chorioretinitis (e.g., choroid tubercles) may be similar to that caused by other congenital infectious agents.[17] In a review by Abughal and coworkers,[17] positive sites of culture for tuberculosis included liver (8 of 9), gastric aspirate (18 of 23), tracheal aspirate (7 of 7), ear (5 of 6), and cerebrospinal fluid (3 of 10).

Treponema pallidum is the spirochete most commonly associated with transplacental hepatic infection (see Chapter 16). Pathologic changes in the liver, which may be found in 95% of infants dying with congenital syphilis,[18] include diffuse hepatitis or focal areas of inflammation, both frequently accompanied by increased connective tissue and enlargement of the liver.[18,19] Involvement of liver has also been documented, on the basis of isolation of organisms or their identification in histologic sections, in newborns with intrauterine infection caused by various *Leptospira* spp.[20,21] Transplacental infection of the fetus with *Borrelia recurrentis* causes little or no inflammation of liver parenchyma or biliary epithelium despite the presence of numerous spirochetes in the sinusoids.[22,23]

With increasing use of broad-spectrum antibiotics, candidal sepsis has emerged as a serious complication in newborn intensive care units, and liver abscesses can develop during the course of disseminated infection.[24] Use of umbilical venous catheters and total parenteral nutrition was reported in the majority of such cases.

PATHOGENESIS

Infectious agents may reach the liver of the fetus or newborn by one of several pathways: transplacental or transoral intrauterine infection; extension of thrombophlebitis of the umbilical vein, through the hepatic artery during the course of a systemic bacteremia; pyelophlebitis caused by a focus of infection in the drainage of the portal vein (mesenteric or splenic veins); direct invasion from contiguous structures or because of trauma or surgical inoculation; and extension up the biliary passages in cases of suppurative cholangitis. Abscesses with no apparent focus of infection seem to be common in newborns compared with older children.[25] In one such case of solitary liver abscess, the nature of the lesion suggested that an umbilical vein infection, obscured by the large collection of purulent material in the abscess, was the probable pathogenesis.[26]

The mode of infection usually determines the pattern of hepatic involvement. Intense and prolonged seeding of the liver parenchyma, such as that which occurs in conjunction with intrauterine infection or neonatal sepsis, almost invariably results in diffuse hepatocellular damage or multiple small inflammatory lesions.[3-5] Umbilical vein thrombophlebitis may cause an abscess of the falciform ligament[27] or extend into a single branch of the portal vein to produce a solitary pyogenic abscess,[5,28,29] or it can lead to disseminated foci of infection through dislodgment of septic emboli.[5,30]

The frequent use of umbilical catheters has been associated with an increase in the numbers of infants with solitary[4,5,28,29,31] or multiple[4,32,33] hepatic abscesses. In three large series, including almost 500 infants who died after placement of umbilical vein catheters, 29 infants were found to have purulent infections of hepatic vessels or parenchyma.[33-35] Use of venous catheters for infusion of hypertonic or acidic solutions may provide a necrotic focus for abscess formation,[28,31,32,35,36] and prolonged or repeated[4,29,31,35] catheterization of a necrotic umbilical stump provides an ideal pathway for introduction of pathogenic organisms.

Although neonatal liver abscesses usually are caused by hematogenous dissemination of bacteria through the hepatic artery or umbilical vein, examples of infection arising from various other sources have been described. Solitary abscesses have followed a presumed portal vein bacteremia caused by amebic colitis.[37,38] Direct invasion of adjacent liver parenchyma from purulent cholecystitis[39] or postoperative perihepatic abscesses[4] also has been observed. Ascending cholangitis, the most frequent cause of hepatic purulent infections in adults,[25] has not been implicated in the causes of newborn infections.

Descriptions of "umbilical sepsis" and "acute interstitial hepatitis" recorded by Morison[40] seem to indicate that his patients had acquired bacterial infections of umbilical vessels with widespread extension into portal tracts. Although mild periportal parenchymal necrosis was observed in a few infants, hepatocellular damage was minimal or absent in most. Similar lesions have been found in infants dying with sepsis[41] and infantile diarrhea.[42]

CLINICAL MANIFESTATIONS

Multiple hepatic abscesses and diffuse hepatitis related to neonatal sepsis or transplacental fetal infection are usually recognized only at autopsy. Very few clinical manifestations referable to hepatocellular damage are evident before death. The signs and symptoms associated with these conditions are those of the underlying sepsis or of secondary metastatic complications, such as meningitis, pneumonitis, or peritonitis. Solitary abscesses are indolent in terms of their development and clinical presentation. Although the suppurative umbilical focus or umbilical catheterization responsible for the introduction of microorganisms can usually be traced to the first week of life, evidence of hepatic involvement is usually not apparent before the second or third week. The abscess frequently becomes a source for the hematogenous dissemination of microorganisms so that most infants have signs and symptoms of a bacteremia. Despite intense infection of the underlying vessels, the umbilical stump usually shows no evidence of inflammation or purulent discharge. The presence of hepatomegaly, a finding commonly associated with neonatal sepsis, also offers little aid in establishing a definitive diagnosis. In one half of infants for whom physical findings are clearly described, a well-delineated, often fluctuant or tender mass could be palpated in the epigastrium or right upper quadrant. On a few occasions, the infant's mother noticed a mass, often several days before the onset of systemic symptoms. Abscesses occur in the right or left lobe of the liver with almost equal frequency and are generally 3 cm or greater in diameter at the time of surgical exploration.

DIAGNOSIS

Hematologic studies are of little value in establishing a diagnosis; leukocyte counts and sedimentation rates may be normal or elevated. The serum levels of liver enzymes may also be normal[43] or elevated.[4,44] Abdominal radiographs are usually normal or show nonspecific displacement of the lower edge of the liver. In five infants, diagnosis was suspected from plain radiographs by the presence of gas within the hepatic shadow.[31,45] Radiologic findings that commonly accompany hepatic abscess in older children, such as an altered contour of the diaphragm, right pleural effusion, and platelike atelectasis,[46] are rarely present in neonates.

Ultrasonography should be the initial imaging study in newborns with clinical evidence of a hepatic abscess.[47,48] If ultrasonography is negative and the diagnosis is still strongly suspected, more sensitive techniques, such as computed tomography (CT) or magnetic resonance imaging (MRI), should be performed.[48-50] Enhancement with contrast agents may increase the definition of smaller abscesses. Because congenital cysts, arteriovenous malformations, and tumors with central necrosis or hemorrhage can mimic hepatic abscess, the diagnosis should always be confirmed by aspiration of purulent material at laparotomy or by means of percutaneous drainage with ultrasound or CT guidance.[51-54]

PROGNOSIS

The prognosis for infants with diffuse liver involvement related to fetal or neonatal sepsis depends on the underlying condition because hepatic function is rarely compromised sufficiently to determine the outcome. In most cases, pathologic changes in the liver are unsuspected before postmortem examination.

Of 28 infants with solitary hepatic abscesses whose course was described, 6 died. Four newborns died with sepsis caused by organisms that were identical to the organisms isolated from the abscess,[28,43,55,56] and the death of another was ascribed to cecal perforation.[38] Prematurity was undoubtedly a major contributing factor in two of these deaths.[28,43]

TREATMENT

Newborns with a solitary hepatic abscess have traditionally been treated with open surgical drainage in conjunction with antibiotic therapy. Percutaneous catheter drainage is less invasive and often is the preferred first treatment. Several investigators have described the use of percutaneous drainage of intrahepatic abscesses and cysts, guided by CT or ultrasonography, in neonates.[8,33,53] When combined with antibiotic therapy and monitored by ultrasonography to ensure resolution, this treatment has been highly effective. It is questionable whether drainage contributed to recovery other than by aiding the selection of antibiotic coverage. Subsequently, patients have been successfully treated with empirical antibiotic therapy alone.[57-59]

The risk of bacteremia and disseminated infection is high in neonates, and the need to identify infecting organisms to guide antibiotic coverage is of greater urgency in the first weeks of life. It is appropriate to ascertain a microbiologic diagnosis with radiographically guided aspiration or drainage of hepatic abscess in a newborn. When proper equipment (e.g., CT, ultrasonography) and experienced personnel are available, this can be attempted percutaneously.[52,53] When they are unavailable, open surgical drainage should be performed. Empirical antibiotic therapy should be reserved only for infants for whom it is believed that the risk of open or closed drainage would exceed the potential benefits.

If purulent material is obtained, initial antibiotic therapy can be selected on the basis of Gram stain. In addition to *S. aureus* and the aerobic enteric organisms commonly associated with hepatic abscesses, anaerobic bacteria have been suspected as the cause of infection in numerous patients. If foul-smelling pus is aspirated or if Gram-stained smears show organisms with the characteristic morphology of anaerobes, metronidazole, β-lactam and β-lactamase inhibitor combinations (e.g., piperacillin and tazobactam), clindamycin, or imipenem should be included in the initial regimen. Cultures of blood, cerebrospinal fluid, and urine should also be considered before initiation of therapy.

If empirical antibiotic therapy is required, it must be adequate for infections caused by *S. aureus*, enteric organisms, and anaerobic bacteria. The combination oxacillin, gentamicin, and clindamycin is appropriate. In nurseries where methicillin-resistant *S. aureus* (MRSA) or methicillin-resistant *Staphylococcus epidermidis* infections have been a problem, substitution of vancomycin for oxacillin can provide coverage for these organisms. Gentamicin (and other aminoglycosides) and vancomycin levels must be monitored and dosages adjusted as necessary. Extended-spectrum cephalosporins (e.g., cefotaxime, cefepime, ceftazidime) and carbapenems (e.g., meropenem) may be used for enteric organisms and *Pseudomonas* spp., often obviating the need for aminoglycosides. β-Lactam and β-lactamase inhibitor combination drugs (e.g., piperacillin and tazobactam or ampicillin and sulbactam) may provide coverage for many enteric organisms and anaerobic bacteria.

Definitive therapy is based on results of bacteriologic cultures that identify the bacteria and its antibiotic susceptibility. Adequate anaerobic transport and culture techniques must be available if meaningful information is to be obtained. Duration of treatment is based on clinical response, cessation of drainage, and resolution of the abscess cavity as determined by serial ultrasound examinations. Parenteral therapy should be maintained for at least 2 weeks, and longer-term therapy may be administered when necessary. In older children with multiple abscesses or in children for whom surgery is not feasible, therapy for 6 weeks or more has been recommended.

Splenic Abscess

Similar to hepatic abscesses, splenic abscesses have been rarely described in infants.[60] Only 1 of 55 splenic abscesses occurred in an infant younger than 6 months. *S. aureus, Candida* spp., and streptococci were the most frequent causes. In 20 of 48 cases, hepatic abscesses coexisted with splenic abscess. In the single infant case, torsion of the splenic vessels was present, whereas in older children, other distant infections of hematologic conditions (e.g., hemoglobinopathy, hematogenous malignancy) were the associated comorbid conditions. Rare etiologies of splenic abscess reported in the neonatal period include tuberculosis,[61] with accompanying thrombocytopenia, and *Entamoeba histolytica*, complicated by fatal colonic perforation.[62]

Infections of the Biliary Tract

The development of ultrasonography has provided a safe and rapid means for evaluating the neonatal biliary tract. Consequently, an increasing number of reports have appeared describing ultrasound changes seen in the first month of life, with hydrops,[63] cholelithiasis,[64-67] and transient distention of the gallbladder associated[63,66,68-70] or unassociated[66,69-71] with sepsis. Ultrasound criteria for separating normal from pathologically enlarged gallbladders and biliary tracts in neonates have also been described.[72,73]

Despite advanced technology and increased surveillance, cholecystitis in the neonate is observed infrequently. The literature has documented a few dozen cases, of which 9 were seen in association with an epidemic of neonatal enteritis caused by *Salmonella enteritidis*.[74] Two cases of acute necrotizing cholecystitis caused by *E. coli* infection were described in a preterm and term neonate.[75] The pathogenesis of this condition is uncertain; and the great majority of cases in the newborn period have been acalculous. It is postulated that sepsis, dehydration, prolonged fasting (e.g., total parenteral nutrition), congenital obstruction, or a stone impacted in the cystic duct leads to biliary stasis and acute distention of the gallbladder. In most cases, resolution of the primary process permits restoration of the flow of bile and relief of distention. In some cases, prolonged obstruction leads to hydrops.[63] Cholecystitis rarely follows, perhaps because of a direct toxic effect of retained bile or because of ischemia related to elevated intraluminal pressure. Bacterial invasion by fecal flora is probably a secondary phenomenon.[76,77] Other organisms that have been isolated from gallbladder contents or tissue include *Serratia marcescens, Pseudomonas* spp., *Enterococcus faecalis*, viridans streptococci, *S. aureus*, and *Clostridium welchii*.

Infants with cholecystitis may become ill at any time during the first weeks of life; most cases are diagnosed in the third or fourth week. The typical clinical picture is one of sepsis together with signs of peritoneal inflammation and a palpable tender right upper quadrant or epigastric mass. Diarrhea frequently accompanies these findings. Although ultrasonography and radionuclide scintigraphy are helpful in suggesting the presence of gallbladder enlargement or inflammation, diagnosis can be confirmed only by surgical exploration.[63,69] Treatment consists of cholecystectomy or tube cholecystotomy combined with systemic antimicrobial therapy based on Gram stain, culture, and susceptibility studies. If a T tube is placed in the gallbladder, a cholangiogram should be obtained to confirm patency of the biliary system before the tube is removed.

Changes compatible with a diagnosis of ascending cholangitis have been described in histologic sections of liver specimens from infants who died with diarrhea accompanied by hepatocellular injury with cholestasis.[57] Bacteria were also identified in the biliary tree of 2 of 178 premature infants who died after placement of an umbilical venous catheter for an exchange transfusion or for delivery of parenteral fluids.[33] The reasons for this association, if any, are unclear. An infant with spontaneous cholangitis caused by *Enterobacter agglomerans*, presenting as a fever of unknown origin at 3 weeks of age, has also been reported.[78] Severe inflammation and fibrosis of extrahepatic bile ducts and diffuse changes in the portal tracts, resembling changes found in biliary atresia, were found in a premature infant who died 3 hours after birth of listeriosis.[79] The investigator postulated that occult prenatal infections with *L. monocytogenes* might be a rare cause of ascending cholangitis manifesting as idiopathic biliary atresia at birth.

Infections of the Adrenal Glands

Multiple adrenal microabscesses are occasionally found as metastatic lesions associated with neonatal sepsis. These abscesses are particularly characteristic of neonatal listeriosis (see Chapter 13). Solitary adrenal abscesses are rare, however; only a few dozen such cases have been described.[9,80] The spectrum of organisms responsible for adrenal abscesses is the same as that seen in neonatal sepsis and includes *E. coli*,[9,81,82] group B streptococci (GBS),[83,84] *Proteus mirabilis*,[85] *S. aureus*,[86] *Bacteroides* spp.,[87] and *Peptostreptococcus*.[88]

About three fourths of neonatal cases are male, and adrenal abscesses are more commonly located on the right side (approximately two thirds of patients); bilateral lesions are uncommon.[80,83,89,90] The same sex and laterality predominance are seen with adrenal hemorrhage in the newborn,[90] and it has been postulated that formation of an adrenal abscess requires a preexisting hematoma as a nidus for bacterial seeding.[89] This theory of pathogenesis is supported further by clinical observations and by objective evidence (e.g., curvilinear calcifications) documenting the presence of hemorrhage before development of an abscess.[86,87,89]

Most infants with adrenal abscess have presented in the third or fourth week of life with signs of sepsis and an abdominal or flank mass. A history of difficult delivery or intrapartum asphyxia was observed in about one half of these infants, and significant maternal fever or infection during labor was observed in about one fourth.[84,89] Although a few infants are afebrile when first evaluated, a palpable mass is almost always present. Abscesses are usually 6 to 8 cm in diameter, with some containing 200 mL of pus[91] and measuring 12 cm in diameter[91] or crossing the midline.[87]

Laboratory studies are helpful in the evaluation of a possible adrenal abscess. Most infants exhibit a leukocytosis; about one third are anemic and with a history of prolonged neonatal jaundice, both of which are features associated with adrenal hemorrhage. Urinary excretion of catecholamines and their metabolites (particularly vanillylmandelic acid and homovanillic acid), which is usually increased with neuroblastoma, is normal. Because most infants with adrenal abscess are seen for evaluation of possible sepsis, a blood culture, lumbar puncture, urine culture, and chest radiograph should be obtained.

Ultrasonography has become a widely accepted modality for initial evaluation of all neonatal abdominal masses. With the presence of an adrenal abscess, ultrasound examination can help to define the extent and cystic nature of the lesion and often can show movable necrotic debris in the abscess cavity.[86-89]

With serial examinations, abscesses can be distinguished from masses associated with liquefying hematoma, adrenal cyst, hydronephrosis of an obstructed upper pole duplication, or necrotic neuroblastoma.[60,84,89,92] Intravenous pyelography shows downward displacement of the kidney and compression of the upper calyces, which confirms the presence of a suprarenal mass.[82,86-89] A round, suprarenal, radiopaque halo or rim with central lucency, which is characteristic of adrenal abscess, may also be seen on early films[83] but is not pathognomonic.[89] Intravenous pyelography adds little diagnostic information to that provided by ultrasound studies. Experience with radionuclide scanning, CT, and MRI in this condition is limited, but these modalities are likely to be as useful as ultrasonography.[84,86,89]

Whatever diagnostic methods are used, concern about persisting signs of sepsis and the possible presence of an adrenal neoplasm usually encourage early efforts to establish a diagnosis. In the past, recommended management has been incision and drainage or resection of the abscess.[89,92,93] Needle aspiration under ultrasound guidance, combined with placement of a catheter for drainage and irrigation, has proved to be a useful alternative method[85,94] and is likely to supplant open drainage as the preferred method. Antibiotic therapy should be based on Gram stain, culture, and susceptibility studies of abscess fluid and should be continued for 10 to 14 days, provided that drainage can be established.

The adrenals are infected in about 15% of infants with congenital syphilis.[18] In addition to the presence of spirochetes, the most frequent and characteristic change is an extraordinary amount of cellular connective tissue in the capsule.

Appendicitis

Acute appendicitis is extremely rare in infants younger than 4 weeks of age. Reviews of more than 25,000 cases of appendicitis in infants and children in Great Britain,[95] Ireland,[96] Germany,[97] and the United States[98-104] revealed only 8 infants who presented during the neonatal period. Since the condition was first described by Albrecht in 1905[105,106] and Diess in 1908,[107] sufficient cases of neonatal suppurative appendicitis have been reported in the literature details that permit characterization of the clinical features.[98,99,101,108-131] Infants with appendicitis caused by other conditions, such as Hirschsprung disease,[132] necrotizing enterocolitis (NEC),[133] or incarceration in an inguinal hernia,[134] have not been included in this discussion.

Inflammation of the appendix is more common in newborn boys than newborn girls. In reports in which the sex was stated, 40 cases occurred in boys, and 17 cases occurred in girls. Prematurity also seems to be a predisposing factor: 23 of the 49 infants whose birth weights were recorded weighed less than 2500 g at birth. The incidence of appendicitis in infants of multiple births (six twins and one triplet) seems to be higher than would be expected on the basis of low birth weight alone.

Although rare, neonatal appendicitis is likely to occur with greater frequency, as perinatal conditions associated with appendicitis, such as prematurity and survival after severe hypoxia, are increasingly common with advances in neonatal care.[135]

MICROBIOLOGY

Because obstruction of the appendiceal lumen is responsible for almost all cases of appendicitis,[135] it is intuitive that gram-negative enteric organisms resident in the bowel are usually isolated from the peritoneal fluid or periappendiceal pus of about 75% of infants. Specific etiologic agents include *E. coli*, *Klebsiella* spp., *Enterobacter* spp., *Pseudomonas* spp., *Proteus* spp., untyped streptococci, *S. aureus*, and *Bacteroides* spp. These bacterial species have also been isolated from the peritoneal fluid of older children with appendicitis.[103,136] Attempts at isolation of anaerobic bacteria have been rarely described.

A case of perforated amebic appendicitis with secondary bacterial peritonitis and multiple hepatic abscesses in a premature infant born in Great Britain has been reported. *E. histolytica* observed in the wall of the necrotic appendix was presumably acquired from the infant's father, who was a carrier.[38] A patient with gangrenous appendicitis associated with *Rhizopus oryzae* has also been reported.[137] It was postulated that the fungus colonized the infant's gut by transfer from an adhesive bandage used to secure an endotracheal tube.

PATHOGENESIS

Obstruction of the appendiceal lumen has been generally accepted as the primary cause of appendicitis in all age groups. The relative rarity of this condition in the first month of life is probably related to factors that serve to decrease the likelihood of obstruction, including a wide-based, funnel-shaped appendix; the predominantly liquid and soft solid diet given to infants; the absence of prolonged periods in the upright position; and the infrequency of infections that cause hyperplasia of the appendiceal lymphoid tissue.[103,138,139] The causes of luminal obstruction in the newborn period, when recognized, are often extrinsic to the appendix itself. Reports of appendicitis caused by the presence of ectopic pancreatic tissue,[98] a fecalith,[108] or meconium plug[104] are unusual exceptions.

Inflammation of the appendix with perforation has been described as the presenting illness in several infants with neonatal Hirschsprung disease.[133,140] The association of these two conditions has been attributed to functional obstruction, increased intraluminal pressure, and fecal trapping that occur proximal to aganglionic segments. Suppurative appendicitis related to incarceration and strangulation of the cecum within an inguinal or scrotal hernia has been found in numerous infants.[134,141]

CLINICAL MANIFESTATIONS

The onset of neonatal appendicitis generally occurs during the first 2 weeks of life. Only 3 of 54 infants with this condition presented between the 1st and 10th day. The reasons for this phenomenon are unclear, particularly in view of the relatively even distribution of cases during the remainder of the first year of life.[101] At least five cases of "prenatal" appendicitis have been described.[95,142-145] Of the four available for analysis, only one showed definite evidence of a suppurative process in the appendix and signs of bowel obstruction clearly present at birth[143]; however, cultures and Gram stain of the pus found at surgery were free of bacteria. Poisoning by mercuric chloride was suspected in one[145] of the remaining three cases, and the other two, who were said to have prenatal rupture of the appendix, were asymptomatic until the 2nd[143] and 12th[142] days of life.

The signs of neonatal appendicitis correspond to the signs of any of the various forms of intestinal obstruction that occur during the newborn period (Table 10-1).[142] Prominent early findings include abdominal distention; progressive and frequently bilious vomiting; and evidence of pain, as manifested by persistent crying, irritability, or "colic." Clinical features such as diarrhea, constipation, lethargy, or refusal to feed may also be evident but are too nonspecific to be helpful in establishing a diagnosis. The presence or absence of fever is an unreliable sign in appendicitis as in other forms of neonatal infection; temperature has been recorded as normal or subnormal in greater than 50% of newborns with this condition. Abdominal tenderness and guarding are inconsistent findings and, when present, are rarely localized to the appendiceal area. Physical signs of sufficient specificity to indicate acute inflammation of the appendix are generally absent until late in the course of the illness, when gangrene and rupture may result in the formation of a localized intraabdominal abscess or cellulitis of the anterior abdominal wall. Erythema or edema, or both, of the right lower quadrant has been observed in several patients. The presence of this finding, particularly when accompanied by a palpable mass in the right iliac fossa, indicates bowel perforation with peritonitis and should suggest a preoperative diagnosis of NEC or appendicitis (see "Necrotizing Enterocolitis").

Table 10-1 Signs of Intraabdominal Neonatal Appendicitis in 55 Infants

Sign	Incidence (%)
Abdominal distention	90
Vomiting	60
Refusal of feedings	40
Temperature ≥38° C	40
Temperature 37-38° C	30
Temperature ≤37° C	30
Pain (crying, restlessness)	30
Lethargy	30
Erythema/edema of right lower quadrant	25
Mass in right lower quadrant	20
Diarrhea	20
Passage of bloody stools	20

DIAGNOSIS

The diagnosis of appendicitis in a neonate is usually determined at surgery performed for evaluation of abdominal distention and suspected peritonitis. With the high incidence of prematurity associated with early appendicitis, bowel perforation from NEC has been a common preoperative consideration.[146] The two conditions can coexist, and in some cases, the appendix may participate in the process of ischemic necrosis and perforation.[128,133]

Laboratory studies are of little value in establishing a diagnosis of appendicitis in a newborn. White blood cell counts of less than 10,000/mm^3 were found in 10 of 30 infants. Urinalyses are usually normal, although ketonuria, which reflects diminished caloric intake, and hematuria and proteinuria may be seen. Because bacteremia may accompany appendiceal perforation and peritonitis, a blood culture and evaluation for metastatic infection with lumbar puncture and chest radiography should be performed. The value of paracentesis for diagnosis of bowel perforation and peritoneal infection is discussed later (see "Necrotizing Enterocolitis").

Radiologic examinations are occasionally helpful but, in most cases, serve only to confirm a clinical impression of small bowel obstruction. The presence of an increased soft tissue density displacing loops of intestine from the right iliac fossa generally indicates appendiceal perforation with abscess formation and is perhaps the most reliable sign of acute appendicitis in the neonate. Extraluminal gas may be localized briefly to the right lower quadrant after rupture of the appendix.[140] The rapid development of an extensive pneumoperitoneum obscures the site of origin of the escaping gas in most infants within a short time.[147] Ultrasonography may aid in detection of a periappendiceal abscess[47] but is not helpful in establishing an early diagnosis of appendicitis because it lacks sensitivity and specificity.

PROGNOSIS

The overall mortality rate from appendicitis in the newborn is high but is improving. Eight of the newborns in the last 12 reported cases have survived, whereas of 60 infants with this condition for whom the outcome was recorded, 38 (64%) died. Survival was unrelated to birth weight. Among factors responsible for mortalities, three seem to be of primary importance: delay in diagnosis, a high incidence of perforation, and the rapid onset of diffuse peritonitis after appendiceal rupture.

Perforation has been identified at surgery or autopsy in 70% of newborns with acute appendicitis. The relative frequency of this complication has been attributed to delays in establishing a diagnosis and to certain anatomic features of the appendix in young infants that predispose it to early necrosis and rupture. These features include a meager blood supply that renders the organ more vulnerable to ischemia; a cecum that is relatively smaller and less distensible than that of adults, forcing a greater intraluminal pressure on the appendix; and the presence of a thin muscularis and serosa that readily lose their structural integrity under the combined effects of ischemia and increased internal pressure.[113,118]

After the appendix ruptures, infants are unable to contain infection efficiently at the site of origin. Rapid dissemination of spilled intestinal contents produces a diffuse peritonitis within hours because of the small size of the infant's omentum, which fails to provide an efficient envelope for escaping material; the relatively longer and more mobile mesenteries, which favor widespread contamination; and the small size of the peritoneal cavity, which also permits access of infected material to areas distant from the site of perforation.[98,113] Peritonitis, accompanied by sepsis and by the massive outpouring of fluids, electrolytes, and proteins from inflamed serosal surfaces, is generally the terminal event in neonatal appendicitis. Deterioration of the infant's condition is often extremely rapid; failure to recognize the underlying illness and to institute appropriate therapy promptly is inevitably followed by a fatal outcome.

TREATMENT

Surgical intervention is essential for survival of young infants with appendicitis. Because vomiting, diarrhea, and anorexia frequently accompany this condition, restoration of fluid and electrolyte balance is a major factor in ensuring a favorable outcome. Loss of plasma into the bowel wall and lumen of the dilated intestine may require additional replacement with whole blood, plasma, or an albumin equivalent. Optimal preparation often necessitates a delay of several hours but is a major determining factor in the success of any surgical procedure done during the neonatal period.

The preoperative use of antibiotics has been recommended in infants with intestinal obstruction to achieve therapeutic blood levels of drug before the time of incision and possible contamination.[104,148] Perforation, fecal spillage, and peritonitis occur so early in the course of neonatal appendicitis that almost all infants with this condition require treatment before surgery. After the diagnosis of gangrenous or perforated appendicitis has been established and surgery has been performed, parenteral antibiotic therapy should be continued for a minimum of 10 days. The combination of clindamycin (or metronidazole), gentamicin (or extended-spectrum cephalosporins), and ampicillin provides adequate coverage against most enteric pathogens and can be used for initial empirical therapy. Alternatively, β-lactam and β-lactamase inhibitor combinations, such as piperacillin and tazobactam or carbapenem antibiotics (e.g., imipenem or meropenem), can be used alone for broad coverage of enteric bacteria, *Pseudomonas* spp., and anaerobic bacteria. Until the infant is able to tolerate alimentation, careful attention to postoperative maintenance of body fluids, electrolyte balance, nutrition, and correction of blood and plasma losses is vital to survival (see "Peritonitis" and "Necrotizing Enterocolitis").

Peritonitis

Peritonitis in the newborn is most commonly associated with perforation of the gastrointestinal tract, ruptured omphaloceles, or wound infections that follow abdominal surgery.[149] It has been estimated that 20% to 40% of gastrointestinal surgical problems in the neonatal period are complicated by bacterial peritonitis (see "Necrotizing Enterocolitis").[149] At pediatric surgical centers in the United States,[150-152] Great Britain,[153] Hungary,[154] Germany,[155,156] France,[157] and Zimbabwe,[158] 1 to 10 cases per year have been reported in retrospective analyses of peritonitis diagnosed during the first month of life. Among almost 3000 infants admitted to a neonatal intensive care unit (NICU) in Liverpool from 1981 to 1982, there were 6 cases of peritonitis, all from NEC perforation of the gastrointestinal tract.[159] Peritonitis was present in 4 (all of low birth weight) of 501 infants on whom consecutive autopsies were performed from 1960 to 1966 at St. Christopher's Hospital for Children in Philadelphia. These cases represented approximately 3% of all patients with inflammatory lesions associated with death in this age group.[160] Potter[12] considered the peritoneum "one of the most frequent points of localization" in infants dying with sepsis.

A preponderance of boys (2.5:1[158,159] and a high incidence of prematurity (33%)[152-155] have been found in unselected series of infants with this condition. These features are probably less a characteristic of bacterial peritonitis in the newborn than of the primary surgical and septic conditions that are responsible for its occurrence (particularly NEC). There seems to be a female preponderance among newborns with primary peritonitis.[153] A high incidence of congenital anomalies not involving the intestinal tract has also been observed among neonates with peritonitis.[152,155,161]

MICROBIOLOGY

The condition that permits bacteria to colonize the peritoneal surface determines the nature of the infecting organisms. Most infants in whom rupture of a viscus and fecal spillage have caused peritonitis are infected by bacteria considered to be part of the normal enteric microflora; however, prior use of antimicrobial agents and colonization patterns within a nursery are important factors in determining which organisms predominate. Although a mixed flora of two to five species can often be recovered,[161] single isolates have been reported in a third of infants with peritonitis.[162] The predominant aerobic organisms usually include *E. coli*, *Klebsiella* spp., *Enterobacter* spp., *Pseudomonas* spp., *Proteus* spp., coagulase-negative and coagulase-positive staphylococci, ungrouped streptococci, *Enterococcus*, and *Candida*.[152,158,162]

Techniques adequate for the isolation of anaerobic organisms have been used infrequently. In a series of 43 consecutive infants with gastrointestinal perforation and bacterial growth from peritoneal fluid, a mixed aerobic-anaerobic flora was isolated, with *Bacteroides* spp. as the predominant anaerobes[161]; remaining specimens grew aerobic or facultative organisms alone, and no culture yielded only anaerobes. In that series and others, the same organisms were frequently isolated from the peritoneal cavity and blood.[150,161]

In contrast to fecal flora isolated from infants with gastrointestinal perforation, gram-positive organisms predominated among neonates with "idiopathic primary peritonitis." This condition is caused by sepsis in most cases, but it also has often been associated with omphalitis. Specific organisms in one representative series included *Streptococcus pneumoniae* (three cases); ungrouped β-hemolytic streptococcus (three cases); and *S. aureus*, *Pseudomonas* spp., and *E. coli* (one case each).[152] Gram-positive cocci were also the major isolates in other reports of peritonitis associated with hematogenous dissemination of organisms or extension from a peripheral suppurative focu.s[55,162-164]

Rarely, peritonitis may be caused by *Candida albicans* in pure culture or mixed with gram-negative enteric organisms.[165] Because clinical findings in this condition are not different from the findings of bacterial peritonitis, the diagnosis is usually established by blood or peritoneal fluid culture. Severe hypothermia has been described as a possible predisposing cause of bowel perforation and peritonitis caused by *Candida*.[166] In addition to well-recognized risk factors, such as prematurity, antibiotic therapy, and parenteral nutrition with deep venous catheters, NEC may be a significant risk factor for systemic candidiasis, in which it was observed in 37% of 30 infants.[167] Only a single infant in this series had a positive culture for *Candida* spp. from the peritoneum, however. Peritoneal catheters or peritoneal dialysis may also be a risk for direct inoculation of *Candida* organisms into the peritoneal space, which occurred in 1 of 26 children[168] (see Chapter 33).

PATHOGENESIS

Acute bacterial peritonitis may occur whenever bacteria gain access to the peritoneal cavity, through intestinal perforation, by extension from a suppurative focus, or by the hematogenous route. Cases of "fetal peritonitis" described in earlier reports were actually examples of meconium peritonitis caused by intrauterine intestinal perforation.[169] Although bacterial colonization of the gastrointestinal tract in the first days of life may lead to infection in this condition, it is an aseptic peritonitis in its initial stages. A similar condition with focal perforation of the ileum or colon occurring postnatally has been described in infants with very low birth weight. Blue-black discoloration of the abdomen, caused by meconium staining of the tissues of the underlying skin, may be the first physical finding in these infants. Clinical, radiographic, and histopathologic evidence of infection or inflammation was notably absent in most cases.

Conditions that predispose to neonatal peritonitis are outlined in Box 10-1. Among almost 400 newborns with peritonitis studied from 1959 to 1978, perforation of the intestinal tract was responsible for 72% of cases, with ruptured omphaloceles or gastroschisis responsible for 12%, hematogenous dissemination or "primary" peritonitis responsible for 12%, and omphalitis and postoperative complications responsible for 2% each.[149,155,170] In a comprehensive review of neonatal peritonitis, Bell[149,161] described common sites and causes of gastrointestinal perforation and their relative frequencies (Figs. 10-1 and 10-2).

Box 10-1 Etiology of Bacterial Peritonitis in the Neonatal Period

- Gastrointestinal perforation
- Necrotizing enterocolitis
- Ischemic necrosis
- Spontaneous focal gastrointestinal perforation
- Volvulus
- Hirschsprung disease
- Meconium ileus (cystic fibrosis)
- Postoperative complications
- Congenital anomalies
- Internal hernia
- Catheter-associated vascular thrombosis
- Indomethacin therapy (enteral or parenteral)
- Trauma
  - Feeding tubes
  - Rectal thermometers, catheters, enema
- Intrauterine exchange transfusion
- Paracentesis of ascites fluid
- Meconium peritonitis with postnatal bacterial contamination
- Peptic ulcer: stomach, duodenum, ectopic gastric mucosa
- Acute suppurative appendicitis
- Infection
  - *Shigella* or *Salmonella* enterocolitis
  - Prenatal sepsis: listeriosis, syphilis, tuberculosis
  - Neonatal sepsis
  - Suppurative omphalitis transmural migration (theory)
  - Congenital luetic enteritis with necrosis
- Ruptured omphalocele or gastroschisis
- Postoperative: anastomotic leaks, wound dehiscence, wound contamination

CLINICAL MANIFESTATIONS

Neonatal peritonitis is a disease primarily of the first 10 days of life; numerous infants have evidence of peritoneal infection within the first 24 hours.[150,152,158] An analysis of etiologic factors responsible for peritonitis in the newborn provides a ready explanation for this observation (see Box 10-1). Most cases of NEC[161,171,172] and spontaneous gastric perforation[150,161,170] occur within the first week. Ruptured omphaloceles and gastroschisis often develop early infections, and in infants with congenital obstruction, the onset of alimentation during the first 12 to 24 hours accentuates distention and ischemic necrosis of the bowel wall, which leads to early intestinal perforation. Exchange transfusions are performed most frequently within the first 1 or 2 days of life and may be followed by enterocolitis within 4 to 24 hours in infants in whom perforation ultimately occurs.[107,173] Neonatal sepsis, with potential peritoneal seeding of microorganisms, is more frequent during the first 48 hours of life than during any subsequent period.[174]

The various signs and symptoms present in a young infant with peritonitis were summarized most succinctly by Thelander[175] in 1939:

> *"The little patient looks sick. He is cyanotic; the respirations are rapid and grunting; the abdomen is distended, and the abdominal wall, the flanks and the scrotum or vulva are usually edematous. Frequently brawny induration of the edematous area, which may resemble erysipelas, is also present. Food is taken poorly or not at all. Vomiting is frequent and persistent. The vomitus contains bile and may contain blood. The stools are either absent or scant; some mucus or blood may be passed. The temperature may be subnormal, but varying degrees of fever have been reported. The blood count is of little or no value. The hemoglobin content may be very high, which probably indicates only dehydration. The leukocytes may or may not respond with a rise."*

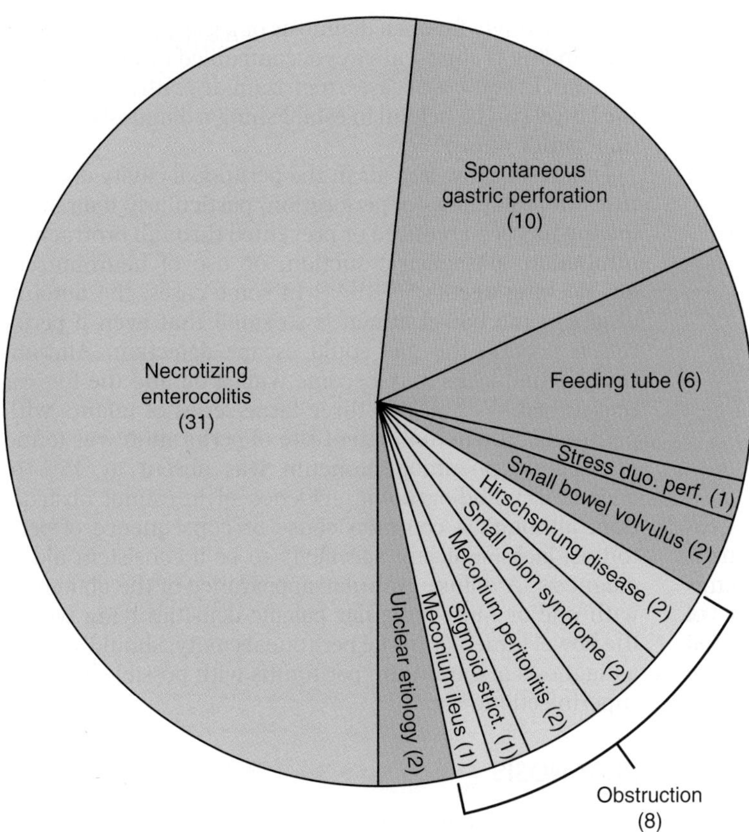

Figure 10-1 Causes of perforation in 60 neonates. *duo. perf.,* Duodenal perforation; *strict.,* stricture. (From Bell MJ: Peritonitis in the newborn—current concepts, *Pediatr Clin North Am* 32:1181-1201, 1985.)

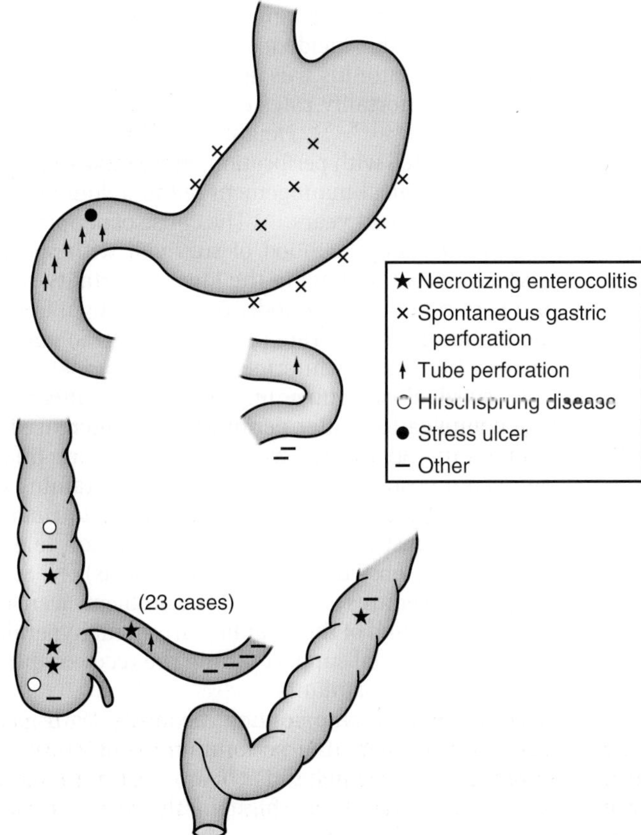

Figure 10-2 Sites of perforation in 60 neonates. (From Bell MJ: Peritonitis in the newborn—current concepts, *Pediatr Clin North Am* 32:1181-1201, 1985.)

Table 10-2 Signs of Bacterial Peritonitis in the Neonate*

Sign	Incidence (%)
Abdominal distention	85
Shock	80
Vomiting	70
Constipation	60
Hypothermia	60
Respiratory distress	55
Fever	15
Diarrhea	15

*Data are based on patients described in references 232, 240, and 243. Redness, edema, and induration of the anterior abdominal wall, noted in only one series, reference 243, are also recognized as characteristic signs.

Although the review by Thelander[175] was limited to neonates with perforation of the intestinal tract, subsequent reports have corroborated the presence of these findings in infants with peritonitis resulting from a wide variety of causes.[151-154,158,161] Not all of the symptoms described may be encountered in any one patient; however, some are always present (Table 10-2).

The large overlap between signs of neonatal peritonitis and sepsis can make it difficult to differentiate the two on the basis of clinical findings. Signs of intestinal obstruction, such as abdominal distention and vomiting, which are seen in 10% to 20% of newborns with sepsis,[9] may reflect a coexistent unrecognized peritonitis. Because the early use of antibiotics often cures hematogenous peritonitis in infants with septicemia, the diagnosis may be missed in infants who survive. Peritonitis unassociated with perforation was found at postmortem examination in 9 of 121 infants with septicemia dying from 1976 to 1988.[149]

DIAGNOSIS

Ultrasonography[47] or abdominal radiographs taken in the erect and recumbent positions showing free intraperitoneal fluid can be helpful in the diagnosis of peritonitis, and sometimes the only evidence of perforation is apparent on these imaging studies. Absence of definition of the right inferior hepatic margin, increased density of soft tissue, and the presence of "floating" loops of bowel have been recorded as positive signs of ascites.[147] Diagnostic paracentesis can be useful in determining whether the fluid is caused by bacterial peritonitis,[163,176] hemoperitoneum, chylous ascites,[177] or bile peritonitis.[178]

The left lateral ("left-side down") decubitus film is of great value in showing small amounts of intraperitoneal gas.[161] Although pneumoperitoneum can be caused by mediastinal air dissecting from the chest into the abdomen,[179] free gas in the peritoneal cavity usually indicates intestinal perforation. An associated pneumatosis intestinalis should suggest the diagnosis of NEC but is not specific for this condition. Several patterns of intraperitoneal gas distribution have been described[47,107,180,181]: the air-dome sign, falciform ligament sign, football sign, lucent-liver sign, saddlebag sign, and gas in the scrotum. Absence of a gastric air-fluid level on an erect abdominal radiograph, with a normal or decreased amount of gas in the small and large bowel, strongly favors a diagnosis of gastric perforation.[180] This finding is almost always accompanied by pneumoperitoneum. In equivocal cases, metrizamide contrast studies of the bowel can be helpful in establishing a diagnosis of intestinal perforation.[182]

Failure to show free air in the peritoneal cavity does not rule out a diagnosis of perforation, particularly if air swallowing has been reduced or prevented through orotracheal intubation, nasogastric suction, or use of neuromuscular blocking agents.[176,182,183] In some cases, the amount of gas in the bowel lumen is so small that even if perforation occurs, the gas could escape detection. Alternatively, small leaks may become walled off and the free air reabsorbed.[182,184,185] In three large series of infants with peritonitis in whom a patent site of perforation was found at surgery, pneumoperitoneum was absent in 35% to 75%.[152,161] Radiographic evidence of intestinal obstruction, although a common cause or consequence of peritonitis, lacks sufficient specificity to be a consistent aid to diagnosis. A diffuse granular appearance of the abdomen, with one or more irregular calcific densities lying within the bowel lumen or in the peritoneal cavity, should suggest a diagnosis of meconium peritonitis with possible bacterial superinfection.[169]

PROGNOSIS

Prematurity, pulmonary infections, shock, and hemorrhage related to perforation of the intestinal tract, sepsis, and disseminated intravascular coagulopathy are often the factors responsible for the death of neonates, who may concurrently have peritonitis diagnosed at surgery or at postmortem examination. For this reason, case-fatality rates often represent the mortality rate among newborns dying with, rather than because of, infection of the peritoneal cavity.[155,161] Before 1970, the incidence of fatalities was exceedingly high when peritonitis was associated with gastrointestinal perforation; mortality rates of 70% were observed in large series.[152-154,157,158,185] Heightened awareness of conditions associated with perforation, more rapid diagnosis, and improved surgical management led to a doubling of survivors in subsequent years.[155] The cause of perforation seems to influence the likelihood of survival, with spontaneous gastric perforation having the lowest mortality rate (10%) and perforation of the duodenum caused by a feeding tube the highest mortality rate (50%); NEC (40%) and all other causes (25%) occupy intermediate positions.[161]

As survival rates have improved, the number of nonlethal complications after perforation has increased proportionally. In one review, two thirds of surviving infants had significant postoperative complications pertaining to infection (e.g., bacteremia, wound infection, intraabdominal abscess) or gastrointestinal tract dysfunction (e.g., esophageal reflux, obstruction, stomal stenosis).[161] Secondary surgical procedures to correct these problems were required in more than half of the infants. Parenteral hyperalimentation for nutritional support during the recovery period was required in 60% of infants.

The mortality rate among neonates with peritonitis from causes other than perforation of the bowel, such as sepsis,[152,154,158] omphalitis,[158] or a ruptured omphalocele,[152,155,158] although high in the past, has not been reassessed in many years.[161] Early diagnosis and institution of appropriate surgical therapy are major factors in reducing the mortality rate.[161] Factors with an apparent adverse influence on prognosis include low birth weight[152,153,155,158,161] and congenital malformations.[155]

TREATMENT

The treatment of bacterial peritonitis is directed primarily toward correction of the causative condition. Careful attention to preoperative preparation of the infant is essential to survival. As soon as bowel obstruction or perforation is diagnosed, continuous nasogastric suction should be instituted for decompression and prevention of aspiration pneumonitis. Diagnostic needle paracentesis is also useful for relief of pneumoperitoneum and may facilitate exchange of gas by reducing the intraabdominal pressure. Shock, dehydration, and electrolyte disturbances should be corrected through parenteral administration of appropriate electrolyte solutions, plasma, or plasma substitutes. If blood is discovered in fluid recovered by gastric suction or abdominal paracentesis, use of whole blood, packed red blood cells, or other fluids may be necessary to correct hypovolemia. Persistent bleeding must be evaluated for disseminated intravascular coagulation or thrombocytopenia, or both, and treated accordingly. Hypothermia, which frequently accompanies neonatal peritonitis, should be corrected before induction of anesthesia. Infants who are unable to tolerate oral or tube feedings within 2 or 3 postoperative days should be started on parenteral hyperalimentation.

If a diagnosis of peritonitis is established at the time of paracentesis or surgery, aerobic and anaerobic cultures of peritoneal contents should be taken before initiation of antibiotic therapy. Parenteral administration of a combination of gentamicin or an extended-spectrum cephalosporin and clindamycin and ampicillin should be continued for 7 to 10 days.[141,148] Other antibiotics that provide a broad spectrum against enteric organisms, *Pseudomonas* spp., enterococci, and anaerobic organisms include β-lactam and β-lactamase inhibitor compounds and carbapenems. In the event of a poor clinical response, culture and susceptibility studies of the infecting organisms should be used as guides for modifying therapy.

Leakage of intestinal contents sometimes results in formation of a localized abscess, rather than contamination of the entire peritoneal cavity. Management of infants with such an abscess should include antimicrobial therapy and surgical drainage of the abscess by the most convenient route.

Necrotizing Enterocolitis

Necrotizing enterocolitis with necrosis of the bowel wall is a severe disease that is one of the most common and devastating infections of the NICU.[186-191] The risk of NEC is inversely related to gestational age, with prematurity and low birth weight the most important risk factors. NEC may develop in approximately 5% of newborns born earlier than 32 weeks of gestation and 10% of infants born earlier than 28 weeks of gestation[192]; for infants between 500 and 1500 g birth weight born between 2000 and 2009, the incidence of NEC ranged from 4.6% to 6.1%.[193] Less than 10% of NEC cases occur in term infants; in these cases, the disease developed in those already admitted to a NICU for some other reason and thus as a complication of treatment, not as a primary diagnosis.[194,195] The overall mortality rate for NEC exceeds 20% and is significantly higher in those infants requiring surgical interventions.[196] The financial cost of caring for infants with NEC in the United States alone may approach $1 billion.[186]

PATHOLOGY AND PATHOGENESIS

Bowel wall necrosis of variable length and depth is the characteristic feature of NEC, with perforation in one third of affected infants generally in the terminal ileum or cecum, where microcirculation is poor. The pathogenesis of NEC is not definitively established, but the etiology is de facto multifactorial with a confluence of predisposing factors contributed by intestinal immaturity, ischemia, infection, and inflammatory response. The preterm infant possesses an immature gastrointestinal tract supplied by a precarious vasculature prone to imbalances in vascular tone. An additional stress, or multiple additional stresses, may trigger the cascade of events that leads to the pathognomonic findings of NEC: disruption of the mucosal barrier, bacterial invasion and proliferation, and gas formation within the bowel wall (Fig. 10-3). Potential triggers may include the increased intestinal metabolic demand of enteral feeding, disturbance in the normal ecologic balance of the gut microflora, and the exaggerated inflammatory response of the highly immunoreactive neonatal intestinal mucosa.[186,191,197] Surgical specimens from early stages of the disease show mucosal edema, hemorrhage, and superficial ulceration with very little inflammation or cellular response. By the second or third day, after progression to pneumatosis and transmural necrosis of the bowel wall, bacterial proliferation and the acute inflammatory reaction become more prominent.[198]

Limited data available from twin studies or candidate gene association studies (e.g., cytokine genes) have yet to establish any specific genetic risk factors for development of NEC.[199,200] Maternal complications of pregnancy, labor, and delivery and neonatal respiratory distress syndrome are thought to be unrelated to the development of NEC, whereas evidence linking NEC to birth asphyxia, hypotension, hypothermia, use of vascular catheters, exchange transfusion, feeding history, abnormalities of gut motility, neonatal achlorhydria, and the presence of patent ductus arteriosus is often contradictory. Each of these conditions, singly or together, may act as a stress leading to mucosal injury, but none has been consistently associated with NEC. NEC has occurred among apparently healthy infants with no known predisposing risk factors.[194]

A number of studies suggest that the incidence of NEC could be higher in NICUs in which enteral feedings are introduced early or in which increased feeding volumes are pushed aggressively[201,202]; however, no absolute consensus has emerged on the ideal protocol for feeding advancement with respect to risk of NEC, especially in very-low-birth-weight infants, where delayed weight gain itself is associated with counterbalancing medical risks.[203]

Infants fed maternal milk have a lower risk of NEC, but the absolute level of protection can be difficult to quantify

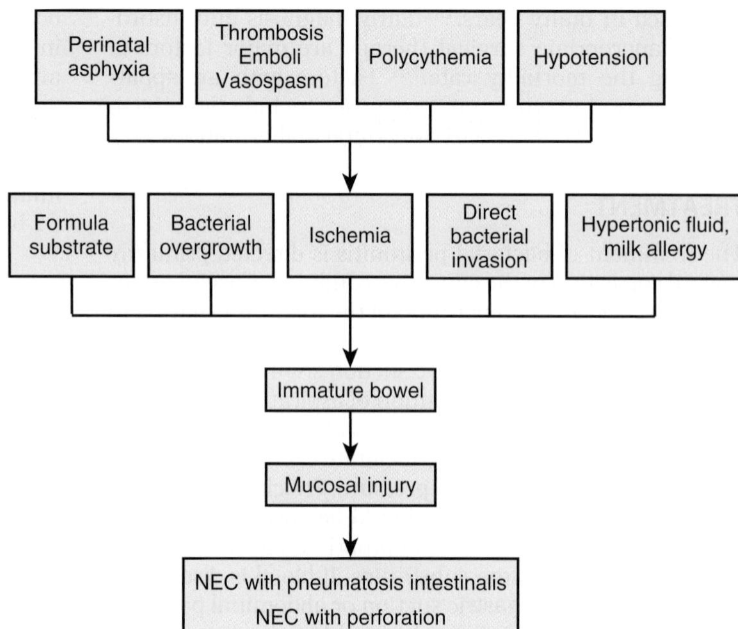

Figure 10-3 Pathogenesis of mucosal injury leading to necrotizing enterocolitis (NEC). (Modified from Walsh MC, Kliegman RM: Necrotizing enterocolitis. *Pediatr Basics* 40:5, 1985.)

because independent risk factors for NEC may also reduce the likelihood of receiving breast milk. However, a recent study indicated that a diet exclusively based on human milk was associated with a lower rate of NEC than a mixed diet of human milk and bovine milk–based products.[204] A recent meta-analysis of clinical trials of formula versus donor breast-milk feeding identified a lower risk of NEC in the human milk–fed infants.[205] In a neonatal rat model of NEC, maternal milk was protective compared with artificial formulas; similar to human NEC, artificial feeding of maternal milk reduced the incidence and severity of NEC injury, and interleukin-10 expression was significantly increased when neonates were fed maternal milk.[206]

MICROBIOLOGY

A long-standing hypothesis postulates that aberrant intestinal microbial colonization in preterm infants is an important contributing factor to the development of NEC.[207,208] Potential microbial etiologies of NEC have been pursued for decades, based on circumstantial evidence including common findings of bacteremia and/or endotoxemia in affected infants and the concept that the pathognomonic imaging finding of pneumatosis intestinalis is suggestive of a gas-forming organism proliferating in submucosal bowel tissue.[186]

The analogous pathology of necrotizing enteritis caused by *Clostridium septicum* and *Clostridium perfringens* in domestic animals, older children, and adults favored suggestions that *Clostridium* spp. (e.g., *C. perfringens, C. difficile, C. butyricum*) might act as a primary pathogen in NEC.[209,210] Subsequent studies have indicated, however, that these species can often be acquired from the nursery environment and could frequently be recovered from healthy neonates.[211,212] Clostridial cytotoxin, which had been recovered from the stool of infants involved in an outbreak of NEC,[213] has also been found in the stool of 90% of normal infants.[211,212] The role of *Clostridium* spp. in NEC thus remains unclear.

The δ-toxins, hemolysins of coagulase-negative staphylococci and *S. aureus*, have also been proposed as possible primary toxins capable of producing NEC in infants. Frequent colonization by δ-toxin staphylococci and higher levels of toxin production by associated strains causing NEC and one outbreak with δ-toxin–producing *S. aureus* strains have been reported.[214,215] Prospective studies have documented significant shifts in aerobic bacterial bowel flora within 72 hours before onset of clinical NEC[216]; the observed shift results from preclinical changes in the intestinal environment. This shift suggests that bacteria isolated at the time of onset were present because of possible intraluminal changes and are not directly involved in NEC. Pending further experimental or epidemiologic observations, the weight of evidence indicates that although bacteria or bacterial toxins may play a primary or secondary role in the pathogenesis of NEC, the occasional association of this condition with a single organism probably reflects patterns of intestinal colonization prevalent in the nursery at the time of an outbreak. Despite intensive efforts to identify a specific infectious agent or toxin in the cause of NEC, convincing reports implicating the same pathogen in more than one outbreak have not appeared.

The advent of 16S ribosomal RNA technology and high-throughput methods for metagenomic analysis should facilitate comprehensive studies of the gut microbes of very-low-birth-weight infants and their disease associations.[208] Smaller preliminary studies using such molecular methods suggest that NEC may be associated with the presence of unusual intestinal microbial species and an overall reduction in the diversity of microbiota; the latter finding may reduce resistance to pathogen colonization, a normal function of the healthy intestinal microbiome.[186]

CLINICAL MANIFESTATIONS

Signs of NEC usually develop in the first 7 days of life, and 50% or greater of cases are recognized within 5 days of

Table 10-3 Modified Bell Staging Criteria and Recommendations for Therapy for Necrotizing Enterocolitis

Stage	Systemic Signs	Intestinal Signs	Radiologic Findings	Treatment
IA (suspected)	Temperature instability Apnea and bradycardia Lethargy	Elevated residuals Mild abdominal distension Emesis Guaiac plus stools	Normal Mild ileus	NPO Antibiotics × 3 days
1B (suspected)	Same as IA	Frank rectal blood	Same as IA	Same as IA
IIA (definite), mild	Same as IA and IB	Same as IB, plus absent bowel sounds ± Abdominal tenderness	Dilation Ileus Pneumatosis intestinalis	NPO; Antibiotics for 7-14 days if examination normal in 24-48 hr
IIB (definite), moderate	Same as IIA with Mild metabolic acidosis Mild thrombocytopenia	Same as IIA with definite abdominal tenderness ± abdominal cellulitis or right lower quadrant mass	Same as IIA with Portal gas ± ascites	NPO Antibiotics × 14 days
IIIA (advanced), bowel intact	Same as IIB plus Hypotension Bradycardia Severe apnea Respiratory/metabolic acidosis Disseminated intravascular coagulation Neutropenia	Same as IIB plus Peritonitis Marked tenderness Abdominal distension	Same as IIB with ascites	Same as IIB plus 200 mL/kg fluid Inotropic agents Assisted ventilation Paracentesis
IIIB (advanced), bowel perforated	Same as IIIA	Same as IIIA	Same as IIIA plus pneumoperitoneum	Same as IIIa plus surgery; NPO

Modified from Walsh MC, Kliegman RM: Necrotizing enterocolitis: treatment based on staging criteria, *Pediatr Clin North Am* 33:179-201, 1986.
NPO, Nothing by mouth.

birth.[171,172] Small immature newborns often develop illness later, during the second to eighth week, whereas low-risk term infants may become ill shortly after delivery, as early as the first 24 hours.

NEC is a disease with a wide spectrum of manifestations, ranging from a mild gastrointestinal disturbance to a fulminant course characterized by early bowel perforation, peritonitis, sepsis, and shock.[217,218] A staging system (Table 10-3) taking these clinical variations into account may be useful in guiding patient evaluation and therapy.[219] The apparent stage of disease for an individual infant usually can be defined on the second day of illness. An infant who exhibits only mild systemic and intestinal signs 24 to 48 hours after onset is unlikely to develop a more serious illness.[220]

The classic presentation of NEC includes a triad of abdominal distention, retention of gastric contents, and gastrointestinal bleeding.[186,197,219,220] These findings are often preceded or accompanied by signs consistent with sepsis, such as lethargy, poor feeding, temperature instability, apnea, and bradycardia; diarrhea is a variable finding. Progression of bowel wall necrosis leading to perforation, peritonitis, and sepsis is reflected in deteriorating vital signs, accompanied by persistent acidosis, clotting disorders, and circulatory collapse. Redness, induration, and edema of the anterior abdominal wall are commonly described in the advanced stages of NEC. In the absence of aggressive medical and surgical intervention, the course is rapidly downhill when late signs appear.

DIAGNOSIS

Radiographic signs of NEC are largely nonspecific,[221] and interobserver variability in the interpretation of films is substantial.[222,223] Radiographic examination of the abdomen remains the most reliable aid, however, in establishing a diagnosis of NEC. Ileus with generalized bowel dilatation and abdominal distention are the earliest radiologic findings.[221] Increasing distention, separation of loops by peritoneal fluid or edema of the bowel wall, a gasless abdomen, pneumatosis intestinalis, and hepatic or portal air occur as NEC worsens.[221] A persistent single dilated loop of bowel remaining relatively unchanged in shape and position in serial films is strongly suggestive,[224] but not diagnostic, of localized bowel ischemia with impending perforation.[225]

If free air or ascites is absent on initial abdominal examination, supine and left lateral decubitus films should be obtained every 6 to 8 hours until improvement or definitive surgery or invasive diagnostic measures have ruled out the presence of perforation. When perforation occurs, it is usually within 1 day after diagnosis[226] but may be delayed for 5 or 6 days.[227,228] Although the presence of pneumoperitoneum or intraperitoneal fluid generally indicates perforation, its absence does not exclude perforation. In one study,[226] only 63% of infants with NEC and proven perforation had free air, 21% had ascites, and 16% had neither free air nor ascites.

When plain films are normal or equivocal, other studies may be diagnostic. A metrizamide gastrointestinal series may show intestinal perforation or abnormalities of the bowel wall, mucosa, or lumen.[229] Real-time ultrasonography may reveal portal venous and hepatic parenchymal gas in standard radiographs.[230,231] Changes on abdominal magnetic resonance imaging may offer a potential for diagnosis early in the course of NEC.[232]

A rapid and direct means of establishing the presence of intestinal necrosis or perforation is by abdominal paracentesis.[233] This procedure is unnecessary in infants to rule out NEC or in infants improving on medical therapy. The procedure is generally reserved for infants suspected, on the basis of clinical, radiographic, and laboratory findings, to have intestinal gangrene. Paracentesis has an accuracy of greater than 90% in determining the need for an operation in NEC.[233] False-positive results are rare; false-negative results are quite common. Patients with a dry tap should be closely observed under medical therapy with continuing serial paracenteses until indications for or against surgical intervention are clearly defined. Infants with a positive result should undergo exploratory surgery immediately.

Thrombocytopenia and disseminated intravascular coagulation are the most common hematologic complications,[234,235] particularly in the presence of bowel gangrene or perforation. Platelet-activating factor has been used to assist in the staging of NEC[236]; a cutoff level of 10.2 ng/mL had a positive predictive value of 100% in identifying infants with stage II or III NEC. Leukopenia and absolute granulocytopenia, apparently caused by margination of white blood cells rather than bone marrow depletion,[237] also have occurred during early stages of the illness.[234,235] A low absolute granulocyte count persisting for 2 to 3 days is associated with a poor prognosis. No consistent urinary abnormalities have been described for NEC, although increased lactate excretion, reflecting heightened enteric bacterial activity, may occur.[238] Increased amounts of fecal-reducing substances have been found in almost three fourths of formula-fed premature infants during early stages of NEC, before the onset of abdominal distention, poor feeding, or emesis.[239]

The evaluation of patients with NEC should include culture of blood and, when appropriate and clinically safe, cerebrospinal fluid, urine, and stool. The likelihood of bacteremia accompanying NEC depends on the severity of bowel involvement; the reported incidence has ranged from 10% to 67% among symptomatic infants. Combined data from several large studies showed positive blood cultures in about one third of newborns with NEC.[227,228,240] The usual organisms have been *E. coli, Klebsiella* spp., *S. aureus*, and *Pseudomonas* spp., whereas enterococci and anaerobic bacteria were isolated occasionally. A spectrum of organisms similar to those causing neonatal sepsis has been isolated from the peritoneal fluid. Meningitis may accompany bacteremia, occurring in approximately 1% of NEC cases.[241]

TREATMENT

Early and aggressive treatment must be initiated for any infant suspected to have NEC. The modified Bell staging system of NEC may guide diagnostic studies, management, antibiotics, and surgical consultation and intervention (see Table 10-3). Umbilical catheters should be removed whenever possible, oral feedings should be stopped, and nasogastric tube drainage should be instituted. Fluid and electrolyte deficits and maintenance require rigorous attention; blood, plasma, or colloid infusions are often necessary for volume expansion and maintenance of tissue perfusion.

After appropriate cultures are obtained, broad-spectrum parenteral antibiotic therapy should be started.[242] Historically, antibiotic coverage has consisted of ampicillin, gentamicin, and either clindamycin or metronidazole. More recently, initial therapy with meropenam or β-lactam and β-lactamase inhibitor combinations (e.g., piperacillin plus tazobactam) with gentamicin may provide coverage against anaerobic, gram-negative enteric aerobic, and many gram-positive pathogens. Vancomycin may be required for resistant gram-positive species, including MRSA. Gentamicin and vancomycin dosages should be modified as necessary on the basis of serum levels. The need for inclusion of clindamycin to provide activity against anaerobic bacteria in the management of NEC has been questioned,[243] based on the observation that anaerobic bacteria are late bowel colonizers, present in relatively much lower numbers in infants than in adult subjects, and that anaerobes other than *Clostridium* spp. have been infrequently identified in NEC.

After immediate treatment has been started, follow-up studies should be instituted. These include serial examinations with measurement of abdominal girth; testing of stools for blood; levels of serum electrolytes, blood glucose, and arterial blood gases; complete blood cell count and platelet count; urine-specific gravity; and supine and left lateral decubitus abdominal radiographs. These tests should be considered every 6 to 8 hours until the infant's clinical condition stabilizes. Attention to vital functions should be provided as necessary on the basis of clinical, laboratory, or radiographic studies. Parenteral nutritional support through a central or peripheral vein must be started as soon as possible.

Early recognition and prompt initiation of medical therapy may reduce the need for surgery. Generally accepted criteria for surgical exploration are a deteriorating clinical condition despite appropriate medical therapy, signs of peritonitis, presence of free air within the abdomen, or a positive paracentesis result. The principles of surgical preparation and management have been discussed by several investigators.[244-246] In addition to laparotomy with removal of necrotic bowel, closed peritoneal drainage has been proposed as an alternative in very small infants, with a resultant survival of greater than 50%.[247]

PREVENTION

Initial observations implicating bacterial proliferation as a factor in pathogenesis of NEC prompted efforts at suppression of gut flora with topical antibiotics in the hope of preventing NEC. Attempts to prevent NEC by giving oral kanamycin or gentamicin prophylactically generated contradictory data. In controlled clinical trials, a significant reduction in the incidence of NEC in treated premature infants was shown in some trials,[248,249] whereas in others, investigators were unable to show any protective effect.[250] Previous studies revealed selective growth of resistant organisms in bowel flora[251] and evidence of significant systemic absorption of aminoglycoside antibiotics in neonates,[252] suggesting that oral aminoglycoside prophylaxis is not free of potential risks. Potential risk factors have not been examined in vancomycin trials, however. Until additional evidence is presented indicating clear-cut benefits from the use of oral aminoglycosides or vancomycin, it does not seem that either agent should be used routinely for prevention of NEC in premature infants.

A number of recent studies have indicated that oral probiotics may alter the bowel flora of the very-low-birth-weight infant to reduce the incidence and severity of NEC.[253,254] Lin and colleagues[255] determined the incidence of NEC (stage II or greater) was significantly lower in the probiotic treatment group (2 of 180) when compared with the control group (10 of 187). Bin-Nun and colleagues[256] reported a reduction in the incidence of NEC with probiotic supplementation from 16% to 4%, with a further reduction in severity of disease among affected infants by Bell's criteria. A meta-analysis of 11 trials of probiotics concluded that the risk for NEC and death was significantly lower, but the risk for sepsis did not differ significantly from those neonates not receiving probiotics.[257]

Excessive or accelerated feedings have been associated with increased frequency of endemic NEC,[258] and some clinicians have recommended a schedule of slow advancement of daily feeding volumes limited to about 20 mL/kg/day. Infants with NEC are more likely to have been fed earlier, to have received full-strength formulas sooner, and to have received larger feeding volumes and increments, and stress and associated respiratory problems may make such infants more vulnerable to NEC.[259] The duration of feeding and rate of advancement of feed volumes may be modifiable risk factors for NEC in preterm infants.[202,203]

Carrion and Egan[260] suggested that relative hypochlorhydria of the neonate may contribute to NEC and found that hydrochloric acid supplements (0.01-0.02 mL of a 1.0-N solution of HCl per mL of formula) significantly reduced NEC rates and lowered gastric pH. Another study has showed that standardized feedings begun at a median of 4 days after onset of NEC can be associated with an abbreviated time until institution of full enteral feedings, a reduced incidence of the use of central catheters and catheter infections, and, ultimately, a shorter hospital stay.[261] Reports of prevention of necrotizing enterocolitis in low-birth-weight infants by IgA-IgG feeding[262,263] are likely functionally correlated to the benefits of breast milk in reducing incidence of the syndrome.[204]

PROGNOSIS

The mortality rate of NEC is difficult to determine because mild cases of suspected NEC are probably more common than is recognized.[264] In studies in which analysis has been limited to infants with "definite NEC," mortality figures range from 20% to 40%,[196] and a longitudinal study over 25 years.[265] A poor prognosis has been linked with very low birth weight, associated congenital defects, bacterial sepsis, disseminated intravascular coagulation, intestinal perforation, and persistent hemodynamic or respiratory instability.[227,266] Surgical intervention, generally reserved for the sickest infants with more extensive bowel involvement, is also associated with higher mortality rates.[196,265]

Infants who survive the acute phase of illness generally do well, although NEC may recur in 5% to 10%.[265,267] In addition to surgical complications (e.g., short bowel syndrome, anastomotic leaks, fistula formation), enteric strictures are probably the most common delayed complication in surviving infants, occurring in 4% to 20%. Usually found at sites of ischemia and necrosis in terminal ileum or colon,[268] these strictures often become apparent within a few weeks but may be delayed 18 months. When multiple strictures occur, the intervening normal bowel may form an enterocyst.[269] Clinically, strictures manifest as frequent episodes of abdominal distention, often with vomiting, obstipation, or hematochezia. Diagnosis is confirmed by gastrointestinal contrast studies. Surgery with removal of the stenotic site is necessary to achieve a cure. The need for bowel resection is one of the most common severe complications of NEC and the major cause of the short bowel syndrome in pediatric patients.

Long-term follow-up of low-birth-weight infants with severe NEC (i.e., Bell stages II and III) has documented higher rates of subnormal body weight (15%-39%) and head circumference (30%) in addition to significant neurodevelopmental impairment (83%).[270] Premature infants with NEC have longer NICU stays, acquire more nosocomial infections, have lower nutrient intake, grow slower, and have higher rates of retinopathy of prematurity and bronchopulmonary dysplasia than age-matched controls.[271] A synergistic effect of NEC and invasive infection can predispose to more severe neurodevelopmental outcomes, including cerebral palsy.[272]

Endocarditis

Neonatal bacterial endocarditis, previously uncommon, has been recognized more frequently in recent years. About 60 cases that meet clinical and bacteriologic criteria sufficient to establish this diagnosis were reported in the literature before the mid-1980s.[35,273-279] The prolonged survival of critically ill infants, including infants with complex congenital heart disease, and the increased use of intravascular catheters, together with advances in the diagnostic sensitivity and availability of echocardiography, may be responsible for an increased recognition of endocarditis. In a 35-year review of 76 cases of endocarditis in children, 10% of patients were younger than 1 year; the youngest patient was 1 month old.[280] Of patients, 62 (83%) had congenital heart disease, and 77% had had prior surgery. Central venous catheters were additional significant risk factors.

At the Mercy Hospital for Women in Melbourne, of more than 12,000 infants admitted to the special care nursery, 8 infants with endocarditis were identified; gestation less than 32 weeks, birth weight less than 1500 g, thrombocytopenia and neutropenia, or increased neutrophil count were common features. The tricuspid valve (8 cases) and mitral valve (2 cases) were most frequently involved. *S. aureus* was isolated from 3 infants and coagulase-negative *Staphylococcus*, *Bacteroides fragilis*, *E. faecalis*, and *E. coli* were isolated 1 each among the infants.[281] In a NICU in Manchester, United Kingdom, between 1990 and 1992, 12 cases of ultrasound-proven endocarditis in newborn infants with structurally normal hearts were identified[282]; two thirds were premature, low-birth-weight infants, whereas the other one third had surgical problems with indwelling central catheters. Among these patients, 10 had coagulase-negative staphylococci identified from blood cultures, 1 had *Streptococcus sanguinis*, and 1 had *C. albicans*.

Etiologic agents of bacterial endocarditis in newborns, which have been identified by isolation from blood cultures or morphologic characteristics of organisms entrapped within valvular vegetations examined at autopsy, include most commonly *S. aureus*, coagulase-negative staphylococci, viridans streptococci, and group B streptococci; less common agents that have been reported include *P. aeruginosa*, *Serratia marcescens*, *Streptococcus pneumoniae*, *Neisseria gonorrhoeae*, *K. pneumoniae*, and *Proteus mirabilis*. Despite widespread cardiovascular involvement associated with congenital syphilis, there is no conclusive evidence that this disease produces valvular heart lesions in infected infants.

Factors that predispose a newborn to endocarditis are not well understood, although intravascular catheters are associated with endocarditis. In contrast to older children, in whom congenital heart disease is often associated with endocarditis,[283] cardiac anomalies are more unusual in neonatal infection.[275,277,282] Bacteremias arising from an infected umbilical stump[273] or skin lesions[284] are presumed sources of valvular involvement in other infants; the invasive organisms associated with these conditions and with neonatal endocarditis in general can infect normal heart valves.[285] Nevertheless, the greater frequency of bacterial and fungal endocarditis in newborns in recent years, particularly in association with prematurity or placement of central vessel catheters, or both, indicates that other, more complex mechanisms may also be operative in some cases.

Damage to the intracardiac endothelium with formation of a sterile platelet-fibrin thrombus at the site of the injury are often the initiating events in a patient with endocarditis. Endocardial trauma caused by placement of cardiac catheters, disseminated intravascular coagulation, and various nonspecific stresses associated with prematurity, such as hypotension and hypoxia, has been implicated in the genesis of thrombi.[285-288] Nonbacterial thrombotic endocarditis or verrucous endocarditis usually remains uninfected and is described as an incidental finding at autopsy.[288] With bacteremia, implantation of organisms may lead to valvular infection. Whether this mechanism or direct bacterial invasion is primarily responsible for valvulitis is unknown. A similar pathogenesis has been postulated for formation of mycotic aortic aneurysms in newborns.[289]

Endocarditis should be suspected in any neonate, particularly a premature infant, with an indwelling vascular catheter, evidence of sepsis, and new or changing heart murmurs. When these findings are accompanied by persistent bacteremia, or by signs of congestive heart failure without underlying heart disease, the diagnosis must be considered seriously. Although Janeway lesions, a generalized petechial rash, and splinter hemorrhages have been seen, murmurs characteristic of semilunar valve insufficiency, Osler nodes, Roth spots, arthritis, and other findings typical of valvular infection in adults and older children have not been observed in neonates. Multiple septic emboli with involvement of the skin, bones, viscera, and central nervous system are common findings, however.[277-279,283,285,287]

Two-dimensional echocardiography stands as an invaluable rapid, noninvasive method for diagnosing endocarditis.[276-278] Although it cannot differentiate between infected and sterile vegetations and other valvular lesions (discussed later), imaging is quite specific, and false-positive readings are uncommon. Less certainty can be placed on a negative report. Despite detection of vegetations 2 mm in diameter with echocardiography, the number of false-negative examinations is significant.[278,290] A diagnosis of bacterial endocarditis should be considered in any infant with a compatible history and physical findings regardless of the results obtained by echocardiography. Use of transesophageal echocardiography, which provides detailed views of the mitral and tricuspid valves, and application of color flow Doppler imaging, which can identify areas of turbulence as blood passes over vegetations or through narrowed valve leaflets, improves diagnostic accuracy.[291]

When endocarditis is suspected, specimens of blood, cerebrospinal fluid, and urine obtained by catheterization or suprapubic aspiration should be sent for bacterial and fungal culture. Because blood drawn from a central catheter often contains organisms colonizing the line but not present in the systemic circulation, at least two peripheral venous blood cultures should be obtained before antimicrobial therapy is initiated. Volumes of 1 to 5 mL, depending on the infant's size, should be adequate. Routine laboratory studies are helpful in supporting a diagnosis of endocarditis in the newborn. The leukocyte count, differential count, and platelet count are usually indicative of sepsis, rather than cardiac valve infection in particular. Microhematuria has been reported, although rarely. A chest radiograph should be obtained to determine signs of cardiac failure or pulmonary or pleural space infection. CT or MRI of the brain can be helpful in an infant with neurologic signs, particularly if left-sided endocarditis or a right-to-left shunt exists. Baseline determinations of inflammatory markers are useful and can be used for assessing the efficacy of the therapy; erythrocyte sedimentation rate and C-reactive protein level have been used.

Intravenous therapy with a penicillinase-resistant penicillin and an aminoglycoside should be started after appropriate cultures have been obtained. In nurseries where MRSA or methicillin-resistant *S. epidermidis* infections have been a problem, vancomycin should be substituted initially for the penicillin antibiotic.[290,291] If endocarditis caused by susceptible *Enterococcus* spp. is suspected, ampicillin should be added or substituted for the penicillinase-resistant penicillin. After the infecting organism is isolated and antibiotic susceptibilities have been determined, specific antimicrobial therapy can be instituted.

Four to 8 weeks of parenteral treatment is usually adequate, depending on the susceptibility of the organism, response to therapy assessed clinically by reduction or elimination of the observed vegetations, and laboratory response. C-reactive protein level often normalizes 2 to 3 weeks before erythrocyte sedimentation rate, and blood cultures are usually sterile after 3 to 5 days of effective therapy. *Candida* spp. may persist for weeks, however, despite the use of active antifungal drugs. Dosage and efficacy should be monitored weekly with clinical and bacteriologic response with or without serum antibiotic and bactericidal levels.[291] Determination of serum bactericidal titers (Schlichter test) is of uncertain value and has never been validated in neonatal endocarditis.[291] Efficacy of treatment may also be monitored with serial echocardiograms taken until vegetations remain stable in size or disappear.[278,292,293]

Intravascular catheters must be removed whenever possible, and the tip of the removed catheter should be cultured. Extremely large or mobile vegetations occluding an outflow tract or posing a high risk of embolism may have to be removed surgically.[278,292] In infants with right-sided endocarditis, demonstration of decreased pulmonary blood flow through the use of ventilation-perfusion scan can be valuable in confirming the presence of emboli, particularly if there is clinical evidence of increasing respiratory effort and diminished peripheral oxygen saturation.

With the availability of echocardiography, improved clinical awareness, and early diagnosis, prognosis has improved. Although there were infrequent survivors before 1973, the first survivors with proven endocarditis were reported in 1983.[278,293] Approximately two thirds of subsequent cases have been cured. Death is usually the result of overwhelming sepsis, often in conjunction with cardiac failure. Early reconstructive surgery for infants who fail medical management may be helpful but has been reported in only a few cases.[294,295]

Inspection of the heart at autopsy has shown the mitral valve to be infected, alone or in combination with other valves, in about half of patients. The tricuspid valve was involved in 12 infants, the pulmonary valve in 7, the aortic valve in 6, infected mural thrombi in 12, and an unspecified site in 3. Microscopic examination of valve cusps has revealed the characteristic lesions of endocarditis, with multiple small, confluent, friable vegetations composed principally of bacteria and thrombi surrounded by inflammatory exudate.[35,279] On gross inspection, these vegetations are easily confused with noninflammatory lesions, such as those of nonbacterial thrombotic endocarditis, blood cysts, developmental valvular defects, or hemangiomas or other vascular anomalies. Cases described as fetal endocarditis in the literature are almost certainly examples of these types of lesions.[296,297]

Pericarditis

Purulent pericarditis is a very unusual complication of neonatal sepsis. Approximately 20 cases of proven infectious origin have been reported within the past 60 years. *S. aureus*[298] and *E. coli*[299] have been the etiologic agents reported most commonly, but cases caused by *Haemophilus influenzae*, *Salmonella* spp., *Klebsiella*, *P. aeruginosa*, *Candida* spp., and *Mycoplasma hominis* have also been described.

Virtually every infant with pericarditis has associated septic foci; pneumonia and multiple pulmonary abscesses are the most common sites. Involvement of pericardium may occur by direct extension from adjoining lung abscesses or by hematogenous spread of bacteria. The presence of infectious processes elsewhere is sufficiently frequent to warrant the suggestion that pericarditis should be suspected in all infants who develop clinical signs of "heart failure" or a sudden increase in the size of the cardiac silhouette during the course of a purulent infection, such as meningitis, pneumonia, or omphalitis.[300]

Neonates with bacterial pericarditis generally present with signs and symptoms suggesting sepsis and respiratory distress. Poor feeding, listlessness, emesis, or abdominal distention may be seen in the presence of tachypnea, tachycardia, and cyanosis of various degrees. More specific signs of cardiac involvement become apparent with the accumulation of increasing amounts of pericardial effusion. The clinical findings of cardiac tamponade are extremely subtle and difficult to differentiate from the findings of myocardial disease with right-sided heart failure. A rapid pulse, quiet precordium, muffled heart sounds, neck vein distention, and hepatomegaly are findings common to both entities. More specific signs of tamponade, such as narrow pulse pressure or respiratory variations in pulse volume of greater than 20 mm Hg (i.e., pulsus paradoxus), are technically difficult to obtain in neonates without an arterial catheter in place. A pericardial friction rub is absent in greater than 50% of older infants and children and in most neonates with purulent pericarditis.

Rapid enlargement of the cardiac silhouette, a globular heart shape with widening of the base on tilting, and diminished cardiac pulsation on fluoroscopic examination are of little value in differentiating pericardial effusion from cardiac dilatation.[301] The early ST segment elevation and subsequent T wave inversion seen on electrocardiogram reflect subepicardial damage or inflammation and are similar to changes seen with primary myocarditis. Diminution in the amplitude of the QRS complex by fluid surrounding the heart is not a constant finding. Confirmation of the presence of a pericardial effusion is usually obtained by two-dimensional echocardiography.[301] In some cases, CT or MRI can also be helpful in delineating the extent of a pericardial effusion[302]; on occasion, pericardial fluid is found incidental to the chest or abdominal scanning. Additional causes of neonatal pericardial effusion other than purulent disease include viral pericarditis, intrapericardial teratoma, maternal lupus, immune and nonimmune fetal hydrops, congenital diaphragmatic defects, chylopericardium, and central venous catheter perforation of the right atrium.

A definitive diagnosis of purulent pericarditis can be made only by obtaining fluid at surgery or through needle aspiration. Care and experience are necessary to facilitate aspiration while avoiding the risks of cardiac puncture or laceration.[300] Accurate monitoring of needle position can usually be obtained through CT guidance, with echocardiographic or fluoroscopic imaging, or by attaching the exploring electrode (V lead) of an electrocardiograph to the needle and by looking for injury current if contact is made with the epicardial surface of the heart.

When fluid is obtained, it should be sent for analysis to the laboratory in a laboratory-approved container appropriate for aerobic and anaerobic culture, mycobacteria, and fungi. In addition to cell count and protein and glucose levels, Gram and acid-fast stains should be performed with cultures for bacteria, viruses, mycobacteria, and fungi. Rapid identification of bacterial antigens by latex agglutination or by counterimmunoelectrophoresis of pericardial fluid, urine, or serum may also help to establish an etiologic diagnosis. Specialized testing for rare bacterial, viral, or fungal organisms by molecular methods may be available by request in specialized (research) or reference laboratories.

Purulent pericarditis is a medical and surgical emergency. Therapy must be directed toward relief of the cardiac tamponade through adequate pericardial drainage and toward resolution of the infection. Both modes of treatment are essential for successful therapy for bacterial pericarditis in the newborn; recovery cannot be expected from treatment with antibiotics alone. Although repeated needle aspirations or catheter drainage[303] may be sufficient, the frequent occurrence of loculations of pus, particularly with staphylococcal infection, suggests that open surgical pericardiostomy is the method of choice to achieve adequate drainage.

Initial therapy should be based on results of Gram stain or antigen detection tests of the pericardial fluid. If no organisms can be identified, treatment can be started with penicillinase-resistant penicillin and an aminoglycoside (or extended-spectrum cephalosporin) until definitive culture and susceptibility data are available. In nurseries where MRSA infection has been a problem, vancomycin should be substituted for penicillin. Despite aggressive management, the prognosis of neonatal purulent pericarditis remains very poor.

Mediastinitis

Purulent mediastinitis abscess in the neonate is a very rare condition that can be acquired through bloodborne dissemination of organisms, or by direct extension from a focus of infection in an adjacent retropharyngeal abscess, pleural or pulmonary abscess, vertebral osteomyelitis, or a complication of thoracic surgery.[304-307] *S. aureus* is the most frequently identified pathogen, but mediastinal infections with *S. pneumoniae, Clostridium* spp., and *E. coli* have also been reported.

Traumatic perforation of the posterior pharynx or esophagus, often the result of resuscitative efforts in infants involving endotracheal or gastric intubation, produces a potential site for entry of microorganisms.[308,309] Retropharyngeal abscess,[310] an infected pseudodiverticulum, or pyopneumothorax may occur as a consequence; purulent mediastinitis has been reported as a complication.[311] At least one case of mediastinitis has occurred as the result of overly vigorous passage of a nasogastric tube through an atretic esophageal pouch.[312] Low (intrathoracic) perforations are said to have a higher risk of mediastinitis and abscess formation than perforations in the cervical region.[308]

Early symptoms are nonspecific and are similar to symptoms of any septic process in a neonate. As purulent fluid accumulates in the mediastinum, it places increasing pressure on the esophagus, trachea, and tributaries of the superior vena cava and thoracic duct, bringing about rapid development of dysphagia, dyspnea, neck vein distention, and facial cyanosis or edema. To maintain a patent tracheal airway, an affected infant lies in an arched position with head extended in a manner very similar to that seen in neonates with congenital vascular ring. A halting, inspiratory, staccato type of breathing, probably because of pain, is also characteristic. Ultimately, the abscess may point on the anterior chest wall or in the suprasternal notch.

Usually, mediastinitis is first suspected when widening of the mediastinum is observed on a chest radiograph obtained for evaluation of respiratory distress. Forward displacement of the trachea and larynx may accompany these findings when retropharyngeal abscess is associated with mediastinitis. Infection after traumatic perforation of the esophagus or pharynx is often accompanied by pneumomediastinum with or without a pneumothorax.[308,312]

Contrast studies performed to define the cause of respiratory or feeding difficulties in infants with mediastinitis may result in flow of radiopaque fluid into an esophageal laceration, mimicking the findings of an atresia, duplication, or diverticulum of the esophagus.[308,309] In such cases, endoscopy often shows a mucosal tear, confirming the diagnosis.[309]

Treatment should be directed toward establishment of drainage and relief of pressure on vital structures through a mediastinotomy and placement of drainage tubes. A tracheostomy or endotracheal tube may be necessary for maintenance of an adequate airway. Initial empirical antimicrobial therapy with clindamycin (or metronidazole), ampicillin, and an aminoglycoside (or extended-spectrum cephalosporin) and a β-lactam plus β-lactamase inhibitor combination should be started after cultures of the blood and all other clinically indicated cultures have been obtained. More limited empirical antibiotic therapy can be provided with a β-lactam and β-lactamase inhibitor combination alone, such as piperacillin plus tazobactam, ampicillin plus sulbactam, ticarcillin plus clavulanate, or meropenem. Specific therapy can subsequently be determined by the results of bacteriologic studies of the cultures or purulent fluid obtained at surgery.

Esophagitis

The esophagus is infrequently a focus for infection of the fetus or newborn. Esophageal atresia is associated with congenital rubella (see Chapter 29). Severe esophagitis has also been reported in neonates with congenital cytomegalovirus infection.[313] The esophagus may be involved in infants with congenital Chagas disease, identified by signs of dysphagia, regurgitation, and megaesophagus.[314] Esophageal disease may follow mediastinitis in the neonate (discussed earlier). Only occasional cases of bacterial esophagitis in a neonate have been reported; a 940-g infant boy developed signs of sepsis on the fifth day of life and died 5 hours later.[315] Premortem blood cultures were positive for *Bacillus* spp. Examination at autopsy revealed histologic evidence of esophagitis with pseudomembranous necrosis of squamous epithelium and many gram-positive bacilli. No other focus of infection was evident.

Infections of Endocrine Organs

Endocrine glands other than the adrenal are rarely involved in fetal or neonatal infection. Nelson[316] reported neonatal suppurative thyroiditis in a term Laotian infant. The infant presented with a left anterior neck mass at 3 days of age. At surgery, a cystic mass within the left lobe of the thyroid was identified. Purulent material within the mass grew viridans streptococci and nonhemolytic streptococci.

Orchitis caused by *S. enteritidis* was described in a 10-week-old neonate.[317] The infant presented with symptoms of sepsis and diarrhea, subsequently developing unilateral scrotal swelling and erythema on the fifth day after onset of illness. Ultrasound examination of the testis showed a patchy increased echo intensity; the diagnosis was confirmed at exploratory surgery to rule out testicular torsion.

Infections of the Salivary Glands

Neonatal infections of salivary glands are uncommon; although rare, involvement of the parotid is the most frequent,[318,319] and submandibular gland infection is infrequent.[320] Most infections are caused by *S. aureus*, but *E. coli*, *P. aeruginosa*, and GBS have also been implicated in suppurative parotitis. Oral anaerobic bacteria, including *Bacteroides* spp. and *Peptostreptococcus* spp., may be found in mixed or isolated infections in more than half of cases.[318] Infections of the salivary glands occur more frequently in premature and male infants[319] and most commonly manifest during the second week of life. The oral cavity is the probable portal of entry for the infecting organism. Bloodborne bacteria may invade the salivary glands, however. Dehydration with resultant decreased salivary flow may be a predisposing cause in some infants.

The clinical manifestations of salivary gland infection include fever, anorexia, irritability, and failure to gain weight. There may be swelling, tenderness, or erythema over the involved gland. Purulent material may be expressed from the ductal opening with or without gentle pressure over the gland.

The diagnosis is made by culture or Gram stain of the pus exuding from the duct or by percutaneous aspiration of a fluctuant area. If microscopic examination of the Gram stain does not suggest a responsible pathogen, initial antibiotic therapy should be directed against *S. aureus*, *E. coli*, and *P. aeruginosa* (i.e., penicillinase-resistant penicillin or vancomycin plus an aminoglycoside or extended-spectrum cephalosporin with activity against *Pseudomonas* organisms). If there is a strong suspicion of involvement with anaerobic bacteria (i.e., negative aerobic cultures or failure to respond to therapy directed at aerobic pathogens), consideration should be given to adding or substituting antibiotics appropriate for anaerobic bacteria (e.g., clindamycin, metronidazole in combination with other antibiotics, or a β-lactam and β-lactamase antibiotic combination alone). The duration of therapy should extend throughout the period of inflammation and 3 to 5 days after signs of local inflammation have disappeared. Incision and drainage often may be required; surgical drainage should be considered if there is not a prompt response to therapy within 72 hours or if the gland becomes fluctuant. When considering incision and drainage, careful attention to preservation of the function of overlying motor branches of cranial nerve VII is important.

Infections of the Skin and Subcutaneous Tissue

Bacterial infections of the skin of the newborn may manifest as maculopapular rash, vesicles, pustules, bullae, abscesses, cellulitis, impetigo, erythema multiforme, and petechiae or purpura. In a review of 2836 neonatal infections in Finland, only 6 were characterized as cellulitis.[321] Most infections of skin, including bullous impetigo, chronic furunculosis, scalded skin syndrome, and breast abscesses, are caused by *S. aureus* and often MRSA (see Chapter 14). Cellulitis frequently accompanied by adenitis and bacteremia may be caused by GBS (see Chapter 12). Cutaneous infections caused by many other bacteria are discussed in this section; however, most microorganisms that cause disease in the neonate may produce cutaneous infections, and those infections are discussed in other chapters when relevant. For additional information on bacterial infections of the neonatal skin the reader is referred to a textbook, *Neonatal Dermatology* by Eichenfield and colleagues,[322] the chapter of Swartz and Weinberg,[323] and a review by Frieden.[324] Excellent color photographs are included in the *Color Atlas of Pediatric Dermatology* by Weinberg and coworkers.[325]

PATHOGENESIS

The skin of the newborn has unique characteristics, including absent microflora at birth; the presence of vernix caseosa; a less acid pH than that of older children; and often the presence of surgical wounds, including the severed umbilical cord, a circumcision site, and catheter wounds. Cutaneous bacterial infection may be a primary event or the result of systemic infection. Septicemic embolic infection may occur at widely separated sites, whereas local infections often occur at a site with an identifiable predisposing cause. Procedures resulting in breaks in the cutaneous continuity, such as forceps abrasions or wounds at fetal electrodes or at venipuncture sites, may be readily identified. The necrotic umbilical cord is a site for proliferation of microorganisms that may invade local tissues.

Infection of the circumcision site remains a concern because it is the most common surgical procedure in infants in the United States. Speert[326] found that many circumcision practitioners in the 19th century frequently disregarded cleanliness. Operators were frequently uneducated, were dirty, and often spat on their instruments. Erysipelas, tetanus, and diphtheria have long been recognized as complications of unsterile surgical technique performed on newborns. In a now obsolete and prohibited part of the Orthodox Jewish circumcision ritual, the operator applied his lips to the fresh circumcision wound and sucked a few drops of blood. Such practices were responsible for transmission of syphilis and tuberculosis in neonates in the past. In one report,[327] a 4-month-old infant presented with a penile ulcer, bilateral inguinal adenopathy, and a draining inguinal sinus caused by *Mycobacterium tuberculosis* after the "barber" spat on his razor before circumcision. Subsequent case reports of severe infection after circumcision include bacteremia related to GBS,[328] staphylococcal scalded skin syndrome,[329] necrotizing fasciitis,[330] and bullous impetigo.[331] Circumcision infection is uncommon, but local spread of infection may be devastating and lead to systemic infection.

Intrapartum fetal monitoring with scalp electrodes and intrauterine pressure catheters and measurements of fetal blood gases through scalp punctures have been associated with infections related to herpesvirus (see Chapter 27), *Mycoplasma* (see Chapter 20), and various aerobic and anaerobic bacteria. Bacterial infections have included pustules, abscesses, and fasciitis.[331-334] Infection rates are relatively low (0.1%-4.5%)[332,333]; however, severe infections, including fasciitis, meningitis, and osteomyelitis, have occurred as severe complications.[335,336] A review[334] of causative organisms in fetal scalp monitor infections found that 61% of infections were polymicrobial, involving anaerobic bacteria, aerobic gram-positive cocci, and gram-negative bacilli.

A multitude of specific virulence factors may be important determinants of disease. Some phage types of *S. aureus* are responsible for local tissue damage and systemic disease; other staphylococci elaborate toxins that result in bullae and other cutaneous pathology. Groups A and B streptococci are responsible for cellulitis and impetigo in infants. *P. aeruginosa* may invade and proliferate in small blood vessels, causing local necrosis and eschar formation (i.e., ecthyma gangrenosum). Infections with *Clostridium* spp. cause disease in devitalized tissues such as the umbilical stump.[337]

MICROBIOLOGY

The skin of the infant is colonized initially by microorganisms present in the maternal birth canal. The skin of infants delivered by cesarean section is usually sterile at birth. After birth, microorganisms may be transferred to the skin during handling by the parents and nursery personnel. The prevalent organisms on the skin during the first few days of life include coagulase-negative staphylococci, diphtheroids, and gram-negative enteric bacilli (including *E. coli*).[338] The umbilicus, genitalia, and adjacent skin areas (groin and abdomen) are colonized first; organisms then spread to the nose, throat, conjunctivae, and other body sites. Organisms present in the nursery environment colonize neonatal skin after a few days in the nursery. *S. aureus*, GBS, and various species of gram-negative bacilli may be present, but the microbiologic flora differs among nurseries and from time to time in the same nursery. Use of soaps and antiseptic solutions modifies the flora on the skin of the newborn. Hexachlorophene decreases colonization with staphylococci and diphtheroids, but gram-negative organisms are unaffected or may increase after use of this agent.[339]

In a 4-year survey (2001-2005) of staphylococcal infections in one center, 89 neonates were infected with staphylococci, and 61 (68.5%) infections were caused by MRSA; 30% of MRSA and methicillin-susceptible *S. aureus* infections manifested with pustular lesions, most often in the groin.[340] Cellulitis or abscess developed with 20% of MRSA and 32% of methicillin-susceptible *S. aureus* lesions, and 13% of lesions developed into an invasive infection (bacteremia, urinary tract infection). Also, infants with MRSA were more likely to have a mother with a history of skin infection (21% vs. 4%). Other investigators have attempted to eradicate high colonization and disease rates in neonatal nurseries with the use of bacteriostatic agents applied to the umbilical cord. In one study with a high rate of MRSA impetigo, 0.3% triclosan (Bacti-Stat) was not effective in slowing the progress of the epidemic.[341] In this epidemic, 22 infants were affected, and all but 2 of the affected infants were circumcised, suggesting that the colonization of the surgical site facilitated invasion of the skin.

EPIDEMIOLOGY

Infant boys are more susceptible to skin infections caused by *S. aureus* than girls. Thompson and coworkers[342] showed that boys were colonized more frequently in every body site cultured, including the nose, groin, rectum, and umbilicus. Their review of studies indicated that in England, the United States, and Australia, approximately 50% more boys had skin lesions than girls. Although the incidence of breast abscesses is equal in boys and girls during the first 2 weeks of life, such abscesses are more frequent thereafter in girls.[343] Hormone production in the female infant after the second week might account for the increase in abscesses of the breast.

Infections caused by MRSA that involve the skin of children and neonates have markedly increased. The *mecA* gene responsible for resistance to oxacillin and nafcillin is often closely linked to a gene responsible for skin invasion. Before 1997, epidemic MRSA infections occurred in neonatal units involving infections of the respiratory tract, nasopharynx, gastrointestinal tract, eye, blood, wounds, or umbilicus.[344] These infections were usually restricted to single nurseries and involved a single genetic variant of MRSA. Since 1990, MRSA infections acquired in the community have been reported with increased frequency,[345] including in infants 2 weeks of age. Of these infections, 91% have involved the skin and soft tissues.

Seasonal variation in the frequency of neonatal skin infections has been reported by Evans and coworkers,[346] who conducted a series of studies at Harlem Hospital in New York. The prevalence of *S. aureus*, *E. coli*, and streptococci in the nares and umbilicus of infants was lowest in the autumn and usually highest in the summer or spring. No seasonal variation was observed for *S. epidermidis* or *Enterobacter* spp. The investigators concluded that seasonal differences must be considered in investigations of bacterial colonization of the newborn skin and that high humidity may favor gram-negative colonization.

The time of onset of skin lesions associated with sepsis may be early (during the first week of life) or late (several weeks or months after birth). Disease acquired in the nursery usually becomes apparent after 5 days of age. Many skin lesions do not appear until after the infant has left the nursery; the observed incidence of skin disease caused by bacteria should include surveillance of infants in the home during the first month of life. Physicians responsible for neonatal care must be alert to the unusual occurrence of skin lesions. The introduction of a new and virulent bacterium, an alteration in technique, or the use of contaminated materials must be considered as possible causes of an increased incidence of such infections.

CLINICAL MANIFESTATIONS

Infants who have skin infections that remain localized that are not invasive or part of a systemic infection have few general signs of disease, such as fever, alteration in feeding habits, vomiting, or diarrhea. These signs may be present when significant tissue invasion occurs, as in abscesses or extensive cellulitis. Cutaneous manifestations that result from infectious diseases are listed in Table 10-4.

Among the common and least specific lesions are maculopapular rashes; these rashes may be caused by viruses (measles, rubella, or enteroviruses), fungi (*Candida* spp.), or bacteria (streptococci or staphylococci), or they may be unassociated with any infectious process. Erythema multiforme lesions have been observed in cases of sepsis related to *S. aureus*[347] and *P. aeruginosa*.[348] Cellulitis, erysipelas, and impetigo are usually associated with streptococcal infection (group A or B),[349] although impetigo caused by *S. aureus* or *E. coli* has also been reported in infants. Vesicles, commonly associated with infections by herpesviruses, also are seen occasionally during early stages of skin lesions caused by *S. aureus*, *H. influenzae*[350] and *P. aeruginosa*. GBS,[351] *S. aureus*, *P. aeruginosa*, herpes simplex virus, and *T. pallidum* may also be responsible for bullous lesions. Pustules

Table 10-4 Manifestations and Etiologies of Infections of the Skin in Newborns

Clinical Manifestation	ETIOLOGIC AGENT	
	Bacterial	**Nonbacterial**
Maculopapular rash	*Treponema pallidum**† *Listeria monocytogenes* *Streptococcus** *Staphylococcus*	Measles virus* Rubella virus* Enteroviruses* Molluscum contagiosum *Candida* spp.*
Cellulitis (erysipelas)	β-Hemolytic streptococci *Achromobacter* spp.	
Impetigo	β-Hemolytic streptococci *Staphylococcus aureus** *Escherichia coli*	
Erythema multiforme	β-Hemolytic streptococci *S. aureus** *Pseudomonas aeruginosa*	
Vesicular or bullous lesions	*S. aureus** *P. aeruginosa* *T. pallidum* *L. monocytogenes*	Herpes simplex virus*† Cytomegalovirus* Varicella virus*† Coxsackieviruses* *Candida* spp.* *Aspergillus* spp.* *Drosophila* larvae *Sarcoptes scabiei*
Pustular rashes	*S. aureus** *L. monocytogenes** *Haemophilus influenzae*	
Ecthyma gangrenosum	*P. aeruginosa*	
Abscesses and wound infections	*S. aureus** *Mycoplasma hominis** *Staphylococcus epidermidis** β-Hemolytic streptococci *E. coli* *Klebsiella* spp. *Proteus mirabilis* *P. aeruginosa* *Salmonella* spp. *Serratia marcescens* *H. influenzae* *Haemophilus parainfluenzae* *Neisseria gonorrhoeae* *Gardnerella vaginalis* *Bacteroides* spp.	*Candida* spp.*
Petechiae, purpura, and ecchymoses	Gram positive and gram-negative bacteria with sepsis *L. monocytogenes* *Streptococcus pneumoniae* *T. pallidum**†	Rubella virus*† Cytomegalovirus*† Herpes simplex virus*† Coxsackievirus B*† *Toxoplasma gondii**†

*See appropriate chapter for further discussion.
†Including infections acquired in utero.

commonly occur in staphylococcal diseases but also occur in infections caused by *L. monocytogenes* and, rarely, in skin infections with *H. influenzae*.

Ecthyma gangrenosum is typically a local manifestation of infection with *P. aeruginosa*.[352-354] Lesions begin as a vesicular eruption on a wide erythematous base. Vesicles rupture and form an indurated black eschar, followed by larger, sharply demarcated, painless necrotic areas, resulting from a small vessel vasculitis with necrosis of the adjacent tissue. The organisms are present in purulent material underlying the necrotic membrane. These lesions are particularly more common adjacent to nose, lip, ear, mouth, and perineum, resulting in avascular necrosis and loss of tissue. *P. aeruginosa* may be grown in pure culture from blood and lesions. Ecthyma is relatively specific for *Pseudomonas* infections, but similar or identical lesions have rarely been described in infections caused by *S. aureus*, *Aeromonas hydrophila*, *E. coli*, *Aspergillus* spp., or *Mucor* spp.[355]

Many infants with *Candida* infections have cutaneous manifestations. Baley and Silverman[356] described 18 infants with systemic candidiasis; 8 had a burnlike truncal erythema, and 9 other infants had typical candidal diaper rashes or maculopapular rashes of the axillae or neck. A case of ecthyma gangrenosum caused by *Candida* infection in a 12-day-old neonate was reported.[357]

Abscesses of the skin and subcutaneous tissue are usually caused by *S. aureus* and, less frequently, by group A streptococci, GBS, or gram-negative enteric bacilli. Community-acquired MRSA organisms are even more likely to produce skin infections with abscess formation. Organisms that colonize the skin over an area that has been disrupted by an abrasion or other wound may invade the subcutaneous tissue and produce an abscess. *Haemophilus* spp., *Gardnerella vaginalis*, *Bacteroides* spp., molluscum contagiosum, *Drosophila* myiasis, scabies, and *Candida* are examples of diverse causes of cutaneous abscesses; virtually any bacterial, fungal, or parasitic agent that is normally or transiently on skin may become a pathogen. *E. coli*, *Klebsiella* spp., *P. aeruginosa*, *N. gonorrhoeae*, and *B. fragilis* have caused wound infections in infants whose scalps were lacerated by forceps, fetal electrodes, or instruments used for obtaining blood from the scalp in utero.

A cephalhematoma may become infected during sepsis or from manipulation of the cephalhematoma,[358,359] such as through diagnostic or therapeutic needle puncture or by puncture from a fetal monitor. The infection may be associated with meningitis[360] or with osteomyelitis of the underlying skull.[361]

S. aureus is the most frequent etiologic agent in breast abscess, but gram-negative enteric bacilli are occasionally identified. Of 36 cases with mastitis seen in Dallas, Texas, during a 16-year period, 32 cases were caused by *S. aureus*, 1 was caused by *E. coli*, and 2 were caused by *Salmonella* spp.; both *E. coli* and *S. aureus* were isolated from one abscess.[343] At Children's Hospital in Boston from 1947 to 1983, 41 cases of mastitis in neonates were managed.[362] *S. aureus* was responsible for 29 of 34 cases with an identifiable bacterial pathogen. All cases occurred in term infants during weeks 1 to 5 of life. Bilaterality and extramammary foci were rare. One third of infants were febrile, and most had elevated white blood cell counts (>15,000 cells/mm^3). Brook[363] found that 5 of 14 breast abscesses contained anaerobic bacteria (i.e., *Bacteroides* spp. and *Peptostreptococcus*), but *S. aureus*, GBS, or enteric bacteria predominated; anaerobic bacteria occurred alone in only 2 of 14 cases.

Omphalitis is defined by the presence of erythema or serous or purulent discharge from the umbilical stump or periumbilical tissues. A review by Cushing[364] provided a useful discussion of the pathophysiology, microbiology, diagnosis, and management of omphalitis. The incidence of infection is more frequent in infants with low birth weight and infants with complications of delivery. A survey of infants born at the Royal Women's Hospital in Brisbane, Australia,[365] identified an incidence of approximately 2% among term infants. The mean age of infants at presentation of omphalitis was 3.2 days. Perhaps because hexachlorophene bathing was used, gram-negative bacilli were more frequently associated with infection than gram-positive cocci. Microbiologic results are difficult to interpret, however, because swabs of the site of infection do not exclude surface contaminants, unless cultures are taken with extreme care and precision.

A series from the United States[366] found that periumbilical fasciitis was more frequent in boys but did not find that umbilical catheterization, low birth weight, or septic delivery was associated with a high risk; overall, the incidence of omphalitis was equal in boys and girls. In this series, omphalitis manifested as discharge, cellulitis, or fasciitis; gram-positive organisms were found in 94% of cultures, and gram-negative bacteria were found in 64%. *S. aureus* was the most frequent isolate, with *E. coli* and *Klebsiella* spp. the next most common. Group A streptococci have been responsible for nursery outbreaks that may include an indolent form of omphalitis characterized by erythema and oozing of the umbilical stump for days to weeks, accompanied by pustular lesions of the abdominal wall in some cases.[367] Neonatal tetanus usually occurs as a result of contamination of the umbilical wound by *Clostridium tetani* at delivery.

Acute necrotizing fasciitis is a bacterial infection of subcutaneous tissue and fascial sheath.[368-370] Infection can arise in an operative wound or in a focal infection, such as a breast abscess, after a procedure such as circumcision or insertion of a fetal monitor, or there may be no apparent predisposing cause. The trunk and extremities are the areas most commonly involved; inflammation spreads rapidly along fascial planes, producing thrombosis and extensive necrosis, with infarcts developing in overlying skin. Vesicles and bullae appear, and the skin may become blue-gray or black. Myositis and bacteremia may accompany fasciitis. Staphylococci, GBS,[371] *E. coli, P. aeruginosa,* anaerobic bacteria,[372] and mixed infections of gram-positive and gram-negative bacteria have been associated with this disease. The bacteria are present in skin lesions, deep fascia, and, in some cases, blood. The mortality remains high despite the use of fasciotomy, wide débridement, and antibiotics.

Perirectal abscesses may occur in newborns. In contrast to older children, most newborns with perirectal abscess do not have underlying immunodeficiency, although infants with acquired or congenital immunodeficiency often present with this condition. The most common causes of perirectal abscess are *S. aureus, E. coli,* or other enteric bacilli[373,374]; however, anaerobic bacteria can also be involved. *S. aureus* and enteric bacilli may be more common in infants and newborns.[373] Recent rectal surgery for conditions such as Hirschsprung disease or imperforate anus (myotomy or rectal dilatation) may be predisposing causes in infants; as in older children, neutropenia may be associated with an increased risk for perirectal abscess.

Otitis externa is uncommon in newborns. Victorin[375] described an outbreak of neonatal infections in which *P. aeruginosa* was cultured from seven infants with suppuration of the auditory canal. The author suggested that this outbreak was caused by contaminated bath water used in the nursery.

DIAGNOSIS

The appearance of a skin lesion alone may be sufficiently typical to suspect certain etiologic agents (e.g., ecthyma gangrenosum), but more often, the appearance is nonspecific. A microbiologic diagnosis should be sought to provide specific therapy. The lesion and the surrounding tissue should be cleaned with 70% ethanol to prevent contamination from organisms that colonize the surface. If crusts are present, they should be lifted with a sterile swab to provide drainage, and cultures should be obtained from the base of the lesion.

Vesicles and pustules can be aspirated with a needle (20 gauge–25 gauge) attached to a syringe, or they can be opened and exudate can be collected on a sterile swab. In general, swabs are not preferred for specimen collection because swab materials bind or inactivate bacterial organisms. Aspiration of abscesses is important; more than one aspiration may be required because the suppurative focus may not be easily distinguished from the surrounding inflammatory tissue. Aspiration of the leading edge or point of maximal inflammation of an area of cellulitis may be valuable and should be performed if no other suppurative or purulent sites are available for culture. A small needle (25 gauge or 26 gauge) should be attached to a tuberculin or other small-volume syringe filled with 0.25 to 0.50 mL of sterile nonbacteriostatic saline; the needle should be inserted into the area of soft tissue to be sampled, with continuous, gentle aspiration applied to the syringe. If no fluid is returned to the syringe, a small amount of fluid should be injected and immediately aspirated back into the syringe. Collected material may be sent to the laboratory in the syringe for Gram stain and culture, or, alternatively, the contents may be washed into a tube of bacteriologic broth medium for transport and subsequent culture.

If swabs are used, care must be taken that the material does not dry before it is plated on bacteriologic media. Swabs preferentially should be directly inoculated or rinsed in bacteriologic media and immediately transported to the microbiology laboratory. Alternatively, they may be refrigerated or placed in appropriate transport media if more than a few hours will elapse before inoculation of media in the laboratory. Whenever sufficient material is available, on swabs or in liquid, several slides should be prepared for Gram staining.

It is often difficult to distinguish petechiae from vascular dilatation. Pressure with a glass slide on the border of the lesion is a simple and reliable method for detecting extravasation of red blood cells. If the lesion disappears on pressure, it is probably caused by dilation of small vessels, whereas persistence of the lesion after application of pressure indicates extravasation of red blood cells. Bacteria may be present in petechial lesions that occur in infants with bacterial sepsis. Blood obtained by aspiration or gentle scraping with a scalpel at the center of the petechiae may reveal the causative organism on Gram stain or culture.

DIFFERENTIAL DIAGNOSIS

Sclerema neonatorum, milia, and erythema toxicum are noninfectious lesions that are often confused with infections of the skin.[376] Bullous and purpuric lesions may be caused by noninfectious disorders, including mast cell diseases (e.g., urticaria pigmentosa), histiocytosis X, acrodermatitis enteropathica, dermatitis herpetiformis, epidermolysis bullosa, congenital porphyria, and pemphigus vulgaris. A syndrome of generalized erythroderma, failure to thrive, and diarrhea has been associated with various forms of immunodeficiency.[377]

Sclerema neonatorum is a diffuse, spreading, waxy hardness of the skin and subcutaneous tissue that occurs during the first weeks of life.[378] The subcutaneous tissue seems to be bound to underlying muscle and bone. This condition is usually seen on the thighs, buttocks, and trunk. Although associated with sepsis in some infants, sclerema also affects infants with dehydration, acidosis, and shock. Most evidence supports the hypothesis that sclerema is a manifestation of shock and insufficiency of the peripheral circulation. Skin biopsy histology shows trabecular thickening between adipocytes and a sparse inflammatory infiltrate of lymphocytes, histiocytes, and multinucleate giant cells. When it occurs in infants with generalized infection, sclerema is associated with a very poor prognosis; exchange transfusion may be one intervention associated with improved survival.

Milia are yellow or pearly white papules that are 1 mm in diameter and usually found on the face (especially the nose), scalp, upper aspect of trunk, and upper extremities, without significant racial or sex difference.[379,380] The lesion is a small cyst formed from retention of sebum in sebaceous glands, and because the cyst is capped by a shiny surface of epidermis, it may be confused with a small pustule. Congenital milia occur in 40% to 50% of newborns, present with a few or numerous lesions, and tend to resolve spontaneously within weeks to several months.[379,380] Milia may be less common and of delayed onset in premature newborns. These cysts may be distinguished from staphylococcal pustules by aspiration and Gram stain of the material.

Erythema toxicum consists of several types of lesions, including 1- to 3-mm, yellow-white papules or pustules on an erythematous base, erythematous macules, or diffuse erythema.[381,382] These lesions are usually present on the trunk but may involve the head and neck and extremities as well. Most lesions appear within the first hours of life and are uncommon after 2 days of age. Erythema toxicum is uncommon in low-birth-weight or premature infants. Affected infants have no signs of systemic illness or local irritation. A smear of the contents of pustules reveals the presence of eosinophils and an absence of bacteria. Other noninfectious pustular lesions of newborns include neonatal pustular melanosis, which is marked by a mixed infiltrate that has a predominance of neutrophils,[383] and infantile acropustulosis, which is characterized by an eosinophilic infiltration of the skin.[384]

Bullae may occur on the skin of the wrist or forearm and usually are caused by trauma.[385] Sucking of the extremity by the infant is believed to cause the bullae, which contain sterile serous fluid. Purpura may be caused by noninfectious conditions, including trauma; erythroblastosis fetalis; or, less frequently, coagulation disorders, maternal drug ingestion, congenital leukemia, and congenital Letterer-Siwe disease.

Diaper rash is primarily a contact dermatitis associated with soilage of the skin by urine and stool and is the most common cutaneous diagnosis in infants, although the incidence is decreasing in the era of disposable diapers.[386,387] The rash may occur as a mild erythema or scaling, a sharply demarcated and confluent erythema, or discrete shallow ulcerations. A beefy red, confluent rash with raised margins, satellite (e.g., folliculitis) oval lesions, or discrete vesicular-pustular lesions indicates secondary invasion by *C. albicans*; risk factors include antibiotic use and diarrhea. Streptococcal and staphylococcal disease accounts for the majority of bacterial causes of diaper dermatitis. Because of its occluded, warm, and moist environment, the diaper area is a common site for the scabies mite in populations at risk. Systemic infectious illnesses, such as herpes simplex or syphilis, that manifest as disseminated neonatal rashes may be characterized early by typical lesions in the diaper area. Persistent diaper rash in the face of standard interventions should raise a concern of infantile psoriasis.

TREATMENT

The treatment of localized skin lesions consists of the use of local antiseptic materials, systemic antimicrobial agents, and appropriate incision and drainage or débridement. Hexachlorophene (3% detergent emulsion) and chlorhexidine (4% solution) are valuable in cleaning small, abraded areas and discrete pustular lesions. Because of concern over its neurotoxicity and cutaneous absorption, hexachlorophene should not be used on large open areas of skin. Topical bacitracin or polysporin are additional options.

Systemic antibiotics should be considered for therapy whenever there is significant soft tissue infection with abscess or cellulitis. The specific antibiotic choice should be made on the basis of the microbiology of the lesion; streptococci may be treated effectively with penicillin G, ampicillin, or extended-spectrum cephalosporins (i.e., cefotaxime or ceftriaxone), whereas staphylococci generally must be treated with penicillinase-resistant penicillins or vancomycin. Infections caused by gram-negative enteric bacilli may be treated with aminoglycosides or extended-spectrum cephalosporins, based on the results of susceptibility testing. Infections caused by *Pseudomonas* organisms can be effectively treated with aminoglycosides or ceftazidime.

Local heat and moist dressings over areas of abscess formation may facilitate localization or spontaneous drainage. Indications for incision and drainage of abscesses in infants are the same as for the indications in older children and adults.

PREVENTION

Prevention of local skin infections is best provided by appropriate routine hygiene, maintenance of the integrity of skin (i.e., avoidance of drying, trauma, or chemical contact), frequent diaper changes, and hygienic care of the umbilicus or other wounds or noninfectious skin inflammation. The following measures of skin care are recommended by the Committee of the Fetus and Newborn of the American Academy of Pediatrics[388] to prevent infection:

1. The first bath should be postponed until the infant is thermally stable.
2. Nonmedicated soap and water should be used; sterile sponges (not gauze) soaked in warm water may be used.
3. The buttocks and perianal should be cleaned with fresh water and cotton or with mild soap and water at diaper changes.

4. Ideally, agents used on the newborn skin should be dispensed in single-use containers.
5. No single method of cord care has proved to be superior, and none is endorsed.

Cord care may include application of alcohol, triple dye (i.e., brilliant green, proflavine hemisulfate, and crystal violet), or antimicrobial agents such as bacitracin. Alcohol hastens drying of the cord but is probably not effective in preventing cord colonization and omphalitis. A randomized study of triple dye, povidone-iodine, silver sulfadiazine, and bacitracin ointment showed comparability in antimicrobial control.[389] In a recent systematic review,[390] evidence supports topical application of chlorhexidine to reduce neonatal mortality and omphalitis in community and primary care settings in developing countries; although cord separation time may be increased, there is no evidence that it increases risk of subsequent morbidity or infection.

During nursery outbreaks of staphylococcal disease, daily hexachlorophene bathing of the diaper area[391] and umbilical cord care with 4% chlorhexidine solution[392] have shown efficacy for preventing further transmission.

Conjunctivitis and Other Eye Infections

Conjunctivitis in the newborn usually results from one of four causes: infection with *N. gonorrhoeae*, infection with *S. aureus*, inclusion conjunctivitis caused by *Chlamydia trachomatis*, or chemical conjunctivitis caused by silver nitrate solution.[393,394] Less commonly, other microorganisms have been implicated as a cause of conjunctivitis, including group A streptococci, GBS, *S. pneumoniae*, *H. influenzae*, *P. aeruginosa*, *Moraxella (Neisseria) catarrhalis*, *Neisseria meningitidis*, *Neisseria cinerea*, *Corynebacterium diphtheriae*, *Pasteurella multocida*, *Clostridium* spp., herpes simplex virus, echoviruses, *M. hominis*, and *Candida* spp. Gonococcal and chlamydial conjunctivitis are reviewed in Chapters 15 and 19, respectively.

An epidemic of erythromycin-resistant *S. aureus* conjunctivitis affected 25 of 215 newborns during a 10-month period; control of the epidemic was achieved by identification of staff carriers and substitution of silver nitrate prophylaxis for erythromycin.[395] Cultures of the conjunctivae of neonates with purulent conjunctivitis and from the comparable eyes of a similar number of infants chosen as control subjects revealed significant differences, suggesting causality for viridans streptococci, *S. aureus*, *E. coli*, and *Haemophilus* spp.[396,397] MRSA infections may have an increased propensity to infect the eye. Conjunctivitis caused by MRSA was reported as the first case in an epidemic that eventually involved 14 neonates in a NICU, including multiple invasive infections and two deaths.[398] MRSA has also caused dacrocystitis[399] and keratitis[400] in neonates.

Infections related to *P. aeruginosa* warrant special attention. Although uncommon, pseudomonal conjunctivitis may be a devastating disease if not recognized and treated appropriately.[401] The infection is usually acquired in the nursery, and the first signs of conjunctivitis appear between the 5th and 18th days of life. At first, the clinical manifestations are localized to the eye and include edema and erythema of the lid and purulent discharge. In some children, the conjunctivitis progresses rapidly, with denuding of the corneal epithelium and infiltration with neutrophils. With extension of the corneal infiltration, perforation of the cornea may occur. The anterior chamber may fill with fibrinous exudate, and the iris can adhere to the cornea. Subsequent invasion of the cornea by small blood vessels (pannus) is characteristic of pseudomonal conjunctivitis. The late ophthalmic complications may be followed by bacteremia and septic foci in other organs.[402]

A review by Lohrer and Belohradsky[403] of 16 cases of serious invasive eye infections in neonates included 13 caused by *P. aeruginosa*, whereas the others were cases of endophthalmitis caused by GBS and *S. pneumoniae*. Other opportunistic gram-negative pathogens associated with outbreaks of infections in nurseries may also include conjunctivitis as a part of the infection syndrome. Multiply antibiotic-resistant *S. marcescens* was responsible for 15 cases of pneumonia, sepsis, and meningitis and for 20 cases of conjunctivitis, cystitis, and wound infection over a 9-month period in a NICU.[404]

Dacryocystitis may complicate a congenital lacrimal sac distention (i.e., dacryocystocele) which may appear as early as the first week of life with edema and erythema of the lower lid. Purulent material emerged from the puncta after moderate pressure over the lacrimal sac; *S. marcescens* was grown from the material.

The physician responsible for management of a child with purulent conjunctivitis must consider the major causes of the disease and must be alert to rare pathogens. In hospitals that practice Credé method (i.e., silver nitrate application), purulent conjunctivitis during the first 48 hours of life is almost always caused by chemical toxicity.[405] After the first 2 days, the pus of an exudative conjunctivitis must be carefully examined by Gram stain for the presence of gram-negative intracellular diplococci, gram-positive cocci in clusters, and gram-negative bacilli. Appropriate cultures should be used for isolation of the organisms concerned. If smears are inconclusive and no pathogens are isolated on appropriate media, with persistent conjunctivitis, a diagnosis of inclusion or chlamydial infection is likely.[405,406]

The treatment approaches to staphylococcal and gonococcal conjunctivitis are discussed in Chapters 14 and 15. Chlamydial conjunctivitis is reviewed in Chapter 19. If infection with *Pseudomonas* spp. is suspected, treatment should be started at once with an effective parenteral antibiotic, such as an aminoglycoside (e.g., tobramycin, amikacin, or gentamicin) with or without an antipseudomonal penicillin or ceftazidime (see Chapter 37) and with a locally applied ophthalmic ointment. The use of subconjunctival gentamicin or other antipseudomonal aminoglycoside is of uncertain value; however, if the cornea seems to be extensively involved, there is a risk of rapid development of endophthalmitis, and the subconjunctival injection of antibiotics should be considered in consultation with an ophthalmologist. If the diagnosis is confirmed, this regimen is continued until the local signs of *Pseudomonas* infection resolve.

Recommendations for ocular chemoprophylaxis are discussed in Chapters 15 and 19. Additional information is available in the 2012 edition of the *Red book: report of the Committee on Infectious Diseases* published by the American Academy of Pediatrics.[407]

References

1. Murphy FM, Baker CJ: Solitary hepatic abscess: a delayed complication of neonatal bacteremia, *Pediatr Infect Dis J* 7:414-416, 1988.
2. Guillois B, Guillemin MG, Thoma M, et al: Neonatal pleuropulmonary staphylococcal infection with multiple abscesses of the liver, *Ann Pediatr (Paris)* 36:681-684, 1989.
3. Dehner LP, Kissane JM: Pyogenic hepatic abscesses in infancy and childhood, *J Pediatr* 74:763-773, 1969.
4. Moss TJ, Pysher TJ: Hepatic abscess in neonates, *Am J Dis Child* 135:726-728, 1981.
5. Chusid MJ: Pyogenic hepatic abscess in infancy and childhood, *Pediatrics* 62:554-559, 1978.
6. Dineen P: Personal communication, New York, 1978, Cornell University College of Medicine.
7. Simeunovic E, Arnold M, Sidler D, et al: Liver abscess in neonates, *Pediatr Surg Int* 25:153-156, 2009.
8. Anagnostakis D, Kamba A, Petrochilou V, et al: Risk of infection associated with umbilical vein catheterization. A prospective study in 75 newborn infants, *J Pediatr* 86:759-765, 1975.
9. Smith RT, Platou ES, Good RA: Septicemia of the newborn; current status of the problem, *Pediatrics* 17:549-575, 1956.
10. Madsen CM, Secouris N: Solitary liver abscess in a newborn, *Surgery* 47:1005-1009, 1960.
11. Sabbaj J, Sutter VL, Finegold SM: Anaerobic pyogenic liver abscess, *Ann Intern Med* 77:627-638, 1972.
12. Potter E: *Pathology of the fetus and infant*, ed 3, Chicago, 1975, Year Book Medical Publishers.
13. Meyer WW, Lind J: Postnatal changes in the portal circulation, *Arch Dis Child* 41:606-612, 1966.
14. Hageman J, Shulman S, Schreiber M, et al: Congenital tuberculosis: critical reappraisal of clinical findings and diagnostic procedures, *Pediatrics* 66:980-984, 1980.
15. Hughesdon MR: Congenital tuberculosis, *Arch Dis Child* 21: 121-138, 1946.
16. Cantwell MF, Shehab ZM, Costello AM, et al: Brief report: congenital tuberculosis, *N Engl J Med* 330:1051-1054, 1994.
17. Abughali N, Van der Kuyp F, Annable W, et al: Congenital tuberculosis, *Pediatr Infect Dis J* 13:738-741, 1994.
18. Oppenheimer EH, Hardy JB: Congenital syphilis in the newborn infant: clinical and pathological observations in recent cases, *Johns Hopkins Med J* 129:63-82, 1971.
19. Venter A, Pettifor JM, Duursma J, et al: Liver function in early congenital syphilis: does penicillin cause a deterioration? *J Pediatr Gastroenterol Nutr* 12:310-314, 1991.
20. Lindsay S, Luke IW: Fatal leptospirosis (Weil's disease) in a newborn infant; case of intrauterine fetal infection with report of an autopsy, *J Pediatr* 34:90-94, 1949.
21. Chung HL, Tsao WC, Mo PS, et al: Transplacental or congenital infection of leptospirosis. Clinical and experimental observations, *Chin Med J (Engl)* 82:777-782, 1963.
22. Fuchs PC, Oyama AA: Neonatal relapsing fever due to transplacental transmission of *Borrelia*, *JAMA* 208:690-692, 1969.
23. Yagupsky P, Moses S: Neonatal *Borrelia* species infection (relapsing fever), *Am J Dis Child* 139:74-76, 1985.
24. Cascio A, Pantaleo D, Corona G, et al: Neonatal liver abscesses associated with candidemia: three cases and review of literature, *J Matern Fetal Neonatal Med* 27:743-749, 2014.
25. Pyrtek LJ, Bartus SA: Hepatic pyemia, *N Engl J Med* 272:551-554, 1965.
26. Sharma K, Kumar R: Solitary abscess of the liver in a newborn infant, *Surgery* 61:812-813, 1967.
27. Lipinski JK, Vega JM, Cywes S, et al: Falciform ligament abscess in the infant, *J Pediatr Surg* 20:556-558, 1985.
28. Brans YW, Ceballos R, Cassady G: Umbilical catheters and hepatic abscesses, *Pediatrics* 53:264-266, 1974.
29. Cohen HJ, Dresner S: Liver abscess following exchange transfusion for erythroblastosis fetalis, *Q Rev Pediatr* 16:148-149, 1961.
30. Elliott RI: The ductus venosus in neonatal infection, *Proc R Soc Med* 62:321-323, 1969.
31. Williams JW, Rittenberry A, Dillard R, et al: Liver abscess in newborn. Complication of umbilical vein catheterization, *Am J Dis Child* 125:111-113, 1973.
32. Santerne B, Morville P, Touche D, et al: Diagnosis and treatment of multifocal neonatal hepatic abscesses using echography, *Presse Med* 16:12-14, 1987.
33. Sarrut S, Alain J, Alison F: The early complications of umbilical vein perfusion in the premature infant, *Arch Fr Pediatr* 26:651-667, 1969.
34. Wiedersberg H, Pawlowski P: Pylephlebitis after umbilical vein catheterization {author's transl}, *Monatsschr Kinderheilkd* 128:128-135, 1980.
35. Scott JM: Iatrogenic lesions in babies following umbilical vein catheterization, *Arch Dis Child* 40:426-429, 1965.
36. Tariq AA, Rudolph N, Levin EJ: Solitary hepatic abscess in a newborn infant: a sequel of umbilical vein catheterization and infusion of hypertonic glucose solutions, *Clin Pediatr (Phila)* 16:577-578, 1977.
37. Axton JH: Amoebic proctocolitis and liver abscess in a neonate, *S Afr Med J* 46:258-259, 1972.
38. Botman T, Ruys PJ: Amoebic appendicitis in a newborn infant, *Trop Geogr Med* 15:221-224, 1963.
39. Heck W, Rehbein F, Reismann B: Pyogenic liver abscess in infancy, *Z Kinderchir*(suppl 1)49, 1966.
40. Morison JE: Umbilical sepsis and acute interstitial hepatitis, *J Pathol Bacteriol* 56:531, 1944.
41. Bernstein J, Brown AK: Sepsis and jaundice in early infancy, *Pediatrics* 29:873-882, 1962.
42. Parker RG: Jaundice and infantile diarrhoea, *Arch Dis Child* 33: 330-334, 1958.
43. Kandall SR, Johnson AB, Gartner LM: Solitary neonatal hepatic abscess, *J Pediatr* 85:567-569, 1974.
44. Cushman P, Ward OC: Solitary liver abscess in a neonate: complication of umbilical vein catheterisation, *Ir J Med Sci* 147:374-375, 1978.
45. Nars PW, Klco L, Fliegel CP: Successful conservative management of a solitary liver abscess in a premature baby, *Helv Paediatr Acta* 38:489-493, 1983.
46. Gwinn JL, Lee FA, Baker CJ, et al: Pyogenic liver abscess, *Am J Dis Child* 123:49-50, 1972.
47. Martin DJ: Neonatal disorders diagnosed with ultrasound, *Clin Perinatol* 12:219-242, 1985.
48. Halvorsen RA Jr, Foster WL Jr, Wilkinson RH Jr, et al: Hepatic abscess: sensitivity of imaging tests and clinical findings, *Gastrointest Radiol* 13:135-141, 1988.
49. Caron KH: Magnetic resonance imaging of the pediatric abdomen, *Semin Ultrasound CT MR* 12:448-474, 1991.
50. Weinreb JC, Cohen JM, Armstrong E, et al: Imaging the pediatric liver: MRI and CT, *AJR Am J Roentgenol* 147:785-790, 1986.
51. Pineiro-Carrero VM, Andres JM: Morbidity and mortality in children with pyogenic liver abscess, *Am J Dis Child* 143:1424-1427, 1989.
52. Diament MJ, Stanley P, Kangarloo H, et al: Percutaneous aspiration and catheter drainage of abscesses, *J Pediatr* 108:204-208, 1986.
53. Rubinstein Z, Heyman Z, Morag B, et al: Ultrasound and computed tomography in the diagnosis and drainage of abscesses and other fluid collections, *Isr J Med Sci* 19:1050-1055, 1983.
54. Lee SH, Tomlinson C, Temple M, et al: Imaging-guided percutaneous needle aspiration or catheter drainage of neonatal liver abscesses: 14-year experience, *AJR Am J Roentgenol* 190:616-622, 2008.
55. Beaven DW: Staphylococcal peritonitis in the newborn, *Lancet* 1:869-871, 1958.
56. Fraga JR, Javate BA, Venkatessan S: Liver abscess and sepsis due to *Klebsiella pneumoniae* in a newborn. A complication of umbilical vein catheterization, *Clin Pediatr (Phila)* 13:1081-1082, 1974.
57. Reynolds TB: Medical treatment of pyogenic liver abscess, *Ann Intern Med* 96:373-374, 1982.
58. Loh R, Wallace G, Thong YH: Successful non-surgical management of pyogenic liver abscess, *Scand J Infect Dis* 19:137-140, 1987.
59. Shaw A, Pierog S: 'Ectopic' liver in the umbilicus: an unusual focus of infection in a newborn infant, *Pediatrics* 44:448-450, 1969.
60. Eklof O, Mortensson W, Sandstedt B: Suprarenal haematoma versus neuroblastoma complicated by haemorrhage. A diagnostic dilemma in the newborn, *Acta Radiol Diagn (Stockh)* 27:3-10, 1986.
61. Amodio J, Biskup D, Rivera R, et al: Tuberculous splenic abscess in a neonate with thrombocytopenia, *Pediatr Radiol* 35:887-890, 2005.
62. Kruger C, Malleyeck I, Naman N: Amoebic abscess of the spleen and fatal colonic perforation, *Pediatr Infect Dis J* 30:91-92, 2011.
63. Bowen A: Acute gallbladder dilatation in a neonate: emphasis on ultrasonography, *J Pediatr Gastroenterol Nutr* 3:304-308, 1984.
64. Brill PW, Winchester P, Rosen MS: Neonatal cholelithiasis, *Pediatr Radiol* 12:285-288, 1982.
65. Callahan J, Haller JO, Cacciarelli AA, et al: Cholelithiasis in infants: association with total parenteral nutrition and furosemide, *Radiology* 143:437-439, 1982.

66. Schirmer WJ, Grisoni ER, Gauderer MW: The spectrum of cholelithiasis in the first year of life, *J Pediatr Surg* 24:1064-1067, 1989.
67. Debray D, Pariente D, Gauthier F, et al: Cholelithiasis in infancy: a study of 40 cases, *J Pediatr* 122:385-391, 1993.
68. Neu J, Arvin A, Ariagno RL: Hydrops of the gallbladder, *Am J Dis Child* 134:891-893, 1980.
69. Peevy KJ, Wiseman HJ: Gallbladder distension in septic neonates, *Arch Dis Child* 57:75-76, 1982.
70. Saldanha RL, Stein CA, Kopelman AE: Gallbladder distention in ill preterm infants, *Am J Dis Child* 137:1179-1180, 1983.
71. Modi N, Keay AJ: Neonatal gallbladder distension, *Arch Dis Child* 57:562, 1982.
72. McGahan JP, Phillips HE, Cox KL: Sonography of the normal pediatric gallbladder and biliary tract, *Radiology* 144:873-875, 1982.
73. Haller JO: Sonography of the biliary tract in infants and children, *AJR Am J Roentgenol* 157:1051-1058, 1991.
74. Guthrie KJ, Montgomery GL: Infections with bacterium enteritidis in infancy with a triad of enteritis, cholecystitis, and meningitis, *J Pathol Bacteriol* 49:393, 1939.
75. Mateos-Corral D, Garza-Luna U, Gutierrez-Martin A: Two reports of acute neonatal acalculous cholecystitis (necrotizing cholecystitis) in a 2-week-old premature infant and a term neonate, *J Pediatr Surg* 41:e3-e5, 2006.
76. Arnspiger LA, Martin JG, Krempin HO: Acute noncalculous cholecystitis in children. Report of a case in seventeen day old infant, *Am J Surg* 100:103-106, 1960.
77. Ternberg JL, Keating JP: Acute acalculous cholecystitis. Complication of other illnesses in childhood, *Arch Surg* 110:543-547, 1975.
78. Wyllie R, Fitzgerald JF: Bacterial cholangitis in a 10-week-old infant with fever of undetermined origin, *Pediatrics* 65:164-167, 1980.
79. Becroft DM: Biliary atresia associated with prenatal infection by *Listeria monocytogenes*, *Arch Dis Child* 47:656-660, 1972.
80. Arena F, Romeo C, Manganaro A, et al: Bilateral neonatal adrenal abscess. Report of two cases and review of the literature, *Pediatr Med Chir* 25:185-189, 2003.
81. Ratnavel N, Farrer K, Sharland M, et al: Neonatal adrenal abscess revisited: the importance of raised inflammatory markers, *Ann Trop Paediatr* 25:63-66, 2005.
82. Blankenship WJ, Bogren H, Stadalnik RC, et al: Suprarenal abscess in the neonate: a case report and review of diagnosis and management, *Pediatrics* 55:239-243, 1975.
83. Carty A, Stanley P: Bilateral adrenal abscesses in a neonate, *Pediatr Radiol* 1:63-64, 1973.
84. Walker KM, Coyer WF: Suprarenal abscess due to group B *Streptococcus*, *J Pediatr* 94:970-971, 1979.
85. Francois A, Berterottiere D, Aigrain Y, et al: Neonatal *Proteus mirabilis* adrenal gland abscess, *Arch Fr Pediatr* 48:559-561, 1991.
86. Rajani K, Shapiro SR, Goetzman BW: Adrenal abscess: complication of supportive therapy of adrenal hemorrhage in the newborn, *J Pediatr Surg* 15:676-678, 1980.
87. Ohta S, Shimizu S, Fujisawa S, et al: Neonatal adrenal abscess due to *Bacteroides*, *J Pediatr* 93:1063-1064, 1978.
88. Bekdash BA, Slim MS: Adrenal abscess in a neonate due to gas-informing organisms: a diagnostic dilemma, *Z Kinderchir* 32:184-187, 1981.
89. Atkinson GO Jr, Kodroff MB, Gay BB Jr, et al: Adrenal abscess in the neonate, *Radiology* 155:101-104, 1985.
90. Gross M, Kottmeier PK, Waterhouse K: Diagnosis and treatment of neonatal adrenal hemorrhage, *J Pediatr Surg* 2:308-312, 1967.
91. Torres Simon JM, Figueras Aloy J, Vilanova Juanola JM, et al: Adrenal abscess in a neonate, *An Esp Pediatr* 31:601-602, 1989.
92. Mittelstaedt CA, Volberg FM, Merten DF, et al: The sonographic diagnosis of neonatal adrenal hemorrhage, *Radiology* 131:453-457, 1979.
93. Zamir O, Udassin R, Aviad I, et al: Adrenal abscess, *Pediatr Surg Int* 2:117-119, 1987.
94. Cohen MD: Clinical utility of magnetic resonance imaging in pediatrics, *Am J Dis Child* 140:947-956, 1986.
95. Etherington-Wilson W: Appendicitis in the newborn. Report on case 16 days old, *Proc R Soc Med* 38:186-187, 1945.
96. Puri P, O'Donnell B: Appendicitis in infancy, *J Pediatr Surg* 13:173-174, 1978.
97. Reuter G, Krause I: Appendicitis of the newborn infant, *Kinderarztl Prax* 43:289-292, 1975.
98. Parsons JM, Miscall BG, McSherry CK: Appendicitis in the newborn infant, *Surgery* 67:841-843, 1970.
99. Schaupp W, Clausen EG, Ferrier PK: Appendicitis during the first month of life, *Surgery* 48:805-811, 1960.
100. Stanley-Brown EG: Acute appendicitis during first five years of life, *Am J Dis Child* 108:134-138, 1964.
101. Fields IA, Naiditch MJ, Rothman PE: Acute appendicitis in infants; ten-year survey at the Los Angeles County Hospital and report of a case of perforated appendicitis in a fifteen-day-old infant with survival, *AMA J Dis Child* 93:287-305, 1957.
102. Norris WJ: Appendicitis in children; review of one thousand cases taken from the records of the Children's Hospital, Los Angeles, *West J Surg Obstet Gynecol* 54:183-192, 1946.
103. Snyder WH Jr, Chaffin L: Appendicitis during first two years of life; report on twenty-one cases and review of four hundred forty-seven cases from the literature, *AMA Arch Surg* 64:549-560, 1952.
104. Grosfeld JL, Weinberger M, Clatworthy HW Jr: Acute appendicitis in the first two years of life, *J Pediatr Surg* 8:285-293, 1973.
105. Massad M, Srouji M, Awdeh A, et al: Neonatal appendicitis: case report and a revised review of the English literature, *Z Kinderchir* 41:241-243, 1986.
106. Schorlemmer GR, Herbst CA Jr: Perforated neonatal appendicitis, *South Med J* 76:536-537, 1983.
107. Caralps-Riera JM, Cohn BD: Bowel perforation after exchange transfusion in the neonate: review of the literature and report of a case, *Surgery* 68:895-898, 1970.
108. Broadbent NR, Jardine JL: Acute appendicitis in a premature infant: a case report, *Aust N Z J Surg* 40:362-364, 1971.
109. Bryant LR, Trinkle JK, Noonan JA, et al: Appendicitis and appendiceal perforation in neonates, *Am Surg* 36:523-525, 1970.
110. Creery RD: Acute appendicitis in the newborn, *Br Med J* 1:871, 1953.
111. Hardman RP, Bowerman D: Appendicitis in the newborn, *Am J Dis Child* 105:99-101, 1963.
112. Kolb G, Schaeffer E: Perforating appendicitis in the first weeks of life, *Kinderarztl Prax* 23:1-4, 1955.
113. Meigher SC, Lucas AW: Appendicitis in the newborn; case report, *Ann Surg* 136:1044-1047, 1952.
114. Neve R, Quenville NF: Appendicitis with perforation in a 12-day-old infant, *Can Med Assoc J* 94:447-448, 1966.
115. Niforoushan MA: Fever and ascites in a newborn, *Clin Pediatr (Phila)* 14:878, 1975.
116. Parkhurst GF, Wagoner SC: Neonatal acute appendicitis, *N Y State J Med* 69:1929-1930, 1969.
117. Smith AL, MacMahon RA: Perforated appendix complicating rhesus immunization in a newborn infant, *Med J Aust* 2:602-603, 1969.
118. Walker RH: Appendicitis in the newborn infant, *J Pediatr* 51:429-434, 1957.
119. Trojanowski JQ, Gang DL, Goldblatt A, et al: Fatal postoperative acute appendicitis in a neonate with congenital heart disease, *J Pediatr Surg* 16:85-86, 1981.
120. Ayalon A, Mogilner M, Cohen O, et al: Acute appendicitis in a premature baby, *Acta Chir Scand* 145:285-286, 1979.
121. Golladay ES, Roskes S, Donner L, et al: Intestinal obstruction from appendiceal abscess in a newborn infant, *J Pediatr Surg* 13:175-176, 1978.
122. Hemalatha V, Spitz L: Neonatal appendicitis, *Clin Pediatr (Phila)* 18:621-622, 1979.
123. Tucci P, Holgersen L, Doctor D, et al: Congenital ureteropelvic junction obstruction associated with unsuspected acute perforated appendicitis in a neonate, *J Urol* 120:247-248, 1978.
124. Kwong MS, Dinner M: Neonatal appendicitis masquerading as necrotizing enterocolitis, *J Pediatr* 96:917-918, 1980.
125. Shaul WL: Clues to the early diagnosis of neonatal appendicitis, *J Pediatr* 98:473-476, 1981.
126. Lassiter HA, Werner MH: Neonatal appendicitis, *South Med J* 76:1173-1175, 1983.
127. Carol J, Creixell S, Hernandez JV, et al: Neonatal appendicitis. Report of a new case, *An Esp Pediatr* 20:807-810, 1984.
128. Bax NM, Pearse RG, Dommering N, et al: Perforation of the appendix in the neonatal period, *J Pediatr Surg* 15:200-202, 1980.
129. Heydenrych JJ, Du Toit DF: Unusual presentations of acute appendicitis in the neonate. A report of 2 cases, *S Afr Med J* 62:1003-1005, 1982.
130. Pathania OP, Jain SK, Kapila H, et al: Fatal neonatal perforation of appendix, *Indian Pediatr* 26:1166-1167, 1989.

131. Arora NK, Deorari AK, Bhatnagar V, et al: Neonatal appendicitis: a rare cause of surgical emergency in preterm babies, *Indian Pediatr* 28:1330-1333, 1991.
132. Arliss J, Holgersen LO: Neonatal appendiceal perforation and Hirschsprung's disease, *J Pediatr Surg* 25:694-695, 1990.
133. Kliegman RM, Fanaroff AA: Necrotizing enterocolitis, *N Engl J Med* 310:1093-1103, 1984.
134. Srouji MN, Buck BE: Neonatal appendicitis: ischemic infarction in incarcerated inguinal hernia, *J Pediatr Surg* 13:177-179, 1978.
135. Jancelewicz T, Kim G, Miniati D: Neonatal appendicitis: a new look at an old zebra, *J Pediatr Surg* 43:e1-e5, 2008.
136. Gross RE: *The surgery of infancy and childhood: its principles and techniques*, Philadelphia, 1953, WB Saunders.
137. Dennis JE, Rhodes KH, Cooney DR, et al: Nosocomical *Rhizopus* infection (zygomycosis) in children, *J Pediatr* 96:824-828, 1980.
138. Buschard K, Kjaeldgaard A: Investigation and analysis of the position, fixation, length and embryology of the vermiform appendix, *Acta Chir Scand* 139:293-298, 1973.
139. Jones WR, Kaye MD, Ing RM: The lymphoid development of the fetal and neonatal appendix, *Biol Neonate* 20:334-345, 1972.
140. Srouji MN, Chatten J, David C: Pseudodiverticulitis of the appendix with neonatal Hirschsprung disease, *J Pediatr* 93:988-990, 1978.
141. Charif P: Perforated appendicitis in premature infants. A case report and review of the literature, *Johns Hopkins Med J* 125:92-94, 1969.
142. Martin LW, Glen PM: Prenatal appendiceal perforation: a case report, *J Pediatr Surg* 21:73-74, 1986.
143. Hill WB, Mason CC: Prenatal appendicitis with rupture and death, *Am J Dis Child* 29:86, 1925.
144. Corcoran WJ: Prenatal rupture of the appendix, *Am J Dis Child* 39:277, 1930.
145. Jackson WF: A case of prenatal appendicitis, *Am J Med Sci* 127:710, 1904.
146. Buntain WL: Neonatal appendicitis mistaken for necrotizing enterocolitis, *South Med J* 75:1155, 1982.
147. Wilkinson RH, Bartlett RH, Eraklis AJ: Diagnosis of appendicitis in infancy. The value of abdominal radiographs, *Am J Dis Child* 118:687-690, 1969.
148. Chang JH: The use of antibiotics in pediatric abdominal surgery, *Pediatr Infect Dis* 3:195-198, 1984.
149. Bell MJ: Peritonitis in the newborn—current concepts, *Pediatr Clin North Am* 32:1181-1201, 1985.
150. Lloyd JR: The etiology of gastrointestinal perforations in the newborn, *J Pediatr Surg* 4:77-84, 1969.
151. McDougal WS, Izant RJ Jr, Zollinger RM Jr: Primary peritonitis in infancy and childhood, *Ann Surg* 181:310-313, 1975.
152. Fonkalsrud EW, Ellis DG, Clatworthy HW Jr: Neonatal peritonitis, *J Pediatr Surg* 1:227-239, 1966.
153. Rickham PP: Peritonitis in the neonatal period, *Arch Dis Child* 30:23-31, 1955.
154. Denes J, Leb J: Neonatal peritonitis, *Acta Paediatr Acad Sci Hung* 10:297-302, 1969.
155. Daum R, Schutze U, Hill E, et al: Mortality of preoperative peritonitis in newborn infants without intestinal obstruction, *Prog Pediatr Surg* 13:267-271, 1979.
156. Schutze U, Fey KH, Hess G: Peritonitis in the neonate, in infancy and childhood {author's transl}, *MMW Munch Med Wochenschr* 116:1201-1207, 1974.
157. Prevot J, Grosdidier G, Schmitt M: Fatal peritonitis, *Prog Pediatr Surg* 13:257-266, 1979.
158. Singer B, Hammar B: Neonatal peritonitis, *S Afr Med J* 46:987-993, 1972.
159. Hensey OJ, Hart CA, Cooke RW: Serious infection in a neonatal intensive care unit: a two-year survey, *J Hyg (Lond)* 95:289-297, 1985.
160. Valdes-Dapena MA, Arey JB: The causes of neonatal mortality: an analysis of 501 autopsies on newborn infants, *J Pediatr* 77:366-375, 1970.
161. Bell MJ: Perforation of the gastrointestinal tract and peritonitis in the neonate, *Surg Gynecol Obstet* 160:20-26, 1985.
162. Mollitt DL, Tepas JJ 3rd, Talbert JL: The microbiology of neonatal peritonitis, *Arch Surg* 123:176-179, 1988.
163. Chadwick EG, Shulman ST, Yogev R: Peritonitis as a late manifestations of group B streptococcal disease in newborns, *Pediatr Infect Dis* 2:142-143, 1983.
164. Serlo W, Heikkinen E, Kouvalainen K: Group A streptococcal peritonitis in infancy, *Ann Chir Gynaecol* 74:183-184, 1985.
165. Johnson DE, Conroy MM, Foker JE, et al: *Candida* peritonitis in the newborn infants, *J Pediatr* 97:298-300, 1980.
166. Kaplan M, Eidelman AI, Dollberg L, et al: Necrotizing bowel disease with *Candida* peritonitis following severe neonatal hypothermia, *Acta Paediatr Scand* 79:876-879, 1990.
167. Butler KM, Rench MA, Baker CJ: Amphotericin b as a single agent in the treatment of systemic candidiasis in neonates, *Pediatr Infect Dis J* 9:51-56, 1990.
168. MacDonald L, Baker C, Chenoweth C: Risk factors for candidemia in a children's hospital, *Clin Infect Dis* 26:642-645, 1998.
169. Pan EY, Chen LY, Yang JZ, et al: Radiographic diagnosis of meconium peritonitis. A report of 200 cases including six fetal cases, *Pediatr Radiol* 13:199-205, 1983.
170. Holgersen LO: The etiology of spontaneous gastric perforation of the newborn: a reevaluation, *J Pediatr Surg* 16:608-613, 1981.
171. Wilson R, Kanto WP Jr, McCarthy BJ, et al: Age at onset of necrotizing enterocolitis: an epidemiologic analysis, *Pediatr Res* 16:82-85, 1982.
172. Wilson R, Kanto WP Jr, McCarthy BJ, et al: Age at onset of necrotizing enterocolitis. Risk factors in small infants, *Am J Dis Child* 136:814-816, 1982.
173. Touloukian RJ, Kadar A, Spencer RP: The gastrointestinal complications of neonatal umbilical venous exchange transfusion: a clinical and experimental study, *Pediatrics* 51:36-43, 1973.
174. Freedman RM, Ingram DL, Gross I, et al: A half century of neonatal sepsis at Yale: 1928 to 1978, *Am J Dis Child* 135:140-144, 1981.
175. Thelander HE: Perforation of the gastrointestinal tract of the newborn infant, *Am J Dis Child* 58:371, 1939.
176. Kosloske AM, Lilly JR: Paracentesis and lavage for diagnosis of intestinal gangrene in neonatal necrotizing enterocolitis, *J Pediatr Surg* 13:315-320, 1978.
177. Gerstein MC, Lindsay WK, McKendry JB: Congenital defects of lymphatics in infancy, *Pediatrics* 19:21-35, 1957.
178. Lees W, Mitchell JE: Bile peritonitis in infancy, *Arch Dis Child* 41: 188-192, 1966.
179. Rosenfeld DL, Cordell CE, Jadeja N: Retrocardiac pneumomediastinum: radiographic finding and clinical implications, *Pediatrics* 85:92-97, 1990.
180. Pochaczevsky R, Bryk D: New roentgenographic signs of neonatal gastric perforation, *Radiology* 102:145-147, 1972.
181. Wind ES, Pillari GP: Lucent liver in the newborn. A roentgenographic sign of pneumoperitoneum, *JAMA* 237:2218-2219, 1977.
182. Cohen MD, Weber TR, Grosfeld JL: Bowel perforation in the newborn: diagnosis with metrizamide, *Radiology* 150:65-69, 1984.
183. Thomas S, Sainsbury C, Murphy JF: Pancuronium belly, *Lancet* 2:870, 1984.
184. Ein SH, Stephens CA, Reilly BJ: The disappearance of free air after pediatric laparotomy, *J Pediatr Surg* 20:422-424, 1985.
185. Emanuel B, Zlotnik P, Raffensperger JG: Perforation of the gastrointestinal tract in infancy and childhood, *Surg Gynecol Obstet* 146: 926-928, 1978.
186. Neu J, Walker WA: Necrotizing enterocolitis, *N Engl J Med* 364: 255-264, 2011.
187. Patel BK, Shah JS: Necrotizing enterocolitis in very low birth weight infants: a systemic review, *ISRN Gastroenterol* 2012:562594, 2012.
188. Wu SF, Caplan M, Lin HC: Necrotizing enterocolitis: old problem with new hope, *Pediatr Neonatol* 53:158-163, 2012.
189. Dominguez KM, Moss RL: Necrotizing enterocolitis, *Clin Perinatol* 39:387-401, 2012.
190. Berman L, Moss RL: Necrotizing enterocolitis: an update, *Semin Fetal Neonatal Med* 16:145-150, 2011.
191. Kim JH: Necrotizing enterocolitis: the road to zero, *Semin Fetal Neonatal Med* 19:39-44, 2014.
192. Stoll BJ, Hansen NI, Bell EF, et al: Neonatal outcomes of extremely preterm infants from the NICHD neonatal research network, *Pediatrics* 126:443-456, 2010.
193. Horbar JD, Carpenter JH, Badger GJ, et al: Mortality and neonatal morbidity among infants 501 to 1500 grams from 2000 to 2009, *Pediatrics* 129:1019-1026, 2012.
194. de Gamarra E, Helardot P, Moriette G, et al: Necrotizing enterocolitis in full-term newborns, *Biol Neonate* 44:185-192, 1983.

195. Christensen RD, Lambert DK, Baer VL, et al: Necrotizing enterocolitis in term infants, *Clin Perinatol* 40:69-78, 2013.
196. Fitzgibbons SC, Ching Y, Yu D, et al: Mortality of necrotizing enterocolitis expressed by birth weight categories, *J Pediatr Surg* 44:1072-1075, discussion 1075–1076, 2009.
197. Morgan JA, Young L, McGuire W: Pathogenesis and prevention of necrotizing enterocolitis, *Curr Opin Infect Dis* 24:183-189, 2011.
198. Santulli TV, Schullinger JN, Heird WC, et al: Acute necrotizing enterocolitis in infancy: a review of 64 cases, *Pediatrics* 55:376-387, 1975.
199. Bhandari V, Bizzarro MJ, Shetty A, et al: Familial and genetic susceptibility to major neonatal morbidities in preterm twins, *Pediatrics* 117:1901-1906, 2006.
200. Henderson G, Craig S, Baier RJ, et al: Cytokine gene polymorphisms in preterm infants with necrotising enterocolitis: genetic association study, *Arch Dis Child Fetal Neonatal Ed* 94:F124-F128, 2009.
201. Patole SK, de Klerk N: Impact of standardised feeding regimens on incidence of neonatal necrotising enterocolitis: a systematic review and meta-analysis of observational studies, *Arch Dis Child Fetal Neonatal Ed* 90:F147-F151, 2005.
202. Henderson G, Craig S, Brocklehurst P, et al: Enteral feeding regimens and necrotising enterocolitis in preterm infants: a multicentre case-control study, *Arch Dis Child Fetal Neonatal Ed* 94:F120-F123, 2009.
203. Morgan J, Young L, McGuire W: Slow advancement of enteral feed volumes to prevent necrotising enterocolitis in very low birth weight infants, *Cochrane Database Syst Rev*, (3), CD001241, 2013.
204. Sullivan S, Schanler RJ, Kim JH, et al: An exclusively human milk-based diet is associated with a lower rate of necrotizing enterocolitis than a diet of human milk and bovine milk-based products, *J Pediatr* 156:562-567, 2010.
205. Quigley MA, Henderson G, Anthony MY, et al: Formula milk versus donor breast milk for feeding preterm or low birth weight infants, *Cochrane Database Syst Rev*, (4)CD002971, 2007.
206. Dvorak B, Halpern MD, Holubec H, et al: Maternal milk reduces severity of necrotizing enterocolitis and increases intestinal il-10 in a neonatal rat model, *Pediatr Res* 53:426-433, 2003.
207. Claud EC, Walker WA: Hypothesis: inappropriate colonization of the premature intestine can cause neonatal necrotizing enterocolitis, *FASEB J* 15:1398-1403, 2001.
208. Morowitz MJ, Poroyko V, Caplan M, et al: Redefining the role of intestinal microbes in the pathogenesis of necrotizing enterocolitis, *Pediatrics* 125:777-785, 2010.
209. Kliegman RM: The role of clostridia in the pathogenesis of neonatal necrotizing enterocolitis. In Borriello SP, editor: *Clostridia in gastrointestinal disease*, Boca Raton, Fla, 1985, CRC Press, pp 68-92.
210. Pedersen PV, Hansen FH, Halveg AB, et al: Necrotising enterocolitis of the newborn—is it gas-gangrene of the bowel? *Lancet* 2:715-716, 1976.
211. Westra-Meijer CM, Degener JE, Dzoljic-Danilovic G, et al: Quantitative study of the aerobic and anaerobic faecal flora in neonatal necrotising enterocolitis, *Arch Dis Child* 58:523-528, 1983.
212. Lishman AH, Al Jumaili IJ, Elshibly E, et al: *Clostridium difficile* isolation in neonates in a special care unit. Lack of correlation with necrotizing enterocolitis, *Scand J Gastroenterol* 19:441-444, 1984.
213. Cashore WJ, Peter G, Lauermann M, et al: Clostridia colonization and clostridial toxin in neonatal necrotizing enterocolitis, *J Pediatr* 98:308-311, 1981.
214. Scheifele DW, Bjornson GL: Delta toxin activity in coagulase-negative staphylococci from the bowels of neonates, *J Clin Microbiol* 26:279-282, 1988.
215. Scheifele DW, Bjornson GL, Dyer RA, et al: Delta-like toxin produced by coagulase-negative staphylococci is associated with neonatal necrotizing enterocolitis, *Infect Immun* 55:2268-2273, 1987.
216. Hoy C, Millar MR, MacKay P, et al: Quantitative changes in faecal microflora preceding necrotising enterocolitis in premature neonates, *Arch Dis Child* 65:1057-1059, 1990.
217. Richmond JA, Mikity V: Benign form of necrotizing enterocolitis, *Am J Roentgenol Radium Ther Nucl Med* 123:301-306, 1975.
218. Barnard JA, Cotton RB, Lutin W: Necrotizing enterocolitis. Variables associated with the severity of disease, *Am J Dis Child* 139:375-377, 1985.
219. Bell MJ, Ternberg JL, Feigin RD, et al: Neonatal necrotizing enterocolitis. Therapeutic decisions based upon clinical staging, *Ann Surg* 187:1-7, 1978.
220. Walsh MC, Kliegman RM: Necrotizing enterocolitis: treatment based on staging criteria, *Pediatr Clin North Am* 33:179-201, 1986.
221. Daneman A, Woodward S, de Silva M: The radiology of neonatal necrotizing enterocolitis (NEC). A review of 47 cases and the literature, *Pediatr Radiol* 7:70-77, 1978.
222. Rehan VK, Seshia MM, Johnston B, et al: Observer variability in interpretation of abdominal radiographs of infants with suspected necrotizing enterocolitis, *Clin Pediatr (Phila)* 38:637-643, 1999.
223. Mata AG, Rosengart RM: Interobserver variability in the radiographic diagnosis of necrotizing enterocolitis, *Pediatrics* 66:68-71, 1980.
224. Johnson JF, Robinson LH: Localized bowel distension in the newborn: a review of the plain film analysis and differential diagnosis, *Pediatrics* 73:206-215, 1984.
225. Leonard T Jr, Johnson JF, Pettett PG: Critical evaluation of the persistent loop sign in necrotizing enterocolitis, *Radiology* 142:385-386, 1982.
226. Frey EE, Smith W, Franken EA Jr, et al: Analysis of bowel perforation in necrotizing enterocolitis, *Pediatr Radiol* 17:380-382, 1987.
227. Kliegman RM, Fanaroff AA: Neonatal necrotizing enterocolitis: a nine-year experience. II. Outcome assessment, *Am J Dis Child* 135:608-611, 1981.
228. Kliegman RM, Fanaroff AA: Neonatal necrotizing enterocolitis: a nine-year experience, *Am J Dis Child* 135:603-607, 1981.
229. Keller MS, Chawla HS: Neonatal metrizamide gastrointestinal series in suspected necrotizing enterocolitis, *Am J Dis Child* 139:713-716, 1985.
230. Lindley S, Mollitt DL, Seibert JJ, et al: Portal vein ultrasonography in the early diagnosis of necrotizing enterocolitis, *J Pediatr Surg* 21: 530-532, 1986.
231. Malin SW, Bhutani VK, Ritchie WW, et al: Echogenic intravascular and hepatic microbubbles associated with necrotizing enterocolitis, *J Pediatr* 103:637-640, 1983.
232. Caplan MS, Jilling T: New concepts in necrotizing enterocolitis, *Curr Opin Pediatr* 13:111-115, 2001.
233. Ricketts RR: The role of paracentesis in the management of infants with necrotizing enterocolitis, *Am Surg* 52:61-65, 1986.
234. Patel CC: Hematologic abnormalities in acute necrotizing enterocolitis, *Pediatr Clin North Am* 24:579-584, 1977.
235. Hutter JJ Jr, Hathaway WE, Wayne ER: Hematologic abnormalities in severe neonatal necrotizing enterocolitis, *J Pediatr* 88: 1026-1031, 1976.
236. Rabinowitz SS, Dzakpasu P, Piecuch S, et al: Platelet-activating factor in infants at risk for necrotizing enterocolitis, *J Pediatr* 138: 81-86, 2001.
237. Christensen RD, Rothstein G, Anstall HB, et al: Granulocyte transfusions in neonates with bacterial infection, neutropenia, and depletion of mature marrow neutrophils, *Pediatrics* 70:1-6, 1982.
238. Garcia J, Smith FR, Cucinell SA: Urinary d-lactate excretion in infants with necrotizing enterocolitis, *J Pediatr* 104:268-270, 1984.
239. Book LS, Herbst JJ, Jung AL: Carbohydrate malabsorption in necrotizing enterocolitis, *Pediatrics* 57:201-204, 1976.
240. Virnig NL, Reynolds JW: Epidemiological aspects of neonatal necrotizing enterocolitis, *Am J Dis Child* 128:186-190, 1974.
241. Kliegman RM, Walsh MC: The incidence of meningitis in neonates with necrotizing enterocolitis, *Am J Perinatol* 4:245-248, 1987.
242. Shah D, Sinn JK: Antibiotic regimens for the empirical treatment of newborn infants with necrotising enterocolitis, *Cochrane Database Syst Rev*, (8), CD007448, 2012.
243. Faix RG, Polley TZ, Grasela TH: A randomized, controlled trial of parenteral clindamycin in neonatal necrotizing enterocolitis, *J Pediatr* 112:271-277, 1988.
244. Burrington JD: Necrotizing enterocolitis in newborn infant, *Clin Perinatol* 5:29-44, 1978.
245. Ghory MJ, Sheldon CA: Newborn surgical emergencies of the gastrointestinal tract, *Surg Clin North Am* 65:1083-1098, 1985.
246. Kastenberg ZJ, Sylvester KG: The surgical management of necrotizing enterocolitis, *Clin Perinatol* 40:135-148, 2013.
247. Ein SH, Shandling B, Wesson D, et al: A 13-year experience with peritoneal drainage under local anesthesia for necrotizing enterocolitis perforation, *J Pediatr Surg* 25:1034-1036, discussion 1036–1037, 1990.
248. Egan EA, Nelson RM, Mantilla G, et al: Additional experience with routine use of oral kanamycin prophylaxis for necrotizing enterocolitis in infants under 1,500 grams, *J Pediatr* 90:331-332, 1977.

249. Grylack LJ, Scanlon JW: Oral gentamicin therapy in the prevention of neonatal necrotizing enterocolitis. A controlled double-blind trial, *Am J Dis Child* 132:1192-1194, 1978.
250. Rowley MP, Dahlenburg GW: Gentamicin in prophylaxis of neonatal necrotising enterocolitis, *Lancet* 2:532, 1978.
251. Boyle R, Nelson JS, Stonestreet BS, et al: Alterations in stool flora resulting from oral kanamycin prophylaxis of necrotizing enterocolitis, *J Pediatr* 93:857-861, 1978.
252. Bhat AM, Meny RG: Alimentary absorption of gentamicin in preterm infants, *Clin Pediatr (Phila)* 23:683-685, 1984.
253. AlFaleh K, Anabrees J: Efficacy and safety of probiotics in preterm infants, *J Neonatal Perinatal Med* 6:1-9, 2013.
254. Chen CC, Allan Walker W: Probiotics and the mechanism of necrotizing enterocolitis, *Semin Pediatr Surg* 22:94-100, 2013.
255. Lin HC, Su BH, Chen AC, et al: Oral probiotics reduce the incidence and severity of necrotizing enterocolitis in very low birth weight infants, *Pediatrics* 115:1-4, 2005.
256. Bin-Nun A, Bromiker R, Wilschanski M, et al: Oral probiotics prevent necrotizing enterocolitis in very low birth weight neonates, *J Pediatr* 147:192-196, 2005.
257. Deshpande G, Rao S, Patole S, et al: Updated meta-analysis of probiotics for preventing necrotizing enterocolitis in preterm neonates, *Pediatrics* 125:921-930, 2010.
258. Anderson DM, Kliegman RM: The relationship of neonatal alimentation practices to the occurrence of endemic necrotizing enterocolitis, *Am J Perinatol* 8:62-67, 1991.
259. McKeown RE, Marsh TD, Amarnath U, et al: Role of delayed feeding and of feeding increments in necrotizing enterocolitis, *J Pediatr* 121:764-770, 1992.
260. Carrion V, Egan EA: Prevention of neonatal necrotizing enterocolitis, *J Pediatr Gastroenterol Nutr* 11:317-323, 1990.
261. Bohnhorst B, Muller S, Dordelmann M, et al: Early feeding after necrotizing enterocolitis in preterm infants, *J Pediatr* 143:484-487, 2003.
262. Eibl MM, Wolf HM, Furnkranz H, et al: Prophylaxis of necrotizing enterocolitis by oral IgA-IgG: review of a clinical study in low birth weight infants and discussion of the pathogenic role of infection, *J Clin Immunol* 10:72S-77S, discussion 77S-79S, 1990.
263. Eibl MM, Wolf HM, Furnkranz H, et al: Prevention of necrotizing enterocolitis in low-birth-weight infants by IgA-IgG feeding, *N Engl J Med* 319:1-7, 1988.
264. Leonidas JC, Hall RT: Neonatal pneumatosis coli: a mild form of neonatal necrotizing enterocolitis, *J Pediatr* 89:456-459, 1976.
265. Schullinger JN, Mollitt DL, Vinocur CD, et al: Neonatal necrotizing enterocolitis. Survival, management, and complications: a 25-year study, *Am J Dis Child* 135:612-614, 1981.
266. Dykes EH, Gilmour WH, Azmy AF: Prediction of outcome following necrotizing enterocolitis in a neonatal surgical unit, *J Pediatr Surg* 20:3-5, 1985.
267. Abbasi S, Pereira GR, Johnson L, et al: Long-term assessment of growth, nutritional status, and gastrointestinal function in survivors of necrotizing enterocolitis, *J Pediatr* 104:550-554, 1984.
268. Janik JS, Ein SH, Mancer K: Intestinal stricture after necrotizing enterocolitis, *J Pediatr Surg* 16:438-443, 1981.
269. Ball TI, Wyly JB: Enterocyst formation: a late complication of neonatal necrotizing enterocolitis, *AJR Am J Roentgenol* 147:806-808, 1986.
270. Walsh MC, Kliegman RM, Hack M: Severity of necrotizing enterocolitis: influence on outcome at 2 years of age, *Pediatrics* 84:808-814, 1989.
271. Leviton A, Dammann O, Engelke S, et al: The clustering of disorders in infants born before the 28th week of gestation, *Acta Paediatr* 99:1795-1800, 2010.
272. Martin CR, Dammann O, Allred EN, et al: Neurodevelopment of extremely preterm infants who had necrotizing enterocolitis with or without late bacteremia, *J Pediatr* 157:751-756, 2010.
273. Macaulay D: Acute endocarditis in infancy and early childhood, *AMA Am J Dis Child* 88:715-731, 1954.
274. Johnson DH, Rosenthal A, Nadas AS: A forty-year review of bacterial endocarditis in infancy and childhood, *Circulation* 51:581-588, 1975.
275. Johnson DH, Rosenthal A, Nadas AS: Bacterial endocarditis in children under 2 years of age, *Am J Dis Child* 129:183-186, 1975.
276. Edwards K, Ingall D, Czapek E, et al: Bacterial endocarditis in 4 young infants. Is this complication on the increase? *Clin Pediatr (Phila)* 16:607-609, 1977.
277. McGuinness GA, Schieken RM, Maguire GF: Endocarditis in the newborn, *Am J Dis Child* 134:577-580, 1980.
278. Kramer HH, Bourgeois M, Liersch R, et al: Current clinical aspects of bacterial endocarditis in infancy, childhood, and adolescence, *Eur J Pediatr* 140:253-259, 1983.
279. Oelberg DG, Fisher DJ, Gross DM, et al: Endocarditis in high-risk neonates, *Pediatrics* 71:392-397, 1983.
280. Gossius G, Gunnes P, Rasmussen K: Ten years of infective endocarditis: a clinicopathologic study, *Acta Med Scand* 217:171-179, 1985.
281. Opie GF, Fraser SH, Drew JH, et al: Bacterial endocarditis in neonatal intensive care, *J Paediatr Child Health* 35:545-548, 1999.
282. Mecrow IK, Ladusans EJ: Infective endocarditis in newborn infants with structurally normal hearts, *Acta Paediatr* 83:35-39, 1994.
283. Soo SS, Bosman DL: *Streptococcus faecalis* in neonatal infective endocarditis, *J Infect* 23:209-210, 1991.
284. Lewis IC: Bacterial endocarditis complicating septicaemia in an infant, *Arch Dis Child* 29:144-146, 1954.
285. Prandstraller D, Marata AM, Picchio FM: *Staphylococcus aureus* endocarditis in a newborn with transposition of the great arteries: successful treatment, *Int J Cardiol* 14:355-358, 1987.
286. Millard DD, Shulman ST: The changing spectrum of neonatal endocarditis, *Clin Perinatol* 15:587-608, 1988.
287. Symchych PS, Krauss AN, Winchester P: Endocarditis following intracardiac placement of umbilical venous catheters in neonates, *J Pediatr* 90:287-289, 1977.
288. Morrow WR, Haas JE, Benjamin DR: Nonbacterial endocardial thrombosis in neonates: relationship to persistent fetal circulation, *J Pediatr* 100:117-122, 1982.
289. Bergsland J, Kawaguchi A, Roland JM, et al: Mycotic aortic aneurysms in children, *Ann Thorac Surg* 37:314-318, 1984.
290. Baltimore RS: Infective endocarditis in children, *Pediatr Infect Dis J* 11:907-912, 1992.
291. Bullaboy CA, Coulson JD, Jennings RB Jr, et al: Neonatal mitral valve endocarditis: diagnosis and successful management, *Clin Pediatr (Phila)* 29:398-400, 1990.
292. Nakayama DK, O'Neill JA Jr, Wagner H, et al: Management of vascular complications of bacterial endocarditis, *J Pediatr Surg* 21: 636-639, 1986.
293. Kavey RE, Frank DM, Byrum CJ, et al: Two-dimensional echocardiographic assessment of infective endocarditis in children, *Am J Dis Child* 137:851-856, 1983.
294. Perelman MJ, Sugimoto J, Arcilla RA, et al: Aortic root replacement for complicated bacterial endocarditis in an infant, *J Pediatr Surg* 24:1121-1123, 1989.
295. Tulloh RM, Silove ED, Abrams LD: Replacement of an aortic valve cusp after neonatal endocarditis, *Br Heart J* 64:204-205, 1990.
296. Favara BE, Franciosi RA, Butterfield LJ: Disseminated intravascular and cardiac thrombosis of the neonate, *Am J Dis Child* 127:197-204, 1974.
297. Begg JG: Blood-filled cysts in the cardiac valve cusps in foetal life and infancy, *J Pathol Bacteriol* 87:177-178, 1964.
298. Gersony WM, McCracken GH Jr: Purulent pericarditis in infancy, *Pediatrics* 40:224-232, 1967.
299. Wynn RJ: Neonatal *E. coli* pericarditis, *J Perinat Med* 7:23-26, 1979.
300. Cayler GC, Taybi H, Riley HD Jr, et al: Pericarditis with effusion in infants and children, *J Pediatr* 63:265-272, 1963.
301. Noren GR, Kaplan EL, Staley NA: Nonrheumatic inflammatory diseases. In Adams FH, Emmanouilides GC, editors: *Moss' heart disease in infants, children and adolescents*, Baltimore, 1983, Williams & Wilkins, pp 585-594.
302. Kanarek KS, de Brigard T, Coleman J, et al: Purulent pericarditis in a neonate, *Pediatr Infect Dis J* 10:549-550, 1991.
303. Zeevi B, Perry SB, Keane JF, et al: Interventional cardiac procedures in neonates and infants: state of the art, *Clin Perinatol* 15:633-658, 1988.
304. Chen TH, Chen CC, Hwang KP, et al: Retropharyngeal abscess with extensive mediastinitis in a 2-day-old neonate, *J Paediatr Child Health* 44:154-155, 2008.
305. Tortoriello TA, Friedman JD, McKenzie ED, et al: Mediastinitis after pediatric cardiac surgery: a 15-year experience at a single institution, *Ann Thorac Surg* 76:1655-1660, 2003.
306. Weichsel M: Mediastinitis in a newborn, *Proc Rudolf Virchow Med Soc City N Y* 22:67-73, 1963.
307. Merriman TE, Taylor RG, Nattrass GR: Vertebral osteomyelitis in an infant presenting with a posterior mediastinal mass, *Pediatr Surg Int* 12:541-543, 1997.

308. Krasna IH, Rosenfeld D, Benjamin BG, et al: Esophageal perforation in the neonate: an emerging problem in the newborn nursery, *J Pediatr Surg* 22:784-790, 1987.
309. Topsis J, Kinas HY, Kandall SR: Esophageal perforation—a complication of neonatal resuscitation, *Anesth Analg* 69:532-534, 1989.
310. Coulthard M, Isaacs D: Neonatal retropharyngeal abscess, *Pediatr Infect Dis J* 10:547-549, 1991.
311. Talbert JL, Rodgers BM, Felman AH, et al: Traumatic perforation of the hypopharynx in infants, *J Thorac Cardiovasc Surg* 74:152-156, 1977.
312. Grunebaum M, Horodniceanu C, Wilunsky E, et al: Iatrogenic transmural perforation of the oesophagus in the preterm infant, *Clin Radiol* 31:257-261, 1980.
313. Azimi PH, Willert J, Petru A: Severe esophagitis in a newborn infant, *Pediatr Infect Dis J* 15:385, 1996.
314. Bittencourt AL: Congenital Chagas disease, *Am J Dis Child* 130: 97-103, 1976.
315. Walsh TJ, Belitsos NJ, Hamilton SR: Bacterial esophagitis in immunocompromised patients, *Arch Intern Med* 146:1345-1348, 1986.
316. Nelson AJ: Neonatal suppurative thyroiditis, *Pediatr Infect Dis* 2: 243-244, 1983.
317. Berner R, Schumacher RF, Zimmerhackl LB, et al: *Salmonella enteritidis* orchitis in a 10-week-old boy, *Acta Paediatr* 83:992-993, 1994.
318. Leake D, Leake R: Neonatal suppurative parotitis, *Pediatrics* 46: 202-207, 1970.
319. David RB, O'Connel EJ: Suppurative parotitis in children, *Am J Dis Child* 119:332-335, 1970.
320. Banks WW, Handler SD, Glade GB, et al: Neonatal submandibular sialadenitis, *Am J Otolaryngol* 1:261-263, 1980.
321. Saarinen M, Takala AK, Koskenniemi E, et al: Spectrum of 2,836 cases of invasive bacterial or fungal infections in children: results of prospective nationwide five-year surveillance in Finland. Finnish Pediatric Invasive Infection Study Group, *Clin Infect Dis* 21:1134-1144, 1995.
322. Eichenfield LF, Frieden IJ, Esterly NB: *Neonatal dermatology*, ed 2, Philadelphia, 2008, Saunders.
323. Swartz MN, Weinberg AN: Bacterial diseases with cutaneous involvement. In Fitzpatrick TB, editor: *Dermatology in general medicine*, New York, 1971, McGraw Hill.
324. Frieden IJ: Blisters and pustules in the newborn, *Curr Probl Pediatr* 19:549-614, 1989.
325. Weinberg S, Prose NS, Kristal L: *Color atlas of pediatric dermatology*, ed 4, New York, 2011, McGraw Hill.
326. Speert H: Circumcision of the newborn; an appraisal of its present status, *Obstet Gynecol* 2:164-172, 1953.
327. Annobil SH, al-Hilfi A, Kazi T: Primary tuberculosis of the penis in an infant, *Tubercle* 71:229-230, 1990.
328. Cleary TG, Kohl S: Overwhelming infection with group B beta-hemolytic *Streptococcus* associated with circumcision, *Pediatrics* 64: 301-303, 1979.
329. Annunziato D, Goldblum LM: Staphylococcal scalded skin syndrome. A complication of circumcision, *Am J Dis Child* 132:1187-1188, 1978.
330. Woodside JR: Necrotizing fasciitis after neonatal circumcision, *Am J Dis Child* 134:301-302, 1980.
331. Stranko J, Ryan ME, Bowman AM: Impetigo in newborn infants associated with a plastic bell clamp circumcision, *Pediatr Infect Dis* 5:597-599, 1986.
332. Siddiqi SF, Taylor PM: Necrotizing fasciitis of the scalp. A complication of fetal monitoring, *Am J Dis Child* 136:226-228, 1982.
333. Okada DM, Chow AW, Bruce VT: Neonatal scalp abscess and fetal monitoring: factors associated with infection, *Am J Obstet Gynecol* 129:185-189, 1977.
334. Cordero L, Anderson CW, Zuspan FP: Scalp abscess: a benign and infrequent complication of fetal monitoring, *Am J Obstet Gynecol* 146:126-130, 1983.
335. Wagener MM, Rycheck RR, Yee RB, et al: Septic dermatitis of the neonatal scalp and maternal endomyometritis with intrapartum internal fetal monitoring, *Pediatrics* 74:81-85, 1984.
336. Brook I, Frazier EH: Microbiology of scalp abscess in newborns, *Pediatr Infect Dis J* 11:766-768, 1992.
337. Bogdan JC, Rapkin RH: Clostridia infection in the newborn, *Pediatrics* 58:120-122, 1976.
338. Sarkany I, Gaylarde CC: Skin flora of the newborn, *Lancet* 1: 589-590, 1967.
339. Sarkany I, Arnold L: The effect of single and repeated applications of hexachlorophane on the bacterial flora of the skin of the newborn, *Br J Dermatol* 82:261-267, 1970.
340. Fortunov RM, Hulten KG, Hammerman WA, et al: Community-acquired *Staphylococcus aureus* infections in term and near-term previously healthy neonates, *Pediatrics* 118:874-881, 2006.
341. Zafar AB, Butler RC, Reese DJ, et al: Use of 0.3% triclosan (bacti-stat) to eradicate an outbreak of methicillin-resistant *Staphylococcus aureus* in a neonatal nursery, *Am J Infect Control* 23:200-208, 1995.
342. Thompson DJ, Gezon HM, Rogers KD, et al: Excess risk of staphylococcal infection and disease in newborn males, *Am J Epidemiol* 84:314-328, 1966.
343. Rudoy RC, Nelson JD: Breast abscess during the neonatal period. A review, *Am J Dis Child* 129:1031-1034, 1975.
344. Reboli AC, John JF Jr, Levkoff AH: Epidemic methicillin-gentamicin-resistant *Staphylococcus aureus* in a neonatal intensive care unit, *Am J Dis Child* 143:34-39, 1989.
345. Purcell K, Fergie J: Epidemic of community-acquired methicillin-resistant *Staphylococcus aureus* infections: a 14-year study at Driscoll Children's Hospital, *Arch Pediatr Adolesc Med* 159:980-985, 2005.
346. Evans HE, Akpata SO, Baki A, et al: Flora in newborn infants: annual variation in prevalence of *Staphylococcus aureus, Escherichia coli*, and streptococci, *Arch Environ Health* 26:275-276, 1973.
347. Starr HJ, Holliday PB Jr: Erythema multiforme as a manifestation of neonatal septicemia, *J Pediatr* 38:315-319, 1951.
348. Washington JL, Fowler RE, Guarino GJ: Erythema multiforme in a premature infant associated with sepsis due to *Pseudomonas, Pediatrics* 39:120-122, 1967.
349. Belgaumkar TK: Letter: Impetigo neonatorum congenita due to group B beta-hemolytic *Streptococcus* infection, *J Pediatr* 86:982-983, 1975.
350. Halal F, Delorme L, Brazeau M, et al: Congenital vesicular eruption caused by *Haemophilus influenzae* type b, *Pediatrics* 62:494-496, 1978.
351. Kline A, O'Donnell E: Group B streptococcus as a cause of neonatal bullous skin lesions, *Pediatr Infect Dis J* 12:165-166, 1993.
352. Bray DA: Ecthyma gangrenosum: full thickness nasal slough, *Arch Otolaryngol* 98:210-211, 1973.
353. Heffner RW, Smith GF: Ecthyma gangrenosum in *Pseudomonas* septicemia, *AMA J Dis Child* 99:524-528, 1960.
354. Basu S, Kumar A: Ecthyma gangrenosum in a premature low-birth-weight newborn, *J Wound Care* 20:587-589, 2011.
355. Pathak A, Singh P, Yadav Y, et al: Ecthyma gangrenosum in a neonate: not always *Pseudomonas, BMJ Case Rep* 27:2013, 2013. pii:bcr2013009287.
356. Baley JE, Silverman RA: Systemic candidiasis: cutaneous manifestations in low birth weight infants, *Pediatrics* 82:211-215, 1988.
357. Agarwal S, Sharma M, Mehndirata V: Solitary ecthyma gangrenosum (EG)-like lesion consequent to *Candida albicans* in a neonate, *Indian J Pediatr* 74:582-584, 2007.
358. Nakwan N, Wannaro J, Dissaneevate P, et al: Septicemia, meningitis, and skull osteomyelitis complicating infected cephalhematoma caused by ESBL-producing *Escherichia coli, Southeast Asian J Trop Med Public Health* 42:148-151, 2011.
359. Mohon RT, Mehalic TF, Grimes CK, et al: Infected cephalhematoma and neonatal osteomyelitis of the skull, *Pediatr Infect Dis* 5:253-256, 1986.
360. Cohen SM, Miller BW, Orris HW: Meningitis complicating cephalhematoma, *J Pediatr* 30:327-329, 1947.
361. Ellis SS, Montgomery JR, Wagner M, et al: Osteomyelitis complicating neonatal cephalhematoma, *Am J Dis Child* 127:100-102, 1974.
362. Walsh M, McIntosh K: Neonatal mastitis, *Clin Pediatr (Phila)* 25:395-399, 1986.
363. Brook I: The aerobic and anaerobic microbiology of neonatal breast abscess, *Pediatr Infect Dis J* 10:785-786, 1991.
364. Cushing AH: Omphalitis: a review, *Pediatr Infect Dis* 4:282-285, 1985.
365. McKenna H, Johnson D: Bacteria in neonatal omphalitis, *Pathology* 9:111-113, 1977.
366. Mason WH, Andrews R, Ross LA, et al: Omphalitis in the newborn infant, *Pediatr Infect Dis J* 8:521-525, 1989.
367. Geil CC, Castle WK, Mortimer EA Jr: Group A streptococcal infections in newborn nurseries, *Pediatrics* 46:849-854, 1970.
368. Pandey A, Gangopadhyay AN, Upadhyaya VD: Necrotising fasciitis in children and neonates: current concepts, *J Wound Care* 17:5-10, 2008.
369. Hsieh WS, Yang PH, Chao HC, et al: Neonatal necrotizing fasciitis: a report of three cases and review of the literature, *Pediatrics* 103:e53, 1999.

370. Goldberg GN, Hansen RC, Lynch PJ: Necrotizing fasciitis in infancy: report of three cases and review of the literature, *Pediatr Dermatol* 2:55-63, 1984.
371. Lang ME, Vaudry W, Robinson JL: Case report and literature review of late-onset group B streptococcal disease manifesting as necrotizing fasciitis in preterm infants: is this a new syndrome? *Clin Infect Dis* 37:e132-135, 2003.
372. Brook I: Microbiology of necrotizing fasciitis associated with omphalitis in the newborn infant, *J Perinatol* 18:28-30, 1998.
373. Arditi M, Yogev R: Perirectal abscess in infants and children: report of 52 cases and review of literature, *Pediatr Infect Dis J* 9:411-415, 1990.
374. Krieger RW, Chusid MJ: Perirectal abscess in childhood. A review of 29 cases, *Am J Dis Child* 133:411-412, 1979.
375. Victorin L: An epidemic of otitis in newborns due to infection with *Pseudomonas aeruginosa*, *Acta Paediatr Scand* 56:344-348, 1967.
376. LaVoo EJ, Paller AS: Common skin problems during the first year of life, *Pediatr Clin North Am* 41:1105-1119, 1994.
377. Glover MT, Atherton DJ, Levinsky RJ: Syndrome of erythroderma, failure to thrive, and diarrhea in infancy: a manifestation of immunodeficiency, *Pediatrics* 81:66-72, 1988.
378. Zeb A, Darmstadt GL: Sclerema neonatorum: a review of nomenclature, clinical presentation, histological features, differential diagnoses and management, *J Perinatol* 28:453-460, 2008.
379. Berk DR, Bayliss SJ: Milia: a review and classification, *J Am Acad Dermatol* 59:1050-1063, 2008.
380. Gordon I: Miliary sebaceous cysts and blisters in the healthy newborn, *Arch Dis Child* 24:286-288, 1949.
381. Morgan AJ, Steen CJ, Schwartz RA, et al: Erythema toxicum neonatorum revisited, *Cutis* 83:13-16, 2009.
382. Schwartz RA, Janniger CK: Erythema toxicum neonatorum, *Cutis* 58:153-155, 1996.
383. Merlob P, Metzker A, Reisner SH: Transient neonatal pustular melanosis, *Am J Dis Child* 136:521-522, 1982.
384. Lucky AW, McGuire JS: Infantile acropustulosis with eosinophilic pustules, *J Pediatr* 100:428-429, 1982.
385. Murphy WF, Langley AL: Common bullous lesions—presumably self-inflicted—occurring in utero in the newborn infant, *Pediatrics* 32:1099-1101, 1963.
386. Ravanfar P, Wallace JS, Pace NC: Diaper dermatitis: a review and update, *Curr Opin Pediatr* 24:472-479, 2012.
387. Erasala GN, Romain C, Merlay I: Diaper area and disposable diapers, *Curr Probl Dermatol* 40:83-89, 2011.
388. American Academy of Pediatrics: *American College of Obstetricians and Gynecologists: Guidelines for perinatal care*, ed 7, Chicago, 2013, American Academy of Pediatrics.
389. Gladstone IM, Clapper L, Thorp JW, et al: Randomized study of six umbilical cord care regimens. Comparing length of attachment, microbial control, and satisfaction, *Clin Pediatr (Phila)* 27:127-129, 1988.
390. Imdad A, Bautista RM, Senen KA, et al: Umbilical cord antiseptics for preventing sepsis and death among newborns, *Cochrane Database Syst Rev*, (5), CD008635, 2013.
391. Gezon HM, Schaberg MJ, Klein JO: Concurrent epidemics of *Staphylococcus aureus* and group A *Streptococcus* disease in a newborn nursery. Control with penicillin G and hexachlorophene bathing, *Pediatrics* 51:383-390, 1973.
392. Seeberg S, Brinkhoff B, John E, et al: Prevention and control of neonatal pyoderma with chlorhexidine, *Acta Paediatr Scand* 73:498-504, 1984.
393. de Toledo AR, Chandler JW: Conjunctivitis of the newborn, *Infect Dis Clin North Am* 6:807-813, 1992.
394. Whitcher JP: Neonatal ophthalmia: have we advanced in the last 20 years? *Int Ophthalmol Clin* 30:39-41, 1990.
395. Hedberg K, Ristinen TL, Soler JT, et al: Outbreak of erythromycin-resistant staphylococcal conjunctivitis in a newborn nursery, *Pediatr Infect Dis J* 9:268-273, 1990.
396. Prentice MJ, Hutchinson GR, Taylor-Robinsin D: A microbiological study of neonatal conjunctivae and conjunctivitis, *Br J Ophthalmol* 61:601-607, 1977.
397. Sandstrom KI, Bell TA, Chandler JW, et al: Microbial causes of neonatal conjunctivitis, *J Pediatr* 105:706-711, 1984.
398. Regev-Yochay G, Rubinstein E, Barzilai A, et al: Methicillin-resistant *Staphylococcus aureus* in neonatal intensive care unit, *Emerg Infect Dis* 11:453-456, 2005.
399. Rutar T: Vertically acquired community methicillin-resistant *Staphylococcus aureus* dacryocystitis in a neonate, *J AAPOS* 13:79-81, 2009.
400. Kim JH, Kim MK, Oh JY, et al: Outbreak of gram-positive bacterial keratitis associated with epidemic keratoconjunctivitis in neonates and infants, *Eye (Lond)* 23:1059-1065, 2009.
401. Stenson S, Newman R, Fedukowicz H: Conjunctivitis in the newborn: observations on incidence, cause, and prophylaxis, *Ann Ophthalmol* 13:329-334, 1981.
402. Burns RP, Rhodes DHJ: *Pseudomonas* eye infection as a cause of death in premature infants, *Arch Ophthalmol* 65:517-525, 1961.
403. Lohrer R, Belohradsky BH: Bacterial endophthalmitis in neonates, *Eur J Pediatr* 146:354-359, 1987.
404. Christensen GD, Korones SB, Reed L, et al: Epidemic *Serratia marcescens* in a neonatal intensive care unit: importance of the gastrointestinal tract as a reservoir, *Infect Control* 3:127-133, 1982.
405. Nishida H, Risemberg HM: Silver nitrate ophthalmic solution and chemical conjunctivities, *Pediatrics* 56:368-373, 1975.
406. Kripke SS, Golden B: Neonatal inclusion conjunctivitis. A report of three cases and a discussion of differential diagnosis and treatment, *Clin Pediatr (Phila)* 11:261-263, 1972.
407. Pickering LK, editor: *Red book: report of the Committee of Infectious Diseases*, Elk Grove Village, Ill, 2012, American Academy of Pediatrics.

11 Microorganisms Responsible for Neonatal Diarrhea

YALDA C. LUCERO, JORGE J. VELARDE, and MIGUEL L. O'RYAN

CHAPTER OUTLINE

Diarrheal disease continues to be a significant cause of morbidity and mortality in children worldwide in the 21st century. The World Health Organization (WHO) estimates about 2 billion cases and 1.9 million deaths yearly by acute diarrhea in children younger than 5 years. Most of these cases occur in infants from developing countries, mainly in Africa and Southeast Asia.[1] These estimates are a decrease from the more than 3 million annual deaths from diarrhea reported 20 years ago,[2] indicating progress in prevention and treatment of acute diarrhea.

Diarrheal disease is less frequent in newborns than in older infants and children, but a higher risk of complications and eventually death exists in this age group. A reduced incidence in newborns probably results from low exposure to enteropathogens and protection associated with breastfeeding.[3-6] Nevertheless, nearly 3 million newborns die every year, among whom 2.7% of deaths are associated with diarrhea.[7] These deaths are concentrated in countries with neonatal mortality rates of 30 or more per 1000 live births, mainly in Africa and Southeast Asia.[7,8] Higher risk of complications in neonatal diarrhea can be explained by a relative state of immunosuppression, inability to take fluids by themselves, and because most cases develop in hospitalized newborns with concomitant pathologies. For infants with very low birth weight (<1500 g), the death rate from diarrhea is 100-fold greater than for infants with higher birth weight.[9]

This chapter discusses the pathogenesis, diagnosis, treatment, and prevention of infectious gastroenteritis in newborns based on the available knowledge. Pathogens that rarely or never cause acute diarrhea in neonates are mentioned and discussed briefly. After an overview of host defense mechanisms and protective factors in human milk, the remainder of the chapter is devoted to specific pathogens that cause inflammatory or noninflammatory diarrhea.

Enteric Host Defense Mechanisms

The gastrointestinal (GI) tract is the first line of contact with a myriad of ingested antigens and microorganisms. Discrimination between potentially harmless and harmful antigens is essential to maintain GI homeostasis. The mechanisms, cells, and molecules involved in microorganism-intestinal interactions are numerous, increasingly complex, and only partially understood. A complete review of this topic is beyond the scope of this chapter, and thus a general view of the main aspects of host defense will be provided.

Components of the enteric immune system include both cells and molecules representing the innate and adaptive immune system. Innate immunity in the GI tract comprises the epithelial barrier, intraepithelial lymphocytes, gastric acidity, mucous layer, antimicrobial peptides, dendritic cells, and macrophages.[10-13] GI adaptive immunity is represented by different lineages of antigen-specific lymphocytes, including B cells, Th1 cells, Th2 cells, Th17 cells, and regulatory T cells.[12,14,15]

It is generally accepted that although most of the constituents required for an intestinal immune response against microorganisms are present in the neonatal gut at birth, they are "immature," principally because neonates have had contact with only few antigens and have not had the opportunity to develop local or systemic immune responses. The amniotic fluid may contain bacteria capable of colonizing the GI tract of the neonate after ingestion.[16] Bacterial DNA has been isolated in meconium of preterm newborns.[17,18] However, this phenomenon seems to be insufficient to robustly prime the GI immune system.

Newborns acquire commensal microorganisms from their surroundings immediately after birth. During delivery, newborns are colonized by multiple strains belonging to the maternal microbiota: after vaginal birth by maternal vaginal and intestinal microbiota (predominantly Lactobacillaceae, Bifidobacteriaceae, Bacterioidaceae, and Enterobacteriaceae) and after cesarean section by maternal skin microbiota (mainly Clostridiaceae, Pseudomonadaceae, and Staphylococcaceae).[19-21] Feeding patterns (human milk vs. milk formula) also influence the microbiota.[21] The establishment of a predetermined intestinal microbiota at birth can influence the correct ontogenesis of gut barrier, as well as motor and immune functions, through a complex neuroendocrine crosstalk.[13] The consequences of alterations in both the acquisition or composition of commensal bacterial communities may contribute to GI diseases in the future, such as food allergy, food intolerance, and inflammatory bowel disease.[13,22]

The gastric acid barrier seems to be at its lowest level of effectiveness during the first months of life. The average gastric pH level of the newborn is high (pH 4 to 7, mean 6).[23,24] Although the pH falls to low levels by the end of the first day of life (pH 2-3),[23] it subsequently rises again; by 7 to 10 days of life, the hydrochloric acid output of the neonatal stomach is far less than that of older infants and children.[24,25] The buffering action of frequent milk feedings and the short gastric emptying time[26-29] introduce additional factors in the neonate that likely allow viable ingested organisms to reach the small intestine.

The intestinal epithelium is much more than a mechanical barrier. It also serves as a nutrient absorptive machine, a regulator of antigen presentation and inflammation, and is critical in maintaining immune homeostasis of the gut.[30,31] Intestinal epithelial cells have receptors, including Toll-like receptors (TLR), for bacterial products and molecular patterns and produce chemokines (e.g., interleukin-8 (IL-8), monocyte chemotactic protein type 1, granulocyte-macrophage colony-stimulating factor), and proinflammatory cytokines (e.g., IL-6, tumor necrosis factor-α, IL-1) in response to invasion by enteropathogens. As a consequence, the gut epithelium orchestrates the immune response.[30,31] The thick mucin-rich glycocalix surrounded by mucus forms a physical barrier embedded with antimicrobial peptides and enzymes.[13] The different composition of adult and neonatal glycocalix may influence susceptibility to GI colonization and infection.[13] Paneth cells in crypts also express TLRs that can be activated by microorganisms, leading to the release of potent antimicrobial agents including lysozyme and cryptidins.[32]

The neonatal T-cell response is predominantly Th2, favoring antibody adaptive responses with an increased potential for hypersensitivity. B-lymphocyte and T-lymphocyte functions are skewed to preferential immunoglobulin M (IgM) production, instead of the more efficient secretory IgA production, in response to antigenic stimulation. IgG is actively transferred from mother to infant across the placenta beginning at about 32 weeks of gestation and peaks by about 37 weeks. Premature neonates, especially infants born before 28 weeks of gestation, are deficient in these maternally derived serum antibodies and cannot secrete IgA.[13,32,33]

Protective Factors in Human Milk

The importance of breastfeeding in the prevention of diarrheal disease has been extensively studied.[34-42] Published studies reporting an association between breastfeeding and diarrhea suggest that infants who are breastfed have fewer and milder episodes of diarrhea than infants who are formula fed. This protection is greatest during the first 3 months of life and declines progressively with increasing age. Partial breastfeeding during weaning confers intermediate protection somewhere in between that provided by exclusive breastfeeding and exclusive formula-feeding.

More than 50 years ago, Mata and Urrutia[43,44] provided a striking demonstration of the protection afforded by breastfeeding in newborns born in a rural Guatemalan village. Despite extremely poor sanitation conditions, accompanied by the demonstration that fecal organisms were present in the colostrum and milk of almost one third of mothers, diarrheal disease did not occur in any of the newborns. The incidence of diarrhea increased significantly only after these infants reached 4 to 6 months of age, when solid food and other fluids were used to supplement human milk. *Escherichia coli* and gram-negative anaerobes (e.g., *Bacteroides* spp.) were found to colonize the intestinal tract during this age period.[43] In contrast, urban infants of a similar ethnic background who were partly or totally artificially fed frequently acquired diarrheal disease caused by enteropathogenic *E. coli* (EPEC). Protection against diarrhea afforded by breastfeeding during the first months of life has also been observed in more industrialized societies such as the United Kingdom.[45] A recent meta-analysis reported a significant benefit of breastfeeding—protecting against morbidity and mortality resulting from acute diarrhea in infants. Specifically, lack of breastfeeding resulted in a relative risk (RR) of 10.5 for diarrhea mortality compared with exclusive breastfeeding among infants 0 to 5 months of age, and a RR of 2.18 compared with any breastfeeding among children aged 6 to 23 months.[42]

Multiple mechanisms by which breastfeeding protects against diarrhea have been postulated. Breastfeeding confers protection by active components in milk and by decreased exposure to organisms present on or in contaminated bottles, food, or water. Many protective components have been identified in human milk and generally are classified as belonging to the major categories of immune cells, antibodies, glycoconjugates, and antiinflammatory factors.[13,46-49]

For any given pathogen, multiple breast-milk factors may help protect the infant. Redundancy of milk protective factors and targeting of complex virulence machinery together create a formidable barrier to enteropathogens. Despite the fact that pathogens can rapidly replicate and mutate, milk continues to protect infants. As an example, human milk has secretory antibodies to *Shigella* virulence antigens and lipopolysaccharides (LPSs).[50,51] Neutral glycolipid Gb3 binds to Shiga toxin.[52,53] and lactoferrin chelates iron, making it unavailable for bacterial metabolism. These antibodies disrupt and degrade the surface-expressed virulence antigens and stimulate phagocytosis.[54-56] Lysozyme in human milk breaks β1,4 bonds between *N*-acetylmuramic acid and *N*-acetylglucosamine, a critical linkage in the peptidoglycans of bacterial cell walls.[13]

The protective effect of human milk antibodies against enteropathogen-specific disease has been described for enteropathogenic *E. coli*,[57] *Vibrio cholerae*,[58] *Campylobacter jejuni*,[59] enterotoxigenic *E. coli* (ETEC),[60] *Shigella* spp.,[50] and *Giardia lamblia*.[61]

In 1960, Montreuil and Mullet[62] determined that oligosaccharides constituted 2.4% of colostrum and 1.3% of mature milk. Only water, lactose, and lipids are present in greater amounts than oligosaccharides. Human milk contains a larger quantity of oligosaccharides than milk from other mammals, and its composition is singularly complex.[63] Despite the fact that substantial energy must be expended by the mother to synthesize the many hundreds of different milk oligosaccharides, the infant does not use them as food. Most of the oligosaccharides pass through the gut undigested.[64,65] Oligosaccharides in breast milk can participate as prebiotics for beneficial microbiota and as decoy receptors, interfering with the attachment of enteric pathogens (virus and bacteria) and toxins.[6,13,66-69] Glycoconjugates contribute to initiate and maintain the growth of *Bifidobacterium* spp. and low pH in the feces of newborn infants, creating an environment antagonistic to the growth of *E. coli*. Human milk oligosaccharides also inhibit leukocyte endothelial adhesion and help explain the low rate of inflammatory disorders in breastfed infants.[70]

In vitro and in vivo assays have demonstrated that lactadherin present in human milk binds rotavirus, inhibits viral replication, and protects against symptomatic infection.[71] Free fatty acids and monoglyceride products of lingual and gastric lipase activity in human milk triglycerides may have antiviral and antiparasitic activity.[13]

Bacterial Pathogens

ESCHERICHIA COLI

E. coli are gram-negative bacilli that promptly colonize the lower intestinal tracts of healthy infants in the first few days of life[72-75] and constitute the predominant aerobic coliform fecal flora throughout life in humans and in many animals. The concept that this species might cause enteric disease was first suggested in the late 19th and early 20th centuries, when several veterinary workers described the association of diarrhea (i.e., scours) in newborn calves infected with certain strains of *E. coli*.[76-81]

In 1905, Moro[82] observed that *Bacterium* (now *Escherichia*) *coli* was found more often in the small intestines of children with diarrhea than in children without diarrhea. Adam[82,83] confirmed these findings and noted the similarity with Asiatic cholera and calf scours. He extended these observations further by suggesting that *E. coli* strains from patients with diarrhea could be distinguished from normal coliform flora by certain sugar fermentation patterns. Although Adam called these disease-producing organisms "dyspepsicoli" and introduced the important concept that *E. coli* could cause enteric disease, biochemical reactions have not proved to be a reliable means of distinguishing nonpathogenic from pathogenic *E. coli* strains. There are now at least six recognized enteric pathotypes of *E. coli*.[84] The pathotypes can be distinguished clinically, epidemiologically, and pathogenetically (Table 11-1).[84-91]

ETEC organisms are defined by their ability to secrete heat-labile (LT) or heat-stabile (ST) enterotoxin, or both.[92,93] LT is closely related to cholera toxin and similarly acts by means of intestinal adenylate cyclase,[94,95] prostaglandin synthesis,[96,97] and possibly platelet-activating factor.[98,99] ST (particularly the variant STa) causes secretion by specifically activating intestinal mucosal guanylate

Table 11-1 Predominant Serogroups, Mechanisms, and Gene Codes Associated with Enterotoxigenic, Enteroinvasive, Enteropathogenic, Enterohemorrhagic, and Enteroaggregative *Escherichia coli*

ETEC	EIEC	EPEC	EHEC	EAEC
SEROGROUPS				
Tremendous variablity, multiple serogroups	O28ac, O29, O112, O115, O124, O136, O143, O144, O147, O152, O164, O167	Typical: O55, O111, O119, O26, O86, O114, O125, O126, O127, O128, O142, O158 Atypical: Serogroups above and many more	O157 (including O157:H7), O26, O128, O103, O39, O91, O111, O113, O121, O145, O103, O138, rough, many others	O3, O44, O78, O15, O77, O51, O104, many others
MECHANISMS				
Adenylate or guanylate cyclase activation	Colonic invasiveness (e.g., *Shigella*)	Localized attachment and effacement	Shiga toxins block protein synthesis; attachment and effacement	Aggregative adherence and toxins
GENE CODES				
Plasmid	Chromosomal and plasmid	Chromosomal and plasmid	Chromosomal and phage	Chromosomal and plasmid

EAEC, Enteroaggregative E. coli; EHEC, enterohemorrhagic E. coli; EIEC, enteroinvasive E. coli; EPEC, enteropathogenic E. coli; ETEC, enterotoxigenic E. coli.

cyclase.[100-102] STb toxin stimulates noncyclic, nucleotide-mediated bicarbonate secretion and seems to be important only in animals.[103-105] Enteroinvasive *E. coli* (EIEC) has the capacity to invade the intestinal mucosa, causing inflammatory enteritis similar to shigellosis.[106-108] EPEC pathogenesis is characterized by a signal transduction mechanism,[84-90,109,110] which is accompanied by a characteristic attaching-and-effacing (A/E) histopathologic lesion in the small intestine.[93,111] Enterohemorrhagic *E. coli* (EHEC) also induces an A/E lesion, but in the colon.[84,92,93] EHEC secretes Shiga toxin, which gives rise to the dangerous sequela of hemolytic-uremic syndrome (HUS). Enteroaggregative *E. coli* (EAEC) adheres to the intestinal mucosa and elaborates enterotoxins and cytotoxins.[84,91,93,112]

A major problem in the recognition of ETEC, EIEC, EPEC, and EHEC strains of *E. coli* is that they are indistinguishable from normal coliform flora of the intestinal tract by the usual bacteriologic methods. Serotyping is valuable in recognizing typical EPEC serotypes[113,114] and EIEC because these organisms tend to fall into a few specific serogroups (see Table 11-1).[115,116] The ability of organisms to produce enterotoxins (LT or ST) is encoded by a transmissible plasmid that can be lost by one strain of *E. coli* or transferred to a previously unrecognized strain.[117-119] Although the enterotoxin plasmids seem to prefer certain serogroups (different from EPEC or invasive serogroups),[120] ETEC is not expected to be strictly limited to a particular set of serogroups. Instead, such strains can only be recognized by identifying production of the enterotoxins or presence of the encoding genes. Enterotoxins can be assayed in ligated animal loops,[121] in tissue culture,[122,123] or by enzyme-linked immunosorbent assay (ELISA)[124] for LT, or in a suckling mouse model for ST.[125,126] Specific DNA probes and, more important, polymerase chain reaction (PCR) assays are available to detect LT and ST genes.[84-86,127] The various *E. coli* pathotypes are generally associated with a broad array of primary and accessory virulence factors, as discussed subsequently[128-130]; additional pathotypes have been suggested based on unique virulence mechanisms but have not yet been widely adopted.[93]

Enterotoxigenic *Escherichia coli*

Nature of the Organism. Although early work on the recognition of *E. coli* as a potential enteric pathogen focused on biochemical or serologic distinctions, there followed a shift in emphasis to the enterotoxins produced by previously recognized and entirely "new" strains of *E. coli*. Beginning in the mid-1950s, with work by De and colleagues[131,132] in Calcutta, *E. coli* strains from patients with diarrhea were found to cause a fluid secretory response in ligated rabbit ileal loops, analogous to that seen with *Vibrio cholerae*. Work by Taylor and associates[133,134] showed that the viable *E. coli* strains did not always produce this secretory response and that enterotoxin production correlated poorly with classically recognized EPEC serotypes. In São Paulo, Trabulsi[135] made similar observations with *E. coli* isolated from children with diarrhea, and several veterinary workers showed that ETEC was associated with diarrhea in piglets and calves.[136-139] A similar pattern was described in 1971, when *E. coli* strains were isolated from upper small bowel samples of adults with acute undifferentiated diarrhea in Bengal.[140,141] Such strains of *E. coli* produced a heat-labile nondialyzable ammonium sulfate–precipitable enterotoxin.[142] Analogous to the usually short-lived diarrheal illnesses of *E. coli* reported by several workers, a short-lived course of the secretory response to *E. coli* culture filtrates was described.[143] Similar to responses to cholera toxin, secretory responses to *E. coli* were associated with activation of intestinal mucosal adenylate cyclase that paralleled the fluid secretory response.[144,145]

Virulence Factors and Pathogenic Mechanisms. The two types of enterotoxins produced by enterotoxigenic *E. coli*[146-148] have been found to be plasmid-encoded but genetically unlinked. The effects of LT follow a lag period required by its intracellular site of action.[94,95,122] LT is internalized into target epithelial cells by retrograde vesicular transport. Once inside the cytoplasm, the toxin acts by adenosine diphosphate ribosylation of the $G_{s\alpha}$ signaling protein.[84,94] The resulting activation of adenylate cyclase leads to accumulation of cyclic adenosine monophosphate (cAMP), which activates the cystic fibrosis transmembrane conductance regulator(CFTR) chloride channel and inhibits sodium reabsorption by the Na^+/H^+ exchanger 3 (NHE3), leading to a net secretion of electrolytes and water.[149] The antigenic similarity of LT and cholera toxin and their apparent binding to the monosialoganglioside GM_1 have enabled the development of ELISAs for detection of LT and cholera toxin.[126,150-152] ST causes an immediate and reversible secretory response.[121] It is a much smaller molecule and is distinct antigenically from LT and cholera toxin.[122,125,126] ST increases intracellular intestinal mucosal cyclic guanosine monophosphate (cGMP) concentrations and specifically activates apical plasma membrane–associated intestinal guanylate cyclase.[100-102] An increase in cGMP leads to activation of the CFTR and inhibition of phosphodiesterase 3, which results in increased concentrations of cAMP.[149] The sum effect for LT is net secretion of electrolytes and water. The receptor for STa responds to an endogenous ligand called guanylin, of which STa is a structural homologue.[153] Both LT and ST may additionally exert some effects on the enteric nervous system that contribute to diarrhea.[149] Because the capacity to produce an enterotoxin may be transmissible between different organisms by a plasmid or even a bacteriophage,[117-119] interstrain gene transfer is likely to be responsible for occasional toxigenic non–*E. coli*. Enterotoxigenic *Klebsiella* and *Citrobacter* strains have been associated with diarrhea in a few reports, often in patients coinfected with ETEC.[154,155]

The plasmids encoding LT and ST also encode the colonization factor antigens (CFAs), adhesins required for intestinal colonization, and the regulator that controls CFA expression.[117-119,156] At least 25 CFAs have been described for human *E. coli* isolates,[84,157-159] against which local IgA antibody may be produced. CFAs are proteinaceous hairlike fimbriae on the bacterial surface that serve as a bridge between the bacterium and the epithelial membrane. Despite the number of CFAs described, a few appear to be most common, including CFA/1, CS1, CS2, CS3, CS4, CS5, CS6, CS7, CS14, CS17, and CS21.[159,160]

The contribution of additional virulence factors to ETEC pathogenesis continues to be investigated. For example, recently, an adhesin found at the tip of the ETEC flagella, EtpA, was found to be important for initial binding to the epithelial cell surface.[161-163] EtpA may be useful in vaccine development as an immunoreactive antigen inducing protective immunity.[161]

Epidemiology and Transmission. ETEC are important diarrheal pathogens among infants in developing countries, predominantly affecting children younger than 2 years,[160,164] This pathogen is estimated to cause 200 million episodes of diarrhea and between 170,000 and 380,000 deaths yearly.[165] Breastfeeding seems to provide some protection to infants. One study from Mexico suggested that breast milk with high LT-ETEC–specific antibodies reduced symptomatic infections by up to 90%.[166] A study in Bangladesh found a relative risk of 0.51 for ETEC-associated diarrhea among infants exclusively breastfed.[167] This effect seems to decrease when additional foods are introduced.[160,168] ETEC have also been recognized among adults with endemic, cholera-like diarrhea in Calcutta, India, and in Dacca, Bangladesh,[94,140] and among travelers to areas such as Central and South America, Africa, and South Asia, although rates in Southeast Asia are significantly lower.[169-173]

The isolation of ETEC is uncommon in sporadic diarrheal illnesses in temperate climates where sanitation facilities are good and where winter viral patterns of diarrhea predominate. ETEC is commonly isolated from infants and children with acute watery summer diarrhea in areas where sanitary facilities are suboptimal,[154,171,174-186] such as Africa,[154] Brazil,[171,178,183,184,187] Argentina,[176] Bengal,[179,180] Mexico,[186] and Native American reservations in the southwestern United States.[181,185] In a multicenter study of acute diarrhea in 3640 infants and children in China, India, Mexico, Myanmar, and Pakistan, 16% of cases had ETEC compared with 5% among 3279 control subjects.[177] A case-control study from northwestern Spain showed a highly significant association of ETEC with neonatal diarrhea (26.5% positivity), often acquired in the hospital.[182] A study conducted at seven sites in Africa and Asia found ETEC to be the most common bacterial pathogen overall in infants younger than 12 months with diarrhea, although the attributable fraction varied by site. The study also noted that the incidence of diarrhea attributed to ETEC decreased with age at all sites.[188] ETEC constitute a major cause of dehydrating diarrhea in infants and young children in these areas.[160,164] Peaks of illnesses tend to occur in the summer or rainy season, and dehydrating illnesses may be life threatening, especially in infants and young children.[160,164,174,178,184] Humans are probably the major reservoirs for the human strains of ETEC, and contaminated food and water constitute the principal vectors.[189,190]

The association of ETEC with outbreaks of diarrhea in newborn nurseries has been documented. Ryder and colleagues[191] isolated ST-producing *E. coli* from 72% of infants with diarrhea, from the environment, and in one instance from an infant's formula during a 7-month period in a prolonged outbreak in a special-care nursery in Texas. Another ST-producing *E. coli* outbreak was reported in 1976 by Gross and associates[192] from a maternity hospital in Scotland.

Clinical Manifestations. The clinical manifestations of ETEC diarrhea tend to be mild and self-limited except in small or undernourished infants, in whom dehydration may be severe and constitute a major threat to life.[193] In many parts of the developing world, acute diarrheal illnesses are the leading recognized causes of death. There is some suggestion that diarrheal illnesses associated with ST-producing ETEC may be more severe than LT-ETEC.[179,194,195] Probably the best definition of the clinical manifestations of ETEC infection comes from volunteer studies with adults. In a recent review that identified 27 studies with doses of 10^8 to 10^{10} ETEC organisms, symptoms included diarrhea, abdominal pain, nausea, headache, and low-grade fever; symptoms were dependent on ETEC strain and dose. Vomiting was less common, occurring after challenge with a few selected strains tested. Incubation periods ranged from 6.8 to 50 hours.[195] Although illness usually resolves spontaneously within 3 to 5 days, it occasionally may persist for 1 week or longer.[160,194] Diarrhea is noninflammatory, without fecal leukocytes or blood.[160] A study in Spain, including children younger than 3 years with ETEC, of whom 9 of 19 were infants younger than 1 month of age, reported 94.7% of children with diarrhea, 31.6% with fever, 63.7% with vomiting, and 42.1% with dehydration.[182] During outbreaks affecting infants and neonates, diarrhea duration has been similar, with a mean of approximately 4 days.[191]

Pathology. As in cholera, the pathologic changes associated with ETEC infection are minimal. From animal experiments in which intestinal loops were infected with these organisms, and at a time when the secretory and adenylate cyclase responses were present, there was only a mild discharge of mucus from goblet cells and otherwise no significant pathologic change in the intestinal tract.[95] Unless terminal complications associated with severe hypotension occur, ETEC organisms rarely disseminate beyond the intestinal tract. Similar to *V. cholerae*, ETEC infection is exclusively intraluminal.[160]

Diagnosis. The preliminary diagnosis of ETEC diarrhea can be suspected by the epidemiologic setting and the noninflammatory nature of stool specimens, which reveal few or no leukocytes. ETEC serotypes vary tremendously, and serology is not typically used for diagnosis.[160] The traditional diagnosis of ETEC relies on enterotoxin detection by bioassays, such as tissue culture or ileal loop assays for LT, or the suckling mouse assay for ST; ELISA methods are available for detection of both LT and ST.[196]

More recently, detection of enterotoxin-encoding genes has superseded detection of the toxins themselves. Gene probes and PCR technologies are available.[85,86,127,196] The presence of *E. coli* genes encoding enterotoxins in patients with diarrhea is generally considered diagnostic, although asymptomatic carriage is known to occur.[160] In epidemiologic studies, it is common to test only three colonies per stool for the presence of ETEC, but it is generally considered that testing additional colonies increases diagnostic sensitivity.[190,197,198]

Therapy and Prevention. The cornerstone of treatment for any diarrheal infection is rehydration.[199] This principle especially pertains to ETEC diarrhea, which is an intraluminal infection with high output of fluid and electrolytes. The glucose absorptive mechanism remains intact in *E. coli* enterotoxin–induced secretion, much as it does in cholera, a concept that has resulted in the major advance of oral glucose–electrolyte therapy. This regimen can usually provide fully adequate rehydration in infants and children capable of tolerating oral fluids, replacing the need for parenteral rehydration in most cases.[200,201] Use of oral glucose–electrolyte therapy is particularly critical in rural areas and developing nations, where early application before dehydration becomes severe may be lifesaving. The current recommended WHO solution contains 2.6 g of sodium chloride, 1.5 g of potassium chloride, 2.9 g of trisodium citrate dihydrate (or 2.5 g sodium bicarbonate), and 20 g of glucose per 1 L of clean or boiled drinking water.[199,202,203] This corresponds to the following concentrations: 75 mmol/L of sodium, 20 mmol/L of potassium, 10 mmol/L of citrate, 65 mmol/L of chloride, and 75 mmol/L of glucose. In a multicenter trial involving 447 children in four countries, a reduced osmolality solution, compared with recommendations before 2002, was found to reduce stool output by 28% and illness duration by 18%.[204] A Cochrane review also found that an oral rehydration solution (ORS) with a total osmolarity of 250 mmol/L or less resulted in decreased stool volume and decreased vomiting.[205] Various recipes for homemade preparations have been described,[203] but unless the cost is prohibitive, the premade standard solution is preferred. Parenteral fluids should be used in cases with severe dehydration and/or if ORS is not tolerated. Zinc supplementation improves outcomes in patients with diarrhea living in resource-limited regions.[203,206,207]

The role of antimicrobial agents in the treatment or prevention of ETEC is controversial. This infection usually resolves within 3 to 5 days in the absence of antibacterial therapy.[199] There is concern about the potential for coexistence of enterotoxigenicity and antibiotic resistance on the same plasmid, and cotransfer of multiple antibiotic resistance and enterotoxigenicity has been well documented.[208] Prophylaxis is not recommended except in specific situations for prevention of traveler's diarrhea.[209] When antibiotic therapy is considered, cefixime, azithromycin, rifaximin, and, in adults, ciprofloxacin are recommended,[199,210,211] emphasizing, although, that in infants, antimicrobials are not routinely recommended.

The prevention and control of ETEC infections are similar to those discussed later for EPEC. Breastfeeding should be encouraged. Vaccine development for the different *E. coli* pathovars has been mostly studied for ETEC. Most promising was a candidate including a mixture of five formalin-inactivated strains expressing different CFAs mixed with recombinant B subunit of cholera toxin (CTb).[212,213] Unfortunately, in a study among Egyptian children, it was not efficacious in preventing ETEC diarrhea.[214] Investigators are now working on increasing the expression of CFAs in this construct and using a hybrid of LT and cholera toxin with the hope of increasing antigenicity and achieving better protective efficacy.[215,216] Other approaches have included an LT toxoid dermal patch and the use of attenuated *Shigella* vectors.[214] A recent Cochrane review concluded that there was insufficient evidence for a benefit from any current vaccine, and thus no current vaccine recommendation can be made.[217] Research is ongoing.

Enteroinvasive *Escherichia coli*

Virulence factors and pathogenic mechanisms. Enteroinvasive *E. coli* is similar genetically, pathogenetically, epidemiologically, and clinically to shigellosis, although the clinical syndrome associated with EIEC may be milder. EIEC causes diarrhea by means of *Shigella*-like intestinal epithelial invasion (discussed later).[84,106-108] The somatic antigens of these invasive strains have been identified and seem to fall into a few recognized O groups (see Table 11-1). Most, if not all, of these bacteria share cell wall antigens with various *Shigella* serotypes and react with antisera against cross-reacting antigen.[107] Not all strains of *E. coli* belonging to the serogroups associated with dysentery-like illness are pathogenic because a large (140 MDa) invasive plasmid designated pINV is also required.[218] Additional biologic tests, including the guinea pig conjunctivitis test (Sereny),[106] gene probes for the pINV plasmid,[84] or PCR diagnosis for virulence factors (IpaH, which also detects *Shigella* spp.)[219,220] are used to confirm the property of invasiveness.

Epidemiology and Transmission. Little is known about the epidemiology and transmission of this organism in newborns and infants; it is more frequently found in children older than 2 years.[221] Investigations in children with diarrhea often yield a low prevalence of EIEC,[222-226] although this can vary by geographic area.[227-230] The pathogen is often associated with outbreaks, and transmission is mostly food- or waterborne.[107] Studies of adult volunteers suggest that attack rates may be lower even after ingestion of inoculums larger than those required to develop *Shigella*-associated disease. Expression of virulence factors may be decreased in EIEC compared with *Shigella*.[231]

Clinical Manifestations. Symptoms often include watery diarrhea, although a dysentery-like syndrome with an inflammatory exudate in stool, invasion and disruption of colonic mucosa has been well described.[84,107]

Descriptions of extensive and severe ileocolitis in infants dying with *E. coli* diarrhea indicate that neonatal disease also can be caused by invasive strains capable of mimicking the pathologic features of shigellosis.[232] The immunofluorescent demonstration of *E. coli* together with an acute inflammatory infiltrate[233] in the intestinal tissue of infants tends to support this impression, although it has been suggested that the organisms may have invaded the bowel wall in the postmortem period.[106] Direct evidence for a pathogenic role of invasive strains of *E. coli* as a cause of neonatal diarrhea is currently lacking.[171] The infrequency with which newborns manifest a dysentery-like syndrome makes it unlikely that this pathogen is responsible for a significant proportion of the diarrheal disease that occurs during the first month of life.

Diagnosis. Enteroinvasive *E. coli* should be suspected in infants who have an inflammatory diarrhea, as evidenced by fecal neutrophils or bloody dysenteric syndromes from which no other invasive pathogens, such as *Campylobacter*, *Shigella*, *Salmonella*, *Vibrio*, or *Yersinia*, can be isolated. In this instance, it may be appropriate to have the fecal *E. coli* isolated and serotyped or tested for invasiveness in the Sereny test and/or for identification of pINV with genetic probes or by nucleic acid amplification techniques.[84]

Therapy and Prevention. The management and prevention of EIEC diarrhea should be similar to that of acute

Shigella or other *E. coli* enteric infections. Ampicillin has been used in adults, but increasing rates of antibiotic resistance have been documented.[106]

Enteropathogenic *Escherichia coli*

Typical EPEC has been a classic cause of severe infant diarrhea in industrialized countries, although its incidence has decreased dramatically in recent years. The serologic distinction of *E. coli* strains associated with epidemic and sporadic infantile diarrhea was first suggested by Goldschmidt[234] in 1933 and confirmed by Dulaney and Michelson[235] in 1935. These researchers found that certain strains of *E. coli* associated with institutional outbreaks of diarrhea would agglutinate with sera from diarrhea patients in other outbreaks. In 1943, Bray[236] isolated a serologically homogeneous strain of *E. coli* (subsequently identified as serogroup O111) from 95% of infants with summer diarrhea in England. He subsequently summarized a larger experience with this organism, isolated from only 4% of asymptomatic control subjects but from 88% of infants with diarrhea, one half of which were hospital-acquired.[237] This strain (initially called *E. coli-gomez* by Varela in 1946) also was associated with infantile diarrhea in Mexico.[238]

An elaborate serotyping system for certain *E. coli* strains that were clearly associated with infantile diarrhea developed from this early work primarily with epidemic diarrhea in infants.[239-241] These strains were first named enteropathogenic *E. coli* by Neter and colleagues[242] in 1955, and the association with particular serotypes can still be observed.[243]

Epidemiology and Transmission. Based on the molecular identification of two virulence factors, EPEC is now classified as either typical, usually associated with classic serotypes, or atypical, which includes a greater diversity of serotypes harboring the characteristic virulence factor. The presence of *eaeA*, the intimin gene, is a genetic determinant for the EPEC pathotype. Typical EPEC (tEPEC) strains also harbor a functional *bfp*A gene, which encodes a bundle-forming pilus (BFP), whereas this is absent in atypical EPEC (aEPEC).[114]

Historically, tEPEC have been an important cause of diarrhea in infants in both industrialized and developing countries.[84,113,244,245] However, more recently, outbreaks have become rare.[246] It is unclear why there has been a decrease in the incidence of tEPEC. Some have attributed the change to an increase in breastfeeding, which is thought to be protective. Alternatively, our current diagnostic methods and definition of EPEC rely less heavily on serology but rather on molecular characteristics. Strains diagnosed as EPEC in earlier studies may not have been pathogenic. Noteworthy are the results of the recent comprehensive Global Enteric Multicenter Study (GEMS) performed in seven sites in Africa, India, Pakistan, and Bangladesh, in which infants 0 to 11 months of age had a 2.6-fold increased risk of death 60 days after the diarrheal episode if their presenting diarrhea was associated with typical EPEC infection.[188] The actual cause of death in these children although was unknown.

Socioeconomic conditions play a significant role in determining the incidence of this disease in different populations.[247] It is unusual for newborn infants born in a rural environment to manifest diarrheal disease caused by EPEC; most infections of the GI tract in these infants occur after the first 6 months of life.[44,248] When living conditions are poor and overcrowding of susceptible infants exists, there is an increase in the incidence of neonatal diarrhea in general[249] and EPEC gastroenteritis in particular.[250-252]

Newborns can acquire typical EPEC during the first days of life by one of several routes: (1) organisms from the mother ingested at the time of birth; (2) bacteria from other infants or toddlers with diarrheal disease or from asymptomatic adults colonized with the organism, commonly transmitted on the hands of nursery personnel or parents in close and prolonged contact with the infant; (3) airborne or droplet infection; (4) fomites; or (5) organisms present in formulas or solid food supplements.[253] Only the first two routes have been shown conclusively to be of significance in the transmission of disease or the propagation of epidemics. The contours of the epidemiologic curves in nursery[251,254-259] and community[251,260,261] outbreaks are in keeping with a contact mode of spread. Transmission of organisms from infant to infant occurs by the fecal-oral route in almost all cases, most likely via the hands of individuals attending to their care.[73,257,259,262] Ill infants represent the greatest risk to individuals around them because of the large numbers of organisms found in their stools[263-266] and vomitus.[267-269] Cross-infection has also been initiated by infants who were healthy at the time of nursery admission.[254,264,270-272] A respiratory mode of transmission has been suggested but not proven.[251]

Historically, studies into the epidemiology of classic EPEC serotypes have dealt with events that occurred during outbreaks in newborn nurseries. Investigations of this sort frequently regard the epidemic as an isolated phenomenon and ignore the strong interdependence that exists between community-acquired and hospital-acquired illness.[272-274] The direction of spread is most often from the reservoir of disease within the community to the hospital. When the original source of a nursery outbreak can be established, frequently it turns out to be an infant born of a carrier mother who recently acquired EPEC infection from a toddler living in the home. Cross-infection epidemics also can be initiated by infected newborns that have been admitted directly into a clean nursery unit from the surrounding district[262,264,275] or have been transferred from a nearby hospital.[270,272,276]

After a nursery epidemic has begun, it generally follows one of two major patterns. Some epidemics are explosive, with rapid involvement of all susceptible infants and a duration that seldom exceeds 2 or 3 months.[254,255,267,277] The case-fatality rate in these epidemics may be very high. Other nursery outbreaks have an insidious onset with a few mild, unrecognized cases; the patients may not even develop illness until after discharge from the hospital. During the next few days to weeks, neonates with an increased number of loose stools are reported by the nurses; shortly thereafter, the appearance of the first severely ill infants makes it apparent that an epidemic has begun.

The nursery can be a source of infection for the community. The release of infants who are in the incubation stages of illness or are convalescent carriers about to relapse may lead to secondary cases of diarrheal disease among young siblings living in widely scattered areas.[251,260,278] These children further disseminate infection to neighboring households, involving playmates of their own age, young infants, and mothers[251,260,279] As the sickest of these contact cases are admitted to different hospitals, they contaminate new susceptible persons, completing the cycle and compounding the outbreak. This feedback mechanism has proved to be a means of spreading infantile gastroenteritis through entire cities,[251,260,279] counties,[260,275,280] and provinces.[261] One major epidemic of diarrhea related to EPEC O111:B4 that occurred in the metropolitan Chicago and northwestern Indiana region during the winter of 1961 involved more than 1300 children and 29 community hospitals during a period of 9 months.[261,281] Almost all of the patients were younger than 2 years, and 10% were younger than 1 month, producing an age-specific attack rate of nearly 4% of neonates in the community. The importance of the hospital as a source of cross-infection in this epidemic was shown through interviews with patients' families, indicating that a minimum of 40% of infants had direct or indirect contact with a hospital shortly before the onset of illness.

It has been suggested, but not proven, that asymptomatic carriers of EPEC in close contact with a newborn infant, such as nursery personnel or family members, might play an important role in the transmission of the bacterium.[272,274,282] Stool culture surveys have shown that at any one time about 1% to 2% of adults[279,283,284] and 1% to 5% of young children[251,278,285] who are free of illness harbor EPEC strains. Higher percentages have been recorded during community epidemics.[251,278] Because this intestinal carriage is transitory,[251,272] the number of individuals who excrete EPEC at one time or another during the year is far higher than the 1% figure recorded for single specimens.[272,284]

The association of atypical EPEC with acute diarrhea is less well established. Multiple studies have found no association, whereas others have found higher rates of aEPEC identified from symptomatic patients in both industrialized countries and the developing world. GEMS did not identify a statistically significant difference for the isolation of aEPEC from symptomatic children or controls.[188] A study in Baltimore, Maryland and New Haven, Connecticut, was similarly unable to establish a relationship between aEPEC and symptomatic infection.[286] On the other hand, a study in Cincinnati, Ohio, found a higher prevalence of aEPEC (6.5% vs. 3.9%) in children younger than 5 years who were brought to the emergency department.[287] Higher rates of aEPEC compared with tEPEC have additionally been reported from Norway, Denmark, and Australia, among others, and have been associated with outbreaks among school-aged children.[283,288,289]

Some of the discrepancy leading to confusion about the significance of aEPEC in diarrheal disease may be due to its significant heterogeneity. By definition, aEPEC must contain *eaeA* and should be capable of causing typical A/E lesions (see later). However, several studies have described marked heterogeneity in serotypes, with fewer strains belonging to the classic serotypes recognized by the WHO, and heterogeneity in identifiable virulence factors.[114,290] Of note, there are reports that aEPEC may be associated with prolonged diarrhea (>14 days).[291] Further studies are required for a more complete understanding of the current epidemiology of both typical and atypical EPEC.[292]

Pathogenesis. Bacterial cultures of the meconium and feces of newborns indicate that EPEC can effectively colonize the intestinal tract in the first days of life.[72-75] Breastfeeding is felt to be protective.[293] Investigators in Misiones, Argentina, noted a lower incidence of EPEC infection, symptomatic or asymptomatic, in breastfed infants younger than 20 months.[294] Similarly, in a recent outbreak in Botswana, where EPEC was commonly isolated from children younger than 5 years, breastfeeding was felt to contribute to improved outcomes.[295] A study in Brazil reported an odds ratio (OR) of 0.1 for breastfeeding in infants with EPEC, suggesting a protective effect.[296] The use of breastfeeding or human milk provided by bottle has shown to be effective in ending nursery epidemics caused by EPEC O111:B4, probably by reducing the incidence of cross-infections among infants.[297,298]

Although dose-effect studies have not been performed among newborns, severe diarrhea has occurred after ingestion of 10^8 EPEC organisms in very young infants.[299,300] The high incidence of cross-infection outbreaks in newborn nurseries suggests that a far lower inoculum can often affect spread in this setting. Inocula of 10^{10} *E. coli* O142 or O127 organisms caused diarrhea in 8 of 10 adult volunteers.[301]

The mechanism by which EPEC causes diarrhea involves a complex array of plasmid and chromosomally encoded traits. Only uncommonly do EPEC strains invade the bloodstream or disseminate.[302] An A/E lesion is characteristic of EPEC; the lesion is manifested by intimate (about 10 nm) apposition of the EPEC to the plasma membrane of the enterocytes, with dissolution of the normal brush border and rearrangement of the cytoskeleton.[111,303] In some instances, the bacteria are observed to rise up on pedestal-like structures, which are diagnostic of the infection.[111] Villus blunting, crypt hypertrophy, histiocytic infiltration in the lamina propria, and a reduction in brush border enzyme expression may also be observed.[303,304]

Two major EPEC virulence factors have been described; strains with both factors are designated as typical EPEC.[84,87,305] One such factor is the locus of enterocyte effacement (LEE), a pathogenicity island encoding a type III secretion system.[306-308] The LEE secretion apparatus injects proteins directly from the cytoplasm of the infecting bacterium into the cytoplasm of the target enterocytes.[307] The injected proteins constitute cytoskeletal toxins, which together elicit the close apposition of the bacterium to the cell and cause the effacement of microvilli.[84,87,111,309] One critical secreted protein, called translocated intimin receptor (Tir),[110] inserts into the plasma membrane of the epithelial cell, where it serves as the receptor for an LEE-encoded EPEC outer membrane protein called intimin, encoded by *eaeA*.[111] The second major virulence factor of typical EPEC is the BFP,[310] which is encoded on a partially conserved 60-MDa virulence plasmid called EPEC adherence factor (EAF).[311] BFP, a member of the type IV pilus family, mediates aggregation of the bacteria to one another and probably to enterocytes themselves, facilitating mucosal colonization.[312] A BFP mutant was attenuated for virulence in adult volunteers.[313] An array of additional virulence factors have been proposed, including effectors encoded both within and outside of the LEE pathogenicity island.[314] A complete understanding of how the coordination of these virulence mechanisms leads to diarrhea remains somewhat elusive.

More recent epidemiologic data suggest that some virulent EPEC may lack the BFP, although still possessing the *eaeA* gene and capable of causing A/E lesions; such strains are termed atypical EPEC (aEPEC).[291,315] These strains exhibit marked variability in serotype and expression of additional virulence factors. Although a complete understanding of virulence mechanisms for aEPEC is still unclear, the presence of some additional virulence factors such as Efa1/LifA, which have adhesive properties and may inhibit lymphocyte proliferation, may be associated with symptomatic infection.[316] Another mechanism for initial attachment to enterocytes is presumed to exist for aEPEC given the absence of BFP.

The role of circulating immunity in the prevention of GI tract disease related to EPEC has not been clearly established. Animal models suggest that a humoral immune response may be protective against subsequent EPEC infection.[317,318] Such a response to LEE-encoded virulence factors has similarly been noted in human infections but not directly correlated with protection.[319,320] EPEC is more common in children, although it is unclear whether this is due to an immune response or innate host factors associated with age. In human infants, the frequency of bacteriologic and clinical relapse related to EPEC of the same serotype[254,255,271] and the capacity of one strain of EPEC to superinfect a patient already harboring a different strain[252,258,321] cast some doubt on the ability of mucosal antibodies to inhibit or alter the course of intestinal infection. Ultimately, the role of an immune response and the potential for an EPEC vaccine continue to be investigated.

Pathology. The principal pathologic lesion in EPEC infection is the A/E lesion, manifest by electron microscopy but not light microscopy. In chronic cases, villus blunting, crypt hypertrophy, histiocytic infiltration of the lamina propria, and reduced brush border enzymes may be seen. Rothbaum and colleagues[303] described similar findings, with dissolution of the glycocalyx and flattened microvilli with the nontoxigenic EPEC strain O119:B14. A wide range of pathologic findings has been reported in infants dying with EPEC gastroenteritis. Most newborns dying with diarrheal disease caused by EPEC show no morphologic changes of the GI tract by gross or microscopic examination of tissues.[234,235] Bray[236] described such "meager" changes in the intestinal tract that "the impression received was that the term gastroenteritis is incorrect." At the other extreme, extensive and severe involvement of the intestinal tract, although distinctly unusual among neonates with EPEC diarrhea, has been discussed in several reviews of the pathologic anatomy of this disease.[321-323] Changes virtually identical to those found in infants dying with necrotizing enterocolitis have been reported.[323] Drucker and coworkers[322] found that among 17 infants with EPEC diarrhea who were dying, "intestinal gangrene, and/or perforation, and/or peritonitis were present in five, and intestinal pneumatosis in five." The reasons for such wide discrepancies in reported EPEC disease pathology are unclear.

The nonspecific pathologic picture described by some researchers includes capillary congestion and edema of the bowel wall and an increase in the number of eosinophils, plasma cells, macrophages, and mononuclear cells in the mucosa and submucosa.[322,324,325] Villous patterns are generally well preserved, although some flattening and broadening of the villi are seen in more severe cases. Almost complete absence of villi and failure of regeneration of small bowel mucosa have been reported in one extreme case.[326] Edema in and around the myenteric plexuses of Auerbach, a common associated finding, may cause the GI tract dilation often seen at autopsy in infants with EPEC infections.[321,325,327] In general, the distal small intestine shows the most marked alterations; however, the reported pathologic findings may be found at all levels of the intestinal tract.

Several complications of EPEC infection have been reported. Candidal esophagitis accounted for significant morbidity in two series collected before[235] and during[321] the antibiotic era. Oral thrush has been seen in 50% of EPEC-infected infants treated with oral or systemic antibiotics.[254,325,328] A measure of fatty metamorphosis of the liver has been reported by several investigators[235,250,325]; however, these changes are nonspecific and probably result from the poor caloric intake associated with persistent diarrhea or vomiting. Some degree of bronchopneumonia, probably a terminal event in most cases, exists in a large proportion of newborns dying of EPEC infection.[235,250,327] In one reported series of fatal infant cases, EPEC was shown by immunofluorescent staining to be present in the bronchi, alveoli, and interalveolar septa.

Mesenteric lymph nodes are often swollen and congested with reactive germinal centers in the lymphoid follicles.[250,284,324] Severe lymphoid depletion, unrelated to the duration or severity of the antecedent illness, also has been described.[275] The kidneys frequently show tubular epithelial toxic changes. Various degrees of tubular degeneration and cloudy swelling of convoluted tubules are common findings.[250,275,325] Renal vein thrombosis or cortical necrosis may be observed in infants with disseminated intravascular coagulation in the terminal phases of the illness. The heart is grossly normal in most instances but may show minimal vacuolar changes of nonspecific toxic myocarditis on microscopic examination.[325,327] Candidal abscesses of the heart[327] and kidneys[275,325,327] have been described. With the exception of mild congestion of the pia arachnoid vessels and some edema of the meninges, examination of the central nervous system reveals few changes.[250,324]

Clinical Manifestations. The incubation period after EPEC exposure is quite variable. Its duration has been calculated mostly from evidence in outbreaks in newborn nurseries, where the time of first exposure can be clearly defined in terms of birth or admission dates. In these circumstances, almost all infants show signs of illness 2 to 12 days after exposure, and most cases show signs within the first 7 days.[250,254,329] In some naturally acquired[72,73] and experimental[300] infections with heavy exposure, the incubation period may be only 24 hours; the stated upper limit is 20 days.[330,331] In adult volunteers fed a high inoculum, the incubation period was less than 3 hours. The first positive stool culture and the earliest recognizable clinical signs of disease occur simultaneously in most infants,[254,256] although colonization may precede symptoms by 7 to 14 days.[255,256,332]

Gastroenteritis associated with typical EPEC infection in the newborn is notable for its marked variation in clinical pattern. Clinical manifestations vary from mild illness manifest only by transient anorexia and failure to gain weight to a sudden explosive fulminating diarrhea causing death within 12 hours of onset. Prematurity, underlying diseases and congenital anomalies often are associated with the more severe forms of illness.[333-336] The onset of illness is usually insidious, with vague signs such as reluctance to feed, lethargy, spitting up of formula, mild abdominal distention, or weight loss that may occur for 1 or 2 days before the first loose stool is passed. Diarrhea usually begins abruptly. It may be continuous and violent, or in milder infections, it may run an intermittent course with 1 or more days of normal stools, followed by 1 or more days of diarrhea. Prominent and persistent vomiting can be an early finding. Fever is an inconstant feature, and when it occurs, the patient's temperature rarely is higher than 39° C (>102.2° F).[337] Prolonged hematochezia, distention, edema, and jaundice are ominous signs and suggest an unfavorable prognosis.[250,261,275]

The clinical relevance of infection compared with colonization with atypical EPEC is controversial. Clinical symptoms have been described in outbreaks of aEPEC. In a study completed in Melbourne, Australia, the clinical presentation included vomiting in 44% and abdominal pain in 20%, along with diarrhea. A low-grade fever was detected in 24% of patients. No patients had macroscopic blood in their stool, but 16% were Hemoccult positive, whereas 20% were found to have fecal leukocytes.[291]

Prolonged diarrhea has been observed for typical EPEC. Infants with mild illness who receive no treatment can continue to have intermittent loose stools for 1 to 3 weeks. In one outbreak related to EPEC O142:K86, more than one third of untreated or inappropriately treated infants had diarrhea for more than 14 days in the absence of a recognized enteric pathogen on repeated culturing.[257] Recurrence can occur, even after adequate treatment.* Atypical EPEC has also been associated with prolonged diarrhea lasting more than 14 days.[289,291] A study in Norway found that 31.6% of patients younger than 2 years with aEPEC had symptoms lasting more than 2 weeks.[289]

Dehydration is the most common and serious complication of gastroenteritis caused by EPEC or a toxin-producing *E. coli*. Virtually all deaths directly attributable to the intestinal infection are caused by disturbances in fluids and electrolytes. When stools are frequent in number, large in volume, and violent in release, as they often are in severe infections with abrupt onset, a neonate can lose 15% of body weight within a few hours.[267,330] Rarely, fluid excretion into the lumen of the bowel proceeds so rapidly that reduction of circulating blood volume and shock may intervene before passage of a single loose stool.[324] Before the discovery of the etiologic agent, epidemic diarrhea of the newborn was also known by the term *cholera infantum*. Even mild disease, however, can lead to fluid and electrolyte imbalance along with nutritional deficiencies.[255,264,295,326] These should be monitored closely, particularly in infants, during the course of illness.[264]

Diagnosis. In 1987, the WHO came to a consensus that O serogroups of *E. coli* should be classified as EPEC: O26, O55, O86, O111, O114 O119, O125, O126, O127, O128, O142, and O158.[113] Serotyping can be used to identify likely EPEC strains, especially in outbreaks.[240] *E. coli*, similar to other Enterobacteriaceae members, possesses cell wall somatic antigens (O), envelope or capsular antigens (K), and, if motile, flagellar antigens (H). Many O groups may be divided further into two or more subgroups (a, b, c), and the K antigens are divisible into at least three varieties (B, L, A) based on their physical behavior. Organisms that do not possess flagellar antigens are nonmotile (designated NM). The EPEC B capsular surface antigen prevents agglutination by antibodies directed against the underlying O antigen. Heating at 100° C for 1 hour inactivates the agglutinability and antigenicity of the B antigen. Slide agglutination tests with polyvalent O or OB antiserum may be performed on suspensions of colonies typical of *E. coli* that have been isolated from infants with diarrhea, especially in nursery outbreaks. Diagnosis by serotyping must be used with caution because it can result in false positives and false negatives. *E. coli* strains that fall into the above serogroups do not necessarily harbor virulence factors essential for pathogenicity.[338] In addition, aEPEC, which are emerging as a more common etiology of childhood diarrhea than tEPEC, have greater serotype variability and may not fall into the above serogroups.[114] Patients at times have been noted to harbor multiple EPEC serogroups and can be asymptomatic carriers. It is important to consider all possible etiologies of diarrhea because the isolation of one of the above serogroups does not necessarily imply it is the cause of diarrhea.

Classic EPEC has been recovered from the vomitus, stool, or bowel contents of infected newborns. Isolation from bile[334] and the upper respiratory tract[70,251,260] has been described in instances in which a specific search has been made. Less commonly, EPEC is isolated from ascitic fluid[339] or purulent exudates[234,250,340]; on occasion, the organism has been recovered from blood cultures,[255,270] urine,[255] and cerebrospinal fluid.

Stool cultures are generally more reliable than rectal swabs in detecting the presence of enteric pathogens, although a properly obtained swab should be adequate to show EPEC in most cases.[241,341,342] Specimens should be obtained as early in the course of the illness as possible because organisms are present in virtually pure culture during the acute phase of the enteritis but rapidly diminish in numbers during convalescence.

After a stool specimen is received, it should be plated as quickly as possible onto noninhibiting media or placed in a preservative medium if it is to be held for longer periods. Deep freezing of specimens preserves viable EPEC when a prolonged delay in isolation is necessary.[239] No biochemical assays readily differentiate between EPEC and nonpathogenic commensal *E. coli*.

Microscopic examination of stools of infants with acute diarrheal illness caused by these organisms usually, but not always, has revealed an absence of fecal neutrophils,[291,301,333,343,344] although data on fecal lactoferrin in human volunteers suggest that an inflammatory process may be important in EPEC diarrhea.[345,346] Serologic methods have not proven to be useful in attempting to establish a retrospective diagnosis of EPEC infection in neonates. Increasing or significantly elevated agglutinin titers rarely could be shown in early investigations[235,250,329];

*References 192, 250, 260, 261, 275, 330.

hemagglutinating antibodies showed a significant response in only 10% to 20% of cases.[328,347]

Before widespread use of molecular methods, the human epithelial type-2 (HEp-2) cell adherence assay was proposed for EPEC diagnosis.[109] The presence of a focal or localized adherence[109] pattern on the surface of HEp-2 or HeLa cells after 3-hour coincubation is a highly sensitive and specific test for detection of EPEC.[348] The requirement for cell culture and expertise in reading this assay limits its utility to the research setting. An ELISA for BFP has been described but is not readily available.[349] The capacity of localized adherence plus EPEC to polymerize F-actin can be detected in tissue culture cells stained with rhodamine-labeled phalloidin.[350] This fluorescence-actin staining test is cumbersome and impractical for routine clinical use.

The current standard for identification of EPEC is the use of molecular techniques to identify specific virulence factors. By definition, EPEC require the LEE pathogenicity island (*eae* gene) and must not produce shiga toxin (*stx* gene). Strains that additionally harbor the EPEC EAF plasmid, identified by the presence of the *bfpA* gene, are considered tEPEC, whereas those missing this gene are considered aEPEC. Specific gene probes and PCR primers for these genes are available.[84] PCR and gene probe analysis can be performed directly on the stools of suspect infants; isolation of the organism should also be attempted. It is important to note that although molecular identification of these genes is the best diagnostic method currently available for EPEC, it is not perfect. *E. coli* strains that harbor *eae* may be missing accessory virulence factors needed to cause diarrhea, as evidenced by multiple studies identifying aEPEC in asymptomatic carriers.[292] In addition, the presence of a gene may not ultimately translate to expression of its virulence factor. Experts suggest that whole-genome sequencing may eventually play a role in a more complete understanding of virulence markers associated with symptomatic infection.[292]

Prognosis. The mortality rate recorded previously in epidemics of typical EPEC gastroenteritis is impressive for its variability. During the 1930s and 1940s, when organisms later recognized as classic enteropathogenic serotypes were infecting infants, the case-fatality ratio among neonates was about 50%.[234,235] During the 1950s and 1960s, about one of every four infected infants still died in many nursery epidemics, but several outbreaks involving the same serotypes under similar epidemiologic circumstances had fatality rates of less than 3%.[351-353] In the 1970s, reports appeared in the literature of a nursery epidemic with a 40% neonatal mortality rate[275] and of an extensive outbreak in a nursery for premature infants with 4% fatalities[255]; another report stated that among "243 consecutive infants admitted to the hospital for EPEC diarrheal disease, none died of diarrheal disease per se."[354] As indicated above, in the GEMS study, the presence of typical EPEC resulted in a 2.6-fold increased risk of death at 60 days not necessarily because of the acute diarrhea episode.[188]

A significant proportion of the infants who died during or shortly after an episode of gastroenteritis already were compromised by preexisting disease[273,310,334] or by congenital malformations[261,329,333] at the time they acquired gastroenteritis. The overall mortality rate among premature infants with EPEC gastroenteritis has not differed significantly over the years from the mortality recorded for term infants.[254,324,334]

Therapy. The management of EPEC gastroenteritis should be directed primarily toward prevention or correction of problems caused by loss of fluids and electrolytes.[199] Most neonates have a relatively mild illness that can be treated with oral rehydration. Infants who appear toxic, infants with voluminous diarrhea and persistent vomiting, and infants with increasing weight loss should be hospitalized for observation and treatment with oral and/or parenteral fluids to carefully maintain fluid and electrolyte balance, and possibly with antimicrobial therapy. The use of atropine-like drugs, paregoric, or loperamide to reduce intestinal motility or cramping should be avoided. Inhibition of peristalsis interferes with an efficient protective mechanism designed to rid the body of intestinal pathogens.

The value of antimicrobial therapy in management of neonatal EPEC gastroenteritis, if any, is uncertain. There are no adequately controlled studies defining the benefits of any antibiotic in eliminating EPEC from the GI tract, reducing the risk of cross-infection in community or nursery outbreaks, or modifying the severity of the illness. Proponents of the use of antimicrobial agents have based their claims for efficacy on anecdotal observations or comparative studies[328]; some postulate that antimicrobial therapy may shorten the length of illness and aid in the control of nursery outbreaks by decreasing length of shedding.[254,352,355] Antibiotic therapy has been used during classic outbreaks and seems to more quickly eradicate EPEC. Oral nonabsorbable antibiotics, such as neomycin,[328,334,352,353] colistin,[257,275,328,356] gentamicin,[255,357] and polymixin,[279] have been used with some success and apparent decrease in mortality, although not well studied. In the past, oral neomycin[328] has been recommended as initial therapy, when resistance is not a concern, until stools are culture negative for EPEC, often within 2 to 4 days.[254,328] Parenteral antibiotics can be considered in patients who are systemically ill with concern for sepsis. Relapses can occur, although they do not require therapy, unless they are associated with illness or high epidemiologic risks to other young infants in the household.[328]

When antimicrobial therapy is considered, it is important to consider local patterns of antibiotic susceptibility because EPEC has frequently been found to be resistant to commonly used antibiotics. During an outbreak in Nairobi among preterm neonates, a high resistance level was identified to trimethoprim-sulfamethoxazole (TMP-SMX), chloramphenicol, oxytetracycline, and ampicillin.[357] A recent study in Iran that identified mostly aEPEC strains isolated from children younger than 5 years found all strains to be resistant to ampicillin, chloramphenicol, streptomycin, ciprofloxacin, trimethroprim, and tetracycline, whereas only 7% were resistant to gentamicin.[358] A study in Mexico including 430 children with acute diarrhea found that both tEPEC and aEPEC frequently were multidrug resistant (three or more antimicrobials were tested, including tetracycline, ampicillin, TMP-SMX, and chloramphenicol). All EPEC isolates were sensitive to gentamicin.[359] In Peru, a study of 557 stool samples from children younger than 1 year found EPEC resistance to ampicillin (72%), cotrimoxazole (72%), and tetracycline (50%). Nalidixic acid resistance was 22%

among EPEC from symptomatic patients. All strains were susceptible to gentamicin, ciprofloxacin, cefotaxime, and ceftazidime.[360] Empirical choice of antibiotics can be guided by local resistance patterns, and antibiotics should be tailored once the EPEC strain is identified and specific antibiotic susceptibilities are characterized.

Prevention. The transmission for EPEC is fecal-oral. Therefore strict adherence to infection control and appropriate hygiene can help prevent spread. Recommendations for controlling nursery outbreaks come from reported experience,[361] although nursery outbreaks have become rare. Stool cultures can be obtained from infected infants, bearing in mind that most clinical microbiology laboratories do not routinely test for EPEC. If necessary, samples can be sent to a reference laboratory such as the Centers for Disease Control and Prevention (CDC). Infants who are symptomatic or shedding EPEC should be isolated or cohorted to a section of the nursery, and hand hygiene should be scrupulous. Enteral antibiotics can be considered and are thought to have helped curtail spread of the infection in past nursery outbreaks,[361] although this is not well studied. Surveillance of hospital personnel who come into contact with the infants can be undertaken. When the involved infants are discharged, thorough disinfection of the area is warranted.[362] The use of prophylactic antibiotics has been shown to be of no value and can select for increased resistance.[363-365] An EPEC vaccine is not currently available; research is ongoing.

Enterohemorrhagic *Escherichia coli*

Since a multistate outbreak of enterohemorrhagic colitis was associated with *E. coli* O157:H7,[366] Shiga toxin–producing *E. coli* (STEC) have been recognized as emerging GI pathogens in most of the industrialized world. A particularly virulent subset of STEC, EHEC, causes frequent and severe outbreaks of GI disease[84,367]; the most virulent EHEC organisms belong to serotype O157:H7. EHEC has a bovine reservoir and is transmitted through undercooked meat, unpasteurized milk, and contaminated vegetables, such as lettuce, alfalfa sprouts, and radish sprouts (as occurred in more than 9000 schoolchildren in Japan)[368,369]. It also spreads directly from person to person.[369,370] The clinical syndrome is characterized by bloody, noninflammatory (sometimes voluminous) diarrhea that is distinct from febrile dysentery with fecal leukocytes seen in shigellosis or EIEC infections.[84] HUS, defined by the occurrence of hemolytic anemia, thrombocytopenia (<150,000/mm^3) and renal insufficiency, is reported to occur as a sequela of EHEC infection in up to 15% to 20% of culture-proven cases.[371] Most cases of EHEC infections have been recognized in outbreaks of bloody diarrhea or HUS in daycare centers, schools, nursing homes, and communities.[370,372,373]

The capacity of EHEC to cause disease is related to the phage-encoded capacity of the organism to produce a Vero cell cytotoxin, subsequently shown to be one of the Shiga toxins (first identified in strains of *Shigella dysenteriae* serotype 1).[374-376] EHEC Shiga toxin 1 is neutralized by antiserum against the Shiga toxin of *S. dysenteriae*, whereas Shiga toxin 2, although biologically similar, is not neutralized by anti–Shiga toxin.[377,378] Similar to Shiga toxin made by *S. dysenteriae*, both EHEC Shiga toxins act by inhibiting protein synthesis by cleaving an adenosine residue from position 4324 in the 28S ribosomal RNA (rRNA) to prevent elongation factor-1–dependent aminoacyl transfer RNA (tRNA) from binding to the 60S rRNA.[374,375] The bacteria intimately adhere to epithelial cells and form A/E lesions, mediated by the LEE pathogenicity island, as described for EPEC.[379,380] EHEC additionally expresses three described systems for stomach acid resistance, which may contribute to its very low infectious dose (1-100 colony-forming units [CFU]).[381] Finally, virulence factors encoded on the pO157 or pO157-like plasmid of EHEC may contribute to adherence; the effects on pathogenesis of its products are an area of ongoing research.[379]

EHEC and other STEC infections should be suspected in neonates who have bloody diarrhea or who may have been exposed in the course of an outbreak among older individuals. Because most cases are caused by ingestion of contaminated food, neonates have a degree of epidemiologic protection from the illness. However, there are case reports of STEC infection and HUS in infants of only a few days of age,[382,383] and FoodNet surveillance in 2011 reports an incidence of 1.69 cases of STEC O157 and 4.07 of non-O157 per 100,000 children younger than 1 year.[384] In vitro data suggest that breast milk may have properties that prevent STEC infection.[385,386] STEC diarrhea is diagnosed by isolation and identification of the pathogen in the feces. *E. coli* O157:H7 does not ferment sorbitol, and this biochemical trait is commonly used in the detection of this serotype.[84,387] Because some nonpathogenic *E. coli* share this characteristic, confirmation of the serotype by slide agglutination is required. These techniques can be performed in most clinical laboratories. Detection of non-O157 serotypes relies on detection of the Shiga toxin; available methods include Shiga toxin ELISA, latex agglutination, and molecular methods.[84,387,388] Current CDC recommendations are to perform both culture and Shiga toxin detection methods simultaneously for the detection of STEC from stools.[388] Stool cultures should be sent as early in the course of illness as possible because recovery of EHEC decreases significantly 7 days after the onset of diarrhea, usually by the time of onset of HUS (5-13 days of illness).[371,389]

Antimicrobial therapy should not be administered to patients who may have STEC infection because it may increase expression of Shiga toxin and rates of HUS.[371,390-392] Management of diarrhea and possible sequelae is supportive, with proper emphasis on fluid and electrolyte replacement. Aggressive parenteral rehydration with isotonic fluids offers some protection from oligoanuric renal failure.[371,393] The use of additional treatment modalities, such as eculizumab[394] and plasma exchange, for the management of HUS has been suggested. However, the benefit from these therapies has not been definitively demonstrated.[371,395] Antimotility agents are contraindicated because they may prolong the duration of STEC-associated bloody diarrhea.[396]

Enteroaggregative *Escherichia coli*

The HEp-2 adherence assay is useful for the detection of EPEC organisms, which exhibit a classic localized adherence pattern.[109] Two other adherence patterns can be discerned in this assay: aggregative and diffuse. These two patterns may define additional pathotypes of diarrheogenic *E. coli*.[84] Strains exhibiting the aggregative adherence pattern (i.e., EAEC) are common pathogens of infants.[112]

EAEC cause diarrhea by colonization of the intestinal mucosa and elaboration of enterotoxins and cytotoxins.[112,397] Many strains induce secretion of inflammatory cytokines in vitro, which may contribute to growth retardation associated with prolonged but otherwise asymptomatic colonization.[91] Several virulence factors in EAEC are under the control of the virulence gene activator AggR.[397] The presence of the AggR regulator or its effector genes has been proposed as a means of detecting truly virulent EAEC strains (called typical EAEC),[397,398] and an empirical gene probe long used for EAEC detection corresponds to one gene under AggR control.[399,400] An EAEC strain (O104:H4) that caused an outbreak in Germany, mostly in adults, expressed Shiga toxin that likely had been horizontally acquired, resulting in high rates of HUS.[401,402] EAEC do not typically elaborate Shiga toxin.

Epidemiology and Transmission. The mode of transmission of EAEC is not well established. In adult volunteer studies, the infectious dose is high (>10^8 CFU), suggesting that at least in adults, person-to-person transmission is unlikely.[403,404] Several outbreaks have been linked to consumption of contaminated food.[405,406] The largest of these outbreaks involved almost 2700 schoolchildren in Japan[405]; a contaminated school lunch was the source implicated in the outbreak of EAEC. Some studies have shown contamination of condiments or milk, which could represent vehicles of foodborne transmission.[407]

A nursery outbreak of EAEC involved 19 infants in Nis, Serbia in 1995.[408] Because these infants did not ingest milk from a common source, it is presumed that horizontal transmission by environmental contamination or hands of health care personnel was possible. Most of the infants were full term and previously well, and they were housed in two separate nursery rooms.

The earliest epidemiologic studies of EAEC implicated this organism as a cause of endemic diarrhea in developing countries.[409-411] In this setting, EAEC as defined by the aggregative pattern of adherence to HEp-2 cells can be found in upward of 30% of the population at any one time.[412] Newer molecular diagnostic modalities have revised this figure downward, although the organism remains highly prevalent in many areas. Several studies from the Indian subcontinent implicated EAEC among the most frequent enteric pathogens.[409,410,413] Other sites reproducibly reporting high incidence rates include Mexico[411] and Brazil.[412,414] There is evidence that EAEC may be increasing in incidence. A study from São Paulo, Brazil, identified EAEC as the prevalent *E. coli* pathotypes in infants,[414] replacing EPEC in this community. Many other sites in developing countries of Africa,[415] Asia,[398,416] and South America[417] have described high endemic rates. A meta-analysis of 41 studies showed an association between EAEC and acute diarrhea in both the developed and developing world.[418]

Several studies have suggested that EAEC is also a common cause of infant diarrhea in industrialized countries.[419-421] Using molecular diagnostic methods, a large prospective study in the United Kingdom identified EAEC as the second most common enteric bacterial pathogen after *Campylobacter*.[422] A similar survey from Switzerland found EAEC to be the most common bacterial enteropathogen.[420] Studies from the United States also have shown a high rate of EAEC diarrhea in infants. Using molecular diagnostic methods, a study in Cincinnati implicated EAEC in 10% and 4.7% of outpatient and inpatient diarrhea cohorts, respectively, of infants younger than 1 year, compared with less than 2% of asymptomatic control infants ($P < .05$).[287] Although epidemiologic studies have shown that EAEC can cause diarrhea in all age groups, several studies suggest that the infection is particularly common in infants and children younger than 2 years.[398,417,418,423]

Clinical Manifestations. Descriptions from outbreaks and volunteer studies suggest that EAEC diarrhea is most often watery, with mucus and accompanied by abdominal pain/cramping.[403,404,408,424] Fever, bloody stools, and fecal leukocytes have been reported but are less common.[424]

Early reports of EAEC infection suggested that this pathogen may be associated with persistent diarrhea (>14 days).[409-411] Later studies suggest, however, that persistent diarrhea may occur in a subset of infected infants[405] and may be linked to malnutrition.[425] In the Serbian outbreak of 19 infected infants, the mean duration of diarrhea was 5.2 days[408]; diarrhea persisted more than 14 days in only 3 patients. Infants in this outbreak had frequent, green, odorless stools. In 3 cases, the stools had mucus, but none had visible blood. Eleven infants developed temperatures higher than 38° C (>100.4° F); only one had vomiting.

Several clinical studies have suggested that EAEC is associated with subclinical inflammation, including the shedding of fecal cytokines and lactoferrin.[91,426,427] Studies in Fortaleza, Brazil suggest that children asymptomatically excreting EAEC may exhibit stunting, compared with uninfected peers.[91] A study from Germany reported an association between EAEC isolation and colic in infants without diarrhea,[419] although this observation has not been reproduced. EAEC should be considered in the differential diagnosis of persistent diarrhea and failure to thrive in infants.

Diagnosis and Therapy. Diagnosis of EAEC requires identification of the organism in the patient's feces. The HEp-2 adherence assay can be used for this purpose, although the specificity of this assay is decreased compared with molecular diagnosis.[109,287] Some reports suggest that the adherence phenotype can be observed using formalin-fixed cells,[428,429] obviating the need to cultivate eukaryotic cells for each assay. PCR for typical EAEC, based on identification of virulence factors, is available in the research setting and is the preferred diagnostic test .[86,430]

Antibiotic therapy using fluoroquinolones in adult patients has been successful.[431] Studies suggest that azithromycin[432] or rifaximin[433] also may be effective in adults with traveler's diarrhea. In addition, a small study of azithromycin treatment during the O104:H4 outbreak was associated with decreased length of shedding; fluoroquinolones carry the risk of increased expression of Shiga toxin.[434,435]

Therapy for infected infants has not been well studied and, if deemed necessary, should be guided by the results of susceptibility testing because EAEC organisms are frequently antibiotic resistant.[415,436]

Other *Escherichia coli* Pathotypes

Additional *E. coli* pathotypes have been described, including diffusely adherent *E. coli* (DAEC)[437] and cytodetaching *E. coli*.[438] The association between DAEC and symptomatic infections in neonates and young infants is not strong.[439] Cytodetaching *E. coli* represent organisms that secrete the *E. coli* hemolysin.[440] It is unclear whether these latter organisms are true enteric pathogens.

SALMONELLA

Nature of the Organism

The genus *Salmonella* comprises two species: *enterica* and *bongori*.[441] *S. bongori* isolates are rare. *S. enterica* is subsequently divided into subspecies and serotypes. Six subspecies have been designated (I: *enterica*, II: *salamae*, IIIa: *arizonae*, IIIb: *diarizonae*, IV: *houtenae*, VI: *indica*). Subspecies I (99% in the United States) and IV encompass the majority of human isolates. These subspecies are then divided by serogroups (i.e., A, B, D, etc.) and serotypes. More than 2500 serotypes have been described. The most common isolated in human infections are listed in Table 11-2. Appropriate designation of a *Salmonella* strain includes its serotype name, as for *S. enterica* serotype Typhimurium or *S.* serotype (or ser.) Typhimurium.[441,442] Biochemical and serologic traits are used routinely by hospital laboratories to differentiate *Salmonella* serovars. *S.* ser. Typhi is different from other salmonellae because it does not produce gas from glucose.[443] Serotyping of *S. enterica* is usually performed by state health departments rather than by hospital laboratories.

There are differences in invasiveness of *Salmonella* strains related to serotype.[444] *S.* ser. Typhi and Paratyphi (enteric fever), *S.* ser. Typhimurium,[445] *S.* ser. Choleraesuis, *S.* ser. Heidelberg,[446,447] *S.* ser. Dublin,[448] *S.* ser. Enteritidis,[445] and *S.* ser. Schwarzengrund[445] are particularly invasive, with bacteremia and extraintestinal focal infections occurring frequently. A study analyzing data collected from *Salmonella* infections in the United States (FoodNet, 1996-1999) found that the proportion of invasive infections was highest for serotypes Dublin, Typhi, Paratyphi A, and Choleraesuis.[445]

The pathogenesis of *Salmonella* is a striking display of a pathogen adapting to and subverting host cellular mechanisms for survival. Salmonellae harbor two pathogenicity islands designated *Salmonella* pathogenicity island-1 and -2 (SPI-1 and SPI-2). Both harbor type III secretion systems (T3SS), similar to EPEC and EHEC.[449] Mediated by SPI-1 T3SS effectors, when *Salmonella* comes into contact with epithelial cells, they induce membrane ruffling and endocytosis, allowing the bacteria to invade the cells. SPI-1 effectors also result in a significant inflammatory response, including upregulation of IL-8, IL-1β, and recruitment of neutrophils.[449,450] This inflammatory process is thought to play a major role in the development of clinical diarrhea. Within a few hours, the majority of bacteria can be found in the lamina propria, where they are engulfed by mononuclear cells.[451] Within these cells, they are eventually found in *Salmonella*-containing vacuoles (SCV), where they are capable of dividing. Survival within SCV is thought to be mediated by the T3SS and effectors of SPI-2; this pathogenicity island can also mediate an inflammatory response.[449,450] Intracellular survival has major clinical significance, accounting for relapse after antibiotic therapy and the inadequacy of some antimicrobial agents that do not effectively penetrate phagolysosomes. It is also perhaps the reason for prolonged febrile courses that occur even in the face of appropriate therapy. Although both humoral immunity and cell-mediated immunity are stimulated during *Salmonella* infections, it is believed that cell-mediated immunity plays a greater role in eradication of the bacteria.[452] T-cell activation of macrophages seems to be important in killing intracellular *Salmonella*.[453] Defective interferon-γ (IFN-γ) production by monocytes of newborns in response to *S.* ser. Typhimurium LPS may explain, in part, the unusual susceptibility of infants to *Salmonella* infection.[454] Studies in mice suggest that T-helper type 1 cell responses in Peyer patches and mesenteric lymph nodes may be central to protection of the intestinal mucosa.[455] Humans who lack the IL-12 receptor and have impaired T-helper type 1 cell responses and IFN-γ production are at increased risk for *Salmonella* infection.[450,456]

S. ser. Typhi strains comprise almost entirely a single global clone, recognized by serologic and biochemically distinct characteristics. Differences between *S.* ser. Typhi and

Table 11-2 Common Serotypes and Serogroups of *Salmonella*

Serogroups	Serotypes
A	Paratyphi A
B	Agona Derby Heidelberg Paratyphi B *(schottmuelleri)* Saint-paul Typhimurium
C_1	Choleraesuis Eimsbuettel Infantis Montevideo Oranienburg Paratyphi C *(hirschfeldii)* Thompson
C_2	Blockley Hadar Muenchen Newport
C_3	Kentucky
D_1	Dublin Enteritidis Javiana Panama Typhi
D_2	Maarssen
E_1	Anatum
E_2	London Newington
E_3	Illinois
E_4	Krefeld Senftenberg

nontyphoidal *Salmonella* (NTS) are an active area of investigation. *S.* ser. Typhi are thought to either decrease or escape the inflammatory response early in infection, consistent with the prolonged incubation period and frequently a lack of diarrhea.[451] This may be due to decreased expression of flagella and the presence of the Vi capsular antigen, which decrease Toll-like receptor 4 (TLR4)- and TLR5-mediated responses.[451] The bacteria additionally elaborate A/B type toxins that may preferentially affect rapidly dividing immune cells.[451,457] Patients who develop classic enteric fever have positive stool cultures early after ingestion of the organism and again late in the course after a period of bacteremia. This course reflects early colonization of the gut, penetration of gut epithelium with infection of mesenteric lymph nodes, and reseeding of the gut during a subsequent bacteremic phase.[458]

Regarding pathologic changes secondary to *Salmonella* infection, ulcer formation is less striking,[459] although villus tip cells are sometimes sloughed. Acute crypt abscesses can be seen in the stomach and small intestine, but the most dramatic changes occur in the colon, where acute diffuse inflammation with mucosal edema and crypt abscesses are the most consistent findings.[460,461] With *S.* ser. Typhi, there also is hyperplasia of Peyer patches in the ileum, with ulceration of overlying tissues.

Epidemiology and Transmission

Worldwide, nontyphoidal *Salmonella* strains are estimated to cause 93.8 million cases of gastroenteritis and 155,000 deaths.[462] In the United States, the CDC estimates 1 million illnesses yearly, with more than 19,000 hospitalizations and 378 deaths.[463] *Salmonella* strains, with the exception of *S.* ser. Typhi and Paratyphi, are carried by various vertebrate animal hosts; human infection often can be traced to infected meat, contaminated milk and infant formula,[464,465] contact with a specific animal,[466] or contamination of vegetables. *S.* ser. Enteritidis is the most common serotype and causes outbreaks most frequently because of contaminated poultry and eggs.[467,468] *S.* ser. Typhimurium, the second most common serotype in the United States, has been associated with outbreaks from a broader range of vehicles, including dairy, vine-stalk vegetables, pork, and beef.[467,468] Despite the 1975 ban by the U.S. Food and Drug Administration (FDA) on interstate commercial distribution of small turtles, these animals continue to be associated with infection, as illustrated by a series of cases in Puerto Rico.[469] Reptiles and amphibians are a significant source of *Salmonella*.[470,471] Up to 90% of these animals harbor *Salmonella* in their GI tract.[466] These organisms are hardy and capable of prolonged survival; organisms have been documented to survive in flour for nearly a year.[472] They have also been demonstrated to survive for several months in powdered infant formula.[465,473] Contaminated food or water is often the source of *Salmonella* infection in older patients; the limited diet of the infant makes contaminated food a less likely source of infection. Although human milk,[474-478] raw milk,[479] powdered milk,[480-482] formula,[483] and cereal[484] have been implicated in transmission to infants, more often fomites, such as delivery room resuscitators,[485] rectal thermometers,[486,487] oropharyngeal suction devices,[488-490] water baths for heating formula,[490] soap dispensers,[491] scales,[492-494] "clean" medicine tables,[492] air-conditioning filters,[492] mattresses, radiant warmers,[495] and dust, serve as reservoirs during nursery outbreaks. One unusual outbreak involving 394 premature and 122 term infants was traced to faulty plumbing, which caused massive contamination of environment and personnel.[483]

Infants are disproportionately affected by both gastroenteritis and invasive nontyphoidal *Salmonella* infections. Recent data from the CDC suggest rates (per 100,000) of *Salmonella* in children younger than 1 year of 133, compared with 16.4 across all age groups.[468] Similar rates are reported in infants younger than 3 months.[496] Rates of invasive *Salmonella*, including ser. Typhi and Paratyphi, in children younger than 1 year were estimated to be 7.8 per 100,000 infants.[445] In children older than 5 years and adults younger than 60 years, rates were less than 1 per 100,000.[445] Children are also less likely to have underlying conditions leading to invasive disease. In one study from Israel, 15% of children younger than 6.5 years with bacteremia had a predisposing condition as opposed to 95% of adults.[497] Additional predisposing factors to *Salmonella* infection in infants include daycare attendance, travel outside the United States, reptile exposure, and riding in a shopping cart next to meat or poultry.[496] Studies where breastfeeding has been addressed have found it to be protective. One case-control study found an OR of 0.5 (95% confidence interval [CI], 0.3 to 0.6) for breastfeeding when assessing infants with salmonellosis versus matched control subjects.[496] Gastric acidity is an important barrier to *Salmonella* infection. Patients with anatomic or functional achlorhydria are at increased risk of developing salmonellosis.[498,499] The hypochlorhydria[25] and rapid gastric emptying typical of early life[28] may partly explain the susceptibility of infants to *Salmonella*.

Adult volunteer studies suggest that large numbers of *Salmonella* (10^5 to 10^9 organisms) need to be ingested to cause disease.[500] It is likely, however, that lower doses cause illness in infants. The occurrence of nursery outbreaks[483,485,486,492,501-522] and intrafamilial spread[523] suggests that organisms are easily spread from person to person; this pattern is typical of low-inoculum diseases transmitted by the fecal-oral route. Although the index case in an outbreak can often be traced to a mother or family member,[477,501-503,505,520,522] subsequent cases may result from contaminated objects in the nursery environment[495,524] serving as a reservoir coming in contact with hands of attending personnel.[492,510,522] The mother of an index case may be symptomatic[506,507,525,526] or asymptomatic with preclinical infection,[511] convalescent infection,[505,508,527] or chronic carriage.[528] The risk of a newborn becoming infected when *Salmonella* is introduced into a nursery has been reported to be 20% to 27%.[483,513] After *Salmonella* enters a nursery, it is difficult to eradicate. Epidemics lasting 6 to 7 weeks,[486,517] 17 weeks,[492] 6 months,[512,516] 1 year,[507] and 27 to 30 months[483,513] have been reported. Spread to nearby pediatric wards has occurred.[514,519] With improvement in infection control practices, the number of nosocomial nursery outbreaks has decreased over several decades, although they continue to be reported.[522,529-531]

The incubation period in nursery outbreaks has varied widely in several studies where careful attention has been paid to this variable. In one outbreak of *S.* ser. Oranienburg involving 35 newborns, 97% of cases occurred within

4 days of birth.[513] In an outbreak of *S.* ser. Typhimurium, each of the ill infants presented within 6 days of birth.[505] These incubation periods are similar to those reported for *Salmonella* ser. Newport in older children and adults, 95% of whom have been reported to be ill within 8 days of exposure.[532,533] Conversely, one outbreak of *Salmonella* ser. Nienstedten involving newborns was characterized by incubation periods of 7 to 18 days.[514]

S. ser. Typhi or Paratyphi is rare in neonates and when diagnosed, children younger than 2 years often have milder illness than school-aged children or adults.[534-536] Nevertheless, there are reported cases in neonates and infants of significant illness.[535,536] Transmission can be from the environment but can also be vertical from a symptomatic or asymptomatic mother.[535,536] It has been suggested that transplacental transmission can occur, but this has not been rigorously studied.[535] Neonates who acquire *S.* ser. Typhi or Paratyphi may either become asymptomatic or develop a neonatal sepsis syndrome with or without meningitis and a short incubation period.[536] Although considered infrequent, *S.* ser. Typhi and Paratyphi should still be considered in neonatal sepsis and sepsis in infants, especially in areas of endemicity. A study in Pakistan found an incidence of Typhi bacteremia in children younger than 12 months to be 506 per 100,000 child-years, unique as a high rate for this age group.[537] Of note, most cases in the United States, where enteric fever is not endemic, are associated with recent travel to endemic regions.[466]

Clinical Manifestations

Several major syndromes occur with nontyphoidal *Salmonella* infection in young infants. Colonization without illness may be a common outcome after ingestion of *Salmonella* by the neonate. A case control-study of 442 infants that involved the Foodborne Diseases Active Surveillance Network documented that symptoms were more common with sporadic non-Typhi *Salmonella* infection.[496] Diarrhea was present in 98%, fever in 73%, and vomiting in 33% of infants with *Salmonella*. The mean duration of diarrhea was 7 days, with a range of 1 to 31 days. A study in Israel[444] found 65% of patients (<3 years of age) with bloody dysentery-like stools and in Taiwan 38% (<2 years of age) had grossly bloody stools.

Nursery outbreaks are instructive in understanding symptoms in neonates, which vary widely and seem to depend on the serotype that is isolated. In one epidemic of *S.* ser. Oranienburg[513] involving 46 newborns, 76% had grossly bloody stools, 11% were febrile, 26% had mucus in their stools, and only 11% were healthy. In a series of *S.* ser. Newport infections involving 11 premature infants,[501] 90% of infants with gastroenteritis had blood in their stools, 10% had fever, 10% had mucus in their stools, and 9% were asymptomatic. In an outbreak of *S.* ser. Typhimurium[505] involving 11 ill and 5 healthy infants, none had bloody stools; all of the symptomatic infants were febrile and most commonly had loose green stools. Of 26 infants infected by *Salmonella* ser. Virchow, 42% were asymptomatic; the rest had mild diarrhea.[509] Seals and colleagues[514] described 12 infants with *S.* ser. Nienstedten, all of whom had watery diarrhea and low-grade fever; none had bloody stools. In a large outbreak in Zimbabwe of *S.* ser. Heidelberg infection reported by Bannerman,[512] 38% of 100 infants were asymptomatic, 42% had diarrhea, 16% had fever, 15% had pneumonia, and 2% developed meningitis. An outbreak of *S.* ser. Worthington was characterized primarily by diarrhea, fever, and jaundice, although 3 of 18 infants developed meningitis, and 17% died.[488] Fifty percent of infants had bloody stools in an outbreak of *S.* ser. Tennessee,[522] whereas none of 27 infants with positive stool cultures had an illness in a different nursery found to be contaminated with the same serovar.[538] Protracted diarrhea caused by *Salmonella* has been reported, although this relationship is not well proven[539]; diarrhea is usually self-limiting.[442] Children younger than 5 years of age may shed *Salmonella* for several weeks. The median was 7 weeks in one study, and 2.6% of children shed the pathogen for 1 year or longer.[540] The use of antibiotics may prolong shedding.[541]

Major extraintestinal complications of *Salmonella* infection may develop in a neonate or infant who becomes bacteremic. Systemic spread may develop in infants who initially present with diarrhea and in some who have no GI tract findings. Bacteremia seems to be more common in neonates. A study of more than 800 children with *Salmonella* infection showed that extraintestinal infection occurred significantly more often (8.7% vs. 3.6%) in the first 3 months of life.[542] Prospective studies of infants in the first year of life suggest that the risk of bacteremia is 1.8% to 6%.[543,544] Recent epidemiologic data are consistent with the above observations from previous studies.[445,496] *Salmonella* bacteremia is often not suspected clinically because the syndrome may be nonspecific and consistent with gram-negative sepsis.[446,447] Even afebrile, well-appearing children with *Salmonella* gastroenteritis have been documented to have bacteremia that persists for several days.[545]

Although infants with bacteremia may have spontaneous resolution without therapy,[546] a sufficient number develop complications to warrant empirical antimicrobial therapy when bacteremia is suspected. The frequency of complications is highest in the first month of life. Meningitis is the most feared complication of bacteremic *Salmonella* disease. Of all cases of nontyphoidal *Salmonella* meningitis, the majority occur in the first 6 months of life.[547,548] Meningitis has a high mortality rate, in part because of high relapse rates. Relapse has been reported in 8% to 60% of cases and may be affected by the choice of antibiotic.[549,550] Recent mortality rates reported vary slightly by region. From Thailand, *Salmonella* bacteremia with meningitis had a mortality of 11.8%[548]; a report from Malawi indicated a near-50% mortality.[550] In some older studies, greater than 90% of patients with meningitis died.[551] The survivors may experience the expected complications of gram-negative neonatal meningitis, including hydrocephalus, seizures, ventriculitis, abscess formation, subdural empyema, and permanent neurologic impairment.[550] Neurologic sequelae have included retardation, hemiparesis, epilepsy, visual impairment, and athetosis.[547]

Salmonella infections can also be complicated by pneumonia,[512] osteomyelitis,[552,553] or septic arthritis.[510,512] Other rare complications of salmonellosis include pericarditis,[554] pyelitis,[555] peritonitis,[505] otitis media,[505] mastitis,[556] cholecystitis,[557] endophthalmitis,[558] cutaneous abscesses,[518] and infected cephalhematoma.[552] Reported mortality rates in nursery outbreaks range from 0% to 20%.[512,520-522,531]

Enteric fever, most often related to *S.* ser. Typhi but also occurring with *S.* ser. Paratyphi A, *S.* ser. Paratyphi B, *Salmonella* ser. Paratyphi C, and other *Salmonella* spp., is reported much less commonly in infants and neonates than in older patients.[534,535] Of 1500 cases of typhoid fever that Osler and McCrae[559] reported, only 2 were in the first year of life. Infected infants may remain asymptomatic or develop typical findings of neonatal sepsis.[536] Enteric fever is often associated with constipation in older patients but is more likely to cause diarrhea in children.[534] Respiratory symptoms and nonspecific febrile illness have also been described.[534,537]

Typhoid fever[491,560] and nontyphoidal *Salmonella* infections[561] during pregnancy put women at risk of aborting the fetus and of premature delivery.[562] Historically, 14% of pregnant women with typhoid fever died.[563] The outlook for carrying the pregnancy to term and delivering a healthy infant seems to have improved dramatically during the antibiotic era.

Diagnosis

The current practice of early discharge of newborns, although potentially decreasing the risk of exposure, can make recognition of a nursery outbreak difficult. Diagnosis of neonatal salmonellosis should trigger an investigation for other cases. Signs of neonatal *Salmonella* infection can be similar to the nonspecific findings seen in most neonatal infections and in neonatal sepsis as described above. Enlarged liver and spleen are common in neonates with positive blood cultures. Fecal leukocyte examination reveals neutrophils in 36% to 82%[344,564] of persons with *Salmonella* infection. Twenty-five percent of children younger than 2 years with *Salmonella* in a small study had fecal leukocytes.[565]

Cultures remain the gold standard for diagnosis of *Salmonella.*[442,566,567] Routine stool cultures usually detect *Salmonella* if two or three different enteric media (i.e., MacConkey, eosin–methylene blue, *Salmonella-Shigella,* Tergitol 7, xylose-lysine-deoxycholate, brilliant green, or bismuth sulfite agar) are used. Stool, rather than rectal swab material, is preferable for culture, particularly if the aim of culture is to detect carriers.[568] Infants who are bacteremic often do not appear sufficiently toxic to raise the suspicion of bacteremia.[569] Blood cultures should be obtained as a routine part of evaluation of neonates with suspected or documented *Salmonella* infection. Ill neonates with *Salmonella* infection should have a cerebrospinal fluid examination performed. Bone marrow cultures also may be indicated when enteric fever is suspected; the sensitivity of bone marrow culture is higher than blood culture,[566,567] especially in a neonate in whom the volume of blood that can be used is limited. Focal invasive infections should be cultured from the site of infection.[570]

The Widal serologic test for *S.* ser. Typhi has been available for more than a century.[567] Additional serologic tests are available. However, the sensitivity and specificity are problematic, and results can be difficult to interpret.[566,567,571,572] These methods have not surpassed culture as the best way to diagnose *Salmonella* infections.

PCR detection in clinical samples is available in the research setting and continue to be investigated and developed.[567,573,574] However, no single molecular detection test is generally available.

If an outbreak of salmonellosis is suspected, further characterization of the organism is imperative.[575] Determination of somatic and flagellar antigens to characterize the specific serotype may be crucial to investigate an outbreak. When the serotype found during investigation of an outbreak is a common one (e.g., *S.* ser. Typhimurium), antimicrobial resistance testing[502,576] and use of molecular techniques, such as plasmid characterization,[576] can be helpful in determining whether a single-strain, common-source outbreak is in progress and for guidance on proper management.

Therapy

As in all enteric infections, attention to fluid and electrolyte abnormalities is the first issue that must be addressed by the physician. Specific measures to eradicate *Salmonella* intestinal infection have met with little success. Multiple studies show that antibiotic treatment of *Salmonella* gastroenteritis prolongs the excretion of *Salmonella.*[541,577-584] Almost half of infected children in the first 5 years of life continue to excrete *Salmonella* 12 weeks after the onset of infection; greater than 2.6% to 5% have positive cultures at 1 year.[540] No benefit of therapy has been shown in comparisons of ampicillin or neomycin versus placebo,[581] chloramphenicol versus no antibiotic treatment,[580] neomycin versus placebo,[582] ampicillin or TMP-SMX versus no antibiotic,[579] and ampicillin or amoxicillin versus placebo.[583] A Cochrane meta-analysis reached similar conclusions regarding the lack of evidence for any efficacy of antibiotic treatment.[541]

Because these studies have few data regarding the risk-benefit ratio of therapy in the neonate, it is uncertain whether they should influence treatment decisions in neonates. Studies that have included a few neonates suggest little benefit from antimicrobial therapy.[505,513,579,585,586] However, because bacteremia is common in neonates, antimicrobial therapy for infants younger than 3 months who have *Salmonella* gastroenteritis is often recommended,[543,544,569,570,587] especially if the infant appears toxic. Premature infants and infants who have other significant debilitating or predisposing conditions (immunocompromised, sickle cell anemia, acquired immunodeficiency syndrome [AIDS]) also merit treatment. The duration of therapy is debatable but should probably be no more than 3 to 5 days if the infant is not seriously ill and if blood cultures are sterile.[587] If toxicity, clinical deterioration, or documented bacteremia complicates gastroenteritis, prolonged treatment is indicated. Even with antimicrobial therapy, some infants develop complications. An infant with typhoid fever should be treated with an appropriate antimicrobial agent; relapses sometimes occur after therapy. Colonized healthy infants discovered by stool cultures to harbor non-Typhi *Salmonella* during evaluation of an outbreak ought to be isolated, but probably should not receive antimicrobial therapy. These infants should be discharged from the nursery as early as possible and followed carefully as outpatients.

Antimicrobial treatment of neonates who have documented extraintestinal dissemination must be prolonged. *Salmonella* bacteremia without localization is generally treated with at least a 10- to 14-day course of therapy.[570,587] Therapy for meningitis must be given for at least 4 to 6 weeks to lessen the risk of relapse.[570,588] About three fourths of patients who have relapses have been treated for 3 weeks or less.[547] Similar to meningitis, treatment for osteomyelitis and other invasive infections must be prolonged to be adequate. Although cures have been reported with 3 weeks of therapy, 4 to 6 weeks of therapy is recommended.[570,587]

Resistance to antibiotics has long been a problem with *Salmonella* infection[577,589] and has been steadily increasing in the United States.[590-592] Resistance has been selected and transmitted partly because therapy has been given for mild illness that should not have been treated[577] and partly because of use of antibiotics in animal feeds.[587] *Salmonella* infections, including enteric fever, have classically been treated with chloramphenicol, ampicillin, or TMP-SMX. However, resistance to these agents has been increasing.[591,593] A recent study conducted with data from the National Antimicrobial Resistance Monitoring System (NARMS) evaluated resistance patterns for non-Typhi *Salmonella* spp. isolated from blood in the United States from 1996 to 2007. This study reported that 8.2 % of isolates were resistant to ampicillin, 7.3% to chloramphenicol, and 7.6% to TMP-SMX.[591] In the developing world, the problem is even more significant. Between 16% and 37.5% of *S.* ser. Typhi isolates from eight Asian countries showed resistance to these antibiotics.[594] Resistance to extended-spectrum cephalosporins and to fluoroquinolones, although still relatively low in the United States, is also an increasing problem. Rates of ceftriaxone resistance among *S. enterica* are reported from NARMS to be 5.3%.[591] Ciprofloxacin resistance was not found. However, 9.6% of strains were resistant to nalidixic acid,[591] which is an indication of decreased effectiveness and higher minimal inhibitory concentrations (MICs) for ciprofloxacin.[595]]. This rate has been increasing over the past several decades.[592] The prevalence of extended spectrum β-lactamases and decreased susceptibility to fluoroquinolones (nalidixic acid and ciprofloxacin) reported in other developed and developing countries are also concerning.[594,596,597]

Antibiotics that are efficacious for the treatment of susceptible *Salmonella* infections include chloramphenicol, ampicillin, TMP-SMX, ceftriaxone or cefotaxime, and fluoroquinolones, among others.[587,598] TMP-SMX, although useful in older children and adults, is not used in neonates because of the risk of kernicterus. Because of the risk of gray baby syndrome, chloramphenicol should not be used in neonates unless other effective agents are unavailable. Recommendations for gastroenteritis in children given by the AAP are to use ampicillin or TMP-SMX unless there is concern for resistance, in which case a fluoroquinolone or azithromycin may be effective.[570] A third-generation cephalosporin can also be considered and may be optimal empirically in neonates if antibiotic susceptibility is not known.[587,599] Therapy should be tailored based on local susceptibility patterns and resistance testing for the isolated strain. The third-generation cephalosporins (cefotaxime, ceftriaxone) represent drugs of choice for invasive salmonellosis, including for meningitis with either ampicillin or ceftriaxone for continued therapy once susceptibilities are known.[570,588] Foci of infection should be drained appropriately.[442,587] Recommendations for treatment of enteric fever are cefotaxime/ceftriaxone or a fluoroquinolone empirically with adjustment of therapy based on susceptibilities.[570,598] A careful history should be taken to ascertain possible exposures, such as a visiting relative, to resistant strains. Difficult-to-treat infections, recurrent or resistant, have been successfully treated with carbapenems.[600]

Fluoroquinolones have been typically avoided because of concerns of possible adverse effects in the cartilage of children. However, a recent review of the literature suggests that the use of fluoroquinolones may be safe in children.[601] Routine use, however, continues to be not recommended and not approved by the FDA for the treatment of *Salmonella* in infants and neonates. However, they should be considered when other options are unavailable due to antimicrobial resistance.[601]

Prevention

Early recognition and intervention of nursery outbreaks of *Salmonella* are critical to achieve appropriate outbreak control. When a neonate develops salmonellosis, a search for other infants who have been in the same nursery should be undertaken. When two or more cases are recognized, environmental cultures, cultures of all infants, cohorting and contact isolation of infected infants, rigorous enforcement of hand hygiene, early discharge of infected infants, and thorough cleaning of all possible fomites in the nursery and delivery rooms are important elements of control.[522] If cases continue to occur, the nursery should be closed to further admissions.

Two vaccines for *S* ser. Typhi are licensed for older children. One is a live-attenuated vaccine, and the second is a Vi polysaccharide vaccine. Neither is recommended for children younger than 2 years.[466]

SHIGELLA

Nature of the Organism

On the basis of DNA relatedness, shigellae and *E. coli* organisms belong to the same species.[602] For historical reasons and because of their medical significance, shigellae have been maintained as separate species, however. Shigellae are gram-negative bacilli that differ from typical *E. coli* because they do not metabolize lactose or do so slowly, are nonmotile, and generally produce no gas during carbohydrate metabolism.[603,604]

Shigellae are classically divided into four species (serogroups) on the basis of metabolic and antigenic characteristics (Table 11-3). The mannitol nonfermenters usually are classified as *S. dysenteriae*.[603] Although the LPS antigens of the 15 recognized members of this group are not related to each other antigenically, these serotypes are grouped together as serogroup A.[605] Serogroup D (*Shigella sonnei*) strains are ornithine decarboxylase positive and slow lactose fermenters.[603] All *S. sonnei* share the same LPS (O antigen), comprising a single seroroup.[606] Shigellae that ferment mannitol (in contrast to *S. dysenteriae*) but do not decarboxylate ornithine or ferment lactose belong to serogroups B and C.[603] Of these, the strains that have LPS antigens immunologically related to each other are grouped together as serogroup B (*Shigella flexneri*), whereas strains harboring O antigens not related to each other or to other shigellae are included in serogroup C (*Shigella boydii*). There

Table 11-3 *Shigella* Serogroups

Serogroups	Serogroup Name	No. Serotypes
A	*S. dysenteriae*	15
B	*S. flexneri*	15 (including subtypes)
C	*S. boydii*	20
D	*S. sonnei*	1

are six major serotypes of *S. flexneri* and 15 subserotypes, and there are 20 antigenically distinct serotypes of *S. boydii*.[606]

The virulence of shigellae has been studied extensively since their recognition as major pathogens at the beginning of the 20th century.[607,608] The major determinants of virulence are encoded by a 120- to 140-MDa plasmid.[609-611] This plasmid, which is found in all virulent shigellae, encodes the synthesis of proteins that are required for invasion of mammalian cells and for the vigorous inflammatory response that is characteristic of the disease.[612,613] Shigellae that have lost this plasmid, have deletions of genetic material from the region involved in synthesis of these proteins, or have the plasmid inserted into the chromosome lose the ability to invade eukaryotic cells and become avirulent[614]; maintenance of the plasmid can be detected in the clinical microbiology laboratory by ability to bind Congo red. The ability to invade cells is the basic pathogenic property shared by all shigellae[615,616] and by *Shigella*-like enteroinvasive *E. coli*, which also possesses the *Shigella* virulence plasmid.[218,612,613,617,618] In the laboratory, *Shigella* invasiveness is studied in tissue culture (HeLa cell invasion), in animal intestine, or in rabbit or guinea pig eye, where instillation of the organism causes keratoconjunctivitis (Sereny test).[619]

Shigella invasiveness is mediated by a set of toxins injected into host cells by virtue of a type III secretion system, which injects the proteins directly from the bacterial cytoplasm to the host cell cytoplasm.[611,620] *Shigella* follows an unusual pathogenetic course. The bacteria invade the epithelial cell via pathogen-directed endocytosis, initially at M cells.[611] They are subsequently introduced into the epithelium, where they are taken up by macrophages. The organisms are able to escape the phagosome and kill the macrophages.[611,621] They additionally invade epithelial cells from the basolateral side and again force lysis of the endocytic vacuole, gaining entry into the host cell cytoplasm, where they are able to divide. The bacteria nucleate actin at one pole and use it to propel them into adjacent cells.[611] Of interest, they are able to avoid autophagy in the host cells.[621] This sequence promotes lateral spread through the mucosa. The process of invasion results in a significant inflammatory response giving rise to the destructive nature of shigellosis.[611,621] There is evidence that they additionally dampen the inflammatory response to promote a favorable environment.[621]

Most key *Shigella* virulence factors are encoded on the virulence plasmid, but several chromosomal loci also enhance virulence.[622,623] This phenomenon has been best studied in *S. flexneri*, in which multiple virulence-enhancing regions of the chromosome have been defined.[610,622,623,624] The specific gene products of some of the chromosomal loci are unknown; one chromosomal virulence segment encodes for synthesis of the O repeat units of LPS. Intact LPS is necessary but not sufficient to cause virulence.[622,625] At least two cell-damaging cytotoxins that also are chromosomally encoded are produced by shigellae. One of these toxins (Shiga toxin) is made in large quantities by *S. dysenteriae* serotype 1 (the Shiga bacillus) and is made infrequently by other shigellae.[626] Shiga toxin is a major virulence factor in *S. dysenteriae*, enhancing virulence at the colonic mucosa and giving rise to sequelae similar to those caused by STEC (discussed earlier). This toxin kills cells by interfering with peptide elongation during protein synthesis.[627-629] Additional toxins, such as (*Shigella* enterotoxin) Shet-1 (chromosomally encoded and limited to *S. flexneri* 2a) and Shet-2 (plasmid-encoded by all serotypes), may also be secreted by shigellae and mediate an initial secretory diarrhea from the small bowel.[605,630-632]

Epidemiology

Similar to other organisms transmitted by the fecal-oral route, Shigellae are commonly spread by food and water, but the low infecting inoculum allows person-to-person spread. Because of this low inoculum, *Shigella* is one of the few enteric pathogens that can infect swimmers.[633] The dose required to cause illness in adult volunteers is 10 organisms for *S. dysenteriae* serotype 1,[634] about 200 organisms for *S. flexneri*,[635] and 500 organisms for *S. sonnei*.[636] Person-to-person transmission of infection probably explains the continuing occurrence of *Shigella* in the developed world. Enteropathogens that require large inocula and are best spread by food or drinking water are less common in industrialized societies because of sewage disposal facilities, water treatment, and food-handling practices. In the United States, daycare centers are a major focus for acquisition of shigellosis.[637] Numerous outbreaks of shigellosis related to crowding, poor sanitation, and the low dose required for diseases have occurred in this setting.[638]

Given the ease of transmission, it is not surprising that the peak incidence of disease occurs during the first 4 years of life. It is, however, paradoxical that symptomatic infection is uncommon in the first year of life.[639-642] The best data on the age-related incidence of shigellosis come from Mata's[639] prospective studies of Guatemalan infants. In these studies, stool cultures were performed weekly on a group of children followed from birth to 3 years of age. The rate of infection was more than 60-fold lower in the first 6 months of life than between 2 and 3 years.[639] The same age-related incidence has been described in the United States[642] and other settings.[641,643-645] A review of three large case series[646-648] suggests that about 1.6% (35 of 2225) of shigellosis cases occur in infants during the neonatal period. The largest series of neonatal shigellosis[645] suggests that the course, complications, and etiologic serogroups are different in neonates than in older children. Although newborns are routinely contaminated by maternal feces, neonatal shigellosis is rare.

In the United States, data from 2005 suggested the incidence of *Shigella* is 4.5 per 100,000. The highest rates are in children 1 to 4 years of age (22/100,000). Most *Shigella* infections are caused by *S. sonnei* (75%) or, less commonly, *S. flexneri* (18%).[649] In most of the developing world, *S. flexneri* is isolated at higher rates as well as *S. dysenteriae* serotype 1.[650] As hygiene and gross domestic product increases, the proportion of *S. sonnei* increases, and that of *S. flexneri* and *S. dysenteriae* decreases.[650,651] Data from Bangladesh suggest that *S. dysenteriae* is less common in neonates, but *S. sonnei* and *S. boydii* are more common.[645]

Clinical Manifestations

The incubation period of shigellosis is related to the number of organisms ingested, but in general, it is 12 to 48 hours. Volunteer studies have shown that after ingestion, illness may be delayed for 1 week or more.[635] Neonatal shigellosis seems to have a similar incubation period. Frequently neonatal cases occur within 3 days of birth, suggestive of fecal-oral transmission during delivery.[646] Mothers of infected neonates are sometimes carriers, although, more typically, they are symptomatic during the perinatal period. Intrauterine infection is rare, although it has been reported.[652] In an older child, the initial signs are usually high fever, abdominal pain, vomiting, toxicity, and large-volume watery stools; diarrhea may be bloody or may become bloody. Painful defecation and severe, crampy abdominal pain associated with frequent passage of small-volume stools with gross blood and mucus are characteristic findings in older children or adults who develop severe colitis.[606,630,653] Many children never develop bloody diarrhea, however.[630] Adult volunteer studies have shown that variations in presentation and course are not related to the dose ingested because some patients develop colitis with dysentery, but others develop only watery diarrhea after ingestion of the same inoculum.[635]

The neonate with shigellosis may have a mild diarrheal syndrome or a severe colitis.[645,646,654-662] Fever in neonates is usually low grade (<38.8° C [<102° F]) if the course is uncomplicated. The neonate has less bloody diarrhea, more dehydration, more bacteremia, and a greater likelihood of death than the older child with shigellosis.[645] Physical examination of the neonate may show signs of toxicity and dehydration, although fever, abdominal tenderness, and rectal findings are less striking than in the older child.[647]

Complications of shigellosis are common.[663] Although the illness is self-limited in the normal host, resolution may be delayed for 1 week or more. In neonates and malnourished children, chronic diarrhea may follow a bout of shigellosis.[654,662] In hospitalized children with *Shigella*, seizure rates up to 45% have been reported.[663-665] Usually, the seizures are brief, generalized, and associated with high fever. Additional risk factors, such as dehydration and electrolyte abnormalities, are often identified.[666,667] Rates when including outpatient cases are likely lower.[666,667] Seizures are uncommon in the first 6 months of life, although neonates have been described with seizures.[656,668] The cerebrospinal fluid generally reveals normal values in these children, but a few have mild cerebrospinal fluid pleocytosis.[667] The neurologic outcome generally is good even with focal or prolonged seizures, but fatalities occasionally occur, often associated with toxic encephalopathy.[669] Although the seizures had been postulated to result from the neurotoxicity of Shiga toxin, this explanation was proved to be incorrect because most shigellae make little or no Shiga toxin, and strains isolated from children with neurologic symptoms often do not produce Shiga toxin.[626,666,670] Hemolysis with or without development of uremia is a complication primarily of *S. dysenteriae* serotype 1 infection.[671]

Sepsis during the course of shigellosis may be caused by the *Shigella* itself or by other gut flora that gain access to the bloodstream through damaged mucosa.[645,672,673] The risk of sepsis is higher in the first year of life, particularly in neonates,[645,654-656,668,674] in malnourished infants, and in infants with *S. dysenteriae* ser. 1 infection.[673] Sepsis may occur in 4% to 12% of neonates with shigellosis.[663,672,675-677] Given the infrequency of neonatal shigellosis, it is striking that a review of the literature suggests 9% of reported cases of *Shigella* sepsis have involved infants in the first month of life.[678] One of the infants with bacteremia[679] reportedly had no discernible illness. Disseminated intravascular coagulation may develop in patients whose course is complicated by sepsis.[677] Meningitis has been described in a septic neonate and infant, although it is extremely rare.[668,680] Colonic perforation has occurred in neonates,[681,682] older children,[683] and adults.[684] Although this complication of toxic megacolon is rare, it seems to be more common in neonates than in older individuals. Bronchopneumonia may complicate the course of shigellosis, but shigellae are rarely isolated from lungs or tracheal secretions.[685] The syndrome of sudden death in the setting of extreme toxicity with hyperpyrexia and convulsions but without dehydration or sepsis (i.e., Ekiri syndrome)[686-688] is rare in neonates. In a nonbacteremic child, other extraintestinal foci of infection, including the vagina[689,690] and eye,[691] rarely occur. Reactive arthritis (formerly known as Reiter syndrome), which rarely complicates the illness in children, has not been reported in neonates.

Although infection is less common in infants than in toddlers, case-fatality rates are highest in infants and are reported to be twice that in older children.[645,692,693] In industrialized societies, less than 1% of children with shigellosis die.[694] In developing countries, case fatality rates are decreasing. In 1999, Kotloff and colleagues[694] reported overall rates of 13.9% in infants 0 to 11 months of age. By 2010, a study in Bangladesh estimated rates of 0.89%.[695] The authors ascribe this trend to improvements in nutrition in addition to improved measles vaccination rates and vitamin A levels.[695] All of these factors may affect severity of *Shigella* infections. *S. dysenteriae* ser. 1 infection in the less-developed world is additionally a more frequent and severe cause of shigellosis.[673]

Diagnosis

Although the diagnosis of shigellosis can be suspected on clinical grounds, other enteropathogens can cause illnesses that are impossible to distinguish clinically. Shigellosis in neonates is rare, as described above. A neonate with watery diarrhea is more likely to be infected with *E. coli*, *Salmonella*, or rotavirus than *Shigella*. Infants presenting with bloody diarrhea may have necrotizing enterocolitis or infection with *Salmonella*, EIEC, *Yersinia enterocolitica*, *C. jejuni*, or *Entamoeba histolytica*. Before cultures establish a diagnosis, clinical and laboratory data may aid in making a presumptive diagnosis. Abdominal radiographs showing pneumatosis intestinalis suggest the diagnosis of necrotizing enterocolitis. A history of several weeks of illness without fever and with few fecal leukocytes suggests *E. histolytica*, rather than *Shigella* infection.[696]

The definitive diagnosis of shigellosis depends on isolation of the organism from stool. Culture may be insensitive, however.[697] In volunteer studies, stool culture failed to detect shigellae in about 20% of symptomatic subjects[635] and has a reported 50% sensitivity when compared with PCR methods.[698] Optimal recovery is achieved by immediate inoculation of stool (as opposed to rectal swabs) onto culture media[630]; shigellae are sensitive to environmental stress. Use of transport media generally decreases the yield of cultures positive for *Shigella*[699] compared with immediate inoculation.

Examination of stool for leukocytes as an indication of colitis can support the clinical suspicion of shigellosis. Abnormalities of white blood cell count and differential count also are used as supporting evidence for the diagnosis. Leukemoid reactions (white blood cells > 50,000/mm^3) occur in almost 15% of children with *S. dysenteriae* serotype 1 but in less than 2% of children with other shigellae.[670] Leukemoid reactions are more frequent in infants than in older children.[671] Even when the total white blood cell count is not dramatically elevated, there may be a striking left shift. Almost 30% of children with shigellosis have greater than 25% bands on the differential cell count.[700-702] Few reports address the white blood cell count in newborns, but those that do suggest that normal or low rather than elevated counts are more common. Although serum and fecal antibodies develop to LPSs and virulence plasmid–associated polypeptides,[703] serologic studies are not useful in the diagnosis of shigellosis. PCR can identify *Shigella* and EIEC in feces[704] and is reported to have increased sensitivity compared with culture.[698] Colonoscopy typically shows inflammatory changes that are most severe in the distal segments of colon.[705]

Therapy

Because dehydration is particularly common in neonatal shigellosis, unlike with older children, attention to correction of fluid and electrolyte disturbances is always the first concern when the illness is suspected. The benefits of antimicrobial therapy in neonates generally seem to outweigh the risks. The chief disadvantages of antimicrobial therapy include cost, drug toxicity, and emergence of antibiotic-resistant shigellae. Because of the self-limited nature of shigellosis, the AAP recommends that less severe illness in normal hosts should not be treated.[570] The WHO recommends empirical treatment of all cases.[606] Children can feel quite ill during the typical bout of shigellosis, however, and appropriate antimicrobial therapy shortens the duration of illness and eliminates shigellae from stool, decreasing secondary spread.[606,706] Complications are probably decreased by antibiotics. Given the higher mortality rates of neonatal shigellosis, therapy should be considered.

The empirical choice of an antimicrobial agent is dictated by susceptibility data for strains circulating in the community at the time the patient's infection occurs. Cefaclor,[707] furazolidone,[708] cephalexin,[709] amoxicillin,[710] kanamycin,[711] and cefamandole[712] all are relatively ineffective agents. In the past, empirical treatment of *Shigella* was recommended with ampicillin or TMP-SMX. High levels of resistance to these antibiotics are now encountered, and these are no longer recommended for empirical therapy. In the United States, a review of data from FoodNet and NARMS from 2000 to 2010 demonstrated 74% resistance to ampicillin and 36% resistance to TMP-SMX for all *Shigella* spp.[713] Rates are higher in the developing world. For instance, a recent study from Pakistan reports 85% resistance to TMP-SMX and 57.7% resistance to ampicillin over a 12-year period.[714] In older children, the AAP recommends parenteral azithromycin, ceftriaxone, or a fluoroquinolone for 3 to 5 days.[570] The WHO recommends ciprofloxacin 15 mg/kg twice daily for 3 days as first-line empirical therapy in patients of all ages. Recommended second-line agents include ceftriaxone (50-100 mg/kg daily for 2-5 days), pivmecillinam (20 mg/kg orally [PO] four times daily for 5 days), or azithromycin (6-20 mg/kg PO daily for 1-5 days).[606] Resistance to these agents is low in the United States.[713] Of note, a recent report documented decreased susceptibility to azithromycin in a strain isolated in Los Angeles.[715] Resistance to ceftriaxone and fluoroquinolones is more commonly reported in the developing world.[716-719] Therapy should be tailored based on antibiotic susceptibilities of individual isolated strains.

Optimal doses for newborns with shigellosis have not been established. For the rare newborn who acquires shigellosis, appropriate therapy often is delayed until susceptibility data are available. This delay occurs because shigellosis is so rare in newborns that it is almost never the presumptive diagnosis in a neonate with watery or bloody diarrhea. Given the higher risk of complications, however, it should remain on the clinician's differential diagnosis. For the neonate infected with *Shigella*, there are few data on which to base a recommendation. A third-generation parenteral cephalosporin is a reasonable choice. Quinolones, such as ciprofloxacin and ofloxacin, have been shown to be effective agents for treating shigellosis.[706,720,721] Although not approved by the FDA, it is generally felt that short courses are safe for children.[601] Other drugs occasionally used to treat diarrhea pose special risks to the infant with shigellosis. Antimotility agents, in addition to their intoxication risk, may pose a special danger in dysentery. In adults, diphenoxylate hydrochloride with atropine has been shown to prolong fever and excretion of the organism.[722]

The response to appropriate antibiotic therapy is generally gratifying, with improvement often apparent in 24 to 48 hours.[606] Complete resolution of diarrhea may not occur until 1 week or more after the start of treatment. In patients who have severe colitis and patients infected by *S. dysenteriae* ser. 1, the response to treatment is delayed.

Prevention

For most of the developing world, the best strategy for prevention of shigellosis during infancy is prolonged breastfeeding. Specific antibodies in milk seem to prevent symptomatic shigellosis[50,51]; nonspecific modification of gut flora and the lack of bacterial contamination of human milk also may be important. Breastfeeding, even when other foods are consumed, decreases the risk of shigellosis; children who continue to consume human milk into the third year of life are still partially protected from illness.[723] In the United States, the best means of preventing infection in the infant is good hand hygiene when an older sibling or parent develops diarrhea. Even in unsanitary environments, secondary spread of shigellae can be dramatically decreased by hand hygiene after defecation and before meals.[606,724]

Spread of shigellae in the hospital nursery can presumably be prevented by the use of contact isolation for infants with diarrhea and attention to thorough hand hygiene. Although nursery personnel have acquired shigellosis from infected newborns,[725] further transmission to other infants in the nursery, although described,[726] is rare. In contrast to *Salmonella*, large outbreaks of nosocomial shigellosis in neonates are rare.

Good hygiene is a particularly difficult problem in daycare centers. The gathering of susceptible children, breakdown in hand hygiene, failure to use different personnel for food preparation and diaper changing, and difficulty controlling the behavior of toddlers all contribute to daycare-focused outbreaks of shigellosis.[638]

Immunization strategies have been studied since the turn of the 20th century. Strategies have included killed vaccines, attenuated strains, and conjugate vaccines, but no vaccine is currently available.[605] Even if immunizations are improved, a role in managing neonates seems unlikely.

CAMPYLOBACTER

Campylobacter is a genus of zoonotic, gram-negative, spiral, microaerophilic, motile bacteria.[727] *Campylobacter* was first recognized in an aborted sheep fetus in the early 1900s[728] and was named *Vibrio fetus* by Smith and Taylor in 1919.[729] This organism subsequently was identified as a major cause of abortion, sterility, and scours in cattle, sheep, and goats.[730,731] It was not until 1947, when it was isolated from the blood culture of a pregnant woman who subsequently aborted at 6 months of gestation, that the significance of *Campylobacter* as a relatively rare cause of bacteremia and perinatal infections in humans was appreciated.[732-734]

This group of bacteria was initially included in the genus *Vibrio*. In 1963, *V. fetus* and related organisms were separated from the vibrios (e.g., *V. cholerae* and *Vibrio parahaemolyticus*) and placed in a new genus, *Campylobacter* (Greek word for "curved rod").[735] Currently, the genus *Campylobacter* contains 15 species, most of which are recognized as animal and human pathogens. The most commonly considered causes of human disease are *C. jejuni, C. coli, C. fetus, C. lari,* and *C. upsaliensis*.[736-738] DNA hybridization studies have shown that these species are genetically diverse, sharing less than 35% DNA homology under stringent hybridization conditions.[739]

Campylobacter has been recognized not only as an opportunistic pathogen in debilitated patients[740,741] but also as a common cause of endemic enteritis, foodborne gastroenteritis outbreaks, extraintestinal infections and postinfectious inflammatory complications (Guillain-Barré syndrome, reactive arthritis, and irritable bowel syndrome).[727,738,741-746] In human fetus and newborn, *C. fetus* can cause perinatal and neonatal infections that result in abortion, premature delivery, bacteremia, and meningitis.[732-734,747-754] Outside the newborn period, *Campylobacter* is a relatively infrequent cause of bacteremia, usually infecting patients with impaired host defenses.[742,755]

Virulence Factors and Pathogenic Mechanisms

Campylobacter harbors different virulence mechanisms acquired from other bacteria; the bacteria does not have genes codifying for secretor systems, and it has only one identifiable cytotoxin (cytolethal distending toxin, CDT). *Campylobacter* has the ability to invade and persist inside epithelial and reticuloendothelial cells, can mimic human epitopes evading the immune system, and can use particular metabolic substrates, different than those required by other bacteria (amino acids and fucose), that confer an adaptive advantage.[756]

C. jejuni, the most common and better known *Campylobacter* sp., can invade and induce a proinflammatory response in the host,[742,756] similar to *Shigella* and *Salmonella*. Although the mechanisms of these effects are not well understood, the main virulence factors involved are discussed in the following paragraphs.

Campylobacter have flagella-mediated motility, and their flagella have structural differences from other bacteria, with 7 rather than 11 protofilaments, formed by glycosylated proteins; this particular structure evades innate immunity recognition through TLR5. In addition, glycosylation of flagella confers strength, rigidity, and charge that facilitate access to more viscous environments and induce agglutination and microcolony formation.[757] Capsular polysaccharide and lipooligosaccharide may promote adhesion to and invasion of host cells, trigger inflammatory processes and mimic host gangliosides, contributing to the development of autoimmune diseases.[757]

Campylobacter secretes molecules involved in adhesion, invasion, toxicity, motility, autoagglutination, biofilm formation, and resistance to host defense mechanisms. Particularly relevant is cytotoxin CDT, a heat-labile protein with a molecular mass of 60 to 70 MDa that shares functional and immunologic properties with cholera toxin and *E. coli* LT.[757,758] This toxin is internalized by host cells and translocated to the nucleus, where it induces cell-cycle arrest and a proinflammatory response.[757]

After ingestion, *C. jejuni* reaches the intestine, penetrates the mucous layer, attaches to epithelial host cells, and is endocytosed by epithelial cells through a flagella-mediated process. Inside the host cell, *C. jejuni* remains in endocytic vacuoles, where it can replicate and induce cytoskeleton rearrangement, which promotes its trafficking to basolateral membrane domains and subepithelial tissue. In addition, *C. jejuni* can invade via a paracellular route, disrupting tight junctions or by intestinal M cells. Once in the subepithelial compartment, *C. jejuni* is phagocytosed by macrophages and dendritic cells, inducing a Th1 response that can control the infection but also cause tissue damage. *C. jejuni* survival and replication inside macrophages remains controversial.[757]

Epidemiology and Transmission

Campylobacter spp. infection is a zoonosis and a leading cause of foodborne/waterborne enteritis.[727] Most symptomatic cases of *Campylobacter* infections are sporadic acute gastroenteritis, occurring mostly in children younger than 5 years.[727,758] The pathogen has been isolated from 2% to 20% of fecal cultures from patients with diarrheal illnesses in various parts of the world.[727,759-763] Most isolates associated with diarrhea (61%-100%) are identified as *C. jejuni*,[764-767] and in some cases, individuals have been shown to be simultaneously infected with *C. jejuni* and *C. coli*.[765] There is a tendency for *C. jejuni* enteritis to occur in the summer in countries with temperate climates.[727,758]

More recently, *Campylobacter* has been recognized as a major cause of foodborne/waterborne gastroenteritis outbreaks, ranking second in bacterial frequency after *Salmonella* spp. in the United States.[758] The frequency of asymptomatic carriage of *C. jejuni* ranges from 0% to 85%, depending on the sanitary condition and food habits of the studied population.[768] In a cohort study in Mexico, 66% of all infections related to *C. jejuni* were asymptomatic.[738]

Campylobacter is a commensal bacterium of the GI tract of many farm animals (mainly poultry) and pets. A majority of chickens from several different geographic locations had high quantities (mean, 4 × 106/g) of *C. jejuni* in the lower intestinal tract or feces. Colonization occurred in some instances despite the use of tetracycline in the chicken feed, to which *Campylobacter* was susceptible in vitro.[769] The internal cavities of chickens remain positive for *Campylobacter* even after they have been cleaned, packaged, and frozen.[770] Cow's milk is probably contaminated from fecal shedding of the organism, and not through udder infection. In contrast to *Salmonella, C. jejuni* organisms that survive usually do not multiply to high concentrations.[771] Such organisms are killed through adequate heating; thus transmission to human hosts occurs through ingestion of undercooked contaminated food (meat), unpasteurized milk, or contaminated water.[727,745,772-775] Domestic puppies or kittens with *C. jejuni* diarrhea also can provide a source for spread, especially to infants or small children.[776] Anecdotal reports of intrafamilial and nursery outbreaks suggest that *C. jejuni* infection may occur after person-to-person transmission.[777,778]

Volunteer studies have shown a variable range in the infecting dose (from 500 to 1 billion), without a clear illness-dose response and with an attack rate of 40% to 60%.[727,779,780] The potential for low-inoculum disease has significant implications, including the need for adoption of strict enteric precautions when infected persons are hospitalized, particularly in maternity and nursery areas. When sporadic diarrhea in neonates caused by *C. jejuni* has been reported, maternal-infant transmission during labor has generally been documented, even in absence of maternal diarrhea during pregnancy.[781-790] In diarrhea outbreaks from neonatal intensive care units (NICUs) person-to-person spread has been documented through molecular typing methods.[791] Fecal excretion may last for a mean of 14 days after diarrhea, reaching up to 4 weeks in untreated children.[792,793]

C. fetus infections occur mostly in older men with a history of farm or animal exposure and in pregnant women during their third trimester.[743] Symptomatically or asymptomatically infected women may have recurrent abortions or premature deliveries and are the source of organisms associated with life-threatening perinatal infections of the fetus or newborn infant.[747-750,794] In several instances of neonatal sepsis and meningitis, *C. fetus* has been isolated from culture of maternal cervix or vagina.[753] Nosocomial nursery outbreaks have been associated to spread from infected infants with different clinical presentations, ranging from asymptomatic carriage to sepsis and meningitis.[795]

Clinical Manifestations

Campylobacter-associated clinical manifestations depend on the species involved. The most common syndrome caused by *C. jejuni* and *C. coli* is acute enteritis, which develops within 1 to 7 days after ingestion of contaminated food or water, associated with watery or bloody diarrhea, fever, and severe abdominal pain (mimicking acute appendicitis).[767] Bacteremia with *C. jejuni* enteritis is an uncommon complication of GI infection, occurring mostly in malnourished children.[767,790] Extraintestinal infections related to *C. jejuni* other than bacteremia are rare, but include cholecystitis,[796] urinary tract infection,[797] and meningitis.[7844] Postinfectious complications in older children and adults that have been associated with *C. jejuni* enteritis include Guillain-Barré syndrome, reactive arthritis, and irritable bowel syndrome.[767,798] Persistent *C. jejuni* infections have been described in patients infected with human immunodeficiency virus (HIV).[799] Maternal symptoms considered to be related to *C. jejuni* infection generally are mild and include fever (75%) and diarrhea (30%). Third-trimester infection related to *C. fetus* or *C. jejuni* may result in abortion or stillbirth. *Campylobacter* is an uncommon infection in neonates, who generally develop mild gastroenteritis when infected[763,781-790]; however, neonatal meningitis caused by *C. jejuni* has been reported.[783,789]

Human infections with *C. fetus* are rare and generally are limited to bacteremia in patients with predisposing conditions or to bacteremia or uterine infections with prolonged fever and pneumonitis that last for several weeks in women during the third trimester of pregnancy.[755] Unless appropriately treated, symptoms usually resolve only after abortion or delivery of an infected infant.[734,747-750] These infected neonates, who are often premature, develop signs suggesting sepsis, including fever, cough, respiratory distress, vomiting, diarrhea, cyanosis, seizures, and jaundice. The condition typically progresses to meningitis, which may be rapidly fatal or may result in serious neurologic sequelae.[734] Additional systemic manifestations include pericarditis, pneumonia, peritonitis, salpingitis, septic arthritis, and abscesses.[800] *C. lari* has caused chronic diarrhea and bacteremia in a neonate.[801]

Pathology

The pathologic findings of *C. fetus* infection in the perinatal period include placental necrosis and, in the neonate, widespread endothelial proliferation, intravascular fibrin deposition, perivascular inflammation, and hemorrhagic necrosis of the brain.[733] A trend for intravascular location and hepatosplenomegaly in adults infected with *C. fetus* has been shown.[741] The pathologic findings in infants and children infected with *Campylobacter* spp. include an acute inflammatory process in the colon or rectum, as evidenced by the clinical presentation of patients who have bloody diarrhea with numerous fecal leukocytes.[802] There also can be crypt abscess formation and an ulcerative colitis or pseudomembranous colitis–like appearance or a hemorrhagic jejunitis or ileitis.[803-805] Mesenteric lymphadenitis, ileocolitis, and acute appendicitis have also been described.

Diagnosis

Fecal culture, microscopic analysis, enzyme immunoassay, and molecular biology are available for detection of *Campylobacter* in feces from patients with enteric infections.[806,807] *C. fetus* and *C. jejuni* are fastidious and may be overlooked on routine fecal cultures. *C. jejuni* grows best in a microaerobic environment of 5% oxygen and 10% carbon dioxide at 42° C. It grows on various media, including *Brucella* and

Mueller-Hinton agars, but optimal isolation requires the addition of selective and nutritional supplements. Growth at 42° C in the presence of cephalosporins may be used to culture selectively for *C. jejuni* from fecal specimens. In a study of six media, charcoal-based selective media and a modified charcoal cefoperazone deoxycholate agar were the most selective for identification of *Campylobacter* spp. Extending the incubation time from 48 to 72 hours led to an increase in the isolation rate regardless of the medium used.[806] The typical darting motility of *Campylobacter* may provide a clue to identification, even in fresh fecal specimens, when viewed by phase-contrast microscopy.[808]

Campylobacter measures 0.2 to 0.5 femtometer (fm) wide and 0.5 to 8 fm long. A curved, motile gram-negative bacillus with a single polar flagellum, the pathogen is oxidase and catalase positive except for *C. upsaliensis*, which is generally catalase negative or weakly positive. *Campylobacter* is distinguished from *Vibrio* organisms by its carbohydrate fermentation characteristics and by its different nucleotide base composition.[809,810] *C. jejuni* and *C. fetus* are distinguished by growth temperature (*C. fetus* grows best at 25° C but can be cultured at 37° C; *C. jejuni* grows best at 42° C) and by nalidixic acid and cephalosporin susceptibilities because *C. jejuni* is susceptible to nalidixic acid and resistant to cephalosporins.

The diagnosis of *C. fetus* infection should be considered when there is an unexplained febrile illness in the third trimester of pregnancy or in the event of recurrent abortion, prematurity, or neonatal sepsis with or without meningitis. A high index of suspicion and prompt, appropriate antimicrobial therapy may prevent the potentially serious neonatal complications that may follow maternal *C. fetus* infection. Isolation of *Campylobacter* from blood or other sterile body sites does not represent the same problem as isolation from stool. Growth occurs with standard blood culture media, but it may be slow. In the case of *C. fetus* infecting the bloodstream or central nervous system, blood culture flasks should be blindly subcultured and held for at least 7 days, otherwise the organism may be missed because of slow or inapparent growth.[750]

Enzyme immunoassay kits have been developed for detection of *Campylobacter* in stool samples. Commercial kits have demonstrated sensitivity and specificity greater than 95% compared with fecal culture and PCR.[807] Detection of *C. jejuni* and *C. coli* by specific PCR or multiplex PCR, together with other enteric pathogens, has been reported.[807,811] Genotyping has been applied to determine the source of infection in *Campylobacter* outbreaks.[811-813]

Therapy and Prevention

Campylobacter enteritis is usually a mild-to-moderate, self-limited acute gastroenteritis in immunocompetent individuals and does not require antimicrobial therapy in this context. In infants with *C. jejuni* gastroenteritis, limited data suggest that appropriate, early antimicrobial therapy results in improvement and rapid clearance of the organism from stool.[814] Severe cases, especially in immunocompromised hosts and systemic infections, are an indication for antimicrobial use. The prognosis is grave in newborns with sepsis or meningitis caused by *C. fetus*.

Antibiotic resistance in *Campylobacter* spp. has emerged during the last 3 decades, related to indiscriminate use of antibiotics in humans and farm animals, especially poultry. *Campylobacter* spp. are often resistant to β-lactams and fluoroquinolones.[815-817] Most strains are susceptible to macrolides, gentamicin, tetracycline, and chloramphenicol.[815-817] In enteric infection, macrolides, mainly azithromycin, are the first-line choice. Strains that are erythromycin resistant often are resistant to azithromycin.[818] *Campylobacter* tends to have higher MICs for clarithromycin than for azithromycin.[819] If erythromycin therapy is initiated within the first 4 days of illness, a reduction in excretion of the organism and resolution of symptoms occur.[820] Nevertheless, controversy remains on the best empirical antimicrobial option of sepsis and meningitis. Successful outcomes have been reported with parenteral administration of aminoglycosides plus fluoroquinolones or third-generation cephalosporins plus macrolides/chloramphenicol or monotherapy with carbapenems.[821] Adjustments may be necessary after obtaining results of in vitro susceptibility studies.

Although data regarding treatment of asymptomatic or convalescent carriers are not unavailable, it seems appropriate to treat colonized pregnant women in the third trimester of pregnancy when there is a risk of perinatal or neonatal infection. The failure of prophylactic parenteral gentamicin in a premature infant has been documented, followed by successful resolution of symptoms and fecal shedding with macrolides.

Contact precautions should be used during any acute diarrheal illness and until the diarrhea has subsided. Hand hygiene after handling raw poultry and washing cutting boards and utensils with soap and water after contact with raw poultry may decrease risk of infection. Pasteurization of milk and chlorination of water are critical. Infected food handlers and hospital employees who are asymptomatic pose no known hazard for disease transmission if proper personal hygiene measures are maintained. Ingestion of human milk that contains anti–*C. jejuni* antibodies has been shown to protect infants from diarrhea caused by *C. jejuni*.[822]

Ongoing research on vaccine development against *Campylobacter* has followed two strategies: to prevent infection in humans, especially food handlers, and to prevent infection in poultry. Phase I/II clinical trials have reported appropriate safety profiles but variable efficacy results of these vaccine prototypes.[727,823,824]

CLOSTRIDIUM DIFFICILE

Virulence Factors and Pathogenic Mechanisms

C. difficile is a spore-forming, gram-positive, anaerobic bacillus that produces two toxins: toxin A, an enterotoxin that causes fluid loss, and toxin B, a cytotoxin recognized for its cytopathic effects in tissue culture.[122,825] Both toxin genes have been cloned and sequenced, encoding proteins with estimated molecular masses of 308 kDa for toxin A and 270 kDa for toxin B.[826] These toxins bind receptors in the apical membrane of colonocytes, enter the cells, and trigger colonocyte fluid secretion and apoptosis. An intense inflammatory reaction develops in the lamina propria underneath the damaged epithelia. Evidence suggests that absence of *C. difficile* toxin receptors in neonates may explain the characteristic lack of symptoms upon infection in this age group.

Breast milk and the commensal microbiota have also been proposed as protective factors.[827]

In the presence of antibiotic pressure, *C. difficile* colonic overgrowth and toxin production occurs. A wide variety of antibacterial, antifungal, antituberculosis, and antineoplastic agents have been associated with *C. difficile* colitis, although penicillins, clindamycin, and cephalosporins are associated most frequently. *C. difficile* and its toxins can be identified in one third of patients with antibiotic-associated diarrhea and in about 98% of patients with pseudomembranous colitis.[828]

Epidemiology

C. difficile can be isolated from soil and frequently exists in the hospital environment. Spores of *C. difficile* are quite persistent in the environment; they have been reported persist for up to 5 months on floor surfaces.[829] Spores of *C. difficile* can be ingested through contact with environmental surfaces, from items such as thermometers and feeding tubes, and from other colonized individuals by fecal-oral transmission.[829-834] Nosocomial spread is related to organisms on the hands of personnel,[829,831,835] and to contaminated surfaces, which may serve as reservoirs.[828,836]

Although all groups are susceptible to infection, newborns represent a special problem. Less than 5% of healthy children older than 2 years[837] and healthy adults carry *C. difficile*,[838] but 35% to 50% of neonates can harbor *C. difficile* and its cytotoxin in their stools, usually in the absence of clinical findings.[839-841]

Infants in NICUs have high rates of colonization, in part because of frequent use of antimicrobial agents in these units.[840,841] Clustering of infected infants suggests that much of the colonization of newborn infants represents nosocomial spread,[836] rather than acquisition of maternal flora. The number of *C. difficile* organisms present in stools of well infants is similar to that found in older patients with pseudomembranous colitis.[839,841] The high frequency of colonization has led to justified skepticism about the pathogenic potential of this organism in very young patients.[842] Although some episodes of diarrhea in early infancy may be caused by *C. difficile*,[843] the high frequency of asymptomatic carriage in this age group suggests that neither colonization nor detection of toxin production is sufficient to establish the diagnosis of *C. difficile* diarrhea in an infant. Rather, other etiologies should be comprehensively sought, and *C. difficile* should be implicated in the absence of another pathogen.

Clinical Manifestations

The usual manifestations of *C. difficile* disease in older children and adults include watery diarrhea, abdominal pain and tenderness, nausea, vomiting, and low-grade fever. Grossly bloody diarrhea is unusual, although occult fecal blood is common. Leukocytosis, elevation of acute phase reactants, and hypoalbuminemia are present during severe illness. Diarrhea usually begins 4 to 9 days into a course of antimicrobial therapy but may be delayed until several weeks after completion of the therapeutic course. Usually, the illness is mild and self-limited if the offending drug is discontinued.[828] Severe colitis with pseudomembranes is less common now than in previous years because the risk of diarrhea developing during antimicrobial therapy is recognized, and the antimicrobial agent typically is stopped.

It is currently controversial whether *C. difficile* causes disease in newborns.[827]

Diagnosis

Isolation of *C. difficile* by stool culture does not distinguish between toxigenic and nontoxigenic isolates. Several techniques for detection of toxins in stool samples have been developed, including enzyme immunoassay (EIA) and PCR.[828,843-845] There are multiple commercially available EIAs that detect either toxin A or both toxins A and B.[843,844,846] These assays are sensitive and easy to perform. Other assays are available for epidemiologic investigation of *C. difficile*–associated outbreaks.[846] Colonoscopy and histologic analysis is indicated in dysenteric cases in which differential diagnosis with inflammatory bowel disease and infection by other agents is necessary. The findings of pseudomembranes and hyperemic, friable rectal mucosa suggest the diagnosis of pseudomembranous colitis by *C. difficile*. Pseudomembranes are not always present; mild cases are often described as nonspecific colitis.[846]

In neonates, the isolation of the bacteria or detection of its toxins is not enough to prove that an illness is related to *C. difficile*. When the clinical picture is consistent, the stool studies are positive for *C. difficile*, and no other cause for illness is found, a diagnosis of "possible" *C. difficile* is made. A favorable response to eradication of *C. difficile* is supportive evidence that the diagnosis is correct.[847] Because of the uncertainty implicit in the ambiguity of neonatal diagnostic criteria, other diagnoses must be considered.

Therapy

Appropriate rehydration, withdrawal of offending antibiotics and oral metronidazole are the first-line treatment of colitis by *C. difficile*. In severe cases, lack of response to metronidazole, or recurrence, oral vancomycin is the second-line option.[846,848] Drugs that decrease intestinal motility should not be administered.

When the decision is made that a neonate's illness might be related to *C. difficile*, the initial approach should include fluid and electrolyte therapy and discontinuation of the offending antimicrobial agent. If the illness persists or worsens, or if the patient has severe diarrhea, oral metronidazole should be instituted. Orally administered vancomycin rarely needs to be considered in neonates.

Breastfeeding should be maintained because evidence suggests a protective role. Neutralizing antibody against *C. difficile* cytotoxin A has been shown in human colostrum. The secretory component of IgA binds to toxin A, inhibiting its binding to receptors.[849-851]

Prevention

In addition to standard precautions, contact precautions are recommended for the duration of illness. Meticulous hand hygiene techniques, proper handling of contaminated waste and fomites, disinfection of surfaces with hypochlorite solution, and limiting the use of antimicrobial agents are the best available methods for control of *C. difficile* infection.[852] A recent meta-analysis including 23 studies concluded that probiotics are effective for preventing *Clostridium difficile*–associated diarrhea in children and adults; these trials did not include neonatal cases.[853]

VIBRIO CHOLERAE

Nature of the Organism

V. cholerae is a gram-negative, curved rod with a polar flagellum. Of the more than 200 serotypes identified, only enterotoxin-producing organisms of serotype O1 and O139 may cause epidemics. *V. cholerae* O1 is divided into two serotypes, Inaba and Ogawa, and two biotypes, classic and El Tor; the latter is the predominant biotype. Nontoxigenic O1 strains and non-O1/O139 strains of *V. cholerae* can cause diarrhea and sepsis, but do not cause outbreaks.[854-856]

Virulence Factors and Pathogenic Mechanisms

V. cholerae O group 1 is the classic example of an enteropathogen whose virulence is caused by enterotoxin production. Cholera toxin is an 84-MDa protein composed of one A subunit and five B subunits. After ingestion, most strains of *V. cholerae* are killed by gastric acidity. Surviving organisms reach the duodenum, where B subunit pentamers bind to host cell receptor gangliosides GM_1 on the enterocyte apical membrane. Then, the A subunit is translocated to the cytoplasm, where it can mediate adenylate cyclase activation, increasing intracellular cAMP concentration. The elevated cAMP levels stimulate an active secretion process of the enterocytes by the opening of chloride channels on the apical membrane. The final effect is a secretory diarrhea.[855,856]

Two other toxins are also encoded within the virulence cassette that encodes cholera toxin. These toxins, zona occludens toxin (zot) and accessory cholera entero toxin (ace), are consistently found in illness-causing strains O1 and O139 but not usually in *V. cholerae* organisms that are less virulent.[854-856]

Epidemiology and Transmission

Since 1960, *V. cholerae* O1, biotype El Tor, has spread as a pandemic from India and Southeast Asia to Africa; the Middle East; southern Europe; and the southern, western, and central Pacific islands (Oceania). In late January 1991, toxigenic *V. cholerae* O1, serotype Inaba, biotype El Tor, appeared in several coastal cities of Peru.[855,857] It rapidly spread to most countries in South and North America. In reported cases, travel from the United States to Latin America or Asia and ingestion of contaminated food transported from Latin America or Asia were incriminated. *V. cholerae* O139 (Bengal) emerged on the Indian subcontinent as a new cause of epidemic cholera in 1993.[858-861] It rapidly spread through Asia and continues to reemerge periodically as a cause of epidemic cholera.

In the United States, an endemic focus of a unique strain of toxigenic *V. cholerae* O1 exists on the Gulf Coast of Louisiana and Texas.[854, 862] This strain is different from the one associated with the epidemic in South America. Most cases of disease associated with the strain endemic to the U.S. Gulf Coast have resulted from the consumption of raw or undercooked shellfish.

In resource-limited countries, *V. cholerae* remains a leading cause of acute diarrhea in neonates, accounting for 5% to 17% of episodes that require hospitalization.[863-865] In developed countries and developing countries where cholera is not endemic, it is extremely rare.

Humans are the only documented natural host, but free-living *V. cholerae* organisms can exist in the aquatic environment. The usual reported vehicles of transmission have included contaminated water or ice; contaminated food, particularly raw or undercooked shellfish; moist grains held at ambient temperature; and raw or partially dried fish. The usual mode of infection is ingestion of contaminated food or water. Boiling water or treating it with chlorine or iodine and adequate cooking of food kill the organism.[856] Asymptomatic infection of family contacts is common, but direct person-to-person transmission of disease has not been documented. Individuals with low gastric acidity are at increased risk for cholera infection. The infectious dose of *V. cholerae* O1 has been estimated to be 10^5 to 10^8 organisms in human volunteers but may be as low as 10^3 organisms in the presence of achlorhydria. The incubation period ranges between 12 hours and 5 days.[856]

Clinical Manifestations

The classic clinical presentation of cholera during an epidemic is profuse secretory diarrhea of up to 1 liter per hour, which can lead to hypovolemic shock in hours if left untreated. Vomiting may be present early in the illness course. Abdominal pain is absent or mild, and patients usually remain afebrile. In endemic cases, the disease may be milder or even asymptomatic.[856]

Cholera acquired during pregnancy, particularly in the third trimester, is associated with a high incidence of fetal death.[866] Miscarriage can be attributed to fetal acidosis and hypoxemia resulting from the marked metabolic and circulatory changes that this disease induces in the mother. The likelihood of delivering a stillborn infant is closely correlated with the severity of the maternal illness. The inability to culture *V. cholerae* from stillborn infants of infected mothers, together with the usual absence of bacteremia in cholera, suggests that transplacental fetal infection is not a cause of intrauterine death.

In neonates, the clinical spectrum of *V. cholerae* is wide and can range from asymptomatic infection to severe diarrhea.[863-865,867] Even infants born to mothers with active diarrheal disease may escape infection, despite evidence that rice-water stools, almost certain to be ingested during the birth process, may contain 10^9 organisms/mL.[867] The reason for this apparently low attack rate among newborns is unknown; however, it probably can be attributed in large part to protection conferred by breastfeeding.[868] Human milk contains antibodies and receptor-like glycoproteins that inhibit adherence of *V. cholerae* and gangliosides that bind cholera toxin.[58-60] The role of transplacentally acquired vibriocidal maternal antibodies has not been determined. Because *V. cholerae* causes neither bacteremia nor intestinal invasion, protection against illness is more likely to be a function of mucosal rather than serum antibodies.[869, 870] Additional factors that may reduce the incidence of neonatal cholera include the large inoculum required for infection and the limited exposure of the newborn to contaminated food and water.

Diagnosis

The WHO has developed a suspected case definition for *V. cholerae* for individuals older than 2 years: "a patient aged 2 years or more who develops acute watery diarrhea in an area known to have cholera" or "a patient aged 5 years or more who develops severe dehydration or dies from acute watery diarrhea, even in an area where cholera is not known to be present." These definitions are not applicable to neonatal infections. Clinicians should request fecal culture from patients suspected to have cholera. Stool specimens can be plated on thiosulfate citrate bile salts sucrose agar directly or after enrichment in alkaline peptone water. Isolates of *V. cholerae* should be confirmed by biochemical test, serogrouping, and serotyping and sent to a reference laboratory to test for cholera toxin production.[856] For rapid detection, a fresh stool sample can be analyzed by dark-field microscopy under 400× magnification, which allows visualization of *Vibrio*-shaped cells with darting motility; the sensitivity of this technique is approximately 50% compared with culture.

More recently, immunologic-based dipstick assays have been developed for rapid detection in settings with limited laboratory capacity. Rapid results of these tests facilitate detection of cases early during an outbreak.[871-873] PCR amplification and oligonucleotide probes have been developed for detection of the cholera toxin gene.[856,874,875]

Therapy and Prevention

The cornerstone of therapy is rehydration by administration of oral or parenteral fluids to correct hydric and electrolyte imbalance. Antimicrobial therapy can eradicate vibrios, reduce the duration of diarrhea, and reduce requirements for fluid replacement. Tetracycline, ciprofloxacin, erythromycin, or azithromycin can be used as first-line options, depending on local resistance.[856,857]

Two oral killed cholera vaccines are in use in developing countries. These vaccines have an excellent safety profile, offering moderate (near 60%) protection for up to 5 years. However, protection seems to be lower in young children.[856,876]

YERSINIA ENTEROCOLITICA

Nature of the Organism, Virulence Factors, and Pathogenic Mechanisms

Yersinia spp. are non–spore forming, gram-negative or gram-variable, rod-shaped or coccoid cells of 0.5- to 0.8-µm width and 1- to 3-µm length. *Y. enterocolitica* has multiple peritrichous flagella that are responsible for motility at 22° to 30° C. Expression of flagella proteins is temperature dependent, being suppressed at 37° C. This mechanism seems intended to evade innate immunity because flagella proteins are potent stimulants of the innate immune system.[877] Yersiniae grow under aerobic and anaerobic culture conditions between 0° and 45° C, and optimally at 25° to 28° C on nonselective and certain selective media.

Y. enterocolitica has a wide range of virulence factors, coded both on the chromosome and on a plasmid.[953,954] They include LPS and proteins related to adhesion, invasion, and flagellar structure; a type III secretion system; genes involved in immune evasion; intracellular persistence; and cytotoxicity (including an enterotoxin closely related to ST of ETEC).[877-880]

The primary event in *Y. enterocolitica* infection is terminal ileum and proximal colon colonization. These bacteria preferentially bind to and penetrate M cells of Peyer patches. After crossing epithelia, they reach the lamina propria, where they are phagocytosed by macrophages. *Y. enterocolitica* can persist and replicate inside macrophages and are transported by these immune cells to mesenteric lymph nodes and eventually to the liver and spleen. Inflammation and microabcesses can develop in the Peyer patches, mesenteric lymph nodes, liver, and spleen. Diarrhea and dysentery associated to this infection is related to intestinal inflammation.[877]

Epidemiology

Y. enterocolitica is a pharyngeal commensal of pigs, the major animal reservoir and constitutes a zoonosis, transmitted to human through ingestion of contaminated food or water. A history of recent consumption of chitterlings (prepared pig intestine) is common in symptomatic individuals.[881] Anecdotally, transmission has been reported after infusion of contaminated blood products.[882]

Y. enterocolitica is a major cause of enteritis/dysentery in much of the industrialized world. Enteritis caused by this organism primarily occurs in children younger than 5 years, with incidence peaking in the winter.[881,883-886] Enteritis by *Y. enterocolitica* in neonates is infrequent, but has occasionally been associated with extraintestinal involvement and sepsis.[887,888]

Clinical Manifestations

There are no distinguishable features of *Y. enterocolitica* enteocolitis compared with other invasive enteric pathogens such as *Shigella* or *Salmonella*. Infants present with febrile watery diarrhea or with stools containing mucus with streaks of blood. In older children and adults, fever, diarrhea, and right lower quadrant pain mimicking appendicitis are often found. In immunocompetent hosts, this represents a self-limited GI infection lasting 3 to 28 days. Extraintestinal involvement can include the microabscesses in the liver, spleen, or lungs; pharyngitis and pneumonia can occasionally be observed. Primary cutaneous *Yersinia* infections with cellulitis, bulla, and abscess formation have also been reported.[877,887]

Sepsis has been commonly reported in neonates (infants, particularly in the first 3 months of life), and immunocompromised patients. Fever is an inconsistent finding in children with bacteremia, and meningitis is rare.[888-892] Postinfectious complications such as reactive arthritis and erythema nodosum may appear a few weeks after enteritis.[877,893]

Diagnosis

Y. enterocolitica can be cultured from throat swabs, mesenteric lymph nodes, peritoneal fluid, blood, and stool. Because laboratory identification of organisms requires special techniques and culture in selective media (CIN agar: cefsulodin, Irgasan, novobiocin), laboratory personnel should be alerted when *Yersinia* is suspected. The most significant traits for identification are the following: motility at 25° C but not at 37° C, urease production, absence of oxidase activity and of production of gas or hydrogen sulphide on Kligler iron agar.[877] Biotyping and serotyping are useful to differentiate pathogenic from nonpathogenic strains, especially in isolates from the environment.[877] More recently, PCR (as a single-pathogen or multiplex platform) and matrix-assisted laser desorption/ionization time-of-flight mass spectrometry analysis have been added as diagnostic possibilities.[893,894,895]

Therapy

The vast majority of enteric infections caused by *Y. enterocolitica* in immunocompetent hosts are self-limited, and antibiotics are not indicated. Antibiotics have to be reserved for severe cases of enterocolitis, sepsis, and extraintestinal abscesses.[877,892]

Most strains of *Y. enterocolitica* are susceptible in vitro to TMP-SMX, aminoglycosides, chloramphenicol, tetracycline, fluoroquinolones, third-generation cephalosporins, and carbapenems.[877,896,897] Therapy in individual cases should be guided by in vitro susceptibility testing, although cefotaxime has been used successfully in bacteremic infants.[898]

AEROMONAS SPECIES

Nature of the Organism, Virulence Factors, and Pathogenic Mechanisms

The genus *Aeromonas* consists of environmental, facultative anaerobic, mesophilic, gram-negative rods that are predominantly motile because of a single polar flagellum, and they produce oxidase, catalase, nitrate reductase, and an array of exoenzymes. Although there are at least 21 species described in this genus, only *A. hydrophila, A. caviae, A. veronii* biovar sobria, and *A. trota* are important human pathogens.[899,900]

Aeromonads may produce a variety of potential virulence factors, including heat-stable and heat-labile enterotoxins, hemolysins, proteases, leukocidin, elastase, fibrinolysin, DNase, lecithinase, lipases, amylase, adhesins, agglutinins, pili, and an array of outer membrane proteins.[899,901,902] Participation of some of these proteins in virulence has been determined in animal models but not consistently in human volunteer studies. Recent reports of endemic diarrhea associated with *Aeromonas* suggest that clinical severity is related to the expression of a specific combination of enterotoxins.[899,903]

Epidemiology

Aeromonas spp. are ubiquitous organisms that can be isolated from almost any environmental niche. Most of the environmental isolates come from fresh- or brackish water sources; aeromonad contamination of chlorinated tap water has been occasionally reported. Aeromonads colonize and can cause disease in cold-blooded animals, including fish, amphibians, and reptiles, which may act as reservoirs.[899,904,905]

Humans acquire infection mostly during warm weather months through contaminated food or water, mainly unpasteurized milk, red meats, poultry, vegetables, fish or other seafoods, or by swimming or bathing in contaminated bodies of water.[899,904-906]

Aeromonas spp.–associated disease burden is difficult to determine because of underreporting and lack of routine diagnosis. Specific diagnostic tests are required to differentiate pathogenic aeromonads from normal flora and other pathogenic gram-negative bacilli such as *Vibrio* spp. and *Plesiomonas* spp.[899,900,906]

Asymptomatic fecal carriage is observed in approximately 1% to 2% of healthy individuals residing in nontropical regions. By contrast, up to 27% of healthy adults residing in tropical areas of Asia carry *Aeromonas* spp. asymptomatically in their stools.[903,907,908]

The first report of a human *Aeromonas* infection occurred in 1954 in a woman with myositis from Jamaica. In 1961, the first strain from human feces was isolated, after which aeromonads have been incriminated as agents of diarrhea, although unequivocal evidence of their pathogenic role in the intestine remains controversial.[903,909] *Aeromonas* have been implicated in 1% to 13% and 2% to 7% of endemic diarrhea in children and adults, respectively. These pathogens have also been associated with 1% to 4% of traveler's diarrhea, especially in people travelling to Southeast Asia.[899]

A recent prospective multicenter in-hospital–based 6-month surveillance study from France reported 78 *Aeromonas* spp.–associated infections, of which 44% were skin and soft tissue infections, 26% bacteremia, 19% gastroenteritis, 6% respiratory tract infection, and 5% miscellaneous.[905]

Aeromonas is an infrequent cause of gastroenteritis in neonates. According to a Brazilian study, 2.4% of stool samples obtained from neonates hospitalized by diarrhea were positive for *Aeromonas*.[910] Diarrhea outbreaks in neonatal units have been reported.

Clinical Manifestations

Although the pathogenic role of *Aeromonas* spp. is still controversial, gastroenteritis is the most common clinical illness attributed to *Aeromonas* infection in humans.[903,905] Both the small and large intestine can be compromised by this infection. A self-limited watery diarrhea is the most common clinical manifestation of *Aeromonas* enteritis, although a cholera-like illness has been reported.[911-914] Fever and vomiting are common in children. One third of patients have a dysentery-like syndrome with bloody mucoid diarrhea associated with colitis[915]; malaise and fever are more common in this form of presentation. In contrast to other causes of dysenteric bacterial gastroenteritis, stool leukocytes are uncommon. Chronic or intermittent diarrhea that lasts for weeks has been described in one third of patients infected by *A. caviae*.[899,915] Complications associated with *Aeromonas* gastroenteritis include bacteremia, intussusception, failure to thrive, HUS, and strangulated intestinal hernia.[899,916]

Other clinical presentations include skin and soft tissue infections, septicemia, intraabdominal infections (peritonitis, pancreatitis, cholangitis, hepatic abscesses), pneumonia (aspiration associated with a near-drowning episode), lung abscess, endophthalmitis, tonsillitis, otitis media, urinary tract infection, endocarditis, meningitis, osteomyelitis, pyogenic arthritis, and suppurative thrombophlebitis.[899,905,914] Sepsis is particularly relevant for its high lethality (up to 60%) in neonates and immunocompromised patients.

Diagnosis

Although a variety of transport media can be used to identify *Aeromonas* in stools, Cary-Blair media is most commonly used. Samples should be transported at room temperature to increase recovery yield. *Aeromonas* grow easily on routine enteric isolation media, such as

MacConkey, xylose lysine deoxycholate (XLD), Hektoen enteric (HE), *Salmonella-Shigella* (SS), and deoxycholate-citrate (DC); however, because they are nonlactose fermenters, they can be misclassified as normal enteric flora. Use of a selective media such as sheep blood agar containing ampicillin is recommended. DNase-toluidine blue agar can be used to detect nonhemolytic and ampicillin-susceptible strains that represent less than 10% of pathogenic strains. CIN agar has been shown to be more cost effective because it allows concomitant isolation of *Yersinia* and *Plesiomonas*. Another highly selective medium is *Aeromonas* agar, which contains Irgasan and d-xylose.[899]

Aeromonas can be differentiated from other gram-negative bacilli by biochemical testing. This genus is oxidase positive, indole positive, and urease negative. The presence of oxidase activity helps to differentiate *Aeromonas* from Enterobacteriaceae. In general, *Aeromonas* spp. can be separated from vibrios by their ability to grow in nutrient broth without sodium chloride supplementation, their inability to grow on thiosulfate–citrate-bile salts–sucrose (TCBS) agar, and their resistance to the vibriostatic agent 2,4-diamino-6,7-diisopropyl-pteridine (O/129).

DNA probes have been developed for *Aeromonas* spp. identification. These techniques have been used in epidemiologic and environmental surveillances but have not proven useful for clinical practice to date. Commercial tests designed for detection of gram-negative bacilli have been used for *Aeromonas* characterization, but major errors in genus and species identification have been reported.[917] 16S rRNA sequencing has not been useful for species discrimination; however, partial sequence analysis of housekeeping genes, such as *gyrB* and *rpoD*, have been more promising for use in epidemiologic studies.[918,919]

Therapy

A 3-day treatment with azithromycin or ceftriaxone in children, and ciprofloxacin or azithromycin in adults, is recommended for treatment of *Aeromonas*-associated gastroenteritis. Ciprofloxacin or third-generation cephalosporin, alone or in combination with an aminoglycoside, is a reasonable initial empirical therapy for skin and soft tissue infections and bacteremia. Although induction of β-lactamases in the clinical setting is rare, clinicians should monitor the patient closely for a potential relapse when using cephalosporins for a serious *Aeromonas* infection.[899]

PLESIOMONAS SHIGELLOIDES

Plesiomonas shigelloides is a gram-negative, facultative anaerobic bacillus that, similar to *Aeromonas*, is a member of the Vibrionaceae family. It is widely disseminated in the environment; outbreaks of disease are usually related to ingestion of contaminated water or seafood.[920] Although it has been associated with outbreaks of diarrheal disease[921] and has been found more commonly in ill than well controls, the role of *P. shigelloides* in GI disease has remained controversial.[922] If it is a true enteropathogen, the mechanism by which it causes disease is unclear.[923,924]

Typical illness consists of watery diarrhea and cramps; sometimes, fever, bloody stools, and emesis occur and last 3 to 42 days.

The role of this organism in neonatal diarrhea has not been extensively investigated. Systemic infections of neonates with sepsis and meningitis have been reported.[925-929]

Diagnosis is not usually made by clinical microbiology laboratory testing because, as with *Aeromonas*, coliforms can be confused with *P. shigelloides* unless an oxidase test is performed.[930] The true frequency of infection is unknown.

The organism has antibiotic susceptibilities similar to *Aeromonas*.[931,932]

Other Bacterial Agents and Fungi

Listeria monocytogenes, a classic cause of neonatal sepsis and meningitis, has been linked to outbreaks of febrile diarrheal disease in immunocompetent adults and children.[933-937] Fever has been reported to occur in up to 72% of ill individuals.[938] Outbreaks have been related to ingestion of contaminated foods. *Listeria* has rarely been described as a cause of neonatal gastroenteritis.[939-941]

The recovery of *Klebsiella* or *Enterobacter* in pure culture from diarrheal stools has led several investigators to suggest that these bacteria may occasionally play a causative role in infantile gastroenteritis and enterocolitis.[942-945] Ingestion of infant formula contaminated with *Enterobacter sakazakii* has been associated with development of bloody diarrhea and sepsis.[946] *Klebsiella* spp. also may be isolated in pure culture from stools of newborns with no enteric symptoms, however.[947-949] Later work has shown that *Klebsiella pneumoniae*, *Enterobacter cloacae*, and *Citrobacter* spp. are capable of producing enterotoxins.[950,951] Reports of isolation of *Citrobacter* spp., describe associations with enteric illnesses in 7% of cases.[952,953] There is inadequate evidence to define the roles of *Klebsiella*, *Enterobacter*, and *Citrobacter* spp. as etiologic agents of enteric illnesses.

Infection with enterotoxin-producing *Bacteroides fragilis* has been associated with mild watery diarrhea.[954] These infections have a peak incidence in children 2 to 3 years of age.[955] These toxin-producing organisms cannot be detected in routine hospital laboratories.

An association between *Providencia* and neonatal enteritis has been substantiated largely by anecdotal reports of nursery outbreaks.[953] These bacteria are rarely isolated from infants with sporadic or community-acquired diarrheal disease.[956-958]

Candida albicans usually is acquired during passage through the birth canal and is considered a normal, although minor, component of the fecal flora of the neonate.[959] Intestinal overgrowth of these organisms frequently accompanies infantile gastroenteritis,[959,960] particularly after antimicrobial therapy.[960-963] The upper small gut may become colonized with *Candida* in malnourished children with diarrhea[964]; whether the presence of the organism is cause or effect is unclear. Stool cultures obtained from infants with diarrheal disease are inconclusive, and although *Candida* enteritis has been reported in adults,[965] the importance of this organism as a primary cause of neonatal gastroenteritis has been difficult to prove. Clinical descriptions of nursery epidemics of candidal enteritis are poorly documented, generally preceding the recognition of EPEC and rotaviruses as a cause of neonatal diarrhea. Even well-studied cases of intestinal involvement add little in the way of substantive proof because secondary invasion of *Candida* has been shown to be a complication of coliform enteritis.[334]

Although diarrhea has sometimes been described as a finding in neonatal disseminated candidiasis, more typically, GI tract involvement with disseminated *Candida* is associated with abdominal distention and bloody stools, mimicking necrotizing enterocolitis.[964-968] Typically, affected infants are premature and have courses complicated by antibiotic administration, intravascular catheter use, and surgical procedures during the first several weeks of life. A trial of oral anticandidal therapy may be helpful in neonates with diarrhea in the presence of oral or cutaneous candidiasis. If the therapy is appropriate, a response should be forthcoming within 2 to 5 days.

Diarrhea sometimes occurs as a manifestation of a systemic infection. Patients with staphylococcal toxic shock syndrome often have diarrhea. Loose stools sometimes occur in sepsis, but it is unclear whether the diarrhea is a cause or an effect. The organisms isolated from blood cultures in a group of Bangladeshi infants and children with diarrhea included *Staphylococcus aureus, Haemophilus influenzae, Streptococcus pneumoniae, Pseudomonas aeruginosa,* and various gram-negative enteric bacilli.[969] It is unknown whether the bacteriology of sepsis associated with diarrhea is similar in the well-nourished infants seen in industrialized countries.

Parasites

Acute diarrhea associated with intestinal parasites is infrequently reported during the neonatal period. In areas with high endemicity, infection of the newborn is likely to be associated with inadequate maternal and delivery care, insufficient environmental sanitation, and poor personal hygiene standards. The occurrence of symptomatic intestinal parasitic infection during the first month of life requires acquisition of the parasite during the first days or weeks; the incubation period for *Entamoeba* is 2 to 4 weeks; for *Giardia intestinalis,* 1 to 3 weeks; and for *Cryptosporidium,* 3 to 14 days.[970,971] The newborn could be infected during delivery by contact with maternal feces,[972] in the hospital through contact with the mother or personnel, or in the household through contact with infected individuals in close contact with the infant. Contaminated water can be an important source of infection for all three parasites, especially for *Cryptosporidium. Giardia* and *Cryptosporidium* can also be acquired by ingestion of contaminated animal stools, a situation that occurs in many underdeveloped settings worldwide where animals reside together with humans. In more developed areas, this situation can occur if indoor pets are present. Nevertheless, infection through these sources is unlikely to occur during the newborn period.

ENTAMOEBA

The genus *Entamoeba* includes six species living in the human intestine, of which three are morphologically identical but genetically distinct and of potential relevance to date: *E. histolytica, E. dispar,* and *E. moshkovskii.* The first species can cause acute nonbloody and bloody diarrhea, necrotizing enterocolitis, ameboma, and liver abscess; the second is currently considered a noninvasive parasite that does not cause disease but can be misclassified as *E. histolytica* by microscopy; and the third, thought also to be nonpathogenic, has been recently postulated as a possible pathogen causing diarrhea in infants.[971,973] Early acquisition of disease tends to be more severe in young infants; rarely, amebic liver abscess and rapidly fatal colitis have been reported in infants.[974-982] A 19-day-old infant from India who presented with 10 to 12 episodes of watery and mucous diarrhea, lethargy, jaundice, and mildly elevated liver enzymes has been described; the child recovered completely after 10 days of intravenous imidazole.[974] More recently, a 14-day-old girl from India who received tap water soon after birth presented with mucoid stools, decreased bowel sounds, abdominal distension, and stool occult blood. Her stool was positive for *E. histolytica* trophozoites. The child received fluids with antibiotics, vitamin K, and intravenous tinidazole from the fifth day of hospital stay and recovered fully.[983] Amebic liver abscess can be preceded by diarrhea or have a clinical presentation of fulminant neonatal sepsis.[975] Asymptomatic colonization of neonates with various species of amebas is common in areas of high endemicity.[984]

Diagnosis can be established by stool examination for cysts and trophozoites (the most common diagnostic technique used in developing countries), by serologic studies, antigen detection assays, and by PCR (common in industrialized countries).[985-988] Microscopy does not readily differentiate the nonpathogenic *E. dispar* from *E. histolytica,* although this can be done in expert hands. Antigen-detection ELISAs specific for *E. histolytica* are a good alternative for developing countries, and PCR is the best method to differentiate all three species.[988,989] Serum antibody assays may be helpful in establishing the diagnosis of amebic dysentery and extraintestinal amebiasis with liver involvement. Persons positive for *E. histolytica* (ELISA, PCR, or expert microscopy) should be treated irrespective of symptoms. The efficacy of treatment with metronidazole for colitis or liver abscess has not been established for the newborn period, although this therapy has been used successfully.[976] Tinidazole was used successfully in one 14-day-old girl.[983] Patients with colitis or liver abscess caused by *E. histolytica* should also receive iodoquinol or paramomycin, as should asymptomatic carriers.[971]

GIARDIA INTESTINALIS

*Giardia intestinalis (*formerly *G. lamblia* and *Giardia duodenalis*) is a binucleate, flagellated protozoan parasite with trophozoite and cyst stages. It is spread by the fecal-oral route through ingestion of cysts. Daycare center outbreaks reflecting person-to-person spread have shown its high infectivity potential.[990-993] Humans are the main reservoir of the parasite, although several animal species can be infected, including cats, dogs, sheep, and cattle, among others, which possibly serve as vehicles of transmission.[971,994] Foodborne transmission and waterborne transmission also occur. *G. duodenalis* is commonly detected in asymptomatic children, especially in resource-deprived settings, most probably because of the intensity of human contact with stools of animal and human origin. In these regions, the overall role of the pathogen as a cause of acute diarrhea has been questioned.[995] Nevertheless, in these settings, *Giardia* may play a significant role in causing acute diarrhea in young infants during a primary infection and as a cause of persistent diarrhea.[996] Even in the poorest world regions, there may be internal area-specific differences in incidence of acute diarrhea associated with *Giardia*, as suggested by a recent case-control study from Madagascar, where the pathogen was clearly more common in cases than control subjects in 2 out of 14 community setting–based sites throughout the country.[997] It is also possible that specific genotypes are causing disease, whereas others are more common in asymptomatic infections.[998] In industrialized regions, the presence of *G. intestinalis* is much more likely to be associated with GI disease.[996] Cases of severe symptomatic infection during the immediate newborn period have not been reported. One report from Portugal describes a premature baby boy who developed vomiting, abdominal distension, and eosinophilia apparently after receiving a nonhydrolized milk formula. He was diagnosed with milk allergy (grade II/III) and giardiasis, based on stool positivity established by microscopy, ELISA, and PCR. Symptoms and eosinophilia subsided after metronidazole treatment and a formula change to hydrolized milk.[999]

Symptoms in giardiasis are related to the age of the patient: Diarrhea, vomiting, anorexia, and failure to thrive are more common in younger children. Seroprevalence studies showed evidence of past or current *G. lamblia* infection in 40% of Peruvian children by the age of 6 months.[1000] In a study of lactating Bangladeshi mothers and their infants, 82% of women and 42% of infants excreted *Giardia* once during the study; in some infants, this occurred before they were 3 months of age.[1001] Of these infected infants, 86% had diarrhea, suggesting that the early exposure to the parasite resulted in disease. In a prospective study of diarrhea conducted in Mexico, infants frequently were infected with *Giardia* from birth to 2 months, with a crude incidence rate of first *Giardia* infection of 1.4 infections per child-year in this age group.[3] The symptom status of these children was not reported, but this study strongly suggests that *G. lamblia* may be more common than currently recognized among newborns living in developing areas.

The diagnosis of giardiasis can be made by microscopy of direct or concentrated stool, repeated on different days because of the fluctuating nature of parasite excretion. Direct fluorescence assays (DFA), EIA assays, solid-phase immunochromatography, and gene amplification by PCR have been developed for detection of both *Giardia* and *Cryptosporidium*.[1002-1004] As expected, PCR and immune-based techniques are more sensitive but less specific than microscopy. Breastfeeding protects against symptomatic giardiasis[3,996,1005] protection that may be mediated by cellular and humoral immunity, especially anti-*Giardia* secretory IgA,[996,1006,1007] and nonspecifically by the antigiardial effects of unsaturated fatty acids.[1008] *Giardia* infections convincingly associated with acute diarrhea should be treated with metronidazole, tinidazole, or nitazoxanide, which are currently considered first-line drugs.[971] Furazolidone and quinacrine are currently considered for refractory disease. Experience with these drugs in neonates is extremely limited, mostly with metronidazole (for treatment of conditions other than giardiasis) and less with tinidazole.[983,1003,1009]

CRYPTOSPORIDIUM

Cryptosporidium spp. are coccidian protozoon related to *Toxoplasma gondii, Cystospora belli,* and *Plasmodium* spp.[1010,1011] The life cycle involves ingestion of thick-walled oocysts; release of sporozoites, which penetrate intestinal epithelium; and development of merozoites. Asexual reproduction and sexual reproduction occur, with the latter resulting in formation of new oocysts that can be passed in stools.

Cryptosporidium spp. are ubiquitous and known for decades to be epidemiologically relevant in immune-compromised individuals (mostly AIDS patients) and in young children from resource-deprived settings, especially those suffering from severe malnutrition.[2012] This pathogen has recently emerged as the second most common cause of moderate-to-severe acute diarrhea in young children from resource-deprived regions.[995] Greater than 90% of cases are caused by *C. parvum* or *C. hominis*, although rarely, infections can occur with other species and genotypes, such as *C. meleagridis, C. felis, C. canis, C. ubiquotum, C. cuniculus*.[1013]

Acquisition of infection is mainly by ingestion of oocysts, either during direct contact with human or animal feces, or from indirect exposure via a transmission vehicle such as contaminated water, food, or fomites. Intestinal cryptosporidiosis occurs most commonly in young children, persons who have contact with animals, travelers returning from high-prevalence regions, and/or those exposed to potentially contaminated drinking or bathing waters.[1012] Because *Cryptosporidium* infects a wide variety of animal species, a history of animal contact among infected persons is common.[1014] Person-to-person spread, particularly in household contacts[1015-1018] and daycare centers,[1019,1020] has been well documented. Waterborne outbreaks of cryptosporidiosis occur and can be of massive proportions.[1021,1022]

The clinical spectrum can vary from asymptomatic infection to life-threatening diarrhea. The clinical manifestations of cryptosporidiosis in immunocompetent children is characterized by watery diarrhea that may be profuse and/or prolonged, vomiting, abdominal pain, myalgia, fever, and weight loss.[1012-1014,1019,1020,1023,1024] Bloody diarrhea is uncommon. Infection can occur in all age groups but is largely concentrated in children younger than 5 years, with increase severity in children younger than 2 years.[2012] In one study from Bangladesh, a significant recovery rate for cryptosporidia in diarrhea cases versus healthy control subjects was found only in infants younger than 12 months.[1025] Infection in the first month of life has been rarely described.[1026,1027] Because symptoms resolve before excretion of oocysts ceases, a newborn whose mother has been ill with cryptosporidiosis in the month before delivery might be at risk even if the mother is asymptomatic at the time of the child's birth.[1028] With the increasing frequency of HIV infection, it is likely that women with symptomatic cryptosporidiosis may deliver an infant who will become infected. Infants infected early in life may develop chronic diarrhea and malnutrition.[1029]

As for *Giardia*, the diagnosis of cryptosporidiosis is typically made by microscopy; for *Cryptosporidium*, Giemsa stain, Ziehl-Neelsen stain, auramine-rhodamine stain, and/or Sheather sugar flotation are used. However, newer techniques include DFA, EIA assays, solid-phase immunochromatography, and gene amplification by

PCR.[995,1004,1030,1031] Multiplex real-time PCR for *E. histolytica*, *G. lamblia*, and *C. parvum* and *C. hominis* remain on the horizon.[1032,1033] Nitazoxanide is effective therapy for immunocompetent adults and children 1 year of age and older with cryptosporidiosis.[971,1034] Treatment of neonates has not been reported, to our knowledge. Because illness is usually self-limited in the normal host, attention to fluid, electrolyte, and nutritional status is usually sufficient. Enteric isolation of hospitalized infants with this illness is appropriate because of the high infectivity. Several studies suggest that the risk of infection early in life may be decreased by breastfeeding.[1027,1035] Using appropriate filtration systems in areas where water treatment is minimal can have a significant impact in decreasing cases of cryptosporidiosis.[1036] The most important measure is to avoid, whenever possible, exposure of newborns and infants to potentially contaminated water or close contact with potentially contaminated animals. At sea level, boiling water 1 minute is useful if water quality is uncertain.[971]

Viruses

ENTERIC VIRUSES

Viruses that infect the intestinal mucosa and cause primarily gastroenteritis are referred to as enteric viruses; they should not be confused with enteroviruses, members of the Picornaviridae family that are associated primarily with systemic illnesses. Enteric viruses include rotaviruses, enteric adenoviruses, human caliciviruses (norovirus and sapovirus), and astroviruses. Other viruses, such as coronaviruses, Breda viruses, pestiviruses, parvoviruses, toroviruses, picobirnaviruses, and bocaviruses, have been sporadically associated with acute diarrhea but are currently considered of uncertain relevance.[1037] Extensive reviews on the role of enteric viruses in childhood diarrhea can be found elsewhere.[1038-1042]

All four enteric viruses could conceivably infect the newborn, but the extent of exposure and clinical manifestations are largely unknown for astrovirus, enteric adenovirus, and human caliciviruses, which include norovirus and sapovirus. Rotavirus and, more recently, norovirus are the most extensively studied enteric viruses. Neonatal rotavirus and norovirus infections can have similar virologic and clinical characteristics of infection in older children, although some differences exist.

ROTAVIRUS

Rotavirus is a 75-nm, nonenveloped virus composed of three concentric protein shells: a segmented genome (11 segments), an RNA-dependent polymerase, and enzymes required for messenger RNA synthesis are located within the inner core. Each segment encodes at least one viral protein (VP). The VP can be part of the structure of the virus, or it may be a nonstructural protein (NSP) required for replication, viral assembly, budding, determination of host range, or viral pathogenesis.[1040]

Six distinct rotavirus groups (A through F) have been identified serologically based on common group antigens,[1043,1044] of which three (A, B, and C) have been identified in humans.[1038] Because group A rotaviruses represent greater than 95% of isolated strains in humans worldwide, further discussion focuses on this group. Group A rotaviruses are subclassified into serotypes based on neutralization epitopes located on the outer capsid. Both rotavirus surface proteins, VP4 and VP7, can induce production of neutralizing antibodies.[1045,1046] At least 10 VP7 types out of a total of 19 identified and 11 VP4 types out of a total of 28 identified have been detected among human rotaviruses.[1047-1049] By sequencing the VP4-coding gene, 8 genomic P types (genotypes) have been identified that correspond to one or more of the described P antigenic types (genotype 8 to antigenic type P1A, 4 to P1B, 6 to P2A, 9 to P3, 13 to P3B, 10 to P4, 3 to P5, and 11 to P8).[1040] Combining G antigenic with P antigenic and genetic typing, a specific rotavirus strain can be identified: P antigenic type (P genetic type), G type. As an example, the human neonatal M37 strain is described as P2A[6], G1. Five combined GP types—P1A[8], G1; P1B[4], G2; P1A[8], G3; P1A[8], G4; P1A[8], G9—account for greater than 95% of the organisms isolated from children, and of these, P1A[8], G1 represents the most common type.[1050] G12 strains, mostly in combination with P1A[8], representing a reassortant between an animal and human strain (as the P1A[8], G9 strain), may be emerging as a sixth common serotype.[1051] Reassortants among human genotypes infecting children less commonly currently include strains G1P[4], G2P[8], and G4P[4], whereas reassortants between animal and human genotypes, which are also less common, include G1P[9] and G4P[6]; probable zoonotic introductions include serotypes G9[P6], G9P[11], G10P[11], and G12P[6]).[1049]

Isolation of less common types seems to be more frequent among neonates with nosocomial rotavirus infections.[1052-1058] Some of these strains may be associated with occurrence of asymptomatic infections, although the existence of naturally acquired asymptomatic strains is controversial. Strains P2A[6], G9; P2A[6], G4; P2A[6], G2; P2A[6], G8; and P8[11], G10 have been reported[1056-1058] from newborn nurseries, some of which seem to be endemic to the newborn units with high rates of asymptomatic infection,[1057-1060] and, less commonly, outbreaks of symptomatic infection.[1052] These findings suggest that specific conditions of the newborn environment (e.g., child, nursery, personnel) may increase the possibility of reassortants among human strains; such strains may persist in these settings, possibly through constant transmission involving asymptomatic newborns, adults, and contaminated surfaces. Neonates can also be symptomatically infected with unusual animal-human reassorted strains in areas of poor sanitary conditions.[1061]

Pathogenesis

Although mechanisms involved in rotavirus pathogenesis have been extensively studied, current understanding of the exact mechanisms involved in human disease remains incomplete. Nevertheless, clinical manifestations are a result of a number of different processes occurring during viral infection.[1062] Rotavirus primarily infects mature enterocytes located in the middle and upper villous epithelium.[1063-1067] Lactase, which is present only on the brush border of the differentiated epithelial cells at these sites, may act as a combined receptor and uncoating enzyme for the virus, permitting transfer of the particles into the cell.[1068] Perhaps for this reason, infection is limited to the mature columnar enterocytes; crypt cells and crypt-derived cuboidal cells, which lack a brush border and are spared from infection.[1049,1068,1069] This concept also may explain why rotavirus infection is less common in infants younger than 32 weeks of gestation than in more mature infants[1070]; at 26 to 34 weeks of gestation, lactase activity is approximately 30% of that found in term infants.[1071]

The upper small intestine is most commonly involved in rotavirus enteritis, although lesions may extend to the distal ileum and rarely to the colon.[1072,1073] Interaction between intestinal cell and rotavirus structural and nonstructural proteins occurs, triggering the death of infected villous enterocytes.[1074] When infected, the villous enterocyte is sloughed, resulting in an altered mucosal architecture that becomes stunted and flattened. The gross appearance of the bowel is usually normal; however, under the dissecting microscope, scattered focal lesions of the mucosal surface are apparent in most cases. Light microscopy also shows patchy changes in villous morphology, compatible with a process of infection, inflammation, and accelerated mucosal renewal. The villi take on a shortened and blunt appearance as tall columnar cells are shed and replaced by less mature cuboidal enterocytes.[1064,1066,1075] Ischemia may also play a role in the loss and stunting of villi[1076] and activation of the enteric nervous system; active secretion of fluid and electrolytes may be another pathogenic mechanism.[1077] Unlike bacterial infections of the gut, rotavirus infections lack of a significant inflammatory host response.[1062]

During the recovery phase, the enteroblastic cells mature and reconstruct the villous structure. Because of the loss of mature enterocytes on the tips of the villi, the surface area of the intestine is reduced. Diarrhea that occurs may be a result of this decrease in surface area, disruption in epithelial integrity, transient disaccharidase deficiency, or altered countercurrent mechanisms and net secretion of water and electrolytes.[1064,1071,1077-1079] The destruction of mature enterocytes does not seem to be a critical element in the pathogenesis of rotavirus infection. The role of nonstructural protein 4 (NSP4) as a "viral enterotoxin," after the initial report of an age-dependent diarrhea in CD1 mice, by triggering calcium-dependent chloride and water secretion,[1080] has been supported by new studies.[1049,1081] The exact mechanism of action of this protein at the intestinal level has been better characterized during the past 5 years. NSP4 does not cause morphologic damage; it impairs glucose absorption and produces moderate calcium-mediated chloride secretion.[1081] Experimental studies have demonstrated that NSP4 products can be secreted from cells and then bind to integrin $\alpha 2\beta 1$ receptors, leading to increased levels of intracellular calcium and subsequent chloride secretion through activation or regulation of specific channels.[1049] The precise contribution of this purported "viral enterotoxin" in human rotavirus–associated diarrhea is unclear.[1082,1083]

It is currently clear that all individuals infected with rotavirus have at least a short period of viremia,[1062] a concept that has enriched our understanding of this infection.[1084] These events could partly explain the sporadic reports of systemic disease associated with rotavirus intestinal infections mentioned later. An association between viremia and more severe disease has been suggested but not sufficiently studied to date.[1084-1087]

Infection and Immunity

Infants with asymptomatic rotavirus infections in the nursery are less likely than uninfected nursery mates to experience severe rotavirus infection later in life[1088,1089]; this finding suggested protective immunity and supported vaccine development. Most studies have indicated that serum and intestinal antirotaviral antibody levels are correlated with protection against infection,[1089-1097] although this correlation has not been universal.[1098,1099] Breastfeeding protects against diarrhea and, specifically, rotavirus disease during the first year of life,[45,56] probably including newborns.[1077] The high prevalence of antirotaviral antibodies in colostrum and human milk has been shown by numerous investigators in widely diverse geographic areas.[3] Maternal rotavirus infection or immunization is accompanied by the appearance of specific antibodies in milk, probably through stimulation of the enteromammary immune system.[1100-1105] Of women examined in London, Bangladesh, Guatemala, Costa Rica, and the United States, 90% to 100% had antirotaviral IgA antibodies in their milk for 2 years of lactation.[12,1100-1106] Rotavirus-specific IgG antibodies have been found during the first few postpartum days in about one third of human milk samples assayed,[1100,1103] whereas IgM antibodies were detectable in about half.[1103]

Glycoproteins in human milk have been shown to prevent rotavirus infection in vitro and in an animal model.[1106] The concentration of one milk glycoprotein, lactadherin, was found to be significantly higher in human milk ingested by infants who developed asymptomatic rotavirus infection than in milk ingested by infants who developed symptomatic infection.[42]

Epidemiology

Rotaviruses probably infect neonates more commonly than previously recognized; most infections seem to be asymptomatic or mildly symptomatic, although symptomatic infections, including severe life-threatening infections, may be more common than previously considered, especially in developing countries.[1056-1059,1107-1123] In a study from India, rotavirus positivity was detected in 56% of symptomatic neonates compared with 45% of asymptomatic neonates.[1121] Rotavirus has a mean incubation period of 2 days, with a range of 1 to 3 days in children and in adults experimentally infected. Fecal excretion of virus often begins a day or so before illness, and maximal excretion usually occurs during the third and fourth days and generally diminishes by the end of the first week, although low concentrations of virus have been detected in neonates for 8 weeks.[1119,1124,1125]

Rotavirus infections are markedly seasonal (autumn and winter) in many areas of the world, although in some countries, seasonality is less striking; the reason for this is unclear.[1126-1131] In nurseries in which persisting endemic infection has permitted long-term surveillance of numerous neonates, rotavirus excretion can follow the seasonal pattern of the community but can also show no seasonal fluctuation.[1132-1134] It is unclear how units in which infection remains endemic for months or years differ from units with a low incidence of rotavirus. Some nurseries are free of rotavirus infection[1134-1136] or minimally affected,[1137] whereas others have rotavirus diarrheal disease throughout the year or in outbreaks that involve 10% to 40% of neonates.[1113,1038,1138]

Low birth weight does not seem to be an important factor in determining the attack rate among infants at risk but may be important in mortality.[1139] Infants in premature or special-care nurseries, despite their prolonged stays and the increased handling necessary for their care, do not exhibit a higher susceptibility to infection; data regarding shedding of the virus are inconsistent.[1136]

After infection is introduced into a nursery, rotavirus is likely to spread steadily and remain endemic until the nursery is closed to new admissions or nursing practices permit interruption of the cycle.[1140] Exactly how the virus is introduced and transmitted is uncertain, although limited observations and experience with other types of enteric disease in maternity units suggest several possibilities. The early appearance of virus in stools of some neonates indicates that infection probably was acquired at delivery. Virus particles can be detected on the first[42,1119] or second[1134] day of life in many infected infants. By day 3 or 4, most infected infants who will shed virus, with or without signs of illness, are doing so.[1108,1119,1134] The numerous virus particles excreted[1119,1134] suggest a fairly large and early oral inoculum. It is unlikely that contamination from any source other than maternal feces could provide an inoculum large enough to cause infection by the second day of life. Transfer of particles from infant to infant on the hands of nursing and medical staff is probably the most important means of viral spread. With 10^8 to 10^{11} viral particles usually present in 1 g of stool, the hands of personnel easily could become contaminated after infection is introduced into a nursery. There are numerous reports of nosocomial and daycare center rotavirus gastroenteritis outbreaks, which attests to the ease with which this agent spreads through a hospital or institutional setting.[1038,1141]

Admission of a symptomatic infant usually is the initiating event, although transfer of a neonate with unapparent infection from one ward to another also has been incriminated. The most important factors influencing the incidence of rotavirus diarrhea in a nursery are the proximity to other newborns and the frequency of hand washing.[1120] During a 4-month study, infants cared for by nursing staff and kept in communal nurseries experienced three epidemics of diarrhea, with attack rates of 20% to 50%. During the same period, only 2% of infants rooming in with their mothers became ill, even though they had frequent contact with adult relatives and siblings.

There is no clear evidence of airborne or droplet infection originating in the upper respiratory tract or spread by aerosolization of diarrheal fluid while diapers are changed. Indirect evidence of airborne transmission includes the high infection rate in closed settings, the isolation of the virus from respiratory secretions,[1107] and the experimental observation of transmission by aerosol droplets in mice.[1108] The respiratory isolation achieved by placing an infant in a closed incubator is not fully protective, however.[1120] No evidence indicates that transplacental or ascending intrauterine infection occurs. Transmission of virus through contaminated fomites, formula, or food is possible, but has not been documented in newborns. Rotavirus particles have not been found in human milk or colostrum.[1103,1106]

Clinical Manifestations

Exposure of a newborn to rotavirus can result in asymptomatic infection or cause mild or severe gastroenteritis.[†] Outbreaks with high attack rates, as measured by rotavirus excretion, have been described, but the extent of symptomatic infection varies.[1109,1111,1119,1121,1138] Severe rotavirus infection is seldom reported during the newborn period,[1019,1138] but the extent of underreporting of severe disease, especially in the less developed areas of the world, has not been evaluated.

It has been hypothesized that asymptomatic infections during the newborn period can be, in part, the result of naturally attenuated strains circulating in this environment. RNA electrophoretic patterns of rotaviruses found in certain nurseries have shown uniform patterns,[1114,1116,1118] and it has been suggested that these strains may be attenuated. The presence of unusual antigenic types, such as P2A[6] type, within nurseries also suggests "less virulent strains." At least 10 rotavirus strains were documented to cocirculate in a tertiary care center during a 2-month period,[1142] and in a different setting, the same rotavirus strains by electropherotype produced asymptomatic infection in neonates and symptomatic infection in older infants.[1201] Newborns within a nursery exposed to a given rotavirus strain can develop symptomatic or asymptomatic infection.[1058,1143,1144] P8[11], G10 was the most common genotype associated with symptomatic and asymptomatic infections in a tertiary care hospital in India.[1121] Because newborns routinely have frequent, relatively loose stools, it is possible that mild diarrhea episodes caused by rotavirus are being wrongly labeled as asymptomatic episodes.

No clinical feature is pathognomonic of rotaviral gastroenteritis. Early signs of illness, such as lethargy, irritability, vomiting, and poor feeding, usually are followed in a few hours by the passage of watery yellow or green stools free of blood but sometimes containing mucus.[1120,1145-1147] Diarrhea usually decreases by the second day of illness and is much improved by the third or fourth day. On occasion, intestinal fluid loss and poor weight gain may continue for 1 or 2 weeks, particularly in low-birth-weight infants.[1109] Although reducing substances frequently are present in early fecal samples,[1070,1110,1120] this finding is not abnormal in neonates, particularly infants who are breastfed.[1148] Nevertheless, infants with prolonged diarrhea should be investigated for monosaccharide or disaccharide malabsorption or intolerance to cow's milk protein, or both.[1149] In a prospective study,[1150] 49% of newborns with GI symptoms in an NICU had rotavirus detected in their stools. Frequent stool emissions (present in 60%), bloody mucoid stool (42%), and watery stools (24%) were risk factors for a rotavirus infection. Bloody mucoid stools, intestinal dilation, and abdominal distention were significantly more common in preterm infants, but severe outcomes, such as necrotizing enterocolitis and death, did not differ among infected term and preterm infants. A more recent study from South Korea suggests that rotavirus may be more

†References 1057, 1058, 1107, 1109, 1133, 1137.

commonly associated with poor feeding and neutropenia in preterm compared with term newborns.[1151]

Longitudinal studies in newborn nurseries and investigations of outbreaks among neonates rarely describe a severe adverse outcome or death.[1070,1104,1120] Because these infants are under constant observation, early detection of excessive fluid losses and the availability of immediate medical care are probably major factors in determining outcome. Rotavirus gastroenteritis caused almost 400,000 infant deaths every year before implementation of national vaccination programs,[1152] concentrated largely in the poorest regions of the world. It is likely that in places where hospital-based care is uncommon, rotavirus causes neonatal deaths secondary to dehydration.

Group A rotavirus has been associated with a wide array of nondiarrheal diseases in infants and children; Reye syndrome, encephalitis–aseptic meningitis, sudden infant death syndrome, inflammatory bowel disease, and Kawasaki syndrome have been described but not systematically studied.[1038] Case reports and small case series have associated neonatal rotavirus infection with necrotizing enterocolitis.[1153,1154] This association may be more common than previously considered, according to more recent reports.[1123] Rotavirus infection may be playing a role in a proportion of cases of necrotizing enterocolitis, although it probably represents one of many potential triggering factors.[1121] A significant association between neonatal rotavirus infection and bradycardia-apnea episodes was detected in one prospective study.[1155] The possible association between natural rotavirus infection and intussusception[1156-1158] gained support after the association was made between the human-simian reassortant vaccine and intussusception in infants older than 2 months (attributable risk, approximately 1:10,000).[1159] Epidemiologic studies have not shown a temporal correlation between peaks of rotavirus infection and increase in cases of intussusception.[1160] Intussusception is extremely uncommon in the newborn; it is highly unlikely that rotavirus or rotavirus vaccination would trigger this disease in neonates.

Diagnosis

There are many methods used for detection of rotavirus in stool specimens, including electron microscopy, immune electron microscopy, ELISA, latex agglutination, gel electrophoresis, culture of the virus, and reverse-transcriptase PCR. ELISA and latex agglutination currently are the most widely used diagnostic techniques for detection of rotavirus in clinical samples. Many commercial kits are available that differ in specificity and sensitivity.[1161-1165] Latex agglutination assays generally are more rapid than ELISAs but are less sensitive. The sensitivity and specificity of commercially available ELISAs surpass 90%. Checking the results of ELISA by another method, such as gel electrophoresis or PCR amplification, may be desirable if there is concern about false-positive results.

Fecal material for detection of rotavirus infection should be obtained during the acute phase of illness. Whole-stool samples are preferred, although suspensions of rectal swab specimens have been adequate for detection of rotavirus by ELISA.[1166,1167] Rotavirus is relatively resistant to environmental temperatures, even tropical temperatures,[1168] although 4° C is desirable for short-term storage and −70° C for prolonged storage.[1038] Excretion of viral particles may precede signs of illness by several days[1126]; maximal excretion by older infants and children usually occurs 3 to 4 days after onset of symptoms.[1169] Neonates can shed virus for 1 to 2 weeks after onset of symptoms.

Therapy and Prevention

The primary goal of therapy is restoration and maintenance of fluid and electrolyte balance. Despite the documented defect in carbohydrate digestion with rotavirus diarrhea, rehydration often can be accomplished with glucose-electrolyte or sucrose-electrolyte solutions given orally.[1170-1172] Intravenous fluids may be needed in neonates who are severely dehydrated, who have ileus, or who refuse to feed. Persistent or recurrent diarrhea after introduction of milk-based formulas or human milk warrants investigation for secondary carbohydrate or milk protein intolerance.[1070,1152] Disaccharidase levels and xylose absorption return to normal within a few days[1075] to weeks after infection.[1064]

Intractable diarrhea related to severe morphologic and enzymatic changes of the bowel mucosa is possible, although rare in the newborn; it may require an elemental diet or parenteral nutrition. Efficacy of antirotavirus antibodies (e.g., hyperimmune colostrum, antibody-supplemented formula, and human serum immunoglobulin) has been postulated, although not convincingly shown.[1173-1176] Regarding use of probiotics, one study suggests that use of lactobacilli during the diarrheal episode may decrease the duration of rotavirus-associated hospital stays, especially when used early in the course of the disease.[1176] A more recent systematic review concluded that probiotics may shorten the duration of acute diarrhea (by a mean of approximately 24 hours), reduce the probability of developing a more prolonged episode (>4 days), and reduce the number of stool emissions (specifically, on day 2).[1177] Several uncertainties persist, such as potential differences associated with different probiotic strains, identification of the best dosage scheme, and differential effects/benefits according to etiology of the diarrhea episode, in order to make a definite recommendation. In any case, if considered, probiotics should be used as a coadjuvant to effective hydration methods. Hand hygiene before and after contact with each infant is the most important means of preventing the spread of infection. Because rotavirus is often excreted several days before illness is recognized, isolation of an infant with diarrhea may occur too late to prevent cross-infection, unless all nursing personnel and medical staff have adhered to this fundamental precaution. Infants who develop gastroenteritis should be moved out of the nursery area if adequate facilities are available and the infant's condition permits transfer. The use of an incubator is valuable in reducing transmission of disease only by serving as a reminder that proper hand hygiene and glove techniques are required, but an incubator per se is of little value as a physical barrier to the spread of virus.[1120] Encouraging rooming-in of infants with their mothers has been shown to be helpful in preventing or containing nursery epidemics.[1178] Temporary closure of the nursery may be required for clinically significant outbreaks that cannot be controlled with other measures.[1056]

Vaccines

Development of rotavirus vaccines began in the early 1980s. Candidate vaccines included bovine and rhesus monkey attenuated strains, human attenuated strains, and bovine-human and rhesus-human reassortant strains.[1039] In August 1998, the first licensed rotavirus vaccine, Rotashield, an oral formulation of a simian-human quadrivalent reassortant vaccine, was recommended for use in children in a three-dose regimen to be received at 2, 4, and 6 months of age. After approximately 500,000 children were vaccinated with more than 1 million doses, a significantly increased risk of intussusceptions (ISs) was observed among vaccinated children, with an overall OR of 1.8.[1179] Use of this vaccine was terminated in the United States, although the license of this vaccine has not been revoked. Two new vaccines proved not to be associated with IS at the risk level observed for Rotashield and proved effective in large phase III trials: a vaccine including five bovine-human reassortant strains that included human G types G1 to G4 and P type P1A[8], and a vaccine that included one human attenuated P1A[8], G1.[1180,1181]

These vaccines showed a protective efficacy against moderate-to severe rotavirus gastroenteritis, which ordinarily led to hospitalizations that surpassed 85% in middle-high income countries and nearly 60% in the poorest world regions with the highest mortality rates.[1182] Protection was broad against the most common serotypes. Key articles and reviews summarizing the studies that support these vaccines can be found elsewhere.[1180-1181] The impact of vaccination in countries that have incorporated the vaccine into national immunization programs has been impressive in terms of a rapid reduction of diarrhea-associated hospitalizations and deaths; rotavirus vaccines are currently considered a priority by the WHO.[1183,1184] A low-level risk for IS in the range of 1:20,000 to 1:100,000—occurring mostly during the first week after the first and, to a lesser degree, second dose—has been observed for both vaccines.[1185,1186] The benefits far outweigh this small risk and thus rotavirus vaccines continue to be highly recommended worldwide.[1187]

Impact of universal vaccination programs on neonatal infections is likely and will depend on the effect of herd immunity in decreasing circulation of rotavirus strains. Indirect protection in nonvaccinated individuals has been observed, suggesting that this phenomenon is occurring. Future strategies for improving protective efficacy in young infants in resource-limited settings may include neonatal vaccination.[1188]

HUMAN CALICIVIRUSES (NOROVIRUS AND SAPOVIRUS), ASTROVIRUS, AND ENTERIC ADENOVIRUSES

All four enteric viruses cause childhood diarrhea, mostly in children younger than 5 years, with a spectrum of disease that can range from asymptomatic infection to severe diarrhea leading to hospitalization and death.[1189] Norovirus has emerged as the second most common virus detected in stools of symptomatic infants, although it is also commonly detected in asymptomatic children, resulting from, in part, prolonged shedding and possibly acquisition of protective immunity from first infections against symptomatic disease but not asymptomatic infection.[1190] In countries that have introduced rotavirus vaccination, norovirus is emerging as the most common pathogen associated with childhood gastroenteritis.[1191] It is likely that enteric adenovirus, astrovirus, and other less common viruses will also increase in their relative (not absolute) proportion because of the reduction of rotavirus disease.[1192]

The role that these viruses may play in neonatal disease is being elucidated. Norovirus has been detected in stools of 5% of preterm newborn babies in whom association with disease was unclear.[1193] Outbreaks have been reported affecting preterm newborns presenting with a myriad of symptoms, of which abdominal distension seems to be common.[1194] Diarrhea and vomiting may be present in low or high proportions of norovirus-positive neonates, and a few neonates may present with sepsis-like symptoms.[1195] As for rotavirus, norovirus may also be a trigger for necrotizing enterocolitis outbreaks in susceptible newborns, some of which may have severe outcomes.[1196] Because neonatal stool samples positive for norovirus by antigen detection methods commonly have not been positive by PCR, the specificity of these tests has been questioned in this population.[1197] Because false-positive results by antigen detection tests seem to occur in neonates, it seems advisable to validate a positive ELISA or immunochromatography test with an appropriate PCR method before reporting a norovirus outbreak.[1198]

Astrovirus has been convincingly associated with a gastroenteritis outbreak in a Chinese neonatal unit.[1199] The outbreak lasted 4 months; diarrhea with a mean of eight stool emissions per day was the most common symptom, and low hygiene standards were implicated as the main cause for the prolonged duration of the outbreak. The outbreak strain was sequenced and corresponded to one of the most common circulating strains, HAstV-1. In another report based on the antigen detection method applied to stools of symptomatic preterm newborns from Italy, positive astrovirus detection was associated with GI symptoms, including bloody stools and necrotizing enterocolitis.[1200] Adenoviruses, not specifically enteric adenoviruses, have been rarely described as causing severe disseminated disease in newborn babies. The most recent report suggests transmission from a mother with diarrhea to the newborn was associated with water-birth delivery.[1201]

Differential Diagnosis

Stools from breastfed neonates are typically watery and yellow, green, or brown. The frequency of stool emissions can vary from one every other day to eight evacuations per day. In an active, healthy infant who is feeding well, has no vomiting, and has a soft abdomen, these varied patterns of stooling are not a cause for concern. Physicians need to consider the infant's previous frequency and consistency of stools and establish a diagnosis of acute diarrhea on an individual basis. Close follow-up of weight increase in infants with nonformed stools can help confirm the clinical impression. A normal weight gain should direct medical action away from stool examinations or treatment.

Diarrhea during the neonatal period is a clinical manifestation of a wide variety of disorders (Table 11-4). The most

Table 11-4 Differential Diagnosis of Neonatal Infectious Diarrhea

Group of Causes	Diagnosis	Reference (s)
Anatomic disorders	Microvillous inclusion disease	1205
	Hirschsprung disease	1206
	Massive intestinal resection (short bowel syndrome)	1207
	Congenital short bowel syndrome	1208
	Intestinal lymphangiectasis	1209
Metabolic and Enzymatic disorders	Congenital disaccharidase deficiency (lactase, sucrase-isomaltase deficiency)	1210, 1211
	Congenital glucose-galactose malabsorption	1212
	Secondary disaccharide, monosaccharide malabsorption:	1213-1219
	After gastrointestinal surgery	
	After infection	
	With milk–soy protein sensitivity	
	Cystic fibrosis	1220
	Syndrome of pancreatic insufficiency and bone marrow dysfunction (Shwachman syndrome)	1221
	Physiologic deficiency of pancreatic amylase	1222
	Intestinal enterokinase deficiency	1223
	Congenital bile acid deficiency syndrome	1224
	α/β-lipoproteinemia	1225
	Acrodermatitis enteropathica	1226, 1227
	Congenital chloride diarrhea	1228-1230
	Primary hypomagnesemia	1231
	Congenital adrenal hyperplasia	1232
	Intestinal hormone hypersecretion	1233,1234
	Non-β islet cell hyperplasia (Wolman disease)	1235
	Transcobalamin II deficiency	1236
	Congenital iron storage	1237
	Hartnup disease	1238
	Congenital Na^+ diarrhea	1239
	Congenital pseudohypoparathyroidism	1240
Inflammatory disorders	Cow's milk protein intolerance	1241, 1242
	Soy protein intolerance	1243, 1244
	Crohn disease	1245
	Ulcerative colitis	1246, 1247
Primary immunodeficiency disorders	Wiskott-Aldrich syndrome	1248
	AIDS	1249
Miscellaneous	Irritable colon of childhood (chronic nonspecific diarrhea)	1250
	Phototherapy for hyperbilirubinemia	1251
	Neonatal Kawasaki disease	1252

AIDS, Acquired immunodeficiency syndrome.

common initiating factor is a primary infection of the GI tract that is mild to moderate in severity, self-limited, and responsive to supportive measures. Acute diarrhea can also be an initial manifestation of a systemic infection, including bacterial and viral neonatal sepsis. Infants with moderate-to-severe diarrhea require close monitoring until the etiologic diagnosis and the clinical evolution are clarified. Noninfectious diseases leading to chronic intractable diarrhea may result in severe hydroelectrolytic and nutritional disturbances, or even death, unless the specific underlying condition is identified and treated appropriately.

The differential diagnosis of a diarrheal illness requires a careful clinical examination to determine whether the child has a localized or a systemic process. Lethargy, abnormalities in body temperature (hypothermia or hyperthermia), decreased feeding, abdominal distention, vomiting, pallor, respiratory distress, apnea, cyanosis, hemodynamic instability, hypotension, hepatomegaly or splenomegaly, coagulation or bleeding disorders, petechiae, and exanthems should initiate an intense laboratory investigation directed at systemic viral or bacterial infection. If the process is deemed a localized intestinal infection, initial evaluation can be focused on differentiating an inflammatory-invasive pathogen from pathogens that cause a noninflammatory process. For this, stool examination for fecal leukocytes, red blood cells, and lactoferrin can be a helpful indicator of the former.

Inflammatory diarrhea can be caused by *Shigella, Salmonella, Campylobacter, V. parahaemolyticus, Y. enterocolitica,* EIEC, EAEC, *C. difficile,* necrotizing enterocolitis, antibiotic-associated colitis, and allergic colitis (i.e., milk or soy intolerance). Noninflammatory causes of diarrhea include ETEC, EPEC, rotaviruses, enteric adenoviruses, norovirus, astrovirus, *G. lamblia,* and *Cryptosporidium. V. cholerae* can cause severe life-threatening neonatal diarrhea in regions where the infection is endemic.[1202] Cytomegalovirus can cause mild-to-severe enteritis that may result in ileal stricture.[1203] Enteroviruses can cause outbreaks of fever, diarrhea, and respiratory symptoms in newborn units.[1204] Although supportive fluid therapy is mandatory for all types of diarrhea, the brief examination for fecal leukocytes and red blood cells can direct the diagnostic and therapeutic approach. Pathogens such as *Shigella, Salmonella,* and EHEC can cause watery or bloody diarrhea, depending on the specific host-pathogen interaction and the pathogenic mechanisms involved.

Fecal cultures should be obtained when an infectious etiology has to be ruled out. The physician has to communicate to the laboratory if uncommon or fastidious bacteria are suspected, because selective and enriched media may be necessary depending on the clinical suspicion.

EIA and PCR are useful for rapid and accurate identification of specific agents. More recently, multiplex PCR allows simultaneous detection of the most frequent enteric pathogens as indicated earlier for specific pathogens.

References

1. Farthing M, Salam MA, Lindberg G, et al: Acute diarrhea in adults and children: a global perspective, *J Clin Gastroenterol* 47:12, 2013.
2. Guerrant RL: Lessons from diarrheal diseases: demography to molecular pharmacology, *J Infect Dis* 169:1206, 1994.
3. Morrow AL, Reves RR, West MS, et al: Protection against infection with *Giardia lamblia* by breast-feeding in a cohort of Mexican infants, *J Pediatr* 121:363, 1992.
4. Morrow AL, Pickering LK: Human milk protection against diarrheal disease, *Semin Pediatr Infect Dis* 5:236, 1994.
5. Mihrshahi S, Ichikawa N, Shuaib M, et al: Prevalence of exclusive breastfeeding in Bangladesh and its association with diarrhoea and acute respiratory infection: results of the multiple indicator cluster survey 2003, *J Health Popul Nutr* 25:195, 2007.
6. Lamberti LM, Fischer Walker CL, Noiman A, et al: Breastfeeding and the risk for diarrhea morbidity and mortality, *BMC Public Health* 11(Suppl 3):S15, 2011.
7. Lozano R, Naghavi M, Foreman K, et al: Global and regional mortality from 235 causes of death for 20 age groups in 1990 and 2010: a systematic analysis for the Global Burden of Disease Study 2010, *Lancet* 380:2095, 2012.
8. Lawn JE, Cousens S, Zupan J: 4 million neonatal deaths: when? where? why? *Lancet* 365:891, 2005.
9. Parashar UD, Kilgore PE, Holman RC, et al: Diarrheal mortality in US infants. Influence of birth weight on risk factors for death, *Arch Pediatr Adolesc Med* 152:47, 1998.
10. McElroy SJ, Weitkamp JH: Innate immunity in the small intestine of the preterm infant, *Neoreviews* 12:517, 2011.
11. Cuenca AG, Wynn JL, Moldawer LL, et al: Role of innate immunity in neonatal infection, *Am J Perinatol* 30:105, 2013.
12. Mezoff EA, Aly H: The winding road to understanding the neonatal origins of inflammatory gastrointestinal disorders, *J Pediatr Gastroenterol Nutr* 57:543, 2013.
13. Newburg DS, Walker WA: Protection of the neonate by the innate immune system of developing gut and of human milk, *Pediatr Res* 61:2, 2007.
14. Fagarasan S, Kawamoto S, Kanagawa O, et al: Adaptive immune regulation in the gut: T cell-dependent and T cell-independent IgA synthesis, *Annu Rev Immunol* 28:243, 2010.
15. Lundell A-C, Björnsson V, Ljung A, et al: Infant B cell memory differentiation and early gut bacterial colonization, *J Immunol* 188:4315, 2012.
16. DiGiulio DB, Romero R, Amogan HP, et al: Microbial prevalence, diversity and abundance in amniotic fluid during preterm labor: a molecular and culture-based investigation, *PLoS One* 3:e3056, 2008.
17. DiGiulio DB: Diversity of microbes in amniotic fluid, *Semin Fetal Neonatal Med* 17:2, 2012.
18. Mshvildadze M, Neu J, Shuster J, et al: Intestinal microbial ecology in premature infants assessed with non-culture based techniques, *J Pediatr* 156:20, 2010.
19. Bettelheim KA, Lennox-King SM: The acquisition of *Escherichia coli* by new-born babies, *Infection* 4:174, 1976.
20. Adlerberth I, Wold AE: Establishment of the gut microbiota in Western infants, *Acta Paediatra* 98:229, 2009.
21. Dominguez-Bello MG, Costello EK, Contreras M, et al: Delivery mode shapes the acquisition and structure of the initial microbiota across multiple body habitats in newborns, *Proc Natl Acad Sci U S A* 107:11971, 2010.
22. Isolauri E: Development of healthy gut microbiota early in life, *J Paediatr Child Health* 48(Suppl 3):1, 2012.
23. Avery GB, Randolph JG, Weaver T: Gastric acidity in the first day of life, *Pediatrics* 37:1005, 1966.
24. Harries JT, Fraser AJ: The acidity of the gastric contents of premature babies during the first fourteen days of life, *Biol Neonat* 12:186, 1968.
25. Agunod M, Yamaguchi N, Lopez R, et al: Correlative study of hydrochloric acid, pepsin, and intrinsic factor secretion in newborns and infants, *Am J Dig Dis* 14:400, 1969.
26. Cavell B: Gastric emptying in preterm infants, *Acta Paediatr Scand* 68:725, 1979.
27. Pildes RS, Blumenthal I, Ebel A: Stomach emptying in the newborn, *Pediatrics* 66:482, 1980.
28. Silverio J: Gastric emptying time in the newborn and the nursling, *Am J Med Sci* 247:732-738, 1964.
29. Cavell B: Gastric emptying in infants, *Acta Paediatr Scand* 60:370, 1971.
30. Rimoldi M, Chieppa M, Vulcano M, et al: Intestinal epithelial cells control dendritic cell function, *Ann NY Acad Sci* 1029:66, 2004.
31. Artis D: Epithelial-cell recognition of commensal bacteria and maintenance of immune homeostasis in the gut, *Nat Rev Immunol* 8:411, 2008.
32. Tanabe H, Ayabe T, Bainbridge B, et al: Mouse paneth cell secretory responses to cell surface glycolipids of virulent and attenuated pathogenic bacteria, *Infect Immun* 73:2312, 2005.
33. Bernt KM, Walker WA: Human milk as a carrier of biochemical messages, *Acta Paediatr Suppl* 88:27, 1999.
34. Fallot ME, Boyd JL, Oski FA: Breast-feeding reduces incidence of hospital admissions for infection in infants, *Pediatrics* 65:1121, 1980.
35. Larsen SA Jr, Homer DR: Relation of breast versus bottle feeding to hospitalization for gastroenteritis in a middle-class U.S. population, *J Pediatr* 92:417, 1978.
36. Cushing AH, Anderson L: Diarrhea in breast-fed and non-breast-fed infants, *Pediatrics* 70:921, 1982.
37. Myers MG, Fomon SJ, Koontz FP, et al: Respiratory and gastrointestinal illnesses in breast- and formula-fed infants, *Am J Dis Child* 138:629, 1984.
38. Feachem RG, Koblinsky MA: Interventions for the control of diarrhoeal diseases among young children: promotion of breast-feeding, *Bull World Health Organ* 62:271, 1984.
39. Forman MR, Graubard BI, Hoffman HJ, et al: The Pima Infant Feeding Study: breast feeding and gastroenteritis in the first year of life, *Am J Epidemiol* 119:335, 1984.
40. Rubin DH, Leventhal JM, Krasilnikoff PA, et al: Relationship between infant feeding and infectious illness: a prospective study of infants during the first year of life, *Pediatrics* 85:464, 1990.
41. Victora CG, Smith PG, Vaughan JP, et al: Infant feeding and deaths due to diarrhea. A case-control study, *Am J Epidemiol* 129:1032, 1989.
42. Newburg DS, Peterson JA, Ruiz-Palacios GM, et al: Role of human-milk lactadherin in protection against symptomatic rotavirus infection, *Lancet* 351:1160, 1998.
43. Wyatt RG, Mata LJ: Bacteria in colostrum and milk of Guatemalan Indian women, *J Trop Pediatr* 15:159, 1969.
44. Mata LJ, Urrutia JJ: Intestinal colonization of breast-fed children in a rural area of low socioeconomic level, *Ann NY Acad Sci* 176:93, 1971.
45. Quigley MA, Kelly YJ, Sacker A: Breastfeeding and hospitalization for diarrheal and respiratory infection in the United Kingdom Millennium Cohort Study, *Pediatrics* 119:837, 2007.
46. Pickering LK, Granoff DM, Erickson JR, et al: Modulation of the immune system by human milk and infant formula containing nucleotides, *Pediatrics* 101:242, 1998.
47. Garofalo R: Cytokines in human milk, *J Pediatr* 156:S36, 2010.
48. Walker A: Breast milk as the gold standard for protective nutrients, *J Pediatr* 156:S3, 2010.
49. Iyengar SR, Walker WA: Immune factors in breast milk and the development of atopic disease, *J Pediatr Gastroenterol Nutr* 55:641, 2012.
50. Hayani KC, Guerrero ML, Morrow AL, et al: Concentration of milk secretory immunoglobulin A against *Shigella* virulence plasmid-associated antigens as a predictor of symptom status in *Shigella*-infected breast-fed infants, *J Pediatr* 121:852, 1992.
51. Hayani KC, Guerrero ML, Ruiz-Palacios GM, et al: Evidence for long-term memory of the mucosal immune system: milk secretory immunoglobulin A against *Shigella* lipopolysaccharides, *J Clin Microbiol* 29:2599, 1991.
52. Newburg DS, Ashkenazi S, Cleary TG: Human milk contains the Shiga toxin and Shiga-like toxin receptor glycolipid Gb3, *J Infect Dis* 166:832, 1992.

53. Herrera-Insua I, Gomez HF, Diaz-Gonzalez VA, et al: Human milk lipids bind Shiga toxin, *Adv Exp Med Biol* 501:333, 2001.
54. Gomez HF, Ochoa TJ, Carlin LG, et al: Human lactoferrin impairs virulence of *Shigella flexneri*, *J Infect Dis* 187:87, 2003.
55. Gomez HF, Ochoa TJ, Herrera-Insua I, et al: Lactoferrin protects rabbits from *Shigella flexneri*-induced inflammatory enteritis, *Infect Immun* 70:7050, 2002.
56. Gomez HF, Herrera-Insua I, Siddiqui MM, et al: Protective role of human lactoferrin against invasion of *Shigella flexneri* M90T, *Adv Exp Med Biol* 501:457, 2001.
57. Cravioto A, Tello A, Villafán H, et al: Inhibition of localized adhesion of enteropathogenic *Escherichia coli* to HEp-2 cells by immunoglobulin and oligosaccharide fractions of human colostrum and breast milk, *J Infect Dis* 163:1247, 1991.
58. Glass RI, Svennerholm AM, Stoll BJ, et al: Protection against cholera in breast-fed children by antibodies in breast milk, *N Engl J Med* 308:1389, 1983.
59. Ruiz-Palacios GM, Calva JJ, Pickering LK, et al: Protection of breast-fed infants against *Campylobacter* diarrhea by antibodies in human milk, *J Pediatr* 116:707, 1990.
60. Laegreid A, Otnaess AB, Fuglesang J: Human and bovine milk: comparison of ganglioside composition and enterotoxin-inhibitory activity, *Pediatr Res* 20:416, 1986.
61. Miotti PG, Gilman RH, Pickering LK, et al: Prevalence of serum and milk antibodies to *Giardia lamblia* in different populations of lactating women, *J Infect Dis* 152:1025, 1985.
62. Montreuil J, Mullet S: Study of the variations of the glucide constituents of human milk during lactation, *Bull Soc Chim Biol (Paris)* 42:365, 1960.
63. Kobata A: Milk glycoproteins and oligosaccharides. In Horowitz MI, Pigman WW, editors: *The glycoconjugates*, New York, 1978, Academic Press, pp 423.
64. Gnoth MJ, Kunz C, Kinne-Saffran E, et al: Human milk oligosaccharides are minimally digested in vitro, *J Nutr* 130:3014, 2000.
65. Chaturvedi P, Warren CD, Buescher CR, et al: Survival of human milk oligosaccharides in the intestine of infants, *Adv Exp Med Biol* 501:315, 2001.
66. Newburg DS, Pickering LK, McCluer RH, et al: Fucosylated oligosaccharides of human milk protect suckling mice from heat-stabile enterotoxin of *Escherichia coli*, *J Infect Dis* 162:1075, 1990.
67. Hong P, Ninonuevo MR, Lee B, et al: Human milk oligosaccharides reduce HIV-1-gp120 binding to dendritic cell-specific ICAM3-grabbing non-integrin (DC-SIGN), *Br J Nutr* 101:482, 2009.
68. Huang P, Farkas T, Marionneau S, et al: Noroviruses bind to human ABO, Lewis, and secretor histo-blood group antigens: identification of 4 distinct strain-specific patterns, *J Infect Dis* 188:19, 2003.
69. Lindesmith L, Moe C, Marionneau S, et al: Human susceptibility and resistance to Norwalk virus infection, *Nat Med* 9:548, 2003.
70. Bode L, Kunz C, Muhly-Reinholz M, et al: Inhibition of monocyte, lymphocyte, and neutrophil adhesion to endothelial cells by human milk oligosaccharides, *Thromb Haemost* 92:1402, 2004.
71. Yolken RH, Peterson JA, Vonderfecht SL, et al: Human milk mucin inhibits rotavirus replication and prevents experimental gastroenteritis, *J Clin Invest* 90:1984, 1992.
72. Cooper ML, Keller HM, Walters EW, et al: Isolation of enteropathogenic *Escherichia coli* from mothers and newborn infants, *Am J Dis Child* 97:266, 1959.
73. Ocklitz HW, Schmidt EF: Enteropathogenic *Escherichia coli* serotypes: infection of newborn through mother, *Br Med J* 2:1036, 1957.
74. Gareau FE, Mackel DC, Boring 3rd JR, et al: The acquisition of fecal flora by infants from their mothers during birth, *J Pediatr* 54:313, 1959.
75. Rosner R: Antepartum culture findings of mothers in relation to infantile diarrhea, *Am J Clin Pathol* 45:732, 1966.
76. Nocard E, Leclainche E: *Les malaides microbiennes des animeux*, ed 2, Paris, 1898, Mason.
77. Joest E: Untersuchungen uber Kalberruhr, *Z Tiermed* 7:377, 1903.
78. Titze C, Weichel A: Die Atiologie der Kalberruhr, *Berl Tierarztl Wochenschr* 26:457, 1908.
79. Jensen CO: *Handbuch der pathogenen Mikroorganismen*, Jena, 1913, G. Fischer.
80. Smith T, Orcutt ML: The bacteriology of the intestinal tract of young calves with special reference to the early diarrhea ("scours"), *J Exp Med* 41:89, 1925.
81. Neonatal enteric infections caused by *Escherichia coli*, *Ann NY Acad Sci* 176:1, 1971.
82. Adam A: Uber die Biologie der Dyspepsiecoli und ihre Beziehungen zur Pathogenese der Dyspepsie und Intoxikation, *Jahrb Kinderheilkd* 101: 295, 1923.
83. Adam A: Zur Frage der bakteriellen atiologie der sogenannten alimentaren Intoxikation, *Jahrb Kinderheilkd* 116:8, 1927.
84. Nataro JP, Kaper JB: Diarrheagenic *Escherichia coli*, *Clin Microbiol Rev* 11:142, 1998.
85. Reischl U, Youssef MT, Wolf H, et al: Real-time fluorescence PCR assays for detection and characterization of heat-labile I and heat-stable I enterotoxin genes from enterotoxigenic *Escherichia coli*, *J Clin Microbiol* 42:4092, 2004.
86. Kimata K, Shima T, Shimizu M, et al: Rapid categorization of pathogenic *Escherichia coli* by multiplex PCR, *Microbiol Immunol* 49:485, 2005.
87. Donnenberg MS, Kaper JB: Enteropathogenic *Escherichia coli*, *Infect Immun* 60:3953, 1992.
88. Levine MM: *Escherichia coli* that cause diarrhea: enterotoxigenic, enteropathogenic, enteroinvasive, enterohemmorrhagic, and enteroadherent, *J Infect Dis* 155:377, 1987.
89. Guerrant RL, Thielman NM: Types of *Escherichia coli* enteropathogens. In Blaser MJ, Smith PD, Ravdin JI, editors: *Infections of the gastrointestinal tract*, New York, 1995, Raven Press, p 687.
90. Schlager TA, Guerrant RL: Seven possible mechanisms for *Escherichia coli* diarrhea, *Infect Dis Clin North Am* 2:607, 1988.
91. Steiner TS, Lima AA, Nataro JP, et al: Enteroaggregative *Escherichia coli* produce intestinal inflammation and growth impairment and cause interleukin-8 release from intestinal epithelial cells, *J Infect Dis* 177:88, 1998.
92. Kaper JB, Nataro JP, Mobley HL: Pathogenic *Escherichia coli*, *Nat Rev Microbiol* 2:123, 2004.
93. Clements A, Young JC, Constantinou N, et al: Infection strategies of enteric pathogenic *Escherichia coli*, *Gut Microbes* 3:87, 2012.
94. Spangler BD: Structure and function of cholera toxin and the related *Escherichia coli* heat-labile enterotoxin, *Microbiol Rev* 56:622, 1992.
95. Guerrant RL, Ganguly U, Casper AG, et al: Effect of *Escherichia coli* on fluid transport across canine small bowel. Mechanism and time-course with enterotoxin and whole bacterial cells, *J Clin Invest* 52:1707, 1973.
96. Peterson JW, Reitmeyer JC, Jackson CA, et al: Protein synthesis is required for cholera toxin-induced stimulation of arachidonic acid metabolism, *Biochim Biophys Acta* 1092:79, 1991.
97. Peterson JW, Ochoa LG: Role of prostaglandins and cAMP in the secretory effects of cholera toxin, *Science* 245:857, 1989.
98. Thielman NM, Marcinkiewicz M, Sarosiek J, et al: Role of platelet-activating factor in Chinese hamster ovary cell responses to cholera toxin, *J Clin Invest* 99:1999, 1997.
99. Guerrant RL, Fang GD, Thielman NM, et al: Role of platelet activating factor in the intestinal epithelial secretory and Chinese hamster ovary cell cytoskeletal responses to cholera toxin, *Proc Natl Acad Sci U S A* 91:9655, 1994.
100. Hughes JM, Murad F, Chang B, et al: Role of cyclic GMP in the action of heat-stable enterotoxin of *Escherichia coli*, *Nature* 271:755, 1978.
101. Field M, Graf LH Jr, Laird WJ, et al: Heat-stable enterotoxin of *Escherichia coli*: in vitro effects on guanylate cyclase activity, cyclic GMP concentration, and ion transport in small intestine, *Proc Natl Acad Sci U S A* 75:2800, 1978.
102. Guerrant RL, Hughes JM, Chang B, et al: Activation of intestinal guanylate cyclase by heat-stable enterotoxin of *Escherichia coli*: studies of tissue specificity, potential receptors, and intermediates, *J Infect Dis* 142:220, 1980.
103. Kennedy DJ, Greenberg RN, Dunn JA, et al: Effects of *Escherichia coli* heat-stable enterotoxin STb on intestines of mice, rats, rabbits, and piglets, *Infect Immun* 46:639, 1984.
104. Weikel CS, Tiemens KM, Moseley SL, et al: Species specificity and lack of production of STb enterotoxin by *Escherichia coli* strains isolated from humans with diarrheal illness, *Infect Immun* 52:323, 1986.

105. Weikel CS, Nellans HN, Guerrant RL: In vivo and in vitro effects of a novel enterotoxin, STb, produced by *Escherichia coli*, *J Infect Dis* 153:893, 1986.
106. DuPont HL, Formal SB, Hornick RB, et al: Pathogenesis of *Escherichia coli* diarrhea, *N Engl J Med* 285:1, 1971.
107. Tulloch EF Jr, Ryan KJ, Formal SB, et al: Invasive enteropathic *Escherichia coli* dysentery. An outbreak in 28 adults, *Ann Intern Med* 79:13, 1973.
108. Parsot C: *Shigella* spp. and enteroinvasive *Escherichia coli* pathogenicity factors, *FEMS Microbiol Lett* 252:11, 2005.
109. Nataro JP, Kaper JB, Robins-Browne R, et al: Patterns of adherence of diarrheagenic *Escherichia coli* to HEp-2 cells, *Pediatr Infect Dis J* 6:829, 1987.
110. Kenny B, DeVinney R, Stein M, et al: Enteropathogenic *E. coli* (EPEC) transfers its receptor for intimate adherence into mammalian cells, *Cell* 91:511, 1997.
111. Nougayrede JP, Fernandes PJ, Donnenberg MS: Adhesion of enteropathogenic *Escherichia coli* to host cells, *Cell Microbiol* 5:359, 2003.
112. Okeke IN, Nataro JP: Enteroaggregative *Escherichia coli*, *Lancet Infect Dis* 1:304, 2001.
113. Trabulsi LR, Keller R, Tardelli Gomes TA: Typical and atypical enteropathogenic *Escherichia coli*, *Emerg Infect Dis* 8:508, 2002.
114. Ochoa TJ, Contreras CA: Enteropathogenic *Escherichia coli* infection in children, *Curr Opin Infect Dis* 24:478, 2011.
115. Rowe B, Scotland SM, Gross RJ: Enterotoxigenic *Escherichia coli* causing infantile enteritis in Britain, *Lancet* 1:90, 1977.
116. Trabulsi LR, Fernandes MR, Zuliani ME: Novas bacterias patogenicas para o intestino do homen, *Rev Inst Med Trop São Paulo* 9:31, 1967.
117. Skerman FJ, Formal SB, Falkow S: Plasmid-associated enterotoxin production in a strain of *Escherichia coli* isolated from humans, *Infect Immun* 5:622, 1972.
118. Takeda Y, Murphy JR: Bacteriophage conversion of heat-labile enterotoxin in *Escherichia coli*, *J Bacteriol* 133:172, 1978.
119. Lathe R, Hirth P, DeWilde M, et al: Cell-free synthesis of enterotoxin of *E. coli* from a cloned gene, *Nature* 284:473, 1980.
120. Merson MH, Rowe B, Black RE, et al: Use of antisera for identification of enterotoxigenic *Escherichia coli*, *Lancet* 2:222, 1980.
121. Evans DG, Evans DJ Jr, Pierce NF: Differences in the response of rabbit small intestine to heat-labile and heat-stable enterotoxins of *Escherichia coli*, *Infect Immun* 7:873, 1973.
122. Sears CL, Kaper JB: Enteric bacterial toxins: mechanisms of action and linkage to intestinal secretion, *Microbiol Rev* 60:167, 1996.
123. Donta ST, Moon HW, Whipp SC: Detection of heat-labile *Escherichia coli* enterotoxin with the use of adrenal cells in tissue culture, *Science* 183:334, 1974.
124. Yolken RH, Greenberg HB, Merson MH, et al: Enzyme-linked immunosorbent assay for detection of *Escherichia coli* heat-labile enterotoxin, *J Clin Microbiol* 6:439, 1977.
125. Dean AG, Ching YC, Williams RG, et al: Test for *Escherichia coli* enterotoxin using infant mice: application in a study of diarrhea in children in Honolulu, *J Infect Dis* 125:407, 1972.
126. Giannella RA: Suckling mouse model for detection of heat-stable *Escherichia coli* enterotoxin: characteristics of the model, *Infect Immun* 14:95, 1976.
127. Barletta F, Ochoa TJ, Cleary TG: Multiplex real-time PCR (MRT-PCR) for diarrheagenic, *Methods Mol Biol* 943:307, 2013.
128. Klipstein FA, Holdeman LV, Corcino JJ, et al: Enterotoxigenic intestinal bacteria in tropical sprue, *Ann Intern Med* 79:632, 1973.
129. Smith HW, Halls S: Observations by the ligated intestinal segment and oral inoculation methods on *Escherichia coli* infections in pigs, calves, lambs and rabbits, *J Pathol Bacteriol* 93:499, 1967.
130. Evans DG, Silver RP, Evans DJ Jr, et al: Plasmid-controlled colonization factor associated with virulence in *Esherichia coli* enterotoxigenic for humans, *Infect Immun* 12:656, 1975.
131. De SN, Chatterje DN: An experimental study of the mechanism of action of *Vibrio cholerae* on the intestinal mucous membrane, *J Pathol Bacteriol* 66:559, 1953.
132. De SN, Bhattacharya K, Sarkar JK: A study of the pathogenicity of strains of *Bacterium coli* from acute and chronic enteritis, *J Pathol Bacteriol* 71:201, 1956.
133. Taylor J, Bettelheim KA: The action of chloroform-killed suspensions of enteropathogenic *Escherichia coli* on ligated rabbit-gut segments, *J Gen Microbiol* 42:309, 1966.
134. Taylor J, Wilkins MP, Payne JM: Relation of rabbit gut reaction to enteropathogenic *Escherichia coli*, *Br J Exp Pathol* 42:43, 1961.
135. Trabulsi LR: Detection of colibacilli associated with infantile diarrheas by the experimental infection of ligated loops of rabbit intestine, *Rev Inst Med Trop São Paulo* 6:197, 1964.
136. Moon HW, Sorensen DK, Sautter JH, et al: Association of *Escherichia coli* with diarrheal disease of the newborn pig, *Am J Vet Res* 27:1007, 1966.
137. Smith HW, Halls S: Studies on *Escherichia coli* enterotoxin, *J Pathol Bacteriol* 93:531, 1967.
138. Truszczynski M, Pilaszek J: Effects of injection of enterotoxin, endotoxin or live culture of *Escherichia coli* into the small intestine of pigs, *Res Vet Sci* 10:469, 1969.
139. Gyles CL, Barnum DA: A heat-labile enterotoxin from strains of *Eschericha coli* enteropathogenic for pigs, *J Infect Dis* 120:419, 1969.
140. Gorbach SL, Banwell JG, Chatterjee BD, et al: Acute undifferentiated human diarrhea in the tropics. I. Alterations in intestinal micrflora, *J Clin Invest* 50:881, 1971.
141. Banwell JG, Gorbach SL, Pierce NF, et al: Acute undifferentiated human diarrhea in the tropics. II. Alterations in intestinal fluid and electrolyte movements, *J Clin Invest* 50:890, 1971.
142. Sack RB, Gorbach SL, Banwell JG, et al: Enterotoxigenic *Escherichia coli* isolated from patients with severe cholera-like disease, *J Infect Dis* 123:378, 1971.
143. Pierce NF, Wallace CK: Stimulation of jejunal secretion by a crude *Escherichia coli* enterotixin, *Gastroenterology* 63:439, 1972.
144. Guerrant RL, Carpenter CC, Pierce NF: Experimental *E. coli* diarrhea: effects of viable bacteria and enterotoxin, *Trans Assoc Am Physicians* 86:111, 1973.
145. Kantor HS, Tao P, Gorbach SL: Stimulation of intestinal adenyl cyclase by *Escherichia coli* enterotoxin: comparison of strains from an infant and an adult with diarrhea, *J Infect Dis* 129:1, 1974.
146. Smith HW, Gyles CL: The effect of cell-free fluids prepared from cultures of human and animal enteropathogenic strains of *Escherichia coli* on ligated intestinal segments of rabbits and pigs, *J Med Microbiol* 3:403, 1970.
147. Kohler EM: Observations on enterotoxins produced by enteropathogenic *Escherichia coli*, *Ann NY Acad Sci* 176:212, 1971.
148. Moon HW, Whipp SC: Systems for testing the enteropathogenicity of *Escherichia coli*, *Ann NY Acad Sci* 176:197, 1971.
149. Dubreuil JD: The whole shebang: the gastrointestinal tract, *Escherichia coli* enterotoxins and secretion, *Curr Issues Mol Biol* 14:71, 2012.
150. Holmgren J, Svennerholm AM: Enzyme-linked immunosorbent assays for cholera serology, *Infect Immun* 7:759, 1973.
151. Svennerholm AM, Holmgren J: Identification of *Escherichia coli* heat-labile enterotoxin by means of a ganglioside immunosrobent assay (Gm1 ELISA) procedure, *Curr Microbiol* 1:19, 1978.
152. Sack DA, Huda S, Neogi PK, et al: Microtiter ganglioside enzyme-linked immunosorbent assay for *Vibrio* and *Escherichia coli* heat-labile enterotoxins and antitoxin, *J Clin Microbiol* 11:35, 1980.
153. Currie MG, Fok KF, Kato J, et al: Guanylin: an endogenous activator of intestinal guanylate cyclase, *Proc Natl Acad Sci U S A* 89:947, 1992.
154. Wadstrom T, Aust-Kettis A, Habte D, et al: Enterotoxin-producing bacteria and parasites in stools of Ethiopian children with diarrhoeal disease, *Arch Dis Child* 51:865, 1976.
155. Wachsmuth K, Wells J, Shipley P, et al: Heat-labile enterotoxin production in isolates from a shipboard outbreak of human diarrheal illness, *Infect Immun* 24:793, 1979.
156. Smith HW, Linggood MA: Observations on the pathogenic properties of the K88, Hly and Ent plasmids of *Escherichia coli* with particular reference to porcine diarrhoea, *J Med Microbiol* 4:467, 1971.
157. Wolf MK: Occurrence, distribution, and associations of O and H serogroups, colonization factor antigens, and toxins of enterotoxigenic *Escherichia coli*, *Clin Microbiol Rev* 10:569, 1997.
158. Cassels FJ, Wolf MK: Colonization factors of diarrheagenic *E. coli* and their intestinal receptors, *J Ind Microbiol* 15:214, 1995.
159. Isidean SD, Riddle MS, Savarino SJ, et al: A systematic review of ETEC epidemiology focusing on colonization factor and toxin expression, *Vaccine* 29:6167, 2011.
160. Qadri F, Svennerholm AM, Faruque AS, et al: Enterotoxigenic *Escherichia coli* in developing countries: epidemiology, microbiology, clinical features, treatment, and prevention, *Clin Microbiol Rev* 18:465, 2005.

161. Fleckenstein JM, Munson GM, Rasko D: Enterotoxigenic *Escherichia coli*: Orchestrated host engagement, *Gut Microbes* 4:392, 2013.
162. Roy K, et al: The EtpA exoprotein of enterotoxigenic *Escherichia coli* promotes intestinal colonization and is a protective antigen in an experimental model of murine infection, Infect, *Immun* 76:2106, 2008.
163. Fleckenstein JM, et al: Molecular mechanisms of enterotoxigenic *Escherichia coli* infection, *Microbes Infect* 12:89, 2010.
164. Wenneras C, Erling V: Prevalence of enterotoxigenic *Escherichia coli*-associated diarrhoea and carrier state in the developing world, *J Health Popul Nutr* 22:370, 2004.
165. World Health Organization: Initiative for Vaccine Research, Diarrhoeal Diseases, 2009. Available from http://www.who.int/vaccine_research/diseases/diarrhoeal/en/index4.html.
166. Long K, Vasquez-Garibay E, Mathewson J, et al: The impact of infant feeding patterns on infection and diarrheal disease due to enterotoxigenic *Escherichia coli*, *Salud Publica Mex* 41:263, 1999.
167. Clemens JD, Rao MR, Chakraborty J, et al: Breastfeeding and the risk of life-threatening enterotoxigenic *Escherichia coli* diarrhea in Bangladeshi infants and children, *Pediatrics* 100:E2, 1997.
168. Long KZ, Wood JW, Vasquez Gariby E, et al: Proportional hazards analysis of diarrhea due to enterotoxigenic *Escherichia coli* and breast feeding in a cohort of urban Mexican children, *Amer J Epidemiol*, 139:193, 1994.
169. Sack DA, Kaminsky DC, Sack RB, et al: Enterotoxigenic *Escherichia coli* diarrhea of travelers: a prospective study of American Peace Corps volunteers, *Johns Hopkins Med J* 141:63, 1977.
170. Guerrant RL, Rouse JD, Hughes JM, et al: Turista among members of the Yale Glee Club in Latin America, *Am J Trop Med Hyg* 29:895, 1980.
171. Guerrant RL, Moore RA, Kirschenfeld PM, et al: Role of toxigenic and invasive bacteria in acute diarrhea of childhood, *N Engl J Med* 293:567, 1975.
172. Hill DR, Beeching NJ: Travelers' diarrhea, *Curr Opin Infect Dis* 23:481, 2010.
173. Shah N, DuPont HL, Ramsey DJ: Global etiology of travelers' diarrhea: systematic review from 1973 to the present, *Am J Trop Med Hyg* 80:609, 2009.
174. Guerrant RL, Kirchhoff LV, Shields DS, et al: Prospective study of diarrheal illnesses in northeastern Brazil: patterns of disease, nutritional impact, etiologies, and risk factors, *J Infect Dis* 148:986, 1983.
175. Echeverria P, Blacklow NR, Smith DH: Role of heat-labile toxigenic *Escherichia coli* and Reovirus-like agent in diarrhoea in Boston children, *Lancet* 2:1113, 1975.
176. Viboud GI, Binsztein N, Svennerholm AM: Characterization of monoclonal antibodies against putative colonization factors of enterotoxigenic *Escherichia coli* and their use in an epidemiological study, *J Clin Microbiol* 31:558, 1993.
177. Huilan S, Zhen LG, Mathan MM, et al: Etiology of acute diarrhoea among children in developing countries: a multicentre study in five countries, *Bull World Health Organ* 69:549, 1991.
178. McLean M, Brennan R, Hughes JM, et al: Etiology of childhood diarrhea and oral rehydration therapy in northeastern Brazil, *Bull Pan Am Health Organ* 15:318, 1981.
179. Nalin DR, McLaughlin JC, Rahaman M, et al: Enterotoxigenic *Escherichia coli* and idiopathic diarrhoea in Bangladesh, *The Lancet* 2:1116, 1975.
180. Ryder RW, Sack DA, Kapikian AZ, et al: Enterotoxigenic *Escherichia coli* and reovirus-like agent in rural Bangladesh, *Lancet* 1:659, 1976.
181. Sack RB, Hirschhorn N, Brownlee I, et al: Enterotoxigenic *Escherichia coli*-associated diarrheal disease in Apache children, *N Engl J Med* 292:1041, 1975.
182. Blanco J, González EA, Blanco M, et al: Enterotoxigenic *Escherichia coli* associated with infant diarrhoea in Galicia, north-western Spain, *J Med Microbiol* 35:162, 1991.
183. Korzeniowski OM, Dantas W, Trabulsi LR, et al: A controlled study of endemic sporadic diarrhoea among adult residents of southern Brazil, *Trans R Soc Trop Med Hyg* 78:363, 1984.
184. Nations MK, de Sousa MA, Correia LL, et al: Brazilian popular healers as effective promoters of oral rehydration therapy (ORT) and related child survival strategies, *Bull Pan Am Health Organ* 22:335, 1988.
185. Hughes JM, Rouse JD, Barada FA, et al: Etiology of summer diarrhea among the Navajo, *Am J Trop Med Hyg* 29:613, 1980.
186. Lopez-Vidal Y, Calva JJ, Trujillo A, et al: Enterotoxins and adhesins of enterotoxigenic *Escherichia coli*: are they risk factors for acute diarrhea in the community? *J Infect Dis* 162:442, 1990.
187. Guerrant R, Kirchhoff LV, Shields DS, et al: Prospective study of diarrheal illnesses in northeastern Brazil: patterns of disease, nutritional impact, etiologies and risk factors, *J Infect Dis* 148:986, 1983.
188. Kotloff KL, Nataro JP, Blackwelder WC, et al: Burden and aetiology of diarrhoeal disease in infants and young children in developing countries (the Global Enteric Multicenter Study, GEMS): a prospective, case-control study, *Lancet* 382:209, 2013.
189. Kudoh Y, Zen-Yoji H, Matsushita S, et al: Outbreaks of acute enteritis due to heat-stable enterotoxin-producing strains of *Escherichia coli*, *Microbiol Immunol* 21:175, 1977.
190. Rosenberg ML, Koplan JP, Wachsmuth IK, et al: Epidemic diarrhea at Crater Lake from enterotoxigenic *Escherichia coli* A large waterborne outbreak, *Ann Intern Med* 86:714, 1977.
191. Ryder RW, Wachsmuth IK, Buxton AE, et al: Infantile diarrhea produced by heat-stable enterotoxigenic *Escherichia coli*, *N Engl J Med* 295:849, 1976.
192. Gross RJ, Rowe B, Henderson A, et al: A new *Escherichia coli* O-group, O159, associated with outbreaks of enteritis in infants, *Scand J Infect Dis* 8:195, 1976.
193. Mondal D, Minak J, Alam M, et al: Contribution of enteric infection, altered intestinal barrier function, and maternal malnutrition to infant malnutrition in Bangladesh, *Clin Infect Dis* 54:185, 2012.
194. Gupta SK, Keck J, Ram PK, et al: Part III. Analysis of data gaps pertaining to enterotoxigenic *Escherichia coli* infections in low and medium human development index countries, 1984-2005, *Epidemiol Infect* 136:721, 2008.
195. Porter CK, Riddle MS, Tribble DR, et al: A systematic review of experimental infections with enterotoxigenic *Escherichia coli* (ETEC), *Vaccine* 29:5869, 2011.
196. Sjoling A, Wiklund G, Savarino SJ, et al: Comparative analyses of phenotypic and genotypic methods for detection of enterotoxigenic *Escherichia coli* toxins and colonization factors, *J Clin Microbiol* 45:3295, 2007.
197. Abe A, Komase K, Bangtrakulnonth A, et al: Trivalent heat-labile- and heat-stable-enterotoxin probe conjugated with horseradish peroxidase for detection of enterotoxigenic *Escherichia coli* by hybridization, *J Clin Microbiol* 28:2616, 1990.
198. Sommerfelt H, Svennerholm AM, Kalland KH, et al: Comparative study of colony hybridization with synthetic oligonucleotide probes and enzyme-linked immunosorbent assay for identification of enterotoxigenic *Escherichia coli*, *J Clin Microbiol* 26:530, 1988.
199. Guerrant RL, Van Gilder T, Steiner TS, et al: Practice guidelines for the management of infectious diarrhea, *Clin Infect Dis* 32:331, 2001.
200. Pizarro D, Posada G, Mata L, et al: Oral rehydration of neonates with dehydrating diarrhoeas, *Lancet* 2:1209, 1979.
201. Santosham M, Daum RS, Dillman L, et al: Oral rehydration therapy of infantile diarrhea: a controlled study of well-nourished children hospitalized in the United States and Panama, *N Engl J Med* 306:1070, 1982.
202. World Health Organization: New formula oral rehydration salts, *WHO Drug Information* 16:121, 2002.
203. King CK, Glass R, Bresee JS, et al: Managing acute gastroenteritis among children: oral rehydration, maintenance, and nutritional therapy, *MMWR Recomm Rep* 52(RR-16):1, 2003.
204. Multicentre evaluation of reduced-osmolarity oral rehydration salts solution: International Study Group on Reduced-osmolarity ORS solutions, *Lancet* 345:282, 1995.
205. Hahn S, Kim S, Garner P: Reduced osmolarity oral rehydration solution for treating dehydration caused by acute diarrhoea in children, *Cochrane Database Syst Rev* (1):CD002847, 2002.
206. Bhandari N, Bahl R, Taneja S, et al: Substantial reduction in severe diarrheal morbidity by daily zinc supplementation in young north Indian children, *Pediatrics* 109:e86, 2002.
207. Bhatnagar S, Wadhwa N, Aneja S, et al: Zinc as adjunct treatment in infants aged between 7 and 120 days with probable serious bacterial infection: a randomised, double-blind, placebo-controlled trial, *Lancet* 379:2072, 2012.
208. Echeverria P, Verhaert L, Ulyangco CV, et al: Antimicrobial resistance and enterotoxin production among isolates of *Escherichia coli* in the Far East, *Lancet* 2:589, 1978.

209. DuPont HL, Ericsson CD, Farthing MJ, et al: Expert review of the evidence base for prevention of travelers' diarrhea, *J Travel Med* 16:149, 2009.
210. Nataro JP: Treatment of bacterial enteritis, *Pediatr Infect Dis J* 17:420, 1998.
211. DuPont HL, Ericsson CD, Farthing MJ, et al: Expert review of the evidence base for self-therapy of travelers' diarrhea, *J Travel Med* 16:161, 2009.
212. Sack DA, Shimko J, Torres O, et al: Randomised, double-blind, safety and efficacy of a killed oral vaccine for enterotoxigenic *E. coli* diarrhoea of travellers to Guatemala and Mexico, *Vaccine* 25:4392, 2007.
213. Svennerholm AM, Tobias J: Vaccines against enterotoxigenic *Escherichia coli*, *Expert RevVaccines* 7:795, 2008.
214. Walker RI, Steele D, Aguado T: Analysis of strategies to successfully vaccinate infants in developing countries against enterotoxigenic *E. coli* (ETEC) disease, *Vaccine* 25:2545, 2007.
215. Holmgren J, Bourgeois L, Carlin N, et al: Development and preclinical evaluation of safety and immunogenicity of an oral ETEC vaccine containing inactivated *E. coli* bacteria overexpressing colonization factors CFA/I, CS3, CS5 and CS6 combined with a hybrid LT/CT B subunit antigen, administered alone and together with dmLT adjuvant, *Vaccine* 31:2457, 2013.
216. Lundgren A, Leach S, Tobias J, et al: Clinical trial to evaluate safety and immunogenicity of an oral inactivated enterotoxigenic *Escherichia coli* prototype vaccine containing CFA/I overexpressing bacteria and recombinantly produced LTB/CTB hybrid protein, *Vaccine* 31:1163, 2013.
217. Ahmed T, Bhuiyan TR, Zaman K, et al: Vaccines for preventing enterotoxigenic *Escherichia coli* (ETEC) diarrhoea, *Cochrane Database Syst Rev* (7):CD009029, 2013.
218. Harris JR, Wachsmuth IK, Davis BR, et al: High-molecular-weight plasmid correlates with *Escherichia coli* enteroinvasiveness, *Infect Immun* 37:1295, 1982.
219. Aranda KR, Fabbricotti SH, Fagundes-Neto U, et al: Single multiplex assay to identify simultaneously enteropathogenic, enteroaggregative, enterotoxigenic, enteroinvasive and Shiga toxin-producing *Escherichia coli* strains in Brazilian children, *FEMS Microbiol Lett* 267:145, 2007.
220. Liu J, Gratz J, Maro A, et al: Simultaneous detection of six diarrhea-causing bacterial pathogens with an in-house PCR-Luminex assay, *J Clin Microbiol* 50:98, 2011.
221. Echeverria P, Sethabutr O, Pitarangsi C: Microbiology and diagnosis of infections with *Shigella* and enteroinvasive *Escherichia coli*, *Rev Infect Dis* 13(Suppl 4):S220, 1991.
222. Garcia PG, Silva VL, Diniz CG: Occurrence and antimicrobial drug susceptibility patterns of commensal and diarrheagenic *Escherichia coli* in fecal microbiota from children with and without acute diarrhea, *J Microbiol* 49:46, 2011.
223. Ratchtrachenchai OA: Prevalence of childhood diarrhoea-associated *Escherichia coli* in Thailand, *J Med Microbiol* 53:237, 2004.
224. Moyo SJ, Maselle SY, Matee MI, et al: Identification of diarrheagenic *Escherichia coli* isolated from infants and children in Dar es Salaam, Tanzania, *BMC Inf Dis* 7:92, 2007.
225. Olesen B, Neimann J, Böttiger B, et al: Etiology of diarrhea in young children in denmark: a case-control study, *J Clin Microbiol* 43:3636, 2005.
226. Hien BT, Scheutz F, Cam PD, et al: Diarrheagenic *Escherichia coli* and *Shigella* strains isolated from children in a hospital case control study in Hanoi, Vietnam, *J Clin Microbiol* 46:996, 2008.
227. Yang JR, Wu FT, Tsai JL, et al: Comparison between O serotyping method and multiplex real-time PCR to identify diarrheagenic *Escherichia coli* in Taiwan, *J Clin Microbiol* 45:3620, 2007.
228. Al-Gallas N, Bahri O, Bouratbeen A, et al: Etiology of acute diarrhea in children and adults in Tunis, Tunisia, with emphasis on diarrheagenic *Escherichia coli*: prevalence, phenotyping, and molecular epidemiology, *Am J Trop Med Hyg* 77:571, 2007.
229. Vieira N, Bates SJ, Solberg OD, et al: High prevalence of enteroinvasive *Escherichia coli* isolated in a remote region of northern coastal Ecuador, *Am J Trop Med Hyg* 76:528, 2007.
230. Perez C, Gomez-Duarte OG, Arias ML: Diarrheagenic *Escherichia coli* in children from Costa Rica, *Am J Trop Med Hyg* 83:292, 2010.
231. Moreno AC, Ferreira LG, Martinez MB: Enteroinvasive *Escherichia coli* vs. *Shigella flexneri*: how different patterns of gene expression affect virulence, *FEMS Microbiol Lett* 301:156, 2009.
232. De Assis A: *Shigella* guanabara, seconded serological type of group B. ceylonensis-dispar, *Hospital Rio J* 33:505, 1948.
233. Lapatsanis PD, Irving IM: A study of specific *E. coli* infections occurring in a unit for surgical neonates, *Acta Paediatr* 52:436, 1963.
234. Goldschmidt R: Untersuchungen zur Atiologie der Durchfallserkrankungen des Sauglings, *Jahrb Kinderheilkd* 139:318, 1933.
235. Dulaney AD, Michelson ID: A Study of B. coli mutabile from an outbreak of diarrhea in the newborn, *Am J Public Health Nations Health* 25:1241, 1935.
236. Bray J: Isolation of antigenically homogeneous strains of *Bact coli neopolitanum* from summer diarrhea of infants, *J Pathol Bacteriol* 60:395, 1945.
237. Bray J, Beaven TED: Slide agglutination of *Bacterium coli* var. *neopolitanum* in summer diarrhea, *J Pathol Bacteriol* 60:395, 1948.
238. Olarte J, Varela G: A complete somatic antigen common to *Salmonella* adelaide, *Escherichia coli*-gomez, and *Escherichia coli* 0111:B4, *J Lab Clin Med* 40:252, 1952.
239. Neter E, Korns RF, Trussel RE: Association of *Escherichia coli* serogroup 0111 with two hospital outbreaks of epidemic diarrhea of the newborn infant in New York State during 1947, *Pediatrics* 12:377, 1953.
240. Kaufman F, DuPont A: *Escherichia* strains from infantile epidemic gastroenteritis, Acta Pathol, *Microbiol Scand* 27:552, 1950.
241. Edwards PR, Ewing WH: *Identification of Enterobacteriaceae*, ed 3, Minneapolis, Minn, 1972, Burgess Publishing.
242. Neter E, Westphal O, Luderitz O, et al: Demonstration of antibodies against enteropathogenic *Escherichia coli* in sera of children of various ages, *Pediatrics* 16:801, 1955.
243. Gronroos JA: Investigations on certain *Escherichia coli* serotypes, with special reference to infantile diarrhoea, *Ann Med* 32:9, 1954.
244. Donnenberg MS, Whittam TS: Pathogenesis and evolution of virulence in enteropathogenic and enterohemorrhagic *Escherichia coli*, *J Clin Invest* 107:539, 2001.
245. Moyenuddin M, Rahman KM: Enteropathogenic *Escherichia coli* diarrhea in hospitalized children in Bangladesh, *J Clin Microbiol* 22:838, 1985.
246. Bower JR, Congeni BL, Cleary TG, et al: *Escherichia coli* O114:nonmotile as a pathogen in an outbreak of severe diarrhea associated with a day care center, *J Infect Dis* 160:243, 1989.
247. Gordon JE: Diarrheal disease of early childhood-worldwide scope of the problem, *Ann NY Acad Sci* 176:9, 1971.
248. Gordon JE, Chitkara ID, Wyon JB: Weanling diarrhea, *Am J Med Sci* 245:345, 1963.
249. Kahn E: The aetiology of summer diarrhoea, *S Afr Med J* 31:47, 1957.
250. Giles C, Sangster G, Smith J: Epidemic gastro-enteritis of infants in Aberdeen during 1947, *Arch Dis Child* 24:45, 1949.
251. Boris M, Thomason BM, Hines VD, et al: A community epidemic of enteropathogenic *Escherichia coli* O126:B16:Nm gastroenteritis associated with asymptomatic respiratory infection, *Pediatrics* 33:18, 1964.
252. Taylor J: The diarrhoeal diseases in England and Wales, with special reference to those caused by *Salmonella, Escherichia* and *Shigella*, *Bull World Health Organ* 23:763, 1960.
253. Epidemiological Research Laboratory of the Public Health Laboratory Service, United Kingdom and Republic of Ireland, *E. coli* gastroenteritis from food, *Br Med J* 1:911, 1976.
254. Stulberg CS, Zuelzer WW, Nolke AC: An epidemic of diarrhea of the newborn cause by *Escherichia coli* O-111, B4, *Pediatrics* 14:133, 1954.
255. Farmer K, Hassall IB: An epidemic of *E. coli* type 055:K59(B5) in a neonatal unit, *N Z Med J* 77:372, 1973.
256. Hugh-Jones K, Ross GI: Epidemics of gastro-enteritis associated with *Esch coli* 0119 infection, *Arch Dis Child* 33:543, 1958.
257. Senerwa D, Olsvik O, Mutanda LN, et al: Colonization of neonates in a nursery ward with enteropathogenic *Escherichia coli* and correlation to the clinical histories of the children, *J Clin Microbiol* 27:2539, 1989.
258. Wright J, Roden AT: *Escherichia coli* O 55 B 5 infection in a gastroenteritis ward; epidemiological applications of H antigen type determinations, *Am J Hyg* 58:133-147, 1953.
259. Balassanian N, Wolinsky E: Epidemiologic and serologic studies of *E. coli* 04:H5 in a premature nursery, *Pediatrics* 41:463-472, 1968.

260. Kessner DM, Shaughnessy HJ, Googins J, et al: An extensive community outbreak of diarrhea due to enteropathogenic *Escherichia coli* O111:B4. I. Epidemiologic studies, *Am J Hyg* 76:27, 1962.
261. Severs D, Fardy P, Acres S, et al: Epidemic gastroenteritis in Newfoundland during 1963 associated with *E. coli* O111:4, *Can Med Assoc J* 94:373, 1966.
262. Jameson JE, Mann TP, Rothfield NJ: Hospital gastro-enteritis: an epidemiological survey of infantile diarrhoea and vomiting contracted in a children's hospital, *Lancet* 267:459, 1954.
263. Thomson S: The role of certain varieties of *Bacterium coli* in gastroenteritis of babies, *J Hyg (Lond)* 53:357, 1955.
264. Page RH, Stulberg CS: Immunofluorescence in epidemiologic control of *E. coli* diarrhea. Incidence, cross-infections, and control in a children's hospital, *Am J Dis Child* 104:149, 1962.
265. Bertrams J, Kuwert E: Leukocyte isoantibodies. Formation, changes of specificity, and persistance of antibodies in women (in relation to pregnancy and labor), *Munch Med Wochenschr* 112:1386, 1970.
266. Thomson S: The numbers of pathogenic bacilli in faeces in intestinal diseases, *J Hyg (Lond)* 53:217, 1955.
267. Belnap WD, O'Donnell JJ: Epidemic gastroenteritis due to *Escherichia coli* O–111;a review of the literature, 1955 a review of the literature, with the epidemiology, bacteriology, and clinical findings of a large outbreak, *J Pediatr* 47:178, 1955.
268. Herweg JC, Middelkamp JN, Thornton HK: *Escherichia coli* diarrhea; the relationship of certain serotypes of *Escherichia coli* to sporadic and epidemic cases of infantile diarrhea, *J Pediatr* 49:629, 1956.
269. Rogers KB, Koegler SJ: Inter-hospital cross-infection of epidemic infantile gastro-enteritis associated with type strains of *Bacterium coli*, *J Hyg (Lond)* 49:152, 1951.
270. Stock AH, Shuman ME: Gastroenteritis in infants associated with specific serotypes of *Escherichia coli*. II. An epidemic of *Escherichia coli* O111:B4 gastroenteritis involving multiple institutions, *Pediatrics* 17:196, 1956.
271. Stulberg CS, Zuelzer WW, Nolke AC, et al: *Escherichia coli* O127:B8, a pathogenic strain causing infantile diarrhea. I. Epidemiology and bacteriology of a prolonged outbreak in a premature nursery, *AMA Am J Dis Child* 90:125, 1955.
272. Thomson S, Watkins AG, Grapy PO: *Escherichia coli* gastroenteritis, *Arch Dis Child* 31:340, 1956.
273. Buttiaux R, Gaudier B, Le Minor L, et al: Epidemiologic research on gastroenteritis due to *Escherichia coli* in a hospital in northern France, *Arch Mal Appar Dig Mal Nutr* 45:225, 1956.
274. Harris AH, Greene DC, Harris AH, et al: Control of epidemic diarrhea of the newborn in hospital nurseries and pediatric wards, *Ann NY Acad Sci* 66:118, 1956.
275. Jacobs SI, Holzel A, Wolman B, et al: Outbreak of infantile gastroenteritis caused by *Escherichia coli* O114, *Arch Dis Child* 45:656, 1970.
276. Clifford SH, Curtin M: Incidence of pathogenic serologic types of *Escherichia coli* among neonatal patients in the New England area, *N Engl J Med* 255:1090, 1956.
277. Greene DC, Albrecht RM: Recent developments in diarrhea of the newborn, *N YState J Med* 55:2764, 1955.
278. Hutchinson RI: *Escherichia coli* (O-types 111, 55 and 26) and their association with infantile diarrhoea; a five-year study, *J Hyg (Lond)* 55:27, 1957.
279. Hinton NA, Macgregor RR: A study of infections due to pathogenic serogroups of *Escherichia coli*, *Can Med Assoc J* 79:359, 1958.
280. Love WC, Gordon AM, Gross RJ, et al: Infantile gastroenteritis due to *Escherichia coli* O142, *Lancet* 2:355, 1972.
281. Shaughnessy HJ, Lesko M, Dorigan F, et al: An extensive community outbreak of diarrhea due to enteropathogenic *Escherichia coli* O111:B4. II. A comparative study of fluorescent antibody identification and standard bacteriologic methods, *Am J Hyg* 76:44, 1962.
282. Kendall N, Vaughan VC, Kusakcioglu A: A study of preparation of infant formulas. A medical and sociocultural appraisal, *Am J Dis Child* 122:215, 1971.
283. Robins-Browne RM, Bordun AM, Tauschek M, et al: *Escherichia coli* and community-acquired gastroenteritis, Melbourne, Australia, *Emerg Infect Dis* 10:1797, 2004.
284. Gamble DR, Rowson KE: The incidence of pathogenic *Escherichia coli* in routine faecal specimens, *Lancet* 273:619, 1957.
285. Bernet CP, Graber CD, Anthony CW: Association of *Escherichia coli* O127:B8 with an outbreak of infantile gastroenteritis and its concurrent distribution in the pediatric population, *J Pediatr* 47:287, 1955.
286. Nataro JP, Mai V, Johnson J, et al: Diarrheagenic *Escherichia coli* infection in Baltimore, Maryland, and New Haven, Connecticut, *Clin Infect Dis* 43:402, 2006.
287. Cohen MB, Nataro JP, Bernstein DI, et al: Prevalence of diarrheagenic *Escherichia coli* in acute childhood enteritis: a prospective controlled study, *J Pediatr* 146:54, 2005.
288. Viljanen MK, Peltola T, Junnila SY, et al: Outbreak of diarrhoea due to *Escherichia coli* O111:B4 in schoolchildren and adults: association of Vi antigen-like reactivity, *Lancet* 336:831, 1990.
289. Afset JE, Bergh K, Bevanger L: High prevalence of atypical enteropathogenic *Escherichia coli* (EPEC) in Norwegian children with diarrhoea, *J Med Microbiol* 52:1015, 2003.
290. Hernandes RT, Elias WP, Vieira MA, et al: An overview of atypical enteropathogenic *Escherichia coli*, *FEMS Microbiol Lett* 297:137, 2009.
291. Nguyen RN, Taylor LS, Tauschek M, et al: Atypical enteropathogenic *Escherichia coli* infection and prolonged diarrhea in children, *Emerg Infect Dis* 12:597, 2006.
292. Donnenberg MS, Finlay BB: Combating enteropathogenic *Escherichia coli* (EPEC) infections: the way forward, *Trends Microbiol* 21:317, 2013.
293. Effect of breastfeeding on infant and child mortality due to infectious diseases in less developed countries: a pooled analysis. WHO Collaborative Study Team on the Role of Breastfeeding on the Prevention of Infant Mortality, *Lancet* 355:451, 2000.
294. Quiroga M, Oviedo P, Chinen I, et al: Asymptomatic infections by diarrheagenic *Escherichia coli* in children from Misiones, Argentina, during the first twenty months of their lives, *Rev Inst Med Trop São Paulo* 42:9, 2000.
295. Creek TL, Kim A, Lu L, et al: Hospitalization and mortality among primarily nonbreastfed children during a large outbreak of diarrhea and malnutrition in Botswana, 2006, *J Acquir Immune Defic Syndr* 53:14, 2010.
296. Blake PA, Ramos S, MacDonald KL, et al: Pathogen-specific risk factors and protective factors for acute diarrheal disease in urban Brazilian infants, *J Infect Dis* 167:627, 1993.
297. Svirsky-Gross S: Pathogenic strains of coli (O,111) among prematures and the use of human milk in controlling the outbreak of diarrhea, *Ann Paediatr* 190:109, 1958.
298. Tassovatz B, Kotsitch A: Le lait de femme et son action de protection contre les infections intestinales chez le nouveau-né, *Ann Paediatr* 8:285, 1961.
299. Adam A: Fortschritte in der Pathogenese und Therapie der Ernahrungs-storungen, *Arztl Forschung* 6:59, 1952.
300. Neter E, Shumway CN: *E. coli* serotype D433: occurrence in intestinal and respiratory tracts, cultural characteristics, pathogenicity, sensitivity to antibiotics, *Proc Soc Exp Biol Med* 75:504, 1950.
301. Levine MM, Bergquist EJ, Nalin DR, et al: *Escherichia coli* strains that cause diarrhoea but do not produce heat-labile or heat-stable enterotoxins and are non-invasive, *Lancet* 1:1119, 1978.
302. Wheeler WE: Spread and control of *Escherichia coli* diarrheal disease, *Ann NY Acad Sci* 66:112, 1956.
303. Rothbaum R, McAdams AJ, Gianella R, Partin JC: A clinicopathologic study of enterocyte-adherent Escherichia coli: a cause of protracted diarrhea in infants. *Gastroenterology* 83:441, 1982.
304. Polotsky YE, Dragunskaya EM, Seliverstova VG, et al: Pathogenic effect of enterotoxigenic *Escherichia coli* and *Escherichia coli* causing infantile diarrhoea, *Acta Microbiol Acad Sci Hung* 24:221, 1977.
305. Vallance BA, Chan C, Robertson ML, et al: Enteropathogenic and enterohemorrhagic *Escherichia coli* infections: emerging themes in pathogenesis and prevention, *Can J Gastroenterol* 16:771, 2002.
306. McDaniel TK, Jarvis KG, Donnenberg MS, et al: A genetic locus of enterocyte effacement conserved among diverse enterobacterial pathogens, *Proc Natl Acad Sci U S A* 92:1664, 1995.
307. McDaniel TK, Kaper JB: A cloned pathogenicity island from enteropathogenic *Escherichia coli* confers the attaching and effacing phenotype on *E. coli* K-12, *Mol Microbiol* 23:399, 1997.
308. Elliott SJ, Wainwright LA, McDaniel TK, et al: The complete sequence of the locus of enterocyte effacement (LEE) from enteropathogenic *Escherichia coli* E2348/69, *Mol Microbiol* 28:1, 1998.
309. Sal-Man N, Biemans-Oldehinkel E, Finlay BB: Structural microengineers: pathogenic *Escherichia coli* redesigns the actin cytoskeleton in host cells, *Structure* 17:15, 2009.
310. Giron JA, Ho AS, Schoolnik GK: An inducible bundle-forming pilus of enteropathogenic *Escherichia coli*, *Science* 254:710, 1991.

311. Stone KD, Zhang HZ, Carlson LK, et al: A cluster of fourteen genes from enteropathogenic *Escherichia coli* is sufficient for the BFP ultrastructure, *MolMicrobiol* 20:325, 1996.
312. Knutton S, Shaw RK, Anantha RP, et al: The type IV bundle-forming pilus of enteropathogenic *Escherichia coli* undergoes dramatic alterations in structure associated with bacterial adherence, aggregation and dispersal, *Mol Microbiol* 33:499, 1999.
313. Bieber D, Ramer SW, Wu CY, et al: Type IV pili, transient bacterial aggregates, and virulence of enteropathogenic *Escherichia coli*, *Science* 280:2114, 1998.
314. Chen HD, Frankel G: Enteropathogenic *Escherichia coli*: unravelling pathogenesis, *FEMS Microbiol Rev* 29:83, 2005.
315. Nataro JP: Atypical enteropathogenic *Escherichia coli*: typical pathogens? *Emerg Infect Dis* 12:696, 2006.
316. Afset JE, Bruant G, Brousseau R, et al: Identification of virulence genes linked with diarrhea due to atypical enteropathogenic *Escherichia coli* by DNA microarray analysis and PCR, *J Clin Microbiol* 44:3703, 2006.
317. Boullier S, Nougayrède JP, Marchès O, et al: Genetically engineered enteropathogenic *Escherichia coli* strain elicits a specific immune response and protects against a virulent challenge, *Microbes Infect* 5:857, 2003.
318. Ghaem-Maghami M, Simmons CP, Daniell S, et al: Intimin-specific immune responses prevent bacterial colonization by the attaching-effacing pathogen *Citrobacter rodentium*, *Infect Immun* 69:5597, 2001.
319. Sanches MI, Keller R, Hartland EL, et al: Human colostrum and serum contain antibodies reactive to the intimin-binding region of the enteropathogenic *Escherichia coli* translocated intimin receptor, *J Pediatr Gastroenterol Nutr* 30:73, 2000.
320. Parissi-Crivelli A, Parissi-Crivelli JM, Giron JA: Recognition of enteropathogenic *Escherichia coli* virulence determinants by human colostrum and serum antibodies, *J Clin Microbiol* 38:2696, 2000.
321. Rozansky R, Rosenmann E, Ben-Ari Y, et al: Enteropathogenic *Escherichia coli* Infections in Infants during the Period from 1957 to 1962, *J Pediatr* 64:521, 1964.
322. Drucker MM, Polliack A, Yeivin R, et al: Immunofluorescent demonstration of enteropathogenic *Escherichia coli* in tissues of infants dying with enteritis, *Pediatrics* 46:855, 1970.
323. Hopkins GB, Gould VE, Stevenson JK, et al: Necrotizing enterocolitis in premature infants. A clinical and pathologic evaluation of autopsy material, *Am J Dis Child* 120:229, 1970.
324. Kirby AC, Hall EG, Coackley W: Neonatal diarrhoea and vomiting; outbreaks in the same maternity unit, *Lancet* 2:201, 1950.
325. Rho YM, Josephson JE: Epidemic enteropathogenic *Escherichia coli*, Newfoundland, 1963: autopsy study of 16 cases, *Can Med Assoc J* 96:392, 1967.
326. Handforth CP, Sorger K: Failure of regeneration of small bowel mucosa following epidemic infantile gastroenteritis, *Can Med Assoc J* 84:425, 1961.
327. McKay DG, Wahle GH Jr: Epidemic gastroenteritis due to *Escherichia coli* O111 B4. II. Pathologic anatomy, with special reference of the presence of the local and generalized Shwartzman phenomena, *AMA Arch Pathol* 60:679, 1955.
328. Nelson JD: Duration of neomycin for enteropathogenic *Escherichia coli* diarrheal disease: a comparative study of 113 cases, *Pediatrics* 48:248, 1971.
329. Cooper ML, Walters EW, Keller HM, et al. Epidemic diarrhea among infants associated with the isolation of a new serotype of *Escherichia coli*: *E. coli* 0127:B8, *Pediatrics* 16:215, 1955.
330. Laurell G, Magnusson JH, Frisell E, et al: Epidemic infantile diarrhea and vomiting, *Acta Paediatr* 40:302, 1951.
331. Rogers KB, Cracknell VM: Epidemic infantile gastroenteritis due to *Escherichia coli* O 114, *J Pathol Bacteriol* 72:27, 1956.
332. Todd RM, Hall EG: Chloramphenicol in prophylaxis of infantile gastro-enteritis, *Br Med J* 1:1359, 1953.
333. Giles C, Sangster G: An outbreak of infantile gastro-enteritis in Aberdeen; the association of a special type of Bact. coli with the infection, *J Hyg (Lond)* 46:1, 1948.
334. Martineau B, Raymond R, Jeliu G: Bacteriological and clinical study of gastro-enteritis with enteropathogenic *Escherichia coli* 0127:B8, *Can Med Assoc J* 79:351, 1958.
335. Gastroenteritis due to *Escherichia coli*, [editorial], *Lancet* 1:32, 1968.
336. Senerwa D, Olsvik O, Mutanda LN, et al: Enteropathogenic *Escherichia coli* serotype O111:HNT isolated from preterm neonates in Nairobi, Kenya, *J Clin Microbiol* 27:1307, 1989.
337. Essers B, Burnens AP, Lanfranchini FM, et al: Acute community-acquired diarrhea requiring hospital admission in Swiss children, *Clin Infect Dis* 31:192, 2000.
338. Campos LC, Franzolin MR, Trabulsi LR: Diarrheagenic *Escherichia coli* categories among the traditional enteropathogenic *E. coli* O serogroups—a review, *Mem Inst Oswaldo Cruz* 99:545, 2004.
339. Riley HD Jr, Start AH, Bracken EC, et al: Enteropathogenic *E. coli* gastroenteritis, *Clin Pediatr (Phila)* 3:93, 1964.
340. Taylor J, Powell BW, Wright J: Infantile diarrhoea and vomiting; a clinical and bacteriological investigation, *Br Med J* 2:117, 1949.
341. Rogers KB: The spread of infantile gastroenteritis in a cubicled ward, *J Hyg* 49:140, 1951.
342. Garcia de Olarte D, Trujillo H, Agudelo N, et al: Treatment of diarrhea in malnourished infants and children. A double-blind study comparing ampicillin and placebo, *Am J Dis Child* 127:379, 1974.
343. Coetzee M, Leary PM: Gentamicin in *Esch coli* gastroenteritis, *Arch Dis Child* 46:646, 1971.
344. Harris JC, Dupont HL, Hornick RB: Fecal leukocytes in diarrheal illness, *Ann Intern Med* 76:697, 1972.
345. Guerrant RL, Araujo V, Soares E, et al: Measurement of fecal lactoferrin as a marker of fecal leukocytes, *J Clin Microbiol* 30:1238, 1992.
346. Miller JR, Barrett LJ, Kotloff K, et al: A rapid test for infectious and inflammatory enteritis, *Arch Intern Med* 154:2660, 1994.
347. Mossel DA, Weijers HA: Results of bacteriological analysis of human milk and its significance for pediatric practice, *Maandschr Kindergeneeskd* 25:37, 1957.
348. Vial PA, Mathewson JJ, DuPont HL, et al: Comparison of two assay methods for patterns of adherence to HEp-2 cells of *Escherichia coli* from patients with diarrhea, *J Clin Microbiol* 28:882, 1990.
349. Albert MJ, Ansaruzzaman M, Faruque SM, et al: An ELISA for the detection of localized adherent classic enteropathogenic *Escherichia coli* serogroups, *J Infect Dis* 164:986, 1991.
350. Knutton S, et al: Actin accumulation at sites of bacterial adhesion to tissue culture cells: basis of a new diagnostic test for enteropathogenic and enterohemorrhagic *Escherichia coli*, *Infect Immunol* 57:1290, 1989.
351. Cooper ML, Keller HM, Walters EW: Comparative frequency of detection of enteropathogenic *E. coli*, *Salmonella* and *Shigella* in rectal swab cultures from infants and young children, *Pediatrics* 19:411, 1957.
352. Wheeler WE, Wainerman B: The treatment and prevention of epidemic infantile diarrhea due to *E. coli* O-111 by the use of chloramphenicol and neomycin, *Pediatrics* 14:357, 1954.
353. Ironside AG, Tuxford AF, Heyworth B: A survey of infantile gastroenteritis, *Br Med J* 3:20, 1970.
354. Nelson JD: Comment. In Gellis S, editor: *Yearbook of pediatrics*, St Louis, 1973, Mosby-Year Book.
355. Valman HB, Wilmers MJ: Use of antibiotics in acute gastroenteritis among infants in hospital, *Lancet* 1:1122, 1969.
356. Murray WA, Kheder J, Wheeler WE: Colistin suppression of *Escherichia coli* in stools. I. Control of a nosocomial outbreak of diarrhea caused by neomycin-resistant *Escherichia coli* O111 B4, *Am J Dis Child* 108:274, 1964.
357. Senerwa D, Mutanda LN, Gathuma JM, et al: Antimicrobial resistance of enteropathogenic *Escherichia coli* strains from a nosocomial outbreak in Kenya, *APMIS* 99:728, 1991.
358. Bakhshi B, Fallahzad S, Pourshafie MR: The occurrence of atypical enteropathogenic *Escherichia coli* strains among children with diarrhea in Iran, *J Infect Chemother* 19:615, 2013.
359. Estrada-Garcia T, Cerna JF, Paheco-Gil L, et al: Drug-resistant diarrheogenic *Escherichia coli*, Mexico, *Emerg Infect Dis* 11:1306, 2005.
360. Ochoa TJ, Ruiz J, Molina M, et al: High frequency of antimicrobial drug resistance of diarrheagenic *Escherichia coli* in infants in Peru, *Am J Trop Med Hyg* 81:296, 2009.
361. Kaslow RA, Taylor A Jr, Dweck HS, et al: Enteropathogenic *Escherichia coli* infection in a newborn nursery, *Am J Dis Child* 128:797, 1974.
362. Sprunt K, Redman W, Leidy G: Antibacterial effectiveness of routine hand washing, *Pediatrics* 52:264, 1973.
363. Kunin CM: Resistance to antimicrobial drugs–a worldwide calamity, *Ann Intern Med* 118:557, 1993.

364. Silver LL, Bostian KA: Discovery and development of new antibiotics: the problem of antibiotic resistance, *Antimicrob Agents Chemother* 37:377, 1993.
365. Nelson JD: Commentary, *J Pediatr* 89:471, 1976.
366. Update: multistate outbreak of *Escherichia coli* O157:H7 infections from hamburgers—western United States, 1992-1993, *MMWR Morb Mortal Wkly Rep* 42:258, 1993.
367. MacDonald KL, Osterholm MT: The emergence of *Escherichia coli* O157:H7 infection in the United States. The changing epidemiology of foodborne disease, *JAMA* 269:2264, 1993.
368. Watanabe H, Wada A, Inagaki Y, et al: Outbreaks of enterohaemorrhagic *Escherichia coli* O157:H7 infection by two different genotype strains in Japan, 1996, *Lancet* 348:831, 1996.
369. Ochoa TJ, Cleary TG: Epidemiology and spectrum of disease of *Escherichia coli* O157, *Curr Opin Infect Dis* 16:259, 2003.
370. Hemolytic-uremic syndrome associated with *Escherichia coli* O 157:H7 enteric infections—United States, 1984, *MMWR Morb Mortal Wkly Rep* 34:20, 1985.
371. Davis TK, McKee R, Schnadower D, et al: Treatment of Shiga toxin-producing *Escherichia coli* Infections, *Infect Dis Clin North Am* 27:577, 2013.
372. Belongia EA, Osterholm MT, Soler JT, et al: Transmission of *Escherichia coli* O157:H7 infection in Minnesota child day-care facilities, *JAMA* 269:883, 1993.
373. Besser RE, Lett SM, Weber JT, et al: An outbreak of diarrhea and hemolytic uremic syndrome from *Escherichia coli* O157:H7 in fresh-pressed apple cider, *JAMA* 269:2217, 1993.
374. Sandvig K: Shiga toxins, *Toxicon* 39:1629, 2001.
375. Ray PE, Liu XH: Pathogenesis of Shiga toxin-induced hemolytic uremic syndrome, *Pediatr Nephrol* 16:823, 2001.
376. Schmidt H: Shiga-toxin-converting bacteriophages, *Res Microbiol* 152:687, 2001.
377. Scotland SM, Smith HR, Rowe B: Two distinct toxins active on Vero cells from *Escherichia coli* O157, *Lancet* 2:885, 1985.
378. Karmali MA, Petric M, Louie S, et al: Antigenic heterogeneity of *Escherichia coli* verotoxins, *Lancet* 1:164, 1986.
379. Lim JY, Yoon J, Hovde CJ: A brief overview of *Escherichia coli* O157:H7 and its plasmid O157, *J Microbiol Biotechnol* 20:5, 2010.
380. Nguyen Y, Sperandio V: Enterohemorrhagic *E. coli* (EHEC) pathogenesis, *Front Cell Infect Microbiol* 2:90, 2012.
381. Welinder-Olsson C, Kaijser B: Enterohemorrhagic *Escherichia coli* (EHEC), *Scandinavian J Inf Dis* 37:405, 2005.
382. Ulinski T, Lervat C, Ranchin B, et al: Neonatal hemolytic uremic syndrome after mother-to-child transmission of *Escherichia coli* O157, *Pediatr Nephrol* 20:1334, 2005.
383. Stritt A, Tschumi S, Kottanattu L, et al: Neonatal hemolytic uremic syndrome after mother-to-child transmission of a low-pathogenic stx2b harboring shiga toxin-producing *Escherichia coli*, *Clin Infect Dis* 56:114, 2013.
384. FoodNet 2011 surveillance report. Available at http://www.cdc.gov/foodnet/PDFs/2011_annual_report_508c.pdf. Accessed September 2013.
385. Adachi E, Tanaka H, Toyoda N, et al: Detection of bactericidal antibody in the breast milk of a mother infected with enterohemorrhagic *Escherichia coli* O157:H7, *Kansenshogaku Zasshi* 73:45, 1999.
386. Noguera-Obenza M, Ochoa TJ, Gomez HF, et al: Human milk secretory antibodies against attaching and effacing *Escherichia coli* antigens, *Emerg Infect Dis* 9:545, 2003.
387. Paton JC, Paton AW: Methods for detection of STEC in humans. An overview, *Methods Mol Med* 73:9, 2003.
388. Gould LH, Bopp C, Strockbine N, et al: Recommendations for diagnosis of shiga toxin–producing *Escherichia coli* infections by clinical laboratories, *MMWR Recomm Rep* 58(RR-12):1, 2009.
389. Tarr PI, Neill MA, Clausen CR, et al: *Escherichia coli* O157:H7 and the hemolytic uremic syndrome: importance of early cultures in establishing the etiology, *J Infect Dis*, 162:553, 1990.
390. Wong CS, Jelacic S, Habeeb RL, et al: The risk of the hemolytic-uremic syndrome after antibiotic treatment of *Escherichia coli* O157:H7 infections, *N Engl J Med* 342:1930, 2000.
391. Safdar N, Said A, Gangnon RE, et al: Risk of hemolytic uremic syndrome after antibiotic treatment of Escherichia coli O157:H7 enteritis: a meta-analysis, *JAMA* 288:996, 2002.
392. Wong CS, Mooney JC, Brandt JR, et al: Risk factors for the hemolytic uremic syndrome in children infected with *Escherichia coli* O157:H7: a multivariable analysis, *Clin Infect Dis* 55:33, 2012.
393. Ake JA, Jelacic S, Ciol MA, et al: Relative nephroprotection during *Escherichia coli* O157:H7 infections: association with intravenous volume expansion, *Pediatrics* 115:e673, 2005.
394. Lapeyraque AL, Malina M, Fremeaux-Bacchi V, et al: Eculizumab in severe Shiga-toxin-associated HUS, *N Engl J Med* 364:2561, 2011.
395. Page AV, Liles WC: Enterohemorrhagic *Escherichia coli* Infections and the Hemolytic-Uremic Syndrome, *Med Clin North Am* 97:681, 2013.
396. Bell BP, Griffin PM, Lozano P, et al: Predictors of hemolytic uremic syndrome in children during a large outbreak of *Escherichia coli* O157:H7 infections, *Pediatrics* 100:E12, 1997.
397. Nataro JP: Enteroaggregative *Escherichia coli*. In Hughes J, editor: *Emerging infections*, vol. 6. Washington, DC, 2003, American Society for Microbiology Press.
398. Sarantuya J, Nishi J, Wakimoto N, et al: Typical enteroaggregative *Escherichia coli* is the most prevalent pathotype among *E. coli* strains causing diarrhea in Mongolian children, *J Clin Microbiol* 42:133, 2004.
399. Baudry B, Savarino SJ, Vial P, et al: A sensitive and specific DNA probe to identify enteroaggregative *Escherichia coli*, a recently discovered diarrheal pathogen, *J Infect Dis* 161:1249, 1990.
400. Nishi J, Sheikh J, Mizuguchi K, et al: The export of coat protein from enteroaggregative *Escherichia coli* by a specific ATP-binding cassette transporter system, *J Biol Chem* 278:45680, 2003.
401. Rasko DA, Webster DR, Sahl JW, et al: Origins of the *E. coli* strain causing an outbreak of hemolytic-uremic syndrome in Germany, *N Engl J Med* 365:709, 2011.
402. Bielaszewska M, Mellmann A, Zhang W, et al: Characterisation of the *Escherichia coli* strain associated with an outbreak of haemolytic uraemic syndrome in Germany, 2011: a microbiological study, *Lancet Infect Dis* 11:671, 2011.
403. Mathewson JJ, Johnson PC, DuPont HL, et al: Pathogenicity of enteroadherent *Escherichia coli* in adult volunteers, *J Infect Dis* 154:524, 1986.
404. Nataro J, Deng Y, Cookson S, et al: Heterogeneity of enteroaggregative *Escherichia coli* virulence demonstrated in volunteers, *J Infect Dis* 171:465, 1995.
405. Itoh Y, Nagano I, Kunishima M, et al: Laboratory investigation of enteroaggregative *Escherichia coli* O untypeable:H10 associated with a massive outbreak of gastrointestinal illness, *J Clin Microbiol* 35:2546, 1997.
406. Smith HR, Cheasty T, Rowe B: Enteroaggregative *Escherichia coli* and outbreaks of gastroenteritis in UK, *Lancet* 350:814, 1997.
407. Adachi JA, Mathewson JJ, Jiang ZD, et al: Enteric pathogens in Mexican sauces of popular restaurants in Guadalajara, Mexico, and Houston, Texas, *Ann Intern Med* 136:884, 2002.
408. Cobeljic M, Miljković-Selimović B, Paunović-Todosijević D, et al: Enteroaggregative *Escherichia coli* associated with an outbreak of diarrhoea in a neonatal nursery ward, *Epidemiol Infect* 117:11, 1996.
409. Bhan MK, Raj P, Levine MM, et al: Enteroaggregative *Escherichia coli* associated with persistent diarrhea in a cohort of rural children in India, *J Infect Dis* 159:1061, 1989.
410. Bhan MK, Khoshoo V, Sommerfelt H, et al: Enteroaggregative *Escherichia coli* and *Salmonella* associated with nondysenteric persistent diarrhea, *Pediatr Infect Dis J* 8:499, 1989.
411. Cravioto A, Tello A, Navarro A, et al: Association of *Escherichia coli* HEp-2 adherence patterns with type and duration of diarrhoea, *Lancet* 337:262, 1991.
412. Lima AA, Fang G, Schorling JB, et al: Persistent diarrhea in northeast Brazil: etiologies and interactions with malnutrition, *Acta Paediatr Suppl* 381:39, 1992.
413. Dutta S, Pal S, Chakrabarti S, et al: Use of PCR to identify enteroaggregative *Escherichia coli* as an important cause of acute diarrhoea among children living in Calcutta, India, *J Med Microbiol* 48:1011, 1999.
414. Scaletsky IC, Fabbricotti SH, Silva SO, et al: HEp-2-adherent *Escherichia coli* strains associated with acute infantile diarrhea, São Paulo, Brazil, *Emerg Infect Dis* 8:855, 2002.
415. Okeke IN, Lamikanra A, Czeczulin J, et al: Heterogeneous virulence of enteroaggregative *Escherichia coli* strains isolated from children in Southwest Nigeria, *J Infect Dis* 181:252, 2000.
416. Bouzari S, Jafari A, Farhoudi-Moghaddam AA, et al: Adherence of non-enteropathogenic *Escherichia coli* to HeLa cells, *J Med Microbiol* 40:95, 1994.

417. Gonzalez R, Díaz C, Mariño M, et al: Age-specific prevalence of *Escherichia coli* with localized and aggregative adherence in Venezuelan infants with acute diarrhea, *J Clin Microbiol* 35:1103, 1997.
418. Huang DB, Nataro JP, DuPont HL, et al: Enteroaggregative *Escherichia coli* is a cause of acute diarrheal illness: a meta-analysis, *Clin Infect Dis* 43:556, 2006.
419. Huppertz HI, Rutkowski S, Aleksic S, et al: Acute and chronic diarrhoea and abdominal colic associated with enteroaggregative *Escherichia coli* in young children living in western Europe, *Lancet* 349:1660, 1997.
420. Pabst WL, Altwegg M, Kind C, et al: Prevalence of enteroaggregative *Escherichia coli* among children with and without diarrhea in Switzerland, *J Clin Microbiol* 41:2289, 2003.
421. Presterl E, Nadrchal R, Wolf D, et al: Enteroaggregative and enterotoxigenic *Escherichia coli* among isolates from patients with diarrhea in Austria, *Eur J Clin Microbiol Infect Dis* 18:209, 1999.
422. Tompkins DS, Hudson MJ, Smith HR, et al: A study of infectious intestinal disease in England: microbiological findings in cases and controls, *Commun Dis Public Health* 2:108, 1999.
423. Nguyen TV, Le Van P, Le Huy C, et al: Detection and characterization of diarrheagenic *Escherichia coli* from young children in Hanoi, Vietnam, *J Clin Microbiol* 43:755, 2005.
424. Huang DB, Mohanty A, DuPont HL, et al: A review of an emerging enteric pathogen: enteroaggregative *Escherichia coli*, *J Med Microbiol* 55:1303, 2006.
425. Estrada-Garcia T, Navarro-Garcia F: Enteroaggregative *Escherichia coli* pathotype: a genetically heterogeneous emerging foodborne enteropathogen, FEMS Immunol, *Med Microbiol* 66:281, 2012.
426. Bouckenooghe AR, Dupont HL, Jiang ZD, et al: Markers of enteric inflammation in enteroaggregative *Escherichia coli* diarrhea in travelers, *Am J Trop Med Hyg* 62:711, 2000.
427. Opintan JA, Newman MJ, Ayeh-Kumi PF, et al: Pediatric diarrhea in southern Ghana: etiology and association with intestinal inflammation and malnutrition, *Am J Trop Med Hyg* 83:936, 2010.
428. Miqdady MS, Jiang ZD, Nataro JP, et al: Detection of enteroaggregative *Escherichia coli* with formalin-preserved HEp-2 cells, *J Clin Microbiol* 40:3066, 2002.
429. Spencer J, Chart H, Smith HR, et al: Improved detection of enteroaggregative *Escherichia coli* using formalin- fixed HEp-2 cells, *Lett Appl Microbiol* 25:325, 1997.
430. Huang DB, Mohamed JA, Nataro JP, et al: Virulence characteristics and the molecular epidemiology of enteroaggregative *Escherichia coli* isolates from travellers to developing countries, *J Med Microbiol* 56:1386, 2007.
431. Wanke CA, Gerrior J, Blais V, et al: Successful treatment of diarrheal disease associated with enteroaggregative *Escherichia coli* in adults infected with human immunodeficiency virus, *J Infect Dis* 178:1369, 1998.
432. Adachi JA, Ericsson CD, Jiang ZD, et al: Azithromycin found to be comparable to levofloxacin for the treatment of US travelers with acute diarrhea acquired in Mexico, *Clin Infect Dis* 37:1165, 2003.
433. DuPont HL, Jiang ZD, Ericsson CD, et al: Rifaximin versus ciprofloxacin for the treatment of traveler's diarrhea: a randomized, double-blind clinical trial, *Clin Infect Dis* 33:1807, 2001.
434. Vonberg RP, Höhle M, Aepfelbacher M, et al: Duration of fecal shedding of Shiga toxin-producing *Escherichia coli* O104:H4 in patients infected during the 2011 outbreak in Germany: a multicenter study, *Clin Infect Dis* 56:1132, 2013.
435. Nitschke M, Sayk F, Härtel C, et al: Association between azithromycin therapy and duration of bacterial shedding among patients with Shiga toxin-producing enteroaggregative *Escherichia coli* O104:H4, *JAMA* 307:1046, 2012.
436. Raju B, Ballal M: Multidrug resistant enteroaggregative *Escherichia coli* diarrhoea in rural southern Indian population, *Scandinavian J Infect Dis* 41:105, 2009.
437. Bilge SS, Clausen CR, Lau W, et al: Molecular characterization of a fimbrial adhesin, F1845, mediating diffuse adherence of diarrhea-associated *Escherichia coli* to HEp-2 cells, *J Bacteriol* 171:4281, 1989.
438. Gunzburg ST, Chang BJ, Elliott SJ, et al: Diffuse and enteroaggregative patterns of adherence of enteric *Escherichia coli* isolated from aboriginal children from the Kimberley region of Western Australia, *J Infect Dis* 167:755, 1993.
439. Ochoa Theresa J, Ecker L, Barletta F, et al: Age–related susceptibility to infection with diarrheagenic *Escherichia coli* among infants from periurban areas in Lima, Peru, *Clin Infect Dis* 49:1694, 2009.
440. Elliott SJ, Srinivas S, Albert MJ, et al: Characterization of the roles of hemolysin and other toxins in enteropathy caused by alpha-hemolytic *Escherichia coli* linked to human diarrhea, *Infect Immun* 66:2040, 1998.
441. Centers for Disease Control and Prevention: National enteric disease surveillance: *Salmonella* surveillance overview, Available at http://www.cdc.gov/nationalsurveillance/PDFs/NationalSalmSurveillOverview_508.pdf. Accessed October 2013.
442. Sanchez-Vargas FM, Abu-El-Haija MA, Gomez-Duarte OG: *Salmonella* infections: an update on epidemiology, management, and prevention, *Travel Med Infect Dis* 9:263, 2011.
443. . Ewing WH: *Edwards and Ewing's identification of enterobacteriaceae*, ed 4, New York, 1986, Elsevier.
444. Shkalim V, Amir A, Samra Z, et al: Characteristics of non-Typhi *Salmonella* gastroenteritis associated with bacteremia in infants and young children, *Infection* 40:285, 2012.
445. Vugia DJ, Samuel M, Farley MM, et al: Invasive *Salmonella* infections in the United States, FoodNet, 1996-1999: incidence, serotype distribution, and outcome, *Clin Infect Dis* 38(Suppl 3):S149, 2004.
446. Meadow WL, Schneider H, Beem MO: *Salmonella* enteritidis bacteremia in childhood, *J Infect Dis* 152:185, 1985.
447. Hyams JS, Durbin WA, Grand RJ, et al: *Salmonella* bacteremia in the first year of life, *J Pediatr* 96:57, 1980.
448. Taylor DN, Bied JM, Munro JS, et al: *Salmonella* dublin infections in the United States, 1979-1980, *J Infect Dis* 146:322, 1982.
449. Haraga A, Ohlson MB, Miller SI: *Salmonellae* interplay with host cells, *Nat Rev Microbiol* 6:53, 2008.
450. Coburn B, Grassl GA, Finlay BB: *Salmonella*, the host and disease: a brief review, *Immunol Cell Biol* 85:112, 2007.
451. Andrews-Polymenis HL, Bäumler AJ, McCormick BA, et al: Taming the elephant: *Salmonella* biology, pathogenesis, and prevention, *Infect Immun* 78:2356, 2010.
452. Mackaness GB: Resistance to intracellular infection, *J Infect Dis* 123:439, 1971.
453. Mackaness GB, Blanden RV, Collins FM: Host-parasite relations in mouse typhoid, *J Exp Med* 124:573, 1966.
454. McKenzie SE, Kline J, Douglas SD, et al: Enhancement *in vitro* of the low interferon-gamma production of leukocytes from human newborn infants, *J Leukoc Biol* 53:691, 1993.
455. George A: Generation of gamma interferon responses in murine Peyer's patches following oral immunization, *Infect Immun* 64:4606, 1996.
456. de Jong R, Altare F, Haagen IA, et al: Severe mycobacterial and *Salmonella* infections in interleukin-12 receptor-deficient patients, *Science* 280:1435, 1998.
457. Spano S, Ugalde JE, Galan JE: Delivery of a *Salmonella* Typhi exotoxin from a host intracellular compartment, *Cell Host Microbe* 3:30, 2008.
458. Hornick RB, Greisman SE, Woodward TE, et al: Typhoid fever: pathogenesis and immunologic control. 2, *N Engl J Med* 283:739, 1970.
459. Giannella RA, Formal SB, Dammin GJ, et al: Pathogenesis of salmonellosis. Studies of fluid secretion, mucosal invasion, and morphologic reaction in the rabbit ileum, *J Clin Invest* 52:441, 1973.
460. Boyd JF: Pathology of the alimentary tract in *Salmonella* Typhimurium food poisoning, *Gut* 26:935, 1985.
461. Day DW, Mandal BK, Morson BC: The rectal biopsy appearances in *Salmonella* colitis, *Histopathology* 2:117, 1978.
462. Majowicz SE, Musto J, Scallan E, et al: The global burden of non-typhoidal *Salmonella* gastroenteritis, *Clin Infect Dis* 50:882, 2010.
463. Scallan E, Hoekstra RM, Angulo FJ, et al: Foodborne illness acquired in the United States–major pathogens, *Emerg Infect Dis* 17:7, 2011.
464. Cahill SM, Wachsmuth IK, Costarrica Mde L, et al: Powdered infant formula as a source of *Salmonella* infection in infants, *Clin Infect Dis* 46:268, 2008.
465. Day JB, Sharma D, Siddique N, et al: Survival of *Salmonella* Typhi and *Shigella dysenteriae* in dehydrated infant formula, *J Food Sci* 76:M324, 2011.
466. Linam WM, Gerber MA: Changing epidemiology and prevention of *Salmonella* infections, *Pediatr Infect Dis J* 26:747, 2007.
467. Gould LH, Walsh KA, Vieira AR, et al: Surveillance for foodborne disease outbreaks - United States, 1998-2008, *MMWR Surveill Summ* 62:1, 2013.

468. Centers for Disease Control and Prevention: Foodborne Diseases Active Surveillance Network (FoodNet): FoodNet surveillance report for 2011, U.S. Department of Health and Human Services, Centers for Disease Control and Prevention. Atlanta, 2012.
469. Pet-turtle-associated salmonellosis–Puerto Rico, *MMWR Morb Mortal Wkly Rep* 33:141, 1984.
470. Aiken AM, Lane C, Adak GK: Risk of *Salmonella* infection with exposure to reptiles in England, 2004-2007, *Euro Surveill* 15:19581, 2010.
471. Mermin J, Hutwagner L, Vugia D, et al: Reptiles, amphibians, and human *Salmonella* infection: a population-based, case-control study, *Clin Infect Dis* 38(Suppl 3):S253, 2004.
472. Thomson S: Paratyphoid fever and bakers' confectionery; an analysis of an epidemic in South Wales, 1952, *Mon Bull Minist Health Public Health Lab, Serv* 12:187, 1953.
473. Barron JC, Forsythe SJ: Dry stress and survival time of *Enterobacter sakazakii* and other Enterobacteriaceae in dehydrated powdered infant formula, *J Food Prot* 70:2111, 2007.
474. Fleischhacker G, Vutue C, Werner HP: Infektion eines Neugeborenen durch *S* Typhimurium-haltige Muttermilch, *Wien Klin Wochenschr* 24:394, 1972.
475. Ryder RW, Crosby-Ritchie A, McDonough B, et al: Human milk contaminated with *Salmonella* kottbus. A cause of nosocomial illness in infants, *JAMA* 238:1533, 1977.
476. Revathi G, Mahajan R, Faridi MM, et al: Transmission of lethal *Salmonella* senftenberg from mother's breast-milk to her baby, *Ann Trop Paediatr* 15:159, 1995.
477. Cooke FJ, Ginwalla S, Hampton MD, et al: Report of neonatal meningitis due to *Salmonella enterica* serotype Agona and review of breast milk-associated neonatal *Salmonella* infections, *J Clin Microbiol* 47:3045, 2009.
478. Chen TL, Thien PF, Liaw SC, et al: First report of *Salmonella* enterica serotype panama meningitis associated with consumption of contaminated breast milk by a neonate, *J Clin Microbiol* 43:5400, 2005.
479. Small RG, Sharp JC: A milk-borne outbreak due to *Salmonella* dublin, *J Hyg (Lond)* 82:95, 1979.
480. Weissman JB, Deen AD, Williams M, et al: An island-wide epidemic of salmonellosis in Trinidad traced to contaminated powdered milk, *West Indian Med J* 26:135, 1977.
481. *Salmonella* anatum infection in infants linked to dried milk, *Commun Dis Rep CDR Wkly* 7:33, 1997.
482. Usera MA, Echeita A, Aladueña A, et al: Interregional foodborne salmonellosis outbreak due to powdered infant formula contaminated with lactose-fermenting *Salmonella* virchow, *Eur J Epidemiol* 12:377, 1996.
483. Mendis NM, De La Motte PU, Gunatillaka PD, et al: Protracted infection with *Salmonella* bareilly in a maternity hospital, *J Trop Med Hyg* 79:142, 1976.
484. Silverstope L, Plazikowski U, Kjellander J, et al: An epidemic among infants caused by *S muenchen*, *J Appl Bacteriol* 24:134, 1961.
485. Rubenstein AD, Fowler RN: Salmonellosis of the newborn with transmission by delivery room resuscitators, *Am J Public Health Nations Health* 45:1109, 1955.
486. McAllister TA, Roud JA, Marshall A, et al: Outbreak of *Salmonella* eimsbuettel in newborn infants spread by rectal thermometers, *Lancet* 1:1262, 1986.
487. Im SW, Chow K, Chau PY: Rectal thermometer mediated cross-infection with *Salmonella* wandsworth in a paediatric ward, *J Hosp Infect* 2:171, 1981.
488. Khan MA, Abdur-Rab M, Israr N, et al: Transmission of *Salmonella* Worthington by oropharyngeal suction in hospital neonatal unit, *Pediatr Infect Dis J* 10:668, 1991.
489. Umasankar S, Mridha EU, Hannan MM, et al: An outbreak of *Salmonella* Enteritidis in a maternity and neonatal intensive care unit, *J Hosp Infect* 34:117, 1996.
490. Riley LW, Cohen ML: Plasmid profiles and *Salmonella* epidemiology, *Lancet* 1:573, 1982.
491. Michel J, Malpuech G, Godenèche P, et al: Clinical and bacteriological study of a salmonellosis epidemic in a hospital (*Salmonella* Oranienburg), *Pediatrie* 25:13, 1970.
492. Watt J, Wegman ME, Brown OW, et al: Salmonellosis in a premature nursery unaccompanied by diarrheal disease, *Pediatrics* 22:689, 1958.
493. Bate JG, James U: *Salmonella* Typhimurium infection dust-borne in a children's ward, *Lancet* 2:713, 1958.
494. Adler JL, Anderson RL, Boring 3rd JR, et al: A protracted hospital-associated outbreak of salmonellosis due to a multiple-antibiotic-resistant strain of *Salmonella* indiana, *J Pediatr* 77:970, 1970.
495. Newman MJ: Multiple-resistant *Salmonella* group G outbreak in a neonatal intensive care unit, *West Afr J Med* 15:165, 1996.
496. Jones TF, Ingram LA, Fullerton KE, et al: A case-control study of the epidemiology of sporadic *Salmonella* infection in infants, *Pediatrics* 118:2380, 2006.
497. Shimoni Z, Lüdtke A, Rahlff I, et al: Nontyphoid *Salmonella* bacteremia: age-related differences in clinical presentation, bacteriology, and outcome, *Clin Infect Dis* 28:822, 1999.
498. Kunz LJ, Waddell WR: Association of *Salmonella* enteritis with operations on the stomach, *N Engl J Med* 255:555, 1956.
499. Gray JA, Trueman AM: Severe *Salmonella* gastroenteritis associated with hypochlorhydria, *Scott Med J* 16:255, 1971.
500. Blaser MJ, Newman LS: A review of human salmonellosis: I. Infective dose, *Rev Infect Dis* 4:1096, 1982.
501. Lamb VA, Mayhall CG, Spadora AC, et al: Outbreak of *Salmonella* Typhimurium gastroenteritis due to an imported strain resistant to ampicillin, chloramphenicol, and trimethoprim-sulfamethoxazole in a nursery, *J Clin Microbiol* 20:1076, 1984.
502. Abroms IF, Cochran WD, Holmes LB, et al: A *Salmonella* newport outbreak in a premature nursery with a one-year follow-up. Effect of ampicillin following bacteriologic failure of response to kanamycin, *Pediatrics* 37:616, 1966.
503. Epstein HC, Hochwald A, Ashe R: *Salmonella* infections of the newborn infant, *J Pediatr* 38:723, 1951.
504. Leeder FS: An epidemic of *Salmonella* Panama infections in infants, *Ann NY Acad Sci* 66:54, 1956.
505. Abramson H: Infection with *Salmonella* Typhimurium in the newborn: epidemiologic and clinical considerations, *Am J Dis Child* 74:576, 1947.
506. Watt J, Carlton E: Studies of the acute diarrheal diseases. XVI. An outbreak of *S* Typhimurium infection among newborn premature infants, *Public Health Rep* 60(Pt 1):734, 1945.
507. Foley AR: An outbreak of paratyphoid B fever in the nursery of a small hospital, *Can J Public Health* 38:73, 1947.
508. Seligmann E: Mass invasion of *Salmonellae* in a babies' ward, *Ann Paediatr* 172:406, 1949.
509. Rowe B, Giles C, Brown GL: Outbreak of gastroenteritis due to *Salmonella* Virchow in a maternity hospital, *Br Med J* 3:561, 1969.
510. Sasidharan CK, Rajagopal KC, Panicker CK: *Salmonella* Typhimurium epidemic in newborn nursery, *Indian J Pediatr* 50:599, 1983.
511. Borecka J, Hocmannova M, van Leeuwen WJ: Nosocomial infection of nurslings caused by multiple drug-resistant strains of *S* Typhimurium—utilization of new typing method based on lysogeny of strains, *Z Bakteriol* 2336:262, 1976.
512. Bannerman CH: *Salmonella* Heidelberg enteritis—an outbreak in the neonatal unit Harare Central Hospital, *Cent Afr J Med* 31:1, 1985.
513. Szanton VL: Epidemic salmonellosis; a 30-month study of 80 cases of *Salmonella* Oranienburg infection, *Pediatrics* 20:794, 1957.
514. Seals JE, Parrott PL, McGowan JE Jr, et al: Nursery salmonellosis: delayed recognition due to unusually long incubation period, *Infect Control* 4:205, 1983.
515. Hering E, Fuenzalida O, Lynch B, et al: Clinico-epidemiological analysis of an outbreak of *Salmonella* Bredeney infection in newborn infants, *Rev Chil Pediatr* 50:81, 1979.
516. Kumari S, Gupta R, Bhargava SK: A nursery outbreak with *Salmonella* newport, *Indian Pediatr* 17:11, 1980.
517. Omland T, Gardborg O: *Salmonella* enteritidis infections in infancy with special reference to a small nosocomial epidemic, *Acta Paediatr* 49:583, 1960.
518. Puri V, Thirupuram S, Khalil A, et al: Nosocomial *Salmonella* Typhimurium epidemic in a neonatal special care unit, *Indian Pediatr* 17:233, 1980.
519. Marzetti G, Laurenti F, De Caro M, et al: *Salmonella* Munchen infections in newborns and small infants. An analysis of the clinical expressions and manner of spread, as studied in two outbreaks, *Clin Pediatr (Phila)* 12:93, 1973.
520. Baine WB, Gangarosa EJ, Bennett JV, et al: Institutional salmonellosis, *J Infect Dis* 128:357, 1973.

521. Schroeder SA, Aserkoff B, Brachman PS: Epidemic salmonellosis in hospitals and institutions. A five-year review, *N Engl J Med* 279:674, 1968.
522. Boehmer TK, Bamberg WM, Ghosh TS, et al: Health care-associated outbreak of *Salmonella* Tennessee in a neonatal intensive care unit, *Am J Infect Control* 37:49, 2009.
523. Wilson R, Feldman RA, Davis J, et al: Salmonellosis in infants: the importance of intrafamilial transmission, *Pediatrics* 69:436, 1982.
524. Mahajan R, Mathur M, Kumar A, et al: Nosocomial outbreak of *Salmonella* Typhimurium infection in a nursery intensive care unit (NICU) and paediatric ward, *J Commun Dis* 27:10, 1995.
525. Jones DM, Pantin CG: Neonatal diarrhoea due to *Salmonella* paratyphi B, *J Clin Pathol* 9:128, 1956.
526. Rubenstein AD, Feemster RF, Smith HM: Salmonellosis as a Public Health Problem in Wartime, *Am J Public Health Nations Health* 34:841, 1944.
527. Neter E: Observations on the transmission of salmonellosis in man, *Am J Public Health Nations Health* 40:929, 1950.
528. Sanders DY, Sinal SH, Morrison L: Chronic salmonellosis in infancy, *Clin Pediatr (Phila)* 13:640, 1974.
529. Bouallegue-Godet O, Ben Salem Y, Fabre L, et al: Nosocomial outbreak caused by *Salmonella enterica* serotype Livingstone producing CTX-M-27 extended-spectrum beta-lactamase in a neonatal unit in Sousse, Tunisia, *J Clin Microbiol* 43:1037, 2005.
530. Cartolano GL, Moulies ME, Seguier JC, et al: A parent as a vector of *Salmonella* brandenburg nosocomial infection in a neonatal intensive care unit, *Clin Microbiol Infect* 9:560, 2003.
531. Vaagland H, Blomberg B, Krüger C, et al: Nosocomial outbreak of neonatal *Salmonella enterica* serotype Enteritidis meningitis in a rural hospital in northern Tanzania, *BMC Infect Dis* 4:35, 2004.
532. Bille B, Mellbin T, Nordbring F: An extensive outbreak of gastroenteritis caused by *Salmonella* Newport. I. Some Observations of 745 Known Cases, *Acta Med Scand* 175:557, 1964.
533. Horwitz MA, Pollard RA, Merson MH, et al: A large outbreak of foodborne salmonellosis on the Navajo Nation Indian Reservation, epidemiology and secondary transmission, *Am J Public Health* 67:1071, 1977.
534. Mahle WT, Levine MM: *Salmonella* Typhi infection in children younger than five years of age, *Pediatr Infect Dis J* 12:627, 1993.
535. Mohanty S, Gaind R, Sehgal R, et al: Neonatal sepsis due to *Salmonella* Typhi and Paratyphi A, *J Infect Dev Ctries* 3:633, 2009.
536. Reed RP, Klugman KP: Neonatal typhoid fever, *Pediatr Infect Dis J* 13:774, 1994.
537. Owais A, Sultana S, Zaman U, et al: Incidence of typhoid bacteremia in infants and young children in southern coastal Pakistan, *Pediatr Infect Dis J* 29:1035, 2010.
538. Hargrett-Bean NT, Pavia AT, Tauxe RV: *Salmonella* isolates from humans in the United States, 1984-1986, *MMWR CDC Surveill Summ* 37:25, 1988.
539. Guarino A, Spagnuolo MI, Russo S, et al: Etiology and risk factors of severe and protracted diarrhea, *J Pediatr Gastroenterol Nutr* 20:173, 1995.
540. Buchwald DS, Blaser MJ: A review of human salmonellosis: II. Duration of excretion following infection with non-Typhi *Salmonella*, *Rev Infect Dis* 6:345, 1984.
541. Onwuezobe IA, Oshun PO, Odigwe CC: Antimicrobials for treating symptomatic non-typhoidal *Salmonella* infection, *Cochrane Database Syst Rev* (11): CD001167, 2012.
542. Schutze GE, Schutze SE, Kirby RS: Extraintestinal salmonellosis in a children's hospital, *Pediatr Infect Dis J* 16:482, 1997.
543. Davis RC: *Salmonella* sepsis in infancy, *Am J Dis Child* 135:1096, 1981.
544. Torrey S, Fleisher G, Jaffe D: Incidence of *Salmonella* bacteremia in infants with *Salmonella* gastroenteritis, *J Pediatr* 108:718, 1986.
545. Katz BZ, Shapiro ED: Predictors of persistently positive blood cultures in children with "occult" *Salmonella* bacteremia, *Pediatr Infect Dis* 5:713, 1986.
546. Yamamoto LG, Ashton MJ: *Salmonella* infections in infants in Hawaii, *Pediatr Infect Dis J* 7:48, 1988.
547. Cohen JI, Bartlett JA, Corey GR: Extra-intestinal manifestations of *Salmonella* infections, *Medicine (Baltimore)* 66:349, 1987.
548. Punpanich W, Netsawang S, Thippated C: Invasive salmonellosis in urban Thai children: a ten-year review, *Pediatr Infect Dis J* 31:e105, 2012.
549. West SE, Goodkin R, Kaplan AM: Neonatal *Salmonella* meningitis complicated by cerebral abscesses, *West J Med* 127:142, 1977.
550. Molyneux EM, Mankhambo LA, Phiri A, et al: The outcome of non-typhoidal *Salmonella* meningitis in Malawian children, 1997-2006,, *Ann Trop Paediatr* 29:13, 2009.
551. Appelbaum PC, Scragg J: *Salmonella* meningitis in infants, *Lancet* 1:1052, 1977.
552. Diwan N, Sharma KB: Isolation of *Salmonella* Typhimurium from cephalhematoma and osteomyelitis, *Indian J Med Res* 67:27, 1978.
553. Konzert W: *Salmonella* osteomyelitis in reference to *Salmonella* Typhimurium epidemics in a newborn infant ward, *Wien Klin Wochenschr* 81:713, 1969.
554. McKinlay B: Infectious diarrhea of the newborn caused by an unclassified species of *Salmonella*, *Am J Dis Child* 54:1252, 1937.
555. Szmuness W, Sikorska J, Szymanek E, et al: The microbiological and epidemiological properties of infections caused by *Salmonella* Enteritidis, *J Hyg (Lond)* 64:9, 1966.
556. Nelson JD: Suppurative mastitis in infants, *Am J Dis Child* 125:458, 1973.
557. Guthrie KJ, Montgomery GI: Infections with *Bacterium enteritidis* in infancy with the triad of enteritis, cholecystitis, and meningitis, *J Path Bact* 49:393, 1939.
558. Corman LI, Poirier RH, Littlefield CA, et al: Endophthalmitis due to *Salmonella* Enteritidis, *J Pediatr* 95:1001, 1979.
559. Osler W, McCrae T: Typhoid fever. In Osler W, editor: *Principles and practice of medicine*, New York, 1912, D Appleton, pp 1-46.
560. Stuart BM, Pullen RL: Typhoid; clinical analysis of 360 cases, *Arch Intern Med (Chic)* 78:629, 1946.
561. Sengupta BS, Ramachander N, Zamah N: *Salmonella* septic abortion, *Int Surg* 65:183, 1980.
562. Diddle AW, Stephens RL: Typhoid fever in pregnancy, *Am J Obstet Gynecol* 38:300, 1939.
563. Hicks HT, French H: Typhoid fever and pregnancy with special references to fetal infection, *Lancet* 1:1491, 1905.
564. Pickering LK, DuPont HL, Olarte J, et al: Fecal leukocytes in enteric infections, *Am J Clin Pathol* 68:562, 1977.
565. Huicho L, Sanchez D, Contreras M, et al: Occult blood and fecal leukocytes as screening tests in childhood infectious diarrhea: an old problem revisited, *Pediatr Infect Dis J* 12:474, 1993.
566. Baker S, Favorov M, Dougan G: Searching for the elusive typhoid diagnostic, *BMC Infect Dis* 10:45, 2010.
567. Wain J, Hosoglu S: The laboratory diagnosis of enteric fever, *J Infect Dev Ctries* 2:421, 2008.
568. McCall CE, Martin WT, Boring JR: Efficiency of cultures of rectal swabs and faecal specimens in detecting *Salmonella* carriers: correlation with numbers of *Salmonellas* excreted, *J Hyg (Lond)* 64:261, 1966.
569. Raucher HS, Eichenfield AH, Hodes HL: Treatment of *Salmonella* gastroenteritis in infants. The significance of bacteremia, *Clin Pediatr (Phila)* 22:601, 1983.
570. Pickering LK, editor: *Red book: report of the Committee on Infectious Diseases*, Elk Grove Village, Ill, 2012, American Academy of Pediatrics.
571. Gotoff SP, Cochran WD: Antibody response to the somatic antigen of *Salmonella* newport in premature infants, *Pediatrics* 37:610, 1966.
572. Hodes HL, Zepp HD, Ainbender E, et al: Production of O and H agglutinins by a newborn infant infected with *Salmonella* Saintpaul, *J Pediatr* 68:780, 1966.
573. Nga TV, Karkey A, Dongol S, et al: The sensitivity of real-time PCR amplification targeting invasive *Salmonella* serovars in biological specimens, *BMC Infect Dis* 10:125, 2010.
574. Gomez-Duarte OG, Bai J, Newell E: Detection of *Escherichia coli*, *Salmonella* spp., *Shigella* spp. *Yersinia enterocolitica*, *Vibrio cholerae*, and *Campylobacter* spp., enteropathogens by 3-reaction multiplex polymerase chain reaction, *Diagn Microbiol Infect Dis* 63:1, 2009.
575. Sanyal D, Douglas T, Roberts R: *Salmonella* infection acquired from reptilian pets, *Arch Dis Child* 77:345, 1997.
576. Rivera MJ, Rivera N, Castillo J, et al: Molecular and epidemiological study of *Salmonella* clinical isolates, *J Clin Microbiol* 29:927, 1991.
577. Aserkoff B, Bennett JV: Effect of antibiotic therapy in acute salmonellosis on the fecal excretion of *Salmonellae*, *N Engl J Med* 281:636, 1969.
578. Dixon JM: Effect of antibiotic treatment on duration of excretion of *Salmonella* Typhimurium by children, *Br Med J* 2:1343, 1965.

579. Kazemi M, Gumpert TG, Marks MI: A controlled trial comparing sulfamethoxazole-trimethoprim, ampicillin, and no therapy in the treatment of *Salmonella* gastroenteritis in children, *J Pediatr* 83:646, 1973.
580. Neill MA, Opal SM, Heelan J, et al: Failure of ciprofloxacin to eradicate convalescent fecal excretion after acute salmonellosis: experience during an outbreak in health care workers, *Ann Intern Med* 114:195, 1991.
581. Pettersson T, Klemola E, Wager O: Treatment of acute cases of *Salmonella* infection and *Salmonella* carriers with ampicillin and neomycin, *Acta Med Scand* 175:185, 1964.
582. Effect of neomycin in non-invasive *Salmonella* infections of the gastrointestinal tract. Joint Project by Members of the Association for the Study of Infectious Disease, *Lancet* 2:1159, 1970.
583. Nelson JD, Kusmiesz H, Jackson LH, et al: Treatment of *Salmonella* gastroenteritis with ampicillin, amoxicillin, or placebo, *Pediatrics* 65:1125, 1980.
584. Asperilla MO, Smego RA, Scott LK: Quinolone antibiotics in the treatment of *Salmonella* infections, *Rev Infect Dis* 12:873, 1990.
585. Edgar WM, Lacey BW: Infection with *S.* Heidelberg: an outbreak presumably not foodborne, *Lancet* 1:161, 1963.
586. Rice PA, Craven C, Wells JG: *Salmonella* Heidelberg enteritis and bacteremia. An epidemic on two pediatric wards, *Am J Med* 60:509, 1976.
587. Ruiz M, Rodríguez JC, Escribano I, et al: Available options in the management of non-Typhi *Salmonella*, *Expert Opin Pharmacother* 5:1737, 2004.
588. Price EH, de Louvois J, Workman MR: Antibiotics for *Salmonella* meningitis in children, *J Antimicrob Chemother* 46:653, 2000.
589. MacDonald KL, Cohen ML, Hargrett-Bean NT, et al: Changes in antimicrobial resistance of *Salmonella* isolated from humans in the United States, *JAMA* 258:1496, 1987.
590. Lee LA, Puhr ND, Maloney EK, et al: Increase in antimicrobial-resistant *Salmonella* infections in the United States, 1989-1990, *J Infect Dis* 170:128, 1994.
591. Crump JA, Medalla FM, Joyce KW, et al: Antimicrobial resistance among invasive nontyphoidal *Salmonella enterica* isolates in the United States: National Antimicrobial Resistance Monitoring System, 1996 to 2007, *Antimicrob Agents Chemother* 55:1148, 2011.
592. Stevenson JE, Gay K, Barrett TJ, et al: Increase in nalidixic acid resistance among non-Typhi *Salmonella enterica* isolates in the United States from 1996 to 2003, *Antimicrob Agents Chemother* 51:195, 2007.
593. Zaki SA, Karande S: Multidrug-resistant typhoid fever: a review, *J Infect Dev Ctries* 5:324, 2011.
594. Chau TT, Campbell JI, Galindo CM, et al: Antimicrobial drug resistance of *Salmonella enterica* serovar Typhi in Asia and molecular mechanism of reduced susceptibility to the fluoroquinolones, *Antimicrob Agents Chemother* 51:4315, 2007.
595. Humphries RM, Fang FC, Aarestrup FM, et al: In vitro susceptibility testing of fluoroquinolone activity against *Salmonella*: recent changes to CLSI standards, *Clin Infect Dis* 55:1107, 2012.
596. Arlet G, Barrett TJ, Butaye P, et al: *Salmonella* resistant to extended-spectrum cephalosporins: prevalence and epidemiology, *Microbes Infect* 8:1945, 2006.
597. Chuang CH, Su LH, Perera J, et al: Surveillance of antimicrobial resistance of *Salmonella enterica* serotype Typhi in seven Asian countries, *Epidemiol Infect* 137:266, 2009.
598. Stephens I, Levine MM: Management of typhoid fever in children, *Pediatr Infect Dis J* 21:157, 2002.
599. Hohmann EL: Nontyphoidal salmonellosis, *Clin Infect Dis* 32:263, 2001.
600. Jean SS, Lee YT, Guo SM, et al: Recurrent infections caused by cefotaxime- and ciprofloxacin-resistant *Salmonella enterica* serotype Choleraesuis treated successfully with imipenem, *J Infect* 51:e163, 2005.
601. Bradley JS, Jackson MA: The use of systemic and topical fluoroquinolones, *Pediatrics* 128:e1034, 2011.
602. Brenner DJ, Fanning GR, Skerman FJ, et al: Polynucleotide sequence divergence among strains of *Escherichia coli* and closely related organisms, *J Bacteriol* 109:953, 1972.
603. Brooks GF, Carroll Karen C, Butel Janet S, et al: *Jawetz, Melnick and Adelberg's medical microbiology*, ed 25, New York, 2010, McGraw-Hill.
604. van den Beld MJ, Reubsaet FA: Differentiation between *Shigella*, enteroinvasive *Escherichia coli* (EIEC) and noninvasive *Escherichia coli*, *Eur J Clin Microbiol Infect Dis* 31:899, 2012.
605. Levine MM, Kotloff KL, Barry EM, et al: Clinical trials of *Shigella* vaccines: two steps forward and one step back on a long, hard road, *Nat Rev Microbiol* 5:540, 2007.
606. World Health Organization: Guidelines for the control of shigellosis, including epidemics due to Shigella dysenteriae type 1, Geneva, 2005, WHO Document Production Services.
607. Phalipon A, Sansonetti PJ: *Shigella*'s ways of manipulating the host intestinal innate and adaptive immune system: a tool box for survival? *Immunol Cell Biol* 85:119, 2007.
608. Sansonetti PJ: The bacterial weaponry: lessons from *Shigella*, *Ann NY Acad Sci* 1072:307, 2006.
609. Sansonetti PJ, Kopecko DJ, Formal SB: Involvement of a plasmid in the invasive ability of *Shigella flexneri*, *Infect Immun* 35:852, 1982.
610. Sansonetti P: Host-pathogen interactions: the seduction of molecular cross talk, *Gut* 50(Suppl 3):1112, 2002.
611. Schroeder GN, Hilbi H: Molecular pathogenesis of *Shigella* spp.: controlling host cell signaling, invasion, and death by type III secretion, *Clin Microbiol Rev* 21:134, 2008.
612. Fernandez MI, Sansonetti PJ: *Shigella* interaction with intestinal epithelial cells determines the innate immune response in shigellosis, *Int J Med Microbiol* 293:55, 2003.
613. Hale TL, Oaks EV, Formal SB: Identification and antigenic characterization of virulence-associated, plasmid-coded proteins of *Shigella* spp. and enteroinvasive *Escherichia coli*, *Infect Immun* 50:620, 1985.
614. Sasakawa C, Kamata K, Sakai T, et al: Molecular alteration of the 140-megadalton plasmid associated with loss of virulence and Congo red binding activity in *Shigella flexneri*, *Infect Immun* 51:470, 1986.
615. Labrec EH, Schneider H, Magnani TJ, et al: Epithelial cell penetration as an essential step in the pathogenesis of bacillary dysentery, *J Bacteriol* 88:1503, 1964.
616. Ogawa H: Experimental approach in studies on pathogenesis of bacillary dysentery—with special references to the invasion of bacilli into intestinal mucosa, *Acta Pathol Jpn* 20:261, 1970.
617. Sansonetti PJ, d'Hauteville H, Formal SB, et al: Plasmid-mediated invasiveness of "*Shigella*-like" *Escherichia coli*, *Ann Microbiol (Paris)* 133:351, 1982.
618. Sansonetti PJ, d'Hauteville H, Ecobichon C, et al: Molecular comparison of virulence plasmids in *Shigella* and enteroinvasive *Escherichia coli*, *Ann Microbiol (Paris)* 134A:295, 1983.
619. Sereny B: Experimental *Shigella* keratoconjunctivitis; a preliminary report, *Acta Microbiol Acad Sci Hung* 2:293, 1955.
620. Marteyn B, Gazi A, Sansonetti P: *Shigella*: a model of virulence regulation in vivo, *Gut Microbes* 3:104, 2012.
621. Ashida H, Ogawa M, Mimuro H, et al: *Shigella* are versatile mucosal pathogens that circumvent the host innate immune system, *Curr Opin Immunol* 23:448, 2011.
622. Sansonetti PJ, Hale TL, Dammin GJ, et al: Alterations in the pathogenicity of *Escherichia coli* K-12 after transfer of plasmid and chromosomal genes from *Shigella flexneri*, *Infect Immun* 39:1392, 1983.
623. Wei J, Goldberg MB, Burland V, et al: Complete genome sequence and comparative genomics of *Shigella flexneri* serotype 2a strain 2457T, *Infect Immun* 71:2775, 2003.
624. Okada N, Sasakawa C, Tobe T, et al: Virulence-associated chromosomal loci of *Shigella flexneri* identified by random Tn5 insertion mutagenesis, *Mol Microbiol* 5:187, 1991.
625. Okamura N, Nagai T, Nakaya R, et al: HeLa cell invasiveness and O antigen of *Shigella flexneri* as separate and prerequisite attributes of virulence to evoke keratoconjunctivitis in guinea pigs, *Infect Immun* 39:505, 1983.
626. Bartlett AV, Prado D, Cleary TG, et al: Production of Shiga toxin and other cytotoxins by serogroups of *Shigella*, *J Infect Dis* 154:996, 1986.
627. Olenick JG, Wolfe AD: *Shigella* toxin inhibition of binding and translation of polyuridylic acid by *Escherichia coli* ribosomes, *J Bacteriol* 141:1246, 1980.
628. Brown JE, Rothman SW, Doctor BP: Inhibition of protein synthesis in intact HeLa cells by *Shigella dysenteriae* 1 toxin, *Infect Immun* 29:98, 1980.
629. Al-Hasani K, Henderson IR, Sakellaris H, et al: The sigA gene which is borne on the she pathogenicity island of *Shigella flexneri* 2a encodes an exported cytopathic protease involved in intestinal fluid accumulation, *Infect Immun* 68:2457, 2000.
630. Ashkenazi S: *Shigella* infections in children: new insights, *Semin Pediatr Infect Dis* 15:246, 2004.

631. Niyogi SK, Vargas M, Vila J: Prevalence of the sat, set and sen genes among diverse serotypes of *Shigella flexneri* strains isolated from patients with acute diarrhoea, *Clin Microbiol Infect* 10:574, 2004.
632. Faherty CS, Harper JM, Shea-Donohue T, et al: Chromosomal and plasmid-encoded factors of *Shigella flexneri* induce secretogenic activity ex vivo, *PLoS One* 7:e49980, 2012.
633. Makintubee S, Mallonee J, Istre GR: Shigellosis outbreak associated with swimming, *Am J Public Health* 77:166, 1987.
634. Levine MM, DuPont HL, Formal SB, et al: Pathogenesis of *Shigella dysenteriae* 1 (Shiga) dysentery, *J Infect Dis* 127:261, 1973.
635. DuPont HL, Hornick RB, Dawkins AT, et al: The response of man to virulent *Shigella flexneri* 2a, *J Infect Dis* 119:296, 1969.
636. Levine MM: Shigella infections and vaccines: experiences from volunteer and controlled field studies. In Rahaman MM, Greenough WB, Novae N, et al, editors: *Shigellosis: a continuing global problem, International Centre for Diarrhoeal Disease Research*, Dacca, 1983, Bangladesh, p 208.
637. Wikswo ME, Hall AJ: Outbreaks of acute gastroenteritis transmitted by person-to-person contact—United States, 2009-2010, *MMWR Surveill Summ* 61:1, 2012.
638. Arvelo W, Hinkle CJ, Nguyen TA, et al: Transmission risk factors and treatment of pediatric shigellosis during a large daycare center-associated outbreak of multidrug resistant *Shigella sonnei*: implications for the management of shigellosis outbreaks among children, *Pediatr Infect Dis J* 28:976, 2009.
639. Mata LG: *The children of Santa Maria Cauque: a prospective field study of health and growth*, Cambridge, Mass, 1978, MIT Press.
640. Stoll BJ, Glass RI, Huq MI, et al: Surveillance of patients attending a diarrhoeal disease hospital in Bangladesh, *Br Med J (Clin Res Ed)* 285:1185, 1982.
641. Floyd TM, Higgins AR, Kader MA: Studies in shigellosis. V. The relationship of age to the incidence of *Shigella* infections in Egyptian children, with special reference to shigellosis in the newborn and in infants in the first six months of life, *Am J Trop Med Hyg* 5:119, 1956.
642. Summary of notifiable diseases: United States—-1991, *MMWR Morb Mortal Wkly Rep* 40:1, 1992.
643. Abu-Elyazeed RR, Wierzba TF, Frenck RW, et al: Epidemiology of *Shigella*-associated diarrhea in rural Egyptian children, *Am J Trop Med Hyg* 71:367, 2004.
644. Viner Y, Miron D, Gottfried E, et al: Neonatal shigellosis, *Isr Med Assoc J* 3:964, 2001.
645. Huskins WC, Griffiths JK, Faruque AS, et al: Shigellosis in neonates and young infants, *J Pediatr* 125:14, 1994.
646. Haltalin KC: Neonatal shigellosis. Report of 16 cases and review of the literature, *Am J Dis Child* 114:603, 1967.
647. Scragg JN, Rubidge CJ, Appelbaum PC: *Shigella* infection in African and Indian children with special reference to *Shigella* septicemia, *J Pediatr* 93:796, 1978.
648. Burry VF, Thurn AN, Co TG: Shigellosis: an analysis of 239 cases in a pediatric population, *Mo Med* 65: 671, 1968.
649. Marcus R: New information about pediatric foodborne infections: the view from FoodNet, *Curr Opin Pediatr* 20:79, 2008.
650. Ram PK, Crump JA, Gupta SK, et al: Part II. Analysis of data gaps pertaining to *Shigella* infections in low and medium human development index countries, 1984-2005, *Epidemiol Infect* 136:577, 2008.
651. WHO Scientific Working Group: Enteric infections due to *Campylobacter, Yersinia, Salmonella*, and *Shigella*, *Bull World Health Organ* 58:519, 1980.
652. Rebarber A, Star Hampton B, Lewis V, et al: Shigellosis complicating preterm premature rupture of membranes resulting in congenital infection and preterm delivery, *Obstet Gynecol* 100:1063, 2002.
653. von Seidlein L, Kim DR, Ali M, et al: A multicentre study of *Shigella* diarrhoea in six Asian countries: disease burden, clinical manifestations, and microbiology, *PLoS Med* 3:e353, 2006.
654. Kraybill EN, Controni G: Septicemia and enterocolitis due to *Shigella sonnei* in a newborn infant, *Pediatrics* 42:529, 1968.
655. Moore EE: *Shigella sonnei* septicaemia in a neonate, *Br Med J* 1:22, 1974.
656. Aldrich JA, Flowers RP, Hall FK: *Shigella sonnei* septicemia in a neonate: a case report, *J Am Osteopath Assoc* 79:93, 1979.
657. Barton LL, Pickering LK: Shigellosis in the first week of life, *Pediatrics* 52:437, 1973.
658. Landsberger M: Bacillary dysentery in a newborn infant, *Arch Pediatr* 59:330, 1942.
659. Neter E: *Shigella sonnei* infection at term and its transfer to the newborn, *Obstet Gynecol* 17:517, 1961.
660. McIntire MS, Jahr HM: An isolated case of shigellosis in the newborn nursery, *Nebr State Med J* 39:425, 1954.
661. Greenberg M, Frant S, Shapiro R: Bacillary dysentery acquired at birth, *J Pediatr* 17:363, 1940.
662. Emanuel B, Sherman JO: Shigellosis in a neonate: successful treatment with an oral elemental diet, *Clin Pediatr (Phila)* 14:725, 1975.
663. Barrett-Connor E, Connor JD: Extraintestinal manifestations of shigellosis, *Am J Gastroenterol* 53:234, 1970.
664. Fischler E: Convulsions as a complication of shigellosis in children, *Helv Paediatr Acta* 17:389, 1962.
665. Ashkenazi S, Dinari G, Zevulunov A, et al: Convulsions in childhood shigellosis. Clinical and laboratory features in 153 children, Am, *J Dis Child* 141:208, 1987.
666. Galanakis E, Tzoufi M, Charisi M, et al: Rate of seizures in children with shigellosis, *Acta Paediatr* 91:101, 2002.
667. Khan WA, Dhar U, Salam MA, et al: Central nervous system manifestations of childhood shigellosis: prevalence, risk factors, and outcome, *Pediatrics* 103:E18, 1999.
668. Whitfield C, Humphries JM: Meningitis and septicemia due to *Shigellae* in a newborn infant, *J Pediatr* 70:805, 1967.
669. Goren A, Freier S, Passwell JH: Lethal toxic encephalopathy due to childhood shigellosis in a developed country, *Pediatrics* 89:1189, 1992.
670. Ashkenazi S, Cleary KR, Pickering LK, et al: The association of Shiga toxin and other cytotoxins with the neurologic manifestations of shigellosis, *J Infect Dis* 161:961, 1990.
671. Rahaman MM, JamiulAlam AK, Islam MR, et al: Shiga bacillus dysentery associated with marked leukocytosis and erythrocyte fragmentation, *Johns Hopkins Med J* 136:65, 1975.
672. Neglia TG, Marr TJ, Davis AT: *Shigella* dysentery with secondary *Klebsiella* sepsis, *J Pediatr* 89:253, 1976.
673. Struelens MJ, Patte D, Kabir I, et al: *Shigella* septicemia: prevalence, presentation, risk factors, and outcome, *J Infect Dis* 152:784, 1985.
674. Levin SE: *Shigella* septicemia in the newborn infant, *J Pediatr* 71:917, 1967.
675. Mata LJ, Urrutia JJ, García B, et al: *Shigella* infection in breast-fed Guatemalan indian neonates, *Am J Dis Child* 117:142, 1969.
676. Haltalin KC, Nelson JD: Coliform septicemia complicating shigellosis in children, *JAMA* 192:441, 1965.
677. Beigelman A, Leibovitz E, Sofer S: Septic shock associated with *Shigella flexneri* dysentery, *Scand J Infect Dis* 34:692, 2002.
678. Martin T, Habbick BF, Nyssen J: Shigellosis with bacteremia: a report of two cases and a review of the literature, *Pediatr Infect Dis* 2:21, 1983.
679. Ruderman JW, Stoller KP, Pomerance JJ: Bloodstream invasion with *Shigella sonnei* in an asymptomatic newborn infant, *Pediatr Infect Dis* 5:379, 1986.
680. Langman G: *Shigella sonnei* meningitis, *S Afr Med J* 86:91, 1996.
681. Clemens JD, Stanton B, Stoll B, et al: Breast feeding as a determinant of severity in shigellosis. Evidence for protection throughout the first three years of life in Bangladeshi children, *Am J Epidemiol* 123:710, 1986.
682. Starke JR, Baker CJ: Neonatal shigellosis with bowel perforation, *Pediatr Infect Dis* 4:405, 1985.
683. Azad MA, Islam M, Butler T: Colonic perforation in *Shigella dysenteriae* 1 infection, *Pediatr Infect Dis* 5:103, 1986.
684. O'Connor HJ, O'Callaghan U: Fatal *Shigella sonnei* septicaemia in an adult complicated by marrow aplasia and intestinal perforation, *J Infect* 3:277, 1981.
685. Alam AN, Chowdhury AA, Kabir IA, et al: Association of pneumonia with undernutrition and shigellosis, *Indian Pediatr* 21:609, 1984.
686. Hoefnagel D: Fulminating, rapidly fatal shigellosis in children, *N Engl J Med* 258:1256, 1958.
687. Sakamoto A, Kamo S: Clinical, statistical observations on ekiri and bacillary dysentery; a study of 785 cases, *Ann Paediatr* 186:1, 1956.
688. Dodd K, Buddingh J, Rapoport S: The etiology of ekiri, a highly fatal disease of Japanese children, *Pediatrics* 3:9, 1949.
689. Davis TC: Chronic vulvovaginitis in children due to *Shigella flexneri*, *Pediatrics* 56:41, 1975.
690. Murphy TV, Nelson JD: *Shigella* vaginitis: report of 38 patients and review of the literature, *Pediatrics* 63:511, 1979.

691. Tobias JD, Starke JR, Tosi MF: *Shigella* keratitis: a report of two cases and a review of the literature, *Pediatr Infect Dis J* 6:79, 1987.
692. Butler T, Dunn D, Dahms B, et al: Causes of death and the histopathologic findings in fatal shigellosis, *Pediatr Infect Dis J* 8:767, 1989.
693. Bennish ML, Harris JR, Wojtyniak BJ, et al: Death in shigellosis: incidence and risk factors in hospitalized patients, *J Infect Dis* 161:500, 1990.
694. Kotloff KL, Winickoff JP, Ivanoff B, et al: Global burden of *Shigella* infections: implications for vaccine development and implementation of control strategies, *Bull World Health Organ* 77:651, 1999.
695. Bardhan P, Faruque AS, Naheed A, et al: Decrease in shigellosis-related deaths without *Shigella* spp.-specific interventions, *Asia, Emerg Infect Dis* 16:1718, 2010.
696. Speelman P, McGlaughlin R, Kabir I, et al: Differential clinical features and stool findings in shigellosis and amoebic dysentery, *Trans R Soc Trop Med Hyg* 81:549, 1987.
697. Taylor WI, Harris B: Isolation of *Shigellae*. II. Comparison of plating media and enrichment broths, *Am J Clin Pathol* 44:476, 1965.
698. Lindsay B, Ochieng JB, Ikumapayi UN, et al: Quantitative PCR for detection of *Shigella* improves ascertainment of *Shigella* burden in children with moderate-to-severe diarrhea in low-income countries, *J Clin Microbiol* 51:1740, 2013.
699. Stypulkowska-Misiurewics H: Problems in bacteriological diagnosis of shigellosis. In Rahaman MM, Greenough WB, Novae N, editors: *Shigellosis: a continuing global problem, International Centre for Diarrhoeal Disease Research*, Dacca, 1983, Bangladesh, p 87.
700. Haltalin KC, Nelson JD, Ring 3rd R, et al: Double-blind treatment study of shigellosis comparing ampicillin, sulfadiazine, and placebo, *J Pediatr* 70:970, 1967.
701. Haltalin KC, Nelson JD, Kusmiesz HT, et al: Optimal dosage of ampicillin for shigellosis, *J Pediatr* 74:626, 1969.
702. Haltalin KC, Nelson JD, Kusmiesz HT: Comparative efficacy of nalidixic acid and ampicillin for severe shigellosis, *Arch Dis Child* 48:305, 1973.
703. Oaks EV, Hale TL, Formal SB: Serum immune response to *Shigella* protein antigens in rhesus monkeys and humans infected with *Shigella* spp, *Infect Immun* 53:57, 1986.
704. Frankel G, Riley L, Giron JA, et al: Detection of *Shigella* in feces using DNA amplification, *J Infect Dis* 161:1252, 1990.
705. Speelman P, Kabir I, Islam M: Distribution and spread of colonic lesions in shigellosis: a colonoscopic study, *J Infect Dis* 150:899, 1984.
706. Christopher PR, David KV, John SM, et al: Antibiotic therapy for *Shigella* dysentery, *Cochrane Database Syst Rev* (8): CD006784, 2010.
707. Ostrower VG: Comparison of cefaclor and ampicillin in the treatment of shigellosis, *Postgrad Med J* 55(Suppl 4):82, 1979.
708. Haltalin KC, Nelson JD: Failure of furazolidone therapy in shigellosis, *Am J Dis Child* 123:40, 1972.
709. Nelson JD, Haltalin KC: Comparative efficacy of cephalexin and ampicillin for shigellosis and other types of acute diarrhea in infants and children, *Antimicrob Agents Chemother* 7:415, 1975.
710. Nelson JA, Haltalin KC: Amoxicillin less effective than ampicillin against *Shigella* in vitro and in vivo: relationship of efficacy to activity in serum, *J Infect Dis* 129(Suppl):S222, 1974.
711. Tong MJ, Martin DG, Cunningham JJ, et al: Clinical and bacteriological evaluation of antibiotic treatment in shigellosis, *JAMA* 214:1841, 1970.
712. Orenstein WA, Ross L, Overturf GD, et al: Antibiotic treatment of acute shigellosis: failure of cefamandole compared with trimethoprim/ sulfamethoxazole and ampicillin, *Am J Med Sci* 282:27, 1981.
713. Shiferaw B, Solghan S, Palmer A, et al: Antimicrobial susceptibility patterns of *Shigella* isolates in Foodborne Diseases Active Surveillance Network (FoodNet) sites, 2000-2010, *Clin Infect Dis* 54(Suppl 5):S458, 2012.
714. Khan E, Jabeen K, Ejaz M, et al: Trends in antimicrobial resistance in *Shigella* species in Karachi, Pakistan, *J Infect Dev Ctries* 3:798, 2009.
715. Sjolund Karlsson M, Bowen A, Reporter R, et al: Outbreak of infections caused by *Shigella sonnei* with reduced susceptibility to azithromycin in the United States, *Antimicrob Agents Chemother* 57:1559, 2013.
716. Ahmed SF, Riddle MS, Wierzba TF, et al: Epidemiology and genetic characterization of *Shigella flexneri* strains isolated from three paediatric populations in Egypt (2000-2004), *Epidemiol Infect* 134:1237, 2006.
717. Tau NP, Smith AM, Sooka A, et al: Molecular characterization of extended-spectrum beta-lactamase-producing *Shigella* isolates from humans in South Africa, 2003-2009, *J Med Microbiol* 61:162, 2012.
718. Taneja N, Mewara A, Kumar A, et al: Cephalosporin-resistant *Shigella flexneri* over 9 years (2001-09) in India, *J Antimicrob Chemother* 67:1347, 2012.
719. Khatun F, Faruque AS, Koeck JL, et al: Changing species distribution and antimicrobial susceptibility pattern of *Shigella* over a 29-year period (1980-2008), *Epidemiol Infect* 139:446, 2011.
720. Bennish ML, Salam MA, Khan WA, et al: Treatment of shigellosis: III. Comparison of one- or two-dose ciprofloxacin with standard 5-day therapy. A randomized, blinded trial, *Ann Intern Med* 117:727, 1992.
721. John JF Jr, Atkins LT, Maple PA, et al: Activities of newer fluoroquinolones against *Shigella sonnei*, *Antimicrob Agents Chemother* 36:2346, 1992.
722. DuPont HL, Hornick RB: Adverse effect of lomotil therapy in shigellosis, *JAMA* 226:1525, 1973.
723. Ahmed F, Clemens JD, Rao MR, et al: Community-based evaluation of the effect of breast-feeding on the risk of microbiologically confirmed or clinically presumptive shigellosis in Bangladeshi children, *Pediatrics* 90:406, 1992.
724. Khan MU: Interruption of shigellosis by hand washing, *Trans R Soc Trop Med Hyg* 76:164, 1982.
725. Salzman TC, Scher CD, Moss R: *Shigellae* with transferable drug resistance: outbreak in a nursery for premature infants, *J Pediatr* 71:21, 1967.
726. Farrar WE Jr, Eidson M, Guerry P, et al: Interbacterial transfer of R factor in the human intestine: in-vivo acquisition of R-factor-mediated kanamycin resistance by a multiresistant strain of *Shigella sonnei*, *J Infect Dis* 126:27, 1972.
727. Kirkpatrick B, Tribble D: Update on human *Campylobacter jejuni* infections, *Curr Opin Gastroenterol* 27:1, 2010.
728. McFadyean F, Stockman S: *Report of the Departmental Committee Appointed by the Board of Agriculture and Fisheries to inquire into epizootic abortion*, vol. 3. London, 1909, His Majesty's Stationery Office.
729. Smith T, Taylor MS: Some morphological and biochemical characters of the spirilla (*Vibrio fetus*, n. spp.) associated with disease of the fetal membranes in cattle, *J Exp Med* 30:200, 1919.
730. Jones FS, Orcutt M, Little RB: Vibrios (*Vibrio jejuni*, n. spp.) associated with intestinal disorders of cows and calves, *J Exp Med* 53:853, 1931.
731. Bryner JH, Estes PC, Foley JW, et al: *1971* Infectivity of three *Vibrio fetus* biotypes for gallbladder and intestines of cattle, sheep, rabbits, guinea pigs, and mice, *Am J Vet Res* 32:465, 1971.
732. Vinzent R, Dumas J, Picard N: Septicémie grave au cours de la grossesse due à un vibrion. Avortement consécutif, *Bull Acad Natl Med* 131:90, 1947.
733. Eden AN: Perinatal mortality caused by *Vibrio fetus*: review and analysis, *J Pediatr* 68:297, 1966.
734. Torphy DE, Bond WW: *Campylobacter fetus* infections in children, *Pediatrics* 64:898, 1979.
735. Sebald M, Veron M: Teneur en bases de l'ADN et classification des vibrions, *Ann Inst Pasteur* 105:897, 1963.
736. Walker RI, Caldwell MB, Lee EC, et al: Pathophysiology of *Campylobacter* enteritis, *Microbiol Rev* 50:81, 1986.
737. Penner JL: The genus *Campylobacter*: a decade of progress, *Clin Microbiol Rev* 1:157, 1988.
738. Calva JJ, Ruiz-Palacios GM, Lopez-Vidal AB, et al: Cohort study of intestinal infection with *Campylobacter* in Mexican children, *Lancet* 1:503, 1988.
739. Owen RJ: Nucleic acids in the classification of campylobacters, *Eur J Clin Microbiol* 2:367, 1983.
740. Bokkenheuser V: *Vibrio fetus* infection in man. I. Ten new cases and some epidemiologic observations, *Am J Epidemiol* 91:400, 1970.
741. Guerrant RL, Lahita RG, Winn WC Jr, et al: Campylobacteriosis in man: pathogenic mechanisms and review of 91 bloodstream infections, *Am J Med* 65:584, 1978.
742. Zilbauer M, Dorrell N, Wren BW, et al: *Campylobacter jejuni*-mediated disease pathogenesis: an update, *Trans R Soc Trop Med Hyg* 102:123, 2008.
743. Skirrow MB: *Campylobacter* enteritis: a "new" disease, *BMJ* 2:9, 1977.

744. Lindquist B, Kjellander J, Kosunen T: *Campylobacter* enteritis in Sweden, *BMJ* 1:303, 1978.
745. Blaser MJ, Berkowitz ID, LaForce FM, et al: *Campylobacter* enteritis: clinical and epidemiologic features, *Ann Intern Med* 91:179, 1979.
746. Guandalini S, Cucchiara S, de Ritis G, et al: *Campylobacter* colitis in infants, *J Pediatr* 102:72, 1983.
747. Wong SN, Tam YC, Yeun KY: *Campylobacter* infection in the neonate: case report and review of the literature, *Pediatr Infect Dis J* 9:665, 1990.
748. Hood M, Todd JM: *Vibrio fetus*—a cause of human abortion, *Am J Obstet Gynecol* 80:506, 1960.
749. van Wering RF, Esseveld H: Vibrio fetus, *Ned Tijdschr Geneeskd* 107:119, 1963.
750. Burgert W Jr, Hagstrom JWC: *Vibrio fetus* meningoencephalitis, *Arch Neurol* 10:196, 1964.
751. Smith JP, Marymont JH, Schweers J Jr: Septicemia due to *Campylobacter fetus* in a newborn infant with gastroenteritis, *Am J Med Technol* 43:38, 1977.
752. West SE, Houghton DJ, Crook S, et al: *Campylobacter* spp. isolated from the cervix during septic abortion: case report, *Br J Obstet Gynaecol* 89:771, 1982.
753. Simor AE, Karmali MA, Jadavji T, et al: Abortion and perinatal sepsis associated with *Campylobacter* infection, *Rev Infect Dis J* 8:397, 1986.
754. Forbes JC, Scheifele DW: Early onset *Campylobacter* sepsis in a neonate, *Pediatr Infect Dis J* 6:494, 1987.
755. Francioli P, Herzstein J, Grob JP, et al: *Campylobacter fetus* subspecies *fetus* bacteremia, *Arch Intern Med* 145:289, 1985.
756. Szymanski CM, Gaynor EC: How a sugary bug gets through the day: recent developments in understanding fundamental processes impacting *Campylobacter jejuni* pathogenesis, *Gut Microbes* 3:135, 2012.
757. van Putten JP, van Alphen LB, Wösten MM, et al: Molecular mechanisms of Campylobacter infection, *Curr Top Microbiol Immunol* 337:197, 2009.
758. Centers for Disease Control: Preliminary FoodNet data on the incidence of infection with pathogens transmitted commonly through food: 10 states 2008, *MMWR Morb Mortal Wkly Rep* 59:418, 2009.
759. Communicable Disease Surveillance Centre and the Communicable Diseases (Scotland) Unit, 1978 *Campylobacter* infections in Britain, *BMJ* 1:1357, 1977.
760. De Mol P, Bosmans E: *Campylobacter* enteritis in Central Africa, *Lancet* 1:604, 1978.
761. Lindquist B, Kjellander J, Kosunen T: *Campylobacter* enteritis in Sweden, *BMJ* 1:303, 1978.
762. Blaser MJ, Reller LB: *Campylobacter* enteritis, *N Engl J Med* 305:1444, 1981.
763. Steele TW, McDermott S: *Campylobacter* enteritis in South Australia, *Med J Aust* 2:404, 1978.
764. Albert MJ, Leach A, Asche V, et al: Serotype distribution of *Campylobacter jejuni* and *Campylobacter coli* isolated from hospitalized patients with diarrhea in Central Australia, *J Clin Microbiol* 30:207, 1992.
765. Riley LW, Finch MJ: Results of the first year of national surveillance of *Campylobacter* infections in the United States, *J Infect Dis* 151:956, 1985.
766. Georges-Courbot MC, Baya C, Beraud AM, et al: Distribution and serotypes of *Campylobacter jejuni* and *Campylobacter coli* in enteric *Campylobacter* strains isolated from children in the Central African Republic, *J Clin Microbiol* 23:592, 1986.
767. Galanis E: *Campylobacter* and bacterial gastroenteritis, *CMAJ* 177:570, 2007.
768. Karmali MA, Fleming PC: Campylobacter enteritis in children, *J Pediatr* 94:527, 1979.
769. Ribeiro CD: *Campylobacter* enteritis, *Lancet* 2:270, 1978.
770. Smith MV, Muldoon AJ: *Campylobacter fetus* subspecies *jejuni (Vibrio fetus)* from commercially processed poultry, *Appl Microbiol* 27:995, 1974.
771. Butzler JP, Skirrow MB: *Campylobacter* enteritis, *Clin Gastroenterol* 8:737, 1979.
772. Gill CO, Harris LM: Contamination of red meat carcasses by *Campylobacter fetus* subsp, *Jejuni Appl Environ Microbiol* 43:977, 1982.
773. Palmer SR, Gully PR, White JM, et al: Water-borne outbreak of *Campylobacter* gastroenteritis, *Lancet* 1:287, 1983.
774. Hood AM, Pearson AD, Shahamat M: The extent of surface contamination of retailed chickens with *Campylobacter jejuni* serogroups, *Epidemiol Infect* 100:17, 1988.
775. Klein BS, Vergeront JM, Blaser MJ, et al: *Campylobacter* infection associated with raw milk, *JAMA* 255:361, 1986.
776. Gras LM, Smid JH, Wagenaar JA, et al: Increased risk for *Campylobacter jejuni* and *C coli* infection of pet origin in dog owners and evidence for genetic association between strains causing infection in humans and their pets, *Epidemiol Infect* 141:2526, 2013.
777. Blaser MJ, Waldman RJ, Barrett T, et al: Outbreaks of *Campylobacter* enteritis in two extended families: evidence for person-to-person transmission, *J Pediatr* 98:254, 1981.
778. Cadranel S, Rodesch P, Butzler JP, et al: Enteritis due to "related *Vibrio*" in children, *Am J Dis Child* 126:152, 1973.
779. Black RE, Levine MM, Clements ML, et al: Experimental *Campylobacter jejuni* infection in humans, *J Infect Dis* 157:472, 1988.
780. Tribble DR, Baqar S, Scott DA, et al: Assessment of the duration of protection in *Campylobacter jejuni* experimental infection in humans, *Infect Immun* 78:1750, 2010.
781. Mawer SL, Smith BAM: *Campylobacter* infection of premature baby, *Lancet* 1:1041, 1979.
782. Karmali MA, Tan YC: Neonatal *Campylobacter* enteritis, *Can Med Assoc J* 122:192, 1980.
783. Thomas K, Chan KN, Riberiro CD: *Campylobacter jejuni/coli* meningitis in a neonate, *Br Med J* 280:1301, 1980.
784. Anders BJ, Lauer BA, Paisley JW: *Campylobacter* gastroenteritis in neonates, *Am J Dis Child* 135:900, 1981.
785. Vesikari T, Huttunen L, Maki R: Perinatal *Campylobacter fetus* ss. *jejuni* enteritis, *Acta Paediatr Scand* 70:261, 1981.
786. Buck GE, Kelly MT, Pichanick AM, et al: *Campylobacter jejuni* in newborns: a cause of asymptomatic bloody diarrhea, *Am J Dis Child* 136:744, 1982.
787. Karmali MA, Norrish B, Lior H, et al: *Campylobacter* enterocolitis in a neonatal nursery, *J Infect Dis* 149:874, 1984.
788. Terrier A, Altwegg M, Bader P, et al: Hospital epidemic of neonatal *Campylobacter jejuni* infection, *Lancet* 2:1182, 1985.
789. Goossens H, Henocque G, Kremp L, et al: Nosocomial outbreak of *Campylobacter jejuni* meningitis in newborn infants, *Lancet* 2:146, 1986.
790. Hershkowici S, Barak M, Cohen A, et al: An outbreak of *Campylobacter jejuni* infection in a neonatal intensive care unit, *J Hosp Infect* 9:54, 1987.
791. Llovo J, Mateo E, Muñoz A, et al: Molecular typing of *Campylobacter jejuni* isolates involved in a neonatal outbreak indicates nosocomial transmission, *J Clin Microbiol* 41:3926, 2003.
792. Figueroa G, Galeno H, Troncoso M, et al: Prospective study of *Campylobacter jejuni* infection in Chilean infants evaluated by culture and serology, *Infect Immun* 27:1040, 1989.
793. Rao MR, Naficy AB, Savarino SJ, Abu-elyazeed R, Wierzba TF, et al: Pathogenicity and convalescent excretion of *Campylobacter* in rural Egyptian, children, *Am J Epidemiol* 154:166, 2001.
794. Gribble MJ, Salit IE, Isaac-Renton J, et al: *Campylobacter* infections in pregnancy: case report and literature review, *Am J Obstet Gynecol* 140:423, 1981.
795. Morooka T, Umeda A, Fujita M, et al: Epidemiologic application of pulsed-field gel electrophoresis to an outbreak of *Campylobacter fetus* meningitis in a neonatal intensive care unit, *Scand J Infect Dis* 28:269, 1996.
796. Darling WM, Peel RN, Skirrow MB: *Campylobacter* cholecystitis, *Lancet* 1:1302, 1979.
797. Davis JS, Penfold JB: *Campylobacter* urinary tract infection, *Lancet* 1:1091, 1979.
798. Kuroki S, Haruta T, Yoshioka M, et al: Guillain-Barré syndrome associated with *Campylobacter* infection, *Pediatr Infect Dis J* 10:149, 1991.
799. Perlman DM, Ampel NM, Schifman RB, et al: Persistent *Campylobacter jejuni* infections in patients infected with human immunodeficiency virus (HIV), *Ann Intern Med* 108:540, 1988.
800. Rettig PJ: *Campylobacter* infections in human beings, *J Pediatr* 94:855, 1979.
801. Chiu CH, Kuo CY, Ou JT: Chronic diarrhea and bacteremia caused by *Campylobacter lari* in a neonate, *Clin Infect Dis* 21:700, 1995.
802. Maki M, Maki R, Vesikari T: Fecal leucocytes in *Campylobacter*-associated diarrhoea in infants, *Acta Paediatr Scand* 68:271, 1979.

803. Lambert ME, Schofield PF, Ironside AG, et al: *Campylobacter* colitis, *Br Med J* 1:857, 1979.
804. Blaser MJ, Parsons RB, Wang WL: Acute colitis caused by *Campylobacter fetus* spp. *jejuni*, *Gastroenterology* 78:448, 1980.
805. King EO: The laboratory recognition of *Vibrio fetus* and a closely related *Vibrio* isolated from cases of human vibriosis, *Ann N Y Acad Sci* 78:700, 1962.
806. Endtz HP, Ruijs GJ, Zwinderman AH, et al: Comparison of six media, including a semisolid agar for the isolation of various *Campylobacter* species from stool specimens, *J Clin Microbiol* 29:1007, 1991.
807. Granato PA, Chen L, Holiday I, et al: Comparison of premier CAMPY enzyme immunoassay (EIA), ProSpecT *Campylobacter* EIA, and ImmunoCard STAT! CAMPY tests with culture for laboratory diagnosis of *Campylobacter* enteric infections, *J Clin Microbiol* 48:4022, 2010.
808. Paisley JW, Mirrett S, Lauer BA, et al: Darkfield microscopy of human feces for presumptive diagnosis of *Campylobacter fetus* subsp. *jejuni* enteritis, *J Clin Microbiol* 15:61, 1982.
809. Harvey SM, Greenwood JR: Relationships among catalase-positive campylobacters determined by deoxyribonucleic acid-deoxyribonucleic acid hybridization, *Int J Syst Bacteriol* 33:275, 1983.
810. Owen RJ: Nucleic acids in the classification of campylobacters, *Eur J Clin Microbiol* 2:367, 1983.
811. Oyofo BA, Thornton SA, Burr DH, et al: Specific detection of *Campylobacter jejuni* and *Campylobacter coli* by using polymerase chain reaction, *J Clin Microbiol* 30:2613, 1992.
812. Eberle KN, Kiess AS: Phenotypic and genotypic methods for typing *Campylobacter jejuni* and *Campylobacter coli* in poultry, *Poult Sci* 91:255, 2012.
813. Ahmed MU, Dunn L, Ivanova EP: Evaluation of current molecular approaches for genotyping of *Campylobacter jejuni* strains, *Foodborne Pathog Dis* 9:375, 2012.
814. Salazar-Lindo E, Sack RB, Chea-Woo E, et al: Early treatment with erythromycin of *Campylobacter jejuni* associated dysentery in children, *J Pediatr* 109:355, 1986.
815. Kiehlbauch JA, Baker CN, Wachsmuth IK: In vitro susceptibilities of aerotolerant *Campylobacter* isolates to 22 antimicrobial agents, *Antimicrob Agents Chemother* 36:717, 1992.
816. LaChance N, et al: Susceptibilities of β-lactamase-positive and -negative strains of *Campylobacter coli* to β-lactam agents, *Antimicrob Agents Chemother* 37:1174, 1993.
817. Iovine NM: Resistance mechanisms in *Campylobacter jejuni*, *Virulence* 4:230, 2013.
818. Rautelin H, Renkonen OV, Kosunen TU: Azithromycin resistance in *Campylobacter jejuni* and *Campylobacter coli*, *Eur J Clin Microbiol Infect Dis* 12:864, 1993.
819. Endtz HP, Broeren M, Mouton RP: In vitro susceptibility of quinolone-resistant *Campylobacter jejuni* to new macrolide antibiotics, *Eur J Clin Microbiol Infect Dis* 12:48, 1993.
820. Salazar-Lindo E, Sack RB, Chea-Woo E, et al: Early treatment with erythromycin of *Campylobacter jejuni* associated dysentery in children, *J Pediatr* 109:355, 1986.
821. Dronda F, García-Arata I, Navas E, et al: Meningitis in adults due to *Campylobacter fetus* subspecies *fetus*, *Clin Infect Dis* 27:906, 1998.
822. Nachamkin I, Fischer SH, Yang XH, et al: Immunoglobulin A antibodies directed against *Campylobacter jejuni* flagellin present in breast-milk, *Epidemiol Infect* 112:359, 1994.
823. Jagusztyn-Krynicka EK, Łaniewski P, Wyszyńska A: Update on *Campylobacter jejuni* vaccine development for preventing human campylobacteriosis, *Expert Rev Vaccines* 8:625, 2009.
824. Garcia AB, Bahrndorff S, Hald B, et al: Design and data analysis of experimental trials to test vaccine candidates against zoonotic pathogens in animals: the case of a clinical trial against *Campylobacter* in broilers, *Expert Rev Vaccines* 11:1179, 2012.
825. Borriello SP, Davies HA, Kamiya S, et al: Virulence factors of *Clostridium difficile*, *Rev Infect Dis* 12:S185, 1990.
826. Wren BW: Molecular characterisation of *Clostridium difficile* toxins A and B, *Rev Med Microbiol* 3:21, 1992.
827. Jangi S, Lamont JT: Asymptomatic colonization by *Clostridium difficile* in infants: implications for disease in later life, *J Pediatr Gastroenterol Nutr* 51:2, 2010.
828. Kelly CP, LaMont JT: *Clostridium difficile*—more difficult than ever, *N Engl J Med* 359:1932, 2008.
829. Tabaqchali S: Epidemiologic markers of *Clostridium difficile*, *Rev Infect Dis* 12:S192, 1990.
830. Kim KH, Fekety R, Batts DH, et al: Isolation of *C difficile* from the environment and contacts of patients with antibiotic-associated colitis, *J Infect Dis* 143:42, 1981.
831. Sheretz RJ, Sarubb FA: The prevalence of *C difficile* and toxin in a nursery population: a comparison between patients with necrotizing enterocolitis and an asymptomatic group, *J Pediatr* 100:435, 1982.
832. Clabots CR, Johnson S, Olson MM, et al: Acquisition of *Clostridium difficile* by hospitalized patients: evidence for colonized new admissions as a source of infection, *J Infect Dis* 166:561, 1992.
833. Bliss DZ, Johnson S, Savik K, et al: Acquisition of *Clostridium difficile* and *Clostridium difficile*-associated diarrhea in hospitalized patients receiving tube feeding, *Ann Intern Med* 129:1012, 1998.
834. Jernigan JA, Siegman-Igra Y, Guerrant RC, et al: A randomized crossover study of disposable thermometers for prevention of *Clostridium difficile* and other nosocomial infections, *Infect Control Hosp Epidemiol* 19:494, 1998.
835. Johnson S, Gerding DN, Olson MM, et al: Prospective controlled study of vinyl glove use to interrupt *Clostridium difficile* transmission, *Am J Med* 88:137, 1990.
836. Johnson S, Gerding DN: *Clostridium difficile*-associated diarrhea, *Clin Infect Dis* 26:1027, 1998.
837. Fekety R, Shah AB: Diagnosis and treatment of *Clostridium difficile* colitis, *JAMA* 269:71, 1993.
838. Hafiz S, Oakley CL: Clostridium difficile: isolation and characterisitics, *J Med Microbiol* 9:129, 1976.
839. Donta ST, Myers MG: *C difficile* toxin in asymptomatic neonates, *J Pediatr* 100:431, 1982.
840. Al-Jumaili I, Shibley M, Lishman AH, et al: Incidence and origin of *C difficile* in neonates, *J Clin Microbiol* 19:77, 1984.
841. Welch DF, Marks MT: Is *C difficile* pathogenic in infants? *J Pediatr* 100:393, 1982.
842. Donta ST, Stuppy MS, Myers MG: Neonatal antibiotic-associated colitis, *Am J Dis Child* 135:181, 1981.
843. Lyerly DM, Neville LM, Evans DT, et al: Multicenter evaluation of the *Clostridium difficile* TOX A/B TEST, *J Clin Microbiol* 36:184, 1998.
844. Kato H, Kato N, Watanabe K, et al: Identification of toxin A-negative, toxin B-positive *Clostridium difficile* by PCR, *J Clin Microbiol* 36, 1998. 2178.
845. Rafferty ME, Baltch AL, Smith RP, et al: Comparison of restriction enzyme analysis, arbitrarily primed PCR, and protein profile analysis typing for epidemiologic investigation of an ongoing *Clostridium difficile* outbreak, *J Clin Microbiol* 36:2957, 1998.
846. McCollum DL, Rodriguez JM: Detection, treatment, and prevention of *Clostridium difficile* infection, *Clin Gastroenterol Hepatol* 10:581, 2012.
847. Hyams JS, Berman MM, Helgason H: Nonantibiotic-associated enterocolitis caused by *Clostridium difficile* in an infant, *J Pediatr* 99:750, 1981.
848. Wenisch C, Parschalk B, Hasenhündl M, et al: Comparison of vancomycin, teicoplanin, metronidazole, and fusidic acid for the treatment of *Clostridium difficile*-associated diarrhea, *Clin Infect Dis* 22:813, 1996.
849. Wada N, Nishida N, Iwaki S, et al: Neutralizing activity against *C difficile* toxin in the supernatants of cultures of colostral cells, *Infect Immun* 29:545, 1980.
850. Dallas S, Rolfe R: Binding of *Clostridium difficile* toxin A to human milk secretory component, *J Med Microbiol* 47:879, 1998.
851. Kim K, Pickering LK, DuPont HL, et al: In vitro and in vivo neutralizing activity of *C difficile* purified toxins A and B by human colostrum and milk, *J Infect Dis* 150:57, 1984.
852. Weber DJ, Anderson DJ, Sexton DJ, et al: Role of the environment in the transmission of *Clostridium difficile* in health care facilities, *Am J Infect Control* 41:S105, 2013.
853. Goldenberg JZ, Ma SS, Saxton JD, et al: Probiotics for the prevention of *Clostridium difficile*-associated diarrhea in adults and children, *Cochrane Database Syst Rev* (5): CD006095, 2013.
854. Levine WC, Griffin PM, Coast Gulf, *Vibrio* Working Group: *Vibrio* infections on the Gulf Coast: results of first year of regional surveillance, *J Infect Dis* 167:479, 1993.
855. Glass RI, Libel M, Brandling-Bennett AD: Epidemic cholera in the Americas, *Science* 256:1524, 1992.
856. Harris JB, LaRocque RC, Qadri F, et al: Cholera, *Lancet* 379:2466, 2012.

857. Swerdlow DL, Ries AA: Cholera in the Americas: guidelines for the clinician, *JAMA* 267:1495, 1992.
858. Siddique AK, Zaman K, Akram K, et al: Emergence of a new epidemic strain of *Vibrio cholerae* in Bangladesh: an epidemiological study, *Trop Geogr Med* 46:147, 1994.
859. Fisher-Hoch SP, Khan A, Inam-ul-Haq, et al: *Vibrio cholerae* O139 in Karachi, Pakistan, *Lancet* 342:1422, 1993.
860. Chongsa-Nguan M, Chaicumpa W, Moolasart P, et al: *Vibrio cholerae* O139 Bengal in Bangkok, *Lancet* 342:430, 1993.
861. Cholera Working Group, International Centre for Diarrhoeal Diseases Research: Bangladesh Large epidemic of cholera-like disease in Bangladesh caused by *Vibrio cholerae* O139 synonym Bengal, *Lancet* 342:387, 1993.
862. Blake PA, Allegra DT, Snyder JD, et al: Cholera—a possible endemic focus in the United States, *N Engl J Med* 302:305, 1980.
863. Sethi NK, Sethi SK: *Vibrio cholerae* diarrhoea in a three-day-old breastfed neonate, *Indian J Pediatr* 68:791, 2001.
864. Khan AM, Faruque AS, Hossain MS: Isolation of *Vibrio cholerae* from neonates admitted to an urban diarrhoeal diseases hospital in Bangladesh, *Ann Trop Paediatr* 25:179, 2005.
865. Khan AM, Hossain MS, Khan AI, et al: Bacterial enteropathogens of neonates admitted to an urban diarrhoeal hospital in Bangladesh, *J Trop Pediatr* 2009(55):122, 2009.
866. Hirschhorn N, Chowdhury A, Lindenbaum J: Cholera in pregnant women, *Lancet* 1:1230, 1969.
867. Haider R, Kabir I, Fuchs GJ, et al: Neonatal diarrhea in a diarrhea treatment center in Bangladesh: clinical presentation, breastfeeding management and outcome, *Indian Pediatr* 37:37, 2000.
868. Gunn RA, Kimball AM, Pollard RA, et al: Bottle feeding as a risk factor for cholera in infants, *Lancet* 2:730, 1979.
869. Merson MH, Black RE, Sack DA, et al: Maternal cholera immunisation and secretory IgA in breast milk, *Lancet* 1:931, 1980.
870. Cash RA, Music SI, Libonati JP, et al: Response of man to infection with *Vibrio cholerae* I. Clinical, serologic and bacteriologic responses to a known inoculum, *J Infect Dis* 129:45, 1974.
871. Yam WC, Lung ML, Ng MH: Evaluation and optimization of a latex agglutination assay for detection of cholera toxin and *Escherichia coli* heat-labile toxin, *J Clin Microbiol* 30:2518, 1992.
872. Hasan JA, Huq A, Tamplin ML, et al: A novel kit for rapid detection of *Vibrio cholerae* O1, *J Clin Microbiol* 32:249, 1994.
873. Bhuiyan NA, Qadri F, Faruque AS, et al: Use of dipsticks for rapid diagnosis of cholera caused by *Vibrio cholerae* O1 and O139 from rectal swabs, *J Clin Microbiol* 41:3939, 2003.
874. Yoh M, Miyagi K, Matsumoto Y, et al: Development of an enzyme-labeled oligonucleotide probe for the cholera toxin gene, *J Clin Microbiol* 31:1312, 1993.
875. Dick MH, Guillerm M, Moussy F, et al: Review of two decades of cholera diagnostics—how far have we really come? *PLoS Negl Trop Dis* 6:e1845, 2012.
876. von Seidlein L, Jiddawi M, Grais RF, et al: The value of and challenges for cholera vaccines in Africa, *J Infect Dis* 208(Suppl 1):S8, 2013.
877. Fabrega A, Vila J: *Yersinia enterocolitica*: pathogenesis, virulence and antimicrobial resistance, *Enferm Infecc Microbiol Clin* 30:24, 2012.
878. Kapperud G, Namork E, Skurnik M, et al: Plasmid-mediated surface fibrillae of *Y pseudotuberculosis* and *Y enterocolitica*: relationship to the outer membrane protein YOP1 and possible importance for pathogenesis, *Infect Immun* 55:2247, 1987.
879. Brubaker RR: Factors promoting acute and chronic diseases caused by yersiniae, *Clin Microbiol Rev* 4:309, 1991.
880. Takao T, Tominaga N, Shimonishi Y, et al: Primary structure of heat-stable enterotoxin produced by *Y enterocolitica*, *Biochem Biophys Res Commun* 125:845, 1984.
881. Ong KL, Gould LH, Chen DL, et al: Changing epidemiology of *Yersinia enterocolitica* infections: markedly decreased rates in young black children, Foodborne Diseases Active Surveillance Network (FoodNet), 1996-2009, *Clin Infect Dis* 54(Suppl 5):S385, 2012.
882. Pietersz RNI, Reesink HW, Pauw W, et al: Prevention of *Yersinia enterocolitica* growth in red blood cell concentrates, *Lancet* 340:755, 1992.
883. Lee LA, Gerber AR, Lonsway DR, et al: *Yersinia enterocolitica* O:3 infections in infants and children, associated with the household preparation of chitterlings, *N Engl J Med* 322:984, 1990.
884. Lee LA, Taylor J, Carter GP, et al: *Yersinia enterocolitica* O:3: an emerging cause of pediatric gastroenteritis in the United States, *J Infect Dis* 163:660, 1991.
885. Morris JG Jr, Prado V, Ferreccio C, et al: *Yersinia enterocolitica* isolated from two cohorts of young children in Santiago, Chile: incidence of and lack of correlation between illness and proposed virulence factors, *J Clin Microbiol* 29:2784, 1991.
886. Metchock B, Lonsway DR, Carter GP, et al: *Yersinia enterocolitica*: a frequent seasonal stool isolate from children at an urban hospital in the southeast United States, *J Clin Microbiol* 29:2868, 1991.
887. Thompson EC: *Yersinia enterocolitica* sepsis in a 3-week-old child, *J Natl Med Assoc* 86:783, 1994.
888. Paisley JW, Lauer BA: Neonatal *Yersinia enterocolitica* enteritis, *Pediatr Infect Dis J* 11:331, 1992.
889. Challapalli M, Cunningham DG: *Yersinia enterocolitica* septicemia in infants younger than three months of age, *Pediatr Infect Dis J* 12:168, 1993.
890. Antonio-Santiago MT, Kaul A, Lue Y, et al: *Yersinia enterocolitica* septicemia in an infant presenting as fever of unknown origin, *Clin Pediatr* 25:213, 1986.
891. Sutton JM, Pasquariell PS: *Yersinia enterocolitica* septicemia in a normal child, *Am J Dis Child* 137:305, 1983.
892. Kohl S, Jacobson JA, Nahmias A: *Yersinia enterocolitica* infections in children, *J Pediatr* 89:77, 1976.
893. Townes JM, Deodhar AA, Laine ES, et al: Reactive arthritis following culture-confirmed infections with bacterial enteric pathogens in Minnesota and Oregon: a population-based study, *Ann Rheum Dis* 67:1689, 2008.
894. Wiemer D, Loderstaedt U, von Wulffen H, et al: Real-time multiplex PCR for simultaneous detection of *Campylobacter jejuni, Salmonella, Shigella* and *Yersinia* species in fecal samples, *Int J Med Microbiol* 301:577, 2011.
895. Ayyadurai S, Flaudrops C, Raoult D, et al: Rapid identification and typing of *Yersinia pestis* and other *Yersinia* species by matrix-assisted laser desorption/ionization time-of-flight (MALDI-TOF) mass spectrometry, *BMC Microbiol* 10:285, 2010.
896. Stolk-Engelaar VM, Meis JF, Mulder JA, et al: In-vitro antimicrobial susceptibility of *Yersinia enterocolitica* isolates from stools of patients in the Netherlands from 1982-1991, *J Antimicrob Chemother* 36:839, 1995.
897. Alzugaray R, Gonzalez Hevia MA, Landeras E, et al: *Yersinia enterocolitica* O:3: antimicrobial resistance patterns, virulence profiles and plasmids, *New Microbiol* 18:215, 1995.
898. Abdel-Haq N, Asmar BI, Abuhammour WM, et al: *Yersinia enterocolitica* infection in children, *Pediatr Infect Dis J* 19:954, 2000.
899. Janda J, Abbott S: The genus *Aeromonas*: taxonomy, pathogenicity, and infection, *Clin Microbiol Rev* 23:35, 2010.
900. Abbott L, Cheung W, Janda J: The genus *Aeromonas*: biochemical characteristics, atypical reactions, and phenotypic identification schemes, *J Clin Microbiol* 41:2348, 2003.
901. Kirov S, Castrisios M, Shaw J: *Aeromonas* flagella (polar and lateral) are enterocyte adhesins that contribute to biofilm formation on surfaces, *Infect Immun* 72:1939, 2004.
902. Sha J, Kozlova E, Chopra A: Role of various enterotoxins in *Aeromonas hydrophila*-induced gastroenteritis: generation of enterotoxin gene-deficient mutants and evaluation of their enterotoxic activity, *Infect Immun* 70:1924, 2002.
903. von Graevenitz A: The role of *Aeromonas* in diarrhea: a review, *Infection* 35:59, 2007.
904. McMahon M, Wilson I: The occurrence of enteric pathogens and *Aeromonas* species in organic vegetables, *Int J Food Microbiol* 70:155, 2001.
905. Lamy B, Kodjo A, colBVH Study Group: Prospective nationwide study of *Aeromonasi* in France, *J Clin Microbiol* 47:1234, 2009.
906. Llopis F, Grau I, Tubau F, et al: Epidemiological and clinical characteristics of bacteraemia caused by *Aeromonas* spp. as compared with *Escherichia coli* and Pseudomonas aeruginosa, *Scand J Infect Dis* 36:335, 2004.
907. Figura N, Marri L, Verdiani S, et al: Prevalence, species differentiation, and toxigenicity of *Aeromonas* strains in cases of childhood gastroenteritis and in controls, *J Clin Microbiol* 23:595, 1986.
908. Pazzaglia G, Sack RB, Salazar E, et al: High frequency of coinfecting enteropathogens in *Aeromonas*-associated diarrhea of hospitalized Peruvian infants, *J Clin Microbiol* 29:1151, 1991.

909. von Graevenitz A, Mensch AH: The genus *Aeromonas* in human bacteriology. Report of 30 cases and review of the literature, *N Engl J Med* 278:245, 1968.
910. Pereira CS, Amorim SD, Santos AF, et al: Characterization of *Aeromonas* spp isolates from newborns hospitalized, *Rev Soc Bras Med Trop* 41:179, 2008.
911. Holmberg S, Farmer J: *Aeromonas hydrophila* and *Plesiomonas shigelloides* as causes of intestinal infection, *Rev Infect Dis* 6:633, 1984.
912. Vila J, Ruiz J, Gallardo F, et al: *Aeromonas* spp. and traveler's diarrhea: clinical features and antimicrobial resistance, *Emerg Infect Dis* 9:552, 2003.
913. Sinha S, Shimada T, Ramamurthy T, et al: Prevalence, serotype distribution, antibiotic susceptibility and genetic profiles of mesophilic *Aeromonas* species isolated from hospitalized diarrhoeal cases in Kolkata, India, *J Med Microbiol* 53:527, 2004.
914. Figueras M: Clinical relevance of *Aeromonas* sM503, *Rev Med Microbiol* 16:145, 2005.
915. Chan S, Ng KC, Lyon DJ, et al: Acute bacterial gastroenteritis: a study of adult patients with positive stool cultures treated in the emergency department, *Emerg Med* 20:335, 2003.
916. Figueras M, Aldea MJ, Fernández N, et al: *Aeromonas* hemolytic uremic syndrome. A case and a review of the literature, *Diagn Microbiol Infect Dis* 58:231, 2007.
917. O'Hara C: Evaluation of the Phoenix 100 ID/AST system and NID panel for identification of Enterobacteriaceae, Vibrionaceae, and commonly isolated nonenteric gram-negative bacilli, *J Clin Microbiol* 44:928, 2006.
918. Alperi A, Figueras MJ, Inza I, et al: Analysis of 16S rRNA gene mutations in a subset of *Aeromonas* strains and their impact in species delineation, *Int Microbiol* 11:185, 2008.
919. Kupfer M, Kuhnert P, Korczak BM, et al: Genetic relationships of *Aeromonas* strains inferred from 16S rRNA, *gyrB* and *rpoB* gene sequences, *Int J Syst Evol Microbiol* 56:2743, 2006.
920. Holmberg SD, Wachsmuth IK, Hickman-Brenner FW, et al: *Plesiomonas* enteric infections in the United States, *Ann Intern Med* 105:690, 1986.
921. Tsukamoto T, Kinoshita Y, Shimada T, et al: Two epidemics of diarrhoeal disease possibly caused by *P shigelloides*, *J Hyg* 80:275, 1978.
922. Holmberg SD, Farmer JJ: A. hydrophila and *P shigelloides* as causes of intestinal infections, *Rev Infect Dis* 6:633, 1984.
923. Herrington DA, Tzipori S, Robins-Browne RM, et al: In vitro and in vivo pathogenicity of *P shigelloides*, *Infect Immun* 55:979, 1987.
924. Brenden RA, Miller MA, Janda JM: Clinical disease spectrum and pathogenic factors associated with *P shigelloides* infections in humans, *Rev Infect Dis* 10:303, 1988.
925. Pathak A, Custer JR, Levy J: Neonatal septicemia and meningitis due to *Plesiomonas shigelloides*, *Pediatrics* 71:389, 1983.
926. Fujita K, Shirai M, Ishioka T, et al: Neonatal *Plesiomonas shigelloides* septicemia and meningitis: a case review, *Acta Paediatr Jpn* 36:450, 1994.
927. Terpeluk C, Goldmann A, Bartmann P, et al: *Plesiomonas shigelloides* sepsis and meningoencephalitis in a neonate, *Eur J Pediatr* 151:499, 1992.
928. Billiet J, Kuypers S, Van Lierde S, et al: *Plesiomonas shigelloides* meningitis and septicaemia in a neonate: report of a case and review of the literature, *J Infect* 19:267, 1989.
929. Ozdemir O, Sari S, Terzioglu S, et al: *Plesiomonas shigelloides* sepsis and meningoencephalitis in a surviving neonate, *J Microbiol Immunol Infect* 43:344, 2010.
930. Alabi SA, Odugbemi T: Biochemical characteristics and a simple scheme for the identification of *Aeromonas* species and *Plesiomonas shigelloides*, *J Trop Med Hyg* 93:166, 1990.
931. Reinhardt JF, George WL: Comparative in vitro activities of selected antimicrobial agents against *Aeromonas* species *and P shigelloides*, *Antimicrob Agents Chemother* 27:643, 1985.
932. Visitsunthorn N, Komolpis P: Antimicrobial therapy in *Plesiomonas shigelloides*–associated diarrhea in Thai children, *Southeast Asian J Trop Med Public Health* 26:86, 1995.
933. Heitmann M, Gerner-Smidt P, Heltberg O: Gastroenteritis caused by *Listeria monocytogenes* in a private day-care facility, *Pediatr Infect Dis J* 16:827, 1997.
934. Sim J, Hood D, Finnie L, et al: Series of incidents of *Listeria monocytogenes* non-invasive febrile gastroenteritis involving ready-to-eat meats, *Lett Appl Microbiol* 35:409, 2002.
935. Schlech W: *Listeria* gastroenteritis—old syndrome, new pathogen, *N Engl J Med* 336:130, 1997.
936. Wing E, Gregory S: *Listeria monocytogenes*: clinical and experimental update, *J Infect Dis* 185:S18, 2002.
937. Aureli P, Fiorucci GC, Caroli D, et al: An outbreak of febrile gastroenteritis associated with corn contaminated by *Listeria monocytogenes*, *N Engl J Med* 342:1236, 2000.
938. Dalton C, Austin CC, Sobel J, et al: An outbreak of gastroenteritis and fever due to *Listeria monocytogenes* in milk, *N Engl J Med* 336:100, 1997.
939. Hof H, Lampidis R, Bensch J: Nosocomial *Listeria gastroenteritis* in a newborn, confirmed by random amplification of polymorphic DNA, *Clin Microbiol Infect* 6:683, 2000.
940. Larsson S, Cederberg A, Ivarsson S, et al: *Listeria monocytogenes* causing hospital-acquired enterocolitis and meningitis in newborn infants, *Br Med J* 2:473, 1978.
941. Edelbroek M, De Nef J, Rajnherc J: *Listeria* meningitis presenting as enteritis in a previously healthy infant: a case report, *Eur J Pediatr* 153:179, 1994.
942. Walcher DN: "*Bacillus mucosus capsulatus*" in infantile diarrhea, *J Clin Invest* 25:103, 1946.
943. Cass JM: *Bacillus lactis aerogenes* infection in the newborn, *Lancet* 1:346, 1941.
944. Sternberg SD, Hoffman C, Zweifler BM: Stomatitis and diarrhea in infants caused by *Bacillus mucosus capsulatus*, *J Pediatr* 38:509, 1951.
945. Worfel MT, Ferguson WW: A new *Klebsiella* type (capsular type 15) isolated from feces and urine, *Am J Clin Pathol* 21:1097, 1951.
946. Simmons BP, Gelfand MS, Haas M, et al: *Enterobacter sakazakii* infections in neonates associated with intrinsic contamination of a powdered infant formula. Infect, *Control Hosp Epidemiol* 10:398, 1989.
947. Ayliffe GAJ, Collins BJ, Pettit F: Contamination of infant feeds in a Milton milk kitchen, *Lancet* 1:559, 1970.
948. Adler JL, Shulman JA, Terry PM, et al: Nosocomial colonization with kanamycin-resistant *Klebsiella pneumoniae*, types 2 and 11, in a premature nursery, *J Pediatr* 77:376, 1970.
949. Hill HR, Hunt CE, Matsen JM: Nosocomial colonization with *Klebsiella*, type 16, in a neonatal intensive-care unit associated with an outbreak of sepsis, meningitis, and necrotizing enterocolitis, *J Pediatr* 85:415, 1974.
950. Panigrahi D, Roy P, Chakrabarti A: Enterotoxigenic *Klebsiella pneumoniae* in acute childhood diarrhea, *Indian J Med Res* 93:293, 1991.
951. Guarino A, Capano G, Malamisura B, et al: Production of *E. coli* STa-like heat stable enterotoxin by *Citrobacter freundii* isolated from humans, *J Clin Microbiol* 25:110, 1987.
952. Lipsky BA, Hook 3rd EW, Smith AA, et al: *Citrobacter* infections in humans: experience at the Seattle Veterans Administration Medical Center and a review of the literature, *Rev Infect Dis* 2:746, 1980.
953. Parida SN, Verma IC, Deb M, et al: An outbreak of diarrhea due to *Citrobacter freundii* in a neonatal special care nursery, *Indian J Pediatr* 47:81, 1980.
954. Sack R, Albert MJ, Alam K, et al: Isolation of enterotoxigenic *Bacteroides fragilis* from Bangladeshi children with diarrhea: a controlled study, *J Clin Microbiol* 32:960, 1994.
955. Sack R, Myers LL, Almeido-Hill J, et al: Enterotoxigenic *Bacteroides fragilis*: epidemiologic studies of its role as a human diarrhoeal pathogen, *J Diarrhoeal Dis Res* 10:4, 1992.
956. Kohler H, Kite P: Neonatal enteritis due to *Providencia* organisms, *Arch Dis Child* 45:709, 1970.
957. Ridge LEL, Thomas MEM: Infection with the Providence type of paracolon bacillus in a residential nursery, *J Pathol Bacteriol* 69:335, 1955.
958. Bhat P, Myers RM, Feldman RA: Providence group of organisms in the aetiology of juvenile diarrhoea, *Indian J Med Res* 59:1010, 1971.
959. Bishop RF, Barnes GL, Townley RRW: Microbial flora of stomach and small intestine in infantile gastroenteritis, *Acta Paediatr Scand* 63:418, 1974.
960. Klingspor L, Stitzing G, Johansen K, et al: Infantile diarrhea and malnutrition associated with *Candida* in a developing community, *Mycoses* 36:19, 1993.
961. Chaudhury A, Nath G, Shukla B, et al: Diarrhoea associated with *Candida* spp.: incidence and seasonal variation, *J Diarrhoeal Dis Res* 14:110, 1996.

962. Enweani I, Obi C, Jokpeyibo M: Prevalence of *Candida* species in Nigerian children with diarrhea, *J Diarrhoeal Dis Res* 12:133, 1994.
963. Ponnuvel K, Rajkumar R, Menon T, et al: Role of *Candida* in indirect pathogenesis of antibiotic associated diarrhea in infants, *Mycopathologia* 135:145, 1996.
964. Omoike IU, Abiodun PO: Upper small intestine microflora in diarrhea and malnutrition in Nigerian children, *J Pediatr Gastroenterol Nutr* 9:314, 1989.
965. Kane JG, Chretien JH, Garagusi VF: Diarrhea caused by *Candida*, *Lancet* 1:335, 1976.
966. Hill HR, Mitchell TG, Matsen JM, et al: Recovery from disseminated candidiasis in a premature neonate, *Pediatrics* 53:748, 1974.
967. Faix RG: Systemic *Candida* infections in infants in intensive care nurseries: high incidence of central nervous system involvement, *J Pediatr* 105:616, 1984.
968. Baley JE, Kliegman RM, Fanaroff AA: Disseminated fungal infections in very low birth weight infants: clinical manifestations and epidemiology, *Pediatrics* 73:144, 1984.
969. Struelens MJ, Bennish ML, Mondal G, et al: Bacteremia during diarrhea: incidence, etiology, risk factors, and outcome, *Am J Epidemiol* 133:451, 1991.
970. Pickering LK: Cryptosporidium. In Pickering LK, Baker CJ, Kimberlin DW, Long SS, editors: *Red book: 2012 report of the Committee on Infectious Diseases*, Elk Grove Village, Ill: 2012, American Academy of Pediatrics, p 296.
971. Red book: *Report of the Committee on Infectious Diseases*, Elk Grove Village, Ill, 2012, American Academy of Pediatrics. 2012:296.
972. Rodriguez-García R, Rodríguez-Guzmán LM, Sánchez-Maldonado MI, et al: Prevalence and risk factors associated with intestinal parasitoses in pregnant women and their relation to the infant's birth weight, *Ginecol Obstet Mex* 70:338, 2002.
973. Shimokawa C, Kabir M, Taniuchi M, et al: *Entamoeba moshkovskii* is associated with diarrhea in infants and causes diarrhea and colitis in mice, *J Infect Dis* 206:744, 2012.
974. Guven A: Amebiasis in the newborn, *Indian J Pediatr* 70:437, 2003.
975. Nazir Z, Qazi SH: Amebic liver abscesses among neonates can mimic bacterial sepsis, *Pediatr Infect Dis J* 24:464, 2005.
976. Axton JHM: Amoebic proctocolitis and liver abscess in a neonate, *S Afr Med J* 46:258, 1972.
977. Botman T, Rusy PJ: Amoebic appendicitis in a newborn infant, *Trop Geogr Med* 15:221, 1963.
978. Hsiung CC: Amebiasis of the newborn: report of three cases, *Chin J Pathol* 4:14, 1958.
979. Dykes AC, Ruebush TK 2nd, Gorelkin L, et al: Extraintestinal amebiasis in infancy: report of three patients and epidemiologic investigations of their families, *Pediatrics* 65:799, 1980.
980. Gomez NA, Cozzarelli R, Alvarez LR, et al: Amebic liver abscess in newborn: report of a case, *Acta Gastroenterol Latinoam* 29:115, 1999.
981. Rao S, Solaymani-Mohammadi S, Petri WA Jr, et al: Hepatic amebiasis: a reminder of the complications, *Curr Opin Pediatr* 21:145, 2009.
982. Rennert W, Ray C: Fulminant amebic colitis in a ten-day-old infant, *Arch Pediatr* 4:92, 1997.
983. Magon P: Neonatal amoebiasis, *Indian J Pediatr* 77:903, 2010.
984. Kotcher E, Mata LJ, Esquivel R, Redmond DL: Acquisition of intestinal parasites in newborn human infants, *Fed Proc* 24:442, 1965.
985. Ravdin JI: Amebiasis, *Clin Infect Dis* 20:1453, 1995.
986. Mirelman D, Nuchamowitz Y, Stolarsky T: Comparison of use of enzyme-linked immunosorbent assay-based kits and PCR amplification of rRNA genes for simultaneous detection of *Entamoeba histolytica* and *E dispar*, *J Clin Microbiol* 35:2405, 1997.
987. Haque R, Ali IKM, Petri WA Jr: Comparison of PCR, isoenzyme analysis, and antigen detection for diagnosis of *Entamoeba histolytica* infection, *J Clin Microbiol* 36:449, 1998.
988. Chacín-Bonilla L: Amebiasis: aspectos clínicos, terapéuticos y de diagnóstico de la infección, *Rev Med Chile* 141:609, 2013.
989. ElBakr A, Samie A, Ezzedine S, et al: Differential detection of *Entamoeba histolytica*, *Entamoeba dispar* and *Entamoeba moshkovskii* in fecal samples by nested PCR in the United Arab Emirates (UAE), *Acta Parasitol* 58:185, 2013.
990. Black RE, Dykes AC, Sinclair SP, et al: Giardiasis in day care centers: evidence of person-to-person transmission, *Pediatrics* 60:486, 1977.
991. Keystone JS, Krajden S, Warren MR: Person-to-person transmission of *G lamblia* in day care nurseries, *Can Med Assoc J* 119:241, 1978.
992. Pickering LK, Evans DG, DuPont HL, et al: Diarrhea caused by *Shigella*, rotavirus, and *Giardia* in day care centers: prospective study, *J Pediatr* 99:51, 1981.
993. Pickering LK, Woodward WE, DuPont HL, et al: Occurrence of *G lamblia* in children in day care centers, *J Pediatr* 104:522, 1984.
994. Coles CL, Levy A, Dagan R, Deckelbaum RJ, Fraser D: Risk factors for the initial symptomatic *Giardia* infection in a cohort of young Arab-Bedouin children, *Ann Trop Paediatr* 29:291, 2009.
995. Kotloff KL, Nataro JP, Blackwelder WC, et al: Burden and aetiology of diarrhoeal disease in infants and young children in developing countries (the Global Enteric Multicenter Study, GEMS): a prospective, case-control study, *Lancet* 382:209, 2013.
996. Muhsen K, Levine MM: A systematic review and meta-analysis of the association between *Giardia lamblia* and endemic pediatric diarrhea in developing countries, *Clin Infect Dis* 55:S271, 2012.
997. Randremanana R, Randrianirina F, Gousseff M, et al: Case-control study of the etiology of infant diarrheal disease in 14 districts in Madagascar, *PLoS One* 7:e44533, 2012.
998. Haque R, Mondal D, Karim A, et al: Prospective case-control study of the association between common enteric protozoal parasites and diarrhea in Bangladesh, *Clin Infect Dis* 48:1191, 2009.
999. Aguiar A, Saraiva S, Pontes M, et al: Eosinophilia in a newborn: a case of giardiasis and milk allergy, *Acta Med Port* 24:463, 2011.
1000. Miotti PG, Gilman RH, Santosham M, et al: Age-related rate of seropositivity and antibody to *Giardia lamblia* in four diverse populations, *J Clin Microbiol* 24:972, 1986.
1001. Islam A, Stoll BJ, Ljungström I, et al: *Giardia lamblia* infections in a cohort of Bangladeshi mothers and infants followed for one year, *J Pediatr* 103:996, 1983.
1002. Adam RD: The biology of *Giardia* spp, *Microbiol Rev* 55:706, 1991.
1003. Pickering LK, Engelkirk PG: Giardia lamblia, *Pediatr Clin North Am* 35:565, 1988.
1004. Elsafi SH, Al-Maqati TN, Hussein MI, et al: Comparison of microscopy, rapid immunoassay, and molecular techniques for the detection of *Giardia lamblia* and *Cryptosporidium parvum*. *Parasitol Res* 112:1641, 2013.
1005. Gendrel D, Richard-Lenoble D, Kombila M, et al: Giardiasis and breastfeeding in urban Africa, *Pediatr Infect Dis J* 8:58, 1989.
1006. Stevens DP, Frank DM: Local immunity in murine giardiasis: is milk protective at the expense of maternal gut? *Trans Assoc Am Physicians* 91:268, 1978.
1007. Andrews JS Jr, Hewlett EL: Protection against infection with *Giardia muris* by milk containing antibody to *Giardia*, *J Infect Dis* 143:242, 1981.
1008. Rohrer L, Winterhalter KH, Eckert J, et al: Killing of *G lamblia* by human milk mediated by unsaturated fatty acids, *Antimicrob Agents Chemother* 30:254, 1986.
1009. Cohen-Wolkowiez M, Ouellet D, Smith PB, et al: Population pharmacokinetics of metronidazole evaluated using scavenged samples from preterm infants, *Antimicrob Agents Chemother* 56: 1828, 2012.
1010. Current WL, Garcia LS: Cryptosporidiosis, *Clin Microbiol Rev* 4:325, 1991.
1011. Heyworth MF: Immunology of *Giardia* and *Cryptosporidium* infections, *J Infect Dis* 166:465, 1992.
1012. Chalmers RM, Davies AP: Minireview: clinical cryptosporidiosis, *Exp Parasitol* 124:138, 2010.
1013. Chalmers RM, Elwin K, Hadfield SJ, et al: Sporadic human cryptosporidiosis caused by *Cryptosporidium cuniculus*, United Kingdom, 2007-2008, *Emerg Infect Dis* 17:536, 2011.
1014. Tzipori S: Cryptosporidiosis in animals and humans, *Microbiol Rev* 47:84, 1983.
1015. Stehr-Green JK, McCaig L, Remsen HM, et al: Shedding of oocysts in immunocompetent individuals infected with Cryptosporidium, *Am J Trop Med Hyg* 36:338, 1987.
1016. Soave R, Ma P: Cryptosporidiosis travelers'diarrhea in two families, *Arch Intern Med* 145:70, 1985.
1017. Collier AC, Miller RA, Meyers JD: Cryptosporidiosis after marrow transplantation, person-to-person transmission and treatment with spiramycin, *Ann Intern Med* 101:205, 1984.

1018. Navin TR: Cryptosporidiosis in humans: review of recent epidemiologic studies, *Eur J Epidemiol* 1:77, 1985.
1019. Alpert G, Bell LM, Kirkpatrick CE, et al: Outbreak of cryptosporidiosis in a day care center, *Pediatrics* 77:152, 1986.
1020. Taylor JP, Perdue JN, Dingley D, et al: Cryptosporidiosis outbreak in a day care center, *Am J Dis Child* 139:1023, 1986.
1021. Hoxie NJ, Davis JP, Vergeront JM, et al: Cryptosporidiosis-associated mortality following a massive waterborne outbreak in Milwaukee, Wisconsin, *Am J Public Health* 87:2032, 1997.
1022. Yoder JS, Harral C, Beach MJ: Centers for Disease Control and Prevention: Cryptosporidiosis surveillance—United States, 2006-2008, *MMWR Surveill Summ* 11:1, 2010.
1023. Jokipii L, Pohiola S, Jokipii AM: *Cryptosporidium*: a frequent finding in patients with gastrointestinal symptoms, *Lancet* 2:358, 1983.
1024. Current WL, Reese NC, Ernst JV, et al: Human cryptosporidiosis in immunocompetent and immunodeficient persons: studies of an outbreak and experimental transmission, *N Engl J Med* 308:1252, 1983.
1025. Haque R, Mondal D, Karim A, et al: Prospective case-control study of the association between common enteric protozoal parasites and diarrhea in Bangladesh, *Clin Infect Dis* 48:1191, 2009.
1026. Enriquez FJ, Avila CR, Ignacio Santos J, et al: *Cryptosporidium* infections in Mexican children: clinical, nutritional, enteropathogenic, and diagnostic evaluations, *Am J Trop Med Hyg* 56:254, 1997.
1027. Mata L, Bolaños H, Pizarro D, et al: Cryptosporidiosis in children from some highland Costa Rican rural and urban areas, *Am J Trop Med Hyg* 33:24, 1984.
1028. Jokipii L, Jokipii AMM: Timing of symptoms and oocyst excretion in human cryptosporidiosis, *N Engl J Med* 313:1643, 1986.
1029. Sallon S, Deckelbaum RJ, Schmid II , et al: *Cryptosporidium*, malnutrition and chronic diarrhea in children, *Am J Dis Child* 142:312, 1988.
1030. Garcia LS, Shimizu RY: Evaluation of nine immunoassay kits (enzyme immunoassay and direct fluorescence) for detection of *Giardia lamblia* and *Cryptosporidium parvum* in human fecal specimens, *J Clin Microbiol* 35:1526, 1997.
1031. MacPherson DW, McQueen R: Cryptosporidiosis: multiattribute evaluation of six diagnostic methods, *J Clin Microbiol* 31:198, 1993.
1032. ten Hove R, Schuurman T, Kooistra M, et al: Detection of diarrhoea-causing protozoa in general practice patients in The Netherlands by multiplex real-time PCR, *Clin Microbiol Infect* 13:1001, 2007.
1033. Taniuchi M, Verweij JJ, Noor Z, et al: High throughput multiplex PCR and probe-based detection with Luminex beads for seven intestinal parasites, *Am J Trop Med Hyg* 84:332, 2011.
1034. Rossignol FJ, Ayoub A, Ayers MS: Treatment of diarrhea caused by *Cryptosporidium parvum*: a prospective of randomized, double-blind, placebo-controlled study of nitazoxanide, *J Infect Dis* 184:103, 2001.
1035. Agnew DG, Lima AA, Newman RD, et al: Cryptosporidiosis in northeastern Brazilian children: association with increased diarrhea morbidity, *J Infect Dis* 177:754, 1998.
1036. Pollock K, Young D, Smith HV, et al: Cryptosporidiosis and filtration of water from Loch Lomond, Scotland, *Emerg Infect Dis* 14:115, 2008.
1037. Cheng WX, Jin Y, Duan ZJ, et al: Human bocavirus in children hospitalized for acute gastroenteritis: a case-control study, *Clin Infect Dis* 47:161, 2008.
1038. Matson DO, O'Ryan ML, Jiang X, et al: Rotavirus, enteric adenoviruses, caliciviruses, astroviruses, and other viruses causing gastroenteritis. In Spector S, Hodinka RL, Young SA, editors: *Clinical virology manual*, ed 3, Washington, DC, 2000, American Society for Microbiology Press, p 270.
1039. Kapikian AZ, Chanock RM: Rotaviruses. In Fields BN, editor: *Fields virology*, ed 3, Philadelphia, 1996, Lippincott-Raven Press, p 1657.
1040. Estes MK: Rotaviruses and their replication. In Fields BN, editor: *Fields virology*, ed 3, Philadelphia, 1996, Lippincott-Raven Press, p 1625.
1041. Wilhelmi I, Roman E, Sanchez-Fauquier A: Viruses causing gastroenteritis, *Clin Microbiol Infect* 9:247, 2003.
1042. Ramani S, Kang G: Viruses causing childhood diarrhoea in the developing world, *Curr Opin Infect Dis* 22:477, 2009.
1043. Bridger JC: Non-group A rotavirus. In Farthing M, editor: *Viruses in the gut*, Welwyn Garden City, UK, 1988, Smith Kline & French, p 79.
1044. Desselberger U: Molecular epidemiology of rotavirus. In Farthing M, editor: *Viruses in the gut*, Welwyn Garden City, UK, 1988, Smith Kline & French, p 55.
1045. Hoshino Y, Saif LJ, Sereno MM: Infection immunity of piglets to either VP3 or VP7 outer capsid protein confers resistance to challenge with a virulent rotavirus bearing the corresponding antigen, *J Virol* 62:74, 1988.
1046. Offit PA, Clark HF, Blavat G: Reassortant rotavirus containing structural proteins VP3 and VP7 from different parents are protective against each parental strain, *J Virol* 57:376, 1986.
1047. Zhou Y, Li L, Okitsu S, et al: Distribution of human rotaviruses, especially G9 strains, in Japan from 1996 to 2000, *Microbiol Immunol* 47:591, 2003.
1048. O'Ryan ML, Matson DO, Estes MK, et al: Molecular epidemiology of rotavirus in children attending day care centers in Houston, *J Infect Dis* 162:810, 1990.
1049. Hyser JM, Estes MK: Rotavirus vaccines and pathogenesis: 2008, *Curr Opin Gastroenterol* 25:36, 2009.
1050. Santos N, Hoshino Y: Global distribution of rotavirus serotypes/genotypes and its implication for the development and implementation of an effective rotavirus vaccine, *Rev Med Virol* 5:29, 2005.
1051. Ndze VN, Papp H, Achidi EA, et al: One year survey of human rotavirus strains suggests the emergence of genotype G12 in Cameroon, *J Med Virol* 85:1485, 2013.
1052. Kilgore P, Unicomb LE, Gentsch JR, et al: Neonatal rotavirus infection in Bangladesh strain characterization and risk factors for nosocomial infection, *Pediatr Infect Dis J* 15:672, 1996.
1053. Tam JS, Zheng BJ, Lo SK, et al: Distinct populations of rotaviruses circulating among neonates and older infants, *J Clin Microbiol* 28:1033, 1990.
1054. Jain V, Parashar UD, Glass RI, et al: Epidemiology of rotavirus in India, *Indian J Pediatr* 68:855, 2001.
1055. Mascarenhas JD, Linhares AC, Gabbay YB, et al: Detection and characterization of rotavirus G and P types from children participating in a rotavirus vaccine trial in Belém, Brazil, *Mem Inst Oswald Cruz* 97:113, 2002.
1056. Widdowson MA, van Doornum GJ, van der Poel WH, et al: An outbreak of diarrhea in a neonatal medium care unit caused by a novel strain of rotavirus: investigation using both epidemiological and microbiological methods, *Infect Control Hosp Epidemiol* 23:665, 2002.
1057. Steele D, Reynecke E, de Beer M, et al: Characterization of rotavirus infection in a hospital neonatal unit in Pretoria, South Africa, *J Trop Pediatr* 48:161, 2002.
1058. Linhares AC, Mascarenhas JD, Gusmão RH, et al: Neonatal rotavirus infection in Belém, northern Brazil: nosocomial transmission of a P[6] G2 strain, *J Med Virol* 67:418, 2002.
1059. Cunliffe NA, Rogerson S, Dove W, et al: Detection and characterization of rotaviruses in hospitalized neonates in Blantyre, Malawi, *J Clin Microbiol* 40:1534, 2002.
1060. Banerjee I, Gladstone BP, Le Fevre AM, et al: Neonatal infection with G10P[11] rotavirus did not confer protection against subsequent rotavirus infection in a community cohort in Vellore, South India, *J Infect Dis* 195:611, 2007.
1061. Mascarenhas JD, Leite JP, Lima JC, et al: Detection of a neonatal human rotavirus strain with VP4 and NSP4 genes of porcine origin, *J Med Microbiol* 56:524, 2007.
1062. Greenberg HB, Estes MK: Rotaviruses: from pathogenesis to vaccination, *Gastroenterology* 136:1939, 2009.
1063. Davidson GP, Bishop RF, Townley RR, et al: Importance of a new virus in acute sporadic enteritis in children, *Lancet* 1:242, 1975.
1064. Bishop RF, Davidson GP, Holmes IH, et al: Virus particles in epithelial cells of duodenal mucosa from children with acute nonbacterial gastroenteritis, *Lancet* 2:1281, 1973.
1065. Holmes IH, Ruck BJ, Bishop RF, et al: Infantile enteritis viruses: morphogenesis and morphology, *J Virol* 16:937, 1975.
1066. Suzuki H, Konno T: Reovirus-like particles in jejunal mucosa of a Japanese infant with acute infectious nonbacterial gastroenteritis, *Tohoku J Exp Med* 115:199, 1975.

1067. Graham DY, Estes MK: Comparison of methods for immunocytochemical detection of rotavirus infections, *Infect Immun* 26:686, 1979.
1068. Holmes IH, Rodger SM, Schnagl RD, et al: Is lactase the receptor and uncoating enzyme for infantile enteritis (rota) viruses? *Lancet* 1:1387, 1976.
1069. Shepherd RW, Butler DG, Cutz E, et al: The mucosal lesion in viral enteritis: extent and dynamics of the epithelial response to virus invasion in transmissible gastroenteritis of piglets, *Gastroenterology* 76:770, 1979.
1070. Cameron DJS, Bishop RF, Veenstra AA, et al: Noncultivable viruses and neonatal diarrhea: fifteen-month survey in a newborn special care nursery, *J Clin Microbiol* 8:93, 1978.
1071. Lebenthal E: Lactose malabsorption and milk consumption in infants and children, *Am J Dis Child* 133:21, 1979.
1072. Philipps AD: Mechanisms of mucosal injury: human studies. In Farthing M, editor: *Viruses in the gut*, Welwyn Garden City, UK, 1988, Smith Kline & French, p 30.
1073. Shepherd RW, Gall DG, Butler DG, et al: Determinants of diarrhea in viral enteritis: the role of ion transport and epithelial changes in the ileum in transmissible gastroenteritis in piglets, *Gastroenterology* 76:20, 1979.
1074. Hoshino Y, Saif LJ, Kang SY, et al: Identification of group A rotavirus genes associated with virulence of a porcine rotavirus and host range restriction of a human rotavirus in the gnotobiotic piglet model, *Virology* 209:274, 1995.
1075. Saulsbury FT, Winklestein JA, Yolken RH: Chronic rotavirus infection in immunodeficiency, *J Pediatr* 97:61, 1980.
1076. Stephen J: Functional abnormalities in the intestine. In Farthing M, editor: *Viruses in the gut*, Welwyn Garden City, UK, 1988, Smith Kline & French, p 41.
1077. Lundgren O, Peregrin AT, Persson K, et al: Role of the enteric nervous system in the fluid and electrolyte secretion of rotavirus diarrhea, *Science* 287:491, 2000.
1078. Kerzner B, Kelly MH, Gall DG, et al: Transmissible gastroenteritis: sodium transport and the intestinal epithelium during the course of viral gastroenteritis, *Gastroenterology* 72:457, 1977.
1079. Gall DG, Chapman D, Kelly M, et al: Na+ transport in jejunal crypt cells, *Gastroenterology* 72:452, 1977.
1080. Ball JM, Tian P, Zeng CQ, et al: Age-dependent diarrhea induced by a rotaviral nonstructural glycoprotein, *Science* 272:101, 1996.
1081. Lorrot M, Vasseur M: How do the rotavirus NSP4 and bacterial enterotoxins lead differently to diarrhea? *Virol J* 4:1, 2007.
1082. Ward RL, Mason BB, Bernstein DI, et al: Attenuation of a human rotavirus vaccine candidate did not correlate with mutations in the NSP4 protein gene, *J Virol* 71:6267, 1997.
1083. Zhang M, Zeng CQ, Dong Y, et al: Mutations in nonstructural glycoprotein NSP4 are associated with altered virus virulence, *J Virol* 72:3666, 1998.
1084. Blutt SE, Matson DO, Crawford SE, et al: Rotavirus antigenemia in children is associated with viremia, *PLoS Med* 4:e121, 2007.
1085. Fischer TK, Ashley D, Kerin T, et al: Rotavirus antigenemia in patients with acute gastroenteritis, *J Infect Dis* 192:913, 2005.
1086. Chiappini E, Galli L, de Martino M: Viremia and clinical manifestations in children with rotavirus infection, *J Infect Dis* 193:1333, 2006.
1087. Huang XL, Chen J, Yu YP, et al: Viraemia and extraintestinal involvement after rotavirus infection, *Zhejiang Da Xue Xue Bao Yi Xue Ban* 35:69, 2006.
1088. Bishop RF, Barnes GL, Cipriani E, et al: Clinical immunity after neonatal rotavirus infection: a prospective longitudinal study in young children, *N Engl J Med* 309:72, 1983.
1089. Bhan MK, Lew JF, Sazawal S, et al: Protection conferred by neonatal rotavirus infection against subsequent rotavirus diarrhea, *J Infect Dis* 168:282, 1993.
1090. Chiba S, Yokoyama T, Nakata S, et al: Protective effect of naturally acquired homotypic and heterotypic rotavirus antibodies, *Lancet* 1:417, 1986.
1091. Greene KY, Kapikian AZ: Identification of VP7 epitopes associated with protection against human rotavirus illness or shedding in volunteers, *J Virol* 66:548, 1992.
1092. Hjelt K, Grauballe PC, Paerregaard A, et al: Protective effect of pre-existing rotavirus-specific immunoglobulin A against naturally acquired rotavirus infection in children, *J Med Virol* 21:39, 1987.
1093. Matson DO, O'Ryan ML, Pickering LK, et al: Characterization of serum antibody responses to natural rotavirus infections in children by VP7-specific epitope-blocking assays, *J Clin Microbiol* 30:1056, 1992.
1094. Ward RL, Knowlton DR, Schiff GM, et al: Relative concentrations of serum neutralizing antibody to VP3 and VP7 protein in adults infected with human rotavirus, *J Virol* 62:1543, 1988.
1095. Clemens JD, Ward RL, Rao MR, et al: Seroepidemiologic evaluation of antibodies to rotavirus as correlates of the risk of clinically significant rotavirus diarrhea in rural Bangladesh, *J Infect Dis* 165:161, 1992.
1096. Matson DO, O'Ryan ML, Herrera I, et al: Fecal antibody responses to symptomatic and asymptomatic rotavirus infections, *J Infect Dis* 167:557, 1993.
1097. O'Ryan M, Matson DO, Estes MK, et al: Anti-rotavirus G type-specific and isotype-specific antibodies in children with natural rotavirus infections, *J Infect Dis* 169:504, 1994.
1098. Zheng BJ, Lo SK, Tam JS, et al: Prospective study of community-acquired rotavirus infection, *J Clin Microbiol* 27, 1989. 2083.
1099. Ward RL, Clemens JD, Knowlton DR, et al: Evidence that protection against rotavirus diarrhea after natural infection is not dependent on serotype-specific neutralizing antibody, *J Infect Dis* 166:1251, 1992.
1100. Totterdell BM, Chrystie IL, Banatvala JE: Cord blood and breast milk antibodies in neonatal rotavirus infection, *Br Med J* 1:828, 1980.
1101. Yolken RH, Wyatt RG, Zissis G, et al: Epidemiology of human rotavirus types 1 and 2 as studied by enzyme-linked immunosorbent assay, *N Engl J Med* 299:1156, 1978.
1102. McLean B, Holmes IH: Transfer of anti-rotaviral antibodies from mothers to their infants, *J Clin Microbiol* 12:320, 1980.
1103. McLean BS, Holmes IH: Effects of antibodies, trypsin, and trypsin inhibitors on susceptibility of neonates to rotavirus infection, *J Clin Microbiol* 13:22, 1981.
1104. Brussow H, Sidoti J, Lerner L, et al: Antibodies to seven rotavirus serotypes in cord sera, maternal sera, and colostrum of German women, *J Clin Microbiol* 29:2856, 1991.
1105. Brussow H, Benitez O, Uribe F, et al: Rotavirus-inhibitory activity in serial milk samples from Mexican women and rotavirus infections in their children during their first year of life, *J Clin Microbiol* 31:593, 1993.
1106. Yolken RH, Wyatt RG, Mata L, et al: Secretory antibody directed against rotavirus in human milk—measurement by means of enzyme-linked immunosorbent assay, *J Pediatr* 93:916, 1978.
1107. Santosham M, Pathak A, Kottapalli S, et al: Neonatal rotavirus infection, *Lancet* 1:1070, 1982.
1108. Madeley CR, Cosgrove BP, Bell EJ: Stool viruses in babies in Glasgow. 2. Investigation of normal newborns in hospital, *J Hyg* 81:285, 1978.
1109. Glasgow JFT, McClure BG, Connolly JH, et al: Nosocomial rotavirus gastroenteritis in a neonatal nursery, *Ulster Med J* 47:50, 1978.
1110. Cameron DJS, Bishop RF, Davidson GP, et al: New virus associated with diarrhoea in neonates, *Med J Aust* 1:85, 1976.
1111. Bryden AS, Thouless ME, Hall CJ, et al: Rotavirus infections in a special-care baby unit, *J Infect* 4:43, 1982.
1112. Grillner L, Broberger U, Chrystie I, et al: Rotavirus infections in newborns: an epidemiological and clinical study, *Scand J Infect Dis* 17:349, 1985.
1113. Tufvesson B, Polberger S, Svanberg L, et al: A prospective study of rotavirus infections in neonatal and maternity wards, *Acta Paediatr Scand* 75:211, 1986.
1114. Hoshino Y, Wyatt RG, Flores J, et al: Serotypic characterization of rotaviruses derived from asymptomatic human neonatal infections, *J Clin Microbiol* 21:425, 1985.
1115. Crewe E, Murphy AM: Further studies on neonatal rotavirus infection, *Med J Aust* 1:61, 1980.
1116. Perez-Schael I, Daoud G, White L, et al: Rotavirus shedding by newborn children, *J Med Virol* 14:127, 1984.
1117. Vial PA, Kotloff KL, Losonsky GA: Molecular epidemiology of rotavirus infection in a room for convalescing newborns, *J Infect Dis* 157:668, 1988.
1118. Haffejee IE: Neonatal rotavirus infections, *Rev Infect Dis* 13:957, 1991.
1119. Jesudoss ES, John TJ, Maiya PP, et al: Prevalence of rotavirus infection in neonates, *Indian J Med Res* 70:863, 1979.

1120. Bishop RF, Cameron DJ, Veenstra AA, et al: Diarrhea and rotavirus infection associated with differing regimens for postnatal care of newborn babies, *J Clin Microbiol* 9:525, 1979.
1121. Ramani S, Sowmyanarayanan TV, Gladstone BP, et al: Rotavirus infection in the neonatal nurseries of a tertiary care hospital in India, *Pediatr Infect Dis J* 27:719, 2008.
1122. Civardi E, Tzialla C, Baldanti F, et al: Viral outbreaks in neonatal intensive care units: what we do not know, *Am J Infect Control* 41:854, 2013.
1123. de Villiers FP, Driessen M: Clinical neonatal rotavirus infection: association with necrotising enterocolitis, *S Afr Med J* 102:620, 2012.
1124. Pickering LK, Bartlett 3rd AV, Reves RR, et al: Asymptomatic rotavirus before and after rotavirus diarrhea in children in day care centers, *J Pediatr* 112:361, 1988.
1125. Vesikari T, Sarkkinen HK, Maki M: Quantitative aspects of rotavirus excretion in childhood diarrhoea, *Acta Paediatr Scand* 70:717, 1981.
1126. Konno T, Suzuki H, Katsushima N, et al: Influence of temperature and relative humidity on human rotavirus infection in Japan, *J Infect Dis* 147:125, 1983.
1127. Bartlett 3rd AV, Reeves RR, Pickering LK: Rotavirus in infant-toddler day care centers: epidemiology relevant to disease control strategies, *J Pediatr* 113:435, 1988.
1128. Matson DO, Estes MK, Burns JW, et al: Serotype variation of human group A rotaviruses in two regions of the United States, *J Infect Dis* 162:605, 1990.
1129. Ryan MJ, Ramsay M, Brown D, et al: Hospital admissions attributable to rotavirus infection in England, *J Infect Dis* 174(Suppl 1): S12, 1996.
1130. Glass R, Kilgore PE, Holman RC, et al: The epidemiology of rotavirus diarrhea in the United States: surveillance and estimates of disease burden, *J Infect Dis* 74(Suppl 1):S5, 1996.
1131. O'Ryan M, Pérez-Schael I, Mamani N, et al: Rotavirus-associated medical visits and hospitalizations in South America: a prospective study at three large sentinel hospitals, *Pediatr Infect Dis J* 20:685, 2001.
1132. Duffy LC, Riepenhoff-Talty M, Byers TE, et al: Modulation of rotavirus enteritis during breast-feeding, *Am J Dis Child* 140:1164, 1986.
1133. van Renterghem L, Borre P, Tilleman J: Rotavirus and other viruses in the stool of premature babies, *J Med Virol* 5:137, 1980.
1134. Murphy AM, Albrey MB, Crewe EB: Rotavirus infections in neonates, *Lancet* 2:1149, 1977.
1135. Soenarto Y, Sebodo T, Ridho R, et al: Acute diarrhea and rotavirus infection in newborn babies and children in Yogyakarta, Indonesia from June 1978 to June 1979, *J Clin Microbiol* 14:123, 1981.
1136. Appleton H, Buckley M, Robertson MH, et al: A search for faecal viruses in newborn and other infants, *J Hyg* 81:279, 1978.
1137. Schnagl RD, Morey F, Holmes IH: Rotavirus and coronavirus-like particles in aboriginal and non-aboriginal neonates in Kalgoorlie and Alice Springs, *Med J Aust* 2:178, 1979.
1138. Dearlove J, Latham P, Dearlove B, et al: Clinical range of neonatal rotavirus gastroenteritis, *Br Med J* 286:1473, 1983.
1139. Parashar UD, Holman RC, Bresee JS, et al: Epidemiology of diarrheal disease among children enrolled in four West Coast health maintenance organizations, *Pediatr Infect Dis J* 17:605, 1998.
1140. Leece JC, King MW, Dorsey WE: Rearing regimen producing piglet diarrhea (rotavirus) and its relevance to acute infantile diarrhea, *Science* 199:776, 1978.
1141. Herruzo R, Omeñaca F, García S, et al: Identification of risk factors associated with nosocomial infection by rotavirus P4G2, in a neonatal unit of a tertiary-care hospital, *Clin Microbiol Infect* 15:280, 2009.
1142. Rodriguez WJ, Kim HW, Brandt CD, et al: Use of electrophoresis of RNA from human rotavirus to establish the identity of stains involved in outbreaks in a tertiary care nursery, *J Infect Dis* 148:34, 1983.
1143. Srivinasan G, Azarcon E, Muldoon MR, et al: Rotavirus infection in a normal nursery: epidemic and surveillance, *Infect Control* 5:478, 1984.
1144. Gerna G, Forster J, Parea M, et al: Nosocomial outbreak of neonatal gastroenteritis caused by a new serotype 4, subtype 4B human rotavirus, *J Med Virol* 31:175, 1990.
1145. Tallet S, MacKenzie C, Middleton P, et al: Clinical, laboratory, and epidemiologic features of a viral gastroenteritis in infants and children, *Pediatrics* 60:217, 1977.
1146. Hieber JP, Shelton S, Nelson JD, et al: Comparison of human rotavirus disease in tropical and temperate settings, *Am J Dis Child* 132:853, 1978.
1147. Mutanda LN: Epidemiology of acute gastroenteritis in early childhood in Kenya. VI. Some clinical and laboratory characteristics relative to the aetiological agents, *East Afr Med J* 57:599, 1980.
1148. Whyte RK, Homes R, Pennock CA: Faecal excretion of oligosaccharides and other carbohydrates in normal neonates, *Arch Dis Child* 53:913, 1978.
1149. Hyams JS, Krause PJ, Gleason PA: Lactose malabsorption following rotavirus infection in young children, *J Pediatr* 99:916, 1981.
1150. Rodriguez WJ, Kim HW, Brandt CD, et al: Rotavirus: a cause of nosocomial infection in a nursery, *J Pediatr* 101:274, 1982.
1151. Shim JO, Son DW, Shim SY, et al: Clinical characteristics and genotypes of rotaviruses in a neonatal intensive care unit, *Pediatr Neonatol* 53:18, 2012.
1152. Prashar UD, Hummelman EG, Bresee JS, et al: Global illness and deaths caused by rotavirus disease in children, *Emerg Infect Dis* 9:565, 2003.
1153. Dani C, Trevisanuto D, Cantarutti F, et al: A case of neonatal necrotizing enterocolitis due to rotavirus, *Pediatr Med Chir* 16:185, 1994.
1154. Goma Brufau AR, Vega Romero M, Martínez Ubieto P, et al: Epidemic outbreak of necrotizing enterocolitis coincident with an epidemic of neonatal rotavirus gastroenteritis, *An Esp Pediatr* 29:307, 1988.
1155. Riedel F, Kroener T, Stein K, et al: Rotavirus infection and bradycardia-apnoea-episodes in the neonate, *Eur J Pediatr* 155:36, 1996.
1156. Konno T, Suzuki H, Kutsuzawa T, et al: Human rotavirus infection in infants and young children with intussusception, *J Med Virol* 2:265, 1978.
1157. Mulcahy DL, Kamath KR, de Silva LM, et al: A two-part study of the aetiological role of rotavirus in intussusception, *J Med Virol* 9:51, 1982.
1158. Nicolas JC, Ingrand D, Fortier B, et al: A one-year virological survey of acute intussusception in childhood, *J Med Virol* 9:267, 1982.
1159. Murphy TV, Gargiullo PM, Massoudi MS, et al: Intussusception among infants given an oral rotavirus vaccine, *N Engl J Med* 22:564, 2001.
1160. Rennels MB, Parashar UD, Holman RC, et al: Lack of an apparent association between intussusception and wild or vaccine virus rotavirus infection, *Pediatr Infect Dis J* 17:924, 1998.
1161. Dennehy P, Hartin M, Nelson SM, et al: Evaluation of the inmunocardstat: rotavirus assay for detection of group A rotavirus in fecal specimens, *J Clin Microbiol* 37:1977, 1999.
1162. Gilchrist MJR, Bretl TS, Moultney K, et al: Comparison of seven kits for detection of rotavirus in fecal specimens with a sensitive, specific enzyme immunoassay, *Diagn Microbiol Infect Dis* 8:221, 1987.
1163. Knisley CV, Bednarz-Prashad A, Pickering LK: Detection of rotavirus in stool specimens with monoclonal and polyclonal antibody-based assay systems, *J Clin Microbiol* 23:897, 1986.
1164. Thomas EE, Puterman ML, Kawano E, et al: Evaluation of seven immunoassays for detection of rotavirus in pediatric stool samples, *J Clin Microbiol* 26:1189, 1988.
1165. Miotti PG, Eiden J, Yolken RH: Comparative efficacy of commercial immunoassays for the diagnosis of rotavirus gastroenteritis during the course of infection, *J Clin Microbiol* 22:693, 1985.
1166. Brandt CD, Kim HW, Rodriguez WJ, et al: Comparison of direct electron microscopy, immune electron microscopy, and rotavirus enzyme-linked immunosorbent assay for detection of gastroenteritis viruses in children, *J Clin Microbiol* 13:976, 1981.
1167. Yolken RH, Kim HW, Clem T, Wyatt RG, et al: Enzyme-linked immunosorbent assay (ELISA) for detection of human reovirus-like agent of infantile gastroenteritis, *Lancet* 2:263, 1977.
1168. Fischer TK, Steinsland H, Valentiner-Branth P: Rotavirus particles can survive storage in ambient tropical temperatures for more than 2 months, *J Clin Microbiol* 40:4763, 2002.
1169. Viera de Torres B, Mazzali de Ilja R, Esparza J: Epidemiological aspects of rotavirus infection in hospitalized Venezuelan children with gastroenteritis, *Am J Trop Med Hyg* 27:567, 1978.

1170. Provisional Committee on Quality Improvement: Subcommittee on Acute Gastroenteritis. Practice parameter: the management of acute gastroenteritis in young children, *Pediatrics* 97:424, 1996.
1171. Sack DA, Chowdhury AM, Eusof A, et al: Oral hydration in rotavirus diarrhoea: a double-blind comparison of sucrose with glucose electrolyte solution, *Lancet* 2:280, 1978.
1172. Black RE, Merson MH, Taylor PR, et al: Glucose vs. sucrose in oral rehydration solutions for infants and young children with rotavirus-associated diarrhea, *Pediatrics* 67:79, 1981.
1173. Ebina T, Ohta M, Kanamaru Y, et al: Passive immunizations of suckling mice and infants with bovine colostrum containing antibodies to human rotavirus, *J Med Virol* 38:117, 1992.
1174. Guarino A, Guandalini S, Albano F, et al: Enteral immunoglobulins for treatment of protracted rotaviral diarrhea, *Pediatr Infect Dis J* 10:612, 1991.
1175. Brunser O, Espinoza J, Figueroa G, et al: Field trial of an infant formula containing anti-rotavirus and anti-*Escherichia coli* milk antibodies from hyperimmunized cows, *J Pediatr Gastroenterol Nutr* 15:63, 1992.
1176. Rosenfeldt V, Michaelsen KF, Jakobsen M, et al: Effect of probiotic *Lactobacillus* strains in young children hospitalized with acute diarrhea, *Pediatr Infect Dis J* 21:411, 2002.
1177. Allen SJ, Martinez EG, Gregorio GV, et al: Probiotics for treating acute infectious diarrhoea, *Cochrane Database Syst Rev* (11): CD003048, 2010.
1178. Birch CJ, Lewis FA, Kennett ML, et al: A study of the prevalence of rotavirus infection in children with gastroenteritis admitted to an infectious disease hospital, *J Med Virol* 1:69, 1977.
1179. Kombo LA, Gerber MA, Pickering LK, et al: Intussusception, infection, and immunization: summary of a workshop on rotavirus, *Pediatrics* 108:E37, 2001.
1180. Vesikari T, Matson DO, Dennehy P, et al: Safety and efficacy of a pentavalent human-bovine (WC3) reassortant rotavirus vaccine, *N Engl J Med* 5:23, 2006.
1181. Ruiz-Palacios GM, Pérez-Schael I, Velázquez FR, et al: Safety and efficacy of an attenuated vaccine against severe rotavirus gastroenteritis, *N Engl J Med* 5:11, 2006.
1182. Soares-Weiser K, Maclehose H, Bergman H, et al: 2012 Vaccines for preventing rotavirus diarrhoea: vaccines in use, *Cochrane Database Syst Rev* (11): CD008521, 2012.
1183. O'Ryan M, Lucero Y, Linhares AC: Rotarix: vaccine performance 6 years postlicensure, *Expert Rev Vaccines* 10:1645, 2011.
1184. Centers for Disease Control and Prevention: Delayed onset and diminished magnitude of rotavirus activity—United States, November 2007-May 2008, *MMWR Morb Mortal Wkly Rep* 57:697, 2008.
1185. Haber P, Patel M, Pan Y, et al: Intussusception after rotavirus vaccines reported to US VAERS, 2006-2012, *Pediatrics* 131:1042, 2013.
1186. Carlin JB, Macartney KK, Lee KJ, et al: Intussusception risk and disease prevention associated with rotavirus vaccines in Australia's national immunization program, *Clin Infect Dis* 57:1427-1434, 2013.
1187. Schwartz JL: Rotavirus vaccines, intussusception, and risk-benefit assessments, *JAMA Pediatr* 167:1093, 2013.
1188. Armah GE, Kapikian AZ, Vesikari T, et al: Efficacy, immunogenicity, and safety of two doses of a tetravalent rotavirus vaccine RRV-TV in Ghana with the first dose administered during the neonatal period, *J Infect Dis* 208:423, 2013.
1189. Ramani S, Kang G: Viruses causing childhood diarrhoea in the developing world, *Curr Opin Infect Dis* 22:477, 2009.
1190. O'Ryan ML, Lucero Y, Prado V, et al: Symptomatic and asymptomatic rotavirus and norovirus infections during infancy in a Chilean birth cohort, *Pediatr Infect Dis J* 28:879, 2009.
1191. Payne DC, et al: Norovirus and medically attended gastroenteritis in U.S. children, *N Engl J Med* 368:1121, 2013.
1192. Chhabra P, Payne DC, Szilagyi PG, et al: Etiology of viral gastroenteritis in children <5 years of age in the United States, 2008-2009, *J Infect Dis* 208:790, 2013.
1193. Naing Z, Rayner B, Killikulangara A, et al: Prevalence of viruses in stool of premature neonates at a neonatal intensive care unit, *J Paediatr Child Health* 49:E221, 2013.
1194. Armbrust S, Kramer A, Olbertz D, et al: Norovirus infections in preterm infants: wide variety of clinical courses, *BMC Res Notes* 2:96, 2009.
1195. Armbrust S, Mueller W, Resch B: Two nosocomial norovirus outbreaks in the neonatal intensive and intermediate care unit, *Eur J Clin Microbiol Infect Dis* 28:1133, 2009.
1196. Turcios-Ruiz RM, Axelrod P, St John K, et al: Outbreak of necrotizing enterocolitis caused by norovirus in a neonatal intensive care unit, *J Pediatr* 153:339, 2008.
1197. Wiechers C, Bissinger AL, Hamprecht K, et al: Apparently nonspecific results found using a norovirus antigen immunoassay for fecal specimens from neonates, *J Perinatol* 28:79, 2008.
1198. Armbrust S, Obinata K, Ikari H, et al: False positive of an immunochromatography kit for detection of norovirus in neonatal feces, *J Infect Chemother* 19:171, 2013.
1199. Li CY, Liu N, Guo WD, et al: Outbreak of neonatal gastroenteritis associated with astrovirus serotype 1 at a hospital in Inner Mongolia, China, *J Clin Microbiol* 48:4306, 2010.
1200. Chappé C, Minjolle S, Dabadie A, et al: Astrovirus and digestive disorders in neonatal units, *Acta Paediatr* 101:e208, 2012.
1201. Soileau SL, Schneider E, Erdman DD, et al: Case report: severe disseminated adenovirus infection in a neonate following water birth delivery, *J Med Virol* 85:667, 2013.
1202. Khan AM, Faruque AS, Hossain MS: Isolation of *Vibrio cholerae* from neonates admitted to an urban diarrhoeal diseases hospital in Bangladesh, *Ann Trop Paediatr* 25:179, 2005.
1203. Srinivasjois RM, Kava MP, Thomas A, et al: Cytomegalovirus-associated ileal stricture in a preterm neonate, *J Pediatr Child Health* 44:80, 2008.
1204. Bina Rai S, Wan Mansor H, Vasantha T, et al: An outbreak of echovirus 11 amongst neonates in a confinement home in Penang, Malaysia, *Med J Malaysia* 62:223, 2007.
1205. Wilson W, Scott RB, Pinto A, et al: Intractable diarrhea in a newborn infant: microvillous inclusion disease, *Can J Gastroenterol* 15:61, 2001.
1206. Stockdale EM, Miller CA: Persistent diarrhea as the predominant symptom of Hirschsprung's disease (congenital dilatation of colon), *Pediatrics* 19:91, 1957.
1207. Wilmore DW: Factors correlating with a successful outcome following extensive intestinal resection in newborn infants, *J Pediatr* 80:88, 1972.
1208. Hasosah M, Lemberg DA, Skarsgard E, et al: Congenital short bowel syndrome: a case report and review of the literature, *Can J Gastroenterol* 22:71, 2008.
1209. Fried D, Gotlieb A, Zaidel L: Intractable diarrhea of infancy due to lymphangiectasis, *Am J Dis Child* 127:416, 1974.
1210. Lebenthal E: Small intestinal disaccharidase deficiency, *Pediatr Clin North Am* 22:757, 1975.
1211. Ament ME, Perera DR, Esther LJ: Sucrase-isomaltose deficiency—a frequently misdiagnosed disease, *J Pediatr* 83:721, 1973.
1212. Marks JF, Norton JB, Fordtran JS: Glucose-galactose malabsorption, *J Pediatr* 69:225, 1969.
1213. Burke V, Anderson CM: Sugar intolerance as a cause of protracted diarrhea following surgery of the gastrointestinal tract in neonates, *Aust Paediatr J* 2:219, 1966.
1214. Bishop RF, Davidson GP, Holmes IH, et al: Virus particles in epithelial cells of duodenal mucosa from children with acute nonbacterial gastroenteritis, *Lancet* 2:1281, 1973.
1215. Coello-Ramirez P, Lifshitz F, Zuniga V: Enteric microflora and carbohydrate intolerance in infants with diarrhea, *Pediatrics* 49:233, 1972.
1216. Akesode F, Lifshitz F, Hoffman KM: Transient monosaccharide intolerance in a newborn infant, *Pediatrics* 51:891, 1973.
1217. Iyngkaran N, Davis K, Robinson MJ, et al: Cow's milk protein—sensitive enteropathy: an important contributing cause of secondary sugar intolerance in young infants with acute infective enteritis, *Arch Dis Child* 54:39, 1979.
1218. Ament ME: Malabsorption syndromes in infancy and childhood. I; II, *J Pediatr* 81(685):867, 1972.
1219. Whyte RK, Homer R, Pennock CA: Faecal excretion of oligosaccharides and other carbohydrates in normal neonates, *Arch Dis Child* 53:913, 1978.
1220. Schwachman H, Redmond A, Khaw KT: Studies in cystic fibrosis: report of 130 patients diagnosed under 3 months of age over a 20 year period, *Pediatrics* 46:335, 1970.
1221. Aggett PJ, Cavanagh NP, Matthew DJ, et al: Schwachman's syndrome: a review of 21 cases, *Arch Dis Child* 55:331, 1980.

1222. Lilibridge CB, Townes PL: Physiologic deficiency of pancreatic amylase in infancy: a factor in iatrogenic diarrhea, *J Pediatr* 82:279, 1973.
1223. Lebenthal E, Antonowicz I, Schwachman H: Enterokinase and trypsin activities in pancreatic insufficiency and diseases of the small intestine, *Gastroenterology* 70:508, 1979.
1224. Powell GK, Jones LA, Richardson J: A new syndrome of bile acid deficiency—a possible synthetic defect, *J Pediatr* 83:758, 1973.
1225. Lloyd JK: Disorders of the serum lipoproteins. I. Lipoprotein deficiency states, *Arch Dis Child* 43:393, 1968.
1226. Cash R, Berger CK: Acrodermatitis enteropathica: defective metabolism of unsaturated fatty acids, *J Pediatr* 74:717, 1969.
1227. Garretts M, Molokhia M: Acrodermatitis enteropathica without hypozincemia, *J Pediatr* 91:492, 1977.
1228. McReynolds EW, Roy III S, Etteldorf JN: Congenital chloride diarrhea, *Am J Dis Child* 127:566, 1974.
1229. Minford AMB, Barr DGD: Prostaglandin synthetase inhibitor in an infant with congenital chloride diarrhea, *Arch Dis Child* 55:70, 1980.
1230. Hihnala S, Höglund P, Lammi L, et al: Long-term clinical outcome in patients with congenital chloride diarrhea, *J Pediatr Gastroenterol Nutr* 42:369, 2006.
1231. Woodard JC, Webster PD, Carr AA: Primary hypomagnesemia with secondary hypocalcemia, diarrhea and insensitivity to parathyroid hormone, *Am J Dig Dis* 17:612, 1972.
1232. Iversen T: Congenital adrenal hyperplasia with disturbed electrolyte regulation, *Pediatrics* 16:875, 1955.
1233. Iida Y, Nose O, Kai H, et al: Watery diarrhoea with a vasoactive intestinal peptide-producing ganglioneuroblastoma, *Arch Dis Child* 55:929, 1980.
1234. Ghishan FK, Soper RT, Nassif ED, et al: Chronic diarrhea of infancy: nonbeta islet cell hyperplasia, *Pediatrics* 64:46, 1979.
1235. Storm W, Wendel U, Sprenkamp M, et al: Wolman's disease in an infant, *Monatsschr Kinderheilkd* 138:88, 1990.
1236. Hakami N, Neiman PE, Canellos GP, et al: Neonatal megaloblastic anemia due to inherited transcobalamin II deficiency in 2 siblings, *N Engl J Med* 285:1163, 1971.
1237. Verloes A, Lombet J, Lambert Y, et al: Tricho-hepato-enteric syndrome: further delineation of a distinct syndrome with neonatal hemochromatosis phenotype, intractable diarrhea, and hair anomalies, *Am J Med Genet* 68:391, 1997.
1238. Jonas AJ, Butler IJ: Circumvention of defective neutral amino acid transport in Hartnup disease using tryptophan ethyl ester, *J Clin Invest* 84:200, 1989.
1239. Holmberg C, Perheentipa J: Congenital Na+ diarrhea: a new type of secretory diarrhea, *J Pediatr* 106:56, 1985.
1240. Makita N, Sato J, Rondard P, et al: Human Gss mutant causes pseudohypoparathyroidism type Ia/neonatal diarrhea, a potential cell-specific role of the palmitoylation cycle, *Proc Natl Acad Sci U S A* 104:17424, 2007.
1241. Bayna SL, Heiner DC: Cow's milk allergy: manifestations, diagnosis and management, *Adv Pediatr* 25:1, 1978.
1242. Hwang JB, Lee SH, Kang YN, et al: Indexes of suspicion of typical cow's milk protein-induced enterocolitis, *J Korean Med Sci* 22:993, 2007.
1243. Halpin TC, Byrne WJ, Ament ME: Colitis, persistent diarrhea, and soy protein intolerance, *J Pediatr* 91:404, 1977.
1244. Powell GK: Milk- and soy-induced enterocolitis of infancy: clinical features and standardization of challenge, *J Pediatr* 93:553, 1978.
1245. Miller RC, Larsen E: Regional enteritis in early infancy, *Am J Dis Child* 122:301, 1971.
1246. Avery GB, Harkness M: Bloody diarrhea in the newborn infant of a mother with ulcerative colitis, *Pediatrics* 34:875, 1964.
1247. Ein SH, Lynch MJ, Stephens CA: Ulcerative colitis in children under one year: a twenty-year review, *J Pediatr Surg* 6:264, 1971.
1248. Sunshine P, Sinatra FR, Mitchell CH: Intractable diarrhoea of infancy, *Clin Gastroenterol* 6:445, 1977.
1249. Scott GB, Buck BE, Leterman JG, et al: Acquired immunodeficiency syndrome in infants, *N Engl J Med* 310:76, 1984.
1250. Davidson M, Wasserman R: The irritable colon of childhood (chronic nonspecific diarrhea syndrome), *J Pediatr* 69:1027, 1966.
1251. Ochoa TJ, Salazar-Lindo E, Cleary TG: Management of children with infection-associated persistent diarrhea, *Semin Pediatr Infect Dis* 15:229, 2004.
1252. Bhatt M M, Anil SR, Sivakumar K, et al: Neonatal Kawasaki disease, *Indian J Pediatr* 71:353, 2004.

12

Group B Streptococcal Infections

MORVEN S. EDWARDS, VICTOR NIZET, and CAROL J. BAKER

CHAPTER OUTLINE

Lancefield group B β-hemolytic streptococci were first recorded as a cause of human infection in 1938, when Fry[1] described three patients with fatal puerperal sepsis. Sporadic cases were reported until the 1970s, when a dramatic increase in the incidence of septicemia and meningitis in neonates caused by group B streptococci (GBS) was documented from geographically diverse regions.[2-4] Emergence of GBS infections in neonates was accompanied by an increasing number of these infections in pregnant women and nonpregnant adults. In pregnant women, infection commonly manifested as localized uterine infection or chorioamnionitis, often with bacteremia, and had an almost uniformly good outcome with antimicrobial therapy. The incidence of perinatal infection associated with GBS remained stable through the early 1990s. Case-fatality rates had declined by then but remained substantial compared with case-fatality rates reported for other invasive bacterial infections in infants. The implementation of the consensus guidelines published in 2002 that are designed to prevent early-onset disease in neonates through universal antenatal culture-based screening at 35 to 37 weeks of gestation, and accompanying intrapartum antibiotic prophylaxis was associated with a substantial decline in the incidence of early-onset neonatal infection by 2008 and has reached a plateau since then.[5]

In recent years, the genomes of several GBS types have been sequenced, opening new avenues for the identification of novel potential vaccine targets.[6,7] The discovery that surface-associated pili are widely distributed among GBS and that a vaccine based on combinations of the three pilus-island variants protects mice against lethal challenge with a wide variety of GBS strains paves the way for the design of pilus-based and perhaps other putative surface protein vaccines for testing in humans.[8-10]

Testing of glycoconjugate GBS candidate vaccines in healthy adults and in pregnant women is ongoing, offering promise that immunization to prevent maternal and infant invasive GBS disease could become a reality.

Organism

Streptococcus agalactiae is the species designation for streptococci belonging to Lancefield group B. This bacterium is a facultative gram-positive diplococcus with an ultrastructure similar to that of other gram-positive cocci. Before

Lancefield's classification of hemolytic streptococci in 1933,[11] this microorganism was identified by its characteristic colonial morphology, its narrow zone of β-hemolysis surrounding colonies on blood agar plates, and its double zone of hemolysis that appeared when plates were refrigerated an additional 18 hours beyond the initial incubation. Occasional strains (1%-4%) are α-hemolytic or nonhemolytic. GBS are readily cultivated in various bacteriologic media. Isolation from respiratory, genital, and gastrointestinal tracts can be enhanced by use of selective enrichment broth containing antimicrobial agents that inhibit growth of other bacterial species indigenous to these sites.[12,13]

COLONIAL MORPHOLOGY AND IDENTIFICATION

Colonies of GBS grown on sheep blood agar are 3 to 4 mm in diameter, produce a narrow zone of β-hemolysis, are gray-white, and are flat and mucoid. β-Hemolysis for some strains is apparent only when colonies are removed from the agar.

Tests for presumptive identification include bacitracin and trimethoprim-sulfamethoxazole disk susceptibility testing (92%-98% of strains are resistant), hydrolysis of sodium hippurate broth (99% of strains are positive), hydrolysis of bile esculin agar (99%-100% of strains fail to react), pigment production during anaerobic growth on certain media (96%-98% of strains produce an orange pigment), and CAMP (Christie-Atkins-Munch-Petersen) testing (98%-100% of strains are CAMP positive).[14] The CAMP factor is a thermostable extracellular protein that, in the presence of the β toxin of *Staphylococcus aureus*, produces synergistic hemolysis when grown on sheep blood agar. Hippurate hydrolysis is an accurate method for presumptive identification of GBS, but the incubation time required limits its usefulness. Definitive identification of GBS requires detection of the group B antigen common to all strains. Lancefield's original method required acid treatment of broth-grown cells to extract the group B antigen from the cell wall.[15] Supernatants brought to neutral pH were mixed with hyperimmune rabbit antiserum prepared by immunization with the group B–variant strain, and precipitins in capillary tubes were recorded. Less time-consuming techniques are now used. Conventional means for presumptive identification of isolates subcultured to blood-agar plates include use of the CAMP test or latex agglutination with GBS antisera. Chromogenic agars that undergo color change in the presence of β-hemolytic colonies of GBS have become available. Most of these do not detect the small percentage of strains that are nonhemolytic. In addition, more rapid techniques have been developed for identifying GBS directly from enrichment broth or after subculture. These include DNA probes and nucleic acid amplification tests (NAAT), such as polymerase chain reaction (PCR).[16] The sensitivity of NAAT, when an enrichment step is included, ranges from 93% to 100%.

Strains of Human and Bovine Origin

Group B streptococci were known to cause bovine mastitis before they were appreciated as pathogenic in humans.[17] Modern veterinary practices have largely controlled epidemics of bovine mastitis, but sporadic cases still occur. Substantial biochemical, serologic, and molecular differences exist between human and bovine isolates.[18] Among typeable bovine strains, patterns of distribution distinct from the patterns of human isolates are noted. Other distinguishing characteristics for bovine strains include their unique fermentation reactions, decreased frequency of pigment production, and susceptibility to bacitracin. Protein X, rarely found in human strains, is commonly present in pathogenic bovine isolates.[19]

The relationship between GBS strains of human and bovine origin has been queried for years. There is no compelling evidence that cattle serve as a reservoir for human disease, and transmission from cows to humans is exceedingly rare. In addition, during the decades when GBS has been a dominant human pathogen, the risk of exposure through direct contact with dairy cattle or ingestion of unpasteurized milk has been unlikely. Application of molecular techniques to strains from bovine sources and those infecting human neonates supports the assertion that these lineages are unrelated. Phylogenetic lineage determination does indicate, however, that some clonal complexes of invasive or colonizing strains in humans are related to ancestral lineages of bovine GBS.[20]

CLASSIFICATION

Lancefield defined two cell wall carbohydrate antigens by using hydrochloric acid–extracted cell supernatants and hyperimmune rabbit antisera: the group B–specific, or "C," substance common to all strains and the type-specific, or "S," substance that allowed classification into types—initially types I, II, and III.[21-23] Strains designated as type I were later shown to have cross-reactive and antigenically distinct polysaccharides designated type Ia and type Ib.[22] GBS historically designated type Ic possessed type Ia capsular polysaccharide (CPS) and a protein antigen common to type Ib, most type II, and rare type III strains.[24] This protein now is designated C protein. Rabbit antibodies directed against CPS protected mice against lethal challenge with homologous, but not heterologous, GBS types, and cross-protection was also afforded when antibodies against C protein were tested.

Current nomenclature designates polysaccharide antigens as type antigens and protein antigens as additional markers for characterization.[25,26] The former type Ic now is designated type Ia/c. Type IV was identified as a new type in 1982, when 62 strains were described that possessed type IV polysaccharide alone or with additional protein antigens.[27] Antigenically distinct types, V through IX, now are characterized. Strains not expressing one of the CPS-specific antigens are designated as nontypeable by serologic methods but often can be assigned a GBS type by PCR-based methods.

C protein is composed of two unrelated components, the trypsin-resistant α C protein and the trypsin-sensitive β C protein. α C protein is expressed on many type Ia, Ib, and II strains.[28] Strains expressing α C protein are more opsonoresistant than are α C–negative strains. α C protein consists of a series of tandem repeating units, and in naturally occurring strains, the repeat numbers can vary. The number of repeating units expressed alters antigenicity and influences the repertoires of antibodies elicited.[29] The use of one or two repeat units of α C proteins elicits antibodies that bind all α C proteins with equal affinity, suggesting its potential as a vaccine candidate.[30,31] β C protein is a single protein with a molecular mass of 124 to 134 kDa that is present in about 10% of isolates. β C protein binds the Fc region of human IgA.[32,33] Strains bearing α and β C proteins possess increased resistance to opsonization in vitro.

GBS express numerous additional surface proteins. Designation of additional α-like repetitive proteins (Alp) numerically (e.g., Alp2 and Alp3) is being considered. Most strains have the gene for just one Alp family protein. Genes encoding Alp1 (also designated "epsilon") are associated with type Ia, and genes encoding Alp3 are associated with type V strains.[34] Alp also are referred to as R proteins, with R1 and R4 as the major ones found on clinical isolates.[34] Rib protein, expressed by most type III strains, has an identical sequence to R4. The gene sequence of a protein initially designated R5 has been renamed group B protective surface protein (BPS).[35] In one large collection, BPS was found in 3.5% of invasive or colonizing isolates, most often in type Ia, II, or V GBS and never in type III.[36] Some GBS contain surface proteins designated as X antigens.[37] The X and R antigens are immunologically cross-reactive. A laddering protein from type V GBS shares sequence homology with α C protein.[38] A protein designated Sip (surface immunogenic protein) is distinct from other known surface proteins. It is produced by all GBS types and confers protection against experimental infection; its role in human infection is unknown.[39]

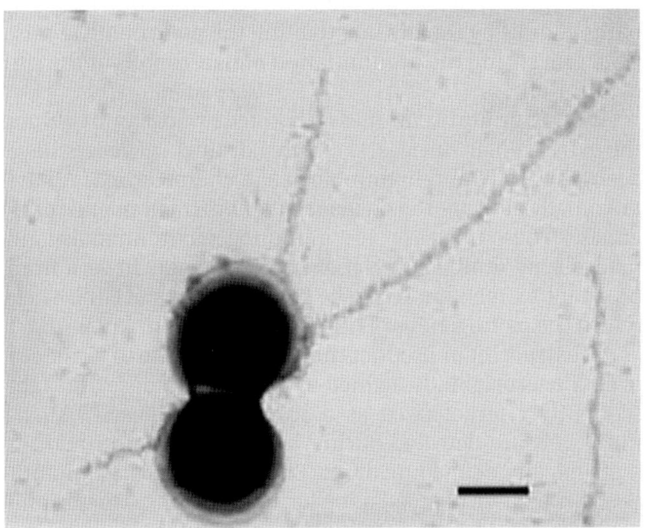

Figure 12-1 Immunogold labeling and transmission electron microscopy of group B streptococcal organisms showing long pilus-like structures extending from the cell surface. (From Lauer P, Rinaudo CD, Soriani M, et al: Genome analysis reveals pili in group B streptococcus, *Science* 309:105, 2005.)

Genome analysis has shown that GBS produce long pilus-like structures. These structures extend from the bacterial surface and beyond CPS (Fig. 12-1).[8] Formed by proteins with adhesive functions, these structures are implicated in host colonization, attachment, and invasion.[40] The pilus-like structures are encoded in genomic pilus islands that have an organization similar to that of pathogenicity islands. Three types of pilus islands have been identified through genomic analysis; these are composed of partially homogeneous covalently linked proteins (pilus islands 1, 2a, and 2b). These pilus proteins are highly surface-expressed and are involved in paracellular translocation through epithelial cells. At least one pilus island is present on all GBS clinical strains tested to date.

ULTRASTRUCTURE

Early concepts suggested a thick, rigid peptidoglycan layer external to the cytoplasmic membrane surrounded by concentric layers of cell wall antigens. Evidence now supports a model in which the group B carbohydrate and the CPS are linked independently to cell wall peptidoglycan.[41] Immunoelectron techniques reveal abundant capsule on Lancefield prototype strains Ia, II, and III, whereas less dense capsules are found on type Ib strains (Fig. 12-2).[42] Similarly, incubation of the reference strains with homologous type-specific antisera reveals a thick capsular layer on types IV, V, and VI.[43,44] Ultrastructural studies show that the C protein also has a surface location.[42] CPS capsule expression can be

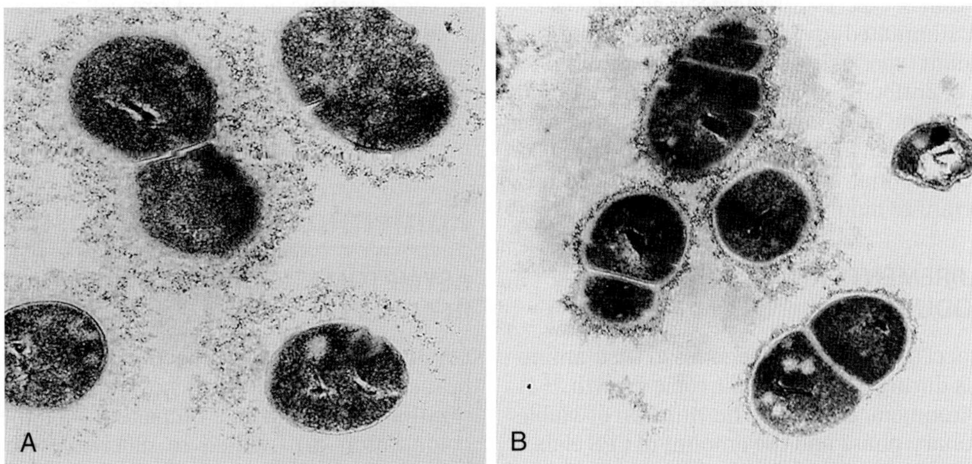

Figure 12-2 Electron micrographs of thin sections of type Ia group B streptococcal prototype strains. **A,** Type Ia strain 090. **B,** Type Ia/c strain A909. Both are stained with ferritin-conjugated type Ia–specific rabbit antibodies. The larger capsule is representative of those found also in Lancefield prototype II strain (18RS21) and type III isolates from infants with meningitis, whereas the smaller capsule is representative of that also found on Lancefield prototype strain Ib (H36B). (Micrographs courtesy Dennis L. Kasper, MD.)

regulated by altering cell growth rate.[45] Immunogold labeling and transmission electron microscopy show that the GBS pilus-like structures extend from the bacterial surface.[8]

IMMUNOCHEMISTRY OF POLYSACCHARIDE ANTIGENS

Lancefield's initial serologic definition used hydrochloric acid and heat treatment, resulting in degraded antigens of small molecular mass. Gentler techniques isolated large molecular mass or "native" polysaccharides that contained sialic acid. Human immunity correlates with antibody to the sialic acid–containing type III structure.[46] With the use of contemporary methods for determination, L-rhamnose, D-galactose, 2-acetamido-2-deoxy-D-glucose, and D-glucitol have been identified as the constituent monosaccharides of the group B antigen. It is composed of four different oligosaccharides, designated I though IV, and linked by a phosphodiester bond to form a complex, highly branched multiantennary structure.[47]

The repeating unit structures of the type-specific CPSs are schematically represented in Figure 12-3. Types Ia, Ib, and III have a five-sugar repeating unit containing galactose, glucose, *N*-acetylglucosamine, and sialic acid in a ratio of 2:1:1:1.[46,48-50] Type II and type V have a seven-sugar repeating unit, type IV and type VII have six-sugar repeats, and type VIII polysaccharide has a four-sugar repeating unit.[43,51-55] Molar ratios vary, but the component monosaccharides are the same among the polysaccharide types except that type VI lacks *N*-acetylglucosamine and type VIII contains rhamnose in the backbone structure.[56]

Each antigen has a backbone repeating unit of two (Ia, Ib), three (III, IV, V, VII, VIII), or four (II) monosaccharides to which one or two side chains are linked. Sialic acid is the exclusive terminal side chain sugar except for the type II polysaccharide, which also has a terminal galactose. The structures of the type Ia and type Ib polysaccharides differ only in a single side-chain linkage, although there are differences in the tertiary configuration of the molecules.[57] These linkages are critical to immunologic specificity and explain the observed immunologic cross-reactivity.[22,58] The desialylated type III polysaccharide is immunologically identical to that of type 14 *Streptococcus pneumoniae*.[59] This observation stimulated investigations concerning the immunodeterminant specificity of human immunity to type III GBS and of antibody recognition of conformational epitopes as a facet of the host immune response.[60] The type III polysaccharide also can form extended helices. The position of the conformational epitope along these helices is potentially important to binding site interactions.[61]

GROWTH REQUIREMENTS AND BACTERIAL PRODUCTS

Group B streptococci are quite homogeneous in their amino acid requirements during aerobic or anaerobic growth.[62] A glucose-rich environment enhances the number of viable GBS during stationary phase and the amount of CPS elaborated.[63] In a modified chemically defined medium, the expression of capsule during continuous growth is regulated by the growth rate.[45] Invasiveness is enhanced by a fast growth rate and is optimal in the presence of at least 5% oxygen.[64,65]

GBS elaborate many products during their growth. Among these is the hemolysin that produces the β-hemolysis surrounding colonies on blood agar. Hemolysin is a surface-associated toxin active against the erythrocytes from several mammalian species. The GBS hemolysin recently has been characterized as the ornithine rhamnolipid pigment and shown to function as a virulence factor, promoting invasion of placental cells.[66] GBS can hydrolyze hippuric acid to benzoic acid and glycine. The hippuricase of GBS is cell associated and is trypsin and heat labile.[67] It is antigenic in rabbits, but its relationship to bacterial virulence, if any, has not been studied.

Most strains of GBS have an enzyme that inactivates complement component C5a by cleaving a peptide at the carboxyl terminus.[68] GBS C5a-ase seems to be a serine esterase; it is distinct from the C5a-cleaving enzyme produced by group A streptococci,[69] although the genes that encode these enzymes are similar.[70] C5a-ase contributes to pathogenesis by rapidly inactivating the neutrophil agonist C5a, preventing the accumulation of neutrophils at the site of infection.[71]

Another group of enzymes elaborated by nearly all GBS are the extracellular nucleases.[72] Three distinct nucleases have been physically and immunologically characterized. All are maximally activated by divalent cations of calcium plus manganese. These nucleases are immunogenic in animals, and neutralizing antibodies to them are detectable in sera from pregnant women known to be genital carriers of GBS. Their role in the pathogenesis of human infection is unknown.

An extracellular product that can contribute to virulence of GBS was originally defined as a neuraminidase and subsequently characterized as a hyaluronate lyase.[73] Maximal levels are detected during late exponential growth in a chemically defined medium. Elaboration of large quantities can be a virulence factor for type III GBS. Musser and coworkers[74] identified a high neuraminidase–producing subset of type III strains that were responsible for most serious GBS infections. Later studies indicated that these were from a single clonal complex, designated ST 17, that has been designated as "hypervirulent." ST 17 is almost exclusively found in type III strains.

GBS synthesize acylated (lipoteichoic) and deacylated glycerol teichoic acids that are cell associated and can be readily extracted and purified.[75] Strains from infants with early- or late-onset disease have higher levels of cell-associated and native deacylated lipoteichoic acid, and this product seems to contribute to attachment to human cells.[76]

Epidemiology and Transmission

ASYMPTOMATIC INFECTION (COLONIZATION) IN ADULTS

Group B streptococcal infection limited to mucous membrane sites is designated as asymptomatic infection, colonization, or carriage. Comparisons of the prevalence of colonization are related to differences in ascertainment techniques. Factors that influence the accuracy of colonization detection include density of colonization, choice of bacteriologic media, body sites sampled, number of culture specimens obtained, and time interval of study.

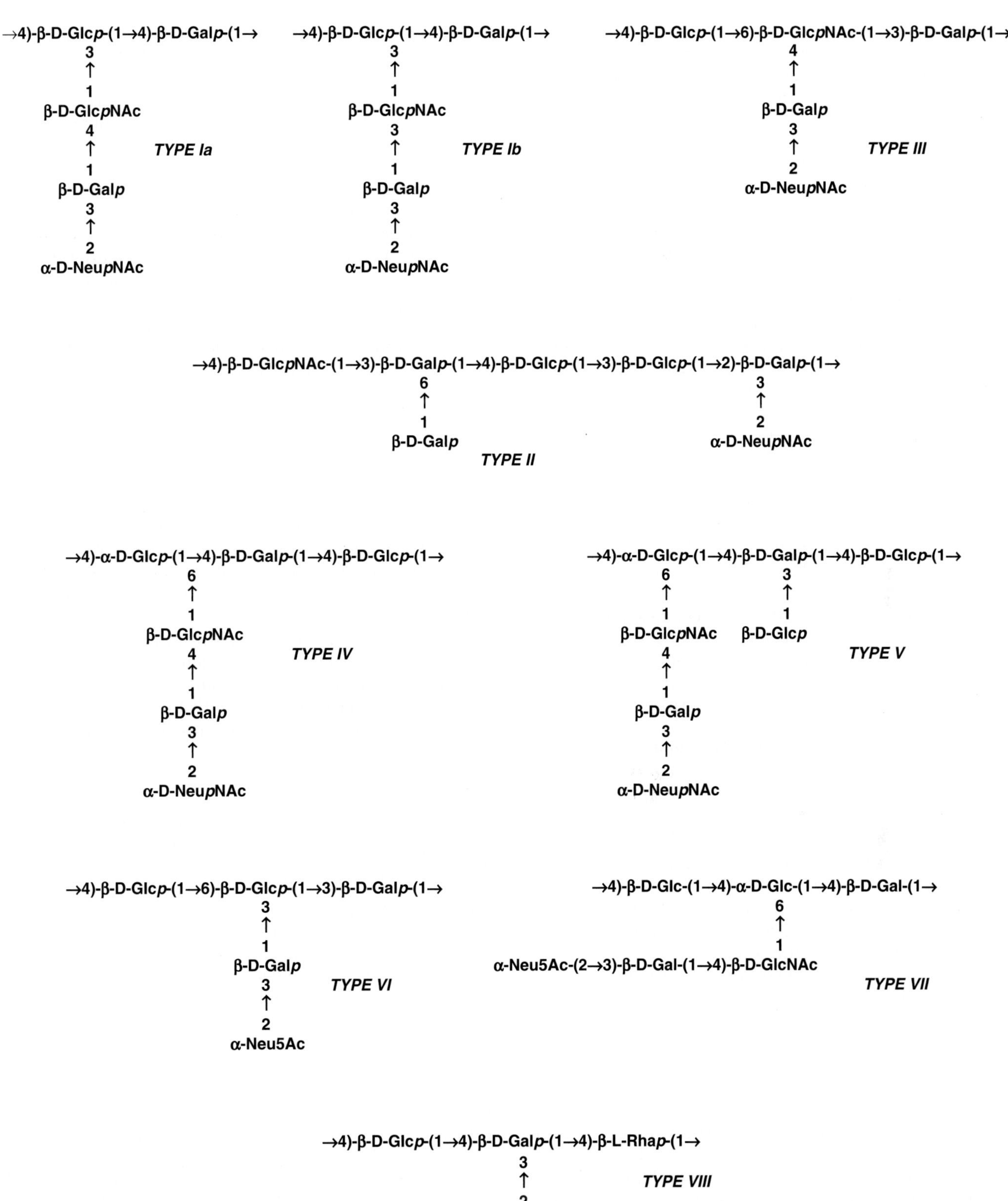

Figure 12-3 Repeating unit structures of group B streptococcal capsular polysaccharides type Ia,[57] type Ib,[57,58] type II,[53,55] type III,[49,50] type IV,[54] type V,[51] type VI,[568] type VII,[52] and type VIII.[56]

Isolation rates are higher with use of an enrichment broth, rather than solid agar media, and with enrichment broth containing substances inhibitory for normal flora (usually antimicrobials). Selective enrichment broths, include Todd-Hewitt broth supplemented either with gentamicin (8 μg/mL) and nalidixic acid (15 μg/mL; TransVag broth) or with colistin (10 μg/mL) and nalidixic acid (15 μg/mL; Lim broth). Addition of 5% sheep blood to TransVag broth or Lim broth can increase the recovery of GBS. Such media inhibit the growth of most gram-negative enteric bacilli and other normal flora that make isolation of streptococci from these sites difficult. Use of selective enrichment broth promotes detection of low numbers of organisms that escape detection when inoculation of swabs is directly onto solid agar.

Isolation rates also are influenced by body sites selected for culture. Female genital culture isolation rates double with progression from the cervical os to the vulva. In addition, culture sampling of lower genital tract and rectal sites increases GBS colonization rates 10% to 15% beyond that found if a single site is cultured. The urinary tract is an important site of infection, especially during pregnancy, which usually manifests as asymptomatic bacteriuria. To predict accurately the likelihood of neonatal exposure to GBS at delivery, maternal culture specimens from the lower vagina and rectum (not perianal area) should be collected.

The prevalence of GBS colonization is influenced by the number of cultures obtained from a site and the interval of sampling. Vaginal colonization patterns can be chronic, transient, or intermittent. A longitudinal cohort study of nonpregnant young women found that almost one half of those who are culture negative at enrollment acquired vaginal colonization during three 4-month intervals of assessment.[77] The duration of colonization among college students is estimated to be 14 weeks for women and 9 weeks for men.[78] The predictive value of a positive second trimester vaginal or rectal culture for colonization at delivery is only 67%.[79] The predictive value of a positive prenatal culture result is highest (73%) in women with vaginal and rectal colonization and lowest (60%) in women with rectal colonization only. Cultures performed 1 to 5 weeks before delivery have a positive predictive value of 87% (95% confidence interval [CI], 83 to 92) for colonization status at delivery in term parturients. The negative predictive value is 96% (95% CI, 95 to 98). Culture specimens collected within this interval perform significantly better than specimens collected 6 or more weeks before delivery.[80]

The primary reservoir for GBS is the lower gastrointestinal tract.[3] The recovery of GBS from the rectum is three to five times more common than recovery from the vagina, and the rectal site predicts persistence or chronicity of carriage.[81] GBS in the gastrointestinal tract is a risk factor for vaginal GBS. Additional support for the lower gastrointestinal tract as the primary reservoir is the association of GBS with infections resulting from gastrointestinal tract surgical procedures. Several factors influence genital carriage of GBS. Among healthy young men and women living in a college dormitory, sexually experienced subjects had colonization rates twice those of sexually inexperienced subjects.[82] In a longitudinal cohort study of nonpregnant young women, African-American ethnicity, having multiple sex partners during a preceding 4-month interval, having frequent sexual intercourse within the same interval, and having sexual intercourse within the 5 days before a follow-up visit were independently associated with vaginal acquisition of GBS.[77] These latter findings suggest either that the organism is sexually transmitted or that sexual activity alters the microenvironment to make it more permissive to colonization. In another study of college women, GBS were isolated significantly more often from sexually experienced women, women studied during the first half of the menstrual cycle, women with an intrauterine device, and women 20 years of age or younger.[83] Colonization with GBS also occurs at a high rate in healthy college students and is associated with having engaged in sexual activity, tampon use, milk consumption, and hand washing done four times daily or less.[84] Fish consumption increased the risk of acquiring some, but not all, capsular types.[85]

A higher prevalence of colonization with GBS is found among pregnant diabetic patients than among nondiabetic controls.[86] Carriage over a prolonged interval reportedly occurs more often in women who use tampons than women who do not.[87] Colonization is more frequent among teenage women than among women 20 years of age or older[83] and among women with three or fewer pregnancies than in women with more than three pregnancies. Hispanic women of Caribbean origin have a high rate of colonization, and African-American women have a higher rate of colonization at delivery than do other racial or ethnic groups.[77,88,89] A large inoculum of vaginal GBS colonization also is more common among African-American than among Hispanic or non-Hispanic white women.[90] Factors that do *not* influence the prevalence of genital colonization in nonpregnant women include use of oral contraceptives[83]; marital status; presence of vaginal discharge or other gynecologic signs or symptoms[83]; carriage of *Chlamydia trachomatis*, *Ureaplasma urealyticum*, *Trichomonas vaginalis*, or *Mycoplasma hominis*; and infection with *Neisseria gonorrhoeae*.

Colonization with GBS can elicit an immune response. In a group of pregnant women evaluated at admission for delivery, vaginal or rectal colonization with types Ia, II, III, or V was associated with significantly higher serum concentrations of immunoglobulin (IgG) specific for the colonizing type compared with noncolonized women.[88] Moderate concentrations of Ia, Ib, II, III, and V CPS-specific IgG also were found in association with colonization during pregnancy.[91] Maternal colonization with type III was least likely to be associated with these CPS-specific antibodies. In contrast to infection with organisms such as *N. gonorrhoeae* or genital mycoplasmas, genital infection with GBS is not related to genital symptoms.[83]

GBS have been isolated from vaginal or rectal sites or both in 15% to 40% of pregnant women. The range in colonization rates relates to intrinsic differences in populations (age, ethnicity, parity, socioeconomic status, geographic location) and to lack of standardization in culture methods used for ascertainment. True population differences account for some of the disparity in reported prevalence rates. When selective enrichment broth is used and vaginal and rectal sites are sampled, the prevalence of maternal colonization with GBS by region is 12% in India and Pakistan, 19% in Asia and the Pacific Islands, 19% in sub-Saharan Africa, 22% in the Middle East and North Africa, 14% in Central and South America, and 26% in the United States.[88,92] The rates of colonization among pregnant women range from 20% to 29% in Eastern Europe, 11% to 21% in Western Europe, 21% to 36% in Scandinavia, and 7% to 32% in Southern Europe.[93] The rate of recurrence of GBS colonization in a subsequent pregnancy is higher compared with women negative for colonization in their prior pregnancy.[94] Pharyngeal carriage rates are low and are similar among pregnant and nonpregnant women and heterosexual men[95,96]; however, rates approach 20% in men who have sex with men.[97] No definite relationship between isolation of GBS from throat cultures and symptoms of pharyngitis has been proved,[98] but some investigators have suggested that these organisms can cause acute pharyngitis.[96]

ASYMPTOMATIC INFECTION IN INFANTS AND CHILDREN

Cultures from the throat and rectum are the best sites for detection of GBS during childhood and until the start of sexual activity.[99,100] In a study of 100 girls ranging in age from 2 months to 16 years, Hammerschlag and coworkers[99] isolated GBS from pharyngeal, rectal or vaginal sites, or both, in 20% of children. The prevalence of positive pharyngeal cultures resembled the prevalence of adults in girls 11 years or older (5%) but approached the prevalence reported for neonates in younger girls (15%). Rectal colonization was detected frequently in girls younger than 3 or older than 10 years of age (about 25%), but was uncommon in girls 3 to 10 years of age. Mauer and colleagues[100] isolated GBS from cultures of vaginal, anal, or pharyngeal specimens or all three in 11% of prepubertal boys and girls. Pharyngeal (5% each) and rectal (10% and 7%) isolation rates were similar for boys and for girls. Persson and coworkers[101] detected fecal carriage of GBS in 4% of healthy boys and girls, and Cummings and Ross[102] found that 2% of English schoolchildren had pharyngeal carriage. Genital colonization in girls is uncommon before puberty.[103] Whether this relates to environmental influences in the prepubertal vagina or to lack of sexual experience before puberty, or both, awaits further study.

TRANSMISSION OF GROUP B STREPTOCOCCI TO NEONATES

The presence of GBS in the maternal genital tract at delivery is the major determinant of colonization and infection in the neonate. Exposure of the neonate to the organism occurs by the ascending route in utero through translocation through intact membranes, through ruptured membranes, or by contamination during passage via the birth canal. Prospective studies have indicated vertical transmission rates of 29% to 85%, with a mean rate of approximately 50% among neonates born to women from whom GBS were isolated from cultures of vagina or rectum or both at delivery. Conversely, only about 5% of healthy infants delivered to culture-negative women become colonized at one or more sites during the first 48 hours of life.

The risk of a neonate acquiring colonization by the vertical route correlates directly with the density of colonization (inoculum size). Neonates born to heavily colonized women are more likely to acquire carriage at mucous membrane sites than neonates born to women with low colony counts of GBS in vaginal cultures at delivery.[104] Boyer and associates [79] found that rates of vertical transmission were substantially higher in women with heavy than in women with light colonization (65% vs. 17%) and that colonization at multiple sites and development of early-onset disease were more likely among infants born to heavily colonized mothers. The likelihood of colonization in a neonate born to a woman who is culture-positive at delivery is unrelated to maternal age, race, parity, or blood type or to duration of labor or method of delivery.[79] It is unclear whether preterm or low-birth-weight neonates are at higher risk for colonization from maternal sources than term infants.

Most neonates exposed to GBS by their mothers have infection that is limited to surface or mucous membrane sites (colonization), which results from contamination of the oropharynx, gastric contents, or gastrointestinal tract by swallowing of infected amniotic fluid or maternal vaginal secretions. In neonates, external auditory canal cultures are more likely to yield GBS than cultures from anterior nares, throat, umbilicus, or rectum in first 24 hours of life,[3,105] and isolation of organisms from the ear canal is a surrogate for the degree of contamination from amniotic fluid and vaginal secretions sequestered during the birth process. After the first 48 hours of life, throat and rectal sites are the best sources for detection of GBS, and positive cultures indicate true colonization (multiplication of organisms at mucous membrane sites), not just maternal exposure.[106]

Other sources for acquisition of GBS in neonates have been established. Horizontal transmission from hospital or community sources is an important, albeit uncommonly proved, mode for transmission of infection.[105,107,108] Acquisition can occur from hands of nursery personnel. In contrast to group A streptococci, which can cause epidemic disease in nurseries, GBS rarely exhibits this potential, and isolation of colonized neonates is not routinely indicated. An epidemic cluster of five infants with late-onset bacteremia infection caused by type Ib GBS occurred among very-low-birth-weight infants in a neonatal intensive care unit in the 1980s.[109] None of the index cases was colonized at birth, establishing that acquisition during hospitalization had occurred. Epidemiologic analysis suggested infant-to-infant spread by means of the hands of personnel, although acquisition from two nurses colonized with the same phage type Ib strain was not excluded. The infection control measures instituted, including cohorting of culture-positive infants and strict hand hygiene, prevented additional cases. Community sources afford a likely potential for transmission of GBS to the neonate. Indirect evidence has suggested that this mode of infection is infrequent.[107] Only 2 of 46 neonates culture negative for GBS when discharged from the newborn nursery acquired mucous membrane infection at 2 months of age.[110] The mode of transmission likely is fecal-oral. Healthy infants colonized from a maternal source or postnatally show persistence of infection at mucous membrane sites for weeks or months.[107,111]

SEROTYPE DISTRIBUTION OF ISOLATES

The differentiation of GBS into CPS types has provided a valuable tool in defining the epidemiology of human infection. In the 1970s and 1980s, virtually all evaluations of GBS isolated from healthy neonates, children, or adults revealed an even distribution into types Ia or Ib, II, and III. This distribution also was reported for isolates from neonates with early-onset infection without meningitis and their mothers.[112] In the 1990, types other than I, II, or III accounted for less than 5% of all isolates.

In the early 1990s, GBS type V emerged as a frequent cause of colonization and invasive disease in neonates and adults.[113-115] Most type V isolates have one pulse-field gel electrophoresis pattern that has been present in the United

States since 1975.[116] Type V now causes a substantial proportion of cases of invasive early-onset disease and infection during pregnancy. Type Ia has increased in prevalence and a corresponding decline has occurred in type II strains causing perinatal disease.[114] Type III strains account for about 70% of isolates from infants with meningitis and continue to be isolated from at least two thirds of infants with late-onset disease globally.[117,118,119] Type IV, which accounts for occasional cases, could be emerging as a more important cause of early-onset infection.[120] Types VI, VII, VIII, and IX rarely cause human disease in the United States or the United Kingdom, but types VI and VIII are the most common serotypes isolated from healthy Japanese women.[121,122]

The contemporary CPS type distribution of GBS from different patient groups is shown in Figure 12-4. Prospective population-based surveillance through the Active Bacterial Core Surveillance/Emerging Infections Program Network of the U.S. Centers for Disease Control and Prevention (CDC) defined the epidemiology of invasive GBS disease in the United States from 1999-2005.[123] The GBS types represented in 528 early-onset disease cases were Ia (30%), III (28%), V (18%), and II (13%). The distribution for 172 pregnancy-associated cases was similar. The type distribution among 469 late-onset cases was Ia (24%), III (51%), and V (14%). Type V predominated among cases in nonpregnant adults, accounting for 31%, followed by Ia (24%), II (12%), and III (12%).

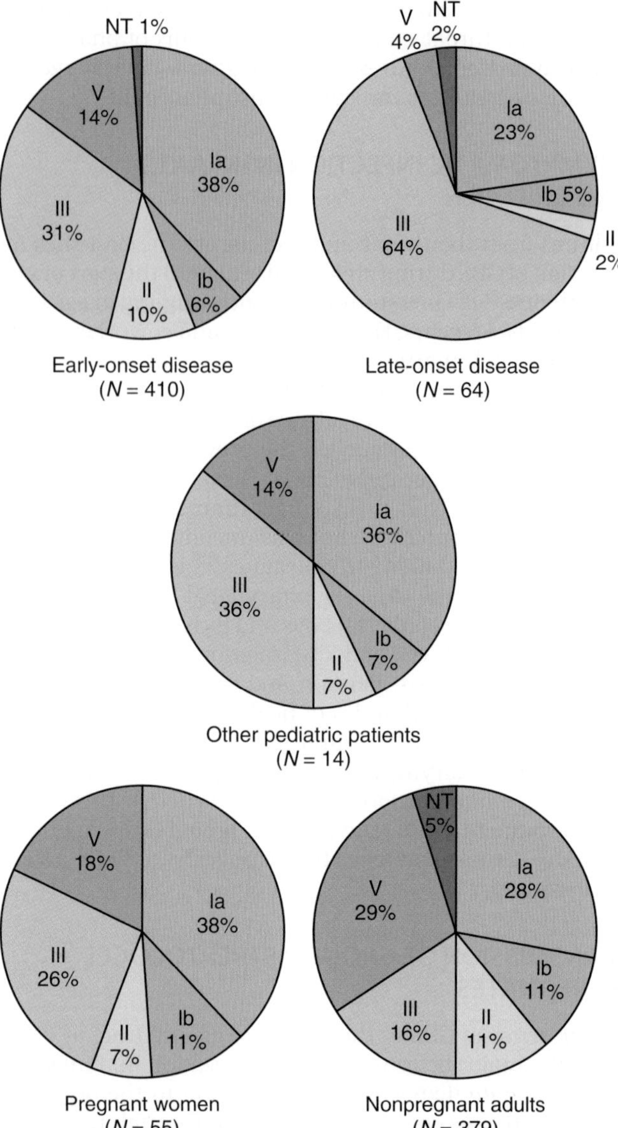

Figure 12-4 Schematic representation of group B streptococcal serotypes isolated from various patient groups. *N*, Number of patient isolates studied; *NT*, nontypeable strains. (Data from Blumberg HM, Stephens DS, Modansky M, et al: Invasive group B streptococcal disease: the emergence of serotype V, *J Infect Dis* 173:365-373. 1996; Zaleznik DF, Rench MA, Hillier S, et al: Invasive disease due to group B *Streptococcus* in pregnant women and neonates from diverse population groups, *Clin Infect Dis* 30:276-281, 2000; and Lin FY, Clemens JD, Azimi PH, et al: Capsular polysaccharide types of group B streptococcal isolates from neonates with early-onset systemic infection, *J Infect Dis* 177:790-792, 1998.)

MOLECULAR EPIDEMIOLOGY

Tools such as multilocus enzyme electrophoresis,[74,124] restriction-enzyme fragment-length polymorphism analysis, pulsed-field gel electrophoresis (PFGE),[125] random-amplified polymorphic DNA assay[126] and multiplex PCR[127] have been used for molecular characterization of GBS isolates. Multilocus sequence typing (MLST) and PFGE are reportedly more appropriate than a semiautomated repetitive sequence-based PCR DiversiLab system (bioMérieux, Durham, NC) for determining the relatedness of invasive GBS strains.[128] These molecular typing techniques have indicated that some geographically and epidemiologically distinct GBS isolates have identical patterns, suggesting dissemination of a limited number of clones in the United States. Molecular techniques also have confirmed the molecular relatedness of mother and infant strains, strains from twins and those from sexual partners.[121,126] Multilocus sequence typing and capsular gene cluster (*cps*) genotyping have been used to investigate the dynamics of perinatal colonization. Changes in capsule expression and recolonization with antigenically distinct GBS clones were detected in culture-positive women over time by applying MLST.[129]

Molecular characterization has been used to explore the role of virulence clones in contributing to invasive disease. Type III strains were classified into three major phylogenetic lineages, with most cases of invasive neonatal disease caused by strains with one restriction digest pattern (type III-3) on the basis of bacterial DNA restriction digest patterns.[130] The genetic variation that distinguishes restriction digest pattern type III-3 strains seems to occur within localized areas of the genome that contain known or putative virulence genes.[131,132] Using genomic subtractive hybridization to identify regions of the genome unique to virulent restriction fragment digest pattern type III-3 strains, a surface protein was identified that mediates epithelial cell invasion.[133] Using MLST, 10 allelic profiles that converged into three groups on concatenation were identified among type III isolates recovered from neonates with invasive disease and from colonized pregnant women.[134] One PFGE group bearing a gene from the capsular synthesis operon has been shown in type III strains causing neonatal meningitis, but not in type III colonizing strains.[135] Clustering of most invasive neonatal isolates into major PFGE groups also has been noted.[136] Among type III strains evaluated by MLST, a single clone, ST17, is reported to be hypervirulent. Additional studies are required to elucidate the differences in virulence among clones identified by these techniques.[137] However, genetic analysis of GBS isolates from worldwide sources demonstrates that epidemic clones, such as clonal complex 17 (CC17) have adapted specifically to the human host.[138] The finding that isolates with different capsular serotypes have the same sequence type suggests that capsular switching can occur.[134,139] Bellais and colleagues[140] have demonstrated that capsular switching from CPS type III to IV does occur within the highly homogeneous CC17 hypervirulent clone. Sequence analysis showed that this capsular switch was due to the exchange of a DNA fragment containing the whole *cps* operon.

INCIDENCE OF INFECTION IN NEONATES AND PARTURIENTS

Two clinical syndromes occur among young infants with GBS disease that are epidemiologically distinct and relate to age at onset.[2,3] The attack rate for the first of these syndromes, designated early onset, because it occurs within the first 6 days of life (mean onset, 12-18 hours), ranged historically from 0.7 to 3.7 per 1000 live births. The attack rate for late-onset infection (onset 7-89 days of age) ranged from 0.5 to 1.8 per 1000 live births. The burden of early-onset disease is disproportionately high in African-American infants for reasons that are not well defined but might include higher maternal colonization rates, higher density of colonization, and higher rates of preterm deliveries compared with white women.[141] There has been a dramatic decline in the incidence of early-onset disease in the United States in association with implementation of universal antenatal screening and use of intrapartum antibiotic prophylaxis (IAP). From 1993 to 1998, when risk-based and GBS culture-based methods were in use, incidence of early-onset disease declined by 65%, from 1.7 to 0.6 per 1000 live births.[5] Comparison of the two approaches showed the superiority of a culture-based approach.[142] The incidence of early-onset disease declined further in association with implementation of guidelines, published in 2002 and revised in 2010, that advocate a culture-based approach for prevention of early-onset disease.[16,123] The national estimate of early-onset invasive disease in 2012 was 0.24 per 1000 live births, but this represented a plateau since 2008.[143] Despite the decline in incidence, GBS remains the most commonly reported pathogen causing early-onset disease, accounting for approximately 40% of cases in the United States.[144] In contrast to its impact on early-onset disease, IAP has had no impact on the incidence of late-onset disease, which has remained stable at approximately 0.3 per 1000 live births since 2002.[123]

Globally, GBS is a leading cause of neonatal sepsis in developed countries, but the burden of disease in the developing world is less clear, and more high-quality studies are needed. The reported incidence of neonatal GBS disease in developing countries ranges from 0 to 3.1 per 1000 live births, with variation within and between geographic regions.[145] Incidence rates are higher when automated culture methods are used. A systemic review and meta-analysis to examine the global burden reported a mean incidence of GBS in infants from birth to 89 days of age of 0.53 per 1000 live births.[146] Substantial heterogeneity existed between studies. Studies that reported use of any intrapartum antibiotic prophylaxis were associated with a lower incidence of early-onset GBS (0.23/1000 live births [95% CI, 0.13 to 0.59]) than those in which prophylaxis was not used (0.75/1000 live births [95% CI, 0.58 to 0.089]).

The male-to-female ratio for early-onset and late-onset GBS disease is equal. Before 1996, 20% to 25% of all infants with GBS disease had onset after the first 6 days of life. In 2012, 57% of infants had disease with onset after 6 days of life.[143] Infants born prematurely constitute approximately one fourth of the total with early-onset disease and one half of the total with late-onset disease.

The importance of GBS as a common pathogen for the perinatal period relates to the pregnant woman as well as her infant. The risk of intraamniotic infection is greater in women with heavy colonization. Implementation of IAP has been associated with a significant decline in the incidence of invasive disease in pregnant women, from 0.29 per 1000 live births in 1993 to 0.23 per 1000 live births in 1998, and a further decline to 0.12 per 1000 live births during 1999 to 2005.[123,142] One half of these infections were associated with infection of the upper genital tract, placenta, or amniotic sac and resulted in fetal death. Among the other infections, bacteremia without a focus (31%), endometritis without fetal death (8%), and chorioamnionitis without fetal death (4%) were the most common manifestations.

Immunology and Pathogenesis

HOST-BACTERIAL INTERACTIONS RELATED TO PATHOGENESIS

The prevalence and severity of GBS diseases in neonates have stimulated intensive investigation to elucidate the pathogenesis of infection. The unique epidemiologic and clinical features of GBS disease pose several basic questions that provide a framework for hypothesis development and experimental testing: How does the organism colonize pregnant women and gain access to the infant before or during delivery? Why are newborns, especially infants born prematurely, uniquely susceptible to infection? What allows GBS to evade host innate immune defenses? How do these organisms gain entry to the bloodstream and then cross the blood-brain barrier to produce meningitis? What specific GBS factors injure host tissues or induce the sepsis syndrome?

Advances in knowledge of pathogenesis have been achieved through analysis of GBS behavior in cell-culture systems and animal models. Advanced molecular genetic techniques have yielded isogenic mutant strains varying solely in the production of a particular component (e.g., capsular polysaccharide). Such mutants are important in establishing the biologic relevance of a given trait and its requirement for virulence in vivo. The sequencing of numerous complete GBS genomes has provided additional context for interpretation of experimental data and comparison with other well-studied pathogens.[6,7]

Although GBS have adapted well to asymptomatic colonization of healthy adults, they remain a potentially devastating pathogen to susceptible infants. This section reviews

Table 12-1 Group B Streptococcal Virulence Factors in Pathogenesis of Neonatal Infection

Virulence Factor	Molecular or Cellular Action(s)	Proposed Role in Pathogenesis
HOST CELL ATTACHMENT/INVASION		
C surface protein	Binds glycosaminoglycans	Epithelial/endothelial invasion
Fibrinogen receptor, FbsA	Binds fibrinogen in extracellular matrix	Epithelial cell attachment
Lipoteichoic acid	Binds host cell surfaces	Epithelial cell attachment
C5a peptidase, ScpB	Binds fibronectin in extracellular matrix	Epithelial cell adherence, invasion
Surface protein Lmb	Binds laminin in extracellular matrix	Epithelial cell attachment
Spb1 surface protein	Promotes epithelial cell uptake	Invasion of epithelial barriers
iagA gene	?Alteration in bacterial cell surface	Blood-brain barrier invasion
Glycoprotein Srr1	Binds fibronectin in extracellular matrix	Vaginal and brain capillary binding
CovRS two-component regulator	Global transcriptional regulator	Regulation of adherence factors
Surface protein HgvA	Endothelial cell binding/uptake	Promotes blood-brain barrier invasion
Pili	Promotes cell surface binding	Epithelial and endothelial cell invasion
INJURY TO HOST TISSUES		
β-Hemolysin/cytolysin	Lyses epithelial and endothelial cells	Damage and spread through tissues causes neuronal apoptosis
Hyaluronate lyase	Cleaves hyaluronan or chondroitin sulfate	Promotes spread through host tissues
CAMP factor	Lyses host cells (co-hemolysin)	Direct tissue injury
RESISTANCE TO IMMUNE CLEARANCE		
Exopolysaccharide capsule	Impairs C3 deposition/activation	Blocks opsonophagocytic clearance
C5a peptidase, ScpB	Cleaves and inactivates human C5a	Inhibits neutrophil recruitment
CAMP factor	Binds to Fc portion of IgG, IgM	Impairment of antibody function
Serine protease, CspA	Cleaves fibrinogen, coats GBS surface with fibrin	Blocks opsonophagocytosis
Fibrinogen receptor, FbsA	? Steric interference with C3 function	Blocks opsonophagocytosis
C protein	Nonimmune binding of IgA	Blocks opsonophagocytosis
β-Hemolysin/cytolysin	Lyses neutrophils macrophages, proapoptotic	Impairment of phagocyte killing
Superoxide dismutase	Inactivates superoxide	Impairment of oxidative burst killing
Carotenoid pigment	Antioxidant effect blocks H_2O_2, singlet oxygen	Impairment of oxidative burst killing
dlt operon genes	Alanylation of lipoteichoic acid	Blocks antimicrobial peptides
Penicillin-binding protein 1a	Alteration in cell wall composition	Blocks antimicrobial peptides
Nuclease A	Degrades DNA	Escape neutrophil extracellular taps
CovRS two-component regulator	Global transcriptional regulator	Phagolysomal survival
ACTIVATION OF INFLAMMATORY MEDIATORS		
Cell wall lipoteichoic acid	Binds pattern recognition receptors (TLRs)	Cytokine activation
Cell wall peptidoglycan	Binds pattern recognition receptors (TLRs)	Cytokine activation
β-Hemolysin/cytolysin	Activation of host cell stress response pathways, inflammasome	iNOS, IL-10, IL-1β release
GAPDH	Triggers IL-10 release	Suppression of neutrophil migration

CAMP, Christie-Atkins-Munch-Petersen; *GAPDH*, glyceraldehyde-3-phosphate dehydrogenase; *GBS*, group B streptococci; H_2O_2, hydrogen peroxide; *IgG, IgM*, and *IgA*, immunoglobulin G, M, and A, respectively; *IL*, interleukin; *iNOS*, inducible nitric oxide synthase.

the current understanding of virulence mechanisms, many of which are revealed or magnified by the unique circumstances of the birth process and the deficiencies of neonatal immune defense. Many of the GBS virulence factors defined to date, with mode of action and proposed role in pathogenesis, are summarized in Table 12-1. Key stages in the molecular, cellular, and immunologic pathogenesis of newborn infection are summarized schematically in Figure 12-5.

Maternal Colonization

The presence of GBS in the genital tract of the mother at delivery determines whether or not a newborn is at risk for invasive disease. Among infants born to colonized women, the risk of early-onset disease is approximately 30-fold that for infants born to women with a negative result on prenatal cultures.[147] A direct relationship exists between the degree (inoculum size) of GBS vaginal colonization, the risk of vertical transmission, and the likelihood of serious disease in the newborn.[104] Consequently, a crucial step in the pathogenesis of invasive disease in the newborn caused by GBS is colonization of pregnant women.

To establish colonization of the female genital tract, GBS must adhere successfully to the vaginal epithelium. Compared with other microorganisms, GBS bind very efficiently to exfoliated human vaginal cells or vaginal tissue culture cells,[148,149] with maximal biofilm formation at the acidic pH characteristic of vaginal mucosa.[150] A low-affinity interaction with epithelial cells is mediated by its amphiphilic cell wall–associated lipoteichoic acid, whereas higher-affinity interactions with host cells are mediated by hydrophobic

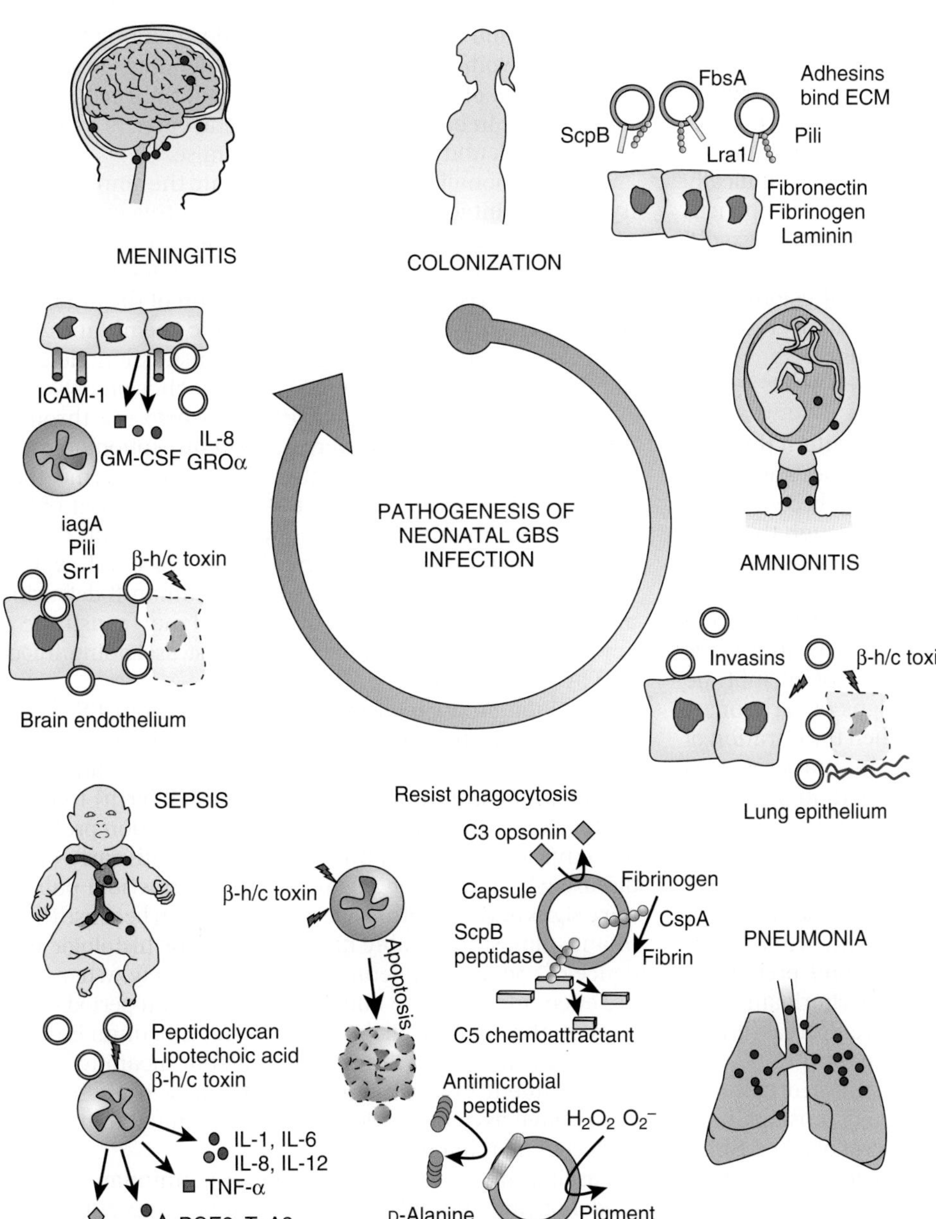

Figure 12-5 Pathologic mechanisms for different types of neonatal group B streptococcal (GBS) infection. *ECM,* Extracellular matrix; *GM-CSF,* granulocyte-macrophage colony-stimulating factor; *GROα,* growth-regulated protein α; *β-h/c,* β-hemolysin/cytolysin; *ICAM-1,* intercellular adhesion molecule-1; *IL-8,* interleukin-8; *PBP1a,* penicillin-binding protein 1a; *PGE2,* prostaglandin E2; *SOD,* superoxide dismutase; *TNF-α,* tumor necrosis factor-α; *TxA2,* thromboxane A2. (Modified from Doran KS, Nizet V: Molecular pathogenesis of neonatal group B streptococcal infection: no longer in its infancy, *Mol Microbiol* 54:23-31, 2004.)

surface proteins. Soluble lipoteichoic acid competitively inhibits epithelial cell adherence[151,152] and decreases vaginal colonization of pregnant mice.[153]

High-affinity protein-mediated interactions of GBS with epithelium are mediated largely through extracellular matrix components, such as fibronectin, fibrinogen, and laminin, which interact with host cell–anchored proteins such as integrins. Binding occurs to immobilized but not soluble fibronectin, suggesting that this interaction requires close proximity of multiple fibronectin molecules and GBS adhesins.[154] For example, a genome-wide phage display technique revealed a fibronectin-binding property associated with the surface-anchored GBS C5a peptidase ScpB, a dual functionality confirmed by decreased fibronectin binding of isogenic ScpB mutants and the direct interaction of recombinant ScpB with solid-phase fibronectin.[155,156] Similar targeted mutagenesis studies showed that adherence of GBS to laminin involves a protein adhesin called Lmb,[157] attachment to fibrinogen is mediated by repetitive motifs within the surface-anchored protein FbsA,[158] and binding to human keratin 4 is carried out by the serine-rich repeat domain protein Srr-1.[159]

Group B streptococci express filamentous cell surface appendages known as pili.[8] Group B streptococcal pili contain three subunits: a backbone pilin protein (PilB), a pilus-associated adhesion (PilA) and a component anchoring the protein assembly to the cell wall (PilC); these components are encoded by two distinct loci in the genome, called pilus islands 1 and 2 (PI-1 and PI-2), the latter presenting two distinct variants, PI-2a and PI-2b.[160,161] Epithelial cell adherence was reduced in isogenic GBS mutants lacking PilA or PilC, but not mutants lacking the PilB backbone.[161] Elucidation of the crystal structure of PilC reveals a specific IgG-like fold domain (N2) required for epithelial cell binding.[162] In a mouse model of GBS vaginal colonization, both pili and Srr-1 protein are required for efficient colonization.[163] The regulation of these and other GBS adherence factors that determine vaginal epithelial cell and extracellular matrix binding is dynamically controlled by environmental pH and the two-component gene regulation system CovRS (CsrRS).[164] Deletion of CovRS results in increased bacterial adherence but decreased invasion of vaginal epithelial cells. In the vaginal colonization model, the host mounts a more robust inflammatory response to the GBS CovRS mutant, accelerated clearance.[165]

Ascending Amniotic Infection

Group B streptococci can reach the fetus in utero through ascending infection of the placental membranes and amniotic fluid. Alternatively, the newborn may become contaminated with the organism on passage through the birth canal. Infection by the ascending route plays a pivotal role in early-onset disease. A direct relationship exists between the duration of membrane rupture before delivery and attack rate for early-onset disease,[166] whereas an inverse relationship exists between the duration of membrane rupture and the age at which clinical signs of early-onset pneumonia and sepsis first appear.[167] When the duration of membrane rupture was 18 hours or less, the attack rate was 0.7 per 1000 live births; when it was more than 30 hours, the attack rate increased to 18.3 per 1000,[166] Histologic examination of placentas from women with GBS chorioamnionitis showed bacterial infiltration along a choriodecidual course, implying that ascending infection may be a primary trigger in many instances of premature rupture.[168]

GBS may promote membrane rupture and premature delivery by several mechanisms. Isolated chorioamniotic membranes exposed to the organism have decreased tensile strength and elasticity and are prone to rupture.[169] GBS also can modify the arachidonic acid metabolism of cultured human amnion cells, favoring production of prostaglandin E2,[170] which is known to stimulate the onset of labor. Stimulation of placental release of macrophage inflammatory protein-lα (MIP-lα), interleukin-8 (IL-8), tumor necrosis factor-α (TNF-α), and matrix metalloproteases can recruit inflammatory cell and trigger alternative molecular signaling pathways that may provoke infection-associated preterm labor.[171,172]

This GBS β-hemolysin/cytolysin (β-h/c) toxin is responsible for the characteristic β-hemolytic phenotype displayed by the organism when grown on sheep blood agar. Mutagenesis and heterologous expression studies have identified the *cyl* gene locus to encode β-h/c and production of an orange carotenoid pigment; a single gene within this locus, *cylE*, is necessary for GBS β-h/c expression and sufficient to confer β-hemolysis when cloned in *E. coli*,[173,174] and one group has recently suggested that the pigment itself may function to form pores in target cell membranes.[175] The β-h/c activity targets a wide variety of host epithelial, endothelial, and immune cell membranes, provoking cellular dysfunction and, ultimately, a necrotic or apoptotic cell death.[176] GBS mutants lacking the CovRS regulator overexpress the toxin and penetrate isolated human chorioamniotic membranes more aggressively in a β-h/c–dependent manner, a finding which appears to correlate with increased hemolysis (and frequent CovRS mutation) among GBS isolated from women in preterm labor.[175] Findings in a novel mouse model of GBS chorioamniotis confirm a critical role for the β-h/c in breaching maternal-fetal barriers to trigger preterm birth and intrauterine fetal demise.[177]

GBS occasionally seem to penetrate into the amniotic cavity through intact membranes. Clinically, this mechanism of entry is suggested by reports of neonates with fulminant early-onset infection after cesarean section and no identifiable obstetric risk factors.[133,178] Migration of the organism through freshly isolated chorioamniotic membranes has been documented by scanning and transmission electron microscopy,[179] and GBS invade primary chorion cells efficiently in vitro and are capable of transcytosing through intact chorion cell monolayers without disruption of intracellular junctions.[180] They also secrete an enzyme that degrades hyaluronic acid, an important component of the extracellular matrix that is abundant in placental tissues and may facilitate amniotic invasion.[73] Placental expression of antimicrobial peptides such as human β-defensins and lactoferrins are induced by GBS and may constitute a key aspect of innate host defense against ascending infection by the pathogen.[181]

Amniotic fluid supports the proliferation of GBS,[182,183] such that when the organism gains access to the uterine cavity, a large inoculum can be delivered to the fetal lung; this results in a continuum of intrapartum (stillbirth) to early postpartum infant death.[183,184] In utero infection probably accounts for the 40% to 60% of newborns with early-onset disease who have poor Apgar scores and in whom pulmonary signs develop within a few hours of birth because these infants almost invariably display clinical or histologic evidence of congenital pneumonia.[183] Conversely, when GBS are encountered in the immediate peripartum period or on passage through the birth canal, a lesser inoculum is delivered to the neonate. Although a small but meaningful risk of subsequent invasive disease exists, most of these newborns have asymptomatic colonization limited to mucosal surfaces and remain healthy.

Fascinating new data collected in a nonhuman primate model of GBS choriodecidual inoculation suggest that the bacterium can induce fetal lung injury without ever crossing the placenta to produce intraamniotic infection or preterm delivery. Proinflammatory cytokines, including TNF-α and IL-8, elicited during transient choriodecidual infection appear to mediate this pathology, which included influx of neutrophils into the fetal intraalveolar space and thickening of the pulmonary interstitium.[185] Analysis of the gene expression profile in these primate fetal lung tissues showed an upregulation in immune response genes but downregulation of key genes associated with cellular growth, angiogenesis, morphogenesis, and development.[186]

Pulmonary and Bloodstream Entry

Early-onset GBS disease is heralded by respiratory symptoms, including tachypnea, hypoxia, cyanosis, and pulmonary hypertension.[187] One third to more than half of infants are symptomatic at birth or within 4 to 6 hours after delivery. Autopsies in fatal early-onset cases reveal that 80% have histologic evidence of lobar or multilobar pneumonia,[188] characterized by dense bacterial infiltration, epithelial cell damage, alveolar hemorrhage, interstitial inflammatory exudate, and hyaline membrane formation.[189] When pneumonia develops in newborn primates exposed by intraamniotic injection of GBS, bacterial density reaches 10^9 to 10^{11} organisms per gram of lung tissue.[190] As shown in rabbits, the poorer resolution of pneumonia in preterm versus term newborns reflects quantitative deficiency of pulmonary alveolar macrophages, mandating the recruitment of neutrophils as a secondary phagocytic defense mechanism.[191]

Group B streptococcal disease rarely is limited to the initial pulmonary focus but spreads to the bloodstream and is circulated through other organs and tissues. The capacity of GBS to cause disruption of the lung epithelial and endothelial barrier evidently involves the process of intracellular invasion, direct cytolytic injury, and damage induced by the inflammatory response of the newborn host. Intracellular invasion of alveolar epithelial and pulmonary endothelial cells by GBS was first noted in newborn macaques after intraamniotic challenge[190] and later confirmed in human tissue culture lines derived from both cellular barriers.[192,193] In vivo and in vitro electron microscopy studies show that host cytoskeletal changes are triggered that lead to endocytotic uptake of the bacterium within a membrane-bound vacuole. Uptake requires induction of signal transduction pathways in the host cell that are mediated by Rho-family guanosine triphosphatases[194] and phosphatidylinositol-3-kinase.[195]

Cellular invasion is correlated with virulence potential. Clinical isolates of GBS from infants with bloodstream infections invade epithelial cells better than strains from the vaginal mucosa of asymptomatic women.[196] FbsA, a GBS fibrinogen-binding protein[197]; Lmb, which mediates laminin binding[198]; and ScpB, which interacts with fibronectin,[156] each play a role in promoting efficient epithelial or endothelial cell invasion. In addition, surface-anchored α C protein specifically interacts with host cell glycosaminoglycan on the epithelial cell surface to promote GBS internalization.[195-199] By contrast, CPS decreases intracellular invasion, presumably through steric interference of certain receptor-ligand interactions.[200] Finally, a specific role for pilus proteins in GBS lung epithelial cell adherence and invasion was recently identified.[201]

Although cellular invasion may play a principal role in bloodstream penetration in late-onset GBS infection, damage to the lung barrier often is evident in severe early-onset infection. Alveolar exudate and hemorrhage in autopsy studies of infants with GBS pneumonia attest to significant pulmonary epithelial and endothelial cell injury.[202] Recent studies in a fetal rat lung explant model show GBS profoundly alters lung morphology and caspase-dependent macrophage apoptosis within the lung interstitium.[203] The cellular damage may result largely from the actions of the pore-forming β-h/c that can lyse lung epithelial and endothelial cells and compromises their barrier function.[204,205] At subcytolytic doses, it promotes intracellular invasion and triggers the release of IL-8, the principal chemoattractant for human neutrophils.[206] Mutants lacking hemolysin expression are less virulent than the corresponding wild-type strains in a rabbit model of GBS pneumonia.[207]

The cytolytic, proinvasive, and proinflammatory effects of GBS β-h/c all are neutralized by dipalmitoyl phosphatidylcholine, the major phospholipid constituent of human lung surfactant.[204,206] This finding may partly explain the increased risk in premature, surfactant-deficient neonates for severe lung injury and invasive disease from GBS infection. Treatment with exogenous surfactant reduces histologic evidence of lung inflammation, improves lung compliance, and mitigates bacterial growth in preterm rabbits infected with GBS.[208,209] Clinical studies exploring the effect of surfactant administration on human infants with GBS sepsis also suggest a beneficial effect.[210,211]

Capsular Polysaccharide and Immune Resistance

On penetration of GBS into the lung tissue or bloodstream of the newborn infant, an immunologic response is recruited to clear the organism. Central to this response are host phagocytic cells, including neutrophils and macrophages. Effective uptake and killing by these cells require opsonization of the bacterium by specific antibodies in the presence of complement.[212-214] Neonates are particularly prone to invasive disease because of their quantitative or qualitative deficiencies in phagocytic cell function, specific antibody, or classical and alternative complement pathways. In addition to these newborn host susceptibilities, GBS possess numerous virulence determinants that seek to thwart each of the key components of effective opsonophagocytic killing. Chief among these factors is the sialylated GBS polysaccharide capsule.

The serotype-specific epitopes of group B streptococcal CPS are created by different arrangements of four monosaccharides (glucose, galactose, *N*-acetylglucosamine, and sialic acid) into a unique repeating unit (see "Immunochemistry of Polysaccharide Antigens"), but unfailingly, these structures contain a terminal sialic acid bound to galactose in an α2→3 linkage. The enzymatic machinery for capsule biosynthesis is encoded in the single long transcript of a 16-gene operon. Heterologous expression of a single polymerase gene (*cpsH*) from this operon can cause a GBS type Ia strain to express type III capsule epitopes, and vice versa.[215]

The conserved GBS terminal α2→3 sialic acid capsular component is identical to a sugar epitope widely displayed on the surface of all mammalian cells.[216] The terminal α2→3-linked sialic acid is overexpressed in humans, who in evolution have lost the genes to produce the alternative sialic acid, *N*-glycolylneuraminic acid (Neu5Gc). It is suggested that GBS may be a particularly troublesome human pathogen because its sialylated capsule has undergone selection to resemble host "self" and avoid immune recognition. Compared with wild-type strains, isogenic capsule-deficient mutants of GBS elicit greater degrees of proinflammatory cytokine release from human cells.[217] Group B streptococci can use this molecular mimicry to engage a sialic acid–binding surface receptor, Siglec-9, expressed on human neutrophils, leading to negative cell signaling cascades that dampen the oxidative burst and bactericidal activities of phagocytic cell.[218]

The properties of group B streptococcal CPS have been studied most thoroughly in serotype III organisms. Sialic acid is a critical element in the epitope of the type III capsule that confers protective immunity. After treatment with sialidase, the altered CPS fails to elicit protective antibodies against GBS infection. Protective antibodies derived from native type III capsule do not bind to the altered (asialo) capsule backbone structure.[219] Sialidase-treated type III

GBS are opsonized more effectively by complement through the alternative pathway and are more readily phagocytosed by human neutrophils in vitro, and exhibits diminished lethality in neonatal rats.[220,221]

Definitive evidence for the role of type III capsule in virulence is provided by the study of isogenic capsule-deficient mutants.[222,223] Compared with the parent strains, isogenic capsule mutants are susceptible to opsonophagocytosis in the presence of complement and healthy adult neutrophils.[224] Opsonization by complement is a pivotal element in host defense against invasive infections; however, the extent of C3 deposition on GBS by the alternative complement pathway is inversely related to the size and density of their polysaccharide capsule present.[224] C3 fragments bound to the acapsular mutant are predominantly in the active form, C3b, whereas the inactive form, C3bi, is predominantly bound to the surface of the parent strain. Moreover, by limiting phagocytic uptake into dendritic cells, GBS capsule decreases release of proinflammatory cytokines important in the bridge between innate and adaptive immunity.[225]

The type III GBS acapsular mutants lose virulence in animal models of infection. In a model of pneumonia and bacteremia, neonatal rats were inoculated with either the parent strain or an acapsular mutant by intratracheal injection. In animals that received the acapsular mutant, fewer GBS were recovered per gram of lung, more bacteria were associated with resident alveolar macrophages, and the animals became significantly less bacteremic than animals that received the parent strain.[226] Subcutaneous injection of the acapsular mutants in neonatal rats resulted in 50% lethal dose (LD_{50}) values that were at least 100-fold greater than the values obtained with the parent strain.[222,227] Mouse passage of various serotypes of GBS was followed by increases in sialylated capsule content that correlated with increased virulence.[228] Taken together, these data provide compelling evidence that the capsule protects the organism from phagocytic clearance during the initial pulmonary phase and the later bacteremic phase of early-onset infection.

Noncapsular Factors That Interfere with Immune Clearance

The ability of GBS to avoid opsonophagocytosis is enhanced by surface proteins that can act in concert with CPS. Serotype II strains displaying both components of the C protein antigen are more resistant to phagocytic killing than are serotype II strains lacking C protein.[229,230] The β antigen of C protein binds human IgA,[231,232] and IgA deposited nonspecifically on the bacterial surface probably inhibits interactions with complement or IgG.[233] A cell surface protease, CspA, targets host fibrinogen, producing adherent fibrin-like cleavage products that coat the bacterial surface and interfere with opsonophagocytic clearance.[234] The GBS BibA protein binds human C4bp, a component of the classical complement pathway, and increases resistance to phagocytic killing.[235] Finally, certain type Ia GBS strains can also use the surface-anchored β protein to engage Siglec-5 on macrophages and neutrophils and downregulate their innate immune function, a unique example of protein-mediated subversion of a host lectin receptor.[236]

After phagocytic uptake of pathogens, neutrophils and macrophages seek to kill the engulfed bacteria by generation of reactive oxygen products and other antimicrobial substances. Streptococci are often thought of as "extracellular pathogens," but these organisms can survive for prolonged periods within the phagolysosome of macrophages.[237,238] Although GBS lack the neutralizing enzyme catalase, they are 10 times more resistant to killing by hydrogen peroxide than is catalase-positive *Staphylococcus aureus*.[239] Several mechanisms for enhanced intracellular survival have been identified. The organism possesses an endogenous source of the oxygen metabolite scavenger glutathione.[239] Another defense against oxidative burst killing is the enzyme superoxide dismutase (SodA), as evidenced by the fact that a SodA mutant is highly susceptible to macrophage killing and survives poorly in vivo.[240] Finally, the orange carotenoid pigment genetically linked to the *cyl* operon encoding β-h/c can scavenge free radicals and neutralize hydrogen peroxide, superoxide, hypochlorite, and singlet oxygen, providing a shield against several elements of phagocyte oxidative burst killing.[176] The antioxidant effects of glutathione, SodA, and carotenoid pigment apparently compensate for the lack of catalase and explain the unexpected persistence of GBS within host phagolysosomes. The acid-responsive CovRS regulator is central to regulation of these phenotypes because CovR knockout mutants are unable to survive inside the phagosome of the macrophage.[241]

Cationic antimicrobial peptides, such as defensins and cathelicidins produced by host phagocytes, also are an important component of innate immune defense against invasive bacterial infection.[242] The GBS *ponA* gene encodes an extracytoplasmic penicillin-binding protein (PBP1a) that promotes resistance to phagocytic killing independent of capsule.[243] GBS mutants with deletion of the *PBP1a* gene are less virulent after lung and systemic challenge, and this is correlated to an increased susceptibility to defensins and cathelicidins.[244] Another way in which the organism avoids antimicrobial peptide clearance is through the D-alanylation of lipoteichoic acid in the bacterial cell wall; this requires activity of gene products that are encoded by the *dlt* operon. A *dltA* mutant exhibits decreased negative surface charge, which impedes cationic host defense peptides from reaching their cell membrane target of action.[245]

Direct cytotoxicity to host phagocytes represents another important virulence mechanism for immune resistance. The GBS β-h/c toxin produces direct cytolytic injury to macrophages and induces macrophage apoptosis over a longer interval. With highly hemolytic strains or with a large bacterial inoculum, killing of the phagocyte seems to outpace the phagocyte's microbicidal mechanisms, allowing bacterial proliferation in vitro in a murine bacteremia model.[241] Addition of an inhibitor of β-h/c blocks cytolysis and reduces apoptosis of macrophages, restoring phagocytic killing.[241] Signaling pathways involved in GBS-induced programmed cell death of macrophages seem to involve either caspase-3 or calpain activation.[246,247]

Deficiencies in the neutrophil response to GBS have been documented in newborn infants. Neutropenia and depletion of the marrow neutrophil storage pool are frequent findings in infants with septicemia[248] and are correlated with poor clinical outcome.[187] Although neutrophilia and an increase in granulocytic stem cells develop in adult rats infected with GBS, severe neutropenia without a change in stem cell counts develops in neonatal rats.[249] Fatal infection in neonatal rats is associated with failure of recovery of depleted myeloid storage pools.[250] The explanation for this finding may be that the proliferative rate of neutrophils in noninfected neonatal animals already is maximal or near-maximal and cannot increase further in response to bacterial challenge[251] Recent data show that extracellular release of glyceraldehyde-3-phosphate dehydrogenase (GAPDH) by GBS induces macrophage IL-10 production, blunting neutrophil recruitment to infected organs.[252] The pathogen also produces an extracellular nuclease that degrades DNA-based neutrophil extracellular traps (NETs), increasingly recognized as a key component of neutrophil antibacterial function.[253]

GBS actively contribute to poor mobilization of neutrophils by production of an enzyme that cleaves and inactivates human C5a, a complement component that stimulates neutrophil chemotaxis.[71] Expression of C5a peptidase reduces the acute neutrophil response to sites of infection in C5a knockout mice reconstituted with human C5a.[254] Expression of GBS C5a peptidase is induced in normal human serum[255]; however, its enzymatic activity is often neutralized, in large part because of naturally occurring IgG antibodies present in many adults.[71] IgG also neutralizes C5a peptidase on the surface of a capsule-deficient GBS mutant but fails to neutralize the enzyme on the surface of the intact encapsulated type III parent strain. The capsule serves to protect the cell-associated C5a peptidase from inactivation by naturally occurring antibodies.

Inflammatory Mediators and Sepsis

When failures in epithelial barrier function and immunologic clearance allow GBS to establish bacteremia in the neonate, sepsis or septic shock develops. Intravenous infusion of GBS in animal models produces similar pathophysiologic changes to human newborn infection, including hypotension, persistent pulmonary hypertension, tissue hypoxemia and acidosis, temperature instability, disseminated intravascular coagulation, neutropenia, and, ultimately, multiple–organ system failure. These similarities have allowed in vivo experiments to elucidate the patterns in which the organism activates host inflammatory mediators to induce sepsis and circulatory shock.

Animal models in which GBS are infused intravenously exhibit a biphasic host inflammatory response.[256-258] The acute phase (≤1 hour after infusion) is manifested by increased pulmonary artery pressure and decreased arterial oxygenation and is associated with an increase in serum levels of thromboxanes. Pulmonary hypertension and hypoxemia persist through the late phase (2-4 hours), in which a progressive pattern of systemic hypotension, decreased cardiac output, and metabolic acidosis develops together with hematologic abnormalities; organ-system dysfunction; and increase in inflammatory markers, such as thromboxanes, TNF-α, and prostacyclins. If production of thromboxane and prostacyclin is blocked by inhibition of the cyclooxygenase pathway in rabbits or lambs infused with GBS, decreased myocardial dysfunction and a significant increase in systemic blood pressure are observed.[259-261]

Infusion of GBS produces pulmonary hypertension in piglets and isolated piglet lung preparations, suggesting a direct interaction of the organism with target cells in lung microvasculature.[262,263] GBS induce release of vasoactive eicosanoids prostacyclin and prostaglandin E2 from lung microvascular cells[264] and stimulate the host inflammatory mediators leukotriene D4[265] and thromboxane A2.[266]

The cytokine IL-12 has an important role in the systemic response to GBS infection. Elevation of IL-12 occurs 12 to 72 hours after challenge in the neonatal rat. Pretreatment with a monoclonal antibody against IL-12 results in greater mortality and intensity of bacteremia, whereas therapeutic administration of IL-12 is associated with a lower mortality rate and bloodstream replication of the organism.[267] By contrast, IL-1β, a known stimulator of cyclooxygenase and lipoxygenase pathways, has a more complex role depending on the stage and magnitude of infection. Activation of the inflammasome by the GBS β-h/c stimulated macrophage IL-1β release, and mice deficient in inflammasome components or the IL-1 receptor were considerably more susceptible to infection than wild-type mice.[268] In contrast, treatment with an IL-1 receptor antagonist improved cardiac output and mean arterial pressure, and increased duration of survival in piglets receiving a continuous infusion of GBS.[269]

TNF-α often is detected in the blood, urine, or cerebrospinal fluid (CSF) of infants with invasive GBS disease.[270] Although infusion of GBS in piglets is associated with TNF-α release during the late phase of hemodynamic response, the TNF-α inhibitor pentoxifylline has only modest effects on pulmonary hypertension, hypoxemia, and systemic hypotension.[271] Marked improvement in these hemodynamic parameters is seen only when pentoxifylline treatment is combined with indomethacin inhibition of thromboxane and prostacyclin synthesis.[272] Serum TNF-α also rises after challenge in rodent models; however, administration of polyclonal or monoclonal anti–TNF-α antibody does not affect overall mortality rate in these animal models.[272,273]

Inhibitor studies have shown that the mitogen-activated protein kinase (MAPK)/Jun *N*-terminal kinase (JNK) signaling pathway is required for the nuclear factor kappa B (NF-κB)–dependent inflammatory response of phagocytes to GBS.[274] Knockout mouse studies indicate that cell wall peptidoglycan–induced activation of p38 and NF-κB depends on the cytoplasmic Toll-like receptor (TLR) adapter protein myeloid differentiation primary response protein 88 (MyD88) but does not require the pattern recognition receptor TLR2 or TLR4.[275] The nitric oxide pathway is implicated in overproduction of proinflammatory cytokines, such as IL-6, and initiation of cellular injury during GBS lung infection.[276] Inducible cyclooxygenase-2 is also stimulated on GBS infection in human monocytes, likely through the MAPK pathway.[277] Infection also stimulates cyclooxygenase-2 and prostaglandin E2 expression in lung tissue in vitro and in vivo. GBS-induced cyclooxygenase-2 and prostaglandin E2 inflammatory response is reduced on treatment with an inducible nitric oxide synthase inhibitor and restored by addition of a nitric oxide donor, showing at least partial regulation by the nitric oxide pathway.[278]

The β-h/c toxin has several immunomodulatory properties that strongly influence the host response to GBS. β-H/c stimulates inducible nitric oxide synthase in macrophages, leading to release of nitric oxide.[279] In a mouse model of bacteremia and arthritis, β-h/c expression is associated with higher mortality, increased bacterial loads, greater degrees of joint injury, and release of the proinflammatory cytokines IL-6 and IL-1α systemically and intraarticularly.[280] Challenge of rabbits with isogenic GBS mutants showed that β-h/c production was associated with significantly higher degrees of hypotension, increased mortality, and evidence of liver necrosis with hepatocyte apoptosis.[281] Partially purified β-h/c preparations produce significant hypotensive actions when infused in rats and rabbits, including death from shock.[282] β-H/c also contributes directly to cardiomyocyte dysfunction and apoptosis, which may magnify its role in the pathophysiology of GBS sepsis.[283] Finally, recent data reveal that p38 MAPK activation by β-h/c contributes to evasion of host defense through induction of the antiinflammatory cytokine IL-10, thereby blunting macrophage activation and immune resistance.[284]

Blood-Brain Barrier Penetration and Meningitis

The pathophysiology of GBS meningitis varies according to age at onset. In early-onset disease, autopsy studies show little or no evidence of leptomeningeal inflammation, despite the presence of abundant bacteria, vascular thrombosis, and parenchymal hemorrhage.[2,204] By contrast, infants with late-onset disease usually have diffuse purulent arachnoiditis with prominent involvement of the base of the brain.[285] Similar age-related differences in central nervous system (CNS) pathology are evident in the infant rat model of invasive disease.[286] These histopathologic differences reflect underdevelopment of the host immunologic response in the immediate neonatal period, with a higher proportion of deaths resulting from overwhelming septicemia.

To produce meningitis, GBS must penetrate human brain microvascular endothelial cells, the single-cell layer constituting the blood-brain barrier. Intracellular invasion and transcytosis of human brain microvascular endothelial cell tissue culture monolayers have been shown in vitro.[287] A number of specific virulence factors have been implicated in blood-brain barrier invasion. At high bacterial densities, invasion by GBS of brain microvascular endothelial cells is accompanied by evidence of β-h/c–induced cellular injury.[206] Correspondingly, β-h/c knockout mutants show decreased blood-brain barrier penetration and decreased lethality from meningitis in vivo.[206] Mutants with a defect in a diglucosyldiacylgycerol synthase (IagA) required for lipoteichoic acid anchoring to the cell wall show decreased brain endothelial invasion and are attenuated in their ability to produce meningitis in mice.[288]

Furthermore, GBS mutants lacking the fibrinogen receptor FbsA, laminin-binding protein Lmb, or pilus backbone subunit protein PilB also showed reduced adherence or invasion of human brain microvascular endothelial cells in vitro.[40,198,289] The pilus adhesin PilA binds collagen and allows GBS to interact with brain endothelial cell integrins, triggering chemokine expression and neutrophil recruitment; a GBS PilA-knockout mutant is associated with reduced neutrophil infiltration and diminished bacterial dissemination into the central nervous system.[290]

More recently, a GBS mutant lacking the surface-anchored, serine-rich repeat motif glycoprotein Srr-1 was attenuated for brain endothelial cell invasion and for production of meningitis in the murine model.[291,292] Similarly, the α C protein expressed by certain GBS strains binds to glycosaminoglycans on brain endothelium, promoting invasion and central nervous system entry.[293] Finally, a newly described surface protein, HgvA, characteristic of the hypervirulent ST-17 GBS clone binds brain capillary cells and choroid plexus and promotes the development of meningitis in these strains.[294]

The host inflammatory response to GBS contributes significantly to the pathogenesis of meningitis and CNS injury. The initiation of the inflammatory response is triggered through the sentinel function of the blood-brain barrier endothelium, which activates a specific pattern of gene transcription for neutrophil recruitment, including production of chemokines (e.g., IL-8, Groα), endothelial receptors (intercellular adhesion molecule-1), and neutrophil activators (granulocyte-macrophage colony-stimulating factor), with the β-h/c representing a major provocative factor.[206] A vascular distribution of cortical lesions in neonatal rats with GBS meningitis indicates that disturbances of cerebral blood flow contribute to neuronal damage.[295] Inflammation of individual brain vessels can lead to focal lesions, whereas diffuse alterations of cerebral blood flow could cause generalized hypoxic-ischemic injury and cerebral edema.[295]

TNF-α production by astrocytes, microglial cells, and infiltrating leukocytes seems to contribute to apoptosis of hippocampal neurons.[296] Intraventricular inoculation of newborn piglets with GBS results in an early sharp increase in CSF TNF-α levels, followed shortly by prostaglandin release and neutrophil influx.[297] GBS signal through TLR2 to activate and stimulate nitric oxide production by microglia cells, resulting in neuronal destruction.[298] In the course of experimental GBS meningitis, microglial apoptosis is triggered via the cysteine protease caspase-8 and is hypothesized to represent a self-dampening mechanism that prevents overstimulation of brain inflammation.[299] However, the GBS β-h/c toxin provokes neuronal apoptosis independently of caspase activation, which worsens clinical outcome in a neonatal rat intracisternal injection model.[300]

Risk Factors for Early-Onset Infection

Infant and maternal factors that increase risk for early-onset GBS infection are listed in Table 12-2. The most important risk determinant is exposure through maternal colonization at delivery. Maternal race or ethnicity correlates significantly with early-onset GBS disease, with enhanced risk for infants

Table 12-2 Risk Factors for Early-Onset Group B Streptococcal Disease

Risk Factor	Representative References
Maternal colonization at delivery	3, 83
High-density maternal colonization	104, 184
Rupture of membranes before onset of labor	184, 301
Preterm delivery < 37-wk gestation	301
Prolonged rupture of membranes ≥ 18 hr	301, 569
Chorioamnionitis	546
Intrapartum fever ≥38° C ≥100.4° F)	301
Intrauterine monitoring	301, 569
Maternal postpartum bacteremia	304
Multiple pregnancy	302, 303
Group B streptococcal bacteriuria or urinary tract infection	301
Cesarean section	3, 184
Low level of antibody to infecting CPS type	310
Young maternal age (<20 yr)	301, 569
Previous infant with invasive group B streptococcal infection	570
Maternal race/ethnicity	84, 114

CPS, Capsular polysaccharide.

born to African-American and Hispanic mothers compared with infants born to white mothers.[88,114,301] Risk correlates directly with density of maternal genital inoculum.[104] Symptomatic early-onset disease develops in 1% to 2% of infants born to colonized women who do not receive IAP, and the rate increases if there is premature onset of labor (before 37 weeks of gestation), chorioamnionitis or interval between rupture of membranes and delivery longer than 18 hours (11%),[184] twin pregnancy (35%),[302,303] or maternal postpartum bacteremia (10%).[304]

Maternal GBS bacteriuria and urinary tract infection are markers for high-inoculum ("heavy") colonization, which enhances infant risk for invasive infection.[305] Heavy colonization in the second trimester of pregnancy also is associated with increased risk of delivering a preterm infant.[306] Among infants born to mothers with premature rupture of membranes at term gestation, maternal chorioamnionitis and colonization with GBS enhance risk for neonatal infection.[307] Vaginal colonization with GBS is an independent risk factor for the development of chorioamnionitis.[308]

Prolonged interval after rupture of membranes (≥18 hours) before delivery and preterm delivery (<37 weeks of gestation) often are concomitant risk factors in neonates with early-onset GBS infection. The estimated incidence of early-onset GBS infection is 10 times higher in preterm than in term neonates.[184] The increased risk in twins likely relates to genetic factors regulating host susceptibility, lack of specific antibody to the infecting strain in the mother, similar density of maternal colonization, and virulence of disease-producing strains.[302,303]

Antibody to Capsular Polysaccharide

Lancefield showed that antibodies directed against capsular type-specific surface antigens of GBS protected mice from lethal challenge.[309] Baker and Kasper[310] showed in 1976 that neonatal risk for type III GBS disease correlated with a deficiency of antibody to type III CPS in maternal sera. Women with type III GBS genital colonization at delivery whose infants remained well more often had antibody concentrations exceeding 2 μg/mL of type III–specific antibodies in their sera than women whose infants developed type III early-onset disease.[311] These antibodies were predominantly IgG.[312] A similar correlation exists between low concentrations of type Ia– and type II–specific antibodies in maternal delivery sera and susceptibility of infants to invasive infection.[313,314] Approximately 15% to 20% of pregnant women have a concentration of IgG to CPS in their delivery serum presumed to protect against invasive disease. These higher concentrations are present significantly more often in sera of women colonized with the homologous GBS type than in sera of noncolonized women.[88,91]

Attempts have been made to quantify the concentration of antibody to group B streptococcal CPS in maternal serum conferring protection against invasive disease in infants. A prospective, multicenter, hospital-based, case-control study of mothers delivering infants with type Ia, III, or V early-onset sepsis and matched colonized control mothers delivering healthy infants quantified the maternal serum concentrations of type Ia, III, and V CPS-specific IgG at delivery that protected neonates from early-onset disease. For types Ia and III, maternal IgG concentrations of 0.5 μg/mL or greater corresponded to a 90% risk reduction. For type V, the same antibody concentration corresponded to 70% risk reduction.[315] The findings of Lin and colleagues[316,317] agreed in principle but described a higher concentration of CPS-specific IgG as the correlate for protection against type Ia or III GBS. Neonates whose mothers had at least a 5 μg/mL concentration of IgG to type Ia CPS in their sera had an 88% lower risk of developing early-onset disease compared with neonates whose mothers had concentrations less than 0.5 μg/mL. Neonates whose mothers had at least a 10 μg/mL concentration of IgG to type III CPS in their sera by enzyme-linked immunosorbent assay had a 91% lower risk for early-onset disease compared with neonates whose mothers had concentrations less than 2 μg/mL. Low concentrations of antibody to type III CPS are uniformly found in acute sera of infants with late-onset type III infection. Among 28 infants with late-onset bacteremia and 51 with meningitis, low levels of antibodies to type III CPS were found in acute sera from all infants. These low levels in term infants with late-onset type III GBS infection correlated with maternal levels at delivery.[311,318]

Antigens with "native" or intact type III polysaccharide specificity must be used to accurately assess human immunity to GBS.[319] Kasper and colleagues[219] used gently extracted (native) and acid-extracted (core) type III GBS and pneumococcal type 14 antigens to study sera from infants with invasive type III infection and their mothers. Concentrations of type III–specific antibodies in sera of sick infants and their mothers had uniformly low binding to intact polysaccharide. Opsonic immunity and immune responses during recovery from invasive disease correlated with antibodies to the native, fully sialylated, but not to the core, desialylated type III polysaccharide or to type 14 pneumococcal antigen.

Mucosal Immune Response

Genital colonization with GBS may elicit antibody responses in cervical secretions. Women with GBS type Ia, II, or III rectal or cervical colonization have elevated levels of IgA and IgG to the colonizing serotype in their cervical secretions compared with cervical secretions from noncolonized women. Elevated amounts of IgA and IgG to the protein antigen R4 also have been found in women colonized with type III strains (most type III strains contain R4 antigen) compared with noncolonized women.[320,321] These findings suggest that a mucosal immune response occurs in response to colonization with GBS. Induction of mucosal antibodies to surface GBS polysaccharide or protein antigens may prevent genital colonization, diminishing vertical transmission of infection from mothers to infants.

Complement and Antibody Interactions

Specific antibody is required, and the classical complement pathway maximizes opsonization of types I, II, and III GBS and facilitates alternative complement pathway–mediated opsonization of type III GBS.[220] A linear relationship exists between antibody concentration and the rate constant of killing of type III strains that is determined, at least in part, by the number of antibody molecules bound per organism.[322,323] IgG subclasses 1, 2, and 3 and IgM support opsonic activity in vitro,[324-327] and an IgA monoclonal antibody activated C3 and conferred protection against lethal infection.[328] Encapsulated and genetically derived acapsular mutants of type III GBS deposit C3 and support its degradation, but an inverse correlation exists between extent of encapsulation and C3 deposition by the alternative pathway.[224,329] Among infants surviving type III GBS meningitis, transient development of specific IgM antibodies supported opsonophagocytosis during convalescence.[330] Clinical isolates of type Ia GBS can be efficiently opsonized by the classical complement pathway in the absence of antibodies.[331] Surface-bound CPS of type Ia strains mediates C1 binding and activation.[332,333] For type Ib GBS, a role for capsule size and density in modulating C3 deposition is reported. Variability among these strains in their capacity for C3 deposition by the alternative pathway also has been shown.[334]

Type II strains possessing both components of the C protein antigen are more resistant to opsonization than strains lacking both components.[229] Strains lacking type II polysaccharide but having C protein are readily opsonized. R protein or an IgA-mediated blocking effect may modulate phagocytosis of some type II strains. Despite the complexity of type II opsonins, it is clear that complement is essential and that integrity of the classical complement pathway is critical. Evaluation of neutrophil-mediated killing of types IV and V GBS also reveals the importance of complement and CPS-specific antibodies.[335,336] When complement is limited, type-specific antibodies facilitate killing. In sufficient concentration, agammaglobulinemic serum promotes opsonization, phagocytosis, and killing of types IV and V GBS.

During the course of septic shock caused by GBS, complement components are consumed. Cairo and associates[337] found a significant association between low levels of total hemolytic complement and fatal outcome from neonatal bacterial sepsis, including GBS. A critical role for C3 activation through the alternative pathway has been shown for potent GBS-induced TNF-α release.[338] This finding and the observation that complement-dependent uptake of CPS by marginal zone B cells seems necessary for an effective immune response to CPS[339] may partially explain this finding.

Pathology

Pathologic findings in early-onset infection depend on the duration of exposure to GBS before or during birth. Intrauterine death has been attributed to GBS infection[180,340] and is considered to be a contributing cause to midgestational fetal loss in women who have experienced either vaginal hemorrhage or septic abortion.[340,341] Fetal membrane infection with GBS can result in spontaneous abortion or premature rupture of membranes, or both, as suggested by Hood and associates in 1961 and others.[342-344]

Becroft and colleagues[345] noted histologic changes consistent with congenital pneumonia in live-born neonates whose autopsy lung cultures yielded GBS. Placentas showed amnionitis in mothers whose infants had fulminant pneumonia and died within 36 hours after birth. Findings were sufficient in stillborn infants to indicate that death occurred as a direct consequence of GBS intraamnionitis infection and intrauterine pneumonia. deSa and Trevenen[341] described pneumonitis with pulmonary interstitial and intraalveolar inflammatory exudates in 15 infants weighing less than 1000 g who had intraamniotic infection; 6 infants were stillborn, and 9 died within hours of birth. Placental examination revealed chorioamnionitis. In a primate model of infection, intraamniotic inoculation of GBS elicited fulminant early-onset neonatal infection.[186] Microscopy of lung tissue revealed organisms within membrane-bound vacuoles of alveolar epithelial cells; interstitial fibroblasts; and organisms present within tissue macrophages of the liver, spleen, and brain, documenting their rapid dissemination.

Amnionitis in association with early-onset GBS sepsis is more frequently detected when death occurs shortly after birth, is a common finding when membranes have been ruptured 24 hours or longer before delivery,[182,341,342] and can be clinically silent in some women. GBS can enter the amniotic fluid cavity through ruptured or intact membranes, allowing fetal aspiration of infected fluid and subsequent pulmonary lesions or bacteremia, without eliciting a local inflammatory response or maternal signs of intraamniotic infection.

Among neonates with fatal early-onset GBS disease, pulmonary lesions are the predominant pathologic feature. The association between pulmonary inflammation and formation of hyaline membranes was first noted by Franciosi and coworkers.[2] Subsequently, autopsy findings in early-onset disease cases revealed “atypical” pulmonary hyaline membranes, and these corresponded with radiographic features consistent with respiratory distress syndrome in some neonates. GBS were frequently present within these membranes, and in some infants these were composed almost entirely of streptococci. Katzenstein and colleagues[189] postulated that invasion of alveolar cells and capillary endothelial cells by GBS resulted in exudation of plasma proteins into the alveoli, deposition of fibrin, and hyaline membrane formation. Immune complex–mediated injury to the lung was proposed as a mechanism for this hyaline membrane formation.

Evidence for pneumonia was found historically in most infants with fatal early-onset GBS congenital pneumonia. The typical histologic features of congenital pneumonia (i.e., alveolar exudates composed of neutrophils, erythrocytes, and aspirated squamous cells, with edema and congestion) were observed either independently or in association with hyaline membrane formation. In neonates with fulminant, rapidly fatal GBS infection, the cellular inflammatory response was less pronounced. An interstitial inflammatory exudate is a common feature of fatal infection, as is pulmonary hemorrhage, which can range from focal interstitial to extensive intraalveolar bleeding.

In central nervous system infection, age at onset predicts distinctive morphologic findings in the brain and meninges. In early-onset meningitis, little or no evidence of leptomeningeal inflammation is seen in three quarters of infants, although purulent meningitis can be observed occasionally. This lack of inflammatory response can be the result of rapidly progressive infection, with an interval of only a few hours from onset of clinical illness until death, or can reflect inadequate host response to infection, or both. Bacteria generally are found in large numbers, and perivascular inflammation, thrombosis of small vessels, and parenchymal hemorrhage frequently are noted. In some preterm infants surviving septic shock caused by early-onset GBS infection, periventricular leukomalacia, a condition characterized by infarction of the white matter surrounding the lateral ventricles, develops.[346] Infants with fatal late-onset meningitis almost always have a diffuse purulent leptomeningitis, especially prominent at the base of the brain, with or without perivascular inflammation and hemorrhage.[2,347] Infants surviving severe meningitis often have multiple areas of infarction or encephalomalacia.

The age-related inflammatory response in infants with GBS infection has a parallel in an experimental model of meningitis.[286] Young infant rats 5 to 10 days of age have numerous bacteria distributed in a perivascular pattern, and organisms can extend transmurally into vessel lumina. These animals generally have no evidence of acute leptomeningeal inflammation or edema. By contrast, 11- to 15-day-old animals have leptomeningitis and cerebritis with a pronounced infiltration of neutrophils and macrophages around meningeal vessels and in perivascular spaces within the cerebral cortex. Because response to infection becomes more efficient within a few weeks after birth, the absence of inflammation in the brain and meninges of infant rats and of human neonates with early-onset GBS infection may relate to chemotactic defects, exhaustion of neutrophil stores, reticuloendothelial system immaturity, or to other deficits in the host response to infection.

Clinical Manifestations and Outcome

EARLY-ONSET INFECTION

When the incidence of neonatal infection caused by GBS increased dramatically in the 1970s, a bimodal distribution became apparent. Two syndromes related to age were described by Franciosi and associates[2] (acute and delayed) and by Baker and Barrett[3] (early and late). Early-onset infection typically manifests within 24 hours of birth (an estimated 85% of cases; median age, 12 hours), but it can become evident during the second 24 hours of life (an estimated 10% of cases) or at any time during the subsequent 5 days. Premature infants often experience onset at or within 6 hours of birth; infants with onset after the first 24 hours of life usually are of term gestation. Late-onset infections occur at 7 to 89 days of age (median age, 37 days). Classification of syndromes by age at onset is useful, but there also is a continuum in age at onset. A few patients with early-onset disease can present at 5 or 6 days of age, and late late-onset infection can affect 3- to 6-month-old infants, especially infants with gestational age of less than 28 weeks. Onset beyond 6 months of age can herald the presentation of human immunodeficiency virus infection or other immune system abnormalities.[348]

Early-onset GBS infection often affects neonates whose mothers have obstetric complications associated with risk for neonatal sepsis: onset of labor before 37 weeks of gestation, prolonged interval at any gestation between rupture of membranes and delivery, rupture of membranes greater than or equal to 18 hours before delivery, intrapartum fever greater than 38° C (>100.4° F), intraamniotic infection, early postpartum febrile morbidity, and twin births (Table 12-3). A nearly threefold increase in risk of early-onset infection has been observed when six or more vaginal examinations are performed before delivery.[349] The incidence of infection correlates inversely with the degree of preterm birth, and GBS is the most frequent pathogen associated with early-onset sepsis in neonates with very low birth weight (<1500 g).[350] One fourth of infants with early-onset disease historically were born before 37 weeks of gestation, but this number has increased since the introduction of prenatal culture screening and IAP for women colonized with GBS.[123] Nevertheless, approximately three fourths of infants with early-onset GBS sepsis are born at term.[351]

Early-onset GBS infection in term neonates often occurs among infants with no defined maternal risk factors other than colonization. In such cases, recognition is often delayed until the appearance of definite signs of sepsis (e.g., tachypnea, apnea, hypotension), but more subtle signs usually precede these overt manifestations. One report found that one third of healthy term neonates with early-onset GBS infection were identified solely on the basis of evaluation for maternal intrapartum temperature exceeding 38° C (100.4° F).[352]

The three most common expressions of early-onset infection are bacteremia without a defined focus of infection, pneumonia, and meningitis. In the 21st century, bacteremia without a focus occurs in 80% to 85%, pneumonia

Table 12-3 Features of Group B Streptococcal Disease in Neonates and Infants

Feature	Early Onset (<7 days)	Late Onset (7-89 days)	Late–Late Onset (>89 days)
Median age at onset	1 day	37 days	>3 months
Incidence of prematurity	Increased	Increased	Common
Maternal obstetric complications	Frequent (70%)	Preterm delivery	Varies
Common manifestations	Septicemia (80%-85%)	Meningitis (25%-30%)	Bacteremia without focus (common)
	Meningitis (5%-10%)	Bacteremia without focus (65%)	Bacteremia with focus (uncommon)
	Pneumonia (10%-15%)	Soft tissue, bone/joint (5%-10%)	
CPS types isolated	Ia (≈30%)	III (≈60%)	Several
	II (≈15%)	Ia (≈25%)	
	III (30%)	V (≈15%)	
	V (20%)		
Case-fatality rate	3%-10%	1%-6%	Low

CPS, Capsular polysaccharide.

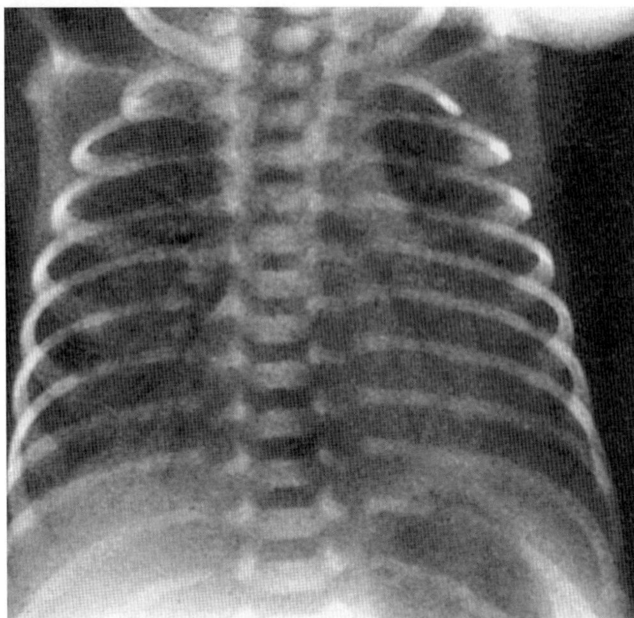

Figure 12-6 Chest radiograph from an infant with early-onset group B streptococcal septicemia shows features consistent with respiratory distress syndrome of the newborn.

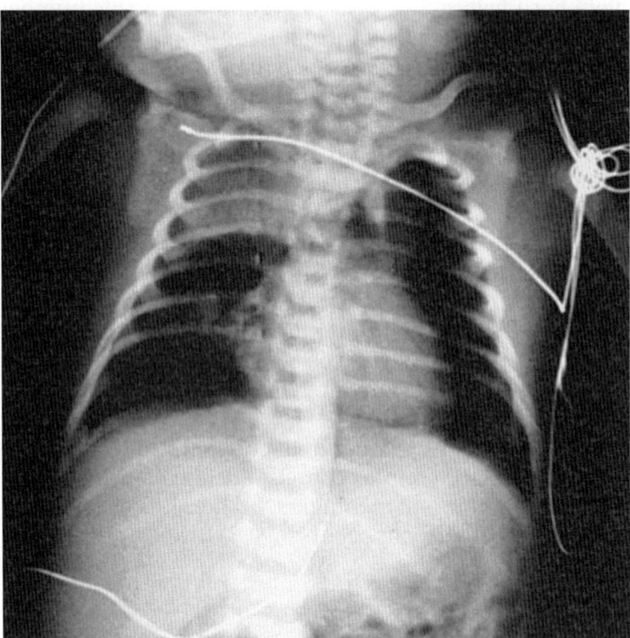

Figure 12-7 Chest radiograph shows right upper and lower lobe infiltrates as manifestations of early-onset group B streptococcal pneumonia in an infant.

occurs in 10% to 15%, and meningitis occurs in 5% to 10% of infants.[123] Bacteremia is often detected in neonates with the latter two presentations, but not always. Regardless of site of involvement, respiratory signs (apnea, grunting respirations, tachypnea, or cyanosis) are the initial clinical findings in more than 80% of neonates. Hypotension is an initial finding in approximately 25%. Infants with fetal asphyxia related to GBS infection in utero can have shock and respiratory failure at delivery.[353] Additional signs include lethargy, poor feeding, hypothermia or fever, abdominal distention, pallor, tachycardia, and jaundice.

Pneumonia occurs in 10% to 15% of infants with early-onset infection, and virtually all of these infants have acute respiratory signs. Most have these respiratory findings in the first few hours of life, many at birth. Among 19 infants with GBS congenital pneumonia at autopsy, 89% had 1-minute Apgar scores of 4 or less, indicating in utero onset of infection. Radiographic features consistent with and indistinguishable from those of surfactant deficiency are commonly found (Fig. 12-6). Treatment with surfactant improves gas exchange in most, although the response is slower than in noninfected infants, and repeated surfactant doses often are needed.[210] Infiltrates suggesting congenital pneumonia (Fig. 12-7) are present in one third of infants. Increased vascular markings suggesting the diagnosis of transient tachypnea of the newborn or pulmonary edema can occur. On occasion, respiratory distress is present in the absence of radiographic abnormalities, appearing as persistent fetal circulation and pulmonary hypertension. Small pleural effusions and cardiomegaly can occur.

Meningitis occurs in 5% to 10% of neonates with early-onset infection. Neonates with meningitis often have a clinical presentation early in the course that is identical to presentation of neonates without meningeal involvement. Respiratory distress can be the most common initial sign, and in 27 infants with early-onset meningitis, seizures were never a presenting feature.[354] Examination of CSF is the only means to exclude meningitis, a finding that requires modification of supportive and specific chemotherapy (see "Treatment" later). Seizures occur during the first 24 hours of therapy in nearly 50% of infants with meningitis. Persistent seizures, semicoma or coma, and a CSF protein concentration greater than 300 mg/dL are associated with a poor prognosis.[355,356]

The case-fatality rate for early-onset infection in the 1970s approached 50%. Current data indicate much lower rates of 2% to 10%. Features associated with fatal outcome include a low 5-minute Apgar score, shock, neutropenia, pleural effusion, apnea, and delay in treatment after onset of symptoms.[353,357] Fatal infection also occurs significantly more often among premature than term neonates (Table 12-4).

Table 12-4 Fatality Rates in Early-Onset Group B Streptococcal Infection

	CASE-FATALITY RATE (%) BY BIRTH WEIGHT (G) OR GESTATIONAL AGE (WK)				
Study	**500-1000**	**1001-1500**	**1501-2000**	**2001-2500**	**<2500**
Boyer et al[571] (1973-1981)	90	25	29	33	3
Baker[504] (1982-1989)	60	25	26	18	5
Weisman et al[353] (1987-1989)	75	40	20	15	6
Schrag et al[5] (1993-1998)		30 (≤33 wk)		10 (34-36 wk)	2 (≥37 wk)
Phares et al[123] (1999-2005)		20 (<37wk)			3 (≥37 wk)

Contemporary data document that the risk of death among preterm cases is 20%, nearly eightfold that of term infants for whom infection was fatal in 3% of cases.[123]

LATE-ONSET INFECTION

Late-onset GBS infection historically affected term infants 7 to 89 days of age who had had an unremarkable maternal obstetric and early neonatal history. Contemporary data indicate that at least half of infants with late-onset disease are born before 37 weeks of gestation.[123] Term infants are younger at presentation for late-onset disease (mean, 30 days) than are preterm infants (mean, 41 days).[358] Late-onset disease has a lower fatality rate (1%-6%) than early-onset disease. Clinical expressions of late-onset disease include bacteremia without a focus of infection (65% of infants), meningitis (25%) and cellulitis or osteoarthritis (2%-3% each) (see Table 12-3).[123]

Bacteremia without a detectable focus of infection is the most common clinical expression of late-onset GBS disease. Bacteremia without a focus typically manifests with nonspecific signs (i.e., fever, poor feeding, irritability). Diagnosis results from the practice of obtaining a blood culture in febrile infants during the first few weeks of life to exclude serious bacterial infection. These infants often are mildly ill, but failure to initiate antimicrobial therapy in a timely manner can result in progression to shock, especially in preterm infants, or extension of infection to distant sites such as the CNS. Either transient or persistent bacteremia can occur. Approximately 3% of infants with late-onset bacteremia without a focus die; survivors typically recover without sequelae after treatment.

The presenting signs in infants with late-onset meningitis almost always include fever; irritability or lethargy, or both; poor feeding; and tachypnea. Upper respiratory tract infection precedes late-onset meningitis in 20% to 30% of infants, suggesting that alteration of mucosal barrier by respiratory viral illness might facilitate entry of GBS into the bloodstream.[2,3] In contrast to early-onset infection, grunting respirations and apnea are less frequent initial findings, and their presence suggests rapidly progressive, fulminant infection. Apnea or hypotension is observed in less than 15% of patients, but there is a spectrum in clinical severity of illness at presentation. Some infants appear clinically well a few hours before initial evaluation and present with seizures, poor perfusion, neutropenia, and large numbers of gram-positive cocci in the CSF. These patients often have a rapidly fatal course, or, if they survive, they are left with devastating neurologic sequelae. Leukopenia or neutropenia at the time of diagnosis has been correlated with fatal outcome in these infants.[357]

Other initial findings associated with increased risk for fatal outcome or permanent neurologic sequelae include seizures at admission, coma or semicoma, need for pressor support, and CSF protein level greater than 300 mg/dL.[356,357,359] These findings most likely reflect a high bacterial inoculum in the CSF and cerebritis. Subdural effusions, which usually are small, unilateral, and asymptomatic, are found in some infants, but these are not associated with permanent sequelae. Subdural empyema, obstructive ventriculitis, large infarctions, and encephalomalacia are uncommon complications.

LATE LATE–ONSET INFECTION

Infections in infants older than 89 days of age account for approximately 10% of cases in infancy.[360] Most of these infants have a gestational age of less than 35 weeks. The need for prolonged hospitalization and the immature host status probably contribute to infection beyond the interval for term neonates. Bacteremia without a focus is a common presentation. On occasion, a focus for infection, such as the CNS, intravascular catheter, or soft tissues, is identified (see Table 12-3). In the outpatient setting, infants older than 89 days of age are likely to have a temperature greater than 39° C (>102.2° F) and a white blood cell count exceeding 15,000/mm^3.[361] A viral infection can precede the onset of bacteremia.[362] When there are no other apparent risk factors for late late–onset infection in a term infant, immunodeficiency should be considered.[363-365]

SEPTIC ARTHRITIS AND OSTEOMYELITIS

The clinical features of 20 infants with GBS septic arthritis alone and 45 infants with osteomyelitis (with or without concomitant septic arthritis) are shown in Table 12-5. The mean age at diagnosis of osteomyelitis (31 days) is greater than that for septic arthritis (20 days). The mean duration of clinical sign is shorter for septic arthritis than for osteomyelitis (2 vs. 9 days). In some infants with osteomyelitis, failure to move the involved extremity since hospital discharge after birth, or shortly thereafter, may be noted; this lack of movement can persist for weeks before the diagnosis is established.[366]

Decreased motion of the involved extremity and evidence of pain with manipulation, such as lifting or diaper changing, are common signs of bone infection. Warmth or erythema can occur occasionally; a history of fever is uncommon. The paucity of signs suggesting infection and the finding of pseudoparalysis have led to an initial diagnosis of Erb palsy and to assessment for possible child abuse.[366,367] In some infants, osteomyelitis of the proximal humerus has been associated with findings on nerve conduction studies consistent with brachial plexus neuropathy,[368,369] and in one infant, sciatic nerve injury at the level of the pelvis caused footdrop in association with iliac osteomyelitis.[370]

Physical findings include fixed flexion of the involved extremity, mild swelling, evidence of pain with passive

Table 12-5 Clinical Features of Group B Streptococcal Bone and Joint Infections

Feature	Septic Arthritis without Osteomyelitis	Osteomyelitis
Mean age at diagnosis (days)	20	31
Mean duration of symptoms (days)	2	9
Most common site	Hip	Humerus
Other common sites	Knee, ankle	Femur, tibia
Usual duration of parenteral therapy (range)	2 weeks (2-3)	3 weeks (2-6)

motion, decreased spontaneous movement, and, in a few infants, erythema and warmth. Most infants with osteomyelitis of the humerus have concomitant infection in the shoulder joint. Lack of associated systemic involvement is the rule, although osteomyelitis can occur in association with sepsis and in infants with other foci of infection such as meningitis.

Infants with septic arthritis often have lower extremity involvement, with the hip joint predominating. By contrast, more than half of the reported infants with osteomyelitis have had involvement of the humerus, and in infants for whom the location was specified, the proximal humerus predominated.[366] Involvement of the femur, vertebrae, or small bones occurs occasionally.[371,372] Usually, only one bone is affected, although infection involving two adjacent bones or multiple nonadjacent bones can occur rarely.[373] GBS bone and joint infections have a good prognosis. At evaluation months to years after diagnosis, most infants with osteomyelitis have had normal function in the affected extremity.

Residual shortening and limitation of motion of the humerus can be observed after osteomyelitis. Growth disturbance can result as a consequence of subluxation of the hip joint after septic arthritis.

Osteomyelitis seems to represent a clinically silent early-onset bacteremia with seeding of a bone and then later onset of clinical expression of infection. An episode of asymptomatic bacteremia with a birth trauma–induced nidus in the proximal humerus could allow localization of bacteria to the bone. Because lytic lesions take more than 10 to 14 days to become radiographically visible, the presence of such lesions on radiographs obtained at hospital admission suggests long-standing infection (Fig. 12-8).

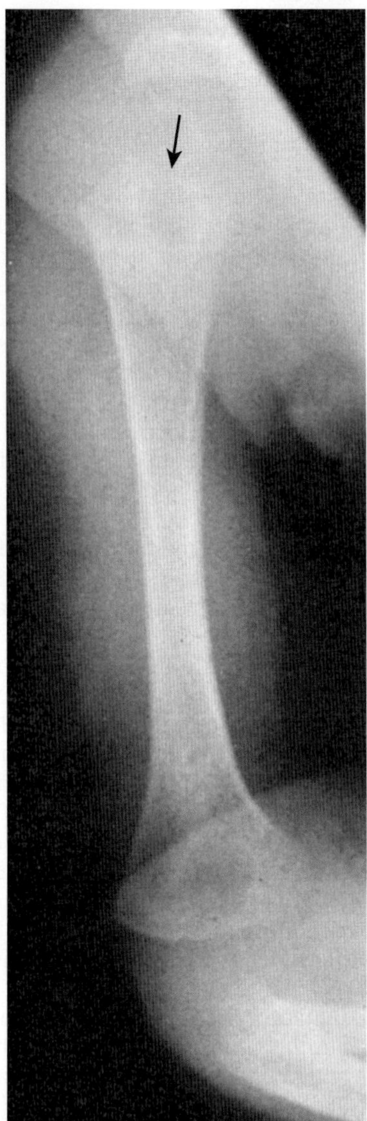

Figure 12-8 Radiograph shows lytic lesion *(arrow)* of the proximal humerus in an infant whose bone biopsy showed osteomyelitis caused by type III group B streptococci.

CELLULITIS OR ADENITIS

The manifestation of late-onset GBS infection, designated as facial cellulitis,[374] submandibular cellulitis,[375] cellulitis/adenitis syndrome,[376] or lymphadenitis,[377] has been reported in at least 25 infants.[378-381] Presenting signs include poor feeding; irritability; fever; and unilateral facial, preauricular, or submandibular swelling, usually, but not always, accompanied by erythema. The mean age at onset is 5 weeks (range, 2-11 weeks), and in contrast to all other expressions of late-onset infection, there is a striking male predominance. The most common sites are the submandibular and parotid, and enlarged adjacent nodes become palpable within 2 days after onset of the soft tissue infection. Four of the five infants with facial or submandibular cellulitis described by Baker[376] had ipsilateral otitis media at the time of diagnosis. Less common sites of involvement with cellulitis are the face, preauricular or inguinal areas, scrotum, anterior neck region, and prepatellar spaces (Fig. 12-9).[376,380,381] In one patient, cellulitis of the neck occurred in association with an infected thyroglossal duct cyst.[376]

Bacteremia almost always is detected in these infants, and cultures of soft tissue or lymph node aspirates have yielded GBS in approximately 90% of infants in whom this procedure was performed. These infants usually are not seriously ill, few have associated meningitis, and recovery within a few days of initiation of appropriate antimicrobial therapy is the rule.[382] Fulminant and fatal facial cellulitis has been described in a 7-hour-old neonate,[4] however, and associated meningitis has been described.[383]

UNUSUAL MANIFESTATIONS OF INFECTION

Numerous uncommon clinical manifestations of early-onset and late-onset GBS infection have been recorded (Table 12-6). Peritonitis[384] and adrenal abscess[385-387] have been described as abdominal manifestations of early- and late-onset infection. Adrenal abscess is thought to result from bacteremic seeding associated with adrenal hemorrhage and subsequent abscess formation. One neonate thought to have neuroblastoma underwent en bloc resection of a large mass with nephrectomy before the diagnosis of adrenal abscess was established.[386] Gallbladder distention is a nonspecific manifestation of early-onset sepsis that usually resolves with medical management of the infection.[388] Late-onset bacteremia can occur in association with

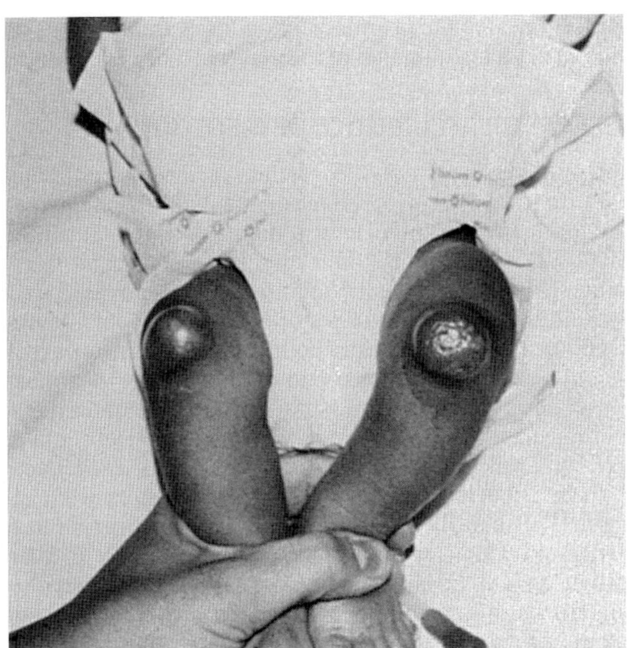

Figure 12-9 Prepatellar bursitis of both knees in an infant who had abraded his knees on the bed sheets. Aspiration of purulent material from the prepatellar space yielded type III group B streptococci. The knee joints were not affected.

jaundice, elevated levels of liver enzymes, and increased direct-reacting bilirubin fraction. Hemolysis and hepatocellular inflammation possibly contribute to the development of jaundice.

Brain abscess rarely occurs in association with recurrence of GBS meningitis. One infant recovered after craniotomy and excision of a well-encapsulated frontal mass but had neurologic sequelae.[389] Another infant presented at 5 weeks of age with a cerebellar cyst believed to represent an astrocytoma.[390] This infant proved to have obstructive hydrocephalus and chronic GBS ventriculitis. Rarely, anterior fontanelle herniation can complicate severe meningitis. The presence of a noncystic doughy mass over the fontanelle indicates that brain herniation may have occurred, and cranial imaging can confirm this diagnosis. One patient with cervical myelopathy initially had absence of extremity movement, but made a good recovery and was able to walk at age 3 years.[391]

Subdural empyema is another unusual complication of GBS meningitis described in patients with early- and late-onset infections.[392,393] The diagnosis is established by needle aspiration of the subdural space.[393] Irritability, vomiting, seizures, increasing head circumference, focal neurologic signs, a tense anterior fontanelle, or a combination of these should prompt evaluation.[392,394] Sterilization of the subdural space was accomplished by open or closed drainage in conjunction with antimicrobial therapy. Basal ganglia and massive cerebral infarction also have been described.[395]

Cardiovascular manifestations of GBS infection are rare. Endocarditis,[109,396,397] pericarditis,[398] myocarditis,[399] and mycotic aneurysm of the aorta[400] have been documented. Echocardiography can be useful in delineating the nature of cardiac involvement, and this technique was used

Table 12-6 Unusual Clinical Manifestations of Group B Streptococcal Infections

Site and Manifestation	Associated with Early-Onset or Late-Onset Infection	Reference
ABDOMEN		
Peritonitis	Both	384
Adrenal abscess	Both	385-387
Gallbladder distention	Early	388
BRAIN		
Abscess	Late	389
Anterior fontanelle herniation	Both	571
Chronic meningitis	Late	390
Subdural empyema	Both	392, 393
Cerebritis	Late	395
Myelopathy/myelitis	Early	391, 573
Ventriculitis of myelomeningocele	Both	574
Oculomotor nerve paralysis	Late	575
Ventriculoperitoneal shunt infection	Late	576
CARDIOVASCULAR		
Asymptomatic bacteremia	Both	4, 577, 578
Endocarditis	Both	109, 396, 397
Pericarditis	Not specified	398
Myocarditis	Late	399
Mycotic aneurysm	Late	400
EAR AND SINUS		
Ethmoiditis	Late	4
Otitis media/mastoiditis	Both	401-404
EYE		
Conjunctivitis/ophthalmia neonatorum	Early	2, 405, 579
Endophthalmitis	Late	406
Retrobulbar abscess	Early	580
RESPIRATORY TRACT		
Diaphragmatic hernia	Both	411
Supraglottitis	Late	407
Pleural empyema	Both	4, 409, 410
Tracheitis	Late	408
SKIN AND SOFT TISSUE		
Abscess of cystic hygroma	Late	425
Breast abscess	Late	428, 581
Bursitis	Late	582
Cellulitis/adenitis	Both	4, 374-381, 583
Dactylitis	Late	584
Fasciitis	Late	418-420
Impetigo neonatorum	Early	421, 422
Purpura fulminans	Both	415-417
Omphalitis	Both	423
Rhabdomyolysis	Late	585
Retropharyngeal cellulitis	Late	426, 427
Scalp abscess	Both	424
Urinary Tract Infection	Both	429

successfully to detect a 0.7-cm vegetation on the anterior leaflet of the mitral valve in a 4-week-old infant with endocarditis caused by a type III strain.[396] Paroxysmal atrial tachycardia can be a presenting feature of GBS septicemia in the absence of focal infection of the heart.[133]

GBS are an uncommon cause of otitis media in the first few weeks of life (2%-3% of cases).[401] Otitis media is more often associated with late-onset disease manifesting as meningitis or submandibular cellulitis.[402-404] The finding of acute mastoiditis at autopsy in one infant with otitis media and meningitis suggests that the middle ear can serve as a portal of entry in a few patients.[404]

Conjunctivitis related to GBS occurs only rarely. Exudative conjunctivitis has been reported, however, in association with early-onset bacteremia.[405] More severe ocular involvement is rare, but endophthalmitis has been noted in infants with septicemia and meningitis.[406] As is the case for other agents producing endophthalmitis, high-grade bacteremia is a likely prelude to this unusual metastatic focus of GBS infection.

Supraglottitis was described in a 3-month-old infant with acute onset of stridor.[407] Swelling of the left aryepiglottic fold, but not the epiglottis, was noted at laryngoscopy. An infant with bacterial tracheitis had a similar presentation.[408] Although pulmonary infection caused by GBS is common, pleural involvement is rare, but it has been reported as a complication of early-onset[409] and late-onset[410] pneumonia. An interesting but unexplained association is delayed development of right-sided diaphragmatic hernia and early-onset GBS sepsis.[411] In affected infants, the onset of respiratory distress invariably occurs at or within 48 hours after birth, whereas the mean age at diagnosis of right-sided diaphragmatic hernia in the 40 reported cases is 11 days (range, 4-91 days). One speculation is that GBS pneumonia causes necrosis of the adjacent diaphragm and results in herniation of viscera into the pleural space. Another is that ventilation increases intrathoracic pressure to mask or delay herniation through a congenital diaphragmatic defect. This phenomenon should be a consideration in an infant whose condition deteriorates despite appropriate management for early-onset disease. Radiographic features include increased density in the right lower lung or irregular aeration or both, followed by progression to elevation of right bowel gas and liver shadow.

In addition to cellulitis and adenitis, GBS uncommonly can produce various unusual skin and soft tissue manifestations, including violaceous cellulitis,[412] perineal cellulitis and septicemia after circumcision,[413] scrotal ecchymosis as a sign of intraperitoneal hemorrhage,[414] purpura fulminans,[415-417] necrotizing fasciitis,[418-420] impetigo neonatorum,[421,422] omphalitis,[423] scalp abscess secondary to fetal scalp electrode,[424] abscess complicating cystic hygroma,[425] retropharyngeal cellulitis,[426,427] and breast abscess.[428] In patients with impetiginous lesions and abscess formation, bacteremia is unusual, but it is a frequent accompaniment to omphalitis and necrotizing fasciitis.

Among infants with early-onset bacteremia, isolation of GBS from the urine is frequent when this body fluid is cultured, but primary urinary tract infection with these organisms is rare. An infant with severe bilateral ureterohydronephrosis and GBS in his urine has been described.[429] The isolation of GBS from a urine culture of a patient without bacteremia is an indication for evaluation for possible structural anomalies of the genitourinary tract.

RELAPSE OR RECURRENCE OF INFECTION

Relapse or recurrence of GBS infection occurs in an estimated 0.5% to 3% of term or preterm infants.[430,431] Signs can develop during treatment for the initial episode or at an interval of 3 days to 3 months after completion of therapy.[432-434] In one review, eight of nine infants with a recurrence were born at 25 to 36 weeks of gestation, and male infants predominated.[433] The first episode occurred at a mean age of 10 days (range, 1-27 days) and the recurrence at a mean age of 42 days (range, 23-68 days) of life. In another report that included a set of fraternal twins, seven of eight infants were preterm (mean, 30 weeks of gestation), each had a birth weight of less than 2500 g, and all infections were late onset.[434] The mean age at initial presentation was 38 days (range, 13-112 days), and at recurrence, it was 57 days (range, 34-130 days). Recurrence often occurs within days after discontinuing antibiotic treatment. Two relapses in one infant have been documented.[430,431,435,436]

Relapse or recurrence of infection can be the result of an undrained focus of infection, such as a brain abscess, or can occur in association with congenital heart disease. Identical isolates recovered from maternal genital and breast milk cultures suggest that breast milk can serve as a source of repeated infant exposure.[437,438] Recurrent infection can have a clinical expression similar to that of the initial episode or can involve new sites (meninges, ventricular or subdural fluid, or both; brain parenchyma; and soft tissue). In most instances, the second episode of GBS disease responds to retreatment with penicillin or ampicillin, but typically the duration of treatment for the recurrence is extended empirically; evidence for longer duration of therapy in this circumstance is lacking.[434]

Because infants who receive treatment for invasive infection often remain colonized with GBS at mucous membrane sites, pharyngeal or gastrointestinal colonization can be the source for recurrence. In addition, infants recovering from invasive infection with type III strains usually lack protective levels of antibody during convalescence. Moylett and colleagues[434] and others[435] used pulsed-field gel electrophoresis to document that isolates from patients with recurrent episodes were identical and were derived from a single clone. Sets of isolates analyzed from first and second episodes and from maternal and infant-colonizing and invasive strains were genotypically identical.[433,434] Recurrent infection in most infants likely is a consequence of reinvasion from persistently colonized mucous membrane sites or from reexposure to a household carrier. Association with transient hypoglobulinemia of infancy has been described.[439] Uncommonly, infants have had a second infection with a strain that is genetically unrelated to the original isolate.

MATERNAL INFECTIONS

In 1938, Fry[1] described three fatal cases of endocarditis in postpartum women. This was the initial insight that GBS was a human pathogen and could cause puerperal infection. Postpartum infections, including septic abortion, bacteremia, chorioamnionitis, endometritis, pneumonia, and septic arthritis, were recorded sporadically, but infections in postpartum women, as in neonates, were uncommonly reported before 1970.[342,440,441] The dramatic increase in incidence of neonatal infections in the 1970s was paralleled by an increased incidence of infections in pregnant women.

Before the institution of IAP in the 1990s, GBS accounted for 10% to 20% of blood culture isolates from febrile women on obstetric services.[442] In the IAP era, GBS is infrequently documented as a cause of maternal peripartum bacteremia, accounting for only 4% of cases in one retrospective cohort study.[443] The clinical presentation of GBS bacteremic infection is characterized by fever, malaise, uterine tenderness with normal lochia, and occasionally chills. Among 40 women with GBS endometritis and endoparametritis described by Faro,[304] GBS were isolated from the endometrium in pure culture in one third of cases, and one third of the women had concomitant bacteremia. In most, signs of infection developed within 24 hours after cesarean section. Clinical features included chills, tachycardia, abdominal distention, and exquisite uterine, parametrial, or adnexal tenderness. Higher fever correlated with risk for concomitant bacteremia. Six infants born to these women developed GBS septicemia, and infection was fatal to three. Contemporary data continue to support the concept that maternal febrile morbidity from chorioamnionitis often is associated with early-onset infection.[444]

The incidence of invasive disease in pregnant women now is 0.12 per 1000 live births, having declined significantly in association with implementation of IAP.[5,114,123] Half of the 409 pregnancy-associated disease cases identified in the United States from 1999 to 2005 by an active population-based surveillance system were associated with infection of the upper genital tract, placenta, or amniotic sac and resulted in fetal death. Among the remainder, manifestations of disease included bacteremia without a focus (31%), endometritis without fetal death (8%), chorioamnionitis without fetal death (4%), pneumonia (2%), and puerperal sepsis (2%). Isolates in pregnancy-associated infections were obtained from blood in 52% of women and from the placenta, amniotic fluid, or conceptus in most of the remainder. When pregnancy outcome was known, most of the women (61%) had a spontaneous abortion or stillborn infant, 5% had infants who developed clinical infection, 4% had induced abortions, and 30% had infants who remained clinically well.[123]

Most obstetric patients with GBS infection, even in the presence of bacteremia, show a rapid response after initiation of antimicrobial therapy. Potentially fatal complications can occur, however, including meningitis,[445] ventriculoperitoneal shunt infection,[446] abdominal abscess,[447] endocarditis,[113,448-450] vertebral osteomyelitis,[451] epidural abscess,[452] or necrotizing fasciitis.[453]

Group B streptococcal bacteriuria during pregnancy is a risk factor for intrauterine or neonatal infection. Asymptomatic bacteriuria, cystitis, or pyelonephritis occurs in 6% to 8% of women during pregnancy. In women with asymptomatic bacteriuria, approximately 20% are caused by GBS.[454] Bacteriuria is a marker for heavy vaginal colonization and indicates enhanced risk for maternal and neonatal infection.[79] In a report series of cases that predated IAP, a cohort of 68 women with asymptomatic GBS bacteriuria had significantly increased risk of preterm delivery compared with nonbacteriuric controls.[343] Stillbirth because of congenital GBS infection can occur even in the current IAP era, and all women with GBS bacteriuria during pregnancy should receive IAP.[455]

Diagnosis

ISOLATION AND IDENTIFICATION OF THE ORGANISM

The definitive diagnosis of invasive GBS infection is established by isolation of the organism from culture of blood, CSF, or a site of suppurative focus (e.g., bone, joint fluid, empyema fluid). Isolation of GBS from surfaces, such as the skin or umbilicus or from mucous membranes, is of no clinical significance.

Lumbar puncture is required to exclude meningeal involvement in infants with invasive GBS infection because clinical features cannot reliably distinguish between meningeal and nonmeningeal involvement. GBS often are isolated from blood at the time of initial evaluation of infants with meningitis, but the blood culture is sterile in 20% to 30%. Wiswell and colleagues[456] found that if lumbar puncture were omitted as part of the sepsis evaluation, the diagnosis of meningitis was missed or delayed in more than one third of infants. Infants with late-onset infection can have meningitis even when focal infection, such as cellulitis, is apparent. If lumbar puncture must be deferred because an infant is clinically unstable, penicillin G or ampicillin at the doses recommended for treatment of GBS meningitis (see "Treatment") should be administered until meningeal involvement can be assessed.

Antigen Detection Methods

Antigen detection is not a substitute for appropriately performed bacterial cultures and now is rarely used to establish a provisional diagnosis. A positive result indicates that GBS antigen is detectable, but not that viable organisms are present. Serum and CSF are the only specimens recommended for testing.[457] In neonates with meningitis, the sensitivity of antigen detection is 72% to 89%. The estimated sensitivity for serum is 30% to 40%. False-positive results have been encountered. The estimated specificity of commercial assays ranges from 95% to 98%. Antigen assays should not be used to assess treatment efficacy.

NAAT such as PCR can have a role in intrapartum testing of vaginal-rectal samples from women with unknown GBS colonization status (see "Prevention"), but they are not routinely used for the diagnosis of infant infection. As a research tool however, a PCR assay targeting the *cylB* gene was shown to be superior to culture methods for detecting GBS in CSF and blood samples from infants with probable GBS sepsis or meningitis.[458] The use of PCR to exclude GBS colonization in neonates, allowing for early discharge of infants, also has been proposed.[459] A fluorescent PCR assay was sensitive and specific for early detection within 4 hours of incubation of GBS in neonatal blood cultures, but such testing is not available commercially.[460]

Other Laboratory Tests

A single measurement of an acute-phase reactant, such as C-reactive protein (CRP), can be elevated during GBS infection, but its usefulness is limited because CRP can be elevated in a number of noninfectious inflammatory conditions. Sequential assessment of CRP values is useful in supporting a diagnosis of sepsis and in excluding sepsis if levels remain persistently normal. The return to normal of the CRP level can be helpful in guiding the duration of antibiotic exposure in suspected GBS infection, minimizing antibiotic exposure in the nursery setting. Levels of inflammatory cytokines, such as IL-6, are elevated acutely during GBS sepsis. In one report, production of IL-6 was noted in all 16 neonates with bacteremic early- or late-onset GBS infection when samples were collected within 48 hours of initiation of antimicrobial therapy.[461] These assays are not routinely used because of the cost of testing, and they are not generally available in clinical laboratories.

Abnormalities in the white blood cell count, including leukopenia, neutropenia, leukocytosis, increase in band forms, or decline in the total white blood cell count in the first 24 hours of life, can be suggestive of GBS infection.[462] A multicenter study found that a low white blood cell count, absolute or relative neutropenia, or an elevated immature to total neutrophil count was more helpful as a predictor of sepsis when the complete blood cell count is obtained after 4 hours of age.[463] Fatal early-onset GBS sepsis can occur with normal leukocyte parameters, however.[464] Measurements of peripheral blood leukocyte parameters generally have a low sensitivity and should be used only as an adjunct to results from blood and CSF cultures.

DIFFERENTIAL DIAGNOSIS

The clinical features in neonates with early-onset GBS infection mimic the features in infants with sepsis caused by other etiologic agents and by some noninfectious illnesses. Radiographic findings of pneumonia are present in some neonates with early-onset GBS sepsis. Neonates with early-onset pneumonia can have apnea and shock within the first 24 hours of life, a 1-minute Apgar score of 5 or less, and an unusually rapid progression of pulmonary disease.[183] Infection also should be considered in neonates with persistent fetal circulation associated with respiratory distress, neutropenia, and systemic hypotension.[357]

The differential diagnosis for late-onset GBS infection depends on the clinical presentation. For infants with meningitis, the characteristic CSF Gram-stain findings can provide a presumptive diagnosis. When this method is inconclusive, other bacteria, including *S. pneumoniae, Escherichia coli, Listeria monocytogenes, Neisseria meningitidis,* as well as viruses must be considered. Fever usually is a presenting feature in term infants, and empirical therapy with broad-spectrum antibiotics customarily is used until culture results are available. Finally, the lengthy list of uncommon manifestations of infection between 1 week and 3 months of age and beyond indicates that GBS should be suspected as an etiologic agent, regardless of site of infection, for infants in this age group.

Treatment

GBS have been a frequent cause of infection in neonates for 4 decades, resulting in increased awareness of associated risk factors and need for prompt and aggressive therapy. Despite striking declines, however, death and disability from these infections still occur. In addition, relapses or reinfections, although uncommon, occur in the face of optimal therapy. These facts should prompt efforts to develop improved treatment modalities.

IN VITRO SUSCEPTIBILITY

Uniform susceptibility of GBS to penicillin G has continued for more than 50 years of use.[465-470] Recently, reduced susceptibility of certain strains of GBS to penicillin and other β-lactam antibiotics has been documented in the United States[471] and Japan[472] and traced to point mutations in penicillin-binding proteins reminiscent of first-step mutations in the evolution of pneumococcal penicillin resistance decades ago. The clinical implications of this finding are as yet unclear. None among almost 2000 isolates of GBS from 2008 to 2009 were penicillin nonsusceptible.[473] In vitro susceptibility of GBS to ampicillin, semisynthetic penicillins, vancomycin, teicoplanin, linezolid, quinopristin/dalfopristin, gatifloxacin, levofloxacin, tigecycline and cephalosporins also is the rule, although the degree of in vitro activity varies.[468,469,474,475] Ceftriaxone is the most active of the cephalosporins in vitro. Imipenem and meropenem are highly active.[466] Resistance to quinolones can occur through mutations in the gyrase and topoisomerase IV genes, usually in patients who have received prior quinolone therapy.[476]

Resistance to erythromycin and clindamycin is increasing. Contemporary data from multiple studies indicate that 20% to 40% of isolates are erythromycin-resistant, and 10% to 30% are resistant to clindamycin.[468,469,477] Rates of resistance in colonizing isolates can be 40% for erythromycin and clindamycin.[478] These high rates of resistance are reported from geographically diverse regions.[479-481]

Macrolide resistance mechanisms include ribosomal modification by a methylase encoded by *erm* genes and drug efflux by a membrane-bound protein encoded by the *mef* gene.[482] The presence of *erm* genes results in the macrolide–lincosamide–streptogramin B resistance phenotype.[483] Erythromycin-resistant isolates that are constitutively resistant, inducibly resistant, or susceptible to clindamycin are described.[484] Alone or in combination, *ermA, ermB,* and *mefA* genes are responsible for resistance in GBS. An *ermT* gene has been identified in a few strains of GBS inducibly resistant to clindamycin.[485] The presence of a composite transposon in GBS and pneumococci suggests that *ermB*-mediated macrolide resistance could be due to the horizontal transfer of a mobile transposable element.[486] A particularly high proportion of strains resistant to erythromycin has been reported for type V.[469,487] Tigecycline and telithromycin are active in vitro against macrolide-resistant GBS, but data confirming their clinical effectiveness are scant.[488,489] The percentage of tetracycline-resistant strains is 75% to nearly 90%. Resistance of GBS to bacitracin, nalidixic acid, trimethoprim-sulfamethoxazole, metronidazole, and aminoglycosides is uniform.

Despite resistance of most GBS strains to aminoglycosides, synergy often is observed when an aminoglycoside (especially gentamicin) and penicillin or ampicillin are used in combination.[490] The best combination theoretically to accelerate the killing of GBS in vivo is penicillin or ampicillin plus gentamicin. Therapeutic concentrations of gentamicin in the serum are not required to achieve synergy.

By contrast, the rapid and predictable bactericidal effect of penicillin or ampicillin on GBS in vitro is ablated by the addition of rifampin.[491] Although in vivo data are lacking, the in vitro antagonism of rifampin when combined with penicillins suggests that they should not be used concurrently in the treatment of proven or suspected GBS disease.

Among the newer β-lactam antibiotics reputed to attain high concentrations of drug in the CSF, only cefotaxime, ceftriaxone, meropenem, and imipenem achieve minimal bactericidal concentrations (MBCs) comparable with MBCs of penicillin G and ampicillin (0.01-0.4 μg/mL),[466,482] and limited data suggest that their efficacy is equivalent to that of penicillin G.[492,493] Despite their uniform susceptibility to penicillin G, GBS require higher concentrations for growth inhibition in vitro than strains belonging to group A. The minimal inhibitory concentration (MIC) of penicillin G to GBS is 4-fold to 10-fold greater than the MIC for group A strains (range, 0.003-0.4 μg/mL).[465] This observation, combined with the observation indicating the significant influence of inoculum size on in vitro susceptibility to penicillin G, may have clinical relevance.[465,494]

When the inoculum of GBS is reduced from 10^5 to 10^4 colony-forming units (CFU)/mL, a twofold lower concentration of penicillin G is sufficient to inhibit in vitro growth. Similarly, if the inoculum is increased from 10^4 to 10^7 CFU/mL, the MBC of ampicillin is increased from 0.06 to 3.9 μg/mL. Such in vitro observations may have in vivo correlates because some infants with GBS meningitis have CSF bacterial inocula of 10^7 to 10^8 CFU/mL.[494] At the initiation of therapy for meningitis, achievable CSF levels of penicillin G or ampicillin may be only one tenth of serum levels. This inoculum effect also has been noted with cefotaxime and imipenem. The dose chosen to treat GBS meningitis can be crucial to the prompt sterilization of CSF.

ANTIMICROBIAL THERAPY

Penicillin G is the drug of choice for treatment of GBS infections. The recommended dosage for treatment of meningitis is high because of the relatively high MIC of penicillin G for GBS (median, 0.06 μg/mL) with respect to attainable levels of this drug in the CSF, the high inoculum in the CSF of some infants, reports of relapse in infants with meningitis treated for 14 days with 200,000 U/kg/day of penicillin G, and the safety of high doses of penicillin G in the newborn. To ensure rapid bactericidal effects, particularly in the CSF, we recommend penicillin G (450,000-500,000 U/kg/day) or ampicillin (300-400 mg/kg/day) for the treatment of meningitis (Table 12-7). There is no evidence to suggest increased risk for adverse reactions at these higher doses even in premature infants.

In the usual clinical setting, antimicrobial therapy is initiated before definitive identification of the organism. Initial therapy should include ampicillin and an aminoglycoside appropriate for the treatment of early-onset neonatal pathogens, including GBS. Such a combination is more effective than penicillin G or ampicillin alone for killing of GBS.[490] We continue combination therapy until the isolate has been identified as GBS and, in patients with meningitis, until a CSF specimen obtained 24 to 48 hours into therapy is sterile. MIC and MBC determinations may be considered in the following settings: (1) a poor bacteriologic response to antimicrobial therapy, (2) relapse or recurrence of infection without a discernible cause, and (3) infections manifested as meningitis or endocarditis.[495] For an infant with late-onset disease in whom CSF reveals gram-positive cocci in pairs or short chains, initial therapy should include ampicillin and gentamicin or ampicillin and cefotaxime. GBS is a frequent cause of meningitis in infants 1 to 8 weeks of age, and combination therapy can improve efficacy early in the course of infection. If pneumococcal meningitis is a consideration, cefotaxime and vancomycin would be a reasonable regimen pending culture confirmation. Because GBS meningitis is uncommon beyond 8 weeks of age, no change is suggested from the use of conventional agents as the initial treatment of meningitis in term infants older than 2 months. For preterm infants remaining hospitalized from birth, empirical therapy can include vancomycin and an aminoglycoside. If meningitis is suspected, cefotaxime should be included in the regimen because vancomycin achieves low CSF concentrations and has a substantially higher MBC against GBS than ceftriaxone or cotaxime.

When the diagnosis of GBS infection is confirmed, and CSF for patients with meningitis obtained 24 to 48 hours into therapy is sterile, treatment can be completed with penicillin G monotherapy. Good outcomes have been achieved

Table 12-7 Antimicrobial Regimens Recommended for Treatment of Group B Streptococcal Infections in Infants*

Manifestation of Infection	Drug	Daily Dose (Intravenous)	Duration
Bacteremia without meningitis	Ampicillin plus gentamicin	150-200 mg/kg plus 7.5 mg/kg	Initial treatment before culture results (48-72 hr)
	Penicillin G	200,000 units/kg	Complete a total treatment course of 10 days
Meningitis	Ampicillin plus gentamicin	300-400 mg/kg plus 7.5 mg/kg	Initial treatment (until cerebrospinal fluid is sterile)
	Penicillin G	450,000-500,000 units/kg	Complete a minimum total treatment course of 14 days†
Septic arthritis	Penicillin G	200,000 units/kg	2-3 wk
Osteomyelitis	Penicillin G	200,000 units/kg	3-4 wk
Endocarditis	Penicillin G	400,000 units/kg	4 wk‡

*No modification of dose by postnatal age is recommended. Oral therapy is never indicated.
†In combination with gentamicin for the first 14 days.
‡Longer treatment (up to 4 wk) may be required for ventriculitis.

when parenteral therapy is given for 10 days for bacteremia without a focus or with most soft tissue infections, 2 to 3 weeks for meningitis or pyarthrosis, and 3 to 4 weeks for osteomyelitis or endocarditis (see Table 12-7). Limited evidence suggests that a 7-day course of therapy can suffice for uncomplicated bacteremia, but additional data would be required to support a change in current recommendations.[496] For infants with meningitis, failure to achieve CSF sterility suggests an unsuspected suppurative focus (subdural empyema, brain abscess, obstructive ventriculitis, septic thrombophlebitis) or failure to administer an appropriate drug in sufficient dosage.

At the completion of therapy in an infant with complicated meningitis, a lumbar puncture should be considered to evaluate whether the CSF findings are compatible with resolution of the inflammatory process or are of sufficient concern to warrant extending treatment or additional diagnostic evaluation. Neutrophils counted as greater than 30% of the total cells and a protein concentration greater than 200 mg/dL warrant consideration of an additional week of treatment. Cranial imaging by magnetic resonance imaging with contrast enhancement toward the end of a planned course of therapy is advisable to document adequate resolution of cerebritis, subdural empyema, and so forth, and for prognostic purposes (see "Prognosis"). Infants with septic arthritis should receive at least 2 weeks and those with osteomyelitis 3 to 4 weeks of parenteral therapy to optimize an uncomplicated outcome. Drainage of the suppurative focus is an adjunct to antibiotic therapy. In infants with septic arthritis, excluding the hip, one-time needle aspiration of the involved joint usually achieves adequate drainage. With hip involvement, immediate open drainage is warranted. For most infants with osteomyelitis, aspiration assists in diagnosis because blood cultures typically are sterile. Diagnostic procedures must be performed early in the course of therapy to optimize isolation of the infecting organism.

With recurrent infection, three points should be considered. First, appropriate antimicrobial therapy fails to eliminate mucous membrane colonization with GBS in 50% of infants. Second, community exposure can result in colonization with a new strain that subsequently invades the bloodstream. Systemic infection in neonates does not elicit protective levels of CPS type-specific antibodies. Recurrent infections do occur in healthy infants. In this event, an evaluation to exclude an immune abnormality can be considered, but detection of abnormalities is rare. Therapy for recurrent infection need not be extended beyond that appropriate to the clinical expression of the recurrent infection. Finally, although it is desirable to eliminate colonization, an efficacious regimen has not been identified. One small prospective study revealed that administration of oral rifampin (20 mg/kg/day for 4 days) to infants after completion of parenteral therapy eliminated mucous membrane colonization in some subjects.[497] Further study is needed to identify a more reliable approach to eliminating colonization.

SUPPORTIVE CARE

Supportive care is important to the successful outcome of most GBS infections. It is imperative that all infants with suspected or proven meningitis receive intensive care observation at least for 24 hours, irrespective of the initial stable presentation, because clinical deterioration is frequent in this circumstance. When early-onset disease is accompanied by respiratory distress, the need for ventilatory assistance should be anticipated before onset of apnea. Early treatment of shock, often not suspected during its initial phase, when systolic pressure is maintained by peripheral vasoconstriction, is crucial. Persistent metabolic acidosis and reasonably normal color are characteristic of this early phase. Persistent perfusion abnormalities after initial attempts to achieve adequate volume expansion warrant placement of a central venous pressure monitoring device and treatment with appropriate inotropic agents. This concept applies also to patients with late-onset meningitis. In patients with meningitis, effective seizure control is required to achieve proper oxygenation, to decrease metabolic demands, prevent additional cerebral edema, and optimize cerebral blood flow. Monitoring of urine output and attention to electrolyte balance and osmolality are needed to detect and manage the early complications of meningitis, such as inappropriate secretion of antidiuretic hormone and increased intracranial pressure. Such intense and careful supportive management requires treatment in an intensive care unit of a tertiary care facility.

Prognosis

Clinical scoring systems have attempted to predict at the time of initial evaluation infants likely to die as a consequence of neonatal GBS infection.[356,357,498] One such score derived from five variables, together with an initial blood pH of less than 7.25, predicted outcome accurately in 93% of infants with early-onset GBS infection. These features were birth weight less than 2500 g, absolute neutrophil count less than 1500 cells/mm^3, hypotension, apnea, and pleural effusion on the initial chest radiograph.[357]

One group at potential risk for sequelae from GBS sepsis is preterm infants with septic shock, who can develop periventricular leukomalacia. Among survivors, substantial neurodevelopmental sequelae have been identified at evaluation during the second year of life. The correlates of severity and duration of shock with periventricular leukomalacia and with long-term morbidity have not been assessed. Prospective, active surveillance of neonatal GBS infections in Germany conducted from 2001 to 2003 found that 14% of 347 infants had neurologic sequelae of infection at the time of discharge from the hospital.[499]

Long-term outcomes for survivors of GBS meningitis are guarded. Among neonates cared for in the 1970s and 1980s, one quarter died in the hospital and 20% of survivors had major neurologic sequelae.[354,355,356] The death rate has declined but outcomes have not improved in the intervening years. Among 41 survivors from a cohort born in 1996 to 1997 in England and Wales, 34% had moderate or severe disability, 27% had mild disability, and 39% were functioning normally at 5 years of age.[500] Stoll and colleagues[501] showed for extremely-low-birth-weight infants that meningitis with or without sepsis was associated with poor neurodevelopmental and growth outcomes and impairment of vision and hearing in early childhood.

Features predictive of death or adverse outcome from GBS meningitis as assessed at hospital discharge include

seizures within hours of hospital admission, coma or semicoma, pressor support, and initial CSF protein of 300 mg/dL or greater and CSF glucose of less than 20 mg/dL.[359] Among 90 term and near-term infants diagnosed with GBS meningitis from 1998 through 2006, five died acutely and five died at 6 months to 3 years of age. Twenty-four of 43 survivors were evaluated at a mean of 7 years of age. Fifty-six percent were functioning normally. Among the remainder, 25% had mild-to-moderate impairment and 19% had severe neurodevelopmental impairment.[502] Because subtle deficits, such as delayed language development and mild hearing loss, may not be detected by routine examination meningitis survivors should undergo audiometric testing during convalescence as well as careful long-term neurologic and developmental assessments.

Prevention

Theoretically, early- and late-onset GBS disease could be prevented if susceptible hosts were not exposed to the microorganism or if exposure occurred in the setting of protective immunity. Several approaches to prevention have been advocated; conceptually, these are directed at eliminating exposure or enhancing host resistance by chemoprophylaxis or immunoprophylaxis. Both strategies have limitations with respect to implementation but could be targeted for the prevention of maternal and neonatal infections and are theoretically achievable.[503,504]

CHEMOPROPHYLAXIS

Historical Precedents

Because maternal genital colonization was recognized to expose infants to the organism, oral penicillin treatment for colonized women was proposed in the early 1970s. Approximately 20% to 30% of third-trimester GBS carriers remained colonized after this treatment, and in most of these women, GBS were isolated from vaginal cultures at delivery.[505-507] Reacquisition from colonized sexual partners was suggested as an explanation for these high failure rates, but failure rates remained high when colonized pregnant women and their spouses received concurrent treatment with penicillin by the oral or the parenteral route.[2,505,508] Yow and colleagues[509] gave intravenous ampicillin at hospital admission to 34 GBS vaginally colonized women and successfully interrupted vertical transmission of GBS to all neonates. In 1986, Boyer and Gotoff[510] provided the first documentation that IAP could prevent invasive early-onset neonatal infection. Women colonized with GBS were randomly assigned to receive routine labor and delivery care or routine care plus intrapartum ampicillin intravenously until delivery. Group B streptococcal sepsis developed in 5 of 79 neonates in the routine care group (1 died), whereas 85 infants born to women in the ampicillin treatment group remained well. Intrapartum ampicillin prophylaxis for GBS carriers also resulted in reduced maternal morbidity.[511] These data established the efficacy of IAP for prevention of early-onset neonatal disease and reduction of GBS-associated febrile maternal morbidity. The cost-effectiveness of this approach subsequently was validated.[512]

In 1992, the American College of Obstetricians and Gynecologists (ACOG)[513] and the American Academy of Pediatrics (AAP)[514] published separate documents regarding maternal IAP for the prevention of early-onset GBS infection. The ACOG technical bulletin was educational, whereas the AAP guidelines were directive. The AAP guidelines specified that if culture screening was performed antenatally, specimens should be obtained from lower vaginal and rectal sites, and GBS culture-positive women should be given intravenous penicillin G or ampicillin intrapartum. The ACOG proposed that culture screening could be avoided by providing treatment for all women with risk factors. Neither the AAP nor ACOG approach was widely implemented, and although invasive disease rates began to diminish, they remained unacceptably high.

Rapid Assays for Antenatal Detection of Group B Streptococci

Bergeron and colleagues[515] described a fluorogenic real time (RT)-PCR technique for rapid identification of women colonized with GBS at admission for delivery. The sensitivity of RT-PCR and of conventional PCR was 97%, the negative predictive value was 99%, and the specificity and positive predictive value were 100%. Results were available from RT-PCR in 45 minutes; by comparison, conventional PCR required 100 minutes, and conventional cultures required 36 hours minimum. Field testing of commercially available assays, such as the Xpert GBS Assay (Cepheid, Sunnyvale, Calif), which uses automated rapid RT-PCR technology has been conducted.[516-518] The performance of RT-PCR in one study was deemed sufficiently robust for possible use in point-of-care settings.[519] One cost-benefit analysis suggested that widespread implementation of RT-PCR would afford benefit over the current culture-based strategy (decrease antimicrobial use), but another concluded that molecular point-of-care testing was cost neutral compared with recommended culture techniques.[520,521]

More recent studies evaluating RT-PCR versus antenatal cultures suggest that PCR testing is superior to antenatal testing, but typically the investigators have sampled only the vaginal without the recommended rectal site or have put swabs directly onto agar media without preceding inoculation into enrichment broth, or both. Studies that use recommended site sampling (vaginal and rectal specimens) and compare RT-PCR with culture processing that includes placing swabs into enrichment broth media, with incubation and then inoculation onto agar media, indicate equivalent sensitivity and specificity of antenatal culture screening and intrapartum PCR testing.[522-524]

There continue to be benefits and difficulties inherent to ascertainment of GBS colonization using RT-PCR even when assays can be processed rapidly 24 hours a day. Currently, RT-PCR detection of GBS colonization should be considered an adjunct to antenatal culture screening at 35 to 37 weeks of gestation.[16]

Intrapartum Antibiotic Prophylaxis

The current era of IAP dates from 1996, when consensus recommendations for the prevention of early-onset GBS disease were endorsed by the CDC, AAP, and ACOG.[457,525,526] These recommendations indicated that obstetric care

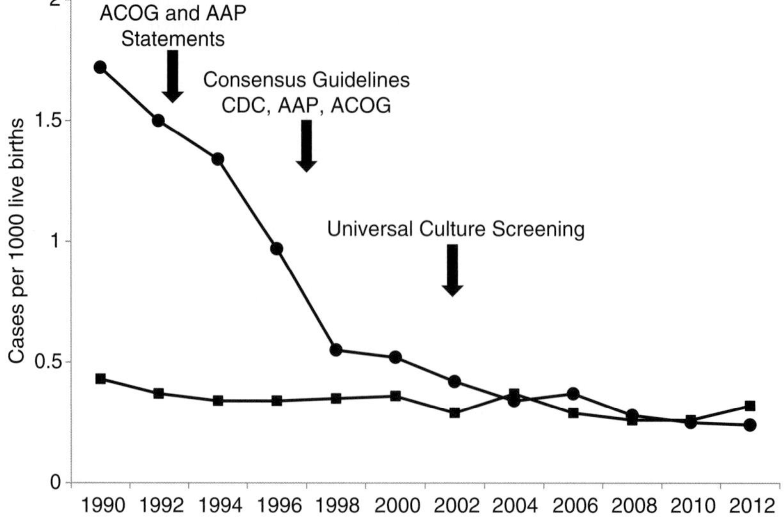

Figure 12-10 Incidence of early-onset *(solid black bullet)* and late-onset *(solid black square)* group B streptococcal disease from 1990 to 2012. The dates of the initial prevention statements from the American College of Obstetricians and Gynecologists (ACOG) and the American Academy of Pediatrics (AAP),[513,514] the 1996 consensus guidelines from the Centers for Disease Control and Prevention (CDC),[525] and the revised 2002 CDC guidelines for universal culture screening[503] are shown.

providers and hospitals should adopt a culture-based or a risk-based policy to identify women to receive IAP. The culture-based approach used lower vaginal and rectal cultures obtained at 35 to 37 weeks of gestation to identify candidates for IAP. The risk-based strategy identified IAP recipients by factors known to increase the likelihood of neonatal GBS disease: labor onset or membrane rupture before 37 weeks of gestation, intrapartum fever greater than or equal to 38° C (±100.4° F), or rupture of membranes 18 or more hours before delivery. In both strategies, women with GBS bacteriuria or previous delivery of an infant with GBS disease were to receive IAP. These strategies each resulted in the administration of IAP to approximately one in four pregnant women.

The incidence of early-onset disease declined by 70% from 1.7 per 1000 live births to 0.5 per 1000 live births by 1999 in association with implementation of one of these two IAP methods[503,527] (Fig. 12-10). A resulting 3900 to 4500 early-onset infections and 200 to 225 neonatal deaths were estimated to be prevented annually.[503,528] By contrast, the rate of late-onset disease remained constant at 0.5 to 0.6 per 1000 live births. Also, the incidence of invasive GBS disease, primarily bacteremia with or without intraamniotic infection or endometritis among pregnant women declined significantly, from 0.29 per 1000 live births in 1993 to 0.23 in 1998.[503,528] By 1999, two thirds of U.S. hospitals in a multistate survey had a formal prevention policy, and numerous individual practitioners had adopted one of the two strategies proposed in 1996.[503,529]

By 2002, it was evident that further reduction in the incidence of early-onset disease could be accomplished by adoption of universal culture screening. A direct comparison in 5144 births showed that the culture-based strategy was 50% more effective than the risk-based strategy in preventing early-onset disease in neonates.[142] Culture-based screening more often resulted in administration of IAP for at least 4 hours before delivery. The 2002 revised CDC guidelines recommending a universal culture-based approach to prevention of perinatal GBS disease are endorsed by the AAP and the ACOG.[503] Early-onset disease incidence declined an additional 29% after issuance of the revised guidelines in 2002, to 0.34 cases per 1000 live births from 2003 to 2007.[141] An additional reduction in incidence occurred in 2008, but since then, as of 2012, incidence has reached a plateau at 0.25 per 1000 live births.

Currently, all pregnant women should be screened in each pregnancy for GBS carriage at 35 to 37 weeks of gestation. The risk-based approach is an acceptable alternative *only* in circumstances in which the culture has not been performed or results are unavailable before delivery. The 2010 revised recommendations from CDC, ACOG, and AAP are essentially the same as those from 2002, but further clarifications have been given for six topics: (1) expanded information on laboratory methods for GBS identification, (2) definition of colony-count threshold for reporting GBS bacteriuria, (3) algorithms for GBS screening and IAP for women with preterm labor or preterm premature rupture of membranes, (4) a minor change in the second dose of penicillin from 3 million U to 2.5 to 3 million U intravenously, (5) updated prophylaxis regimens for women with allergy to penicillin, and (6) a simplified algorithm for management of neonates with respect to risk for early-onset GBS disease. Culture specimens from pregnant women should be obtained from the lower vagina and the rectum using the same or two different swabs. These swabs should be placed in a nonnutritive transport medium, transferred to a laboratory where the swabs are incubated overnight in a selective enrichment broth, and subcultured onto suitable agar medium for isolation of GBS.[16] At the time of labor or rupture of membranes, IAP should be given to all pregnant women identified antenatally as carriers of GBS. The indications for IAP are shown in Figure 12-11. Group B streptococcal bacteriuria during the current pregnancy or prior delivery of an infant with invasive GBS disease always is an indication for IAP, so antenatal screening is unnecessary for these women.[16] If culture results are unknown at the onset of labor or rupture of membranes, the risk factors listed in Figure 12-11 should be used to determine the need to institute IAP. Women who present with preterm labor before antenatal GBS screening should have cultures obtained and IAP initiated. If labor ceases and cultures are negative, IAP is discontinued, and antenatal screening is performed at 35 to 37 weeks of gestation. If labor ceases and cultures are positive, some experts recommend oral amoxicillin for another 5 to 7 days.

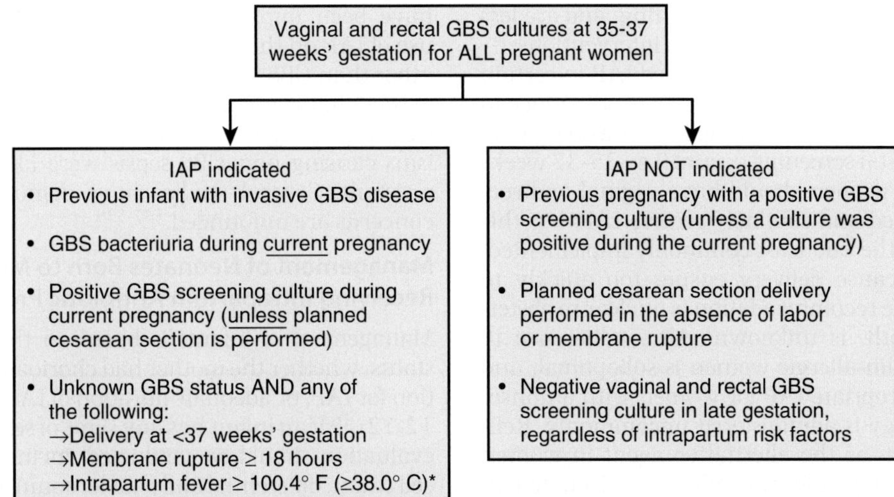

Figure 12-11 Recommendations for culture-based screening for maternal colonization with group B streptococci (GBS) and administration of intrapartum antibiotic prophylaxis (IAP). *If chorioamnionitis is suspected, broad-spectrum antibiotic therapy that includes an agent known to be active against GBS should replace GBS IAP. (Modified from Centers for Disease Control and Prevention: Prevention of perinatal group B streptococcal disease: revised guidelines from CDC, *MMWR Morb Mortal Wkly Rep* 59[RR-10]:1-32, 2010.)

Planned cesarean section before rupture of membranes and onset of labor constitute an exception to the need for IAP for women colonized with GBS. These women are at extremely low risk for having an infant with early-onset disease. Culture-negative women who are delivered at 37 weeks of gestation or later need not receive IAP routinely. Therapeutic use of broad-spectrum antibiotics in labor should be used as is appropriate for maternal indications, such as intraamniotic infection.

The recommended maternal IAP regimen consists of penicillin G (5 million U initially, then 2.5-3 million U every 4 hours thereafter until delivery).[16] Penicillin or ampicillin given 4 or more hours before delivery reliably prevents vertical transmission and early-onset disease.[530] Ampicillin administered as a 2-g intravenous loading dose and then 1 g every 4 hours until delivery is an alternative to penicillin.[503] The rationale for the high initial dose of the β-lactam antibiotic relates to the desired drug concentrations needed in the amniotic and vaginal fluids (peak approximately 3 hours after completion of the initial dose) to reduce substantially the number of GBS at either site. IAP "failures" typically occur when penicillin or ampicillin has been initiated 2 or less hours before delivery; clindamycin has been given without susceptibility testing, and clindamycin-resistant early-onset GBS neonatal sepsis ensued; or appropriate IAP is given in the setting of clinically apparent or silent intraamniotic infection.

Prophylaxis for penicillin-allergic women must take into account increasing resistance among GBS to erythromycin and clindamycin. Women *not* at high risk for anaphylaxis (e.g., a rash without anaphylaxis or respiratory compromise) should receive cefazolin, 2 g intravenously as an initial dose and then 1 g every 8 hours until delivery. Cefazolin has pharmacokinetics similar to penicillin with respect to peak concentrations in serum and amniotic fluid of pregnant women. Women whose GBS isolates are tested and found to be clindamycin susceptible by a D test and who are at high risk for anaphylaxis with penicillin can receive clindamycin at a dose of 900 mg every 8 hours. However, the efficacy of clindamycin in preventing early-onset GBS disease is not known, and clindamycin prophylaxis failures have occurred.[531] If susceptibility testing is unavailable or the results are unknown, or when isolates are resistant to clindamycin, vancomycin, 1 g intravenously every 12 hours until delivery, is an alternative for women with serious penicillin hypersensitivity reactions. Neither the pharmacokinetics of vancomycin in amniotic nor vaginal fluids nor its efficacy in preventing early-onset disease has been investigated.

The risk of anaphylaxis from administration of penicillin is low. Estimates range from 4 events per 10,000 to 4 per 100,000 patients. Anaphylaxis associated with administration of a β-lactam antibiotic as IAP for the prevention of early-onset GBS infection has been reported but is rare.[142,532,533] Most pregnant women reporting a penicillin allergy that is not anaphylaxis have negative testing for hypersensitivity and are able to receive IAP with penicillin safely.[534] A fetal demise in association with new-onset penicillin allergy during IAP has been reported in a woman with rheumatoid arthritis.[535] No adult fatalities in association with IAP are reported, and the risk of a fatal event is low because the antimicrobials are administered in a hospital setting where medical intervention is readily available. Despite these data and the 2010 guidelines, adherence to appropriate use of IAP in penicillin-allergic women is poor.[536]

Numerous residual problems, barriers to implementation, and missed opportunities must be overcome to achieve maximal benefit from IAP. Procedural issues, such as suboptimal culture processing and collection of cultures earlier than 5 weeks before delivery, constitute one set of problems. Laboratories may not adhere to recommended methods for isolation of GBS, a problem that remains despite the 2010 consensus recommendations and one that results in colonized women delivering infants with early-onset disease. Even optimal antenatal culture methods miss some women who are colonized at delivery, exposing their neonate to GBS and resulting in colonization or illness. Another problem is that women who are not screened adequately more often are medically underserved; women in their teens, blacks, and Hispanics are more likely than whites to receive inadequate prenatal care and prenatal testing, and are less likely to receive recommended prevention interventions.

Problems surround lack of recommended IAP in certain circumstances. The most prominent is lack of adherence to the 2010 recommendation for routine IAP in women who deliver before antenatal screening occurs (i.e., 35-37 weeks of gestation). These women should have vaginal and rectal cultures performed and routinely receive IAP, but this recommendation is the one least commonly implemented. Whether this is because delivery ensues too quickly to administer IAP or the recommendation is unclear to obstetric providers, or both, is unknown. Also, adherence to guidelines in penicillin-allergic women is suboptimal, and cefazolin as the appropriate IAP for women with a nonserious penicillin allergy is administered uncommonly. Reliance on clindamycin as the alternative agent in women without serious penicillin allergy results in inadequate IAP in at least 20% of patients when antimicrobial susceptibility testing of colonizing isolates is not performed antenatally.[16]

A final issue is a need for increased awareness of perinatal GBS infection. In one report, only 47% of women younger than 50 years reported having heard of GBS. Women with a high school education or less; with low household income; or reporting black, Asian/Pacific Islander, or "other" race had lower awareness than that noted in other women. Efforts to raise awareness should target women from groups that traditionally are medically underserved. Hospital infection control teams can contribute to these efforts by spearheading educational efforts toward effective implementation among hospital obstetric staff and laboratory personnel.[528]

Impact of Intrapartum Antibiotic Prophylaxis on Neonatal Sepsis

The efficacy of IAP in preventing early-onset GBS infection has been shown in numerous observational studies and in countries other than the United States when guidelines have been implemented.[142,349] The impact of increased use of IAP on the occurrence of sepsis caused by organisms other than GBS is a subject of ongoing evaluation. Concern existed that neonatal sepsis caused by organisms other than GBS, especially *E. coli*, would increase and that the organisms causing non–GBS sepsis were likely to be ampicillin resistant. Several studies have demonstrated that these concerns are unfounded.[537-539]

Management of Neonates Born to Mothers Receiving Intrapartum Antibiotic Prophylaxis

Management of infants is based on the neonate's clinical status, whether the mother had chorioamnionitis, an indication for IAP, or adequate duration of IAP, and gestation (Fig. 12-12).[16] If an infant has any signs of sepsis, a full diagnostic evaluation should be conducted, including complete blood cell count, differential and platelet count, blood culture; chest radiograph if the neonate has respiratory signs; and if the infant is clinically stable, a lumbar puncture. Then empirical therapy should be initiated pending laboratory results.[16] Although published reports vary, a minimum of 10% and a maximum of nearly 40% of infants with meningitis have a negative blood culture.[456] If lumbar puncture is deferred and therapy is continued for more than 48 hours because of suspected infection, CSF should be obtained for routine studies and culture. Depending on the CSF results, therapy appropriate for sepsis or presumed meningitis is given.

If a woman has suspected chorioamnionitis, her healthy appearing infant should have a limited diagnostic evaluation, including a blood culture at birth and complete blood count, differential and platelet count at birth or 6 to 12 hours later. Most experts would then initiate empirical therapy pending culture results. This approach is based on the infant's exposure to suspected or established infection. The duration of therapy is based on results of cultures and the infant's clinical course (see "Treatment"). If the mother was

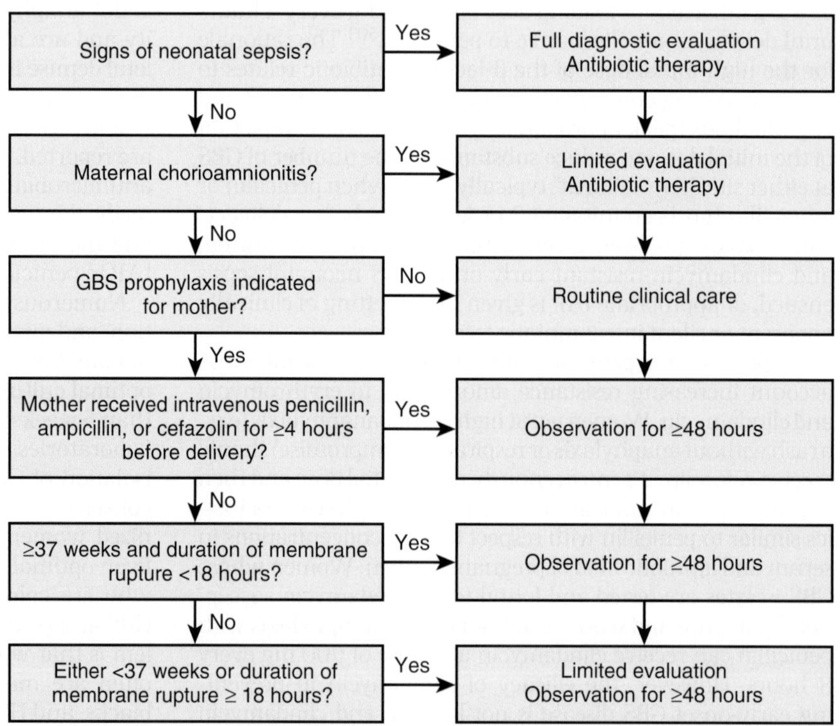

Figure 12-12 Algorithm for prevention of early-onset GBS disease among newborns. (Modified from Centers for Disease Control and Prevention: Prevention of perinatal group B streptococcal disease: revised guidelines from CDC, *MMWR Morb Mortal Wkly Rep* 59[RR-10]:1-32, 2010.)

a candidate for IAP and received adequate IAP (4 or more hours of penicillin, ampicillin, or cefazolin) before delivery, her healthy appearing infant should receive routine clinical care with 48 hours observation. If the mother has not received adequate IAP and the rupture of membranes has been less than 18 hours, the healthy appearing infant who has a gestational age of 37 weeks or more should receive observation in the hospital for a minimum of 48 hours. However, if the infant is either less than 37 weeks of gestation or delivery occurs 18 or more hours before delivery, the infant should have a limited evaluation and observation in the hospital for 48 hours. If in any of these circumstances, the neonate develops signs of sepsis, a full diagnostic evaluation should be performed and empirical broad-spectrum antibiotic therapy initiated, typically with ampicillin and gentamicin. The approach presented in Figure 12-12 is not to be taken as an exclusive management pathway. Hospital discharge at 24 hours of age can be reasonable under certain circumstances, specifically when the infant is born after the mother has received a β-lactam as IAP for 4 hours or longer before delivery, has a gestational age of 37 weeks or more, and is healthy appearing. Other discharge criteria also should be met, and the infant should be under the care of a person able to comply with instructions for home observation, with ready access to medical care.[16] The risk of bacterial infection in healthy appearing newborns is low. The revised 2010 CDC guidelines for prevention of early-onset GBS disease[16] also were endorsed by ACOG and AAP.[540] Because some recommendations from neonatologists were in conflict with the 2010 recommended infant management guidelines,[463] further clarification was needed to establish Figure 12-12 as the optimal care pathway.[541]

The influence of maternal IAP on the clinical spectrum of early-onset infection in term infants has been evaluated.[542,543] Exposure to antibiotics in labor does not change the clinical spectrum of disease or the onset of clinical signs of infection within 24 to 48 hours of birth for infants with early-onset GBS infection. Infants whose mothers have received IAP are less likely to be ill, to require assisted ventilation, or to have proven bacterial infection. These infants are not more likely to undergo invasive procedures or to receive antibiotics.[542] The number of infants undergoing evaluation for sepsis has decreased in association with implementation of IAP guidelines, and among GBS-negative women, ordering of laboratory tests diminished by almost 40% after the 2002 guidelines[544] and are anticipated to decrease even more if the 2010 infant management recommendations are fully implemented.[541]

Chemoprophylaxis for the Neonate

In the special circumstance of an apparently nonaffected sibling in a twin or multiple birth with early-onset[302,303] or late-onset[303] GBS disease, the well appearing sibling of a neonate with invasive infection is at increased risk of developing GBS disease. At the time of diagnosis of GBS disease in the index patient of a multiple birth, the other infant or infants should be assessed clinically.[303] If signs of infection are noted, cultures of blood and CSF should be obtained, and empirical antimicrobial treatment should be initiated until laboratory results become available. If cultures yield GBS, a full course of treatment is appropriate. If findings from the clinical assessment are unremarkable, management should be undertaken on a case-by-case basis. The risk for a poor outcome when the second twin is not evaluated until clinical signs of infection are apparent warrants caution in this circumstance. Even when empirical therapy is given and invasive infection is excluded, later onset is possible.[545]

IMMUNOPROPHYLAXIS

A promising approach to prevention of GBS disease is immunoprophylaxis.[504,546] The underlying principle is that IgG directed against CPS of GBS, critical for protection against invasive disease, is provided by active or passive immunization. Human sera containing a sufficient concentration of CPS-specific antibody have been shown in animal models of infection to protect against lethal challenge with each of the major group B streptococcal CPS types.[547] Provision of protective levels of CPS type-specific immunity to the newborn could be achieved by active maternal immunization with passive protection of the neonate.

The first candidate GBS vaccine, a purified type III CPS, underwent testing in healthy adults in 1978.[319] Subsequently, types Ia and II CPS vaccines were studied. Although these vaccines were well tolerated and elicited a primarily IgG class response within 2 to 4 weeks, the immunogenicity was variable. It was discovered that nearly 90% of healthy young adults had very low preimmunization serum concentrations of CPS-specific antibodies in association with presumed immunologic naïveté. These low levels predicted a poor immune response in many so that only 40% and 60% developed significant type-specific antibody responses after immunization with type Ia and type III CPS vaccines, respectively. By contrast, 88% of adults immunized with type II CPS vaccine responded with fourfold or greater increases in type II CPS–specific antibodies. These early trials verified the feasibility of immunization as an approach to prevent GBS disease and revealed the need to develop candidate vaccines with enhanced immunogenicity. The first study conducted in pregnant women was an encouragement to the ultimate potential success of a GBS vaccine program. Among 25 pregnant responders to a type III CPS GBS vaccine, 90% delivered infants with substantial levels of specific antibody to the type III CPS in cord sera that promoted functional activity in vitro throughout the first 3 months of life in most instances.

Development of the first group B streptococcal CPS conjugate vaccine, type III CPS–tetanus toxoid, was driven by the prominence of type III among infants with early and late-onset disease and by its dominance as a cause of meningitis. Type III CPS was linked covalently to monomeric tetanus toxoid by reductive amination coupling chemistry.[548] Group B streptococcal CPS–protein conjugate vaccines of all clinically important types in developed countries (Ia, Ib, II, III, and V) subsequently were developed and found to be immunogenic and protective in experimental animals.[548-552] The first clinical evaluation of the type III CPS–tetanus toxoid conjugate showed greater than fourfold increases in postimmunization CPS-specific IgG in 90% of healthy nonpregnant women.[553] The vaccine was well tolerated, and the antibodies, predominantly of the IgG class, were functional in vitro and protective in a murine model of infection.

Conjugate vaccines to each of the clinically relevant group B streptococcal CPS types causing invasive disease have been tested in nearly 500 healthy adults 18 to 50 years of age.[553-556] Systemic responses, such as low-grade fever, chills, headache or myalgias, always short-lived, were observed in less than 2% of volunteers. Local reactions were frequent but mild, typically consisting of pain without erythema or swelling, and resolved within 48 to 72 hours. Immune responses to each of the conjugate vaccines, with the exception of type V, are dose dependent. Doses of 4 to 15 μg of the CPS component have elicited greater than fourfold increases in CPS-specific IgG in 80% to 93% of recipients of type Ia, Ib, II, III, and V conjugates at 8 weeks after immunization. Evaluation of a vaccine combining type II and type III CPS, each conjugated to tetanus toxoid, showed no immune interference compared with response after administration of one of the monovalent vaccines.[557]

A phase I randomized placebo-controlled, double-blinded trial of type III CPS–tetanus toxoid conjugate vaccine was conducted in 30 healthy pregnant women at 30 to 32 weeks of gestation.[558] Immunization was well tolerated. Geometric mean concentrations of IgG elicited to type III CPS from immunized women were significantly increased from preimmunization values and correlated well with infant cord values. Sera from the infants of vaccinated women collected at 1 and 2 months of age promoted in vitro opsonization and killing of type III GBS by human neutrophils.

Although glycoconjugates are the most likely first GBS vaccine candidates, the precise formulation will be challenging. Currently, the most prevalent types causing global GBS perinatal disease are III and Ia. Bellais and colleagues[140] identified the presence of the CC17-specific surface protein encoding the *hvgA* gene of a type III GBS strain from France. Using a variety of molecular techniques, they were able to demonstrate a CPS switch from type III to type IV that used the entire *cps* operon. Use of surface proteins that are conserved across most GBS serotypes offers another strategy for vaccine development. The C protein could be an alternative to tetanus toxoid as the protein component of a conjugate vaccine.[547,551,559] Invasive disease, but not colonization, elicits α C–specific and β C–specific IgM and IgG in adults.[560,561] A type III polysaccharide–C protein conjugate vaccine theoretically could prevent most systemic infections. A recombinant β C protein modified to eliminate its IgA-binding site conjugated to type III CPS has been shown to be immunogenic in mice, inducing polysaccharide and C protein–specific functional IgG.[562] The GBS surface proteins, Rib, Sip, and C5a peptidase, each have been shown to elicit antibodies that are protective in experimental models of GBS infection.[563-565] Their roles in human infection are not established, however.

The discovery that surface-associated pilus-like islands are distributed widely among GBS clinical isolates potentially paves the way for the development of pilus island–based vaccines. An entire pilus island has been transferred from group B *Streptococcus* to a nonpathogenic species. Mucosally delivered *Lactococcus*-expressing pilus island 1 protected mice from challenge with pilus 1–containing GBS strains.[9] Pilus islands 1, 2a, and 2b, alone or in combination, were identified on each of 289 GBS isolates from infants and adults with invasive disease, and most were highly surface expressed.[10] A combination of the three pilus-island components conferred protection against all tested GBS challenge strains. A vaccine exclusively constituted by pilus components in concept could be broadly efficacious in preventing infections caused by GBS.[10,566]

Recent studies emphasize the importance of perinatal GBS disease not only in resource-rich but also developing countries, with a substantial impact on global neonatal mortality.[145,146] IAP is not feasible in many countries and does not prevent late-onset disease. Maternal immunization, which has eliminated maternal and neonatal tetanus, is an attractive prevention method. In the United States and some European countries, which now recommend routine influenza and tetanus and diphtheria toxoids plus acellular pertussis vaccine for pregnant women, the platform for a GBS vaccine appears to be growing. Recent phase I and II trials of a trivalent Ia, Ib, III GBS glycoconjugate in pregnant women conducted by Novartis Vaccines (Basel) is encouraging and it is hoped that further industry development will progress. Meanwhile, physicians, their patients and pharmaceutical industry leaders must perceive this mode of prevention to be of high benefit and negligible risk, especially when pregnant women are the target population for immunization. The cost of developing suitable vaccines, although substantial, is considerably less than the death, disability, and treatment associated with these infections.[512,567] If the prevention of GBS disease is to become a reality, however, physicians, public health officials, parents, and patients must join together as advocates for pregnant women, neonates, and young infants.

References

1. Fry RM: Fatal infections by haemolytic streptococcus group B, *Lancet* 1:199-201, 1938.
2. Franciosi RA, Knostman JD, Zimmerman RA: Group B streptococcal neonatal and infant infections, *J Pediatr* 82:707-718, 1973.
3. Baker CJ, Barrett FF: Transmission of group B streptococci among parturient women and their neonates, *J Pediatr* 83:919-925, 1973.
4. Howard JB, McCracken GH Jr: The spectrum of group B streptococcal infections in infancy, *Am J Dis Child* 128:815-818, 1974.
5. Schrag SJ, Zywicki S, Farley MM, et al: Group B streptococcal disease in the era of intrapartum antibiotic prophylaxis, *N Engl J Med* 342:15-20, 2000.
6. Tettelin H, Masignani V, Cieslewicz MJ, et al: Complete genome sequence and comparative genomic analysis of an emerging human pathogen, serotype V *Streptococcus agalactiae*, *Proc Natl Acad Sci U S A* 99:12391-12396, 2002.
7. Glaser P, Rusniok C, Buchrieser C, et al: Genome sequence of *Streptococcus agalactiae*, a pathogen causing invasive neonatal disease, *Mol Microbiol* 45:1499-1513, 2002.
8. Lauer P, Rinaudo CD, Soriani M, et al: Genome analysis reveals pili in group B *Streptococcus*, *Science* 309:105, 2005.
9. Buccato S, Maione D, Rinaudo CD, et al: Use of *Lactococcus lactis* expressing pili from group B *Streptococcus* as a broad-coverage vaccine against streptococcal disease, *J Infect Dis* 194:331-340, 2006.
10. Margarit I, Rinaudo CD, Galeotti CL, et al: Preventing bacterial infections with pilus-based vaccines: the group B streptococcus paradigm, *J Infect Dis* 199:108-115, 2009.
11. Lancefield RC: A serological differentiation of human and other groups of hemolytic streptococci, *J Exp Med* 57:571-595, 1933.
12. Baker CJ, Clark DJ, Barrett FF: Selective broth medium for isolation of group B streptococci, *Appl Microbiol* 26:884-885, 1973.
13. Lim DV, Morales WJ, Walsh AF: Lim group B Strep Broth and coagglutination for rapid identification of group B streptococci in preterm pregnant women, *J Clin Microbiol* 25:452-453, 1987.
14. Christie R, Atkins NE, Munch-Petersen E: A note on a lytic phenomenon shown by group B streptococci, *Aust J Exp Biol Med Sci* 22: 197-200, 1944.

15. Lancefield RC: A microprecipitin technic for classifying hemolytic streptococci, and improved methods for producing antisera, *Proc Soc Exp Biol Med* 38:473-478, 1938.
16. Centers for Disease Control and Prevention: Prevention of perinatal group B streptococcal disease—revised guidelines from CDC, *MMWR Recomm Rep* 59(RR-10):1-32, 2010.
17. Stableforth AW: Incidence of various serological types of *Streptococcus agalactiae* in herds of cows in Great Britain, *J Pathol Bacteriol* 46:21-119, 1938.
18. Finch LA, Martin DR: Human and bovine group B streptococci: two distinct populations, *J Appl Bacteriol* 57:273-278, 1984.
19. Wibawan IWT, Lämmler C: Properties of group B streptococci with protein surface antigens X and R, *J Clin Microbiol* 282:834-2836, 1990.
20. Bohnsack JF, Whiting AA, Martinez G, et al: Serotype III *Streptococcus agalactiae* from bovine milk and human neonatal infections, *Emerg Infect Dis* 10:1412-1419, 2004.
21. Lancefield RC, Hare R: The serological differentiation of pathogenic and non-pathogenic strains of hemolytic streptococci from parturient women, *J Exp Med* 61:335-349, 1935.
22. Lancefield RC: Two serological types of group B hemolytic streptococci with related, but not identical, type-specific substances, *J Exp Med* 67:25-40, 1938.
23. Freimer EH: Type-specific polysaccharide antigens of group B streptococci. II. The chemical basis for serological specificity of the type II HCl antigen, *J Exp Med* 125:381-392, 1967.
24. Wilkinson HW, Eagon RG: Type-specific antigens of group B type Ic streptococci, *Infect Immun* 4:596-604, 1971.
25. Jelínková J, Motlová J: The nomenclature of GBS, *Antibiot Chemother* 35:49-52, 1985.
26. Henrichsen J, Ferrieri P, Jelinkova J, et al: Nomenclature of antigens of group B streptococci, *Int J Syst Bacteriol* 34:500, 1984.
27. Perch B, Kjems E, Henrichsen J: New serotypes of group B streptococci isolated from human sources, *J Clin Microbiol* 10:109-110, 1979.
28. Johnson DR, Ferrieri P: Group B streptococcal Ibc protein antigen: distribution of two determinants in wild-type strains of common serotypes, *J Clin Microbiol* 19:506-510, 1984.
29. Madoff LC, Michel JL, Gong EW, et al: Group B streptococci escape host immunity by deletion of tandem repeat elements of the alpha C protein, *Proc Natl Acad Sci U S A* 93:4131-4136, 1996.
30. Kling DE, Gravekamp C, Madoff LC, et al: Characterization of two distinct opsonic and protective epitopes within the alpha C protein of the group B *Streptococcus*, *Infect Immun* 65:1462-1467, 1997.
31. Gravekamp C, Horensky DS, Michel JL, et al: Variation in repeat number within the alpha C protein of group B streptococci alters antigenicity and protective epitopes, *Infect Immun* 64:3576-3583, 1996.
32. Jerlström PG, Chhatwal GS, Timmis KN: The IgA-binding 3 antigen of the C protein complex of group B streptococci: sequence determination of its gene and detection of two binding regions, *Mol Microbiol* 54:843-849, 1991.
33. Jerlström PG, Talay SR, Valentin-Weigand P, et al: Identification of an immunoglobulin A binding motif located in the beta-antigen of the c protein complex of group B streptococci, *Infect Immun* 64: 2787-2793, 1996.
34. Ferrieri P, Baker CJ, Hillier SL, et al: Diversity of surface protein expression in group B streptococcal colonizing and invasive isolates, *Indian J Med Res* 119(Suppl):191-196, 2004.
35. Erdogan S, Fagan PK, Talay SR, et al: Molecular analysis of group B protective surface protein, a new cell surface protective antigen of group B streptococci, *Infect Immun* 70:803-811, 2002.
36. Flores AE, Chhatwal GS, Hillier SL, et al: Expression of group B protective surface protein (BPS) by invasive and colonizing isolates of group B streptococci, *Curr Microbiol* 69:894-898, 2014.
37. Pattison IH, Matthews PRJ, Howell DG: The type classification of group B streptococci with special reference to bovine strains apparently lacking in type polysaccharide, *J Pathol Bacteriol* 69:41-50, 1955.
38. Lachenauer CS, Madoff LC: A protective surface protein from type V group B streptococci shares N-terminal sequence homology with the alpha C protein, *Infect Immun* 64:4255-4260, 1996.
39. Rioux S, Martin D, Ackermann HW, et al: Localization of surface immunogenic protein on group B *Streptococcus*, *Infect Immun* 69:5162-5265, 2001.
40. Maisey HC, Hensler M, Nizet V, et al: Group B streptococcal pilus proteins contribute to adherence to and invasion of brain microvascular endothelial cells, *J Bacteriol* 189:1464-1467, 2007.
41. Deng L, Kasper DL, Krick TP, et al: Characterization of the linkage between the type III capsular polysaccharide and the bacterial cell wall of group B *Streptococcus*, *J Biol Chem* 275:7497-7504, 2000.
42. Kasper DL, Baker CJ: Electron microscopic definition of surface antigens of group B *Streptococcus*, *J Infect Dis* 139:147-151, 1979.
43. von Hunolstein C, D'Ascenzi S, Wagner B, et al: Immunochemistry of capsular type polysaccharide and virulence properties of type VI *Streptococcus agalactiae* (group B streptococci), *Infect Immun* 61:1272-1280, 1993.
44. Ráyc M, Jelínková J, Motlová J, et al: Immuno-electronmicroscopic demonstration of capsules on group-B streptococci of new serotypes and type candidates, *J Med Microbiol* 25:147-149, 1988.
45. Paoletti LC, Ross RA, Johnson KD: Cell growth rate regulates expression of group B *Streptococcus* type III capsular polysaccharide, *Infect Immun* 64:1220-1226, 1996.
46. Baker CJ, Kasper DL, Davis CE: Immunochemical characterization of the native type III polysaccharide of group B *Streptococcus*, *J Exp Med* 143:258-270, 1976.
47. Michon F, Brisson JR, Dell A, et al: Multiantennary group-specific polysaccharide of group B *Streptococcus*, *Biochemistry* 27: 5341-5351, 1988.
48. Tai JY, Gotschlich EC, Lancefield RC: Isolation of type-specific polysaccharide antigen from group B type Ib streptococci, *J Exp Med* 149:58-66, 1979.
49. Jennings HJ, Rosell KG, Kasper DL: Structural determination and serology of the native polysaccharide antigen of the type III group B *Streptococcus*, *Can J Biochem* 58:112-120, 1980.
50. Wessels MR, Pozsgay V, Kasper DL, et al: Structure and immunochemistry of an oligosaccharide repeating unit of the capsular polysaccharide of type III group B *Streptococcus*, *J Biol Chem* 262:8262-8267, 1987.
51. Wessels MR, DiFabio JL, Benedì VJ, et al: Structural determination and immunochemical characterization of the type V group B *Streptococcus* capsular polysaccharide, *J Biol Chem* 266:6714-6719, 1991.
52. Kogan G, Brisson JR, Kasper DL, et al: Structural elucidation of the novel type VII group B *Streptococcus* capsular polysaccharide by high resolution NMR spectroscopy, *Carbohydr Res* 277:1-9, 1995.
53. Kasper DL, Baker CJ, Galdes B, et al: Immunochemical analysis and immunogenicity of the type II group B streptococcal capsular polysaccharide, *J Clin Invest* 72:260-269, 1983.
54. Wessels MR, Benedí WJ, Jennings HJ, et al: Isolation and characterization of type IV group B *Streptococcus* capsular polysaccharide, *Infect Immun* 57:1089-1094, 1989.
55. Jennings HJ, Rosell KG, Katzenellenbogen E, et al: Structural determination of the capsular polysaccharide antigen of type II group B *Streptococcus*, *J Biol Chem* 258:1793-1798, 1983.
56. Kogan G, Uhrín D, Brisson JR, et al: Structural and immunochemical characterization of the type VIII group B *Streptococcus* capsular polysaccharide, *J Biol Chem* 271:8786-8790, 1996.
57. Jennings HJ, Katzenellenbogen E, Lugowski C, et al: Structure of native polysaccharide antigens of type Ia and type Ib group B *Streptococcus*, *Biochemistry* 22:1258-1264, 1983.
58. Schifferle RE, Jennings HJ, Wessels MR, et al: Immunochemical analysis of the types Ia and Ib group B streptococcal polysaccharides, *J Immunol* 135:4164-4170, 1985.
59. Lindberg B, Lönngren J, Powell DA: Structural studies of the specific type 14 pneumococcal polysaccharide, *Carbohydr Res* 58:117-186, 1977.
60. Wessels MR, Paoletti LC, Guttormsen HK, et al: Structural properties of group B streptococcal type III polysaccharide conjugate vaccines that influence immunogenicity and efficacy, *Infect Immun* 66: 2186-2192, 1998.
61. Zou W, Jennings HJ: The conformational epitope of type III group B *Streptococcus* capsular polysaccharide, *Adv Exp Med Biol* 491: 473-484, 2001.
62. Milligan TW, Doran TI, Straus DC, et al: Growth and amino acid requirements of various strains of group B streptococci, *J Clin Microbiol* 7:28-33, 1978.
63. Baker CJ, Kasper DL: Microcapsule of type III strains of group B *Streptococcus*: production and morphology, *Infect Immun* 13:189-194, 1976.

64. Malin G, Paoletti LC: Use of a dynamic in vitro attachment and invasion system (DIVAS) to determine influence of growth rate on invasion of respiratory epithelium by group B *Streptococcus*, *Proc Natl Acad Sci U S A* 98:13335-13340, 2001.
65. Johri AK, Padilla J, Malin G, et al: Oxygen regulates invasiveness and virulence of group B *Streptococcus*, *Infect Immun* 71:6707-6711, 2003.
66. Whidbey C, Harrell MI, Burnside K, et al: A hemolytic pigment of group B *Streptococcus* allows bacterial penetration of human placenta, *J Exp Med* 210:1265-1281, 2013.
67. Ferrieri P, Wannamaker LW, Nelson J: Localization and characterization of the hippuricase activity of group B streptococci, *Infect Immun* 7:747-752, 1973.
68. Bohnsack JF, Mollison KW, Buko AM, et al: Group B streptococci inactivate complement component C5a by enzymic cleavage at the C-terminus, *Biochem J* 273:635-640, 1991.
69. Bohnsack JF, Zhou XN, Williams PA, et al: Purification of a protease from group B streptococci that inactivates human C5a, *Biochim Biophys Acta* 1079:222-228, 1991.
70. Cleary PP, Handley J, Suvorov AN, et al: Similarity between the group B and A streptococcal C5a peptidase genes, *Infect Immun* 60:4239-4244, 1992.
71. Hill HR, Bohnsack JF, Morris EZ, et al: Group B streptococci inhibit the chemotactic activity of the fifth component of complement, *J Immunol* 141:3551-3556, 1988.
72. Ferrieri P, Gray ED, Wannamaker LW: Biochemical and immunological characterization of the extracellular nucleases of group B streptococci, *J Exp Med* 151:56-68, 1980.
73. Pritchard DG, Lin B, Willingham TR, et al: Characterization of the group B streptococcal hyaluronate lyase, *Arch Biochem Biophys* 315:431-437, 1994.
74. Musser JM, Mattingly SJ, Quentin R, et al: Identification of a high-virulence clone of type III *Streptococcus agalactiae* (group B *Streptococcus*) causing invasive neonatal disease, *Proc Natl Acad Sci U S A* 86:4731-4735, 1989.
75. Nealon TJ, Mattingly SJ: Association of elevated levels of cellular lipoteichoic acids of group B streptococci with human neonatal disease, *Infect Immun* 39:1243-1251, 1983.
76. Goldschmidt JC Jr, Panos C: Teichoic acids of *Streptococcus agalactiae*: chemistry, cytotoxicity, and effect on bacterial adherence to human cells in tissue culture, *Infect Immun* 43:670-677, 1984.
77. Meyn L, Moore DM, Hillier SL, et al: Association of sexual activity with colonization and vaginal acquisition of group B *Streptococcus* in nonpregnant women, *Am J Epidemiol* 155:949-957, 2002.
78. Foxman B, Gillespie B, Manning SD, et al: Incidence and duration of group B *Streptococcus* by serotype among male and female college students living in a single dormitory, *Am J Epidemiol* 163:544-551, 2006.
79. Boyer KM, Gadzala CA, Kelly PD, et al: Selective intrapartum chemoprophylaxis of neonatal group B streptococcal early-onset disease. II. Predictive value of prenatal cultures, *J Infect Dis* 148:802-809, 1983.
80. Yancey MK, Schuchat A, Brown LK, et al: The accuracy of late antenatal screening cultures in predicting genital group B streptococcal colonization at delivery, *Obstet Gynecol* 88:811-815, 1996.
81. Persson K, Bjerre B, Elfström L, et al: Longitudinal study of group B streptococcal carriage during late pregnancy, *Scand J Infect Dis* 19:325-329, 1987.
82. Manning SD, Neighbors K, Tallman PA, et al: Prevalence of group B *Streptococcus* colonization and potential for transmission by casual contact in healthy young men and women, *Clin Infect Dis* 39: 380-388, 2004.
83. Baker CJ, Goroff DK, Alpert S, et al: Vaginal colonization with group B *Streptococcus*: a study in college women, *J Infect Dis* 135:392-397, 1977.
84. Bliss SJ, Manning SD, Tallman P, et al: Group B *Streptococcus* colonization in male and non-pregnant female university students: a cross-sectional prevalence study, *Clin Infect Dis* 34:184-190, 2002.
85. Foxman B, Gillespie BW, Manning SD, et al: Risk factors for group B streptococcal colonization: potential for different transmission systems by capsular type, *Ann Epidemiol* 17:854-862, 2007.
86. Ramos E, Gaudier FL, Hearing LR, et al: Group B *Streptococcus* colonization in pregnant diabetic women, *Obstet Gynecol* 89:257-260, 1997.
87. Christensen KK, Dykes AK, Christensen P: Relation between use of tampons and urogenital carriage of group B streptococci, *BMJ* 289:731-732, 1984.
88. Campbell JR, Hillier SL, Krohn MA, et al: Group B streptococcal colonization and serotype-specific immunity in pregnant women at delivery, *Obstet Gynecol* 96:498-503, 2000.
89. Hickman ME, Rench MA, Ferrieri P, et al: Changing epidemiology of group B streptococcal (GBS) colonization, *Pediatrics* 104:203-209, 1999.
90. Newton ER, Butler MC, Shain RN: Sexual behavior and vaginal colonization by group B *Streptococcus* among minority women, *Obstet Gynecol* 88:577-582, 1996.
91. Davies HD, Adair C, McGeer A, et al: Antibodies to capsular polysaccharides of group B *Streptococcus* in pregnant Canadian women: relationship to colonization status and infection in the neonate, *J Infect Dis* 184:285-291, 2001.
92. Stoll BJ, Schuchat A: Maternal carriage of group B streptococci in developing countries, *Pediatr Infect Dis J* 17:499-503, 1998.
93. Barcaite E, Bartusevicius A, Tameliene R, et al: Prevalence of maternal group B streptococcal colonisation in European countries, *Acta Obstet Gynecol Scand* 87:260-271, 2008.
94. Turrentine MA, Ramirez MM: Recurrence of group B streptococci colonization in subsequent pregnancy, *Obstet Gynecol* 112:259-264, 2008.
95. Ferrieri P, Blair LL: Pharyngeal carriage of group B streptococci: detection by three methods, *J Clin Microbiol* 6:136-139, 1977.
96. Chretien JH, McGinniss CG, Thompson J, et al: Group B beta-hemolytic streptococci causing pharyngitis, *J Clin Microbiol* 10:263-266, 1979.
97. Sackel SG, et al: *Isolation of group B Streptococcus from 18th Interscience Conference on Antimicrobial Agents and Chemotherapy*, Atlanta, 1978, [abstract 467]. October 1-4, 1978.
98. Hayden GF, Murphy TF, Hendley JO: Non-group A streptococci in the pharynx. Pathogens or innocent bystanders? *Am J Dis Child* 143:794-797, 1989.
99. Hammerschlag MR, Baker CJ, Alpert S, et al: Colonization with group B streptococci in girls under 16 years of age, *Pediatrics* 60:473-477, 1977.
100. Mauer M, Thirumoorthi MC, Dajani AS: Group B streptococcal colonization in prepubertal children, *Pediatrics* 64:65-67, 1979.
101. Persson KS, Bjerre B, Elfström L, et al: Faecal carriage of group B streptococci, *Eur J Clin Microbiol* 5:156-159, 1986.
102. Cummings CG, Ross PW: Group B streptococci (GBS) in the upper respiratory tract of schoolchildren, *Health Bull* 40:81-86, 1982.
103. Shafer MA, Sweet RL, Ohm-Smith MJ, et al: Microbiology of the lower genital tract in postmenarchal adolescent girls: differences by sexual activity, contraception, and presence of nonspecific vaginitis, *J Pediatr* 107:974-981, 1985.
104. Ancona RJ, Ferrieri P, Williams PP: Maternal factors that enhance the acquisition of group B streptococci by newborn infants, *J Med Microbiol* 13:273-280, 1980.
105. Ferrieri P, Cleary PP, Seeds AE: Epidemiology of group B streptococcal carriage in pregnant women and newborn infants, *J Med Microbiol* 10:103-114, 1976.
106. Anthony BF, Okada DM, Hobel CJ: Epidemiology of the group B *Streptococcus*: maternal and nosocomial sources for infant acquisitions, *J Pediatr* 95:431-436, 1979.
107. Paredes A, Wong P, Mason EO Jr, et al: Nosocomial transmission of group B streptococci in a newborn nursery, *Pediatrics* 59:679-682, 1976.
108. Easmon CSF, Hastings MJ, Clare AJ, et al: Nosocomial transmission of group B streptococci, *BMJ* 283:459-461, 1981.
109. Noya FJD, Rench MA, Metzger TG, et al: Unusual occurrence of an epidemic of type Ib/c group B streptococcal sepsis in a neonatal intensive care unit, *J Infect Dis* 155:1135-1144, 1987.
110. Gardner SE, Mason EO Jr, Yow MD: Community acquisition of group B *Streptococcus* by infants of colonized mothers, *Pediatrics* 66: 873-875, 1980.
111. Hansen SM, Uldbjerg N, Kilian M, et al: Dynamics of *Streptococcus agalactiae* colonization in women during and after pregnancy and in their infants, *J Clin Microbiol* 42:83-89, 2004.
112. Baker CJ, Barrett FF: Group B streptococcal infection in infants: the importance of the various serotypes, *JAMA* 230:1158-1160, 1974.
113. Blumberg HM, Stephens DS, Modansky M, et al: Invasive group B streptococcal disease: the emergence of serotype V, *J Infect Dis* 173:365-373, 1996.

114. Zaleznik DF, Rench MA, Hillier S, et al: Invasive disease due to group B *Streptococcus* in pregnant women and neonates from diverse population groups, *Clin Infect Dis* 30:276-281, 2000.
115. Davies HD, Raj S, Adair C, et al: Population-based active surveillance for neonatal group B streptococcal infections in Alberta, Canada: implications for vaccine formulation, *Pediatr Infect Dis J* 20:879-884, 2001.
116. Elliott JA, Farmer KD, Facklam RR: Sudden increase in isolation of group B streptococci, serotype V, is not due to emergence of a new pulsed-field gel electrophoresis type, *J Clin Microbiol* 36:2115-2116, 1998.
117. Fluegge K, Supper S, Siedler A, et al: Serotype distribution of invasive group B streptococcal isolates in infants: results from a nationwide active laboratory surveillance study over 2 years in Germany, *Clin Infect Dis* 40:760-763, 2005.
118. Madzivhandila M, Adrian PV, Cutland CL, et al: Serotype distribution and invasive potential of group B *Streptococcus* isolates causing disease in infants and colonizing maternal-newborn dyads, *PLoS One* 6:e17861, 2011.
119. Lamagni TL, Keshishian C, Efstratiou A, et al: Emerging trends in the epidemiology of invasive group B streptococcal disease in England and Wales, 1991-2010, *Clin Infect Dis* 57:682-688, 2013.
120. Ferrieri P, Lynfield R, Creti R, et al: Serotype IV and invasive group B *Streptococcus* disease in neonates, Minnesota, USA, 2000-2010, *Emerg Infect Dis* 19:551-558, 2013.
121. Matsubara K, Katayama K, Baba K, et al: Seroepidemiologic studies of serotype VIII group B *Streptococcus* in Japan, *J Infect Dis* 186: 855-858, 2002.
122. Matsubara K, Mikamo H, Numa M, et al: Three fatal cases of invasive serotype VI group B streptococcal infection, *J Infect* 53:e139-e142, 2006.
123. Phares CR, Lynfield R, Farley MM, et al: Epidemiology of invasive group B streptococcal disease in the United States, 1999–2005, *JAMA* 299:2056-2065, 2008.
124. Quentin R, Huet H, Wang FS, et al: Characterization of *Streptococcus agalactiae* strains by multilocus enzyme genotype and serotype: identification of multiple virulent clone families that cause invasive neonatal disease, *J Clin Microbiol* 33:2576-2581, 1995.
125. Gordillo ME, Singh KV, Baker CJ, et al: Comparison of group B streptococci by pulsed field gel electrophoresis and by conventional electrophoresis, *J Clin Microbiol* 31:1430-1434, 1993.
126. Limansky AS, Sutich EG, Guardati MC, et al: Genomic diversity among *Streptococcus agalactiae* isolates detected by a degenerate oligonucleotide-primed amplification assay, *J Infect Dis* 177: 1308-1313, 1998.
127. Imperi M, Pataracchia M, Alfarone G, et al: A multiplex PCR assay for the direct identification of the capsular type (Ia to IX) of *Streptococcus agalactiae*, *J Microbiol Meth* 80:212-214, 2010.
128. Al Nakib M, Longo M, Tazi A, et al: Comparison of the Diversilab system with multi-locus sequence typing and pulsed-gel electrophoresis for the characterization of *Streptococcus agalactiae* invasive strains, *J Microbiol Meth* 85:137-142, 2011.
129. Luan SL, Granlund M, Sellin M, et al: Multilocus sequence typing of Swedish invasive group B streptococcus isolates indicates a neonatally associated genetic lineage and capsule switching, *J Clin Microbiol* 43:3727-3733, 2005.
130. Adderson EE, Takahashi S, Bohnsack JF: Bacterial genetics and human immunity to group B streptococci, *Mol Genet Metab* 71: 451-454, 2000.
131. Bohnsack JF, Whiting AA, Bradford RD, et al: Long-range mapping of the *Streptococcus agalactiae* phylogenetic lineage restriction digest pattern type III-3 reveals clustering of virulence genes, *Infect Immun* 70:134-139, 2002.
132. Takahashi S, Detrick S, Whiting AA, et al: Correlation of phylogenetic lineages of group B streptococci, identified by analysis of restriction-digestion patterns of genomic DNA, with *infB* alleles and mobile genetic elements, *J Infect Dis* 186:1034-1038, 2002.
133. Adderson EE, Takahashi S, Wang Y, et al: Subtractive hybridization identifies a novel predicted protein mediating epithelial cell invasion by virulent serotype III group B *Streptococcus agalactiae*, *Infect Immun* 71:6857-6863, 2003.
134. Davies HD, Jones N, Whittam TS, et al: Multilocus sequence typing of serotype III group B *Streptococcus* and correlation with pathogenic potential, *J Infect Dis* 189:1097-1102, 2004.
135. Bidet P, Brahimi N, Chalas C, et al: Molecular characterization of serotype III group B *Streptococcus* isolates causing neonatal meningitis, *J Infect Dis* 188:1132-1137, 2003.
136. von Both U, John A, Fluegge K, et al: Molecular epidemiology of invasive neonatal *Streptococcus agalactiae* isolates in Germany, *Pediatr Infect Dis J* 27:903-906, 2008.
137. Dore N, Bennett D, Kaliszer M, et al: Molecular epidemiology of group B streptococci in Ireland: associations between serotype, invasive status and presence of genes encoding putative virulence factors, *Epidemiol Infect* 131:823-833, 2003.
138. Sørensen UBS, Poulsen K, Ghezzo C, et al: Emergence and global dissemination of host-specific *Streptococcus agalactiae* clones, *mBio* 1: 1-9, 2010.
139. Jones N, Bohnsack JF, Takahashi S, et al: Multilocus sequence typing system for group B Streptococcus, *J Clin Microbiol* 41:2530-2536, 2003.
140. Bellais S, Six A, Fouet A, et al: Capsular switching in group B *Streptococcus* CC17 hypervirulent clone: a future challenge for polysaccharide vaccine development, *J Infect Dis* 206:1745-1752, 2012.
141. Perinatal group B streptococcal disease after universal screening recommendations—United States, 2003–2005, *MMWR Morb Mortal Wkly Rep* 56:701-705, 2007.
142. Schrag SJ, Zell ER, Lynfield R, et al: A population-based comparison of strategies to prevent early-onset group B streptococcal disease in neonates, *N Engl J Med* 34:7233-7239, 2002.
143. Centers for Disease Control and Prevention: Active bacterial core surveillance report, emerging infections program network, group B streptococcus, 2012. Available at http://www.cdc.gov/abcs/reports-findings/survreports/gbs12.pdf. Accessed Feb. 24, 2014.
144. Weston EJ, Pondo T, Lewis MM, et al: The burden of invasive early-onset neonatal sepsis in the United States, 2005-2008, *Pediatr Infect Dis J* 30:937-941, 2011.
145. Dagnew AF, Cunnington MC, Dube Q, et al: Variation in reported neonatal group B streptococcal disease incidence in developing countries, *Clin Infect Dis* 55:91-102, 2012.
146. Edmond KM, Kortsalioudaki C, Scott S, et al: Group B streptococcal disease in infants aged younger than 3 months: systemic review and meta-analysis, *Lancet* 379:547-556, 2012.
147. Boyer KM, Gotoff SP: Strategies for chemoprophylaxis of GBS early-onset infections, *Antibiot Chemother* 35:267-280, 1985.
148. Sobel JD, Myers P, Levison ME, et al: Comparison of bacterial and fungal adherence to vaginal exfoliated epithelial cells and human vaginal epithelial tissue culture cells, *Infect Immun* 35:697-701, 1982.
149. Jelínková J, Grabovskaya KB, Ryc M, et al: Adherence of vaginal and pharyngeal strains of group B streptococci to human vaginal and pharyngeal epithelial cells, *Zentralbl Bakteriol Mikrobiol Hyg [A]* 262:492-499, 1986.
150. Hoet YR, Li CM, Yu CH, et al: The enhancement of biofilm formation in group B streptococcal isolates at vaginal pH, *Med Microbiol Immunol* 202:105-115, 2013.
151. Nealon TJ, Mattingly SJ: Role of cellular lipoteichoic acids in mediating adherence of serotype III strains of group B streptococci to human embryonic, fetal, and adult epithelial cells, *Infect Immun* 43:523-530, 1984.
152. Teti G, Tomasello F, Chiofalo MS, et al: Adherence of group B streptococci to adult and neonatal epithelial cells mediated by lipoteichoic acid, *Infect Immun* 55:3057-3064, 1987.
153. Cox F: Prevention of group B streptococcal colonization with topically applied lipoteichoic acid in a maternal-newborn mouse model, *Pediatr Res* 16:816-819, 1982.
154. Tamura GS, Rubens CE: Group B streptococci adhere to a variant of fibronectin attached to a solid phase, *Mol Microbiol* 15:581-589, 1995.
155. Beckmann C, Waggoner JD, Harris TO, et al: Identification of novel adhesins from group B streptococci by use of phage display reveals that C5a peptidase mediates fibronectin binding, *Infect Immun* 70:2869-2876, 2002.
156. Cheng Q, Stafslien D, Purushothaman SS, et al: The group B streptococcal C5a peptidase is both a specific protease and an invasin, *Infect Immun* 70:2408-2413, 2002.
157. Spellerberg B, Rozdzinski E, Martin S, et al: Lmb, a protein with similarities to the LraI adhesin family, mediates attachment of *Streptococcus agalactiae* to human laminin, *Infect Immun* 67:871-878, 1999.
158. Schubert A, Zakikhany K, Schreiner M, et al: A fibrinogen receptor from group B *Streptococcus* interacts with fibrinogen by repetitive units with novel ligand binding sites, *Mol Microbiol* 46:557-569, 2002.

159. Samen U, Eikmanns BJ, Reinscheid DJ, et al: The surface protein Srr-1 of *Streptococcus agalactiae* binds human keratin 4 and promotes adherence to epithelial HEp-2 cells, *Infect Immun* 75:5405-5414, 2007.
160. Rosini R, Rinaudo CD, Soriani M, et al: Identification of novel genomic islands coding for antigenic pilus-like structures in *Streptococcus agalactiae*, *Mol Microbiol* 61:126-141, 2006.
161. Dramsi S, Caliot E, Bonne I, et al: Assembly and role of pili in group B streptococci, *Mol Microbiol* 60:1401-1413, 2006.
162. Krishnan V, Gaspar AH, Ye N, et al: An IgG-like domain in the minor pilin GBS52 of *Streptococcus agalactiae* mediates lung epithelial cell adhesion, *Structure* 15:893-903, 2007.
163. Sheen Jimenez A, Wang NY, et al: Serine-rich repeat proteins and pili promote *Streptococcus agalactiae* colonization of the vaginal tract, *J Bacteriol* 193:6834-6842, 2011.
164. Park Jiang S, Wessels MR: CsrRS and environmental pH regulate group B streptococcus adherence to human epithelial cells and extracellular matrix, *Infect Immun* 80:3975-3984, 2012.
165. Patras Wang NY, Fletcher EM, et al: Group B *Streptococcus* CovR regulation modulates host immune signalling pathways to promote vaginal colonization, *Cell Microbiol* 15:1154-1167, 2013.
166. Stewardson-Krieger PB, Gotoff SP: Risk factors in early-onset neonatal group B streptococcal infections, *Infection* 6:50-53, 1978.
167. Tseng PI, Kandall SR: Group B streptococcal disease in neonates and infants, *N Y State J Med* 74:2169-2173, 1974.
168. Evaldson GR, Malmborg AS, Nord CE: Premature rupture of the membranes and ascending infection, *Br J Obstet Gynaecol* 89:793-801, 1982.
169. Schoonmaker JN, Lawellin DW, Lunt B, et al: Bacteria and inflammatory cells reduce chorioamniotic membrane integrity and tensile strength, *Obstet Gynecol* 74:590-596, 1989.
170. Bennett PR, Rose MP, Myatt L, Elder MG: Preterm labor: stimulation of arachidonic acid metabolism in human amnion cells by bacterial products, *Am J Obstet Gynecol* 156:649-655, 1987.
171. Dudley DJ, Edwin SS, Van Wagoner J, et al: Regulation of decidual cell chemokine production by group B streptococci and purified bacterial cell wall components, *Am J Obstet Gynecol* 177:666-672, 1997.
172. Estrada-Gutierrez G, Gomez-Lopez N, Zaga-Clavellina V, et al: Interaction between pathogenic bacteria and intrauterine leukocytes triggers alternative molecular signaling cascades leading to labor in women, *Infect Immun* 78:4792-4799, 2010.
173. Spellerberg B, Martin S, Franken C, et al: Identification of genetic determinants for the hemolytic activity of *Streptococcus agalactiae* by ISS1 transposition, *J Bacteriol* 181:3212-3219, 1999.
174. Pritzlaff CA, Chang JC, Kuo SP, et al: Genetic basis for the beta-haemolytic/cytolytic activity of group B *Streptococcus*, *Mol Microbiol* 39:236-247, 2001.
175. G. Whidbey, Harrell MI, Burnside K, et al: A hemolytic pigment of group B *Streptococcus* allows bacterial penetration of human placenta, *J Exp Med* 210:1265-1281, 2013.
176. Liu GY, Doran KS, Lawrence T, et al: Sword and shield: linked group B streptococcal beta-hemolysin/cytolysin and carotenoid pigment act synergistically to subvert host phagocyte defenses, *Proc Natl Acad Sci USA* 10:14491-14496, 2004.
177. Randis TM, Gelber SE, Hooven TA, et al: Group B *Streptococcus* β-hemolysin/cytolysin breaches maternal fetal barriers to cause preterm birth and intrauterine demise in vivo, *J Infect Dis* 210:265-273, 2014.
178. Ferrieri P, Cleary PP, Seeds AE: Epidemiology of group B streptococcal carriage in pregnant women and newborn infants, *J Med Microbiol* 10:103-114, 1977.
179. Galask RP, Varner MW, Petzold CR, et al: Bacterial attachment to the chorioamniotic membranes, *Am J Obstet Gynecol* 148:915-928, 1984.
180. Winram SB, Jonas M, Chi E, et al: Characterization of group B streptococcal invasion of human chorion and amnion epithelial cells in vitro, *Infect Immun* 66:4932-4941, 1998.
181. Boldenow E, Jones S, Lieberman RW, et al: Antimicrobial peptide response to group B *Streptococcus* in human extraplacental membranes in culture, *Pediatrics* 34:480-485, 2013.
182. Hemming VG, Nagarajan K, Hess LW, et al: Rapid in vitro replication of group B *Streptococcus* in term human amniotic fluid, *Gynecol Obstet Invest* 19:124-129, 1985.
183. Baker CJ: Early onset group B streptococcal disease, *J Pediatr* 93: 124-125, 1978.
184. Pass MA, Gray BM, Khare S, et al: Prospective studies of group B streptococcal infections in infants, *J Pediatr* 95:437-443, 1979.
185. Adams-Waldorf KM, Gravett MG, McAdams RM, et al: Choriodecidual group B streptococcal inoculation induces fetal lung injury without intra-amniotic infection and preterm labor in *Macaca nemestrina*, *PLoS One* 6:e28972, 2011.
186. McAdams RM, Vanderhoeven J, Beyer RP, et al: Choriodecidual infection downregulates angiogenesis and morphogenesis pathways in fetal lungs from *Macaca nemestrina*, *PLoS One* 7:e46863, 2012.
187. Payne NR, Burke BA, Day DL, et al: Correlation of clinical and pathologic findings in early onset neonatal group B streptococcal infection with disease severity and prediction of outcome, *Pediatr Infect Dis J* 7:836-847, 1988.
188. Hemming VG, McCloskey DW, Hill HR: Pneumonia in the neonate associated with group B streptococcal septicemia, *Am J Dis Child* 130:1231-1233, 1976.
189. Katzenstein A, Davis C, Braude A: Pulmonary changes in neonatal sepsis due to group B beta-hemolytic streptococcus: relation to hyaline membrane disease, *J Infect Dis* 133:430-435, 1976.
190. Rubens CE, Raff HV, Jackson JC, et al: Pathophysiology and histopathology of group B streptococcal sepsis in *Macaca nemestrina* primates induced after intraamniotic inoculation: evidence for bacterial cellular invasion, *J Infect Dis* 164:320-330, 1991.
191. Sherman MP, Johnson JT, Rothlein R, et al: Role of pulmonary phagocytes in host defense against group B streptococci in preterm versus term rabbit lung, *J Infect Dis* 166:818-826, 1992.
192. Rubens CE, Smith S, Hulse M, et al: Respiratory epithelial cell invasion by group B streptococci, *Infect Immun* 60:5157-5163, 1992.
193. Gibson RL, Lee MK, Soderland C, et al: Group B streptococci invade endothelial cells: type III capsular polysaccharide attenuates invasion, *Infect Immun* 61:478-485, 1993.
194. Burnham CA, Shokoples SE, Tyrrell GJ: Rac1, RhoA, and Cdc42 participate in HeLa cell invasion by group B streptococcus, *FEMS Microbiol Lett* 272:8-14, 2007.
195. Shin S, Paul-Satyaseela M, Lee JS, et al: Focal adhesion kinase is involved in type III group B streptococcal invasion of human brain microvascular endothelial cells, *Microb Pathog* 4:168-173, 2006.
196. Valentin-Weigand P, Chhatwal GS: Correlation of epithelial cell invasiveness of group B streptococci with clinical source of isolation, *Microb Pathog* 19:83-91, 1995.
197. Schubert A, Zakikhany K, Pietrocola G, et al: The fibrinogen receptor FbsA promotes adherence of *Streptococcus agalactiae* to human epithelial cells, *Infect Immun* 72:6197-6205, 2004.
198. Tenenbaum T, Spellerberg B, Adam R, et al: *Streptococcus agalactiae* invasion of human brain microvascular endothelial cells is promoted by the laminin-binding protein, *Lmb Microbes Infect* 9:714-720, 2007.
199. Baron MJ, Bolduc GR, Goldberg MB, et al: Alpha C protein of group B *Streptococcus* binds host cell surface glycosaminoglycan and enters cells by an actin-dependent mechanism, *J Biol Chem* 279: 24714-24723, 2004.
200. Hulse ML, Smith S, Chi EY, et al: Effect of type III group B streptococcal capsular polysaccharide on invasion of respiratory epithelial cells, *Infect Immun* 61:4835-4841, 1993.
201. Sharma P, Lata H, Arya DK, et al: Role of pilus proteins in adherence and invasion of *Streptococcus agalactiae* to the lung and cervical epithelial cells, *J Biol Chem* 288:4023-4034, 2013.
202. Quirante J, Ceballos R, Cassady G: Group B beta-hemolytic streptococcal infection in the newborn. I. Early onset infection, *Am J Dis Child* 128:659-665, 1974.
203. Kling DE, Tsvang I, Murphy MP, et al: Group B *Streptococcus* induces a caspase-dependent apoptosis in fetal rat lung interstitium, *Microb Pathogen* 61-62:1-10, 2013.
204. Nizet V, Gibson RL, Chi EY, et al: Group B streptococcal beta-hemolysin expression is associated with injury of lung epithelial cells, *Infect Immun* 64:3818-3826, 1996.
205. Gibson RL, Nizet V, Rubens CE: Group B streptococcal beta-hemolysin promotes injury of lung microvascular endothelial cells, *Pediatr Res* 45:626-634, 1999.
206. Doran KS, Chang JC, Benoit VM, et al: Group B streptococcal beta-hemolysin/cytolysin promotes invasion of human lung epithelial cells and the release of interleukin-8, *J Infect Dis* 185:196-203, 2002.
207. Hensler ME, Liu GY, Sobczak S, et al: Virulence role of group B *Streptococcus* beta-hemolysin/cytolysin in a neonatal rabbit model of early-onset pulmonary infection, *J Infect Dis* 191:1287-1291, 2005.

208. Herting E, Jarstrand C, Rasool O, et al: Experimental neonatal group B streptococcal pneumonia: effect of a modified porcine surfactant on bacterial proliferation in ventilated near-term rabbits, *Pediatr Res* 36:784-791, 1994.
209. Herting E, Sun B, Jarstrand C, et al: Surfactant improves lung function and mitigates bacterial growth in immature ventilated rabbits with experimentally induced neonatal group B streptococcal pneumonia, *Arch Dis Child Fetal Neonatal Ed* 76:F3-F8, 1997.
210. Auten RL, Notter RH, Kendig JW, et al: Surfactant treatment of full-term newborns with respiratory failure, *Pediatrics* 87:101-107, 1991.
211. Herting E, Gefeller O, Land M, et al: Surfactant treatment of neonates with respiratory failure and group B streptococcal infection, *Pediatrics* 106:957-964, 2000.
212. Shigeoka AO, Hall RT, Hemming VG, et al: Role of antibody and complement in opsonization of group B streptococci, *Infect Immun* 21:34-40, 1978.
213. Anderson DC, Hughes BJ, Edwards MS, et al: Impaired chemotaxigenesis by type III group B streptococci in neonatal sera: relationship to diminished concentration of specific anticapsular antibody and abnormalities of serum complement, *Pediatr Res* 17:496-502, 1983.
214. Edwards MS, Nicholson-Weller A, Baker CJ, et al: The role of specific antibody in alternative complement pathway-mediated opsonophagocytosis of type III, group B *Streptococcus*, *J Exp Med* 151: 1275-1287, 1980.
215. Chaffin DO, Beres SB, Yim HH, et al: The serotype of type Ia and III group B streptococci is determined by the polymerase gene within the polycistronic capsule operon, *J Bacteriol* 182:4466-4477, 2000.
216. Angata T, Varki A: Chemical diversity in the sialic acids and related alpha-keto acids: an evolutionary perspective, *Chem Rev* 102: 439-469, 2002.
217. Doran KS, Liu GY, Nizet V: Group B streptococcal beta-hemolysin/cytolysin activates neutrophil signaling pathways in brain endothelium and contributes to development of meningitis, *J Clin Invest* 112:736-744, 2003.
218. Carlin AF, Uchiyama S, Chang YC, et al: Molecular mimicry of host sialylated glycans allows a bacterial pathogen to engage neutrophil Siglec-9 and dampen the innate immune response, *Blood* 113: 3333-3336, 2009.
219. Kasper DL, Baker CJ, Baltimore RS, et al: Immunodeterminant specificity of human immunity to type III group B streptococcus, *J Exp Med* 149:327-339, 1979.
220. Edwards MS, Kasper DL, Jennings HJ, et al: Capsular sialic acid prevents activation of the alternative complement pathway by type III, group B streptococci, *J Immunol* 128:1278-1283, 1982.
221. Shigeoka AO, Rote NS, Santos JI, et al: Assessment of the virulence factors of group B streptococci: correlation with sialic acid content, *J Infect Dis* 147:857-863, 1983.
222. Rubens CE, Wessels MR, Heggen LM, et al: Transposon mutagenesis of type III group B *Streptococcus*: correlation of capsule expression with virulence, *Proc Natl Acad Sci U S A* 84:7208-7212, 1987.
223. Yim HH, Nittayarin A, Rubens CE: Analysis of the capsule synthesis locus, a virulence factor in group B streptococci, *Adv Exp Med Biol* 418:995-997, 1997.
224. Marques MB, Kasper DL, Pangburn MK, et al: Prevention of C3 deposition by capsular polysaccharide is a virulence mechanism of type III group B streptococci, *Infect Immun* 60:3986-3993, 1992.
225. Lemire P, Houde M, Lecours MP, et al: Role of capsular polysaccharide in group B *Streptococccus* interactions with dendritic cells, *Microb Infect* 14:1064-1076, 2012.
226. Martin TR, Ruzinski JT, Rubens CE, et al: The effect of type-specific polysaccharide capsule on the clearance of group B streptococci from the lungs of infant and adult rats, *J Infect Dis* 165:306-314, 1992.
227. Wessels MR, Rubens CE, Benedí VJ, et al: Definition of a bacterial virulence factor: sialylation of the group B streptococcal capsule, *Proc Natl Acad Sci USA* 86:8983-8987, 1989.
228. Orefici G, Recchia S, Galante L: Possible virulence marker for Streptococcus agalactiae (Lancefield group B), *Eur J Clin Microbiol Infect Dis* 7:302-305, 1988.
229. Payne NR, Ferrieri P: The relation of the Ibc protein antigen to the opsonization differences between strains of type II group B streptococci, *J Infect Dis* 151:672-681, 1985.
230. Baker CJ, Webb BJ, Kasper DL, et al: The role of complement and antibody in opsonophagocytosis of type II group B streptococci, *J Infect Dis* 154:47-54, 1986.
231. Russell-Jones GJ, Gotschlich EC, Blake MS: A surface receptor specific for human IgA on group B streptococci possessing the Ibc protein antigen, *J Exp Med* 160:1467-1475, 1984.
232. Jerlström PG, Chhatwal GS, Timmis KN: The IgA-binding beta antigen of the C protein complex of group B streptococci: sequence determination of its gene and detection of two binding regions, *Mol Microbiol* 5:843-849, 1991.
233. Payne NR, Kim YK, Ferrieri P: Effect of differences in antibody and complement requirements on phagocytic uptake and intracellular killing of "C" protein-positive and -negative strains of type II group B streptococci, *Infect Immun* 55:1243-1251, 1987.
234. Harris TO, Shelver DW, Bohnsack JF, et al: A novel streptococcal surface protease promotes virulence, resistance to opsonophagocytosis, and cleavage of human fibrinogen, *J Clin Invest* 111:61-70, 2003.
235. Santi I, Scarselli M, Mariani M, et al: BibA: a novel immunogenic bacterial adhesin contributing to group B *Streptococcus* survival in human blood, *Mol Microbiol* 63:754-767, 2007.
236. Carlin AF, Chang YC, Areschoug T, et al: Group B *Streptococcus* suppression of phagocyte functions by protein-mediated engagement of human Siglec-5, *J Exp Med* 206:1691-1699, 2009.
237. Cornacchione P, Scaringi L, Fettucciari K, et al: Group B streptococci persist inside macrophages, *Immunology* 93:86-95, 1998.
238. Teixeira CF, Azevedo NL, Carvalho TM, et al: Cytochemical study of *Streptococcus agalactiae* and macrophage interaction, *Microsc Res Tech* 54:254-259, 2001.
239. Wilson CB, Weaver WM: Comparative susceptibility of group B streptococci and *Staphylococcus aureus* to killing by oxygen metabolites, *J Infect Dis* 152:323-329, 1985.
240. Poyart C, Pellegrini E, Gaillot O, et al: Contribution of Mn-cofactored superoxide dismutase (SodA) to the virulence of *Streptococcus agalactiae*, *Infect Immun* 69:5098-5106, 2001.
241. Cumley NJ, Smith LM, Anthony M, et al: The CovS/CovR acid response regulator is required for intracellular survival of group B *Streptococcus* in macrophages, *Infect Immun* 80:1650-1661, 2012.
242. Nizet V, Ohtake T, Lauth X, et al: Innate antimicrobial peptide protects the skin from invasive bacterial infection, *Nature* 414:454-457, 2001.
243. Jones AL, Needham RH, Clancy A, et al: Penicillin-binding proteins in *Streptococcus agalactiae*: a novel mechanism for evasion of immune clearance, *Mol Microbiol* 4:7247-7256, 2003.
244. Hamilton A, Popham DL, Carl DJ, et al: Penicillin-binding protein 1a promotes resistance of group B streptococcus to antimicrobial peptides, *Infect Immun* 74:6179-6187, 2006.
245. Poyart C, Pellegrini E, Marceau M, et al: Attenuated virulence of *Streptococcus agalactiae* deficient in D-alanyl-lipoteichoic acid is due to an increased susceptibility to defensins and phagocytic cells, *Mol Microbiol* 49:1615-1625, 2003.
246. Ulett GC, Maclean KH, Nekkalapu S, et al: Mechanisms of group B streptococcal-induced apoptosis of murine macrophages, *J Immunol* 175:2555-2562, 2005.
247. Fettucciari K, Fetriconi I, Mannucci R, et al: Group B *Streptococcus* induces macrophage apoptosis by calpain activation, *J Immunol* 176:7542-7556, 2006.
248. Wheeler JG, Chauvenet AR, Johnson CA, et al: Neutrophil storage pool depletion in septic, neutropenic neonates, *Pediatr Infect Dis* 3:407-409, 1984.
249. Christensen RD, MacFarlane JL, Taylor NL, et al: Blood and marrow neutrophils during experimental group B streptococcal infection: quantification of the stem cell, proliferative, storage and circulating pools, *Pediatr Res* 16:549-553, 1982.
250. Zeligs BJ, Armstrong CD, Walser JB, et al: Age-dependent susceptibility of neonatal rats to group B streptococcal type III infection: correlation of severity of infection and response of myeloid pools, *Infect Immun* 37:255-263, 1982.
251. Christensen RD, Hill HR, Rothstein G: Granulocytic stem cell (CFUc) proliferation in experimental group B streptococcal sepsis, *Pediatr Res* 17:278-280, 1983.
252. Madureira P, Andrade EB, Gama B, et al: Inhibition of IL-10 production by maternal antibodies against group B *Streptococcus* GAPDH confers immunity to offspring by favoring neutrophil recruitment, *PLoS Pathog* 7:e1002363, 2011.
253. Derre-Bobillot A, Cortes-Perez NG, Yamamoto Y, et al: Nuclease A (Gbs0661), an extracellular nuclease of *Streptococcus agalactiae*, attacks the neutrophil extracellular traps and is needed for full virulence, *Mol Microbiol* 89:518-531, 2013.

254. Bohnsack JF, Widjaja K, Ghazizadeh S, et al: A role for C5 and C5a-ase in the acute neutrophil response to group B streptococcal infections, *J Infect Dis* 175:847-855, 1997.
255. Gleich-Theurer U, Aymanns S, Haas G, et al: Human serum induces streptococcal c5a peptidase expression, *Infect Immun* 77: 3817-3825, 2009.
256. Rojas J, Larsson LE, Hellerqvist CG, et al: Pulmonary hemodynamic and ultrastructural changes associated with group B streptococcal toxemia in adult sheep and newborn lambs, *Pediatr Res* 17: 1002-1008, 1983.
257. Hemming VG, O'Brien WF, Fischer GW, et al: Studies of short-term pulmonary and peripheral vascular responses induced in oophorectomized sheep by the infusion of a group B streptococcal extract, *Pediatr Res* 18:266-269, 1984.
258. Gibson Truog WE, Henderson WRRL, Redding GJ: Group B streptococcal sepsis in piglets: effect of combined pentoxifylline and indomethacin pretreatment, *Pediatr Res* 31:222-227, 1992.
259. Peevy KJ, Chartrand SA, Wiseman HJ, et al: Myocardial dysfunction in group B streptococcal shock, *Pediatr Res* 19:511-513, 1985.
260. Peevy KJ, Panus P, Longenecker GL, et al: Prostaglandin synthetase inhibition in group B streptococcal shock: hematologic and hemodynamic effects, *Pediatr Res* 20:864-866, 1986.
261. O'Brien WF, Golden SM, Bibro MC, et al: Short-term responses in neonatal lambs after infusion of group B streptococcal extract, *Obstet Gynecol* 65:802-806, 1985.
262. Gibson RL, Redding GJ, Truog WE, et al: Isogenic group B streptococci devoid of capsular polysaccharide or beta-hemolysin: pulmonary hemodynamic and gas exchange effects during bacteremia in piglets, *Pediatr Res* 26:241-245, 1989.
263. Bowdy BD, Aziz SM, Marple SL, et al: Organ-specific disposition of group B streptococci in piglets: evidence for a direct interaction with target cells in the pulmonary circulation, *Pediatr Res* 27:344-348, 1990.
264. Gibson RL, Soderland C, Henderson WR Jr, et al: Group B streptococci (GBS) injure lung endothelium in vitro: GBS invasion and GBS-induced eicosanoid production is greater with microvascular than with pulmonary artery cells, *Infect Immun* 63:271-279, 1995.
265. Schreiber MD, Covert RF, Torgerson LJ: Hemodynamic effects of heat-killed group B beta-hemolytic streptococcus in newborn lambs: role of leukotriene D4, *Pediatr Res* 31:121-126, 1992.
266. Pinheiro JM, Pitt BR, Gillis CN: Roles of platelet-activating factor and thromboxane in group B *Streptococcus*-induced pulmonary hypertension in piglets, *Pediatr Res* 26:420-424, 1989.
267. Mancuso G, Cusumano V, Genovese F, et al: Role of interleukin 12 in experimental neonatal sepsis caused by group B streptococci, *Infect Immun* 65:3731-3735, 1997.
268. Costa A, Gupta R, Signorino G, et al: Activation of the NLRP3 inflammasome by group B streptococci, *J Immunol* 188, 1953-1960.
269. Vallette JD, Goldberg RN, Suguihara C, et al: Effect of an interleukin-1 receptor antagonist on the hemodynamic manifestations of group B streptococcal sepsis, *Pediatr Res* 38:704-708, 1995.
270. Williams PA, Bohnsack JF, Augustine NH, et al: Production of tumor necrosis factor by human cells in vitro and in vivo, induced by group B streptococci, *J Pediatr* 123:292-300, 1993.
271. Gibson RL, Redding GJ, Henderson WR, et al: Group B streptococcus induces tumor necrosis factor in neonatal piglets: effect of the tumor necrosis factor inhibitor pentoxifylline on hemodynamics and gas exchange, *Am Rev Respir Dis* 143:598-604, 1991.
272. Teti G, Mancuso G, Tomasello F, et al: Production of tumor necrosis factor-alpha and interleukin-6 in mice infected with group B streptococci, *Circ Shock* 38:138-144, 1992.
273. Teti G, Mancuso G, Tomasello F: Cytokine appearance and effects of anti-tumor necrosis factor alpha antibodies in a neonatal rat model of group B streptococcal infection, *Infect Immun* 61:227-235, 1993.
274. Kenzel S, Mancuso G, Malley R, et al: c-Jun kinase is a critical signaling molecule in a neonatal model of group B streptococcal sepsis, *J Immunol* 176:3181-3188, 2006.
275. Henneke P, Takeuchi O, Malley R, et al: Cellular activation, phagocytosis, and bactericidal activity against group B streptococcus involve parallel myeloid differentiation factor 88-dependent and independent signaling pathways, *J Immunol* 169:3970-3977, 2002.
276. Raykova VD, Glibetic M, Ofenstein JP, et al: Nitric oxide-dependent regulation of pro-inflammatory cytokines in group B streptococcal inflammation of rat lung, *Ann Clin Lab Sci* 33:62-67, 2003.
277. Maloney CG, Thompson SD, Hill HR, et al: Induction of cyclooxygenase-2 by human monocytes exposed to group B streptococci, *J Leukoc Biol* 67:615-621, 2000.
278. Natarajan G, Glibetic M, Raykova V, et al: Nitric oxide and prostaglandin response to group B streptococcal infection in the lung, *Ann Clin Lab Sci* 37:170-176, 2007.
279. Ring A, Braun JS, Nizet V, et al: Group B streptococcal beta-hemolysin induces nitric oxide production in murine macrophages, *J Infect Dis* 182:150-157, 2000.
280. Puliti M, Nizet V, von Hunolstein C, et al: Severity of group B streptococcal arthritis is correlated with beta-hemolysin expression, *J Infect Dis* 182:824-832, 2000.
281. Ring A, Depnering C, Pohl J, et al: Synergistic action of nitric oxide release from murine macrophages caused by group B streptococcal cell wall and beta-hemolysin/cytolysin, *J Infect Dis* 186:1518-1521, 2002.
282. Griffiths BB, Rhee H: Effects of haemolysins of groups A and B streptococci on cardiovascular system, *Microbios* 69:17-27, 1992.
283. Hensler ME, Miyamoto S, Nizet V: Group B streptococcal beta-hemolysin/cytolysin directly impairs cardiomyocyte viability and function, *PLoS One* 3:e2446, 2008.
284. Bebien M, Hensler ME, Davanture S, et al: The pore-forming toxin beta hemolysin/cytolysin triggers p38 MAPK-dependent IL-10 production in macrophages and inhibits innate immunity, *PLoS Pathog* 8:e1002812, 2012.
285. Berman PH, Banker BQ: Neonatal meningitis: a clinical and pathological study of 29 cases, *Pediatrics* 38:6-24, 1966.
286. Ferrieri P, Burke B, Nelson J: Production of bacteremia and meningitis in infant rats with group B streptococcal serotypes, *Infect Immun* 27:1023-1032, 1980.
287. Nizet V, Kim KS, Stins M, et al: Invasion of brain microvascular endothelial cells by group B streptococci, *Infect Immun* 65:5074-5081, 1997.
288. Doran KS, Engelson EJ, Khosravi A, et al: Blood-brain barrier invasion by group B *Streptococcus* depends upon proper cell-surface anchoring of lipoteichoic acid, *J Clin Invest* 115:2499-2507, 2005.
289. Tenenbaum T, Bloier C, Adam R, et al: Adherence to and invasion of human brain microvascular endothelial cells are promoted by fibrinogen-binding protein FbsA of *Streptococcus agalactiae*, *Infect Immun* 73:4404-4409, 2005.
290. Banerjee A, Kim BJ, Carmona EM, et al: Bacterial pili exploit integrin machinery to promote immune activation and efficient blood-brain barrier penetration, *Nat Comm* 2:462, 2011.
291. van Sorge NM, Quach D, Gurney MA, et al: The group B streptococcal serine-rich repeat 1 glycoprotein mediates penetration of the blood-brain barrier, *J Infect Dis* 199:1479-1487, 2009.
292. Seo HS, Mu R, Kim BJ, et al: Binding of glycoprotein Srr1 of *Streptococcus agalactiae* to fibrinogen promotes attachment to brain endothelium and the development of meningitis, *PLoS Pathog* 10:e1002947, 2013.
293. Chang YC, Wang Z, Flax LA, et al: Glycosaminoglycan binding facilitates entry of a bacterial pathogen into central nervous systems, *PLoS Pathog* 7:e1002082, 2011.
294. Tazi A, Disson O, Bellais S, et al: The surface protein HvgA mediates group B streptococcus hypervirulence and meningeal tropism in neonates, *J Exp Med* 207:2313-2322, 2010.
295. Kim YS, Sheldon RA, Elliott BR, et al: Brain injury in experimental neonatal meningitis due to group B streptococci, *J Neuropathol Exp Neurol* 54:531-539, 1995.
296. Bogdan I, Leib SL, Bergeron M, et al: Tumor necrosis factor-alpha contributes to apoptosis in hippocampal neurons during experimental group B streptococcal meningitis, *J Infect Dis* 176:693-697, 1997.
297. Ling EW, Noya FJ, Ricard G, et al: Biochemical mediators of meningeal inflammatory response to group B streptococcus in the newborn piglet model, *Pediatr Res* 38:981-987, 1995.
298. Lehnardt S, Henneke P, Lien E, et al: A mechanism for neurodegeneration induced by group B streptococci through activation of the TLR2/MyD88 pathway in microglia, *J Immunol* 177:583-592, 2006.
299. Lehnardt S, Wennekamp J, Freyer D, et al: TLR2 and caspase-8 are essential for group B *Streptococcus*-induced apoptosis in microglia, *J Immunol* 179:6134-6143, 2007.
300. A. Reiss Braun JS, Jäger K, et al: Bacterial pore-forming cytolysins induce neuronal damage in a rat model of neonatal meningitis, *J Infect Dis* 203:393-400, 2011.

301. Schuchat A, Deaver-Robinson K, Plikaytis BD, et al: Multistate case-control study of maternal risk factors for neonatal group B streptococcal disease, *Pediatr Infect Dis J* 13:623-629, 1994.
302. Pass MA, Khare S, Dillon HC: Twin pregnancies: incidence of group B streptococcal colonization and disease, *J Pediatr* 97:635-637, 1980.
303. Edwards MS, Jackson CV, Baker CJ: Increased risk of group B streptococcal disease in twins, *JAMA* 245:2044-2046, 1981.
304. Faro S: Group B beta-hemolytic streptococci and puerperal infections, *Am J Obstet Gynecol* 139:686-689, 1981.
305. Schuchat A: Group B *Streptococcus*, *Lancet* 353:51-56, 1999.
306. Regan JA, Klebanoff MA, Nugent RP, et al: Colonization with group B streptococci in pregnancy and adverse outcome, *Am J Obstet Gynecol* 174:1354-1360, 1996.
307. Seaward PG, Hannah ME, Myhr TL, et al: International multicenter term PROM study: evaluation of predictors of neonatal infection in infants born to patients with premature rupture of membranes at term, *Am J Obstet Gynecol* 179:635-639, 1998.
308. Yancey MK, Duff P, Clark P, et al: Peripartum infection associated with vaginal group B streptococcal colonization, *Obstet Gynecol* 84:816-819, 1994.
309. Lancefield RC, McCarty M, Everly WN: Multiple mouse-protective antibodies directed against group B streptococci, *J Exp Med* 142: 165-179, 1975.
310. Baker CJ, Kasper DL: Correlation of maternal antibody deficiency with susceptibility to neonatal group B streptococcal infection, *N Engl J Med* 294:753-756, 1976.
311. Baker CJ, Edwards MS, Kasper DL: Role of antibody to native type III polysaccharide of group B *Streptococcus* in infant infection, *Pediatrics* 68:544-549, 1981.
312. Guttormsen HK, Baker CJ, Edwards MS, et al: Quantitative determination of antibodies to type III group B streptococcal polysaccharide, *J Infect Dis* 173:142-150, 1996.
313. Gray BM, Pritchard DG, Dillon HC Jr: Seroepidemiological studies of group B *Streptococcus* type II, *J Infect Dis* 151:1073-1080, 1985.
314. Gotoff SP, Papierniak CK, Klegerman ME, et al: Quantitation of IgG antibody to the type-specific polysaccharide of group B *Streptococcus* type 1b in pregnant women and infected infants, *J Pediatr* 105:628-630, 1984.
315. Baker CJ, Carey VJ, Rench MA, et al: Maternal antibody at delivery protects neonates from early-onset group B streptococcal disease, *J Infect Dis* 209:781-788, 2014.
316. Lin FY, Weisman LE, Azimi PH, et al: Level of maternal IgG anti-group B streptococcus type III antibody correlated with protection of neonates against early-onset disease caused by this pathogen, *J Infect Dis* 190:928-934, 2004.
317. Lin FY, Philips JB 3rd, Azimi PH, et al: Level of maternal antibody required to protect neonates against early-onset disease caused by group B *Streptococcus* type Ia: a multicenter, seroepidemiology study, *J Infect Dis* 184:1022-1028, 2001.
318. Baker CJ, Kasper DL, Tager IRAB, et al: Quantitative determination of antibody to capsular polysaccharide in infection with type III strains of group B *Streptococcus*, *J Clin Invest* 59:810-818, 1977.
319. Baker CJ, Edwards MS, Kasper DL: Immunogenicity of polysaccharides from type III group B *Streptococcus*, *J Clin Invest* 61:1107-1110, 1978.
320. Hordnes K, Tynning T, Kvam AI, et al: Cervical secretions in pregnant women colonized rectally with group B streptococci have high levels of antibodies to serotype III polysaccharide capsular antigen and protein, *R Scand J Immunol* 47:179-188, 1998.
321. Hordnes K, Tynning T, Kvam AI, et al: Colonization in the rectum and uterine cervix with group B streptococci may induce specific antibody responses in cervical secretions of pregnant women, *Infect Immun* 64:1643-1652, 1996.
322. De Cueninck BJ, Eisenstein TK, McIntosh TS, et al: Quantitation of in vitro opsonic activity of human antibody induced by a vaccine consisting of the type III-specific polysaccharide of group B streptococcus, *Infect Immun* 39:1155-1160, 1983.
323. Pincus SH, Shigeoka AO, Moe AA, et al: Protective efficacy of IgM monoclonal antibodies in experimental group B streptococcal infection is a function of antibody avidity, *J Immunol* 140:2779-2785, 1988.
324. Givner LB, Baker CJ, Edwards MS: Type III group B *Streptococcus*: functional interaction with IgG subclass antibodies, *J Infect Dis* 155:532-539, 1987.
325. Kim JS, Kim KS, Wass CA, et al: A human IgG 3 is opsonic in vitro against type III group B streptococci, *J Clin Immunol* 10:154-159, 1990.
326. Anthony BF, Concepcion NF: Opsonic activity of human IgG and IgM antibody for type III group B streptococci, *Pediatr Res* 26: 383-387, 1989.
327. Campbell JR, Baker CJ, Metzger TG, et al: Functional activity of class-specific antibodies to type III, group B *Streptococcus*, *Pediatr Res* 23:31-34, 1988.
328. Bohnsack JF, Hawley MM, Pritchard DG, et al: An IgA monoclonal antibody directed against type III antigen on group B streptococci acts as an opsonin, *J Immunol* 143:3338-3342, 1989.
329. Campbell JR, Baker CJ, Edwards MS: Deposition and degradation of C3 on type III group B streptococci, *Infect Immun* 59:1978-1983, 1991.
330. Edwards MS, Hall MA, Rench MA, Baker CJ: Patterns of immune response among survivors of group B streptococcal meningitis, *J Infect Dis* 161:65-70, 1990.
331. Baker CJ, Edwards MS, Webb BJ, Kasper DL: Antibody-independent classical pathway-mediated opsonophagocytosis of type Ia, group B *Streptococcus*, *J Clin Invest* 69:394-404, 1982.
332. Levy NJ, Kasper DL: Surface-bound capsular polysaccharide of type Ia group B *Streptococcus* mediates C1 binding and activation of the classic complement pathway, *J Immunol* 136:4157-4162, 1986.
333. Levy NJ, Kasper DL: Antibody-independent and -dependent opsonization of group B *Streptococcus* requires the first component of complement C1, *Infect Immun* 49:19-24, 1985.
334. Smith CL, Smith AH: Strain variability of type Ib group B streptococci: unique strains are resistant to C3 deposition by the alternate complement pathway, *Clin Res* 40:823A, 1992.
335. Hall MA, Edwards MS, Baker CJ: Complement and antibody participation in opsonophagocytosis of type IV and V group B streptococci, *Infect Immun* 60:5030-5035, 1992.
336. Hall MA, Hickman ME, Baker CJ, et al: Complement and antibody in neutrophil-mediated killing of type V group B *Streptococcus*, *J Infect Dis* 170:88-93, 1994.
337. Cairo MS, Worcester C, Rucker R, et al: Role of circulating complement and polymorphonuclear leukocyte transfusion in treatment and outcome in critically ill neonates with sepsis, *J Pediatr* 110: 935-941, 1987.
338. Levy O, Jean-Jacques RM, Cywes C, et al: Critical role of the complement system in group B *Streptococcus*-induced tumor necrosis factor alpha release, *Infect Immun* 71:6344-6353, 2003.
339. Pozdnyakova O, Guttormsen HK, Lalani FN, et al: Impaired antibody response to group B streptococcal type III capsular polysaccharide in C3- and complement receptor 2-deficient mice, *J Immunol* 170: 84-90, 2003.
340. Singer DB, Campognone P: Perinatal group B streptococcal infection in midgestation, *PediatrPathol* 52:71-276, 1986.
341. deSa DJ, Trevenen CL: Intrauterine infections with group B beta-haemolytic streptococci, *Br J Obstet Gynaecol* 91:237-239, 1984.
342. Hood M, Janney A, Dameron G: Beta-hemolytic *Streptococcus* group B associated with problems of perinatal period, *Am J Obstet Gynecol* 82:809-818, 1961.
343. Moller M, Thomsen AC, Borch K, et al: Rupture of fetal membranes and premature delivery associated with group B streptococci in urine of pregnant women, *Lancet* 2:69-70, 1984.
344 Novak RW, Platt MS: Significance of placental findings in early-onset group B streptococcal neonatal sepsis, *Clin Pediatr* 24: 256-258, 1985.
345. Becroft DMO, Farmer K, Mason GH, et al: Perinatal infections by group B 4-hemolytic streptococci, *Br J Obstet Gynaecol* 83:960-965, 1976.
346. Faix RG, Donn SM: Association of septic shock caused by early-onset group B streptococcal sepsis and periventricular leukomalacia in the preterm infant, *Pediatrics* 76:415-419, 1985.
347. Van Peenen PF, Cannon RE, Seibert DJ: Group B beta-hemolytic streptococci causing fatal meningitis, *Mil Med* 130:65-67, 1965.
348. DiJohn D, Krasinski K, Lawrence R, et al: Very late onset of group B streptococcal disease in infants infected with the human immunodeficiency virus, *Pediatr Infect Dis J* 9:925-928, 1990.
349. Schuchat A, Zywicki SS, Dinsmoor MJ, et al: Risk factors and opportunities for prevention of early-onset neonatal sepsis: a multicenter case-control study, *Pediatrics* 105:21-26, 2000.

350. Stoll BJ, Gordon T, Korones SB, et al: Early-onset sepsis in very low birth weight neonates: a report from the National Institute of Child Health and Human Development Neonatal Research Network, *J Pediatr* 129:72-80, 1996.
351. Stoll BJ, Hansen NI, Sánchez PJ, et al: Early onset neonatal sepsis: the burden of group B streptococcal and *E. coli* disease continues, *Pediatrics* 127:817-826, 2011.
352. Chen KT, Ringer S, Cohen AP, et al: The role of intrapartum fever in identifying asymptomatic term neonates with early-onset neonatal sepsis, *J Perinatol* 22:653-657, 2002.
353. Weisman LE, Stoll BJ, Cruess DF, et al: Early-onset group B streptococcal sepsis: a current assessment, *J Pediatr* 121:428-433, 1992.
354. Chin KC, Fitzhardinge PM: Sequelae of early-onset group B streptococcal neonatal meningitis, *J Pediatr* 106:819-822, 1985.
355. Haslam RHA, Allen JR, Dorsen MM, et al: The sequelae of group B beta-hemolytic streptococcal meningitis in early infancy, *Am J Dis Child* 131:845-849, 1977.
356. Edwards MS, Rench MA, Haffar AA, et al: Long-term sequelae of group B streptococcal meningitis in infants, *J Pediatr* 106:717-722, 1985.
357. Payne NR, Burke BA, Day DL, et al: Correlation of clinical and pathologic findings in early onset neonatal group B streptococcal infection with disease severity and prediction of outcome. *Pediatr Infect Dis J* 7:836-847, 1988.
358. Berardi A, Rossi C, Lugli L, et al: Group B *Streptococcus* late-onset disease, *Pediatrics* 131:e361-e368, 2013.
359. Levent F, Baker CJ, Rench MA, et al: Early outcomes of group B streptococcal meningitis in the 21st century, *Pediatr Infect Dis J* 29:1009-1012, 2010.
360. Yagupsky P, Menegus MA, Powell KR: The changing spectrum of group B streptococcal disease in infants: an eleven-year experience in a tertiary care hospital, *Pediatr Infect Dis J* 10:801-808, 1991.
361. Garcia Peña BM, Harper MB, Fleisher GR: Occult bacteremia with group B streptococci in an outpatient setting, *Pediatrics* 102:67-72, 1998.
362. Raymond J, Armengaud JB, Lambe C, et al: Late-onset neonatal infections caused by group B *Streptococcus* associated with viral infection, *Pediatr Infect Dis J* 26:963-1955, 2007.
363. Hussain SM, Luedtke GS, Baker CJ, et al: Invasive group B streptococcal disease in children beyond early infancy, *Pediatr Infect Dis J* 14:278-281, 1995.
364. De Witt CC, Ascher DP, Winkelstein J: Group B streptococcal disease in a child beyond early infancy with a deficiency of the second component of complement (C2), *Pediatr Infect Dis J* 18:77-78, 1999.
365. Krause JC, Ghandil P, Chrabieh M, et al: Very late-onset group B streptococcus meningitis, sepsis, and systemic shigellosis due to interleukin-1 receptor-associated kinase-4 deficiency, *Clin Infect Dis* 49:1393-1396, 2009.
366. Edwards MS, Baker CJ, Wagner ML, et al: An etiologic shift in infantile osteomyelitis: the emergence of the group B *Streptococcus*, *J Pediatr* 93:578-583, 1978.
367. Baevsky RH: Neonatal group B beta-hemolytic *Streptococcus* osteomyelitis, *Am J Emerg Med* 17:619-622, 1999.
368. Clay SA: Osteomyelitis as a cause of brachial plexus neuropathy, *Am J Dis Child* 136:1054-1056, 1982.
369. Sadleir LG, Connolly MB: Acquired brachial-plexus neuropathy in the neonate: a rare presentation of late-onset group-B streptococcal osteomyelitis, *Dev Med Child Neurol* 40:496-499, 1998.
370. Ammari LK, Offit PA, Campbell AB: Unusual presentation of group B *Streptococcus* osteomyelitis, *Pediatr Infect Dis J* 11:1066-1067, 1992.
371. Obando I, Martin E, Alvarez-Aldean J, et al: Group B *Streptococcus* pelvic osteomyelitis presenting as footdrop in a newborn infant, *Pediatr Infect Dis J* 10:703-705, 1991.
372. Barton LL, Villar RG, Rice SA: Neonatal group B streptococcal vertebral osteomyelitis, *Pediatrics* 98:459-461, 1996.
373. Broughton RA, Edwards MS, Haffar A, et al: Unusual manifestations of neonatal group B streptococcal osteomyelitis, *Pediatr Infect Dis J* 1:410-412, 1982.
374. Hauger SB: Facial cellulitis: an early indicator of group B streptococcal bacteremia, *Pediatrics* 67:376-377, 1981.
375. Patamasucon P, Siegel JD, McCracken GH Jr: Streptococcal submandibular cellulitis in young infants, *Pediatrics* 67:378-380, 1981.
376. Baker CJ: Group B streptococcal cellulitis/adenitis in infants, *Am J Dis Child* 136:631-633, 1982.
377. Fluegge K, Greiner P, Berner R: Late onset group B streptococcal disease manifested by isolated cervical lymphadenitis, *Arch Dis Child* 88:1019-1020, 2003.
378. Pathak A, Hwu HH: Group B streptococcal cellulitis, *South Med J* 78:67-68, 1985.
379. Haque KN, Bashir O, Kambal AMM: Delayed recurrence of group B streptococcal infection in a newborn infant: a case report, *Ann Trop Paediatr* 6:219-220, 1986.
380. Rand TH: Group B streptococcal cellulitis in infants: a disease modified by prior antibiotic therapy or hospitalization? *Pediatrics* 81: 63-65, 1988.
381. Brady MT: Cellulitis of the penis and scrotum due to group B *Streptococcus*, *J Urol* 137:736-737, 1987.
382. Shetty SK, Hindley D: Late onset group B streptococcal disease manifests as submandibular cellulitis, *BMJ Case Rep*, 2010. pii:bcr0220102726.
383. Albanyan EA, Baker CJ: Is lumbar puncture necessary to exclude meningitis in neonates and young infants: lessons from group B *Streptococcus* cellulitis-adenitis syndrome, *Pediatrics* 102:985-986, 1998.
384. Chadwick EG, Shulman ST, Yogev R: Peritonitis as a late manifestation of group B streptococcal disease in newborns, *Pediatr Infect Dis J* 2:142-143, 1983.
385. Walker KM, Coyer WF: Suprarenal abscess due to group B streptococcus, *J Pediatr* 94:970-971, 1979.
386. Atkinson GO Jr, Kodroff MB, Gay BB Jr, et al: Adrenal abscess in the neonate, *Radiology* 155:101-104, 1985.
387. Carty A, Stanley P: Bilateral adrenal abscesses in a neonate, *Pediatr Radiol* 1:63-64, 1973.
388. Peevy KJ, Wiseman HJ: Gallbladder distension in septic neonates, *Arch Dis Child* 57:75-76, 1982.
389. Siegel JD, Shannon KM, De Passe BM: Recurrent infection associated with penicillin-tolerant group B streptococci: a report of two cases, *J Pediatr* 99:920-924, 1981.
390. Sokol DM, Demmler GJ, Baker CJ: Unusual presentation of group B streptococcal ventriculitis, *Pediatr Infect Dis J* 9:525-527, 1990.
391. Coker SB, Muraskas JK, Thomas C: Myelopathy secondary to neonatal bacterial meningitis, *Pediatr Neurol* 10:259-261, 1994.
392. Ferguson L, Gotoff SP: Subdural empyema in an infant due to group B beta-hemolytic *Streptococcus*, *Am J Dis Child* 131:97, 1977.
393. McReynolds EW, Shane R: Diabetes insipidus secondary to group B beta streptococcal meningitis, *J Tenn Med Assoc* 67:117-120, 1974.
394. Dorand RD, Adams G: Relapse during penicillin treatment of group B streptococcal meningitis, *J Pediatr* 89:188-190, 1976.
395. Kim KS, Kaye KL, Itabashi HH, et al: Cerebritis due to group B *Streptococcus*, *Scand J Infect Dis* 14:305-308, 1982.
396. Barton CW, Crowley DC, Uzark K, et al: A neonatal survivor of group B beta-hemolytic streptococcal endocarditis, *Am J Perinatol* 1: 214-215, 1984.
397. Horigome H, Okada Y, Hirano T, et al: Group B streptococcal endocarditis in infancy with a giant vegetation on the pulmonary valve, *Eur J Pediatr* 153:140-142, 1994.
398. Harper IA: The importance of group B streptococci as human pathogens in the British Isles, *J Clin Pathol* 244:38-441, 1971.
399. Ancona RJ, McAuliffe J, Thompson TR, et al: Group B streptococcal sepsis with osteomyelitis and arthritis, *Am J Dis Child* 133:919-920, 1979.
400. Agarwala BN: Group B streptococcal endocarditis in a neonate, *Pediatr Cardiol* 9:51-53, 1988.
401. Shurin PA, Howie VM, Pelton SI, et al: Bacterial etiology of otitis media during the first six weeks of life, *J Pediatr* 92:893-896, 1978.
402. Sapir-Ellis S, Johnson A, Austin TL: Group B streptococcal meningitis associated with otitis media, *Am J Dis Child* 130:1003-1004, 1976.
403. Tetzlaff TR, Ashworth C, Nelson JD: Otitis media in children less than 12 weeks of age, *Pediatrics* 59:827-832, 1977.
404. Ermocilla R, Cassady G, Ceballos R: Otitis media in the pathogenesis of neonatal meningitis with group B beta-hemolytic *Streptococcus*, *Pediatrics* 54:643-644, 1974.
405. Armstrong JH, Zacarias F, Rein MF: Ophthalmia neonatorum: a chart review, *Pediatrics* 57:884-892, 1976.
406. Sparks JR, Recchia FM, Weitkamp JH: Endogenous group B streptococcal endophthalmitis in a preterm infant, *J Perinatol* 27:392-394, 2007.
407. Lipson A, Kronick JB, Tewfik L, et al: Group B streptococcal supraglottitis in a 3-month-old infant, *Am J Dis Child* 140:411-412, 1986.
408. Park JW: Bacterial tracheitis caused by *Streptococcus agalactiae*, *Pediatr Infect Dis J* 9:450-451, 1990.
409. Sokal MM, Nagaraj A, Fisher BJ, et al: Neonatal empyema caused by group B beta-hemolytic *Streptococcus*, *Chest* 81:390-391, 1982.

410. LeBovar Y, Trung PH, Mozziconacci P: Neonatal meningitis due to group B streptococci, *Ann Pediatr* 17:207-213, 1970.
411. Strunk T, Simmer K, Kikiros C, et al: Late-onset right-sided diaphragmatic hernia in neonates—case report and review of the literature, *Eur J Pediatr* 166:521-526, 2007.
412. Nudelman R, Bral M, Sakhai Y, et al: Violaceous cellulitis, *Pediatrics* 70:157-158, 1982.
413. Barton LL, Kapoor NK: Recurrent group B streptococcal infection, *Clin Pediatr* 21:100-101, 1982.
414. Amoury RA, Barth GW, Hall RT, et al: Scrotal ecchymosis: sign of intraperitoneal hemorrhage in the newborn, *South Med J* 75: 1471-1478, 1982.
415. Isaacman SH, Heroman WM, Lightsey A: Purpura fulminans following late-onset group B beta-hemolytic streptococcal sepsis, *Am J Dis Child* 138:915-916, 1984.
416. Lynn NJ, Pauly TH, Desai NS: Purpura fulminans in three cases of early-onset neonatal group B streptococcal meningitis, *J Perinatol* 11:144-146, 1991.
417. Zenciroglu A, Karagol BS, Ipek MS, et al: Neonatal purpura fulminans secondary to group B streptococcal infection, *Pediatr Hematol Oncol* 8:620-625, 2010.
418. Ramamurthy RS, Srinivasan G, Jacobs NM: Necrotizing fasciitis and necrotizing cellulitis due to group B *Streptococcus*, *Am J Dis Child* 131:1169-1170, 1977.
419. Goldberg GN, Hansen RC, Lynch PJ: Necrotizing fasciitis in infancy: report of three cases and review of the literature, *Pediatr Dermatol* 2:55-63, 1984.
420. Lang ME, Vaudry W, Robinson JL: Case report and literature review of late-onset group B streptococcal disease manifesting as necrotizing fasciitis in preterm infants. Is this a new syndrome? *Clin Infect Dis* 37:e132-e135, 2003.
421. Lopez JB, Gross P, Boggs TR: Skin lesions in association with beta-hemolytic *Streptococcus* group B, *Pediatrics* 58:859-860, 1976.
422. Belgaumkar TK: Impetigo neonatorum congenita due to group B beta-hemolytic *Streptococcus* infection, *J Pediatr* 86:982-983, 1975.
423. Jacobs MR, Koornhof HJ, Stein H: Group B streptococcal infections in neonates and infants, *S Afr Med J* 54:154-158, 1978.
424. Feder AM Jr, MacLean WC, Moxon R: Scalp abscess secondary to fetal scalp electrode, *J Pediatr* 89:808-809, 1976.
425. Wiswell TE, Miller JA: Infections of congenital cervical neck masses associated with bacteremia, *J Pediatr Surg* 21:173-174, 1986.
426. Bourgeois FT, Shannon MW: Retropharyngeal cellulitis in a 5-week-old infant, *Pediatrics* 109:e51-e53, 2002.
427. Kelly CP, Isaacman DJ: Group B streptococcal retropharyngeal cellulitis in a young infant: a case report and review of the literature, *J Emerg Med* 23:179-182, 2002.
428. Nelson JD: Bilateral breast abscess due to group B *Streptococcus*, *Am J Dis Child* 130:567, 1976.
429. St. Laurent-Gagnon T, Weber ML: Urinary tract *Streptococcus* group B infection in a 6-week-old infant, *JAMA* 240:1269, 1978.
430. Shoda T, Miyagi N, Shirai K, et al: Double recurrence of group B streptococcus bacteremia in an immunocompetent infant, *Pediatr International* 54:701-703, 2012.
431. Soukka H, Rantakokko-Jalava K, Vähäkuopus S, et al: Three distinct episodes of GBS septicemia in a healthy newborn during the first month of life, *Eur J Pediatr* 169:1275-1277, 2010.
432. Atkins JT, Heresi GP, Coque TM, et al: Recurrent group B streptococcal disease in infants: who should receive rifampin? *J Pediatr* 132:537-539, 1998.
433. Green PA, Singh KV, Murray BE, Baker CJ: Recurrent group B streptococcal infections in infants: clinical and microbiologic aspects, *J Pediatr* 125:931-938, 1994.
434. Moylett EH, Fernandez M, Rench MA, et al: A 5-year review of recurrent group B streptococcal disease: lessons from twin infants, *Clin Infect Dis* 30:282-287, 2000.
435. Denning DW, Bressack M, Troup NJ, et al: Infant with two relapses of group B streptococcal sepsis documented by DNA restriction enzyme analysis, *Pediatr Infect Dis J* 7:729-732, 1988.
436. Simón JL, Bosch J, Puig A, et al: Two relapses of group B streptococcal sepsis and transient hypogammaglobulinemia, *Pediatr Infect Dis J* 8:729-730, 1989.
437. Kotiw M, Zhang GW, Daggard G, et al: Late-onset and recurrent neonatal group B streptococcal disease associated with breast-milk transmission, *Pediatr Dev Pathol* 6:251-256, 2003.
438. Wang LY, Chen CT, Liu WH, et al: Recurrent neonatal group B streptococcal disease associated with infected breast milk, *Clin Pediatr (Phila)* 46:547-549, 2007.
439. Jones SM, Steele RW: Recurrent group B streptococcal bacteremia, *Clin Pediatr* 51:884-887, 2012.
440. Ramsay AM, Gillespie M: Puerperal infection associated with haemolytic streptococci other than Lancefield's group A, *J Obstet Gynaecol Br Emp* 48:569-585, 1941.
441. Butter MNW, de Moor CE: *Streptococcus agalactiae* as a cause of meningitis in the newborn, and of bacteremia in adults, *Antonie van Leeuwenhoek* 33:439-450, 1967.
442. Ledger WJ, Norman M, Gee C, et al: Bacteremia on an obstetric-gynecologic service, *Am J Obstet Gynecol* 121:205-212, 1975.
443. Cape A, Tuomala RE, Taylor C, et al: Peripartum bacteremia in the era of group B *Streptococcus* prophylaxis, *Obstet Gynecol* 121: 812-818, 2013.
444. Tudela CM, Stewart RD, Roberts SW, et al: Intrapartum evidence of early-onset group B *Streptococcus*, *Obstet Gynecol* 119:626-629, 2012.
445. Aharoni A, Potasman I, Levitan Z, et al: Postpartum maternal group B streptococcal meningitis, *Rev Infect Dis* 12:273-276, 1990.
446. Kane JM, Jackson K, Conway JH: Maternal postpartum group B beta-hemolytic streptococcus ventriculoperitoneal shunt infection, *Arch Gynecol Obstet* 269:139-141, 2004.
447. Sexton DJ, Rockson SG, Hempling RE, et al: Pregnancy-associated group B streptococcal endocarditis: a report of two fatal cases, *Obstet Gynecol* 66:44-47S, 1985.
448. Backes RJ, Wilson WR, Geraci JE: Group B streptococcal infective endocarditis, *Arch Intern Med* 145:693-696, 1985.
449. Seaworth BJ, Durack DT: Infective endocarditis in obstetric and gynecologic practice, *Am J Obstet Gynecol* 154:180-188, 1986.
450. Vartian CV, Septimus EJ: Tricuspid valve group B streptococcal endocarditis following elective abortion, *Rev Infect Dis* 13:997-998, 1991.
451. Lischke JH, McCreight PHB: Maternal group B streptococcal vertebral osteomyelitis: an unusual complication of vaginal delivery, *Obstet Gynecol* 76:489-491, 1990.
452. Jenkin G, Woolley IJ, Brown GV, et al: Postpartum epidural abscess due to group B *Streptococcus*, *Clin Infect Dis* 25:1249, 1997.
453. Sutton GP, Smirz LR, Clark DH, et al: Group B streptococcal necrotizing fasciitis arising from an episiotomy, *Obstet Gynecol* 66:733-736, 1985.
454. Wood EG, Dillon HC: A prospective study of group B streptococcal bacteriuria in pregnancy, *Am J Obstet Gynecol* 140:515-520, 1981.
455. Gibbs RS, Roberts DJ: Case records of the Massachusetts General Hospital. Case 27-2007. A 30-year-old pregnant woman with intrauterine fetal death, *N Engl J Med* 357:918-925, 2007.
456. Wiswell TE, Baumgart S, Gannon CM, et al: No lumbar puncture in the evaluation for early neonatal sepsis. Will meningitis be missed? *Pediatrics* 95:803-806, 1995.
457. American Academy of Pediatrics Committee on Infectious Diseases and Committee on Fetus and Newborn: revised guidelines for prevention of early-onset group B streptococcal (GBS) infection, *Pediatrics* 99:489-496, 1997.
458. de Zoysa A, Edwards K, Gharbia S, et al: Non-culture detection of *Streptococcus agalactiae* (Lancefield group B *Streptococcus*) in clinical samples by real-time PCR, *J Clin Microbiol* 61:1086-1090, 2012.
459. Natarajan G, Johnson YR, Zhang F, et al: Real-time polymerase chain reaction for the rapid detection of group B streptococcal colonization in neonates, *Pediatrics* 118:14-22, 2006.
460. Golden SM, Stamilio DM, Faux BM, et al: Evaluation of a real-time fluorescent PCR assay for rapid detection of group B streptococci in neonatal blood, *Diagn Microbiol Infect Dis* 50:7-13, 2004.
461. Vallejo JG, Baker CJ, Edwards MS: Interleukin-6 production by human neonatal monocytes stimulated by type III group B streptococci, *J Infect Dis* 174:332-337, 1996.
462. Greenberg DN, Yoder BA: Changes in the differential white blood cell count in screening for group B streptococcal sepsis, *Pediatr Infect Dis J* 9:886-889, 1990.
463. Polin RA; Committee on Fetus and Newborn: Management of neonates with suspected or proven early-onset bacterial sepsis, *Pediatrics* 129:1006-1015, 2012.
464. Christensen RD, Rothstein G, Hill HR, et al: Fatal early onset group B streptococcal sepsis with normal leukocyte counts, *Pediatr Infect Dis J* 4:242-245, 1985.

465. Baker CJ, Webb BJ, Barrett FF: Antimicrobial susceptibility of group B streptococci isolated from a variety of clinical sources, *Antimicrob Agents Chemother* 10:128-131, 1976.
466. Fernandez M, Hickman ME, Baker CJ: Antimicrobial susceptibilities of group B streptococci isolated between 1992 and 1996 from patients with bacteremia or meningitis, *Antimicrob Agents Chemother* 42:1517-1519, 1998.
467. Meyn LA, Hillier SL: Ampicillin susceptibilities of vaginal and placental isolates of group B *Streptococcus* and *Escherichia coli* obtained between 1992 and 1994, *Antimicrob Agents Chemother* 41: 1173-1174, 1997.
468. Biedenbach DJ, Stephen JM, Jones RN: Antimicrobial susceptibility profile among β-haemolytic *Streptococcus* spp. collected in the SENTRY Antimicrobial Surveillance Program-North America, 2001, *Diag Microbiol Infect Dis* 46:291-294, 2003.
469. Manning SD, Foxman B, Pierson CL, et al: Correlates of antibiotic-resistant group B *Streptococcus* isolated from pregnant women, *Obstet Gynecol* 101:74-79, 2003.
470. Chen KT, Puopolo KM, Eichenwald EC, et al: No increase in rates of early-onset neonatal sepsis by antibiotic-resistant group B *Streptococcus* in the era of intrapartum antibiotic prophylaxis, *Am J Obstet Gynecol* 192:1167-1171, 2005.
471. Dahesh S, Hensler ME, Van Sorge NM, et al: Point mutation in the group B streptococcal pbp2x gene conferring decreased susceptibility to beta-lactam antibiotics, *Antimicrob Agents Chemother* 52: 2915-2918, 2008.
472. Nagano N, Nagano Y, Kimura K, et al: Genetic heterogeneity in pbp genes among clinically isolated group B streptococci with reduced penicillin susceptibility, *Antimicrob Agents Chemother* 52: 4258-4267, 2008.
473. Kasahara K, Baltus AJ, Lee SH, et al: Prevalence of non-penicillin-susceptible group B *Streptococcus* in Philadelphia and specificity of penicillin resistance screening methods, *J Clin Microbiol* 48: 1468-1469, 2010.
474. Manning SD, Pearlman MD, Tallman P, et al: Frequency of antibiotic resistance among group B *Streptococcus* isolated from healthy college students, *Clin Infect Dis* 33:e137-e139, 2001.
475. Brandon M, Dowzicky MJ: Antimicrobial susceptibility among gram-positive organisms collected from pediatric patients globally between 2004 and 2011: results from the tigecycline evaluation and surveillance trial, *J Clin Microbiol* 51:2371-2378, 2013.
476. Wehbeh W, Rojas-Diaz R, Li X, et al: Fluoroquinolone-resistant *Streptococcus agalactiae*: epidemiology and mechanism of resistance, *Antimicrob Agents Chemother* 49:2495-2497, 2005.
477. Capanna F, Emonet SP, Cherkaoui A, et al: Antibiotic resistance patterns among group B *Streptococcus* isolates: implications for antibiotic prophylaxis for early-onset neonatal sepsis, *Swiss Med Wkly* 143:w13778, 2013.
478. Borchardt SM, DeBusscher JH, Tallman PA, et al: Frequency of antimicrobial resistance among invasive and colonizing group B streptococcal isolates, *BMC Infect Dis* 6:57, 2006.
479. Fitoussi F, Loukil C, Gros I, et al: Mechanisms of macrolide resistance in clinical group B streptococci isolated in France, *Antimicrob Agents Chemother* 45:1889-1891, 2001.
480. Betriu C, Culebras E, Gómez M, et al: Erythromycin and clindamycin resistance and telithromycin susceptibility in Streptococcus agalactiae, *Antimicrob Agents Chemother* 47:1112-1114, 2003.
481. Acikgoz ZC, Almayanlar E, Gamberzade S, et al: Macrolide resistance determinants of invasive and noninvasive group B streptococci in a Turkish hospital, *Antimicrob Agents Chemother* 48:1410-1412, 2004.
482. de Azavedo JCS, McGavin M, Duncan C, et al: Prevalence and mechanisms of macrolide resistance in invasive and noninvasive group B *Streptococcus* isolates from Ontario, Canada, *Antimicrob Agents Chemother* 45:3504-3508, 2001.
483. Marimón JM, Valiente A, Ercibengoa M, et al: Erythromycin resistance and genetic elements carrying macrolide efflux genes in Streptococcus agalactiae, *Antimicrob Agents Chemother* 49:5069-5074, 2005.
484. Heelan JS, Hasenbein ME, McAdam AJ: Resistance of group B *Streptococcus* to selected antibiotics, including erythromycin and clindamycin, *J Clin Microbiol* 42:1263-1264, 2004.
485. DiPersio LP, DiPersio JR: Identification of an *erm(T)* gene in strains of inducibly clindamycin-resistant group B *Streptococcus*, *Diagn Microbiol Infect Dis* 57:189-193, 2007.
486. Puopolo KM, Klinzing DC, Lin MP, et al: A composite transposon associated with erythromycin and clindamycin resistance in group B *Steptococcus*, *J Med Microbiol* 56:947-955, 2007.
487. Lin FY, Azimi PH, Weisman LE, et al: Antibiotic susceptibility profiles for group B streptococci isolated from neonates, 1995–1998, *Clin Infect Dis* 31:76-79, 2000.
488. Betriu C, Culebras E, Rodríguez-Avial I, et al: In vitro activities of tigecycline against erythromycin-resistant *Streptococcus pyogenes* and *Streptococcus agalactiae*: mechanisms of macrolide and tetracycline resistance, *Antimicrob Agents Chemother* 48:323-325, 2004.
489. Bingen E, Doit C, Bidet P, et al: Telithromycin susceptibility and genomic diversity of macrolide-resistant serotype III group B streptococci isolated in perinatal infections, *Antimicrob Agents Chemother* 48:677-680, 2004.
490. Swingle HM, Bucciarelli RL, Ayoub EM: Synergy between penicillins and low concentrations of gentamicin in the killing of group B streptococci, *J Infect Dis* 152:515-520, 1985.
491. Maduri-Traczewski M, Szymczak EG, Goldmann DA: In vitro activity of penicillin and rifampin against group B streptococci, *Rev Infect Dis* 5:S586-S592, 1983.
492. Hall MA, Ducker DA, Lowes JA, et al: A randomized prospective comparison of cefotaxime versus netilmicin/penicillin for treatment of suspected neonatal sepsis, *Drugs* 35:169-188, 1988.
493. Bradley JS, Ching DL, Wilson TA, et al: Once-daily ceftriaxone to complete therapy of uncomplicated group B streptococcal infection in neonates, *Clin Pediatr* 31:274-278, 1992.
494. Feldman WE: Concentrations of bacteria in cerebrospinal fluid of patients with bacterial meningitis, *J Pediatr* 88:549-552, 1976.
495. Kim KS: Clinical perspectives on penicillin tolerance, *J Pediatr* 112:509-514, 1988.
496. Poschl JM, Hellstern G, Dertlioglou N, et al: Six day antimicrobial therapy for early-onset group B streptococcal infection in near-term and term neonates, *Scand J Infect Dis* 35:302-305, 2003.
497. Fernandez M, Rench MA, Albanyan EA, et al: Failure of rifampin to eradicate group B streptococcal colonization in infants, *Pediatr Infect Dis J* 20:371-376, 2001.
498. Lannering B, Larsson LE, Rojas J, et al: Early onset group B streptococcal disease: seven year experience and clinical scoring system, *Acta Paediatr Scand* 72:597-602, 1983.
499. Fluegge K, Siedler A, Heinrich B, et al: Incidence and clinical presentation of invasive neonatal group B streptococcal infections in Germany, *Pediatrics* 117:e1139-e1145, 2006.
500. de Louvois J, Halket S, Harvey D: Neonatal meningitis in England and Wales: sequelae at 5 years of age, *Eur J Pediatr* 164:730-734, 2005.
501. Stoll BJ, Hansen NI, Adams-Chapman I, et al: Neurodevelopmental and growth impairment among extremely low-birth-weight infants with neonatal infection, *JAMA* 292:2357-2365, 2004.
502. Libster R, Edwards KM, Levent F, et al: Long-term outcomes of group B streptococcal meningitis, *Pediatrics* 130:e8-e15, 2012.
503. Centers for Disease Control and Prevention: Prevention of perinatal group B streptococcal disease: revised guidelines from CDC, *MMWR Morb Mortal Wkly Rep* 51:1-22, 2002.
504. Baker CJ: Immunization to prevent group B streptococcal disease: victories and vexations, *J Infect Dis* 161:917-921, 1990.
505. Gardner SE, Yow MD, Leeds LJ, et al: Failure of penicillin to eradicate group B streptococcal colonization in the pregnant woman, *Am J Obstet Gynecol* 135:1062-1065, 1979.
506. Gordon JS, Sbara AJ: Incidence, technique of isolation, and treatment of group B streptococci in obstetric patients, *Am J Obstet Gynecol* 126:1023-1026, 1976.
507. Hall RT, Barnes W, Krishnan L, et al: Antibiotic treatment of parturient women colonized with group B streptococci, *Am J Obstet Gynecol* 124:630-634, 1976.
508. Lewin EB, Amstey MS: Natural history of group B *Streptococcus* colonization and its therapy during pregnancy, *Am J Obstet Gynecol* 139:512-515, 1981.
509. Yow MD, Mason EO, Leeds LJ, et al: Ampicillin prevents intrapartum transmission of group B *Streptococcus*, *JAMA* 241:1245-1247, 1979.
510. Boyer KM, Gotoff SP: Prevention of early-onset neonatal group B streptococcal disease with selective intrapartum chemopraxis, *N Engl J Med* 314:1665-1669, 1986.
511. Matorras R, García-Perea A, Madero R, et al: Maternal colonization by group B streptococci and puerperal infection; analysis of intrapartum chemoprophylaxis, *Eur J Obstet Gynecol Reprod Biol* 38:203-207, 1990.

512. Mohle-Boetani JC, Schuchat A, Plikaytis BD, et al: Comparison of prevention strategies for neonatal group B streptococcal infection: an economic analysis, *JAMA* 270:1442-1448, 1993.
513. ACOG technical bulletin: Group B streptococcal infections in pregnancy, *ACOG Tech Bull* 170:1-5, 1992.
514. American Academy of Pediatrics Committee on Infectious Diseases: Committee on Fetus and Newborn: Guidelines for prevention of group B streptococcal (GBS) infection by chemoprophylaxis, *Pediatrics* 90:775-778, 1992.
515. Bergeron MG, Ke D, Ménard C, et al: Rapid detection of group B streptococci in pregnant women at delivery, *N Engl J Med* 343:175-179, 2000.
516. Edwards RK, Novak-Weekley SM, Koty PP, et al: Rapid group B streptococci screening using a real-time polymerase chain reaction assay, *Obstet Gynecol* 111:1335-1341, 2008.
517. Davies HD, Miller MA, Faro S, et al: Multicenter study of a rapid molecular-based assay for the diagnosis of group B *Streptococcus* colonization in pregnant women, *Clin Infect Dis* 39:1129-1135, 2004.
518. Gavino M, Wang E: A comparison of a new rapid real-time polymerase chain reaction system to traditional culture in determining group B streptococcus colonization, *Am J Obstet Gynecol* 197:388, 2007.
519. Honest H, Sharma S, Khan KS: Rapid tests for group B *Streptococcus* colonization in laboring women: a systematic review, *Pediatrics* 117:1055-1066, 2006.
520. Poncelet-Jasserand E, Forges F, Varlet MN, et al: Reduction of the use of antimicrobial drugs following the rapid detection of *Streptococcus agalactiae* in the vagina at delivery by real-ltime PCR assay, *Brit J Obstet Gynaec* 120:1098-1109, 2013.
521. El Helali N, Giovangrandi Y, Guyot K, et al: Cost and effectiveness of intrapartum group B *Streptococcus* polymerase chain reaction screening for term deliveries, *Obstet Gynec* 119:822-829, 2012.
522. Riedlinger J, Beqaj SH, Milish MA, et al: Multicenter evaluation of the BD Max GBS assay for detection of group B streptococci in prenatal vaginal and rectal screening swab specimens from pregnant women, *J Clin Microbiol* 48:4239-4241, 2010.
523. Martinez de Tejada B, Pfister RE, Renzi G, et al: Intrapartum group B streptococcus detection by rapid polymerase chain reaction assay for the prevention of neonatal sepsis, *Clin Micro Infect* 17:1786-1791, 2011.
524. Berg B, Houseman JL, Garrasi MA, et al: Culture-based method with performance comparable to that of PCR-based methods for detection of group B *Streptococcus* in screening samples from pregnant women, *J Clin Microbiol* 51:1253-1255, 2013.
525. Centers for Disease Control and Prevention: Prevention of perinatal group B streptococcal disease: a public health perspective, *MMWR Morb Mortal Wkly Rep* 45:1-24, 1996.
526. American College of Obstetricians and Gynecologists Committee on Obstetric Practice: Prevention of early-onset group B streptococcal disease in newborns, Washington, DC, 1996, American College of Obstetricians and Gynecologists.
527. Schuchat A: Group B streptococcal disease: from trials and tribulations to triumph and trepidation, *Clin Infect Dis* 33:751-756, 2001.
528. Schrag SJ, Whitney CG, Schuchat A: Neonatal group B streptococcal disease: how infection control teams can contribute to prevention efforts, *Infect Control Hosp Epidemiol* 21:473-483, 2000.
529. Centers for Disease Control and Prevention: Hospital-based policies for prevention of perinatal group B streptococcal disease—United States, 1999, *MMWR Morb Mortal Wkly Rep* 49:936-940, 2000.
530. Fairlie T, Zell E, Schrag S: Effectiveness of intrapartum antibiotic prophylaxis for prevention of early-onset group B streptococcal disease, *Obstet Gynec* 121:570-577, 2013.
531. Blaschke A, Pulver LS, Korgenski EK, et al: Clindamycin-resistant group B *Streptococcus* and failure of intrapartum prophylaxis to prevent early-onset disease, *J Pediatr* 156:501-503, 2010.
532. Dunn AB, Blomquist J, Khousami V: Anaphylaxis in labor secondary to prophylaxis against group B streptococcus: a case report, *J Reprod Med* 44:381-384, 1999.
533. Heim K, Alge A, Marth C: Anaphylactic reaction to ampicillin and severe complication in the fetus, *Lancet* 337:859-860, 1991.
534. Philipson EH, Lang DM, Gordon SJ, et al: Management of group B *Streptococcus* in pregnant women with penicillin allergy, *J Reprod Med* 52:480-484, 2007.
535. Sheikh J: Intrapartum anaphylaxis to penicillin in a woman with rheumatoid arthritis who had no prior penicillin allergy, *Ann Allergy Asthma Immunol* 99:287-289, 2007.
536. Paccione K, Wiesenfeld H: Guideline adherence for intrapartum group B streptococci prophylaxis in penicillin-allergic patients, *Infect Dis Obstet Gynec* 917304, 2013.
537. Pinto NM, Soskolne EI, Pearlman MD, et al: Neonatal early-onset group B streptococcal disease in the era of intrapartum chemoprophylaxis: residual problems, *J Perinatol* 23:265-271, 2003.
538. Cárdenas V, Davis RL, Hasselquist MB, et al: Barriers to implementing the group B streptococcal prevention guidelines, *Birth* 29: 285-290, 2002.
539. Puopolo K, Eichenwald E: No change in the incidence of ampicillin-resistant, neonatal early-onset sepsis over 18 years, *Pediatrics* 125:e1031-e1038, 2010.
540. Baker C, Byington C, Polin R: Policy statement—recommendations for the prevention of perinatal group B streptococcal disease, *Pediatrics* 128:611-616, 2011.
541. Brady M, Polin R: Prevention and management of infants with suspected or proven neonatal sepsis, *Pediatrics* 132:166-168, 2013.
542. Balter S, Zell ER, O'Brien KL, et al: Impact of intrapartum antibiotics on the care and evaluation of the neonate, *Pediatr Infect Dis J* 22: 853-857, 2003.
543. Bromberger P, Lawrence JM, Braun D, et al: The influence of intrapartum antibiotics on the clinical spectrum of early-onset group B streptococcal infection in term infants, *Pediatrics* 106:244-250, 2000.
544. Davis RL, Hasselquist MB, Cardenas V, et al: Introduction of the new Centers for Disease Control and Prevention group B streptococcal prevention guideline at a large West Coast health maintenance organization, *Am J Obstet Gynecol* 184:603-610, 2001.
545. Rubin EE, McDonald JC: Group B streptococcal disease in twins: failure of empiric therapy to prevent late onset disease in the second twin, *Pediatr Infect Dis J* 10:921-923, 1991.
546. Schuchat A: Epidemiology of group B streptococcal disease in the United States: shifting paradigms, *Clin Microbiol Rev* 11:497-513, 1998.
547. Madoff LC, Michel JL, Gong EW, et al: Protection of neonatal mice from group B streptococcal infection by maternal immunization with beta C protein, *Infect Immun* 60:4989-4994, 1992.
548. Wessels MR, Paoletti LC, Kasper DL, et al: Immunogenicity in animals of a polysaccharide-protein conjugate vaccine against type III group B *Streptococcus*, *J Clin Invest* 86:1428-1433, 1990.
549. Wessels MR, Paoletti LC, Pinel J, et al: Immunogenicity and protective activity in animals of a type V group B streptococcal polysaccharide-tetanus toxoid conjugate vaccine, *J Infect Dis* 171:879-884, 1995.
550. Paoletti LC, Wessels MR, Rodewald AK, et al: Neonatal mouse protection against infection with multiple group B streptococcal (GBS) serotypes by maternal immunization with a tetravalent GBS polysaccharide-tetanus toxoid conjugate vaccine, *Infect Immun* 62:3236-3243, 1994.
551. Madoff LC, Paoletti LC, Tai JY, et al: Maternal immunization of mice with group B streptococcal type III polysaccharide-beta C protein conjugate elicits protective antibody to multiple serotypes, *J Clin Invest* 94:286-292, 1994.
552. Paoletti LC, Madoff LC: Vaccines to prevent neonatal GBS infection, *Semin Neonatol* 7:315-323, 2002.
553. Kasper DL, Paoletti LC, Wessels MR, et al: Immune response to type III group B streptococcal polysaccharide-tetanus toxoid conjugate vaccine, *J Clin Invest* 98:2308-2314, 1996.
554. Baker CJ, Paoletti LC, Wessels MR, et al: Safety and immunogenicity of capsular polysaccharide-tetanus toxoid conjugate vaccines for group B streptococcal types Ia and Ib, *J Infect Dis* 179:142-150, 1999.
555. Baker CJ, Paoletti LC, Rench MA, et al: Use of capsular polysaccharide-tetanus toxoid conjugate vaccine for type II group B *Streptococcus* in healthy women, *J Infect Dis* 182:1129-1138, 2000.
556. Baker CJ, Paoletti LC, Rench MA, et al: Immune response of healthy women to 2 different group B streptococcal type V capsular polysaccharide-protein conjugate vaccines, *J Infect Dis* 189:1103-1112, 2004.
557. Baker CJ, Rench MA, Fernandez M, et al: Safety and immunogenicity of a bivalent group B streptococcal conjugate vaccine for serotypes II and III, *J Infect Dis* 188:66-73, 2003.
558. Baker CJ, Rench MA, McInnes P: Immunization of pregnant women with group B streptococcal type III capsular polysaccharide-tetanus toxoid conjugate vaccine, *Vaccine* 21:3468-3472, 2003.

559. Michel JL, Madoff LC, Kling DE, et al: Cloned alpha and beta C-protein antigens of group B streptococci elicit protective immunity, *Infect Immun* 59:2023-2028, 1991.
560. Pannaraj PS, Kelly JK, Madoff LC, et al: Group B *Streptococcus* bacteremia elicits beta C protein-specific IgM and IgG in humans, *J Infect Dis* 195:353-356, 2007.
561. Pannaraj PS, Kelly JK, Rench MA, et al: Alpha C protein-specific immunity in humans with group B streptococcal colonization and invasive disease, *Vaccine* 26:502-508, 2008.
562. Yang HH, Madoff LC, Guttormsen HK, et al: Recombinant group B streptococcus beta C protein and a variant with the deletion of its immunoglobulin A-binding site are protective mouse maternal vaccines and effective carriers in conjugate vaccines, *Infect Immun* 75:3455-3461, 2007.
563. Larsson C, Holmgren J, Lindahl G, et al: Intranasal immunization of mice with group B streptococcal protein Rib and cholera toxin B subunit confers protection against lethal infection, *Infect Immun* 72:1184-1187, 2004.
564. Martin D, Rioux S, Gagnon E, et al: Protection from group B streptococcal infection in neonatal mice by maternal immunization with recombinant Sip protein, *Infect Immun* 70:4897-4901, 2002.
565. Cheng Q, Debol S, Lam H, et al: Immunization with C5a peptidase or peptidase-type III polysaccharide conjugate vaccines enhances clearance of group B streptococci from lungs of infected mice, *Infect Immun* 70:6409-6415, 2002.
566. Martins E, Melo-Cristino J, Ramirez M: Distribution of pilus islands in *Streptococcus agalactiae* that cause human infections: insights into evolution and implication for vaccine development, *Clin Vaccine Immunol* 20:313-316, 2013.
567. Stratton KR, Durch JS, Lawrence RS, editors: Committee to Study Priorities for Vaccine Development, Division of Health Promotion and Disease Prevention, Institute of Medicine: Vaccines for the 21st century: a tool for decisionmaking, Washington, DC, 1999, National Academy of Sciences.
568. Kogan G, Uhrín Dusan, Brisson Jean-Robert, et al: Structure of the type VI group B *Streptococcus* capsular polysaccharide determined by high resolution NMR spectroscopy, *J Carbohydr Chem* 13: 1071-1078, 1994.
569. Adair CE, Kowalsky L, Quon H, et al: Risk factors for early-onset group B streptococcal disease in neonates: a population-based case-control study, *Can Med Assoc J* 169:198-203, 2003.
570. Baker CJ, Webb BJ, Kasper DL, et al: The natural history of group B streptococcal colonization in the pregnant woman and her offspring. II. Determination of serum antibody to capsular polysaccharide from type III group B *Streptococcus*, *Am J Obstet Gynecol* 137:39-42, 1980.
571. Boyer KM, Gadzala CA, Burd LI, et al: Selective intrapartum chemoprophylaxis of neonatal group B streptococcal early-onset disease. I. Epidemiologic rationale, *J Infect Dis* 148:795-801, 1983.
572. Cueva JP, Egel RT: Anterior fontanel herniation in group B *Streptococcus* meningitis in newborns, *Pediatr Neurol* 10:332-334, 1994.
573. Schimmel MS, Schlesinger Y, Berger I, et al: Transverse myelitis: unusual sequelae of neonatal group B streptococcus disease, *J Perinatol* 22:580-581, 2002.
574. Ellenbogen RG, Goldmann DA, Winston KR: Group B streptococcal infections of the central nervous system in infants with myelomeningocele, *Surg Neurol* 29:237-242, 1988.
575. Mukherjee S, Askwith JK: Transient isolated oculomotor nerve paralysis in neonatal group B streptococcal meningitis, *J Paediatr Child Health* 44:231-232, 2008.
576. McAdams RM, Simone S, Grant G, et al: Ventricular peritoneal shunt infection resulting from group B streptococcus, *Pediatr Crit Care Med* 7:586-588, 2006.
577. Ramsey PG, Zwerdling R: Asymptomatic neonatal bacteremia, *N Engl J Med* 295:225, 1977.
578. Roberts KB: Persistent group B *Streptococcus* bacteremia without clinical "sepsis" in infants, *J Pediatr* 88:1059-1060, 1976.
579. Poschl JM, Hellstern G, Ruef P, et al: Ophthalmia neonatorum caused by group B *Streptococcus*, *Scand J Infect Dis* 34:921-922, 2002.
580. Klusmann A, Engelbrecht V, Unsöld R, et al: Retrobulbar abscess in a neonate, *Neuropediatrics* 32:219-220, 2001.
581. Rench MA, Baker CJ: Group B streptococcal breast abscess in a mother and mastitis in her infant, *Obstet Gynecol* 73:875-877, 1989.
582. Brian MJ, O'Ryan M, Waagner D: Prepatellar bursitis in an infant caused by group B *Streptococcus*, *Pediatr Infect Dis J* 11:502-503, 1992.
583. Ruiz-Gomez D, Tarpay MM, Riley HD: Recurrent group B streptococcal infections: report of three cases, *Scand J Infect Dis* 11:35-38, 1979.
584. Frieden IJ: Blistering dactylitis caused by group B streptococci, *Pediatr Dermatol* 6:300-302, 1989.
585. Turner MC, Naumburg EG: Acute renal failure in the neonate: two fatal cases due to group B streptococci with rhabdomyolysis, *Clin Pediatr (Phila)* 26:189-190, 1987.

13 Listeriosis

TOBIAS R. KOLLMANN, TIMOTHY L. MAILMAN, and ROBERT BORTOLUSSI

CHAPTER OUTLINE

Listeria monocytogenes is a serious and sometimes lethal pathogen, especially for pregnant women and their fetuses, the newborn, and for older adults and immunocompromised individuals.[1]

The pathogen was first described in 1926 by Murray and colleagues[2] during an investigation of an epizootic outbreak of infection in laboratory rabbit and guinea pigs. Human disease caused by *L. monocytogenes* was identified in 1929 by Nyfeldt.[3] The present name is derived from the fact that monocytosis develops in less than 24 hours after intravenous infection in experimental animals.[4] Although there is some controversy over the name *"Listeria,"* it is commonly believed that it was named in honor of British surgeon Joseph Lister.[5,6] Although Burn already recognized *L. monocytogenes* as a serious pathogen for human newborns in 1936,[7] the first confirmed transmission from animals to humans was only documented in 1983.[8] A recent upsurge in outbreaks in the human population has refocused attention on this organism.[1]

The Organism

Listeria organisms are regular, short, facultatively anaerobic, non–spore-forming, gram-positive rods that are motile and form bluish gray colonies on nutrient agar. They are non–acid fast, catalase-positive but do not branch or form capsules.[9] Of six *Listeria* spp. (*L. monocytogenes, Listeria innocua, Listeria grayi, Listeria welshimeri, Listeria seeligeri,* and *Listeria ivanovii*), *L. monocytogenes* is the most important human pathogen[10,11]; the few case reports regarding other species causing infection typically involve immunocompromised hosts.[12] Peritrichous flagella enable most *Listeria* species to exhibit tumbling motility at 25° C to 30° C; this motility helps clinical laboratories distinguish *Listeria* from morphologically similar microbes, such as *Corynebacterium* and *Erysipelothrix*.[9] Inoculated semisolid motility media reveal a distinctive "umbrella" or "swarming" pattern at room temperature.[13] Expression of flagellin (and thus motility) in most clinical isolates is turned off at 37° C.[13,14] On sheep blood agar, *L. monocytogenes* exhibits a narrow zone of β-hemolysis (nonhemolytic strains exist) and a rectangular area of increased hemolysis when streaked on blood agar in proximity to *Staphylococcus aureus* (the Christie, Atkins, Munch-Peterson [CAMP] test).[9] *Listeria* tolerate low temperatures, high salt concentrations, and high (alkaline) pH, which allows replication in soil, water, sewage, manure, animal feed, and, most importantly, refrigerated foods.[10,15-17] The entire genome of *L. monocytogenes* has been sequenced.[18,19]

TYPING

Historically, *L. monocytogenes* strain typing has been based on somatic (O) and flagellar (H) antigens. This system discriminates 13 serotypes, many of which represent genetically diverse groups of strains. Only four serotypes (1/2a, 1/2b, 1/2c, and 4b) cause most human listeriosis.[20-22] Multilocus sequence typing (MLST) is emerging as a genotyping tool, with both the power to discriminate different lineages and the ability to provide a standardized global approach to defining clones and clonal complexes. Epidemic clones (ECs) of *L. monocytogenes* are typically defined as isolates of a presumably common ancestor that are genetically related and involved in temporally and geographically unrelated outbreaks.[23] Recent application of MLST to 300 isolates from five continents revealed a partitioning of genotypic diversity between clinical isolates, on one hand, and food or environmental isolates, on the other, while simultaneously identifying the existence of a few prevalent and globally distributed clones.[24]

Epidemiology

The United States Department of Agriculture projects approximately 2500 cases of serious *Listeria* infection per year in the United States, with a mortality of approximately 20% (compared with 13,000 cases of salmonellosis [0.4% mortality], *Campylobacter* [0.1% mortality], and *Yersinia* [0.01% mortality]).[25] In the United States alone, illness caused by *L. monocytogenes* costs $2.6 billion annually and leads to loss of 9400 quality-adjusted life-years.[26] Most infections are sporadic and have no known epidemiologic explanation,[27] but *Listeria* is the leading cause of death resulting from foodborne infection in the United States as well as several European countries.[28-31] Although promotion of preventative measures, as well as monitoring and voluntary recall of contaminated food products, has resulted in a reduction in the prevalence of listeriosis over recent decades, risk for foodborne infection remains high,[1] and the incidence in older adults has in fact increased again.[32-34]

NATURAL RESERVOIR AND TRANSMISSION TO HUMANS

Listeria species are ubiquitous in nature, with their natural habitat in decaying plant matter.[35] Spoiled silage appears to be a source of infection for ruminant animals.[36] Although direct transmission of *L. monocytogenes* to humans from infected animals has been described,[37,38] most human infections are acquired through ingestion of contaminated food.[39,40] *L. monocytogenes* isolates from clinical and food specimens are highly heterogenous; this suggests that infection does not simply reflect a few highly virulent subtypes of *Listeria*.[41]

Asymptomatic fecal carriage in healthy humans after ingestion of contaminated foods in nonoutbreak settings has been reported, with a prevalence of 2% to 10%, but is higher during outbreaks[1,42-45]; carriage may be as high as 26% in household contacts of patients with listeriosis.[40] Dissemination of *L. monocytogenes* from colonized humans can also occasionally play a role in transmission.[46] Maternal colonization does not invariably lead to invasive illness of the fetus or newborn,[47] but transmission of *L. monocytogenes* from mother to fetus is believed to occur in utero via infected amniotic fluid or the maternal circulation.[1]

NOSOCOMIAL TRANSMISSION

Although most cases of listeriosis occur in the community, nosocomial listeriosis in both neonates and adults has been described.[48-58] Person-to-person transmission caused by suboptimal infection control is likely to be responsible for most of these small clusters. Among clusters reported in newborns, the index case may manifest as early-onset infection, and subsequent cases appear as late-onset listeriosis. Multiple cases of early-onset disease in the same hospital unit would suggest the possibility of foodborne or another common source.[59]

RISK FACTORS FOR SEVERE LISTERIOSIS

Community-acquired listeriosis may occur spontaneously in adult subjects with no known underlying predisposing conditions[60] but only at a relatively low frequency, ranging from 0.1 to 11 per 1,000,000 persons.[61-65] In high-risk populations, such as the newborn, the elderly, and adults with immunocompromised function, incidence of infection and associated morbidity and mortality is high (Box 13-1). The list of specific immune defects associated with an increased risk for severe *Listeria* infection is long and includes defects in gastrointestinal defense, cell-autonomous immunity, and innate as well as adaptive systemic immunity.[66-77] Among patients with human immunodeficiency virus (HIV) infection in the era before antiretroviral therapy, a 400- to 1000-fold increased risk of suffering systemic invasive listeriosis, compared with HIV-negative subjects, has been documented.[16] The clinical use of anti–tumor necrosis factor (TNF) or TNF receptor antibodies has more recently been identified as a risk factor for severe infection with *L. monocytogenes*.[78,79] Alcoholism, diabetes, and cirrhosis[80] also increase risk for infection.

Listeriosis is 18 times more common in pregnant (12/100,000) than nonpregnant women (0.7/100,000), and overall 16% to 27% of all infections with *L. monocytogenes* occur in pregnancy.[1,47,81,82] This occurs despite no differences in carriage rates of fecal or vaginal specimens between pregnant and nonpregnant individuals.[83] The underlying factors leading to an increase in susceptibility to listeriosis during pregnancy remain unknown.

Box 13-1 People at High Risk of Listeriosis

Pregnant Women[1,47,81-83]

- The risk of listeriosis is about 20 times higher among pregnant women than among nonpregnant healthy adults.
- About one third of listeriosis cases are diagnosed in pregnant women.
- Pregnant women with listeriosis are at increased risk of spontaneous abortion, preterm delivery, or stillbirth.

Newborns[1,63,70-72,75,82,84-92]

- Newborns are at greater risk of developing severe infection than pregnant women.
- Newborns may present clinically with
  - Early-onset listeriosis (transmitted via placenta and usually diagnosed as sepsis in the first day of life).
  - Late-onset infection (≥7 days of life).

Nonpregnant Adults[16,66-77,80]

- About 50% of all cases occur at age 60 years or older.
- Immunocompromised patients.
- People with cancer, diabetes, or kidney disease.
- People with human immunodeficiency virus/acquired immunodeficiency syndrome: Listeriosis is up to 300 times more likely to occur in this group than in healthy adults.
- Patients receiving immunosuppressive drug therapy (e.g., high-dose glucocorticosteroid, tumor necrosis factor inhibitor).
- Transplant patients receiving antirejection drug therapy.

The most common and thus relevant predisposition to severe listeriosis, however, is age, in that the very young and very old are at highest risk.[1,84-86] Perinatal and newborn infections represent 30% to 40% of the total caseload in humans.[87,88] Furthermore, symptomatic listeriosis has an exceptionally high mortality rate in the unborn, the newborn, and the elderly, ranging from 20% to greater than 60%.[63,82] The annual incidence of reported perinatal and neonatal listeriosis in nonoutbreak settings ranges between 2 to 13 per 100,000 live births[72,89-91]; during outbreaks, incidence can be as high 1% to 2% of all deliveries.[70,71] However, the true incidence is probably much higher because abortion and stillbirth caused by *Listeria* go largely unrecognized because bacterial cultures are not obtained routinely in these cases. The reasons for this increased susceptibility at the extreme ends of the age spectrum have only partially been delineated.[75,92]

Pathogenesis

As for most infectious pathogens, the risk of developing clinical disease depends on intensity of the exposure, virulence of the organism, and the ability of the host to defend against infection.

EXPOSURE

Infection with *L. monocytogenes* begins with the ingestion of the bacteria. Bacterial load, measured as a function of the inoculum of *L. monocytogenes*, has been mathematically linked to increased risk for infection and confirmed by finding of a significantly elevated concentration of *Listeria* in contaminated foods during outbreaks.[93] All of this suggests that dose likely matters.[8,94] The infectious dose is estimated to be 10^4 to 10^6 organisms (colony forming units [CFU])/g of ingested food, but may be as low as 10 CFU/g in immunocompromised hosts and patients who have diminished gastric acidity or have an injured intestinal lining.[43,45,70,95-99]

VIRULENCE

Clinical risk for invasive listeriosis is influenced by the pathogenic potential of the infecting strain. For example, among the many *L. monocytogenes* strains, serovars 1/2a, 1/2b, and 4b are responsible for 95% of human infections, and most outbreaks are caused by strains of serovar 4b.[100] In tracing the journey of the organism from ingestion through to successful replication in the host, an array of virulence factors comes into play.[101] Survival of *Listeria* in the human gastrointestinal tract has been tightly linked to bacterial sigma factor σ^B.[102,103] σ^B drives expression of enzymes that permit bacterial survival in the acidic upper gastrointestinal tract[104,105]; the alkaline, bilious environment of the proximal small intestine,[106-110] as well as the high salt concentrations throughout the gastrointestinal tract.[111-113] The transit across the mucosal barrier begins with adhesion of *L. monocytogenes* to the mucosal lining via the Ami surface protein.[114,115] After adhesion, *L. monocytogenes* enters intestinal target cells either through phagocytosis (for M cells) or through actions of additional listerial surface proteins (for intestinal epithelial cells) called internalins.[116,117] Among the 25 internalin-like proteins,[118-120] InlA and InlB are the most important. InlA binds to the host adhesion protein E-cadherin. E-cadherin is transiently exposed to the luminal surface of the intestinal villi during remodeling of epithelial junctions and goblet cells (GCs), thereby offering an entry point to *L. monocytogenes* in the gut.[121,122] In addition to its established role in crossing of the intestinal barrier, InlA also appears to be involved in the crossing of the maternofetal placental barrier by binding to E-cadherin–expressing syncytiotrophoblasts.[123] *Listeria* rapidly transcytoses across the intestinal epithelium and is released in the lamina propria by exocytosis, from where it disseminates systemically[122] without histologic evidence of significant inflammation in the bowel wall.[85]

Infection of the liver is facilitated by the bacterial adhesin FbpA,[124] which binds to human fibronectin expressed on the surface hepatocytes.[125] Listerial internalin B (InlB) then engages the host hepatocyte growth factor receptor (a tyrosine kinase receptor, Met) and complement component C1q receptor,[126,127] which mediates hepatocyte entry via endocytosis.[20,116,128-134] In addition to intestinal enterocytes and hepatocytes, *Listeria* can also infect, grow, and spread in fibroblasts, epithelial cells, vascular endothelial cells, and renal tubular epithelial cells.[116,135] However, although invasion efficiency varies with host cell type, it never reaches the entry rate observed in phagocytes.[20] M cells, monocytes, macrophages, and dendritic cells are infected in all organs and are the main carriers of *L. monocytogenes* during its systemic spread.[66,136] Entry of *L. monocytogenes* into these cells occurs via phagocytosis,[68] initiated after lipoteichoic acid, a component of the listerial cell wall, is bound by type I/II scavenger receptors and/or complement receptors.[137]

During the early course of infection, *L. monocytogenes* resides within a vacuole (for nonphagocytic cells) or a phagosome (in monocyte/macrophage-derived cells) (Fig. 13-1).[135,138,139] The escape of *L. monocytogenes* from the single-layer membrane vacuoles/phagosomes is assisted by two virulence-associated bacterial molecules: listeriolysin O (LLO) and phosphatidylinositol–phospholipase C (PlcA).[140] LLO is encoded in the *hly* gene cluster, and in mice, but not humans, is essential for bacterial escape from vacuoles.[141,142] LLO is a secreted cholesterol–dependent cytolysin (CDC) toxin that binds the phagosomal membrane as cholesterol-associated monomers that oligomerize into large complexes and then penetrate the membrane, forming a pore.[143,144] The pores also lead to increased pH and decreased calcium ion (Ca^{2+}) concentration within the phagosomal compartment, inhibiting phagosome maturation.[145] Because the activity of LLO is optimal at the acidic pH of the phagosome, it is less active at the neutral pH of the cytoplasm, preventing excessive cell damage. As with other CDCs, LLO is a potent signaling protein that can activate important pathways, such as nuclear factor kappa B,[146] mitogen-activated protein kinase,[147] and protein kinase C.[146,148] In animal models, LLO is required in vivo for bacterial growth in placental trophoblastic cells and for subsequent fetal invasion.[149]

The C-type phospholipases, phosphatidylinositol-specific (PI-PLC) and a broad-range phosphatidylcholine (PC-PLC), mediate *L. monocytogenes* escape from the vacuole/phagosome by digesting the phagosomal membrane.[150-154] Although the two phospholipases act synergistically with LLO to lyse primary and secondary vacuoles, allowing *L.*

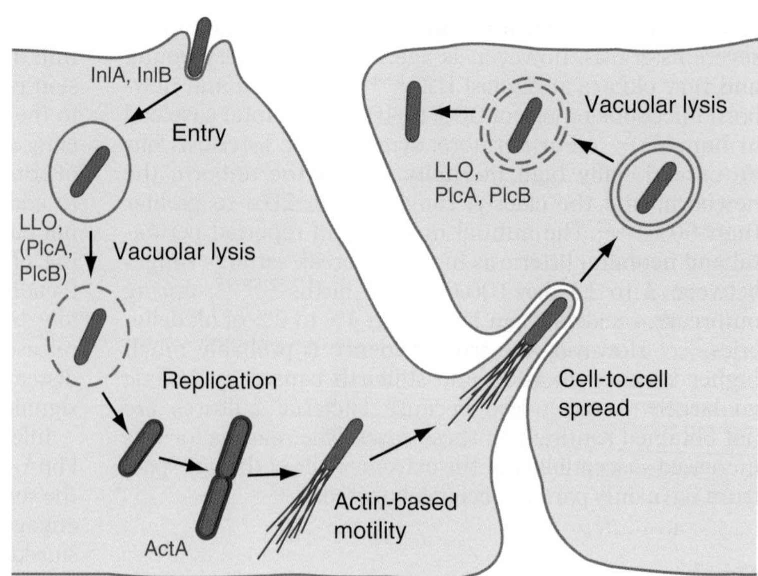

Figure 13-1 Intracellular cell cycle of *Listeria monocytogenes. L. monocytogenes* binds to epithelial host cells and promotes its own uptake in a process mediated by the two bacterial surface proteins InlA and InlB. The secreted pore-forming toxin listeriolysin O (LLO) (together with the bacterial phospholipases PlcA and PlcB, depending on the cell type and species) promotes vacuolar rupture and bacterial escape to the cytoplasm, where *L. monocytogenes* can replicate efficiently. Surface expression of ActA allows intracellular bacteria to polymerize host cell actin and to generate actin comet tails, which propel *L. monocytogenes* through the cytoplasm and through membrane protrusions into neighboring cells. There, bacteria localize in a double-membrane vacuole, which can be lysed by LLO, PlcA, and PlcB to start a new infection cycle. (From Pizarro-Cerda J, Kuhbacher A, Cossart P: Entry of *Listeria monocytogenes* in mammalian epithelial cells: an updated view, *Cold Spring Harb Perspect Med* 2:pii:a010009, 2012.)

monocytogenes to escape into the cytoplasm.[155-157] The C-type phospholipase PlcB promotes lysis of the human primary vacuole even in the absence of LLO[156,158] and directly inhibits downstream signaling.[159-161] *L. monocytogenes* also requires host factors to assist in bacterial escape from the phagosome.[139] Although *Listeria* activates host antimicrobial nitric oxide (NO), normally important in the degradation of phagocytosed bacteria, in the case of *L. monocytogenes* infection, NO instead leads to downregulation of the vacuolar-type H^+–adenosine triphosphatase (ATP)ase (V-ATPase), which in turn inhibits maturation of the secondary phagolysosome and aids bacterial escape into the cytoplasm.[162]

Once free in the cytoplasm, *L. monocytogenes* co-opts host-provided nutrients necessary for its intracellular multiplication. In the cytoplasm *L. monocytogenes* also induces polymerization of host actin filaments to move within the cytoplasm and to spread from cell to cell.[163-166] The bacterial surface protein ActA is the only bacterial determinant necessary for host actin-based motility of *L. monocytogenes.*[167,168] It binds and activates the host Arp2/3 complex, inducing actin polymerization.[169-171] ActA is primarily involved in driving *Listeria* toward the cytoplasmic membrane, where the bacterium is then enveloped in filopodium-like structures (also termed a listeriopod) that are engulfed by adjacent cells, leading to the formation of secondary double-layer membrane vacuoles.[172-175] In human cells, PlcB-mediated lysis of the secondary (now double-layer membrane) vacuoles initiates a new cycle of infection.[176] *L. monocytogenes* does not always have to escape the phagosome but can replicate inside modified vacuoles called SLAPs (spacious *Listeria*-containing phagosomes)[177,178]; however, the rate of bacterial replication inside SLAPs is reduced (>8 hours) compared with bacterial replication in the cytosol (<30 minutes).[173]

Invasion of the placenta is a crucial element in the pathogenesis of congenital listeriosis. E-cadherin is expressed on villous cytotrophoblasts and in localized areas of the basal plasma membrane of syncytiotrophoblasts.[123] Syncytiotrophoblasts are directly exposed to maternal blood in the intervillous space and are considered a form of specialized endothelium. InlA is required for *L. monocytogenes* to cross the human maternofetal barrier,[123,179-181] which in part explains the specific tropism of the organism for the placenta.[123] InlB facilitates the transfer of *L. monocytogenes* across placenta,[123,182,183] a process that also involves ActA[149] and the host mannose receptor C type 1.[184]

The mechanisms by which *Listeria* accesses the central nervous system (CNS) remain poorly understood, but two major routes of infection have been proposed.[185] A retrograde neural route is likely to occur in ruminants upon crossing of the oral epithelium, and this probably accounts for the observation that *Listeria* induces almost exclusively rhombencephalitis in these animals.[186] In contrast, the hematogenous route is likely the more frequent in humans, in whom bacteria circulating in the blood, either free or associated with phagocytes, are thought to breach the blood-brain barrier. Only In1B and In1A have been clearly implicated in facilitating the transfer of *L. monocytogenes* across the blood–brain barrier.[187]

Regulation of Bacterial Virulence Gene Expression

The genes that encode the most prominent virulence-associated proteins—LLO, ActA, PlcA, and PlcB—are situated adjacent to each other in a 9.6 kb virulence gene cluster [188] that is principally regulated by a pleiotropic virulence regulator PrfA. [189] PrfA's function is regulated by temperature[190]: At a temperature lower than 30° C, the untranslated region of *prfA* mRNA adopts a stable secondary structure that prevents binding of the ribosome and blocks translation. In the host, the temperature of 37° C induces melting of the secondary structure; consequently, PrfA is translated and activates virulence gene expression.[191] There are yet other mechanisms involved in regulating the virulence of *Listeria;* for most of these, the mechanisms are not fully understood.[46,192]

HOST RESPONSE

Although human exposures to *Listeria* are common occurrences,[193] most infections are sporadic and have no epidemiologic explanation[27]; this suggests that casual exposure to the same strains of *Listeria* can lead to severe infection only if a host exhibits particular vulnerabilities.[70,71] The fact that specific age groups suffer a much higher risk of severe outcome suggests that inherent deficiencies of defense against *L. monocytogenes* exist in the host defense of the pregnant, the newborn, and the older versus the young adult.[92] However, the mechanisms leading to this susceptibility are incompletely understood.[75] *L. monocytogenes* has been used extensively in mouse infection models to elucidate the inner workings of the host response to pathogenic challenge. And although mice mimic certain aspects of human immunity and pathogen susceptibility, the model has limitations for *L. monocytogenes*.[194-198] Knowledge about the human response to *Listeria* infection is confined primarily to results obtained from in vitro experiments.[75] Differences between the neonatal and adult innate and adaptive host immune response to *L. monocytogenes* infection undoubtedly contribute to their difference in clinical response.[92,199] However, from plants to humans, the ability to control infection at the level of an individual cell equates firmly with survival of the host[200]; this capacity for cell intrinsic self-defense is called cell-autonomous immunity.[200-202] Elegant experiments conducted in mice decades ago already clearly identified that age-dependent susceptibility to primary infection with *L. monocytogenes* correlates best with age-dependent differences in the function of monocytes and macrophages.[203,204] Since then, we have learned that for the host not to succumb to *L. monocytogenes*, monocytes and macrophages have to rapidly trap and kill the ingested bacteria.[20,66,68]

Cell Autonomous Immunity

From the moment *L. monocytogenes* adheres to a target host cell, a response is set into motion that aims to restrict bacterial invasion and survival. In macrophages, *L. monocytogenes* activates at least three pathways[67]: (1) a MyD88-dependent pathway emanating from the cell surface and phagosome, leading to expression of cytokines and reactive oxygen species; (2) a stimulator of interferon genes (STING)/interferon regulatory factor (IRF)3–dependent pathway emanating from the cytosol, leading to the expression of type 1 interferon (IFN) and coregulated genes; and (3) an absent in melanoma 2 (AIM2)/caspase-1–dependent inflammasome pathway, resulting in proteolytic activation and secretion of interleukin (IL)-1 and IL-18 and pyroptotic cell death. The outcome of the host-cell pathogen molecular tug of war depends on the speed of phagosome maturation versus listerial escape from the phagosome.[205] Phagosomal escape can occur as rapidly as 30 minutes after bacterial cell entry[139]; this does not leave much time for the host cell autonomous immune response. Despite their central importance to host defense, the molecular mechanisms involved in the human cell autonomous response are currently unknown.[75]

Systemic Immunity

Molecules released by the infected and dying cells recruit neutrophils, which in turn destroy extracellular bacteria and digest dying cells.[206] This process also leads to formation of granulomas at sites of infection, thereby "walling off the infection."[68] These innate immune effector cascades limit the spread of *L. monocytogenes* during the early phase of infection. In the immune-competent host-adaptive person, T-cell immune responses peak about 1 week after primary infection, leading to complete clearance of infected cells; this process also leads to acquired resistance to subsequent infection (immune memory).[207] Acquired immunity is not dependent on clinical symptomatic infection because T cells specific for *L. monocytogenes* are frequently present in healthy individuals without history of listeriosis.[71,208-212]

Innate Immune Response. The first line of defense against *Listeria* is the gastrointestinal barrier.[213] Within intestinal crypts, Paneth cells produce antimicrobial effectors, including lysozyme, phospholipase A2, and α-defensins, whereas squamous mucosal keratinocytes express calprotectin.[214] Ménard and colleagues[215] described an antimicrobially active form of a host defense peptide, called CRAMP (cathelin-related antimicrobial peptide), in the epithelium of neonatal mice, which is expressed constitutively during the first weeks of life only and provides significant protection against listerial growth in the gut.

Within infected tissues, bacteria are initially taken up by resident macrophages, which produce chemokines to promote recruitment of blood monocytes and neutrophils to the site of infection.[216] After migration into the tissues, neutrophils kill extracellular bacteria through secretion of bactericidal granules, lipocalin,[217] and neutrophil extracellular traps (NETs).[218-220] Monocytes/macrophages are also the main source of TNF-α and reactive oxygen and nitrogen species, which are crucial for a protective response.[221-223] In mice, neonatal susceptibility correlates with delayed systemic production of innate cytokines and activation of natural killer cells.[203,204,224] Innate cytokine responses of human neonates also markedly differ from those of adults, but their exact role in the increased susceptibility of the human neonate to systemic listeriosis remains to be determined.[92]

Adaptive Immune Response. Several diseases or medications that interfere with cell-mediated immunity are known to increase susceptibility to systemic listeriosis[71]; disorders of the adaptive humoral immune system (immunoglobulin) are, however, not associated with excessive prevalence of listeriosis.[1] This suggests a central role of the adaptive cell-mediated immune system in defense against *L. monocytogenes* in the human host. Cytotoxic T lymphocytes (CD8 phenotype) can destroy *Listeria*-infected cells,[225,226] and the development of T-helper (Th; CD4 phenotype) cell subsets during the immune response is pivotal as they produce IFNγ, which makes tissue resident macrophages more effective at killing ingested bacteria.[68,224] Some crucial mediators of adaptive immune defense against *Listeria* appear to differ qualitatively or quantitatively in neonates.[199] Neonatal $CD4^+$ T cells are less prone to produce IFNγ.[199,227] In addition, neonatal $CD4^+$ Th1 cells undergo apoptosis when reexposed to antigen.[228] Finally, the reduced production of innate IL-12p70 and increased production of IL-10 by neonatal innate cells upon stimulation is expected to lead to suboptimal activation of T cells and thus increased susceptibility to listeriosis.[92]

Host Response to *Listeria* During Pregnancy

Pregnant females have an approximately 20-fold greater risk of acquiring listeriosis.[229,230] Although the duration of listeriosis is almost twice as long in gestating animals than in control groups,[231] immune memory to *Listeria* in pregnant mice is not reduced in spleen or liver but only locally at the placental interphase, suggesting that local immunosuppressive effects that also play a role in prevention of rejection of the fetal graft, play a role in the increased susceptibility to *Listeria* infection during pregnancy.[232] Perhaps not surprising then was the finding that similar immune memory responses can be found among mothers and infants surviving natural *Listeria* infection.[233] In mice, *L. monocytogenes* infection induces reductions in maternal Foxp3$^+$ regulatory T-cell suppression, with ensuing disruptions in fetal tolerance, which play critical roles in pathogenesis of immune-mediated fetal wastage.[234]

Pathology

The gross and microscopic appearance of the placenta in listeriosis, although not pathognomic, is sufficiently distinct to enable a presumptive diagnosis by the experienced pathologist (Fig. 13-2)[235] Massive involvement of the liver, covered in grayish yellow nodules is typical.[86] Analogous findings are observed in the spleen, adrenal glands, lungs, esophagus, posterior pharyngeal wall, tonsils, lymph nodes, thymus, bone marrow, myocardium, testes, and skeletal muscles. The intestinal tract is affected to a variable degree, with a preference for the lymphatic structures of the small intestine and appendix. Cutaneous lesions of neonatal listeriosis occur most commonly on the back and lumbar region[236] (Figs.13-3 and 13-4). In listeriosis of the central nervous system, granuloma formation is also typical.[237] Histologically, the granuloma's *(listerioma)* center is necrotic, and the periphery contains an abundance of chronic inflammatory cells. *Listeria* is present in variable numbers within these necrotic foci and can be demonstrated with a Gram stain or Levaditi silver impregnation.

Listeria placentitis is characterized grossly by multiple minute white or gray necrotic areas within the villous parenchyma and deciduas, the largest tending to occur in basal villi and the decidua basalis.[235,238,239] Typically, localized collections of polymorphonuclear leukocytes are

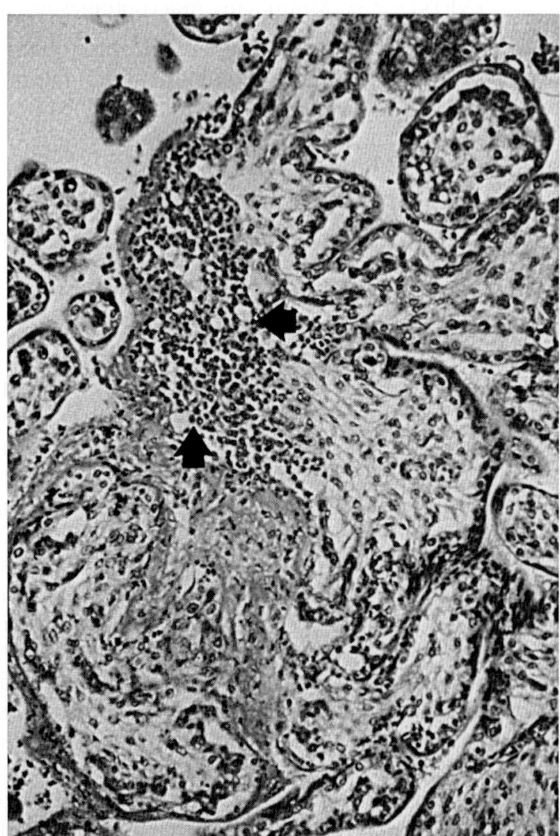

Figure 13-2 *Listeria* placentitis. Note the microabscess between the necrotic villous trophoblast and the stroma *(arrows)*. Chorionic villi are enmeshed by intervillous and inflammatory material. (Courtesy IWK Health Centre, Pathology Department, Halifax, Nova Scotia, Canada.)

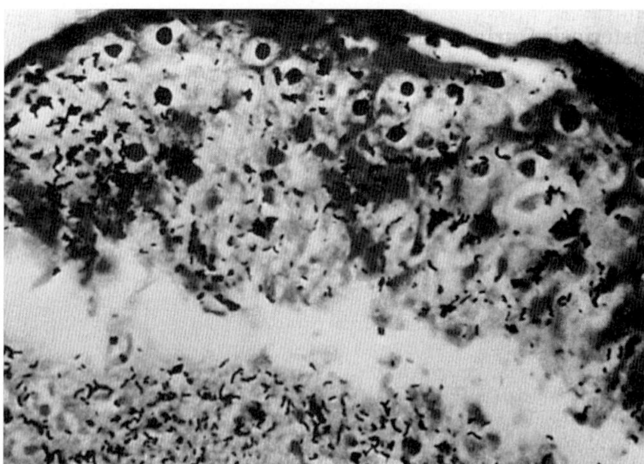

Figure 13-3 Cutaneous listeriosis. Note the numerous gram-positive rods that extend from the dermis below into the epidermis above. (Courtesy IWK Health Centre, Pathology Department, Halifax, Nova Scotia, Canada.)

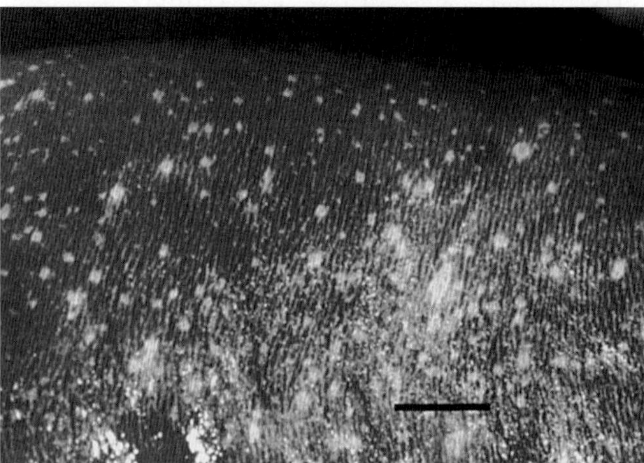

Figure 13-4 Rash of neonatal *Listeria monocytogenes* infection. Areas of small, elevated, pale pustules surrounded by a deep-red erythematous base seen on the abdomen of a premature neonate. (Horizontal bar: ≈1 cm.) (Courtesy Dr. Robert Bortolussi, IWK Health Centre, Halifax, Nova Scotia, Canada.)

found between the villous trophoblast and stroma, and inflamed or necrotic chorionic villi are enmeshed in intervillous inflammatory material and fibrin. Chorioamnionitis, deciduitis, villitis, and funisitis (in order of frequency) are seen. Cord lesions may be confined to superficial foci. Gram-positive rods are usually demonstrable within the necrotic centers of villous and decidual microabscesses, as well as within the membranes and umbilical cord.

Clinical Manifestations

Clinical symptomatic infection with *L. monocytogenes* is called listeriosis[95] and exists in two forms, depending on the immunologic status of the host: noninvasive gastrointestinal listeriosis and invasive listeriosis.[63,70,176] In immunocompetent children and adults, noninvasive listeriosis develops as a febrile gastroenteritis.[45,95] However, in vulnerable groups, such as the pregnant female and her unborn fetus, newborns, infants up to approximately 2 months of age,[240] adults older than 60 years, and some immune compromised children and adults,[63,70] *L. monocytogenes* can enter into the systemic circulation and spread to other parts of the body.[70] The main target organs are the placenta, liver, and spleen as well as the central nervous system.[46,71] This clinical pattern of invasive listeriosis derives from the unique capacity of *L. monocytogenes* to cross three barriers: the intestinal, blood-brain, and placental barriers.[180]

LISTERIOSIS IN PREGNANCY

Although maternal symptoms of infection may be pronounced at the time of delivery, symptoms in the mother usually subside with delivery, with or without antibiotic treatment. Clinically identified cases of maternal listeriosis become more readily identifiable after the fifth month of pregnancy; yet even then, approximately one third of infected patients remain clinically asymptomatic.[82,241] In two thirds of infected pregnancies, symptoms precede onset of labor by 2 to 14 days. Of those symptomatic, 65% have fever, 30% a "flulike" illness, 20% back pain (which may be mistaken for a urinary tract infection), 10% headache, 7% vomiting/diarrhea, and 4% muscle pains or sore throat.[1] Spontaneous abortion occurs in 10% to 20% of clinically symptomatic listeriosis cases during pregnancy; the prognosis for stillbirth is worse if infection occurs early in pregnancy (overall 11% end in intrauterine fetal demise).[241] Another approximately 50% deliver preterm (average length of gestation < 35 weeks in approximately 70% of cases).[82] Thirty-four percent of infected pregnancies demonstrate fetal distress, and 75% display meconium-stained amniotic fluid.[1] However, early treatment of *Listeria* sepsis in pregnancy can prevent infection and sequelae in the fetus and newborn.[242]

Neonatal Listeriosis

The first descriptions of neonatal listeriosis were published in the 1930s by Burn.[7,243,244] Since then, neonatal infection has been recognized as the most common clinical form of human listeriosis. As with group B streptococcal (GBS)infection, neonatal listeriosis is divided into two clinical forms, defined by age at onset: early-onset (≤1 week of age) and late-onset (>1 week of age) infection. However, in contrast to GBS infection, fecal carriage of *Listeria* does not lead to colonization of the genital tract.[245,246] Clinical and laboratory manifestations of neonatal listeriosis are outlined in Table 13-1, based on clinical cases in which early and late onset of the disease could be differentiated.[21,50,88,90,247-254]

Early-Onset Neonatal Listeriosis

Early onset infection (<7 days of life) accounts for the majority of cases (62%).[82] *L. monocytogenes* was responsible for 6% of all sepsis cases presenting in the first 48 hours of life in a network of U.K. neonatal units and for 4% of early-onset neonatal meningitis in Australasia.[82]

Approximately two thirds of newborns born to mothers infected late in pregnancy develop early-onset disease.[82] The association of early-onset listeriosis with prematurity and maternal infection suggests the presence of intrauterine infection. The frequent presence of chorioamnionitis in the absence of ruptured membranes[90,255] supports the hypothesis of *Listeria* infection occurring by a transplacental route. However, because the heaviest foci for neonatal infection are lung and gut, the fetus may also be infected by swallowing contaminated amniotic fluid.[256] In 50% to 74% of early-onset cases, the mother reports a history of an influenza-like illness; blood cultures are often positive for *Listeria* from such mothers.[70]

Although early-onset disease may occur up to 7 days of age, most cases are clinically apparent at delivery or develop within 1 or 2 days of life and appear with bacteremia (37%), meningitis (33%), pneumonia (6%) and other (focal) infections (15%). At birth, such cases demonstrate meconium staining, cyanosis, apnea, respiratory distress, and pneumonia; meconium-stained amniotic fluid is a common feature of in utero *Listeria*-infected infants and may occur at any gestational age; meconium staining in infants younger than 32 weeks of age is, in fact, rare except in presence of *Listeria* infection. Although respiratory distress and pneumonia occur frequently, radiographic features are entirely nonspecific, with patchy bronchopneumonic infiltrates that are probably caused by aspiration of infected amniotic fluid; only after days of infection, a more coarse, mottled, or nodular pattern has been described.[70] Assisted ventilation is frequently necessary in such infants; persistent hypoxia despite ventilator assistance is often seen in severely affected infants. The more severe the cases, the more prominent CNS involvement can become. Diarrhea,

Table 13-1 Clinical and Laboratory Findings of Early-Onset and Late-Onset Neonatal Listeriosis

Feature	Early-Onset	Late-Onset
Mortality (%)	25	15
Median age in days (range)	1 (0-6)	14 (7-35)
Male (%)	60	67
Preterm (%)	65	20
Respiratory involvement (%)	50	10
Meningitis (%)	25	95
Blood isolate (%)	75	20
Maternal perinatal illness (%)	50	0

Data for early-onset disease are from references 70, 82, 90, and 255, and for late-onset disease, the data are from references 17, 50, 58, 82, 266, and 267.

conjunctivitis, and myocarditis also have been described.[70] Other unusual forms of listeriosis, such as isolated endocarditis,[257,258] endophthalmitis,[259,260] liver abscesses,[86] peritonitis,[261,262] osteomyelitis, and septic arthritis[263] have been described in adults but are rare in infants. Papular cutaneous and mucocutaneous lesions are sometimes observed in newborns when listeriosis is disseminated.[264] On the skin, they appear as slightly elevated pale patches (1-2 mm in diameter) with a bright erythematous base. Biopsy of these areas demonstrates microabscesses and abscesses with leukocytic infiltrates and culturable *L. monocytogenes* (see Fig. 13-3). This rash has been termed *granulomatosis infantiseptic*um (see Fig. 13-4). These are to be distinguished from the primary skin lesions caused by *Listeria* that are observed in adults[37,265] as the result of direct contact, such as handling a cow's placenta by a veterinarian or farmer after abortion.[38]

Laboratory features of early-onset listeriosis are entirely nonspecific. A leukocytosis with presence of immature cells may be seen, or, with severe infection, neutropenia. Thrombocytopenia and anemia may also occur.[248,251] These laboratory and clinical features fail to distinguish listeriosis from early-onset GBS or other neonatal bacterial infection. Early onset-neonatal listeriosis has a high mortality rate (20%-60%). Even in those who survive, a significant number (12.7%) develop long-term neurologic sequelae.[1,82]

Late-Onset Neonatal Listeriosis

Neonatal listerial infection that occurs after 7 days of life is termed *late-onset* infection. Most late-onset disease occurs within weeks (mean age, 14 days), and only rarely past the first month of life.[82] The precise epidemiologic factors contributing to late-onset infection of the newborn are still unknown. Although it is presumed that similar to late-onset GBS infection, transmission during delivery may be one source of late-onset infection,[70,71,241] the maternal history in these cases is usually negative, suggesting perinatal or postnatal, possibly even nosocomial, exposure in affected infants.[17]

The late-onset form of neonatal listeriosis is less common than the early-onset form and usually affects term infants, who appear healthy until the onset of meningitis (67%-93%) or, less commonly, septicemia (approximately one third of cases).[50,58,82,266,267] Although there is some overlap between early- and late-onset forms of listeriosis, the clinical patterns are usually distinct. Clinical features alone do not distinguish listerial meningitis in this age group because they are subtle, including fever, irritability, lethargy, and poor feeding.[17,267] Often, infants do not appear excessively ill and may therefore elude diagnosis for several days. Other clinical forms of disease at this age are less common but may include *Listeria*-induced colitis with associated diarrhea and sepsis without meningitis.[268,269]

Laboratory features of late-onset infection are nonspecific as well. Cell counts in cerebrospinal fluid (CSF) are usually high, with a predominance of neutrophils and band forms, but not all infections have the polymorphonuclear cell predominance. On occasion, a high number of monocytes, as in tuberculous meningitis, may be seen. Gram stain of CSF may not always suggest a diagnosis because the organism may be rare and/or the morphology atypical. The appearance of organisms as illustrated in Figure 13-5 is characteristic of listeriosis in the early phase of severe meningitis. The case fatality rate is about 25%[82]; long-term sequelae are uncommon.[70,71]

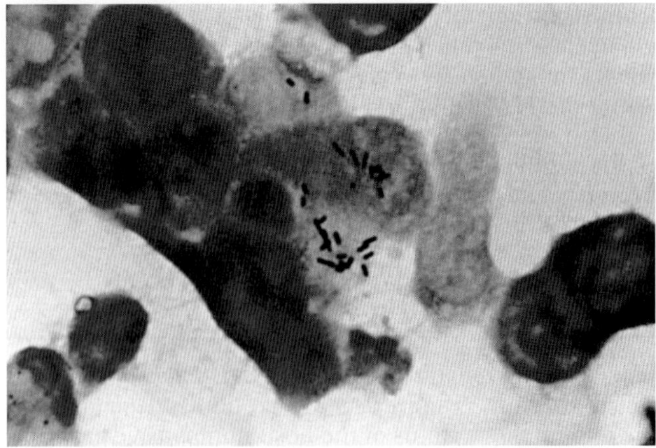

Figure 13-5 Short, gram-positive, intracellular organisms with variable length and rounded ends are arranged irregularly. (Courtesy IWK Health Centre, Pathology Department, Halifax, Nova Scotia, Canada.)

LISTERIOSIS IN THE OLDER CHILD AND ADULT

Most infections with *L. monocytogenes* in the healthy adult host remain entirely asymptomatic.[70] However, a self-limiting febrile gastroenteritis syndrome can occur even in healthy adults and children.[270] Although symptoms overlap considerably, children are more likely to have fever and vomiting, whereas adults typically have arthromyalgias and nonbloody diarrhea. Other symptoms may include sore throat and profound fatigue. The incubation period after ingestion of contaminated food is usually less than 24 hours but has ranged from 6 hours to 10 days.[270,271]

In immunocompromised adult patients and the elderly, bacteremia and/or meningitis may occur, with an associated mortality of 30% to 60%.[87,88] Presenting signs and symptoms are indistinguishable from other causes and typically include fever and myalgias after a prodromal illness of nausea and diarrhea. During the bacteremic phase, an accompanying conjunctivitis is sometimes observed.[272] Although the incidence of listeriosis in immunocompromised children is higher than in immune competent children, the clinical features of listeriosis are similar to those in nonimmunosuppressed patients. These commonly include meningitis or septicemia, but rhombencephalitis, brain abscess, arthritis, osteomyelitis, endocarditis, endophthalmitis, liver abscess, and peritonitis may occur as well.[17,74,17,273] Meningitis caused by *Listeria* can also lead to delayed cerebral thrombosis, indicative of the intense inflammatory response elicited during infection.[274]

Diagnosis

The clinical signs and symptoms of listeriosis overlap considerably with other fetal and neonatal infections, making a specific diagnosis based solely on clinical grounds difficult. Supportive laboratory tests are thus of tremendous help. Appropriate specimens for staining, culture, or molecular detection vary with the clinical syndrome.

MICROSCOPY AND GRAM STAIN

In clinical specimens, Gram stains typically demonstrate short intracellular as well as extracellular gram-positive rods.[149] Finding short, sometimes coccoid, gram-positive rods in meconium suggests possible listeriosis. The morphology of *L. monocytogenes* can vary with culture condition and age of the culture (older cultures [>72hrs] are notorious for being gram variable), and over-decolorized *Listeria* can lead to misdiagnosis as *Haemophilus influenzae*.[275] Confusion with pneumococcal meningitis is also possible in primary culture, where early listerial growth may yield coccobacillus-like morphology with occasional short chains.

CULTURE AND IDENTIFICATION

Cultures of blood, cerebrospinal fluid, placenta, amniotic fluid, lochia and meconium, and tissues at biopsy or autopsy samples offer the best chances for identifying *Listeria*. Stool culture is not done routinely because special media are required, and 2% to 10% of healthy adults are colonized with *Listeria*.[1,40,42-45]

L. monocytogenes grows well on common media; including sheep blood agar, brain-heart infusion, trypticase soy, and thioglycollate broths. Growth in ambient air occurs between 4° C and 37° C, with fastest growth rates occurring between 30° C and 37° C. Selective media can be used for isolation from nonsterile sites but are primarily applied in epidemiologic studies. Cold enrichment techniques were used historically but are rarely required in the clinical laboratory setting.[276,277]

After 48 hours at 37° C on 5% sheep blood agar, typical colonies are 0.2 to 1.5 mm in diameter. Narrow zones of β-hemolysis may be visualized, often only by removing the colony. Catalase test is usually positive.[278] *L. seeligeri* and *L. ivanovii* are also β-hemolytic but generally nonpathogenic in humans. Speciation is aided by the CAMP test. *Staphylococcus aureus* gives a positive CAMP reaction for *L. monocytogenes* and *L. seeligeri*, whereas *Rhodococcus equi* gives a positive reaction for *L. ivanovii*.[279] Discrimination is further aided by sugar fermentation patterns. *L. monocytogenes* produces acid from L-rhamnose and α-methyl-D-mannoside but not from xylose. *L. ivanovii* and *L. seeligeri* produce acid from D-xylose only. Automated systems (e.g., Vitek, bioMérieux, Durham, NC; Microscan Walkaway, Dade Behring, West Sacramento, CA), commercial biochemical strips (e.g., API *Listeria* bioMérieux, Durham, NC; MICRO-ID Listeria, Organon Teknika, Durham, NC), and DNA probes (e.g., AccuProbe *Listeria* Culture Identification Test, Hologic Gen-Probe, San Diego, CA) may further aid identification in many clinical microbiology laboratories.

MOLECULAR AND OTHER DETECTION METHODS

Increasingly, polymerase chain reaction (PCR)-based methods are used to detect *Listeria* in clinical samples, such as cerebrospinal fluid[280,281] Spurred by the food industry's need for rapid and sensitive *Listeria* screening, approved kits for real-time PCR[282] and amplification with sequencing of *Listeria* 16S ribosomal RNA genes[283] have been adopted. Although approval of clinical diagnostic kits has lagged behind the food industry, broad-range 16S PCR has become widely accepted for detecting bacterial pathogens from sterile clinical sites.[284,285] Compared with culture, 16S PCR offers the advantage of being able to detect nonviable organisms when antibiotics have been given to a patient before collection of the sample.

SEROLOGY

The classic agglutination reaction (Widal test) demonstrates antibodies against O and H antigens of the various *Listeria* serovars. Unfortunately, the antigenic complexity of *L. monocytogenes* has prevented agreement on interpretation of agglutination reactions for diagnostic purposes. Complement-fixing titers of greater than 1:8 for *Listeria* have a sensitivity and specificity of 78% and 91%, respectively; however, the positive predictive value is only 75%.[286,287] Detection of antibodies to LLO has also been used to diagnose human listeriosis.[288] The sensitivity and specificity of the test is greater than 90%, and during a febrile gastroenteritis outbreak, it correlated well with clinical illness.[269] Although these results are impressive, the technique is not commercially available. A precipitin test,[289] indirect hemagglutination reaction,[290] and antigen fixation test[291] have also been described, showing apparent success but remain commercially unavailable.

Therapy

Intravenous ampicillin used in combination with an aminoglycoside, typically gentamicin, remains the treatment of choice for invasive *L. monocytogenes* infections. However, there are no randomized controlled trials to provide sound evidence for the choice and duration of antibiotic therapy.

Susceptibility testing for *Listeria* has become more standardized with the publication of guidelines both in North America and in Europe. In North America, minimal inhibitory concentrations (MIC) are based on the Clinical Laboratory Standards Institute guidelines, and susceptibility of *L. monocytogenes* to ampicillin is defined as an MIC less than or equal to 2mg/L[292]; in Europe, MICs are based on the European Committee on Antimicrobial Susceptibility Testing guidelines, with susceptibility to ampicillin defined as an MIC less than or equal to 1 mg/L.[293] Clinical strains show nearly universal susceptibility to ampicillin, penicillin, vancomycin, erythromycin, and tetracycline,[294-297] although cases of transferable plasmid-mediated antibiotic resistance have been reported.[82,296,298-302] Of more concern, penicillin and gentamicin resistance has been increasingly reported in isolates from commercial farms.[299,303] Although ampicillin may be used alone in immunocompetent patients with less severe infections or once clinical response has occurred, it is important to recognize that ampicillin is only bacteriostatic for *L. monocytogenes* at the concentrations that can be achieved in blood or CSF.[304-307] An aminoglycoside is thus often added for synergy, a phenomenon supported only by in vitro studies and partially replicated in animal models.[308] Of note, if gentamicin were to be used as a single agent, *L. monocytogenes* would survive intracellularly where gentamicin penetration is poor; single gentamicin therapy is thus never recommended.[309-311]

For penicillin-allergic patients, trimethoprim-sulfamethoxazole (TMP-SMX) has been used successfully,[312] with and without the addition of rifampin.[308,310,313-315] However, TMP-SMX cannot be recommended for use in perinatal infections because of the concern of bilirubin toxicity.[313] For patients with both penicillin and sulfa allergies, vancomycin has been used successfully, albeit based on scant clinical experience. *Listeria* infections have also been treated successfully with linezolid.[310,316] The use of ciprofloxacin in animal models has not suggested any therapeutic advantage over ampicillin.[317,318] The activity of newer fluoroquinolines against *L. monocytogenes* appears better, with moxifloxacin being effective for eradication of the organism from the intracellular compartment.[319,320] However, moxifloxacin was equivalent to ampicillin plus gentamicin in animal model and thus does not offer an obvious advantage over standard therapy.[321]

Cephalosporins are not active against *L. monocytogenes*.[258,304,311] In fact, cephalosporins are incorporated into selective media to inhibit other bacteria and enhance *Listeria* recovery.[15] Similarly, inherent resistance to clindamycin, tetracyclines, and macrolides is common. Antagonism also seems to occur between certain antibiotic combinations, for instance, erythromycin and penicillins, erythromycin and aminoglycosides, penicillin and chloramphenicol, and penicillin and tetracycline.[304,305]

Duration of therapy depends on the clinical syndrome, the presence of underlying disease, and the response to treatment. For most invasive infections without meningitis, 10 to 14 days of therapy appears sufficient. When meningitis is present, many experts recommend 2 to 3 weeks of therapy. Longer courses may be necessary for endocarditis, rhombencephalitis, and severe complicated infections. When treating CNS infections, diagnostic imaging of the brain near the end of anticipated therapy may be used to evaluate the possibility of parenchymal involvement and determine the need for an extended duration of therapy.

Listeria gastroenteritis, in otherwise healthy individuals, is generally a self-limited illness, and no data exist with regard to the efficacy of antimicrobial therapy. In high-risk individuals, such as pregnant women and those with immunocompromise, who have either symptomatic illness or who are known to have ingested a contaminated food, it may be prudent to administer treatment/prophylaxis with a course of oral amoxicillin or TMP-SMX.[270]

SUGGESTED MANAGEMENT

Listeriosis in Pregnant Women

If amnionitis is present, initial treatment should be given by the intravenous route to ensure adequate tissue levels (ampicillin, 4-6 g/day divided into four equal doses plus an aminoglycoside). If amnionitis is not present or if acute symptoms of amnionitis have subsided, oral antibiotics are an option (amoxicillin, 2-3 g/day divided into four equal doses). In both situations, treatment should continue for 14 days. If the patient has a significant β-lactam allergy, therapeutic options are limited. Erythromycin may be given (the estolate form should be avoided because of increased liver toxicity during pregnancy), although there are no universal susceptibility guidelines for erythromycin and *Listeria*. TMP-SMX is an active agent, but theoretical risks of use in pregnancy must be balanced against potential benefits.[313]

Early-Onset Neonatal Listeriosis

Ampicillin in combination with an aminoglycoside is the preferred management for early-onset infection. For infants with body weight less than 2000 g, ampicillin at 100 mg/kg/day (divided into two equal doses) should be administered for the first week of life. For infants with body weight of greater than 2000 g, 150 mg/kg/day (divided into three equal doses) should be administered for the first week of life. For the second week of life, the appropriate dosages are 150 mg/kg/day and 200 mg/kg/day for infants weighing less than and greater than 2000 g body weight, respectively. Aminoglycoside doses vary with the agent chosen. For gentamicin, the suggested dosages are 5 mg/kg/day (divided into two equal doses) for the first week of life and 7.5 mg/kg/day (divided into three equal doses) for the second week of life. Ten to 14 days of treatment is recommended for early-onset neonatal sepsis caused by *L. monocytogenes*; however, a longer course of treatment should be given in the uncommon event of early-onset neonatal listeriosis with meningitis.

Late-Onset Neonatal Listeriosis

Meningitis is commonly present in late-onset listeriosis. Delayed eradication of the organism may be seen in such cases. Ampicillin (200-400 mg/kg/day divided into four to six equal doses) in combination with an aminoglycoside is recommended. Lumbar puncture should be repeated in 48 to 72 hours to assess effectiveness of therapy. In the event of delayed clearance (>2 days), further investigations are indicated, including computed tomography or cranial ultrasonography to assess for the presence of cerebritis or intracranial hemorrhage. If the organism remains present in the cerebrospinal fluid after several days, the addition of vancomycin, rifampin, or TMP-SMX may be considered. However, experience with such combination therapy for listeriosis in neonates is limited.[322] Length of treatment is generally 14 to 21 days, depending on the clinical course.

Prognosis

Maternal listeriosis may result in abortion, stillbirth, or early neonatal death.[1] Although the relative risk of fetal death is difficult to determine, spontaneous abortion rates of 10% to 20% and stillborn rates of 11% have been quoted.[1] Fetal distress and/or meconium staining of amniotic fluid are estimated to occur in 75% of perinatal cases.[1] Convincing evidence that *L. monocytogenes* is associated with repeated abortions is lacking.[323] Fetal loss with early gestational infection is a recognized complication of maternal infection. In late-gestational maternal infection, sparing of the fetus has been reported,[324] but it is probably uncommon unless antepartum antibiotics have been administered to the mother.[325,326]

Early-onset neonatal listeriosis accounts for the largest recognizable group of infections caused by *L. monocytogenes*. Although fetal or neonatal infection with *L. monocytogenes* is known to have a high fatality (40%),[248,251] the impact of infection on long-term morbidity is less clear. Most survivors appear to be fine and remain without sequelae.[251,327,328] If present, sequelae are likely related to the associated complications of prematurity, pneumonia, and sepsis; hydrocephalus and cerebral palsy also have been reported.[325,327] Rotheberg[329] found an increased incidence of developmental delay assessed at a mean age of 29.5 months among small-for-age (<1250 g at birth) *Listeria*-infected infants who required assisted ventilation. Naege,[330] who studied children 4 to 7 years after they recovered from early-onset listeriosis, also found increased neurodevelopmental handicaps, including increased risk for hydrocephalus.[331] In contrast, Evans and coworkers[327] found no evidence of neurodevelopmental sequelae in six of eight survivors studied at a mean age of 15 months and again at 32 months. The two infants with neurodevelopmental sequelae had severe acute perinatal sepsis with meningitis; both had spastic diplegia. The authors concluded that long-term sequelae after neonatal early-onset listeriosis were uncommon. If meningitis is not present, the outcome may be generally good. Early treatment of maternal disease affects fetal and neonatal outcome favorably.[251,325]

Late-onset *Listeria* meningitis has a mortality rate of less than 10%. The outcome after *Listeria* meningitis may be more favorable than the outcome associated with other types of bacterial meningitis.[254,267] Long-term sequelae of late-onset listeriosis are uncommon,[70,71] except in cases of treatment failures, where the subsequent increased risk of relapse (in some cases, weeks or months elapse between episodes) can lead to high mortality rate and long-term sequelae. Here the major sequelae appear as hydrocephalus and possibly mental retardation.[332]

Beyond the newborn period, the outcome of listeriosis depends on the nature of any underlying disease and the availability of intensive medical care. Among adults with no underlying malignancy, the long-term outcome of *Listeria* meningitis is excellent.[333]

Prevention and Outbreak Management

Foodborne outbreaks of listeriosis are unpredictable and may occur in a wide geographic area.[15,16] Therefore reporting of all cases of listeriosis to public health authorities is important to identify outbreaks early (i.e., listeriosis is a notifiable disease).[22,334-336] Case-control studies and environmental sampling are important aspects of outbreak investigations.[17,334] Strains of *Listeria* from clinical and environmental isolates should be forwarded to a reference laboratory for appropriate epidemiologic typing. Serotyping and multifocus enzyme electrophoresis typing should be performed to characterize the epidemic strain.

During an outbreak of listeriosis, pregnant women presenting with a sepsis syndrome or flulike illness should be empirically treated with ampicillin and an aminoglycoside after appropriate cultures of blood, rectum, and vagina have been obtained. Amniocentesis for diagnosis of chorioamnionitis may be indicated, depending on the clinical presenation.[337] If membranes have ruptured and contamination is suspected, use of selective media may enhance the isolation of *Listeria* from these patients.

Box 13-2 Recommendations for Reducing the Risk of Listeriosis[30,338]

General Recommendations

- Thoroughly cook raw food from animal sources, such as beef, pork, and poultry.
- Wash raw vegetables thoroughly before eating.
- Keep uncooked meats separate from vegetables, from cooked foods, and ready-to-eat foods.
- Avoid raw (unpasteurized) milk or foods made from unpasteurized milk.
- Wash hands, knives, and cutting boards after handling uncooked foods.
- Consume perishable and ready-to-eat foods as soon as possible.

Additional Recommendations for High-Risk Groups

- Do not eat hot dogs or ready-to-eat foods, such as delicatessen meats, unless they are reheated until steaming hot.
- Wash hands after handling hot dogs and ready-to-eat foods.
- Do not eat soft cheeses (e.g., feta, brie, and camembert) or blue-veined cheeses unless they have labels that clearly state they are made from pasteurized milk.
- Do not eat refrigerated pâtés or meat spreads; canned or "shelf-stable" (pasteurized) pâtés and meat spreads may be eaten.
- Do not eat refrigerated smoked seafood unless it is contained in a cooked dish, such as a casserole; canned or shelf-stable smoked seafood may be eaten.

The recognition that sporadic cases of listeriosis are foodborne has prompted dissemination of preventive guidelines (Box 13-2).[30,338] The guidelines for preventing listeriosis are similar to those for preventing other foodborne illnesses and include thorough cooking of raw food from animals and thorough washing of vegetables and utensils. Persons at high risk, such as pregnant women, should also avoid soft cheeses and prepared salads, meats and cheeses from delicatessen counters.[27] Thoroughly heating leftover foods until they are steaming hot has also been recommended.[339] Adherence to these food guidelines by pregnant women unfortunately appears limited. Improved education of pregnant women regarding risk of listeriosis in pregnancy thus appears necessary.[340,341] For example, a decrease in the rates of listeriosis in some geographic areas in the United States has been temporally associated with the publication of these guidelines and industry efforts directed at removing foodborne pathogens from the food chain.[342]

References

1. Lamont RF, Sobel J, Mazaki-Tovi S, et al: Listeriosis in human pregnancy: a systematic review, *J Perinatal Med* 39:227-236, 2011.
2. Murray EDG, Webb RA, Swann MBR: A disease of rabbits characterized by a large monouclear leucocytosis, caused by a hitherto undescribed *Bacillus: Bacterium monocytogenes*, *J Pathol Bacteriol* 29:407, 1926.
3. Nyfeldt A: Etiologie de la mononucleose infectieuse, *Compt Rend Soc Biol* 101:590-591, 1929.
4. Bortolussi R, Burbridge S, Durnford P, Schellekens H: Neonatal *Listeria monocytogenes* infection is refractory to interferon, *Pediatr Res* 29(4 Pt 1):400-402, 1991.
5. Pirie JHH: A new disease of veld rodents, *"Tiger River disease." Publ S Afr Inst Med Res* 3:163-186, 1927.

6. Pirie JHH: Chage of name for a genus of bacteria, *Nature* 145:264, 1940.
7. Burn CG: Clinical and pathological features of an infection reused by new pathogen of the genus *Listerella*, *Am J Pathol* 12:341-348, 1936.
8. Schlech WF 3rd, Lavigne PM, Bortolussi RA, et al: Epidemic listeriosis—evidence for transmission by food, *N Engl J Med* 308:203-206, 1983.
9. Seeliger HPR: *Listeriosis*, New York, 1961, Karger.
10. Holt JG, Krieg NR, Sneath PHA: *Bergey's manual of determinative bacteriology*, Baltimore, 1994, Williams & Wilkins, pp 566-567.
11. Lessing MP, Curtis GD, Bowler IC: *Listeria ivanovii* infection, *J Infect* 29:230-231, 1994.
12. Salimnia H, Patel D, Lephart PR, Fairfax MR, Chandrasekar PH: *Listeria grayi*: vancomycin-resistant, gram-positive rod causing bacteremia in a stem cell transplant recipient, *Transpl Infect Dis* 12: 526-528, 2010.
13. Way SS, Thompson LJ, Lopes JE, et al: Characterization of flagellin expression and its role in *Listeria monocytogenes* infection and immunity, *Cell Microbiol* 6:235-242, 2004.
14. Peel M, Donachie W, Shaw A: Temperature-dependent expression of flagella of *Listeria monocytogenes* studied by electron microscopy, SDS-PAGE and western blotting, *J Gen Microbiol* 134:2171-2178, 1988.
15. Bortolussi R: An ongoing problem: perinatal infection due to *Listeria monocytogenes*, an old pathogen reborn, *Clin Invest Med* 7:213-215, 1984.
16. Gellin BG, Broome CV: Listeriosis, *JAMA* 261:1313-1320, 1989.
17. Schuchat A, Swaminathan B, Broome CV: Epidemiology of human listeriosis, *Clin Microbiol Rev* 4:169-183, 1991.
18. Hain T, Ghai R, Billion A, et al: Comparative genomics and transcriptomics of lineages I, II, and III strains of *Listeria monocytogenes*, *BMC Genomics* 13:144, 2012.
19. Kuenne C, Billion A, Mraheil MA, et al: Reassessment of the *Listeria monocytogenes* pan-genome reveals dynamic integration hotspots and mobile genetic elements as major components of the accessory genome, *BMC Genomics* 14:47, 2013.
20. Cossart P: Illuminating the landscape of host-pathogen interactions with the bacterium *Listeria monocytogenes*, *Proc Natl Acad Sci U S A* 108:19484-19491, 2011.
21. McLauchlin J: Distribution of serovars of *Listeria monocytogenes* isolated from different categories of patients with listeriosis, *Eur J Clinical Microbiol Infect Dis* 9:210-213, 1990.
22. Pinner RW, Schuchat A, Swaminathan B, et al: Role of foods in sporadic listeriosis. II. Microbiologic and epidemiologic investigation. The *Listeria* Study Group, *JAMA* 267:2046-2050, 1992.
23. Lomonaco S, Verghese B, Gerner-Smidt P, et al: Novel epidemic clones of *Listeria monocytogenes*, United States, 2011, *Emerg Infect Dis* 19:147-150, 2013.
24. Koopmans MM, Brouwer MC, Bijlsma MW, et al: Listeria monocytogenes sequence type 6 and increased rate of unfavorable outcome in meningitis: epidemiological cohort study, *Clin Infect Dis* 57: 247-253, 2014.
25. Wing EJ, Gregory SH: *Listeria monocytogenes*: clinical and experimental update, *J Infect Dis* 185(Suppl 1):S18-S24, 2002.
26. Hoffmann S, Batz MB, Morris JG Jr: Annual cost of illness and quality-adjusted life year losses in the United States due to 14 foodborne pathogens, *J Food Protect* 75:1292-1302, 2012.
27. Varma JK, Samuel MC, Marcus R, et al: *Listeria monocytogenes* infection from foods prepared in a commercial establishment: a case-control study of potential sources of sporadic illness in the United States, *Clin Infect Dis* 44:521-528, 2007.
28. Multistate outbreak of listeriosis associated with Jensen Farms cantaloupe—United States, August-September 2011, *MMWR Morb Mortal Wkly Rep* 60:1357-1358, 2011.
29. Vaillant V, de Valk H, Baron E, et al: Foodborne infections in France, *Foodborne Pathog Dis* 2:221-232, 2005.
30. Lynch M, Painter J, Woodruff R, Braden C: Surveillance for foodborne-disease outbreaks—United States, 1998-2002, *Morb Mortal Wkly Rep Surveill Summ* 55:1-42, 2006.
31. Werber D, Hille K, Frank C, et al: Years of potential life lost for six major enteric pathogens, Germany, 2004-2008, *Epidemiol Infect* 141:961-968, 2013.
32. Cartwright EJ, Jackson KA, Johnson SD, et al: Listeriosis outbreaks and associated food vehicles, United States, 1998-2008, *Emerg Infect Dis* 19:1-9, 2013.
33. Pouillot R, Hoelzer K, Jackson KA, Henao OL, Silk BJ: Relative risk of listeriosis in Foodborne Diseases Active Surveillance Network (FoodNet) sites according to age, pregnancy, and ethnicity, *Clin Infect Dis* 54(Suppl 5):S405-S410, 2012.
34. Pontello M, Guaita A, Sala G, et al: *Listeria monocytogenes* serotypes in human infections (Italy, 2000-2010), *Ann Ist Super Sanita* 48:146-150, 2012.
35. Welshimer HJ: Isolation of *Listeria monocytogenes* from vegetation, *J Bacteriol* 95:300-303, 1968.
36. Low JC, Renton CP: Septicaemia, encephalitis and abortions in a housed flock of sheep caused by *Listeria monocytogenes* type 1/2, *Vet Rec* 116:147-150, 1985.
37. Owen CR, Meis A, Jackson JW, Stoenner HG: A case of primary cutaneous listeriosis, *N Engl J Med* 262:1026-1028, 1960.
38. McLauchlin J, Low JC: Primary cutaneous listeriosis in adults: an occupational disease of veterinarians and farmers, *Vet Rec* 135: 615-617, 1994.
39. Elischerova K, Stupalova S: Proceedings: listeriosis in professionally exposed persons, *Acta Microbiol Acad Sci Hung* 19:379-384, 1972.
40. Bojsen-Moller J: Human listeriosis. Diagnostic, epidemiological and clinical studies, *Acta Path Microbiol Scand B Microbiol Immunol* (Suppl 229):1-157, 1972.
41. Houhoula DP, Peirasmaki D, Konteles SJ, et al: High level of heterogeneity among *Listeria monocytogenes* isolates from clinical and food origin specimens in Greece, *Foodborne Pathog Dis* 9:848-852, 2012.
42. Mascola L, Sorvillo F, Goulet V, et al: Fecal carriage of *Listeria monocytogenes*—observations during a community-wide, common-source outbreak, *Clin Infect Dis* 15:557-558, 1992.
43. Schlech WF 3rd: Foodborne listeriosis, *Clin Infect Dis* 31:770-775, 2000.
44. Kampelmacher EH, Huysinga WT, van Noorle Jansen LM. The presence of *Listeria monocytogenes* in feces of pregnant women and neonates, *Zentralbl Bakteriol Orig A* 222:258-262, 1972.
45. Schlech WF 3rd, Schlech WF 4th, Haldane H, et al: Does sporadic *Listeria* gastroenteritis exist? A 2-year population-based survey in Nova Scotia, Canada, *Clin Infect Dis* 41:778-784, 2005.
46. Dussurget O: New insights into determinants of Listeria monocytogenes virulence, *Int Rev Cell Mol Biol.* 270:1-38, 2008.
47. Jackson KA, Iwamoto M, Swerdlow D: Pregnancy-associated listeriosis, *Epidemiol Infect* 138:1503-1509, 2010.
48. Florman AL, Sundararajan V: Listeriosis among nursery mates, *Pediatrics* 41:784-788, 1968.
49. Larson S: *Listeria monocytogenes* causing hospital-acquired entercolitis and meningitis in newborn infants, *Br Med J* 2:473-474, 1978.
50. Filice GA, Cantrell HF, Smith AB, et al: *Listeria monocytogenes* infection in neonates: investigation of an epidemic, *J Infect Dis* 138:17-23, 1978.
51. Campbell AN, Sill PR, Wardle JK: *Listeria* meningitis acquired by cross infection in a delivery suite, *Lancet* 2:752-753, 1981.
52. Nelson KE, Warren D, Tomasi AM, Raju TN, Vidyasagar D: Transmission of neonatal listeriosis in a delivery room, *Am J Dis Child* 139:903-905, 1985.
53. Simmons MD, Cockcroft PM, Okubadejo OA: Neonatal listeriosis due to cross-infection in an obstetric theatre, *J Infect* 13:235-239, 1986.
54. Graham JC, Lanser S, Bignardi G, Pedler S, Hollyoak V: Hospital-acquired listeriosis, *J Hosp Infect* 51:136-139, 2002.
55. Guevara RE, Tormey MP, Nguyen DM, Mascola L: *Listeria monocytogenes* in platelets: a case report, *Transfusion* 46:305-309, 2006.
56. Facinelli B, Varaldo PE, Casolari C, Fabio U: Cross-infection with *Listeria monocytogenes* confirmed by DNA fingerprinting, *Lancet* 2:1247-1248, 1988.
57. Green HT, Macaulay MB: Hospital outbreak of *Listeria monocytogenes* septicaemia: a problem of cross infection? *Lancet* 2:1039-1040, 1978.
58. Larsson S, Cederberg A, Ivarsson S, Svanberg L, Cronberg S: *Listeria monocytogenes* causing hospital-acquired enterocolitis and meningitis in newborn infants, *Br Med J* 2:473-474, 1978.
59. Schuchat A, Lizano C, Broome CV, et al: Outbreak of neonatal listeriosis associated with mineral oil, *Pediatr Infect Dis J* 10:183-189, 1991.
60. Nieman RE, Lorber B: Listeriosis in adults: a changing pattern. Report of eight cases and review of the literature, 1968-1978, *Rev Infect Dis* 2:207-227, 1980.
61. Davies JW, Ewan EP, Varughese P, Acres SE: *Listeria monocytogenes* infections in Canada, *Clin Invest Med* 7:315-320, 1984.

62. Bowmer EJ, McKiel JA, Cockcroft WH, Schmitt N, Rappay DE: *Listeria monocytogenes* infections in Canada, *Can Med Assoc J* 109:125-129, 1973.
63. Ruzante JM, Majowicz SE, Fazil A, Davidson VJ: Hospitalization and deaths for select enteric illnesses and associated sequelae in Canada, 2001-2004, *Epidemiol Infect* 139:937-945, 2011.
64. Gaulin C, Ramsay D, Bekal S: Widespread listeriosis outbreak attributable to pasteurized cheese, which led to extensive cross-contamination affecting cheese retailers, Quebec, Canada, 2008, *J Food Protect* 75:71-78, 2012.
65. Taillefer C, Boucher M, Laferrière C, Morin L: Perinatal listeriosis: Canada's 2008 outbreaks, *J Obstet Gynaecol Can* 32:45-48, 2010.
66. Unanue ER, Carrero JA: Studies with *Listeria monocytogenes* lead the way, *Adv Immunol* 113:1-5, 2012.
67. Witte CE, Archer KA, Rae CS, et al: Innate immune pathways triggered by *Listeria monocytogenes* and their role in the induction of cell-mediated immunity, *Adv Immunol* 113:135-156, 2012.
68. Serbina NV, Shi C, Pamer EG: Monocyte-mediated immune defense against murine *Listeria monocytogenes* infection, *Adv Immunol* 113:119-134, 2012.
69. Condotta SA, Richer MJ, Badovinac VP, Harty JT: Probing CD8 T cell responses with *Listeria monocytogenes* infection, *Adv Immunol* 113:51-80, 2012.
70. Bortolussi R: Listeriosis: a primer, *CMAJ* 179:795-797, 2008.
71. Posfay-Barbe KM, Wald ER: Listeriosis, *Semin Fetal Neonatal Med* 14:228-233, 2009.
72. Doorduyn Y, de Jager CM, van der Zwaluw WK, et al: Invasive *Listeria monocytogenes* infections in the Netherlands, 1995-2003, *Eur J Clin Microbiol Infect Dis* 25:433-442, 2006.
73. Hugin AW, Cerny A, Wrann M, Hengartner H, Zinkernagel RM: Effect of cyclosporin A on immunity to *Listeria monocytogenes*, *Infect Immun* 52:12-17, 1986.
74. Skogberg K, Syrjanen J, Jahkola M, et al: Clinical presentation and outcome of listeriosis in patients with and without immunosuppressive therapy, *Clin Infect Dis* 14:815-821, 1992.
75. Sherrid AM, Kollmann TR: Age-dependent differences in systemic and cell-autonomous immunity to *L. monocytogenes*, *Clin Dev Immunol* 2013:917198, 2013.
76. Schlech WF 3rd, Chase DP, Badley A: A model of food-borne *Listeria monocytogenes* infection in the Sprague-Dawley rat using gastric inoculation: development and effect of gastric acidity on infective dose, *Int J Food Microbiol.* 18:15-24, 1993.
77. Ho JL, Shands KN, Friedland G, Eckind P, Fraser DW: An outbreak of type 4b *Listeria monocytogenes* infection involving patients from eight Boston hospitals, *Arch Intern Med* 146:520-524, 1986.
78. Bruminhent J, Lynch TK, Gefen J, Santoro J: *Listeria monocytogenes* cholecystitis: a possible new syndrome, *Am J Med Sci* 345:414-417, 2012.
79. Bodro M, Paterson DL: Listeriosis in patients receiving biologic therapies, *Eur J Clin Microbiol Infect Dis* 32:1225-1230, 2013.
80. Cabellos C, Viladrich PF, Ariza J, et al: Community-acquired bacterial meningitis in cirrhotic patients, *Clin Microbiol Infect* 14:35-40, 2008.
81. Goulet V, Hebert M, Hedberg C, et al: Incidence of listeriosis and related mortality among groups at risk of acquiring listeriosis, *Clin Infect Dis* 54:652-660, 2012.
82. Okike IO, Lamont RF, Heath PT: Do we really need to worry about *Listeria* in newborn infants? *Pediatr Infect Dis J* 32:405-406, 2013.
83. Lamont RJ, Postlethwaite R: Carriage of *Listeria monocytogenes* and related species in pregnant and non-pregnant women in Aberdeen, Scotland, *J Infect* 13:187-193, 1986.
84. Ireton K: Entry of the bacterial pathogen *Listeria monocytogenes* into mammalian cells, *Cell Microbiol.* 9:1365-1375, 2007.
85. Ramaswamy V, Cresence VM, Rejitha JS, et al: *Listeria*—review of epidemiology and pathogenesis, *J Microbiol Immunol Infect* 40:4-13, 2007.
86. Scholing M, Schneeberger PM, van den Dries P, Drenth JP: Clinical features of liver involvement in adult patients with listeriosis. Review of the literature, *Infection* 35:212-218, 2007.
87. Gellin BG, Broome CV, Bibb WF, et al: The epidemiology of listeriosis in the United States—-1986. Listeriosis Study Group, *Am J Epidemiol* 133:392-401, 1991.
88. Siegman-Igra Y, Levin R, Weinberger M, et al: *Listeria monocytogenes* infection in Israel and review of cases worldwide, *Emerg Infect Dis* 8:305-310, 2002.
89. Schmidt-Wolf G, Seeliger HP, Schretten-Brunner A: Menschilishe listeroisise-erkrankungen in der Bundesrepublik Deutschland 1969-1985, *Zentralbl Bakteriol Mikrobiol Hyg* 265:472, 1985.
90. Nolla-Salas J, Bosch J, Gasser I, et al: Perinatal listeriosis: a population-based multicenter study in Barcelona, Spain (1990-1996), *Am J Perinatol* 15:461-467, 1998.
91. McLaughlin J: Human listeriosis in Britain, 1967-85, a summary of 722 cases: 1. Listeriosis during pregnancy and the newborn, *Epidemiol Infect* 104:191-201, 1990.
92. Kollmann TR, Levy O, Montgomery RR, Goriely S: Innate immune function by Toll-like receptors: distinct responses in newborns and the elderly, *Immunity* 37:771-783, 2012.
93. Farber JM, Ross WH, Harwig J: Health risk assessment of *Listeria monocytogenes* in Canada, *Int J Food Microbiol* 30:145-156, 1996.
94. Smith MA, Takeuchi K, Anderson G, et al: Dose-response model for *Listeria monocytogenes*-induced stillbirths in nonhuman primates, *Infect Immun* 76:726-731, 2008.
95. Schlech WF 3rd: *Listeria* gastroenteritis—old syndrome, new pathogen, *N Engl J Med* 336:130-132, 1997.
96. DeCherney AP, Pernoll ML, editors: *Current obstetric and gynecologic diagnosis and treatment*, ed 8, Boston, 1994, McGraw-Hill.
97. Gillespie IA, McLauchlin J, Little CL, et al: Disease presentation in relation to infection foci for non-pregnancy-associated human listeriosis in England and Wales, 2001 to 2007, *J Clin Microbiol* 47:3301-3307, 2009.
98. Morgan M: Control of intragastric pH and volume, *Br J Anaesth* 56:47-57, 1984.
99. Miclat NN, Hodgkinson R, Marx GF: Neonatal gastric pH, *Anesth Analg* 57:98-101, 1978.
100. Swaminathan B, Gerner-Smidt P: The epidemiology of human listeriosis, *Microb Infect* 9:1236-1243, 2007.
101. Gray MJ, Freitag NE, Boor KJ: How the bacterial pathogen *Listeria monocytogenes* mediates the switch from environmental Dr. Jekyll to pathogenic Mr. Hyde, *Infect Immun* 74:2505-2512, 2006.
102. Sleator RD, Gahan CG, Hill C: A postgenomic appraisal of osmotolerance in *Listeria monocytogenes*, *Appl Environ Microbiol* 69:1-9, 2003.
103. Kim H, Marquis H, Boor KJ: SigmaB contributes to *Listeria monocytogenes* invasion by controlling expression of inlA and inlB, *Microbiology* 151:3215-3222, 2005.
104. Cotter PD, Gahan CG, Hill C: A glutamate decarboxylase system protects *Listeria monocytogenes* in gastric fluid, *Mol Microbiol* 40: 465-475, 2001.
105. Cotter PD, Ryan S, Gahan CG, Hill C: Presence of GadD1 glutamate decarboxylase in selected *Listeria monocytogenes* strains is associated with an ability to grow at low pH, *Appl Environ Microbiol* 71: 2832-2839, 2005.
106. Dussurget O, Cabanes D, Dehoux P, et al: *Listeria monocytogenes* bile salt hydrolase is a PrfA-regulated virulence factor involved in the intestinal and hepatic phases of listeriosis, *Mol Microbiol* 45: 1095-1106, 2002.
107. Kazmierczak MJ, Mithoe SC, Boor KJ, Wiedmann M: *Listeria monocytogenes* sigma B regulates stress response and virulence functions, *J Bacteriol* 185:5722-5734, 2003.
108. Sue D, Boor KJ, Wiedmann M: Sigma(B)-dependent expression patterns of compatible solute transporter genes *opuCA* and *lmo1421* and the conjugated bile salt hydrolase gene *bsh* in *Listeria monocytogenes*, *Microbiology* 149:3247-3256, 2003.
109. Begley M, Sleator RD, Gahan CG, Hill C: Contribution of three bile-associated loci, *bsh*, *pva*, and *btlB*, to gastrointestinal persistence and bile tolerance of *Listeria monocytogenes*, *Infect Immun* 73:894-904, 2005.
110. Sleator RD, Wemekamp-Kamphuis HH, Gahan CG, Abee T, Hill C: A PrfA-regulated bile exclusion system (BilE) is a novel virulence factor in *Listeria monocytogenes*, *Mol Microbiol* 55:1183-1195, 2005.
111. Sleator RD, Gahan CG, Hill C: Identification and disruption of the *proBA* locus in *Listeria monocytogenes*: role of proline biosynthesis in salt tolerance and murine infection, *Appl Environ Microbiol* 67:2571-2577, 2001.
112. Wemekamp-Kamphuis HH, Wouters JA, Sleator RD, et al: Multiple deletions of the osmolyte transporters BetL, Gbu, and OpuC of *Listeria monocytogenes* affect virulence and growth at high osmolarity, *Appl Environ Microbiol* 68:4710-4716, 2002.
113. Borezee E, Pellegrini E, Berche P: OppA of *Listeria monocytogenes*, an oligopeptide-binding protein required for bacterial growth at low temperature and involved in intracellular survival, *Infect Immun* 68:7069-7077, 2000.

114. Milohanic E, Pron B, Berche P, Gaillard JL: Identification of new loci involved in adhesion of *Listeria monocytogenes* to eukaryotic cells. European *Listeria* Genome Consortium, *Microbiology* 146:731-739, 2000.
115. Milohanic E, Jonquieres R, Cossart P, Berche P, Gaillard JL: The autolysin Ami contributes to the adhesion of *Listeria monocytogenes* to eukaryotic cells via its cell wall anchor, *Mol Microbiol* 39: 1212-1224, 2001.
116. Pizarro-Cerda J, Kuhbacher A, Cossart P: Entry of *Listeria monocytogenes* in mammalian epithelial cells: an updated view, *Cold Spring Harb Perspect Med* 2, 2012. pii:a010009.
117. Bou Ghanem EN, Jones GS, Myers-Morales T, et al: InlA promotes dissemination of *Listeria monocytogenes* to the mesenteric lymph nodes during foodborne infection of mice, *PLoS Pathog* 8:e1003015, 2012.
118. Glaser P, Frangeul L, Buchrieser C, et al: Comparative genomics of *Listeria* species, *Science* 294:849-852, 2001.
119. Nelson KE, Fouts DE, Mongodin EF, et al: Whole genome comparisons of serotype 4b and 1/2a strains of the food-borne pathogen *Listeria monocytogenes* reveal new insights into the core genome components of this species, *Nucleic Acids Res* 32:2386-2395, 2004.
120. Hamon M, Bierne H, Cossart P: *Listeria monocytogenes*: a multifaceted model, *Nat Rev Microbiol* 4:423-434, 2006.
121. Pentecost M, Otto G, Theriot JA, Amieva MR: *Listeria monocytogenes* invades the epithelial junctions at sites of cell extrusion, *PLoS Pathog* 2:e3, 2006.
122. Nikitas G, Deschamps C, Disson O, et al: Transcytosis of *Listeria monocytogenes* across the intestinal barrier upon specific targeting of goblet cell accessible E-cadherin, *J Exp Med* 208:2263-2277, 2011.
123. Lecuit M, Nelson DM, Smith SD, et al: Targeting and crossing of the human maternofetal barrier by *Listeria monocytogenes*: role of internalin interaction with trophoblast E-cadherin, *Proc Natl Acad Sci U S A* 101:6152-6157, 2004.
124. Osanai A, Li SJ, Asano K, et al: Fibronectin-binding protein, FbpA, is the adhesin responsible for pathogenesis of *Listeria monocytogenes* infection, *Microbiol Immunol* 57:253-262, 2013.
125. Dramsi S, Bourdichon F, Cabanes D, et al: FbpA, a novel multifunctional I virulence factor, *Mol Microbiol.* 53:639-649, 2004.
126. Bierne H, Cossart P: InlB, a surface protein of *Listeria monocytogenes* that behaves as an invasin and a growth factor, *J Cell Sci* 115 (Pt 17):3357-3367, 2002.
127. Jiwani S, Wang Y, Dowd GC, et al: Identification of components of the host type IA PI 3-kinase pathway that promote internalization of *Listeria monocytogenes*, *Infect Immun* 80:1252-1256, 2012.
128. Chatterjee SS, Hossain H, Otten S, et al: Intracellular gene expression profile of Listeria monocytogenes, *Infect Immun* 74:1323-1338, 2006.
129. Veiga E, Cossart P: The role of clathrin-dependent endocytosis in bacterial internalization, *Trends Cell Biol* 16:499-504, 2006.
130. Khelef N, Lecuit M, Bierne H, Cossart P: Species specificity of the *Listeria monocytogenes* InlB protein, *Cell Microbiol* 8:457-470, 2006.
131. Bonazzi M, Cossart P: Bacterial entry into cells: a role for the endocytic machinery, *FEBS Lett* 580:2962-2967, 2006.
132. Veiga E, Cossart P: *Listeria* hijacks the clathrin-dependent endocytic machinery to invade mammalian cells, *Nat Cell Biol.* 7:894-900, 2005.
133 Veiga E, Guttman JA, Bonazzi M, et al: Invasive and adherent bacterial pathogens co-opt host clathrin for infection, *Cell Host Microbe* 2:340-351, 2007.
134. Martins M, Custodio R, Camejo A, et al: *Listeria monocytogenes* triggers the cell surface expression of Gp96 protein and interacts with its N terminus to support cellular infection, *J Biol Chem* 287: 43083-43093, 2012.
135. Seveau S, Pizarro-Cerda J, Cossart P: Molecular mechanisms exploited by *Listeria monocytogenes* during host cell invasion, *Microb Infect* 9:1167-1175, 2007.
136. Edelson BT: Dendritic cells in *Listeria monocytogenes* infection, *Adv Immunol* 113:33-49, 2012.
137. Flannagan RS, Cosio G, Grinstein S: Antimicrobial mechanisms of phagocytes and bacterial evasion strategies, *Nat Rev Microbiol* 7:355-366, 2009.
138. Liu D: Identification, subtyping and virulence determination of *Listeria monocytogenes*, an important foodborne pathogen, *J Med Microbiol* 55:645-659, 2006.
139. Lam GY, Czuczman MA, Higgins DE, Brumell JH: Interactions of *Listeria monocytogenes* with the autophagy system of host cells, *Adv Immunol* 113:7-18, 2012.
140. Hamon MA, Ribet D, Stavru F, Cossart P: Listeriolysin O: the Swiss army knife of *Listeria*, *Trends Microbiol* 20:360-368, 2012.
141. Gedde MM, Higgins DE, Tilney LG, Portnoy DA: Role of listeriolysin O in cell-to-cell spread of *Listeria monocytogenes*, *Infect Immun* 68: 999-1003, 2000.
142. Portnoy DA, Jacks PS, Hinrichs DJ: Role of hemolysin for the intracellular growth of *Listeria monocytogenes*, *J Exp Med* 167:1459-1471, 1988.
143. Beauregard KE, Lee KD, Collier RJ, Swanson JA: pH-dependent perforation of macrophage phagosomes by listeriolysin O from *Listeria monocytogenes*, *J Exp Med* 186:1159-1163, 1997.
144. Higgins DE, Shastri N, Portnoy DA: Delivery of protein to the cytosol of macrophages using *Escherichia coli* K-12, *Mol Microbiol* 31: 1631-1641, 1999.
145. Shaughnessy LM, Hoppe AD, Christensen KA, Swanson JA: Membrane perforations inhibit lysosome fusion by altering pH and calcium in *Listeria monocytogenes* vacuoles, *Cell Microbiol* 8:781-792, 2006.
146. Kayal S, Lilienbaum A, Poyart C, et al: Listeriolysin O-dependent activation of endothelial cells during infection with *Listeria monocytogenes*: activation of NF-κB and upregulation of adhesion molecules and chemokines, *Mol Microb* 31:1709-1722, 1999.
147. Tang P, Sutherland CL, Gold MR, Finlay BB: *Listeria monocytogenes* invasion of epithelial cells requires the MEK-1/ERK-2 mitogen-activated protein kinase pathway, *Infect Immun* 66:1106-1112, 1998.
148. Wadsworth SJ, Goldfine H: Mobilization of protein kinase C in macrophages induced by *Listeria monocytogenes* affects its internalization and escape from the phagosome, *Infect Immun* 70:4650-4660, 2002.
149. Le Monnier A, Autret N, Join-Lambert OF, et al: ActA is required for crossing of the fetoplacental barrier by *Listeria monocytogenes*, *Infect Immun* 75:950-957, 2007.
150. Goldfine H, Bannam T, Johnston NC, Zuckert WR: Bacterial phospholipases and intracellular growth: the two distinct phospholipases C of *Listeria monocytogenes*, *Symp Ser Soc Appl Microbiol* 27:7S-14S, 1998.
151. Leimeister-Wachter M, Domann E, Chakraborty T: Detection of a gene encoding a phosphatidylinositol-specific phospholipase C that is co-ordinately expressed with listeriolysin in *Listeria monocytogenes*, *Mol Microbiol* 5:361-366, 1991.
152. Mengaud J, Braun-Breton C, Cossart P: Identification of phosphatidylinositol-specific phospholipase C activity in *Listeria monocytogenes*: a novel type of virulence factor? *Mol Microbiol* 5:367-372, 1991.
153. Geoffroy C, Raveneau J, Beretti JL, et al: Purification and characterization of an extracellular 29-kilodalton phospholipase C from *Listeria monocytogenes*, *Infect Immun* 59:2382-2388, 1991.
154. Vazquez-Boland JA, Kocks C, Dramsi S, et al: Nucleotide sequence of the lecithinase operon of *Listeria monocytogenes* and possible role of lecithinase in cell-to-cell spread, *Infect Immun* 60:219-230, 1992.
155. Camilli A, Tilney LG, Portnoy DA: Dual roles of plcA in *Listeria monocytogenes* pathogenesis, *Mol Microbiol* 8:143-157, 1993.
156. Grundling A, Gonzalez MD, Higgins DE: Requirement of the *Listeria monocytogenes* broad-range phospholipase PC-PLC during infection of human epithelial cells, *J Bacteriol* 185:6295-6307, 2003.
157. Smith GA, Marquis H, Jones S, et al: The two distinct phospholipases C of *Listeria monocytogenes* have overlapping roles in escape from a vacuole and cell-to-cell spread, *Infect Immun* 63:4231-4237, 1995.
158. Marquis H, Doshi V, Portnoy DA: The broad-range phospholipase C and a metalloprotease mediate listeriolysin O-independent escape of *Listeria monocytogenes* from a primary vacuole in human epithelial cells, *Infect Immun* 63:4531-4534, 1995.
159. Poussin MA, Leitges M, Goldfine H: The ability of *Listeria monocytogenes* PI-PLC to facilitate escape from the macrophage phagosome is dependent on host PKCbeta, *Microb Pathog* 46:1-5, 2009.
160. Wadsworth SJ, Goldfine H: *Listeria monocytogenes* phospholipase C-dependent calcium signaling modulates bacterial entry into J774 macrophage-like cells, *Infect Immun* 67:1770-1778, 1999.
161. Poussin MA, Goldfine H: Involvement of *Listeria monocytogenes* phosphatidylinositol-specific phospholipase C and host protein kinase C in permeabilization of the macrophage phagosome, *Infect Immun* 73:4410-4413, 2005.

162. Cole C, Thomas S, Filak H, Henson PM, Lenz LL: Nitric oxide increases susceptibility of Toll-like receptor-activated macrophages to spreading *Listeria monocytogenes*, *Immunity* 36:807-820, 2012.
163. Mounier J, Ryter A, Coquis-Rondon M, Sansonetti PJ: Intracellular and cell-to-cell spread of *Listeria monocytogenes* involves interaction with F-actin in the enterocytelike cell line Caco-2, *Infect Immun* 58:1048-1058, 1990.
164. Theriot JA, Mitchison TJ, Tilney LG, Portnoy DA: The rate of actin-based motility of intracellular *Listeria monocytogenes* equals the rate of actin polymerization, *Nature* 357:257-260, 1992.
165. Tilney LG, Portnoy DA: Actin filaments and the growth, movement, and spread of the intracellular bacterial parasite, *Listeria monocytogenes*, *J Cell Biol* 109:1597-1608, 1989.
166. Tilney LG, Connelly PS, Portnoy DA: Actin filament nucleation by the bacterial pathogen, *Listeria monocytogenes*, *J Cell Biol* 111: 2979-2988, 1990.
167. Domann E, Wehland J, Rohde M, et al: A novel bacterial virulence gene in *Listeria monocytogenes* required for host cell microfilament interaction with homology to the proline-rich region of vinculin, *EMBO J* 11:1981-1990, 1992.
168. Kocks C, Hellio R, Gounon P, Ohayon H, Cossart P: Polarized distribution of *Listeria monocytogenes* surface protein ActA at the site of directional actin assembly, *J Cell Sci* 105:699-710, 1993.
169. Boujemaa-Paterski R, Gouin E, Hansen G, et al: *Listeria* protein ActA mimics WASp family proteins: it activates filament barbed end branching by Arp2/3 complex, *Biochemistry* 40:11390-11404, 2001.
170. Skoble J, Portnoy DA, Welch MD: Three regions within ActA promote Arp2/3 complex-mediated actin nucleation and *Listeria monocytogenes* motility, *J Cell Biol* 150:527-538, 2000.
171. Skoble J, Auerbuch V, Goley ED, Welch MD, Portnoy DA: Pivotal role of VASP in Arp2/3 complex-mediated actin nucleation, actin branch-formation, and *Listeria monocytogenes* motility, *J Cell Biol* 155:89-100, 2001.
172. Rajabian T, Gavicherla B, Heisig M, et al: The bacterial virulence factor InlC perturbs apical cell junctions and promotes cell-to-cell spread of *Listeria*, *Nat Cell Biol* 11:1212-1218, 2009.
173. Mostowy S, Cossart P: Virulence factors that modulate the cell biology of listeria infection and the host response, *Adv Immunol* 113: 19-32, 2012.
174. Leung N, Gianfelice A, Gray-Owen SD, Ireton K: Impact of the *Listeria monocytogenes* protein InlC on infection in mice, *Infect Immun* 81:1334-1340, 2013.
175. Gouin E, Adib-Conquy M, Balestrino D, et al: The *Listeria monocytogenes* InlC protein interferes with innate immune responses by targeting the IκB kinase subunit IKKα, *Proc Natl Acad Sci U S A* 107:17333-17338, 2010.
176. Vazquez-Boland JA, Kuhn M, Berche P, Chakraborty T, et al: *Listeria* pathogenesis and molecular virulence determinants, *Clin Microbiol Rev* 14:584-640, 2001.
177. Birmingham CL, Canadien V, Kaniuk NA, et al: Listeriolysin O allows *Listeria monocytogenes* replication in macrophage vacuoles, *Nature* 451:350-354, 2008.
178. Lam GY, Cemma M, Muise AM, Higgins DE, Brumell JH: Host and bacterial factors that regulate LC3 recruitment to *Listeria monocytogenes* during the early stages of macrophage infection, *Autophagy* 9:985-995, 2013.
179. Bonazzi M, Veiga E, Pizarro-Cerda J, Cossart P: Successive post-translational modifications of E-cadherin are required for InlA-mediated internalization of *Listeria monocytogenes*, *Cell Microbiol* 10: 2208-2222, 2008.
180. Lecuit M: Understanding how *Listeria monocytogenes* targets and crosses host barriers, *Clin Microbiol Infect* 11:430-436, 2005.
181. Jacquet C, Doumith M, Gordon JI, et al: A molecular marker for evaluating the pathogenic potential of foodborne *Listeria monocytogenes*, *J Infect Dis* 189:2094-2100, 2004.
182. Greiffenberg L, Goebel W, Kim KS, et al: Interaction of *Listeria monocytogenes* with human brain microvascular endothelial cells: InlB-dependent invasion, long-term intracellular growth, and spread from macrophages to endothelial cells, *Infect Immun* 66:5260-5267, 1998.
183. Shen Y, Naujokas M, Park M, Ireton K: InlB-dependent internalization of *Listeria* is mediated by the Met receptor tyrosine kinase, *Cell* 103:501-510, 2000.
184. Hashino M, Tachibana M, Shimizu T, Watarai M: Mannose receptor, C type 1 contributes to bacterial uptake by placental trophoblast giant cells, *FEMS Immunol Med Microbiol* 66:427-435, 2012.
185. Disson O, Lecuit M: Targeting of the central nervous system by *Listeria monocytogenes*, *Virulence* 3:213-221, 2012.
186. Rocha PR, Lomonaco S, Bottero MT, et al: Ruminant rhombencephalitis-associated *Listeria monocytogenes* strains constitute a genetically homogeneous group related to human outbreak strains, *Appl Environ Microbiol* 79:3059-3066, 2013.
187. Grundler T, Quednau N, Stump C, et al: The surface proteins InlA and InlB are interdependently required for polar basolateral invasion by *Listeria monocytogenes* in a human model of the blood-cerebrospinal fluid barrier, *Microb Infect* 15:291-301, 2013.
188. Gouin E, Mengaud J, Cossart P: The virulence gene cluster of *Listeria monocytogenes* is also present in *Listeria ivanovii*, an animal pathogen, and *Listeria seeligeri*, a nonpathogenic species, *Infect Immun* 62:3550-3553, 1994.
189. Kazmierczak MJ, Wiedmann M, Boor KJ: Contributions of *Listeria monocytogenes* sigmaB and PrfA to expression of virulence and stress response genes during extra- and intracellular growth, *Microbiology* 152:1827-1838, 2006.
190. Johansson J, Mandin P, Renzoni A, et al: An RNA thermosensor controls expression of virulence genes in *Listeria monocytogenes*, *Cell* 110:551-561, 2002.
191. Deshayes C, Bielecka MK, Cain RJ, et al: Allosteric mutants show that PrfA activation is dispensable for vacuole escape but required for efficient spread and *Listeria* survival in vivo, *Mol Microbiol* 85: 461-477, 2012.
192. Mellin JR, Cossart P: The non-coding RNA world of the bacterial pathogen, *Listeria monocytogenes*, *RNA Biol* 9:372-378, 2012.
193. Grif K, Patscheider G, Dierich MP, Allerberger F: Incidence of fecal carriage of *Listeria monocytogenes* in three healthy volunteers: a one-year prospective stool survey, *Eur J Clin Microbiol Infect Dis* 22: 16-20, 2003.
194. Seok J, Warren HS, Cuenca AG, et al: Genomic responses in mouse models poorly mimic human inflammatory diseases, *Proc Natl Acad Sci U S A* 110:3507-3512, 2013.
195. Reimer T, Schweizer M, Jungi TW: Type I IFN induction in response to *Listeria monocytogenes* in human macrophages: evidence for a differential activation of IFN regulatory factor 3 (IRF3), *J Immunol* 179:1166-1177, 2007.
196. Stockinger S, Kastner R, Kernbauer E, et al: Characterization of the interferon-producing cell in mice infected with *Listeria monocytogenes*, *PLoS Pathog* 5:e1000355, 2009.
197. Guzman CA, Rohde M, Chakraborty T, et al: Interaction of *Listeria monocytogenes* with mouse dendritic cells, *Infect Immun* 63: 3665-3673, 1995.
198. Darji A, Chakraborty T, Wehland J, Weiss S: TAP-dependent major histocompatibility complex class I presentation of soluble proteins using listeriolysin, *Eur J Immunol* 27:1353-1359, 1997.
199. Wilson CB, Kollmann TR: Induction of antigen-specific immunity in human neonates and infants, *Nestlé Nutr Workshop Ser Paediatr Program* 61:183-195, 2008.
200. Kim BH, Shenoy AR, Kumar P, Bradfield CJ, MacMicking JD: IFN-inducible GTPases in host cell defense, *Cell Host Microbe* 12: 432-444, 2012.
201. Beutler B, Jiang Z, Georgel P, et al: Genetic analysis of host resistance: Toll-like receptor signaling and immunity at large, *Ann Rev Immunol* 24:353-389, 2006.
202. MacMicking JD: Interferon-inducible effector mechanisms in cell-autonomous immunity, *Nat Rev Immunol* 12:367-382, 2012.
203. Wirsing von König CH, Finger H, Hof H, Emmerling P: Postnatal development of resistance against infection in an experimental model, *Zentralbl Bakteriol* 242:547-554, 1978.
204. Wirsing von König CH, Heymer B, Finger H, Emmerling P, Hof H: Alteration of non-specific resistance to infection with *Listeria monocytogenes*, *Infection* 16(Suppl 2):S112-S117, 1988.
205. Diacovich L, Gorvel JP: Bacterial manipulation of innate immunity to promote infection, *Nat Rev Microbiol* 8:117-128, 2010.
206. Kobayashi SD, Braughton KR, Whitney AR, et al: Bacterial pathogens modulate an apoptosis differentiation program in human neutrophils, *Proc Natl Acad Sci U S A* 100:10948-10953, 2003.
207. Pamer EG: Immune responses to *Listeria monocytogenes*, *Nat Rev Immunol* 4:812-823, 2004.

208. Darji A, Mohamed W, Domann E, Chakraborty T: Induction of immune responses by attenuated isogenic mutant strains of *Listeria monocytogenes*, *Vaccine* 21(Suppl 2):S102-S109, 2003.
209. Goossens PL, Milon G, Cossart P, Saron MF: Attenuated *Listeria monocytogenes* as a live vector for induction of CD8+ T cells in vivo: a study with the nucleoprotein of the lymphocytic choriomeningitis virus, *Int Immunol* 7:797-805, 1995.
210. Kollmann TR, Reikie B, Blimkie D, et al: Induction of protective immunity to *Listeria monocytogenes* in neonates, *J Immunol* 178:3695-3701, 2007.
211. Reikie BA, Smolen KK, Fortuno ES 3rd, et al: A single immunization near birth elicits immediate and lifelong protective immunity, *Vaccine* 29:83-90, 2010.
212. Munk ME, Kaufmann SH: *Listeria monocytogenes* reactive T lymphocytes in healthy individuals, *Microb Pathog* 5:49-54, 1988.
213. Williams DR, Chanos P: Application of anti-listerial bacteriocins: monitoring enterocin expression by multiplex relative reverse transcription-PCR, *Biochem Soc Trans* 40:1544-1548, 2012.
214. Zaia AA, Sappington KJ, Nisapakultorn K, et al: Subversion of antimicrobial calprotectin (S100A8/S100A9 complex) in the cytoplasm of TR146 epithelial cells after invasion by *Listeria monocytogenes*, *Mucosal Immunol* 2:43-53, 2009.
215. Ménard S, Forster V, Lotz M, et al: Developmental switch of intestinal antimicrobial peptide expression, *J Exp Med* 205:183-193, 2008.
216. Williams MA, Schmidt RL, Lenz LL: Early events regulating immunity and pathogenesis during *Listeria monocytogenes* infection, *Trends Immunol* 33:488-495, 2012.
217. Liu S, Takala TM, Wan X, Reunanen J, Saris PE: Cell-mediated killing of *Listeria monocytogenes* by leucocin C producing *Escherichia coli*, *Microbiol Res* 168:300-304, 2013.
218. Conlan JW, North RJ: Neutrophils are essential for early anti-*Listeria* defense in the liver, but not in the spleen or peritoneal cavity, as revealed by a granulocyte-depleting monoclonal antibody, *J Exp Med* 179:259-268, 1994.
219. Carr KD, Sieve AN, Indramohan M, et al: Specific depletion reveals a novel role for neutrophil-mediated protection in the liver during *Listeria monocytogenes* infection, *Eur J Immunol* 41:2666-2676, 2011.
220. Shi C, Hohl TM, Leiner I, et al: Ly6G+ neutrophils are dispensable for defense against systemic *Listeria monocytogenes* infection, *J Immunol* 187:5293-5298, 2011.
221. Serbina NV, Salazar-Mather TP, Biron CA, Kuziel WA, Pamer EG: TNF/iNOS-producing dendritic cells mediate innate immune defense against bacterial infection, *Immunity* 19:59-70, 2003.
222. Havell EA: Evidence that tumor necrosis factor has an important role in antibacterial resistance, *J Immunol* 143:2894-2899, 1989.
223. Shiloh MU, MacMicking JD, Nicholson S, et al: Phenotype of mice and macrophages deficient in both phagocyte oxidase and inducible nitric oxide synthase, *Immunity* 10:29-38, 1999.
224. Bortolussi R, Rajaraman K, Serushago B: Role of tumor necrosis factor-alpha and interferon-gamma in newborn host defense against *Listeria monocytogenes* infection, *Pediatr Res* 32:460-464, 1992.
225. Harty JT, Lenz LL, Bevan MJ: Primary and secondary immune responses to *Listeria monocytogenes*, *Curr Opin Immunol* 8:526-530, 1996.
226. Conlan JW, North RJ: Roles of *Listeria monocytogenes* virulence factors in survival: virulence factors distinct from listeriolysin are needed for the organism to survive an early neutrophil-mediated host defense mechanism, *Infect Immun* 60:951-957, 1992.
227. Adkins B: Peripheral CD4+ lymphocytes derived from fetal versus adult thymic precursors differ phenotypically and functionally, *J Immunol* 171:5157-5164, 2003.
228. Li L, Lee HH, Bell JJ, et al: IL-4 utilizes an alternative receptor to drive apoptosis of Th1 cells and skews neonatal immunity toward Th2, *Immunity* 20:429-440, 2004.
229. Poulsen KP, Czuprynski CJ: Pathogenesis of listeriosis during pregnancy, *Anim Health Res Rev* 14:30-39, 2013.
230. Poulsen KP, Faith NG, Steinberg H, Czuprynski CJ: Bacterial load and inflammation in fetal tissues is not dependent on IL-17a or IL-22 in 10-14 day pregnant mice infected with *Listeria monocytogenes*, *Microb Pathog* 56:47-52, 2013.
231. Abram M, Doric M: Primary *Listeria monocytogenes* infection in gestating mice, *Folia Microbiol (Praha)* 42:65-71, 1997.
232. Redline RW, Lu CY: Role of local immunosuppression in murine fetoplacental listeriosis, *J Clin Invest* 79:1234-1241, 1987.
233. Issekutz TB, Evans J, Bortolussi R: The immune response of human neonates to *Listeria monocytogenes* infection, *Clin Invest Med* 7:281-286, 1984.
234. Rowe JH, Ertelt JM, Xin L, Way SS: *Listeria monocytogenes* cytoplasmic entry induces fetal wastage by disrupting maternal Foxp3+ regulatory T cell-sustained fetal tolerance, *PLoS Pathog* 8:e1002873, 2012.
235. Klatt EC, Pavlova Z, Teberg AJ, Yonekura ML: Epidemic perinatal listeriosis at autopsy, *Human Pathol* 17:1278-1281, 1986.
236. Reiss HJ: Pathologic anatomy of *Listeria* infection in children, *Kinderarztl Prax* 92-100, 1953.
237. Armstrong RW, Fung PC: Brainstem encephalitis (rhombencephalitis) due to *Listeria monocytogenes*: case report and review, *Clin Infect Dis* 16:689-702, 1993.
238. Steele PE, Jacobs DS: *Listeria monocytogenes*. Macroabscesses of placenta, *Obstet Gynecol* 53:124-127, 1979.
239. Topalovski M, Yang SS, Boonpasat Y: Listeriosis of the placenta: clinicopathologic study of seven cases, *Amer J Obstet Gynecol* 169:616-620, 1993.
240. Wilson CB: Immunologic basis for increased susceptibility of the neonate to infection, *J Pediatr* 108:1-12, 1986.
241. Kaur S Malik SV, Vaidya VM Barbuddhe SB: *Listeria monocytogenes* in spontaneous abortions in humans and its detection by multiplex PCR, *J Appl Microbiol* 103:1889-1896, 2007.
242. Bubonja-Sonje M, Mustac E, Brunn A, Deckert M, Abram M: Listeriosis in pregnancy: case report and retrospective study, *J Matern Fetal Neonat Med* 26:321-323, 2013.
243. Burn CG: Unidentified gram-positive bacillus associated with meningo-encephalitis, *Proc Soc Exp Biol Med* 31:1095, 1934.
244. Burn CG: Characteristics of a new species of the genus *Listerella* obtained from human sources, *J Bacteriol* 30:573, 1935.
245. Bortolussi R: Neonatal listeriosis, *Semin Perinatol* 14(4 Suppl 1): 44-48, 1990.
246. Silver HM: Listeriosis during pregnancy, *Obst Gynecol Surv* 53: 737-740, 1998.
247. Lorber B: Listeriosis, *Clin Infect Dis* 24:1-9, 1997.
248. Ahlfors CE, Goetzman BW, Halsted CC, Sherman MP, Wennberg RP: Neonatal listeriosis, *Am J Dis Child* 131:405-408, 1977.
249. Loeb MB, Ford-Jones EL, Styliadis S, et al: Perinatal listeriosis, *J Soc Obstet Gynecol Can.* 18:164-170, 1996.
250. Albritton WL, Wiggins GL, Feeley JC: Neonatal listeriosis: distribution of serotypes in relation to age at onset of disease, *J Pediatr* 88:481-483, 1976.
251. Evans JR, Allen AC, Stinson DA, Bortolussi R, Peddle LJ: Perinatal listeriosis: report of an outbreak, *Pediatr Infect Dis J* 4:237-241, 1985.
252. Lennon D, Lewis B, Mantell C, et al: Epidemic perinatal listeriosis, *Pediatr Infect Dis J* 3:30-34, 1984.
253. Becroft DM, Farmer K, Seddon RJ, et al: Epidemic listeriosis in the newborn, *Br Med J* 3:747-751, 1971.
254. Visintine AM, Oleske JM, Nahmias AJ: *Listeria monocytogenes* infection in infants and children, *Am J Dis Child* 131:339, 1977.
255. McLauchlin J: Human listeriosis in Britain, 1967-85, a summary of 722 cases. 2. Listeriosis in non-pregnant individuals, a changing pattern of infection and seasonal incidence, *Epidemiol Infect* 104:191-201, 1990.
256. Chaudhuri K, Chang QC, Tan EK, Yong EL: Listeriosis in pregnancy with placental abruption, *J Obstet Gynaecol* 32:594, 2012.
257. Spyrou N, Anderson M, Foale R: *Listeria* endocarditis: current management and patient outcome—world literature review, *Heart* 77:380-383, 1997.
258. Miguel-Yanes JM, Gonzalez-Ramallo VJ, Pastor L: Outcome of *Listeria monocytogenes* prosthetic valve endocarditis: as bad as it looks? *Scand J Infect Dis* 36:709-711, 2004.
259. Jackson TL, Eykyn SJ, Graham EM, Stanford MR: Endogenous bacterial endophthalmitis: a 17-year prospective series and review of 267 reported cases, *Surv Ophthalmol* 48:403-423, 2003.
260. Betriu C, Fuentemilla S, Mendez R, Picazo JJ, Garcia-Sanchez J: Endophthalmitis caused by *Listeria monocytogenes*, *J Clin Microbiol* 39:2742-2744, 2001.
261. Sivalingam JJ, Martin P, Fraimow HS, Yarze JC, Friedman LS: *Listeria monocytogenes* peritonitis: case report and literature review, *Am J Gastroenterol* 87:1839-1845, 1992.
262. Dylewski JS: Bacterial peritonitis caused by *Listeria monocytogenes*: case report and review of the literature, *Can J Infect* 7:59-62, 1996.
263. Nadarajah K, Pritchard C: *Listeria monocytogenes* septic arthritis in a patient treated with etanercept for rheumatoid arthritis, *J Clin Rheumatol* 11:120-122, 2005.

264. Benitez-Segura I, Fiol-Jaume M, Balliu PR, Tejedor M: *Listeria monocytogenes*: generalised maculopapular rash may be the clue, *Arch Dis Child Fetal Neonat* 98:F64, 2013.
265. Felsenfeld O: Diseases of poultry transmissible to man, *Iowa State Coll Vet* 13:89, 1951.
266. Hood M: Listeriosis as an infection of pregnancy manifested in the newborn, *Pediatrics* 27:390-396, 1961.
267. Kessler SL, Dajani AS: *Listeria* meningitis in infants and children, *Pediatr Infect Dis J* 9:61-63, 1990.
268. Pron B, Boumaila C, Jaubert F, et al: Comprehensive study of the intestinal stage of listeriosis in a rat ligated ileal loop system, *Infect Immun* 66:747-755, 1998.
269. Dalton CB, Austin CC, Sobel J, et al: An outbreak of gastroenteritis and fever due to *Listeria monocytogenes* in milk, *N Engl J Med* 336:100-105, 1997.
270. Ooi ST, Lorber B: Gastroenteritis due to *Listeria monocytogenes*, *Clin Infect Dis* 40:1327-1332, 2005.
271. Goulet V, King LA, Vaillant V, de Valk H: What is the incubation period for listeriosis? *BMC Infect Dis* 13:11, 2013.
272. Krittisch AW: Experimenteller Beitrag zur Biologie des *Bacterium-monocytogens* mit besenderer Berucksichtigung seiner Bezehung zur infektiosen Mononukleose des Menschen, *Zentralbl Bakteriol Hyg* 131:89, 1934.
273. Massarotti EM, Dinerman H: Septic arthritis due to *Listeria monocytogenes*: report and review of the literature, *J Rheumatol* 17:111-113, 1990.
274. Lucas MJ, Brouwer MC, van de Beek D: Delayed cerebral thrombosis in bacterial meningitis: a prospective cohort study, *Intensive Care Med* 39:866-871, 2013.
275. Bille J, Doyle MP: Listeria and erysipelothrix. In Ballows A, Hausler WJ Jr, Hermann KL, et al: *Manual of clinical microbiology*, ed 5, Washington DC, 1991, American Society of Microbiology, pp 287-295.
276. van Netten P, Perales I, van de Moosdijk A, Curtis GD, Mossel DA: Liquid and solid selective differential media for the detection and enumeration of *L. monocytogenes* and other *Listeria* spp, *Int J Food Microbiol* 8:299-316, 1989.
277. Gray ML, Stafseth HJ, Thorp F, Sholl LB, Riley WF: A new technique for isolating listerellae from the bovine brain, *J Bacteriol* 55:471, 1948.
278. Cepeda JA, Millar M, Sheridan EA, et al: Listeriosis due to infection with a catalase-negative strain of *Listeria monocytogenes*, *J Clin Microbiol* 44:1917-1918, 2006.
279. Seeliger HPR, Jones D: *The genus Listeria*, Baltimore, 1986, Williams and Wilkins.
280. Backman A, Lantz P, Radstrom P, Olcen P: Evaluation of an extended diagnostic PCR assay for detection and verification of the common causes of bacterial meningitis in CSF and other biological samples, *Mol Cell Probes* 13:49-60, 1999.
281. Lohmann CP, Gabel VP, Heep M, Linde HJ, Reischl U: *Listeria monocytogenes*-induced endogenous endophthalmitis in an otherwise healthy individual: rapid PCR-diagnosis as the basis for effective treatment, *Eur J Ophthal* 9:53-57, 1999.
282. Huijsdens XW, Linskens RK, Taspinar H, et al: *Listeria monocytogenes* and inflammatory bowel disease: detection of *Listeria* species in intestinal mucosal biopsies by real-time PCR, *Scand J Gastroenterol* 38:332-333, 2003.
283. Chiba M, Kono M, Hoshina S, et al: Presence of bacterial 16S ribosomal RNA gene segments in human intestinal lymph follicles, *Scand J Gastroenterol* 35:824-831, 2000.
284. Boving MK, Pedersen LN, Moller JK: Eight-plex PCR and liquid-array detection of bacterial and viral pathogens in cerebrospinal fluid from patients with suspected meningitis, *J Clin Microbiol.* 47:908-913, 2009.
285. Le Monnier A, Abachin E, Beretti JL, Berche P, Kayal S: Diagnosis of *Listeria monocytogenes* meningoencephalitis by real-time PCR for the hly gene, *J Clin Microbiol* 49:3917-3923, 2011.
286. Hudak AP, Lee SH, Issekutz AC, Bortolussi R: Comparison of three serological methods—enzyme-linked immunosorbent assay, complement fixation, and microagglutination—in the diagnosis of human perinatal *Listeria monocytogenes* infection, *Clin Invest Med* 7:349-354, 1984.
287. Winblad S: Studies of antibodies in human listeriosis. 1. Antibodies in cases of bacteriologically verified human listeriosis, *Acta Pathol Microbiol Scand* 58:123-132, 1963.
288. Berche P, Reich KA, Bonnichon M, et al: Detection of anti-listeriolysin O for serodiagnosis of human listeriosis, *Lancet* 335:624-627, 1990.
289. Drew RM: Occurrence of two immunological groups within the genus *Listeria;* studies based upon precipitation reactions, *Proc Soc Exp Biol Med* 61:30-33, 1946.
290. Schierz G, Burger A: *The detection of Listeria antibodies by passive hemagglutination. Proceedings of the Third International Symposium on Listeriosis*, Netherlands, 1966, Bilthoven. 77.
291. Njoku-Obi AN: An antigen-fixation test for the serodiagnosis of *Listeria monocytogenes* infections, *Cornell Vet* 52:415-430, 1962.
292. Jorgensen JH, Hindler JA, Bernard K, et al: *Methods for antimicrobial dilution and disk susceptibility testing of infrequently isolated or fastidious bacteria; approved guideline*, ed 2, Wayne, Pa, 2010, Clinical and Laboratory Standards Institute, pp 30.
293. European Committee on Antimicrobial Susceptibility Testing (EUCAST): EUCAST clinical breakpoint table v. 3.1. July 23, 2013. Available at http://www.eucast.org/fileadmin/src/media/PDFs/EUCAST_files/Breakpoint_tables/Breakpoint_table_v_3.1.pdf.
294. MacGowan AP: Listeriosis—the therapeutic options, *J Antimicrob Chemother* 26:721-722, 1990.
295. Suarez MM, Bautista RM, Almela M, et al: *Listeria monocytogenes* bacteremia: analysis of 110 episodes, *Med Clin (Barc)* 129:218-221, 2007.
296. Charpentier E, Gerbaud G, Jacquet C, Rocourt J, Courvalin P: Incidence of antibiotic resistance in *Listeria* species, *J Infect Dis* 172: 277-281, 1995.
297. Espaze EP, Roubeix YG, Le Berre JY, Courtieu AI: In vitro susceptibility of *Listeria monocytogenes* to some antibiotics and their combinations, *Zentralbl Bakteriol* 240:76-85, 1978.
298. Poyart-Salmeron C, Carlier C, Trieu-Cuot P, Courtieu AL, Courvalin P: Transferable plasmid-mediated antibiotic resistance in *Listeria monocytogenes*, *Lancet* 335:1422-1426, 1990.
299. Srinivasan V, Nam HM, Nguyen LT, et al: Prevalence of antimicrobial resistance genes in *Listeria monocytogenes* isolated from dairy farms, *Foodborne Pathog Dis* 2:201-211, 2005.
300. Walsh D, Duffy G, Sheridan JJ, Blair IS, McDowell DA: Antibiotic resistance among *Listeria*, including *Listeria monocytogenes*, in retail foods, *J Appl Microbiol* 90:517-522, 2001.
301. Hansen JM, Gerner-Smidt P, Bruun B: Antibiotic susceptibility of *Listeria monocytogenes* in Denmark 1958-2001, *Acta Pathol Microbiol Scand* 113:31-36, 2005.
302. Soriano F, Zapardiel J, Nieto E: Antimicrobial susceptibilities of *Corynebacterium* species and other non-spore-forming gram-positive bacilli to 18 antimicrobial agents, *Antimicrob Agents Chemother* 39:208-214, 1995.
303. Prazak MA, Murano EA, Mercado I, Acuff GR: Antimicrobial resistance of *Listeria monocytogenes* isolated from various cabbage farms and packing sheds in Texas, *J Food Protect* 65:1796-1799, 2002.
304. Espaze EP, Reynaud AE: Antibiotic susceptibilities of *Listeria*: in vitro studies, *Infection* 16(Suppl 2):S160-S164, 1988.
305. Gordon RC, Barrett FF, Clark DJ: Influence of several antibiotics, singly and in combination, on the growth of *Listeria monocytogenes*, *J Pediatr* 80:667-670, 1972.
306. Gordon RC, Barrett FF, Yow MD: Ampicillin treatment of listeriosis, *J Pediatr* 77:1067-1070, 1970.
307. Vischer WA, Rominger C: Rifampicin against experimental listeriosis in the mouse, *Chemotherapy* 24:104-111, 1978.
308. Hawkins AE, Bortolussi R, Issekutz AC: In vitro and in vivo activity of various antibiotics against *Listeria monocytogenes* type 4b, *Clin Invest Med* 7:335-341, 1984.
309. Edmiston CE Jr, Gordon RC: Evaluation of gentamicin and penicillin as a synergistic combination in experimental murine listeriosis, *Antimicrob Agents Chemother* 16:862-863, 1979.
310. Morosi S, Francisci D, Baldelli F: A case of rhombencephalitis caused by *Listeria monocytogenes* successfully treated with linezolid, *J Infect* 52:e73-e75, 2006.
311. Traub WH: Perinatal listeriosis. Tolerance of a clinical isolate of *Listeria monocytogenes* for ampicillin and resistance against cefotaxime, *Chemotherapy* 27:423-431, 1981.
312. Stamm AM: Chloramphenicol: ineffective for treatment of *Listeria* meningitis, *Am J Med* 72:830, 1982.
313. Forna F, McConnell M, Kitabire FN, et al: Systematic review of the safety of trimethoprim-sulfamethoxazole for prophylaxis in HIV-infected pregnant women: implications for resource-limited settings, *AIDS Rev* 8:24-36, 2006.

314. Hof H, Waldenmeier G: Therapy of experimental listeriosis—an evaluation of different antibiotics, *Infection* 16(Suppl 2):S171-S174, 1988.
315. Scheld WM: Evaluation of rifampin and other antibiotics against *Listeria monocytogenes* in vitro and in vivo, *Rev Infect Dis* 5(Suppl 3): S593-S599, 1983.
316. Munoz P, Ferreira L, Marin M, et al: First report of *Listeria monocytogenes* endocarditis treated with linezolid, *Int J Antimicrob Agents* 28:480-481, 2006.
317. van Ogtrop ML, Mattie H, Sekh BR, van Strijen E, van Furth R: Comparison of the antibacterial efficacies of ampicillin and ciprofloxacin against experimental infections with *Listeria monocytogenes* in hydrocortisone-treated mice, *Antimicrob Agents Chemother* 36:2375-2380, 1992.
318. Cherubin CE, Appleman MD, Heseltine PN, Khayr W, Stratton CW: Epidemiological spectrum and current treatment of listeriosis, *Rev Infect Dis* 13:1108-1114, 1991.
319. Carryn S, Van Bambeke F, Mingeot-Leclercq MP, Tulkens PM: Comparative intracellular (THP-1 macrophage) and extracellular activities of beta-lactams, azithromycin, gentamicin, and fluoroquinolones against *Listeria monocytogenes* at clinically relevant concentrations, *Antimicrob Agents Chemother* 46:2095-2103, 2002.
320. Martinez-Martinez L, Joyanes P, Suarez AI, Perea EJ: Activities of gemifloxacin and five other antimicrobial agents against *Listeria monocytogenes* and coryneform bacteria isolated from clinical samples, *Antimicrob Agents Chemother* 45:2390-2392, 2001.
321. Sipahi OR, Turhan T, Pullukcu H, et al: Moxifloxacin versus ampicillin + gentamicin in the therapy of experimental *Listeria monocytogenes* meningitis, *J Antimicrob Chemother* 61:670-673, 2008.
322. Fanos V, Dall'Agnola A: Antibiotics in neonatal infections: a review, *Drugs* 58:405-427, 1999.
323. Gray ML: Epidemiological aspects of listeriosis, *Am J Publ Health* 53:554-563, 1963.
324. Hune OS: Maternal *Listeria monocytogenes* septicemia with sparing of the fetus, *Obstet Gynecol* 48:335, 1976.
325. Katz VL, Weinstein L: Antepartum treatment of *Listeria monocytogenes* septicemia, *South Med J* 75:1353-1354, 1982.
326. Fuchs S, Hochner-Celnikier D, Shalev O: First trimester listeriosis with normal fetal outcome, *Eur J Clin Microbiol Infect Dis* 13:656-658, 1994.
327. Evans JR, Allen AC, Bortolussi R, Issekutz TB, Stinson DA: Follow-up study of survivors of fetal and early onset neonatal listeriosis, *Clin Invest Med* 7:329-334, 1984.
328. Teberg AJ, Yonekura ML, Salminen C, Pavlova Z: Clinical manifestations of epidemic neonatal listeriosis, *Pediatr Infect Dis J* 6:817-820, 1987.
329. Rotheberg AD, Maisels MJ, Bagnato S, et al: Outcome for surviviors of mechanical ventilation weighing less than 1200 gm at birth, *J Pediatr* 98:106, 1981.
330. Naege RL: Amnionic fluid infections, neonatal hyperbilirubinemia and psychomotor impairment, *Pediatrics* 62:497, 1978.
331. Line FG, Cherry WB: Meningitis due to *Listeria monocytogenes*; report of two cases, *J Am Med Assoc* 148:366-369, 1952.
332. Watson GW, Fuller TJ, Elms J, Kluge RM: *Listeria* cerebritis: relapse of infection in renal transplant patients, *Arch Intern Med* 138:83-87, 1978.
333. Roed C, Engsig FN, Omland LH, Skinhoj P, Obel N: Long-term mortality in patients diagnosed with *Listeria monocytogenes* meningitis: a Danish nationwide cohort study, *J Infect* 64:34-40, 2012.
334. Tappero JW, Schuchat A, Deaver KA, Mascola L, Wenger JD: Reduction in the incidence of human listeriosis in the United States. Effectiveness of prevention efforts? The Listeriosis Study Group, *JAMA* 273:1118-1122, 1995.
335. Furyk JS, Swann O, Molyneux E: Systematic review: neonatal meningitis in the developing world, *Trop Med Int Health* 16:672-679, 2011.
336. Goulet V, de Valk H, Pierre O, et al: Effect of prevention measures on incidence of human listeriosis, France, 1987-1997, *Emerg Infect Dis* 7:983-989, 2001.
337. Petrilli ES, D'Ablaing G, Ledger WJ: *Listeria monocytogenes* chorioamnionitis: diagnosis by transabdominal amniocentesis, *Obstet Gynecol* 55(Suppl 3):5S-8S, 1980.
338. Centers for Disease Control and Prevention: Listeria (listeriosis). Atlanta, 2011 (updated September 21, 2011). Available at http://www.cdc.gov/listeria/prevention.html. Accessed June 24, 2013.
339. Centers for Disease Control and Prevention: Outbreak of listeriosis—northeastern United States, 2002, *MMWR Morb Mortal Wkly Rep* 51:950-951, 2002.
340. Ogunmodede F, Jones JL, Scheftel J, et al: Listeriosis prevention knowledge among pregnant women in the USA, *Infect Dis Obstet Gynecol* 13:11-15, 2005.
341. Bondarianzadeh D, Yeatman H, Condon-Paoloni D: *Listeria* education in pregnancy: lost opportunity for health professionals, *Aust N Z J Public Health* 31:468-474, 2007.
342. Voetsch AC, Angulo FJ, Jones TF, et al: Reduction in the incidence of invasive listeriosis in foodborne diseases active surveillance network sites, 1996-2003, *Clin Infect Dis* 44:513-520, 2007.

14 Staphylococcal Infections

JOHN S. BRADLEY and VICTOR NIZET

CHAPTER OUTLINE

Staphylococcal disease has been recognized in neonates for centuries and reported at least as early as 1773, when pemphigus neonatorum was described.[1] Outbreaks of staphylococcal disease in nurseries were first noted in the late 1920s,[2] and the memorable term "cloud baby" was subsequently coined to describe index cases, often asymptomatic, who contaminated the nursery atmosphere with *Staphylococcus aureus* that colonized their respiratory tract, skin, or umbilical cord.[3] Until the late 1970s, staphylococcal disease in newborn infants was caused most often by *S. aureus*.[4] However, in the recent decades, coagulase-negative staphylococci (CoNS) have assumed an equally important role, especially in premature infants in neonatal intensive care units (NICUs),[5-7] often responsible for half or more of all cases of clinically significant bacterial disease. Management of staphylococcal disease in infants has become increasingly more complicated, reflecting the increasing incidence of methicillin resistance and the threat of vancomycin resistance among isolates of *S. aureus* and CoNS. This chapter summarizes current information about *S. aureus* and CoNS and the diseases these organisms produce in newborns and young infants.

Epidemiology and Transmission

STAPHYLOCOCCUS AUREUS

Many factors influence transmission of staphylococci among newborns, including nursery design, density of the infant population, and obstetric and nursing practices. Other factors influencing transmission include virulence properties of the individual *S. aureus* strains and immunogenetic factors characteristic of the newborn host. A particular factor that is critical in one epidemic may not be a driving factor under different circumstances.

Quantitative culture studies demonstrate that very small numbers of *S. aureus* are capable of establishing colonization in the newborn. Fewer than 10 bacteria can initiate umbilical colonization in 50% of newborns, whereas approximately 250 organisms can produce the same effect on the nasal mucosa.[8] Colonization of the newborn umbilicus, nares, and skin takes place early in life. By the fifth day in the nursery, the colonization rate among nursery inhabitants may be as high as 90%.[9] The umbilicus or rectum usually is colonized before the nares are.[10,11]

Most evidence indicates that the initial and perhaps major source of *S. aureus* infection is medical and nursing personnel.[8] A *S. aureus* strain common among medical attendants is far more likely than a maternal strain to colonize a given infant in the nursery[12]; in 85% of cases, infant colonization with *S. aureus* is likely to originate from an attendant's touch.[13] Persons with overt cutaneous lesions or disease often are highly contagious, but asymptomatic carriers can also be contagious,[14] and carriage on the skin, in the anterior nares, and in the perineal area is relevant.[15,16] The frequency of intestinal carriage of the pathogen may be greatly underestimated.[17]

Soon after the introduction of methicillin in 1960, methicillin-resistant *S. aureus* (MRSA) emerged as an important nosocomial pathogen.[18] For MRSA, resistance is mediated through the *mecA* gene, which encodes an altered penicillin-binding protein (PBP2a) with markedly reduced affinity for most β-lactam antibiotics.[19] MRSA isolates frequently harbor additional antibiotic resistance determinants, further limiting treatment options. Risk factors for MRSA infection include prior antimicrobial treatment, prolonged hospitalization, and stay within an intensive care unit.[20] Since the mid-1990s, infection with community-acquired MRSA (CA-MRSA) has been reported increasingly in patients without hospital contact or traditional risk factors for MRSA.[21,22] CA-MRSA strains typically have a distinct antibiotic susceptibility pattern, and more frequently cause skin and soft tissue infections or necrotizing pneumonias compared with methicillin-susceptible *S. aureus* (MSSA). CA-MRSA isolates are readily transmitted between family members and close contacts.[22]

The National Institute of Child Health and Human Development (NICHD) Neonatal Research Network reported that from 2006 to 2008, approximately 3.7% of initial episodes of late-onset sepsis (LOS) or meningitis among very-low-birth-weight (VLBW) infants (<1500 g) were caused by *S. aureus*, with 28% of these attributable to MRSA; outcomes were similar in the two groups.[23] Carey and colleagues[24] reported the epidemiology of MSSA and MRSA in the NICU at Columbia University Medical Center. During the study period, there were 123 infections caused by MSSA and 49 infections caused by MRSA (28%). Overall, the clinical presentations and the crude mortality rates (16%-17%) were similar in both groups, although infants with MRSA infections were significantly younger at clinical presentation than infants with MSSA infections. The most common manifestations were bacteremia (36%), skin/soft tissue/wound infection (31%), bacteremia plus skin/soft tissue infection (15%), endocarditis (7%), and rare cases of tracheitis, osteomyelitis, meningitis, or mediastinitis. The risk of developing MSSA or MRSA infection was inversely related to birth weight, with 53% of infections occurring in VLBW infants and the majority of infections in infants weighing greater than 2500 g associated with surgical procedures. Reports of small outbreaks of community-acquired MRSA in NICUs and well-baby nurseries have appeared with increasing frequency.[25-27]

When clusters of staphylococcal disease associated with hospital exposure occur, temporal clustering of cases suggests the possibility of an outbreak caused by a single strain.[28] In these situations, strain identity requires characterization based on a molecular technique, such as pulsed-field gel electrophoresis (PFGE) or multilocus sequence typing (MLST). MLST is a sequence-based typing system that uses the sequence of seven or more housekeeping genes to evaluate the genetic relatedness of strains of staphylococci.[29] The discriminatory power of this approach is less than that of PFGE, so the usefulness for the evaluation of local outbreaks is less.[30] Next-generation whole-genome sequencing has recently been applied to investigate MRSA transmission in the NICU setting and identified an increased risk of transmission from infants with as yet undiscovered MRSA colonization, in contrast to known MRSA-positive infants.[31]

COAGULASE-NEGATIVE STAPHYLOCOCCI

Coagulase-negative staphylococci are common inhabitants of human skin and mucous membranes. *Staphylococcus epidermidis* is the species found most commonly as a member of the normal flora of the nasal mucosa and the umbilicus of the newborn.[32] With sensitive culture techniques, the nose, umbilicus, and chest skin are colonized with CoNS in up to 83% of neonates by 4 days of age.[33] Rates of colonization with *S. epidermidis* in one study of infants in a large academic NICU were as follows: nose, 89%; throat, 84%; umbilicus, 90%; and stool, 86%; simultaneous percentages for *S. aureus* were 17%, 17%, 21%, and 10%, respectively.[32] Although most infants acquire CoNS from environmental sources, including hospital personnel, a small percentage are colonized by vertical transmission.[34,35] Isolates of *S. epidermidis* and other CoNS resistant to multiple antibiotic agents are common. In a study involving premature neonates, D'Angio and associates[36] demonstrated that the incidence of strains resistant to multiple antibiotics rose from 32% to 82% by the end of the first week of life.

The observation that CoNS are important nosocomial pathogens among newborns, especially low-birth-weight (LBW) infants in NICUs, is explained by the prevalence of colonization with these organisms at multiple sites and the widespread use of invasive therapeutic modalities that subvert normal host epithelial barrier defenses. Examples of invasive treatments include endotracheal intubation, mechanical ventilation, placement of umbilical and other central venous catheters, urinary bladder catheters, and ventriculoperitoneal shunts, and the use of feeding tubes. In recent epidemiology, CoNS account for greater than half of bloodstream isolates obtained from neonates with LOS.[5-7] An inverse relationship exists between the rate of infection with CoNS and both birth weight and gestational age. Additional risk factors that are associated with CoNS bacteremia among VLBW neonates include respiratory distress syndrome, bronchopulmonary dysplasia, patent ductus arteriosus, severe intraventricular hemorrhage, and necrotizing enterocolitis (NEC).[5,7]

Certain nutritional factors are associated with the development of LOS, including delayed initiation of enteral feeding, prolonged period to reach full enteral feeding status, delayed re-attainment of birth weight, and prolonged parenteral hyperalimentation.[5] Administration of intralipids through a Teflon catheter has also been shown in a case-control study to be associated with an increased risk of bacteremia caused by CoNS.[37] Most experts feel the clinical and experimental data suggest that CoNS have not become more virulent over time. Rather, these ubiquitous organisms have become more common pathogens because therapeutic approaches have become increasingly invasive and because VLBW premature infants with compromised immunity are surviving longer. Indeed, the very interventions sustaining the hospitalized LBW neonate concurrently expose them to serious nosocomial infections, with CoNS at the forefront of causative agents.[7]

Microbiology

Staphylococci are members of the family Micrococcaceae and are nonmotile, non–spore-forming bacteria that are catalase-negative. Species of staphylococci are separated into two large groups on the basis of ability to produce the extracellular enzyme coagulase. Organisms that produce coagulase are known as coagulase-positive staphylococci, primarily *S. aureus*,[38] and organisms that produce no coagulase are referred to as CoNS. The presence of coagulase can be evaluated either by assessing broth medium for secreted enzyme, which reacts with coagulase-reacting factor in plasma and results in formation of a fibrin clot, or by testing for cell-bound enzyme, which results in clumping when a suspension of organisms is incubated with plasma.

Staphylococci grow best in an aerobic environment but can proliferate under anaerobic conditions as well. They grow readily on most routine laboratory media, including Luria broth, and usually are isolated from clinical specimens by using sheep blood agar. Gram stain reveals gram-positive cocci ranging from 0.7 to 1.2 mM in diameter, usually visible in irregular grapelike clusters (Fig. 14-1A). Growth in liquid culture often results in a predominance of single cocci, pairs, tetrads, and chains of three or four cells. Of note, dying organisms and bacteria in stationary phase or ingested by phagocytes may appear to be gram-negative. Growth on blood agar results in round, convex, shiny opaque colonies that are 1 to 2 mm in diameter after 24 hours of incubation. *S. aureus* colonies often are deep yellow or golden in color and typically are surrounded by a zone of β-hemolysis (see Fig. 14-1B). By contrast, colonies of CoNS usually are chalk-white, often lacking surrounding hemolysis.

STAPHYLOCOCCUS AUREUS

The staphylococcal cell wall is composed of two major components, peptidoglycan and teichoic acid.[39,40] *S. aureus* peptidoglycan is composed of chains of N-acetylglucosamine, N-acetylmuramic acid, alanine, glutamic acid, and lysine or diaminopimelic acid, with pentaglycine bridges that cross-link these chains. Four transpeptidases, or penicillin-binding proteins called PBP1, PBP2, PBP3, and PBP4 play an important role in peptidoglycan biosynthesis and are inactivated by β-lactams.[41] A mutated form of PBP2 (PBP2a) encoded by the *mecA* gene is the basis of methicillin resistance in the current epidemic of hospital- and community-acquired MRSA. Teichoic acid is a polymer of ribitol phosphate that is held in the cell wall by covalent attachment to the insoluble peptidoglycan. Staphylococcal teichoic acid is antigenic, and antibodies to this substance cause agglutination of isolated staphylococcal cell walls.[42] Antibodies to teichoic acid enhance opsonophagocytic killing of nonencapsulated strains of *S. aureus* but have little effect on encapsulated isolates.[43] By way of contrast, antibodies to peptidoglycan play a key role in the opsonization of encapsulated *S. aureus*.[44] Antibodies to both *S. aureus* teichoic acid and peptidoglycan are widespread in screens of the human population.[44]

In addition to peptidoglycan and teichoic acid, other components of the *S. aureus* cell wall include protein A, an immunoglobulin Fc-binding protein, and a number of other surface-expressed proteins. Similar to the situation with other gram-positive bacteria, many *S. aureus* proteins anchored in the cell wall possess a carboxy-terminal LP(X)TG motif, which serves as a sorting signal for a membrane enzyme called sortase (SrtA).[45,46] This enzyme cleaves polypeptides between the threonine and the glycine of the LP(X)TG motif and catalyzes formation of an amide bond between the carboxy group of threonine and the amino group of peptidoglycan cross-bridges.[46] These include several proteins involved in extracellular matrix binding and promoting *S. aureus* adherence to host epithelium.[47]

S. aureus produces a polysaccharide capsular layer external to the cell wall. Capsular antigens are limited in antigenic specificity and highly conserved among clinical isolates, where the predominant capsules identified are serotype 5 and serotype 8.[48] The serotype 5 *S. aureus* capsule has the structure (→4)-3-*O*-Ac-β-D-ManNAcA-(1→4)-α-l-FucNAc-(1→3)- β-D-FucNAc-(1→)$_n$ while serotype 8 capsule has the structure (→3)-4-*O*-Ac-β-D-ManNAcA-(1→3)- α-l-FucNAc-(1→3)- β-D-FucNAc-(1→)$_n$.[49,50] Although these two capsular polysaccharides differ only in the sugar linkages the sites of *O*-acetylation of the mannosaminuronic acid residues, they remain serologically distinct. Capsule plays a role in the pathogen's resistance to phagocyte

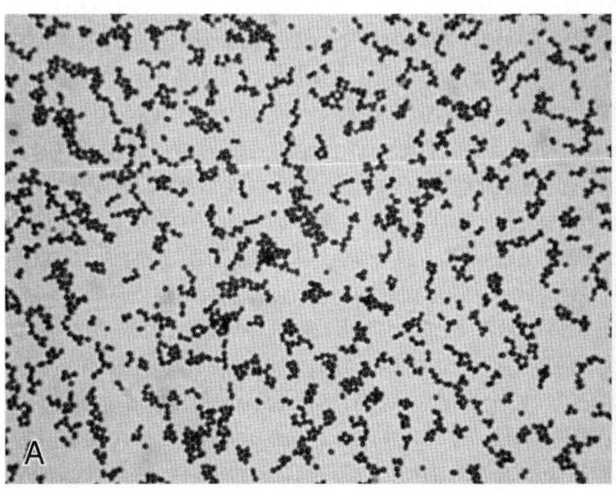

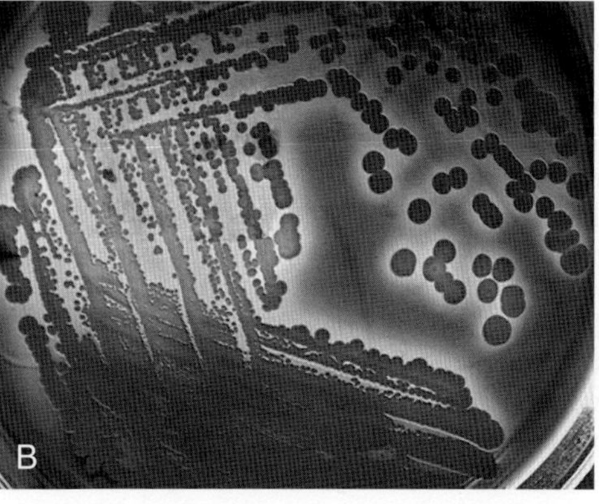

Figure 14-1 A, Gram stain of *Staphylococcus aureus* showing characteristic clusters. **B,** Blood-agar plate showing growth of *S. aureus* with zone of β-hemolysis surrounding colonies.

clearance.[48] Loss of capsule expression may be associated with bacterial persistence during chronic infections.[51]

Small colony variants (SCVs) of *S. aureus* isolated from clinical specimens have been recognized for nearly a century. SCVs have now been linked to persistent and relapsing *S. aureus* infections, including chronic osteomyelitis and soft tissue abscesses.[52,53] These phenotypes can be traced to biochemical defects in electron transport, which are associated with the slow growth and reduced α-toxin production and which promote survival and persistence within endothelial cells. It is hypothesized that the intercellular location represents a privileged niche against the actions of host innate defense molecules and antibiotics.[54] Because they can be overlooked in the laboratory because of their fastidious growth, extra efforts to identify SCVs should be undertaken in the setting of persistent or relapsing *S. aureus* infection despite antibiotic therapy.[52,53]

Nucleotide sequencing of the whole genome for several isolates of *S. aureus*, including MRSA strains,[55,56] have established that the genome is 2.8 to 2.9 Mb in size, with approximately 2600 to 2700 open reading frames (ORFs) and an overall guanine:cytosine content of approximately 33%.[57,58] Much of the *S. aureus* genome appears to have been acquired by lateral gene transfer.[55] Most antibiotic resistance genes are carried on mobile genetic elements, including a unique resistance island. Pathogenicity islands belonging to at least three different classes have been identified, including toxic shock syndrome (TSS) toxin islands, exotoxin islands, and enterotoxin islands. Of interest, the exotoxin and enterotoxin islands are closely linked to other gene clusters encoding putative virulence factors. Historically, phage typing and serologic typing were the most common systems for differentiating strains of *S. aureus* for epidemiologic purposes.[59] Later, molecular approaches such as PFGE and MLST became the standard for defining strain identity in a patient with multiple isolates or in a possible outbreak involving multiple patients.[60,61] Next-generation high-throughput genotyping technologies are now becoming the standard to understand the geographic origin and intrahospital spread of important microbial pathogens such as *S. aureus*,[62] including the analysis of NICU outbreaks.[31]

COAGULASE-NEGATIVE STAPHYLOCOCCI

Coagulase-negative staphylococci are a heterogeneous group of organisms divided into 32 species.[38] The following 15 species of CoNS are found as members of the normal human flora: *S. epidermidis, S. haemolyticus, S. saprophyticus, S. capitis, S. warnerii, S. hominis, S. xylosus, S. cohnii, S. simulans, S. auricularis, S. saccharolyticus, S. caprae, S. pasteuri, S. lugdunensis*, and *S. schleiferi*.[38,63] Among these species, several occupy very specific niches on the skin. For example, *S. capitis* is most abundant on the head, where sebaceous glands are plentiful. *S. auricularis* has a striking predilection for the external auditory canal. *S. hominis* and *S. haemolyticus* are most common in the axillae and the pubic area, where apocrine glands are numerous.

Speciation of CoNS is accomplished on the basis of a series of biochemical characteristics, simplified in recent years by the commercial availability of available miniaturized kits.[38] Differentiation of two strains belonging to the same species (subspeciation) represents a more difficult problem, however. Analogous to the situation with *S. aureus*, techniques for distinguishing strains of a given species include PFGE, MLST, and next-generation sequencing.[64,65] The composition of CoNS is quite similar to the makeup of *S. aureus*, except that the teichoic acid contains glycerol in place of ribose and the cell wall lacks protein A. Determination of the genome of *S. epidermidis* strain ATCC 12228 (a commensal isolate not associated with disease) revealed a genome approximately 2.5 Mb in size, with 2419 ORFs, greater than 10% smaller than the published genomes of *S. aureus* isolates.[66] In comparison with the available *S. aureus* genomes, ATCC 12228 contains fewer antibiotic resistance genes and lacks pathogenicity islands and a capsule locus. A homologue of the *S. aureus srtA* gene is present, along with nine proteins predicted to contain an LP(X)TG motif.

Pathogenesis of Disease

VIRULENCE MECHANISMS OF *STAPHYLOCOCCUS AUREUS*

The pathogenic process of *S. aureus* infection begins with colonization of host skin or mucosal surfaces and involves bacterial attachment to host cells, often via components of the extracellular matrix. To persist, the organism produces molecules that decrease the effectiveness of complement and antibody-mediated opsonophagocytosis and block effectors of host immune cell killing, such as reactive oxygen species and antimicrobial peptides. Ultimately, the organism expresses specific factors that damage host cells and degrade components of the extracellular matrix, thus contributing to persistence and facilitating spread within normally sterile sites of the host.

Epithelial Attachment and Invasion

S. aureus initiated adherence by binding to components of the extracellular matrix of the host. This adherence is mediated by protein adhesins known as MSCRAMMs (microbial surface components recognizing adhesive matrix molecules), which are typically covalently anchored to the cell wall peptidoglycan through the action of sortase enzymes that recognize an LP(X)TG motif in the *C*-terminal region of the protein.[67,68] *S. aureus* MSCRAMMs can promote binding to fibronectin, fibronogen, and collagen. Most strains express two related fibronectin-binding proteins, FnBPA and FnBPB, which mediate bacterial attachment to immobilized fibronectin in vitro and contribute to *S. aureus* binding to plasma clots and foreign bodies removed from the host.[69] *S. aureus* also expresses the fibrinogen-binding proteins, or "clumping factors" ClfA and ClfB.[70] Each Clf protein recognizes a different part of the fibrinogen model, and together, may synergistically act to allow *S. aureus* to attach more firmly to vascular thrombi under flow stress within the bloodstream. A fibronectin bridge from surface-anchored *S. aureus* ClfA to integrins in the epithelial cell surface promotes intracellular invasion by the pathogen.[71] In rat endocarditis studies, ClfA mutant *S. aureus* strains have reduced virulence.[72] Finally, the collagen-binding MSCRAMM Cna allows *S. aureus* to adhere to collagenous tissues such as cartilage[73]; a Cna-null mutant strain of *S. aureus* is significantly attenuated for virulence in a murine septic arthritis model.[74] The *icaADBC*-encoded polysaccharide intercellular adhesin (PIA) or polymeric *N*-acetyl-glucosamine (PNAG) contributes to *S. aureus* biofilm development[75]; these genes and a resultant phenotype shared by *S. epidermidis* are discussed in more detail later.

Innate Immune Resistance

The propensity of *S. aureus* to produce systemic infections, even in otherwise healthy infants, children, and adults, reflects the capacity of this pathogen to resist host innate immune clearance mechanisms that normally function to prevent microbial dissemination beyond epithelial surfaces. The multiple mechanisms used by this preeminent disease agent are summarized schematically in Figure 14-2.

Cationic antimicrobial peptides, such as cathelicidins and defensins, produced by epithelial cells and phagocytes are an important first line of defense against invasive bacterial infection. By incorporating positively charged residues into its cell wall lipoteichoic and teichoic acid, *S. aureus* increases electrostatic repulsion of these defense peptides. D-alanylation of teichoic acids mediated by the *dlt* operon is present in both pathogens, promoting resistance to adenosine monophosphate and neutrophil killing by increasing surface charge.[76,77] In addition, positively-charged lysyl-phosphatidylglycerol modifications of teichoic acids are encoded in the functions of the *S. aureus mprF* or *lysC* genes, and contribute to human antimicrobial peptide resistance.[78,79] *S. aureus* mutants defective in *dlt* or *mprF genes* show reduced virulence in small animal infection models.[77,80] The secreted proteases V8 and aureolysin of *S. aureus* function to degrade antimicrobial peptides, which could contribute further to *S. aureus* resistance to this important branch of the innate defense system.[81,82]

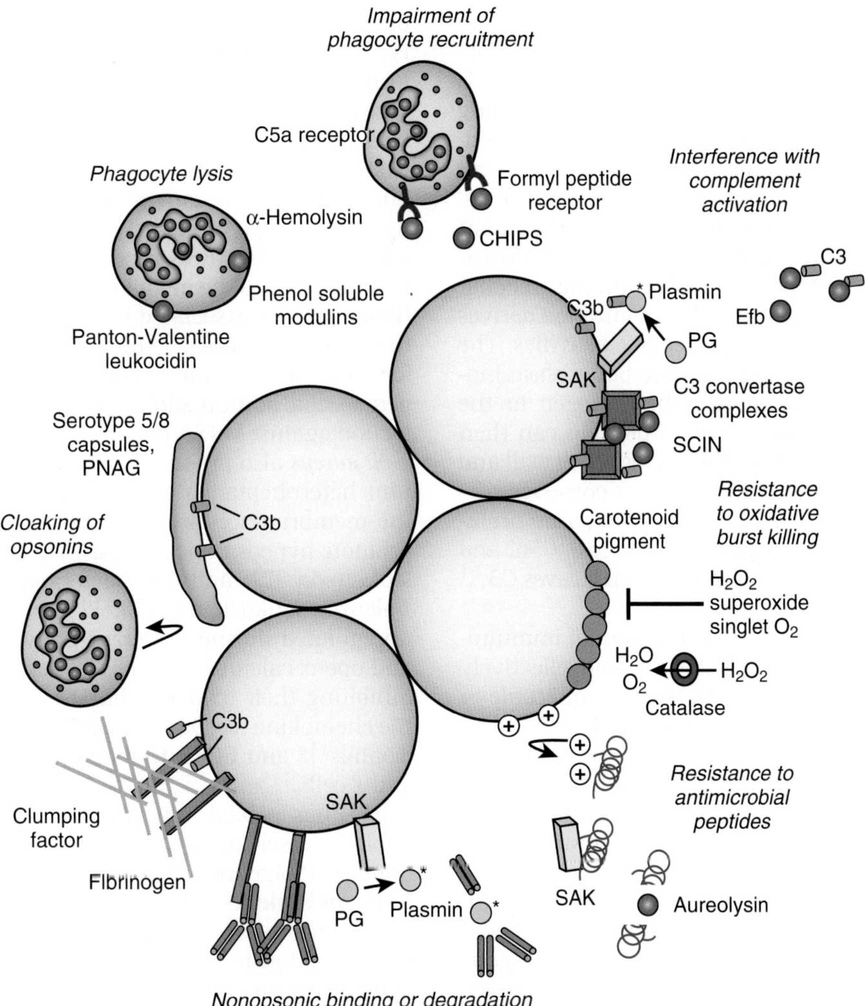

Figure 14-2 *Staphylococcus aureus* possesses multiple virulence mechanisms to resist clearance by host phagocytic cells. Phagocyte recruitment is restricted by chemotaxis inhibitory protein of staphylococci (CHIPS) binding to chemokine receptors. Complement activation is blocked by protein Efb binding of soluble C3 and inhibition of the both the classical/lectin and alternative C3 convertases by staphylococcal complement inhibitor (SCIN). Staphyloxanthin pigment provides an antioxidant shield, whereas catalase detoxifies hydrogen peroxide (H_2O_2). Resistance to cationic antimicrobial peptides is afforded by positive charge modifications of the cell wall, aureolysin-mediated proteolysis, and binding/inactivation by staphylokinase (SAK). Protein A binds the Fc domain of immunoglobulin G in a nonopsonic manner, whereas fibrinogen-binding clumping factor and the surface polysaccharide capsule and poly-*N*-acetylglucosamine (PNAG) cloak surface-bound opsonins from phagocyte recognition. The heptameric pore-forming toxins α-hemolysin and Panton-Valentine leukocidin and phenol-soluble modulins target leukocyte membranes. The plasminogen (PG)-binding protein staphylokinase (SAK) activates the zymogen to the active protease plasmin, which can degrade complement opsonin C3b and the immunoglobulin Fc domain.

Many *S. aureus* strains produce the chemotaxis inhibitory protein of staphylococci (CHIPS), which binds with high avidity to the leukocyte receptors for C5a and *N*-formyl peptides, thereby blocking functional engagement of the respective chemoattractants, and delaying neutrophil recruitment to the site of infection.[83] *S. aureus* also expresses the extracellular adherence protein (Eap), which binds and inhibits intercellular adhesion molecule-1 (ICAM-1), the endothelial receptor required to initiate leukocyte adhesion and diapedesis.[84]

S. aureus expresses multiple factors to interfere with host complement-mediated clearance.[85] Cleavage of C3 to opsonically active C3b is accomplished after assembly of C3 convertase complexes: C4bC2a (classical/lectin pathways) or C3bBb (alternative pathway) on the bacterial surface. The secreted approximately 10-kD *S. aureus* protein known as staphylococcal complement inhibitor (SCIN) binds and stabilizes both convertases on the bacterial surface, preventing generation of additional convertases, impairing their enzymatic activities, and effectively inhibiting all three complement pathways.[86] *S. aureus* clumping factor binds the host complement inhibitory protein factor 1, which subsequently cleaves C3b into iC3b,[87] preventing further amplification of the complement cascade or its activation via the alternative pathway. The secreted *S. aureus* fibrinogen-binding protein Efb-C can bind free C3, altering the solution conformation of this critical complement component such that it is unable to participate in its downstream opsonization functions.[88] Finally, another mechanism of interference with complement opsonization derives from bacterial cooptation of host proteolytic activities. The *S. aureus* surface receptor staphylokinase binds plasminogen from host serum and converts the zymogen to the active protease plasmin. Surface-bound plasmin can then cleave human C3b and C3bi from the bacterial cell wall and impair neutrophil phagocytosis.[89] *S. aureus* possesses several broad-spectrum proteases, including the serine protease V8, which is capable of degrading C3a, C3b, C5a, and C5b,[90] and aureolysin, a metalloprotease that cleaves C3,[91] among other substrates.

S. aureus is able to inhibit effector function of immunoglobulin when the pathogen binds its Fc region, effectively decorating the bacterial surface with the host molecule in a "backwards," nonopsonic orientation.[92] Most notably, protein A, the most abundant protein on the surface of *S. aureus*, binds to the Fc region of IgM and IgG to inhibit opsonophagocytic killing.[93] In addition, the majority of *S. aureus* clinical isolates express surface capsules composed of serotype 5 or 8 polysaccharide.[48] The presence of *S. aureus* capsule is associated with reduced opsonophagocytic uptake of the pathogen by neutrophils and increased virulence in a mouse bacteremia model.[94,95] Analogous functions can be ascribed to an additional *S. aureus* surface polysaccharide, poly-*N*-acetylglucosamine.[96] Neither of the *S. aureus* exopolysaccharides directly inhibit deposition of complement factors on the bacterial surface; rather they appear to serve as a superficial "cloak" that restricts access of phagocytes to the opsonins.[92]

Catalase production is a diagnostic tool used to distinguish staphylococci from streptococci in the clinical laboratory, and the ability of staphylococcal catalase to detoxify hydrogen peroxide (H_2O_2) generated during oxidative burst may promote phagocyte resistance and virulence.[97] The golden pigment for which *S. aureus* is named is a carotenoid molecule with potent antioxidant properties that are necessary and sufficient to promote bacterial neutrophil resistance and virulence in a subcutaneous infection model.[98,99] The superoxide-driven Fenton reaction between H_2O_2 and an appropriate transition metal (e.g., iron) catalyst generates highly toxic hydroxyl radicals important in phagocyte killing. However, *S. aureus* expression of bacterial nitric oxide (NO) synthase generates NO that inhibits Fenton chemistry.[100,101] *S. aureus* also resists oxidative stress through superoxide dismutases, as confirmed by diminished in vivo survival of mutants lacking these enzymes.[102]

Secreted Toxins

A number of *S. aureus* secreted factors possess cytolytic activity against host cells and can serve to facilitate tissue spread, promote inflammatory responses and, especially when the target is a phagocytic cell, promote bacterial innate immune evasion. Perhaps the best-studied is *S. aureus* α-toxin (also referred to as α-hemolysin), which forms heptamers in the membranes of a variety of cell types, creating large pores.[103,104] Pore formation induced by *S. aureus* α-toxin is associated with release of nitric oxide from endothelial cells and stimulation of apoptosis in lymphocytes.[105,106] *S. aureus* production of α-toxin may also promote escape from the phagolysome after macrophage engulfment.[107] MRSA production of α-toxin, which binds to and activates the metalloprotease ADAM-10 in lung epithelial cells, is associated with high lethality in the mouse model of pneumonia.[108] Immunization with an inactivated form of α-toxin, which cannot form pores, generates antigen-specific immunoglobulin G responses and provides protection against MRSA pneumonia.[109]

S. aureus also produces an additional family of two-subunit heteroheptameric toxins capable of oligomerizing in the membrane of target leukocytes to produce pores and promote hypoosmotic cell lysis. These include γ-hemolysin, leukotoxin ED, and the bacteriophage-encoded Panton-Valentine leukocidin (PVL).[110] The γ-hemolysin is strongly upregulated during *S. aureus* growth in human blood[111] and opens calcium channels in neutrophil membranes,[112] inhibiting their oxidative burst.[113] Leukotoxin ED targets the chemokine receptors CXCR1 and CXCR2 to deplete neutrophils[114] and CCR5 to damage other myeloid cell types and T cells.[115]

PVL has gained notoriety because of its strong epidemiologic association with severe cases of CA-MRSA infections.[116] Phage transduction of PVL into a previously naïve *S. aureus* background was reported to increase virulence in murine necrotizing pneumonia model,[117] but an inadvertent mutation in the accessory gene regulator *(agr)* locus of the test strain probably led to spurious interpretations of the PVL linkage to disease pathogenesis.[118] A more direct test of isogenic deletion of PVL in the epidemic USA300 and USA400 clones associated with severe CA-MRSA infections had no effect on neutrophil lysis nor virulence in murine skin abscess and systemic infection models[119] but did contribute to proinflammatory cytokine release and muscle necrosis at higher inoculums and in certain mouse genetic backgrounds.[120] Of note, mouse neutrophils are more resistant to PVL action than human or rabbit neutrophils.[121] In a rabbit pneumonia model, PVL enhanced the capacity of USA300 MRSA to cause severe necrotic lung infection and death, and purified PVL administered directly into the lung caused severe lung injury by recruiting and lysing neutrophils, which caused lung damage by release of cytotoxic granule contents.[122]

Phenol-soluble modulins (PSMs) are a recently recognized group of small peptides produced by *S. aureus* with important roles in immune evasion and virulence.[123] PSMs possess an amphipathic α-helical structure and membrane destabilizing properties that can recruit, activate, and lyse neutrophils by signaling through formyl peptide receptor-2,[124] inducing a marked proinflammatory response while promoting bacterial survival. PSMs allow *S. aureus* to escape the phagolysosome and replicate intracellularly[125] and can synergistically exaggerate the cytolytic effect of PVL on human neutrophils.[126] Other *S. aureus*–secreted toxins include β-hemolysin, a sphingomyelinase enzyme.[127] Through targeted mutagenesis, β-hemolysin was recently found to contribute to *S. aureus*–induced lung injury, neutrophilic inflammation, and vascular leakage of serum proteins into the alveolar spaces, in part mediated by the ability of the toxin to promote ectodomain shedding of syndecan-1, a major proteoglycan coating lung epithelial cells.[128]

S. aureus elaborates a number of toxins with superantigenic capacity, able to promote aberrant interaction between MHC class II on the surface of antigen-presenting cells (e.g., macrophages) with the β-chain of the T-cell receptor, leading to polyclonal T-cell activation and potentially staphylococcal TSS.[129] As many as 20 distinct *S. aureus* superantigens are known, prominently including TSS toxin-1, and staphylococcal enterotoxins A to E and G to J. The genes encoding the *S. aureus* superantigens are present on accessory genetic elements, such as prophages, transposons, plasmids, or chromosomal pathogenicity islands. The contribution of the superantigens to the severe disease manifestations of *S. aureus* is well demonstrated, but the potential evolutionary advantage of superantigen production to the pathogen is not clear. One possible advantage of T-cell activation at the site of infection might be dysregulated cytokine expression patterns that suppress effective local inflammatory responses.[129]

Certain strains of *S. aureus* express the exfoliative (epidermolytic) toxins ETA, ETB, ETC, and/or ETD. These toxins have recently been identified as glutamate-specific serine proteases that specifically and efficiently cleave a single peptide bond in the extracellular region of human and mouse desmoglein 1 (Dsg1), a desmosomal intercellular adhesion molecule, leading to the exfoliative phenotype of scalded skin syndrome and bullous impetigo.[130,131]

Quorum Sensing and Regulation of Virulence Factor Expression

S. aureus appears to impose tight regulation on the differential expression of specific sets of virulence determinants at different stages of growth or the pathogenic process. For example, cell wall–associated adhesive factors that facilitate the initial stages of infection are selectively produced during the exponential phase of in vitro growth.[132] Conversely, almost all *S. aureus* extracellular proteins and secreted toxins presumed to play a greater role in evasion of the immune system and tissue spread are synthesized predominantly in the postexponential phase of growth.[132] These processes are under the cell-density (quorum sensing)–dependent control of the *agr* locus.[133,134] Like other bacterial quorum sensing systems, *agr* encodes an autoactivating peptide (AIP) that is the inducing ligand for the *agr* signal receptor (AgrC). The unique effector of global gene regulation in the *agr* system is the regulatory RNA molecule RNAIII.[134] Agr mutants show decreased virulence in murine infection models.[135]

VIRULENCE MECHANISMS OF COAGULASE-NEGATIVE STAPHYLOCOCCI

Until recently, the pathogenic potential of CoNS received little attention. With the emergence of these organisms as prominent pathogens in neonates and hospitalized patients with intravascular devices, investigation has intensified in an effort to identify important virulence factors and to inform new approaches to treatment and prevention.[136] Two main reasons for the increasing rate of CoNS infections are spreading antibiotic resistance among CoNS and the ever-increasing development and use of medical devices.[137] Attention has centered primarily on *S. epidermidis*, the species most commonly associated with clinical disease, usually in association with central intravenous catheters. Other species that have been examined, although to a lesser extent, include *S. saprophyticus*, *S. lugdunensis*, and *S. schleiferi*.

When CoNS infections are initiated on intravascular catheters and other prosthetic devices, the ability of the bacterium to adhere to the hydrophobic surface of the foreign body is a first critial step in the pathogenic process (Fig. 14-3). CoNS are able to colonize virtually any plastic surface.[138] In addition, plastic objects in the human body soon become coated with host extracellular matrix proteins,[139] such that CoNS can colonize the devices either by direct attachment to the plastic or by binding to the host extracellular matrix, and both processes are likely to play a role in the initial establishment of infection. Overall surface hydrophobicity of varies among CoNS strains, and increased hydrophobicity can be correlated to better plastic binding[140]; however, no linkage between surface hydrophobicity and clinical infectivity has been established.[137]

Transposon mutagenesis identified AltE, a putative CoNS autolysin protein, as promoting adherence to plastic surfaces[141]; an *S. epidermidis* AltE mutant shows diminished pathogenicity in a rat model of catheter-associated infection.[142] Two large surface proteins present in some *S. epidermidis* strains, SSP-1 and SSP-2—one likely a degradation product of the other—are present in fibrillar structures on the bacterial surface and promote binding to polystyrene.[143]

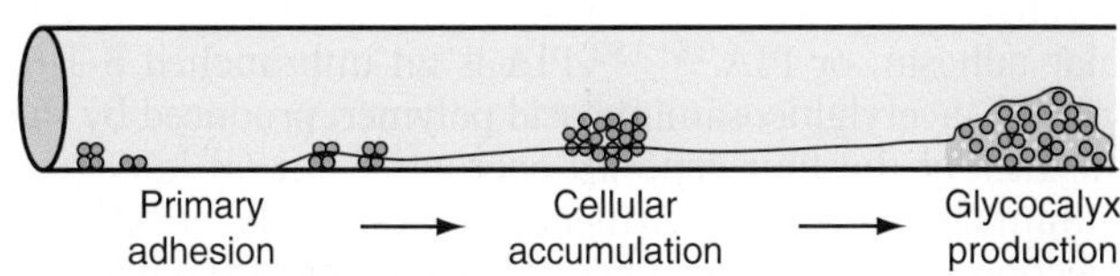

Figure 14-3 Schematic model of the phases involved in *Staphylococcus epidermidis* biofilm formation.

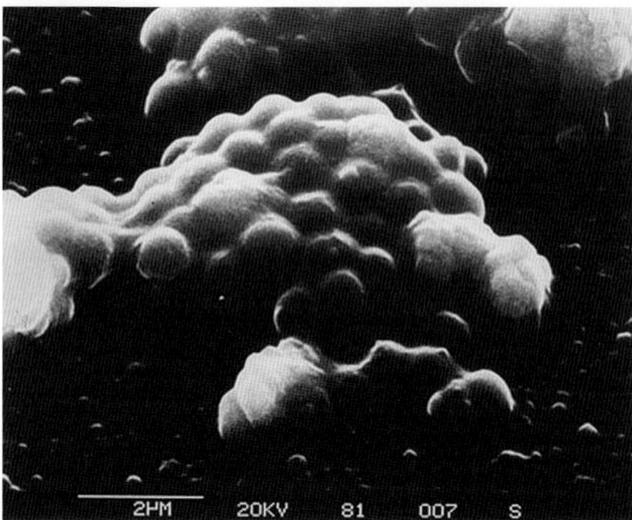

Figure 14-4 Scanning electron micrograph showing the presence of a *Staphylococcus epidermidis* biofilm on an explanted intravascular catheter. The biofilm is characterized by multilayered cell clusters embedded in an extracellular polysaccharide. (From von Eiff C, Peters G, Heilmann C: Pathogenesis of infections due to coagulase-negative staphylococci, *Lancet Infect Dis* 2:677–685, 2002.)

Following in the pattern of *S. aureus*, extracellular matrix binding surface components or MSCRAMMs are beginning to be well characterized in CoNS. The fibrinogen-binding protein Fbe (also known as SdrG) of *S. epidermidis* resembles *S. aureus* clumping factor, with the presence of multiple serine/aspartate repeat domains and a capacity to bind to the β-chain of the host matrix protein.[144-146] *S. epidermidis* cell wall teichoic acid enhances overall adherence to fibronectin, perhaps serving as a bridging molecule between bacterial MSCRAMMs and fibronectin-coated surfaces.[147] Phage-display technology was used to identify an *S. epidermidis* protein, EmbP, capable of mediating binding to fibronectin, whereas GehD, an *S. epidermidis* lipase enzyme, appears to promote collagen attachment.[148] Finally, the above-mentioned AltE also contains a domain with vitronectin-binding capacity that may contribute to its virulence phenotype in the rate model.[141]

After initial attachment to a biomaterial, organisms multiply and form complex multilayered aggregates that involve intercellular adhesion and are referred to as biofilms (Fig. 14-4; see also Fig. 14-3). Historically, isolates of CoNS were often described as elaborating "slime" and "slime-associated antigen," terms that we now realize refer to biofilms and the presence of abundant quantities of a specific polysaccharide molecule. Significant degrees of slime production were reported in greater than 80% of CoNS isolates from infants with invasive disease.[149,150] The main virulence factor responsible for the formation of these cellular aggregates in certain *S. epidermidis* strains is now recognized to be a secreted exopolysaccharide called polysaccharide intercellular adhesin, or PIA.[151,152] PIA is an unbranched β-1,6-linked N-acetylglucosaminic acid polymer, produced by the enzymes of the four-gene *ica* operon.[153] An *ica* knockout mutant shows reduced virulence in a rat model of catheter infection,[142] and *S. epidermidis* strains isolated from patients with foreign infections were more likely to possess the *ica* genes and form robust biofilms in vitro than strains from asymptomatic individuals.[154] Expression of the PIA is subject to on-off phase-switching that may be attributable to reversible insertion and excision of mobile genetic element (IS*256*) in the *ica* operon.[155] A 140-kD CoNS extracellular protein known as accumulation-associated protein (AAP) appears to cooperate with PIA in promoting biofilm growth.[156]

CoNS biofilm formation provides a nonspecific physical barrier to cellular and humoral defense mechanisms.[152,157] The formation of CoNS biofilms is dependent upon the regulatory control exerted by a homologue of the *S. aureus agr* locus.[158] *S. epidermidis* embedded within biofilms binds less complement C3b and IgG and is therefore less susceptible to neutrophil killing.[159] CoNS biofilm-associated polysaccharide also is capable of inhibiting the antimicrobial action of both vancomycin and teichoplanin.[160] In the clinical setting, formation of biofilms on the catheter surface has been shown to make eradication of CoNS infection more problematic.[161,162]

S. epidermidis expresses a 27-kD serine protease called GluSE that is expressed during biofilm formation and has been shown to degrade fibrinogen and the complement-derived chemoattractant C5, suggesting a potential role in immune evasion.[163] *S. epidermidis* also express a group of secreted amphiphilic peptides called phenol-soluble modulins (PSM), which have neutrophil chemotactic ability and generate other proinflammatory effects, including activating neutrophil oxidative burst and degranulation.[164]

ROLE OF HOST DEFENSES

Even under the most ideal conditions, infants in the hospital are surrounded by staphylococci. Physical barriers such as the skin and mucous membranes represent a major defense against staphylococcal disease. Bacteremic disease most often develops when organisms colonizing the skin gain access to the bloodstream through the portal created by an intravascular catheter. Other routes for entry into the bloodstream include the intestinal tract after injury to the epithelial barrier, the respiratory tract in patients receiving mechanical ventilation, and the umbilicus when the umbilical cord remains in place. Newborn innate immunity demonstrates several distinct deficits predisposing to staphylococcal infection, including diminished skin integrity, impaired cytokine responses, low complement levels, and reduced expression of innate antimicrobial peptides, all of which are exaggerated in preterm or LBW neonates.[165]

The presence of intact neutrophil phagocytic function is a critical factor involved in controlling replication and spread of staphylococci.[166] The bone marrow's ability to respond to infection with rapidly enhanced production and maturation of neutrophil precursors is limited compared with adults.[167] Neutrophils from newborns have relatively diminished motility toward chemoattractants compared with that in cells from older children and adults,[168] in part the result of diminished chemotactic factors, such as the complement-derived C5a and the CXC chemokine interleukin-8 (IL-8).[169,170] Neutrophils from young infants also exhibit decreased diapedesis across endothelium, possibly because of impaired capacity to upregulate endothelial cell expression of the CR3 receptor.[171] Beyond decreases in neutrophil number, chemotaxis, and transepithelial migration, the capacity for neutrophil adherence and phagocytosis is reduced in neonates, largely because of deficiencies in opsonins, including complement and specific antibody.[166] Compared with adult cells, neonatal neutrophils are less able to produce DNA-based extracellular traps (NETs) important for capturing and killing extracellular bacteria.[172]

Phagocytic killing appears to be intact in normal-term newborns but may be compromised in stressed infants, at least in part because of reduced production of reactive oxygen species.[173,174] A defective oxidative burst of neutrophils from preterm neonates on exposure to CoNS has been documented.[175,176] The multifaceted antioxidant capacities of *S. aureus*, including catalase and the carotenoid staphyloxanthin pigment likely underpin its prominent role as an opportunistic pathogen in such settings, as well as in patients with marginal patients with chronic granulomatous disease (CGD), where defects in reduced nicotinamide adenine dinucleotide phosphate oxidase lead to marginal oxidative burst function. CGD may occasionally present with *S. aureus*, *Serratia* spp., or *Aspergillus* spp. in the neonatal period.[177]

Specific antibody is less important than complement in opsonization of *S. aureus* and plays a limited role in defense against neonatal staphylococcal disease.[178] For example, in general, there is no correlation between antibody titers against *S. aureus* and the likelihood of asymptomatic carriage versus clinical disease.[179,180] Consistent with this information, an attempt many years ago to protect the newborn from staphylococcal disease by immunizing the mother near term was unsuccessful.[181]

CoNS-induced cytokine production from human neonatal monocytes varies with gestational age,[182,183] and preterm newborn monocytes show reduced IL-1β, IL-6, IL-8, and tumor necrosis factor-α (TNF-α) production despite adult-level expression of Toll-like receptor 2.[184] The block in TNF-α production may contribute to impaired antistaphylococcal neutrophil responses because TNF-α plays an important role in neutrophil activation.[165]

In most cases of neonatal staphylococcal disease, the role of T cells is unclear. In animal models, T cells are found to contribute to the development of abscesses during *S. aureus* infection.[185] T cells are centrally involved, however, in the immune response to several *S. aureus* toxins, including toxic shock syndrome toxin-1 (TSST-1), the staphylococcal enterotoxins, and the staphylococcal exfoliative toxins (ETA, ETB, ETC, and ETD), and thus in associated pathogenesis. The consequence of this dysregulated T-cell overactivation is proliferation of a large proportion of T cells and release of a number of cytokines, including TNF-α, IL-1, and interferon-γ.[186] These molecules are major contributors to the systemic manifestations of staphylococcal scalded skin syndrome (SSSS), TSS, and food poisoning.

Pathology

The most characteristic pathologic lesion associated with *S. aureus* infection is a local abscess, consisting of necrotic tissue, fibrin, and a large number of live and dead neutrophils. Similarly, CoNS infection is characterized by infiltration of neutrophils, usually with moderate necrosis. Other pathologic findings are described next in the sections on clinical manifestations.

Clinical Manifestations

Staphylococci are capable of producing a profound variety of clinical syndromes in the newborn infant, including those with high mortality rates, as was reviewed more than 50 years ago.[187] The clinical manifestations of staphylococcal infection are most prominently a function of two factors: the gestational age of the infants, with extremely LBW infants at highest risk of infection and subsequent complications, and the strain of staphylococcus causing the infection, with the CoNS generally causing more mild infection compared with *S. aureus*, particularly relevant to recent CA-MRSA. As noted in earlier sections of this chapter, staphylococci are armed with an impressive array of virulence factors. They may merely colonize skin, respiratory or gastrointestinal tract mucosa without apparent harm to the host, or cause invasive, lethal disease. CoNS are most often benign colonizers of skin and gastrointestinal tract in the newborn, causing frequent but relatively mild infections in the hospitalized premature infant. In contrast, coagulase-positive strains (*S. aureus*) are more commonly associated with clinically aggressive, invasive infections. The subsequent sections provide both a general overview of clinical manifestations as well as organ-specific manifestations.

BACTEREMIA/SEPSIS

The most common manifestations of invasive staphylococcal infection are bacteremia/sepsis. Studies describing symptomatic bacteremia in neonates, both community-acquired and hospital-acquired, provide an overall framework in which CoNS and *S. aureus* infection can be defined and include both early-onset sepsis (EOS) and LOS syndromes.[7,23,26,188-201]

EOS is most often related to acute infectious complications of late pregnancy and delivery, or colonization of the infant at birth and subsequent development of clinical symptoms within the first 48 to 72 hours of life. The signs and symptoms associated with staphylococcal septicemia usually are nonspecific and include disturbances of temperature regulation, respiration, circulation, gastrointestinal function, and central nervous system (CNS) activity. Hypothermia is more common than fever and often is observed as the initial sign. Respiratory distress frequently manifests as episodes of apnea and bradycardia, particularly in infants who weigh less than 1500g. Other abnormalities related to respiration include tachypnea, retractions, and cyanosis. In 20% to 30% of infants, gastrointestinal abnormalities develop, including poor feeding, regurgitation, abdominal distention, diarrhea, and bloody stools. Evidence of poor perfusion can include mottling, poor capillary refill, and metabolic acidosis. In some infants, lethargy, irritability, or poor suck may also be noted.

The incidence of EOS caused by *S. aureus* appears to reflect the characteristics of circulating strains and varies by year and region of the world (see "Epidemiology and Transmission"). Clinical descriptions of staphylococcal sepsis include a positive blood culture, usually in the context of nonspecific clinical signs and symptoms that may include apnea, bradycardia, irritability, poor feeding, abdominal distention, lethargy, hypotonia, hypothermia or hyperthermia, hypotension with poor tissue perfusion, and cyanosis and increased oxygen requirement with respiratory distress. In a 75-year collection of data from Yale-New Haven Hospital,[6] *S. aureus* represented the etiology of EOS from 28% (1928-1932) to 3% (1979-1988), with a rate in the present era (1989-2003) of 7%. In the Yale experience, mortality from all causes of EOS dropped from about 90% with the earliest data set to approximately 5% of all inborn infants from 1989 to 2003. In NICHD Neonatal Research Network data from 2006 to 2008, approximately 3.7% of initial episodes of LOS or meningitis among VLBW infants (<1500 g) were caused by *S. aureus*, with roughly one third of cases being MRSA[23]; similar findings were reported in a study based at Columbia University Medical Center.[24]

EOS caused by CoNS is reported extremely infrequently, likely because of the noninvasive nature of most strains. These reports may reflect true infection, particularly in VLBW infants,[193,202] although the extent of symptoms attributable to infection in these infants is difficult to assess. Otherwise, particularly for term infants, a positive culture of blood for CoNS may represent a contaminant unrelated to the underlying illness. True CoNS infection is very uncommon in infants with birth weight greater than 2000 g and gestation longer than 34 weeks.[203]

When considering neonatal LOS syndrome, occurring after the fifth day of life in hospitalized infants, both *S. aureus* and CoNS are well-documented pathogens. In the NICHD Neonatal Research Network, *S. aureus* was the second most common pathogen to cause LOS in VLBW (401-1500 g) infants.[5] CA-MRSA produces particularly devastating infection, with 7 of 8 infants hospitalized in the NICU of Texas Children's Hospital in Houston presenting in septic shock; the case-fatality ratio was 38% in this series, despite appropriate support and antimicrobial therapy.[204] In a maternity hospital in Houston during the same period, mortality attributable to the invasive *S. aureus* infection was 6%, with infection-attributable late sequelae of 12%.[204] In this report, only 3 of 39 *S. aureus* infections were caused by MRSA; all 3 infants recovered without sequelae. In a retrospective review of 12 neonates with bacteremia caused by MSSA, compared with 11 neonates infected by CA-MRSA, collected from 1993 to 2003 in Tel Aviv, mortality rates were virtually identical: 25% versus 27%, respectively.[198] In a larger series of 90 infants from Taiwan with bacteremia caused by MRSA, 75% of infants were premature, 54% of infections were thought to be catheter related, 21% were associated with skin and soft tissue infections, 17% associated with pneumonia, 8% with bone and joint infection, 3% with meningitis, and 3% with peritonitis.[205] This rate of metastatic infection attributed to MRSA appears greater than that noted with MSSA and is clearly greater than rates seen with CoNS bacteremia. Of those infants with resolved MRSA infection, 10% had at least one recurrence. At Duke University Medical Center, mortality and neurodevelopmental outcomes in infants with bacteremia caused by MSSA (median age, 26.5 days) were compared with MRSA (median age, 26 days).[206] Although the duration of staphyloccocal bacteremia was shorter in neonates with MSSA (1 vs. 4.5 days), the mortality and neurodevelopmental outcomes were statistically similar to infants infected with MRSA. Similar clinical outcomes were reported comparing MSSA and MRSA infection in the NICHD Neonatal Research Network data from 2006 to 2008.

The largest burden of disease in LOS caused by staphylococci is catheter-related CoNS bacteremia in premature infants. In the NICU, CoNS cause between 40% and 60% of all bacteremic episodes.[5,7,207-209] Rates of catheter-associated bacteremia have been tracked by the U.S. Centers for Disease Control and Prevention (CDC),[210] and other collaborative groups, including the Pediatric Prevention Network[188] and the Vermont Oxford National Evidence-Based Quality Improvement Collaborative for Neonatology.[211] Clinical manifestations of infection are frequently related to the gestational and chronologic age of the newborn but are most often nonspecific. In a retrospective review of invasive staphylococcal infections in a maternity hospital in Houston from 2000 to 2002, bacteremia was present in 94% of 108 infants with invasive CoNS infection, resulting in a wide range of nonspecific symptoms, including apnea and bradycardia in 52%, an increased oxygen requirement in 90%, lethargy in 31%, abdominal distention in 30%, increased blood pressure support requirement in 22%, and temperature instability in 18%.[202] Similar findings were published by investigators in the NICHD Neonatal Research Network,[23] highlighting the burden of disease in the VLBW infants.

CoNS infections have often been associated with many risk factors (see "Epidemiology and Transmission"), but the ultimate outcome of infants infected with CoNS may more closely follow their comorbidities than be linked to bacterial pathogenicity. In a review of data collected by the Pediatrix Medical Group (Winchester, VA), Benjamin and colleagues[191] noted that the survival of LBW infants (≤1250 g) after a positive blood culture for CoNS was virtually identical (8%) to that of infants evaluated for sepsis yielding sterile blood cultures, in contrast to much higher rates of mortality with gram-negative organisms or *Candida*.[191] Similar findings suggesting lack of attributable mortality to CoNS bacteremia documented that, for infants who ultimately died of any cause, death occurred more than 7 days after the positive blood culture for CoNS in 75% of infants.[5] These findings were also confirmed in VLBW infants in Israel when reporting on 3462 episodes of LOS, documenting a mortality within 72 hours of CoNS bacteremia of only 1.8%.[212] Others have suggested that persisting positive blood cultures for CoNS, despite appropriate antibiotic coverage, are associated with an increase in overall complications, with a mortality as high as 7%.[190]

Treatment of catheter-associated CoNS infections remains controversial. Karlowicz and colleagues[213] prospectively evaluated treatment with vancomycin versus catheter removal. In those treated with vancomycin who experienced clearing of bacteremia within 1 to 2 days, success without catheter removal occurred in 79%, whereas in those with persisting bacteremia of 3 to 4 days, the success rate declined to 44%, and in those with bacteremia persisting beyond 4 days, none were successfully treated with medical therapy alone, a finding similar to that by Benjamin and colleagues[214] in a retrospective review, in which the rate of metastatic infection increased significantly after four or more positive cultures. Others have attempted to limit the empirical use of vancomycin in the NICU by comparing outcomes using vancomycin-containing empirical regimens during one period of study, with cloxacillin-containing regimens during another. When all-cause mortality was assessed at 14 days after positive blood culture,

0 of 45 infants receiving vancomycin versus 4 of 37 infants not receiving vancomycin had died. When examined on an individual case basis, only one of the deaths was possibly attributed to CoNS sepsis.[215]

TOXIC SHOCK SYNDROMES

In addition to clinical manifestations related to bacteremia, toxin-mediated clinical disease may also occur, including SSSS (see later), TSS,[216] and neonatal TSS-like exanthematous disease.[217] TSS is caused by pyrogenic toxin superantigens produced by *S. aureus*. These superantigens include TSST-1 and several enterotoxins, most commonly staphylococcal enterotoxin serotype B or C.[218,219] TSS has been described in a 4-day-old term infant male, with poor feeding and vomiting at 3 days of age, followed by hypotension, respiratory distress, and multiorgan failure on day 4 of life. Generalized erythema developed at 6 days of age. This infant was colonized on the umbilicus with a methicillin-susceptible strain that produced staphylococcal enterotoxins C, G, and I.[216]

A similar disease caused by MRSA has been described in Japan, producing erythema in association with either thrombocytopenia, elevated C-reactive protein (CRP), or fever[217]; this presentation has been termed neonatal toxic shock syndrome–like exanthematous disease (NTED) (Fig. 14-5).[217] Since the time of the first description, surveys in Japan have shown that up to 70% of Japanese hospitals have reported a similar illness in neonates.[220] The causative strains all carried the TSST-1 gene, as well as the staphylococcal enterotoxin C gene.[221] The pathophysiology of NTED begins with colonization with MRSA, a common occurrence among Japanese newborns. Typically, the colonizing strain of MRSA produces TSST-1,[221] and the symptoms of the disease are related to the overactivation of TSST-1–reactive T cells.[222] NTED does not develop in all infants who are colonized with TSST-1–producing MRSA, suggesting that protection from this illness may be mediated by the transplacental transfer of maternal antibody directed against TSST-1.[217]

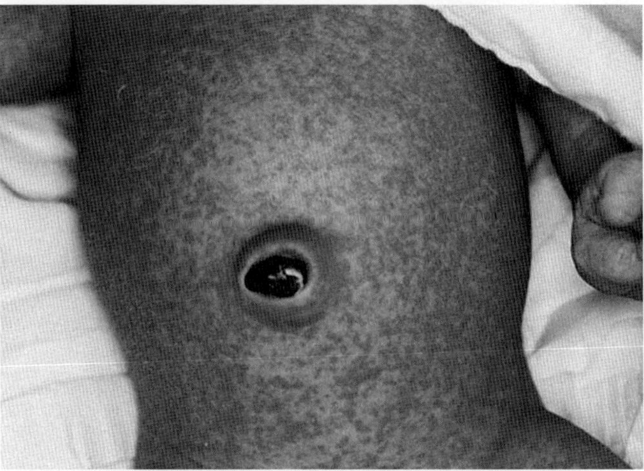

Figure 14-5 Typical exanthem in a full-term infant with neonatal toxic shock syndrome–like exanthematous disease. (From Takahashi N, Nishida H, Kato H, et al: Exanthematous disease induced by toxic shock syndrome toxin 1 in the early neonatal period, *Lancet* 351:1614–1619, 1998.)

ENDOCARDITIS

Although endocarditis in the neonate is a rare entity, autopsy studies from the 1970s revealed unsuspected endocarditis in 0.2% to 3% of neonates who came to autopsy.[223,224] Historically, *S. aureus* has been the predominant bacterial pathogen among neonates with endocarditis,[225] but more recent reports indicate that CoNS is now most common.[226-229] Premature infants with prolonged central catheter bacteremia and infants with congenital heart disease are most likely to develop *S. aureus* endocarditis in association with bacteremia.[227,229-233] Endocarditis has also been described in infants infected by CA-MRSA.[234]

The signs and symptoms of endocarditis in neonates often are nonspecific and similar to those of other conditions such as sepsis or congenital heart disease, including poor feeding, tachycardia, and respiratory distress.[225] Clinical features, in general, may not be able to distinguish bacteremia with endocarditis from infants with bacteremia without endocarditis.[229] Murmurs can be appreciated in up to 75% of neonates with endocarditis, with hepatosplenomegaly present in up to 50%, skin abscesses in 44%, arthritis in 12%, and petechiae in 12%. Blood cultures and echocardiography are the most important diagnostic tests, although urine cultures may be positive in up to 38%.[227,232] The yield of a single blood culture has been reported to be between 77% and 97%. When three blood cultures are obtained, the yield approaches 100%.[232] When persistence of CoNS bacteremia occurs in VLBW infants, it is critical to perform echocardiography such that endocarditis be excluded.[235]

All neonates with *S. aureus* bacteremia should be evaluated by echocardiogram. The thin chest wall of the neonates makes echocardiography a highly sensitive tool for diagnosis of endocarditis in this age group. The limitations of this technique include the inability to detect lesions less than 2mm in diameter and to differentiate between vegetations and other masses, such as thrombi.[227] In all age groups of children, up to 12% of those bacteremic with *S. aureus* may have clear evidence of endocarditis; children with underlying congenital heart disease and *S. aureus* bacteremia demonstrate a much greater risk of endocarditis compared with those with no cardiac malformations (53% vs. 3%).[230] Mortality in children with *S. aureus* bacteremia and endocarditis has been reported as high as 40%.[230]

In the Australasian Study Group for Neonatal Infections, bacteremia caused by CoNS in 1281 infants during 1991 to 2000 was associated with endocarditis in 3 (0.2%); in those with bacteremia caused by *S. aureus*, endocarditis occurred in 3 of 223 (1.3%) infants infected with methicillin-susceptible strains and in 1 of 65 (2%) infants infected with CA-MRSA strains. Historically, the prognosis for neonates with endocarditis has been grave. Series published in recent years report disease-specific survival rates ranging from 40% to 70%.[227,229,232]

PUSTULOSIS, CUTANEOUS ABSCESS, CELLULITIS

For infants presenting to Texas Children's Hospital in Houston, skin infection was the most common manifestation of staphylococcal disease (88%) in term or late preterm infants (≥36 weeks gestation). Of those with skin infection, about two thirds presented with cellulitis or abscess, whereas one third presented with pustulosis, a localized, nonsystemic, invasive cutaneous form of infection. Of interest, two thirds of all *S. aureus* infections were caused by CA-MRSA, with both CA-MRSA and MSSA presenting with skin or invasive infection in roughly equal percentages; the proportion of infections caused by CA-MRSA increased over the period of observation, from 2001 to 2006.[236,237] A similar experience was reported from Chicago, in which 11 infants younger than 1 month were culture positive for CA-MRSA, with cutaneous lesions consisting of pustules and vesicles, most commonly present in the diaper area. Resolution of cutaneous infection occurred with the use of mupirocin ointment. No infant required surgical drainage, and no infant developed systemic manifestations of disease or required hospitalization with intravenous antibiotic therapy.[238] Similar clusters of skin-only pustules and vesicles have been reported from other centers.[239]

Evaluation of newborn infants discharged from the hospital, but readmitted within 30 days of age, provided a somewhat different profile of clinical disease caused by staphylococci.[236] Infants infected with MRSA presented at 7 to 12 days of age, in contrast to those infected with MSSA, whose presentations occurred evenly spaced over the first month of life. The majority of these infants (87% for MRSA and 86% for MSSA) presented with skin and soft tissue infection. Cellulitis with or without abscess was responsible for about two thirds of hospitalizations. Pustulosis,[240] primarily involving skin covered by a diaper, was the most prominent sign in approximately one third of infections. Invasive disease occurred in about 10% of infants, including bacteremia, urinary tract infection, osteomyelitis, myositis, and empyema.

A study of the clinical characteristics of neonates hospitalized in a level 3 NICU (40 beds) and cultured weekly from the nose and inguinal areas, to assess ongoing colonization status, demonstrated that of 152 infants known to be colonized over the study period of 2002 to 2004, 6 (3.9%) developed MRSA sepsis, 3 (2.0%) developed conjunctivitis, 2 (1.3%) developed chest tube–site wound infections, and 2 (1.3%) developed cellulitis.[241]

ADENITIS AND PAROTITIS

In the newborn, *S. aureus* cervical adenitis can be another manifestation of nursery colonization. At least two outbreaks of cervical adenitis resulting from nurseries were reported in 1972. One outbreak involving 25 infants had an attack rate of 1.9%, and another involving 9 infants had an attack rate of 5.6%.[242,243] As with other manifestations of nursery-associated *S. aureus* disease, illness usually appears after discharge from the hospital. The mean incubation periods in the two outbreaks in England were 86 and 72 days, respectively. Because of the delay in onset of disease, confirmation of a nursery as the source of the infection may be difficult and would necessitate careful epidemiologic investigation. Deep neck abscesses have been reported secondary to MSSA or MRSA.[244,245] Neonatal suppurative parotitis is an uncommon infection among newborns, occurring with an incidence of 13.8 per 10,000 admissions.[246,247] Premature neonates (one third of cases) and males appear to be at highest risk for suppurative parotitis, which is most frequently caused by *S. aureus*.[248,249] Fever was seen in less than half of them (47%). Premature babies constituted a third of the patients. Diagnosis of suppurative parotitis relies on the clinical findings of parotid swelling, fever, and pus expressed from Stensen's duct on compression of the parotid gland.[247,250]

BREAST INFECTION

A series of 39 neonatal breast abscesses caused by *S. aureus* were reported by Rudoy and Nelson[251] from Dallas in 1975. These infants developed infection most commonly during the second week of life, when neonatal breast tissue is still enlarged in response to transplacental estrogens. The infection is clinically easy to detect, with acute onset of swelling, erythema, and tenderness of the affected breast, with progression of the infection over several hours, occasionally spreading to surrounding tissues (Fig 14-6). Spontaneous drainage of purulent material from the infant's breast

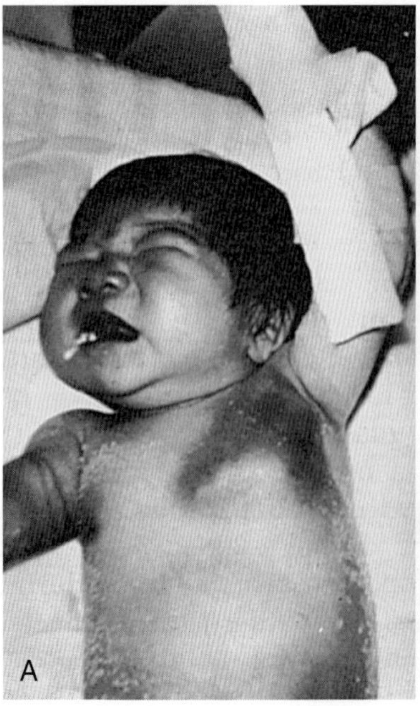

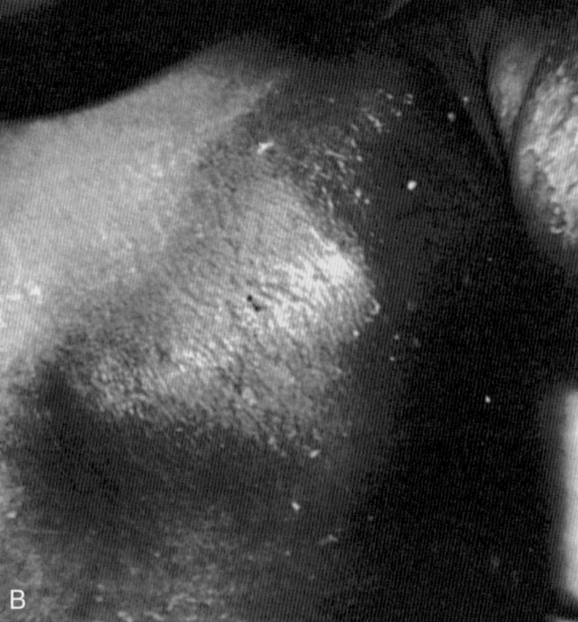

Figure 14-6 A and **B,** Left breast abscess in a 12-day-old infant. The abscess extends toward the right side of chest and up over the arm. The infant responded well to incision and drainage and antibiotic treatment.

may or may not occur. Culture and Gram stain of purulent discharge is diagnostic. Management includes systemic antistaphylococcal antimicrobials as well as careful surgical drainage of abscessed tissue within the breast, particularly in female infants. In the report from Dallas, one third of infant girls followed into early adolescence were documented to have decreased breast size as a complication of the infection.[251]

In other series of cases in which follow-up histories were obtained, a decrease in breast size was noted in two of six individuals who were examined at the ages of 8 and 15 years, respectively.[251,252] A series of three female neonates with necrotizing fasciitis as a complication of breast infection/abscess were collected from the Hôpital Necker in Paris over a 30-year period, all caused by MSSA, with no infant having a concurrently positive blood culture. All infants survived after extensive surgery and prolonged antibiotic therapy. In one of three cases followed through puberty, breast development did not occur on the affected side.[253] Antimicrobial therapy should be provided intravenously until a clear and substantial response can be documented. In locations with a high prevalence of CA-MRSA, therapy should include clindamycin or vancomycin.

FUNISITIS, OMPHALITIS, NECROTIZING FASCIITIS

Funisitis, mild inflammation of the umbilical stump with minimal drainage and minimal erythema in the surrounding tissue, is a local, noninvasive entity. However, infections of the umbilical stump may become invasive, and occur in a full spectrum of clinical presentations from funisitis, to massive abdominal wall inflammation with erythema and indurative edema associated with necrotizing fasciitis. In an attempt to define the stages of the spectrum of infection, some experts have separated the infection into distinct categories: category 1, funisitis/umbilical discharge (shaggy unhealthy umbilical stump, malodorous, and/or purulent discharge); category 2, omphalitis with abdominal wall cellulitis (periumbilical erythema, superficial tenderness besides findings in category 1); category 3, omphalitis with systemic sepsis; category 4, omphalitis with fasciitis (umbilical necrosis with extensive local disease, periumbilical ecchymosis, crepitus bullae, and evidence of involvement of superficial and deep fascia).[254]

Cultures of umbilical tissue in all categories of infection often yield several organisms, including *S. aureus* and CA-MRSA.[237,255] Management of categories 1 to 3 is usually with aggressive local care and systemic, broad-spectrum antibiotic therapy active against enteric bacilli, anaerobes, and *S. aureus*, with an option to provide oral therapy only for infants in category 1, if close observation and frequent reexamination can be arranged.

The most life-threatening entity, necrotizing fasciitis, requires immediate administration of broad-spectrum antibiotics and supportive care, with aggressive surgical débridement. As *S. aureus* may be just one of several pathogens cultured, the exact role of *S. aureus* in the overall clinical disease process cannot be accurately assessed. Of 7 infants presenting at 4 to 14 days of age with necrotizing fasciitis in Los Angeles, 4 were culture-positive for *S. aureus* in a mixed infection.[256] In Muscat, Oman, 10 of 14 neonates had *S. aureus* cultured from umbilical tissue, including 1 infant positive for MRSA, with 3 of these 10 infants having concurrent staphylococcal bacteremia.[257] Despite aggressive management, the mortality rates of polymicrobial necrotizing fasciitis have been 60% to 70% from sites in the United States,[256,257] suggesting that earlier recognition with aggressive surgical management and critical care support, antimicrobial therapy that includes activity against *S. aureus*, or CA-MRSA if appropriate, may be necessary to improve outcomes. A report of three cases of MRSA necrotizing fasciitis from the Chang Gung Children's Hospital in Taiwan was published in 1999.[258] Mastitis was a nidus for extension to necrotizing fasciitis in another series of neonatal patients.[253] Single cases of neonates from San Diego and Chicago were also reported.[259,260]

Neonates present for medical attention between 5 and 16 days of age with acute development of symptoms over 24 to 48 hours and rapid spread of erythema with indurative edema of infected tissues that have not been known to be previously traumatized. The infants may appear systemically ill with fever, irritability, and a laboratory evaluation suggesting acute inflammation with an elevated peripheral white blood count, CRP, and frequently a blood culture that is positive for *S. aureus*. Although imaging should not delay emergent surgical débridement, magnetic resonance imaging (MRI) is the preferred modality in adults and presumably infants, to define the characteristic soft tissue characteristics of necrotizing fasciitis.[261,262] In addition to broad-spectrum antimicrobials outlined above and surgical débridement, the role of hyperbaric oxygen treatment is poorly defined, with no prospective, randomized clinical trial data, and only single cases or small case series that may or may not support adjunctive hyperbaric oxygen therapy.[258,262,263]

STAPHYLOCOCCAL SCALDED SKIN SYNDROME AND BULLOUS IMPETIGO

Staphylococcal scalded skin syndrome has been reported in both full-term and premature infants,[264-268] with the first reported series of patients in 1878 from Prague by Ritter von Rittershain of a clinical infection that is likely to have included patients with SSSS.[269] Clinical characteristics in neonates are similar to those in infants and older children[270] with acute onset of infection associated with erythema, either macular or generalized, usually starting on the face and moving to the trunk within 24 hours. Erythema is accentuated in the flexor creases of the extremities, similar to streptocococcal toxin disease but with minimal mucus membrane erythema. Within 48 hours, the involved tender skin, primarily on the face, diaper area, and extremities, begins to form superficial, clear, flaccid bullae that subsequently break, revealing bright red, moist skin. These lesions demonstrate a separation of tissue layers within the epidermis, at the junction of the stratum spinosum and stratum granulosum, because of the effect of staphylococcal exfoliative toxins A and B on desmoglein-1 (see "Pathogenesis of Disease"). The characteristic histologic feature of SSSS is intraepidermal cleavage through the granular layer, without evidence of epidermal necrosis or inflammatory cell infiltrate (Fig. 14-7).[271] This appearance is distinct from that in toxic epidermal necrolysis, characterized by a subepidermal split- and full-thickness necrosis of the epidermis. Desquamation may be local, under the bullae, or generalized (Fig. 14-8). Before formation of bullae, erythematous skin will demonstrate intraepidermal separation when gentle tangential pressure is applied (Nikolsky sign), resulting in blister formation. These cutaneous findings may occur in the context of low-grade fever in about 20% of infants. Given the relatively high layer of epidermis involved, no major clinical sequelae occur as there are no substantial fluid, electrolyte, or protein losses, in contrast to erythema multiforme involving the dermal-epidermal junction. After appropriate antimicrobial therapy, the denuded skin dries within the subsequent few days, and in the absence of superinfection, heals completely within a few weeks with no scar formation.

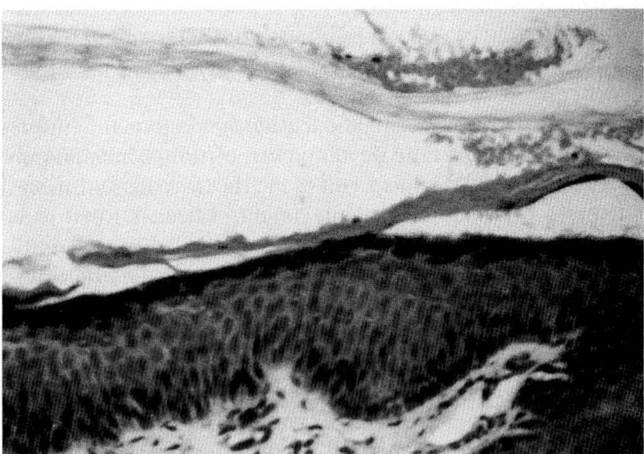

Figure 14-7 Photomicrograph of a skin biopsy from a patient with staphylococcal scalded skin syndrome, stained with hematoxylin and eosin. The histologic appearance is characterized by epidermal splitting at the granular layer of the epidermis. Magnification is approximately ×200. (From Hardwick N, Parry CM, Sharpe GR: Staphylococcal scalded skin syndrome in an adult. Influence of immune and renal factors, *Br J Dermatol* 132:468–471, 1995.)

In a recent 8-year (2004-2012) retrospective review of 39 neonates diagnosed with SSSS, mean patient age was 17 days, boys were more commonly affected (64%), the face was the most common body part affected and the area most frequently initially affected, and pneumonia the most common complication (three fourths of cases).[272] Fever, leukocytosis, or elevated CRP levels were uncommon; the median length of hospitalization was 9 days; and all neonates were cured without scarring after antibiotic treatment.[272]

Localized staphylococcal infection complicated by SSSS may also occur with the presence of wound infections, cutaneous abscesses, or conjunctivitis.[266,268,273] Bacteremia is very uncommon with SSSS but has been reported.[274,275] Although infection is most commonly described in full-term neonates during the first few months of life, infections in premature infants, including those with extremely low birth weight, have also been described.[264-267] Scarlatina, as the only clinical manifestation of infection caused by an epidemic strain of SSSS-causing *S. aureus*, has also been observed.[268]

Congenital SSSS infection, acquired before delivery as a function of maternal amnionitis, has been reported in both term[275,276] and preterm[277] infants, with a mortality rate that may be higher than the extremely low rate documented for disease acquired postnatally. Outbreaks of disease among hospitalized infants in nurseries have occurred, but most have been effectively stopped with standard infection-control practices.[268,278]

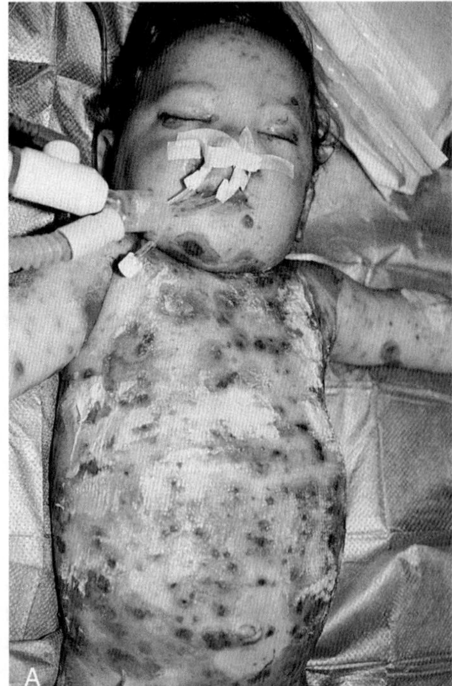

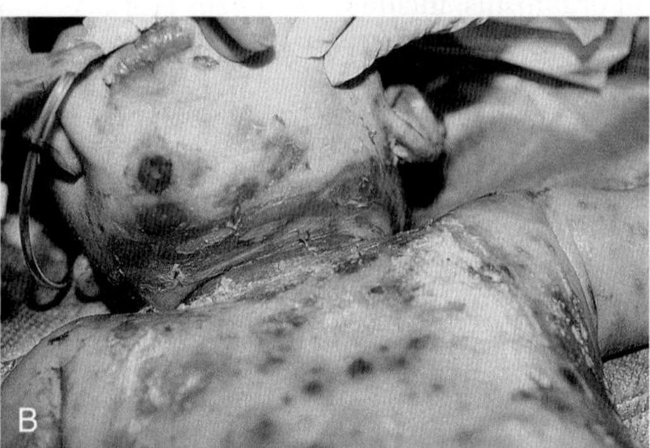

Figure 14-8 Generalized staphylococcal scalded skin syndrome in a previously well newborn infant. **A** and **B,** The characteristic well-demarcated erythematous superficial exfoliation, with areas of skin sparing, can be seen. (From Ladhani S, Joannou CL, Lochrie DP, et al: Clinical, microbial, and biochemical aspects of the exfoliative toxins causing staphylococcal scalded-skin syndrome, *Clin Microbiol Rev* 12:224–242, 1999.)

PNEUMONIA

Neonatal pneumonia caused by *S. aureus* has been described for decades, often reported to occur in community epidemics in infants during the first month of life. These infections, even before the advent of CA-MRSA, have been known to cause severe disease with a high mortality rate that may reflect virulence of strains circulating at that time.[187,279,280]

A lower respiratory tract infection may occur as a primary pneumonia as the sole clinical manifestation of infection caused by *S. aureus*, with acquisition of the organism after contact with family members or hospital staff. Pneumonia may also occur as part of more generalized, invasive, disseminated staphylococcal infection. In a recently reported large series of neonatal sepsis/bacteremia cases, pneumonia caused by either CoNS or *S. aureus* is only rarely listed as a primary diagnosis, or a complication, without details provided about the clinical presentation of lower respiratory tract disease.[5,188,189,201,209] The infection is often hospital acquired in a neonate with underlying lung disease, most commonly chronic lung disease (bronchopulmonary dysplasia), especially in those receiving concurrent mechanical ventilation.

An early study of neonatal staphylococcal pneumonia was reported from New Zealand in 1956 during an epidemic of primarily cutaneous infections. Eight infants died of pneumonia in this epidemic, and they presented at 2 to 3 weeks of age with irritability and poor feeding, followed by dyspnea, cough, and fever.[279] Death occurred in these infants between 1 and 5 days after admission, with autopsy findings documenting empyema, consolidation, and abscess formation. In a study of community-acquired *S. aureus* infection in neonates from Houston between 2001 and 2005, infants were described who had no underlying disease, no indwelling catheters, and no previous hospitalization. Of 89 neonates identified with *S. aureus* infection, only 1 had a primary lung infection, caused by CA-MRSA, producing a necrotizing pneumonia complicated by pneumothorax and empyema, requiring video-assisted thoracoscopic surgery and chest tube drainage. Other cases of severe CA-MRSA neonatal pneumonia have been reported, including hospital-acquired infections in premature neonates.[26,194,281] In hospitalized, bacteremic neonates with CA-MRSA in Houston, 2 of 8 had lung involvement: a 24-week gestation 14-day-old infant with empyema, pneumatocoeles, and concurrent endocarditis, and a 28-week gestation infant had multiple comorbidities, including bronchopulmonary dysplasia with infection acquired at 411 days of age, characterized by lung abscess. Both infants died. Two fatal cases of MRSA pneumonia complicated by pleural empyema in neonates from Quebec were also reported.[282]

In a point-prevalence survey of neonatal infections in 29 Pediatric Prevention Network NICUs in the United States and Canada, 116 NICU-acquired infections were reported, with 15 (13%) respiratory associated, virtually all in infants with birth weights of 501 to 1500 g, with only 2 infections associated with CoNS, and only 1 associated with *S. aureus*.[188] In a review of invasive staphylococcal infections of hospitalized neonates admitted to level 2 or level 3 nurseries in Houston, 3 of 41 infants with *S. aureus* infection and 14 of 108 with CoNS infection were documented to have pneumonia.[202] In this population of infants, many had comorbidities, including respiratory distress syndrome in 85% of neonates ultimately diagnosed with any invasive *S. aureus* infection and in 95% of those with CoNS. Similarly, bronchopulmonary dysplasia was documented in 65% of *S. aureus* infected infants and 75% of those infected by CoNS. The Australasian Study Group for Neonatal Infections collected data on infants with documented bacteremia, occurring at between 48 hours and 30 days of age. Of 1281 episodes of CoNS bacteremia, only 6 (0.5%) were documented to have pneumonia,[209] in contrast to 223 with MSSA bacteremia associated with 9 (4%) cases of pneumonia, and 65 cases of MRSA bacteremia associated with 8 (12%) cases of pneumonia.[189]

MENINGITIS

Meningitis is infrequently encountered in neonates with *S. aureus* bacteremia[202,236,237] but may be found when a lumbar puncture is performed after empirical antibiotic therapy has been started. In a large series of 90 episodes of MRSA bacteremia in neonates in a Taiwanese NICU, 2 infants were noted to have meningitis.[205] In a report from Australia and New Zealand, meningitis was reported in 5 of 223 infants with MSSA bacteremia (2.2%), and 3 of 65 infants had MRSA bacteremia (5%).[209] However, in most reports where cerebrospinal fluid (CSF) white blood cell counts are provided, they are often below 200 cells/mm^3, suggesting that these infants with a CSF pleocytosis and negative CSF cultures may not have true staphylococcal bacterial meningitis. Virtually no infant from any series had a positive CSF culture for *S. aureus*, including 12 bacteremic infants with a documented pleocytosis from Texas Children's Hospital.[237] It is possible that the pleocytosis represents the entry of staphylococcal cell wall components or inflammatory mediators into CSF during bacteremia, perhaps facilitated by capillary leak that often accompanies staphylococcal sepsis. Other possibilities include very early bacterial meningitis or a staphylococcal parameningeal focus of infection that was not identified in infants nor included in the reports.

Among 1281 episodes of CoNS sepsis, 5 (0.4%) were reported to be associated with meningitis.[209] An additional 2 cases of CoNS meningitis were reported in premature infants from a single institution, born at 24 and 25 weeks of gestation, 1 with a grade IV intraventricular hemorrhage on the fifth day of life, developing symptomatic disease at 20 days of age the second premature infant did not have an intraventricular hemorrhage, but developed disease at 18 days of age, Multiple cultures in both infants confirmed infection, caused by *S. epidermidis* in 1 infant, and *S. capitis*/*S. warneri* in the other.[283] A major risk factor for CoNS meningitis is prior neurosurgery, in particular ventriculoperitoneal shunt insertion.[284]

BRAIN ABSCESS

Brain abscesses caused by *S. aureus* have been described in neonates, most often as a complication of sepsis.[285-287] Clinical presentation includes nonspecific symptoms of systemic infection, a bulging fontanel, and may not include focal neurologic deficits. The key to diagnosis includes ultrasonography or computed tomography (CT) imaging of the head, with the administration of an intravenous contrast agent, and if not contraindicated, an evaluation of lumbar CSF.

Surgical drainage of the abscess is usually performed after prolonged antistaphylococcal therapy. Long-term outcome has included neurologic deficits of varying degrees. A case of multiple brain abscesses caused by complicating MRSA bacteremia in a 29-week–gestation premature infant was successfully treated and recently reported.[288]

Neonates with intraventricular hemorrhage, acute hydrocephalus, congenital malformation, or CNS parenchymal injury, will often require management of increased intracranial pressure by repeated lumbar puncture, or by placement of a shunt originating in the CSF ventricles.[289,290] CoNS clearly represent the most common organisms to infect shunt material, producing mild-to-moderate inflammation and systemic signs and symptoms of infection[289-293]; occasional infection caused by *S. aureus* has also been reported.[290,293] Shunt removal is the preferred method of treatment because sterilization of in situ shunt material is often quite difficult.[291] Treatment with high-dose systemic antimicrobials active against the isolated pathogens, usually vancomycin, from 3 to 10 days post–shunt removal is recommended, depending on the clinical status and the microbiologic response to treatment. Some authors also recommend using intraventricular vancomycin therapy if therapeutic ventricular CSF concentrations cannot be achieved with systemic therapy.[291,294,295] The role of linezolid in the treatment of shunt infections remains to be defined but may represent an option for CA-MRSA strains that are not fully susceptible to vancomycin.[296] Although the CoNS infections are seldom associated with acute toxicity or mortality, management with long-term antibiotic therapy and repeated surgical interventions for removal and placement of shunts each carry risks to the neonate.

OSTEOMYELITIS AND SEPTIC ARTHRITIS

Bone and joint infections have long been known to occur with invasive staphylococcal infection in the neonate, with rates of late sequelae as high as 50%.[297-302] In contrast to infections in older children, the usual distinction between infection of the bone and infection of the joint in the neonate is not as easily made given the unique neonatal anatomy, with easy spread of organisms initially inoculated into metaphyseal bone, through transphyseal vessels into the epiphysis and subsequently into the joint.[303,304] In addition to decompression of metaphyseal bone infection into the adjacent joint, erosion through the thin cortical bone may also occur, creating subperiosteal abscesses and subsequent involvement of the soft tissues of the extremity.[297,303,305] Virtually all reported cases have been caused by *S. aureus*, with recent reports now documenting the occurrence of CA-MRSA as a cause of neonatal osteomyelitis.[302,306]

The clinical presentation of neonatal bone and joint infections appears to take three general forms. First, the infection may be secondary to that of staphylococcal sepsis with bacteremia in which the focal bone and joint findings may not be the most prominent presenting symptom, but bone and joint sequelae of bacteremia become more apparent as the systemic infection is treated.[189,302] Second, and probably most common, an occult bacteremic inoculation of bone may occur, leading to either a single site, or in up to 50% of infants, multiple sites of infection.[301,302,306] In these infants, the clinical findings may be subtle, with signs of irritability, with or without fever, with swelling around the affected bone and/or joint, and occasionally failure to move the limb (pseudoparalysis).[302,307,308] Risk factors for bacteremia in these infants include umbilical artery catheterization and prematurity.[300-302,309] In bacteremic disease, the femur and tibia are the most prominently involved bones, infected in approximately 80% of all cases of osteomyelitis.[300-302] Adjacent joints may be involved clinically in 25% to 50% of cases, although in an autopsy review of staphylococcal osteomyelitis, all infants with bone infection were documented on pathology to have adjacent arthritis.[300,302-304] Because most of the data are from small case series, accurate data on the presenting signs and symptoms may reflect strains circulating in a region at a particular point in time or may be related to outbreaks of specific strains.[189] Because of delays in the diagnosis of osteomyelitis, the location of the infection, which often involves bone on both sides of the physis and frequent involvement of the adjacent joint, late sequelae are common after bacteremic infection, with up to 50% of infants described to have long-term sequelae, including limb shortening, and decreased range of motion.[299-301]

A third clinical scenario leading to a bone or joint may be specifically linked to trauma. Osteomyelitis of the calcaneus has been documented to occur as a complication of heelstick blood sampling, most often presenting with focal swelling, erythema, and drainage.[310] Recent reports cite continuing problems secondary to a single heelstick that is used for metabolic screening in all newborns.[311] Fetal scalp monitoring has been associated with skull osteomyelitis.[312] Pyogenic arthritis of the hip is a reported complication of femoral vein venipuncture.[313]

Bone radiographs can show destructive changes in the bone, becoming apparent in the second week of infection. In the case of arthritis, widening of the joint space and bulging of the soft tissues may be seen as a clue to diagnosis. Ultrasonography may identify collections of pus that are subperiosteal or in the soft tissues. Although radionuclide bone scanning with technetium may provide additional useful information regarding the involvement of multiple bones, the normal increased vascularity of the neonatal metaphysis, may blur the differentiation between infection and increased uptake that is commonly seen in osteomyelitis in older children. Decreased blood flow from necrotic injury to the bone may lead to false-negative test results in the newborn. MRI is becoming the preferred imaging modality, based on excellent visualization of both soft tissues and bone, with a lack of ionizing radiation. However, MRI may be too sensitive in assessment of tissue inflammation in bones and soft tissues adjacent to the infected site, suggesting a greater extent of infection than is actually present. MRI with contrast provides additional information on inflammation in both bones and soft tissues and may be particularly helpful when imaging the spine to detect vertebral osteomyelitis/diskitis. CT imaging of neonatal bones and joints has a more limited role in diagnosis of acute infection.

GASTROINTESTINAL

S. aureus is a common colonizer of the gastrointestinal tract of newborns, present in up to 93% of asymptomatic infants.[314] The prevalence of colonization is not surprising, considering that large numbers of *S. aureus* can be recovered from samples of breast milk expressed from normal breasts of lactating and nonlactating women.[315] Recent metagenomic analyses indicate that in VLBW premature infants, meconium is not sterile and is less diverse from birth in infants who will develop nosocomial LOS, a phenotype severely worsened by prolonged empirical antibiotics.[316] Low diversity and redominance of *Staphylococcus* was seen in infants who developed sepsis, whereas healthy infants had more diversity and predominance of *Clostridium*, *Klebsiella*, and *Veillonella*.[316] Genetic studies confirm the gastrointestinal tract as a reservoir of CoNS associated with LOS.[317]

S. aureus disease in the gastrointestinal tract can be caused by one of the enterotoxins produced by the organism or can be a manifestation of bacterial invasion of the mucosa resulting in enterocolitis.[318] Although *S. aureus* has been described to colonize the gastrointestinal tract in the absence of clinical disease,[314] certain poorly defined risk factors may place colonized infants at risk of invasive disease, including feeding tubes and previous antibiotic therapy that may have facilitated colonization with *S. aureus*.[319] Clinical presentation includes signs and symptoms of generalized sepsis, in association with frequent, blood-tinged, thin, mucus-containing diarrheal stools. A recent report of neonatal staphylococcal enterocolitis, caused by MRSA, described a need for therapy with both intravenous and oral vancomycin to establish a microbiologic cure for both the systemic infection and colonization; the infant ultimately developed colonic stricture as a late complication of infection.[320] Delta-toxin–producing CoNS[321] and MRSA[322] have not been confirmed to play a major role in the pathogenesis of neonatal NEC, although they may play a supporting role in the disease process in some infants.

Diagnosis

In the previously cited reports on clinical manifestations of staphylococcal infection, diagnosis is most often made by direct culture of the infected tissues or abscesses if the disease is focal, or by cultures of blood, urine, or CSF for diagnosis of sepsis/bacteremia, pyelonephritis, and meningitis/shunt infection, respectively. Organism identification and susceptibility testing are essential in understanding both the organism-specific severity of disease, as well as provide information on appropriate antimicrobial therapy. In addition, having the laboratory save the neonate's isolate allows one to compare subsequent episodes of infection by that organism in that infant or compare episodes of infection by the organism that may have spread to or from other neonates.

The diagnosis of infection by nonspecific laboratory tests that assess inflammation in the infant being evaluated can provide supportive evidence for infection. A detailed evaluation of specific tests, such as the total white blood count, the immature neutrophil (band-form) count, the mature:immature white blood cell ratio, the CRP, procalcitonin, cytokines[323-327] (IL-6, IL-8, IL-10, TNF-α), and chemokines[328,329] (interferon-γ–inducible protein-10, monocyte chemoattractant protein-1, RANTES [regulated on activation, normal T-cell expressed and secreted], epithelial neutrophil-activating peptide-78), is beyond the scope of this chapter. The sensitivity, specificity, and positive predictive values vary with investigating institution and the population of neonates studied, with some laboratory test results increasing within a few hours of the onset of infection, whereas others may not increase for 1 to 2 days. Rather than a single test, a set of tests may offer the best hope for diagnosing early infection and tracking the response to therapy.[329,330] At the present time, CRP and procalcitonin appear to be among the most useful and the most widely available tests for assessment of neonatal sepsis. Some studies have suggested the usefulness of an elevated immature-to-total neutrophil ratio in identifying infants with CoNS septicemia.[331-333] No test has the ability to identify all infected infants, with the responsibility for decisions on further investigation and empirical antimicrobial therapy still requiring clinical judgment. The more premature and younger the infant, the greater is the interval from the time of infection to the time of a positive nonspecific test for inflammation. *S. aureus*, both MSSA and MRSA, appear to generate far more vigorous responses than CoNS. Therefore these nonspecific tests of inflammation cannot play a decisive role in the determination of whether a single positive blood culture for CoNS represents a true positive culture, or a contaminant.

Multiple positive blood cultures for the same strain of CoNS in a relatively asymptomatic infant may provide evidence of true infection that is more reliable than the white blood count or any cytokine concentration. Polymerase chain reaction techniques to detect 16S ribosomal RNA in plasma, followed by specific probes for *S. aureus* and CoNS, show promise but cannot currently be used as the sole diagnostic test for staphylococcal infection.[334] The evaluation of emerging nonculture-based diagnostic methodologies for neonatal infection are discussed in detail in Chapter 36.

Antibiotic Treatment (see also Chapter 37)

GENERAL PRINCIPLES

Optimal treatment for staphylococcal infections in neonates is designed to achieve both an appropriate antimicrobial exposure at the site of infection, as well as surgical control of the infection by drainage of any abscess and removal of any potentially infected foreign material. As with all neonatal bacterial infections, cultures of appropriate samples, based on signs and symptoms of infection, physical examination, and imaging, should provide the necessary information regarding the identity and susceptibility pattern of the pathogen.[335] The choice of empirical therapy, before susceptibility test results are known, depends on the local antibiotic resistance patterns for coagulase-positive and -negative staphylococci, the severity of infection, and the toxicity profile of the antibiotic for that infant.

For CoNS, susceptibility patterns are quite varied and are often based on the particular species isolated. For coagulase-positive strains, it is essential to know the susceptibility to β-lactamase stable penicillins. Culture and susceptibility information directly impacts selection of definitive therapy, allowing the use of the most narrow spectrum, least toxic antimicrobial regimens.

Although β-lactam agents are preferred for treatment of methicillin-susceptible staphylococcal infections in the neonate because of their bactericidal activity and overall safety, several other clinically useful classes may also show in vitro activity, including glycopeptides, aminoglycosides, lipopeptides, oxazolidinones, lincosamides, rifamycins, and trimethoprim-sulfamethoxazole (TMP-SMX). Unfortunately, as with so many other drugs for neonates, adequate prospective data on the safety and efficacy of these antimicrobials for the various tissue sites of infection caused by CoNS, MSSA, and MRSA are not available. Therefore extrapolation from other pediatric and adult data is necessary, with cautions for the neonate on both outcomes at dosages suggested, as well as on the safety of these antimicrobials.

Antimicrobial therapy of *S. aureus* infections should be separated into those that are susceptible to methicillin (MSSA) and those that are resistant (MRSA). Among MRSA, further differentiation should be made between the more antibiotic-resistant hospital-acquired strains (HA-MRSA) from those that are community acquired (CA-MRSA). No MRSA strains can be killed by penicillin or ampicillin, by the β-lactamase–stable, antistaphylococcal penicillins (methicillin, nafcillin, oxacillin, dicloxacillin), by the currently available cephalosporins (cephalexin, cephalothin, cefazolin, cefuroxime, cefotaxime, ceftriaxone), or by the carbapenems (meropenem, imipenem, ertapenem, doripenem). The HA-MRSA strains carry relatively large antibiotic resistance gene cassettes with concurrent resistance to clindamycin, macrolides (erythromycin, clarithromycin, and azithromycin), and aminoglycosides, a resistance profile that is usually not seen in CA-MRSA strains.

For mild-to-moderate invasive staphylococcal infections in neonates in areas of the world where methicillin resistance is still minimal, empirical therapy with first-generation cephalosporins (parenteral cefazolin, oral cephalexin) or antistaphylococcal penicillins (parenteral methicillin, oxacillin, nafcillin) is preferred. In some cases of mild skin infection, topical antibiotic therapy with mupirocin may suffice. For mild-to-moderate infections in those areas where CA-MRSA occurs at substantial rates (5%-10% or greater), clindamycin or vancomycin intravenously should be used empirically until susceptibility data are available. If clindamycin is used, caution should be exercised in treating erythromycin-resistant, clindamycin-susceptible strains of *S. aureus* with clindamycin, because those strains may display inducible clindamycin resistance (see "Clindamycin" later). The role of oral therapy for neonatal staphylococcal infections is not yet well defined. For MRSA strains that are susceptible, erythromycin, azithromycin, and clindamycin may be considered for mild infections, or step-down therapy in newborns who have responded well initially to intravenous therapy. TMP-SMX may be considered for mild infections in infants who no longer exhibit physiologic jaundice.

For serious infections in neonates in regions of the world in which CA-MRSA is routinely isolated, empirical therapy with vancomycin is preferred over clindamycin, given the bactericidal nature of killing and extensive experience with vancomycin in the newborn. For suspected *S. aureus* infections that are nosocomially acquired within institutions in which MRSA is present in other neonates, empirical therapy with vancomycin for presumed MRSA is also recommended. Furthermore, with data suggesting that the most common pathogen responsible for bloodstream infections in LOS in hospitalized neonates is CoNS, most often resistant to β-lactam antibiotics, vancomycin is likely to provide effective therapy. For situations in which cultures demonstrate MSSA or methicillin- or penicillin-susceptible CoNS, it is imperative that therapy be switched back to traditional β-lactam antibiotics to minimize antibiotic pressure on staphylococcal species from vancomycin or clindamycin and thus to delay the emergence of resistance to these antibiotics. β-Lactam antibiotics are, in general, less toxic to the neonate, compared with vancomycin and clindamycin, and are better tolerated.

VANCOMYCIN

Vancomycin is a first-generation, bactericidal glycopeptide antibiotic. Vancomycin normally inhibits growth of the organism by binding to cell wall precursors, inhibiting transglycosylase function, and cell wall synthesis. Complete resistance to vancomycin is relatively recent and quite limited, with the first cases of complete resistance being reported in 2002. However, of great importance is the observation that within every population of *S. aureus*, a very low frequency of vancomycin intermediately-resistant organisms exist, which may become selected in infants with prolonged exposure to vancomycin.[335] By contrast, complete vancomycin resistance is still exceedingly rare and created by a different mechanism that parallels vancomycin resistance in enterococci.

Dosing of vancomycin is classically designed to achieve an area under the curve:minimal inhibitory concentration (AUC:MIC) ratio of greater than or equal to 250, and this is associated with microbiologic cure in experimental in vitro and in vivo animal models, as well as in retrospective analyses of infections in adults. In neonates, many dosing recommendations exist, including both intermittent dosing as well as continuous infusion, primarily based on chronologic and gestational age, as well as based on serum creatinine.[336-341] An initial loading dose of 15 mg/kg is most often recommended,[342] followed by repeated dosing every 8 to 24 hours, reflecting longer dosing intervals for the youngest, most premature infants. Each dose should be administered over 60 minutes. In neonates, data on continuous infusion of vancomycin are scant, and there is no randomized controlled study available on the efficacy and safety of continuous or intermittent infusions.[342] Close monitoring of renal function and serum concentrations of vancomycin are recommended in all neonates receiving therapy, allowing for adjustment of vancomycin dosing regardless of the initial empirical dosing regimen chosen. Intraventricular vancomycin has been used to treat CNS infections, primarily ventriculoperitoneal shunt infections caused by CoNS,[294,295] although CSF concentrations may be therapeutic after intravenous administration.[337] Newer analysis in the pediatric population suggests that targeted exposure using the vancomycin AUC:MIC, compared with trough concentrations, is a more realistic target in children. Depending on age, serum creatinine, and MIC distribution, vancomycin at a dosage of 60 to 70 mg/kg/day was necessary to achieve AUC:MIC greater than or equal to 400 in 75% of patients[343]; such monitoring requires Bayesian estimation based on both peak and trough levels to ensure accuracy in predicting drug exposure.[344]

CLINDAMYCIN AND ERYTHROMYCIN

Both clindamycin, a lincosamide, and erythromycin, a macrolide, inhibit ribosomal function and produce a primarily bacteriostatic effect by binding to sites on the ribosome. Most strains of MSSA remain susceptible to clindamyin and erythromycin; many strains of CA-MRSA remain susceptible, but most strains of HA-MRSA and CoNS are resistant to these antibiotics. Staphylococcal resistance to erythromycin may occur by two mechanisms: by methylase-mediated dimethylation of the 23S ribosomal binding site of the macrolides and by the presence of an efflux pump that expels the macrolide from the intracellular environment of the pathogen. The methylase gene *erm* is usually inducible, but in any large population of organisms, mutants will occur that constitutively produce methylase, providing complete resistance to all macrolides (erythromycin, azithromycin, clarithromycin), clindamycin, and the streptogramins (quinupristin/dalfopristin). By contrast, the most prevalent macrolide efflux pump for staphylococci, *msrA*, does not recognize, bind to, or eliminate clindamycin from within the bacteria, allowing these strains to remain susceptible to clindamycin. Any strain that demonstrates in vitro erythromycin resistance and clindamycin susceptibility must also be tested for methylase-mediated clindamycin resistance by an additional assay, the D-test. Current laboratory reporting guidelines suggest that hospitals report erythromycin-resistant, D-test–positive strains as clindamycin resistant, on the basis of reported clinical failures of clindamycin in treating infections caused by inducible organisms. Because the true clinical significance of inducible *erm*-mediated resistance for clindamycin is not well defined at present, it is prudent to use other antibiotic options for the seriously ill neonate with infection caused by a D-test positive strain.

Erythromycin is associated with the occurrence of pyloric stenosis in the newborn infant,[345] a side effect that is likely to be less prevalent in clarithromycin and azithromycin. Clindamycin, erythromycin, and azithromycin are available in oral and intravenous formulations, but little prospective, comparative data exist for their use in the neonate.

LINEZOLID

Of the newer approved antibiotics with activity against MRSA, linezolid is the only one currently approved by the United States Food and Drug Administration (FDA) for use in the neonate.[346] As might be predicted, resistance to linezolid has been documented to develop in adults receiving therapy for a bacteremic MRSA infection, although to date, resistance remains rare.[347] Linezolid is an oxazolidinone-class protein synthesis inhibitor, the first of this new class of antibiotics. Linezolid is a ribosome-inhibiting, bacteriostatic agent, active against both *S. aureus* and CoNS.[348] Data on pharmacokinetics are available for all pediatric age groups, including premature neonates younger than 34 weeks of age. Linezolid can be administered both intravenously and orally, with virtually 100% of the agent absorbed by the oral route. Protein binding in plasma is approximately 30%, and the drug is well distributed in tissues. Linezolid is cleared by the kidneys, both unchanged and after oxidation of the parent compound. Because oxidation of linezolid is not dependent on renal function, no dose reduction is needed for renal insufficiency. Linezolid has been studied in neonates and older children for nosocomial and community-acquired pneumonia and for complicated and uncomplicated skin and skin structure infections.[349,350] The clinical response rates for each of these tissue specific infections were equivalent to comparator agents, usually vancomycin. The pathogen-specific response rates for infections caused by *S. aureus*, for both methicillin-sensitive and methicillin-resistant strains, and response rates in infections caused by coagulase-negative staphylococci were also statistically equivalent to vancomycin. Similarly, the rates for clinical and laboratory adverse events were equivalent to those in vancomycin-treated control patients. In neonates and children enrolled in these registration trials, the hematologic toxicity profiles for both neutropenia and thrombocytopenia were equivalent to vancomycin.[348] These data suggest that hematologic toxicity of thrombocytopenia and neutropenia seen in adults may not be seen as frequently in neonates and children.

Recommendations for the dosage regimen for preterm neonates less than 7 days of age (gestational age younger than 34 weeks) are based on data from registration trials involving very few neonates. Preterm neonates should be initially given 10 mg/kg every 12 hours. For neonates with a poor response to infection caused by a susceptible organism, an increased dose of 10 mg/kg every 8 hours can be provided. However, by 7 days of age, all neonates, regardless of gestational age, should receive 10 mg/kg every 8 hours. The interpatient variability in neonates was noted to be greater than that seen in adults and may reflect variation in the rate of maturation of mechanisms of elimination.

Unfortunately, in studies of CSF, linezolid concentrations in infants with ventriculoperitoneal shunts receiving systemic therapeutic dosing, adequate concentrations were not consistently achieved. Although a case report exists for the treatment of a staphylococcal CNS infection in a neonate,[296] the routine use of linezolid for the treatment of CNS infections cannot be recommended at this time. Similarly, case reports on the treatment of neonatal endocarditis caused by MRSA exist, but the safety and efficacy of linezolid for this indication remains to be defined. The role of combination therapy using linezolid is also not defined. A new anti-staphylococcal oxazolidinone, tedixolid (Sivextro, Cubist Pharmaceuticals, Lexington, Mass), was approved by the FDA in 2014 for use in adults, but has yet to be studied in the newborn population.

DAPTOMYCIN

An antibiotic approved only for use in adults, daptomycin is a novel lipopeptide bactericidal agent for gram-positive organisms, including *S. aureus* and CoNS. Structurally, daptomycin is a 13–amino acid cyclic peptide with a lipophilic tail that inserts into the cell membrane, leading to depolarization of the membrane; inhibition of protein, DNA, and RNA synthesis; and cell death. Daptomycin shows concentration-dependent killing pharmacodynamics. It is available only in an intravenous formulation. The prolonged half-life in adults of 8 to 9 hours allows for once-daily dosing. The antibiotic is highly protein bound (90%) and is excreted primarily by the kidney with little degradation of the parent compound. In renal insufficiency, the dose is decreased according to the degree of renal failure. In adults, daptomycin is approved by the FDA for the treatment of complicated skin and skin structure infections (caused by *S. aureus*, including MRSA), as well as for bacteremia and endocarditis. Daptomycin also shows in vitro activity against vancomycin-resistant *S. aureus* and should represent an effective agent should these strains become more widespread. Daptomycin is not indicated for the treatment of pneumonia because surfactant binding to the antibiotic is associated with inactivation. A recent study of single-dose pharmacokinetics in young infants showed clearance similar to older children and higher than seen in adolescents and adults.[351] Neurologic toxicity has been demonstrated in a neonatal beagle pup animal model at doses similar to those proposed for human infants, suggesting that daptomycin not be used in neonates until additional data are available. Myopathy is a potential adverse event noted in early phase I studies but with once-daily dosing in adults, and in the preliminary newborn data,[351] no muscle toxicity (elevated creatinine phosphokinase) was documented.

QUINUPRISTIN-DALFOPRISTIN

The streptogramins are antibiotic derivatives of natural products of *Streptomyces pristinaespiralis*. Two of the streptogramins, quinupristin and dalfopristin, when used together in a fixed combination, have been shown to be bactericidal against many gram-positive organisms, including staphylococci and certain enterococci. Each antibiotic is bacteriostatic, but, when used together in a 30:70 ratio, the combination is bactericidal. The combination is approved by the FDA as Synercid for adults, for the treatment of vancomycin-resistant *Enterococcus faecium* infections and for the treatment of skin and skin structure infections caused by *S. aureus* (only methicillin-susceptible strains were isolated from study patients). In vitro, quinupristin-dalfopristin is also active against MRSA and vancomycin-resistant *S. aureus*, although no clinical data are available for treatment of these infections. Quinupristin-dalfopristin is available only in an intravenous preparation. Both drugs are primarily eliminated through biliary excretion, with minimal metabolism. Inflammation and pain at the infusion site are substantial problems. Furthermore, many mechanisms of bacterial resistance have been documented, ultimately limiting the clinical usefulness of this combination.

COMBINATION ANTIMICROBIAL THERAPY

Although many combinations of antibiotics have been used in adults, few have been studied prospectively, with virtually no prospective comparative evaluations available for children and neonates. For invasive *S. aureus* disease, infective endocarditis in adults has resulted in some of the highest mortality rates, resulting in guidelines that recommend aggressive combination therapy based on animal model in vitro data, data from CoNS infections, and in the absence of human data for *S. aureus*.[352] For MSSA endocarditis, combination therapy with a β-lactam penicillin (oxacillin or nafcillin), with the addition of rifampin plus the addition of gentamicin for the first 2 weeks of therapy, is believed to result in optimal microbiologic efficacy. For MRSA, vancomycin plus rifampin, with gentamicin for the first 2 weeks of therapy, should be considered.[352] A report on vancomycin plus rifampin combination therapy of persisting CoNS bacteremia after removal of a central catheter provides some support to this approach.[353]

A Cochrane review of intravenous immunoglobulin therapy of suspected or documented neonatal sepsis evaluated nine clinical trials. Although substantial heterogeneity existed across studies in immune globulin preparations, dosing regimens, and populations studied, no substantial benefit was derived from treatment, particularly with respect to mortality in infants with either documented infection suspected or subsequently proven infection.[354]

CATHETER REMOVAL

The decision to remove an indwelling catheter from a neonate with bacteremia often is difficult, especially when securing subsequent intravascular access may be challenging. Delayed removal of a central catheter in the setting of bacteremia may be associated with an increased risk of infection-related complications.[214] For infants with CoNS bacteremia, successful treatment of bacteremia may be possible with the central venous catheter in situ.[214] However, if bacteremia persists for longer than 4 days, the chance for subsequent clearance is reduced,[213] and the risk of end-organ damage may be increased.[190,214] The presence of a ventricular reservoir or ventriculoperitoneal shunt increases the chance of the development of meningitis in the setting of prolonged catheter-related bacteremia. Thus prompt removal of an indwelling central venous catheter should be considered in infants with CNS hardware.[213] A relationship between the dwell time of peripherally inserted central catheters and risk of line-associated bacteremias has been calculated,[355] so the true need for central access in support of individual patients should be assessed daily.

Prevention

HYGIENIC MEASURES

Major efforts to prevent staphylococcal infections in neonates, rather than being required to treat them, are of great value. General principles underlying nosocomial infection in the NICU and measures to reduce their occurrence that apply broadly to staphylococcal infections are discussed in detail in Chapter 35. Some specific considerations relevant to staphylococci are discussed briefly here.

Staphylococci may be spread through the fomites; thus overcrowding of infants in an NICU may increase the risk of colonization and the potential for disease. In an outbreak situation, attempts to control the spread of staphylococci through remediation of overcrowding and isolation of infected or colonized patients have been shown effective in helping to curtail the outbreak, even in the case of MRSA.[356]

A primary determinant of infant colonization is nursing care. Maintaining an appropriate nurse-to-infant ratio is an important factor in reducing disease once a disease-associated *S. aureus* strain gains entrance to a nursery, especially in an NICU.[357] In addition, there are a variety of preventive maneuvers directed at those with direct infant contact, including frequent mask, gown, and glove changes before handling infants[358,359]; application of antimicrobial or antiseptic ointment or spray[360,361]; and elimination of carriers from the nursery area.[362,363] In some situations, control of an epidemic requires removal of the nurse carrier from the nursery.[364]

Currently, the Centers for Disease Control and Prevention recommends contact isolation for patients colonized or infected with MRSA.[365] This practice was shown to reduce nosocomial transmission of MRSA by 16-fold during an outbreak of MRSA in a NICU.[366] Several recent publications have focused on nursery infection control measures, documented to be effective in preventing the entry of CA-MRSA into a nursery, and its spread within the nursery.[367-370]

In the early 1960s, attempts were made to stop virulent *S. aureus* epidemics in 10 NICUs throughout the United States by using the technique of bacterial interference.[371,372] This technique involved deliberate implantation of an *S. aureus* strain of low virulence (502A) on the nasal mucosa and umbilicus of newborns to prevent colonization with the virulent *S. aureus* strain. Although this procedure was successful in curtailing epidemics,[373] it is not widely used or recommended currently.

Proper hand hygiene among nursery health care providers is a fundamental factor in reducing colonization rates. Mortimer and associates[374] achieved a reduction in infant colonization from 92% to 53% by insisting that attendants wash their hands. Proper education and monitoring of hand-hygiene practices are critical to the effectiveness of this intervention.[375,376] Hands must be cleansed before and after patient contact or contact with equipment that is used for patient care. Hands also should be cleansed after glove removal. Proper hand hygiene involves applying alcohol-based waterless rubs if hands are not soiled,[377] or washing the hands for at least 10 to 15 seconds with either chlorhexidine gluconate or triclosan hand-washing agents.[378]

With the rise in prominence of CoNS as nosocomial pathogens, strategies for disease prevention have become increasingly important. As with *S. aureus,* strict hand hygiene is of primary importance in minimizing staff-to-patient and patient-to-patient spread of CoNS. In addition, meticulous surgical technique to limit intraoperative bacterial contamination is critical in minimizing infection related to foreign bodies. Strict attention to protocols for the insertion and management of intravenous and intraarterial catheters may decrease the risk of catheter-related infections.[379] In patients who require intravenous access for prolonged periods of time, percutaneous placement of a small diameter silastic catheter is preferred when possible. In one study, these catheters were maintained for as long as 80 days, with an infection rate of less than 10% in infants weighing less than 1500g.[380]

ANTIBIOTIC PROPHYLAXIS

Investigational therapies to reduce neonatal bacteremia caused by staphylococci have been directed at the use of antibiotic prophylaxis, for instance, antibiotic-impregnated devices. Given the large burden of CoNS catheter infections in premature infants, investigations of prophylactic antibiotics to prevent infection were undertaken by a number of institutions, as recently reviewed.[381-385] Vancomycin was documented to be successful in significantly decreasing the rate of suspected or documented sepsis caused by CoNS. Antibiotic-based methods to prevent bacteremic infection have included the use of a vancomycin solution (25 μg/mL) to dwell inside the infant's central venous catheter two to three times daily for up to 60 minutes[384]; the administration of low-dose vancomycin at 5 mg/kg twice daily[383]; or the addition of vancomycin to hyperalimentation solutions to a concentration of 25 μg/mL for routine administration. Although all three methods were successful at decreasing episodes of sepsis, the overall mortality in treatment versus control groups was not affected. Because of concerns for the emergence of vancomycin-resistant organisms, routine use of prophylactic vancomycin for all neonates at risk of CoNS bacteremia is not currently recommended. Potential risks associated with prophylactic vancomycin, including ototoxicity, nephrotoxicity, and selection for resistant bacteria, have not been well evaluated.

IMMUNE PROPHYLAXIS

Studies evaluating the effectiveness of immune globulin preparations have, in general, not documented convincing, substantial benefits for the populations of premature infants studied.[386] This may, however, reflect the lack of effectiveness of a specific biologic preparation or suggest that particular subpopulations may benefit more from treatment than others, rather than proving the immune globulins have no potential role in prophylaxis or treatment. Other polyclonal antibody approaches to prophylaxis in premature infants have used high-titer anti–*S. aureus* immune globulin (Altastaph; Nabi Biopharmaceuticals, Rockville, MD), prepared from adult volunteers immunized with a staphylococcal vaccine. Pharmacokinetic, safety, and clinical outcome data in neonates randomized to receive either immune globulin or placebo did not show benefit in the limited trials performed to date.[386,387]

Studies of monoclonal antibodies directed against specific staphylococcal epitopes are ongoing. A randomized, placebo-controlled trial was recently conducted in premature infants to prevent staphylococcal infection, using an intravenous immunoglobulin preparation selected from donors with high activity against specific staphylococcal fibrinogen-binding protein, clumping-factor A, and Ser-Asp dipeptide repeat G (INH-A21 [Veronate]; Inhibitex, Alpharetta, Ga). No benefit to prophylaxis was noted in the recipients of this staphylococcal-specific immune globulin.[388,389] An antistaphylococcal monoclonal antibody, BSYX-A110 (Biosynexus, Gaithersburg, Md), has been developed for the prevention of CoNS sepsis. This antibody targets staphylococcal lipoteichoic acid and has been shown to be safe and well tolerated when administered by intravenous infusion to high-risk neonates.[390] The efficacy of any monocolonal antibody therapeutics in preventing CoNS infections and related morbidity and mortality has not been established and, as such, they are not currently recommended.[391]

Lactoferrin is an iron-binding glycoprotein present in breast milk that is believed to contribute to innate antibacterial immunity of the intestinal barrier through a combination of restricting pathogen access to iron, cell wall lytic activity of its component peptides, and promotion of epithelial barrier maturation.[392] Human recombinant lactoferrin may synergize with vancomycin and nafcillin in terms of in vitro activity against CoNS.[393] A recent randomized study of bovine lactoferrin supplementation in VLBW premature infants demonstrated a promising reduction in the rate of LOS in the treatment group (risk ratio, 0.34; 95% confidence interval, 0.17 to 0.70).[394]

Conclusion

Staphylococcal infections result in significant morbidity and mortality in the neonate. Although CoNS are frequent causes of less severe infections, the continuing relatively high rate of community-associated and hospital-associated infections caused by more aggressive *S. aureus* and the recent emergence of CA-MRSA with exceptionally high mortality rates has created an unprecedented need to understand the biology and mechanisms of virulence of staphylococci. In this way, we can generate improved approaches to both prevent and treat infections. A profound need exists to develop more safe and effective antimicrobials and immune therapies to mitigate the substantial morbidity and mortality caused by these pathogens.

Acknowledgment

The authors are indebted to Rachel C. Orscheln, Henry R. Shinefield, and Joseph W. St. Geme III, whose previous contributions to this chapter and clinical images provided the strong baseline framework and inspiration for the current version.

References

1. Fox T: Epidemic pemphigus of newly born (impetigo contagiosa et bullosa neonatorum), *Lancet* 1:1323, 1935.
2. Rulison ET: Control of impetigo neonatorum: advisability of a radical departure in obstetrical care, *JAMA* 93:903, 1929.
3. Eichenwald HF, Kotsevalov O, Fasso LA: The "cloud baby": an example of bacterial-viral interaction, *Am J Dis Child* 100:161-173, 1960.
4. Dixon RE, Kaslow RA, Mallinson GF, et al: Staphylococcal disease outbreaks in hospital nurseries in the United States—December 1971 through March 1972, *Pediatrics* 51:413-417, 1973.
5. Stoll BJ, Hansen N, Fanaroff AA, et al: Late-onset sepsis in very low birth weight neonates: the experience of the nichd neonatal research network, *Pediatrics* 110:285-291, 2002.
6. Bizzarro MJ, Raskind C, Baltimore RS, et al: Seventy-five years of neonatal sepsis at Yale: 1928-2003, *Pediatrics* 116:595-602, 2005.
7. Marchant EA, Boyce GK, Sadarangani M, et al: Neonatal sepsis due to coagulase-negative staphylococci, *Clin Dev Immunol* 2013:586076, 2013.
8. Shinefield HR, Ribble JC, Boris M, et al: Bacterial interference: its effect on nursery-acquired infection with *Staphylococcus aureus*: I. Preliminary observations, *Am J Dis Child* 105:646-654, 1963.
9. Fairchild JP, Graber CD, Vogel EH, et al: Flora of the umbilical stump: 2479 cultures, *J Pediatr* 53:538-546, 1958.
10. Gillespie WA, Simpson K, Tozer RC: Staphylococcal infection in a maternity hospital: epidemiology and control, *Lancet* 2:1075-1080, 1958.
11. Hurst V: Transmission of hospital staphylococci among newborn infants: II. Colonization of the skin and mucous membranes of the infants, *Pediatrics* 25:204-214, 1960.
12. Schaffer TE, Sylvester RF, Baldwin JN, et al: Staphylococcal infections in newborn infants: II. Report of 19 epidemics caused by an identical strain of *Staphylococcus pyogenes*, *Am J Public Health* 47:990-994, 1957.
13. Wolinsky E, Lipsitz PJ, Mortimer EA Jr : Acquisition of staphylococci by newborns: direct versus indirect transmission, *Lancet* 2:620-622, 1960.
14. Shinefield HR, Ribble JC, Sutherland JM, et al: Bacterial interference: its effect on nursery-acquired infection with *Staphylococcus aureus*: II. The Ohio epidemic, *Am J Dis Child* 105:655-662, 1963.
15. Hare R, Thomas CGA: The transmission of *Staphylococcus aureus*, *Br Med J* 2:840-844, 1956.
16. Ridely M: Perineal carriage of *Staphylococcus aureus*, *Br Med J* 1:270-273, 1959.
17. Acton DS, Plat-Sinnige MJ, van Wamel W, et al: Intestinal carriage of *Staphylococcus aureus*: how does its frequency compare with that of nasal carriage and what is its clinical impact? *Eur J Clin Microbiol Infect Dis* 28:115-127, 2009.
18. Thompson RL, Cabezudo I, Wenzel RP: Epidemiology of nosocomial infections caused by methicillin-resistant *Staphylococcus aureus*, *Ann Intern Med* 97:309-317, 1982.
19. Hiramatsu K, Cui L, Kuroda M, et al: The emergence and evolution of methicillin-resistant *Staphylococcus aureus*, *Trends Microbiol* 9:486-493, 2001.
20. Boyce JM: Methicillin-resistant *Staphylococcus aureus*. Detection, epidemiology, and control measures, *Infect Dis Clin North Am* 3:901-913, 1989.
21. Salgado CD, Farr BM, Calfee DP: Community-acquired methicillin-resistant *Staphylococcus aureus*: a meta-analysis of prevalence and risk factors, *Clin Infect Dis* 36:131-139, 2003.
22. Eady EA, Cove JH: Staphylococcal resistance revisited: community-acquired methicillin resistant *Staphylococcus aureus*—an emerging problem for the management of skin and soft tissue infections, *Curr Opin Infect Dis* 16:103-124, 2003.
23. Shane AL, Hansen NI, Stoll BJ, et al: Methicillin-resistant and susceptible *Staphylococcus aureus* bacteremia and meningitis in preterm infants, *Pediatrics* 129:e914-e922, 2012.
24. Carey AJ, Duchon J, Della-Latta P, et al: The epidemiology of methicillin-susceptible and methicillin-resistant *Staphylococcus aureus* in a neonatal intensive care unit, 2000-2007, *J Perinatol* 30:135-139, 2009.
25. Gould IM, Girvan EK, Browning RA, et al: Report of a hospital neonatal unit outbreak of community-associated methicillin-resistant *Staphylococcus aureus*, *Epidemiol Infect* 137:1242-1248, 2009.
26. McAdams RM, Ellis MW, Trevino S, et al: Spread of methicillin-resistant *Staphylococcus aureus* USA300 in a neonatal intensive care unit, *Pediatr Int* 50:810-815, 2008.
27. Heinrich N, Mueller A, Bartmann P, et al: Successful management of an MRSA outbreak in a neonatal intensive care unit, *Eur J Clin Microbiol Infect Dis* 30:909-913, 2011.
28. Saiman L, Jakob K, Holmes KW, et al: Molecular epidemiology of staphylococcal scalded skin syndrome in premature infants, *Pediatr Infect Dis J* 17:329-334, 1998.
29. Enright MC, Day NP, Davies CE, et al: Multilocus sequence typing for characterization of methicillin-resistant and methicillin-susceptible clones of *Staphylococcus aureus*, *J Clin Microbiol* 38:1008-1015, 2000.
30. Diep BA, Perdreau-Remington F, Sensabaugh GF: Clonal characterization of *Staphylococcus aureus* by multilocus restriction fragment typing, a rapid screening approach for molecular epidemiology, *J Clin Microbiol* 41:4559-4564, 2003.
31. Nubel U, Nachtnebel M, Falkenhorst G, et al: MRSA transmission on a neonatal intensive care unit: epidemiological and genome-based phylogenetic analyses, *PLoS One* 8:e54898, 2013.
32. Goldmann DA: Bacterial colonization and infection in the neonate, *Am J Med* 70:417, 1981.
33. Simpson RA, Spencer AF, Speller DCE, et al: Colonization by gentamicin-resistant *Staphylococcus epidermidis* in a special care baby unit, *J Hosp Infect* 7:108-120, 1986.
34. Hall SL, Riddell SW, Barnes WG, et al: Evaluation of coagulase-negative staphylococcal isolates from serial nasopharyngeal cultures of premature infants, *Diagn Microbiol Infect Dis* 13:17-23, 1990.
35. Patrick CH, John JF, Levkoff A, et al: Relatedness of strains of methicillin-resistant coagulase-negative *Staphylococcus* colonizing hospital personnel and producing bacteremias in a neonatal intensive care unit, *Pediatr Infect Dis J* 11:935-940, 1992.
36. D'Angio CT, McGowan KL, Baumgart S, et al: Surface colonization with coagulase-negative staphylococci in premature neonates, *J Pediatr* 114:1029-1034, 1989.
37. Freeman J, Goldmann DA, Smith NE, et al: Association of intravenous lipid emulsion and coagulase negative staphylococcal bacteremia in neonatal intensive care units, *N Engl J Med* 323:301-308, 1990.
38. Kloos W: *Taxonomy and systemics of staphylococci indigenous to humans*, New York, 1997, Churchill Livingstone.
39. Giesbrecht P, Wecke J, Reinicke B: On the morphogenesis of the cell wall of staphylococci, *Int Rev Cytol* 44:225-318, 1976.
40. Braddiley J, Brock JH, Davidson AL, et al: The wall composition of micrococci, *J Gen Microbiol* 54:393-396, 1968.
41. Labischinski H: Consequences of interaction of β-lactam antibiotics with penicillin binding proteins from sensitive and resistant *Staphylococcus aureus* strains, *Med Microbiol Immunol (Berl)* 181:241-265, 1992.

42. Juergens WG, Sanderson AR, Strominger JL: Chemical basis for the immunological specificity of a strain of *Staphylococcus aureus*, *J Exp Med* 117:925-935, 1963.
43. Lee JC, Pier GB: *Vaccine-based strategies for prevention of staphylococcal diseases*, New York, 1997, Churchill Livingstone.
44. Verburgh HA, Peters R, Rozenberg-Arska M, et al: Antibodies to cell wall peptidoglycan of *Staphylococcus aureus* in patients with serious staphylococcal infections, *J Infect Dis* 144:1-9, 1981.
45. Fischetti VA, Pancholi V, Schneewind O: Conservation of a hexapeptide sequence in the anchor region of surface proteins from gram-positive cocci, *Mol Microbiol* 4:1603-1605, 1990.
46. Mazmanian SK, Ton-That H, Schneewind O: Sortase-catalysed anchoring of surface proteins to the cell wall of *Staphylococcus aureus*, *Mol Microbiol* 40:1049-1057, 2001.
47. Foster TJ, Hook M: Surface protein adhesins of *Staphylococcus aureus*, *Trends Microbiol* 6:484-488, 1998.
48. O'Riordan K, Lee JC: *Staphylococcus aureus* capsular polysaccharides, *Clin Microbiol Rev* 17:218-234, 2004.
49. Moreau M, Richards JC, Fournier JM, et al: Structure of the type 5 capsular polysaccharide of *Staphylococcus aureus*, *Carbohydr Res* 201:285-297, 1990.
50. Fournier JM, Vann WF, Karakawa WW: Purification and characterization of *Staphylococcus aureus* type 8 capsular polysaccharide, *Infect Immun* 45:87-93, 1984.
51. Tuchscherr L, Loffler B, Buzzola FR, et al: *Staphylococcus aureus* adaptation to the host and persistence: role of loss of capsular polysaccharide expression, *Future Microbiol* 5:1823-1832, 2010.
52. von Eiff C: *Staphylococcus aureus* small colony variants: a challenge to microbiologists and clinicians, *Int J Antimicrob Agents* 31:507-510, 2008.
53. Proctor RA, von Eiff C, Kahl BC, et al: Small colony variants: a pathogenic form of bacteria that facilitates persistent and recurrent infections, *Nat Rev Microbiol* 4:295-305, 2006.
54. Garcia LG, Lemaire S, Kahl BC, et al: Antibiotic activity against small-colony variants of *Staphylococcus aureus*: review of in vitro, animal and clinical data, *J Antimicrob Chemother* 68:1455-1464, 2013.
55. Holden MT, Feil EJ, Lindsay JA, et al: Complete genomes of two clinical *Staphylococcus aureus* strains: evidence for the rapid evolution of virulence and drug resistance, *Proc Natl Acad Sci U S A* 101:9786-9791, 2004.
56. Diep BA, Gill SR, Chang RF, et al: Complete genome sequence of USA300, an epidemic clone of community-acquired meticillin-resistant *Staphylococcus aureus*, *Lancet* 367:731-739, 2006.
57. Baba T, Takeuchi F, Kuroda M, et al: Genome and virulence determinants of high virulence community-acquired MRSA, *Lancet* 359:1819-1827, 2002.
58. Kuroda M, Ohta T, Uchiyama I, et al: Whole genome sequencing of methicillin-resistant *Staphylococcus aureus*, *Lancet* 357:1225-1240, 2001.
59. Parker MT, Roundtree PM: Report (1966-1970) of the subcommittee on phage typing of staphylococci to the international committee on nomenclature of bacteria, *Int J Syst Bacteriol* 21:167, 1971.
60. Prevost G, Jaulhoc B, Piedmont Y: DNA fingerprinting of pulsed-field gel electrophoresis is more effective than ribotyping in distinguishing among methicillin-resistant *Staphylococcus aureus* isolates, *J Clin Microbiol* 30:967-973, 1992.
61. Tenover FC, Arbeit R, Archer G, et al: Comparison of traditional and molecular methods of typing isolates of *Staphylococcus aureus*, *J Clin Microbiol* 32:407-415, 1994.
62. Aziz RK, Nizet V: Pathogen microevolution in high resolution, *Sci Transl Med* 2, 2010. 16ps14.
63. Pfaller MA, Herwaldt LA: Laboratory, clinical and epidemiological aspects of coagulase-negative staphylococci, *Clin Microbiol Rev* 1:281-299, 1988.
64. Wu F, Della-Latta P: Molecular typing strategies, *Semin Perinatol* 26:357-366, 2002.
65. Donkor ES: Sequencing of bacterial genomes: principles and insights into pathogenesis and development of antibiotics, *Genes (Basel)* 4:556-572, 2013.
66. Zhang YQ, Ren SX, Li HL, et al: Genome-based analysis of virulence genes in a non-biofilm-forming *Staphylococcus epidermidis* strain (ATCC 12228), *Mol Microbiol* 49:1577-1593, 2003.
67. Heilmann C: Adhesion mechanisms of staphylococci, *Adv Exp Med Biol* 715:105-123, 2011.
68. Speziale P, Pietrocola G, Rindi S, et al: Structural and functional role of *Staphylococcus aureus* surface components recognizing adhesive matrix molecules of the host, *Future Microbiol* 4:1337-1352, 2009.
69. Clarke SR, Foster SJ: Surface adhesins of *Staphylococcus aureus*, *Adv Microb Physiol* 51:187-224, 2006.
70. Rivera J, Vannakambadi G, Hook M, et al: Fibrinogen-binding proteins of gram-positive bacteria, *Thromb Haemost* 98:503-511, 2007.
71. Fowler T, Wann ER, Joh D, et al: Cellular invasion by *Staphylococcus aureus* involves a fibronectin bridge between the bacterial fibronectin-binding mscramms and host cell β1 integrins, *Eur J Cell Biol* 79:672-679, 2000.
72. Moreillon P, Entenza JM, Francioli P, et al: Role of *Staphylococcus aureus* coagulase and clumping factor in pathogenesis of experimental endocarditis, *Infect Immun* 63:4738-4743, 1995.
73. Patti JM, Jonsson H, Guss B, et al: Molecular characterization and expression of a gene encoding a *Staphylococcus aureus* collagen adhesin, *J Biol Chem* 267:4766-4772, 1992.
74. Patti JM, Bremell T, Krajewska-Pietrasik D, et al: The *Staphylococcus aureus* collagen adhesin is a virulence determinant in experimental septic arthritis, *Infect Immun* 62:152-161, 1994.
75. O'Gara JP: Ica and beyond: biofilm mechanisms and regulation in *Staphylococcus epidermidis* and *Staphylococcus aureus*, *FEMS Microbiol Lett* 270:179-188, 2007.
76. Peschel A, Otto M, Jack RW, et al: Inactivation of the *dlt* operon in *Staphylococcus aureus* confers sensitivity to defensins, protegrins, and other antimicrobial peptides, *J Biol Chem* 274:8405-8410, 1999.
77. Collins LV, Kristian SA, Weidenmaier C, et al: *Staphylococcus aureus* strains lacking d-alanine modifications of teichoic acids are highly susceptible to human neutrophil killing and are virulence attenuated in mice, *J Infect Dis* 186:214-219, 2002.
78. Staubitz P, Neumann H, Schneider T, et al: MprF-mediated biosynthesis of lysylphosphatidylglycerol, an important determinant in staphylococcal defensin resistance, *FEMS Microbiol Lett* 231:67-71, 2004.
79. Nishi H, Komatsuzawa H, Fujiwara T, et al: Reduced content of lysyl-phosphatidylglycerol in the cytoplasmic membrane affects susceptibility to moenomycin, as well as vancomycin, gentamicin, and antimicrobial peptides, in *Staphylococcus aureus*, *Antimicrob Agents Chemother* 48:4800-4807, 2004.
80. Weidenmaier C, Peschel A, Kempf VA, et al: DltABCD- and MprF-mediated cell envelope modifications of *Staphylococcus aureus* confer resistance to platelet microbicidal proteins and contribute to virulence in a rabbit endocarditis model, *Infect Immun* 73:8033-8038, 2005.
81. Selsted ME, Tang YQ, Morris WL, et al: Purification, primary structures, and antibacterial activities of beta-defensins, a new family of antimicrobial peptides from bovine neutrophils, *J Biol Chem* 268:6641-6648, 1993.
82. Sieprawska-Lupa M, Mydel P, Krawczyk K, et al: Degradation of human antimicrobial peptide LL-37 by *Staphylococcus aureus*-derived proteinases, *Antimicrob Agents Chemother* 48:4673-4679, 2004.
83. Postma B, Poppelier MJ, van Galen JC, et al: Chemotaxis inhibitory protein of *Staphylococcus aureus* binds specifically to the C5a and formylated peptide receptor, *J Immunol* 172:6994-7001, 2004.
84. Haggar A, Ehrnfelt C, Holgersson J, et al: The extracellular adherence protein from *Staphylococcus aureus* inhibits neutrophil binding to endothelial cells, *Infect Immun* 72:6164-6167, 2004.
85. Rooijakkers SH, van Kessel KP, van Strijp JA: Staphylococcal innate immune evasion, *Trends Microbiol* 13:596-601, 2005.
86. Rooijakkers SH, Ruyken M, Roos A, et al: Immune evasion by a staphylococcal complement inhibitor that acts on C3 convertases, *Nat Immunol* 6:920-927, 2005.
87. Hair PS, Echague CG, Sholl AM, et al: Clumping factor a interaction with complement factor i increases C3b cleavage on the bacterial surface of *Staphylococcus aureus* and decreases complement-mediated phagocytosis, *Infection Immun* 78:1717-1727, 2010.
88. Hammel M, Sfyroera G, Ricklin D, et al: A structural basis for complement inhibition by *Staphylococcus aureus*, *Nat Immunol* 8:430-437, 2007.
89. Jin T, Bokarewa M, Foster T, et al: *Staphylococcus aureus* resists human defensins by production of staphylokinase, a novel bacterial evasion mechanism, *J Immunol* 172:1169-1176, 2004.
90. Jusko M, Potempa J, Kantyka T, et al: Staphylococcal proteases aid in evasion of the human complement system, *J Innate Immun* 6:31-46, 2014.

91. Laarman AJ, Ruyken M, Malone CL, et al: *Staphylococcus aureus* metalloprotease aureolysin cleaves complement C3 to mediate immune evasion, *J Immunol* 186:6445-6453, 2011.
92. Foster TJ: Immune evasion by staphylococci, *Nat Rev Microbiol* 3:948-958, 2005.
93. Kim HK, Thammavongsa V, Schneewind O, et al: Recurrent infections and immune evasion strategies of *Staphylococcus aureus*, *Curr Opin Microbiol* 15:92-99, 2012.
94. Thakker M, Park JS, Carey V, et al: *Staphylococcus aureus* serotype 5 capsular polysaccharide is antiphagocytic and enhances bacterial virulence in a murine bacteremia model, *Infect Immun* 66:5183-5189, 1998.
95. Luong TT, Lee CY: Overproduction of type 8 capsular polysaccharide augments *Staphylococcus aureus* virulence, *Infect Immun* 70:3389-3395, 2002.
96. Kropec A, Maira-Litran T, Jefferson KK, et al: Poly-*N*-acetylglucosamine production in *Staphylococcus aureus* is essential for virulence in murine models of systemic infection, *Infect Immun* 73:6868-6876, 2005.
97. Mandell GL: Catalase, superoxide dismutase, and virulence of *Staphylococcus aureus*. In vitro and in vivo studies with emphasis on staphylococcal-leukocyte interaction, *J Clin Invest* 55:561-566, 1975.
98. Liu GY, Essex A, Buchanan JT, et al: *Staphylococcus aureus* golden pigment impairs neutrophil killing and promotes virulence through its antioxidant activity, *J Exp Med* 202:209-215, 2005.
99. Clauditz A, Resch A, Wieland KP, et al: Staphyloxanthin plays a role in the fitness of *Staphylococcus aureus* and its ability to cope with oxidative stress, *Infect Immun* 74:4950-4953, 2006.
100. Gusarov I, Shatalin K, Starodubtseva M, et al: Endogenous nitric oxide protects bacteria against a wide spectrum of antibiotics, *Science* 325:1380-1384, 2009.
101. van Sorge NM, Beasley FC, Gusarov I, et al: Methicillin-resistant *Staphylococcus aureus* bacterial nitric-oxide synthase affects antibiotic sensitivity and skin abscess development, *J Biol Chem* 288: 6417-6426, 2013.
102. Karavolos MH, Horsburgh MJ, Ingham E, et al: Role and regulation of the superoxide dismutases of *Staphylococcus aureus*, *Microbiology* 149:2749-2758, 2003.
103. Gouaux JE, Braha O, Hobaugh MR, et al: Subunit stoichiometry of staphylococcal alpha-hemolysin in crystals and on membranes: a heptameric transmembrane pore, *Proc Natl Acad Sci U S A* 91:12828-12831, 1994.
104. Bhakdi S, Tranum-Jensen J: Alpha-toxin of *Staphylococcus aureus*, *Microbiol Rev* 55:733-751, 1991.
105. Suttorp N, Fuhrmann M, Tannert-Otto S, et al: Pore-forming bacterial toxins potently induce release of nitric oxide in porcine endothelial cells, *J Exp Med* 178:337-341, 1993.
106. Jonas D, Waley I, Berger T, et al: Novel path to apoptosis: small transmembrane pores created by staphylococcal alpha-toxin in T lymphocytes evoke internucleosomal DNA degradation, *Infect Immun* 62:1304-1312, 1994.
107. Jarry TM, Memmi G, Cheung AL: The expression of alpha-haemolysin is required for *Staphylococcus aureus* phagosomal escape after internalization in CFT-1 cells, *Cell Microbiol* 10:1801-1814, 2008.
108. Inoshima I, Inoshima N, Wilke GA, et al: A *Staphylococcus aureus* pore-forming toxin subverts the activity of ADAM10 to cause lethal infection in mice, *Nat Med* 17:1310-1314, 2011.
109. Bubeck Wardenburg J, Schneewind O: Vaccine protection against *Staphylococcus aureus* pneumonia, *J Exp Med* 205:287-294, 2008.
110. Kaneko J, Kamio Y: Bacterial two-component and hetero-heptameric pore-forming cytolytic toxins: structures, pore-forming mechanism, and organization of the genes, *Biosci Biotechnol Biochem* 68:981-1003, 2004.
111. Malachowa N, DeLeo FR: Staphylococcus aureus survival in human blood, *Virulence* 2:567-569, 2011.
112. Staali L, Monteil H, Colin DA: The staphylococcal pore-forming leukotoxins open Ca2+ channels in the membrane of human polymorphonuclear neutrophils, *J Membr Biol* 162:209-216, 1998.
113. Colin DA, Monteil H: Control of the oxidative burst of human neutrophils by staphylococcal leukotoxins, *Infect Immun* 71:3724-3729, 2003.
114. Reyes-Robles T, Alonzo F 3rd, Kozhaya L, et al: *Staphylococcus aureus* leukotoxin ED targets the chemokine receptors CXCR1 and CXCR2 to kill leukocytes and promote infection, *Cell Host Microbe* 14:453-459, 2013.
115. Alonzo F 3rd, Kozhaya L, Rawlings SA, et al: CCR5 is a receptor for *Staphylococcus aureus* leukotoxin ED, *Nature* 493:51-55, 2013.
116. Gillet Y, Issartel B, Vanhems P, et al: Association between *Staphylococcus aureus* strains carrying gene for Panton-Valentine leukocidin and highly lethal necrotising pneumonia in young immunocompetent patients, *Lancet* 359:753-759, 2002.
117. Labandeira-Rey M, Couzon F, Boisset S, et al: *Staphylococcus aureus* Panton-Valentine leukocidin causes necrotizing pneumonia, *Science* 315:1130-1133, 2007.
118. Villaruz AE, Wardenburg JB, Khan BA, et al: A point mutation in the *agr* locus rather than expression of the Panton-Valentine leukocidin caused previously reported phenotypes in *Staphylococcus aureus* pneumonia and gene regulation, *J Infect Dis* 200:724-734, 2009.
119. Bubeck Wardenburg J, Palazzolo-Ballance AM, Otto M, et al: Panton-Valentine leukocidin is not a virulence determinant in murine models of community-associated methicillin-resistant *Staphylococcus aureus* disease, *J Infect Dis* 198:1166-1170, 2008.
120. Tseng CW, Kyme P, Low J, et al: *Staphylococcus aureus* Panton-Valentine leukocidin contributes to inflammation and muscle tissue injury, *PLoS One* 4:e6387, 2009.
121. Loffler B, Hussain M, Grundmeier M, et al: *Staphylococcus aureus* Panton-Valentine leukocidin is a very potent cytotoxic factor for human neutrophils, *PLoS Pathog* 6:e1000715, 2010.
122. Diep BA, Chan L, Tattevin P, et al: Polymorphonuclear leukocytes mediate *Staphylococcus aureus* Panton-Valentine leukocidin-induced lung inflammation and injury, *Proc Natl Acad Sci U S A* 107:5587-5592, 2010.
123. Wang R, Braughton KR, Kretschmer D, et al: Identification of novel cytolytic peptides as key virulence determinants for community-associated MRSA, *Nat Med* 13:1510-1514, 2007.
124. Kretschmer D, Gleske AK, Rautenberg M, et al: Human formyl peptide receptor 2 senses highly pathogenic *Staphylococcus aureus*, *Cell Host Microbe* 7:463-473, 2010.
125. Grosz M, Kolter J, Paprotka K, et al: Cytoplasmic replication of *Staphylococcus aureus* upon phagosomal escape triggered by phenol-soluble modulin α, *Cell Microbiol* 16:451-465, 2014.
126. Hongo I, Baba T, Oishi K, et al: Phenol-soluble modulin α3 enhances the human neutrophil lysis mediated by Panton-Valentine leukocidin, *J Infect Dis* 200:715-723, 2009.
127. Wadstrom T, Mollby R: Studies on extracellular proteins from *Staphylococcus aureus*: VII. Studies on beta-hemolysin, *Biochim Biophys Acta* 242:308, 1972.
128. Hayashida A, Bartlett AH, Foster TJ, et al: *Staphylococcus aureus* β-toxin induces lung injury through syndecan-1, *Am J Pathol* 174:509-518, 2009.
129. Fraser JD, Proft T: The bacterial superantigen and superantigen-like proteins, *Immunol Rev* 225:226-243, 2008.
130. Nishifuji K, Sugai M, Amagai M: Staphylococcal exfoliative toxins: "molecular scissors" of bacteria that attack the cutaneous defense barrier in mammals, *J Dermatol Sci* 49:21-31, 2008.
131. Plano LR: *Staphylococcus aureus* exfoliative toxins: how they cause disease, *J Invest Dermatol* 122:1070-1077, 2004.
132. Björklind A, Arvidson S: Mutants of *Staphylococcus aureus* affected in the regulation of exoprotein synthesis, *FEMS Microbiol Lett* 7:203-206, 1980.
133. Novick RP: Autoinduction and signal transduction in the regulation of staphylococcal virulence, *Mol Microbiol* 48:1429-1449, 2003.
134. Novick RP, Geisinger E: Quorum sensing in staphylococci, *Annu Rev Genet* 42:541-564, 2008.
135. Abdelnour A, Arvidson S, Bremell T, et al: The accessory gene regulator (*agr*) controls *Staphylococcus aureus* virulence in a murine arthritis model, *Infect Immun* 61:3879-3885, 1993.
136. Rogers KL, Fey PD, Rupp ME: Coagulase-negative staphylococcal infections, *Infect Dis Clin North Am* 23:73-98, 2009.
137. Otto M: Virulence factors of the coagulase-negative staphylococci, *Front Biosci* 9:841-863, 2004.
138. Ludwicka A, Locci R, Jansen B, et al: Microbial colonization of prosthetic devices. V. Attachment of coagulase-negative staphylococci and "slime"-production on chemically pure synthetic polymers, *Zentralbl Bakteriol Mikrobiol Hyg B* 177:527-532, 1983.
139. Gristina A: Biomaterial-centered infection: microbial adhesion versus tissue integration, *Clin Orthop Relat Res* 2004:4-12, 1987.
140. Kristinsson KG: Adherence of staphylococci to intravascular catheters, *J Med Microbiol* 28:249-257, 1989.

141. Heilman C, Hussain M, Peters G, et al: Evidence for autolysin-mediated primary attachment of *Staphylococcus epidermidis* to a polystrene surface, *Mol Microbiol* 24:1013-1024, 1997.
142. Rupp ME, Fey PD, Heilman C, et al: Characterization of the importance of *Staphylococcus epidermidis* autolysin and polysaccharide intercellular adhesin in the pathogenesis of intravascular catheter-associated infection in a rat model, *J Infect Dis* 183:1038-1042, 2001.
143. Timmerman CP, Fleer A, Besnier JM, et al: Characterization of a proteinaceous adhesion of *Staphylococcus epidermidis* which mediates attachment to polystrene, *Infect Immun* 59:4187-4192, 1991.
144. McCrea KW, Hartford O, Davis S, et al: The serine-aspartate repeat (Sdr) protein family in *Staphylococcus epidermidis*, *Microbiology* 146:1535-1546, 2000.
145. Pei L, Flock JI: Lack of *Fbe*, the gene for a fibrinogen-binding protein from *Staphylococcus epidermidis*, reduces its adherence to fibrinogen coated surfaces, *Microb Pathog* 31:185-193, 2001.
146. Nilsson M, Frykberg L, Flock JI, et al: A fibrinogen-binding protein of *Staphylococcus epidermidis*, *Infect Immun* 66:2666-2673, 1998.
147. Hussain M, Heilman C, Peters G, et al: Teichoic acid enhances adhesion of *Staphylococcus epidermidis* to immobilized fibronectin, *Microb Pathog* 31:261-270, 2001.
148. Bowden MG, Visai L, Longshaw CM, et al: Is the gehd lipase from *Staphylococcus epidermidis* a collagen binding adhesin? *J Biol Chem* 277:43017-43023, 2002.
149. Hall RT, Hall SL, Barnes WG, et al: Characteristics of coagulase-negative staphylococci from infants with bacteremia, *Pediatr Infect Dis J* 6:377-383, 1987.
150. Gruskay JA, Nachamkin I, Baumgart S, et al: Predicting the pathogenicity of coagulase-negative *Staphylococcus* in the neonate: slime production, antibiotic resistance, and predominance of *Staphylococcus epidermidis* species, *Pediatrics* 20:397-399, 1986.
151. Mack D, Nedelmann M, Krokotsch A, et al: Characterization of transposon mutants of biofilm-producing *Staphylococcus epidermidis* impaired in the accumulative phase of biofilm production: genetic identification of a hexosamine-containing polysaccharide intercellular adhesion, *Infect Immun* 62:3244-3253, 1994.
152. Rohde H, Frankenberger S, Zahringer U, et al: Structure, function and contribution of polysaccharide intercellular adhesin (PIA) to *Staphylococcus epidermidis* biofilm formation and pathogenesis of biomaterial-associated infections, *Eur J Cell Biol* 89:103-111, 2010.
153. McKenney D, Hubner J, Muller E, et al: The *ica* locus of *Staphylococcus epidermidis* encodes production of the capsular polysaccharide/adhesin, *Infect Immun* 66:4711-4720, 1998.
154. Galdbart JO, Allignet J, Tung HS, et al: Screening for *Staphylococcus epidermidis* markers discriminating between skin-flora strains and those responsible for infections of joint prostheses, *J Infect Dis* 182:351-355, 2000.
155. Ziebuhr W, Krimmer V, Rachid S, et al: A novel mechanism of phase variation of virulence in *Staphylococcus epidermidis*: evidence for control of the polysaccharide intercellular adhesin synthesis by alternating insertion and excision of the insertion sequence element IS256, *Mol Microbiol* 32:345-356, 1999.
156. Hussain M, Herrmann M, von Eiff C, et al: A 140-kilodalton extracellular protein is essential for the accumulation of s *Staphylococcus epidermidis* strains on surfaces, *Infect Immun* 65:519-524, 1997.
157. Kocianova S, Vuong C, Yao Y, et al: Key role of poly-gamma-DL-glutamic acid in immune evasion and virulence of *Staphylococcus epidermidis*, *J Clin Invest* 115:688-694, 2005.
158. Vuong C, Götz F, Otto M: Construction and characterization of an *agr* deletion mutant of *Staphylococcus epidermidis*, *Infect Immun* 68:1048-1053, 2000.
159. Kristian SA, Birkenstock TA, Sauder U, et al: Biofilm formation induces C3a release and protects *Staphylococcus epidermidis* from IgG and complement deposition and from neutrophil-dependent killing, *J Infect Dis* 197:1028-1035, 2008.
160. Farber BF, Kaplan MH, Clogston AG: *Staphylococcus epidermidis* extracted slime inhibits the antimicrobial action of glycopeptide antibodies, *J Infect Dis* 161:37-40, 1990.
161. Kristinsson KG, Spencer RC: Slime production as a marker for clinically significant infection with coagulase-negative staphylococci, *J Infect Dis* 154:728-729, 1986.
162. Younger JJ, Christensen GD, Bartley DL, et al: Coagulase-negative staphylococci isolated from cerebrospinal fluid shunts: importance of slime production, species identification, and shunt removal to clinical outcome, *J Infect Dis* 156:548-554, 1987.
163. Ohara-Nemoto Y, Ikeda Y, Kobayashi M, et al: Characterization and molecular cloning of a glutamyl endopeptidase from *Staphylococcus epidermidis*, *Microb Pathog* 33:33-41, 2002.
164. Liles WC, Thomsen AR, O'Mahony DS, et al: Stimulation of human neutrophils and monocytes by staphylococcal phenol-soluble modulin, *J Leukoc Biol* 70:96-102, 2001.
165. Power Coombs MR, Kronforst K, Levy O: Neonatal host defense against staphylococcal infections, *Clin Dev Immunol* 2013:826303, 2013.
166. Koenig JM, Yoder MC: Neonatal neutrophils: the good, the bad, and the ugly, *Clin Perinatol* 31:39-51, 2004.
167. Mease AD: Tissue neutropenia: the newborn neutrophil in perspective, *J Perinatol* 10:55-59, 1990.
168. Anderson DC, Hughes B, Smith CW: Abnormality motility of neonatal polymorphonuclear leukocytes, *J Clin Invest* 68:863-874, 1981.
169. Schibler KR, Trautman MS, Liechty KW, et al: Diminished transcription of interleukin-8 by monocytes from preterm neonates, *J Leukoc Biol* 53:399-403, 1993.
170. Yoshimura TK, Matsuskima K, Tanaka S, et al: Purification of a human monocyte derived neutrophil chemotactic factor that shares sequence homology with other host defense cytokines, *Proc Natl Acad Sci U S A* 84:9233-9237, 1987.
171. Zimmerman GA, Prescott SM, McIntyre TM: Endothelial cell, interactions with granulocytes: tethering and signaling molecules, *Immunol Today* 13:93-100, 1992.
172. Yost CC, Cody MJ, Harris ES, et al: Impaired neutrophil extracellular trap (NET) formation: a novel innate immune deficiency of human neonates, *Blood* 113:6419-6427, 2009.
173. Shigeoka AO, Charette RP, Wyman ML, et al: Defective oxidative metabolic responses of neutrophils from stressed infants, *J Pediatr* 98:392-398, 1981.
174. Strauss RG, Snyder EL: Activation and activity of the superoxide-generating system of neutrophils from human infants, *Pediatr Res* 17:662-664, 1983.
175. Gessler P, Nebe T, Birle A, et al: Neutrophil respiratory burst in term and preterm neonates without signs of infection and in those with increased levels of C-reactive protein, *Pediatr Res* 39:843-848, 1996.
176. Bjorkqvist M, Jurstrand M, Bodin L, et al: Defective neutrophil oxidative burst in preterm newborns on exposure to coagulase-negative staphylococci, *Pediatr Res* 55:966-971, 2004.
177. Herman TE, Siegel MJ: Chronic granulomatous disease of childhood: Neonatal serratia, hepatic abscesses, and pulmonary aspergillosis, *J Perinatol* 22:255-256, 2002.
178. Banffer JRJ, Franken JF: Immunization with leucocidin toxoid against staphylococcal infection, *Pathol Microbiol (Basel)* 30:166-174, 1967.
179. Lack CH, Towers AG: Serological tests for staphylococcal infection, *Br Med J* 2:1227-1231, 1962.
180. Florman AL, Lamberston GH, Zepp H, et al: Relation of 7S and 19S staphylococcal hemagglutinating antibody to age of individual, *Pediatrics* 32:501, 1963.
181. Lavoipierre GJ, Newell KW, Smith MHD, et al: A vaccine trial for neonatal staphylococcal disease, *Am J Dis Child* 122:377-385, 1971.
182. Peoples JD, Cheung S, Nesin M, et al: Neonatal cord blood subsets and cytokine response to bacterial antigens, *Am J Perinatol* 26:647-657, 2009.
183. Tatad AM, Nesin M, Peoples J, et al: Cytokine expression in response to bacterial antigens in preterm and term infant cord blood monocytes, *Neonatology* 94:8 15, 2008.
184. Strunk T, Prosser A, Levy O, et al: Responsiveness of human monocytes to the commensal bacterium *Staphylococcus epidermidis* develops late in gestation, *Pediatr Res* 72:10-18, 2012.
185. McLoughlin RM, Solinga RM, Rich J, et al: CD4+ T cells and CXC chemokines modulate the pathogenesis of *Staphylococcus aureus* wound infections, *Proc Natl Acad Sci U S A* 103:10408-10413, 2006.
186. Marrach P, Kappler J: The staphylococcal enterotoxin and their relatives, *Science* 248:705-711, 1990.
187. Eichenwald HF, Shinefield HR: The problem of staphylococcal infection in newborn infants, *J Pediatr* 56:665-674, 1960.
188. Sohn AH, Garrett DO, Sinkowitz-Cochran RL, et al: Prevalence of nosocomial infections in neonatal intensive care unit patients: results from the first national point-prevalence survey, *J Pediatr* 139:821-827, 2001.
189. Isaacs D, Fraser S, Hogg G, et al: *Staphylococcus aureus* infections in Australasian neonatal nurseries, *Arch Dis Child Fetal Neonatal Ed* 89:F331-F335, 2004.

190. Chapman RL, Faix RG: Persistent bacteremia and outcome in late-onset infection among infants in a neonatal intensive care unit, *Pediatr Infect Dis J* 22:17-21, 2003.
191. Benjamin DK, DeLong E, Cotten CM, et al: Mortality following blood culture in premature infants: increased with gram-negative bacteremia and candidemia, but not gram-positive bacteremia, *J Perinatol* 24:175-180, 2004.
192. Ronnestad A, Abrahamsen TG, Medbo S, et al: Septicemia in the first week of life in a Norwegian national cohort of extremely premature infants, *Pediatrics* 115:e262-e268, 2005.
193. Stoll BJ, Hansen NI, Higgins RD, et al: Very low birth weight preterm infants with early onset neonatal sepsis: the predominance of gram-negative infections continues in the National Institute of Child Health and Human Development Neonatal Research Network, 2002-2003, *Pediatr Infect Dis J* 24:635-639, 2005.
194. Regev-Yochay G, Rubinstein E, Barzilai A, et al: Methicillin-resistant *Staphylococcus aureus* in neonatal intensive care unit, *Emerg Infect Dis* 11:453-456, 2005.
195. Huang YC, Chou YH, Su LH, et al: Methicillin-resistant s *Staphylococcus aureus* colonization and its association with infection among infants hospitalized in neonatal intensive care units, *Pediatrics* 118:469-474, 2006.
196. Khashu M, Osiovich H, Henry D, et al: Persistent bacteremia and severe thrombocytopenia caused by coagulase-negative *Staphylococcus* in a neonatal intensive care unit, *Pediatrics* 117:340-348, 2006.
197. Gomez-Gonzalez C, Alba C, Otero JR, et al: Long persistence of methicillin-susceptible strains of *Staphylococcus aureus* causing sepsis in a neonatal intensive care unit, *J Clin Microbiol* 45:2301-2304, 2007.
198. Kuint J, Barzilai A, Regev-Yochay G, et al: Comparison of community-acquired methicillin-resistant *Staphylococcus aureus* bacteremia to other staphylococcal species in a neonatal intensive care unit, *Eur J Pediatr* 166:319-325, 2007.
199. Hira V, Sluijter M, Estevao S, et al: Clinical and molecular epidemiologic characteristics of coagulase-negative staphylococcal bloodstream infections in intensive care neonates, *Pediatr Infect Dis J* 26:607-612, 2007.
200. Seybold U, Halvosa JS, White N, et al: Emergence of and risk factors for methicillin-resistant *Staphylococcus aureus* of community origin in intensive care nurseries, *Pediatrics* 122:1039-1046, 2008.
201. Carey AJ, Saiman L, Polin RA: Hospital-acquired infections in the NICU: epidemiology for the new millennium, *Clin Perinatol* 35:223-249, 2008.
202. Healy CM, Palazzi DL, Edwards MS, et al: Features of invasive staphylococcal disease in neonates, *Pediatrics* 114:953-961, 2004.
203. Healy CM, Baker CJ, Palazzi DL, et al: Distinguishing true coagulase-negative *Staphylococcus* infections from contaminants in the neonatal intensive care unit, *J Perinatol* 33:52-58, 2013.
204. Healy CM, Hulten KG, Palazzi DL, et al: Emergence of new strains of methicillin-resistant *Staphylococcus aureus* in a neonatal intensive care unit, *Clin Infect Dis* 39:1460-1466, 2004.
205. Chuang YY, Huang YC, Lee CY, et al: Methicillin-resistant *Staphylococcus aureus* bacteraemia in neonatal intensive care units: an analysis of 90 episodes, *Acta Paediatr* 93:786-790, 2004.
206. Cohen-Wolkowiez M, Benjamin DK Jr, Fowler VG Jr, et al: Mortality and neurodevelopmental outcome after *Staphylococcus aureus* bacteremia in infants, *Pediatr Infect Dis J* 26:1159-1161, 2007.
207. Sanghvi KP, Tudehope DI: Neonatal bacterial sepsis in a neonatal intensive care unit: a 5 year analysis, *J Paediatr Child Health* 32:333-338, 1996.
208. Beck-Sague CM, Azimi P, Fonseca SN, et al: Bloodstream infections in neonatal intensive care unit patients: results of a multicenter study, *Pediatr Infect Dis J* 13:1110-1116, 1994.
209. Isaacs D: A ten year, multicentre study of coagulase negative staphylococcal infections in Australasian neonatal units, *Arch Dis Child Fetal Neonatal Ed* 88:F89-F93, 2003.
210. Edwards JR, Peterson KD, Andrus ML, et al: National healthcare safety network (NHSN) report, data summary for 2006 through 2007, issued November 2008, *Am J Infect Control* 36:609-626, 2008.
211. Kilbride HW, Powers R, Wirtschafter DD, et al: Evaluation and development of potentially better practices to prevent neonatal nosocomial bacteremia, *Pediatrics* 111:e504-e518, 2003.
212. Makhoul IR, Sujov P, Smolkin T, et al: Pathogen-specific early mortality in very low birth weight infants with late-onset sepsis: a national survey, *Clin Infect Dis* 40:218-224, 2005.
213. Karlowicz MG, Furigay PJ, Croitoru DP, et al: Central venous catheter removal versus *in situ* treatment in neonates with coagulase-negative staphylococcal bacteremia, *Pediatr Infect Dis J* 21:22-27, 2002.
214. Benjamin DK Jr, Miller W, Garges H, et al: Bacteremia, central catheters, and neonates: when to pull the line, *Pediatrics* 107:1272-1276, 2001.
215. Lawrence SL, Roth V, Slinger R, et al: Cloxacillin versus vancomycin for presumed late-onset sepsis in the neonatal intensive care unit and the impact upon outcome of coagulase negative staphylococcal bacteremia: a retrospective cohort study, *BMC Pediatr* 5:49, 2005.
216. Powell C, Bubb S, Clark J: Toxic shock syndrome in a neonate, *Pediatr Infect Dis J* 26:759-760, 2007.
217. Takahashi N, Uehara R, Nishida H, et al: Clinical features of neonatal toxic shock syndrome-like exanthematous disease emerging in Japan, *J Infect* 59:194-200, 2009.
218. Schlievert PM: Alteration of immune function by staphylococcal pyrogenic exotoxin type C: possible role in toxic-shock syndrome, *J Infect Dis* 147:391-398, 1983.
219. Schlievert PM: Staphylococcal enterotoxin B and toxic-shock syndrome toxin-1 are significantly associated with non-menstrual TSS, *Lancet* 1:1149-1150, 1986.
220. Takahashi N, Kato H, Imanishi K, et al: Immunopathophysiological aspects of an emerging neonatal infectious disease induced by a bacterial superantigen, *J Clin Invest* 106:1409-1415, 2000.
221. Kikuchi K, Takahashi N, Piao C, et al: Molecular epidemiology of methicillin-resistant *Staphylococcus aureus* strains causing neonatal toxic shock syndrome-like exanthematous disease in neonatal and perinatal wards, *J Clin Microbiol* 41:3001-3006, 2003.
222. Takahashi N, Nishida H, Kato H, et al: Exanthematous disease induced by toxic shock syndrome toxin 1 in the early neonatal period, *Lancet* 351:1614-1619, 1998.
223. Symchych PS, Krauss AN, Winchester P: Endocarditis following intracardiac placement of umbilical venous catheters in neonates, *J Pediatr* 90:287-289, 1977.
224. Johnson DH, Rosenthal A, Nadas AS: A forty-year review of bacterial endocarditis in infancy and childhood, *Circulation* 51:581-588, 1975.
225. Millard DD, Shulman ST: The changing spectrum of neonatal endocarditis, *Clin Perinatol* 15:587-608, 1988.
226. Mecrow IK, Ladusans EJ: Infective endocarditis in newborn infants with structurally normal hearts, *Acta Paediatr* 83:35-39, 1994.
227. Daher AH, Berkowitz FE: Infective endocarditis in neonates, *Clin Pediatr (Phila)* 34:198-206, 1995.
228. Pearlman SA, Higgins S, Eppes S, et al: Infective endocarditis in the premature neonate, *Clin Pediatr (Phila)* 37:741-746, 1998.
229. Opie GF, Fraser SH, Drew JH, et al: Bacterial endocarditis in neonatal intensive care, *J Paediatr Child Health* 35:545-548, 1999.
230. Valente AM, Jain R, Scheurer M, et al: Frequency of infective endocarditis among infants and children with *Staphylococcus aureus* bacteremia, *Pediatrics* 115:e15-e19, 2005.
231. Milazzo AS Jr, Li JS: Bacterial endocarditis in infants and children, *Pediatr Infect Dis J* 20:799-801, 2001.
232. O'Callaghan C, McDougall P: Infective endocarditis in neonates, *Arch Dis Child* 63:53-57, 1988.
233. Armstrong D, Battin MR, Knight D, et al: *Staphylococcus aureus* endocarditis in preterm neonates, *Am J Perinatol* 19:247-251, 2002.
234. Sung TJ, Kim HM, Kim MJ: Methicillin-resistant *Staphylococcus aureus* endocarditis in an extremely low-birth-weight infant treated with linezolid, *Clin Pediatr (Phila)* 47:504-506, 2008.
235. Linder N, Hernandez A, Amit L, et al: Persistent coagulase-negative staphylococci bacteremia in very-low-birth-weight infants, *Eur J Pediatr* 170:989-995, 2011.
236. Fortunov RM, Hulten KG, Hammerman WA, et al: Community-acquired *Staphylococcus aureus* infections in term and near-term previously healthy neonates, *Pediatrics* 118:874-881, 2006.
237. Fortunov RM, Hulten KG, Hammerman WA, et al: Evaluation and treatment of community-acquired *Staphylococcus aureus* infections in term and late-preterm previously healthy neonates, *Pediatrics* 120:937-945, 2007.
238. James L, Gorwitz RJ, Jones RC, et al: Methicillin-resistant *Staphylococcus aureus* infections among healthy full-term newborns, *Arch Dis Child Fetal Neonatal Ed* 93:F40-F44, 2008.
239. Nguyen DM, Bancroft E, Mascola L, et al: Risk factors for neonatal methicillin-resistant *Staphylococcus aureus* infection in a well-infant nursery, *Infect Control Hosp Epidemiol* 28:406-411, 2007.

240. Mogre DA: Generalised staphylococcal pustulosis in a neonate: a case report, *Australas Med J* 6:532-535, 2013.
241. Kim YH, Chang SS, Kim YS, et al: Clinical outcomes in methicillin-resistant *Staphylococcus aureus*-colonized neonates in the neonatal intensive care unit, *Neonatology* 91:241-247, 2007.
242. Ayliffe GA, Brightwell KM, Ball PM, et al: Staphylococcal infection in cervical glands of infants, *Lancet* 2:479-480, 1972.
243. Dewar J, Porter IA, Smylie GH: Staphylococcal infection in cervical glands of infants, *Lancet* 2:712, 1972.
244. Falup-Pecurariu O, Leibovitz E, Pascu C, et al: Bacteremic methicillin-resistant *Staphylococcus aureus* deep neck abscess in a newborn—case report and review of literature, *Int J Pediatr Otorhinolaryngol* 73:1824-1827, 2009.
245. Mutlu M, Dereci S, Aslan Y: Deep neck abscess in neonatal period: case report and review of literature, *Int J Pediatr Otorhinolaryngol* 78:577-582, 2014.
246. Sabatino G, Verrotti A, de Martino M, et al: Neonatal suppurative parotitis: a study of five cases, *Eur J Pediatr* 158:312-314, 1999.
247. Ismail EA, Seoudi TM, Al-Amir M, et al: Neonatal suppurative parotitis over the last 4 decades: report of three new cases and review, *Pediatr Int* 55:60-64, 2013.
248. Spiegel R, Miron D, Sakran W, et al: Acute neonatal suppurative parotitis: case reports and review, *Pediatr Infect Dis J* 23:76-78, 2004.
249. Raad II , Sabbagh MF, Caranasos GJ: Acute bacterial sialadenitis: a study of 29 cases and review, *Rev Infect Dis* 12:591-601, 1990.
250. David RB, O'Connel EJ: Suppurative parotitis in children, *Am J Dis Child* 119:332, 1970.
251. Rudoy RC, Nelson JD: Breast abscess during the neonatal period. A review, *Am J Dis Child* 129:1031-1034, 1975.
252. Kalwbow H: Über mastitis neonatorum und ihre folgen, *Zentralbl Gynakol* 60:1821, 1936.
253. Bodemer C, Panhans A, Chretien-Marquet B, et al: Staphylococcal necrotizing fasciitis in the mammary region in childhood: a report of five cases, *J Pediatr* 131:466-469, 1997.
254. Sawardekar KP: Changing spectrum of neonatal omphalitis, *Pediatr Infect Dis J* 23:22-26, 2004.
255. Mason WH, Andrews R, Ross LA, et al: Omphalitis in the newborn infant, *Pediatr Infect Dis J* 8:521-525, 1989.
256. Lally KP, Atkinson JB, Woolley MM, et al: Necrotizing fasciitis. A serious sequela of omphalitis in the newborn, *Ann Surg* 199:101-103, 1984.
257. Samuel M, Freeman NV, Vaishnav A, et al: Necrotizing fasciitis: a serious complication of omphalitis in neonates, *J Pediatr Surg* 29:1414-1416, 1994.
258. Hsieh WS, Yang PH, Chao HC, et al: Neonatal necrotizing fasciitis: a report of three cases and review of the literature, *Pediatrics* 103:e53, 1999.
259. Dehority W, Wang E, Vernon PS, et al: Community-associated methicillin-resistant *Staphylococcus aureus* necrotizing fasciitis in a neonate, *Pediatr Infect Dis J* 25:1080-1081, 2006.
260. Hayani KC, Mathew R, Oyedele T, et al: Neonatal necrotizing fasciitis due to community-acquired methicillin resistant *Staphylococcus aureus*, *Pediatr Infect Dis J* 27:480-481, 2008.
261. Yu JS, Habib P: MR imaging of urgent inflammatory and infectious conditions affecting the soft tissues of the musculoskeletal system, *Emerg Radiol* 16:267-276, 2009.
262. Edlich RF, Cross CL, Dahlstrom JJ, et al: Modern concepts of the diagnosis and treatment of necrotizing fasciitis, *J Emerg Med* 39:261-265, 2010.
263. Brown DR, Davis NL, Lepawsky M, et al: A multicenter review of the treatment of major truncal necrotizing infections with and without hyperbaric oxygen therapy, *Am J Surg* 167:485-489, 1994.
264. Kapoor V, Travadi J, Braye S: Staphylococcal scalded skin syndrome in an extremely premature neonate: a case report with a brief review of literature, *J Paediatr Child Health* 44:374-376, 2008.
265. Makhoul IR, Kassis I, Hashman N, et al: Staphylococcal scalded-skin syndrome in a very low birth weight premature infant, *Pediatrics* 108:E16, 2001.
266. Peters B, Hentschel J, Mau H, et al: Staphylococcal scalded-skin syndrome complicating wound infection in a preterm infant with postoperative chylothorax, *J Clin Microbiol* 36:3057-3059, 1998.
267. Rieger-Fackeldey E, Plano LR, Kramer A, et al: Staphylococcal scalded skin syndrome related to an exfoliative toxin A- and B-producing strain in preterm infants, *Eur J Pediatr* 161:649-652, 2002.
268. Curran JP, Al-Salihi FL: Neonatal staphylococcal scalded skin syndrome: massive outbreak due to an unusual phage type, *Pediatrics* 66:285-290, 1980.
269. Ritter von Rittershain G: Die exfoliative dermatitis jüngerer säuglinge, *Zentralztg Kinderheilkd* 2:3-23, 1878.
270. Melish ME, Glasgow LA: Staphylococcal scalded skin syndrome: the expanded clinical syndrome, *J Pediatr* 78:958-967, 1971.
271. Farrell AM: Staphylococcal scalded-skin syndrome, *Lancet* 354:880-881, 1999.
272. Li MY, Hua Y, Wei GH, et al: Staphylococcal scalded skin syndrome in neonates: an 8-year retrospective study in a single institution, *Pediatr Dermatol* 31:43-47, 2014.
273. Farroha A, Frew Q, Jabir S, et al: Staphylococcal scalded skin syndrome due to burn wound infection, *Ann Burns Fire Disasters* 25:140-142, 2012.
274. Hoffmann R, Lohner M, Bohm N, et al: Staphylococcal scalded skin syndrome (SSSS) and consecutive septicaemia in a preterm infant, *Pathol Res Pract* 190:77-81, 1994; discussion 81-73.
275. Lo WT, Wang CC, Chu ML: Intrauterine staphylococcal scalded skin syndrome: report of a case, *Pediatr Infect Dis J* 19:481-482, 2000.
276. Loughead JL: Congenital staphylococcal scaled skin syndrome: report of a case, *Pediatr Infect Dis J* 11:413-414, 1992.
277. Haveman LM, Fleer A, de Vries LS, et al: Congenital staphylococcal scalded skin syndrome in a premature infant, *Acta Paediatr* 93:1661-1662, 2004.
278. Dancer SJ, Simmons NA, Poston SM, et al: Outbreak of staphylococcal scalded skin syndrome among neonates, *J Infect* 16:87-103, 1988.
279. Beaven DW, Burry AF: Staphylococcal pneumonia in the newborn; an epidemic with 8 fatal cases, *Lancet* 271:211-215, 1956.
280. Shinefield HR, Ruff NL: Staphylococcal infections: a historical perspective, *Infect Dis Clin North Am* 23:1-15, 2009.
281. Yee-Guardino S, Kumar D, Abughali N, et al: Recognition and treatment of neonatal community-associated MRSA pneumonia and bacteremia, *Pediatr Pulmonol* 43:203-205, 2008.
282. Rougemont AL, Buteau C, Ovetchkine P, et al: Fatal cases of *Staphylococcus aureus* pleural empyema in infants, *Pediatr Dev Pathol* 12:390-393, 2009.
283. Drinkovic D, Pottumarthy S, Knight D, et al: Neonatal coagulase-negative staphylococcal meningitis: a report of two cases, *Pathology* 34:586-588, 2002.
284. Bauer F, Huttova M, Rudinsky B, et al: Nosocomial meningitis caused by *Staphylococcus* other than *S. aureus* in children: multicentre study, *Neuro Endocrinol Lett* 28(Suppl 2):34-35, 2007.
285. de Oliveira RS, Pinho VF, Madureira JF, et al: Brain abscess in a neonate: an unusual presentation, *Childs Nerv Syst* 23:139-142, 2007.
286. Regev RH, Dolfin TZ, Zamir C: Multiple brain abscesses in a premature infant: complication of *Staphylococcus aureus* sepsis, *Acta Paediatr* 84:585-587, 1995.
287. Vartzelis G, Theodoridou M, Daikos GL, et al: Brain abscesses complicating *Staphylococcus aureus* sepsis in a premature infant, *Infection* 33:36-38, 2005.
288. Arora P, Kalra VK, Pappas A: Multiple brain abscesses in a neonate after blood stream infection with methicillin-resistant *Staphylococcus aureus*, *J Pediatr* 161:563-563.e1 2012.
289. Vinchon M, Dhellemmes P: Cerebrospinal fluid shunt infection: risk factors and long-term follow-up, *Childs Nerv Syst* 22:692-697, 2006.
290. Reinprecht A, Dietrich W, Berger A, et al: Posthemorrhagic hydrocephalus in preterm infants: long-term follow-up and shunt-related complications, *Childs Nerv Syst* 17:663-669, 2001.
291. Anderson EJ, Yogev R: A rational approach to the management of ventricular shunt infections, *Pediatr Infect Dis J* 24:557-558, 2005.
292. Sciubba DM, Noggle JC, Carson BS, et al: Antibiotic-impregnated shunt catheters for the treatment of infantile hydrocephalus, *Pediatr Neurosurg* 44:91-96, 2008.
293. Filka J, Huttova M, Tuharsky J, et al: Nosocomial meningitis in children after ventriculoperitoneal shunt insertion, *Acta Paediatr* 88:576-578, 1999.
294. James HE, Bradley JS: Aggressive management of shunt infection: combined intravenous and intraventricular antibiotic therapy for twelve or less days, *Pediatr Neurosurg* 44:104-111, 2008.
295. Nava-Ocampo AA, Mojica-Madera JA, Villanueva-Garcia D, et al: Antimicrobial therapy and local toxicity of intraventricular administration of vancomycin in a neonate with ventriculitis, *Ther Drug Monit* 28:474-476, 2006.

296. Cook AM, Ramsey CN, Martin CA, et al: Linezolid for the treatment of a heteroresistant *Staphylococcus aureus* shunt infection, *Pediatr Neurosurg* 41:102-104, 2005.
297. Potter CM: Osteomyelitis in the newborn, *J Bone Joint Surg Br* 36-B:578-583, 1954.
298. Walsh SZ, Craig JD: Generalized osteomyelitis in a newborn infant, *J Pediatr* 52:313-318, 1958.
299. Bergdahl S, Ekengren K, Eriksson M: Neonatal hematogenous osteomyelitis: risk factors for long-term sequelae, *J Pediatr Orthop* 5:564-568, 1985.
300. Frederiksen B, Christiansen P, Knudsen FU: Acute osteomyelitis and septic arthritis in the neonate, risk factors and outcome, *Eur J Pediatr* 152:577-580, 1993.
301. Williamson JB, Galasko CS, Robinson MJ: Outcome after acute osteomyelitis in preterm infants, *Arch Dis Child* 65:1060-1062, 1990.
302. Wong M, Isaacs D, Howman-Giles R, et al: Clinical and diagnostic features of osteomyelitis occurring in the first three months of life, *Pediatr Infect Dis J* 14:1047-1053, 1995.
303. Ogden JA: Pediatric osteomyelitis and septic arthritis: the pathology of neonatal disease, *Yale J Biol Med* 52:423-448, 1979.
304. Ogden JA, Lister G: The pathology of neonatal osteomyelitis, *Pediatrics* 55:474-478, 1975.
305. Offiah AC: Acute osteomyelitis, septic arthritis and discitis: differences between neonates and older children, *Eur J Radiol* 60:221-232, 2006.
306. Korakaki E, Aligizakis A, Manoura A, et al: Methicillin-resistant *Staphylococcus aureus* osteomyelitis and septic arthritis in neonates: diagnosis and management, *Jpn J Infect Dis* 60:129-131, 2007.
307. Waseem M, Devas G, Laureta E: A neonate with asymmetric arm movements, *Pediatr Emerg Care* 25:98-99, 2009.
308. Parmar J: Case report: septic arthritis of the temporomandibular joint in a neonate, *Br J Oral Maxillofac Surg* 46:505-506, 2008.
309. Lim MO, Gresham EL, Franken EA Jr, et al: Osteomyelitis as a complication of umbilical artery catheterization, *Am J Dis Child* 131:142-144, 1977.
310. Lilien LD, Harris VJ, Ramamurthy RS, et al: Neonatal osteomyelitis of the calcaneus: complication of heel puncture, *J Pediatr* 88:478-480, 1976.
311. Yuksel S, Yuksel G, Oncel S, et al: Osteomyelitis of the calcaneus in the newborn: an ongoing complication of guthrie test, *Eur J Pediatr* 166:503-504, 2007.
312. Overturf GD, Balfour G: Osteomyelitis and sepsis: severe complications of fetal monitoring, *Pediatrics* 55:244-247, 1975.
313. Asnes RS, Arendar GM: Septic arthritis of the hip: a complication of femoral venipuncture, *Pediatrics* 38:837-841, 1966.
314. Barrie D: Staphylococcal colonization of the rectum in the newborn, *Br Med J* 1:1574-1576, 1966.
315. Ottenheimer EJ, Minchew IBH, Cohen LS, et al: Studies of the epidemiology of staphylococcal infection, *Bull Johns Hopkins Hosp* 109:114, 1961.
316. Madan JC, Salari RC, Saxena D, et al: Gut microbial colonisation in premature neonates predicts neonatal sepsis, *Arch Dis Child Fetal Neonatal Ed* 97:F456-F462, 2012.
317. Soeorg H, Huik K, Parm U, et al: Genetic relatedness of coagulase-negative staphylococci from gastrointestinal tract and blood of preterm neonates with late-onset sepsis, *Pediatr Infect Dis J* 32:389-393, 2013.
318. Christie CD, Lynch-Ballard E, Andiman WA: Staphylococcal enterocolitis revisited: cytotoxic properties of *Staphylococcus aureus* from a neonate with enterocolitis, *Pediatr Infect Dis J* 7:791-795, 1988.
319. Gutman LT, Idriss ZH, Gehlbach S, et al: Neonatal staphylococcal enterocolitis: association with indwelling feeding catheters and *S. aureus* colonization, *J Pediatr* 88:836-839, 1976.
320. Masunaga K, Mazaki R, Endo A, et al: Colonic stenosis after severe methicillin-resistant *Staphylococcus aureus* enterocolitis in a newborn, *Pediatr Infect Dis J* 18:169-171, 1999.
321. Scheifele DW, Bjornson GL, Dyer RA, et al: Delta-like toxin produced by coagulase-negative staphylococci is associated with neonatal necrotizing enterocolitis, *Infect Immun* 55:2268-2273, 1987.
322. Overturf GD, Sherman MP, Scheifele DW, et al: Neonatal necrotizing enterocolitis associated with delta toxin-producing methicillin-resistant *Staphylococcus aureus*, *Pediatr Infect Dis J* 9:88-91, 1990.
323. Mehr S, Doyle LW: Cytokines as markers of bacterial sepsis in newborn infants: a review, *Pediatr Infect Dis J* 19:879-887, 2000.
324. Mishra UK, Jacobs SE, Doyle LW, et al: Newer approaches to the diagnosis of early onset neonatal sepsis, *Arch Dis Child Fetal Neonatal Ed* 91:F208-F212, 2006.
325. Makhoul IR, Yacoub A, Smolkin T, et al: Values of C-reactive protein, procalcitonin, and *Staphylococcus*-specific PCR in neonatal late-onset sepsis, *Acta Paediatr* 95:1218-1223, 2006.
326. Vazzalwar R, Pina-Rodrigues E, Puppala BL, et al: Procalcitonin as a screening test for late-onset sepsis in preterm very low birth weight infants, *J Perinatol* 25:397-402, 2005.
327. Sherwin C, Broadbent R, Young S, et al: Utility of interleukin-12 and interleukin-10 in comparison with other cytokines and acute-phase reactants in the diagnosis of neonatal sepsis, *Am J Perinatol* 25:629-636, 2008.
328. Harris MC, D'Angio CT, Gallagher PR, et al: Cytokine elaboration in critically ill infants with bacterial sepsis, necrotizing enterocolitis, or sepsis syndrome: correlation with clinical parameters of inflammation and mortality, *J Pediatr* 147:462-468, 2005.
329. Lam HS, Ng PC: Biochemical markers of neonatal sepsis, *Pathology* 40:141-148, 2008.
330. Lopez Sastre JB, Perez Solis D, Roques Serradilla V, et al: Procalcitonin is not sufficiently reliable to be the sole marker of neonatal sepsis of nosocomial origin, *BMC Pediatr* 6:16, 2006.
331. Patrick CC, Kaplan SL, Baker CJ, et al: Persistent bacteremia due to coagulase-negative staphylococci in low birthweight neonates, *Pediatrics* 84:977-985, 1989.
332. Baumgart S, Hall SE, Campos JM, et al: Sepsis with coagulase-negative staphylococci in critically ill newborns, *Am J Dis Child* 137:461-463, 1983.
333. Schmidt BK, Kirpalani HM, Corey M, et al: Coagulase-negative staphylococci as true pathogens in newborn infants: a cohort study, *Pediatr Infect Dis J* 6:1026-1031, 1987.
334. Ohlin A, Backman A, Bjorkqvist M, et al: Real-time PCR of the 16S-rRNA gene in the diagnosis of neonatal bacteraemia, *Acta Paediatr* 97:1376-1380, 2008.
335. Bradley JS: Which antibiotic for resistant gram-positives, and why? *J Infect* 68(Suppl 1):S63-S75, 2014.
336. Capparelli EV, Lane JR, Romanowski GL, et al: The influences of renal function and maturation on vancomycin elimination in newborns and infants, *J Clin Pharmacol* 41:927-934, 2001.
337. Reiter PD, Doron MW: Vancomycin cerebrospinal fluid concentrations after intravenous administration in premature infants, *J Perinatol* 16:331-335, 1996.
338. de Hoog M, Mouton JW, van den Anker JN: Vancomycin: pharmacokinetics and administration regimens in neonates, *Clin Pharmacokinet* 43:417-440, 2004.
339. Rodvold KA, Everett JA, Pryka RD, et al: Pharmacokinetics and administration regimens of vancomycin in neonates, infants and children, *Clin Pharmacokinet* 33:32-51, 1997.
340. Plan O, Cambonie G, Barbotte E, et al: Continuous-infusion vancomycin therapy for preterm neonates with suspected or documented gram-positive infections: a new dosage schedule, *Arch Dis Child Fetal Neonatal Ed* 93:F418-F421, 2008.
341. Sanchez P, Bradley JS, Nelson JD: Antiinfective therapy for newborns. In Bradley JS, Nelson JD, editors: *Nelson's pocket book of pediatric antimicrobial therapy: 2008-2009*. Buenos Aires, Argentina, 2008, Alliance for World-Wide Editing, pp 16-29.
342. Jacqz-Aigrain E, Zhao W, Sharland M, et al: Use of antibacterial agents in the neonate: 50 years of experience with vancomycin administration, *Semin Fetal Neonatal Med* 18:28-34, 2013.
343. Le J, Bradley JS, Murray W, et al: Improved vancomycin dosing in children using area under the curve exposure, *Pediatr Infect Dis J* 32:e155-e163, 2013.
344. Le J, Ngu B, Bradley JS, et al: Vancomycin monitoring in children using Bayesian estimation, *Ther Drug Monit* 36:510-518, 2014.
345. Lozada LE, Royall MJ, Nylund CM, et al: Development of pyloric stenosis after a 4-day course of oral erythromycin, *Pediatr Emerg Care* 29:498-499, 2013.
346. Gostelow M, Gonzalez D, Smith PB, et al: Pharmacokinetics and safety of recently approved drugs used to treat methicillin-resistant *Staphylococcus aureus* infections in infants, children and adults, *Expert Rev Clin Pharmacol* 7:327-340, 2014.
347. Meka VG, Gold HS: Antimicrobial resistance to linezolid, *Clin Infect Dis* 39:1010-1015, 2004.
348. Dotis J, Iosifidis E, Ioannidou M, et al: Use of linezolid in pediatrics: a critical review, *Int J Infect Dis* 14:e638-e648, 2010.
349. Deville JG, Adler S, Azimi PH, et al: Linezolid versus vancomycin in the treatment of known or suspected resistant gram-positive infections in neonates, *Pediatr Infect Dis J* 22:S158-S163, 2003.

350. Jungbluth GL, Welshman IR, Hopkins NK: Linezolid pharmacokinetics in pediatric patients: an overview, *Pediatr Infect Dis J* 22:S153-S157, 2003.
351. Cohen-Wolkowiez M, Watt KM, Hornik CP, et al: Pharmacokinetics and tolerability of single-dose daptomycin in young infants, *Pediatr Infect Dis J* 31:935-937, 2012.
352. Baddour LM, Wilson WR, Bayer AS, et al: Infective endocarditis: diagnosis, antimicrobial therapy, and management of complications, *Circulation* 111:e394-e434, 2005.
353. Soraisham AS, Al-Hindi MY: Intravenous rifampicin for persistent staphylococcal bacteremia in premature infants, *Pediatr Int* 50:124-126, 2008.
354. Ohlsson A, Lacy JB: Intravenous immunoglobulin for suspected or subsequently proven infection in neonates, *Cochrane Database Syst Rev*: CD001239, 2004.
355. Milstone AM, Reich NG, Advani S, et al: Catheter dwell time and clabsis in neonates with PICCs: a multicenter cohort study, *Pediatrics* 132:e1609-e1615, 2013.
356. Andersen BM, Lindemann R, Bergh K, et al: Spread of methicillin-resistant *Staphylococcus aureus* in a neonatal intensive unit associated with understaffing, overcrowding and mixing of patients, *J Hosp Infect* 50:18-24, 2002.
357. Haley RW, Cushion NB, Tenover FC, et al: Eradication of endemic methicillin-resistant *Staphylococcus aureus* infections from a neonatal intensive care unit, *J Infect Dis* 171:614-624, 1995.
358. Rountree PM, Heseltine M, Rheuben J, et al: Control of staphylococcal infection of newborn by treatment of nasal carriers in staff, *Med J Aust* 1:528-532, 1956.
359. Gillespie WA, Adler VG: Control of an outbreak of staphylococcal infection in a hospital, *Lancet* 1:632-634, 1957.
360. Martin WJ, Nichols DR, Henderson ED: The problem of management of nasal carriers of staphylococci, *Proc Mayo Clinic* 35:282-292, 1960.
361. Williams JD, Waltho CA, Ayliffe GAJ, et al: Trials of five antibacterial creams in the control of nasal carriage of *Staphylococcus aureus*, *Lancet* 2:390-392, 1967.
362. Smith RT: The role of the chronic carrier in an epidemic of staphylococcal disease in a newborn nursery, *Am J Dis Child* 95:461-468, 1958.
363. Wysham DN, Mulhern ME, Navarre GC, et al: Staphylococcal infections in an obstetric unit: I. Epidemiologic studies of pyoderma neonatorum, *N Engl J Med* 257:295-303, 1957.
364. Belani A, Sherertz RJ, Sullivan ML, et al: Outbreak of staphylococcal infection in two hospital nurseries traced to a single nasal carrier, *Infect Control* 7:487-490, 1986.
365. Garner JS: Guideline for isolation precautions in hospitals. The hospital infection control practices advisory committee, *Infect Control Hosp Epidemiol* 17:53-80, 1996.
366. Jernigan JA, Titus MG, Groschel DH, et al: Effectiveness of contact isolation during a hospital outbreak of methicillin-resistant *Staphylococcus aureus*, *Am J Epidemiol* 143:496-504, 1996.
367. Gerber SI, Jones RC, Scott MV, et al: Management of outbreaks of methicillin-resistant *Staphylococcus aureus* infection in the neonatal intensive care unit: a consensus statement, *Infect Control Hosp Epidemiol* 27:139-145, 2006.
368. Bertin ML, Vinski J, Schmitt S, et al: Outbreak of methicillin-resistant *Staphylococcus aureus* colonization and infection in a neonatal intensive care unit epidemiologically linked to a healthcare worker with chronic otitis, *Infect Control Hosp Epidemiol* 27:581-585, 2006.
369. Otter JA, Klein JL, Watts TL, et al: Identification and control of an outbreak of ciprofloxacin-susceptible EMRSA-15 on a neonatal unit, *J Hosp Infect* 67:232-239, 2007.
370. McDonald JR, Carriker CM, Pien BC, et al: Methicillin-resistant *Staphylococcus aureus* outbreak in an intensive care nursery: potential for interinstitutional spread, *Pediatr Infect Dis J* 26:678-683, 2007.
371. Shinefield HR, Ribble JC, Boris M: Bacterial interference between strains of *Staphylococcus aureus*, 1960 to 1970, *Am J Dis Child* 121:148-152, 1971.
372. Light IJ, Sutherland JM, Schott JE: Control of a staphylococcal outbreak in a nursery—use of bacterial interference, *JAMA* 193:699-704, 1965.
373. Shinefield HR: Bacterial interference, *Ann N Y Acad Sci* 236:444-455, 1974.
374. Mortimer EA Jr, Lipsitz PJ, Wolinsky E, et al: Transmission of staphylococci between newborns: importance of the hands of personnel, *Am J Dis Child* 104:289-295, 1962.
375. Kretzer EK, Larson EL: Behavioral interventions to improve infection control practices, *Am J Infect Control* 26:245-253, 1998.
376. Tibballs J: Teaching hospital medical staff to handwash, *Med J Aust* 164:395-398, 1996.
377. Pittet D: Improving compliance with hand hygiene in hospitals, *Infect Control Hosp Epidemiol* 21:381-386, 2000.
378. Ehrenkranz NJ, Alfonso BC: Failure of bland soap handwash to prevent hand transfer of patient bacteria to urethral catheters, *Infect Control Hosp Epidemiol* 12:654-662, 1991.
379. Aly H, Herson V, Duncan A, et al: Is bloodstream infection preventable among premature infants? A tale of two cities, *Pediatrics* 115:1513-1518, 2005.
380. Durand M, Ramanathan R, Martinelli B, et al: Prospective evaluation of percutaneous central venous silastic catheters in newborn infants with birth weights of 510 to 3,920 grams, *Pediatrics* 78:245-250, 1986.
381. Lodha A, Furlan AD, Whyte H, et al: Prophylactic antibiotics in the prevention of catheter-associated bloodstream bacterial infection in preterm neonates: a systematic review, *J Perinatol* 28:526-533, 2008.
382. Spafford PS, Sinkin RA, Cox C, et al: Prevention of central venous catheter-related coagulase-negative staphylococcal sepsis in neonates, *J Pediatr* 125:259-263, 1994.
383. Cooke RW, Nycyk JA, Okuonghuae H, et al: Low-dose vancomycin prophylaxis reduces coagulase-negative staphylococcal bacteraemia in very low birthweight infants, *J Hosp Infect* 37:297-303, 1997.
384. Garland JS, Alex CP, Henrickson KJ, et al: A vancomycin-heparin lock solution for prevention of nosocomial bloodstream infection in critically ill neonates with peripherally inserted central venous catheters: a prospective, randomized trial, *Pediatrics* 116:e198-e205, 2005.
385. Jardine LA, Inglis GD, Davies MW: Prophylactic systemic antibiotics to reduce morbidity and mortality in neonates with central venous catheters, *Cochrane Database Syst Rev*: CD006179, 2008.
386. Ohlsson A, Lacy JB: Intravenous immunoglobulin for preventing infection in preterm and/or low birth weight infants, *Cochrane Database Syst Rev*: CD000361, 2013.
387. Benjamin DK, Schelonka R, White R, et al: A blinded, randomized, multicenter study of an intravenous *Staphylococcus aureus* immune globulin, *J Perinatol* 26:290-295, 2006.
388. DeJonge M, Burchfield D, Bloom B, et al: Clinical trial of safety and efficacy of INH-A21 for the prevention of nosocomial staphylococcal bloodstream infection in premature infants, *J Pediatr* 151:260-265, 2007.
389. de la Morena MT: Specific immune globulin therapy for prevention of nosocomial staphylococcal bloodstream infection in premature infants: not what we hoped for!, *J Pediatr* 151:232-234, 2007.
390. Weisman LE, Thackray HM, Cracia-Prats JA: Phase I/II double blind, placebo controlled, dose escalation, safety and pharmacokinetics study in very low birth weight neonates of BSYX-A110, an anti-staphylococcal monoclonal antibody for the prevention of staphylococcal bloodstream infections, *Antimicrob Agents Chemother* 53:2879-2886, 2009.
391. Shah PS, Kaufman DA: Antistaphylococcal immunoglobulins to prevent staphylococcal infection in very low birth weight infants, *Cochrane Database Syst Rev*: CD006449, 2009.
392. Orsi N: The antimicrobial activity of lactoferrin: current status and perspectives, *Biometals* 17:189-196, 2004.
393. Venkatesh MP, Rong L: Human recombinant lactoferrin acts synergistically with antimicrobials commonly used in neonatal practice against coagulase-negative staphylococci and *Candida albicans* causing neonatal sepsis, *J Med Microbiol* 57:1113-1121, 2008.
394. Manzoni P, Rinaldi M, Cattani S, et al: Bovine lactoferrin supplementation for prevention of late-onset sepsis in very low-birth-weight neonates: a randomized trial, *JAMA* 302:1421-1428, 2009.

15 Gonococcal Infections

JOANNE E. EMBREE

CHAPTER OUTLINE

Infections of the fetus and newborn infant caused by *Neisseria gonorrhoeae* are restricted primarily to mucosal surfaces of the newborn infant, although scalp abscess and systemic infections, including bacteremia, meningitis, and septic arthritis, can occasionally occur.[1,2] The most common condition related to infection by this organism during the neonatal period is ophthalmia neonatorum, or neonatal conjunctivitis. *N. gonorrhoeae* produces purulent conjunctivitis in the newborn, which may lead to blindness if untreated. Ophthalmia neonatorum is therefore the primary disease entity discussed in this chapter.

Ophthalmia neonatorum had been a well-recognized entity, affecting 1% to 15% of newborns, in Europe and North America when Hirschberg and Krause[3] first described neonatal infection caused by *N. gonorrhoeae* in an infant with purulent conjunctivitis in 1881. Shortly thereafter, the topical instillation of silver nitrate into the newborn's eyes immediately after birth dramatically reduced the incidence of this disease caused by *N. gonorrhoeae*.[4-6] Maternal systemic infection during pregnancy also is rare, and transplacental congenital infection of the fetus has not been described. Maternal genital mucosal infection may result in an ascending infection, however, with chorioamnionitis leading to premature rupture of the placental membranes and preterm delivery.[7] In developed countries, screening and treatment of pregnant women for gonococcal infections with tracing of named contacts, along with the use of neonatal ophthalmic prophylaxis, have substantially reduced the incidence of gonococcal ophthalmia neonatorum.[2] In developing countries, improvements in access to medical care and aggressive programs for prevention and treatment of sexually transmitted diseases (STDs) are additional relevant public health measures. In conjunction with prevention strategies for human immunodeficiency virus (HIV) infection and acquired immunodeficiency syndrome (AIDS), such programs have continued to reduce the incidence of gonococcal infection and its complications, such as ophthalmia neonatorum, in areas where these interventions have been introduced.[8] However, despite the overall decreasing prevalence of *N. gonorrhoeae* infection worldwide, gonococcal ophthalmia neonatorum remains a significant illness.

Epidemiology and Transmission

The incidence of neonatal gonococcal illness is related to the prevalence of *N. gonorrhoeae* colonization among women of childbearing age and to the rates of gonococcal acquisition during pregnancy. These numbers are quite variable worldwide. In general, when antibiotic treatment for gonorrhea became available in the mid-20th century, rates of infection among women decreased worldwide as these agents became more readily accessible and health care programs improved. However, with the emergence of chromosomal resistance to penicillin, the production of penicillinase by some strains, and the expansion of the AIDS epidemic in the 1990s, rates began to increase again. In response, efforts to control this infection, which some authorities had hoped could ultimately be eliminated by the middle of the 21st century, have needed to be strengthened.

The World Health Organization published estimates of the burden of gonorrheal disease in various regions at the end of the 20th century.[9] Although these estimates are useful in highlighting regions of high burden of disease, such as sub-Saharan Africa and South/Southeast Asia, with an estimated 17 million and 27 million infections, respectively, considerable variation within regions exists. This variation is clearly reflected in the differences seen in the reported cases of gonorrhea the United States in 2011, the most recent year for which this data has been compiled.[10] In the United States during that year, the prevalence was 104.1 per 100,000. Rates varied across the country, with Vermont having the lowest prevalence at 7.7 per 100,000 and the District of Columbia having the highest at 429.9 per 100,000. Overall, the prevalence among women was higher than men (108.9/100,000 vs. 98.7/100,000, respectively). The highest rates were seen among women 15 to 19 years of age (556.5/100,000) and 20-to 24-year-olds (584.2/100,000). Further significant differences are noted among specific populations. The United States has set a goal of reducing the national prevalence of gonorrhea to less than 19 cases per 100,000 among adults; however, that goal is unlikely to be met in the near future.

Canada has placed an emphasis on STD control also and has an exclusively publicly funded health care system that in theory reduces a number of health care access barriers. Gonorrhea prevalence rates have decreased from 1980, when the prevalence among women was 166/100,000 population.[11] The highest rates at that time were among women 15 to 19 years of age and 20 to 24 years of age, which were similar to the United States prevalence at 510 versus 598 per 100,000, respectively, in 2011. In 2008, the prevalence among women in Canada was approximately 34 per 100,000, which represents a significant increase from 1997, when rates were the lowest at 11 per 100,000. The increase has occurred primarily among women 15 to 19 years of age and 20 to 24 years of age; in these age groups, rates rose from 69 and 60 per 100,000, respectively, in 1997 to 186.6 and 166.3 per 100,000, respectively. Also, as in the United States, rates in Canada vary considerably among the different provinces and territories. In 1997, Canada set as its goal the elimination of endemic transmission of *N. gonorrhoeae* by 2010. Similar to the United States, Canada has not met its goals. The reasons for the rate increases in Canada and the failure to eliminate endemic transmission are complex, but a proportion of the increase is likely related to the almost universal change in diagnostic procedures in Canada from culture to nucleic acid–based testing, which includes the use of urine specimens. Nucleic acid–based testing is considerably more sensitive than culture, thereby increasing the number of infected individuals identified and is more acceptable to patients, thereby increasing the number of infected individuals who present for testing.

Factors that increase a pregnant woman's risk of acquiring *N. gonorrhoeae* infection are similar to the factors that increase the risk of acquisition of any other sexually transmitted infection. The prevalence of *N. gonorrhoeae* in the population or network in which a woman socializes and chooses her sexual partners determines the likelihood of exposure to this pathogen. Women who have multiple sexual partners or whose partners have multiple sexual contacts markedly increase their risk of exposure to *N. gonorrhoeae*. Women who do not use condoms or other barrier protection increase their risk of acquisition of *N. gonorrhoeae* infection on exposure to the organism. Women and their partners who do not have convenient access to medical care or who do not seek available care for diagnosis and treatment of STIs will have higher rates of infection. It is unknown whether women who are HIV positive have an increased risk of infection by *N. gonorrhoeae* on exposure to it. Factors that are markers for an increased likelihood of gonococcal infection among pregnant women include younger age, unmarried status, homelessness, problems with drug or alcohol abuse, prostitution, low-income professions, and, in the United States, being black. Gonococcal infections are diagnosed more frequently in the summer months in the United States, probably reflecting transient changes in social behavior during vacations.[12]

N. gonorrhoeae is primarily transmitted from the infected maternal cervix during vaginal delivery. It has been estimated that colonization and infection of the neonate occur in only one third of instances in which the mother is infected.[13] The infant's mucous membranes become colonized on swallowing contaminated fluid during labor and delivery. In instances of an ascending infection, the consequences include premature rupture of the membranes with early onset of labor with premature delivery or septic abortion.[7,14] This association was dramatically shown in one study in which premature rupture of membranes occurred in 6 (43%) of 14 women with untreated gonococcal infection during pregnancy, compared with 4 (3%) of 144 women whose infection had been appropriately treated.[14] Thus screening and treatment programs for gonococcal infections during pregnancy are appropriate to reduce the risk of adverse pregnancy outcomes related to maternal infection in addition to prevention of ophthalmia neonatorum.

Worldwide, there has been concern about the development and transmission of antibacterial resistance among isolates of *N. gonorrhoeae*. Newer testing protocols that involve nonculture techniques have made tracking the development of antibiotic resistance more difficult. Fortunately, in the United States, antibiotic resistance among gonococci has been monitored systematically since 1986 by using selected STD clinics through the Gonococcal Isolate Surveillance Project.[10] In 2011, 31.1% of gonococcal isolates in the United States were resistant to at least one antimicrobial agent; 11.8% were resistant to penicillin and 16.9% were resistant to tetracycline. Once the resistance rate to an antibiotic is 5% or more, the involved drug is not recommended for general use to treat gonococcal infections. As a result, in the United States penicillin is no longer recommended for primary therapy for gonococcal disease, and tetracycline ointment is not recommended for newborn ocular prophylaxis.[2]

Microbiology

N. gonorrhoeae is a gram-negative diplococcus. It uses glucose for growth but not maltose, sucrose, or lactose. This is one of the characteristics used to distinguish *N. gonorrhoeae* isolates from *Neisseria meningitidis* and other colonizing *Neisseria* species, such as *N. cinerea, N. flava, N. subflava, N. lactamica, N. mucosa*, and *N. sicca*. *N. gonorrhoeae* produces acid only when grown in glucose. In addition, the organism is oxidase positive, hydroxyprolyl aminopeptidase positive, nitrate negative, DNase negative, catalase positive, strongly superoxol positive, and colistin resistant.[15] *N. gonorrhoeae* is an obligate aerobe but lacks superoxide dismutase, which moderates the effects of oxygen radicals in most other aerobic bacteria. When grown in anaerobic conditions, virulent strains express a lipoprotein called Pan 1. Its function is unknown, but it elicits an immunoglobulin M (IgM) antibody response in acute infection.

When cultured in the laboratory, *N. gonorrhoeae* forms three different colony types. Pinpoint colonies, classified as P^+ and P^{++}, usually are seen only on primary isolation. These colony types are distinguished from the large granular colonies, classified as P^-, by the presence of pili, which are thin bacterial appendages on the cell surface that are involved in attachment to mammalian cells and which confer resistance to killing of the bacteria by neutrophils. *N. gonorrhoeae* has the genetic capacity to turn on and turn off pilus expression. With repeated subculturing at 37° C, the genes are no longer expressed, and the pili disappear, resulting in colonial-type changes. Associated with this change is a reduction in virulence. *N. gonorrhoeae* also may form colonies that are either opaque or clear. This characteristic is related to the expression of a specific surface protein called Opa. Clinical isolates from mucosal surfaces tend to express Opa and form opaque colonies, whereas gonococci isolated from systemic infections tend not to express Opa, and the colonies are more transparent on culture media.

Colonial morphology is of no use in differentiating gonococcal types or strains. Typing of gonococcal isolates for epidemiologic purposes has changed significantly over the past decade with the introduction of newer technologies. The older typing schemes using a combination of auxotyping (use of growth requirements) and serotyping of porins (proteins on the cell membrane that provide channels to allow substances into the bacterial cell) has been replaced with hybridization patterns of *porB* or DNA sequencing of *porB* (one of the genes that code for porins). Use of pulse-field gel electrophoresis of bacterial DNA and multilocus sequence typing are very helpful for epidemiologic studies.

Pathogenesis

To produce infection, *N. gonorrhoeae* first attaches to epithelial cells, penetrates, and then destroys the infected cells.[1,15] Attachment to epithelial cells is related to the presence of pili and Opa. Penetration of the gonococcus into cells occurs through either phagocytosis or endocytosis. Several bacteria usually are found within each infected cell, but whether this represents invasion of the cell by multiple organisms or growth and multiplication of organisms within the infected cell is unknown. Gonococci possess a cytotoxic lipopolysaccharide and produce proteases, phospholipases, and elastases that ultimately destroy the infected cells. Some strains of gonococci seem to be relatively less susceptible to phagocytosis and are thought to be more capable of causing disseminated infection. Gonococci are found in the subepithelial connective tissue very quickly after infection. This dissemination may be due to the disruption of the integrity of the epidermal surface with cell death, or the gonococci may migrate into this area by moving between cells. Epithelial cell death triggers a vigorous inflammatory response with the development of small abscesses below the mucosal surface and the production of pus. Initially, this is primarily due to neutrophils but is then replaced over time by macrophages and lymphocytes if the individual is not treated.

Human serum contains IgM antibody directed against lipopolysaccharide antigens on the gonococcus, which inhibits invasion. An IgG antibody directed against a surface protein antigen present on some gonococci (classified as serum-resistant gonococci) will block the bactericidal action of the antilipopolysaccharide IgM antibody.[16] These serum-resistant strains are the most common ones involved in systemic infections in adults and probably in neonates as well. Infants' sera, in which maternal IgM antibody is absent, do not show serum bactericidal activity against *N. gonorrhoeae*[17]; in theory, infants should be highly susceptible to invasive infection. Because such infection does not occur frequently, additional protective factors must function to prevent it.

N. gonorrhoeae produces an IgA1 protease, which inactivates secretory IgA by cleaving it at the hinge region. This inactivation facilitates mucosal colonization and probably plays a role in the poor mucosal protection seen against subsequent gonococcal reinfection. IgA1 protease is also a proinflammatory factor and can trigger the release of proinflammatory cytokines from human monocytic subpopulations and a dose-dependent T-helper type 1 T-cell response.[18] Although symptomatic gonococcal infection stimulates a brisk inflammatory response, it does not produce a significant immunologic response.[19] There is very little immunologic memory; as a result, recurrent infections occur easily on reexposure. In general, antibody responses are modest after initial infection, however, and no evidence of a boosting effect has been found when antibody levels are studied in response to subsequent infections.

Adults with mucosal gonococcal infections have a discernible decreased $CD4^+$ count, which recovers with treatment or clearance of the infection and has led to speculation that gonococci actually have a suppressive effect on the host immune response. In support of this theory, *N. gonorrhoeae* Opa proteins have shown to be able to bind carcinoembryonic antigen–related cell adhesion molecule 1, expressed by primary $CD4^+$ T lymphocytes, and to suppress their activation and proliferation.[20] This immunosuppressive effect may have significant consequences in populations with coexisting epidemics of gonorrhea and HIV/AIDS.

Because only approximately one third of neonates exposed to *N. gonorrhoeae* during vaginal delivery become colonized and infected, additional protective innate factors are in effect. Significant antibacterial polypeptide activity has been shown in human amniotic fluid and within the vernix caseosa.[21,22] The presence of numerous antibacterial polypeptides in the vernix may be important for surface defense against gonococcal infection, but specific studies have not yet been done.

As stated previously, antibiotic resistance in *N. gonorrhoeae* to penicillin, tetracycline, quinolones, cephalosporins, macrolides, and spectinomycin has become problematic in many regions.[2,10,11,23] Penicillin resistance can be a result either of alterations in the penicillin-binding proteins or changes in antibiotic efflux (which are encoded on the bacterial chromosome) or the production of a penicillinase. At present, chromosomally-mediated resistance is the predominant mechanism for penicillin resistance in North America. The alterations responsible for chromosomal resistance to penicillin include the *mtr* gene mutation, which increases efflux of antibiotics out of the bacterial cell and which affects several other antibiotics in addition to penicillin; the *penA* gene mutation, which alters the penicillin binding proteins; and the *penB* gene mutation, which affects the antibiotic transit through the bacterial membranes. *N. gonorrhoeae* can accumulate several mutations, resulting in resistance to multiple classes of antibiotics. Of recent concern has been the effect of these mutations (which may have been transferred to *N. gonorrhoeae* from nonpathogenic oral *Neisseria* on a DNA cassette that contained multiple *penA* mutations) on increasing the minimal inhibitory concentrations (MICs) of third-generation cephalosporins.[23] This has resulted in an increase of the recommended dosage of these antibiotics for treatment of gonococcal infections. Although not applicable to the pediatric population for systemic use, high levels of resistance rapidly developed for both tetracycline and quinolone classes of antibiotics and eliminated their potential for topical use to prevent infection.

Pathology

In most affected infants, gonococcal disease manifests as infection of mucosal membranes. The eye is most frequently involved, but funisitis and infant vaginitis, rhinitis, and urethritis also have been observed.[24-27] Primary mucosal infection by *N. gonorrhoeae* involves the columnar and transitional epithelia. When pharyngeal colonization is evaluated, it is found in 35% of ophthalmia neonatorum cases.[28] Systemic infection is rarely observed among neonates, but cases of meningitis and arthritis have been described[29-31] along with gonococcal scalp abscesses attributed to intrauterine fetal monitoring[32] and, in one instance, a gingival abscess.[33] One case of gonococcal ventriculitis has been reported in an infant who received a ventriculoamniotic shunt in utero.[34]

Clinical Manifestations

Ophthalmia neonatorum caused by *N. gonorrhoeae* is classically an acute purulent conjunctivitis that appears 2 to 5 days after birth. On occasion, the initial presentation is more subacute or the onset may be delayed beyond 5 days of life.[1] Infants who become infected in utero may have symptoms at or shortly after birth. Asymptomatic colonization has been documented.[35] Typically, early in the illness, tense edema of both lids develops, followed by profuse purulent conjunctival exudates (Fig. 15-1). If treatment is delayed, the infection progresses beyond the superficial epithelial layers of the eye to involve the subconjunctival connective tissue of the palpebral conjunctivae and the cornea. Infection of the cornea can lead to ulcerations, perforation, or rarely panophthalmitis, which may result in loss of the eye. Neonatal sepsis, arthritis, and skin abscesses caused by *N. gonorrhoeae* are not clinically distinguishable from conditions caused by other bacterial pathogens more commonly associated with these syndromes in this age group.

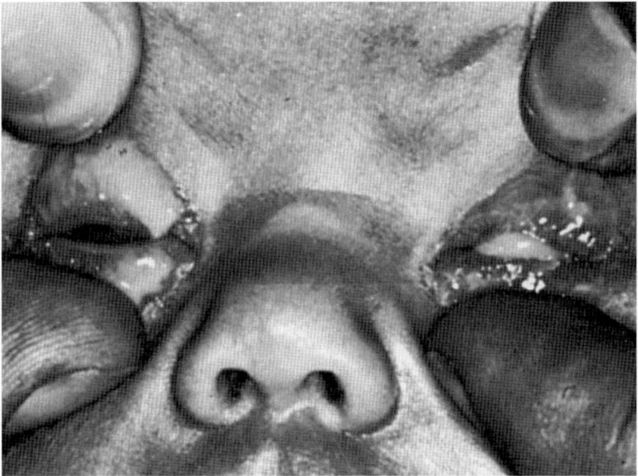

Figure 15-1 Bilateral acute gonococcal ophthalmia neonatorum. Appearance after inappropriate topical therapy for 2 weeks with neomycin-polymyxin B-bacitracin (Neosporin), sulfonamide, and chloramphenicol ophthalmic ointments.

Diagnosis

Clinicians should suspect gonococcal ophthalmia neonatorum in an infant in whom purulent conjunctivitis develops during the first week of life or if what was thought to be chemical conjunctivitis is prolonged beyond 24 to 48 hours. Gram stain of the exudate usually reveals the gram-negative, intracellular, bean-shaped diplococci typical of *N. gonorrhoeae*, which provide a presumptive diagnosis. Other *Neisseria* species—in particular, *N. meningitidis*—cannot be distinguished from the gonococcus by Gram stain appearance. *N. gonorrhoeae* must be isolated and tested for antibiotic susceptibility before a definitive diagnosis is made. A definitive diagnosis is important because of the public health and social consequences of the diagnosis of gonorrhea in an infant. If gonococcal ophthalmia neonatorum is suspected on the basis of the Gram stain appearance, cultures should be obtained from additional mucosal sites in the infant. The mother and her sexual partner or partners also should be tested for gonorrhea, along with additional testing of the infant, mother, and sexual partners for other sexually transmitted infections, including HIV infection.[2,36]

Isolation of *N. gonorrhoeae* from the exudate by culture is the diagnostic gold standard. Samples of the exudate should be collected by swabbing and should be inoculated directly onto blood agar, MacConkey agar, and chocolate agar or chocolate-inhibitory media. The inhibitory medium, which contains antibiotics to inhibit other bacteria, should be placed in a commercial carbon dioxide incubator or candle jar to provide an adequate concentration of carbon dioxide and should be incubated at 36° C. Cultures are examined daily for the presence of typical colonies. Colonies resembling *N. gonorrhoeae* are identified further by Gram stain, by a positive oxidase test, and by use of glucose, but not maltose, sucrose, or lactose. Antibiotic sensitivity and penicillinase production should be tested.

Further testing to confirm the identification of the isolate may be done in a reference laboratory if desired. DNA-based and polymerase chain reaction–based technologies have replaced gonococcal cultures in many laboratories.[2,36] These assays have a high degree of sensitivity and detect more true cases of gonorrheal infection in adults than can be achieved by current culture methods. When correctly used, they also are very specific. Their suitability for diagnosis of gonorrheal infections in children without the additional use of culture methods, with the associated legal implications in older children, has not been extensively studied, however. In addition, extensive use of these methods for primary diagnosis impairs the tracking of antimicrobial resistance patterns unless there is a surveillance system such as that in place in the United States.[10]

If gonococcal ophthalmia neonatorum is presumptively or definitively diagnosed, testing should also be conducted for other sexually transmitted pathogens, in particular, *Chlamydia trachomatis*, because the two organisms frequently are found to coinfect pregnant women.[2,36] Also, the diagnosis of gonococccal infection in the neonate should trigger an investigation of the infant's mother and her sexual partner or partners for STDs.

Differential Diagnosis

At present, *N. gonorrhoeae* causes less than 1% of cases of ophthalmia neonatorum in North America, western Europe, Australia, and New Zealand and in areas and communities elsewhere where there is access to prenatal care and STD prevention programs. In other areas, the risk of gonococcal ophthalmia is higher depending on the prevalence of gonococcal infection among the pregnant women in the population. Even in areas with high prevalence rates, however, ophthalmia caused by *N. gonorrhoeae* accounts for less than 5% of cases of neonatal conjunctivitis. Table 15-1 shows other organisms that can produce conjunctivitis in the newborn period and the relative overall frequency of resultant infections, the usual time of presentation since birth, and relative severity.

In general, conjunctivitis seen within 24 hours of birth usually is assumed to be a reaction to silver nitrate, if this has been used for prophylaxis. As described previously, however, in the instance of prolonged rupture of membranes and premature delivery, symptomatic gonococcal ophthalmia may be observed during this period as well. Also, some infants have a less acute course, with appearance of symptoms after 5 days of age. Reliance on the timing between 2 and 5 days after delivery of the onset of symptoms may be an unreliable clinically distinguishing feature. The possibility of gonococcal infection should be considered in every neonate with conjunctivitis present after 24 hours of birth, and appropriate diagnostic testing to detect the organism should be done. In some instances, neonates with gonococcal ophthalmia neonatorum may be infected by additional pathogens, in particular, *C. trachomatis*. The differential diagnosis of cutaneous or systemic gonococcal infection of the neonate includes the bacterial or fungal pathogens that are frequently involved in these types of infections during this time period and are discussed in more detail in Chapters 6, 10, 33, and 34.

Table 15-1 Differential Diagnosis of Ophthalmia Neonatorum

Etiologic Condition/Agent	Percentage of Cases	Relative Severity	Usual Time of Onset After Delivery
Chemical conjunctivitis	Dependent on use	+	6-24 hr
Neisseria gonorrhoeae	<1	+++	2-5 days
Neisseria meningitidis	<1	++	2 days-2 wk
Neisseria cinerea	<1	+	2 days-2 wk
Herpes simplex virus	<1	++	2-14 days
Chlamydia trachomatis	2-40	+	5 days-2 wk
Other bacteria	30-50	++	2 days-2 wk
Group A and B streptococci			
Staphylococcus aureus			
Haemophilus species			
Klebsiella pneumoniae			
Escherichia coli			
Pseudomonas aeruginosa			
Enterococcus			
Pneumococcus			

Treatment

The principles of management of STDs in any age group apply when a neonate is determined to have a suspected or confirmed gonococcal infection. As stated previously, investigation and treatment of the mother and her sexual contacts for *N. gonorrhoeae* are essential, as is the investigation of the infant, the mother, and her sexual contacts for other sexually transmitted infections, including recent acquisition of HIV. STDs are like wolves—they travel in packs.

As discussed previously, because a significant proportion of gonococci worldwide is resistant to penicillin, either by decreased penicillin binding or by penicillinase production, this antibiotic is no longer recommended for therapy, unless the infecting isolate has been tested and found to be sensitive. Most recommendations and guidelines for the treatment of gonococcal ophthalmia neonatorum identify ceftriaxone at a dose of 25 to 50 mg/kg (not to exceed 125 mg) intramuscular (IM) or intravenous (IV) in a single dose as the agent of choice (Table 15-2).[2,36,37] Ceftriaxone must be administered cautiously to infants with hyperbilirubinemia, especially infants born prematurely. In that instance, cefotaxime at a dose of 100 mg/kg IV or IM can be used as an alternative. One dose of ceftriaxone or cefotaxime is adequate therapy for gonococcal conjunctivitis. The addition of either erythromycin or azithromycin for additional coverage for *Chlamydia* infection is also recommended unless the mother has been shown not to be coinfected. Use of this additional antibiotic will provide dual antibiotic treatment for gonorrhea, because most isolates are susceptible to macrolide antibiotics.[2,36] Irrigation of the eye with saline drops hourly until

Table 15-2 Recommended Treatment for Neonatal Gonococcal Infections

Condition	Recommended Therapy
Ophthalmia neonatorum	Ceftriaxone 25-50 mg/kg IV or IM in a single dose, not to exceed 125 mg *or* cefotaxime 100 mg/kg IV or IM; topical antibiotic therapy alone is inadequate and is unnecessary if systemic treatment is administered
Gonococcal meningitis, sepsis, arthritis, or scalp lesions	Ceftriaxone 25-50 mg/kg/day IV or IM in a single daily dose for 7 days *or* cefotaxime 25 mg/kg IV or IM every 12 hr for 7 days, with a duration of 10-14 days if meningitis is documented; 14 days if arthritis is documented or 28 days if endocarditis is documented
Known exposure at birth but asymptomatic	Ceftriaxone 25-50 mg/kg IV or IM in a single dose, not to exceed 125 mg *or* cefotaxime 100 mg/kg IV or IM

IM, Intramuscularly; *IV*, intravenously.

the eye discharge has abated is also important to reduce the long-term consequences of the infection. Instillation of topical antibiotics into the eyes in addition to systemic therapy does not improve outcome and is not necessary.

Infants who have gonococcal ophthalmia should be hospitalized and evaluated for signs of disseminated infection (e.g., sepsis, arthritis, meningitis). Disseminated infection in the neonate should be treated either with ceftriaxone (50 mg/kg/day) or with cefotaxime (100 mg/kg/day) in consultation with an expert in infectious diseases. The duration of the recommended treatment course varies depending on the clinical presentation, with a suggested duration of 7 days for scalp infections, 10 to 14 days for sepsis/meningitis, 14 days for arthritis, and 28 days for endocarditis. Because of the rarity of these situations, there are no results from clinically controlled trials to help guide therapy.

Asymptomatic infants born to mothers who have documented untreated infection are at high risk of developing disseminated disease and therefore should also receive treatment with ceftriaxone at a dose of 25 to 50 mg/kg (not to exceed 125 mg) IM or IV in a single dose or cefotaxime at a dose of 100 mg/kg IV or IM as soon as the mother's infection is diagnosed.

Prognosis

With early recognition, effective antibiotic treatment and appropriate management of the eye discharge, cure rates for gonococcal ophthalmia and other neonatal manifestations of gonococcal infection in the newborn are close to 100%. By contrast, permanent corneal damage after gonococcal ophthalmia neonatorum was the usual clinical outcome in the preantibiotic era.

Prevention

Prevention of gonococcal infection of the fetus and neonate is best achieved by preventing gonococcal infection of the mother. One way to accomplish this goal is by the reduction of the prevalence of *N. gonorrhoeae* in the core high-risk populations that serve as its reservoir for pregnant women. Targeted treatment and prevention campaigns among commercial sex workers, sexually active adolescents and young adults who have multiple partners, and groups with high prevalence of gonococcal infection or who have other risk factors that result in increased high-risk sexual activity, such as individuals with street drug and alcohol abuse problems and homosexual men who have multiple contacts, would reduce the prevalence in the general population. Education of youth before sexual maturity about the risks of STDs and about ways in which they can protect themselves from acquiring these diseases does not increase the rates of sexual activity among adolescents and should be encouraged as a joint responsibility of parents or primary care providers, the schools, and health care providers. Provision of accessible health care with readily available antibiotics that are appropriate and effective against circulating strains of *N. gonorrhoeae* also is imperative for this purpose. Finally, to support optimal health behaviors, persons of all ages need to be able to feel confident that they will not be stigmatized for seeking health care for an STD.

Because infection with *N. gonorrhoeae* during pregnancy may result in adverse pregnancy outcomes, such as premature rupture of membranes and preterm delivery, screening of pregnant women for infection in early pregnancy is advisable. Women identified as having gonococcal infection should receive prompt treatment.[2,36] Recommended treatment now includes the use of a higher dose of ceftriaxone (250 mg rather than 125 mg IM) in a single dose, along with azithromycin 1 g orally. Women for whom a third-generation cephalosporin is contraindicated should receive azithromycin at a dose of 2 g orally. Use of the oral drug cefixime as an alternative is not recommended for treatment in the United States.[38] In Canada, ceftriaxone is the recommended treatment of choice, but use of cefixime at an increased dosage of 800 mg rather than the previously recommended 400-mg dosage is suggested for those situations where IM administration would not be advised. Follow-up testing to ensure eradication of the infection and to detect reinfection is imperative.[39]

Testing for other STDs should be done, and the mother should be offered HIV testing. In addition, counseling related to avoidance of further infection is an important component of management. Tracing and treatment of sexual contacts are necessary to reduce the risk of subsequent infection. In one study in Louisiana of 751 pregnant women whose charts were reviewed retrospectively, 5.1% were diagnosed with gonorrhea at the first prenatal visit, and 2.5% acquired the infection during their pregnancy.[40] Women whose sexual behavior or social circumstances place them at risk of acquiring sexually transmitted infection during pregnancy should be retested for gonorrhea (and other STDs) in the third trimester. Retesting is most conveniently accomplished at the time of screening for group B streptococci.

Since the late 1800s, eye prophylaxis has been the hallmark of prevention of gonococcal ophthalmia neonatorum. Currently, many jurisdictions mandate the use of ocular prophylaxis for newborns through legislation. Most others recommend and encourage its use. The issue is controversial in areas of low prevalence of *N. gonorrhoeae* infection and among populations with extremely low risk of the disease. In these situations, the concerns regarding the complications of the use of the prophylactic agents must be balanced against the actual risk of the disease and the ability, or the wish, to provide an alternative management approach involving close observation of the infant with early therapy if necessary.

At present, data from clinical trials support the use of 1% silver nitrate, 0.5% erythromycin, 1% tetracycline, or 2.5% povidone-iodine for prophylaxis against gonococcal ophthalmia neonatorum.* All of these agents are less effective against chlamydial conjunctivitis, however, and to date, there is no truly effective ocular agent to prevent that infection. Most agents are well tolerated, although a chemical conjunctivitis commonly is seen after instillation of silver nitrate. This reaction involves epithelial desquamation and a polymorphonuclear leukocytic exudate [41] and usually appears within 6 to 8 hours and disappears within 24 to 48 hours. A mild chemical conjunctivitis may be seen in 10% to 20% of infants who

*References 1, 2, 5, 6, 36, 37.

received povidone-iodine prophylaxis and, as well, there is a mild transient brownish discoloration of the sclera.[5,42] Use of antibiotic agents has the potential to lead to increased antibiotic resistance in other colonizing bacteria, which could lead to outbreaks of infection in the nursery.[43] Studies have been done looking at the effectiveness of fusidic acid for prophylaxis of ophthalmia neonatorum to which *N. gonorrhoeae* is susceptible in vitro. Studies done to date show it to be promising, but the incidence of gonorrheal infection has been too low in the populations studied to assess its effectiveness against this organism in the clinical context.[6]

Failure of prophylaxis can occur. If the illness is established by the time of delivery, ocular prophylaxis is ineffective. In extremely rare instances, infection may be acquired after prophylaxis had been provided. Some experts have suggested that irrigation of the eyes with saline too soon after silver nitrate application is the cause of such treatment failures. On occasion, the erythromycin eye ointment may not have penetrated to the eye itself as a result of difficulties in keeping the infant's eye exposed during application of ointment by inexperienced health care providers.[44]

At present, specific prophylaxis given immediately (minimum delay of 1 hour) after birth, using any of the following regimens, is recommended by most professional societies and government bodies: (1) 1% silver nitrate in single-dose ampules, (2) 0.5% erythromycin ophthalmic ointment in single-use tubes, or (3) 1% tetracycline ophthalmic ointment in single-use tubes. Of note, only 0.5% erythromycin ophthalmic ointment is available for this use in the United States. Povidone-iodine also is considered to be a safe and effective alternative in resource-poor countries.

If the membranes have been ruptured, if the infant is premature, or if close follow-up cannot be ensured, treatment for ophthalmia neonatorum with ceftriaxone or cefotaxime, rather than use of eye prophylaxis, is recommended. Also, in instances where there is a disruption in the supply of eye prophylaxis, use of ceftriaxone or cefotaxime treatment is recommended rather than use of other ophthalmic preparations developed for older children or adults.[2]

References

1. Woods CR: Gonococcal infections in neonates and young children, *Semin Pediatr Infect Dis* 16:258-270, 2005.
2. Centers for Disease Control and Prevention: Sexually transmitted diseases treatment guidelines 2010, *MMWR Morb Mortal Wkly Rep* 59:1-110, 2010.
3. Hirschberg J, Krause F: *Zentralbl Prakt Augen* 5:39, 1881.
4. Forbes G, Forbes GM: Silver nitrate and the eyes of the newborn, *Am J Dis Child* 121:1-3, 1971.
5. Darling EK, McDonald H: A meta-analysis of the efficacy of ocular prophylactic agents used for the prevention of gonococcal and chlamydial ophthalmia neonatorum, *J Midwifery Womens Health* 55:319-327, 2010.
6. Zuppa AA, D'Andrea V, Catenazzi P, et al: Ophthalmia neonatorum: what kind of prophylaxis? *J Maternal Fetal Neonatal Med* 24:769-773, 2011.
7. Elliott B, Brunham RC, Laga M, et al: Maternal gonococcal infection as a preventable risk factor for low birth weight, *J Infect Dis* 161: 531-553, 1990.
8. Moses S, Ngugi EN, Costigan A, et al: Response of a sexually transmitted infection epidemic to a treatment and prevention programme in Nairobi, Kenya, *Sex Transm Infect* 78:114-120, 2002.
9. World Health Organization (WHO): Global prevalence and incidence of selected curable sexually transmitted infections: overview and estimates, Geneva, 2001, WHO/Communicable Disease Surveillance and Response/Educational Development Center.
10. Centers for Disease Control and Prevention: Sexually transmitted disease surveillance, 2011. Available at http://www.cdc.gov/std/stats11/gonorrhea.htm. Accessed July 2, 2014.
11. Public Health Agency of Canada: Report on sexually transmitted infections in Canada, 2008. Available at http://www.phac-aspc.gc.ca/std-mts/report/sti-its2008/04-eng.php. Accessed July 2, 2014.
12. Cornelius CE 3rd: Seasonality of gonorrhea in the United States, *HSMHA Health Rep* 86:157-160, 1971.
13. Rothenberg R: Ophthalmia neonatorum due to *Neisseria gonorrhoeae*: prevention and treatment, *Sex Transm Dis* 6:187-191, 1979.
14. Charles AG, Cohen S, Kass MB, Richman R: Asymptomatic gonorrhea in prenatal patients, *Am J Obstet Gynecol* 108:595-599, 1970.
15. Marrazzo JM, Handsfield HH, Sparling PF: 1995 Neisseria gonorrhoeae. In Mandell GL, Bennett JE, Dolin R, editors: *Mandell, Douglas, and Bennett's principles and practice of infectious diseases*, ed 7, Philadelphia, 2010, Churchill Livingstone/Elsevier, pp 2753-2770.
16. Joiner KA, Scales R, Warren KA, et al: Mechanism of action of blocking immunoglobulin G for *Neisseria gonorrhoeae*, *J Clin Invest* 76:1765-1772, 1985.
17. Schoolnik GK, Ochs HD, Buchanan TM: Immunoglobulin class responsible for bactericidal activity of normal human sera, *J Immunol* 122:1771-1779, 1979.
18. Tsirpouchtsidis A, Hurwitz R, Brinkmann V, et al: Neisserial immunoglobulin A1 protease induces specific T-cell responses in humans, *Infect Immunol* 70:335-344, 2002.
19. Hedges SR, Mayo MS, Mestecky J, et al: Limited local and systemic antibody responses to *Neisseria gonorrhoeae* during uncomplicated genital infections, *Infect Immun* 67:3937-3946, 1999.
20. Boulton IC, Gray-Owen SD: Neisserial binding to CEACAM1 arrests the activation and proliferation of CD4+ T lymphocytes, *Nat Immunol* 3:229-236, 2002.
21. Yoshio H, Tollin M, Gudmundsson GH, et al: Antimicrobial polypeptides of human vernix caseosa and amniotic fluid: implications for newborn innate defense, *Pediatr Res* 53:211-216, 2003.
22. Marchini G, Lindow S, Brismar H, et al: The newborn infant is protected by an innate antimicrobial barrier: peptide antibiotics are present in the skin and vernix caseosa, *Br J Dermatol* 147:127-134, 2002.
23. Bolan GA, Sparling F, Wasserheit JN: The emerging threat of untreatable gonococcal infection, *N Engl J Med* 366:485-487, 2012.
24. Hunter GW, Fargo ND: Specific urethritis (gonorrhea) in a male newborn, *Am J Obstet Gynecol* 38:520-521, 1939.
25. Stark AR, Glode MP: Gonococcal vaginitis in a neonate, *J Pediatr* 94:298-299, 1979.
26. Barton LL, Shuja M: Neonatal gonococcal vaginitis, *J Pediatr* 98: 171-172, 1981.
27. Kirkland H, Storer RV: Gonococcal rhinitis in an infant, *BMJ* 1: 263-267, 1931.
28. Fransen L, Nsanze H, Klauss V, et al: Ophthalmia neonatorum in Nairobi, Kenya: the roles of *Neisseria gonorrhoeae* and *Chlamydia trachomatis*, *J Infect Dis* 153:862-869, 1986.
29. Bradford WL, Kelley HW: Gonococcal meningitis in a newborn infant, *Am J Dis Child* 46:543-549, 1933.
30. Kohen DP: Neonatal gonococcal arthritis: three cases and review of the literature, *Pediatrics* 53:436-440, 1974.
31. Babl FE, Ram S, Barnett ED, et al: neonatal gonococcal arthritis after negative prenatal screening and despite conjunctival prophylaxis, *Pediatr Infect Dis J* 19:346-349, 2000.
32. D'Auria A, Tan L, Kreitzer M, et al: Gonococcal scalp wound infection, *MMWR Morb Mortal Wkly Rep* 24:115-116, 1975.
33. Urban MN, Heruada AR: Gonococcal gum abscess in a 10-week old infant, *Clin Pediatr* 16:193-194, 1977.
34. Bland RS, Nelson LH, Meis PJ, et al: Gonococcal ventriculitis associated with ventriculoamniotic shunt placement, *Am J Obstet Gynecol* 147:781-784, 1983.
35. Wald ER, Woodward CL, Marston G, Gilbert LM: Gonorrheal disease among children in a university hospital, *Sex Transm Dis* 7:41-43, 1980.
36. Public Health Agency of Canada: Canadian guidelines on sexually transmitted infections—updated January 2010. Available at http://www.phac.aspc.gc.ca/std-mts/sti-its/cgsti-1dcits/section-5-6-eng.php, 2010. Accessed July 2, 2014.
37. American Academy of Pediatrics: Prevention of neonatal ophthalmia. In Pickering LK, Baker CJ, Kimberlin DW, Long SS, editors: *Redbook 2012, Report of the Committee on Infectious Diseases*, ed 29, Elk Grove Village, Ill, 2012, American Academy of Pediatrics, pp 880-882.

38. Centers for Disease Control and Prevention: Update to CDC's sexually transmitted diseases treatment guidelines, 2010: oral cephalosporins no longer recommended treatment for gonococcal infections, *MMWR Morb Mortal Wkly Rep* 61:590-594, 2010.
39. Public Health Agency of Canada: Important notice—public health information update on the treatment for gonococcal infection. Available at http://www.phac-aspc.gc.ca/std-mts/sti-its/alert/2011/alert-gono-eng.php, 2011. Accessed July 2, 2014.
40. Miller JM Jr, Maupin RT, Mestad RE, Nsuami M: Initial and repeated screening for gonorrhea during pregnancy, *Sex Transm Dis* 30: 728-730, 2003.
41. Norn MS: Cytology of the conjunctival fluid in newborn with references to Credé's prophylaxis, *Acta Ophthalmol* 38:491-495, 1960.
42. Isenberg SJ, Apt L, Wood M: A controlled trial of povidone-iodine as prophylaxis against ophthalmia neonatorum, *N Engl J Med* 332:562-566, 1995.
43. Hedberg K, Ristinen TL, Soler JT, et al: Outbreak of erythromycin-resistant staphylococcal conjunctivitis in a newborn nursery, *Pediatr Infect Dis J* 9:268-273, 1990.
44. Laga M, Plummer FA, Piot P, et al: Prophylaxis of gonococcal and chlamydial ophthalmia neonatorum: a comparison of silver nitrate and tetracycline, *N Engl J Med* 17:653-657, 1988.

16 Syphilis

TOBIAS R. KOLLMANN and SIMON R.M. DOBSON

CHAPTER OUTLINE

Syphilis is a sexually transmitted disease caused by infection with the bacterium *Treponema pallidum*. Congenital syphilis results when the infection is transmitted from a pregnant mother to her fetus. Syphilis has been known for a long time to cause serious infections in the newborn of an infected mother.[1] The horror syphilis causes is best encapsulated in its other old name "lues," which means "plague" in Latin. Unfortunately, this is the most appropriate name still, because a staggering number of adults and newborn infants in both developed and developing countries are suffering and dying as a consequence of infection with *T. pallidum*.[2] The World Health Organization (WHO) estimates that each year more than 2 million pregnant women suffer from syphilis; two thirds of these will suffer a serious adverse pregnancy outcome.[3-5] The 2012 Report on Global Burden of Disease estimates that congenital syphilis is responsible for greater than 2% of all deaths among live-born infants.[6] Furthermore, the excess cost per case of congenital syphilis in the United States is approximately $10,000 (in 2009 U.S. dollars.)[7] Consequently, the elimination of congenital syphilis is an extremely important objective.[8-10]

Organism

The name *Treponema* (Greek) meaning "turning thread," is based on its twisting motion, and *pallidum* (Latin) derives from its pale yellow color. *T. pallidum* belongs to the order Spirochaetales, family Spirochaetaceae, and genus *Treponema. Borrelia, Spirochaeta, Leptospira,* and *Cristispira* are other genera of this order, grouped together primarily based on their morphologic characteristics, that is, being helix shaped (Fig. 16-1). *T. pallidum* has approximately 8 to 14 helices per cell.[11] Despite greater than 95% sequence homology, complete DNA sequencing has allowed the human disease-causing *Treponema* to be identified as subspecies, namely, *T. pallidum* subsp. *pallidum* (syphilis), *T. pallidum* subsp. *pertenue* (yaws), *T. pallidum* subsp. *carateum* (pinta), and *T. pallidum* subsp. *endemicum* (bejel).[12-14] Only *T. pallidum* and possibly *T. pertenue*[15] can cause congenital infection.[16-18] There are also several other nonpathogenic treponemes that inhabit the oral cavity and intestinal tract of humans.[19]

T. pallidum has finely tapered ends, lacking the hook shape found in several human commensal

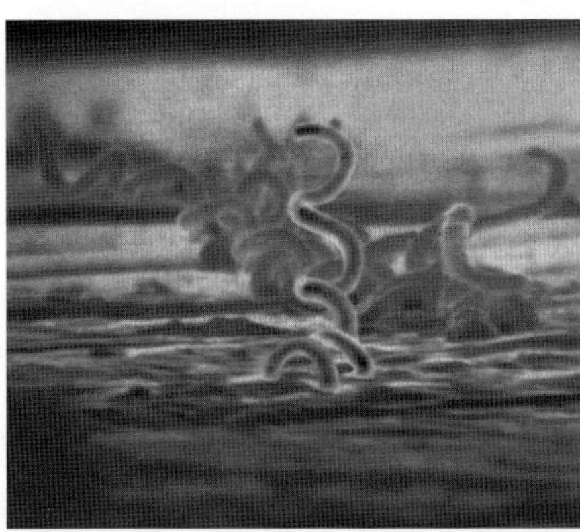

Figure 16-1 Electron micrograph of *Treponema pallidum* on cultures of cotton-tail rabbit epithelium cells, displaying the characteristic helical structure of treponemes. (Courtesy Centers for Disease Control and Prevention/Dr. David Cox, Public Health Image Library #1977.)

spirochetes.[12,13] An outer membrane consisting of a lipid bilayer surrounds the endoflagella, cytoplasmic membrane, and protoplasmic cylinder. The spirochete's corkscrew motility results from the action of these endoflagella and can readily be observed in fresh preparations examined via darkfield microscopy.[20] The genome of *T. pallidum* (Nichols strain, maintained in rabbits since 1912) has been sequenced in its entire length. It represents an approximately 1-Mb circular chromosome with just more than 1000 predicted open reading frames encoding all factors necessary for replication, transcription, translation, and mobility. Although *T. pallidum* does not appear to rely on iron acquisition from the host,[21-23] the presence of only a minimal number of genes encoding molecules important in metabolism indicates a metabolically close interaction with the infected host cell.[14,22-25] Genetic polymorphisms at two loci have enabled strain typing of clinical isolates of *T. pallidum*, providing tools for the investigation of syphilis transmission and epidemiology.[26,27]

T. pallidum is a macroaerophilic gram-negative bacterium that is primarily dependent on glycolysis for energy production. It is highly sensitive to oxygen and temperature and thus not readily maintained in culture.[17] It can be passaged for a limited number of replicative cycles with a generation time of 30 to 33 hours in rabbit epithelial cell monolayers.[27] *T. pallidum* can also be propagated by intratesticular inoculation of rabbits, where it displays a replicative cycle of approximately 30 hours. From infected rabbit testes, *T. pallidum* can be purified through density centrifugation. Such purified organisms retain their antigenicity but not their motility nor their virulence. Outside of humans, only rabbits and primates infected with *T. pallidum* develop primary and secondary but not tertiary syphilis, and neither animal has been demonstrated to pass *T. pallidum* on vertically.[16,28,29] Although *T. pallidum* can be passed on vertically in pigs, no good animal model for congenital syphilis exists that recapitulates the clinical findings of the transplacentally infected human.[30-33] This lack of a good animal model and the inability to culture and manipulate these organisms in vitro has prevented a detailed mechanistic understanding of virulence mechanisms or host-pathogen interactions in congenital syphilis.[34,35]

Transmission

Syphilis can be passed horizontally from person to person through direct contact, such as during sexual activity, resulting in acquired syphilis, or vertically from mother to baby, resulting in congenital syphilis. *T. pallidum* does not survive outside of its human host, and is easily killed by heat, drying, and soap and water. Syphilis is thus unlikely to be spread through casual contact or through contact with fomites.[36]

Acquired Syphilis

Humans are the only known natural host of *T. pallidum*. Horizontal transmission results primarily from sexual activity, although anecdotal reports cite kissing as a potential route as well.[37] Because of the low survival rate of *T. pallidum* outside of its host, direct contact with an infected person's bodily secretions containing spirochetes is necessary for transmission. Although sexual transmission depends on many factors, such as stage of the disease, overall, about half of those who have sexual contact with an infected partner will acquire the disease, with an estimated 50% infective dose of 50 bacteria.[38,39] Because sexual contact is the most common mode of transmission for acquired disease, the sites of inoculation usually are the genital organs, but lips, tongue, and abraded areas of the skin have been described as well. Such an entry point is identified as the site of the initial ulcerating sore, or chancre.[37] Health care providers (HCPs) or laboratory workers have apparently become infected with *T. pallidum* through accidental contact with infected secretions when appropriate personal protective equipment (e.g., gloves) was not worn.[37]

Congenital Syphilis

Although transmission of syphilis to the fetus can occur throughout pregnancy (spirochetes have been visualized in tissue at gestational ages as early as 9 weeks),[40-42] the likelihood of vertical transmission increases with advancing gestation. The organism is isolated with increasing frequency during gestation from umbilical cord blood, amniotic fluid,[43-47] and placenta.[48-50] A newborn occasionally may be infected perinatally, that is, at delivery by contact with an infectious lesion present in the birth canal or perineum. Postnatal transmission from mother to child is exceedingly rare, and there are no data that indicate breast milk itself as being associated with mother to child transmission.[51,52]

The likelihood of vertical transmission is directly related to the maternal stage of syphilis, with early primary syphilis resulting in significantly higher transmission rates than late latent infection (known as the "Kassowitz law").[53,54] This may relate to maternal spirochetemia in early syphilis.[55] Among pregnant women who had untreated primary or secondary early syphilis, the rate of transmission is 60% to

100% but decreases with later stages of maternal infection to approximately 40% with early latent infection and 8% with late latent infection. In one study, where *T. pallidum* was passed on from mother to fetus during early primary or secondary (<4-years duration) untreated syphilis, approximately one half of the infants were born prematurely, stillborn, or died as neonates, and congenital syphilis developed in the other half, that is, approximately 100% were affected. In contrast, in women with early latent syphilis, 20% to 60% of their infants were healthy at birth, 20% premature, and 16% were stillborn; 4% died as neonates, and 40% of those appearing healthy at birth developed the stigmata of congenital syphilis later in life. In the case of untreated late syphilis, about 70% of the newborns appeared healthy, 10% were stillborn, and approximately 9% were premature; about 1% died as neonates, and about 10% of those appearing healthy at birth developed signs of congenital syphilis later in life.[53,54,56]

SYPHILIS AND HUMAN IMMUNODEFICIENCY VIRUS

Despite the recognition that syphilis and human immunodeficiency virus (HIV) are a deadly combination, limited conclusive data exist to describe the interaction between the two infections or their impact on vertical transmission.[57,58] Potential interactions include acceleration of the natural history of either disease, alterations in the clinical or laboratory manifestations, increased risk for syphilitic complications, and diminished response to syphilis therapy.[27,37,59,60] Genital sores, for instance, chancres caused by syphilis, make it easier to sexually transmit and acquire HIV infection, with an estimated two- to fivefold increased risk of acquiring HIV if exposed to that infection when a syphilitic chancre is present.[36] This is likely caused by the breaks in the skin or mucous membranes in a syphilitic chancre, which bleed easily. *T. pallidum* also promotes the induction of HIV replication in infected cells.[61] Increasing proportions of newborns that are infected with congenital syphilis also are born to mothers with HIV.[62] Immune dysfunction associated with HIV infection may also permit a greater degree of treponemal proliferation and lead to a higher rate of fetal infection. HIV-infected women who acquire syphilis during pregnancy may also not respond adequately to currently recommended penicillin therapy, thereby increasing the risk of fetal infection with *T. pallidum*.[63] However, available data suggest that if the natural history of acquired syphilis is modified by HIV, the difference shows considerable overlap with the course of syphilitic disease progression in persons without HIV.[27]

SYPHILIS IN SEXUALLY ABUSED CHILDREN

Identification of syphilis in young children raises the question of possible sexual abuse. Fortunately, it is an uncommon complication among sexually abused children, found in 1% or less in a case series from the United States.[64] The clinical manifestations may provide insight into the timing of acquisition of infection, but this information may not always help to resolve the potential dilemma of whether the clinical findings are those of previously unrecognized congenital syphilis versus postnatally acquired syphilis. Evaluation of children by specialists in the area of child sexual abuse is highly recommended.[64] Children diagnosed with syphilis also should be evaluated for HIV infection and other sexually transmitted diseases.

INFECTION CONTROL

Standard precautions are recommended for all patients, including infants with suspected or proven congenital syphilis. Infected infants and adults with infectious lesions should be placed in contact isolation for the first 24 hours of therapy, and appropriate personal protective equipment (e.g., gloves) should be worn by staff for all patient contact during this time period. Once antimicrobial therapy has been initiated, the risk of transmission is virtually nonexistent because penicillin in sufficient dosage causes a complete disappearance of viable treponemes from syphilitic lesions within a few hours.[65] All people, including hospital personnel, who have had unprotected close contact with a patient with early congenital syphilis before identification of the disease or within the first 24 hours of therapy should be examined clinically for the presence of lesions 2 to 3 weeks after contact. Close unprotected contact is defined as skin (intact or abraded) contact with infectious bodily fluids. Serology in the exposed should be assessed at time 0 and again at 1 month and 3 to 6 months postexposure, or sooner if symptoms occur. If the degree of exposure is considered substantial, immediate treatment should be considered, as outlined later under postexposure prophylaxis in the "Therapy" section.[64,66] All exposures should also be reported to the responsible occupational health officer.

Epidemiology

The epidemiologic curve of syphilis has consistently reflected societal transitions.[67-69] After major public health successes in the early 1990s, the incidence of acquired syphilis shows an alarming resurgence all across the globe, including the United States and Canada.[70-72] Local outbreaks of primary and secondary syphilis have occurred in North America and Canada in almost cyclic patterns roughly every 7 to 10 years.[73-75] These cycles underscore the need for syphilis elimination rather than only control.

CONGENITAL SYPHILIS

The trends for congenital syphilis follow those of acquired syphilis in the adult female population.[76] The dramatic increase in the number of cases of congenital syphilis in 1990 to 1991 was due both to an increase in actual cases and to the use of revised reporting guidelines beginning in 1989.[73,77,78] Previous criteria for reporting cases of congenital syphilis had been based on a clinical case definition.[79] Because of the high incidence of congenital disease in infants born to inadequately treated mothers, current definitions of congenital syphilis for a probable case (which should be reported and treated) require only (1) that the infant be born to a mother with untreated or inadequately treated syphilis or (2) that the child has physical or laboratory signs of congenital syphilis. Use of these guidelines increased the number of reported cases of congenital syphilis almost fourfold in the 1990s.[80,81] Of importance, this current definition by the Centers for Disease Control and Prevention (CDC) acknowledges the public health burden of the disease because these infants require medical and public health interventions. Using this new surveillance-based case definition, until the year 2005, the rate of congenital syphilis in the United States had declined every year over 14 consecutive years, with an overall reduction of 74.2%. But between 2005 and 2006, for the first time, the rate of congenital syphilis increased again (3.7% from 8.2 to 8.5 cases/100,000 live births). In 2006, 349 cases were reported in the United States, compared with 339 in 2005. In 2006, 26 states, the District of Columbia, and one outlying area had rates of congenital syphilis that exceeded the Healthy People 2010 target of 1 case per 100,000 live births,[82] indicating how widespread the resurgence of congenital syphilis is in the United States. In Canada, the rates of congenital syphilis followed a similar trend.[71] Delayed access to prenatal care has been identified as the main issue in North America; for example; nearly all mothers in an outbreak in downtown Vancouver who delivered a child with congenital syphilis had histories of substance abuse or street involvement.[67]

GLOBAL PERSPECTIVE

Worldwide, syphilis has grown into a staggering public health problem.[83-85] The WHO estimates that 12 million people are infected with syphilis each year, 90% of whom are in developing countries. In sub-Saharan Africa, syphilis is a serious problem among women in the fertile age group, with national surveys reporting rates ranging from 3.1% in Uganda to 4.2% in Madagascar, 6.6% in Ghana, and 8.3% in Zambia.[86,87] In southern Africa an estimated quarter of all stillbirths and 10% of all neonatal deaths are due to congenital syphilis.[88]

Recent data from the WHO indicate that only 68% of women in the world currently receive antenatal care; in consequence, congenital syphilis has a higher impact than any other major neonatal infection, including HIV infection and tetanus.[89,90] With that, considerable burden is placed on the already limited health services in many developing countries.[91,92] For example, newborns with congenital syphilis are more likely to be admitted to a neonatal intensive care unit, to stay longer in hospital, and to receive care costing three times more than those without the disease. In one large South African referral hospital, on average, 1 in 12 pediatric intensive care beds is occupied by a baby with congenital syphilis.[8,10]

Pathogenesis

Understanding the pathogenesis of *T. pallidum* in pregnancy will rely on understanding the complex relationships between the unique ability of this particular treponeme to cross the placental barrier and its ability to cause fetal demise or the many early and late manifestations of congenital syphilis in a live-born infant.[27] These complex and changing host-pathogen relationships are superimposed on the genetic background of both mother and fetus.[27] The complexity and rapid changes of these host-pathogen relationships has made gathering mechanistic insights into the molecular, cellular, and organismal pathogenesis extremely difficult.

TREPONEMAL VIRULENCE-ASSOCIATED FACTORS

As reviewed by Woods,[93] congenital syphilis starts with *T. pallidum* bacteria crossing from mother to fetus. Transplacental transmission during maternal spirochetemia can occur as early as 9 to 10 weeks of gestation and at any subsequent time during pregnancy. Viable spirochetes in amniotic fluid obtained by amniocentesis from a woman with early syphilis have been reported as early as 14 weeks of gestation, proving that the fetus can sustain replication of viable treponemes after infection with *T. pallidum* very early in pregnancy.[45] Transmission in utero causes the wide dissemination of the organism in the fetus (analogous to secondary acquired syphilis). Untreated congenital syphilis can progress through the same stages as postnatally acquired syphilis. Infection begins when virulent *T. pallidum* attach to host cells via the proximal hook. There appears to be a ligand-receptor adherence mechanism involving the treponemal outer membrane proteins. Virulent strains attach to metabolically active mammalian cells, and treponemes are capable of multiplication only while attached. Highly replicative fetal and infant cells appear to support treponemal growth maximally, with endothelial cells the prime target. Virulent treponemal strains produce hyaluronidase, which may facilitate the perivascular infiltration. *T. pallidum* is coated with fibronectin of host origin; this coating appears to protect the organism from antibody-mediated phagocytosis and allows the organism to adhere to the surface of host phagocytes with only limited ingestion. This coating may also block complement-mediated lysis of the coated treponemes. Treponemes also acquire other host proteins, such as ceruloplasmin and transferrin.[93,94]

HOST RESPONSE

Pathologic changes in congenital syphilis are similar to those that occur in acquired syphilis, except for the absence of a primary or chancre stage. Because infection involves the placenta[40] and spreads hematogenously to the fetus, widespread involvement is characteristic. No matter which organ is involved, the essential microscopic appearance of lesions is that of perivascular infiltration of lymphocytes, plasma cells, and histiocytes, with obliterative endarteritis and extensive fibrosis.[16,95] These typical histopathologic features of the inflammatory response to invasion by *T. pallidum* suggest an important role for immune-mediated injury in the pathogenesis of congenital syphilis.[96]

T. pallidum infection simultaneously elicits local as well as systemic innate and adaptive immune responses.[97,98] It is generally believed that a strong Th1 response to any infection during pregnancy may compromise pregnancy outcome. In pregnancy, a gradual dampening of the intensity of immune responses to favor the maintenance and growth of the fetus may thus result in incomplete clearance of *T. pallidum* from lesions, hence allowing the development of a chronic infection and the resulting multitude of clinical findings in congenital syphilis.[99] The increased production of inflammatory cytokines interleukin-2 (IL-2), interferon-γ (IFN- γ), tumor necrosis factor-α (TNF- α), and prostaglandins induced by fetal infection, together with the intense inflammatory responses associated with activation of macrophages by treponemal lipoproteins, may be responsible for fetal death or preterm delivery.[23] Resolution of both the primary and the secondary manifestations of infection correlate with the development of cellular immune responses.[27]

Host Innate Immune Response

Although *T. pallidum* does not contain lipopolysaccharide, the lipoproteins and glycolipids present under the outer membrane have been shown to activate the innate inflammatory response via Toll-like receptor 4 (TLR4).[100] These lipoproteins are not surface exposed; live *T. pallidum* thus elicits a lesser inflammatory response than *T. pallidum* lysates.[27,96,101] This feature may explain how live treponemes can persist in extracellular loci yet elicit little or no inflammatory response, and may also account for the pronounced systemic (Jarisch-Herxheimer) reaction observed soon after the initiation of penicillin therapy, where dying treponemes release proinflammatory mediators in large quantities. Polymorphonuclear leukocytes (neutrophils) ingest *T. pallidum*, incorporating them into phagocytic vacuoles, where they are killed and digested. Overall, phagocytosis occurs relatively slowly and is facilitated by the presence of immune serum.[102] However, relatively large numbers of treponemes are needed to activate the phagocytic response, and small numbers of treponemes may escape recognition.[103] Activation of TLR4 on macrophages by treponemal lipoproteins induces production of TNF-α[103,104] and IL-12),[105] which favors the development of Th1-type immunity. A 47-kDa treponemal lipoprotein can activate human vascular endothelial cells directly to upregulate cell surface expression of intercellular adhesion molecule-1 and procoagulant activity.[104,106] These actions may contribute to the fibrin deposition and perivasculitis that are characteristic histopathologic findings in syphilis.[27]

Host Adaptive Immune Response

In acquired syphilis, IgM and IgG antibodies are detectable by the time the primary chancre appears, yet humoral immunity is insufficient to control the infection. Furthermore, T-cell–mediated immunity appears to be suppressed during the primary and secondary stages of infection.[93] Nevertheless, ultimate eradication of acute infection only occurs when T cells infiltrate syphilitic lesions, which leads to activation of macrophages and phagocytosis of antibody-opsonized treponemes.

Host Cell-Mediated Immune Response. The lack of cell surface targets has led *T. pallidum* to be labeled a "stealth pathogen."[27] But the importance of cellular immunity in containing the infection and in its immune pathology is shown by the presence of granulomata, which, in the case of gummatous disease (see later), assume a necrotizing character.[93] In primary chancres, CD4+ T cells and macrophages predominate, whereas in the lesions of secondary syphilis, the majority of the cellular infiltrate is composed of CD8+ T cells. This is surprising because *T. pallidum* is believed to be mostly an extracellular pathogen. Increased expression of the Th1 cytokines IL-2 and IFN-γ are seen in lesions of both primary and secondary syphilis.[101,107,108] Circulating T lymphocytes responsive to treponemal antigens can already be detected in late primary syphilis, but cell-mediated immune responses peak in the secondary stage. Clinically measureable delayed-type hypersensitivity to treponemal antigens appears only late in secondary syphilis and may be related to the onset of latency. Increased apoptosis of peripheral blood lymphocytes and CD4+ T cells by a Fas-mediated pathway in patients with secondary early syphilis could account for the incomplete clearance of *T. pallidum* from the lesions, leading to the establishment of chronic infection.[109] Overall, the mechanisms that lead to latency are, however, not well understood.[27]

Host Antibody-Mediated Humoral Immune Response. Humoral immunity has been a subject of study in syphilis since the serendipitous discovery of antibody to cardiolipin by Wassermann early in the 19th century. Circulating immunoglobulin G (IgG) and IgM antibodies to *T. pallidum* are detectable by the time the chancre appears (i.e., with the onset of primary syphilis), with antibodies to *T. pallidum* detected in 90% and antibody to cardiolipin in 75% of cases.[110] Antibodies to *T. pallidum* recognize a wide range of treponemal proteins.[111,112]. Higher titers are reached as the infection disseminates in the secondary stage.[113,114] In primary syphilis, the main IgG subclass is IgG1, whereas in secondary syphilis, IgG1 and IgG3 predominate.[115] If the patient is treated adequately, IgM antibody declines during the next 1 to 2 years, but IgG antibody usually persists through the lifetime of the patient.[27]

The overall antibody response of congenitally infected infants parallels that in acquired syphilis. IgM antibodies to specific *T. pallidum* proteins can often be detected in neonatal serum obtained at birth.[116-119] The range of IgM antibody responses to the proteins of *T. pallidum* in the sera of overtly infected newborns is comparable to that for disseminated (secondary) infection in adults.[120] The IgM response of the infant, however, is distinct from that of the mother and is uniformly directed against the 47-kDa immunodominant membrane lipoprotein antigen. As would be expected based on the transplacental transfer of IgG, the IgG levels and antigen specificity of infected infants largely match those of their mothers.[118-120]

Human sera containing antibodies can immobilize *T. pallidum* in the presence of complement —the basis of the old *T. pallidum* immobilization test for diagnosing syphilis—and can block attachment of the organism to eukaryotic cells. Also, human immune serum facilitates uptake of *T. pallidum* by human polymorphonuclear leukocytes.[103] Only a small percentage of primary syphilis patients have immobilizing antibodies,[16,121] but *T. pallidum*–immobilizing antibody is present in the majority of patients with active secondary syphilis.[18]

Immune-Mediated Protection

Rabbits immunized with irradiated *T. pallidum* display complete protective immunity to challenge.[122] This argues that it should be possible to achieve protective immunity, possibly through vaccination.[123] Although patients who have been previously treated for syphilis can be reinfected, untreated patients appear to have at least a degree of immunity to repeated infection. In the 19th century in Dublin, Colles[124,125] observed that wet nurses who breastfed infants with congenital syphilis often developed chancres of the nipple, whereas the mothers of such infants did not, implying that they were somehow protected from repeated infection; this has become known as the Colles law. Subsequent studies in which prison volunteers in the United States were inoculated with *T. pallidum* likewise demonstrated that men with untreated syphilis did not develop chancres at the site of cutaneous inoculation, whereas those who had been treated for syphilis in the past (especially those that had been treated early during primary or secondary stages), as well as those who had not had the infection, did develop infection.[38] This suggests that persons with untreated secondary syphilis or true latent infection are resistant to rechallenge with *T. pallidum,* as are those with untreated congenital syphilis.[38] This state has been referred to as "chancre immunity" or "chancre fast." But such protection from untreated previous disease only represents a relative resistance to reinfection such that the development of a chancre with reinfection is unusual but may, in fact, simply depend on the challenge inoculum. This state of relative resistance applies to persons who maintain a reactive nontreponemal antibody test ("serofast"), as well as to those who become sero–nonreactive[126,127] (see later).

Nineteenth-century physicians knew that a degree of maternal immunity is acquired during infection. In 1846, Kassowitz observed that the longer syphilis exists untreated in a woman before pregnancy occurs, the more likely it is that when she does become pregnant, her treponemes will be held in check, and the less likely it is that her fetus will be affected (the Kassowitz law).[124,128] It remains unclear what factors determine which mothers, particularly those in the latent stage of infection, will pass disease to their fetuses. It also is not clear why some infants who are infected in utero are born without any clinical manifestations, with the subsequent development of overt disease in the first weeks or months of life or even later at puberty. In summary, although active or prior syphilis modifies the response of the patient to subsequent reinfection, protection is unpredictable.[27]

Pathology

Although there are many similarities between the pathology of acquired and congenital syphilis, there also are some key differences. Acquired syphilis is a lifelong infection that progresses in three clear characteristic stages[93,123]: after initial invasion through mucous membranes or skin, the organism undergoes rapid multiplication and disseminates widely. Spread through the perivascular lymphatics and then through the systemic circulation occurs even before the clinical development of the primary lesion. Ten to 90 days later (usually within 3 to 4 weeks), the patient manifests an inflammatory response to the infection at the site of the inoculation. The resulting lesion, the chancre, is characterized by the profuse discharge of spirochetes, accumulation of mononuclear leukocytes and the swelling of capillary endothelia. The regional lymph nodes become enlarged as well, with the cellular infiltrate in the lymph node resembling that of the primary chancre lesions. Resolution of the primary lesion eventually occurs via fibrosis (scarring) at the primary chancre site, and reconstruction of the normal architecture in the lymph node. Secondary lesions develop when tissues of ectodermal origin, such as skin, mucous membranes, and central nervous system, become infected, resulting in vasculitis. The cellular infiltrate resembles that of the primary lesion, with the predominance of plasma cells but with CD8 T cells instead of CD4 T cells. There is little or no necrosis, and healing of secondary lesions occurs without scarring. Tertiary syphilis appears to be the result of chronic swelling of the capillary endothelium, resulting in tissue fibrosis or necrosis and may involve any organ system. It often is asymmetric. Gummata are lesions typified by extensive necrosis, a few giant cells, and a paucity of organisms. They commonly occur in internal organs, bone, and skin. The other major form of tertiary lesion is a diffuse chronic perivascular inflammation, with plasma cells and lymphocytes but without caseation, that may result in an aortic aneurysm, paralytic dementia, or tabes dorsalis.

Congenital syphilis cannot as readily be divided into these three stages.[129] Because it is a result of hematogenous infection, dissemination is wide. Of note, most pathologic studies were done on stillborn infants or infants who died early in life, producing significant heterogeneity in the findings secondary to varying length of infection before pathologic examination. Similar to the acquired form, in congenital syphilis, an intense inflammatory response is also focused on the perivascular environment rather than distributed throughout the parenchyma.[124] Bone, liver, pancreas, intestine, kidney, and spleen are involved most severely. Other tissues, such as the brain, pituitary gland, lymph nodes, and lungs, may be infected as well.[130]

Erythroblastosis involving the placenta has been frequently observed.[131] Live- or stillborn, the placenta of infants with congenital syphilis is often large, thick, and pale. Spirochetes may be identified in placental tissue by using conventional staining, although they may be difficult to visualize,[40,48,132] whereas nucleic acid amplification methods readily identify *T. pallidum* genome in involved placental specimens.[133] Three histopathologic features commonly are seen in an infected placenta (Fig. 16-2): enlarged and hypercellular villi, proliferative fetal vascular changes, and both acute and chronic inflammation of the villi.[133,134] The umbilical cord may exhibit significant inflammation with abscess-like foci of necrosis located within the Wharton jelly, centered around the umbilical vessels, resulting in what is termed necrotizing funisitis.[135] Macroscopically, the umbilical cord resembles a "barber's pole"; the edematous portions have a spiral striped zone of red and pale blue discoloration, interspersed with streaks of chalky white.[134,136,137] Histochemical staining as well as nucleic acid amplification approaches have demonstrated spirochetes within the wall of the umbilical vessels.[138] Given these typical findings, placental and umbilical cord histopathology should be performed on every case of suspected syphilis, especially if the placenta is unexpectedly large.* Sheffield and colleagues[134] showed that the addition of histologic evaluation to conventional diagnostic evaluations improved the detection rate for

*References 48, 132, 134, 136, 137, 139.

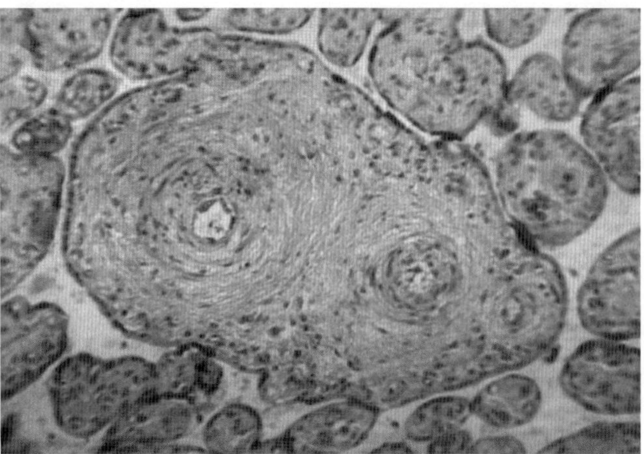

Figure 16-2 Photomicrograph revealing cytoarchitectural changes seen in congenital syphilis of the placenta. The chorionic villi are enlarged and contain dense laminated connective tissue, and the capillaries distributed throughout the villi are compressed by this connective tissue proliferation. (Hematoxylin and eosin stain; magnification ×450) (Courtesy Centers for Disease Control and Prevention/Susan Lindsley, 1971, Public Health Image Library #2347.)

congenital syphilis from 67% to 89% in live-born infants and 91% to 97% in stillborn infants.

The gastrointestinal tract shows a pattern of mononuclear cell infiltration in the mucosa and submucosa, with subsequent thickening resulting from the ensuing fibrosis. This is most prominent in the small bowel.[140-142] An intense pancreatitis is often present, with a perivascular inflammatory infiltrate, obliteration of ductules and acini, reduction in the number of islets, and extensive fibrosis.[140] Oppenheimer and Hardy[140] found that 15 of 16 livers from infants who died before 9 weeks of age were abnormal; lesions varied considerably in severity but included inflammation in the interstitial stroma and perivascular network, especially in the area of the portal triads, with diffuse hepatitis and excessive extramedullary hematopoiesis.[140] Gummas have rarely been described in the liver of infants with congenital syphilis; cirrhosis also appears to be an uncommon complication.[140]

Renal involvement appears to be the consequence of injury to the glomeruli by immune complex deposition,[143] just as has been described for the glomerulitis of secondary syphilis in adults.[144] An epimembranous glomerulopathy[145] is common and is associated with two different forms of immune complex injury: one involving complement deposition in addition to IgA, IgM, and IgG and the other involving immune complexes without complement deposition along the basement membrane.[143] A perivascular inflammatory infiltrate, consisting of plasma cells and lymphocytes involving the interstitial tissues, is also prominent.[143,145] Elution studies have demonstrated the presence of antitreponemal antibodies in the eluate as well as treponemal antigen.[146]

The "pneumonia alba" of congenital syphilis is characterized by yellow-white, heavy, firm, and grossly enlarged lungs.[95] A marked increase in the amount of connective tissue in the interalveolar septa and the interstitium associated with collapse and loss of alveolar spaces explains the increased weight and density of the lung. This obliterative fibrosis of the lung is now reported only rarely.[140]

Widespread involvement of bones is characteristic of congenital syphilis. Radiographs of long bones show evidence of osteochondritis and periostitis, especially in the long bones and ribs. The excessive fibrosis occurring at the osseous-cartilaginous junction is referred to as "syphilitic granulation tissue" and contains numerous blood vessels surrounded by the inflammatory infiltrate.[95] Small islands of cartilage may persist in the ossified bone.[140] A subperiosteal deposit of osteoid, which can completely encircle the shaft of the long bone, is a feature of the periostitis.[124] An associated osteomyelitis (osteitis) usually is present and, when it involves the long bones, is called diaphysitis.[147] Microscopically, an inflammatory infiltrate with erosion of the trabeculae and prominent fibrosis is seen.[148] In the skull, the periosteal reaction eventually can lead to the radiographic feature of frontal bossing. The basic process of the osseous disturbance seems to involve a failure to convert cartilage in the normal sequence to mature bone.[144]

The skin may show vesicular or bullous lesions, which have fluid rich in treponemes. Guarner and associates[141] reported that a constant feature throughout the dermal tissues was concentric macrophage infiltrate around vessels, giving an onionskin appearance.

The neuropathologic features of congenital syphilis are comparable with those of acquired syphilis, except that the parenchymatous processes (general paresis, tabes dorsalis) are rare. Meningeal involvement is apparent as a discoloration and thickening of the basilar meninges,[95] especially around the brainstem and the optic chiasm. Microscopically, endarteritis typically is present, depending on the severity and chronicity of the infection as well as on the blood vessels involved. Various degrees of neuronal injury can ensue. As the infection resolves, fibrosis can occur, with formation of adhesions that obliterate the subarachnoid space, leading to an obstructive hydrocephalus or to a variety of cranial nerve palsies. Interstitial inflammation and fibrosis of the anterior lobe of the pituitary gland, at times accompanied by focal necrosis, also have been reported among infants with congenital syphilis.[149] The posterior lobe remains unaffected. An evolving anterior pituitary gumma was noted at autopsy in a 3-day-old infant with congenital syphilis that did not respond to treatment.[130]

Clinical Manifestations

Because of the protean clinical manifestations, syphilis, both acquired and congenital, has been described as one of the "great imitators."[27,150] Thus a high index of suspicion is needed for the clinician to consider syphilis in both the pregnant female and the newborn infant.

SYPHILIS IN PREGNANCY

Two caveats should be heeded by the clinician caring for pregnant women: any ulcer, regardless of location, that is painless, indurated, and indolent and fails to heal within 2 weeks warrants exclusion of syphilis as a diagnosis. Similarly, any generalized skin eruption, regardless of its morphology, should be viewed as secondary (disseminated) syphilis until proven otherwise.[151]

Whether pregnant or not, it is characteristic for the course of untreated acquired syphilis to progress through three or four stages over a period of many years. Most clinical definitions of acquired *T. pallidum* infection categorize early syphilis as including primary and secondary syphilis as well as early latent syphilis with a latency of less than 1 year[62] or less than 2 years (WHO) after infection. Late syphilis, on the other hand, consists of late latent, tertiary, and, depending on nomenclature, quaternary syphilis (or "metalues").

Primary Syphilis in Pregnancy

The time between infection with syphilis and the start of the first symptom can range from 10 to 90 days (average, 21 days), at which point a dark red macule or papule develops at the site of inoculation and rapidly progresses to an erosion called a chancre. It usually occurs as a single lesion, but there may be multiple lesions.[152] The size of the chancre increases to 0.5 to 2cm over the course of 1 to 2 weeks, until a typical, indolent, well-circumscribed, flat ulcer with a yellow-coated base and an indurated, nonundermined wall results. This is followed by edema and bilateral painless lymphadenopathy. Chancres often are unrecognized in women because they cause no symptoms and because their location on the labia minora, within the vagina, or on the cervix or perineum makes detection difficult. As a result, only 30% to 40% of infected women are diagnosed in the primary stage.[57,85] Two thirds of extragenital chancres occur orally or periorally; most of the rest occur perianally. Chancres rarely occur on the lips, tongue, tonsil, nipple, or fingers. Because the chancre can appear 1 to 3 weeks before a serologic response, direct detection of the pathogen (e.g., by darkfield microscopy) is vital in this phase of the disease.[153] The chancre lasts 3 to 8 weeks and then heals without treatment. The mechanism for healing is obscure; it is believed that local immunity is partly responsible because secondary lesions appear during or after the regression of the primary one. However, if adequate treatment is not administered, the infection progresses to the secondary stage.

Secondary Syphilis in Pregnancy

Two to 10 weeks after the primary lesions, an infected woman may experience secondary disease, characterized by fever, fatigue, weight loss, anorexia, pharyngitis, myalgia, arthralgia, and generalized lymphadenopathy. These constitutional symptoms are accompanied by various exanthems and alopecia. Because of the protean clinical manifestations, secondary syphilis is often misdiagnosed.[154-156] Lesions of secondary syphilis result from the dissemination of *T. pallidum* from syphilitic chancres, and the term *disseminated syphilis* probably would be more appropriate.[157]

The rash of secondary syphilis,[158] often the first clinical manifestation noticed, develops symmetrically in approximately 75% of untreated subjects and appears as rough, red, or reddish brown spots (syphilids); they occur most often on the palms, soles, and trunk, where they tend to follow skin lines. However, rashes with a different appearance may occur on any part of the body, and pustular, papular, lichenoid, nodular, ulcerative, plaquelike, annular, and even urticarial and granulomatous forms can occur. The vesiculobullous eruption that is common in congenital syphilis rarely occurs in adults. Contrary to a widely held belief, the exanthema can itch, especially in dark-skinned patients. Often the rash is very faint and not recognized at all. Rashes associated with secondary syphilis can already appear as the chancre is healing (in approximately 15%, the chancre is still present) or several weeks after the chancre has healed. Various mucosal manifestations can be of diagnostic importance and are present in one third to one half of patients. Mucosal plaques (representing superficial mucosal erosions) and syphilitic angina are the most frequent and can involve the oral cavity, vulva, vagina, or cervix. Localized enanthems or perlèche-like lesions are also possible. Expansive, smooth lesions (plaques lisses) and gray-white plaques (plaques opalines) are rare. Erythematous, moist plaques can occur in warm, moist, intertriginous regions, where initial papules enlarge and become exuberant, raised, wartlike lesions termed condylomata lata (often confused with condyloma acuminata, which are caused by human papillomavirus infection). Papules of the scalp can lead to "moth-eaten" alopecia. This hair loss can occasionally also affect eyebrows and eyelashes. Secondary lesions of the skin and mucous membranes are contagious.[158]

Generalized lymphadenopathy, fever, malaise, splenomegaly, sore throat, headache, and arthralgia (with a noticeable nocturnal pattern) can be present.[153] Other organ involvement may include gastritis, hepatitis,[159,160] glomerulonephritis or nephrotic syndrome,[161,162] periostitis,[163-165] uveitis, iritis, and meningitis.[157] *T. pallidum* has been isolated from the cerebrospinal fluid (CSF) of 30% of adults with untreated secondary syphilis.[63] The signs and symptoms of secondary syphilis usually resolve with or without treatment. But without treatment, the infection will progress to the latent and possibly late stages of disease.[55]

Latent Syphilis in Pregnancy

Subclinical or latent syphilis is defined as the period after infection when patients are seroreactive but demonstrate no clinical manifestations of disease. This latent phase can last for years.[166,167] It is sometimes interrupted during the first few (<4) years by recurrences of symptoms of secondary syphilis. Of note, treponemes can still be present in the blood intermittently and be passed across the placenta to the fetus. The first year after infection is considered "early latent," and the subsequent period "late latent" syphilis. This classification is based on the time period of communicability (not just to the fetus), which is higher in the first year after infection compared with later time points.[36] If the duration of syphilis infection cannot be determined, then the disease is classified as "latent syphilis of unknown duration." Approximately 60% of untreated patients in the late latent stage continue to have an asymptomatic course, whereas 30% to 40% develop symptoms of late or tertiary disease. Progress of disease from late latent to late symptomatic syphilis usually is prevented if appropriate antimicrobial therapy is given.[36]

Late Stages (Tertiary Disease) in Pregnancy

Knowledge about the clinical appearances of these late stages of acquired syphilis comes from two prospective and one retrospective study conducted with infected patients who did not receive therapy.[27] Mortality from untreated syphilis has been described to be about 8% to 14%.[124] After 15 years, three quarters of infected subjects show evidence of tertiary syphilis, 50% to 80% of whom have cardiovascular complications.[168,169] Cardiovascular involvement of tertiary syphilis most commonly involves the great vessels of the heart, where syphilitic aortic and pulmonary arteritis develop. One of the complications of this is aortic regurgitation. The inflammatory reaction also may cause stenosis of the coronary ostia, with resulting angina, myocardial insufficiency, and death.[170] The gummata of tertiary disease found in 9% of untreated subjects, are nonprogressive, localized nodules that can have central necrosis. Because these lesions are relatively quiescent, the term *benign tertiary syphilis* often is used. Spirochetes are extremely sparse or absent.

Approximately 15% of untreated infected subjects develop neurosyphilis in the tertiary stage, but in persons infected with HIV, manifestations of neurosyphilis can occur at any stage. Neurosyphilis may be asymptomatic or, if symptomatic, may occur in a variety of ways. Classic presentations include paralytic dementia, tabes dorsalis, amyotrophic lateral sclerosis, meningovascular syphilis, seizures, optic atrophy, and gummatous changes of the spinal cord. Neurosyphilis may resemble virtually any other neurologic disease.[170]

ACQUIRED SYPHILIS IN CHILDREN

Most recognized syphilitic disease in children is congenital (see later). Acquired syphilis in prepubertal children often resembles the clinical course of acquired syphilis in adults. Children with acquired syphilis should be assumed to have been infected through sexual abuse, unless another method of transmission can clearly be identified.[171-175]

CONGENITAL SYPHILIS

The spectrum of congenital syphilis is similar in many ways to that of other congenital infections in which the infecting organism spreads hematogenously from the pregnant woman to her fetus.[129] The extent of damage to the fetus depends on the stage of development when infection occurs and the elapsed time before treatment is initiated. With infection early in pregnancy and in the absence of therapy, fetal demise with spontaneous abortion (often after the first trimester) or late-term stillbirth occurs, but premature delivery or neonatal death also may occur.† In live-born infants, infection can be clinically recognizable or silent at birth (approximately two thirds of live-born cases are asymptomatic at birth but then develop signs and symptoms sometimes up to decades later).[93,178,179]

The postnatal clinical course of congenitally acquired syphilis has been divided somewhat arbitrarily into early and late stages.[27,93] Clinical manifestations appearing within the first 2 years of life are designated early, and those occurring after this time are called late. The clinical manifestations of early congenital syphilis appear as a direct result of active infection with resulting inflammation. Infants can have hepatosplenomegaly, lymphadenopathy, mucocutaneous lesions, osteochondritis and pseudoparalysis, edema, rash, hemolytic anemia, or thrombocytopenia, all of which usually appear within the first 2 to 8 weeks of life (Box 16-1). The clinical manifestations of late congenital syphilis represent the scars induced by initial lesions of early congenital syphilis or reactions to persistent and ongoing inflammation. These so-called stigmata of late congenital syphilis reflect the delayed expression of a prenatal insult. Manifestations of late congenital syphilis may involve the central nervous system (CNS), bones and joints, teeth, eyes, and skin and may not become apparent until many years after birth (Table 16-1).[180-182]

†References 4, 40, 66, 124, 176, 177.

Box 16-1 Clinical Manifestations of Early Congenital Syphilis*

- Osteochondritis, periostitis
- Snuffles, hemorrhagic rhinitis
- Condylomata lata
- Bullous lesions, palmar and plantar rash
- Mucous patches
- Hepatomegaly, splenomegaly
- Jaundice
- Nonimmune hydrops fetalis
- Generalized lymphadenopathy
- Central nervous system signs
  - Elevated cell count or protein in cerebrospinal fluid
- Hematologic findings
  - Hemolytic anemia
  - Diffuse intravascular coagulation
  - Thrombocytopenia
- Pneumonitis
- Nephrotic syndrome
- Placental villitis or vasculitis (unexplained enlarged placenta)
- Intrauterine growth restriction

Data from Rathbun KC: Congenital syphilis: a proposal for improved surveillance, diagnosis and treatment, Sex Transm Dis *10:102-107, 1983.*
**Arranged in decreasing order of importance.*

Table 16-1 Clinical Manifestations of Late Congenital Syphilis

Dentition	Hutchinson teeth, mulberry molars (Moon's or Fournier's molars)
Eye	Interstitial keratitis, healed chorioretinitis, secondary glaucoma (uveitis), corneal scarring
Ear	Eighth nerve deafness
Nose and face	"Saddle nose," protuberant mandible
Skin	Rhagades
Central nervous system	Mental retardation, arrested hydrocephalus, convulsive disorders, optic nerve atrophy, juvenile general paresis, cranial nerve palsies
Bones and joints	"Saber shins," Higouménakis sign, Clutton joints

Early Congenital Syphilis

After fetal infection occurs, any organ system can be affected because of the transplacental hematogenous spirochetal dissemination (see Box 16-1). The onset of most clinical findings of early congenital syphilis occurs between birth and about 3 months of age, with most cases occurring within the first 5 weeks of age.[138,140,143,148,183-187]

Intrauterine Growth Restriction. Intrauterine growth restriction of prenatally infected infants may be noted at birth.[168] The effect of syphilis on the growth of the fetus in utero is likely to be related to the timing and severity of the fetal infection.[188] Case reports describe newborns with congenital syphilis as small for gestational age (SGA).[189] Whether SGA was the result of syphilitic infection or other cofactors (e.g., use of illicit intravenous [IV] drugs by the mother)[190] that affected fetal growth was not known. Historically, severely infected infants with congenital syphilis have been described as a premature infant with marasmus, a pot belly, "old man" facies, and withered skin.[124] The degree of extreme early-onset failure to thrive (FTT) has been correlated with the frequently encountered pathologic finding of intense pancreatitis and inflammation of the gastrointestinal tract.[140] Rectal bleeding caused by syphilitic ileitis with ulcer formation and associated intestinal obstruction has also been reported to be linked to this appearance.[143] Last, involvement of the anterior pituitary gland in congenital syphilis can manifest as persistent hypoglycemia beyond the early neonatal period and through such endocrine abnormalities contribute to the FTT.[149]

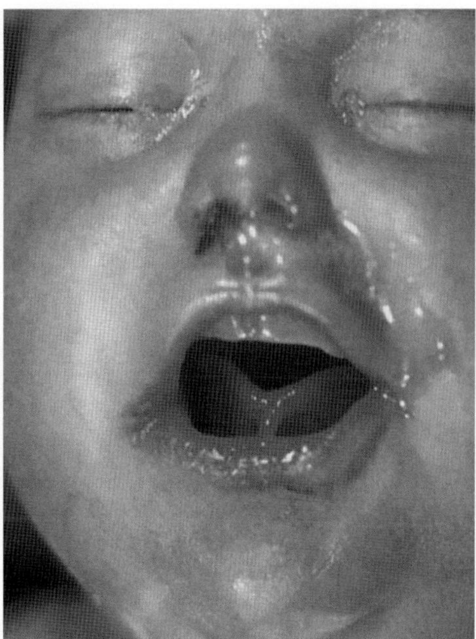

Figure 16-3 The face of a newborn infant with congenital syphilis displaying snuffles. (Courtesy Centers for Disease Control and Prevention/Dr. Norman Cole, 1963, Public Health Image Library #2246.)

Mucocutaneous Manifestations. Mucous patches may be seen in the mouth and genital tract[168,191] and are more prevalent in infants with severe systemic disease.[192] After the first 2 or 3 months of life, condylomata can arise on such affected mucous membranes or other areas of skin affected by moisture or friction, for instance, the perioral area, especially the nares and the angles of the mouth, as well as the perianal area.[193,194] These highly contagious areas are flat or wartlike and moist. The condylomata can be single or multiple and may occur in the absence of other signs of infection. Rhinitis, coryza, or snuffles (Fig. 16-3) indicate involvement of the upper respiratory tract mucosa. This manifestation usually appears in the first week of life and seldom later than the third month. It was reported in two thirds of patients in the early literature[195] but now appears less common.[191] A mucus discharge develops, with character similar to that of discharge during viral upper respiratory tract infections, but it is more severe and persists longer. The discharge can become progressively more profuse and occasionally is blood-tinged. Snuffles also has been associated with laryngitis and an aphonic cry.[191,196]

A syphilitic rash appears in as many as 70% of infected infants.[197] It may be apparent at birth or develop during the first few weeks of life.[191,196] The typical skin eruption consists of small, oval, copper-red maculopapular lesions, reminiscent of secondary acquired syphilitic lesions that subsequently become coppery brown.[194] The hands and feet often are most severely affected. As the rash changes color, very fine superficial desquamation or scaling can occur, particularly on the palms and soles (Fig. 16-4). If the rash is present at birth, it often is widely disseminated and bullous and is called pemphigus syphiliticus, typically involving the palms and soles (Fig. 16-5).[194,198] The lesions vary in size and can contain a cloudy hemorrhagic fluid that teems with treponemes. When these bullae rupture, they leave a denuded area that can undergo extensive maceration and crusting. Pemphigus syphiliticus evolves over 1 to 3 weeks, and is followed by desquamation and crusting. As the rash fades, the lesions become coppery or dusky red,

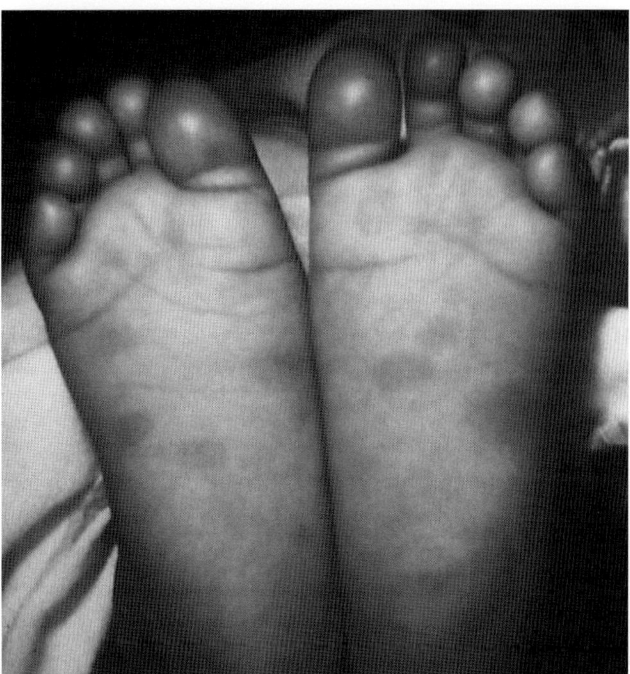

Figure 16-4 This newborn presented with symptoms of congenital syphilis that included lesions on the soles of both feet. (Courtesy Centers for Disease Control and Prevention, 1970, Public Health Image Library #4148.)

and pigmentation may persist. Other maculopapular types of eruptions are also found in early congenital syphilis. The lesions can be annular or circinate or can have the appearance of any other kind of lesion seen in acquired secondary syphilis. Petechial lesions can result from thrombocytopenia. Ectodermal changes in syphilitic infants include suppuration and exfoliation of the nails, loss of hair and eyebrows, choroiditis, and iritis.[199] Fissures develop about the lips,

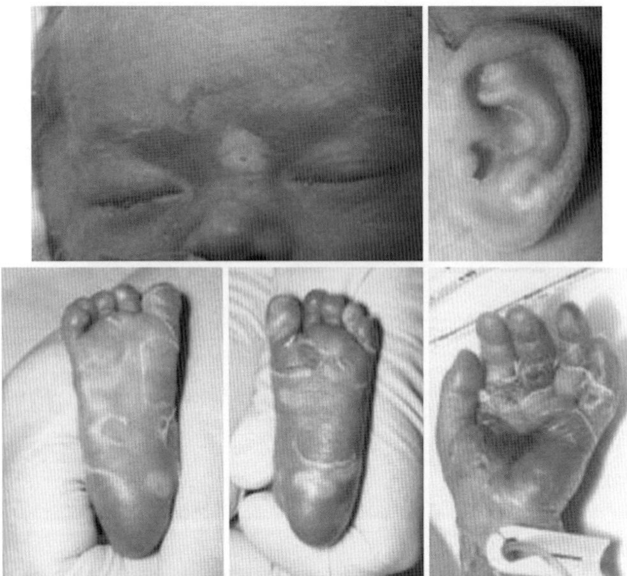

Figure 16-5 This newborn infant with congenital syphilis displays multiple, punched-out, pale, blistered lesions on the ear and the bridge of the nose; also shown is an associated desquamation of palms and plantar surfaces of the feet. (From Battin M, Voss L: Beware of infants with respiratory distress, rash, and hepatomegaly at birth: a case of congenital syphilis, *N Z Med J* 120:U2448, 2007.)

nares, and anus. They bleed readily and heal with scarring. A cluster of scars radiating around the mouth is named rhagades and is a characteristic of late congenital syphilis. Comparable eruptions also can be found in other body folds or intertriginous areas. Healing, with possible desquamation and crusting of the various skin lesions, occurs over the course of 1 to 3 weeks.[200,201] All mucocutaenous lesions and discharges contain abundant spirochetes and are contagious.[195]

Hepatomegaly, Hepatitis, Splenomegaly, and Lymphadenopathy. Hepatomegaly is present in nearly all infants with congenital syphilis and may occur in the absence of splenomegaly, although the reverse is not true (unlike congenital cytomegalovirus [CMV] infection).[191] Hepatomegaly and ascites are attributed largely to heart failure but may be caused in part by hepatic infection and extramedullary hematopoiesis.[202] Hepatitis appears to be an early manifestation and can be detected as elevation of aminotransferase levels even in fetal blood. Neonatal syphilitic hepatitis is associated with visible spirochetes on biopsy of liver tissue. Jaundice, which has been recorded in 33% of patients,[191] can be caused by syphilitic hepatitis or by the hemolytic component of the disease and thus be associated with elevation predominantly of direct or indirect bilirubin levels, respectively. Jaundice may, in fact, be the only initial manifestation of the disease. Hepatic dysfunction in the form of elevated serum aminotransferases, alkaline phosphatase, and direct bilirubin initially can worsen with initiation of penicillin therapy and can persist for several weeks irrespective of treatment.[203-205] The prothrombin time may also be delayed.[204] Splenomegaly is present in half of such cases. Generalized nonsuppurative adenopathy, including epitrochlear sites, may be present in some cases.[168,191] These lymph nodes can be as large as 1cm in diameter but typically are nontender and firm. If an infant has palpable epitrochlear nodes, the diagnosis of syphilis is highly probable.[93] However, generalized enlargement of the lymph nodes is quite uncommon in congenital syphilis.

Hematologic Manifestations. Anemia, thrombocytopenia, and leukopenia or leukocytosis are common findings in congenital syphilis.[183] A characteristic feature in the immediate newborn period is that of a Coombs-negative hemolytic anemia. The hemolytic process is often accompanied by cryoglobulinemia, immune complex formation, and macroglobulinemia. The hemolysis, like the liver disease, is refractory to therapy and may persist for weeks. After the neonatal period, chronic nonhemolytic anemia can develop.[206,207] Other findings include polychromasia and erythroblastemia. Although the leukocyte counts usually are within the normal range,[206] leukopenia, leukocytosis, or a leukemoid reaction can all occur.[191] Lymphocytosis and monocytosis may also be features. Thrombocytopenia, related to decreased platelet survival rather than to insufficient production of platelets, often is present and can be the only manifestation of early congenital syphilis. Hemophagocytosis has been described and may play an important role in the pathogenesis of anemia and thrombocytopenia.[208] Hydrops fetalis, or diffuse edema, results from anemia-related congestive heart failure, and a negative Coombs test in the setting of hydrops strongly suggests the etiology of congenital syphilis.[209]

Bone Involvement. Bone findings[210] are a frequent manifestation of early congenital syphilis and occur in 60% to 80% of untreated cases. They usually occur as multiple symmetric lesions. Overall, the bone abnormalities are due to periostitis and cortical demineralization, mostly in the metaphyseal and diaphyseal portions of long bones, as well as osteochondritis, which affects the joints.[210] The changes are nonspecific and variable, ranging from radiopaque bands to actual fragmentation and apparent destruction with mottled areas of radiolucency. Frequently, an enhanced zone of provisional calcification (radiopaque band) is associated with osteoporosis immediately beneath the dense zone.[147] The Wegner sign represents points of calcified cartilage along the nutrient cartilage canal. The demineralization and osseous destruction of the upper medial tibial metaphysis is called the Wimberger sign (Fig. 16-6).[196] Epiphyseal separation may occur as a result of a fracture of the brittle layer of calcified cartilage. In severe cases, the radiolucent areas that probably represent a growth arrest abnormality can appear as columns, giving a "celery stick" appearance of alternating bands of longitudinal translucency and relative density.[196] Solomon and Rosen[211, 212] reported that in more than one third of 112 infants with congenital syphilis, radiographic findings were consistent with trauma of bone made more fragile by syphilitic infection. Whereas the above described findings of periostitis require about 16 weeks for radiographic diagnosis, osteochondritic events in the major joints already can be evident radiographically 5 weeks after fetal infection has occurred.[213]

Obstetric radiography may allow for the in utero diagnosis of fetal syphilis by demonstrating periosteal cloaking.[214] Maternal treatment has been associated with radiologic

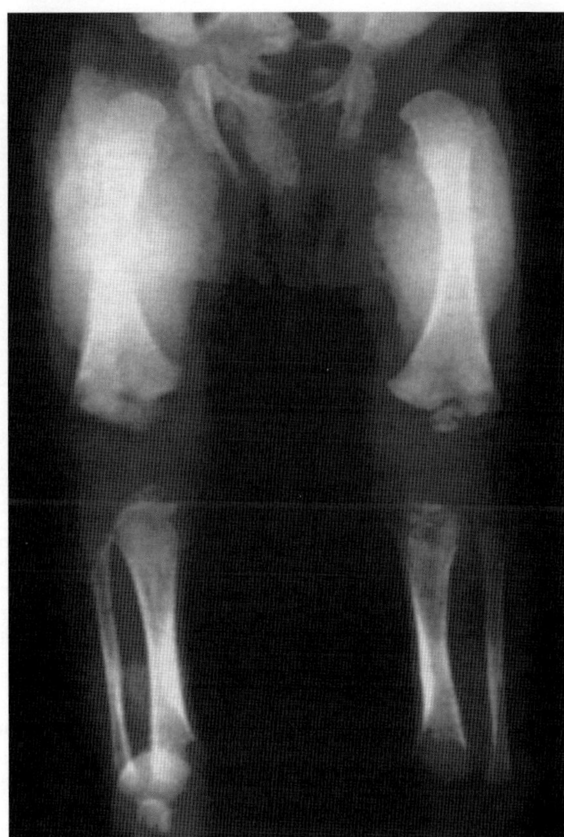

Figure 16-6 Anteroposterior film of both lower extremities of a 1-month-old infant with congenital syphilis showing demineralization and osseous destruction of the proximal medial tibial metaphysis bilaterally (Wimberger sign).

resolution of these lesions. Bone scans have been performed in very few patients; they reveal diffuse abnormalities when performed, but such scans are neither helpful nor recommended.[215-217] Because of their frequency and early appearance, the radiographic changes in the bones, both osteochondritis and periostitis, are of diagnostic value.[148]

Most bone lesions are not clinically discernible, except in the pseudoparalysis of Parrot,[218,219] where the bony changes or a superimposed fracture, or both, lead to pain, causing the infant to refuse to move the involved extremity. Clinically, it can manifest as irritability in an infant of a few weeks of age, who does not move one of the limbs.[189] The upper extremities are affected more frequently than lower extremities, and unilateral involvement predominates. This clinical picture can mimic Erb palsy but rarely is present at birth.[220] Bony involvement usually resolves spontaneously (i.e., even without therapy) during the first 6 months of life.[168,189,218,221]

Nervous System and Ocular Manifestations. Without therapy, approximately 15% of infants with congenital syphilis develop findings such as meningitis, meningeal irritation, bulging fontanelle, cranial nerve palsies, seizures, hydrocephalus, or abnormal pituitary function.[168,222] Of note, neurosyphilis may occur in the absence of any other overt sign or symptom of congenital syphilis.[223]

There are two primary clinical presentations of neurosyphilis, although overlap may be considerable. Acute syphilitic leptomeningitis appears during the first year of life, usually between the ages of 3 and 6 months of untreated infants. Signs can suggest acute bacterial meningitis, including a stiff neck, progressive vomiting, Kernig sign, bulging fontanelles, separation of the suture, and hydrocephalus.[222] In contrast with this clinical picture, CSF reveals abnormalities consistent with an aseptic meningitis, with up to 200 mononuclear cells per mm,[224] a modest increase in protein (50 to 200 mg/dL), and a normal glucose value. The CSF Venereal Disease Research Laboratory (VDRL) test is positive. This is the one form of CNS involvement that responds to specific therapy.[168,196,222]

Chronic meningovascular syphilis, on the other hand, generally presents toward the end of the first year of life and can have a protracted course, resulting in progressive hydrocephalus, cranial nerve palsies or vascular lesions of the brain, and gradual intellectual deterioration.[222] The hydrocephalus is of low grade, progressive, and communicating as a result of obstruction in the basilar cisterns. Cranial nerve palsies and seizures can complicate the picture. The seventh nerve most often is involved, but the third, fourth, and sixth cranial nerves also can be affected. Optic atrophy can be preceded by papilledema.

A variety of cerebrovascular syndromes have been described, but they are rare. Cerebral infarction results from syphilitic endarteritis and can occur between the first and second years of life, commonly manifesting as acute hemiplegia or later in life, manifesting as multiple intracranial aneurysm.[225] Convulsions frequently complicate this clinical picture early in life. In addition, involvement of the pituitary gland in congenital syphilis is relatively common, occurring in approximately 40% of autopsy cases, and consists of interstitial inflammation and fibrosis with gumma formation in the anterior lobe. Clinical disease in affected infants is manifested by persistent hypoglycemia and diabetes insipidus.[149,226]

The occurrence of syphilitic involvement of the eye in early congenital syphilis is rare. Chorioretinitis, salt-and-pepper fundus, glaucoma, uveitis, cataract,[227] and chancres of the eyelid have been described.[124] The young infant rarely manifests the signs of photophobia and diminution in vision that occur in older patients. Congenital glaucoma can occur and should be a diagnostic consideration in the presence of blepharospasm, cloudy cornea, enlarged cornea (diameter exceeding 12 mm), and excessive tearing. Inflammation of the uveal tract, including the iris and ciliary body anteriorly and the choroid posteriorly, affects the retina because of the close anatomic relationship of the cornea to the structures of the uveal tract.[124] In consequence, chorioretinitis, rather than uveitis, is the more commonly diagnosed ocular problem in infancy.[227] Rarely, a chancre of the eyelid appears 4 weeks after birth, presumably resulting from recently developed syphilitic lesions of the maternal genitalia.[124]

Other Findings. *Fever* has been reported to accompany other signs of congenital syphilis in infants beyond the immediate newborn period.[203,228] *Pneumonia alba,* a fibrosing pneumonitis, occurs in a minority of cases in the developed world but still represents a frequent finding in developing countries.[93] The classic radiographic appearance is one of complete opacification of both lung fields and is thus termed pneumonia alba. More commonly, a diffuse infiltrate involving all lung areas is seen on chest radiographs. Follow-up evaluation of children who have recovered from congenital syphilis has shown that at least 10% may develop chronic pulmonary disease, particularly if premature and required mechanical ventilation.[93] The clinical picture of *nephrotic syndrome* may appear at 2 or 3 months of age, the predominant manifestation being generalized edema, including pretibial, scrotal, and periorbital areas, together with ascites.[229-233] Rarely, the infant can have hematuria with less severe proteinuria but more profound azotemia, which suggests that a glomerulitis predominates. *Myocarditis*[140] has been found at autopsy in approximately 10% of infants who die, although the clinical significance of this finding is not clear. *Gastrointestinal* presentations include rectal bleeding caused by syphilitic ileitis, necrotizing enterocolitis, malabsorption secondary to fibrosis of the gastrointestinal tract, and fetal bowel dilatation seen on antenatal ultrasonography. Some children with symptomatic congenital syphilis also may present with sepsis caused by other bacteria, including *Escherichia coli*, group B streptococci, and *Yersinia* species, presumed to be secondary to the breakdown of the gastrointestinal mucosal barrier.[184,234]

Late Congenital Syphilis

In patients older than 2 years, late congenital syphilis can manifest as (1) the stigmata of the disorder that represent the scars of initial lesions or developmental changes induced by the early infection; (2) ongoing inflammation, although *T. pallidum* is not demonstrable; or (3) a persistently positive result on treponemal serologic tests for syphilis in the absence of apparent disease (see Table 16-1).[62,66,178] Treatment of neonates with congenital syphilis has nearly eliminated these consequences in developed countries, but late manifestations occur in approximately 40% of untreated survivors. Many of these manifestations appear not to be reversible with antibiotic treatment.[93,235]

Mucocutaneous Manifestations. An infrequent sign of late congenital syphilis is linear scars that become fissured or ulcerated, resulting in deeper scars called rhagades.[236] These scars are located around body orifices, including the mouth, nostrils, genitalia and anus.[124] The sequelae of syphilitic rhinitis include failure of the maxilla to grow fully, resulting in a concave configuration in the middle section of the face with relative protuberance of the mandible and an associated high palatal arch. Inflammation of the nasal mucosa can affect the cartilage, leading to destruction of the underlying bone and perforation of the nasal septum. The resulting depression of the roof of the septum gives the appearance of a "saddle nose."[124]

Bone and Joint Findings. Bone involvement in late congenital syphilis is relatively infrequent in comparison with the frequent occurrence of abnormalities in early congenital syphilis.[51,124] The sequelae of prolonged periosteal reactions can involve the skull and result in frontal bossing (olympian brow), anterior bowing of the midtibia (saber shin), perforation of the palate,[237] or thickening of the sternoclavicular portion of the clavicle (Higouménakis sign; for unknown reasons, this tends to occur on the side of dominant handedness).[180] Joint involvement is rare. Clutton joints are symmetric, painless, sterile, synovial effusions, usually localized to the knees.[238,239] Perforation of the hard palate almost is pathognomic of congenital syphilis.[124,240]

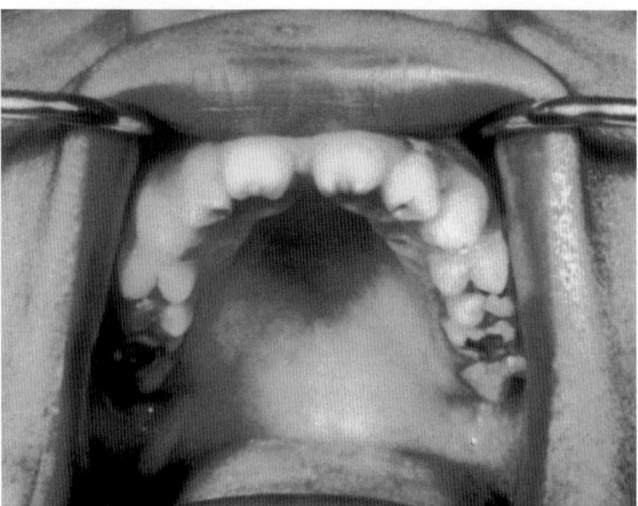

Figure 16-7 Photograph of Hutchinson teeth resulting from congenital syphilis. Hutchinson teeth are a congenital anomaly in which the permanent incisor teeth are narrow and notched. Note the notched edges and "screwdriver" shape of the central incisors. (Courtesy Centers for Disease Control and Prevention/Susan Lindsley, 1971, Public Health Image Library #2385.)

Dental Involvement. Syphilitic vasculitis around the time of birth can damage the developing tooth buds and lead to dental anomalies called Hutchinson teeth—abnormal permanent upper central incisors that are peg shaped and notched, usually with obvious thinning and discoloration of enamel in the area of the notching. They are widely spaced and shorter than the lateral incisors; the width of the biting surface is less than that of the gingival margin[241] (Fig. 16-7), and mulberry molars (also known as a Moon or Fournier molar), which are multicuspid first molars where the tooth's grinding surface (narrower than that at the gingival margin), has many small cusps instead of the usual four well-formed cusps[236] (Fig. 16-8). The enamel itself tends to be poorly developed.[124,180] Radiographic studies can lead to the diagnosis even while deciduous teeth are in place. Deciduous teeth are largely unaffected except for a possible predisposition to dental caries.[124] Early treatment (<3-4 months of age) may prevent these dental changes of syphilis.[235]

Nervous System, Ear, and Ocular Manifestations. The same manifestations of neurosyphilis seen in acquired syphilis may occur in congenital syphilis and can include mental retardation, arrested hydrocephalus, convulsive disorders, juvenile general paresis, and cranial nerve abnormalities, including deafness and blindness, which is due to optic nerve atrophy.[222] Paresis is seen more frequently and tabes dorsalis less frequently in the congenital form than in the acquired form of the disease.[80,124,195] Overall, these findings are relatively uncommon.[242] However, eighth nerve deafness develops in approximately 3% of untreated cases. Together, Hutchinson teeth, interstitial keratitis, and eighth nerve deafness comprise the Hutchinson triad,[80] with eighth nerve deafness the least common component of

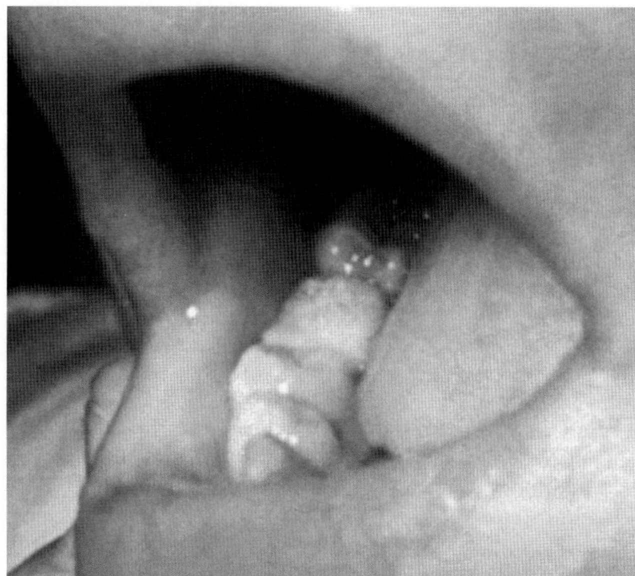

Figure 16-8 Photograph of mulberry molar resulting from congenital syphilis. Mulberry molar is a condition where the first lower molar tooth has become dome shaped because of malformation caused by congenital syphilis. (Courtesy Centers for Disease Control and Prevention/Susan Lindsley, 1971, Public Health Image Library #2386.)

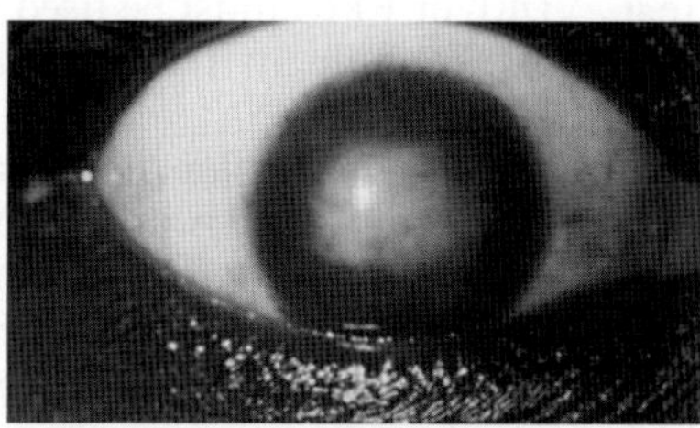

Figure 16-9 Photograph depicts the presence of a diffuse stromal haze in the cornea of a child, known as interstitial keratitis, which was due to late-stage congenital syphilis. Interstitial keratitis, which is an inflammation of the connective tissue structure of the cornea, usually affects both eyes and can occur as a complication to congenital or acquired syphilis. Interstitial keratitis usually occurs in children older than 2 years. (Courtesy Centers for Disease Control and Prevention/Susan Lindsley, 1973, Public Health Image Library #6837.)

the triad. [243] Osteochondritis affecting the otic capsule can lead to cochlear degeneration and fibrous adhesions, resulting in eighth nerve deafness as well as vertigo. Although the deafness usually occurs in the first decade, it may not appear until the third or fourth decade of life. It often starts with sudden loss of high-frequency hearing, with normal conversational tones affected later.[180,244,245]

Eye involvement can lead to interstitial keratitis, secondary glaucoma, or corneal scarring. In keratitis, a severe inflammatory reaction begins in one eye, detectable as a ground-glass appearance of the cornea (Fig. 16-9), accompanied by vascularization of the adjacent sclera, then generally becomes bilateral over the ensuing weeks to months. Spirochetes are not detectable in these lesions.[246] Symptoms include photophobia, pain, excessive lacrimation, and blurred vision. Patients can have conjunctival injection, miosis, keratitis, or anterior uveitis, or a combination of these findings. Interstitial keratitis is considered preventable if treatment is given before age 3 months.[235] Interstitial keratitis usually appears at puberty and is not affected by penicillin therapy but responds transiently to corticosteroid treatment.[247] It often has a relapsing course that can result in secondary glaucoma or corneal clouding. Early retinal involvement or hydrocephalus can lead to optic atrophy.[80]

Diagnosis

The diagnosis of syphilis, whether congenital or acquired, is usually suspected based on clinical and epidemiologic findings and ideally then confirmed by direct identification of treponemes in clinical specimens, supported by positive serologic findings.[248] In clinical practice, however, diagnosis is most often made by clinical findings supported by serologic methods alone.[249,250]

DIRECT IDENTIFICATION

Currently available methods to identify *T. pallidum* in clinical specimens obtained from a primary chancre or active secondary lesions in the mother or any lesion, body fluid, or tissue biopsy in an infant are (1) darkfield microscopy, (2) direct fluorescent antibody (DFA) staining, (3) demonstration of the organism by special stains on histopathologic examination, (4) the rabbit infectivity test, and (5) detection of *T. pallidum* DNA.[251] Ideal starting material is lesion exudate or tissue material, including placenta or umbilical cord. Specimens can also be scraped from moist mucocutaneous lesions or aspirated from a regional lymph node. The scaly skin eruption of syphilis is not a good source of material for darkfield microscopy. Bullae should be aspirated with a sterile syringe and needle. Papules or condylomata should be cleaned thoroughly with physiologic saline solution with no additives, then abraded with gauze until oozing occurs to collect serum rather than blood. For darkfield microscopy, a sterile glass slide is applied to the exudate, which then is covered by a drop of normal saline and a coverslip. Evaluation of these slides requires much experience and must be done immediately (within 5-10 minutes) on freshly obtained tissue because these corkscrew-shaped organisms are identified by their characteristic movements. Because about 10^5organisms/mL are required for visualization, a negative darkfield examination does not rule out syphilis. Nonpathogenic commensal spirochetes, for instance, of the oral flora, can be confused with *T. pallidum*, even by experienced examiners. Darkfield microscopy of oral lesions should not be performed for this reason, unless direct fluorescent antibody techniques are used that allow the examiner to distinguish *T. pallidum* from nonpathogenic treponemes. For experienced examiners, the sensitivity of darkfield microscopy ranges from 79% to 97%, specificity from 77% to 100%. If the result of the initial darkfield examination is negative, it should be repeated on at least 2 successive days to confirm a negative result. If a darkfield microscope is unavailable, a DFA stain for *T. pallidum* can be used[138]: Exudate is collected in capillary tubes or slides and stained with specific antibody in a DFA or indirect fluorescent antibody (IFA) tests for *T. pallidum*. These tests use either monoclonal or polyclonal antibodies against *T. pallidum* that are directly fluorescein tagged or use a second fluorescein-tagged antibody (IFA) to detect the primary antibody-antigen complex.[252]

Polymerase chain reaction (PCR)-based tests have replaced the rabbit infectivity test (RIT) as the reference standard for syphilis diagnostic tests. The PCR assay is capable of detecting an amount of purified treponemal DNA equivalent to that of only a few organisms (about 0.01 pg).[43] Compared with isolation of the organism by rabbit infectivity testing, the sensitivity and specificity of PCR on CSF is 65% to 71% and 97% to 100%, respectively.[119,253-257] *T. pallidum* DNA has been detected by PCR in such body fluids as amniotic fluid and infant blood, cerebrospinal fluid, and endotracheal aspirate.[119,253,256] The RIT involves intratesticular inoculation of the specimen into a rabbit and awaiting serologic seroconversion and orchitis, with subsequent visualization of motile spirochetes by darkfield microscopy in testicular tissue; it has a sensitivity of less than 10 organisms.[258] RIT, however, is performed only in research laboratories and may take several months for identification of the organism.

INDIRECT IDENTIFICATION

Serologic assays have played a prominent role in the clinical diagnosis of syphilis since the early 1900s.[259] Nontreponemal antibody tests detect a nonspecific immune reaction and consist of the rapid plasma reagin (RPR) and VDRL assay. Treponemal antibody tests are serologic tests that detect a specific interaction between serum immunoglobulins and surface antigens of *T. pallidum*. Both nontreponemal and treponemal tests have their advantages and disadvantages. In most circumstances, both need to be used in conjunction, to make the serodiagnosis of infection with syphilis.

Nontreponemal Tests

Nontreponemal tests for syphilis detect antibodies to cardiolipin (diphosphatidylglycerol), a component of normal cell membranes in mammalian tissue. The original test, as described by Wassermann, used syphilitic tissue as complement-fixing antigen to detect the presence of antibody (i.e., reagin, a term that should not be used anymore because it is easily confused with IgE), which is induced by *T. pallidum*. Extracts of other normal tissue, such as beef heart, had similar properties, and purification and standardization of these materials led to the use as antigen of preparations containing cardiolipin.[259] Diphosphatidylglycerol constitutes only a small proportion of the lipids of *T. pallidum*, and these organisms may in fact be unable to synthesize this substance at all; it is possible that they incorporate it from damaged host tissues.[260] Thus production of anticardiolipin antibody could reflect an autoimmune host response to a slightly altered or a differently presented cardiolipin. In this context, it is interesting that anticardiolipin antibody reflects ongoing tissue damage, its detection correlating closely with the amount of activity in the early stages of syphilis infection. These observations may explain why patients with autoimmune diseases, such as systemic lupus erythematosus, characteristically have positive nontreponemal test results as well.[259]

The currently available nontreponemal tests, the RPR and the VDRL slide test, all use purified cardiolipin in lecithin-cholesterol liposomes; both nontreponemal tests measure both IgG and IgM antibodies.[111,261,262] The RPR test is positive in approximately 85% of cases of primary syphilis and in 98% of cases of secondary syphilis. VDRL is positive in approximately 80% of primary cases and in 95% of secondary cases (Table 16-2). The VDRL is the only serologic assay approved for testing reactivity of cerebrospinal fluid.[110,240] RPR and VDRL results are reported as dilutions or titers so that a relative degree of reactivity can be determined. Changes of two dilutions (i.e., a fourfold change from, e.g., 1:2 to 1:8) are considered significant when assessing disease activity. The RPR titer is often one to two dilutions higher than the VDRL test.[62] When nontreponemal tests are used to monitor treatment response, the same specific test (e.g., VDRL or RPR) must be used throughout the follow-up period, preferably by the same laboratory, to ensure comparability of results.[153]

Table 16-2 Seroreactivity of Common Tests for Untreated Syphilis

	% POSITIVE			
Test	**Primary Stage**	**Secondary Stage**	**Latent Stage**	**Tertiary Stage**
VDRL or RPR	80-85	95-98	75	<66
FTA-ABS, TP-PA	75-85	100	100	100

FTA-ABS, Fluorescent treponemal antibody, absorbed with non–*Treponema pallidum* treponemes; *RPR*, rapid plasma reagin; *TP-PA*, *T. pallidum* particle agglutination; *VDRL*, Venereal Disease Research Laboratory.

These quantitative titers help define disease activity and monitor response to therapy, that is, a fourfold decrease suggests adequate therapy, whereas a fourfold increase indicates active disease (treatment failure or reinfection). The quantitative nontreponemal test usually decreases fourfold within 6 months after adequate therapy for primary or secondary syphilis and usually becomes nonreactive within 1 year after successful therapy if the infection was treated during the early stages (primary or secondary syphilis). The patient usually becomes seronegative within 2 years, even if the initial titter was high or the infection was congenital.[62,263,264] But even without treatment, the VDRL titer slowly declines and is in fact negative in one third of patients with late syphilis.[110] Of importance, mothers with persistently negative nontreponemal test results do not pass the infection on to their offspring.[265] A small minority of patients will remain serofast, with persisting low positive titers despite receiving adequate therapy. This serofast state is more common in patients treated for latent or tertiary syphilis.

These tests occasionally produce positive results in patients for whom there is no evidence of syphilitic infection, called "biologic false-positive" (BFP; this term is meant to distinguish BFPs from positive reactions resulting from technical errors (e.g., Wharton jelly contamination in cord blood specimens leads to technical false-positive reactions).[240,266] Nontreponemal antibody cross reacts with more than 200 non–*T. pallidum* spirochetal antigens (but not with the agents of Lyme disease), and thus can produce false-positive results. Usually, BFP test results have titers less than 1:8 and a negative confirmatory treponemal test but are reported with a frequency of 1% to 20%.[153,259,267] They are classified as either acute (<6 months) or chronic.

Acute BFP reactions can be associated with other infections (Epstein-Barr virus, varicella, measles, malaria, tuberculosis, brucellosis, mumps, lymphogranuloma venereum, and hepatitis, among others). Chronic BFP reactions are often associated with advancing age, autoimmune diseases and chronic inflammatory processes (e.g., systemic lupus erythematosus, polyarteritis nodosa, antiphospholipid syndrome, chronic liver disease, endocarditis), and malignancy (especially if associated with production of excess IgM), or, rarely, with pregnancy itself.[153,267] Among HIV-positive patients, 10% to 30% demonstrate false-positive nonspecific reactions.[268] The antibody detected by the VDRL test in chronic BFP reactions predominantly is IgM, whereas in syphilis, it mainly is IgG; patients with chronic BFP reactions and systemic lupus erythematosus commonly also have a reactive fluorescent treponemal antibody absorption (FTA-ABS) test (see later).

False-negative results can occur when a high concentration of antibody inhibits agglutination (the prozone phenomenon), which can be avoided with serial dilutions of the serum. This occurs in approximately 1% to 2% of individuals, usually those with secondary syphilis.[269-271] Failure to recognize a prozone effect in maternal serum tested during pregnancy has resulted in failure to diagnose congenital syphilis.[271] Nontreponemal test results may also be falsely negative (i.e., nonreactive) in early (prechancre state) primary syphilis, latent syphilis of long duration, and late congenital syphilis, because, over the course of time, even some untreated patients may revert to seronegative nontreponemal status.[153,272-274] In summary, nontreponemal tests are used primarily for screening (i.e., to establish a presumptive diagnosis) and monitoring of therapy.[275] In most instances, a nontreponemal positive reaction is followed up with a treponemal specific test for confirmation.

Treponema-Specific Serologic Tests

Infection with *T. pallidum* causes the host to produce antitreponemal antibodies, which are detected by specific assays, including the FTA-ABS test and the treponemal-specific microhemagglutination test (MHA-TP), now replaced by the *T. pallidum* particle agglutination test (TP-PA). FTA-ABS and TP-PA tests measure both IgG and IgM antibodies directed against lyophilized *T. pallidum*–Nichols strain antigen. For the FTA-ABS test, antigen is fixed on a slide, the patient's serum allowed to react with antigen, and the bound antibody is then detected with fluorescent-labeled antihuman immunoglobulin antibody, identified by fluorescent microscopy. Test sera are usually preabsorbed with extracts from nonpathogenic *Treponema phagedenis* to eliminate group-reactive antibody, rendering the FTA-ABS relatively specific for disease with virulent treponemal species. However, the FTA-ABS test is expensive, time consuming, and requires a fluorescence microscope and a highly trained technician. It is not recommended for general screening but for confirmation of positive nontreponemal tests and the diagnosis of later stages of syphilis in which the results of nontreponemal tests may be negative. Microhemagglutination tests, and specifically, the TP-PA test, depend on the passive hemagglutination of erythrocytes or latex particles that have been coated with Nichols strain *T. pallidum* antigen. These tests have been automated, are easy to perform, and relative inexpensive.[276-283] *Treponema*-specific tests are positive in 75% (TP-PA) to 85% (FTA-ABS) of patients with primary syphilis and in 100% of patients with secondary syphilis (see Table 16-2).[115,276] Of note, unlike the nontreponemal tests, titers of the treponemal tests are irrelevant because they do not correlate with disease activity. False-positive results of specific treponemal tests rarely occur but may do so in patients with other spirochetal diseases, including Lyme disease, leptospirosis, rat-bite fever, relapsing fever, and diseases caused by other pathogenic *Treponema* spp. (e.g., yaws, pinta).[93] A few disease states, such as systemic lupus erythematosus, polyarteritis, or related conditions, and, in one report, even pregnancy, are said to cause a false-positive FTA-ABS result.[284] Nontreponemal tests can be used to differentiate Lyme disease from syphilis because, for instance, the VDRL test is nonreactive in Lyme disease. Although treponemal-specifc tests are unlikely to revert to a nonreactive state after treatment of the infected patient, unless treatment was given very early in infected adults, the majority of successfully treated early congenital syphilis cases will serorevert (become negative) their treponemal tests by 18 months.[285]

Other Serologic Tests

Specific treponemal IgM tests have been developed and shown great promise in small studies. Unlike IgG, IgM does not cross the placenta, and detection of specific IgM in a baby would thus be a strong indication of infection.[93] Efforts to produce a more sensitive and more specific test are ongoing, for instance, using recombinant *T. pallidum* antigens.[119,286,287] These treponemal enzyme immunoassays (EIAs) have advantages such as automation, lack of prozone phenomena, and increased sensitivity in late stages of disease.[288-290] Such reactive screening tests need to be confirmed with another treponemal test that is different from the one used for screening, for example, TP-HA if an EIA is used for screening, as well as a quantitative test to assess disease activity (RPR or VDRL).

Rapid or Point-of-Care (POC) Tests. Several rapid or POC tests have been developed.[291,292] Most of these tests are immunochromatographic strip-based assays that detect specific antibodies to *T. pallidum* antigen. They adhere to the WHO Sexually Transmitted Diseases Diagnostic Initiative (SDI) established ASSURED criteria: *A*ffordable, *S*ensitive, *S*pecific, *U*ser-friendly, *R*apid and robust, *E*quipment free, and *D*eliverable to those who need them. Rapid and POC tests can therefore be performed on one patient at a time, with results communicated to the patient within minutes, thus saving time, preventing loss to follow-up, and allowing same-day treatment administration. In trials, rapid and POC tests have been shown to have the potential to interrupt vertical transmission.[86,293-295] Overall, rapid and POC tests perform well in both sensitivity and specificity compared with laboratory-based specific treponemal tests.[291,292] Given that these tests detect treponemal antibodies that persist even after cure, most rapid and POC tests do not allow the clinician to distinguish between active and past successfully treated infection. When possible, rapid and POC tests should thus be coupled with nontreponemal tests (RPR, VDRL). However, the rapid and POC tests were designed mainly for resource-limited settings with no access to a laboratory, where the risk of overtreatment resulting from persistent positive tests appears more readily acceptable than the risk of nontreatment.[86,293-295]

Cerebrospinal Fluid Tests. For evaluation of possible neurosyphilis, the VDRL test should be performed on CSF.[296-298] As in evaluating a patient for neurosyphilis, a CSF specimen without contamination by peripheral blood is needed.[299] In addition to VDRL testing of CSF, evaluation of CSF protein and white blood cell (WBC) count is used to assess the likelihood of CNS involvement.[300] Fewer data exist for the TP-PA test for CSF, and none exist for the RPR test; these two tests should not be used for CSF evaluation. Results from the VDRL test should be interpreted cautiously because a negative result on a VDRL test of CSF does not exclude a diagnosis of neurosyphilis.

Because of the wide range of normal values for CSF, red blood cells, and WBCs in the neonatal period, it has been difficult to unequivocally define the proportion of infants with congenital syphilis who have abnormalities of these laboratory values. The American Academy of Pediatrics[66] identifies an abnormal CSF WBC count in infants being evaluated for possible congenital syphilis as greater than 25 cells/mm^3 and protein as greater than 150 mg/dL (>170 mg/dL if the infant is premature). A reactive CSF VDRL test is considered to be specific for neurosyphilis in older children and adults. However, in neonates, the significance of a reactive CSF VDRL test is suspect because maternal nontreponemal IgG antibodies can pass from maternal serum to fetal and neonatal serum and then diffuse into CSF. Moreover, children may fail to have a reactive VDRL test on initial examination and still develop signs of neurosyphilis later. Using rabbit infectivity testing to determine the presence of the spirochete in the CSF specimen, Michelow and coworkers[253] found that central nervous system invasion with *T. pallidum* occurs in 41% of infants who have clinical, laboratory, or radiographic abnormalities of congenital syphilis. None of these infants had clinical signs of neurologic disease. When compared with isolation of spirochetes in CSF by rabbit inoculation, the sensitivity and specificity in CSF of a reactive VDRL test, elevated WBC count, and elevated protein were 54% and 90%; 38% and 88%; and 56% and 78%, respectively. CSF findings consistent with neurosyphilis are very common findings among infants with other clinical signs of congenital syphilis but are also present in approximately 8% of asymptomatic infants born to mothers with untreated early syphilis.[151,168,253]

Approach to the Diagnosis of Acquired Syphilis in Pregnancy

All women should be screened serologically for syphilis early in pregnancy with a nontreponemal test (e.g., VDRL or RPR). In areas of high prevalence of syphilis and in patients considered at high risk of syphilis, a nontreponemal serum test at the beginning of the third trimester (28 weeks of gestation) and again at delivery are also indicated.[62,301,302] The RPR test is most commonly used to screen pregnant women for possible infection with *T. pallidum*.[185,303] However, in areas of the world without access to laboratory-based testing, rapid and POC tests are to be recommended, ideally before 28 weeks.[295,304]

A definitive laboratory diagnosis of syphilis in pregnancy can be made when the presence of *T. pallidum* is confirmed by direct tests of clinical specimens. A probable or presumptive diagnosis of syphilis can be made when (1) nonspecific serologic tests are reactive in the presence of clinical findings compatible with syphilis or (2) CSF is reactive by VDRL testing.[62] Specific treponemal serologic tests should be used to confirm diagnoses suspected on the basis of clinical findings or positive nontreponemal tests. Use of only one type of serologic test is insufficient for a probable diagnosis because false-positive nontreponemal test results occur with various medical conditions, and false-positive treponemal test results occur with other spirochetal diseases (see earlier). Low-titer, false-positive, nontreponemal antibody test results occasionally occur even in pregnancy. When a pregnant woman has a reactive nontreponemal test result and a persistently negative treponemal test result, a false-positive test result is confirmed.

Differentiating syphilis treated in the past from reinfection often is difficult unless the nontreponemal titer is increasing. For women who tested positive and were treated during pregnancy, follow-up serologic testing is necessary to assess the efficacy of therapy. A woman who had been adequately treated with penicillin and followed with quantitative serologic testing and who has no evidence of reinfection does not need retreatment with each subsequent pregnancy. However, up to one third of congenital syphilis infections appear to be due to repeat infections,[305] indicating that any pregnant woman with syphilis, past or present, should be reevaluated carefully, and if any doubt exists about the adequacy of previous treatment or the presence of active infection or risk for reinfection, a course of treatment should be given to prevent congenital syphilis. This is especially true in areas of the world that do not have access to nontreponemal tests such as RPR or VDRL. All pregnant women who have syphilis should also be tested for other sexually transmitted diseases, including HIV infection. Any woman who delivers a stillborn infant after 20 weeks of gestation should also be tested for syphilis.[62,66]

The above approach of serologic screening is a poor diagnostic approach during the incubation or early primary stage of syphilis, and cases of congenital syphilis have occurred in women who were incubating syphilis at the time of delivery, that is, at a time their screening serologic tests were still negative. During those times, results of the nontreponemal (RPR or VDRL) tests may not show reactivity because reactivity occurs up to 4 to 8 weeks after the infection is acquired and several days to 1 week after the development of a chancre.[306] In fact, in primary syphilis during pregnancy, nonreactivity on nontreponemal testing is reported to occur in one fourth to one third of cases.[270,271] Nonreactivity on the treponemal tests occurs in as many as 36% of cases of primary syphilis.[259] Thus the clinician caring for pregnant women has to maintain a high level of suspicion in cases of a sexually active pregnant female. Detection of the spirochete from active lesions is the only means to establish the diagnosis in this scenario; this requires careful physical examination at multiple time points during pregnancy.[62]

Usually, HIV infection in women does not alter serology, but atypical results must be expected.[153] Frequent false-negative serology in primary and secondary syphilis,[307,308] prozone phenomenon,[309] "serofast" reactions,[310] and treponemal-specific antibodies becoming negative after therapy[311] have all been reported. Despite such varying serologic responses, workup for syphilis in HIV-infected women should not be different than that for HIV-negative cases[307]

Approach to the Diagnosis of Congenital Syphilis

Several diagnostic categories for congenital syphilis have been proposed, and minor differences among case definitions formulated by several agencies and experts still exist.[62,312-314] In Box 16-2, we have attempted to reconcile several of these with the CDC guidelines. A *"definitive"* diagnosis of congenital syphilis can be made in the rare situation in which the organism can be identified directly in the infant. A *"highly probable"* diagnosis is suggested if there are clinical findings consistent with congenital syphilis (see Box 16-1 and Table 16-1), if the infant has a fourfold higher nontreponemal serologic titer than the mother, or if the infant has a positive CSF VDRL test result. The diagnostic category of *"probable"* describes clinically asymptomatic infants who have a nontreponemal serologic titer that is equal to or less than that of the mother but where the maternal treatment either did not occur at all, was inadequate, was not documented, or failed (i.e., did not lead to a sufficient drop in maternal nontreponemal titers). The diagnosis of *"possible"* congenital syphilis is made when the nontreponemal serologic test result of an asymptomatic infant is reactive but equal to or less than that of a mother who did receive adequate treatment either during or before this pregnancy. The diagnosis of congenital syphilis is *"unlikely"* if the nontreponemal serologic test result of an asymptomatic infant born to an adequately treated mother is nonreactive. Given the difficulty of diagnosis and the severity of untreated congenital syphilis, the "evaluate and treat when uncertain" approach to congenital syphilis is the most prudent (see "Therapy").

Overall, the decision to evaluate and ultimately treat an infant for congenital syphilis has to be based upon clinical, serologic, as well as epidemiologic considerations. The evaluation includes an assessment of the mother for general risk factors, followed by an evaluation of the mother's current known serologic status. No newborn infant should be discharged from the hospital without determination of the mother's serologic status for syphilis during this pregnancy, no matter if both mother and infant are asymptomatic.[315] Cord blood should not be tested because it frequently yields false-positive or false-negative results. Tests of postnatal infant serum can be nonreactive if maternal titers are low or the mother was infected late in pregnancy. Conversely, transplacental transmission of nontreponemal and treponemal antibodies to the fetus can occur in a mother who has been treated appropriately for syphilis during pregnancy, resulting in positive test results in the uninfected newborn infant.

Taken together, this means that the optimal starting point for the serologic evaluation of a suspected case of congenital syphilis is maternal serum.[62,139,234] An infant's serologic titer often is one to two dilutions less than that of the mother's; thus an infant may have a nonreactive umbilical cord VDRL test but have a mother with a reactive serologic test for syphilis at delivery.[316] When the only evidence of congenital syphilis is a newly positive maternal nontreponemal test, the maternal diagnosis should be confirmed with a treponemal test before an otherwise well, asymptomatic infant undergoes further evaluation and treatment for congenital syphilis, unless the time to wait for results would unduly delay providing appropriate care for the infant or there is significant risk for loss to follow-up.[66,93]

All infants born to seropositive mothers require a careful examination and a quantitative nontreponemal syphilis test.[317] The test performed on the infant should be the same as that performed on the mother to enable comparison of titer results.[119]

Infants who have

1. Normal physical findings AND
2. A serum quantitative nontreponemal antibody titer that is less than fourfold greater than the maternal titer do not require further laboratory or clinical evaluation IF maternal treatment adequate for the stage of syphilis was administered more than 4 weeks before delivery (including before pregnancy) AND either
   a. If the mother had early syphilis at the time of treatment, her nontreponemal titers decreased at least fourfold and have remained low and stable through the time of delivery, *or*

Box 16-2 Modified Diagnostic Categories of Infants Born to Mothers With Clinical or Serologic Evidence of Syphilis

Definite Diagnosis (CDC Scenario 1)

1. Confirmation of presence of *Treponema pallidum* by darkfield microscopic or histologic examination or RIT; positive PCR

Highly Probable Diagnosis (CDC Scenario 1)

1. STS (RPR, VDRL) titer 4-fold greater than maternal STS titer
2. STS (RPR, VDRL) reactive in presence of clinical findings consistent with syphilis
3. STS (VDRL) reactive in cerebrospinal fluid
4. Reactive treponemal antibody test after age 15 mo

Probable Diagnosis (CDC Scenario 2)

1. Infant STS (RPR, VDRL) titer reactive, but same or less than fourfold maternal titer in absence of clinical disease, but in the face of inadequate* maternal therapy

Possible Diagnosis (CDC Scenario 3 and 4)

1. Asymptomatic infant STS (RPR, VDRL) reactive, but adequate maternal therapy

Unlikely Diagnosis

1. Asymptomatic infant STS (RPR, VDRL) nonreactive and adequate maternal therapy
2. STS nonreactive before age 6 mo

Modified from Centers for Disease Control and Prevention. http://www.cdc.gov/mmwr/preview/mmwrhtml/mm5914a1.htm. Accessed July 4, 2014.

CDC, Centers for Disease Control and Prevention; *PCR,* polymerase chain reaction; *RIT,* rabbit infectivity test; *RPR,* rapid plasma reagin (test); *STS,* serologic test for syphilis; *VDRL,* Venereal Disease Research Laboratory (test).

*Mother was not treated, inadequately treated (i.e., was treated with a nonpenicillin regimen or was treated less than 30 days before delivery or titers did not fall appropriately) or has no documentation of having received treatment.

b. If the mother had late syphilis at the time of treatment, her nontreponemal titers have remained low and stable, and there is no evidence of relapse and no risk for reinfection.[93,303]

If these requirements are not completely met, or even the slightest doubt exists, evaluation for syphilis in an infant should occur and include the following[36,66]:

1. Physical examination.
2. A quantitative nontreponemal serologic test for syphilis using serum from the infant (not cord blood, because false-positive and false-negative results can occur); a specific treponemal test, such as the FTA-ABS test, is not necessary in the newborn period if the mother is known to have a reactive result.
3. Long-bone radiographs, unless the diagnosis has been established otherwise. Long-bone radiographs are one of the most sensitive clinical investigations for detection of physical evidence of congenital syphilis in otherwise asymptomatic infants[318]; they are abnormal in approximately 65% of infants with clinical findings of syphilis but only in a minority of asymptomatic infants, that is, if osteochondritis or periostitis is found in an infant born to a mother with a reactive serologic tests for syphilis, this is indicative of congenital syphilis, and the infant requires a full course of IV penicillin therapy. The value of long-bone radiographs and CSF examinations in the diagnosis of congenital syphilis has been questioned during a time when syphilis was of low prevalence in the study population,[319,320] but the recommendations for long-bone radiographs and CSF VDRL determinations are based on their sensitivity and specificity from previous epidemics,[318] and thus most relevant again today.
4. Complete blood cell count, including hematocrit and hemoglobin, red blood cell count, reticulocyte count, platelet count, WBC count with differential, and direct Coombs test.
5. Other clinically indicated tests (e.g., chest radiography, liver function tests, cranial ultrasonography, ophthalmologic examination, and auditory brainstem response).
6. Pathologic examination of the placenta or umbilical cord by using specific fluorescent antitreponemal antibody staining or PCR.[119]
7. A VDRL test of CSF and analysis of CSF for cells and protein concentration (specific indications explained later).

Cerebrospinal fluid should be examined in all infants who are evaluated for congenital syphilis if the infant has any of the following: (1) abnormal physical examination findings consistent with congenital syphilis, (2) a serum quantitative nontreponemal titer that is fourfold greater than the mother's titer, or (3) a positive darkfield or fluorescent antibody test result on body fluid(s).[62,66,119,321] These infants are considered to have proven disease, and spirochetemia with invasion of the central nervous system occurs in approximately 40% to 50% of these infants; therefore they must receive a full 10-day course of IV penicillin therapy.[119,253] Leukocytosis (25 WBCs/mm or more)[224] and elevated protein content (greater than 150mg/dL in full-term and greater than 170mg/dL in preterm infants) in the CSF in an infant who exhibits any features suggestive of congenital syphilis should be regarded as supportive of the diagnosis. Also, an infant with reactive CSF on VDRL testing should receive presumptive treatment for neurosyphilis.[300] Specific treponemal tests should not be done using CSF in infants suspected of having congenital syphilis because the results cannot be interpreted properly.[296-298] Given that the diagnosis of congenital neurosyphilis is difficult to establish without a positive direct test and because findings such as the presence of red blood cells in the CSF as a result of a traumatic lumbar puncture can produce a false-positive serologic reaction, and other markers in the CSF of newborns and infants (CSF WBC counts and protein concentrations) vary widely as well, it is generally agreed that any infant with proven or probable congenital syphilis requires 10 days of parenteral treatment with penicillin G regardless of CSF test results.[62,66]

In summary, the problem of unequivocally identifying the infected infant underscores the need for an "evaluate and treat when uncertain" approach to congenital syphilis in general and to congenital neurosyphilis in particular. Given this paradigm, although preferred for optimal planning of care, a complete evaluation may be not necessary if a full 10-day course of parenteral penicillin is provided because such therapy would treat congenital central nervous system infection.[318,319]

In poorly resourced settings, the major difficulties in making a diagnosis of congenital syphilis are identifying the potentially large number of babies who have congenital syphilis as their mother's infection has remained undetected during pregnancy and confirming clinical suspicion without sophisticated laboratory tests. In these situations, confirmation of clinical suspicion is restricted to the VDRL or RPR or the newer rapid tests.[292] The value of undertaking a lumbar puncture or bone radiographs in asymptomatic infants in resource-poor settings in an attempt to confirm the diagnosis is questionable. In instances where infection is probable or suspected, the baby should simply be treated for congenital syphilis with a full 10-day course of IV penicillin G.[86]

Differential Diagnosis

The typical findings of congenital syphilis, such as snuffles, vesiculobullous eruption, hepatosplenomegaly, generalized lymphadenopathy, symmetrical bony lesions closely resemble features of other diseases in neonates that are unrelated to syphilis. For example, congenital infections caused by cytomegalovirus, *Toxoplasma gondii*, herpes simplex virus, and rubella virus; bacterial sepsis; as well as blood group incompatibility, battered child syndrome, and periostitis of prematurity are among numerous neonatal conditions that have to be considered in the differential diagnosis. This is largely due to the fact that most findings in syphilis are due to the inflammatory reaction to a widely disseminated pathogen, and this pathogenesis unites many of the above listed entities.[93,322-324]

DERMATOLOGIC MANIFESTATIONS

The vesiculobullous manifestations of congenital syphilis may be confused with other infections or with congenital disorders of the skin that can present as vesiculobullous eruptions.[325]

Infection caused by *Staphylococcus aureus* can produce vesicles or bullae on any part of the body. Severe infection may result in confluent bullae with erythema and desquamation (Ritter disease). Examination of aspirated fluid reveals many polymorphonuclear leukocytes and, on occasion, gram-positive cocci in clusters and culture will yield the organism. *Pseudomonas aeruginosa* septicemia can be accompanied by a cutaneous eruption consisting of clustered pearly vesicles on an erythematous background, which rapidly becomes purulent green or hemorrhagic.[326] When the lesion ruptures, a circumscribed ulcer with a necrotic base appears and may persist, surrounded by a purplish cellulitis. Culture of the lesion and the blood confirms the diagnosis. In the septicemic early-onset form of listeriosis, a cutaneous eruption consisting of miliary lesions resembling papules, pustules, or papulopustules can occur over the entire body, with a predilection for the back.[327] Culture of these lesions and blood usually reveals *Listeria monocytogenes* as the etiologic agent. Additional infectious causes of vesicular or bullous lesions of the skin of the newborn include group B streptococci,[328] *Haemophilus influenzae* type b,[329] *Mycobacterium tuberculosis*,[330] and cytomegalovirus.[331]

In virus-induced eruptions, the vesicles are located in the midepidermis. In herpesvirus infection, vesicles are the most common dermatologic manifestation. They tend to be sparsely disseminated throughout the body, or they may occur in crops or clusters. Involvement of the palms and soles has been recorded, as has the formation of bullae. Recurrence of these skin lesions is not unusual. Culture, fluorescent staining, or PCR on scrapings from the base of these lesions would reveal herpes simplex virus. Varicella-zoster infection also appears to have a similar pattern but rarely occurs in the newborn period, and the diagnosis may be discarded on epidemiologic or clinical grounds. Variola and vaccinia can affect the fetus or newborn and cause vesicular eruptions. Appropriate epidemiologic evidence should be sought to exclude these diagnoses.

Mucocutaneous candidiasis may manifest as a vesicular dermatitis at the end of the first week of life. The vesicles usually become confluent and rupture, leaving a denuded area surrounded by satellite vesicles or pustules. Congenital candidiasis with skin manifestations also has been described, and severe systemic involvement may accompany this intrauterine infection.[332]

A variety of hereditary disorders of the skin appear at birth or in early infancy as vesiculobullous eruptions.[325] Epidermolysis bullosa is a group of specific genetic disorders. Erythema toxicum, miliaria rubra, incontinentia pigmenti, urticaria pigmentosa, epidermolytic hyperkeratosis, acrodermatitis enteropathica, Langerhans cell histiocytosis (histiocytosis X), transient neonatal pustular melanosis, infantile acropustulosis, and aplasia cutis congenita should all be included in the differential diagnosis.[325]

SNUFFLES

Increased neonatal nasal discharge is not an uncommon phenomenon but has not been well studied. It is described as mucoid rhinorrhea with nasal mucosal edema in the afebrile newborn that results in stertor, poor feeding, and respiratory distress. The etiology is most often not identified but presumed to be allergic in nature. The recognition and treatment of this condition is important because neonates are obligate nasal breathers. Recommended is a diagnostic-therapeutic trial consisting of conservative therapy (suctioning) and corticosteroid. An important alternate consideration not to be missed is infection with *Chlamydia trachomatis*, but this entity should be recognized by the associated clinical findings.[330]

LYMPHADENOPATHY

Lymph node size varies with age and the location, but in neonates, lymph nodes are normally barely palpable. Localized lymphadenopathy can be found in one third of neonates and infants, usually in nodes that drain areas with skin irritation or localized infections. Generalized adenopathy is rare in the neonate, and if present can be seen with other congenital infections such as cytomegalovirus.[333]

HEPATOSPLENOMEGALY

When the clinical presentation is hepatosplenomegaly with or without jaundice, the list of possibilities in the differential diagnosis is extensive and includes all causes of elevated direct and indirect bilirubin. The physician should consider isoimmunization (e.g., Rh incompatibility, ABO incompatibility), other infectious diseases (early-onset sepsis, CMV infection, congenital rubella, herpes simplex infection, coxsackievirus B or other enteroviral infections, toxoplasmosis), neonatal hepatitis, diseases of the biliary tract (e.g., extrahepatic biliary atresia or choledochal cyst), and genetic and metabolic disorders (e.g., cystic fibrosis, galactosemia, and α1-antitrypsin deficiency).[333]

HYDROPS FETALIS

Hydrops fetalis can be caused by chronic anemia (isoimmunization disorder, homozygous α-thalassemia, fetomaternal, or fetofetal transfusions), cardiac or pulmonary failure resulting from causes other than anemia (large arteriovenous malformations, premature closure of the foramen ovale, cystic adenomatoid malformation, pulmonary lymphangiectasia), perinatal tumors (neuroblastoma, chorioangioma), achondroplasia, renal disorders (congenital nephrosis, renal vein thrombosis), and infections, such as congenital CMV infection, toxoplasmosis, parvovirus B19 infection,[334] and congenital hepatitis.[335] Most cases of hydrops are caused by isoimmunization disorders, which can be excluded as a cause by a negative direct Coombs test result. A normal hemoglobin electrophoresis pattern excludes the diagnosis of α-thalassemia. The Kleihauer-Betke technique of acid elution for identifying fetal cells in the maternal circulation can aid in ruling out the diagnosis of fetomaternal transfusion. Other diagnostic considerations can be discarded on the basis of appropriate radiographic studies, placental examination, urinalysis with microscopy, biopsy, and immunologic studies.[333]

RENAL DISEASE

In the neonate and young infant, the nephrotic syndrome and acute nephritis occur infrequently. The former more often is associated with infantile microcystic disease, minimal-lesion nephrotic syndrome, or renal vein thrombosis than with congenital syphilis.[333] Neonatal nephritis can occur as a manifestation of congenital syphilis, hereditary nephritis, hemolytic-uremic syndrome, and, rarely, pyelonephritis. The clinical signs that distinguish syphilitic renal involvement from the other conditions mentioned include the presence of other manifestations of early congenital syphilis, a positive result on serologic tests for syphilis, elevated levels of IgG (in infantile microcystic disease, the levels of IgG are low), and the response to specific therapy for syphilis.[240]

OPHTHALMOLOGIC INVOLVEMENT

Neonatal glaucoma, an uncommon finding in syphilis, occurs as an isolated genetic disorder and may be associated with a variety of syndromes (e.g., aniridia, Hallermann-Streiff syndrome, Rieger anomaly, Lowe syndrome, Sturge-Weber syndrome, oculodentodigital syndrome, Pierre Robin syndrome); it also is associated with congenital rubella.[336] Nasolacrimal duct obstruction is a more frequent cause of excessive lacrimation in the newborn period and early infancy.

BONY INVOLVEMENT

Periostitis of congenital syphilis usually occurs during the early months of life and must be distinguished from that seen in healing rickets, battered child syndrome, infantile cortical hyperostosis, a variety of poorly understood disorders presumed to be related to nutritional deficiencies, occasionally pyogenic osteomyelitis,[148] and prostaglandin-induced periostitis.[337] Although the Wimberger sign formerly was thought to be pathognomonic of congenital syphilis, it has been described in other disease states, including osteomyelitis, hyperparathyroidism, and infantile generalized fibromatosis.[196,338] And the "celery stick" appearance of alternating bands of longitudinal translucency and relative density is a finding also seen in congenital rubella and CMV infection.[148]

Therapy

Parenteral penicillin is the preferred drug for treatment of syphilis at any stage.[36] Recommendations for specific types of penicillin and duration of therapy vary, depending on the stage of disease and clinical manifestations.[339] However, parenteral penicillin G is the only documented effective therapy for patients who have neurosyphilis, congenital syphilis, or syphilis during pregnancy and is also recommended for HIV-infected patients. Such patients always should be treated with parenteral penicillin G, even if desensitization for penicillin allergy is necessary.[36] Penicillin resistance has not been described in *T. pallidum*, which is exquisitely sensitive, with a penicillin minimal inhibitory concentration of 0.004 U (or 0.0025 μg/mL).[340-342] However, effective therapy for syphilis has to be maintained for at least 7 to 10 days because of the slow replication of *T. pallidum* (every 30 hours).[343]

TREATMENT OF ACQUIRED SYPHILIS IN PREGNANCY

Regardless of the stage of pregnancy, infected patients should be treated with penicillin according to the dosage schedules appropriate for the stage of syphilis.[36,250] Early syphilis, that is, primary, secondary, and early latent infection, is treated with benzathine penicillin G, 50,000 units (U)/kg up to the maximum dose of 2.4 million U intramuscularly (IM) in a single dose.[36,342-344] Many experts recommend that an additional dose of benzathine penicillin G be provided 1 week after the initial dose.[36] Late latent syphilis requires benzathine penicillin administered as 50,000 U/kg up to the adult dose of 2.4 million U at 1 week intervals for 3 consecutive weeks (i.e., total combined dose of 150,000 U/kg up to the maximum dose of 7.2 million U), but only if the CSF examination has excluded neurosyphilis. When the duration of infection is not known, then the patient should be treated as for late latent disease (i.e., 3 weeks). Management and treatment decisions may be guided further by the use of fetal ultrasonography.[346] Evidence of fetal infection may require additional doses of benzathine penicillin G until resolution of fetal abnormalities can be documented.[240]

Benzathine penicillin G has been shown to be safe during pregnancy.[347] A pregnant woman with a history of penicillin allergy should be treated with penicillin after desensitization (see later for instructions) because no proven alternative therapy has been established. In some patients, skin testing may be helpful. In the pregnant woman, desensitization should be performed in consultation with a specialist and only in facilities in which emergency assistance is available.[348] Pregnant women who received therapy for gonorrhea with ceftriaxone have a high rate of cure of primary syphilis, but failures have occurred, and efficacy in pregnancy is not well studied.[349] This regimen therefore cannot be assumed to provide adequate therapy for syphilis in pregnancy. To emphasize: Any therapy other than penicillin is considered inadequate therapy during pregnancy.[50,350] Nonetheless, failure rates of penicillin for prevention of fetal infection range from 2% to as high as 14%.[351] The majority of fetal treatment failures seem to occur after maternal treatment for secondary syphilis[352]; treatment failure in such cases may be explained in part by the marked spirochetemia that occurs during secondary syphilitic infection.[353,354]

Treatment of Neurosyphilis in the Pregnant Patient

Invasion of the CNS by *T. pallidum* can occur during any stage of syphilis.[63] Benzathine penicillin does not reliably produce inhibitory CSF levels of penicillin,[355] and a number of reports describe the persistence of treponemes in the CSF after benzathine penicillin therapy for syphilis.[42,356-362] The recommended regimen for pregnant adults with neurosyphilis is aqueous crystalline penicillin G, 18 to 24 million U/day, administered IM as 3 to 4 million U every 4 hours or continuous infusion for 10 to 14 days. If adherence to therapy can be ensured, patients may be treated with an alternative regimen of IM penicillin G, 2.4 million U once daily plus probenecid, 500 mg orally four times per day, both for 10 to 14 days. Because these regimens are shorter than that used for late latent syphilis, some experts recommend following both of these regimens with benzathine penicillin G 2.4 million U (or 50,000 U/kg per dose), IM, weekly for 1 to 3 doses.[62]

Human Immunodeficiency Virus

For HIV-infected pregnant women with primary or secondary syphilis, some authorities recommend up to three once-weekly doses of 2.4 million U of benzathine penicillin

G, in addition to the single IM dose of benzathine penicillin G. HIV-infected patients who have either late latent syphilis or syphilis of unknown duration require a CSF examination before treatment. If nontreponemal antibody titers have not declined fourfold by 6 months with primary or secondary syphilis, or by 6 to 12 months in early latent syphilis, or if the titer has increased fourfold at any time, a CSF examination should be performed and the patient re-treated with 7.2 million U of benzathine penicillin G (administered as three once-weekly doses of 2.4 million U each) if CSF examination findings are normal. HIV-infected pregnant patients who have CSF abnormalities consistent with neurosyphilis should receive treatment for neurosyphilis as described earlier.[57,62]

Postexposure Prophylaxis

Recommendations for postexposure prophylaxis for syphilis for exposed or possibly exposed HCPs are based on guidelines for the epidemiologic treatment of suspected sexual contacts[363-366]: IM benzathine penicillin G 2.4 million U in one dose; alternatively, doxycycline, 100 mg PO bid for 2 weeks can be considered, but only for the proven nonpregnant HCP.

TREATMENT OF CONGENITAL SYPHILIS

Infants should be treated for congenital syphilis if they have definite, highly probable, probable, or possible disease. Even infants in the "unlikely" category (for definitions of these terms, see Box 16-2) are recommended to receive therapy, as are infants born to mothers with either clinical or serologic evidence of syphilis infection, for whom test results cannot exclude infection, who cannot be evaluated completely, or for whom adequate follow-up cannot be ensured.[62,366] The difference between these categories is only the type of therapy that is recommended. Infants in the *definitive* and *highly probable* category should be treated with IV aqueous crystalline penicillin G for a total of 10 to 14 days at 50,000 U/kg per dose every 12 hours (100,000 U/kg/day) during the first 7 days of life and every 8 hours during days of life 8 to 30 (150,000 U/kg/day). IM procaine penicillin G, 50,000 U/kg/day as a single daily dose for 10 to 14 days, has also been proposed by some experts as an alternative.[62,318,367] Although no treatment failures have yet been documented with IM procaine penicillin, optimal CSF concentrations are not achieved; the more conservative approach thus would require an unequivocally negative CSF examination available before initiating this form of therapy.[368] Of note, a full 10-day course of penicillin is preferred even if the infant received ampicillin initially for possible sepsis. Also, if more than 1 day of therapy is missed, the entire course needs to be restarted.[62]

Clinically Asymptomatic Infants

Treatment decisions of *clinically "asymptomatic" infants* (i.e., in the probable, possible, or unlikely category) are based on (1) the maternal history of syphilis and past treatment and (2) the infant serologic evaluation. Maternal treatment for syphilis is deemed inadequate if (1) the mother's penicillin dose is unknown, undocumented, or inadequate; (2) the mother received a nonpenicillin regimen during pregnancy for syphilis; (3) treatment was given within less than 30 days of the infant's birth; or (4) the mother has early syphilis and has a nontreponemal titer that has increased fourfold.[369,370] For the asymptomatic infant of a mother with a positive serologic screen, three possible scenarios thus need to be considered[62,119,367]:

1. If the mother's treatment was inadequate, and the asymptomatic infant's nontreponemal test is reactive, the infant is deemed to have *probable* congenital syphilis.[62] If medical follow-up is certain, this infant may be treated with a single IM dose of benzathine penicillin G, 50,000 U/kg. Single-dose benzathine penicillin G therapy has been widely used in the past, and its use allows for earlier hospital discharge of the infant, with subsequent improved maternal-infant interaction and decrease in hospitalization costs.[371] This regimen has also been supported by two small clinical studies.[372,373] If the infant is to receive such a single IM injection of benzathine penicillin G, then a complete evaluation, including a lumbar puncture, is mandatory.[62,367] Given the difficulty of ruling out neurosyphilis unequivocally, many experts prefer the 10-day intravenous course with aqueous crystalline penicillin G for all infants in this category.[253,348] In summary, if any part of the evaluation is abnormal, unavailable, or uninterpretable (e.g., CSF contaminated by blood), a full 10- to 14-day regimen is recommended.[367] If the meaning of a positive RPR test result in an otherwise normal infant is in doubt and the results of all other tests are negative, repeat quantitative RPR testing should be undertaken.[62,367]
2. If the mother's treatment was adequate, but the asymptomatic infant's nontreponemal serum test reactive, the infant is said to have *possible* congenital syphilis. Some experts recommend that a single dose of benzathine penicillin be administered as described above.[62,367,372,373] Failure of such therapy in three infants, however, has been reported.[355,374,375] Given these concerns, most experts suggest that all infants with possible congenital syphilis receive parenteral penicillin therapy for 10 days, especially if the mother had secondary syphilis at delivery or seroconverted during the pregnancy.[45,131,351]
3. If the mother was treated adequately during the pregnancy, and the asymptomatic infant's serologic assessment is nonreactive, the infant is *unlikely* to have congenital syphilis. But because of the inability to rule out possible transmission to the fetus in these cases, we do recommend a single IM dose of benzathine penicillin even for infants falling into this "unlikely" group. If the choice is made not to treat an infant in this category, close follow-up has to be certain, and such an infant needs to undergo a second RPR test within 3 to 4 weeks of birth. Finally, the appearance of secondary or tertiary syphilis in a mother within the year after delivery should prompt a thorough reevaluation of the infant.[203,316]

Internationally Adopted Children

Congenital syphilis sometimes is undiagnosed and often inadequately treated in developing countries. Syphilis testing, therefore, is recommended as part of the evaluation of *internationally adopted children*, regardless of history or report of evaluation and treatment abroad.[93,376] When congenital syphilis of any stage and site is identified beyond the neonatal period, the treatment regimen for acquired neurosyphilis should be used: 200,000 to 300,000 U/kg/day of aqueous crystalline penicillin G, given as 50,000 U/kg every 4 to 6 hours for a minimum of 10 to 14 days. Some experts would follow this regimen with IM doses of benzathine penicillin G, 50,000 U/kg weekly for 3 weeks. If the patient has no clinical manifestations of disease, the CSF examination is normal, and the result of the VDRL test of CSF is negative, some experts would treat only with three weekly doses of benzathine penicillin G (50,000 U/kg, IM). When IV or IM penicillin preparations are unavailable (see later) or cannot be tolerated, IV ampicillin or parenteral ceftriaxone can be considered as alternative therapy, but careful clinical and serologic follow-up is essential when these regimens are used because data for efficacy are insufficient.[62,93,367]

FOLLOW-UP FOR THE SYPHILIS-INFECTED PREGNANT WOMAN

Treated pregnant women with syphilis should have quantitative nontreponemal serologic tests repeated at 28 to 32 weeks of gestation, at delivery, and following the recommendations for the stage of disease. Serologic titers may be repeated monthly in women at high risk of reinfection or in geographic areas where the prevalence of syphilis is high. The clinical and antibody response should be appropriate for stage of disease. In practice, however, most women will deliver before their serologic response to treatment can definitively be assessed. All pregnant women with acquired syphilis and all of their recent sexual contacts should be evaluated for syphilis and other sexually transmitted infections. For pregnant HIV-infected women with syphilis, careful follow-up is essential, because higher rates of treatment failure have been reported.[62,367]

In the pregnant woman with primary/secondary syphilis, re-treatment should be considered necessary, if clinical signs or symptoms persist or recur, if a fourfold increase in titer of a nontreponemal test occurs (also evaluate CSF and HIV status), or if the nontreponemal titer fails to decrease fourfold within 6 months after therapy (also evaluate for HIV and re-treat unless follow-up for continued clinical and serologic assessment can be ensured). In the pregnant woman with latent syphilis, perform a CSF evaluation and re-treat if titers increase fourfold, if an initially high titer (>1:32) fails to decrease at least fourfold within 12 to 24 months, or if signs or symptoms attributable to syphilis develop at any time. In all these instances, re-treatment should be performed with 3 weekly injections of IM benzathine penicillin G, 2.4 million U, unless CSF examination indicates that neurosyphilis is present, at which time treatment for neurosyphilis should be initiated. In general, only one re-treatment course is indicated. The possibility of reinfection or concurrent HIV infection always should be considered when re-treating pregnant patients with syphilis. Pregnant patients with neurosyphilis must have periodic serologic testing, clinical evaluation at 6-month intervals, and repeated CSF examinations. If the CSF cell count has not decreased after 6 months or CSF is not entirely normal after 2 years of therapy, re-treatment should be considered.[62,367]

FOLLOW-UP FOR THE SYPHILIS-INFECTED INFANT

Infants should be reevaluated after treatment for definite, probable, or possible congenital syphilis during regular scheduled well-child care visits, that is, multiple times during the first year of life.[66] Nontreponemal serologic tests should be incorporated into routine pediatric care after conclusion of treatment or until results become nonreactive or the titer has decreased fourfold.[66] When nontreponemal antibodies are of maternal origin, titers usually become negative within 3 months and should be negative by 6 months of age if the infant was not infected.[377] The serologic response after therapy may decline slower for infants treated after the neonatal period. If the choice was made not to treat an infant in the unlikely category, a nontreponemal test has to be performed at 3 to 4 weeks of age; untreated infants who are not seronegative by 6 months of age should be fully reevaluated clinically and treated. If titers of nontreponemal antibodies remain stable or increase after ages 6 to 12 months in any infant, the child should be reevaluated (including CSF analysis) and treated with a 10-day parenteral course of penicillin G, even if they had been treated previously.[62,367] Treponemal-specific antibodies of maternal origin may persist for as long as 12 to 15 months in 15% of uninfected infants,[378] rendering these tests of little help during infancy. However, reactivity at 18 months or beyond is indicative of congenital infection.[379,380] The recommendation of a second treponemal test beyond 15 months as a way of retrospectively diagnosing congenital syphilis is not merely for epidemiologic use. An established diagnosis can help in medical and developmental follow-up evaluation of the child.[185]

All infants and children should be evaluated thoroughly for the extent of disease if there is serologic evidence of treatment failure or of recurrent disease. Such evaluation should, at a minimum, consist of CSF examination and complete blood count and platelet count. Other tests, such as long-bone radiographs, liver function tests, hearing evaluation, and ophthalmologic evaluation, should be performed as clinically indicated. Infants with congenital neurosyphilis (or unavailable, abnormal, or uninterpretable CSF WBC count or protein concentration or positive CSF VDRL) should have repeat clinical and CSF evaluations every 6 months until their CSF indices are normal. A reactive CSF VDRL test at any time represents indication for re-treatment with a full 10- to 14-day course. If CSF WBC counts do not steadily decline at each examination or remain abnormal at 2 years, re-treatment also is indicated.[62,93,367]

Although treatment can cure the infection, the prognosis in treated congenital syphilis depends on the degree of damage before the initiation of therapy. In general, the earlier treatment is initiated, the more likely it is that a satisfactory response can be obtained.[186] If marked damage to the fetus has occurred, treatment in utero may not prevent abortion, stillbirth, or neonatal death, and even if treatment keeps the newborn infant alive, stigmata can remain. If the treatment is provided prenatally or within the first 3 months of life, and such stigmata have not yet become apparent, they generally can be prevented.[235] Interstitial keratitis is an exception; this complication does not seem to be responsive to specific antibiotic therapy. On occasion, dramatic relief has been afforded by the use of corticosteroids and mydriatics, although relapses have occurred with cessation of corticosteroid therapy. The osseous lesions seem to heal independently of specific therapy. Treatment of congenital syphilis in the late stage does not reverse the stigmata.[381]

PROBLEMS ASSOCIATED WITH PENICILLIN THERAPY

Penicillin Hypersensitivity

Skin testing for *penicillin hypersensitivity* is recommended for those with a history of known or presumed penicillin allergy.[382] Testing with the major and minor determinants can reliably identify people at high risk of reacting to penicillin; currently, only the major determinant (benzylpenicilloyl poly-L-lysine) and penicillin G skin tests are available commercially. Testing with the major determinant of penicillin G is estimated to miss 3% to 6% of penicillin-allergic patients who are at risk of serious or fatal reactions. Thus a cautious approach (i.e., hospitalization) to penicillin therapy is advised when a patient with a history of known or presumed allergic reactions to penicillin cannot be tested with all of the penicillin skin test reagents. An oral or intravenous desensitization protocol for patients with a positive skin test result is available (www.cdc.gov/nchstp/dstd/penicillinG.htm) and should be performed in a hospital setting.[367,383] Oral desensitization is regarded as safer and easier to perform. Desensitization usually can be completed in approximately 4 hours, after which the first therapeutic dose of penicillin can be given.[62,383]

Jarisch-Herxheimer Reaction

The *Jarisch-Herxheimer reaction,* a common occurrence in the treatment of acquired early syphilis in adults,[384] consists of chills, fever (38° C or higher), generalized malaise, hypotension, tachycardia, tachypnea, accentuation of the cutaneous lesions, leukocytosis, and, exceedingly rarely, death. It begins within 2 hours of treatment, peaks at approximately 8 hours, and disappears in 24 to 36 hours. The cause of the reaction is not known,[385] although release of *T. pallidum* membrane lipoproteins that stimulate proinflammatory cytokines likely explains this clinical phenomenon.[386] Approximately 40% of pregnant women who receive treatment for syphilis demonstrate a Jarisch-Herxheimer reaction.[334,387] In addition, these women may experience the onset of uterine contractions and preterm labor, with decreased fetal activity and fetal heart rate changes, including late decelerations, which last up to 24 to 48 hours and may lead to fetal death. No prophylactic measure or treatment is currently available. Abnormal ultrasonographic findings in the fetus, as well as fetal monitoring for 24 hours, may identify pregnancies at highest risk, but concern for its occurrence should not delay treatment.[388,389] Of note, β-lactam antibiotics for group B *Streptococcus* intrapartum prophylaxis can trigger the Jarisch-Herxheimer reaction in patients with undiagnosed syphilis.[390]

In congenital syphilis, the incidence of the Jarisch-Herxheimer reaction is low, although it may be more common when treatment occurs later in infancy[203]; when it does occur, it varies in severity, ranging from fever to cardiovascular collapse and seizures.[119,195]

Penicillin Shortage

During periods of *penicillin shortage,* see www.cdc.gov/nchstp/dstd/penicillinG.htm for updates. Currently, the following is recommended[36]:

1. For infants with clinical definitive or highly probable congenital syphilis, check local sources for aqueous crystalline penicillin G (potassium or sodium). If IV penicillin G is limited, substitute some or all daily doses with procaine penicillin G (50,000 U/kg/dose/day, IM, in a single daily dose for 10 days). If aqueous or procaine penicillin G is not available, ceftriaxone (in doses according to age and weight) may be considered with careful clinical and serologic follow-up. Ceftriaxone must be used with caution in infants with jaundice. For infants younger than 30 days, use 75 mg/kg/day, IV/IM, in a single daily dose for 10 to 14 days; however, dose adjustment might be necessary based on birth weight. For older infants, the dose should be 100 mg/kg/day in a single daily dose. Studies that strongly support ceftriaxone for the treatment of congenital syphilis have not been conducted. Therefore ceftriaxone should be used in consultation with a specialist in the treatment of infants with congenital syphilis. Management may include a repeat CSF examination at age 6 months if the initial examination was abnormal.
2. For infants at risk with probable or possible congenital syphilis, use procaine penicillin G, 50,000 U/kg/dose/day, IM, in a single dose for 10 days, or benzathine penicillin G, 50,000 U/kg IM as a single dose. If any part of the evaluation for congenital syphilis is abnormal, CSF examination is not interpretable, CSF examination was not performed, or follow-up is uncertain, procaine penicillin G is recommended. A single dose of ceftriaxone is not considered adequate therapy.
3. For premature infants with probable or possible congenital syphilis, and who might not tolerate IM injections because of decreased muscle mass, IV ceftriaxone may be considered with careful clinical and serologic follow-up. Ceftriaxone dosing must be adjusted to age and birth weight.[36]

Prevention

The cornerstone of congenital syphilis control is prenatal screening and treatment of infected mothers with penicillin, which is a cost-effective intervention in high- as well as low-endemic settings.[10,86,391,392] Although universal syphilis screening for pregnant women is recommended in the national reproductive health strategies of almost every nation of the world,[393] actual rates of screening vary widely between and within countries from, for instance, less than 5% to 40% in Mozambique and 32% to 83% in the United States.[10,305,394] Ideally, every woman who becomes pregnant should undergo at least one serologic test for syphilis during the first trimester.[139,266,301,395] For communities and populations in which the prevalence of syphilis is high or for women in high-risk groups, repeated testing at the beginning of the third trimester (at 28 weeks of gestation)[396] and at delivery is recommended.[36] It is a national policy in the United States that no infant should be discharged from the nursery before results of maternal serologic screening during the current pregnancy have been documented.[36] With the practice of early discharge at 48 hours or less, it becomes the responsibility of the HCP to arrange for adequate follow-up in infants who are discharged before the result of the maternal serologic test is known.[89,394,397-399] In fact, for the majority of cases, it is the medical providers who are responsible for missing well-defined opportunities to prevent congenital syphilis.[400,401]

Successful strategies in the control of congenital syphilis[402,403] have to

- Promote early attendance for antenatal care and educating women (and men) about the benefits of syphilis screening and treatment; this is especially important for women at high risk, who are most often among society's marginalized groups[67,404-406]
- Promote education about and modification of high-risk sexual behavior[36,82]
- Implement decentralized same-day screening and treatment and use of rapid point-of-care screening tests[407,408]
- Provide testing free of charge[88]
- For high-risk groups, include a second test late in pregnancy, at delivery, and again in the month after birth[203,316,409]
- Carry out contact tracing and treatment of infected partners[203,316,409]
- Provide prompt treatment of all babies who have confirmed, probable, or suspected congenital syphilis

When enhancements of standard public health measures, such as contact tracing, education of at-risk groups and physicians, increased diagnostic and treatment services, and intensified screening cannot control outbreaks, an alternative used both in developing and developed countries with some success is targeted mass treatment. For example, the British Columbia Centre for Disease Control implemented a mass treatment/prophylaxis program with good short-term success, delivering over 7000 treatment doses of azithromycin (1.8 g orally in a single dose) in two rounds over 5 weeks to adults at high risk for syphilis.[410-412] However, a later rebound in numbers of cases occurred, which is presumed to have been caused by incomplete coverage of "high-frequency transmitters."[411,413] A similar program in Rinakai, Uganda delivered more than 20,000 1-g treatment doses of azithromycin.[414-416] The use of azithromycin and oral forms of penicillin offers advantages over the traditional use of injectable penicillin in terms of compliance.[250,417] However, recent reports of azithromycin-resistant *T. pallidum* in the United States, where the use of azithromycin is far higher than in sub-Saharan Africa, indicate the potential problems associated with its use for syphilis.[418,419] Two smaller-scale mass treatment programs in North America have been conducted using benzathine penicillin G, and both were judged successful.[420,421] Of note, there currently is no evidence to suggest that oral treatment is sufficient for the treatment of syphilis in pregnancy.[417,422]

Globally, newly developed rapid POC tests now allow women to be screened for syphilis exposure at their primary care visit and, if positive, treated on the spot at a cost of \$0.19 to \$1.00.[291,292,393,423] The availability of these simple tests, coupled with the low cost of a single penicillin injection, means that it is now possible for any woman attending antenatal care, no matter how remote the setting, to be tested and promptly treated for syphilis as part of basic health services.[393] Rapid testing and same-day treatment of those infected has been shown to reduce the incidence of perinatal death and stillbirth attributable to syphilis by approximately 50%.[295] On March 1, 2012, the Global Congenital Syphilis Partnership, with members including the Bill and Melinda Gates Foundation, Save the Children, the WHO, and the Centers for Disease Control and Prevention, was launched in response to data demonstrating the cost-effectiveness and practicability of rapid syphilis testing.[424] This well-organized global effort now offers the hope to finally turn the tide against this deadly scourge.[425]

References

1. Obladen M: Curse on two generations: a history of congenital syphilis, *Neonatology* 103:274-280, 2013.
2. Gomez GB, Kamb ML, Newman LM, et al: Untreated maternal syphilis and adverse outcomes of pregnancy: a systematic review and meta-analysis, *Bull World Health Organ* 91:217-226, 2013.
3. Schmid G: Economic and programmatic aspects of congenital syphilis prevention, *Bull World Health Organ* 82:402-409, 2004.
4. Ingraham NR: The value of penicillin alone in the prevention and treatment of congenital syphilis, *Acta Derm Venereol* 31(Suppl):60-87, 1951.
5. McDermott J, Steketee R, Larsen S, et al: Syphilis-associated perinatal and infant mortality in rural Malawi, *Bull World Health Organ* 71:773-780, 1993.
6. Lozano R, Naghavi M, Foreman K, et al: Global and regional mortality from 235 causes of death for 20 age groups in 1990 and 2010: a systematic analysis for the Global Burden of Disease Study 2010, *Lancet* 380:2095-2128, 2012.
7. Owusu-Edusei K Jr, Introcaso CE, Chesson HW: Hospitalization cost of congenital syphilis diagnosis from insurance claims data in the United States, *Sex Transm Dis* 40:226-229, 2013.
8. Saloojee H, Velaphi S, Goga Y, et al: The prevention and management of congenital syphilis: an overview and recommendations, *Bull World Health Organ* 82:424-430, 2004.
9. Hossain M, Broutet N, Hawkes S: The elimination of congenital syphilis: a comparison of the proposed World Health Organization action plan for the elimination of congenital syphilis with existing national maternal and congenital syphilis policies, *Sex Transm Dis* 34(Suppl 7):S22-S30, 2007.
10. Schmid GP, Stoner BP, Hawkes S, et al: The need and plan for global elimination of congenital syphilis, *Sex Transm Dis* 34(Suppl 7):S5-S10, 2007.
11. Lafond RE, Lukehart SA: Biological basis for syphilis, *Clin Microbiol Rev* 19:29-49, 2006.
12. Hovind-Hougen K: Determination by means of electron microscopy of morphological criteria of value for classification of some spirochetes in particular treponemes, *Acta Pathol Microbiol Scand B (Suppl)* 225:1-41, 1976.
13. Canale-Parola E: Physiology and evolution of spirochetes treponemal infection, *Bacteriol Rev* 157:32, 1977.
14. Fraser CM, Morris SJ, Weinstock GM: Complete genome sequence of *Treponema pallidum*, the syphilis spirochete, *Science* 281:375-378, 1998.
15. Roman GC, Roman LN: Occurrence of congenital, cardiovascular, visceral, neurologic, and neuro-ophthalmologic complications in late yaws: a theme for future research, *Rev Infect Dis* 8:760-770, 1986.
16. Turner TB, Hollander DHH: Biology of the treponematoses based on studies carried out at the International Treponematosis Laboratory Center of the Johns Hopkins University under the auspices of the World Health Organization, *Monogr Ser World Health Organ* 35:3-266, 1957.
17. Wilcox RR, Guthe T: *Treponema pallidum*: a bibliographical review of the morphology, culture and survival of *T. pallidum* and associated organisms, *Bull World Health Organ* 35:1-169, 1966.
18. Turner TB: Syphilis and the treponematoses. In Mudd S, editor: *Infectious agents and host reactions*, Philadelphia, 1970, WB Saunders.

19. Bruckner DA: Nomenclature for aerobic and anaerobic bacteria. In Feigin RD, Cherry JD, Demmler GJ, et al, editors: *Textbook of pediatric infectious diseases*, ed 5, Philadelphia, 2004, WB Saunders, pp 1082-1099.
20. Walker AN: Rapid plasma reagin (RPR) card test. A screening method for treponemal disease, *Br J Vener Dis* 47:259-262, 1971.
21. Flood JM, Weinstock HS, Guroy ME, et al: Neurosyphilis during the AIDS epidemic, San Francisco, 1985-1992, *J Infect Dis* 177:931-940, 1998.
22. Weinstock GM, Smajs D, Hardham J, et al: From microbial genome sequence to applications, *Res Microbiol* 151:151-158, 2000.
23. Radolf JD, Steiner B, Shevchenko D: Treponema pallidum: doing a remarkable job with what it's got, *Trends Microbiol* 7:7-9, 1999.
24. Pennisi E: Genome reveals wiles and weak points of syphilis, *Science* 281:324-325, 1998.
25. Norris SJ, Fraser CM, Weinstock GM: Illuminating the agent of syphilis: the *Treponema pallidum* genome project, *Electrophoresis* 19:551-553, 1998.
26. Pillay A, Liu H, Chen CY, et al: Molecular subtyping of *Treponema pallidum* subspecies *pallidum*, *Sex Transm Dis* 25:408-414, 1998.
27. Peeling RW, Hook EW 3rd: The pathogenesis of syphilis: the Great Mimicker, revisited, *J Pathol* 208:224-232, 2006.
28. Klein JO: Current concepts of infectious diseases in the newborn infant, *Adv Pediatr* 31:405-446, 1984.
29. Hook EW3rd, Marra CM: Acquired syphilis in adults, *N Engl J Med* 326:1060-1069, 1992.
30. Fitzgerald TJ: Experimental congenital syphilis in rabbits, *Can J Microbiol* 31:757-762, 1985.
31. Wicher K, Baughn RE, Wicher V, et al: Experimental congenital syphilis: guinea pig model, *Infect Immun* 60:271-277, 1992.
32. Kajdacsy-Balla A, Howeedy A, Bagasra O: Experimental model of congenital syphilis, *Infect Immun* 61:3559-3561, 1993.
33. Wicher K, Baughn RE, Abbruscato F, et al: Vertical transmission of *Treponema pallidum* to various litters and generations of guinea pigs, *J Infect Dis* 179:1206-1212, 1999.
34. Fieldsteel AH, Becker FA, Stout JG: Prolonged survival of virulent *Treponema pallidum* (Nichols strain) in cell-free and tissue culture systems, *Infect Immun* 18:173-182, 1977.
35. Fieldsteel AH, Cox DL, Moeckli RA: Cultivation of virulent *Treponema pallidum* in tissue culture, *Infect Immun* 32:908-915, 1981.
36. Centers for Disease Control and Prevention, Workowski KA, Berman SM: Sexually transmitted diseases treatment guidelines, 2006 [erratum in *MMWR Recomm Rep* 55:997, 2006], *MMWR Recomm Rep* 55(RR-11):1-94, 2006.
37. Singh AE, Romanowski B: Syphilis: review with emphasis on clinical, epidemiologic, and some biologic features, *Clin Microbiol Rev* 12:187-209, 1999.
38. Magnuson HJ, Eagle H, Fleischman R: The minimal infectious inoculum of Spirochaeta pallida (Nichols strain), and a consideration of its rate of multiplication in vivo, *Am J Syphilis Gonorrhea Vener Dis* 32:1-18, 1948.
39. Cates W Jr, Rothenberg RB, Blount JH: Syphilis control. The historic context and epidemiologic basis for interrupting sexual transmission of *Treponema pallidum*, *Sex Transm Dis* 23:68-75, 1996.
40. Dorman HG, Sahyun BF: Identification and significance of spirochetes in placenta: report of 105 cases with positive findings, *Am J Obstet Gynecol* 33:954-967, 1937.
41. Harter CA, Benirschke K: Fetal syphilis in the first trimester, *Am J Obstet Gynecol* 124:705-711, 1976.
42. Silverstein AM: Congenital syphilis and the timing of immunogenesis in the human foetus, *Nature* 194:196-197, 1962.
43. Burstain JM, Grimprel E, Lukehart SA: Sensitive detection of *Treponema pallidum* by using the polymerase chain reaction, *J Clin Microbiol* 29:62-69, 1991.
44. Nathan L, Twickler DM, Peters MT, et al: Fetal syphilis: correlation of sonographic findings and rabbit infectivity testing of amniotic fluid, *J Ultrasound Med* 12:97-101, 1993.
45. Nathan L, Bohman VR, Sánchez PJ, et al: In utero infection with *Treponema pallidum* in early pregnancy, *Prenat Diagn* 17:119-123, 1997.
46. Sánchez PJ, Wendel GD, Grimprel E: Evaluation of molecular methodologies and rabbit infectivity testing for the diagnosis of congenital syphilis and central nervous system invasion by *Treponema pallidum*, *J Infect Dis* 167:148-157, 1993.
47. Wendel GD Jr, Sánchez PJ, Peters MT, et al: Identification of *Treponema pallidum* in amniotic fluid and fetal blood from pregnancies complicated by congenital syphilis, *Obstet Gynecol* 78(5 Pt 2):890-895, 1991.
48. Qureshi F, Jacques SM, Reyes MP: Placental histopathology in syphilis, *Hum Pathol* 24:779-784, 1993.
49. Fojaca RM, Hensely GT, Moskowitz L: Congenital syphilis and necrotizing funisitis, *JAMA* 261:1788-1790, 1989.
50. Fenton LJ: Light IJ: Congenital syphilis after maternal treatment with erythromycin, *Obstet Gynecol* 47:492-494, 1976.
51. Nabarro JND: *Congenital syphilis*, Baltimore, 1954, Williams & Wilkins.
52. Ballantyne JW: *Manual of antenatal pathology and hygiene*, Edinburgh, 1902, William Green & Son.
53. Fiumara NJ: The incidence of prenatal syphilis at the Boston City Hospital, *N Engl J Med* 247:48-52, 1952.
54. Ingraham NR: The value of penicillin alone in the prevention and treatment of congenital syphilis, *Acta Derm Venereol* 31(Suppl 24):60-87, 1951.
55. Baughn RE, Musher DM: Secondary syphilitic lesions, *Clin Microbiol Rev* 18:205-216, 2005.
56. Sheffield JS, Wendel GD, Zeray F: Congenital syphilis: the influence of maternal stage of syphilis on vertical transmission, *Am J Obstet Gynecol* 180:85-88, 1999.
57. Lynn WA, Lightman S: Syphilis and HIV: a dangerous combination, *Lancet Infect Dis* 4:456-466, 2004.
58. Erbelding EJ: Syphilis rates climb again, *Hopkins HIV Rep* 16:8-9, 2004.
59. Golden MR, Marra CM, Holmes KK: Update on syphilis: resurgence of an old problem, *JAMA* 290:1510-1514, 2003.
60. Poulton M, Curtis S, McElborough D, et al: Syphilis: mimicking yet another disease!, *Sex Transm Infect* 77:325, 2001.
61. Theus SA, Harrich DA, Gaynor R: *Treponema pallidum*, lipoproteins, and synthetic lipoprotein analogues induce human immunodeficiency virus type 1 gene expression in monocytes via NF-κB activation, *J Infect Dis* 177:941-950, 1998.
62. Centers for Disease Control and Prevention, Available at http://www.cdc.gov/mmwr/preview/mmwrhtml/mm5914a1.htm. Accessed July 4, 2014.
63. Lukehart SA, Hook EW, Baker-Zander SA 3rd, et al: Invasion of the central nervous system by *Treponema pallidum*: implications for diagnosis and treatment, *Ann Intern Med* 109:855-862, 1988.
64. Woods CR: Syphilis in children: congenital and acquired, *Semin Pediatr Infect Dis* 16:245-257, 2005.
65. Tucker HA: Robinson RC: Disappearance time of *T. pallidum* from lesions of early syphilis following administration of crystalline penicillin G, *Bull Johns Hopkins Hosp* 80:169-173, 1947.
66. Pickering LK: Syphilis. In Pickering LK, editor: *Red book: report of the Committee on Infectious Diseases*, ed 29, Elk Grove Village, Ill, 2012, American Academy of Pediatrics, pp 690-703.
67. Zenilman JM: Congenital syphilis in immigrants–are politics and nativism driving us in reverse? *Sex Transm Dis* 35:344-345, 2008.
68. Tucker JD, Chen XS, Peeling RW: Syphilis and social upheaval in China, *N Engl J Med* 362:1658-1661, 2010.
69. Tucker JD, Cohen MS: China's syphilis epidemic: epidemiology, proximate determinants of spread, and control responses, *Curr Opin Infect Dis* 24:50-55, 2011.
70. CentersforDiseaseControlandPrevention:Congenitalsyphilis–United States, 2003-2008, *MMWR Morb Mortal Wkly Rep* 59:413-417, 2010.
71. Singh AE, Sutherland K, Lee B, et al: Resurgence of early congenital syphilis in Alberta, *CMAJ* 177:33-36, 2007.
72. Jones H, Taylor D, Montgomery CA, et al: Prenatal and congenital syphilis in British Columbia, *J Obstet Gynaecol Can* 27:467-472, 2005.
73. Dunn RA, Webster LA, Nakashima AK, et al: Surveillance for geographic and secular trends in congenital syphilis—United States, 1983-1991, *MMWR CDC Surveill Summ* 42:59-71, 1993.
74. St. Louis ME, Wasserheit JM: Elimination of syphilis in the United States, *Science* 281:353-354, 1998.
75. Hahn RA, Magder LS, Aral SO, et al: Race and the prevalence of syphilis seroreactivity in the United States population: a national sero-epidemiologic study, *Am J Public Health* 79:467-470, 1989.
76. Follett T, Clarke DF: Resurgence of congenital syphilis: diagnosis and treatment, *Neonatal Netw* 30:320-328, 2011.
77. Zenker P: New case definition for congenital syphilis reporting, *Sex Transm Dis* 18:44-45, 1991.

78. Ikeda MK, Jenson HB: Evaluation and treatment of congenital syphilis, *J Pediatr* 117:843-852, 1990.
79. Mascola L, Pelosi R, Blount JH: Congenital syphilis revisited, *Am J Dis Child* 139:575-580, 1985.
80. Sánchez PJ: Congenital syphilis, *Adv Pediatr Infect Dis* 7:161-180, 1992.
81. Cohen DA, Boyd D, Prabhudas I, et al: The effects of case definition in maternal screening and reporting criteria on rates of congenital syphilis, *Am J Public Health* 80:316-317, 1990.
82. Centers for Disease Control and Prevention: Sexually transmitted disease surveillance 2006 supplement: syphilis surveillance report. *MMWR Morb Mortal Wkly Rep* 59:413-417, 2010.
83. Nicoll A, Hamers FF: Are trends in HIV, gonorrhoea, and syphilis worsening in western Europe? *BMJ* 324:1324-1327, 2002.
84. Marcus U, Hamouda O: Syphilis in Germany, 2004: diagnoses increasing, particularly in smaller cities and rural areas, *Euro Surveill* 10:E050728.3, 2005.
85. Lautenschlager S: Sexually transmitted infections in Switzerland: return of the classics, *Dermatology* 210:134-142, 2005.
86. Walker GJ, Walker DG: Congenital syphilis: a continuing but neglected problem, *Semin Fetal Neonatal Med* 12:198-206, 2007.
87. Chi BH, Wang L, Read JS, et al: Predictors of stillbirth in sub-Saharan Africa, *Obstet Gynecol* 110:989-997, 2007.
88. Gloyd S, Chai S, Mercer MA: Antenatal syphilis in sub-Saharan Africa: missed opportunities for mortality reduction, *Health Policy Plan* 16:29-34, 2001.
89. Finelli L, Berman SM, Koumans EH, et al: Congenital syphilis, *Bull World Health Organ* 76(Suppl 2):126-128, 1998.
90. Schmid G: Economic and programmatic aspects of congenital syphilis prevention, *Bull World Health Organ* 82:402-409, 2004.
91. Mbopi Keou FX, Mbu R, Mauclère P, et al: Antenatal HIV prevalence in Yaounde, Cameroon, *Int J STD AIDS* 9:400-402, 1998.
92. Gichangi P, Renterghem LV, Karanja J, et al: Congenital syphilis in a Nairobi maternity hospital, *East Afr Med J* 81:589-593, 2004.
93. Woods CR: Syphilis in children: congenital and acquired, *Semin Pediatr Infect Dis* 16:245-257, 2005.
94. Peterson K, Baseman JB, Alderete JF: *Treponema pallidum* receptor binding proteins interact with fibronectin, *J Exp Med* 157:1958-1970, 1983.
95. Robbins SL: *Pathologic basis of disease*, Philadelphia, 1974, WB Saunders.
96. Radolf JD: Role of outer membrane architecture in immune evasion by *Treponema pallidum* and *Borrelia burgdorferi*, *Trends Microbiol* 2:307-311, 1994.
97. Salazar JC, Cruz AR, Pope CD, et al: *Treponema pallidum* elicits innate and adaptive cellular immune responses in skin and blood during secondary syphilis: a flow-cytometric analysis, *J Infect Dis* 195:879-887, 2007.
98. Sellati TJ, Waldrop SL, Salazar JC, et al: The cutaneous response in humans to *Treponema pallidum* lipoprotein analogues involves cellular elements of both innate and adaptive immunity, *J Immunol* 166:4131-4140, 2001.
99. Wicher V, Wicher K: Pathogenesis of maternal-fetal syphilis revisited, *Clin Infect Dis* 33:354-363, 2001.
100. Schroder NW, Eckert J, Stübs G, et al: Immune responses induced by spirochetal outer membrane lipoproteins and glycolipids, *Immunobiology* 213:329-340, 2008.
101. Salazar JC, Hazlett KR, Radolf JD: The immune response to infection with *Treponema pallidum*, the stealth pathogen, *Microbes Infect* 4:1133-1140, 2002.
102. Alder JD, Friess L, T.M.: Phagocytosis of opsonized *Treponema pallidum* subsp. *pallidum* proceeds slowly, *Infect Immun* 58:1167-1173, 1990.
103. Musher DM, Hague-Park M, Gyorkey F, et al: The interaction between *Treponema pallidum* and human polymorphonuclear leukocytes, *J Infect Dis* 147:77-86, 1983.
104. Thomas DD, Navab M, Haake DA, et al: *Treponema pallidum* invades intercellular junctions of endothelial cell monolayers, *Proc Natl Acad Sci U S A* 85:3608-3612, 1988.
105. Brightbill HD, Libraty DH, Krutzik SR, et al: Host defense mechanisms triggered by microbial lipoproteins through toll-like receptors, *Science* 285:732-736, 1999.
106. Riley BS, Oppenheimer-Marks N, Hansen EJ, et al: Virulent *Treponema pallidum* activates human vascular endothelial cells, *J Infect Dis* 165:484-493, 1992.
107. Podwinska J, Lusiak M, Zaba R, et al: The pattern and level of cytokines secreted by Th1 and Th2 lymphocytes of syphilitic patients correlate to the progression of the disease, *FEMS Immunol Med Microbiol* 28:1-14, 2000.
108. Van Voorhis WC, Barrett LK, Koelle DM, et al: Primary and secondary syphilis lesions contain mRNA for Th1 cytokines, *J Infect Dis* 173:491-495, 1996.
109. Fan Y-M, Zeng WJ, Wu ZH, et al: Immunophenotypes, apoptosis, and expression of Fas and Bcl-2 from peripheral blood lymphocytes in patients with secondary early syphilis, *Sex Transm Dis* 31:221-224, 2004.
110. Olansky S: Serodiagnosis of syphilis, *Med Clin North Am* 56:1145-1150, 1972.
111. Swancott MA, Radolf JD, Norgard MV: The 34-kilodalton membrane immunogen of *Treponema pallidum* is a lipoprotein, *Infect Immun* 58:384-392, 1990.
112. Willcox RR: Changing patterns of treponemal disease, *Br J Vener Dis* 50:169-178, 1974.
113. Baker-Zander SA, Hook EW 3rd, Bonin P, et al: Antigens of *Treponema pallidum* recognized by IgG and IgM antibodies during syphilis in humans, *J Infect Dis* 151:264-272, 1985.
114. Gerber A, Krell S, Morenz J: Recombinant *Treponema pallidum* antigens in syphilis serology, *Immunobiology* 196:535-549, 1996.
115. Baughn RE, Jorizzo JL, Adams CB, et al: Ig class and IgG subclass responses to *Treponema pallidum* in patients with syphilis, *J Clin Immunol* 8:128-139, 1988.
116. Lewis LL, Taber LH, Baughn RE: Evaluation of immunoglobulin M Western blot analysis in the diagnosis of congenital syphilis, *J Clin Microbiol* 28:296-302, 1990.
117. Morgan CA, Lukehart SA, Van Voorhis WC: Protection against syphilis correlates with specificity of antibodies to the variable regions of *Treponema pallidum* repeat protein K, *Infect Immun* 71:5605-5612, 2003.
118. Sánchez PJ, McCracken Jr GH, Wendel GD, et al: Molecular analysis of the fetal IgM response to *Treponema pallidum* antigens: implications for improved serodiagnosis of congenital syphilis, *J Infect Dis* 159:508-517, 1989.
119. Sánchez PJ, Wendel GD Jr, Grimprel E, et al: Evaluation of molecular methodologies and rabbit infectivity testing for the diagnosis of congenital syphilis and neonatal central nervous system invasion by *Treponema pallidum*, *J Infect Dis* 167:148-157, 1993.
120. Dobson SR, Taber LH, Baughn RE: Recognition of *Treponema pallidum* antigens by IgM and IgG antibodies in congenitally infected newborns and their mothers, *J Infect Dis* 157:903-910, 1988.
121. Garner MF, Backhouse JL, Daskalopoulos G, Walsh JL: *Treponema pallidum* haemagglutination test for syphilis. Comparison with TPI and FTA-ABS tests, *Br J Vener Dis* 48:470-473, 1972.
122. Miller JN: Value and limitations of nontreponemal and treponemal tests in the laboratory diagnosis of syphilis, *Clin Obstet Gynecol* 18:191-203, 1975.
123. Peeling RW, Hook EW: The pathogenesis of syphilis: the great mimicker, revisted, *J Pathol* 208:224-232, 2006.
124. Nabarro D: *Congenital syphilis*, London, 1954, E Arnold.
125. Dennie CC: The dying syphilologist, *AMA Arch Derm Syphilol* 62:615-621, 1950.
126. Fiumara NJ: Acquired syphilis in three patients with congenital syphilis, *N Engl J Med* 290:1119-1120, 1974.
127. Pavithran K: Acquired syphilis in a patient with late congenital syphilis, *Sex Transm Dis* 14:119-121, 1987.
128. Rosebury T: *Microbes and morals: the strange story of venereal disease*, New York, 1971, Viking Press.
129. Dobson S: Congenital syphilis resurgent, *Adv Exp Med Biol* 549:35-40, 2004.
130. Benzick AE, Wirthwein DP, Weinberg A, et al: Pituitary gland gumma in congenital syphilis after failed maternal treatment: a case report, *Pediatrics* 104:e4, 1999.
131. Sheffield JS, Sánchez PJ, Morris G, et al: Congenital syphilis after maternal treatment for syphilis during pregnancy, *Int J STD AIDS* 13:569-573, 2002.
132. Russell P, Altshuler G: Placental abnormalities of congenital syphilis. A neglected aid to diagnosis, *Am J Dis Child* 128:160-163, 1974.
133. Genest DR, Choi-Hong SR, Tate JE, et al: Diagnosis of congenital syphilis from placental examination: comparison of histopathology, Steiner stain, and polymerase chain reaction for *Treponema pallidum* DNA, *Hum Pathol* 27:366-372, 1996.

134. Sheffield JS, Sánchez PJ, Wendel GD Jr, et al: Placental histopathology of congenital syphilis, *Obstet Gynecol* 100:126-133, 2002.
135. Wendel GD: Gestational and congenital syphilis, *Clin Perinatol* 15:287-303, 1988.
136. Fojaco RM, Hensley GT, Moskowitz L: Congenital syphilis and necrotizing funisitis, *JAMA* 261:1788-1790, 1989.
137. Jacques SM, Qureshi F: Necrotizing funisitis: a study of 45 cases, *Hum Pathol* 23:1278-1283, 1992.
138. Bromberg K, Rawstron S, Tannis G: Diagnosis of congenital syphilis by combining *Treponema pallidum*-specific IgM detection with immunofluorescent antigen detection for *T. pallidum*. *J Infect Dis* 168:238-242, 1993.
139. Reyes MP, Hunt N, Ostrea EM Jr, et al: Maternal/congenital syphilis in a large tertiary-care urban hospital, *Clin Infect Dis* 17:1041-1046, 1993.
140. Oppenheimer EH, Hardy JB: Congenital syphilis in the newborn infant: clinical and pathological observations in recent cases, *Johns Hopkins Med J* 129:63-82, 1971.
141. Guarner J, Greer PW, Bartlett J, et al: Congenital syphilis in a newborn: an immunopathologic study, *Mod Pathol* 12:82-87, 1999.
142. Ajayi NA, Marven S, Kaschula RO, et al: Intestinal ulceration, obstruction, and haemorrhage in congenital syphilis, *Pediatr Surg Int* 15:391-393, 1999.
143. Kaplan BS, Wiglesworth FW, Marks MI, et al: The glomerulopathy of congenital syphilis–an immune deposit disease, *J Pediatr* 81:1154-1156, 1972.
144. Gamble CN, Reardan JB: Immunopathogenesis of syphilitic glomerulonephritis. Elution of antitreponemal antibody from glomerular immune-complex deposits, *N Engl J Med* 292:449-454, 1975.
145. Hill LL, Singer DB, Falletta J, et al: The nephrotic syndrome in congenital syphilis: an immunopathy, *Pediatrics* 49:260-266, 1972.
146. Losito A, Bucciarelli E, Massi-Benedetti F, et al: Membranous glomerulonephritis in congenital syphilis, *Clin Nephrol* 12:32-37, 1979.
147. Cremin BJ, Draper R: The value of radiography in perinatal deaths, *Pediatr Radiol* 11:143-146, 1981.
148. Cremin BJ, Fisher RM: The lesions of congenital syphilis, *Br J Radiol* 43:333-341, 1970.
149. Daaboul JJ, Kartchner W, Jones KL: Neonatal hypoglycemia caused by hypopituitarism in infants with congenital syphilis, *J Pediatr* 123:983-985, 1993.
150. Chakraborty R, Luck S: Syphilis is on the increase: the implications for child health, *Arch Dis Child* 93:105-109, 2008.
151. Nathan L, Twickler DM, Peters MT, et al: Fetal syphilis: correlation of sonographic findings and rabbit infectivity testing of amniotic fluid, *J Ultrasound Med* 12:97-101, 1993.
152. Chapel TA: The variability of syphilitic chancres, *Sex Transm Dis* 5:68-70, 1978.
153. Lautenschlager S: Diagnosis of syphilis: clinical and laboratory problems, *J Dtsch Dermatol Ges* 4:1058-1075, 2006.
154. Blair EK, Sedlack RE, Snyder JP, et al: Unsuspected syphilitic hepatitis in a patient with low-grade proteinuria and abnormal liver function, *Mayo Clin Proc* 65:1365-1367, 1990.
155. Drusin LM, Topf-Olstein B, Levy-Zombek E: Epidemiology of infectious syphilis at a tertiary hospital, *Arch Intern Med* 139:901-904, 1979.
156. Manton SL, Egglestone SI, Alexander I, et al: Oral presentation of secondary syphilis, *Br Dent J* 160:237-238, 1986.
157. Musher DM: Syphilis, *Infect Dis Clin North Am* 1:83-95, 1987.
158. Lautenschlager S: Cutaneous manifestations of syphilis: recognition and management, *Am J Clin Dermatol* 7:291-304, 2006.
159. Feher J, Somogyi T, Timmer M, et al: Syphilitic hepatitis: clinical, immunological and morphological aspects, *Acta Med Acad Sci Hung* 32:155-161, 1975.
160. Józsa L, Timmer M, Somogyi T, et al: Hepatitis syphilitica. A clinico-pathological study of 25 cases, *Acta Hepatogastroenterol (Stuttg)* 24:344-347, 1977.
161. Braunstein GD, Lewis EJ, Galvanek EG, et al: The nephrotic syndrome associated with secondary syphilis. An immune deposit disease, *Am J Med* 48:643-648, 1970.
162. Bhorade MS, Carag HB, Lee HJ, et al: Nephropathy of secondary syphilis. A clinical and pathological spectrum, *JAMA* 216:1159-1166, 1971.
163. Dismukes WE, Delgado DG, Mallernee SV, et al: Destructive bone disease in early syphilis, *JAMA* 236:2646-2648, 1976.
164. Tight RR, Warner JF: Skeletal involvement in secondary syphilis detected by bone scanning, *JAMA* 235:2326, 1976.
165. Shore RN, Kiesel HA, Bennett HD: Osteolytic lesions in secondary syphilis, *Arch Intern Med* 137:1465-1467, 1977.
166. Sánchez PJ, Wendel GD: Syphilis in pregnancy, *Clin Perinatol* 24:71-90, 1997.
167. Holder WR, Knox JM: Syphilis in pregnancy, *Med Clin North Am* 56:1151-1160, 1972.
168. Ingall D, Sánchez PJ: Syphilis. In Remington JS, Klein JO, editors: *Infectious diseases of the fetus and newborn infant*, Philadelphia, 2001, WB Saunders, pp 643-681.
169. Roy B: The Tuskegee Syphilis Experiment: biotechnology and the administrative state, *J Natl Med Assoc* 87:56-67, 1995.
170. Goh BT: Syphilis in adults, *Sex Transm Infect* 81:448-452, 2005.
171. Bays J, Chadwick D: The serologic test for syphilis in sexually abused children and adolescents, *Adolesc Pediatr Gynecol* 4:148-151, 1991.
172. Knight J, Richardson AC, White KC: The role of syphilis serology in the evaluation of suspected sexual abuse, *Pediatr Infect Dis* 11:125-127, 1992.
173. Lande MB, Richardson AC, White KC: The role of syphilis serology in the evaluation of suspected sexual abuse, *Pediatr Infect Dis J* 11:125-127, 1992.
174. Shew ML, Fortenberry JD: Syphilis screening in adolescents, *J Adolesc Health* 13:303-305, 1992.
175. Silber TJ, Niland NF: The clinical spectrum of syphilis in adolescence, *J Adolesc Health Care* 5:112-116, 1984.
176. Gust DA, Levine WC, St Louis ME, et al: Mortality associated with congenital syphilis in the United States, 1992-1998, *Pediatrics* 109:E79, 2002.
177. Fiumara NJ: A legacy of syphilis, *Arch Dermatol* 92:676-678, 1965.
178. Lago EG, Vaccari A, Fiori RM: Clinical features and follow-up of congenital syphilis, *Sex Transm Dis* 40:85-94, 2013.
179. Ortiz-Lopez N, Diez M, Diaz O, et al: Epidemiological surveillance of congenital syphilis in Spain, 2000-2010, *Pediatr Infect Dis J* 31:988-990, 2012.
180. Fiumara NJ, Lessell S: Manifestations of late congenital syphilis, *Arch Dermatol* 102:78-83, 1970.
181. Brown WJ, Moore MB Jr: Congenital syphilis in the United States, *Clin Pediatr (Phila)* 2:220-222, 1963.
182. Sever JL: Effects of infections on pregnancy risk, *Clin Obstet Gynecol* 16:225-234, 1973.
183. Lascari AD, Diamond J, Nolan BE: Anemia as the only presenting manifestation of congenital syphilis, *Clin Pediatr (Phila)* 15:90-91, 1976.
184. Ricci JM, Fojaco RM, O'Sullivan MJ: Congenital syphilis: the University of Miami/Jackson Memorial Medical Center experience, 1986-1988, *Obstet Gynecol* 74:687-693, 1989.
185. Taber LH, Huber TW: Congenital syphilis, *Prog Clin Biol Res* 3:183-190, 1975.
186. Tan KL: The re-emergence of early congenital syphilis, *Acta Paediatr Scand* 62:601-607, 1973.
187. Murali MV, Nirmala C, Rao JV: Symptomatic early congenital syphilis: a common but forgotten disease, *Case Rep Pediatr* 2012:934634, 2012.
188. Naeye RL: Fetal growth with congenital syphilis: a quantitative study, *Am J Clin Pathol* 55:228-231, 1971.
189. Teberg A, Hodgman JE: Congenital syphilis in newborn, *Calif Med* 118:5-10, 1973.
190. Webber MP, Lambert G, Bateman DA, et al: Maternal risk factors for congenital syphilis: a case-control study, *Am J Epidemiol* 137:415-422, 1993.
191. Saxoni F, Lapaanis P, Pantelakis SN: Congenital syphilis: a description of 18 cases and re-examination of an old but ever-present disease, *Clin Pediatr (Phila)* 6:687-691, 1967.
192. Leao JC, Gueiros LA, Porter SR: Oral manifestations of syphilis, *Clinics* 61:161-166, 2006.
193. Willcox RR: Venereal diseases in the newborn; some recent developments, *Br J Clin Pract* 11:868-870, 1957.
194. King AJ: Advances in the study of venereal disease, *Br J Clin Pract* 25:295-301, 1971.
195. Platou RV, Kometani JT: Penicillin therapy of late congenital syphilis, *Pediatrics* 1:601-616, 1948.
196. Woody NC, Sistrunk WF, Platou RV: Congenital syphilis: a laid ghost walks, *J Pediatr* 64:63-67, 1964.
197. Lugo A, Sánchez S, Sánchez JL: Congenital syphilis, *Pediatr Dermatol* 23:121-123, 2006.

198. Tana M, Lio A, Vento G: Early congenital syphilis in a premature newborn: typical cutaneous manifestations in atypical skin areas, *Arch Dis Child Fetal Neonatal* 97:F471, 2012.
199. Reddy S, Bushore D, Levy A, et al: Early diffuse alopecia in a neonate with congenital syphilis, *Pediatr Dermatol* 23:564-566, 2006.
200. Olansky S, Rogers WG, Anthony WC: Diagnosis of anogenital ulcers, *Cutis* 17:705-708, 1976.
201. Gutman LT: Congenital syphilis. In Mandell GL, editor: *Atlas of infectious disease*, Philadelphia, 1996, Current Medicine.
202. Hollier LM, Harstad TW, Sánchez PJ, et al: Fetal syphilis: clinical and laboratory characteristics, *Obstet Gynecol* 97:947-953, 2001.
203. Dorfman DH, Glaser JH: Congenital syphilis presenting in infants after the newborn period, *N Engl J Med* 323:1299-1302, 1990.
204. Shah MC, Barton LL: Congenital syphilitic hepatitis, *Pediatr Infect Dis J* 8:891-892, 1989.
205. Long WA, Ulshen MH, Lawson EE: Clinical manifestations of congenital syphilitic hepatitis: implications for pathogenesis, *J Pediatr Gastroenterol Nutr* 3:551-555, 1984.
206. Whitaker JA, Sartain P, Shaheedy M: Hematological aspects of congenital syphilis, *J Pediatr* 66:629-636, 1965.
207. Sartain P: The anemia of congenital syphilis, *South Med J* 58:27-31, 1965.
208. Pohl M, Niemeyer CM, Hentschel R, et al: Haemophagocytosis in early congenital syphilis, *Eur J Pediatr* 158:553-555, 1999.
209. Bulova SI, Schwartz E, Harrer WV: Hydrops fetalis and congenital syphilis, *Pediatrics* 49:285-287, 1972.
210. Toohey JS: Skeletal presentation of congenital syphilis: case report and review of the literature, *J Pediatr Orthop* 5:104-106, 1985.
211. Solomon A, Rosen E: The aspect of trauma in the bone changes of congenital lues, *Pediatr Radiol* 3:176-178, 1975.
212. Solomon A, Rosen E: Focal osseous lesions in congenital lues, *Pediatr Radiol* 7:36-39, 1978.
213. Rose EK, Gyorgy P, Ingraham NR Jr: Treatment of infantile congenital syphilis; results with aqueous penicillin alone in 60 infants followed for an average of 2 years after treatment, *Am J Dis Child* 77:729-735, 1949.
214. Cremin BJ, Shaff MI: Congenital syphilis diagnosed in utero, *Br J Radiol* 48:939-941, 1975.
215. Heyman S, Mandell GA: Skeletal scintigraphy in congenital syphilis, *Clin Nucl Med* 8:531-534, 1983.
216. Wolpowitz A: Osseous manifestations of congenital syphilis, *S Afr Med J* 50:675-676, 1976.
217. Siegel D, Hirschman SZ: Syphilitic osteomyelitis with diffusely abnormal bone scan, *Mt Sinai J Med* 46:320-322, 1979.
218. Wilkinson RH, Heller RM: Congenital syphilis: resurgence of an old problem, *Pediatrics* 47:27-30, 1971.
219. Brion LP, Manuli M, Rai B, et al: Long-bone radiographic abnormalities as a sign of active congenital syphilis in asymptomatic newborns, *Pediatrics* 88:1037-1040, 1991.
220. Fan P, Fu M, Liao W, et al: Early congenital syphilis presented with exclusive bending pain of extremity: case report, *J Dermatol* 34:214-216, 2007.
221. Szalay GC, Teberg A: Congenital syphilis in newborn, *Calif Med* 119:75, 1973.
222. Wolf B, Kalangu K: Congenital neurosyphilis revisited, *Eur J Pediatr* 152:493-495, 1993.
223. Silva S, Henriques R, Gomes JP, et al: Could we miss congenital neurosyphilis? *Lancet Infect Dis* 12:816, 2012.
224. Dennie CC: *A history of syphilis*, Springfield, Ill, 1962, Charles C Thomas.
225. Opina AD, Tafur A: A night with Venus, a lifetime with Mercury: a case of multiple intracranial aneurysms, *Am J Med Sci* 343:498-500, 2012.
226. Nolt D, Saad R, Kouatli A, et al: Survival with hypopituitarism from congenital syphilis, *Pediatrics* 109:e63, 2002.
227. Contreras F, Pereda J: Congenital syphilis of the eye with lens involvement, *Arch Ophthalmol* 96:1052-1053, 1978.
228. Berry MC, Dajani AS: Resurgence of congenital syphilis, *Infect Dis Clin North Am* 6:19-29, 1992.
229. Papaioannou AC, Asrow GG, Schuckmell NH: Nephrotic syndrome in early infancy as a manifestation of congenital syphilis, *Pediatrics* 27:636-641, 1961.
230. Pollner P: Nephrotic syndrome associated with congenital syphilis, *JAMA* 198:263-266, 1966.
231. Rosen EU, Abrahams C, Rabinowitz L: Nephropathy of congenital syphilis, *S Afr Med J* 47:1606-1609, 1973.
232. Yuceoglu AM, Sagel I, Tresser G, et al: The glomerulopathy of congenital syphilis. A curable immune-deposit disease, *JAMA* 229:1085-1089, 1974.
233. McDonald R, Wiggelinkhuizen J, Kaschula RO: The nephrotic syndrome in very young infants, *Am J Dis Child* 122:507-512, 1971.
234. Rawstron SA, Bromberg K: Comparison of maternal and newborn serologic tests for syphilis, *Am J Dis Child* 145:1383-1388, 1991.
235. Putkonen T: Does early treatment prevent dental changes in congenital syphilis? *Acta Derm Venereol* 43:240-249, 1963.
236. Khetarpal S, Kempf E, Mostow E: Congenital syphilis: early- and late-stage findings of rhagades and dental anomalies, *Pediatr Dermatol* 28:401-403, 2011.
237. Bagri NK, Gupta V: Palatal perforation due to late congenital syphilis, *Indian J Pediatr* 81:216-217, 2014.
238. Fiumara NJ, Lessell S: Manifestations of late congenital syphilis. An analysis of 271 patients, *Arch Dermatol* 102:78-83, 1970.
239. Borella L, Goobar JE, Clark GM: Synovitis of the knee joints in late congenital syphilis. Clutton's joints, *JAMA* 180:190-192, 1962.
240. Sánchez MR: Infectious syphilis, *Semin Dermatol* 13:234-242, 1994.
241. Fiumara NJ: A retrospective approach to syphilis in the 1970s, *Int J Dermatol* 21:400-403, 1982.
242. Fiumara NJ, Fleming WL, Downing JG: The incidence of prenatal syphilis at the Boston City Hospital. *N Engl J Med* 247:48-52, 1970.
243. Pessoa L, Galvao V: Clinical aspects of congenital syphilis with Hutchinson's triad, *BMJ Case Rep*, 2011. pii:bcr1120115130, 2011.
244. Hendershot EL: Luetic deafness, *Otolaryngol Clin North Am* 11:43-47, 1978.
245. Rothenberg R, Becker G, Wiet R: Syphilitic hearing loss, *South Med J* 72:118-120, 1979.
246. Ashley D, Greenwood R, McCaw-Binns A, et al: Medical conditions present during pregnancy and risk of perinatal death in Jamaica, *Paediatr Perinat Epidemiol* 8(Suppl 1):66-85, 1994.
247. Azimi PH: Interstitial keratitis in a five-year-old, *Pediatr Infect Dis J* 18:299-311, 1999.
248. Herremans T, Kortbeek L, Notermans DW: A review of diagnostic tests for congenital syphilis in newborns, *Eur J Clin Microbiol Infect Dis* 29:495-501, 2010.
249. Lewis LL: Congenital syphilis. Serologic diagnosis in the young infant, *Infect Dis Clin North Am* 6:31-39, 1992.
250. Wendel GD, Sheffield JS, Hollier LM, et al: Treatment of syphilis in pregnancy and prevention of congenital syphilis, *Clin Infect Dis* 35(Suppl 2):S200-S209, 2002.
251. Gayet-Ageron A, Lautenschlager S, Ninet B, et al: Sensitivity, specificity and likelihood ratios of PCR in the diagnosis of syphilis: a systematic review and meta-analysis, *Sex Transm Infect* 89:251-256, 2013.
252. Yobs AR, Rockwell DH, Clark JW Jr: Treponemal survival in humans after penicillin therapy: a preliminary report, *Br J Vener Dis* 40:248-253, 1964.
253. Michelow IC, Wendel GD Jr, Norgard MV, et al: Central nervous system infection in congenital syphilis, *N Engl J Med* 346:1792-1798, 2002.
254. Palmer HM, Higgins SP, Herring AJ, et al: Use of PCR in the diagnosis of early syphilis in the United Kingdom, *Sex Transm Infect* 79:479-483, 2003.
255. Liu H, Rodes B, Chen CY, et al: New tests for syphilis: rational design of a PCR method for detection of *Treponema pallidum* in clinical specimens using unique regions of the DNA polymerase I gene, *J Clin Microbiol* 39:1941-1946, 2001.
256. Grimprel E, Sánchez PJ, Wendel GD, et al: Use of polymerase chain reaction and rabbit infectivity testing to detect *Treponema pallidum* in amniotic fluid, fetal and neonatal sera, and cerebrospinal fluid, *J Clin Microbiol* 29:1711-1718, 1991.
257. Marra CM: Neurosyphilis, *Curr Neurol Neurosci Rep* 4:435-440, 2004.
258. Turner TB, Hardy PH, Newman B: Infectivity tests in syphilis, 1969, *Sex Transm Infect* 76(Suppl 1):S7, 2000.
259. Larsen SA, Steiner BM, Rudolph AH: Laboratory diagnosis and interpretation of tests for syphilis, *Clin Microbiol Rev* 8:1-21, 1995.
260. Matthews TG, O'Herlihy C: Significance of raised immunoglobulin M levels in cord blood of small-for-gestational-age infants, *Arch Dis Child* 53:895-898, 1978.
261. Moskophidis M, Muller F: Molecular analysis of immunoglobulins M and G immune response to protein antigens of *Treponema pallidum* in human syphilis, *Infect Immun* 43:127-132, 1984.

262. Muller F: Specific immunoglobulin M and G antibodies in the rapid diagnosis of human treponemal infections, *Diagn Immunol* 4:1-9, 1986.
263. Schroeter AL, Lucas JB, Price EV, et al: Treatment for early syphilis and reactivity of serologic tests, *JAMA* 221:471-476, 1972.
264. Fiumara NJ: Reinfection primary, secondary, and latent syphilis: the serologic response after treatment, *Sex Transm Dis* 7:111-115, 1980.
265. Peterman TA, Newman DR, Davis D, et al: Do women with persistently negative nontreponemal test results transmit syphilis during pregnancy? *Sex Transm Dis* 40:311-315, 2013.
266. Chhabra RS, Brion LP, Castro M, et al: Comparison of maternal sera, cord blood, and neonatal sera for detecting presumptive congenital syphilis: relationship with maternal treatment, *Pediatrics* 91:88-91, 1993.
267. Nandwani R, Evans DT: Are you sure it's syphilis? A review of false positive serology, *Int J STD AIDS* 6:241-248, 1995.
268. Kuznetsov AV, Burgdorf WH, Prinz JC: Latent syphilis confirmed by polymerase chain reaction in 2 HIV-positive patients with inconclusive serologic test results, *Arch Dermatol* 141:1169-1170, 2005.
269. Felman YM, Nikitas JA: Sexually transmitted diseases. Secondary syphilis, *Cutis* 29:322, 1982.
270. Sparling PF: Diagnosis and treatment of syphilis, *N Engl J Med* 284:642-653, 1971.
271. Levine Z, Sherer DM, Jacobs A, et al: Nonimmune hydrops fetalis due to congenital syphilis associated with negative intrapartum maternal serology screening, *Am J Perinatol* 15:233-236, 1998.
272. Smith G, Holman RP: The prozone phenomenon with syphilis and HIV-1 co-infection, *South Med J* 97:379-382, 2004.
273. Taniguchi S, Osato K, Hamada T: The prozone phenomenon in secondary syphilis, *Acta Derm Venereol* 75:153-154, 1995.
274. Taniguchi Y, Shan E, Ohyanagi S, et al: Syphilis in old age, *Int J Dermatol* 34:38-39, 1995.
275. Sánchez PJ: Laboratory tests for congenital syphilis, *Pediatr Infect Dis J* 17:70-71, 1998.
276. Garner MF: The IgM FTA test for syphilis in the newborn, *Aust N Z J Obstet Gynaecol* 12:179-181, 1972.
277. Rudolph AH: The microhemagglutination assay for *Treponema pallidum* antibodies (MHA-TP), a new treponemal test for syphilis: where does it fit? *J Am Vener Dis Assoc* 3:3-8, 1976.
278. Rudolph AH: Serologic diagnosis of syphilis: an update, *South Med J* 69:1196-1197, 1203, 1976.
279. Larsen SA, Hambie EA, Pettit DE, et al: Specificity, sensitivity, and reproducibility among the fluorescent treponemal antibody-absorption test, the microhemagglutination assay for *Treponema pallidum* antibodies, and the hemagglutination treponemal test for syphilis, *J Clin Microbiol* 14:441-445, 1981.
280. Fiumara NJ: Treatment of primary and secondary syphilis. Serological response, *JAMA* 243:2500-2502, 1980.
281. O'Neill P, Warner RW, Nicol CS: *Treponema pallidum* haemagglutination assay in the routine serodiagnosis of treponemal disease, *Br J Vener Dis* 49:427-431, 1973.
282. Lesinski J, Krach J, Kadziewicz E: Specificity, sensitivity, and diagnostic value of the TPHA test, *Br J Vener Dis* 50:334-340, 1974.
283. Larsen SA, Farshy CE, Pender BJ, et al: Staining intensities in the fluorescent treponemal antibody-absorption (FTA-Abs) test: association with the diagnosis of syphilis, *Sex Transm Dis* 13:221-227, 1986.
284. Musher D: An unusual cause of FUO, *Hosp Pract* 13:134-135, 1978.
285. Singh AE, Guenette T, Gratrix J, et al: Seroreversion of treponemal tests in infants meeting Canadian surveillance criteria for confirmed early congenital syphilis, *Pediatr Infect Dis J* 32:199-202, 2013.
286. Isaacs RD, Radolf JD: Molecular approaches to improved syphilis serodiagnosis, *Serodiagn Immunother Infect Dis* 3:299-306, 1989.
287. Van Voorhis WC, Barrett LK, Lukehart SA, et al: Serodiagnosis of syphilis: antibodies to recombinant Tp0453, Tp92, and Gpd proteins are sensitive and specific indicators of infection by *Treponema pallidum*, *J Clin Microbiol* 41:3668-3674, 2003.
288. Egglestone SI, Turner AJ: Serological diagnosis of syphilis. PHLS Syphilis Serology Working Group, *Commun Dis Public Health* 3:158-162, 2000.
289. Young H: Guidelines for serological testing for syphilis, *Sex Transm Infect* 76:403-405, 2000.
290. Young H, Aktas G, Moyes A: Enzywell recombinant enzyme immunoassay for the serological diagnosis of syphilis, *Int J STD AIDS* 11:288-291, 2000.
291. Jafari Y, Peeling RW, Shivkumar S, et al: Are *Treponema pallidum* specific rapid and point-of-care tests for syphilis accurate enough for screening in resource limited settings? Evidence from a meta-analysis, *PLoS One* 8:e54695, 2013.
292. Pai NP, Kurji J, Singam A, et al: Simultaneous triple point-of-care testing for HIV, syphilis and hepatitis B virus to prevent mother-to-child transmission in India, *Int J STD AIDS* 23:319-324, 2012.
293. Herring A, Ballard R, Mabey D, et al: Evaluation of rapid diagnostic tests: syphilis, *Nat Rev Microbiol* 4(Suppl 12):S33-S40, 2006.
294. Peeling RW, Holmes KK, Mabey D, et al: Rapid tests for sexually transmitted infections (STIs): the way forward, *Sex Transm Infect* 82(Suppl 5):v1-v6, 2006.
295. Hawkes S, Matin N, Broutet N, et al: Effectiveness of interventions to improve screening for syphilis in pregnancy: a systematic review and meta-analysis, *Lancet Infect Dis* 11:684-691, 2011.
296. Leclerc G, Giroux M, Birry A, et al: Study of fluorescent treponemal antibody test on cerebrospinal fluid using monospecific anti-immunoglobulin conjugates IgG, IgM, and IgA, *Br J Vener Dis* 54:303-308, 1978.
297. Muller F: Immunological and laboratory aspects of treponematoses, *Dermatol Monatsschr* 170:357-366, 1984.
298. Lee JB, Farshy CE, Hunter EF, et al: Detection of immunoglobulin M in cerebrospinal fluid from syphilis patients by enzyme-linked immunosorbent assay, *J Clin Microbiol* 24:736-740, 1986.
299. Izzat NN, Bartruff JK, Glicksman JM, et al: Validity of the VDRL test on cerebrospinal fluid contaminated by blood, *Br J Vener Dis* 47:162-164, 1971.
300. Thorley JD, Kaplan JM, Holmes RK, et al: Passive transfer of antibodies of maternal origin from blood to cerebrospinal fluid in infants, *Lancet* 1:651-653, 1975.
301. Monif GR, Williams BR Jr, Shulman ST, et al: The problem of maternal syphilis after serologic surveillance during pregnancy, *Am J Obstet Gynecol* 117:268-270, 1973.
302. Bellingham FR: Syphilis in pregnancy: transplacental infection, *Med J Aust* 2:647-648, 1973.
303. Stoll BJ, Lee FK, Larsen S, et al: Clinical and serologic evaluation of neonates for congenital syphilis: a continuing diagnostic dilemma, *J Infect Dis* 167:1093-1099, 1993.
304. Hawkes SJ, Gomez GB, Broutet N: Early antenatal care: does it make a difference to outcomes of pregnancy associated with syphilis? A systematic review and meta-analysis, *PLoS One* 8:e56713, 2013.
305. Warner L, Rochat RW, Fichtner RR, et al: Missed opportunities for congenital syphilis prevention in an urban southeastern hospital, *Sex Transm Dis* 28:92-98, 2001.
306. Felman Y: How useful are the serologic tests for syphilis? *Int J Dermatol* 21:79-81, 1982.
307. Augenbraun M, Rolfs R, Johnson R, et al: Treponemal specific tests for the serodiagnosis of syphilis. Syphilis and HIV Study Group, *Sex Transm Dis* 25:549-552, 1998.
308. Hicks CB, Benson PM, Lupton GP, et al: Seronegative secondary syphilis in a patient infected with the human immunodeficiency virus (HIV) with Kaposi sarcoma. A diagnostic dilemma, *Ann Intern Med* 107:492-495, 1987.
309. Haslett P, Laverty M: The prozone phenomenon in syphilis associated with HIV infection, *Arch Intern Med* 154:1643-1644, 1994.
310. Malone JL, Wallace MR, Hendrick BB, et al: Syphilis and neurosyphilis in a human immunodeficiency virus type-1 seropositive population: evidence for frequent serologic relapse after therapy, *Am J Med* 99:55-63, 1995.
311. Janier M, Chastang C, Spindler E, et al: A prospective study of the influence of HIV status on the seroreversion of serological tests for syphilis, *Dermatology* 198:362-369, 1999.
312. Risser WL, Hwang LY: Problems in the current case definitions of congenital syphilis, *J Pediatr* 129:499-505, 1996.
313. Rathbun KC: Congenital syphilis: a proposal for improved surveillance, diagnosis, and treatment, *Sex Transm Dis* 10:102-107, 1983.
314. Rathbun KC: Congenital syphilis, *Sex Transm Dis* 10:93-99, 1983.
315. Zetola NM, Engelman J, Jensen TP, et al: Syphilis in the United States: an update for clinicians with an emphasis on HIV coinfection, *Mayo Clin Proc* 82:1091-1102, 2007.
316. Sánchez PJ, Wendel GD, Norgard MV: Congenital syphilis associated with negative results of maternal serologic tests at delivery, *Am J Dis Child* 145:967-969, 1991.
317. Talati AJ, Koneru P: Neonates at risk for congenital syphilis: radiographic and cerebrospinal fluid evaluations, *South Med J* 104: 827-830, 2011.

318. Moyer VA, Schneider V, Yetman R, et al: Contribution of long-bone radiographs to the management of congenital syphilis in the newborn infant, *Arch Pediatr Adolesc Med* 152:353-357, 1998.
319. Beeram MR, Chopde N, Dawood Y, et al: Lumbar puncture in the evaluation of possible asymptomatic congenital syphilis in neonates, *J Pediatr* 128:125-129, 1996.
320. Risser WL, Hwang LY: Problems in the current case definitions of congenital syphilis, *J Pediatr* 129:499-505, 1996.
321. Coles FB, Hipp SS, Silberstein GS, et al: Congenital syphilis surveillance in upstate New York, 1989-1992: implications for prevention and clinical management, *J Infect Dis* 171:732-735, 1995.
322. Lee G, Ball C, Sellars M, et al: Congenital syphilis as a differential diagnosis of non-accidental injury, *Eur J Pediatr* 167:1071-1072, 2008.
323. Lee MC, Robinson JL, Lee BE, et al: An infant with seizures, rash, and hepatosplenomegaly, *Clin Infect Dis* 46:451, 2008.
324. Lee V, Kinghorn G: Syphilis: an update, *Clin Med* 8:330-333, 2008.
325. Esterly NB, Solomon LM: Neonatal dermatology. II. Blistering and scaling dermatoses, *J Pediatr* 77:1075-1088, 1970.
326. Geppert LJ, Baker HJ, Copple BI, et al: *Pseudomonas* infections in infants and children, *J Pediatr* 41:555-561, 1952.
327. Ray CG, Wedgwood RJ: Neonatal listeriosis. Six case reports and a review of the literature, *Pediatrics* 34:378-392, 1964.
328. Lopez JB, Gross P, Boggs TR: Skin lesions in association with beta-hemolytic *Streptococcus* group B, *Pediatrics* 58:859-861, 1976.
329. Halal F, Delorme L, Brazeau M, et al: Congenital vesicular eruption caused by *Haemophilus influenzae* type b, *Pediatrics* 62:494-496, 1978.
330. Hageman J, Shulman S, Schreiber M, et al: Congenital tuberculosis: critical reappraisal of clinical findings and diagnostic procedures, *Pediatrics* 66:980-984, 1980.
331. Blatt J, Kastner O, Hodes DS: Cutaneous vesicles in congenital cytomegalovirus infection, *J Pediatr* 92:509, 1978.
332. Dvorak AM, Gavaller B: Congenital systemic candidiasis. Report of a case, *N Engl J Med* 274:540-543, 1966.
333. Oski FA, Naiman JL: *Hematologic problems in the newborn*, ed 2, Philadelphia, 1972, WB Saunders.
334. Anand A, Gray ES, Brown T, et al: Human parvovirus infection in pregnancy and hydrops fetalis, *N Engl J Med* 316:183-186, 1987.
335. Klein VR, Cox SM, Mitchell MD, et al: The Jarisch-Herxheimer reaction complicating syphilotherapy in pregnancy, *Obstet Gynecol* 75(3 Pt 1): 375-380, 1990.
336. Weiss DI, Cooper LZ, Green RH: Infantile glaucoma. A manifestation of congenital rubella, *JAMA* 195:725-727, 1966.
337. Ringel RE, Brenner JI, Haney PJ, et al: Prostaglandin-induced periostitis: a complication of long-term PGE1 infusion in an infant with congenital heart disease, *Radiology* 142:657-658, 1982.
338. Mannelli L, Perez FA, Parisi MT, et al: A case of congenital syphilis, *Emerg Radiol*, 2013.
339. De Santis M, De Luca C, Mappa I, et al: Syphilis infection during pregnancy: fetal risks and clinical management, *Infect Dis Obstet Gynecol* 2012:430585, 2012.
340. Eagle H, Fleischman R, Musselman AD: Effect of schedule of administration on the therapeutic efficacy of penicillin; importance of the aggregate time penicillin remains at effectively bactericidal levels, *Am J Med* 9:280-299, 1950.
341. Eagle H, Fleischman R, Musselman AD: The effective concentrations of penicillin in vitro and in vivo for streptococci, pneumococci, and Treponema pallidum, *J Bacteriol* 59:625-643, 1950.
342. Eagle H, Fleischman R, Musselman AD: The bactericidal action of penicillin in vivo: the participation of the host, and the slow recovery of the surviving organisms, *Ann Intern Med* 33:544-571, 1950.
343. Idsoe O, Guthe T, Willcox RR: Penicillin in the treatment of syphilis. The experience of three decades, *Bull World Health Organ* 47:1-68, 1972.
344. Augenbraun MH, Rolfs R: Treatment of syphilis, 1998: nonpregnant adults, *Clin Infect Dis* 28(Suppl 1):S21-S28, 1999.
345. Musher DM: How much penicillin cures early syphilis? *Ann Intern Med* 109:849-851, 1988.
346. Araujo Junior E, Martins Santana EF, Rolo LC, Nardozza LM, Moron AF: Prenatal diagnosis of congenital syphilis using two- and three-dimensional ultrasonography: case report, *Case Rep Infect Dis* 2012:478436, 2012.
347. Galvao TF, Silva MT, Serruya SJ, et al: Safety of benzathine penicillin for preventing congenital syphilis: a systematic review, *PLoS One* 8:e56463, 2013.
348. Wendel GD, Stark BJ, Jamison RB, Molina RD, Sullivan TJ: Penicillin allergy and desensitization in serious infections during pregnancy, *N Engl J Med* 312:1229-1232, 1985.
349. Hook EW, Roddy RE, Hardsfield HH: Ceftriaxone therapy for incubating and early syphilis, *J Infect Dis* 158:881-884, 2001.
350. Philipson A, Sabeth LD, Charles D: Transplacental passage of erythromycin and clindamycin. *N Engl J Med* 288:1219-1221, 1973.
351. Harris VJ, Jimenez CA, Vidyasagar D: Value of bone roentgenograms in diagnosis. Congenital syphilis with unusual clinical presentations, *IMJ Ill Med J* 151:371-374, 1977.
352. Alexander JM, Sheffield JS, Sánchez PJ, et al: Efficacy of treatment for syphilis in pregnancy, *Obstet Gynecol* 93:5-8, 1999.
353. Conover CS, Rend CA, Miller GB Jr, et al: Congenital syphilis after treatment of maternal syphilis with a penicillin regimen exceeding CDC guidelines, *Infect Dis Obstet Gynecol* 6:134-137, 1998.
354. Nathan L, Bawdon RE, Sidawi E: Penicillin levels following administration of benzathine penicillin G in pregnancy, *Obstet Gynecol* 82: 338-342, 1993.
355. Speer ME, Taber LH, Clark DB, et al: Cerebrospinal fluid levels of benzathine penicillin G in the neonate, *J Pediatr* 91:996-997, 1977.
356. Goldman JN, Girard KF: Intraocular treponemes in treated congenital syphilis, *Arch Ophthalmol* 78:47-50, 1967.
357. Dunlop EM, King AJ, Wilkinson AE: Study of late ocular syphilis. Demonstration of treponemes in aqueous humour and cerebrospinal fluid. 3. General and serological findings, *Trans Ophthalmol Soc U K* 88:275-294, 1969.
358. Ryan SJ, Hardy PH, Hardy JM, et al: Persistence of virulent *Treponema pallidum* despite penicillin therapy in congenital syphilis, *Am J Ophthalmol* 73:258-261, 1972.
359. Hardy JB, Hardy PH, Oppenheimer EH, et al: Failure of penicillin in a newborn with congenital syphilis, *JAMA* 212:1345-1349, 1970.
360. Bayne LL, Schmidley JW, Goodin DS: Acute syphilitic meningitis. Its occurrence after clinical and serologic cure of secondary syphilis with penicillin G, *Arch Neurol* 43:137-138, 1986.
361. Jorgensen J, Tikjob G, Weismann K: Neurosyphilis after treatment of latent syphilis with benzathine penicillin, *Genitourin Med* 62:129-131, 1986.
362. Markovitz DM, Beutner KR, Maggio RP, et al: Failure of recommended treatment for secondary syphilis, *JAMA* 255:1767-1768, 1986.
363. Franco A, Aprea L, Dell'Isola C, et al: Clinical case of seroconversion for syphilis following a needlestick injury: why not take a prophylaxis? *Infez Med* 15:187-190, 2007.
364. De Baets AJ, Sifovo S, Pazvakavambwa IE: Access to occupational postexposure prophylaxis for primary health care workers in rural Africa: a cross-sectional study, *Am J Infect Control* 35:545-551, 2007.
365. Meyer GS: Occupational infection in health care. The century-old lessons from syphilis, *Arch Intern Med* 153:2439-2447, 1993.
366. Hart G: Epidemiologic treatment for syphilis and gonorrhea, *Sex Transm Dis* 7:149-152, 1980.
367. Sivakumaran M, Murphy PT, Booker DJ, et al: Paroxysmal cold haemoglobinuria caused by non-Hodgkin's lymphoma, *Br J Haematol* 105:278-279, 1999.
368. Azimi PH, Janner D, Berne P, et al: Concentrations of procaine and aqueous penicillin in the cerebrospinal fluid of infants treated for congenital syphilis, *J Pediatr* 124:649-653, 1994.
369. Radcliffe M, Meyer M, Roditi D, et al: Single-dose benzathine penicillin in infants at risk of congenital syphilis—results of a randomised study. *S Afr Med J* 87:62-65, 1997.
370. Benzick AE, Wirthwein DP, Weinberg A: Pituitary gland gumma in congenital syphilis after failed maternal treatment: a case report, *Pediatrics* 104:e1-e4, 1999.
371. Bateman DA, Phibbs CS, Joyce T, et al: The hospital cost of congenital syphilis, *J Pediatr* 130:752-758, 1997.
372. Paryani SG, Vaughn AJ, Crosby M, et al: Treatment of asymptomatic congenital syphilis: benzathine versus procaine penicillin G therapy, *J Pediatr* 125:471-475, 1994.
373. Radcliffe M, Meyer M, Roditi D, et al: Single-dose benzathine penicillin in infants at risk of congenital syphilis—results of a randomised study, *S Afr Med J* 87:62-65, 1997.
374. Beck-Sague C, Alexander ER: Failure of benzathine penicillin G treatment in early congenital syphilis, *Pediatr Infect Dis J* 6:1061-1064, 1987.
375. Woolf A, Wilfert CM, Kelsey DB: Childhood syphilis in North Carolina, *N C Med J* 41:443-449, 1980.

376. Staat MA: Infectious disease issues in internationally adopted children, *Pediatr Infect Dis J* 21:257-258, 2002.
377. Chang SN, Chung KY, Lee MG, et al: Seroreversion of the serological tests for syphilis in the newborns born to treated syphilitic mothers, *Genitourin Med* 71:68-70, 1995.
378. Rawstron SA, Mehta S, Marcellino L, et al: Congenital syphilis and fluorescent treponemal antibody test reactivity after the age of 1 year, *Sex Transm Dis* 28:412-416, 2001.
379. Ikeda MK, Jenson HB: Evaluation and treatment of congenital syphilis, *J Pediatr* 117:843-852, 1990.
380. Rathburn KC: Congenital syphilis, *Sex Transm Dis* 10:93-99, 1983.
381. Pendergrass EP, Bromer RS: Congenital bone syphilis: preliminary report: roentgenologic study with notes on the histology and pathology of the condition, *AJR Am J Roentgenol* 22:1, 1929.
382. Centers for Disease Control and Prevention: Management of persons who have a history of penicillin allergy. Sexually transmitted treatment guidelines, 2010. Available at http://www.cdc.gov/std/treatment/2010/penicillin-allergy.htm. Accessed August 30, 2013.
383. Wendel GD Jr, Stark BJ, Jamison RB, et al: Penicillin allergy and desensitization in serious infections during pregnancy, *N Engl J Med* 312:1229-1232, 1985.
384. Gelfand JA, Elin RJ, Berry FW Jr, et al: Endotoxemia associated with the Jarisch-Herxheimer reaction, *N Engl J Med* 295:211-213, 1976.
385. Young EJ, Weingarten NM, Baughn RE, et al: Studies on the pathogenesis of the Jarisch-Herxheimer reaction: development of an animal model and evidence against a role for classical endotoxin, *J Infect Dis* 146:606-615, 1982.
386. Radolf JD, Arndt LL, Akins DR, et al: *Treponema pallidum* and *Borrelia burgdorferi* lipoproteins and synthetic lipopeptides activate monocytes/macrophages, *J Immunol* 154:2866-2877, 1995.
387. Myles TD, Elam G, Park-Hwang E, et al: The Jarisch-Herxheimer reaction and fetal monitoring changes in pregnant women treated for syphilis, *Obstet Gynecol* 92:859-864, 1998.
388. Klein VR, Cox SM, Mitchell MD, et al: The Jarisch-Herxheimer reaction complicating syphilotherapy in pregnancy, *Obstet Gynecol* 92:375-380, 1990.
389. Myles TD, Elam G, Park-Hwang E, et al: The Jarisch-Herxheimer reaction and fetal monitoring changes in pregnant women treated for syphilis, *Obstet Gynecol* 92:859-864, 1998.
390. Rac MW, Greer LG, Wendel GD Jr: Jarisch-Herxheimer reaction triggered by group B streptococcus intrapartum antibiotic prophylaxis, *Obstet Gynecol* 116(Suppl 2):552-556, 2010.
391. Rydzak CE, Goldie SJ: Cost-effectiveness of rapid point-of-care prenatal syphilis screening in sub-Saharan Africa, *Sex Transm Dis* 35:775-784, 2008.
392. Terris-Prestholt F, Watson-Jones D, Mugeye K, et al: Is antenatal syphilis screening still cost effective in sub-Saharan Africa, *Sex Transm Infect* 79:375-381, 2003.
393. Kamb M: Congenital syphilis: not gone and all too forgotten, *World J Pediatr* 6:101-102, 2010.
394. Tikhonova L, Salakhov E, Southwick K, et al: Congenital syphilis in the Russian Federation: magnitude, determinants, and consequences, *Sex Transm Infect* 79:106-110, 2003.
395. Hurtig AK, Nicoll A, Carne C, et al: Syphilis in pregnant women and their children in the United Kingdom: results from national clinician reporting surveys 1994-7, *BMJ* 317:1617-1619, 1998.
396. Southwick KL, Blanco S, Santander A, et al: Maternal and congenital syphilis in Bolivia, 1996: prevalence and risk factors, *Bull World Health Organ* 79:33-42, 2001.
397. Knight J, Richardson S, Petric M, et al: Contributions of suboptimal antenatal care and poor communication to the diagnosis of congenital syphilis, *Pediatr Infect Dis J* 14:237-240, 1995.
398. Finelli L, Crayne EM, Spitalny KC: Treatment of infants with reactive syphilis serology, New Jersey: 1992 to 1996, *Pediatrics* 102:e27, 1998.
399. Finelli L, Levine WC, Valentine J, et al: Syphilis outbreak assessment, *Sex Transm Dis* 28:131-135, 2001.
400. Patel SJ, Klinger EJ, O'Toole D, et al: Missed opportunities for preventing congenital syphilis infection in New York City, *Obstet Gynecol* 120:882-888, 2012.
401. Introcaso CE, Bradley H, Gruber D, et al: Missed opportunities for preventing congenital syphilis infection, *Sex Transm Dis* 40:431, 2013.
402. Hawkes S: Congenital syphilis: the story of a Greek tragedy, *Sex Transm Dis* 40:95-96, 2013.
403. Peeling RW, Mabey D, Ballard RC: Introducing new diagnostics into STI control programmes: the importance of programme science, *Sex Transm Infect* 89:115-119, 2013.
404. Hotez PJ: Neglected infections of poverty in the United States of America, *PLoS Negl Trop Dis* 2:e256, 2008.
405. Costa CC, Freitas LV, Sousa DM, et al: Congenital syphilis in Ceara: epidemiological analysis of one decade, *Rev Esc Enferm USP* 47:152-159, 2013.
406. Domingues RM, Saracen V, Hartz ZM, Leal Mdo C: Congenital syphilis: a sentinel event in antenatal care quality, *Rev Saude Publica* 47:147-157, 2013.
407. Montoya PJ, Lukehart SA, Brentlinger PE, et al: Comparison of the diagnostic accuracy of a rapid immunochromatographic test and the rapid plasma reagin test for antenatal syphilis screening in Mozambique, *Bull World Health Organ* 84:97-104, 2006.
408. Fonck K, Claeys P, Bashir F, et al: Syphilis control during pregnancy: effectiveness and sustainability of a decentralized program, *Am J Public Health* 91:705-707, 2001.
409. Nakashima AK, Rolfs RT, Flock ML, et al: Epidemiology of syphilis in the United States, 1941–1993, *Sex Transm Dis* 23:16-23, 1996.
410. Rekart M, Patrick D, Jolly A, et al: Mass treatment/prophylaxis during an outbreak of infectious syphilis in Vancouver, British Columbia, *Can Commun Dis Rep* 26:101-105, 2000.
411. Rekart ML, Patrick DM, Chakraborty B, et al: Targeted mass treatment for syphilis with oral azithromycin, *Lancet* 361:313-314, 2003.
412. Rekart ML, Wong T, Wong E, et al: The impact of syphilis mass treatment one year later: self-reported behaviour change among participants, *Int J STD AIDS* 16:571-578, 2005.
413. Pourbohloul B, Rekart ML, Brunham RC: Impact of mass treatment on syphilis transmission: a mathematical modeling approach, *Sex Transm Dis* 30:297-305, 2003.
414. Wawer MJ, Sewankambo NK, Serwadda D, et al: Control of sexually transmitted diseases for AIDS prevention in Uganda: a randomised community trial. Rakai Project Study Group, *Lancet* 353:525-535, 1999.
415. Kiddugavu MG, Kiwanuka N, Wawer MJ, et al: Effectiveness of syphilis treatment using azithromycin and/or benzathine penicillin in Rakai, Uganda, *Sex Transm Dis* 32:1-6, 2005.
416. Riedner G, Rusizoka M, Todd J, et al: Single-dose azithromycin versus penicillin G benzathine for the treatment of early syphilis, *N Engl J Med* 353:1236-1244, 2005.
417. Riedner G, Hoffmann O, Rusizoka M, et al: Decline in sexually transmitted infection prevalence and HIV incidence in female barworkers attending prevention and care services in Mbeya Region, Tanzania, *AIDS* 20:609-615, 2006.
418. Holmes KK: Azithromycin versus penicillin G benzathine for early syphilis, *N Engl J Med* 353:1291-1293, 2005.
419. Ballard RC, Berman SM, Fenton KA: Azithromycin versus penicillin for early syphilis, *N Engl J Med* 354:203-205, 2006.
420. Jaffe HW, Rice DT, Voigt R, et al: Selective mass treatment in a venereal disease control program, *Am J Public Health* 69:1181-1182, 1979.
421. Hibbs JR, Gunn RA: Public health intervention in a cocaine-related syphilis outbreak, *Am J Public Health* 81:1259-1262, 1991.
422. Zhou P, Qian Y, Xu J, et al: Occurrence of congenital syphilis after maternal treatment with azithromycin during pregnancy, *Sex Transm Dis* 34:472-474, 2007.
423. Mabey DC, Sollis KA, Kelly HA, et al: Point-of-care tests to strengthen health systems and save newborn lives: the case of syphilis, *PLoS Med* 9:e1001233, 2012.
424. Testing for syphilis during pregnancy, *Lancet Infect Dis* 12:255, 2012.
425. Limb M: New scheme aims to eradicate congenital syphilis in three years, *BMJ* 344:e1616, 2012.

17 Borrelia *Infections: Lyme Disease and Relapsing Fever*

HENRY M. FEDER, JR.

CHAPTER OUTLINE

Lyme Disease

Lyme disease, caused by the spirochete *Borrelia burgdorferi*, is the most common vector-borne illness in the United States. Although, in retrospect, a form of the illness had been recognized in Scandinavia in the early 1900s, modern awareness of Lyme disease began in the mid-1970s after a group of parents living on one small street reported a cluster of cases of "juvenile rheumatoid arthritis" in their children. Investigation of this unexplained "epidemic" of arthritis led to the description of "Lyme arthritis" in 1977 by Steere and colleagues.[1] This original description included 39 children and 12 adults from three bordering Connecticut communities (Lyme, Old Lyme, and East Haddam) and ultimately led to the discovery of its bacterial etiology.[1-3] The reported incidence of Lyme disease and its geographic range have increased dramatically in recent years, with approximately 30,000 cases reported annually. In 2013, the Centers for Disease Control and Prevention (CDC) announced, based on ongoing studies, that the 30,000 cases may represent an underestimate by a factor of ten.[4]

Several spirochetes are known to cause transplacental infections in various animals and in humans.[5] *Treponema pallidum* has been the most thoroughly investigated spirochete with respect to transplacental transmission in humans. Infection of the mother with *Treponema pallidum* during pregnancy is frequently associated with transplacental infection, resulting in congenital syphilis in the offspring. Congenital syphilis is often associated with clinically significant neurologic disease, such as hydrocephalus, cerebral palsy, deafness, blindness, convulsive disorders, and mental retardation. Adverse fetal outcomes also have been documented in gestational infections with *Leptospira canicola*, an etiologic agent of leptospirosis, and with other *Borrelia* species, including the etiologic agents of relapsing fever (discussed later). Because *B. burgdorferi* is a spirochete, whether it too can cause congenital infection is naturally of considerable interest.

EPIDEMIOLOGY AND TRANSMISSION

B. burgdorferi is transmitted by species of ticks of the *Ixodes* genus. In the United States, the usual vector in the Northeast and the upper Midwest is *Ixodes scapularis* (the deer tick or black-legged tick), whereas *Ixodes pacificus* (the western black-legged tick) is the usual vector on the Pacific Coast.[6] In Europe, the most important vector for the spirochete is *Ixodes ricinus*, which commonly feeds on sheep and cattle.

The life cycle of *I. scapularis* consists of three stages—larva, nymph, and adult—that develop during a 2-year period.[6] Ticks feed once during each stage of the life cycle. The larvae emerge in the early summer from eggs laid in the spring by the adult female tick. Greater than 95% of the larvae are born uninfected with *B. burgdorferi* because transovarial transmission rarely occurs. The larvae feed on a wide variety of small mammals, such as the white-footed mouse, that are natural reservoirs for *B. burgdorferi*. Tick larvae become infected by feeding on animals that are infected with the spirochete. The tick emerges the following spring in the nymphal stage. This stage of the tick is most likely to transmit infections to humans,[7] presumably because it is active at times during which humans are most likely to be in tick-infested areas and because it is very small and difficult to see. Consequently, the tick is more likely to be able to feed for a relatively long time, which increases the likelihood of transmission. If the nymphal tick is not infected with *B. burgdorferi*, it may subsequently become infected if it feeds on an infected animal during this stage of its development. The nymphs molt in the late summer or early fall and reemerge as adults. If the adult is infected, it also may transmit *B. burgdorferi* to humans. The adult deer tick may breed and spend the winter on a white-tailed deer (hence its name). In areas of abundant deer, decreasing the deer population may result in a parallel decrease of the deer tick population. In the spring, the females lay their eggs and die, completing the 2-year life cycle. The density of the deer tick population varies based on geography, the deer population, and the weather.

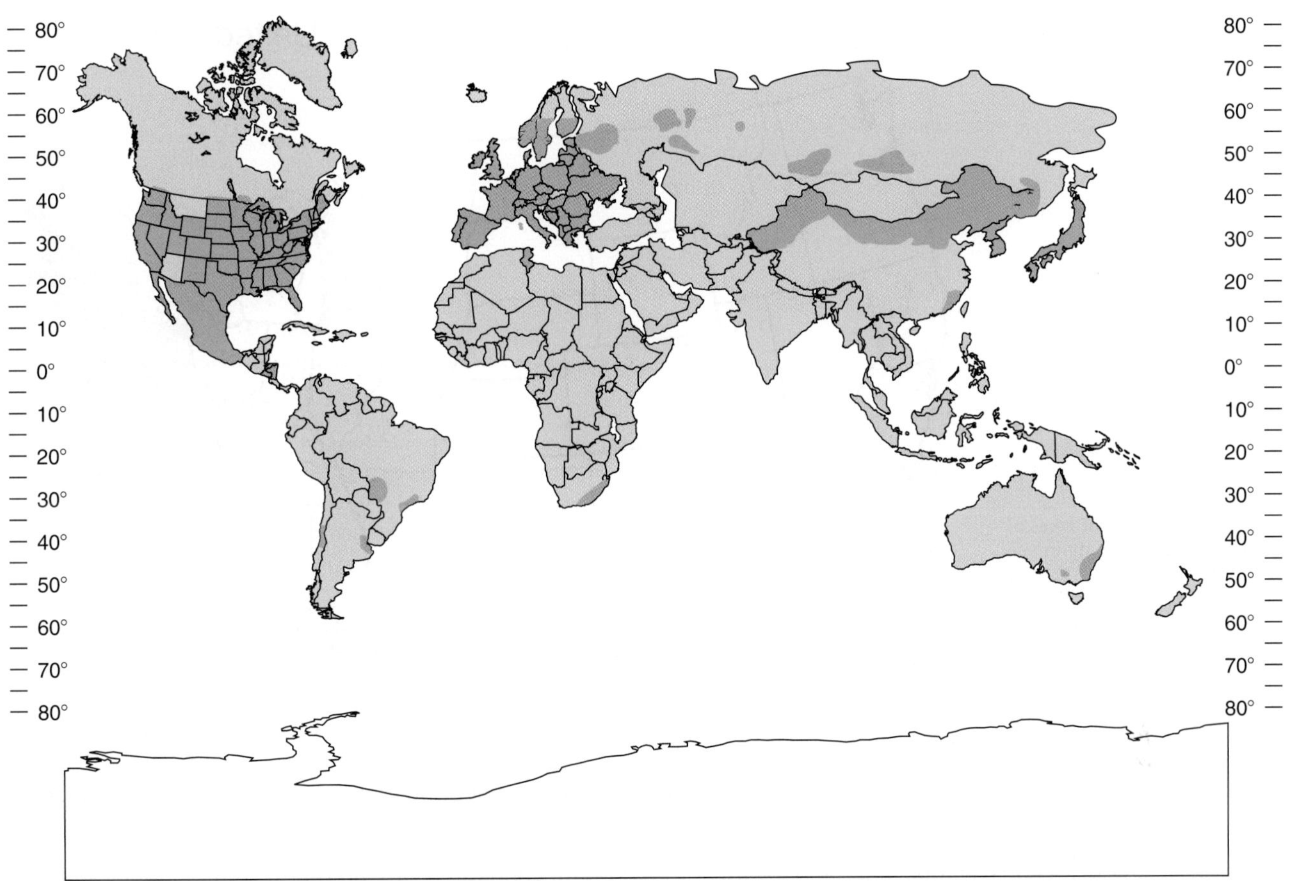

Figure 17-1 Worldwide geographic distribution of reported Lyme disease.

Numerous factors are associated with the risk of transmission of *B. burgdorferi* from infected ticks to humans. The proportion of infected ticks varies greatly by geographic area and by the stage of the tick in its life cycle. *I. pacificus* often feeds on lizards, which are not a competent reservoir for *B. burgdorferi*. Consequently, less than 5% of these ticks are infected with *B. burgdorferi*, so Lyme disease is rare in the Pacific states. By contrast, *I. scapularis* feeds on small mammals (usually field mice), which are competent reservoirs for *B. burgdorferi*. As a result, in highly endemic areas, the rates of infection for different stages of deer ticks are, approximately, 2% for larvae, 15% to 30% for nymphs, and 30% to 50% for adults.

B. burgdorferi is transmitted when an infected tick inoculates saliva into the blood vessels of the skin of its host. The risk of transmission of *B. burgdorferi* from infected deer ticks is related to the duration of feeding. It takes hours for the mouthparts of ticks to implant in the host, and much longer (days) for the tick to become fully engorged from feeding. *B. burgdorferi* is found primarily in the midgut of the tick, but as the tick feeds and becomes engorged, the bacteria migrate to the salivary glands, from which they can be transmitted. Experiments with animals have shown that infected nymph-stage ticks must feed for 48 hours or longer, and infected adult ticks must feed for 72 hours or longer before the risk of transmission of *B. burgdorferi* becomes substantial.[8] Results of a study of transmission of Lyme disease to humans are consistent with these experimental results.[7] Among persons bitten by nymph-stage ticks, for which the duration of feeding could be estimated, the risk of Lyme disease was 0% among persons bitten by nymphs that had fed for less than 72 hours but was 25% among persons bitten by nymphs that had fed for 72 hours or more. Approximately 75% of persons who recognize that they have been bitten by a deer tick remove the tick within 48 hours after it has begun to feed,[9] which may explain why only a small proportion of persons who recognize that they have been bitten by deer ticks subsequently develop Lyme disease. The risk of Lyme disease is greater from unrecognized bites because, in such instances, the tick is able to feed until fully engorged.

Substantial evidence indicates that the risk of Lyme disease after a recognized deer tick bite, even in hyperendemic areas, is only 1% to 3%.[7,10,11] The expertise to identify the species, stage, and degree of engorgement of a tick and to assess the degree of risk is rarely available to individuals who are bitten. The dog or wood tick, which does not transmit Lyme disease, is more than twice as large as the deer tick; however, subjects frequently misidentify dog ticks as deer ticks. Many "ticks" submitted for identification by physicians turned out actually to be spiders, lice, scabs, or dirt, none of which can transmit Lyme disease. In addition, estimates by patients of the duration for which the tick fed or degree of engorgement are unreliable.[12]

Lyme disease occurs throughout the world (Fig. 17-1). In the United States, greater than 95% of cases of Lyme disease occur in 12 eastern states—Maine, New Hampshire, Vermont, Massachusetts, Rhode Island, Connecticut,

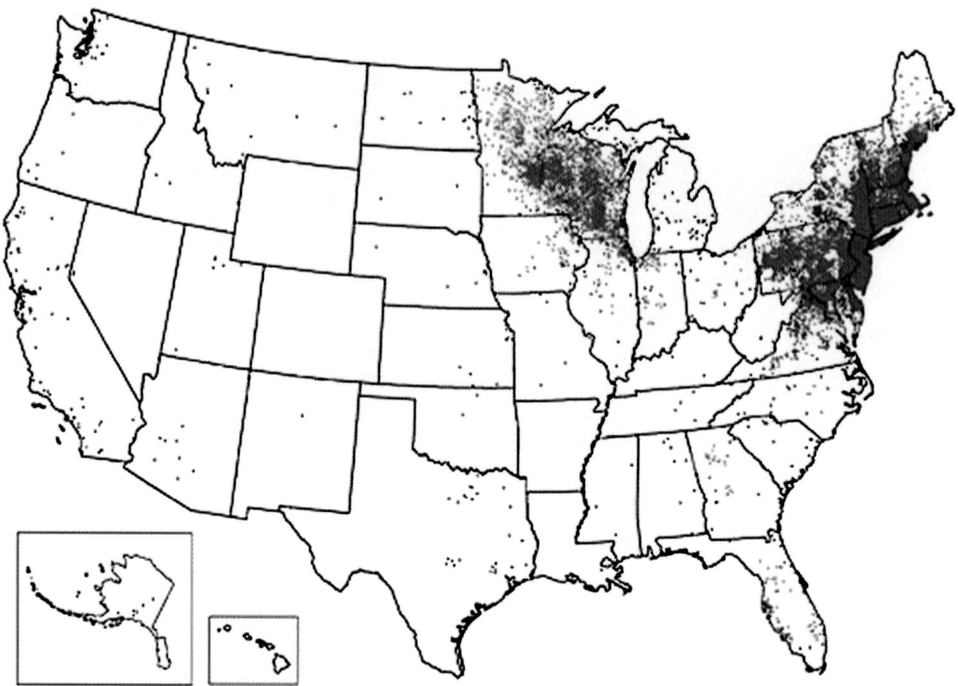

Figure 17-2 Number of cases of Lyme disease, by county in the United States, 2011. (From Centers for Disease Control and Prevention: Reported cases of Lyme disease–United States, 2011; reported cases of Lyme disease by year. Available at http://www.cdc.gov/MedicalDevices/Safety/AlertsandNotices/PublicHealthNotifications/ucm062429.htm. Accessed July 31, 2014.)

New York, New Jersey, Pennsylvania, Maryland, Delaware, and Virginia—and two Midwestern states—Minnesota and Wisconsin (Fig. 17-2).[13] In Europe, most cases occur in the Scandinavian countries and in central Europe (especially in Germany, Austria, and Switzerland), although cases have been reported from throughout the region.

Although an increase in frequency and an expansion of the geographic distribution of Lyme disease in the United States have occurred in recent years, the incidence of Lyme disease even in endemic areas varies substantially from region to region and within local areas. Information about the incidence of the disease is complicated by reliance, in most instances, on passive reporting of cases and by the high frequency of misdiagnosis of the disease. From 2003 through 2012, approximately 30,000 cases of Lyme disease were reported to the CDC each year (Fig. 17-3),[13] but ongoing studies suggest that the true number of Americans diagnosed with Lyme disease approaches 300,000 yearly.[4]

MICROBIOLOGY

The spirochetal bacterium *B. burgdorferi* is a fastidious, microaerophilic organism that in vitro must be grown on special media. It is slow growing, with a cell membrane that is covered by flagella and a loosely associated outer membrane. Major antigens of the bacteria include the outer surface lipoproteins OspA, OspB, and OspC (highly charged basic proteins of molecular masses of about 31 kDa, 34 kDa, and 23 kDa, respectively) and the 41-kDa flagellar protein. The organism is more properly classified as the *Borrelia burgdorferi* sensu lato ("in the broad sense") species complex, which has been subclassified into several genomospecies, among which the major ones that cause human diseases are *Borrelia burgdorferi* sensu stricto ("in the strict sense"), *Borrelia garinii*, and *Borrelia afzelii*. In the United States, only *B. burgdorferi* sensu stricto has been isolated from humans. By contrast, substantial variability exists in the species of *B. burgdorferi* isolated from humans in Europe, most of which are either *B. garinii* or *B. afzelii*. The complete genome of the organism has been sequenced.[14] The biology of *B. burgdorferi* is complex, as might be expected in view of the complicated life cycle of this vector-borne bacterium, part of which is spent in ticks (with a primitive immune system) and part of which is spent in mammals, which have a highly evolved immune system. The reader is referred to other sources for detailed discussion of the genetics and physiology of this organism.[15]

PATHOGENESIS AND PATHOLOGY

In approximately 90% of patients in the United States, Lyme disease begins with the characteristic expanding skin lesion, erythema migrans, at the site of the tick bite.[16,17] During the development of the initial erythema migrans, the spirochete disseminates via the bloodstream; this may be asymptomatic or may be characterized by malaise, fatigue, headache, arthralgia, myalgia, fever, and regional lymphadenopathy. Days to weeks after the tick bite, infection may be clinically manifested in the skin as multiple erythema migrans. Then weeks to months after the initial infection clinical infection may involve the nervous system, heart, and/or the joints. The ability of the spirochete to spread through skin and other tissues may be facilitated by the binding of human plasminogen and its activators to the surface of the organism.[18] During dissemination, *B.*

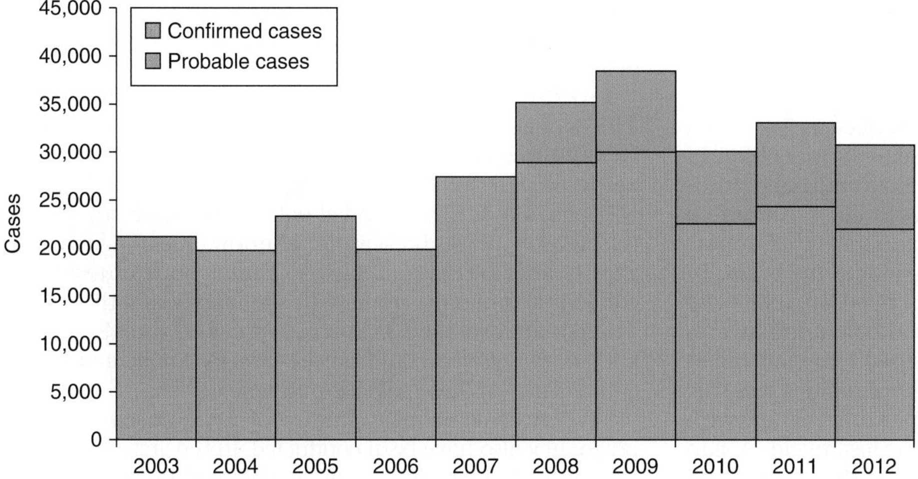

Figure 17-3 Reported cases of Lyme disease by year in the United States, 2003 to 2012. (Modified from Centers for Disease Control and Prevention: Reported cases of Lyme disease by year. Available at **http://www.cdc.gov/media/releases/2013/p0819-lyme-disease.html**. Accessed July 31, 2014.)

burgdorferi attaches to certain host integrins,[19,20] matrix glycosaminoglycans,[21] and extracellular matrix proteins,[22] which may explain the organism's particular tissue tropisms (e.g., collagen fibrils in the extracellular matrix in the heart, nervous system, and joints).[21] In addition, the sequences of OspC vary considerably among strains, and only a few groups of sequences are associated with disseminated disease.[23]

Studies in mice have shown the importance of inflammatory innate immune responses in controlling early disseminated Lyme disease. In humans with erythema migrans, infiltrates of macrophages and T cells produce inflammatory and antiinflammatory cytokines.[24] In addition, evidence suggests that in disseminated infections, adaptive T-cell and B-cell responses in lymph nodes produce antibodies against many components of the spirochete.[25,26]

The mechanism by which *B. burgdorferi* interacts with the host immune responses to produce Lyme neuroborreliosis or Lyme arthritis is not fully understood.[27-30] In the initial attempt to eliminate *B. burgdorferi*, the innate immune response to the organism results in the release of cytokines, chemokines, and other immune mediators that produce an inflammatory response. This inflammatory response damages host tissues in the process of attempting to eradicate the *Borrelia* organisms. Subsequently, an adaptive immune response is initiated through the processing and presentation of *B. burgdorferi* antigens by macrophages and dendritic cells. This response results in the release of additional immune mediators, which further exacerbate the damage produced by the inflammatory response.[27-30]

Several spirochetes have the ability to cause transplacental infections in various animals and in humans.[5] Transplacental transmission of *B. burgdorferi* has been documented in several animal studies, including case reports, case series, and transmission studies. *B. burgdorferi* has been cultured from fetal tissues of a coyote and a white-footed mouse and from the blood of a newborn calf.[31-33] The presence of *B. burgdorferi* in fetal tissues of a white-footed mouse and a house mouse also has been shown by polymerase chain reaction (PCR) assay.[34] Serologic evaluations also have been used to document in utero fetal infection with *B. burgdorferi* in an aborted calf, a newborn foal, and four beagle pups.[32,33,35] Several animal studies have linked infection with *B. burgdorferi* during pregnancy with fetal wastage and reproductive failure in cows and beagles.[33,35] Infection with *B. burgdorferi* during pregnancy also has been associated with reproductive failure and severe fetal infection in horses[36] and with increased fetal loss in mice.[37]

In animal experiments, transplacental transmission of *B. burgdorferi* was documented by PCR assay in 19 of 40 pups born to female beagles that had been intradermally inoculated with this spirochete multiple times during pregnancy.[35] Only 4 of the 19 pups had culture-positive tissues, and none of the pups had any evidence of inflammation. In other studies, neither female rats inoculated with *B. burgdorferi* intraperitoneally at 4 days of gestation nor pregnant hamsters infected by tick bite just before gestation showed any culture evidence of transplacental transmission of *B. burgdorferi* to their offspring.[38,39] In another study, offspring of naturally infected white-footed mice were unable to transmit *B. burgdorferi* to spirochete-free deer ticks allowed to feed on them.[40]

Transplacental transmission of *B. burgdorferi* in humans has been shown in association with adverse fetal outcome in several case reports. The first was a report by Schlesinger and coworkers[41] in 1985 that described a 28-year-old woman with untreated Lyme disease during the first trimester of pregnancy and who gave birth at 35 weeks of gestation to an infant with widespread cardiovascular abnormalities. The infant died during the first week of life, and postmortem examination showed spirochetes morphologically compatible with *B. burgdorferi* in the infant's spleen, kidneys, and bone marrow but not in the heart. In contrast with the mononuclear cell infiltrate and proliferation of fibroblasts usually seen with congenital syphilis,[42] there was no evidence of inflammation, necrosis, or granuloma formation in the infant's heart or other organs. In 1987, MacDonald and coworkers[43] described a 24-year-old woman with untreated Lyme disease in the first trimester of pregnancy who gave birth at term to a stillborn infant weighing 2500 g. *B. burgdorferi* was cultured from the liver, and spirochetes were seen in the heart, adrenal glands, liver, brain, and placenta with immunofluorescence and silver staining techniques. No evidence of inflammation was seen, however, and no abnormalities were noted except for a small ventricular septal defect.

Weber and colleagues[44] in 1988 described a 37-year-old woman who received penicillin orally for 1 week for erythema migrans during the first trimester of pregnancy. She subsequently gave birth to a 3400-g at-term infant who died at 23 hours of age of what was described as "perinatal brain damage." *B. burgdorferi* was subsequently identified in the newborn's brain by using immunochromogenic staining with monoclonal antibodies. However, on postmortem examination, no significant inflammation or other abnormalities were found in any organ, including the brain. In 1997, Trevisan and associates[45] described an otherwise healthy infant who presented with multiple annular erythematous lesions, fever, and generalized lymphadenopathy at 3 weeks of age. These clinical abnormalities recurred throughout the first 3 years of life despite oral therapy with amoxicillin and the macrolide antibiotic josamycin. A skin biopsy specimen revealed spirochetes by silver stain and was positive for *B. burgdorferi* by PCR assay. In addition, serologic studies were positive for infection with *B. burgdorferi*. The patient's mother had no history of either a tick bite or Lyme disease, but she had been involved in outdoor activities in an endemic area and had a weakly positive serologic test for Lyme disease.

Several case reports have described pregnant women with either erythema migrans or neuroborreliosis who received appropriate antimicrobial therapy at different stages of their pregnancies.[46-50] In none of these reports was there an association between Lyme disease in the mother and an adverse outcome of the pregnancy.

Transplacental transmission of *B. burgdorferi* also has been investigated in a study of 60 placentas from asymptomatic women who lived in an area endemic for Lyme disease and whose results on serologic testing by enzyme-linked immunosorbent assay (ELISA) were either positive or equivocal for antibodies to *B. burgdorferi*.[51] All 60 placentas were examined with a Warthin-Starry silver stain for evidence of infection with *B. burgdorferi*; 3 (5%) were positive for spirochetes. PCR assays for *B. burgdorferi* nucleotide sequences were performed on 2 of these 3 placentas and were positive in both. The women from whom these 3 placentas were obtained all had equivocal results on ELISAs and negative results on Western blot analysis for Lyme disease and negative results on serologic tests for syphilis. In addition, none of these women had a history of either a tick bite or a clinical course consistent with Lyme disease. All of these pregnancies had entirely normal outcomes.

In addition to the individual case reports, several published case series have assessed the relationship between Lyme disease in pregnant women and fetal outcomes. Two of these case series were conducted by the CDC. The first was a retrospective investigation conducted in 19 women with Lyme disease during pregnancy and who were identified by the investigators without knowing the fetal outcomes.[52] The adverse outcomes included prematurity, cortical blindness, intrauterine fetal death, syndactyly, and a generalized neonatal rash. Infection with *B. burgdorferi* could not be directly implicated as the cause of any of these outcomes. The second case series included 17 women who acquired Lyme disease during pregnancy and were evaluated prospectively.[53] One woman had a spontaneous abortion with no evidence of an infection with *B. burgdorferi* on either stains or cultures of the fetal tissue, 1 woman had an infant with isolated syndactyly, and 15 women were delivered of normal infants with no clinical or serologic evidence of infection with *B. burgdorferi*.

In 1999, Maraspin and coworkers[54] reported a series of 105 women with erythema migrans during pregnancy. Ninety-three (88.6%) of the 105 women had healthy infants delivered at term, 2 (1.9%) pregnancies ended with a miscarriage, and 6 (5.7%) ended with a preterm birth. One of the preterm infants had cardiac abnormalities, and two died shortly after birth. Four (3.8%) infants born at term had congenital anomalies (one with syndactyly and three with urologic abnormalities). As with a previous study, infection with *B. burgdorferi* could not be directly implicated as the cause of any of these adverse outcomes.

Several epidemiologic studies of Lyme disease during pregnancy also have been conducted. In the first, Williams[55] examined 421 serum specimens obtained from cord blood and found no association between the presence of immunoglobulin G (IgG) antibodies to *B. burgdorferi* and congenital malformations. In another study, Nadal and associates[56] investigated outcomes in 1434 infants of 1416 women for the presence of antibodies to *B. burgdorferi* at the time of delivery. Of the women, 12 (0.85%) were found to be seropositive, but only 1 woman had a history consistent with Lyme disease during pregnancy. Of the infants born to the 12 seropositive women, 2 had transient hyperbilirubinemia, 1 had transient hypotonia, 1 was postterm and small for gestational age with evidence of chronic placental insufficiency, 1 had transient macrocephaly, and 1 had transient supraventricular extra beats. The infant born to the woman with a clinical history of Lyme disease during pregnancy had a ventricular septal defect. At follow-up evaluations, approximately 9 to 17 months later, all of the children, except for the child with the cardiac defect, were entirely well, and none had serologic evidence of infection with *B. burgdorferi*.

In 1994, Gerber and Zalneraitis[57] surveyed neurologists in areas of the United States in which Lyme disease was endemic at that time to determine how many had seen a child with clinically significant neurologic disease whose mother had been diagnosed as having Lyme disease during pregnancy. None of the 162 pediatric and 37 adult neurologists who responded to the survey had ever seen a child whose mother had been diagnosed with Lyme disease during pregnancy. The investigators concluded that congenital neuroborreliosis was either not occurring or occurring at an extremely low frequency in areas endemic for Lyme disease. In a retrospective case-control study carried out in an area endemic for Lyme disease, 796 "case" children with congenital cardiac anomalies were compared with 704 "control" children without cardiac defects with respect to Lyme disease in their mothers either during or before the pregnancy.[58] No association was found between congenital heart defects and either a tick bite or Lyme disease in the mothers either within 3 months of conception or during pregnancy.

Investigators in New York performed two studies of the relationship between Lyme disease in pregnant women and adverse outcomes of the pregnancies. The first was an unselected, prospective, population-based investigation in an area endemic for Lyme disease in which approximately 2000 women in Westchester County, New York, were evaluated for clinical and serologic evidence of Lyme disease at the first prenatal visit and again at delivery.[59] Of these women, 11 (0.7%) were seropositive, and 79 (4%) reported at the first prenatal visit that they had had Lyme disease sometime in the past. One woman with an untreated influenza-like illness in the second trimester had a negative result on serologic testing for Lyme disease at the prenatal visit but a positive result at delivery. In addition, during the study period, clinical Lyme disease was diagnosed in 15 pregnant women. No association was found between exposure of the mother to *B. burgdorferi* either before conception or during pregnancy and fetal death, prematurity, or congenital malformations. In the second study, the researchers compared 5000 infants, half from an area in which Lyme disease was endemic and half from an area without Lyme disease, who served as control subjects. The researchers found no significant difference in the overall incidence of congenital malformations between the two groups.[60] Although there was a statistically significant higher rate of cardiac malformations in the endemic area compared with that in the control area, no relationship was noted between a cardiac malformation and either a clinical history or serologic evidence of Lyme disease. The researchers concluded from the findings of these two studies that a pregnant woman with a past infection with *B. burgdorferi*, either treated or untreated, did not have an increased risk of early fetal loss or of having a low-birth-weight infant or an infant with congenital malformations.[60]

Two reports have documented the presence of *B. burgdorferi* in cow's milk. In 1988, Burgess[33] cultured *B. burgdorferi* from 1 of 3 samples of colostrum from cows but from none of 44 samples of cow's milk. Lischer and colleagues[61] used a PCR assay to identify nucleotide sequences of *B. burgdorferi* in the milk of a cow with clinical Lyme disease. In a similar investigation of human milk, Schmidt and coworkers[62] examined breast milk from two lactating women with erythema migrans and from three lactating women with no clinical evidence of Lyme disease. The breast milk samples from both women with erythema migrans tested positive for *B. burgdorferi* by PCR assay, whereas the breast milk samples from all three healthy women tested negative. No other reports have corroborated these findings in human milk. *B. burgdorferi* has never been cultured from breast milk, and transmission of Lyme disease through breastfeeding has never been documented.

CLINICAL MANIFESTATIONS

The clinical manifestations of Lyme disease depend on the stage of the illness: early localized disease, early disseminated disease, or late disease. Erythema migrans, the manifestation of early localized Lyme disease, appears at the site of the tick bite, 3 to 30 days (typically 7-10 days) after the bite. Erythema migrans is found in about 90% of patients with objective evidence of infection with *B. burgdorferi*.[63,64] In a prospective study of 10,936 subjects given Lyme vaccine versus placebo, 147 subjects developed definite Lyme disease and 142 of 147 (97%) presented with erythema migrans.[17] Erythema migrans begins as a red macule or papule and expands for days to weeks to form a large, annular erythematous lesion that ranges from 5 to 70 cm in diameter (median, 15 cm). This rash may be uniformly erythematous, or it may appear as a target lesion with a variable degree of central clearing or central purpura (target lesion). It can vary greatly in shape and, occasionally, may have vesicular or necrotic areas in the center. Erythema migrans is usually asymptomatic but may be pruritic or painful, and it may be accompanied by systemic findings, such as fever, malaise, headache, regional lymphadenopathy, stiff neck, myalgia, or arthralgia. In a large prospective study of erythema migrans in adults,[65] the erythema migrans rashes included homogenous erythema (59%), central erythema (30%), central clearing (9%), or central purpura (2%). In addition, 7% of lesions had central vesicles or ulcerations. Thus target lesions occurred in 41% of patients.

The most common manifestation of early disseminated Lyme disease in the United States is multiple erythema migrans. The secondary skin lesions, which usually appear 3 to 5 weeks after the tick bite, consist of multiple annular erythematous lesions similar to, but usually smaller than, the primary lesion. Other common manifestations of early disseminated Lyme disease are cranial nerve palsies, especially facial nerve palsy, and meningitis. Systemic symptoms such as fever, myalgia, arthralgia, headache, and fatigue also are common in this stage of Lyme disease. Carditis, which usually is manifested by third-degree heart block and/or myocarditis, is a rare manifestation of early disseminated disease.[63,64]

The most common manifestation of late Lyme disease, which occurs weeks to months after the initial infection, is arthritis. The arthritis is usually monarticular and affects the large joints, particularly the knee. The affected joint often is swollen and mildly tender; the intense pain associated with a septic arthritis usually is not present. Encephalitis, encephalopathy, and polyneuropathy also are manifestations of late Lyme disease, but each is very rare.[63]

The clinical manifestations of Lyme disease also may depend on which subspecies of *B. burgdorferi* is causing the infection.[31] The differences in subspecies found in Europe and in North America may account for differences in the frequencies of certain clinical manifestations of Lyme disease in these areas. Neurologic manifestations of Lyme disease are more common in Europe, whereas rheumatologic manifestations are more common in North America. In addition, certain skin and soft tissue manifestations of Lyme disease, such as acrodermatitis chronica atrophicans and lymphocytomas, occur in Europe but are extremely rare in the United States.

There has been substantial controversy about an entity that has been called "chronic Lyme disease." There is no evidence that persistent *B. burgdorferi* infection unresponsive to an appropriate antibiotic exists.[66] Nonspecific symptoms (e.g., fatigue, irritability, forgetfulness, arthralgia, or myalgia) may persist for weeks or months in patients who are successfully treated for early Lyme disease; the presence of these subjective symptoms should not be regarded as an indication for additional antimicrobial therapy. These symptoms may respond to nonsteroidal antiinflammatory drugs. Within 6 months of completion of the initial course of antimicrobial therapy, these nonspecific symptoms usually resolve with or without any therapies. For the unusual patients who have symptoms that persist longer than 6 months after the completion of antimicrobial therapy, an attempt should be made to determine if there exists a non–Lyme disease explanation or if there has been reinfection. Most likely these are post–Lyme disease symptoms and the cause is unknown.[66] A parallel example is persistent fatigue after mononucleosis, which was initially thought to be secondary to persistent Epstein-Barr virus (EBV) infection (and was called chronic mononucleosis). Later it was shown that the EBV viremia had resolved in these patients, and the cause of the persistent fatigue was unknown.

There is a network of doctors that diagnose many patients with "chronic Lyme disease," including patients from non–Lyme endemic areas. Many of these patients diagnosed with "chronic Lyme disease" have no evidence of either current or past infection with *B. burgdorferi*.[67] There have been four double-blind randomized clinical trials of long-term antibiotic treatment for patients with evidence of past infection with *B. burgdorferi* and subsequent symptoms that persist for at least 6 months after conventional (or longer) treatment with antibiotics.[66] The results of all of these studies showed that long-term treatment provided little or no benefit but was associated with substantial risks to the patient.[68] In addition, prolonged use of antibiotics encourages selection of antibiotic-resistant bacteria that pose risks to the patients and to the community. These results add to the already substantial data that "chronic Lyme disease" is not a persistent infection but more likely should be classified as a syndrome of medically unexplained symptoms[69] or post–Lyme disease symptoms.

Ixodes ticks may transmit other pathogens in addition to *B. burgdorferi*, including *Babesia*, *Anaplasma*, other *Borrelia* species, and viruses. These agents may be transmitted either separately from or simultaneously with *B. burgdorferi*. The frequency with which coinfection occurs is unknown. The impact of coinfection on the clinical presentation and the response to treatment of Lyme disease, although well documented and important in rare selected cases, seems to be of minor significance in most instances. In the south-central United States, in areas such as Missouri, another tick-borne infection that causes erythema migrans has been recognized.[70] Southern tick-associated rash illness (STARI) is transmitted by the tick *Amblyomma americanum*, the Lone Star tick. The cause of STARI was originally thought to be *Borrelia lonestari*, but this has not been confirmed. In contrast to Lyme disease, it does not seem to cause systemic disease. Similar to Lyme disease, there is no evidence that STARI is associated with congenital disease in children. STARI causes a rash similar to erythema migrans and in areas where the deer tick and Lone Star tick cohabitate, the skin manifestations of these two diseases overlap.[71]

DIAGNOSIS

The CDC clinical case definition for Lyme disease initially was intended for epidemiologic surveillance purposes. When used in conjunction with CDC and U.S. Food and Drug Administration (FDA) guidelines for diagnostic tests,[72] however, this case definition has been widely accepted as a means to standardize the clinical diagnosis of Lyme disease (Box 17-1).

For patients in locations endemic for Lyme disease who present with the characteristic lesion of erythema migrans, the diagnosis of Lyme disease should be based on the clinical presentation alone. In such situations, laboratory testing is neither necessary nor recommended. With the exception of erythema migrans, however, the clinical manifestations of Lyme disease are nonspecific. For patients who do not have erythema migrans, the diagnosis of Lyme disease should usually be based on objective clinical findings and positive laboratory tests. These laboratory tests may consist of either direct identification of *B. burgdorferi* in the patient or demonstration of a serologic response to the organism.

Methods for identifying the presence of *B. burgdorferi* in a patient (e.g., culture, histopathologic examination, antigen detection) generally have poor sensitivity or specificity or both and may require invasive procedures (e.g., a biopsy of the skin) to obtain an appropriate specimen for testing. Isolation of *B. burgdorferi* from a symptomatic patient should be considered diagnostic of Lyme disease. *B. burgdorferi* has been isolated from blood, skin biopsy specimens, cerebrospinal fluid (CSF), myocardial biopsy specimens, and the synovium of patients with Lyme disease. *B. burgdorferi* can take 6 weeks to grow in culture. The best chance of culturing *B. burgdorferi* from a patient is when erythema migrans is present,[73] although at this stage of the disease, the diagnosis should be largely clinical. During the later stages of Lyme disease, culture is much less sensitive. In addition, it is necessary for patients to undergo an invasive procedure, such as a biopsy, to obtain appropriate tissue or fluid for culture. Culture is indicated only in rare circumstances.

Box 17-1 **CDC Lyme Disease Case Definition for Public Health Surveillance Purposes**

Erythema migrans: Single primary red macule or papule, expanding over days to weeks to large round lesion ≥5 cm diameter (physician confirmed), ± central clearing, ± secondary lesions, ± systemic symptoms (fever, fatigue, headache, mild neck stiffness, arthralgia, myalgia)

Plus

Known exposure ≤30 days before onset to endemic area (in which ≥2 confirmed cases have been acquired, or in which *Borrelia burgdorferi*–infected tick vectors are established)

Or

One or more late manifestations without other etiology

1. Musculoskeletal: Recurrent brief episodes of monarticular or pauciarticular arthritis with objective joint swelling, ± chronic arthritis
2. Neurologic: Lymphocytic meningitis, facial palsy, other cranial neuritis, radiculoneuropathy, encephalomyelitis (confirmed by CSF *B. burgdorferi* antibody > serum *B. burgdorferi* antibody)
3. Cardiovascular: Acute second-degree or third-degree atrioventricular conduction defects lasting days to weeks, ± myocarditis

Plus

Laboratory confirmation by either

1. Isolation of *B. burgdorferi* from patient specimen
2. Diagnostic levels of *B. burgdorferi* IgM or IgG antibodies in serum or CSF (initial ELISA or IFA screen, followed by Western blot of positive or equivocal results)

Modified from Centers for Disease Control and Prevention: Case definitions for infectious conditions under public health surveillance, MMWR Recomm Rep *46(RR-10):20-21, 1997.*

CDC, Centers for Disease Control and Prevention; *CSF,* cerebrospinal fluid; *ELISA,* enzyme-linked immunosorbent assay; *IFA,* immunofluorescence assay; *IgG, IgM,* immunoglobulin G, M, respectively.

B. burgdorferi has been identified with silver stains (Warthin-Starry or modified Dieterle) and with immunohistochemical stains (with monoclonal or polyclonal antibodies) in skin, synovial, and myocardial biopsy specimens. *B. burgdorferi* can be confused with normal tissue structures, however, or it may be missed because it often is present in low concentrations. Considerable training and experience are needed for skill in identifying spirochetes in tissues. Direct detection of *B. burgdorferi* in tissue is of limited practical value.

Attempts have been made to develop antigen-based diagnostic tests for Lyme disease, but no convincing data indicating the accuracy of any of these tests are available. All of these tests should be considered experimental until additional studies confirm their validity and reproducibility. Assays to detect *B. burgdorferi* antigens in CSF or urine have poor specificity and poor sensitivity and are not recommended.[74]

Tests that use PCR techniques to identify *B. burgdorferi* are sometimes helpful. Results of such tests may be positive for some time after the spirochetes are no longer viable, however. In addition, the risk of false-positive results on PCR assays is great, especially when they are performed in commercial laboratories. If a PCR test is done, it should be performed in a reference laboratory that meets the highest standards of quality control for diagnostic PCR assays. Because of its limited availability, expense, and insufficient evidence of its value in the management of most patients, PCR is at present reserved for special situations. Use of PCR assay may be appropriate in testing of specimens such as synovial tissue or fluid from patients with persistent arthritis after a course of appropriate antibiotic therapy for late Lyme disease; samples of abnormal CSF from patients who are seropositive for antibodies to *B. burgdorferi* and have a neurologic illness that is compatible with, but not typical of, Lyme disease. At present, there is insufficient evidence of the accuracy, predictive value, or clinical significance of a PCR test of urine for *B. burgdorferi*, and its use for decisions regarding the management of patients has been strongly discouraged.[75]

In most cases, the confirmation of Lyme disease in patients without erythema migrans usually is based on the demonstration of antibodies to *B. burgdorferi* in the serum. The normal antibody response to acute infection with *B. burgdorferi* is well described.[76] Specific IgM antibodies appear first, usually 3 to 4 weeks after the infection begins. These antibodies peak after 6 to 8 weeks and usually decline. A prolonged elevation of IgM antibodies sometimes is seen, however, even after effective antimicrobial treatment.[77] Consequently, the results of serologic tests for specific IgM antibodies should not be used as the sole indicator of the timing of an infection. Specific IgG antibodies usually appear 6 to 8 weeks after the onset of the infection. These antibodies peak in 4 to 6 months. The IgG antibody titer may decline after treatment, but even after the patient is clinically cured, these antibodies usually remain detectable for many years.[78,79]

The immunofluorescent antibody test was the initial serologic test for diagnosing Lyme disease. It requires subjective interpretation and is time consuming to perform. It has largely been replaced by the ELISA. The ELISA method may give false-positive results because of cross-reactive antibodies in patients with other spirochetal infections (e.g., syphilis, leptospirosis, relapsing fever), certain viral infections (e.g., varicella), and autoimmune diseases (e.g., systemic lupus erythematosus). In contrast to patients with syphilis, patients with Lyme disease do not have positive results on nontreponemal tests for syphilis, such as the Venereal Disease Research Laboratory or rapid plasma reagin (RPR). In addition, antibodies directed against bacteria in the normal oral flora may cross react with antigens of *B. burgdorferi* to produce a false-positive ELISA result.

The first-generation ELISA method used either whole cells of *B. burgdorferi* or the supernatant of sonicated spirochetes as the antigen. To improve the specificity of the ELISA, new assays have been developed that use less complex fractions of the spirochetes, such as the bacterial membrane, or purified native or recombinant proteins, alone or in combination.[76]

Immunoblot (western blot) analysis for serum antibodies to *B. burgdorferi* also is used as a serologic test for Lyme disease. Some investigators have suggested that immunoblot is more sensitive and more specific than ELISA, but this is debatable. Immunoblot is most useful for validating a positive or equivocal ELISA result, especially in patients with a low clinical likelihood of having Lyme disease. For serologic testing for Lyme disease, it is recommended that a sensitive ELISA be performed, and, if results are either positive or equivocal, that a western blot analysis be done to confirm the specificity of the result. Specimens that give a negative result on a sensitive ELISA do not require immunoblot.

One reason for the poor sensitivity of serologic tests for Lyme disease is that erythema migrans, which is the clinical finding that usually brings patients to medical attention, usually appears within 2 to 3 weeks of onset of infection with *B. burgdorferi*. Antibodies to *B. burgdorferi* often are not detected at this early stage of the disease. The antibody response to *B. burgdorferi* also may be abrogated in patients with early Lyme disease who receive prompt treatment with an effective antimicrobial agent; in these patients, antibodies against *B. burgdorferi* may never develop, at least as a result of that exposure. Most patients with early, disseminated Lyme disease and virtually all patients with late Lyme disease have serum antibodies to *B. burgdorferi*, however. Seropositivity may persist for years, even after successful antimicrobial therapy. Ongoing seropositivity, even persistence of IgM, is not a marker of active infection. Likewise, serologic tests should not be used to assess the adequacy of antimicrobial therapy.

Serologic tests for Lyme disease have not been adequately standardized. The accuracy and the reproducibility of currently available serologic tests, especially widely used, commercially produced kits, are poor.[80] Use of these commercial diagnostic test kits for Lyme disease would result in a high rate of misdiagnosis. As with any diagnostic test, the predictive value of serologic tests for Lyme disease depends primarily on the probability that the patient has Lyme disease based on the clinical and epidemiologic history and the physical examination (the "pretest probability" of Lyme disease). Use of serologic tests to "rule out" Lyme disease in patients with a low probability of the illness would result in a very high proportion of test results that are falsely positive. Antibody tests for Lyme disease should not be used as screening tests.[72,81,82]

With few exceptions, the probability that a patient has Lyme disease would be very low in areas in which Lyme disease is rare. Even in areas with a high prevalence of Lyme disease, patients with only nonspecific signs and symptoms, such as fatigue, headache, and arthralgia, are not likely to have Lyme disease. Although such nonspecific symptoms are common in patients with Lyme disease, they are almost always accompanied by more specific objective findings, such as erythema migrans, facial nerve palsy, or arthritis. Even when more accurate tests performed by reference laboratories are available, clinicians should order serologic tests for Lyme disease selectively, reserving them for patients from populations with a relatively high prevalence of Lyme disease who have specific objective clinical findings that are suggestive of Lyme disease so that the predictive value of a positive result is high.[81,82]

If a symptomatic patient is positive for antibodies to *B. burgdorferi*, Lyme disease may or may not be the cause of that patient's symptoms. The positive test may be a false-positive result (a common occurrence), or the patient may have been infected with *B. burgdorferi* previously. When serum antibodies to *B. burgdorferi* do develop, they may persist for many years despite adequate treatment and clinical cure of the illness. In addition, there is a background rate of seropositivity among patients in endemic areas who have never had clinically apparent Lyme disease.[78]

The diagnosis of an infection of the central nervous system (CNS) with *B. burgdorferi* is made by showing the presence of inflammation in the CSF and *Borrelia*-specific intrathecal antibodies.[83] Most patients with typical cases of Lyme neuroborreliosis have antibodies to *B. burgdorferi* in serum, and testing for the presence of antibodies in the CSF usually is unnecessary.[75] In some instances, examination of the CSF for antibodies to *B. burgdorferi* may be indicated. Because antibodies to *B. burgdorferi* may be present in the CSF as the result of passive transit through a leaky blood-brain barrier, detection of antibodies in the CSF is not proof of infection. Better evidence of CNS disease is the demonstration of intrathecal production of antibodies. This can be accomplished by simultaneously measuring the antibodies in the serum and CSF by ELISA and calculating the "CSF index." PCR assay of the CSF is usually not helpful because of low sensitivity for confirming the diagnosis of CNS Lyme disease.[75,84]

A lymphoproliferative assay that assesses the cell-mediated immune response to *B. burgdorferi* has been developed as a diagnostic test for Lyme disease. This assay has not been standardized, however, and is not approved by the FDA. The indications for this lymphoproliferative assay are few, if any.[85]

The diagnosis of Lyme disease in a pregnant woman should be made in accordance with the currently accepted CDC case definition (see Box 17-1). There is no indication for routine prenatal serologic screening of asymptomatic healthy women. Serosurveys have shown that the seroprevalence rates among pregnant women were comparable to those in the general population and that asymptomatic seroconversion during pregnancy was unusual.[59,60,86]

MANAGEMENT AND TREATMENT

Pediatricians are sometimes confronted with the challenge of how to manage an infant born to a woman who was diagnosed with Lyme disease during her pregnancy. The difficulty arises because of the paucity of evidence that congenital Lyme disease is a clinical problem. In addition, for reasons cited earlier, the diagnosis in the mother often is inaccurate. First, parents should be reassured that there is no evidence that the infant is at increased risk of any problem from maternal Lyme disease. Next, an attempt should be made to ascertain the accuracy of the diagnosis in the mother; if the mother did not have objective signs of Lyme disease (e.g., erythema migrans) or if the diagnosis was based on nonspecific symptoms (e.g., fatigue, myalgia) and a positive serologic test result, then it is likely that the diagnosis is inaccurate.

There is no reason to order serologic tests for Lyme disease in infants who are asymptomatic (even if diagnosis of Lyme disease in the mother is accurate). If such tests are ordered, it is important to remember that if the mother did have Lyme disease and is seropositive, the infant may have passively acquired antibodies from the mother and so may remain seropositive for many months, even in the absence of infection. Because of the high frequency of false-positive test results, a positive test result for IgM antibodies against *B. burgdorferi* in an asymptomatic child should be interpreted with a high degree of skepticism.

The choice of antibiotic and the duration of treatment for Lyme disease depend on the stage of the disease that is being treated (Box 17-2). In general, pregnant women should receive the same treatment as other patients, except that use of doxycycline is not recommended during pregnancy.[87]

Early Localized Disease

Doxycycline is the drug of choice for children 8 years and older with early localized Lyme disease.[87] Individuals who are taking doxycycline should avoid sun exposure because a rash develops in sun-exposed areas 20% to 30% of the time; use of sunscreen may decrease this risk. Amoxicillin is recommended for children younger than 8 years, for pregnant women, and for patients who cannot tolerate doxycycline. For patients allergic to penicillin, cefuroxime axetil is an alternative drug. Erythromycin or azithromycin may also be used, but they are less effective than the other agents. Most experts recommend a 14- to 21-day course of therapy for early localized Lyme disease, although evidence indicates that 10 days of doxycycline constitutes adequate treatment in adults with uncomplicated infection.[87,88] Courses shorter than 14 to 21 days have not been studied for amoxicillin or cefuroxime axetil therapy.

A prompt clinical response to treatment is usual, with resolution of erythema migrans within several days of initiating therapy. On occasion, a Jarisch-Herxheimer reaction, which usually consists of an elevated temperature and worsening myalgia, develops shortly after antimicrobial treatment is initiated. Jarisch-Herxheimer reactions are more common in patients with multiple erythema migrans. These reactions do not constitute an indication to discontinue antimicrobial therapy, and symptoms respond to nonsteroidal antiinflammatory drugs. Appropriate treatment of erythema migrans almost always prevents development of the later stages of Lyme disease, except these later manifestations may develop during the first 1 to 2 weeks of antibiotic therapy.

Box 17-2 Antimicrobial Treatment of Lyme Disease

Early Disease

Localized Erythema Migrans

Doxycycline, 2-4 mg/kg/day twice daily (maximum 100 mg/dose) for 14-21 days (do not use in children younger than 8 years), or amoxicillin, 50 mg/kg/day three times daily (maximum 500 mg/dose) for 14-21 days. Preferred alternative agent for patients who cannot take either amoxicillin or doxycycline is cefuroxime axetil, 30 mg/kg/day twice daily (maximum 500 mg/dose) for 14-21 days. Erythromycin and azithromycin are less effective alternatives for patients who cannot take other recommended agents.

Neurologic Disease

Isolated seventh cranial nerve or other cranial nerve palsy: Treat as for localized erythema migrans, but for 14-21 days (doxycycline preferred if possible).

Meningitis (with or without encephalitis or radiculoneuritis): Ceftriaxone, 50-75 mg/kg once daily (maximum 2 g/dose) for 14-28 days. Alternatives include penicillin G, 200,000-400,000 U/kg/day (maximum 18-24 million U/day) every 4 hr, or cefotaxime 150 mg/kg/day (maximum 2 g/dose) divided every 8 hr for 14-28 days, and oral doxycycline, 4 mg/kg/day twice daily (maximum 200 mg/dose) for 14-21 days.

Carditis

First-degree or second-degree heart block: Treat as for localized erythema migrans.

Third-degree heart block or other evidence of severe carditis: Treat as for meningitis.

Late Disease

Arthritis

Doxycycline, 2-4 mg/kg/day twice daily (maximum 100 mg/dose) for 28 days (do not use in children younger than 8 yr), or amoxicillin, 50 mg/kg/day twice daily (maximum 500 mg/dose) for 28 days. Preferred alternative agent for patients who cannot take either amoxicillin or doxycycline is cefuroxime axetil, 30 mg/kg/day twice daily (maximum 500 mg/dose) for 28 days. For recurrent or persistent arthritis for which oral treatment has failed, either a second course of one of the orally administered agents for 28 days or a course of parenteral treatment for 14 to 28 days (as for meningitis) is indicated.

Neurologic Disease

Treat as for meningitis above for 14-28 days.

Early Disseminated and Late Disease

Multiple erythema migrans and initial episodes of arthritis should be treated with orally administered antimicrobial agents. If peripheral facial nerve palsy is the only neurologic manifestation of Lyme disease, the patient can be given an oral regimen of antimicrobials. If facial nerve palsy is accompanied by clinical evidence of CNS involvement (e.g., nuchal rigidity), a lumbar puncture should be performed. If there is pleocytosis (usually lymphocytic), parenteral antimicrobials may be prescribed. In the United States, meningitis is usually treated with ceftriaxone; however, there is data from Europe that Lyme meningitis can be successfully treated with oral doxycycline.[89]

Some experts prescribe a second course of an orally administered antimicrobial agent for recurrent or persistent arthritis. Nonsteroidal antiinflammatory drugs are a useful adjunct to antimicrobial therapy for patients with arthritis or tapping the knee effusion and injecting steroids. Parenteral antibiotics versus oral antibiotics for recurrent/persistent Lyme arthritis have not been studied.

Although mild carditis is usually treated orally with either doxycycline or amoxicillin, most experts recommend parenterally administered therapy for severe carditis (third-degree heart block). When the heart block resolves, patients can then be treated orally. Other neurologic manifestations of late Lyme disease (e.g., encephalitis, encephalopathy) are very rare and should be treated with antimicrobials administered parenterally.

The optimal duration of antimicrobial therapy for the various stages of Lyme disease is not well established, but there is no evidence that children with any manifestation of Lyme disease benefit from prolonged (>4 weeks) courses of either orally or parenterally administered antimicrobial agents. Lyme disease, similar to other infections (mononucleosis), may trigger a fatigue/fibromyalgia syndrome that does not respond to additional courses of antimicrobials but may be managed with symptomatic therapy.

PROGNOSIS

Attempts to determine the potential impact of gestational Lyme disease on the outcome of the pregnancy have been limited for several reasons.[90] First, the prevalence of Lyme disease among pregnant women, even in highly endemic areas, is low, making it difficult to perform studies with sufficient statistical power. Second, diagnoses of gestational Lyme disease that are based on seropositivity, a history of a tick bite, or even a retrospective clinical history are often unreliable. Finally, because of increased awareness and concern about Lyme disease, it is difficult to find women with suspected gestational Lyme disease who did not receive antimicrobial treatment.

Despite these limitations, *B. burgdorferi* can cross the placenta, presumably during a period of spirochetemia. The frequency and clinical significance of transplacental transmission of *B. burgdorferi* are unclear. Although a temporal relationship between Lyme disease during pregnancy and adverse outcomes has been documented, a causal relationship has not been established. Claims for the existence of a congenital Lyme disease syndrome are undermined by the absence of an inflammatory response in fetal tissue, absence of a fetal immunologic response, and lack of a consistent clinical outcome in affected pregnancies. Analysis of the current data indicates that there is no evidence of increased risk of abnormal outcomes with Lyme disease during pregnancy.

It is difficult to conduct high-quality studies of clinical outcome in patients with Lyme disease. On the basis of the available data, the long-term prognosis for adults or children who receive appropriate antimicrobial therapy for Lyme disease, regardless of the stage of the disease, seems to be excellent.[91] The most common reason for a lack of response to appropriate antimicrobial therapy for Lyme disease is misdiagnosis (i.e., the patient actually does not have Lyme disease).

In approximately 10% of adults and less than 5% of children with Lyme arthritis, inflammatory joint disease develops that typically affects one knee for months to years and does not respond to antimicrobial therapy. An increased frequency of certain HLA-DR4 and HLA-DR2 alleles has been noted among these patients. Initially, these patients have a positive PCR for *Borrelia burgdorferi* in the joint fluid, but the fluid becomes negative after antibiotic therapy. These patients may be treated with synovectomy.[92] Thus the cause of recurrent/persistent arthritis is not persistent infection but rather infection-induced autoimmunity and/or retained spirochetal antigens.[93]

PREVENTION

Reducing the risk of tick bites is one strategy to prevent Lyme disease. In endemic areas, clearing brush and trees, removing leaf litter and woodpiles, and keeping grass mowed and mulch separating grass from woods may reduce exposure to ticks. Application of pesticides to residential properties is effective in suppressing populations of ticks but may be harmful to other wildlife and to people. Erecting fences to exclude deer from residential yards and maintaining tick-free pets also may reduce exposure to ticks.

Tick and insect repellents that contain *N,N*-diethyl-*m*-toluamide (DEET) applied to the skin provide additional protection. DEET-containing repellents can be used in infants 2 months of age and older. Products with 20% to 30% concentrations of DEET can be effective for 6 to 8 hours. DEET should be applied sparingly only to exposed skin but not to a child's face, hands, or skin that is either irritated or abraded. After the child returns indoors, skin that was treated should be washed with soap and water. Permethrin (a synthetic pyrethroid) is available in a spray for application to clothing only and is particularly effective because it kills ticks on contact.

Most people who recognize a tick bite remove the tick within 48 hours[9]; the risk of Lyme disease from recognized deer tick bites is low—approximately 1% to 3% in areas with a high incidence of Lyme disease. The risk of Lyme disease probably is higher from unrecognized bites because, in those cases, the tick feeds for a longer time. A large study of antimicrobial prophylaxis after tick bites among adults found that a single, 200-mg dose of doxycycline was 87% effective in preventing Lyme disease.[7] Amoxicillin (250 mg tid for 10 days) is also effective to prevent Lyme disease after tick bites.[92]

There is no evidence that pregnant women are at increased risk of Lyme disease after a deer tick bite. The only drug that has been shown to be effective in preventing Lyme disease after a tick bite, doxycycline, is not recommended for use during pregnancy because of its possible effect on the developing fetus. Consequently, antimicrobial prophylaxis is not recommended for pregnant women.

Serologic testing for Lyme disease after a recognized tick bite also is not recommended. Antibodies to *B. burgdorferi* that are present at the time that the tick is removed likely would be due either to a false-positive test result or to an earlier infection with *B. burgdorferi*, rather than to a new infection from the recent bite. Likewise, in this setting, the predictive value of a positive result is very low.

Ascertainment of whether the tick is infected, using tests such as PCR, is also not recommended. Although testing ticks with PCR may provide important epidemiologic information, the predictive values for infection of humans of either a positive or a negative PCR test result is unknown. The result may be positive even if only very few organisms are present, and it provides no information about the duration of feeding, a key determinant of the risk of transmission. In addition, the problems of false-positive results caused by contamination with amplification products and false-negative results caused by inhibition of PCR by substances in the sample (e.g., blood) limit the test's validity.

People should be taught to inspect themselves and their children's bodies and clothing daily after possible deer tick exposure. An attached tick should be grasped with medium-tipped tweezers as close to the skin as possible and removed by gently pulling the tick straight out. If some of the mouthparts remain embedded in the skin, they should be left alone or removed aseptically like a splinter.

Relapsing Fever

Relapsing fever is an arthropod-borne zoonosis caused by various *Borrelia* species. There are two forms of relapsing fever. Tick-borne relapsing fever (TBRF), or endemic relapsing fever, is caused by various *Borrelia* species associated with soft ticks of the genus *Ornithodoros*. Louse-borne relapsing fever (LBRF), or epidemic relapsing fever, is caused by *Borrelia recurrentis*, which is associated with the human body louse (*Pediculus humanus*).[94]

The distribution and occurrence of TBRF depend on the enzootic cycle of the transmitting tick vector. In contrast, the distribution and occurrence of LBRF depend on socioeconomic and ecologic factors. LBRF usually occurs in epidemics that are associated with catastrophic events (e.g., war, famine, natural disasters) that result in overcrowding and dissemination of body lice.[94] LBRF is endemic in the highlands of East Africa (Ethiopia, Sudan, Somalia, Chad) and in the South American Andes (Bolivia, Peru). TBRF has been reported worldwide, with the exception of a few areas in the South Pacific. In North America, *Borrelia hermsii* and *Borrelia turicatae* are the major causes of TBRF.[85]

LBRF is transmitted when there is contamination of abraded or normal skin with hemolymph of an infected crushed louse. In TBRF, human infection occurs when saliva or coxal fluid containing the *Borrelia* organisms are released in the feeding puncture.

After an incubation period of approximately 7 days (range, 4 to ≥18 days), the onset of disease is signaled by fever. The fever coincides with large numbers of *Borrelia* organisms in the blood. The relapsing pattern is due to variation of lipoproteins that results in new antigenic variants of major surface lipoproteins and the recurrence of large numbers of *Borrelia* organisms in the blood.[85,94] The most common clinical manifestations of relapsing fever are splenomegaly (41%-77%), hepatomegaly (17%-66%), jaundice (7%-36%), rash (8%-28%), respiratory symptoms (16%-34%), and CNS involvement (9% 30%).[94] Other complaints include nausea, vomiting, cough, dizziness, and epistaxis.[95] The findings on physical examination may be normal, but tachycardia, tachypnea, jaundice, purpura, or hepatosplenomegaly may be present. The clinical manifestations of LBRF and TBRF are similar, although LBRF is usually associated with a single relapse, whereas multiple relapses are more common with TBRF.

The definitive diagnosis of relapsing fever is established by the demonstration of *Borrelia* organisms in the peripheral blood of febrile patients. In approximately 70% of cases, spirochetes can be seen in the initial blood smear, and the yield increases with multiple smears. Serologic tests are not generally available and, if performed, are of limited diagnostic value because of antigenic variation of strains and the complexity of the relapsing phenomenon. Molecular methods are highly effective in detecting and identifying *Borrelia* species.[96,97]

Several antibiotics, including tetracyclines, penicillin, ampicillin, erythromycin, and chloramphenicol, are known to be effective for treating relapsing fever. TBRF has an overall case-fatality rate of 2% to 5%, but the rate is greater than 20% in infants younger than 1 year.[94]

In some areas of Africa, relapsing fever during pregnancy is associated with a 30% risk of pregnancy loss and fetal and infant mortality rates of 15% and 44%, respectively. Common complications of relapsing fever during pregnancy are low birth weight, preterm delivery, spontaneous abortion, and neonatal death. Most pregnancy and perinatal complications have been reported from sub-Saharan Africa, although there are reports from developed countries as well. Pregnant women showed significantly higher densities of spirochetes than nonpregnant women, and a correlation has been seen between density of spirochetes and risk of birth during the attack and risk of complications.[95,98,99]

Maternal-infant transmission of relapsing fever has been reported primarily from sub-Saharan Africa, but cases from developed countries, such as the United States and Israel, have also been reported. Transplacental transmission in humans has been established and seems to be the most likely explanation for most of the neonatal cases. In many of these neonatal cases, infections after or during the birth could not be definitively excluded.[98]

The clinical signs of relapsing fever in the newborn are those of neonatal sepsis and are nonspecific: apathy, vomiting, tachypnea, acidosis, and bleeding tendency. An unusually high concentration of *Borrelia* organisms is found in the peripheral blood smears in affected neonates. The overall mortality in this age group is higher (>40%) than in any other age group.[98]

References

1. Steere AC, Malawista SE, Snydman DR, et al: Lyme arthritis: an epidemic of oligoarticular arthritis in children and adults in three Connecticut communities, *Arthritis Rheum* 20:7-17, 1977.
2. Burgdorfer W, Barbour AG, Hayes SF, et al: Lyme disease-a tick-borne spirochetosis? *Science* 216:1317-1319, 1982.
3. Tugwell P, Dennis DT, Weinstein A, et al: Laboratory evaluation in the diagnosis of Lyme disease, *Ann Intern Med* 127:1109-1123, 1997.
4. Centers for Disease and Control and Prevention: CDC provides estimate of Americans with Lyme disease each year. 2013. Media relations. Available at http://www.cdc.gov/media/releases/2013/p0819-lyme-disease.html. Accessed July 31, 2014.
5. Kollmann D, Dobson S: Treponema pallidum. In Remington JS, Klein JO, Wilson CB, et al, editors: *Infectious diseases of the fetus and newborn infant*, ed 7, Philadelphia, 2010, Saunders.
6. Lane RS, Piesman J, Burgdorfer W: Lyme borreliosis: relation of its causative agent to its vectors and hosts in North America and Europe, *Annu Rev Entomol* 36:587-609, 1991.
7. Nadelman RB, Nowakowski J, Fish D, et al: Prophylaxis with single-dose doxycycline for the prevention of Lyme disease after an *Ixodes scapularis* tick bite, *N Engl J Med* 345:79-84, 2001.
8. Piesman J: Dynamics of *Borrelia burgdorferi* transmission by nymphal *Ixodes dammini* ticks, *J Infect Dis* 167:1082-1085, 1993.
9. Falco RC, Fish D, Piesman J: Duration of tick bites in a Lyme disease-endemic area, *Am J Epidemiol* 143:187-192, 1996.
10. Shapiro ED, Gerber MA, Holabird NB, et al: A controlled trial of antimicrobial prophylaxis for Lyme disease after deer-tick bites, *N Engl J Med* 327:1769-1773, 1992.
11. Shapiro ED: Doxycycline for tick bites—not for everyone, *N Engl J Med* 345:133-134, 2001.
12. Schwartz BS, Nadelman RB, Fish D, et al: Entomologic and demographic correlates of anti-tick saliva antibody in a prospective study of tick bite subjects in Westchester County, New York, *Am J Trop Med Hyg* 48:50-57, 1993.
13. Centers for Disease Control and Prevention: Reported cases of Lyme disease—United States, 2011; reported cases of Lyme disease by year, United States. Available at http://www.cdc.gov, 2003-2012. Accessed July 31, 2014.
14. Fraser CM, Casjens S, Huang WM, et al: Genomic sequence of a Lyme disease spirochaete, *Borrelia burgdorferi*, *Nature* 390:580-586, 1997.
15. Bergström S, Noppa L, Gylfe A, Östberg Y: Molecular and cellular biology of *Borrelia burgdorferi sensu lato*, In Gray JS, Kahl O, Lane RS, Stanek G, editors: *Lyme borreliosis: biology, epidemiology, and control*, Wallingford, UK, 2002, CABI Publishing, pp 47-90.
16. Gerber MA, Shapiro ED, Burke GS, et al: Lyme disease in children in southeastern Connecticut. Pediatric Lyme Disease Study Group, *N Engl J Med* 335:1270-1274, 1996.
17. Steere AC, Sikand VK, Meurice F, et al: Vaccination against Lyme disease with recombinant *Borrelia burgdorferi* outer-surface lipoprotein A with adjuvant. Lyme Disease Vaccine Study Group, *N Engl J Med* 339:209-215, 1998.
18. Coleman JL, Gebbia JA, Piesman J, et al: Plasminogen is required for efficient dissemination of *B. burgdorferi* in ticks and for enhancement of spirochetemia in mice, *Cell* 89:1111-1119, 1997.
19. Coburn J, Leong LM, Erban JK: Integrin alpha IIb beta 3 mediates binding of the Lyme disease agent *Borrelia burgdorferi* to human platelets, *Proc Natl Acad Sci U S A* 90:7059-7063, 1993.
20. Coburn J, Magoun L, Bodary SC, et al: Integrins alpha(v)beta3 and alpha5beta1 mediate attachment of lyme disease spirochetes to human cells, *Infect Immun* 66:1946-1952, 1998.
21. Guo BP, Brown EL, Dorward DW, et al: Decorin-binding adhesins from *Borrelia burgdorferi*, *Mol Microbiol* 30:711-723, 1998.
22. Probert WS, Johnson BJ: Identification of a 47 kDa fibronectin-binding protein expressed by *Borrelia burgdorferi* isolate B31, *Mol Microbiol* 30:1003-1015, 1998.
23. Seinost G, Dykhuizen DE, Dattwyler RJ, et al: Four clones of *Borrelia burgdorferi* sensu stricto cause invasive infection in humans, *Infect Immun* 67:3518-3524, 1999.
24. Mullegger RR, McHugh G, Ruthazer R, et al: Differential expression of cytokine mRNA in skin specimens from patients with erythema migrans or acrodermatitis chronica atrophicans, *J Invest Dermatol* 115:1115-1123, 2000.
25. Krause A, Brade V, Schoerner C, et al: T cell proliferation induced by *Borrelia burgdorferi* in patients with Lyme borreliosis. Autologous serum required for optimum stimulation, *Arthritis Rheum* 34: 393-402, 1991.
26. Akin E, McHugh GL, Flavell RA, et al: The immunoglobulin (IgG) antibody response to OspA and OspB correlates with severe and prolonged Lyme arthritis and the IgG response to P35 correlates with mild and brief arthritis, *Infect Immun* 67:173-181, 1999.
27. Nardelli DT, Callister SM, Schell RFl: Lyme arthritis: current concepts and a change in paradigm, *Clin Vaccine Immunol* 15:21-34, 2008.
28. Hu L: Lyme arthritis, *Infect Dis Clin North Am* 19:947-961, 2005.
29. Pachner AR, Steiner I: Lyme neuroborreliosis: infection, immunity, and inflammation, *Lancet Neurol* 6:544-552, 2007.
30. Rupprecht TA, Koedel U, Fingerle V, et al: The pathogenesis of Lyme neuroborreliosis: from infection to inflammation, *Mol Med* 14: 205-212, 2008.
31. Anderson JF, Johnson RC, Magnarelli LA: Seasonal prevalence of *Borrelia burgdorferi* in natural populations of white-footed mice, *Peromyscus leucopus*, *J Clin Microbiol* 25:1564-1566, 1987.
32. Burgess EC, Windberg LA: *Borrelia* sp. infection in coyotes, black-tailed jack rabbits and desert cottontails in southern Texas, *J Wildl Dis* 25:47-51, 1989.
33. Burgess EC: *Borrelia burgdorferi* infection in Wisconsin horses and cows, *Ann N Y Acad Sci* 539:235-243, 1988.

34. Burgess EC, Wachal MD, Cleven TD: *Borrelia burgdorferi* infection in dairy cows, rodents, and birds from four Wisconsin dairy farms, *Vet Microbiol* 35:61-77, 1993.
35. Gustafson JM, Burgess EC, Wachal MD, et al: Intrauterine transmission of *Borrelia burgdorferi* in dogs, *Am J Vet Res* 54:882-890, 1993.
36. Burgess EC, Gendron-Fitzpatrick A, Mattison M: Borrelia burgdorferi. Proceedings of the 5th international conference on equine infectious diseases, 1989, pp 217–220.
37. Silver RM, Yang L, Daynes RA, et al: Fetal outcome in murine Lyme disease, *Infect Immun* 63:66-72, 1995.
38. Moody KD, Barthold SW: Relative infectivity of *Borrelia burgdorferi* in Lewis rats by various routes of inoculation, *Am J Trop Med Hyg* 44:135-139, 1991.
39. Woodrum JE, Oliver JH Jr: Investigation of venereal, transplacental, and contact transmission of the Lyme disease spirochete, *Borrelia burgdorferi*, in Syrian hamsters, *J Parasitol* 85:426-430, 1999.
40. Mather TN, Telford SR 3rd, Adler GH: Absence of transplacental transmission of Lyme disease spirochetes from reservoir mice *(Peromyscus leucopus)* to their offspring, *J Infec Dis* 164:564-567, 1991.
41. Schlesinger PA, Duray PH, Burke BA, et al: Maternal-fetal transmission of the Lyme disease spirochete, *Borrelia burgdorferi*, *Ann Intern Med* 103:67-68, 1985.
42. Oppenheimer EH, Hardy JB: Congenital syphilis in the newborn infant: clinical and pathological observations in recent cases, *Johns Hopkins Med J* 129:63-82, 1971.
43. MacDonald AB, Benach JL, Burgdorfer W: Stillbirth following maternal Lyme disease, *N Y State J Med* 87:615-616, 1987.
44. Weber K, Bratzke HJ, Neubert U, et al: *Borrelia burgdorferi* in a newborn despite oral penicillin for Lyme borreliosis during pregnancy, *Pediatr Infect Dis J* 7:286-289, 1988.
45. Trevisan G, Stinco G, Cinco M: Neonatal skin lesions due to a spirochetal infection: a case of congenital Lyme borreliosis? *Int J Dermatol* 36:677-680, 1997.
46. Grandsaerd MJ, Meulenbroeks AA: Lyme borreliosis as a cause of facial palsy during pregnancy, *Eur J Obstet Gynecol Reprod Biol* 91:99-101, 2000.
47. Mikkelsen AL, Palle C: Lyme disease during pregnancy, *Acta Obstet Gynecol Scand* 66:477-478, 1987.
48. Schaumann R, Fingerle V, Buchholz K, et al: Facial palsy caused by *Borrelia* infection in a twin pregnancy in an area of nonendemicity, *Clin Infect Dis* 29:955-956, 1999.
49. Schutzer SE, Janniger CK, Schwartz RA: Lyme disease during pregnancy, *Cutis* 47:267-268, 1991.
50. Stiernstedt G: Lyme borreliosis during pregnancy, *Scand J Infect Dis Suppl* 71:99-100, 1990.
51. Figueroa R, Bracero LA, Aguero-Rosenfeld M, et al: Confirmation of *Borrelia burgdorferi* spirochetes by polymerase chain reaction in placentas of women with reactive serology for Lyme antibodies, *Gynecol Obstet Invest* 41:240-243, 1996.
52. Markowitz LE, Steere AC, Benach JL, et al: Lyme disease during pregnancy, *JAMA* 255:3394-3396, 1986.
53. Ciesielski CA, Russell H, Johnson S, et al: Prospective study of pregnancy outcome in women with Lyme disease. In Program and Abstracts of Twenty-Seventh International Conference of Antimicrobial Agents and Chemotherapy, New York, 1987, abstract 39.
54. Maraspin V, Cimperman J, Lotric-Furlan S, et al: Erythema migrans in pregnancy, *Wien Klin Wochenschr* 111:933-940, 1999.
55. Williams CL: Lyme disease during pregnancy: a cord blood serosurvey, *Ann N Y Acad Sci* 539:504-506, 1988.
56. Nadal D, Hunziker UA, Bucher HU, et al: Infants born to mothers with antibodies against *Borrelia burgdorferi* at delivery, *Eur J Pediatr* 148:426-427, 1989.
57. Gerber MA, Zalneraitis EL: Childhood neurologic disorders and Lyme disease during pregnancy, *Pediatr Neurol* 11:41-43, 1994.
58. Strobino B, Abid S, Gewitz M: Maternal Lyme disease and congenital heart disease: a case-control study in an endemic area, *Am J Obstet Gynecol* 180:711-716, 1999.
59. Strobino BA, Williams CL, Abid S, et al: Lyme disease and pregnancy outcome: a prospective study of two thousand prenatal patients, *Am J Obstet Gynecol* 169:367-374, 1993.
60. Williams CL, Strobino B, Weinstein A, et al: Maternal Lyme disease and congenital malformations: a cord blood serosurvey in endemic and control areas, *Paediatr Perinat Epidemiol* 9:320-330, 1995.
61. Lischer CJ, Leutenegger CM, Braun U, et al: Diagnosis of Lyme disease in two cows by the detection of *Borrelia burgdorferi* DNA, *Vet Rec* 146:497-499, 2000.
62. Schmidt BL, Aberer E, Stockenhuber C, et al: Detection of *Borrelia burgdorferi* DNA by polymerase chain reaction in the urine and breast milk of patients with Lyme borreliosis, *Diagn Microbiol Infect Dis* 21:121-128, 1995.
63. Nadelman RB, Wormser GP: Lyme borreliosis, *Lancet* 352:557-565, 1998.
64. Shapiro ED, Gerber MA: Lyme disease, *Clin Infect Dis* 31:533-542, 2000.
65. Smith RP, Schoen RT, Rahn DW, et al: Clinical characteristics and treatment outcomes of early Lyme disease in patients with microbiologically confirmed erythema migrans, *Ann Intern Med* 236: 421-428, 2002.
66. Feder HM Jr, Johnson BJ, O'Connell S, et al: A critical appraisal of "chronic Lyme disease," *N Engl J Med* 357:1422-1430, 2007.
67. Johnson M, Feder HM Jr: Chronic Lyme disease: a survey of Connecticut primary care physicians, *J Pediatr* 157:1025-1029, 2010.
68. Halperin JJ: Prolonged Lyme disease treatment: enough is enough, *Neurology* 70:986-987, 2008.
69. Hatcher S, Arroll B: Assessment and management of medically unexplained symptoms, *BMJ* 336:1124-1128, 2008.
70. Wormser GP, Masters E, Nowakowski J, et al: Prospective clinical evaluation of patients from Missouri and New York with erythema migrans-like skin lesions, *Clin Infect Dis* 41:958-965, 2005.
71. Feder HM Jr, Hoss DM, Zemel L, et al: Southern tick-associated rash illness (STARI) in the North: STARI following a tick bite in Long Island, New York, *Clin Infect Dis* 53:e142-e146, 2011.
72. Food and Drug Administration: FDA Public Health Advisory: assays for antibodies to Borrelia burgdorferi, 1997. Limitations, use, and interpretation for supporting a clinical diagnosis of Lyme disease. July 7. Available at http://www.fda.gov/MedicalDevices/Safety/AlertsandNotices/PublicHealthNotifications/ucm062429.htm. Accessed July 31, 2014.
73. Wormser GP, Forseter G, Cooper D, et al: Use of a novel technique of cutaneous lavage for diagnosis of Lyme disease associated with erythema migrans, *JAMA* 268:1311-1313, 1992.
74. Klempner MS, Schmid CH, Hu L, et al: Intralaboratory reliability of serologic and urine testing for Lyme disease, *Am J Med* 110:217-219, 2001.
75. Bunikis J, Barbour AG: Laboratory testing for suspected Lyme disease, *Med Clin North Am* 86:311-340, 2002.
76. Craft JE, Grodzicki RL, Steere AC: Antibody response in Lyme disease: evaluation of diagnostic tests, *J Infect Dis* 149:789-795, 1984.
77. Hilton E, Tramontano A, DeVoti J, et al: Temporal study of immunoglobin M seroreactivity to *Borrelia burgdorferi* in patients treated for Lyme borreliosis, *J Clin Microbiol* 35:774-776, 1997.
78. Feder HM Jr, Gerber MA, Luger SW, et al: Persistence of serum antibodies to *Borrelia burgdorferi* in patients treated for Lyme disease, *Clin Infect Dis* 15:788-793, 1992.
79. Kalish RA, Kaplan RF, Taylor E, et al: Evaluation of study patients with Lyme disease, 10-20-year follow-up, *J Infect Dis* 183:453-460, 2001.
80. Bakken LL, Case KL, Callister SM, et al: Performance of 45 laboratories participating in a proficiency testing program for Lyme disease serology, *JAMA* 268:891-895, 1992.
81. Seltzer EG, Shapiro ED: Misdiagnosis of Lyme disease: when not to order serologic tests, *Pediatr Infect Dis J* 15:762-763, 1996.
82. Nichol G, Dennis DT, Steere AC, et al: Test-treatment strategies for patients suspected of having Lyme disease: a cost-effectiveness analysis, *Ann Intern Med* 128:37-48, 1998.
83. Steere AC, Berardi VP, Weeks KE, et al: Evaluation of the intrathecal antibody response to *Borrelia burgdorferi* as a diagnostic test for Lyme neuroborreliosis, *J Infect Dis* 161:1203-1209, 1990.
84. Avery RA, Frank G, Eppes SC: Diagnostic utility of *Borrelia burgdorferi* cerebrospinal fluid polymerase chain reaction in children with Lyme meningitis, *Pediatr Infect Dis J* 24:705-708, 2005.
85. Nordstrand A, Bunikis I, Larsson C, et al: Tickborne relapsing fever diagnosis obscured by malaria, Togo, *Emerg Infect Dis* 13:117-123, 2007.
86. Bracero LA, Wormser GP, Leikin E, et al: Prevalence of seropositivity to the Lyme disease spirochete during pregnancy in an epidemic area: a preliminary report, *J Matern Fetal Investig* 2:265-268, 1992.
87. Wormser GP, Dattwyler RJ, Shapiro ED, et al: The clinical assessment, treatment, and prevention of lyme disease, human granulocytic anaplasmosis, and babesiosis: clinical practice guidelines by the Infectious Diseases Society of America, *Clin Infect Dis* 43:1089-1134, 2006.

88. Wormser GP, Ramanathan R, Nowakowski J, et al: Duration of antibiotic therapy for early Lyme disease. A randomized, double-blind, placebo-controlled trial, *Ann Intern Med* 138:697-704, 2003.
89. Dotevall L, Hagberg L: Successful oral doxycycline treatment of Lyme disease-associated facial palsy and meningitis, *Clin Infect Dis* 28:569-574, 1999.
90. Elliott DJ, Eppes SC, Klein JD: Teratogen update: Lyme disease, *Teratology* 64:276-281, 2001.
91. Shapiro ED: Long-term outcomes of persons with Lyme disease, *Vector Borne Zoonotic Dis* 2:279-281, 2002.
92. Feder HM Jr: Lyme disease in children, *Infect Dis Clin North Am* 22:315-326, 2008.
93. Steere AC: Reinfection versus relapse in Lyme disease, *New Engl J Med* 367:1950-1951, 2012.
94. Southern PM, Sanford JP: Relapsing fever: a clinical and microbiological review, *Medicine* 48:129-149, 1969.
95. Dupont HT, La Scola B, Williams R, et al: A focus of tick-borne relapsing fever in southern Zaire, *Clin Infect Dis* 25:139-144, 1997.
96. Le CT: Tick-borne relapsing fever in children, *Pediatrics* 66:963-966, 1980.
97. Wyplosz B, Mihaila-Amrouche L, Baixench MT, et al: Imported tick-borne relapsing fever, France, *Emerg Infect Dis* 11:1801-1803, 2005.
98. Larsson C, Andersson M, Guo BP, et al: Complications of pregnancy and transplacental transmission of relapsing-fever borreliosis, *J Infect Dis* 194:1367-1374, 2006.
99. Jongen VH, van Roosmalen J, Tiems J, et al: Tick-borne relapsing fever and pregnancy outcome in rural Tanzania, *Acta Obstet Gynecol Scand* 76:834-838, 1997.

18 Tuberculosis

WILLEM A. HANEKOM, LUCY L. LINLEY, JAMES NUTTALL, and THOMAS R. HAWN

CHAPTER OUTLINE

Mycobacterium tuberculosis (Mtb) may spread by aerosol when an adult with pulmonary tuberculosis (TB) coughs. Ninety percent of newly infected adults never develop disease; in the other 10%, TB most commonly manifests as lung disease.

Infants and young children appear to have a 5- to 10-fold increased risk of progressing to TB disease after infection, compared with adults[1,2] The young could be viewed as epidemiologic sentinels of Mtb spread because the paucibacillar and noncavitory nature of their lung disease usually precludes transmission. The young are also at increased risk of disseminated forms of disease, such as TB meningitis and miliary disease. Approximately 4% of the global TB burden occurs in persons younger than 15 years; this may be as high as 15% in endemic areas.[3] The relative neglect of childhood TB was highlighted on World TB Day in 2013, when the World Health Organization (WHO) released a roadmap for intervention in the childhood epidemic.[4]

In this chapter, each section will first address TB beyond the newborn period, defined as the first 28 days of life, followed by a specific focus on the pregnant woman and the newborn. Finally, special considerations in human immunodeficiency virus (HIV) infection and in the setting of drug resistance are discussed.

Brief History

Recent studies suggest that Mtb comigrated with humans from Africa during the Neolithic expansion, approximately 70,000 years ago.[5] The pathogen has therefore evolved with humans and did not emerge as a zoonosis, as was previously thought.

TB has been termed "phthisis," "consumption," and the "white plague" over the ages. The disease caused up to 20% of all deaths in Europe between the 17th and 19th centuries. Incidence and death rates decreased dramatically during the 20th century, only to be followed by resurgence in the 1980s,[6] resulting in the WHO declaring TB a global health emergency in 1993.

Robert Koch was the first to identify the pathogen, in 1882.[7] Koch also developed tuberculin, a purified protein derivative (PPD) of Mtb, which was initially, albeit unsuccessfully, tested as a vaccine. Charles Mantoux later adapted PPD as a skin test to diagnose Mtb infection; this test remains the most commonly used test of infection. Microscopy and culture have been the mainstays for identification of the organism since the pathogen's discovery, until the advent of direct ex vivo molecular detection techniques in the 21st century.

Bacillus Calmette-Guérin (BCG), still the only commercially available vaccine to prevent TB, was first used in 1921.[8,9] Early strategies to treat TB disease involved isolation in sanatoria. Streptomycin was the first antimicrobial used against Mtb, in the 1940s, whereas the current cornerstones of therapy, isoniazid (INH) and rifampin (RIF), were introduced in the 1950s and 1970s, respectively.

Epidemiology

IN THE ADULT AND OLDER CHILD

The TB epidemic remains a global health crisis. One third of the world's population is infected with Mtb, and approximately 1% become newly infected every year[3] In 2012, 8.6 million people developed TB disease; 1.3 million died of the disease.[3]

The epidemiology of TB may be divided into three stages, for simplicity: exposure, infection, and disease. Exposure occurs when a person comes into close contact with an adult with untreated pulmonary TB who coughs up the pathogen. Adults with more severe disease, for instance, those with large pulmonary cavities, are more likely to spread the bacterium. After coughing, organisms are contained within microdroplets, which "hang" in the air, particularly within poorly ventilated, enclosed environments. (In contrast, most common respiratory viruses spread via macrodroplets, which rapidly drop to surfaces.) Exposed persons may inhale the pathogen, and approximately 35% will become infected; risk of infection varies according to duration and proximity of exposure.

Established infection is defined by a host T-cell response to Mtb, detected by the tuberculin skin test (TST), or by an interferon-γ (IFN-γ) release assay (IGRA).[10] In a TST, membrane proteins of the bacterium are injected intradermally, and skin induration caused by influx of mycobacteria-specific CD4 T cells is measured 48 to 72 hours later. In an IGRA, whole blood or peripheral blood mononuclear cells are exposed to Mtb-specific antigens, which are taken up by monocytes and dendritic cells and presented to Mtb-specific T cells, which, in turn, produce IFN-γ measurable in the plasma/supernatant. The TST or IGRA will turn positive between 2 and 10 weeks after exposure. Evidence of infection should be regarded as a sentinel event for identifying persons that transmit in a community. (Recommendations and interpretation of TSTs and IGRAs, and intervention, are discussed later.)

Approximately 90% of persons infected with Mtb never develop disease, reflecting successful host control of the pathogen. About half of those who do become diseased do so within 2 years of infection, whereas disease may manifest much later in life in the other 50%. Overt or relative immune compromise increases risk of progression from infection to disease; immune compromise may be due to HIV infection,[11] diabetes mellitus,[12] malnutrition,[13] immunomodulatory drug therapy,[14] smoking,[15] silicosis,[16] malignancy,[17] renal disease,[18] older age, alcoholism,[19] and overcrowding and poverty.[20] The risk of progression to disease after infection in infants and young children appears to be fivefold to 10-fold higher than that of adults: This risk may therefore be as high as 50% in the first year of life.[1]

In reality, because of access to care and intervention, the transition from susceptibility to cure is much more complex than exposure, infection, and disease (Fig. 18-1). Further, the American Thoracic Society (ATS) and Centers for Disease Control and Prevention (CDC) have introduced a classification system for use in public health communication, reporting, and contact investigations: class 0: no TB exposure; class 1: TB exposure, no evidence of infection; class 2: latent TB infection, no disease; class 3: TB, clinically active; class 4: TB, not clinically active; class 5: TB suspect, diagnosis pending.[21]

Most of the world's TB cases occur in Southeast Asia, whereas the incidence of disease is highest in southern Africa, where rates are about 1% per year.[3] Southern Africa contributes the highest burden of TB patients coinfected with HIV; for instance, in South Africa, 62% of all patients with TB are HIV infected.[3] Untreated HIV infection had been a major driver of an uncontrolled TB epidemic in this region for more than a decade, although this appears to be changing now. The southern African incidence is approximately 200-fold higher than that in the United States, where disease is most common in urban, low-income areas, and where greater than 60% of adults and greater than 25% of children with TB are foreign-born.[22]

The global prevalence of TB has been declining since the year 2000, whereas the incidence has been falling since 2002. Regardless, in 2013, many countries with a high burden of TB disease had not demonstrated a decrease in incidence.[3] In contrast, great progress has been made in reducing mortality from TB: This rate has decreased by 41% since 1990. The WHO Stop TB Partnership goal of halving

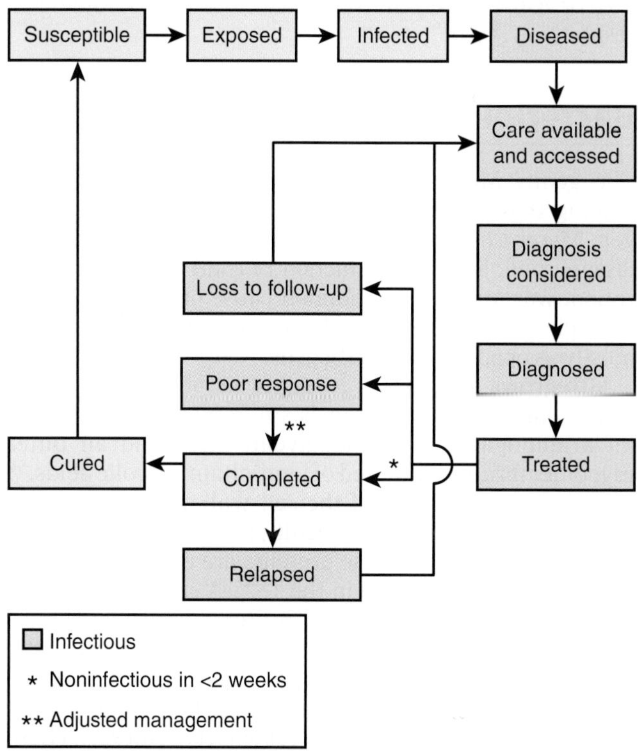

Figure 18-1 Interaction of tuberculosis susceptibility, exposure, infection, disease, and intervention.

prevalence and mortality by 2015, compared with 1990, is therefore likely to be achieved; however, a second goal of eradication by 2050 (incidence of $<1/10^6$) is not achievable, given current trends.[3]

IN PREGNANCY

A series of 24 cases of TB during pregnancy reported in 1850 strongly suggested that the disease is more severe during pregnancy.[23] However, the largest series of TB in pregnancy, published in the mid-20th century, refuted the notion.[23] Some studies have shown an increased risk of disease in the mother during the immediate postpartum period,[24,25] but this has not been confirmed in all studies.[26-30]

IN THE NEWBORN

The epidemiology of fetal and newborn exposure to TB has not been studied extensively; most information has emerged from case reports.[31-47] TB disease manifesting within the first 28 days of life is most commonly the result of aerosol transmission, after early postnatal exposure to an adult with pulmonary TB, most commonly the mother. In exceedingly rare cases, infants may be infected in utero, manifesting so-called congenital TB.

The risk of the asymptomatic newborn acquiring TB infection or disease after exposure to a mother or health care worker with active TB disease has not been quantified in a systematic manner. It is also not known how long it takes for the TST or IGRA to turn positive after exposure in the newborn. Very few cases of nosocomial transmission to the newborn in health care settings have been reported: The proportions of exposed newborns that converted their TST or IGRA were relatively small, 0% to 2.9% and 9%, respectively.[40,48,49]

Bacteriology

The genus *Mycobacterium* has more than 100 species. Among these, Mtb is the most successful human pathogen. *Mycobacterium bovis* is the commonest cause of animal disease, and, before introduction of routine milk pasteurization, was a relatively common cause of human disease. Multiple other species are able to cause disease in humans, mostly as opportunistic pathogens.

Mtb grows slowly and is highly aerobic. The bacterium's complex cell wall consists of a plasma membrane, an arabinogalactan-peptidoglycan layer and an outer mycomembrane composed of long-chain mycolic acids.[50] The high lipid content of the cell wall affords the property of acid-fast staining. Multiple proteins are found within the cell wall. These proteins are extracted to generate PPD, which is used in the TST. A capsule, comprising polysaccharides, secreted proteins, and glycolipids, surrounds the wall.[51] The capsule has received little attention until recently because this structure may be destroyed altogether by detergents, such as Tween, or by physical shaking, used in mycobacterial culture. These and other structural and secreted components of the wall and capsule are virulence determinants.

Mtb was first sequenced in 1998.[52] About 4 million base pairs encode approximately 4000 proteins. About 10% of genes are from a unique PE_PGRS family (the proline–glutamic acid superfamily—PE–contains the PGRS family, which is characterized by guanine-cytosine–rich sequences), which appear to be important virulence factors.[53] Sequencing has revealed existence of seven major lineages of Mtb globally, each with distinct geographic distributions.[5] Among the lineages, the so-called Beijing strain appears hypervirulent, because global spread has been the most successful of all strains.[54] Sequencing has also revealed that variation in immunodominant proteins among global strains is minimal, compared with greater diversity among other proteins, suggesting that preferential immune recognition of immunodominant proteins affords evolutionary advantage for the pathogen.[55]

Pathogenesis and Pathology

IN THE ADULT AND OLDER CHILD

Mtb is inhaled into distal airways, which are lined with alveolar macrophages, the primary cells that take up the pathogen[56,57] Uptake is mediated through specific receptors, such as the mannose receptor. Within the macrophage, Mtb is contained within a phagosome, although escape from the phagosome into the cytoplasm may also occur.[58]

The macrophage recognizes Mtb as foreign through a range of pathogen recognition receptors, such as Toll-like receptors, each of which binds specific bacterial components.[59] Engagement of these receptors results in an inflammatory response. An early component of inflammation is macrophage release of mediators to recruit other immune cells, such as neutrophils and NK cells. These cells may aid bacterial control; for instance, NK cells may produce IFN-γ, which can activate macrophages for better intracellular control of the bacteria. Intracellular control may be mediated by molecules contained within lysosomes, after the latter organelle fuses with an Mtb-containing phagosome. Autophagy, a process of engulfment of the phagosome containing Mtb, or of the pathogen within the cytoplasm, thereby enveloping it within a double membrane, is one of multiple other mechanisms of intracellular control described.[60] Established infection after exposure is an indication of failure of first-line innate responses; it appears that, by far, the majority of persons will become infected when exposure is proximal and constant.

Poor control of Mtb may result in death of the infected macrophage. The released Mtb may be then taken up by other macrophages or by dendritic cells. The latter cells are critical for initiation of adaptive immunity: They migrate to regional lymph nodes, where T cells are encountered. The dendritic cells present peptides of Mtb, generated through intraphagosomal processing of bacterial components, on their surface, in association with major histocompatibility complex (MHC) class II molecules. Naïve or antigen-experienced CD4 T cells that are specific for the presented peptide antigen will bind and start replicating. These activated CD4 T cells then migrate back to the lung, attracted by molecules released during the inflammatory process. Here, CD4 T cells bind local macrophages, which also present antigen on their surface. The CD4 T cells activate these macrophages through production of cytokines, such as IFN-γ and tumor necrosis factor-α, or through binding of surface activating molecules. Macrophage activation results in greater efficiency in intracellular control of Mtb. Animal models suggest that initiation of adaptive immunity in the lung is the most important determinant of control of Mtb infection.

At the disease site, cells organize to form a granuloma. This histologic structure consists of macrophages and macrophage-derived cells at the center and a ring of CD4 T cells on the periphery. T cell subsets other than CD4 cells, as well as B cells, may also be present, implying a potential role in mycobacterial control. The primary role of the granulomas appears to be isolation of Mtb, although recent evidence in experimental models suggests that the pathogen may exploit granuloma organization to allow spread from cell to cell.[61] The latter is one example of a hallmark of host-pathogen interaction in TB: The pathogen has evolved multiple strategies to exploit host control mechanisms for its own gain, or to evade host control.[62] Evasion mechanisms include a 10- to 14-day delay in migration of dendritic cells from the disease site to the lymph nodes, allowing ongoing bacterial replication and establishment of infection before adaptive immunity arrives to control the infection.[63] Other evasion mechanisms include arrest of the phagosome in an early stage, preventing its fusion with lysosomes, subversion of acidification of phagolysosomes (acidification is critical for function of lysosomal effectors), inhibition of autophagy and inhibition of antigen presentation on the cellular surface.[62]

In most humans, host immune mechanisms control the infection and therefore prevent clinical disease manifestations. However, even if this is the case, Mtb appears not to be eradicated because serial imaging in nonhuman primate models of clinical latency show sporadic reactivation of granulomas without resulting disease. Further, reactivation disease may manifest many years after the primary infection. Finally, manifestation of disease at organs distal to the lung, often after prolonged latency, suggests that asymptomatic granuloma breakdown with a bacteremia may occur early in Mtb pathogenesis, allowing infection to establish in meninges, kidney, and bone, for example.

The determinants of progression from controlled infection to disease, or later reactivation, remain incompletely understood. The infecting strain, dose and repetitive exposure may be important. On the host side, either an inadequate immune response or an excessive inflammatory response appears to increase risk of TB disease.[56,64] Inadequate immunity may place HIV-infected persons or persons with diabetes mellitus, for example, at risk of TB disease, whereas excessive inflammation may be in response to repeated Mtb infection or perhaps other respiratory pathogen exposure, which trigger a prolonged inflammatory process. Heterogeneity in inflammatory capacity may be important; ultimately, individual host-pathogen interactions are important.[65]

The histologic hallmark of disease is granuloma breakdown or inadequate organization of this structure. Adolescents and adults characteristically have a greater inflammatory response, compared with children, with greater breakdown, often resulting in cavities in the lung. This is why adolescents and adults have higher bacterial loads and spread the pathogen. Children often have limited parenchymal involvement but marked lymph node involvement, which can cause airway compression and other complications. Breakthrough of granulomas into blood vessels, the pleura, and the pericardium may result in miliary disease, pleural effusions, and pericarditis, respectively.

IN PREGNANCY

The pathogenesis in pregnancy is similar to that described above, except that TB of the genital tract may be particularly relevant because direct dissemination to the fetus may occur.[66] Genitourinary TB most commonly involves the fallopian tubes in greater than 90% of women, followed by the uterus, ovaries, and cervix. Infertility is a common manifestation.

TB may involve the placenta, but this appears to be very rare (Fig. 18-2). For example, only 9 cases of placental TB were found in a cases series of 2000 placentas examined in a report from 1904, whereas the incidence of other forms of TB was much higher at that time.[67] Granulomas in villi and in the intervillous space appear most common, although decidual and chorionic involvement was also observed (see Fig. 18-2). Placental involvement is likely to reflect hematogenous dissemination, which may be due to severe disease or due to the "silent" bacteremia mentioned earlier. It is important to note that placental involvement may occur without affecting the fetus.[68]

Similarly, fetal involvement may occur without any placental lesions; however, intrauterine dissemination of Mtb to the fetus is very rare. This may occur via hematogenous dissemination, when blood flow to the fetus results in

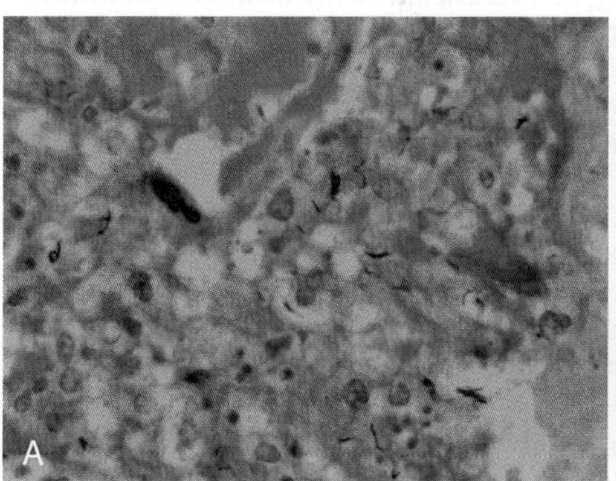

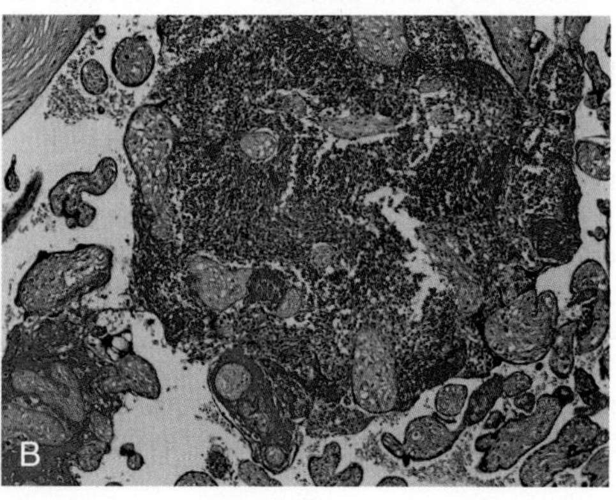

Figure 18-2 A, Acid-fast bacilli in a placenta. **B,** Tuberculosis granulomas in the perivillous space. (Courtesy Department of Pathology, Groote Schuur Hospital, Cape Town, South Africa.)

primary involvement of the liver; however, multiple organ systems may be involved.

Alternatively, the fetus may inspire infected amniotic fluid, resulting from infection of the endometrium and chorioamnionitis.

IN THE NEWBORN

The pathogenesis of TB in the newborn is similar to that at older ages, except, as mentioned earlier, in rare cases of congenital TB. Therefore the majority of newborns are infected via the aerosol route. Breastfeeding is not recognized as a route of Mtb transmission.

The immune system of the young newborn is relatively immature (reviewed in Chapter 4), which may result in the substantially increased risk of progression to TB disease after infection, or in greater risk of disseminated disease, compared with older ages. Relatively immature myeloid cells, such as macrophages and dendritic cells, as well as relatively immature T cells in the newborn, may contribute to this risk.

The pathology of TB in the newborn depends on the route of transmission. For example, aerosol transmission after birth is more likely to be associated with pulmonary disease in the newborn, as would be inhalation of infected amniotic fluid. In contrast, liver disease is prominent when infection occurs via the umbilical vein, although lung, bone marrow, bone, adrenal, gastrointestinal, kidney, spleen, skin, and lymph node involvement have also been described. Any mechanism of intrauterine infection would occur when the fetal immune system is likely to be immature and risk of disseminated disease is likely to be high. The histologic lesions are similar in appearance to those of older children or adults.

Clinical Presentation

IN THE ADULT AND OLDER CHILD

Latent TB infection (LTBI) is by definition asymptomatic.

As mentioned earlier, the lung is by far the most common site of symptomatic disease. Early symptoms of pulmonary TB may be constitutional, such as loss of appetite, malaise, and fatigue, often lasting for weeks. Classic symptoms include chronic cough, low-grade fever, weight loss or failure to thrive, night sweats, and chest pain. Dyspnea and hemoptysis may manifest but occur in a small fraction of cases only. Symptoms develop insidiously, and patients often present to health care facilities only after an acute bacterial pulmonary superinfection.

On physical examination of the lungs, signs reflect the many possible underlying structural effects, for instance, consolidation, cavitation, pleural effusion, and complications from airway obstruction, such as collapse and hyperinflation. Clubbing, erythema nodosum, and phlyctenular conjunctivitis may be found but are rare. Up to 25% of persons with radiographic evidence of pulmonary disease are asymptomatic.[69]

Pulmonary disease in children manifests as does adult lung disease, although some features, such as night sweats, are less common.[70]

TB may affect virtually any extrapulmonary organ, although these manifestations are much rarer than those of lung disease. Of importance, up to 35% of children with TB may have extrapulmonary disease manifestations, making a comprehensive physical examination mandatory. The symptoms and signs reflect the organ system involved. In children, lymph node involvement, usually presenting as palpable or even visible glands in the neck, is relatively common. Less than 5% of TB disease in children younger than 2 years manifests as meningitis, often presenting with altered levels of consciousness, nuchal rigidity, and seizures. Even fewer young children present with miliary disease, when widespread bacterial dissemination commonly results in hepatosplenomegaly, lymphadenopathy, and significant weight loss. In adults, and more rarely in children, other sites that may be involved include the pericardial space, genitourinary tract, bones and joints, and skin. Again, symptoms and signs will follow underlying structural involvement.

IN PREGNANCY

As mentioned earlier, there is little evidence to support a dogma that pregnancy places women at increased risk of TB disease after infection. However, some studies have shown that extrapulmonary disease appears as common as pulmonary disease in pregnancy, which is not the case in the general population.[71,72]

Symptoms of TB in pregnancy are similar to those in the nonpregnant person, with some caveats: malaise and fatigue and other nonspecific symptoms may be ascribed to pregnancy itself, by both patients and care providers. In addition, weight loss may be masked by pregnancy.[71]

IN THE NEWBORN

As for older persons, active TB disease may be symptomatic or asymptomatic in newborns. Symptoms are usually nonspecific and may include poor feeding, poor weight gain, lethargy, and nonresolving or recurrent pneumonia. Duration of symptoms often depends on the clinical setting: If an index case is known during pregnancy or the peripartum period, alert clinicians would recognize symptoms early, whereas absence of such a case may result in presence of symptoms for weeks before a diagnosis of TB is made in the infant. The diagnosis of TB as a cause of nonresolving or recurrent pneumonia may also be delayed. In congenital TB caused by intrauterine infection, signs and symptoms may be present at birth; however, manifestations more commonly appear in the second or third week of life.[73-75]

Peng and colleagues[76] reviewed 170 cases of congenital TB published in the literature. The mean age of onset was day 20 of life. The mothers of 162 patients were diagnosed with active tuberculosis during pregnancy or after parturition. Nonspecific signs and symptoms were common and included fever, respiratory distress, and hepatosplenomegaly. Skin lesions, seizures, jaundice, ear discharge, paravertebral abscess and hematologic abnormalities also occurred. Schaaf and colleagues[47] also reviewed congenital TB and classified symptoms according to frequency (Table 18-1).

Table 18-1 Most Frequent Signs and Symptoms of Congenital Tuberculosis

Symptoms and Signs	Occurrence
Respiratory distress, including tachypnea Hepatomegaly, splenomegaly Fever (usually low grade) Prematurity/low birth weight	Common (i.e., >40%)
Cough, may be acute or chronic Poor feeding Failure to thrive Abdominal distension (including ascites)	Frequent (i.e., 25%-40%)
Irritability Peripheral lymphadenopathy Sepsis syndrome	Infrequent (i.e., 10%-25%)
Skin papular/pustular or ulcerative lesions Tuberculosis meningitis Jaundice (obstructive) Otorrhea/mastoiditis Wheeze or stridor Apnea or cyanosis attacks Facial nerve palsy Shock	Rare (i.e., <10%)

From Schaaf HS, Collins A, Bekker A, Davies PD: Tuberculosis at extremes of age, *Respirology* 15:747-763, 2010.

Diagnosis

IN THE ADULT AND OLDER CHILD

A primary component of the diagnosis of LTBI or TB disease is *epidemiologic history* of exposure, either by identification of an index case (a coughing adult with pulmonary disease) or by membership of, or origin from, a community with a high incidence of disease. It is important to note that in high-prevalence settings, molecular epidemiology studies suggest that greater than 50% of new infections occur outside the immediate household.[77] Risk factors that should be noted are those mentioned in the epidemiology section above. In high-prevalence areas, particularly in settings where HIV is prevalent, integration of HIV and TB care is recommended and should involve routine screening for either infections/diseases.[78]

Chest radiographs are commonly used for diagnosis. Adults most commonly present with upper lobe consolidation and may manifest cavitation. Pleural effusions are relatively common. In contrast, pulmonary cavitation is uncommon in paucibacillary childhood TB, whereas intrathoracic lymph node enlargement is characteristic, with complications of bronchial or bronchiolar obstruction, such as segmental collapse or hyperinflation. Miliary disease in small children manifests with multiple small (<5 mm) lesions in the parenchymal space. Overall, chest radiographs are relatively insensitive because only gross pathology will be visible. Remarkable variability in expert interpretations of radiographs is also common.[79] High-resolution chest computed tomography (CT) has greater sensitivity in identifying lung lesions.

Immunologic tests are also used for diagnosis. LTBI is diagnosed by a TST or an IGRA. The tests can also be helpful when active, symptomatic disease is present but cannot differentiate LTBI from active disease and may be negative in up to 40% of patients with active TB disease. In the United States, high-risk persons are screened with a TST or an IGRA; the American Academy of Pediatrics (AAP) has made specific recommendations for when testing for LTBI should occur (Box 18-1).[80] In other settings, different recommendations may apply. For instance, in many high-prevalence settings, routine testing of all persons exposed to TB disease cannot be delivered because the primary focus is on finding and treating active TB disease.

The most commonly used TST is the Mantoux test. The AAP interpretation of Mantoux test results is shown in Box 18-2; again, interpretation may differ in other settings, based on the tuberculin used and local epidemiology. BCG vaccination is the most common cause of a false positive TST; however, results are usually interpreted without taking into account BCG vaccination, particularly if this occurred at birth because epidemiologic studies in high-prevalence areas have shown that a positive result is most likely to be attributable to Mtb infection. False-negative Mantoux tests may be caused by inappropriate administration; the test may also be negative during the 2 to 10 weeks that it takes for conversion after exposure in children younger than 3 months; in the presence of poor nutrition and acute viral infections, such as influenza and measles; in HIV-infected persons; and in patients with disseminated TB disease.[80]

The two commercially available IGRAs are the Quanti-FERON Gold In-Tube test (Celletis/Qiagen, Chadstone, Australia) and the T Spot TB test (Oxford Immunotec, Abingdon,

Box 18-1 Recommendation for Testing for *Mycobacterium tuberculosis* Infection in the United States

Children for Whom Immediate TST or IGRA is Indicated

Contacts of people with confirmed or suspected contagious tuberculosis (contact investigation)

Children with radiographic or clinical findings suggesting tuberculosis disease

Children immigrating from countries with endemic infection (e.g., Asia, Middle East, Africa, Latin America, countries of the former Soviet Union), including international adoptees

Children with travel histories to countries with endemic infection and substantial contact with indigenous people from such countries. If the child is well and has no history of exposure, the TST or IGRA should be delayed for up to 10 weeks after return

Children Who Should Have Annual TST or IGRA

Children infected with human immunodeficiency virus (TST only)

Children at increased risk of progression of LTBI to tuberculosis disease, that is, those with medical conditions such as diabetes mellitus, chronic renal failure, malnutrition, congenital or acquired immunodeficiencies, and children receiving tumor necrosis factor (TNF) antagonists. (Without recent exposure, these people are not at increased risk of acquiring tuberculosis infection and should be evaluated for other disease processes.) An initial TST or IGRA should be performed before initiation of immunosuppressive therapy, including prolonged steroid administration, use of TNF-α antagonists, or other immunosuppressive therapy.

From American Academy of Pediatrics; Pickering LK, editor: Red book: 2012 report of the Committee on Infectious Diseases, *ed 29, Elk Grove Village, Ill, 2012, American Academy of Pediatrics.*

IGRA, Interferon-γ release assay; *LTBI,* latent tuberculosis infection; *TST,* tuberculin skin test.

Box 18-2 Definitions of a Positive Mantoux Skin Test

Induration 5 mm or Greater

Children in close contact with known or suspected contagious people with tuberculosis disease
Children suspected to have tuberculosis disease:
- Findings on chest radiograph consistent with active or previous tuberculosis disease
- Clinical evidence of tuberculosis disease

Children receiving immunosuppressive therapy or with immunosuppressive conditions, including human immunodeficiency virus (HIV) infection

Induration 10 mm or greater

Children at increased risk of disseminated tuberculosis disease:
- Children younger than 4 years of age
- Children with other medical conditions, including Hodgkin disease, lymphoma, diabetes mellitus, chronic renal failure, or malnutrition

Children with likelihood of increased exposure to tuberculosis disease:
- Children born in high-prevalence regions of the world
- Children who travel to high-prevalence regions of the world
- Children frequently exposed to adults who are HIV infected, homeless, users of illicit drugs, residents of nursing homes, incarcerated or institutionalized

Induration 15 mm or Greater

Children age 4 years or older

From American Academy of Pediatrics; Pickering LK, editor: Red book: 2012 report of the Committee on Infectious Diseases, *ed 29, Elk Grove Village, Ill, 2012, American Academy of Pediatrics.*

Box 18-3 Use of TST versus IGRA in Children

TST Preferred, IGRA Acceptable

Children <5 years of age

IGRA Preferred, TST Acceptable

Children ≥5 years of age who have received BCG vaccine
Children ≥5 years of age who are unlikely to return for TST reading

Performing Both TST and IGRA Should be Considered When

An initial and repeat IGRA are indeterminate
The initial test (TST or IGRA) is *negative* and
- Clinical suspicion for TB disease is moderate to high
- Risk of progression and poor outcome is high

The initial TST is *positive* and
- >5 years of age and history of BCG vaccination
- Additional evidence needed to increase compliance
- Nontuberculous mycobacterial disease is suspected

From American Academy of Pediatrics; Pickering LK, editor: Red book: 2012 report of the Committee on Infectious Diseases, *ed 29, Elk Grove Village, Ill, 2012, American Academy of Pediatrics.*
BCG, Bacillus Calmette-Guérin; *IGRA,* interferon-γ release assay; *TST,* tuberculin skin test.

United Kingdom).[10] These are validated tests, where a specific quantitative value is regarded as positive; however, these results are interpreted in conjunction with results from the negative and positive controls, which may lead to an "indeterminate" result; in this case, the test should be repeated. The main advantage over the TST is that antigens contained in IGRAs are present in Mtb but not in *M. bovis;* therefore BCG vaccination will not affect results. The antigens may be present in some nontuberculous mycobacteria (*Mycobacteria kansasii, Mycobacteria szulgai,* and *Mycobacteria marinum*), which, as with TSTs, may cause false-positive results. The AAP has made some recommendations for use of either or both an IGRA and TST (Box 18-3)[80]; the group points out that IGRAs should not be used in children younger than 2 years unless TB disease is suspected. In children aged 2 to 4 years, there are limited data about the usefulness of IGRAs in determining Mtb infection, but IGRA testing can be performed if TB disease is suspected. Extensive clinical evidence questions the usefulness of IGRA versus TST for diagnosis of Mtb infection or TB disease in developing-country clinical settings.[10]

Microbiologic tests are commonly performed on sputum, collected from a productive cough, after induction of cough with hypertonic saline nebulization, or from aspiration of gastric contents of the young child upon awaking and before ambulation or feeding. As a first step, direct visualization of the acid-fast organism through microscopy is attempted: this may be up to 90% sensitive in adults, when multiple specimens are examined, but is usually less than 5% sensitive in infants and children, an indication of differential bacterial loads in different age groups. For culture, liquid media is preferred over solid media because of shorter times to positive results. Liquid cultures are often positive between 1 and 6 weeks, mostly in less than 3 weeks. These delays confound programmatic implementation in low-resource settings. Time-to-positive culture reflects bacterial load in the specimens; therefore, time-to-positive results is expected to be longer in children. The sensitivity of culture in children is much lower than in adults and usually in the range of 40%.

Newer, direct ex vivo nucleic acid amplification techniques for detection of Mtb in sputum, such as Xpert MTB/RIF assay (Cepheid, Sunnyvale, Calif), may revolutionize early detection of Mtb. A recent Cochrane review of 15 studies showed that Xpert, an easy-to-use, enclosed assay system, had a pooled sensitivity and specificity of 88% and 98%, respectively, for replacement of smear microscopy.[81] The sensitivity was 67% when used in addition to smear microscopy, with culture as the denominator. Xpert has shown sensitivity in children with smear-negative TB disease that approaches that of adults.[82] Of interest, a pilot study of children with suspected TB disease showed that stool might be useful for detection of Mtb by using nucleic acid amplification techniques.[83] Other new first-line detection methods have also shown promise; for instance, sensitivity of the microscopic observation drug sensitivity (MODS) assay appears similar to that of Xpert, although MODS is more labor intensive and results appear operator dependent.[84] MODS is used to detect, by microscopy, the characteristic cording behavior of the pathogen within 5 to 10 days of incubation in culture medium; isoniazid and RIF resistance can also be detected with this assay, hence the name.

Drug susceptibility testing should be done as a routine, where resources are available. Conventional methods, using egg- or agar-based media are still in wide use, and the cumulative sensitivity for first-line drugs (see later) is invariantly greater than 90%, whereas performance for detection of resistance among second-line drugs (see later) is generally not as optimal.[85] The disadvantage is that assay completion takes at least 3 weeks; therefore there has been a shift toward more rapid techniques, including phenotypic assays such as MODS and liquid culture in the presence of antimicrobials, with sensitivities that approach those of solid culture. Detection of common Mtb genomic markers of drug resistance has recently been incorporated into molecular probes of the bacterium after culture or directly ex vivo in sputum, such as in XpertTB.[86] Performance of these assays depends on the rate of occurrence of specific genotypic resistance determinants; for instance, presence of *katG* and *inhA* will detect approximately 50% and approximately 25% of INH resistance, whereas *rpoB* will detect approximately 95% of RIF resistance.

At present, no reliable *peripheral blood or urine tests* are available for detection of TB disease, although these are the focus of intensive current research. In addition, large-scale investigation into prospective peripheral blood markers of risk of TB disease is currently underway. Prospective use of the IGRA may be useful in the latter setting: In a high-prevalence setting, conversion of the QuantiFERON Gold In-Tube test from negative to positive was associated with an eightfold higher risk of progression to TB disease.[87]

Extrapulmonary disease is generally diagnosed by site-specific pathologic specimens or imaging. These include examination of cerebrospinal fluid and brain magnetic resonance imaging for meningitis, ultrasonography for abdominal disease, and biopsy and radiographs for bone disease. Classic granulomas seen on histology, especially when containing acid-fast organisms, are pathognomonic in the presence of epidemiologic and other clinical support of the diagnosis.

Multiple classifications of TB disease have emerged, including the commonly used terms "definite," "probable," and "possible" disease. "Definite" TB is usually defined by identification of Mtb in clinical specimens, whereas "probable" disease refers to very strong clinical, epidemiologic, and laboratory features suggestive of TB, in absence of identification of the pathogen. "Possible" TB refers to a likely diagnosis but with features that are not as convincing as for "probable" disease. In practice, these terms are of limited use because, almost invariably, management of "possible" disease is similar to that of "definite" or "probable" disease.

The *differential diagnosis* of pulmonary TB includes community-acquired pneumonia, although the latter classically has a more acute presentation over days rather than the chronic nature of TB presenting over weeks to months. In adults, lung cancer, sarcoidosis, and disease caused by nontuberculous bacteria, *Nocardia, Actinomyces,* endemic fungi (e.g., *Cryptococcus,* Coccidioides immitis, and *Histoplasma* spp.), and *Paragonimus* should also be considered. In children, other causes of intrathoracic lymph node enlargement, such as hematologic malignancies, should be considered. The differential diagnosis in children also includes sarcoidosis, malnutrition, connective tissue disorders, and disease caused by *Mycoplasma* and nontuberculous mycobacteria.

IN PREGNANCY

Diagnosis is often delayed because symptoms may be masked as those of pregnancy itself, such as fatigue and malaise; disease is commonly diagnosed during the third trimester only. Because extrapulmonary disease is relatively more common, classic pulmonary manifestations of TB would have lesser sensitivity in diagnosis of disease in pregnancy.

Antenatal care during pregnancy presents an ideal opportunity to screen and evaluate women at risk of TB, using risk factors as mentioned earlier. The focus is on early diagnosis of active tuberculosis to limit morbidity and mortality in the mother, the fetus, and the newborn. Routine testing for LTBI in pregnant women is not indicated unless treatment will be initiated if the test is positive, which is not common in high-prevalence settings.

Diagnostic approaches are similar to those in nonpregnant women. The TST appears not to be affected by pregnancy and is safe. It is not clear how pregnancy affects the IGRA; in clinical practice, this test continues to be used. Radiographic evaluation of pregnant patients should allow shielding of the fetus from potentially damaging effects of radiation.

Suspected or confirmed TB disease in the newborn (see later) may lead to a diagnosis of previously unrecognized TB in the mother.[88] Delayed diagnosis of TB in the mother may result in prolonged exposure of multiple newborns in a nursery, as well as family members, visitors to hospital, and health care workers. A similar situation arises when a health care worker involved in the care of newborns is found to have active TB disease.

IN THE NEWBORN

TB should be considered in cases when other infections are contemplated, particularly when there is poor response to antibiotic therapy and serologic and microbiologic tests for other infections are negative. *The differential diagnosis* includes HIV infection; syphilis; cytomegalovirus infection; herpes infection; causes of atypical pneumonia, such as *Chlamydia trachomatis* and *Mycoplasma pneumoniae;* nontuberculous mycobacterial disease; disseminated *M. bovis* BCG disease; congenital pulmonary malformations, such as lobar emphysema; and gastroesophageal reflux.

Diagnostic evaluation should also be initiated when clinical features suggest TB disease or when the newborn is exposed to a source case with TB infection or disease, such as the mother, another household or other close contact, or a health care worker. Close communication between the physician caring for the pregnant or postpartum woman with TB and the physician caring for the exposed or infected newborn is essential.

Laboratory investigation for suspected newborn TB is similar to that of older patients. A TST or IGRA is usually indicated, although interpretation is difficult in the newborn, particularly when BCG was given at birth. Chest radiography is essential (Fig. 18-3). Abnormal chest radiographs were found in 133 infants with congenital TB, of whom 83 cases showed miliary tuberculosis and multiple pulmonary nodules.[89] Abdominal ultrasonography is recommended to identify lymph node enlargement or, more rarely, hepatic, renal, or splenic involvement. Repeated gastric aspirates are indicated for detection of acid-fast bacilli and for culture and detection of Mtb DNA by nuclear amplification techniques. Tracheal aspirates or bronchoalveolar lavage should be examined if the infant is mechanically ventilated, or pleural fluid should be evaluated if a pleural effusion is present. Evaluation of cerebrospinal fluid

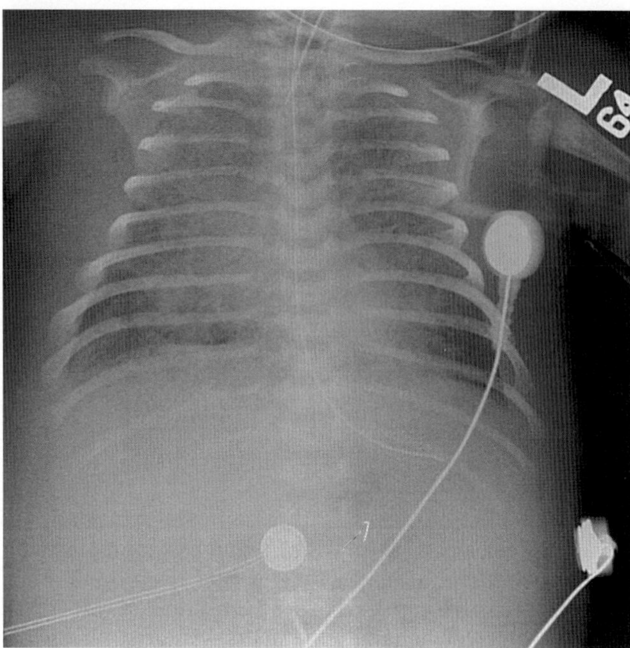

Figure 18-3 Chest radiograph from a 1-month-old infant with congenital tuberculosis.

is indicated in newborns with features of disseminated disease, although culture is positive in less than 20% of cases where meningitis is present. Fine-needle aspiration of subcutaneous lymph nodes or liver biopsy for histology, as well as TB microscopy and culture, should be considered. Some experts recommend examination of middle ear fluid and of bone marrow. No specific data exist on the performance of most tests in the newborn because of small sample sizes in series; however, Hageman[90] described positive cultures for Mtb in 10 of 12 gastric aspirates, in all 3 bone marrow and all 3 lymph node biopsies, and in 2 of 4 bone marrow aspirates.

Cantwell and colleagues[89] have listed specific criteria for diagnosis of congenital TB. One or more of the following should be present: tuberculous lesions evident in the first week of life, primary hepatic complex or caseating hepatic granulomas, evidence of tuberculous infection of the maternal genital tract. In addition, the possibility of postnatal transmission should be excluded by a thorough investigation of contacts. It should be pointed out that this definition is not often practical in the clinical setting because time of acquisition of disease does not influence management of the newborn.

Management

IN THE ADULT AND OLDER CHILD

The goals of treatment are not only to decrease morbidity and mortality from active TB disease but also to prevent progression from latent to active disease and to interrupt and prevent transmission of the tubercle bacilli to contacts of an infectious patient. In this section, treatment of active drug-sensitive TB disease and of LTBI is addressed; special considerations in HIV-TB coinfection and MDR-TB are addressed later. It should be pointed out that recommendations may differ in different countries, often dictated by local resources.

Active pulmonary TB disease caused by drug-sensitive strains is treated by a combination of four bactericidal drugs: INH, RIF, pyrazinamide (PZA), and ethambutol (EMB).[91,92] All four drugs are given for 2 months, termed the induction phase, followed by INH and RIF alone for another 4 months, termed the continuation phase (Tables 18-2 and 18-3). If the strain is fully sensitive to INH, RIF, and PZA, the fourth drug EMB may be omitted. All four drugs have excellent oral bioavailability and penetrate most tissues well. PZA achieves excellent intramacrophage concentrations. Second-line therapy, which may be introduced when adverse events occur or drug resistance is present (see later), most commonly includes fluoroquinolones and streptomycin (see Table 18-2).

A number of factors influence the total duration of therapy for lung disease. For patients who do not have radiographic evidence of cavitation and have a susceptible organism and a negative sputum culture at 2 months, standard 6-month therapy is adequate. This duration is often termed "short course," based on previous regimens that took longer to complete. Patients with cavitary lesions and a positive sputum culture at 2 months should be treated for 9 months because relapse rates after 6 months of therapy are high. In this setting, adherence should be assessed and drug resistance considered, whereas monthly sputum testing should continue until the culture becomes negative. If a drug regimen lacks RIF, for instance, because of adverse effects or resistance, the duration of therapy is lengthened to 12 to 18 months. If a drug regimen lacks PZA, the duration of therapy is often lengthened for up to 24 months. In refractory cases of pulmonary disease or in the presence of complications, surgical removal of diseased lung may be indicated.

The duration of treatment for extrapulmonary disease depends on the site of infection. For meningeal and disseminated TB, the continuation phase is extended for a total of 9 to 12 months of therapy. For lymphadenitis and most other sites of infection, 6 months total duration is sufficient.

In certain categories of TB disease, such as meningitis and pericardial disease, corticosteroids are used as adjunctive immunomodulatory therapy. Steroid therapy improves outcome in TB pericarditis in multiple ways (when compared with placebo in a randomized controlled trial): more rapid decrease in the mean pulse rate and jugular venous pressure, earlier recovery of physical activity, and lower rates of pericardectomy and death.[93] In this trial, the dose of oral prednisolone in adults and children older than 15 years was 60 mg daily for weeks 1 through 4, followed by 30 mg for weeks 5 through 8; 15 mg for weeks 9 to 10; and then 5 mg for week 11. A Cochrane analysis of seven randomized controlled trials that evaluated outcome of steroid use in TB meningitis concluded that death is decreased but not disability.[94] There was variation in dose and schedule of steroid administration in the different trials; no current consensus recommendation exists.[95] Expert consultation is advised for all cases of pericardial and meningeal TB and for possible steroid use in extrapulmonary TB.

First-line anti-TB drugs are safe in the majority of patients (see Table 18-2). Regardless, adverse events will result in a

Table 18-2 Chemotherapeutic Agents Commonly Used to Treat Tuberculosis

	Dose	Side Effects	Interactions	Remarks
FIRST LINE				
Isoniazid	*Daily:* Adults: 5-10 mg/kg PO Children: 10-15 mg/kg PO Maximum dose: 300 mg *Twice weekly:* 20-30 mg/kg PO Maximum dose: 900 mg	Hepatitis, peripheral neuritis, rash, dizziness	Potentiation of phenytoin, Antabuse	Inexpensive Used in treatment of TB infection and TB disease
Rifampin	*Daily and twice weekly:* Adults: 10-15 mg/kg PO Children: 10-20 mg/kg PO Maximum dose, regardless of interval: 600 mg	Hyperbilirubinemia, fever, purpura	Inhibition of many drugs: oral contraceptives, quinidine, coumarin drugs, digoxin, oral hypoglycemics, HIV protease inhibitors, certain nonnucleoside reverse-transcriptase inhibitors	Colors urine and other body secretions orange
Ethambutol	*Daily:* Adults: 15-25 mg/kg PO Children: 20 mg/kg PO *Twice weekly:* 50 mg/kg PO Maximum dose, regardless of interval: 2.5 g	Optic neuritis (rare at 15 mg/kg), reversible, rash		Use with caution in patients with renal disease and in children when eye testing is not possible
Pyrazinamide	*Daily:* Adults: 20-25 mg/kg PO Children: 30-40 mg/kg *Twice weekly:* 50 mg/kg PO Maximum dose, regardless of interval: 2g	Hyperuricemia, rash, hepatitis		When used for the first 2 months with isoniazid and rifampin, can shorten total duration of therapy to 6 months
SECOND LINE				
Moxifloxacin	Adults: 400 mg qd PO	Tendonopathy/rupture, QT prolongation	Cardiac medications	Not recommended for routine use in those younger than18 yr
Streptomycin	*Daily and twice weekly:* Adults: 15-20 mg/kg IM Children: 20-40 mg/kg IM Maximum dose: 1g	Ototoxicity (auditory and vestibular) and renal toxicity	Potentiation of neuromuscular blocking agents	Use with caution in older patients and in those with renal disease

HIV, Human immunodeficiency disease; *IM,* intramuscularly; *PO,* orally.

Table 18-3 Drug Regimens for Culture-Positive Pulmonary Tuberculosis Caused by Drug-Susceptible Organisms

*	INITIAL PHASE: DRUGS AND DURATION†		CONTINUATION PHASE: DRUGS AND MINIMAL DURATION*		**Total Duration (months)**	**Rating HIV⁻**	**Rating HIV⁺**
1.	INH, RIF, PZA, EMB	Daily or 5×/wk for 8 wk	1a. INH/RIF	Daily or 5×/wk for 18 wk	6	A(I)	A(II)
			1b. INH/RIF	2×/wk for 18 wk	6	A(I)	A(II)
			1c. INH/RPT	1×/wk for 18 wk	6	B(I)	E(I)
2	INH/RIF/PZA/EMB	Daily for 2 wk, then 2×/wk for 6 wk OR 5×/wk for 2 wk, then 2×/wk for 6 wk	2a. INH/RIF	2×/wk for 18 wk	6	A(II)	B(II)
			2b. INH/RPT	Daily for 18 wk	6	B(I)	E(I)
3.	INH/RIF/PZA/EMB	3×/wk for 8 wk	3a. INH/RIF	3×/wk for 18 wk	6	B(I)	B(II)
4.	INH/RIF/EMB	Daily or 5×/wk for 8 wk	4a. INH/RIF	Daily or 5×/wk for 31 wk	9	C(I)	C(II)
			4b. INH/RIF	2×/wk for 31 wk	9	C(I)	C(II)

Modified from guidelines developed and published as follows: American Thoracic Society, Centers for Disease Control and Prevention, Infectious Diseases Society of America: Treatment of tuberculosis, *MMWR Recomm Rep* 52:(RR-11) 1-77, 2003. [Erratum in *MMWR Recomm Rep* 53:1203, 2005. Dosage error in article text].

EMB, Ethambutol; *HIV,* human immunodeficiency virus; *INH,* isoniazid; *PZA,* pyrazinamide; *RIF,* rifampin; *RPT,* rifapentine.

Definitions of evidence ratings: A, Preferred; B, acceptable alternative; C, offer when A and B cannot be given; E, should never be given; I, randomized clinical trial; II, data from clinical trials that were not randomized or were conducted in other populations; III, expert opinion.

*A 4-month continuation phase is used for the majority of patients. The 7-month continuation phase is only recommended for three groups: patients with cavitary pulmonary tuberculosis caused by drug-susceptible organisms and whose sputum culture obtained at the time of completion at 2 months of treatment is positive; patients whose initial phase of treatment did not include PZA; and patients being treated with once weekly INH and rifapentine and whose sputum culture obtained at completion of the initial phase is positive. In addition, some authorities recommend 7-month continuation phase for HIV-infected children.

†Ethambutol is not routinely used in young children because of difficulties in eye monitoring.

Box 18-4 Recommendations for Therapy of Tuberculosis in Children in the United States

Latent Tuberculosis Infection

Mycobacterium tuberculosis (Mtb) strain from index case is isoniazid susceptible
- 9 months of isoniazid, once daily; if daily therapy is not possible, directly observed therapy (DOT) twice weekly can be used

Mtb strain from index case is isoniazid resistant
- 6 months of rifampin, once daily; if daily therapy is not possible, DOT twice weekly can be used

Mtb strain from index case is isoniazid and rifampin resistant
- Consult a tuberculosis specialist

Pulmonary and Extrapulmonary Disease (Except Meningitis)

Mtb strain from index case or patient is drug susceptible
- 2 months of isoniazid, rifampin, pyrazinamide, and ethambutol daily or twice weekly, followed by 4 months of isoniazid and rifampin by DOT
- If hilar adenopathy only, a 6-month course of isoniazid and rifampin is sufficient

If drug resistance is a concern
- Add at least two drugs to match the presumed drug susceptibility pattern and consult a tuberculosis expert

Mycobacterium bovis, which is drug susceptible
- 9-12 months of isoniazid and rifampin

Meningitis

Mtb strain from index case or patient is drug susceptible
- 2 months of isoniazid, rifampin, pyrazinamide, and an aminoglycoside or ethambutol or ethionamide, once daily, followed by 7-10 months of isoniazid and rifampin, once daily or twice weekly (9-12 months total)
- For patients who may have acquired tuberculosis in geographic areas where resistance to streptomycin is common, kanamycin, amikacin, or capreomycin can be used instead of streptomycin

M. bovis, which is drug susceptible
- At least 12 months of therapy without pyrazinamide

Modified from American Academy of Pediatrics; Pickering LK, editor: Red book: 2012 report of the Committee on Infectious Diseases, *ed 29, Elk Grove Village, Ill, 2012, American Academy of Pediatrics.*

change of drug regimens in up to 10% of diseased patients. Major toxicities of INH include increased hepatic aminotransferase concentrations and neuropathy. INH-associated neuropathy is prevented by routine co-administration of pyridoxine. RIF may cause increased hepatic aminotransferase concentrations, nausea, and orange discoloration of body fluids, which is harmless but uniformly noticed. PZA is the most common cause of hepatitis. Despite overlapping liver toxicities of INH, RIF, and PZA, routine monitoring of hepatic aminotransferases is not indicated unless a patient has underlying liver disease. EMB may cause optic neuritis. Although this adverse effect is uncommon, baseline and follow-up visual acuity and red-green color discrimination testing is recommended.

Treatment is usually administered within a strategy called DOTS—"directly observed treatment, short-course"— which means that an independent observer watches the patient swallow his/her anti-TB therapy. The WHO advises that all TB patients should have at least the first two months of their therapy observed because ultimate outcomes have been shown to be better.[91] Several regimens that do not require daily medication are available, particularly for the continuation phase (see Table 18-3).

Treatment of active disease in children is mostly similar to that in adults, except that pyridoxine is not routinely used with INH, except in children with diets likely to be deficient in pyridoxine and in those who experience paresthesias while on INH (Box 18-4). Further, EMB use is limited in children in whom visual acuity cannot be assessed reliably. Because of the lower bacillary burden in pediatric TB and difficulty of monitoring for visual adverse side effects, a three-drug induction regimen that excludes EMB is often sufficient; however, the drug may be needed if there is evidence of cavitary disease, with higher bacillary burdens.

In most countries, TB is a notifiable disease. Reporting to the local health department should result in investigation of all household members or other contacts for TB.

Various treatment options are available for treating adults with LTBI (Table 18-4).[96] Nine months of INH therapy is highly efficacious in preventing progression to active

Table 18-4 Drug Regimens Recommended by the American Thoracic Society and the Centers for Disease Control and Prevention for the Treatment of Latent Tuberculosis Infection in Adults

Drug(s)	Duration	Rating HIV$^-$	Rating HIV$^+$	Comments
Isoniazid	9 months, daily*†	A(II)	A(II)	Preferred regimen
Isoniazid-rifapentine	12 weeks, weekly with DOT	A(I)		Recommended for age ≥ 12 yr; unknown for age < 12 yr or HIV$^+$
Isoniazid	9 months, 2×/wk*†	B(II)	B(II)	Must use DOT
Isoniazid	6 months, daily	B(I)	C(I)	Not for HIV$^+$, children, or those with fibrotic lesions
Rifampin	4 months, daily	B(II)	B(III)	For HIV$^+$, rifabutin may be substituted to avoid drug interactions
Rifampin-PZA	2 months, daily	D(II)	D(II)	Avoid this regimen because of liver toxicity

DOT, Directly observed treatment; *HIV,* human immunodeficiency virus; *PZA,* pyrazinamide.

*Recommended for persons < age 18 yr. *Strength of recommendation: A, Preferred; B, acceptable alternative; C, offer when A and B cannot be given; D, moderate evidence for lack of efficacy or for adverse outcome supports a recommendation against use and should generally not be offered; E, good evidence for lack of efficacy or for adverse outcome supports a recommendation against use and should never be offered.

†Recommended for pregnant women. †Quality of evidence: I, Randomized clinical trial data; II, data from clinical trials that are not randomized or were conducted in other populations; III, expert opinion.

TB disease in low-prevalence settings.[97,98] In higher-prevalence settings, risk of reinfection compromises efficacy of this therapy.[99] Further, some countries recommend 6 months of INH because of greater adherence, while efficacy remains relatively high. INH treatment of LTBI is also efficacious and recommended in immune-suppressed populations, including HIV-infected and solid-organ transplant patients.[100,101] In 2011, the PREVENT TB randomized study in adults demonstrated that a 12-week course of weekly rifapentine and INH was as efficacious as 9 months of INH.[102] Based on this data, the CDC recommends this regimen as an alternative to 9 months of INH for HIV-negative patients greater than or equal to 12 years of age.[103]

Treatment of LTBI in children takes into account the higher risk of progressing from latent to active disease, the risk of the most serious forms of active disease, and lesser availability of data on newer LTBI regimens.[96] Therefore only the 9-month course of INH (either daily or 2 times/week with directly observed therapy) is recommended (see Table 18-4). If INH cannot be given because of adverse side effects, RIF has been used successfully in children. The INH-rifapentine regimen may be considered on a case by case basis in 2- to 11-year-olds but is not recommended for children younger than 2 years.

Current research into TB therapy includes discovery of new compounds and a focus on shorter regimens, which could increase adherence, reduce recurrence, and reduce emergence of drug resistance.

IN PREGNANCY

Treatment of active TB in pregnancy is important for the benefit of the mother, the fetus, and the community. In addition to the risk to the pregnant woman, untreated TB may result in low birth weight and, rarely, congenital tuberculosis. According to WHO recommendations, the treatment of TB in pregnant women should be the same as for nonpregnant women.[91] In contrast, the American Thoracic Society guidelines discourage use of PZA in pregnancy because detailed teratogenicity data are not available; in this case, INH and RIF should be given for 9 months.[92]

INH, RIF, and EMB all cross the placenta, but there have been no reports linking either INH or RIF to excess fetal malformations. Isoniazid-induced increases in hepatic aminotransferases during pregnancy are rare. Pyridoxine supplementation should be given to pregnant women treated with INH. Streptomycin is the only anti-TB drug that has been shown to have harmful effects on the human fetus, ranging from mild hearing loss to congenital deafness, and should not be used in pregnancy. There are similar concerns about neonatal deafness related to use of other aminoglycosides (amikacin, kanamycin, and capreomycin) in pregnancy.[92]

IN THE NEWBORN

A newborn with possible, probable, or confirmed TB disease should immediately start treatment with daily INH, RIF, and PZA and, in case of disseminated disease, an aminoglycoside, for 2 months.[47,80,90] As for adults, INH and RIF are continued for a further 4 months. Dose adjustment may be considered if toxicity develops; in this case, expert opinion should be sought. Pyridoxine supplementation should be given. Corticosteroids are indicated for TB meningitis (2 mg/kg/day of prednisone, maximum 60 mg/day, for 4-6 weeks and tapered thereafter) and may be considered for newborns with pleural or pericardial effusions, severe miliary disease, endobronchial disease causing airway obstruction or atelectasis, and abdominal TB. Drug susceptibility testing of the organism isolated from the mother or household contact, newborn, or both should be performed and therapy adjusted if drug resistance is present (see later).

Although placental disease does not necessarily occur in all cases of congenital TB, every effort should be made to identify the strain by microbiologic testing of the placenta.

The AAP recommended management of the newborn possibly exposed to Mtb is based on the disease status of the source case[80]:

1. Source case has a positive TST or IGRA but a normal chest radiograph.
   If the source case is the mother and she is asymptomatic, the newborn and mother should remain together. There is no contraindication to breastfeeding, and the newborn does not require specific clinical evaluation, investigation, or therapy. The mother or household contact may be a candidate for treatment of LTBI after the initial postpartum period, because a positive TST or IGRA in the mother or household contact may indicate possible exposure to other contagious persons. Other household members should therefore be evaluated by history and physical examination and receive a TST or an IGRA test; however, this should not delay discharge of the newborn after delivery.
2. Source case has clinical signs and symptoms, or an abnormal chest radiograph, consistent with TB disease.
   The infant should be evaluated for TB disease. If the latter is diagnosed, therapy as delineated earlier should be initiated. If TB disease is excluded, INH is given, with supplemental pyridoxine. At 3 to 4 months of age, a TST should be performed; if positive, the infant should be reassessed for TB disease. If disease is excluded, INH should be continued for a total of 9 months, with monthly follow up. If the TST result is negative at 3 to 4 months of age and the source has good adherence and response to treatment and is no longer contagious, INH is discontinued. BCG vaccination of the newborn should be considered if the source case has MDR TB or does not receive DOT; HIV-infected infants should not receive BCG (see "Prevention," later). As for all treatment recommendations, different approaches may apply in different geographies.

Separation of the mother or other source case from the newborn is recommended until the diagnostic evaluation has been completed and prophylactic chemotherapy or treatment has been initiated, if required. Adherence of the mother or household contact to infection control measures may allow the newborn to be reintroduced to the family. Once INH has been started in the newborn, separation is no longer required, unless drug resistance is suspected or confirmed, adherence to treatment is poor, or supervision of treatment is poor. Women with TB disease who have received 2 or more weeks of appropriate anti-TB therapy are not considered contagious and may breastfeed.

Feeding with breast milk is recommended irrespective of the TB status of the mother.[80] First-line anti-TB drugs cross into breast milk in small amounts, but these have not been linked to adverse events or development of drug resistance. Breastfeeding is not recommended for babies of mothers receiving treatment with rifabutin or fluoroquinolones or other second-line anti-TB drugs; expert advice should be sought.[92,104]

Prognosis

Most TB disease and most strains of Mtb are eminently treatable. It has been estimated that 87% of all cases of TB in the world in 2012 were treated successfully. Treatment success primarily depends on severity of disease, resistance pattern of the offending strain, and patient adherence.

Overall, mortality rates vary according to region. In the Americas, this rate was 1.9 per 100,000 in 2012, whereas, in Africa, it was 26 per 100,000. The WHO has estimated that 8% of all deaths caused by TB among HIV-uninfected persons are in children younger than 15 years. In low-prevalence countries, risk factors for death in adults include increased age, delay in diagnosis of TB, extensive radiographic involvement, the need for mechanical ventilation, end-stage renal disease, diabetes, and immunosuppression.

Complications of TB include immune reconstitution inflammatory syndrome in HIV-infected persons (see later), adult respiratory distress syndrome, pneumothorax, bronchiectasis, empyema, extensive lung destruction, right middle lobe syndrome, and hemoptysis. In children, complications resulting from lymph node obstruction of the large airways are relatively common.

Recurrent disease may be due to relapse; that is, the same strain causes disease again in an inadequately treated person, or due to reinfection with another strain, particularly in high-prevalence settings. It is estimated that the risk of recurrent disease in high-prevalence settings is at least 5% within the first year after completion of therapy; a high index of suspicion within the first year of completion of therapy is therefore warranted. Overall, approximately 10% of all TB cases in the world are retreatment cases.

IN PREGNANCY

Untreated TB in pregnancy has the same morbidity as TB in the general population. Fetuses and babies born to mothers with untreated active TB are at increased risk of intrauterine growth restriction, low birth weight, low Apgar scores, and early fetal demise.[105-107] Their mothers are at increased risk of preeclampsia and antepartum hemorrhage.

TB in women is linked to subsequent infertility.[66] The World Bank has estimated that TB kills more women each year than all other causes of maternal mortality combined.[108]

IN THE NEWBORN

No systematic data are available regarding the outcomes of TB in newborns. In the case series of 170 congenital TB cases referred to earlier, 68 patients died, often before therapy was instituted, whereas the death rate among those on therapy was 21.7%.[76] A low leukocyte count, younger age of onset, and presence of intracranial granulomas were associated with poor outcome.

Infection Control

As mentioned earlier, adolescents or adults with untreated TB are much more likely to be infectious than infants or children. Factors associated with infectiousness in adults include presence of a cough, lung cavities, acid-fast bacilli on sputum smear, disease of the lungs, airway or larynx, and less than 2 weeks of adherent treatment.[109] In general, patients can be considered noninfectious when they have had three consecutive negative sputum smears collected within 8- to 24-hour intervals and their symptoms have improved clinically.

Spread of Mtb has been shown to be higher when the concentration of infectious bacilli in the air is high, within small, enclosed spaces, when ventilation is poor (particularly when recirculation of air containing infectious droplet nuclei occurs), when improper specimen handling procedures generate infectious droplet nuclei and when positive air pressure in an infectious patient's room causes spread to surrounding areas.

The goals of effective TB infection control programs are to detect TB disease early and promptly, to isolate those who have or are suspected of having TB disease by using airborne precautions and to treat people who have or who are suspected of having TB disease. The CDC has published recommendations for infection control of TB in health care settings, in public and at home. In practice, availability of resources in diverse settings and stigma (such as identification of a person wearing a mask in a community as having TB) drive effectiveness of implemented procedures.

Prevention

Prevention of TB disease in the newborn period may be achieved either by vaccination or by chemoprophylaxis (addressed earlier).

BCG is the only currently available vaccine to prevent TB disease.[9] BCG was developed early in the 20th century and is a live-attenuated strain of *M. bovis*. The vaccine has approximately 80% efficacy in preventing disseminated forms of TB early in childhood, that is, meningitis and miliary disease, and is therefore, throughout the world, given to most newborns soon after birth.[9,110-112] BCG has some efficacy in preventing pulmonary disease in early childhood, but this effect is variable.[9] Multiple uncontrolled observational studies have recently suggested that BCG may prevent Mtb infection.[113-115] The efficacy of BCG may depend on the geographic environment where it is used; for instance, the vaccine appears more protective at latitudes farther from the equator.[9] This may be due to immune priming with environmental mycobacteria, more abundant in tropical regions, leading to inadequate BCG intake, or masking of BCG's effects.[116] BCG is safe, although local skin reactions are common.[9] Severe vaccine adverse events, such as disseminated BCG disease, occur in less than 5 per million vaccinations, usually in the context of congenital cellular immune deficiency.[9] The use of BCG in HIV-exposed and -infected infants is discussed later.

It is not clear whether BCG would have any protective efficacy if given after exposure of a newborn to Mtb. In this setting, the infant will be on antimycobacterial therapy (see earlier), which would compromise taking the live BCG vaccine. BCG vaccination should therefore be deferred until 2 weeks after chemoprophylaxis has been completed and after an evaluation for TB has been completed, also because BCG may result in a false-positive TST. However, when BCG is not given at birth, it is important that the vaccine be administered after completion of chemotherapy, to allow protective effects of BCG for possible future Mtb exposure.

Novel vaccination approaches against TB, currently in the experimental stage, include the use of recombinant BCG and Mtb vaccines.[117,118] The parental strain is modified either to circumvent immune evasion mechanisms of the bacterium, to be safer (also in HIV-infected infants), or to overexpress antigens thought to be important for immune control of Mtb. Other novel vaccination approaches involve so-called boost vaccines, which would be given after priming with BCG, Mtb infection, or environmental mycobacterial infection. These vaccines include viral vectored constructs and adjuvanted subunits and contain antigens thought to be important for control of mycobacteria.[117,118]

Special Considerations in Human Immunodeficiency Virus Infection or Exposure

Human immunodeficiency infection is an important risk factor for developing TB disease. Mtb and HIV coinfected adults and children not on antiretroviral therapy (ART) have an annual TB disease risk of approximately 10%, although this risk may be reduced dramatically by ART.[119] No specific data exist about this risk in the HIV-infected newborn population.

All persons who present with TB disease should be tested for HIV infection. Disease presentation in HIV-infected persons may follow the same pattern as that in noncompromised persons or may be atypical.[120-122] HIV-infected adults with more advanced immune compromise often present with disease that resembles that of children, with lesser pulmonary cavitation and increased risk of disseminated disease.

Most patients with HIV infection who contract TB respond well to routine treatment. Indeed, TB is the most treatable of all the life-threatening opportunistic infections associated with acquired immunodeficiency syndrome. In adults, the treatment regimens are identical to those for HIV-negative patients (see Table 18-2; see Box 18-4).[123,124] In contrast, in HIV-infected children, some authorities recommend extending the total duration of therapy for tuberculosis in such patients by providing an additional 3 months of continuation therapy (for a total of 9 months) because of the possibility of relapse resulting from failing immunity.[80]

Immune reconstitution inflammatory syndrome (IRIS) can occur after initiating ART in patients with TB.[122,125,126] IRIS can present in patients who begin ART with occult TB, so-called unmasking IRIS, or in those with known TB, paradoxic IRIS. The incidence of paradoxic IRIS may be as high as 54%, with an overall 15.7% shown in a meta-analysis.[126] Risk factors include a low CD4 count, a short duration between initiation of TB treatment and ART, and disseminated TB. The median onset is 14 days after starting ART, and focal and systemic inflammatory features are prominent, including fever, pulmonary infiltrates, pleural effusions, lymphadenopathy, and involvement of any organ where Mtb is located. IRIS may be severe, requiring hospitalization in nearly 50%. Diagnosis of IRIS is critically important because the treatment includes the addition of antiinflammatory and/or immunosuppressive medications.[127] Large studies have addressed the optimal time to initiate ART in patients with TB and have uniformly shown that delay in initiating ART in a person with low CD4 counts (<50/μL) is associated with increased mortality.[128-130] In persons with CD4 counts greater than 50, ART may be deferred for about 8 weeks, except if other indicators of poor outcome are present, such as multiorgan disease.

Drug interaction between anti-TB drugs and ART is another major consideration in the management of coinfected patients, particularly when the patient is on a protease inhibitor–containing regimen.[123,131] Extensive recommendations for managing these interactions exist.[123,131] Treatment of TB in persons with HIV infection is often complicated and requires individualization with close monitoring throughout the course of treatment to ensure that the response has been satisfactory.

Fetal and newborn exposure to TB has increased significantly in communities with high HIV infection rates because of the concurrent HIV/TB epidemics. Presentation, evaluation, and management of the HIV-exposed or -infected newborn for TB are similar to that of HIV-uninfected newborns.[80,122]

BACILLUS CALMETTE-GUÉRIN IN HUMAN IMMUNODEFICIENCY–EXPOSED AND –INFECTED INFANTS

Epidemiologic evidence of efficacy of BCG vaccination in protecting HIV-infected infants or children against TB, including disseminated TB, is lacking. HIV infection among infants is known to severely impair the immune response after BCG vaccination.[132] Further, the risk of disease caused by live-attenuated *M. bovis* BCG in HIV-infected infants not on ART approaches, or exceeds, the risk of TB disease in high-prevalence settings.[133,134]

A classification system for BCG vaccine–associated disease in HIV-infected infants has been devised.[135] Local disease is defined as a BCG injection site abscess, scar, or ulceration; regional disease includes ipsilateral regional lymph node involvement, including enlargement, suppuration, and fistula formation; distant disease involves any site beyond local or regional disease, with microbiologic confirmation of the vaccine strain from pulmonary secretions, cerebrospinal fluid, bone, or distant skin, for example. Disseminated BCG disease is defined as *M. bovis* BCG confirmed from more than one distant site and/or from at least one blood or bone marrow culture.

In infants born to HIV-infected mothers, BCG disease should be considered when local or regional BCG adverse events occur. The most specific diagnostic result is a positive mycobacterial culture (e.g., from sputum, biopsy material, or blood), where the BCG strain is confirmed by polymerase chain reaction assay. This differs from routine microbiologic laboratory procedures, which detect the Mtb complex that includes both Mtb and *M. bovis.* Isolating *M. bovis* BCG does not eliminate the possibility of coexisting Mtb disease, for instance, concurrent BCG lymphadenitis and pulmonary TB. Management of severe BCG-vaccine associated disease typically involves multidrug regimens incorporating INH, RIF, ethambutol, and a fluoroquinolone, tailored to drug susceptibility results and continued for at least 9 months, in addition to ART.[136] PZA is not effective against *M. bovis.* The case fatality rate of distant or disseminated BCG disease is reported to be as high as 75% in infants not treated with ART.[135]

BCG should not be used in infants or children known to be infected with HIV.[137] In developing countries, BCG is usually given at birth, regardless of HIV exposure. In this setting, close follow-up is recommended to identify and treat BCG-related complications. Early introduction of ART in infants infected with HIV lessens the chance and severity of BCG disease; regardless, BCG-IRIS still does occur. In settings where good health care infrastructure, including early diagnosis of HIV infection and ART, are routinely available, BCG vaccination should not be given to infants born to HIV-infected mothers until these infants have been shown to be HIV-uninfected.

Special Considerations in Drug-Resistant Tuberculosis (DR-TB)

Drug resistance is increasing globally. Approximately 4% of primary Mtb isolates are multidrug resistant (MDR), defined as resistant to INH and RIF, compared with 20.2% of organisms isolated during re-treatment.[3] Among MDR strains, nearly 10% are extensively drug resistant (XDR), that is, additional fluoroquinolone and injectable aminoglycoside resistance is present. XDR strains have been isolated in 92 countries. Totally drug-resistant (TDR) strains of Mtb have also been described.

In addition to MDR and XDR, Mtb strains may also be monoresistant. Resistance is a laboratory diagnosis, based on drug susceptibility testing during/after culture. Newer sputum nuclear amplification tests, such as Xpert, may detect resistance strains earlier through identification of common genotypic determinants of resistance.[86]

Drug-resistant (DR) strains should be managed in consultation with experts because of changes in duration of therapy and management of side effects with use of the second-line agents: fluoroquinolones such as moxifloxacin, streptomycin, capreomycin, kanamycin, ethionamide, and cycloserine.[138] With the exception of moxifloxacin, these second-line drugs are generally less potent and more difficult to administer because of potentially dangerous side effects.

With rising levels of drug resistance worldwide, there has been renewed interest in repurposing drugs for treating TB or discovering new TB drugs. Examples of repurposed drugs include the fluoroquinolones and linezolid. Linezolid, a drug developed for gram-positive bacterial infections, was found to induce culture conversion in 87% of patients with XDR-TB.[139] In December 2012, the U.S. Food and Drug Administration approved bedaquiline, the first drug developed exclusively for TB in more than 50 years.[140] Bedaquiline targets the adenosine triphosphate synthase of MTB and is effective against MDR-TB.

Exposure of the fetus or newborn to DR-TB and to the drugs used for its treatment during pregnancy or postpartum is an emerging problem. These problems should again be managed in consultation with an expert. Certain drugs used in the treatment of DR-TB should preferably be avoided during pregnancy and breastfeeding.[104] However, in the setting of MDR-TB or XDR-TB with limited treatment options, the use of drugs with potential toxicity to the fetus may be unavoidable; in this setting, the mother should be counseled carefully. Aminoglycosides may cause infant deafness and should be avoided during pregnancy if possible. Cycloserine, *p*-aminosalicylic acid, ethionamide, and fluoroquinolones should be used in pregnancy only where there are no suitable alternatives. Despite concerns about teratogenicity and fetal toxicity, multiple reports of no adverse effects on the newborn infant related to MDR-TB treatment during pregnancy have emerged.[141-144] Further, DR-TB may coexist with HIV infection, and overlapping drug toxicities and interactions may lead to poor compliance with treatment.

If the mother or household source case is diagnosed with MDR-TB or XDR-TB, separation of the source case and newborn is recommended. The diagnostic evaluation of the newborn and transmission precautions are the same as for drug-sensitive TB disease. As stated earlier, most anti-TB drugs are excreted in breast milk in very small amounts, when compared with doses used in the treatment of infants. However, the effect of long-term exposure to breast milk in this context is not known, and replacement feeding with infant formula may be rational in this setting, unless infant formula is not safe or feasible.

There are no evidence-based recommendations on chemoprophylaxis for the asymptomatic newborn exposed to MDR-TB or XDR-TB. Universal use of second-line drugs for chemoprophylaxis in asymptomatic MDR-TB contacts is not recommended; INH prophylaxis should be used, with close follow-up for at least 2 years, with initiation of empiric MDR-TB treatment if TB disease develops. Regardless of these recommendations, transmission of MDR-TB to children who had been in contact with adult MDR-TB cases and who received INH chemoprophylaxis has been reported, and multidrug chemoprophylactic regimens based on three drugs selected according to the mother's or household contact's drug susceptibility pattern have been successfully used in children. High-dose INH (15-20 mg/kg/day), ethionamide or ethambutol, and a quinolone, with prolonged careful clinical follow-up, may be recommended, based on expert guidance (also see Box 18-4).

Because of the adverse side effects of tendinopathy, quinolones are not widely used in children and not recommended for routine use in those younger than 18 years. Streptomycin was the first drug developed for TB treatment and is currently a second-line agent that is injectable and administered intramuscularly. With ototoxicity, both vestibular and auditory, and renal toxicity and a requirement for parenteral administration, streptomycin is not widely used.

References

1. Marais BJ, Gie RP, Schaaf HS, et al: The natural history of childhood intra-thoracic tuberculosis: a critical review of literature from the pre-chemotherapy era, *Int J Tuberc Lung Dis* 8:392-402, 2004.
2. Marais BJ, Gie RP, Schaaf HS, et al: Childhood pulmonary tuberculosis: old wisdom and new challenges, *Am J Respir Crit Care Med* 173:1078-1090, 2006.
3. World Health Organization: Global tuberculosis report, 2013 (including supplement). Available at http://apps.who.int/iris/bitstream/10665/91355/1/9789241564656_eng.pdf. Accessed Sept. 2, 2014.
4. World Health Organization: Roadmap for childhood TB: toward zero deaths Geneva, 2013, World Health Organization. Available at http://apps.who.int/iris/bitstream/10665/89506/1/9789241506137_eng.pdf?ua=1. Accessed Sept. 2, 2014.
5. Comas I, Coscolla M, Luo T, et al: Out-of-Africa migration and Neolithic coexpansion of *Mycobacterium tuberculosis* with modern humans, *Nat Genet* 45:1176-1182, 2013.
6. Brudney K, Dobkin J: Resurgent tuberculosis in New York City. Human immunodeficiency virus, homelessness, and the decline of tuberculosis control programs, *Am Rev Respir Dis* 144:745-749, 1991.
7. Koch R: Die Aetiologie der Tuberculose, *Berliner Klinischen Wochenschrift* 15:221-230, 1882.
8. Fine PEM, Carneiro IAM, Milstien JB, et al: Issues relating to the use of BCG in immunization programmes: a discussion document, Geneva, 1999, World Health Organization.
9. Fine PEM: BCG vaccines and vaccination. In Reichman LB, Hershfield ES, editors: *Tuberculosis: a comprehensive international approach*, New York, 2000, Marcel Dekker, pp 503–522.
10. Pai M, Denkinger CM, Kik SV, et al: Gamma interferon release assays for detection of *Mycobacterium tuberculosis* infection, *Clin Microbiol Rev* 27:3-20, 2014.
11. Lawn SD, Kranzer K, Wood R: Antiretroviral therapy for control of the HIV-associated tuberculosis epidemic in resource-limited settings, *Clin Chest Med* 30:685-699, 2009.
12. Restrepo BI: Convergence of the tuberculosis and diabetes epidemics: renewal of old acquaintances, *Clin Infect Dis* 45:436-438, 2007.
13. Lonnroth K, Raviglione M: Global epidemiology of tuberculosis: prospects for control, *Semin Respir Crit Care Med* 29:481-491, 2008.
14. Keane J, Gershon S, Wise RP, et al: Tuberculosis associated with infliximab, a tumor necrosis factor alpha-neutralizing agent, *N Engl J Med* 345:1098-1104, 2001.
15. Davies PD, Yew WW, Ganguly D, et al: Smoking and tuberculosis: the epidemiological association and immunopathogenesis, *Trans R Soc Trop Med Hyg* 100:291-298, 2006.
16. Calvert GM, Rice FL, Boiano JM, et al: Occupational silica exposure and risk of various diseases: an analysis using death certificates from 27 states of the United States, *Occup Environ Med* 60:122-129, 2003.
17. Kuo SC, Hu YW, Liu CJ, et al: Association between tuberculosis infections and non-pulmonary malignancies: a nationwide population-based study, *Br J Cancer* 109:229-234, 2013.
18. Andrew OT, Schoenfeld PY, Hopewell PC, et al: Tuberculosis in patients with end-stage renal disease, *Am J Med* 68:59-65, 1980.
19. Kolappan C, Gopi PG, Subramani R, et al: Selected biological and behavioural risk factors associated with pulmonary tuberculosis, *Int J Tuberc Lung Dis* 11:999-1003, 2007.
20. Spence DP, Hotchkiss J, Williams CS, et al: Tuberculosis and poverty, *BMJ* 307:759-761, 1993.
21. Diagnostic standards and classification of tuberculosis in adults and children. This official statement of the American Thoracic Society and the Centers for Disease Control and Prevention was adopted by the ATS Board of Directors, July 1999. This statement was endorsed by the Council of the Infectious Disease Society of America, September 1999, *Am J Respir Crit Care Med* 161(4 Pt 1):1376-1395, 2000.
22. Centers for Disease Control and Prevention: Reported tuberculosis in the United States, 2012, Atlanta, 2013, U.S. Department of Health and Human Services.
23. Hedvall E: Pregnancy and tuberculosis, *Acta Med Scand Suppl* 286: 1-101, 1953.
24. Cromie JB: Pregnancy and pulmonary tuberculosis, *Br J Tuberc Dis Chest* 48:97-101, 1954.
25. Zenner D, Kruijshaar ME, Andrews N, et al: Risk of tuberculosis in pregnancy: a national, primary care-based cohort and self-controlled case series study, *Am J Respir Crit Care Med* 185:779-784, 2012.
26. Cohen JD, Patton EA, Badger TL: The tuberculous mother; a five- to twenty-year follow-up of 149 women with 401 full-term pregnancies, *Am Rev Tuberc* 65:1-23, 1952.
27. Edge JR: Pulmonary tuberculosis and pregnancy, *Br Med J* 1: 845-847, 1952.
28. Rosenbach LM, Gangemi CR: Tuberculosis and pregnancy, *J Am Med Assoc* 161:1035-1038, 1956.
29. Stewart CJ, Simmonds FA: Child-bearing and pulmonary tuberculosis, *Br Med J* 2:726-729, 1947.
30. Stewart CJ, Simmonds FA: Prognosis of pulmonary tuberculosis in married women, *Tubercle* 35:28-30, 1954.
31. Bekker A, Du Preez K, Schaaf HS, et al: High tuberculosis exposure among neonates in a high tuberculosis and human immunodeficiency virus burden setting, *Int J Tuberc Lung Dis* 16:1040-1046, 2012.
32. Berkowitz FE, Severens JL, Blumberg HM: Exposure to tuberculosis among newborns in a nursery: decision analysis for initiation of prophylaxis, *Infect Control Hosp Epidemiol* 27:604-611, 2006.
33. Crockett M, King SM, Kitai I, et al: Nosocomial transmission of congenital tuberculosis in a neonatal intensive care unit, *Clin Infect Dis* 39:1719-1723, 2004.
34. Isaacs D, Jones CA, Dalton D, et al: Exposure to open tuberculosis on a neonatal unit, *J Paediatr Child Health* 42:557-559, 2006.
35. Laartz BW, Narvarte HJ, Holt D, et al: Congenital tuberculosis and management of exposures in a neonatal intensive care unit, *Infect Control Hosp Epidemiol* 23:573-579, 2002.
36. Lee LH, LeVea CM, Graman PS: Congenital tuberculosis in a neonatal intensive care unit: case report, epidemiological investigation, and management of exposures, *Clin Infect Dis* 27:474-477, 1998.
37. Light IJ, Saidleman M, Sutherland JM: Management of newborns after nursery exposure to tuberculosis, *Am Rev Respir Dis* 109: 415-419, 1974.
38. Millership SE, Anderson C, Cummins AJ, et al: The risk to infants from nosocomial exposure to tuberculosis, *Pediatr Infect Dis J* 28:915-916, 2009.
39. Nair PM, Narang A: Management of a baby of tuberculous mother, *Indian Pediatr* 29:797-801, 1992.
40. Perry A, Angoulvant F, Chadelat K, et al: Neonatal exposure to active pulmonary tuberculosis in a maternity ward: screening and clinical course of a cohort of exposed infants, *Arch Pediatr* 19:396-403, 2012.
41. Raucher HS, Gribetz I: Care of the pregnant woman with tuberculosis and her newborn infant: a pediatrician's perspective, *Mt Sinai J Med* 53:70-76, 1986.
42. Saengnipanthkul S, Jirapradittha J, Kiatchoosakun P: Outcome of neonates exposed to active pulmonary tuberculosis, *J Med Assoc Thai* 95:756-760, 2012.
43. Saitoh M, Ichiba H, Fujioka H, et al: Connatal tuberculosis in an extremely low birth weight infant: case report and management of exposure to tuberculosis in a neonatal intensive care unit, *Eur J Pediatr* 160:88-90, 2001.
44. Skevaki CL, Kafetzis DA: Tuberculosis in neonates and infants: epidemiology, pathogenesis, clinical manifestations, diagnosis, and management issues, *Paediatr Drugs* 7:219-234, 2005.
45. Steiner P, Rao M, Victoria MS, et al: Miliary tuberculosis in two infants after nursery exposure: epidemiologic, clinical, and laboratory findings, *Am Rev Respir Dis* 113:267-271, 1976.
46. Winters A, Agerton TB, Driver CR, et al: Congenital tuberculosis and management of exposure in three neonatal intensive care units, *Int J Tuberc Lung Dis* 14:1641-1643, 2010.
47. Schaaf HS, Collins A, Bekker A, et al: Tuberculosis at extremes of age, *Respirology* 15:747-763, 2010.
48. Borgia, P., Cambieri A, Chini F, et al., Suspected transmission of tuberculosis in a maternity ward from a smear-positive nurse: preliminary results of clinical evaluations and testing of neonates potentially exposed, Rome, Italy, 1 January to 28 July 2011, *Euro Surveill* 16:40, 2011.
49. Dubrulle S, Vervel C, Boutignon H, et al: Exposure of a cohort of newborn infants to tuberculosis in a neonatology service, *Arch Pediatr* 17:1491-1494, 2010.
50. Niederweis M, Danilchanka O, Huff J, et al: Mycobacterial outer membranes: in search of proteins, *Trends Microbiol* 18:109-116, 2010.
51. Sani M, Houben EN, Geurtsen J, et al: Direct visualization by cryo-EM of the mycobacterial capsular layer: a labile structure containing ESX-1-secreted proteins, *PLoS Pathog* 6:e1000794, 2010.
52. Cole ST, Brosch R, Parkhill J, et al: Deciphering the biology of *Mycobacterium tuberculosis* from the complete genome sequence, *Nature* 393:537-544, 1998.

53. Copin R, Coscollá M, Seiffert SN, et al: Sequence diversity in the pe_pgrs genes of *Mycobacterium tuberculosis* is independent of human T cell recognition, *MBio* 5, 2014. e00960-e13.
54. van der Spuy GD, Kremer K, Ndabambi SL, et al: Changing *Mycobacterium tuberculosis* population highlights clade-specific pathogenic characteristics, *Tuberculosis (Edinb)* 89:120-125, 2009.
55. Comas I, Chakravartti J, Small PM, et al: Human T cell epitopes of *Mycobacterium tuberculosis* are evolutionarily hyperconserved, *Nat Genet* 42:498-503, 2010.
56. Nunes-Alves C, Booty MG, Carpenter SM, et al: In search of a new paradigm for protective immunity to TB, *Nat Rev Microbiol* 12: 289-299, 2014.
57. Dorhoi A, Reece ST, Kaufmann SH: For better or for worse: the immune response against *Mycobacterium tuberculosis* balances pathology and protection, *Immunol Rev* 240:235-251, 2011.
58. Welin A, Lerm M: Inside or outside the phagosome? The controversy of the intracellular localization of *Mycobacterium tuberculosis*, *Tuberculosis (Edinb)* 92:113-120, 2012.
59. Kleinnijenhuis J, Oosting M, Joosten LA, et al: Innate immune recognition of *Mycobacterium tuberculosis*, *Clin Dev Immunol* 2011:405310, 2011.
60. Bradfute SB, Castillo EF, Arko-Mensah J, et al: Autophagy as an immune effector against tuberculosis, *Curr Opin Microbiol* 16: 355-365, 2013.
61. Davis JM, Ramakrishnan L: The role of the granuloma in expansion and dissemination of early tuberculous infection, *Cell* 136:37-49, 2009.
62. Gupta A, Kaul A, Tsolaki AG, et al: *Mycobacterium tuberculosis*: immune evasion, latency and reactivation, *Immunobiology* 217: 363-374, 2012.
63. Urdahl KB, Shafiani S, Ernst JD: Initiation and regulation of T-cell responses in tuberculosis, *Mucosal Immunol* 4:288-293, 2011.
64. Kaufmann SH, Dorhoi A: Inflammation in tuberculosis: interactions, imbalances and interventions, *Curr Opin Immunol* 25:441-449, 2013.
65. Di Pietrantonio T, Schurr E: Host-pathogen specificity in tuberculosis, *Adv Exp Med Biol* 783:33-44, 2013.
66. Abbara A, . Davidson RN: Medscape: etiology and management of genitourinary tuberculosis, *Nat Rev Urol* 8:678-688, 2011.
67. Warthin SA, Murray Cowie D: A contribution to the casuistry of placental and congenital tuberculosis: miliary tuberculosis of the other in seventh month of pregnancy; tuberculosis of placenta; agglutination thrombi, containing many tubercle bacilli, in placenta and fetus, *J Infect Dis* 1:140-169, 1904.
68. Rich AR, Rich AR, Follis RH Jr: Effect of low oxygen tension upon the development of experimental tuberculosis, *Johns Hopkins Hosp* 71:345-357, 1942.
69. Hoa NB, Sy DN, Nhung NV, et al: National survey of tuberculosis prevalence in Viet Nam, *Bull World Health Organ* 88:273-280, 2010.
70. Perez-Velez CM, Marais BJ: Tuberculosis in children, *N Engl J Med* 367:348-361, 2012.
71. Kothari A, Mahadevan N, Girling J: Tuberculosis and pregnancy—results of a study in a high prevalence area in London, *Eur J Obstet Gynecol Reprod Biol* 126:48-55, 2006.
72. Knight M, Kurinczuk JJ, Nelson-Piercy C, et al: Tuberculosis in pregnancy in the UK, *BJOG* 116:584-588, 2009.
73. Adhikari M, Pillay T, Pillay DG: Tuberculosis in the newborn: an emerging disease, *Pediatr Infect Dis J* 16:1108-1112, 1997.
74. Manji KP, Msemo G, Tamim B, et al: Tuberculosis (presumed congenital) in a neonatal unit in Dar-es-Salaam, Tanzania, *J Trop Pediatr* 47:153-155, 2001.
75. Pillay T, Adhikari M, Mokili J, et al: Severe, rapidly progressive human immunodeficiency virus type 1 disease in newborns with coinfections, *Pediatr Infect Dis J* 20:404-410, 2001.
76. Peng W, Yang J, Liu E: Analysis of 170 cases of congenital TB reported in the literature between 1946 and 2009, *Pediatr Pulmonol* 46:1215-1224, 2011.
77. Verver S, Warren RM, Munch Z, et al: Proportion of tuberculosis transmission that takes place in households in a high-incidence area, *Lancet* 363:212-214, 2004.
78. Schulz SA, Draper HR, Naidoo P: A comparative study of tuberculosis patients initiated on ART and receiving different models of TB-HIV care, *Int J Tuberc Lung Dis* 17:1558-1563, 2013.
79. Andronikou S, Brauer B, Galpin J, et al: Interobserver variability in the detection of mediastinal and hilar lymph nodes on CT in children with suspected pulmonary tuberculosis, *Pediatr Radiol* 35:425-428, 2005.
80. American Academy of Pediatrics: In Pickering LK, editor: *Red book: 2012 report of the Committee on Infectious Diseases*, ed 29, Elk Grove Village, Ill, 2012, American Academy of Pediatrics.
81. Steingart, KR, Schiller I, Horne DJ, et al., Xpert(R) MTB/RIF assay for pulmonary tuberculosis and rifampicin resistance in adults. *Cochrane Database Syst Rev* (1):CD009593, 2014.
82. Nicol MP, Workman L, Isaacs W, et al: Accuracy of the Xpert MTB/RIF test for the diagnosis of pulmonary tuberculosis in children admitted to hospital in Cape Town, South Africa: a descriptive study, *Lancet Infect Dis* 11:819-824, 2011.
83. Nicol MP, Spiers K, Workman L, et al: Xpert MTB/RIF testing of stool samples for the diagnosis of pulmonary tuberculosis in children, *Clin Infect Dis* 57:e18-e21, 2013.
84. Leung E, Minion J, Benedetti A, et al: Microcolony culture techniques for tuberculosis diagnosis: a systematic review, *Int J Tuberc Lung Dis* 16:16-23, 2012.
85. Rodriguez JC, García-Pachon E, Ruiz M, et al: Drug susceptibility of the *Mycobacterium* genus: in vitro tests and clinical implications, *Curr Clin Pharmacol* 1:277-289, 2006.
86. Lawn SD: Diagnosis of pulmonary tuberculosis, *Curr Opin Pulm Med* 19:280-288, 2013.
87. Machingaidze S, Verver S, Mulenga H, et al: Predictive value of recent QuantiFERON conversion for tuberculosis disease in adolescents, *Am J Respir Crit Care Med* 186:1051-1056, 2012.
88. Spark RP, Pock NA, Pedron SL, et al: Perinatal tuberculosis and its public health impact: a case report, *Tex Med* 92:50-53, 1996.
89. Cantwell MF, Shehab ZM, Costello AM, et al: Brief report: congenital tuberculosis, *N Engl J Med* 330:1051-1054, 1994.
90. Hageman JR: Congenital and perinatal tuberculosis: discussion of difficult issues in diagnosis and management, *J Perinatol* 18: 389-394, 1998.
91. World Health Organization: Treatment of tuberculosis guidelines—4th ed, 2010. Available at http://whqlibdoc.who.int/publications/2010/9789241547833_eng.pdf?ua=1. Accessed Sept. 2, 2014.
92. American Thoracic Society: Centers for Disease Control and Prevention, Infectious Diseases Society of America: Treatment of tuberculosis, *MMWR Recomm Rep* 52(RR-11):1-77, 2003.
93. Strang JI, Kakaza HH, Gibson DG, et al: Controlled trial of prednisolone as adjuvant in treatment of tuberculous constrictive pericarditis in Transkei, *Lancet* 2:1418-1422, 1987.
94. Prasad K, Singh MB: Corticosteroids for managing tuberculosis meningitis, *Cochrane Database System Rev* 1:CD002244, 2008.
95. Thwaites G, Fisher M, Hemingway C, et al: British Infection Society guidelines for the diagnosis and treatment of tuberculosis of the central nervous system in adults and children, *J Infect* 59:167-187, 2009.
96. Centers for Disease Control and Prevention: Latent tuberculosis infection: a guide for primary care providers, 2013. Available at http://www.cdc.gov/tb/publications/LTBI/default.htm, Accessed April 9, 2014.
97. Targeted tuberculin testing and treatment of latent tuberculosis infection. This official statement of the American Thoracic Society was adopted by the ATS Board of Directors, July 1999. This is a Joint Statement of the American Thoracic Society (ATS) and the Centers for Disease Control and Prevention (CDC). This statement was endorsed by the Council of the Infectious Diseases Society of America. (IDSA), September 1999, and the sections of this statement, *Am J Respir Crit Care Med* 161(4 Pt 2):S221-S247, 2000.
98. Comstock GW, Baum C, Snider DE Jr: Isoniazid prophylaxis among Alaskan Eskimos: a final report of the bethel isoniazid studies, *Am Rev Respir Dis* 119:827-830, 1979.
99. Churchyard GJ, Fielding KL, Lewis JJ, et al: A trial of mass isoniazid preventive therapy for tuberculosis control, *N Engl J Med* 370: 301-310, 2014.
100. Gordin KFM, Matts JP, Miller C, et al: A controlled trial of isoniazid in persons with anergy and human immunodeficiency virus infection who are at high risk for tuberculosis. Terry Beirn Community Programs for Clinical Research on AIDS, *N Engl J Med* 337:315-320, 1997.
101. Whalen CC, Johnson JL, Okwera A, et al: A trial of three regimens to prevent tuberculosis in Ugandan adults infected with the human immunodeficiency virus. Uganda–Case Western Reserve University Research Collaboration, *N Engl J Med* 337:801-808, 1997.
102. Sterling TR, Villarino ME, Borisov AS, et al: Three months of rifapentine and isoniazid for latent tuberculosis infection, *N Engl J Med* 365:2155-2166, 2011.

103. Centers for Disease Control and Prevention: Recommendations for use of an isoniazid-rifapentine regimen with direct observation to treat latent *Mycobacterium tuberculosis* infection, *MMWR Morb Mortal Wkly Rep* 60:1650-1653, 2011.
104. Briggs G, Freeman R, Yaffe SJ: *Drugs in pregnancy and lactation: a reference guide to fetal and neonatal risk*, Philadelphia, 2005, Lippincott Williams & Wilkins.
105. Davidson PT: Managing tuberculosis during pregnancy, *Lancet* 346:199-200, 1995.
106. Jana N, Barik S, Arora N: Increased risk of low birthweight and small for gestational age infants among women with tuberculosis, *BJOG* 117:1432-1433, 2010. author reply 1433-4.
107. Snider DE Jr, Layde PM, Johnson MW, et al: Treatment of tuberculosis during pregnancy, *Am Rev Respir Dis* 122:65-79, 1980.
108. Connolly M, Nunn P: Women and tuberculosis, *World Health Stat Q* 49:115-119, 1996.
109. World Health Organization. WHO policy on TB infection control in health-care facilities, congregate settings and households, 2009. Available at http://whqlibdoc.who.int/publications/2009/9789241598323_eng.pdf?ua=1. Accessed Sept. 2, 2014.
110. Abubakar I, Ariti C, Beynon R, et al: Systematic review and meta-analysis of the current evidence on the duration of protection by bacillus Calmette-Guérin vaccination against tuberculosis, *Health Technol Assess* 17:1-372, 2013. v-vi.
111. Trunz BB, Fine P, Dye C: Effect of BCG vaccination on childhood tuberculous meningitis and miliary tuberculosis worldwide: a meta-analysis and assessment of cost-effectiveness, *Lancet* 367: 1173-1180, 2006.
112. Mangtani P, Abubakar I, Ariti C, et al: Protection by BCG vaccine against tuberculosis: a systematic review of randomized controlled trials, *Clin Infect Dis* 58:470-480, 2014.
113. Basu Roy R, Sotgiu G, Altet-Gómez N, et al: Identifying predictors of interferon-gamma release assay results in pediatric latent tuberculosis: a protective role of bacillus Calmette-Guérin? A pTB-NET collaborative study, *Am J Respir Crit Care Med* 186:378-384, 2012.
114. Eisenhut M, Paranjothy S, Abubakar I, et al: BCG vaccination reduces risk of infection with *Mycobacterium tuberculosis* as detected by gamma interferon release assay, *Vaccine* 27:6116-6120, 2009.
115. Soysal A, Millington KA, Bakir M, et al: Effect of BCG vaccination on risk of *Mycobacterium tuberculosis* infection in children with household tuberculosis contact: a prospective community-based study, *Lancet* 366:1443-1451, 2005.
116. Barreto ML, Pereira SM, Pilger D, et al: Evidence of an effect of BCG revaccination on incidence of tuberculosis in school-aged children in Brazil: second report of the BCG-REVAC cluster-randomised trial, *Vaccine* 29:4875-4877, 2011.
117. Kaufmann SH: Tuberculosis vaccine development: strength lies in tenacity, *Trends Immunol* 33:373-379, 2012.
118. Kaufmann SH, Hussey G, Lambert PH: New vaccines for tuberculosis, *Lancet* 375:2110-2119, 2010.
119. Lawn SD, Badri M, Wood R: Tuberculosis among HIV-infected patients receiving HAART: long term incidence and risk factors in a South African cohort, *AIDS* 19:2109-2116, 2005.
120. Elliott AM, Halwiindi B, Hayes RJ, et al: The impact of human immunodeficiency virus on presentation and diagnosis of tuberculosis in a cohort study in Zambia, *J Trop Med Hyg* 96:1-11, 1993.
121. Gilks CF, Brindle RJ, Otieno LS, et al: Extrapulmonary and disseminated tuberculosis in HIV-1-seropositive patients presenting to the acute medical services in Nairobi, *AIDS* 4:981-985, 1990.
122. Walters E, Cotton MF, Rabie H, et al: Clinical presentation and outcome of tuberculosis in human immunodeficiency virus infected children on anti-retroviral therapy, *BMC Pediatr* 8:1, 2008.
123. Lawn SD, MeKintjes G, McIlleron H, et al: Management of HIV-associated tuberculosis in resource-limited settings: a state-of-the-art review, *BMC Med* 11:253, 2013.
124. Chang KC, Yew WW: Management of difficult multidrug-resistant tuberculosis and extensively drug-resistant tuberculosis: update 2012, *Respirology* 18:8-21, 2013.
125. Meintjes G, Rabie H, Wilkinson RJ, et al: Tuberculosis-associated immune reconstitution inflammatory syndrome and unmasking of tuberculosis by antiretroviral therapy, *Clin Chest Med* 30:797-810, 2009. x.
126. Muller M, Wandel S, Colebunders R, et al: Immune reconstitution inflammatory syndrome in patients starting antiretroviral therapy for HIV infection: a systematic review and meta-analysis, *Lancet Infect Dis* 10:251-261, 2010.
127. Meintjes G, Wilkinson RJ, Morroni C, et al: Randomized placebo-controlled trial of prednisone for paradoxical tuberculosis-associated immune reconstitution inflammatory syndrome, *AIDS* 24: 2381-2390, 2010.
128. Abdool Karim SS, Naidoo K, Grobler A, et al: Timing of initiation of antiretroviral drugs during tuberculosis therapy, *N Engl J Med* 362:697-706, 2010.
129. Abdool Karim SS, Naidoo K, Grobler A, et al: Integration of antiretroviral therapy with tuberculosis treatment, *N Engl J Med* 365: 1492-1501, 2011.
130. Naidoo K, Baxter C, Abdool Karim SS: When to start antiretroviral therapy during tuberculosis treatment? *Curr Opin Infect Dis* 26: 35-42, 2013.
131. Lee SS, Meintjes G, Kamarulzaman A, et al: Management of tuberculosis and latent tuberculosis infection in human immunodeficiency virus-infected persons, *Respirology* 18:912-922, 2013.
132. Mansoor N, Scriba TJ, de Kock M, et al: HIV-1 infection in infants severely impairs the immune response induced by Bacille Calmette-Guérin vaccine, *J Infect Dis* 199:982-990, 2009.
133. Hesseling AC, Marais BJ, Gie RP, et al: The risk of disseminated Bacille Calmette-Guérin (BCG) disease in HIV-infected children, *Vaccine* 25:14-18, 2007.
134. Hesseling AC, Johnson LF, Jaspan H, et al: Disseminated bacille Calmette-Guérin disease in HIV-infected South African infants, *Bull World Health Organ* 87:505-511, 2009.
135. Hesseling AC, Rabie H, Marais BJ, et al: Bacille Calmette-Guérin vaccine-induced disease in HIV-infected and HIV-uninfected children, *Clin Infect Dis* 42:548-558, 2006.
136. Rabie H, Violari A, Duong T, et al: Early antiretroviral treatment reduces risk of bacille Calmette-Guérin immune reconstitution adenitis, *Int J Tuberc Lung Dis* 15:1194-1200, 2011. i.
137. Global Advisory Committee on Vaccine Safety, 29-30 November 2006, *Wkly Epidemiol Rec* 82:18-24, 2007.
138. Seddon JA, Furin JJ, Gale M, et al: Caring for children with drug-resistant tuberculosis: practice-based recommendations, *Am J Respir Crit Care Med* 186:953-964, 2012.
139. Lee M, Lee J, Carroll MW, et al: Linezolid for treatment of chronic extensively drug-resistant tuberculosis, *N Engl J Med* 367: 1508-1518, 2012.
140. Cohen J: Infectious disease. Approval of novel TB drug celebrated—with restraint, *Science* 339:130, 2013.
141. Drobac PC, del Castillo H, Sweetland A, et al: Treatment of multidrug-resistant tuberculosis during pregnancy: long-term follow-up of 6 children with intrauterine exposure to second-line agents, *Clin Infect Dis* 40:1689-1692, 2005.
142. Nitta AT, Milligan D: Management of four pregnant women with multidrug-resistant tuberculosis, *Clin Infect Dis* 28:1298-1304, 1999.
143. Palacios E, Dallman R, Muñoz M, et al: Drug-resistant tuberculosis and pregnancy: treatment outcomes of 38 cases in Lima, Peru, *Clin Infect Dis* 48:1413-1419, 2009.
144. Shin S, Guerra D, Rich M, et al: Treatment of multidrug-resistant tuberculosis during pregnancy: a report of 7 cases, *Clin Infect Dis* 36:996-1003, 2003.

19 Chlamydia *Infections*

TONI DARVILLE

CHAPTER OUTLINE

In 1911, Lindner and colleagues[1] identified typical intracytoplasmic inclusions in infants with a nongonococcal form of ophthalmia neonatorum called *inclusion conjunctivitis of the newborn* (ICN) or inclusion blennorrhea, leading to the elucidation of the epidemiology of sexually transmitted chlamydial infections. Mothers of affected infants were found to have inclusions in their cervical epithelial cells, and fathers of affected infants had inclusions in their urethral cells. For 50 years, cytologic demonstration of chlamydial inclusions in epithelial cells was the only diagnostic procedure available. When chlamydial isolation procedures were developed, first in the yolk sac of the embryonated hen's egg and later in tissue culture, studies again showed *Chlamydia trachomatis* as the etiology of conjunctivitis in the index case and then confirmed the genital tract reservoir of the agent.[2] Although ICN was studied for 60 years, an appreciation of the importance of chlamydial infection of the respiratory tract in infants did not evolve until the late 1970s, with the impetus of the report by Beem and Saxon.[3]

C. trachomatis is now recognized as the most common sexually transmitted bacterial pathogen in Western industrialized society. Although most *C. trachomatis* infections in men and women are asymptomatic, infection can lead to severe reproductive complications in women. The infection can be transmitted from an infected mother to her newborn during delivery, producing conjunctivitis or pneumonia or both. *C. trachomatis* is likely the most common cause of conjunctivitis in infants younger than 1 month and is a common cause of afebrile pneumonia in infants younger than 3 months.

Epidemiology and Transmission

Reported chlamydial prevalence rates in the United States include 2% to 7% among female college students, 4% to 12% among women attending a family planning clinic, and 6% to 20% among men and women attending a clinic for sexually transmitted diseases or persons entering correctional facilities.[4,5] Many men and most women infected with *C. trachomatis* are either asymptomatic or minimally symptomatic, and presentation for diagnosis is a result of screening or referral after a contact develops symptoms. Regional estimates are hampered by underdiagnosis and underreporting of cases. Because symptoms are absent or minimal in most women and many men, a large reservoir of asymptomatic infection is present that can sustain the pathogen within a community.

Young age (<20 years) is the sociodemographic factor most strongly associated with chlamydial infection (relative risk among women <25 years of age compared with older women is 2 to 3.5).[6] Although the prevalence of chlamydial infection is increased in the black population and in socioeconomically disadvantaged individuals, there is broad socioeconomic and geographic distribution of infection.[7,8] Other risk factors for cervical chlamydial infection in women are anatomic or hormonal (i.e., use of depotmedroxyprogesterone acetate injections or ectopy after use of oral contraceptives),[9] and behavioral (i.e., number of sexual partners).

For purposes relevant to this chapter, the major method of transmission of *C. trachomatis* is sexual. Partner transmission rates are approximately 65% and appear to be similar for female-male and male-female transmission.[10] The child-to-child and intrafamilial infecting patterns that predominate in trachoma endemic areas have not been proven to cause disease in newborns. Chlamydiae cause one third to one half of nongonococcal urethritis in men, and concomitant infections with gonococci are common in both men and women.

An infant born to a mother with a chlamydial infection of the cervix is at 60% to 70% risk of acquiring the infection during passage through the birth canal.[11] Of exposed infants, 20% to 50% develop conjunctivitis, and 5% to 20% develop pneumonia. The rectum and vagina of infants exposed during delivery may also be infected, but a clear-cut relationship with disease in these sites has yet to be elucidated.[12] In utero transmission is not known to occur. Infection after cesarean section is seen rarely, usually after premature rupture of the membranes. No evidence supports postnatal transmission from the mother or other family members.

Studies in the 1980s identified *C. trachomatis* in 14% to 46% of infants younger than 1 month with conjunctivitis.[13] The prevalence of neonatal chlamydial inclusion conjunctivitis has decreased in areas where screening and treatment of chlamydial infection in pregnant women is a regular practice. In the Netherlands, prenatal screening for *C. trachomatis* is not routine. Evaluation of infants younger than 3 months referred to a Dutch children's hospital or to an ophthalmologist for evaluation of persistent conjunctivitis from 1996 to 2002 revealed *C. trachomatis* infection in 63%.[14]

There is no evidence to suggest that infants with chlamydial infections should be isolated. Transmission of the organism to other infants in nurseries or intensive care units has not been reported. Standard precautions consisting of hand hygiene between patient contacts are recommended. Use of protective gloves, masks or face shields, and nonsterile gowns is recommended when performing procedures likely to generate splashes of body fluids, secretions, or excretions.

Microbiology

PATHOGEN

Chlamydiae are obligate intracellular parasites that cause various diseases in animal species at virtually all phylogenetic levels. Traditionally, the order Chlamydiales has contained one genus with four recognized species: *C. trachomatis, Chlamydia psittaci, Chlamydia pneumoniae,* and *Chlamydia pecorum.* More recent taxonomic analysis involving the 16S and 23S ribosomal RNA genes has found that the order Chlamydiales contains at least four distinct groups at the family level and provides a potential rationale for splitting the genus *Chlamydia* into two genera, *Chlamydia* and *Chlamydophila.*[15] The genus *Chlamydophila* would contain *C. pneumoniae, C. pecorum,* and *C. psittaci.* The scientific community has not to date accepted this split of the genus, and for the purposes of this chapter, these organisms are referred to as *Chlamydia.*

C. psittaci is responsible for psittacosis, a chlamydial infection contracted by humans from infected birds and characterized by interstitial pneumonitis. This infection should be suspected in any patient with atypical pneumonia who has contact with birds. *C. pneumoniae* causes pneumonia, pharyngitis, and bronchitis in humans and may accelerate atherosclerosis. Epidemiologic studies have revealed that *C. pneumoniae* is a common cause of infection in school-age children and young adults; along with *Mycoplasma,* it is probably the most common cause of community-acquired pneumonia in this age group. It is not known to cause disease in newborns and is not discussed further here. *C. trachomatis* is associated with a spectrum of diseases. The species *C. trachomatis* contains 18 serologically distinct variants known as serovars. Serovars A, B, Ba, and C cause ocular trachoma, a major cause of blindness in many developing countries, particularly in Africa, Asia, and the Middle East. Ocular trachoma is considered the most common cause of preventable blindness in the world. Three serovars, L_1, L_2, and L_3, are associated with lymphogranuloma venereum, a sexually transmitted disease that is rare in the United States but is still quite prevalent in many developing countries and is more common among men who have sex with men. Perinatal transmission is rare with lymphogranuloma venereum. Serovars D through K produce infections of the genital tract—urethritis and epididymitis in men and cervicitis and salpingitis in women—the most prevalent chlamydial diseases. Major complications of female genital tract disease include acute pelvic inflammatory disease, ectopic pregnancy, infertility, and infant pneumonia and conjunctivitis.

Similar to gram-negative bacteria, chlamydiae have an outer membrane that contains lipopolysaccharide and membrane proteins, but their outer membrane contains no detectable peptidoglycan, despite the presence of genes encoding proteins for its synthesis. This genomic finding is the basis for the so-called chlamydial peptidoglycan paradox because it has been known for years that β-lactam antibiotics inhibit chlamydial development. Although chlamydiae contain DNA, RNA, and ribosomes, during growth and replication, they obtain high-energy phosphate compounds from the host cell. Consequently, they are considered energy parasites. The chlamydial genome size is only 660 kDa, which is smaller than that of any other prokaryote except *Mycoplasma* species. All chlamydiae encode an abundant protein, the major outer membrane protein (MOMP) that is surface exposed in *C. trachomatis* and is the primary determinant of serologic classification.

CHLAMYDIAL DEVELOPMENTAL CYCLE

The biphasic developmental cycle of chlamydiae is unique among microorganisms and involves two highly specialized morphologic forms, as shown in Figure 19-1. The extracellular form or elementary body (EB) contains extensive disulfide cross-links within and between outer membrane proteins, giving it an almost sporelike structure that is stable outside of the cell. The small (350 nm in diameter) infectious EB is inactive metabolically. The developmental cycle is initiated when an EB attaches to a susceptible epithelial cell. Numerous candidate adhesins have been proposed, but their identity and that of associated epithelial cell receptors remain uncertain. One documented mechanism of entry into the epithelial cell is by receptor-mediated endocytosis via clathrin-coated pits,[16] but evidence exists that chlamydiae may exploit multiple mechanisms of entry. The process of EB internalization is very efficient, suggesting that EBs trigger their own internalization by cells that are not considered professional phagocytes.

When inside the cell, surface antigens of the EB seem to prevent fusion of the endosome with lysosomes, protecting the pathogen from enzymatic destruction. Hiding from host attack by antibody or cell-mediated defenses, the EB

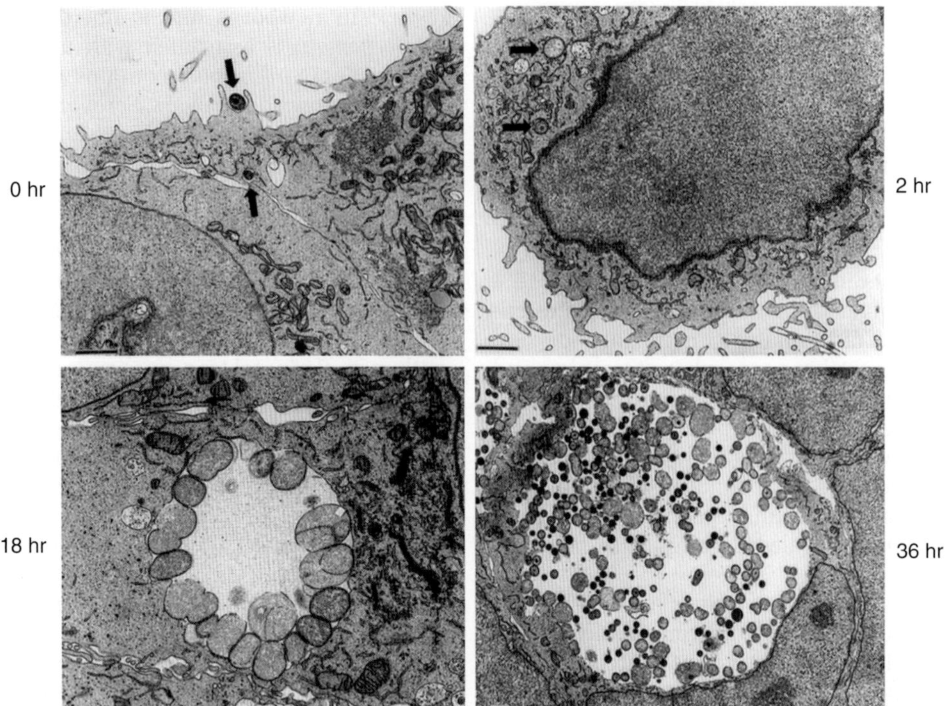

Figure 19-1 *Chlamydia trachomatis* developmental cycle. Infection is initiated by elementary bodies (EBs). *0 hr,* Immediately after endocytosis. EBs are found within tightly associated membrane vesicles. *2 hr,* Within a few hours, EBs differentiate into larger, metabolically active reticulate bodies (RBs). *18 hr,* As RBs multiply, inclusion increases in size to accommodate bacterial progeny. RBs are typically observed juxtaposed to inclusion membrane. *36 hr,* As infection progresses, increasing numbers of chlamydiae are observed unattached in interior of inclusion. These unattached organisms are, for the most part, EBs and intermediate developmental forms. EBs accumulate within inclusion even as RBs, still associated with inclusion membrane, continue to multiply, until cell undergoes lysis at 40 to 48 hours after infection. (From Hackstadt T, Fischer ER, Scidmore MA, Rockey DD, Heinzen RA: Origins and functions of the chlamydial inclusion [review], *Trends Microbiol* 5:288-293, 1997.)

reorganizes into the replicative form, the reticulate body (RB). RBs successfully parasitize the host cell and divide and multiply. As the RB divides by binary fission, it fills the endosome, now a cytoplasmic inclusion, with its progeny. After 48 to 72 hours, multiplication ceases, and nucleoid condensation occurs as the RBs transform to new infectious EBs. The EBs are released from the cell by cytolysis,[17] by a process of exocytosis, or by extrusion of the whole inclusion,[18] leaving the host cell intact. The last-mentioned process may explain the frequency of asymptomatic or subclinical chlamydial infections. Release of the infectious EBs allows infection of new host cells to occur.

Pathogenesis

CONJUNCTIVITIS

Chlamydiae replicate extensively in epithelial cells of the conjunctiva and cause considerable cell damage. The inflammatory reaction consists mostly of neutrophils. Conjunctivitis in most untreated patients resolves spontaneously during the first few months of life. On occasion, infants maintain persistent conjunctivitis, and pannus formation (neovascularization of the cornea) and scarring typical of trachoma have been reported. Loss of vision is rare. Micropannus and some scarring may occur in infants if they are not treated within the first 2 weeks of the disease.[19] If treated early, no ocular sequelae develop.

PNEUMONIA

The nasopharynx is the most frequent site of perinatally acquired chlamydial infection, with approximately 70% of infected infants having positive cultures at that site.[20] Most of these infections are asymptomatic and may persist for 29 months.[21] Chlamydial pneumonia develops in only about 30% of infants with nasopharyngeal infection. Conjunctivitis is not a prerequisite for development of pneumonia.

Pathology

In ICN, the affected conjunctiva is highly vascularized and edematous. Inclusions are found in the conjunctival epithelial cells. There is a massive infiltration of polymorphonuclear leukocytes, and pseudomembrane formation may occur. Lymphoid follicles, such as are seen in adults or older children with chlamydial infection of the conjunctiva, are not usually observed until the disease has been active for 1 or 2 months. Because ICN spontaneously resolves by that time in most infants, lymphoid follicles are not commonly observed.

Because pneumonia is rarely fatal, and in most infants follows a relatively benign course, there has been little occasion to obtain lung specimens. When such specimens have been obtained, no characteristic pathologic features have been described. Biopsy material has shown pleural congestion and alveolar and bronchiolar mononuclear cell infiltrates with eosinophils and focal aggregations of neutrophils.[22]

Clinical Manifestations

The principal clinical manifestations in infants are ICN, occurring in the first 3 weeks of life, and pneumonia, which occurs within the first 3 months.

CONJUNCTIVITIS

Inclusion conjunctivitis of the newborn usually follows an incubation period of 5 to 14 days after delivery, or earlier if amniotic membranes ruptured prematurely. Disease manifestations vary widely and range from mild conjunctival injection with scant watery or mucoid discharge to severe mucopurulent conjunctivitis with chemosis and pseudomembrane formation. The eyelids swell, and the conjunctivae become injected and swollen (Fig. 19-2). The "pseudomembrane" consists of inflammatory exudate that adheres to the inflamed surface of the conjunctiva. Except for micropannus formation, the cornea is usually spared. Evaluation of 37 Dutch infants who tested positive for *Chlamydia* revealed mucopurulent eye discharge as the presenting symptom for 35 (95%), swelling of the eyelids for 27 (73%), and conjunctival erythema for 24 (65%); bilateral eye involvement was observed in 27 infants (73%). Presenting symptoms were similar in a group of 22 infants diagnosed with other bacterial pathogens.[14]

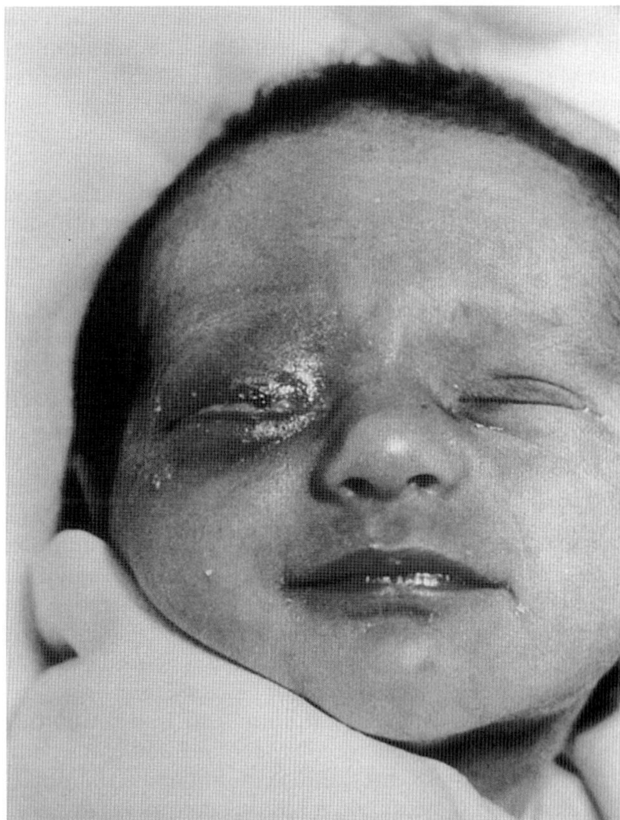

Figure 19-2 Infant with chlamydial conjunctivitis. (From Long S, Pickering LK, Prober CG, editors: *Principles and practice of pediatric infectious diseases*, New York, 2003, Churchill Livingstone, p 904.)

PNEUMONIA

Most infants with chlamydial pneumonia are symptomatic before the eighth week of life, with the insidious development of nasal obstruction or discharge or both, tachypnea, and a repetitive staccato cough.[3,23] Some infants may have symptoms the second week of life, initially involving the upper respiratory tract. Characteristically, infants have been symptomatic for 3 or more weeks before presentation. Most are only moderately ill and are afebrile. A history or presence of conjunctivitis can be elicited in half the cases. Some infants may develop apnea. Crepitant inspiratory rales are commonly heard. Expiratory wheezes are distinctly uncommon.

Hyperinflation of the lungs usually accompanies the infiltrates seen on chest radiographs. Infiltrates are most commonly bilateral and interstitial; reticulonodular patterns and atelectasis have also been described.[24] Possible laboratory findings include a distinctive peripheral eosinophilia (>400 cells/mm^3), mild arterial hypoxemia, and elevated serum immunoglobulins. Untreated disease can linger or recur. In very young infants, respiratory symptoms may occur early and be associated with feeding problems and apnea.

PERINATAL INFECTIONS AT OTHER SITES

Infants born to mothers infected with *C. trachomatis* may also become infected in the rectum and urogenital tract.[25] Although these infections are generally asymptomatic, they may persist for 3 years. Consequently, differentiating infection acquired perinatally from infection resulting from sexual abuse can be particularly difficult in young children.

Diagnosis

CONJUNCTIVITIS

Several nonculture methods are approved by the U.S. Food and Drug Administration (FDA) for diagnosis of ICN. These include enzyme immunoassays, specifically, Chlamydiazyme (Abbott Diagnostics, Chicago); MicroTrak EIA (Genetic Systems, Seattle); and direct fluorescent antibody assays using fluorescein-conjugated monoclonal antibodies to stain chlamydial EBs in a smear, including Syva MicroTrak (Genetic Systems) and Pathfinder (Sanofi-Pasteur, Chaska, Minn). These tests perform well on conjunctival specimens, with sensitivities of greater than 90% and specificities of 95% or greater compared with culture.[26,27] Nucleic acid amplification tests (NAATs) have not yet been FDA approved for testing of conjunctival specimens from infants. However, sensitivity and specificity are expected to be as high as the often less available FDA-approved direct immunodetection methods.

For resource-poor settings, a useful diagnostic method is examination of Giemsa-stained conjunctival scrapings for the presence of blue-stained intracytoplasmic inclusions within epithelial cells. The sensitivity of the test varies from 22% to

95%, depending on the technique of specimen collection and the examiner's expertise. This method also allows visualization of other bacteria, such as gonococci, or cytologic findings suggesting viral infection. Isolation of chlamydiae from conjunctival scrapings inoculated into tissue cell culture is a more reliable, although more costly, method of diagnosis. Serologic diagnosis of chlamydial conjunctivitis (in contrast to pneumonia) is unreliable because of the presence of maternally transmitted immunoglobulin G (IgG) antibody and the inconsistent appearance of IgM antibody in this infection.

Even if a firm diagnosis of chlamydial conjunctivitis is established, one must be mindful of the possibility of a dual infection, particularly with *Neisseria gonorrhoeae*. For this reason, appropriate stain and culture of the conjunctival exudate should be obtained.

PNEUMONIA

Enzyme immunoassays and direct fluorescent antibody assays for *Chlamydia* do not perform well with nasopharyngeal specimens and are not approved for this purpose. The definitive diagnosis of pneumonia can be made by culture of the organism from the respiratory tract. *Chlamydia* culture has been defined by the Centers for Disease Control and Prevention (CDC) as isolation of the organism in tissue culture and confirmation by microscopic identification of the characteristic inclusions by fluorescent antibody staining.[28] The likelihood of obtaining a positive culture is enhanced by deep suction of the trachea or by collecting a nasopharyngeal aspirate, rather than obtaining a specimen with a swab.[29] An acute microimmunofluorescence serum titer of *C. trachomatis*–specific IgM of 1:32 or greater is also diagnostic. In contrast, IgG is not diagnostic because passively transferred maternal antibody may persist at high titers for months. The serologic test of choice is the microimmunofluorescence procedure of Wang and colleagues,[30] in which EBs are used as antigen. Only a few clinical reference laboratories perform this test.

Indirect evidence of chlamydial pneumonia includes hyperinflation and bilateral diffuse infiltrates on chest radiographs, eosinophilia of 0.3 to 0.4 × 10^9/L (300 to 400/μL) or more in peripheral blood counts, and increased total serum IgG (>5 g/L [>500 mg/dL]) and IgM (>1.1 g/L [>110 mg/dL]) concentrations. The absence of any or all of these findings does not exclude the diagnosis, however.

Highly sensitive NAATs are commercially available for diagnosis of genital chlamydial infection in adolescents and adults. NAATs have FDA approval for vaginal and cervical swabs from women, urethral swabs from men, and urine from men and women. Information on the use of NAATs in children is limited, but PCR is likely to prove as reliable as culture for the detection of *C. trachomatis* in conjunctival, nasopharyngeal, tracheal aspirate, and lung biopsy specimens.

Differential Diagnosis

CONJUNCTIVITIS

Inclusion conjunctivitis of the newborn must be distinguished from conjunctivitis produced by pyogenic bacteria, particularly *N. gonorrhoeae*. Gonococcal ophthalmia usually occurs earlier, about 2 to 5 days after birth, although overlap in age at onset can occur. Gonococcal disease is usually more rapidly progressive than disease caused by *C. trachomatis*. Gonococcal infection can be diagnosed presumptively by examination of the Gram-stained smear of the exudate and confirmed by culture of the exudate. Staphylococcal conjunctivitis is usually acquired nosocomially from the nursery environment and is characterized more by purulent discharge than by redness. This and other forms of pyogenic conjunctivitis—which may be due to *Streptococcus pneumoniae*, *Haemophilus* species, or gram-negative bacteria such as *Pseudomonas aeruginosa*—can be appropriately diagnosed by Gram stain and culture of the exudate.

Of viral infections, neonatal herpes simplex (see Chapter 26) is the most important. This disease is characterized by involvement of the skin and the eye, vesicle formation, and occasional corneal involvement. Adenovirus infection of the newborn is very rare but has been described.

Chemical conjunctivitis related to instillation of silver nitrate at birth may also produce marked redness and a purulent discharge. These symptoms start on the first day of life and disappear after a few days, however, distinguishing this entity from a chlamydial infection.

PNEUMONIA

An afebrile, tachypneic infant presenting with a staccato cough in the first 3 months of life is very likely to have chlamydial disease. Cytomegalovirus may produce an interstitial pneumonia in preterm newborns that receive transfusions from cytomegalovirus-positive donors; however, it often produces signs and symptoms in other organ systems. Congenital infections with the rubella virus and *Toxoplasma gondii* also produce multiorgan involvement, as does perinatal infection with herpes simplex virus. Adenovirus or parainfluenza virus infection may produce an interstitial pneumonia but without the characteristic staccato cough or eosinophilia. Respiratory syncytial virus is a common cause of pneumonia in early infancy, but it often produces fever in the early stages, and wheezing because of airway obstruction is common with this illness. Respiratory syncytial virus is not associated with eosinophilia. Respiratory syncytial virus infection can be rapidly diagnosed by performing an enzyme immunoassay on a nasopharyngeal wash specimen.

Many pyogenic bacteria may produce lower respiratory tract infections in infancy. Group B streptococci, *S. pneumoniae*, *Staphylococcus aureus*, *H. influenzae*, and coliform bacteria are the most common. These patients are generally more toxic and febrile, and have pulmonary consolidation rather than an interstitial infiltrate. *Bordetella pertussis* classically causes a paroxysmal cough with an inspiratory whoop and posttussive emesis. Lymphocytosis is seen with whooping cough, and apnea occurs in infants younger than 6 months. Infants with *Pneumocystis jirovecii* pneumonia develop a characteristic syndrome of subacute diffuse pneumonitis with dyspnea at rest, tachypnea, oxygen desaturation, nonproductive cough, and fever.

Prognosis

CONJUNCTIVITIS

If untreated, ICN may persist for many weeks, but it usually resolves spontaneously without complications. The scarring that occurs in trachoma that leads to lid deformities is not seen. Superficial corneal vascularization and conjunctival scar formation can occur, however.[19]

PNEUMONIA

Untreated infants are usually ill for several weeks, with frequent cough, poor feeding, and poor weight gain. A few infants require oxygen, and fewer require ventilatory support. Beem and colleagues[31] found in a series of 11 infants that the total course of illness is 24 to 61 days, with an average of 43 days; mortality is exceptionally rare. Follow-up evaluation of a small cohort of children who had *C. trachomatis* pneumonia in infancy showed an increased prevalence of chronic cough and abnormal lung function compared with age-matched controls.[32]

Therapy

Topical treatment of inclusion conjunctivitis is not recommended primarily because of failure to eliminate concurrent nasopharyngeal infection. Recommended therapy for conjunctivitis is oral erythromycin, 50 mg/kg/day in four divided doses for 14 days. The failure rate is around 20%, and a second course of therapy may be required.[20] Problems with compliance and tolerance are frequent. In one small study, azithromycin suspension given at a dose of 20 mg/kg/day, one dose daily for 3 days, was safe and effective for ICN.[33] Oral sulfonamides may be used after the immediate neonatal period for infants who do not tolerate erythromycin.

Chlamydial pneumonia is treated with erythromycin, 50 mg/kg/day in four divided doses for 14 days. An oral sulfonamide is an alternative for infants who do not tolerate macrolides. There is convincing evidence that this treatment shortens the clinical course of pneumonia and eliminates the organism from the respiratory tract. Beyond specific antimicrobial therapy, infants require standard support measures, with attention to nutrition and to fluid status. Oxygen and ventilatory therapy may be required in a few cases. A specific diagnosis of *C. trachomatis* infection in an infant should prompt treatment of the mother and sexual partners.

An association between orally administered erythromycin and infantile hypertrophic pyloric stenosis (IHPS) has been reported in infants younger than 6 weeks who were given the drug for prophylaxis after nursery exposure to pertussis.[34] The risk of IHPS after treatment with other macrolides (e.g., azithromycin dihydrate and clarithromycin) is unknown. Because confirmation of erythromycin as a contributor to cases of IHPS requires additional investigation and because alternative therapies are not as well studied, the American Academy of Pediatrics continues to recommend use of erythromycin for treatment of *C. trachomatis* in infants. Parents of infants treated with erythromycin should be informed about the signs and potential risks of developing IHPS. Cases of pyloric stenosis after use of oral erythromycin should be reported to the FDA as an adverse drug reaction.

Prophylactic therapy of infants born to mothers known to have untreated chlamydial infection is not indicated because the efficacy of such prophylaxis is unknown. Infants should be monitored for signs of infection and to ensure appropriate treatment if infection develops. If adequate follow-up cannot be ensured, prophylaxis may be considered.

Prevention

Because *C. trachomatis* infections are transmitted vertically from mother to infant during delivery, an effective prevention measure is screening and treatment of pregnant women for *C. trachomatis* infection before delivery. The CDC currently recommends screening all pregnant women during their first prenatal visit and during the third trimester if high-risk (<25 years of age or other risk factors, such as new or multiple sexual partners).[28] Azithromycin (1 g orally as a single dose) and amoxicillin (1.5 g/day orally in three divided doses for 7 days) are recommended treatment regimens for pregnant women. Erythromycin base (2 g/day orally in four divided doses for 7 days) or erythromycin ethylsuccinate (3.2 g/day in four divided doses for 7 days) are alternatives. Half doses of erythromycin daily for 14 days may be given in pregnant women who are intolerant of the full-dose regimen. Because these regimens are not highly efficacious, a second course of therapy may be needed. Doxycycline and ofloxacin are contraindicated during pregnancy.

Ocular prophylaxis with topical erythromycin or tetracycline has reduced the incidence of gonococcal ophthalmia but does not seem to be effective against *C. trachomatis*.[35] The only means of preventing chlamydial infection of the newborn is treatment of infected mothers before delivery.

Ongoing efforts to develop a *C. trachomatis* vaccine to protect persons from genital tract infection have concentrated primarily on the use of peptides derived from MOMP or recombinant synthetic MOMP polypeptides as immunogens. Future work may incorporate molecular technology and our increasing understanding of the host response to chlamydiae to develop one or more new vaccines. Stimulation of long-term mucosal immunity in the genital tract is a challenge; it is unclear whether all genital infections could be prevented, or whether only more invasive disease, such as salpingitis, might be preventable using vaccine technology.

References

1. Lindner K: Gonoblennorrhoe, einschlussblennorrhoe und trachoma, *Albrecht von Graefes Arch Ophthalmol* 78:380-390, 1911.
2. Jones BR, Al-Hussaini MK, Dunlop EMC: Genital infection in association with TRIC virus infection of the eye: I. Isolation of virus from urethra, cervix, and eye: preliminary report, *Br J Vener Dis* 40:19-24, 1964.
3. Beem MO, Saxon EM: Respiratory-tract colonization and a distinctive pneumonia syndrome in infants infected with *Chlamydia trachomatis*, *N Eng J Med* 296:306-310, 1977.

4. Hardick J, Hsieh YH, Tulloch S, et al: Surveillance of *Chlamydia trachomatis* and *Neisseria gonorrhoeae* infections in women in detention in Baltimore, *Maryland. Sex Transm Dis* 30:64-70, 2003.
5. Weinstock H, Berman S, Cates W Jr: Sexually transmitted diseases among American youth: incidence and prevalence estimates 2000, *Perspect Sex Reprod Health* 36:6-10, 2004.
6. Gaydos CA, Howell MR, Quinn TC, et al: Sustained high prevalence of *Chlamydia trachomatis* infections in female army recruits, *Sex Transm Dis* 30:539-544, 2003.
7. Burstein GR, Gaydos CA, Diener-West M, et al: Incident *Chlamydia trachomatis* infections among inner-city adolescent females [see comments], *JAMA* 280:521-526, 1998.
8. Gaydos CA, Howell MR, Pare B, et al: *Chlamydia trachomatis* infections in female military recruits, *N Eng J Med* 339:739-744, 1998.
9. Jacobson DL, Peralta L, Farmer M, et al: Relationship of hormonal contraception and cervical ectopy as measured by computerized planimetry to chlamydial infection in adolescents, *Sex Transm Dis* 27:313-319, 2000.
10. Quinn TC, Gaydos C, Shepherd M, et al: Epidemiologic and microbiologic correlates of *Chlamydia trachomatis* infection in sexual partnerships, *JAMA* 276:1737-1742, 1996.
11. Hammerschlag MR, Anderka M, Semine DZ, et al: Prospective study of maternal and infantile infection with *Chlamydia trachomatis*, *Pediatrics* 64:142-148, 1979.
12. Schachter J, Grossman M, Holt J, et al: Infection with *Chlamydia trachomatis*: involvement of multiple anatomic sites in neonates, *J Infect Dis* 139:232-234, 1979.
13. Rapoza PA, Quinn TC, Kiessling LA, et al: Assessment of neonatal conjunctivitis with a direct immunofluorescent monoclonal antibody stain for *Chlamydia*, *JAMA* 255:3369-3373, 1986.
14. Rours IG, Hammerschlag MR, Ott A, et al: *Chlamydia trachomatis* as a cause of neonatal conjunctivitis in Dutch infants, *Pediatrics* 121: e321-e326, 2008.
15. Everett KD, Bush RM, Andersen AA: Emended description of the order Chlamydiales, proposal of Parachlamydiaceae fam. Nov. and Simkaniaceae fam. Nov., each containing one monotypic genus, revised taxonomy of the family Chlamydiaceae, including a new genus and five new species, and standards for the identification of organisms, *Int J Syst Bacteriol* 49(Pt 2):415-440, 1999.
16. Wyrick PB, Choong J, Davis CH, et al: Entry of genital *Chlamydia trachomatis* into polarized human epithelial cells, *Infect Immun* 57: 2378-2389, 1989.
17. De La Maza LM, Peterson EM: Scanning electron microscopy of Mccoy cells infected with *Chlamydia trachomatis*, *Exp Mol Pathol* 36:217-226, 1982.
18. Todd WJ, Caldwell HD: The interaction of *Chlamydia trachomatis* with host cells: ultrastructural studies of the mechanism of release of a biovar II strain from HeLa 229 cells, *J Infect Dis* 151:1037-1044, 1985.
19. Mordhorst CH, Dawson C: Sequelae of neonatal inclusion conjunctivitis and associated disease in parents, *Am J Ophthalmol* 71:861-867, 1971.
20. Hammerschlag MR, Chandler JW, Alexander ER, et al: Longitudinal studies on chlamydial infections in the first year of life, *Pediatr Infect Dis* 1:395-401, 1982.
21. Bell TA, Stamm WE, Wang SP, et al: Chronic *Chlamydia trachomatis* infections in infants, *JAMA* 267:400-402, 1992.
22. Frommell GT, Bruhn FW, Schwartzman JD: Isolation of *Chlamydia trachomatis* from infant lung tissue, *N Eng J Med* 296:1150-1152, 1977.
23. Schachter J, Lum L, Gooding CA, et al: Pneumonitis following inclusion blennorrhea, *J Pediatr* 87:779-780, 1975.
24. Radkowski MA, Kranzler JK, Beem MO, et al: *Chlamydia* pneumonia in infants: radiography in 125 cases, *AJR Am J Roentgenol* 137:703-706, 1981.
25. Schachter J, Grossman M, Sweet RL, et al: Prospective study of perinatal transmission of *Chlamydia trachomatis*, *JAMA* 255:3374-3377, 1986.
26. Hammerschlag MR, Roblin PM, Cummings C, et al: Comparison of enzyme immunoassay and culture for diagnosis of chlamydial conjunctivitis and respiratory infections in infants, *J Clin Microbiol* 25:2306-2308, 1987.
27. Judson BA, Lambert PP: Improved Syva MicroTrak *Chlamydia trachomatis* direct test method, *J Clin Microbiol* 26:2657-2658, 1988.
28. Workowski KA, Berman SM: Centers for Disease Control and Prevention sexually transmitted disease treatment guidelines, *Clin Infect Dis* 53(Suppl 3):S59-S63, 2011.
29. Harrison HR, English MG, Lee CK, et al: *Chlamydia trachomatis* infant pneumonitis: comparison with matched controls and other infant pneumonitis, *N Eng J Med* 298:702-708, 1978.
30. Wang SP, Grayston JT: Human serology in *Chlamydia trachomatis* infection with microimmunofluorescence, *J Infect Dis* 130:388-397, 1974.
31. Beem MO, Saxon E, Tipple MA: Treatment of chlamydial pneumonia of infancy, *Pediatrics* 63:198-203, 1979.
32. Harrison HR, Taussig LM, Fulginiti VA: *Chlamydia trachomatis* and chronic respiratory disease in childhood, *Pediatr Infect Dis* 1:29-33, 1982.
33. Hammerschlag MR, Gelling M, Roblin PM, et al: Treatment of neonatal chlamydial conjunctivitis with azithromycin, *Pediatr Infect Dis J* 17:1049-1050, 1998.
34. Centers for Disease Control and Prevention: Hypertrophic pyloric stenosis in infants following pertussis prophylaxis with erythromycin—Knoxville, Tennessee, 1999, *JAMA* 283:471-472, 2000.
35. Hammerschlag MR, Cummings C, Roblin PM, et al: Efficacy of neonatal ocular prophylaxis for the prevention of chlamydial and gonococcal conjunctivitis, *N Eng J Med* 320:769-772, 1989.

20 Mycoplasmal Infections

R. DOUG HARDY and OCTAVIO RAMILO

CHAPTER OUTLINE

Mycoplasmas are prokaryotes of the class Mollicutes and represent the smallest known free-living organisms. Their small size of 150 to 350 nm is more on the order of viruses than of bacteria. They lack a cell wall and are bound by a cell membrane. Many of the biologic properties of mycoplasmas are due to the absence of a rigid cell wall, including resistance to β-lactam antibiotics and marked pleomorphism among individual cells. The mycoplasmal cell membrane contains phospholipids, glycolipids, sterols, and various proteins. Mycoplasmas are able to grow in cell-free media and possess RNA and DNA. The entire genomes of many of the *Mycoplasma* species have been sequenced and have been found to be among the smallest of prokaryotic genomes; the *Mycoplasma genitalium* genome consists of only 580,070 DNA base pairs and only 470 predicted coding regions.[1] The elimination of genes related to synthesis of amino acids, fatty acid metabolism, and cholesterol necessitates a parasitic dependence on their host for exogenous nutrients, such as nucleic acid precursors, amino acids, fatty acids, and sterols. In mammals, *Mycoplasma* species most commonly colonize mucosal surfaces, such as the respiratory and genital tracts. At least 16 different species of Mollicutes colonize the mucosa of humans.

Ureaplasma species and *Mycoplasma hominis* are the mycoplasmas most commonly isolated from the genital tract of women and are associated with maternal and fetal infection. This chapter focuses on these two species in the maternal and fetal, neonatal, and very young infant populations. Mycoplasmal illnesses in other populations, such as immunocompromised older children and nonpregnant adults, are not discussed. *Mycoplasma pneumoniae, M. genitalium*, and *Mycoplasma fermentans* are mentioned briefly.

The originally identified species *Ureaplasma urealyticum* has been divided into two species, *Ureaplasma parvum* and *Ureaplasma urealyticum*, based on 16S ribosomal RNA sequences; the 14 described serovars were reassigned, with *U. parvum* containing 4 serovars (1, 3, 6, and 14) and *U. urealyticum* containing the remaining 10 serovars (2, 4, 5, 7, 8, 9, 10, 11, 12, and 13). Most of the available literature simply refers to *U. urealyticum* without differentiation into *U. parvum* or *U. urealyticum*. A few more recent investigations distinguish between *U. parvum* and *U. urealyticum* in their results, although not enough data are available to fully determine if the two species or 14 serovars differ in pathogenicity; initial data suggest that *Ureaplasma* virulence is species and serovar independent.[2] In this chapter, *Ureaplasma* is used to refer to *U. parvum* and *U. urealyticum* without differentiation.

Ureaplasma and *Mycoplasma hominis*: Colonization and Diseases of the Urinary and Reproductive Tracts in Adults

COLONIZATION

Ureaplasma and *M. hominis* are commensal organisms in the lower female genital tract. Colonization of the female lower urogenital tract by *Ureaplasma* and *M. hominis* generally occurs as a result of sexual activity. Sexual contact is the major mode of transmission of these organisms, and colonization increases dramatically with increasing numbers of sexual partners.[3-5]

In an asymptomatic woman, these mycoplasmas may be found throughout the lower urogenital tract, including the external cervical os, vagina, labia, and urethra.[6,7] The vagina yields the largest number of organisms, followed by the periurethral area and the cervix.[7] *Ureaplasma* is isolated less often from urine than from the cervix, but *M. hominis* is present in the urine and in the cervix with approximately the same frequency. In asymptomatic men, mycoplasmas also have been isolated from urine, semen, and the distal urethra.[8]

Ureaplasma can be isolated from the vagina of 40% to 80% of sexually active, asymptomatic women; *M. hominis* is found in 21% to 70%. Both microorganisms can be found concurrently in 31% to 60% of women.[9,10] In men, colonization with each is less prevalent. In women, colonization has been linked to younger age, lower socioeconomic status, multiple sexual partners, black ethnicity, oral contraceptive use, and recent antimicrobial therapy.[5,10,11] In addition, mycoplasmas are prevalent in the lower genital tract of pregnant women.[9,12,13] When genital mycoplasmas are present at the first prenatal visit, usually they persist throughout the pregnancy. Studies suggest that postmenopausal women are infrequently colonized with genital mycoplasmas.[14]

URINARY TRACT

Three disease associations have been established for *Ureaplasma* and *M. hominis* in the urinary tract: urethritis in men caused by *Ureaplasma*, urinary calculi caused by *Ureaplasma*, and pyelonephritis caused by *M. hominis*.[15] Intraurethral inoculation of human volunteers and nonhuman primates with *Ureaplasma* produces urethritis.[15] Serologic studies and clinical responsiveness in antimicrobial treatment trials also support a causative role of this organism in urethritis.[15] The common presence of ureaplasmas in the urethra of asymptomatic men suggests either that only certain serovars of ureaplasmas are pathogenic or that predisposing factors, such as lack of mucosal immunity, must exist in individuals in whom symptomatic infection develops. Alternatively, disease may develop only on initial exposure to ureaplasmas. *Ureaplasma* also has been implicated in urethroprostatitis and epididymitis.[16]

Ureaplasma has been shown to have a limited role in the production of urinary calculi. *Ureaplasma* produces urease, which splits urea into ammonia and carbon dioxide, and has been shown to induce crystallization of struvite and calcium phosphates in artificial urine in vitro, indicating a capacity of the pathogen to induce stone formation.[17,18] Renal calculi have been induced experimentally by inoculation of pure cultures of *Ureaplasma* directly into the bladder and renal pelvis of rats. *Ureaplasma* has been isolated from stones recovered by surgery in 6 of 15 patients. In 4 of the 6 patients, no other urease-producing organisms were isolated either in the stone or in urine sampled from the renal pelvis. *Proteus mirabilis* is the most common infectious cause of similar stones in humans. The frequency with which *Ureaplasma* reaches the kidney, the predisposing factors that allow this to occur, and the relative frequency of renal calculi induced by this organism compared with that of calculi induced by other organisms are unknown.

Even with the high incidence of *M. hominis* in the lower urogenital tract, this organism has been isolated from the upper urinary tract only in patients with symptoms of acute infection.[19] In one study, *M. hominis* was recovered from samples of ureteral urine collected during surgery from 7 of 80 patients (4 in pure culture) with acute pyelonephritis, and in a second study from 3 of 18 patients with acute exacerbation of chronic pyelonephritis. *M. hominis* was not found in the upper urinary tract of 22 patients with chronic pyelonephritis without acute exacerbation or in 60 patients with noninfectious urinary tract disease.

REPRODUCTIVE TRACT

M. hominis is considered an etiologic agent of pelvic inflammatory disease.[20-23] Inoculation of *M. hominis* into fallopian tubes of primates induces parametritis and salpingitis within 3 days,[24] whereas inoculation of human fallopian tube explants produces ciliostasis.[25] The organism has been isolated in pure cultures from the fallopian tubes of approximately 8% of women with salpingitis diagnosed by laparoscopy but not in any women without salpingitis.[20] The organism also can be isolated from the endometrium. A role for this organism in cases of pelvic inflammatory disease not associated with either *Neisseria gonorrhoeae* or *Chlamydia trachomatis* is supported by significant increases in specific antibodies to *M. hominis*.[22] *Ureaplasma* is not considered to be a cause of pelvic inflammatory disease.[16]

Chorioamnionitis, Clinical Amnionitis, and Maternal Septicemia

HISTOLOGIC CHORIOAMNIONITIS

Isolation of *Ureaplasma*, but not *M. hominis*, from the chorioamnion uniformly has shown a significant association with histologic chorioamnionitis.[26-32] Studies in which extensive culture for other agents was performed reported that women whose amniotic membranes contained *Ureaplasma* were more likely to have histologic evidence of chorioamnionitis than women without *Ureaplasma*, even after adjusting for duration of labor, premature rupture of membranes, duration of membrane rupture, and presence of other bacteria.[29] *Ureaplasma* in the chorioamnion was found to be significantly associated with histologic chorioamnionitis in the presence of intact membranes when delivery was by cesarean section.[33] In some cases, *Ureaplasma* was the only organism isolated. Case reports[27,34,35] indicate that *Ureaplasma* can persist in the amniotic fluid for 7 weeks in the presence of an intense inflammatory response and in the absence of ruptured membranes or labor and can be isolated as a single microorganism when cultures for multiple agents are performed. These findings show that ureaplasmas can produce histologic changes consistent with chorioamnionitis.

INFECTION OF THE AMNIOTIC FLUID AND CLINICAL AMNIONITIS

Although *Ureaplasma* and *M. hominis* can invade the amniotic fluid at 16 to 20 weeks of gestation in the presence of intact membranes and in the absence of other microorganisms, these infections tend to be clinically silent and chronic (Fig. 20-1).[27,34] *Ureaplasma* and *M. hominis* have been isolated more frequently from the chorioamnion than from the amniotic fluid. Isolation of organisms from the chorioamnion or amniotic fluid has been significantly associated with histologic evidence of chorioamnionitis but not with clinical amnionitis.[33] Ureaplasmas can be detected in the amniotic fluid in 50% of asymptomatic and symptomatic individuals.[36] Based on these reports, the role of *Ureaplasma* in clinical amnionitis remains unclear.

In an investigation by Yoon and colleagues,[37] amniocentesis was performed in 154 patients with preterm premature rupture of membranes. Amniotic fluid was cultured for aerobic and anaerobic bacteria and for mycoplasmas. Polymerase chain reaction (PCR) assay for *Ureaplasma* also was performed on the fluid. These investigators found that amniotic fluid culture for mycoplasmas missed 42% of cases identified as positive by *Ureaplasma* PCR assay. Patients with a negative result on amniotic fluid culture for *Ureaplasma* but a positive result on PCR assay had a significantly shorter interval from amniocentesis to delivery, higher amniotic fluid interleukin-6 (IL-6) concentrations, and higher white blood cell counts compared with patients without detection of *Ureaplasma* by culture or PCR assay. Subsequently, in a similar investigation by the same group[38] in 257 patients with preterm labor and intact membranes, significant findings were similar except that the prevalence of *Ureaplasma* was lower.

The detection of *M. hominis* does not correlate with clinical symptoms. *M. hominis* commonly invades the chorioamnion and amniotic fluid, but such invasion rarely occurs in the absence of other organisms, particularly ureaplasmas. It is unclear whether this organism alone is a cause of histologic chorioamnionitis or clinical amnionitis[33]

POSTPARTUM AND POSTABORTAL FEVER

M. hominis[39-42] and *Ureaplasma*[43,44] have been isolated from blood cultures from women with postpartum fever and septic abortion. Serologic investigations indicate that *M. hominis* is a common cause of postpartum fever, as shown by a fourfold or greater increase in mycoplasmacidal antibody titer.[45] In a study at Boston City Hospital,[46] blood was obtained from 327 women shortly after vaginal delivery. Of these 327 women, 10 had blood cultures that grew *M. hominis*, *Ureaplasma* grew in 15, and *M. hominis* and *Ureaplasma* were isolated in 1 woman. The frequency of isolation of mycoplasmas was inversely related to the interval between delivery and the time at which the blood was obtained for culture. Twenty women whose blood culture grew mycoplasmas at the time of delivery were reevaluated with a second culture 1 or more days later; a positive result

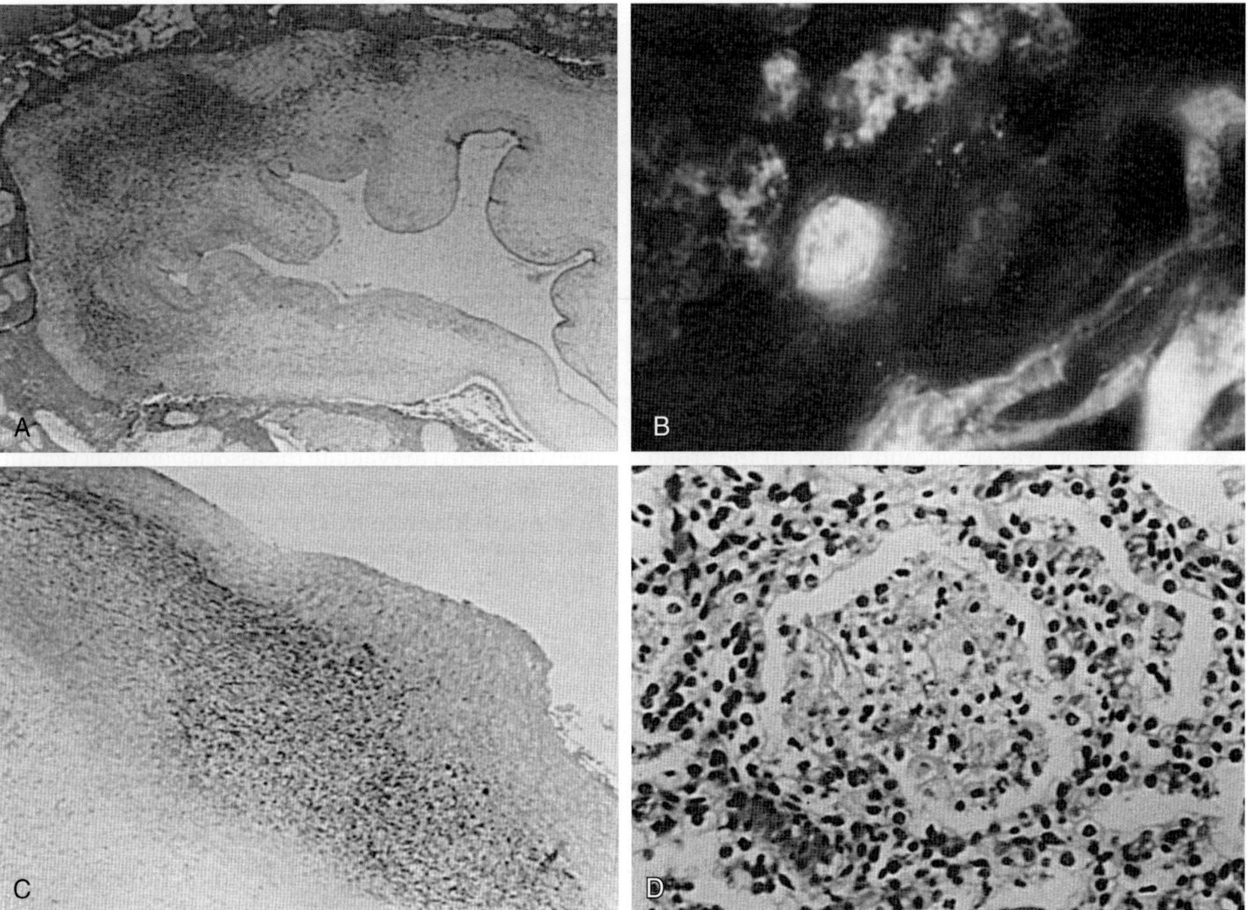

Figure 20-1 A, Section of placenta at 24 weeks of gestation showing extensive inflammation in amnion and chorion (magnification 25×). *Ureaplasma* was isolated from amniotic fluid 7 weeks before delivery and from multiple fetal organs at postmortem examination. **B,** Adjacent section of placenta stained with rabbit anti–*Ureaplasma* serovar 1 serum and reacted with fluorescein-labeled goat anti–rabbit immunoglobulin G (magnification 750×). **C,** Photomicrograph of umbilical cord from same case as in **A** and **B** shows extensive inflammation (magnification 25×). **D,** Photomicrograph of lung tissue shows histologic evidence of pneumonia (magnification 50×).

was obtained on the second blood culture in only 1 of the 20 women. Pathogenic bacteria were cultured from the blood of 16 of the 327 women, including 4 of the 11 women with *M. hominis* but none from the women with *Ureaplasma*.

In a prospective study of 620 blood cultures from febrile obstetric patients,[47] *Ureaplasma* was the second and *M. hominis* the third most common microorganism isolated. All specimens were obtained during febrile postpartum or postabortum episodes. Mycoplasmas were isolated on numerous occasions from blood drawn more than 2 days after the procedure. Endometritis or histologically documented chorioamnionitis was present in half of the patients, and fever persisted after delivery or abortion in many of the cases despite administration of antibiotics directed at organisms other than mycoplasmas. Fever resolved after tetracycline therapy.

It has been shown that colonization of the chorioamnion with ureaplasmas in women with intact membranes undergoing cesarean delivery is a significant and independent predictor of ensuing endometritis.[48] Endometritis occurred in 28% of women with ureaplasmas isolated from the chorioamnion at cesarean delivery, compared with only 8.4% if the culture result was negative and 8.8% if only bacteria but no ureaplasmas were isolated.

Roberts and associates[49] found ureaplasmas to be the most common microorganism isolated from postcesarean wound infections. Of 47 cultures with a positive result from 939 wounds, ureaplasmas were recovered from 29. In addition, one third of the cultures positive for ureaplasmas yielded no other microorganisms. *M. hominis* has been recovered from the joint fluid of women postpartum. These women had been febrile during the immediate postpartum period, and signs of arthritis developed 7 days to 3 weeks after delivery.[50] Cases of postpartum pneumonia with isolation of *M. hominis* from pleural fluid and cases of *M. hominis* wound infections after cesarean section also have been reported.[51-54]

Andrews and coworkers[55] performed a randomized, double-blind, placebo-controlled trial in 597 women to compare rates of postcesarean endometritis after prophylaxis with cefotetan versus cefotetan plus doxycycline and azithromycin. The frequency of postcesarean endometritis and wound infection was significantly lower in the group that received cefotetan plus doxycycline and azithromycin. The investigators concluded that this extended-spectrum antibiotic prophylaxis regimen, with activity against mycoplasmas, reduced the frequency of postcesarean endometritis and wound infection. *Mycoplasma* cultures were not obtained in this investigation, however, so it is unclear that the improved outcome was specifically due to the addition of doxycycline and azithromycin prophylaxis aimed at *Mycoplasma* infections versus other synergistic antibacterial or immunomodulatory effects of these agents.

Adverse Pregnancy Outcome

FETAL LOSS

Although studies have found the presence of *Ureaplasma* and *M. hominis* in the genital tract to be significantly associated with spontaneous abortion and early pregnancy loss,[56] their actual role in these events is uncertain. Both organisms have been isolated from the lungs, brain, heart, and viscera of aborted fetuses and stillborn infants, in some cases in the presence of an inflammatory response and in the absence of other organisms.[27,31,57,58] In these cases, it was unclear whether death of the fetus occurred before these organisms "invaded." *Ureaplasma* has been found more frequently in the products of early abortions and midtrimester fetal losses than in products of induced abortions.[59,60] *Ureaplasma* has been isolated more frequently from the placentas of aborted fetuses than from controls.[28,30]

Although rates of isolation of ureaplasmas from the lower genital tract of women with habitual abortion are not different from those of normal controls, ureaplasmas are isolated more frequently from the endometrium of women with habitual abortion.[59,60] When only patients with a positive result on cervical culture are considered, no higher endometrial colonization rates are found.[61] Antibody titers to *Ureaplasma* are higher in mothers with a history of fetal loss.[62] These epidemiologic studies are difficult to interpret, however, because the comparability of the various groups of women is uncertain, and the role of other potential infectious agents was not always taken into account.

Isolation of *Ureaplasma* from amniotic fluid in pure culture from women with intact membranes and subsequent fetal loss in the presence of histologic chorioamnionitis has been reported.[27,34,35] Berg and associates[63] performed a retrospective analysis of 2718 amniocentesis specimens obtained for genetic indications and cultured for *Ureaplasma* and *M. hominis*. Of the 2718 patients, 49 (1.8%) patients were found to be positive for one or both organisms. Of 43 patients who could be evaluated, 35 were given oral erythromycin at the discretion of the physician caring for the patient. Rates of midtrimester loss were 11.4% and 44.4% ($P = .04$) in the treated and untreated groups. This study showed that treatment of amniotic mycoplasmal colonization with erythromycin may decrease midtrimester losses. Prospective controlled trials are necessary to validate this hypothesis.

PRETERM BIRTH

Multiple studies involving almost 12,000 patients have been conducted to evaluate the association of cervical ureaplasmal infection with prematurity.[64,65] The evidence fails to establish a consistent relationship between the presence of *Ureaplasma* in the lower genital tract of the mother and prematurity or low birth weight in the infant.

At least six prospective studies have evaluated the role of ureaplasmal infection of the amniotic fluid in the etiology of prematurity. Three of these studies investigated the outcome of pregnancy when ureaplasmas were detected at the time of genetic amniocentesis at 12 to 20 weeks of gestation, when membranes were intact, and when labor had not begun.[27,34,66] In an investigation by Cassell and colleagues,[27] two infants with *Ureaplasma* isolated from amniotic fluid were born preterm; both infants died, and both had evidence of pneumonia. *Ureaplasma* was isolated in pure culture at postmortem examination in both cases. In a study by Gray and associates,[34] 7 of 10 patients from whom ureaplasmas were isolated by culture of the amniotic fluid subsequently aborted within 4 to 7 weeks after amniocentesis and at less than 25 weeks of gestation. The three remaining infants were born at less than 37 weeks of gestation, and two of these died. Histologic evidence of chorioamnionitis was present in all 10 placentas, and histologic evidence of pneumonia was present in all eight fetuses. Placentas grew *Ureaplasma*, but results were negative for cultures of all other microorganisms in six of seven evaluated at delivery and in four of the six fetal lungs that were evaluated.

The third and largest investigation by Gerber and coworkers[66] used PCR assay and detected *Ureaplasma* in 29 of 254 (11.4%) amniotic fluid specimens. As might be expected, a higher percentage of *Ureaplasma*-positive amniotic fluid samples were found in this study that used PCR than in previous investigations that relied solely on culture. Subsequent preterm labor occurred in 17 (58.6%) *Ureaplasma*-positive women compared with 10 (4.4%) women whose cultures were *Ureaplasma* negative ($P < .0001$). Preterm birth occurred in 7 (24.1%) *Ureaplasma*-positive women compared with 1 (0.4%) *Ureaplasma*-negative woman ($P < .0001$). *Ureaplasma*-positive women had a higher prevalence of preterm labor in a prior pregnancy (20.7%) than the *Ureaplasma*-negative women (2.7%; $P < .0008$).

In contrast to the above-mentioned studies, in the remaining three studies, culture of amniotic fluid was performed on women hospitalized with preterm labor and intact membranes. *Ureaplasma* in the amniotic fluid was not consistently associated with preterm birth in these studies.[67-69]. In these later studies of women with preterm labor, the mean gestation was 31.5 weeks, compared with 12 to 20 weeks of gestation in the previous studies of women with no labor.

A significant relationship between isolation of *Ureaplasma* from the chorioamnion and preterm birth has been documented in three of six prospective studies.[28-30,70-72] In most patients in these investigations, membrane rupture had occurred, however, which could have led to intrapartum microbial invasion of the chorioamnion, potentially confounding the results even if the duration of membrane rupture is taken into account.

As noted previously, Berg and associates[63] performed a retrospective analysis of 2718 genetic amniocentesis specimens cultured for *Ureaplasma* and *M. hominis*. Of the 2718 specimens, 49 (1.8%) were found to be positive for either organism. Of 43 patients who could be evaluated in this study, 35 received treatment with oral erythromycin. Preterm delivery rates were similar in the treated and untreated groups (19.4% and 20%). The investigators speculated that the lack of a treatment effect may have been due to recolonization with mycoplasmas.

The sum of the evidence suggests that the risk of preterm labor and delivery is increased when ureaplasmas are detected at amniocentesis at 12 to 20 weeks of gestation in women with intact membranes before onset of labor. Otherwise, the association between preterm birth and ureaplasmas is uncertain.

Transmission of *Ureaplasma* and *Mycoplasma hominis* to the Fetus and Newborn

Ureaplasma and *M. hominis* can be transmitted to a fetus from an infected woman either in utero or at the time of delivery by passage through a colonized birth canal. The isolation of *Ureaplasma* in pure culture from the chorioamnion, amniotic fluid, and internal fetal organs in the presence of funisitis and pneumonia[27] and a specific IgM response[73] can be taken as evidence that fetal infection can occur in utero. Investigators[74,75] also have found that *Ureaplasma* and *M. hominis* can be isolated from endotracheal specimens collected within 30 minutes to 24 hours after birth from infants who were delivered by cesarean section with intact membranes. It is thought that the acquisition of *Ureaplasma* and *M. hominis* can occur in utero either by an ascending route secondary to colonization of the mother's genital tract or transplacentally from the mother's blood. Each of these organisms has been isolated from maternal and umbilical cord blood at the time of delivery.[76,77]

The rate of vertical transmission of *Ureaplasma* and *M. hominis* ranges from 18% to 88%.[77-81] Chua and colleagues[81] prospectively investigated the transmission and colonization of *Ureaplasma* and *M. hominis* from mothers to term and preterm newborns delivered by the vaginal route. The rates of maternal cervical colonization with *Ureaplasma* and *M. hominis* were 57.5% and 15.8%, respectively, whereas the rates for isolation of *Ureaplasma* and *M. hominis* from nasopharyngeal secretions of the newborns were 50.8% and 6.6%, respectively. The vertical transmission rates were 88.4% for *Ureaplasma* and 42.1% for *M. hominis*. Maternal transmission was not associated with gestational age. In preterm neonates, the isolation of mycoplasmas was not associated with gestational age or birth weight. There was a tendency for *Ureaplasma* to persist in preterm newborns, especially in neonates with birth weight less than 2 kg. Colonization of full-term infants seems to be transient, with a sharp decrease in isolation rates after 3 months of age.[82] In premature infants with ureaplasmal infection, persistence of the organism in the lower respiratory tract and cerebrospinal fluid (CSF) has been documented for weeks to months.[74,83]

Perinatal *Ureaplasma* and *Mycoplasma hominis* Infection

Many prospective studies based on direct culture of the affected site indicate that *Ureaplasma* and *M. hominis* can cause invasive disease in infants, particularly in infants born prematurely. The presence of mycoplasmas in the chorioamnion or amniotic fluid does not always result in infection of the fetus, however. Similarly, the isolation of mycoplasmas from surface cultures (e.g., eyes, ears, nose, throat, gastric aspirates, vagina) is not indicative of invasive disease.

PNEUMONIA

Case reports,[34,84,85] retrospective studies,[86] and prospective studies[27,31,34] indicate an association of *Ureaplasma* with congenital and neonatal pneumonia. The organism has been isolated from affected lungs in the absence of other pathogens, such as chlamydiae, viruses, fungi, and bacteria, in the presence of chorioamnionitis and funisitis[27] and has been shown within fetal membranes by immunofluorescence[27] and in lung lesions by electron and immunofluorescence microscopy.[73] A specific IgM response has been shown in some cases of neonatal pneumonia.[73]

In a study of 98 infants,[74] respiratory distress syndrome, the need for assisted ventilation, severe respiratory insufficiency, and death were significantly more common in infants born at less than 34 weeks of gestation from whom *Ureaplasma* was recovered from endotracheal aspirates at delivery than in infants with a negative culture result. In another series of 292 infants with birth weights less than 2500 g who were studied by follow-up evaluation for 4 weeks after birth, isolation of *Ureaplasma* from the endotracheal aspirate within 1 week of birth (mean age, 1.3 days) was significantly associated with radiographic pneumonia, whereas no such association was found for uninfected infants.[87] *Ureaplasma* was the most common organism isolated (15% of infants) among these 292 patients, and it was isolated in pure culture in 71%.

Cultrera and colleagues[88] investigated for molecular evidence of *U. urealyticum* or *U. parvum* respiratory colonization in preterm infants with or without respiratory distress syndrome. Significantly, 15 of 24 preterm neonates with respiratory distress syndrome and 4 of 26 without respiratory distress syndrome were PCR positive for *Ureaplasma* ($P < .001$). Of the 15 preterm infants PCR positive for *Ureaplasma*, 5 had *U. urealyticum* and 10 had *U. parvum* isolated. In this investigation, *Ureaplasma* culture was positive in 5 of 50 subjects, compared with 19 of 50 subjects by PCR method ($P < .05$).

Conversely, other investigators have found a possible protective effect associated with the isolation of *Ureaplasma* from preterm infants. In a prospective consecutive investigation of 143 ventilated newborns born at less than 28 weeks of gestation, Hannaford and coworkers[89] isolated *Ureaplasma* from endotracheal aspirates of 39 (27%) infants. Respiratory distress syndrome occurred significantly less often in infants from whom *Ureaplasma* was isolated than in infants from whom it was not isolated ($P = .002$). In addition, a trend for lower mortality rates in the first 28 days of life was identified among *Ureaplasma*-positive infants. Berger and associates[90] also found an apparently protective effect of *Ureaplasma* isolated from the amniotic cavity at the time of delivery against hyaline membrane disease in infants with a mean gestational age of 29 to 30 weeks, although this was nonsignificant. No increase in acute morbidity or mortality was found to be associated with *Ureaplasma* isolation.

The baboon model of prematurity has been used to investigate the pathogenicity of *Ureaplasma*. At age 140 days, baboons show physiologic and pathologic characteristics similar to those of human neonates of 30 to 32 weeks of gestation (e.g., they have hyaline membrane disease).[91] Endotracheal inoculation of premature baboons with *Ureaplasma* isolated from human infants results in histologic pulmonary lesions, including acute bronchiolitis with epithelial ulceration and polymorphonuclear cell infiltration, indistinguishable from those of hyaline membrane disease.[92]

Yoder and colleagues[93] performed an investigation in premature baboons that offers an explanation for the divergent findings in human studies of *Ureaplasma* and respiratory status in preterm infants. Premature baboon infants were delivered 48 to 72 hours after maternal intraamniotic inoculation with *Ureaplasma*. Two distinct patterns of disease were observed in the baboon infants. Baboons with persistent *Ureaplasma* tracheal colonization manifested worse lung function and prolonged elevated tracheal cytokines. Conversely, colonized baboons that subsequently cleared *Ureaplasma* from tracheal cultures showed improved lung function compared with unexposed control animals.

In addition, pneumonia with persistent pulmonary hypertension has been described in newborn infants with *Ureaplasma* isolated from the lower respiratory tract.[84,85] Although cases of ureaplasmal pneumonia have been documented in full-term infants, pneumonia resulting from this agent is thought to occur much less frequently than in premature neonates. Case reports indicate that *M. hominis* can be a cause of pneumonia in newborns, but it has not been implicated as a common etiologic agent in prospective studies. These mycoplasmas are not thought to be a significant cause of acute respiratory disease in otherwise healthy infants after the first month of life.[33]

CHRONIC LUNG DISEASE

Ureaplasma frequently colonizes the neonatal respiratory tract. Although most investigations support a significant association between ureaplasmas and chronic lung disease (CLD) in preterm infants, its role in causation of CLD is uncertain. CLD is most often defined as a requirement for supplemental oxygen at 28 days of age or at 36 weeks of postconceptional age. Presence of concurrent chest radiographic changes compatible with CLD sometimes is included in this definition.

In a meta-analysis of 17 investigations published before 1995, Wang and coworkers[94] explored the association between *Ureaplasma* and CLD. The studies in this analysis included preterm and term neonates. CLD was defined as a requirement for oxygen at 28 to 30 days of age, and diagnosis of *Ureaplasma* colonization required the recovery of *Ureaplasma* from a respiratory or surface specimen. The estimates of relative risk exceeded 1 in all of the investigations; however, the lower confidence interval (CI) included 1 in 7 (41%). The meta-analysis concluded that the relative risk (RR) for the development of CLD in colonized infants was 1.72 (95% CI, 1.5 to 1.96) times that for noncolonized infants. In the analysis, investigations that focused on extremely premature, very-low-birth-weight (VLBW) neonates did not identify a significantly different RR from that for investigations that included all neonates. Also, the RR did not differ significantly between studies in which only endotracheal aspirates were used to define colonization and other studies.

Subsequent to this meta-analysis, the association of *Ureaplasma* with chronic pulmonary disease, including bronchopulmonary dysplasia (or CLD), has been confirmed in multiple studies[89,90,95-103] but not in others.[104-110] Perzigian and colleagues[96] prospectively investigated a cohort of 105 VLBW (<1500 g) infants; in 22 (21%) infants, results of tracheal aspirate cultures were positive for *Ureaplasma* at birth. At 28 days of age, *Ureaplasma*-positive patients were significantly more likely to have CLD than were *Ureaplasma*-negative patients, despite routine use of exogenous surfactant. *Ureaplasma*-positive infants also required significantly longer duration of oxygen therapy and of mechanical ventilation. No significant differences were found for CLD at 36 weeks of postconceptional age or for duration of hospitalization.

Another meta-analysis appraisal of the association between *Ureaplasma* and CLD was undertaken by Schelonka and coworkers[111] with investigations published before 2005. This analysis included 23 studies of infants colonized or infected with *Ureaplasma*, with an aggregate of 2216 infants in whom CLD was defined as persisting oxygen requirement at 28 days of age, and included 8 studies of 751 infants in whom CLD was defined at 36 weeks of postconceptional age. A significant association between respiratory *Ureaplasma* and CLD was shown at 28 days of age (odds ratio [OR], 2.8; 95% CI, 2.3 to 3.5) and 36 weeks of postconceptional age (OR, 1.6; 95% CI, 1.1 to 2.3).

Because neither the relationship of *Ureaplasma* species nor the concentration of ureaplasmas with the development of CLD had yet been investigated, a prospective study was designed to look for such an association. In 175 VLBW infants, endotracheal aspirates were obtained at birth for quantitative culture; the results were analyzed for correlation with the development of CLD.[108] Ureaplasmas were isolated from 66 (38%) of the 175 infants. No statistically significant associations were identified between the development of CLD and the *Ureaplasma* species isolated (*U. urealyticum* or *U. parvum*) or the concentration of ureaplasmas in the lower respiratory tract secretions.

Because the observed disparities in these studies might be explained in part by the variable persistence of *Ureaplasma* colonization of the infant respiratory tract, a prospective longitudinal study was performed to investigate this possibility. In 125 VLBW infants, culture and PCR assay were used to sample for *Ureaplasma* in the respiratory tract frequently over the course of their neonatal intensive care unit stay. It was found that the pattern of colonization was predictive for the development of CLD.[97] In this study, 40 (32%) of 125 infants had at least one specimen positive for *Ureaplasma*; however, only 18 (45%) of the 40 had persistent colonization throughout their hospitalization. Only persistent *Ureaplasma* colonization was associated with a significantly increased risk of development of CLD at 28 days of age and at 36 weeks after conception. Neither early transient colonization nor late acquisition of *Ureaplasma* was associated with CLD. The study by Yoder and colleagues[93] in premature baboons similarly found that the pattern of tracheal colonization was important in the manifestations of respiratory disease.

Inadequate detection of *Ureaplasma* in neonates can be another confounding factor in CLD research. False-negative results for isolation of *Ureaplasma* from respiratory specimens could weaken the calculated association with CLD. Using in situ hybridization for *Ureaplasma* on lung autopsy tissue from 7 infants with positive cultures and 7 infants with negative cultures for *Ureaplasma* from the lower respiratory tract, Benstein and coworkers[95] found all 7 culture-positive infants were positive for *Ureaplasma* by in situ hybridization; 2 of the culture-negative infants were positive by in situ hybridization. The in situ hybridization results had 100% correlation with the presence of histopathologic evidence of bronchopulmonary dysplasia at autopsy of these 14 infants.

Although properly conducted antimicrobial agent trials showing reduction in CLD incidence and severity in neonates with *Ureaplasma* would support a causal role for this microorganism, failure of amelioration with effective therapy does not indicate that *Ureaplasma* does not have some role in the development of CLD. Initial small trials of therapy with erythromycin or clarithromycin failed to provide evidence that therapy, predicted by in vitro testing to be effective, decreases CLD severity or produces clinical improvement in neonates with *Ureaplasma*.[90,100,109,112-115] Two randomized, controlled trials using erythromycin, together involving 37 VLBW infants with *Ureaplasma* isolated from the respiratory tract, failed to show a reduction in the incidence of CLD after 7 to 10 days of erythromycin therapy.[112] In one of these trials, erythromycin treatment significantly reduced the isolation of *Ureaplasma* from the respiratory tract, but it did not significantly alter required length of time with supplemental oxygen.[109]

However, larger more recent randomized, placebo-controlled trials have yielded results indicating a reduction in CLD with macrolide treatment of preterm infants with *Ureaplasma* isolated from the respiratory tract. In 74 preterm infants with *Ureaplasma* isolated from nasopharyngeal swab culture and then randomized to receive intravenous clarithromycin or placebo for 10 days, clarithromycin treatment resulted in eradication of *Ureaplasma* in 68.5% of the patients, and the incidence of CLD was significantly lower in the clarithromycin group than in the placebo group (2.9% vs. 36.4%; $P < .001$). Multivariate logistic regression analysis confirmed the independent preventive effect of clarithromycin for the development of CLD (OR, 27.2 [95% CI, 2.5 to 296.1]; $P = .007$).[116] In another investigation, preterm infants were randomized to azithromycin (10 mg/kg/day for 7 days, followed by 5 mg/kg/day for a maximum of 6 weeks) or placebo. The primary end points were incidence of CLD or mortality without regard to *Ureaplasma*. A total of 220 infants were enrolled ($n = 111$ with azithromycin and 109 with placebo). Incidence of CLD without regard to *Ureaplasma* was 76% for the azithromycin group versus 84% for the placebo group ($P = .2$). However, the incidence of CLD in the *Ureaplasma*-positive subgroup was 73% in the azithromycin group versus 94% in the placebo group ($P = .03$). Analysis of patients in the *Ureaplasma* subgroup only, using the exact logistic model demonstrated a decrease in CLD or death in the azithromycin group, with an estimated OR of 0.026 (95% CI, 0.001 to 0.618).[117] It appears that further clinical trials are to be conducted.[118]

Debate over the concept that initiating therapy after birth may be too late to influence the outcome of an inflammatory process with possible onset in utero was partially addressed in the ORACLE (Overview of Role of Antibiotics in the Curtailment of Labour and Early Delivery) I and ORACLE II prenatal trials (erythromycin or amoxicillin–clavulanic acid, or both, in a randomized double-blind, placebo-controlled design) involving a combined total of 11,121 women with preterm, prelabor rupture of fetal membranes or spontaneous preterm labor.[119,120] One of the primary outcomes of these trials was CLD, defined as the need for daily supplementary oxygen at age 36 weeks after conception; the other primary outcomes were neonatal death and major cerebral abnormality. ORACLE I and ORACLE II revealed no statistically significant reduction in any primary outcome. *Ureaplasma* colonization was not specifically addressed in these trials, however, so the results should not be generalized to address *Ureaplasma* and CLD directly.

To investigate for the presence of a long-term detrimental effect of perinatal *Ureaplasma* infection, a cohort of 40 preterm infants was prospectively followed for 12 months.[121] In 22 (55%) infants, *Ureaplasma* was present in samples obtained from the trachea or blood, or both, at birth. Infants with perinatal *Ureaplasma* required significantly more days of hospitalization than infants without *Ureaplasma*. The difference was attributed to an increase in respiratory tract disease among the infants with perinatal *Ureaplasma*. In addition, CLD was associated with significantly more admissions in infants with perinatal *Ureaplasma* than in infants without it. Syrogiannopoulos and associates[77] monitored 108 full-term infants during the first 3 months of life. These researchers were unable to show an increased risk of lower respiratory illness during this period of observation in 51 of 108 infants with persistent pharyngeal *Ureaplasma* colonization compared with infants who were not pharyngeally colonized at 3 months of life.

Although *Ureaplasma* has not been definitively shown to cause CLD, investigations have identified possible pathogenic mechanisms through which it may contribute to CLD. *Ureaplasma* has been hypothesized to induce lung injury through immunopathogenic mechanisms involving the release of pulmonary cytokines and chemokines after exposure to this microorganism either in utero or postnatally. It also has been proposed that *Ureaplasma* infection potentiates oxygen-induced lung injury.[95,97,122]

Although much effort has been expended to define the role of *Ureaplasma* in CLD, no clear conclusions can be made at the present time, although most of the investigations seem to indicate a significant association. Novel strategies need to be instituted to explore the link between these entities further.

BLOODSTREAM INFECTIONS

Ureaplasmas have been isolated from blood cultures from neonates.[47,75,76,83,123-126] Case reports also have described the isolation of ureaplasmas from the bloodstream of neonates with pneumonia.[74,85] Cassell and associates[75] found that 26% of preterm infants with endotracheal aspirates that grew *Ureaplasma* also had a positive result on blood cultures for this organism, suggesting that bacteremia with ureaplasmas can be common in preterm infants. Cases of *M. hominis* bacteremia with systemic symptoms accompanied by an antibody response also have been reported.[127,128]

Not all investigations have been successful in recovering mycoplasmas from the blood of infants.[123,129,130] Mycoplasmas were not isolated from blood cultures obtained within 30 minutes of birth from 146 preterm infants in Israel.[123] In addition, investigators did not isolate mycoplasmas from the 191 blood cultures in a prospective study of older infants hospitalized for possible sepsis.[130]

Goldenberg and coworkers[131] evaluated the frequency of umbilical cord blood infections with *Ureaplasma* and *M. hominis* in 351 mother-infant pairs with deliveries between 23 and 32 weeks of gestational age, to determine their association with various obstetric conditions, markers of placental inflammation, and newborn outcomes. *Ureaplasma* or *M. hominis*, or both, were present in 82 (23%) cord blood cultures. Of the women with a positive cord blood culture for *Ureaplasma* or *M. hominis*, or both, 43 (52%) had *Ureaplasma* only, 21 (26%) had *M. hominis* only, and 18 (22%) had *Ureaplasma* and *M. hominis*. Positive cultures for *Ureaplasma* or *M. hominis*, or both, were more common in infants of nonwhite women (27.9% vs. 16.8%; $P = .016$), in women younger than 20 years of age, in women undergoing a spontaneous compared with an indicated preterm delivery (34.7% vs. 3.2%; $P = .0001$), and in women delivering at earlier gestational ages. Intrauterine infection and inflammation were more common among infants with a positive cord blood culture for *Ureaplasma* or *M. hominis*, or both, as evidenced by positive placental cultures for these and other bacteria, elevated cord blood IL-6 levels, and placental histology. Infants with positive cord blood cultures for *Ureaplasma* or *M. hominis*, or both, were more likely to have neonatal systemic inflammatory response syndrome (41.3% vs. 25.7%; adjusted OR, 1.86; 95% CI, 1.08 to 3.21), but were not significantly different for other neonatal outcomes, including CLD (26.8% vs. 10.1%; adjusted OR, 1.99; 95% CI, 0.91 to 4.37), respiratory distress syndrome, intraventricular hemorrhage, or death.

CENTRAL NERVOUS SYSTEM INFECTIONS

In general, the clinical significance of recovering *Ureaplasma* or *M. hominis* from a central nervous system (CNS) specimen from a neonate is uncertain. In some situations, an association with a disease process seems plausible, whereas in others, no corresponding disease state is apparent. Multiple cases of *M. hominis* CNS infection (meningitis, brain abscess) have been described in full-term and preterm infants.[132-142] *Ureaplasma* also has been isolated from the CSF of infants with suspected sepsis and meningitis.[5,74,83,129,143-144]

In a prospective trial in 100 mostly premature infants, *Ureaplasma* was isolated from the CSF of 8, and *M. hominis* was isolated from the CSF of 5 who were undergoing investigation for suspected sepsis or treatment of hydrocephalus.[83] Of the eight neonates with *Ureaplasma*, six had severe intraventricular hemorrhage, three had hydrocephalus, and four had ureaplasmas isolated several times in the CSF. *Ureaplasma* infection was significantly associated with severe intraventricular hemorrhage ($P < .001$). *Ureaplasma* was isolated from the respiratory tract of four of the eight infants with CSF infections. Five infants received treatment with erythromycin or doxycycline. Three infants with *Ureaplasma* infection died. All five of the neonates from whom *M. hominis* was isolated from the CSF were being investigated for suspected sepsis; prominent neurologic signs and CSF pleocytosis were noted in only one neonate. This infant received doxycycline treatment and improved but had substantial neurologic sequelae (Fig. 20-2).[83] No infants infected with *M. hominis* died. A subsequent study by the same group of investigators in 318 infants isolated *Ureaplasma* from the CSF of 5 and *M. hominis* from the CSF of 9. Spontaneous clearance of the organisms was documented in 5 of the infants, and 12 infants had a good outcome.[145]

Shaw and colleagues[146] performed a prospective study of 135 preterm infants undergoing lumbar puncture and found *Ureaplasma* in the CSF of 1 neonate and *M. hominis* in none. *Ureaplasma* continued to be isolated from this 1 infant over the course of 16 weeks, despite treatment with erythromycin. The organism maintained in vitro susceptibility to

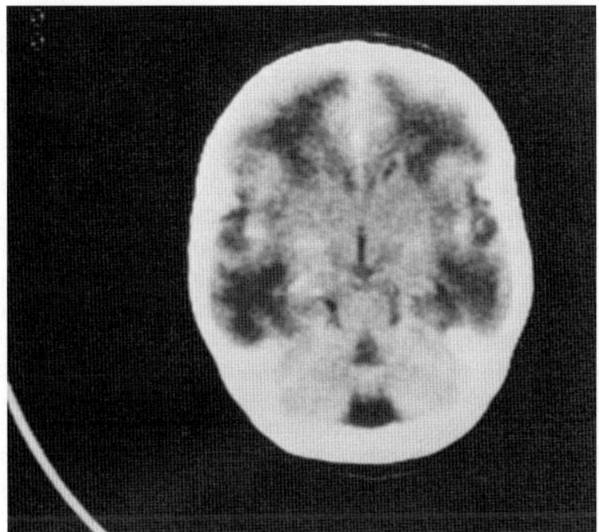

Figure 20-2 A 37-week gestation newborn who had hypothermia, hypotonia, and lethargy noted at age 3 days. Computed tomography showed decreased attenuation predominantly of supratentorial white matter symmetrically with punctate early calcified lesions. Examination of cerebrospinal fluid showed mononuclear pleocytosis, and *Mycoplasma hominis* was isolated. Cerebrospinal fluid culture was sterile after 5 days of doxycycline treatment, but the infant had spastic quadriplegia at 6 months of age.

erythromycin. Doxycycline treatment was associated with the disappearance of the organism.

In a prospective study by Ollikainen and coworkers,[74] *Ureaplasma* was isolated from the CSF of four of six infants born at less than 34 weeks of gestation. None had pleocytosis or hypoglycorrhachia in the CSF. Three had the organism also isolated from blood, and one had *Ureaplasma* isolated from a tracheal sample. One infant died and had a postmortem brain culture positive for *Ureaplasma*. None had intracranial hemorrhage.

Valencia and associates[129] isolated *M. hominis* from 9 and *Ureaplasma* from 1 of 69 consecutive infants in whom CSF was cultured within the first 3 months of life for suspected sepsis. The CSF indices, except for bloody specimens, were considered to be normal for newborns. Only 1 of the infants whose CSF culture grew *M. hominis* had clinical signs compatible with systemic infection. The other infants were healthy but were evaluated secondary to maternal fever and prolonged rupture of membranes. All 10 infants received ampicillin and gentamicin, antimicrobial agents without good activity against these organisms, and had a good clinical outcome.

In cultures of CSF from 920 infants in a neonatal intensive care unit, *Ureaplasma* was isolated from 2 (0.2%), and *M. hominis* was isolated from none.[113] Likitnukul and colleagues[130] and Mårdh[132] failed to recover mycoplasmas from CSF of infants in prospective investigations. The study by Likitnukul's group[130] involved infants who had been previously discharged from the hospital and had returned because of suspected sepsis. No mycoplasmas were recovered from the CSF of 47 preterm infants cultured within the first week of life by Izraeli and coworkers.[123] The reason for the frequent isolation of mycoplasmas in some studies but not in others is uncertain. Possible technical reasons are discussed by Waites and colleagues[147] and Heggie and associates.[148]

The question of whether mycoplasmas are linked to abnormalities on CNS imaging also has been investigated, although in an indirect manner. Perzigian and associates[96] prospectively investigated a cohort of 105 VLBW infants in whom 22 (21%) results of tracheal aspirate culture were positive for *Ureaplasma* at birth. No differences were found between the groups for intraventricular hemorrhage or cystic periventricular leukomalacia. Similarly, in a study of 464 VLBW infants, Dammann and coworkers[149] addressed the question of whether *Ureaplasma* or *M. hominis* cultured from the placenta was associated with an increased risk of cerebral white matter echolucency on ultrasonography as a measure of white matter damage. The cranial ultrasound studies were performed up to a median of 22 days of life. Culture results were as follows: 139 of 464 (30%) were positive for *Ureaplasma*, 27 (6%) were positive for *M. hominis*, and 21 (5%) were positive for *Ureaplasma* and *M. hominis*. It was found that with a positive result on culture for *Ureaplasma*, the infants were not at increased risk of cerebral white matter damage. The presence of *M. hominis* was associated with a trend toward an increased risk of echolucency ($P = .08$).

The clinical findings in newborns with *Ureaplasma* and *M. hominis* isolated from the CSF are variable. *Ureaplasma* and *M. hominis* may produce abnormal CSF indices with pleocytosis, or an inflammatory reaction in CSF may be absent.[74,83,129,134] In some infants, mycoplasmas are cleared spontaneously from the CSF, whereas in others, the organisms have been shown to persist for weeks to months even after appropriate treatment.[33,139,150-152]

OTHER SITES OF INFECTION IN THE NEONATE

M. hominis also has been isolated from pericardial fluid,[153] subcutaneous abscesses,[154-156] and the submandibular lymph node of neonates.[157] The first reported case of *M. hominis* endocarditis in a child was published more recently.[158] *Ureaplasma* and *M. hominis* have been isolated from the urine, but the clinical significance was uncertain.[130]

Other Mycoplasmas

The role of other mycoplasmas, such as *M. genitalium*, *M. fermentans*, and *M. pneumoniae*, in maternal and fetal and neonatal infections is not thought to be prominent, although investigations are limited. *M. genitalium* was not isolated by culture of the chorioamnion of 609 women or by culture or PCR assay of 232 amniotic fluid samples tested.[159] To evaluate the impact of *M. genitalium* on the outcome of pregnancy, cervical samples from 1014 women were assayed by PCR techniques for the presence of *M. genitalium*.[160] Among those women, *M. genitalium* was isolated in 6.2%, but its isolation was not significantly associated with adverse outcomes of pregnancy (preterm delivery, small for gestational age, spontaneous abortion, stillbirth). Taylor-Robinson[161] more recently reviewed disease associations with *M. genitalium*.

M. fermentans was detected in amniotic fluid collected at the time of cesarean section from 4 of 232 women with intact membranes.[159] Placental tissue also was positive for *M. fermentans* on PCR assay in three women. Villitis and chorioamnionitis were present in two of the four positive specimens, and no other organisms were detected.

Diagnosis

Culture and PCR assay are appropriate methods for the diagnosis of *Mycoplasma* and *Ureaplasma* infections. Culture of *Ureaplasma* and *M. hominis* requires special handling, however, with techniques and media generally unavailable outside major medical centers or reference laboratories. Detailed laboratory techniques for culture and identification of mycoplasmas and ureaplasmas have been reviewed by others.[33,162]

Ureaplasmas and mycoplasmas are extremely susceptible to adverse environmental conditions. Correct methods of collecting, processing, and transporting specimens are important for reliable and interpretable culture results. A specific ureaplasmal transport medium, such as Shepard 10B broth,[163,164] for *Ureaplasma* and *M. hominis* should be available for direct inoculation of clinical specimens and swabs at the time of collection. If specimens are allowed to sit at room temperature and are not inoculated into appropriate media, the recovery of these organisms is unlikely. Only swabs tipped with calcium alginate or Dacron with plastic or wire shafts should be used for sampling of mucosal surfaces. Blood should be collected free of anticoagulants and immediately inoculated into the transport medium in a 1:5 to 1:10 ratio.[33]

Specimens should be refrigerated at 4° C and protected from drying in a sealed container until transported to the laboratory. If transport to a suitable laboratory is not possible within 6 to 12 hours after collection, the specimen in appropriate transport medium should be stored at −70° C and shipped frozen on dry ice. Ureaplasmas and mycoplasmas are stable for long periods when kept frozen at −70° C in a protein-containing support medium, such as Shepard 10B broth. Storage at −20° C is less reliable and results in a significant loss in number of organisms in a relatively short time.[33] Before collecting a clinical sample for culture, it is appropriate to arrange processing of samples with the microbiology laboratory.

Ureaplasma and *M. hominis* grow within 2 to 5 days. Broth cultures are incubated at 37° C under atmospheric conditions; agar plates are incubated under 95% nitrogen and 5% carbon dioxide. Colonies of *Ureaplasma* can be identified on A8 agar by urease production. The colonies often are amorphous. Colonies of other mycoplasmas are urease negative and have a typical "fried egg" appearance (Fig. 20-3).

PCR assays for the detection of *Ureaplasma* and *M. hominis*[106,165-167] have been developed. These assays seem to have greater sensitivity than culture in most studies.[37,38,97,168,169] A combination of PCR assay and culture should give the most reliable results. Although enzyme-linked immunosorbent assays have been developed to detect *Ureaplasma*- and *M. hominis*–specific antibodies in sera, serologic testing is not recommended for the routine diagnosis of *Ureaplasma* and *M. hominis* infections. The use of these assays is limited to the research setting. Because of the fastidiousness and slow growth of *M. genitalium* and *M. fermentans*, PCR assay, in situ hybridization, and immunohistochemistry are recommended for detection of these mycoplasmas.[159,170,171]

Treatment of Neonatal Infections

A positive result on culture or PCR assay for *Ureaplasma* or *M. hominis* from a normally sterile site, particularly in the absence of other microorganisms, is justification to

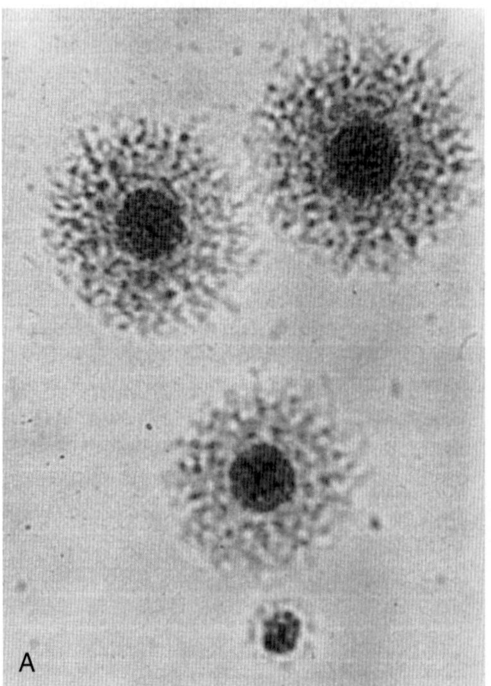

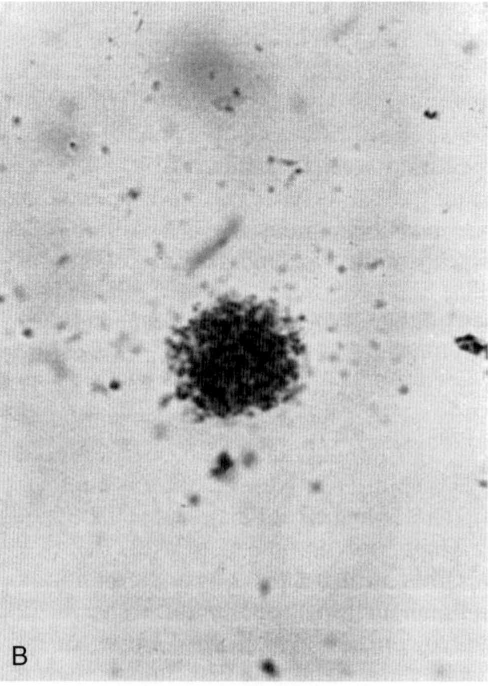

Figure 20-3 A, *Mycoplasma hominis* (original magnification 100×). **B,** *Ureaplasma* (original magnification 1000×). (Modified from Klein JO: Mycoplasmas, genitourinary tract infection, and reproductive failure, *Hosp Pract* 6:127-133, 1971.)

consider treatment for infants with evidence of infectious inflammation. On the basis of the current understanding of these organisms, however, the isolation of *Ureaplasma* or *M. hominis* in the absence of disease generally does not warrant treatment.

Formulation of guidelines for treatment when these organisms are isolated from a maternal or fetal or neonatal specimen is difficult, in view of the following considerations as reviewed in this chapter:

- Causation has not been clearly established for many conditions associated with *Ureaplasma* and *M. hominis* (all maternal and fetal and neonatal associations except postpartum and postabortal fever).
- Organisms are often present (e.g., in CSF, bloodstream, respiratory tract, amniotic fluid, or lower genital tract) with little or no adverse clinical outcome.
- Organisms are often spontaneously cleared (e.g., from CSF, bloodstream, or respiratory tract) without treatment.
- No definitive controlled trials have been performed for many sites of infection (e.g., CSF, bloodstream, amniotic fluid, lung in acute pneumonia).
- Evidence that treatment can be useful comes from uncontrolled case reports for which the outcome without treatment is unknown.
- Comparative clinical trials among antimicrobials have not been performed to assess their relative efficacy.
- Often the clinical indication for culture or PCR assay has resolved before the positive result is reported.
- However, recent randomized, placebo-controlled trials have yielded results indicating a reduction in CLD with macrolide treatment of preterm infants with *Ureaplasma* isolated from the respiratory tract. Nonetheless, more investigation is likely needed.

Treatment may be warranted in some situations, so decisions must be made on a case-by-case basis to ensure full consideration of the risk-benefit ratio related to disease and treatment. The relative contribution of *Ureaplasma* and *M. hominis* infection to morbidity and mortality is difficult to establish because most cases have been reported in VLBW preterm infants with multiple complications or in infants with clinical problems that probably contribute to the poor outcome. A recent Cochrane review concluded that there is insufficient evidence to assess whether pregnant women who have vaginal colonization with *Ureaplasma* should be treated with antibiotics to prevent preterm birth.[172] An authoritative reference suggests that definitive efficacy of antimicrobial agents in the treatment of CNS *Ureaplasma* infections in infants is lacking.[173]

The treatment of some nonneonatal *Ureaplasma* and *M. hominis* infections is better established. *Ureaplasma* urethritis and *M. hominis* pyelonephritis, pelvic inflammatory disease, postabortal fever, and postpartum fever and infections with either organism in immunocompromised patients (especially patients with hypogammaglobulinemia) generally are considered to warrant treatment.

Erythromycin generally has been considered the antimicrobial agent of choice for neonatal ureaplasmal infections (not involving the CNS), although clinical superiority over other agents has not been investigated.[174] Erythromycin has been used in most clinical trials in infants with *Ureaplasma*.[100,109,112-115] Other agents with in vitro activity against *Ureaplasma* and variable clinical experience include clarithromycin, azithromycin, doxycycline, and chloramphenicol.[90,175-178] In vitro activities of newer agents, such as quinolones and ketolides, against *Ureaplasma* have been reported; clinical experience is largely lacking.[174,179-182] Resistance to macrolides, doxycycline, fluoroquinolones, and chloramphenicol has been reported.[174,183-185] *M. hominis* is resistant to erythromycin and to other macrolides and azolides.[174-177] Doxycycline is the drug of choice for treatment of *M. hominis* infections, although resistance has been reported.[15,139,186-188] Clindamycin and chloramphenicol also are generally active in vitro against *M. hominis*.[174] In vitro activity of newer antimicrobials against *M. hominis* has been reported; clinical experience is lacking, however.[174,179-182]

Antimicrobial susceptibility testing should be considered when it is deemed necessary to treat *Ureaplasma* or *M. hominis* infection in a neonate, especially for the persistent isolation of either organism from a normally sterile site because resistance to commonly used antibiotics is not rare. Some tetracycline-resistant strains of *Ureaplasma* can be erythromycin resistant, but high-level erythromycin resistance in *Ureaplasma* is uncommon.[168] Penetration of the blood-brain barrier by antimicrobials should be considered in treating a CNS infection, as should the safety and pharmacokinetics of antimicrobials in newborns in making treatment decisions.

References

1. Fraser CM, Gocayne JD, White O, et al: The minimum gene compliment of *Mycoplasma genitalum*, *Science* 230:397-404, 1995.
2. Sung TJ, Xiao L, Duffy L, et al: Frequency of *Ureaplasma* serovars in respiratory secretions of preterm infants at risk for bronchopulmonary dysplasia, *Pediatr Infect Dis J* 30:379-383, 2011.
3. McCormack WM, Xiao L, Duffy L, et al: Sexual experience and urethral colonization with genital mycoplasmas, *Ann Intern Med* 78:696-698, 1973.
4. McCormack WM, Almeida PC, Bailey PE, et al: Sexual activity and vaginal colonization with genital mycoplasmas, *JAMA* 221: 1375-1377, 1972.
5. McCormack WM: *Ureaplasma urealyticum*: ecologic niche and epidemiologic considerations, *Pediatr Infect Dis J* 5:S232-S233, 1986.
6. McCormack WM, Rankin JS, Lee YH: Localization of genital mycoplasmas in women, *Am J Obstet Gynecol* 112:920-923, 1972.
7. Braun P, Klein JO, Lee YH, et al: Methodologic investigations and prevalence of genital mycoplasmas in pregnancy, *J Infect Dis* 121:391-400, 1970.
8. Taylor-Robinson D, McCormack WM: The genital mycoplasmas, *N Engl J Med* 302:1003-1010, 1980.
9. Faye-Kette H, La Ruche G, Ali-Napo L, et al: Genital mycoplasmas among pregnant women in Cote d'Ivoire, West Africa: prevalence and risk factors, *Int J STD AIDS* 11:599-602, 2000.
10. Clegg A, Passey M, Yoannes M, et al: High rates of genital *Mycoplasma* infection in the highlands of Papua New Guinea determined both by culture and by a commercial detection kit, *J Clin Microbiol* 35:197-200, 1997.
11. McCormack WM, Rosner B, Alpert S, et al: Vaginal colonization with *Mycoplasma hominis* and *Ureaplasma urealyticum*, *Sex Transm Dis* 134:67-70, 1986.
12. McCormack WM, Rosner B, Lee YH: Colonization with genital mycoplasmas in women, *Am J Epidemiol* 97:240-245, 1973.
13. Braun P, Lee YH, Klein JO, et al: Birth weight and genital mycoplasmas in pregnancy, *N Engl J Med* 284:167-171, 1971.
14. Mårdh PA, Weström L: T-mycoplasmas in the genitourinary tract of the female, *Acta Pathol Microbiol Scand* 78B:367-374, 1970.

15. Cassell GH, Davis JK, Waites KB, et al: Pathogenesis and significance of urogenital mycoplasmal infections. In Bondi A, editor: *Urogenital infections: new developments in laboratory diagnosis and treatment*, New York, 1987, Plenum Publishing, pp 93-115.
16. Taylor-Robinson D: *Ureaplasma urealyticum, Mycoplasma hominis*, and *Mycoplasma genitalium*. In Mandell GL, Bennett JE, Dolan R, editors: *Principles and practice of infectious diseases*, Philadelphia, 2000, Churchill Livingstone, pp 2027-2032.
17. Becopoulos T, Tsagatakis E, Constantinides C, et al: *Ureaplasma urealyticum* and infected renal calculi, *J Chemother* 3:39-41, 1991.
18. Grenabo L, Hedelin H, Pettersson S: Urinary stones caused by *Ureaplasma urealyticum*: a review, *Scand J Infect Dis Suppl* 53: 46-49, 1988.
19. Thomsen AC, Taylor-Robinson D, Brogaard Hansen K, et al: The infrequent occurrence of mycoplasmas in amniotic fluid from women with intact fetal membranes, *Acta Obstet Gynecol Scand* 3:425-429, 1983.
20. Mårdh PA, Weström L: Tubal and cervical cultures in acute salpingitis with special reference to *Mycoplasma hominis* and T-strain mycoplasmas, *Br J Vener Dis* 46:179-186, 1970.
21. Mårdh PA: Mycoplasmal PID: a review of natural and experimental infections, *Yale J Biol Med* 56:529, 1983.
22. Miettinen A, Paavonen J, Jansson E, et al: Enzyme immunoassay for serum antibody to *Mycoplasma hominis* in women with acute pelvic inflammatory disease, *Sex Transm Dis* 10(Suppl 4):289, 1983.
23. Henry-Suchet J, Catalan F, Loffredo V, et al: Microbiology of specimens obtained by laparoscopy from controls and from patients with pelvic inflammatory disease or infertility with tubal obstruction: *Chlamydia trachomatis* and *Ureaplasma urealyticum*, *Am J Obstet Gynecol* 138:1022-1925, 1980.
24. Moller BR, Freundt EA, Black FT, et al: Experimental infection of the genital tract of female grivet monkeys by Mycoplasma hominis, *Infect Immun* 20:248-257, 1978.
25. Mårdh PA, Weström L, Mecklenburg C: Studies on ciliated epithelia of the human genital tract. I. Swelling of the cilia of fallopian tube epithelium in organ cultures infected with *Mycoplasma hominis*, *Br J Vener Dis* 52:52-57, 1976.
26. Ureaplasmas of humans: with emphasis on maternal and neonatal infections. Proceedings of an international symposium of the International Organization for Mycoplasmology. Seattle, Washington, October 10-12, 1985. Tribute to Dr. Maurice Charles Shepard, *Pediatr Infect Dis* 5(Suppl 6):S221-S354, 1986.
27. Cassell GH, Davis RO, Waites KB, et al: Isolation of *Mycoplasma hominis* and *Ureaplasma urealyticum* from amniotic fluid at 16–20 weeks gestation: potential effect on pregnancy outcome, *Sex Transm Dis* 10:294-302, 1983.
28. Embree JE, Krause VW, Embil JA, et al: Placental infection with *Mycoplasma hominis* and *Ureaplasma urealyticum*: clinical correlation, *Obstet Gynecol* 56:475-481, 1980.
29. Hillier SL, Martius J, Krohn M, et al: A case-control study of chorioamnionic infection and histologic chorioamnionitis in prematurity, *N Engl J Med* 319:972-978, 1988.
30. Kundsin RB, Driscoll SG, Monson RR, et al: Association of *Ureaplasma urealyticum* in the placenta with perinatal morbidity and mortality, *N Engl J Med* 310:941-945, 1984.
31. Quinn PA, Butany J, Chipman M, et al: A prospective study of microbial infection in stillbirths and early neonatal death, *Am J Obstet Gynecol* 151:238-249, 1985.
32. Quinn PA, Butany J, Taylor J, et al: Chorioamnionitis: its association with pregnancy outcome and microbial infection, *Am J Obstet Gynecol* 156:379-387, 1987.
33. Cassell GH, Waites KB, Crouse DT: Mycoplasmal infections. In Remington JS, Klein JO, editors: *Infectious diseases of the fetus and newborn infant*, ed 5, Philadelphia, 2001, Saunders, pp 733-767.
34. Gray DJ, Robinson HB, Malone J, et al: Adverse outcome in pregnancy following amniotic fluid isolation of *Ureaplasma urealyticum*, *Prenat Diagn* 12:111-117, 1992.
35. Foulon W, Naessens A, Dewaele M, et al: Chronic *Ureaplasma urealyticum* amnionitis associated with abruptio placentae, *Obstet Gynecol* 68:280-282, 1986.
36. Cassell GH, Waites KB, Gibbs RS, et al: The role of *Ureaplasma urealyticum* in amnionitis, *Pediatr Infect Dis J* 5:247-252, 1986.
37. Yoon BH, Romero R, Kim M, et al: Clinical implications of detection of *Ureaplasma urealyticum* in the amniotic cavity with the polymerase chain reaction, *Am J Obstet Gynecol* 183:1130-1137, 2000.
38. Yoon BH, Romero R, Lim JH, et al: The clinical significance of detecting *Ureaplasma urealyticum* by the polymerase chain reaction in the amniotic fluid of patients with preterm labor, *Am J Obstet Gynecol* 189:919-924, 2003.
39. Stokes EJ: Human infection with pleuropneumonia-like organisms, *Lancet* 1:276-279, 1955.
40. Harwick HJ, Purcell RH, Iuppa JB, et al: *Mycoplasma hominis* and abortion, *J Infect Dis* 121:260-268, 1970.
41. Harwick HJ, Iuppa JB, Purcell RH, et al: *Mycoplasma hominis* septicemia associated with abortion, *Am J Obstet Gynecol* 99:725-727, 1967.
42. Tully JG, Brown MS, Sheagren JN, et al: Septicemia due to *Mycoplasma hominis* type 1, *N Engl J Med* 273:648-650, 1965.
43. Caspi E, Herczeg E, Solomon F, et al: Amnionitis and T strain mycoplasmemia, *Am J Obstet Gynecol* 111:1102-1106, 1971.
44. Sompolinsky D, Solomon F, Leiba H, et al: Puerperal sepsis due to T-strain *Mycoplasma*, *Isr J Med Sci* 7:745-748, 1971.
45. Edelin KC, McCormack WM: Infection with *Mycoplasma hominis* in postpartum fever, *Lancet* 2:1217-1221, 1980.
46. McCormack WM, Rosner B, Lee YH, et al: Isolation of genital mycoplasmas from blood obtained shortly after vaginal delivery, *Lancet* 1:596-599, 1975.
47. Neman-Simha V, Renaudin H, de Barbeyrac B, et al: Isolation of genital mycoplasmas from blood of febrile obstetrical-gynecologic patients and neonates, *Scand J Infect Dis* 24:317-321, 1992.
48. Andrews W, Shah SR, Goldenberg RL, et al: Post-cesarean endometritis: role of asymptomatic antenatal colonization of the chorioamnion with *Ureaplasma urealyticum*, *Am J Obstet Gynecol* 170:416, 1994.
49. Roberts S, Maccato M, Faro S, et al: The microbiology of post-cesarean wound morbidity, *Obstet Gynecol* 81:383-386, 1993.
50. Mycoplasma hominis. Newsnotes, *BMJ* 2:816, 1974.
51. Word BM, Baldridge A: *Mycoplasma hominis* pneumonia and pleural effusion in a postpartum adolescent, *Pediatr Infect Dis J* 9:295-296, 1990.
52. Young MJ, Cox RA: Near fatal puerperal fever due to *Mycoplasma hominis*, *Postgrad Med J* 66:147-149, 1990.
53. Phillips LE, Faro S, Pokorny SF, et al: Postcesarean wound infection by *Mycoplasma hominis* in a patient with persistent postpartum fever, *Diagn Microbiol Infect Dis* 7:193-197, 1987.
54. Maccato M, Faro S, Summers KL: Wound infections after cesarean section with *Mycoplasma hominis* and *Ureaplasma urealyticum*: a report of three cases, *Diagn Microbiol Infect Dis* 13:363-365, 1990.
55. Andrews WW, Hauth JC, Cliver SP, et al: Randomized clinical trial of extended spectrum antibiotic prophylaxis with coverage for *Ureaplasma urealyticum* to reduce post-cesarean delivery endometritis, *Obstet Gynecol* 101:1183-1189, 2003.
56. Donders GG, Van Bulck B, Caudron J, et al: Relationship of bacterial vaginosis and mycoplasmas to the risk of spontaneous abortion, *Am J Obstet Gynecol* 183:431-437, 2000.
57. Cassell GH, Cole BC: Mycoplasmas as agents of human disease, *N Engl J Med* 304:80-89, 1981.
58. McCormack WM, Taylor-Robinson D: The genital mycoplasmas. In Holmes KK, editor: *Sexually transmitted diseases*, New York, 1984, McGraw-Hill, pp 408-419.
59. Sompolinsky D, Solomon F, Elkina L, et al: Infections with Mycoplasma and bacteria in induced midtrimester abortion and fetal loss, *Am J Obstet Gynecol* 121:610-616, 1975.
60. Stray-Pederson B, Engard J, Reikvam TM: Uterine T-*Mycoplasma* colonization in reproductive failure, *Am J Obstet Gynecol* 130:307, 1978.
61. Naessens A, Foulon W, Cammu H, et al: Epidemiology and pathogenesis of *Ureaplasma urealyticum* in spontaneous abortion and early preterm labor, *Acta Obstet Gynecol Scand* 66:513-516, 1987.
62. Quinn PA, Shewchuk AB, Shuber J, et al: Serologic evidence of *Ureaplasma urealyticum* infection in women with spontaneous pregnancy loss, *Am J Obstet Gynecol* 145:245-250, 1983.
63. Berg TG, Philpot KL, Welsh MS, et al: *Ureaplasma/Mycoplasma*-infected amniotic fluid: pregnancy outcome in treated and nontreated patients, *J Perinatol* 19:275-277, 1999.
64. Cassell GH, Waites KB, Watson HL, et al: *Ureaplasma urealyticum* intrauterine infection: role in prematurity and disease in newborns, *Clin Microbiol Rev* 6:69-87, 1993.
65. Romero R, Mazor M, Oyarzun E, et al: Is genital colonization with *Mycoplasma hominis* or *Ureaplasma urealyticum* associated with prematurity/low birth weight? *Obstet Gynecol* 73:532-536, 1989.

66. Gerber S, Vial Y, Hohlfeld P, et al: Detection of *Ureaplasma urealyticum* in second-trimester amniotic fluid by polymerase chain reaction correlates with subsequent preterm labor and delivery, *J Infect Dis* 187:518-521, 2003.
67. Gravett MG, Hummel D, Eschenbach DA, et al: Preterm labor associated with subclinical amniotic fluid infection and with bacterial vaginosis, *Obstet Gynecol* 67:229-237, 1986.
68. Romero R, Sirtori M, Oyarzun E, et al: Infection and labor. V. Prevalence, microbiology, and clinical significance of intraamniotic infection in women with preterm labor and intact membranes, *Am J Obstet Gynecol* 161:817-824, 1989.
69. Watts DH, Krohn MA, Hillier SL, et al: The association of occult amniotic fluid infection with gestational age and neonatal outcome among women in preterm labor, *Obstet Gynecol* 79:351-357, 1992.
70. Hillier SL, Krohn MA, Kiviat NB, et al: Microbiologic causes and neonatal outcomes associated with chorioamnion infection, *Am J Obstet Gynecol* 165:955-961, 1991.
71. Naessens A, Foulon W, Breynaert J, et al: Postpartum bacteremia and placental colonization with genital mycoplasmas and pregnancy outcome, *Am J Obstet Gynecol* 160:647-650, 1989.
72. Zlatnik FJ, Gellhaus TM, Benda JA, et al: Histologic chorioamnionitis, microbial infection, and prematurity, *J Obstet Gynaecol* 76:355-359, 1990.
73. Quinn PA, Gillan JE, Markestad T, et al: Intrauterine infection with *Ureaplasma urealyticum* as a cause of fatal neonatal pneumonia, *Pediatr Infect Dis J* 4:538-543, 1985.
74. Ollikainen J, Hiekkaniemi H, Korppi M, et al: *Ureaplasma urealyticum* infection associated with acute respiratory insufficiency and death in premature infants, *J Pediatr* 122:756-760, 1993.
75. Cassell GH, Waites KB, Crouse DT, et al: Association of *Ureaplasma urealyticum* infection of the lower respiratory tract with chronic lung disease and death in very low birthweight infants, *Lancet* 2:240-245, 1988.
76. Kelly VN, Garland SM, Gilbert GL: Isolation of genital mycoplasmas from the blood of neonates and women with pelvic infection using conventional SPS-free blood culture media, *Pathology* 19:277-280, 1987.
77. Syrogiannopoulos GA, Kapatais-Zoumbos K, Decavalas GO, et al: *Ureaplasma urealyticum* colonization of full term infants: perinatal acquisition and persistence during early infancy, *Pediatr Infect Dis J* 9:236-240, 1990.
78. Sanchez P, Regan JA: Vertical transmission of *Ureaplasma urealyticum* in full term infants, *Pediatr Infect Dis J* 6:825-828, 1988.
79. Sanchez P, Regan JA: Vertical transmission of *Ureaplasma urealyticum* from mothers to preterm infants, *Pediatr Infect Dis J* 9:398-401, 1990.
80. Dinsmoor MJ, Ramamurthy RS, Gibbs RS: Transmission of genital mycoplasmas from mother to neonate in women with prolonged membrane rupture, *Pediatr Infect Dis J* 8:483-487, 1989.
81. Chua KB, Ngeow YF, Lim CT, et al: Colonization and transmission of *Ureaplasma urealyticum* and *Mycoplasma hominis* from mothers to full and preterm babies by normal vaginal delivery, *Med J Malaysia* 54:242-246, 1999.
82. Foy HM, Kenny GE, Levinsohn EM, et al: Acquisition of mycoplasmata and T-strains during infancy, *J Infect Dis* 121:579-587, 1970.
83. Waites KB, Rudd PT, Crouse DT, et al: Chronic *Ureaplasma urealyticum* and *Mycoplasma hominis* infections of central nervous systems in preterm infants, *Lancet* 2:17-21, 1988.
84. Waites KB, Crouse DT, Philips JB 3rd, et al: *Ureaplasma* pneumonia and sepsis associated with persistent pulmonary hypertension of the newborn, *Pediatrics* 83:84-89, 1991.
85. Brus F, van Waarde WM, Schoots C, et al: Fatal ureaplasmal pneumonia and sepsis in a newborn infant, *Eur J Pediatr* 150:782-783, 1991.
86. Tafari N, Ross S, Naeye RL, et al: *Mycoplasma* "T" strains and perinatal death, *Lancet* 1:108-109, 1976.
87. Crouse DT, Odrezin GT, Cutter GR, et al: Radiographic changes associated with tracheal isolation of *Ureaplasma urealyticum* from neonates, *Clin Infect Dis* 17(Suppl 1):S122-S130, 1993.
88. Cultrera R, Seraceni S, Germani R, et al: Molecular evidence of *Ureaplasma urealyticum* and *Ureaplasma parvum* colonization in preterm infants during respiratory distress syndrome, *BMC Infect Dis* 6:166, 2006.
89. Hannaford K, Todd DA, Jeffery H, et al: Role of *Ureaplasma urealyticum* in lung disease of prematurity, *Arch Dis Child Fetal Neonatal* 81:F162-F167, 1999.
90. Berger A, Witt A, Haiden N, et al: Microbial invasion of the amniotic cavity at birth is associated with adverse short-term outcome of preterm infants, *J Perinat Med* 31:115-121, 2003.
91. Escobedo MB, Hilliard JL, Smith F, et al: A baboon model of bronchopulmonary dysplasia, *Exp Mol Pathol* 37:323-324, 1982.
92. Walsh WF, Butler J, Coalson J, et al: A primate model of *Ureaplasma urealyticum* infection in the premature infant with hyaline membrane disease, *Clin Infect Dis* 17:S158-S162, 1993.
93. Yoder BA, Coalson JJ, Winter VT, et al: Effects of antenatal colonization with *Ureaplasma urealyticum* on pulmonary disease in the immature baboon, *Pediatr Res* 54:797-807, 2003.
94. Wang EEL, Ohlsson A, Kellner JD: Association of *Ureaplasma urealyticum* colonization with chronic lung disease of prematurity: results of a metaanalysis, *J Pediatr* 127:640-644, 1995.
95. Benstein BD, Crouse DT, Shanklin DR, et al: *Ureaplasma* in lung. 2. Association with bronchopulmonary dysplasia in premature newborns, *Exp Mol Pathol* 75:171-177, 2003.
96. Perzigian RW, Adams JT, Weiner GM, et al: *Ureaplasma urealyticum* and chronic lung disease in very low birth weight infants during the exogenous surfactant era, *Pediatr Infect Dis J* 17:620-625, 1998.
97. Castro-Alcaraz S, Greenberg EM, Bateman DA, et al: Patterns of colonization with *Ureaplasma urealyticum* during neonatal intensive care unit hospitalizations of very low birth weight infants and the development of chronic lung disease, *Pediatrics* 110:e45, 2002.
98. Garland SM, Bowman ED: Role of *Ureaplasma urealyticum* and *Chlamydia trachomatis* in lung disease in low birth weight infants, *Pathology* 28:266-269, 1996.
99. Iles R, Lyon A, Ross P, McIntosh N: Infection with *Ureaplasma urealyticum* and *Mycoplasma hominis* and the development of chronic lung disease in pre-term infants, *Acta Paediatr* 85:482-484, 1996.
100. Pacifico L, Panero A, Roggini M, et al: *Ureaplasma urealyticum* and pulmonary outcome in a neonatal intensive care population, *Pediatr Infect Dis J* 16:579-586, 1997.
101. Kafetzis DA, Skevaki CL, Skouteri V, et al: Maternal genital colonization with *Ureaplasma urealyticum* promotes preterm delivery: association of the respiratory colonization of premature infants with chronic lung disease and increased mortality, *Clin Infect Dis* 39:1113-1122, 2004.
102. Abele-Horn M, Genzel-Boroviczény O, Uhlig T, et al: *Ureaplasma urealyticum* colonization and bronchopulmonary dysplasia: a comparative prospective multicentre study, *Eur J Pediatr* 157:1004-1011, 1998.
103. Agarwal P, Rajadurai VS, Pradeepkumar VK, et al: *Ureaplasma urealyticum* and its association with chronic lung disease in Asian neonates, *J Paediatr Child Health* 36:487-490, 2000.
104. Da Silva, O, Gregson D, Hammerberg O: Role of *Ureaplasma urealyticum* and *Chlamydia trachomatis* in development of bronchopulmonary dysplasia in very low birth weight infants, *Pediatr Infect Dis J* 16:364-369, 1997.
105. Van Waarde WM, Brus F, Okken A, et al: *Ureaplasma urealyticum* colonization, prematurity and bronchopulmonary dysplasia, *Eur Respir J* 10:886-890, 1997.
106. Couroucli XI, Welty SE, Ramsay PL, et al: Detection of microorganisms in the tracheal aspirates of preterm infants by polymerase chain reaction: association of adenovirus infection with bronchopulmonary dysplasia, *Pediatr Res* 47:225-232, 2000.
107. Cordero L, Coley BD, Miller RL, et al: Bacterial and *Ureaplasma* colonization of the airway: radiologic findings in infants with bronchopulmonary dysplasia, *J Perinatol* 17:428-433, 1997.
108. Heggie AD, Bar-Shain D, Boxerbaum B, et al: Identification and quantification of ureaplasmas colonizing the respiratory tract and assessment of their role in the development of chronic lung disease in preterm infants, *Pediatr Infect Dis J* 20:854-859, 2001.
109. Jonsson B, Rylander M, Faxelius G: *Ureaplasma urealyticum*, erythromycin and respiratory morbidity in high-risk preterm neonates, *Acta Paediatr* 87:1079-1084, 1998.
110. Ollikainen J, Korppi M, Heiskanen-Kosma T, et al: Chronic lung disease of the newborn is not associated with *Ureaplasma urealyticum*, *Pediatr Pulmonol* 32:303-307, 2001.
111. Schelonka RL, Katz B, Waites KB, et al: Critical appraisal of the role of *Ureaplasma* in the development of bronchopulmonary dysplasia with metaanalytic techniques, *Pediatr Infect Dis J* 24:1033-1039, 2005.
112. Buhrer C, Hoehn T, Hentschel J: Role of erythromycin for treatment of incipient chronic lung disease in preterm infants colonised with Ureaplasma urealyticum, *Drugs* 61:1893-1899, 2001.

113. Heggie AD, Jacobs MR, Butler VT, et al: Frequency and significance of isolation of *Ureaplasma urealyticum* and *Mycoplasma hominis* from cerebrospinal fluid and tracheal aspirate specimens from low birth weight infants, *J Pediatr* 124:956-961, 1994.
114. Lyon AJ, McColm J, Middlemist L, et al: Randomised trial of erythromycin on the development of chronic lung disease in preterm infants, *Arch Dis Child Fetal Neonatal Ed* 78:F10-F14, 1998.
115. Bowman ED, Dharmalingam A, Fan WQ, et al: Impact of erythromycin on respiratory colonization of *Ureaplasma urealyticum* and the development of chronic lung disease in extremely low birth weight infants, *Pediatr Infect Dis J* 17:615-620, 1998.
116. Ozdemir R, Erdeve O, Dizdar EA, et al: Clarithromycin in preventing bronchopulmonary dysplasia in *Ureaplasma urealyticum*–positive preterm infants, *Pediatrics* 128:e1496-e1501, 2011.
117. Ballard HO, Shook LA, Bernard P, et al: Use of azithromycin for the prevention of bronchopulmonary dysplasia in preterm infants: a randomized, double-blind, placebo controlled trial, *Pediatr Pulmonol* 46:111-118, 2011.
118. Viscardi RM, Othman AA, Hassan HE, et al: Azithromycin to prevent bronchopulmonary dysplasia in *Ureaplasma*-infected preterm infants: pharmacokinetics, safety, microbial response, and clinical outcomes with a 20-milligram-per-kilogram single intravenous dose, *Antimicrob Agents Chemother* 57:2127-2133, 2013.
119. Kenyon SL, Taylor DJ, Tarnow-Mordi W: Broad-spectrum antibiotics for preterm, prelabour rupture of fetal membranes: the ORACLE I randomised trial. ORACLE Collaborative Group, *Lancet* 357: 979-988, 2001.
120. Kenyon SL, Taylor DJ, Tarnow-Mordi W: Broad-spectrum antibiotics for spontaneous preterm labour: the ORACLE II randomised trial. ORACLE Collaborative Group, *Lancet* 357:989-994, 2001.
121. Ollikainen J: Perinatal *Ureaplasma urealyticum* infection increases the need for hospital treatment during the first year of life in preterm infants, *Pediatr Pulmonol* 30:402-405, 2000.
122. Viscardi RM, Atamas SP, Luzina IG, et al: Antenatal *Ureaplasma urealyticum* respiratory tract infection stimulates proinflammatory, profibrotic responses in the preterm baboon lung, *Pediatr Res* 60:141-146, 2006.
123. Izraeli S, Samra Z, Sirota L, et al: Genital mycoplasmas in preterm infants: prevalence and clinical significance, *Eur J Pediatr* 150: 804-807, 1991.
124. Taylor-Robinson D, Furr PM, Liberman MM: The occurrence of genital mycoplasmas in babies with and without respiratory diseases, *Acta Paediatr Scand* 73:383-386, 1984.
125. Steytler JG: Statistical studies on mycoplasma-positive human umbilical cord blood cultures, *S Afr J Obstet Gynecol* 8:10-13, 1970.
126. Ollikainen J, Hiekkaniemi H, Korppi M, et al: *Ureaplasma urealyticum* cultured from brain tissue of preterm twins who died of intraventricular hemorrhage, *Scand J Infect Dis* 25:529-531, 1993.
127. Dan M, Tyrrell DL, Stemke GW, et al: *Mycoplasma hominis* septicemia in a burned infant, *J Pediatr* 99:743-744, 1981.
128. Unsworth PF, Taylor-Robinson D, Shoo EE, Furr PM: Neonatal mycoplasmemia. *Mycoplasma hominis* as a significant cause of disease? *J Infect* 10:163-168, 1985.
129. Valencia GB, Taylor-Robinson D, Shoo EE, et al: *Mycoplasma hominis* and *Ureaplasma urealyticum* in neonates with suspected infection, *Pediatr Infect Dis J* 12:571-573, 1993.
130. Likitnukul S, Kusmiesz H, Nelson JD, et al: Role of genital mycoplasmas in young infants with suspected sepsis, *J Pediatr* 109:971-974, 1986.
131. Goldenberg RL, Andrews WW, Goepfert AR, et al: The Alabama preterm birth study: umbilical cord blood *Ureaplasma urealyticum* and *Mycoplasma hominis* cultures in very preterm newborn infants, *Am J Obstet Gynecol* 198:43.e1-43.e5, 2008.
132. Mårdh PA: *Mycoplasma hominis* infections of the central nervous system in newborn infants, *Sex Transm Dis* 10:331-334, 1983.
133. McDonald JC: *Mycoplasma hominis* meningitis in a premature infant, *Pediatr Infect Dis J* 7:795-798, 1988.
134. Wealthall SR: *Mycoplasma* meningitis in infants with spina bifida, *Dev Med Child Neurol* 17:117-122, 1975.
135. Siber GR, Alpert S, Smith AL, et al: Neonatal central nervous system infection due to *Mycoplasma hominis*, *J Pediatr* 90:625-627, 1977.
136. Kirk N, Kovar I: *Mycoplasma hominis* meningitis in a preterm infant, *J Infect* 15:109-110, 1987.
137. Hjelm E, Jonsell G, Linglöf T, et al: Meningitis in a newborn infant caused by *Mycoplasma hominis*, *Acta Paediatr Scand* 69:415-418, 1980.
138. Gewitz M, Dinwiddie R, Rees L, et al: *Mycoplasma hominis*: a cause of neonatal meningitis, *Arch Dis Child* 54:231-233, 1979.
139. Gilbert GL, Law F, Macinnes SJ: Chronic *Mycoplasma hominis* infection complicating severe intraventricular hemorrhage, in a premature neonate, *Pediatr Infect Dis J* 7:817-818, 1988.
140. Boe O, Diderichsen J, Matre R: Isolation of *Mycoplasma hominis* from cerebrospinal fluid, *Scand J Infect Dis* 5:285-288, 1973.
141. Rao RP, Ghanayem NS, Kaufman BA, et al: *Mycoplasma hominis* and *Ureaplasma* species brain abscess in a neonate, *Pediatr Infect Dis J* 21:1083-1085, 2002.
142. Knausz M, Niederland T, Dósa E, et al: Meningo-encephalitis in a neonate caused by maternal *Mycoplasma hominis* treated successfully with chloramphenicol, *J Med Microbiol* 51:187-188, 2002.
143. Waites KB, Duffy LB, Crouse DT, et al: Mycoplasmal infection of cerebrospinal fluid in newborn infants from a community hospital population, *Pediatr Infect Dis J* 9:241-245, 1990.
144. Waites KB, Crouse DT, Cassell GH: Systemic neonatal infection due to *Ureaplasma urealyticum*, *Clin Infect Dis*(Suppl 1)S131-S135, 1993.
145. Waites KB, Duffy LB, Crouse DT, et al: Mycoplasmal infections of cerebrospinal fluid in newborn infants from a community hospital population, *Pediatr Infect Dis J* 9:241-245, 1990.
146. Shaw NJ, Pratt BC, Weindling AM: *Ureaplasma* and *Mycoplasma* infections of central nervous systems in preterm infants, *Lancet* 2:1530-1531, 1989.
147. Waites KB, Cassell GH, Duffy LB, et al: Isolation of *Ureaplasma urealyticum* from low birth weight infants, *J Pediatr* 126:502-504, 1995.
148. Waites KB, Cassell GH, Duffy LB, et al: Isolation of *Ureaplasma urealyticum* from low birth weight infants, *J Pediatr* 126:502-504, 1995.
149. Heggie AD, et al: Antenatal *Mycoplasma* infection, the fetal inflammatory response and cerebral white matter damage in very-low-birthweight infants, *Paediatr Perinat Epidemiol* 17:49-57, 2003.
150. Shaw NJ, Pratt BC, Weindling AM: *Ureaplasma* and *Mycoplasma* infections of the central nervous system in preterm infants, *Lancet* 23:1530-1531, 1989.
151. Waites KB, Brown MB, Stagno S, et al: Association of genital mycoplasmas with exudative vaginitis in a 10 year old: a case of misdiagnosis, *Pediatrics* 71:250-252, 1983.
152. Garland SM, Murton LJ: Neonatal meningitis caused by Ureaplasma urealyticum, *Pediatr Infect Dis J* 6:868-870, 1987.
153. Miller TC, Baman SI, Albers WH: Massive pericardial effusion due to *Mycoplasma hominis* in a newborn, *Am J Dis Child* 136:271-272, 1982.
154. Glaser JB, Engelbert M, Hamerschlag M: Scalp abscess associated with *Mycoplasma hominis* infection complicating intrapartum monitoring, *Pediatr Infect Dis J* 2:468-470, 1983.
155. Sacker I, Brunell PA: Abscess in newborn infants caused by *Mycoplasma*, *Pediatrics* 46:303-304, 1970.
156. Abdel-Haq N, Asmar B, Brown W: *Mycoplasma hominis* scalp abscess in the newborn, *Pediatr Infect Dis J* 21:1171-1173, 2002.
157. Powell DA, Miller K, Clyde WA Jr: Submandibular adenitis in a newborn caused by Mycoplasma hominis, *Pediatrics* 63:789-799, 1979.
158. Dominguez SR, Littlehorn C, Nyquist AC: *Mycoplasma hominis* endocarditis in a child with a complex congenital heart defect, *Pediatr Infect Dis J* 25:851-852, 2006.
159. Blanchard A, Hamrick W, Duffy L, et al: Use of the polymerase chain reaction for detection of *Mycoplasma fermentans* and *Mycoplasma genitalium* in the urogenital tract and amniotic fluid, *Clin Infect Dis* 17(Suppl 1):S272-S279, 1993.
160. Labbe AC, Frost E, Deslandes S, et al: *Mycoplasma genitalium* is not associated with adverse outcomes of pregnancy in Guinea-Bissau, *Sex Transm Infect* 78:289-291, 2002.
161. Taylor-Robinson D: *Mycoplasma genitalium*—an up-date, *Int J STD AIDS* 13:145-151, 2002.
162. Cassell GH, Blanchard A, Duffy L, et al: Mycoplasmas. In Howard BJ, editor: *Clinical and pathogenic microbiology*, St. Louis, 1994, Mosby-Year Book, pp 491-502.
163. Shepard MC, Masover GK: Special features of ureaplasmas. In Barile MF, Razin S, editors: *The mycoplasmas. I. Cell biology*, New York, 1979, Academic Press, pp 452-494.
164. Shepard MC: Culture media for ureaplasmas. In Razin S, Tully JG, editors: *Methods in mycoplasmology*, New York, 1983, Academic Press.
165. Blanchard A, Hentschel J, Duffy L, et al: Detection of *Ureaplasma urealyticum* by polymerase chain reaction in the urogenital tract of adults, in amniotic fluid, and in the respiratory tract of newborns, *Clin Infect Dis* 17(Suppl 1):S148-S153, 1993.

166. Blanchard A, Yáñez A, Dybvig K, et al: Evaluation of intraspecies genetic variation within the 16S rRNA gene of *Mycoplasma hominis* and detection by polymerase chain reaction, *J Clin Microbiol* 31:1358-1361, 1993.
167. Luki N, Lebel P, Boucher M, et al: Comparison of polymerase chain reaction assay with culture for detection of genital mycoplasmas in perinatal infections, *Eur J Clin Microbiol Infect Dis* 17:255-263, 1998.
168. Abele-Horn M, Wolff C, Dressel P, et al: Polymerase chain reaction versus culture for detection of *Ureaplasma urealyticum* and *Mycoplasma hominis* in the urogenital tract of adults and the respiratory tract of newborns, *Eur J Clin Microbiol Infect Dis* 15:595-598, 1996.
169. Cunliffe NA, Fergusson S, Davidson F, et al: Comparison of culture with the polymerase chain reaction for detection of *Ureaplasma urealyticum* in endotracheal aspirates of preterm infants, *J Med Microbiol* 45:27-30, 1996.
170. de Barbeyrac B, Bernet-Poggi C, Fébrer F, et al: Detection of *Mycoplasma pneumoniae* and *Mycoplasma genitalium* in clinical samples by polymerase chain reaction, *Clin Infect Dis* 17(Suppl 1):S83-S89, 1993.
171. Lo SC, Dawson MS, Wong DM, et al: Identification of *Mycoplasma incognitus* infection in patients with AIDS: an immunohistochemistry, in situ hybridization and ultrastructural study, *Am J Trop Med Hyg* 41:601-616, 1989.
172. Raynes Greenow CH, Roberts CL, Bell JC, et al: Antibiotics for *Ureaplasma* in the vagina in pregnancy, *Cochrane Database Syst Rev*(9): CD003767, 2011.
173. American Academy of Pediatrics: *Ureaplasma urealyticum* infections. In Pickering LK, editor: *Red Book: 2012 Report of the Committee on Infectious Diseases*, Elk Grove Village, Ill, 2012, American Academy of Pediatrics, pp 772-774.
174. Taylor-Robinson D, Bebear C: Antibiotic susceptibilities of mycoplasmas and treatment of *Mycoplasma* infections, *J Antimicrob Chemother* 40:622-630, 1997.
175. Waites KB, Crouse DT, Cassell GH: Antibiotic susceptibilities and therapeutic options for *Ureaplasma urealyticum* infections in neonates, *Pediatr Infect Dis J* 11:23-29, 1992.
176. Waites KB, Crouse DT, Cassell GH: Therapeutic consideration for *Ureaplasma urealyticum* infections in neonates, *Clin Infect Dis* 17(Suppl 1):S208-S214, 1993.
177. Waites KB, Cassell GH, Canupp KC, et al: In vitro susceptibilities of mycoplasmas and ureaplasmas to new macrolides and aryl-fluoroquinolones, *Antimicrob Agents Chemother* 32:1500-1502, 1988.
178. Kober MB, Mason BA: Colonization of the female genital tract by resistant *Ureaplasma urealyticum* treated successfully with azithromycin, *Clin Infect Dis* 278:401-402, 1998.
179. Waites KB, Crabb DM, Bing X, et al: In vitro susceptibilities to and bactericidal activities of garenoxacin (BMS-284756) and other antimicrobial agents against human mycoplasmas and ureaplasmas, *Antimicrob Agents Chemother* 47:161-165, 2003.
180. Kenny GE, Cartwright FD: Susceptibilities of *Mycoplasma hominis, M. pneumoniae*, and *Ureaplasma urealyticum* to GAR-936, dalfopristin, dirithromycin, evernimicin, gatifloxacin, linezolid, moxifloxacin, quinupristin-dalfopristin, and telithromycin compared to their susceptibilities to reference macrolides, tetracyclines, and quinolones, *Antimicrob Agents Chemother* 45:2604-2608, 2001.
181. Waites KB, Crabb DM, Duffy LB: In vitro activities of ABT-773 and other antimicrobials against human mycoplasmas, *Antimicrob Agents Chemother* 47:39-42, 2003.
182. Bebear CM, Renaudin H, Charron A, et al: In vitro activity of trovafloxacin compared to those of five antimicrobials against mycoplasmas including *Mycoplasma hominis* and *Ureaplasma urealyticum* fluoroquinolone-resistant isolates that have been genetically characterized, *Antimicrob Agents Chemother* 44:2557-2560, 2000.
183. Braun P, Klein JO, Kass EH: Susceptibility of *Mycoplasma hominis* and T-strains to 14 antimicrobial agents, *Appl Microbiol* 19:62-70, 1970.
184. Thornsberry C, Barry AJ: *1988 Methods for dilution-anti-microbial susceptibility tests for bacteria that grow aerobically. Tentative standards*, ed 2, Villanova, PA, 1988, National Committee for Clinical Laboratory Standards.
185. Duffy L, Glass J, Hall G, et al: Fluoroquinolone resistance in *Ureaplasma parvum* in the United States, *J Clin Microbiol* 44:1590-1591, 2006.
186. Mardh PA: *Mycoplasma hominis* infection of the central nervous system in newborn infants, *Sex Transm Dis* 10:332-334, 1983.
187. Koutsky LA, Stamm WE, Brunham RC, et al: Persistence of *Mycoplasma hominis* after therapy: importance of tetracycline resistance and of co-existing vaginal flora, *Sex Transm Dis* 10:374-381, 1983.
188. Cummings MC, McCormack WM: Increase in resistance of *Mycoplasma hominis* to tetracyclines, *Antimicrob Agents Chemother* 34:2297-2299, 1990.

21 Bordetella pertussis *and Other* Bordetella *spp. Infections*

DELMA J. NIEVES, ULRICH HEININGER, and JAMES D. CHERRY

CHAPTER OUTLINE

Pertussis, commonly known as "whooping cough," is an acute infectious illness of the respiratory tract causing disease in all age groups but taking its worst toll in unprotected infants and neonates too young to benefit from immunization.[1-12] It is caused by *Bordetella pertussis* and, less frequently, by *Bordetella parapertussis* and *Bordetella holmesii*.[1,3,11,13-16] The first epidemic of pertussis was noted in Paris in 1578 and described by Guillaume de Baillou in 1640.[3,10,17] Isolation of *B. pertussis* was reported in 1906 by Bordet and Gengou.[18,19] By the 1940s and 1950s, whole-cell pertussis vaccines were demonstrated to be efficacious in children.[1,3,10,20,21] However, because of concerns relating to serious temporally related adverse events with whole-cell vaccines, acellular pertussis vaccines were developed and came into widespread use in the late 1990s.[1,3,22,23]

It is clear that *B. pertussis* infections cause their most severe illness in unprotected neonates and young infants and that the major source of infection is unrecognized pertussis in the mother or another family member.[1,4,5,11,12,24-39]

Organisms

Bordetella is a gram-negative, pleomorphic, aerobic bacillus that is grouped together on the basis of genotypic characteristics, and species is differentiated by phenotypic characteristics. Most *Bordetella* species have relatively simple requirements, but *B. pertussis* is quite fastidious and is inhibited by constituents in common laboratory media, such as fatty acids, metal ions, sulfides, and peroxides.[11,40,41]

The genus *Bordetella* today consists of nine species, four of which cause human respiratory illness (*B. pertussis, B. parapertussis, B. bronchiseptica,* and *B. holmesii*). *B. pertussis* and *B. parapertussis* are the usual etiologic agents of pertussis, but 86% to 95% of illnesses are caused by *B. pertussis*.[7,11,14,42,43] *B. pertussis* infects exclusively humans. A separate lineage of *B. parapertussis* has been recovered from sheep as well as humans.[44] In rare instances, *B. bronchiseptica*, which normally is enzootic in pigs, dogs, cats, rodents, and other animals, has been isolated from humans with pertussis-like cough illnesses.[45-53] *B. holmesii* is an occasional cause of pertussis-like illness in adolescents and young adults.[16,54]

B. pertussis expresses approximately 3121 proteins, many of which are antigenic or biologically active. Since the isolation of *B. pertussis* in 1906, its microbiologic characteristics have been determined using animal-model and organ-culture systems. The use of these systems has led to many views that are incorrect.[55] Fimbriae (FIM), of which there are two serotypes (types 2 and 3), are protein projections on the surface of *B. pertussis* that are highly immunogenic.[11,43,56-59] Antibody to FIM causes agglutination of the organism. FIM function as adhesins but may also serve to sustain the attachment established by other adherence factors.[3,59-61] Data from two trials in which serologic correlates of immunity were studied indicated that antibody to FIM is important for protection.[62,63]

Filamentous hemagglutinin (FHA) is a component of the cell wall of all *Bordetella* spp.[3,11,60,64-70] It is highly immunogenic and is the dominant attachment factor for *Bordetella* in animal-model systems.[11,71,72] FHA is a component of most diphtheria, tetanus, and acellular component pertussis combination (DTaP and Tdap) vaccines.[6] However, the importance of antibody to FHA and protection from disease is not clear. In the two serologic correlates of immunity studies, FHA did not contribute to protection.[62,63]

Pertactin (PRN) is an outer membrane protein of *B. pertussis* that allows it to resist neutrophil-mediated clearance.[11,65,73-77] Vaccine efficacy trials conducted in the 1990s revealed that DTaP vaccines containing PRN in addition to pertussis toxin (PT) and FHA were more effective.[11,78-80] Another study revealed that anti-PRN antibodies were required for efficient phagocytosis of *B. pertussis* by host immune cells.[77] In addition to PRN, there are a number of other similar proteins (autotransporters) that interfere with the host innate immune system.[55]

PT is a critical factor related to mortality in young infants. PT is an adenosine diphosphate (ADP)-ribosylating toxin synthesized and secreted exclusively by *B. pertussis.* It is an A-B toxin with an enzymatically active A subunit (S1) and a B oligomer (S2-S5) binding portion.[3,11,66,74,81-91] PT inactivates G proteins, a process resulting in disruption of signaling pathways and leading to histamine sensitization, enhancement of insulin secretion in response to regulatory signals, and both suppressive and stimulatory immunologic effects in animal model systems.[11] PT also is responsible for leukocytosis with lymphocytosis in *B. pertussis* infections.[3,11] In mouse and rat models, PT inhibits chemotaxis and migration of neutrophils, monocytes/macrophages, and lymphocytes to infection sites, and PT also functions as an adhesin in the adherence of *B. pertussis* to human macrophages and ciliated respiratory epithelial cells. PT is not expressed by *B. parapertussis.*[14,92] PT contributes to morbidity in *B. pertussis* infections, as indicated by the severity of illness, which tends to be greater than that caused by *B. parapertussis* infection. The A promoter of PT catalyzes ADP-ribosylation of the α subunit of trimeric G proteins, which disturbs metabolic functions of many host cells and leads to a variety of biologic activities, including the lymphocytosis-promoting effect.[11,88]

Adenylate cyclase toxin (ACT) is an extracytoplasmic enzyme that impairs host immune cell function.[3,11,66,70,93-96] Dermonecrotic toxin (DNT) is a cytoplasmic protein that causes skin necrosis in laboratory animals,[97] and tracheal cytotoxin (TCT) causes local damage to respiratory epithelium in hamster tracheal organ cultures and in cultured hamster tracheal epithelial cells.[98,99]

The type III secretion system (TTSS) allows *Bordetella* to translocate effector proteins directly into the plasma membrane or cytoplasm of host cells.[100,127]

The lipopolysaccharide (LPS) of *B. pertussis* is similar to the endotoxins of other gram-negative bacteria.[3,11,66,101] Its function in disease is unknown, but it may act as an adhesin. LPS is a major cause of reactions to whole-cell pertussis vaccines.[102] LPS is a significant agglutinogen. Antibody to LPS reduces colonization of *B. pertussis* in the lungs and trachea of mice after aerosol challenge.[103]

In summary, human infections with *B. pertussis* are due to a number of proteins that are adhesins (mainly FIM but also the B oligomer of PT and LPS) or that interfere with innate immunity (PRN and other autotransporters, ACT and PT). Clinical disease is due to the A subunit of PT and an as yet unidentified toxin or process that causes the cough. *B. pertussis* infection and clinical illness in humans is noninflammatory in nature, unless there is a concomitant viral or secondary bacterial infection.[55]

Epidemiology and Transmission

Pertussis caused by *B. pertussis* is an extremely infectious disease, with an estimated 12 to 17 secondary cases produced by a typical primary case in an entirely susceptible population.[104-106] Attack rates in susceptible household contacts range from 70% to 100%.[1,3] In the prevaccine era in the United States, the average attack rate of reported pertussis was 157 per 100,000 population.[1] Previous studies, however, suggested that reported cases represent only between 15% and 25% of cases that actually occur.[107-110] With the introduction and widespread use of whole-cell pertussis vaccines, the attack rate of reported pertussis in the United States fell approximately 150-fold from 1943 to 1976. For the 7-year period from 1976 to 1982, the attack rate in the United States remained between 0.5 and 1.0 per 100,000 population. From 1982 to 2012, the attack rate curve shifted modestly upward and reached a rate of 15.2 per 100,000 in 2012.[111] Possible reasons for the resurgence of reported pertussis that have been suggested are (1) increased vaccine failures resulting from genetic changes in *B. pertussis,* (2) increased vaccine failures related to vaccines of lessened potency (in general, DTaP [diphtheria-tetanus–acellular pertussis; childhood] vaccines are less efficacious than are DTP vaccines), (3) waning immunity, (4) greater awareness of pertussis, and (5) the availability of better laboratory tests (the use of polymerase chain reaction [PCR] for diagnosis).[2,80,106,112-116] Pertussis epidemics in the prevaccine era occurred at 2- to 5-year intervals, and these cycles have continued in the vaccine era. As noted by Fine and Clarkson,[117,118] this continuation of the characteristic cycling during the vaccine era as occurred in the prevaccine era indicates that, although immunization has controlled disease, it has not reduced transmission of the organism in the population.[1,113,119,120]

In the prevaccine era, the following percentages of cases by age were noted in Massachusetts: younger than 1 year, 7.5%; 1 to 4 years, 41.1%; 5 to 9 years, 46.0%; 10 to 14 years, 4.1%; and 15 years and older, 0.9%. Associated with the marked reduction in reported cases of pertussis in the United States resulting from widespread pediatric immunization, a major shift occurred in the percentages by age category.[4] During the period from 1978 to 1981, the age distributions were as follows: younger than 1 year, 53.%; 1 to 4 years, 26.5%; 5 to 9 years, 8.2%; 10 to 14 years, 5.4%; and 15 years or older, 6.5%. In contrast, U.S. data for 2010 revealed the following: younger than 1 year, 15%; 1 to 6 years, 22%; 7 to 10 years, 18%; 10 to 19 years, 20%; and 20 years or older, 25%. Today, pertussis in adolescents and adults is an important source of *B. pertussis* infection in unimmunized or partially immunized children.* *B. pertussis* infections are endemic in adults, are often not diagnosed as pertussis, and are responsible for cyclic outbreaks in susceptible children.[2,57,112,113,129-135]

Transmission is thought to occur by respiratory droplets from a coughing patient that reach the upper respiratory tract of a susceptible person or contaminate environmental

*References 2, 26, 39, 112, 113, 121-128.

surfaces, which then a new host touches and autoinoculates.[3] Transmissibility is greatest early in the illness, that is, during the catarrhal and early paroxysmal phases.

Pathogenesis

After the patient is exposed to *B. pertussis*, the pathogenesis of infection depends on four important steps: mucosal attachment, evasion of host defenses, local damage, and systemic disease.[†] Although much has been learned about the biologically active and antigenic components of the organism, the exact mechanisms of pathogenesis in human disease are not fully understood. Infection is initiated in the respiratory tract by the attachment of *B. pertussis* organisms to the cilia of ciliated epithelial cells.[61] Adhesins (PT, FIM, LPS) facilitate this attachment.[11,55] PRN as well as other autotransporters, often mislabeled as adhesins, have specific biologic activities.[11,77,138-143] Antibody to PRN is associated with lack of attachment. Two household contact studies of serologic correlates of protection both found antibody to PRN to be the most important in preventing pertussis.[62,63]

Both ACT and PT adversely affect immune cell function and, therefore, allow infection, once initiated, to continue.[‡] PT prevents migration of lymphocytes and macrophages to areas of infection and adversely affects phagocytosis and intracellular killing. ACT enters phagocytic cells and catalyzes excessive production of cyclic adenosine monophosphate, which intoxicates neutrophils and results in a decrease in phagocytosis. Clinical experience and recent studies indicate that PT is the major causative factor in deaths in young infants.[12,37,144] PT inhibits G proteins, and this is the cause of the leukocytosis with lymphocytosis. It has been suggested that the extreme leukocytosis results in obstruction in small pulmonary vessels, and this leads to severe pulmonary hypertension.[37] However, it is possible that the inhibition of G proteins in other cells in the lung or heart is the cause of death.[12,144] In contrast to the situation in *B. pertussis* infection, leukocytosis with lymphocytosis is not a characteristic of *B. parapertussis* infection because this organism does not liberate PT.

TCT, DNT, and ACT all have been implicated as contributors to local tissue damage in the respiratory tract.[3,97,99] However, there are no data indicating tissue damage in human infections caused by these three toxins.

The cause of the hallmark paroxysmal cough of disease caused by *B. pertussis* infection is unknown. The paroxysmal cough is unique because of its long duration and memory, returning when people have subsequent respiratory viral infections. PT has been suggested to be the cause of the prolonged cough in pertussis. However, because persistent cough is a major manifestation of *B. bronchiseptica* infection in dogs and of *B. parapertussis* infection in children, and because neither organism expresses PT, this hypothesis should be refuted.[11,14,76] Recently, Hewitt and Canning[145] have suggested that bradykinin plays a role in the initiation of the cough. During *B. pertussis* infection, bradykinin production is increased, exhibits a prolonged half-life in the airways, and responsiveness to bradykinin reception activation is increased. Bradykinin activates sensory nerves implicated in cough. However, the *Bordetella* protein(s) or processes that stimulate the unique coughing in pertussis remain unknown.[55]

Cell-mediated immune function is altered by *B. pertussis* infection. In some studies, cell-mediated immunity was depressed, whereas in others it was augmented.[146]

Various antibodies develop after exposure of the human host to infection with *B. pertussis*. The development of agglutinins, hemagglutination-inhibiting antibodies, and bactericidal antibodies has been described.[1] Enzyme-linked immunosorbent (ELISA) techniques have demonstrated class-specific antibodies (immunoglobulin A [IgA], IgE, IgG, and IgM) to many of the specific proteins of *B. pertussis*.[147-149] These antibodies develop after infection and, with the exception of IgA antibodies, also after immunization. Neutralizing antibody to PT likewise develops after both infection and immunization.[149,150] Specific IgA antibodies to PT and FHA can also be demonstrated in nasopharyngeal (NP) secretions and saliva.[151,152]

At present, both *B. pertussis* infection and immunization with whole-cell (DTwP) or acellular pertussis (DTaP) vaccines clearly elicit protection of varying degrees and duration against pertussis, neither providing life-long protection.[§] Studies in young German and American men looking at the rate and mean values of IgA antibodies to pertussis antigens (which result from infection and not from primary vaccination) demonstrated no difference, suggesting that rates of adult infection were the same regardless of personal history of childhood immunization.[153] In Germany, routine childhood immunization was not carried out during the 1970s and 1980s, and pertussis was epidemic.

The nature of immunity in pertussis remains poorly understood. The consensus has been that serum antibodies greater than some unknown concentration to one or more of the pertussis antigens are responsible for protection.[130] However, no serologic correlate of immunity has been accepted. Although several large vaccine trials were carried out in the late 1980s and early 1990s, only two were done in a manner that allowed the study of possible serologic correlates of immunity.[62,63] In a nested household contact study looking at the roles of IgG antibodies to PT, FHA, PRN, and FIM 2 in children at the time of household exposure to *B. pertussis*, it was shown that geometric mean antibody values to PT, PRN, and FIM 2 were higher in noncases than in cases; however, in the classification tree and regression analyses, only antibodies against PRN contributed significantly to protection.[62] Similarly, a Swedish study found that higher antibody values to PRN and FIM 2/3 correlated with protection.[63] However, some children get pertussis despite large amounts of antibody to either or both PRN and FIM.[164,165] Data from a study by Weiss and colleagues[166] suggested that high antibody values to PT can block the protective effect of antibody to PRN and perhaps FIM.

Cell-mediated immune responses to PT, FHA, and PRN also occur.[167-176] Studies in a murine respiratory infection model suggest that cellular immunity plays an important role in bacterial clearance and augments the effects of antibody by predominantly T-helper 1 (TH1) cell stimulation.[169,170] Human studies demonstrate a cellular immune response shortly after natural infection with

†References 3, 11, 43, 61, 66, 97, 99, 103, 136, 137.

‡References 3, 70, 81, 82, 93, 94, 137.

§References 4, 11, 22, 55, 106, 113, 114, 132, 153-163.

B. pertussis, with PT, FHA, and PRN preferentially inducing the synthesis of TH1 cells.[175] Immunization with a whole-cell pertussis vaccine resulted in a TH1 response, whereas the response to acellular vaccines is more heterogeneous and involves both TH1 and TH2 cells. Persistent memory T and B cells and anamnestic antibody responses are important in long-term immunity.[168]

Immunity developed after having *B. pertussis* infection or receiving vaccination with a whole-cell pertussis vaccine does not protect against illness caused by *B. parapertussis*, and, similarly, infection with *B. parapertussis* does not induce protection against disease caused by *B. pertussis*.[177,178] However, in a vaccine efficacy trial in Germany, the results showed some evidence that the acellular pertussis multicomponent vaccine, which contained a large amount of FHA, offered some protection against *B. parapertussis* infections, whereas the whole-cell vaccine, which contained minimal amounts of FHA, did not.[179]

Pathology

Data on pathology of *B. pertussis* infections have been determined mainly by postmortem study in fatal cases.[‖] In a study of autopsy material from 15 infants (≤4 months of age), the consistent histopathologic features were necrotizing bronchiolitis and pneumonia, intraalveolar hemorrhage and fibrinous edema, and abundant intraalveolar macrophages.[37] Angiolymphatic aggregates of mixed leukocytes in the intralobular septa and pleurae were seen in 86% of the specimens. Intact *Bordetella* organisms were noted in cilia of the trachea, bronchi, and bronchioles and within airways and alveoli. The pathogen was also noted intracellularly in alveolar macrophages and respiratory epithelium. Despite the fact that all patients had severe pneumonia, the ciliated respiratory epithelial cells appeared relatively normal. Six of the patients had evidence of coinfections with one or more other agents (cytomegalovirus, 1 child; respiratory syncytial virus [RSV], 2 children; *Streptococcus pneumoniae*, 2 children; *Streptococcus pyogenes*, 2 patients; *Moraxella catarrhalis*, 1 child; and viridans streptococci, 1 child).

Pathologic changes in the brain and liver have also been described.[1,3,11] Microscopic or gross cerebral hemorrhage may be noted, and cortical atrophy has been observed. These changes most likely are the result of anoxic brain damage. In some studies of pertussis encephalopathy, findings suggested meningoencephalitis with perivascular cuffs of lymphocytes within cerebral gray matter and pleocytosis.[183] However, the studies in which inflammation was demonstrated were performed before modern virologic techniques became available. Therefore the neurologic findings in these instances may have been caused by interactions with neurotropic viruses or other infectious agents and were not the result of *B. pertussis* infection.[3] Fatty infiltration of the liver has been noted in patients with pertussis encephalopathy.

Although *B. pertussis* infection is a localized infection involving ciliated cells of the respiratory tract, bacteremia has been noted in immunocompromised adults.[184-186]

‖References 1, 3, 10, 37, 45, 180-182.

Clinical; *Bordetella pertussis* Infections

ADULTS, INCLUDING PREGNANT WOMEN AND MOTHERS

The clinical presentation in adults, including pregnant women, can be nonspecific, including findings of coryza and cough without the characteristic whoop. Several studies have found that from 12% to 30% or more of persons with acute illness with cough of at least 1 to 2 weeks of duration have evidence of *B. pertussis* infection, whereas it varies from 21% to 86% in those with classic pertussis symptoms, such as paroxysmal cough, whoop, and posttussive vomiting.[¶] Three important points relating to pertussis in adults (including pregnant women) and older children are the occurrence of coryza that does not become purulent, the lack of fever, and the lack of leukocytosis with lymphocytosis that is seen in primary infections in young children. Also important in pertussis in adults is the occurrence of sweating episodes between paroxysms of coughing. Whereas complications of pertussis in adolescents and adults are less common than in young children, hospitalization, pneumonia, and seizures do occur.[11] In addition, urinary incontinence, fractured ribs, herniated intervertebral disc, hearing loss, angina attack, carotid artery dissection and encephalopathy may occur.[4,11,113,156,188]

In 2008, the Advisory Committee on Immunization Practices (ACIP) presented their recommendations for the prevention of pertussis among pregnant and postpartum women and their infants.[195] In this report, they reviewed the literature relating to pertussis in pregnancy.[196-199] They concluded that the morbidity of pertussis was not increased among pregnant women compared with nonpregnant women. Granström and associates[197] reported 32 women who had pertussis in late pregnancy. These illnesses were not associated with obstetric complications, and all pregnancies went to term. Reports of adverse effects upon the fetus are rare,[198,199] and no causal relationship with abnormal fetal development or fetal morbidity has been established. The fetus of one woman with pertussis had an extradural hematoma and the fetus of another woman had tracheal obstruction.[198,199]

McGregor and associates[200] described three cases of maternal-infant pairs in which the mother-to-newborn transmission of pertussis led to severe pertussis in the child. Each of the mothers described had prolonged severe paroxysmal cough associated with posttussive emesis. In the first case, the mother developed a severe nonproductive whooping-like cough 5 days after delivery, with development of paroxysm and posttussive emesis. In the second case, the mother and a sibling had begun coughing 1 day before delivery. In the third case, immediately postpartum, the mother complained of coryza-like symptoms with a gradually increasing cough with paroxysm.

In another instance, a 22 year-old mother was hospitalized 6 days before delivery because of severe paroxysms of

¶References 2, 4, 11, 113, 123, 125, 129, 130, 132, 134, 154a, 187, 192, 193.

TABLE 21-1 Clinical Characteristics of Pertussis in Young Infants

	Smith and Vyas, 2000	Castagnini and Munoz, 2010	Taffarel et al, 2012	Murray et al, 2013	Berger et al, 2013	Rocha et al, 2013
Number of points	9	33	41	31	127	18
Age	<7 weeks (all PICU)	≤30 days	Mean age, 2.38 months	≤90 days (all PICU)	105 (83%) were <3 months	≤2 months
Cough	9 (100%)	32 (97%)	N/A	N/A	125 (98%)	16 (89%)
Apnea	5 (56%)	19 (58%)	N/A	N/A	62 (49%)	N/A
Cyanotic spell	N/A	30 (91%)	N/A	N/A	92 (72%)	2 (11%)
Seizures	5 (56%)	1 (3%)	N/A	4 (13%)	14 (11%)	1 (6%)
O_2 need	N/A	27 (82%)	24 (59%)	N/A	104 (82%)	18 (100%)
Mechanical ventilation	9 (100%)	9 (27%)	31 (76%)	8 (26%)	55 (43%)	6 (33%)
Hyper/hypotension	7 (78%)	N/A	27 (66%)	4 (13%)	45 (35%)	4 (22%)
Pulmonary hypertension	1 (11%)	N/A	16 (39%)	6 (19%)	16 (13%)	4 (22%)
Need for dialysis	N/A	N/A	4 (10%)	3 (10%)	20 (16%)	N/A
Died	6 (67%)	0 (0%)	17 (41%)	4 (13%)	12 (9%)	3 (17%)

Data from references 12, 25, 182, 211, 232, and 233.
N/A, Not available; *PICU*, pediatric intensive care unit.

coughing with posttussive emesis.[24] The neonate had the onset of cough on the seventh day of life and subsequently died of the illness.

Multiple studies have demonstrated that the source of infection in infants is usually a family member.[#] In a study of 616 infant cases, the source was identified in 43%.[26] A family member was the source 75% of the time, and the mother was the most common source (32%). Of the source persons, 56% were adults, and 20% were 10 to 19 years of age. In studies of household contacts, asymptomatic infections in family members are common occurrences.[130,204,205] Deen and associates[130] found that 52 (46%) of 114 household contacts who remained well had laboratory evidence of *B. pertussis* infection. In another study, 21 of 399 healthy infants who were controls in a study of sudden infant death syndrome (SIDS) had PCR-positive NP samples.[206] In a study at one hospital during the California pertussis epidemic of 2009 to 2010, 32 infants younger than 3 months were hospitalized with pertussis, and household coughing contacts were reported for 24 out of the 32 patients with pertussis (75%); the patient's mother was the contact in 10 patients (42%), and a sibling was the contact in 11 patients (46%).[36]

A study of pregnant women in the Netherlands from January 2004 to January 2006 looked at the seroprevalence of *Bordetella pertussis* infection during pregnancy.[207] Specific antibodies against pertussis toxin were measured in umbilical cord blood samples, maternal blood samples at 12 weeks of gestation, delivery, and 2 months after delivery. In total, 20 (6.3%) of 315 pregnant women in the study had serologic evidence of *B. pertussis* infection during or shortly before pregnancy, which was much higher than the incidence of reported cases for that age group. They concluded that their findings emphasized that *B. pertussis* infection often remains unreported, possibly because of a subclinical course of infection or the failure to recognize or report the disease by a general practitioner.

NEONATES AND YOUNG INFANTS

Pertussis in neonates and young infants is a unique experience.[4,11] Its spectrum of clinical manifestations varies by age, immunization status, and the presence or absence of transplacentally acquired antibody.[*a] Most deaths resulting from *B. pertussis* infection occur in neonates and early infancy, and morbidity is most severe in infants.[†a] From 1997 through 2000, 8276 cases of pertussis were reported in infants in the United States.[231] Of this group, 59% were hospitalized, 11% had pneumonia, 1% had seizures, 0.2% had encephalopathy, and 0.7% died. Eighty-seven percent of these infant cases occurred in children younger than 6 months. Clinical characteristics of pertussis in young infants as described in several recent studies are presented in Table 21-1.[‡a]

B. pertussis infection in neonates is particularly severe, with a death rate of between 1% and 3%.[§a] Clinical characteristics of pertussis in early infancy are summarized in Box 21-1. A common initial finding is apnea, and typical coughing may not be observed. Seizures in association with apnea caused by hypoxia occur frequently. Severe pulmonary hypertension is a relatively common problem in pertussis in the first 4 months of life.[‖a] The severity of disease and the risk of death correlate directly with the white blood cell (WBC) count and, in particular, the number of lymphocytes.[¶a] WBC counts in the range of 30,000 to more than 100,000 cells/mm³ are common findings.

#References 5, 26, 39, 130, 166, 201-203.

*aReferences 1, 3, 24, 27, 121, 200, 202, 203, 208-210.
†aReferences 5, 11, 12, 24, 30-34, 37, 38, 105, 120, 121, 144, 182, 200, 201, 206, 209-230.
‡aReferences 12, 25, 182, 211, 232, 233.
§aReferences 24, 27, 34, 200, 209, 215, 217, 234.
‖aReferences 12, 28, 30, 31, 33, 37, 213, 215, 221, 227, 230, 232.
¶aReferences 5, 11, 24, 31-34, 37, 120, 200, 209, 211-213, 215, 216, 218, 219, 221.

Box 21-1 Clinical Features of Pertussis in Young Infants

1. Initially, infant looks deceptively well; coryza, sneezing, throat clearing, no fever, mild cough
2. Paroxysmal stage: gagging, gasping, eye bulging, bradycardia (tachycardia occurs in severe illness), cyanosis, vomiting
3. No or minimal fever unless complicated by a secondary bacterial infection or a concomitant viral infection
4. Leukocytosis with lymphocytosis
5. Apneic episodes
6. Seizures
7. Respiratory distress
8. Pneumonia and pulmonary hypertension
9. Shock/hypotension with renal failure
10. Death associated with pulmonary hypertension and pneumonia
11. Adenovirus or respiratory syncytial virus coinfection can confuse picture

Data from references 4, 11, 187, and 194.

A recent California Department of Public Health study has provided useful information relating to risk factors for pulmonary hypertension and death.[12] This study involved 31 infants younger than or equal to 90 days of age with pertussis admitted to a pediatric intensive care unit (PICU) in Southern California. Infants with pulmonary hypertension or who died had higher WBC counts (>30,000 cells/mm^3), more rapid pulse (>170) and respiratory rates (>70), and were more likely to have pneumonia than those who did not have pulmonary hypertension or die. In addition, in those with pulmonary hypertension or who died, the WBC count rose more rapidly, and the pulse and respiratory rates attained higher levels sooner than in those without pulmonary hypertension or death.

Coinfections with respiratory viruses (RSV, adenovirus, influenza viruses) and respiratory bacterial pathogens (*S. pneumoniae, Haemophilus influenzae*) are relatively frequent.[#a]

A recent study by Berger and associates[25] described 127 children hospitalized with critical pertussis and again found worse severity of illness in patients younger than 3 months. Eighty-three percent of patients were younger than 3 months. The median WBC count was significantly higher in those requiring mechanical ventilation (35,200/mm^3 vs. 26,100/mm^3), those with pulmonary hypertension (68,400/mm^3 vs. 25,100/mm^3), and nonsurvivors (66,300/mm^3 vs. 26,100/ mm^3).

B. pertussis infection has been noted in association with SIDS, but whether a cause-and-effect relationship exists is not clear.[206,210,217,234] Nicoll and Gardner,[210] in a study in England, found that many deaths attributed to SIDS were, in fact, related to *B. pertussis* infection. Using PCR, *B. pertussis* DNA was noted in NP specimens from 9 (18%) of 51 infants who had sudden, unexpected deaths.[217] In a subsequent study, specimens were collected for PCR from 254 infants who experienced sudden, unexplained deaths and from 441 healthy matched control subjects.[206] The rate of PCR-positive results in the sudden death cases was 5.1%; it was 5.3% in the control group. In a careful follow-up histopathologic study with unique immunohistochemical staining of specimens from a subset of these fatal cases, no evidence of specific *B. pertussis* pulmonary infection or pathologic features was found.[240]

Aside from prevention of disease, early detection can make a difference in outcomes. However, early and/or presenting symptoms in neonates are not often obvious. A recent study comparing hospitalized patients younger than 3 months with confirmed pertussis versus RSV or influenza indicated several features that should alert clinicians to pertussis, including paroxysmal cough, posttussive emesis, lack of congestion, and lack of fever.[36]

#a References 5, 24, 36, 37, 182, 218, 235-239.

Other *Bordetella* Infections

BORDETELLA PARAPERTUSSIS

B. parapertussis infection in children can cause unrecognized infection, mild pertussis, or typical pertussis.[11] In a study of 38 children with *B. parapertussis* illnesses compared with 76 children with *B. pertussis* illnesses, the results were as follows: *B. pertussis*/*B. parapertussis*, in percentages—cough for longer than 4 weeks, 57%/37% (P = .06); whooping, 80%/59% (P = .07); whooping for longer than 2 weeks, 26%/18% (P = .05); paroxysms, 90%/83%; posttussive vomiting, 47%/42%; and mean leukocyte and lymphocyte counts, 12,500/mm^3 and 7600 per mm^3/7800 per mm^3 and 3500/mm^3 ($P < .0001$), respectively.[14] In another study in Italy, children with *B. parapertussis* infection had the following rates of findings: cough, 100%; paroxysms, 76%; whooping, 33%; posttussive vomiting, 42%; apnea, 29%; and cyanosis, 12%.[241] All of these rates, except cough and paroxysms, were lower in children with *B. parapertussis* infections than in children with *B. pertussis* infections. Concomitant infections with *B. pertussis* and *B. parapertussis* are not rare.[242-244] Deaths in 3 infants have been described, but it is likely that in all three instances, the infants also had *B. pertussis* infections.[192]

During the period 2008 to 2010, clinical specimens from nine states were tested by PCR for *B. pertussis* and *B. parapertussis* in a commercial laboratory.[42] Of the positive samples, 13.99% were identified as *B. parapertussis*. The *B. parapertussis* positive samples had no seasonal periodicity, whereas the *B. pertussis* positives occurred between weeks 22 and 38 each year. Neither neonatal *B. parapertussis* cases nor *B. parapertussis* cases in pregnant women have been described.

BORDETELLA BRONCHISEPTICA

B. bronchiseptica causes respiratory infections in at least 18 different mammals.[66] Most notable are atrophic rhinitis in pigs, kennel cough (rhinotracheitis) in dogs, and bronchopneumonia in rabbits and other laboratory animals.

In 1911, McGowan[245] observed that laboratory workers exposed to various animals with *B. bronchiseptica* infections on occasion had respiratory illness. In 1926, a 5-year-old girl with a pertussis-like illness was found to be infected with *B. bronchiseptica*.[246] Her illness commenced about 10 to 12 days after she had been given a rabbit with mild "snuffles."

Otherwise healthy children who became infected with *B. bronchiseptica* after being exposed to farm animals or pets usually have pertussis-like illnesses.[11]

In 2008, Rath and coworkers[247] described an infant who had recurrent episodes of pertussis-like illness caused by *B. bronchiseptica* that cleared after imipenem therapy. In another recent study, another immunocompetent infant with recurrent pertussis-like illness was described.[248]

Occasional infections in humans have been noted during the last 40 years, with the majority occurring in immunocompromised adults, including patients with acquired immunodeficiency syndrome (AIDS).[52,249-251] Respiratory infections have ranged from mild upper respiratory illnesses to pneumonia. In patients with AIDS, the pneumonia frequently is cavitary. Sinusitis and bronchitis also occur.

No *B. bronchiseptica* infections in neonates or pregnant women have been described.

BORDETELLA HOLMESII

In 1999, Yih and associates[16] reported the isolation of *B. holmesii* from the NP specimens of 33 patients suspected of having pertussis. Twenty-three of the cases were investigated further, and 19 (82%) of these patients were adolescents, 2 (9%) were adults, and 2 (9%) were children. All had cough; 61% had paroxysms, 26% had posttussive vomiting, and 9% had whoop. More recently, *B. holmesii* has been isolated from NP specimens from patients with pertussis-like illnesses in the United States, France, Canada, and the Netherlands.[15,252,253] The incidence of pertussis-like illness caused by *B. holmesii* is unknown. *B. holmesii* contains IS*481* (insertion sequence *481*) and IS*1001*. These two ISs are routinely used to diagnose *B. pertussis* and *B. parapertussis*, respectively, by PCR.[42,88,254,296] If both IS*481* and IS*1001* are positive, then it is thought the illness is due to *B. holmesii*. However, because infection with both *B. pertussis* and *B. parapertussis* can occur, dual positives can be either *B. holmesii* or mixed infections with *B. pertussis* and *B. parapertussis*.[42]

No *B. holmesii* infections in neonates or pregnant women have been described.

Diagnosis

DIFFERENTIAL DIAGNOSIS

In typical pertussis, the clinical diagnosis should be apparent based on the paroxysmal cough with posttussive vomiting and whooping and lack of significant fever. However, the cause of the illness can be *B. pertussis, B. parapertussis, B. holmesii*, and perhaps *B. bronchiseptica*. A history of contact with a known case will help to establish the diagnosis in a patient with mild or atypical illness. The presence of leukocytosis with lymphocytosis in a child with a cough illness or the presence of apnea in an infant is a strong indication that the illness is caused by *B. pertussis* and not another *Bordetella* spp.[14] Lymphocytosis of 10,000 or more cells/mm^3 is observed in few other cough illnesses.

Many other infectious agents cause illnesses with prolonged and repetitive cough that can be confused with *B. pertussis* infections.[11] In particular, *Mycoplasma pneumoniae, Chlamydia pneumoniae*, adenoviruses, bocavirus, and other respiratory viruses all can cause prolonged cough illnesses.[1,3,255-262] In addition, coughing episodes may be seen in asthma, bronchiolitis, bacterial pneumonia, cystic fibrosis, *Coccidioides immitis* infection, and other fungal pulmonary infections and tuberculosis.[4] Another problem is the cough associated with sinusitis, which can be confused with *B. pertussis* infection. The cough associated with gastroesophageal reflux also can be confused with pertussis, as can cough associated with an airway foreign body.

SPECIFIC DIAGNOSIS

A laboratory diagnosis of pertussis caused by *B. pertussis* or other *Bordetella* spp. can be made by culturing the organisms on appropriate media, by PCR, and by demonstrating the presence of specific antibodies. *Bordetella* spp. can be recovered from NP specimens, with the highest rate of isolation occurring within the first 3 weeks of cough.[4,187,263,264] Specimens for culture can be collected either by swabbing the nasopharynx, by NP washing, or by NP aspiration.[3,265] In general, NP aspiration gives the highest yield of positive cultures, and NP wash is the least sensitive.

B. pertussis and *B. parapertussis* are recovered most easily by direct plating of the specimen from the patient onto selective media.[3,266,267,267a] Specific swabs (calcium alginate or Dacron) and media (Regan-Lowe or Bordet-Gengou agar and modified Stainer-Scholte broth) are required, and laboratory personnel should be experienced in isolating the organisms. If cultures cannot be inoculated directly, the use of Regan-Lowe transport medium is recommended. In classic disease in children, the culture will be positive in approximately 80% of cases if the specimen is obtained within 2 weeks of the onset of cough and antibiotics have not been administered previously.[149,268,268a]

Since the late 1980s, numerous PCR assays with primers derived from many different chromosomal regions have been developed for the diagnosis of *B. pertussis, B. parapertussis, B. holmesii*, and *B. bronchiseptica* infections, and they have been evaluated in multiple studies by comparison with culture and clinically typical pertussis.[*b]

PCR has the advantage of having much higher sensitivity than that of conventional culture. At present, the most commonly used primers for the diagnosis of pertussis include IS*481* and IS*1001*.[11,187,254,296] IS*481* occurs in the genomes of *B. pertussis* (>50 copies) and *B. holmesii* (8-10 copies) but not in *B. parapertussis*. IS*1001* occurs in the genomes of *B. parapertussis* and *B. holmesii* (≈20 copies) but not in *B. pertussis*. The genome of *B. bronchiseptica* generally contains neither IS*481* nor IS*1001*. However, in recent studies, *B. bronchiseptica* strains were found to contain IS*1001* in their genomes (in the form of an IS*1001*-like element, called hIS*1001*).[254,286,297] False-positive results are a potential problem with the use of PCR for establishing the diagnosis of pertussis.[284,298,299] False-positive results can occur if specimens are opened in the pertussis laboratory before transport to the PCR laboratory.[11] False-positive results also can result from contamination of the air in a room in which the previous patient had pertussis and in a room where pertussis vaccine was administered.[282,292]

*bReferences 41, 42, 165, 187, 254, 268, 268a, 269-296.

Moreover, as noted earlier, *B. bronchiseptica* can be mistaken for *B. parapertussis* when the IS*1001* primer is used.[286,297] Therefore rigorous internal and external laboratory controls are necessary. In addition, because ISs are somewhat promiscuous, nucleic acid amplification tests should, whenever possible, be accompanied with conventional culture.

Obtaining a routine laboratory diagnosis of *B. pertussis* infection in adults or in other atypical cases is hampered by the problem that medical care usually is not sought until the third or fourth week of the illness, and antibiotics frequently have been administered before the possibility of pertussis was considered.[114,132,189] During the last 25 years, the most significant advance in the diagnosis of pertussis has been the development of ELISA.[11]

Natural infection with *B. pertussis* is followed by a rise in serum concentrations of IgA, IgG, and IgM antibodies to specific antigens of the organism.[148,149,189,300-305] In contrast to natural infection, primary immunization of children induces mainly IgM and IgG, but not IgA, antibodies.

Serologic testing for *B. pertussis* infection in the clinical setting is not well standardized but is widely available in Europe and North America.[187] In the research setting, the use of ELISA contributed significantly to establishing the diagnosis of *B. pertussis* infection in many patients with negative cultures.[†b] Most useful is the determination of IgG and IgA antibodies to PT and FHA. The most reliable proof of acute infection is the demonstration of a significant increase in antibody values between acute-phase and convalescent-phase serum specimens. Frequently, because collection of acute-phase specimens is delayed and, therefore the acute-phase values already are elevated, significant increases between first and second serum specimens cannot be demonstrated. However, a diagnosis can usually be established on the basis of a high value or values on a single serum specimen.[130,132,134,189,307] Because *B. parapertussis* infection induces cross-reacting antibodies to *B. pertussis* FHA, the use of this antigen alone cannot differentiate *B. pertussis* from *B. parapertussis* infection.[304,308]

Today in clinical practice, the laboratory diagnosis of pertussis should be approached as follows: In all cases in which the cough illness is of less than 2 weeks of duration in adolescents and adults or 3 weeks of duration in children, a NP specimen should be obtained for culture or PCR. In adults who have had cough for greater than 2 weeks of duration, single-serum ELISA is the preferred method, provided they have not been immunized against pertussis in the previous 12 months.[114] This method also can be used in children if they have not been immunized within a year. At present, many commercial laboratories offer single-serum diagnostic tests for *B. pertussis,* and almost all the offered tests lack specificity. Any test that uses the whole organism in the test is fraught with false-positive results. Tests that report specific IgM antibodies also are unreliable. The greatest sensitivity and specificity for the serologic diagnosis of *B. pertussis* infection are achieved by an ELISA or ELISA-like test with the measurement of IgG and IgA antibodies to PT. Single high values of IgG or IgA antibodies to PT are indicative of infection.[11] In our opinion, a sensitive and specific test in North America is available from Focus Diagnostics, Cypress, California.[309] The performance of a number of European commercial serum ELISA kits for the diagnosis of *B. pertussis* illness has been evaluated by Riffelmann and associates.[310] They found that three kits that used PT as the antigen had specificities and sensitivities in the 80% to 90% range.

Not all infected persons develop antibody responses to PT. In children, approximately 25% lack an adequate response, as do approximately 10% of adolescents and adults.[194,304]

[†b]References 56, 131, 132, 134, 189, 204, 205, 306, 306a.

Treatment

ANTIBIOTICS

Several antibiotics have in vitro efficacy against *B. pertussis*.[256,311-319] The first choice for treatment since the 1970s has been oral erythromycin; this ameliorates the symptoms if it is given early during the course of the illness and eliminates the organism from the nasopharynx within a few days, thereby shortening the period of contagiousness.[314] The dose for children is 40 to 50 mg/kg/day given every 6 hours for 14 days. A 7-day course of erythromycin estolate was shown in a large study in Canada to be as efficacious as 14 days of treatment.[320]

The newer macrolides, azithromycin (10 mg/kg on day 1 and 5 mg/kg on days 2-5 as a single dose for 5 days) for children or clarithromycin (15 to 20 mg/kg/day in two divided doses for 7 days) for children also can be expected to be effective.[319,321] Although rare, the use of erythromycin in young infants is associated with hypertrophic pyloric stenosis, so parents need to be educated about the symptoms of this potential risk.[322-324] Because of this risk, the Centers for Disease Control and Prevention (CDC) and several European authorities recommend treating neonates with azithromycin rather than erythromycin.[319] The CDC and the American Academy of Pediatrics (AAP) recommend an azithromycin dose of 10 mg/kg for 5 days.[321] However, we could find nothing in the literature to support this recommendation rather than what we suggest (10 mg/kg on day 1, followed by 5 mg/kg on days 2-5). Furthermore, because two neonates developed pyloric stenosis on the 10 mg/kg for 5-day dosing regimen, and because there are no data relating to failure on our dose, we believe that our dosing regimen should be used in neonates.[323] Trimethoprim-sulfamethoxazole can be used as an alternative agent in those who cannot tolerate erythromycin.[317] The first erythromycin-resistant strain of *B. pertussis* was isolated from a 2-month-old male infant in Yuma County, Arizona, in June 1994.[218] Four more resistant *B. pertussis* strains were recovered from cases in California, Utah, and Minnesota.[325-327] In France, macrolide resistance developed during illness in a neonate. In Japan, six *B. pertussis* strains were found to have high level resistance to nalidixic acid and decreased susceptibilities to fluoroquinolones.[328] At present, no evidence of a pattern of emerging macrolide resistance has been seen, but because PCR rather than culture is becoming the diagnostic method of choice in many laboratories, the chance of missing resistant strains is a problem.

Patients infected with *B. parapertussis* and *B. holmesii* also can be treated with macrolides, but *B. bronchiseptica* usually is resistant to erythromycin so that alternative therapy is necessary.[11] *B. bronchiseptica* strains usually are sensitive to aminoglycosides, extended-spectrum, third-generation penicillins, tetracyclines, quinolones, and trimethoprim-sulfamethoxazole.

SUPPORTIVE CARE

Historically, no infectious disease has a greater list of remedies lauded as beneficial but without objective evidence of effectiveness.[20,329] Supportive care includes avoidance of factors that provoke attacks of coughing and maintenance of hydration and nutrition. In the hospital, gentle suction to remove secretions and well-humidified oxygen may be required, particularly in infants with pneumonia and significant respiratory distress. In severe infections in neonates and young infants, assisted ventilation is often necessary.

However, infants who develop pulmonary hypertension with respiratory and cardiovascular failure respond poorly to aggressive therapy (pulmonary artery vasodilators and extracorporeal membrane oxygenation [ECMO]) and have high mortality rates. Because data suggest that the refractory pulmonary hypertension results from the extreme leukocytosis with lymphocytosis, which is always present in fatal cases, our opinion is that leukocyte-reducing measures, such as exchange transfusion (ET), should be implemented.[‡b] ET may be better than leukofiltration because it removes PT, which inhibits other G proteins that might also contribute to cardiac or pulmonary failure, as well as reducing the WBC count.

Because data on the effectiveness of ET is lacking, members of our group reported findings of 10 young infants in California (2005-2011) who underwent ET for the treatment of pertussis: 5 died and 5 survived.[35] All infants had WBC counts greater than or equal to 62,000 cells/mm^3, and all were intubated. Nine of the 10 cases had pneumonia. The median WBC count among fatal cases was 76,000/mm^3, and it was 82,000/mm^3 among survivors. All 5 infants who died had pulmonary hypertension, shock/hypotension, and pneumonia; 4 of 5 had organ failure; 3 of 5 received extracorporeal membrane oxygenation; and none had seizures.

A literature review notes six reports with sufficient data related to timing of events on 13 young infants who received ET for the treatment of severe pertussis.[35] Eleven of the 13 survived. Of the survivors, 5 were reported to have been in cardiogenic shock before ET, but none had organ failure. Both infants who died had renal failure before ET. More recently, Taffarel and colleagues[233] in Argentina reviewed 41 infants with pertussis, cared for in their PICU between January 2003 and March 2011. Nine of the infants received ET in their management. The four ETs that were carried out before 2011 were done as "rescue therapy in very ill patients"; all of these infants died. The five ETs performed in 2011 were done preemptively, and the ET was based on a WBC count greater than 95,000/mm^3 without requiring severe cardiopulmonary compromise; 4 of 5 of this group survived.

The study of 127 patients by Berger and colleagues[25] included 14 patients who received leukoreduction therapy (12 ETs, 1 leukopheresis, 1 both). Of the 25 patients with initial WBC values greater than 50,000 WBC/mm^3, 13 received leukoreduction. Of the 13, 8 survived compared with 9 survivors in the 12 who did not receive leukoreduction. They concluded that survival benefit could not be established with leukoreduction. However, there was no analysis with regards to timing of the leukoreduction therapy. They note that 8 of the 13 patients had pulmonary hypertension. Overall, 12 patients died, 9 of whom had pulmonary hypertension. Among 115 survivors, only 7 had pulmonary hypertension. Hence it appears that leukoreduction therapy was performed in patients already suffering significant complications and, at which point, presumably very little could change the course of illness. In our opinion, ET for management of very severe pertussis in young infants is a biologically sound procedure, and the decision for ET should be based on the early appearance of pneumonia, the presence of pulmonary hypertension, and the rapidity in the rise of the WBC count.

The use of corticosteroids has received attention in the treatment of pertussis.[329,330] Cortisone treatment in the murine model of pertussis increased the mortality rate.[331] In a study by Roberts and associates,[332] dexamethasone treatment did not shorten the course of hospitalization compared with untreated control subjects.

The use of salbutamol has also been suggested as having some value, but no benefit was noted in three studies reviewed by Bettiol and coworkers.[329,333] Pillay and Swingler[334] reviewed the symptomatic treatment of pertussis and found no statistically significant benefit for the use of diphenhydramine, dexamethasone, or salbutamol.

Prognosis

The prognosis in pertussis is related to the patient's age. In older children and adults, the prognosis is good, but infants (and particularly neonates) have a significant risk of death and development of encephalopathy.[§b] In addition, long-term follow-up suggests that apnea or seizures at the time of disease in children may be associated with subsequent intellectual impairment.[336] The present availability of PICUs and assisted ventilation has reduced the rate of mortality in infants who receive medical care. Unfortunately, many deaths occur outside the hospital. No evidence has shown that pertussis impairs ventilatory function later in life.[337]

Prevention

Only a summary of pertussis vaccines and pertussis immunizations will be presented here. For more complete information, the reader is referred to the 29th edition of the Report of the Committee on Infectious Diseases of the AAP[321]; the CDC (www.cdc.gov); the pertussis chapters in Cherry and Feigin, *Textbook of Pediatric Infectious Diseases*[4]; or the pertussis chapter in the sixth edition of Plotkin and colleagues, *Vaccines*.[6]

WHOLE-CELL VACCINES (DTWP)

The first pertussis vaccines were developed in the 1920s, and effective vaccines have enjoyed worldwide use since the late 1940s.[1,3,11] From 1943 to 1976, a 150-fold reduction in the

‡bReferences 12, 29, 31, 35, 221, 223.

§bReferences 5, 12, 24, 27, 31, 34, 38, 120, 144, 182, 200, 201, 208, 212, 214, 215, 219, 220, 222-225, 228, 229, 335.

pertussis attack rate was noted in association with widespread childhood pertussis immunization in the United States.

As pertussis was brought under control in many countries, attention shifted to concern about severe temporally related events (SIDS and so-called "vaccine encephalopathy") attributed to the whole-cell pertussis component in diphtheria-tetanus-pertussis combination vaccines (DTwP). This concern led to the disruption of successful immunization programs in many countries. Many controlled studies in the latter part of the 20th century have demonstrated that DTwP vaccines do not cause SIDS or "vaccine encephalopathy".[4,11,338] However, DTwP immunization is associated with many local and systemic side effects. These reactions include redness and induction at the injection site, fever, drowsiness, fretfulness, vomiting, anorexia, and persistent crying. In addition, as noted in one study, 0.1% of DTwP recipients had high-pitched, unusual crying, 0.06% had convulsions, and 0.06% had hypotonic-hyporesponsive episodes.[102]

ACELLULAR VACCINES (DTAP AND TDAP)

The adverse reactions associated with whole-cell pertussis component vaccines led to the development of acellular pertussis component combination (DTaP) vaccines. Research in the 1970s showed that three *B. pertussis* antigens (PT, FHA, LPS) were released into the medium during culture and that these antigens could be concentrated and separated by density gradient centrifugation.[3,136,339] This finding allowed for the development and production of acellular vaccines by six manufacturers in Japan.[23,339-341] All six vaccines had minimal or no endotoxin (LPS) but different amounts of PT and FHA. Subsequently, the vaccines were found to contain varying amounts of FIM 2 and PRN.

DTaP vaccines were put into routine use in Japan in 1981. However, in Japan in 1981, the first dose of vaccine was administered at 2 years of age, and no efficacy data existed relating to efficacy in young infants. Therefore efficacy trials for a number of candidate DTaP vaccines were planned and carried out in Europe and Africa in the early 1990s.

A World Health Organization (WHO) committee met in Geneva in January 1991 to develop a primary case definition for the efficacy trials.[342] The WHO case definition was as follows: (1) an illness with 21 days or more of spasmodic cough and either culture-confirmed infection with *B. pertussis* or serologic evidence of infection with *B. pertussis* as indicated by a significant rise in IgA or IgG antibody by ELISA against PT or FHA in paired sera or (2) contact with a case of culture-confirmed pertussis in the household with onset within 28 days before or after the onset of cough in the study vaccinee. Even though it was noted by some committee members that this definition would inflate efficacy (by eliminating many laboratory confined cases with less severe cough illnesses), it was used in all eight trials that evaluated nine candidate vaccines.

When efficacy was calculated using a clinical definition that included all cough illnesses of greater than or equal to 7 days, it was found that three- and four-component vaccines (containing PRN and FIM, as well as PT and FHA) had greater efficacy than PT or PT/FHA vaccines.[4,6,11] Of the nine candidate DTaP vaccines studied, only two are presently routinely used in the United States and throughout much of the world. It should be noted that in five of the trials, the comparative DTwP vaccine had greater efficacy than the trial DTaP vaccines.

Because DTaP vaccines do not contain LPS, they are less reactogenic than DTwP vaccines. Temporally related persistent crying, hypotonic-hyporesponsive episodes, and seizures were rare events after receipt of immunization with DTaP vaccines in the efficacy trials.[6] In a large active surveillance program (IMPACT), researchers found that risks of having febrile seizures and hypotonic-hyporesponsive episodes after receiving pertussis-containing vaccines decreased significantly after the introduction of DTaP vaccines in Canada.[343] In a Vaccine Safety Datalink study, Huang and coworkers[344] did not observe an increased risk for seizures in children 6 weeks to 23 months of age after DTaP vaccination.

In about 2005, two acellular pertussis component, diphtheria, and tetanus toxoid vaccines (Tdap vaccines) became available for use in adolescents and adults.[128,345-349] Both these vaccines elicit vigorous antibody responses to the antigens that they contain after a single dose.

DTaP vaccines were adopted for routine use in infants and young children in many countries in the late 1990s, and the use of DTwP vaccines was discontinued. In many of these same countries, Tdap vaccines have been put into routine use in preadolescents and adolescents and selectively used in adults.

The pertussis epidemics in the United States in 2010 and 2012, as well as epidemic diseases in Australia and other countries using DTaP vaccines has led to many recent studies relating to vaccine failure.[55,106,111,157-163,350,351] The reasons for DTaP and Tdap vaccine failure were recently reviewed by one of us (JDC), and subsequent studies in California, other states, and Australia support many of the suggestions about DTaP and Tdap failure in contrast with DTwP vaccines.[106]

SCHEDULES AND CONTRAINDICATIONS

Although there are many different schedules in use throughout the world for both DTaP and DTP, the most frequently used is a primary series at 2, 4, and 6 months. In the United States and some other countries, booster doses of DTaP are given during the first half of the second year of life and at 4 to 6 years of age. Other primary schedules used in some countries rely on two doses in the first year of life (given at 2 and 3, 2 and 4, or 3 and 5 months of age), followed by a third dose at 12 months of age.

Tdap schedules vary considerably throughout the world and are also changing. The most common recommendation is for universal immunization of preadolescents and adolescents and the selective immunization of adults. Various cocooning programs have been or are being established.[321,352-359] These programs include postpartum immunization of the mother, the father, grandparents, siblings, and immunization of mothers-to-be during the second or third trimesters of pregnancy.

In 2012, the ACIP voted to recommend use of Tdap during every pregnancy.[360] Newer data indicate that maternal antipertussis antibodies are short lived, repeat vaccines are safe and well tolerated, and vaccinating during the third trimester (optimally at weeks 30-32 of pregnancy) would provide the highest concentration of maternal antibodies to be transferred to the newborn.[361-363] Moreover, one recent study showed lower median cord blood PT, FHA, and PRN IgG antibody values in 20 infants with PCR-confirmed pertussis before 6 months of age when compared with 80 age-matched control infants (10.5 vs. 13.5 anti-PT IU/mL, 14.5 vs. 18.0 anti-FHA, 6.0 vs. 9.0 anti-PRN, respectively). These findings support the concept of infant protection by maternal antibodies and the strategy of pertussis booster immunization in pregnant women.[362]

If not administered during pregnancy, Tdap should be given immediately postpartum. Present DTaP and Tdap vaccines available in the United States are presented in Table 21-2.

It should be recognized that deaths in neonates and young infants are due to the effects of PT, and antibody to PT will prevent these deaths. This is the reason for immunization of pregnant women in the third trimester. Another approach is to start immunization at birth.[114,360,364-368]

There is concern regarding maternal Tdap immunization and the blunting of the immune response of the infant to the primary immunization series. This was addressed in a recent study by Hardy-Fairbanks and colleagues.[369] They studied 16 pregnant women who chose to receive Tdap to determine whether prenatal Tdap vaccination reduces the infant immune response to routine DTaP immunization. Compared with control infants, more newborns in the Tdap group demonstrated pertussis antibody concentrations at or above the defined benchmark levels. At 2 months of age (before the first infant vaccination), pertussis antibody in infants of mothers vaccinated with Tdap during pregnancy remained higher than those of control infants (3.2- to 22.8-fold greater). After the primary series, antibody concentrations to pertussis antigens were modestly lower in the Tdap group (0.7- to 0.8-fold lower), except for FIM (1.5-fold greater). However, antibody concentrations before and after the booster dose of DTaP at 12 to 18 months of life showed no notable differences between groups. They concluded that maternal Tdap immunization resulted in higher concentrations of pertussis antibodies in their infants during the period between birth and the first vaccine dose, compared with infants of unvaccinated mothers. Therefore this offered protection during the most vulnerable time period, when morbidity and mortality associated with infant pertussis is the greatest.

TABLE 21-2 *Bordetella pertussis* Antigens in DTaP and Tdap Vaccines

	INFANTS AND CHILDREN				PREADOLESCENT, ADOLESCENT, AND ADULT	
Antigen	**Infanrix***	**Pediarix†**	**Daptacel**	**Pentacel‡**	**Boostrix**	**Adacel**
PT (μg)	25	25	10	20	8	2.5
FHA (μg)	25	25	5	20	8	5
PRN (μg)	8	8	3	3	2.5	3
FIM 2/3 (μg)	—	—	5	5	—	5
D (Lf)	25	25	15	15	2.5	2
T (Lf)	10	10	5	5	5	5

DTaP, Diphtheria-tetanus–acellular pertussis (childhood) vaccine; *Tdap,* tetanus-diphtheria-acellular pertussis (adult) vaccine.
*This vaccine is also available (in countries other than the United States) with various further antigens, including *Haemophilus influenzae* type B, hepatitis B surface antigen, and inactivated polio.
†This vaccine also contains hepatitis B surface antigen and inactivated polio.
‡This vaccine also contains *H. influenzae* type B and inactivated polio.

Similar to immunization in pregnancy, there is also concern that immunization at birth also blunts the subsequent immune response of the infant after the routine schedule at 2, 4, and 6 months.[364,366,368,370,371]

The immunization of infants at birth, followed by an accelerated schedule, should provide some early protection and prevent deaths. Because some studies of early immunization have shown a suppression of the overall response to the vaccine antigens compared with a more delayed schedule, early immunization has, in recent years, not been looked upon favorably.[364,366] However, recent epidemics suggest that there may be reason for change.

Over the years, pertussis vaccine recommendations have undergone many changes. In particular, contraindications to pertussis immunization are evolving continually. An important note, however, is that few scientific data support any of the present contraindications. The primary goal of national immunization programs is to vaccinate all infants, children, and now adolescents and adults. In the United States, the most recent recommendations of the Committee on Infectious Diseases of the AAP and the ACIP generally should be followed.[321,352,360] However, individual case-by-case decisions often need to be made.

ISOLATION AND PROPHYLACTIC MEASURES

Erythromycin, azithromycin, or clarithromycin treatment of an index case shortens the duration of communicability of the organisms and thus limits spread of the disease. During the first few days of treatment, contact with susceptible persons should be avoided. In general, close contacts (household members, those in daycare centers, playmates) of the index case should be protected from infection. Such protection can be implemented by the prophylactic use of erythromycin for 14 days, azithromycin for 5 days, or clarithromycin for 7 days.[11,319,321,372] Active immunization of all exposed persons (children, adolescents, and adults) who are not adequately vaccinated also should be conducted.

The use of prophylactic antibiotics in adolescents and adults in exposure situations, such as classrooms and hospital settings, frequently is recommended. This approach often involves many people and considerable expense.

In our experience, the side effects of erythromycin (but less so with other macrolides) are such that adult compliance is poor. Therefore our opinion is that erythromycin and other macrolides should generally not be used prophylactically in these large group settings but only recommended for those in close contact with young infants and for all others for treatment at the first sign of respiratory illness in those exposed.

Acknowledgments

We greatly appreciate the help of Amabelle Aguelo in the preparation of this manuscript.

References

1. Cherry JD: The epidemiology of pertussis and pertussis immunization in the United Kingdom and the United States: a comparative study, *Curr Prob Pediatr* 14:1-78, 1984.
2. Cherry JD: The epidemiology of pertussis: a comparison of the epidemiology of the disease pertussis with the epidemiology of *Bordetella pertussis* infection, *Pediatrics* 115:1422-1427, 2005.
3. Cherry JD, Brunell PA, Golden GS, et al: Report of the task force on pertussis and pertussis immunization: 1988, *Pediatrics* 81:939-984, 1988.
4. Cherry JD, Heininger U: Pertussis and other *Bordetella* infections. In Cherry JD, Feigin RD, Demmler-Harrison GJ, Kaplan SL, editors: *Textbook of pediatric infectious diseases*, ed 7, Philadelphia, 2013, Saunders.
5. Crowcroft NS, Booy R, Harrison T, et al: Severe and unrecognised: pertussis in U.K. infants, *Arch Dis Child* 88:802-806, 2003.
6. Edwards K, Decker MD: Pertussis vaccines. In Plotkin S, Orenstein WA, Offit PA, editors: *Vaccines*, Philadelphia, 2013, Saunders, pp 447-492.
7. Gordon JE, Hood RI: Whooping cough and its epidemiological anomalies, *Am J Med Sci* 222:333-361, 1951.
8. Heininger U, Klich K, Stehr K, et al: Clinical findings in *Bordetella pertussis* infections: results of a prospective multicenter surveillance study, *Pediatrics* 100:E10, 1997.
9. Holmes WH: *Bacillary and rickettsial infections acute and chronic, a textbook: black death to white plague*, New York, 1940, Macmillan. 395–414.
10. Lapin JH: *Whooping cough*, Springfield, Ill, 1943, Charles C Thomas.
11. Mattoo S, Cherry JD: Molecular pathogenesis, epidemiology, and clinical manifestations of respiratory infections due to *Bordetella pertussis* and other *Bordetella* subspecies, *Clin Microbiol Rev* 18: 326-382, 2005.
12. Murray E, Nieves D, Bradley JS, et al: Characteristics of severe pertussis infections among infants ≤90 days of age admitted to pediatric intensive care units—Southern California, September 2009-June 2011, *J Pediatr Infect Dis* 2:1-6, 2013.
13. Dorbecker C, Licht C, Korber F, et al: Community-acquired pneumonia due to *Bordetella holmesii* in a patient with frequently relapsing nephrotic syndrome, *J Infect* 54:e203-e205, 2007.
14. Heininger U, Stehr K, Schmitt-Grohe S, et al: Clinical characteristics of illness caused by *Bordetella parapertussis* compared with illness caused by *Bordetella pertussis*, *Pediatr Infect Dis J* 13:306-309, 1994.
15. Njamkepo E, Bonacorsi S, Debruyne M, et al: Significant finding of *Bordetella holmesii* DNA in nasopharyngeal samples from french patients with suspected pertussis, *J Clin Microbiol* 49:4347-4348, 2011.
16. Yih WK, Silva EA, Ida J, et al: *Bordetella holmesii*-like organisms isolated from Massachusetts patients with pertussis-like symptoms, *Emerg Infect Dis* 5:441-443, 1999.
17. Cone TC Jr: Whooping cough is first described as a disease sui generis by Baillou in 1640, *Pediatrics* 46:522, 1970.
18. Bordet J, Gengou O: Le microbe de la coqueluche, *Ann Inst Pasteur (Paris)* 20:48-68, 1906.
19. Bordet J, Gengou O: L'endotoxin coquelucheuse, *Ann Inst Pasteur (Paris)* 23:415-419, 1909.
20. Cherry JD: Historical perspective on pertussis and use of vaccines to prevent it, *Microbe* 2:139-144, 2007.
21. Medical Research Council: Vaccination against whooping cough: relation between protection in children and results of laboratory tests, *Br Med J* 2:454-462, 1956.
22. Cherry JD: Historical review of pertussis and the classical vaccine, *J Infect Dis* 174:259-263, 1996.
23. Kimura M, Kuno-Sakai H: Pertussis vaccines in Japan, *Acta Paediatr Jap* 30:143-153, 1988.
24. Beiter A, Lewis K, Pineda EF, et al: Unrecognized maternal peripartum pertussis with subsequent fatal neonatal pertussis, *Obstet Gynecol* 82:691-693, 1993.
25. Berger JT, Carcillo JA, Shanley TP, et al: Critical pertussis illness in children: a multicenter prospective cohort study, *Pediatr Crit Care Med* 14:356-365, 2013.
26. Bisgard KM, Pascual FB, Ehresmann KR, et al: Infant pertussis: who was the source? *Pediatr Infect Dis J* 23:985-989, 2004.
27. Christie CD, Baltimore RS: Pertussis in neonates, *Am J Dis Child* 143:1199-1202, 1989.
28. Donoso A, Leon J, Ramirez M, et al: Pertussis and fatal pulmonary hypertension: a discouraged entity, *Scand J Infect Dis* 37:145-148, 2005.
29. Donoso AF, Cruces PI, Camacho JF, et al: Exchange transfusion to reverse severe pertussis-induced cardiogenic shock, *Pediatr Infect Dis J* 25:846-848, 2006.
30. Goulin GD, Kaya KM, Bradley JS: Severe pulmonary hypertension associated with shock and death in infants infected with *Bordetella pertussis*, *Crit Care Med* 21:1791-1794, 1993.
31. Grzeszczak MJ, Churchwell KB, Edwards KM, et al: Leukopheresis therapy for severe infantile pertussis with myocardial and pulmonary failure, *Pediatr Crit Care Med* 7:580-582, 2006.
32. Hackman R, Perrin DG, Karmali M, et al: Fatal *bordetella pertussis* infection: report of two cases with novel pathologic findings, *Pediatr Pathol Lab Med* 16:643-653, 1996.
33. Halasa NB, Barr FE, Johnson JE, et al: Fatal pulmonary hypertension associated with pertussis in infants: does extracorporeal membrane oxygenation have a role? *Pediatrics* 112:1274-1278, 2003.
34. Hoppe JE: Neonatal pertussis, *Pediatr Infect Dis J* 19:244-247, 2000.
35. Nieves D, Bradley JS, Gargas J, et al: Exchange blood transfusion in the management of severe pertussis in young infants, *Pediatr Infect Dis J* 32:698-699, 2013.
36. Nieves DJ, Singh J, Ashouri N, et al: Clinical and laboratory features of pertussis in infants at the onset of a California epidemic, *J Pediatr* 159:1044-1046, 2011.
37. Paddock CD, Sanden GN, Cherry JD, et al: Pathology and pathogenesis of fatal *Bordetella pertussis* infection in infants, *Clin Infect DIs* 47:328-338, 2008.
38. Rowlands HE, Goldman AP, Harrington K, et al: Impact of rapid leukodepletion on the outcome of severe clinical pertussis in young infants, *Pediatr* 126:e816-e827, 2010.
39. Wendelboe AM, Njamkepo E, Bourillon A, et al: Transmission of *Bordetella pertussis* to young infants, *Pediatr Infect Dis J* 26:293-299, 2007.
40. Vancanneyt M, Vandamme P, Kersters K: Differentiation of *Bordetella pertussis*, *B. parapertussis*, and *B. bronchiseptica* by whole-cell protein electrophoresis and fatty acid analysis, *Int J Syst Bacteriol* 45:843-847, 1995.
41. Wirsing von Konig CH, Riffelmann M, Coenye T: *Bordetella* and related genera. In Versalovic J, editor: *Manual of clinical microbiology*, vol. 1. Washington, DC, 1970, American Society for Microbiology Press.
42. Cherry JD, Seaton BL: Patterns of *Bordetella parapertussis* respiratory illnesses: 2008-2010, *Clin Infect Dis* 54:534-537, 2012.
43. Preston NW: Pertussis today. In Wardlaw AC, Parton R, editors: *Pathogenesis and immunity in pertussis*, New York, 1988, John Wiley & Sons, pp 1-18.
44. Porter JF, Connor K, Donachie W: Isolation and characterization of *Bordetella parapertussis*-like bacteria from ovine lungs, *Microbiology* 140(Pt 2):255-261, 1994.
45. Choy KW, Wulffraat NM, Wolfs TF, et al: *Bordetella bronchiseptica* respiratory infection in a child after bone marrow transplantation, *Pediatr Infect Dis J* 18:481-483, 1999.
46. Decker GR, Lavelle JP, Kumar PN, et al: Pneumonia due to *Bordetella bronchiseptica* in a patient with AIDS, *Rev Infect Dis* 13:1250-1251, 1991.
47. Gueirard P, Weber C, Le Coustumier A, et al: Human *Bordetella bronchiseptica* infection related to contact with infected animals: persistence of bacteria in host, *J Clin Microbiol* 33:2002-2006, 1995.
48. Ng VL, Boggs JM, York MK, et al: Recovery of *Bordetella bronchiseptica* from patients with AIDS, *Clin Infect Dis* 15:376-377, 1992.
49. Stefanelli P, Mastrantonio P, Hausman SZ, et al: Molecular characterization of two *Bordetella bronchiseptica* strains isolated from children with coughs, *J Clin Microbiol* 35:1550-1555, 1997.
50. Switzer WP, Mare CJ, Hubbard ED. Incidence of *Bordetella bronchiseptica* in wildlife and man in Iowa, *Am J Vet Res* 27:1134-1136, 1966.
51. Tamion F, Girault C, Chevron V, et al: *Bordetella bronchoseptica* pneumonia with shock in an immunocompetent patient, *Scand J Infect Dis* 28:137-138, 1996.
52. Woolfrey BF, Moody JA: Human infections associated with *Bordetella bronchiseptica*, *Clin Microbiol Rev* 4:243-255, 1991.
53. Borras Sans M, Bonal J, Bonet J, et al: *Bordetella bronchiseptica* septicemia in a hemodialysis patient, *Nephron* 59:676, 1991.
54. Mazengia E, Silva EA, Peppe JA, et al: Recovery of *Bordetella holmesii* from patients with pertussis-like symptoms: use of pulsed-field gel electrophoresis to characterize circulating strains, *J Clin Microbiol* 38:2330-2333, 2000.
55. Cherry JD: Pertussis: challenges today and for the future, *PLoS Pathog* 9:e1003418, 2013.
56. Mink CM, O'Brien CH, Wassilak S, et al: Isotype and antigen specificity of pertussis agglutinins following whole-cell pertussis vaccination and infection with *Bordetella pertussis*, *Infect Immun* 62:1118-1120, 1994.

57. Mooi FR, van Loo IH, van Gent M, et al: *Bordetella pertussis* strains with increased toxin production associated with pertussis resurgence, *Emerg Infect Dis* 15:1206-1213, 2009.
58. Robinson A, Ashworth LA, Irons LI: Serotyping *Bordetella pertussis* strains, *Vaccine* 7:491-494, 1989.
59. Robinson A, Irons LI, Seabrook RN, et al: Structure-function studies of *Bordetella pertussis* fimbriae. In Manclark CR, editor: *Proceedings of the Sixth International Symposium on Pertussis, DHHS publication no. (FDA) 90*, Bethesda, MD, 1990, Department of Health and Human Services, U.S. Public Health Service, pp 126-135.
60. Tuomanen E: *Bordetella pertussis* adhesins. In Wardlaw AC, Parton R, editors: *Pathogenesis and immunity in pertussis*, New York, 1988, John Wiley & Sons, pp 75-94.
61. Weiss AA, Hewlett EL: Virulence factors of *Bordetella pertussis*, *Ann Rev Microbiol* 40:661-686, 1986.
62. Cherry JD, Gornbein J, Heininger U, et al: A search for serologic correlates of immunity to *Bordetella pertussis* cough illnesses, *Vaccine* 16:1901-1906, 1998.
63. Storsaeter J, Hallander HO, Gustafsson L, et al: Levels of anti-pertussis antibodies related to protection after household exposure to *Bordetella pertussis*, *Vaccine* 16:1907-1916, 1998.
64. Abramson T, Kedem H, Relman DA: Proinflammatory and proapoptotic activities associated with *Bordetella pertussis* filamentous hemagglutinin, *Infect Immun* 69:2650-2658, 2001.
65. Bhargava A, Leininger E, Roberts M, et al: Filamentous hemagglutinin and the 69-kDa protein, pertactin, promote adherence of *Bordetella pertussis* to epithelial cells and macrophages. Paper presented at the Sixth International Symposium on Pertussis, Bethesda, Md, September 26-28, 1990, pp 137–138.
66. Cotter PA, Miller JF: Bordetella. In Groisman EA, editor: *Principles of bacterial pathogenesis*, San Diego, 2001, Academic Press, pp 619-674.
67. Henderson MW, Inatsuka CS, Sheets AJ, et al: Contribution of *Bordetella* filamentous hemagglutinin and adenylate cyclase toxin to suppression and evasion of interleukin-17-mediated inflammation, *Infect Immun* 80:2061-2075, 2012.
68. Kimura A, Mountzouros KT, Relman DA, et al: *Bordetella pertussis* filamentous hemagglutinin: evaluation as a protective antigen and colonization factor in a mouse respiratory infection model, *Infect Immun* 58:7-16, 1990.
69. Makhov AM, Hannah JH, Brennan MJ, et al: Filamentous hemagglutinin of *Bordetella pertussis*. A bacterial adhesin formed as a 50-nm monomeric rigid rod based on a 19-residue repeat motif rich in beta strands and turns, *J Mol Biol* 241:110-124, 1994.
70. Vidakovics MLA, Lamberti Y, van der Pol WL, et al: Adenylate cyclase influences filamentous haemagglutinin-medicated attachment of *Bordetella pertussis* to epithelial alveolar cells, *FEMS Immunol Med Microbiol* 48:140-147, 2006.
71. Sato H, Sato Y: *Bordetella pertussis* infection in mice: correlation of specific antibodies against two antigens, pertussis toxin, and filamentous hemagglutinin with mouse protectivity in an intracerebral or aerosol challenge system, *Infect Immun* 46:415-421, 1984.
72. Shahin RD, Amsbaugh DF, Leef MF: Mucosal immunization with filamentous hemagglutinin protects against *Bordetella pertussis* respiratory infection, *Infect Immun* 60:1482-1488, 1992.
73. Inatsuka CS, Xu Q, Vujkovic-Cvijin I, et al: Pertactin is required for *Bordetella* species to resist neutrophil-mediated clearance, *Infect Immun* 78:2901-2909, 2010.
74. Leininger E, Kenimer JG, Brennan MJ: Surface proteins of *Bordetella pertussis*: role in adherence. Paper presented at the Sixth International Symposium on Pertussis. Bethesda, Md, September 26-28, 1990, pp 25–26.
75. Novotny P: Pathogenesis in *Bordetella* species, *J Infect Dis* 161: 581-583, 1990.
76. Novotny P, Chubb AP, Cownley K, et al: Biologic and protective properties of the 69-kDa outer membrane protein of *Bordetella pertussis*: a novel formulation for an acellular pertussis vaccine, *J Infect Dis* 164:114-122, 1991.
77. Hellwig SM, Rodriguez ME, Berbers GA, et al: Crucial role of antibodies to pertactin in *Bordetella pertussis* immunity, *J Infect Dis* 188: 738-742, 2003.
78. Cherry JD: Comparative efficacy of acellular pertussis vaccines: an analysis of recent trials, *Pediatr Infect Dis* 16:90-96, 1997.
79. Cherry JD, Olin P: Commentaries: the science and fiction of pertussis vaccines, *Pediatrics* 104:1381-1383, 1999.
80. Gustafsson L, Hallander HO, Olin P, et al: A controlled trial of a two-component acellular, a five-component acellular, and a whole-cell pertussis vaccine, *N Engl J Med* 334:349-355, 1996.
81. Andreasen C, Carbonetti NH: Pertussis toxin inhibits early chemokine production to delay neutrophil recruitment in response to *Bordetella pertussis* respiratory tract infection in mice, *Infect Immun* 76:5139-5148, 2008.
82. Andreasen C, Powell DA, Carbonetti NH: Pertussis toxin stimulates il-17 production in response to *Bordetella pertussis* infection in mice, *PLoS One* 4:e7079, 2009.
83. Arciniega JL, Shahin RD, Burnette WN, et al: Contribution of the B oligomer to the protective activity of genetically attenuated pertussis toxin, *Infect Immun* 59:3407-3410, 1991.
84. Arico B, Rappuoli R: *Bordetella parapertussis* and *Bordetella bronchiseptica* contain transcriptionally silent pertussis toxin genes, *J Bacteriol* 169:2847-2853, 1987.
85. Carbonetti NH, Artamonova GV, Van Rooijen N, et al: Pertussis toxin targets airway macrophages to promote *Bordetella pertussis* infection of the respiratory tract, *Infect Immun* 75:1713-1720, 2007.
86. Furman BL, Sidey FM, Smith M: Metabolic disturbances produced by pertussis toxin. In Wardlaw AC, Parton R, editors: *Pathogenesis and immunity in pertussis*, New York, 1988, John Wiley & Sons, pp 147-172.
87. Irons LI, Gorringe AR: Pertussis toxin: production, purification, molecular structure, and assay. In Wardlaw AC, Parton R, editors: *Pathogenesis and immunity in pertussis*, New York, 1988, John Wiley & Sons, pp 95-120.
88. Locht C, Coutte L, Mielcarek N: The ins and outs of pertussis toxin, *FEBS J* 278:4668-4682, 2011.
89. Pittman M: Pertussis toxin: the cause of the harmful effects and prolonged immunity of whooping cough. A hypothesis, *Rev Infect Dis* 1:401-412, 1979.
90. Pittman M: The concept of pertussis as a toxin-mediated disease, *Pediatr Infect Dis J* 3:467-486, 1984.
91. Ui M: The multiple biological activities of pertussis toxin. In Wardlaw AC, Parton R, editors: *Pathogenesis and immunity in pertussis*, New York, 1988, John Wiley & Sons, pp 121-146.
92. Cherry JD: Pertussis: the trials and tribulations of old and new pertussis vaccines, *Vaccine* 10:1033-1038, 1992.
93. Carbonetti NH: Pertussis toxin and adenylate cyclase toxin: key virulence factors of *Bordetella pertussis* and cell biology tools, *Future Microbiol* 5:455-469, 2010.
94. Hewlett EL, Gordon VM: Adenylate cyclase toxin of *Bordetella pertussis*. In Wardlaw AC, Parton R, editors: *Pathogenesis and immunity in pertussis*, New York, 1988, John Wiley & Sons, pp 193-209.
95. Khelef N, Sakamoto H, Guiso N: Both adenylate cyclase and hemolytic activities are required by *Bordetella pertussis* to initiate infection, *Microbial Pathog* 12:227-235, 1992.
96. Weiss AA, Hewlett EL, Myers GA, et al: Pertussis toxin and extracytoplasmic adenylate cyclase as virulence factors of *Bordetella pertussis*, *J Infect Dis* 150:219-222, 1984.
97. Nakase Y, Endoh M: Heat-labile toxin of *Bordetella pertussis*. In Wardlaw AC, Parton R, editors: *Pathogenesis and immunity in pertussis*, New York, 1988, John Wiley & Sons, pp 217-229.
98. Cundell DR, Kanthakumar K, Taylor GW, et al: Effect of tracheal cytotoxin from *Bordetella pertussis* on human neutrophil function in vitro, *Infect Immun* 62:639-643, 1994.
99. Goldman WE: Tracheal cytotoxin of *Bordetella pertussis*. In Wardlaw AC, Parton R, editors: *Pathogenesis and immunity in pertussis*, New York, 1988, John Wiley & Sons, pp 237-246.
100. Fennelly NK, Sisti F, Higgins SC, et al: *Bordetella pertussis* expresses a functional type III secretion system that subverts protective innate and adaptive immune responses, *Infect Immun* 76:1257-1266, 2008.
101. Chaby R, Caroff M: Lipopolysaccharides of *Bordetella pertussis* endotoxin. In Wardlaw AC, Parton R, editors: *Pathogenesis and immunity in pertussis*, New York, 1988, John Wiley & Sons, pp 247-272.
102. Cody CL, Baraff LJ, Cherry JD, et al: Nature and rates of adverse reactions associated with DTP and DT immunizations in infants and children, *Pediatrics* 68:650-660, 1981.
103. Mountzouros KT, Kimura A, Cowell JL: A bactericidal monoclonal antibody specific for the lipooligosaccharide of *Bordetella pertussis* reduces colonization of the respiratory tract of mice after aerosol infection with *B. pertussis*, *Infect Immun* 60:5316-5318, 1992.
104. Anderson RM, May RM: Vaccination and herd immunity to infectious diseases, *Nature* 318:323-329, 1985.
105. Fine PE: Herd immunity: history, theory, practice, *Epidemiol Rev* 15:265-302, 1993.

106. Cherry JD, Harriman K, Why do vaccine-preventable disease outbreaks occur in the United States? *Infect Dis Special Ed* 15:53-57, 2012.
107. Haward RA: Scale of undernotification of infectious diseases by general practitioners, *Lancet* 1:873-874, 1973.
108. Jenkinson D: Whooping cough: what proportion of cases is notified in an epidemic? *BMJ* 287:183-185, 1983.
109. Stocks P: *Studies in the population of England and Wales 1944-47. Studies on medical and population subjects. No. 2*, London, 1949, His Majesty's Stationery Office.
110. Joint Committee on Vaccination and Immunisation: The whooping cough epidemic, 1977-79. In *Whooping cough: reports from the Committee on Safety in Medicine and the Joint Committee on Vaccination and Immunisation*, London, 1981, Department of Health and Social Security, Her Majesty's Stationery Office, p 170.
111. Center for Disease Control and Prevention: Summary of notifiable diseases—United States, 2010, *MMWR Morb Mortal Wkly Rep* 59: 1-111, 2012.
112. Cherry JD: Epidemiology of pertussis, *Pediat Infect Dis J* 25:361-362, 2006.
113. Cherry JD: Epidemiological, clinical, and laboratory aspects of pertussis in adults, *Clin Infect Dis* 28:112-117, 1999.
114. Cherry JD: Epidemic pertussis in 2012—the resurgence of a vaccine-preventable disease, *N Engl J Med* 367:785-787, 2012.
115. Christie CD, Marx ML, Marchant CD, et al: The 1993 epidemic of pertussis in Cincinnati. Resurgence of disease in a highly immunized population of children, *N Engl J Med* 331:16-21, 1994.
116. Greco D, Salmaso S, Mastrantonio P, et al: A controlled trial of two acellular vaccines and one whole-cell vaccine against pertussis. Progetto Pertosse Working Group, *N Engl J Med* 334:341-348, 1996.
117. Fine PE, Clarkson JA: The recurrence of whooping cough: possible implications for assessment of vaccine efficacy, *Lancet* 1:666-669, 1982.
118. Fine PEM: Epidemiological considerations for whooping cough eradication. In Wardlaw AC, Parton R, editors: *Pathogenesis and immunity in pertussis*, New York, 1988, John Wiley & Sons, pp 451-467.
119. Cherry JD: *Strategies for diphtheria, tetanus, and pertussis (DTP) immunization: report of the 104th Ross Conference on Pediatric Research*, Columbus, Ohio, 1994, Ross Products Division, Abbott Laboratories. 218–225.
120. McEniery JA, Delbridge RG, Reith DM: Infant pertussis deaths and the management of cardiovascular compromise, *J Paediatr Child Health* 40:230-232, 2004.
121. Nelson JD: The changing epidemiology of pertussis in young infants. The role of adults as reservoirs of infection, *Am J Dis Child* 132: 371-373, 1978.
122. Valenti WM, Pincus PH, Messner MK: Nosocomial pertussis: possible spread by a hospital visitor, *Am J Dis Child* 134:520-521, 1980.
123. Cherry JD, Baraff LJ, Hewlett E: The past, present, and future of pertussis. The role of adults in epidemiology and future control, *West J Med* 150:319-328, 1989.
124. Mortimer EA Jr: Pertussis and its prevention: a family affair, *J Infect Dis* 161:473-479, 1990.
125. Linnemann CC Jr, Nasenbeny J: Pertussis in the adult, *Ann Rev Med* 28:179-185, 1977.
126. Kurt TL, Yeager AS, Guenette S, et al: Spread of pertussis by hospital staff, *JAMA* 221:264-267, 1972.
127. Linnemann CC Jr, Ramundo N, Perlstein PH, et al: Use of pertussis vaccine in an epidemic involving hospital staff, *Lancet* 2:540-543, 1975.
128. Centers for Disease Control and Prevention: Preventing tetanus, diphtheria, and pertussis among adolescents: use of tetanus toxoid, reduced diphtheria toxoid and acellular pertussis vaccines recommendations of the Advisory Committee on Immunization Practices (ACIP), *MMWR Recomm Rep* 55(RR-3):1-34, 2006.
129. Birkebaek NH, Kristiansen M, Seefeldt T, et al: *Bordetella pertussis* and chronic cough in adults, *Clin Infect Dis* 29:1239-1242, 1999.
130. Deen JL, Mink CA, Cherry JD, et al: Household contact study of *Bordetella pertussis* infections, *Clin Infect Dis* 21:1211-1219, 1995.
131. Deville JG, Cherry JD, Christenson PD, et al: Frequency of unrecognized *Bordetella pertussis* infections in adults, *Clin Infect Dis* 21: 639-642, 1995.
132. Schmitt-Grohe S, Cherry JD, Heininger U, et al: Pertussis in German adults, *Clin Infect Dis* 21:860-866, 1995.
133. Wirsing von Konig CH, Postels-Multani S, Bock HL, et al: Pertussis in adults: frequency of transmission after household exposure, *Lancet* 346:1326-1329, 1995.
134. Wright SW, Edwards KM, Decker MD, et al: Pertussis infection in adults with persistent cough, *JAMA* 273:1044-1046, 1995.
135. de Melker HE, Versteegh FG, Schellekens JF, et al: The incidence of *Bordetella pertussis* infections estimated in the population from a combination of serological surveys, *J Infect* 53:106-113, 2006.
136. Hewlett EL, Cherry JD: New and improved vaccines against pertussis. In Woodrow GC, Levine MM, editors: *New generation vaccines*, New York, 1990, Marcel Dekker, pp 231-250.
137. Munoz JJ: Action of pertussigen (pertussis toxin) on the host immune system. In Wardlaw AC, Parton R, editors: *Pathogenesis and immunity in pertussis*, New York, 1988, John Wiley & Sons, pp 173-192.
138. Barnes MG, Weiss AA: BrkA protein of *Bordetella pertussis* inhibits the classical pathway of complement after C1 deposition, *Infect Immun* 69:3067-3072, 2001.
139. Marr N, Oliver DC, Laurent V, et al: Protective activity of the *Bordetella pertussis* BrkA autotransporter in the murine lung colonization model, *Vaccine* 26:4306-4311, 2008.
140. Marr N, Shah NR, Lee R, et al: *Bordetella pertussis* autotransporter Vag8 binds human C1 esterase inhibitor and confers serum resistance, *PLoS One* 6:e20585, 2011.
141. Noofeli M, Bokhari H, Blackburn P, et al: Bapc autotransporter protein is a virulence determinant of *Bordetella pertussis*, *Microb Pathogen* 51:169-177, 2011.
142. Oliver DC, Fernandez RC: Antibodies to BrkA augment killing of *Bordetella pertussis*, *Vaccine* 20:235-241, 2001.
143. Williams CL, Haines R, Cotter PA: Serendipitous discovery of an immunoglobulin-binding autotransporter in *Bordetella* species, *Infect Immun* 76:2966-2977, 2008.
144. Zipprich J, Murray E, Kong D, et al: *Risk factors associated with infant death from pertussis: preliminary results from a case-control study*, Boston, 2012, Pediatric Academic Societies.
145. Hewitt M, Canning BJ: Coughing precipitated by *Bordetella pertussis* infection, *Lung* 188(suppl 1):S73-S79, 2010.
146. Olsen LC: Pertussis, *Medicine (Baltimore)* 54:427-469, 1975.
147. Hedenskog S, Bjorksten B, Blennow M, et al: Immunoglobulin E response to pertussis toxin in whooping cough and after immunization with a whole-cell and an acellular pertussis vaccine, *Intl Arch Allergy Appl Immunol* 89:156-161, 1989.
148. Manclark CR, Meade BD, Burstyn DG: Serological response to *Bordetella pertussis*. In Rose NR, Friedman H, Fahey JL, editors: *Manual of clinical laboratory immunology*, Washington, DC, 1986, American Society for Microbiology, pp 388-394.
149. Onorato IM, Wassilak SG: Laboratory diagnosis of pertussis: the state of the art, *Pediatr Infect Dis J* 6:145-151, 1987.
150. Halperin SA, Bortolussi R, Kasina A, et al: Use of a Chinese hamster ovary cell cytotoxicity assay for the rapid diagnosis of pertussis, *J Clin Microbiol* 28:32-38, 1990.
151. Granstrom G, Askelof P, Granstrom M: Specific immunoglobulin a to *Bordetella pertussis* antigens in mucosal secretion for rapid diagnosis of whooping cough, *J Clin Microbiol* 26:869-874, 1988.
152. Zackrisson G, Lagergard T, Trollfors B, et al: Immunoglobulin a antibodies to pertussis toxin and filamentous hemagglutinin in saliva from patients with pertussis, *J Clin Microbiol* 28:1502-1505, 1990.
153. Cherry JD, Beer T, Chartrand SA, et al: Comparison of values of antibody to *Bordetella pertussis* antigens in young German and American men, *Clin Infect Dis* 20:1271-1274, 1995.
154. Cherry JD: Pertussis in the preantibiotic and prevaccine era, with emphasis on adult pertussis, *Clin Infect Dis* 28(Suppl 2):107-111, 1999.
154a. Cherry JD: The present and future control of pertussis, *Clin Infect Dis* 51:663-667, 2010.
155. Versteegh FG, Schellekens JF, Nagelkerke AF, et al: Laboratory-confirmed reinfections with *Bordetella pertussis*, *Acta Paediatr* 91: 95-97, 2002.
156. Cherry JD: Why do pertussis vaccines fail?, *Pediatrics* 129:968-970, 2012.
157. Klein NP, Bartlett J, Rowhani-Rahbar A, et al: Waning protection after fifth dose of acellular pertussis vaccine in children, *N Engl J Med* 367:1012-1019, 2012.
158. Liko J, Robison SG, Cieslak PR: Priming with whole-cell versus acellular pertussis vaccine, *N Engl J Med* 368:581-582, 2013.
159. Misegades LK, Winter K, Harriman K, et al: Association of childhood pertussis with receipt of 5 doses of pertussis vaccine by time since last vaccine dose, California, 2010, *JAMA* 308:2126-2132, 2012.
160. Sheridan SL, Ware RS, Grimwood K, et al: Number and order of whole cell pertussis vaccines in infancy and disease protection, *JAMA* 308:454-456, 2012.

161. Skoff TH, Cohn AC, Clark TA, et al: Early impact of the U.S. Tdap vaccination program on pertussis trends, *Arch Pediatr Adolesc Med* 166:344-349, 2012.
162. Tartof SY, Lewis M, Kenyon C, et al: Waning immunity to pertussis following 5 doses of DTAP, *Pediatrics* 131:e1047-e1052, 2013.
163. Witt MA, Arias L, Katz PH, et al: Reduced risk of pertussis among persons ever vaccinated with whole cell pertussis vaccine compared to recipients of acellular pertussis vaccines in a large U.S. cohort, *Clin Infect Dis* 56:1248-1254, 2013.
164. Cherry JD, Heininger U, Richards DM, et al: Antibody response patterns to *Bordetella pertussis* antigens in vaccinated (primed) and unvaccinated (unprimed) young children with pertussis, *Clin Vaccine Immunol* 17:741-747, 2010.
165. Tondella ML, Carlone GM, Messonnier N, et al: International *Bordetella pertussis* assay standardization and harmonization meeting report. Centers for Disease Control and Prevention, Atlanta, Georgia, United States, 19-20 July 2007, *Vaccine* 27:803-814, 2009.
166. Weiss AA, Patton AK, Millen SH, et al: Acellular pertussis vaccines and complement killing of *Bordetella pertussis*, *Infect Immun* 72:7346-7351, 2004.
167. Ausiello CM, Lande R, Urbani F, et al: Cell-mediated immunity and antibody responses to *Bordetella pertussis* antigens in children with a history of pertussis infection and in recipients of an acellular pertussis vaccine, *J Infect Dis* 181:1989-1995, 2000.
168. Mahon BP, Brady MT, Mills KH: Protection against *Bordetella pertussis* in mice in the absence of detectable circulating antibody: implications for long-term immunity in children, *J Infect Dis* 181:2087-2091, 2000.
169. Mills KH, Redhead K: Cellular immunity in pertussis, *J Med Microbiol* 39:163-164, 1993.
170. Mills KH, Barnard A, Watkins J, et al: Cell-mediated immunity to *Bordetella pertussis*: role of Th1 cells in bacterial clearance in a murine respiratory infection model, *Infect Immun* 61:399-410, 1993.
171. Minh NNT, He Q, Edelman K, et al: Cell-mediated immune responses to antigens of *Bordetella pertussis* and protection against pertussis in school children, *Pediatr Infect Dis J* 18:366-370, 1999.
172. Ryan M, Murphy G, Ryan E, et al: Distinct T-cell subtypes induced with whole cell and acellular pertussis vaccines in children, *Immunology* 93:1-10, 1998.
173. Ryan M, Murphy G, Gothefors L, et al: *Bordetella pertussis* respiratory infection in children is associated with preferential activation of type 1 T helper cells, *J Infect Dis* 175:1246-1250, 1997.
174. Tomoda T, Ogura H, Kurashige T: Immune responses to *Bordetella pertussis* infection and vaccination, *J Infect Dis* 163:559-563, 1991.
175. Wiertz EJ, Loggen HG, Walvoort HC, et al: In vitro induction of antigen specific antibody synthesis and proliferation of T lymphocytes with acellular pertussis vaccines, pertussis toxin and filamentous haemagglutinin in humans, *J Biol Standard* 17:181-190, 1989.
176. Zepp F, Knuf M, Habermehl P, et al: Pertussis-specific cell-mediated immunity in infants after vaccination with a tricomponent acellular pertussis vaccine, *Infect Immun* 64:4078-4084, 1996.
177. Lautrop H: Observations on parapertussis in Denmark, 1950-1957, *Acta Pathol Microbiol Scand* 43:255-266, 1958.
178. Taranger J, Trollfors B, Lagergard T, et al: Parapertussis infection followed by pertussis infection, *Lancet* 344:1703, 1994.
179. Heininger U, Stehr K, Christenson P, et al: Evidence of efficacy of the Lederle/Takeda acellular pertussis component diphtheria and tetanus toxoids and pertussis vaccine but not the Lederle whole-cell component diphtheria and tetanus toxoids and pertussis vaccine against *Bordetella parapertussis* infection, *Clin Infect Dis* 28:602-604, 1999.
180. Linnemann CC Jr: Host-parasite interactions in pertussis. In Manclark CR, Hill JC, editors: *International Symposium on Pertussis, publication no. (NIH) 79-1830*, Washington, DC, 1979, U.S. Dept. of Health, Education, and Welfare, U.S. Government Printing Office, pp 3-18.
181. Mallory FB, Hornor AA: Pertussis: the histological lesion in the respiratory tract, *J Med Res* 27:115-123, 1912.
182. Smith C, Vyas H: Early infantile pertussis; increasingly prevalent and potentially fatal, *Eur J Pediatr* 159:898-900, 2000.
183. Woolf AL, Caplin H: Whooping cough encephalitis, *Arch Dis Child* 31:87-91, 1956.
184. Janda WM, Santos E, Stevens J, et al: Unexpected isolation of *Bordetella pertussis* from a blood culture, *J Clin Microbiol* 32:2851-2853, 1994.
185. Troseid M, Jonassen TO, Steinbakk M: Isolation of *Bordetella pertussis* in blood culture from a patient with multiple myeloma, *J Infect* 52:e11-e13, 2006.
186. Centers for Disease Control and Prevention: Fatal case of unsuspected pertussis diagnosed from a blood culture: Minnesota, 2003, *MMWR Morb Mortal Wkly Rep* 53:131-132, 2004.
187. Cherry JD, Tan T, Wirsing von Konig CH, et al: Clinical definitions of pertussis: summary of a global pertussis initiative roundtable meeting, February 2011, *Clin Infect Dis* 54:1756-1764, 2012.
188. De Serres G, Shadmani R, Duval B, et al: Morbidity of pertussis in adolescents and adults, *J Infect Dis* 182:174-179, 2000.
189. Mink CM, Cherry JD, Christenson P, et al: A search for *Bordetella pertussis* infection in university students, *Clin Infect Dis* 14:464-471, 1992.
190. Nennig ME, Shinefield HR, Edwards KM, et al: Prevalence and incidence of adult pertussis in an urban population, *JAMA* 275:1672-1674, 1996.
191. Postels-Multani S, Schmitt HJ, Wirsing von Konig CH, et al: Symptoms and complications of pertussis in adults, *Infection* 23:139-142, 1995.
192. Linnemann CC, Perry EB: *Bordetella parapertussis*. Recent experience and a review of the literature, *Am J Dis Child* 131:560-563, 1977.
193. Cherry JD: Pertussis in the preantibiotic and prevaccine era, with emphasis on adult pertussis, *Clin Infect Dis* 28:107-111, 1999.
194. Cherry JD: Unpublished observations.
195. Murphy TV, Slade BA, Broder KR, et al: Prevention of pertussis, tetanus, and diphtheria among pregnant and postpartum women and their infants: recommendations of the Advisory Committee on Immunization Practices (ACIP), *MMWR* 57:1-51, 2008.
196. MacLean DW, Calder MA: Pertussis in pregnancy, *Scottish Med J* 26:250-253, 1981.
197. Granström G, Granström M, Sterner G: Whooping cough in late pregnancy, *Scand J Infect Dis Suppl* 71:27-29, 1990.
198. Bonnefoy O, Maugey-Laulom B, Diris B, et al: Fetal extradural hematoma: prenatal diagnosis and postmortem examination, *Fetal Diagn Ther* 20:262-265, 2005.
199. Haugen G, Jenum PA, Scheie D, et al: Prenatal diagnosis of tracheal obstruction: possible association with maternal pertussis infection, *Ultrasound Obstetr Gynecol* 15:69-73, 2000.
200. McGregor J, Ogle JW, Curry-Kane G: Perinatal pertussis, *Obstet Gynecol* 68:582-586, 1986.
201. Baron S, Njamkepo E, Grimprel E, et al: Epidemiology of pertussis in French hospitals in 1993 and 1994: thirty years after a routine use of vaccination, *Pediatr Infect Dis J* 17:412-418, 1998.
202. Elliott E, McIntyre P, Ridley G, et al: National study of infants hospitalized with pertussis in the acellular vaccine era, *Pediatr Infect Dis J* 23:246-252, 2004.
203. Kowalzik F, Barbosa AP, Fernandes VR, et al: Prospective multinational study of pertussis infection in hospitalized infants and their household contacts, *Pediatr Infect Dis J* 26:238-242, 2007.
204. Long SS, Welkon CJ, Clark JL: Widespread silent transmission of pertussis in families: antibody correlates of infection and symptomatology, *J Infect Dis* 161:480-486, 1990.
205. Long SS, Lischner HW, Deforest A, et al: Serologic evidence of subclinical pertussis in immunized children, *Pediatr Infect Dis J* 9:700-705, 1990.
206. Heininger U, Kleemann WJ, Cherry JD: A controlled study of the relationship between *Bordetella pertussis* infections and sudden unexpected deaths among German infants, *Pediatrics* 114:e9-e15, 2004.
207. Nooitgedagt JE, de Greeff SC, Elvers BH, et al: Seroprevalence of *Bordetella pertussis* infection during pregnancy measured by IgG antibodies against pertussis toxin, *Clin Infect Dis* 49:1086-1089, 2009.
208. Farizo KM, Cochi SL, Zell ER, et al: Epidemiological features of pertussis in the United States, 1980-1989, *Clin Infect Dis* 14:708-719, 1992.
209. Heininger U, Stehr K, Cherry JD: Serious pertussis overlooked in infants, *Eur J Pediatr* 151:342-343, 1992.
210. Nicoll A, Gardner A: Whooping cough and unrecognised postperinatal mortality, *Arch Dis Child* 63:41-47, 1988.
211. Castagnini LA, Munoz FM: Clinical characteristics and outcomes of neonatal pertussis: a comparative study, *J Pediatr* 156:498-500, 2010.
212. Crowcroft NS, Andrews N, Rooney C, et al: Deaths from pertussis are underestimated in England, *Arch Dis Child* 86:336-338, 2002.
213. De Berry BB, Lynch JE, Chung DH, et al: Pertussis with severe pulmonary hypertension and leukocytosis treated with extracorporeal membrane oxygenation, *Pediatr Surg Intl* 21:692-694, 2005.

214. Gil A, Oyaguez I, Carrasco P, et al: Hospital admissions for pertussis in Spain, 1995-1998, *Vaccine* 19:4791-4794, 2001.
215. Guris D, Strebel PM, Bardenheier B, et al: Changing epidemiology of pertussis in the United States: increasing reported incidence among adolescents and adults, 1990-1996, *Clin Infect Dis* 28:1230-1237, 1999.
216. Haberling DL, Holman RC, Paddock CD, et al: Infant and maternal risk factors for pertussis-related infant mortality in the United States, 1999 to 2004, *Pediatr Infect Dis J* 28:194-198, 2009.
217. Heininger U, Stehr K, Schmidt-Schlapfer G, et al: *Bordetella pertussis* infections and sudden unexpected deaths in children, *Eur J Pediatr* 155:551-553, 1996.
218. Lewis K, Saubolle MA, Tenover FC, et al: Pertussis caused by an erythromycin-resistant strain of *Bordetella pertussis*, *Pediatr Infect Dis J* 14:388-391, 1995.
219. Mikelova LK, Halperin SA, Scheifele D, et al: Predictors of death in infants hospitalized with pertussis: a case-control study of 16 pertussis deaths in Canada, *J Pediatr* 143:576-581, 2003.
220. Namachivayam P, Shimizu K, Butt W: Pertussis: severe clinical presentation in pediatric intensive care and its relation to outcome, *Pediatr Crit Care Med* 8:207-211, 2007.
221. Pierce C, Klein N, Peters M: Is leukocytosis a predictor of mortality in severe pertussis infection? *Intensive Care Med* 26:1512-1514, 2000.
222. Pooboni S, Roberts N, Westrope C, et al: Extracorporeal life support in pertussis, *Pediatr Pulmonol* 36:310-315, 2003.
223. Romano MJ, Weber MD, Weisse ME, et al: Pertussis pneumonia, hypoxemia, hyperleukocytosis, and pulmonary hypertension: improvement in oxygenation after a double volume exchange transfusion, *Pediatrics* 114:e264-e266, 2004.
224. Sawal M, Cohen M, Irazuzta JE, et al: Fulminant pertussis: a multicenter study with new insights into the clinico-pathological mechanisms, *Pediatr Pulmonol* 44:970-980, 2009.
225. Skladal D, Horak E, Fruhwirth M, et al: Successful treatment of ARDS and severe pulmonary hypertension in a child with *Bordetella pertussis* infection, *Wien Klin Wochenschr* 116:760-762, 2004.
226. Somerville RL, Grant CC, Grimwood K, et al: Infants hospitalised with pertussis: estimating the true disease burden, *J Paediatr Child Health* 43:617-622, 2007.
227. Sreenan CD, Osiovich H: Neonatal pertussis requiring extracorporeal membrane oxygenation, *Pediatr Surg Intl* 17:201-203, 2001.
228. Tanaka M, Vitek CR, Pascual FB, et al: Trends in pertussis among infants in the United States, 1980-1999, *JAMA* 290:2968-2975, 2003.
229. Vitek CR, Pascual FB, Baughman AL, et al: Increase in deaths from pertussis among young infants in the United States in the 1990s, *Pediatr Infect Dis J* 22:628-634, 2003.
230. Williams GD, Numa A, Sokol J, et al: ECLS in pertussis: does it have a role? *Intensive Care Med* 24:1089-1092, 1998.
231. Centers for Disease Control and Prevention: Pertussis: United States, 1997-2000, *MMWR Morb Mortal Wkly Rep* 51:73-76, 2002.
232. Rocha G, Flor-de-Lima F, Soares P, et al: Severe pertussis in newborns and young vulnerable infants, *Pediatr Infect Dis J* 32:1152-1154, 2013.
233. Taffarel P, Bonetto G, Haimovich A: Severe pertussis, progression and exchange transfusion as an alternative treatment. Case reports, *Arch Argent Pediatr* 110:327-330, 2012.
234. Lindgren C, Milerad J, Lagercrantz H: Sudden infant death and prevalence of whooping cough in the Swedish and Norwegian communities, *Eur J Pediatr* 156:405-409, 1997.
235. Aoyama T, Ide Y, Watanabe J, et al: Respiratory failure caused by dual infection with *Bordetella pertussis* and respiratory syncytial virus, *Acta Paediatr Japon* 38:282-285, 1996.
236. Cosnes-Lambe C, Raymond J, Chalumeau M, et al: Pertussis and respiratory syncytial virus infections, *Eur J Pediatr* 167:1017-1019, 2008.
237. Dagan R, Hall CB, Menegus MA: Atypical bacterial infections explained by a concomitant virus infection, *Pediatrics* 76:411-414, 1985.
238. Korppi M, Hiltunen J: Pertussis is common in nonvaccinated infants hospitalized for respiratory syncytial virus infection, *Pediatr Infect Dis J* 26:316-318, 2007.
239. Miron D, Srugo I, Kra-Oz Z, et al: Sole pathogen in acute bronchiolitis: is there a role for other organisms apart from respiratory syncytial virus? *Pediatr Infect Dis J* 29:e7-e10, 2010.
240. Cherry JD, Paddock CD, Greer PW, et al: The respiratory pathology in infants with sudden unexpected deaths in whom respiratory specimens were initially PCR-positive or PCR-negative for *Bordetella pertussis*, *Infection* 39:545-548, 2011.
241. Mastrantonio P, Stefanelli P, Giuliano M, et al: *Bordetella parapertussis* infection in children: epidemiology, clinical symptoms, and molecular characteristics of isolates, *J Clin Microbiol* 36:999-1002, 1998.
242. Hoppe JE: Update on respiratory infection caused by *Bordetella parapertussis*, *Pediatr Infect Dis J* 18:375-381, 1999.
243. Iwata S, Aoyama T, Goto A, et al: Mixed outbreak of *Bordetella pertussis* and *Bordetella parapertussis* in an apartment house, *Dev Biol Standard* 73:333-341, 1991.
244. Mertsola J: Mixed outbreak of *Bordetella pertussis* and *Bordetella parapertussis* infection in Finland, *Eur J Clin Microbiol* 4:123-128, 1985.
245. McGowan JP: Some observations on a laboratory epidemic, principally among dogs and cats, in which the animals affected presented the symptoms of the disease called "distemper", *J Pathol Bacteriol* 15:372-430, 1911.
246. Brown JH: *Bacillus bronchisepticus* infection in a child with symptoms of pertussis, *Bull Johns Hopkins Hosp* 38:147-153, 1926.
247. Rath BA, Register KB, Wall J, et al: Persistent *Bordetella bronchiseptica* pneumonia in an immunocompetent infant and genetic comparison of clinical isolates with kennel cough vaccine strains, *Clin Infect Dis* 46:905-908, 2008.
248. de la Torre MJ, de la Fuente CG, de Alegria CR, et al: Recurrent respiratory infection caused by *Bordetella bronchiseptica* in an immunocompetent infant, *Pediatr Infect Dis J* 31:981-983, 2012.
249. Amador C, Chiner E, Calpe JL, et al: Pneumonia due to *Bordetella bronchiseptica* in a patient with AIDS, *Rev Infect Dis* 13:771-772, 1991.
250. Dworkin MS, Sullivan PS, Buskin SE, et al: *Bordetella bronchiseptica* infection in human immunodeficiency virus-infected patients, *Clin Infect Dis J* 28:1095-1099, 1999.
251. Wernli D, Emonet S, Schrenzel J, et al: Evaluation of eight cases of confirmed *Bordetella bronchiseptica* infection and colonization over a 15-year period, *Clin Microbiol Infect* 17:201-203, 2010.
252. Mooi FR, Bruisten S, Linde I, et al: Characterization of *Bordetella holmesii* isolates from patients with pertussis-like illness in the Netherlands, *FEMS Immunol Med Microbiol* 64:289-291, 2012.
253. Rodgers L, Martin SW, Cohn A, et al: Epidemiologic and laboratory features of a large outbreak of pertussis-like illnesses associated with cocirculating *Bordetella holmesii* and *Bordetella pertussis*—Ohio, 2010-2011, *Clin Infect Dis* 56:322-331, 2013.
254. Tatti KM, Sparks KN, Boney KO, et al: Novel multitarget real-time PCR assay for rapid detection of *Bordetella* species in clinical specimens, *J Clin Microbiol* 49:4059-4066, 2011.
255. Arnold JC, Singh KK, Spector SA, et al: Human bocavirus: prevalence and clinical spectrum at a children's hospital, *Clin Infect Dis* 43:283-288, 2006.
256. Baraff LJ, Wilkins J, Wehrle PF: The role of antibiotics, immunizations, and adenoviruses in pertussis, *Pediatrics* 61:224-230, 1978.
257. Collier AM, Connor JD, Irving WR Jr: Generalized type 5 adenovirus infection associated with the pertussis syndrome, *J Pediatr* 69: 1073-1078, 1966.
258. Connor JD: Evidence for an etiologic role of adenoviral infection in pertussis syndrome, *N Engl J Med* 283:390-394, 1970.
259. Davis SF, Sutter RW, Strebel PM, et al: Concurrent outbreaks of pertussis and *Mycoplasma pneumoniae* infection: clinical and epidemiological characteristics of illnesses manifested by cough, *Clin Infect Dis* 20:621-628, 1995.
260. Hallander HO, Gnarpe J, Gnarpe H, et al: *Bordetella pertussis*, *Bordetella parapertussis*, *Mycoplasma pneumoniae*, *Chlamydia pneumoniae* and persistent cough in children, *Scand J Infect Dis* 31:281-286, 1999.
261. Nelson KE, Gavitt F, Batt MD, et al: The role of adenoviruses in the pertussis syndrome, *J Pediatr* 86:335-341, 1975.
262. Wirsing von Konig CH, Rott H, Bogaerts H, et al: A serologic study of organisms possibly associated with pertussis-like coughing, *Pediatr Infect Dis J* 17:645-649, 1998.
263. Heininger U, Cherry JD, Eckhardt T, et al: Clinical and laboratory diagnosis of pertussis in the regions of a large vaccine efficacy trial in Germany, *Pediatr Infect Dis J* 12:504-509, 1993.
264. Strebel PM, Cochi SL, Farizo KM, et al: Pertussis in Missouri: evaluation of nasopharyngeal culture, direct fluorescent antibody testing, and clinical case definitions in the diagnosis of pertussis, *Clin Infect Dis* 16:276-285, 1993.
265. Hallander HO, Reizenstein E, Renemar B, et al: Comparison of nasopharyngeal aspirates with swabs for culture of *Bordetella pertussis*, *J Clin Microbiol* 31:50-52, 1993.

266. Hoppe JE: Methods for isolation of *Bordetella pertussis* from patients with whooping cough, *Eur J Clin Microbiol Infect Dis* 7:616-620, 1988.
267. Loeffelholz MJ: Bordetella. In Murray PR, Baron EJ, Jorgensen JH, editors: *Manual of clinical microbiology*, Washington, DC, 2003, American Society for Microbiology, pp 780-788.
267a. Cherry JD, Grimprel E, Guiso N, et al: Defining pertussis epidemiology: clinical, microbiologic and serologic perspectives, *Pediatr Infect Dis J* 24(Suppl 5):S25-S34, 2005.
268. Heininger U, Schmidt-Schlapfer G, Cherry JD, et al: Clinical validation of a polymerase chain reaction assay for the diagnosis of pertussis by comparison with serology, culture, and symptoms during a large pertussis vaccine efficacy trial, *Pediatrics* 105:E31, 2000.
268a. Heininger U, Cherry JD, Lugauer S, et al. Reactogenicity data following fourth and fifth doses of the Wyeth-Lederle Takeda acellular pertussis component vaccine: the Erlangen trial. Paper presented at Acellular Pertussis Vaccine Conference, Bethesda, Md, November 12-14, 2000.
269. Andre P, Caro V, Njamkepo E, et al: Comparison of serological and real-time PCR assays to diagnose *Bordetella pertussis* infection in 2007, *J Clin Microbiol* 46:1672-1677, 2008.
270. Douglas E, Coote JG, Parton R, et al: Identification of *Bordetella pertussis* in nasopharyngeal swabs by PCR amplification of a region of the adenylate cyclase gene, *J Med Microbiol* 38:140-144, 1993.
271. Erlandsson A, Backman A, Nygren M, et al: Quantification of *Bordetella pertussis* in clinical samples by colorimetric detection of competitive PCR products, *APMIS* 106:1041-1048, 1998.
272 Farrell DJ, McKeon M, Daggard G, et al: Rapid-cycle PCR method to detect *Bordetella pertussis* that fulfills all consensus recommendations for use of PCR in diagnosis of pertussis, *J Clin Microbiol* 38: 4499-4502, 2000.
273. Glare EM, Paton JC, Premier RR, et al: Analysis of a repetitive DNA sequence from *Bordetella pertussis* and its application to the diagnosis of pertussis using the polymerase chain reaction, *J Clin Microbiol* 28:1982-1987, 1990.
274. Grimprel E, Begue P, Anjak I, et al: Comparison of polymerase chain reaction, culture, and Western immunoblot serology for diagnosis of *Bordetella pertussis* infection, *J Clin Microbiol* 31:2745-2750, 1993.
275. Guthrie JL, Robertson AV, Tang P, et al: Novel duplex real-time PCR assay detects *Bordetella holmesii* in specimens from patients with pertussis-like symptoms in Ontario, Canada, *J Clin Microbiol* 48: 1435-1437, 2010.
276. He Q, Mertsola J, Soini H, et al: Sensitive and specific polymerase chain reaction assays for detection of *Bordetella pertussis* in nasopharyngeal specimens, *J Pediatr* 124:421-426, 1994.
277. Houard S, Hackel C, Herzog A, et al: Specific identification of *Bordetella pertussis* by the polymerase chain reaction, *Res Microbiol* 140:477-487, 1989.
278. Knorr L, Fox JD, Tilley PAG, et al: Evaluation of real-time PCR for diagnosis of *Bordetella pertussis* infection, *BMC Infect Dis* 6:1-12, 2006.
279. Li Z, Jansen DL, Finn TM, et al: Identification of *Bordetella pertussis* infection by shared-primer PCR, *J Clin Microbiol* 32:783-789, 1994.
280. Lichtinghagen R, Diedrich-Glaubitz R, von Horsten B: Identification of *Bordetella pertussis* in nasopharyngeal swabs using the polymerase chain reaction: evaluation of detection methods, *Eur J Clin Chem Biochem* 32:161-167, 1994.
281. Lind-Brandberg L, Welinder-Olsson C, Lagergard T, et al: Evaluation of PCR for diagnosis of *Bordetella pertussis* and *Bordetella parapertussis* infections, *J Clin Microbiol* 36:679-683, 1998.
282. Mandal S, Tatti KM, Woods-Stout D, et al: Pertussis pseudo-outbreak linked to specimens contaminated by *Bordetella pertussis* DNA from clinic surfaces, *Pediatrics* 129:e424-e430, 2012.
283. Mastrantonio P, Stefanelli P, Giuliano M: Polymerase chain reaction for the detection of *Bordetella pertussis* in clinical nasopharyngeal aspirates, *J Med Microbiol* 44:261-266, 1996.
284. Meade BD, Bollen A: Recommendations for use of the polymerase chain reaction in the diagnosis of *Bordetella pertussis* infections, *J Med Microbiol* 41:51-55, 1994.
285. Olcen P, Backman A, Johansson B, et al: Amplification of DNA by the polymerase chain reaction for the efficient diagnosis of pertussis, *Scand J Infect Dis* 24:339-345, 1992.
286. Register KB, Sanden GN: Prevalence and sequence variants of is481 in *Bordetella bronchiseptica*: implications for IS481-based detection of *Bordetella pertussis*, *J Clin Microbiol* 44:4577-4583, 2006.
287. Reizenstein E, Johansson B, Mardin L, et al: Diagnostic evaluation of polymerase chain reaction discriminative for *Bordetella pertussis*, *B. parapertussis*, and *B. bronchiseptica*, *Diagn Microbiol Infect Dis* 17: 185-191, 1993.
288. Reizenstein E, Lindberg L, Mollby R, et al: Validation of nested *Bordetella* PCR in pertussis vaccine trial, *J Clin Microbiol* 34:810-815, 1996.
289. Roorda L, Buitenwerf J, Ossewaarde JM, et al: A real-time PCR assay with improved specificity for detection and discrimination of all clinically relevant *Bordetella* species by the presence and distribution of three insertion sequence elements, *BMC Res Notes* 4:11, 2011.
290. Schlapfer G, Cherry JD, Heininger U, et al: Polymerase chain reaction identification of *Bordetella pertussis* infections in vaccinees and family members in a pertussis vaccine efficacy trial in Germany, *Pediatr Infect Dis J* 14:209-214, 1995.
291. Schlapfer G, Senn HP, Berger R, et al: Use of the polymerase chain reaction to detect *Bordetella pertussis* in patients with mild or atypical symptoms of infection, *Eur J Clin Microbiol Infect Dis* 12:459-463, 1993.
292. Tatti KM, Slade B, Patel M, et al: Real-time polymerase chain reaction detection of *Bordetella pertussis* DNA in acellular pertussis vaccines, *Pediatr Infect Dis J* 27:73-74, 2008.
293. van der Zee A, Agterberg C, Peeters M, et al: A clinical validation of *Bordetella pertussis* and *Bordetella parapertussis* polymerase chain reaction: comparison with culture and serology using samples from patients with suspected whooping cough from a highly immunized population, *J Infect Dis* 174:89-96, 1996.
294. van der Zee A, Agterberg C, Peeters M, et al: Polymerase chain reaction assay for pertussis: simultaneous detection and discrimination of *Bordetella pertussis* and *Bordetella parapertussis*, *J Clin Microbiol* 31:2134-2140, 1993.
295. van Kruijssen AM, Templeton KE, van der Plas RN, et al: Detection of respiratory pathogens by real-time PCR in children with clinical suspicion of pertussis, *Eur J Pediatr* 166:1189-1191, 2007.
296. Loeffelholz M: Towards improved accuracy of *Bordetella pertussis* nucleic acid amplification tests, *J Clin Microbiol* 50:2186-2190, 2012.
297. Friedman LE, Messina MT, Santoferrara L, et al: Characterization of *Bordetella bronchiseptica* strains using phenotypic and genotypic markers, *Vet Microbiol* 117:313-320, 2006.
298. Aintablian N, Walpita P, Sawyer MH: Detection of *Bordetella pertussis* and respiratory syncytial virus in air samples from hospital rooms, *Infect Contr Hosp Epidemiol* 19:918-923, 1998.
299. Muller FM, Hoppe JE, Wirsing von Konig CH: Laboratory diagnosis of pertussis: state of the art in 1997, *J Clin Microbiol* 35:2435-2443, 1997.
300. Conway SP, Balfour AH, Ross H: Serologic diagnosis of whooping cough by enzyme-linked immunosorbent assay, *Pediatr Infect Dis J* 7:570-574, 1988.
301. Friedman RL: Pertussis: the disease and new diagnostic methods, *Clin Microbiol Rev* 1:365-376, 1988.
302. Halperin SA, Bortolussi R, MacLean D, et al: Persistence of pertussis in an immunized population: results of the Nova Scotia enhanced pertussis surveillance program, *J Pediatr* 115:686-693, 1989.
303. Mertsola J, Ruuskanen O, Kuronen T, et al: Serologic diagnosis of pertussis: evaluation of pertussis toxin and other antigens in enzyme-linked immunosorbent assay, *J Infect Dis* 161:966-971, 1990.
304. Stehr K, Cherry JD, Heininger U, et al: A comparative efficacy trial in Germany in infants who received either the Lederle/Takeda acellular pertussis component DTP (DTAP) vaccine, the Lederle whole-cell component DTP vaccine, or DT vaccine, *Pediatrics* 101:1-11, 1998.
305. Viljanen MK, Ruuskanen O, Granberg C, et al: Serological diagnosis of pertussis: IgM, IgA and IgG antibodies against *Bordetella pertussis* measured by enzyme-linked immunosorbent assay (ELISA), *Scand J Infect Dis* 14:117-122, 1982.
306. Hallander HO, Storsaeter J, Mollby R: Evaluation of serology and nasopharyngeal cultures for diagnosis of pertussis in a vaccine efficacy trial, *J Infect Dis* 163:1046-1054, 1991.
306a. Mink CA, Sirota NM, Nugent S: Outbreak of pertussis in a fully immunized adolescent and adult population, *Arch Pediatr Adolesc Med* 148:153-157, 1994.
307. Wirsing von Konig CH, Gounis D, Laukamp S, et al: Evaluation of a single-sample serological technique for diagnosing pertussis in unvaccinated children, *Eur J Clin Microbiol Infect Dis* 18:341-345, 1999.

308. Granstrom M, Lindberg AA, Askelof P, et al: Detection of antibodies in human serum against the fimbrial haemagglutinin of *Bordetella pertussis* by enzyme-linked immunosorbent assay, *J Med Microbiol* 15:85-96, 1982.
309. Prince HE, Lape-Nixon M, Matud J: Evaluation of a tetraplex microsphere assay for *Bordetella pertussis* antibodies, *Clin Vaccine Immunol* 13:266-270, 2006.
310. Riffelmann M, Thiel K, Schmetz J, et al: Performance of commercial enzyme-linked immunosorbent assays for detection of antibodies to *Bordetella pertussis*, *J Clin Microbiol* 48:4459-4463, 2010.
311. Bass JW: Pertussis: current status of prevention and treatment, *Pediatr Infect Dis J* 4:614-619, 1985.
312. Bass JW: Erythromycin for treatment and prevention of pertussis, *Pediatr Infect Dis J* 5:154-157, 1986.
313. Bass JW, Klenk EL, Kotheimer JB, et al: Antimicrobial treatment of pertussis, *J Pediatr* 75:768-781, 1969.
314. Bergquist SO, Bernander S, Dahnsjo H, et al: Erythromycin in the treatment of pertussis: a study of bacteriologic and clinical effects, *Pediatr Infect Dis J* 6:458-461, 1987.
315. Hoppe JE: State of art in antibacterial susceptibility of *Bordetella pertussis* and antibiotic treatment of pertussis, *Infection* 26:242-246, 1998.
316. Hoppe JE, Eichhorn A: Activity of new macrolides against *Bordetella pertussis* and *Bordetella parapertussis*, *Eur J Clin Microbiol Infect Dis* 8:653-654, 1989.
317. Hoppe JE, Halm U, Hagedorn HJ, et al: Comparison of erythromycin ethylsuccinate and co-trimoxazole for treatment of pertussis, *Infection* 17:227-231, 1989.
318. Hoppe JE, Haug A: Antimicrobial susceptibility of *Bordetella pertussis* (part I), *Infection* 16:126-130, 1988.
319. Centers for Disease Control and Prevention: Recommended antimicrobial agents for the treatment and postexposure prophylaxes of pertussis: 2005 CDC guidelines, *MMWR* 54:1-16, 2005.
320. Halperin SA, Bortolussi R, Langley JM, et al: Seven days of erythromycin estolate is as effective as fourteen days for the treatment of *Bordetella pertussis* infections, *Pediatrics* 100:65-71, 1997.
321. American Academy of Pediatrics: Pertussis (whooping cough). In Pickering L, Baker C, Kimberlin D, Long S, editors: *Red book: 2012 report of the Committee on Infectious Diseases*, Elk Grove Village, Ill, 2012, American Academy of Pediatrics.
322. Honein MA, Paulozzi LJ, Himelright IM, et al: Infantile hypertrophic pyloric stenosis after pertussis prophylaxis with erythromcyin: a case review and cohort study, *Lancet* 354:2101-2105, 1999.
323. Morrison W: Infantile hypertrophic pyloric stenosis in infants treated with azithromycin, *Pediatr Infect Dis J* 26:186-188, 2007.
324. Centers for Disease Control and Prevention: Hypertrophic pyloric stenosis in infants following pertussis prophylaxis with erythromycin—Knoxville, Tennessee, 1999, *MMWR Morb Mortal Wkly Rep* 48:1117-1120, 1999.
325. Guillot S, Descours G, Gillet Y, et al: Macrolide-resistant *Bordetella pertussis* infection in newborn girl, France, *Emerg Infect Dis* 18: 966-968, 2012.
326. Korgenski EK, Daly JA: Surveillance and detection of erythromycin resistance in *Bordetella pertussis* isolates recovered from a pediatric population in the intermountain west region of the United States, *J Clin Microbiol* 35:2989-2991, 1997.
327. Lee B: Progressive respiratory distress in an infant treated for presumed pertussis, *Pediatr Infect Dis J* 19: 475, 492-493, 2000.
328. Ohtsuka M, Kikuchi K, Shimizu K, et al: Emergence of quinolone-resistant *Bordetella pertussis* in Japan, *Antimicrob Agents Chemother* 53:3147-3149, 2009.
329. Bettiol S, Thompson MJ, Roberts NW, et al: Symptomatic treatment of the cough in whooping cough, *Cochrane Database Syst Rev* (1): CD003257, 2010.
330. Zoumboulakis D, Anagnostakis D, Albanis V, et al: Steroids in treatment of pertussis. A controlled clinical trial, *Arch Dis Child* 48:51-54, 1973.
331. Iida T, Kunitani A, Komase Y, et al: Studies on experimental infection with *Bordetella pertussis*: effect of cortisone on the infection and immunity in mice, *Jpn J Exp Med* 33:283-295, 1983.
332. Roberts I, Gavin R, Lennon D: Randomized controlled trial of steroids in pertussis, *Pediatr Infect Dis J* 11:982-983, 1992.
333. Broomhall J, Herxheimer A: Treatment of whooping cough: the facts, *Arch Dis Child* 59:185-187, 1984.
334. Pillay V, Swingler G: Symptomatic treatment of the cough in whooping cough, *Cochrane Database Syst Rev* (3):CD003257, 2003.
335. Falcon M, Rafael M, Garcia C, et al: Increasing infant pertussis hospitalization and mortality in South Texas, 1996 to 2006, *Pediatr Infect Dis J* 29:265-267, 2010.
336. Swansea Research Unit of the Royal College of General Practitioners: Study of intellectual performance of children in ordinary schools after certain serious complications of whooping cough, *BMJ* 295:1044-1047, 1987.
337. Johnston ID, Strachan DP, Anderson HR: Effect of pneumonia and whooping cough in childhood on adult lung function, *N Engl J Med* 338:581-587, 1998.
338. Cherry JD: 'Pertussis vaccine encephalopathy': it is time to recognize it as the myth that it is, *JAMA* 263:1679-1680, 1990.
339. Sato Y, Kimura M, Fukumi H: Development of a pertussis component vaccine in Japan, *Lancet* 1:122-126, 1984.
340. Cherry JD, Mortimer EA Jr: Acellular and whole-cell pertussis vaccines in Japan: report of a visit by US scientists, *JAMA* 257: 1375-1376, 1987.
341. Noble GR, Bernier RH, Esber EC, et al: Acellular and whole-cell pertussis vaccines in Japan. Report of a visit by US scientists, *JAMA* 257:1351-1356, 1987.
342. World Health Organization: *World Health Organization meeting on case definition of pertussis, Geneva*, Geneva, 1991, World Health Organization. January 10-11, 1991, MIM/EPI/PERT/9.1.
343. Le Saux N, Barrowman NJ, Moore DL, et al: Decrease in hospital admissions for febrile seizures and reports of hypotonic-hyporesponsive episodes presenting to hospital emergency departments since switching to acellular pertussis vaccine in Canada: a report from impact, *Pediatrics* 112:348-353, 2003.
344. Huang WT, Gargiullo PM, Broder KR, et al: Lack of association between acellular pertussis vaccine and seizures in early childhood, *Pediatrics* 126:263-269, 2010.
345. Centers for Disease Control and Prevention: Preventing tetanus, diphtheria, and pertussis among adults: use of tetanus toxoid, reduced diphtheria toxoid and acellular pertussis vaccine, *MMWR Morb Mortal Wkly Rep* 55:1-33, 2006.
346. Cherry JD: Pertussis vaccines for adolescents and adults, *Pediatrics* 116:755-756, 2005.
347. Food and Drug Administration: Product approval information-licensing action, package insert: Boostrix. Tetanus toxoid, reduced diphtheria toxoid and acellular pertussis vaccine, adsorbed. Glaxosmithkline Biologicals, Rockville, Md, 2005, U.S. Department of Health and Human Services, Food and Drug Administration, Center for Biologics Evaluation and Research. Available at http://www.Fda.Gov/cber/label/tdapgla122905lb.pdf. Accessed November 1, 2008.
348. Food and Drug Administration: Product approval information-licensing action, package insert: tetanus toxoid, reduced diphtheria toxoid and acellular pertussis vaccine adsorbed Adacel. Sanofi Pasteur, Rockville, Md, 2006, U.S. Department of Health and Human Services, Food and Drug Administration, Center for Biologics Evaluation and Research. Available at http://www.fda.gov/cber/label/tdapave012306lb.pdf. Accessed November 1, 2008.
349. Heininger U, Cherry JD: Pertussis immunization in adolescents and adults: *Bordetella pertussis* epidemiology should guide vaccination recommendations, *Expert Opin Biol Ther* 6:1-13, 2006.
350. Queenan AM, Cassiday PK, Evangelista A: Pertactin-negative variants of *Bordetella pertussis* in the United States, *N Engl J Med* 368:583-584, 2013.
351. Winter K, Harriman K, Zipprich J, et al: California pertussis epidemic, 2010, *J Pediatr* 368:583-584, 2012.
352. Centers for Disease Control and Prevention: Updated recommendations for use of tetanus toxoid, reduced diphtheria toxoid and acellular pertussis vaccine (Tdap) in pregnant women and persons who have or anticipate having close contact with an infant aged < 12 months—Advisory Committee on Immunization Practices (ACIP), 2011, *MMWR Morb Mortal Wkly Rep* 60:1424-1426, 2011.
353. Grizas AP, Camenga D, Vazquez M: Cocooning: a concept to protect young children from infectious diseases, *Curr Opin Pediatr* 24:92-97, 2012.
354. Castagnini LA, Healy CM, Rench MA, et al: Impact of maternal postpartum tetanus and diphtheria toxoids and acellular pertussis immunization on infant pertussis infection, *Clin Infect Dis* 54:78-84, 2012.
355. Healy CM, Rench MA, Castagnini LA, et al: Pertussis immunization in a high-risk postpartum population, *Vaccine* 27:5599-5602, 2009.

356. Libster R, Edwards KM: How can we best prevent pertussis in infants? *Clin Infect Dis* 54:85-87, 2012.
357. Prato R, Martinelli D, Marchetti F, et al: Feasibility of a cocoon strategy for the prevention of pertussis in Italy: a survey of prevention department healthcare providers, *Pediatr Infect Dis J* 31:1304-1307, 2012.
358. Walter EB, Allred N, Rowe-West B, et al: Cocooning infants: Tdap immunization for new parents in the pediatric office, *Acad Pediatr* 9:344-347, 2009.
359. Wiley KE, Zuo Y, Macartney KK, et al: Sources of pertussis infection in young infants: a review of key evidence informing targeting of the cocoon strategy, *Vaccine* 31:618-625, 2013.
360. Centers for Disease Control and Prevention: Tdap for pregnant women: information for providers, Available at http://www.cdc.gov/vaccines/vpd-vac/pertussis/tdap-pregnancy-hcp.htm. Accessed September 1, 2013.
361. Gall SA, Myers J, Pichichero M: Maternal immunization with tetanus-diphtheria-pertussis vaccine: effect on maternal and neonatal serum antibody levels, *Am J Obstet Gynecol* 204:334.e331-334.e335, 2011.
362. Heininger U, Riffelmann M, Bar G, et al: The protective role of maternally derived antibodies against *Bordetella pertussis* in young infants, *Pediatr Infect Dis J* 32:695-698, 2013.
363. Heininger U, Riffelmann M, Leineweber B, et al: Maternally derived antibodies against *Bordetella pertussis* antigens pertussis toxin and filamentous hemagglutinin in preterm and full term newborns, *Pediatr Infect Dis J* 28:443-445, 2009.
364. Baraff LJ, Leake RD, Burstyn DG, et al: Immunologic response to early and routine dtp immunization in infants, *Pediatrics* 73:37-42, 1984.
365. Belloni C, De Silvestri A, Tinelli C, et al: Immunogenicity of a three-component acellular pertussis vaccine administered at birth, *Pediatrics* 111:1042-1045, 2003.
366. Burstyn DG, Baraff LJ, Peppler MS, et al: Serological response to filamentous hemagglutinin and lymphocytosis-promoting toxin of *Bordetella pertussis*, *Infect Immun* 41:1150-1156, 1983.
367. Halasa NB, O'Shea A, Shi JR, et al: Poor immune responses to a birth dose of diphtheria, tetanus, and acellular pertussis vaccine, *J Pediatr* 153:327-332, 2008.
368. Wood N, McIntyre P, Marshall H, et al: Acellular pertussis vaccine at birth and one month induces antibody responses by two months of age, *Pediatr Infect Dis J* 29:209-215, 2010.
369. Hardy-Fairbanks AJ, Pan SJ, Decker MD, et al: Immune responses in infants whose mothers received Tdap vaccine during pregnancy, *Pediatr Infect Dis J* 32:1257-1260, 2013.
370. Knuf M, Schmitt HJ, Wolter J, et al: Neonatal vaccination with an acellular pertussis vaccine accelerates the acquisition of pertussis antibodies in infants, *J Pediatr* 152:655-660, 2008. 660.e651.
371. Ulloa-Gutierrez R: Pertussis vaccination in newborns, *Exp Rev Vaccine* 8:153-157, 2009.
372. Steketee RW, Wassilak SG, Adkins WN Jr, et al: Evidence for a high attack rate and efficacy of erythromycin prophylaxis in a pertussis outbreak in a facility for the developmentally disabled, *J Infect Dis* 157:434-440, 1988.

SECTION III

VIRAL INFECTIONS

SECTION OUTLINE

22 Human Immunodeficiency Virus/Acquired Immunodeficiency Syndrome in the Infant

AVINASH K. SHETTY and YVONNE A. MALDONADO

CHAPTER OUTLINE

The human immunodeficiency virus type 1 (HIV-1) pandemic remains one of the greatest public health challenges in the 21st century.[1] More than 3 decades after the initial descriptions of acquired immunodeficiency syndrome (AIDS) in adults and children, the epidemiology of HIV has evolved significantly in high-income as well as low- and middle-income countries (LMIC) because of extraordinary biomedical advances in prevention, coupled with programmatic scale-up of antiretroviral treatment (ART).[2-12] Mother-to child transmission (MTCT) of HIV is the most common source of HIV infection among infants and children.[13] Although HIV infection in children has been acquired in the past by the transfusion of contaminated blood or coagulation products, this mode of transmission has been virtually eliminated in the United States.[14-17] In the United States and other high-income countries, widespread implementation of universal antenatal HIV testing, combination antiretroviral treatment (cART) during pregnancy, elective cesarean section, and avoidance of breastfeeding has led to virtual elimination of MTCT.[18-22] Dramatic declines in the number of HIV-infected children who acquired the infection perinatally have been reported, and new pediatric infections are exceedingly rare.[18] Rates of MTCT in the United States are less than 2%, and most new infections occur because of missed prevention opportunities.[23,24] Availability of cART has led to improved survival of HIV-infected children into adolescence and adulthood, changing most HIV infections into a treatable chronic illness rather than a fatal disease.[10,25-30]

In contrast, prevention of mother-to-child transmission of HIV (PMTCT) remains a major public health challenge in LMIC.[9] It is estimated that more than 900 infections occur daily worldwide in children younger than 15 years, of which 90% occur via MTCT.[31] More than 90% of these affected children reside in sub-Saharan Africa, where prolonged breastfeeding is the cultural norm.[31-33] In these settings, postnatal transmission through breastfeeding accounts for 30% to 40% of new pediatric HIV infections.[34] In recent years, remarkable advances have been made in the development of effective antiretroviral (ARV) interventions to reduce the risk of postnatal transmission of HIV during breastfeeding.[35-38] In response to new evidence from clinical trials, the World Health Organization (WHO) has issued new HIV and PMTCT guidelines.[39,40] In addition, progress has been made in increasing access to ART for people living with HIV/AIDS in LMIC.[31] The possibility that success of PMTCT interventions in high-income countries could be extended to LMIC has led to an ambitious global plan toward virtual elimination of MTCT worldwide by 2015, developed by the Joint United Nations Programme on HIV/AIDS (UNAIDS).[41-45]

This chapter reviews the epidemiology and prevention of HIV infection in infants; discusses evaluation and management of HIV-exposed infants; and highlights certain unique features of HIV infection in infants, with a focus on early diagnosis and treatment.

Epidemiology

GLOBAL SCOPE OF THE PROBLEM

The HIV pandemic is a major public health problem, with cases reported to the WHO from virtually every country.[1,7,8,46] At the end of December 2011, an estimated 34 million people (31.4-35.9 million) were living with HIV (an increase from 29.4 million in 2001), including 15.7 million women and 3.3 million children younger than 15 years.[46] Nearly 97% of people living with HIV live in LMICs, and the adult HIV prevalence worldwide is estimated at 0.8%.[46] Sub-Saharan Africa bears the brunt of the epidemic, accounting for 69% of HIV infections; approximately 23.5 million HIV-infected people live in sub-Saharan Africa, including more than 3 million children younger than 15 years, representing more than 90% of all children with HIV.[42,46,47] South and Southeast Asia account for 4 million HIV-infected people, followed by 3 million people living with HIV in the Americas, including the Caribbean.[48]

The complex and diverse epidemiology of HIV worldwide has evolved significantly after the peak of HIV incidence around 1997.[7,8,46,49,50] Recent data from UNAIDS indicate an encouraging trend, with rates of new HIV infections continuing to decline among general populations. Overall, a greater than 20% decline in new HIV infections was noted in 2011 (when compared with 2001 incidence rates), with the most significant declines in the Caribbean and sub-Saharan Africa.[48] In 2011, an estimated 2.5 million people became newly infected with HIV, including 330,000 children younger than 15 years.[46] Although HIV testing centers have increased in many countries, approximately 50% of people living with HIV do not know their HIV status.[48] In 2011, an estimated 1.7 million people died because of AIDS-related illness (24% fewer than in 2005), including 230,000 children younger than 15 years (20% less than in 2005).[46]

Primary HIV infection among women of childbearing age fuels the perinatal HIV epidemic. Women constitute nearly one half of all HIV/AIDS infections worldwide, and more than one half of these (58%) living in sub-Saharan Africa.[51] Young women and adolescent females are at highest risk of HIV acquisition because of a myriad of complex biologic, behavioral, and structural factors.[51] In LMIC, antenatal HIV prevalence rates can vary considerably, ranging from less than 5% to greater than 35% in some high–HIV-burden countries.[13,31] Although HIV prevalence among young pregnant women has declined in Kenya, Malawi, and Zimbabwe, most countries in Southern Africa have antenatal prevalence rates between 20% to 30%; rates can reach 35% to 40% in some antenatal clinics in South Africa, Swaziland, Lesotho, and Botswana.[13,31,47] In 2009, an estimated 1.4 million HIV-infected women became pregnant, 90% of whom lived in 22 countries in sub-Saharan Africa and India.[42] Approximately 900 HIV-infected infants are born each day.[31,44]

In LMIC, children constitute 14% of new HIV infections worldwide and nearly a fifth of annual HIV deaths.[31] Without access to combination ART, greater than 50% of HIV-infected children in sub-Saharan Africa die by their second birthday.[52] In the absence of rapid identification and early access to ART, 26% of postnatal and 52% of perinatal HIV infections result in child mortality 1 year after acquiring HIV.[53] Based on UNAIDS estimates, 17.3 million children have been orphaned by the AIDS epidemic.[46]

UNITED STATES

Human Immunodeficiency Virus in Women

Currently, approximately 1.2 million individuals in the United States are living with HIV/AIDS, including approximately 280,000 women.[49,54] In 2010, an estimated 47,500 people became newly infected with HIV.[55] Since the beginning of the HIV epidemic in the United States, men accounted for the majority of new HIV infections and AIDS diagnoses. However, the incidence of HIV infection among women increased gradually until the late 1980s but then declined in the early 1990s and has remained relatively stable over the past decade.[56,57] Of reported AIDS cases in adults, women accounted for 8% in 1985, 13% in 1993, 20% in 1995, 23% in 1999, and 27% in 2000; at the end of 2010, an estimated 25% of adults and adolescent females aged 13 years or older and living with HIV were women; 15% of HIV-positive women are unaware of their infection.[55] In 2010, there were 9500 new HIV infections among women, acquired mostly (84%) via heterosexual contact with an individual known to have or at high risk for HIV infection.[55] Young women (25-44 years of age) accounted for the majority of new HIV infections among women.

Women of color, especially black/African-American, and Hispanic/Latina women are disproportionately affected by HIV infection compared with women of other races or ethnicities.[55] Of the total number of new HIV diagnosis among women in 2010, 64% occurred in black/African-American females (representing 12% of the U.S. female population), followed by 15% in Hispanic/Latina females (representing ≈14% of the population). In contrast, white females (representing 68% of the female adult and adolescent population) accounted for only 18% of new HIV diagnosis among females.[55] In 2010, the rate of new HIV infections (per 100,000 population) is estimated to be 20 times higher among black/African-American women compared with rate of white women, whereas the rate among Hispanic/Latina women was four times higher compared with white women; however, recent data from the Centers for Disease Control and Prevention (CDC) indicate a decrease in new HIV infections among black/African-American women (n = 6100; 21% decrease between 2008 and 2010).[55] Greater than 75% of women with AIDS are in the reproductive age group at the time of diagnosis. In 2009, 4693 deaths occurred among women with AIDS.[56] In 2010, HIV infection was among the top 10 leading causes of death for black/African-American females aged 10 to 64 years and Hispanic/Latina females aged 25 to 44 years.[55]

Regional HIV seroprevalence rates vary, with the highest rates found among women residing in the Northeast and southern states. In 2009, the top 10 states with the highest number of women/girls living with AIDS were New York (n = 23,859), followed by Florida (n = 15,081), California (n = 7817), Texas (n = 6795), New Jersey (n = 6312), Maryland (n = 6080), Pennsylvania (n = 4961), Georgia (n = 4679), Illinois (n = 3638) and Puerto Rico (n = 3326).[54,58] During 2010, the highest rates of new AIDS diagnoses (per 100,000 population) among adult and adolescent females were in the District of Columbia (79.9), Maryland (18.5), and Louisiana (15.5), followed by Florida (14.7), the U.S. Virgin Islands (14.3), New York (14.1), New Jersey (11.6), Delaware (10.9), and Mississippi (10.3).[54,58]

For women living with HIV, the most common mode of transmission is high-risk heterosexual exposure and intravenous drug use (IDU). Among black and Latina women, heterosexual transmission accounts for 85% and 82% of new HIV/AIDS diagnosis, respectively, compared with white women (72%).[56] Injection drug use accounts for a greater proportion (28%) of new infections among white women.[56] A number of social factors, such as poverty, tight social networks, and assortative mixing as well as lack of prenatal care, antenatal HIV testing, and early access to combination ART, contribute to the high rates of HIV infection among black women in the United States.[59]

Human Immunodeficiency Virus/Acquired Immunodeficiency Syndrome in Infants and Children

At the end of 2009, using a confidential name-based HIV infection reporting mechanism, an estimated 10,834 children younger than 13 years were diagnosed with HIV in 46 states in the United States; of these, 9522 (88%) were infected via MTCT.[60] In the United States, almost all new diagnosis of HIV/AIDS in children younger than 13 years resulted from MTCT. In 2006, approximately 8700 pregnant women with HIV gave birth, compared with 6000 to 7000 births in 2000, representing an increase of 30%.[61] However, since the mid-1990s, the annual number of diagnoses of perinatally acquired HIV/AIDS cases has declined by greater than 90% in the United States as a result of routine antenatal HIV testing in conjunction with implementation of effective interventions to prevent transmission.[61-63] In 1991, the annual number of perinatally acquired HIV infections peaked at 1650 infants but significantly declined to an estimated 215 to 370 cases in 2005, 182 cases in 2008, and 131 cases in 2009.[17,62,63] In 2010, an estimated 217 children younger than 13 years were diagnosed with HIV in the 46 states using a confidential name-based HIV infection reporting mechanism; of these, 162 (75%) acquired HIV perinatally.[61]

Cases of AIDS in children have accounted for less than 1% of all reported AIDS cases in the United States.[17] An estimated 9898 cumulative AIDS diagnoses have been reported among children; 91% of those children acquired HIV perinatally.[60] Since the beginning of the HIV/AIDS epidemic through 2009, an estimated 5626 children younger than 13 years who were diagnosed with AIDS have died in the 50 states and the District of Columbia; of these, 4986 (89%) were infected via the perinatal route.[61]

The racial and ethnic and geographic distribution of AIDS cases in children parallels that of women with AIDS. Racial/ethnic disparities in perinatal HIV/AIDS incidence have persisted since the early part of the epidemic; 78% of children with AIDS were black or Hispanic in 1981 to 1986.[64] Of the 9522 perinatal HIV cases at the end of 2009, 63% were in black/African Americans, 22% were in Hispanics/Latinos, and 13% were in whites; these figures include persons of all ages who acquired HIV via MTCT.[61] Of the perinatally infected children born during 2007 through 2009, the CDC estimated that black/African-American children had the highest HIV rate per 100,000 live births annually; however, the annual rate had declined from 15.2 in 2007 to 9.9 in 2009. Among Hispanic/Latino children, HIV rates had remained stable from 2007 through 2009.[61]

Although significant declines in the rate of perinatally acquired HIV infection among infants have been documented in the United States, the rate of acquisition of HIV/AIDS among adolescents and young adults continues to increase, occurring primarily among populations of minority race or ethnicity. Young black men who have sex with men (MSM) are at highest risk; new HIV cases increased by 48% in young MSM from 2006 to 2009.[57] Recent data from the CDC indicated a continued increase (22%) in new infections among young gay and bisexual men from 2007 to 2010.[55] Infection among adolescent women is acquired primarily through heterosexual contact.[57] In 2007, 31% of adolescents and youth aged 13 to 19 years diagnosed with HIV were females, compared with 23% of individuals aged 20 to 24 years and 26% of adults aged 25 years or older.[17,65] In 2007, cases of AIDS in adolescents and young adults aged 13 to 24 years accounted for 4% of people living with HIV infection in the United States.[17,65]

Although a dramatic decline (<2%) in the rate of perinatal HIV transmission has been documented, because of the relatively stable incidence of HIV among women of childbearing age, perinatal HIV infection will continue to occur each year, primarily among young black women, warranting continued surveillance.[13,56] In addition to MTCT, transmission of HIV to infants, children, and adolescents can occur via sexual contact (vaginal, anal, or orogenital), mucous membrane exposure to contaminated blood or other body fluids, IDU, and percutaneous blood exposure from contaminated needles or other sharp objects, such as tattooing.[17,66,67] Probable HIV transmission from HIV-infected caregivers to their infants via feeding blood-tinged prechewed food has been reported, but no transmission of HIV infection to household contacts through casual contact has occurred in the United States.[17,68,69] Other modes of transmission of HIV, such as exposure to contaminated blood products, have declined significantly and almost eliminated because of effective screening methods.[14-17]

Transmission

MOTHER-TO-CHILD HIV TRANSMISSION: RATES, TIMING, RISK FACTORS, AND MECHANISMS

Mother-to-child transmission of HIV can occur in utero, during labor and delivery, or postnatally through breastfeeding.[34,70,71] In the United States, the transmission rate without PMTCT interventions is estimated to be 25% to 30%; in European studies, it was found to be lower, at 15% to 20%.[72,73] A higher transmission rate of 25% to 45% has been observed among breastfeeding populations in sub-Saharan Africa.[34] These variations in transmission rates likely reflect differences in infant feeding patterns, maternal and obstetric risk factors, viral factors, and methodologic differences among studies. Data suggest that most children are infected during the intrapartum period.[34] Studies based on cord blood or newborn HIV polymerase chain reaction (PCR) testing indicate that 50% to 60% of the perinatal HIV transmission occurs around the time of labor and delivery.[74]

An infant is considered to have been infected in utero if the HIV-1 genome can be detected by PCR or cultured from blood within 48 hours of birth. In contrast, a child is considered to have intrapartum infection if diagnostic assays, such as culture, PCR, and serum p24 antigen, are negative in blood samples obtained during the first week of life but became positive during the period from day 7 to 90 of life and the infant has not been breastfed.[75] In the breastfed infant, 20% to 25% of HIV transmission occurs during pregnancy, 35% to 50% during labor and delivery, and another 25% to 35% during lactation.[34]

INTRAUTERINE TRANSMISSION

In utero transmission may occur through HIV infection in the placenta or fetal exposure to cell-free or cell-associated HIV in the amniotic fluid. In early studies using PCR and in situ hybridization technology, the virus was detected in some aborted fetuses of 8 to 20 weeks of gestational age and in amniotic fluid.[76-80] Maternal decidual leukocytes, placental villous macrophages (Hofbauer cells), and endothelial cells stain positive for gp41 antigen and HIV nucleic acids.[80] The placenta can be infected through $CD4^+$ trophoblasts or through the occasional occurrence of chorioamnionitis.[81,82] However, subsequent studies in animals and human fetuses reported almost no transmission during the first and second trimester of pregnancy.[83,84] There is no clear predictive value for the identification of HIV in the placenta and the infection of the fetus or newborn, and important technical limitations exist in studies conducted on fetal or placenta tissues, particularly because of the difficulty in excluding contamination with maternal blood.[85] Based on viral detection during the first 48 hours of birth, intrauterine transmission occurs in about 20% to 25% of infections.[34] Statistical modeling data also suggest that most in utero HIV transmission occurs during the last few weeks before delivery when the vascular integrity of the placenta is disrupted.[13,71]

INTRAPARTUM INFECTION

Intrapartum transmission may occur because of direct exposure of the fetus or infant with infected maternal secretions during birth or maternal-to-fetal microtransfusions during uterine contractions.[86,87] Intrapartum transmission is supported by studies failing to detect HIV in the first month of life in infants born to HIV-infected women but with subsequent detection of virus after 1 to 3 months of life.[88-92] In a study by the French Collaborative Study Group, timing of transmission was estimated with a mathematical model.[93] Data for 95 infected infants (infants seropositive at 18 months and infants who died of HIV disease before this age and who were exclusively bottle-fed) were used in the model, which indicated that one third of the infants were infected in utero less than 2 months before delivery (95th percentile). In the remaining 65% of cases (95% confidence interval [CI], 22% to 92%), the date of infection was estimated as the day of birth. The estimated median period between birth and the positivity of viral markers (HIV PCR or HIV culture) was 10 days (95% CI, 6% to 14%), and the 95th percentile was estimated at 56 days.[93]

Additional evidence to support mucosal exposure to maternal virus during delivery as a likely route of transmission includes findings of increased HIV infection rates in first-born twins, increased risk associated with prolonged rupture of membranes, and the protective effect, although incomplete, of cesarean delivery before onset of labor.[94-97] Some reports have documented an increased risk of MTCT associated with placental malaria infection, but not others.[98,99]

Although numerous maternal, obstetric, infant, host genetic, and viral factors may modify perinatal HIV transmission risk, maternal plasma HIV RNA level is the strongest predictor of intrauterine and intrapartum transmission (Box 22-1).[20,100-104] Transmission can occur rarely, however, among pregnant women with low or undetectable serum levels of HIV around the time of labor and delivery.[105] Other maternal risk factors associated with higher rates of perinatal HIV infection include women with advanced clinical disease, acute HIV infection during pregnancy, and low $CD4^+$ counts.[106-109] HIV viral load in cervicovaginal secretions is an independent risk factor for perinatal HIV transmission.[110] Maternal genital ulcer diseases, especially herpes simplex virus (HSV) and syphilis and other coinfections (such as hepatitis C virus, hepatitis B virus, malaria, tuberculosis), may increase the risk.[111-114] Behavioral risk factors including maternal substance abuse, cigarette smoking during pregnancy, and noncompliance to ART may also increase the risk of transmission.[115]

Box 22-1 Risk Factors Contributing to Perinatal Human Immunodeficiency Virus (HIV) Transmission

Maternal

- High maternal viral load in plasma (and breast milk in breastfeeding populations)
- Low maternal CD4 T-lymphocyte count
- High vaginal/cervical shedding of HIV
- Advanced maternal clinical disease
- Concurrent genital ulcer disease resulting from STIs (syphilis, genital HSV)
- Coinfections (TB, malaria, HBV, HCV)
- Behavioral (cigarette smoking, substance abuse, poor adherence to combination ART)

Obstetric

- Instrumentation (amniocentesis, invasive monitoring)
- Chorioamnionitis
- Prolonged rupture of membranes
- Vaginal delivery (VL > 1000 copies/mL)

Fetal/Infant

- Prematurity
- Twin gestation (higher infection rate in first born twin)
- Low birth weight
- Infant feeding choice (breastfeeding duration, mixed infant feeding)
- Maternal breast disease (mastitis, abscess, cracked or bleeding nipples)

Genetic/Immunologic

- Maternal-infant HLA concordance
- Upregulation of CCR5 receptor expression in placenta
- Toll-like receptor 9 polymorphisms
- β-Defensin polymorphisms
- Mannose-binding lectin polymorphisms

ART, Antiretroviral therapy; *HBV,* hepatitis B virus; *HCV,* hepatitis C virus; *HLA,* human leukocyte antigen; *HSV,* herpes simplex virus; *STIs,* sexually transmitted infections; *TB,* tuberculosis; *VL,* viral load.

Obstetric risk factors associated with increased risk of transmission include vaginal delivery, prolonged rupture of membranes, chorioamnionitis, and invasive obstetric procedures.[101,116,117] Premature infants born to HIV-infected women have a higher rate of perinatal HIV infection than full-term infants.[109,118] Data from a large international meta-analysis of 15 prospective cohort studies and a randomized controlled trial from Europe have shown that cesarean section performed before labor and rupture of membranes reduces perinatal transmission of HIV-1 by 50% to 87%, independent of the use of ART or zidovudine (ZDV) prophylaxis.[95,96]

Viral and host genetic factors may also influence MTCT.[37,38,119-124] Besides maternal viral load, other factors affecting transmission include viral subtype, circulating recombinant forms, resistance viral strains and replication kinetics, and fitness.[37,38] Genetic and phylogenetic studies indicate that infant quasi-species are highly homogeneous and generally represent minor maternal variants, confirming that vertical transmission of clade B HIV occurs across a selective bottleneck.[120,121] In one study, infant clones did not differ from the maternal clones in *env* length or glycosylation, and all infant variants used the CCR5 co-receptor but were not macrophage tropic.[121] Preferential in utero transmission of HIV subtype C, compared with subtype A or D, has been reported.[122]

Host genetic factors including maternal-infant human leukocyte antigen (HLA) concordance and maternal HLA class I homozygosity have been associated with increased risks of MTCT, whereas genetic variants of chemokine and chemokine receptors have yielded conflicting results.[123,124] Genetic variants of Toll-like receptors (TLRs) and defensins (e.g., TLR9 and β-defensin 1), crucial determinants of innate immune response, may also influence host-virus interactions and MTCT.[119]

POSTNATAL INFECTION

In LMIC, where prolonged breastfeeding (>6 months) is the cultural norm and safe replacement feeding is not affordable, feasible, sustainable, or safe, postnatal transmission of HIV through breast milk remains a significant challenge.[33,35,36] In the absence of interventions, postnatal transmission of HIV through breastfeeding can account for one third to one half of all HIV infections globally and carries an estimated transmission risk of about 15% when breastfeeding is prolonged and continued into the second year of life.[34,125,126]

Studies show that the highest risk of breast-milk HIV transmission occurs during the first 4 to 6 weeks of life, varying from 0.7% to 1% per week, with a lower but continued risk thereafter.[37,126-129] In studies from sub-Saharan Africa, the risk of late postnatal HIV transmission after 4 to 6 weeks of age was 8.9 infections per 100 child-years of breastfeeding and relatively constant at approximately 0.7% per month of breastfeeding.[126,129] Acute HIV infection in the mother during breastfeeding confers a higher risk of MTCT because of high levels of viral replication in maternal plasma and breast milk.[130-132] In one report, the cumulative risk of breast-milk HIV transmission was 14% for chronic maternal infection compared with 25% to 30% for maternal infections acquired during late pregnancy or lactation.[129]

Risk factors for breast-milk HIV transmission include women seroconverting during lactation, high HIV DNA or RNA level in maternal plasma and breast milk, low maternal $CD4^+$ cell count, maternal symptomatic disease or AIDS, prolonged duration of breastfeeding, mixed infant feeding (breast milk plus formula milk) in the initial few months of life, oral lesions in the infant (e.g., candidiasis), abrupt weaning, and maternal breast problems (e.g., bleeding or cracked nipples, subclinical and clinical mastitis, and breast abscesses).[37, 38, 133-140]

HIV has been isolated from cell-associated (DNA) and cell-free fractions of human breast milk from HIV-infected women and has been detected by culture or PCR in varying frequencies (39%-89%) in many studies.[141-145] Breast-milk viral load levels are very high soon after birth.[141] However, viral shedding may be intermittent, and variation in breast-milk viral load between left and right breasts during the first 3 months of lactation has been reported.[145]

MECHANISMS OF TRANSMISSION

The mechanisms of MTCT are complex, requiring the virus to breach a mucosal barrier (placenta, the oral mucosa, or gastrointestinal [GI] tract).[70,146-149] Mucosal transmission may be enhanced via the interaction of HIV with several C-type lectins, including dendritic cell–specific intercellular adhesion molecule-3–grabbing nonintegrin (DC-SIGN), expressed on dendritic cells located beneath the mucosal epithelium.[147] DC-SIGN serves as an HIV-1 receptor, mediates virus adhesion to DCs, and recognizes pathogen-associated molecular patterns (PAMPs).[147] DC-SIGN heightens HIV capture at mucosal entry sites, allowing its transport to CD4 T lymphocytes through transinfection.[147] DC-SIGN is expressed on placental macrophages (Hofbauer cells), and genetic polymorphisms of this molecule have been associated with risk of MTCT.[150]

In general, most infants escape infection despite an immature immune system and continued repetitive exposure to the virus (e.g., breastfeeding).[146] Of the various routes of MTCT, transplacental HIV transmission is the least efficient.[146] Some experts have hypothesized that fetal T-regulatory (Treg) cells may curb intrauterine transmission, given the ability of these cells to suppress inflammatory responses.[146] Treg cells have been shown to suppress immune responses when exposed to maternal antigens in utero.[151] Exposure to certain antigens (e.g., placental malarial infection) in the intrauterine period has been associated with increased Treg cells at birth.[152] In addition, robust HIV-specific T-cell responses have been demonstrated in HIV-exposed, uninfected infants after depletion of Treg cells in vitro.[153] Further, placental inflammation is associated with in utero.[104,154] The gut of newborn infants has an abundance of memory $CD4^+CCR5^+$ T cells, which are targets for HIV infection and facilitate MTCT.[155] Likewise, fetal tissues and cells are more susceptible to HIV infection than adult cells.[156] Thus other amniotic and/or placental factors may play a role in suppression of fetal gut inflammatory responses in utero.[146,157,158]

Most intrapartum MTCT likely occurs via mucosal exposure.[146] This is supported by studies demonstrating the protective effect of cesarean section, presence of HIV in infant gastric aspirates, and presence of $CD4^+CCR5^+$ T cells in the neonatal gut.[95,96,155,159] In addition, inflammatory cytokines and chemokines found in placentas of transmitting mothers are absent in placentas of mothers who transmit during intrapartum period.[154] MTCT generally occurs in the presence of HIV-specific antibody transferred across the placenta during the third trimester of pregnancy.[146,160] The role of maternal neutralizing and/or nonneutralizing antibodies in influencing MTCT risk is unclear, although in simian immunodeficiency models, broadly neutralizing antibodies can prevent infection and modify immune responses in infected neonatal macaques.[146,161,162]

The mechanisms of breast-milk HIV transmission are poorly understood.[70,71,149] A complex interplay of factors, including the nature and size of HIV reservoirs in breast milk, host susceptibility, various immune and nonimmune breast-milk factors, may be responsible for postnatal transmission during breastfeeding.[149] Only a minority of breast-fed infants born to HIV-infected mothers acquire postnatal infection by unknown mechanisms, despite prolonged and repeated daily exposure to HIV in breast milk.[148,163] The reported probability of breast-milk transmission of HIV is extremely low, at 0.00064/L ingested and 0.00028/day of breastfeeding.[164] Prolonged breastfeeding over a period of several months to years can result in postnatal transmission rates of greater than 15%.[125,126]

The primary HIV reservoirs in human milk are RNA (as cell-free virus), DNA (as cell-associated virus integrated in latent T cells, and intracellular RNA (as cell-associated virus in activated T cells).[143,149] HIV can gain entry into breast milk via passive transfer from the vascular compartment or through local replication in mammary gland tissues and breast milk.[149,163,164] The mammary epithelium serves as an effective barrier to HIV entry.[148] Compared with plasma, the concentration of cell-free HIV RNA in breast milk is approximately 2 logarithms lower.[165] Cell-free, as well as cell-associated, viruses are associated with breast-milk HIV transmission.[142-144] However, recent studies suggest that cell-associated virus (either latently infected or activated virus-producing T cells) in breast milk may be a stronger predictor for transmission of HIV to the infant than cell-free virus.[149,166] cART administered during pregnancy or postpartum can suppress cell-free HIV RNA but not cell-associated HIV DNA load in breast milk.[167] Another recent report found that cell-associated virus level (per mL) is more important for early postpartum HIV transmission (at 6 weeks) than cell-free virus.[168]

Inflammatory breast conditions (e.g., mastitis or abscess) can result in increased mammary epithelial cell (MEC) permeability (rise in breast-milk sodium levels), viral shedding, and transmission.[135,143,169] Subclinical mastitis (defined by elevated breast-milk sodium levels in asymptomatic women) can occur in mothers who do not breastfeed exclusively or during weaning. In such instances, infrequent breast emptying can lead to ductal inflammation and increased MEC permeability. Subclinical mastitis has been associated with increased breast-milk HIV loads and a higher risk of postnatal HIV transmission through breast milk.[170] However, a study from Zimbabwe found that laboratory indicators of mastitis (e.g., sodium levels and cell counts) were not predictive of increased breast-milk HIV RNA levels.[171]

The origin and evolution of HIV in breast milk is an area of ongoing research.[172,173] HIV variants found in breast milk are genetically indistinguishable from those present in plasma.[172-174] Studies indicate that viral evolution is limited in breast milk, reflecting restricted replication.[174-176] A recent report demonstrated that breast milk may be initially seeded by an early HIV variant differing from the viral variants present in maternal plasma. Thereafter exchange of distinct viral sequences between plasma and breast milk results in multiple independent lineages of HIV without compartmentalization.[173]

Although the virus enters through the infant's mouth during breastfeeding, the precise portal of entry of HIV at various mucosal targets (e.g., oral mucosa, tonsils, GI tract) is unclear.[149] HIV in breast milk may enter the submucosal layer of the infant gut because of breaks in the intestinal epithelial cell layer, which may occur from inflammation caused by nonexclusive breastfeeding or other coexisting pathogens.[163,177] Low gastric acidity in neonates may facilitate entry of cell-free or cell-associated virus into intestinal epithelial cells.[178] Mixed infant feeding may result in mucosal inflammation and immune activation in the infant GI tract, possibly facilitating HIV transfer across the gut lumen.[13,146,179]

Although mucosal breaches facilitate viral entry, transmission of HIV may also occur through intact fetal oral and intestinal mucosal membranes.[180] Transmission of HIV across the intestinal mucosal barrier is believed to occur after the virus attaches to immature dendritic cells of the infant gut, which then transport antigen to Peyer patches of the intestinal mucosa. Once the mucosal barrier is breached, HIV infects CD4$^+$ T cells and disseminates to the draining lymph nodes and the lymphoid system.[181]

Breast milk contains myriad factors with immunologic, antimicrobial, and antiinflammatory properties that may reduce the risk of transmission of HIV during breastfeeding among infants, despite repeated daily exposure to the virus.[146,182] Some innate factors (e.g., mucin, polyanionic proteins, lysozyme, lactoferrin, bile salt–stimulated lipase, and secretory leucocyte protease inhibitor) in human milk exhibit strong HIV inhibitory activity in vitro.[146,183-185] For example, bile salt–stimulated lipase can bind DC-SIGN and differentially inhibit viral capture and infection of CD4 T lymphocytes.[184,185] Increased concentration of long-chain n-6 polyunsaturated fatty acids, human milk oligosaccharides, α-defensins, and erythropoietin in breast milk has been correlated with decreased risk of postnatal transmission of HIV during breastfeeding.[186-189]

Breast milk also contains soluble/humoral and cellular factors that mediate innate and adaptive immune effects, including cytokines (interferon-γ [IFN-γ]), chemokines (regulated on activation, normal T-cell expressed and secreted [RANTES]), HIV-specific antibodies, CD8$^+$ HIV-specific cytotoxic T lymphocytes, CD4$^+$ HIV-specific helper T lymphocytes, natural killer (NK) cells, and macrophages.[190-192] The source of HIV in breast milk is likely infected T cells or macrophages derived from gut-associated lymphoid tissue (GALT) via the enteromammary axis.[163,193-197] CCR5-expressing memory CD4 T cells represent the majority of lymphocytes in breast milk.[190,192] Compared with peripheral blood CD4 T$^+$ cells, breast-milk T lymphocytes exhibit primarily an effector memory phenotype (CD45RO$^+$), express more activation markers, display stronger expression of HIV co-receptors, and demonstrate mucosal homing receptors, identical to B cells located in GALT.[149] The presence of breast-milk cellular immune responses against HIV has also been studied, but their significance in decreasing transmission is unclear.[163,190,192,193] In recent studies, HIV–Gag-specific IFN-γ responses were detected among HIV-exposed breastfeeding infants and have been associated with early protection from MTCT.[198,199]

Activated latently infected CD4 T$^+$ cells favor viral replication and release from the persistent stable HIV reservoirs in breast milk.[149] Recent studies indicate that latently infected CD4 cells and spontaneously activated CD4 T$^+$ cells are not affected by maternal ART and may play an important role in residual breast-milk HIV transmission.[200] Breast-milk cellular reservoirs and possible cell-to-cell HIV transfer from breast milk to the infant's intestinal mucosae remain a concern regarding the feasibility of elimination of breastfeeding transmission of HIV.[149] The biologic relevance of HIV-specific T cells in breast milk needs future research.[192] Although breast milk contains maternal HIV-specific antibodies (secretory immunoglobulin A [IgA], secretory IgM, and IgG), their role in protection against postnatal HIV infection is uncertain.[163,194,201,202] Likewise, the role of functionally effective neutralizing antibodies in preventing breast-milk HIV transmission is unknown and warrants future studies.[37,163,191]

Molecular Biology

Significant progress has been made in understanding the structural and molecular biology of HIV.[203,204] Based on the sequence homology of the envelope proteins, two types of HIV viruses, HIV-1 and HIV-2, can cause AIDS in humans.[204] HIV-1 and HIV-2 are lentiviruses belonging to the Retroviridae family and have a complex genomic structure.[205] The HIV viruses are closely related to the simian immunodeficiency viruses (SIVs), which are agents in African green monkeys and sooty mangabey monkeys *(Cercocebus atys)*.[206] In 1989, the virus closely related to HIV-1 (SIVcpz) was found in chimpanzees *(Pan troglodytes)*, whose natural range is in West-Central Africa (Cameroon, Equatorial Guinea, Congo, and Central African Republic), whereas the virus closely related to HIV-2 (SIVsm) was found in sooty mangabey monkeys, whose natural range is in West Africa.[207-209] Although HIV-1 and HIV-2 share similar transmission routes, cellular targets, and AIDS-defining manifestations, HIV-2 infection is characterized by lower transmission rates, slower disease progression, and a lower mortality rate compared with HIV-1.[209]

HIV-1 variants are classified into four distinct groups: group M (main), group O (outlier), group N (new), and a recently described group P, each representing an independent cross-species transmission event from chimpanzees and/or gorillas to humans.[210] Group M accounts for most HIV-1 infections globally and is divided further into 10 subtypes or clades (A to K), sub-subtypes, and inter-subtype circulating recombinant forms (CRFs).[211] The HIV-1 subtypes and CRFs vary considerably from region to region. Subtype B is the predominant HIV-1 subtype in North America, the Caribbean, Latin America, and Australia, whereas subtypes C predominate in Southern Africa, Ethiopia, and India.[212] There is considerable genetic diversity in Central Africa, Western and Central Europe, where all subtypes and many CRFs are implicated.[212] In Western and Central Europe, all major subtypes and many CRFs and unique recombinant forms (URFs) are detected. In Eastern Europe and Central Asia, the HIV-1 epidemic is dominated by subtype A and subtype B.[212] The majority of infections in South and Southeast Asia are caused by CRF01_AE subtype.[212]

HIV-1 is an enveloped cytopathic virus with a diameter of approximately 110 to 150 nm. The outer coat of the virus is composed of a lipid bilayer membrane envelope surrounding a cylindric, electrodense core of structural proteins.[204,213] The HIV core includes the replication enzymes, viral genomic RNA, and is encased by a cone-shaped shell consisting of the viral capsid protein.[204] Embedded throughout the outer coat of the virus are host cellular proteins, as well as trimeric envelope (Env) spikes that protrude through the surface of the HIV virion.[204,214] Each Env spike is composed of three surface glycoproteins gp120, each of which is noncovalently anchored by the transmembrane glycoprotein gp41 molecule.[215,216] The outer subunits of gp120 and gp41 are derived from a common precursor, gp160, and remain primary targets for vaccine development.[213]

The bullet-shaped retroviral core or capsid consists of 2000 copies of the viral protein p24 and contains two copies of the single-stranded HIV RNA, each of which possesses a copy of viral genes.[217] Both ends of the HIV RNA strands contain an RNA sequence called the long terminal repeat (LTR). Viral or host cellular proteins can activate certain regions of the LTR, which act as molecular switches to control production of new viruses. Similar to all retroviruses, HIV-1 contains structural and regulatory genes and accessory proteins.[217] The structural genes include *gag*, which encodes the core nucleocapsid polypeptides (gp24, p17, p9); *env*, which encodes for the surface-coated proteins of the virus (gp120 and gp41); and *pol*, which encodes for the viral replication enzymes (reverse transcriptase, integrase, and protease) involved in the later steps of the virus life cycle. In addition, there are two regulatory (Tat and Rev) and four accessory proteins (Vif, Vpr, Vpu, and Nef) that are essential for viral replication and pathogenicity.[217]

The regulatory proteins Tat and Rev are expressed early during cellular infection, whereas virion-associated proteins, such as Env, Pol, and Gag are expressed later. The accessory proteins often play an important role in modulating the host immune response and are major determinants of HIV-1 species tropism. For example, Vif, a cytoplasmic phosphoprotein encoded by the *vif* gene during the late stage of the HIV life cycle, acts by preventing viral encapsidation of a potent restriction factor in host cells (apolipoprotein B messenger RNA [mRNA]-editing enzyme-catalytic APOBEC3G/F protein), resulting in inactivation of the antiviral effect and enhancing HIV replication.[218] Besides Vif-APOBEC proteins, other major viral and cellular determinants for HIV-1 species tropism include Gag-CA/CypA, Gag-CA/tripartite motif (TRIM) proteins, and Vpu-Tetherin/BST-2.[217,219] More recently, two studies showed that the SIV Vpx protein can counteract inhibition of HIV-1 infection of macrophages mediated by the sterile alpha motif and histidine-aspartic (HD) domain–containing protein-1 (SAMHD1), a myeloid-cell–specific HIV-1 restriction factor.[220,221]

The life cycle of HIV-1 is characterized by several distinct steps, beginning with viral entry into host cells engaging cell surface receptors, uncoating and integration, viral mRNA biogenesis and transport, and ending with viral egress and maturation of nascent particles into infectious virions.[204,222-224] A wide array of host proteins are involved in the replication cycle, whereas certain host restriction factors counteract to suppress viral replication.[217,219-221] HIV-1 primarily infects CD4 T-lymphocyte cells, macrophages, and other host cells (e.g., dendritic cells).[225] During sexual transmission of HIV, dendritic cells located at or near mucosal sites are the first target cells for initiation of HIV infection.[226]

Members of the chemokine receptor family are coreceptors for HIV-1 entry into target cells. The main HIV coreceptors are CC chemokine receptor 5 (CCR5) or CXC chemokine receptor 4 (CXCR4).[227] Early reports described two classes of HIV-1 based on their ability to infect $CD4^+$ T cells (T tropic) or macrophages (M tropic). Subsequently, it was discovered that T-tropic viruses use the CXCR4 chemokine coreceptor (called X4 viruses), whereas M-tropic viruses use the CCR5 chemokine co-receptor (called R5 viruses).[228-230] HIV-1 may use CCR5 (R5) or CXCR4 (X4) co-receptors either individually or in combination (R5X4).[231] HIV-1 phenotype (co-receptor usage and tropism) is determined by genetic sequences within gp120 molecule, especially in the highly variable envelope V3 residues.[232]

The first step in the entry process of HIV into a cell is the binding of virion Env glycoprotein gp120 to the host cell-surface receptor CD4, followed by interactions with a co-receptor CC chemokine receptor (CCR5) or CXC chemokine receptor type 4 (CXCR4).[233-237] This binding results in a cascade of conformational change in the Env that exposes a fusion domain in gp41, resulting in fusion of the viral and host cell membranes, allowing the viral genome to gain entry into the cell.[222,223,238-240] HIV virions enter the cell and are partially uncoated, facilitating the process of reverse transcription, an essential step in retroviral replication.[241] The viral reverse-transcriptase enzyme transforms the single-stranded viral RNA into linear double-stranded DNA, whereas the less specific ribonuclease H (RNase H) degrades and removes the viral genomic RNA template.[241] This linear viral DNA molecule is circularized, yielding the preintegration complex (PIC).[204] After nuclear import, the retroviral PIC is inserted into a host cell chromosome by the viral integrase at random sites as an integrated provirus, aided by the host chromatin-binding protein lens epithelium-derived growth factor.[242,243] Proviral transcription by host RNA polymerase II, aided by the viral transactivator protein (Tat) and positive transcription elongation factor b (P-TEFb) results in production of viral mRNAs of varying sizes.[244] The smaller viral mRNAs are exported easily from the nucleus into the cytoplasm, whereas the export of full length (unspliced) and partially spliced mRNAs is regulated by the viral Rev protein and aided by the host nuclear export factor CRM1 protein.[204,245] mRNA templates serve as templates for Gag, Pol, and Env proteins, and genome-length RNA is packaged into viral particles with protein components.[246]

HIV-1 becomes enveloped while budding through the plasma membrane. During or after retroviral budding, the precursor polypeptide Gag and Gag-Pol is cleaved by the viral protease, resulting in synthesis of retroviral structural proteins capsid (CA), matrix (MA), and nucleocapsid (NC) proteins and the enzymes reverse transcriptase, integrase, and protease, leading to the formation of the mature conical core.[247] Virus maturation is crucial for particle infectivity.[248] Proteins of the ESCRT (endosomal sorting complex required for transport) complex and ALG-2-interacting proteinX (ALIX) mediate viral particle budding, separation of the viral envelope from the plasma membrane, and release of infectious virions.[249]

Although integration is a central event in the replication cycle of retroviruses, it is also a common feature of all retroviruses to accumulate large amounts of unintegrated viral DNA in cells that are fully competent templates for HIV-1 core and envelope antigen production.[250] The latent proviral DNA represents a viral reservoir that is unaffected by ART and can be activated by host-cell responses to antigens, mitogens, or cytokines.[251,252] Latently infected cells, primarily resting memory CD4 T cells, remain a major hurdle to achieving a sterilizing or a functional HIV-1 cure.[253]

Immunopathogenesis

Research conducted over the past 2 decades has yielded significant insights into understanding of the viral and immunopathogenesis of HIV infection.[146,254-258] Dendritic cells or macrophages are initially targeted by HIV, an interaction that transmits the virus to $CD4^+$ T cells.[224] The activation and direct infection of $CD4^+$ T cells result in high rates of viral production and eventually severe immune deficiency resulting from $CD4^+$ T-cell depletion.[224,259,260] $CD4^+$ T-cell loss in HIV infection occurs because of direct viral-induced cell killing as well as immune activation–induced cell death.[261-263]

It is well established that the mucosal immune system plays a vital role in the transmission and pathogenesis of AIDS.[264,265] After an early burst of viremia and dissemination, rapid and profound loss of "activated" memory $CD4^+$ T cells (mostly Th17 phenotype) in the GALT, particularly in the intestine, is a hallmark of early HIV infection in adults.[266-268] In acute infection, CD4 depletion and impairment of the intestinal barrier from enteropathy and subsequent microbial translocation result in chronic immune activation.[261,262,265] Recent evidence suggests that HIV-induced chronic immune activation via activation of the innate and adaptive immune system plays a central role in the immunopathogenesis of HIV/AIDS.[261,262] Although progress has been made in the immunology of pediatric HIV infection, the true correlates of immune protection and immune failure and mechanisms of infection in neonatal target cells in the context of extreme viral and HLA diversity are poorly understood.[146,147,254,257]

VIRAL REPLICATION IN EARLY INFANT INFECTION

Human immunodeficiency virus strains transmitted from mother to child are typically minor maternal variants, predominantly macrophage-tropic and nonsyncytium-inducing R5 strains, that use CCR5 co-receptor to infect $CD4^+$ T cells, although use of CXCR4 (X4) has been reported.[146,254,258] Compared with adult cells, HIV replicates more readily in neonatal T lymphocytes and monocytes or macrophages, and this increased susceptibility is influenced by differential mRNA expression of several host genes associated with the virus life cycle.[254,269] In vitro studies suggest that integration of HIV into highly conserved host genes in neonatal (cord blood) cells may contribute to increased gene expression and viral replication compared with adult cells.[254,270] Analysis of many HIV structural, regulatory (*tat* and *rev*), and accessory (*vif, vpr, vpu, nef*) genes, has revealed conservation of functional domains of these genes during vertical transmission.[271,272] In addition, the *vif* and *vpr* sequences of transmitting mothers were more heterogeneous and more functional than sequences of nontransmitting mothers.[254,272]

Other HIV genes may also play a crucial role in virus transmission and pathogenesis. Functional domains in the HIV-1 functional LTR are conserved during vertical transmission, suggesting that a functional LTR sequence is crucial in viral gene expression, transmission, and pathogenesis.[273] Other properties exhibited by vertically transmitted viruses include enhanced replication kinetics and fitness compared with nontransmitted viruses.[195,274]

A recent study showed that fetal and neonatal intestine have a large subset of memory $CD4^+CCR5^+$ T cells with predominantly a Th1 and Th17 phenotype, suggesting that the neonatal gut may be a primary target for HIV infection and replication, as observed in adults.[146,155] A study in neonatal rhesus macaques demonstrated a rapid and profound loss of intestinal $CD4^+$ T cells after acute SIV infection.[275] Compared with adult macaques, intestinal $CD4^+$ T-cell turnover and proliferation are markedly increased in infant macaques and may result in a more sustained pool of selective target cells for HIV replication.[276] Increased viral replication may lead to a more rapid exhaustion of a finite precursor $CD4^+$ T-cell pool, resulting in faster disease progression in infants.[277]

Perinatal HIV infection is characterized by plasma RNA levels that rapidly reach very high levels, often exceeding 10^5 to 10^7 copies/mL during the first year of life, decreasing only slowly with age to a "setpoint" by approximately 5 years of age.[277-281] In a study of 106 HIV-infected infants, the median plasma HIV RNA value at 1 month of age was 318,000 copies/mL, and it was common to see viral levels that exceeded 10^6 copies/mL.[282] In the absence of ART, HIV replication is very efficient, and plasma HIV RNA levels exceeding 1 million copies/mL are not unusual, with levels declining gradually over the first 24 to 36 months of life.[282] A continued decrease in plasma HIV-1 RNA levels (mean, −0.2 to −0.3 logarithm decline/year) has been noted in vertically infected children through 5 to 6 years of age.[281,282] Compared with adults, peak and setpoint viral load are usually greater than 1 logarithm greater in perinatal HIV infection.[283] Viral loads are higher among infants who acquire HIV infection during the peripartum period, compared with those infected postnatally through breast milk.[283] In contrast, the viral setpoint in many adults is attained within weeks of acute infection because of HIV-specific T-cell responses, remains relatively steady for several years during clinical latency, and is an important predictor for subsequent disease progression.[284,285]

As in adults, higher infant viral loads correlate with a more rapid disease progression and high risk of mortality in the absence of ART,[278,280,285-288] whereas lower levels of plasma HIV RNA with combination ART are associated with clinical benefit.[26,289,290] These data indicate that high viral load is a critical determinant of pediatric disease progression and provide a strong argument for early and aggressive intervention with ART.[291] In one study, significant age-related differences in HIV disease progression were noted in vertically infected children younger than 5 years.[292] Younger children were at higher risk for disease progression or mortality compared with older children, irrespective of plasma viral load or CD4 lymphocyte count.[292] In children older than 5 years, the risk of disease progression and mortality was similar to that noted in young adults; viral load and CD4 lymphocyte level were important predictors of HIV progression.[292] In contrast, the clinical course of HIV infection in adolescents and adults is relatively slow, with progression to AIDS or death within 10 years among untreated patients.[293]

The very high plasma HIV RNA levels in infants with HIV infection may be related to many factors, including the increased susceptibility of neonatal target cells to HIV-1 infection, a large and renewable CD4 T-cell pool size, presence of an active thymus, and delayed or ineffective HIV-specific immune responses.[146,254,257,294-297]

HUMAN IMMUNODEFICIENCY VIRUS–SPECIFIC IMMUNE CONTROL

Vertically infected infants face many challenges in mounting a specific immune response to HIV.[146,257,295,298] Perinatal HIV transmission occurs before the immune system is fully developed in an infant, allowing for more efficient viral replication and less efficient immunologic containment of the virus.[146,254,257,298] The immunologic milieu in the neonate is tolerogenic, characterized by enhanced regulatory T-cell activity and increased interleukin 10 (IL-10) production.[257] The adaptive immune response in early months of life is characterized by the preferential induction of Th17- and Th2-type immunity, which facilitates clearance of extracellular pathogens rather than intracellular pathogens (e.g., viruses).[257] In addition, there is decreased production of type I IFNs and Th1 decrease in cytokines, such as IL-12 and IFN-γ.

In adults with acute HIV infection, HLA class I–restricted CD8$^+$ (cytotoxic) T lymphocytes (CTL) play a crucial role in generation of HIV-specific immune responses to reduce viral load.[299,300] CTL lyse HIV-infected cells through the recognition of virus-derived peptides (or "epitopes") presented on the surface of the infected cells by HLA class I molecules.[301] HLA-restricted CTL responses drive the evolution of HIV through selection of viral sequence polymorphisms ("immune escape mutations").[301]

Although HIV-specific CTL activity can be shown at a very early age, even in the fetus, the response is weak and less broad to optimally reduce viral load in infants.[302-306] In addition, vertically transmitted maternal virus may be preadapted to the infant's HLA alleles, affecting the infant's ability to mount an early CTL response restricted by shared HLA alleles.[296,307-310] HIV-specific CTL responses become more frequent and broad in infected infants with age.[304-307,311] In one study, the Gag-specific CD8 T-cell response at 3 months of age correlated with clinical outcome and survival at 12 months.[312] Another study found that robust functional CD8 T-cell responses are not detected until 3 years of age in vertically acquired children, primarily among those with adequate CD4 T-cell compartment.[313] Polyfunctional HIV-specific CD8 T-cell responses are associated with slower disease progression in children as in adult HIV infection.[314] Immune activation and the upregulation of programmed cell-death protein 1 (PD1), an inhibitory molecule produced by CD8 T cells, have been noted during the course of HIV infection in children.[315,316] The narrow CTL responses in infants can result in viral escape mutants within the first year of life.[296,310,317-319] In addition, persistent viral replication may lead to the selection of compensatory mutations that increase viral fitness.[257] Certain HLA alleles (HLA-B*27, HLA-B*57, Cw-2, or DQB1-2) are associated with slower disease progression, indicating that CTL responses can have an important role in suppression of viral replication in pediatric HIV infection.[320-325]

Compared with adults, HIV-specific CD4 T-cell responses are not detected initially in most vertically infected infants; subsequent responses remain narrow and low magnitude but increase with age.[257,305,307,326-328] Studies in infant SIV-macaque model suggest that increased regulatory T-cell activity in early life may contribute to the suppression of viral specific CD4 T-cell responses.[257,329] HIV-specific CD4 T-cell responses may also be important for T-cell–mediated viral control and enhance the capacity of HIV-specific CD8 T cells to suppress viral replication.[257,316,330,331] In one study, the frequency of Gag-specific CD4 T cells in infected infants at 3 and 6 months of age correlated inversely with viral load.[312] In another study, the magnitude of Gag-specific CD4 T-cell responses was associated with control of viral replication in ARV-naïve children.[311]

The passive transfer of maternal, nonneutralizing antibodies could inhibit development of HIV-specific immune responses.[328] Detection of antibodies mediating HIV-specific antibody-dependent, cell-mediated cytotoxicity (ADCC) is delayed in most vertically infected infants until after 1 year of age.[332] Defective ADCC activity against HIV-infected target cells in neonates may also result in poor control of HIV.[333,334] After the decline of passively transferred maternal antibody-dependent, cell-mediated cytotoxicity antibodies, the production of HIV-envelope cytotoxic antibodies is delayed in vertically infected infants.[335] Although neutralizing antibodies can be generated during early infection,[336-338] the precise role of neutralizing antibodies in limiting mother-to-child transmission of HIV is unclear and warrants further investigation.[339-341]

The viral load in perinatally acquired HIV infection eventually decreases over time, although the precise mechanisms remain unknown.[257] In the absence of ART, less than 10% of vertically infected children are well by 8 years of age, referred to as HIV long-term nonprogressors (LTNPs).[342] There are fewer reports of LTNPs or "slow progressors" in children.[342-344] In one study, lower levels of immune activation were noted among LTNP in the first weeks of perinatally acquired HIV infection.[342] In adult HIV infection, immune activation results in CD4$^+$ T-cell loss and is an important prognosis marker for disease progression than viral load.[263,345] In contrast, CD8 T-cell activity may not be significant in the neonate given the tolerogenic regulatory T-cell environment and low-magnitude Th-cell responses.[257] In pediatric slow progressors, the decline of HIV viremia eventually occurs because of increase in the breadth and magnitude of HIV-specific adaptive immune responses over time.[304-307,311,326]

IMMUNE CONSEQUENCES IN HUMAN IMMUNODEFICIENCY VIRUS INFECTION

Untreated HIV infection results in profound deficiencies in cell-mediated and humoral immunity caused by quantitative and qualitative defects.[346] Progressive dysfunction of the immune system with selective depletion of CD4+ T cells occurs because of direct infection and immune activation.[261-263] Increased immune activation can occur in HIV-infected children in association with decreased naïve T-cell numbers, increased apoptosis, and accelerated T-cell differentiation.[347,348] In infants, thymic dysfunction associated with HIV infection may also have a significant impact on the developing immune system, leading to progressive depletion of thymic CD4 T-lymphocyte cells, dramatic decrease in cortical CD4/CD8 double-positive cells, and an increased percentage of CD8 cells.[254,349,350]

Compared with adults, CD4+ T-cell depletion may be less striking in children because of their relative lymphocytosis. Flow cytometric analysis of lymphocyte subpopulations in healthy children revealed age-related changes in many of the different subgroups.[351-353] Comparison of lymphocyte subsets in HIV-infected versus noninfected children younger than 2 years showed no difference for absolute CD8+ counts but clearly decreased levels of CD4+ cells.[354] HIV-specific CD4 T-cell responses are crucial for B-cell antibody formation in addition to generation of HIV-specific CD8 T-cell responses to control viremia.[257,316,330,331]

Abnormalities of the humoral immune system can precede or accompany abnormalities of the cellular immune system in HIV infection and consist of polyclonal B lymphocyte activation, resulting in hypergammaglobulinemia (especially IgG and IgA), abnormal primary or secondary antibody responses (T-lymphocyte–dependent and –independent antigens), decreased lymphocyte proliferation in response to an antigen; in addition, impaired function of other immune cells (monocytes/macrophages, NK lymphocytes, dendritic cells, and neutrophils) has been reported.[346, 355-358] Panhypogammaglobulinemia is noted in less than 10% of patients and is associated with poor prognosis.[17]

Several studies indicate that HIV-infected children have reduced antibody responses to certain childhood vaccines (e.g., diphtheria, acellular pertussis vaccine).[335,359-361] Reduced antibody responses after immunization and vaccine failures in HIV-infected infants may result from a poor primary immune response, failure to generate memory responses, or loss of memory cells.[335] Most vertically infected infants who receive cART before 3 months of age develop antibody and lymphoproliferative responses to routine infant vaccines, although persistent HIV-specific immune responses are not detected.[302,328,335] More recent studies have reported a sustained increase in peripheral blood CD5 cell counts and robust immune reconstitution among HIV-infected children after prolonged cART,[362,363] permitting discontinuation of prophylactic therapy for opportunistic infections (OIs).[364]

HUMAN IMMUNODEFICIENCY VIRUS RESERVOIRS

In individuals receiving suppressive ART, HIV can establish a state of latent infection in resting memory CD4+ T cells during development of immunologic memory responses.[365-367] The size and distribution of the viral reservoir may be affected by chronic immune activation, inflammation, and immune dysfunction even in patients receiving potent ART.[365] Although early initiation of ART in HIV-infected individuals can significantly reduce the size of the replication-competent resting CD4+ T-cell latent HIV reservoir, a stable pool of long-lived latently infected CD4+ T cells persists, representing a formidable challenge to HIV cure.[365,368,369] The CD4+ T-cell latent HIV reservoir is established in vertically infected infants despite initiation of ART by 8 weeks of age.[370] However, the size of the replication-competent resting CD4+ T cell in infants is associated with time to first undetectable viral load, suggesting that starting ART very early in infants may prevent establishment of a long-lived latent HIV reservoir.[370] The recent finding of detectable viral load (relapse) after an earlier report of a "functional" cure in a perinatally infected infant who received cART within hours of birth is disappointing and warrants further studies.[371]

Diagnosis

EARLY INFANT DIAGNOSIS

Many advances have been made in the area of laboratory diagnosis of HIV infection.[372-374] Routine HIV antibody testing (e.g., enzyme immunoassays, Western blot) cannot be used in infants for the diagnosis of HIV infection because of transplacental passage of maternal IgG antibodies to the virus that are present in infants up to 18 months of age.[374] The diagnosis of HIV infection in infants warrants the use of PCR-based DNA or RNA assays (referred to as HIV nucleic acid amplification tests [NAATs]) that are highly sensitive and specific and now widely available in developed countries.[374-376]

The HIV DNA PCR assay detects cell-associated proviral DNA and is the preferred test for early infant HIV diagnosis in the United States; approximately 30% to 40% of HIV-infected neonates will test positive by HIV DNA PCR assay by 48 hours of life, whereas 93% of infected infants will have a positive HIV DNA PCR assay result by 2 weeks of age.[377] By 1 month of age, the sensitivity and specificity of HIV DNA PCR assays for detection of HIV subtype B are 90% to 100% and 95% to 100%, respectively.[378-380] However, the HIV DNA PCR assay is less sensitive for identifying non–B subtype virus and has been associated with false-negative tests in patients with non–B subtype HIV infection.[372]

HIV RNA PCR assay detects plasma viral RNA and can also be used for early infant diagnosis.[372] The newer HIV RNA assay is as sensitive or more sensitive and as specific for detection of HIV subtype B compared with HIV DNA PCR assay.[381-383] False-positive HIV RNA results can occur in HIV-exposed neonates, warranting the need to repeat any positive test for confirmation.[17,384,385] In addition, a false-negative result can occur in neonates receiving ARV prophylaxis.[17] In contrast, HIV DNA PCR assay can detect proviral DNA in peripheral blood mononuclear cells and will be positive in HIV-infected patients on ART with undetectable viral loads.[17] The choice of NAATs also depends on the HIV subtype because of the genetic variability of HIV globally. HIV RNA PCR may be more sensitive than HIV DNA PCR test for detection of non–B subtype virus, such as subtype C, which is highly prevalent in sub-Saharan Africa.[386] Therefore it is prudent to use HIV RNA PCR for diagnosis of infants born to women known or suspected to have non–B subtype HIV infection.[372,374,375] In many studies, the sensitivity of HIV-1 RNA PCR is not affected by the presence of maternal or infant ZDV or nevirapine (NVP) prophylaxis.[385,387]

HIV DNA or RNA PCR testing is recommended by the U.S. Public Health Service (PHS) at 14 to 21 days of age, and if test results are negative, repeat testing at 1 to 2 months of age and again at 4 to 6 months of age.[17,372,375] Virologic testing is recommended at birth by some experts to diagnose in utero infection if mothers did not receive ART or prophylaxis during pregnancy or in other high-risk scenarios, but cord blood specimen should not be used because of possible contamination with maternal blood.[375] It is assumed that children who have a positive HIV PCR result within the first 48 hours after birth were infected in utero, whereas those who are infected during the intrapartum period might become positive 2 to 6 weeks after birth.[75] An infant is diagnosed with HIV infection if two separate blood samples test positive for HIV DNA or RNA PCR.[372] If infection is confirmed, the infant should be promptly referred to a pediatric HIV specialist for consideration of cART and care[220] to prevent rapid disease progression noted in some vertically infected infants.[277,278,291,372,388]

HIV infection can be *presumptively excluded* in nonbreastfeeding HIV-exposed children younger than 18 months if (1) two negative HIV DNA or RNA PCR tests result from separate specimens, both of which were obtained at or after 2 weeks of age and one of which was obtained at or after 4 weeks of age; *or* (2) one negative HIV RNA or DNA PCR test results from a specimen obtained at or after 8 weeks of age; *or* (3) one negative HIV antibody test is obtained at or after 6 months of age; *and* no other laboratory (e.g., no subsequent positive PCR test results, if performed) or clinical (e.g., no AIDS-defining illness) evidence of HIV infection is obtained.[17,372]

HIV infection can be *definitively excluded* in nonbreastfeeding HIV-exposed children younger than 18 months if (1) two negative HIV DNA or RNA PCR tests result from separate specimens, both of which were obtained at or after 1 month of age and one of which was obtained at or after 4 months of age; (2) two negative HIV antibody tests from separate specimens, both of which were obtained at or after 6 months of age; *and* no other laboratory (e.g., no subsequent positive PCR test results, if performed) or clinical (e.g., no AIDS-defining illness) evidence of HIV infection is obtained.[17,372]

In children with two negative HIV DNA PCR test results, many physicians confirm the absence of HIV infection by documenting a negative HIV antibody test result at 12 to 18 months of age ("seroreversion").[372] A nonbreastfed infant is considered HIV negative if two antibody test samples drawn at least 1 month apart, and both obtained after 6 months of age, are negative.[17] If HIV antibody testing is performed at 12 months of age in an HIV-exposed infant not known to be infected, and if the infant is still antibody positive, repeat testing at 18 months of age is recommended. Detection of HIV antibody in a child 18 months of age or older is diagnostic of HIV infection. Documentation of seroreversion may be more important when non–subtype B HIV is possible or present. In breastfed infants, definite exclusion of HIV infection is based on negative diagnostic test obtained at greater than 6 weeks after cessation of breastfeeding.[376] Table 22-1 provides a diagram outlining the initial evaluation and clinical care of the HIV-exposed infant, as recommended by the American Academy of Pediatrics (AAP).[372]

Table 22-1 Evaluation and Management of Infants Exposed to Human Immunodeficiency Virus (HIV)

	INFANT AGE											
Test	**Birth**	**2 wk**	**3 wk**	**4 wk**	**6 wk**	**2 mo**	**4 mo**	**6 mo**	**9 mo**	**12 mo**	**15 mo**	**18 mo**
History, physical examination (including weight, height, head circumference)*	+	+	+	+	+	+	+	+	+	+	+	+
Assess risk of other infections	+											
Antiretroviral prophylaxis	+				+†							
Complete blood cell count	+			+		+‡						
HIV DNA or RNA PCR§	+¶	+			+		+					
PCP prophylaxis (with TMP-SMX)					+‖							
HIV antibody testing												+#
Immunizations	HIV-exposed infants should receive all routine childhood immunizations, including hepatitis B vaccine, inactivated polio vaccine, diphtheria–tetanus toxoids–acellular pertussis vaccine, *Haemophilus influenzae* type b vaccine, pneumococcal conjugate vaccine, and rotavirus vaccine.[17] If infant HIV infection is confirmed, then recommendations for the HIV-infected must be followed. Readers are referred to the 2012 edition of the American Academy of Pediatrics' *Red Book* for guidance regarding immunization practices in HIV-infected children.[17]											

ARV, Antiretroviral; *cART*, combination antiretroviral therapy; *PCP*, *Pneumocystis jirovecii* (formerly *carinii*) pneumonia; *PCR*, polymerase chain reaction; *TMP-SMX*, trimethoprim-sulfamethoxazole; *ZDV*, zidovudine.

*Review maternal history for possible exposure to coinfections (e.g., tuberculosis, syphilis, herpes simplex virus, cytomegalovirus, or hepatitis B virus).

†ZDV to prevent perinatal transmission should be started soon after birth but certainly within 12 hr. ZDV is discontinued at 6 wk of age; combination ARV prophylaxis is recommended for infants whose mothers have not received antepartum ARVs; cART should be started in a child who is proved to be infected according to pediatric treatment guidelines, with close laboratory monitoring.

‡Complete blood cell count is measured at baseline before starting ZDV, at 4 wk, and rechecked at 8 wk if severe anemia was noted at the 4-wk visit.

§Repeat PCR immediately if positive to confirm infection. If the initial test at 2-3 wk of age is negative, repeat test at 4 wk-2 mo and at 4-6 mo of age to identify or exclude HIV-1 infection as early as possible.

‖PCP prophylaxis can be avoided if or discontinued if HIV infection is presumptively or definitely excluded on the basis of negative HIV virologic tests at 2 and 4-6 wk; if infant is diagnosed with HIV, PCP prophylaxis should be continued for 1 yr.

¶Some experts recommend obtaining an HIV PCR test at birth to exclude intrauterine HIV infection if the mother did not receive cART during pregnancy or in other high-risk situations.

#HIV-1 antibody testing may be performed to confirm loss of passively transferred maternal antibody in infants already determined to be definitely HIV uninfected on the basis of serial negative virologic tests.

HIV isolation by culture is not recommended for routine diagnosis because culture is less sensitive, more expensive, needs a specialized laboratory, and results are not available for up to 28 days.[389] Use of HIV-1 p24 antigen detection is not recommended for diagnosis of infant HIV-1 because of its poor sensitivity compared with HIV DNA PCR or culture.[17,390]

Nonspecific laboratory parameters may also suggest HIV infection. Hypergammaglobulinemia, a nonspecific but early finding of HIV infection, is noted in up to 90% of perinatally infected infants by 6 months of age.[391,392] CD4 counts must be interpreted within the bounds of the age-dependent normal range, and changes in counts may result in a decrease in the normal CD4 to CD8 T-lymphocyte count ratio of greater than or equal to 1.0 in vertically infected infants by 1 to 2 months of age, compared with HIV-exposed, uninfected infants.[17,393]

Classification of Human Immunodeficiency Virus Infection in Children

Human immunodeficiency virus infection in children and adolescents causes a wide range of clinical manifestations, from asymptomatic infection to AIDS resulting from progressive immunodeficiency. The CDC has classified HIV infection in children to determine the severity of disease. The AIDS case definitions developed by the CDC in 1987, and subsequently revised in 1993, 1994, and 2008, are intended primarily for public health surveillance and reporting purposes for monitoring the HIV epidemic.[394-397]

The revised 1994 CDC classification system for HIV infection in children younger than 13 years is based on (1) HIV infection status, (2) clinical disease, and (3) immunologic status (Table 22-2).[396] Clinical categories are stratified from N, indicating no signs or symptoms, through A, B, and C, for mild, moderate, and severe (AIDS-defining) symptoms, respectively. The revised 2008 pediatric AIDS case definitions did not make any changes in the HIV infection classification system, the 24 AIDS-defining conditions for children younger than 13 years, or the AIDS case definition for children younger than 18 months.[397] Diagnosis is established if an AIDS-defining disease occurs (Table 22-3).[396]

In the pre–highly active antiretroviral treatment (HAART)-era, *Pneumocystis jirovecii* (formerly *carinii*) pneumonia (PCP) was the leading AIDS-defining illness diagnosed during the first year of life and associated with a high mortality rate.[398] Other common AIDS-defining conditions in U.S. children with vertically acquired infection include lymphoid interstitial pneumonitis (LIP), multiple or recurrent serious bacterial infections, HIV encephalopathy, wasting syndrome, *Candida* esophagitis, cytomegalovirus (CMV) disease, and *Mycobacterium avium-intracellulare* complex (MAC) infection (see Table 22-3).[399] In the post-HAART period, a significant decrease in the number of OIs was noted in HIV-infected children.[28,400] Likewise, significant decline in mortality was noted between 1994 and 2000, from 7.2 to 0.8 deaths/100 person-years.[26]

The case definitions are similar for adults and children, with some important exceptions.[396] LIP and multiple or recurrent serious bacterial infections are AIDS-defining illness only for children. Also, certain herpes virus infections (cytomegalovirus, herpes simplex virus) and toxoplasmosis of the central nervous system (CNS) are AIDS-defining conditions only for adults and children older than 1 month.[396]

The immunologic categories place emphasis on the CD4 T-cell lymphocyte count and percentages for age and include stage 1, no evidence of immunosuppression; stage 2, moderate immunosuppression; and stage 3, indicating severe immunosuppression.[396,397] Once classified, a child cannot be reclassified into a less severe category, even if the child's clinical status or immune function improves in response to ART or resolution of clinical events. HIV-exposed infants whose HIV infection status is indeterminate (unconfirmed) are classified by placing a prefix E (for perinatally exposed) before the appropriate classification code (e.g., EN2).[397]

HIV infection in infants and children has a different presentation from that in adults.[298] Children are more likely than adults to have serious bacterial infections, and LIP is almost entirely restricted to the pediatric age group. OIs such as PCP often manifest as primary diseases with a more aggressive course because of lack of prior immunity.[398] Toxoplasmosis, cryptococcal infection, and the occurrence of cancer, especially Kaposi sarcoma, are less common in HIV-infected children.[298,399]

Clinical Manifestations and Pathology

The early clinical manifestations of HIV infection in infants are highly variable and often nonspecific.[401] Infants with perinatally acquired HIV infection are often asymptomatic, and physical examination is usually normal in the neonatal period. Although a distinctive craniofacial dysmorphism characterized by microcephaly, hypertelorism, flattened nasal bridge, triangular philtrum, and patulous lips was suggested as a possible congenital HIV syndrome,[402] these findings reported during the early AIDS epidemic have not been confirmed in subsequent reports.[403] In a prospective cohort study of 200 perinatally acquired HIV-1 infections, the median age of onset of any HIV-related symptom or sign was 5.2 months; the probability of remaining asymptomatic was 19% at 1 year and 6.1% at 5 years.[404] In another large prospective cohort study, AIDS-defining conditions developed in approximately 23% and 40% of perinatally infected infants by 1 and 4 years.[405]

Growth delay is an early and frequent finding of untreated perinatal HIV infection, and linear growth is most severely affected in children with high viral loads.[406] Other features of infection in early infancy could include unexplained persistent or recurrent fevers, generalized lymphadenopathy, often associated with hepatosplenomegaly and recurrent or persistent otitis media. Also commonly encountered are oral or diaper candidiasis, developmental delay, parotitis, and nonspecific dermatitis.[17]

Before the widespread use of pediatric ART and use of prophylaxis, PCP was a common AIDS-defining illness in infancy, accounting for approximately 50% of all AIDS-defining conditions. Other clinical manifestations noted during the course of HIV infection in infants and children

Table 22-2 1994 Centers for Disease Control and Prevention Revised Classification System for Human Immunodeficiency Virus Infection in Children Younger Than 13 Years

Using this system, children are classified according to three parameters: infection status, clinical status, and immunologic status. The categories are mutually exclusive. When classified in a more severe category, a child is not reclassified in a less severe category, even if the clinical or immunologic status improves.*

PEDIATRIC HIV CLASSIFICATION

	CLINICAL CATEGORIES			
Immune Categories	**No Symptoms (N)**	**Mild Symptoms (A)**	**Moderate Symptoms (B)†**	**Severe Symptoms (C)†**
No suppression (1)	N1	A1	B1	C1
Moderate suppression (2)	N2	A2	B2	C2
Severe suppression (3)	N3	A3	B3	C3

IMMUNOLOGIC CATEGORIES BASED ON AGE-SPECIFIC CD4+ T-LYMPHOCYTE COUNTS AND PERCENTAGE OF TOTAL LYMPHOCYTES

The immunologic category classification is based on age-specific CD4+ T-lymphocyte count or percentage of total lymphocytes and is designed to determine severity of immunosuppression attributable to HIV for age. If either CD4+ count or percent results in classification into a different category, the child should be classified into the more severe category. A value should be confirmed before the child is reclassified into a less severe category.

	AGE GROUPS		
Immunologic Category	**0-11 mo**	**1-5 yr**	**>6 yr**
No suppression (1)	>1500 cells/μL (>25%)	>1000 cells/μL (>25%)	>500 cells/μL (>25%)
Moderate suppression (2)	750-1499 cells/μL (15%-24%)	500-999 cells/μL (15%-24%)	200-499 cells/μL (15%-24%)
Severe suppression (3)	<750 cells/μL (<15%)	<500 cells/μL (<15%)	<200 cells/μL (<15%)

CLINICAL CATEGORIES FOR CHILDREN WITH HIV INFECTION

Category N: Not Symptomatic

Children who have no signs or symptoms considered to be the result of HIV infection or who have only one of the conditions listed in category A

Category A: Mildly Symptomatic

Children with two or more of the following conditions but none of the conditions listed in categories B and C:

Lymphadenopathy (>0.5 cm at more than two sites; bilateral = one site)

Hepatomegaly

Splenomegaly

Dermatitis

Parotitis

Recurrent or persistent respiratory infection, sinusitis, or otitis media

Category B: Moderately Symptomatic

Children who have symptomatic conditions other than those listed for category A or C that are attributed to HIV infection

Examples of conditions in clinical category B include but are not limited to:

Anemia (<8 g/dL), neutropenia (<1000/mm^3), or thrombocytopenia (<100,000/mm^3) persisting >30 days

Bacterial meningitis, pneumonia, or sepsis (single episode)

Candidiasis, oropharyngeal thrush, persisting for >2 mo in children >6 mo of age

Cardiomyopathy

Cytomegalovirus infection, with onset before 1 mo of age

Diarrhea, recurrent or chronic

Hepatitis

Herpes simplex virus stomatitis, recurrent (more than two episodes within 1 yr)

Herpes simplex virus bronchitis, pneumonitis, or esophagitis with onset before 1 mo of age

Herpes zoster (shingles) involving at least two distinct episodes or more than one dermatome

Leiomyosarcoma

Lymphoid interstitial pneumonia or pulmonary lymphoid hyperplasia complex

Nephropathy

Nocardiosis

Persistent fever (lasting >1 mo)

Toxoplasmosis, onset before 1 mo of age

Varicella, disseminated (complicated chickenpox)

Category C: Severely Symptomatic

Children who have any condition listed in the 1987 surveillance case definition for AIDS, with the exception of lymphoid interstitial pneumonia

Serious bacterial infections, multiple or recurrent (i.e., any combination of at least two culture-confirmed infections within a 2-yr period of the following types: septicemia, pneumonia, meningitis, bone or joint infection, or abscess of an internal body organ or body cavity [excluding otitis media], superficial skin or mucosal abscesses, and indwelling catheter-related infections)

Table 22-2 1994 Centers for Disease Control and Prevention Revised Classification System for Human Immunodeficiency Virus Infection in Children Younger Than 13 Years—cont'd

AGE GROUPS
Candidiasis, esophageal or pulmonary (bronchi, trachea, lungs)
Coccidioidomycosis, disseminated (at site other than or in addition to lungs or cervical or hilar nodes)
Cryptosporidiosis or isosporidiosis with diarrhea persisting >1 mo
Cytomegalovirus disease with onset of symptoms at age >1 mo (other than liver, spleen, or lymph nodes)
Encephalopathy (at least one of the following progressive findings present for at least 2 mo in the absence of a concurrent illness, other than HIV infection, that could explain the findings): (1) failure to attain or loss of developmental milestones or loss of intellectual ability verified by standard developmental scale or neuropsychological tests; (2) impaired brain growth or acquired microcephaly shown by head circumference measurements or brain atrophy shown by CT or MRI (serial imaging is required for children <2 yr of age); (3) acquired symmetrical motor deficit manifested by two or more of the following: paresis, pathologic reflexes, ataxia, or gait disturbance
Herpes simplex virus infection causing a mucocutaneous ulcer that persists for more than 1 mo or bronchitis, pneumonitis, or esophagitis for any duration affecting a child >1 mo of age
Histoplasmosis, disseminated (other than or in addition to lungs or cervical lymph nodes)
Kaposi sarcoma
Lymphoma, primary, in brain
Lymphoma, small, noncleaved cell (Burkitt), or immunoblastic or large cell lymphoma of B cell or unknown immunologic phenotype
Mycobacterium tuberculosis, disseminated or extrapulmonary
Mycobacterium, other species or unidentified species, disseminated (other than or in addition to lungs, skin, or cervical or hilar lymph nodes)
Mycobacterium avium-intracellulare complex or *Mycobacterium kansasii,* disseminated (other than or in addition to lungs, skin, or cervical or hilar lymph nodes)
Pneumocystis jirovecii (formerly *carinii*) pneumonia
Progressive multifocal leukoencephalopathy
Salmonella (nontyphoid) septicemia, recurrent
Toxoplasmosis of the brain with onset >1 mo of age
Wasting syndrome in the absence of a concurrent illness, other than HIV infection, that could explain the following findings: persistent weight loss >10% of baseline *or* downward crossing of at least two of the following percentiles on weight-for-height chart on two consecutive measurements >30 days apart *plus* chronic diarrhea (i.e., at least two loose stools per day for >30 days) *or* documented fever (for >30 days, intermittent or constant)

From Centers for Disease Control and Prevention: Recommendations of the U.S. Public Health Service Task Force on the use of zidovudine to reduce perinatal transmission of human immunodeficiency virus, *MMWR Morb Mortal Wkly Rep* 43:1-20, 1994.
AIDS, Acquired immunodeficiency syndrome; *HIV,* human immunodeficiency virus.
*Children whose HIV infection status is not confirmed are classified by using the grid with a letter *E* (for vertically exposed) placed before the appropriate classification code (e.g., *EN2*).
†Category C and lymphoid interstitial pneumonitis in category B are reportable to state and local health departments as AIDS.

Table 22-3 AIDS Indicator Diseases Diagnosed in 8086 Children Younger Than 13 Years Reported to the Centers for Disease Control and Prevention Through 1997

Disease	No. Children Diagnosed	Percent of Total*
Pneumocystis jirovecii (formerly *carinii*) pneumonia	2700	33
Lymphocytic interstitial pneumonitis	1942	24
Recurrent bacterial infections	1619	20
Wasting syndrome	1419	18
Encephalopathy	1322	16
Candida esophagitis	1266	16
Cytomegalovirus disease	658	8
Mycobacterium avium infection	639	8
Severe herpes simplex infection	370	5
Pulmonary candidiasis	307	4
Cryptosporidiosis	291	4
Cancer	162	2

From Centers for Disease Control and Prevention: U.S. HIV and AIDS cases reported through December 1997. HIV/AIDS Surveillance report: year-end edition, *MMWR Morb Mortal Wkly Rep* 9:1-44, 1997.
AIDS, Acquired immunodeficiency syndrome.
*The sum of percentages is greater than 100 because some patients have more than one disease.

who remain undiagnosed or receive ineffective ART include encephalopathy, recurrent and chronic otitis media and sinusitis, recurrent invasive bacterial infections, other OIs, chronic diarrhea, cardiomyopathy, and nephropathy.[407]

INFECTIOUS COMPLICATIONS

Infections in HIV-infected infants not receiving combination ART can be serious or life threatening. The difficulty in treating these infectious episodes, their chronicity, and their tendency to recur distinguish them from the normal infections of early infancy. It is helpful to document each episode and to evaluate the course and frequency of their recurrences. In the pre-HAART era, the frequency of OIs varied by age, immune status, prior history of OI, and pathogen.[408,409] With early infant HIV diagnosis and linkage to care and an ART program, the frequency of historically reported AIDS-defining illness and OIs has dramatically decreased among children living with HIV in the United States and other resource-rich countries.[400] During the pre-ART era, the most common OIs (event rate, > 1.0/100 child-years) reported among U.S. children with vertically acquired infection included serious bacterial infections (e.g., pneumonia, bacteremia), PCP, disseminated MAC, herpes zoster, esophageal and tracheobronchial candidiasis, and CMV disease.[28,399,400] Other rare OIs (event rate, <1.0/100 child-years) included CMV disease, cryptosporidiosis, tuberculosis (TB), systemic fungal infections, and toxoplasmosis.[408] In the post-ART era, the rate of OI decreased from 12.5 to 0.8 cases per 100,000 person-years pre-ART and post-ART, respectively.[400] Despite these impressive declines, HIV-infected children continue to experience the same types of OIs, even in the era of combination ART, highlighting the need for early recognition, treatment, and prevention.[408]

Bacterial Infections

Recurrent and serious bacterial infections (SBI), such as pneumonia, bloodstream infection (BSI), urinary tract infection, meningitis, bone and joint infections, and abscess, are so typical of untreated HIV infection in children that they were included in the revised CDC definition of 1987.[394,409] In the pre-ART era, SBI was the most common OI in HIV-infected children (event rate, 15/100 child-years.[409] Recurrent bacterial infections accounted for 21% of all pediatric AIDS-defining conditions reported to the CDC through 2007.[410] Perinatally infected infants with low CD4 lymphocyte counts are at highest risk for developing SBI.[411] The occurrence of minor bacterial infections, such as otitis media and sinusitis, were very common (17-85/100 child-years) in untreated HIV-infected children.[412]

Streptococcus pneumoniae is the most frequent cause of SBI in children infected with HIV worldwide, accounting for greater than 50% of bacterial BSI.[400,409,413,414] In a study of vertically infected children younger than 6 months, pneumococcal bacteremia occurred at an annual rate of 11.3 episodes per 100 patient-years.[411] In the post-ART era, the incidence of invasive pneumococcal disease in HIV-infected children declined by greater than 80%, from 1.9 to 0.3 cases per 100 patient-years pre-ART and post-ART era, respectively.[415]

Other commonly implicated bacteria included *Salmonella* species, *Staphylococcus aureus*, and *Neisseria meningitidis*.[416] In children with central venous catheters, infection caused by coagulase-negative staphylococci, gram-negative enteric bacilli, *S. aureus*, *Pseudomonas aeruginosa*, and *Candida* species is common.[417] Very-late-onset group B streptococcal disease (at 3.5-5 months of age) and other rare infections, such as congenital syphilis, may also occur given the higher prevalence of untreated or inadequately treated syphilis among HIV-positive pregnant women.[418,419]

Mycobacterial infections have assumed an increasingly important role in the pathology of HIV-infected infants and children. Although unusual, congenital TB has been described in children born to HIV-infected mothers with TB.[420] An important issue for the neonatologist is whether the mother is infected with *M. tuberculosis* and may transmit the disease to her child. Studies have documented an increased rate of TB in HIV-infected children, but unlike other OIs, the risk of acquiring TB is not predicted by the CD4 T-lymphocyte count.[421,422] Infants remain at highest risk of disease progression, including development of serious complications, such as miliary TB and tuberculous meningitis.[408] Atypical radiographic findings, such as multilobar infiltrates and diffuse interstitial disease, may be noted in HIV-infected children with TB. The diagnosis and treatment of *M. tuberculosis* disease in HIV-infected infants is complex, given the multiple drug interactions between ARVs, antimycobacterial agents, and prophylactic antimicrobials (e.g., macrolides, azoles). The emergence and effective transmission of multidrug-resistant and extensively drug-resistant tuberculosis is a major challenge to control of TB worldwide.[423] Consultation with a pediatric infectious disease specialist must be sought, and the reader is referred to published CDC guidelines and expert reviews.[408,424]

MAC was the second most frequently reported OI in HIV-infected children in the United States after PCP in the pre-ART era. However, the incidence of MAC disease in HIV-infected children significantly declined from 1.3 to 1.8 episodes during the pre-ART era to 0.14 to 0.2 episodes per 100 person-years during the post-ART era.[28,400] Disseminated infection with MAC is very unusual during the first year of life. In the absence of prophylaxis, infection with MAC complex occurs in almost 20% of HIV-infected children with advanced disease (CD4 count < 50 cells/mm^3) and manifests as nonspecific symptoms, such as night sweats, weight loss, and low-grade fevers.[408] Treatment usually consists of a minimum of two drugs (e.g., clarithromycin or azithromycin plus ethambutol). Prophylaxis with clarithromycin or azithromycin should be initiated in HIV-infected infants younger than 1 year with a CD4$^+$ count less than 750 cells/mm^3.[408]

Viral Infections

Viral infections are important causes for morbidity and mortality in HIV-infected children. Primary varicella can be unusually severe and can recur as zoster, often manifesting with very few, atypical lesions, but the disease course is less complicated in the era of combination ART.[425] The varicella-zoster virus (VZV) may become resistant to standard treatment with acyclovir.[426] MTCT of VZV has not been reported among HIV-positive pregnant women infected with varicella.[408] CMV infection can result in esophagitis, hepatitis, enterocolitis, or retinitis.[427,428] HIV-infected women coinfected with CMV may carry a higher risk for MTCT of CMV.[429] CMV can become resistant to treatment with ganciclovir, necessitating the use of foscarnet or combination regimens.[408]

Other encountered viruses in HIV-infected infants and children are herpes simplex virus, influenza, human herpes virus 8, and hepatitis B and C virus.[408,429] Perinatal hepatitis C transmission rates of 6% to 23% have been reported in infants born to HIV/HCV coinfected mothers.[430] The effect of hepatitis C coinfection on HIV disease progression is unclear in children.[431] Infection with the measles virus is associated with a high mortality in HIV-infected children and often manifests without the typical rash and can result in fatal giant cell pneumonia.[432,433] Infection with respiratory syncytial virus can also result in rapid and sometimes fatal respiratory compromise and in chronic or persistent viral shedding or infection.[434]

Fungal and Protozoal Infections

Oral candidiasis is common even in healthy, non–HIV-infected newborns and infants. Infection beyond infancy, involvement of pharynx and esophagus, and persistence despite treatment with antifungal agents are more typical for immunocompromised children.[28,409] Disseminated candidiasis is uncommon, however, in the absence of predisposing factors, such as central venous catheters or total parenteral nutrition.[435]

Although infection with *Cryptococcus neoformans* is common in adults with HIV infection, it is less common in children.[436,437] Likewise, invasive disease caused by *Aspergillus* species is very rare in children with perinatally acquired HIV infection.[438] The incidence of other fungal infections varies with the prevalence of the organism in the specific geographic area. Disseminated histoplasmosis as the AIDS-defining illness has been described in a few infants.[439,440]

Early in the HIV epidemic, PCP was the most common AIDS indicator disease in almost 40% of the pediatric cases reported to the CDC.[398] This situation has changed dramatically, however, since the implementation of perinatal HIV prevention guidelines, combination ART, and PCP chemoprophylaxis.[408] The incidence rate of PCP in HIV-infected children dramatically declined from 1.3 cases per 100 child-years during the pre-ART era to less than 0.5 cases per 100 child-years during the ART era.[28] The peak incidence of PCP in infancy occurs during the first year of life, with more than 50% of cases between 3 to 6 months of life, often as the first symptom of HIV infection.[398] Presumably, PCP represents primary infection in these infants. Maternal-to-fetal transmission of PCP has also been documented.[441] PCP is a leading cause of death among HIV-infected infants and children in sub-Saharan Africa.[442]

Most children with PCP present with an acute febrile illness, with cough, tachypnea, and hypoxemia; chest radiographs typically reveal diffuse interstitial and alveolar infiltrates but may be normal in some cases.[408,443] A significant decrease in CD4 T-lymphocyte (CD4) cell count and percentage is a risk factor for PCP. The diagnosis in infants is usually made by performing a bronchoscopy with bronchoalveolar lavage (sensitivity, 55%-97%) and demonstration of the organism in pulmonary tissues or fluids.[408] Obtaining an induced sputum is difficult in young children, and an open lung biopsy is only rarely necessary.[408] PCR assays to detect the organism have been developed but are not widely available in most centers. Empirical therapy should be initiated promptly while awaiting results.

The treatment of choice for PCP includes high-dose intravenous (IV) trimethoprim-sulfamethoxazole (TMP-SMX); IV pentamidine isethionate is an alternative agent if patients are intolerant to TMP-SMX or experience clinical treatment failure after 5 to 7 days of TMP-SMX.[408] Early adjunctive treatment with corticosteroids has been beneficial in adults and children with moderate-to-severe PCP and is commonly recommended for patients with an initial arterial oxygen pressure of less than 70 mm Hg or an arterial-alveolar gradient of greater than 35 mm Hg.[408,444,445]

PCP has been associated with a mortality of 39% to 65% in infants despite improved diagnosis and treatment.[446,447] Chemoprophylaxis is highly effective in preventing PCP and is recommended for all HIV-infected infants younger than 12 months, regardless of CD4 count or percentage.[448-450] Prophylaxis is also recommended for HIV-exposed infants with indeterminate HIV infection status until they are determined to be HIV-uninfected or presumptively HIV-uninfected on the basis of negative virologic tests at 2 and 4 weeks of life.[374,397,451,452] Breakthrough infections can occur despite prophylaxis.[453,454]

Encephalitis caused by *Toxoplasma gondii* is common in adults with HIV infection but only rarely seen in children.[408] Several case reports of *T. gondii* encephalitis in infants 5 weeks to 18 months of age have been published, however. Some of these infants probably acquired *Toxoplasma* infection in utero, but the overall MTCT of *T. gondii* in HIV-infected pregnant women is unknown.[408,455-457] Toxoplasmosis is an important differential diagnosis in an HIV-infected patient with an intracerebral mass.

Protozoal infections of the GI tract often represent difficult diagnostic and therapeutic problems and can be associated with an intractable diarrhea. Opportunistic pathogens such as *Giardia, Microsporidium, Isospora belli (Cystoisospora belli)*, and *Cryptosporidium* usually occur with advanced disease. Infection with *Cryptosporidium* has a prevalence of 3% to 3.6% among children with diarrhea.[458] HIV-infected children are at risk for prolonged diarrheal disease, with often severe wasting warranting aggressive nutritional support.

ENCEPHALOPATHY

Encephalopathy, often with early onset, was a frequent and typical manifestation of untreated HIV infection in children, accounting for approximately 15% of all AIDS-defining events.[410,459] In the post-ART era, the incidence of overt and rapidly progressive HIV encephalopathy has dramatically decreased, but it may be associated with more subtle and insidious CNS manifestations.[460-462]

Symptoms of encephalopathy in the newborn or young infant initially include delayed head control or delayed acquisition of a social smile and variable degrees of truncal hypotonia.[463] Subsequently, impairment of cognitive, behavioral, and motor functions becomes apparent. Typical findings include a loss of or failure to attain normal developmental milestones, weakness, secondary or acquired microcephaly, intellectual deficits, or neurologic symptoms such as ataxia and pyramidal tract signs, including spasticity or rigidity.[464] Computed tomographic scan of the brain may show cerebral atrophy (85% of cases), calcifications in the basal ganglia and periventricular frontal white matter, and decreased attenuation in the white matter (Fig. 22-1).[465,466] The cerebrospinal

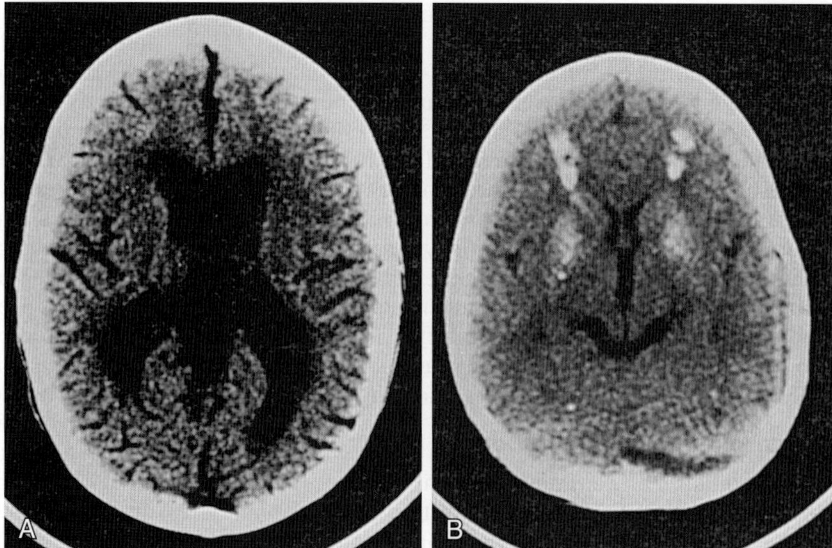

Figure 22-1 CT scans of the brains of two infants with HIV-associated encephalopathy. **A,** Cerebral atrophy with enlarged ventricles and widened sulci. **B,** Calcifications in basal ganglia and frontal white matter.

fluid profile is often normal; however, mild pleocytosis and elevated protein concentrations may be present.[467]

The neuropathogenesis of HIV encephalopathy is poorly understood.[460,468] Studies have shown that HIV enters the CNS soon after primary infection and may persist in this compartment during the course of HIV infection.[468] CNS targets of HIV infection may be different in children and adults. In contrast to terminally differentiated cells of the mature nervous system of adults, the immature nervous system of children has mitotically active cells. Blood-derived macrophages, microglial cells, and their derivatives harbor HIV in the CNS.[460,468] The neuropathogenesis of HIV encephalopathy appears to involve a cascade of viral proteins, various cytokines (i.e., tumor necrosis factor [TNF-α]) and chemokines, and neurotransmitters that promote ongoing inflammation, excitation, and overstimulation of the *N*-methyl-D-aspartate–type receptor (NMDAR) system.[460,469] This subsequently leads to neuronal injury and death secondary to apoptosis or necrosis, astrocytosis, as well as dendritic and synaptic damage.[470] Neural progenitor cells may also be involved in the neuropathgenesis of HIV encephalopathy.[471] Neuropathologic evidence of pediatric HIV-related CNS disease includes decreased brain weight, cortical atrophy, symmetrical intracerebral calcifications, white-matter changes, reactive astrocytosis, and subcortical gray-matter abnormalities of the basal ganglia, thalamus, claustrum, caudate, putamen, globus pallidus, and hippocampus.[472-474] HIV has been isolated from the brain of aborted fetuses from HIV-infected women and from the brain and cerebrospinal fluid of HIV-infected children and adults.[472,473]

The optimal HAART regimen to treat HIV encephalopathy has not been established.[475] The rate of progression and severity of HIV encephalopathy are highly variable. HAART in children may prevent, reduce, or improve neurologic manifestations of HIV infection.[460,462,468,476] In early studies, ZDV continuous therapy improved cognitive performance and reduced brain atrophy in a small study of symptomatic HIV-infected children.[477,478] Combination therapy with ZDV and didanosine (ddI) was more effective than monotherapy with either agent in improving age-appropriate neurocognitive scores in young children with symptomatic HIV.[478-481] CNS penetration differs substantially among current ARVs.[462,482] Of the available agents, ZDV has the best penetration into the CSF, followed by stavudine (d4T) and high-dose abacavir (ABC).[475] In one report, a 74% reduction in the risk of death was noted with high CNS-penetrating ART regimens compared with low CNS-penetrating regimens.[462]

Children infected with HIV display a range of neuropsychological problems, including learning and attention disorders, emotional and behavioral problems, depression, autistic behavior, and social withdrawal.[479,483,484] One study examined the effects of perinatal HIV infection, in combination with other health and social factors, on cognitive development. The investigators found that an early AIDS-defining illness increased the risk of chronic static encephalopathy during the preschool and early school-age years.[485]

INTERSTITIAL LUNG DISEASE

Lymphocytic interstitial pneumonitis, or pulmonary lymphoid hyperplasia (PLH), is seen almost exclusively in the pediatric patient with HIV infection and is still included into the CDC definition of AIDS-defining diseases for children younger than 13 years (see Table 22-2). The incidence of LIP is difficult to assess but may affect 50% of HIV-infected children.[486] The illness is often characterized by an insidious onset with cough and tachypnea, but fever is absent; other findings may include generalized lymphadenopathy, hepatomegaly, splenomegaly, salivary gland enlargement, and digital clubbing. Clinically, there is a wide spectrum in the severity of this disease; a child may be asymptomatic with only radiologic changes or can become severely compromised with exercise intolerance or with oxygen dependency and the need for high-dose corticosteroid therapy. Children with LIP are at higher risk to develop frequent bacterial and viral infections.[487]

A diffuse, interstitial, often reticulonodular infiltrative process is typically observed on radiologic examination and is sometimes associated with hilar or mediastinal lymphadenopathy, often confused with miliary TB (Fig. 22-2).[486,488] On lung biopsy, peribronchiolar lymphoid aggregates, or a diffuse lymphoid infiltration of the alveolar septa and peribronchiolar areas is seen.[489] Recent reports have suggested

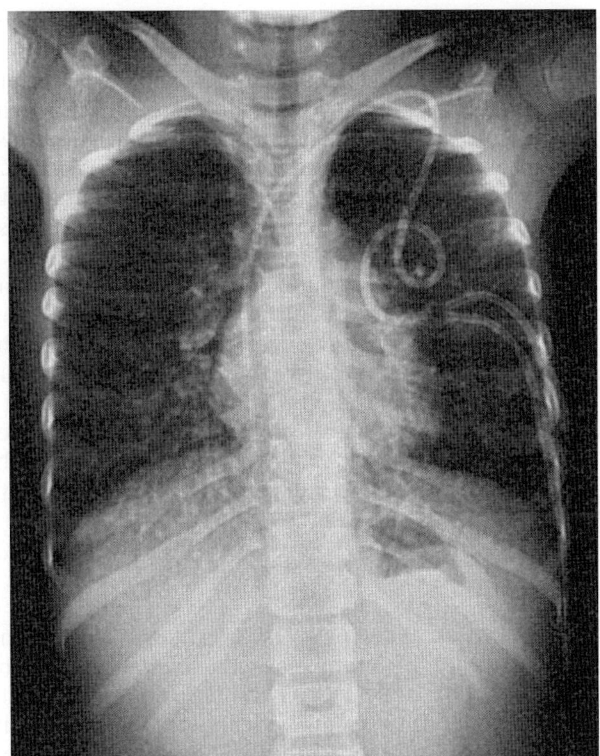

Figure 22-2 Chest radiograph of an 8-year-old girl with severe lymphocytic interstitial pneumonitis who is oxygen and steroid dependent.

a possible role of Epstein-Barr virus (EBV) in the pathogenesis of LIP/PLH.[490] Treatment of LIP is indicated only in a symptomatic child with hypoxia and consists of oral therapy with corticosteroids to suppress the lymphocytic proliferation.[491] Receipt of ART can result in clinical improvement and complete resolution of LIP.[492] LIP has been associated in some studies with a better prognosis than other HIV-related manifestations, such as encephalopathy or PCP, with a median survival of 72 months after diagnosis, compared with 1 month for encephalopathy and 11 months for PCP.[401]

CARDIOVASCULAR COMPLICATIONS

Cardiovascular complications typically occur in the advanced stage of HIV disease.[493,494] During the pre-ART era, chronic cardiovascular disease resulted in mortality in 25% of HIV-infected children younger than 10 years; 28% developed serious cardiac events after AIDS-defining illness.[494,495] In a recent review, 2- to 5-year incidence of symptomatic heart failure varied from 4% to 28% in HIV patients.[493] Cardiac abnormalities complicating the course of HIV disease may include progressive left ventricular (LV) diastolic dysfunction, pericardial effusion, lymphocytic interstitial myocarditis, dilated cardiomyopathy, infective endocarditis, premature myocardial infarction or stroke, and rarely malignancy.[493,496] Risk factors for mortality include abnormalities in LV structure and function.[497] Patients with cardiovascular abnormalities may be asymptomatic.[493] Echocardiographic abnormalities detected in patients receiving cART therapy were LV systolic dysfunction (18%), LV hypertrophy (6.5%), and left atrial dilation (40%). Receipt of long-term cART appears to be cardioprotective for HIV-infected children and adolescents.[498]

The pathogenesis of cardiovascular disease in HIV-infected patients is not well elucidated; endomyocardial biopsy specimens from patients with myocarditis during the pre-ART era have revealed EBV, cytomegalovirus, adenovirus, and HIV in myocytes, suggesting a possible etiologic role.[493] Microscopically, hypertrophy of the myocardium with only rare foci of inflammatory lymphocytic infiltrates is usually present.[494,499] Myocyte injury may occur as a result of proteolytic enzymes or high levels of TNF-α, inducible nitric oxide synthase, and IL-6 from infected myocardial interstitial cells.[493,494,499,500] Metabolic complications, including lipodystrophy, insulin resistance, lactic acidosis, bone loss, are well-described adverse effects of ARVs; dyslipidemia and accelerated atherosclerosis are a major concern with long-term use of protease inhibitors.[452,493,499]

GASTROINTESTINAL DISEASE

Dysfunction of the digestive tract is a frequent problem in untreated infants and young children with AIDS, characterized by persistent diarrhea, malabsorption, and malnutrition or growth failure.[501] Progressive weight loss, anorexia, and sometimes pathogen-negative diarrhea characterize the wasting syndrome often seen in association with HIV disease.[502] Wasting can result from decreased oral intake (resulting from primary cachexia, OIs of upper GI tract, or medication adverse effects), malabsorption, or metabolic imbalance caused by a proinflammatory condition with chronic HIV infection.[501] In an Italian study of 200 HIV-infected children, Galli and colleagues[503] observed a higher incidence of hepatitis and diarrhea, with onset during the first year of life (occurring in 20%-50% of cases) than at any later time. Commonly encountered pathogens that may cause severe diarrhea are *Cryptosporidium, M. avium-intracellulare* complex, *Microsporidium, Salmonella,* and *Shigella.*[504] Wasting is an independent risk factor for death among HIV-infected infants who present with severe acute malnutrition in sub-Saharan Africa.[505]

Liver enlargement and moderate rise in hepatic enzymes are common findings in HIV-infected children but usually not associated with clinical manifestations. Hepatitis can result from an infection, including cytomegalovirus, EBV, the hepatitis viruses, HIV-1, *M. avium-intracellulare* complex, fungi or protozoans, and can evolve into a chronic hepatitis or cholangitis.[408,506] Side effects of ARVs (e.g., NVP), antimicrobial agents (e.g., sulfonamides), and malignancy can also cause hepatitis.[408] In HIV-infected adults, coinfection with hepatitis B virus (HBV) or hepatitis C virus (HCV) can lead to progression of liver disease and hepatic fibrosis and cirrhosis, but data on the prevalence, natural history, and impact of HIV/HBV or HIV/HCV coinfection in vertically infected children is limited, warranting further research.[408,507-510]

Candida albicans and the herpes viruses are often the cause of infections of the oral cavity and of esophagitis. Esophagitis in the HIV-infected child does not manifest with typical symptoms or dysphagia but may be the cause of poor appetite and weight loss. Pancreatitis is a rare complication of HIV infection in children and may occur as a result of OIs, such as CMV, or as a side effect of ARVs.[511,512]

NEPHROPATHY

Renal disease in children with perinatal HIV infection can range from glomerular diseases to acute renal injury, urinary tract infections, electrolyte imbalances, and drug-induced nephrotoxicity.[513] The spectrum of glomerular disease includes immune-mediated chronic kidney diseases, HIV immune complex kidney disease (HIVICK), HIV-associated nephropathy (HIVAN), thrombotic microangiopathies, disorders of proximal tubular function, and acute kidney injury.[514] The histopathologic finding of HIVAN in children consists of classic focal segmental glomerulosclerosis (FSGS) with or without mesangial hyperplasia in association with microcystic tubular dilatation and interstitial inflammation.[514,515] Mesangial proliferative lesions secondary to immune complex deposits have been reported in some children with HIVAN.[516] The advent of cART has dramatically decreased the incidence of HIVAN, but the impact on the outcome of other types of renal disease has not been impressive.[513]

HEMATOLOGIC PROBLEMS

Hematologic manifestations are common and well described in HIV-infected children.[517-520] Anemia is the most common manifestation and can occur because of chronic disease, adverse effects of ARVs (e.g., ZDV), nutritional causes (e.g., iron deficiency anemia), hemoglobinopathies, red cell enzyme defects, or infections (e.g., chronic parvovirus B19, cytomegalovirus, disseminated MAC infection).[408,517-520] Therapy with recombinant erythropoietin can be helpful in cases of ZDV-associated macrocytic anemia when use of alternative ARVs is not an option.[521] The use of high-dose intravenous immune globulin (IVIG) may be beneficial in some patients with persistent parvovirus B19 infection.[522] Leukopenia (white blood cell count < 3000 cells/mm^3), and neutropenia (absolute neutrophil count < 1500 cells/mm^3) has been noted in 26% to 38% and 43% of untreated pediatric patients, respectively.[519] Causes of neutropenia include HIV infection, infection with opportunistic pathogens, such as *M. avium-intracellulare* complex or cytomegalovirus, or medication side effects (e.g., ZDV, TMP-SMX, ganciclovir). Therapy with granulocyte colony-stimulating factor can result in resolution of neutropenia and prevention of infections.[523]

Thrombocytopenia (<150000 cells/mm^3) can occur because of underproduction or shortened platelet survival and has been reported in 19% of the children; thrombocytopenia has also been described in HIV-infected infants as well as children receiving cART.[524-526] Resolution of thrombocytopenia is often noted with cART. Other treatment options include corticosteroids, intravenous gamma globulins, and intravenous anti–D immunoglobulin, but recurrence of thrombocytopenia may be noted after initial improvement. Splenectomy is an option for HIV-infected children with refractory thrombocytopenia.[527] Rituximab use in chronic, recurrent immune-mediated thrombocytopenia has been reported.[528]

SKIN

Mucocutaneous disease is very common in pediatric HIV infection but often manifests in an unusual or atypical or severe form.[529,530] Cutaneous manifestations can be caused by infections and infestations, inflammatory conditions, tumors, and reactions to ARV agents.[529] The most common lesions with an infectious cause are oral thrush and diaper rash (*C. albicans*), chickenpox (acute or chronic), recurrent shingles (VZV), and molluscum contagiosum.[531] Bacterial infections and a highly contagious form of scabies have also been reported with some frequency. Severe seborrheic dermatitis or a nonspecific, intensely pruritic eczematous dermatitis can pose difficult and frustrating clinical problems, necessitating prolonged therapy. Pruritic papular eruption (PPE) is a major cause of morbidity among HIV-infected adults and children living in resource-limited settings.[532-534] PPE is characterized by bilateral, symmetrical, pruritic papules on the extremities, with duration longer than 1 month. The mechanism of disease in PPE is unknown but believed to represent a hypersensitivity reaction to arthropod bites and is associated with immunodeficiency.[534,535] Drug eruptions seem to be more common in HIV-infected patients and can occur with TMP-SMX or ARVs, especially NVP or efavirenz (EFV).[452]

MALIGNANCIES

Malignancies associated with HIV infection in infants and children are rare, but the incidence is higher than in the general population.[517,536] The most common cancer in HIV-infected children is non-Hodgkin lymphoma (Burkitt or immunoblastic type) as a systemic disease or as a primary CNS tumor.[517,537] Kaposi sarcoma (KS) has been described in a few children, including a 6-day-old infant, but is relatively uncommon in the United States.[537-540] Reports from sub-Saharan Africa indicate that KS occurs commonly in HIV-infected children, where the prevalence of human herpesvirus 8 infection is high.[541] In young children, HIV-associated KS is characterized by lymph node involvement, and mortality is high among those with severe immunosuppression.[542] An association with EBV and AIDS-associated non-Hodgkin lymphoma, leiomyomas and leiomyosarcomas, and soft tissue tumors has been reported.[543,544]

IMMUNE CONSTITUTION INFLAMMATORY SYNDROME

An excessive inflammatory response referred to as immune reconstitution inflammatory syndrome (IRIS), resulting in a paradoxic clinical deterioration, may be experienced by HIV-infected infants and children with severe immune deficiency soon after starting ART.[545] Reports of IRIS are limited in children. In one report from South Africa, 21% of children developed IRIS at a median of 16 days (range, 7-115 days) post-HAART initiation.[545] IRIS has been observed after various OIs, with pathogens such as mycobacteria, including bacillus Calmette-Guérin, *M. tuberculosis*, cryptococci, herpes viruses, and progressive multifocal encephalopathy.[545-547] Early ART may reduce the risk of occurrence of IRIS.[548]

Prognosis

Infants with perinatally acquired HIV infection have widely variable clinical courses and durations of survival.[†] Studies from developed countries and sub-Saharan Africa indicate

[†]References 26, 27, 52, 53, 388, 401, 549.

that HIV disease often progresses more rapidly in infants than in adults.[52,401] Without ART, the risk of mortality in HIV-infected children residing in the United States and Europe is 10% to 20%.[298] In contrast, data from Africa showed that about a third of children with HIV infection die by their first birthday and more than half by the age of 2 years.[52]

Natural history studies of perinatal HIV infection were performed before the routine use of cART.[401,549] Early reports suggest a bimodal disease expression, with 15% to 20% of untreated HIV infected infants rapidly progressing to AIDS or death during the first year of life ("rapid progressors"), whereas others exhibiting late onset of symptoms with long-term survival ("slow progressors") had a better prognosis, some surviving into young adulthood.[342-344,401,549,550] In a study from North America enrolling 128 HIV-infected children, disease progression to clinical classes A, B, and C occurred at a median age of 5, 11, and 48 months, respectively.[551] In another study, the overall median survival time for children with perinatal HIV infection was 30 months, but onset of AIDS-defining illness in infancy resulted in a median survival time of approximately 7 months.[401] In a European study of 392 HIV-infected children, Blanche and colleagues[388] found that 20% of children developed an AIDS-defining illness (class C disease) or died within the first year of life, followed by disease progression in 4.7% per year, reaching a cumulative incidence of 26% mortality by 6 years of age.

Certain clinical and laboratory findings may predict disease progression in perinatally-acquired HIV-infected children who have not received cART. Factors associated with poor prognosis for untreated vertically infected infants include a high virus load (>100,000 copies/mL), severe immunosuppression, onset of hepatosplenomegaly and lymphadenopathy (<3 months of life), and occurrence of AIDS-defining conditions during infancy, such as PCP pneumonia, HIV encephalopathy, or severe wasting.[401,465,549,551] In contrast, slow loss of CD4 count, late onset of clinical symptoms, and occurrence of LIP are associated with improved survival.[552]

Infants with intrauterine or intrapartum acquisition of infection have the fastest disease progression.[52,553] Children born to mothers with advanced disease, low CD4 counts and high viral load tend to progress more rapidly to category C disease or death, emphasizing the importance of diagnosis and adequate treatment of HIV-infected pregnant women.[554] Children with HIV infection acquired through a transfusion during the neonatal period tend to have a prolonged asymptomatic period.[555]

With the introduction of cART in the late 1990s, the natural history of HIV infection in children has changed significantly; HIV has evolved into a chronic illness, and perinatally infected children treated with long-term cART are maturing into adolescents and adults worldwide.[10,25,26,290]

In resource-rich countries, increasing use of cART between 1994 and 2006 has resulted in dramatic decreases (81%-93%) in morbidity and mortality rates in HIV-infected children.[26,27,556] In the United States, mortality in HIV-infected children decreased from 7.2 per 100 person-years in 1993 to 0.8 per 100 person-years in 2006, but the mortality rate is 30 times higher compared with other children, even in the cART era.[26] Between 1994 and 2006, hospitalization rates and HIV-related morbidity also decreased significantly.[556,557]

With early infant HIV diagnosis and linkage to care and treatment programs, the frequency of historically reported AIDS-defining illness and OIs have dramatically decreased among HIV-infected children in resource-rich countries.[400] Although deaths related to OIs have decreased significantly, mortality can result from non–AIDS-defining infections and multiorgan failure.[26] Other challenges for physicians are related to provision of lifelong care to HIV-infected children, addressing issues related to ART compliance and toxicity, resistance and treatment failure, transition through adolescence and adult care, and quality of life.[10,25]

Treatment

Treatment of pediatric HIV infection with cART is associated with reduction in mortality, OIs, HIV encephalopathy and other complications, improvement in growth and neurodevelopment, improvement in virologic and immunologic parameters, and better quality of life.[557-561] HAART has evolved from simple nucleoside reverse-transcriptase inhibitor (NRTI) regimens of the 1980s and early 1990s to current complex regimens of NRTIs in combination with protease inhibitors (PIs) or nonnucleoside reverse-transcriptase inhibitors (NNRTIs), or both.[290,562-564] cART with three or more ARVs is currently recommended for the treatment of HIV infection in infants and children.[375] The goal of ART is maximally suppressing HIV replication in the blood, preferably to undetectable levels; immune reconstitution; restoring and preserving immune function; minimizing ARV-related side effects; and preventing emergence of drug-resistant viral mutations.[375]

ANTIRETROVIRAL DRUGS

As of 2013, 24 ARVs were approved for use in the United States in HIV-infected adolescents and adults; of those, 19 have approved pediatric treatment indication, and 16 are available as a pediatric formulation or capsule or tablet.[565] Therapeutic drugs fall into five major classes based on mechanism of action: NRTIs, NNRTIs, protease inhibitors (PIs), entry inhibitors (fusion inhibitor and CCR5 antagonist), and integrase inhibitors.[375,562,564] More detailed and updated information about ARV agents can be obtained at the United States federal AIDS information website (http://aidsinfo.nih.gov/guidelines).

The most commonly used ARVs in newborns and infants— the NRTIs ZDV, lamivudine (3TC), emtricitabine (FTC), and ddI; the NNRTI NVP; and the PIs, lopinavir-ritonavir (LPV/r)—are briefly reviewed in Table 22-4. All are available in a liquid formulation. Neonates and young infants have immature liver metabolism and delayed renal clearance of drugs, and these factors can result in varying ARV dose requirements between infants and older children and incorrect drug dosing.[566-569] Subtherapeutic drug concentrations resulting from underdosing or poor adherence can result in emergence of ARV drug resistance, especially in vertically infected infants who tend to have high viral load. The most pediatric dosing experience with NRTIs is limited to very few ARV drugs, including ZDV, 3TC, ddI, d4T, NVP, and LPV/r. In preterm infants, pharmacokinetic and dosing data are available only for ZDV.[569]

Table 22-4 Antiretroviral Drugs and Recommended Dosages in Neonates and Infants Younger Than 3 Months

Drug	Preparations	Dosage	Adverse Effects
NUCLEOSIDE REVERSE-TRANSCRIPTASE INHIBITORS			
Zidovudine (ZDV)	Syrup: 10 mg/mL	Neonatal/infant dose (age <6 wk) <30 weeks' gestation: Oral ZDV 2 mg/kg (or 1.5 mg/kg IV), 2× daily for the first 4 wk of age, followed by 3 mg/kg PO (or 2.3 mg/kg IV), 2× daily after age 4 wk >30 to <35 weeks' gestation: Oral ZDV 2 mg/kg (or 1.5 mg/kg IV), 2× daily for the first 2 wk of age, followed by 3 mg/kg PO (or 2.3 mg/kg IV), 2× daily after age >15 days ≥35 weeks' gestation: Oral ZDV 4 mg/kg (or 3 mg/kg IV), 2× daily *Pediatric dose (6 wk-<18 yr):* 180-240 mg/m^2 of BSA PO q12hr *or* 160 mg/m^2 PO q8hr; twice-daily dosing preferred in clinical practice. *Body weight–based dosing:* 12 mg/kg PO q12hr (4 to <9 kg); 9 mg/kg PO q12hr (9 to <30 kg)	Macrocytic anemia, neutropenia, nausea, vomiting, headache, hepatotoxicity, myopathy, nail pigmentation, hyperlipidemia, insulin resistance/diabetes mellitus, lipoatrophy, lactic acidosis, hepatomegaly with steatosis
Lamivudine (3TC)	Pediatric oral solution: 10 mg/mL	*Neonatal/infant dose (age < 4 wk):* 2 mg/kg of body weight PO q12hr *Pediatric dose (age ≥ 4 wk):* 4 mg/kg of body weight PO q12hr	Headache, fatigue, reduced appetite, nausea, diarrhea, rash, pancreatitis, peripheral neuropathy, anemia, neutropenia, lactic acidosis, hepatomegaly with steatosis
Didanosine (ddI)	Pediatric powder for oral solution: 10 mg/mL (reconstituted)	*Premature:* No data *Neonatal/infant dose (age 2 wk-<3 mo):* 50 mg/m^2 of BSA q12hr *Infant dose (≥3-8 mo of age):* 100 mg/m^2 of BSA PO q12hr *Pediatric dose (age > 8 mo):* 120 mg/m^2 (range, 90-150 mg/m^2) of BSA PO q12hr	Peripheral neuropathy, electrolyte abnormalities, diarrhea, abdominal pain, nausea, vomiting, lactic acidosis, hepatomegaly with steatosis (risk increased with combination of d4T with ddI), pancreatitis, retinitis, insulin resistance/diabetes mellitus
Stavudine (d4T)	Solution: 1 mg/mL	*Neonatal/infant dose (age birth-13 days):* 0.5 mg/kg of body weight PO q12hr *Pediatric dose (age≥14 days up to weight of 30 kg):* 1 mg/kg of body weight PO q12hr	Headache, gastrointestinal upsets, rash, lipoatrophy peripheral neuropathy, pancreatitis, mitochondrial toxicity, lactic acidosis, hepatomegaly with steatosis (combination of d4T with ddI may result in enhanced toxicity), increased liver enzymes, insulin resistance/diabetes mellitus, ascending neuromuscular weakness (unusual)
Abacavir (ABC)	Solution: 20 mg/mL	*Neonatal/infant dose (age <3 mo):* Not approved for infants<3 mo of age *Pediatric dose (age ≥ 3 mo):* 8 mg/kg PO twice daily	*Hypersensitivity reaction (HSR) that may be fatal; HSR symptoms may include fever; rash; nausea; vomiting; malaise or fatigue; loss of appetite; respiratory symptoms (e.g. sore throat, cough, dyspnea)
NONNUCLEOSIDE REVERSE-TRANSCRIPTASE INHIBITORS			
Nevirapine (NVP)	Suspension: 10 mg/mL	*Neonatal/infant dose (age ≤14 days):* Treatment dose not defined in this age group *Pediatric dose (age >15 days to < 8 yr):* 200 mg/m^2 of BSA/dose twice daily (Start treatment with once daily for the first 14 days. If no rash or adverse effects, give the drug twice daily.)	Skin rash, including Stevens-Johnson syndrome and toxic epidermal necrolysis, fever, headache, nausea, symptomatic hepatitis, including fatal hepatic necrosis, severe systemic hypersensitivity reactions
PROTEASE INHIBITORS			
Lopinavir-ritonavir (LPV/r)	Pediatric oral solution: 80 mg/20 mg LPV/r/mL)	*Neonatal/infant dose (age <14 days):* No safety/dosing data available; not recommended for use *Neonatal/infant dose (age 14 days-12 mo):* 300 mg/75 mg LPV/r per m^2 of BSA *or* 16 mg/4 mg LPV/r per kg body weight twice daily. Because dosage data is not available for LPV/r administered with NVP in infants ≤6 mo of age, LPV/r should not be administered in combination with NVP in these infants.	Diarrhea, nausea, vomiting, headache, skin rash in patients receiving other antiretroviral agents, lipid abnormalities, fat redistribution, new-onset diabetes mellitus, hyperglycemia, ketoacidosis, hemolytic anemia, pancreatitis, and life-threatening hepatitis Risk of cardiac toxicity, adrenal dysfunction and overdose, especially in premature infants

Data from Panel on Antiretroviral Therapy and Medical Management of HIV-Infected Children: Guidelines for the use of antiretroviral agents in pediatric HIV infection. Available at http://aidsinfonihgov/Content Files/Pediatric Guidelinespdf. Accessed November 22, 2013.

BSA, Body surface area; *GA,* gestational age; *IV,* intravenous.

*Before starting ABC, patients must be tested for the HLA-B*5701 allele to screen for risk of hypersensitivity; patients with the HLA-B*5701 allele should not receive ABC. Patients with no prior HLA-B*5701 testing who are tolerating ABC do not need to be tested.

Dual NRTI combinations are the backbone of cART in children. Added to this dual NRTI backbone is an NNRTI or a PI. The combinations of NRTIs with the most data available include ZDV and 3TC, ZDV and ddI, and d4T and 3TC. The ZDV-3TC combination is the most widely used dual NRTI because of its extensive safety data in children.[375] Bone marrow suppression (macrocytic anemia, neutropenia) may be noted with ZDV use. Mitochondrial toxicity and associated effects (e.g., peripheral neuropathy, myopathy, pancreatitis, lactic acidosis, cardiomyopathy) are major adverse effects of NRTIs in adults but have been reported in children.[570] Thus NRTIs such as ddI and d4T are generally not recommended as first-line drugs in infants and children.[564] The combination of d4T and ZDV is not recommended because of virologic antagonism; in addition, 3TC plus FTC is not recommended because of similar structure and associated resistance with a single-gene mutation (M184V), and d4T plus ddI is not recommended because of significant toxic effects.[375]

The acceptable NNRTI for infant use is NVP, whereas EFV is approved only for children younger than 3 years. Compared with PIs, NNRTIs are associated with fewer adverse effects.[375] Rarely, NVP is associated with serious hepatic toxicity or rash that can progress to Stevens-Johnson syndrome, but these adverse effects are more common in adults than in children.[375,564] The one available NRTI, tenofovir (TDF), is not approved for use in neonates and children younger than 2 years.[375] The most commonly used PI in infants is LPV/r. Most PIs are coformulated with low-dose ritonavir (pharmacokinetic "booster"), which inhibits cytochrome P450 3A4 (CYP3A4) isoenzyme, resulting in increased concentrations of the second, boosted PI. Based on pharmacokinetic studies of LPV/r in neonates, a higher dose (300 mg/m^2/dose) is recommended in younger infants compared with older children (230 mg/m^2/dose), with the need for frequent dose adjustments during the first year of life.[567] Serious cardiac (atrioventricular block, bradycardia, cardiomyopathy), metabolic (lactic acidosis) and central CNS (depression) adverse effects have been reported in neonates receiving LPV/r.[562,571] Therefore LPV/r is U.S. Food and Drug Administration (FDA) approved for use in term neonates after a postmenstrual age of 42 weeks and a postnatal age older than 14 days.[375] Although fosamprenavir boosted with low-dose ritonavir is FDA approved for use in infants older than 4 weeks and older children, the U.S. expert panel limits the use of this agent only in infants older than 6 months.[375] ARVs can cause drug interactions, especially NVP and PIs.[375] Metabolic complications (dyslipidemia, fat maldistribution, insulin resistance) are a major concern with long-term ART.[572]

Several promising second-generation agents as well as new classes of ARVs have been FDA approved for adult use and are currently being evaluated in pediatric clinical trials. These agents include etravirine (newer NNRTI), duranavir (PI), maraviroc (CCR5 antagonist), and raltegravir (integrase inhibitor). However, pharmacokinetic and safety data are limited in children, and none of these agents have been approved for use in neonates and infants.[375] More detailed and updated information about ARV agents can be obtained at the U.S. federal AIDS information website (http://aidsinfo.nih.gov/guidelines).[375]

Pediatricians and neonatologists should consult a pediatric infectious disease specialist for evaluation and treatment of HIV-infected infants. Close collaboration between the child's primary health care provider and a pediatric HIV specialist is strongly recommended. Whenever possible, children should be enrolled in clinical trials; access and information can be obtained by calling 1-800-TRIALS-A (AIDS Clinical Trials Group [ACTG]) or 301-402-0696 (HIV and AIDS Malignancy Branch, National Cancer Institute).

TIMING OF cART INITIATION

The optimal timing of cART initiation in HIV-infected children has been a subject of debate and controversy.[563] In the past several years, many randomized clinical trials (RCTs) have investigated ART strategies in children younger than 2 years.[573-578] Compared with older children and adults, treatment of HIV infection in young infants is a major challenge because laboratory markers (e.g., CD4 cell count) cannot reliably predict disease progression in infants, and choice of ARVs is limited.[579,580] The consideration of early treatment for asymptomatic infants is based on the rationale that untreated infants are at highest risk of rapid disease progression to AIDS or death, even when immune degradation and virus replication are moderately well contained.[550,551,573,580-582]

Observational studies from the United States and Europe indicated that early initiation of cART in HIV-infected infants may enhance survival.[583-590] In 2007, a RCT conducted in South Africa (Children with HIV Early Antiretroviral Therapy [CHER] study) addressed the critical question of when to begin cART in asymptomatic HIV-1–infected infants who are diagnosed early in life.[573] CHER found that initiation of cART before 12 weeks of age in asymptomatic infants with normal immune function resulted in 76% reduction in mortality (95% CI, 49% to 89%; $P < .001$) and 75% reduction in HIV disease progression (95% CI, 59% to 85%; $P < .001$), compared with infants starting cART until they met clinical or CD4 criteria (CD4 percentages < 25%) for initiation of ART.[573] In 2013, final results from the South African CHER study at 4 years follow-up showed better clinical and immunologic outcomes in children receiving early intensive ART in infancy, followed by treatment interruption compared with children in the deferred ART arm; treatment interruption was safe with no evidence of excess disease progression but warrants close monitoring.[591] Early cART can result in complete cessation of viral replication and the preservation of normal immune function in some infants.[584,592] A CHER neurologic substudy showed better neurodevelopmental outcomes reported among children in the early ART group compared with the delayed treatment group at 11 months of age, although the differences were relatively small.[593]

Although the benefit of immediate cART in HIV-infected infants younger than 12 months is well established, the optimum time to initiate ART in asymptomatic children older than 1 year is unclear, and warrants a careful consideration of risks and benefits because ART may need to be continued lifelong.[594,595] Primary concerns include long-term adverse effects to ARVs and treatment failure, especially in LMIC, where access to pediatric ART may be limited.[594] In a recently conducted randomized, open-label trial in Cambodia and Thailand (PREDICT), no significant benefit of early treatment was observed in children aged 1 to 12 years with CD4 counts of 15% to 24% randomized to immediate versus deferred ART.[596] In addition, a substudy of the PREDICT trial revealed no differences in neurodevelopmental outcomes in HIV-infected children older than 1 year randomized to early versus deferred ART.[597] However, observational studies suggest that delayed ART in children until older than 7 years or at low CD4 counts may not achieve immune reconstitution.[594,598]

TREATMENT RECOMMENDATIONS

Based on the CHER study results, reporting a fourfold reduction of mortality and disease progression among infected infants receiving early treatment with cART compared with delayed treatment, the U.S. Panel on Antiretroviral Therapy and Medical Management of HIV-Infected Children recommends immediate initiation of ART for all HIV-infected infants younger than 12 months, regardless of clinical status, CD4+ percentage, or HIV RNA level findings.[375,573] The CHER study findings changed policy in all settings.[573] In 2008, the Paediatric European Network for Treatment of AIDS (PENTA) and the WHO guidelines were revised to recommend immediate ART for all infants younger than 12 months.[599,600] In 2010, the WHO increased the age for immediate initiation of ART to all children younger than 2 years, irrespective of their clinical or immunologic status, based on programmatic considerations and an increased risk of disease progression and mortality in infants 1 to 2 years of age.[581,582,601]

In 2013, the WHO consolidated guidelines, recommending immediate initiation of lifelong cART in all children younger than 5 years, regardless of their clinical or immune status, with the goal to simplify criteria for ART initiation, improve treatment access, and reduce mortality in LMIC.[39] For programmatic considerations and the fact that disease progression in older children is similar to that of young adults, the 2013 WHO guidelines recommended initiation of cART at a CD4 count of less than or equal to 500 for children aged 5 years and older, aligning with adult treatment initiation criteria.[39] In contrast, U.S. and European guidelines recommend initiation of cART in older HIV-infected children based on clinical, immunologic, and virologic criteria.[375,599] ART is recommended for all symptomatic children (with AIDS or CDC clinical category C or most clinical category B conditions).[375]

CHOICE OF INITIAL ANTIRETROVIRAL REGIMEN

If perinatal HIV infection is confirmed, the infant should be promptly referred to a pediatric HIV specialist for care and treatment.[375,602] Monotherapy should never be offered to HIV-infected children. The only exception is the use of ZDV monotherapy in infants with indeterminate HIV status during the first 6 weeks of life, as part of the prophylaxis regimen to prevent perinatal transmission. As soon as an infant is proved to be infected while on ZDV prophylaxis, therapy should be changed to a standard triple ARV therapy.[22]

Several factors may influence the choice of initial ART regimen, including age; availability of formulations; pharmacokinetic drug dosing data; potential short- and long-term toxicity; viral resistance; drug interactions; and presence of concomitant illnesses, such as TB, hepatitis B or C, and chronic hepatic or renal disease.[375,562,564] A triple-drug cART, consisting of two NRTIs plus a third agent from a different class (either a ritonavir-boosted PI or a NNRTI) as the initial regimen is recommended by U.S., European, and WHO pediatric ART guidelines.[375,599,601] Suppression of virus to undetectable levels, long-term preservation of immune function, and minimal ARV-related toxicity are the desired goals.[375]

The choice of NNRTI- versus PI-based cART regimen for initial therapy is complicated in LMIC, where infants often have prior exposure to peripartum single-dose nevirapine (sdNVP) prophylaxis for PMTCT.[579] In this setting, treatment failure resulting from NVP resistance is a major concern.[603-605] Data from the P1060 RCT conducted in seven African countries offer some insights for choice of NNRTI- versus PI-based regimen for initial ART. The study results demonstrated that a LPV/r-based cART regimen is superior to a NVP-based regimen among vertically infected infants and children aged 2 to 35 months, regardless of prior perinatal NVP exposure.[576,577] However, data from a European/U.S. trial (PENPACT 1) showed no significant difference in virologic outcome between PI- and NNRTI-based ART in children without perinatal NVP exposure.[606]

In the United States, the preferred ART regimen for children older than 14 days to younger than 3 years includes two NRTIs plus LPV/r.[375] The genetic barrier for resistance for LPV/r is high, whereas a single gene mutation can confer high-level resistance to NVP. However, liquid LPV/r is not palatable and can result in high triglyceride concentrations in young children.[607] In some studies (NEVEREST, P1060), infants receiving a NVP-based regimen exhibited better immune responses and growth compared with infants receiving a LPV/r-based regimen.[574,576,577] Thus a combination of two NRTIs plus liquid NVP is listed in the U.S. guidelines as an acceptable alternative for infants without prior peripartum exposure to NVP and who are intolerant to LPV/r.[375]

The preferred dual-NRTI combination for initial therapy in infants younger than 3 months is ZDV-3TC or ZDV-FTC, whereas ABC plus 3TC (or FTC) is recommended for children aged 3 months or older across all guidelines.[375,599,601] Given the risk of ABC-associated hypersensitivity reaction, prescreening for HLA-B*5701 must be performed before ABC administration. Alternative dual-NRTI backbone options include ddI plus (3TC or FTC) and, only in special circumstances, a combination of d4T plus (3TC or FTC) may be used.[375]

In the 2013 WHO guidelines, the preferred dual NRTI backbone options for initial therapy in infants and children under age 3 years includes ABC-3TC or ZDV-3TC.[601] LPV/r is recommended as the preferred PI for HIV-infected infants and children younger than 3 years of age, regardless of prior exposure to NNRTI; if LPV/r use is not feasible, treatment with NVP is a recommended NNRTI option.[601]

ARV resistance testing (viral genotyping) is recommended before starting cART in newly diagnosed treatment-naïve infants younger than 12 months, especially if the mother has known or suspected infection with drug-resistant virus.[375] Drug-resistant virus may be transmitted from mother to infant during peripartum or breastfeeding; resistance can also emerge in infants exposed to ARV prophylaxis for PMTCT.[375] A change in ART regimen should be considered if there is evidence of treatment failure (virologic, immunologic, or clinical), ART side effects, or a new superior regimen becomes available.[375]

CLINICAL AND LABORATORY MONITORING

HIV-infected infants started on cART should be monitored closely for evaluation of adherence, efficacy and medication side effects. Baseline laboratory assessments must be performed before starting ART, including a complete blood count (CBC), comprehensive metabolic panel (CMP), viral load, and CD4 T-lymphocyte count/percentage. The infant must be assessed within 1 to 2 weeks of starting therapy to ensure appropriate administration of ARV, discuss clinical concerns, and support adherence.

After the initial treatment initiation visit, the next follow-up is recommended at 4 to 8 weeks, with subsequent follow-ups every 3 to 4 months to measure effectiveness of ART regimen (as measured by viral load, CD4 count/percentage), assess potential medication adverse events (as measured by CBC and CMP), and adherence. In infected infants and children with suppressed immune function, cART can result in recovery of CD4 lymphocyte count of at least 50 cells/mm^3 or an increase of at least 5% at the end of 12 months of treatment.[375] HIV-infected mothers must be linked to care and treatment, psychosocial support, and counseling regarding family planning.

CHALLENGES

Treatment of infected infants with cART is complex, and response to cART in infants may be slower compared with older children and adults.[608,609] Viral suppression rates ranging from 70% to 80% have been reported among infants who received cART before 12 months of age.[610,611] In another study of perinatally infected children receiving early ART, 98% had normal immune function, and 78% achieved viral suppression at the end of 5-year follow-up.[587] Infants are less likely to achieve viral suppression because of very high viral loads, inadequate ARV drug concentrations, and poor adherence because of demanding regimens or unpleasant tasting suspensions (e.g., ritonavir) or adverse effects.[579]

Other challenges include limited availability of pediatric ARV formulations, need for frequent dose adjustments in infancy, need for refrigeration and cold chain supply (e.g., LPV), drugs with short shelf life (e.g., ddI), immature drug metabolism, and lack of age-specific pharmacokinetic data to guide pediatric dosing.[375,579] Long-term toxicity and emergence of drug resistance, resulting in treatment failures, are other serious concerns.[375,612-614]

Resistance to NNRTI is common in HIV-infected infants who are exposed to NVP prophylaxis during antepartum/intrapartum period or during breastfeeding.[615,616] Extended NVP prophylaxis during breastfeeding also confers a high rate of NVP resistance in infants who acquire infection after 6 weeks of age.[617] Despite prior exposure to NNRTI, NVP is still included in first regimens for treatment of maternal and infant HIV infection in LMIC because of the low cost, availability in generic formulation/fixed-dose combinations (FDCs), ease of administration, and poor access to resistance testing.[579] Access to second-line ARVs and development of appropriate formulations of PIs in FDCs and increasing access to ART for HIV-infected children is a major priority in LMIC.[579]

Despite the scale-up of pediatric HIV care and treatment services in LMIC in recent years, only 23% of children in need of ART were receiving treatment in 2010.[31] Barriers to treatment in LMIC include delay in identification of infected infants because of lack of diagnostic testing for early infant diagnosis of HIV infection; poor health systems and linkages, resulting in high drop-out rates in the PMTCT cascade; and lack of prioritization and advocacy for pediatric treatment.[31,579]

Studies indicate that good clinical, immunologic, and virologic outcomes can be achieved using cART in HIV-infected children living in sub-Saharan Africa and other LMIC, and outcomes are comparable to infected children living in high-income countries.[618,619] Other important issues related to ART that warrant investigation include long-term effects on growth and development; neurocognitive function; bone growth; metabolic abnormalities; and the relationship between pediatric ART and interventions for malaria, tuberculosis, and malnutrition.[620]

PRIMARY CARE

A family-centered approach involving a specialist pediatric HIV multidisciplinary team (including an HIV social worker) in collaboration with a primary care physician is crucial for long-term successful management. Other crucial aspects of HIV management include careful monitoring of growth and development, assessment of organ system involvement, development and psychosocial assessments and intervention.[602]

Immunizations

HIV-infected children are at highest risk for developing vaccine-preventable diseases compared with HIV-uninfected.[408] Therefore the AAP recommends routine immunizations with some modifications for all HIV-exposed infants, whether they are infected or not.[17] Similar to other newborns, children born to HIV-infected mothers should receive hepatitis B vaccinations, but if the mother is positive for the hepatitis B surface antigen, the child should also receive hepatitis B immune globulin within 12 hours after birth. Readers are referred to expert guidelines and the most recent edition of the AAP's *Red Book* for recommendations regarding immunization practices in HIV-infected children.[17,408]

Infants infected with HIV should be vaccinated at the appropriate age with inactivated vaccines (diphtheria, tetanus toxoids, acellular pertussis, *Haemophilus influenzae* type b, hepatitis B, hepatitis A, and pneumococcal conjugate vaccines).[17,621] HIV-infected children who have received the PCV vaccine series should also receive a single dose of 23-valent polysaccharide pneumococcal vaccine at 24 months of age or older, with a minimum interval of 8 weeks since the last PCV.[17]

Live-virus vaccine (oral poliovirus) or live bacterial vaccines (bacillus Calmette-Guérin) should not be given to patients with HIV infection because of the potential risk of disseminated disease from vaccine virus. The exception is measles-mumps-rubella (MMR) vaccine and varicella-zoster immunization, which can be given to asymptomatic HIV-infected children aged 12 months or older who do not have current evidence of severe immunosuppression (defined as CD4 percentages ≥15% for ≥6 months for children younger than 5 years). Two doses of MMR vaccine are recommended: first dose at age 12 through 15 months and second dose at 4 through 6 years.

Individuals with perinatal HIV infection who were vaccinated before establishment of effective cART should be revaccinated with two appropriately spaced doses of MMR vaccine, once effective ART has been established.[622] Children who are eligible must receive two doses of monovalent varicella vaccine at an interval of 3 months.[17] The oral rotavirus vaccine may be administered in HIV-exposed and HIV-infected infants, regardless of CD4 T-cell count, according to age-recommended guidelines.[17,408] Beginning at 6 months of age, all HIV-infected children must receive the inactivated influenza vaccine annually.

In general, immunosuppressed children vaccinated before receiving cART have low levels of protective immunity. Although most children on cART may respond to revaccination after immune reconstitution, waning immunity remains a concern.[623] In areas of high HIV prevalence, children at increased risk for VPD may potentially benefit from revaccination.[623]

Passive immunization of children with HIV infection is recommended in certain circumstances, especially after exposure to measles, varicella, or tetanus.[17,408] In the past, studies have documented the beneficial effects of IVIG in reducing the morbidity associated with serious bacterial infections in some children with HIV infection.[624-626] However, the role of IVIG is very limited in the current era of cART and use of chemoprophylaxis to prevent OIs. The current recommendation is to use prophylactic IVIG (400 mg/kg body weight every 2 to 4 weeks) in HIV-infected children with hypogammaglobulinemia (IgG < 400 mg/dL) or who develop recurrent serious infections (such as bacteremia, meningitis, or pneumonia), despite receipt of vaccines and antibiotic prophylaxis.[408]

Chemoprophylaxis

The CDC has published guidelines for prevention and treatment of OIs in HIV-infected infants and children.[408] Chemoprophylaxis is highly effective in preventing PCP and is recommended for all HIV-infected infants younger than 12 months, regardless of CD4 count or percentage.[448-450] In addition, HIV-exposed infants with indeterminate HIV infection status should receive chemoprophylaxis until they are determined to be HIV-uninfected or presumptively HIV-uninfected.[374,397,451,452] Secondary chemoprophylaxis is recommended for infants and children who have suffered from an episode of PCP.

The recommended prophylactic regimen is TMP-SMX (TMP 2.5 to 5 mg/kg body weight/dose with SMX 12.5 to 25 mg/kg body weight/dose) given orally in two divided doses each day on 3 consecutive days per week.[408] The alternative regimen is TMP-SMX given once daily for 3 days per week or twice daily 7 days per week.[408] If TMP-SMX is not tolerated, alternative regimens are dapsone taken orally or atovaquone or intravenous pentamidine.[408] Breakthrough infections can occur with every regimen, however, and seem to be most frequent with intravenous pentamidine and least common with TMP-SMX.[453,454] Based on adult studies, many experts recommend stopping primary or secondary prophylaxis for PCP in children older than 1 year and receiving cART for more than 6 months and who have evidence of immune reconstitution.[408]

Prophylaxis for MAC infection with clarithromycin or azithromycin orally once weekly should be offered to infants younger than 12 months with $CD4^+$ counts less than 750 cells/μL, children 1 to 2 years of age with $CD4^+$ counts less than 500 cells/μL, children 2 to 6 years of age with $CD4^+$ counts less than 75 μL, and children older than 6 years with $CD4^+$ counts less than 50 cells/μL.[408,627,628] Rifabutin is an alternative agent for MAC prophylaxis if patients are intolerant to macrolide therapy.[408] Primary prophylaxis for prevention of candidiasis is not recommended for HIV-infected infants and children.[408]

Prevention

Major advances have been made in prevention of perinatal transmission of HIV, resulting in near elimination of MTCT in the United States and other resource-rich countries.[18,22,23] Perinatal HIV transmission rates have decreased to less than 2% in the United States and Europe because of widespread implementation of routine antenatal HIV testing ("opt-out" approach), use of ARV prophylaxis and cART, elective cesarean delivery, and avoidance of breastfeeding (Box 22-2).[19,20,629,630] Guidelines and recommendations for use of ARV in pregnant women for maternal health and perinatal HIV prevention are available from the U.S. PHS (http://www.aidsinfo.nih.gov) and other professional societies (AAP and the American College of Obstetricians and Gynecologists).[22]

Box 22-2 Strategies to Prevent Perinatal Human Immunodeficiency Virus (HIV) Transmission

- Primary prevention of HIV infection in women of childbearing age
- Prevention of unintended pregnancies in HIV-infected women
- Prevention of perinatal HIV infection
  - Universal antenatal ("opt-out") HIV testing
  - Combination antiretroviral therapy early in pregnancy
  - Elective cesarean delivery*
  - Provision of neonatal antiretroviral prophylaxis
  - Avoidance of breastfeeding
- Provision of treatment, care, and support to HIV-positive women and their families

*Before labor and before rupture of membranes and if maternal viral load is greater than 1000 copies/mL near the time of delivery.

Efforts to prevent perinatal HIV transmission have been pursued since the initial reports of AIDS in infants in 1983.[5,6] In 1985, the CDC issued guidelines recommending that HIV-infected women in the United States should not breastfeed.[631] Before 1994, MTCT rates were approximately 20% to 25% in the absence of ARV interventions.[72] A landmark study published in 1994 by the Pediatric AIDS Clinical Trials Group (PACTG; 076 protocol) showed that a long course of ZDV prophylaxis given to HIV infected mother starting at 14 to 34 weeks of gestation and intravenously during labor, and to the newborn for 6 weeks, reduced in utero and intrapartum HIV transmission by nearly 70% in a nonbreastfeeding population (Table 22-5).[632]

The success of the PACTG 076 protocol in 1994 has had a major impact on the prevention of perinatal transmission of HIV and resulted in the formulation of CDC prevention guidelines.[22,633,634] Widespread implementation of these recommendations and the introduction of initially dual and then triple ART regimens, including treatment of pregnant women, since the late 1990s has led to a dramatic decrease in the number of newly HIV-infected infants in industrialized countries.[19,20,629,630,633-635] In 1992, approximately 2000 infants in the United States acquired perinatal HIV infection annually, whereas currently fewer than 200 infants acquire HIV infection yearly.[636-638]

PRENATAL HUMAN IMMUNODEFICIENCY VIRUS COUNSELING AND TESTING

Human immunodeficiency virus testing during pregnancy is the gateway to access effective interventions to prevent perinatal HIV transmission and link HIV-positive women to care and treatment.[13] In 1995, the CDC issued guidelines that all pregnant women should be offered HIV testing and recommended ZDV for all pregnant HIV-infected women according to the PACTG 076 regimen.[633,639] In 1998, the Institute of Medicine released a report recommending

Table 22-5 Pediatric AIDS Clinical Trials Group 076 Zidovudine Regimen

Time of Zidovudine Administration	Route	Regimen
Antepartum	Oral	100 mg zidovudine 5× daily, initiated at 14-34 wk of gestation and continued throughout pregnancy
Intrapartum	Intravenous	During labor and delivery, intravenous administration of zidovudine in a 1-hr initial dose of 2 mg/kg, followed by continuous infusion of 1 mg/kg/hr until delivery
Postpartum	Oral	Oral zidovudine to newborn (zidovudine syrup at 2 mg/kg/dose q6hr) for the first 6 wk of life, beginning at 8-12 hr after birth; if infant cannot tolerate oral zidovudine, it can be given intravenously at a dosage of 1.5 mg/kg q6hr

From Centers for Disease Control and Prevention: Public Health Service task force recommendations for the use of antiretroviral drugs in pregnant women infected with HIV-1 for maternal health and for reducing perinatal HIV-1 transmission in the United States, *MMWR Morb Mortal Wkly Rep* 47:1-31, 1998.

universal HIV screening with right of refusal for all pregnant women.[640] In 1999, the U.S. Congress provided target funding for prevention of perinatal HIV infection in states with high prevalence.[13] In 2001, CDC issued revised HIV counseling and testing guidelines for pregnant women recommending strategies to reduce barriers to offering antenatal HIV testing, including routine opt-out HIV screening for all pregnant women, offering rapid HIV testing during labor/delivery period for women with unknown HIV status.[641] In 2003 to 2006, the CDC reported high uptake of screening of pregnant women using the "opt-out" strategy.

In 2006, the CDC expanded the use of the "opt-out" strategy to include routine HIV testing in health care facilities to all patients 13 to 64 years of age and all pregnant women as part of the routine panel of antenatal tests, a second HIV test in the third trimester for women living in areas with high incidence of HIV or women at high risk, and rapid testing for women with unknown status at the time of labor and delivery.[642] In some states, routine HIV testing during pregnancy is mandated by law.[17] Health care providers should provide routine education about HIV infection and testing as part of comprehensive care for all women of reproductive age.

ANTIRETROVIRAL PROPHYLAXIS TO PREVENT MOTHER-TO-CHILD HUMAN IMMUNODEFICIENCY VIRUS TRANSMISSION

Over the past decade, innovative PMTCT clinical trials conducted in both high-income countries and LMIC have yielded important observations (Tables 22-6, 22-7, and 22-8).[13,22,35,643-671] Observational studies have demonstrated that combination ARV regimens during pregnancy are more effective for prevention of perinatal HIV transmission than ZDV alone.[20,22] A number of short-course ARV regimens (ZDV alone, ZDV plus 3TC, sdNVP, sdNVP plus short-course ZDV or ZDV/3TC) have been effective in reducing MTCT.[643-654] Combination ARV regimens administered over a prolonged period are more efficacious in reducing transmission compared with short-course single-drug regimens.[22]

Combination ARVs are very effective in reducing perinatal transmission even among women with advanced disease.[659,665] Longer duration (28 weeks of gestation) of antepartum ARV prophylaxis is more effective than shorter duration (36 weeks of gestation) of ARV prophylaxis, indicating that a significant proportion of intrauterine transmission occurs from 28 through 36 weeks.[648] A prolonged duration of infant postexposure prophylaxis does not substitute for longer duration of maternal ARV prophylaxis.[652]

Some women may not receive any prenatal care and may present in labor without receiving any antepartum ARV prophylaxis. In this setting, several efficacious intrapartum and postpartum regimens may be effective in reducing transmission based on data from international trials.[647,649,650,653] A longer three-part antepartum, intrapartum, and postpartum ARV prophylaxis is more effective in reducing transmission than ARV prophylaxis taken only during antepartum/intrapartum periods or intrapartum/postpartum periods.[647,651,652] Intrapartum preexposure prophylaxis with NNRTIs (ZDV/3TC) alone is not effective in reducing transmission without the addition of infant postexposure prophylaxis.[647] Another trial conducted in South Africa comparing the efficacy of intrapartum/newborn sdNVP versus intrapartum/postpartum ZDV/3TC showed similar efficacy in the two groups.[653]

Several trials conducted in formula-fed and breastfed populations in LMIC have shown that addition of maternal/infant sdNVP to maternal short-course ZDV or ZDV/3TC regimen provided increased efficacy for reducing perinatal HIV transmission compared with short-course maternal regimen alone.[651,654,672] In contrast, an international, blinded, placebo-controlled phase III trial conducted in the United States, Europe, Brazil, and the Bahamas (PACTG 316) found no additional benefit from addition of single-dose intrapartum/newborn NVP among nonbreastfeeding populations in high-income settings when women received combination ARV prophylaxis during pregnancy and elective cesarean section was made available.[655] All neonates received the standard 6-week ZDV course, and the overall risk of perinatal HIV transmission was very low (1.5%).[655] In the PACTG 316 study, NVP resistance developed in 15% of the women who received single-dose intrapartum NVP.[655,673] Thus addition of intrapartum NVP doses is not recommended for HIV-infected women in the United States who have received cART throughout pregnancy.[22]

When the mother has not received any ARV prophylaxis during pregnancy or during the intrapartum period (because of late HIV diagnosis in the mother or infant, often after labor and delivery), observational data from the United States suggest that administration of 6-week course of oral ZDV prophylaxis to the infant (started within 24 hours after birth) was effective in reducing transmission.[674] A study conducted in a breastfeeding population in Malawi showed that the addition of 1 week of ZDV to infant sdNVP had a superior efficacy at 6 to 8 weeks of age, compared with infant sdNVP alone (MTCT rate 7.7% in sdNVP plus ZDV arm vs. 12.1% in sdNVP arm; 36% efficacy).[662]

Table 22-6 Antiretroviral Prophylaxis for Prevention of Mother-to-Child HIV Transmission During Antenatal and Intrapartum Period

NONBREASTFEEDING POPULATIONS				
Trial/Site/Year (Reference)	**Study Details/Infant Feeding Choice**	**Maternal ARV Prophylaxis**	**Infant ARV Prophylaxis**	**Transmission Rate and Efficacy**
LONG-COURSE ZDV PROPHYLAXIS VERSUS PLACEBO				
PACTG 076/ United States, France/1994 (632)	Randomized trial; $n = 477$ pregnant women enrolled; 409 delivered; 415 live births; ZDV (180 infants) vs. placebo (183 infants) FF	AP: Oral ZDV 100 mg 5× daily starting at 14 wk gestation IP: IV ZDV during delivery PP: None	Oral ZDV for 6 wk	MTCT rate: At 18 mo: 8.3% ZDV vs. 25.5% placebo (68% efficacy)
SHORT-COURSE ARV PROPHYLAXIS VERSUS PLACEBO				
CDC/Thailand/ 1999 (643)	$n = 397$ randomized women; 393 delivered; 395 live births ZDV vs. placebo FF	AP: Oral ZDV 300 mg q12hr starting at 36 wk gestation IP: Oral ZDV 300 mg q3hr PP: None	None	MTCT rate: At 6 mo: 9.4% ZDV vs. 18.9% placebo (50% efficacy)
RETRO- CI/Ivory Coast/1999 (644)	Randomized trial; $n = 280$ women enrolled; 230 infants with HIV infection status ZDV vs. placebo BF	AP: Oral ZDV 300 mg q12hr starting at 36 wk gestation until onset of labor IP: Oral ZDV 300 mg at onset of labor and q3hr until delivery PP (mother): none	None	MTCT rate: At 4 wk: 12.2% ZDV vs. 21.7% placebo (44% efficacy) At 3 mo: 16.5% ZDV vs. 26.1% placebo (37% efficacy)
DITRAME (ANRS 049a)/Ivory Coast/Burkina Faso/1999, 2002 (645,646)	Randomized trial; $n = 421$ women; 400 live births ZDV vs. placebo BF	AP: Oral ZDV 300 mg q12hr starting at 36 wk gestation until labor IP: Oral ZDV 600 mg at onset of labor PP (mother): Oral ZDV 300 mg q12hr for 1 wk	None	MTCT rate: At 6 mo: 18% ZDV vs. 27.5% placebo (38% efficacy) At 15 mo: 21.5% ZDV vs. 30.6% placebo (30% efficacy) Pooled analysis of data from DITRAME and RETRO-CI: MTCT rate at 24 mo: 22.5% ZDV vs. 30.2% placebo (26% efficacy)
PETRA/Tanzania, Uganda, South Africa/2002 (647)	Randomized trial; $n = 1457$ women randomized; 1501 infants AP/IP/PP ZDV/3TC vs. IP/PP ZDV/3TC vs. IP-only ZDV/3TC vs. placebo BF and FF	ZDV/3TC (regimen A) AP: Oral ZDV 300 mg q12hr plus 3TC 150 mg q12hr from 36 wk gestation IP: Oral ZDV 300 mg q3hr plus 3TC 150 mg q12hr PP (mother): Oral ZDV 300 mg q12hr plus 3TC 150 mg q12hr for 1 wk ZDV/3TC (regimen B) AP: None IP: Oral ZDV 300 mg q3hr plus 3TC 150 mg q12hr PP (mother): Oral ZDV 300 mg q12hr plus 3TC 150 mg q12hr for 1 wk ZDV/3TC (regimen C) AP: None IP: Oral ZDV 300 mg q3hr plus 3TC 150 mg q12hr PP (mother): None PP (infant): None	ZDV, 4 mg/kg + 3TC, 2 mg/kg twice daily for 7 days	MTCT rate at 6 wk: 5.7% regimen A 8.9% regimen B 14.2 regimen C 15.3% placebo; efficacy compared with placebo is 63%, 42%, and 0%, respectively MTCT rate at 18 mo: 14.9% regimen A 18.1% regimen B 20% regimen C 22.2% placebo Efficacy compared with placebo is 34%, 18%, and 0%, respectively
LONGER VERSUS SHORTER ZDV REGIMENS				
PHPT-1/Thailand/2000 (648)	Randomized trial; $n = 1437$ Four ZDV regimens with varying durations of AP and infant PP dosing, no placebo FF	ZDV (long-long, LL) AP: Oral ZDV 300 mg q12hr starting at 28 wk gestation IP: Oral ZDV 300 mg q3hr PP (mother): None ZDV (long-short, LS) AP: Oral ZDV 300 mg q12hr starting at 28 wk gestation IP: Oral ZDV 300 mg q3hr PP (mother): None ZDV (short-long, SL) AP: Oral ZDV 300 mg q12hr starting at 36 wk gestation IP: Oral ZDV 300 mg q3hr PP (mother): None ZDV (short-short, SS) AP: Oral ZDV 300 mg q12hr starting at 36 wk gestation IP: Oral ZDV 300 mg q3hr PP (mother): None	ZDV (LL) Oral ZDV 2 mg/kg q6hr for 6 wk ZDV (LS) Oral ZDV 2 mg/kg q6hr for 3 days ZDV (SL) Oral ZDV 2 mg/kg q6hr for 6 wk ZDV (SS) Oral ZDV 2 mg/kg q6hr for 3 days	MTCT rate: At 6-mo final analysis: 6.5% (LL) vs. 4.7% (LS) vs. 8.6% SL (no statistical difference) In utero transmission: 1.6% (LL + LS) vs. 5.1% (SL +SS) (difference statistically significant) At 6-mo interim analysis: 4.1% (LL) vs. 10.5% (SS) (SS arm stopped at interim analysis)

Table 22-6 Antiretroviral Prophylaxis for Prevention of Mother-to-Child HIV Transmission During Antenatal and Intrapartum Period—cont'd

NONBREASTFEEDING POPULATIONS

Trial/Site/Year (Reference)	Study Details/Infant Feeding Choice	Maternal ARV Prophylaxis	Infant ARV Prophylaxis	Transmission Rate and Efficacy
ULTRA-SHORT-COURSE ANTIRETROVIRAL PROPHYLAXIS: SDNVP DURING INTRAPARTUM PERIOD				
HIVNET 012/ Uganda/2003 (649,650)	Randomized trial; $n = 626$ sdNVP vs. ZDV BF	NVP arm: AP: None IP: sdNVP 200 mg × 1 PP (mother): None ZDV arm: AP: None IP: Oral ZDV 600 mg, then 300 mg q3hr PP (mother): None	PP (infant): sdNVP 2 mg/kg × 1 at birth PP (infant): ZDV 4 mg/kg q12hr for 1 wk	MTCT rate: At 6-8 wk: 11.8% NVP vs. 20.2% ZDV (42% efficacy) At 18 mo: 15.7% NVP vs. 25.8 ZDV (41% efficacy)
SAINT/South Africa/2003 (664)	Randomized trial; $n = 1317$ Intrapartum maternal/ infant NVP vs. maternal/infant ZDV/3TC BF and FF	NVP arm: AP: None IP: sdNVP 200 mg × 1 PP (mother): sdNVP 200 mg × 1 ZDV/3TC arm: AP: None IP: Oral ZDV 300 mg q3hr plus 3TC 150 mg q12hr PP (mother): ZDV 300 mg q12hr plus 3TC 150 mg q12hr for 1 wk	NVP arm: sdNVP 2 mg/kg × 1 at birth ZDV arm: ZDV 4 mg/kg q12hr plus 3TC 2 mg/kg q12hr for 1 wk	MTCT rate: At 8 wk: 12.3% NVP vs. 9.3% ZDV/3TC (not statistically significant, $P = .11$)
ZDV PLUS sdNVP PROPHYLAXIS				
PHPT-2/ Thailand/ 2004 (654)	Randomized trial; $n = 1844$ ZDV alone vs. ZDV + maternal and infant sdNVP vs. ZDV + maternal sdNVP RF	AP: ZDV from 28 wk gestation IP: Oral ZDV alone or ZDV + sdNVP PP: ZDV for 1 wk with or without sdNVP, infant only	sdNVP	MTCT rate: At 6 mo: 1.1% NVP-NVP vs. 6.3% placebo-placebo ZDV-alone arm terminated during an interim analysis (inferiority) because of higher MTCT compared with NVP-NVP arm (6.3% vs. 1.1%); No statistical difference in MTCT rate between the infant receiving or not receiving sdNVP (2.0% vs. 2.8%, respectively)
DITRAME Plus (ANRS 1201.0) Trial/Ivory Coast/2005 (651)	Open label, ZDV + sdNVP BF and FF	AP: ZDV from 36 wk gestation IP: oral ZDV + sdNVP	sdNVP + ZDV for 1 wk	MTCT rate at 6 wk: 6.5% (95% CI, 3.9% to 9.1%) MTCT rate (historical control group receiving short-course ZDV, 98% breastfed infants) 12.8%
DITRAME Plus (ANRS 1201.1) Trial/Ivory Coast/2005 (651)	Open label, ZDV + 3TC + sdNVP BF and FF	AP: ZDV + 3TC from 32 wk gestation (stopped at 3 days PP) IP: Oral ZDV + 3TC + sdNVP	sdNVP + ZDV for 1 wk	MTCT rate at 6 wk: 4.7% (95% CI, 2.4% to 7.0%) MTCT rate (historical control group receiving short-course ZDV, 98% breastfed infants) 12.8%
COMBINATION ARVS				
PACTG 316/ United States, Europe, Brazil, Bahamas/2002 (655)	Observational study; $n = 1248$ sdNVP vs. placebo among women receiving ZDV alone or dual- or triple-combination ARV regimens FF	NVP arm: AP: Standard ART starting from 14 wk gestation (77% combination, 23% ZDV alone) IP: IV ZDV 2 mg/kg, then 1 mg/kg/hr plus NVP 200 mg × 1 PP: ART if needed Placebo arm: AP: Standard ART starting from 14 wk gestation (77% combination, 23% ZDV alone) IP: IV ZDV 2 mg/kg, then 1 mg/kg/hr plus NVP placebo PP: ART if needed	NVP arm: ZDV 2 mg/kg for 6 wk plus NVP 2 mg/kg × 1 at birth Placebo arm: ZDV 2 mg/kg q6hr for 6 wk plus NVP placebo at birth	MTCT rate: At 6 mo: 1.4% NVP vs. 1.6% NVP placebo Trial terminated early because of very low MTCT in both arms 23% women received ZDV alone; 77 women received dual- or triple-combination ARV regimens

Data from Panel on Treatment of HIV-Infected Pregnant Women and Prevention of Perinatal Transmission: *Recommendations for use of antiretroviral drugs in pregnant HIV-1 infected women for maternal health and interventions to reduce perinatal HIV transmission in the United States, 2013.* Available at http://aidsinfo.nih.gov/contentfiles/lvguidelines/PerinatalGL.pdf. Accessed August 2, 2013.

AP, Antepartum; *ART*, antiretroviral therapy; *ARVs*, antiretrovirals; *BF*, breastfeeding; *CDC*, Centers for Disease Control and Prevention; *FF*, formula feeding; *IP*, intrapartum; *IV*, intravenous; *MTCT*, mother-to-child human immunodeficiency virus transmission; *NVP*, nevirapine; *PACTG*, Pediatric AIDS Clinical Trials Group; *PP*, postpartum; *RF*, replacement feeding; *sd*, single dose; *3TC*, lamivudine; *ZDV*, zidovudine.

Table 22-7 Maternal Antiretroviral Postpartum Regimens to Prevent Mother-to-Child Human Immunodeficiency Virus Transmission During Breastfeeding

		MATERNAL TRIPLE ANTIRETROVIRAL INTERVENTION		
Trial/Site/Year (Reference)	**Study Details/Infant Feeding Choice**	**Maternal ARV Regimen**	**Infant ARV Regimen**	**Results**
OBSERVATIONAL STUDIES				
KiBS/ Kenya/2011 (656)	Observational; enrolled women regardless of CD4 count; $n = 497$ infants BF	AP: ZDV + 3TC + NVP (or LPV/r in mid-2005 if CD4 count > 250) from 34-36 wk gestation IP: Continue above regimen PP: Continue triple ART for 6 mo postpartum if maternal CD4 count > 200 Continue triple ART for life if CD4 < 200	sdNVP	No comparison group MTCT rate: 2.5% at birth; 4.2% at 6 wk, 5% at 6 mo, 5.7% at 12 mo, 7% at 24 mo
MITRA PLUS/ Tanzania/ 2008 (657)	Open-label, nonrandomized, prospective cohort study; enrolled women, regardless of CD4 count; $n = 441$ infants ZDV/3TC/NVP (NVP replaced by NLV after reports of hepatotoxicity with NVP use in women with higher CD4 counts) BF	AP: ZDV + 3TC + NVP (or NLF in 10/2005 if CD4 count > 200) from 34 wk gestation (earlier if CD4 < 200) IP: Continue above regimen PP: Continue triple ART for 6 mo postpartum if CD4 count > 200 Continue triple ART for life if CD4 < 200 or WHO stage 3/4 disease	ZDV + 3TC for 1 wk after birth	No comparison group MTCT rate: 4.1% at 6-8 wk; 5% at 6 mo; HIV or death: 8.6% at 6 mo; 12.8% at 12 mo
RANDOMIZED TRIALS				
Kesho Bora/ Burkina Faso, Kenya, South Africa/ 2009 (658)	Randomized trial Enrolled women with CD4 200-500 824 women enrolled; 805 infants BF	AP: Starting at 28-36 wk gestation; Arm 1: ZDV/3TC/LPV/r Arm 2: ZDV IP: Arm 1: ZDV/3TC/LPV/r Arm 2: ZDV + sdNVP PP: Arm 1: Continue triple ART through 6.5 mo postpartum Arm 2: ZDV/3TC for 1 wk (no postnatal prophylaxis)	Arm 1: sdNVP + ZDV for 1 wk Arm 2: sdNVP + ZDV for 1 wk (no postnatal prophylaxis)	MTCT rate: At birth: 1.8% in triple ART prophylaxis arm vs. 2.5% in ZDV/sdNVP arm At 6 wk: 3.3% in triple ART prophylaxis arm vs. 5.5% in ZDV/sdNVP arm At 6 mo: 4.9% in triple ART prophylaxis arm vs. 8.2% in ZDV/sdNVP arm At 12 mo: 5.4% in triple ART prophylaxis arm vs. 9.5% in ZDV/sdNVP arm
Mma Bana/ Botswana/ 2009 (659)	Randomized trial, $n = 1200$ Enrolled women with CD4 > 200; 560 women enrolled and randomized to PI-based regimen or triple-nucleoside regimen; 553 infants BF	AP: Starting at 26-34 wk gestation Arm 1: ZDV/3TC/LPV/r Arm 2: ZDV/3TC/ABC IP: Arm 1: ZDV/3TC/LPV/r Arm 2: ZDV/3TC/ABC PP: Arm 1: Continue ZDV/3TC/LPV/r through 6 mo postpartum Arm 2: Continue ZDV/3TC/ABC through 6 mo postpartum	Arm 1: sdNVP + ZDV for 4 wk Arm 2: sdNVP + ZDV for 4 wk	MTCT rate: Overall transmission rate of 1.1% at 6 mo Mortality rate: 2.5% at 6 mo
BAN/ Malawi/2010 (660,661)	Randomized trial; Postpartum maternal triple-ARV drug prophylaxis arm vs. infant NVP vs. control group (no ART); Women with CD4 > 250 cells/mm³; 2369 mother-infant pairs randomized BF	AP: All mothers received ZDV from 28 wk of gestation IP: All mothers received sdNVP + ZDV for 1 wk PP: Mothers randomized to maternal triple ARV prophylaxis (ZDV/3TC + NVP/NFV/LPV/r twice daily) through 28 wk; control group did not receive extended ARV prophylaxis	PP regimen: All infants received sdNVP + ZDV for 1 wk Infants randomized to extended NVP prophylaxis through 28 wk Control group did not receive extended ARV prophylaxis	MTCT at age 28 wk was 5.7% in control group; 2.9% in maternal triple-drug prophylaxis arm ($P = .009$ vs. control); 1.7% in infant NVP arm ($P < .001$ vs. control group)

Data from Panel on Treatment of HIV-Infected Pregnant Women and Prevention of Perinatal Transmission: *Recommendations for use of antiretroviral drugs in pregnant HIV-1 infected women for maternal health and interventions to reduce perinatal HIV transmission in the United States, 2013.* Available at http://aidsinfo.nih.gov/contentfiles/lvguidelines/PerinatalGL.pdf. Accessed August 2, 2013.

ABC, Abacavir; *AP,* antepartum; *ART,* antiretroviral therapy; *BAN,* Breastfeeding, Antiretroviral, and Nutrition Study; *BF,* breastfeeding; *FF,* formula feeding; *IP,* intrapartum; *KiBS,* Kisumu Breastfeeding Study; *LPV/r,* lopinavir/ritonavir; *MTCT,* mother-to-child HIV transmission; *NFV,* nelfinavir; *NVP,* nevirapine; *PP,* postpartum; *sd,* single dose; *3TC,* lamivudine; *WHO,* World Health Organization; *ZDV,* zidovudine.

Table 22-8 Infant Antiretroviral Prophylaxis to Prevent Mother-to-Child Human Immunodeficiency Virus Transmission During Breastfeeding

		MATERNAL AND INFANT ANTIRETROVIRAL INTERVENTION		
Trial/Site/Year (Reference)	**Study Details/Infant Feeding Choice**	**Maternal ARV Regimen**	**Infant ARV Regimen**	**Results**
SHORT-COURSE INFANT ARV PROPHYLAXIS				
NVAZ/ Malawi/ 2003 (662)	*n* = 1119 infants (484 sdNVP/ZDV vs. 468 sdNVP) BF	AP or IP: None (late presenters) PP: None	sdNVP ± ZDV for 1 wk	MTCT rate: 15.3% at 6-8 wk in sdNVP + ZDV arm vs. 20.9% in sdNVP-only arm (*P* = .03) MTCT rate among infants HIV uninfected at birth: 7.7% at 6-8 wk in sdNVP + ZDV arm vs. 12.1% in sdNVP-only arm (36% efficacy)
Postnatal NVP/ ZDV/ Malawi/ 2004 (663)	*n* = 894 infants (446 sdNVP/ZDV vs. 448 sdNVP) BF	AP: None IP: sdNVP PP: None	sdNVP ± ZDV for 1 wk	MTCT rate: 16.3% at 6-8 wk in sdNVP + ZDV arm vs. 14.1% in sdNVP-only arm (*P* = .30) MTCT rate among infants HIV uninfected at birth: 6.5% at 6-8 wk in sdNVP + ZDV arm vs. 16.9% in sdNVP-only arm
LONG-COURSE INFANT ARV PROPHYLAXIS				
PEP infant prophylaxis/ South Africa/2005 (664)	BF and FF	AP: None IP: None	sdNVP vs. ZDV for 6 wk	MTCT rate for formula-fed infants: 14.3% at 6 wk in sdNVP arm vs. 14.1% in ZDV arm (*P* = .30) MTCT rate for breastfed infants: 12.2% at 6 wk in sdNVP arm vs. 19.6% in ZDV arm (*P* = .03)
MASHI/Botswana/ 2006 (668)	Phase I, randomized, double-blind, placebo-controlled, multicenter trial; *n* = 1200 (short-course) ZDV + neonatal sdNVP ± maternal sdNVP and ± BF BF (median duration, 5.9 mo) and FF	First randomization: AP: ZDV from 34 wk IP: Oral ZDV + either sdNVP vs. placebo Women with CD4 T-cell counts <200 cells/mm³ receive combination ART	Second randomization: BF/ZDV for 6 mo + sdNVP vs. FF/ZDV for 1 mo + sdNVP	MTCT rate: 9.1% at 7 mo in BF/ZDV arm vs. 5.6% in FF arm Mortality rate: 4.9% at 7 mo in BF/ZDV arm vs. 9.3% in FF arm HIV-free survival: 15.6% at 18 mo in BF/ZDV arm vs. 14.2% in FF arm
PEPI/ Malawi/ 2008 (667)	Randomized clinical trial; *n* = 3016 sdNVP + ZDV for 1 wk (control) vs. two extended infant regimens (NVP or NVP/ZDV) for 14 wk BF (90% at 6 mo and 29%-32% at 9 mo)	AP: None IP: sdNVP (if mothers present in time)	sdNVP + ZDV or 1 wk (control) vs. control + NVP for 14 wk vs. control + NVP/ZDV for 14 wk	MTCT rate among infants HIV uninfected at birth: 5.1% at 6 wk in control arm vs. 1.7% in extended NVP arm (67% efficacy) and 1.6% in extended NVP/ZDV arm (69% efficacy) MTCT rate among infants HIV uninfected at birth: 10.6% at 9 mo in control arm vs. 5.2% in extended NVP arm (51% efficacy) and 6.4% in extended NVP/ZDV arm (45% efficacy)
SWEN/ Uganda, Ethiopia, India/ 2008 (666)	Randomized clinical trials (combined analysis of three studies); *n* = 2024 Infant sdNVP vs. NVP for 6 wk BF (73% at 14 wk and 31% at 6 mo)	AP: None IP: sdNVP	sdNVP vs. NVP for 6 wk	MTCT rate among infants HIV uninfected at birth: 5.3% at 6 wk in sdNVP arm vs. 2.5% in extended NVP arm (RR, 0.54; *P* = .009) MTCT rate among infants HIV uninfected at birth: 9% at 6 mo in sdNVP arm vs. 6.9% in extended NVP arm (RR, 0.80; *P* = .16) Risk of HIV infection or death: Significantly lower in extended NVP arm at both 6 wk (RR = 0.58) and 6 mo of age (RR = 0.78)
MITRA/ Tanzania/ 2008 (669)	Open-label, nonrandomized study (observational); *n* = 398 Infant 3TC for 6 mo BF (median duration, 18 wk)	AP: ZDV/3TC from 36 wk through labor IP: ZDV/3TC PP: ZDV/3TC for 1 wk	3TC for 6 mo	MTCT rate at 6 mo: 4.9% (postnatal MTCT rate among infants aged 6 wk to 6 mo was 1.2%)
BAN/ Malawi/2010 (660,661)	Postpartum maternal triple-ARV drug prophylaxis vs. infant NVP in women with CD4 counts ≥ 250 cells/mm³ BF	AP: None IP regimens: Arm 1 (control): ZDV/3TC + sdNVP Arm 2 (control): ZDV/3TC + sdNVP Arm 3 (control): ZDV/3TC + sdNVP	PP regimen: Arm 1 (control): Maternal ZDV/3TC for 1 week; infant sdNVP + ZDV/3TC for 1 wk Arm 2: Control as above, then maternal ZDV/3TC/LPV/r for 6 mo Arm 3 (control): Control as above, then infant NVP for 6 mo	Postnatal infection rate in infants HIV uninfected at age 2 wk: MTCT at age 28 wk was 5.7% in control arm 1; 2.9% in maternal triple-drug prophylaxis arm 2 (*P* = .009 vs. control); 1.7% in infant NVP arm 3 (*P* < .001 vs. control) No significant difference between maternal triple-drug prophylaxis arm 2 and infant NVP arm 3 (*P* = .12)

Continued

Table 22-8 Infant Antiretroviral Prophylaxis to Prevent Mother-to-Child Human Immunodeficiency Virus Transmission During Breastfeeding—cont'd

		MATERNAL AND INFANT ANTIRETROVIRAL INTERVENTION		
Trial/Site/Year (Reference)	**Study Details/Infant Feeding Choice**	**Maternal ARV Regimen**	**Infant ARV Regimen**	**Results**
HPTN 046/ South Africa, Tanzania, Uganda, Zimbabwe/ 2012 (670)	Phase III, randomized, double-blind, placebo-controlled multicenter study; *n* = 1527 Infant NVP prophylaxis 6 wk vs. 6 mo to prevent postnatal MTCT BF	AP: If indicated for maternal health, HIV-positive mothers received AP drugs	All infants received daily NVP from birth through age 6 wk Infant randomization at age 6 wk Arm 1: Daily infant NVP from age 6 wk to 6 mo Arm 2: Daily infant placebo from age 6 wk to 6 mo	Postnatal infection at 6 mo among infants HIV uninfected at age 6 wk: 1.1% (0.3%-1.8%) in the extended NVP arm 1 and 2.4% (1.3%-3.6%) in the placebo arm 2 (*P* = .049), equating to a 54% reduction in transmission For mothers who were receiving triple ARV drugs at infant randomization, the infant HIV infection rate was 0.2% at 6 mo among uninfected infants at age 6 wk; no statistical difference was noted between extended NVP arm (0.5%) vs. placebo arm (0%) Among infants uninfected at age 6 weeks born to mothers with CD4 T-lymphocyte counts >350 cells/mm³ who were not receiving triple ARV drugs, postnatal HIV infection rate at 6 mo was 0.7% (0%-1.5%) in the extended NVP arm compared with placebo arm (2.8%) [*P* = .014]
NICHD-HPTN 040/ PACTG 1043/ United States, Argentina, Brazil, South Africa/ 2012 (675)	Infant prophylaxis with 6 wk ZDV vs. 6 wk infant ZDV + NVP (three doses in the first wk of life) vs. 6-wk infant ZDV + 3TC/NFV for 2 wk FF	AP: None IP: IV ZDV during labor and delivery if mothers presented early	Arm 1 (control): Infant ZDV for 6 wk Arm 2: Control as above plus NVP with first dose within 48 hr of birth, second dose 48 hr later, and third dose 96 hr after the second dose Arm 3: Control as above, plus 3TC and NFV from birth through 2 wk of life	Intrapartum HIV transmission among infants HIV uninfected at birth: 4.8% (3.2%-7.1%) ZDV arm 1 vs. 2.2% (1.2%-3.9%) in ZDV + NVP arm 2 (*P* = .046 compared with arm 1) vs. 2.4% (1.4%-4.3%) in ZDV + 3TC/NVP arm 3 (*P* = .046 compared with arm 1)

Data from Panel on Treatment of HIV-Infected Pregnant Women and Prevention of Perinatal Transmission: *Recommendations for use of antiretroviral drugs in pregnant HIV-1 infected women for maternal health and interventions to reduce perinatal HIV transmission in the United States, 2013.* Available at http://aidsinfo.nih.gov/contentfiles/lvguidelines/PerinatalGL.pdf. Accessed August 2, 2013.

AP, Antepartum; *ART*, antiretroviral therapy; *BF*, breastfeeding; *FF*, formula feeding; *HIV*, human immunodeficiency virus; *HPTN*, HIV Prevention Trials Network; *IP*, intrapartum; *IV*, intravenous; *LPV/r*, lopinavir/ritonavir; *MTCT*, mother-to-child HIV transmission; *NFV*, nelfinavir; *NVP*, nevirapine; *PEP*, postexposure prophylaxis; *PP*, postpartum; *RR*, risk ratio; *sd*, single dose; *3TC*, lamivudine; ZDV, zidovudine.

A recent study (NICHD-HPTN 040/P1043) conducted in formula-fed infant populations in the United States, Argentina, Brazil, and South Africa compared the efficacy of three neonatal ARV regimens in infants born to HIV-positive mothers, who did not receive any ARV drugs during pregnancy and before labor.[675] This study enrolled 1735 formula-fed infants and demonstrated that combination infant ARV prophylaxis regimens, consisting of ZDV for 6 weeks plus three doses of NVP during the first week of life (birth, 48 hours, and 96 hours of life) or ZDV plus 3TC plus nelfinavir given from birth to 2 weeks of life, decreased the risk of intrapartum transmission by approximately 50% compared with the standard ZDV-alone regimen.[675] Thus combination ARV prophylaxis is recommended for infants born to HIV-infected women in the United States who have not received ARV medications during pregnancy.[22]

The mechanisms of action of ARV prophylaxis in reducing perinatal transmission of HIV is likely multifactorial, including reducing maternal viral load in blood and genital secretions during antepartum period and provision of infant preexposure and postexposure prophylaxis during labor and delivery.[‡] A high maternal plasma concentration of HIV is a crucial risk factor for intrauterine and intrapartum transmission to the infant.[100,102] Thus decreasing viral load during pregnancy is an important mechanism of action of ARVs.

Studies have reported low levels of genital tract HIV RNA or DNA shedding among women with undetectable plasma viral load.[676-678] In addition, perinatal transmission can occur across the entire range of maternal viral load among pregnant women, including those with very low or undetectable serum levels of HIV on ART.[679-681] Thus other factors besides maternal viral load may influence MTCT.[682] Studies have documented that levels of maternal viral load at delivery and antenatal ART are independently associated with perinatal HIV transmission, and receipt of maternal cART was associated with the lowest rates of transmission.[29] Therefore combination ARV drugs are recommended for all HIV-infected pregnant women to reduce the risk of perinatal transmission, irrespective of maternal viral load.[22]

In the PACTG 076 study, ZDV reduced maternal HIV RNA only modestly, and change in maternal HIV RNA levels accounted for only 17% of the reported efficacy of ZDV.[105] In addition, ZDV reduced transmission at all levels of maternal HIV RNA levels. The continued efficacy of ZDV

‡References 22, 647, 650, 653, 662, 664, 675.

Box 22-3 U.S. Public Health Service Guidelines for Preventing Perinatal Human Immunodeficiency Virus (HIV) Transmission

HIV-Positive Women Currently on ART Who Became Pregnant

Mother

- Continue current combination ART during antepartum and intrapartum period if the regimen is safe and effective in achieving optimal viral suppression
- ARV resistance testing if maternal viral load > 500-1000 copies/mL
- Continuous intravenous ZDV infusion during labor for women with viral load > 400 copies/mL (or unknown viral load) near delivery, regardless of antepartum regimen or mode of delivery
- Scheduled cesarean delivery at 38 wk of gestation if maternal plasma viral load > 1000 copies/mL near the time of delivery

Neonate

- Oral ZDV should be prescribed to the neonate as soon as possible after delivery (preferably within 6-12 hr of birth) and then continued for 6 wk.

HIV-Positive Pregnant Women Who Have Never Received ART

Mother

- ARV resistance testing before starting ARV prophylaxis or therapy, but treatment must not be delayed pending results of resistance testing if maternal HIV diagnosis is made late in pregnancy
- Combination ART during antepartum and intrapartum period
- Continuous intravenous ZDV infusion during labor for women with viral load >400 copies/mL (or unknown viral load) near delivery, regardless of antepartum regimen or mode of delivery
- Scheduled cesarean delivery at 38 wk of gestation if maternal plasma viral load > 1000 copies/mL near the time of delivery
- Linkage to care and treatment program to evaluate the need for continuation of combination ART postpartum

Neonate

- Oral ZDV should be prescribed to the neonate as soon as possible after delivery (preferably within 6-12 hr of birth) and then continued for 6 wk.

HIV-Positive Pregnant Women Who Are ART Experienced but Not Currently on ART

Mother

- ARV resistance testing before restarting ARV prophylaxis or therapy, but treatment must not be delayed pending results of resistance testing if maternal HIV diagnosis is made late in pregnancy.
- Combination ART during antepartum and intrapartum period
- Continuous intravenous ZDV infusion during labor for women with viral load >400 copies/mL (or unknown viral load) near delivery, regardless of antepartum regimen or mode of delivery
- Scheduled cesarean delivery at 38 wk of gestation if maternal plasma viral load > 1000 copies/mL near the time of delivery
- Linkage to care and treatment program to evaluate the need for continuation of combination ART postpartum

Neonate

- Oral ZDV should be prescribed to the neonate as soon as possible after delivery (preferably within 6-12 hr of birth) and then continued for 6 wk.

HIV-Positive Women Who Have Received No ART Before Labor

Mother

- Continuous intravenous ZDV infusion during labor

Neonate

- Combination ARV drug regimen as soon as possible after birth (oral ZDV for 6 wk to the infant plus three doses of oral NVP in the first week of life (at birth, 48 hr later, and 96 hr after the second dose)

Data from Panel on Treatment of HIV-Infected Pregnant Women and Prevention of Perinatal Transmission: Recommendations for use of antiretroviral drugs in pregnant HIV-1 infected women for maternal health and interventions to reduce perinatal HIV transmission in the United States, *2013. Available at http://aidsinfo.nih.gov/contentfiles/lvguidelines/PerinatalGL.pdf. Accessed August 2, 2013.*

ART, Antiretroviral therapy; *ARV,* antiretroviral; *NVP,* nevirapine; *ZDV,* zidovudine.

in reducing transmission, even in women with low viral loads, suggests that preexposure and postexposure prophylaxis of the infant during labor and delivery may have been a substantial component of protection.[§]

COMBINATION ANTIRETROVIRAL DRUGS DURING PREGNANCY

Current U.S. PHS task force recommendations regarding use of ARVs by pregnant HIV-infected women and prevention of perinatal HIV transmission are summarized in Box 22-3.[22] A multidisciplinary approach involving HIV specialists, obstetricians, pediatricians, social workers, and patient navigators is recommended to optimize care for HIV-infected pregnant women.[683] Initial prenatal assessment of infected women should include staging of HIV disease (clinical manifestations, measurements of plasma viral load and CD4 cell count); history of prior and current ARV use and genotypic resistance testing; determination of the need for prophylaxis of OIs; evaluation of general health, including comorbid conditions (such as hepatitis C, hepatitis B, or TB); immunizations; and baseline laboratory investigations (CBC, renal and liver function tests).[22]

After counseling regarding the potential risks and benefits of ART, all HIV-infected pregnant women must receive fully suppressive combination ARV regimens, including at least three ARV agents, for either treatment of maternal HIV infection or PMTCT, regardless of plasma viral load and CD4 cell count.[22] In general, the criteria for initiation of cART in pregnant HIV-infected women or women of childbearing age are the same as for HIV-infected adults and adolescents.[684] The choice of treatment regimen must be individualized based on prior ARV history and presence of comorbidities. The selection of ARVs should be based on known efficacy data, pregnancy-specific pharmacokinetic and pharmacodynamic data to guide dosing, good placental passage, potential maternal and fetal adverse effects, and teratogenicity.[22] Drug-resistance testing should

§References 647, 650, 653, 662, 664, 675.

be performed for all women before starting ART and for women who are already receiving ART without fully suppressed viral load (>500-1000 copies/mL). However, decisions regarding initiating ARV prophylaxis must not be delayed, especially when women present late in pregnancy or need ART for their own health.[22]

HIV-infected women already receiving a fully suppressive cART regimen for their own health and presenting for antenatal care should continue their regimen.[22] For ARV-naïve women who need treatment for their own health, cART must be initiated immediately, even during the first trimester. For women who need cART for PMTCT only, immediate initiation of therapy is a consideration, but some experts suggest delaying therapy until after 10 to 12 weeks of gestation because of potential risk of short- and long-term drug toxicity for the fetus or newborn.[685] The guidelines also recommend that ZDV (used in the PACTG 076 study) should be included in the maternal ARV regimen, although a woman already receiving cART with fully suppressed viral load should continue her regimen.[22]

A triple-drug combination ART, consisting of two NRTIs plus either a PI or a NNRTI is recommended for ARV-naïve women (Table 22-9). Use of single or dual NRTIs alone is not recommended for therapy of HIV infection.[22] The preferred dual NRTI regimen of choice is ZDV and 3TC, based on data from clinical trials and established safety during pregnancy.[28] LPV/r and atazanavir with low-dose ritonavir are the preferred PIs for use during pregnancy.[22]

For women who have documented resistance to ZDV or cannot tolerate the drug because of toxicity, an alternative ARV drug with good placental passage may be selected to provide preexposure prophylaxis to the fetus.[22] Alternative NRTIs include ABC, FTC, and the NRTI TDF.[22,686] Alternative PIs include ritonavir-boosted darunavir (DRV/r) and saquinavir. Limited experience exists for the use of integrase inhibitor raltegravir during pregnancy and is a consideration when preferred and alternative drugs cannot be used.[22,687,688] Data are currently insufficient for the newer NNRTIs (etravirine and rilpivirine), PIs (fosamprenavir, tipranavir), and entry inhibitors (enfurvitide and maraviroc).

Adverse events related to the use of ARV agents during pregnancy must be closely monitored. Hyperglycemia, new-onset diabetes mellitus, exacerbation of existing diabetes mellitus and ketoacidosis may be associated with PI therapy, requiring standard glucose screening at 24 to 28 weeks of gestation.[22] Although NVP is the preferred NNRTI during pregnancy, the drug is not recommended for pregnant HIV-positive women with CD4 counts greater than 250 cells/μL because of the increased risk of potentially life-threatening hepatic toxicity noted in women with higher CD4 counts.[22,689] The combination of d4T and ddI is not recommended during pregnancy because of potential risk of mitochondrial toxicity and lactic acidosis, resulting in fatal outcomes.[690,691] Another NNRTI, EFV, is not recommended during the first trimester of pregnancy as part of the maternal cARV regimen because of concerns of teratogenicity but may be continued if the woman is already receiving an EFV-based regimen with undetectable viral load.[22,692]

During the intrapartum period, ART must be administered to all HIV-infected pregnant women, irrespective of viral load or CD4 cell count. The U.S. guidelines recommend intravenous ZDV as part of intrapartum ARV prophylaxis. If an elective cesarean section is planned, ZDV infusion should begin 3 hours before surgery. All other ARVs must be continued during the intrapartum period with the only exception of d4T, which should not be given during ZDV infusion because of known antagonism.[22]

Maternal cART must be continued postpartum if indicated for maternal health or discontinued if ARVs were used solely for PMTCT, but these decisions must be made in close consultation with an HIV specialist.[22] Many factors must be taken into consideration about continuing ART postpartum, including current recommendations for initiating ART, current and nadir CD4 T-lymphocyte counts and trends, maternal viral load, adherence issues, seronegative sexual partner, and patient preference.[22] Expert guidelines recommend continuation of ART postpartum in women with nadir CD4 counts less than the currently recommended threshold for initiation of ART and/or symptomatic HIV infection.[22] The risks versus benefits of discontinuing ART in postpartum HIV women with higher CD4 counts is unknown and is the subject of a future clinical trial, entitled Promoting Maternal and Infant Survival Everywhere (PROMISE).[693]

A recent landmark study (HPTN 052) involving serodiscordant couples demonstrated that early institution of ART among HIV-infected individuals results in a substantial reduction in sexual transmission of HIV to their uninfected partners.[694] Therefore, in serodiscordant couples, continued administration of ARVs may be recommended in postpartum HIV-positive women with CD4 counts between 350 to 550 cells/μL and can be considered for women with CD4 counts greater than 550 cells/μL to prevent sexual transmission of HIV to the uninfected male partner.[22] Health care providers caring for HIV-infected women and their infants can seek free consultation from a federally funded service program: the National Perinatal HIV Hotline at 1-888-448-8765.

SAFETY OF ANTIRETROVIRAL PROPHYLAXIS IN PREGNANCY

With widespread use of ARV prophylaxis to prevent perinatal HIV transmission in LMIC and the increasing availability of cART for HIV-infected mothers during pregnancy and postpartum during breastfeeding, an increasing number of infants are being exposed to ARVs in utero and during the postnatal period.[695] However, limited data exist on the long-term consequences of ART exposure on the fetus and newborn. Animal data have shown that nucleoside analogues may be carcinogenic and can cause mitochondrial dysfunction.[570] An extensive review of short- and medium-term data from several studies indicates, however, that ART during pregnancy has been well tolerated by mothers and infants.[33] Except for mild, transient anemia, no serious short-term maternal or infant adverse effects have been noted with prophylactic ZDV regimens.[22]

Many studies have reported the link between ART exposure during pregnancy and adverse effects on the fetus and newborn, including stillbirth, preterm delivery, and small-for-gestational age, compared with ZDV monotherapy.[696-699] In a study from France, in utero exposure to nucleoside analogues has been associated with mitochondrial dysfunction in HIV-exposed uninfected infants; however, this association was not found in studies from the United States

Table 22-9 Preferred and Alternative Antiretroviral Agents During Pregnancy

Antiretroviral Drug	FDA Pregnancy Category	Experience During Pregnancy and PK Data	Adverse Effects and Concerns
PREFERRED NUCLEOSIDE/NUCLEOTIDE REVERSE-TRANSCRIPTASE INHIBITORS (NRTIS): ZIDOVUDINE, LAMIVUDINE			
Zidovudine (ZDV), Azidothymidine (AZT)	C	Extensive experience; PK not significantly altered in pregnancy; no change in dosing indicated High placental transfer to the fetus	Anemia, neutropenia, mitochondrial toxicity (neuropathy, myopathy, cardiomyopathy, pancreatitis, lactic acidosis, hepatomegaly with steatosis) No evidence of human teratogenicity Well tolerated during pregnancy and safe for mothers and infants in the short term
Lamivudine (3TC)[†]	C	Extensive experience; PK not significantly altered in pregnancy; no change in dosing indicated High placental transfer to the fetus	Headache, fatigue, reduced appetite, nausea, diarrhea, rash, anemia, neutropenia mitochondrial toxicity (neuropathy, myopathy, cardiomyopathy, pancreatitis, lactic acidosis, hepatomegaly with steatosis) No evidence of human teratogenicity Well tolerated during pregnancy and safe for mothers and infants in the short-term
Alternative NRTIs: Abacavir (ABC),* emtricitabine (FTC), tenofovir (TDF)[‡]			
Use in special circumstances because of toxicity concerns: Didanosine (ddI), stavudine (d4T)[†]			
PREFERRED NONNUCLEOSIDE REVERSE-TRANSCRIPTASE INHIBITORS (NNRTIS)			
Nevirapine (NVP)	B	Extensive experience; PK not significantly altered; no change in dosing indicated High placental transfer to the fetus	Skin rash, including Stevens-Johnson syndrome and toxic epidermal necrolysis, fever, headache, nausea, and abnormal liver enzymes Severe life-threatening hepatotoxicity and rash in women with a CD4 T-cell count >250 cells/mL, hypersensitivity reactions For pregnant HIV-positive women with CD4 T-cell count >250, NVP should be started only if benefit clearly outweighs the risk of rash associated hepatotoxicity Women who are already receiving NVP at the beginning of pregnancy and are tolerating the drug may continue NVP, regardless of CD4 count Elevated baseline liver enzymes may increase risk of NVP toxicity No evidence of human teratogenicity
Use in special circumstances: Efavirenz (EFV), classified as FDA Pregnancy Class D; case reports of neural tube defects with first trimester exposure; relative risk unclear			
Insufficient data to recommend use in pregnancy: Etravirine (ETR), rilpivirine (RPV)			
PROTEASE INHIBITORS (PIS)			
Lopinavir-ritonavir (LPV/r)	C	AUC decreased in second and third trimester with standard dosing; PK studies suggest increase in dosing to 600 mg/150 mg 2× daily in second and third trimester, especially in PI-experienced patients Low placental transfer to the fetus	*More frequent*: Diarrhea, nausea, vomiting, headache, skin rash in patients receiving other ARVs, lipid abnormalities *Less frequent*: Fat redistribution *Rare:* New onset diabetes mellitus, hyperglycemia, ketoacidosis, hemolytic anemia, pancreatitis, and life-threatening hepatitis No evidence of human teratogenicity Well tolerated during pregnancy and safe for mothers and infants in the short term
Atazanavir boosted with low-dose ritonavir (ATV/r)	C	Standard dosing of ATV/r results in decreased plasma concentrations of the drug in pregnancy Low placental transfer to the fetus	Generally safe Hyperbilirubinemia may need to be monitored No evidence of human teratogenicity
Alternative PIs: Darunavir/ritonavir (DRV/r), saquinavir/ritonavir (SQV/r)			
Use in special circumstances: Indinavir/ritonavir (IDV/r), nelfinavir (NFV)			
Insufficient data to recommend use in pregnancy: Fosamprenavir (FPV), tipranavir (TPV)			
Entry inhibitors: Enfuvirtide (T20), maraviroc (MVC) Insufficient data to recommend use in pregnancy			
Integrase inhibitors: Raltegravir (RAL) Use in special circumstances			

Data from Panel on Treatment of HIV-Infected Pregnant Women and Prevention of Perinatal Transmission: *Recommendations for use of antiretroviral drugs in pregnant HIV-1 infected women for maternal health and interventions to reduce perinatal HIV transmission in the United States, 2013.* Available at http://aidsinfo.nih.gov/contentfiles/lvguidelines/PerinatalGL.pdf. Accessed August 2, 2013.

ABC, Abacavir; *AUC,* area under the curve; *FDA,* Food and Drug Administration; *HIV,* human immunodeficiency virus; *HLA,* human leukocyte antigen; *PK,* pharmacokinetics.

*Risk of hypersensitivity reaction with ABC (5%-8% of nonpregnant individuals; check HLA B*5701 before starting ABC.

[†]Combinations of ddI and 3TC and ddI and d4T should not be used with one another because of the association with severe life-threatening lactic acidosis during pregnancy.

[‡]Limited experience in pregnancy; potential fetal bone effects; tenofovir plus 3TC or FTC is the preferred NRTI pair for HIV-infected women with chronic hepatitis B coinfection.

and Europe.[700-703] Renal damage and effects on fetal growth and bone mineralization have been concerns related to the use of TDF during pregnancy.[22] However, recent reports indicate no increase in adverse pregnancy outcomes or birth defects in infants exposed to TDF-based ART compared with those receiving a non-TDF regimen.[704-706]

PI-based cART regimens initiated early during pregnancy may be associated with an increased risk of preterm births.[697] However, the benefits of PI-based ART for maternal health and PMTCT seem to outweigh the small risk of prematurity and, in general, most PIs can be considered safe for use during pregnancy.[22] Transient adrenal dysfunction in HIV-exposed uninfected infants has been associated with prenatal and postnatal exposure to LPV/r.[707]

Safety of EFV in pregnancy has been a concern because of animal studies and case reports suggesting an association between CNS defects (neural tube defects) and EFV exposure during pregnancy.[692,708-710] A recent observational study has reported an increased risk of birth defects with use of EFV in the first trimester.[711] However, data from a systematic review and meta-analysis found no increased risk of birth defects or neural tube defects in infants exposed to EFV in utero.[712] The FDA lists EFV as a pregnancy category D drug, and the U.S. guidelines recommend the use of alternative regimen, when possible.[28]

Neonatal anemia can result from prophylactic maternal and infant ZDV regimens.[22,713,714] Many studies have found no association between in utero ARV exposure and neurodevelopmental function.[702,703,715-717] The long-term effects on infants exposed to ARVs in utero are unknown, warranting development of surveillance systems and further research.[695,696] Health care providers who treat maternal/pediatric HIV-infected patients should report instances of prenatal exposure to ARVs to the Antiretroviral Pregnancy Registry (1-800-258-4263) or online at http://www.apregistry.com.

ELECTIVE CESAREAN DELIVERY

The role of elective cesarean section delivery in reducing perinatal HIV transmission was recognized before the advent of cART during pregnancy.[95,96] Data from a randomized controlled trial from Europe and a large international meta-analysis of 15 prospective cohort studies have shown that cesarean section performed before labor and rupture of membranes reduces perinatal transmission of HIV by 50% to 80%, independent of the use of ART or ZDV prophylaxis.[95,96] Both these studies were performed before the advent of HAART during pregnancy, and there was no information on maternal serum HIV RNA level.

Because the level of maternal serum HIV RNA level is an important predictor of perinatal HIV transmission, it is debatable if any additional benefit would be conferred by an elective cesarean section among women successfully treated with cART and who have a very low or undetectable viral load.[100-102,718] In the Women and Infant Transmission Study, no transmission occurred among women with a plasma viral load of less than 1000 copies/mL, but the results were limited by a small sample size.[100] A recent observational cohort study demonstrated a significantly lower risk of transmission in women with delivery viral load of less than 400 copies/mL and who underwent elective cesarean section, compared with vaginal delivery.[719]

The American College of Obstetrics and Gynecology and U.S. guidelines recommend scheduled cesarean section at 38 weeks of gestation for women with viral load greater than 1000 copies/mL or unknown viral load near the time of delivery, to reduce the risk of perinatal HIV transmission.[22,720] Given the low rate of transmission in women receiving ART with plasma viral load of less than 1000 copies/mL, it is unclear if elective cesarean section would offer any additional benefit and therefore is not routinely recommended.[22] Because of the increased risk of infectious disease complications in HIV-infected women after cesarean delivery, prophylactic antibiotics are recommended during the perioperative period.[720,721] The U.S. PHS task force recommendations regarding mode of delivery to reduce perinatal HIV transmission are summarized in Box 22-4.

NEONATAL ANTIRETROVIRAL PROPHYLAXIS

All HIV-exposed infants must receive ARV prophylaxis as soon as possible after birth, preferably within 6 to 12 hours of life, to reduce the risk of perinatal HIV transmission (Table 22-10).[22] When the mother has received cART during pregnancy, neonatal ZDV at gestational age–appropriate dosing for 6 weeks is the recommended ARV prophylaxis regimen in the United States. When the mother has not received antepartum ARV during pregnancy, combination ARV prophylaxis, including ZDV for 6 weeks plus three doses of NVP during the first week of life (birth, 48 hours, and 96 hours of life), is recommended for the HIV-exposed infant (Box 22-5; see Table 22-10).[22,675]

In these scenarios, a pediatric HIV specialist should be consulted and mothers be counseled regarding the potential benefits and risk of combination infant ARV prophylaxis. In premature infants, only ZDV and NVP are recommended for ARV prophylaxis because data on pharmacokinetics, dosing, and safety of alternative ARV drugs are lacking. Infant ARV prophylaxis initiated after 48 hours of birth is not effective.[674]

Social services should be involved before the mother and baby are discharged from the hospital to ensure compliance to follow-up visits. Newborns should be discharged with a supply of oral ZDV syrup. A CBC is recommended at birth and at 4 weeks of age (after starting infant ZDV prophylaxis) to monitor for potential hematologic toxicity (anemia and neutropenia).[22] Some experts recommend serum chemistry and liver function tests at birth and when HIV PCR testing is done in infants exposed to combination ARV drug regimens during pregnancy or during the neonatal period.[22]

Virologic tests (HIV DNA or RNA assays) are needed for early infant HIV diagnosis and should be performed at 14 to 21 days of life, 1 to 2 months of age, and 4 to 6 months of age.[22] For any positive HIV DNA PCR result, the infant should be re-tested immediately for confirmatory PCR testing. If infection is confirmed by two positive virologic tests, ARV prophylaxis must be discontinued, and a pediatric infectious disease consultation should be requested for confirming the diagnosis and initiation of cART if the infant is found to be HIV infected.[17,372,373]

All HIV-exposed infants with indeterminate HIV status should receive TMP-SMX to prevent PCP, starting at

Box 22-4 U.S. Public Health Service Guidelines Related to Mode of Delivery for Preventing Perinatal Human Immunodeficiency Virus (HIV) Transmission

HIV-Positive Women Presenting Late In Pregnancy (>36 wk of Gestation), Not Currently on ART and Results of Viral Load and CD4 T-Lymphocyte Count Are Unavailable Before Delivery

- Start combination ART.
- Counsel women on the beneficial effect of scheduled cesarean delivery in reducing perinatal HIV transmission, if viral suppression cannot be documented before 38 weeks' gestation.
- Scheduled cesarean delivery at 38 weeks' gestation, as determined by best obstetric dating.
- Administer a loading dose of intravenous (IV) ZDV, followed by continuous IV infusion before scheduled cesarean section.
- Continue other ARV drugs per schedule during the perioperative period.
- Follow standard cesarean delivery management procedures, including use of prophylactic antibiotics.

HIV-Positive Women Presenting in the Third Trimester, Currently on ART but Viral Load Remains >1000 Copies/mL at 36 wk of Gestation

- Consult HIV specialist for recommendations regarding appropriate ART regimen.
- Continue the current combination ART regimen if optimal virus suppression is achieved.
- Recommend scheduled cesarean section if optimal viral load suppression not documented by 38 weeks of gestation given the additional beneficial effect in reducing perinatal HIV transmission. Discuss the potential risks of operative delivery with woman (e.g., anesthesia, surgery and postoperative infection).
- Perform scheduled cesarean delivery at 38 wk of gestation as determined by best obstetric dating.
- Administer a loading dose of IV ZDV, followed by continuous IV infusion before scheduled cesarean section.
- Continue other ARV drugs per schedule during the perioperative period.
- Follow standard cesarean delivery management procedures, including use of prophylactic antibiotics.

HIV-Positive Pregnant Women Who Are Currently Receiving Combination ART and Have Undetectable Viral Load at 36 wk of Gestation

- Counsel mothers on the very low risk (<1%) of perinatal HIV with undetectable viral load, even with a vaginal delivery and lack of evidence of additional benefit of scheduled cesarean section in such circumstances.
- Discuss the potential risks and uncertain benefits of cesarean delivery compared with vaginal delivery in women with undetectable viral load.

HIV-Positive Pregnant Women With Viral Load >1000 Copies/mL Who Have Opted for Scheduled Cesarean Delivery But Present After Membrane Rupture or Onset of Labor at >37 wk of Gestation

- Immediate initiation of IV Zidovudine.
- Decisions regarding mode of delivery should be individualized taking into consideration several factors affecting perinatal transmission of HIV including duration of membrane rupture and/or labor, maternal viral load, and current ART regimen.
- Vaginal delivery management (if selected) should be individualized; invasive procedures (such as scalp electrodes, invasive monitoring and operative delivery); If clinically indicated, some experts recommend oxytocin to expedite delivery.
- Cesarean section (if selected), if feasible, loading dose of IV ZDV must be administered and completed before the procedure.

Data from Panel on Treatment of HIV-Infected Pregnant Women and Prevention of Perinatal Transmission: Recommendations for use of antiretroviral drugs in pregnant HIV-1 infected women for maternal health and interventions to reduce perinatal HIV transmission in the United States, 2013. *Available at http://aidsinfo.nih.gov/contentfiles/lvguidelines/PerinatalGL.pdf. Accessed August 2, 2013.*

ART, Antiretroviral therapy; *ARV,* antiretroviral; *ZDV,* zidovudine.

Box 22-5 Indications for Combination Antiretroviral Prophylaxis to Human Immunodeficiency Virus (HIV)-Exposed Infants

- HIV-positive mothers who have not received antepartum and intrapartum ARV drugs
- HIV-positive mothers who have only received intrapartum antiretroviral (ARV) drugs
- HIV-positive mothers who received antepartum and intrapartum ARV drugs but have not achieved optimal viral suppression at delivery
- Mothers infected with ARV drug-resistant virus

Data from Panel on Treatment of HIV-Infected Pregnant Women and Prevention of Perinatal Transmission: Recommendations for use of antiretroviral drugs in pregnant HIV-1 infected women for maternal health and interventions to reduce perinatal HIV transmission in the United States, 2013. *Available at http://aidsinfo.nih.gov/contentfiles/lvguidelines/PerinatalGL.pdf. Accessed August 2, 2013.*

6 weeks of age after completion of infant ARV prophylaxis regimen.[22] Prophylaxis for PCP need not be initiated or can be stopped when infant HIV infection is presumptively or definitely excluded.

AVOIDANCE OF BREASTFEEDING

The risk of postnatal HIV transmission through breastfeeding is well documented.[37,38] In the United States and resource-rich countries where infant formulas are affordable, feasible, acceptable, safe, and readily available, HIV-infected mothers should be advised not to breastfeed their infants.[22,722] In addition, physicians must ask mothers about premastication of foods for infant feeding, counsel HIV-infected caregivers to avoid this practice, and discuss safe feeding options.[17,22,68,723]

In recent years, several open-label observational studies and RCTs have evaluated the efficacy of maternal or infant ARV prophylaxis during breastfeeding to decrease postnatal HIV transmission(see Tables 22-7 and 22-8).[22,656-671] Administration of maternal triple ARV prophylaxis to breastfeeding HIV-positive mothers for 6 months postpartum results in MTCT rates ranging from 1.2% to 4.1% at

Table 22-10 Antiretroviral Strategies to Prevent Perinatal Human Immunodeficiency Virus Transmission

MATERNAL COMBINATION ARV REGIMEN	
Antepartum	Combination ARV* (may include oral ZDV, 200 mg 3× daily or 300 mg, 2× daily as part of maternal ARV regimen)
Intrapartum	IV ZDV 2 mg/kg during the first hr, followed by continuous infusion of 1 mg/kg/hr until delivery; continue other ARVs during intrapartum period
NEONATAL PROPHYLAXIS†	
ZDV Prophylaxis for Infants Whose Mothers Have Received Antepartum/Intrapartum ARVs	
≥35 weeks' gestation	Oral ZDV 4 mg/kg (or 3 mg/kg IV if unable to tolerate oral agents), 2× daily until 6 wk of age
≥30 to <35 weeks' gestation	Oral ZDV 2 mg/kg (or 1.5 mg/kg IV), 2× daily for the first 2 weeks of age, followed by 3 mg/kg PO (or 2.3 mg/kg IV), 2× daily for the next 4 wk of life
<30 weeks' gestation	Oral ZDV 2 mg/kg (or 1.5 mg/kg IV), 2× daily for the first 4 weeks of age, followed by 3 mg/kg PO (or 2.3 mg/kg IV), 2× daily for the next 2 wk of life
Additional ARV Prophylaxis for Infants Whose Mothers Have Not Received Antepartum ARVs	
Combination	Oral ZDV as shown above *Plus* Oral NVP 8 mg/dose (birth weight 1.5-2 kg) or 12 mg/dose (birth weight > 2 kg), given as a three-dose regimen‡

Data from Panel on Treatment of HIV-Infected Pregnant Women and Prevention of Perinatal Transmission: *Recommendations for use of antiretroviral drugs in pregnant HIV-1 infected women for maternal health and interventions to reduce perinatal HIV transmission in the United States, 2013.* Available at http://aidsinfo.nih.gov/contentfiles/lvguidelines/PerinatalGL.pdf. Accessed August 2, 2013.

ARV, Antiretroviral prophylaxis; *IV*, intravenous; *NVP*, nevirapine; *ZDV*, zidovudine.

*For maternal treatment or perinatal HIV prevention prophylaxis.

†ARV prophylaxis must begin as soon after birth as possible, and preferably within 6-12 hr of delivery; if infant is unable to tolerate oral ZDV, intravenous administration is recommended.

‡NVP dosing regimen: Dose 1, birth-48 hr; dose 2, 48 hr after first; and dose 3, 96 hr after second.

4 to 6 weeks of age and 1.4% to 5% at 6 months of age.[655,656-660] Likewise, administration of extended ARV prophylaxis to breastfeeding infants born to HIV-positive mothers results in postnatal transmission rates of 1.2% to 4.4% (from 1-6 weeks until 6-7 months of infant age).[660,666,667,669,670]

Despite significant efficacy, maternal or infant ARV cannot fully eliminate breast-milk HIV transmission. In addition, emergence of multiclass drug resistance in breastfeeding infants who acquire infection despite maternal triple-drug or extended NVP prophylaxis is a major concern.[617,724,725] Therefore breastfeeding by HIV-infected mothers is not recommended in the United States, regardless of maternal viral load and receipt of cART.[22]

ANTICIPATORY GUIDANCE AND PRIMARY CARE FOR HUMAN IMMUNODEFICIENCY VIRUS–EXPOSED INFANTS

The clinical care of the HIV-exposed infant is depicted in Table 22-1. Age-appropriate anticipatory guidance must be provided to all HIV-exposed infants similar to the guidance provided for non–HIV-exposed infants. In addition, mothers and caregivers of HIV-exposed infants must receive anticipatory guidance around all components of care for the HIV-exposed infant. In addition, HIV education related to modes of transmission must be provided to mothers and other caregivers, stressing the fact that touching, hugging, or kissing their infants is safe. HIV-exposed infants should receive all routine childhood immunizations, including hepatitis B vaccine, inactivated polio vaccine, diphtheria–tetanus toxoids–acellular pertussis vaccine, *H. influenzae* type b vaccine, pneumococcal conjugate vaccine, and rotavirus vaccine.[17] If infant HIV infection is confirmed, then immunization recommendations for the HIV-infected must be followed. Readers are referred to the most recent edition of the AAP's *Red Book* for guidance regarding immunization practices in HIV-infected children.[17]

CHALLENGES TO ELIMINATION OF PERINATAL HUMAN IMMUNODEFICIENCY VIRUS TRANSMISSION IN THE UNITED STATES

Despite significant advances in perinatal HIV prevention, approximately 150 HIV-infected babies are now born annually in the United States, primarily because of missed opportunities to implement effective interventions.[18,24] Reported barriers to elimination of MTCT include inadequate prenatal care, especially in women with substance abuse, lack of antenatal HIV testing, acquisition of new infection in women later in pregnancy and during breastfeeding, and poor maternal adherence to ART during pregnancy.[9,13,726]

Knowledge of a woman's HIV status during labor is crucial for providing ARV prophylaxis for those who test positive and their HIV-exposed infants, to prevent perinatal transmission.[727] Routine antenatal HIV testing ("opt-out" approach) is recommended for all women as soon as pregnancy is confirmed. To reduce missed prevention opportunities, repeat testing in the third trimester of pregnancy is recommended for high-risk women, to detect new infections as well as rapid HIV testing of women who present in labor with unknown HIV status.[641,642]

Other challenges include preventing new-incident HIV infections in women of childbearing age, especially adolescent girls of minority race or ethnicity, and addressing delayed diagnosis of HIV in some pregnant women.[13] The

CDC has collaborated with four national organizations, forming the National Organizations' Collaborative to Eliminate Perinatal HIV in the United States. Reaching challenging populations of HIV-infected women and investigation of "prophylaxis failures" is crucial to meet the goal of elimination of PMTCT.[43]

WORLD HEALTH ORGANIZATION REVISED GUIDELINES FOR PREVENTION OF MOTHER-TO-CHILD TRANSMISSION

Postnatal transmission of HIV during breastfeeding is a major concern in LMIC, particularly in sub-Saharan Africa, where breastfeeding is the cornerstone of child survival and remains the only feasible, safe, and culturally acceptable infant feeding choice.[38,43,728] Decreasing the duration of breastfeeding by early weaning may reduce postnatal transmission but results in high rates of morbidity and mortality in infants because of malnutrition or infectious diseases.[729] Although exclusive breastfeeding can decrease the risk of postnatal transmission, compared with mixed infant feeding, the risk is not eliminated.[730] Thus development of innovative strategies to make prolonged breastfeeding safer was a crucial priority for LMIC.

In the past few years, there has been remarkable progress in the discovery of effective ARV drug regimens to prevent postnatal transmission of HIV during breastfeeding.[8-11] Randomized trials have shown that triple-drug ART administered to the mother or provision of extended ARV prophylaxis to the infant during breastfeeding can significantly reduce postnatal transmission of HIV.[35,36,728] In 2010, after a review of the available evidence, the WHO published revised PMTCT guidelines recommending provision of lifelong triple-drug ART for HIV-infected pregnant women who require ART for their own health (CD4 count ≤ 350 cells/mm^3 and/or WHO stage 3 or 4 disease).[41]

The recommended regimen for cART includes ZDV plus 3TC plus NVP or EFV; other alternative choices include TDF plus 3TC or FTC plus NVP or TDF plus 3TC or FTC plus EFV. Breastfed infants of HIV-positive women receiving combination ART should receive daily NVP prophylaxis from birth and continued until 6 weeks of age, whereas nonbreastfed HIV-exposed infants should receive daily NVP or ZDV prophylaxis from birth until 6 weeks of age.[41]

For pregnant women who do not require ART for their own health (CD4 count >350 cells/mm^3 and/or WHO stage 1 or 2 disease), the 2010 guidelines offer two prophylaxis options: *Option A*—maternal daily ZDV from 14 weeks of gestation, single–dose NVP and ZDV/3TC during labor and delivery, a 7-day course of ZDV/3TC "tail" postpartum, and daily infant NVP prophylaxis from birth and continued until 1 week after complete cessation of breastfeeding—or *Option B*—maternal triple-drug ARV prophylaxis given to the mother during pregnancy, starting from 14 weeks of gestation and continued until 1 week after complete cessation of breastfeeding, and daily infant NVP or ZDV prophylaxis after birth until 6 weeks of age. The choices of recommended maternal triple-drug ARV regimens include ZDV/3TC plus LPV/r, ZDV/3TC plus ABC, ZDV/3TC plus EFV, or TDF/3TC or FTC plus EFV. HIV-exposed infants who are breastfeeding should receive daily NVP prophylaxis from birth and continued until 6 weeks of age.[41]

In April 2012, the WHO issued guidance for LMIC, describing the programmatic and operational benefits of using a single, universal, lifelong triple ART regimen for HIV-infected pregnant and breastfeeding women, regardless of their CD4 T-lymphocyte counts (Option B+).[40] The rationale for this new guidance is to simplify and harmonize complex PMTCT regimens, enable additional women to access HAART (without CD4 testing), confer additional maternal health benefits, and prevent sexual transmission of HIV to discordant male partners.[40,694] Some countries (e.g., Malawi) have successfully implemented the WHO Option B+ strategy, resulting in a sixfold increase in the number of pregnant and lactating HIV-positive women starting ART.[731]

Despite the enthusiasm and strong advocacy of many international organizations for LMIC to consider implementation of Option B+ approach, many concerns remain, especially those related to ethical, medical, programmatic, and economic issues.[732,733] Suboptimal adherence to ART during pregnancy and postpartum remains a significant problem in LMIC.[734] In a systematic review and meta-analysis of 51 studies involving 20,153 HIV-infected pregnant women, only 73.5% of women achieved optimal ART adherence.[734] In addition, emergence of resistance in HIV-infected infants exposed to ARV prophylaxis for PMTCT is a major concern.[615-617,732] Recent reports have documented high risk of NVP resistance in breastfeeding infants, who become infected after 6 weeks of age, despite receiving extended postnatal NVP prophylaxis.[617]

In 2013, the WHO consolidated guidelines based on scientific evidence and programmatic experience, with the goal of simplifying delivery of ART.[39,735] The 2013 guidelines for ART recommended earlier initiation of ART at CD4 cell counts less than or equal to 500 cells/mm^3 for all adults and children older than 5 years.[39] In addition, based on clinical benefits, programmatic, and prevention considerations, immediate initiation of cART is recommended for all pregnant women, individuals in discordant partnerships, and children younger than 5 years.[39] The rationale for recommending lifelong ART to all pregnant and breastfeeding HIV-infected women is to harmonize with adult guidelines and to link and retain more pregnant women in care and treatment programs.[735]

WORLD HEALTH ORGANIZATION REVISED GUIDELINES FOR INFANT FEEDING

In 2010, the WHO also revised infant feeding guidelines, allowing national governmental authorities and ministries of health to principally counsel and support HIV-infected mothers to breastfeed their infants and receive maternal or infant ARV prophylaxis *or* completely avoid all exposure to breast milk based on the local environmental context (personal, household, and health service), costs, and careful consideration of the expected risk versus benefits of replacement feeding.[736] The revised WHO guidance aims to achieve HIV-free survival among infants as well as increasing maternal life expectancy.[41,736] The revised infant feeding recommendations evolved from several studies that showed that early weaning (at age 6 months or earlier) was associated with increased risk of infant morbidity and mortality among HIV-exposed but infected infants.[729,737,738]

The WHO recommends exclusive breastfeeding for the first 6 months of life in resource-limited settings where breastfeeding is the norm and replacement feeding is not acceptable, feasible, affordable, sustainable, and safe (AFASS). In such instances, complementary foods may be introduced at 6 months, with continued breastfeeding for the first 12 months of life. Weaning must be gradual over a period of 1 month, and maternal or infant ARV prophylaxis must be continued until 1 week after complete cessation of breastfeeding.[736]

Research has shown that heat treatment of expressed breast milk can inactivate HIV and could reduce postnatal transmission of HIV during breastfeeding.[739-741] In 2010, the WHO recommended the use of expressed heat-treated breast milk as an interim feeding strategy in selected circumstances: (1) low-birth-weight or ill infants unable to feed, (2) mothers temporarily unable to breastfeed because of mastitis or other illness, (3) need of assisting mothers to stop breastfeeding, (4) temporary unavailability of ARV drugs.[736]

Future Goals

In 2011, the UNAIDS announced a call for the virtual elimination of new HIV infections among children by 2015.[42] The two overall global targets are (1) to reduce the number of new pediatric HIV infections by 90% by 2015 and (2) to reduce the number of HIV-associated deaths to women during the antepartum, intrapartum, and postpartum periods by 50% in 2015.[42] The targets related to the four prongs of PMTCT are (1) reducing new HIV infections in women aged 15 to 49 years by 50%, (2) reducing the unmet needs for family planning (FP) among HIV-infected women to zero, (3) reducing the risk of MTCT to less than 5%, and (4) providing ART to 90% of eligible HIV-infected women in 2015.[42]

Key strategies to achieve the goal of virtual elimination of MTCT include strengthening maternal and child health systems, instituting high levels of coverage and retention in the PMTCT cascade, and providing for universal access and large-scale implementation of the revised WHO PMTCT guidelines by using decentralized family-centered approaches and strong linkages to HIV care and treatment of infants, their mothers, and families.[742-744] Other important strategies include prevention of new HIV infections in young women and prevention of unintended pregnancy among women living with HIV by strengthening and integrating FP services in HIV service delivery programs.[745,746]

Pharmacovigilance studies are urgently needed to determine long-term ARV drug safety for both mother and infant.[695] Development of a safe and effective vaccine and the use of passive immunization strategies for PMTCT, especially during breastfeeding, remains a top priority for elimination of residual transmission that is not prevented by ARV strategies.[747,748] HIV cure strategies focused on elimination of viral reservoirs through very early cART in neonates is currently being studied.[371,749,750] Rapid translation of scientific discoveries into policy and practice in conjunction with financial and technical resources, political will, country ownership, and accountability are paramount to eliminate new pediatric HIV infection worldwide.

References

1. Piot P, Quinn TC: Response to the AIDS pandemic, *N Engl J Med* 368:2210-2218, 2013.
2. Centers for Disease Control and Prevention: *Pneumocystis* pneumonia—Los Angeles, *MMWR Morb Mortal Wkly Rep* 30:250-252, 1981.
3. Centers for Disease Control and Prevention: Kaposi's sarcoma and *Pneumocystis* pneumonia among homosexual men—New York City and California, *MMWR Morb Mortal Wkly Rep* 30 :305-308, 1981.
4. Centers for Disease Control and Prevention: Unexplained immunodeficiency and opportunistic infections in infants—New York, New Jersey, California, *MMWR Morb Mortal Wkly Rep* 31:665-667, 1982.
5. Ammann AJ, Cowan MJ, Wara DW, et al: Acquired immunodeficiency in an infant: possible transmission by means of blood products, *Lancet* 1:956-958, 1983.
6. Oleske J, Minnefor A, Cooper R Jr, et al: Immune deficiency syndrome in children, *JAMA* 249:2345-2349, 1983.
7. Beyrer C, Karim QA: The changing epidemiology of HIV in 2013, *Curr Opin Infect Dis* 8:306-310, 2013.
8. De Cock KM, Jaffe HW, Curran JW: The evolving epidemiology of HIV/AIDS, *AIDS* 26:1205-1213, 2012.
9. Govender T, Coovadia SH: Eliminating mother-to-child HIV transmission and keeping mothers alive: recent progress, *J Infect* 68: S57-S62, 2014.
10. Sohn AH, Hazra R: The changing epidemiology of the global paediatric HIV epidemic: keeping track of perinatally HIV-infected adolescents, *J Int AIDS Soc* 167:18555, 2013.
11. Forbes JC, Alimenti AM, Singer J, et al: A national review of vertical HIV transmission, *AIDS* 26:757-763, 2012.
12. Moodley P, Parboosing R, Moodley D: Reduction in perinatal HIV infections in Kwazulu-Natal, South Africa in the era of more effective prevention of mother to child transmission interventions (2004-2012), *J Acquir Immune Defic Syndr* 63:410-415, 2013.
13. Fowler MG, Gable AR, Lampe MA, et al: Perinatal HIV and its prevention: progress towards an HIV-free generation, *Clin Perinatol* 37:699-719, 2010.
14. Selik RM, Ward JW, Buehler JW: Trends in transfusion-associated acquired immune deficiency syndrome in the United States, 1982 through 1991, *Transfusion* 33:890-893, 1993.
15. Jones DS, Perez-Padilla R, del-Rio C, et al: Epidemiology of transfusion-associated acquired immune deficiency syndrome in the United States, 1981 through 1998, *Pediatrics* 89:123-127, 1992.
16. Schreiber GB, Busch MP, Kleinman SH, et al: The risk of transfusion-transmitted viral infections, *N Engl J Med* 334:1685-1690, 1996.
17. American Academy of Pediatrics: Human immunodeficiency virus infection. In Pickering LK, Baker CJ, Kimberlin DW, et al: *Red book*, ed 28, Elk Grove Village, Ill, 2012, American Academy of Pediatrics, pp 418-437.
18. Nesheim S, Taylor A, Lampe MA, et al: A framework for elimination of perinatal HIV infection in the United States, *Pediatrics* 130: 738-744, 2012.
19. Townsend CL, Cortina-Borja M, Peckham CS, et al: Low rates of mother-to-child transmission of HIV following effective pregnancy interventions in the United Kingdom and Ireland, 2000-2006, *AIDS* 22:973-981, 2008.
20. Cooper ER, Charurat M, Mofenson L, et al: Combination antiretroviral strategies for the treatment of pregnant HIV-1 infected women and prevention of perinatal HIV-1 transmission, *J Acquir Immune Defic Syndr Hum Retroviral* 29:484-494, 2002.
21. Read JS: Prevention of mother-to-child transmission of HIV: antiretroviral strategies, *Clin Perinatol* 37:765-776, 2010.
22. Panel on Treatment of HIV-Infected Pregnant Women and Prevention of Perinatal Transmission: Recommendations for use of antiretroviral drugs in pregnant HIV-1 infected women for maternal health and interventions to reduce perinatal HIV transmission in the United States, 2013. Available at http://aidsinfo.nih.gov/contentfiles/lvguidelines/PerinatalGL.pdf. Accessed August 2, 2013.
23. Kelly Paul CE, Paul SM, Vali FM, et al: Towards elimination of perinatal HIV transmission: New Jersey hospital barriers to rapid HIV testing in labor and delivery, 2005, *Public Health Rep* 126:145-152, 2011.
24. Whitmore SK, Taylor AW, Espinoza L, et al: Correlates of mother-to-child transmission of HIV in the United States and Puerto Rico, *Pediatrics* 129:e74-e81, 2012.

25. Hazra R, Siberry GK, Mofenson LM: Growing up with HIV: children, adolescents and young adults with perinatally acquired HIV infection, *Annu Rev Med* 61:169-185, 2010.
26. Brady MT, Oleske JM, Williams PL, et al: Decline in mortality rates and changes in causes of death in HIV-1 infected children during the HAART era, *J Acquir Immune Defic Syndr* 53:86-94, 2010.
27. Kapogiannis BG, Soe MM, Nesheim SR, et al: Mortality trends in the US perinatal AIDS collaborative transmission study (1986-2004), *Clin Infect Dis* 53:1024-1034, 2011.
28. Gona P, Van Dyke RB, Williams PL, et al: Incidence of opportunistic and other infections in HIV-infected children in the HAART era, *JAMA* 296:292-300, 2006.
29. Mofenson LM, Cotton MF: The challenges of success: adolescents with perinatal HIV infection, *J Int AIDS Soc* 16:18650, 2013.
30. Patel K, Hernán MA, Williams PL, et al: Long-term effectiveness of highly active antiretroviral therapy on the survival of children and adolescents with HIV infection: a 10-year follow-up study, *Clin Infect Dis* 46:507-515, 2008.
31. Joint United Nations Program on HIV/AIDS (UNAIDS): Global HIV/AIDS response: epidemic update and health sector progress towards universal access, Geneva, 2011, UNAIDS, July 29, 2013. Available at http://whqlibdoc.who.int/publications/2011/9789241502986_eng.pdf. Accessed July 30, 2013.
32. Becquet R, Dabis F: Turning the tide on HIV in women and children: preventing breast-milk HIV transmission while increasing maternal life expectancy, *Clin Infect Dis* 56:140-142, 2012.
33. McIntyre J: Use of antiretrovirals during pregnancy and breastfeeding in low-income and middle-income countries, *Curr Opin HIV AIDS* 5:48-53, 2010.
34. DeCock KM, Fowler MG, Mercier E, et al: Prevention of mother-to-child HIV transmission in resource-poor countries: translating research into policy and practice, *JAMA* 283:1175-1182, 2000.
35. Mofenson LM: Antiretroviral drugs to prevent breastfeeding HIV transmission, *Antivir Ther* 15:537-553, 2010.
36. Kourtis AP, de Vincenzi I, Jamieson DJ, et al: Antiretroviral drugs during breastfeeding for the prevention of postnatal transmission of HIV-1, *Adv Exp Med Biol* 743:173-183, 2012.
37. Bulterys M, Ellington S, Kourtis AP: HIV-1 and breastfeeding: biology of transmission and advances in prevention, *Clin Perinatol* 37:807-824, 2010.
38. Fowler MG, Kourtis AP, Aizire J, et al: Breastfeeding and transmission of HIV-1: epidemiology and global magnitude, *Adv Exp Med Biol* 743:3-25, 2012.
39. World Health Organization: Consolidated guidelines on the use of antiretroviral drugs for treating and preventing HIV infection. Recommendations for a public health approach, Geneva, 2013, World Health Organization. Available at http://www.who.int/hiv/pub/guidelines/arv2013/download/en/index.html. Accessed July 31, 2013.
40. World Health Organization: Programmatic update: use of antiretroviral drugs for treating pregnant women and preventing HIV infection in infants—executive summary, Geneva, 2012, World Health Organization. Available at http://www.who.int/hiv/pub/mtct/programmatic_update2012/en/index.html. Accessed July 25, 2013.
41. World Health Organization: Antiretroviral drugs for treating pregnant women and preventing HIV infections in infants: recommendations for a public health approach, 2010 version, Geneva, 2010, World Health Organization. Available at http://www.who.int/hiv/pub/mtct/guidelines/en/. Accessed July 25, 2012.
42. Joint United Nations Program on HIV/AIDS (UNAIDS): Global plan towards the elimination of new HIV infections among children by 2015 and keeping their mothers alive, 2011-2015, July 28, 2013. Available at http://www.unaids.org/en/media/unaids/contentassets/documents/unaidspublication/2011/20110609_jc2137_global-plan-elimination-hiv-children_en.pdf. Accessed July 30, 2013.
43. Mofenson LM: Prevention of mother-to-child HIV transmission: can we meet the goal of global elimination of new pediatric infections? *Curr Opin HIV AIDS* 8:443-446, 2013.
44. Abrams EJ, Myer L: Can we achieve an AIDS-free generation? Perspectives on the global campaign to eliminate new pediatric infections, *J Acquir Immune Defic Syndr* 63:S208-S212, 2013.
45. Mofenson LM: Protecting the next generation: eliminating perinatal HIV-1 infection, *N Engl J Med* 362:2316-2318, 2010.
46. Joint United Nations Program on HIV/AIDS (UNAIDS): UNAIDS 2012 report on the global AIDS epidemic, Geneva. Available at http://www.unaids.org/en/media/unaids/contentassets/documents/epidemiology/2012/gr2012/20121120_unaids_global_report_2012_with_annexes_en.pdf. Accessed July 30, 2013.
47. Joint United Nations Program on HIV/AIDS (UNAIDS): UNAIDS 2012. Together we will end AIDS, Geneva. Available at http://www.unaids.org/en/media/unaids/contentassets/documents/epidemiology/20122/20120718_togetherwewillendaids_en.pdf. Accessed July 30, 2013.
48. Joint United Nations Program on HIV/AIDS (UNAIDS): UNAIDS 2012 World AIDS Day report, Geneva. Available at http://www.unaids.org/en/media/unaids/contentassets/documents/epidemiology/2012/gr2012/jc2434_worldaidsday_results_en.pdf. Accessed July 30, 2013.
49. Fauci AS, Folkers GK: Towards an AIDS-free generation, *JAMA* 308:343-344, 2012.
50. Reynolds SJ, Quinn TC: Setting the stage: current state of affairs and major challenges, *Clin Infect Dis* 50(Suppl 3):S71-S76, 2010.
51. Karim QA, Sibeko S, Baxter C: Preventing HIV infection in women: a global health imperative, *Clin Infect Dis* 50(Suppl 3):S122-S129, 2010.
52. Newell ML, Coovadia H, Cortina-Borja M, et al: Mortality of infected and uninfected infants born to HIV-infected mothers in Africa: a pooled analysis, *Lancet* 364:1236-1243, 2004.
53. Becquet R, Marston M, Dabis F, et al: Children who acquire HIV infection perinatally are at higher risk of early death than those acquiring infection through breast milk: a meta-analysis, *PLoS One* 7:28510, 2012.
54. Centers for Disease Control and Prevention, HIV surveillance report, 2011, Atlanta, February 23, 2013. Available at http://www.cdc.gov/hiv/topics/surveillance/resources/reports. Accessed July 30, 2013.
55. Centers for Disease Control and Prevention: Estimated HIV incidence among adults and adolescents in the United States, 2007-2010, *HIV Surveill Suppl Rep* 17(No 4), 2012. Available at http://www.cdc.gov/hiv/topics/surveillance/resources/reports/#supplemental. Accessed July 28, 2013.
56. Centers for Disease Control and Prevention: HIV surveillance—United States, 1981-2008, *MMWR Morb Mortal Wkly Rep* 60:689-693, 2011.
57. Prejean J, Song R, Hernandez A, et al: Estimated HIV incidence in the United States, 2006–2009, *PLoS One* 6:e17502, 2011.
58. Centers for Disease Control and Prevention: Fact sheet: estimates of new HIV infections in the United States, 2007–2010; December 2012. Available at http://www.cdc.gov/nchhstp/newsroom/docs/2012/hiv-infections-2007-2010.pdf. Accessed July 30, 2013.
59. Aral SO, Adimora AA, Fenton KA: Understanding and responding to the HIV and other sexually transmitted infections in African Americans, *Lancet* 372:337-340, 2008.
60. Centers for Disease Control and Prevention: HIV surveillance report, 22 Atlanta, 2010. Available at http://www.cdc.gov/hiv/topics/surveillance/resources/reports/. Accessed July 30, 2013.
61. CentersforDiseaseControlandPrevention.Factsheet:HIVamongpregnant women, infants, and children in the United States, 2007–2010, December 2012. Available at http://www.cdc.gov/hiv/pdf/risk_WIC.pdf. Accessed July 30, 2013.
62. Taylor AW, Zhang X, Whitmore SK, et al: Estimated number of perinatal HIV infections in the United States, 2005–2009. In *Programs and abstracts of the National HIV Prevention Conference 2009*, Atlanta, August 23–29, 2009; Abstract 109M.
63. Centers for Disease Control and Prevention: Racial/ethnic disparities among children with diagnoses of perinatal HIV infection—34 states, 2004–2007, *MMWR Morb Mortal Wkly Rep* 59:97-101, 2010.
64. Lindegren ML, Steinberg S, Byers RH Jr: Epidemiology of HIV/AIDS in children, *Pediatr Clin N Am* 47:1-20, 2000.
65. Centers for Disease Control and Prevention, HIV surveillance report, 20, 2008, Atlanta. Available at http://www.cdc.gov/hiv/topics/surveillance/resources/reports/. Published June 2010. Accessed July 30, 2013.
66. Farrow JA, Schwartz RH, Vanderleeuw J: Tatooing behavior in adolescents: a comparison study, *Am J Dis Child* 145:184-187, 1991.
67. Reed J: Epidemiology and prevention of HIV infection in children and adolescents. In Long SS, Pickering LK, Prober CG, editors: *Principles and practice of pediatric infectious diseases*, ed 4, Philadelphia, 2012, Elsevier, pp 641-648.

68. Gaur AH, Dominguez KL, Kalish ML, et al: Practice of feeding premasticated food to infants: a potential risk factor for HIV transmission, *Pediatrics* 124:658-666, 2010.
69. Centers for Disease Control and Prevention: Human immunodeficiency virus transmission in household settings—United States, *MMWR Mor Mortal Wkly Rep* 43:353-356, 2004.
70. Kourtis AP, Bulterys M: Mother-to-child transmission of HIV-1: pathogenesis, mechanisms and pathways, *Clin Perinatol* 37: 721-738, 2010.
71. Kourtis AP, Lee FK, Abrams EJ, et al: Mother-to-child transmission of HIV-1: timing and implications for prevention, *Lancet Infect Dis* 6:726-732, 2006.
72. Working Group on Mother-to-Child Transmission of HIV: Rates of mother-to-child transmission of HIV-1 in Africa, America, and Europe: results from 13 perinatal studies, *J Acquir Immune Defic Syndr Hum Retrovirol* 8:506-510, 1995.
73. The European Collaborative Study: Vertical transmission of HIV-1: maternal immune status and obstetric factors, *AIDS* 10:1675-1681, 1996.
74. Simonon A, Lepage P, Karita E, et al: An assessment of the timing of mother-to child transmission of human immunodeficiency virus type 1 by means of polymerase chain reaction, *J Acquir Immune Defic Syndr* 7:952-957, 1994.
75. Bryson YJ, Luzuriaga K, Sullivan JL, et al: Proposed definitions for in utero versus intrapartum transmission of HIV-1, *N Engl J Med* 327:1246-1247, 1992.
76. Sprecher S, Soumenkoff G, Puissant F, et al: Vertical transmission of HIV in 15-week fetus, *Lancet* 2:288-289, 1986.
77. Jovaisas E, Koch MA, Schäfer A, et al: 1985 LAV/HTLV-III in 20-week fetus, *Lancet* 2:1129, 1985.
78. Mano H, Chermann JC: Fetal human immunodeficiency virus type 1 infection of different organs in the second trimester, *AIDS Res Hum Retroviruses* 7:83-88, 1991.
79. Mundy DC, Schinazi RF, Gerber AR, et al: Human immunodeficiency virus isolated from amniotic fluid, *Lancet* 2:459-460, 1987.
80. Lewis SH, Reynolds-Kohler C, Fox HE, et al: HIV-1 in trophoblastic and villous Hofbauer cells, and haematological precursors in eight-week fetuses, *Lancet* 335:565-568, 1990.
81. Amirhessami-Aghili N, Spector SA: Human immunodeficiency virus type 1 infection of human placenta: potential route for fetal infection, *J Virol* 65:2231-2236, 1991.
82. Zachar V, Thomas RA, Jones T, et al: Vertical transmission of HIV: detection of proviral DNA in placental trophoblasts, *AIDS* 8: 129-130, 1994.
83. Brossard Y, Aubin JT, Mandelbrot L, et al: Frequency of early in utero HIV-1 infection: a blind DNA polymerase chain reaction study on 100 fetal thymuses, *AIDS* 9:359-366, 1995.
84. Van Dyke RB, Korber BT, Popek E, et al: The Ariel Project: a prospective cohort study of maternal-child transmission of human immunodeficiency virus type 1 in the era of maternal antiretroviral therapy, *J Infect Dis* 179:319-328, 1999.
85. Mattern CFT, Murray K, Jensen A, et al: Localization of human immunodeficiency virus core antigen in term human placentas, *Pediatrics* 89:207-209, 1992.
86. Newell ML: Mechanisms and timing of mother-to-child transmission of HIV-1, *AIDS* 12:831-837, 1998.
87. Kaneda T, Shiraki K, Hirano K, et al: Detection of maternofetal transfusion by placental alkaline phosphatase levels, *J Pediatr* 130: 730-735, 1997.
88. Krivine A, Yakudima A, Le May M, et al: A comparative study of virus isolation, polymerase chain reaction, and antigen detection in children of mothers infected with human immunodeficiency virus, *J Pediatr* 116:372-376, 1990.
89. Rogers MF, Ou CY, Rayfield M, et al: Use of the polymerase chain reaction for early detection of the proviral sequences of human immunodeficiency virus in infants born to seropositive mothers, *N Engl J Med* 320:1649-1654, 1989.
90. Weiblen BJ, Lee FK, Cooper ER, et al: Early diagnosis of HIV infection in infants by detection of IgA HIV antibodies, *Lancet* 335:988-990, 1990.
91. Quinn TC, Kline RL, Halsey N, et al: Early diagnosis of perinatal HIV infection by detection of viral-specific IgA antibodies, *JAMA* 266:3439-3942, 1991.
92. Krivine A, Firtion G, Cao L, et al: HIV replication during the first weeks of life, *Lancet* 339:1187-1189, 1992.
93. Rouzioux C, Costagliola D, Burgard M, et al: Estimated timing of mother-to-child human immunodeficiency virus type 1 (HIV-1) transmission by use of a Markov model. The HIV Infection in Newborns French Collaborative Study Group, *Am J Epidemiol* 142: 1330-1337, 1995.
94. Goedert JJ, Duliège AM, Amos CI, et al: High risk of HIV-1 infection for firstborn twins, *Lancet* 338:1471-1475, 1991.
95. European Mode of Delivery Collaboration: Elective caesarean-section versus vaginal delivery in prevention of vertical HIV-1 transmission: a randomised clinical trial, *Lancet* 353:1035-1039, 1999.
96. The International Perinatal HIV Group: The mode of delivery and the risk of vertical transmission of human immunodeficiency virus type 1—a meta-analysis of 15 prospective cohort studies, *N Engl J Med* 340:977-987, 1999.
97. Boer K, England K, Godfried MH, Thorne C: Mode of delivery in HIV-infected pregnant women and prevention of mother-to-child transmission: changing practices in Western Europe, *HIV Med* 11:368-378, 2010.
98. Brahmbhatt H, Sullivan D, Kigozi G, et al: Association of HIV and malaria with mother-to-child transmission, birth outcomes, and child mortality, *J Acquir Immune Defic Syndr* 47:472-476, 2008.
99. Inion I, Mwanyumba F, Gaillard P, et al: Placental malaria and perinatal transmission of human immunodeficiency virus type 1, *J Infect Dis* 188:1675-1678, 2003.
100. Garcia PM, Kalish LA, Pitt J, et al: Maternal levels of plasma human immunodeficiency virus type 1 RNA and the risk of perinatal transmission. Women and Infants Transmission Study Group, *N Engl J Med* 341:394-402, 1999.
101. Mofenson LM, Lambert JS, Stiehm ER, et al: Risk factors for perinatal transmission of human immunodeficiency virus type 1 in women treated with zidovudine, *N Engl J Med* 341:385-393, 1999.
102. Magder LS, Mofenson L, Paul ME, et al: Risk factors for in utero and intrapartum transmission of HIV, *J Acquir Immune Defic Syndr* 38: 87-95, 2005.
103. Ioannidis JP, Abrams EJ, Ammann A, et al: Perinatal transmission of human immunodeficiency virus type 1 by pregnant women with RNA virus loads < 1000 copies/ml, *J Infect Dis* 183:539-545, 2001.
104. St Louis ME, Kamenga M, Brown C, et al: Risk for perinatal HIV-1 transmission according to maternal immunologic, virologic, and placental factors, *JAMA* 269:2853-2859, 1993.
105. Sperling RS, Shapiro DE, Coombs RW, et al: Maternal viral load, zidovudine treatment, and the risk of transmission of human immunodeficiency virus type 1 from mother to infant. Pediatric AIDS Clinical Trials Group Protocol 076 Study Group, *N Engl J Med* 335: 1621-1629, 1996.
106. Newell ML, Peckham C: Risk factors for vertical transmission of HIV-1 and early markers of HIV-1 infection in children, *AIDS* 7(Suppl 1):S591-S597, 1993.
107. Magder LS, Mofenson L, Paul ME, et al: Risk factors for in utero and intrapartum transmission of HIV, *J Acquir Immune Defic Syndr* 38: 87-95, 2005.
108. Mayers MM, Davenny K, Schoenbaum EE, et al: A prospective study of infants of human immunodeficiency virus seropositive and seronegative women with a history of intravenous drug use or of intravenous drug-using sex partners, in the Bronx, New York City, *Pediatrics* 88:1248-1256, 1991.
109. European Collaborative Study: Risk factors for mother-to-child transmission of HIV-1, *Lancet* 339:1007-1012, 1992.
110. Chuachoowong R, Shaffer N, Siriwasin W, et al: Short-course antenatal zidovudine reduces both cervicovaginal human immunodeficiency virus type 1 RNA levels and risk of perinatal transmission. Bangkok Collaborative Perinatal HIV Transmission Study Group, *J Infect Dis* 181:99-106, 2000.
111. Mepham SO, Bland RM, Newell ML: Prevention of mother-to-child transmission of HIV in resource-rich and -poor settings, *BJOG* 118:202-218, 2011.
112. Cowan FM, Humphrey JH, Ntozini R, et al: Maternal herpes simplex virus type 2 infection, syphilis and risk of intra-partum transmission of HIV-1: results of a case control study, *AIDS* 22:193-201, 2008.
113. England K, Thorne C, Newell M: Vertically acquired paediatric coinfection with HIV and hepatitis C virus, *Lancet* 6:83-90, 2006.
114. Vogler MA, Singh R, Wright R: Complex decisions in managing HIV infection during pregnancy, *Curr HIV/AIDS Rep* 8:122-131, 2011.

115. Galli L, Puliti D, Chiappini E, et al: Is the interruption of antiretroviral treatment during pregnancy an additional major risk factor for mother-to-child transmission of HIV type 1? *Clin Infect Dis* 48:1310-1317, 2009.
116. Landesman SH, Kalish LA, Burns DN, et al: Obstetrical factors and the transmission of human immunodeficiency virus type 1 from mother-to-child, *N Engl J Med* 334:1617-1623, 1996.
117. European Collaborative Study: Vertical transmission of HIV-1: maternal immune status and obstetric factors, *AIDS* 10:1675-1681, 1996.
118. Tovo PA, de Martino M, Gabiano C, et al: Mode of delivery and gestational age influence perinatal HIV-1 transmission, *J Acquir Immune Defic Syndr Hum Retrovirol* 11:88-94, 1996.
119. Freguja R, Gianesin K, Zanchetta M, et al: Cross-talk between virus and host innate immunity in pediatric HIV-1 infection and disease progression, *New Microbiol* 35:249-257, 2012.
120. Wolinsky SM, Wike CM, Korber BT, et al: Selective transmission of human immunodeficiency virus type-1 variants from mothers to infants, *Science* 255:1134-1137, 1992.
121. Kishko M, Somasundaran M, Brewster F, et al: Genotypic and functional properties of early infant HIV-1 envelopes, *Retrovirology* 8:67, 2011.
122. Renjifo B, Gilbert P, Chaplin B, et al: Preferential in-utero transmission of HIV-1 subtype C as compared to HIV-1 subtype A or D, *AIDS* 18:1629-1636, 2004.
123. Mackelprang RD, John-Stewart G, Carrington M, et al: Maternal HLA homozygosity and mother-child HLA concordance increase the risk of vertical transmission of HIV-1, *J Infect Dis* 197:1156-1161, 2008.
124. Contopoulos-Ioannidis DG, O'Brien TR, Goedert JJ, et al: Effect of CCR5-delta32 heterozygosity on the risk of perinatal HIV-1 infection: a meta-analysis, *J Acquir Immune Defic Syndr* 32:70-76, 2003.
125. Kuhn L, Sinkala M, Kankasa C, et al: High uptake of exclusive breastfeeding and reduced early post-natal HIV transmission, *PLoS One* 2:e1363, 2007.
126. Coutsoudis A, Dabis F, Fawzi W, et al: Late postnatal transmission of HIV-1 in breast-fed children: an individual patient data meta-analysis, *J Infect Dis* 189:2154-2166, 2004.
127. Nduati R, John G, Mbori-Ngacha D, et al: Effect of breastfeeding and formula feeding on transmission of HIV-1: a randomized controlled trial, *JAMA* 283:1167-1174, 2000.
128. Moodley D, Moodley J, Coovadia H, et al: South African Intrapartum Nevirapine Trial (SAINT) investigators. A multicenter randomized controlled trial of nevirapine versus a combination of zidovudine and lamivudine to reduce intrapartum and early postpartum mother-to-child transmission of human immunodefiency virus type 1, *J Infect Dis* 187:725-735, 2003.
129. Humphrey JH, Marinda E, Mutasa K, et al: ZVITAMBO Study Group. Mother to child transmission of HIV among Zimbabwean women who seroconverted postnatally: prospective cohort study, *BMJ* 341:c6580, 2010.
130. Lockman S, Creek T: Acute maternal HIV infection during pregnancy and breastfeeding: substantial risk to infants, *J Infect Dis* 200:667-689, 2009.
131. John GC, Nduati RW, Mbori-Ngacha DA, et al: Correlates of mother-to-child human immunodeficiency virus type 1 (HIV-1) transmission: association with maternal plasma HIV-1 RNA load, genital HIV-1 DNA shedding, and breast infections, *J Infect Dis* 183:206-212, 2001.
132. Jamieson DJ, Sibailly TS, Sadek R, et al: HIV-1 viral load and other risk factors for mother-to-child transmission of HIV-1 in a breastfeeding population in Côte d'Ivoire, *J Acquir Immune Defic Syndr* 34:430-436, 2003.
133. Shetty AK, Maldonado Y: Antiretroviral drugs to prevent mother-to-child transmission of HIV during breastfeeding, *Curr HIV Res* 11:102-125, 2013.
134. Mmiro FA, Aizire J, Mwatha AK, et al: Predictors of early and late mother-to-child transmission of HIV-1 in a breastfeeding population: HIV-1 network for prevention trials 012 experience, Kampala, Uganda, *J Acquir Immune Defic Syndr* 52:32-39, 2009.
135. Semba RD, Kumwenda N, Hoover DR, et al: Human immunodeficiency virus load in breast milk, mastitis, and mother-to-child transmission of human immunodeficiency virus type 1, *J Infect Dis* 180:93-98, 1999.
136. Coutsoudis A, Pillay K, Spooner E, et al: Influence of infant-feeding patterns on early mother-to-child transmission of HIV-1 in Durban, South Africa: a prospective cohort study. South African Vitamin A Study Group, *Lancet* 354:471-476, 1999.
137. Iliff PJ, Piwoz EG, Tavengwa NV, et al: Early exclusive breastfeeding reduces the risk of postnatal HIV-1 transmission and increases HIV-1-free survival, *AIDS* 19:699-708, 2005.
138. Cournil A, De Vincenzi I, Gaillard P, et al: Kesho Bora Study Group. Relationship between mortality and feeding modality among children born to HIV-infected mothers in a research setting: the Kesho Bora Study, *AIDS* 27:1621-1630, 2013.
139. Homsy J, Moore D, Barasa A, et al: Breastfeeding, mother-to-child HIV transmission, and mortality among infants born to HIV-infected women on highly active antiretroviral therapy in rural Uganda, *J Acquir Immune Defic Syndr* 53:28-35, 2010.
140. Kafulafula G, Hoover DR, Taha TE, et al: Frequency of gastroenteritis and gastroenteritis associated mortality with early weaning in HIV-1-uninfected children born to HIV-infected women in Malawi, *J Acquir Immune Defic Syndr* 53:6-13, 2010.
141. Rousseau CM, Nduati RW, Richardson BA, et al: Longitudinal analysis of human immunodeficiency virus type 1 RNA in breast milk and of its relationship to infant infection and maternal disease, *J Infect Dis* 187:741-747, 2003.
142. Lewis P, Nduati R, Kreiss JK, et al: Cell-free HIV type 1 in breast milk, *J Infect Dis* 177:34-39, 1998.
143. Koulinska IN, Villamor E, Chaplin B, et al: Transmission of cell-free and cell-associated HIV-1 through breastfeeding, *J Acquir Immune Defic Syndr* 41:93-99, 2006.
144. Slyker JA, Chung MH, Lehman DA, et al: Incidence and correlates of HIV-1 RNA detection in the breast milk of women receiving HAART for the prevention of HIV-1 transmission, *PLoS One* 7:e29777, 2012.
145. Willumsen JF, Newell ML, Filteau SM, et al: Variation in breastmilk HIV-1 viral load in left and right breasts during the first 3 months of lactation, *AIDS* 15:1896-1898, 2001.
146. Tobin NH, Aldrovandi GM: Immunology of pediatric HIV infection, *Immunol Rev* 254:143-169, 2013.
147. Da Silva RC, Segat L, Crovella S: Role of DC-SIGN and LC-SIGN receptors in HIV-1 vertical transmission, *Hum Immunol* 72:305-311, 2011.
148. Aldrovandi GM, Kuhn L: What infants and breasts teach us about natural protection from HIV infection, *J Infect Dis* 202(Suppl 3):S366-S370, 2010.
149. Van de Peere P, Rubbo PA, Viljoen J, et al: HIV-1 reservoirs in breast milk and challenges to elimination of breast-feeding transmission of HIV, *Sci Transl Med* 18:143sr3, 2012.
150. Boily-Larouche G, Milev MP, Zijenah LS, et al: Naturally-ocurring genetic variants in human DC-SIGN increase HIV-1 capture, cell-transfer and risk of mother-to-child transmission, *PLoS One* 7:e40706, 2012.
151. Mold JE, Michaëlsson J, Burt TD, et al: Maternal alloantigens promote the development of tolerogenic fetal regulatory T cells in utero, *Science* 322:1562-1565, 2008.
152. Flanagan KL, Halliday A, Burl S, et al: The effect of placental malaria infection on cord blood and maternal immunoregulatory responses at birth, *Eur J Immunol* 40:1062-1072, 2010.
153. Legrand FA, Nixon DF, Loo CP, et al: Strong HIV-1-specific T-cell responses in HIV-1 exposed uninfected infants and neonates revealed after regulatory T-cell removal, *PLoS One* 1:e102, 2006.
154. Kumar SB, Rice CE, Milner DA Jr, et al: Elevated cytokine and chemokine levels in the placenta are associated with in-utero HIV-1 mother-to-child transmission, *AIDS* 26:685-694, 2012.
155. Bunders MJ, van der Loos CM, Klarenbeek PL, et al: Memory CD4(+) CCR5(+) T cells are abundantly present in the gut of newborn infants to facilitate mother-to-child transmission of HIV-1, *Blood* 120:4383-4390, 2012.
156. Steiner K l, Malhotra I, Mungai PL, et al: In utero activation of fetal memory T cells alters host regulatory gene expression and affects HIV susceptibility, *Virology* 425:23-30, 2012.
157. Johnson EL, Chakraborty R: Placental Hofbauer cells limit HIV-1 replication and potentially offset mother to child transmission (MTCT) by induction of immunoregulatory cytokines, *Retrovirology* 9:101, 2012.
158. Joubert BR, Franceschini N, Mwapasa V, et al: Regulation of CCR5 expression in human placenta: insights from a study of mother-to-child transmission of HIV in Malawi, *PLoS One* 5:e9212, 2010.
159. Mandelbrot L, Burgard M, Teglas JP, et al: Frequent detection of HIV-1 in the gut aspirates of neonates born to HIV-infected mothers, *AIDS* 13:2143-2149, 1999.

160. Stiehm ER, Lambert JS, Mofenson LM, et al: Efficacy of zidovudine and human immunodeficiency virus (HIV) hyperimmune immunoglobulin for reducing perinatal HIV transmission from HIV-infected women with advanced disease: results of a pediatric AIDS Clinical Trials Group protocol 185, *J Infect Dis* 179:567-575, 1999.
161. Ng CT, Jaworski JP, Jayaraman P, et al: Passive neutralizing antibody controls SHIV viremia and enhances B cell responses in infant macaques, *Nat Med* 16:1117-1119, 2010.
162. Hessell AJ, Poignard P, Hunter M, et al: Effective, low-titer antibody protection against low-dose repeated mucosal SHIV challenge in macaques, *Nat Med* 15:951-954, 2009.
163. Kourtis AP, Butera S, Ibegbu C, et al: Breast milk and HIV-1: vector of transmission or vehicle of protection? *Lancet Infect Dis* 3: 786-793, 2003.
164. Toniolo A, Serra C, Conaldi PG, et al: Productive HIV-1 infection of normal human mammary epithelial cells, *AIDS* 9:859-866, 1995.
165. Richardson BA, John-Stewart GC, Hughes JP, et al: Breast-milk infectivity in human immunodeficiency virus type 1-infected mothers, *J Infect Dis* 187:736-740, 2003.
166. Bulterys M, Chao A, Dushimimana A, et al: HIV-1 seroconversion after 20 months of age in a cohort of breastfed children born to HIV-1-infected women in Rwanda, *AIDS* 9:93-94, 1995.
167. Shapiro RL, Ndung'u T, Lockman S, et al: Highly active antiretroviral therapy started during pregnancy or postpartum suppresses HIV-1 RNA, but not DNA, in breast milk, *J Infect Dis* 192:713-719, 2005.
168. Ndirangu J, Viljoen J, Bland RM, et al: Cell-free (RNA) and cell-associated (DNA) HIV-1 and postnatal transmission through breastfeeding, *PLoS One* 7:e51493, 2012.
169. Kantarci S, Koulinska IN, Aboud S, et al: Subclinical mastitis, cell-associated HIV-1 shedding in breast milk, and breast-feeding transmission of HIV, *J Acquir Immune Defic Syndr* 46:651-654, 2007.
170. Walter J, Kuhn L, Aldrovandi GM: Advances in basic science understanding of mother-to-child HIV-1 transmission, *Curr Opin HIV AIDS* 3:146-150, 2008.
171. Gantt S, Shetty AK, Seidel KD, et al: Laboratory indicators of mastitis are not associated with elevated HIV-1 DNA loads or predictive of HIV-1 RNA loads in breast milk, *J Infect Dis* 196:570-576, 2007.
172. Salazar-Gonzalez JF, Salazar MG, Learn GH, et al: Origin and evolution of HIV-1 in breast milk determined by single-genome amplification and sequencing, *J Virol* 85:2751-2763, 2011.
173. Gray RR, Salemi M, Lowe A, et al: Multiple independent lineages of HIV-1 persist in breast milk and plasma, *AIDS* 25:143-152, 2011.
174. Heath L, Conway S, Jones L, et al: Restriction of HIV-1 genotypes in breast milk does not account for the population transmission genetic bottleneck that occurs following transmission, *PLoS One* 5:e10213, 2010.
175. Gantt S, Carlsson J, Heath L, et al: Genetic analysis of HIV-1 env sequences demonstrate limited compartmentalization in breast milk and suggest viral replication within the breast that increases with mastitis, *J Virol* 84:10812-10819, 2010.
176. Gray L, Fiscus S, Shugars D: HIV-1 variants from a perinatal transmission pair demonstrate similar genetic and replicative properties in tonsillar tissues and peripheral blood mononuclear cells, *AIDS Res Human Retroviruses* 23:1095-1104, 2007.
177. Van De Perre P: Mother-to-child transmission of HIV-1: the "all mucosal" hypothesis as a predominant mechanism of transmission, *AIDS* 13:1133-1138, 1999.
178. Meng G, Wei X, Wu X, et al: Primary intestinal epithelial cells selectively transfer R5 HIV-1 to CCR5+ cells, *Nat Med* 8:150-156, 2002.
179. Kourtis AP, Jamieson DJ, de Vincenzi I, et al: Prevention of human immunodeficiency virus-1 transmission to the infant through breastfeeding: new developments, *Am J Obstet Gynecol* 197(Suppl 3): S113-S122, 2007.
180. Tugizow SM, Herrera R, Veluppillai P, et al: Differential transmission of HIV traversing fetal oral/intestinal epithelia and adult oral epithelia, *J Virol* 86:2556-2570, 2012.
181. Belyakov IM, Berzofsky JA: Immunobiology of mucosal HIV infection and the basis for development of a new generation of mucosal AIDS vaccines, *Immunity* 20:247-253, 2004.
182. Lepage P, Van de Perre P: The immune system of breast milk: antimicrobial and anti-inflammatory properties, *Adv Exp Med Biol* 743:121-137, 2012.
183. Saeland E, de Jong MA, Nabatov AA, et al: MUC1 in human milk blocks transmission of human immunodeficiency virus from dendritic cells to T cells, *Mol Immunol* 46:2309-2316, 2009.
184. Naarding MA, Dirac AM, Ludwig IS, et al: Bile salt-stimulated lipase from human milk binds DC-SIGN and inhibits human immunodeficiency virus type 1 transfer to CD4+T cells, *Antimicrob Agents Chemother* 50:3367-3374, 2006.
185. Stax MJ, Naarding MA, Tanck MW, et al: Binding of human milk to pathogen receptor DC-SIGN varies with bile salt stimulated lipase (BSSL) gene polymorphism, *PLoS One* 6:e17316, 2011.
186. Villamor E, Koulinska IN, Furtado J, et al: Long-chain n-6 polyunsaturated fatty acids in breast milk decrease the risk of HIV transmission through breastfeeding, *Am J Clin Nutr* 86:682-689, 2007.
187. Bode L, Kuhn L, Kim HY, et al: Human milk oligosaccharide concentration and risk of postnatal transmission of HIV through breastfeeding, *Am J Clin Nutr* 96:831-839, 2012.
188. Kuhn L, Trabattoni D, Kankasa C, et al: Alpha-defensins in the prevention of HIV transmission among breastfed infants, *J Acquir Immune Defic Syndr* 39:138-142, 2005.
189. Arsenault JE, Webb AL, Koulinska IN, et al: Association between breast milk erythropoietin and reduced risk of mother-to-child transmission of HIV, *J Infect Dis* 202:370-373, 2010.
190. Becquart P, Petitjean G, Tabaa YA, et al: Detection of a large T-cell reservoir able to replicate HIV-1 actively in breast milk, *AIDS* 20:1453-1462, 2006.
191. Bélec L, Kourtis AP: B lymphocyte-derived humoral immune defenses in breast milk transmission of the HIV-1, *Adv Exp Med Biol* 743:139-160, 2012.
192. Sabbaj S, Ibegbu CC, Kourtis AP: Cellular immunity in breast milk: implications for postnatal transmission of HIV-1 to the infant, *Adv Exp Med Biol* 743:161-169, 2012.
193. Sabbaj S, Edwards BH, Ghosh MK, et al: Human immunodeficiency virus-specific CD8R T cells in human breast milk, *J Virol* 76: 7365-7373, 2002.
194. Tuaillon E, Valea D, Becquart P, et al: Human milk-derived B cells: a highly activated switched memory cell population primed to secrete antibodies, *J Immunol* 182:7155-7162, 2009.
195. Kong X, West JT, Zhang H, et al: The human immunodeficiency virus type 1 envelope confers higher rates of replicative fitness to perinatally transmitted viruses than to nontransmitted viruses, *J Virol* 82:11609-11618, 2008.
196. Zhang H, Rola M, West JT, et al: Functional properties of the HIV-1 subtype C envelope glycoprotein associated with mother-to-child transmission, *Virology* 400:164-174, 2010.
197. Roux M, McWilliams M, Phillips-Quagliata JM, et al: Origin of IgA-secreting plasma cells in the mammary gland, *J Exp Med* 146: 1311-1322, 1977.
198. Lohman-Payne B, Slyker JA, Moore S, et al: Breast milk cellular HIV-specific interferon γ responses are associated with protection from peripartum HIV transmission, *AIDS* 26:2007-2016, 2012.
199. Farquhar C, Lohman-Payne B, Overbaugh J, et al: Breast milk HIV-1 RNA levels and female sex are associated with HIV-1-specific CD8+ T-cell responses in HIV-1-exposed, uninfected infants in Kenya, *J Infect Dis* 204:1806-1810, 2011.
200. Valea D, Tuaillon E, Al Tabaa Y, et al: CD4+ T cells spontaneously producing human immunodeficiency virus type I in breast milk from women with or without antiretroviral drugs, *Retrovirology* 8:34, 2011.
201. Becquart P, Hocini H, Lévy M, et al: Secretory anti-human immunodeficiency virus (HIV) antibodies in colostrum and breast milk are not a major determinant of the protection of early postnatal transmission of HIV, *J Infect Dis* 181:532-539, 2000.
202. Yu X, Pollock D, Duval M, et al: Neutralization of HIV by milk expressed antibody, *J Acquir Immune Defic Syndr* 62:10-16, 2013.
203. Ganser-Pornillos B, Yeager M, Sundquist WI: The structural biology of HIV assembly, *Curr Opin Struct Biol* 18:1-24, 2008.
204. Engelman A, Cherepanov P: The structural biology of HIV-1: mechanistic and therapeutic insights, *Nat Rev Microbiol* 10:279-290, 2012.
205. Merk A, Subramaniam S: HIV-1 envelope glycoprotein structure, *Curr Opin Struct Biol* 23:268-276, 2013.
206. Sharp PM, Hahn BH: The evolution of HIV-1 and the origin of AIDS, *Phil Trans R Soc B* 365:2487-2494, 2010.
207. Peeters M, Fransen K, Delaporte E, et al: Isolation and characterization of a new chimpanzee lentivirus (simian immunodeficiency virus isolate cpz-ant) from a wild captured chimpanzee, *AIDS* 3:625-630, 1992.
208. Hitsch VM, Olmsted RA, Murphey-Corb M, et al: An African primate lentivirus (SIVsm) closely related to HIV-2, *Nature* 339:389-392, 1989.

209. Lemey P, Pybus OG, Wang B, et al: Tracing the origin and history of the HIV-1 epidemic, *Proc Natl Acad Sci U S A* 100:6588-6592, 2003.
210. Plantier JC, Leoz M, Dickerson JE, et al: A new human immunodeficiency virus derived from gorillas, *Nat Med* 15:871-872, 2009.
211. Robertson DL, Anderson JP, Bradac JA, et al: HIV-1 nomenclature proposal, *Science* 288:55-56, 2000.
212. Hemelaar J, Gouws E, Ghys PD, et al: Global trends in molecular epidemiology of HIV-1 during 2000-2007, *AIDS* 25:679-689, 2011.
213. Kwong PD, Mascola JR, Nabel GJ: The changing face of HIV vaccine research, *J Int AIDS Soc* 15:17407, 2012.
214. Liu J, Bartesaghi A, Borgnia MJ, et al: Molecular architecture of native HIV-1 gp120 trimers, *Nature* 455:109-113, 2008.
215. Checkley MA, Luttge BG, Freed EO: HIV-1 envelope glycoprotein biosynthesis, trafficking, and incorporation, *J Mol Biol* 410:582-608, 2011.
216. Wyatt R, Sodroski J: The HIV-1 envelope glycoproteins: fusogens, antigens, and immunogens, *Science* 280:1884-1888, 1998.
217. Nomaguchi M, Doi N, Matsumoto Y, et al: Species tropism of HIV-1 modulated by viral accessory proteins, *Front Microbiol* 3:1-6, 2013.
218. Wissing SL, Galloway NL, Greene WC: HIV-1 Vif versus the APOBEC3 ctidine deaminases: an intracellular duel between pathogen and host restriction factors, *Mol Aspects Med* 31:383-397, 2010.
219. Neil SJ, Zang T, Bieniasz PD: Tether inhibits retrovirus release and is antagonized by HIV-1 vpu, *Nature* 451:425-430, 2008.
220. Laguette N, Sobhian B, Casartelli N, et al: SAMDH1 is the dendritic- and myeloid-cell-specific HIV-1 restriction factor counteracted by Vpx, *Nature* 474:654-657, 2011.
221. Hrecka K, Hao C, Gierszewska M, et al: Vpx relieves inhibition of HIV-1 infection of macrophages mediated by SAMDH1 protein, *Nature* 474:658-661, 2011.
222. Weiss RA: Thirty years on: HIV receptor gymnastics and the prevention of infection, *BMC Biol* 11:57, 2013.
223. Klasse PJ: The molecular basis of HIV entry, *Cell Microbiol* 14: 1183-1192, 2012.
224. Fauci AS, Pantaleo G, Stanley S, et al: Immunopathogenic mechanisms of HIV infection, *Ann Intern Med* 124:654-663, 1996.
225. Dalgleish AG, Beverley PC, Clapham PR, et al: The CD4 (T4) antigen is an essential component of the receptor for the AIDS retrovirus, *Nature* 312:763-767, 1984.
226. Pope M, Haase AT: Transmission, acute HIV-1 infection and the quest for strategies to prevent infection, *Nat Med* 9:847-852, 2003.
227. Soulie C, Calvez V, Marcelin AG: Coreceptor usage in different reservoirs, *Curr Opin HIV AIDS* 5:450-455, 2012.
228. Dragic T, Litwin V, Allaway GP, et al: HIV-1 entry into CD4+ cells is mediated by the chemokine receptor CC-CKR-5, *Nature* 381: 667-673, 1996.
229. Deng H, Liu R, Ellmeier W, et al: Identification of a major co-receptor for primary isolates of HIV-1, *Nature* 381:661-666, 1996.
230. Feng Y, Broder CC, Kennedy PE, et al: HIV-1 entry cofactor: functional cDNA cloning of a seven-transmembrane, G protein-coupled receptor, *Science* 272:872-877, 1996.
231. Berger EA, Doms RW, Fenyö EM, et al: A new classification for HIV-1, *Nature* 391:240, 1998.
232. Jensen MA, van't Wout AB: Predicting HIV-1 coreceptor usage with sequence analysis, *AIDS Rev* 5:104-112, 2003.
233. Kwong PD, Wyatt R, Robinson J, et al: Structure of an HIV gp120 envelope glycoprotein in complex with the CD4 receptor and a neutralizing human antibody, *Nature* 393:648-659, 1998.
234. Wu L, Gerard NP, Wyatt R, et al: CD4-induced interaction of primary HIV-1 gp120 glycoproteins with the chemokine receptor CCR-5, *Nature* 384:179-183, 1996.
235. Wilen CB, Tilton JC, Doms RW: Molecular mechanisms of HIV entry. Viral molecular machines, *Adv Exp Med Biol* 726:223-242, 2012.
236. Wu X, Chien EY, Mol CD, et al: Structures of the CXCR4 chemokine GPCR with small-molecule and cyclic peptide antagonists, *Science* 330:1066-1071, 2010.
237. Tan Q, Zhu Y, Li J, et al: Structure of the CCR5 chemokine receptor-HIV entry inhibitor maraviroc complex, *Science* 341:1387-1390, 2013.
238. Buzon V, Natrajan G, Schibli D, et al: Crystal structure of HIV-1 gp41 including both fusion peptide and membrane proximal external regions, *PLoS Pathog* 6:e10000880, 2010.
239. Chan DC, Fass D, Berger JM, et al: Core structure of gp41 from the HIV envelope glycoprotein, *Cell* 89:263-273, 1997.
240. Weissenhorn W, Dessen A, Harrison SC, et al: Atomic structure of the ectodomain from HIV-1 gp41, *Nature* 387:426-430, 1997.
241. Le Grice SF: Human immunodeficiency virus reverse transcriptase: 25 years of research, drug discovery, and promise, *J Biol Chem* 287:40850-40857, 2012.
242. Matreyek KA, Engelman A: Viral and cellular requirements for the nuclear entry of retroviral preintegration nucleoprotein complexes, *Viruses* 5:2483-2511, 2013.
243. Vandegraaff N, Engelman A: Molecular mechanisms of HIV integration and therapeutic intervention, *Expert Rev Mol Med* 9:1-19, 2007.
244. Peterlin BM, Price DH: Controlling the elongation phase of transcription with P-TEFb, *Mol Cell* 23:297-305, 2006.
245. Daugherty MD, Liu B, Frankel AD: Structural basis for cooperative RNA binding and export complex assembly by HIV Rev, *Nature Struct Mol Biol* 17:1337-1442, 2010.
246. Freed EO, Martin MA: HIVs and their replication. In Knipe DM, Howley PM, editors: *Fields virology*, ed 5, New York, 2007, Lippincott, pp 2107-2186.
247. Jacks T, Power MD, Masiarz FR, et al: Characterization of ribosomal frameshifting in HIV-1 gag-pol expression, *Nature* 331:280-283, 1988.
248. Adamson CS, Salzwedel K, Freed EO: Virus maturation as a new HIV-1 therapeutic target, *Expert Opin Ther Targets* 13:895-908, 2009.
249. Jouvenet N: Dynamics of ESCRT proteins, *Cell Mol Life Sci* 69: 4121-4133, 2012.
250. Sloan RD, Wainberg MA: The role of unintegrated DNA in HIV infection, *Retrovirology* 8:52, 2011.
251. Chun TW, Nickle DC, Justement JS, et al: HIV-infected individuals receiving effective antiviral therapy for extended periods of time continually replenish their viral reservoir, *J Clin Invest* 115: 3250-3255, 2005.
252. Unutmaz D, KewalRamani VN, Marmon S, et al: Cytokine signals are sufficient for HIV-1 infection of resting human T lymphocytes, *J Exp Med* 189:1735-1746, 1999.
253. Siliciano JD, Kajdas J, Finzi D, et al: Long-term follow-up studies confirm the stability of the latent reservoir for HIV-1 in resting CD4+ T cells, *Nat Med* 9:727-728, 2003.
254. Ahmad N: Molecular mechanisms of HIV-1 mother-to-child transmission and infection in neonatal target cells, *Life Sci* 88: 980-986, 2011.
255. Beima-Sofie KM, Bigham AW, Lingappa JR, et al: Toll-like receptor variants are associated with infant HIV-1 acquisition and peak plasma HIV-1 level, *AIDS* 27:2431-2439, 2013.
256. Singh KK, Wang Y, Gray KP, et al: Genetic variants in the host restriction factor APOBEC3G are associated with HIV-1 related disease progression and central nervous system impairment in children, *J Acquir Immune Defic Syndr* 62:197-203, 2013.
257. Prendergast AJ, Klenerman P, Goulder PJ: The impact of differential antiviral immunity in children and adults, *Nature Rev* 12:636-648, 2012.
258. van't Wout AB, Kootstra NA, Mulder-Kampinga GA, et al: Macrophage-tropic variants initiate human immunodeficiency virus type 1 infection after sexual, parenteral, and vertical transmission, *J Clin Invest* 94:2060-2067, 1994.
259. Perelson AS, Essunger P, Cao Y, et al: Decay characteristics of HIV-1 infected compartments during combination therapy, *Nature* 387:188-191, 1997.
260. Luzuriaga K, Wu H, McManus M, et al: Dynamics of HIV-1 replication in vertically infected infants, *J Virol* 73:362-367, 1999.
261. Miedema F, Hazenberg MD, Tesselaar K, et al: Immune activation and collateral damage in AIDS pathogenesis, *Frontiers Immunol* 4: 1-14, 2013.
262. Douek DC, Roederer M, Koup RA: Emerging concepts in the immunopathogenesis of AIDS, *Annu Rev Med* 60:471-484, 2009.
263. Hazenberg MD, Otto SA, van Benthem BH, et al: Persistent immune activation in HIV-1 infection is associated with progression to AIDS, *AIDS* 17:1881-1888, 2003.
264. Paiardini M, Frank I, Pandrea I, et al: Mucosal immune dysfunction in AIDS pathogenesis, *AIDS Rev* 10:36-46, 2008.
265. Marchetti G, Tincati C, Silvestri G: Microbial translocation in the pathogenesis of HIV infection and AIDS, *Clin Microbiol Rev* 26: 2-18, 2013.
266. Mehandru S, Poles MA, Tenner-Racz K, et al: Primary HIV-1 infection is associated with preferential depletion of CD4+ T lymphocytes from effector sites in the gastrointestinal tract, *J Exp Med* 200: 761-770, 2004.

267. Veazey RS, Lackner AA: HIV swiftly guts the immune system, *Nat Med* 11:469-470, 2005.
268. Mehandru S, Dandekar S: Role of the gastrointestinal tract in establishing infection in primates and humans, *Curr Opin HIV AIDS* 3: 22-27, 2008.
269. Sundaravaradan V, Mehta R, Harris DT, et al: Differential expression and interaction of host factors augment HIV-1 gene expression in neonatal mononuclear cells, *Virology* 400:32-43, 2010.
270. Wellensiek BP, Ramakrishnan R, Sundaravaradan V, et al: Differential HIV-1 integration targets more actively transcribed host genes in neonatal than adult blood mononuclear cells, *Virology* 385:28-38, 2009.
271. Hahn T, Ramakrishnan R, Ahmad N: Evaluation of genetic diversity of human immunodeficiency virus type 1 NEF gene associated with vertical transmission, *J Biomed Sci* 10:436-450, 2003.
272. Ramakrishnan R, Hussain M, Holzer A, et al: Evaluations of HIV type 1 rev gene diversity and functional domains following perinatal transmission, *AIDS Res Hum Retroviruses* 21:1035-1045, 2005.
273. Mehta R, Sundaravaradan V, Ahmad N: Mutations generated in human immunodeficiency virus type 1 long terminal repeat during vertical transmission correlate with viral gene expression, *Virology* 375:170-181, 2008.
274. Kliks SC, Wara DW, Landers DV, et al: Features of HIV-1 that could influence maternal-child transmission, *JAMA* 272:467-474, 1994.
275. Wang X, Das A, Lackner AA, et al: Intestinal double-positive CD4+CD8+ T cells of neonatal rhesus macaques are proliferating, activated memory cells and primary targets for SIVMAC251 infection, *Blood* 112:4981-4990, 2008.
276. Wang X, Xu H, Pahar B, et al: Simian immunodeficiency virus selectively infects proliferating CD4+ T cells in neonatal rhesus macaques, *Blood* 116:4168-4174, 2010.
277. Abrams EJ, Weedon J, Steketee RW, et al: Association of human immunodeficiency virus (HIV) load early in life with disease progression among HIV-infected infants. New York City Perinatal HIV Transmission Collaborative Study Group, *J Infect Dis* 178:101-108, 1998.
278. Shearer WT, Quinn TC, LaRussa P, et al: Viral load and disease progression in infants infected with human immunodeficiency virus type 1, *N Engl J Med* 336:1337-1342, 1997.
279. European Collaborative Study: Level and pattern of HIV-1 RNA viral load over age: differences between girls and boys, *AIDS* 16:97-104, 2002.
280. Mofenson LM, Korelitz J, Meyer WA 3rd, et al: The relationship between serum human immunodeficiency virus type 1 (HIV-1) RNA level, CD4 lymphocyte percent, and long-term mortality risk in HIV-1-infected children, *J Infect Dis* 175:1029-1038, 1997.
281. Dunn D: Short-term risk of disease progression in HIV-1 infected children receiving no antiretroviral therapy or zidovudine monotherapy: a meta-analysis, *Lancet* 362:1605-1611, 2003.
282. McIntosh K, Shevitz A, Zaknun D, et al: Age- and time-related changes in extracellular viral load in children vertically infected by human immunodeficiency virus, *Pediatr Infect Dis J* 15: 1087-1091, 1996.
283. Richardson BA, Mbori-Ngacha D, Lavreys L, et al: Comparison of human immunodeficiency virus type 1 viral loads in Kenyan women, men, and infants during primary and early infection, *J Virol* 77:7120-7123, 2003.
284. Geskus RB, Prins M, Hubert JB, et al: The HIV RNA setpoint theory revisited, *Retrovirology* 4:65, 2007.
285. Mellors JW, Rinaldo CR Jr, Gupta P, et al: Prognosis of HIV-1 infection predicted by the quantity of virus in plasma, *Science* 272: 1167-1170, 1996.
286. Dickover RE, Dillon M, Leung KM, et al: Early prognostic indicators in primary perinatal human immunodeficiency virus type 1 infection: importance of viral RNA and the timing of transmission on long-term outcome, *J Infect Dis* 178:375-387, 1998.
287. Mellors JW, Kingsley LA, Rinaldo CR Jr, et al: Quantitation of HIV-1 RNA in plasma predicts outcome after seroconversion, *Ann Intern Med* 122:573-579, 1995.
288. Rich KC, Fowler MG, Mofenson LM, et al: Maternal and infant factors predicting disease progression in human immunodeficiency virus type 1-infected infants. Women and Infants Transmission Study Group, *Pediatrics* 105:e8, 2000.
289. Palumbo PE, Raskino C, Fiscus S, et al: Predictive value of quantitative plasma HIV RNA and CD4 lymphocyte count in HIV-infected infants and children, *JAMA* 279:756-761, 1998.
290. Gortmaker SL, Hughes M, Cervia J, et al: Effect of combination therapy including protease inhibitors on mortality among children and adolescents infected with HIV-1, *N Engl J Med* 345:1522-1528, 2001.
291. Goetghebuer T, Le Chenadec J, Haelterman E, et al: Short- and long-term immunological and virological outcome in HIV-infected infants according to the age at antiretroviral treatment initiation, *Clin Infect Dis* 54:878-881, 2012.
292. Dunn D, Woodburn P, Duong T, et al: Current CD4 cell count and the short-term risk of AIDS and death before the availability of effective antiretroviral therapy in HIV-infected children and adults, *J Infect Dis* 197:398-404, 2008.
293. Walker BD, Yu XG: Unravelling the mechanisms of durable control of HIV-1, *Nat Rev Immunol* 13:487-498, 2013.
294. Sperduto AR, Bryson YJ, Chen IS: Increased susceptibility of neonatal monocyte/macrophages to HIV-1 infection, *AIDS Res Hum Retroviruses* 9:1277-1285, 1993.
295. Luzuriaga K, Newell ML, Dabis F, et al: Vaccines to prevent transmission of HIV-1 via breastmilk: scientific and logistical priorities, *Lancet* 368:511-521, 2006.
296. Pillay T, Zhang HT, Drijfhout JW, et al: Unique acquisition of cytotoxic T-lymphocyte escape mutants in infant human immunodeficiency virus type 1 infection, *J Virol* 79:1277-1285, 2005.
297. Thobakgale CF, Prendergast A, Crawford H, et al: Impact of HLA in the mother and infant on disease progression of pediatric human immunodeficiency virus type 1 infection, *J Virol* 83:10234-10244, 2009.
298. Prendergast A, Tudor-Williams G, Jeena P, et al: International perspectives, progress, and future challenges of paediatric HIV infection, *Lancet* 370:68-80, 2007.
299. Borrow P, Lewicki H, Hahn BH, et al: 1994 Virus-specific CD8+ cytotoxic T-lymphocyte activity associated with control of viremia in primary human immunodeficiency virus type 1 infection, *J Virol* 68:6103-6110, 1994.
300. Streeck H, Nixon DF: T cell immunity in acute HIV-1 infection, *J Infect Dis* 202:S302-S308, 2010.
301. Carlson JM, Brumme ZL: HIV evolution in response to HLA-restricted CTL selection pressures: a population-based perspective, *Microbes Infect* 10:455-461, 2008.
302. Luzuriaga K, Holmes D, Hereema A, et al: HIV-1-specific cytotoxic T lymphocyte responses in the first year of life, *J Immunol* 154: 433-443, 1995.
303. Scott ZA, Beaumier CM, Sharkey M, et al: HIV-1 replication increases HIV-specific CD4+ T cell frequencies but limits proliferative capacity in chronically infected children, *J Immunol* 170:5786-5792, 2003.
304. Shalekoff S, Meddows-Taylor S, Gray GE, et al: Identification of human immunodefiency virus-1 specific CD8+ and CD4+ T cell responses in perinatally infected infants and their mothers, *AIDS* 23:789-798, 2009.
305. Thobakgale CF, Ramduth D, Reddy S, et al: Human immunodeficiency virus-specific CD8+ T-cell activity is detectable from birth in the majority of in utero-infected infants, *J Virol* 81:12775-12784, 2007.
306. Lohman BL, Slyker JA, Richardson BA, et al: Longitudinal assessment of human immunodeficiency virus type-1 (HIV-1)-specific γ interferon responses during the first year of life in HIV-1 infected infants, *J Virol* 79:8121-8130, 2005.
307. Huang S, Dunkley-Thompson J, Tang Y, et al: Deficiency of HIV-gag-specific T cells in early childhood correlates with poor viral containment, *J Immunol* 181:8103-8111, 2008.
308. Goulder BJ, Brander C, Tang Y, et al: Evolution and transmission of stable CTL escape mutations in HIV infection, *Nature* 412:334-338, 2001.
309. Kuhn L, Abrams EJ, Palumbo P, et al: Maternal versus paternal inheritance of HLA class I alleles among HIV-infected children: consequences for clinical disease progression, *AIDS* 18:1281-1289, 2004.
310. Sanchez-Merino V, Nie S, Luzuriaga K: HIV-1-specific CD8 T cell responses and viral evolution in women and infants, *J Immunol* 175:6976-6986, 2005.
311. Prendergast A, Goodliffe H, Clapson M, et al: Gag-specific CD4 T-cell responses are associated with virological control of paediatric HIV-1 infection, *AIDS* 25:1329-1331, 2011.
312. Nqoko B, Day CL, Mansoor N, et al: HIV-specific Gag responses in early infancy correlate with clinical outcome and inversely with viral load, *AIDS Res Hum Retroviruses* 27:1311-1316, 2011.
313. Sandberg JK, Fast NM, Jordan KA, et al: HIV-specific CD8+ T cell function in children with vertically acquired HIV-1 infection is critically influenced by age and the state of the CD4+ Tcell compartment, *J Immunol* 170:4403-4410, 2003.

314. Thobakgale CF, Streeck H, Mkhwanazi N, et al: CD8+ T cell polyfunctionality profiles in progressive and nonprogressive pediatric HIV type 1 infection, *AIDS Res Hum Retroviruses* 28:1005-1012, 2011.
315. Prendergast A, O'Callaghan M, Menson E, et al: Factors influencing T cell activation and programmed death 1 expression in HIV-infected children, *AIDS Res Hum Retroviruses* 28:465-468, 2012.
316. Ssewanyana I, Baker CA, Ruel T, et al: The distribution and immune profile of T cell subsets in HIV-infected children from Uganda, *AIDS Res Hum Retroviruses* 25:65-71, 2009.
317. Leslie A, Kavanagh D, Honeyborne I, et al: Transmission and accumulation of CTL escape variants drive negative associations between HIV polymorphisms and HLA, *J Exp Med* 201:891-902, 2005.
318. Feeney ME, Tang Y, Pfafferott K, et al: HIV-1 viral escape in infancy followed by emergence of a variant-specific CTL response, *J Immunol* 174:7524-7530, 2005.
319. Prado JG, Prendergast A, Thobakgale C, et al: Replicative capacity of human immunodeficiency virus type 1 transmitted from mother to child is associated with pediatric disease progression rate, *J Virol* 84:492-502, 2010.
320. Singh KK, Gray PK, Wang Y, et al: HLA alleles are associated with altered risk for disease progression and central nervous system impairment of HIV-infected children, *J Acqui Immune Defic Syndr* 57:32-39, 2011.
321. Feeney ME, Tang Y, Roosevelt KA, et al: Immune escape precedes breakthrough human immunodeficiency virus type 1 viremia and broadening of the cytotoxic T-lymphocyte response in an HLA-B27-positive long-term-nonprogressing child, *J Virol* 78: 8927-8930, 2004.
322. Salgado M, Simón A, Sanz-Minguela B, et al: An additive effect of protective host genetic factors correlates with HIV-non progression status, *J Acquir Immune Defic Syndr* 56:300-305, 2011.
323. Kaslow RA, Carrington M, Apple R, et al: Influence of combinations of human major histocompatibility complex genes on the course of HIV-1 infection, *Nat Med* 2:405-411, 1996.
324. Gao X, O'Brien TR, Welzel TM, et al: HLA-B alleles associate consistently with HIV heterosexual transmission, viral load, and progression to AIDS, but not susceptibility to infection, *AIDS* 24:1835-1840, 2010.
325. Gillespie GM, Kaul R, Dong T, et al: Cross-reactive cytotoxic T lymphocytes against a HIV-1 p24 epitope in slow progressors with B-57, *AIDS* 16:961-972, 2002.
326. Feeney ME, Draenert R, Roosevelt KA, et al: Reconstitution of virus-specific CD4 proliferative responses in pediatric HIV-1 infection, *J Immunol* 171:6968-6975, 2003.
327. Ramduth D, Thobakgale CF, Mkhwanazi NP, et al: Detection of HIV type 1 gag-specific CD4(+) T cell responses in acutely infected infants, *AIDS Res Hum Retroviruses* 24:265-270, 2008.
328. Luzuriaga K, McManus M, Catalina M, et al: Early therapy of vertical human immunodeficiency virus type 1 (HIV-1) infection: control of viral replication and absence of persistent HIV-1-specific immune responses, *J Virol* 74:6984-6991, 2000.
329. Hartigan-O'Connor DJ, Abel K, McCune JM: Suppression of SIV-specific CD4+T cells by infant but not adult macaque regulatory T cells: implications for SIV disease progression, *J Exp Med* 204: 2679-2692, 2007.
330. Porichis F, Kauffman DE: HIV-specific CD4 T cells and immune control of viral replication, *Curr Opin HIV AIDS* 6:174-180, 2011.
331. Ssewanyana I, Elrelaei M, Dorsey G, et al: Profile of T cell immune responses in HIV-infected children from Uganda, *J Infect Dis* 196:1667-1670, 2007.
332. Pugatch D, Sullivan JL, Pikora CA, et al: Delayed generation of antibodies mediating HIV-1 specific antibody-dependent cellular cytotoxicity in vertically-infected infants, *J Infect Dis* 176:643-648, 1997.
333. Ziegner U, Campbell D, Weinhold K, et al: Deficient antibody-dependent cellular cytotoxicity against human immunodeficiency virus (HIV)-expressing target cells in perinatal HIV infection, *Clin Diagn Lab Immunol* 6:718-724, 1999.
334. Farquhar C, John-Stewart G: The role of infant immune responses and genetic factors in preventing HIV-1 acquisition and disease progression, *Clin Exp Immunol* 134:367-377, 2003.
335. Obaro SK, Pugatch D, Luzuriaga K: Immunogenicity and efficacy of childhood vaccines in HIV-1-infected children, *Lancet Infect Dis* 4:510-518, 2004.
336. Wei X, Decker JM, Wang S, et al: Antibody neutralization and escape by HIV-1, *Nature* 422:307-312, 2003.
337. Braibant M, Barin F: The role of neutralizing antibodies in prevention of HIV-1 infection: what can we learn from the mother-to-child transmission context? *Retrovirology* 10:103, 2013.
338. Baan E, de Ronde A, Stax M, et al: HIV-1 autologous antibody neutralization associated with mother to child transmission, *PLOS One* 8, e69274, 2013.
339. Lynch JB, Nduati R, Blish CA, et al: The breadth and potency of passively acquired human immunodeficiency virus type 1-specific neutralizing antibodies do not correlate with the risk of infant infection, *J Virol* 85:5252-5261, 2011.
340. Mabuka J, Goo L, Omenda MM, et al: HIV-1 maternal and infant variants show similar sensitivity to broadly neutralizing antibodies, but sensitivity varies by subtype, *AIDS* 27:1535-1544, 2013.
341. Chaillon A, Wack T, Braibant M, et al: The breadth and titer of maternal HIV-1 specific heterologous neutralizing antibodies are not associated with a lower rate of mother-to-child transmission of HIV-1, *J Virol* 86:10540-10546, 2012.
342. Paul ME, Mao C, Charurat M, et al: Predictors of immunologic long-term nonprogression in HIV-infected children: implications for initiating therapy, *J Allergy Clin Immunol* 115:848-855, 2005.
343. Ananworanich J, Apornpong T, Kosalaraksa P, et al: Characteristics of lymphocyte subsets in HIV-infected, long-term non-progressor, and healthy Asian children through 12 years of age, *J Allergy Clin Immunol* 126:1294-1301, 2010.
344. Hofer CB, Oliveira RH, Machado ES, et al: Neonatal factors associated with HIV long term non-progressors in a cohort of vertically infected children in Rio de Janeiro, Brazil ('Peixe' Project), *Braz J Infect Dis* 13:276-279, 2009.
345. Deeks SG, Kitchen CM, Liu L, et al: Immune activation set point during early HIV infection predicts subsequent CD4+ T-cell changes independent of viral load, *Blood* 104:942-947, 2004.
346. Aldrovandi GC, Cerini C: Immunopathogenesis of HIV-1 infection. In Long SS, Pickering LK, Prober CG, editors: *Principles and practice of pediatric infectious diseases*, ed 4, Philadelphia, 2012, Elsevier.
347. Douek DC, McFarland RD, Keiser PH, et al: Changes in thymic function with age and during the treatment of HIV infection, *Nature* 396:690-695, 1998.
348. Plaeger-Marshall S, Isacescu V, O'Rourke S, et al: T cell activation in pediatric AIDS pathogenesis: three color immunophenotyping, *Clin Immunol Immunopathol* 71:19-26, 1994.
349. Nahmias AJ, Clark WS, Kourtis AP, et al: Thymic dysfunction and time of infection predict mortality in human immunodeficiency virus-infected infants. CDC Perinatal AIDS Collaborative Transmission Study Group, *J Infect Dis* 178:680-685, 1998.
350. Kourtis AP, Ibegbu C, Nahmias AJ, et al: Early progression of disease in HIV-infected infants with thymus dysfunction, *N Engl J Med* 335:1431-1436, 1996.
351. Erkeller-Yuksel FM, Deneys V, Yuksel B, et al: Age-related changes in human blood lymphocyte subpopulations, *J Pediatr* 120:216-222, 1992.
352. European Collaborative Study: Age-related standards for T lymphocyte subsets based on uninfected children born to human immunodeficiency virus 1-infected mothers, *Pediatr Infect Dis J* 11:1018-1026, 1992.
353. Comans-Bitter WM, de Groot R, van den Beemd R, et al: 1997 Immunophenotyping of blood lymphocytes in childhood: reference values for lymphocyte subpopulations, *J Pediatr* 130:388-393, 1997.
354. McKinney RE, Wilfert CM: Lymphocyte subsets in children younger than 2 years old: normal values in a population at risk for human immunodeficiency virus infection and diagnostic and prognostic application to infected children, *Pediatr Infect Dis J* 11:639-644, 1992.
355. Ghosh S, Feyen O, Jebran AF, et al: Memory B cell function in HIV-infected children: decreased memory B cells despite ART, *Pediatr Res* 66:185-190, 2009.
356. Luzuriaga K, Koup RA, Pikora CA, et al: Deficient human immunodeficiency virus type 1-specific cytotoxic T cell responses in vertically infected children, *J Pediatr* 119:230-236, 1991.
357. Bekker V, Scherpbier H, Pajkrt D, et al: Persistent humoral immune defect in highly active antiretroviral therapy-treated children with HIV-1 infection: loss of specific antibodies against vaccine strains and natural viral infection, *Pediatrics* 118:e315-e322, 2006.
358. Borkowsky W, Rigaud M, Krasinski K, et al: Cell-mediated and humoral immune responses in children infected with human immunodeficiency virus during the first four years of life, *J Pediatr* 120:371-375, 1992.

359. Ching N, Deville JG, Nielsen KA, et al: Cellular and humoral immune responses to a tetanus toxoid booster in perinatally HIV-1-infected children and adolescents receiving highly active antiretroviral therapy (HAART), *Eur J Pediatr* 166:51-56, 2007.
360. Melvin AJ, Mohan KM: Response to immunization with measles, tetanus, and *Haemophilus influenzae* type b vaccines in children who have human immunodeficiency virus type 1 infection and are treated with highly active antiretroviral therapy, *Pediatrics* 111:e641-644, 2003.
361. De Martino M, Podda A, Galli L, et al: Acellular pertussis vaccine in children with perinatal human immunodeficiency virus-type 1 infection, *Vaccine* 15:1235-1238, 1997.
362. Patel K, Hernán MA, Williams PL, et al: Long-term effects of highly active antiretroviral therapy on CD4 cell evolution among children and adolescents infected with HIV: 5 years and counting, *Clin Infect Dis* 46:1751-1760, 2008.
363. Weinberg A, Dickover R, Britto P, et al: Continuous improvement in the immune system of HIV-infected children on prolonged antiretroviral therapy, *AIDS* 22:2267-2277, 2008.
364. Centers for Disease Control and Prevention: Guidelines for the prevention and treatment of opportunistic infections among HIV-exposed and HIV-infected children: recommendations from the Centers for Disease Control and Prevention, the HIV Medicine Association of the National Institutes of Health, Infectious Disease Society of America, *MMWR Recomm Rep* 55(RR-14):1-17, 2008.
365. Katlama C, Deeks SG, Autran B, et al: Barriers to a cure for HIV: new ways to target and eradicate HIV-1 reservoirs, *Lancet* 381: 2109-2117, 2013.
366. Siliciano JD, Siliciano RF: Biomarkers of HIV replication, *Curr Opin HIV AIDS* 5:491-497, 2010.
367. Blankson JN, Persaud D, Siliciano RF: The challenge of viral reservoirs in HIV-1 infection, *Annu Rev Med* 53:557-593, 2002.
368. von Wyl V, Gianella S, Fischer M, et al: Early antiretroviral therapy during primary HIV-1 infection results in a transient reduction of the viral setpoint upon treatment interruption, *PLoS One* 6:e27463, 2011.
369. Ananworanich J, Schuetz A, Vandergeeten C, et al: Impact of multi-targeted antiretroviral treatment on gut T cell depletion and HIV reservoir seeding during acute HIV infection, *PLoS One* 7:e33948, 2012.
370. Persaud D, Palumbo PE, Ziemniak C, et al: Dynamics of the resting CD4+ T-cell latent HIV reservoir in infants initiating HAART less than 6 months of age, *AIDS* 26:1483-1490, 2012.
371. Persaud D, Gay H, Ziemniak C, et al: Absence of HIV-1 detectable viremia after treatment cessation in an infant, *N Engl J Med* 369:1828-1835, 2013.
372. Havens PL, Mofenson LM: American Academy of Pediatrics, Committee on Pediatric AIDS: HIV testing and prophylaxis to prevent mother-to-child transmission in the United States, *Pediatrics* 122:1127-1134, 2008.
373. King SM: American Academy of Pediatrics, Committee on Pediatric AIDS: Evaluation and treatment of the human immunodeficiency virus-1-exposed infant, *Pediatrics* 114:497-505, 2004.
374. Read JS: American Academy of Pediatrics, Committee on Pediatric AIDS: Diagnosis of HIV infection in children younger than 18 months in the United States, *Pediatrics* 120:e1547-e1562, 2007.
375. Panel on Antiretroviral Therapy and Medical Management of HIV-Infected Children: Guidelines for the use of antiretroviral agents in pediatric HIV infection. Available at http://aidsinfonihgov/Content Files/Pediatric Guidelinespdf. Accessed November 22, 2013.
376. World Health Organization: *WHO recommendation on the diagnosis of HIV infection in infants and children*, Geneva, 2010, World Health Organization, pp 1–52.
377. Dunn DT, Brandt CD, Krivine A, et al: The sensitivity of HIV-1 DNA polymerase chain reaction in the neonatal period and the relative contributions of intra-uterine and intra-partum transmission, *AIDS* 9:7-11, 1995.
378. Bremer JW, Lew JF, Cooper E, et al: Diagnosis of infection with human immunodeficiency virus type 1 by a DNA polymerase chain reaction assay among infants enrolled in the Women and Infants' Transmission Study, *J Pediatr* 129:198-207, 1996.
379. Kline MW, Lewis DE, Hollinger FB, et al: A comparative study of human immunodeficiency virus culture, polymerase chain reaction and anti-human immunodeficiency virus immunoglobulin A antibody detection in the diagnosis during early infancy of vertically acquired human immunodeficiency virus infection, *Pediatr Infect Dis J* 13:90-94, 1994.
380. Kovacs A, Xu J, Rasheed S, et al: Comparison of a rapid nonisotopic polymerase chain reaction assay with four commonly used methods for the early diagnosis of human immunodeficiency virus type 1 infection in neonates and children, *Pediatr Infect Dis J* 14:948-954, 1995.
381. Lambert JS, Harris DR, Stiehm ER, et al: Performance characteristics of HIV-1 culture and HIV-1 DNA and RNA amplification assays for early diagnosis of perinatal HIV-1 infection, *J Acquir Immune Defic Syndr* 34:512-519, 2003.
382. Simonds RJ, Brown TM, Thea DM, et al: Sensitivity and specificity of a qualitative RNA detection assay to diagnose HIV infection in young infants. Perinatal AIDS Collaborative Transmission Study, *AIDS* 12:1545-1549, 1998.
383. Steketee RW, Abrams EJ, Thea DM, et al: Early detection of perinatal human immunodeficiency virus (HIV) type 1 infection using HIV RNA amplification and detection. New York City Perinatal HIV Transmission Collaborative Study, *J Infect Dis* 175:707-711, 1997.
384. Rouet F, Montcho C, Rouzioux C, et al: Early diagnosis of paediatric HIV-1 infection among African breast-fed children using a quantitative plasma HIV RNA assay, *AIDS* 15:1849-1856, 2001.
385. Nesheim S, Palumbo P, Sullivan K, et al: Quantitative RNA testing for diagnosis of HIV-infected infants, *J Acquir Immune Defic Syndr* 32:192-195, 2003.
386. Kline NE, Schwarzwald H, Kline MW: False negative DNA polymerase chain reaction in an infant with subtype C human immunodeficiency virus 1 infection, *Pediatr Infect Dis J* 21:885-886, 2002.
387. Young NL, Shaffer N, Chaowanachan T, et al: Early diagnosis of HIV-1-infected infants in Thailand using RNA and DNA PCR assays sensitive to non-B subtypes, *J Acquir Immune Defic Syndr* 24:401-407, 2000.
388. Blanche S, Newell ML, Mayaux MJ, et al: Morbidity and mortality in European children vertically infected by HIV-1. The French Pediatric HIV Infection Study Group and European Collaborative Study, *J Acquir Immune Defic Syndr Hum Retrovirol* 14:442-450, 1997.
389. McIntosh K, Pitt J, Brambilla D, et al: Blood culture in the first 6 months of life for the diagnosis of vertically transmitted human immunodeficiency virus infection. The Women and Infants Transmission Study Group, *J Infect Dis* 170:996-1000, 1994.
390. Krivine A, Yakudima A, Le May M, et al: A comparative study of virus isolation, polymerase chain reaction, and antigen detection in perinatally acquired human immunodeficiency virus, *J Pediatr* 116:372-376, 1990.
391. Kline MW, Hollinger FB, Rosenblatt HM, et al: Sensitivity, specificity and predictive value of physical examination, culture and other laboratory studies in the diagnosis during early infancy of vertically acquired human immunodeficiency virus infection, *Pediatr Infect Dis J* 12:33-36, 1993.
392. Vigano A, Principi N, Crupi L, et al: Elevation of IgE in HIV-infected children and its correlation with the progression of disease, *J Allergy Clin Immunol* 95:627-632, 1995.
393. W, Shearer T, Rosenblatt HM, Schluchter MD, et al: Immunologic targets of HIV infection: T cells. NICHD IVIG Clinical Trials Group, and the NHLBI P2C2 Pediatric Pulmonary and Cardiac Complications of HIV Infection Study Group, *Ann N Y Acad Sci* 693:35-51, 1993.
394. Centers for Disease Control and Prevention: Revision of the CDC surveillance case definition for acquired immunodeficiency syndrome. Council of State and Territorial Epidemiologists; AIDS Program, Center for Infectious Diseases, *MMWR Morb Mortal Wkly Rep* 36(Suppl 1): 1-15, 1987.
395. Centers for Disease Control and Prevention: 1993 Revised classification system for HIV infection and expanded surveillance case definition for AIDS among adolescents and adults, *MMWR Recomm Rep* 41(RR-17):1-19, 1992.
396. Centers for Disease Control and Prevention: Revised classification system for human immunodeficiency virus infection in children less than 13 years of age, *MMWR Recomm Rep* 43(RR-12):1-7, 1994.
397. Centers for Disease Control and Prevention: Revised surveillance case definitions for HIV infection among adults, adolescents, and children aged <18 months and for HIV infection and AIDS among children aged 18 months to <13 years—United States, 2008, *MMWR Recomm Rep* 57(RR-10):1-12, 2008.
398. Simonds RJ, Oxtoby MJ, Caldwell MB, Gwinn ML, Rogers MF: *Pneumocystis carinii* pneumonia among US children with perinatally acquired HIV infection, *JAMA* 270:470-473, 1993.

399. Mofenson LM, Oleske J, Serchuck L, et al: Treating opportunistic infections among HIV-exposed and infected children: recommendations from CDC, the National Institutes of Health, and the Infectious Diseases Society of America, *MMWR Recomm Rep* 53(RR-14):1-92, 2004.
400. Nesheim SR, Kapogiannis BG, Soe MM, et al: Trends in opportunistic infections in the pre- and post-highly active antiretroviral therapy eras among HIV-infected children in the perinatal AIDS Collaborative Transmission Study, 1986-2004, *Pediatrics* 120:100-109, 2007.
401. Scott GB, Hutto C, Makuch RW, et al: Survival in children with perinatally acquired human immunodeficiency virus type 1 infection, *N Engl J Med* 321:1791-1796, 1989.
402. Marion RW, Wiznia AA, Hutcheon G, et al: Human T-cell lymphotropic virus type III (HTLV- III) embryopathy: a new dysmorphic syndrome associated with intrauterine HTLV-III infection, *Am J Dis Child* 140:638-640, 1986.
403. Qazi QH, Sheikh TM, Fikrig S, et al: Lack of evidence for craniofacial dysmorphism in perinatal human immunodeficiency virus infection, *J Pediatr* 112:7-11, 1998.
404. Galli L, de Martino M, Tovo PA, et al: Italian Register for HIV Infection in Children. Onset of clinical signs with HIV-1 perinatal infection, *AIDS* 9:455-461, 1995.
405. Natural history of vertically-acquired human immunodeficiency virus-1 infection. The European Collaborative Study, *Pediatrics* 94:815-819, 1994.
406. Pollack H, Glasberg H, Lee E, et al: Impaired early growth of infants perinatally infected with human immunodeficiency virus: correlation with viral load, *J Pediatr* 130:915-922, 1997.
407. Kline MW: Vertically acquired human immunodeficiency virus infection, *Semin Pediatr Infect Dis* 10:147-153, 1999.
408. Mofenson LM, Brady MT, Danner SP, et al: Guidelines for the Prevention and Treatment of Opportunistic Infections among HIV-exposed and HIV-infected children: recommendations from CDC, the National Institutes of Health, the HIV Medicine Association of the Infectious Diseases Society of America, the Pediatric Infectious Diseases Society, and the American Academy of Pediatrics. and the Infectious Diseases Society of America, *MMWR Recomm Rep* 58(RR-11): 1-166, 2009.
409. Danker WM, Lindsey JC, Levin MJ: Correlates of opportunistic infections in children infected with the human immunodeficiency virus managed before highly active antiretroviral therapy, *Pediatr Infect Dis J* 20:40-48, 2001.
410. Centers for Disease Control and Prevention. Pediatric HIV/AIDS surveillance. Available at http://www.cdc.gov/hiv/topics/surveillance/resources/slides/pediatric/index.htm. Accessed December 10, 2013.
411. Farley JJ, King JC Jr, Nair P, et al: Invasive pneumococcal disease among infected and uninfected children of mothers with human immunodeficiency virus infection, *J Pediatr* 124:853-858, 1994.
412. Mofenson LM, Korelitz J, Pelton S, et al: Sinusitis in children infected with human immunodeficiency virus: clinical characteristics, risk factors, and prophylaxis. National Institute of Child Health and Human Development Intravenous Immunoglobulin Clinical Trial Study Group, *Clin Infect Dis* 21:1175-1181, 1995.
413. Kapogiannis BG, Soe MM, Nesheim SR, et al: Trends in bacteremia in the pre- and post-highly active antiretroviral therapy era among HIV-infected children in the US Perinatal AIDS Collaborative Transmission Study (1986–2004), *Pediatrics* 121:e1229-1239, 2008.
414. Lichenstein R, King JC Jr, Farley JJ, et al: Bacteremia in febrile human immunodeficiency virus-infected children presenting to ambulatory care settings, *Pediatr Infect Dis J* 17:381-385, 1998.
415. Steenhoff AP, Wood SM, Rutstein RM, et al: Invasive pneumococcal disease among human immunodeficiency virus-infected children, 1989-2006, *Pediatr Infect Dis J* 27:886-891, 2008.
416. Cohen C, Singh E, Wu HM, et al: Increased incidence of meningococcal disease in HIV-infected individuals associated with higher case-fatality ratios in South Africa, *AIDS* 24:1351-1360, 2010.
417. Roilides E, Marshall D, Venzon D, et al: Bacterial infections in human immunodeficiency virus type 1-infected children: the impact of central venous catheters and antiretroviral agents, *Pediatr Infect Dis J* 10:813-819, 1991.
418. Di John D, Krasinski K, Lawrence R, et al: Very late onset of group B streptococcal disease in infants infected with the human immunodeficiency virus, *Pediatr Infect Dis J* 9:925-928, 1990.
419. Schulte JM, Burkham S, Hamaker D, et al: Syphilis among HIV-infected mothers and their infants in Texas from 1988 to 1994, *Sex Transm Dis* 28:315-320, 2001.
420. Pillay T, Sturm AW, Khan M, et al: Vertical transmission of *Mycobacterium tuberculosis* in KwaZulu Natal: impact of HIV-1 co-infection, *Int J Tuberc Lung Dis* 8:59-69, 2004.
421. Marais BJ, Graham SM, Cotton MF, et al: Diagnostic and management challenges for childhood tuberculosis in the era of HIV, *J Infect Dis* 196(Suppl 1):S76-S85, 2007.
422. Hesseling AC, Cotton MF, Jennings T, et al: High incidence of tuberculosis among HIV-infected infants: evidence from a South African population-based study highlights the need for improved tuberculosis control strategies, *Clin Infect Dis* 48:108-114, 2009.
423. Gandhi NR, Nunn P, Dheda K, et al: Multidrug-resistant and extensively drug-resistant tuberculosis: a threat to global control of tuberculosis, *Lancet* 375:1830-1843, 2010.
424. Starke JR, Correa AG: Management of mycobacterial infection and disease in children, *Pediatr Infect Dis J* 14:455-470, 1995.
425. Kelley R, Mancao M, Lee F, et al: Varicella in children with perinatally acquired human immunodeficiency virus infection, *J Pediatr* 124:271-273, 1994.
426. Lyall EG, Ogilvie MM, Smith NM, et al: Acyclovir resistant varicella zoster and HIV infection, *Arch Dis Child* 70:133-135, 1994.
427. Doyle M, Atkins JT, Rivera-Matos IR: Congenital cytomegalovirus infection in infants infected with human immunodeficiency virus type 1, *Pediatr Infect Dis J* 15:1102-1106, 1996.
428. Kitchen BJ, Engler HD, Gill VJ, et al: Cytomegalovirus infection in children with human immunodeficiency virus infection, *Pediatr Infect Dis J* 16:358-363, 1997.
429. Kovacs A, Schluchter M, Easley K, et al: Cytomegalovirus infection and HIV-1 disease progression in infants born to HIV-1-infected women. Pediatric Pulmonary and Cardiovascular Complications of Vertically Transmitted HIV Infection Study Group, *N Engl J Med* 341:77-84, 1999.
430. Toussi SS, Abadi J, Rosenberg M, et al: Prevalence of hepatitis B and C virus infections in children infected with HIV, *Clin Infect Dis* 45:795-798, 2007.
431. Pappalardo BL: Influence of maternal human immunodeficiency virus (HIV) co-infection on vertical transmission of hepatitis C virus (HCV): a meta-analysis, *Int J Epidemiol* 32:727-734, 2003.
432. Kaplan LJ, Daum RS, Smaron M, et al: Severe measles in immunocompromised patients, *JAMA* 267:1237-1241, 1992.
433. Nadel S, McGann K, Hodinka RL, et al: Measles giant cell pneumonia in a child with human immunodeficiency virus infection, *Pediatr Infect Dis J* 10:542-544, 1991.
434. King JC, Burke AR, Clemens JD, et al: Respiratory syncytial virus illnesses in human immunodeficiency virus- and noninfected children, *Pediatr Infect Dis J* 12:733-739, 1993.
435. Gonzales CE, Venzon D, Lee S, et al: Risk factors for fungemia in children infected with human immunodeficiency virus: a case control study, *Clin Infect Dis* 23:515-521, 1996.
436. Leggiadro RJ, Kline MW, Hughes WT: Extrapulmonary cryptococcosis in children with acquired immunodeficiency syndrome, *Pediatr Infect Dis J* 10:658-662, 1991.
437. Gonzales GE, Shetty D, Lewis LL, et al: Cryptococcosis in human immunodeficiency virus-infected children, *Pediatr Infect Dis J* 15:796-800, 1996.
438. Shetty D, Giri N, Gonzalez CE, et al: Invasive aspergillosis in human immunodeficiency virus-infected children, *Pediatr Infect Dis* 16:216-221, 1997.
439. Sarosi GA, Johnson PC: Disseminated histoplasmosis in patients infected with human immunodeficiency virus, *Clin Infect Dis* 14(Suppl 1):S60-S67, 1992.
440. Byers M, Feldman S, Edwards J: Disseminated histoplasmosis as the acquired immunodeficiency syndrome-defining illness in an infant, *Pediatr Infect Dis J* 11:127-128, 1992.
441. E. Mortier, Pouchot J, Bossi P, et al., Maternal-fetal transmission of *Pneumocystis carinii* in human immunodeficiency virus infection, *N Engl J Med* 332:825, 1995.
442. Chintu C, Mudenda V, Lucas S, et al: Lung diseases at necropsy in African children dying from respiratory illnesses: a descriptive necropsy study, *Lancet* 360:985-990, 2002.
443. Connor E, Bagarazzi M, McSherry G, et al: Clinical and laboratory correlates of *Pneumocystis carinii* pneumonia in children infected with HIV, *JAMA* 265:1693-1697, 1991.

444. The National Institutes of Health–University of California Expert Panel for Corticosteroids as Adjunctive Therapy for *Pneumocystis* Pneumonia: 1990 consensus statement on the use of corticosteroids as adjunctive therapy for *Pneumocystis* pneumonia in the acquired immunodeficiency syndrome, *N Engl J Med* 323:1500-1504, 1990.
445. McLaughlin GE, Virdee SS, Schleien CL, et al: Effect of corticosteroids on survival of children with acquired immunodeficiency syndrome and *Pneumocystis carinii*-related respiratory failure, *J Pediatr* 126:821-824, 1995.
446. Bernstein LJ, Bye MR, Rubinstein A: Prognostic factors and life expectancy in children with acquired immunodeficiency syndrome and *Pneumocystis carinii* pneumonia, *Am J Dis Child* 143:775-778, 1989.
447. Kovacs A, Frederick T, Church J, et al: CD4 T-lymphocyte counts and *Pneumocystis carinii* pneumonia in pediatric HIV infection, *JAMA* 265:1698-1703, 1991.
448. Centers for Disease Control and Prevention: Guidelines for prophylaxis against *Pneumocystis carinii* pneumonia for children infected with human immunodeficiency virus, *MMWR Morb Mortal Wkly Rep* 40:1-13, 1991.
449. Simonds RJ, Lindegren ML, Thomas P, et al: Prophylaxis against *Pneumocystis carinii* pneumonia among children with perinatally acquired human immunodeficiency virus infection in the United States, *N Engl J Med* 332:786-790, 1995.
450. Thea DM, Lambert G, Weedon J, et al: Benefit of primary prophylaxis before 18 months of age in reducing the incidence of Pneumocystis carinii pneumonia and early death in a cohort of 112 human immunodeficiency virus-infected infants, *Pediatrics* 97:59-64, 1996.
451. Centers for Disease Control and Prevention: 1995 revised guidelines for prophylaxis against *Pneumocystis carinii* pneumonia for children infected with or perinatally exposed to human immunodeficiency virus. National Pediatric and Family HIV Resource Center and National Center for Infectious Diseases, Centers for Disease Control and Prevention, *MMWR Recomm Rep* 44(RR-4):1-11, 1995.
452. Pyrgos V, Shoham S, Roilides E, et al: *Pneumocystis* pneumonia in children, *Paediatr Respir Rev* 10:192-198, 2009.
453. Mueller BU, Butler KM, Husson RN, et al: *Pneumocystis carinii* pneumonia despite prophylaxis in children with human immunodeficiency virus infection, *J Pediatr* 119:992-994, 1991.
454. Nachman SA, Mueller BU, Mirochnick M, et al: High failure rate of dapsone and pentamidine as *Pneumocystis carinii* pneumonia prophylaxis in human immunodeficiency virus-infected children, *Pediatr Infect Dis J* 13:1004-1006, 1994.
455. Minkoff H, Remington JS, Holman S, et al: Vertical transmission of *Toxoplasma* by human immunodeficiency virus-infected women, *Am J Obstet Gynecol* 176:555-559, 1997.
456. Mitchell CD, Erlich SS, Mastrucci MT, et al: Congenital toxoplasmosis occurring in infants infected with human immunodeficiency virus 1, *Pediatr Infect Dis J* 9:512-518, 1990.
457. Medlock MD, Tilleli JT, Pearl GS: Congenital cardiac toxoplasmosis in a newborn with acquired immunodeficiency syndrome, *Pediatr Infect Dis J* 9:129-132, 1990.
458. Cordell RL, Addiss DG: Cryptosporidiosis in child care settings: a review of the literature and recommendations for prevention and control, *Pediatr Infect Dis J* 13:310-317, 1994.
459. Lobato MN, Caldwell MB, Ng P, et al: Encephalopathy in children with perinatally acquired human immunodeficiency virus infection, *J Pediatr* 126:710-715, 1995.
460. Mitchell CD: HIV-1 encephalopathy among perinatally infected children: neuropathogenesis and response to highly active antiretroviral therapy, *Ment Retard Dev Disabil Res Rev* 12:216-222, 2006.
461. Nachman SA, Chernoff M, Gona P, et al: Incidence of noninfectious conditions in perinatally HIV-infected children and adolescents in the HAART era, *Arch Pediatr Adoles Med* 163:164-171, 2009.
462. Patel K, Ming X, Williams PL, et al: Impact of HAART and CNS-penetrating antiretroviral regimens on HIV encephalopathy among perinatally infected children and adolescents, *AIDS* 23:1893-1901, 2009.
463. Cooper ER, Hanson C, Diaz C, et al: Encephalopathy and progression of human immunodeficiency virus disease in a cohort of children with perinatally acquired human immunodeficiency virus infection. Women and Infants Transmission Study Group, *J Pediatr* 132:808-812, 1998.
464. European Collaborative Study: Neurologic signs in young children with human immunodeficiency virus infection, *Pediatr Infect Dis J* 9:402-406, 1990.
465. Epstein LG, Sharer LR, Oleske JM, et al: Neurologic manifestations of human immunodeficiency virus infection in children, *Pediatrics* 78:678-687, 1986.
466. DeCarli C, Civitello LA, Brouwers P, et al: The prevalence of computed tomographic abnormalities of the cerebrum in 100 consecutive children symptomatic with the human immunodeficiency virus, *Ann Neurol* 34:198-205, 1993.
467. Hollander H, Levy JA: Neurologic abnormalities and recovery of human immunodeficiency virus from cerebrospinal fluid, *Ann Intern Med* 106:692-695, 1987.
468. Van R, Harrington PR, Dow A, et al: Neurologic and neurodevelopmental manifestations of pediatric HIV/AIDS: a global perspective, *Eur J Paediatr Neurol* 11:1-9, 2007.
469. Kaul M, Zheng J, Okamoto S, et al: HIV-1 infection and AIDS: consequences for the CNS, *Cell Death* 12:878-892, 2005.
470. Epstein LG, Gelbard HA: HIV-1 induced neuronal injury in the developing brain, *J Leukoc Biol* 65:453-457, 1999.
471. Schwartz L, Major EO: Neural progenitors and HIV-1 associated central nervous system disease in adults and children, *Curr HIV Res* 4:319-327, 2006.
472. Lyman YD, Kress Y, Kure K, et al: Detection of HIV in fetal central nervous tissue, *AIDS* 4:917-920, 1990.
473. Kozlowski PB, Brudkowska J, Kraszpulski M, et al: Microencephaly in children congenitally infected with human immunodeficiency virus: a gross-anatomical morphometric study, *Acta Neuropathol* 93:136-145, 1997.
474. Mirza A, Rathore MH: Human immunodeficiency virus and the central nervous system, *Semin Pediatr Neurol* 19:119-123, 2012.
475. Saavedra-Lozano J, Ramos JT, Sanz F, et al: Salvage therapy with abacavir and other reverse transcriptase inhibitors for human immunodeficiency-associated encephalopathy, *Pediatr Infect Dis J* 25:1142-1152, 2006.
476. Sanchez-Ramon S, Resino S, Bellón Cano JM, et al: Neuroprotective effects of early antiretrovirals in vertical HIV infection, *Pediatr Neurol* 29:218-221, 2003.
477. DeCarli C, Fugate L, Falloon J, et al: Brain growth and cognitive improvement in children with human immunodeficiency virus-induced encephalopathy after 6 months of continuous zidovudine infusion, *J Acquir Immune Defic Syndr* 4:585-592, 1991.
478. Pizzo PA, Eddy J, Falloon J, et al: Effect of continuous intravenous infusion of zidovudine (AZT) in children with symptomatic HIV infection, *N Engl J Med* 319:889-896, 1988.
479. Raskino C, Pearson DA, Baker CJ, et al: Neurologic, neurocognitive and brain growth outcomes in human immunodeficiency virus-infected children receiving different nucleoside antiretroviral regimens, *Pediatrics* 104:e32, 1999.
480. Portegies P: HIV-1, the brain and combination therapy, *Lancet* 346:1244-1245, 1995.
481. McCoig C, Castrejón MM, Castaño E, et al: Effects of combination antiretroviral therapy on cerebrospinal fluid HIV RNA, HIV resistance, and clinical manifestations of encephalopathy, *J Pediatr* 141:36-44, 2002.
482. Wynn HE, Brundage RC, Fletcher CV: Clinical implications of CNS penetration of antiretroviral drugs, *CNS Drugs* 16:595-609, 2002.
483. Brouwers P, DeCarli C, Civitello L, et al: Correlation between computed tomographic brain scan abnormalities and neuropsychological function in children with symptomatic human immunodeficiency virus disease, *Arch Neurol* 52:39-44, 1995.
484. Brouwers P, Tudor-Williams G, DeCarli C, et al: Relation between stage of the disease and neurobehavioral measures in children with symptomatic HIV disease, *AIDS* 9:713-720, 1995.
485. Smith R, Malee K, Leighty R, et al: Effects of perinatal HIV infection and associated risk factors on cognitive development among young children, *Pediatrics* 117:851-862, 2006.
486. Connor EM, Andiman WA: Lymphoid interstitial pneumonitis. In Pizzo PA, Wilfert CA, editors: *Pediatric AIDS. The challenge of HIV infection in infants, children, and adolescents*, Baltimore, 1994, Williams & Wilkins, pp 467-482.
487. Sharland M, Gibb DM, Holland F: Respiratory morbidity from lymphocytic interstitial pneumonitis (LIP) in vertically acquired HIV infection, *Arch Dis Child* 76:334-336, 1997.

488. Zar HJ: Chronic lung disease in human immunodeficiency virus (HIV) infected children, *Pediatr Pulmonol* 43:1-10, 2008.
489. Joshi VV, Kauffman S, Oleske JM, et al: Polyclonal polymorphic B-cell lymphoproliferative disorder with prominent pulmonary involvement in children with acquired immune deficiency syndrome, *Cancer* 59:1455-1462, 1987.
490. Bhoopat L: Relationship of cell bearing EBER and p24 antigens in biopsy-proven lymphocytic interstitial pneumonia in HIV-1 subtype E infected children, *Appl Immunohistochem Mol Morphol* 19: 547-551, 2011.
491. Rubinstein A, Bernstein LJ, Charytan M, et al: Corticosteroid treatment for pulmonary lymphoid hyperplasia in children with the acquired immune deficiency syndrome, *Pediatr Pulmonol* 4:13-17, 1988.
492. Dufour V, Wislez M, Bergot E, et al: Improvement of symptomatic human immunodeficiency virus-related lymphoid interstitial pneumonia in patients receiving highly active antiretroviral therapy, *Clin Infect Dis* 36:e127-130, 2003.
493. Lipshultz SE, Miller TL, Wilkinson JD, et al: Cardiac effects in perinatally HIV-infected and HIV-exposed but uninfected children and adolescents: a view from the United States of America, *J Int AIDS Soc* 16:18597, 2013.
494. Lipshultz SE, Easley KA, Orav EJ, et al: Cardiac dysfunction and mortality in HIV-infected children: the prospective P2C2 HIV multicenter study. Pediatric pulmonary and cardiac complications of vertically transmitted HIV infection (P2C2 HIV) study group, *Circulation* 102:1542-1548, 2000.
495. Morse CG, Kovacs JA: Metabolic and skeletal complications of HIV infection: the price of success, *JAMA* 296:844-854, 2006.
496. Luginbuhl LM, Orav EJ, McIntosh K, et al: Cardiac morbidity and related mortality in children with HIV infection, *JAMA* 269: 2869-2875, 1993.
497. Fisher SD, Easley KA, Orav EJ, et al: Mild dilated cardiomyopathy and increased left ventricular mass predict mortality: the prospective P2C2 HIV Multicenter Study, *Am Heart J* 150:439-447, 2005.
498. Lipshultz SE, Williams PL, Wilkinson JD, et al: Cardiac status of HIV-infected children treated with long-term combination antiretroviral therapy: results from the Adolescent Master Protocol of the NIH multicenter pediatric HIV/AIDS cohort study, *JAMA Pediatr* 1:8, 2013.
499. Lipshultz SE, Mas CM, Henkel JM, et al: HAART to heart: highly active antiretroviral therapy and the risk of cardiovascular disease in HIV-infected or exposed children and adults, *Expert Rev Anti Infect Ther* 10:661-674, 2012.
500. Pozzan G, Pagliari C, Tuon FF, et al: Diffuse-regressive alterations and apoptosis of myocytes: possible causes of myocardial dysfunction in HIV-related cardiomyopathy, *Int J Cardiol* 132:90-95, 2009.
501. Miller TL, Agostoni C, Duggan C, et al: Gastrointestinal and nutritional complications of human immunodeficiency virus infection, *J Pediatr Gastroenterol Nutr* 47:247-253, 2008.
502. Grunfeld C, Feingold KR: Metabolic disturbances and wasting in the acquired immunodeficiency syndrome, *N Engl J Med* 327: 329-337, 1992.
503. Galli L, de Martino M, Tovo PA, et al: Onset of clinical signs in children with HIV-1 perinatal infection, *AIDS* 9:455-461, 1995.
504. Pickering LK: Infections of the gastrointestinal tract. In Pizzo PA, Wilfert CA, editors: *Pediatric AIDS. The challenge of HIV infection in infants, children, and adolescents*, Baltimore, 1994, Williams & Wilkins, pp 377-404.
505. Walker AS, Mulenga V, Sinyinza F, et al: Determinants of survival without antiretroviral therapy after infancy in HIV-1-infected Zambian children in the CHAP Trial, *J Acquir Immune Defic Syndr* 42: 637-645, 2006.
506. Persaud D, Bangaru B, Greco MA, et al: Cholestatic hepatitis in children infected with the human immunodeficiency virus, *Pediatr Infect Dis J* 12:492-498, 1993.
507. Operskalski EA, Kovacs A: HIV/HCV co-infection: pathogenesis, clinical complications, treatment, and new therapeutic technologies, *Curr HIV/AIDS Rep* 8:12-22, 2011.
508. England K, Thorne C, Newell ML: Vertically acquired paediatric coinfection with HIV and hepatitis C virus, *Lancet Infect Dis* 6:83-90, 2006.
509. Healy SA, Gupta S, Melvin AJ: HIV/HBV coinfection in children and antiviral therapy, *Expert Rev Anti Infect Ther* 11:251-263, 2013.
510. Claret-Teruel G, Noguera-Julian A, Esteva C, et al: Impact of human immunodeficiency virus coinfection on the progression of mother-to-child transmitted hepatitis C virus infection, *Pediatr Infect Dis J* 30:801-814, 2011.
511. Miller TL, Winter HS, Luginbuhl LM, et al: Pancreatitis in pediatric human immunodeficiency virus infection, *J Pediatr* 120:223-227, 1992.
512. Butler KM, Venzon D, Henry N, et al: Pancreatitis in human immunodeficiency virus-infected children receiving dideoxyinosine, *Pediatrics* 91:747-751, 1993.
513. Bhimma R, Purswani MU, Kala U, et al: Kidney disease in children and adolescents with perinatal HIV-1 infection, *J Int AIDS Soc* 16:18596, 2013.
514. Ramsuran D, Bhimma R, Ramdial PK, et al: The spectrum of HIV-related nephropathy in children, *Pediatr Nephrology* 27:821-827, 2012.
515. Ray PE: Taking a hard look at the pathogenesis of childhood HIV-associated nephropathy, *Pediatr Nephrol* 24: 2109-2119, 2009.
516. Ingulli E, Tejani A, Fikrig S, et al: Nephrotic syndrome associated with acquired immunodeficiency syndrome in children, *J Pediatr* 119:710-716, 1991.
517. McClain. K: Hematologic manifestations and malignancies of children with AIDS, *Semin Pediatr Infect Dis* 6:26-30, 1995.
518. Nigro G, Gattinara GC, Mattia S, et al: Parvovirus-B19-related pancytopenia in children with HIV infection, *Lancet* 340:115, 1992.
519. Mueller BU: Hematological problems and their management in children with HIV infection. In Pizzo PA, Wilfert CA, editors: *Pediatric AIDS. The challenge of HIV infection in infants, children, and adolescents*, Baltimore, 1994, Williams & Wilkins, pp 591-602.
520. Mueller BU, Tannenbaum S, Pizzo PA: Bone marrow aspirates and biopsies in children with human immunodeficiency virus infection, *J Pediatr Hematol Oncol* 18:266-271, 1996.
521. Henry DH, Beall GN, Benson CA, et al: Recombinant human erythropoietin in the treatment of anemia associated with human immunodeficiency virus (HIV) infection and zidovudine therapy: overview of four clinical trials, *Ann Intern Med* 117:739-748, 1992.
522. Griffin TC, Squires JE, Timmons CF, et al: Chronic human parvovirus B19-induced erythroid hypoplasia as the initial manifestation of human immunodeficiency virus infection, *J Pediatr* 118:899-901, 1991.
523. Mueller BU, Jacobsen F, Butler KM, et al: Combination treatment with azidothymidine and granulocyte colony-stimulating factor in children with human immunodeficiency virus infection, *J Pediatr* 121:797-802, 1992.
524. Ballem PJ, Belzberg A, Devine DV, et al: 1992 Kinetic studies of the mechanism of thrombocytopenia in patients with human immunodeficiency virus infection, *N Engl J Med* 327:1779-1789, 1992.
525. Rigaud M, Leibovitz E, Quee CS, et al: Thrombocytopenia in children infected with human immunodeficiency virus: long-term follow-up and therapeutic considerations, *J Acquir Immune Defic Syndr* 5:450-455, 1992.
526. Vannappagari V, Nkhoma ET, Atashili J, et al: Prevalence, severity, and duration of thrombocytopenia among HIV patients in the era of highly active antiretroviral therapy, *Platelets* 22:611-618, 2011.
527. Ellaurie M, Burns ER, Bernstein LJ, et al: Thrombocytopenia and human immunodeficiency virus in children, *Pediatrics* 82:905-908, 1988.
528. Ahemed HN, Ball C, Height SE, et al: Rituximab in chronic, recurrent HIV-associated immune thrombocytopenia purpura, *Br J Haematol* 127:607, 2004.
529. Mankahla A, Mosam A: Common skin conditions in children with HIV/AIDS, *Am J Clin Dermatol* 13:153-166, 2012.
530. Prose NS: 1994 Skin problems. In Pizzo PA, Wilfert CA, editors: *Pediatric AIDS. The challenge of HIV infection in infants, children, and adolescents*, Baltimore, 1994, Williams & Wilkins, pp 535-546.
531. von Seidlein L, Gillette SG, Bryson Y, et al: Frequent recurrence and persistence of varicella-zoster virus infections in children infected with human immunodeficiency virus type 1, *J Pediatr* 128:52-57, 1996.
532. Umoru D, Oviawe O, Ibadin M, et al: Mucocutaneous manifestation of pediatric human immunodeficiency virus/acquired immunodeficiency syndrome (HIV/AIDS) in relation to degree of immunosuppression: a study of a West African population, *Int J Dermatol* 51:305-312, 2012.
533. Resnick JS, Van Beek M, Furmanski L, et al: Etiology of pruritic papular eruption with HIV infection in Uganda, *JAMA* 292:2614-2621, 2004.

534. Farsani TT, Kore S, Nadol P, et al: Etiology and risk factors associated with a pruritic papular eruption with HIV infection in India, *J Int AIDS Soc* 16:17325, 2013.
535. McCalmont TH, Altemus D, Maurer T, et al: Eosinophilic folliculitis. The histologic spectrum, *Am J Dermatopathol* 17:439-446, 1995.
536. Kest H, Brogly S, McSherry G, et al: Malignancy in perinatally human immunodeficiency virus-infected children in the United States, *Pediatr Infect Dis J* 24:237-242, 2005.
537. Granovsky MO, Mueller BU, Nicholson HS, et al: Cancer in human immunodeficiency virus-infected children: a case series from the Children's Cancer Group and National Cancer Institute, *J Clin Oncol* 16:1729-1735, 1998.
538. Connor E, Boccon-Gibod L, Joshi V, et al: Cutaneous acquired immunodeficiency syndrome-associated Kaposi's sarcoma in pediatric patients, *Arch Dermatol* 126:791-793, 1990.
539. Buck BE, Scott GB, Valdes-Dapena M, et al: Kaposi sarcoma in two infants with acquired immune deficiency syndrome, *J Pediatr* 103:911-913, 1983.
540. Gutierrez-Ortega P, Hierro-Orozco S, Sanchez-Cisneros R, et al: Kaposi's sarcoma in a 6-day-old infant with human immunodeficiency virus, *Arch Dermatol* 125:432-433, 1989.
541. Tukei VJ, Kekitiinwa A, Beasley RP, et al: Prevalence and outcome of HIV-associated malignancies in children, *AIDS* 25:1789-1793, 2011.
542. Cox CM, El-Mallawany NK, Kabue M, et al: Clinical characteristics and outcomes of HIV-infected children diagnosed with Kaposi sarcoma in Malawi and Botswana, *Pediatr Blood Cancer* 60:1274-1280, 2013.
543. Bhatia K, Shiels MS, Berg A, et al: Sarcomas other than Kaposi sarcoma occurring in immunodeficiency: interpretations from a systematic literature review, *Curr Opin Oncol* 24:537-546, 2012.
544. Preciado MV, Fallo A, Chabay P, et al: Epstein-Barr virus-associated lymphoma in HIV infected children, *Pathol Res Pract* 198:327-332, 2002.
545. Smith K, Kuhn L, Coovadia A, et al: Immune reconstitution inflammatory syndrome among HIV-infected South African infants initiating antiretroviral therapy, *AIDS* 23:1097-1107, 2009.
546. Wang ME, Castillo ME, Montano SM, et al: Immune reconstitution inflammatory syndrome in human immunodeficiency virus-infected children in Peru, *Pediatr Infect Dis J* 28:900-903, 2009.
547. Oberdorfer P, Washington CH, Katanyuwong K, et al: Progressive multifocal leukoencephalopathy in HIV-infected children: a case report and literature review, *Int J Pediatr* 2009:348507, 2009.
548. Rabie H, Violari A, Duong T, et al: Early antiretroviral treatment reduces risk of bacille Calmette-Guérin immune reconstitution adenitis, *Int J Tuberc Lung Dis* 15:1194-1200, 2011.
549. Blanche S, Tardieu M, Duliege A, et al: Longitudinal study of 94 symptomatic infants with perinatally acquired human immunodeficiency virus infection: evidence for a bimodal expression of clinical and biological symptoms, *Am J Dis Child* 144:1210-1215, 1990.
550. Gray L, Newell ML, Thorne C, et al: Fluctuations in symptoms in human immunodeficiency virus-infected children: the first 10 years of life, *Pediatrics* 108:116-122, 2001.
551. Diaz C, Hanson C, Cooper ER, et al: Disease progression in a cohort of infants with vertically acquired HIV infection observed from birth: the Women and Infants Transmission Study (WITS), *J Acquir Immune Defic Syndr Hum Retrovirol* 14:442-450, 1997.
552. Features of children perinatally infected with HIV-1 surviving longer than 5 years. Italian Register for HIV infection in Children, *Lancet* 342:191-195, 1994.
553. Mphatswe W, Blanckenberg N, Tudor-Williams G, et al: High frequency of rapid immunological progression in African infants infected in the era of perinatal HIV prophylaxis, *AIDS* 21: 1253-1256, 2007.
554. Abrams EJ, Wiener J, Carter R, et al: Maternal health factors and early pediatric antiretroviral therapy influence the rate of perinatal HIV-1 disease progression in children, *AIDS* 17:867-877, 2003.
555. Frederick T, Mascola L, Eller A, et al: Progression of human immunodeficiency virus disease among infants and children infected perinatally with human immunodeficiency virus or through neonatal blood transfusion, *Pediatr Infect Dis J* 13:1091-1097, 1994.
556. Judd A, Doerholt K, Tookey PA, et al: Morbidity, mortality, and response to treatment by children in the United Kingdom and Ireland with perinatally acquired HIV infection during 1996-2000: planning for teenage and adult care, *Clin Infect Dis* 45:918-924, 2007.
557. Viani RM, Araneta MR, Deville JG, et al: Decrease in hospitalization and mortality rates among children with perinatally acquired HIV type 1 infection receiving highly active antiretroviral therapy, *Clin Infect Dis* 39:725-731, 2004.
558. Lindsey JC, Malee KM, Brouwers P, et al: Neurodevelopmental functioning in HIV-infected infants and young children before and after the introduction of protease-inhibitor-based highly active antiretroviral therapy, *Pediatrics* 119:e681-693, 2007.
559. Nachman SA, Lindsey JC, Moye J, et al: Growth of human immunodeficiency virus-infected children receiving highly active antiretroviral therapy, *Pediatr Infect Dis J* 24:352-357, 2005.
560. Storm DS, Boland MG, Gortmaker SL, et al: Protease inhibitor combination therapy, severity of illness, and quality of life among children with perinatally acquired HIV-1 infection, *Pediatrics* 115: e173-e182, 2005.
561. Guillen S, García San Miguel L, Resino S, et al: Opportunistic infections and organ-specific diseases in HIV-1-infected children: a cohort study (1990-2006), *HIV Med* 11:245-252, 2010.
562. Rakhmanina N, Ryan Phelps B: Pharmacotherapy of pediatric HIV infection, *Pediatr Clin N Am* 59:1093-1115, 2012.
563. Maron G, Gaur AH, Flynn PM: Antiretroviral therapy in HIV-infected infants and children, *Pediatr Infect Dis J* 29:360-363, 2010.
564. Siberry GA, Hazra R: Management of HIV infection. In Long SS, Pickering LK, Prober CG, editors: *Principles and practice of pediatric infectious diseases*, ed 4, Philadelphia, 2012, Elsevier, pp 664-672.
565. Food and Drug Administration: Approved antiretroviral drugs for pediatric treatment of HIV infection. Available at http://wwwfda.gov/ForConsumers/ByAudience/ForPatientAdvocates/HIVandAIDSActivities/ucm118951.htm. Accessed November 18, 2013.
566. Rakhmanina NY, van den Anker JN: Pharmacological research in pediatrics: from neonates to adolescents, *Adv Drug Deliv Rev* 58: 4-14, 2006.
567. Chadwick EG, Yogev R, Alvero CG, et al: Long-term outcomes for HIV-infected infants less than 6 months of age at initiation of lopinavir/ritonavir combination antiretroviral therapy, *AIDS* 25:643-649, 2011.
568. Menson EN, Walker AS, Sharland M, et al: Underdosing of antiretrovirals in UK and Irish children with HIV as an example of problems in prescribing medicines to children 1997-2005: a cohort study, *BMJ* 332:1183-1187, 2006.
569. Capparelli EV, Mirochnick M, Dankner WM, et al: Pharmacokinetics and tolerance of zidovudine in preterm infants, *J Pediatr* 142:47-52, 2003.
570. Foster C, Lyall H: HIV and mitochondrial toxicity in children, *J Antimicrob Chemother* 61:8-12, 2008.
571. McArthur MA, Kalu SU, Foulks AR, et al: Twin preterm neonates with cardiac toxicity related to lopinavir/ritonavir therapy, *Pediatr Infect Dis J* 28:1127-1129, 2009.
572. Barlow-Mosha L, Eckard AR, McComsey GA, et al: Metabolic complications and treatment of perinatally HIV-infected children and adolescents, *J Int AIDS Soc* 16:18600, 2013.
573. Violari A, Cotton MF, Gibb DM, et al: Early antiretroviral therapy and mortality among HIV-infected infants, *N Eng J Med* 359: 2233-2244, 2008.
574. Coovadia A, Abrams EJ, Stehlau R, et al: Reuse of nevirapine in exposed HIV-infected children after protease inhibitor-based viral suppression: a randomized controlled trial, *JAMA* 304:1082-1090, 2010.
575. Kuhn L, Coovadia A, Strehlau R, et al: Switching children previously exposed to nevirapine to nevirapine-based treatment after initial suppression with a protease-inhibitor-based regimen: long-term follow-up of a randomized open-label trial, *Lancet Infect Dis* 12:521-530, 2012.
576. Palumbo P, Lindsey JC, Hughes MD, et al: Antiretroviral treatment for children with peripartum nevirapine exposure, *N Engl J Med* 363:1510-1520, 2010.
577. Violari A, Lindsey JC, Hughes MD, et al: Nevirapine versus ritonavir-boosted lopinavir in HIV-infected children, *N Engl J Med* 366: 2380-2389, 2012.
578. Prendergast A, Mphatswe W, Tudor-Williams G, et al: Early virological suppression with three-class antiretroviral therapy in HIV-infected African infants, *AIDS* 22:1333-1343, 2008.
579. Prendergast AJ, Penazzato M, Cotton M, et al: Treatment of young children with HIV infection: using evidence to inform policymakers, *PLoS Med* 9:e10001273, 2012.
580. HIV Paediatric Prognostic Markers Collaborative Study: Predictive value of absolute CD4 cell count for disease progression in untreated HIV-1 infected children, *AIDS* 20:1289-1294, 2006.

581. HIV Paediatric Prognostic Markers Collaborative Study Group (HPPMCS): Short-term risk of disease progression in HIV-1 infected children receiving no antiretroviral therapy or zidovudine monotherapy: a meta-analysis, *Lancet* 362:1605-1611, 2003.
582. Cross Continents Collaboration for Kids (3Cs4kids) Analysis and Writing Committee: markers for predicting mortality in untreated HIV-infected children in resource-limited settings: a meta-analysis, *AIDS* 22:97-105, 2008.
583. Berk DR, Falkovitz-Halpern MS, Hill DW, et al: Temporal trends in early clinical manifestations of perinatal HIV infection in a population-based cohort, *JAMA* 293:2221-2231, 2005.
584. Faye A, Le Chenadec J, Dollfus C, et al: Early versus deferred antiretroviral multidrug therapy in infants infected with HIV type 1, *Clin Infect Dis* 39:1692-1698, 2004.
585. Luzuriaga K, McManus M, Mofenson L, et al: A trial of three antiretroviral regimens in HIV-1 infected children, *N Engl J Med* 350: 2471-2480, 2004.
586. Judd A: Early antiretroviral therapy in HIV-1-infected infants, 1996-2008: treatment response and duration of first-line regimens, *AIDS* 25:2279-2287, 2011.
587. Chiappini E, Galli L, Tovo PA, et al: Five-year follow-up of children with perinatal HIV-1 infection receiving early highly active antiretroviral therapy, *BMC Infect Dis* 9:140, 2009.
588. Goetghebuer T, Haelterman E, Le Chenadec J, et al: Effect of early antiretroviral therapy on the risk of AIDS/death in HIV-infected infants, *AIDS* 23:597-604, 2009.
589. Newell ML, Patel D, Goetghebuer T, et al: CD4 cell response to antiretroviral therapy in children with vertically acquired HIV infection: is it associated with age at initiation, *J Infect Dis* 193:954-962, 2006.
590. Goetghebuer T, Le Chenadec J, Haelterman E, et al: Short- and long-term immunological and virological outcome in HIV-infected infants according to the age at antiretroviral treatment initiation, *Clin Infect Dis* 54:878-881, 2012.
591. Cotton MF, Violari A, Otwombe K, et al: Early time-limited antiretroviral therapy versus deferred therapy in South African infants infected with HIV: results from children with HIV early antiretroviral (CHER) randomized trial, *Lancet* 382:1555-1563, 2013.
592. Chiappini E, Galli L, Tovo PA, et al: Virologic, immunologic, and clinical benefits from early combined antiretroviral therapy in infants with perinatal HIV-1 infecton, *AIDS* 20:207-215, 2006.
593. Laughton B, Cornell M, Grove D, et al: Early antiretroviral therapy improves neurodevelopmental outcomes in infants, *AIDS* 26: 1685-1690, 2012.
594. Collins IJ, Judd A, Gibb DM: Immediate antiretroviral therapy in young HIV-infected children: benefits and risks, *Curr Opin HIV AIDS* 9:87-94, 2014.
595. Welch SB, Gibb D: When should children with HIV infection be started on antiretroviral therapy, *PLoS Med* 5:e73, 2008.
596. Puthanakit T, Saphonn V, Ananworanich J, et al: Early versus deferred antiretroviral therapy for children older than 1 year infected with HIV (PREDICT): a multicenter, randomized, open-label trial, *Lancet Infect Dis* 12:933-941, 2012.
597. Puthanakit T, Ananworanich J, Vonthanak S, et al: Cognitive function and neurodevelopmental outcomes in HIV-infected children older than 1 year of age randomized to early versus deferred antiretroviral therapy: the PREDICT neurodevelopmental study, *Pediatr Infect Dis J* 32:501-508, 2013.
598. Lewis J, Walker AS, Castro H, et al: Age and CD4 count at initiation of antiretroviral therapy in HIV-infected children: effects on long-term T-cell reconstitution, *J Infect Dis* 205:548-556, 2012.
599. Welch S, Sharland M, Lyall EG, et al: PENTA 2009 guidelines for the use of antiretroviral therapy in paediatric HIV-1 infection, *HIV Med* 10:591-613, 2009.
600. World Health Organization. Report of the WHO technical reference group, paediatric HIV/ART care guideline group meeting. Revised treatment recommendations for infants. Available at http://www.who.int/hiv/pub/paediatric/art_meeting_april2008/en/index.html. Accessed November 18, 2013.
601. World Health Organization. Antiretroviral therapy for HIV infection in infants and children: towards universal access. Recommendations for a public health approach. Available at http://www.who.int/hiv/pub/paediatric/infants2010/en/index.html. Accessed November 18, 2013.
602. Camacho-Gonzalez AF, Ross AC, Chakraborty R: The clinical care of the HIV-1 infected infant, *Clin Perinatol* 37:873-885, 2010.
603. Lockman S, Shapiro RL, Smeaton LM, et al: Response to antiretroviral therapy after a single, peripartum dose of nevirapine, *N Engl J Med* 356:135-147, 2007.
604. Musiime V, Ssali F, Kayiwa J, et al: Response to non-nucleoside reverse transcriptase inhibitor-based therapy in HIV-infected children with perinatal exposure to single-dose nevirapine, *AIDS Res Hum Retroviruses* 25:989-996, 2009.
605. MacLeod IJ, Rowley CF, Thior I, et al: Minor resistant variants in nevirapine-exposed infants may predict virologic failure on nevirapine-containing ART, *J Clin Virol* 48:162-167, 2010.
606. PENPACT-1 (PENTA 9/PACTG 390) Study Team, Babiker A, Castro nee Green H, et al: First-line antiretroviral therapy with a protease inhibitor versus non-nucleoside reverse transcriptase inhibitor and switch at higher versus low viral load in HIV-infected children: an open-label, randomized phase 2/3 trial, *Lancet Infect Dis* 11: 273-283, 2011.
607. Hazra R, Cohen RA, Gonin R, et al: Lipid levels in the second year of life among HIV-infected and HIV-exposed uninfected Latin American children, *AIDS* 26:235-240, 2012.
608. Chadwick EG, Capparelli EV, Yogev R, et al: Pharmacokinetics, safety, and efficacy of lopinavir/ritonavir in infants less than 6 months of age: 24 week results, *AIDS* 22:249-255, 2008.
609. Walker AS, Doerholt K, Sharland M, et al: Response to highly active antiretroviral therapy varies with age: the UK and Ireland Collaborative HIV Paediatric study, *AIDS* 18:1915-1924, 2004.
610. Chadwick EG, Pinto J, Yogev R, et al: Early initiation of lopinavir/ritonavir in infants less than 6 weeks of age: pharmacokinetics and 24-week safety and efficacy, *Pediatr Infect Dis J* 28:215-219, 2009.
611. Van der Linden D, Hainaut M, Goetghebuer T, et al: Effectiveness of early initiation of protease inhibitor-sparing antiretroviral regimens in human immunodeficiency virus-1 vertically infected infants, *Pediatr Infect Dis J* 26:359-361, 2007.
612. Riordan A, Bugembe T: Update on antiretroviral therapy, *Arch Dis Child* 94:70-74, 2009.
613. Kenny J, Musiime V, Judd A, et al: Recent advances in pharmacovigilance of antiretroviral therapy in HIV-infected and exposed children, *Curr Opin HIV AIDS* 7:305-316, 2012.
614. Sigaloff K, Calis JC, Geelen SP, et al: HIV-1 resistance mutations after failure of first-line antiretroviral treatment among children in resource-poor regions: a systematic review, *Lancet* 11:769-779, 2011.
615. Bertagnolio S, Penazzato M, Jordan MR, et al: World Health Organization generic protocol to assess drug-resistant HIV among children < 18 months of age and newly diagnosed with HIV in resource-limited countries, *Clin Infect Dis* 54(Suppl 4):S260-S354, 2012.
616. Arrive E, Newell ML, Ekouevi DK, et al: Prevalence of resistance to nevirapine in mothers and children after single-dose exposure to prevent vertical transmission of HIV-1: a meta-analysis, *Int J Epidemiol* 36:1009-1021, 2007.
617. Fogel JM, Mwatha A, Richardson P, et al: Impact of maternal and infant antiretroviral drug regimens on drug resistance in HIV-infected breastfeeding infants, *Pediatr Infect Dis J* 32:e164-e169, 2013.
618. Sutcliffe CG, van Dijk JH, Bolton C, et al: Effectiveness of antiretroviral therapy among HIV-infected children in sub-Saharan Africa, *Lancet Infect Dis* 8:477-489, 2008.
619. Ciaranello AL, Chang Y, Margulis AV, et al: Effectiveness of pediatric antiretroviral therapy in resource-limited settings: a systematic review and metanalysis, *Clin Infect Dis* 49:1915-1927, 2009.
620. Heidari S, Mofenson LM, Hobbs CV, et al: Unresolved antiretroviral treatment management issues in HIV-infected children, *J Acquir Immune Defic Syndr* 59:161-169, 2012.
621. Nuorti JP, Whitney CG: Prevention of pneumococcal disease among infants and children: use of 13-valent pneumococcal conjugate vaccine and 23-valent pneumococcal polysaccharide vaccine- recommendations of the Advisory Committee on Immunization Practices (ACIP), *MMWR Recomm Rep* 59(RR-11):1-18, 2010.
622. McLean HQ, Fiebelkorn AP, Temte JL, et al: Prevention of measles, rubella, congenital rubella syndrome, and mumps, 2013: summary recommendations of the Advisory Committee on Immunization Practices (ACIP), *MMWR Recomm Rep* 62(RR-04):1-34, 2013.

623. Sutcliffe CG, Moss WJ: Do children infected with HIV receiving HAART need to be revaccinated? *Lancet Infect Dis* 10:630-642, 2010.
624. Mofenson LM, Moye J Jr: Intravenous immune globulin for the prevention of infections in children with symptomatic human immunodeficiency virus infection, *Pediatr Res* 33(Suppl 1):S80-S89, 1993.
625. Spector SA, Gelber RD, McGrath N, et al: A controlled trial of intravenous immune globulin for the prevention of serious bacterial infections in children receiving zidovudine for advanced HIV infection, *N Engl J Med* 331:1181-1187, 1994.
626. National Institute of Child Health and Human Development Intravenous Immunoglobulin Study Group: Intravenous immune globulin for the prevention of bacterial infections in children with symptomatic human immunodeficiency virus infection, *N Engl J Med* 325:73-80, 1991.
627. Pierce M, Crampton S, Henry D, et al: A multicenter trial of clarithromycin as prophylaxis against disseminated *Mycobacterium avium* complex infections with advanced acquired human immunodeficiency syndrome, *N Engl J Med* 335:384-391, 1996.
628. Havlir DV, Dubé MP, Sattler FR, et al: Prophylaxis against disseminated *Mycobacterium avium* complex with weekly azithromycin, daily rifabutin, or both, *N Engl J Med* 335:392-398, 1996.
629. Birkhead GS, Pulver WP, Warren BL, et al: Progress in prevention of mother-to-child transmission of HIV in New York State: 1998-2008, *J Public Health Manag Pract* 16:481-491, 2010.
630. Birkhead GS, Pulver WP, Warren BL, et al: Acquiring human immunodeficiency virus during pregnancy and mother-to-child transmission in New York: 2002-2006, *Obstet Gynecol* 115:1247-1255, 2010.
631. Centers for Disease Control and Prevention: Recommendations for assisting in the prevention of perinatal transmission of human T-lymphotrophic virus type III/lymphadenopathy-associated virus and acquired immunodeficiency, *MMWR Morb Mortal Wkly Rep* 34:721-732, 1985.
632. Connor EM, Sperling RS, Gelber R, et al: Reduction of maternal-infant transmission of immunodeficiency virus type 1 with zidovudine treatment, *N Engl J Med* 331:1173-1180, 1994.
633. Centers for Disease Control and Prevention: Recommendations of the U.S. Public Health Service Task Force on the use of zidovudine to reduce perinatal transmission of human immunodeficiency virus, *MMWR Morb Mortal Wkly Rep* 43:1-20, 1994.
634. Connor EM, Mofenson LK: Zidovudine for the reduction of perinatal human immunodeficiency virus transmission. Pediatric AIDS Clinical Trials Group protocol 076—results and treatment recommendations, *Pediatr Infect Dis J* 14:536-541, 1995.
635. Centers for Disease Control and Prevention: Success in implementing Public Health Service guidelines to reduce perinatal transmission of HIV: Louisiana, Michigan, New Jersey and South Carolina, 1993, 1995, and 1998, *MMWR Morb Mortal Wkly Rep* 47:688-691, 1998.
636. Centers for Disease Control and Prevention: Achievements in public health. Reduction in perinatal transmission of HIV infection—United States, 1985-2005, *MMWR Morb Mortal Wkly Rep* 55:592-597, 2006.
637. Rogers MF, Taylor AW, Nesheim SR: Preventing perinatal transmission of HIV: the national perspective, *J Public Health Manag Pract* 16:505-508, 2010.
638. McKenna MT, Hu X: Recent trends in the incidence and morbidity that are associated with perinatal human immunodeficiency virus infection in the United States, *Am J Obstet Gynecol* 197(Suppl 3): S10-S16, 2007.
639. Centers for Disease Control and Prevention: US Public Health Service recommendations for human immunodeficiency virus counseling and voluntary testing for pregnant women, *MMWR Recomm Rep* 44(RR-7):1-15, 1995.
640. Institute of Medicine, National Research Council: *Reducing the odds: preventing perinatal transmission of HIV in the United States*, Washington, DC, 1999, National Academies Press.
641. Centers for Disease Control and Prevention: Revised guidelines for HIV counseling, testing, and referral and revised recommendations for HIV screening of pregnant women, *MMWR Recomm Rep* 50 (RR-19):1-110, 2001.
642. Branson BM, Handsfield HH, Lampe MA, et al: Revised recommendations for HIV testing of adults, adolescents, and pregnant women in health-care settings, *MMWR Recomm Rep* 55(RR-14):1-17, 2006.
643. Shaffer N, Chuachoowong R, Mock PA, et al: Short-course zidovudine for perinatal HIV-1 transmission in Bangkok, Thailand: a randomised controlled trial. Bangkok Collaborative Perinatal HIV-1 Transmission Study Group, *Lancet* 353:773-780, 1999.
644. Wiktor SZ, Ekpini E, Karon JM, et al: Short-course oral zidovudine for prevention of mother-to-child transmission of HIV-1 in Abidjan, Côte d'Ivoire: a randomized trial, *Lancet* 353:781-785, 1999.
645. Dabis F, Msellati P, Meda N, et al: 6-Month efficacy, tolerance, and acceptability of a short regimen of oral zidovudine to reduce vertical transmission of HIV-1 in breastfed children in Côte d'Ivoire and Burkina Faso: a double-blind placebo-controlled multicentre trial. DITRAME Study Group, *Lancet* 353:786-792, 1999.
646. Leroy V, Karon JM, Alioum A, et al: Twenty-four month efficacy of a maternal short-course zidovudine regimen to prevent mother-to-child transmission of HIV-1 in West Africa, *AIDS* 16:631-641, 2002.
647. The Petra Study Team: Efficacy of three short-course regimens of zidovudine and lamivudine in preventing early and late transmission of HIV-1 from mother to child in Tanzania, South Africa and Uganda [Petra Study]: a randomized, double blind, placebo-controlled trial, *Lancet* 359:1178-1186, 2002.
648. Lallemant M, Jourdain G, Le Coeur S, et al: A trial of shortened zidovudine regimens to prevent mother-to child transmission of human immunodeficiency virus type 1, *N Engl J Med* 343:982-991, 2000.
649. Guay LA, Musoke P, Fleming T, et al: Intrapartum and neonatal single dose nevirapine compared with zidovudine for prevention of mother-to-child transmission of HIV-1 in Kampala, Uganda: HIV-1NET 012 randomized trial, *Lancet* 354:795-802, 1999.
650. Jackson JB, Musoke P, Fleming T, et al: Intrapartum and neonatal single-dose nevirapine compared with zidovudine for prevention of mother-to-child transmission of HIV-1 in Kampala, Uganda: 18-month follow-up of the HIVNET 012 randomised trial, *Lancet* 362:859-868, 2003.
651. Dabis F, Bequet L, Ekouevi DK, et al: Field efficacy of zidovudine, lamivudine and single-dose nevirapine to prevent peripartum HIV transmission, *AIDS* 19:309-318, 2005.
652. Leroy V, Sakarovitch C, Cortina-Borja M, et al: Is there a difference in the efficacy of peripartum antiretroviral regimens in reducing mother-to-child transmission of HIV in Africa? *AIDS* 19:1865-1875, 2005.
653. Moodley D, Moodley J, Coovadia H, et al: A multicenter randomized trial of nevirapine versus a combination of zidovudine and lamivudine to reduce intrapartum and early postpartum mother-to-child transmission of HIV-1, *J Infect Dis* 187:725-735, 2003.
654. Lallemant M, Jourdain G, Le Coeur S, et al: Single-dose perinatal nevirapine plus standard zidovudine to prevent mother-to-child transmission of HIV-1 in Thailand, *N Engl J Med* 351:217-228, 2004.
655. Dorenbaum A, Cunningham CK, Gelber RD, et al: Two-dose intrapartum/newborn nevirapine and standard antiretroviral therapy to reduce perinatal HIV transmission: a randomized trial, *JAMA* 288:189-198, 2002.
656. Thomas TK, Masaba R, Borkowf CB, et al: Triple-antiretroviral prophylaxis to prevent mother-to-child HIV transmission through breastfeeding—the Kisumu Breastfeeding Study, Kenya: a clinical trial, *PLoS Med* 8:e1001015, 2011.
657. Kilewo C, Karlsson K, Ngarina M, et al: Prevention of mother-to-child transmission of HIV-1 through breastfeeding by treating mothers with triple antiretroviral therapy in Dar es Salaam, Tanzania: the Mitra Plus study, *J Acquir Immune Defic Syndr* 52:406-416, 2009.
658. The Kesho Bora Study Group, de Vincenzi I: Triple antiretroviral compared with zidovudine and single-dose nevirapine prophylaxis during pregnancy and breastfeeding for prevention of mother-to-child transmission of HIV-1 (Kesho Bora study): a randomised controlled trial, *Lancet Infect Dis* 11:171-180, 2011.
659. Shapiro RL, Hughes MD, Ogwu A, et al: Antiretroviral regimens in pregnancy and breast-feeding in Botswana, *N Engl J Med* 362: 2282-2294, 2010.
660. Chasela CS, Hudgens MG, Jamieson DJ, et al: Maternal or infant antiretroviral drugs to reduce HIV-1 transmission, *N Engl J Med* 362:2271-2281, 2010.
661. Jamieson DJ, Chasela CS, Hudgens MG, et al: Maternal and infant antiretroviral regimens to prevent postnatal HIV-1 transmission: 48-week follow-up of the BAN randomised controlled trial, *Lancet* 379:2449-2458, 2012.
662. Taha TE, Kumwenda NI, Gibbons A, et al: Short postexposure prophylaxis in newborn babies to reduce mother-to-child transmission of HIV-1: NVAZ randomized clinical trial, *Lancet* 362:1171-1177, 2003.

663. Taha TE, Kumwenda NI, Hoover DR, et al: Nevirapine and zidovudine at birth to reduce perinatal transmission of HIV in an African setting: a randomized controlled trial, *JAMA* 292:202-209, 2004.
664. Gray GE, Urban M, Chersich MF, et al: A randomized trial of two postexposure prophylaxis regimens to reduce mother-to-child HIV-1 transmission in infants of untreated mothers, *AIDS* 19:1287-1289, 2005.
665. Kesho Bora Study Group: Eighteen-month follow-up of HIV-1 infected mothers and their children enrolled in the Kesho Bora study observational cohorts, *J Acquir Immune Defic Syndr* 54:533-541, 2010.
666. Bedri A, Gudetta B, Isehak A, et al: Extended-dose nevirapine to 6 weeks of age for infants to prevent HIV transmission via breastfeeding in Ethiopia, India, and Uganda: an analysis of three randomised controlled trials, *Lancet* 372:300-313, 2008.
667. Kumwenda NI, Hoover DR, Mofenson LM, et al: Extended antiretroviral prophylaxis to reduce breast-milk HIV-1 transmission, *N Engl J Med* 359:119-129, 2008.
668. Thior I, Lockman S, Smeaton LM, et al: Breastfeeding plus infant zidovudine prophylaxis for 6 months vs formula feeding plus infant zidovudine for 1 month to reduce mother–to–child HIV transmission in Botswana: a randomized trial: the Mashi Study, *JAMA* 296: 794-805, 2006.
669. Kilewo C, Karlsson K, Massawe A, et al: Prevention of mother-to-child transmission of HIV-1 through breastfeeding by treating infants prophylactically with lamivudine in Dar es Salaam, Tanzania: the Mitra study, *J Acquir Immune Defic Syndr* 48:315-323, 2008.
670. Coovadia HM, Brown ER, Fowler MG, et al: Efficacy and safety of an extended nevirapine regimen in infant children of breastfeeding mothers with HIV-1 infection for prevention of postnatal HIV-1 transmission (HPTN 046): a randomised, double-blind, placebo-controlled trial, *Lancet* 379:221-228, 2012.
671. Fowler MG, Coovadia H, Herron CM, et al: Efficacy and safety of an extended nevirapine regimen in infants of breastfeeding mothers with HIV-1 infection for prevention of HIV-1 transmission (HPTN 046): 18-month results of a randomized, double-blind, placebo-controlled trial, *J Acquir Immune Defic Syndr* 65:366-374, 2014.
672. Shapiro RL, Thior I, Gilbert PB, et al: Maternal single-dose nevirapine versus placebo as part of an antiretroviral strategy to prevent mother-to-child HIV transmission in Botswana, *AIDS* 20:1281-1288, 2006.
673. Cunningham CK, Chaix ML, Rekacewicz C, et al: Development of resistance mutations in women receiving standard antiretroviral therapy who received intrapartum nevirapine to prevent perinatal human immunodeficiency virus type 1 transmission. A substudy of Pediatric AIDS Clinical Trials Group Protocol 316, *J Infect Dis* 186:181-188, 2002.
674. Wade NA, Birkhead GS, Warren BL, et al: Abbreviated regimens of zidovudine prophylaxis and perinatal transmission of the human immunodeficiency virus, *N Engl J Med* 339:1409-1414, 1998.
675. Nielsen-Saines K, Watts DH, Veloso VG, et al: Three postpartum antiretroviral regimens to prevent intrapartum HIV infection, *N Engl J Med* 366:2368-2379, 2012.
676. Launay O, Tod M, Tschöpe I, et al: Residual HIV-1 RNA and HIV-1 DNA production in the genital tract reservoir of women treated with HAART: the prospective ANRS EP24 GYNODYN study, *Antivir Ther* 16:843-852, 2011.
677. Cu-Uvin S, DeLong AK, Venkatesh KK, et al: Genital tract HIV-1 RNA shedding among women with below detectable plasma viral load, *AIDS* 24:2489-2497, 2010.
678. Henning TR, Kissinger P, Lacour N, et al: Elevated cervical white blood cell infiltrate is associated with genital HIV detection in a longitudinal cohort of antiretroviral therapy-adherent women, *J Infect Dis* 202:1543-1552, 2010.
679. Tubiana R, Le Chenadec J, Rouzioux C, et al: Factors associated with mother-to-child transmission of HIV-1 despite a maternal viral load <500 copies/ml at delivery: a case-control study nested in the French perinatal cohort (EPF-ANRS CO1), *Clin Infect Dis* 50:585-596, 2010.
680. Warszawski J, Tubiana R, Le Chenadec J, et al: Mother-to-child HIV transmission despite antiretroviral therapy in the ANRS French Perinatal Cohort, *AIDS* 22:289-299, 2008.
681. European Collaborative Study: Mother-to-child transmission of HIV infection in the era of highly active antiretroviral therapy, *Clin Infect Dis* 40:458-465, 2005.
682. European Collaborative Study: Maternal viral load and vertical transmission of HIV-1: an important factor but not the only one, *AIDS* 13:1377-1385, 1999.
683. Anderson BL, Cu-Uvin S: Pregnancy and optimal care of HIV-infected patients, *Clin Infect Dis* 48:449-455, 2009.
684. Panel on Antiretroviral Guidelines for Adults and Adolescents: Guidelines for the use of antiretroviral agents in HIV-1 infected adults and adolescents, October 14, 2011, pp 1–167. Available at http://aidsinfo.nih.gov/guidelines. Accessed November 29, 2013.
685. Heidari S, Mofenson L, Cotton MF, et al: Antiretroviral drugs for preventing mother-to-child transmission of HIV: a review of potential effects on HIV-exposed but uninfected children, *J Acquir Immune Defic Syndr* 57:290-296, 2011.
686. Mirochnick M, Taha T, Kreitchmann R, et al: Pharmacokinetics and safety of tenofovir in HIV-infected women during labor and their infants during the first week of life, *J Acquir Immune Defic Syndr* 65:33-41, 2014.
687. McKeown DA, Rosenvinge M, Donaghy S, et al: High neonatal concentrations of raltegravir following transplacental transfer in HIV-1 positive pregnant women, *AIDS* 24:2416-2418, 2010.
688. Croci L, Trezzi M, Allegri MP, et al: Pharmacokinetic and safety of raltegravir in pregnancy, *Eur J Clin Pharmacol* 68:1231-1232, 2012.
689. Stern JO, Robinson PA, Love J, et al: A comprehensive hepatic safety analysis of nevirapine in different populations of HIV-infected patients, *J Acquir Immune Defic Syndr* 34(Suppl 1):S21-S33, 2003.
690. Wohl DA, Pilcher CD, Evans S, et al: Absence of sustained hyperlactatemia in HIV-infected patients with risk factors for mitochondrial toxicity, *J Acquir Immune Defic Syndr* 35:274-278, 2004.
691. Sarner L, Fakoya A: Acute onset lactic acidosis and pancreatitis in the third trimester of pregnancy in HIV-1 positive women taking antiretroviral medications, *Sex Transm Infect* 78:58-59, 2002.
692. Rakhmanina N, van den Anker JN: Efavirenz in the therapy of HIV infection, *Expert Opin Drug Metab Toxicol* 6:95-103, 2010.
693. National Institute of Allergy and Infectious Disease: Evaluating strategies to reduce mother-to-child transmission of HIV-1 infection in populations using formula feeding (PROMISE). Available at http://clinicaltrials.gov/ct/show/NCT01253538. Accessed November 18, 2013.
694. Cohen MS, Chen YQ, McCauley M, et al: HPTN 052 Study Team. Prevention of HIV-1 infection with early antiretroviral therapy, *N Engl J Med* 365:493-505, 2011.
695. Newell ML, Bunders MJ: Safety of antiretroviral drugs in pregnancy and breastfeeding for mother and child, *Curr Opin HIV AIDS* 8:504-510, 2013.
696. Watts DH, Mofenson LM: Antiretrovirals in pregnancy: a note of caution, *J Infect Dis* 206:1639-1641, 2012.
697. Watts DH, Williams PL, Kacanek D, et al: Combination antiretroviral therapy and preterm birth, *J Infect Dis* 207:612-621, 2013.
698. Chen JY, Ribaudo HJ, Souda S, et al: Highly active antiretroviral therapy and adverse birth outcomes in Botswana, *J Infect Dis* 206:1695-1705, 2012.
699. Townsend CL, Tookey PA, Newell ML, et al: Antiretroviral therapy in pregnancy: balancing the risk of preterm delivery with prevention of mother-to-child HIV transmission, *Antivir Ther* 15:775-783, 2010.
700. Barret B, Tardieu M, Rustin P, et al: Persistent mitochondrial dysfunction in HIV-1 exposed but uninfected infants: clinical screening in a large prospective cohort, *AIDS* 17:1769-1785, 2003.
701. Brogly SB, Ylitalo N, Mofenson LM, et al: In utero nucleoside reverse transcriptase inhibitor exposure and signs of possible mitochondrial dysfunction in HIV uninfected children, *AIDS* 21:929-938, 2007.
702. European Collaborative Study: Exposure to antiretroviral therapy in utero or early life: the health of uninfected children born to HIV-infected women, *J Acquir Immune Defic Syndr* 32:380-387, 2003.
703. Alimenti A, Forbes JC, Oberlander TF, et al: A prospective controlled study of neurodevelopment in HIV-uninfected children exposed to combination antiretroviral drugs in pregnancy, *Pediatrics* 118:e1139-e1145, 2006.
704. Siberry GK, Williams PL, Mendez H, et al: Safety of tenofovir use during pregnancy: early growth outcomes in HIV-exposed uninfected infants, *AIDS* 26:1151-1159, 2012.
705. Gibb DM, Kizito H, Russell EC, et al: Pregnancy and infant outcomes among HIV-infected women taking long-term ART with and without tenofovir in the DART trial, *PLoS Med* 9:e1001217, 2012.
706. Colbers A, Hawkins DA, Gingelmaier A, et al: The pharmacokinetics, safety and efficacy of tenofovir and emtricitabine in HIV-1 infected pregnant women, *AIDS* 27:739-748, 2012.

707. Simon A, Warszawski J, Kariyawasam D, et al: Association of prenatal and post-natal exposure to lopinavir-ritonavir and adrenal dysfunction among uninfected infants of HIV-infected mothers, *JAMA* 306:70-78, 2011.
708. Saitoh A, Hull AD, Franklin P, et al: Myelomeningocele in an infant with intrauterine exposure to efavirenz, *J Perinatol* 25:555-556, 2005.
709. Fundaro C, Genovese O, Rendeli C, et al: Myelomeningocele in a child with intrauterine exposure to efavirenz, *AIDS* 16:299-300, 2002.
710. De Santis M, Carducci B, De Santis L, et al: Periconceptional exposure to efavirenz and neural tube defects, *Arch Internal Med* 162:355, 2002.
711. Knapp KM, Brogly SB, Muenz DG, et al: Prevalence of congenital anomalies in infants with in utero exposure of antiretrovirals, *Pediatr Infect Dis J* 31:164-170, 2012.
712. Ford N, Calmy A, Mofenson L: Safety of efavirenz in the first trimester of pregnancy: an updated systematic review and meta-analysis, *AIDS* 25:2301-2304, 2011.
713. Dryden-Peterson S, Shapiro RL, Hughes MD, et al: Increased risk of severe infant anemia after exposure to maternal HAART, Botswana, *J Acquir Immune Defic Syndr* 56:428-436, 2011.
714. Lahoz R, Noguera A, Rovira N, et al: Antiretroviral-related hematologic short-term toxicity in healthy infants: implications of the new neonatal 4-week zidovudine regimen, *Pediatr Infect Dis J* 29:376-379, 2010.
715. Sirois PA, Huo Y, Williams PL, et al: Safety of perinatal exposure to antiretroviral medications: developmental outcomes in infants, *Pediatr Infect Dis J* 32:648-655, 2013.
716. Williams PL, Marino M, Malee K, et al: Neurodevelopment and in utero antiretroviral exposure of HIV-exposed uninfected infants, *Pediatrics* 125:e250-e260, 2010.
717. Brogly SB, Abzug MJ, Watts DH, et al: Birth defects among children born to human immunodeficiency virus-infected women: pediatric AIDS clinical trials protocols 219 and 219C, *Pediatr Infect Dis J* 29:721-727, 2010.
718. Read J, Newell MK, Efficacy and safety of cesarean delivery for prevention of mother-to-child transmission of HIV-1, *Cochrane Database Syst Rev* (4):CD005479, 2005
719. Boer K, England K, Godfried MH, et al: Mode of delivery in HIV-infected pregnant women and prevention of mother-to-child transmission: changing practices in Western Europe, *HIV Med* 11:368-378, 2010.
720. Committee on Obstetric Practice: ACOG committee opinion scheduled cesarean delivery and the prevention of vertical transmission of HIV infection, *Int J Gynaecol Obstet* 73:279-281, 2001.
721. Louis J, Landon MB, Gersnoviez RJ, et al: Perioperative morbidity and mortality among human immunodeficiency virus infected women undergoing cesarean delivery, *Obstet Gynecol* 110:385-390, 2007.
722. Committee on Pediatric AIDS: Infant feeding and transmission of human immunodeficiency virus in the United States, *Pediatrics* 131:391-396, 2013.
723. Ivy W, Landon MB, Gersnoviez RJ, et al: Premastication as a route of pediatric HIV transmission: case-control and cross-sectional investigations, *J Acquir Immune Defic Syndr* 59:207-212, 2012.
724. Zeh C, Weidle PJ, Nafisa L, et al: HIV-1 drug resistance emergence among breastfeeding infants born to HIV-infected mothers during a single-arm trial of triple-antiretroviral prophylaxis for prevention of mother-to-child transmission: a secondary analysis, *PLoS Med* 8:e1000430, 2011.
725. Moorthy A, Gupta A, Bhosale R, et al: Nevirapine resistance and breast-milk HIV transmission: effects of single and extended-dose nevirapine prophylaxis in subtype C HIV-infected infants, *PLoS One* 4:e4096, 2009.
726. Peters V, Liu KL, Dominguez K, et al: Missed opportunities for perinatal HIV prevention among HIV-exposed infants born 1996-2000, pediatric spectrum of HIV disease cohort, *Pediatrics* 111:1186-1191, 2003.
727. Bulterys M, Jamieson DJ, O'Sullivan MJ, et al: Rapid HIV-1 testing during labor: a multicenter study, *JAMA* 292:219-233, 2004.
728. Rollins N, Coovadia H: Breastfeeding and HIV transmission in the developing world: past, present, future, *Curr Opin HIV AIDS* 8:467-473, 2013.
729. Kuhn L, Sinkala M, Semrau K, et al: Elevations in mortality associated with weaning persist into the second year of life among uninfected children born to HIV-infected mothers, *Clin Infect Dis* 50:437-444, 2010.
730. Becquet R, Bland R, Leroy V, et al: Duration, pattern of breastfeeding and postnatal transmission of HIV: pooled analysis from West and South African cohorts, *PLoS Med* 4:e7397, 2009.
731. Schouten EJ, Jahn A, Midiani D, et al: Prevention of mother-to-child transmission of HIV and the health-related Millennium Development Goals: time for a public health approach, *Lancet* 378:282-284, 2011.
732. Ahmed S, Kim MH, E.J Abrams: Risks and benefits of lifelong antiretroviral treatment for pregnant and breastfeeding women: a review of the evidence for the Option B+ approach, *Curr Opin HIV AIDS* 8: 474-489, 2013.
733. Coutsoudis A, Goga A, Desmond C, et al: Is Option B+ the best choice, *Lancet* 381:269-271, 2013.
734. Nachega JB, Uthman OA, Anderson J, et al: Adherence to antiretroviral therapy during and after pregnancy in low-income, middle-income, and high-income countries: a systematic review and meta-analysis, *AIDS* 26:2039-2052, 2012.
735. Doherty M, Ford N, Vitoria M, et al: The 2013 WHO guidelines for antiretroviral therapy: evidence-based recommendations to face new epidemic realities, *Curr Opin HIV AIDS* 8:528-534, 2013.
736. World Health Organization: Guidelines on HIV-1 and infant feeding. Principles and recommendations for infant feeding in the context of HIV-1 and a summary of evidence, 2010, pp 1–49. Available at http://whqlibdoc.who.int/publications/2010/9789241599535_eng.pdf. Accessed January 16, 2013.
737. Onyango-Makumbi C, Bagenda D, Mwatha A, et al: Early weaning of HIV-1 exposed uninfected infants and risk of serious gastroenteritis: findings from two perinatal HIV-1 prevention trials in Kampala, Uganda, *J Acquir Immune Defic Syndr* 53:20-27, 2010.
738. Creek TL, Kim A, Lu L, et al: Hospitalization and mortality among primarily nonbreastfed children during a large outbreak of diarrhea and malnutrition in Botswana, *J Acquir Immune Defic Syndr* 53: 14-19, 2010.
739. Israel–Ballard K, Donovan R, Chantry C, et al: Flash–heat inactivation of HIV–1 in human milk: a potential method to reduce postnatal transmission in developing countries, *J Acquir Immune Defic Syndr* 45:318-323, 2007.
740. Hoque SA, Hoshino H, Anwar KS, et al: Transient heating of expressed breast milk up to 65 degrees C inactivates HIV-1 in milk: a simple, rapid, and cost-effective method to prevent transmission, *J Med Virol* 85:187-193, 2013.
741. Chantry CJ, Young SL, Rennie W, et al: Feasibility of using flash-heated breastmilk as an infant feeding option for HIV-exposed, uninfected infants after 6 months of age in urban Tanzania, *J Acquir Immune Defic Syndr* 60:43-50, 2012.
742. Doherty K, Ciaranello A: What is needed to eliminate new pediatric HIV infections: the contribution of model-based analysis, *Curr Opin HIV AIDS* 8:457-466, 2013.
743. Lyons C, Mushavi A, Ngobeni-Allen F, et al: Ending pediatric AIDS and achieving a generation born HIV-free, *J Acquir Immune Defic Syndr* 60(Suppl 2):S35-S38, 2012.
744. Chi B, Bolton-Moore C, Holmes CB: Prevention of mother-to-child HIV transmission within the continuum of maternal, newborn and child health services, *Curr Opin HIV AIDS* 8:498-503, 2013.
745. Shetty AK: Epidemiology of HIV infection win women and children: a global perspective, *Curr HIV Res* 11:81-92, 2013.
746. Wilcher R, Petruney T, Cates W: The role of family planning in elimination of new pediatric HIV infection, *Curr Opin HIV AIDS* 8:490-497, 2013.
747. Mofenson LM: Prevention of mother-to-child HIV-1 transmission—why we still need a preventive immunization strategy, *J Acquir Immune Defic Syndr* 58:359-362, 2011.
748. Lohman-Payne B, Skyler J, Rowland-Jones SL: Immune approaches for the prevention of breast milk transmission of HIV-1, *Adv Exp Med Biol* 743:185-195, 2012.
749. Hammer SM: Baby steps on the road to HIV eradication, *N Engl J Med* 369:1855-1857, 2013.
750. Eyal N, Kuritzkes DR: Challenges in clinical trial design for HIV-1 cure research, *Lancet* 382:1464-1465, 2013.

23 Varicella, Measles, and Mumps

ANNE A. GERSHON, MONA MARIN, and JANE F. SEWARD

CHAPTER OUTLINE

The viruses that cause varicella, zoster, measles, and mumps may complicate the management of a mother, fetus, or newborn when maternal infection with one of these agents occurs during pregnancy or at term. In the United States and other countries with widespread vaccine use, most women of childbearing years are immune to measles and mumps, and there is little opportunity for exposure to these infections because the current population is highly immunized. These diseases posed more problems during pregnancy during the first half of the 20th century than they do now.

In countries such as the United States, where a licensed varicella vaccine has routinely been used since 1995, the incidence of varicella among women of childbearing age has also declined because of personal and herd immunity with decreased transmission of virus. Varicella-zoster virus (VZV) may still inflict significant fetal damage as the cause of congenital varicella syndrome, especially in locations where the vaccine is not being used. Improved methods for control, including better diagnostic methods, antiviral therapy with acyclovir, passive immunization with varicella-zoster immunoglobulin (VZIG or VariZIG), and use of live-attenuated varicella vaccine, have decreased prenatal and postnatal morbidity from this virus, however. Understanding of this viral infection at the molecular level, including clarification of the cause of zoster by studies of viral DNA, RNA, and proteins in latency and study of specific viral glycoproteins and their importance in the immune response have advanced our knowledge and can be expected to lead to further improved therapeutic modalities.

Varicella and Zoster

Varicella (i.e., chickenpox) is an acute, highly contagious disease that most commonly occurs in childhood. It is characterized by a generalized exanthem consisting of vesicles that develop in successive crops and that rapidly evolve to pustules, crusts, and scabs. Zoster (i.e., herpes zoster, shingles) occurs in persons who have previously had varicella. It is typified by a painful or pruritic (or both) vesicular eruption usually restricted to one or more segmental dermatomes. An abundance of virologic, epidemiologic, and immunologic evidence has been amassed, indicating that these two illnesses are caused by the same etiologic agent,[1] which was designated VZV. Varicella is a manifestation of primary infection with VZV. After the acute infection subsides, VZV, similar to other herpesviruses, persists in a latent form. For VZV, the site of latent infection is in the dorsal root and cranial nerve ganglia and intestinal ganglia, where certain early viral genes and proteins are expressed in latency.[2-5] VZV may subsequently be reactivated with expression of all of its genes as immunity wanes with time. The reactivated infection assumes the segmental distribution of the nerve cells in which latent virus resided, giving rise to zoster. A description of the historical recognition of disease caused by VZV follows.

Varicella is a modernized Latin word used since at least 1764 and intended to connote a diminutive of the more serious variola (i.e., smallpox).[6] The etymology of "chicken" in chickenpox is less clear. It may also be a diminutive derived from the French *pois chiche*, or "chick pea," a dwarf species of pea (*Cicer arietinum*).[6] Other authors doubt this Latin origin and conjecture that the word originated from the farmyard fowl, in which case it has a teutonic ancestry in the Old English *cicen* and the Middle High German *kuchen*.[7] *Herpes* has been used to designate a malady since 1398 ("this euyll callyd Herpes")[8] and derives from the Greek word meaning "to creep"; *zoster* is the Greek and Latin word meaning "girdle" or "belt." Shingles, from the Latin *cingulus* (meaning "girdle"), was also used in the 14th century as *schingles* to describe "icchynge and scabs wett and drye."[8]

ORGANISM

Classification and Morphology

VZV (herpesvirus varicellae) is a member of the Herpesviridae family. In addition to a burgeoning number of animal herpesviruses, this group includes seven additional, closely related viruses that infect humans: herpes simplex viruses (HSV) types 1 and 2 (herpesvirus hominis), cytomegalovirus (CMV), Epstein-Barr virus, and human herpesviruses 6, 7, and 8. Only one antigenic type of VZV has been identified, but molecular studies have revealed some minor differences in VZV that have proved useful for epidemiologic studies.[9,10]

Common properties of the family include a DNA genome and enveloped virions exhibiting icosahedral symmetry with a diameter of 180 to 200 nm.[1] Nucleocapsids, which are assembled in the nucleus, have a diameter of about 100 nm, and consist of a DNA core surrounded by 162 identical subunits, or capsomeres. Nucleocapsids acquire a temporary envelope at the nuclear membrane; they are transported further via the endoplasmic reticulum to the Golgi, where they receive a final envelope. In cell cultures, virions are packaged in vesicles identified as endosomes, which are acidic.[11,12] Virus particles are released from these structures at the cell surface by exocytosis. Extracellular virions are extremely pleomorphic compared with virions of HSV. This pleomorphism, presumably reflecting injury to the envelope possibly caused by exposure to acid or enzymes in endosomes, is believed to account for the lability and lack of cell-free virus that characterizes VZV in tissue culture and in its spread through the body during varicella infection, and it distinguishes VZV from HSV.[11-13] In vivo, enveloped and well-formed VZV is released from cells of the superficial epidermis (strateum corneum), yielding highly infectious virions capable of airborne spread and with a great degree of communicability.[14]

Molecular studies have elucidated details concerning how latent VZV infection is established, maintained, and reactivated. Latent infection comes from virions present in skin during varicella and/or from T-cell associated viremia in varicella.[15] It is unlikely, however, that complete viral replication occurs in the neuron during establishment of latency because the neuron must survive, and replication would be expected to cause cell death. The replication process of VZV is begun during latent infection, but a block in the cascade of viral gene expression probably occurs. Numerous laboratories have found that least six viral genes and their protein gene products are reported to be expressed in latently infected neurons.[15] These proteins are confined to the cell cytoplasm. It seems that when these proteins are transduced into the nucleus by factors still to be determined, reactivation occurs, with formation of all 72 VZV gene products and synthesis of infectious, enveloped virions in tissues such as nerve and skin.[4] Recently, however, a much more restricted gene expression in VZV latency has been proposed.[16] It is currently not yet clear how this controversy regarding VZV latency will eventually be resolved.

Propagation

VZV grows readily in diploid human fibroblasts, such as WI 38 cells, the most commonly used cell type for virus isolation. VZV also can be propagated in certain epithelial cells, such as human embryonic kidney, primary human amnion cells, primary human thyroid cells, and Vero (African green monkey kidney) cells. Similar to CMV, the cytopathic effect of VZV is focal in cell culture because of its cell-associated character, and cytopathic effects develop more slowly (3-7 days) than with HSV. Animal models for varicella (guinea pigs)[17] and for zoster (rats)[18] have been described. An in vitro model of latency and reactivation in guinea pig enteric neurons has also been developed and provides a setting in which to study factors that influence latency and reactivation.[4]

Serologic Tests and Antigenic Properties of Varicella-Zoster Virus

Several serologic tests are available to measure antibodies to VZV, including indirect immunofluorescence, often called fluorescent antibody to membrane antigen (FAMA)[19,20]; latex agglutination[21]; enzyme-linked immunosorbent assay (ELISA)[22-25]; radioimmunoassay[26]; immune adherence hemagglutination[27]; neutralization[22,28]; and complement-enhanced neutralization.[29] All of these methods are more sensitive than the complement fixation assay.[30] Data gathered from these assays show that antibody to VZV develops within a few days after the onset of varicella, persists for many years, and is present before the onset of zoster.

Serologic cross-reactions between HSV and VZV have been described.[31,32] HSV and VZV share common antigens, and similar polypeptides and glycoproteins have been identified for both viruses, but cross-protection has not been observed.[33-35] Rare simultaneous infections with one or more human herpesviruses have been reported.[36,37] Elevations in heterologous antibody titers in apparent HSV or VZV infections may result from cross-reactions of the viruses but also may indicate simultaneous infection by both viruses.

VZV produces at least eight major glycoprotein antigens—B, C, E, H, I, K, L, and M—all of which are on the envelope of the virus and on the surface of infected cells. The glycoproteins and internal antigens, such as the capsid and tegument, stimulate production of neutralizing and other types of antibodies and cellular immunity.[38-40] The most prominent glycoprotein of VZV is glycoprotein E. Antibodies elaborated in varicella and zoster are of the immunoglobulin G (IgG), IgA, and IgM classes.[41,42]

Immunity to Varicella-Zoster Virus

Immunity to VZV is a complex interaction between humoral and cell-mediated immune responses, with the possibility of partial and complete immunity to the virus.

Humoral and cellular immunity are important in the control of primary varicella infection. Cell-mediated immunity is important for viral clearance, providing long-term protection against varicella and preventing symptomatic VZV reactivation. Immunity to varicella usually is long lasting. However, it might wane occasionally; rarely, second episodes of varicella have been reported among immunocompetent persons.

Clinical reinfection with VZV has been observed in some persons despite a positive antibody titer at exposure.[43-46] Most clinical reinfections are mild, however, which suggests that partial immunity to the virus may be present. In a study by Bogger-Goren and colleagues,[47] moreover, seronegative children who had positive cellular immune responses were likely to be protected against varicella after household exposure. In contrast, children with negative cellular immune responses became infected. Secretory IgA against VZV has also been demonstrated after varicella.[48] Although it has not been shown, it is further hypothesized that cellular immunity at the mucosal level may play a role in protection against clinical varicella.

Immunologic evidence consistent with asymptomatic reinfection with VZV, manifested by an increase in VZV-specific IgG or IgA or the production of IgM and an increase in the cell-mediated immune response to VZV (external boosting), has been documented in adults with a household exposure to varicella.[49,50] Subclinical reactivation with possible subsequent boosting of immunity (internal boosting) is also possible.[51-56]

In addition to predisposing to reinfection with the virus, incomplete immunity to VZV is associated with development of zoster.[51] In addition to clinical zoster, silent reactivation of latent VZV in persons who have had previous varicella probably occurs; this may be detected immunologically by an increase in antibody titer or the transient appearance of specific IgM, although it is difficult to rule out the possibility of an exogenous exposure.[42,55,57,58] Sometimes, clinical manifestations of zoster, such as pain, may occur in the absence of a rash—so-called zoster sine herpete. Silent reactivation of VZV in bone marrow transplant patients has been shown by polymerase chain reaction (PCR) assay.[56] Zoster results in patients who have latent VZV infection when specific cell-mediated immunity is depressed.[59-62] Defective antibody responses to VZV glycoproteins have not been associated with development of zoster in immunocompromised persons.[63] Similarly, the increased incidence of zoster in elderly adults has been associated with loss of cell-mediated immunity to VZV,[64,65] whereas antibody to VZV does not wane with age but tends to increase.[66]

It is possible to provide humoral immunity to persons at high risk for developing severe varicella by passive immunization. Although used successfully to prevent severe varicella, passive immunization has not prevented zoster in persons at high risk for it.[67] It is uncertain whether passive immunization of a woman with varicella can prevent infection of her fetus or development of congenital varicella syndrome, although some evidence suggested a benefit to the fetus too.[68,69] It is possible to increase cell-mediated immunity to VZV by immunization, and this approach was demonstrated in several studies.[70-72] Results of a large, double-blind, controlled study in healthy vaccinees older than 60 years indicated that approximately half of more than 15,000 vaccinated individuals were protected from developing zoster.[73]

EPIDEMIOLOGY AND TRANSMISSION

Varicella ranks as one of the most communicable of human diseases. No extrahuman reservoir of VZV is known. Because the supply of susceptible persons, especially in the era before the urbanization of society, would be rapidly exhausted by so contagious a disease, virus latency may have adaptive evolutionary significance in perpetuating infection. In isolated communities, cases of zoster would be responsible for the reintroduction of VZV and its transmission as varicella to new generations of susceptible individuals.[1,51]

Communicability

Patients with varicella are considered to be contagious for 1 to 2 days before rash becomes obvious[74] and for as long as new lesions continue to appear and while they are moist (usually 5-7 days after rash onset). Historically, transfer of VZV was believed to occur via respiratory droplets, and limited epidemiologic evidence suggests that transmission can occur before the onset of rash[74-77] although the question of whether the early onset with few localized lesions went unnoticed is appropriate. It is rare, however, to isolate VZV from the pharynx of infected patients, and isolation has occurred only after the onset of rash. A study using PCR methods showed that VZV DNA is present in the nasopharynx of a high percentage of children during the early stages of clinical varicella,[78] but the presence of VZV DNA does not necessarily indicate the presence of infectious virus. In contrast, VZV can readily be cultured from the vesicular lesions in varicella and zoster. Cell-free VZV virions are known to be produced in large quantities in skin lesions and are the type of particle that could be aerosolized and involved in viral transmission. In a study of leukemic recipients of live-attenuated varicella vaccine, only individuals with skin lesions as a side effect of varicella vaccination spread vaccine-type virus to varicella-susceptible close contacts.[79] Similarly, the rare documented instances of transmission of vaccine virus from healthy vaccinees to other susceptible individuals (9 vaccinees who transmitted the virus to 11 contacts) occurred only when the vaccinee had a rash (including 4 cases from herpes zoster).[80] Therefore the major source of infectious VZV seems to be the skin, although it is possible that transmission from the respiratory tract can also occur. Airborne spread of varicella has been documented,[81,82] but indirect transfer by fomites has not. VZV DNA has been detected in air samples for many hours in hospitals,[83] but the relationship to infectivity of the virus is unclear.

Incubation Period

The usual incubation period for varicella is 14 to 16 days. The range is 10 to 21 days, unless passive immunization has been given, in which case the incubation period may be prolonged to 1 week or more (usually up to 28 days).[76,84-86]

Relationship Between Varicella and Zoster

It is documented that exposure of susceptible persons to zoster may result in varicella. Vesicular fluid from patients with zoster produced varicella when inoculated into susceptible children.[87,88] Other studies have confirmed that a similar relationship exists under conditions of natural exposure.[89] Claims to the contrary notwithstanding,[90,91] it has not been documented that zoster is acquired from other patients with zoster or varicella. There are reports in the literature of occurrence of zoster in persons who happen to have been exposed to varicella or zoster, but these are chance events. The possibility that zoster is acquired from other patients with zoster of varicella was hypothesized in the past, but it is not supported by the current concepts of the pathogenesis of zoster, particularly the strict segmental distribution of lesions and the demonstrated presence of VZV DNA, RNA, and certain viral proteins in ganglia during latency.[2,3,92] Studies have also determined that VZV DNA from zoster isolates is identical to that which caused the primary infection, proving that zoster is caused by reactivation of latent VZV.[93-95]

Transplacental Transmission

In pregnancy, VZV may be transmitted across the placenta, resulting in congenital or neonatal varicella.[96] The consequences of transplacental infection are discussed in a later section.

Epidemiology

Varicella is worldwide in distribution, and, in the absence of a vaccination program, it affects nearly every person by midadulthood. The epidemiology of varicella differs between temperate and tropical/subtropical regions.[97] In temperate climates, infection occurs at younger ages (preschool aged children or children in early elementary school), with most children being infected by 15 years of age and less than 5% of adults remaining susceptible. There is a strong seasonal variation, with more cases and outbreaks occurring in winter and spring. In contrast, in tropical areas, children acquire varicella at older ages and a higher proportion of young adults remain susceptible, leading to a higher proportion of cases occurring among adults. The factors that determine the differences in epidemiology of varicella between temperate and tropical climates are not well understood but may relate to properties of VZV, which is thermolabile; climate influence other than temperature; population density; and the risk for exposure (e.g., differences in urban/rural residence and attendance in child care). Varicella is a more serious disease in young infants, adults, and immunocompromised persons, in whom there are higher rates of complications and deaths than in healthy children.

In the United States, before the introduction of live-attenuated varicella vaccine in 1995, varicella accounted for about 4 million cases, 11,000 to 15,000 hospitalizations, and 100 to 150 deaths every year. With the introduction of the routine one-dose regimen among children, significant changes in the epidemiology of varicella have occurred, with evidence of personal and herd immunity.[98,99] There is less varicella disease occurring in all age groups, and the seasonality of the disease has disappeared. By 2005, varicella had declined approximately 90% compared with prevaccine years in active surveillance sites in which vaccination coverage had reached 90% among young children.[100] The greatest decline (>90%) occurred in children aged 1 to 9 years, and an approximately 80% decline in incidence also occurred in infants not eligible for vaccination. Varicella-related hospitalizations declined greater than 75% to 88% from prevaccine years, and deaths decreased by 88% overall from 1990 to 1994 and from 2005 to 2007[101]; in persons younger than 20 years, there was a 97% decline in deaths. Although the age-specific incidence has declined in all age groups, the median age at infection has increased, and cases occur predominantly in children in upper elementary school rather than in the preschool years.[100] Seroprevalence studies in the early vaccine era (1999-2004) reflect the increased VZV seroprevalence among children (89% of children aged 6-11 years and 97% of those aged 12-19 years had VZV IgG antibodies) with maintenance of high seroprevalence among adults (98% of persons aged 20-49 years had VZV IgG).[102] Cases continued to occur even in settings with high one-dose varicella vaccine coverage, and seropositivity did not always result after one dose.[103] Therefore in 2006, a routine two-dose childhood varicella vaccination program with catch-up vaccination of all individuals without evidence of immunity was adopted in the United States.[104] From 2006 to 2010, varicella incidence declined further (≈70%), and fewer outbreaks have been reported.[105]

Varicella is more contagious than mumps but less so than measles.[85,106] One study that compared all three diseases found that after exposure within households, 61% of susceptible persons of all age groups (without a history of previous disease) developed varicella, compared with 76% for measles and 31% for mumps.[85] Another study found the attack rate for varicella at 87% among susceptible exposed household contacts.[107] Compared with measles, varicella is about 80% as infectious in the household but only 35% to 65% as infectious in the community. The reason probably is that varicella requires closer contact for transmission, such as that occurring in the household, whereas in the community, there are more casual contacts. Measles may infect efficiently even through casual contacts.[106]

Evidence of Immunity to Varicella

In the prevaccine era, a history of varicella was a valid measure of immunity. Because the rash is distinctive and subclinical cases occur rarely, most parents knew if their child had had varicella. Serologic testing has been used to assess the accuracy of reported histories of varicella. In adults, a positive history was highly predictive of serologic immunity; 97% to 99% of persons who reported a history were seropositive.[108-110] However, the majority of adults who had negative or uncertain histories were also seropositive (71%-93%).[108,110,111] This finding is supported by epidemiologic data from one study that found the attack rate after household exposure in parents who reported themselves as being susceptible was 5%.[107]

In the early vaccine era, data indicated that the negative and positive predictive values of a history of varicella among adults were similar to those from the prevaccine era. In a study that included pregnant women attending prenatal care during 2001 to 2004 in Antelope Valley, California, and Philadelphia, who self-reported having had varicella, 98% had serologic evidence of immunity to varicella.[112] Among those who reported a negative or uncertain history of varicella, 7% to 17% were seronegative. In another study, Perella and colleagues[113] found similar predictive values among young adults (aged 15-29 years).

However, this second study indicated that for cohorts born since 1994, the validity of reported varicella history is no longer highly predictive of seropositivity.

Considering the changes in the epidemiology of varicella in the United States, the Advisory Committee on Immunization Practices (ACIP) recommends as evidence of immunity a provider-verified history of disease (of varicella or zoster) rather than a self-reported history. Other criteria indicating evidence of immunity for adults include serologic evidence of immunity or laboratory confirmation of disease, documentation of receipt of two doses of varicella vaccine, and birth in the United States before 1980; however, birth in the United States before 1980 is not considered evidence of immunity for health care personnel, pregnant women, and immunocompromised persons.[104] Table 23-1 presents evidence of immunity to varicella for pregnant women; the same criteria are used for varicella immunity for health care personnel and immunocompromised persons.

As more women of childbearing age have vaccine-induced immunity to varicella, the assessment of the immune status will shift toward documenting that the pregnant woman has received two doses of vaccine. For persons who have documentation of receipt of two doses, serologic testing to document presence of antibodies is not recommended because commercially available serologic assays for VZV IgG yield high rates of false-negative results.[104]

Incidence of Varicella, Mumps, and Measles in Pregnancy

With varicella, mumps, and measles being highly infectious and primarily childhood diseases, a low proportion of adults, and inherently of women of childbearing age, are susceptible (<10%). Only a few studies have addressed the incidence of varicella, mumps, and measles during pregnancy; they were conducted before widespread use of vaccines and are not representative today. In a prospective study of clinically recognized infections that occurred during 30,059 pregnancies in 1958 to 1964, approximately 1600 women with presumed measles, varicella, and mumps were identified.[114] This study's findings suggested the minimum frequency per 10,000 pregnancies was 0.6 case for measles, 5 cases for varicella, and 10 cases for mumps. An estimate in 1992 projected an incidence of 7 cases of varicella per 10,000 pregnancies.[115]

Today, measles and mumps are rare in the United States, and varicella is becoming less common. Given the high seroprevalence of antibodies either through vaccination or natural infection in the adult population and the decrease in circulation of measles, mumps, and VZV after implementation of the vaccination programs, varicella, mumps, and measles all are now unusual during pregnancy in the United States. It is likely that women immigrants from countries with tropical climates have a higher susceptibility to VZV and are at higher risk for contracting varicella during pregnancy than U.S.-born women if exposed; nonetheless, incidence is expected to be low because of low virus circulation.

Incidence and Distribution of Zoster

Zoster is primarily a disease of adults, especially older adults or immunosuppressed patients. Several studies in the United States found the incidence of zoster between 3.2 and 4.2 per 1000 population per year (age-adjusted to the 2000 population), translating into an estimated 1 million cases annually.[116-119] This estimate was confirmed in the studies of Oxman[73] on zoster vaccine. Hope-Simpson,[51] describing patients of all ages in a general practice observed during a 16-year period in the United Kingdom, found an incidence of 3.4 cases per 1000 otherwise healthy people per year.

Adults and children older than 2 years who have zoster usually give a history of a previous episode of varicella; in younger infants with zoster, a history of intrauterine exposure to VZV can often be elicited.[52] The latency period between primary infection and zoster is shorter if varicella occurs prenatally rather than later in childhood.[120] Varicella in the first year of life increases the risk of childhood zoster, with a relative risk roughly between 3 and 21.[121,122] Possibly, this phenomenon is caused by immaturity of the immune response to VZV in young infants, permitting early viral reactivation.[123]

Age is the most important risk factor for the development of zoster. After infancy, the incidence of zoster increases

Table 23-1 Presumptive Evidence of Immunity for Pregnant Women for Varicella, Measles and Mumps, 2013

Disease	Year of Birth as Presumptive Immunity	History of Disease	Laboratory Evidence of Immunity	Laboratory Confirmation of Disease	Documented Vaccination
Varicella	Not accepted	Verified by health care provider (history of varicella or herpes zoster)	VZV IgG	Viral DNA detection by PCR/culture, IgM, rise in IgG,	2 doses
Measles	Before 1957	Not accepted	Measles IgG	IgM, significant rise (usually fourfold) in IgG, virus RNA detection by RT-PCR/culture	1 dose*
Mumps	Before 1957	Not accepted	Mumps IgG	IgM, significant rise (usually fourfold) in IgG, virus detection/culture	1 dose*

From Marin M, Guris D, Chaves SS, Schmid S, Seward JS: Prevention of varicella: recommendations of the Advisory Committee on Immunization Practices (ACIP), *MMWR Recomm Rep* 56(RR-4):1, 2007; and Marin M, Bialek SR, Seward JF: Updated recommendations for use of VariZIG—United States, 2013, *MMWR Morb Mortal Wkly Rep* 62:574, 2013.

IgG, IgM, Immunoglobulin G and M, respectively; *PCR,* polymerase chain reaction; *RT,* reverse transcriptase; *VZV,* varicella-zoster virus.

Note: Criteria for acceptable evidence of immunity were developed to guide vaccination assessment and administration in clinical and public health settings. They provide presumptive, rather than absolute, evidence of immunity. People who meet these criteria have a very high likelihood of immunity.

*One dose is acceptable unless the pregnant female is school aged (<18 years), is attending a post–high-school educational institution, or is a health care provider, in which case two doses are considered acceptable presumptive evidence of immunity.

with age, especially after 50 years of age (greater than two thirds of zoster cases occur in persons aged 50 years and older). The attack rate in octogenarians was 14 times that of children in the series by Hope-Simpson.[51] Most studies have also shown that zoster incidence is higher among women than among men. Second attacks of zoster were historically considered unusual, although recent evidence suggests that the rates are comparable to those of the first episode in immunocompetent individuals.[124] It is possible that some of the recurrent cases might be caused by reactivation of HSV; in one study, HSV was isolated from 13% of a series of 47 immunocompetent patients with clinically diagnosed zoster.[125] Zoster in adults and children occurs with increased frequency in patients with altered cell-mediated immunity: malignant hematopoietic neoplasms (especially Hodgkin disease), patients after organ transplantation, and patients infected with human immunodeficiency virus (HIV).[126-128] Spinal trauma, irradiation, and corticosteroid therapy may also be precipitating factors. The distribution of lesions in varicella, which primarily affects the trunk, head, and neck, is reflected in a proportionately greater representation of these regions in the segmental lesions of zoster.[52]

Incidence of Zoster in Pregnancy

Recent studies on the incidence of zoster in pregnancy are lacking. In 1979, based on the number of live births, fertility rate, and incidence of zoster among persons aged 15 to 44 years, Brazin and colleagues[129] projected approximately 6000 cases annually in pregnant women in the United States, which suggested that gestational zoster might be more common than gestational varicella. This is likely to change with the implementation of the varicella vaccination program. Assuming that there are 3.5 million pregnant women yearly in the United States, this calculates to a rate of 20 cases per 10,000 pregnant women per year. Nevertheless, zoster, similar to varicella, seems to be rare or uncommon in pregnancy. In contrast to varicella, little information exists regarding whether there is an increased severity of zoster in pregnant women compared with the general population. Therefore most experts infer that zoster in pregnancy is no more severe than it is in women who are not pregnant. Implications of gestational zoster for the fetus are discussed in a subsequent section.

Nosocomial Varicella in the Nursery

The precise risk of horizontal transmission in maternity wards or the newborn nursery after VZV has been introduced is unclear, but based on experience, it is very low.[130-143] In reports in which the number of neonates exposed is stated, 249 exposures resulted in only 8 instances of transmission to infants; most of the exposed neonates had mothers with positive or uncertain histories of varicella.[130-133,137-143] This low rate of transmission is likely due in part to the role that maternal immunity plays in protection of the infant and that, in general, most women of childbearing age in the United States are immune, with some higher susceptibility among women from tropical and subtropical areas outside of the United States. Additional factors supporting a low risk of transmission are relatively brief periods of exposure in health care settings compared with the household setting, where 80% to 90% of susceptible persons become clinically infected[52,107]; relative lack of intimacy of contact in the nursery, particularly for infants in isolettes; administration of postexposure prophylaxis; and high varicella immunity among health care workers because of prior disease or vaccination coupled with the requirement that health care workers have evidence of immunity to varicella.

Because IgG antibodies to VZV cross the placenta,[130,144] full-term newborns of immune mothers are generally protected from varicella. Studies using sensitive assays to measure antibodies to VZV in the pre–varicella vaccine era demonstrated that high levels of passively acquired antibodies are present at birth and during the first 3 to 4 months of life; after 6 months of age, it was unusual for VZV antibodies to be detected.[130,145-147] Antibodies to VZV have also been detected (>90%) in premature infants and infants with low birth weight born to mothers with a 25-week gestation or those weighing greater than 1000 g.[131,132,148] Nevertheless, perinatal varicella has been reported rarely in infants born to women with positive histories of varicella or serology.[133,134,149-151] In the study by Newman,[134] varicella developed in a mother and her infant after exposure to a student midwife with varicella. The mother had experienced varicella as a child and had a few remaining skin scars; apparently, she had developed a second episode as an adult. Readett and McGibbon[151] reported two cases of postpartum infection in neonates whose mothers had histories of varicella. After delivery at home, each of these infants was exposed within 24 hours of birth to a sibling with varicella and subsequently developed skin lesions when 12 and 14 days old. Their mothers did not develop varicella in the perinatal period and were found to have serum-neutralizing antibodies to VZV.

In the literature before 1975, VZV antibody titers were not often reported because sensitive tests for measuring these antibodies were not readily available. Since that time, infection of a few seropositive infants after postnatal exposure to VZV has been documented.[133,149] These infants either had mothers with a history of varicella and VZV seropositivity or had VZV antibody that was transplacentally acquired. In one instance, mild varicella developed in a 2-week-old, 1040-g infant who was seropositive at exposure and was passively immunized with VZIG 72 hours after the exposure.[133] In another study, five infants younger than 2 months, all of whom were seropositive at exposure, developed varicella in a children's institution; all disease was mild (<20 lesions).[149] Complete protection of every neonate against varicella is not guaranteed by immunity in the mother. However, when varicella develops in the presence of maternal antibodies, it seems to be modified.

Attenuated disease in young infants was also documented in a community-based study.[152] In this study, clinical disease assessed by the proportion of infants with 50 or more lesions, fever, and varicella-related complications was milder among younger (0-5 months, n = 175) versus older (6-11 months, n = 344) infants, possibly because of the presence of maternal VZV antibodies. Eight infants were younger than 1 month at the time of varicella onset; all of them had fewer than 50 lesions, 1 infant was hospitalized, and 1 had a varicella-related complication (unspecified).

Reports largely confirm the low rate of transmissibility of varicella in neonates. Freud[135] described an infant who had transplacentally acquired disease and developed lesions on the second day of life. None of the other neonates in the nursery became infected, but the index infant had been isolated immediately, so exposure had been very brief. When transferred to another ward, with older children, this same infant transmitted the disease to 2 older children, who were 4 and 7 years of age, respectively. Odessky and associates[136] reported three instances of congenital varicella in which 2 infants were immediately isolated, but the third was not recognized as having varicella and exposed other neonates for 4 days. The number at risk is not stated, but no instances of transmission were observed. In a report by Harris,[137] 35 infants were exposed to 2 infants with congenital varicella for periods of 18 and 10 hours, respectively, before isolation. None subsequently became infected, possibly because all the mothers had positive histories of varicella. In an additional case described by Matseoane and Abler,[138] an infant developed transplacentally acquired varicella at 9 days of age and exposed 13 other neonates in the nursery for periods of 2 to 10 hours before isolation. Six mothers had a positive history of varicella, three did not, and four did not know. None of the exposed mothers or infants developed varicella. Friedman and colleagues[142] report an outbreak in a neonatal intensive care unit (NICU) after a 25-week-gestation infant, whose mother had varicella 2 weeks previously, developed hemorrhagic varicella and exposed 14 infants over several days. None of the infants in isolettes became ill, but 4 who were in open warming units at exposure developed varicella 10 days later. All had received VZIG, and in each instance, the mother gave a history of varicella. The illnesses were mild, with only a few papular skin lesions, but 3 of the 4 infants were positive for VZV on immunofluorescence testing of skin scrapings. Each infant with varicella was treated with intravenous (IV) acyclovir. The incidence of disease was higher in infants of less than 29 weeks of gestation than in infants of longer gestation.

Lack of transmission despite hospital exposure to an adult with varicella in NICUs was also reported.[131,132,139-141,143] In some reports, lack of transmission to the neonate is difficult to explain. In 1965, Newman[134] reported two cases of varicella that occurred in mothers in the same prenatal ward 18 to 19 days after exposure to the index-infected infant and its mother. One mother developed varicella 7 days antepartum, and the other developed the disease 3 days postpartum. Each mother was immediately isolated from the ward but not from her own infant; neither of the infants developed varicella. In all, 139 mothers, excluding the index case, were exposed, and 8 developed infection. Three of 42 staff members also became infected. The index infant was the only neonate infected; all other infants, including those born to the 8 infected mothers, remained free of disease. (*Experiences with nosocomial varicella in the newborn nursery with additional details were presented in the previous editions of this textbook [see Table 22-1 in the 2010, seventh edition]*).

Since introduction of the varicella vaccine in the United States, one experience describing exposure in a neonatal unit has been reported.[143] A neonatal nurse developed varicella after being exposed to her son, who had breakthrough varicella despite a history of two doses of varicella vaccine. The nurse exposed 34 neonates in the NICU. All exposed neonates were given IV immunoglobulin, and those born at less than 28 weeks of gestation (9) also received acyclovir; none developed varicella.

The varicella vaccination program implemented in the United States in 1995 greatly impacted both VZV circulation in the community and the profile of population immunity, which influenced nosocomial varicella, including the nursery. A community-based study found that the incidence of varicella in infants in the United States declined 90% from 1995 to 2008.[152] A similar experience was described from Australia, where there has been a reduction in the frequency of congenital varicella syndrome (100%) and neonatal varicella (85%) in the first years after the introduction of the universal varicella vaccination program.[153] With high population immunity, the risk of exposure will be lowered further. In terms of population immunity, more vaccinated women will enter childbearing age. Similarly to measles, the amount and persistence of VZV maternal antibodies transferred to infants of vaccinated women are likely to be lower than those transferred from naturally infected women. Therefore infants born to vaccinated mothers are likely to have lower levels or more rapid declines of maternal antibodies and may be at an increased risk of varicella and related complications if exposed and infected in the early months of life. Even if low, the risk for nosocomial transmission of varicella in nurseries remains, and measures to prevent transmission should be immediately implemented, considering the potential for severe disease in this population. Maintaining high vaccination coverage among health care personnel caring for these infants and among their household contacts will increase in importance.

PATHOGENESIS OF VARICELLA AND ZOSTER

In the usual case of varicella, the portal of entry and initial site of virus replication is probably the oropharynx, specifically the tonsil.[154] Attempts to show this directly have been unrewarding, however. In five patients whose blood, throat secretions, and skin were cultured repeatedly during the prodromal period and after the appearance of cutaneous lesions, VZV was recovered from a throat swab in only one instance and from the blood in none. In contrast, vesicle fluid from these patients yielded VZV in all instances.[155] Attempts to isolate the virus from the blood of six additional patients were positive in only one instance—on the second day of rash in an immunosuppressed host. Other, more extensive searches for VZV in throat secretions of patients with varicella, even during the incubation period, proved essentially negative.[156,157] In one report, VZV was isolated from nasal swabs in 4 of 11 children on days 2 through 4 after onset of the rash. VZV could not be isolated during the incubation period or even during the first day of the rash. It was unclear whether the virus was multiplying in the nasal mucosa.[158]

VZV has been isolated from blood obtained from patients with varicella. Ozaki and colleagues[159] cultured blood from 7 immunocompetent children; VZV was isolated a few days before the onset of rash or within 1 day after onset. Asano and coworkers[160] similarly isolated VZV from the blood of 7 of 12 otherwise healthy patients with early varicella. The patients from whom virus could not be isolated had been studied after they had the rash for more than 4 days. Both groups of investigators introduced an additional technical step into the blood culture process that might explain why they were successful in isolating VZV when many others before them had not been. The white blood cells were separated on Ficoll-Hypaque gradients and added to cell cultures. Although there was no evidence of viral growth in these cultures, they were blindly passaged onto new cell cultures. Evidence of growth of VZV was present in these second cultures after the blind passage within 2 to 5 days. Before these studies, VZV had been isolated only from blood obtained from immunocompromised patients with varicella or zoster.[156,161,162] The white blood cell infected with VZV is a mononuclear cell, but it is uncertain whether monocytes or lymphocytes, or both, are involved.[159,160] Experiments in the SCID-hu mouse model have shown that VZV is lymphotropic for human $CD4^+$ and $CD8^+$ T lymphocytes and that human T cells release some infectious virus.[163]

Data from PCR studies of patients with varicella have yielded various results. In the study by Koropchak and associates,[164] performed 24 hours after rash onset in 12 patients, 3.3% of oropharyngeal samples, 67% of mononuclear cells, and 75% of skin vesicles were positive for VZV DNA. In the study by Ozaki and coworkers[165] of pharyngeal secretions of varicella patients, 26% were positive during the incubation period, and 90% were positive after clinical onset. Evidence of VZV viremia is indicated by PCR studies, from patients with varicella and also in zoster patients.[166-168] PCR assay is more sensitive than immunofluorescence or viral culture.[169]

Virus is readily recovered from cutaneous lesions soon after the onset of varicella. Isolation of VZV was successful in 23 of 25 cases in which vesicle fluid was cultured within 3 days after the onset of the rash but was successful in only 1 of 7 specimens collected 4 to 8 days after onset.[155] In contrast, the virus apparently persists longer in vesicles of zoster patients, in whom 7 of 10 specimens collected later than 3 days after onset were positive.[139] PCR assay is more sensitive than virus culture. In the study by Koropchak and colleagues,[164] VZV was recovered from only 21% of skin lesions, but 75% were positive by PCR assay. In contrast to smallpox, varicella is no longer communicable by the time the lesions have crusted and scabbed.

The pathogenesis of varicella seems to be as follows: Transmission is probably effected by airborne spread of virus from cutaneous vesicles and to a lesser extent by respiratory droplets from patients with varicella or zoster. After an initial period of virus replication in the oropharynx in the susceptible individual, there is invasion of the local lymph nodes and a primary viremia of low magnitude, delivering virus to the viscera.[170] After several more days of virus multiplication, a secondary viremia of greater magnitude occurs, resulting in widespread cutaneous dissemination of virus and rash. Data in the SCID-hu mouse model alternatively suggest that VZV is targeted to the skin early in varicella and is initially controlled to a great extent by innate immunity.[171] Cropping of the vesicles is thought to represent several viremic phases. In the body, the virus spreads by cell-to-cell contact; viremia also is cell associated. Enveloped, cell-free infectious VZV is present, however, in the vesicular skin vesicles. Crusting and scabbing of the vesicles and pustules occur as host defense mechanisms, particularly as various forms of cell-mediated immunity become active. Latency is achieved from the cell-free VZV particles in the skin that are in proximity to sensory nerve endings and also by viremia.[15]

The pathogenesis of zoster differs from that of varicella. Before development of zoster, latent VZV begins to reactivate and multiply in the sensory ganglion (or ganglia) because of local factors that remain to be clarified.[2,172] Then VZV travels down the axon to the skin supplied by that nerve. Development of a localized rash occurs if there is a deficiency in cell-mediated immunity to VZV.[60-52,173] Visceral herpes zoster, with ulceration, achalasia, and/or pseudoobstruction, has also been reported from reactivation of latent VZV in the enteric nervous system. This may occur with or without accompanying rash.[174,175] Compromise in cell-mediated immunity to VZV leading to herpes zoster may be obvious, as in patients who have undergone transplantation, therapy for malignant disease, or HIV infection,[176] or, presumably, it may be transient, as in healthy persons who develop zoster for no apparent reason. In immunosuppressed patients, a viremic phase with zoster has been documented occasionally,[177,178] and this probably happens after skin involvement has occurred, especially if there continues to be an inadequate immune response to VZV after the virus has reached the skin. The clinical manifestation of this viremia is disseminated zoster, in which vesicular lesions develop outside the original dermatome. A viremic phase in pregnant patients with disseminated zoster has not been documented, but it seems logical to assume that viremia would be a prerequisite for dissemination, as in nonpregnant patients.

PATHOLOGY

Cutaneous Lesions

Histologic changes in the skin leading to the formation of vesicles are essentially identical for varicella, zoster, and HSV infection. The hallmark of each is the presence of multinucleated giant cells and intranuclear inclusions, changes that are not found in the vesicular lesions caused by vaccinia virus and coxsackieviruses. The lesion is primarily localized in the epidermis, where ballooning degeneration of cells in the deeper layers is accompanied by intercellular edema. As edema progresses, the cornified layers are separated from the more basal layers to form a delicate vesicle with a thin roof. An exudate consisting primarily of mononuclear cells is seen in the dermis, but the characteristic nuclear changes of epithelial cells are absent in this region.

The predominant cells in vesicular lesions are polymorphonuclear leukocytes. These cells may play a role in generating interferon in vesicular lesions, which may be important in recovery from the disease.[179] In vitro data also suggest that the polymorphonuclear leukocyte plays a role in host defense against VZV, possibly by mediating antibody-dependent cell-mediated cytotoxicity.[180-182] Cytotoxic T cells play a role in recovery from VZV infections, and recent immunologic information on children with severe varicella or zoster has also implicated natural killer (NK) cells in host defense against the virus.[181-188]

Visceral Lesions in the Fetus and Placenta

Few reports describe the appearance of the placenta in cases of congenital varicella with or without survival. Garcia[189] observed grossly visible necrotic lesions of the placenta in a case of varicella occurring in the fourth month of pregnancy that resulted in spontaneous abortion. Microscopically, central areas of necrosis were surrounded by epithelioid cells and rare giant cells of the foreign body type, giving a granulomatous appearance. Some decidual cells had typical intranuclear inclusions.

Descriptions of the pathology of visceral lesions in fetal or neonatal varicella are restricted to autopsies in fatal cases.[189-194] Grossly, the lesions are small, punctate, and white or yellow and resemble miliary tuberculosis. Microscopically, their appearance resembles the lesions of the placenta: central necrotic areas, often resembling fibrinoid necrosis, surrounded by a few epithelioid cells and a scant infiltrate of mononuclear cells. Intranuclear inclusions are present. The skin, lungs, and liver are uniformly involved (Table 23-2).[189] In the case described by Garcia,[189] the cortical, subependymal, and basilar structures of the cerebrum were totally destroyed and accompanied by extensive calcification. Although a search for *Toxoplasma* was negative, serologic data to rule out dual infection are lacking in the report. The gross and microscopic lesions of fatal perinatal varicella resemble lesions of disseminated HSV infection, including a preference for the liver and adrenal gland, but the provided data suggest that involvement of the brain is more common in neonatal HSV infection than it is in fatal neonatal varicella. A neonate with fatal hemorrhagic varicella with pneumonia and hepatitis is shown in Figure 23-1.

Visceral Lesions in the Mother

In fatal cases of varicella in pregnant women, maternal death is usually caused by pulmonary involvement. The pathologic course of varicella pneumonia in pregnant women is identical to the course in nonpregnant women and in children.[195,196] Interstitial pneumonitis may follow a peribronchiolar distribution of disease. Intranuclear inclusions may be found in alveolar lining cells, macrophages, capillary endothelium, and tracheobronchial mucosa. Necrotic foci may be accompanied by hemorrhage, and hyaline membranes lining the alveoli are often prominent.

Table 23-2 Frequency of Gross and Microscopic Lesions in Seven Autopsied Cases of Fetal and Neonatal Varicella

Organ	No. Cases/No. Examined (%)	References
Skin	7/7 (100)	189-194
Lungs	7/7 (100)	189-194
Liver	7/7 (100)	189-194
Adrenals	6/7 (86)	189, 190, 192-194
Esophagus or intestines	5/6 (83)	178-182, 189
	4/5 (80)	
Thymus	5/7 (71)	189, 190, 192, 194
Kidneys	4/7 (56)	189, 190, 192, 194
Spleen	3/7 (43)	189, 192-194
Pancreas	2/7 (29)	189, 190, 192
Heart	1/5 (20)	189, 193
Brain*		189
Miscellaneous		
Ovaries	1	190
Bone marrow	1	192
Placenta	1	189

*Not well documented; possibility of concomitant toxoplasmosis not definitively excluded.

Zoster

The pathologic picture of cutaneous lesions in zoster is indistinguishable from varicella lesions. The dorsal root ganglion of the affected dermatome exhibits a mononuclear inflammatory infiltrate. There may also be necrosis of ganglion cells and demyelination of the corresponding axon. There are no descriptions of these lesions in pregnant women or in neonates specifically.

CLINICAL MANIFESTATIONS

Varicella Rash

After an incubation period of usually 13 to 17 days,[52,197] varicella is heralded by the approximately simultaneous occurrence of fever and rash. In adults, the exanthem is often preceded by a prodromal fever and constitutional symptoms lasting 2 or 3 days.[7] On occasion, one or more isolated vesicles may precede a generalized exanthem by 1 or 2 days. The rash is characteristically centripetal, beginning on the face or scalp and spreading rapidly to the trunk but with relative sparing of the extremities. The lesions begin as red macules but progress quickly to vesicles

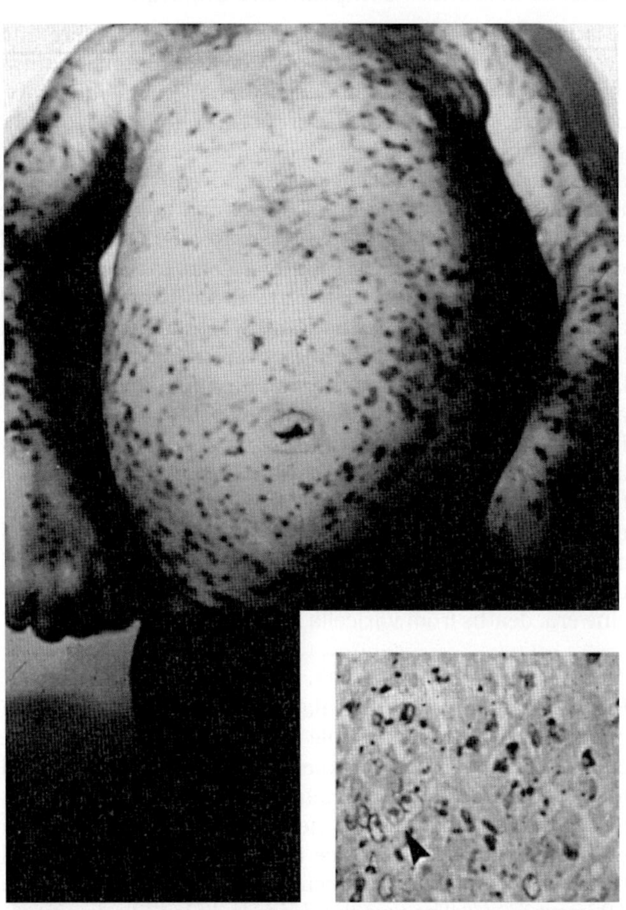

Figure 23-1 Congenital hemorrhagic varicella complicated by pneumonia and hepatitis. The mother of this infant developed varicella a few days before delivery. Zoster immunoglobulin was unavailable at that time. *Inset* shows section of liver with intranuclear inclusion bodies obtained at autopsy.

and crusts. Itching is the rule. There is a tendency for new lesions to occur in crops. In contrast to smallpox, all stages of lesions—vesicles, pustules, and scabs—may occur simultaneously in the same anatomic region. New crops often continue to appear over a 2- to 5-day period. Lesions may be more numerous in skin folds or in the diaper area. The total number of vesicles varies from only two or three in very mild cases, especially in infants, to thousands of lesions that border on confluence, especially in adults.[7] In many cases, one or two mucosal lesions may occur in the mouth or, less commonly, on the vulva. On occasion, the lesions may be bullous or hemorrhagic. Residual scarring is exceptional. Constitutional symptoms tend to be mild, even in the presence of an extensive exanthem.

Complications of Varicella

The most common complication is secondary bacterial infection, usually caused by group A β-hemolytic streptococci or staphylococci. Skin infections may lead to severe sequelae, such as toxic shock syndrome and necrotizing fasciitis.[198-206] Central nervous system (CNS) complications, which are uncommon, include encephalitis, cerebellar ataxia, aseptic meningitis, stroke, and vasculopathy.[207-212] Glomerulonephritis,[213,214] myocarditis,[215,216] and arthritis[217,218] have also been reported.

Varicella in Immunocompromised Children

It is widely appreciated that varicella may be severe and even fatal in children with an underlying malignancy, children with congenital deficits in cellular immunity, children receiving high doses of corticosteroids for any reason,[219] and children with underlying infection with HIV and acquired immunodeficiency syndrome (AIDS).[128,220] Historically, children with leukemia had a mortality rate approaching 10% if untreated[221] and sometimes developed what has been called progressive varicella. Instead of developing new vesicular lesions for several days, they continued to have fever and new lesions for 2 weeks after the onset of illness. Frequently, their skin lesions become hemorrhagic, large, and umbilicated. Varicella pneumonia often ensued and was a major factor contributing to the death of a child. It is believed that this abnormal response to VZV represents a failure of the normal cell-mediated immunity response to eliminate the virus.[221] The cell-mediated immunity response to VZV includes antibody-dependent cell-mediated cytotoxicity; NK cells; cytotoxic T cells, including CD4 and CD8 cells; and NK cells.[38,180-188,222-224] Today, in the vaccine era, deaths from varicella have become rare.[101]

Varicella Pneumonia

Primary varicella pneumonia is a dreaded complication of varicella and is responsible for most fatalities. It is most common in immunocompromised patients, in adults, and in most cases of fatal neonatal varicella,[189-191,225] but it is rarely seen in otherwise healthy children. It has been suggested that the incidence is about 15% in adults and that 90% of cases have occurred in persons older than 19 years.[225,226] The true incidence is difficult to determine because chest radiographs are not performed in most cases of varicella, and extensive radiographic evidence of disease may be present when pulmonary symptoms are only minimal. In male military recruits with varicella, virtually all of whom had been hospitalized and had chest radiographs, radiographic evidence of pneumonia was found in 16.3% of 110 cases.[227]

Two reviews of varicella pneumonia in adults outline the major features.[196,228] The onset of pneumonia usually occurs in 2 to 4 days but sometimes occurs 10 days after the appearance of the exanthem. Fever and cough are present in 87% to 100% of cases, and dyspnea occurs in 70% to 80%. Other symptoms and signs include cyanosis (42%-55%), rales (55%), hemoptysis (35%-38%), and chest pain (21%). Radiographic changes seem to correlate best with the severity of the rash rather than with the physical examination of the lungs. The radiograph typically reveals a diffuse nodular or miliary pattern, most pronounced in the perihilar regions. The radiographic appearance changes rapidly. The white blood cell count ranges from 5000 to 20,000 cells/mm^3 and is of little help in differentiating viral from secondary bacterial pneumonia. Pneumonia is usually self-limiting, and recovery is temporally correlated with clearing of skin lesions. The fatality rate has been variously estimated at 10% to 30%, but it probably approximates the lower of these values if immunocompromised hosts are excluded.[196,228] Blood gas analyses and pulmonary function tests indicate a significant diffusion defect that may persist in some cases for months after clinical recovery.[229] The introduction of antiviral chemotherapy has greatly improved the outcome in this disease.

Maternal Effects of Varicella

Reports from the mid-20th century suggested that when varicella occurred during pregnancy, it was a highly lethal disease. Deaths usually resulted from varicella pneumonia, in some cases accompanied by glomerulitis and renal failure or myocarditis, occurring after the fourth month of gestation.[230,231] Harris and Rhoades[232] reviewed the literature to 1963 and found a reported mortality of 41% for 17 pregnant women with varicella pneumonia compared with 11% for 236 nonpregnant adults with varicella pneumonia. Other reports question, however, whether varicella, especially in the absence of pneumonia, is more serious in pregnant women than in the adult population at large.[193,233,234] Because most cases of gestational varicella with an uncomplicated course are undoubtedly not reported, the denominator of the case-fatality ratio (CFR) is unknown. In a prospective study of 150 cases of varicella in pregnancy in 1966, only one maternal death related to varicella pneumonia was recorded.[235]

In a very large, collaborative, prospective study published in 2002, there were no fatalities in 347 consecutive pregnant women with varicella, although 18 (5.2%) had radiologic evidence of pneumonia.[236,237] Although the data did not reach statistical significance in this study, it seems striking that 16 (89%) of 18 reported cases of pneumonia occurred in women who developed varicella after the 16th week of pregnancy.

Based on case reports and reviews of gestational varicella (with and without pneumonia), 542 cases of varicella in pregnant women have been reported since 1963. There were 16 deaths (3%). All of the deaths occurred among the 75 (14%) women who had varicella pneumonia (21% fatality rate for pneumonia). Deaths occurred in 1 (<1%) of 166 women whose disease occurred during the first trimester, 4 (2%) of 168 women whose disease occurred during the second trimester, and 11 (5%) of 208 women whose disease occurred during the third trimester. Antiviral therapy was used only after 1985. No deaths occurred among an additional 8 women who were exposed to varicella in late pregnancy but did not develop an exanthem until the first few days postpartum.*

It remains uncertain whether varicella pneumonia has a graver prognosis when it occurs during pregnancy. There is no definitive evidence that varicella in the absence of pneumonia is a more serious illness in pregnant women than in other adults; however, the risk of developing pneumonia may be increased after the 16th week of pregnancy. It seems likely that older mortality information on varicella in pregnancy reflected the pre–antiviral therapy era and was biased by selective reporting of fatal cases.

Some patients with varicella during pregnancy who were treated with acyclovir have been reported.[234,236-241,248-256] These reports suggest that acyclovir has improved the outcome of this complication of varicella, although controlled studies have not been performed. Although various dosages have been used, the standard dosage of 30 mg/kg/day given IV would seem appropriate for treatment of pregnant women with varicella pneumonia. Congenital abnormalities from administration of acyclovir to women during pregnancy have not been observed.[257,258]

Controlled studies of the value of corticosteroids in pregnant women with varicella pneumonia have not been performed. Several reports indicate that 2 of 6 pregnant women treated with corticosteroids died, whereas 8 of 17 pregnant women given supportive therapy without corticosteroids died.[232,242-244,259] It seems that administration of an antiviral drug is of greater importance than administration of corticosteroids. Passive immunization may be administered to seronegative women after close exposure to VZV to attempt to modify the infection; although uncertain, this approach may prevent fetal infection.[69,104,260] In a study from 1994, among 97 women who developed varicella after passive immunization with VZIG, there were no observed cases of congenital varicella syndrome.[68] About two abnormal infants could be expected in a series of this magnitude, but the number of women followed is too low to achieve statistical significance.

Effects of Gestational Varicella on the Fetus

Chromosomal Aberrations. Available data on chromosomal aberrations are often difficult to interpret, particularly in the absence of controls, which is often the case. VZV can induce chromosomal abnormalities in vitro and in vivo. When human diploid fibroblasts were infected with the virus, a high proportion of cells observed were in metaphase arrest, as if they were under the influence of colchicine.[261] The incidence of chromatid and chromosomal breaks ranged from 26% to 45% 24 hours after infection compared with 2% for control cultures. In the acute phase of varicella, up to the 5th day of rash, peripheral blood leukocytes show a 17% to 28% incidence of chromosomal breaks compared with 6% in controls, but 1 month after infection, these abnormalities disappeared.[262] A single case report suggested the possibility that chromosomal damage may be more lasting when varicella is acquired in utero. A boy with bird-headed dwarfism, born to a mother who contracted varicella in the 6th month of pregnancy, had a 26% incidence of chromosomal breakage in peripheral blood leukocytes when he was examined at 2 years of age.[263] Chromosomal analyses in four infants with congenital varicella syndrome, whose mothers had varicella at the 8th, 14th, 16th, and 20th week of gestation, were reported as normal.[264-267]

Information on chromosomal aberrations in infants who have no congenital anomalies and are the offspring of mothers with gestational varicella is lacking. Further concern about the possibility of persistent chromosomal abnormalities after intrauterine exposure to VZV is suggested by a prospective survey of deaths among children born in England and Wales from 1950 to 1952 whose mothers had varicella in pregnancy. Two deaths, both from acute leukemia, were reported among the offspring of 270 women; the two children developed acute leukemia at the ages of 3 and 4 years, respectively, after intrauterine exposure at 25 and 23 weeks of gestation, respectively.[268] In the absence of confirmation, it remains questionable whether exposure to varicella in utero is a risk factor for leukemia or other malignancies.

Abortion and Prematurity. Several studies have addressed the question of whether gestational varicella and other viral diseases result in an increased incidence of spontaneous abortion or prematurity. In a retrospective study in 1948, only 4 cases of varicella were identified among 26,353 pregnant women.[269] No stillbirths occurred in these cases. Prospective studies have tended to confirm that maternal varicella during pregnancy is not associated with a significant excess of prematurity[235] or fetal death.[245] Among 826 virus-infected pregnant subjects observed in New York City from 1957 to 1964, 150 women with varicella were followed to term. After exclusion of fetal deaths and multiple births, 5 of 135 live-born infants were found to have birth weights of less than 2500 g. This incidence of prematurity was lower than in the control group of non–virus-infected pregnant women (Table 23-3). Similarly, in the study by Paryani and Arvin,[246] premature delivery occurred in 2 (5%) of 42 pregnancies, with delivery at 31 and 35 weeks of gestation, respectively.

Table 23-3 Frequency of Low Birth Weight Among Infants Born to Mothers With Selected Viral Infections During Pregnancy

	VIRUS-INFECTED GROUP			CONTROL GROUP*		
Disease	No. Live Births	No. with Low Birth Weight†	%	No. Live Births	No. with Low Birth Weight†	%
Rubella	359	50	13.9	402	21	5.2
Varicella	135	5	3.7	146	13	8.9
Mumps	117	9	7.7	122	4	3.3
Measles	60	10	16.7	62	2	3.3

Modified from Siegel M, Fuerst HT: Low birth weight and maternal virus diseases: a prospective study of rubella, measles, mumps, chickenpox, and hepatitis, *JAMA* 197:680, 1966.

*Control group was matched for age, race, and parity of mother and type of obstetric service.

†Low birth weight was defined as <2500 g.

Note: Fetal deaths and multiple births were excluded from the analysis.

*References 134, 189, 193, 232, 234, 237-247.

In a prospective study involving 194 women with gestational varicella and 194 control women, the rate of spontaneous abortion was 3% and 7%, respectively, in the first 20 weeks.[270] In the large prospective series of Enders and associates[68] of 1330 women in England and Germany who developed varicella, 36 (3%) experienced spontaneous abortions after varicella in the first 16 weeks. In the prospective study of Pastuszak and coworkers,[271] involving 106 women with varicella in the first 20 weeks of pregnancy, there were more premature births (14.3%) among women with varicella than among control subjects (5.6%; $P = .05$). There is no question, however, that the congenital varicella syndrome is associated with low birth weight. Approximately one third of reported cases of the syndrome have been premature, had low birth weight, or were small for gestational age.

An accurate assessment of the incidence of fetal mortality after maternal varicella is difficult to obtain. Fetal wastage is probably underreported, in part because some spontaneous abortions occur before prenatal care is sought. In the prospective study of maternal viral diseases in New York City referred to earlier,[245] nine fetal deaths were observed among 144 instances of maternal varicella. Five fetal deaths occurred among 32 pregnancies in the first trimester, four among 60 second-trimester pregnancies, and none among 52 third-trimester pregnancies (Table 23-4). These deaths do not represent significant increases in fetal wastage associated with varicella infection, compared with control groups in which no maternal viral infection occurred. There was a significant excess of fetal deaths only for mumps, and these occurred primarily in the first trimester. Only three of the nine fetal deaths associated with maternal varicella occurred within 2 weeks of the onset of the mother's illness, and two of these were in the first trimester. Two additional deaths occurred 2 to 4 weeks after the onset of maternal varicella, two occurred 5 to 9 weeks after the onset of maternal illness, and two occurred 10 or more weeks after the onset of maternal illness. The absence of a close temporal relationship between most fetal deaths and maternal disease provides further support for the concept that maternal varicella during pregnancy does not commonly result in fetal mortality.

Although the incidence of fetal death is not increased by maternal varicella, fetal deaths have been associated with maternal varicella. Deaths in utero may result from direct invasion of the fetus by VZV[69,189,272-274] or from the presumed toxic effects of high fever, anoxia, or metabolic changes caused by maternal disease.[245] The precise mechanisms of these toxic effects have not been elucidated. When maternal disease is unusually severe, particularly in cases of varicella pneumonia, fetal death may also result from premature onset of labor or death in utero caused by maternal death.[†]

Congenital Malformations. For many years, there was uncertainty about whether gestational varicella led to a symptomatic congenital infection. Intensive investigation from the mid-1970s until the end of the 20th century led to the recognition that VZV can cause fetal malformations. Two types of investigations were done to determine whether varicella during pregnancy leads to a congenital syndrome. The first investigations were retrospective analyses or case reports describing specific anomalies that occurred in the offspring of mothers who had gestational varicella. These reports were necessarily highly selective and did not define the incidence of such anomalies. They consistently described a syndrome of skin scarring, eye and brain damage, and limb hypoplasia, however, that might follow intrauterine varicella.

The second type of analysis consisted of prospective studies of pregnant women followed throughout pregnancy and afterward. The problem was to delineate the coincidence of two events, each of which is itself uncommon—gestational varicella and congenital malformations—to determine the magnitude of risk to the fetus. Siegel,[275] despite an 8-year observation period encompassing approximately 190,000 pregnancies annually in New York City, was able to identify only four malformations among infants born to 135 mothers who had varicella during pregnancy, compared with five malformations among 146 matched controls. The follow-up period was 5 years and included psychomotor and audiometric tests. Varicella occurred during the first trimester in only 27 of the pregnancies complicated by varicella, and of these, 2 (7.4%) were associated with congenital anomalies compared with anomalies in 3 (3.4%) of 87 pregnancies in the control population.

The largest single prospective series is that of Enders and associates.[68] In a joint prospective study in Germany and the United Kingdom from 1980 to 1993, Enders and associates[68] followed 1373 women with varicella and 366 with zoster during pregnancy. Of the women with varicella, 1285 continued to term, and 9 infants had defects attributed to congenital varicella syndrome. The incidence was 2 (0.4%)

[†]References 193, 232, 239, 242, 243, 273.

Table 23-4 Fetal Deaths in Relation to Gestational Age After Selected Virus Infections During Pregnancy

	WEEKS OF GESTATION		
Infection Groups	**0-11**	**12-27**	**>28**
Mumps			
No. cases	33	51	43
No. fetal deaths	9	1	0
%	27.3	2	—
Measles			
No. cases	19	29	17
No. fetal deaths	3	1	1.9
%	15.8	3.4	5.9
Varicella			
No. cases	32	60	52
No. fetal deaths	5	4	0
%	15.6	4.7	—
Controls			
No. cases	1010*	392†	152†
No. fetal deaths	131	15	1
%	13	3.8	0.7

Modified from Siegel M, Fuerst HT, Peress NS: Comparative fetal mortality in maternal virus diseases: a prospective study on rubella, measles, mumps, chickenpox, and hepatitis, *N Engl J Med* 274:768, 1966.

*Subjects were attending prenatal clinic in first trimester without having virus infections.

†Controls were matched for age, race, and parity of the mother and type of obstetric service.

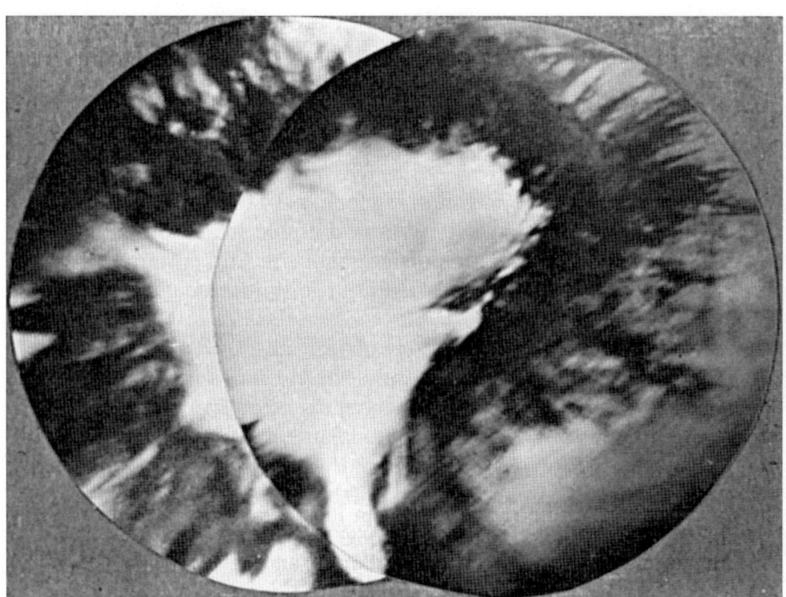

Figure 23-2 Fundus photograph of right eye of a 13-month-old patient shows central gliosis with surrounding ring of black pigment. The child's mother had varicella during the early fourth month of pregnancy. (Modified from Charles N, Bennett TW, Margolis S: Ocular pathology of the congenital varicella syndrome, *Arch Ophthalmol* 95:2034, 1977.)

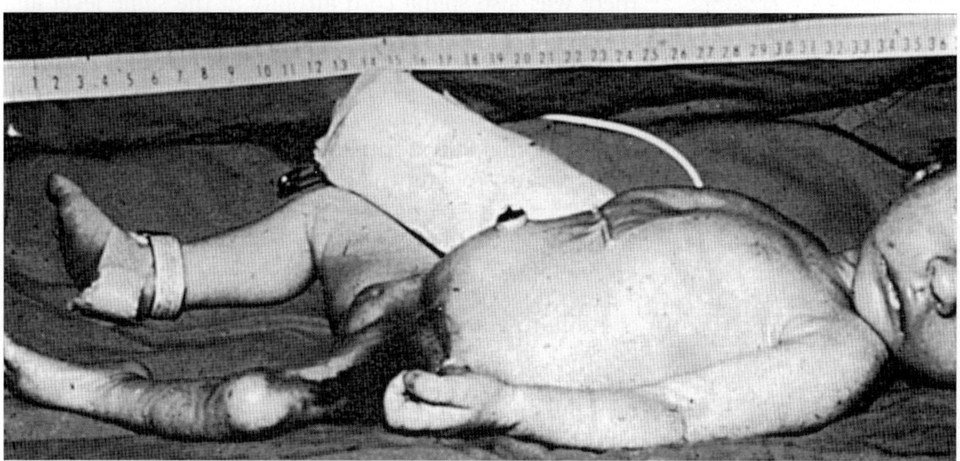

Figure 23-3 This infant, whose mother had varicella during the 13th to 15th weeks of pregnancy, had bilateral microphthalmia with cataracts and an atrophic left leg. The infant died of bronchopneumonia at age 6½ months. (From Srabstein JC, Morris N, Larke RP, et al: Is there a congenital varicella syndrome? *J Pediatr* 84:239, 1974.)

of 472 for infections between 0 and 12 weeks and 7 (2%) of 351 for infections between 13 and 20 weeks. In a collaborative prospective study in the United States, 347 women with gestational varicella were reported, and adequate follow-up of their infants was available in 231.[237] In this cohort, there was one case (0.4%) of the congenital syndrome and two cases of fetal death, including one case of hydrops. If these cases are included, the rate of congenital varicella was 1.3%. The mother of the one child with the syndrome had varicella at 24 weeks; the child had skin, eye, and CNS involvement.

That congenital varicella syndrome is a reality is now widely appreciated. It has become possible to make a tissue diagnosis of congenital varicella syndrome only more recently because affected infants do not chronically shed virus as is seen in congenital infections with rubella virus and CMV.[69,272,274,276,277] Congenital varicella syndrome may be prevented in the future by widespread use of varicella vaccine, analogous to the situation for congenital rubella.

The constellation of developmental abnormalities described in individual case reports of infants born to mothers who had varicella in early pregnancy and in prospective series is sufficiently distinctive to indicate that VZV is a teratogen. In 1947, LaForet and Lynch[278] described an infant with multiple congenital anomalies after maternal varicella in early pregnancy. The infant had hypoplasia of the entire right lower extremity, talipes equinovarus, and absent deep tendon reflexes on the right. Cerebral cortical atrophy, cerebellar aplasia, chorioretinitis, right torticollis, insufficiency of the anal and vesical sphincters, and cicatricial cutaneous lesions of the left lower extremity were present. The syndrome then seemed to be all but forgotten until 1974, when Srabstein and coworkers[279] rekindled interest in the subject by reporting another case and reviewing the literature, concluding that although the virus could not be isolated from the infants, congenital varicella syndrome typically consisted of some combination of cicatricial skin lesions, ocular abnormalities, limb deformities, mental retardation, and early death after maternal varicella in early pregnancy (Figs. 23-2 to 23-4). Numerous additional reports in the literature of the syndrome, encompassing more than 100 cases, indicate there is a wide spectrum of manifestations (Table 23-5).[‡]

Although at one time it was thought that congenital varicella syndrome occurred after maternal VZV infection in the first trimester of pregnancy, current evaluation

‡References 69, 120, 242, 246, 264-274, 276-343.

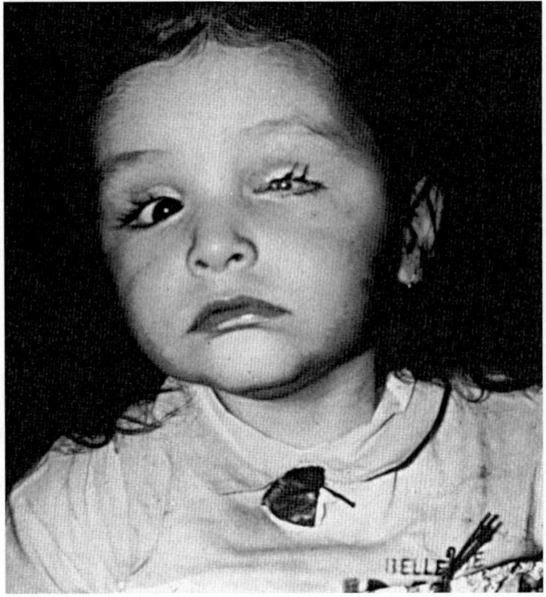

Figure 23-4 A child, whose mother had varicella during the 16th week of pregnancy, had atrophy of the left orbit, with blindness that required cosmetic enucleation. Severe chorioretinitis occurred in the right eye. Except for blindness, the child developed normally. She died of pneumonia when approximately 4 years of age. (Modified from Frey HM, Bialkin G, Gershon A: Congenital varicella: case report of a serologically proved long-term survivor, *Pediatrics* 59:110, 1977.)

Table 23-5 Reported Symptoms and Signs in Infants With Congenital Varicella Syndrome, 1947-2002

Symptom	Estimated Incidence (%)
Skin lesions (cicatricial scars, skin loss)	60-70
Ocular abnormalities (chorioretinitis, Horner syndrome, anisocoria, microphthalmia, cataract, nystagmus)	60
Neurologic abnormalities (cortical atrophy, mental retardation, microcephaly, seizures, dysphagia, limb paresis)	60
Abnormal limbs (hypoplasia, equinovarus, abnormal or absent digits)	50
Prematurity, low birth weight	35
Death in early infancy	25
Abnormalities of gastrointestinal tract	10
Urinary tract abnormalities	10
Zoster in infancy	20

See references 245, 246, 264-344

of the data indicates that cases also occur in the second trimester. Of 82 cases for which data are available, 32 (39%) occurred after maternal varicella that developed before week 13, 47 (59%) occurred after maternal varicella that developed between weeks 13 and 26, and 1 (1%)[319] occurred after maternal varicella that developed during week 28. The average gestation when maternal varicella occurred was 15 weeks. Only 6 cases occurring after maternal zoster have been reported[310,311,339,340,344]; not all of these are well documented virologically. Four occurred after maternal zoster in the first trimester, one followed zoster in the second trimester,[339] and one followed zoster in the third trimester.[344] Of 109 reported affected infants, 103 (95%) cases followed maternal varicella, and 6 (5%) followed maternal zoster (disseminated in one instance).

Scars of the skin, usually cicatricial lesions, are the most prominent stigmata, although a few patients have had no rash at all.[326,329,330,345] Eye abnormalities (i.e., chorioretinitis, microphthalmia, Horner syndrome, cataract, and nystagmus) and neurologic damage are almost as common; other features include a hypoplastic limb, prematurity, and early death. The features of the syndrome are summarized in Table 23-5.

Cutaneous scars were usually observed overlying a hypoplastic limb but also have been seen in the contralateral limb.[278] Characteristically, the skin scars are cicatricial, depressed, and pigmented and often have a zigzag configuration. Such scars are thought to be the result of zoster that occurred before birth. In some patients, large areas of scarred skin have required skin grafting.[291,299] In other patients, the rash was bullous[298] or consisted of multiple, scattered, depressed, white scars.[302,304,319] In one infant, healing zoster was present at the T11 dermatome at birth; there was also spinal cord atrophy at the same level and aganglionosis of the intestine.[318]

Ocular abnormalities include chorioretinitis, Horner syndrome or anisocoria, microphthalmia, cataract, and nystagmus.[§]

Rarely, major abnormalities were confined to the eye. There was no apparent effect of timing of maternal varicella during gestation; the times of infection varied from 9 to 23 weeks in these infants. Figure 23-2 is a photograph showing retinal involvement in one of these patients.[302,313]

Neurologic involvement is about as common as skin and eye abnormalities in infants with congenital varicella syndrome. Patients with cerebral cortical atrophy, diffuse brain involvement, or mental retardation (frequently accompanied by abnormal electroencephalograms and seizures or myoclonic jerks) have been described.[278,279,286-288,321] In a few patients, cerebrospinal fluid (CSF) findings were normal[120,279,288,315]; in others, there were increased numbers of leukocytes or protein levels.[278,285,287] Bulbar palsy is suspected to result in dysphagia and bouts of aspiration pneumonia in some of these children.[‖]

Deep tendon reflexes were reported as normal in one infant[287] and diminished to absent in six,[¶] and they were in some cases accompanied by sensory deficits.[120,279,284,288,315] Electromyography in some patients revealed a denervation pattern with loss of motor units.[279,288,289,311,315] A biopsy specimen in one instance showed replacement of muscle bundles by fat.[279] At least five children with vocal cord paralysis have been reported.[321,329,331,332]

Abnormalities of the limbs can be extremely dramatic in presentation and are seen in about half of affected infants. The most common limb abnormality, which first called attention to this congenital syndrome, is hypoplasia of a limb, most commonly unilateral involvement of a leg or arm (see Table 23-5). Hypoplasia or absence of digits has also

[§]References 69, 246, 264 ,265, 268, 270-272, 274-291, 293-306, 308, 309, 312-315, 318, 319, 339, 340.

[‖]References 246, 279, 283, 285, 288, 295, 296, 301, 302, 305, 308, 321-323.

[¶]References 266, 267, 278, 279, 283, 284.

been observed.[278,280,283,284,287-289] Talipes equinovarus or a calcaneovalgus deformity has also occurred.[#]

This complex of abnormalities in the limbs, including the bony abnormalities, is probably attributable to a neuropathy caused by direct viral invasion of the ganglia and spinal cord.[329]

About one fourth of these infants died within the first 14 months of life. One infant with the obvious syndrome was stillborn.[274] In one infant who died at 6 months, autopsy revealed a necrotizing encephalitis with various degrees of gliosis and inflammatory infiltrates. Focal calcification was observed in white and gray matter of the cerebrum, brainstem, and cerebellum. Atrophy of the anterior columns of the spinal cord and scarring in the ganglion corresponding to the distribution of the skin lesions and an atrophic limb were also present. No inclusion bodies were identified.[279] Among infants with a hypoplastic limb, 40% had evidence of mental retardation or died early. The presence of a hypoplastic limb on an ultrasound examination suggests a poor outcome.

About one third of affected infants were premature or had low birth weight for their gestational ages, and about 10% had various abnormalities of the gastrointestinal tract, including reflux, duodenal stenosis, jejunal dilation, microcolon, atresia of the sigmoid colon, and sphincter malfunction.[*a]

A similar percentage had abnormalities of the urinary tract, often caused by poor or absent bladder sphincter function.[†a]

Involvement of the cervical or lumbar spinal cord and the autonomic nervous system is thought to account for the observed hypoplasia or aplasia of limbs and digits, motor and sensory defects, decrease or absence of deep tendon reflexes, Horner syndrome, and gastrointestinal and urinary tract abnormalities.[341]

Figures 23-3 and 23-4 depict two children with stigmata of congenital varicella syndrome. One has severe[279] and one has relatively mild involvement.[302,313]

ZOSTER AFTER CONGENITAL VARICELLA SYNDROME. Of children with congenital varicella syndrome, 15% develop clinical zoster in infancy or early childhood, almost all in the first year of life.[‡a]

This finding is of particular interest because cell-mediated immunity to VZV in 2 of 10 of children with the syndrome has been reported to be absent as determined by lymphocyte transformation.[246,265] In the series by Enders and associates[68] of 1291 live births (without congenital varicella syndrome), of whom conservatively perhaps 25% were infected with VZV (the attack rate could be as high as 50%), the rate of zoster in childhood was 3%. Zoster seems to be more common in children with congenital varicella syndrome than in infants who were infected with VZV in utero but were asymptomatic at birth.

DIAGNOSIS OF CONGENITAL VARICELLA SYNDROME. During the neonatal period or infancy, attempts to isolate VZV from the skin, CSF, eye, and other tissues in infants with developmental defects were negative.[§a]

[#] References 266, 267, 271, 274, 278, 287, 295, 309, 311, 315, 339.
[*a] References 277, 278, 285, 299, 313, 314, 317, 318, 320.
[†a] References 245, 278, 279, 282, 297, 310, 315, 318.
[‡a] References 69, 276, 277, 282, 296, 301, 304, 305, 315, 319, 321, 322, 325.
[§a] References 264, 279, 287, 295, 296, 301, 302.

Although rubella virus and CMV are commonly isolated from young infants affected by these viruses, failure to isolate VZV in these cases is probably explained by the fact that the period of viral replication occurred during early gestation, and no replicating virus persisted by the time of birth. In children who developed zoster at an early age, it has been possible to isolate VZV from the rash.[245,289,314] In seven infants who died, autopsy results showed apparent dissemination of VZV with varicella-like involvement of the lungs, liver, spleen, adrenals, or pancreas.[265-267,271,288-291]

Total IgM concentrations in the serum or cord blood of six infants were measured.[264,279,288,300-302] In three instances, the levels were clearly increased, with values of 48 to 100 mg/dL found when the infants were 1.5 to 6 weeks of age. Specific VZV antibodies in the IgM fraction were not detected in seven cases in which they were sought,[246,288,302,308,341] but they were detectable in six other cases.[69,265,266,292,300] In one of these cases, VZV IgM was detected prenatally by obtaining blood by cordocentesis.[341] In most infants, a decline of antibodies in the serum was observed, a finding compatible with a fetal or a maternal origin. In 10 instances, persistence of or an increase in antibodies in the infant supported a presumption of intrauterine infection.[‖a]

It has been possible to document some reported cases of congenital varicella syndrome, but not all of them, because antibody titers may be inconclusive even in children with the apparent full-blown and distinctive constellation of abnormalities. Some children were diagnosed even before it was possible to measure antibody titers to VZV. The development of zoster at an early age can be interpreted as substantiating VZV infection in utero. Although many of the cases reported as congenital varicella syndrome lack proof, it has been possible to show that some infants with characteristic stigmata were infected in utero with VZV, although an active, chronic infection does not exist. Modern molecular methods, such as PCR and in situ hybridization, have been useful for proving congenital varicella syndrome in a few reported infants and will undoubtedly be used to prove future cases.[69,272,274-277,321] In the future, it is expected that these will become the methods of choice rather than antibody testing. It is also predicted that with widespread use of varicella vaccine, the incidence of this unusual cause of congenital disease will become rare.

Fetal Malformations and Management of Pregnant Women With Varicella-Zoster Virus Infection. In the 1990s, the incidence of fetal malformations after maternal VZV infection was clarified. Varicella is a significantly greater threat than zoster; 95% of reported cases of congenital varicella syndrome have followed maternal varicella. In the series by Enders and associates[68] of 366 women with zoster in pregnancy, there were no cases of congenital varicella syndrome. This outcome is not unexpected because zoster is probably less likely to be accompanied by a viremia than is varicella; many fetuses may escape VZV infection from maternal zoster. Because zoster is a secondary infection, residual maternal immunity to VZV may at least partially protect the fetus from damage, analogous to that seen when congenital CMV infection is caused by reactivation

[‖a] References 264, 281, 284, 301-303, 313, 315.

rather than primary CMV infection.[345] As with CMV infection, however, it is possible, although rare, for fetal stigmata to follow secondary maternal infection.

The time at which maternal VZV infection occurs during gestation also influences whether the infant is likely to be severely damaged. Infection during the first and early second trimesters seems to be the most critical. Most reported cases of congenital varicella syndrome have occurred when the onset of maternal infection was before the 20th week of pregnancy. Only seven infants with some of the stigmata have been recorded as the result of maternal varicella after the 20th week.[237,272,307-309,317,344] When maternal varicella occurs after the 20th week, the infant may be infected, but usually the only evidence is a positive VZV antibody titer when the infant is older than 1 year and, in some cases, development of zoster at an early age.

Eleven prospective studies of the incidence of congenital varicella syndrome have been published. Data from these studies are presented in Table 23-6. There are 14 cases of congenital varicella syndrome in 858 (1.6%) women who developed varicella in the first 20 weeks of pregnancy. If the entire gestational period is considered, 2245 women who had varicella during pregnancy were delivered of live-born infants; the overall incidence of congenital varicella syndrome was 0.6%. These data indicate that the risk for development of congenital varicella syndrome is mostly confined to the first 20 weeks of pregnancy, and the risk after maternal varicella in the first 20 weeks of pregnancy is extremely low, on the order of 1% to 2%. Weeks 7 to 20 are the time of the greatest risk.[69] The tendency to develop overwhelming forms of VZV infection in the fetus indicates the increased ability of VZV to multiply in fetal tissues, which is similar to that of other viruses, such as rubella virus and CMV.

Counseling of pregnant women who have acquired varicella during pregnancy can be very difficult. Because the congenital syndrome is rare, termination of pregnancy is not routinely recommended, in contrast to recommendations for gestational rubella. When the syndrome does occur, however, it is likely to be severe. It would be helpful if prenatal diagnoses were available, but diagnostic attempts, such as measurement of maternal antibody titers and amniocentesis, have not proved useful. Although blood may be obtained by cordocentesis for antibody testing, the presence of fetal VZV IgM does not mean that the infant has congenital varicella syndrome, but only that infection with VZV has occurred. Similarly, PCR assay may identify an infected fetus, but not one with malformations.[343,346]

Ultrasonography has been used successfully to identify the following fetal abnormalities after maternal varicella: hydrocephalus 12 weeks later[265]; clubfeet and hydrocephalus 13 weeks later[295]; a large, bullous skin lesion originally believed to be a meningocele 15 weeks later[298]; calcifications in the liver and other organs 9, 15, and 18 weeks later[276,296,323]; a hypoplastic limb and clubfoot 11 and 16 weeks later[69,276]; and a lacuna of the skull 25 weeks later.[292] Successful use of ultrasonography as a diagnostic tool to identify this syndrome prenatally has also been reported in cases with evidence of widespread infection.[334-337] Three published reports indicate, however, that ultrasonography is not infallible. In two infants, ultrasound scans were normal 3 weeks after maternal varicella, but the fetuses were later diagnosed as having congenital varicella syndrome.[266,295] One infant was diagnosed with liver calcifications by ultrasonography at 27 weeks and a positive PCR assay for VZV; his mother had varicella at 12.5 weeks. At birth, no obvious anomalies were present, and the infant did well except for development of zoster at age 8 months.[343] Even defects detected by ultrasonography must be interpreted with some caution.

Because about 40% of reported patients with a hypoplastic limb also sustained brain damage or died in early infancy, the presence of a limb abnormality on ultrasonography seems to suggest a poor overall prognosis for the fetus. Two women were reported to have terminated their pregnancies after the diagnosis of congenital varicella syndrome was made based on abnormal limbs on ultrasound scan. At autopsy, the fetuses were found to be severely affected.[69,343] Because abnormalities may not be detected by ultrasonography immediately after maternal varicella, by the time any is noticed, it may be too late to consider interruption of pregnancy, depending on the time of onset of maternal varicella.

Although congenital varicella syndrome varies in severity, most cases are severe. It would be helpful if maternal infection could be identified and appropriate management initiated as early as possible. It is uncertain whether administration of VZIG or acyclovir to a pregnant woman can prevent her fetus from developing the congenital varicella syndrome. Passive immunization may help, however, and will cause no harm.[70] In the study by Enders and associates,[68] there were no cases of the congenital syndrome in 97 women who were given VZIG on exposure; it is unknown how many of these women were in the first 20 weeks of pregnancy.

A syndrome resembling the congenital varicella syndrome may also rarely occur after intrauterine infection with HSV.[347]

Table 23-6 Incidence of Congenital Varicella Syndrome: Results of Prospective Studies, 1960-1997

	INCIDENCE OF SYNDROME	
Year	**First Trimester/ First 20 Weeks**	**Total Gestation**
1960[603]	0/70	0/288
1973[274]	2/27	2/135
1984[292]	0/23	1/38
1986[250]	1/11	
1992[274]	0/40	
1994[272]	1/49	
1994[263]	7/351	7/1291
1994[271]	2/99	2/146
1996[234]	0/26	
1997[252]	0/22	
2002[237]	0/140	1/347
Total reported	13/858 (1.6%)	14/2245 (0.6%)

Perinatal Varicella

Perinatal varicella includes disease that is acquired postnatally by droplet infection and that is transplacentally transmitted or congenital. Varicella is considered to be exclusively transplacentally transmitted when it occurs within 10 days of birth.

Postnatally Acquired Varicella. Postnatally acquired varicella, which can begin 10 to 28 (average, ≈15) days after birth, is generally mild.[348] The experiences with nosocomial varicella infections in the newborn nursery that were described in a previous section further corroborate the benign nature of the disease and the fact that transmission to neonates in this environment is inefficient and rarely reaches epidemic proportions.

Deaths among neonates caused by postnatally acquired disease are rare, but some data indicate an appreciably higher incidence of complications or deaths in neonates than in older children.[133,136-138,348,349] Preblud and associates[348] found that of 92 reported deaths caused by varicella from 1968 to 1978 in children younger than 1 year, only 5 occurred in newborns (8 hours-19 days old). Although mortality was increased by a factor of four for infants younger than 1 year, compared with older children, there was a low calculated death rate for varicella throughout childhood (8/100,000 patients if <1 year and 2/100,000 patients 1-14 years of age).[348] One 15-day-old infant with severe disseminated varicella born to a woman who developed varicella 7 days after delivery has been described.[349] The child survived; acyclovir was administered for 10 days. The only other report in the English literature of severe postnatally acquired varicella in an infant younger than 1 month is that of Gustafson and colleagues.[133] The term infant with Turner syndrome was exposed to varicella when 7 days old, developed more than 200 vesicles, and died of pneumonia; however, the role of VZV in this infant's death was unclear because no autopsy was performed. An infant with vaccine type (Oka strain) varicella was reported.[350] Possibly, this infant was infected by aerosolization of varicella vaccine because the newborn was in the same room with the mother when the vaccination was performed. The illness in the infant was mild.

Congenital Varicella: Maternal Infection Near Term. Congenital varicella is not inevitable when maternal varicella occurs in the 21 days preceding parturition. In only 8 (24%) of 34 reported cases of maternal disease with onset during this period did varicella develop in the neonate within the first 10 days of life.[134,193,233,235] An identical attack rate of 24% for congenital varicella after the occurrence of maternal varicella within 17 days preceding delivery was arrived at by Meyers.[351] He reviewed many cases in the literature and also14 examples that were reported to the Centers for Disease Control and Prevention (CDC) from 1972 to 1973. Attack rates on the order of 50% were reported, however, in two studies on the efficacy of passive immunization to prevent severe neonatal varicella.[352,353] In Meyers' study,[354] there was no statistically significant relationship between day of onset of the rash in the mother and subsequent attack rates of congenital varicella. Seven of 22 neonates born to mothers whose rash appeared less than 5 days antepartum ultimately developed congenital varicella, whereas 4 of 24 infants born to mothers whose rash began 5 to 14 days antepartum had congenital disease.[351] These data indicate that the attack rate in congenital varicella (25%-50%) is lower than after household exposure to VZV (80%-90%) and suggest that bloodborne transmission may be less efficient than transmission by the skin and respiratory routes.

The incubation period in congenital varicella, defined as the interval between the onset of rash in the mother and onset in the fetus or neonate, is usually 9 to 15 days.[352] This interval is slightly shorter than the normal postnatal incubation period, possibly because fetal tissues are more susceptible to VZV than more mature tissues. Rarely, presumably when fetal infection is caused by the primary maternal viremia, the exanthem appears in the mother and neonate within 3 days of each other[136] or even simultaneously.[354] The average incubation period in 36 cases reported in the literature was 11 days, with a maximum of 16 days. In only three instances was the incubation period less than 6 days.[351]

In contrast to postnatally acquired neonatal varicella, congenital varicella can be associated with significant mortality. Severe cases clinically resemble varicella in the immunocompromised host. An infant who died of hemorrhagic varicella with pulmonary and liver involvement is shown in Figure 23-1. The spectrum of illness also includes extremely mild infections with only a handful of vesicles. Erlich and coworkers[190] first observed that infants born with the rash or who had an early onset of rash survived, whereas infants who died had a relatively late onset of rash. It was hypothesized that for neonates with early onset, maternal illness had occurred long enough before parturition to allow antibodies to be elaborated by the mother and to cross the placenta. Subsequent reports offer strong confirmation of these observations. As reviewed by Meyers,[351] there were no deaths among 22 infants with congenital varicella, whose onset of rash occurred between birth and 4 days of age. In contrast, 4 (21%) of 19 neonates in whom the rash began when they were 5 to 10 days of age died (Table 23-7).[351] These 4 deaths occurred among 13 neonates (31%) whose mothers' exanthems developed within 4 days before birth, but no deaths were observed among 23 neonates with congenital varicella whose mothers developed a rash 5 or more days before birth.

Further support for the protective or modifying effect of maternal antibody has come from measurements of placental transfer of IgG to VZV.[144] When varicella occurred more than 1 week before delivery, complement-fixing antibody titers in maternal and cord blood were similar. In contrast, when infection occurred 3 to 5 days before delivery, maternal antibody was present at parturition, and antibodies to VZV in the neonate were absent or at least eightfold lower. These data suggest that a lag of several days occurs before IgG antibodies to VZV cross the placenta and equilibrate with the fetal circulation. The development of mild congenital varicella in the presence of placentally transferred maternal antibody

Table 23-7 Deaths From Congenital Varicella in Relation to Date of Onset of Rash in Mother or Neonate

Onset	Neonatal Deaths	Neonatal Cases	%
Day of onset of rash in neonate			
0-4	0	22	0
5-10	4	19	21
Onset of maternal rash, days antepartum			
≥5	0	23	0
0-4	4	13	31

Data from Meyers JD: Congenital varicella in term infants: risk reconsidered, *J Infect Dis* 129:215, 1974; with permission from the University of Chicago.

has also been shown using the more sensitive FAMA test.[98] The neonate may be at risk for developing severe varicella because the immune system is immature, as has been shown by Kohl[355] with regard to host defense against HSV.

Zoster in Neonates and Older Children

The most characteristic feature of zoster is the localization of the rash. It is nearly always unilateral, does not cross the midline, and is typically limited to an area of skin served by one to three sensory ganglia. In children, prodromes of malaise, fever, headache, and nausea may be observed. Pain and paresthesias in the involved dermatome may precede the exanthem by 4 or 5 days. Involvement of the dermatomes of the head, neck, and trunk is more common than involvement of the extremities, a distribution that also reflects the density of lesions in varicella.[52] Erythematous papules give rise to grouped vesicles, which progress to pustules in 2 to 4 days. New crops of vesicles may keep appearing for 1 week. Pain may be associated with the exanthem and usually abates as the skin lesions scab; in elderly adults, severe and incapacitating neuralgia of the involved nerve may persist for months. Cutaneous dissemination of vesicles to sites distant from the involved dermatome is observed uncommonly and is more frequent in compromised hosts, such as patients with lymphoma or immunologic deficiencies.

Zoster occurs as host defense mechanisms against VZV wane in a person who has previously experienced varicella. Because immunity is relatively durable, this hypothesis presumes that zoster occurs predominantly in older persons and is rare in neonates. Among 192 patients with zoster in a general practice, the attack rate increased progressively with age.[52] Only six patients were younger than 10 years; the youngest was 2 years of age. In two reported series describing zoster in a total of 22 children, only two cases occurred in children younger than 2 years.[233,356] These reports confirm the rarity of zoster among infants. When zoster occurs in children who have not previously had varicella, there is often a history of intrauterine exposure to VZV. In these reports, the mothers contracted varicella during gestation but gave birth to normal infants who, without ever developing varicella despite frequent childhood exposure, developed typical zoster at a young age, many in the first few months of life.[120,322,357-361] In most of these infants, the course of zoster was benign. One infant developed a second attack of zoster when 10 months of age; the first occurred when the infant was 4 months of age.[357]

Although there are six reports of zoster during the neonatal period,[362-367] it is doubtful whether any of these cases diagnosed on clinical grounds is an authentic example of zoster. HSV may produce a vesicular exanthem in the newborn that appears to have a dermatomal distribution. Virus isolation (or demonstration of VZV DNA or antigen from skin lesions) is required before a diagnosis of zoster can be accepted. Serologic studies are not useful in differentiating these diseases.

DIAGNOSIS AND DIFFERENTIAL DIAGNOSIS

Varicella

In a neonate with a widespread, generalized vesicular exanthem and a history of recent maternal varicella or postnatal exposure, a diagnosis of varicella can usually be made with confidence on clinical grounds alone. Greater difficulty is encountered when lesions are few or when there is no history of exposure.

Diagnostic Techniques. If laboratory diagnosis is required, it is best accomplished by showing VZV antigen or DNA in skin lesions or isolating virus from vesicular fluid. VZV antigen may be shown by using immunofluorescence, using a monoclonal antibody to VZV that is conjugated to fluorescein and is commercially available.[169,368,369] For virus isolation, fluid should be promptly inoculated onto tissue cultures because VZV is labile. PCR assay has proved extremely sensitive and accurate for diagnosis of VZV infections.[164,370-376] In situ hybridization is also a useful diagnostic technique.[277,377,378]

VZV infections may be documented by demonstration of a fourfold or greater increase in VZV antibody titer by using a sensitive test such as FAMA or ELISA. The presence of specific IgM in one serum specimen suggests recent VZV infection.[41,42,379] Persistence of VZV antibody beyond the age of 8 months is highly suggestive of intrauterine varicella, provided that there is no history of clinical varicella after birth.[27] Persistence of VZV antibody with no decrease in titer over several months in a young infant (as long as all sera are tested simultaneously) is highly suggestive of intrauterine infection. A FAMA or latex agglutination antibody titer of 1:4 or greater beyond 8 months of life is suggestive of immunity to varicella, provided that the patient has not received gamma globulin or other blood products in the previous 3 to 4 months. Physicians should be aware that no serologic test is 100% accurate for identifying individuals immune to varicella, although these antibody tests are generally reliable.[380]

Differential Diagnosis. Several diseases may be considered in the differential diagnosis of varicella in the newborn, including neonatal HSV, contact dermatitis, hand-foot-and-mouth syndrome and other enterovirus infections, and impetigo. In neonatal HSV, cutaneous lesions may be relatively sparse and may be absent altogether despite widespread visceral dissemination. Vesicles tend to occur in clusters, rather than in the more even distribution seen in varicella. Fever, marked toxicity, and encephalitis are more common in neonates with HSV. Stained smears of vesicle fluid (i.e., Tzanck preparation) are not helpful in differentiating HSV from varicella because both are characterized by multinucleated giant cells and intranuclear inclusion bodies. In cell cultures, HSV typically produces a widespread cytopathic effect in 24 to 48 hours, whereas the cytopathic effect caused by VZV is cell associated and focal and develops more slowly. Indirect immunofluorescence using monoclonal antibodies conjugated to fluorescein can be performed on smears of skin scrapings; if positive, the assay can identify VZV, HSV-1, and HSV-2 within several hours. Paired serum samples can be examined for increasing antibody titers to HSV and VZV antigens. It is exceedingly rare for varicella to develop in a newborn in the absence of any (i.e., infant or mother) exposure to varicella or zoster. In contrast, most infants with neonatal HSV have no recognized exposure to the virus.

Although 95% of cases of perinatal HSV are transmitted during delivery, a syndrome similar to congenital varicella syndrome, with limb and eye abnormalities, skin scarring, and zosteriform rashes, has rarely been observed after the unusual occurrence of intrauterine transmission of HSV.[381,382] In an infant with stigmata of congenital varicella syndrome whose mother has no history of varicella during pregnancy, congenital HSV should be considered. It may be impossible to make a definitive diagnosis immediately, unless the infant develops a vesicular zosteriform rash from which the causative virus can be identified. Determination of antibody titers to HSV and VZV at presentation and when infants are 8 to 12 months of age may be useful to establish a diagnosis.

In some cases of contact dermatitis, papules and vesicles may appear after exposure to specific chemical irritants. Typically, they appear on exposed body surfaces and do not have the characteristic distribution of varicella or smallpox.

In patients with hand-foot-and-mouth syndrome, a vesicular exanthem usually caused by coxsackievirus A16 or A5, may be observed during the enterovirus season (i.e., summer or early autumn). There are rarely more than a dozen vesicles, and they typically occur on the distal extremities, especially the palms and soles. Painful vesicular lesions that ulcerate quickly may also be seen in the oropharynx. The causative virus is readily isolated from vesicle fluid or from feces.

Impetigo may occur in neonates. In bullous impetigo (i.e., pemphigus neonatorum), large blebs are present instead of the smaller vesicles of varicella. This disease, which is caused by *Staphylococcus aureus*, may be associated with high fever, toxicity, septicemia, and death. Alternative diagnoses include syphilis, group B streptococcal infection, and incontinentia pigmenti, which may cause vesiculobullous lesions in a neonate.

Smallpox is traditionally part of the differential diagnosis of vesicular lesions in neonates. Although smallpox was eradicated, there is concern that the disease may reemerge because of bioterrorism. Classically, the vesicles of smallpox appear to be at the same stage of development instead of showing the pattern of crops over several days. A centrifugal distribution of the skin rash is prominent. The best approach in a suspicious situation is to rule out the possibility of VZV or HSV infection as described previously, preferably by immunofluorescence testing. If the test results are negative, a search for smallpox may be indicated, especially if the history of the patient warrants it. Accurate diagnosis may be achieved in hours by electron microscopy of the vesicle fluid or crusts; such microscopic examination reveals virus particles whose morphology is very different from that of viruses of the herpes family. Smallpox modified by exposure to vaccinia in the distant past and alastrim (i.e., variola minor) may be particularly difficult to distinguish from varicella. In suspicious cases, the CDC and local health department should be promptly involved.

Disseminated vaccinia is rare today because smallpox vaccine (i.e., vaccinia virus) is not routinely used, although a bioterrorism attack could change the scenario. Vaccinia can be considered in a neonate exposed postnatally to a person who has been recently vaccinated. The lesions resemble those of smallpox. Impression smears of vesicle fluid do not show intranuclear inclusions or giant cells. Laboratory diagnosis may be achieved by electron microscopy and immunofluorescence.

Zoster

Zoster usually is easily recognized by the typical dermatomal distribution of the vesicular lesions. In the differential diagnosis, the main entity to be distinguished in the neonatal period is HSV appearing in a linear pattern. Identification of VZV or HSV DNA by PCR assay, antigen by immunofluorescence or virus isolation is the only reliable means of differentiating these entities when the distribution of the exanthem is linear. Contact dermatitis should also be considered in the differential diagnosis of zosteriform lesions in the neonatal period.

THERAPY

Treatment of the Mother

Acyclovir is the antiviral drug of choice for treatment of potentially severe or severe VZV infections.[383,384] Acyclovir itself has no antiviral action, but when it is phosphorylated by enzymes produced by cells infected with VZV, it is incorporated as a DNA chain terminator, and it inhibits viral DNA polymerase. Because these actions occur only in virus-infected cells, acyclovir is well tolerated and associated with little toxicity. The drug is available in topical, oral, and IV formulations.

The safety of acyclovir has been shown in the past 35 years, and there is good reason to use this drug liberally in clinical situations for which it is indicated, even during pregnancy. Although most VZV infections in normal hosts are self-limited, there is a low but real fatality rate from varicella in adults. For this reason and because long-term toxicity of acyclovir in the fetus seems unlikely, acyclovir is recommended more often for use during pregnancy in women with varicella than previously. A registry of patients (and their offspring) who have received acyclovir during pregnancy has been established.[257,258] In general, pregnant women who develop varicella should be treated with orally administered acyclovir and observed carefully. Pregnant women who develop severe varicella while receiving oral therapy, especially patients who develop pneumonia, should be promptly treated with IV acyclovir.[385] Supportive respiratory therapy (e.g., nasal oxygen, tracheostomy, ventilatory assistance) should be used as needed. Controlled studies of corticosteroids for varicella pneumonia are unavailable; steroids are not recommended. Antibiotics should be given if there is evidence of bacterial superinfection.

Anecdotal reports on the apparently successful use of acyclovir in pregnant women with varicella have been published, although controlled studies have not been performed. The data suggest that most women who develop varicella in pregnancy ultimately survive without sequelae.[236] This is undoubtedly the result of increasing awareness of the potential seriousness of the illness on the part of medical providers and the more liberal use of acyclovir today.

There is little information on the use of acyclovir for pregnant women with zoster. Presumably, because zoster would be expected to be self-limited in most women of childbearing age, there would be little need for antiviral therapy in this situation. Especially in the setting of an extensive rash or severe pain, use of acyclovir, particularly as oral therapy, should be strongly considered. Alternatively, one of the newer drugs, such as famciclovir or valacyclovir, can be used to treat pregnant women who develop severe zoster. The dose of famciclovir is 500 mg taken orally three times daily; the dose of valacyclovir is 1 g taken orally three times daily. Both medications are administered for 7 days. There is no information on the use of famciclovir or valacyclovir in pregnancy. Although famciclovir and valacyclovir are converted to acyclovir, and acyclovir is the active drug in the blood, there is more safety information on use of acyclovir in pregnancy, and for that reason it is probably preferable.

Acyclovir has been most effective when it is administered within 1 day after the onset of varicella and 3 days after onset of zoster. The usual adult dose for IV acyclovir is 10 mg/kg, given three times daily. Orally administered acyclovir has been found to have a modest effect on the fever and rash of varicella in otherwise healthy populations. A multicenter, double-blind, placebo-controlled, collaborative study involving 815 similarly treated children, who were given 20 mg/kg of acyclovir orally four times daily, shortened the course of illness by about 1 day.[386] The benefit to secondary household cases was not increased beyond that of primary cases. Similar results emerged from a study involving adolescents with varicella.[387] The modest benefit conferred by oral acyclovir therapy is not surprising in view of the self-limited nature of varicella in children and the poor oral absorption of acyclovir. There is a similar benefit for adults with varicella who were given oral acyclovir (800 mg taken five times daily for 5 days) within 24 hours of onset of rash.[388,389]

In the double-blind, placebo-controlled study of Wallace and associates,[389] involving 76 military recruits, the duration of illness was shortened by about 1 day, and the personnel were able to return to work 1 day sooner on average, if they received acyclovir. There is no information regarding treatment of pregnant women, and physicians are reluctant to extrapolate to them from studies involving mainly healthy young men. Given the possibility that acyclovir will help and is unlikely to harm, however, the drug should be strongly considered for most adults today with early varicella, pregnant or not.

Orally administered valacyclovir is now also used to treat varicella, although valacyclovir is considerably more costly than acyclovir. For children with varicella who are older than 2 years, the dose is 20 mg/kg/dose (not to exceed 1 g/dose) three times daily for 5 days. For adults, the dose is 1 g three times daily for 5 days. For treatment of zoster, valacyclovir is usually recommended for 7 days. Famciclovir given orally (500 mg three times daily) is also recommended for treatment of zoster in adults.

Treatment of the Newborn Infant

Although there is little information on the use of acyclovir for varicella in newborns, it has been used to treat many infants with neonatal HSV infection. In a study in which 95 infants received acyclovir (30 mg/kg/day IV), no short-term or long-term toxicity was observed.[384-386] Pharmacokinetic studies have indicated that dose adjustments for acyclovir may be necessary in premature infants and infants with hepatic or renal dysfunction.[390-392] There are no data about the use of oral acyclovir for severe neonatal infections caused by VZV, and acyclovir is poorly absorbed when given by the gastrointestinal route. A dose of 1500 mg/m^2 of acyclovir, given IV in three divided daily doses, is recommended for infants with severe or rapidly progressing varicella. It is not recommended that infants with congenital varicella syndrome receive treatment with acyclovir, except in the unusual setting of active zoster.

PREVENTION

Passive Immunization Against Varicella

Controlled studies have indicated that pooled serum immunoglobulin attenuates but does not prevent varicella when administered to susceptible family contacts[107] and that zoster immunoglobulin (ZIG, prepared from patients recovering from herpes zoster) prevents clinical varicella when given to susceptible healthy children within 72 hours of household exposure.[393] Additional uncontrolled studies of immunocompromised children, such as children with leukemia receiving maintenance chemotherapy, at high risk for developing severe or fatal varicella have indicated that ZIG administered within 72 hours of a household exposure usually modifies varicella so that the infection is mild or subclinical.[87,394,395] VZIG (prepared from plasma obtained from healthy, volunteer blood donors identified by routine screening to have high antibody titers to VZV) became available in 1978. Serologic and clinical evaluations demonstrated that VZIG was similar to ZIG in preventing or modifying clinical illness in susceptible, immunocompromised children if administered within 96 hours of exposure to varicella.[396,397] The VZIG product currently approved in the United States is VariZIG (Cangene Corporation, Winnipeg, Manitoba, Canada).[260] VariZIG can be ordered from the exclusive U.S. distributor, FFF Enterprises (requests at 800 843-7477 or online at http://www.fffenterprises.com). Patients exposed to varicella or zoster who are recommended to receive VariZIG are immunocompromised patients without evidence of immunity,[104] newborn infants whose mothers have signs and symptoms of varicella around the time of delivery (i.e., 5 days before to 2 days after), hospitalized premature infants born at greater than or equal to 28 weeks of gestation whose mothers do not have evidence of immunity to varicella, hospitalized premature infants born at less than 28 weeks of gestation or who weigh less than or equal to 1000 g at birth regardless of their mothers' evidence of immunity to varicella, and pregnant women without evidence of immunity to varicella.[260,398] The recommended dose is 1.25 mL (1 vial or 125 U) for each 10 kg of body weight, with a maximum dosage of 6 mL (5 vials or 625 U) intramuscularly.[260] The minimum dose is 0.5 vial (62.5 IU) for patients weighing less than or equal to 2.0 kg and one vial (125 IU) for patients weighing 2.1 to 10.0 kg. VariZIG should be administered as soon as possible after exposure to VZV and within 10 days.[260,398] Passive immunization may prolong the incubation period of varicella by greater than or equal to 1 week.[86,87]

Evidence indicates that infants born to women who develop varicella 5 days or less before delivery are at risk for developing disseminated or fatal varicella; these infants benefit from passive immunization with VZIG. In an uncontrolled study by Hanngren and coworkers,[352] 41 neonates born to women who developed varicella between

4 days before and 2 days after delivery received 1 mL of ZIG, and the illness was modified. Although the attack rate was 51%, and the incubation period averaged 11 days, there were no fatalities, instead of the expected mortality rate of about 30%, and 13 (62%) of 21 had fewer than 20 vesicles with no fever. Two (10%) had severe infections, and 1 was treated with interferon. In a study of VZIG by Preblud and colleagues,[353] a similar varicella attack rate of 45% was observed in 132 infants. In this study, a dose of 125 U (1.25 mL) of VZIG was administered. The illness also was modified: of 53 infants with varicella, 74% had less than 50 vesicles, and only 10% had more than 100 vesicles. No antiviral therapy was given; there was one death in the group, but it was unclear that it was caused by varicella. The high attack rates of varicella in these studies compared with historical data have not been explained. In previous studies, infant attack rates of 24% in late[351] and overall[246] pregnancy have been reported. Successful passive immunization would, if anything, be expected to decrease the attack rate, rather than increase it. Nevertheless, the mildness of the illness and absence of mortality in these two studies support the recommendation for passive immunization of infants born to women with varicella at term. Since the introduction of ZIG and VZIG for use in appropriate neonates, fatalities from neonatal varicella have become rare. Infants born to women with the onset of varicella more than 5 days before delivery can be expected to have mild infection,[97,190,351,399,400] and passive immunization is not recommended for these infants.

VariZIG should be administered to infants born to mothers with varicella 5 days or less before delivery as soon as possible after birth. Administration of VariZIG to the mother before delivery of the infant is not recommended because a larger dose would be required to provide passive immunization to the infant, and no benefit to the mother would result. Early delivery of the infant of a mother with active varicella is also not recommended; the longer the infant remains in utero, the more likely there will be transplacental transfer of maternal antibody. A diagram of the relationship between maternal and infant varicella, development of maternal antibodies, and transplacental transfer of these antibodies is shown in Figure 23-5. Because women with zoster near term have high antibody titers to VZV, it is unnecessary to administer VariZIG to their infants.

There have been reports of infants ($n = 15$) who developed severe or fatal congenital varicella despite prompt administration of VZIG in the recommended dosage.[401-407] The reason for the severity of these cases is not fully understood, but they seem to be unusual or rare. All but one of these infants were born at term; for most, information on health status at birth was provided, and newborns were described as "healthy." Most of these children were reported from the United Kingdom, and the VZIG used there might have been less potent than that produced in the United States; also, some infants might have received lower antibody titers because, in the United Kingdom, the recommended VZIG dosage was increased over time.

Although it is recommended that VariZIG be administered to infants born to women who develop varicella in the first 2 days after delivery, only a few reports indicate that this timing of birth at onset of maternal varicella is associated with increased risk to the infant. One of the reported infants

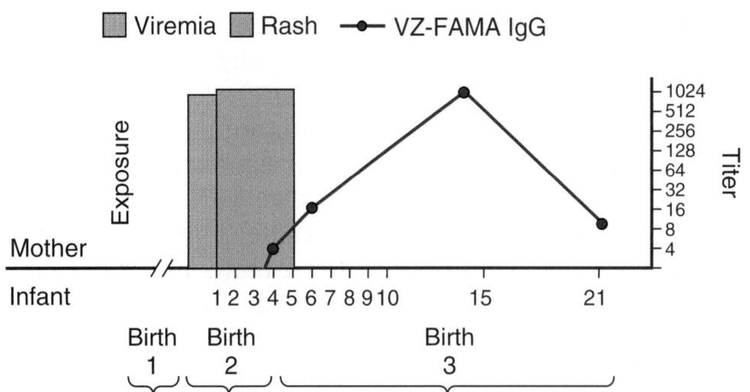

Figure 23-5 Diagrammatic representation of transmission of varicella-zoster virus (VZV) and VZV antibody to a fetus in maternal varicella near term. When the infant is born during the maternal incubation period (1), no varicella occurs unless the infant is exposed postnatally to the infection. When the infant is born 0 to 4 days after onset of maternal varicella (2), disseminated varicella may develop because the infection is not modified by maternal antibody. The onset of varicella occurs when the infant is 5 to 10 days of age. Infants born 5 days or more after maternal varicella (3) receive maternal antibody, which leads to mild infection. This diagram is based on data for 50 newborn infants with varicella. *FAMA,* Fluorescent antibody to membrane antigen; *IgG,* immunoglobulin G. (Modifed from Gershon A: Varicella in mother and infant: problems old and new. In Krugman S, Gershon A, editors: *Infection of the fetus and newborn infant,* New York, 1975, Alan R Liss, p 79.)

with fatal varicella, despite passive immunization, was born to a woman who developed varicella on the second postpartum day.[404] Treatment with acyclovir was initiated after viscerally disseminated disease had already occurred. A child with severe varicella whose mother developed varicella 3 days after delivery has also been reported.[408] This child was treated with a leukocyte transfusion from her mother and thymic hormone and survived. This therapy is not recommended for this purpose at present.

Exposed newborns who did not receive passive immunization should be treated with IV acyclovir if they develop varicella. No precise guidelines exist for management of newborn infants who have been exposed to VZV, received prophylactic VariZIG, and nevertheless developed varicella because no studies of this situation have been performed, possibly because of the unusual occurrence of the problem. Some experts recommend treatment with acyclovir of all infants who develop varicella despite passive immunization.[402,403,409,410] Acyclovir could be administered either orally (20 mg/kg four times daily for 5-7 days) or IV (10 mg/kg three times daily), depending on the condition of the infant. Another option is close observation of the infant, with administration of acyclovir if varicella appears to be progressing beyond a mild illness. Signs of progression would include persistent high fever, rapid evolution of large numbers of vesicles (>50 skin vesicles), hemorrhagic manifestations, and/or respiratory involvement that are indications for IV acyclovir.

Pregnant women who are closely exposed to persons with varicella or zoster and who have no evidence of immunity should be passively immunized with VariZIG. The rationale for passive immunization of the mother is primarily to protect her from developing severe varicella; it is uncertain whether this step modifies infection in the fetus, although some evidence suggests that it may be beneficial for the fetus too, likely by preventing maternal viremia.[69,70]

Because some low-birth-weight infants may have low or absent levels of transplacentally acquired maternal VZV antibody, it is recommended that premature infants of less than 28 weeks of gestation or who weigh less than 1000 g at birth be passively immunized after close exposure to VZV, regardless of their mothers' immune status. Premature infants born at greater than or equal to 28 weeks of gestation are recommended to receive VariZIG if they are exposed and their mothers do not have evidence of immunity to varicella. These premature infants are considered at high risk for severe varicella and are recommended to receive VariZIG during the entire period for which they require hospital care for their prematurity.[260,398]

The data on the beneficial effect of passive immunization presented earlier in the section pertain to administration of passive immunization within 4 days (96 hours) of exposure. Limited experience from outside the United States suggests that, compared with administration of the immune globulins (IGs) within 4 days of exposure, administration more than 4 days (up to 10 days) after exposure results in comparable reductions in incidence of varicella and attenuation of disease.[411-414] However, one study indicated an increase in varicella incidence with increasing time between exposure and administration of ZIG, but disease was attenuated in all cases.[415] Since 2013, it has been recommended in the United States that VariZIG be administered as soon as possible after exposure to VZV and within 10 days.[104,260]

Administration of passive immunization to term infants who are 2 to 7 days of age at the time of exposure is not recommended, but it may be done optionally to decrease morbidity from varicella in this age group.[416] Passive immunization is not useful for prevention of zoster in patients at high risk for zoster or for treatment of patients with varicella or zoster,[417] and should not be used to try to prevent development of varicella pneumonia in the pregnant woman with varicella or dissemination in an already infected infant. Passive immunization should not be used to try to control nosocomial varicella because it does not prevent varicella but, rather, modifies it.

Guidelines for Preventive Measures and Isolation Procedures

Institution of preventive measures to minimize the possibility of transmission of infection to other neonates, mothers, and hospital personnel is needed. Health care institutions should ensure that all health care personnel have evidence of immunity to varicella (see Table 23-1). This information should be documented and readily available at the work location. Health care personnel without evidence of immunity to varicella should receive two doses of varicella vaccine administered 4 to 8 weeks apart. Recently vaccinated health care personnel do not require any restriction in their work activities; however, health care personnel who develop a vaccine-related rash should avoid contact with persons without evidence of immunity to varicella and who are at risk for severe disease and complications until all lesions resolve.[418]

Any hospital patient isolated because of varicella or zoster should be in a separate room with the door closed, preferably in a room with air pressure negative compared with that in the corridor. Visitors and staff should be limited to persons immune to varicella. They should wear a new gown for each entry and wash their hands when leaving. Bedding and tissues soiled with respiratory excreta of the patient should be bagged and autoclaved. Special precautions for feces, urine, and needles or blood products are not required. Terminal disinfection of the room is likewise unnecessary.

Guidelines for preventive measures and isolation procedures are summarized below. In the vaccine era, more emphasis will be on preventive measures, and isolation procedures rarely need to be considered because the incidence of varicella is low. Before discharge from the hospital, mothers without evidence of immunity should receive their first dose of varicella vaccine or the second if they had previously received one dose. Breastfeeding is not a contraindication for vaccination.

If there are siblings or others at home with active VZV infections at the time mother and infant are ready for discharge from the hospital, one of the following alternatives can be used:

1. The mother and neonate may be sent home after boarding the older siblings with immune relatives until the siblings are no longer infectious.
2. The mother can return home while the neonate remains in the nursery.
3. The neonate can be boarded with a surrogate mother until the siblings are no longer infectious.
4. Some experts recommend administration of VariZIG to the newborns in anticipation of imminent exposure and sending the newborn home without separation of family members.

When a pregnant woman without evidence of immunity is exposed to varicella or zoster 6 to 20 days antepartum, she may become infectious before the onset of exanthem, during hospitalization for labor and the puerperium, assuming an average stay of 72 hours. This calculation is based on a minimum incubation period (exposure until onset of rash) of 10 days and a period of communicability preceding the exanthem by 2 days. When maternal exposure occurs less than 6 days before the onset of labor, the mother is unlikely to become infectious until after she has returned home. If a pregnant woman without evidence of immunity to varicella is admitted for delivery after a known varicella or zoster exposure, she should be observed carefully. If she develops symptoms consistent with varicella, she should be isolated immediately, and control efforts should be instituted to prevent transmission, including evaluating hospital contacts (health care personnel, other mothers, and infants) for evidence of immunity to varicella and offering vaccine or VariZIG as appropriate.

The greatest risk of nosocomial varicella exists when a pregnant woman develops varicella lesions less than 5 days before delivery or in the immediate postpartum period. If the neonate is born with lesions (i.e., congenital varicella), the mother and her newborn should be isolated (they can be isolated together) and sent home as soon as they are clinically stable. Other exposed mothers and infants in the nursery may also be sent home at the earliest date possible. If the mothers do not have evidence of immunity, they should be vaccinated before discharge. Passive immunization should be given to exposed infants if they are in the groups recommended for VariZIG. Exposed hospital personnel should also be assessed for evidence of immunity to varicella.[104,418] Those without evidence of immunity should receive post-exposure prophylaxis with varicella vaccine (see "Active

Immunization Against Varicella") or VariZIG if vaccine is contraindicated. If health care personnel received their first dose of varicella vaccine postexposure, they may continue to work in the nursery for 7 days after exposure but should be furloughed from days 8 to 21 after exposure because they are potentially infectious.[418] If an employee received VariZIG, the incubation period may be extended by a week, thus extending the time during which they should be furloughed from 21 to 28 days after exposure. Health care personnel who received their second dose of vaccine within 3 to 5 days postexposure can continue to work but should be monitored daily during days 8 to 21 after exposure for fever, skin lesions, and systemic symptoms suggestive of varicella.[418]

When maternal varicella occurs within approximately 5 days of delivery or immediately postpartum and no lesions are present in the neonate, the infant should be administered VariZIG. In addition, to minimize the possibility of infection of the infant, the mother and the infant should be isolated separately until the mother's varicella vesicles have dried (normally 5-7 days after the onset of maternal rash), even if the infant has been passively immunized. If the infant develops clinical varicella, the mother may care for the infant. Transplacentally acquired varicella, beginning 7 to 15 days after disease appears in the mother, ultimately develops in about one half of these neonates despite administration of passive immunization. Infants who did not develop varicella after exposure in utero are at risk for postnatally acquired varicella unless isolated from their mothers. If no lesions develop in the neonate by the time the mother is noninfectious, both may be sent home. Guidelines for exposed hospital personnel and patients are similar to those described previously.

In congenital varicella, lesions may be absent in the mother at the time of delivery but present in the neonate. This may occur after rare subclinical infection in the mother[134] or because the onset of the exanthem in the infant occurs after the lesions in the mother have already healed. In either circumstance, the newborn should be isolated; the mother is not at risk and may be isolated with her newborn.

Active Immunization Against Varicella

A live-attenuated varicella vaccine was developed in Japan by Takahashi and colleagues.[419] This vaccine was licensed in 1995 by the U.S. Food and Drug Administration (FDA) for varicella-susceptible healthy children older than 1 year, adolescents, and adults. The vaccine is also licensed for use in many countries in Europe, Latin America, and in Asia, including Japan. In the United States, two doses of varicella vaccine are routinely recommended at ages 12 to 15 months and 4 to 6 years.[104,398] The minimum interval between doses for children age younger than 13 years is 3 months. All persons 13 years or older without evidence of immunity should also receive two doses 4 to 8 weeks apart. For exposed persons without evidence of immunity and without contraindications to vaccination, the vaccine is recommended as postexposure prophylaxis within 3 to 5 days after exposure. A second dose of vaccine should be given at the age-appropriate interval after the first dose to individuals who do not develop varicella. The varicella vaccine is contraindicated in pregnancy. Women of childbearing age should be assessed for evidence of varicella immunity and those without evidence of immunity vaccinated before they become pregnant. It is recommended that women avoid pregnancy for 1 month after varicella vaccination. Prenatal assessment of women for evidence of varicella immunity is recommended. Upon completion or termination of their pregnancies women who do not have evidence of varicella immunity should receive the first dose of vaccine before discharge from the health care facility. The second dose should be administered 4 to 8 weeks later.

The vaccine has proved to be safe and highly effective.[420-422] The reported seroconversion rate after two doses of vaccine in healthy adults is about 90%.[219,421] Serologic testing for immunity after immunization is not recommended because negative antibody titer after immunization does not always indicate vaccine failure because commercially available ELISA antibody tests often fail to identify individuals who have responded to the vaccine.[423]

The main adverse effect of vaccination is development of a very mild transient rash about 2 to 3 weeks (ranging from a few days to 6 weeks) after immunization. Originally, there was concern that the vaccine virus could spread to susceptible persons, but spread is extremely rare (9 documented instances with more than130 million doses distributed).[81] Contagion has not been reported in the absence of rash (with one exception below), and contact cases that have resulted from exposure to a vaccinated individual with a rash have uniformly been mild. There is no evidence of clinical reversion to wild-type VZV.[80,81,219,421] One instance of spread occurred when a healthy child was immunized and his pregnant mother developed mild varicella, from which the vaccine-type virus was identified by PCR assay.[424] The mother terminated the pregnancy; the products of conception were negative for VZV by PCR assay. A recent publication reported neonatal varicella with vaccine-strain VZV 22 days after maternal postpartum vaccination; the mother did not have a rash but the newborn was in the room when the mother was vaccinated, and the most plausible mode of transmission was deemed aerosolization when the vaccine-filed syringe was cleared of air bubbles rather than transmission from the mother.[350]

To date, there is no evidence of the Oka vaccine strain causing congenital varicella syndrome. Data from a pregnancy registry that followed the birth outcomes of pregnant women who had inadvertently received varicella vaccine has not detected any cases with features consistent with congenital varicella syndrome in their offspring; however, the sample size was small (860 women enrolled, but only 20% were known VZV seronegative women) and has precluded exclusion of the 1% to 2% risk of congenital varicella syndrome associated with wild VZV infection during pregnancy; to date, the registry data could exclude a maximal theoretical risk of greater than 4%. Nonetheless, these data are reassuring on the low risk for congenital varicella syndrome after inadvertent varicella vaccination.

The Oka strain, like wild-type VZV, may cause latent infection, and can reactivate from latency to cause zoster. A number of vaccinated children have developed zoster, and of interest, the Oka strain has been implicated in only about 50% to 66% of the cases, the remainder being due to wild-type virus.[81,425] Of importance, the incidence of zoster after vaccination is lower than that after natural infection.[61,81]

The risk of immunizing healthy toddlers is calculated to be lower than not immunizing them and risking their development of natural varicella that would expose a varicella-susceptible pregnant mother to the fully virulent virus.[426] Widespread use of vaccine in the United States decreased or may even eliminate the problems of congenital malformations and severe varicella in the neonatal period, as has occurred with rubella.

Measles

Measles (i.e., rubeola) is a highly communicable childhood disease whose hallmarks are fever, coryza, conjunctivitis, cough, and a generalized maculopapular rash that usually appears 1 to 2 days after a specific enanthem (i.e., Koplik spots). The word *measles* means "little spots" and is derived from the Dutch word for the disease, *maeselen,* a diminutive of *maese,* meaning "spot" or "stain."[427] Although measles was described in medieval times, it was not until the 17th century that Sydenham differentiated the disease from smallpox and scarlet fever.

ORGANISM

Classification and Morphology

Measles virus is a paramyxovirus, but some of its properties, such as the lack of neuraminidase, are distinct from properties of other members of this family. Similar to paramyxoviruses, measles virions have a diameter of 100 to 250 nm and consist of a helical ribonucleoprotein core surrounded by a lipid envelope.

In cell culture, virions replicate predominantly in the cytoplasm and are released from the cell surface by budding. The envelope of the virion is composed of at least two glycoproteins: F, which causes membrane fusion and is crucial for infectivity, and H, the hemagglutinin. A nonglycosylated matrix protein, M, also exists on the envelope. Antibodies to glycoprotein F inhibit viral infectivity.[428] Other internal structural proteins are the large protein (L), the phosphoprotein or polymerase (P), and the nucleocapsid protein (N). C and V proteins interact with cellular proteins and play roles in regulation of transcription and replication. The cellular receptors for measles virus are the complement regulatory protein CD46 expressed on human lymphocytes and many other human cell types and the signaling lymphocyte activation molecule (SLAM) CDw150 molecule.[429,430]

Measles virus has been fully sequenced. Genomic data indicate that during the resurgence of measles in 1989 to 1992, only genotype D3 measles viruses were isolated. After enhanced measles control during and after the resurgence, from 1993 onward a variety of different measles genotypes have been detected, reflecting importations from other countries and the absence of an endemic genotype since 1994.[431] The latest data support this contention and indicate that there is no endemic measles in the United States; the few circulating viruses identified are imported from other countries.[432-434]

Propagation and Identification of Measles Virus

Primary cultures of human embryonic kidney and rhesus monkey kidney cells have proved to be superior to all others for the isolation of measles virus, although the agent has been adapted after several passages to numerous continuous cell lines.[430] Cytopathic effect on primary isolation is not generally detected before 5 to 10 days. Rapid identification may be accomplished by reverse-transcriptase (RT) PCR assay and use of immunofluorescence staining with monoclonal antibodies.[430]

Antigenic Properties and Serologic Tests

Measles virus isolates are antigenically homogeneous, although there are numerous genotypes.[434] Some cross-reactivity of soluble ribonucleoprotein antigens and hemagglutinins has been observed among measles and the related viruses of rinderpest and canine distemper, but not with other paramyxoviruses. The hemagglutination inhibition test has essentially been replaced with more modern assays for antibodies.[430]

ELISA presently is the most useful and sensitive method for measuring antibodies to measles virus.[430,435,436] A similar test that identifies specific IgM antibody is useful diagnostically on an acute serum specimen, including using alternative specimens such as dried blood spots and saliva.[430,437,438]

EPIDEMIOLOGY AND TRANSMISSION

Measles is one of the most communicable of the childhood exanthems, with secondary attack rates among exposed susceptible contacts of approximately 90%.[85,106,439,440] The virus is spread chiefly by the airborne route as aerosolized droplet nuclei, especially in persons with a cough.[439,441] Rarely, transmission may occur by means of articles soiled by respiratory secretions. There is some uncertainty concerning the precise portal of entry of the virus. Although the virus may gain access through the nose or the oropharynx, the work of Papp[442] suggests that the conjunctival mucosa is at least a possible portal of entry. Others have, more recently, proposed viral entry at the tonsils.[443]

Before use of measles vaccine, measles occurred worldwide in temperate, tropical, and arctic climates. As recently as 1980, measles was estimated to cause 2.6 million deaths globally.[444] Because of its infectiousness, in populations sufficiently high to support endemic disease transmission, epidemics typically occurred at intervals of 2 to 3 years, especially in urban areas, and almost every person in the population was infected by adolescence. In interepidemic years, few cases of measles occurred, probably because the supply of susceptible persons had been exhausted. Additional births continually added to this pool, permitting epidemic transmission when the pool was sufficiently large.

In the United States, the disease had a peak incidence between March and May. Seasonal variation was attributed to the crowding of children indoors and in schools in the winter, resulting in increased transmission The highest risk of death from measles was in infants younger than 12 months and in adults. Patterns of disease varied with respect to age, incidence, and severity in different geographic regions. In urban areas of industrialized countries, measles infected predominantly school-aged children 5 to 9 years of age, followed by preschool-aged children. In rural areas of the same countries, children tended to be older when they contracted the disease and more likely to reach adulthood without becoming infected. For this reason, measles in pregnant women may be observed more often among women from rural or otherwise geographically isolated localities (see later discussion). A different pattern of disease was seen in less developed areas, such as equatorial Africa, where measles occurred predominantly in children younger than 2 years and had a high fatality rate.[445] Protein deficiency and vitamin A deficiency are associated with an increased incidence of complications, such as bronchopneumonia and death. Still another pattern of infection has been observed in extremely isolated regions of the world, where whole populations may never have experienced measles before its exogenous introduction. In a classic description of such an epidemic in the Faroe Islands in 1846, measles was observed to spread rapidly through an entire population, regardless of age, with an attack rate of virtually 100%.[446] Mortality rates tend to be higher in populations having little experience with measles. An extreme example is the Fiji Islands epidemic of 1875, in which 20,000 people, or about one fourth of the population, are said to have died.[446] Despite advances in treatment and improved access to medical care, measles continues to cause substantial mortality and morbidity globally.[447] A recent review of measles case-fatality rates from community-based studies (median CFR ratio, 3.9%) in developing countries highlighted current severe consequences of measles and the potential for prevention.[448,449]

The use of live-attenuated measles vaccine in the United States since 1963 has decreased the incidence of measles to extremely low levels and has interrupted year-round endemic disease transmission.[450] Before 1963, of the 3 to 4 million measles cases estimated to occur annually, there were about 400,000 cases of measles reported each year. A record low of 1497 cases was reported in 1983, but in the late 1980s and early 1990s, there was an increase in the incidence of measles that eventually came under control.[451] From 1989 to 1991, there were more than 55,000 reported cases with more than 120 measles-associated deaths reported to the CDC, but after 1991, the number of reported cases decreased significantly.[452] Measles occurring despite vaccination may be the result of primary vaccine failure, a "no take" for the vaccine, or secondary vaccine failure because of loss of immunity to measles after vaccination.[453,454] There is little evidence, however, that secondary immune failure (i.e., that protective immunity induced by measles wanes with time) is significant.[453,454] A study of persistence of measles antibody 10 years after receipt of the second dose of measles-mumps-rubella (MMR) vaccine showed that less than 5% of students had low antibody levels and none were seronegative.[455]

In the United States, improved implementation of measles vaccine recommendations, including the two-dose recommendation for children instituted in 1989, has resulted in a decline of the number of annual cases of measles to an all-time low. Interruption of year-round endemic measles transmission (or measles elimination) was declared in the United States in 2000.[449,452] Measles has become a rare disease in the United States, with cases and small outbreaks linked to measles importations. From 2001 to 2008, a median of 56 cases was reported annually.[433] During 2008 and 2011, 140 and 220 cases, respectively, were reported, with the majority of cases associated with measles importations from Europe, Asia, and the Middle East. The vast majority of cases were eligible for immunization but unvaccinated.[433,456,457] Maintaining high vaccine coverage throughout the United States is critical to prevent sustained transmission of measles.[457-459]

Incidence of Measles in Pregnant Women

Because measles is well controlled in the United States by high vaccine coverage[458] it now occurs very rarely during pregnancy. However, a measles outbreak in 2013 among a community in New York City who oppose vaccination highlighted that unvaccinated pregnant women and their infants remain at risk for acquiring measles.[459] In association with large measles outbreaks in Europe from 2010 to 2013 and ongoing measles transmission in Japan, measles cases affecting pregnant women and/or their newborn infants have been also described from France, Switzerland, and Japan.[460-463] It is likely with the changing epidemiology of measles secondary to vaccine program implementation that there may be some immunity gaps in young adults and women of childbearing age. Therefore, in countries where measles remains endemic or where outbreaks are occurring, some pregnant women and their newborns are likely to be affected by measles.

PATHOGENESIS

By analogy with other viral infections whose pathogenesis has been better delineated, the initial multiplication of measles virus is believed to occur in epithelial and lymphoid cells near the portal of entry. A transient viremia delivers virus to the reticuloendothelial system, where further replication occurs. A second viremia, more severe and more sustained, disseminates virus to the skin, gut, respiratory tract, and other affected organs. In monkeys, this viremia may occur for more than 1 week before the appearance of the prodrome or exanthem. Measles virus replicates in and probably destroys lymphocytes in the peripheral blood,[464] giving rise to a circulating lymphopenia. The symptoms of measles are probably attributable to inflammation accompanying necrosis of cells in which the virus is replicating. By the time the exanthem appears, 12 to 14 days after infection, measles virus is actively replicating in the skin, gut, and respiratory mucosa.

Electron microscopy of biopsy specimens of Koplik spots and cutaneous lesions reveals syncytial giant cells whose nuclear and cytoplasmic inclusions contain aggregates of microtubules that are 15 to 20 nm in diameter and characteristic of paramyxovirus infection.[465] This finding and the observation that convalescent measles serum injected into the skin can prevent the local development of the exanthema[466] suggest that replication of virus per se is directly responsible for the lesions. Nevertheless, it is possible that an interaction between viral antigen and antibody is required. The latter hypothesis is supported by the observation that immunosuppressed children who develop giant cell pneumonia caused by measles virus do not develop a rash and do not elaborate antibodies.[467,468] Virus titers in the viscera have already diminished considerably by the time the exanthem appears, and serum antibodies are readily detectable within 24 hours. There is also experimental evidence that T lymphocytes are important in the development of some symptoms of measles, such as the rash, and in recovery from the disease.[469]

Incubation Period for Measles Acquired by Droplet Infection

The usual interval between exposure to measles and onset of first symptoms (i.e., prodrome) is about 10 days; 12 to 14 days usually elapse before the onset of rash. Considerable variation may be observed, however.[426] Intervals between exposure and onset of rash range from 7 to 21 days unless passive immunization has been given, in which case the incubation period may be prolonged by greater than or equal to 1 week to 28 days.[398] The incubation period in modified measles (see "Clinical Manifestations") may last an additional 7 days (to 28 days because of the presence of low levels of measles antibodies).[398,452,470]

Incubation Period for Hematogenously Acquired Measles

It has been claimed that infantile measles may be acquired by transfusion of maternal blood presumably containing measles virus.[471] Two infants developed typical enanthems and exanthems 13 and 14 days after transfusion, and their mothers developed measles exanthems 4 and 2 days after blood donation. The infants had not been visited by their mothers for 4 days and 1 day before transfusion. Hematogenous transmission may not have occurred, however, because the mothers may have been shedding virus from the respiratory tract at the time they last handled their infants.

Intrauterine hematogenous transmission is well documented (discussed later). In these cases, the onset of disease in the infant may occur almost simultaneously with that in the mother or after a variable interval that is less than the minimum time required for extrauterine infection by the respiratory route.

Period of Communicability

Measles is more communicable during the prodrome and catarrhal stage of infection than during the period of the exanthem. Dramatic corroboration of this observation was provided during an epidemic in Greenland in 1962.[472] Deliberate exposure of 400 susceptible persons to disease was achieved by having a patient on the first day of appearance of the exanthem cough twice in the face of each. Not a single transmission resulted. When the experiment was repeated with a patient during the preexanthematous period, measles was readily transmitted.

Patients with measles should be considered infectious from the onset of the prodrome (about 4 days before the appearance of the exanthem) until 4 days after the onset of the exanthema,[398] although the risk of contagion abruptly diminishes several days after the rash appears, concomitant with the appearance of circulating neutralizing antibodies. Measles virus isolation and RNA detection are more likely to be successful when the specimens are collected early (ideally within 3 days of rash onset, but up to 10 days post-rash may be successful.[473]

PATHOLOGY

The replication of measles virus in epithelial cells of the mucous membranes and skin leads to the formation of intranuclear inclusions and syncytial giant cells, which can contain 100 nuclei per cell (i.e., Warthin-Finkeldey cells).[474] Focal hyaline necrosis of epithelial cells is accompanied by a subepithelial exudate containing predominantly mononuclear leukocytes. The pathology of cutaneous lesions and Koplik spots is essentially similar.[475] It is likely that virus replicates simultaneously in the skin and mucous membranes, but Koplik spots are detected earlier than the exanthem, probably because the epithelium that forms the roof of the lesions is thinner and more translucent in the mucous membranes.

Similar lesions containing the characteristic multinucleated giant cells may be widespread throughout the respiratory and gastrointestinal tracts. The pharynx, tonsils, bronchial epithelium, appendix, colon, and lymph nodes have been involved. Viral bronchitis occurs in most cases of measles. Necrotic columnar epithelial cells and giant cells are sloughed into the lumen of the bronchi and bronchioles. When this damage is extensive, the regenerating epithelium frequently undergoes squamous metaplasia and is accompanied by bronchial and peribronchial inflammation. Extension of the process into the alveolar septa results in interstitial pneumonitis. Secondary bacterial infection commonly supervenes, leading to a bronchopneumonia with purulent exudate.

Using immunofluorescence and immunoperoxidase methodology, measles virus has been shown in the placental syncytial trophoblastic cells and decidua in a 25-week fetus of a woman who developed gestational measles. The fetus was spared. It is postulated that placental damage induced by the virus, leading to hypoxia, is responsible for fetal death during maternal measles.[475]

The pathologic signs of measles encephalitis are not readily distinguishable from signs of other postinfectious encephalitides, such as those caused by vaccinia, varicella, and rubella. The characteristic lesion is perivenous demyelination, often accompanied by mild perivascular infiltrates of mononuclear leukocytes, petechial hemorrhages, and microglial proliferation. Neuronal damage and meningeal inflammation are not prominent. Nuclear or cytoplasmic inclusions and giant cells are inconstant. Measles virus has been isolated infrequently from the brain or spinal cord, and it is unclear whether the pathologic changes in the brain are a direct result of measles virus or an allergic response to a virus-induced product or antigen-antibody complexes.[476,477]

Because of the spectrum of pathology, including acute demyelinating encephalitis and acute hemorrhagic leukoencephalitis, it has been postulated that measles encephalitis is an autoimmune process. Myelin basic protein has been shown in the CSF of patients with measles encephalitis, and the pathologic process has been likened to experimental allergic encephalitis as produced in animal models.[478] One theory regarding pathogenesis is that measles virus has an epitope similar to the epitope of the encephalitogenic sequence in CNS myelin (i.e., an instance of molecular mimicry leading to disease).[479] A second form of encephalitis is caused by continued replication of measles virus in the brains of immunocompromised patients.[480]

CLINICAL MANIFESTATIONS

Prodrome and Rash

The prodrome typically begins 10 to 11 days after exposure, with fever and malaise, followed within 24 hours by coryza, sneezing, conjunctivitis, and cough. During the next 2 to

3 days, this catarrhal phase is accentuated, with markedly infected conjunctivae and photophobia. Toward the end of the prodrome, Koplik spots appear. They are tiny (no larger than a pinhead), granular, slightly raised white lesions surrounded by a halo of erythema. Beginning with less than a dozen specks on the lateral buccal mucosa, Koplik spots may multiply during a 24-hour period to affect virtually all the mucous membranes of the cheeks and may extend to the lips and eyelids. Hundreds of spots may be present. At this stage, the lesions may be said to resemble grains of salt on a wet background. Koplik spots appear 1 to 2 days before the exanthem.

The rash, which appears 12 to 14 days after exposure, begins on the head and neck, especially behind the ears and on the forehead. At first, the lesions are red macules 1 to 2 mm in diameter, but over 2 or 3 days, they enlarge and coalesce. By the second day, the exanthem has spread to the trunk and upper extremities. The lower extremities are involved by the third day. The lesions are most prominent in regions where the exanthem appears first—the face and upper trunk. By the third or fourth day, the exanthem begins to fade in the order of its appearance. A brown staining of the lesions often persists for 7 to 10 days and is followed by fine desquamation.

The clinical course of measles may be greatly altered by administration of immunoglobulin during the incubation period. In modified measles, the catarrhal phase may be completely suppressed, and the exanthem may be limited to a few macules on the trunk.

Complications and Mortality

The most frequent complications of measles involve the respiratory tract. Otitis media and mild croup are common in young children during the catarrhal phase, but bacterial or viral pneumonia is the complication that results in death most frequently. If carefully sought, fine rales and radiologic evidence of bronchopneumonia can be found during the early exanthematous phase in most patients. Cough may persist beyond the peak of the exanthem in uncomplicated measles, but when the fever fails to decline or recurs as the rash is fading, a bacterial superinfection is usually present. The chest radiograph may show consolidation. A peripheral blood polymorphonuclear leukocytosis is present. When bacterial superinfection occurs, antimicrobial therapy is indicated and should be directed against the most likely etiologic agents: *Streptococcus pneumoniae, S. aureus,* and *Streptococcus pyogenes*. Smears and cultures of sputum should be obtained, but in young infants, it may be necessary to treat bacterial superinfection without a specific etiologic diagnosis because of the difficulty in obtaining adequate sputum and the potential gravity of the illness (see "Therapy" under "Varicella and Zoster").

After otitis and pneumonia, encephalitis is the most frequent serious complication of measles. It is far less common than pneumonia. Encephalitis, including coma and gross cerebral dysfunction, is estimated to occur with a frequency of 1 per 1000 cases[476] but is probably more common if drowsiness, irritability, and transient electroencephalographic changes are accepted as evidence of encephalitis. This complication occurs in all age groups, including the neonatal period. A fatal outcome has been recorded in an infant, born in the hospital, who developed measles with encephalitis when 27 days old.[477] Measles encephalitis may occur at any stage of the illness but appears most commonly 3 to 7 days after the onset of the exanthem. The initial symptoms are drowsiness and irritability, followed by lethargy, convulsions, and coma. The CSF changes are those of a mild aseptic meningitis. Mental obtundation may clear over 1 to 4 days or may assume a more protracted course that is associated with a higher incidence of such sequelae as severe behavioral abnormalities and mental retardation. Death occurs in about 11% of measles patients who have measles encephalitis.[476]

Other complications of measles that have been described include thrombocytopenic purpura, appendicitis, myocarditis, subacute sclerosing panencephalitis, and reactivation or exacerbation of previously acquired tuberculosis. In a study of 3220 U.S. Air Force recruits with measles, whose mean age was 19 years, from 1976 to 1979, bacterial superinfection and elevated serum aminotransferase levels were observed in 30%, otitis was seen in 29%, sinusitis was seen in 25%, bronchospasm was seen in 17%, and pneumonia was seen in 3%.[481]

The precise CFR in measles is highly variable among different populations and at different periods in the history of the same population. In the United States, measles mortality declined from 25 per 1000 reported cases in 1912 to 1 per 1000 reported cases in 1962, with population level declines (per 100,000 people) reported in the United States, as a whole, and states such as Massachusetts, in particular.[446] Because the decline preceded the widespread use of antibiotics, much of the change is attributed to improved social conditions: less crowding, improved nutrition, and better medical care. In the United States since 1963, the CFR has averaged about 0.1% based on reported cases, but when measles was more common, it may have been closer to 0.01% if estimated unreported cases of measles are included in the calculation.[482] During 2001 to 2008 in the United States, when reporting is considered to be fairly complete, 2 deaths occurred among 557 reported measles cases.[433] The risk is considerably greater, however, in children younger than 1 year and adults.[483] Data obtained during an epidemic in Greenland in 1951 confirmed that death rates were higher for infants and adults. The age-specific death rate (per 1000 cases) was 26 for infants younger than 1 year and 15 for infants 1 to 2 years of age; no deaths were recorded in children 2 to 14 years of age, and then case fatality increased among adults to 24 per 1000 cases from 35 to 54 years of age and was 129 per 1000 cases for persons older than 55 years.[484] In cases for which adequate information was available, all deaths of children younger than 1 year apparently were caused by pneumonia, which occurred during the prodrome or shortly after the onset of the exanthem. Although mortality rates have declined globally since the 1950s, a recent review of measles case-fatality rates from community-based studies in developing countries highlighted that mortality rates are still high in these settings (median CFR, 3.9%; range, 0%-40.2%) and measles still causes deaths in highly developed country settings.[433,485] Children with underlying infection with HIV have been reported to be at risk for developing severe measles, and fatalities have been reported, especially in children who have developed AIDS.[486] In Africa, it has also been observed that infants born to HIV-infected women have lower titers of measles antibodies in cord sera than infants from women not infected with HIV. The outcome has been that these infants are at greater risk for developing measles early in infancy.[487] One adolescent with HIV infection who had previously received measles vaccine developed fatal measles pneumonia after the second vaccine dose.[488] Because the infection was proved to be from the vaccine virus, measles vaccine is no longer recommended for HIV-infected children who have developed AIDS or evidence of severe immunosuppression.[452] Immunocompromised children with underlying malignant diseases who have not been immunized are also at risk for developing severe and fatal measles.[489-491]

Maternal Effects of Measles

Because of the relative rarity of measles among adults, most studies on measles in pregnant women and their offspring involve relatively small numbers, many are case series without comparison groups, and some report on hospitalized cases only, which likely represent the most serious cases. Nevertheless, several studies involving a comparison group provide good evidence that a pregnant woman with measles is at greater risk of serious complications and death than other adults with this disease.[492] Some of the published experiences leading to this conclusion are summarized in the following paragraphs.

In the early part of the 20th century, fatality rates for pregnant women with measles were reported to be approximately 15%, mostly caused by pneumonia in the puerperium.[493,494] In the 1951 Greenland epidemic, 4 deaths (4.9%) occurred among 83 women who had measles during pregnancy or the puerperium. In contrast, 19 deaths (1.7%) occurred among 1099 nonpregnant women between the ages of 15 and 54 years ($\chi^2 = 3.9$, $P = .05$).[484] There was no significant difference in the frequency of pneumonia as a complication of measles among pregnant and nonpregnant women in the same age group, but heart failure was observed far more often in pregnant women with measles. Heart failure was observed in 7 patients with gestational measles. Of these, 3 were in the second half of pregnancy, and 4 were in the puerperium. Although in some patients heart failure occurred during the prodrome, it occurred within 2 weeks after onset of the exanthem in most women.

Additional experience from case series in the United States and Australia since the late 1930s supports the concept that measles during pregnancy is only rarely catastrophic. Among 24 women with gestational measles in an outbreak in rural Oklahoma from 1938 to 1939, no deaths occurred, and serious morbidity was likewise not increased.[495] In another epidemic, reported in 1950 from Australia, 18 hospitalized cases of gestational measles were observed. Complications were reported in only one case—a woman in the third trimester with measles pneumonia.[496]

From 1988 to 1992 in the United States, when there was a resurgence of measles, numerous pregnant women developed this infection. Thirteen such women who were hospitalized in Houston, Texas, were reported because 7 (54%) had respiratory complications that were the basis for their hospitalization. They required supplemental oxygen and monitoring in the intensive care unit, and 1 woman died.[497] These women seemed to have primary measles pneumonia, rather than bacterial superinfection. Nine of these 13 women were treated with aerosolized ribavirin administered by facemask. Hepatitis, shown by elevations of aminotransferases, also occurred frequently in these women, but this is a common finding in nonpregnant adults that seems to be of little clinical importance. During this same period, a comparative study was performed based on review of medical records from 58 pregnant women from Los Angeles with measles and measles cases reported to the notifiable disease surveillance system. Of these women, 35 (60%) were hospitalized for measles, 15 (26%) developed pneumonia, and 2 (3%) died.[498] Compared with 748 cases of measles among women of childbearing age who were not pregnant, pregnant cases were twice as likely to be admitted to hospital, three times more likely to be diagnosed with pneumonia, and six times as likely to die from measles complications.[498] A series of 8 hospitalized cases of measles in pregnant women in Japan in 2000 reported complications in the mothers that included 2 cases of pneumonia and 1 case of hemorrhagic shock.

Effects of Gestational Measles on the Fetus

Chromosomal Aberrations. The possibility that measles occurring in pregnancy may damage the fetus is suggested by the observation that there is a high frequency of chromosomal breaks in leukocyte metaphase preparations between the second and fifth day of the exanthema.[499] Other reports have not fully confirmed the preceding observations, however. Miller[500] found no chromosomal breaks in leukocytes of patients with measles who were examined 1 to 12 days after onset of the rash, but he attributed this discrepancy to methodologic differences involving more gentle treatment of the leukocytes. A report from Japan[501] also failed to show an increased frequency of chromosomal breaks per cell in patients with measles, compared with those in normal subjects. A significant increase in chromosomal breaks was observed, however, in patients with Down syndrome who had measles, and it was inferred that their chromosomes were more sensitive to measles infection.[501]

These chromosomal abnormalities are transient and disappear during convalescence. No studies have examined whether intrauterine exposure of the fetus to measles results in longer-lasting chromosomal aberrations.

Abortion and Prematurity. Studies examining outcomes of pregnancy complicated by measles infection are limited by study design (case reports or series), small numbers, and lack of control groups. The consensus of several reports dealing with the frequency of premature births is that this untoward event occurs more often in association with measles during pregnancy than in the pregnant population at large. In contrast to rubella, in which there is retarded intrauterine development, prematurity caused by measles is associated with normal intrauterine development but premature expulsion of the fetus. There are no studies that demonstrate unequivocally that gestational measles also causes a higher rate of spontaneous abortion, but only small studies have been conducted. It seems possible that measles is responsible for some instances of spontaneous abortion.

Among the retrospective studies is that of Dyer,[495] who reported 24 cases of gestational measles from rural Oklahoma in 1938 to 1939. Uterine contractions, which typically occurred during the illness, were identified in 11 of the 24 women and caused premature delivery of the fetus in 9 (38%). Among 6 women infected before 20 weeks of gestation, premature labor occurred in 3, one of whom had a spontaneous abortion 7 days after onset of measles rash at 18 weeks of gestation. Among 12 pregnancies infected from 20 to 36 weeks of gestation, 2 women developed premature labor and delivery at 33 weeks of gestation. Four women developed measles before delivery at 38 to 40 weeks of gestation, and two of their babies had measles at birth and recovered fully. Two mothers developed measles rash on the third and seventh day after delivery, respectively. Their babies developed measles rash on the second and fourteenth day after delivery, respectively, and although both recovered from their acute infection, the baby with early rash onset died of pneumonia at 1 month of age. (Also see "Congenital Measles".)

Adverse outcomes of gestational measles on the fetus were described in a hospital case series of 18 pregnant women with measles reported in the epidemic in South Australia in 1950.[496] There were three abortions or stillbirths, which occurred in 1 of 7 women who had measles in the first trimester, 1 of 8 women who had measles in the second trimester, and 1 of 3 women who had measles in the third trimester. Abortions followed the onset of the exanthem by 2 to 3 weeks in the patients who became ill in the first and second trimesters. The patient with measles in the third trimester had severe measles pneumonia and expelled a macerated fetus 7 weeks later. One live premature birth was recorded in the third trimester.

In the 1951 Greenland epidemic, birth or abortion occurred in 26 of the 76 pregnant women while they had measles.[484] Thirteen were term pregnancies. Of the remainder, spontaneous abortion at 3 to 5 months of gestation occurred in 7 women (9%). There were six instances of premature delivery (8%), and perinatal death ensued in three. A retrospective analysis of 51 women in Greenland who developed measles during the first 3 months of pregnancy from 1951 to 1962 also suggested a high fetal death rate. One half with measles in the first 2 months and one fifth with measles in the third month experienced spontaneous abortions.[502] The abortion rate in the third month may not be different from uninfected pregnancies. During an outbreak in 1981 to 1982 in Israel, a case series of five hospitalized maternal measles cases and their outcomes were reported.[503] All babies were born prematurely (range, 28-34 weeks) with a mean duration between maternal onset of illness and delivery of 3.5 days and a mean birth weight of 1496 g. None had any signs of measles at birth or in the neonatal period.

Controlled, prospective studies done in New York City during 1957 to 1964 showed a significant association between maternal measles and prematurity but not between maternal measles and abortion. Low birth weight (<2500 g) was identified in 10 (16.7%) of 60 infants born to measles-infected mothers compared with 2 (3.3%) of 62 matched control infants ($\chi^2 = 6.2$; $P < .025$) (see Table 23-3).[245] When fetal mortality was examined in relation to gestational age (see Table 23-4), it was found that three deaths (15.8%) occurred in 19 cases of measles in the first trimester, one (3.4%) occurred in 29 cases in the second trimester, and one (5.9%) occurred in 17 cases in the third trimester.[245] These figures were not significantly different from those for fetal deaths in control pregnancies not involving measles. Of the five fetal deaths that occurred in pregnant women with measles, two of the deaths occurred within 2 weeks of maternal disease.

The resurgence of measles from 1989 to 1991 in the United States resulted in measles in numerous pregnant women. In the experience of Atmar and associates,[497] who summarized a hospitalized case series of complications of measles during pregnancy, there was an adverse fetal outcome in 4 (31%) of 13 affected pregnancies. Two women gave birth in the 34th and 35th weeks, and 1 spontaneously aborted at 16 weeks during measles. One additional woman and her fetus died at 20 weeks. In a report from Los Angeles of 58 women, 18 (31%) of the pregnancies ended before 37 weeks of gestation (5 were abortions, and 13 were preterm deliveries that resulted in two fetal deaths and three neonatal deaths); 16 had labor onset within 14 days of onset of measles rash.[498] There were no comparisons provided with outcomes in pregnant women without measles.

Congenital Defects. The teratogenic potential of gestational measles for the fetus has been challenging to study because of the rarity of the infection during pregnancy, particularly during the first trimester, when the process of organogenesis is most active. In contrast to gestational varicella, no particular constellation of abnormalities has been found among the sporadic instances of congenital defects that have occurred because of measles in the mother during pregnancy. Isolated instances of birth defects, including buphthalmos,[504] congenital heart disease,[502,505] cleft lip,[269] pyloric stenosis,[505] genu valgum,[504] cerebral leukodystrophy,[502] and cyclopia[502] have been reported in infants born to mothers with measles diagnosed during the organogenic period. In a retrospective analysis of 10 measles epidemics in Greenland, the outcomes of 327 women who acquired measles during pregnancy, including 252 of their children who were examined, were described.[502] Among 58 infants with mothers infected in the first trimester, 5 had congenital malformations, three of which were extremely rare and severe (atypical leukodystrophy, cyclopia, and multiple cardiac anomalies) and resulted in death before 10 months of age. Unfortunately, there was no comparison group, although this rate of major malformation is higher than described for the general population.

No congenital malformations were observed in four infants born to mothers who had measles during the first 4 months of pregnancy in the Oklahoma outbreak.[495] Similarly, in the 1951 Greenland epidemic, there were no congenital malformations among the infants of 76 mothers with gestational measles, although the number of cases that occurred in the first trimester is unclear.[484] After the epidemic in South Australia,[496] two infants with congenital defects (one with Down syndrome and one with partial deafness) were recorded among infants whose mothers had measles during the first trimester. No birth defects occurred in infants born to 8 mothers with measles in the second trimester and 3 mothers who had been ill in the third trimester. Although one of the five infants born during the outbreak in 1981 to 1982 in Israel was severely malformed, this was not caused by maternal measles, which had begun only a few days before birth. Five additional reported Israeli infants had no congenital anomalies, but all their mothers had measles just before delivery.[503] In the Houston report of 13 pregnant women, the fetal gestational age at onset of maternal measles ranged from 16 to 35 weeks (mean, 27 weeks). Follow-up of eight of these infants, delivered at a mean of 12 weeks later (range, 1-24 weeks), revealed that no infants had congenital malformations.[497]

Because they were uncontrolled, these analyses are incapable of establishing whether the incidence of congenital defects is increased as a result of gestational measles. One controlled prospective study is inconclusive because only small numbers of pregnant women with measles could be studied. Among 60 children who were born to mothers who had gestational measles and were followed to the age of 5 years, only one congenital malformation was identified, compared with a virtually identical incidence of one defect among 62 control children.[235] The defect in the infected group was bilateral deafness in an infant weighing 1990 g born to a mother who had measles at 6 weeks of gestation.

In summary, scientific evidence is lacking to demonstrate that the risk of congenital anomalies is increased after measles during pregnancy. In some cases, documentation that the maternal illness was measles and not rubella or other exanthems is lacking. Available data are limited by small sample size and lack of control groups. Nevertheless, the fact that no constellation of defects has been described in babies, even after epidemics involving adults, is reassuring. If there is any increased risk of malformations from gestational measles, this risk seems to be small, if it exists at all.

Perinatal Measles

As in varicella, perinatal measles includes transplacental infection and disease acquired postnatally by the respiratory route. Because the shortest incubation period from infection to the first appearance of the exanthem is 7 days, measles exanthems acquired before 7 days of life may be considered transplacental in origin. The most usual incubation period for measles is 10 to 14 days,[506] so most, though not all, disease appearing in infants at 14 days or later is probably acquired outside the uterus.

Postnatally Acquired Measles. Several reports describe cases of measles in which the onset of the exanthem occurred in infants 14 to 30 days of age. The course of the disease in these cases varied from generally mild to severely ill.[495,507-509] In one infant with notably mild illness and little fever, the illness began at 14 days of age. This neonate had been nursed by the mother, in whom the prodrome of measles developed on the first postpartum day. Because circulating and presumably also secretory antibodies appear within 48 hours of the onset of the exanthem, it is possible that the neonate's illness was modified by measles-specific IgA antibodies present in the mother's milk.[495,507,508] In a report of four cases of postnatally acquired measles, two of the three babies with onsets of symptoms at 14, 14, and 30 days, respectively, became seriously ill with pneumonia. Neither of them received convalescent serum. The baby who received IG had a mild course of illness.[509] A report from Japan in 1997 described seven cases of measles in infants during the first month of life. No case was described as severe, although there were three infants with pneumonia, two of whom had received IG at exposure.[510]

There are reports of infants with prolonged presence of the measles genome in their mononuclear cells after vertical transmission of measles.[511,512] Rapidly progressive subacute sclerosing panencephalitis has also been reported after vertically acquired measles infection.[513-518]

Outbreaks of nosocomial measles in the newborn nursery apparently have not been recorded in the 20th century. This is probably because of the low incidence of measles in the United States and other developed countries, nearly universal immunity in mothers in urban areas, and corresponding protection of the newborn by passive antibodies. However, along with changing measles epidemiology and the continued risk of exposure for unvaccinated persons, even in countries with low incidence, recent reports of cases of congenital measles after measles infection in unvaccinated mothers around the time of delivery have underscored the importance of high levels of awareness and appropriate investigation and response to measles cases in nurseries and obstetric wards.[459-463,519] One of these occurrences resulted in nosocomial measles transmission to a member of the medical staff.[463]

Congenital Measles. The historical literature described congenital measles as cases in which the exanthem was present at birth and infections acquired in utero in which the rash appeared during the first 10 days of life. In congenital measles, the incubation period was defined as the interval between onset of exanthem in the mother and in the infant, ranging from 2[495] to 10 days[520] (mean, 6 days). At that time, the incubation period for measles was considered to be 11 to 14 days.[509] However, household studies of measles transmission later defined the measles incubation period, measured from rash onset to rash onset, to be as short as 7 days. Thus some early reports of congenital measles may have been postnatally acquired. Consistent with current guidance, it seems reasonable to now consider that the upper range of the interval between onset of rash in the mother and baby that should be considered unequivocally as transplacentally acquired congenital measles to be less than 7 days. A nearly simultaneous onset in the mother and neonate implies that measles virus in the maternal bloodstream may sometimes cross the placenta in sufficient quantity to cause disease in the fetus without the need for many additional cycles of replication. The placenta may act as a barrier of limited effectiveness, however, as suggested by instances in which disease does not appear in the fetus until 6 days after its appearance in the mother. Early studies also demonstrated that maternal measles immediately preceding parturition by no means invariably involved the fetus. In a historical report of 44 pregnancies in which a maternal rash was present at delivery, exanthematous measles was reported in only 13 neonates (30%).[494] However, with development of improved rapid diagnostic tests such as PCR assay, measles infection without clinical manifestations are being reported.[462,519]

Later reports include 19 instances in which maternal rashes of measles, with onsets ranging from 7 days antepartum to 3 days postpartum, were associated with clinically apparent measles in the infant in only 5 cases (26%).[¶a] Eight of these infants received IG (0.25 mL/kg) at birth, however,

[¶a] References 459, 460, 462, 463, 495, 507, 509, 519, 521.

including the three who developed measles.[503,521] During the Greenland epidemic of 1951, no examples of congenital measles were observed among infants born to 13 women who had measles at parturition.[484] It seems that most of these neonates do not experience subclinical measles without exanthem but simply are not infected. This conclusion is supported by the observation that infants whose mothers had measles late in the third trimester are fully susceptible to infection later in childhood.[494] During the Faroe Islands epidemic of 1846, many pregnant women had measles, and 36 years later, their infants were infected as adults in a new epidemic in 1882.[509] However, some recent examples of measles infections in newborns of mothers with measles around the time of delivery indicate that infections do occur.

As in congenital varicella, the spectrum of illness in congenital measles varies from a mild illness, in which the rash is transient and Koplik spots may be absent, to rapidly fatal disease. The precise CFR is uncertain because the course of measles in different populations has been so variable, even in older children and adults. Reports from early in the 20th century showed that among 22 cases of congenital measles culled from the literature in which IG prophylaxis was not given, there were seven deaths.[494,495,509,520] Approximately the same CFR (30%-33%) was observed whether the rash was present at birth or appeared subsequently. However, because nearly all reports of deaths preceded the antibiotic era, effective clinical management of prematurity and use of measles IG, the current CFR is undoubtedly now significantly lower than it was previously because of improved supportive care and appropriate antimicrobial therapy of bacterial superinfections.[484,494] Recent confirmed cases of congenital measles (illness or infection) from Switzerland, France, Japan, and the United States, in which some of the infants were given intravenous immunoglobulin (IVIG) before rash onset, reported mild illness.[459-463,519]

Insufficient data are available to evaluate whether transplacentally acquired antibodies to measles virus may diminish the CFR in congenital measles when the mother's exanthem appears more than 48 hours antepartum. More precise information on the time of appearance of the maternal rash is needed to answer this question definitively. Although firm data are unavailable, administration of IG at birth may decrease mortality.[497,503,521]

Most reports of death related to congenital measles do not specify the immediate cause, but pneumonia is among the leading complications.[†#ab]

DIAGNOSIS AND DIFFERENTIAL DIAGNOSIS

The diagnosis of measles is easy when there is a history of recent exposure, and the typical catarrhal phase is followed by Koplik spots and a maculopapular exanthem in the characteristic distribution. Koplik spots are pathognomonic. The diagnosis is more difficult, however, during the prodrome (when the illness is maximally communicable) or when the illness and the exanthem are attenuated by passively acquired measles antibodies. Measles antibodies may be contained in transfused plasma or immunoglobulin, or they may cross the placenta to the neonate if the mother develops measles shortly before parturition. The atypical exanthem of measles in subjects who have been previously immunized with inactivated measles vaccine may potentially also cause diagnostic difficulties.

When the diagnosis cannot be made confidently on clinical and epidemiologic grounds, laboratory confirmation is indicated so that appropriate measures can be taken to prevent the occurrence of nosocomial measles among susceptible persons. Detection of measles-specific IgM antibody and measles RNA by RT-PCR assay are the most common methods for confirmation of measles infection.[430,473] Provided adequate specimens are collected during appropriate time intervals, PCR assay is positive in greater than 90% of patients with measles, even at early stages of the infection. Efforts should be made to obtain a serum sample and throat swab (or nasopharyngeal swab) from suspected cases at first contact. Because measles IgM antibodies develop during the first few days after rash onset, a negative IgM test result before 3 days may be a false negative and should be repeated. According to a study at CDC using an in-house–developed capture assay, approximately 23% of measles cases where specimens were collected within 72 hours of rash onset did not have detectable IgM.[523] The diagnosis may also be confirmed by increasing IgG antibody titers in acute and convalescent sera.[436,437,524] Older techniques to rapidly diagnose included examination of exfoliated cells from the pharynx, nasal and buccal mucosa, conjunctiva, or urinary tract by direct staining for epithelial giant cells[525,526] or identification of measles antigens by direct immunofluorescence.[527-529]

The following diseases and conditions are to be considered in the differential diagnosis of measles. None is likely to occur in the newborn.

1. *Drug eruptions and other allergies.* Maculopapular exanthems may be caused by various drugs and chemicals in susceptible persons. A history of exposure is of paramount importance in distinguishing these causes from measles. An urticarial component may be seen in some instances of drug hypersensitivity but is not present in measles.
2. *Kawasaki disease.* This illness is often confused with measles, and vice versa, in children younger than 5 years. Classic signs include conjunctivitis, red cracked lips, strawberry tongue, morbilliform or scarlatiniform rash, induration of the hands and feet, and usually a solitary enlarged cervical lymph node. In confusing cases, viral diagnostic procedures may be necessary to rule measles in or out.
3. *Rubella.* The maculopapular exanthem of rubella is finer and more transient; it undergoes a more rapid evolution and does not assume the blotchy configuration often seen in measles. The posterior cervical and postauricular lymphadenopathies of rubella are not present in measles, and conversely, the prominent catarrhal symptoms in the prodrome of measles are not a feature of rubella.
4. *Scarlet fever.* The rash of scarlet fever is punctate and extremely fine rather than papular. It blanches on pressure and is accentuated in skin folds. The onset is typically abrupt without a prodrome. There is an accompanying sore throat, and the cheeks are flushed. Peripheral blood leukocytosis is usual, in contrast to the leukopenia of measles.

[#a]References 494, 495, 497, 503, 521, 522.

5. *Meningococcemia.* When the early rash of meningococcemia is maculopapular rather than petechial, it may be confused with measles. In contrast to measles, it has no characteristic distribution.
6. *Roseola.* The exanthem of roseola, which usually appears when the patient's temperature decreases to normal, typically appears on the trunk before it is evident on the head. It lasts only 1 or 2 days. Roseola, which is caused by human herpesvirus type 6, is seen most often in children younger than 3 years and is almost never seen in adults.
7. *Atypical measles.* This hypersensitivity disease is related to infection with measles virus in persons who received killed measles vaccine years ago. Killed measles vaccine was removed from the U.S. market in 1968. Extremely high measles hemagglutination inhibition antibody titers (e.g., 1:1 million) have been observed in patients with this disease.
8. *Other infections.* Rocky Mountain spotted fever, toxoplasmosis, enterovirus infections, parvovirus infection, and infectious mononucleosis may cause maculopapular exanthems resembling measles.

THERAPY

The treatment of uncomplicated measles is symptomatic. IG has no proven value in established disease. Antibiotics are not indicated for prophylaxis of bacterial superinfections (i.e., otitis and pneumonia). When these complications develop, antimicrobial therapy should be selected on the basis of Gram stain and culture of appropriate body fluids, such as sputum. If culture specimens cannot be obtained or if the illness is grave, broad-spectrum antibiotics may be selected on the basis of the most likely offending pathogens. The antibiotic regimen for pneumonia, most commonly caused by *S. pneumoniae* or *S. aureus*, should include a penicillinase-resistant penicillin; the drug of choice for otitis media, which is usually caused by *S. pneumoniae* or *Haemophilus influenzae*, is amoxicillin. Vitamin A (200,000 IU orally once daily for 2 days for infants 12 months of age and older, 100,000 IU orally once daily for 2 days for infants 6 to 11 months of age, and 50,000 IU orally once daily for 2 days for infants younger than 6 months) has been used to treat infants with measles and seems to decrease the severity of the infection.[530-532] A third age-specific dose should be given 2 to 4 weeks later to children with vitamin A deficiency. The drug ribavirin has been used experimentally to treat severe measles in immunocompromised and other high-risk patients.[533-535]

PREVENTION

Passive Immunization

Human IG is a blood product used to provide antibodies for short-term prevention of infectious diseases, including measles.[452] IG is prepared from plasma pools derived from thousands of donors. In the United States, potency of IG products have declined as a result of change in the donor population from persons with immunity from natural disease to persons with predominantly vaccine-induced immunity.[452,536] The proportion of mothers with vaccine-induced immunity in the United States and elsewhere has also increased, and offspring of vaccinated women lose transplacentally acquired measles antibodies at an earlier age than infants born to mothers with naturally acquired immunity.[537-539] In 2013, recommendations for use of IG for postexposure prophylaxis were revised to increase the dosage of intramuscularly administered immunoglobulin (IMIG) for healthy persons, to expand the recommendation for use of IGIM to include exposed infants aged birth to 6 months, and to recommend administering IVIG for severely immunocompromised persons and pregnant women without evidence of measles immunity. IVIG is recommended for pregnant women in order to administer doses high enough to achieve estimated protective levels of measles antibody titers. For infants 6 to 11 months of age, MMR vaccine can be administered in place of IG if vaccine is administered within 72 hours.[452]

Passive immunization with IG is recommended for the prevention of measles in exposed persons without evidence of measles immunity, including pregnant women, neonates, and their contacts in the delivery room or newborn nursery (see "Nosocomial Measles in the Nursery"). IMIG should be given as soon as possible after exposure but may be administered within 6 days of exposure to contacts without evidence of measles immunity. MMR vaccine within 72 hours of exposure should be used for exposed contacts eligible for vaccination (see "Active Immunization"). The recommended dose of IMIG is 0.25 mL/kg for "normal" children and 0.5 mL/kg for immunocompromised children (maximum dose, 15 mL), and the recommended dose of IVIG is 400 mg/kg. It is recommended that persons without evidence of measles immunity who receive IG should subsequently receive MMR vaccine no earlier than 6 months after IMIG administration and 8 months after IVIG administration, provided the person is then aged 12 months or older and the vaccine is not otherwise contraindicated.[452]

Active Immunization

Measles vaccine has been used in the United States since 1963. The currently licensed live measles vaccines are derivatives of the Edmonston B strain that have been further attenuated. In the United States, measles vaccine is only available as combined MMR or MMRV vaccine. MMRV vaccine is licensed for use only in children aged 1 to 12 years. Measles vaccines produce a noncommunicable infection, which is mild or inapparent. Clinical trials were conducted in children; a double-blind placebo-controlled trial in twins showed very low rates of adverse effects attributable to measles vaccination.[540] Effects attributed to vaccination were 0.5% to 4.1% more common in vaccinated compared with placebo children, and symptoms and signs most commonly observed 7 to 11 days postvaccination were local reactions; mild, moderate, or high fever; irritability; and generalized rash. Placebo-controlled trials have not been conducted among adults; noncontrolled studies report higher rates of systemic reactions and arthropathy after rubella vaccination in adults.[452]

In the United States, two doses of MMR vaccine are recommended routinely for children at 12 to 15 months and 4 to 6 years of age. All school-aged children in grades K to 12 should be vaccinated with two doses. Two doses are also recommended for adults at high risk of exposure and transmission (i.e., students attending colleges or other post–high-school educational facilities, health care personnel, and international travelers) who do not have other evidence of measles immunity, and one dose is recommended for other adults aged greater than or equal to 18 years who do not have other evidence of measles immunity.[452] Measles vaccine is highly effective, with one dose inducing seroconversion in 95% of recipients greater than or equal to 12 months of age and preventing clinical disease in greater than 90% of exposed susceptible recipients. Two doses provide higher levels of protection.[541] Live-attenuated measles vaccines are contraindicated in pregnant women because of the theoretical risk to the fetus when the mother receives a live-virus vaccine.[452] In one small series, Edmonston B measles vaccine and gamma globulin were administered to seven pregnant women, 18 to 34 years of age, who were in the second to eighth months of pregnancy. There were no serologic data. Three of the seven developed fever (>38.5° C) and rash. All delivered healthy infants at term.[542] Vaccination is not recommended routinely for infants younger than 12 months because the induction of immunity and the elaboration of antibodies may be suppressed by residual transplacentally acquired maternal antibodies. However, infants 6 to 11 months who travel abroad should receive one dose and during a measles outbreak; vaccination may be recommended for infants 6 months and older. If infants receive a vaccine dose before 12 months of age, they need to receive two additional doses, at an appropriate interval, once they reach 12 months of age.[398,452] A single fatality in a young adult with HIV infection resulting from vaccine-associated measles pneumonia after reimmunization has been reported.[488] Therefore MMR vaccine is not recommended for HIV-infected persons aged greater than or equal to 12 months and who have evidence of severe immunosuppression,[452] but it may be administered to other HIV-infected persons who lack evidence of measles immunity.

Although MMR vaccine had an excellent safety record, in 1998 the question was raised about whether this vaccine might result in autism in previously healthy children. Scientific evidence does not support a causal association between vaccines and autism.[543-545] Nevertheless, the public in the United Kingdom became so concerned regarding this possibility that use of measles vaccine decreased significantly, leading to reestablishment of endemic disease transmission and outbreaks affecting adolescents who missed out on vaccination during childhood.[546-548] Although vaccine coverage in children in the United Kingdom has increased, measles outbreaks continue in the United Kingdom, fueled by susceptible adolescents who missed out on vaccination during childhood. Potentially, this development could lead to an increase in measles in pregnant women in the United Kingdom, although the government has initiated a large catch-up campaign to address the immunity gap.[549] In the United States, MMR coverage has remained greater than 90% in young children and adolescents 13 to 17 years of age.[458,550]

Nosocomial Measles in the Nursery: Guidelines for Prevention

Most women of childbearing age in the United States are immune to measles because of previous natural infection or vaccination. Because it is amply documented that infants born to immune mothers are usually protected by transplacentally acquired antibodies, measles outbreaks in newborn nurseries are extraordinarily rare. Studies by Krugman and colleagues[551] indicated that before the introduction of live-attenuated measles vaccine, 94% of infants had passive hemagglutination inhibition antibodies when 1 month of age, 47% had antibodies at 4 months of age, and 26% had antibodies at 6 months of age. Although in the vaccine era measles seroprevalance among women of childbearing age is similar, 7% of U.S.-born infants might lack measles antibodies at birth, and up to 90% may be seronegative by 6 months.[452,552,553] The rarity of measles among mothers, newborns, and hospital staff in the newborn nursery makes it difficult to assess the precise risk when the virus has been introduced. Nonetheless, if measles infection or disease is confirmed in a nursery setting,[459-463] public health response measures designed to prevent disease in individuals exposed and the spread of infection to neonates of uncertain immune status should be instituted immediately.

If any measles cases are confirmed in a hospital or other health care setting, respiratory etiquette and airborne precautions should be instituted immediately. Health care personnel should be checked for evidence of measles immunity. Those without evidence should receive postexposure prophylaxis with the first dose of MMR vaccine or IMIG if vaccine is contraindicated. These health care workers should be excluded from providing care from 5 to 21 days after exposure.[452] Health care personnel who have documentation of one dose of measles or MMR vaccine should receive the second dose and may remain at work.[418,452] Infants born to mothers who have evidence of measles immunity (which includes at least one of the following: documentation of at least one dose of live measles-containing or MMR vaccine, laboratory evidence of measles immunity, laboratory confirmation of disease, or birth before 1957 [history of measles disease is no longer considered acceptable evidence of immunity]) are assumed not to be at risk when exposed to measles in the neonatal period. If siblings at home have measles in a communicable stage, neonates born to mothers with evidence of immunity may be discharged from the hospital with no prophylaxis. In the absence of maternal immunity, the neonate and mother should not have contact with the older siblings until they are no longer infectious (i.e., 4 days after rash onset). The mother and neonate and any older siblings who lack evidence of measles immunity should receive MMR vaccine, if administered within 72 hours of exposure, or IMIG (0.5 mg/kg; maximum dose, 15 mL) within 6 days of exposure.[452]

If a mother without evidence of measles immunity is admitted for delivery after a known measles exposure, she should be observed carefully. If she develops symptoms consistent with measles (including fever and respiratory symptoms), she should be isolated immediately, and control efforts should be instituted to prevent transmission, including evaluating hospital contacts for evidence of measles immunity and offering vaccine or IG, as appropriate.

If a mother develops measles immediately antepartum or postpartum and her infant is born with congenital measles disease or infection, the mother and infant should be isolated together using airborne precautions until 96 hours (4 days) after the appearance of the exanthem. Close observation of the neonate for signs of bronchopneumonia and other complications is warranted. Other exposed mothers and hospital personnel without evidence of measles immunity should receive immediate prophylaxis with vaccine or immunoglobulin, as described previously, followed by vaccination at a later date. Other exposed neonates should receive immediate prophylaxis with IG, as described previously.

If a mother develops perinatal measles, but her infant is born without signs of infection, each should be isolated separately.[554] The infant may have measles infection without rash, may be incubating transplacentally acquired measles, or may be at risk for postnatally acquired infection. Unless measles infection is immediately confirmed in the baby, the infant should receive IG. The mother may be discharged with her infant after the fourth day of exanthem. The neonate should be followed closely and observed for signs of measles for 28 days.[452]

The availability of virus diagnostic facilities varies, and the approach to potential nosocomial spread of measles may differ from place to place. If vaccination records are not available, serologic testing to determine evidence of measles immunity is the ideal approach if test results can be available rapidly. If serologic testing is expensive or unavailable, it may be simpler to administer MMR vaccine or IG to all exposed eligible persons who do not have a history of previous vaccination with live-attenuated measles virus vaccine.

Neonates or mothers isolated because of measles require a separate room with the door closed or a special airborne isolation room with negative-pressure ventilation.[554] Only visitors and staff with documented evidence of measles immunity should enter the room. Gown and hand-washing precautions must be observed; an N95 respirator or a respirator with similar effectiveness in preventing airborne transmission should be worn, and containment of bedding and tissues soiled with respiratory excreta should be double bagged and autoclaved. Because measles virus is excreted in the urine during the early exanthematous phase, it is also advisable to treat the urine as potentially infectious and to disinfect nondisposable bedpans. Terminal disinfection of the room is recommended.

Mumps

Mumps is an acute, generalized, communicable disease whose most distinctive feature is swelling of one or both parotid glands. Involvement of other salivary glands, the meninges, the pancreas, and the testes of postpubertal males is also common. The origin of the name is obscure but probably is related to the Old English verb *to mump*, meaning "to sulk," or to the Scottish verb meaning "to speak indistinctly."

ORGANISM

Properties and Propagation

Mumps virus is a member of the paramyxovirus family and has most of the morphologic and physicochemical properties described for measles. Five antigens have been described: two envelope glycoproteins, a hemagglutinin-neuraminidase (H-N), a hemolysis cell fusion (F) glycoprotein antigen, and a matrix envelope protein. There are two internal antigens: a nucleocapsid protein (NP) and an RNA polymerase protein (P).[555]

Mumps virus is readily isolated after inoculation of appropriate clinical specimens into various host systems. Rapid identification may be accomplished by use of cells grown in shell vials and use of fluorescein-labeled monoclonal antibodies and molecular methods, such as RT-PCR.[556-558] The virus may be recovered during the first few days of illness from saliva, throat washings, and urine and from the CSF of patients with mumps meningitis. Shedding of virus in the urine may persist longer, sometimes 2 weeks. Less commonly, the virus is present in blood, milk, and testicular tissue.[555,557]

PCR tests are widely used to diagnose mumps. ELISA assays are useful for diagnosing (IgM or a significant rise [usually fourfold] in IgG titers) and determining immunity to mumps (mumps IgG).[555,559] All test methods present challenges in vaccinated persons.[559]

EPIDEMIOLOGY AND TRANSMISSION

Period of Communicability

Mumps occurs worldwide and is endemic in most areas where routine vaccination with mumps-containing vaccine is not practiced. In the United States, before widespread vaccination against mumps, the incidence was highest in the winter, reaching a peak in March and April. Mumps was principally a disease of childhood, with most infections occurring between the ages of 5 and 15 years. Mumps in infancy is very uncommon (discussed later). In the prevaccine era, approximately one third of infections were subclinical. Epidemics occurred frequently among school children and outbreaks in confined populations, including in boarding schools, the military, and other institutions, and were frequently described. Live-attenuated mumps vaccine was licensed in the United States in 1967. In 1977, the ACIP recommended universal childhood vaccination with a single dose. In 1989, the ACIP recommended that school-age children receive two doses of MMR vaccine for improved measles control. After use of mumps vaccine, the incidence of clinical mumps declined dramatically in the United States, and mumps remains an extremely uncommon disease. In 2006, there was a resurgence of mumps, however, with 6584 cases reported to the CDC. Many cases occurred on college campuses, and disease occurred in individuals who had received the recommended two doses of vaccine.[560,561] Since 2006, episodic large mumps outbreaks have continued to occur in the United States among adolescents and young adults in high-contact settings in the United States.[562-565] Between 2006 and 2013, several large mumps outbreaks, described in similar settings in highly vaccinated young adults in other countries,[566,567] occurred in the United States and abroad. Most cases occurred among two-dose vaccinated individuals, primarily school-aged children and young adults in high-contact settings.

Incubation Period

The usual incubation period, measured between exposure to infection and onset of parotitis, is 16 to 18 days (range, 12-25 days). Infected persons may shed virus before the onset of clinical disease, and an estimated 15% to 27% of mumps infections are subclinical.[568-570]

Incidence of Mumps in Pregnancy

The incidence of mumps in pregnancy is unknown. Because there is now little opportunity for exposure to mumps and many women are immune, the incidence is expected to be low. The incidence in prospective studies in the prevaccine era was variously estimated as between 0.8 and 10 cases per 10,000 pregnancies.[114,235]

PATHOGENESIS

Mumps is transmitted by droplet nuclei, saliva, and fomites. The precise pathogenesis of infection has not been established; although experimentally infected monkeys may develop parotitis, no animal model closely resembles human disease. After entry into the host, the virus initially replicates in the epithelium of the upper respiratory tract. A viremia ensues, after which there is localization in glandular or CNS tissues. Parotitis is believed to occur as a result of viremia, rather than the reverse, because, in many instances, generalized disease precedes involvement of the parotid gland, which may not be involved at all.

PATHOLOGY

Studies of the pathology of mumps are few because the disease is rarely fatal. The histologic changes that have been observed in the parotid gland and the testis are similar. The inflammatory exudate consists of perivascular and interstitial infiltrates of mononuclear cells accompanied by prominent edema. There is necrosis of acinar and duct epithelial cells in the salivary glands and of the germinal epithelium of the seminiferous tubules.

There are few reports of placental pathology in gestational mumps. Garcia and associates[571] described a 29-year-old Brazilian woman with a history of two bleeding episodes during pregnancy and who developed mumps in her fifth month. A hysterotomy was subsequently performed, yielding a macerated 90-g fetus. Necrotizing villitis and accumulation of necrotic material, mononuclear cells, and nuclear fragments were found in the intervillous spaces of the placenta. Necrotizing granulomas and cytoplasmic inclusions consistent with mumps virus infection were also identified. Two additional women with mumps in the tenth week and second month of pregnancy underwent therapeutic abortions. Typical inclusion bodies were identified in both placentas and in the adrenal cortex of one fetus.[571] No virologic or serologic data were available on these three women, however, so it is possible that their parotitis was caused by an agent other than mumps virus. Transplacental passage of virus should not be assumed to occur invariably, however, because, in several instances, passage could not be documented.[571-573] Live-attenuated mumps virus has been recovered from the placenta of pregnant women (but not from fetal tissues) who were vaccinated 10 days before undergoing saline-induced abortion.[574]

CLINICAL MANIFESTATIONS

The prodrome of mumps consists of fever, malaise, myalgia, and anorexia. Parotitis is the most typical clinical presentation of mumps. Swelling of salivary glands is accompanied by tenderness to palpation and obliteration of the space between the earlobe and the angle of the mandible. The swelling progresses for 2 to 3 days, then gradually subsides, and disappears in 1 week or less. The orifice of Stensen duct is commonly red and swollen. In most cases, parotitis is bilateral, although the onset in each gland may be asynchronous by 1 or more days. The submaxillary glands are involved less often than the parotid and almost never by themselves. The sublingual glands are only rarely affected. In some cases of mumps, parotitis is absent, but other typical symptoms are present.

Orchitis is the most common manifestation other than parotitis in postpubertal males; before use of mumps vaccine, it affected about 20% of postpubertal patients. Sterility, even with bilateral mumps orchitis, occurred infrequently. Orchitis in infancy has been described but is not well documented.[575] Mastitis occurred in 31% of postpubertal women with mumps during the mumps epidemic in a virgin population in Alaska.[568] Oophoritis is far less common. It is associated with lower abdominal pain, and the ovaries rarely may be palpable. Oophoritis does not lead to sterility.

Aseptic meningitis may occur in children and adults. Although pleocytosis of the CSF may occur in 50% of cases of clinical mumps, signs of meningeal irritation occur in a smaller proportion of cases, variably estimated at 5% to 25%. The CSF may contain 1000 cells/mm^3. Within the first 24 hours, polymorphonuclear leukocytes may predominate, but by the second day, most cells are lymphocytes. In the absence of parotitis, the syndrome of aseptic meningitis in mumps is indistinguishable clinically from meningitis caused by enteroviruses and other viruses. The course is almost invariably self-limited. Rarely, cranial nerve palsies have led to permanent sequelae, of which deafness is the most common. In the prevaccine era, permanent unilateral deafness caused by mumps occurred in 1 of 20,000 infected persons; bilateral, severe hearing loss was very rare.[576]

Mumps pancreatitis may cause abdominal pain. The incidence of this manifestation is unclear because reliable diagnostic criteria are difficult to obtain. An elevated serum amylase level may be present in parotitis or pancreatitis. The character of the abdominal pain is rarely sufficiently distinctive to permit unequivocal diagnosis. Other complications of mumps include thyroiditis, myocarditis, nephritis, and arthritis.

The peripheral blood cell count in mumps is not characteristic. The white blood cell count may be elevated, normal, or depressed, and the differential count may reveal a mild lymphocytosis or a polymorphonuclear leukocytosis.

Maternal Effects of Mumps

In contrast to varicella and measles, when mumps occurs in pregnant women, the illness is generally benign and is not appreciably more severe than it is in other women.[568,577-584] In a 1957 "virgin soil" epidemic of mumps among the Inuit, 20 infections occurred in pregnant women. Of these, only 8 (40%) were clinically apparent, compared with an incidence of 57 clinically apparent cases (62%) among 92 nonpregnant women.[568] Some complications, such as mastitis and perhaps thyroiditis, are more frequent in postpubertal women than in men but probably do not occur more commonly in pregnant women than in other women.[568] Mumps virus has been isolated on the third postpartum day from the milk of a woman who developed parotitis 2 days antepartum.[585] Her infant, who was not breastfed, did not develop clinically apparent mumps. Aseptic meningitis, apparently without unduly high incidence or severity, has also been reported in pregnant women.[586] Deaths from mumps are exceedingly rare in pregnant women and in the population as a whole. One death has been reported in a woman who developed mumps complicated by glomerulonephritis at 8 months of gestation.[587]

Effects of Gestational Mumps on the Fetus

Abortion. One study has demonstrated an excessive number of abortions associated with gestational mumps when the disease occurs during the first trimester.[245] However, other studies do not corroborate this finding. In prospective studies of fetal mortality in virus diseases, Siegel and associates[245] observed 9 spontaneous abortions (fetal deaths) (27%) among 33 first-trimester pregnancies complicated by mumps, compared with 131 (13%) of 1010 matched uninfected control subjects (see Table 23-4). This difference is significant ($\chi^2 = 5.6$; $P < .02$). Mumps-associated fetal deaths occurred in only 1 of 51 second-trimester pregnancies and none of 43 third-trimester pregnancies. In contrast to fetal deaths associated with measles, fetal deaths associated with mumps were closely related temporally to maternal infection: 6 of the 10 deaths occurred within 2 weeks after the onset of maternal mumps.[245] The only other study with a comparison group involved very small numbers of pregnant women with mumps during the first trimester, and conclusions cannot be drawn from these data.[568]

Other reports describe isolated cases of abortion associated with gestational mumps. Most cases occurred in the first 4 months of pregnancy.[577,582,584,586,588,589] In one instance, mumps virus was isolated from a 10-week fetus spontaneously aborted 4 days after the mother developed clinical mumps.[586]

Prematurity. In the only prospective study of low birth weight (a surrogate measure of prematurity) in relation to maternal mumps infection, no significant association was found.[245] Nine (7.7%) of 117 pregnant women with mumps gave birth to infants with birth weights of less than 2500 g, compared with 4 (3.3%) of 122 uninfected pregnant women in a control group).

Congenital Malformations. In experimentally infected animals, mumps virus may induce congenital malformations.[590-592] Definitive evidence of a teratogenic potential for mumps virus in humans has not been shown, however. Many reports describe the occurrence of congenital malformations after gestational mumps, but no data are available in most of these studies regarding the incidence of anomalies in uninfected matched control pregnancies. Swan[588] reviewed the literature in 1951 and found 18 anomalies in the offspring of 93 pregnancies complicated by mumps. These included 4 malformations originating in the first trimester (i.e., cutaneous nevus, imperforate anus, spina bifida, and Down syndrome) and 9 originating in the second trimester (i.e., four cases of Down syndrome and miscellaneous other malformations). Other reports have described malformation of the external ear,[578] intestinal atresia,[584] chorioretinitis and optic atrophy in the absence of evidence of congenital toxoplasmosis,[593] corneal cataracts,[504] and urogenital abnormalities.[594] One case of hydrocephalus caused by obstruction of the foramen of Monro in an infant whose mother had serologically proven mumps during the fifth month of pregnancy has been described.[595] A similar phenomenon has been seen after extrauterine mumps with encephalitis[596] and in an animal model.[592] In the only controlled, prospective study, the rate of congenital malformations in children whose mothers had mumps during pregnancy (2/117) was essentially identical to the rate in infants born to uninfected mothers (2/123).[275] The two affected infants, both of whom were mentally retarded, were not born to any of the 24 pregnant women who had mumps in the first trimester. Similarly, no association between gestational mumps and fetal malformations was reported by British investigators, who evaluated the outcomes of 501 pregnancies complicated by maternal mumps and found no significant differences compared with a control series.[597]

Endocardial Fibroelastosis. A postulated association between gestational mumps infection and endocardial fibroelastosis in the offspring was at one time the subject of much debate.[598] An extensive review of evidence for and against an etiologic role for mumps virus in this condition by Finland[599] in the 1970s was inconclusive, and there was little more information in the literature for the next 30 years. The issue remains unresolved. The rarity of mumps during pregnancy and the rarity of endocardial fibroelastosis as a possible sequela in the fetus make it unlikely that conclusive data will ever be obtained.

Molecular approaches, however, seem to have shed new light on the issue. Using PCR assay, mumps virus genome was detected in two of 2 fatal cases of fibroelastosis.[600] In another study of 29 fatal cases of mumps, fragments of the mumps genome were identified in 20 cases.[601] Adenovirus was identified in the remainder. It was hypothesized that endocardial fibroelastosis is the end result of myocarditis. As mumps has become rare because of vaccination, endocardial fibroelastosis has also become rare.[601] The possible role of intrauterine mumps was not addressed in these two modern studies and it may be impossible to evaluate further given the rarity of mumps in developed countries today.

Perinatal Mumps

In contrast to congenital varicella and measles, congenital mumps or even postnatally acquired perinatal mumps has rarely been documented virologically or serologically. Although several cases of parotitis have been reported in women near delivery and in their neonates and infants,[568,602-605] the significance of these reports is often uncertain, especially when clinically apparent parotitis only is present in the mother. Other viral, bacterial, and noninfectious causes are difficult to exclude without laboratory evidence of mumps infection. Among the possible explanations for the rarity of transplacental and postnatally acquired mumps in neonates are the rarity of mumps today, protection of the neonate by passive maternal antibodies, exclusion of mumps virus from the fetus by a hypothetical placental barrier, relative insusceptibility of fetal and neonatal tissues to infection by mumps virus, and occurrence of infections that are predominantly subclinical. Nevertheless, there have been occasional confirmed reports of congenital mumps. Mumps virus was isolated from two infants whose mothers had mumps at delivery. One infant had parotitis, and the other had pneumonia; presumably, transplacental transmission had occurred.[505] With the availability of improved laboratory testing, there have been additional confirmed reports of congenital mumps complicated by pneumonia.[606,607] A recent report from the United States described congenital mumps infection with serious complications in the newborn of a mother infected with mumps 2 weeks before delivery. The baby became febrile on the second day of life and developed tachypnea and cyanosis on day 4, which progressed to severe respiratory distress requiring mechanical ventilation. Mechanical ventilation was provided for 19 days, and the infant was discharged at 55 days of age. Mumps was confirmed by IgM, and mumps virus RNA was identified from buccal smear.[606]

A differentiation between lack of susceptibility and subclinical infection as explanations for failure of the neonate to develop parotitis or other manifestations of mumps can be made only by adequate serologic investigations and viral isolation or identification attempts. These data were often unavailable in early studies. Several investigators have observed that clinically apparent mumps with parotitis[608,609] or orchitis[575] during the first year of life tends to be a very mild disease and that age-specific attack rates for manifest disease related to mumps increase progressively until age 5 years.[610] Antibodies to mumps virus are known to cross the placenta and to persist for several months.[611]

DIAGNOSIS AND DIFFERENTIAL DIAGNOSIS

The diagnosis of mumps is easy when there is acute, bilateral, painful parotitis with a history of recent exposure. More difficulty is encountered when the disease is unilateral, when the manifestations are confined to organs other than the parotid gland, or when there is no history of mumps exposure. In these cases, laboratory confirmation may be obtained by virus identification or isolation or serologic testing. Because there are other causes of parotitis, and mumps is now rare in the United States, most sporadic cases of parotitis will not be due to mumps virus; therefore, except during outbreaks, laboratory confirmation of suspected mumps cases should be sought.[612]

Among neonates, few conditions need be considered in the differential diagnosis. Clinical parotitis in this age group is rare. Suppurative parotitis of the newborn, usually caused by *S. aureus*, is most often unilateral.[613] Pus can be expressed from the parotid duct, and there is a polymorphonuclear leukocytosis of the peripheral blood. Other diagnostic considerations in neonates include infection with parainfluenza viruses and coxsackieviruses, drug-induced parotitis, and facial cellulitis. In addition to these conditions in neonates, the differential diagnosis in pregnant women includes anterior cervical lymphadenitis, idiopathic recurrent parotitis, salivary gland calculus with obstruction, sarcoidosis with uveoparotid fever, and salivary gland tumors.

Other entities should be considered when the manifestations appear in organs other than the parotid. Testicular torsion in infancy may produce a painful scrotal mass resembling mumps orchitis.[575] In countries where mumps still exhibits seasonality, aseptic meningitis related to mumps typically occurs in the winter and early spring, and enterovirus aseptic meningitis is most common in the summer and early autumn. Other viruses may also cause aseptic meningitis that is clinically indistinguishable from mumps.

THERAPY

Treatment of parotitis is symptomatic. Analgesics and application of heat or cold to the parotid area may be helpful. Mumps immunoglobulin has no proven value in the prevention or treatment of mumps. Mastitis may be managed by the application of ice packs and breast binders. Testicular pain may be minimized by the local application of cold and gentle support for the scrotum. In some instances, severe cases of orchitis have seemed to respond to systemic administration of corticosteroids.

PREVENTION

Active Immunization

Live-attenuated mumps virus vaccine is available in the United States as MMR vaccine and MMRV vaccine. MMRV vaccine is only licensed for children aged 1 to 12 years, so MMR vaccine should be used for vaccination of adolescents and adults. Two doses of mumps-containing or MMR vaccine have a median effectiveness of 88% (range, 66%-95%) in preventing mumps. In the United States, for mumps prevention, two doses of MMR vaccine are recommended routinely for children at 12 to 15 months and 4 to 6 years of age, respectively. Older children, adolescents, or adults without evidence of mumps immunity should also be vaccinated (see Table 23-1).[452] Two doses are recommended for adults at high risk of exposure and transmission (students attending colleges or other post–high-school educational facilities, health care personnel, and international travelers), and one dose is recommended for other adults.[452] Vaccination of infants younger than 12 months is not recommended because of possible interference by passive maternal antibodies, unless the child is traveling internationally and is 6 to 11 months of age, when one MMR dose is recommended for measles protection. MMR vaccine is not recommended for pregnant women, for patients receiving systemic corticosteroids, or for other persons with known severe immunodeficiencies (e.g., from hematologic and solid tumors, receipt of chemotherapy, congenital immunodeficiency, or long-term immunosuppressive therapy, or patients with HIV who are severely immunocompromised). Because of the large multistate mumps outbreak in 2006, in which vaccine failure after two doses was documented, needs for booster immunization have been explored.[452,560,561,614] As of 2013, data on use and effectiveness of a third dose of MMR vaccine for mumps outbreak control are limited and are considered insufficient to recommend for or against the use of a third dose of MMR vaccine for mumps outbreak control.[452,564,565] The CDC has issued guidance for consideration for use of a third dose in specifically identified target populations, along with criteria for public health departments to consider for decision making (http://www.cdc.gov/vaccines/pubs/surv-manual/chpt09-mumps.html).

Passive Immunization

Passive immunization for mumps is not effective, and no mumps immune globulin is available.[452]

Prevention of Nosocomial Mumps in the Newborn Nursery

In contrast to varicella and measles, mumps does not seem to be a potentially serious hazard in the newborn nursery. Outbreaks of nosocomial mumps are uncommon[615] although recent outbreaks in hospital settings, including three mumps cases in health care personnel working in a NICU, demonstrate that exposures in these settings can occur with considerable disruption and cost to the institution.[616,617] Most mothers are immune, and neonates born to mothers without evidence of mumps immunity rarely develop clinically apparent mumps. However, prudence dictates that mothers who develop parotitis or other manifestations of mumps in the period immediately antepartum or postpartum should be isolated from other mothers and neonates who lack evidence of mumps immunity, including their own baby. Although one clinical report highlighted that transmission of mumps occurred in a hospital setting, despite isolation of patients with mumps from the time of onset of parotitis,[618] isolation of mumps patients is recommended because mumps virus continues to be shed after parotitis onset.[398,452,559] Infected subjects shed mumps virus in respiratory secretions for several days before and after the onset of parotitis or other manifestations recognizable as mumps.[619] Updated CDC policy recommends that patients with mumps be isolated for 5 days after onset of parotitis.[619,620]

Mumps IG is no longer available. There is no scientific evidence that live-attenuated mumps virus vaccine is protective when administered postexposure. A recent study reported a lower attack rate in exposed two-dose vaccinated family members who received a third dose of MMR vaccine postexposure, compared with those who did not, but the difference was not statistically significant.[621] However, MMR vaccine may theoretically modify or prevent disease by inducing neutralizing antibodies before the onset of illness because of the long incubation period of mumps. It can be considered for exposed hospital personnel and puerperal mothers who lack evidence of mumps immunity, to protect them from future exposures. Some hospitals have the facilities to test for susceptibility to mumps by measurement of antibody titers, whereas others do not. Testing for evidence of immunity on an ongoing basis could eliminate some use of vaccine for the previously described situation.

Isolation procedures for mumps include the use of a single room for a patient with the door closed at all times except to enter. Personnel with evidence of mumps immunity caring for the patient should implement droplet precautions (gown and gloves). Terminal disinfection of the room is desirable.

References

1. Weller TH: Varicella and herpes zoster: changing concepts of the natural history, control, and importance of a not-so-benign virus, *N Engl J Med* 309:1362, 1983.
2. Lungu O, Annunziato PW, Gershon A, et al: Reactivated and latent varicella-zoster virus in human dorsal root ganglia, *Proc Natl Acad Sci U S A* 92:10980, 1995.
3. Lungu O, Panagiotidis CA, Annunziato PW, et al: Aberrant intracellular localization of varicella-zoster virus regulatory proteins during latency, *Proc Natl Acad Sci U S A* 95:780, 1998.
4. Chen J, Gershon AA, Li ZS, et al: Latent and lytic infection of isolated guinea pig enteric and dorsal root ganglia by varicella zoster virus, *J Med Virol* 70:S71, 2003.
5. Mahalingham R, Wellish M, Cohrs R, et al: Expression of protein encoded by varicella-zoster virus open reading frame 63 in latently infected human ganglionic neurons, *Proc Natl Acad Sci U S A* 93:2122, 1996.
6. *Oxford English Dictionary*, ed 1 (Suppl 1), London, 1933, Oxford University Press.
7. Christie AB: Chickenpox. In Christie AB, editor: *Infectious diseases: epidemiology and clinical practice*, Edinburgh, 1969, E & S Livingstone.
8. Angelicus B: *De Propreitatibus Rerum*, Liber septimus, vol XCIII, London, 1398, Trevisa John.
9. Muir WB, Nichols R, Breuer J: Phylogenetic analysis of varicella-zoster virus: evidence of intercontinental spread of genotypes and recombination, *J Virol* 76:1971, 2002.
10. Sengupta N, Taha Y, Scott FT, et al: Varicella-zoster-virus genotypes in East London: a prospective study in patients with herpes zoster, *J Infect Dis* 196:1014, 2007.
11. Gabel C, Dubey L, Steinberg SP, et al: Varicella-zoster virus glycoproteins are phosphorylated during posttranslational maturation, *J Virol* 63:4264, 1989.
12. Gershon A, Cosio L, Brunell PA: Observations on the growth of varicella-zoster virus in human diploid cells, *J Gen Virol* 18:21, 1973.
13. Cook ML, Stevens J: Labile coat: reason for noninfectious cell-free varicella zoster virus in culture, *J Virol* 2:1458, 1968.
14. Chen JJ, Zhu Z, Gershon AA, et al: Mannose 6-phosphate receptor dependence of varicella zoster virus infection in vitro and in the epidermis during varicella and zoster, *Cell* 119:915, 2004.
15. Gershon AA: Varicella zoster vaccines and their implications for development of HSV vaccines, *Virology* 435:29-36, 2013.
16. Ouwendijk WJ, Choe A, Nagel MA, et al: Restricted varicella-zoster virus transcription in human trigeminal ganglia obtained soon after death, *J Virol* 86:10203, 2012.
17. Myers M, Connelly BL: Animal models of varicella, *J Infect Dis* 166:S48, 1992.
18. Sadzot-Delvaux C, Merville-Louis MP, Delrée P, et al: An in vivo model of varicella-zoster virus latent infection of dorsal root ganglia, *J Neurosci Res* 26:83, 1990.
19. Williams V, Gershon A, Brunell P: Serologic response to varicella-zoster membrane antigens measured by indirect immunofluorescence, *J Infect Dis* 130:669, 1974.
20. Zaia J, Oxman M: Antibody to varicella-zoster virus-induced membrane antigen: immunofluorescence assay using monodisperse glutaraldehyde-fixed target cells, *J Infect Dis* 136:519, 1977.
21. Gershon A, Steinberg S, LaRussa P: *Measurement of antibodies to VZV by latex agglutination*, Anaheim, Calif, 1992, Society for Pediatric Research.
22. Forghani B, Schmidt N, Dennis J: Antibody assays for varicella-zoster virus: comparison of enzyme immunoassay with neutralization, immune adherence hemagglutination, and complement fixation, *J Clin Microbiol* 8:545, 1978.
23. Gershon AA, Frey HM, Steinberg SP, et al: Determination of immunity to varicella using an enzyme-linked immunosorbent assay, *Arch Virol* 70:169, 1981.
24. LaRussa P, Steinberg S, Waithe E, et al: Comparison of five assays for antibody to varicella-zoster virus and the fluorescent-antibody-to-membrane-antigen test, *J Clin Microbiol* 25:2059, 1987.
25. Shehab Z, Brunell P: Enzyme-linked immunosorbent assay for susceptibility to varicella, *J Infect Dis* 148:472, 1983.
26. Friedman MG, Leventon-Kriss S, Sarov I: Sensitive solid-phase radioimmunoassay for detection of human immunoglobulin G antibodies to varicella-zoster virus, *J Clin Microbiol* 9:1, 1979.
27. Gershon A, Kalter Z, Steinberg S: Detection of antibody to varicella-zoster virus by immune adherence hemagglutination, *Proc Soc Exp Biol Med* 151:762, 1976.
28. Caunt AE, Shaw DG: Neutralization tests with varicella-zoster virus, *J Hyg (Lond)* 67:343, 1969.
29. Grose C, Edmond BJ, Brunell PA: Complement-enhanced neutralizing antibody response to varicella-zoster virus, *J Infect Dis* 139:432, 1979.
30. Gold E, Godek G: Complement fixation studies with a varicella-zoster antigen, *J Immunol* 95:692, 1965.

31. Schmidt NJ, Lennette EH, Magoffin RL: Immunological relationship between herpes simplex and varicella-zoster viruses demonstrated by complement-fixation, neutralization and fluorescent antibody tests, *J Gen Virol* 4:321, 1969.
32. Schaap GJP, Huisman J: Simultaneous rise in complement-fixing antibodies against herpesvirus hominis and varicella-zoster virus in patients with chickenpox and shingles, *Arch Gesamte Virusforsch* 25:52, 1968.
33. Schmidt NJ: Further evidence for common antigens in herpes simplex and varicella-zoster virus, *J Med Virol* 9:27, 1982.
34. Shiraki K, Okuno T, Yamanishi K, et al: Polypeptides of varicella-zoster virus (VZV) and immunological relationship of VZV and herpes simplex virus (HSV), *J Gen Virol* 61:255, 1982.
35. Kitamura K, Namazue J, Campo-Vera H, et al: Induction of neutralizing antibody against varicella-zoster virus (VZV) by gp 2 and cross-reactivity between VZV gp 2 and herpes simplex viruses gB, *Virology* 149:74, 1986.
36. Lemon SM, Hutt LM, Huang YT, et al: Simultaneous infection with multiple herpesviruses, *Am J Med* 66:270, 1979.
37. Landry ML, Hsiung GD: Diagnosis of dual herpesvirus infection: varicella-zoster virus (VZV) and herpes simplex viruses. In Nahmias AJ, Dowdle WR, Schinazi RF, editors: *The human herpesviruses*, New York, 1981, Elsevier.
38. Arvin AM: Cell-mediated immunity to varicella-zoster virus, *J Infect Dis* 166:S35, 1992.
39. Davison A, Edson CM, Ellis RW, et al: New common nomenclature for glycoprotein genes of varicella-zoster virus and their products, *J Virol* 57:1195, 1986.
40. Arvin AM, Sharp M, Moir M, et al: Memory cytotoxic T cell responses to viral tegument and regulatory proteins encoded by open reading frames 4, 10, 29, and 62 of varicella-zoster virus, *J Virol* 15:507, 2002.
41. Brunell P, Gershon AA, Uduman SA, et al: Varicella-zoster immunoglobulins during varicella, latency, and zoster, *J Infect Dis* 132:49, 1975.
42. Gershon A, Steinberg SP, Borkowsky W, et al: IgM to varicella-zoster virus: demonstration in patients with and without clinical zoster, *Pediatr Infect Dis* 1:164, 1982.
43. Gershon AA, Steinberg SP, Gelb L: Clinical reinfection with varicella-zoster virus, *J Infect Dis* 149:137, 1984.
44. Junker AK, Angus E, Thomas E: Recurrent varicella-zoster virus infections in apparently immunocompetent children, *Pediatr Infect Dis J* 10:569, 1991.
45. Junker AK, Tilley P: Varicella-zoster virus antibody avidity and IgG-subclass patterns in children with recurrent chickenpox, *J Med Virol* 43:119, 1994.
46. Martin KA, Junker AK, Thomas EE, et al: Occurrence of chickenpox during pregnancy in women seropositive for varicella-zoster virus, *J Infect Dis* 170:991, 1994.
47. Bogger-Goren S, Bernstein JM, Gershon AA, et al: Mucosal cell mediated immunity to varicella zoster virus: role in protection against disease, *J Pediatr* 105:195, 1984.
48. Bogger-Goren S, Baba K, Hurley P, et al: Antibody response to varicella-zoster virus after natural or vaccine-induced infection, *J Infect Dis* 146:260, 1982.
49. Gershon AA, Steinberg S: NIAID Collaborative Varicella Vaccine Study Group: Live attenuated varicella vaccine: protection in healthy adults in comparison to leukemic children, *J Infect Dis* 161:661, 1990.
50. Arvin A, Koropchak CM, Wittek AE. Immunologic evidence of reinfection with varicella-zoster virus, *J Infect Dis* 148:200, 1983.
51. Hope-Simpson RE: The nature of herpes zoster: a long-term study and a new hypothesis, *Proc R Soc Med* 58:9, 1965.
52. Mehta SK, Cohrs RJ, Forghani B, et al: Stress-induced subclinical reactivation of varicella zoster virus in astronauts, *J Med Virol* 72:174, 2004.
53. Schunemann S, Mainka C, Wolff MH: Subclinical reactivation of varicella-zoster virus in immunocompromised and immunocompetent individuals, *Intervirology* 41:98, 1998.
54. Luby J, Ramirez-Ronda C, Rinner S, et al: A longitudinal study of varicella zoster virus infections in renal transplant recipients, *J Infect Dis* 135:659, 1977.
55. Ljungman P, Lönnqvist B, Gahrton G, et al: Clinical and subclinical reactivations of varicella-zoster virus in immunocompromised patients, *J Infect Dis* 153:840, 1986.
56. Wilson A, Sharp M, Koropchak CM, et al: Subclinical varicella-zoster virus viremia, herpes zoster, and T lymphocyte immunity to varicella-zoster viral antigens after bone marrow transplantation, *J Infect Dis* 165:119, 1992.
57. Weigle K, Grose C: Molecular dissection of the humoral immune response to individual varicella-zoster viral proteins during chickenpox, quiescence, reinfection, and reactivation, *J Infect Dis* 149:741, 1984.
58. Gilden DH, Wright RR, Schneck SA, et al: Zoster sine herpete, a clinical variant, *Ann Neurol* 35:530, 1994.
59. Arvin AM, Pollard RB, Rasmussen LE, et al: Selective impairment in lymphocyte reactivity to varicella-zoster antigen among untreated lymphoma patients, *J Infect Dis* 137:531, 1978.
60. Hardy IB, Gershon AA, Steinberg SP, et al: The incidence of zoster after immunization with live attenuated varicella vaccine: a study in children with leukemia, *N Engl J Med* 325:1545, 1991.
61. Ruckdesche JC, Schimpff SC, Smyth AC, et al: Herpes zoster and impaired cell-associated immunity to the varicella-zoster virus in patients with Hodgkin's disease, *Am J Med* 62:77, 1977.
62. Hardy IB, Gershon AA, Steinberg SP, et al: *Incidence of zoster after live attenuated varicella vaccine*, Chicago, September 29-October 2, 1991, 31st Interscience Conference on Antimicrobial Agents and Chemotherapy.
63. LaRussa PL, Gershon AA, Steinberg SP, et al: Antibodies to varicella-zoster virus glycoproteins I, II, and III in leukemic and healthy children, *J Infect Dis* 162:627, 1990.
64. Burke BL, Steele RW, Beard OW, et al: Immune responses to varicella-zoster in the aged, *Arch Intern Med* 142:291, 1982.
65. Miller AE: Selective decline in cellular immune response to varicella-zoster in the elderly, *Neurology* 30:582, 1980.
66. Gershon A, Steinberg S: Antibody responses to varicella-zoster virus and the role of antibody in host defense, *Am J Med Sci* 282:12, 1981.
67. Stevens D, Merigan T: Zoster immune globulin prophylaxis of disseminated zoster in compromised hosts, *Arch Intern Med* 140:52, 1980.
68. Enders G, Miller E, Cradock-Watson J, et al: Consequences of varicella and herpes zoster in pregnancy: prospective study of 1739 cases, *Lancet* 343:1548, 1994.
69. Cohen A, Maschopoulos P, Stiehm RE, et al: Congenital varicella syndrome: the evidence for secondary prevention with varicella-zoster immune globulin, *CMAJ* 183:204, 2011.
70. Levin M: Can herpes zoster be prevented? *Eur J Clin Microbiol Infect Dis* 15:1, 1996.
71. Levin M, Murray M, Rotbart HA, et al: Immune response of elderly individuals to a live attenuated varicella vaccine, *J Infect Dis* 166:253, 1992.
72. Levin M, Murray M, Zerbe GO, et al: Immune responses of elderly persons 4 years after receiving a live attenuated varicella vaccine, *J Infect Dis* 170:522, 1994.
73. Oxman MN, Levin MJ, Johnson GR, et al: A vaccine to prevent herpes zoster and postherpetic neuralgia in older adults, *N Engl J Med* 352:2271, 2005.
74. Brunell PA: Transmission of chickenpox in a school setting prior to the observed exanthem, *Am J Dis Child* 143:1451, 1989.
75. Evans P: An epidemic of chickenpox, *Lancet* 2:339, 1940.
76. Gordon JE, Meader FM: The period of infectivity and serum prevention of chickenpox, *JAMA* 93:2013, 1929.
77. Moore DA, Hopkins RS: Assessment of a school exclusion policy during a chickenpox outbreak, *Am J Epidemiol* 133:1161, 1991.
78. Kido S, Ozaki T, Asada H, et al: Detection of varicella-zoster virus (VZV) DNA in clinical samples from patients with VZV by the polymerase chain reaction, *J Clin Microbiol* 29:76, 1991.
79. Tsolia M, Gershon AA, Steinberg SP, et al: Live attenuated varicella vaccine: evidence that the virus is attenuated and the importance of skin lesions in transmission of varicella-zoster virus, *J Pediatr* 116:184, 1990.
80. Gershon A, Takahashi M, Seward J: Live attenuated varicella vaccine. In Plotkin S, Orenstein W, Offit P, editors: *Vaccines*, ed 6, Philadelphia, 2013, Saunders, pp 837-869.
81. Gustafson TL, Lavely GB, Brawner ER Jr, et al: An outbreak of nosocomial varicella, *Pediatrics* 70:550, 1982.
82. Leclair JM, Zaia JA, Levin MJ, et al: Airborne transmission of chickenpox in a hospital, *N Engl J Med* 302:450, 1980.
83. Sawyer M, Chamberlin CJ, Wu YN, et al: Detection of varicella-zoster virus DNA in air samples from hospital rooms, *J Infect Dis* 169:91, 1993.

84. Hope-Simpson RE: Infectiousness of communicable diseases in the household (measles, mumps, and chickenpox), *Lancet* 2:549, 1952.
85. Hanngren K, Falksveden L, Grandien M, et al: Zoster immunoglobulin in varicella prophylaxis: a study among high-risk patients, *Scand J Infect Dis* 15:327, 1983.
86. Gershon A, Steinberg S, Brunell P: Zoster immune globulin: a further assessment, *N Engl J Med* 290:243, 1974.
87. Kundratitz K: Experimentelle Übertragung von Herpes Zoster auf den Menschen und die Beziehungen von Herpes Zoster zu Varicellen, *Monatsschr Kinderheilkd* 29:516, 1925.
88. Bruusgaard E: The mutual relation between zoster and varicella, *Br J Dermatol Syphilis* 44:1, 1932.
89. Seiler HE: A study of herpes zoster particularly in its relationship to chickenpox, *J Hyg (Lond)* 47:253, 1949.
90. Schimpff S, Serpick A, Stoler B, et al: Varicella-zoster infection in patients with cancer, *Ann Intern Med* 76:241, 1972.
91. Berlin BS, Campbell T: Hospital-acquired herpes zoster following exposure to chickenpox, *JAMA* 211:1831, 1970.
92. Mahalingham R, Wellish M, Wolf W, et al: Latent varicella-zoster viral DNA in human trigeminal and thoracic ganglia, *N Engl J Med* 323:627, 1990.
93. Hayakawa Y, Torigoe S, Shiraki K, et al: Biologic and biophysical markers of a live varicella vaccine strain (Oka): identification of clinical isolates from vaccine recipients, *J Infect Dis* 149:956, 1984.
94. Straus SE, Reinhold W, Smith HA, et al: Endonuclease analysis of viral DNA from varicella and subsequent zoster infections in the same patient, *N Engl J Med* 311:1362, 1984.
95. Williams DL, Gershon AA, Gelb LD, et al: Herpes zoster following varicella vaccine in a child with acute lymphocytic leukemia, *J Pediatr* 106:259, 1985.
96. Gershon A: Varicella in mother and infant: problems old and new. In Krugman S, Gershon A, editors: *Infections of the fetus and newborn infant*, New York, 1975, Alan R Liss.
97. Seward JF, Galil K, Wharton M: Epidemiology of varicella. In Arvin AM, Gershon AA, editors: *Varicella-zoster virus: virology and clinical management*, Cambridge, UK, 2000, Cambridge University Press, p 187.
98. Seward JF, Watson BM, Peterson CL, et al: Varicella disease after introduction of varicella vaccine in the United States, 1995–2000, *JAMA* 287:606, 2002.
99. Marin M, Meissner HC, Seward JF: Varicella prevention in the United States: a review of successes and challenges, *Pediatrics* 122:e744, 2008.
100. Guris D, Jumaan AO, Mascola L, et al: Changing varicella epidemiology in active surveillance sites: United States, 1995-2005, *J Infect Dis* 197(Suppl 2):S71, 2008.
101. Marin M, Zhang JX, Seward JF: Near Elimination of varicella deaths in the US after implementation of the vaccination program, *Pediatrics* 128:214, 2011.
102. Reynolds MA, Kruszon-Moran D, Jumaan A, et al: Varicella seroprevalence in the U.S.: data from the National Health and Nutrition Examination Survey, 1999-2004, *Public Health Rep* 125:860, 2010.
103. Michalik DE, Steinberg SP, LaRussa PS, et al: Primary vaccine failure after 1 dose of varicella vaccine in healthy children, *J Infect Dis* 197:944, 2008.
104. Marin M, Guris D, Chaves SS, et al: Prevention of varicella: recommendations of the Advisory Committee on Immunization Practices (ACIP), *MMWR Recomm Rep* 56(RR-4):1, 2007.
105. Bialek SR, Perella D, Zhang J, et al: impact of a routine two-dose varicella vaccination program on varicella epidemiology, *Pediatrics* 132:e1134, 2013.
106. Yorke JA, London WP: Recurrent outbreaks of measles, chickenpox and mumps: II. Systematic differences in contact rates and stochastic effects, *Am J Epidemiol* 98:469, 1973.
107. Ross AH, Lencher E, Reitman G: Modification of chickenpox in family contacts by administration of gamma globulin, *N Engl J Med* 267:369, 1962.
108. Weber DJ, Rutala WA, Hamilton H: Prevention and control of varicella-zoster infections in healthcare facilities [review], *Infect Control Hosp Epidemiol* 17:694, 1996.
109. Alter SJ, Hammond JA, McVey CJ, et al: Susceptibility to varicella-zoster virus among adults at high risk for exposure, *Infect Control* 7:448, 1986.
110. Brunell PA, Wood D: Varicella serological status of healthcare workers as a guide to whom to test or immunize, *Infect Control Hosp Epidemiol* 20:355, 1999.
111. Krasinski K, Holzman RS, LaCouture R, et al: Hospital experience with varicella-zoster virus, *Infect Control* 7:312, 1986.
112. Watson B, Civen R, Reynolds M, et al: Validity of self-reported varicella disease history in pregnant women attending prenatal clinics, *Public Health Rep* 122:499, 2007.
113. Perella D, Fiks AG, Jumaan A, et al: Validity of reported varicella history as a marker for varicella zoster virus immunity among unvaccinated children, adolescents, and young adults in the post-vaccine licensure era, *Pediatrics* 123:e820, 2009.
114. Sever J, White LR: Intrauterine viral infections, *Annu Rev Med* 19:471, 1968.
115. Balducci J, Rodis JF, Rosengren S, et al: Pregnancy outcome following first-trimester varicella infection, *Obstet Gynecol* 79:5, 1992.
116. Yawn BP, Saddier P, Wollan PC, et al: A population-based study of the incidence and complication rates of herpes zoster before zoster vaccine introduction, *Mayo Clin Proc* 82:1341, 2007.
117. Insinga RP, Itzler RF, Pellissier JM, et al: The incidence of herpes zoster in a United States administrative database, *J Gen Intern Med* 20:748, 2005.
118. Donahue JG, Choo PW, Manson JE, et al: The incidence of herpes zoster, *Arch Intern Med* 155:1605, 1995.
119. Mullooly JP, Riedlinger K, Chun C, et al: Incidence of herpes zoster, 1997-2002, *Epidemiol Infect* 133:245, 2005.
120. Brunell PA, Kotchmar GSJ: Zoster in infancy: failure to maintain virus latency following intrauterine infection, *J Pediatr* 98:71, 1981.
121. Baba K, Yabuuchi H, Takahashi M, et al: Increased incidence of herpes zoster in normal children infected with varicella-zoster virus during infancy: community-based follow up study, *J Pediatr* 108:372, 1986.
122. Guess H, Broughton DD, Melton LJ 3rd, et al: Epidemiology of herpes zoster in children and adolescents: a population-based study, *Pediatrics* 76:512, 1985.
123. Terada K, Kawano S, Yoshihiro K, et al: Varicella-zoster virus (VZV) reactivation is related to the low response of VZV-specific immunity after chickenpox in infancy, *J Infect Dis* 169:650, 1994.
124. Yawn BP, Wollan PC, Kurland MJ, et al: Herpes zoster recurrences more frequent than previously reported, *Mayo Clin Proc* 86:88, 2011.
125. Kalman CM, Laskin OL: Herpes zoster and zosteriform herpes simplex virus infections in immunocompetent adults, *Am J Med* 81:775, 1986.
126. Locksley RM, Flournoy N, Sullivan KM, et al: Infection with varicella-zoster virus after marrow transplantation, *J Infect Dis* 152:1172, 1985.
127. Veenstra J, Krol A, van Praag RM, et al: Herpes zoster, immunological deterioration and disease progression in HIV-1 infection, *AIDS* 9:1153, 1995.
128. Gershon A, Mervish N, LaRussa P, et al: Varicella-zoster virus infection in children with underlying HIV infection, *J Infect Dis* 175:1496, 1997.
129. Brazin SA, Simkovich JW, Johnson WT: Herpes zoster during pregnancy, *Obstet Gynecol* 53:175, 1979.
130. Gershon A, Raker R, Steinberg S, et al: Antibody to varicella-zoster virus in parturient women and their offspring during the first year of life, *Pediatrics* 58:692, 1976.
131. Mendez D, Sinclair MB, Garcia S, et al: Transplacental immunity to varicella-zoster virus in extremely low birthweight infants, *Am J Perinatol* 9:236, 1992.
132. Wang E, Prober C, Arvin AM: Varicella-zoster virus antibody titers before and after administration of zoster immune globulin to neonates in an intensive care nursery, *J Pediatr* 103:113, 1983.
133. Gustafson TL, Shehab Z, Brunell P: Outbreak of varicella in a newborn intensive care nursery, *Am Dis Child* 138:548, 1984.
134. Newman CGH: Perinatal varicella, *Lancet* 2:1159, 1965.
135. Freud P: Congenital varicella, *Am J Dis Child* 96:730, 1958.
136. Odessky L, Newman B, Wein GB: Congenital varicella, *N Y State J Med* 54:2849, 1954.
137. Harris LE: Spread of varicella in nurseries, *Am J Dis Child* 105:315, 1963.
138. Matseoane SL, Abler C: Occurrence of neonatal varicella in a hospital nursery, *Am J Obstet Gynecol* 92:575, 1965.
139. Lipton S, Brunell PA: Management of varicella exposure in a neonatal intensive care unit, *JAMA* 261:1782, 1989.
140. Patou G, Midgley P, Meurisse EV, et al: Immunoglobulin prophylaxis for infants exposed to varicella in a neonatal unit, *J Infect* 20:207, 1990.

141. Gold WL, Boulton JE, Goldman C, et al: Management of varicella exposures in the neonatal intensive care unit, *Pediatr Infect Dis J* 12:954, 1993.
142. Friedman CA, Temple DM, Robbins KK, et al: Outbreak and control of varicella in a neonatal intensive care unit, *Pediatr Infect Dis J* 13:152, 1994.
143. Kellie SM, Makvandi M, Muller ML: Management and outcome of a varicella exposure in a neonatal intensive care unit: lessons for the vaccine era, *Am J Infect Control* 39:844, 2011.
144. Brunell P: Placental transfer of varicella-zoster antibody, *Pediatrics* 38:1034, 1966.
145. Pinquier D, Gagneur A, Balu L, et al: Prevalence of anti-varicella-zoster virus antibodies in French infants under 15 months of age, *Clin Vaccine Immunol* 16:484, 2009.
146. Heininger U, Desgrandchamps D, Schaad UB: Seroprevalence of varicella-zoster virus IgG antibodies in Swiss children during the first 16 months of age, *Vaccine* 24:3258, 2006.
147. Leuridan E, Hens N, Hutse V, et al: Kinetics of maternal antibodies against rubella and varicella in infants, *Vaccine* 29:2222, 2011.
148. Raker R, Steinberg S, Drusin LM, et al: Antibody to varicella-zoster virus in low birth weight infants, *J Pediatr* 93:505, 1978.
149. Baba K, Yabuuchi H, Takahashi M, et al: Immunologic and epidemiologic aspects of varicella infection acquired during infancy and early childhood, *J Pediatr* 100:881, 1982.
150. Hyatt HW: Neonatal varicella, *J Natl Med Assoc* 59:32, 1967.
151. Readett MD, McGibbon C: Neonatal varicella, *Lancet* 1:644, 1961.
152. Chaves SS, Lopez AS, Watson TL, et al: Varicella in infants after implementation of the US varicella vaccination program, *Pediatrics* 128:1071, 2011.
153. Khandaker G, Marshall H, Peadon E, et al: Congenital and neonatal varicella: impact of the national varicella vaccination programme in Australia, *Arch Dis Child* 96:453, 2011.
154. Ku CC, Padilla JA, Grose C, et al: Tropism of varicella-zoster virus for human tonsillar CD4(+) T lymphocytes that express activation, memory, and skin homing markers, *J Virol* 76:11425, 2002.
155. Gold E: Serologic and virus-isolation studies of patients with varicella or herpes zoster infection, *N Engl J Med* 274:181, 1966.
156. Myers MG: Viremia caused by varicella-zoster virus: association with malignant progressive varicella, *J Infect Dis* 140:229, 1979.
157. Nelson A, St Geme J: On the respiratory spread of varicella-zoster virus, *Pediatrics* 37:1007, 1966.
158. Trlifajova J, Bryndova D, Ryc M: Isolation of varicella-zoster virus from pharyngeal and nasal swabs in varicella patients, *J Hyg Epidemiol Microbiol Immunol* 28:201, 1984.
159. Ozaki T, Ichikawa T, Matsui Y, et al: Lymphocyte-associated viremia in varicella, *J Med Virol* 19:249, 1986.
160. Asano Y, Itakura N, Hiroishi Y, et al: Viremia is present in incubation period in nonimmunocompromised children with varicella, *J Pediatr* 106:69, 1985.
161. Feldman S, Epp E: Isolation of varicella-zoster virus from blood, *J Pediatr* 88:265, 1976.
162. Feldman S, Epp E: Detection of viremia during incubation period of varicella, *J Pediatr* 94:746, 1979.
163. Moffat JF, Stein MD, Kaneshima H, et al: Tropism of varicella-zoster virus for human CD4+ and CD8+ T lymphocytes and epidermal cells in SCID-hu mice, *J Virol* 69:5236, 1995.
164. Koropchak C, Graham G, Palmer J, et al: Investigation of varicella-zoster virus infection by polymerase chain reaction in the immunocompetent host with acute varicella, *J Infect Dis* 163:1016, 1991.
165. Ozaki T, Miwata H, Asano Y, et al: Varicella-zoster virus DNA in throat swabs of vaccinees, *Arch Dis Child* 267:328, 1993.
166. de Jong MD, Schuurman T, et al: Quantitation of varicella-zoster virus DNA in whole blood, plasma, and serum by PCR and electrochemiluminescence, *J Clin Microbiol* 38:2568, 2000.
167. Quinlivan ML, Ayres KL, Kelly PJ, et al: Persistence of varicella-zoster virus viraemia in patients with herpes zoster, *J Clin Virol* 50:130, 2010.
168. Mainka C, Fuss B, Geiger H, et al: Characterization of viremia at different stages of varicella-zoster virus infection, *J Med Virol* 56:91, 1998.
169. Vazquez M, LaRussa PS, Gershon AA, et al: The effectiveness of the varicella vaccine in clinical practice, *N Engl J Med* 344:955, 2001.
170. Grose CH: Variation on a theme by Fenner, *Pediatrics* 68:735, 1981.
171. Ku CC, Zerboni L, Ito H, et al: Varicella-zoster virus transfer to skin by T cells and modulation of viral replication by epidermal cell interferon-α, *J Exp Med* 200:917, 2004.
172. Ouwendijk WJ, Abendroth A, Traina-Dorge V, et al: T-cell infiltration correlates with CXCL10 expression in ganglia of cynomolgus macaques with reactivated simian varicella virus, *J Virol* 87:2979, 2012.
173. Rand KH, Rasmussen LE, Pollard RB, et al: Cellular immunity and herpesvirus infections in cardiac transplant patients, *N Engl J Med* 296:1372, 1977.
174. Edelman DA, Antaki F, Basson MD, et al: Ogilvie syndrome and herpes zoster: case report and review of the literature, *J Emerg Med* 39:696, 2009.
175. Chen J, Gershon AA, Li Z, et al: Varicella zoster virus (VZV) infects and establishes latency in enteric neurons, *J Neurovirol* 17:578, 2011.
176. Friedman-Kien A, Lafleur FL, Gendler E, et al: Herpes zoster: a possible early clinical sign for development of acquired immunodeficiency syndrome in high-risk individuals, *J Am Acad Dermatol* 14:1023, 1988.
177. Feldman S, Chaudary S, Ossi M, et al: A viremic phase for herpes zoster in children with cancer, *J Pediatr* 91:597, 1977.
178. Gershon A, Steinberg S, Silber R: Varicella-zoster viremia, *J Pediatr* 92:1033, 1978.
179. Stevens D, Ferrington RA, Jordan GW, et al: Cellular events in zoster vesicles: relation to clinical course and immune parameters, *J Infect Dis* 131:509, 1975.
180. Szanton E, Sarov I: Interaction between polymorphonuclear leukocytes and varicella-zoster infected cells, *Intervirology* 24:119, 1985.
181. Ihara T, Starr SE, Ito M, et al: Human polymorphonuclear leukocyte-mediated cytotoxicity against varicella-zoster virus-infected fibroblasts, *J Virol* 51:110, 1984.
182. Ihara T, Ito M, Starr SE: Human lymphocyte, monocyte and polymorphonuclear leucocyte mediated antibody-dependent cellular cytotoxicity against varicella-zoster virus-infected targets, *Clin Exp Immunol* 63:179, 1986.
183. Banovic T, Yanilla M, Simmons R, et al: Disseminated varicella infection caused by varicella vaccine strain in a child with low invariant natural killer T cells and diminished CD1d expression, *J Infect Dis* 204:1893, 2011.
184. Levy O, Orange JS, Hibberd P, et al: Disseminated varicella infection due to vaccine (Oka) strain varicella-zoster virus in a patient with a novel deficiency in natural killer cells, *J Infect Dis* 188:948, 2003.
185. Novakova L, Lehuen A, Novak J: Low numbers and altered phenotype of invariant natural killer T cells in recurrent varicella zoster virus infection, *Cell Immunol* 269:78, 2011.
186. Vossen MT, Biezeveld MH, de Jong MD, et al: Absence of circulating natural killer and primed CD8+ cells in life-threatening varicella, *J Infect Dis* 191:198, 2005.
187. Etzioni A, Eidenschenk C, Katz R, et al: Fatal varicella associated with selective natural killer cell deficiency, *J Pediatr* 146:423, 2005.
188. Terada K, Kawano S, Yagi Y, et al: Alteration of T cells and natural killer cells during chickenpox in infancy, *J Clin Immunol* 16:55, 1996.
189. Garcia AGP: Fetal infection in chickenpox and alastrim, with histopathologic study of the placenta, *Pediatrics* 32:895, 1963.
190. Erlich RM, Turner JAP, Clarke M: Neonatal varicella, *J Pediatr* 53:139, 1958.
191. Lucchesi PF, LaBoccetta AC, Peale AR: Varicella neonatorum, *Am J Dis Child* 73:44, 1947.
192. Oppenheimer EH: Congenital chickenpox with disseminated visceral lesions, *Bull Johns Hopkins Hosp* 74:240, 1944.
193. Pearson HE: Parturition varicella-zoster, *Obstet Gynecol* 23:21, 1964.
194. Steen J, Pederson RV: Varicella in a newborn girl, *J Oslo City Hosp* 9:36, 1959.
195. Ranney EK, Norman MG, Silver MD: Varicella pneumonitis, *Can Med Assoc J* 96:445, 1967.
196. Triebwasser JH, Harris RE, Bryant RE, et al: Varicella pneumonia in adults: report of seven cases and a review of the literature, *Medicine (Baltimore)* 46:409, 1967.
197. Gordon JE: Chickenpox: an epidemiologic review, *Am J Med Sci* 244:362, 1962.
198. Bradley JS, Schlievert PM, Sample TG: Streptococcal toxic shock-like syndrome as a complication of varicella, *Pediatr Infect Dis J* 10:77, 1991.
199. Brogan TV, Nizet V, Waldhausen JH, et al: Group A streptococcal necrotizing fasciitis complicating primary varicella: a series of fourteen patients, *Pediatr Infect Dis J* 14:588, 1995.

200. Centers for Disease Control and Prevention: Outbreak of invasive group A streptococcus associated with varicella in a childcare center—Boston, Mass, 1997, *MMWR Morb Mortal Wkly Rep* 46:944, 1997.
201. Davies HD, McGeer A, Schwartz B, et al: Invasive group A streptococcal infections in Ontario, Canada, *N Engl J Med* 335:547, 1996.
202. Doctor A, Harper MB, Fleischer GR: Group A beta-hemolytic streptococcal bacteremia: historical review, changing incidence, and recent association with varicella, *Pediatrics* 96:428, 1995.
203. Gonzalez-Ruiz A, Ridgway GL, Cohen SL, et al: Varicella gangrenosa with toxic shock-like syndrome due to group A streptococcus infection in an adult, *Clin Infect Dis* 20:1058, 1995.
204. Mills WJ, Mosca VS, Nizet V: Invasive group A streptococcal infections complicating primary varicella, *J Pediatr Orthop* 16:522, 1996.
205. Peterson CL, Vugia DJ, Meyers HB, et al: Risk factors for invasive group A streptococcal infections in children with varicella: a case-control study, *Pediatr Infect Dis J* 15:151, 1996.
206. Wilson G, Talkington DF, Gruber W, et al: Group A streptococcal necrotizing fasciitis following varicella in children: case reports and review, *Clin Infect Dis* 20:1333, 1995.
207. Johnson R, Milbourn PE: Central nervous system manifestations of chickenpox, *Can Med Assoc J* 102:831, 1970.
208. Jenkins RB: Severe chickenpox encephalopathy, *Am J Dis Child* 110:137, 1965.
209. Ciccone S, Faggioli R, Calzolari F, et al: Stroke after varicella-zoster infection: report of a case and review of the literature, *Pediatr Infect Dis J* 29:864, 2010.
210. Miravet E, Danchaivijitr N, Basu H, et al: Clinical and radiological features of childhood cerebral infarction following varicella zoster virus infection, *Dev Med Child Neurol* 49:417, 2007.
211. Nagel MA, Traktinskiy I, Azarkh Y, et al: Varicella zoster virus vasculopathy: analysis of virus-infected arteries, *Neurology* 77:364, 2011.
212. Nagel MA, Choe A, Khmeleva N, et al: Search for varicella zoster virus and herpes simplex virus-1 in normal human cerebral arteries, *J Neurovirol* 19:181, 2013.
213. Minkowitz S, Wenk R, Friedman E, et al: Acute glomerulonephritis associated with varicella infection, *Am J Med* 44:489, 1968.
214. Yuceoglu AM, Berkovich S, Minkowitz S: Acute glomerular nephritis as a complication of varicella, *JAMA* 202:113, 1967.
215. Morales A, Adelman S, Fine G: Varicella myocarditis, *Arch Pathol* 91:29, 1971.
216. Moore CM, Henry J, Benzing G 3rd, et al: Varicella myocarditis, *Am J Dis Child* 118:899, 1969.
217. Priest JR, Groth KE, Balfour HH: Varicella arthritis documented by isolation of virus from joint fluid, *J Pediatr* 93:990, 1978.
218. Ward JR, Bishop B: Varicella arthritis, *JAMA* 212:1954, 1970.
219. Gershon A: Varicella-zoster virus: prospects for control, *Adv Pediatr Infect Dis* 10:93, 1995.
220. Jura E, Chadwick EG, Josephs SH, et al: Varicella-zoster virus infections in children infected with human immunodeficiency virus, *Pediatr Infect Dis J* 8:586, 1989.
221. Feldman S, Hughes W, Daniel C: Varicella in children with cancer: 77 cases, *Pediatrics* 80:388, 1975.
222. Ihara T, Kamiya H, Starr SE, et al: Natural killing of varicella-zoster virus (VZV)-infected fibroblasts in normal children, children with VZV infections, and children with Hodgkin's disease, *Acta Pediatr Jpn* 31:523, 1989.
223. Arvin A, Sharp M, Smith S, et al: Equivalent recognition of a varicella-zoster virus immediate early protein (IE62) and glycoprotein I by cytotoxic T lymphocytes of either CD4+ or CD8+ phenotype, *J Immunol* 146:257, 1991.
224. Cooper E, Vujcic L, Quinnan G: Varicella-zoster virus-specific HLA-restricted cytotoxicity of normal immune adult lymphocytes after in vitro stimulation, *J Infect Dis* 158:780, 1988.
225. Krugman S, Goodrich C, Ward R: Primary varicella pneumonia, *N Engl J Med* 257:843, 1957.
226. Mermelstein RH, Freireich AW: Varicella pneumonia, *Ann Intern Med* 55:456, 1961.
227. Weber DM, Pellecchia JA: Varicella pneumonia: study of prevalence in adult men, *JAMA* 192:572, 1965.
228. Sargent EN, Carson MJ, Reilly ED: Varicella pneumonia: a report of 20 cases with postmortem examination in 6, *Calif Med* 107:141, 1967.
229. Bocles JS, Ehrenkranz NJ, Marks A: Abnormalities of respiratory function in varicella pneumonia, *Ann Intern Med* 60:183, 1964.
230. Fish SA: Maternal death due to disseminated varicella, *JAMA* 173:978, 1960.
231. Hackel DB: Myocarditis in association with varicella, *Am J Pathol* 29:369, 1953.
232. Harris RE, Rhoades ER: Varicella pneumonia complicating pregnancy: report of a case and review of the literature, *Obstet Gynecol* 25:734, 1965.
233. Brunell PA: Varicella-zoster infections in pregnancy, *JAMA* 199:315, 1967.
234. Baren J, Henneman P, Lewis R: Primary varicella in adults: pneumonia, pregnancy, and hospital admission, *Ann Emerg Med* 28:165, 1996.
235. Siegel M, Fuerst HT: Low birth weight and maternal virus diseases: a prospective study of rubella, measles, mumps, chickenpox, and hepatitis, *JAMA* 197:88, 1966.
236. Harger JH, Ernest JM, Thurnau GR, et al: Risk factors and outcome of varicella-zoster virus pneumonia in pregnant women, *J Infect Dis* 185:422, 2002.
237. Harger JH, Ernest JM, Thurnau GR, et al: Frequency of congenital varicella syndrome in a prospective cohort of 347 pregnant women, *Obstet Gynecol* 100:260, 2002.
238. Esmonde TF, Herdman G, Anderson G: Chickenpox pneumonia: an association with pregnancy, *Thorax* 44:812, 1989.
239. Cox SM, Cunningham FG, Luby J: Management of varicella pneumonia complicating pregnancy, *Am J Perinatol* 7:300, 1990.
240. Smego RA, Asperilla MO: Use of acyclovir for varicella pneumonia during pregnancy, *Obstet Gynecol* 78:1112, 1991.
241. Broussard OF, Payne DK, George RB: Treatment with acyclovir of varicella pneumonia in pregnancy, *Chest* 99:1045, 1991.
242. Pickard RE: Varicella pneumonia in pregnancy, *Am J Obstet Gynecol* 101:504, 1968.
243. Mendelow DA, Lewis GC: Varicella pneumonia during pregnancy, *Obstet Gynecol* 33:98, 1969.
244. Geeves RB, Lindsay DA, Robertson TI: Varicella pneumonia in pregnancy with varicella neonatorum: report of a case followed by severe digital clubbing, *Aust N Z J Med* 1:63, 1971.
245. Siegel M, Fuerst HT, Peress NS: Comparative fetal mortality in maternal virus diseases: a prospective study on rubella, measles, mumps, chickenpox, and hepatitis, *N Engl J Med* 274:768, 1966.
246. Paryani SG, Arvin AM: Intrauterine infection with varicella-zoster virus after maternal varicella, *N Engl J Med* 314:1542, 1986.
247. Figueroa-Damian R, Arrendondo-Garcia JL: Perinatal outcome of pregnancies complicated with varicella infection during the first 20 weeks of gestation, *Am J Perinatol* 14:411, 1997.
248. Landsberger EJ, Hager WD, Grossman JH: Successful management of varicella pneumonia complicating pregnancy: a report of 3 cases, *J Reprod Med* 31:311, 1986.
249. Lotshaw RR, Keegan JM, Gordon HR: Parenteral and oral acyclovir for management of varicella pneumonia in pregnancy: a case report with review of literature, *W V Med J* 87:204, 1991.
250. Hockberger RS, Rothstein RJ: Varicella pneumonia in adults: a spectrum of disease, *Ann Emerg Med* 115:931, 1986.
251. Hollingsworth HM, Pratter MR, Irwin RS: Acute respiratory failure in pregnancy, *J Intensive Care Med* 4:11, 1989.
252. Hankins GDV, Gilstrap LC, Patterson AR: Acyclovir treatment of varicella pneumonia in pregnancy, *Crit Care Med* 15:336, 1987.
253. Glaser JB, Loftus J, Ferragamo V, et al: Varicella in pregnancy, *N Engl J Med* 315:1416, 1986.
254. Boyd K, Walker E: Use of acyclovir to treat chickenpox in pregnancy, *BMJ* 296:393, 1988.
255. White RG: Chickenpox in pregnancy, *BMJ* 196:864, 1988.
256. Eder SE, Apuzzio JA, Weiss G: Varicella pneumonia during pregnancy: treatment of 2 cases with acyclovir, *Am J Perinatol* 5:16, 1988.
257. Andrews EB, Tilson HH, Hurn BA, et al: Acyclovir in pregnancy registry, *Am J Med* 85:123, 1988.
258. Centers for Disease Control and Prevention: Acyclovir registry. *MMWR Morb Mortal Wkly Rep* 42:806, 1993.
259. Pearse BM: Characterization of coated-vesicle adaptors: their reassembly with clathrin and with recycling receptors, *Methods Cell Biol* 31:229, 1989.
260. Marin M, Bialek SR, Seward JF: Updated recommendations for use of VariZIG—United States, 2013, *MMWR Morb Mortal Wkly Rep* 62:574, 2013.
261. Benyesh-Melnick M, Stich HF, Rapp F, et al: Viruses and mammalian chromosomes. III. Effect of herpes zoster virus on human embryonal lung cultures, *Proc Soc Exp Biol Med* 117:546, 1964.

262. Aula P: Chromosomes and virus infections, *Lancet* 1:720, 1964.
263. Massimo I, Vianello MG, Dagna-Bricarelli F, et al: Chickenpox and chromosome aberrations, *BMJ* 2:172, 1965.
264. Collier E: Congenital varicella cataract, *Am J Ophthalmol* 86:627, 1978.
265. Cuthbertson G, Weiner CP, Giller RH, et al: Prenatal diagnosis of second-trimester congenital varicella syndrome by virus-specific immunoglobulin M, *J Pediatr* 111:592, 1987.
266. Harding B, Bonner JA: Congenital varicella-zoster: a serologically proven case with necrotizing encephalitis and malformations, *Acta Neuropathol* 76:311, 1988.
267. Hammad E, Helin I, Pasca A: Early pregnancy varicella and associated congenital anomalies, *Acta Paediatr Scand* 78:963, 1989.
268. Adelstein AM, Donovan JW: Malignant disease in children whose mothers had chickenpox, mumps, or rubella in pregnancy, *BMJ* 2:629, 1972.
269. Fox MJ, Krumpiegel ER, Teresi JL: Maternal measles, mumps, and chickenpox as a cause of congenital anomalies, *Lancet* 1:746, 1948.
270. Jones KL, Johnson KA, Chambers CD: Offspring of women infected with varicella during pregnancy: a prospective study, *Teratology* 49:29, 1994.
271. Pastuszak A, Levy M, Schick B, et al: Outcome after maternal varicella infection in the first 20 weeks of pregnancy, *N Engl J Med* 330:901, 1994.
272. Michie CA, Acolet D, Charlton R, et al: Varicella-zoster contracted in the second trimester of pregnancy, *Pediatr Infect Dis J* 10:1050, 1992.
273. Connan L, Ayoubi J, Icart J, et al: Intra-uterine fetal death following maternal varicella infection, *Eur J Obstet Gynecol* 68:205, 1996.
274. Sauerbrai A, Müller D, Eichhorn U, et al: Detection of varicella-zoster virus in congenital varicella syndrome: a case report, *Obstet Gynecol* 88:687, 1996.
275. Siegel M: Congenital malformations following chickenpox, measles, mumps, and hepatitis: results of a cohort study, *JAMA* 226:1521, 1973.
276. Mouly F, Mirlesse V, Mériteт JF, et al: Prenatal diagnosis of fetal varicella-zoster virus infection with polymerase chain reaction of amniotic fluid in 107 cases, *Am J Obstet Gynecol* 177:894, 1997.
277. Ussery XT, Annunziato P, Gershon AA, et al: Congenital varicella-zoster infection and Barrett's esophagus, *J Infect Dis* 178:539, 1998.
278. LaForet EG, Lynch LL: Multiple congenital defects following maternal varicella, *N Engl J Med* 236:534, 1947.
279. Srabstein JC, Morris N, Larke RP, et al: Is there a congenital varicella syndrome? *J Pediatr* 84:239, 1974.
280. Alfonso I, Palomino JA, DeQuesada G, et al: Picture of the month: congenital varicella syndrome, *Am J Dis Child* 138:603, 1984.
281. Alkalay AL, Pomerance JJ, Yamamura JM, et al: Congenital anomalies associated with maternal varicella infections during early pregnancy, *J Perinatol* 7:69, 1987.
282. Borzykowski M, Harris RF, Jones RWA: The congenital varicella syndrome, *Eur J Pediatr* 137:335, 1981.
283. Dietzsch H, Rabenalt P, Trlifajova J: Varizellen-Embryopathie: kliniche und serologische Verlaufsbeobachtungen. Kinderarztl, *Prax* 3:139, 1980.
284. Fuccillo DA: Congenital varicella, *Teratology* 15:329, 1977.
285. Hajdi G, Mészner Z, Nyerges G, et al: Congenital varicella syndrome, *Infection* 14:177, 1986.
286. McKendry JBJ: Congenital varicella associated with multiple defects, *Can Med Assoc J* 108:66, 1973.
287. Rinvik R: Congenital varicella encephalomyelitis in surviving newborn, *Am J Dis Child* 117:231, 1969.
288. Savage MO, Moosa A, Gordon RR: Maternal varicella infection as a cause of fetal malformations, *Lancet* 1:352, 1973.
289. Schlotfeld-Schafer I, Schaefer P, Flatz S, et al: Congenitales Varicellensyndrom, *Monatsschr Kinderheilkd* 131:106, 1983.
290. Dudgeon HA, editor: *Viral diseases of the fetus and newborn*, Philadelphia, 1982, Saunders, p 161.
291. Enders G: Varicella-zoster virus infection in pregnancy, *Prog Med Virol* 29:166, 1984.
292. Essex-Cater A, Heggarty H: Fatal congenital varicella syndrome, *J Infect* 7:77, 1983.
293. Lamy M, Minkowski A, Choucroun J: Embryopathie d'origine infectieuse, *Semaine Med* 27:989, 1951.
294. Konig R, Gutjahr P, Kruel R, et al: Konnatale varizellen-embryofetopathy, *Helv Paediatr Acta* 40:391, 1985.
295. Scharf A, Scherr O, Enders G, et al: Virus detection in the fetal tissue of a premature delivery with a congenital varicella syndrome, *J Perinat Med* 18:317, 1990.
296. DaSilva O, Hammerberg O, Chance GW: Fetal varicella syndrome, *Pediatr Infect Dis J* 9:854, 1990.
297. Magliocco AM, Demetrick DJ, Sarnat HB, et al: Varicella embryopathy, *Arch Pathol Lab Med* 116:181, 1992.
298. Alexander I: Congenital varicella, *BMJ* 2:1074, 1979.
299. Bailie FB: Aplasia cutis congenita of neck and shoulder requiring a skin graft: a case report, *Br J Plast Surg* 36:72, 1983.
300. Brice JEH: Congenital varicella resulting from infection during second trimester at pregnancy, *Arch Dis Child* 51:474, 1976.
301. Dodion-Fransen J, Dekegel D, Thiry L: Maternal varicella infection as a cause of fetal malformations, *Scand J Infect Dis* 5:149, 1973.
302. Frey H, Bialkin G, Gershon A: Congenital varicella: case report of a serologically proved long-term survivor, *Pediatrics* 59:110, 1977.
303. Pettay O: Intrauterine and perinatal viral infections, *Ann Clin Res* 11:258, 1979.
304. Taranger J, Blomberg J, Strannegard O: Intrauterine varicella: a report of two cases associated with hyper-A-immunoglobulinemia, *Scand J Infect Dis* 13:297, 1981.
305. Unger-Koppel J, Kilcher P, Tonz O: Varizellenfetopathie, *Helv Paediatr Acta* 40:399, 1985.
306. White MI, Daly BM, Moffat MA, et al: Connective tissue naevi in a child with intra-uterine varicella infection, *Clin Exp Dermatol* 15:149, 1990.
307. Palmer CGS, Pauli RM: Intrauterine varicella infection, *J Pediatr* 112:506, 1988.
308. Lambert SR, Taylor D, Kriss A, et al: Ocular manifestations of the congenital varicella syndrome, *Arch Ophthalmol* 107:52, 1989.
309. Bai PVA, John TJ: Congenital skin ulcers following varicella in late pregnancy, *J Pediatr* 94:65, 1979.
310. Klauber GT, Flynn FJ, Altman BD: Congenital varicella syndrome with genitourinary anomalies, *Urology* 8:153, 1976.
311. Michon L, Aubertin D, Jager-Schmidt G: Deux observations de malformations congenitales paraissant relever d'embryopathies zosteriennes, *Arch Fr Pediatr* 16:695, 1959.
312. Enders G: Serodiagnosis of varicella-zoster virus infection in pregnancy and standardisation of the ELISA IgG and IgM antibody tests, *Dev Biol Stand* 52:221, 1982.
313. Charles N, Bennett TW, Margolis S: Ocular pathology of the congenital varicella syndrome, *Arch Ophthalmol* 95:2034, 1977.
314. Andreou A, Basiakos H, Hatzikoumi I, et al: Fetal varicella syndrome with manifestations limited to the eye, *Am J Perinatol* 12:347, 1995.
315. Kotchmar G, Grose C, Brunell P: Complete spectrum of the varicella congenital defects syndrome in 5-year-old child, *Pediatr Infect Dis* 3:142, 1984.
316. Grose C: Congenital varicella-zoster virus infection and the failure to establish virus-specific cell-mediated immunity, *Mol Biol Med* 6:453, 1989.
317. Salzman MB, Sood SK: Congenital anomalies resulting from maternal varicella at 25 and a half weeks of gestation, *Pediatr Infect Dis J* 11:504, 1992.
318. Hitchcock R, Birthistle K, Carrington D, et al: Colonic atresia and spinal cord atrophy associated with a case of fetal varicella syndrome, *J Pediatr Surg* 30:1344, 1995.
319. Lloyd KM, Dunne JL: Skin lesions as the sole manifestation of the fetal varicella syndrome, *Clin Exp Dermatol* 15:149, 1990.
320. Scheffer IE, Baraitser M, Brett EM: Severe microcephaly associated with congenital varicella infection, *Dev Med Child Neurol* 33:916, 1991.
321. Randel R, Kearns DB, Sawyer MH: Vocal cord paralysis as a presentation of intrauterine infection with varicella-zoster virus, *Pediatrics* 97:127, 1996.
322. Bennet R, Forsgren M, Herin P: Herpes zoster in a 2-week-old premature infant with possible congenital varicella encephalitis, *Acta Pediatr Scand* 74:979, 1985.
323. Byrne JLB, Ward K, Kochenour NK, et al: Prenatal sonographic diagnosis of fetal varicella syndrome, *Am J Hum Genet* 47:A470, 1990.
324. Mazzella M, Arioni C, Bellini C, et al: Severe hydrocephalus associated with congenital varicella syndrome, *Can Med Assoc J* 168:561, 2003.
325. Huang CS, Lin SP, Chiu NC, et al: Congenital varicella syndrome as an unusual cause of congenital malformation: report of one case, *Acta Paediatr Taiwan* 42:239, 2001.

326. Dimova PS, Karparov AA: Congenital varicella syndrome: case with isolated brain damage, *J Child Neurol* 16:595, 2001.
327. Kent A, Paes B: Congenital varicella syndrome: a rare case of central nervous system involvement without dermatological features, *Am J Perinatol* 17:253, 2000.
328. Liang CD, Yu TJ, Ko SF: Ipsilateral renal dysplasia with hypertensive heart disease in an infant with cutaneous varicella lesions: an unusual presentation of congenital varicella syndrome, *J Am Acad Dermatol* 43:864, 2000.
329. Cooper C, Wojtulewicz J, Ratnamohan VM, et al: Congenital varicella syndrome diagnosed by polymerase chain reaction—scarring of the spinal cord, not the skin, *J Paediatr Child Health* 36:186, 2000.
330. Choong CS, Patole S, Whitehall J: Congenital varicella syndrome in the absence of cutaneous lesions, *J Paediatr Child Health* 36:184, 2000.
331. Forrest J, Mego S, Burgess M: Congenital and neonatal varicella in Australia, *J Paediatr Child Health* 36:108, 2000.
332. Gaynor EB: Congenital varicella and the newborn cry, *Otolaryngol Head Neck Surg* 104:541, 1991.
333. Taylor WG, Walkinshaw SA, Thompson MA: Antenatal assessment of neurological impairment, *Arch Dis Child* 68:604, 1993.
334. Kerkering KW: Abnormal cry and intracranial calcifications: clues to the diagnosis of fetal varicella-zoster syndrome, *J Perinatol* 21:131, 2001.
335. Hartung J, Enders G, Chaoui R, et al: Prenatal diagnosis of congenital varicella syndrome and detection of varicella-zoster virus in the fetus: a case report, *Prenat Diagn* 19:163, 1999.
336. Hofmeyr GJ, Moolla S, Lawrie T: Prenatal sonographic diagnosis of congenital varicella infection—a case report, *Prenat Diagn* 16:1148, 1996.
337. Petignat P, Vial Y, Laurini R, et al: Fetal varicella-herpes zoster syndrome in early pregnancy: ultrasonographic and morphological correlation, *Prenat Diagn* 21:121, 2001.
338. Verstraelen H, Vanzieleghem B, Defoort P, et al: Prenatal ultrasound and magnetic resonance imaging in fetal varicella syndrome: correlation with pathology findings, *Prenat Diagn* 23:705, 2003.
339. Duehr PA: Herpes zoster as a cause of congenital cataract, *Am J Ophthalmol* 39:157, 1955.
340. Webster MH, Smith CS: Congenital abnormalities and maternal herpes zoster, *BMJ* 4:1193, 1977.
341. Grose C, Itani O, Weiner C: Prenatal diagnosis of fetal infection: advances from amniocentesis to cordocentesis—congenital toxoplasmosis, rubella, cytomegalovirus, varicella virus, parvovirus and human immunodeficiency virus, *Pediatr Infect Dis J* 8:459, 1989.
342. Alkalay AL, Pomerance JJ, Rimoin D: Fetal varicella syndrome, *J Pediatr* 111:320, 1987.
343. Lecuru F, Taurelle R, Bernard JP, et al: Varicella-zoster virus infection during pregnancy: the limits of prenatal diagnosis, *Eur J Obstet Gynecol Reprod Biol* 56:67, 1994.
344. West SL, Newton RW, Baildam EM, et al: Recurrent hemiplegia associated with cerebral vasculopathy following third trimester maternal herpes zoster infection, *Dev Med Child Neurol* 48:991, 2006.
345. Fowler KB, Stagno S, Pass RF, et al: The outcome of congenital cytomegalovirus infection in relation to maternal antibody status, *N Engl J Med* 326:663, 1992.
346. Isada NB, Paar DP, Johnson MP, et al: In utero diagnosis of congenital varicella zoster infection by chorionic villus sampling and polymerase chain reaction, *Am J Obstet Gynecol* 165:1727, 1991.
347. Johansson AB, Rassart A, Blum D, et al: Lower-limb hypoplasia due to intrauterine infection with herpes simplex virus type 2: possible confusion with intrauterine varicella-zoster syndrome, *Clin Infect Dis* 38:e57, 2004.
348. Preblud S, Bregman DJ, Vernon LL: Deaths from varicella in infants, *Pediatr Infect Dis* 4:503, 1985.
349. Rubin L, Leggiadro R, Elie MT, et al: Disseminated varicella in a neonate: implications for immunoprophylaxis of neonates postnatally exposed to varicella, *Pediatr Infect Dis* 5:100, 1986.
350. Kluthe M, Herrera A, Blanca H, et al: Neonatal vaccine-strain varicella-zoster virus infection 22 days after maternal postpartum vaccination, *Pediatr Infect Dis J* 31:977, 2012.
351. Meyers J: Congenital varicella in term infants: risk reconsidered, *J Infect Dis* 129:215, 1974.
352. Hanngren K, Grandien M, Granstrom G: Effect of zoster immunoglobulin for varicella prophylaxis in the newborn, *Scand J Infect Dis* 17:343, 1985.
353. Preblud S, Nelson WL, Levin M, et al: *Modification of congenital varicella infection with VZIG*, New Orleans, September 28-October 1, 1986, 26th Interscience Conference on Antimicrobial Agents and Chemotherapy.
354. Nankervis GA, Gold E: Varicella-zoster viruses. In Kaplan AS, editor: *The herpesviruses*, New York, 1973, Academic Press.
355. Kohl S: The neonatal human's immune response to herpes simplex virus infection: a critical review, *Pediatr Infect Dis J* 8:67, 1989.
356. Winkelman RK, Perry HO: Herpes zoster in children, *JAMA* 171:876, 1959.
357. David T, Williams M: Herpes zoster in infancy, *Scand J Infect Dis* 11:185, 1979.
358. Dworsky M, Whitely R, Alford C: Herpes zoster in early infancy, *Am J Dis Child* 134:618, 1980.
359. Helander I, Arstila P, Terho P: Herpes zoster in a 6-month-old infant, *Acta Dermatol* 63:180, 1982.
360. Lewkonia IK, Jackson AA: Infantile herpes zoster after intrauterine exposure to varicella, *BMJ* 3:149, 1973.
361. Lyday JH: Report of severe herpes zoster in a 13 and one-half-year-old boy whose chickenpox infection may have been acquired in utero, *Pediatrics* 50:930, 1972.
362. Adkisson MA: Herpes zoster in a newborn premature infant, *J Pediatr* 66:956, 1965.
363. Bonar BE, Pearsall CJ: Herpes zoster in the newborn, *Am J Dis Child* 44:398, 1932.
364. Counter CE, Korn BJ: Herpes zoster in the newborn associated with congenital blindness: report of a case, *Arch Pediatr* 67:397, 1950.
365. Feldman GV: Herpes zoster neonatorum, *Arch Dis Child* 27:126, 1952.
366. Freud P, Rook GD, Gurian S: Herpes zoster in the newborn, *Am J Dis Child* 64:895, 1942.
367. Music SI, Fine EM, Togo Y: Zoster-like disease in the newborn due to herpes-simplex virus, *N Engl J Med* 284:24, 1971.
368. Gershon A, Steinberg S, LaRussa P: Varicella-zoster virus. In Lennette EH, editor: *Laboratory diagnosis of viral infections*, New York, 1982, Marcel Dekker.
369. Rawlinson WD, Dwyer DE, Gibbons VL, et al: Rapid diagnosis of varicella-zoster virus infection with a monoclonal antibody based direct immunofluorescence technique, *J Virol Methods* 23:13, 1989.
370. Hughes P, LaRussa P, Pearce JM, et al: Transmission of varicella-zoster virus from a vaccinee with underlying leukemia, demonstrated by polymerase chain reaction, *J Pediatr* 124:932, 1994.
371. Ito M, Nishihara H, Mizutani K, et al: Detection of varicella zoster virus (VZV) DNA in throat swabs and peripheral blood mononuclear cells of immunocompromised patients with herpes zoster by polymerase chain reaction, *Clin Diagn Virol* 4:105, 1995.
372. LaRussa P, Lungu O, Hardy I, et al: Restriction fragment length polymorphism of polymerase chain reaction products from vaccine and wild-type varicella-zoster virus isolates, *J Virol* 66:1016, 1992.
373. LaRussa P, Steinberg S, Gershon A: Diagnosis and typing of varicella-zoster virus (VZV) in clinical specimens by polymerase chain reaction (PCR), Orlando, Fla, October 4-7, 1994, 34th Interscience Conference on Antimicrobial Agents and Chemotherapy.
374. Mahalingham R, Wellish M, Cabirac G, et al: Polymerase chain reaction diagnosis of varicella-zoster virus. In Becker Y, Darai G, editors: *Diagnosis of human viruses by polymerase chain reaction technology*, vol. 1, New York, 1992, Springer-Verlag.
375. Puchhammer-Stockl E, Kunz C, Wagner G, et al: Detection of varicella zoster virus (VZV) in fetal tissue by polymerase chain reaction, *J Perinat Med* 22:65, 1994.
376. Sawyer M, Wu YN: Detection of varicella-zoster virus DNA by polymerase chain reaction in CSF of patients with VZV-related central nervous system complications, New Orleans, October 17-20, 1993, 33rd Interscience Conference on Antimicrobial Agents and Chemotherapy.
377. Annunziato P, Lungu O, Gershon A, et al: In situ hybridization detection of varicella zoster virus in paraffin-embedded skin biopsy specimens, *Clin Diagn Virol* 7:69, 1997.
378. Silliman CC, Tedder D, Ogle JW, et al: Unsuspected varicella-zoster virus encephalitis in a child with acquired immunodeficiency syndrome, *J Pediatr* 123:418, 1993.
379. Gershon AA, LaRussa P: Varicella-zoster virus. In Donowitz LG, editor: *Hospital-acquired infection in the pediatric patient*, Baltimore, 1988, Williams & Wilkins.
380. Le CT, Lipson M: Difficulty in determining varicella-zoster immune status in pregnant women, *Pediatr Infect Dis J* 8:650, 1989.

381. Vasileiadis GT, Roukema HW, Romano W, et al: Intrauterine herpes simplex infection, *Am J Perinatol* 20:55, 2003.
382. Grose C: Congenital infections caused by varicella zoster virus and herpes simplex virus, *Semin Pediatr Neurol* 1:43, 1994.
383. Whitley RJ, Straus S: Therapy for varicella-zoster virus infections. Where do we stand? *Infect Dis Clin Pract* 2:100, 1993.
384. Whitley RJ, Gnann JW: Acyclovir: a decade later, *N Engl J Med* 327:782, 1992.
385. Greffe BS, Dooley SL, Deddish RB, et al: Transplacental passage of acyclovir, *J Pediatr* 108:1020, 1986.
386. Dunkel L, Arvin AM, Whitley RJ, et al: A controlled trial of oral acyclovir for chickenpox in normal children, *N Engl J Med* 325:1539, 1991.
387. Balfour HH, Rotbart HA, Feldman S, et al: Acyclovir treatment of varicella in otherwise healthy adolescents, *J Pediatr* 120:627, 1992.
388. Feder H: Treatment of adult chickenpox with oral acyclovir, *Arch Intern Med* 150:2061, 1990.
389. Wallace MR, Bowler WA, Murray NB, et al: Treatment of adult varicella with oral acyclovir: a randomized, placebo-controlled trial, *Ann Intern Med* 117:358, 1992.
390. Whitley RJ, Middlebrooks M, Gnann JW: Acyclovir: the past ten years, *Adv Exp Med Biol* 278:243, 1990.
391. Whitley R, Arvin A, Prober C, et al: A controlled trial comparing vidarabine with acyclovir in neonatal herpes simplex virus infection, *N Engl J Med* 324:444, 1991.
392. Englund J, Fletcher CV, Balfour HH: Acyclovir therapy in neonates, *J Pediatr* 119:129, 1991.
393. Brunell P, Ross A, Miller LH, et al: Prevention of varicella by zoster immune globulin, *N Engl J Med* 280:1191, 1969.
394. Brunell P, Gershon AA, Hughes WT: Prevention of varicella in high-risk children: a collaborative study, *Pediatrics* 50:718, 1972.
395. Orenstein W, Heymann DL, Ellis RJ, et al: Prophylaxis of varicella in high risk children: response effect of zoster immune globulin, *J Pediatr* 98:368, 1981.
396. Zaia J, Levin MJ, Preblud SK, et al: Evaluation of varicella-zoster immune globulin: protection of immunosuppressed children after household exposure to varicella, *J Infect Dis* 147:737, 1983.
397. Levin MJ, Nelson WL, Preblud SR, et al: Clinical trials with varicella-zoster immunoglobulins. In Movell A, Nydegger U, editors: *Clinical use of intravenous immunoglobulins*, London, 1986, Academic Press, p 255.
398. American Academy of Pediatrics: Varicella-zoster infections. In Pickering LK, Baker CJ, Kimberlin DW, Long SS, editors: *Red book: 2012 report of the Committee on Infectious Diseases*, ed 29, Elk Grove Village, Ill, 2012, American Academy of Pediatrics, p 774.
399. Neustadt A: Congenital varicella, *Am J Dis Child* 106:96, 1963.
400. O'Neill RR: Congenital varicella, *Am J Dis Child* 104:391, 1962.
401. Bakshi S, Miller TC, Kaplan M, et al: Failure of VZIG in modification of severe congenital varicella, *Pediatr Infect Dis* 5:699, 1986.
402. Haddad J, Simeoni U, Willard D: Perinatal varicella, *Lancet* 1:494, 1986.
403. Holland P, Isaacs D, Moxon ER: Fatal neonatal varicella infection, *Lancet* 2:1156, 1986.
404. King S, Miller TC, Kaplan M, et al: Fatal varicella-zoster infection in a newborn treated with varicella-zoster immunoglobulin, *Pediatr Infect Dis* 5:588, 1986.
405. Oglivie MM, Stephens JRD, Larkin M: Chickenpox in pregnancy, *Lancet* 1:915, 1986.
406. Williams H, Latif A, Morgan J, et al: Acyclovir in the treatment of neonatal varicella, *J Infect* 15:65, 1987.
407. Reynolds L, Struik S, Nadel S: Neonatal varicella: varicella zoster immunoglobulin (VZIG) does not prevent disease, *Arch Dis Child Fetal Neonatal Ed* 81:F69, 1999.
408. Fried D, Hanukoglu A, Birk O: Leukocyte transfusion in severe neonatal varicella, *Acta Pediatr Scand* 71:147, 1982.
409. Haddad J, Latif A, Morgan J, et al: Acyclovir in prophylaxis and perinatal varicella, *Lancet* 1:161, 1987.
410. Sills JA, Galloway A, Amegavie L, et al: Acyclovir in prophylaxis and perinatal varicella, *Lancet* 1:161, 1987.
411. Evans EB, Pollock TM, Cradock-Watson JE, et al: Human anti-chickenpox immunoglobulin in the prevention of chickenpox, *Lancet* 1:354, 1980.
412. Miller E, Marshall R, Vurdien J: Epidemiology, outcome and control of varicella-zoster infection, *Rev Med Microbiol* 4:222, 1993.
413. Enders G, Miller E: Varicella and herpes zoster in pregnancy and the newborn. In Arvin A, Gershon A, editors: *Varicella-zoster virus: virology and clinical management*, Cambridge, UK, 2000, Cambridge University Press.
414. Koren G, Money D, Boucher M, et al: Serum concentrations, efficacy, and safety of a new, intravenously administered varicella zoster immune globulin in pregnant women, *J Clin Pharmacol* 42:267, 2002.
415. Winsnes R: Efficacy of zoster immunoglobulin in prophylaxis of varicella in high-risk patients, *Acta Paediatr Scand* 67:77, 1978.
416. Gershon A: Commentary on VZIG in infants, *Pediatr Infect Dis J* 6:469, 1987.
417. Gershon A: Immunoprophylaxis of varicella-zoster infections, *Am J Med* 76:672, 1984.
418. Centers for Disease Control and Prevention: Immunization of health-care personnel: recommendations of the Advisory Committee on Immunization Practices (ACIP), *MMWR Recomm Rep* 60(RR-7):1, 2011.
419. Takahashi M, Otsuka T, Okuno Y, et al: Live vaccine used to prevent the spread of varicella in children in hospital, *Lancet* 2:1288, 1974.
420. Sharrar RG, LaRussa P, Galea SA, et al: The postmarketing safety profile of varicella vaccine, *Vaccine* 19:916, 2000.
421. Chaves SS, Haber P, Walton K, et al: Safety of varicella vaccine after licensure in the United States: experience from reports to the vaccine adverse event reporting system, 1995-2005, *J Infect Dis* 197(Suppl 2):S170, 2008.
422. Seward JF, Marin M, Vasquez M: Varicella vaccine effectiveness in the United States program: a review, *J Infect Dis* 197:S82-S89, 2008.
423. Saiman L, Crowley K, Gershon A: Control of varicella-zoster infections in hospitals. In Abrutyn E, editor: *Infection control reference service*, Philadelphia, 1997, Saunders.
424. Salzman MB, Sharrar RG, Steinberg S, et al: Transmission of varicella-vaccine virus from a healthy 12 month old child to his pregnant mother, *J Pediatr* 131:151, 1997.
425. Weinmann S, Chun C, Schmid DS, et al: Incidence and clinical characteristics of herpes zoster among children in the varicella vaccine era, 2005-2009, *J Infect Dis* 208:2013, 1859.
426. Long S: Toddler-to-mother transmission of varicella-vaccine virus. How bad is that? *J Pediatr* 131:10, 1997.
427. Wain H: *The story behind the word*, Springfield, Ill, 1958, Charles C Thomas.
428. Choppin P, Richardson CD, Merz DC, et al: The functions and inhibition of the membrane glycoproteins of paramyxoviruses and myxoviruses and the role of the measles virus M protein in subacute sclerosing panencephalitis, *J Infect Dis* 143:352, 1981.
429. Rota PA, Liffick SL, Rota JS, et al: Molecular epidemiology of measles viruses in the United States, 1997-2001, *Emerg Infect Dis* 8:902, 2002.
430. Bellini WJ, Icenogle J: Measles and rubella virus. In Murray PR, editor: *Manual of clinical microbiology*, Washington, DC, 2007, American Society for Microbiology Press.
431. Rota PA, Rota JS, Redd SB, et al: Genetic analysis of molecular epidemiology of measles virus isolated in the United States between 1989 and 2001: absence of an endemic genotype since 1994, *J Infect Dis* 189:S160, 2004.
432. Collier M, Cierzniewski A, Duszynski T, et al: Measles outbreak associated with international travel, Indiana, 2011, *J Pediatric Infect Dis Soc* 2:110, 2013.
433. Parker Fiebelkorn A, Redd SB, Gallagher K, et al: Measles in the United States during the postelimination era, *J Infect Dis* 202:1520, 2010.
434. Rota PA, Featherstone DA, Bellini WJ: Molecular epidemiology of measles virus [review], *Curr Top Microbiol Immunol* 330:129, 2009.
435. Cohen BJ, Parry RP, Doblas D, et al: Measles immunity testing: comparison of two measles IgG ELISAs with plaque reduction neutralisation assay, *J Virol Methods* 131:209, 2006.
436. Weigle K, Murphy D, Brunell P: Enzyme-linked immunosorbent assay for evaluation of immunity to measles virus, *J Clin Microbiol* 19:376, 1984.
437. Uzicanin A, Lubega I, Nanuynja M, et al: Dried blood spots on filter paper as an alternative specimen for measles diagnostics: detection of measles immunoglobulin M antibody by a commercial enzyme immunoassay, *J Infect Dis* 204(Suppl 1):S564, 2011.

438. Warrener L, Slibinskas R, Chua KB, et al: A point-of-care test for measles diagnosis: detection of measles-specific IgM antibodies and viral nucleic acid, *Bull World Health Organ* 89:675, 2011.
439. Strebel PM, Papania MJ, Fiebelkorn AP, et al: Measles vaccines. In Plotkin S, Orenstein WA, Offit P, editors: *Vaccines*, ed 6, Philadelphia, 2012, Saunders, p 352.
440. Fine PE, Mulholland K: Community immunity. In Plotkin S, Orenstein WA, Offit P, editors: *Vaccines*, ed 6, Philadelphia, 2012, Saunders, p 1395.
441. Perry RT, Halsey NA: The clinical significance of measles: a review, *J Infect Dis* 189(Suppl 1):S4, 2004.
442. Papp K: Experiences prouvant que la voie d'infection de la rougeole est la contamination de la musqueuse conjunctivale, *Rev Immunol* 20:27, 1956.
443. Leonard VH, Sinn PL, Hodge G, et al: Measles virus blind to its epithelial cell receptor remains virulent in rhesus monkeys but cannot cross the airway epithelium and is not shed, *J Clin Invest* 118:2448, 2008.
444. Strebel PM, Cochi SL, Hoekstra E, et al: A world without measles, *J Infect Dis* 204(Suppl 1):S1, 2011.
445. Morley DC, Woodland M, Martin WJ: Measles in Nigerian children: a study of the disease in West Africa, and its manifestations in England and other countries during different epochs, *J Hyg Lond* 61:113, 1963.
446. Babbott FL Jr, Gordon JE: Modern measles, *Am J Med Sci* 225:334, 1954.
447. Simons E, Ferrari M, Fricks J, et al: Assessment of the 2010 global measles mortality reduction goal: results from a model of surveillance data, *Lancet* 379:2173, 2012.
448. Wolfson LJ, Grais RF, Luquero FJ, et al: Estimates of measles case fatality ratios: a comprehensive review of community-based studies, *Int J Epidemiol* 38:192, 2009.
449. Orenstein WA, Hinman AR: Measles: the burden of preventable deaths, *Lancet* 379:2130, 2012.
450. Orenstein WA, Papania MJ, Wharton ME: Measles elimination in the United States, *J Infect Dis* 189(Suppl 1):S1, 2004.
451. Atkinson WL, Orenstein WA, Krugman S: The resurgence of measles in the United States, 1989-1990, *Annu Rev Med* 43:451, 1992.
452. Centers for Disease Control and Prevention, 2013 Prevention of measles, rubella, congenital rubella syndrome and mumps: Summary recommendations of the Advisory Committee on Immunization Practices (ACIP), *MMWR Morb Mortal Wkly Rep* 62(RR-04):1, 2013.
453. Hickman CJ, Hyde TB, Sowers SB, et al: Laboratory characterization of measles virus infection in previously vaccinated and unvaccinated individuals, *J Infect Dis* 204(Suppl 1):S549, 2011.
454. Dine MS, Hutchins SS, Thomas A, et al: Persistence of vaccine-induced antibody to measles 26-33 years after vaccination, *J Infect Dis* 189(Suppl 1):S123, 2004.
455. LeBaron CW, Beeler J, Sullivan BJ, et al: Persistence of measles antibodies after 2 doses of measles vaccine in a postelimination environment, *Arch Pediatr Adolesc Med* 161:294, 2007.
456. Centers for Disease Control and Prevention: Measles—United States, January 1-August 24, 2013, *MMWR Morb Mortal Wkly Rep* 62:741, 2013.
457. Centers for Disease Control and Prevention: Documentation and verification of measles, rubella and congenital rubella syndrome elimination in the region of the Americas. United States Nat Rep March 28, 2012, Available at http://www.cdc.gov/measles/downloads/Report-elimination-measles-rubella-crs.pdf. Accessed May 6, 2014.
458. Centers for Disease Control and Prevention: National, state, and local area vaccination coverage among children aged 19-35 months—United States, 2012, *MMWR Morb Mortal Wkly Rep* 6:733, 2013.
459. Arciuolo RJ, Brantley TR, Asfaw MM, et al: Notes from the field: measles outbreak among members of a religious community—Brooklyn, New York, March-June 2013, *MMWR Morb Mortal Wkly Rep* 62:752, 2013.
460. Peruzzo M, Giannini O, Bianchetti MG: Measles in a mother and her newborn baby, *Arch Dis Child* 97:660, 2012.
461. Biron C, Beaudeax O, Ponge A, et al: Measles in the Nantes teaching hospital during the 2008-2009 epidemic, *Med Mal Infect* 41:415, 2011.
462. Giusti D, Burette J, Nguyen Y, et al: Virological diagnosis and management of two cases of congenital measles, *J Med Virol* 85:2136, 2013.
463. Ohji G, Satoh H, Satoh H, et al: Congenital measles caused by transplacental infection, *Pediatr Infect Dis J* 28:166, 2009.
464. Berg RB, Rosenthal MS: Propagation of measles virus in suspensions of human and monkey leukocytes, *Proc Soc Exp Biol Med* 106:581, 1961.
465. Suringa DWR, Bank LJ, Ackerman AB: Role of measles virus in skin lesions and Koplik's spots, *N Engl J Med* 283:1139, 1970.
466. Debre R, Celers J: Measles: pathogenicity and epidemiology. In Debre R, Celers J, editors: *Clinical virology*, Philadelphia, 1970, Saunders.
467. Mitus A, Enders JF, Craig JM, et al: Persistence of measles virus and depression of antibody formation in patients with giant cell pneumonia after measles, *N Engl J Med* 261:882, 1959.
468. Enders J, McCarthy K, Mitus A, et al: Isolation of measles virus at autopsy in cases of giant cell pneumonia without rash, *N Engl J Med* 261:875, 1959.
469. Lachmann P: Immunopathology of measles, *Proc R Soc Med* 67:12, 1974.
470. Stillerman M, Thalhimer W: Attack rate and incubation period of measles, *Am J Dis Child* 67:15, 1944.
471. Baugess H: Measles transmitted by blood transfusion, *Am J Dis Child* 27:256, 1924.
472. Littauer J, Sorensen K: The measles epidemic at Umanak in Greenland in 1962, *Dan Med Bull* 12:43, 1965.
473. Kutty P, Rota J, Bellini W: Manual for the surveillance of vaccine-preventable diseases, ed 6, Chapter 7, "Measles," 2013. Available at http://www.cdc.gov/vaccines/pubs/surv-manual/chpt07-measles.html. Accessed May 6, 2014.
474. Warthin AS: Occurrence of numerous large giant cells in tonsils and pharyngeal mucosa in prodromal stage of measles: report of four cases, *Arch Pathol* 11:864, 1932.
475. Moroi K, Saito S, Kurata T, et al: Fetal death associated with measles virus infection of the placenta, *Am J Obstet Gynecol* 164:1107, 1991.
476. La Boccetta AC, Tornay AS: Measles encephalitis: report of 61 cases, *Am J Dis Child* 107:247, 1964.
477. Musser JH, Hauser GH: Encephalitis as a complication of measles, *JAMA* 90:1267, 1928.
478. Pearl PL, Abu-Farsakh H, Starke JR, et al: Neuropathology of two fatal cases of measles in the 1988–1989 Houston epidemic, *Pediatr Neurol* 6:126, 1990.
479. Jahnke U, Fischer EH, Alvord EC: Hypothesis—certain viral proteins contain encephalitogenic and/or neuritogenic sequences, *J Neuropathol Exp Neurol* 44:320, 1985.
480. Kipps A, Dick G, Moodie JW: Measles and the central nervous system, *Lancet* 2:1406, 1983.
481. Gremillion DH, Crawford GE: Measles pneumonia in young adults: an analysis of 106 cases, *Am J Med* 71:539, 1981.
482. Centers for Disease Control and Prevention: Measles surveillance, *MMWR Morb Mortal Wkly Rep* 9, 1973.
483. Gindler J, Tinker S, Markowitz L, et al: Acute measles mortality in the United States, 1987-2002, *J Infect Dis* 189(Suppl 1):S69, 2004.
484. Christensen PE, Schmidt H, Bang HO, et al: An epidemic of measles in southern Greenland, 1951, *Acta Med Scand* 144:430, 1953.
485. Mortamet G, Dina J, Freymuth F, et al: Measles in France, *Arch Pediatr* 19:1269, 2012.
486. Krasinski K, Borkowsky W: Measles and measles immunity in children infected with human immunodeficiency virus, *JAMA* 261:2512, 1989.
487. Embree JE, Datta P, Stackiw W, et al: Increased risk of early measles in infants of human immunodeficiency type 1-seropositive mothers, *J Infect Dis* 165:262, 1992.
488. Angel JB, Walpita P, Lerch RA, et al: Vaccine-associated measles pneumonitis in an adult with AIDS, *Ann Intern Med* 129:104, 1998.
489. Kaplan LJ, Daum RS, Smaron M, et al: Severe measles in immunocompromised patients, *JAMA* 267:1237, 1992.
490. Kernahan J, McQuillin J, Craft A: Measles in children who have malignant disease, *BMJ* 295:15, 1987.
491. Breitfeld V, Hashida Y, Sherman FE, et al: Fatal measles infection in children with leukemia, *Lab Invest* 28:279, 1973.
492. Enders M, Biber M, Exler S: Measles, mumps and rubella virus infection in pregnancy. Possible adverse effects on pregnant women, pregnancy outcome and the fetus, *Bundesgesundheitsblatt Gesundheitsforschung Gesundheitsschutz* 50:1393, 2007.
493. Greenhill JP: Acute (extragenital) infections in pregnancy, labor, and the puerperium, *Am J Obstet Gynecol* 25:760, 1933.
494. Nouvat JR: *Rougeole et grossesse [medical thesis]*, Bordeaux, 1904, France.
495. Dyer I: Measles complicating pregnancy: report of 24 cases with three instances of congenital measles, *South Med J* 33:601, 1940.

496. Packer AD: The influence of maternal measles (morbilli) on the newborn child, *Med J Aust* 1:835, 1950.
497. Atmar RL, Englund JA, Hammill H: Complications of measles during pregnancy, *Clin Infect Dis* 14:217, 1992.
498. Eberhart-Phillips JE, Frederick PD, Baron RC, et al: Measles in pregnancy: a descriptive study of 58 cases, *Obstet Gynecol* 82:797, 1993.
499. Nichols WW, Levan A, Hall B, Ostergren G: Measles-associated chromosome breakage. Preliminary communication, *Hereditas* 48:367, 1962.
500. Miller ZB: Chromosome abnormalities in measles, *Lancet* 2:1070, 1963.
501. Higurashi M, Tamura T, Nakatake T: Cytogenic observations in cultured lymphocytes from patients with Down's syndrome and measles, *Pediatr Res* 7:582, 1973.
502. Jespersen CS, Littauer J, Sigild U: Measles as a cause of fetal defects, *Acta Pediatr Scand* 66:367, 1977.
503. Gazala E, Karplus M, Sarov I: The effect of maternal measles on the fetus, *Pediatr Infect Dis* 4:202, 1985.
504. Rones B: The relationship of German measles during pregnancy to congenital ocular defects, *Med Ann DC* 13:285, 1944.
505. Swan C, Tostevin AL, Moore B, et al: Congenital defects in infants following infectious diseases during pregnancy, with special reference to relationship between German measles and cataract, deaf mutism, heart disease and microcephaly, and to period in pregnancy in which occurrence of rubella was followed by congenital abnormalities, *Med J Aust* 2:201, 1943.
506. Stillerman M, Marks HH, Thalhimer W: Prophylaxis of measles with convalescent serum, *Am J Dis Child* 67:1, 1944.
507. Canelli AF: Sur le comportement normal et pathologique de l'immunity antimorbilleuse chez le nourison jeune, *Rev Fr Pediatr* 5:668, 1929.
508. Ronaldson GW: Measles at confinement with subsequent modified attack in the child, *Br J Child Dis* 23:192, 1926.
509. Kohn JL: Measles in newborn infants (maternal infection), *J Pediatr* 23:192, 1933.
510. Narita M, Togashi T, Kikuta H: Neonatal measles in Hokkaido, Japan, *Pediatr Infect Dis J* 16:908, 1997.
511. Betta Ragazzi SL, De Andrade Vaz-de-Lima LR, Rota P, et al: Congenital and neonatal measles during an epidemic in São Paulo, Brazil in 1997, *Pediatr Infect Dis J* 24:377, 2005.
512. Nakata Y, Nakayama T, Ide Y, et al: Measles virus genome detected up to four months in a case of congenital measles, *Acta Paediatr* 91:1263, 2002.
513. Catanzaro A, Jackson M: Rapidly progressive subacute sclerosing panencephalitis in perinatally acquired measles virus infection, *Lancet* 345:8957, 1995.
514. Cruzado D, Masserey-Spicher V, Roux L, et al: Early onset and rapidly progressive subacute sclerosing panencephalitis after congenital measles infection, *Eur J Pediatr* 161:438, 2002.
515. Dasopoulou M, Covanis A: Subacute sclerosing panencephalitis after intrauterine infection, *Acta Paediatr* 93:1251, 2004.
516. Simsek E, Oztürk A, Yavuz C, et al: Subacute sclerosing panencephalitis (SSPE) associated with congenital measles infection, *Turk J Pediatr* 47:58, 2005.
517. Sawaishi Y, Abe T, Yano T, et al: SSPE following neonatal measles infection, *Pediatr Neurol* 20:63, 1999.
518. Zwiauer K, Forstenpointner E, Popow-Kraupp T, et al: Rapid progressive subacute sclerosing panencephalitis after perinatally acquired measles virus infection, *Lancet* 345:1124, 1995.
519. Yoshida M, Matsuda H, Furuya K: Two cases of measles in pregnant women immediately preceding delivery (case reports), *Clin Exp Obstet Gynecol* 38:177, 2011.
520. Richardson DL: Measles contracted in utero, *R I Med J* 3:13, 1920.
521. Muhlbauer B, Berns LM, Singer A: Congenital measles—1982, *Isr J Med Sci* 19:987, 1983.
522. Noren GR, Adams P Jr, Anderson RC: Positive skin reactivity to mumps virus antigen in endocardial fibroelastosis, *J Pediatr* 62:604, 1963.
523. Helfand RF, Heath JL, Anderson LJ, et al: Diagnosis of measles with an IgM capture EIA: the optimal timing of specimen collection after rash onset, *J Infect Dis* 175:195, 1997.
524. Rossier E, Miller H, McCulloch B, et al: Comparison of immunofluorescence and enzyme immunoassay for detection of measles-specific immunoglobulin M antibody, *J Clin Microbiol* 29:1069, 1991.
525. Abreo F, Bagby J: Sputum cytology in measles infection: a case report, *Acta Cytol* 35:719, 1991.
526. Lightwood R, Nolan R: Epithelial giant cells in measles as an aid in diagnosis, *J Pediatr* 77:59, 1970.
527. Llanes-Rodas R, Liu C: Rapid diagnosis of measles from urinary sediments stained with fluorescent antibody, *N Engl J Med* 275:516, 1966.
528. Minnich LL, Goodenough F, Ray CG: Use of immunofluorescence to identify measles virus infections, *J Clin Microbiol* 29:1148, 1991.
529. Smaron MF, Saxon E, Wood L, et al: Diagnosis of measles by fluorescent antibody and culture of nasopharyngeal secretions, *J Virol Methods* 33:223, 1991.
530. Arrieta C, Zaleska M, Stutman HR, et al: Vitamin A levels in children with measles in Long Beach, California, *J Pediatr* 121:75, 1992.
531. Frieden TR, Sowell AL, Henning KJ, et al: Vitamin A levels and severity of measles, *Am J Dis Child* 146:182, 1992.
532. Hussey GD, Klein M: A randomized, controlled trial of vitamin A in children with severe measles, *N Engl J Med* 323:160, 1990.
533. Forni AL, Schluger NW, Roberts RB: Severe measles pneumonitis in adults: evaluation of clinical characteristics and therapy with intravenous ribavirin, *Clin Infect Dis* 19:454, 1994.
534. Mustafa MM, Weitman SD, Winick NJ, et al: Subacute measles encephalitis in the young immunocompromised host: report of two cases diagnosed by polymerase chain reaction and treated with ribavirin and review of the literature, *Clin Infect Dis* 16:654, 1993.
535. Goetz MB, Mathisen GE: Clinical course and treatment of adults with severe measles pneumonitis, *Clin Infect Dis* 21:443, 1995.
536. Audet S, Virata-Theimer ML, Beeler JA, et al: Measles-virus-neutralizing antibodies in intravenous immunoglobulins, *J Infect Dis* 194:781, 2006.
537. Chui LL, Marusyk RG, Pabst HF: Measles virus specific antibody in infants in a highly vaccinated society, *J Med Virol* 33:199, 1991.
538. Pabst HF, Spady DW, Marusyk RG, et al: Reduced measles immunity in infants in a well-vaccinated population, *Pediatr Infect Dis J* 11:525, 1992.
539. Lennon J, Black F: Maternally derived measles immunity in sera of vaccine-protected mothers, *J Pediatr* 108:671, 1986.
540. Peltola H, Heinonen OP: Frequency of true adverse reactions to measles-mumps-rubella vaccine. A double-blind placebo-controlled trial in twins, *Lancet* 1:939, 1986.
541. Uzicanin A, Zimmerman L: Field effectiveness of live attenuated measles-containing vaccines: a review of published literature, *J Infect Dis* 204(Suppl 1):S133, 2011.
542. Gudnadottir M, Black FL: Measles vaccination in adults with and without complicating conditions, *Arch Gesamte Virusforsch* 16:521, 1965.
543. Hornig M, Briese T, Buie T, et al: Lack of association between measles virus vaccine and autism with enteropathy: a case-control study, *PLoS One* 3:e3140, 2008.
544. DeStefano F: Vaccines and autism: evidence does not support a causal association, *Clin Pharmacol Ther* 82:756, 2007.
545. Board of Health Promotion and Disease Prevention: *Institute of Medicine, Immunization Safety Review Committee: Immunization safety review. Vaccines and autism*, Washington, DC, 2004, National Academies Press.
546. Coughlan S, Connell J, Cohen B, et al: Suboptimal measles-mumps-rubella vaccination coverage facilitates an imported measles outbreak in Ireland, *Clin Infect Dis* 35:84, 2002.
547. Editorial team: Measles once again endemic in the United Kingdom. *Euro Surveill* 2008;13:pii:18919. Available at http://www.eurosurveillance.org/ViewArticle.aspx?ArticleId=18919. Accessed May 6, 2014.
548. Vivancos R, Keenan A, Farmer S, et al: An ongoing large outbreak of measles in Merseyside, England, January to June 2012. *Euro Surveill* 2012:17:pii:20226. Erratum in *Euro Surveill* 2012:17: pii:20235.
549. Lacobucci G: Government launches campaign to give MMR vaccine to a million children in England, *BMJ* 346:f2696, 2013.
550. National and state vaccination coverage among adolescents aged 13-17 years—United States, 2012, *MMWR Morb Mortal Wkly Rep* 62:685, 2013.
551. Krugman S, Giles JP, Friedman H: Studies on immunity to measles, *J Pediatr* 66:471, 1965.
552. McQuillan GM, Kruszon-Moran D, Hyde TB, et al: Seroprevalence of measles antibody in the US population, 1999-2004, *J Infect Dis* 196:1459, 2007.
553. Gans HA, Yasukawa LL, Alderson A, et al: Humoral and cell-mediated immune responses to an early 2-dose measles vaccination regimen in the United States, *J Infect Dis* 190:83, 2004.

554. Siegel JD, Rhinehart E, Jackson M, et al: Healthcare Infection Control Practices Advisory Committee: Guideline for isolation precautions: preventing transmission of infectious agents in healthcare settings, 2007. Available at http://www.cdc.gov/hicpac/pdf/isolation/Isolation2007.pdf Accessed May 6, 2014.
555. Orvell C: The reactions of monoclonal antibodies with structural proteins of mumps virus, *J Immunol* 132:2622, 1984.
556. Lennette E: *Laboratory diagnosis of viral infections*, New York, 1992, Marcel Dekker.
557. Boddicker JD, Rota PA, Kreman T, et al: Real-time reverse transcription-PCR assay for detection of mumps virus RNA in clinical specimens, *J Clin Microbiol* 45:2902, 2007.
558. Reid F, Hassan J, Irwin F, et al: Epidemiologic and diagnostic evaluation of a recent mumps outbreak using oral fluid samples, *J Clin Virol* 41:134, 2008.
559. Parker Fiebelkorn A, Barskey AE, Hickman C, et al: Manual for the surveillance of vaccine-preventable diseases. ed 5, Chapter 9, “Mumps,” 2012. Available at http://www.cdc.gov/vaccines/pubs/surv-manual/chpt09-mumps.pdf. Accessed May 6, 2014.
560. Anderson LJ, Seward JF: Mumps epidemiology and immunity: the anatomy of a modern epidemic, *Pediatr Infect Dis J* 27(Suppl 10): S75S79, 2008.
561. Dayan GH, Quinlisk MP, Parker AA, et al: Recent resurgence of mumps in the United States, *N Engl J Med* 358:1580, 2008.
562. Centers for Disease Control and Prevention: Mumps outbreak on a university campus—California, 2011, *MMWR Morb Mortal Wkly Rep* 61:986, 2012.
563. Barskey AE, Schulte C, Rosen JB, et al: Mumps outbreak in Orthodox Jewish communities in the United States, *N Engl J Med* 367:1704, 2012.
564. Nelson GE, Aguon A, Valencia E, et al: Epidemiology of a mumps outbreak in a highly vaccinated island population and use of a third dose of measles-mumps-rubella vaccine for outbreak control—Guam 2009 to 2010, *Pediatr Infect Dis J* 32:374, 2013.
565. Ogbuanu IU, Kutty PK, Hudson JM, et al: Impact of a third dose of measles-mumps-rubella vaccine on a mumps outbreak, *Pediatrics* 130:e1567, 2012.
566. Greenland K, Whelan J, Fanoy E, et al: Mumps outbreak among vaccinated university students associated with a large party, the Netherlands, 2010, *Vaccine* 30:4676, 2012.
567. Bangor-Jones RD, Dowse GK, Giele CM, et al: A prolonged mumps outbreak among highly vaccinated Aboriginal people in the Kimberley region of Western Australia, *Med J Aust* 191:398, 2009.
568. Philip RN, Reinhard KR, Lackman DB: Observations on a mumps epidemic in a “virgin” population, *Am J Epidemiol* 69:91, 1959.
569. Reed D, Brown G, Merrick R, et al: A mumps epidemic on St. George Island, Alaska, *JAMA* 199:113, 1967.
570. Falk WA, Buchan K, Dow M, et al: The epidemiology of mumps in southern Alberta 1980-1982, *Am J Epidemiol* 130:736, 1989.
571. Garcia A, Pereira JM, Vidigal N, et al: Intrauterine infection with mumps virus, *Obstet Gynecol* 56:756, 1980.
572. Chiba Y, Ogra PA, Nakao T: Transplacental mumps infection, *Am J Obstet Gynecol* 122:904, 1975.
573. Monif GR: Maternal mumps infection during gestation: observations on the progeny, *Am J Obstet Gynecol* 121:549, 1974.
574. Yamauchi T, Wilson C, St Geme JW Jr: Transmission of live, attenuated mumps virus to the human placenta, *N Engl J Med* 290:710, 1974.
575. Connolly NK: Mumps orchitis without parotitis in infants, *Lancet* 1:69, 1953.
576. Everberg G: Deafness following mumps, *Acta Otolaryngol* 48:397, 1957.
577. Bowers D: Mumps during pregnancy, *West J Surg Obstet Gynecol* 61:72, 1953.
578. Greenberg MW, Beilly JS: Congenital defects in the infant following mumps during pregnancy, *Am J Obstet Gynecol* 57:805, 1949.
579. Hardy JB: Viral infection in pregnancy: a review, *Am J Obstet Gynecol* 93:1052, 1965.
580. Homans A: Mumps in a pregnant woman: premature labor, followed by the appearance of the same disease in the infant, twenty-four hours after its birth, *Am J Med Sci* 29:56, 1855.
581. Moore JH: Epidemic parotitis complicating late pregnancy: report of a case, *JAMA* 97:1625, 1931.
582. Schwartz HA: Mumps in pregnancy, *Am J Obstet Gynecol* 60:875, 1950.
583. Siddall RS: Epidemic parotitis in late pregnancy, *Am J Obstet Gynecol* 33:524, 1937.
584. Ylinen O, Jervinen PA: Parotitis during pregnancy, *Acta Obstet Gynecol Scand* 32:121, 1953.
585. Kilham L: Mumps virus in human milk and in milk of infected monkey, *Am J Obstet Gynecol* 33:524, 1951.
586. Kurtz J, Tomlinson A, Pearson J: Mumps virus isolated from a fetus, *BMJ* 284:471, 1982.
587. Dutta PC: A fatal case of pregnancy complicated with mumps, *J Obstet Gynaecol Br Emp* 42:869, 1935.
588. Swan C: Congenital malformations associated with rubella and other virus infections. In Banks HS, editor: *Modern practice in infectious fevers*, New York, 1951, PB Hoeber.
589. Hyatt H: Relationship of maternal mumps to congenital defects and fetal deaths, and to maternal morbidity and mortality, *Am Pract Dig Treat* 12:359, 1961.
590. Robertson GG, Williamson AP, Blattner RJ: Origin and development of lens cataracts in mumps-infected chick embryos, *Am J Anat* 115:473, 1964.
591. St Geme JW Jr, Davis CW, Peralta HJ, et al: The biologic perturbations of persistent embryonic mumps virus infection, *Pediatr Res* 7:541, 1973.
592. Johnson RT, Johnson KP, Edmonds CJ: Virus-induced hydrocephalus: development of aqueductal stenosis in hamsters after mumps infection, *Science* 157:1066, 1967.
593. Holowach J, Thurston DL, Becker B: Congenital defects in infants following mumps during pregnancy: a review of the literature and a report of chorioretinitis due to fetal infection, *J Pediatr* 50:689, 1957.
594. Grenvall H, Selander P: Some virus diseases during pregnancy and their effect on the fetus, *Nord Med* 37:409, 1948.
595. Baumann B, Danon L, Weitz R, et al: Unilateral hydrocephalus due to obstruction of the foramen of Monro. Another complication of intrauterine mumps infection, *Eur J Pediatr* 139:158, 1982.
596. Timmons G, Johnson K: Aqueductal stenosis and hydrocephalus after mumps encephalitis, *N Engl J Med* 283:1505, 1970.
597. Manson MM, Logan WPD, Loy RM: *Rubella and other virus infections during pregnancy*, London, 1960, Her Majesty's Stationery Office.
598. St Geme J Jr, Noren GR, Adams P: Proposed embryopathic relation between mumps virus and primary endocardial fibroelastosis, *N Engl J Med* 275:339, 1966.
599. Finland M: Mumps. In Charles D, Finland M, editors: *Obstetric and perinatal infections*, Philadelphia, 1973, Lea & Febiger.
600. Calabrese F, Rigo E, Milanesi O, et al: Molecular diagnosis of myocarditis and dilated cardiomyopathy in children: clinicopathologic features and prognostic implications, *Diagn Mol Pathol* 11:212, 2002.
601. Ni J, Bowles NE, Kim YH, et al: Viral infection of the myocardium in endocardial fibroelastosis: molecular evidence for the role of mumps virus as an etiologic agent, *Circulation* 95:133, 1997.
602. Zardini V: Eccezionale casso di parotite epidemica in neonato da madre convalescente della stessa malattia, *Lattante* 33:767, 1962.
603. Shouldice D, Mintz S: Mumps in utero, *Can Nurse* 51:454, 1955.
604. Jones JF, Ray G, Fulginiti VA: Perinatal mumps infection, *J Pediatr* 96:912, 1980.
605. Reman O, Freymuth F, Laloum D, et al: Neonatal respiratory distress due to mumps, *Arch Dis Child* 61:80, 1986.
606. Sahdev S, Roth P, Arroyo SE: Congenital mumps pneumonia and persistent pulmonary hypertension, *Pediatr Infect Dis J* 30:272, 2011.
607. Groenendaal F, Rothbarth PH, van den Anker JN, et al: Congenital mumps pneumonia: a rare cause of neonatal respiratory distress, *Acta Paediatr Scand* 79:1252, 1990.
608. Meyer MB: An epidemiologic study of mumps: its spread in schools and families, *Am J Hyg* 75:259, 1962.
609. Hoen E: Mumpsinfektion beim jungen Sugling, *Kinderprtzl* 36:27, 1968.
610. Harris RW, Turnbull CD, Isacson P, et al: Mumps in a Northeast metropolitan community: epidemiology of clinical mumps, *Am J Epidemiol* 88:224, 1968.
611. Hodes D, Brunell P: Mumps antibody: placental transfer and disappearance during the first year of life, *Pediatrics* 45:99, 1970.
612. Barskey AE, Juieng P, Whitaker BL, et al: Viruses detected among sporadic cases of parotitis, United States, 2009-2011, *J Infect Dis* 208:2013, 1979.
613. Sanford HN, Shmigelsky II: Purulent parotitis in the newborn, *J Pediatr* 26:149, 1945.
614. Peltola H, Jokinen S, Paunio M, et al: Measles, mumps, and rubella in Finland: 25 years of a nationwide elimination programme, *Lancet Infect Dis* 8:796, 2008.

615. Wharton M, Cochi SL, Hutcheson RH, et al: Mumps transmission in hospitals, *Arch Intern Med* 150:47, 1990.
616. Gilroy SA, Domachowske JB, Johnson L, et al: Mumps exposure of a health care provider working in a neonatal intensive care unit leads to a hospital-wide effort that prevented an outbreak, *Am J Infect Control* 39:697, 2011.
617. Bonebrake AL, Silkaitis C, Monga G, et al: Effects of mumps outbreak in hospital, Chicago, Illinois, USA, 2006, *Emerg Infect Dis* 16:426, 2010.
618. Brunell PA, Brickman A, O'Hare D, et al: Ineffectiveness of isolation of patients as a method of preventing the spread of mumps, *N Engl J Med* 279:1357, 1968.
619. Kutty PK, Kyaw MH, Dayan GH, et al: Guidance for isolation precautions for mumps in the United States: a review of the scientific basis for policy change, *Clin Infect Dis* 50:1619, 2010.
620. Centers for Disease Control and Prevention: Updated recommendations for isolation of persons with mumps, *MMWR Morb Mortal Wkly Rep* 57:1103, 2008.
621. Fiebelkorn AP, Lawler J, Curns AT, et al: Mumps postexposure prophylaxis with a third dose of measles-mumps-rubella vaccine, Orange County, New York, USA, *Emerg Infect Dis* 19:1411, 2013.

24 Cytomegalovirus

WILLIAM BRITT

CHAPTER OUTLINE

Human cytomegaloviruses (HCMV) comprise a group of agents in the herpesvirus family known for their ubiquitous distribution in humans and in numerous other mammals. In vivo and in vitro infections with CMV are highly species specific and result in a characteristic cytopathology of greatly enlarged (cytomegalic) cells containing intranuclear and cytoplasmic inclusions.[1] The strikingly large, inclusion-bearing cells with a typical owl's eye appearance were first reported by Ribbert[2] in 1881 from the kidneys of a stillborn infant with congenital syphilis. Subsequently, Jesionek and Kiolemenoglou[3] reported similar findings for another stillborn infant with congenital syphilis. In 1907, Lowenstein[4] described inclusions in 4 of 30 parotid glands obtained from children from 2 months to 2 years of age. Subsequently, Goodpasture and Talbot[5] noted the similarity of these cells to the inclusion-bearing cells (giant cells) found in cutaneous lesions caused by varicella virus, and they postulated that cytomegaly was the result of a similar agent. The observation of a similar cytopathic effect after infection with herpes simplex virus (HSV) led Lipschutz[6] and then others to suggest that these characteristic cellular changes were a specific reaction of the host to infection with a virus. The observation by Cole and Kuttner[7] that inclusion-bearing salivary glands from older guinea pigs were infectious for younger animals after being passed through a filter in a highly species-specific manner led to the denomination of these agents as *salivary gland viruses*. The cellular changes observed in tissue sections from patients with a fatal infection led to the use of the term *cytomegalic inclusion disease* (CID) years before the causative agent was identified.

In 1954, Smith[8] succeeded in propagating murine cytomegalovirus (MCMV) in explant cultures of mouse embryonic fibroblasts. Use of similar techniques led to the independent isolation of HCMV shortly thereafter by Smith,[9] Rowe and coworkers,[10] and Weller and colleagues.[11] Smith isolated the agent from two infants with CID. Rowe and associates isolated three strains of CMV from adenoidal tissue of children undergoing adenoidectomy, including the commonly used laboratory-adapted strain of CMV *AD169*. Weller and associates isolated the virus from the urine and liver of living infants with generalized CID. The term *cytomegalovirus* was proposed in 1960 by Weller and colleagues[12] to replace the names CID and salivary gland virus, which were misleading because the virus usually infected other organs and because the name salivary gland virus had been used to designate unrelated agents obtained from bats.

The propagation of CMV in vitro led to the rapid development of serologic methods. Using such antibody assays and viral isolation, several investigators quickly established that HCMV was a significant pathogen in humans. This ancient virus, like other members of the herpes virus family, infects almost all humans at some time during their lives.[13,14] Evidence of infection has been found in all populations tested. The age at acquisition of infection differs in various geographic groups and socioeconomic settings, which results in major differences in prevalence among groups. The natural history of HCMV infection is complex. After a primary infection, viral excretion, occasionally from several sites, persists for weeks, months, or even years. Episodes of recurrent infection with renewed viral shedding are common years after the primary infection. These episodes of recurrent infection are thought to be due to reactivation of latent viruses, increased levels of virus production from a source of persistent infection, or reinfections with a genetically different strain of CMV.

In immunocompetent hosts, CMV infections are generally subclinical. However, when infection occurs during pregnancy without consequences for the mother, it can have serious repercussions for the fetus. Even though most immunocompromised hosts tolerate CMV infections without overt clinical symptoms, in some instances, such as in patients with the acquired immunodeficiency syndrome (AIDS) and allograft recipients who have received immunosuppressive agents, CMV can cause end-organ disease of varying severity, and the infection can be life threatening. As a result of a long-standing and close host-parasite relationship, many—probably thousands—genetically different strains of CMV have evolved and circulate in the general population.[15,16] Most recently, the incredible genetic complexity of HCMV derived from infected infants and adults has been demonstrated by next-generation sequencing (deep sequencing).[17] These studies have provided evidence that HCMV in an individual does not exist as a homogenous genetic species but as a mixture of major and minor genetic variants similar to the quasi-species of RNA viruses such as hepatitis C virus.[17]

The Virus

Cytomegalovirus is the largest and structurally most complex member of the family of human herpesviruses. It has been classified as a betaherpesvirus based on several biochemical criteria, such as the genome size, guanosine and cytosine content, slow replicative cycle, and restricted in vivo and in vitro tropism. Other members of this subfamily of herpesviruses include other mammalian cytomegaloviruses and the agents associated with the exanthem roseola, human herpesviruses 6 and 7.[18-20] Early estimates of its size based on electron microscopic studies indicated that the CMV particles were heterogeneous in size, with an estimate of 175 to 200 nm in diameter being a commonly accepted size, a finding consistent with its measurement by more contemporary techniques.[21-23] Intracellular and extracellular particles are heterogeneous in size, likely a reflection of the variability of envelope glycoprotein content. The virus genome consists of more than 230 kilobase pairs of linear double-stranded DNA (dsDNA), making CMV nearly 50% larger than the alphaherpesviruses, HSV, and varicella-zoster virus.[24] In contrast to other betaherpesviruses, including other cytomegaloviruses, HCMV contains both terminal and internal repeated nucleotide sequences that enable the genome to exist in four isomeric forms, similar to HSV and other alphaherpesviruses.[25] The biologic advantage(s) that favor four isomeric forms of the genome of this virus has not been determined but is clearly dependent on replication of the genome in a permissive cell.[26]

The nucleotide sequence of several clinical isolates of CMV has recently been determined and from the analysis of these strains it is estimated that CMVs can encode more than 250 open reading frames (ORFs). More recently, investigators have reported a much larger number of ORFs that potentially encode small polypeptides of as yet undetermined function. Individual viral genes and ORFs are designated by their location in the unique long region (UL), unique short region (US), or the internal or terminal repeat regions (IRS, IRL, TRS, TRL) of the prototypic genome of CMV.[25,27] In addition to the massive size of the genome, other posttranscriptional modifications can also increase the complexity of the coding sequence of CMV. A limited number of CMV genes represent spliced transcripts, primarily those encoding immediate and early gene products. In some cases, multiple proteins can arise from a single gene by use of internal translation initiation sites. Finally, HCMV encodes more than 20 small noncoding regulatory RNAs, viral microRNAs that have critical functions in the replication of this virus.

Although in many cases, experimental verification of viral specific proteins arising from predicted ORFs has not been accomplished, it is nevertheless obvious that the proteome of virus-encoded proteins within the virus infected cell will be exceedingly complex. Consistent with this postulate has been the complexity of the proteome of the virion. Mass spectrometry revealed that the extracellular particle contained more than 100 unique virus-encoded proteins and an indeterminant number of host cell proteins.[28] It is also of interest to note that the organization of the CMV genome is similar to that of other herpesviruses in that conserved gene blocks encoding replicative and virion structural proteins can be found in similar locations.[25,27] The organization of the genome has allowed the assignment of positional homologues between members for different subfamilies of herpesviruses, an approach that has been instrumental in the identification of genomic coding sequences of CMV proteins. Outside of these conserved gene blocks are genes or gene families that are unique to individual betaherpesvirus. These genes are thought to impart specific in vivo tropism and the species restricted growth characteristic of these viruses.[25,29]

The CMV virion consists of three identifiable regions: the capsid containing the dsDNA viral genome, the tegument, and the envelope (Fig. 24-1A). The capsid of CMV consists

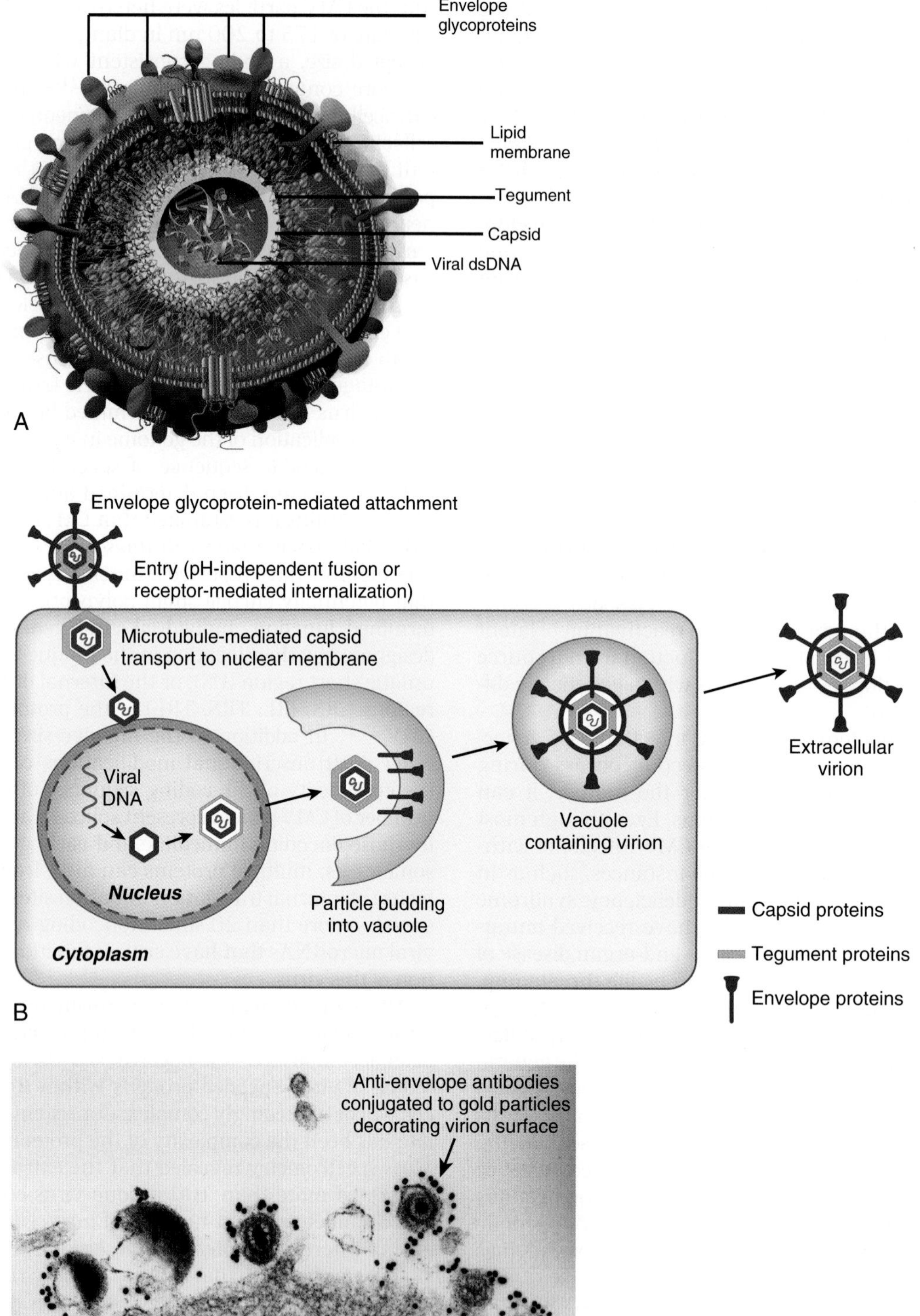

Figure 24-1 **A,** Schematic representation of human cytomegalovirus virion (CMV). Viral double-stranded DNA (dsDNA) is shown encapsulated in protein capsid, which is surrounded by amorphous layer designated the tegument. Surrounding these structures is a lipid envelope into which glycoproteins are embedded. **B,** Proposed pathways of human cytomegalovirus assembly within infected cells. Note tegument particle budding into cytoplasmic vacuoles, where it acquires its final envelope. Virus leaves cells by exocytic mechanism. **C,** Electron microscopic analysis of extracellular virus with envelope glycoprotein gN decorated with gold particles (dark spheres). (Rendering of CMV courtesy Andrew Townsend and Jay Nelson, Oregon Health and Science University, Portland, Ore.)

of six proteins that have functional and structural homologues in other herpesviruses.[30,31]

The capsid of CMV has been studied by high resolution cryoelectron microscopy, and its structure is nearly identical to that of HSV, with the exception that it has slightly larger internal dimensions secondary to the requirement for incorporation of a genome that is about 60% larger than HSV. The capsid consists of 162 capsomere subunits, consisting of 150 hexons and 12 pentons arranged in iscosahedral symmetry.[21] The subunits of the capsid are thought to be partially assembled in the cytoplasm of the infected cell, followed by self-assembly using products of the viral UL80a ORF.[31] Proteins encoded by this ORF serve as a scaffold for the assembly of the individual capsomeres.[31] Once the shell is assembled, newly replicated concatemeric viral DNA enters the capsid shell through a portal generated by the portal protein and the action of virus-encoded protein complex termed the terminase complex, generating the intranuclear capsid.[30-34] This replication strategy is very similar to that of dsDNA bacteriophages.

Several steps in the assembly of the viral DNA-containing capsid are unique to CMV, including the cleavage of unit length DNA by a viral terminase and the formation of the capsid portal. At least one of these steps in virus replication has been demonstrated to be the target of antiviral drugs.[34-36] Capsids containing infectious DNA leave the nucleus by as yet poorly understood pathways and are enveloped in the cytoplasm. Evidence has been presented to suggest that CMVs could leave the nucleus by focal disruption of the nuclear membrane.[37-40] A conserved group of viral proteins—m50 and m53 in MCMV, UL50 and UL53 in HCMV—have been shown to be essential for nuclear egress and have been termed the nuclear egress complex.[41] A mechanism that is consistent with available evidence remains to be presented, although an operational pathway of virus assembly has been suggested by several lines of evidence (Fig. 24-1B).

The tegument of CMV is without doubt the most structurally complex and heterogeneous structure in the virion. An undetermined number of viral proteins and viral RNAs can be found in the tegument of infectious particles.[42] Although it is generally argued that the tegument has no identifiable structure and is usually described as an amorphous layer between the envelope and the capsid, more recent studies have argued that at least the innermost region of the tegument assumes the structure of the underlying icosahedral capsid.[21,43] Proteins within the tegument are characteristically phosphorylated and, in many cases, serve regulatory functions for virus replication. In addition, some tegument proteins also appear to have a primary role in maintenance of the structural integrity of the virion. Tegument proteins have a variety of functions in the infected cell, ranging from blocking intrinsic cellular responses that degrade incoming DNA to effects such as direct stimulation of cell-cycle progression from G_0-G_1 by degradation of the product of the retinoblastoma gene, *Rb*, as well as blocking progression at the G_1/S junction of the cell cycle.[44-52] In addition, other tegument proteins have been shown to enhance transcription from the immediate-early (IE) genes and to accelerate the replication of viral DNA and facilitate export of unspliced viral messenger RNAs (mRNAs) from the nucleus of the infected cell.[53-57] Finally, other tegument proteins have been proposed to modify critical cellular responses to stress, such as in the mammalian target of rapamycin (mTOR) pathway and to alter cellular structures, such as the infected cell nucleus, to facilitate nuclear egress of capsids containing viral DNA.[58-62] A comprehensive review of HCMV tegument proteins has been published.[45]

These examples illustrate the functional complexity of CMV tegument proteins and suggest that it will be difficult, in some cases, to assign a unique function to an individual protein in the replicative cycle of CMV. Finally, the tegument contains the most immunogenic proteins of the virions, including the immunodominant targets of T-lymphocyte responses and antibody responses.[63-66] In the case of one of the most abundant tegument proteins, pp65 (UL83 ORF), studies have shown that up to 2% to 5% of peripheral blood $CD8^+$ lymphocytes from CMV infected hosts are specific for this single protein.[65,67,68] More recent studies have identified a large number of CMV-encoded targets of $CD8^+$ and $CD4^+$ responses and have provided evidence that in some individuals, up to 15% of total T-cell reactivity is directed at antigens encoded by CMV.[65] It remains unclear why the normal host has devoted such a large percentage of peripheral $CD8^+$ lymphocyte reactivity to CMV, although persistence of the virus that is facilitated by immune evasion functions has been argued as an explanation.

The envelope of CMV rivals the tegument in terms of the number of unidentified proteins and the limited amount of information on the function of many envelope proteins. Sequence analysis of the CMV genome indicates that more than 50 viral ORFs exhibit predicted amino acid motifs found in glycoproteins.[15,69,70] The number of glycoproteins that are present in the envelope of CMV is unknown, but at least 12 different glycoproteins have been defined experimentally.[71-73]

Recent studies of laboratory-maintained strains of HCMV have suggested that the gM/gN complex represents the most abundant proteins in the virion envelope, with gB and the gH/gL/gO complex being the second and third most abundant group of glycoproteins in the envelope, respectively.[28] The abundance of these different glycoproteins in the envelope of recent clinical isolates of CMV has not been studied, but it is clear that in some of these viruses, the gH/gL/gO complex is replaced with gH/gL/gUL128-131 complex secondary to the extended cell tropsism provided by the gH/gL/UL128-131 complex.[74-76] The gH/gL/UL128-131 complex has been shown to greatly enhance the entry of HCMV into epithelial, endothelial, and monocytic cells and is thought to be very important for infection and spread in vivo. In contrast this complex is thought to be lost during in vitro passages in human fibroblast cells, perhaps secondary to the fusion activity of this complex.[77] There appears to be a redundancy in function for several of these glycoproteins such that several are thought to be responsible for attachment and fusion; however, it is also likely that these redundancies are a reflection of in vitro assays and that in vivo each of these proposed functions could be essential for virus infectivity, particularly in different cell types. Of importance, in rodent models of HCMV infection, the protein homologues of the gH/gL/UL128-131 complex have been shown to have a major role in in vivo virulence of the infection.[78]

The envelope glycoproteins induce a readily detectable antibody response in the infected hosts, and neutralizing antibodies directed against gB, gH, gM/gN, and the gH/gL/gUL128-131 complex can be demonstrated in HCMV immune serum.[79-84] Moreover, considerable amounts of data from both human and animal studies have indicated that antiviral antibodies directed at proteins of the envelope are a major component of the host protective response to this virus, such as illustrated by the decoration of the viral envelope with antibodies directed at specific glycoproteins (Fig. 24-1C). These results, together with the numerous studies that have demonstrated that envelope glycoproteins play a key role in the early steps of viral infection, including binding to the target cell and entry, argue that these components of the viral envelope are a logical target for the development of prophylactic vaccines that will induce antibody responses.

CYTOMEGALOVIRUS REPLICATION

Virus replication is initiated when CMV attaches to the cell surface (see Fig. 24-1B). Early studies suggested that an initial low-affinity engagement of virion glycoproteins with cell surface proteoglycans was then followed by more specific and higher-affinity receptor interactions and fusion with the plasma membrane, an entry mechanism common to herpesvirus entry.[85,86] The cellular receptor(s) for CMV was initially proposed to be the epidermal growth factor receptor and then later to include integrins.[87-89] More recent findings have argued against the role of the epidermal growth factor receptor as a receptor for CMV and have suggested that the platelet-derived growth factor (PDGF) receptor can function at least as a signaling receptor for CMV.[90,91] Even more recent findings have provided definitive evidence that PDGF does not function as a conventional receptor for CMV entry.[92] Finally, other authors have described a viral entry pathway into fibroblasts that uses macropinocytosis, a pathway that HCMV could easily follow.[93] Regardless of the specific receptor used by CMV, several studies have shown that CMV attachment and possibly fusion with the host cell membrane results in a cascade of cellular responses mediated by signaling pathways.[86,94-97] Signaling pathways can be activated by the attachment of ultraviolet-inactivated, noninfectious virus as well as a single envelope glycoprotein, indicating that the process of binding and fusion with the cell membrane is sufficient to induce these IE cellular responses. More recent studies have suggested that the majority of responses noted in the early studies was secondary to activation of intracellular Toll-like receptor signaling after entry of viral dsDNA into the cytoplasm of the infected cell.[98] After infection with CMV, more than 1400 cellular genes are either induced or repressed, suggesting that infection with this virus elicits a myriad of host cell responses.[96] Included in these early responses are activation of transcription factors, such as nuclear factor kappa B; increases in second messengers, such as PI3 kinase activity; increased expression of type I interferons (IFNs) and interferons-stimulated genes; and induction of responses that inhibit cellular innate responses that block virus infection (RNA-dependent protein kinase) or lead to apoptosis of the infected cell.[99-105] Thus CMV infection prepares the host cell for virus replication as well as inhibiting host cellular responses that could attenuate virus infection.

After attachment and penetration, the DNA-containing viral capsid is rapidly transported to the nucleus, likely using the microtubular network of the cell (see Fig 24-1B).[106-108] Once viral DNA enters the nucleus, the *IE* genes of the virus are expressed in the absence of any de novo viral protein synthesis, suggesting that either host or virion proteins are responsible for their induction. These genes include the abundant *IE-1* and *IE-2* genes. Both gene products arise from the same region of the genome and actually share some amino acid sequences secondary to RNA splicing in the primary transcripts. The *IE-1* gene product is a 72 kDa phosphoprotein (pp72, or IE-1) that is readily detectable throughout infection in permissive cells and is the target of antibody assays for detection of CMV infected cells. IE-2 is a promiscuous transactivating protein and likely is responsible for activating many of the early and late genes of CMV and some cellular genes.[27,109]

Additional *IE* genes include virus encoded inhibitors of cellular apoptotic responses and viral functions that block cellular antiviral responses.[105,110-112] The remaining replication program of CMV is similar to that initially described for bacteriophages and for HSV and involves the coordinated and sequential temporal expression of viral genes as well as the coordinated inhibition of viral gene expression.[27] The regulation of CMV transcription, translation, and replication is exceedingly complex and is well beyond the scope of this chapter and can be found discussed in a recent monograph.[113] It includes conventional modes of regulation, including transactivation and/or silencing of promoter elements, splicing, and regulation of spliced message transport from the nucleus, and recently a role for viral-encoded microRNAs has been identified as a mechanism of viral gene regulation in infected cells.[114-122] A major goal of virus-control of replication is to permit temporally regulated expression of the viral genome. The next set of viral genes expressed during infection are early or β-genes. These genes are primarily genes encoding viral proteins that are required for replication of viral DNA or alteration of cellular responses, such as progression through the cell cycle or cellular apoptotic responses.[27,123] Examples of these genes include the viral DNA polymerase, alkaline exonuclease, ribonucleotide reductase, the viral protein kinase, and other replicative enzymes. Some virion structural proteins are also made during this interval. The final set of viral genes that are expressed are the late or γ-genes. These genes encode virion structural proteins and are required for the assembly of an infectious particle. The entire replicative cycle is estimated to take between 36 and 48 hours in permissive human fibroblast cells. Abortive infections in nonpermissive cells have also been characterized, and, in general, viral gene expression is limited to the *IE* genes and possibly to a limited number of early genes.

After viral DNA replication in the nucleus of infected cells, concatameric DNA is cleaved by a viral protein that exhibits terminase activity during packaging into the procapsid by mechanisms that closely resemble the pathway of bacteriophage assembly. Studies in the assembly of alphaherpesviruses have provided a much greater understanding of the mechanisms and pathways of viral capsid assembly and DNA packaging during herpesvirus replication. The interested reader is referred to these studies and to more complete discussions.[113,124,125] The viral capsid leaves the nucleus by as yet undetermined mechanisms that require function of two tegument proteins, UL50 and UL53, which have been designated as the nuclear egress complex, and enters the cytoplasm as a partially tegumented, subviral particle.[41] Assembly of the mature particle takes place in the cytoplasm of the infected cell in a specialized compartment that has been termed the assembly compartment.[126] It is believed that this is a modified cellular compartment of the distal secretory pathway.[72,126-129] Virion structural proteins are transported to this compartment, and, presumably through a series of protein interactions, the virus is assembled and finally enveloped, possibly through a process of wrapping by envelope glycoprotein containing endosomes. This latter step is of considerable complexity because of the large number of virion glycoproteins that comprise the envelope of infectious virion. Virus is presumably released by cell lysis in cells, such as fibroblasts, and by as yet poorly defined exocytic pathways in certain other cell types.

Latency is a common theme of herpesviruses, particularly of the alphaherpesviruses, such as HSV. The concept of latency with CMV in the human host, and not at a single-cell level, is somewhat more controversial in that virus persistence in the host is more likely associated with chronic low-level productive infection and intermittent excretion. However, latent CMV infection has been demonstrated in macrophages obtained from infected nonimmunocompromised donors and also in in vitro models of infection with CMV.[130-134] The mechanisms that favor the establishment of latent infections are not known, and the viral genome in latently infected cells is thought to be maintained as closed circular viral DNA that persists as an episome in latently infected cells, and not by integration into the host DNA.[135] More definitive information is available on the signals that induce reactivation from latent infection. These include proinflammatory cytokines, such as tumor necrosis factor-α (TNF-α), and possibly INF-γ.[133,136] Several laboratories have reported that latently infected cells of the monocytic lineage express CD34.[137-139] Recent studies have suggested that a transcript arising from UL81-82 (LUNA) is expressed during latency in $CD34^+$ cells, which may provide investigators a better view of the mechanism(s) involved in maintaining latency in these cells.[140-142] HCMV can become activated and replicate CMV after exposure to these cytokines in vivo, such as in the setting of rejection of an allograft. This mechanism could explain aspects of the pathogenesis of CMV infection in uninfected allograft recipients transplanted with an organ from a CMV infected donor.[143-145] It is also likely that such latently infected cells could account for the transmission of CMV from blood products from seronegative host.[146] More recently, arguments for a role of host and viral microRNAs in maintenance of herpesvirus latency have been put forth, raising the possibility for even more complexity in the relationship between these large DNA viruses and their persistently infected host.[114-122,147,148]

CYTOMEGALOVIRUS CELLULAR TROPISM

Cytomegalovirus can be detected in a wide variety of cell types in vivo.[149-151] Studies using tissue from autopsies or biopsies have demonstrated virus in almost every cell type, including epithelial cells, endothelial cells, smooth muscle cells, neuronal cells and supporting cells in the central nervous system (CNS), retinal epithelium, dermal fibroblasts, and cells of the monocyte/macrophage lineage. Thus there appears to be a very limited restriction of the host cellular tropism in vivo. Routine virus isolation and propagation in vitro requires that the host cell be permissive for CMV replication. Although transformed cells are generally not susceptible to CMV infection, primary cells such as astrocytes, endothelial cells, smooth muscle cells, macrophages, and fibroblasts have all been shown to be permissive for CMV replication in vitro. However, the yield of infectious virus from these various cell types is highly variable, ranging from very low (macrophages) to high (fibroblasts). Primary human fibroblasts are the most commonly used cells for the recovery and propagation of CMV, and, if adequately maintained, can yield up to 10^6 to 10^7 infectious particles/mL of supernatant from cultures infected with laboratory strains of CMV. In contrast, recent clinical viral isolates often yield a fraction of this amount of virus, and almost all of the progeny virions are cell associated. The explanation for the differences in replication phenotype is not completely understood, but studies have suggested that it is the presence of a pentameric complex of glycoproteins in the envelope of recent clinical isolates, the gH/gL/gpUL128-131 complex, that allows extended cellular tropism of recent clinical isolates but also results in increased cell fusion of primary fibroblasts and concomitant reduction in virus production.[77] Because the gH/gL/gpUL128-131 complex is not required for in vitro replication in fibroblasts and perhaps even inhibits replication, particularly the production of extracellular virus, viruses with mutations within genomic sequences encoding these proteins are selected against during prolonged in vitro culture in human fibroblasts and must be maintained in endothelial or epithelial cells to maintain expression of the gH/gL/gpUL128-131 complex. The expression of this glycoprotein complex by recent clinical isolates is required for their extended tropism, and these viruses will infect primary endothelial cells, epithelial cells, macrophages, and primary smooth muscle cells, whereas commonly used laboratory strains of CMV will not infect these cell types. Although not understood, studies have provided some inkling as to possible mechanisms that lead to extended cellular tropisms of some recent clinical viral isolates. Assays of virus entry into cells have indicated that CMV can enter human fibroblast cells by direct fusion with the plasma membrane after engagement with a cell surface receptor by a pH-independent mechanism or, alternatively, after attachment to a receptor, internalization by endocytosis, and low-pH fusion with the limiting membrane of the endocytic vesicle in epithelial cells (see Fig. 24-1B).[152] It has been shown that the gH/gL/gpUL128-131 complex is required for the latter mechanism of entry, thus suggesting that cellular receptors may dictate the cellular tropism of CMV in nonhuman fibroblast cells. Of importance, this restriction in entry is only the first level of restriction for permissive replication because other cellular functions can limit CMV replication even if entry can be accomplished. This latter mechanism has not been well defined.

Epidemiology

OVERVIEW

Cytomegalovirus is highly species specific and can replicate only in cells of human origin and in cells from the great apes, and humans are believed to be the only reservoir. CMV infection is endemic and without seasonal variation. Seroepidemiologic surveys have found CMV infection in every human population that has been tested.[14] The prevalence of antibody to CMV increases with age, but, according to geographic and ethnic and socioeconomic backgrounds, the patterns of acquisition of infection vary widely among populations (Fig. 24-2).[153,154] Seroprevalence based on testing of specimens from the Third National Health and Nutrition Examination Survey (NHANES III) ranged from 36% in persons 6 to 11 years of age to 88.8% in persons 70 to 79 years of age, demonstrating a lifelong risk of acquiring CMV infection.[153,154] Overall in the United States, CMV seroprevalence was reported to be 58.9%.[153,154] Racial differences were also apparent from this study, with higher seroprevalence seen in African-American and Hispanic populations than in white populations.[153,154] Of interest, a recent study raised the possibility that the seroprevalence in urban African Americans in the United States may be decreasing such that an increasing number of individuals reach early adulthood without evidence of CMV infection.[155] In addition to age and race, other risk factors for CMV infection included fewer years of formal education, nonprivate health insurance, and being born in another country.[153,154]

In general, the prevalence of CMV infection is higher in developing countries and among the lower socioeconomic strata of the more developed nations. These differences are particularly striking during childhood. For instance, in sub-Saharan Africa, South America, and Asia, the rate of seropositivity was 95% to 100% among preschool children studied, whereas surveys in the United Kingdom and in certain populations in the United States have generally found that less than 20% of children of similar ages are seropositive. Several factors are believed to account for these differences, but likely breastfeeding and exposure to young children are factors that contribute to early acquisition of CMV.

The level of immunity among women of childbearing age, which is an important factor in determining the incidence of congenital and perinatal CMV infections, also varies widely among different populations. Past reports indicated that seropositivity rates in young women in the United States and Western Europe range from less than 50% to 85%. In contrast, in sub-Saharan Africa, Central and South America, and in southern Asia, the rate of seropositivity is greater than 90% by the end of the second decade of life. More important, from the point of view of congenital infection, prospective studies of pregnant women in the United States indicate that the rate of CMV acquisition for childbearing-aged women of middle-to-higher socioeconomic background is approximately 2% per year, whereas it is 6% per year among women of lower socioeconomic background, a finding that suggests a possible relationship between risks of exposure and rates of congenital CMV infection.[156,157]

The modes of transmission from person to person are incompletely understood. The following features of CMV infection make it difficult to study the modes of acquisition. A large reservoir of CMV exists in most populations. Furthermore, in the majority of persons, CMV infections are subclinical, including those acquired in utero and during the perinatal period. Infected persons continuously expose other susceptible persons. Excretion of large amounts of virus persists for years after congenital, perinatal, and early postnatal infections. Prolonged viral shedding from multiple sites, lasting more than 6 months in most persons, is also a feature of primary infection in older children and adults. Because recurrence of existing infections is almost certainly frequent, intermittent excretion of virus can be anticipated in a significant proportion of seropositive adults. Regardless of whether or not CMV is maintained as a latent infection with periodic reactivation or as a chronic persistent infection yielding low titers of infectivity, the virus continually spreads within a population. Finally, normal individuals with existing immunity and infection can be readily reinfected after exposure to a new strain of CMV, providing reservoirs of virus in the community. Transmission occurs by direct or indirect person-to-person contact. Sources of virus include urine, oropharyngeal secretions, cervical and vaginal secretions, semen, milk, tears, blood products, and organ allografts.

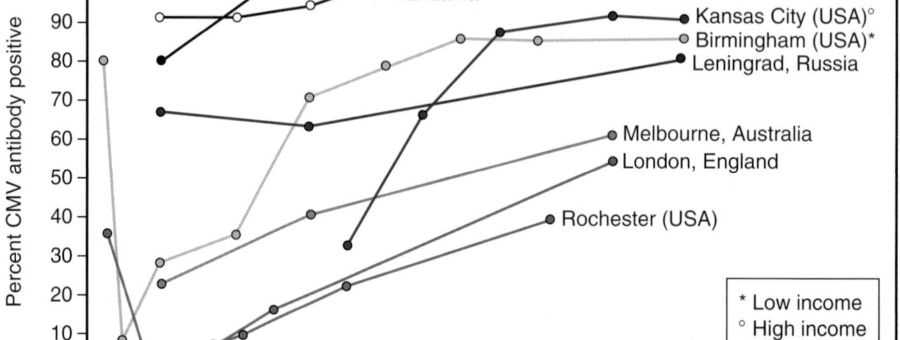

Figure 24-2 Age-related prevalence of antibody to cytomegalovirus (CMV) in various populations. (From Alford CA, et al: Epidemiology of cytomegalovirus. In Nahmias AJ, Dowdle WR, Schinazi RE, editors: *The human herpesviruses,* New York, 1981, Elsevier, p 161, with permission.)

CMV is thought to have limited capacity to infect populations because the spread of infection appears to require close or intimate contact with infected secretions. Although at first glance this would appear to result in the limited exposure of most persons to CMV, the unremitting nature of exposure to persons persistently excreting virus could result in frequent infection, a finding consistent with seroprevalence to CMV exceeding 90% in most populations in the world. Furthermore, in seroimmune populations, rates of reinfection with new strains of CMV have been reported to range from 17% to 30%.[158,159] The prevalence of CMV infection in developed countries appears to be higher in populations of low socioeconomic status, possibly a reflection of factors that account for increased exposure to CMV, such as crowding, sexual practices, and increased exposure to infants and toddlers. Finally, sexual contact also contributes to the spread of CMV, and CMV is considered a sexually transmitted infection (STI). Higher rates of seropositivity have been observed among males and females with multiple sex partners and histories of sexually transmitted diseases, as well as in sexually active homosexual men.[160-164]

BREASTFEEDING

Cytomegalovirus is commonly excreted in milk collected postpartum from seropositive women; the rates of excretion range from 13% to 32% by isolation of virus in tissue cultures to in excess of 70% when tested by polymerase chain reaction (PCR) assay.[165-170] The peak of excretion is between 2 weeks and 2 months postpartum. The risk of transmission of CMV infection to the infants is high, ranging from 39% to 59%. The risk of transmission by lactating mothers has been weakly correlated with viral loads greater than 10^3 genome equivalents/mL; however, there were a significant number of uninfected infants exposed to similar amounts of CMV in breast milk.[171] CMV can be detected in different components of breast milk. There is consensus that milk whey is the material of choice to detect the virus during lactation. Fractions of milk containing milk cells are less likely to have detectable virus by either culture or PCR methods. This may explain why rates of viral isolation are lower in colostrum compared with mature milk. The majority of infants infected after ingestion of virus-containing breast milk begin to excrete CMV between 3 weeks and 3 months of age.

Conservatively, it is estimated that nearly 40% of all infants who have been breastfed for at least 1 month by CMV seropositive mothers become infected postnatally. The majority of these infants chronically excrete CMV in urine and saliva, thus creating a large pool of infected infants who can efficiently spread CMV. Because in most populations of the world the seroprevalence of CMV infection in women of childbearing age is high (80%-100%), and most women breastfeed their infants for more than 1 month, acquisition of CMV through ingestion of breast milk from a seropositive women is quite high and undoubtedly is the most common mode of CMV transmission (Table 24-1).

YOUNG CHILDREN AS A SOURCE OF CYTOMEGALOVIRUS

Certain child-rearing practices influence the spread of CMV among children. In 1971, Weller[1] first suggested that the high rate of seropositivity among Swedish children was probably due to the frequent use of daycare centers. Swedish children had a rate of infection that was three to four times higher than that observed in London or in Rochester, New York. As shown in Table 24-2, high rates of CMV infection among children attending daycare centers were later confirmed in Sweden and have been reported in several studies in the United States.[172-176]

Multiple studies have shown that the rate of CMV infection in children was substantially higher among those in daycare compared with those who remained at home.[172-176] In a study of group of 70 children in daycare of middle- to upper-income background whose ages ranged from 3 to 65 months, the rate of CMV excretion in urine and saliva was 51%.[172] The lowest rate of excretion (9%) occurred in infants younger than 1 year, and the highest rate (88%) was among toddlers in their second year of life. Twelve infants whose mothers were seronegative excreted CMV, which indicated that their infection was not congenitally or perinatally acquired.

Similar results were reported by Adler,[173] who also noted that greater than 50% of initially seronegative children acquired daycare-associated strains of CMV, as determined by restriction fragment polymorphism of viral DNA. In addition, CMV was shown to be very efficiently transmitted from child to child in the daycare setting and it was not unusual to find excretion rates as high as 20% to 40% in young toddlers.[173,177] In many instances, these rates of infection are substantially higher than the seroprevalence rates for the parents of the children and young adults in the cities where the studies were done.[178] Evidence strongly suggests that

Table 24-1 Breastfeeding Patterns and Prevalence of Cytomegalovirus Infections in Young Children of Various Nations

	BREASTFEEDING RATE		% SEROPOSITIVE	
Nation	**Ever**	**At 3 Mo**	**Mothers**	**Children (age)**
Solomon Islands	100	97	100	100 (5 mo to 4 yr)
India				
Vellore	96	64	98	80 (1 yr)
Pondicherry			97	67 (1-5 yr)
Barbados	96	?	77	62 (1-5 yr)
Guatemala	95	?	98	47 (6 mo-1 yr)
Chile	89	?	92	42 (1-2 yr)
Japan				
Sapporo	?	56	67	42 (6 mo-2 yr)
Sendai			85	38 (1 yr)
Finland (Helsinki)	95	50	55	28 (1 yr)
United States				
Houston, Texas	46	?	48	15 (1 yr)
Birmingham, Alabama	8	?	85	8 (1 yr)
France (Paris)	85	?	56	10 (10 mo)
Canada (Nova Scotia)	49	26	34	12 (6 mo-1 yr)
United Kingdom (Manchester)	51	13	59	12 (3-11 mo)

Modified from Pass RF: Transmission of viruses through human milk. In Howell RR, Morris FH Jr, Pickering K, editors: *Role of human milk in infant nutrition and health,* Springfield, Ill, 1986, Charles C Thomas, pp 205-224.

Table 24-2 Prevalence of Cytomegalovirus Excretion Among Children in Daycare Centers

Investigator	Year	Location	% Infected (no.)
Stangert	1976	Stockholm	35 (7/20)
Strom	1979	Stockholm	72 (13/18)
Pass	1982	Birmingham, Alabama	51 (36/70)
Adler	1985	Richmond, Virginia	24 (16/66)
Hutto	1985	Birmingham, Alabama	41 (77/188)
MMWR	1985	Birmingham, Alabama	29 (66/231)
Jones	1985	San Francisco, California	22 (31/140)
Murph	1986	Iowa City, Iowa	22 (9/41)
Adler	1987	Richmond, Virginia	53 (55/104)

From Adler SP: Cytomegalovirus transmission among children in day care, their mothers and caretakers, *Pediatr Infect Dis J* 7:279-285, 1988.
MMWR, Morbidity and Mortality Weekly Report.

the high rate of CMV infection among children in group daycare is caused by horizontal transmission from child to child. The route of transmission that appears most likely is the transfer of virus that occurs through saliva on hands and toys.[179,180] No studies have demonstrated CMV transmission through respiratory droplets.

These observations in daycare centers indicate that transmission of CMV between young children is very efficient. Once infected, these children excrete CMV in large quantities and for extended periods of time. With increasing use of group child care in the United States and the emphasis that has been placed on breastfeeding, changes in the epidemiology of CMV can be expected within the next decades.[178] It is also of interest to note that toddlers infected in group daycare settings can be readily reinfected with new strains of CMV introduced into the group daycare facility by new enrollees, therefore creating additional sources of virus exposure for employees and parents.[181]

An important issue is whether children excreting CMV can become a source of infection for susceptible child care personnel and parents, particularly women who may become pregnant. This type of transmission has been confirmed by crude genetic analysis of CMV DNA.[182-185] Seroepidemiologic studies suggest that parents often acquire CMV from their children, who became infected outside the family. For instance, Yeager[186] first reported that 7 of 15 (47%) seronegative mothers of premature infants who acquired CMV in a nursery seroconverted within 1 year. Dworsky and colleagues[187] reported that the rate of seroconversion for women with at least one child living at home was 5.5%, significantly higher than the 2.3% rate for women from the same clinic who were pregnant for the first time or the rates for susceptible nursery nurses and for physicians in training. A significant association between seroconversion among children and seroconversion among susceptible parents has been demonstrated, and the infection in a child often preceded seroconversion in the parents.[188] There is also compelling evidence linking the acquisition of CMV by children in daycare with subsequent infection in their mothers and caregivers.[189-193] Several studies have demonstrated that CMV-seronegative parents have a significant risk of acquiring CMV infection if their infants and children attend daycare. The highest risk of seroconversion is approximately 20% to 45% in parents with a child shedding CMV at 18 months of age. On average, parents acquired infection within 4.2 months (range, 3-7 months) after their children become infected. For caretakers working with young children in daycare centers, the annual rate of seroconversion is approximately 10%, which is significantly higher than the 2% annual rate occurring in hospital employees matched for age, race, and marital status. These observations provided evidence that parents and women who work with children in daycare centers have an occupational risk of acquiring CMV. It is reasonable to expect that as many as 50% of susceptible children between the age of 1 and 3 years who attend daycare will acquire CMV from their classmates and will become an important source of infection for susceptible parents and caregivers.

MATERNAL INFECTION AND VERTICAL TRANSMISSION

Because maternal CMV infection is the origin of congenital infections and of most perinatal infections, it is important to review the relevant issues that pertain to vertical transmission. As used in the following discussion, vertical transmission implies transmission from mother to infant and not germline transmission.

Congenital Infection

Congenital infection (present at birth) is assumed to be the result of transplacental transmission. In the United States, congenital CMV infection occurs in 0.2% to 2.2% (average, 1%) of all newborns.[156,194] However, as shown in Table 24-3, the incidence of congenital infection is quite variable in different populations.

The natural history of CMV during pregnancy is particularly complex and dependent on several characteristics of the population. Infections such as rubella and toxoplasmosis cannot serve as definitive models, and some aspects of the natural history of congenital CMV infections more closely resemble those of the natural history of congenital syphilis. In the case of rubella and toxoplasmosis, in utero transmission occurs only as a result of a primary infection acquired during pregnancy, whereas the in utero transmission of CMV can occur as a consequence of both primary and nonprimary infections, including both reinfection and reactivation.[195,196] Far from being a rare event, congenital infection resulting from nonprimary maternal CMV infection has been shown to be common, especially in highly immune populations, and increases with increasing maternal seroprevalance (Fig. 24-3; see Table 24-3), a characteristic of congenital CMV infection that distinguishes it from either rubella or toxoplasmosis and follows more closely the natural history of congenital syphilis. The initial clue was provided by three independent reports of congenital CMV infections that occurred in consecutive pregnancies.[13,197] In all three instances, the first infant was severely affected or died, and the second-born infant in each case was subclinically infected. More convincing evidence came from

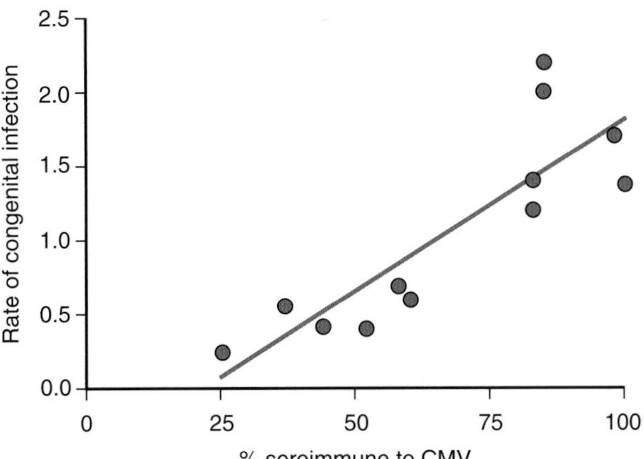

Figure 24-3 Increasing maternal cytomegalovirus (CMV) seroprevalence associated with increasing rates of congenital CMV infections. (Data from Stagno S, Pass RF, Dworsky ME, Alford CA Jr: Maternal cytomegalovirus infection and perinatal transmission, *Clin Obstet Gynecol* 25:563-576, 1982.)

Table 24-3 Rate of Congenital CMV Infection in Relation to Rate of Maternal Immunity in Various Locales

Location and Date	No. of Infants	% Congenital CMV Infection	% Maternal Seropositivity
Manchester, England, 1978	6051	0.24	25
Aarhus-Viborg, Denmark, 1979	3060	0.4	52
Hamilton, Canada, 1980	15,212	0.42	44
Halifax, Canada, 1975	542	0.55	37
Birmingham, Alabama (upper SES), 1981	2698	0.6	60
Houston, Texas (upper SES), 1980	461	0.6	50
London, England, 1973	720	0.69	58
Houston, Texas (low SES), 1980	493	1.2	83
Abidjan, Ivory Coast, 1978	2032	1.38	100
Sendai, Japan, 1970	132	1.4	83
Santiago, Chile, 1978	118	1.7	98
Helsinki, Finland, 1977	200	2.0	85
Birmingham, Alabama (low SES), 1980	1412	2.2	85

From Stagno S, Pass RF, Dworsky ME, Alford CA Jr: Maternal cytomegalovirus infection and perinatal transmission, *Clin Obstet Gynecol* 25:563-576, 1982.
CMV, Cytomegalovirus; *SES*, socioeconomic status.

a prospective study of women known to be seroimmune before conception.[196] The rate of congenital CMV infection was 1.9% among 541 infants born to these seropositive women. Clearly, the 10 congenitally infected infants were not infected as a result of primary maternal CMV infection because all mothers were known to have been infected with CMV from 1 to several years before the onset of pregnancy. Shortly after these studies were published, Schopfer and associates[195] found that in an Ivory Coast population in which virtually all inhabitants are infected in childhood, the prevalence of congenital CMV infection was 1.4%. Additional studies from Africa, Brazil and India have confirmed these early reports and demonstrated again that the rate of congenital CMV infection is directly related to the CMV seroprevalence of the maternal population. In these populations, maternal seroprevalence is nearly 100%, yet the rate of congenital CMV infection was approximately 1%.[195,198-203]

This phenomenon of intrauterine transmission in the presence of substantial maternal immunity (nonprimary infection) has been attributed to reactivation of endogenous virus in some cases and to reinfection with different strains of CMV in other instances. Initially, support for a mechanism of reactivation as an explanation for recurrent infection came from the observation that the viruses isolated from each of three pairs of congenitally infected siblings were identical when examined by restriction endonuclease analysis, a crude method of analysis that can sample only gross differences in genetic complexity.[204] In two of these three pairs, the first-born infant was severely affected, whereas the second-born sibling was subclinically infected, which suggested that virulence of infection was not related to strain and that maternal immunity in some way attenuated the fetal infection. Closer examination of these early data, however, suggested that in at least one of these cases, reinfection with a new strain of virus that differed genetically from the previous maternal isolate could explain the recurrent congenital infection.

More recent studies indicate that women who are CMV seropositive can become reinfected with a different strain of CMV, leading to intrauterine transmission and symptomatic congenital infection.[158,159,205] This important study documented this unique aspect of the biology of CMV and assessed maternal humoral immunity to strain-specific epitopes of CMV glycoprotein H in serum specimens from women with preconceptional immunity who were sampled during previous as well as the current pregnancy. Of the 16 mothers with congenitally infected infants, 10 (67%) had acquired new antibody specificities against glycoprotein H, compared with only 4 of the 30 (12%) mothers of uninfected infants. The observations from this study have been confirmed in other populations, most recently in Brazil, in which reinfection occurred at an annualized rate of nearly 35% in a maternal population, with near-universal seroimmunity to CMV and in normal women during an intrapartum period.[158,159]

Intrauterine transmission of CMV in immune women explains the direct relationship between the incidence of congenital CMV infection and the rate of seropositivity, as shown in Table 24-3. A more recent meta-analysis of a number of studies provided a model of congenital CMV infections that demonstrated the majority of congenital infections in most populations result from nonprimary maternal infections and that primary maternal infections will remain a minor source of congenitally infected infants.[206] At present, it is extremely difficult to define by virologic or serologic markers which patient may undergo a reactivation of CMV or reinfection with a new strain of virus, and it is nearly impossible to define the timing of intrauterine transmission with such reactivations or reinfections during pregnancy. The sites from which CMV reactivates to produce congenital infection are not known and are likely inaccessible to sampling during pregnancy. Although CMV excretion is a relatively common event during and after pregnancy, the simple isolation of virus during pregnancy has not been shown to signal an increased risk of intrauterine infection.

Virus can be shed at variable rates from single or multiple sites after primary or recurrent infections in females, whether pregnant or not. Sites of excretion include the genital tract, cervix, urinary tract, pharynx, and breast. In pregnant women, virus is excreted most commonly from the cervix and, in decreasing order, the urinary tract and the oropharynx. In the immediate postpartum period, the frequency of viral shedding into breast milk is quite high and can reach 40% of seropositive women when assayed by conventional virus isolation and is about 70% to 90% when analyzed by PCR assay. The rates of cervical and urinary tract shedding in nonpregnant women are comparable to those found in pregnant cohorts with similar demographic and socioeconomic characteristics. In general, rates of cervical shedding range from 5.2% for nonpregnant women enrolled in private obstetric practice or family planning clinics to 24.5% among women attending a sexually transmitted disease clinic .[161,163] Pregnancy per se has no discernible effect on the overall prevalence of viral shedding. However, the prevalence of excretion is lower (2.6%) in the first trimester than near term (7.6%).[204] This rate is comparable to the prevalence of genital excretion in nonpregnant women.

The rates of CMV excretion in the genital and urinary tracts of women are inversely related to age after puberty. In one study, the rate of genital CMV excretion fell from 15% in girls between 11 and 14 years of age to undetectable levels in women age 31 years and older.[204] From a peak of 8% in the younger group, urinary excretion fell to 0% in women age 26 years and older. No CMV excretion occurred from either site in postmenopausal women.

A transient depression of cellular immune responses to CMV antigens during the second and third trimesters was reported in early studies, suggesting a role for altered immunity during pregnancy and CMV replication.[207] A number of other studies have failed to confirm these findings and, of importance, none of the mothers in the initial report shed virus during the period of depressed cellular immune response, nor did they transmit the infection to their infants. Increased rates of congenital infections have been reported in maternal populations with a high incidence of human immunodeficiency virus (HIV) infection, suggesting a role of depressed cellular immunity and increased rates of transmission.[208-210]

Lilleri and coworkers[211] identified a cohort of pregnant women with primary CMV infection and analyzed their virus-specific T-cell responses. Several findings of this study are directly relevant to understanding the role of T-lymphocyte responses to CMV in the natural history of congenital CMV. First, there was no difference in the kinetics of $CD4^+$ and $CD8^+$ CMV-specific responses between pregnant and nonpregnant women, a finding that argues against a virus-specific immune deficiency during pregnancy that could increase CMV transmission to the fetus.[211] Moreover, the duration of viremia was similar in women who transmitted virus to their fetuses, compared with women who failed to transmit virus, suggesting that obvious defects in control of virus replication cannot readily explain intrauterine transmission.[211] However, it is also important to note that women with primary infection who did not transmit virus to their offspring developed quantitatively higher CMV-specific $CD4^+$ T-lymphocyte responses and developed these responses sooner than women who transmitted virus to their offspring.[211] This finding is provocative and suggested that the more rapid development of T-cell responses to CMV could in some way alter parameters of the maternal infection and lessen the risk of transmission to the fetus. It has also been shown that antibody responses to glycoprotein B are significantly higher at the time of delivery in women with primary CMV infection who transmitted the infection in utero, compared with those who did not, suggesting that the amount of antiviral antibody is not reflective of protection from transmission.[212] However, analysis of the qualitative antibody response revealed lower neutralizing antibody titers in transmitters, suggesting an association between neutralizing activity and intrauterine transmission. In this study, a significant correlation was found between neutralizing titers and antibody avidity, indicating that antibody avidity maturation is critical for production of high levels of neutralizing antibodies during primary CMV infection, findings that at least superficially parallel those of the findings of Lilleri[211] detailed above. In a separate study, higher levels of transplacentally acquired maternal antibodies against glycoprotein B and neutralizing antibodies were observed in infants with symptomatic infection at birth and who went on to develop sequelae.[213] Unfortunately, these and other studies suffer from the limitations associated with measurement of immunologic functions in specimens from patients in which the timing of maternal infection, placental infection, and/or fetal transmission cannot be ascertained but only defined within large time intervals, such as trimesters of pregnancy. Critical features of protective responses, such as the level of protective immune responses at the time of virus dissemination to the placenta and fetus, cannot be defined by such studies, and only correlation or associations can be inferred from existing data.

Table 24-4 Association Between Maternal Excretion of CMV from Various Sites and Subsequent Infection of the Infant

Only Site of Maternal Excretion	No. of Infants Infected/No. Exposed (%)
Breast Milk	
Breastfed infant	19/30 (63)
Bottle-fed infant	0/9 (0)
Cervix	
Third trimester and postpartum	8/14 (57)
Third trimester	18/68 (26)
First and second trimester	1/8 (12)
Urine*	0/11 (0)
Saliva†	0/15 (0)
Nonexcreting women	
Bottle-fed infant	0/125 (0)
Breastfed infant	0/11 (9)

From Stagno S, Reynolds DW, Pass RF, Alford CA: Breast milk and the risk of cytomegalovirus infection, *N Engl J Med* 302:1073, 1980, with permission.
*Late third trimester.
†Excretion 1 day postpartum.

Perinatal Infection

In contrast to the poor correlation that exists between CMV excretion during pregnancy and congenital infection, there is a good correlation between maternal shedding in the genital tract and milk and perinatal acquisition. As shown in Table 24-4, the two most efficient modes of transmission in the perinatal period were exposure to infected breast milk, which resulted in a 63% rate of perinatal infection, and exposure in the infected genital tract, particularly in late gestation, which was associated with transmission in 26% to 57% of the cases (natal infection). Viral shedding from the pharynx and urinary tract of the mother late in gestation and during the first months postpartum has not been associated with perinatal transmission.

There is considerable variability in perinatal transmission of CMV throughout the world.[214] The age of the mother and her prior experience with CMV, which in turn influence the frequency of viral excretion into the genital tract and breast milk, are certainly important factors. Younger seropositive women who breastfeed have an increased risk for transmitting virus to their offspring, especially in those women from lower socioeconomic groups.[178] In Japan, Guatemala, Finland, and India, where the rates of CMV excretion within the first year of life are extremely high (39%-56%), the practice of breastfeeding is almost universal and the majority of women of childbearing age are seroimmune for CMV likely secondary to perinatal acquisition of CMV. Recent studies from Brazil and India have confirmed these early observations and documented near-universal seroprevalence in maternity populations.[202,215]

SEXUAL TRANSMISSION

A large number of epidemiologic studies support the classification of CMV as an STI. This is consistent with excretion of this virus in cervical secretions, vaginal fluid, and semen. Sexual transmission in most populations in the world likely plays a minor role as a source of primary CMV infection secondary to the high rate of infection during infancy and childhood, but its importance in reinfection in women and subsequent congenital infection is suspected and has not been rigorously examined. In developed countries, the infection is acquired at a lower rate in childhood, resulting in a burst in the prevalence of infection after puberty in some populations, an observation that parallels the acquisition of other herpesviruses, such as Epstein-Barr virus. Several lines of evidence indicate that sexual transmission of CMV is at least partly responsible for this increase in seroprevalence. As noted previously, an increased seroprevalence of CMV and excretion of virus has been found in women attending sexually transmitted disease clinics and in young male homosexuals. Handsfield and colleagues[216] demonstrated that previously infected individuals could be reinfected by a different strain of CMV. More recently, an association between CMV excretion and bacterial vaginosis (BV) has been described together with findings that argued that infection with multiple strains of CMV could be correlated with the presence of bacterial vaginosis, an STI.[164] Evidence has also been provided for sexual transmission in general populations.[217]Among the many variables investigated, significant correlations were found among seropositivity to CMV, greater numbers of lifetime sexual partners, and past or present infection with other sexually transmitted infections.

NOSOCOMIAL TRANSMISSION

Nosocomial CMV infection is an important hazard of blood transfusion and organ transplantation. In immunocompromised hosts, such as small premature newborns and bone marrow transplant recipients, transfusion-acquired CMV infection has been associated with serious morbidity and even fatal infection. The association between the acquisition of CMV infection and blood transfusion was first suggested in 1960 by Kreel and coworkers,[218] who described a syndrome characterized by fever and leukocytosis occurring 3 to 8 weeks after open heart surgery. The reports that followed soon afterward expanded the syndrome to include fever, atypical lymphocytosis, splenomegaly, rash, and lymphadenopathy.[219-222] The term *postperfusion mononucleosis* was then proposed. Prospective studies incriminated blood transfusion as the major risk factor and demonstrated that although the clinical syndrome occurred in approximately 3% of the patients undergoing transfusion, inapparent acquisition of CMV infection ranged from 9% to 58%, depending on the mode of detection. It has been estimated that the percentage of blood donors capable of transmitting CMV ranges from 2.5% to 12%. In a study of seronegative children receiving blood for cardiac surgery, the risk of acquiring CMV was calculated to be 2.7% per unit of unscreened blood, a practice which no longer takes place in most centers.[220] A significant correlation between the risk of acquisition of CMV by patients labeled seronegative and the number of units of blood (total volume) transfused was noted early on.[221] Under conditions found in blood banks, CMV inoculated in whole blood persisted for 28 days and in freshly frozen plasma for 97 days. More recent modifications of blood banking practices have greatly reduced the risk of CMV infection after blood transfusion; however, it is important to note that studies from Europe have demonstrated that up to 15% of serologically negative blood donors, as detected by commercial antibody assays, may in fact harbor CMV DNA in their peripheral blood and therefore potentially transmit virus to a donor, a finding that may also explain that approximately 1% to 2% of recipients of blood transfusions from CMV seronegative donors develop CMV infections.[146]

In very early studies, the observation that two newborns who received large volumes of fresh blood subsequently developed symptomatic CMV infections led McCracken and associates[223] to suggest an association between blood transfusion and clinically apparent postnatal CMV infection. Subsequent reports indicated an association between postnatal CMV infection and exchange transfusions.[224] Intrauterine transfusions have also been implicated in CMV infection of mothers and their infants as well as transmission from cord blood–derived stem cells requiring the screening of cord blood donors for CMV infection. CMV infections resulting from transfusion of blood products have also been shown to cause significant end-organ disease in newborn infants, particularly premature infants and infants born to women without immunity to CMV. Extremely premature infants born to seropositive mothers are also at increased risk because the transplacental transfer of specific antibodies does not occur until the later stages of gestation. Infected infants with passively acquired anti-CMV antibodies develop milder disease than infected infants without passively acquired antibodies.[225] This observation is a compelling argument for the role of antiviral antibodies in protecting the host against severe disease.

Transmission of CMV by transplantation of an allograft from donors previously infected with CMV continues to represent a major clinical problem in allograft transplantation. Transplantation of a kidney from a seropositive donor into a seronegative recipient results in primary CMV infection in 80% of the patients that can often contribute to both acute and chronic graft failure. The clinical manifestations of the infection vary widely, depending principally on immunosuppressive regimens and the use of antivirals as prophylaxis in the early posttransplant period. Many reports have suggested that CMV infection in the posttransplant period has an adverse effect on the survival of the allograft.[226-228] CMV was recognized as a major cause of morbidity and mortality in recipients of hematopoietic allografts and autografts and continues to represent an important opportunistic infection in these populations.[229-234] Interstitial pneumonitis is the most significant manifestation of the infection; its mortality approached 100% before the availability of antiviral agents. From 70% to 100% of recipients of heart transplants excrete CMV.[235-238] Severe disease has traditionally been thought to be more often associated with primary than with reactivated infection. Studies in several transplant populations have documented significant disease after superinfection with strains of CMV derived from the allograft.[239-242] These early findings and subsequent findings argue for a complex relationship between host immunity, infection with new strains of virus, and protective responses. Unfortunately, the precise role of CMV in allograft recipients continues to be undefined secondary to the heterogeneity of transplant recipients and the often transplant center–specific natural history of CMV infections in these patients. The detection of CMV nucleic acid in kidneys of infected donors and of latent CMV in cells of macrophage/monocyte lineage clearly demonstrated that the transplanted organs and hematopoietic allografts can serve as the source of virus in transplant recipients.[143]

Nosocomial transmission is possible in the nursery setting, which suggests that workers' hands or contaminated fomites might be involved. However, the very low rate of CMV infection in newborn infants of seronegative mothers who are not exposed to other important sources such as seropositive blood products indicates that transmission of CMV via fomites or workers' hands is uncommon.

TRANSMISSION TO HOSPITAL WORKERS

Because hospital workers are often women of childbearing age, there has been concern about occupational risk through contact with patients shedding CMV. As illustrated in Table 24-5, the majority of older studies carried out have indicated that the risk was not significantly different from the general population.

The risk for CMV seroconversion among hospital personnel is a function of the prevalence of CMV excretion among patients, the prevalence of susceptible health care workers, and the degree of their exposure to infected patients. In general, among hospitalized infants and children, viruria occurs in approximately 1% of newborns and as great as 5% to 10% of older infants and toddlers. Much of the literature relevant to this topic was generated before institution of universal precautions. Therefore it is nearly impossible to estimate the risks of acquisition of CMV infection by hospital workers in contemporary health care facilities.

Working with hospitalized children inevitably leads to contact with a child shedding CMV; however, it is important that workers who develop a primary infection not assume that

Table 24-5 Rates of Primary Cytomegalovirus Infection Among Health Care Workers and Others

Study (reference no.)	Group	No. in Group	Seroconversions (%/yr)
Yeager, 1975 (776)	Nonnurses	27	0
	Neonatal nurses	34	4.1
	Pediatric nurses	31	7.7
Dworsky et al, 1983 (777)	Medical students	89	0.6
	Pediatric residents	25	2.7
	Neonatal nurses	61	3.3
Friedman et al, 1984* (754)	"High risk": pediatric intensive care unit, blood intravenous team	57	12.3
	"Low risk": pediatric ward nurses, noncontact	151	3.3
Brady et al, 1985 (778)	Pediatric residents	122	3.8
Adler et al, 1986 (779)	Pediatric nurses	31	4.4
	Neonatal nurses	40	1.8
Demmler et al, 1986 (780)	Pediatric nurses	43	0
	Pediatric "therapists"	76	0
Balfour and Balfour, 1986 (781)	Transplant/dialysis nurses	117	1.04
	Neonatal intensive care unit nurses	96	2.28
	Nursing students	139	2.25
	Blood donors	167	1.57
Stagno et al, 1986 (157)	Middle-income pregnant women	4692	2.5
	Low-income pregnant women	507	6.8

Modified from Pass RF, Stagno S: Cytomegalovirus. In Donowitz LG, editor: *Hospital-acquired infection in the pediatric patient,* Baltimore, 1988, Williams & Wilkins.

*Only study in a children's hospital reporting a statistically significant difference in relation to occupational contact.

their occupational exposure or contact with a specific patient is the source of infection. Three old reports illustrate this point. Yow and coworkers,[146] Wilfert and associates,[147] and Adler and associates[148] described health care workers who acquired CMV while pregnant and after attending patients known to be excreting CMV.[191,243,244] In each of these reports, the source of CMV for hospital workers was not from patients. With the implementation of universal precautions in the care of hospitalized patients, the risk of nosocomial transmission of CMV to health care workers is undoubtedly much lower than the risk of acquiring the infection in the community.

Pathogenesis

The disease manifestations of CMV infections can be conveniently divided into those associated with acute infection and productive virus replication and with those associated with chronic infections, in which the relationship between disease and virus replication is not easily defined. Considerably more is known about acute infectious syndromes because acute CMV infections can be temporally related to specific symptoms, specific laboratory abnormalities, and responses to antiviral therapies that target virus replication. Infrequently, acute CMV syndromes can occur in presumably normal individuals and, in these cases, present as an infectious mononucleosis that is indistinguishable clinically from the infectious mononucleosis associated with Epstein-Barr virus infection.[245,246] Of interest, normal individuals with symptomatic infections often have increased viral burdens, as measured by serologic responses, compared with persons with asymptomatic infections, raising the possibility that these normal persons could have as yet undefined deficits in immunity.[66] More commonly, acute CMV infections that result in symptomatic disease occur in immunocompromised hosts.

In general, acute CMV syndromes that are associated with clinical disease often share several common characteristics, including (1) occurrence in hosts with altered cellular immunity, (2) poorly controlled virus replication, (3) multiorgan involvement, (4) end-organ disease secondary to direct viral cytopathic effects, and (5) clinical manifestations of disease that often correlate with virus burden. In patients with invasive CMV infections, such as those in allograft recipients, organ dysfunction and often disease course have been correlated with increasing virus burden.[227,247-252] It is important to note that there is usually not an absolute level of viral replication, as measured by viral genome copy number in the peripheral blood, that is predictive of the onset of an invasive infection and end-organ disease in all persons, indicating that a set point of virus replication does not define disease in all patients. Rather, it appears that finding increasing levels of virus replication (genome copy number) is more useful in the identification of individuals at risk for invasive disease and presumably reflects ongoing viral replication in the absence of efficient host control of virus replication, with an increasing risk of dissemination and end-organ disease. More recent studies in laboratory animal models have argued that conventional models of virus dissemination from secondary targets of infection, such as the liver, may not be reflect the biology of CMV.[253] These authors argued that although the endothelium of the liver can disseminate infectious MCMV and that hepatocytes replicate large amounts of virus that can spread within the liver, this site of virus replication does not appear to be the major source of virus that subsequently is disseminated through the blood.[254,255] The major source of virus that disseminates to distal sites after acute infection thus remains undefined, and other sites of virus replication, such as the spleen, should be considered.[253]

Chronic disease syndromes that have been associated with CMV include a variety of chronic inflammatory diseases of older populations, such as atherosclerotic vascular disease and vascular processes associated with chronic allograft rejection.[236,256-264] In addition, the progressive and late-onset hearing loss associated with congenital CMV infection could be considered in this same category.[265-270] The characteristics of populations experiencing these manifestations of CMV infection are different from those described above and do not include hosts with obvious immune dysfunction. In fact, most individuals have normal immunity, and allograft recipients undergoing chronic graft rejection may have increased immune responsiveness within the allograft. Viral replication may be a prerequisite for disease, but the level of virus replication has not been directly related with disease. The course of the disease in animal models of CMV-associated vascular disease is that of ongoing inflammation that is enhanced and prolonged by the presence of CMV.[271-275] Inhibition of virus replication early in the course of infection in animal models has been shown to dramatically alter the course of disease, suggesting that virus must seed these areas and establish a persistent infection.[273] The presence of the virus in areas of inflammation increases the expression of soluble mediators of inflammation, such as cytokines and chemokines, and in some cases, virus-infected cells actively recruit inflammatory cells, including monocytes, into the area of disease.[276-278] The bidirectional interactions between CMV and the host inflammatory response are unique and appear to favor virus persistence, viral gene expression, and eventual virus dissemination. In fact, it is a peculiarity of the biology of CMV that it can often be recovered from sites of intense inflammation, an observation suggesting that CMV could enhance host inflammatory responses to favor its replication.

CMV INFECTION AND CELL-ASSOCIATED VIREMIA

An important aspect of the pathogenesis of CMV infection is the route of infection and spread within the host. In general, it is believed that virus is either acquired at mucosal sites (community exposures) or by bloodborne transmission, such as after blood transfusion or transplantation of an infected allograft. It is believed that cell-free virus is responsible for community-acquired CMV infection based on recovery of virus from saliva and from cell-free genital tract secretions, yet only limited data directly supports this possibility. More convincing evidence comes from studies in breastfeeding women that have demonstrated that infectious virus is present in the cell-free fraction of breast milk.[170] This finding suggests that cell-free virus can infect a mucosal surface. Animal models of CMV infection have most commonly used either intraperitoneal or subcutaneous inoculations; however, oral infection with cell-free MCMV has been accomplished, and rhesus macaques have been infected by the oral route[279, 280] (personal communication, S. Jonjic, University of Rijeka, Rijeka, Croatia).

After infection, local replication, and amplification of virus titer in regional sites, the spread of CMV within an infected host is likely to be cell associated based on findings from immunocompromised patients and studies in experimental animal models, although cell-free dissemination is also possible, particularly in severely immunocompromised individuals, such as HIV-infected individuals who are not receiving antiretroviral therapy.[130,254,281-284] During infection of mucosal surfaces that occurs after exposures in the community and bloodborne infections in transplant patients, the mode of spread and dissemination of the virus is likely the same, albeit with different kinetics and quantity of infected cells in the vasculature and infected organs. In all but the most severely immunocompromised patients, infectivity that can be demonstrated in the blood compartment is most frequently associated with endothelial cells and leukocytes, including polymorphonuclear leukocytes, from the buffy coat fraction of peripheral blood.[285-287]

Polymorphonuclear leukocytes (PMNs) cannot support virus replication but have been shown to carry infectious virus and viral gene products.[288,289] It has been proposed that CMV-infected endothelial cells or fibroblasts can transfer infectious virus to PMNs, and, in turn, these cells can transmit virus by a microfusion event between virus-containing vesicles and susceptible cells.[288] Although this mechanism of virus transmission has been demonstrated in vitro, it has not been experimentally verified in vivo in animal models of CMV infection, but the role of PMNs in transmission of infectious CMV in vivo is consistent with clinical observations, and the correlation between CMV antigen-positive PMNs (antigenemia assay) and disseminated infection has been shown to be a diagnostic tool for the identification of patients at risk for invasive infection with CMV.[290-295] In addition, antigen-positive PMNs can be detected in normal hosts infected with CMV, but with a drastically reduced frequency compared with immunocompromised patients, suggesting that even in normal hosts, PMNs may be a potential common mode of virus dissemination.

Other cells within the leukocyte fraction of peripheral blood cells support CMV persistence and also transmit infectious virus, including monocyte and macrophages derived by differentiation of blood monocytes[283,296-298] Granulocyte/monocyte progenitor cells have been proposed as sites of latency based on in vitro infections and can be detected as antigen-containing cells in immunocompromised patients with disseminated CMV infection.[131-133,283,284,298-300] Mobilization of granulocyte/monocyte progenitor cells by granulocyte-macrophage colony-stimulating factor (GM-CSF) has been shown to be associated with increased incidence in CMV infections in hematopoietic cell allograft recipients and in a humanized mouse model.[139,301] In animal models of HCMV infection, an important role of myeloid precursors in the spread of MCMV has been demonstrated, including the role of virus-encoded chemokine-like molecules in chemoattraction of myeloid progenitor cells, leading to dissemination of the virus from local sites of replication (see following section). Furthermore, macrophages derived from peripheral blood monocytes have been shown to harbor infectious CMV upon stimulation with specific cytokines, including TNF-α.[130,136,144] Viral replication and expression of a variety of early and late proteins can be demonstrated in macrophages after infection with recently derived CMV clinical isolates. Together, these data have argued for a mechanism of in vivo spread, which includes infection of circulating monocytes that, upon entry into an organ, undergo differentiation into a tissue macrophage that can support productive CMV infection.[136] Another cell lineage believed to be critical for the in vivo spread of CMV is endothelial cells in a variety of microvascular beds. Endothelial cells have been shown to support CMV replication in vitro, and infection of these cells results in a variety of cellular responses, including the release of cytokines and chemokines.[296,302-309] Both lytic and nonlytic productive infections have been described, suggesting that endothelial cells can respond very differently to infection.[302,305,310,311] Virus infection of endothelial cells is thought to be an initial step for infection of various tissues during CMV dissemination, and likewise, endothelial cell infection appears to be critical for the hematogenous spread from infected tissue.[288,296,309] Early studies in transplant populations described viral antigen–containing endothelial cells circulating in the blood of viremic transplant patients.[306,312,313] These cells are believed to be infected endothelial cells that slough into the circulation, presumably secondary to local infection and/or inflammation. A similar role for endothelial cells in spread of CMV in both the murine model and guinea pig CMV model has also been proposed.[314] Finally, in an elegant series of experiments, Sacher and coworkers[253] demonstrated that replication of MCMV within endothelial cells is essential for dissemination of this virus from sites such as the liver.[254]

VIRUS-ENCODED PATHOGENIC FUNCTIONS

To date, specific CMV encoded virulence factors have not been identified. Early studies attempted to correlate differences in restriction fragment lengths of endonuclease-digested DNA of viral isolates from congenitally infected infants with clinical outcome. This genetic analysis proved too crude to allow identification of subtle changes in the viral genome. More recently, numerous studies have reported a possible linkage between polymorphisms in a gene encoding the major envelope glycoprotein gB and disease.[315-318] Almost all of these studies have failed to demonstrate any specific linkage between different gB genotypes and disease, and most recently, studies using other polymorphisms in several viral genes *(UL11, UL18, UL40,UL73, UL74, UL144)* have failed to establish a specific genetic linkage between a unique genotype and disease.[319-327] In fact, recent studies using next-generation sequencing have demonstrated that such CMV "genotypes" actually represent minor genetic variants among the background of CMV genetic variants such that the commonly identified gB genotypes represented less than 5% of the gB sequence variants in CMV isolated from a single individual.[328] Although the explanation for the vast polymorphisms in CMV is unclear, several characteristics of CMV infections, including frequent reinfections with new strains of virus in exposed populations and the potential for recombination between strains of virus, are likely reasons for the variability in the nucleotide sequences of different viral isolates.[205,242,317,329] Yet differences in biologic behavior of CMVs exist such that some strains exhibit extended tropism and can infect endothelial cells, macrophages, and epithelial cells in addition to permissive primary fibroblast cells. This extended tropism is a property of recently derived isolates of CMV, and once these viruses are repeatedly passaged through fibroblast cells, their extended tropism is quickly lost. It is believed that one or more viral genes are responsible for their extended tropism in vivo and that without the selective pressure of replication in vivo, these genes are lost or mutated under in vitro conditions.

Specific genes that permit extended tropism in vitro have been identified and include the most well characterized group encoded by the ORFs UL128-131.[75-77] In addition, the presence of large numbers of genes that modify the immune response to CMV also raise the possibility that these genes will encode a function that inhibits innate responses from cells such as macrophages and could also contribute to the extended tropism of some isolates. Other viral genes encode functional chemokine receptors (US28), viral cytokine-like molecules (vIL10, vIL-8), and viral anti-apoptotic functions (vICA, UL37), all of which have been proposed to contribute to the in vivo replication and virulence of CMV infections.[110,330-338] An interesting observation suggested that different viral genotypes could be found in different tissues from infants with symptomatic congenital CMV infections who died in early infancy, a provocative finding that raises the possibility of as yet undefined viral functions that target different viruses to different tissues in vivo.[339] This finding must be tempered by the more recent findings that have detailed the vast genetic variability of CMVs when analyzed by more sophisticated methods.

Although defining the function of viral genes in the in vivo replication and spread of CMV has been difficult because of the restricted tropism of CMV to cells of human origin, much information has been gathered from studies in animal models. Using the mouse model of CMV infection, several laboratories have identified specific viral genes that appeared to be required for efficient replication and spread in vivo.[281,340-346] Three viral genes encoded by m139, 140, 141 ORFs of MCMV have been shown to play a critical role in viral replication in monocyte/macrophages but have little to no effect on the replication of the virus in mouse fibroblasts.[282,341,347-349] The in vivo phenotype of viruses that lacked these genes indicated these genes were required for in vivo dissemination and spread of MCMV.[333,348] To date, the mechanism that accounts for restricted replication in monocytes of MCMV with deletions in these specific genes is unknown, although it appears that these genes contribute to survival of mononuclear cells infected with MCMV. The CMV gene(s) that permit replication in monocyte/macrophages has not been definitively identified, but of interest, the MCMV genes *m139, m140,* and *m141* are homologous to a family of CMV genes (*US22* gene family). Similarly, the *m38.5* of MCMV has been shown to inhibit the apoptotic function of the intrinsic pathway by binding to the proapoptotic effector, BAX.[350,351] Deletion of the m38.5 results in a virus that replicates poorly in mononuclear cells and, as expected, has decreased capacity to disseminate in vivo. Recent studies have also identified that the m41.1 and m36 proteins encoded by MCMV are also responsible for mononuclear cell tropism in vivo.[111,352] Another example of a viral gene that directly influences in vivo tropism and replication of CMV is the MCMV gene *M45*. Endothelial cell tropism of MCMV can be linked to this single viral gene *(M45)*, and it is believed that expression of this gene limits resistance of endothelial cells to MCMV-induced apoptosis.[314] Of interest, the deletion of the homologous reading frame in CMV *(UL45)* was not associated with the loss of endothelial tropism.[353] More recently, the function of the M45 protein has been redefined by Upton and colleagues.[354] These investigators demonstrated that M45 functions as an inhibitor of RIP3 (receptor-interacting protein kinase 3), which is a component of the RIP1-RIP3 complex, which together initiate programmed cellular necrosis (necroptosis), a response to virus infection.[354,355] Thus it appears that CMVs have developed mechanisms to limit two pathways of cell death after virus infection as a mechanism to permit virus replication.

Other genes in MCMV encode functional chemokines, such as the murine CMV chemokine-1 (MCK-1) encoding by *UL129* that exhibits activity similar to interleukin-8 (IL-8) in humans.[282,333,347] Studies in mice have suggested that the capacity of this gene product to recruit inflammatory cells into a site of virus replication is important for cell-associated virus spread within infected animals.[282,333] In the absence of this virus-encoded function, virus replication remains localized to the site of infection, secondary to a failure to recruit and infect infiltrating inflammatory cells, thus limiting viral dissemination.[282,333] Further characterization of this complex of MCMV viral proteins has determined that in addition to the proposed chemokine-like activity, these viral glycoproteins are required for infection of monocytes and macrophages.[78] A functionally homologous viral gene in CMV *(UL146)* could influence the spread of CMV in vivo.[356] The protein encoded by *UL146* is a secreted protein that appears to function as a CXCL chemokine (*v*-CXCL1) and can induce chemotaxis and degranulation of PMNs.[356] It has been postulated that this viral chemokine can recruit PMNs in vivo and thus promote CMV dissemination.[333] In severely immunocompromised hosts, such as AIDS patients with gastrointestinal and retinal disease secondary to disseminated CMV infection, neutrophil infiltration can be observed in the lamina propria as well as in the retina.[357-359] Infection of lamina propria macrophages with CMV in vitro results in the induction of IL-8 release from these cells, suggesting that CMV can both induce IL-8 release as well as encode a viral IL-8–like molecule.[333, 360] Such findings are consistent with the proposed mechanism of chemokine expression and CMV dissemination from sites of virus replication. This mechanism of dissemination is consistent with the histopathologic findings noted in severely immunocompromised patients; however, it should be noted that a neutrophil infiltrate is not an invariant feature of the histopathology of naturally acquired CMV infections and interactions between other virus-encoded chemokines and chemokine receptors, and peripheral blood leukocytes could contribute to virus dissemination. Finally, recent findings have demonstrated that CMV engages Toll-like receptors, with resultant induction of proinflammatory cytokines and chemokines cascades.[361] This observation raises the possibility that virus infection alone can recruit cells such as monocytes and PMNs to sites of infection without the requirement of a specific viral chemokine.[361] Other viral genes likely induce host cell genes that, in turn, facilitate virus replication. Microarray and differential display experiments have demonstrated that fatty acid metabolism is altered in CMV-infected cells and that expression of cyclooxygenase-2 (COX-2), an enzyme required for prostaglandin synthesis and initiation of early steps in inflammation, is induced. Additional experiments have shown that if COX-2 activity is blocked, CMV replication is blocked.[362] Together, these experiments demonstrated that a CMV-encoded gene(s) could induce a cellular enzyme that, in turn, facilitated its replication, possibly by increasing the inflammatory response to the infection. This host response presumably leads to the recruitment of inflammatory cells into the site of virus replication, thereby promoting infection of infiltrating cells and virus spread.

CMV encodes four G-coupled protein receptor (GPCR)-like molecules in ORFs UL33, UL78, US27 and US28.[276, 363-366]

The *US28* gene encodes a GPCR that is constitutively activated and that can also signal after interaction with chemokines, including RANTES (regulated on activation, normal T-cell expressed and secreted), monocyte chemoattractant protein-1 (MCP-1), and fractalkine.[276,366-368] Reports have detailed possible roles for this molecule in the spread of CMV in vivo, including (1) as a chemokine sink to limit host cell chemotaxis to CMV-infected cells; (2) providing an anti-apoptotic function; (3) recruitment of infected mononuclear cells to the sites of inflammation, leading to dissemination of virus; and (4) perhaps even by binding of virus or virus-infected cells to chemokine-expressing endothelial cells.[366-370] Arterial smooth muscle cells expressing *US28* have been shown to migrate down chemokine gradients, thereby providing a mechanism for the localization of CMV-infected cells to sites containing inflammatory cellular infiltrates.[276] Although the role of US28 in CMV-induced vascular disease has been well described and supported by in vitro models of smooth muscle cell migration, the importance of *US28* in virus dissemination from local site of infection remains to be more completely defined. A recent report has also provided evidence that the *US28* gene can respond to different chemokines depending on the resident cell infected by CMV, a finding that demonstrates the adaptation of this virus to different host cells.[368] Perhaps more provocative have been studies that implicated expression of CMV *US28* in tumorogenesis through induction of cell proliferation and angiogenesis.[371] Together, these and other studies suggest that the large coding sequence of CMV encodes proteins that are essential for efficient replication and for spread within the infected animal but likely have little if any function in in vitro replication of virus.

HOST IMMUNITY AND THE PATHOGENESIS OF CYTOMEGALOVIRUS INFECTIONS

In normal hosts, both innate and adaptive cellular immune responses can limit but not prevent the spread of CMV from secondary sites such as the liver and spleen. The roles of both innate and adaptive cellular immune responses in the control of virus replication and spread to other sites have been extensively investigated in experimental animal models of CMV infection.[372, 373] Increased levels of virus replication follow the loss of either group of cellular immune responses.[373-377] The importance of innate immunity, both natural killer (NK)-cell responses and IFN responses have been repeatedly demonstrated in small-animal models of HCMV infections.[373,378] More recently, an important role of γΔT cells in control of MCMV infection has been demonstrated through depletion of other immune effector functions in a murine model of CMV infection.[379] The loss of virus specific $CD4^+$ or $CD8^+$ cytotoxic T-lymphocyte (CTL) responses is associated with uncontrolled virus replication and lethal disease in these models.[374,376,377,380]

Virus-specific antibodies appear to contribute minimally to control of local virus replication but play a key role in limiting bloodborne dissemination of the virus.[381,382] Antiviral antibody responses can control virus replication even in animals devoid of T lymphocytes, suggesting a critical role of this adaptive response to protective immunity to this virus.[383] A recent study described the role of antiviral antibodies in limiting spread of MCMV to specific organs, thus providing additional evidence for an important function of antiviral antibodies in control of virus dissemination.[382] These findings are of interest because in this model of CMV infection, virus spread is almost entirely by cell-associated virus and not cell-free virus, raising several interesting questions, including the mechanism(s) by which antiviral antibodies restrict virus dissemination.[281,342]

Consistent with the findings in experimental animal models, studies in immunocompromised human hosts have repeatedly demonstrated that deficits in innate immunity and the loss of adaptive immune responses predispose the host to CMV infections and, depending on the severity of the immune deficit, can lead to invasive disease, resulting in significant morbidity and mortality.[233,250,384-390] Several striking examples of the relationship between deficits in adaptive immunity and invasive CMV disease have been documented. These include the development of pneumonitis in bone marrow and cardiac allograft recipients, prolonged CMV viremia, and end-organ disease, such as retinitis in AIDS patients with high viral (HIV) burdens and low $CD4^+$ lymphocyte counts.

Perhaps the most convincing evidence for the critical role of T-lymphocyte responses in host resistance to invasive CMV infection were studies in bone marrow allograft recipients who received ex vivo expanded CMV-specific $CD8^+$ CTL and were transiently protected from invasive CMV infection compared with a group of historical control patients, a finding that suggested that in this case CMV-specific $CD8^+$ effector cells served only to control virus replication but not eliminate virus infection.[386] Additional studies using this therapeutic strategy have been reported.[391-393] Another interesting finding from this study was that patients who failed to generate CMV-specific CD4+ T-lymphocyte responses failed to generate long-term protection from CMV and developed invasive infections late in the course of their transplant.[386,394] Of interest, this observation was confirmed in later studies and demonstrated that patients who failed to develop a sufficiently robust CMV-specific $CD4^+$ T-lymphocyte response developed late-onset invasive CMV disease. It is of interest that these early observations in humans predated more recent studies that have shown that a $CD4^+$ response is required for maintenance of long-term immunity to infectious agents.[395-401]

Effector cells and mediators of the innate immune response have also been shown to be critical for control of CMV infections. Although most studies have been done in murine models of CMV infections, loss of NK-cell activity and invasive CMV infection has been reported.[402-406] Studies have also suggested that individuals with specific defects in innate immune responses, such as those associated with IFN responses and/or deficits in effector molecules (such as perforin), may be at increased risk for herpesvirus infections, although CMV infections have not been consistently identified in these individuals.[407,408] As noted earlier, in murine models, NK cells and IFNs have been shown to play a critical role in resistance to MCMV infection and appear to represent an initial host response that can limit virus replication and spread during the development of more efficient effector functions of the adaptive immune system.[409-410] In contrast to the role of antiviral antibodies in limiting dissemination of MCMV, the importance of antiviral antibodies in protective responses to HCMV infections remains controversial. Numerous studies have demonstrated a correlation between antiviral antibody responses, particularly virus neutralizing antibodies, and patient outcome.[212,225,411-413] In addition, studies in solid-organ transplant patients given intravenous immunoglobulins (IVIGs) containing anti-CMV antibodies have suggested that virus-specific antibodies can provide some degree of protection from invasive infections.[414-419] In other transplant populations, such as bone marrow allograft recipients, the efficacy of anti-CMV immunoglobulins remains unproven, and their use varies between different transplant centers.[233,234,420-426] Animal models other than mice have also indicated that antiviral antibodies could provide some degree of protection. Convincing evidence has been obtained in a guinea pig model of congenital CMV infection in which passive transfer of anti–guinea pig CMV (gpCMV) antibodies limited maternal disease and disease in infected offspring.[382,427,428] Similarly, transplacentally acquired anti-MCMV antibodies have been shown to protect newborn mice from CNS infection associated with perinatal MCMV infection.[429]

A study in pregnant women suggested that passive transfer of antibodies could limit intrauterine transmission of CMV, reduce the incidence of significant disease and, amazingly, lead to resolution of existing CNS defects.[430] The results of this study were provocative and have stirred considerable debate in this field of investigation. Aspects of the study design, clinical outcome measures, and uncertainty surrounding mechanisms of action of the immunoglobulin preparations have all contributed to the lack of a consensus on the validity of the results of this study; however, the results of the study have increased interest in similar therapeutic approaches. However, a recently completed controlled trial using the same immunoglobulin preparation failed to demonstrate any protective effect from transmission to the fetus, suggesting that the positive findings from the first trial were flawed secondary to study design.[431] Thus available data remain inconclusive in terms of the protective role of antiviral antibodies in limiting disease caused by CMV after intrauterine infections, presumably because antiviral antibodies could freely pass into the fetal circulation and, if protective, could alter the outcome of intrauterine infections. The ramifications for the mode of action of antiviral antibodies can be readily appreciated when the design of prophylactic vaccines is undertaken.

MODULATION OF THE HOST IMMUNE RESPONSE TO CYTOMEGALOVIRUS

Over the last 10 years, a host of laboratories have identified multiple viral genes whose products interfere with immune recognition and clearance of virus-infected cells. A description of some of these genes and their mode(s) of action is provided in Table 24-6.

The importance of these genes in the biology of CMV in vivo is not completely understood; however, animal models of CMV infection have allowed investigators to assign the importance of homologous genes during virus infection. The results from these studies have indicated that viral functions can actively interfere with virus clearance during acute infection in experimental animals.[432-436] Although a complete discussion of these viral genes and their mechanisms of immune evasion is outside the scope of this chapter, several pertinent observations can be made as to the importance of these viral genes in the pathogenesis of CMV infections. First, it should be noted that these viral genes do not prevent recognition and control of CMV infections in normal hosts, as evidenced by the limited pathogenicity of this virus in normal individuals and in experimental animal models. Some investigators have argued that the phenotype of these viral genes can only be appreciated in the immunocompromised hosts. Moreover, the vast amount of literature describing the function of immune evasion genes has been carried in experimental animals and during acute infection. In most studies, the function of these viral genes has only been

Table 24-6 Examples of Mechanisms of CMV Modulation of Host Immune Responses

Innate Immune Responses	Viral Gene	Mechanism
↓ Intrinsic cellular response to virus infection	*UL82*	Inhibits function of cellular DAXX function (degradation)
↓ Interferon responses	*UL83 (pp65)*	↓ IRFs, ↓ NF-κB
	TRS1	↓ PKR activity
↓ NK-cell activity	*UL18*	MHC class I decoy
	UL40	↑ HLA-E expression
Adaptive Immune Responses	**Viral Gene**	**Mechanism**
↓ CD8⁺, MHC-restricted CTL	*US2, US3, US11*	↓ Class I expression
↓ CD4⁺ responses	*US2*	HLA-DR degradation
	US6	Blocks TAP transport
↓ Antibody activity	*TRL11*	Viral Fc receptor
Antigenic variation	*UL73, UL55, UL75*	Loss of antibody binding
Blocking antibody recognition	*UL73 (gN)*	Carbohydrate blocks antibody access to glycoproteins (glycan shield)
Cytokines, Chemokine Responses	**Viral Gene**	**Mechanism**
Chemokine receptors (GPCRs)	*US28, US27*	GPCR acts as sink for extracellular chemokines
Chemokines	*UL21.5*	Chemokine receptor decoy inhibits RANTES
Cytokine	*UL111a*	Viral IL-10

Modified from References 45, 333, 434, 444, 768-775.

CTL, Cytotoxic lymphocyte; *DAXX*, death-domain–associated protein; *HLA*, human leukocyte antigen; *IL*, interleukin; *IRFs*, interferon regulatory factors; *MHC*, major histocompatibility complex; *NF-κB*, nuclear factor kappa B; *NK*, natural killer; *PKR*, RNA-dependent protein kinase; *RANTES*, regulated on activation, normal T-cell expressed and secreted; *TAP*, transporter associated with antigen presenting.

evaluated in a limited number of target organs, raising the question of whether some of these genes could be tissue specific. Finally, other investigators have raised the question of whether these genes function to focus the immune response only on a limited number of viral antigens, thus restricting the available antigens for immune recognition. Yet, CMVs have committed a large amount of their genome to immune evasion functions (an estimated 20 genes in the genome of CMV), and many of these genes are conserved in animal and HCMVs. Studies in experimental animals have demonstrated that immune evasion functions facilitate tissue-specific virus replication advantage in vivo.[433,435,436] These observations suggest that these genes almost certainly play a critical role in the in vivo persistence of these viruses.

Immune evasion functions encoded by CMVs have been shown to interfere with innate immune responses and adaptive immune responses to virus infected cells. In addition, mutations in viral structural proteins and in viral proteins recognized by the immune system also appear to allow escape from immunologic control. Mutations in CMV viral genes encoding targets of dominant $CD8^+$ CTL responses have been reported.[437] One of the more interesting observations is that one MCMV gene, *m157*, previously shown to activate NK responses through NK receptor Ly49H in strains of mice that were genetically resistant to MCMV infection, acquired mutations within weeks of infection.[438,439] Viruses with mutations in the *m157* gene were shown to replicate to higher titers in strains of resistant mice. This mutational event appears to be secondary to immune selection because genetically susceptible strains of mice that do not use this NK-cell activation pathway do not generate viruses with mutations in the *m157* gene.[439] Recent studies in mice have also documented that NK cells, through activation of Ly49H by *m157* of MCMV, provide in vivo selective pressure to shape the virologic landscape of mice infected with multiple strains of MCMV obtained from wild mice.[440] These observations provide an in vivo confirmation of the coevolution of CMVs and the host's attempt to control virus infection.

Antigenic variations in virion envelope glycoproteins that are targets of virus neutralizing antibodies have been well described. Strain-specific neutralizing antibody responses to the envelope glycoprotein B have been described.[441,442] In addition, a study of the polymorphic envelope glycoprotein N suggested that immune selection was responsible for the variation in amino acid sequence of gN derived from different virus isolates.[326,443] Further evidence of immune evasion functions has been provided by a recent study of the role of carbohydrate modifications on gN. In this study, the extensive glycosylation of this envelope glycoprotein was shown to provide a shield (glycan shield) that limited antibody recognition of at least three unrelated envelope glycoproteins (gB, gH, gN).[444] Thus CMVs, including HCMV, can evade immune recognition by a variety of active mechanisms, such as immune evasion genes, and by more conventional strategies, such as loss of antigenic determinants or loss of key antigens required for activation and recognition by immune cells.

PATHOGENESIS OF ACUTE INFECTIONS

Very early in the study of CMV infections, disease manifestations associated with congenital and perinatal CMV infections were related to the level of virus excretion, a marker for virus replication.[445] Subsequent studies in allograft recipients and in patients with AIDS have confirmed these findings and have consistently demonstrated that increased CMV replication in these patients was a key predictor of invasive disease. Unchecked virus replication and dissemination lead to multiorgan disease as illustrated by autopsy studies of neonates with congenital CMV infections, allograft recipients, and AIDS patients. Studies in rhesus macaques infected with rhesus CMV (RhCMV) have yielded results consistent with the proposed pathogenesis of human infection and provided a more detailed view of infection with this virus.[446] In these studies, virus given either intravenously (IV) or by a mucosal route resulted in bloodborne dissemination and widespread infection of a number of organs, including the liver and spleen.[446] The kinetics of the virus replication differed between the two groups with a lag in peak virus titers and liver infection noted in animals inoculated by a mucosal route. This result suggested that a local or regional amplification of virus was required after mucosal infection before bloodborne dissemination to the liver and spleen. This finding is consistent with experimental findings in guinea pigs and mice infected with the respective CMVs.[345,447-449]

Of interest, rhesus macaques that were inoculated by mucosal exposure remained asymptomatic and failed to exhibit clinical and laboratory abnormalities observed in animals given virus IV.[446] Together, these findings parallel clinical and laboratory findings in humans infected from community exposures versus those derived from blood products.

The dissemination of CMV from the liver and spleen to distal sites likely occurs in the normal immunocompetent individual as well as in the immunocompromised host. However, it is also quite likely that the quantity and duration of the viral dissemination is different in these two populations. In contrast to community-acquired CMV infections in normal adults, persistent viral DNAemia, as detected by PCR assay, is characteristic of populations with disseminated CMV infections, such as AIDS patients or infants with symptomatic congenital CMV infection.[251,450-455] Although it appears that the natural history of CMV infection includes local replication at mucosal sites, followed by amplification of virus and spread to the viscera, such as liver and spleen, findings in murine models of infection have argued that dissemination occurs very early after infection, and end-organ disease develops after loss of adaptive immunity and may not require dissemination from viral reservoirs. Virus replication in these organs further increases the quantity of viruses, and virus then spreads to distal organs and sites of persistence, such as the salivary glands and renal tubules. Thus, from observations in humans and in experimental models of infection, symptomatic infection appears to be related to the level of virus replication in sites seeded by the primary viremia, such as the liver and spleen. It follows that parenteral exposure from sources such as contaminated blood is associated with symptomatic infections because a larger viral inoculum is delivered to the organs such as the liver, often in the absence of a developing immune response that would normally be present after infection of a mucosal surface. The duration of virus replication likely represents a composite of the level of dissemination and the efficiency of the host immune response in the control of replicating CMV.

PATHOGENESIS OF CENTRAL NERVOUS SYSTEM INFECTIONS IN CONGENITALLY INFECTED INFANTS

The disease manifestations of congenital CMV infections include manifestations seen in adult immunocompromised hosts with disseminated CMV infections, such as hepatitis and, infrequently, pneumonitis and adrenalitis.[456-458] Unique to congenital CMV infection is the presence of CNS disease, a manifestation rarely seen even in the most immunocompromised allograft recipients. CMV encephalitis has been reported in patients with AIDS, but this disease can be distinctly different both clinically and pathologically from CMV infection of the CNS associated with intrauterine infection.[456,459] Furthermore, CNS involvement in infants with congenital CMV infections often is associated with ongoing disease, such as progressive hearing loss during the first few years of life, at a time when there is no apparent progression of structural damage in the CNS.[265-267,269,460-467]

The pathogenesis of CMV CNS infection in the developing fetus is poorly understood for several reasons, including the lack of a sufficiently large number of cases from autopsy studies. In addition, animal models of CNS infection that were developed to study the pathogenesis of congenital CMV infection have thus far received limited interest. The MCMV model is useful for the study of many aspects of CMV infection, but congenital infection with MCMV does not occur in mice. The other widely used small-animal model, the guinea pig, can be used to study intrauterine infections, and early reports suggested that CNS infections developed in these animals.[468,469] However, the usefulness of this model for studying CNS infection has not been defined, and because only a limited number of observational studies have been reported, it has been difficult to assign its value as an informative model. The rhesus macaque offers perhaps the most relevant model for the study of CMV CNS infections for several obvious reasons, including the similarities in brain development shared between macaques and humans. In addition, the rhesus CMV is more closely related to CMV than are the rodent and gpCMVs. However, this model is expensive, and these experimental animals are in limited supply secondary to their use in studies of HIV. For these reasons, our understanding of CNS infection with CMV remains limited.

Infection of the developing CNS is associated with a number of structural abnormalities that are dependent on the age of fetus at the time of CNS infection. Imaging studies of living infants and children with congenital CMV infections and clinical findings consistent with CNS disease have been informative. Commonly noted abnormalities include periventricular calcifications, ventriculomegaly, and loss of white/gray matter demarcation.[470-472] More refined imaging studies have detailed loss of normal brain architecture with loss of normal radial neuronal migration and cerebellar hypoplasia.[473-482] Limited autopsy studies have confirmed these imaging abnormalities and have also demonstrated the presence of inflammatory infiltrates in the parenchyma of the brain.[471] This latter finding is consistent with the presence of increased protein and inflammatory cells in spinal fluid obtained from congenitally infected infants with CNS disease. Together, these findings argue for a pathogenic spectrum that likely includes lytic infection of neuronal progenitor cells in the subventricular gray area, vasculitis with loss of supporting vessels in the developing brain, and meningoencephalitis with release of inflammatory mediators. It is also likely that multiple mechanisms of disease contribute to CNS disease in infants infected in utero depending on the gestational age of the infant. Hopefully, studies in rodent models that can be more easily manipulated will provide insight into the pathogenesis of this CNS infection.

It is unclear why the fetal and newborn brains are susceptible to CMV infection, compared with the adult brain; however, findings from experimental models suggest that the developing cells of the CNS are particularly susceptible to the lytic or possibly the apoptotic effects of CMVs.[483-485] In animal models, including both mouse and rhesus macaques, infection of the developing CNS results in widespread lytic virus replication, including neuronal progenitor cells of the subventricular gray area and endothelium.[486-488] Lytic virus replication in this area would lead to loss of normal neuronal development, radial migration, and vascularity of the developing brain. Extravasation of blood from damaged microvasculature would lead to calcifications that are prominent findings in imaging studies of CMV-infected newborn infants. Virus could spread through the ventricular system and infect additional areas of the subventricular germinal zone. Similar mechanisms of disease in severely immunocompromised AIDS patients with CMV encephalitis have been described. The pathologic descriptions include a more common finding of focal encephalitis with micronodular gliosis and significantly less frequent, but more extensive, infection, described as ventriculoencephalitis associated with CMV ventriculitis.[459] The more severe manifestations of CMV CNS infection can be explained by lytic virus infection of neuronal progenitor cells, glial cells in the CNS, and destruction of supporting vasculature. As indicated above, intracerebral inoculation of fetal rhesus macaques with RhCMV results in similar findings as described in severely affected human infants and suggests that if CMV enters the CNS early in development significant structural damage will ensue.

Other infants infected in utero with CMV exhibit clinical findings consistent with CNS involvement, including developmental delays and loss of perceptual functions, but do not have structural damage of the brain that can be detected by routine imaging techniques. At least one autopsy series has suggested that affected infants without calcifications can have neuronal migration deficits manifest as pachygyri and other abnormalities such as cerebellar hypoplasia.[471,478,482] The mechanisms leading to loss of normal architecture are unknown but could be related to ongoing inflammation in the CNS secondary to intrauterine meningoencephalitis. Various inflammatory mediators have been shown to cause loss of neuron and supporting cells function and can modify vascular permeability and endothelial function. Furthermore, evidence from experimental animal models has suggested that cytokines/chemokines may directly influence neuronal radial migration.[489,490] The results of a study carried out in mice demonstrated that host inflammatory responses, and not virus replication, was not responsible for the neurodevelopmental abnormalities observed in newborn animals infected with MCMV.[491] Thus ongoing inflammation may result in loss of normal brain architecture secondary to delayed or absent radial migration of neurons destined for the cerebral cortex.[492]

PATHOGENESIS OF HEARING LOSS ASSOCIATED WITH CONGENITAL CMV INFECTION

Hearing loss represents the most common long-term sequela of congenital CMV infection, and its pathogenesis is perhaps the least understood of any manifestation of CMV infection. Hearing loss can vary between mild to profound, unilateral or bilateral, and can develop or progress after the perinatal period. Thus it is possible that hearing impairment may represent a common outcome resulting from CMV infections in different parts of the auditory apparatus or, alternatively, secondary to infection at different stages in the developmental program of the auditory system. Besides the potential complexity of the disease, several other reasons likely contribute to the lack of understanding of the pathogenesis of hearing loss that follows congenital CMV infection. One of the most apparent is the lack of adequate histopathologic examinations of affected tissue from infected infants. A previous literature review revealed that only 12 temporal bones from congenitally infected infants have been studied and described in the medical literature.[493] In addition, most of the studies were done without the aid of modern techniques of virus and viral antigen detection and relied almost entirely on conventional histologic examinations. These limitations, together with the lack of adequate information on the maternal and fetal infection, have resulted in the lack of solid clues to the possible mechanisms of virus-induced damage to the auditory system. More recently, a very informative study of temporal bones obtained from a limited number of fetuses terminated secondary to intrauterine CMV infection have detailed several findings, including the infection of the inner ear, inflammatory cell infiltrate, and involvement of the vestibular system, but autolysis prevented an assessment of the hair cells.[494] Hearing loss in CNS infections in adults with AIDS or transplant infections is rare and not well described, presumably because these infections differ significantly from congenital CMV infection in both the extent of CNS involvement and the underlying diseases and treatment that lead to CNS infection in these immunocompromised patients, and perhaps most important, congenital CMV infections occur during development. Last, animal models of CMV hearing loss have been developed and have provided some information regarding selected aspects of the hearing loss associated with CMV. In general, however, they have failed to recapitulate the disease, and in some cases, early findings have been difficult to reproduce. Very recently, a murine model of congenital CMV infection and hearing loss has been developed that could provide some insight into the pathogenesis of the human disease.[495-499]

A comprehensive review of temporal bone pathology in infants with congenital CMV infection was published by Strauss.[500,501] The specimens in this series were from infants who died between 3 weeks and 5 months of age. A single case report of a 14-year-old patient with severe neuromuscular sequelae resulting from congenital CMV was described.[502] Findings in the inner ear, cochlea, vestibular system, and auditory/vestibular neural structures were described in all patients. Five of the original nine specimens had evidence of endolabyrinthitis, and virus was isolated from the endolymph in three of the nine specimens.[501] Viral antigen in the spiral ganglion was detected by immunofluorescence in two cases in which routine histology failed to demonstrate viral inclusions.[265] Cochlear and vestibular findings were variable and ranged from rare inclusion-bearing cells in or adjacent to the sensory neuroepithelium of the cochlea or vestibular system to more extensive involvement of the nonsensory epithelium. Routine histology failed to detect viral inclusions in the auditory/vestibular neural structures, but viral antigens were detected in the spiral ganglion when specimens were examined by immunofluorescence.[265] Of interest, inflammatory infiltrates were minimal and reported in only three patients in this series.[501] Perhaps the most interesting results were those reported in the examination of tissue from the 14-year-old patient with extensive sequelae from congenital CMV infection. In this patient, extensive cellular degeneration, fibrosis, and calcifications were observed in the cochlea and vestibular systems.[502] Several generalizations can be made from this limited data. First, in all but two of these cases, virus, viral antigens, or histopathologic findings consistent with virus infection were present in the cochlea or vestibular apparatus. These findings indicate that virus replication could have occurred in the sensory neuroepithelium and nonsensory epithelium and that cellular damage could be explained by a direct viral cytopathic effect. In addition, viral-induced damage can also result from bystander effects secondary to immune-mediated cytopathology. Thus CMV could induce loss of sensory neuroepithelium in the absence of direct infection of the sensory neuroepithelium, but secondary to infection of supporting epithelium, followed by host immunopathologic responses. However, an inflammatory infiltrate was seen in only three of nine specimens, an unexpected finding based on the role that the inflammatory response is thought to play in CMV end organ disease in other patient populations. Yet, it is well documented that infants with congenital CMV have a delay in the development of immunologic responses to CMV, and it could be argued that findings in the cochlea and vestibular apparatus are consistent with the ineffectual immune responses of congenitally infected infants. An alternative and not exclusive possibility is that infection of the inner ear structures is a late and, in some cases, a postnatal event. The relationship between susceptibility of cells of the sensory neuroepithelium and supporting epithelium to infection with CMV and their developmental status is unknown. Thus these cells could be resistant to CMV infection until late in development. In this case, findings from specimens of the autopsy series described above may reflect recent infection before host inflammatory responses. Such an explanation is, however, inconsistent with the course of fetal CMV infection in other parts of the CNS in most of the patients included in autopsy studies. A third possibility is that hearing loss in some infected infants is related to alterations in the neural networks leading from the cochlea to the eighth nerve. Such a potential mechanism has been demonstrated in rodents, in which synapse formation between efferents from the spiral ganglion and cochlear nuclei in the brain stem must take place during a critical time in development, or hearing circuits are impaired.[503-505] Finally, the findings of extensive degenerative changes, together with fibrosis and calcifications in the temporal bones from the oldest patient, presumably reflect the natural history of CMV labyrinthitis and, depending on the rate at which these changes develop, could also explain the progressive nature of hearing loss associated with congenital CMV infection. The loss of neuroepithelium, either secondary to direct virus-mediated damage or secondary to host-derived inflammation, followed by fibrosis would be consistent with the profound hearing impairment that develops in some children with congenital CMV infection. Of interest, findings in experimental animal models have indicated that exaggerated deposition of extracellular matrix is part of the inflammatory response in the inner ear, and this host response possibly leads to the ossification that is observed in animals inoculated directly into the labyrinth with CMV.[506,507]

Studies in animal models have only recently begun to yield insight into the pathogenesis of hearing loss after congenital CMV infection. Findings in small-animal models have mirrored some of the findings in congenitally infected infants. In these models, a consistent finding has been that both virus and inflammation are required for the development of pathology in the inner ear. In fact, a study in guinea pigs demonstrated that virus infection in immunocompromised animals was not associated with the typical pathologic findings in virus-infected normal animals.[506] Similarly, blocking virus replication with antiviral compounds or pretreating the animals with virus neutralizing antibodies limited the development of inner ear pathology.[508-513] Studies in newly developed murine models have demonstrated hearing loss, including progressive hearing loss, associated with limited histopathologic findings but significant inflammation, suggesting that host-derived responses may be critical in the pathogenesis of hearing loss in CMV infected infants.[497,499] Thus interrupting either virus replication or the local host inflammatory response could offer some therapeutic benefit to these patients.

NATURE OF MATERNAL INFECTION

The nature of the maternal infection is a major pathogenetic factor for congenital CMV infection. Primary infections are more likely to be transmitted to the fetus and are thought to be more frequently associated with fetal damage than recurrent infections.[514] With primary CMV infection, as in other infections during pregnancy, there appears to be some innate barrier against vertical transmission.[156,157,270,515,516] Intrauterine transmission after primary infection occurs in 30% to 40% of cases.[156,270] Contrary to previous findings, more recent findings have argued that gestational age has an important influence on the risk of transmission of CMV in utero such that transmission is more frequent with increasing gestational age.[156,157,270,515,517-519] However, with regard to the role of gestational age on the expression of disease in the fetus and offspring, infection at an earlier gestational age has been associated with more severe disease and worse outcome.* It is, however, important to note that definition of the interval in pregnancy in which maternal seroconversion occurred does not necessarily define a similar time of fetal infection, so the gestational age dependence of transmission and/or virulence must be viewed in the context of this limitation in the current studies.

Congenital infection may also result from recurrences of infection.[156,195-197,202,203,395,521-525] The term *recurrence* is used here to represent either reactivation of infection or reinfection with the same or a different strain of CMV during pregnancy. Despite the inability of maternal immunity to prevent transmission of this virus to the fetus, congenital infections that result from recurrent infections are thought to be less likely to produce clinical evidence of disease in the infected offspring than those resulting from primary infections.[156,526] The relationship between primary infection and clinically apparent congenital infection in the offspring was challenged initially by studies from Sweden and more recently in the United States and other regions of the world.† These studies have shown that clinically apparent congenital infections are frequently observed in infants infected after a recurrent maternal infection and that long-term sequelae, such as hearing loss, can be present in such infants. Thus the dogmatic assumption that more severe symptomatic congenitally infected newborn infants are products of a primary maternal infection is at best controversial. The risk of congenital CMV infection resulting from a recurrence of infection during pregnancy ranges from a high of 1.5% for a U.S. population of low socioeconomic background to 0.19% for women of middle or upper socioeconomic background from the United States, United Kingdom, or Sweden.[156,270,530,531] In the developing world, studies in maternal populations with near-universal seroimmunity have demonstrated congenital infection rates of 1% to 2%, and, of interest, infants with clinically apparent infections and infants who develop long-term sequelae from congenital CMV infections have been described in these populations.[195,200,202,203,395] In fact, the rates of symptomatic congenital infection and subsequent hearing loss in congenitally infected infants from a maternity population with greater than 96% seroimmunity to CMV before pregnancy were similar to those reported in several different large series of infants with congenital CMV infections.[203,532]

In nonprimary maternal infections, it is likely that preexisting maternal immunity could alter the parameters of CMV in the mother and developing fetus at least to some extent. It is unknown if preexisting cellular immunity is more important than humoral immunity; however, maternal immunoglobulin G (IgG) antibodies are transmitted to the fetus, and thus, at a first approximation, could alter the virologic parameters of fetal infection. Cases of symptomatic congenital infection have been reported after therapeutic immune suppression, in women with lupus or AIDS, and even in women with intact immune systems, suggesting that altered maternal immunity either from immunosuppression or from an inability to recognize a recurrent maternal infection (reinfection) can lead to fetal infection and disease.[530,533-538]

The rhesus macaque model of CMV neuropathogenesis requires direct infection of the developing rhesus fetus and disease can be observed even in the presence of maternal T lymphocyte and antiviral antibody immunity to the virus.[487] This result would argue that once virus

*References 157, 270, 515, 516, 518, 520.

†References 164, 202, 203, 509, 523-525, 527-529.

enters the fetus, a critical balance between fetal immunity, maternal immunity that can be transferred to the fetus, and viral inoculum will determine the extent and severity of fetal infection. Such a complex relationship between virus and immunity suggests that analysis of specimens derived from human natural history studies will likely provide only a limited insight into this intrauterine infection. In the rhesus macaque model of CVM infections, investigators have demonstrated that the presence of viral immune evasion function permits reinfection of previously infected monkeys.[539] Deletion of these viral genes that encode functions to degrade major histocompatibility class I molecules, and thus limit T-lymphocyte recognition of virus-infected cells, resulted in an attenuated virus that was incapable of infecting previously immune monkeys.[539]

PERINATAL INFECTION

Naturally acquired perinatal CMV infections result from exposure to infected maternal genital secretions at birth or to breast milk during the first months of postnatal life.[169,170,540,541] The presence of CMV at these two sites may be the result of either primary or recurrent maternal infection. Iatrogenic CMV infections are acquired predominantly from transfusions of blood or blood products and, in the past, banked breast milk from CMV-infected donors. Exposure to CMV in the maternal genital tract can result in a 30% to 50% rate of perinatal infection. The transmission from mother to infant through breast milk occurs in 30% to 70% of cases if nursing lasts for more than 1 month.[167,169-171,542-548] After ingestion of the virus, CMV infection is presumably established at a mucosal surface (buccal, pharyngeal, or esophageal mucosa) or in the salivary glands. Rarely, perinatal CMV infection and, rarely, congenital CMV infections have been associated with pneumonitis, and in early reports, CMV pneumonia was reported to account for significant mortality in congenitally infected infants.[223]

Transmission of CMV by blood transfusion is more likely to occur when large quantities of blood are transfused, providing some clues as to the nature of persistence of CMV in cells of the blood and an indirect assessment of the frequency of CMV-infected cells in the blood. The failure to isolate CMV from the blood or blood elements of healthy seropositive blood donors suggests that the virus exists in a latent state, presumably within leukocytes. It has been suggested that CMV reactivates after transfusion when infected cells encounter the allogeneic stimulus. CMV genomes are activated when transfused to a recipient, particularly if immunologically immature or deficient. As was discussed previously, mobilization of $CD34^+$ myeloid cells by GM-CSF can lead to an increase in the incidence of CMV infection in recipients of such mobilized myeloid cells, suggesting that administration of this growth factor can favor reactivation of latent CMV.[139,301,549]

PERSISTENT VIRAL EXCRETION

Congenitally and perinatally acquired CMV infections are characterized by chronic viral excretion.[457] Virus is consistently shed into the urine for up to 6 years or longer and into saliva for 2 to 4 years. Not only does excretion persist much longer in congenitally infected infants than in infected older children and adults, the quantity of virus excreted is also much greater. Even asymptomatic congenitally or perinatally infected infants excrete quantities of virus that usually exceed those detectable in seriously ill immunocompromised older patients by 1 to 2 logarithms. As illustrated in Figure 24-4, the highest quantities of virus are excreted during the first 6 months of life. Infants with symptomatic congenital CMV infection excrete significantly larger amounts than those with asymptomatic congenitally or perinatally acquired infections (see Fig. 24-4, *A*). The excretion of CMV in various body fluids has been reviewed recently.[550] Similar results have been obtained when peripheral blood of congenitally infected infants has been analyzed by quantitative PCR assay (see Fig. 24-4, *B*).[551] Of interest, a relationship has been identified between the viral DNA copy number in peripheral blood and long-term outcome, suggesting that monitoring congenitally infected infants by this assay could identify those at risk for sequelae and thus select a population of congenitally infected infants that could be considered as potential candidates for treatment with antiviral agents (see following sections).[551,552] More recently, the quantity of CMV in the peripheral blood was quantified by PCR assay in hopes of providing prognostic information on the risk of hearing loss.[553] Unfortunately, the overlap in the results between infants with hearing loss and those without hearing loss was significant and suggested that simply determining viral burden in peripheral blood of congenitally infected infants was not adequate for screening infants to define the risk of hearing loss.

Pathology

Early reports of histopathologic changes associated with CMV infections relied on a demonstration of cytomegaly and nuclear and cytoplasmic inclusions. The distinctive features include large cells 20 to 35 mm in diameter with a large nucleus containing round, oval, or reniform inclusions. These large inclusions are separated from the nuclear membrane by a clear zone, which gives the inclusion the so-called owl's eye appearance. The inclusions within the nucleus show DNA positivity by histochemical staining, whereas the cytoplasmic inclusions contain carbohydrates, as evidenced by periodic acid–Schiff positivity. The cytoplasmic inclusions vary from minute dots to distinct rounded bodies 3 to 4 mm in diameter. The cytoplasmic inclusions are usually aggregated opposite to the eccentrically placed inclusion-bearing nucleus and appear to represent a cytoplasmic site of virus assembly.[127,554] Unfortunately, the classic CMV inclusion-bearing cell may be only scattered throughout involved tissue and missed by routine sectioning. This finding has been confirmed when more refined techniques, such as in situ DNA hybridization and immunofluorescence using CMV-specific monoclonal antibodies, have been used to define the extent of infection with CMV in immunocompromised patients.[555,556]

COMMONLY INVOLVED ORGAN SYSTEMS

Disseminated disease can occur in the infected fetus and congenitally infected infant. CMV can cause a multisystem disease in which almost all major organ systems are involved.[456]

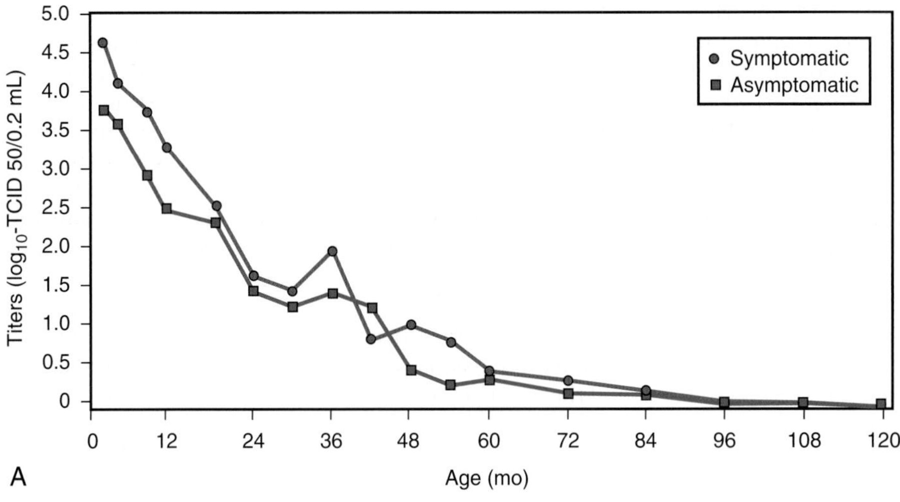

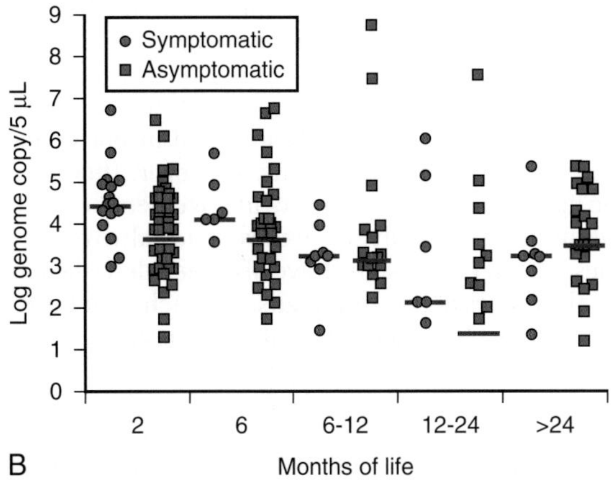

Figure 24-4 A, Viral load detected by urine excretion of infectious virus in infants with symptomatic and asymptomatic congenital human cytomegalovirus infection as a function of age. Titers are expressed as log of tissue culture infectious doses (TCID) in which 50% of wells contained virus. **B,** Genomic copies of human cytomegalovirus in blood from congenitally infected infants with symptomatic (●) and asymptomatic (■) infections. Median values are designated by red horizontal bars.

Central Nervous System

Involvement of the CNS is perhaps the most important consequence of fetal infection with CMV. Most descriptions of the pathology of CNS infection are relevant only to infants with severe CID, which is occasionally fatal.[456,471,557-559] In the vast majority of infected infants, the infection can be described grossly as focal encephalitis and periependymitis. The encephalitis can involve cells of both the gray and white matter, as well as cells within the choroid plexus. Inclusion-bearing cells have been identified in neurons, glia, ependyma, choroid plexus, meninges, vascular endothelium, and in cells lying free in the ventricles. Rarely, inclusion-bearing cells have been identified in the cerebrospinal fluid (CSF).[560] Resolution of acute encephalitis leads to gliosis and calcification. Previous descriptions have emphasized the periventricular location of calcifications; however, these lesions can be located anywhere in the brain.[472,478,482] CMV has been isolated on a few occasions from CSF, and more recently, PCR assay has been used to demonstrate CMV in the CSF.[561,562] Recent studies of brain tissue derived from fetuses terminated at gestational age 21 to 22 weeks because of prenatal detection of CMV infection have extended these findings somewhat.[563,564] Although only 62% of terminated fetuses had evidence of CNS involvement, a smaller group of the terminated fetuses exhibited extensive involvement in most areas of the brain, with areas of focal accumulation of granzyme-positive $CD8^+$ T lymphocytes.[564] The highest copy number of viral DNA was found in the CNS of fetuses with the most extensive involvement, as was the most intense $CD8^+$ T-lymphocyte infiltration.[564] Furthermore, the extent of pathologic findings in the brain was directly related to the degree of damage in the placenta, raising the possibility that significant placental insufficiency contributed to the findings in this group of fetuses. Thus it is difficult to assign either direct virus cytopathology, immunopathology, or placental damage as the primary mechanism of disease in this series of infected fetuses; however, the lack of extensive loss of brain parenchyma associated with viral antigens suggested that virus-mediated tissue destruction was an unlikely mechanism of disease. A very recent study in a murine model of CNS disease in congenital CMV infection clearly demonstrated that inflammation and immunopathology and not direct virus cytopathology were the major cause of disease-induced CNS damage.[491] The only other group of patients with a significant incidence of CMV encephalitis are persons with HIV/AIDS. Infection of the CNS by CMV is well described in these patients and again has been characterized as ventriculoencephalitis in which the virus is thought to spread through the ventricular system and result in widespread disease in the periventricular neuroepithelium and a second more common form described as a focal encephalitis.[459]

CMV infection of structures of the hearing apparatus has been described as noted in the previous sections. Viral inclusion–bearing cells and viral antigen–containing cells can also be found within structures of the inner ear, including the organ of Corti, the spiral ganglion, and in epithelial cells of striae vascularis of the cochleae.[265,565-567] Finally, involvement of the eye, including chorioretinitis, optic neuritis, cataract formation, colobomas, and microphthalmos, has been demonstrated.[265,568-570] The histopathologic changes associated with retinitis begin as an acute vasculitis that spreads into the choroid through the vascular basement membrane. CMV has been isolated from fluid of the anterior chamber of the eye.[571] Anecdotal cases of cataracts have been described in congenitally infected infants. Finally, the clinical findings of infants with CMV chorioretinitis differ from that of HIV/AIDS patients with retinitis in that level of retinal involvement is often less and the cellular infiltrate and retinal edema is also limited when the findings in infants with congenital CMV infections are compared with those of patients with HIV/AIDS. It is of interest that chorioretinitis in congenitally infected infants has been associated with an increased risk of long-term cognitive disorders in congenitally infected infants.[572]

Liver

Involvement of the liver is common in congenital CMV infections. Clinical evidence of hepatitis as manifested by hepatomegaly, elevated levels of serum aminotranferases, and direct hyperbilirubinemia is frequently seen in infants with symptomatic congenital infections. Pathologic descriptions of hepatic involvement include mild cholangitis with CMV infections of bile duct cells, intralobular cholestasis, and obstructive cholestasis secondary to extramedullary hematopoiesis.[456] Liver calcifications have been detected radiologically in infants with congenital infections.[573,574] Clinical and laboratory evidence of liver disease eventually subsides in surviving infants and only anecdotal cases of cirrhosis have been reported.

Hematopoietic System

Hematologic abnormalities, including thrombocytopenia, anemia, and extramedullary hematopoiesis, are common in symptomatically infected infants, but these abnormalities almost invariably resolve within the first year of life. The exact mechanism accounting for these disturbances is not certain, although congestive splenomegaly resulting in platelet and red blood cell trapping certainly must play some part in the overall process. Significant splenomegaly is not uncommon, and congestion, extramedullary hematopoiesis, and diminished size of lymphoid follicles can be seen histologically. Recent studies in MCMV have proposed a mechanism for the development of extramedullary hematopoiesis in CMV infection that involves control of virus spread by NK-cell–mediated cytotoxicity and preservation of the localized inflammation needed to drive this response to CVM infection.[575]

In congenital CMV infections, thrombocytopenia may persist for several months, even years, with or without petechiae. Anemia is another feature of symptomatic congenital CMV infection. The presence of indirect hyperbilirubinemia, extramedullary hematopoiesis, and erythroblastemia indicates active hemolysis, but mechanisms that account for these findings have not been well described.

Kidneys

Macroscopically, the kidneys show no alterations. Microscopically, inclusion-bearing cells are commonly seen, especially in the cells lining the distal convoluted tubules and collecting ducts.[456,576] Affected cells may desquamate into the lumina of the tubules and appear in the urine sediment. Inclusions can be found occasionally in Bowman capsules and proximal tubules. Mononuclear cell infiltration may be present in the peritubular zones of the kidney.

Endocrine Glands

Secretory cells of endocrine glands commonly contain typical CMV inclusions. In the pancreas, both the endocrine and the exocrine cells are affected.[456] Some reports describe intralobular or periductal mononuclear infiltration, suggesting focal pancreatitis. There is no evidence-based association between congenital CMV infection and the development of diabetes mellitus. CMV inclusion–bearing cells have been documented in follicular cells of the thyroid, the adrenal cortex, and the anterior pituitary.

Gastrointestinal Tract

The salivary glands are commonly involved in both congenital and perinatal CMV infections. However, there are no reliable figures on the frequency of involvement because the examination of the salivary glands is not always part of autopsies.[456] CMV inclusions have also been described in the mucosal surfaces of the esophagus, stomach, and intestine and in the vessels of ulcerative intestinal lesions.[456,577]

Lungs

Pulmonary CMV lesions are similar in the newborn and the adult. Microscopically, the majority of the inclusion-bearing cells are alveolar cells that lie free in terminal air spaces. In general, there is little inflammatory reaction; however, in the more severe cases, focal interstitial infiltration by lymphocytes and plasma cells can be found.

Placenta

Abnormalities are present in the placentas of a majority of patients with symptomatic CMV infection and have been reported to be infrequent with subclinical infections.[578,579-582] CMV DNA can be frequently detected in both the decidua and placenta of seropositive women, even though the rate of congenital infection in this population is about 1%, a finding that supported the hypothesis that the placenta represents a barrier for fetal infection.[583-585] Early studies have suggested that placentas are not remarkable in size or macroscopic appearance; however, more recent reports have suggested placenta enlargement in some women who delivered infected infants.[586] The most specific feature histologically is the presence of inclusion-bearing cells, which may be found in endothelial cells, in cells attached to the capillary walls, or in Hofbauer or stromal cells.[579,581] Other lesions include focal necrosis, which in early gestation shows sparse infiltration by lymphocytes, macrophages, and a few plasma cells. The early lesions present as foci of necrosis of the stroma and occasionally of the vessels of the villi. The focus of necrosis is later invaded by inflammatory cells, histiocytes, and fibroblasts. At later gestational ages, these focal lesions become densely cellular, with plasma cells predominating over lymphocytes.

Deposition of intracellular and extracellular hemosiderin can be found in stem and terminal villi and is presumably the result of fetal hemorrhage during the necrotizing phase or of maternal intervillous thrombosis.[587] Calcification within villi or on basement membranes has also been described as a late manifestation of placental CMV infection.

In recent years there has been increased interest in understanding the role the placenta plays in congenital CMV infection.[578,588] In vitro systems have been developed to examine interactions between CMV and the placenta. Studies from these systems have uncovered a complex relationship between maternal immunity and the likelihood of CMV replication in distinct areas of the placenta and the decidua.[309,578,589] In addition, other investigators have noted that the immune tolerance of the placenta could limit efficient clearance of virus. The placenta produces the immunosuppressive chemokine IL-10, and expression of human leukocyte antigen-G in the placenta is thought to limit NK-cell activity.[590-595] These findings have led investigators to suggest that CMV replication in the placenta is poorly controlled and that transmission to the fetus occurs after infection of cytotrophoblasts.[589] More recent studies have suggested that CMV can dysregulate the expression of proteins essential for normal placentation and that CMV infection of the placenta can lead to placental insufficiency and intrauterine growth restriction and potentially other effects on the fetus.[578] This proposed mechanism of disease is consistent with a potential immunomodulatory role of passively transferred IVIG in pregnant women.[430] Of interest, a study in the guinea pig model of congenital infection that demonstrated the protection from perinatal CMV disease by a recombinant virus expressing a gpCMV envelope glycoprotein could be interpreted as reflecting the capacity of antiviral immunity to limit the placental insufficiency induced by gpCMV infection in these pregnant animals.[596] Finally, the placenta can also produce proinflammatory cytokines and chemokines, including TNF and MCP-1, in response to CMV infection.[597-602] Generation of such inflammatory mediators and subsequent recruitment of inflammatory monocytes from both fetal and maternal circulation can alter placental function and contribute to adverse outcomes of pregnancies associated with CMV infection.[587]

Clinical Manifestations

CONGENITAL INFECTION

Approximately 10% of the estimated 20,000 to 40,000 infants (0.5%-1% of all live births) born annually with congenital CMV infection in the United States have signs and symptoms at birth that are consistent with the diagnosis of a congenital infection. Significantly, less than one half of these symptomatic infants have typical generalized CID, characterized mainly by the clinical manifestations given in Table 24-7.[‡] Another 5% of these infants present with milder or atypical involvement, and 90% are born with subclinical congenital infection. Because early studies only emphasized symptomatic infections, congenital CMV was considered a rare and often fatal disease. In the early reports, many patients were referred to the investigators because of abnormalities in normal development; this led to a selection bias of a group of patients at a higher risk for persistent abnormalities and neurologic damage. The use of more sensitive and specific methods of diagnosis, particularly viral isolation and newer methods of rapid virus detection, has allowed prospective longitudinal study of newborns with symptomatic and asymptomatic congenital CMV infections. This has resulted in a more accurate understanding of the infection and its clinical spectrum.

‡References 1, 153, 194, 270, 458, 514, 603.

Symptomatic Infection

Acute Manifestations. Clinically apparent infections or CID is characterized by involvement of multiple organs, in particular, the reticuloendothelial and CNS, with or without ocular and auditory damage. Weller and Hanshaw[604] defined the abnormalities found most frequently in infants with symptomatic congenital infection as hepatomegaly, splenomegaly, microcephaly, jaundice, and petechiae (see Table 24-7).

In addition, the magnitude of the prenatal insult is thought to be reflected by the occurrence of microcephaly with or without cerebral calcification, intrauterine growth retardation, and prematurity, although many of the earlier studies describing symptomatic congenital CMV infections were plagued by enrollment bias of only the most severely affected patients.[§] Inguinal hernia in males and chorioretinitis with

§References 86, 164, 367-370, 470, 472, 478, 482, 515, 605, 606.

Table 24-7 Clinical and Laboratory Findings in 106 Infants with Symptomatic Congenital Cytomegalovirus Infection in the Newborn Period

Abnormality	Positive/Total Examined (%)
Prematurity (<38 wk)	36/106 (34)
Small for gestational age	53/106 (50)
Petechiae	80/106 (76)
Jaundice	69/103 (67)
Hepatosplenomegaly	63/105 (60)
Purpura	14/105 (13)
Neurologic findings	
One or more of the following:	72/106 (68)
Microcephaly	54/102 (53)
Lethargy/hypotonia	28/104 (27)
Poor suck	20/103 (19)
Seizures	7/105 (7)
Elevated alanine aminotransferase (>80 U/L)	46/58 (83)
Thrombocytopenia	
$<100 \times 10^3$/mm^3	62/81 (77)
$<50 \times 10^3$/mm^3	43/81 (53)
Conjugated hyperbilirubinemia	
Direct serum bilirubin > 4 mg/dL	47/68 (69)
Hemolysis	37/72 (51)
Increased cerebrospinal fluid protein (>120 mg/dL)*	24/52 (46)

From Boppana S, Pass RF, Britt WS, et al: Symptomatic congenital cytomegalovirus infection: neonatal morbidity and mortality, *Pediatr Infect Dis J* 11:93-99, 1992, with permission.
*Determinations in the first week of life.

or without optic atrophy are less common. Clinical findings occasionally include hydrocephalus, hemolytic anemia, and pneumonitis. Among the most severely affected infants, mortality rates may be as high as 10% to 30%.[223,458] Most deaths occur in the neonatal period and are usually due to multiorgan disease with severe hepatic dysfunction, bleeding, and disseminated intravascular coagulation. When death occurs after the first month but during the first year, it is usually secondary to severe failure to thrive, possibly secondary to ongoing liver disease and dysfunction combined with severe CNS dysfunction. Death after the first year is usually restricted to the severely neurologically damaged children and is due to malnutrition, aspiration pneumonia, and infections associated with neurologically impaired infants.

HEPATOMEGALY. This clinical finding, along with splenomegaly, is probably the most common abnormality found in the newborn period in infants born with a symptomatic congenital CMV infection.[607] The liver edge is smooth and nontender and usually measures 4 to 7 cm below the right costal margin. Liver function tests are often abnormal and reflect hepatocellular dysfunction and cholestasis. The persistence of hepatomegaly is variable. In some infants, liver enlargement disappears by the age of 2 months. In others, significant enlargement persists throughout the first year of life. However, hepatomegaly extending beyond the first 12 months of life is an uncommon finding in infants with CID.

SPLENOMEGALY. Enlargement of the spleen exists to a greater or lesser degree in all the common human congenital infections and is especially frequent in congenital CMV infections.[458] It may be the only abnormality present at birth. In some instances, splenomegaly and a petechial rash coexist as the only manifestations of the disease. On occasion, the enlargement is such that the spleen may be felt 10 to 15 cm below the costal margin. Splenomegaly usually persists longer than hepatomegaly and is thought to contribute to persistent thrombocytopenia in some patients.

JAUNDICE. Jaundice is a common manifestation of congenital CID. The pattern of hyperbilirubinemia may take several forms, ranging from high levels on the first day to undetectable jaundice on the first day with gradual elevation of the bilirubin level to clinically apparent jaundice. The level of jaundice in the early weeks of life may fluctuate considerably.[458] In some instances, jaundice is a transient phenomenon, beginning on the first day and disappearing by the end of the first week. More often, however, jaundice tends to persist beyond the time of physiologic jaundice. Less commonly, transient jaundice may occasionally occur in early infancy with pronounced elevation of bilirubin levels during the third month. Bilirubin levels are elevated in both the direct and the indirect components. Characteristically, the direct component increases after the first few days of life and may constitute as much as 50% of the total bilirubin level. Hepatic aminotransferases are elevated but abnormalities in coagulation secondary to liver disease are infrequently observed.

PETECHIAE AND PURPURA. There is evidence from experimental animal models that CMV has a direct effect on the megakaryocytes of the bone marrow that results in a depression of the platelets and a localized or generalized petechial rash, although similar studies have not been carried out in humans infected with CMV. In some patients, the rash is purpuric (Fig. 24-5), not unlike that observed in the expanded rubella syndrome.

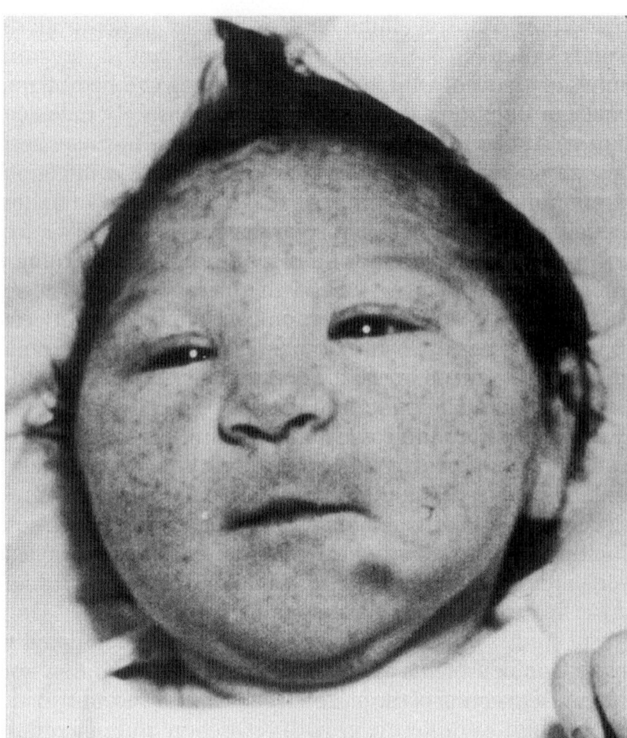

Figure 24-5 Symptomatic congenital cytomegalovirus infection manifested by microcephaly and petechiae.

Unlike the latter infection, however, pinpoint petechiae are a more common manifestation and a blueberry muffin–like rash is not characteristic. These petechiae are rarely present at birth but often appear within a few hours thereafter; they may be transient, disappearing within 48 hours. The petechiae may be the only clinical manifestation of CMV infection. More often, however, enlargement of the spleen and liver is associated with the finding of petechiae. The petechiae may persist for weeks after birth. Crying, coughing, the application of a tourniquet, a lumbar puncture, or restraints of any kind may result in the appearance of petechiae even months after birth. Platelet counts in the first week of life range from less than 10,000 to 125,000, with a majority in the 20,000-to-60,000 range. Some infants with petechial rashes do not have associated thrombocytopenia. Rarely, if ever, is significant bleeding associated with the thrombocytopenia associated with congenital CMV infection.

MICROCEPHALY. Microcephaly, currently defined in epidemiologic studies as a head circumference of less than the third percentile, was found to be present in 14 of 17 patients with CID in the early studies of Medearis[608] in 1964. As tissue culture methods became more widely used and clinical awareness of the infection increased, microcephaly became a less prominent symptom in subsequent series that included mainly infants born with less severe disease. In a more recent examination of 106 surviving patients who were born with symptomatic CMV infection, 53% were microcephalic.[458] As was noted previously, aspects of this study and many other studies that have catalogued the clinical and laboratory findings of infants with symptomatic congenital CMV infections have been limited by enrollment bias of only those children with the most obvious clinical findings.

Table 24-8 Sequelae in Children After Congenital Cytomegalovirus Infection

Sequelae	% Symptomatic (no.)	% Symptomatic Screened Population (no.)*	% Asymptomatic (no.)
Sensorineural hearing loss	58 (58/100)	34(24/70)	7.4 (22/299)
Bilateral hearing loss	37 (37/100)	50 (12/24)	2.7 (8/299)
Speech threshold moderate to profound (60-90 dB)†	27 (27/100)		1.7 (5/299)
Chorioretinitis	20.4 (19/93)	10 (7/20)	2.5 (7/281)
IQ < 70	55 (33/60)	25 (10/40)	3.7 (6/159)
Microcephaly, seizures or paresis/paralysis	51.9 (54/104)		2.7 (9/330)
Microcephaly	37.5 (39/104)	35(25/70)	1.8 (6/330)
Seizures	23.1 (24/104)	1(1/70)	0.9 (3/330)
Paresis/paralysis	12.5 (13/104)		0 (0/330)
Death‡	5.8 (6/104)		0.3 (1/330)

Modified from Pass RF, Fowler KB, Boppana S: Progress in cytomegalovirus research. In Landini MP, editor: *Proceedings of the Third International Cytomegalovirus Workshop,* Bologna, Italy, June 1991, London, 1991, Excerpta Medica, pp 3-10.
IQ, Intelligence quotient.
*Sequelae in only symptomatic infants identified by prospective screening (S.A. Ross, unpublished data).
†For the ear with better hearing.
‡After newborn period.

A more recent study has examined this bias within a large cohort of infants with congenital CMV infection and has refined the estimates of symptoms and laboratory abnormalities in a group of infected infants identified through newborn screening and an unscreened group (referral population) of infants with congenital CMV infections.[194] Remarkable differences were noted between the populations, and it was concluded that the incidence of severe disease was less than originally reported (Table 24-8).[194] Similar findings have been reported by investigators in the United Kingdom and Sweden.[603] These investigators noted that of the total group of 176 infants, 11% had symptomatic congenital CMV infections that were described as mild, and only 6% of the entire cohort had severe CNS sequelae.[603] Finally, it is important to note that not all infants with microcephaly in the perinatal period will continue to have head circumferences of less than the third percentile later in infancy. However, microcephaly is the most specific predictor of future cognitive impairment in congenitally infected infants (this is especially true if the head measurement is close to the fifth percentile in an infant of low birth weight). Intracranial calcifications suggest that the infant will have at least moderate and probably severe delays in cognitive development.[472,609]

Ocular Defects. The principal abnormality related to the eye in CMV infection is chorioretinitis, with strabismus and optic atrophy.[265,472,569] Microphthalmos, cataracts, retinal necrosis and calcification, blindness, anterior chamber and optic disc malformations, and pupillary membrane vestige have also been described in association with generalized congenital CID. Despite this, the presence of abnormalities such as microphthalmos and cataracts is strong presumptive evidence that the disease process is not caused by CMV. Chorioretinitis has been reported to occur in approximately 14% of infants born with symptomatic congenital infection.[472,569] Although chorioretinitis occurs less frequently in symptomatic congenital CMV than in congenital toxoplasmosis, lesions caused by CMV and *Toxoplasma* cannot be differentiated on the basis of location or appearance alone.[265,569] Both *Toxoplasma gondii* and CMV can induce central retinal lesions. On occasion, the appearance of strabismus with subsequent referral to an ophthalmologist will result in the diagnosis of chorioretinitis. Any infant with suspected CMV infection or strabismus in early life should be examined carefully for retinal lesions. Chorioretinitis caused by CMV, however, differs from that caused by *Toxoplasma* in that postnatal progression is rare in infants with congenital CMV.

Fetal Growth Retardation. Intrauterine growth retardation (IUGR), occasionally severe, was reported in 50% of 106 patients with symptomatic congenital CMV infection, whereas prematurity occurred in 34% (see Table 24-7).[472] Infants with asymptomatic congenital infection in general do not exhibit IUGR or prematurity, and CMV has not been considered a common cause of either condition in infants without overt clinical findings of congenital CMV infections. Although frequently included in more recent descriptions of symptomatic congenital CMV infection, original studies of the natural history of congenital CMV infections did not include fetal growth retardation as a finding that defined symptomatic congenital CMV infection.

Pneumonitis. Pneumonitis, a common clinical manifestation of CMV infection after hematopoietic and solid-organ transplantation in adults, is not usually a part of the clinical presentation of congenital CMV infection in newborns. Diffuse interstitial pneumonitis occurs in less than 1% of congenitally infected infants, even when the most severely affected cases are considered. CMV-associated pneumonitis has been described in infants with perinatally acquired CMV infections.[610]

Dental Defects. Congenital CMV infection is also associated with a distinct defect of enamel, which thus far seems to affect mainly primary dentition.[611] This defect is more severe in children with the symptomatic form of the infection than in those born with asymptomatic infections (Fig. 24-6). The mechanism(s) leading to enamel dysplasia in infants with congenital CMV is unknown.

Clinically, this defect appears on all or nearly all of the teeth and is characterized by generalized yellowish discoloration. The enamel is opaque and moderately soft and tends to chip away from dentin. Affected teeth tend to be susceptible to mechanical trauma, leading to dental caries that are

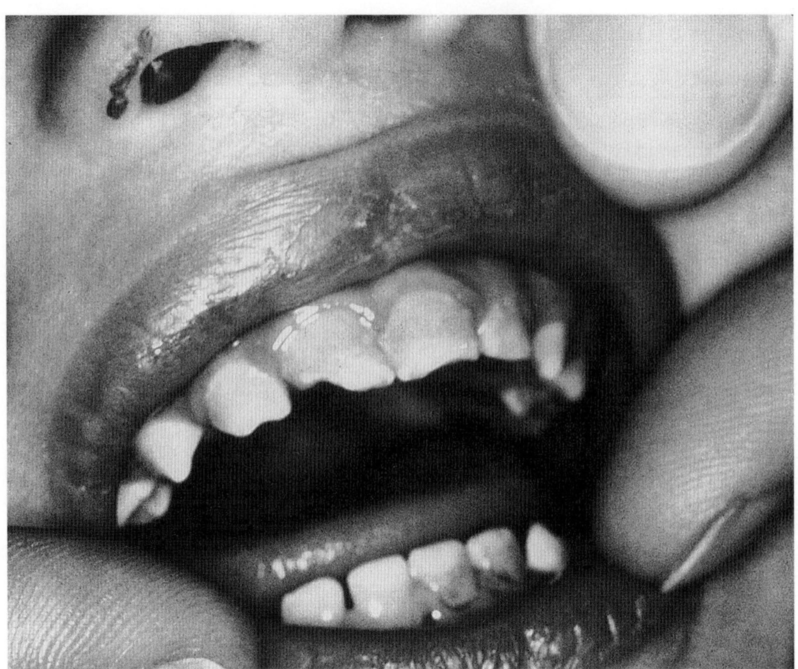

Figure 24-6 Cytomegalovirus (CMV)-affected teeth. This patient had a clinically severe congenital CMV infection. Note fractured borders and opaque and hypocalcified enamel.

frequently seen in these children. In our longitudinal studies, this defect of enamel was documented in 27% of 92 children born with symptomatic congenital CMV infection and in 4% of 267 who were born with the subclinical form and who were observed for at least 2 years. These patients usually require extensive orthodontic therapy. It is evident that these defects do not involve permanent teeth to the same degree.

DEAFNESS. Sensorineural deafness is the most common disorder of neurodevelopmental deficit caused by congenital CMV infection. Medearis[608] was the first investigator to call attention to the presence of deafness in symptomatic congenitally-infected infants. Subsequent reports confirmed this association and provided evidence that CMV can also cause sensorineural hearing loss in children with clinically inapparent congenital infection (see Table 24-8).[‖] In fact, CMV is now considered one of the most important causes of deafness in childhood and, in the United States, is thought to be the most common etiology of nonfamilial sensorimotor hearing loss, causing an estimated 25% of all cases of hearing loss.[269,467,615-618]

The frequency and severity of the hearing impairment is increased in patients with symptomatic infection (58%) compared with asymptomatic infection at birth (7.4%). In general, hearing loss is progressive in 50%, bilateral in 50%, and of late onset in 20% of cases. The predictors of hearing loss in children with symptomatic congenital CMV infection are IUGR, petechiae, hepatosplenomegaly, thrombocytopenia, and intracerebral calcifications. These are similarly the predictors of significantly higher viral loads in newborn infants.[551,552,619,620] However, the presence of microcephaly and other neurologic abnormalities in one study failed to predict hearing loss.[619] Using logistic regression analysis, only petechiae and IUGR were shown to be independent predictors of hearing loss. As noted previously, the viral load measured in peripheral blood does predict the hearing outcome of congenitally infected infants.[551-553,620]

‖References 223, 265-267, 269, 461, 465, 472, 509, 612-614.

Long-Term Outcome. The likelihood of survival with normal intellect and hearing after symptomatic congenital CMV infection is clearly reduced compared with uninfected infants, but previous studies have overestimated the likelihood of significant long-term sequelae in most infants with congenital CMV infections.[223,458,541,569,621-625]

As shown in Table 24-8, in our earlier prospective studies that included a combined population of patients derived from a screened newborn population and referral patients, one or more sequelae have occurred in the vast majority of the patients with symptomatic congenital infection who survived.[458] However, when symptomatically infected infants who were identified through an unbiased screening program in this cohort were analyzed separately, only about 50% suffered any long-term sequelae (see Table 24-8).[194] These more recent results were in surprisingly good agreement with findings from investigators who have described their patients identified by a newborn screening program.[603]

Psychomotor retardation, usually combined with neurologic complications and microcephaly, occurred in nearly 70% of those infants reported in a series of patients that included screened and referral patients. When only infants identified by screening were analyzed, the incidence of psychomotor retardation in infants with symptomatic congenital CMV infection appears to be about 25%, a finding that is consistent with the findings of a recently reported screening study from Europe (see Table 24-8).[194,603] Sensorineural hearing loss was seen in 50%. The hearing loss is bilateral in 67% of patients with hearing loss and is progressive in 54%. Although reflective of the literature, it is also important to note that rates of progressive loss and profound hearing loss are likely overestimates produced by the enrollment bias present in previous reports. Of interest, a single study from Europe reported a significant incidence of vestibular dysfunction in infants with congenital CMV.[626] Chorioretinitis or optic atrophy occurred in 20% of cases. Expressive language delays independent from hearing loss and mental impairment have also been described. Several studies have searched for clinical predictors of intelligence and developmental outcome and found that microcephaly at birth, development of neurologic abnormalities during the first year of life, ocular lesions (chorioretinitis), and microcephaly that became apparent after birth were significantly associated with a low performance on cognitive and developmental testing.[572] A consistent predictor of adverse neurodevelopmental outcome is the presence of cranial computed tomographic (CT) abnormalities detected within the first month of life.[472,609,627] In infants with symptomatic congenital CMV infection, abnormal CT findings, particularly intracerebral calcifications, are common. It has been reported that nearly 90% of children with abnormal newborn CT scans develop at least one sequela compared with 29% among those with a normal study.[472] In this particular study, which included 56 children with symptomatic congenital CMV, only 1 child with a normal CT scan had an intelligence quotient of less than 70, in contrast to 59% of those with imaging abnormalities. Newborn CT abnormalities were also associated with an abnormal hearing screen at birth and hearing loss on follow-up. Of interest, none of the neonatal neurologic findings was predictive of an abnormal CT.[472] Overall, it can be anticipated that about 50% of infants with symptomatic congenital infections who survive will exhibit mild-to-severe long-term sequelae; however, it should again be stressed that this is likely an overestimate secondary to the enrollment bias that was common to many of the early natural history studies of congenital CMV infections.

Asymptomatic Infection

As described in the previous section, nearly 90% of infants with congenital CMV infections have no early clinical manifestations, and their long-term outcome appears much better than infants with clinically apparent infections. Nevertheless, there is now solid evidence derived from controlled prospective studies that at least 10% to 15% of these infants are at risk of developing a number of developmental abnormalities, including sensorineural hearing loss, microcephaly, motor defects (e.g., spastic diplegia or quadriplegia), mental retardation, chorioretinitis, dental defects, and others that were once thought to be limited to infants with symptomatic congenital infections. These abnormalities usually become apparent within the first 2 years of life.[265,460,509,622,628] Table 24-8 shows results based on a prospective longitudinal study of 330 patients with asymptomatic congenital infection who were followed by using serial clinical, psychometric, audiometric, and visual assessments. Follow-up studies of patients with inapparent congenital CMV infection have also been reported.[460,527,609,625,629-634] In general, their findings are consistent with the results of studies from this institution that are presented in Table 24-8.

The most frequent long-term sequelae in children born with subclinical congenital CMV infection is hearing loss. Fowler and associates[460] evaluated 307 children with documented asymptomatic congenital CMV infection and compared their audiometric assessments with 76 uninfected siblings of children with asymptomatic congenital CMV infection and 201 children whose neonatal screen for this infection showed negative results. Sensorineural hearing loss occurred only in children with congenital CMV infection. Among them, 22 (7.2%) had hearing loss. In 11 of the 22 children (50%), the hearing loss was bilateral. Among the children with hearing loss, further deterioration of hearing occurred in 50%, with a median age at first progression of 18 months (range, 2-70 months). Delayed onset of sensorineural hearing loss occurred in 18% of the children, with the median age of detection at 27 months (range, 25-62 months). Also, fluctuating hearing loss was documented in 22.7% of the children with hearing loss. These results are very similar to those obtained by Williamson and coworkers[631] in Houston. A study in Sweden of more than 10,000 newborns screened for both hearing loss and congenital CMV infection found that this congenital infection was the leading cause of sensorineural hearing loss, accounting for 40% of the cases with hearing loss.[509] Hicks[618] found 14 cases of congenital CMV infection with sensorineural hearing loss in 12,371 neonates screened for CMV, a rate of approximately 1.1 per 1,000 live births. The rate was 0.6 per 1000 when only cases with bilateral loss of 50 dB or greater were considered. These results suggest that congenital CMV infection could lead to sensorineural hearing loss in a significant number of young children.[467,615-618] Similar results have been obtained in populations outside of the United States and Northern Europe. In a study from Brazil derived from a population of women with greater than 96% seroprevalence for CMV, congenital infection was detected in 1% of newborn infants, and hearing loss (>60 dB) was present in approximately 8% of infected infants.[203, 532] Taken together, these studies indicate that the universal screening for hearing loss will detect less than half of all the cases of sensorineural hearing loss caused by congenital CMV infection. Because the vast majority of these infants are asymptomatic at birth, they are not recognized as being at high risk for hearing loss and, perhaps more important, are not being further tested to detect late-onset hearing loss. The universal screening of neonates for hearing loss should be combined with screening for congenital CMV infections.

Prospective studies of children with subclinical congenital CMV infections have also revealed a wide but significant spectrum of neurologic complications.[631] It has been estimated that within the first 2 years of life, 2% to 7% of the infants in this group develop microcephaly with various degrees of mental retardation and neuromuscular defects. How often milder forms of brain damage, such as learning or behavioral difficulties, will occur as these patients grow older is unknown and not being investigated. Studies of the intellectual development of children with asymptomatic congenital CMV infections have shown conflicting results. However, one study evaluated 204 prospectively followed children with asymptomatic congenital CMV infections and 177 uninfected siblings ranging in age from 6 to 203 months.[635] Parents were administered a developmental profile, and the children were administered an objective intelligence measure. Results showed that children with asymptomatic congenital CMV infection did not demonstrate intellectual impairment and that they performed similarly to uninfected siblings.

Children with asymptomatic congenital CMV infections have a low risk of chorioretinitis. The current estimate is that it occurs in 2% of these children and, like the hearing loss, may not be present at birth.

In summary, these observations underscore the need for longitudinal follow-up of patients with congenital CMV infection, regardless of the initial clinical presentation. Careful assessments of perceptual functions (hearing, visual acuity), psychomotor development, and learning abilities must be made to recognize the full impact of CMV. With early identification of a problem, corrective measures can be instituted to reduce psychosocial and learning problems.

Effect of Type of Maternal Infection on Symptoms and Long-Term Outcome

Studies have clearly demonstrated that preexisting maternal immunity does not prevent CMV from reactivating during pregnancy or acquiring a new strain of CMV and cannot reliably prevent transmission in utero nor symptomatic congenital infections.¶ A study of young, predominantly African-American women with one or more previous deliveries was carried out to estimate the protection conferred by preconception maternal immunity.[637] In the nearly 3500 multiparous women who had previously delivered newborns screened for congenital CMV infection and who subsequently enrolled in this study, the overall rate of congenital CMV infection was 1.3%. Congenital infection occurred in 18 of 604 newborns (3.0%; 95% confidence interval [CI], 1.8% to 4.7%) born to initially seronegative mothers compared with 29 among the 2857 births (1.0%; 95% CI, 0.7% to 1.4%) to immune mothers. Of the initially seronegative women, 23.5% seroconverted for an annualized seroconversion rate of 7.8% per year, with 12.7% of these seroconversions resulting in congenital CMV infection. One percent of infants born to mothers immune to CMV before conception had congenital infection. These results show that young women who have immunity to CMV from naturally acquired infections have about 60% lower relative risk of delivering a baby with congenital CMV infections within a 3-year period compared with women who were initially seronegative. Although this study confirmed a relative protective effect of preexisting immunity that was first reported nearly 3 decades ago, the absolute protective effect was modest if one considers that nearly twice as many infants with congenital infection were born to women with preexisting serologic immunity than from women with primary infection during pregnancy in this same population.[637] This study, together with studies from maternal populations with high seroprevalence for CMV, suggested that even though maternal immunity to CMV can limit the incidence of congenital infections presumably by decreasing the rate of transmission, the vast majority of infants with congenital CMV will be born to women with serologic immunity before conception in maternal population of high CMV seroprevalence. An informative analysis using modeling of congenital CMV infections has provided support for the importance of nonprimary maternal infections in the overall natural history of this perinatal infection (see later).[206]

It is generally argued that primary maternal infection results in a higher risk of symptomatic infection; however, data that has emerged in recent years, including our own prospective studies, raise the possibility that recurrent maternal infection may result in adverse outcome more frequently than previously thought. In 1999, prospective studies carried out in Sweden and the United States reported the presence of symptomatology at birth and the development of long-term sequelae in children born with congenital CMV infection after a recurrence of maternal infection (Table 24-9).[527,528]

Our study included 246 children with congenital CMV infection from the screening of 20,885 neonates.[528] Of the 246 infants, 47 were symptomatic at birth, and 8 of the 47 (17%) were born to mothers with recurrent CMV infection as defined by seropositive status at the time of a previous pregnancy. Demographically, the women in this study have been characterized as predominantly black (93%), single (96%), young (46% ≤ 20 years of age), and with no private insurance. More recently, a summary of the outcome of congenital CMV infection as function of the type of maternal infection from a screened population has been tabulated, and, from this study, it is apparent that damaging congenital infections are frequent after nonprimary maternal infections (Table 24-10).[270]

A study in this population concluded that in women who are seropositive for CMV, reinfection with different strains of CMV rather than reactivation of the endogenous strain can lead to intrauterine transmission and symptomatic congenital infection, a finding confirmed in a study of a highly seroimmune (>96% CMV immune) women in Brazil.[158,205,638] Most recently, a study that combined the findings from a screened newborn population in the United Kingdom and Sweden reported that more symptomatically infected infants were born to women with nonprimary infections than were born to women with primary infection during pregnancy.[603] In contrast, a smaller study of women who are predominantly white, married, of mid-to-high socioeconomic background, and somewhat older has

Table 24-9 Classification of Maternal Infection and Outcome of Infants With Congenital Cytomegalovirus Infection

Maternal Infection	Symptomatic at Birth	CNS Sequelae
Primary	9/30 (30%)	5/23 (22%)
Nonprimary	9/32 (28%)	8/23 (35%)

From Ahlfors K, Ivarsson SA, Harris S: Report on a long-term study of maternal and congenital cytomegalovirus infection in Sweden: review of prospective studies available in the literature, *Scand J Infect Dis* 31:443-457, 1999.
CNS, Central nervous system.

Table 24-10 Outcome of Congenital Cytomegalovirus Infection in Relation to Classification of Maternal Infection

Sequela	Primary (*N* = 76)	Nonprimary (*N* = 75)	Unknown (*N* = 136)
Hearing loss	9 (12%)	10 (13%)	22 (16%)
IQ < 70	4/37 (11%)	3/33 (9%)	13/76 (17%)
Motor deficits	2	3	5
Seizures	5	1	5
Chorioretinitis	2	1	1
Any sequela	13 (17%)	12 (16%)	31 (23%)

IQ, Intelligence quotient.

¶References 13, 195, 196, 202, 203, 205, 636.

not revealed the occurrence of symptomatic congenital CMV infection as a result of a recurrence of maternal infection. A summary of available data from nearly 4 decades of study of congenital CMV infections from a single institution has been presented as a schematic of the natural history of congenital CMV infections (Fig. 24-7). Finally, a recent report described findings from several computational models of the natural history of congenital CMV that were based on available data. These authors suggested that the contribution of cases of congenital CMV infection that result from primary maternal infection to the overall incidence of congenital CMV infections will remain constant and at a relatively low level secondary to the increasing force of infection in women with previous infection (nonprimary maternal infections), a possible explanation for the consistent observation that the incidence of congenital CMV infections increases dramatically as the incidence of seroimmunity in a maternal population increases.[206]

Public Health Significance

The public health impact of congenital CMV infection in the United States is significant, as shown in Table 24-11. Using models of congenital CMV infection in which the average rate of is 0.5% to 1% and the birth rate is 4 million per year, approximately 20,000 to 40,000 infants are born each year with congenital CMV infections. Of these, as many as 2000 infants present with signs and symptoms of congenital infection. About 200 of them can be expected to die within the first year, and nearly 1000 of the survivors could develop long-term sequelae. Another approximately 2000 to 3000 of subclinically infected (asymptomatic infections) infants develop significant hearing loss and/or deficits in cognition and motor activities. In addition to the personal and family suffering associated with these conditions, the cost to society for caring for these children has been estimated to be more than 1 billion dollars each year.[639]

PERINATAL INFECTION

As discussed in previous sections, perinatal infections can be acquired from exposure to virus in the maternal genital tract at delivery, from breast milk, or through multiple blood transfusions.[167,169,540,545-548,640-648] To establish the diagnosis of perinatal CMV infection, one must first exclude congenital infection by showing an absence of viral excretion during the first 2 weeks of life. Several studies have suggested that PCR assays can detect viral DNA in saliva or blood specimens from infants exposed to CMV after delivery but not congenitally infected, further indicating that confirmation of congenital CMV infections requires isolation of virus within 2 weeks of birth. The incubation period of perinatal CMV infection ranges between 4 and 12 weeks. Although the quantity of virus excreted by infants with perinatal infection is less than that seen with intrauterine acquisition, the infection is also chronic, with viral excretion persisting for years.[457]

The vast majority of infants with naturally acquired perinatal infections remain asymptomatic. Many of these infections result from nonprimary maternal infections, and therefore infants are born with variable levels of maternal antibody. Asymptomatic perinatal CMV infection in full-term and otherwise healthy infants does not appear to have an adverse effect on growth, perceptual functions, or motor or psychosocial development. CMV has been incriminated as a cause of pneumonitis in infants younger than 4 months.[610] In a study undertaken

Table 24-11 Public Health Impact of Congenital CMV Infection in the United States

Parameter	Estimated Figure
No. of live births per year	4,000,000
Rate of congenital CMV infection (average)	0.5%-1%
No. of infected infants	20-40,000
No. of infants symptomatic at birth (5%-7%)	1400-2800
No. with fatal disease (±12%)	168-336
No. with sequelae (50% of survivors)	616-1232
No. of infants asymptomatic at birth (93%-95%)	18,600-37,200
No. with late sequelae (15%)	2790-5580
Total no. with sequelae or fatal outcome	3406-6812

Modified from Fowler KB, Stagno S, Pass RF, et al: The outcome of congenital cytomegalovirus infection in relation to maternal antibody status, *N Engl J Med* 326:663-667, 1992.
CMV, Cytomegalovirus.

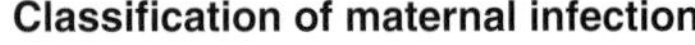

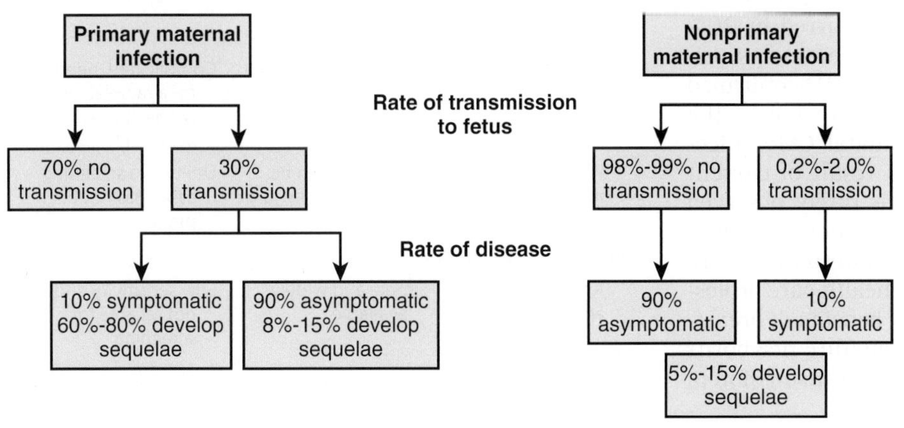

Figure 24-7 Natural history of congenital human cytomegalovirus infection, 1975-1998. The transmission rate varies depending on the population. Women of lower socioeconomic status have rates reported as high as 2.0%, whereas women from middle and upper middle class socioeconomic groups have rates of less than 0.2%.

to define the possible association of CMV and other respiratory pathogens with pneumonitis in young infants, CMV was isolated in 21 of 104 patients (21%) enrolled.[610] Only 3% of 97 hospitalized controls were infected. CMV-associated pneumonitis occurs throughout the year, in contrast to the common respiratory virus infections, which occur most often in winter and early spring. Although still consistent with available data, this study was carried out when diagnostic assays for respiratory viruses were in their infancy, and thus the results from this study remain controversial.

In premature and ill full-term infants, Yeager and colleagues[186] originally reported that naturally acquired CMV infection may pose a greater risk. They found that premature infants weighing less than 1500 g at birth who acquired CMV from a maternal source often developed hepatosplenomegaly, neutropenia, lymphocytosis, and thrombocytopenia, coinciding with the onset of virus excretion. Of interest was the observation that infected newborns required longer treatment with oxygen than uninfected patients. In a later study, Paryani and coworkers[649] from the same group reported a prospective study of 55 premature infants, including control infants, and suggested that there may be a propensity for an increased incidence of neuromuscular impairments, particularly in premature infants with the onset of CMV excretion during the first 2 months of life. However, sensorineural hearing loss, chorioretinitis, and microcephaly occurred with similar frequency in both groups. Similar findings were reported by Vochem[342] and Maschmann.[641,650] In the past, transfusion-acquired perinatal CMV infection has been associated with significant morbidity and mortality, particularly in premature infants with a birth weight of less than 1500 g born to CMV-seronegative mothers.[224,651] The syndrome of posttransfusion CMV infection in premature newborns was characterized by Ballard and coworkers.[652] They isolated CMV from 16 of 51 preterm infants with a mean birth weight of 1000 g and found that 14 of the 16 virus-positive infants had a constellation of symptoms that resembled CID. This recognizable, self-limited syndrome consisted of deterioration of respiratory function, hepatosplenomegaly, unusual gray pallor with disturbing septic appearance, both an atypical and an absolute lymphocytosis, thrombocytopenia, and hemolytic anemia. The syndrome was more severe in low-birth-weight infants and occurred 4 to 12 weeks after the transfusion, when the infants were progressing satisfactorily. Although the course of the disease was generally self-limited (lasting 2-3 weeks), death occurred in 20% of the ill infants. Subsequent work by Yeager and associates,[186] Zhang and associates,[407] and Adler[653] confirmed these observations. As has been discussed previously, the incidence of transfusion-acquired perinatal CMV infections has decreased dramatically as a result of current blood bank practices and fortunately is rarely observed today. Breast milk–acquired perinatal infections continue to occur, and because these infections can result in severe life- and organ-threatening infections, health care professionals must be aware of the risks and benefits of breast-milk supplementation in extremely premature newborns as well as approaches to reduce the risk of transmission of CMV by breast milk.

Diagnosis

DETECTION OF VIRUS

The diagnosis of congenital CMV infection should be entertained in any newborn with signs of congenital infection, if there is a history of maternal seroconversion or a mononucleosis-like illness during pregnancy or if an infant fails a newborn hearing screening examination. The conventional method for the diagnosis of congenital infection is virus isolation in tissue culture, which is generally accomplished with urine and/or saliva or by more contemporary approaches involving demonstration of CMV DNA by PCR assay (Table 24-12).[451,654-659] Combining tissue culture with immunofluorescence detection of antibody reactivity to the CMV-encoded IE-1 or pp72 protein shortens the time to detection of infectious virus in the urine or saliva and has been used to diagnose infants with congenital CMV infections.[660-663]

CMV-IgM serology has never been shown to have adequate sensitivity or specificity for the diagnosis of congenital CMV infection. With diagnostic methods that detect the virus, viral antigens and nucleic acids, it is possible to confirm the diagnosis from blood, CSF, and biopsy material. Of particular interest is the possibility of diagnosis by PCR assay on blood stored on filter paper.[658,664] This approach has been studied by a number of laboratories, and numerous reports have suggested its potential value.[620,664-669] Representative studies include those from Sweden, in which

Table 24-12 Summary of the Available Diagnostic Methods for the Identification of Infants With Congenital CMV Infection

Method	Advantages	Disadvantages
DETECTION OF VIRUS OR VIRAL ANTIGENS		
Standard tube culture method	Standard reference method	Takes 2-4 weeks, not suitable for screening
Shell vial assay	Rapid, sensitive and commercially available	Expensive, not suitable for screening
Microtiter plate immunofluorescent antibody assay	Rapid, sensitive, reliable, simple, inexpensive	Cell culture based, not commercially available
CMV antigenemia	Rapid and simple	Sensitivity and utility to screen newborns is not known, expensive
NUCLEIC ACID AMPLIFICATION METHODS		
DNA hybridization assay	Sensitive and reliable	Complicated, need for a radiolabeled probe; limited availability
PCR amplification methods	Simple and can be used to screen large numbers	Utility as a screening assay has not been proven
SEROLOGIC METHODS		
Anti-CMV IgM antibody assay	Simple and widely available	Low sensitivity and not reliable for screening

CMV, Cytomegalovirus; *IgM,* immunoglobulin M; *PCR,* polymerase chain reaction.

CMV DNA was detected in dried blood specimens from 13 of 16 (81%) infants with congenital CMV infection.[658] Italian investigators using a similar method obtained a sensitivity of 100% and a specificity of 98.5% in a study of 205 neonates, including 14 with congenital infections.[670] Both groups of investigators used a nested PCR method to detect CMV DNA in dried blood specimens, which added complexity to this assay, thus reducing its potential use as a screening assay. In addition, samples selected for many reports that have described the use of dried blood spots for detection of CMV were enriched in infants with congenital CMV and, in some cases, infants with symptomatic congenital CMV infections. Because of the potential bias caused by sample selection, it remained unclear if such an approach could be used to screen newborn populations for congenital CMV infections. Recent results from a large ongoing study of more than 20,000 specimens from screened population clearly demonstrated that dried blood-spot testing using PCR is inferior in terms of sensitivity (20%-35% sensitivity, depending on conditions of the PCR assay) to conventional methodology using inoculation of saliva and/or urine on permissive human fibroblasts, followed by detection of CMV-encoded IE-1 by immunologic approaches.[671] More recently, this same group of investigators reported findings from screening more than 34,000 infants by using a saliva-based PCR assay.[659] The results of this study confirmed the lack of sensitivity of dried blood-spot screening approaches and also reported that the use of saliva in the PCR platform provided a sensitivity of greater than 97%, a sensitivity similar to conventional modes of detection of CMV in saliva that require the use of tissue culture.[659] To confirm a congenital CMV infection, demonstration of virus must be attempted in the first 2 weeks of life because viral excretion after that time may represent an infection acquired at birth (natal) by exposure to an infected birth canal or one acquired in the neonatal period by exposure to breast milk or blood products. In the previous section, it was noted that viral nucleic acid detection by PCR assay in specimens from saliva or blood within the first 2 weeks of life should be confirmed by detection of viral nucleic acids in urine and/or virus isolation from urine. Although isolation of CMV during the first 2 weeks of life proves a congenital CMV infection, it does not necessarily confirm an etiologic relationship with an existing disease. Urine and saliva are the preferred specimens for culture because they contain larger amounts of virus. The viability of CMV is surprisingly good when specimens are properly stored. For instance, when positive urine specimens (without preservatives) are stored at 4° C for 7 days, the rate of isolation drops to only 93%; it drops to only 50% after 1 month of storage.[672] However, storage and transport at ambient temperature or freezing should never be used because infectivity is rapidly lost.

TISSUE CULTURE

Standard tissue culture–based viral isolation requires inoculation of specimen into monolayers of primary human fibroblasts. Typically, 2 to 4 weeks can be required for the appearance of the characteristic cytopathic effect. Since 1980, methods for rapid viral diagnosis became available. Several modifications of the standard tissue culture method combined with immunologic detection of IE CMV-induced antigens have maintained high specificity and sensitivity yet allowed the confirmation of diagnosis within 24 hours of inoculation of the clinical specimen.[661-663]

Typically, this test includes the use of monoclonal antibodies to CMV-specific early antigens with low-speed centrifugation of the clinical specimens onto the monolayer of fibroblasts growing on cover slips inside shell vials.[661-663] When this method was evaluated with clinical specimens (blood; urine; bronchoscopy lavage; lung, liver, and kidney biopsy samples; sputum; and others), obtained primarily from immunosuppressed patients, the sensitivity approached 80%, and the specificity ranged from 80% to 100%. Subsequently, another adaptation of this rapid immunofluorescent assay used 96-well microtiter plates and a monoclonal antibody that is reactive with the major IE HCMV protein that is expressed in the nucleus of infected cells within hours of virus entry.[662] This rapid assay detected all but 1 of 19 specimens identified by standard virus isolation method from 1676 newborn urine specimens, achieving a sensitivity of 94.5% and a specificity of 100%. This test retained high sensitivity and specificity when saliva instead of urine was tested.[660] To date, this microtiter plate method using either saliva or urine samples is the most rapid, simple to perform, and inexpensive alternative to the standard virus isolation method. It is suitable for mass screening, and there is no drop in sensitivity for specimens at 4° C for up to 3 days. This study also showed that the sensitivity of the microtiter plate method declined rapidly for specimens from older infants and children with congenital CMV infection and from virus-infected children attending daycare centers. Thus it is not recommended for either screening or diagnosing CMV infections in older infants and children.

DNA HYBRIDIZATION

Rapid diagnosis of CMV has been accomplished by DNA hybridization.[673-676] The sensitivity and specificity of this method is good when the specimens contain 10^3 or more tissue culture infective doses per milliliter. However, the methodology is rarely, if ever, used in routine settings and was quickly replaced with PCR-based technologies.

DNA AMPLIFICATION

Detection of viral DNA by PCR amplification has proven extremely sensitive and versatile for the detection of CMV genetic material in a variety of clinical samples, including urine, CSF, blood, plasma, saliva, and biopsy material. In one of the earliest applications of this technology for the diagnosis of congenital CMV, Demmler and colleagues[656] identified 41 urine specimens positive by PCR assay from a total of 44 specimens positive by tissue culture. No positive PCR results were found in 27 urine specimens that were negative by tissue culture. In another early study, Warren and coworkers[657] used the PCR technique to detect CMV in saliva from children who were between the ages of 1 month and 14 years and who had either congenital or perinatal CMV infection, and they compared the results with a standard tissue culture method and microtiter plate detection of IE antigen, with tissue culture results as a reference. The sensitivity of PCR was 89.2%, and the specificity was 95.8%. Reproducibility was excellent. If primer selection and amplification conditions are carefully chosen, PCR results are comparable to standard tissue culture isolation of virus, except in extreme cases of very low levels of virus infectivity. Some advantages include the minute amount of specimen and the fact that infectious virus is not required, allowing for retrospective diagnosis of CMV infection if the appropriate specimens are available. Nelson and colleagues[654] showed that PCR detection of CMV DNA in serum is a sensitive, specific, and rapid method for diagnosis of infants with symptomatic congenital CMV infection. The PCR assay detected CMV DNA in the serum of 18 infants with symptomatic infection: 1 of 2 with asymptomatic infection, and 0 of 32 control infants. Virus isolation from blood specimens is often difficult and insensitive compared with PCR detection of viremia. As noted above, Boppana and colleagues[659] have definitively shown that PCR assays using saliva as a substrate are as sensitive as standard tissue culture approaches for the diagnosis of congenital CMV and, in their hands, this assay performed with greater than 97% sensitivity. The use of quantitative PCR (real-time PCR) to detect and quantitate CMV DNA in various clinical specimens, including dried blood spots obtained from a drop of neonatal blood applied to solid support, such as a Guthrie card, at the time of the newborn metabolic screen could offer both diagnostic and prognostic information from a single test. As an example of the value of such an approach that could lead to identification of infants at risk for hearing loss, Boppana and colleagues[677] determined virus burden in the peripheral blood of a group of congenitally infected infants with and without hearing loss. Their findings indicated that it is possible to identify infected infants at higher risk for the development of hearing loss (Fig. 24-8). Advantages of PCR-based methods to screen newborn infants include (1) no need for tissue culture facilities; (2) minute amount of specimens; (3) once dried, the samples on swabs or on filter paper are no longer infectious, thus reducing the biohazard risk; (4) ease of shipment and transport without occupational exposure to infectious material; (5) possibility to quantify CMV DNA in PCR-positive samples; (6) adaptation of robotic automation; (7) retrospective diagnosis when appropriate specimens are available; and (8) simplified storage at room temperature

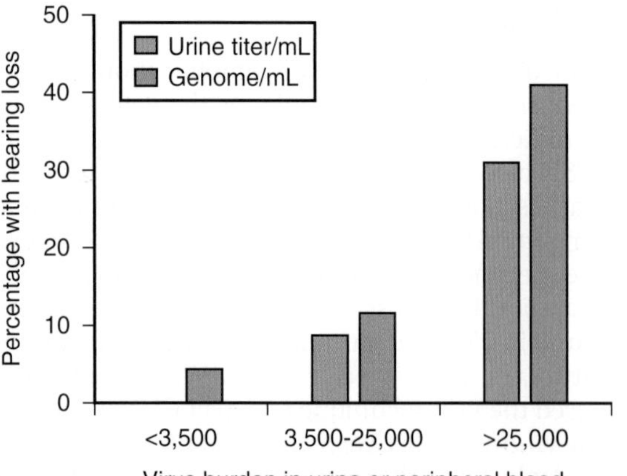

Figure 24-8 Hearing loss in infants with human cytomegalovirus congenital infection as a function of viral genome copy number in urine and blood. Note increasing incidence of hearing loss with increasing genome copy number. (Primary data courtesy Dr. Suresh Boppana, University of Alabama, Birmingham.)

for many years. The ease of sample collection, transport, and sample handling suggest that screening assays such as described by Boppana and colleagues could be readily incorporated into routine newborn screening programs.

ANTIGENEMIA

An assay to detect CMV antigenemia by means of monoclonal antibodies to the tegument protein pp65 encoded by CMV in polymorphonuclear leukocytes has shown good sensitivity and, perhaps more important, good predictive value of the risk of disease when compared with conventional methods (serology, culture) for the diagnosis of CMV disease in immunocompromised adult subjects.[290,678-682] Revello and Gerna[451] assayed pp65 antigenemia, viremia, and DNAemia in peripheral blood leukocytes from 75 infants born to mothers who had primary CMV infection during pregnancy. The results of this study revealed that when compared with the technique of virus isolation from urine, the sensitivity of PCR, antigenemia, and viremia were 100%, 42.5%, and 28%, respectively. The specificity of the three assays was 100%.

DETECTION OF IMMUNE RESPONSE

With congenital CMV infection, antibody production begins in utero and is continued probably during the life span of the host.

Detection of IgG Antibodies

Serologic tests that measure IgG antibody are readily available, easier to perform, and more readily automated than are most virologic methods. However, their correct interpretation is complicated by the presence of antibodies (IgG class) that are normally transmitted from the mother to the fetus.[445] A negative antibody titer in cord and maternal sera is in almost all cases sufficient evidence to exclude the diagnosis of congenital CMV infection. In uninfected infants born to seropositive mothers, IgG antibodies decrease with a half-life of approximately 1 month and become undetectable by most routine assays between 4 and 9 months of age. In contrast, in infected infants, IgG antibody levels persist for long periods at comparable or sometimes higher levels than in their mothers. CMV infections are commonly acquired during the neonatal period mostly from maternal sources (milk, genital secretions) and blood or blood products, and the distinction from congenital infection is not possible by routine serologic means. In both situations, IgG antibody titers tend to remain stable for many months. A neonatal infection in the face of a negative maternal IgG antibody titer should point to transmission from other sources, for example, blood transfusion or nosocomial.

Many serologic assays have been described and evaluated for the detection of CMV IgG antibodies. Among these, enzyme-linked immunosorbent assays (ELISA), are most commonly used.

Detection of IgM Antibodies

Infected fetuses usually produce specific IgM antibodies. IgM antibodies are not transferred by the placenta, and thus their detection in cord or neonatal blood represents a fetal antibody response. There are a number of different assays for IgM antibodies, but before deciding on the use of any particular test, it is important to know its specificity, sensitivity, and reproducibility. None has thus far reached a level of specificity and sensitivity to match the virologic assays described in the previous section.

The solid-phase radioimmunoassay (RIA) described by Griffiths and Kangro[683] remains among the best, with a reported sensitivity of 89% and a specificity of 100% for diagnosis of congenital CMV infections. With the first generation of commercially available IgM ELISA, the specificity was nearly 95% with a sensitivity of approximately 70% when evaluating congenitally infected infants.[684] The IgM capture ELISA and other immunoassays have not fared much better when testing for congenital CMV infection. A Western blot format has been used in the study of IgM antibodies in patients with active CMV infection and was based on antibodies reactive with the viral polypeptides.[685] Clinicians should not rely on IgM assays to diagnose congenital CMV infection. Continued research in this area may provide a simple and generally available method for rapid, definitive diagnosis of congenital infections in both ill and asymptomatic neonates.

DIAGNOSIS OF CYTOMEGALOVIRUS INFECTION DURING PREGNANCY

Clinical Signs and Symptoms

The great majority of primary CMV infections in immunocompetent hosts are subclinical, and infections occurring in pregnant women are no exception. Less than 5% of pregnant women with proven primary CMV infections are symptomatic, with an even smaller percentage manifesting mononucleosis-like syndrome. Clinical manifestations have not been reported with recurrent infections (reactivations or reinfections).

Laboratory Markers

The diagnosis of primary CMV infection can be easily confirmed by documenting seroconversion (i.e., the de novo appearance of virus-specific IgG antibodies in a pregnant woman who was seronegative). In the absence of serologic screening, this is seldom available in clinical practice. The presence of IgG antibodies denotes past infection from 2 weeks to years in duration.

IgM Assays

Of the several tests commercially available, most perform reasonably well, with excellent specificity (95%) and sensitivity (100%).[686-688] The IgM antibody response varies widely from one patient to another. Seropositivity can be detected up to 16 weeks, but it is unusual to last more than 1 year. It is typical to see sharp drops in titers within the first 2 to 3 months of infection. More sensitive assays of IgM antibodies have detected maternal CMV-specific IgM antibodies up to 1 year from enrollment in clinical studies.[212]

IgM assays have been developed based on recombinant CMV proteins and peptides. Both structural and nonstructural CMV-encoded proteins react with IgM antibodies. The detection of specific IgM antibodies can be accomplished by Western blot, immunoblot, or microparticle enzyme immunoassay.[685-688] As noted above, sensitivities approaching 98% with specificities of 98% have been claimed with commercially available assays.

IgG Avidity Assay

This assay is based on the observation that IgG antibodies of low avidity are present during the first months after the onset of infection. With time, IgG antibodies of increasingly higher avidity are produced, and eventually only IgG of high avidity is detected in persons with long-standing CMV infection. An application of this approach was first used to define differences in avidity in women with primary infection who transmitted virus to their offspring.[212] This study demonstrated differences in the avidity of CMV anti-IgG responses that were correlated with the development of virus neutralizing antibodies, suggesting that maturation of the virus neutralizing antibody response was linked to avidity maturation of IgG antibody responses.[212] The results of the currently available avidity test are reported as an index representing the percentage of IgG antibody bound to the antigen after denaturation treatment with 6 M urea.[451,655,688-694] Similar approaches have been reported for other infectious agents, including rubella. In one study, an avidity index value of approximately 20% was obtained in serum samples collected within 3 months after onset of primary infection, in contrast to an avidity index of 78% in sera from persons with remote infection (Fig. 24-9).[695]

In determining the risk of congenital CMV, a moderate-to-high avidity index obtained before the 18th week of

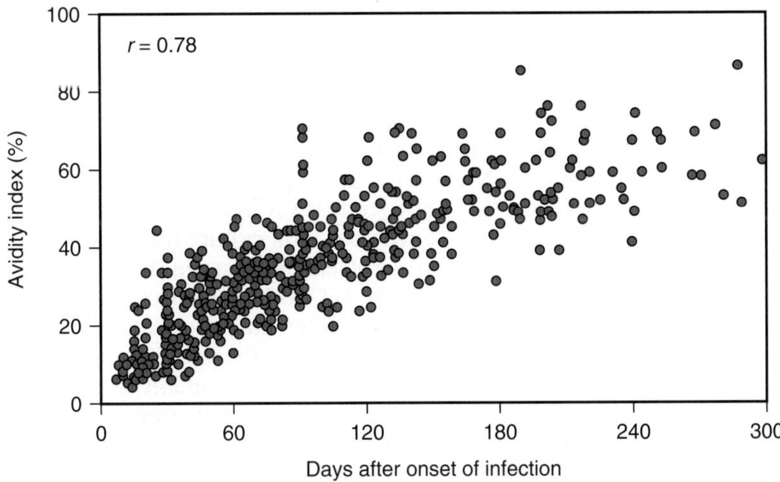

Figure 24-9 Kinetics of immunoglobulin G avidity index. (From Revello MG, Gerna G: Diagnosis and management of human cytomegalovirus infection in the mother, fetus, and newborn infant, *Clin Microbiol Rev* 15:680-715, 2002.)

gestation has a negative predictive value of 100%. When the avidity index is determined between 21 and 23 weeks of gestation, the negative predictive value dropped to 91%.[655,696] The explanation for this observation is that some of the women who transmitted the infection in utero had acquired the infection at a very early gestational age. One important limitation of early studies using the IgG avidity test was the lack of standardization. In one study, the ability of these IgG avidity assays to identify primary CMV infection almost reached 100%, whereas the ability to exclude a recent infection ranged from 20% to 96%. When coupled with the detection of CMV specific IgM antibodies, the avidity test has been used to estimate risk of primary infection and damaging congenital infection.[655,691,694,697,698] This approach has been extensively used in Europe and now represents a component of routine testing in pregnant women, although there remains concern about the standardization of the various assays.[699] However, it is not widely used in the United States, presumably secondary to the lack of widespread screening for CMV infections in pregnant women.

Viral Cultures

Cytomegalovirus excretion from multiple sites, such as urine, saliva, and genital secretions, is common and can last from weeks to several months after a primary infection. Unfortunately, the same occurs with reinfections and reactivations, thus making this diagnostic approach of limited value. Viremia, as determined by conventional tissue culture methods, is too insensitive to confirm the diagnosis of primary infection in immunocompetent hosts.

Other Tests

Other diagnostic methods with greater sensitivity and specificity include the determination of antigenemia (number of pp65-positive peripheral blood leukocytes); PCR quantification of CMV DNA in whole blood (DNAemia), leukocytes (leuko-DNAemia), or plasma; and determination of IE and late mRNA (RNAemia) in blood. Some of these assays are commercially available. The data supporting their diagnostic value derives largely from studies in immunosuppressed patients with primary CMV infections, reactivations, and dissemination of infection and evaluation of antiviral treatments. In many cases, individual assays are center specific and results from one center are often difficult to standardize within other centers. One study of immunocompetent adults, including a large proportion of pregnant women with primary CMV infection, showed that pp65 antigenemia was detected in 57% of patients examined within the first month after the onset of primary infection.[700] The percentage of positive results dropped to 25% a month later and to 0% 5 months later. Viremia was detected in 26% of patients during the first month only. DNAemia (measured by PCR test) was detected in 100% of patients tested during the first month, in 89% of those tested in the second month, and in 47% of those tested 3 months after the onset of primary infection. DNAemia lasted between 4 and 6 months in 26% of patients, whereas no patient remained positive beyond 6 months from the onset of infection. None of these three assays were positive in patients with remote CMV infection, including nine subjects with proven recurrences. The results of this study indicated that antigenemia and DNAemia, when run on blood specimens, rapidly and specifically diagnosed CMV infection, and it was argued that these assays could provide an estimate of the onset for primary infection in pregnant women.[700] In contrast to these findings, CMV DNA was detected in the urine (83% of samples tested) and blood (54% of samples tested) from a group of seroimmune women enrolled in a 3-year observational study.[701] The results from this study demonstrated that CMV viremia and viruria are intermittent but frequent in normal persons with seroimmunity to this virus. Thus it is uncertain whether screening women for viremia or viruria will provide any definitive information that can be easily related to the likelihood of delivering a congenitally infected infant. The detection of IE mRNA was also proposed as a diagnostic tool for primary CMV infection in healthy persons.[288,702] This test was consistently negative in all patients with previous CMV infection, likely because of its poor sensitivity. In contrast, all patients within the first month of a primary infection were reported to be positive. The proportion of positive results declined over time, with all patients testing negative after 6 months of the onset of CMV infection. The kinetics of this test resembled that of DNA detection and, in at least one comparison, the IE mRNA test was slightly more sensitive in the early phase of primary CMV infection.[288]

Maternal Laboratory Tests of Fetal Infection

In utero transmission of CMV infection occurs in approximately 30% to 40% of primary infections acquired during pregnancy.[156] Thus far there are no reliable tests to identify transmission of infection to the fetus. Moreover, there are no maternal prognostic markers of fetal infection with recurrent maternal infections. A recent study has shown that reinfection with a different strain of CMV, as measured by new antibody specificity against epitopes of the virion envelope glycoprotein H, can be associated with symptomatic congenital CMV infection.[158,205,532] The methodology used in these studies does not represent standard laboratory assays and can only identify maternal reinfections and does not define the risk of a damaging fetal infection.

PRENATAL DIAGNOSIS

The prenatal diagnosis of CMV is possible by testing fetal blood obtained by cordocentesis and amniotic fluid obtained by amniocentesis. Fetal blood can be used for both determination of specific IgM antibodies and direct viral markers. IgM antibodies have been reported to be detectable after 20 weeks of gestation. However, because of low sensitivity (≈50%), it has limited diagnostic value.[703-705] On the other hand, studies of viral load in fetal blood show that the sensitivity of antigenemia was approximately 58%, of viremia 55%, and of DNAemia 82%. The specificity was 100% for the three assays.[451] In one study, PCR assay of fetal blood had a sensitivity of 41%, whereas viral culture had a sensitivity of only 7%. With the use of fetal blood, even the most sensitive assays will miss nearly 15% to 20% of infected fetuses. In addition, the risk of fetal loss after fetal blood sampling must be considered and in some precludes the use of this approach.

Results in amniotic fluid are substantially better, and this method can be viewed as the current standard for prenatal diagnosis.[706,707] Viral isolation in tissue culture has a sensitivity of approximately 60%, whereas the sensitivity of PCR can reach 100%. The specificity of both assays is excellent.[451,655,703,708,709] Quantitative PCR has shown that when the amniotic fluid contains greater than or equal to 10^5 genome equivalents of CMV DNA, the risk of symptomatic congenital CMV infection is significantly higher than when the viral load is less than or equal to 10^3 genome equivalents.[655,710-712] Other studies have suggested that viral load in the amniotic fluid may not be predictive of the severity of intrauterine infection but more closely related to the gestational age of the pregnancy.[713]

A confounding factor that remains in prenatal diagnosis of congenital CMV is the gestational age at the time of amniocentesis or cordocentesis. After a primary maternal infection, it may take from weeks to months for transplacental transmission of CMV to occur. An interval of 7 weeks between maternal onset of infection and diagnostic tests for fetal infection has been proposed as a reasonable interval by some investigators.[708,714-716] Gestational age at the time of testing is also important because the sensitivity can be as low as 30% when amniotic fluid is obtained before the 21st week of gestation, whereas it can be 100% if the test is performed after 21 weeks of gestation.[#] More recently, imaging techniques have been applied to the prenatal diagnosis of congenital CMV infections. The improved specificity for the diagnosis of CNS abnormalities as detected by ultrasonography and, more recently, by magnetic resonance imaging suggest that these techniques could contribute significantly to the diagnosis of this intrauterine infection.[525,720]

To counsel pregnant women, it is important to remember that the vast majority (90%-95%) of children with congenital CMV infection escape significant CNS sequelae, whereas about 10% are at risk for some degree of hearing loss. In the absence of specific antiviral treatment for prenatal therapy, the only alternative available after a prenatal diagnosis of congenital CMV infection is to terminate the pregnancy or to observe. The presence or absence of ultrasonographic evidence of fetal abnormalities could represent an important component of the information provided during counseling of women at risk.

DIAGNOSIS OF PERINATALLY ACQUIRED INFECTIONS

For perinatally acquired infections, viral culture or CMV DNA detection by PCR assay from urine and saliva are the preferred diagnostic methods, but CMV excretion usually does not begin until 3 to 12 weeks after exposure. For diagnostic specificity, it is imperative to have a negative result from urine or saliva specimens collected within the first 2 weeks of life. In early infancy, antibody assays have the same limitations described earlier for infants with congenital CMV infection. Differentiation between congenital and perinatal CMV infections are important because of the differences in the risks of long-term sequelae.

Differential Diagnosis

During the newborn period, the constellation of hepatosplenomegaly, petechiae, and direct hyperbilirubinemia with or without pneumonitis, microcephaly, and ocular and neurologic abnormalities that characterize CID is common to several disease entities, including other congenital infections, such as congenital rubella syndrome, toxoplasmosis, syphilis, neonatal HSV infections, and, less likely, hepatitis B and varicella virus infections. The differential diagnosis of symptomatic congenital CMV infection also includes bacterial sepsis and noninfectious disorders, such as hemolytic diseases related to Rh or ABO incompatibilities or red blood cell defects; metabolic disorders, such as galactosemia and tyrosinemia; immune thrombocytopenia; histocytosis X, congenital leukemia; and other diseases in which hepatosplenomegaly is a prominent clinical component. In addition, one should consider the possibility of a rare genetic disease linked to the unregulated production of interferons, the Aicardi-Goutières syndrome.[721-726] The list of diseases that must be considered in the differential diagnosis becomes obviously broader as the clinical manifestations diminish in severity.

In addition, multiple infections may coexist in the same patient. Consequently, the laboratory workup for the differential diagnosis must be complete.

CONGENITAL RUBELLA SYNDROME

Congenital rubella has been virtually eliminated in the United States after the successful immunization program adopted years ago. Yet, as with other vaccine modifiable disease, the resurgence of rubella infections in selected populations will not be unexpected.[727] Although symptomatic congenital rubella and CMV infections share many signs and symptoms, central cataracts, congenital heart defects, raised purpuric rather than petechial rash, salt-and-pepper lesions as opposed to chorioretinitis, and the absence of cerebral calcifications are more likely to occur with congenital rubella syndrome than with CID.

CONGENITAL TOXOPLASMOSIS

Almost all the manifestations observed in CID have been described for symptomatic congenital toxoplasmosis. Some differences are worthy of note. For instance, the calcifications of toxoplasmosis are generally scattered throughout the cerebral cortex, whereas the calcifications of CID tend to occur in the periventricular areas. The rash associated with toxoplasmosis is usually maculopapular but is not petechial or purpuric. Chorioretinitis in the two diseases cannot be differentiated on the basis of appearance or distribution. However, it is more likely that chorioretinitis related to CMV is associated with other major clinical manifestations, such as microcephaly. Not uncommonly, the chorioretinitis of toxoplasmosis is an isolated finding.

CONGENITAL SYPHILIS

The most consistent signs of early congenital syphilis are osteochondritis and epiphysitis on radiography of the long bones. These signs occur in approximately 90% of infected patients and are more likely to appear in patients who become symptomatic in the first week of life. Rhinitis, sometimes associated with laryngitis, is another common manifestation of congenital syphilis; it is often followed by a dark red maculopapular rash. Lesions of the skin and mucous

[#] References 655, 704, 705, 708, 714, 715, 717-719.

membranes are also seen. Hepatosplenomegaly and hepatocellular damage with cholestatic jaundice occurs but is less common in early syphilis than in CID, although either diagnosis should be considered in infants with elevated direct reacting bilirubin and evidence of hepatocellular disease. Calcifications of the brain are not characteristic of congenital syphilis. However, choroiditis may be seen.

NEONATAL HERPES SIMPLEX VIRUS INFECTIONS

Congenital herpes simplex virus infections are less common than neonatal HSV infections and likely account for approximately 5% of cases of perinatal HSV infections, yet they are more likely to pose a diagnostic dilemma because they may resemble CID. Microcephaly, intracranial calcifications, chorioretinitis with and without optic atrophy, and hepatosplenomegaly are common clinical manifestations of intrauterine HSV infections. The presence of skin vesicles or scarring present at birth is valuable for the differential diagnosis. The more common form of HSV infection, neonatal infection, is acquired during parturition and does not usually present as an acute disease until 5 to 21 days of age. Unlike the situation in typical CID, the infant is well during most of the first week of life. When illness does occur, it may be accompanied by seizures, encephalitis, respiratory distress, bleeding disorders, and small vesicular lesions that tend to cluster into crops.

Treatment

CHEMOTHERAPY

A small number of systemically administered antiviral agents have been used in therapeutic trials of serious, life- or sight-threatening CMV disease. Currently, two antiviral agents, ganciclovir and foscarnet, are licensed for this purpose in immunocompromised patients. Foscarnet inhibits viral replication by inhibiting viral DNA polymerase, and ganciclovir acts as a chain terminator during elongation of the newly synthesized viral DNA.

The Collaborative Antiviral Study Group (CASG) under the auspices of the National Institutes of Allergy and Infectious Diseases first conducted a phase II pharmacokinetic/pharmacodynamic study that established the safe dose of ganciclovir to be used in young infants.[728] A phase III randomized, controlled study followed newborn infants with symptomatic congenital infection involving the CNS.[729] A total of 100 patients were enrolled. Those in the ganciclovir treatment arm received 6 mg/kg/dose administered IV every 12 hours for 6 weeks of treatment. The primary end point was improved hearing (as assessed by brainstem-evoked response) between baseline and 6 months follow-up or, for those with normal hearing at enrollment, preservation of normal hearing at follow-up. Twenty-one (84%) of 25 ganciclovir-treated patients had hearing improvement or maintained normal hearing at 6 months, compared with 10 of 17 (59%) in the no-treatment group (P = .06). At 6-months follow-up, none of the ganciclovir-treated infants had hearing deterioration (0/25), compared with 7 of 17 (41%) in the no-treatment group (P <.01). Alternatively, 5 of 24 (21%) of ganciclovir recipients had worsening of hearing in their best ear between baseline and greater than or equal to 1 year, compared with 13 of 19 (68%) in the no-treatment group (P <.01). This study was viewed as evidence of the feasibility of treatment of selected cases of congenital CMV infections with an antiviral agent. Of importance, there were limitations in this study, including a significant number of patients not included in the final analysis and the requirement to treat each ear as a separate data point, a statistically justifiable method but one that may have uncertain rationale from a standpoint of CNS plasticity and neural development. Regardless of these limitations, the information from this study suggested that at least in some patients, treatment of congenital CMV in the perinatal period could alter the long-term morbidity of this infection. This trial was extended once an oral formulation of ganciclovir became available and a comparison trial of 6 weeks versus 6 months of oral ganciclovir has been completed, and the results from this trial will be available in the fall of 2013 (D. Kimberlin, personal communication).

The most significant toxicity in the treated group was neutropenia, with 29 of 46 (63%) patients developing moderate-to-severe neutropenia, compared with 9 of 43 (21%) of the no-treatment group (P <.01). Half the patients with neutropenia required dosage adjustment, and 12% had discontinuation of therapy. This study demonstrates that 6 weeks of IV ganciclovir in symptomatic congenital CMV infected infants prevents worsening of hearing loss at 6 months and 1 year of follow-up. In addition, treated patients had a more rapid resolution of their liver function abnormalities and improvements in short-term growth and head circumference when compared with controls. There are no reports on the therapeutic efficacy of combined therapy (i.e., foscarnet plus ganciclovir). Anecdotal reports have not thus far supported the use of hyperimmune immunoglobulin or antiviral treatment for the purpose of treating the fetus in utero.[430,730]

PASSIVE IMMUNIZATION

Hyperimmune plasma and immunoglobulin have been used with some success as prophylaxis for primary CMV infections in immunosuppressed transplant patients. A meta-analysis of randomized, controlled trials of immunoglobulin as prophylaxis for CMV disease in adult transplant recipients found a significant beneficial effect.[458]

It remains unclear if the effect of CMV immunoglobulins on the improved outcome in transplant patients is directly related to their antiviral effects. Some authors have argued that at least in the case of hematopoietic allograft recipients, any benefit from passive transfer of immune globulins is secondary to immunomodulatory activities of these biologics.

It has been argued for many years that passive immunoprophylaxis would not be effective in the treatment of congenital infections because the cases are identified weeks and months after infection occurred in utero. An uncontrolled trial performed in Italy in 2005, however, has provided data that raised the possibility that such an approach could indeed limit diseases in the infected fetus and perhaps even lessen the risk of transmission from an infected woman. This study used a commercial source of CMV immune globulin to treat women with primary CMV during pregnancy. The passive transfer of antibody reduced the frequency of virus transmission to the offspring and reduced the incidence of disease in infected infants.[430] In addition to being an uncontrolled study, the use of clinical end points that are controversial (head ultrasonography) has led to considerable skepticism of the validity of the findings by many investigators. However, this study did raise several very provocative questions, including the possibility that the beneficial effect of immunoglobulin treatment in this study could be more related to its antiinflammatory effects on the placenta rather than a direct antiviral effect within the infected fetus. More questions were generated by this study than addressed; however, if nothing else, this study has increased interest in passive prophylaxis/therapy with biologics as an alternative to vaccines for the prevention of damaging congenital CMV infections. A follow-up controlled trial using the same preparation of IVIG but carried out by a different group of investigators reported that treatment with IVIG during pregnancy provided no benefit in the prevention of intrauterine CMV transmission in women with primary CMV infection during pregnancy.[431]

VACCINES

In the United States, congenital CMV infection is a significant public health problem. It is the leading cause of sensorineural hearing loss and the leading infectious cause of brain damage in children.[596,731] Not surprisingly, the Institute of Medicine of the National Academy of Sciences concluded that a vaccine to prevent congenital CMV infection should be a top priority. Despite 30 years of research efforts, no such vaccine is available. Virus neutralizing antibody responses have been detected against gB, gH, gM/gN, and the UL128-131/gH/gL pentameric complex, whereas T lymphcyte responses have been detected against peptides from nearly every structural protein of the virus.[65,68,79,732-736] A major hurdle for the design and testing of vaccines is the lack of a relevant animal model. Each model has obvious drawbacks, perhaps the most significant being that HCMV has obvious unique characteristics in terms of its replication, cellular tropism, and pathogenesis in humans that is not precisely recapitulated in any animal model. Thus each animal model can study aspects of HCMV infections but cannot fully reproduce the human disease.

The strategies for vaccine development have included live-attenuated vaccine (Towne strain). This vaccine induces a significant antibody response and cell-mediated immunity, as determined by lymphoproliferative response. In CMV-seronegative recipients of kidneys from seropositive donors, this vaccine reduced disease severity but did not prevent infection.[737] It also protected against a very low-dose virulent CMV challenge in normal volunteers.[738] In a more recent trial, this vaccine failed to decrease the rate of acquisition of CMV in parents of children in daycare. It was noted that the magnitude of the induced immune response was 10-fold lower than that generated by natural infection.[739] The Towne vaccine was not excreted by vaccinees.

Recombinant Virus Vaccine

The genome of the virulent Toledo strain of CMV, divided into four fragments, was inserted in the genetic background of the attenuated Towne strain gene, creating four chimeras. The ability of these four recombinant virus strains to generate antibody and cell-mediated immune responses in the absence of clinical side effects has been evaluated in a phase I study.[740]

Subunit Vaccines

A CMV vaccine based on the envelope glycoprotein gB combined with a novel adjuvant (MF59) was tested in a double-blind placebo-controlled trial of seronegative adult volunteers.[733] Results showed that after three doses, the antibody responses to gB and neutralizing antibodies exceeded the levels in seropositive control subjects. Cell-mediated immunity as measured by lymphocyte proliferation was generated in vaccinees. A recent study carried out in seronegative women suggested that gB subunit vaccine prevented maternal infection, as measured by seroconversion in about 50% of vaccinated women, a surprising finding that must be confirmed but one that does suggest that vaccine immunity against CMV is feasible.[741] The results of this small trial remain controversial, however, because the duration of protection was extremely short lived (<6 months), and the CI that suggested statistical significance for the observed protective effect was large. Furthermore, the lack of outcome measures that could reveal potential differences in counseling between vaccine and control groups remains an important confounder in this study because the role of counseling in limiting CMV acquisition is well documented.[742] For these and other reasons, it is unlikely that such monovalent vaccine will move forward in additional trials in seronegative women. A major target of the cell-mediated immune response is pp65. In an effort to elicit this response, a recent study made use of the nonreplicating canarypox expression vector in which CMV pp65 has been inserted. A phase I trial on seronegative volunteers found that pp65-specific CTLs were elicited after only two vaccinations. In addition, an antibody response to pp65 was also demonstrated. In this preliminary study, the canarypox CMV pp65 recombinant vaccine seems to generate an immune response similar to that provided by natural infection.[734] A canarypox CMV recombinant that contained gB did not induce neutralizing antibodies. Other approaches have included recombinant alphavirus-vectored CMV gB and a fusion protein between pp65 and IE-1.[743] This vectored subunit vaccine induced significant neutralizing antibody and IFN-γ responses in T lymphocytes from immunized adult volunteers.[744] Another approach has been the use of the DNA vaccine platform. A clinical trial using a bivalent DNA vaccine (DNA encoding gB and pp65) induced antibodies and a cellular immune response in adult volunteers that included long-term T-lymphocyte memory.[745] More recent strategies for CMV vaccine development have focused on inclusion of the gH/gL/Ul128-131 pentameric complex in candidate vaccine because of the importance of this glycoprotein complex in the extended cell tropism of CMV. In addition, antibodies against this protein complex have extraordinary virus neutralization activity.[79,736,746] Studies in the rhesus macaque model of HCMV infection suggest that immunization with this pentameric complex could impart protective immunity.[747] Finally, the capacity of CMV to readily reinfect immune individuals has led several investigators to propose CMV as a vaccine vector for other agents. Recent findings in rhesus macaques have validated this strategy and have demonstrated not only reinfection of previously immune animals but induction of immunity against simian immunodeficiency virus, a model of HIV infection in humans.[748] Together with findings in other animal models of CMV infection and the reported frequency of reinfections in immunocompetent humans, these results suggest that the prevention of infection by this virus will be a difficult goal for any vaccine that can induce natural levels of immunity.

Prevention

In general, CMV is not very contagious, and its horizontal transmission requires close direct contact with infected material, namely, secretions that contain the virus and, less likely, fomites. With the exception of studies that were designed to prevent infection through blood and blood products and grafted organs, no broad-based strategies for preventing the transmission of this virus have been tested. Education of susceptible individuals has been shown to significantly reduce the incidence of infection, a finding that must be incorporated into any vaccine or biologic trial with an end point for prevention of maternal infection and/or limiting congenital infections.[749] Two clinical trials illustrated the value of prevention of CMV acquisition during pregnancy. The first was reported by Adler[750] and clearly demonstrated that education alone could result in rates of prevention of infection comparable to any current candidate vaccines. A more recent study in France also demonstrated the effectiveness of counseling in limiting acquisition of CMV during pregnancy.[742] Of importance, counseling could also potentially prevent reinfections of women with existing immunity.

PREGNANT WOMEN

An average of 2% of susceptible pregnant women acquire CMV infection during pregnancy in the United States; the majority of these individuals have no symptoms, and only 40% of the episodes result in fetal infection (see Fig. 24-7).[193,751] Because there is no proven prenatal therapy and the risk of fetal morbidity is low, several investigators have concluded that routine serologic screening of pregnant women for primary CMV infections during pregnancy is of limited value. However, reliable and inexpensive serologic tests are now available so that women of childbearing age can be informed of their immune status. Because of the risk of congenital infection in offspring of immune women, seroimmune women should also be counseled as to risks of virus exposure and routes of virus acquisition. Primary CMV infection should be suspected in pregnant women with symptoms compatible with a heterophil-negative, mononucleosis-like syndrome. To more precisely define a recent asymptomatic primary CMV infection, serologic tests such as IgM capture ELISA, IgG avidity index, and DNAemia (PCR) could be used. At present, there are no reliable means to determine whether intrauterine transmission has occurred after symptomatic or subclinical primary infection in early gestation or to assess the relatively small number of fetuses at risk of disease. The sensitivity and specificity of prenatal diagnosis by testing fetal blood obtained by cordocentesis or amniotic fluid PCR assay and viral culture are good after 20 weeks of gestation. Thus there is still limited information to serve as a basis for recommendations regarding termination of pregnancy after a primary CMV infection acquired in early gestation. Similarly, there is no definitive information regarding how long conception should be delayed after documented primary infection is acquired in a woman of childbearing age. Viral excretion is not a sensitive and specific indicator because virus is shed into saliva for weeks or months after infection and into urine and the cervix for months or years.

The data on which to base recommendations for prevention of congenital CMV infection after recurrent maternal infection are even more incomplete. Preexisting immunity does not prevent the virus from reactivating or reinfection, nor does it effectively control the occasional spread to the fetus. Preexisting maternal immunity affords significant protection to the fetus. However, evidence that, in some high-risk populations, reinfections with an antigenically different virus can cause fetal disease and long-term sequelae may temper this statement. At present, there are no techniques for identifying women with reactivation of CMV that results in intrauterine transmission.

The principal sources of CMV infection among women of childbearing age are exposure to children excreting CMV and sexual contacts. Recommendations for prevention of sexual transmission of CMV are beyond the scope of this review. Suffice it to say, they are similar to those advocated for the prevention of other sexually transmitted infections. As for the risk from exposure to children, at greater risk are susceptible pregnant mothers of CMV-infected children who attend daycare centers. Hand washing and simple hygienic measures that are routine for hospital care can be recommended, but it is unrealistic to expect all mothers to comply.

Because CMV has been found to be endemic in the daycare setting and is found everywhere in hospitals, questions often arise about the occupational risks to pregnant personnel in these facilities. Although hospital workers do not appear to be at increased risk for CMV infection, personnel who work in daycare centers are at increased risk.[*a] In the hospital, universal precautions and routine procedures for hand washing and infection control should make nonparenteral acquisition of CMV infections less likely than in the community. The majority of patients who shed CMV are asymptomatic and go unrecognized when caring for known CMV-excreting patients; thus these routine measures should be combined with a special recommendation that pregnant caretakers be especially careful in handling such patients.[752] In the daycare setting, where hygiene is difficult at best, these preventive measures may be more difficult to implement. Although there is still debate about the need for routine serologic screening of female personnel and daycare workers, some investigators believe that it should be recommended for potentially childbearing women whose occupation exposes them to CMV. Knowing their immune status can be helpful in counseling pregnant women at risk. All personnel should be provided with information on prevention measures and reassured that common sense steps, such as hand washing and avoiding contact with

[*a] References 172, 177, 179, 184, 187, 190, 191, 752, 753.

secretions, should prevent acquisition of infection.[749,752] Attempts to identify all congenitally CMV-infected children and children excreting this virus in the workplace, so that seronegative workers and parents can avoid contact with them, pose serious logistic problems and would require frequent periodic testing.

NOSOCOMIAL INFECTION

Hospitalized patients who receive blood products and organ transplants are at risk for nosocomial CMV infection. Transfusion of blood products, on the other hand, can be an important source of perinatal CMV infections. Early studies demonstrated that the use of blood products from seronegative donors prevents the transmission of CMV and the subsequent risk of disease.[225,653,754,755] However, this approach has obvious drawbacks in areas where a large percentage of the donor population is seropositive. Clearly, the availability of seronegative donors as well as the additional cost involved in serologic screening and processing the blood must be evaluated by regional blood banks.

The use of filters to remove leukocytes is also an effective means of eliminating posttransfusion CMV infection in adult patients and in newborns, even in low-birth-weight infants.[756-761] Filtration results in a significant disruption and depletion of leukocytes and is thought to provide a similar reduction in the rate of CMV transmission after transfusion. Studies have demonstrated a 1% to 2% transmission rate of CMV when exclusively CMV seronegative donor blood has been used, a finding in agreement with a recent finding that up to 15% of antibody-negative persons will have CMV circulating in peripheral blood mononuclear cells, as detected by PCR assay.[146,762] Many hospitals are using one of these approaches to prevent transfusion-acquired perinatal CMV infections. It is a local hospital and blood bank policy to determine whether transfusion-associated CMV disease is a problem and which method to choose based on their donor populations. However, individual nurseries have adopted the policy that all transfusions of blood or blood products should be with seronegative blood, irrespective of the infant's birth weight and maternal immune status.

The absence of CMV infection in premature infants born to seronegative mothers and who receive only seronegative blood products suggests that spread of CMV from hands of personnel or from fomites must be rare. Until more information is available, the only logical recommendation is hand washing and routine infection control measures.

Rarely is perinatal infection through breast milk a cause for concern, at least for full-term newborns who receive their mother's milk.[634] Premature infants, who generally do not receive sufficient quantities of specific transplacental antibodies, are at higher risk for morbidity.[†a] Storage of naturally infected breast milk at −20° C (freezer temperature) significantly reduces but does not eliminate infectivity.[765,766] Heat treatment of breast milk at 72° C for 10 seconds eliminates all infectious viruses without affecting the nutritional and immunologic properties of milk.[167,168,641]

[†a] References 167, 169, 544, 546, 640-642, 647, 648, 763, 764.

References

1. Weller TH: The cytomegaloviruses: ubiquitous agents with protean clinical manifestations, *N Engl J Med* 285:203-214, 1971.
2. Ribbert D: Uber protozoenartige Zellen in der Niereeines syphilitischen Neugoborenen und in der Parotis von Kindern, *Zentralbl Allg Pathol* 15:945-948, 1904.
3. Jesionek A, Kiolemenoglou B: Uber einen befund von protozoenartigen Gebilden in den Organen eines heriditarluetischen Fotus, *Munch Med Wochenschr* 51:1905-1907, 1904.
4. Lowenstein C: Uber protozoenartigen Gebilden in de Organen von Dindern, *Zentralbl Allg Pathol* 18:513-518, 1907.
5. Goodpasture EW, Talbot FB: Concerning the nature of "proteozoan-like" cells in certain lesions of infancy, *Am J Dis Child* 21:415-421, 1921.
6. Lipschutz B: Untersuchungen uber die atiologie der krankheiten der herpesgruppe (herpes zoster, herpes genitalis, herpes febrilis), *Arch Derm Syph (Berl)* 136:428-482, 1921.
7. Cole R, Kuttner AG: A filtrable virus present in the submaxillary glands of guinea pigs, *J Exp Med* 44:855-873, 1926.
8. Smith MG. Propagation in tissue cultures of a cytopathogenic virus from human salivary gland virus disease, *Proc Soc Exp Biol Med* 92:424-430, 1956.
9. Smith MG: Propagation in tissue cultures of cytopathogenic virus from human salivary gland (SVG) virus disease, *Proc Soc Exp Biol Med* 92:424-430, 1956.
10. Rowe WP, Hartley JW, Waterman S, et al: Cytopathogenic agent resembling human salivary gland virus recovered from tissue cultures of human adenoids, *Proc Soc Exp Biol Med* 92:418-424, 1956.
11. Weller TH, Macaulay JC, Craig JM, et al: Isolation of intranuclear inclusion producing agents from infants with illnesses resembling cytomegalic inclusion disease, *Proc Soc Exp Biol Med* 94:4-12, 1957.
12. Weller TH, Hanshaw JB, Scott DE: Serologic differentiation of viruses responsible for cytomegalic inclusion disease, *Virology* 12:130-132, 1960.
13. Krech U, Konjajev Z, Jung M: Congenital cytomegalovirus infection in siblings from consecutive pregnancies, *Helv Paediatr Acta* 26:355-362, 1971.
14. Gold E, Nankervis GA: Cytomegalovirus. In Evans AS, editor: *Viral infections of humans: epidemiology and control*, ed 2, New York, 1982, Plenum Press, pp 167-186.
15. Davison AJ, Dolan A, Akter P, et al: The human cytomegalovirus genome revisited: comparison with the chimpanzee cytomegalovirus genome, *J Gen Virol* 84:17-28, 2003. [Erratum in *J Gen Virol* 2003;84(Pt 4):1053].
16. Bradley AJ, Kovacs IJ, Gatherer D, et al: Genotypic analysis of two hypervariable human cytomegalovirus genes, *J Med Virol* 80: 1615-1623, 2008.
17. Renzette N, Bhattacharjee B, Jenson JD, et al: Extensive genome-wide variability of human cytomegalovirus in congenitally infected infants, *PLoS Pathog* 7:e1001344, 2011.
18. Black JB, Pellett PE: Human herpesvirus 7, *Rev Med Virol* 9:245-262, 1999.
19. Campadelli-Fiume G, Mirandola P, Menotti L: Human herpesvirus 6: an emerging pathogen, *Emerg Infect Dis* 5:353-366, 1999.
20. Clark DA: Human herpesvirus 6, *Rev Med Virol* 10:155-173, 2000.
21. Chen DH, Jiang H, Lee M, et al: Three-dimensional visualization of tegument/capsid interactions in the intact human cytomegalovirus, *Virology* 260:10-16, 1999.
22. Trus BL, Gibson W, Cheng N, et al: Capsid structure of simian cytomegalovirus from cryoelectron microscopy: evidence for tegument attachment sites, *J Virol* 73:2181-2192, 1999. [Erratum in *J Virol* 1999;73:4530].
23. Smith JD, De Harven E: Herpes simplex virus and human cytomegalovirus replication in WI-38 cells. I. Sequence of viral replication, *J Virol* 12:919-930, 1973.
24. Murphy E, Rigoutsos I, Shibuya T, et al: Reevaluation of human cytomegalovirus coding potential, *Proc Natl Acad Sci U S A* 100:13585-13590, 2003.
25. Mocarski ES, Tan Courcelle C: Cytomegaloviruses and their replication. In Howley PM, Griffin DE, editors: *Fields virology*, ed 4, Philadelphia, 2001, Lippincott Williams & Wilkins, pp 2629-2673.
26. Borst EM, Hahn G, Koszinowski UH, et al: Cloning of the human cytomegalovirus (HCMV) genome as an infectious bacterial artificial chromosome in *Escherichia coli*: a new approach for construction of HCMV mutants, *J Virol* 73:8320-8329, 1999.

27. Mocarski E: Betaherpes viral genes and their function. In Arvin A, Campadielli-Fume G, Mocarski E, et al, editors: *Human herpesviruses: biology, therapy, and immunoprophylaxis*, Cambridge, UK, 2007, Cambridge University Press, pp 204-230.
28. Varnum SM, Streblow DN, Monroe ME, et al: Identification of proteins in human cytomegalovirus (HCMV) particles: the HCMV proteome, *J Virol* 78:10960-10966, 2004. [Erratum in *J Virol* 2004:78:13395].
29. Murphy E, Shenk T: Human cytomegalovirus genome. In Shenk T, Stinski MF, editors: *Human cytomegalovirus*, Berlin/Heidelberg, 2008, Springer-Verlag, pp 1-20.
30. Britt W: Maturation and egress. In Arvin A, Campadielli-Fume G, Mocarski E, et al, editors: *Human herpesviruses: biology, therapy, and immunoprophylaxis*, Cambridge, UK, 2007, Cambridge University Press, pp 311-323.
31. Gibson W: Structure and function of the cytomegalovirus virion. In Shenk T, Stinski MF, editors: *Human cytomegalovirus*, Berlin/Heidelberg, 2008, Springer-Verlag, pp 187-204.
32. Bogner E, Radsak K, Stinski MF: The gene product of human cytomegalovirus open reading frame UL56 binds the pac motif and has specific nuclease activity, *J Virol* 72:2259-2264, 1998.
33. Scheffczik H, Savva CG, Holzenburg A, et al: The terminase subunits pUL56 and pUL89 of human cytomegalovirus are DNA-metabolizing proteins with toroidal structure, *Nucleic Acids Res* 30:1695-1703, 2002.
34. Krosky PM, Underwood MR, Turk SR, et al: Resistance of human cytomegalovirus to benzimidazole ribonucleosides maps to two open reading frames: UL89 and UL56, *J Virol* 72:4721-4728, 1998.
35. Kaul DR, Stoelben S, Cober E, et al: First report of successful treatment of multidrug-resistant cytomegalovirus disease with the novel anti-CMV compound AIC246, *Am J Transplant* 11:1079-1084, 2011.
36. Goldner T, Hewlett G, Ettischer N, et al: The novel anticytomegalovirus compound AIC246 (Letermovir) inhibits human cytomegalovirus replication through a specific antiviral mechanism that involves the viral terminase, *J Virol* 85:10884-10893, 2011.
37. Mou F, Wills EG, Park R, et al: Effects of lamin A/C, lamin B1, and viral US3 kinase activity on viral infectivity, virion egress, and the targeting of herpes simplex virus U(L)34-encoded protein to the inner nuclear membrane, *J Virol* 82:8094-8104, 2008.
38. Reynolds AE, Wills EG, Roller RJ, et al: Ultrastructural localization of the herpes simplex virus type 1 UL31, UL34, and US3 proteins suggests specific roles in primary envelopment and egress of nucleocapsids, *J Virol* 76:8939-8952, 2002.
39. Krosky PM, Baek MC, Coen DM: The human cytomegalovirus UL97 protein kinase, an antiviral drug target, is required at the stage of nuclear egress, *J Virol* 77:905-914, 2003.
40. Hamirally S, Kamil JP, Ndassa-Colday YM, et al: Viral mimicry of Cdc2/cyclin-dependent kinase 1 mediates disruption of nuclear lamina during human cytomegalovirus nuclear egress, *PLoS Pathog* 5:e1000275, 2009.
41. Popa M, Ruzsics Z, Lotzerich M, et al: Dominant negative mutants of the murine cytomegalovirus M53 gene block nuclear egress and inhibit capsid maturation, *J Virol* 84:9035-9046, 2010.
42. Bresnahan WA, Shenk T: A subset of viral transcripts packaged within human cytomegalovirus particles, *Science* 288:2373-2376, 2000.
43. Yu X, Shah S, Lee M, et al: Biochemical and structural characterization of the capsid-bound tegument proteins of human cytomegalovirus, *J Struct Biol* 174:451-460, 2011.
44. Hume AJ, Kalejta RF: Regulation of the retinoblastoma proteins by the human herpesviruses, *Cell Div* 4:1, 2009.
45. Kalejta RF: Functions of human cytomegalovirus tegument proteins prior to immediate early gene expression, *Curr Top Microbiol Immunol* 325:101-115, 2008.
46. Hume AJ, Finkel JS, Kamil JP, et al: Phosphorylation of retinoblastoma protein by viral protein with cyclin-dependent kinase function, *Science* 320:797-799, 2008.
47. Fortunato EA, Spector DH: p53 and RPA are sequestered in viral replication centers in the nuclei of cells infected with human cytomegalovirus, *J Virol* 72:2033-2039, 1998.
48. Salvant BS, Fortunato EA, Spector DH: Cell cycle dysregulation by human cytomegalovirus: influence of the cell cycle phase at the time of infection and effects on cyclin transcription, *J Virol* 72:3729-3741, 1998.
49. Hayashi ML, Blankenship C, Shenk T: Human cytomegalovirus UL69 protein is required for efficient accumulation of infected cells in the G1 phase of the cell cycle, *Proc Natl Acad Sci U S A* 97:2692-2696, 2000.
50. Tavalai N, Stamminger T: Intrinsic cellular defense mechanisms targeting human cytomegalovirus, *Virus Res* 157:128-133, 2011.
51. Maul GG: Initiation of cytomegalovirus infection at ND10, *Curr Top Microbiol Immunol* 325:117-132, 2008.
52. Hwang ES, Zhang Z, Cai H, et al: Human cytomegalovirus IE1-72 protein interacts with p53 and inhibits p53-dependent transactivation by a mechanism different from that of IE2-86 protein, *J Virol* 83:12388-12398, 2009.
53. Zielke B, Thomas M, Giede-Jeppe A, et al: Characterization of the betaherpesviral pUL69 protein family reveals binding of the cellular mRNA export factor UAP56 as a prerequisite for stimulation of nuclear mRNA export and for efficient viral replication, *J Virol* 85:1804-1819, 2011.
54. Toth Z, Stamminger T: The human cytomegalovirus regulatory protein UL69 and its effect on mRNA export, *Front Biosci* 13:2939-2949, 2008.
55. Stamminger T, Gstaiger M, Weinzierl K, et al: Open reading frame UL26 of human cytomegalovirus encodes a novel tegument protein that contains a strong transcriptional activation domain, *J Virol* 76:4836-4847, 2002.
56. Lischka P, Toth Z, Thomas M, et al: The UL69 transactivator protein of human cytomegalovirus interacts with DEXD/H-Box RNA helicase UAP56 to promote cytoplasmic accumulation of unspliced RNA, *Mol Cell Biol* 26:1631-1643, 2006.
57. Baldick CJ Jr, Marchini A, Patterson CE, et al: Human cytomegalovirus tegument protein pp71 (ppUL82) enhances the infectivity of viral DNA and accelerates the infectious cycle, *J Virol* 71:4400-4408, 1997.
58. Buchkovich NJ, Maguire TG, Yu Y, et al: Human cytomegalovirus specifically controls the levels of the endoplasmic reticulum chaperone BiP/GRP78, which is required for virion assembly, *J Virol* 82: 31-39, 2008.
59. Buchkovich NJ, Yu Y, Zampieri CA, et al: The TORrid affairs of viruses: effects of mammalian DNA viruses on the PI3K-Akt-mTOR signalling pathway, *Nat Rev Microbiol* 6:266-275, 2008.
60. Kudchodkar SB, Yu Y, Maguire TG, et al: Human cytomegalovirus infection alters the substrate specificities and rapamycin sensitivities of raptor- and rictor-containing complexes, *Proc Natl Acad Sci U S A* 103:14182-14187, 2006.
61. Munger J, Bennett BD, Parikh A, et al: Systems-level metabolic flux profiling identifies fatty acid synthesis as a target for antiviral therapy, *Nat Biotechnol* 26:1179-1186, 2008.
62. Moorman NJ, Cristea IM, Terhune SS, et al: Human cytomegalovirus protein UL38 inhibits host cell stress responses by antagonizing the tuberous sclerosis protein complex, *Cell Host Microbe* 3:253-262, 2008.
63. Landini MP, LaPlaca M: Humoral immune response to human cytomegalovirus proteins: a brief review, *Comp Immunol Microbiol Infect Dis* 14:97-105, 1991.
64. Zaia JA, Forman SJ, Ting YP, et al: Polypeptide-specific antibody response to human cytomegalovirus after infection in bone marrow transplant recipients, *J Infect Dis* 153:780-787, 1986.
65. Sylwester AW, Mitchell BL, Edgar JB, et al: Broadly targeted human cytomegalovirus-specific CD4+ and CD8+ T cells dominate the memory compartments of exposed subjects, *J Exp Med* 202: 673-685, 2005.
66. Hayes K, Alford CA, Britt WJ: Antibody response to virus-encoded proteins after cytomegalovirus mononucleosis, *J Infect Dis* 156: 615-621, 1987.
67. Kern F, Bunde T, Faulhaber N, et al: Cytomegalovirus (CMV) phosphoprotein 65 makes a large contribution to shaping the T cell repertoire in CMV-exposed individuals, *J Infect Dis* 185:1709-1716, 2002.
68. Boppana SB, Britt WJ: Recognition of human cytomegalovirus gene products by HCMV-specific cytotoxic T cells, *Virology* 222:293-296, 1996.
69. Murphy E, Yu D, Grimwood J, et al: Coding capacity of laboratory and clinical strains of human cytomegalovirus, *Proc Natl Acad Sci U S A* 100:14976-14981, 2003.
70. Chee MS, Bankier AT, Beck S, et al: Analysis of the protein-coding content of the sequence of human cytomegalovirus strain AD169, *Curr Top Microbiol Immunol* 154:125-170, 1990.
71. Britt WJ, Boppana S: Human cytomegalovirus virion proteins, *Hum Immunol* 65:395-402, 2004.
72. Eickmann M, Glickhorn D, Radsak K: Glycoprotein trafficking in virion morphogenesis. In Reddehase MJ, editor: *Cytomegaloviruses: molecular biology and immunology*, Norfolk, UK, 2006, Caister, pp 245-264.

73. Mach M: Antibody-mediated neutralization of infectivity. In Reddehase MJ, editor: *Cytomegaloviruses: molecular biology and immunology*, Norfolk, UK, 2006, Caister, pp 265-283.
74. Wang D, Yu QC, Schroer J, et al: Human cytomegalovirus uses two distinct pathways to enter retinal pigmented epithelial cells, *Proc Natl Acad Sci U S A* 104:20037-20042, 2007.
75. Hahn G, Revello MG, Patrone M, et al: Human cytomegalovirus *UL131-128* genes are indispensable for virus growth in endothelial cells and virus transfer to leukocytes, *J Virol* 78:10023-10033, 2004.
76. Ryckman BJ, Rainish BL, Chase MC, et al: Characterization of the human cytomegalovirus gH/gL/UL128-131 complex that mediates entry into epithelial and endothelial cells, *J Virol* 82:60-70, 2008.
77. Wang D, Shenk T: Human cytomegalovirus UL131 open reading frame is required for epithelial cell tropism, *J Virol* 79:10330-10338, 2005.
78. Wagner F, Brizic I, Prager A, et al: The viral chemokine MCK-2 of murine cytomegalovirus promotes infection as part of a gH/gL/MCK-2 complex, *PLoS Pathog* 9:e1003493, 2013.
79. Cui X, Meza BP, Adler SP, et al: Cytomegalovirus vaccines fail to induce epithelial entry neutralizing antibodies comparable to natural infection, *Vaccine* 26:5760-5766, 2008.
80. Britt WJ, Vugler L, Butfiloski EJ, et al: Cell surface expression of human cytomegalovirus (HCMV) gp55-116 (gB): use of HCMV-vaccinia recombinant virus infected cells in analysis of the human neutralizing antibody response, *J Virol* 64:1079-1085, 1990.
81. Meyer H, Masuho Y, Mach M: The gp116 of the gp58/116 complex of human cytomegalovirus represents the amino-terminal part of the precursor molecule and contains a neutralizing epitope, *J Gen Virol* 71:2443-2450, 1990.
82. Rasmussen L, Matkin C, Spaete R, et al: Antibody response to human cytomegalovirus glycoproteins gB and gH after natural infection in humans, *J Infect Dis* 164:835-842, 1991.
83. Marshall GS, Rabalais GP, Stout GG, et al: Antibodies to recombinant-derived glycoprotein B after natural human cytomegalovirus infection correlate with neutralizing activity, *J Infect Dis* 165: 381-384, 1992.
84. Urban M, Klein M, Britt WJ, et al: Glycoprotein H of human cytomegalovirus is a major antigen for the neutralizing humoral immune response, *J Gen Virol* 77:1537-1547, 1996.
85. Compton T: Receptors and immune sensors: the complex entry path of human cytomegalovirus, *Trends Cell Biol* 14:5-8, 2004.
86. Boehme KW, Compton T: Virus entry and activation of innate immunity. In Reddehase MJ, editor: *Cytomegaloviruses: molecular biology and immunology*, Norfolk, UK, 2006, Caister, pp 111-130.
87. Wang X, Huong SM, Chiu ML, et al: Epidermal growth factor receptor is a cellular receptor for human cytomegalovirus, *Nature* 424: 456-461, 2003.
88. Wang X, Huang DY, Huong SM, et al: Integrin alphavbeta3 is a coreceptor for human cytomegalovirus, *Nat Med* 11:515-521, 2005.
89. Feire AL, Koss H, Compton T: Cellular integrins function as entry receptors for human cytomegalovirus via a highly conserved disintegrin-like domain, *Proc Natl Acad Sci U S A* 101:15470-15475, 2004.
90. Soroceanu L, Akhavan A, Cobbs CS: Platelet-derived growth factor-alpha receptor activation is required for human cytomegalovirus infection, *Nature* 455:391-395, 2008.
91. Cobbs CS, Soroceanu L, Denham S, et al: Human cytomegalovirus induces cellular tyrosine kinase signaling and promotes glioma cell invasiveness, *J Neurooncol* 85:271-280, 2007.
92. Vanarsdall AL, Wisner TW, Lei H, et al: PDGF receptor-alpha does not promote HCMV entry into epithelial and endothelial cells but increased quantities stimulate entry by an abnormal pathway, *PLoS Pathog* 8:e1002905, 2012.
93. Yamauchi Y, Helenius A: Virus entry at a glance, *J Cell Sci* 126:1289-1295, 2013.
94. Zhu H, Cong JP, Mamtora G, et al: Cellular gene expression altered by human cytomegalovirus: global monitoring with oligonucleotide arrays, *Proc Natl Acad Sci USA* 95:14470-14475, 1998.
95. Zhu H, Cong JP, Shenk T: Use of differential display analysis to assess the effect of human cytomegalovirus infection on the accumulation of cellular RNAs: induction of interferon-responsive RNAs, *Proc Natl Acad Sci U S A* 94:13985-13990, 1997.
96. Browne EP, Wing B, Coleman D, et al: Altered cellular mRNA levels in human cytomegalovirus-infected fibroblasts: viral block to the accumulation of antiviral mRNAs, *J Virol* 75:12319-12330, 2001.
97. Simmen KA, Singh J, Luukkonen BG, et al: Global modulation of cellular transcription by human cytomegalovirus is initiated by viral glycoprotein B, *Proc Natl Acad Sci U S A* 98:7140-7145, 2001.
98. DeFilippis VR, Sali T, Alvarado D, et al: Activation of the interferon response by human cytomegalovirus occurs via cytoplasmic double-stranded DNA but not glycoprotein B, *J Virol* 84:8913-8925, 2010.
99. Yurochko AD: Human cytomegalovirus modulation of signal transduction, *Curr Top Microbiol Immunol* 325:205-220, 2008.
100. Yu Y, Alwine JC: Human cytomegalovirus major immediate-early proteins and simian virus 40 large T antigen can inhibit apoptosis through activation of the phosphatidylinositide 3′-OH kinase pathway and the cellular kinase Akt, *J Virol* 76:3731-3738, 2002.
101. Sambucetti LC, Cherrington JM, Wilkinson GW, et al: NF-kappa B activation of the cytomegalovirus enhancer is mediated by a viral transactivator and by T cell stimulation, *EMBO J* 8:4251-4258, 1989.
102. Child S, Jarrahian S, Harper V, et al: Complementation of vaccinia virus lacking the double stranded RNA-binding protein gene E3L by human cytomegalovirus, *J Virol* 76:4912-4918, 2002.
103. Hakki M, Geballe AP: Double-stranded RNA binding by human cytomegalovirus pTRS1, *J Virol* 79:7311-7318, 2005.
104. Zimmerman A, Hengel H: Cytomegalovirus interference with interferons. In Reddehase MJ, editor: *Cytomegaloviruses: molecular biology and immunology*, Norfolk, UK, 2006, Caister, pp 321-339.
105. Fliss PM, Brune W: Prevention of cellular suicide by cytomegaloviruses, *Viruses* 4:1928-1949, 2012.
106. Ogawa-Goto K, Tanaka K, Gibson W, et al: Microtubule network facilitates nuclear targeting of human cytomegalovirus capsid, *J Virol* 77:8541-8547, 2003.
107. Radtke K, Dohner K, Sodeik B: Viral interactions with the cytoskeleton: a hitchhiker's guide to the cell, *Cell Microbiol* 8:387-400, 2006.
108. Wolfstein A, Nagel CH, Radtke K, et al: The inner tegument promotes herpes simplex virus capsid motility along microtubules in vitro, *Traffic* 7:227-237, 2006.
109. Stinski MF, Shenk T: Functional roles of the human cytomegalovirus essential IE86 protein. In Shenk T, Stinski MF, editors: *Human cytomegalovirus*, Berlin/Heidelberg, 2008, Springer-Verlag, pp 133-152.
110. McCormick AL: Control of apoptosis by human cytomegalovirus. In Shenk T, Stinski MF, editors: *Human cytomegalovirus*, Berlin/Heidelberg, 2008, Springer-Verlag, pp 281-294.
111. Fleming P, Kvansakul M, Voigt V, et al: MCMV-mediated inhibition of the pro-apoptotic Bak protein is required for optimal in vivo replication, *PLoS Pathog* 9:e1003192, 2013.
112. Handke W, Krause E, Brune W: Live or let die: manipulation of cellular suicide programs by murine cytomegalovirus, *Med Microbiol Immunol* 201:475-486, 2012.
113. Reddehase MJ: *Cytomegaloviruses: from molecular pathogenesis to intervention*, London, 2013, Caister Academic Press.
114. Cullen BR: Viral and cellular messenger RNA targets of viral microRNAs, *Nature* 457:421-425, 2009.
115. Gottwein E, Cullen BR: Viral and cellular microRNAs as determinants of viral pathogenesis and immunity, *Cell Host Microbe* 3: 375-387, 2008.
116. Grey F, Nelson J: Identification and function of human cytomegalovirus microRNAs, *J Clin Virol* 41:186-191, 2008.
117. Grey F, Meyers H, White EA, et al: A human cytomegalovirus-encoded microRNA regulates expression of multiple viral genes involved in replication, *PLoS Pathog* 3:e163, 2007.
118. Nelson JA: Small RNAs and large DNA viruses, *N Engl J Med* 357:2630-2632, 2007.
119. Grey F, Antoniewicz A, Allen E, et al: Identification and characterization of human cytomegalovirus-encoded microRNAs, *J Virol* 79:12095-12099, 2005.
120. Murphy E, Vanicek J, Robins H, et al: Suppression of immediate-early viral gene expression by herpesvirus-coded microRNAs: implications for latency, *Proc Natl Acad Sci U S A* 105:5453-5458, 2008.
121. Dolken L, Krmpotic A, Kothe S, et al: Cytomegalovirus microRNAs facilitate persistent virus infection in salivary glands, *PLoS Pathog* 6:e1001150, 2010.
122. Dolken L, Malterer G, Erhard F, et al: Systematic analysis of viral and cellular microRNA targets in cells latently infected with human gamma-herpesviruses by RISC immunoprecipitation assay, *Cell Host Microbe* 7:324-334, 2010.
123. Pari GS: Nuts and bolts of human cytomegalovirus lytic DNA replication. In Shenk T, Stinski MF, editors: *Human cytomegalovirus*, Berlin/Heidelberg, 2008, Springer, pp 153-167.

124. Newcomb WW, Homa FL, Thomsen DR, et al: In vitro assembly of the herpes simplex virus procapsid: formation of small procapsids at reduced scaffolding protein concentration, *J Struct Biol* 133:23-31, 2001.
125. Heymann JB, Cheng N, Newcomb WW, et al: Dynamics of herpes simplex virus capsid maturation visualized by time-lapse cryo-electron microscopy, *Nat Struct Biol* 10:334-341, 2003.
126. Sanchez V, Greis KD, Sztul E, et al: Accumulation of virion tegument and envelope proteins in a stable cytoplasmic compartment during human cytomegalovirus replication. Characterization of a potential site of virus assembly, *J Virol* 74:975-986, 2000.
127. Alwine JC: The human cytomegalovirus assembly compartment: a masterpiece of viral manipulation of cellular processes that facilitates assembly and egress, *PLoS Pathog* 8:e1002878, 2012.
128. Homman-Loudiyi M, Hultenby K, Britt W, et al: Envelopment of human cytomegalovirus occurs by budding into Golgi-derived vacuole compartments positive for gB, Rab 3, trans-Golgi network 46, and mannosidase II, *J Virol* 77:3191-3203, 2003. [Erratum in *J Virol Arch* 2003;77:8179].
129. Das S, Vasanji A, Pellett PE: Three-dimensional structure of the human cytomegalovirus cytoplasmic virion assembly complex includes a reoriented secretory apparatus, *J Virol* 81:11861-11869, 2007.
130. Taylor-Wiedeman J, Sissons P, Sinclair J: Induction of endogenous human cytomegalovirus gene expression after differentiation of monocytes from healthy carriers, *J Virol* 68:1597-1604, 1994.
131. Kondo K, Xu J, Mocarski ES: Human cytomegalovirus latent gene expression in granulocyte-macrophage progenitors in culture and in seropositive individuals, *Proc Natl Acad Sci USA* 93:11137-11142, 1996.
132. Soderberg-Naucler C, Fish KN, Nelson JA: Reactivation of latent human cytomegalovirus by allogeneic stimulation of blood cells from healthy donors, *Cell* 91:119-126, 1997.
133. Soderberg-Naucler C, Fish KN, Nelson JA: Interferon-gamma and tumor necrosis factor-alpha specifically induce formation of cytomegalovirus-permissive monocyte-derived macrophages that are refractory to the antiviral activity of these cytokines, *J Clin Invest* 100:3154-3163, 1997.
134. Reeves M, Sinclair J: Aspects of human cytomegalovirus latency and reactivation. In Shenk T, Stinski MF, editors: *Human cytomegalovirus*, Berlin/Heidelberg, 2008, Springer-Verlag, pp 297-313.
135. Bolovan-Fritts CA, Mocarski ES, Wiedeman JA: Peripheral blood CD14(+) cells from healthy subjects carry a circular conformation of latent cytomegalovirus genome, *Blood* 93:394-398, 1999.
136. Soderberg-Naucler C, Streblow DN, Fish KN, et al: Reactivation of latent human cytomegalovirus in CD14(+) monocytes is differentiation dependent, *J Virol* 75:7543-7554, 2001.
137. Goodrum F, Caviness K, Zagallo P: Human cytomegalovirus persistence, *Cell Microbiol* 14:644-655, 2012.
138. Jarvis MA, Nelson JA: Molecular basis of persistence and latency. In Arvin A, Campadelli-Fiume G, Mocarski E, et al, editors: *Human herpesviruses: biology, therapy, and immunoprophylaxis*, Cambridge, UK, 2007, Cambridge University Press.
139. Smith MS, Goldman DC, Bailey AS, et al: Granulocyte-colony stimulating factor reactivates human cytomegalovirus in a latently infected humanized mouse model, *Cell Host Microbe* 8:284-291, 2010.
140. Reeves M, Sinclair J: Regulation of human cytomegalovirus transcription in latency: beyond the major immediate-early promoter, *Viruses* 5:1395-1413, 2013.
141. Reeves M, Woodhall D, Compton T, et al: Human cytomegalovirus IE72 protein interacts with the transcriptional repressor hDaxx to regulate LUNA gene expression during lytic infection, *J Virol* 84:7185-7194, 2010.
142. Reeves MB, Sinclair JH: Circulating dendritic cells isolated from healthy seropositive donors are sites of human cytomegalovirus reactivation in vivo, *J Virol* 87:10660-10667, 2013.
143. Gnann JW, Ahlmen J, Svalander C, et al: Inflammatory cells in transplanted kidneys are infected by human cytomegalovirus, *Am J Pathol* 132:239-248, 1988.
144. Hummel M, Zhang Z, Yan S, et al: Allogeneic transplantation induces expression of cytomegalovirus immediate-early genes in vivo: a model for reactivation from latency, *J Virol* 75:4814-4822, 2001.
145. Hummel M, Abecassis MM: A model for reactivation of CMV from latency, *J Clin Virol* 25(Suppl 2):S123-S136, 2002.
146. Roback JD, Hillyer CD, Drew WL, et al: Multicenter evaluation of PCR methods for detecting CMV DNA in blood donors, *Transfusion* 41:1249-1257, 2001.
147. Dolken L, Pfeffer S, Koszinowski UH: Cytomegalovirus microRNAs, *Virus Genes* 38:355-364, 2009.
148. Poole E, McGregor Dallas SR, Colston J, et al: Virally induced changes in cellular microRNAs maintain latency of human cytomegalovirus in CD34(+) progenitors, *J Gen Virol* 92:1539-1549, 2011.
149. Sinzger C, Plachter B, Stenglein S, et al: Immunohistochemical detection of viral antigens in smooth muscle, stromal, and epithelial cells from acute human cytomegalovirus gastritis, *J Infect Dis* 167: 1427-1432, 1993.
150. Sinzger C, Muntefering H, Loning T, et al: Cell types infected in human cytomegalovirus placentitis identified by immunohistochemical double staining, *Virchows Archiv A Pathol Anat Histopathol* 423:249-256, 1993.
151. Sinzger C, Digel M, Jahn G: Cytomegalovirus cell tropism. In Shenk T, Stinski MF, editors: *Human cytomegalovirus*, Berlin/Heidelberg, 2008, Springer-Verlag, pp 63-84.
152. Ryckman BJ, Jarvis MA, Drummond DD, et al: Human cytomegalovirus entry into epithelial and endothelial cells depends on genes *UL128* to *UL150* and occurs by endocytosis and low-pH fusion, *J Virol* 80:710-722, 2006.
153. Colugnati FA, Staras SA, Dollard SC, et al: Incidence of cytomegalovirus infection among the general population and pregnant women in the United States, *BMC Infect Dis* 7:71, 2007.
154. Staras SA, Dollard SC, Radford KW, et al: Seroprevalence of cytomegalovirus infection in the United States, 1988-1994, *Clin Infect Dis* 43:1143-1151, 2006.
155. Wilms IR, Best AM, Adler SP: Cytomegalovirus infections among African-Americans, *BMC Infect Dis* 8:107, 2008.
156. Kenneson A, Cannon MJ: Review and meta-analysis of the epidemiology of congenital cytomegalovirus (CMV) infection, *Rev Med Virol* 17:253-276, 2007.
157. Stagno S, Pass RF, Cloud G, et al: Primary cytomegalovirus infection in pregnancy. Incidence, transmission to fetus, and clinical outcome, *JAMA* 256:1904-1908, 1986.
158. Yamamoto AY, Mussi-Pinhata MM, Boppana SB, et al: Human cytomegalovirus reinfection is associated with intrauterine transmission in a highly cytomegalovirus-immune maternal population, *Am J Obstet Gynecol* 202:297.e1-297.e8, 2010.
159. Ross SA, Arora N, Novak Z, et al: Cytomegalovirus reinfections in healthy seroimmune women, *J Infect Dis* 201:386-389, 2010.
160. Jordan MC, Rousseau WE, Noble GR, et al: Association of cervical cytomegaloviruses with venereal disease, *N Engl J Med* 288:932-934, 1973.
161. Coonrod D, Collier AC, Ashley R, et al: Association between cytomegalovirus seroconversion and upper genital tract infection among women attending a sexually transmitted disease clinic: a prospective study, *J Infect Dis* 177:1188-1193, 1998.
162. Drew WL, Mintz L, Miner RC, et al: Prevalence of cytomegalovirus infection in homosexual men, *J Infect Dis* 143:188-192, 1981.
163. Chandler SH, Holmes KK, Wentworth BB, et al: The epidemiology of cytomegaloviral infection in women attending a sexually transmitted disease clinic, *J Infect Dis* 152:597-605, 1985.
164. Ross SA, Boppana SB: Congenital cytomegalovirus infection: outcome and diagnosis, *Semin Pediatr Infect Dis* 16:44-49, 2005.
165. Hayes D, Danks M, Givas H, et al: Cytomegalovirus in human milk, *N Engl J Med* 287:177, 1972.
166. Hamprecht K, Goelz R, Maschmann J: Breast milk and cytomegalovirus infection in preterm infants, *Early Hum Dev* 81:989-996, 2005.
167. Hamprecht K, Maschmann J, Jahn G, et al: Cytomegalovirus transmission to preterm infants during lactation, *J Clin Virol* 41:198-205, 2008.
168. Hamprecht K, Maschmann J, Muller D, et al: Cytomegalovirus (CMV) inactivation in breast milk: reassessment of pasteurization and freeze-thawing, *Pediatr Res* 56:529-535, 2004.
169. Hamprecht K, Maschmann J, Vochem M, et al: Epidemiology of transmission of cytomegalovirus from mother to preterm infant by breastfeeding, *Lancet* 357:513-518, 2001.
170. Hamprecht K, Vochem M, Baumeister A, et al: Detection of cytomegaloviral DNA in human milk cells and cell free milk whey by nested PCR, *J Virol Methods* 70:167-176, 1998.
171. Yasuda A, Kimura H, Hayakawa M, et al: Evaluation of cytomegalovirus infections transmitted via breast milk in preterm infants with a real-time polymerase chain reaction assay, *Pediatrics* 111: 1333-1336, 2003.

172. Pass RF, August AM, Dworsky ME, et al: Cytomegalovirus infection in a day care center, *N Engl J Med* 307:477-479, 1982.
173. Adler SP: The molecular epidemiology of cytomegalovirus transmission among children attending a day care center, *J Infect Dis* 152:760-768, 1985.
174. Murph JR, Bale JF, Murray JC, et al: Cytomegalovirus transmission in a Midwest day care center: possible relationship to child care practices, *J Pediatr* 109:35-39, 1986.
175. Murph JR, Bale JF Jr: The natural history of acquired cytomegalovirus infection among children in group day care, *Am J Dis Child* 142:843-846, 1988.
176. Hutto SC, Ricks RE, Garvie M, et al: Epidemiology of cytomegalovirus infections in young children: day care vs home care, *Pediatr Infect Dis* 4:149-152, 1985.
177. Pass RF, Little EA, Stagno S, et al: Young children as a probable source of maternal and congenital cytomegalovirus infection, *N Engl J Med* 316:1366-1370, 1987.
178. Stagno S, Cloud GA: Working parents: the impact of day care and breast-feeding on cytomegalovirus infections in offspring, *Proc Natl Acad Sci U S A* 91:2384-2389, 1994.
179. Hutto C, Little EA, Ricks R, et al: Isolation of cytomegalovirus from toys and hands in a day care center, *J Infect Dis* 154:527-530, 1986.
180. Faix RG: Survival of cytomegalovirus on environmental surfaces, *J Pediatr* 106:649-652, 1985.
181. Bale JF Jr, Petheram SJ, Souza IE, et al: Cytomegalovirus reinfection in young children, *J Pediatr* 128:347-352, 1996.
182. Dworsky M, Lakeman A, Stagno S: Cytomegalovirus transmission within a family, *Pediatr Infect Dis* 3:236-238, 1984.
183. Murph JR, Souza IE, Dawson JD, et al: Epidemiology of congenital cytomegalovirus infection: maternal risk factors and molecular analysis of cytomegalovirus strains, *Am J Epidemiol* 147:940-947, 1998.
184. Murph JR, Baron JC, Brown CK, et al: The occupational risk of cytomegalovirus infection among day-care providers, *JAMA* 265:603-608, 1991.
185. Spector SA, Spector DH: Molecular epidemiology of cytomegalovirus infections in premature twin infants and their mother, *Pediatr Infect Dis* 1:405-409, 1982.
186. Yeager AS: Transmission of cytomegalovirus to mothers by infected infants: another reason to prevent transfusion-acquired infections, *Pediatr Infect Dis* 2:295, 1983.
187. Dworsky M, Welch K, Cassady G, et al: Occupational risk for primary cytomegalovirus infection among pediatric health care workers, *N Engl J Med* 309:950-953, 1983.
188. Taber LH, Frank AL, Yow MD, et al: Acquisition of cytomegaloviral infections in families with young children: a serological study, *J Infect Dis* 151:948-952, 1985.
189. Adler SP: Cytomegalovirus and child day care. Evidence for an increased infection rate among day-care workers, *N Engl J Med* 321:1290-1296, 1989.
190. Adler SP: Molecular epidemiology of cytomegalovirus: viral transmission among children attending a day care center, their parents, and caretakers, *J Pediatr* 112:366-372, 1988.
191. Adler SP, Baggett J, Wilson M, et al: Molecular epidemiology of cytomegalovirus in a nursery: lack of evidence for nosocomial transmission, *J Pediatr* 108:117-123, 1986.
192. Pass RF, Hutto SC, Ricks R, et al: Increased rate of cytomegalovirus infection among parents of children attending day care centers, *N Engl J Med* 314:1414-1418, 1986.
193. Marshall BC, Adler SP: The frequency of pregnancy and exposure to cytomegalovirus infections among women with a young child in day care, *Am J Obstet Gynecol* 200:163.e1-163.e5, 2009.
194. Dreher A, Arora N, Fowler K, et al: Changing estimates of disease and outcome in children with symptomatic congenital cytomegalovirus infection, *J Pediatr* 164:855-859, 2014.
195. Schopfer K, Lauber E, Krech U: Congenital cytomegalovirus infection in newborn infants of mothers infected before pregnancy, *Arch Dis Child* 53:536-539, 1978.
196. Stagno S, Reynolds DW, Huang ES, et al: Congenital cytomegalovirus infection: occurrence in an immune population, *N Engl J Med* 296:1254-1258, 1977.
197. Embil JA, Ozere RJ, Haldane EV: Congenital cytomegalovirus infection in two siblings from consecutive pregnancies, *J Pediatr* 77: 417-421, 1970.
198. van der Sande MA, Kaye S, Miles DJ, et al: Risk factors for and clinical outcome of congenital cytomegalovirus infection in a peri-urban West-African birth cohort, *PLoS One* 2:e492, 2007.
199. Manicklal S, Emery VC, Lazzarotto T, et al: The "silent" global burden of congenital cytomegalovirus, *Clin Microbiol Rev* 26:86-102, 2013.
200. Yamamoto AP, Mussi-Pinhata MM, Pinto PC, et al: Congenital cytomegalovirus infection in preterm and full-term newborn infants from a population with a high seroprevalence rate, *Pediatr Infect Dis J* 20:188-192, 2001.
201. Gaytant MA, Steegers EA, Semmekrot BA, et al: Congenital cytomegalovirus infection: review of the epidemiology and outcome, *Obstet Gynecol Surv* 57:245-256, 2002.
202. Dar L, Pati S, Patro A, et al: Congenital cytomegalovirus infection in a highly seropositive semi-urban population in India, *Pediatr Infect Dis J* 27:841-843, 2008.
203. Mussi-Pinhata MM, Yamamoto AY, Moura Brito RM, et al: Birth prevalence and natural history of congenital cytomegalovirus infection in a highly seroimmune population, *Clin Infect Dis* 49:522-528, 2009.
204. Stagno S, Pass RF, Dworsky ME, et al: Maternal cytomegalovirus infection and perinatal transmission, *Clin Obstet Gynecol* 25: 563-576, 1982.
205. Boppana SB, Rivera LB, Fowler KB, et al: Intrauterine transmission of cytomegalovirus to infants of women with preconceptional immunity, *N Engl J Med* 344:1366-1371, 2001.
206. de Vries JJ, van Zwet EW, Dekker FW, et al: The apparent paradox of maternal seropositivity as a risk factor for congenital cytomegalovirus infection: a population-based prediction model, *Rev Med Virol* 23:241-249, 2013.
207. Gehrz RC, Christianson WR, Linner KM, et al: Cytomegalovirus specific humoral and cellular immune responses in human pregnancy, *J Infect Dis* 143:391-395, 1981.
208. Duryea EL, Sanchez PJ, Sheffield JS, et al: Maternal human immunodeficiency virus infection and congenital transmission of cytomegalovirus, *Pediatr Infect Dis J* 29:915-918, 2010.
209. Frederick T, Homans J, Spencer L, et al: The effect of prenatal highly active antiretroviral therapy on the transmission of congenital and perinatal/early postnatal cytomegalovirus among HIV-infected and HIV-exposed infants, *Clin Infect Dis* 55:877-884, 2012.
210. Guibert G, Warszawski J, Le Chenadec J, et al: Decreased risk of congenital cytomegalovirus infection in children born to HIV-1-infected mothers in the era of highly active antiretroviral therapy, *Clin Infect Dis* 48:1516-1525, 2009.
211. Lilleri D, Fornara C, Furione M, et al: Development of human cytomegalovirus-specific T cell immunity during primary infection of pregnant women and its correlation with virus transmission to the fetus, *J Infect Dis* 195:1062-1070, 2007.
212. Boppana SB, Britt WJ: Antiviral antibody responses and intrauterine transmission after primary maternal cytomegalovirus infection, *J Infect Dis* 171:1115-1121, 1995.
213. Boppana SB, Miller J, Britt WJ: Transplacentally acquired antiviral antibodies and outcome in congenital human cytomegalovirus infection, *Viral Immunol* 9:211-218, 1996.
214. Pass RF: Transmission of viruses through human milk. In Howell RR, Morriss FH, Pickering LK, editors: *Role of human milk in infant nutrition and health*, Springfield, Ill, 1986, Charles C Thomas Publishers, pp 205-224.
215. Yamamoto AY, Castellucci RA, Aragon DC, et al: Early high CMV seroprevalence in pregnant women from a population with a high rate of congenital infection, *Epidemiol Infect* 141:2187-2191, 2013.
216. Handsfield HH, Chandler SH, Caine VA, et al: Cytomegalovirus infection in sex partners: evidence for sexual transmission, *J Infect Dis* 151:344-348, 1985.
217. Staras SA, Flanders WD, Dollard SC, et al: Influence of sexual activity on cytomegalovirus seroprevalence in the United States, 1988-1994, *Sex Transm Dis* 35:472-479, 2008.
218. Kreel I, Zaroff LI, Canter JW, et al: A syndrome following total body perfusion, *Surg Gynecol Obstet* 111:317-321, 1960.
219. Seaman AJ, Starr A: Febrile post-cariotomy lymphocytic splenomegaly: a new entity, *Ann Surg* 156:956-960, 1962.
220. Armstrong JA, Tarr GC, Youngblood LA, et al: Cytomegalovirus infection in children undergoing open heart surgery, *Yale J Biol Med* 49:83-91, 1976.
221. Prince AM, Szmuness W, Millian SJ, et al: A serologic study of cytomegalovirus infections associated with blood transfusions, *N Engl J Med* 284:1125-1131, 1971.

222. Stevens DP, Barker LF, Ketcham AS, et al: Asymptomatic cytomegalovirus infection following blood transfusion in tumor surgery, *JAMA* 211:1341-1344, 1970.
223. McCracken GJ, Shinefield HR, Cobb K, et al: Congenital cytomegalic inclusion disease. A longitudinal study of 20 patients, *Am J Dis Child* 117:522-539, 1969.
224. Kumar A, Nankervis GA, Cooper AR, et al: Acquisition of cytomegalovirus infection in infants following exchange transfusion: a prospective study, *Transfusion* 20:327-331, 1980.
225. Yeager AS, Grumet FC, Hafleigh EB, et al: Prevention of transfusion-acquired cytomegalovirus infections in newborn infants, *J Pediatr* 98:281-287, 1981.
226. Tolkoff-Rubin NE, Fishman JA, Rubin RH: The bidirectional relationship between cytomegalovirus and allograft injury, *Transplant Proc* 33:1773-1775, 2001.
227. Razonable RR: Management strategies for cytomegalovirus infection and disease in solid organ transplant recipients, *Infect Dis Clin North Am* 27:317-342, 2013.
228. Atabani SF, Smith C, Atkinson C, et al: Cytomegalovirus replication kinetics in solid organ transplant recipients managed by preemptive therapy, *Am J Transplant* 12:2457-2464, 2012.
229. Boudreault AA, Xie H, Rakita RM, et al: Risk factors for late-onset cytomegalovirus disease in donor seropositive/recipient seronegative kidney transplant recipients who receive antiviral prophylaxis, *Transpl Infect Dis* 13:244-249, 2011.
230. Ljungman P: Beta-herpesvirus challenges in the transplant recipient, *J Infect Dis* 186:S99-S109, 2002.
231. Meyers JD, Flournoy N, Thomas ED: Nonbacterial pneumonia after allogeneic marrow transplantation: a review of ten years' experience, *Rev Infect Dis* 4:1119-1132, 1982.
232. Rubin R: Clinical approach to infection in the compromised host. In Rubin R, Young LS, editors: *Infection in the organ transplant recipient*, New York, 2002, Kluwer Academic Press, pp 573-679.
233. Boeckh M, Nichols WG, Papanicolaou G, et al: Cytomegalovirus in hematopoietic stem cell transplant recipients: current status, known challenges, and future strategies, *Biol Blood Marrow Transplant* 9: 543-558, 2003.
234. Boeckh M: Management of cytomegalovirus infections in blood and marrow transplant recipients, *Adv Exp Med Biol* 458:89-109, 1999.
235. Valantine HA, Luikart H, Doyle R, et al: Impact of cytomegalovirus hyperimmune globulin on outcome after cardiothoracic transplantation: a comparative study of combined prophylaxis with CMV hyperimmune globulin plus ganciclovir versus ganciclovir alone, *Transplantation* 72:1647-1652, 2001.
236. Valantine HA: Role of CMV in transplant coronary artery disease and survival after heart transplantation, *Transpl Infect Dis* 1(Suppl 1):25-30, 1999.
237. Singh N: Cytomegalovirus infection in solid organ transplant recipients: new challenges and their implications for preventive strategies, *J Clin Virol* 35:474-477, 2006.
238. Griffiths PD, Clark DA, Emery VC: Betaherpesviruses in transplant recipients, *J Antimicrob Chemother* 45:29-34, 2000.
239. Grundy JE, Super M, Lui S, et al: The source of cytomegalovirus infection in seropositive renal allograft recipients is frequently the donor kidney, *Transplant Proc* 19:2126-2128, 1987.
240. Grundy JE, Super M, Sweny P, et al: Symptomatic cytomegalovirus infection in seropositive kidney recipients: reinfection with donor virus rather than reactivation of recipient virus, *Lancet* 16:132-135, 1988.
241. Chou SW: Acquisition of donor strains of cytomegalovirus by renal-transplant recipients, *N Engl J Med* 314:1418-1423, 1986.
242. Chou SW: Cytomegalovirus infection and reinfection transmitted by heart transplantation, *J Infect Dis* 155:1054-1056, 1987.
243. Yow MD, Lakeman AD, Stagno S, et al: Use of restriction enzymes to investigate the source of a primary cytomegalovirus infection in a pediatric nurse, *Pediatrics* 70:713-716, 1982.
244. Wilfert CM, Huang ES, Stagno S: Restriction endonuclease analysis of cytomegalovirus deoxyribonucleic acid as an epidemiologic tool, *Pediatrics* 70:717-721, 1982.
245. Klemola E, Kaariainen L: Cytomegalovirus as a possible cause of a disease resembling infectious mononucleosis, *Br Med J* 2:1099-1102, 1965.
246. Andersson J, Stern H: Cytomegalovirus as a possible cause of a disease resembling infectious mononucleosis, *Br Med J* 1:672, 1966.
247. Guerrero A, Riddell SR, Storek J, et al: Cytomegalovirus viral load and virus-specific immune reconstitution after peripheral blood stem cell versus bone marrow transplantation, *Biol Blood Marrow Transplant* 18:66-75, 2012.
248. Hassan-Walker AF, Kidd IM, Sabin C, et al: Quantity of human cytomegalovirus (CMV) DNAemia as a risk factor for CMV disease in renal allograft recipients: relationship with donor/recipient CMV serostatus, receipt of augmented methylprednisolone and antithymocyte globulin (ATG), *J Med Virol* 58:182-187, 1999.
249. Zaia JA, Forman SJ, Gallagher MT, et al: Prolonged human cytomegalovirus viremia following bone marrow transplantation, *Transplantation* 37:315-317, 1984.
250. Lacey SF, Gallez-Hawkins G, Crooks M, et al: Characterization of cytotoxic function of CMV-pp65-specific CD8+ T-lymphocytes identified by HLA tetramers in recipients and donors of stem-cell transplants, *Transplantation* 74:722-732, 2002.
251. Spector SA, Hsia K, Crager M, et al: Cytomegalovirus (CMV) DNA load is an independent predictor of CMV disease and survival in advanced AIDS, *J Virol* 73:7027-7030, 1999.
252. Emery VC, Sabin CA, Cope AV, et al: Application of viral-load kinetics to identify patients who develop cytomegalovirus disease after transplantation, *Lancet* 355:2032-2036, 2000.
253. Sacher T, Podlech J, Mohr CA, et al: The major virus-producing cell type during murine cytomegalovirus infection, the hepatocyte, is not the source of virus dissemination in the host, *Cell Host Microbe* 3:263-272, 2008.
254. Sacher T, Jordan S, Mohr CA, et al: Conditional gene expression systems to study herpesvirus biology in vivo, *Med Microbiol Immunol* 197:269-276, 2008.
255. Sacher T, Mohr CA, Weyn A, et al: The role of cell types in cytomegalovirus infection in vivo, *Eur J Cell Biol* 91:70-77, 2012.
256. Grattan MT, Moreno-Cabral CE, Starnes VA, et al: Cytomegalovirus infection is associated with cardiac allograft rejection and atherosclerosis, *JAMA* 261:3561-3566, 1989.
257. Melnick JL, Petrie BL, Dreesman GR, et al: Cytomegalovirus antigen within human arterial smooth muscle cells, *Lancet* 2:644-647, 1983.
258. Nieto FJ, Szklo M, Sorlie PD: Cytomegalovirus infection and coronary heart disease, *Circulation* 100:e139, 1999.
259. Nieto FJ, Adam E, Sorlie P, et al: Cohort study of cytomegalovirus infection as a risk factor for carotid intimal-medial thickening, a measure of subclinical atherosclerosis, *Circulation* 94:922-927, 1996.
260. Hosenpud JD: Coronary artery disease after heart transplantation and its relation to cytomegalovirus, *Am Heart J* 138:S469-S472, 1999.
261. Koskinen PK, Kallio EA, Tikkanen JM, et al: Cytomegalovirus infection and cardiac allograft vasculopathy, *Transplant Infect Dis* 1:115-126, 1999.
262. Zhu J, Quyyumi AA, Norman JE, et al: Cytomegalovirus in the pathogenesis of atherosclerosis: the role of inflammation as reflected by elevated C-reactive protein levels, *J Am Coll Cardiol* 34:1738-1743, 1999.
263. Evans PC, Soin A, Wreghitt TG, et al: An association between cytomegalovirus infection and chronic rejection after liver transplantation, *Transplantation* 69:30-35, 2000.
264. Soderberg-Naucler C, Emery VC: Viral infections and their impact on chronic renal allograft dysfunction, *Transplantation* 71:SS24-SS30, 2001.
265. Stagno S, Reynolds DW, Amos CS, et al: Auditory and visual defects resulting from symptomatic and subclinical congenital cytomegaloviral and toxoplasma infections, *Pediatrics* 59:669-678, 1977.
266. Dahle AJ, McCollister FP, Stagno S, et al: Progressive hearing impairment in children with congenital cytomegalovirus infection, *J Speech Hear Disord* 44:220-229, 1979.
267. Dahle AJ, Fowler KB, Wright JD, et al: Longitudinal investigation of hearing disorders in children with congenital cytomegalovirus, *J Am Acad Audiol* 11:283-290, 2000.
268. Fowler KB, McCollister FP, Dahle AJ, et al: Progressive and fluctuating sensorineural hearing loss in children with asymptomatic congenital cytomegalovirus infection, *J Pediatr* 130:624-630, 1997.
269. Fowler KB, Boppana SB: Congenital cytomegalovirus (CMV) infection and hearing deficit, *J Clin Virol* 35:226-231, 2006.
270. Boppana S, Fowler KB: Persistence in the population: epidemiology and transmission. In Arvin A, Campadielli-Fume G, Mocarski E, et al, editors: *Human herpesviruses: biology, therapy, and immunoprophylaxis*, Cambridge, UK, 2007, Cambridge University Press, pp 795-813.

271. Koskinen P, Lemstrom K, Bruggeman C, et al: Acute cytomegalovirus infection induces a subendothelial inflammation (endothelialitis) in the allograft vascular wall. A possible linkage with enhanced allograft arteriosclerosis, *Am J Pathol* 144:41-50, 1994.
272. Lemstrom K, Koskinen P, Krogerus L, et al: Cytomegalovirus antigen expression, endothelial cell proliferation, and intimal thickening in rat cardiac allografts after cytomegalovirus infection, *Circulation* 92:2594-2604, 1995.
273. Lemstrom KB, Bruning JH, Bruggeman CA, et al: Triple drug immunosuppression significantly reduces immune activation and allograft arteriosclerosis in cytomegalovirus-infected rat aortic allografts and induces early latency of viral infection, *Am J Pathol* 144:1334-1347, 1994.
274. Li F, Yin M, Van Dam JG, et al: Cytomegalovirus infection enhances the neointima formation in rat aortic allografts: effect of major histocompatibility complex class I and class II antigen differences, *Transplantation* 65:1298-1304, 1998.
275. Zhou YF, Shou M, Guetta E, et al: Cytomegalovirus infection of rats increases the neointimal response to vascular injury without consistent evidence of direct infection of the vascular wall, *Circulation* 100:1569-1575, 1999.
276. Streblow DN, Soderberg-Naucler C, Vieira J, et al: The human cytomegalovirus chemokine receptor US28 mediates vascular smooth muscle cell migration, *Cell* 99:511-520, 1999.
277. Streblow DN, Dumortier J, Moses AV, et al: Mechanisms of cytomegalovirus-accelerated vascular disease: induction of paracrine factors that promote angiogenesis and wound healing, *Curr Top Microbiol Immunol* 325:397-415, 2008.
278. Streblow DN, Kreklywich CN, Andoh T, et al: The role of angiogenic and wound repair factors during CMV-accelerated transplant vascular sclerosis in rat cardiac transplants, *Am J Transplant* 8:277-287, 2008.
279. dela Pena MG, Strelow L, Barry PA, et al: Use of specific-pathogen-free (SPF) rhesus macaques to better model oral pediatric cytomegalovirus infection, *J Med Primatol* 41:225-229, 2012.
280. Sequar G, Britt WJ, Lakeman FD, et al: Experimental coinfection of rhesus macaques with rhesus cytomegalovirus and simian immunodeficiency virus: pathogenesis, *J Virol* 76:7661-7671, 2002.
281. Stoddart CA, Cardin RD, Boname JM, et al: Peripheral blood mononuclear phagocytes mediate dissemination of murine cytomegalovirus, *J Virol* 68:6243-6253, 1994.
282. Noda S, Aguirre SA, Bitmansour A, et al: Cytomegalovirus MCK-2 controls mobilization and recruitment of myeloid progenitor cells to facilitate dissemination, *Blood* 107:30-38, 2006.
283. Taylor-Wiedeman J, Sissons JG, Borysiewicz LK, et al: Monocytes are a major site of persistence of human cytomegalovirus in peripheral blood mononuclear cells, *J Gen Virol* 72(Pt 9):2059-2064, 1991.
284. Sinclair J, Sissons P: Latent and persistent infections of monocytes and macrophages, *Intervirology* 39:293-301, 1996.
285. Gerna G, Zipeto D, Percivalle E, et al: Human cytomegalovirus infection of the major leukocyte subpopulations and evidence for initial viral replication in polymorphonuclear leukocytes from viremic patients, *J Infect Dis* 166:1236-1244, 1992.
286. Schafer P, Tenschert W, Cremaschi L, et al: Cytomegalovirus cultured from different major leukocyte subpopulations: association with clinical features in CMV immunoglobulin G-positive renal allograft recipients, *J Med Virol* 61:488-496, 2000.
287. Liapis H, Storch GA, Hill DA, et al: CMV infection of the renal allograft is much more common than the pathology indicates: a retrospective analysis of qualitative and quantitative buffy coat CMV-PCR, renal biopsy pathology and tissue CMV-PCR, *Nephrol Dial Transplant* 18:397-402, 2003.
288. Gerna G, Percivalle E, Baldanti F, et al: Human cytomegalovirus replicates abortively in polymorphonuclear leukocytes after transfer from infected endothelial cells via transient microfusion events, *J Virol* 74:5629-5638, 2000.
289. Kas-Deelen AM, The TH, Blom N, et al: Uptake of pp65 in in vitro generated pp65-positive polymorphonuclear cells mediated by phagocytosis and cell fusion? *Intervirology* 44:8-13, 2001.
290. The TH, van der Bij W, van den Berg AP, et al: Cytomegalovirus antigenemia, *Rev of Infect Dis* 12:734-744, 1990.
291. van der Bij W, Speich R: Management of cytomegalovirus infection and disease after solid-organ transplantation, *Clin Infect Dis* 33:1, 2001.
292. Singh N, Paterson DL, Gayowski T, et al: Cytomegalovirus antigenemia directed pre-emptive prophylaxis with oral versus I.V. ganciclovir for the prevention of cytomegalovirus disease in liver transplant recipients: a randomized, controlled trial, *Transplantation* 70:717-722, 2000.
293. Nichols WG, Boeckh M: Recent advances in the therapy and prevention of CMV infections, *J Clin Virol* 16:25-40, 2000.
294. Boeckh M, Gooley TA, Myerson D, et al: Cytomegalovirus pp65 antigenemia-guided early treatment with ganciclovir versus ganciclovir at engraftment after allogeneic marrow transplantation: a randomized double-blind study, *Blood* 88:4063-4071, 1996.
295. Nichols WG, Corey L, Gooley T, et al: Rising pp65 antigenemia during preemptive anticytomegalovirus therapy after allogeneic hematopoietic stem cell transplantation: risk factors, correlation with DNA load, and outcomes, *Blood* 97:867-874, 2001.
296. Waldman WJ, Knight DA, Huang EH, et al: Bidirectional transmission of infectious cytomegalovirus between monocytes and vascular endothelial cells: an in vitro model, *J Infect Dis* 171:263-272, 1995.
297. Riegler S, Hebart H, Einsele H, et al: Monocyte-derived dendritic cells are permissive to the complete replicative cycle of human cytomegalovirus, *J Gen Virol* 81:393-399, 2000.
298. Fish KN, Stenglein SG, Ibanez C, et al: Cytomegalovirus persistence in macrophages and endothelial cells, *Scandinavian J Infect Dis Suppl* 99:34-40, 1995.
299. Hahn G, Jores R, Mocarski ES: Cytomegalovirus remains latent in a common precursor of dendritic and myeloid cells, *Proc Natl Acad Sci U S A* 95:3937-3942, 1998.
300. Sinclair J: Human cytomegalovirus: latency and reactivation in the myeloid lineage, *J Clin Virol* 41:180-185, 2008.
301. Holmberg LA, Boeckh M, Hooper H, et al: Increased incidence of cytomegalovirus disease after autologous CD34-selected peripheral blood stem cell transplantation, *Blood* 94:4029-4035, 1999.
302. Fish KN, Soderberg-Naucler C, Mills LK, et al: Human cytomegalovirus persistently infects aortic endothelial cells, *J Virol* 72:5661-5668, 1998.
303. Sinzger C, Grefte A, Plachter B, et al: Fibroblasts, epithelial cells, endothelial cells and smooth muscle cells are major targets of human cytomegalovirus infection in lung and gastrointestinal tissues, *J Gen Virol* 76:741-750, 1995.
304. Plachter B, Sinzger C, Jahn G: Cell types involved in replication and distribution of human cytomegalovirus, *Adv Virus Res* 46:195-261, 1996.
305. Sinzger C, Knapp J, Plachter B, et al: Quantification of replication of clinical cytomegalovirus isolates in cultured endothelial cells and fibroblasts by a focus expansion assay, *J Virol Methods* 63:103-112, 1997.
306. Gerna G, Zavattoni M, Baldanti F, et al: Circulating cytomegalic endothelial cells are associated with high human cytomegalovirus (HCMV) load in AIDS patients with late-stage disseminated HCMV disease, *J Med Virol* 55:64-74, 1998.
307. Evans PC, Coleman N, Wreghitt TG, et al: Cytomegalovirus infection of bile duct epithelial cells, hepatic artery and portal venous endothelium in relation to chronic rejection of liver grafts, *J Hepatol* 31:913-920, 1999.
308. Kas-Deelen AM, de Maar EF, Harmsen MC, et al: Uninfected and cytomegalic endothelial cells in blood during cytomegalovirus infection: effect of acute rejection, *J Infect Dis* 181:721-724, 2000.
309. Maidji E, Percivalle E, Gerna G, et al: Transmission of human cytomegalovirus from infected uterine microvascular endothelial cells to differentiating/invasive placental cytotrophoblasts, *Virology* 304:53-69, 2002.
310. Kahl M, Siegel-Axel D, Stenglein S, et al: Efficient lytic infection of human arterial endothelial cells by human cytomegalovirus strains, *J Virol* 74:7628-7635, 2000.
311. Sinzger C, Kahl M, Laib K, et al: Tropism of human cytomegalovirus for endothelial cells is determined by a post-entry step dependent on efficient translocation to the nucleus, *J Gen Virol* 81:3021-3035, 2000.
312. Percivalle E, Revello MG, Vago L, et al: Circulating endothelial giant cells permissive for human cytomegalovirus (HCMV) are detected in disseminated HCMV infections with organ involvement, *J Clin Invest* 92:663-670, 1993.
313. Grefte A, van der Giessen M, van Son W, et al: Circulating cytomegalovirus (CMV)-infected endoethelial cells in patients with an active CMV infection, *J Infect Dis* 167:270-277, 1993.
314. Brune W, Menard C, Heesemann J, et al: A ribonucleotide reductase homolog of cytomegalovirus and endothelial cell tropism, *Science* 291:303-305, 2001.
315. Fries BC, Chou S, Boeckh M, et al: Frequency distribution of cytomegalovirus envelope glycoprotein genotypes in bone marrow transplant recipients, *J Infect Dis* 169:769-774, 1994.

316. Rasmussen L, Hong C, Zipeto D, et al: Cytomegalovirus gB genotype distribution differs in human immunodeficiency virus-infected patients and immunocompromised allograft recipients, *J Infect Dis* 175:179-184, 1997.
317. Haberland M, Meyer-Konig U, Hufert FT: Variation within the glycoprotein B gene of human cytomegalovirus is due to homologous recombination, *J Gen Virol* 80:1495-1500, 1999.
318. Bale JF Jr, Murph JR, Demmler GJ, et al: Intrauterine cytomegalovirus infection and glycoprotein B genotypes, *J Infect Dis* 182: 933-936, 2000.
319. Lurain NS, Kapell KS, Huang DD, et al: Human cytomegalovirus UL144 open reading frame: sequence hypervariability in low-passage clinical isolates, *J Virol* 73:10040-10050, 1999.
320. Bale JF Jr, Petheram SJ, Robertson M, et al: Human cytomegalovirus a sequence and UL144 variability in strains from infected children, *J Med Virol* 65:90-96, 2001.
321. Rasmussen L, Geissler A, Winters M: Inter- and intragenic variations complicate the molecular epidemiology of human cytomegalovirus, *J Infect Dis* 187:809-819, 2003.
322. Rasmussen L, Geissler A, Cowan C, et al: The genes encoding the gCIII complex of human cytomegalovirus exist in highly diverse combinations in clinical isolates, *J Virol* 76:10841-10848, 2002.
323. Garrigue I, Corte MF, Magnin N, et al: Variability of *UL18, UL40, UL111a* and *US3* immunomodulatory genes among human cytomegalovirus clinical isolates from renal transplant recipients, *J Clin Virol* 40:120-128, 2007.
324. Garrigue I, Faure-Della Corte M, Magnin N, et al: UL40 human cytomegalovirus variability evolution patterns over time in renal transplant recipients, *Transplantation* 86:826-835, 2008.
325. Hitomi S, Kozuka-Hata H, Chen Z, et al: Human cytomegalovirus open reading frame UL11 encodes a highly polymorphic protein expressed on the infected cell surface, *Arch Virol* 142:1407-1427, 1997.
326. Pignatelli S, Dal Monte P, Rossini G, et al: Human cytomegalovirus glycoprotein N (gpUL73-gN) genomic variants: identification of a novel subgroup, geographical distribution and evidence of positive selective pressure, *J Gen Virol* 84:647-655, 2003.
327. Pignatelli S, Dal Monte P, Landini MP: gpUL73 (gN) genomic variants of human cytomegalovirus isolates are clustered into four distinct genotypes, *J Gen Virol* 82:2777-2784, 2001.
328. Renzette N, Bhattacharjee B, Jensen JD, et al: Extensive genome-wide variability of human cytomegalovirus in congenitally infected infants, *PLoS Pathog* 7:e1001344, 2011.
329. Chou SW: Reactivation and recombination of multiple cytomegalovirus strains from individual organ donors, *J Infect Dis* 160:11-15, 1989.
330. Hayajneh WA, Colberg-Poley AM, Skaletskaya A, et al: The sequence and antiapoptotic functional domains of the human cytomegalovirus UL37 exon 1 immediate early protein are conserved in multiple primary strains, *Virology* 279:233-240, 2001.
331. Skaletskaya A, Bartle LM, Chittenden T, et al: A cytomegalovirus-encoded inhibitor of apoptosis that suppresses caspase-8 activation, *Proc Natl Acad Sci U S A* 98:7829-7834, 2001.
332. Goldmacher VS: vMIA, a viral inhibitor of apoptosis targeting mitochondria, *Biochimie* 84:177-185, 2002.
333. Mocarski ES Jr: Immunomodulation by cytomegaloviruses: manipulative strategies beyond evasion, *Trends Microbiol* 10:332-339, 2002.
334. Saederup N, Mocarski ES Jr: Fatal attraction: cytomegalovirus-encoded chemokine homologs, *Curr Top Microbiol Immunol* 269:235-256, 2002.
335. Spencer JV, Lockridge KM, Barry PA, et al: Potent immunosuppressive activities of cytomegalovirus-encoded interleukin-10, *J Virol* 76:1285-1292, 2002.
336. Jenkins C, Garcia W, Godwin MJ, et al: Immunomodulatory properties of a viral homolog of human interleukin-10 expressed by human cytomegalovirus during the latent phase of infection, *J Virol* 82:3736-3750, 2008.
337. Goldmacher VS: Cell death suppression by cytomegaloviruses, *Apoptosis* 10:251-265, 2005.
338. Lockridge KM, Zhou SS, Kravitz RH, et al: Primate cytomegaloviruses encode and express an IL-10-like protein, *Virology* 268: 272-280, 2000.
339. Arav-Boger R, Foster CB, Zong JC, et al: Human cytomegalovirus-encoded alpha-chemokines exhibit high sequence variability in congenitally infected newborns, *J Infect Dis* 193:788-791, 2006.
340. Hanson LK, Slater JS, Karabekian Z, et al: Replication of murine cytomegalovirus in differentiated macrophages as a determinant of viral pathogenesis, *J Virol* 73:5970-5980, 1999.
341. Hanson LK, Slater JS, Karabekian Z, et al: Products of US22 genes M140 and M141 confer efficient replication of murine cytomegalovirus in macrophages and spleen, *J Virol* 75:6292-6302, 2001.
342. Bale JF Jr, O'Neil ME: Detection of murine cytomegalovirus DNA in circulating leukocytes harvested during acute infection of mice, *J Virol* 63:2667-2673, 1989. [erratum appears in *J Virol* 1989;63:4120].
343. Collins TM, Quirk MR, Jordan MC: Biphasic viremia and viral gene expression in leukocytes during acute cytomegalovirus infection of mice, *J Virol* 68:6305-6311, 1994.
344. Mitchell BM, Leung A, Stevens JG: Murine cytomegalovirus DNA in peripheral blood of latently infected mice is detectable only in monocytes and polymorphonuclear leukocytes, *Virology* 223:198-207, 1996.
345. Kern ER: Animal models for cytomegalovirus infection: murine CMV. In Zak O, Sande M, editors: *Handbook of animal models of infection*, London, 1999, Academic Press, pp 927-934.
346. Reddehase MJ, Podlech J, Grzimek NK: Mouse models of cytomegalovirus latency: overview, *J Clin Virol* 25:S23-S36, 2002.
347. Saederup N, Lin YC, Dairaghi DJ, et al: Cytomegalovirus-encoded beta chemokine promotes monocyte-associated viremia in the host, *Proc Natl Acad Sci U S A* 96:10881-10886, 1999.
348. Saederup N, Aguirre SA, Sparer TE, et al: Murine cytomegalovirus CC chemokine homolog MCK-2 (m131-129) is a determinant of dissemination that increases inflammation at initial sites of infection, *J Virol* 75:9966-9976, 2001.
349. Menard C, Wagner M, Ruzsics Z, et al: Role of murine cytomegalovirus *US22* gene family members in replication in macrophages, *J Virol* 77:5557-5570, 2003.
350. Jurak I, Schumacher U, Simic H, et al: Murine cytomegalovirus m38.5 protein inhibits Bax-mediated cell death, *J Virol* 82:4812-4822, 2008.
351. Brune W: Inhibition of programmed cell death by cytomegaloviruses, *Virus Res* 157:144-150, 2011.
352. Ebermann L, Ruzsics Z, Guzman CA, et al: Block of death-receptor apoptosis protects mouse cytomegalovirus from macrophages and is a determinant of virulence in immunodeficient hosts, *PLoS Pathog* 8:e1003062, 2012.
353. Hahn G, Khan H, Baldanti F, et al: The human cytomegalovirus ribonucleotide reductase homolog UL45 is dispensable for growth in endothelial cells, as determined by a BAC-cloned clinical isolate of human cytomegalovirus with preserved wild-type characteristics, *J Virol* 76:9551-9555, 2002.
354. Upton JW, Kaiser WJ, Mocarski ES: Virus inhibition of RIP3-dependent necrosis, *Cell Host Microbe* 7:302-313, 2010.
355. Kaiser WJ, Upton JW, Mocarski ES: Viral modulation of programmed necrosis, *Curr Opin Virol* 3:296-306, 2013.
356. Penfold ME, Dairaghi DJ, Duke GM, et al: Cytomegalovirus encodes a potent alpha chemokine, *Proc Natl Acad Sci U S A* 96:9839-9844, 1999.
357. Pepose JS, Holland GN, Nestor MS, et al: Acquired immune deficiency syndrome. Pathogenic mechanisms of ocular disease, *Ophthalmology* 92:472-484, 1985.
358. Jacobson MA, O'Donnell JJ, Porteus D, et al: Retinal and gastrointestinal disease due to cytomegalovirus in patients with the acquired immune deficiency syndrome: prevalence, natural history and response to ganciclovir therapy, *Q J Med* 67:473-486, 1988.
359. Wilcox CM, Chalasani N, Lazenby A, et al: Cytomegalovirus colitis in acquired immunodeficiency syndrome: a clinical and endoscopic study, *Gastroint Endosc* 48:39-43, 1998.
360. Redman TK, Britt WJ, Wilcox CM, et al: Human cytomegalovirus enhances chemokine production by lipopolysaccharide-stimulated lamina propria macrophages, *J Infect Dis* 185:584-590, 2002.
361. Compton T, Kurt-Jones EA, Boehme KW, et al: Human cytomegalovirus activates inflammatory cytokine responses via CD14 and Toll-like receptor 2, *J Virol* 77:4588-4596, 2003.
362. Zhu H, Cong JP, Bresnahan WA, et al: Inhibition of cyclooxygenase 2 blocks human cytomegalovirus replication, *Proc Natl Acad Sci U S A* 99:3932-3937, 2002.
363. Margulies BJ, Browne H, Gibson W: Identification of the human cytomegalovirus G protein-coupled receptor homologue encoded by *UL33* in infected cells and enveloped virus particles, *Virology* 225:111-125, 1996.

364. Rosenkilde MM, Waldhoer M, Luttichau HR, et al: Virally encoded 7TM receptors, *Oncogene* 20:1582-1593, 2001.
365. Beisser PS, Goh CS, Cohen FE, et al: Viral chemokine receptors and chemokines in human cytomegalovirus trafficking and interaction with the immune system. CMV chemokine receptors, *Curr Top Microbiol Immunol* 269:203-234, 2002.
366. Beisser P, Lavreysen H, Bruggeman C, et al: Chemokines and chemokine receptors encoded by cytomegaloviruses. In Shenk T, Stinski MF, editors: *Human cytomegalovirus*, Berlin/Heidelberg, 2008, Springer-Verlag.
367. Billstrom Schroeder M, Worthen GS: Viral regulation of RANTES expression during human cytomegalovirus infection of endothelial cells, *J Virol* 75:3383-3390, 2001.
368. Vomaske J, Melnychuk RM, Smith PP, et al: Differential ligand binding to a human cytomegalovirus chemokine receptor determines cell type-specific motility, *PLoS Pathog* 5:e1000304, 2009.
369. Billstrom Schroeder M, Christensen R, Worthen GS: Human cytomegalovirus protects endothelial cells from apoptosis induced by growth factor withdrawal, *J Clin Virol* 25:S149-S157, 2002.
370. Randolph-Habecker JR, Rahill B, Torok-Storb B, et al: The expression of the cytomegalovirus chemokine receptor homolog US28 sequesters biologically active CC chemokines and alters IL-8 production, *Cytokine* 19:37-46, 2002.
371. Maussang D, Verzijl D, van Walsum M, et al: Human cytomegalovirus-encoded chemokine receptor US28 promotes tumorigenesis, *Proc Natl Acad Sci U S A* 103:13068-13073, 2006.
372. Wills MR, Carmichael A, Sissons JG: Adaptive cellular immunity to human cytomegalovirus. In Reddehase MJ, editor: *Cytomegaloviruses: molecular biology and immunology*, Norfolk, UK, 2006, Caister, pp 341-367.
373. Jonjic S, Bubic I, Krmpotic A: Innate immunity to cytomegaloviruses. In Reddehase MJ, editor: *Cytomegaloviruses: molecular biology and immunology*, Norfolk, UK, 2006, Caister, pp 285-321.
374. Holtappels R, Munks MW, Podlech J, et al: CD8 T-cell-based immunotherapy of cytomegalovirus disease in the mouse model of the immunocompromised bone marrow transplantation recipient. In Reddehase MJ, editor: *Cytomegaloviruses: molecular biology and immunology*, Norfolk, UK, 2006, Caister, pp 383-419.
375. Steffens HP, Kurz S, Holtappels R, et al: Preemptive CD8 T-cell immunotherapy of acute cytomegalovirus infection prevents lethal disease, limits the burden of latent viral genomes, and reduces the risk of virus recurrence, *J Virol* 72:1797-1804, 1998.
376. Polic B, Hengel H, Krmpotic A, et al: Hierarchical and redundant lymphocyte subset control precludes cytomegalovirus replication during latent infection, *J Exp Med* 188:1047-1054, 1998.
377. Krmpotic A, Bubic I, Polic B, et al: Pathogenesis of murine cytomegalovirus infection, *Microbes Infect* 5:1263-1277, 2003.
378. Lucin P, Pavic I, Polic B, et al: Gamma interferon-dependent clearance of cytomegalovirus infection in salivary glands, *J Virol* 66:1977-1984, 1992.
379. Mach M. Gamma/delta T cells mediate resistance to murine CMV infection. [Manuscript in preparation, 2014.]
380. Bantug GR, Cekinovic D, Bradford R, et al: CD8+ T lymphocytes control murine cytomegalovirus replication in the central nervous system of newborn animals, *J Immunol* 181:2111-2123, 2008.
381. Jonjic S, Pavic I, Polic B, et al: Antibodies are not essential for the resolution of primary cytomegalovirus infection but limit dissemination of recurrent virus, *J Exp Med* 179:1713-1717, 1994.
382. Cekinovic D, Golemac M, Pugel EP, et al: Passive immunization reduces murine cytomegalovirus-induced brain pathology in newborn mice, *J Virol* 82:12172-12180, 2008.
383. Klenovsek K, Weisel F, Schneider A, et al: Protection from CMV infection in immunodeficient hosts by adoptive transfer of memory B cells, *Blood* 110:3472-3479, 2007.
384. Reusser P, Riddell SR, Meyers JD, et al: Cytotoxic T-lymphocyte response to cytomegalovirus after human allogeneic bone marrow transplantation: pattern of recovery and correlation with cytomegalovirus infection and disease, *Blood* 78:1373-1380, 1991.
385. Riddell SR, Gilbert MJ, Li CR, et al: Reconstitution of protective CD8+ cytotoxic T lymphocyte responses to human cytomegalovirus in immunodeficient humans by the adoptive transfer of T cell clones. In Michelson S, Plotkin SA, editors: *Multidisciplinary approach to understanding cytomegalovirus disease*, Amsterdam, 1993, Elsevier Science, pp 155-164.
386. Walter EA, Greenberg PD, Gilbert MJ, et al: Reconstitution of cellular immunity against cytomegalovirus in recipients of allogeneic bone marrow by transfer of T-cell clones from the donor, *N Engl J Med* 333:1038-1044, 1995.
387. Li CR, Greenberg PD, Gilbert MJ, et al: Recovery of HLA-restricted cytomegalovirus (CMV)-specific T-cell responses after allogeneic bone marrow transplant: correlation with CMV disease and effect of ganciclovir prophylaxis, *Blood* 83:1971-1979, 1994.
388. Horn B, Bao L, Dunham K, et al: Infusion of cytomegalovirus specific cytotoxic T lymphocytes from a sero-negative donor can facilitate resolution of infection and immune reconstitution, *Pediatr Infect Dis J* 28:65-67, 2009.
389. Cobbold M, Khan N, Pourgheysari B, et al: Adoptive transfer of cytomegalovirus-specific CTL to stem cell transplant patients after selection by HLA-peptide tetramers, *J Exp Med* 202:379-386, 2005.
390. Reusser P, Cathomas G, Attenhofer R, et al: Cytomegalovirus (CMV)-specific T cell immunity after renal transplantation mediates protection from CMV disease by limiting the systemic virus load, *J Infect Dis* 180:247-253, 1999.
391. Blyth E, Clancy L, Simms R, et al: Donor-derived CMV-specific T cells reduce the requirement for CMV-directed pharmacotherapy after allogeneic stem cell transplantation, *Blood* 121:3745-3758, 2013.
392. Meij P, Jedema I, Zandvliet ML, et al: Effective treatment of refractory CMV reactivation after allogeneic stem cell transplantation with in vitro-generated CMV pp65-specific CD8+ T-cell lines, *J Immunother* 35:621-628, 2012.
393. Bao L, Cowan MJ, Dunham K, et al: Adoptive immunotherapy with CMV-specific cytotoxic T lymphocytes for stem cell transplant patients with refractory CMV infections, *J Immunother* 35:293-298, 2012.
394. Boeckh M, Leisenring W, Riddell SR, et al: Late cytomegalovirus disease and mortality in recipients of allogeneic hematopoietic stem cell transplants: importance of viral load and T-cell immunity, *Blood* 101:407-414, 2003.
395. Kaye S, Miles D, Antoine P, et al: Virological and immunological correlates of mother-to-child transmission of cytomegalovirus in The Gambia, *J Infect Dis* 197:1307-1314, 2008.
396. Aubert G, Hassan-Walker AF, Madrigal JA, et al: Cytomegalovirus-specific cellular immune responses and viremia in recipients of allogeneic stem cell transplants, *Journal of Infectious Diseases* 184:955-963, 2001.
397. Matloubian M, Concepcion RJ, Ahmed R: CD4+ T cells are required to sustain CD8+ cytotoxic T-cell responses during chronic viral infection, *J Virol* 68:8056-8063, 1994.
398. Grakoui A, John Wherry E, Hanson HL, Walker C: Ahmed R: Turning on the off switch: regulation of anti-viral T cell responses in the liver by the PD-1/PD-L1 pathway, *J Hepatol* 45:468-472, 2006.
399. Barber DL, Wherry EJ, Masopust D, et al: Restoring function in exhausted CD8 T cells during chronic viral infection, *Nature* 439:682-687, 2006.
400. Shin H, Blackburn SD, Blattman JN, Wherry EJ: Viral antigen and extensive division maintain virus-specific CD8 T cells during chronic infection, *Journal of Experimental Medicine* 204:941-949, 2007.
401. Sun JC, Bevan MJ: Defective CD8 T cell memory following acute infection without CD4 T cell help.[comment], *Science* 300:339-342, 2003.
402. Biron CA, Byron KS, Sullivan JL: Severe herpesvirus infections in an adolescent without natural killer cells, *N Engl J Med* 320:1731-1735, 1989.
403. Hadaya K, de Rham C, Bandelier C, et al: Natural killer cell receptor repertoire and their ligands, and the risk of CMV infection after kidney transplantation, *Am J Transplant* 8:2674-2683, 2008.
404. Biron CA, Brossay L: NK cells and NKT cells in innate defense against viral infections, *Current Opin Immunol* 13:458-464, 2001.
405. Kuijpers TW, Baars PA, Dantin C, et al: Human NK cells can control CMV infection in the absence of T cells, *Blood* 112:914-915, 2008.
406. Stern M, Elsasser H, Honger G, et al: The number of activating KIR genes inversely correlates with the rate of CMV infection/reactivation in kidney transplant recipients, *Am J Transplant* 8:1312-1317, 2008.
407. Zhang SY, Boisson-Dupuis S, Chapgier A, et al: Inborn errors of interferon (IFN)-mediated immunity in humans: insights into the respective roles of IFN-alpha/beta, IFN-gamma, and IFN-lambda in host defense, *Immunol Rev* 226:29-40, 2008.
408. Zhang SY, Jouanguy E, Ugolini S, et al: TLR3 deficiency in patients with herpes simplex encephalitis, *Science* 317:1522-1527, 2007.

409. Robbins SH, Bessou G, Cornillon A, et al: Natural killer cells promote early CD8 T cell responses against cytomegalovirus, *PLoS Pathog* 3:e123, 2007.
410. Presti RM, Pollock JL, Dal Canto AJ, et al: Interferon gamma regulates acute and latent murine cytomegalovirus infection and chronic disease of the great vessels, *J Exp Med* 188:577-588, 1998.
411. Rasmussen L, Morris S, Wolitz R, et al: Deficiency in antibody response to human cytomegalovirus glycoprotein gH in human immunodeficiency virus-infected patients at risk for cytomegalovirus retinitis, *J Infect Dis* 170:673-677, 1994.
412. Schoppel K, Kropff B, Schmidt C, et al: The humoral immune response against human cytomegalovirus is characterized by a delayed synthesis of glycoprotein-specific antibodies, *J Infect Dis* 175:533-544, 1997.
413. Schoppel K, Schmidt C, Einsele H, et al: Kinetics of the antibody response against human cytomegalovirus-specific proteins in allogeneic bone marrow transplant recipients, *J Infect Dis* 178:1233-1243, 1998.
414. Snydman DR, Werner BG, Heinze-Lacey B, et al: Use of cytomegalovirus immune globulin to prevent cytomegalovirus disease in renal transplant recipients, *N Engl J Med* 317:1049-1054, 1987.
415. Snydman DR, Werner BG, Dougherty NN, et al: Cytomegalovirus immune globulin prophylaxis in liver transplantation. A randomized, double-blind placebo-controlled trial, *Ann Intern Med* 119:984-991, 1993.
416. Bonaros NE, Kocher A, Dunkler D, et al: Comparison of combined prophylaxis of cytomegalovirus hyperimmune globulin plus ganciclovir versus cytomegalovirus hyperimmune globulin alone in high-risk heart transplant recipients, *Transplantation* 77:890-897, 2004.
417. Bonaros N, Mayer B, Schachner T, et al: CMV-hyperimmune globulin for preventing cytomegalovirus infection and disease in solid organ transplant recipients: a meta-analysis, *Clin Transplant* 22: 89-97, 2008.
418. Hoetzenecker K, Hacker S, Hoetzenecker W, et al: Cytomegalovirus hyperimmunoglobulin: mechanisms in allo-immune response in vitro, *Eur J Clin Invest* 37:978-986, 2007.
419. Leroy F, Sechet A, Abou Ayache R, et al: Cytomegalovirus prophylaxis with intravenous polyvalent immunoglobulin in high-risk renal transplant recipients, *Transplant Proc* 38:2324-2326, 2006.
420. Raanani P, Gafter-Gvili A, Paul M, et al: Immunoglobulin prophylaxis in hematopoietic stem cell transplantation: systematic review and meta-analysis, *J Clin Oncol* 27:770-781, 2009.
421. Winston DJ, Ho WG, Lin CH, et al: Intravenous immune globulin for prevention of cytomegalovirus infection and interstitial pneumonia after bone marrow transplantation, *Ann Intern Med* 106:12-18, 1987.
422. Emanuel D, Cunningham I, Jules-Elysee K, et al: Cytomegalovirus pneumonia after bone marrow transplantation successfully treated with the combination of ganciclovir and high-dose intravenous immune globulin, *Ann Intern Med* 109:777-782, 1988.
423. Schmidt GM, Kovacs A, Zaia JA, et al: Ganciclovir/immunoglobulin combination therapy for the treatment of human cytomegalovirus-associated interstitial pneumonia in bone marrow allograft recipients, *Transplantation* 46:905-907, 1988.
424. Zaia JA: Prevention and management of CMV-related problems after hematopoietic stem cell transplantation, *Bone Marrow Transplant* 29:633-638, 2002.
425. Bowden RA, Sayers M, Flournoy N, et al: Cytomegalovirus immune globulin and seronegative blood products to prevent primary cytomegalovirus infection after marrow transplantation, *N Engl J Med* 314:1006-1010, 1986.
426. Bowden RA, Fisher LD, Rogers K, et al: Cytomegalovirus (CMV)-specific intravenous immunoglobulin for the prevention of primary CMV infection and disease after marrow transplantation, *J Infect Dis* 164:483-487, 1991.
427. Bratcher DF, Bourne N, Bravo FJ, et al: Effect of passive antibody on congenital cytomegalovirus infection in guinea pigs, *J Infect Dis* 172:944-950, 1995.
428. Chatterjee A, Harrison CJ, Britt WJ, et al: Modification of maternal and congenital cytomegalovirus infection by anti-glycoprotein b antibody transfer in guinea pigs, *J Infect Dis* 183:1547-1553, 2001.
429. Slavuljica I, Busche A, Babic M, et al: Recombinant mouse cytomegalovirus expressing a ligand for the NKG2D receptor is attenuated and has improved vaccine properties, *J Clin Invest* 120:4532-4545, 2010.
430. Nigro G, Adler SP, La Torre R, et al: Passive immunization during pregnancy for congenital cytomegalovirus infection, *N Engl J Med* 353:1350-1362, 2005.
431. Revello MG, Lazzarotto T, Guerra B, et al: A randomized trial of hyperimmune globulin to prevent congenital cytomegalovirus, *N Engl J Med* 370:1316-1326, 2014.
432. Krmpotic A, Messerle M, Crnkovic-Mertens I, et al: The immunoevasive function encoded by the mouse cytomegalovirus gene m152 protects the virus against T cell control in vivo, *J Exp Med* 190: 1285-1296, 2001.
433. Jonjic S, Babic M, Polic B, et al: Immune evasion of natural killer cells by viruses, *Curr Opin Immunol* 20:30-38, 2008.
434. Reddehase MJ: Antigens and immunoevasins: opponents in cytomegalovirus immune surveillance, *Nat Rev Immunol* 2:831-844, 2002.
435. Reddehase MJ, Simon CO, Seckert CK, et al: Murine model of cytomegalovirus latency and reactivation, *Curr Top Microbiol Immunol* 325:315-331, 2008.
436. Holtappels R, Podlech J, Pahl-Seibert MF, et al: Cytomegalovirus misleads its host by priming of CD8 T cells specific for an epitope not presented in infected tissues, *J Exp Med* 199:131-136, 2004.
437. Zaia JA, Gallez-Hawkins G, Li X, et al: Infrequent occurrence of natural mutations in the pp65(495-503) epitope sequence presented by the HLA A*0201 allele among human cytomegalovirus isolates, *J Virol* 75:2472-2474, 2001.
438. Scalzo AA, Yokoyama WM: Cmv1 and natural killer cell responses to murine cytomegalovirus infection, *Curr Top Microbiol Immunol* 321:101-122, 2008.
439. Voigt V, Forbes CA, Tonkin JN, et al: Murine cytomegalovirus *m157* mutation and variation leads to immune evasion of natural killer cells, *Proc Natl Acad Sci U S A* 100:13483-13488, 2003.
440. McWhorter AR, Smith LM, Masters LL, et al: Natural killer cell dependent within-host competition arises during multiple MCMV infection: consequences for viral transmission and evolution, *PLoS Pathog* 9:e1003111, 2013.
441. Klein M, Schoppel K, Amvrossiadis N, et al: Strain-specific neutralization of human cytomegalovirus isolates by human sera, *J Virol* 73:878-886, 1999.
442. Britt WJ: Recent advances in the identification of significant human cytomegalovirus-encoded proteins, *Transplant Proc* 23:64-69, 1991.
443. Burkhardt C, Himmelein S, Britt W, et al: The glycoprotein N of human cytomegalovirus induce a strain specific antibody response during natural infection, *J Gen Virol* 90(Pt 8):1951-1961, 2009.
444. Kropff B, Burkhardt C, Schott J, et al: Glycoprotein N of human cytomegalovirus protects the virus from neutralizing antibodies, *PLoS Pathog* 8:e1002999, 2012.
445. Stagno S, Reynolds DW, Tsiantos A, et al: Comparative, serial virologic and serologic studies of symptomatic and subclinical congenital and natally acquired cytomegalovirus infection, *J Infect Dis* 132:568-577, 1975.
446. Lockridge KM, Sequar G, Zhou SS, et al: Pathogenesis of experimental rhesus cytomegalovirus infection, *J Virol* 73:9576-9583, 1999.
447. Griffith BP, McCormick SR, Booss J, et al: Inbred guinea pig model of intrauterine infection with cytomegalovirus, *Am J Pathol* 122: 112-119, 1986.
448. Griffith BP, Lucia HL, Bia FJ, et al: Cytomegalovirus-induced mononucleosis in guinea pigs, *Infect Immun* 32:857-863, 1981.
449. Griffith BP, Aquino-de Jesus MJ: Guinea pig model of congenital cytomegalovirus infection, *Transplant Proc* 23:29-31, 1991.
450. Bowen EF, Sabin CA, Wilson P, et al: Cytomegalovirus (CMV) viraemia detected by polymerase chain reaction identifies a group of HIV-positive patients at high risk of CMV disease, *AIDS* 11:889-893, 1997.
451. Revello MG, Gerna G: Diagnosis and management of human cytomegalovirus infection in the mother, fetus, and newborn infant, *Clin Microbiol Rev* 15:680-715, 2002.
452. Boeckh M, Boivin G: Quantitation of cytomegalovirus: methodologic aspects and clinical applications, *Clin Microbiol Rev* 11:533-554, 1998.
453. Pang XL, Fox JD, Fenton JM, et al: Interlaboratory comparison of cytomegalovirus viral load assays, *Am J Transplant* 9:258-268, 2009.
454. Drew WL: Laboratory diagnosis of cytomegalovirus infection and disease in immunocompromised patients, *Curr Opin Infect Dis* 20:408-411, 2007.
455. Spector SA, Merrill R, Wolf D, et al: Detection of human cytomegalovirus in plasma of AIDS patients during acute visceral disease by DNA amplification, *J Clin Microbiol* 30:2359-2365, 1992.

456. Becroft DMO: Prenatal cytomegalovirus infection: epidemiology, pathology, and pathogenesis. In Rosenberg HS, Bernstein J, editors: *Perspectives in pediatric pathology*, New York, 1981, Masson Press, pp 203-241.
457. Stagno S, Pass RF, Dworsky ME, et al: Congenital and perinatal cytomegaloviral infections, *Semin Perinatol* 7:31-42, 1983.
458. Boppana SB, Pass RF, Britt WJ, et al: Symptomatic congenital cytomegalovirus infection: neonatal morbidity and mortality, *Pediatr Infect Dis J* 11:93-99, 1992.
459. Arribas JR, Storch GA, Clifford DB, et al: Cytomegalovirus encephalitis, *Ann Intern Med* 125:577-587, 1996.
460. Fowler KB, McCollister FP, Dahle AJ, et al: Progressive and fluctuating sensorineural hearing loss in children with asymptomatic congenital cytomegalovirus infection, *J Pediatr* 130:624-630, 1997.
461. Williamson WD, Demmler GJ, Percy AK, et al: Progressive hearing loss in infants with asymptomatic congenital cytomegalovirus infection, *Pediatrics* 90:862-866, 1992.
462. Ludwig A, Hengel H: Epidemiological impact and disease burden of congenital cytomegalovirus infection in Europe, *Euro Surveill* 14: 26-32, 2009.
463. Ogawa H, Suzutani T, Baba Y, et al: Etiology of severe sensorineural hearing loss in children: independent impact of congenital cytomegalovirus infection and GJB2 mutations, *J Infect Dis* 195:782-788, 2007.
464. Engman ML, Malm G, Engstrom L, et al: Congenital CMV infection: prevalence in newborns and the impact on hearing deficit, *Scand J Infect Dis* 40:935-942, 2008.
465. Barbi M, Binda S, Caroppo S, et al: Neonatal screening for congenital cytomegalovirus infection and hearing loss, *J Clin Virol* 35:206-209, 2006.
466. Iwasaki S, Yamashita M, Maeda M, et al: Audiological outcome of infants with congenital cytomegalovirus infection in a prospective study, *Audiol Neurootol* 12:31-36, 2007.
467. Grosse SD, Ross DS, Dollard SC: Congenital cytomegalovirus (CMV) infection as a cause of permanent bilateral hearing loss: a quantitative assessment, *J Clin Virol* 41:57-62, 2008.
468. Griffith BP, Lucia HL, Hsiung GD: Brain and visceral involvement during congenital cytomegalovirus infection of guinea pigs, *Pediatr Res* 16:455-459, 1982.
469. Bia FJ, Griffith BP, Fong CKY, et al: Cytomegalovirus infections in the guinea pig: experimental models for human disease, *Rev Infect Dis* 5:177-195, 1983.
470. Bale JF Jr, Bray PF, Bell WE: Neuroradiographic abnormalities in congenital cytomegalovirus infection, *Pediatr Neurol* 1:42-47, 1985.
471. Perlman JM, Argyle C: Lethal cytomegalovirus infection in preterm infants: clinical, radiological, and neuropathological findings, *Ann Neurol* 31:64-68, 1992.
472. Boppana SB, Fowler KB, Vaid Y, et al: Neuroradiographic findings in the newborn period and long-term outcome in children with symptomatic congenital cytomegalovirus infection, *Pediatrics* 99: 409-414, 1997.
473. Boesch C, Issakainen J, Kewitz G, et al: Magnetic resonance imaging of the brain in congenital cytomegalovirus infection, *Pediatr Radiol* 19:91-93, 1989.
474. Barkovich AJ, Lindan CE: Congenital cytomegalovirus infection of the brain: imaging analysis and embryologic considerations, *Am J Neuroradiol* 15:703-715, 1994.
475. Steinlin MI, Nadal D, Eich GF, et al: Late intrauterine Cytomegalovirus infection: clinical and neuroimaging findings, *Pediatr Neurol* 15:249-253, 1996.
476. Picone O, Simon I, Benachi A, et al: Comparison between ultrasound and magnetic resonance imaging in assessment of fetal cytomegalovirus infection, *Prenat Diagn* 28:753-758, 2008.
477. Baskin HJ, Hedlund G: Neuroimaging of herpesvirus infections in children, *Pediatr Radiol* 37:949-963, 2007.
478. de Vries LS, Gunardi H, Barth PG, et al: The spectrum of cranial ultrasound and magnetic resonance imaging abnormalities in congenital cytomegalovirus infection, *Neuropediatrics* 35:113-119, 2004.
479. Hayward JC, Titelbaum DS, Clancy RR, et al: Lissencephaly-pachygyria associated with congenital cytomegalovirus infection, *J Child Neurol* 6:109-114, 1991.
480. Mejaski-Bosnjak V: Congenital CMV infection: a common cause of childhood disability, *Dev Med Child Neurol* 50:403, 2008.
481. Suzuki Y, Toribe Y, Mogami Y, et al: Epilepsy in patients with congenital cytomegalovirus infection, *Brain Dev* 30:420-424, 2008.
482. Sugita K, Ando M, Makino M, et al: Magnetic resonance imaging of the brain in congenital rubella virus and cytomegalovirus infections, *Neuroradiology* 33:239-242, 1991.
483. Tsutsui Y, Kosugi I, Kawasaki H: Neuropathogenesis in cytomegalovirus infection: indication of the mechanisms using mouse models, *Rev Med Virol* 15:327-345, 2005.
484. Cheeran MC, Hu S, Ni HT, et al: Neural precursor cell susceptibility to human cytomegalovirus diverges along glial or neuronal differentiation pathways, *J Neurosci Res* 82:839-850, 2005.
485. Luo MH, Schwartz PH, Fortunato EA: Neonatal neural progenitor cells and their neuronal and glial cell derivatives are fully permissive for human cytomegalovirus infection, *J Virol* 82:9994-10007, 2008.
486. Tarantal AF, Salamat MS, Britt WJ, et al: Neuropathogenesis induced by rhesus cytomegalovirus in fetal rhesus monkeys *(Macaca mulatta)*, *J Infect Dis* 177:446-450, 1998.
487. Chang WL, Tarantal AF, Zhou SS, et al: A recombinant rhesus cytomegalovirus expressing enhanced green fluorescent protein retains the wild-type phenotype and pathogenicity in fetal macaques, *J Virol* 76:9493-9504, 2002.
488. van den Pol AN, Reuter JD, Santarelli JG: Enhanced cytomegalovirus infection of developing brain independent of the adaptive immune system, *J Virol* 76:8842-8854, 2002.
489. Zou YR, Kottmann AH, Kuroda M, et al: Function of the chemokine receptor CXCR4 in haematopoiesis and in cerebellar development, *Nature* 393:595-599, 1998.
490. Zhu Y, Yu T, Zhang XC, et al: Role of the chemokine SDF-1 as the meningeal attractant for embryonic cerebellar neurons, *Nat Neurosci* 5:719-720, 2002.
491. Kosmac K, Bantug GR, Pugel EP, et al: Glucocortiocoid treatment of MCMV infected newborn mice attenuates CNS inflammation and limits deficits in cerebellar development, *PLoS Pathog* 9:e1003200, 2013.
492. Koontz T, Bralic M, Tomac J, et al: Altered development of the brain after focal herpesvirus infection of the central nervous system, *J Exp Med* 205:423-435, 2008.
493. Boppana S, Britt W: Cytomegalovirus. In Newton VE, Vallely PJ, editors: *Infection and hearing impairment*, Sussex, UK, 2006, John Wiley and Sons, pp 67-93.
494. Teissier N, Delezoide AL, Mas AE, et al: Inner ear lesions in congenital cytomegalovirus infection of human fetuses, *Acta Neuropathol* 122:763-774, 2011.
495. Li L, Kosugi I, Han GP, et al: Induction of cytomegalovirus-infected labyrinthitis in newborn mice by lipopolysaccharide: a model for hearing loss in congenital CMV infection, *Lab Invest* 88:722-730, 2008.
496. Wang Y, Patel R, Ren C, et al: A comparison of different murine models for cytomegalovirus-induced sensorineural hearing loss, *Laryngoscope* 123:2801-2806, 2013.
497. Schachtele SJ, Mutnal MB, Schleiss MR, et al: Cytomegalovirus-induced sensorineural hearing loss with persistent cochlear inflammation in neonatal mice, *J Neurovirol* 17:201-211, 2011.
498. Juanjuan C, Yan F, Li C, et al: Murine model for congenital CMV infection and hearing impairment, *Virol J* 8:70, 2011.
499. Bradford R, Yoo Y, Jonjic S, et al: Hearing loss following newborn infection with murine CMV: a model of hearing loss in infants with congenital CMV, *Submitted to PLoS Pathog*, 2013.
500. Strauss M: A clinical pathologic study of hearing loss in congenital cytomegalovirus infection, *Laryngoscope* 95:951-962, 1985.
501. Strauss M: Human cytomegalovirus labyrinthitis, *Am J Otolaryngol* 11:292-298, 1990.
502. Rarey KE, Davis LE: Temporal bone histopathology 14 years after cytomegalic inclusion disease: a case study, *Laryngoscope* 103: 904-909, 1993.
503. Mostafapour SP, Cochran SL, Del Puerto NM, et al: Patterns of cell death in mouse anteroventral cochlear nucleus neurons after unilateral cochlea removal, *J Comp Neurol* 426:561-571, 2000.
504. Mostafapour SP, Del Puerto NM, Rubel EW: bcl-2 Overexpression eliminates deprivation-induced cell death of brainstem auditory neurons, *J Neurosci* 22:4670-4674, 2002.
505. Franklin SR, Brunso-Bechtold JK, Henkel CK: Unilateral cochlear ablation before hearing onset disrupts the maintenance of dorsal nucleus of the lateral lemniscus projection patterns in the rat inferior colliculus, *Neuroscience* 143:105-115, 2006.
506. Harris JP, Fan JT, Keithley EM: Immunologic responses in experimental cytomegalovirus labyrinthitis, *Am J Otolaryngol* 11:304-308, 1990.

507. Chen MC, Harris JP, Keithley EM: Immunohistochemical analysis of proliferating cells in a sterile labyrinthitis animal model, *Laryngoscope* 108:651-656, 1998.
508. Harris JP, Woolf NK, Ryan AF, et al: Immunologic and electrophysiological response to cytomegaloviral inner ear infection in the guinea pig, *J Infect Dis* 150:523-530, 1984.
509. Harris S, Ahlfors K, Ivarsson S, et al: Congenital cytomegalovirus infection and sensorineural hearing loss, *Ear Hear* 5:352-355, 1984.
510. Woolf NK, Koehrn FJ, Harris JP, et al: Congenital cytomegalovirus labyrinthitis and sensorineural hearing loss in guinea pigs, *J Infect Dis* 160:929-937, 1989.
511. Woolf NK: Guinea pig model of congenital CMV-induced hearing loss: a review, *Transplant Proc* 23:32-34, 1991.
512. Woolf NK, Ochi JW, Silva EJ, et al: Ganciclovir prophylaxis for cochlear pathophysiology during experimental guinea pig cytomegalovirus labyrinthitis, *Antimicrob Agents Chemother* 32:865-872, 1988.
513. Fukuda S, Keithley EM, Harris JP: Experimental cytomegalovirus infection: viremic spread to the inner ear, *Am J Otolaryngol* 9: 135-141, 1988.
514. Fowler KB, Stagno S, Pass RF, et al: The outcome of congenital cytomegalovirus infection in relation to maternal antibody status, *N Engl J Med* 326:663-667, 1992.
515. Demmler GJ: Infectious Diseases Society of America and Centers for Disease Control. Summary of a workshop on surveillance for congenital cytomegalovirus disease, *Rev Infect Dis* 13:315-329, 1991.
516. Monif GRG, Egan EA, Held B, et al: The correlation of maternal cytomegalovirus infection during varying stages in gestation with neonatal involvement, *J Pediatr* 80:17-20, 1972.
517. Enders G, Daiminger A, Bader U, et al: Intrauterine transmission and clinical outcome of 248 pregnancies with primary cytomegalovirus infection in relation to gestational age, *J Clin Virol* 52:244-246, 2011.
518. Picone O, Vauloup-Fellous C, Cordier AG, et al: A series of 238 cytomegalovirus primary infections during pregnancy: description and outcome, *Prenat Diagn* 33:751-758, 2013.
519. Yow MD, Williamson DW, Leeds LJ, et al: Epidemiologic characteristics of cytomegalovirus infection in mothers and their infants, *Am J Obstet Gynecol* 158:1189-1195, 1988.
520. Pass RF, Fowler KB, Boppana SB, et al: Congenital cytomegalovirus infection following first trimester maternal infection: symptoms at birth and outcome, *J Clin Virol* 35:216-220, 2006.
521. Ahlfors K, Harris S, Ivarsson S, et al: Secondary maternal cytomegalovirus infection causing symptomatic congenital infection, *N Engl J Med* 305:284, 1981.
522. Ahlfors K, Ivarsson S, Harris S: Report on a long-term study of maternal and congenital cytomegalovirus infection in Sweden. Review of prospective studies available in the literature, *Scand J Infect Dis* 31:443-457, 1999.
523. Ahlfors K, Ivarsson SA, Harris S: Secondary maternal cytomegalovirus infection: a significant cause of congenital disease, *Pediatrics* 107:1227-1228, 2001.
524. Rahav G, Gabbay R, Ornoy A, et al: Primary versus nonprimary cytomegalovirus infection during pregnancy, Israel, *Emerg Infect Dis* 13:1791-1793, 2007.
525. Zalel Y, Gilboa Y, Berkenshtat M, et al: Secondary cytomegalovirus infection can cause severe fetal sequelae despite maternal preconceptional immunity, *Ultrasound Obstet Gynecol* 31:417-420, 2008.
526. Fowler K, McCollister F, Pass R, et al: Childhood deafness: the importance of congenital cytomegalovirus screening, *Am J Epidemiol* 136:954, 1992.
527. Ahlfors K, Ivarsson SA, Harris S: Report on a long-term study of maternal and congenital cytomegalovirus infection in Sweden. Review of prospective studies available in the literature, *Scand J Infect Dis* 31:443-457, 1999.
528. Boppana SB, Fowler KB, Britt WJ, et al: Symptomatic congenital cytomegalovirus infection in infants born to mothers with preexisting immunity to cytomegalovirus, *Pediatrics* 104:55-60, 1999.
529. Ross SA, Fowler KB, Ashrith G, et al: Hearing loss in children with congenital cytomegalovirus infection born to mothers with preexisting immunity, *J Pediatr* 148:332-336, 2006.
530. Ahlfors K, Ivarsson SA, Harris S, et al: Congenital cytomegalovirus infection and disease in Sweden and the relative importance of primary and secondary maternal infections, *Scand J Infect Dis* 16:129-137, 1984.
531. Griffiths PD, Baboonian C: A prospective study of primary cytomegalovirus infection during pregnancy: final report, *Br J Obstet Gynaecol* 91:307-315, 1984.
532. Yamamoto AY, Mussi-Pinhata MM, Isaac Mde L, et al: Congenital cytomegalovirus infection as a cause of sensorineural hearing loss in a highly immune population, *Pediatr Infect Dis J* 30:1043-1046, 2011.
533. Rutter D, Griffiths P, Trompeter RS: Cytomegalic inclusion disease after recurrent maternal infection, *Lancet* 2:1182, 1985.
534. Evans TJ, McCollum JPK, Valdimarsson H: Congenital cytomegalovirus infection after maternal renal transplantation, *Lancet* 1: 1359-1360, 1975.
535. Laifer SA, Ehrlich GD, Huff DS, et al: Congenital cytomegalovirus infection in offspring of liver transplant recipients, *Clin Infect Dis* 20:52-55, 1995.
536. Mussi-Pinhata MM, Yamamoto AY, Figueiredo LT, et al: Congenital and perinatal cytomegalovirus infection in infants born to mothers infected with human immunodeficiency virus, *J Pediatr* 132: 285-290, 1998.
537. Doyle M, Atkins JT, Rivera-Matos IR: Congenital cytomegalovirus infection in infants infected with human immunodeficiency virus type 1, *Pediatr Infect Dis J* 15:1102-1106, 1996.
538. Jones MM, Lidsky MD, Brewer EJ, et al: Congenital cytomegalovirus infection and maternal systemic lupus erythematosus: a case report, *Arthritis Rheum* 29:1402-1404, 1986.
539. Hansen SG, Powers CJ, Richards R, et al: Evasion of CD8+ T cells is critical for superinfection by cytomegalovirus, *Science* 328:102-106, 2010.
540. Reynolds DW, Stagno S, Hosty TS, et al: Maternal cytomegalovirus excretion and perinatal infection, *N Engl J Med* 289:1-5, 1973.
541. Pass RF, Stagno S, Myers GJ, et al: Outcome of symptomatic congenital CMV infection: results of long-term longitudinal follow-up, *Pediatrics* 66:758-762, 1980.
542. Pass RF, Hutto C, Stagno S, et al: Congenital cytomegalovirus infection: prospects for prevention, *Ann N Y Acad Sci* 477:123-127, 1986.
543. Stronati M, Lombardi G, Di Comite A, et al: Breastfeeding and cytomegalovirus infections, *J Chemother* 19(Suppl 2):49-51, 2007.
544. Takahashi R, Tagawa M, Sanjo M, et al: Severe postnatal cytomegalovirus infection in a very premature infant, *Neonatology* 92:236-239, 2007.
545. Alford C: Breast milk transmission of cytomegalovirus (CMV) infection, *Adv Exp Med Biol* 310:293-299, 1991.
546. Capretti MG, Lanari M, Lazzarotto T, et al: Very low birth weight infants born to cytomegalovirus-seropositive mothers fed with their mother's milk: a prospective study, *J Pediatr* 154:842-848, 2009.
547. Lombardi G, Garofoli F, Manzoni P, et al: Breast milk-acquired cytomegalovirus infection in very low birth weight infants, *J Matern Fetal Neonatal Med* 25(Suppl 3):57-62, 2012.
548. Kurath S, Halwachs-Baumann G, Müller W, et al: Transmission of cytomegalovirus via breast milk to the prematurely born infant: a systematic review, *Clin Microbiol Infect* 16:1172-1178, 2010.
549. Shimamura M, Britt WJ: G-CSF and CD34+ progenitor cells in hematopoietic grafts: too fertile for human cytomegalovirus, *Cell Host Microbe* 8:223-224, 2010.
550. Rosenthal LS, Fowler KB, Boppana SB, et al: Cytomegalovirus shedding and delayed sensorineural hearing loss: results from longitudinal follow-up of children with congenital infection, *Pediatr Infect Dis J* 28:515-520, 2009.
551. Boppana SB, Fowler KB, Pass RF, et al: Congenital cytomegalovirus infection: association between virus burden in infancy and hearing loss, *J Pediatr* 146:817-823, 2005.
552. Lanari M, Lazzarotto T, Venturi V, et al: Neonatal cytomegalovirus blood load and risk of sequelae in symptomatic and asymptomatic congenitally infected newborns, *Pediatrics* 117:e76-e83, 2006.
553. Ross SA, Novak Z, Fowler KB, et al: Cytomegalovirus blood viral load and hearing loss in young children with congenital infection, *Pediatr Infect Dis J* 28:588-592, 2009.
554. Sanchez V, Angeletti PC, Engler JA, et al: Localization of human cytomegalovirus structural proteins to the nuclear matrix of infected human fibroblasts, *J Virol* 72:3321-3329, 1998.
555. Myerson D, Hackman RC, Nelson JA, et al: Widespread presence of histologically occult cytomegalovirus, *Hum Pathol* 15:430-439, 1984.

556. Borisch B, Jahn G, Scholl BC, et al: Detection of human cytomegalovirus DNA and viral antigens in tissues of different manifestations of CMV infection, *Virchows Arch B Cell Pathol Incl Mol Pathol* 55:93-99, 1988.
557. Wolf A, Cowden D: Perinatal infections of the central nervous system, *J Neuro Pathol Exp Neurol* 18:191-243, 1959.
558. Naeye RL: Cytomegalic inclusion disease, the fetal disorder, *Am J Clin Pathol* 47:738-744, 1967.
559. Marques Dias MJ, Harmant-van Rijckevorsel G, Landrieu P, et al: Prenatal cytomegalovirus disease and cerebral microgyria: evidence for perfusion failure, not disturbance of histogenesis, as the major cause of fetal cytomegalovirus encephalopathy, *Neuropediatrics* 15:18-24, 1984.
560. Arey LB: Cytomegalic inclusion disease in infancy, *Am J Dis Child* 88:525-526, 1954.
561. Troendle Atkins J, Demmler GJ, Williamson WD, et al: Polymerase chain reaction to detect cytomegalovirus DNA in the cerebrospinal fluid of neonates with congenital infection, *J Infect Dis* 169: 1334-1337, 1994.
562. Balcarek KB, Oh MK, Pass RF: Maternal viremia and congenital CMV infection. In Michelson S, Plotkin SA, editors: *Multidisciplinary approach to understanding cytomegalovirus disease*, New York, 1993, Excerpta Medica, pp 169-173.
563. Gabrielli L, Bonasoni MP, Lazzarotto T, et al: Histological findings in foetuses congenitally infected by cytomegalovirus, *J Clin Virol* 46(Suppl 4):S16-S21, 2009.
564. Gabrielli L, Bonasoni MP, Santini D, et al: Congenital cytomegalovirus infection: patterns of fetal brain damage, *Clin Microbiol Infect* 18:E419-E427, 2012.
565. Keithley EM, Woolf NK, Harris JP: Development of morphological and physiological changes in the cochlear induced by cytomegalovirus, *Laryngoscope* 99:409-414, 1989.
566. Myers EN, Stool S: Cytomegalic inclusion disease of the inner ear, *Laryngoscope* 78:1904-1915, 1968.
567. Davis GL: Cytomegalovirus in the inner ear. Case report and electron microscopic study, *Ann Otol Rhinol Laryngol* 78:1179-1188, 1969.
568. Boppana S, Amos C, Britt W, et al: Late onset and reactivation of chorioretinitis in children with congenital cytomegalovirus infection, *Pediatr Infect Dis J* 13:1139-1142, 1994.
569. Anderson KS, Amos CS, Boppana S, et al: Ocular abnormalities in congenital cytomegalovirus infection, *J Am Optom Assoc* 67: 273-278, 1996.
570. Mets MB: Eye manifestations of intrauterine infections, *Ophthalmol Clin North Am* 14:521-531, 2001.
571. Guyton TB, Ehrlich F, Blanc WA, et al: New observations in generalized cytomegalic-inclusion disease of the newborn: report of a case with chorioretinitis, *N Engl J Med* 257:803-807, 1957.
572. Conboy TJ, Pass RF, Stagno S, et al: Early clinical manifestations and intellectual outcome in children with symptomatic congenital cytomegalovirus infection, *J Pediatr* 111:343-348, 1987.
573. Ansari BM, Davies DB, Jones MR: Calcification in liver associated with congenital cytomegalic inclusion disease, *J Pediatr* 90: 661-662, 1977.
574. Alix D, Castel Y, Gouedard H: Hepatic calcification in congenital cytomegalic inclusion disease, *J Pediatr* 92:856, 1978.
575. Jordan S, Ruzsics Z, Mitrovic M, et al: Natural killer cells are required for extramedullary hematopoiesis following murine cytomegalovirus infection, *Cell Host Microbe* 13:535-545, 2013.
576. Fetterman GH, Sherman FE, Fabizio NS, et al: Generalized cytomegalic inclusion disease of the newborn: localization of inclusions in the kidney, *Arch Pathol* 86:86-94, 1968.
577. Reyes C, Pereira S, Warden MJ, et al: Cytomegalovirus enteritis in a premature infant, *J Pediatr Surg* 32:1545-1547, 1997.
578. Pereira L, Maidji E: Cytomegalovirus infection in the human placenta: maternal immunity and developmentally regulated receptors on trophoblasts converge, *Curr Top Microbiol Immunol* 325: 383-395, 2008.
579. Muhlemann K, Menegus MA, Miller RK: Cytomegalovirus in the perfused human term placenta in vitro, *Placenta* 16:367-373, 1995.
580. Sachdev R, Nuovo GJ, Kaplan C, et al: In situ hybridization analysis for cytomegalovirus in chronic villitis, *Pediatr Pathol* 10:909-917, 1990.
581. Benirschke K, Mendoza GR, Bazeley PL: Placental and fetal manifestations of cytomegalovirus infection, *Virchows Arch* 16:121-139, 1974.
582. Benirschke K, Kaufmann P: *Pathology of the human placenta*, New York, 1990, Springer-Verlag.
583. McDonagh S, Maidji E, Chang HT, et al: Patterns of human cytomegalovirus infection in term placentas: a preliminary analysis, *J Clin Virol* 35:210-215, 2006.
584. Dankner WM, Pass RF, Stagno S, et al: Polymerase chain reaction for the detection of cytomegalovirus in placentas from congenitally infected infants, *Pediatr Res* 31:160A, 1992.
585. Trincado DE, Munro SC, Camaris C, et al: Highly sensitive detection and localization of maternally acquired human cytomegalovirus in placental tissue by in situ polymerase chain reaction, *J Infect Dis* 192:650-657, 2005.
586. La Torre R, Nigro G, Mazzocco M, et al: Placental enlargement in women with primary maternal cytomegalovirus infection is associated with fetal and neonatal disease, *Clin Infect Dis* 43:994-1000, 2006.
587. Iwasenko JM, Howard J, Arbuckle S, et al: Human cytomegalovirus infection is detected frequently in stillbirths and is associated with fetal thrombotic vasculopathy, *J Infect Dis* 203:1526-1533, 2011.
588. Pereira L, Maidji E, McDonagh S, et al: Insights into viral transmission at the uterine-placental interface, *Trends Microbiol* 13:164-174, 2005.
589. Fisher S, Genbacev O, Maidji E, et al: Human cytomegalovirus infection of placental cytotrophoblasts in vitro and in utero: implications for transmission and pathogenesis, *J Virol* 74:6808-6820, 2000.
590. Roth I, Corry DB, Locksley RM, et al: Human placental cytotrophoblasts produce the immunosuppressive cytokine interleukin 10, *J Exp Med* 184:539-548, 1996.
591. Blanco O, Tirado I, Munoz-Fernandez R, et al: Human decidual stromal cells express HLA-G: effects of cytokines and decidualization, *Hum Reprod* 23:144-152, 2008.
592. Kuroki K, Maenaka K: Immune modulation of HLA-G dimer in maternal-fetal interface, *Eur J Immunol* 37:1727-1729, 2007.
593. Hunt JS, Langat DK, McIntire RH, et al: The role of HLA-G in human pregnancy, *Reprod Biol Endocrinol* 4(Suppl 1):S10, 2006.
594. Ishitani A, Sageshima N, Hatake K: The involvement of HLA-E and -F in pregnancy, *J Reprod Immunol* 69:101-113, 2006.
595. McIntire RH, Hunt JS: Antigen presenting cells and HLA-G—a review, *Placenta* 26(Suppl A):S104-S109, 2005.
596. Schleiss MR, Lacayo JC, Belkaid Y, et al: Preconceptual administration of an alphavirus replicon UL83 (pp65 homolog) vaccine induces humoral and cellular immunity and improves pregnancy outcome in the guinea pig model of congenital cytomegalovirus infection, *J Infect Dis* 195:789-798, 2007.
597. Hamilton ST, Scott G, Naing Z, et al: Human cytomegalovirus-induces cytokine changes in the placenta with implications for adverse pregnancy outcomes, *PLoS One* 7:e52899, 2012.
598. Mocarski ES, Upton JW, Kaiser WJ: Viral infection and the evolution of caspase 8-regulated apoptotic and necrotic death pathways, *Nat Rev Immunol* 12:79-88, 2011.
599. Arcuri F, Toti P, Buchwalder L, et al: Mechanisms of leukocyte accumulation and activation in chorioamnionitis: interleukin 1 beta and tumor necrosis factor alpha enhance colony stimulating factor 2 expression in term decidua, *Reprod Sci* 16:453-461, 2009.
600. Arcuri F, Buchwalder L, Toti P, et al: Differential regulation of colony stimulating factor 1 and macrophage migration inhibitory factor expression by inflammatory cytokines in term human decidua: implications for macrophage trafficking at the fetal-maternal interface, *Biol Reprod* 76:433-439, 2007.
601. Lockwood CJ, Matta P, Krikun G, et al: Regulation of monocyte chemoattractant protein-1 expression by tumor necrosis factor-alpha and interleukin-1beta in first trimester human decidual cells: implications for preeclampsia, *Am J Pathol* 168:445-452, 2006.
602. Toti P, Arcuri F, Tang Z, et al: Focal increases of fetal macrophages in placentas from pregnancies with histological chorioamnionitis: potential role of fibroblast monocyte chemotactic protein-1, *Am J Reprod Immunol* 65:470-479, 2011.
603. Townsend CL, Forsgren M, Ahlfors K, et al: Long-term outcomes of congenital cytomegalovirus infection in Sweden and the United Kingdom, *Clin Infect Dis* 56:1232-1239, 2013.
604. Weller TH, Hanshaw JB: Virologic and clinical observations on cytomegalic inclusion disease, *N Engl J Med* 266:1233-1244, 1962.

605. Boppana SB, Fowler KB, Pass RF, et al: Newborn findings and outcome in children with symptomatic congenital CMV infection, *Pediatr Res* 31:158A, 1992.
606. Malm G, Engman ML: Congenital cytomegalovirus infections, *Semin Fetal Neonatal Med* 12:154-159, 2007.
607. Hanshaw JB: Cytomegalovirus infections, *Pediatr Rev* 4:332, 1983.
608. Medearis DN: Observations concerning human cytomegalovirus infection and disease, *Bull Johns Hopkins Med J* 114:181-211, 1964.
609. Noyola DE, Demmler GJ, Nelson CT, et al: Early predictors of neurodevelopmental outcome in symptomatic congenital cytomegalovirus infection, *J Pediatr* 138;325-331, 2001.
610. Stagno S, Brasfield DM, Brown MB, et al: Infant pneumonitis associated with cytomegalovirus, chlamydia, pneumocystis, and ureaplasma: a prospective study, *Pediatrics* 68:322-329, 1981.
611. Stagno S, Pass RF, Thomas JP, et al: Defects of tooth structure in congenital cytomegalovirus infection, *Pediatrics* 69:646-648, 1982.
612. Hickson LMH, Alcock D: Progressive hearing loss in children with congenital cytomegalovirus, *J Paediatr Child Health* 27:105-107, 1991.
613. Foulon I, Naessens A, Foulon W, et al: 10-year prospective study of sensorineural hearing loss in children with congenital cytomegalovirus infection, *J Pediatr* 153:84-88, 2008.
614. Nance WE, Lim BG, Dodson KM: Importance of congenital cytomegalovirus infections as a cause for pre-lingual hearing loss, *J Clin Virol* 35:221-225, 2006.
615. Barbi M, Binda S, Caroppo S, et al: A wider role for congenital cytomegalovirus infection in sensorineural hearing loss, *Pediatr Infect Dis J* 22:39-42, 2003.
616. Karltorp E, Hellström S, Lewensohn-Fuchs I, et al: Congenital cytomegalovirus infection—a common cause of hearing loss of unknown aetiology, *Acta Paediatr* 101:e357-e362, 2012.
617. Misono S, Sie KC, Weiss NS, et al: Congenital cytomegalovirus infection in pediatric hearing loss, *Arch Otolaryngol Head Neck Surg* 137:47-53, 2011.
618. Hicks T, Fowler K, Richardson M, et al: Congenital cytomegalovirus infection and neonatal auditory screening, *J Pediatr* 123:779-782, 1993.
619. Rivera LB, Boppana SB, Fowler KB, et al: Predictors of hearing loss in children with symptomatic congenital cytomegalovirus infection, *Pediatrics* 110:762-767, 2002.
620. Walter S, Atkinson C, Sharland M, et al: Congenital cytomegalovirus: association between dried blood spot viral load and hearing loss, *Arch Dis Child Fetal Neonatal Ed* 93:F280-F285, 2008.
621. Williamson WD, Desmond MM, LaFevers N, et al: Symptomatic congenital cytomegalovirus: disorders of language, learning and hearing, *Am J Dis Child* 136:902-905, 1982.
622. Saigal S, Luynk O, Larke B, et al: The outcome in children with congenital cytomegalovirus infection: a longitudinal follow-up study, *Am J Dis Child* 136:896-901, 1982.
623. Berenberg W, Nankervis G: Long-term follow-up of cytomegalic inclusion disease of infancy, *Pediatrics* 37:403, 1970.
624. Ramsay ME, Miller E, Peckham CS: Outcome of confirmed symptomatic congenital cytomegalovirus infection, *Arch Dis Child* 66: 1068-1069, 1991.
625. Ivarsson SA, Lernmark B, Svanberg L: Ten-year clinical, developmental and intellectual follow-up of children with congenital cytomegalovirus infection without neurologic symptoms at one year of age, *Pediatrics* 99:800-803, 1997.
626. Zagolski O: Vestibular-evoked myogenic potentials and caloric stimulation in infants with congenital cytomegalovirus infection, *J Laryngol Otol* 122:574-579, 2008.
627. Kylat RI, Kelly EN, Ford-Jones EL: Clinical findings and adverse outcome in neonates with symptomatic congenital cytomegalovirus (SCCMV) infection, *Eur J Pediatr* 165:773-778, 2006.
628. Melish ME, Hanshaw JB: Congenital cytomegalovirus infection: developmental progress of infants detected by routine screening, *Am J Dis Child* 126:190-194, 1973.
629. Kumar ML, Nankervis GA, Gold E: Inapparent congenital cytomegalovirus infection: a follow-up study, *N Engl J Med* 288:1370-1377, 1973.
630. Reynolds DW, Stagno S, Stubbs KG, et al: Inapparent congenital cytomegalovirus infection with elevated cord IgM levels: causal relationship with auditory and mental deficiency, *N Engl J Med* 209: 291-296, 1974.
631. Williamson WD, Percy AK, Yow MD, et al: Asymptomatic congenital cytomegalovirus infection, *Am J Dis Child* 144:1365-1368, 1990.
632. Kashden J, Frison S, Fowler K, et al: Intellectual assessment of children with asymptomatic congenital cytomegalovirus infection, *J Dev Behav Pediatr* 19:254-259, 1998.
633. Preece PM, Pearl KN, Peckham CS: Congenital cytomegalovirus infection, *Arch Dis Child* 59:1120-1126, 1984.
634. Pearl KN, Preece PM, Ades A, et al: Neurodevelopmental assessment after congenital cytomegalovirus infection, *Arch Dis Child* 62:323-326, 1986.
635. Conboy TJ, Pass RF, Stagno S, et al: Intellectual development in school-aged children with asymptomatic congenital cytomegalovirus infection, *Pediatrics* 77:801-806, 1986.
636. Yamamoto AY, Mussi-Pinhata MM, Isaac MDL, et al: Congenital cytomegalovirus infection as a cause of sensorineural hearing loss in a highly seropositive population, *Pediatr Infect Dis J* 30:1043-1046, 2011.
637. Fowler KB, Stagno S, Pass RF: Maternal immunity and prevention of congenital cytomegalovirus infection, *JAMA* 289:1008-1011, 2003.
638. Mussi-Pinhata MM, Yamamoto AY, Moura-Britto RM, et al: Birth prevalence and natural history of congenital cytomegalovirus (CMV) infection in highly seroimmune population, *Clin Infect Dis* 49:522-528, 2009.
639. Arvin AM, Fast P, Myers M, et al: Vaccine development to prevent cytomegalovirus disease: report from the National Vaccine Advisory Committee, *Clin Infect Dis* 39:233-239, 2004.
640. Stagno S, Reynolds DW, Pass RF, et al: Breast milk and the risk of cytomegalovirus infection, *N Engl J Med* 302:1073-1076, 1980.
641. Vochem M, Hamprecht K, Jahn G, et al: Transmission of cytomegalovirus to preterm infants through breast milk, *Pediatr Infect Dis J* 17:53-58, 1998.
642. Neuberger P, Hamprecht K, Vochem M, et al: Case-control study of symptoms and neonatal outcome of human milk-transmitted cytomegalovirus infection in premature infants, *J Pediatr* 148:326-331, 2006.
643. Kothari A, Ramachandran VG, Gupta P: Cytomegalovirus infection in neonates following exchange transfusion, *Indian J Pediatr* 73: 519-521, 2006.
644. Nankervis GA, Bhumbra NA: Cytomegalovirus infections of the neonate and infant, *Adv Pediatr Infect Dis* 1:61-74, 1986.
645. Bhumbra NA, Lewandowski P, Lau P, et al: Evaluation of a prescreening blood donor program for prevention of perinatal transfusion-acquired cytomegalovirus (CMV) infection, *J Perinat Med* 16:127-131, 1988.
646. Miron D, Brosilow S, Felszer K, et al: Incidence and clinical manifestations of breast milk-acquired cytomegalovirus infection in low birth weight infants, *J Perinatol* 25:299-303, 2005.
647. Mussi-Pinhata MM, Yamamoto AY, do Carmo Rego MA, et al: Perinatal or early-postnatal cytomegalovirus infection in preterm infants under 34 weeks gestation born to CMV-seropositive mothers within a high-seroprevalence population, *J Pediatr* 145:685-688, 2004.
648. Doctor S, Friedman S, Dunn MS, et al: Cytomegalovirus transmission to extremely low-birthweight infants through breast milk, *Acta Paediatr* 94:53-58, 2005.
649. Paryani SG, Yeager AS, Hosford-Dunn H, et al: Sequelae of acquired cytomegalovirus infection in premature and sick term infants, *J Pediatr* 107:451-456, 1985.
650. Maschmann J, Hamprecht K, Dietz K, et al: Cytomegalovirus infection of extremely low-birth weight infants via breast milk, *Clin Infect Dis* 33:1998-2003, 2001.
651. Yeager AS: Transfusion-acquired cytomegalovirus infection in newborn infants, *Am J Dis Child* 128:478-483, 1974.
652. Ballard RB, Drew WL, Hufnagle KG, et al: Acquired cytomegalovirus infection in pre-term infants, *Am J Dis Child* 133:482-485, 1979.
653. Adler SP: Transfusion-associated cytomegalovirus infections, *Rev Infect Dis* 5:977-993, 1983.
654. Nelson CT, Istas AS, Wilkerson MK, et al: PCR detection of cytomegalovirus DNA in serum as a diagnostic test for congenital cytomegalovirus infection, *J Clin Microbiol* 33:3317-3318, 1995.
655. Lazzarotto T, Guerra B, Lanari M, et al: New advances in the diagnosis of congenital cytomegalovirus infection, *J Clin Virol* 41:192-197, 2008.
656. Demmler GJ, Buffone GJ, Schimbor CM, et al: Detection of cytomegalovirus in urine from newborns by using polymerase chain reaction DNA amplification, *J Infect Dis* 158:1177-1184, 1988.
657. Warren WP, Balcarek K, Smith R, et al: Comparison of rapid methods of detection of cytomegalovirus in saliva with virus isolation in tissue culture, *J Clin Microbiol* 30:786-789, 1992.

658. Johansson PJ, Jonsson M, Ahlfors K, et al: Retrospective diagnostics of congenital cytomegalovirus infection performed by polymerase chain reaction in blood stored on filter paper, *Scand J Infect Dis* 29:465-468, 1997.
659. Boppana SB, Ross SA, Shimamura M, et al: Saliva polymerase-chain-reaction assay for cytomegalovirus screening in newborns, *N Engl J Med* 364:2111-2118, 2011.
660. Balcarek KB, Warren W, Smith RJ, et al: Neonatal screening for congenital cytomegalovirus infection by detection of virus in saliva, *J Infect Dis* 167:1433-1436, 1993.
661. Shuster EA, Beneke JS, Tegtmeier GE, et al: Monoclonal antibody for rapid laboratory detection of cytomegalovirus infections: characterization and diagnostic application, *Mayo Clin Proc* 60:577-585, 1985.
662. Boppana SB, Smith RJ, Stagno S, et al: Evaluation of a microtiter plate fluorescent-antibody assay for rapid detection of human cytomegalovirus infection, *J Clin Microbiol* 30:721-723, 1992.
663. Stirk PR, Griffiths PD: Use of monoclonal antibodies for the diagnosis of cytomegalovirus infection by the detection of early antigen fluorescent foci (DEAFF) in cell culture, *J Med Virol* 21:329-337, 1987.
664. Barbi M, Binda S, Primache V, et al: Diagnosis of congenital cytomegalovirus infection by detection of viral DNA in dried blood spots, *Clin Diagn Virol* 6:27-32, 1996.
665. Yamamoto AY, Mussi-Pinhata MM, Pinto PC, et al: Usefulness of blood and urine samples collected on filter paper in detecting cytomegalovirus by the polymerase chain reaction technique, *J Virol Methods* 97:159-164, 2001.
666. Soetens O, Vauloup-Fellous C, Foulon I, et al: Evaluation of different cytomegalovirus (CMV) DNA PCR protocols for analysis of dried blood spots from consecutive cases of neonates with congenital CMV infections, *J Clin Microbiol* 46:943-946, 2008.
667. Yamagishi Y, Miyagawa H, Wada K, et al: CMV DNA detection in dried blood spots for diagnosing congenital CMV infection in Japan, *J Med Virol* 78:923-925, 2006.
668. Barbi M, Binda S, Caroppo S: Diagnosis of congenital CMV infection via dried blood spots, *Rev Med Virol* 16:385-392, 2006.
669. Barbi M, Binda S, Primache V, et al: Cytomegalovirus DNA detection in Guthrie cards: a powerful tool for diagnosing congenital infection, *J Clin Virol* 17:159-165, 2000.
670. Barbi M, Binda S, Primache V, et al: Congenital cytomegalovirus infection in a northern Italian region. NEOCMV Group, *Eur J Epidemiol* 14:791-796, 1998.
671. Boppana SB, Ross SA, Novak Z, et al: Dried blood spot real-time polymerase chain reaction assays to screen newborns for congenital cytomegalovirus infection, *JAMA* 303:1375-1382, 2010.
672. Reynolds DW, Stagno S, Alford C: Laboratory diagnosis of cytomegalovirus infections. In Lennette E, Schmidt NJ, editors: *Diagnostic procedures for viral, rickettsial, and chlamydial infections*, ed 5, Washington, DC, 1979, American Public Health Association, pp 399-439.
673. Chou S, Merigan TC: Rapid detection and quantitation of human cytomegalovirus in urine through DNA hybridization, *N Engl J Med* 308:921-925, 1983.
674. Spector SA, Rua JA, Spector DH, et al: Detection of human cytomegalovirus in clinical specimens by DNA-DNA hybridization, *J Infect Dis* 150:121-126, 1984.
675. Lurain NS, Thompson KD, Farrand SK: Rapid detection of cytomegalovirus in clinical specimens by using biotinylated DNA probes and anlysis of cross-reactivity with herpes simplex virus, *J Clin Microbiol* 24:724-730, 1986.
676. Schuster V, Matz B, Wiegand H, et al: Detection of human cytomegalovirus in urine by DNA-DNA and RNA-DNA hybridization, *J Infect Dis* 154:309-314, 1986.
677. Bradford RD, Cloud G, Lakeman AD, et al: Detection of cytomegalovirus (CMV) DNA by polymerase chain reaction is associated with hearing loss in newborns with symptomatic congenital CMV infection involving the central nervous system, *J Infect Dis* 191:227-233, 2005.
678. Erice A, Holm MA, Gill PC, et al: Cytomegalovirus (CMV) antigenemia assay is more sensitive than shell vial cultures for rapid detection of CMV in polymorphonuclear blood leukocytes, *J Clin Microbiol* 30:2822-2825, 1992.
679. Percivalle E, Genini E, Chiesa A, et al: Comparison of a new Light Diagnostics and the CMV Brite to an in-house developed human cytomegalovirus antigenemia assay, *J Clin Virol* 43:13-17, 2008.
680. Hernando S, Folgueira L, Lumbreras C, et al: Comparison of cytomegalovirus viral load measure by real-time PCR with pp65 antigenemia for the diagnosis of cytomegalovirus disease in solid organ transplant patients, *Transplant Proc* 37:4094-4096, 2005.
681. Boeckh M: Rising CMV PP65 antigenemia and DNA levels during preemptive antiviral therapy, *Haematologica* 90:439, 2005.
682. Sullivan KM, Dykewicz CA, Longworth DL, et al: Preventing opportunistic infections after hematopoietic stem cell transplantation: the Centers for Disease Control and Prevention, Infectious Diseases Society of America, and American Society for Blood and Marrow Transplantation Practice Guidelines and beyond. *Hematology Am Soc Hematol Educ Program* 392-421, 2001.
683. Griffiths PD, Kangro HO: A user's guide to the indirect solid-phase radioimmunoassay for the detection of cytomegalovirus-specific IgM antibodies, *J Virol Methods* 8:271-282, 1984.
684. Stagno S, Tinker MK, Elrod C, et al: Immunoglobulin M antibodies detected by enzyme-linked immunosorbent assay and radioimmunoassay in the diagnosis of cytomegalovirus infections in pregnant women and newborn infants, *J Clin Microbiol* 21:930-935, 1985.
685. Lazzarotto T, Ripalti A, Bergamini G, et al: Development of a new cytomegalovirus (CMV) immunoglobulin M (IgM) immunoblot for detection of CMV-specific IGM, *J Clin Microbiol* 36:3337-3341, 1998.
686. Gentile M, Galli C, Pagnotti P, et al: Measurement of the sensitivity of different commercial assays in the diagnosis of CMV infection in pregnancy, *Eur J Clin Microbiol Infect Dis* 28:977-981, 2009.
687. Busse C, Strubel A, Schnitzler P: Combination of native and recombinant cytomegalovirus antigens in a new ELISA for detection of CMV-specific antibodies, *J Clin Virol* 43:137-141, 2008.
688. Lagrou K, Bodeus M, Van Ranst M, et al: Evaluation of the new ARCHITECT CMV IgM, IgG and IgG avidity assays, *J Clin Microbiol* 47:1695-1699, 2009.
689. Lazzarotto T, Spezzacatena P, Varani S, et al: Anticytomegalovirus (anti-CMV) immunoglobulin G avidity in identification of pregnant women at risk of transmitting congenital CMV infection, *Clin Diagn Lab Immunol* 6:127-129, 1999.
690. Lazzarotto T, Spezzacatena P, Pradelli P, et al: Avidity of immunoglobulin G directed against human cytomegalovirus during primary and secondary infections in immunocompetent and immunocompromised subjects, *Clin Diagn Lab Immunol* 4:469-473, 1997.
691. Bodeus M, Van Ranst M, Bernard P, et al: Anticytomegalovirus IgG avidity in pregnancy: a 2-year prospective study, *Fetal Diagn Ther* 17:362-366, 2002.
692. Bodeus M, Beulne D, Goubau P: Ability of three IgG-avidity assays to exclude recent cytomegalovirus infection, *Eur J Clin Microbiol Infect Dis* 20:248-252, 2001.
693. Kanengisser-Pines B, Hazan Y, Pines G, et al: High cytomegalovirus IgG avidity is a reliable indicator of past infection in patients with positive IgM detected during the first trimester of pregnancy, *J Perinat Med* 37:15-18, 2009.
694. Enders G, Daiminger A, Bader U, et al: The value of CMV IgG avidity and immunoblot for timing the onset of primary CMV infection in pregnancy, *J Clin Virol* 56:102-107, 2013.
695. Revello MG, Gerna G: Diagnosis and implications of human cytomegalovirus infection in pregnancy, *Fetal Matern Med Rev* 11: 117-134, 1999.
696. Maine GT, Lazzarotto T, Landini MP: New developments in the diagnosis of maternal and congenital CMV infection, *Expert Rev Mol Diagn* 1:19-29, 2001.
697. Vauloup-Fellous C, Berth M, Heskia F, Dugua JM, Grangeot-Keros L: Re-evaluation of the VIDAS((R)) cytomegalovirus (CMV) IgG avidity assay: determination of new cut-off values based on the study of kinetics of CMV-IgG maturation, *J Clin Virol* 56:118-123, 2013.
698. Lagrou K, Bodeus M, Van Ranst M, Goubau P: Evaluation of the new architect cytomegalovirus immunoglobulin M (IgM), IgG, and IgG avidity assays, *J Clin Microbiol* 47:1695-1699, 2009.
699. Revello MG, Genini E, Gorini G, et al: Comparative evaluation of eight commercial human cytomegalovirus IgG avidity assays, *J Clin Virol* 48:255-259, 2010.
700. Revello MG, Zavattoni M, Sarasini A, et al: Human cytomegalovirus in blood of immunocompetent persons during primary infection: prognostic implications for pregnancy, *J Infect Dis* 177:1170-1175, 1998.
701. Arora N, Novak Z, Fowler KB, et al: Cytomegalovirus viruria and DNAemia in healthy seropositive women, *J Infect Dis* 202:1800-1803, 2010.

702. Revello MG, Lilleri D, Zavattoni M, et al: Human cytomegalovirus immediate-early messenger RNA in blood of pregnant women with primary infection and of congenitally infected newborns, *J Infect Dis* 184:1078-1081, 2001.
703. Donner C, Liesnard C, Content J, et al: Prenatal diagnosis of 52 pregnancies at risk for congenital cytomegalovirus infection, *Obstet Gynecol* 82:481-486, 1993.
704. Lamy ME, Mulongo KN, Gadisseux JF, et al: Prenatal diagnosis of fetal cytomegalovirus infection, *Am J Obstet Gynecol* 166:91-94, 1992.
705. Lynch L, Daffos F, Emanuel D, et al: Prenatal diagnosis of fetal cytomegalovirus infection, *Am J Obstet Gynecol* 165:714-718, 1991.
706. Lazzarotto T, Guerra B, Gabrielli L, Lanari M, Landini MP: Update on the prevention, diagnosis and management of cytomegalovirus infection during pregnancy, *Clin Microbiol Infect* 17:1285-1293, 2011.
707. Benoist G, Leruez-Ville M, Magny JF, et al: Management of pregnancies with confirmed cytomegalovirus fetal infection, *Fetal Diagn Ther* 33:203-214, 2013.
708. Lipitz S, Yagel S, Shalev E, et al: Prenatal diagnosis of fetal primary cytomegalovirus infection, *Obstet Gynecol* 89:763-767, 1997.
709. Liesnard CA, Revelard P, Englert Y: Is matching between women and donors feasible to avoid cytomegalovirus infection in artificial insemination with donor semen?, *Hum Reprod* 13:25-31, 1998. discussion 32–34.
710. Lazzarotto T, Varani S, Guerra B, et al: Prenatal indicators of congenital cytomegalovirus infection, *J Pediatr* 137:90-95, 2000.
711. Lazzarotto T, Gabrielli L, Foschini MP, et al: Congenital cytomegalovirus infection in twin pregnancies: viral load in the amniotic fluid and pregnancy outcome, *Pediatrics* 112:e153-e157, 2003.
712. Guerra B, Lazzorotto T, Quarta S, et al: Prenatal diagnosis of symptomatic congenital cytomegalovirus infection, *Am J Obstet Gynecol* 183:476-482, 2000.
713. Goegebuer T, Van Meensel B, Beuselinck K, et al: Clinical predictive value of real-time PCR quantification of human cytomegalovirus DNA in amniotic fluid samples, *J Clin Microbiol* 47:660-665, 2009.
714. Liesnard C, Donner C, Brancart F, et al: Prenatal diagnosis of congenital cytomegalovirus infection: prospective study of 237 pregnancies at risk, *Obstet Gynecol* 95:881-888, 2000.
715. Donner C, Liesnard C, Brancart F, et al: Accuracy of amniotic fluid testing before 21 weeks' gestation in prenatal diagnosis of congenital cytomegalovirus infection, *Prenat Diagn* 14:1055-1059, 1994.
716. Bodeus M, Hubinont C, Bernard P, et al: Prenatal diagnosis of human cytomegalovirus by culture and polymerase chain reaction: 98 pregnancies leading to congenital infection, *Prenat Diagn* 19:314-317, 1999.
717. Grose C, Meehan T, Weiner CP: Prenatal diagnosis of congenital cytomegalovirus infection by virus isolation after amniocentesis, *Pediatr Infect Dis J* 11:605-607, 1992.
718. Pass RF: Commentary: is there a role for prenatal diagnosis of congenital cytomegalovirus infection? *Pediatr Infect Dis J* 11:608-609, 1992.
719. Weiner CP, Grose C: Prenatal diagnosis of congenital cytomegalovirus infection by virus isolation from amniotic fluid, *Am J Obstet Gynecol* 163:1253-1255, 1990.
720. Benoist G, Salomon LJ, Mohlo M, et al: Cytomegalovirus-related fetal brain lesions: comparison between targeted ultrasound examination and magnetic resonance imaging, *Ultrasound Obstet Gynecol* 32:900-905, 2008.
721. Goutières F, Aicardi J, Barth PG, et al: Aicardi-Goutières syndrome: an update and results of interferon-alpha studies, *Ann Neurol* 44:900-907, 1998.
722. Goutières F: Aicardi-Goutières syndrome, *Brain Dev* 27:201-206, 2005.
723. Fazzi E, Cattalini M, Orcesi S, et al: Aicardi-Goutières syndrome, a rare neurological disease in children: a new autoimmune disorder? *Autoimmun Rev* 12:506-509, 2013.
724. Rice GI, Kasher PR, Forte GM, et al: Mutations in ADAR1 cause Aicardi-Goutières syndrome associated with a type I interferon signature, *Nat Genet* 44:1243-1248, 2012.
725. Chahwan C, Chahwan R: Aicardi-Goutières syndrome: from patients to genes and beyond, *Clin Genet* 81:413-420, 2012.
726. Rossler L, Ludwig-Seibold C, Thiels C, et al: Aicardi-Goutières syndrome with emphasis on sonographic features in infancy, *Pediatr Radiol* 42:932-940, 2012.
727. Tookey PA, Bedford H, Peckham CS: Act now to prevent re-emergence of congenital rubella, *BMJ* 347:f4498, 2013.
728. Whitley RJ, Cloud G, Gruber W, et al: A pharmacokinetic and pharmacodynamic evaluation of ganciclovir for the treatment of symptomatic congenital cytomegalovirus infection: results of a phase II study, *J Infect Dis* 175:1080-1086, 1997.
729. Kimberlin DW, Lin CY, Sanchez PJ, et al: Effect of ganciclovir therapy on hearing in symptomatic congenital cytomegalovirus disease involving the central nervous system: a randomized, controlled trial, *J Pediatr* 143:16-25, 2003.
730. Nigro G, Torre RL, Pentimalli H, et al: Regression of fetal cerebral abnormalities by primary cytomegalovirus infection following hyperimmunoglobulin therapy, *Prenat Diagn* 28:512-517, 2008.
731. Pass RF, Burke RL: Development of cytomegalovirus vaccines: prospects for prevention of congenital CMV infection, *Semin Pediatr Infect Dis* 13:196-204, 2002.
732. Pass RF, Duliege AM, Boppana S, et al: A subunit cytomegalovirus vaccine based on recombinant envelope glycoprotein B and a new adjuvant, *J Infect Dis* 180:970-975, 1999.
733. Adler SP, Plotkin SA, Gonczol E, et al: A canarypox vector expressing cytomegalovirus (CMV) glycoprotein B primes for antibody responses to a live attenuated CMV vaccine (Towne), *J Infect Dis* 180:843-846, 1999.
734. Berencsi K, Gyulai Z, Gonczol E, et al: A canarypox vector-expressing cytomegalovirus (CMV) phosphoprotein 65 induces long-lasting cytotoxic T cell responses in human CMV-seronegative subjects, *J Infect Dis* 183:1171-1179, 2001.
735. Shimamura M, Mach M, Britt WJ: Human cytomegalovirus infection elicits a glycoprotein M (gM)/gN-specific virus-neutralizing antibody response, *J Virol* 80:4591-4600, 2006.
736. Macagno A, Bernasconi NL, Vanzetta F, et al: Isolation of human monoclonal antibodies that potently neutralize human cytomegalovirus infection by targeting different epitopes on the gH/gL/UL128-131A complex, *J Virol* 84:1005-1013, 2013.
737. Gonczol E, Plotkin S: Development of a cytomegalovirus vaccine: lessons from recent clinical trials, *Expert Opin Biol Ther* 1:401-412, 2001.
738. Plotkin SA, Starr SE, Friedman HM, et al: Protective effects of Towne cytomegalovirus vaccine against low-passage cytomegalovirus administered as a challenge, *J Infect Dis* 159:860-865, 1989.
739. Adler SP, Starr SE, Plotkin SA, et al: Immunity induced by primary human cytomegalovirus infection protects against secondary infection among women of childbearing age, *J Infect Dis* 171:26-32, 1995.
740. Heineman TC, Schleiss M, Bernstein DI, et al: A phase 1 study of 4 live, recombinant human cytomegalovirus Towne/Toledo chimeric vaccines, *J Infect Dis* 193:1350-1360, 2006.
741. Pass RF, Zhang C, Evans A, et al: Vaccine prevention of maternal cytomegalovirus infection, *N Engl J Med* 360:1191-1199, 2009.
742. Vauloup-Fellous C, Picone O, Cordier AG, et al: Does hygiene counseling have an impact on the rate of CMV primary infection during pregnancy? Results of a 3-year prospective study in a French hospital, *J Clin Virol* 46(Suppl 4):S49-S53, 2009.
743. Reap EA, Dryga SA, Morris J, et al: Cellular and humoral immune responses to alphavirus replicon vaccines expressing cytomegalovirus pp65, IE1, and gB proteins, *Clin Vaccine Immunol* 14:748-755, 2007.
744. Bernstein DI, Reap EA, Katen K, et al: Randomized, double-blind, Phase 1 trial of an alphavirus replicon vaccine for cytomegalovirus in CMV seronegative adult volunteers, *Vaccine* 28:484-493, 2009.
745. Wloch MK, Smith LR, Boutsaboualoy S, et al: Safety and immunogenicity of a bivalent cytomegalovirus DNA vaccine in healthy adult subjects, *J Infect Dis* 197:1634-1642, 2008.
746. Lilleri D, Kabanova A, Revello MG, et al: Fetal human cytomegalovirus transmission correlates with delayed maternal antibodies to gH/gL/pUL128-130-131 complex during primary infection, *PLoS One* 8:e59863, 2013.
747. Wussow F, Yue Y, Martinez J, et al: A vaccine based on the rhesus cytomegalovirus UL128 complex induces broadly neutralizing antibodies in rhesus macaques, *J Virol* 87:1322-1332, 2013.
748. Hansen SG, Vieville C, Whizin N, et al: Effector memory T cell responses are associated with protection of rhesus monkeys from mucosal simian immunodeficiency virus challenge, *Nat Med* 15:293-299, 2009.
749. Cannon MJ, Davis KF: Washing our hands of the congenital cytomegalovirus disease epidemic, *BMC Public Health* 5:70, 2005.

750. Adler SP, Finney JW, Manganello AM, et al: Prevention of child-to-mother transmission of cytomegalovirus among pregnant women, *J Pediatr* 145:485-491, 2004.
751. Stagno S, Whitley RJ: Herpesvirus infections of pregnancy. Part I: cytomegalovirus and Epstein-Barr virus infections, *N Engl J Med* 313:1270-1274, 1985.
752. Pass R, Stagno S: Cytomegalovirus. In Donowitz L, editor: *Hospital-acquired infection in the pediatric patient*, Baltimore, 1988, Williams & Wilkins.
753. Friedman HM, Lewis MR, Nemerofsky DM, et al: Acquisition of cytomegalovirus infection among female employees at a pediatric hospital, *Pediatr Infect Dis J* 3:233-235, 1984.
754. Bowden RA: Cytomegalovirus infections in transplant patients: methods of prevention of primary cytomegalovirus, *Transplant Proc* 23:136-138, 1991.
755. Bowden RA: Transfusion-transmitted cytomegalovirus infection, *Hematol Oncol Clin North Am* 9:155-166, 1995.
756. Lipson SM, Shepp DH, Match ME, et al: Cytomegalovirus infectivity in whole blood following leukocyte reduction by filtration, *Am J Clin Pathol* 116:52-55, 2001.
757. Pietersz RN, van der Meer PF, Seghatchian MJ: Update on leucocyte depletion of blood components by filtration, *Transfus Sci* 19: 321-328, 1998.
758. Xu D, Yonetani M, Uetani Y, et al: Acquired cytomegalovirus infection and blood transfusion in preterm infants, *Acta Paediatr Jpn* 37:444-449, 1995.
759. Gilbert GL, Hayes K, Hudson IL, et al: Prevention of transfusion-acquired cytomegalovirus infection in infants by blood filtration to remove leucocytes. Neonatal Cytomegalovirus Infection Study Group, *Lancet* 1:1228-1231, 1989.
760. Fisk JM, Snyder EL: Universal pre-storage leukoreduction: a defensible use of hospital resources: the Yale-New Haven Hospital experience, *Dev Biol (Basel)* 120:39-44, 2005.
761. Blajchman MA, Goldman M, Freedman JJ, et al: Proceedings of a consensus conference: prevention of post-transfusion CMV in the era of universal leukoreduction, *Transfus Med Rev* 15:1-20, 2001.
762. Larsson S, Soderberg-Naucler C, Wang FZ, et al: Cytomegalovirus DNA can be detected in peripheral blood mononuclear cells from all seropositive and most seronegative healthy blood donors over time, *Transfusion* 38:271-278, 1998.
763. Goelz R, Hihn E, Hamprecht K, et al: Effects of different CMV-heat-inactivation-methods on growth factors in human breast milk, *Pediatr Res* 65:458-461, 2009.
764. Knorr B, Kessler U, Poschl J, et al: A haemophagocytic lymphohistiocytosis (HLH)-like picture following breastmilk transmitted cytomegalovirus infection in a preterm infant, *Scand J Infect Dis* 39:173-176, 2007.
765. Dworsky M, Stagno S, Pass RF, et al: Persistence of cytomegalovirus in human milk after storage, *J Pediatr* 101:440-443, 1982.
766. Maschmann J, Hamprecht K, Weissbrich B, et al: Freeze-thawing of breast milk does not prevent cytomegalovirus transmission to a preterm infant, *Arch Dis Child Fetal Neonatal Ed* 91:F288-F290, 2006.

25 Enterovirus, Parechovirus, and Saffold Virus Infections

JAMES D. CHERRY and PAUL KROGSTAD

CHAPTER OUTLINE

The enteroviruses, parechoviruses, and Saffold viruses are all members of the picornavirus family, a group of small, nonenveloped RNA viruses.[1-4] Enteroviruses, including the polioviruses, coxsackieviruses, echoviruses, and numerically designated types, and parechoviruses constitute two distinct genera among the Picornaviridae, although Saffold viruses are members of the genus *Cardiovirus*, genetically related to Theiler murine encephalomyelitis virus.[5] The enteroviruses, parechoviruses, and Saffold viruses exhibit clear differences in their physical and biochemical properties and mode of replication, but they are discussed together here because of shared features in their epidemiology, pathogenesis and clinical manifestations.[1,3,5-20] Congenital and neonatal infections have been linked with many different enteroviruses and parechoviruses.[1,3,6-17,21-38] At the present time, there are no data on congenital or neonatal infections with Saffold viruses, but the similarity of their clinical manifestations in older infants and children to those of both enteroviruses and parechoviruses suggests that reports will soon appear.

Historical recognition of enterovirus infection began with poliomyelitis.[39] The earliest record is an Egyptian stele of the 18th dynasty (1580-1350 BC), which shows a young man with a withered, shortened leg, the characteristic deformity of paralytic poliomyelitis.[40,41] Underwood,[42] a London pediatrician, published the first medical description in 1789 in his *Treatise on Diseases of Children.* During the 19th century, many reports appeared in Europe and the United States describing small clusters of cases of “infantile paralysis.” The authors were greatly puzzled about the nature of the affliction; not until the 1860s and 1870s was the spinal cord firmly established as the seat of the pathologic process. The contagious nature of poliomyelitis was not appreciated until the latter part of the 19th century. Medin, a Swedish pediatrician, was the first to describe the epidemic nature of poliomyelitis (1890), and his pupil Wickman[43] worked out the basic principles of the epidemiology.

Poliovirus was first isolated in monkeys by Landsteiner and Popper in 1908.[44] The availability of a laboratory animal assay system opened up many avenues of research that in the ensuing 40 years led to the demonstration that an unrecognized intestinal infection was common and that paralytic disease was a relatively uncommon event. In 1949, Enders and associates[45] reported the growth of poliovirus type 2 in tissue culture, leading to the development of poliovirus vaccines in the 1950s and 1960s.

Coxsackieviruses and echoviruses have had a shorter history. Epidemic pleurodynia was first clinically described in northern Germany in 1735 by Hannaeus,[8,46] more than 200 years before the coxsackieviral cause of this disease was discovered. In 1948, Dalldorf and Sickles[47] first reported the isolation of a coxsackievirus by using suckling mouse inoculation. However, the development of tissue culture methods by Enders and his colleagues[45] paved the way for the recovery of a large number of other cytopathic viruses. Most of these "new" viruses failed to produce illness in laboratory animals. Because the relationships of many of these newly recovered agents to human disease were unknown, they were called orphan viruses.[10] Later, several agents were grouped together and called *e*nteric *c*ytopathogenic *h*uman *o*rphan viruses, or *echo*viruses. Enteroviruses were first categorized together and named in 1957 by a committee sponsored by the National Foundation for Infantile Paralysis[48]; the human enteric tract was believed to be the natural habitat of these agents, giving rise to the group nomenclature.

Subsequently, analysis of the replication, genome and protein content[1-4] of echoviruses 22 and 23 found that they were distinctly different from most of the agents designated as enteroviruses, and they were placed in the genus *Parechovirus*. More recently, using molecular detection methods, Saffold viruses were identified in human infections.[5,49] Extensive seroepidemiologic studies indicate that infections with Saffold virus types 2 and 3 are very common in young children. Some clinical associations have been noted, but it would seem that most infections are asymptomatic.[5,18-20,49-59] As noted above, no data on congenital or neonatal infections with Saffold viruses have as yet been presented.

Inactivated polio vaccines (IPV) and live-attenuated oral poliovirus vaccines (OPV) became available in the late 1950s and early 1960s, and there has been a dramatic reduction in worldwide poliomyelitis because of immunization with IPV and OPV and the efforts of the global immunization initiative.[60-66] The last case of confirmed paralytic polio in the Western Hemisphere caused by a nonvaccine type occurred in 1991.[65] Aside from the polio immunization successes, there have been few major advances or new modes of prevention or treatment for enteroviral diseases.[67-70] However, the use of nucleic acid detection systems has progressed over the past 2 decades, and rapid diagnosis of meningitis and other enteroviral and parechoviral illnesses has become possible.[22,71-87]

The Viruses

TAXONOMY[1,2,14,88-103]

Enteroviruses, parechoviruses and Saffold viruses are RNA viruses belonging to the family *Picornaviridae* (pico = small). They are grouped together because they share certain physical, biochemical, and molecular properties. In electron micrographs, the viruses are seen as 27- to 30-nm particles that consist of naked (nonenveloped) protein capsids, constituting approximately 70% to 75% of the mass of particles, and dense central cores containing the single-stranded message-sense genomic RNA.

The original classification of human enteroviruses is shown in Table 25-1. The enteroviruses were originally distributed into four groups based on their different effects in tissue culture and pattern of disease in experimentally infected animals: polioviruses (causal agents of poliomyelitis in humans and nonhuman primates); coxsackie A viruses (coxsackievirus A), associated with herpangina, human central nervous system (CNS) disease, and flaccid paralysis in suckling mice); coxsackie B viruses (coxsackievirus B) (human CNS and cardiac disease, spastic paralysis in mice); and the echoviruses (nonpathogenic in mice and not initially linked to human disease).

Although this scheme was initially useful, many strains were subsequently isolated that do not conform to such rigid specificities. For example, several coxsackievirus A strains replicate and have a cytopathic effect in monkey kidney tissue cultures, and some echovirus strains cause paralysis in mice. For this reason, and to simplify the nomenclature, subsequent enteroviruses were assigned sequential numbers. After this convention, the prototype enterovirus strains Fermon, Toluca-1, J 670/71, and BrCr (identified from 1959-1973) were numerically designated enterovirus (EV) 68 through 71, respectively. Additional enteroviruses continued to be identified that could not be identified using antisera specific for the classic serotypes. More than 50 additional such EV types have been assigned, although not all have been linked to human disease.

Complicating matters somewhat, studies of echoviruses 22 and 23 found that they exhibited genomic and proteomic differences from other enteroviruses, and hence they were reclassified in the new genus *Parechovirus* as parechoviruses types 1 and 2.[2-4] Similarly, hepatitis A virus was

Table 25-1 Original Classification of Human Enteroviruses: Animal and Tissue Culture Spectrum*

		CYTOPATHIC EFFECT		ILLNESS AND PATHOLOGY	
Virus	**Serologic Types**†	**Monkey Kidney Tissue Culture**	**Human Tissue Culture**	**Suckling Mouse**	**Monkey**
Polioviruses	1-3	+	+	—	+
Coxsackieviruses A	1-24‡	—	—	+	—
Coxsackieviruses B	1-6	+	+	+	—
Echoviruses	1-34§	+	±	—	—

*Many enterovirus strains have been isolated that do not conform to these categories , leading to the revised classification scheme shown in Table 25-2.

†Newer types were eventually assigned enterovirus type numbers instead of coxsackievirus A, coxsackievirus B, or echovirus numbers. Types 68 through 71 (EV68-EV71) were initially identified.

‡Coxsackievirus A23 was found to be the same as echovirus 9.

§Echovirus 10 was reclassified as a reovirus: Echoviruses 22 and 23 were made the first members of the *Parechovirus* genus of Picornaviridae, and echovirus 28 was reclassified as a rhinovirus.

initially assigned the designation of EV72 but was reclassified as the sole member of the *Hepatovirus* genus within the picornavirus family because of marked genetic and biologic distinctions from the enteroviruses.

In recent years, genetic, biologic and molecular properties have been used to revise picornavirus taxonomy, leading to a reorganization of the human enteroviruses into four alphabetically designated human enterovirus species (HEV-A, -B, -C, and -D) (Table 25-2). Determining the nucleotide sequence encoding the viral VP1capsid protein now plays a major role in the approach to taxonomy and predictably identifies viruses originally classified by serologic means, leading to the term "molecular serotyping."[98,100,104,105] This approach will, no doubt, dominate future phylogenetic studies. Of interest, the application of molecular phylogenetic approaches has also revealed that recombination between circulating enteroviruses is a frequent event and is likely to increase their genetic diversity. This propensity for recombination has played a role in recent outbreaks of paralytic diseases involving vaccine-derived stains and in well-documented cases of HEV-B infections.[2,106-114]

Similarly, molecular analysis has led to the identification of 16 distinct types of human parechoviruses.[115] Of these, types 1 and 3 have most often been associated with human illness. Substantial recombination among the parechoviruses has also been noted, allowing rapid genetic diversification.[116,117]

MORPHOLOGY AND REPLICATION

The genome of picornaviruses is a single-stranded, positive-sense RNA molecule approximately 7.4 to 8 kb in length.[99] It consists of a 5′ noncoding region, followed by a single long open-reading frame, a short 3′ noncoding region, and a polyA tail. The 5′ noncoding region folds into highly conserved structures that are thought to play a role in the initiation of the replication of the viral genome and contain an internal ribosome entry site, which is essential for the initiation of translation. Similarly, the 3′ noncoding region is well conserved within each picornavirus genus and is thought to be involved in replication of the viral genome. The viral genome is packaged into naked capsids that exhibit icosahedral symmetry with 20 triangular faces and 12 vertices.

Enterovirus replication begins with the adsorption of virions to cell surface receptors, which are typically integrins or immunoglobulin-like proteins (Table 25-3). The virions penetrate the surface of the cell, uncoat, and the viral genome functions as messenger RNA for the viral polyprotein. This polypeptide contains three domains, P1 to P3, which are cleaved into three to four proteins each. The P1 region is liberated from the polyprotein by the viral 2A protein, a chymotrypsin-like protease. P1 is initially split into three proteins—VP0, VP1, and VP3—by the viral 3C protease. VP0 is then further processed into two smaller proteins, VP4 and VP2. Portions of VP1, VP2, and VP3 are exposed at the surface of the virion, whereas VP4 is entirely internal. VP1, VP2, and VP3 have no sequence homology but share the same topology.[2] Specifically, they form an eight-stranded antiparallel β-barrel that is wedge shaped and composed of two antiparallel β-sheets. The amino acid sequences in the loops that connect the β-strands and the N- and C-terminal sequences that extend from the β-barrel domain of VP1, VP2, and VP3 give each enterovirus its distinct antigenicity.

The replication of enteroviruses occurs in the cytoplasm in membrane-associated replication complexes, and is completed rapidly (5-10 hours). Studies of polioviruses and coxsackieviruses have shown that enteroviral replication is associated with disruption of cellular protein secretion, and

Table 25-2 Genomic Classification of Enteroviruses

Species Designation	Types
Human enterovirus A (HEV-A)	Coxsackievirus A2-8, A10, A12, A14, A16
	Enterovirus A71, A76, A89, A90, A91, A114, A119
Human enterovirus B (HEV-B)	Coxsackievirus A9
	Coxsackievirus B 1-6
	Echovirus 1-9, 11-21, 24-27, 29-33
	Enterovirus B69, B73-B75, B77-B88, B93, B97, B98, B100, B101, B106, B107
Human enterovirus C (HEV-C)	Poliovirus 1-3
	Coxsackievirus A1, A11, A13, A17, A19-22, A24
	Enterovirus C95, C96, C99, C102, C104, C105, C109, C113, C116-C118
Human enterovirus D (HEV-D)	Enterovirus D68, D70, D94, D111

From Knowles NJ, Hovi T, Hyypiä T, et al: Picornaviridae. In King AMQ, Adams MJ, Carstens EB, Lefkowitz EJ, editors: *Virus taxonomy: classification and nomenclature of viruses. Ninth report of the International Committee on Taxonomy of Viruses,* San Diego, 2012, Elsevier, pp 855-880.

Coxsackievirus (CV) A15 has been reclassified as a strain of CV A11, and CV A18 as a strain of CVA13. Echovirus 34 has been recognized as a variant of coxsackievirus A24.

Table 25-3 Cellular Receptors and Cofactors for Infection of Representative Enteroviruses

Virus	HEV Species	Receptor	Cofactor for Infection*
Enterovirus 71	HEV-A	PSGL-1, SCARB2	
Coxsackieviruses B1-6	HEV-B	CAR	Some coxsackieviruses B may use CD55 (DAF) or heparin for attachment
Echovirus 9	HEV-B	$\alpha_v\beta_3$ integrin (vitronectin receptor)	MAP-70
Echoviruses 1, 8	HEV-B	VLA-2 ($\alpha_2\beta_1$ integrin)	Heparin sulfate
Coxsackieviruses A13, 17, 20, 21, 24	HEV-C	ICAM-1	
Polioviruses 1-3	HEV-C	CD155 (PVR)	
Enterovirus 70	HEV-D	CD55 (DAF)	

CAR, Coxsackie and adenovirus receptor; DAF, decay accelerating factor; *HEV,* human enterovirus; *ICAM-1,* intercellular adhesion molecule 1; *PSGL-1,* P-selectin glycoprotein ligand 1; *PVR,* poliovirus receptor; *SCARB2,* scavenger receptor class B member 2; *VLA-2,* very late activation antigen-2 (a human integrin).

*The cofactors generally facilitate adhesion to cells, but their sole expression is insufficient to permit infection to occur.

host cell protein synthesis is suppressed because of cleavage of eIF4G by the enteroviral 2A protein. The coxsackievirus 2A protein also cleaves dystrophin, a cytoskeletal protein; this activity has been hypothesized to play a role in damage to the myocardium.[118,119]

The parechoviruses replicate in a similar fashion.[120] Integrins ($\alpha_v\beta_3$ and perhaps $\alpha_v\beta_1$) have been identified as key receptors.[121] In contrast to the enteroviruses, the parechovirus 2A protein does not function as a protease but may function in genome replication.[122] Moreover, parechoviral capsids are composed of three proteins: VP1, VP3, and an uncleaved VP0 protein. In addition, parechovirus replication occurs in small, discrete foci in the cytoplasm, rather than in large accumulations of membranous vesicles like the enteroviruses. Moreover, transcription and translation do not appear to be disrupted by the parechoviruses, perhaps explaining their relatively mild and delayed cytopathic effect when grown in tissue culture.[3]

The replication of Saffold viruses has received little specific study thus far, but they are likely to exhibit features of other members of the *Cardiovirus* genus.[123]

REPLICATION CHARACTERISTICS AND HOST SYSTEMS[1,96,124,125]

Enteroviruses and parechoviruses are relatively stable viruses in that they retain infectivity for several days at room temperature and can be stored indefinitely at ordinary freezer temperatures (−20° C). They are inactivated quickly by heat (>56° C), formaldehyde, chlorination, and ultraviolet light but are refractory to ether, ethanol, and isopropanol.

Enterovirus strains grow rapidly when adapted to susceptible host systems and cause cytopathology in tissue culture in 2 to 7 days. The typical tissue culture cytopathic effect is shown in Figure 25-1; characteristic pathologic findings in mice are shown in Figures 25-2 and 25-3. Final titers of virus recovered in the laboratory vary markedly among different viral strains and the host system used; typically, concentrations of 10^3 to 10^7 infectious doses per 0.1 mL of tissue culture fluid or tissue homogenate are obtained. Unadapted viral strains frequently require long periods of incubation. In both tissue culture and suckling mice, evidence of growth usually is visible. Blind passage occasionally is necessary for the cytopathology to become apparent.

Although many different primary and secondary tissue culture systems support the growth of various enteroviruses, primary rhesus monkey kidney cultures generally are accepted to have the most inclusive spectrum. Other simian kidney tissue cultures, however, also have the same broad spectrum.[126] Tissue cultures of human origin have a more limited spectrum, but several echovirus types have shown more consistent primary isolation in human than in monkey kidney.[127-129] A satisfactory system for the primary recovery of enteroviruses from clinical specimens would include primary rhesus, cynomolgus, or African green monkey kidney tissue cultures; a diploid, human embryonic lung fibroblast cell strain; rhabdomyosarcoma cell line tissue cultures; and intraperitoneal and intracerebral inoculation of suckling mice younger than 24 hours.[93,96,125,128,130,131]

Human parechovirus types 1 to 6 can be isolated in several commonly used tissue culture systems.[115,132] Human parechovirus types 1, 4, and 6 can be recovered in HT29 (primary colorectal adenocarcinoma) cells. Types 1 and 4 can be isolated in Vero (African green monkey kidney), A549 (human lung adenocarcinoma), and RD (rhabdomyosarcoma) cells. Human parechovirus 3 grows in Vero and A549 cells.

ANTIGENIC CHARACTERISTICS[1,14,41,93,96]

Although some minor cross-reactions exist between several coxsackievirus and echovirus types, common group antigens of diagnostic importance have not been defined well. Heat treatment of virions and the use of synthetic peptides

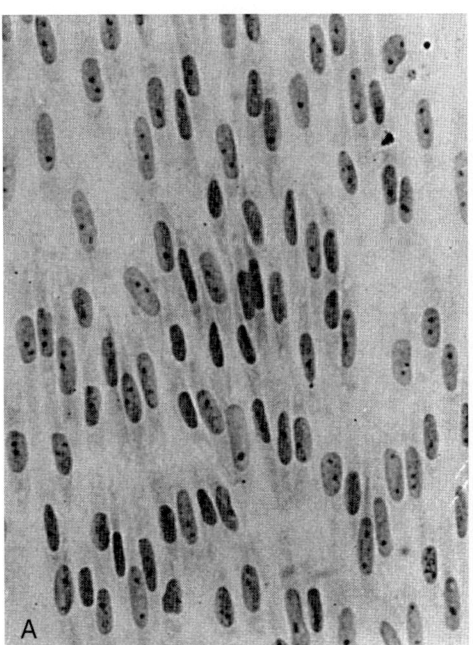

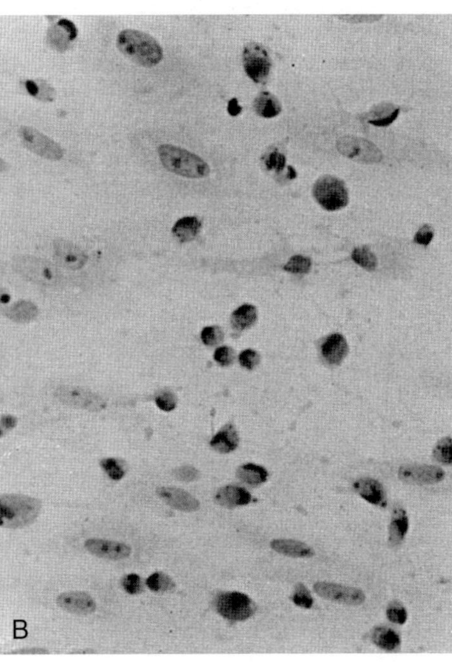

Figure 25-1 Fetal rhesus monkey kidney tissue culture (HL-8). **A,** Uninoculated tissue culture. **B,** Echovirus 11 cytopathic effect.

have produced antigens with broad enteroviral reactivity.[133,134] These antigens have been used in enzyme-linked immunosorbent assay (ELISA) and complement-fixation tests to determine IgG and IgM enteroviral antibodies and for antigen detection. In one study, Terletskaia-Ladwig and colleagues[133] reported the identification of patients infected with enteroviruses by the use of an immunoglobulin M (IgM) enzyme immunoassay (EIA). This test used heat-treated coxsackievirus B5 and echovirus 9 as antigens, and it identified patients infected with echoviruses 4, 11, and 30. The sensitivity of the test was 35%. In another study involving heat-treated virus or synthetic peptides, the respective sensitivities were 67% and 62%.[134] However, both tests lacked specificity. Intratypic strain differences are common findings, and some strains (prime strains) are neutralized poorly by antisera to prototype viruses. However, in animals, these prime strains induce antibodies that neutralize the specific prototype viruses.

The identification of polioviral, coxsackieviral, and echoviral types by neutralization in suckling mice or tissue culture with antiserum pools is relatively well defined. Neutralization is induced by the epitopes on structural proteins VP1, VP2, and VP3; in particular, several epitopes are clustered on VP1. Prime strains do cause diagnostic difficulty because frequently they are not neutralized by the reference antisera, which is a particular problem with echoviruses 4, 9, and 11 and enterovirus 71. If these types are suspected, in some instances, this problem can be overcome

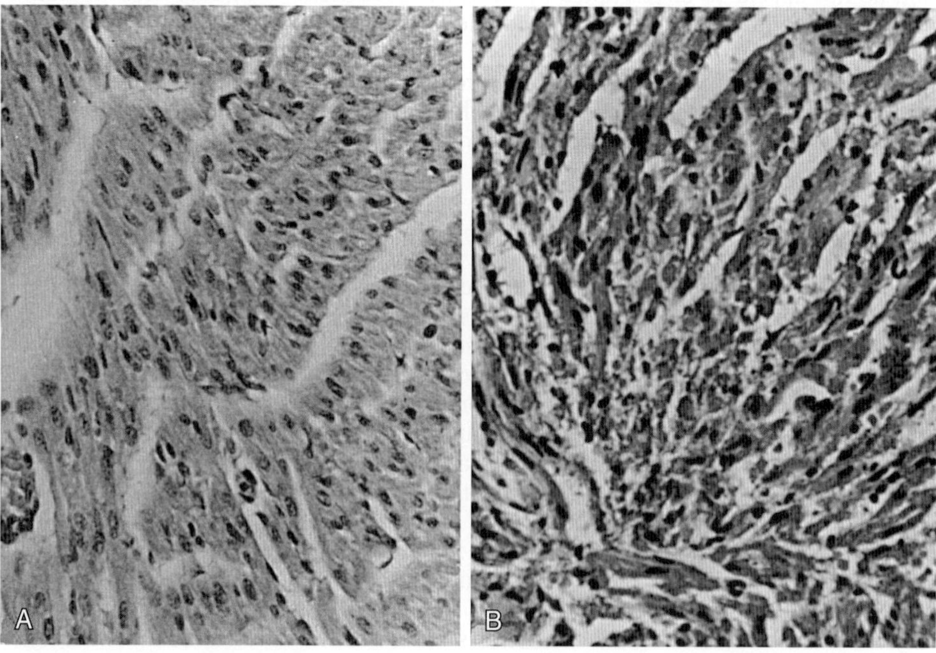

Figure 25-2 Suckling mouse skeletal muscle. **A,** Normal suckling mouse skeletal muscle. **B,** Skeletal muscle of suckling mouse infected with coxsackievirus A16.

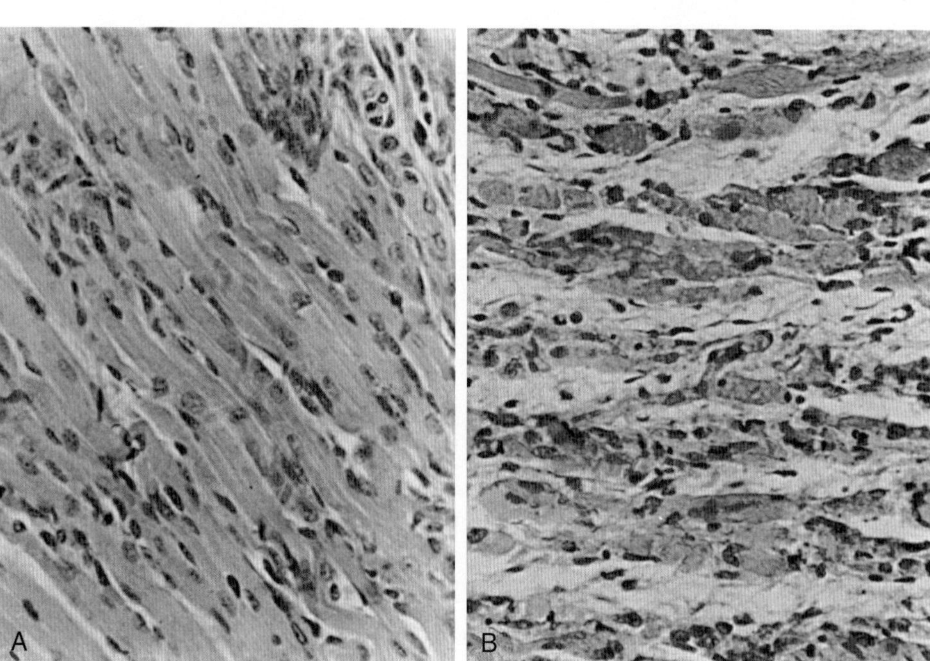

Figure 25-3 Suckling mouse myocardium. **A,** Normal suckling mouse myocardium. **B,** Myocardium of suckling mouse infected with coxsackievirus B1.

by using antisera in less diluted concentrations or antisera prepared against several different strains of problem viruses. Recently, Kubo and associates[92] have been able to type enteroviral isolates not identified through neutralization by nucleotide sequence analysis of the VP4 gene. They specifically identified prime strains of echovirus 18 and enterovirus 71. Sequence analysis of the VP1 gene also is useful for typing enteroviral prime strains not identified by neutralization.[97]

HOST RANGE

It was long believed that humans were the only natural hosts of enteroviruses.[8-10,16,17,135] Enteroviruses have also been recovered in nature from sewage,[136] flies,[136-138] swine,[139,140] dogs,[141,142] a calf,[143] a budgerigar (i.e., small Australian parakeet),[144] a fox,[145] mussels,[146] clams,[147] and oysters.[148] Serologic evidence of infection with enteroviruses similar to human strains has been found in chimpanzees and other nonhuman primates,[149,150] cattle,[151] rabbits,[152] a fox,[152] a chipmunk,[152] and a marmot.[152] It is possible that infection in some of these reports was the result of their direct contact with infected humans or infected human excreta. However, genetically distinct enteroviruses have been identified in cattle, possums, domesticated pigs, sheep, and nonhuman primates.[1,2,14,88-103]

Although enteroviruses do not multiply in flies, they appear to be a possible significant vector in situations of poor sanitation and heavy human infection.[136-138] The contamination of shellfish is also intriguing[145-147,153-156] because, in addition to their possible role in human infection, they offer a source of enteroviral storage during cold weather. Contaminated foods are another possible source of human infection.[157]

Epidemiology and Transmission

GENERAL CONSIDERATIONS

Enteroviruses and parechoviruses are spread from person to person by fecal-oral and possibly by oral-oral (respiratory) routes.[6-10,13-17,135] Swimming and wading pools may serve as a means of spread of enteroviruses during the summer.[158] Children are the main susceptible cohort; they are immunologically susceptible, and their unhygienic habits facilitate spread. Spread is from child to child (by feces to skin to mouth) and then within family groups. Recovery of enteroviruses is inversely related to age; the prevalence of antibodies to common enteroviruses and parechoviruses increases with age. The incidence of infections and the prevalence of antibodies do not differ between boys and girls. Oral-oral transmission by way of the contaminated hands of health care personnel and transmission by fomites have been documented on a long-term care pediatric ward.[159] Echovirus 18 was isolated from human breast milk, and it was possible that enterovirus transmission to the baby occurred through the breast milk.[160] Chang and colleagues[161] detected coxsackievirus B3 in breast milk of two symptomatic mothers, and their babies both suffered severe illnesses with hepatic necrosis and meningitis caused by coxsackievirus B3.

GEOGRAPHIC DISTRIBUTION AND SEASONALITY

Enteroviruses and parechoviruses have a worldwide distribution.* Neutralizing antibodies for specific viral types have been found in serologic surveys throughout the world, and most strains have been recovered in worldwide isolation studies. In any one area, there are frequent fluctuations in predominant types. Epidemics probably depend on new susceptible persons in the population rather than on reinfections; they may be localized and sporadic and may vary in cause from place to place in the same year. Pandemic waves of infection also occur.

In temperate climates, enteroviral infections occur primarily in the summer and fall, but in the tropics, they are prevalent all year.[14,135,164] A basic concept in understanding their epidemiology is the far greater frequency of unrecognized infection than that of clinical disease. This is illustrated by poliomyelitis, which remained an epidemiologic mystery until it was appreciated that unrecognized infections were the main source of contagion. Serologic surveys were instrumental in elucidating the problem. In populations living in conditions of poor sanitation and hygiene, epidemics do not occur, but wide dissemination of polioviruses has been confirmed by demonstrating the presence of specific antibodies to all three types in nearly 100% of children by the age of 5 years.

Epidemics of poliomyelitis first began to appear in Europe and the United States during the latter part of the 19th century; they continued with increasing frequency in the economically advanced countries until the introduction of effective vaccines in the 1950s and 1960s.[39,40,164,165] The evolution from endemic to epidemic follows a characteristic pattern, beginning with collections of a few cases, then endemic rates that are higher than usual, followed by severe epidemics with high attack rates.

The age group attacked in endemic areas and in early epidemics is the youngest one; more than 90% of paralytic cases begin in children younger than 5 years. After a pattern of epidemicity begins, it is irreversible unless preventive vaccination is carried out. Because epidemics recur over a period of years, there is a shift in age incidence such that relatively fewer cases are in the youngest children; the peak often occurs in the 5- to 14-year-old group, and an increasing proportion is in young adults. These changes are correlated with socioeconomic factors and improved standards of hygiene; when children are protected from immunizing infections in the first few years of life, the pool of susceptible persons builds up, and introduction of a virulent strain often is followed by an epidemic.[166] Extensive use of vaccines in the past 5 decades has resulted in elimination of paralytic poliomyelitis from large geographic areas, but the disease remains endemic in various parts of the world. Although seasonal periodicity is distinct in temperate climates, some viral activity does take place during the winter.[167] Infection and acquisition of postinfection immunity occur with greater intensity and at earlier ages among crowded, economically deprived populations with less efficient sanitation facilities.

Molecular techniques have allowed the study of genotypes of specific viral types in populations over time.[167-170]

*References 7, 14, 135, 157, 162, 163, 163a.

For example, Mulders and colleagues[171] studied the molecular epidemiology of wild poliovirus type 1 in Europe, the Middle East, and the Indian subcontinent. They found four major genotypes circulating. Two genotypes were found predominantly in Eastern Europe, a third genotype was circulating mainly in Egypt, and the fourth genotype was widely dispersed. All four genotypes were found in Pakistan.

The epidemiologic behavior of nonpolio enteroviruses and parechoviruses parallels that of polioviruses; unrecognized infections far outnumber those with distinctive symptoms. The agents are disseminated widely throughout the world, and outbreaks related to one or another type of virus occur regularly. These outbreaks tend to be localized, with different agents being prevalent in different years. In the late 1950s, however, echovirus 9 had a far wider circulation, sweeping through a large part of the world and infecting children and young adults. This behavior has been repeated occasionally with other enteroviruses; after a long absence, a particular agent returns and circulates among the susceptible persons of different ages who have been born since the previous epidemic occurred. Other agents remain endemic in a given area, surfacing as sporadic cases and occasionally as small outbreaks. Multiple types are frequently active at the same time, although one agent commonly predominates in a given locality.

There are no available data on the incidence of symptomatic congenital and neonatal enteroviral infections. From the frequency of reports in the literature, it appears that severe neonatal disease caused by enteroviruses decreased slightly during the late 1960s and early 1970s and then became more common again. In 2007, there was an increase in the detection of severe neonatal disease caused by coxsackievirus B1 infection, which has subsequently persisted as the most common enterovirus type reported to the National Enterovirus Surveillance System.[172,173]

Although more than 100 nonpolio enterovirus types and 16 parechovirus types have been identified, only 24 different virus types have been noted in the 48 years from 1961 to 2005. The five most prevalent nonpolio enterovirus isolations per year in the United States are shown in Table 25-4.[11,174-181] Most patients from whom viruses were isolated had neurologic illnesses. It is possible that other enteroviruses were also prevalent but did not produce clinical disease severe enough to cause physicians to submit specimens for study. Many coxsackievirus A infections, even in epidemics, have probably gone undiagnosed because suckling mouse inoculation was not performed. The use of molecular detection methods may better reveal these in the future.

An analysis of the Centers for Disease Control and Prevention (CDC) nonpolio enterovirus data for 14 years found that early isolates in a particular year were predictive of isolates for the remainder of that year.[181] The six most common isolates during March, April, and May were predictive of 59% of the total isolates during July through December of the same year. Khetsuriani and associates[36] at the CDC presented an extensive report on enterovirus surveillance in the United States for the period 1970 to 2005. During this period, the five most common enterovirus isolates, in order, have been echovirus 9, echovirus 11, echovirus 30, coxsackievirus B5, and echovirus 6. During the most recent period (2006-2008), the most common isolates, in order, have been coxsackievirus B1, echovirus 6, echovirus 9, echovirus 18, and coxsackievirus A9.[173] Similar data are available for the most common enteroviral isolates in Spain from 1988 to 1997 and in Belgium from 1980 to 1994.[182,183] The most common enterovirus isolated in both countries was echovirus 30. In 1997 and 1998, major epidemic disease caused by enterovirus 71 occurred in Taiwan, Malaysia, Australia, and Japan[183-187] Similar outbreaks have since continued in other countries such as Australia and in Southeast Asia.[188-197]

Live-attenuated trivalent polioviral vaccine was used until 2000 in the United States and has eliminated epidemic poliomyelitis in the Western Hemisphere. It is unclear if circulation of the polio vaccine strains had any effects on enteroviral ecology. In 1970, polioviruses accounted for only 6% of the total enteroviral isolations from patients with neurologic illnesses.[198] Although the figures are not directly comparable, more than one third of the enteroviral isolations in 1962 from similar patients were polioviruses.[199] However, Horstmann and associates[200] studied specimens from sewage and asymptomatic children during the vaccine era and found that the number of yearly polioviral isolations (presumably vaccine strains) was greater than the number of nonpolio enteroviruses. However, the prevalence of oral polio vaccine viruses did not seem to affect the seasonal epidemiology of other enteroviruses.

TRANSPLACENTAL TRANSMISSION

Polioviruses

Poliovirus infections in pregnancy can result in abortion, stillbirth, neonatal disease, or no evidence of fetal involvement.[201] Gresser and associates[202] have shown that the human amniotic membrane in organ culture can be infected, resulting in a persistent low-grade infection. It has been observed on many occasions that maternal poliomyelitis occurring late in pregnancy has resulted in transplacental transmission of the virus to the fetus in utero.[203-224] The evidence that transplacental passage of virus occurs in early pregnancy is meager. Schaeffer and colleagues[216] were able to recover virus from the placenta and the fetus after a spontaneous abortion in a 24-year-old woman with poliomyelitis.

Although attenuated poliovirus vaccines have been given to pregnant women, there has never been a search for the transplacental passage of vaccine virus.[225-227] Viremia occurs after oral administration of polio vaccine, and, on occasion, this virus probably is passed transplacentally to the fetus.[228-235]

Coxsackieviruses

Several investigators have studied coxsackievirus infections in pregnant animals and the transplacental passage of virus to the fetus. Dalldorf and Gifford[236] studied two strains of coxsackievirus B1 and one of coxsackievirus A8 in gravid mice. In only one instance (coxsackievirus B1) were they able to recover virus from a fetus. They thought that this result was inconclusive because they were unable to recover virus in five other instances. Berger and Roulet[237] observed muscle lesions in the young of gravid mice infected with coxsackieviruses A1 and B1. Selzer[238] studied several

Table 25-4 Predominant Types of Nonpolio Enteroviral Isolations in the United States: 1961-2008*

	FIVE MOST COMMON VIRAL TYPES PER YEAR				
	First	**Second**	**Third**	**Fourth**	**Fifth**
1961	Coxsackievirus B5	Coxsackievirus B2	Coxsackievirus B4	Echovirus 11	Echovirus 9
1962	Coxsackievirus B3	Echovirus 9	Coxsackievirus B2	Echovirus 4	Coxsackievirus B5
1963	Coxsackievirus B1	Coxsackievirus A9	Echovirus 9	Echovirus 4	Coxsackievirus B4
1964	Coxsackievirus B4	Coxsackievirus B2	Coxsackievirus A9	Echovirus 4	Echovirus 6, coxsackievirus B1
1965	Echovirus 9	Echovirus 6	Coxsackievirus B2	Coxsackievirus B5	Coxsackievirus B4
1966	Echovirus 9	Coxsackievirus B2	Echovirus 6	Coxsackievirus B5	Coxsackievirus A9, A16
1967	Coxsackievirus B5	Echovirus 9	Coxsackievirus A9	Echovirus 6	Coxsackievirus B2
1968	Echovirus 9	Echovirus 30	Coxsackievirus A16	Coxsackievirus B3	Coxsackievirus B4
1969	Echovirus 30	Echovirus 9	Echovirus 18	Echovirus 6	Coxsackievirus B4
1970	Echovirus 3	Echovirus 9	Echovirus 6	Echovirus 4	Coxsackievirus B4
1971	Echovirus 4	Echovirus 9	Echovirus 6	Coxsackievirus B4	Coxsackievirus B2
1972	Coxsackievirus B5	Echovirus 4	Echovirus 6	Echovirus 9	Coxsackievirus B3
1973	Coxsackievirus A9	Echovirus 9	Echovirus 6	Coxsackievirus B2	Coxsackievirus B5, echovirus 5
1974	Echovirus 11	Echovirus 4	Echovirus 6	Echovirus 9	Echovirus 18
1975	Echovirus 9	Echovirus 4	Echovirus 6	Coxsackievirus A9	Coxsackievirus B4
1976	Coxsackievirus B2	Echovirus 4	Coxsackievirus B4	Coxsackievirus A9	Coxsackievirus B3, echovirus 6
1977	Echovirus 6	Coxsackievirus B1	Coxsackievirus B3	Echovirus 9	Coxsackievirus A9
1978	Echovirus 9	Echovirus 4	Coxsackievirus A9	Echovirus 30	Coxsackievirus B4
1979	Echovirus 11	Echovirus 7	Echovirus 30	Coxsackievirus B2	Coxsackievirus B4
1980	Echovirus 11	Coxsackievirus B3	Echovirus 30	Coxsackievirus B2	Coxsackievirus A9
1981	Echovirus 30	Echovirus 9	Echovirus 11	Echovirus 3	Coxsackievirus A9, echovirus 5
1982	Echovirus 11	Echovirus 30	Echovirus 5	Echovirus 9	Coxsackievirus B5
1983	Coxsackievirus B5	Echovirus 30	Echovirus 20	Echovirus 11	Echovirus 24
1984	Echovirus 9	Echovirus 11	Coxsackievirus B5	Echovirus 30	Coxsackievirus B2, A9
1985	Echovirus 11	Echovirus 21	Echovirus 6, 7†		Coxsackievirus B2
1986	Echovirus 11	Echovirus 4	Echovirus 7	Echovirus 18	Coxsackievirus B5
1987	Echovirus 6	Echovirus 18	Echovirus 11	Coxsackievirus A9	Coxsackievirus B2
1988	Echovirus 11	Echovirus 9	Coxsackievirus B4	Coxsackievirus B2	Echovirus 6
1989	Coxsackievirus B5	Echovirus 9	Echovirus 11	Coxsackievirus B2	Echovirus 6
1990	Echovirus 30	Echovirus 6	Coxsackievirus B2	Coxsackievirus A9	Echovirus 11
1991	Echovirus 30	Echovirus 11	Coxsackievirus B1	Coxsackievirus B2	Echovirus 7
1992	Echovirus 11	Echovirus 30	Echovirus 9	Coxsackievirus B1	Coxsackievirus A9
1993	Echovirus 30	Coxsackievirus B5	Coxsackievirus A9	Echovirus 7	Coxsackievirus B3
1994	Coxsackievirus B2	Coxsackievirus B3	Echovirus 6	Echovirus 30	Enterovirus 71
1995	Echovirus 9	Echovirus 11	Coxsackievirus A9	Coxsackievirus B2	Echovirus 30, coxsackievirus B5
1996	Coxsackievirus B5	Echovirus 17	Echovirus 6	Coxsackievirus A9	Coxsackievirus B4
1997	Echovirus 30	Echovirus 6	Echovirus 7	Echovirus 11	Echovirus 18
1998	Echovirus 30	Echovirus 9	Echovirus 11	Coxsackievirus B3	Echovirus 6
1999	Echovirus 11	Echovirus 16	Echovirus 9	Echovirus 14	Echovirus 25
2000	Coxsackievirus B5	Echovirus 6	Coxsackievirus A9	Coxsackievirus B4	Echovirus 11
2001	Echovirus 18	Echovirus 13	Coxsackievirus B2	Echovirus 6	Echovirus 4
2002	Echovirus 7	Echovirus 9	Coxsackievirus B1	Echovirus 11	Coxsackievirus B5
2003	Echovirus 9	Echovirus 30	Coxsackievirus B1	Coxsackievirus B4	Coxsackievirus A9
2004	Echovirus 30	Echovirus 9	Coxsackievirus A9	Coxsackievirus B5	Coxsackievirus B4
2005	Coxsackievirus B5	Echovirus 6	Echovirus 30	Echovirus 18	Coxsackievirus B3
2006	Echovirus 6	Echovirus 9	Coxsackievirus A9	Coxsackievirus B5	Coxsackievirus B3
2007	Coxsackievirus B1	Echovirus 18	Echovirus 9	Coxsackievirus B4	Echovirus 11
2008	Coxsackievirus B1	Echovirus 30	Echovirus 6	Echovirus 9	Echovirus 11

Data from references 174, 176-181, and 608 and from personal communication from A. LaMonte-Fowlkes, Epidemiology Branch, Division of Viral Diseases, National Center for Immunization and Respiratory Diseases, Centers for Disease Control and Prevention, Atlanta, for the 2005 data.

*The majority of patients from whom viruses were isolated had neurologic illnesses.

†Third- and fourth-place tie.

viruses in gravid mice; coxsackievirus A9 was found in the placentas of two mice but in no fetuses, and coxsackievirus A18 was not recovered from fetuses or placentas. Selzer[238] found that coxsackieviruses B3 and B4 passed the placental barrier. Soike[239] also observed that in the last week of pregnancy, coxsackievirus B3 reached fetal mice transplacentally. Modlin and Crumpacker[240] reported that infection in late gestational mice was more severe than that occurring in early pregnancy and that transplacental infection of the fetus occurred transiently during the maternal infection. Flamm[241] observed that coxsackievirus A9, when injected intravenously in rabbits, reached the blastocyst early in pregnancy and the amniotic fluid later in pregnancy. He also demonstrated congenital infection in mice with coxsackievirus A1.[242]

Palmer and coworkers[243] studied the gestational outcome in pregnant mice inoculated intravenously with the Theiler murine encephalomyelitis virus, a murine enterovirus. In early gestational infections, they found a high rate of placental and fetal abnormalities. The rates of fetal abnormalities and placental infection were greater than the rate of fetal viral infection, suggesting that the adverse effects of the viral infections were direct and indirect. Gestational infection could result in virus passage to the fetus and fetal damage or in placental compromise with indirect fetal damage.

In another study, using the same murine model with the Theiler murine encephalomyelitis virus, Abzug[244] found that maternal factors (i.e., compromised uteroplacental blood flow, concomitant infection, and advanced age) increased the risk of transplacental fetal infection.

In humans, the transplacental passage of coxsackieviruses at term has been documented on several occasions. Benirschke[245] studied the placentas in three cases of congenital coxsackievirus B disease and could find no histologic evidence of infection. In 1956, Kibrick and Benirschke[246] reported the first case of intrauterine infection with coxsackievirus B3. In this instance, the infant was delivered by cesarean section and had clinical evidence of infection several hours after birth. Brightman and colleagues[247] recovered coxsackievirus B5 from the placenta and rectum of a premature infant. No histologic abnormalities of the placenta were identified. Konstantinidon and associates[248] described the transplacental infection with coxsackievirus B3, which they confirmed using molecular techniques. At fetal autopsy they found mild arthrogryposis, necrotic meningoencephalitis with vascular calcifications, interstitial pneumonitis, mild myocardial hypertrophy, and chronic monocytic placental villitis. Coxsackievirus RNA was detected in placental tissue of six babies who had severe respiratory failure and subsequent nervous system sequelae.[249] Other evidence of intrauterine infection has been presented for coxsackieviruses A4 and B2 through B6.[250-258] More recently, a number of life-threatening cases of coxsackievirus B1 were noted to have their onset during the first day of life, suggesting intrauterine infection.[259,260]

Evidence for intrauterine infection during the first and second trimesters of pregnancy with coxsackieviruses is less clear. Burch and coworkers[261] reported the results of immunofluorescent studies of two fetuses of 5 months of gestation and one fetus of 6 months of gestation; the 6-month-old fetus had evidence of coxsackievirus B4 myocarditis, one 5-month-old fetus showed signs of coxsackievirus B3 infection, and the other 5-month-old fetus showed evidence of coxsackievirus B2, B3, and B4 infections. Basso and associates[250] recovered coxsackievirus B2 from the placenta, liver, and brain of a fetus after a spontaneous abortion at 3 months of gestation. Plager and coworkers[262] found no evidence of intrauterine viral transmission of coxsackievirus B5 infections during the first and second trimesters of pregnancy.

Euscher and associates[263] detected coxsackievirus RNA in placental tissue from six of seven newborn infants with respiratory difficulties and other manifestations at birth. Of these infants, one died shortly after birth, and the other six suffered neurodevelopmental delays. The placentas of 10 normal infants were examined for coxsackievirus RNA, and results of these studies were negative. Three of the placentas from the affected infants showed focal chronic villitis, two showed focal hemorrhagic endovasculitis, and one showed focal calcifications. In addition to respiratory distress, two neonates had rashes, two had seizures, two had thrombocytopenia, and one had intraventricular hemorrhage.

Echoviruses, Numbered Enteroviruses, and Parechoviruses

Less is known about transplacental passage of other enteroviruses than about that of coxsackieviruses and polioviruses. Women in all stages of pregnancy are frequently infected with echoviruses, and viremia is commonly seen in these infections.[264] In particular, epidemic disease related to echovirus 9 has been studied epidemiologically and serologically.[265-267] In these studies, a search for teratogenesis was performed, but no definitive virologic investigations have been carried out; asymptomatic transplacental infection might have occurred. Echoviruses 6, 7, 9, 11, 19, 27, 30, and 33 have been identified in cases of transplacentally acquired infections.[250,268-276] Otonkoski and coworkers[277] reported the occurrence of neonatal type 1 diabetes after a possible maternal echovirus 6 infection. Hughes and colleagues[278] reported a newborn with echovirus 14 infection who had a markedly elevated level of IgM (190mg/dL) on the sixth day of life; it seems likely that this infant was also infected in utero.

Despite these reports, transplacental echoviruses infections seem to be rare: Cherry and colleagues[254] cultured samples from 590 newborns during a period of enteroviral prevalence without isolating an echovirus. Antepartum serologic study of a group of 55 mothers in this study showed that 5 (9%) were actively infected with echovirus 17 during the 6-week period before delivery. In two other large nursery studies, there was no suggestion of intrauterine echovirus infections.[279,280]

Newer, numbered enteroviruses have also been associated with transplacental infection. Chow and associates[281] described a 1300-g fetus, which was stillborn after 26 weeks of gestation, with unilateral hydrocephalus, hepatosplenomegaly, fibrotic peritonitis, and meconium staining. Enterovirus 71 was isolated from the amniotic fluid, and the same virus was identified by polymerase chain reaction (PCR) assay in the cord blood and by immunohistochemical staining in the fetal midbrain and liver.

Berkovich and Smithwick[282] described a newborn without clinical illness and who had specific IgM parechovirus 1 antibody in the cord blood, suggesting intrauterine infection with this virus. In three studies of human parechovirus illnesses in neonates, symptoms have been noted on the first and second days of life, suggesting ascending infection or contact infection during birth.[37,283-285]

ASCENDING INFECTION AND CONTACT INFECTION DURING BIRTH

Definitive evidence is lacking for ascending infection or contact infection with enteroviruses during birth. In prospective studies of genital herpes simplex and cytomegaloviral infections, there have been no enteroviral isolations.[286,287] These results suggest that ascending infections with enteroviruses, if they occur at all, are rare. However, Reyes and associates[288] recovered coxsackievirus B5 from the cervix of four third-trimester pregnant women. Three of the four positive cultures were obtained 3 weeks or more before delivery. In the fourth case, the cervical culture was obtained the day before delivery, and the child was delivered by cesarean section. All of the infants were healthy, but unfortunately, culture for virus was possible only from the infant delivered by cesarean section; the result was negative. In an earlier study, Reyes and colleagues[272] reported a child who died of a disseminated echovirus 11 infection. The illness had its onset on the third day of life, and the virus was recovered from the mother's cervix at that time.

Enteroviral infection during the birth process seems probable.[28,254,289] The fecal carriage rate of enteroviruses in asymptomatic adult patients varies between 0% and 6% or higher in different population groups.[290-292] Cherry and associates[254] found that in 2 (4%) of 55 mothers, enteroviruses were present in the feces shortly after delivery. Katz,[293] in a discussion of a child with neonatal coxsackievirus B4 infection, suggested that the infant might have inhaled maternally excreted organisms during birth. The fact that this child had pneumonia tends to support the contention. Infections occurring 2 to 7 days after birth could have been acquired during passage through the birth canal.

NEONATAL INFECTION

Neonatal infections and illnesses from enteroviruses are relatively common.[294] Transmission of enteroviruses to newborns is similar to that for populations of older people. The main factor in the spread of virus is human-to-human contact. During the summer and fall of 1981 in Rochester, New York, 666 neonates were cultured for enteroviruses within 24 hours of birth and then weekly for 1 month.[272] The incidence of acquisition of nonpolio enteroviral infections during this period was 12.8%. Two risk factors were identified: lower socioeconomic status and lack of breastfeeding.

Polioviruses

Clinical poliomyelitis is rare in neonates, but the infection rate before the vaccine era was never determined. It is probable that the rarity of neonatal poliomyelitis was not related to lack of viral transmission but reflected the protection against clinically evident disease offered by specific, transplacentally transmitted antibodies directed against poliovirus. From experience gained in vaccine studies, it is apparent that infants with passively acquired antibody can be regularly infected.[295-307]

In 1955, Bates[207] reviewed the literature on poliomyelitis in infants younger than 1 month. He described six infants who apparently were not infected by their mothers and who had had other likely contacts. A neighbor was the contact in one case, siblings in two cases, nursery nurses in two cases, and an uncle in the sixth case. In most other infants, the mother had had poliomyelitis shortly before the child was born and probably was the contact. The mode of transmission—intrauterine, during birth, or postnatal contact—is unknown.

Bergeisen and colleagues[308] reported a case of paralytic poliomyelitis from a type 3 vaccine viral strain. They suggested that the source of this virus might have been the child of the neonate's babysitter, who was vaccinated about 2 weeks before the onset of the illness.

Coxsackieviruses

Several epidemics with coxsackieviruses B in newborn nurseries have been studied. Brightman and coworkers [247] observed an epidemic of coxsackievirus B5 in a premature nursery. Their data suggested that the virus was introduced into this nursery by an infant with a clinically inapparent infection who had been infected in utero. Secondary infections occurred in 12 infants and two nurses. The timing of the secondary cases suggested that three generations of infection had occurred and that the nurses had been infected during the second generation. The investigators suggested that the infection had spread from infant to infant and from infant to nurse.

Javett and colleagues[309] documented an acute epidemic of myocarditis associated with coxsackievirus B3 infection in a Johannesburg maternity home. Unfortunately, no epidemiologic investigation or search for asymptomatic infected infants was performed. However, analysis of the onset dates of the illnesses indicated that single infections occurred for five generations, and then five children became ill within a 3-day period.

Kipps and colleagues[310] carried out epidemiologic investigations in two coxsackievirus B3 nursery epidemics. In the first epidemic, the initial infection was probably transmitted from a mother to her child; this infant was then the source of five secondary cases in newborns and one illness in a nurse. Infants with four of the five secondary cases were located on one side of the nursery, but only one cot was close to the cot of the index patient, and this cot did not adjoin the cots of the three other infants with contact cases. In the second outbreak, an infant who also was infected by his mother probably introduced the virus into the nursery. Infants with the three secondary cases were geographically far removed from the one with the primary case of infection.

There have been many other instances of isolated nursery infections and small outbreaks with coxsackieviruses, and it seems that the most consistent source of original nursery infection is transmission from a mother to her child,[309-349] but introduction of virus into the nursery by personnel also occurs.[325,350]

Echoviruses and Parechoviruses

Although many outbreaks of echovirus infections have been observed in newborn nurseries, information on viral transmission is incomplete.[31,351-383] Cramblett and coworkers[354] reported an outbreak of echovirus 11 disease in four infants in an intensive care nursery. All infants were in enclosed incubators, and three patients became ill within 24 hours; the fourth child became ill 4 days later. Echovirus 11 was recovered from two members of the nursery staff. These data suggest that transmission from personnel to infants occurred because of inadequate hand washing. In another outbreak in an intensive care unit (ICU), the initial patient was transferred to the nursery because of severe echovirus 11 disease.[372] After transfer, infection occurred in the senior house officer and a psychologist in the unit. It was inferred by the investigators that spread by respiratory droplets to nine other infants occurred from these infected personnel.

In a maternity unit outbreak of echovirus 11 involving six secondary cases,[368] infection spread through close contact between the infected newborns and the nurses. In another reported nosocomial echovirus 11 outbreak, infants in an intermediate care unit for more than 2 days were more likely to become infected than those who were there for less than 2 days. Illness was also associated with gavage feeding, mouth care, and being a twin.[365]

Modlin[31] reviewed reports of 16 nursery echovirus outbreaks involving 206 ill infants. In only 4 of the 16 outbreaks was the source identified, and in all 4, the primary case was an infant who acquired infection vertically from its mother. After introduction of an infected newborn into a nursery, spread to other infants by personnel is common.[371,375,378,379] Risk factors for nursery transmission as described by Rabkin and coworkers[375] were "lower gestational age or birth weight, antibiotic or transfusion therapy, nasogastric intubation or feeding, proximity in the nursery to the index patient, and care by the same nurse during the same shift as the index patient."

Wilson and associates[378] reported an intensive care nursery epidemic in which respiratory syncytial virus and echovirus 7 infections occurred concurrently. This epidemic persisted from January to June 1984 despite an aggressive isolation cohorting program. A major factor in persistence was asymptomatic infections with both viruses.

Sato and associates[384] reported a point-source outbreak of echovirus 33 infection in nine newborns related to one nursery over a 10-day period. The primary case was born to a mother who was febrile and who had a high echovirus 33 neutralizing antibody titer in a convalescent-phase serum specimen.

Jack and colleagues[363] observed the endemic occurrence of asymptomatic infection with parechovirus 1 in a nursery during an 8-month period. A total of 44 infants were infected during this time, and nursery infection occurred when there was no known activity of parechovirus 1 in the community at large. The investigators believed that the endemic viral infection was spread by fecal contamination of hands of nursery personnel.

Nakao and colleagues[373] and Berkovich and Pangan[352] also documented parechovirus 1 infections in nurseries. Like Jack and colleagues,[363] they observed that the infections seemed to be endemic to the nurseries rather than related to community epidemics. More recently in July 2009, an outbreak of human parechovirus type 1 occurred in a neonatal unit in Croatia.[283] This involved seven neonates with respiratory and/or gastrointestinal symptoms. The source of this outbreak was not discussed.

Pathogenesis

EVENTS DURING PATHOGENESIS

Congenital infections with enteroviruses result from transplacental passage of virus to fetus. The method of transport from mother to fetus is poorly understood. Maternal viremia during enteroviral infections is common, and because virus has been recovered from the placenta on several occasions, it is probable that active infection of the placenta also occurs. Benirschke[245] found no histologic evidence of placental disease in three cases of established transplacentally acquired coxsackievirus B infections. Batcup and associates[385] found diffuse perivillous fibrin deposition with villous necrosis and inflammatory cell infiltration of the placenta in a woman who 2 weeks earlier, at 33 weeks of gestation, had coxsackievirus A9 meningitis. The woman was delivered of a macerated, stillborn infant. At birth, virus was recovered from the placenta but not from the stillborn infant.

It is assumed that infection in the fetus results from hematogenous dissemination initiated in the involved placenta. It is also possible that some in utero infection results from the ingestion of virus contained in amniotic fluid; in this situation, primary fetal infection involves the pharynx and lower alimentary tract. The portal of entry of infection during the birth process and the neonatal period is similar to that for older children and adults.

Figure 25-4 shows a schematic diagram of the events of pathogenesis. After initial acquisition of virus by the oral or respiratory route, implantation occurs in the pharynx and the lower alimentary tract. Within 1 day, the infection extends to the regional lymph nodes. On about the third day, minor viremia occurs, resulting in involvement of many secondary infection sites. In congenital infections, infection is initiated during the minor viremia phase. Multiplication of virus in secondary sites coincides with the onset of clinical symptoms. Illness can vary from minor to fatal infections. Major viremia occurs during the period of multiplication of virus in the secondary infection sites; this period usually lasts from the third to the seventh days of infection. In many echovirus and coxsackievirus infections, CNS involvement apparently occurs at the same time as other secondary organ involvement. This occasionally appears to happen with polioviral infections; however, more commonly, the CNS symptoms of poliomyelitis are delayed, suggesting that seeding occurred later in association with the major viremia.

Cessation of viremia correlates with the appearance of serum antibody. The viral concentration in secondary infection sites begins to diminish on about the seventh day. However, infection continues in the lower intestinal tract for prolonged periods.

FACTORS THAT AFFECT PATHOGENESIS

The pathogenesis and pathology of enterovirus and parechovirus infections depend on the virulence, tropism, and inoculum concentration of virus, as well as on many specific host factors. Enteroviruses have marked differences in tropism and virulence. Although some generalizations can be made in regard to tropism, there are marked differences even among strains of specific viral types.

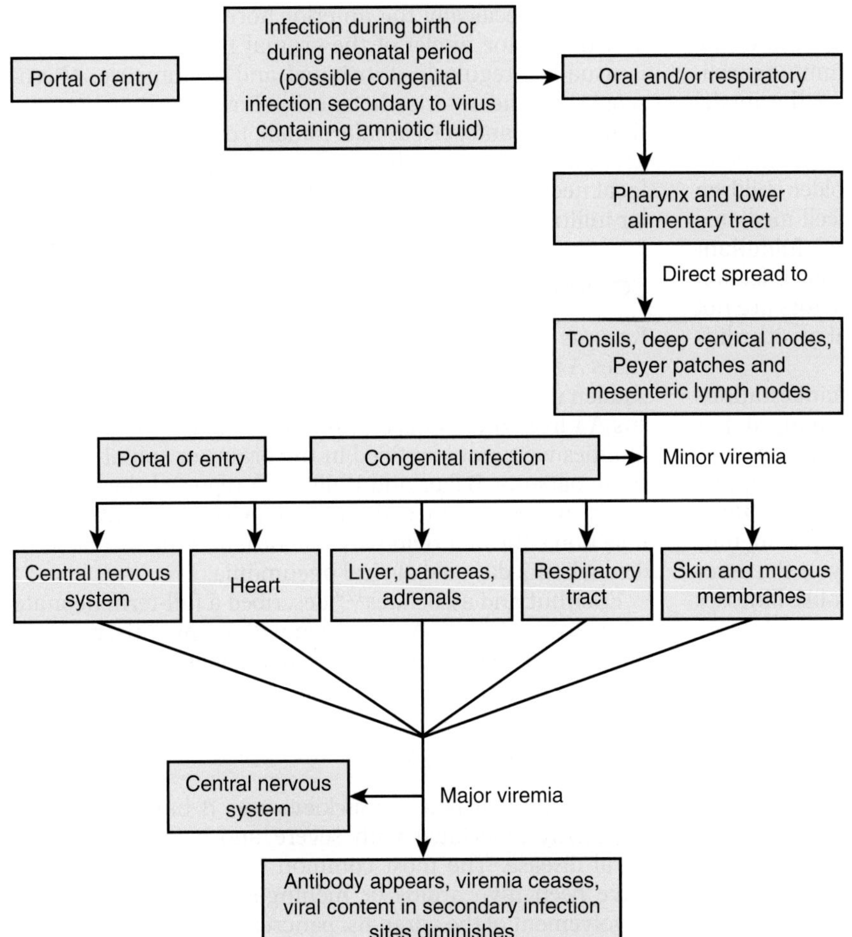

Figure 25-4 Pathogenesis of congenital and neonatal enterovirus infections.

Differences in virulence of specific enteroviral types may be the result of recombination among enteroviruses or point mutations.[385-387]

Enterovirus infections of the fetus and neonate are thought to be more severe than similar infections in older individuals. This is undoubtedly true for coxsackievirus B infections and probably also true for coxsackievirus A, echovirus, and poliovirus infections. Although the reasons for this increased severity are largely unknown, several aspects of neonatal immune mechanisms offer clues. The similarity of coxsackievirus B infections in suckling mice to those in human neonates has provided a useful animal model. Heineberg and coworkers[388] compared coxsackievirus B1 infections in 24-hour-old suckling mice with similar infections in older mice. They observed that adult mice produced interferon (IFN) in all infected tissues, whereas in suckling mice, only small amounts of IFN were identified in the liver. They thought that the difference in outcome of coxsackievirus B1 infections in suckling and older mice could be explained by the inability of the cells of the immature animal to elaborate IFN. Additional studies of abnormalities of innate immunity in neonates may enhance our understanding of the severity of enterovirus infections in newborns.[389]

Others thought that the increased susceptibility of suckling mice to severe coxsackievirus infections was related to the transplacentally acquired, increased concentrations of adrenocortical hormones.[390,391] Kunin[392] suggested that the difference in age-specific susceptibility might be explained at the cellular level. He showed that a variety of tissues of newborn mice bound coxsackievirus B3, whereas tissues of adult mice were virtually inactive in this regard.[392,393] It has been suggested that the progressive loss of receptor-containing cells or of receptor sites on persisting cells with increasing age might be the mechanism that accounts for infections of lesser severity in older animals. Supporting this suggestion, Ito and colleagues[394] showed that expression of the coxsackie and adenovirus receptor (CAR) (see Table 25-3) decreases as rats age. Teisner and Haahr[395] suggested that the increased susceptibility of suckling mice to severe and fatal coxsackievirus infections might be from physiologic hypothermia and poikilothermia during the first week of life.

In the past, it was assumed that specific pathology in various organs and tissues in enteroviral infections was caused by the direct cytopathic effect and tropism of a particular virus. However, a large number of studies using murine myocarditis model systems have suggested that host immune responses contribute to the pathology.[1,386,396-411] These studies suggest that T-cell–mediated processes and virus-induced autoimmunity cause acute and chronic tissue damage. Other studies suggest that the primary viral cytopathic effect is responsible for tissue damage and that various T-cell responses are a response to the damage, not the cause.[412] A review of various murine myocarditis model systems suggests that the genetics of the hosts and of the viral strains determine the likelihood of autoimmune, cell-mediated cellular damage.[†] However, none of the model systems is appropriate for the evaluation of the pathogenesis of neonatal myocarditis. Although available studies suggest that enterovirus-induced myocarditis in older children and adults occasionally may have a delayed cell-mediated component, the short incubation period and fulminant nature of neonatal disease, as well as the similar infection in suckling mice, suggest that autoimmune factors are not major in the pathogenesis of acute enteroviral myocarditis in neonates.

During the last 45 years, the clinical manifestations caused by several enteroviral serotypes have changed. For example, echovirus 11 infection initially was noted in association with an outbreak of upper respiratory infection in a day nursery more than 50 years ago.[413] Then in the 1960s, it was found to be related to exanthem and aseptic meningitis.[314,414] After this, and occurring presently, is the association of echovirus infection and severe sepsis-like illnesses with hepatitis in neonates.[‡]

Another example relates to enterovirus 71 infections. Initially, this virus was noted in association with aseptic meningitis, with only a small number of cases also having exanthem.[421,422] During the last several decades, severe epidemic disease with enterovirus 71 has occurred in Taiwan, Singapore, Australia, Malaysia, Japan, and other countries in Southeast Asia. In these epidemics, hand-foot-and-mouth syndrome is a major finding, and the neurologic disease is more severe than in the past.[188-197]

These phenotypic changes could be the result of point mutations or the result of recombination among enteroviruses.[§] Chan and AbuBakar[107] have presented evidence indicating that a recombination event occurred between enterovirus 71 and coxsackievirus A16.

Pathology

GENERAL CONSIDERATIONS

Great variations in the clinical signs of congenital and neonatal enterovirus infections are paralleled by wide variations in pathology. Because pathologic material usually is available only from patients with fatal illnesses, the discussion in this section considers only the more severe enteroviral manifestations. It is worth emphasizing, however, that these fatal infections account for only a small portion of all congenital and neonatal enterovirus infections. The pathologic findings in infants with milder infections, such as nonspecific febrile illness, have not been described.

POLIOVIRUSES

The pathologic findings in fatal neonatal poliomyelitis are similar to those seen in disease of older children and adults.[32,203,206,210,221] The major findings have involved the CNS, specifically the anterior horns of the spinal cord and the motor nuclei of the cranial nerves. Involvement is usually irregularly distributed and asymmetric. Microscopically, the anterior horn cells show neuronal destruction; gliosis; and perivascular, small, round cell infiltration. Myocarditis has also been observed,[206] characterized by focal necrosis of muscle fibers and various degrees of cellular infiltration.

COXSACKIEVIRUSES A

Records of neonatal illnesses associated with coxsackieviruses A are rare.[426-428] Gold and coworkers,[428] in a study of sudden unexpected death in infants, recovered coxsackievirus A4 from the brains of three children. Histologic abnormalities were not identified in the brains or spinal cords of these patients. Baker and Phillips[426] reported the death of twins in association with coxsackievirus A3 intrauterine infections; the first twin was stillborn, and the second twin died when 2 days old of viral pneumonia.

Eisenhut and associates[429] described a full-term neonate with coxsackievirus A9 infection with meningitis, myocarditis, and disseminated intravascular coagulation who died on the seventh day of life.

COXSACKIEVIRUSES B

Of the enteroviruses, coxsackieviruses B have been most frequently associated with severe and catastrophic neonatal disease. The most common findings in these cases have been myocarditis or meningoencephalitis, or both. Involvement of the adrenals, pancreas, liver, and lungs has occurred.

Brain and Spinal Cord

The meninges are congested, edematous, and occasionally mildly infiltrated with inflammatory cells.[‖] Lesions in the brain and spinal cord are focal rather than diffuse but frequently involve many different areas. The lesions consist of areas of eosinophilic degeneration of cortical cells, clusters of mononuclear and glial cells (Fig. 25-5), and perivascular cuffing. On occasion, areas of liquefaction necrosis unassociated with inflammation are seen.

Heart

Grossly, the heart is usually enlarged, with dilation of the chambers and flabby musculature.[¶] Microscopically, the pericardium frequently contains some inflammatory cells; and thickening, edema, and focal infiltrations of inflammatory cells may be found in the endocardium. The myocardium (Fig. 25-6) is congested and contains infiltrations of inflammatory cells (i.e., lymphocytes, mononuclear cells, reticulum cells, histiocytes, plasma cells, and polymorphonuclear and eosinophil leukocytes). Involvement of the myocardium is often patchy and focal but occasionally is diffuse. The muscle shows loss of striation, edema, and eosinophilic degeneration. Muscle necrosis without extensive cellular infiltration is common.

[†]References 385, 395-398, 400-403, 405, 407, 409.
[‡]References 270-272, 355, 370, 372, 375, 377, 415-420.
[§]Reference 107, 108, 110, 111, 113, 423-425.
[‖]References 246, 257, 293, 319, 322, 335, 430.
[¶]References 109, 246, 257, 309, 319, 322.

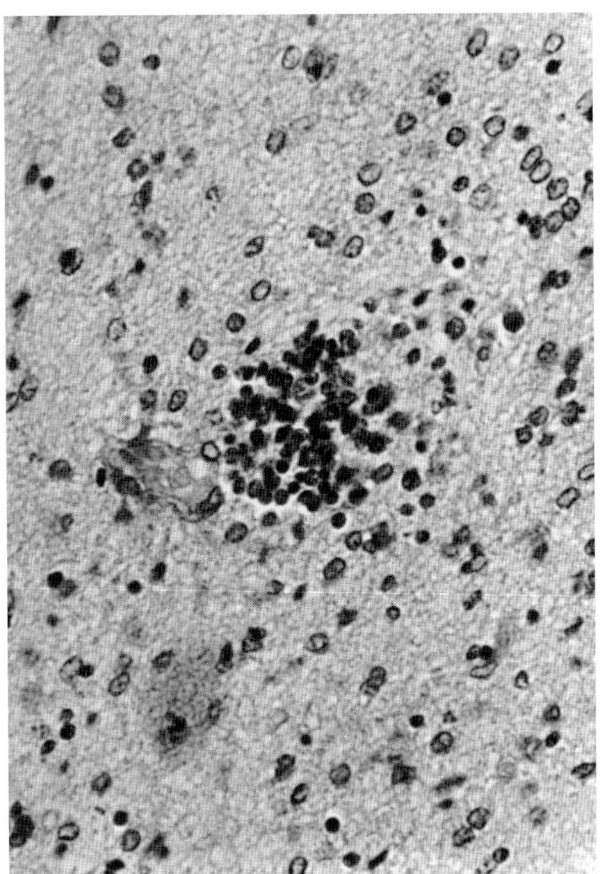

Figure 25-5 Coxsackievirus B4 encephalitis in a 9-day-old infant. Notice focal infiltrate of mononuclear and glial cells.

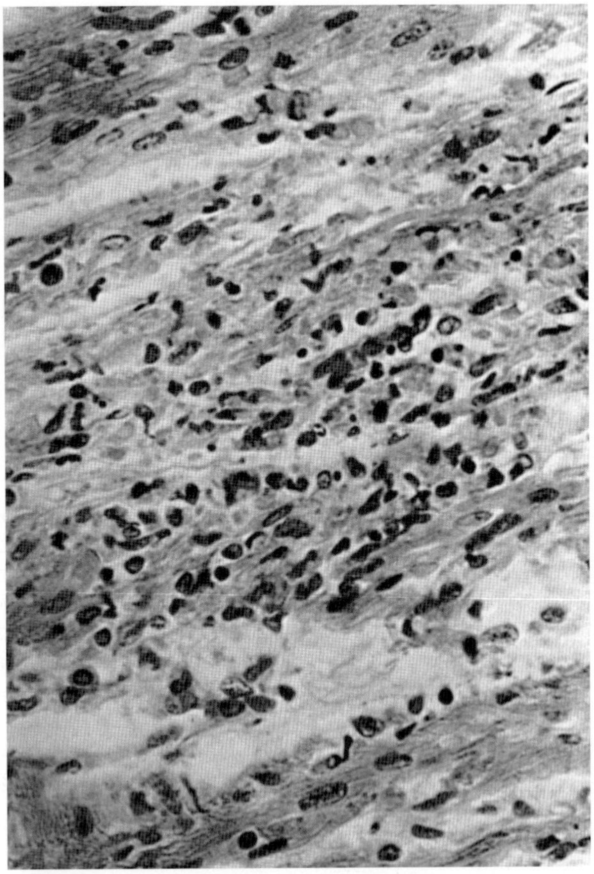

Figure 25-6 Coxsackievirus B4 myocarditis in a 9-day-old infant. Notice myocardial necrosis and mononuclear cellular infiltration.

Other Organs

The lungs commonly have areas of mild focal pneumonitis with peribronchiolar mononuclear cellular infiltrations.[246,293,322,335,431-433] Massive pulmonary hemorrhage has been observed. The liver is frequently engorged and occasionally contains isolated foci of liver cell necrosis and mononuclear cell infiltrations. A neonate with a coxsackievirus B1 infection developed a sepsis-like illness on the fourth day of life with severe hepatitis and subsequently developed progressive liver calcifications.[432] In the pancreas, infiltration of mononuclear cells, lymphocytes, and plasma cells has been observed, and occasional focal degeneration of the islet cells occurs. Congestion has been observed in the adrenal glands, with mild-to-severe cortical necrosis and infiltration of inflammatory cells.

ECHOVIRUSES

In an earlier period, although frequently responsible for neonatal illnesses, echoviruses were rarely associated with fatal infections. During the past 40 years, however, there have been many reports of fatal illnesses in newborns from echovirus type 11.[#] In virtually all cases, the major pathologic finding was massive hepatic necrosis; other findings included hemorrhagic necrosis of the adrenal glands, hemorrhage in other organs, myocardial necrosis, and acute tubular necrosis of the kidneys. Wang and colleagues[420] studied four neonates (three with echovirus 11 and one with echovirus 5 infections) with fulminant hepatic failure and observed two histopathologic patterns associated with minimal inflammation but extensive hemorrhagic necrosis. One pattern indicated ongoing endothelial injury with endotheliitis and fibrinoid necrosis. The second pattern, which was seen in the two neonates who initially survived, was that of venoocclusive disease. Virus has not been identified in hepatocytes. Extensive myositis of the strap muscles of the neck occurred in one case.[417] Massive hepatic necrosis has also occurred in infections with echoviruses 3, 5, 6, 7, 9, 14, 19, 20, and 21.[*a] Wreghitt and associates[438] described a neonate with a fatal echovirus 7 infection. This infant was found to have massive disseminated intravascular coagulation, with bleeding in the adrenal glands, renal medulla, liver, and cerebellum.

At autopsy, one infant with echovirus 6 infection was found to have cloudy and thickened leptomeninges, liver necrosis, adrenal and renal hemorrhage, and mild interstitial pneumonitis.[419] One infant with echovirus 9 infection had an enlarged and congested liver with marked central necrosis,[436] and another with this virus had interstitial pneumonitis without liver involvement.[269] Three infants with echovirus 11 infections had renal and adrenal hemorrhage and small-vessel thrombi in the renal medulla and in

---

#References 31, 270, 273, 368, 415-419, 432.

*aReferences 24, 268, 278, 370, 420, 432, 434-437.

the medulla and the inner cortex of the adrenal glands.[372] In these patients, the livers were normal. Two infants, one with echovirus 6 and the other with echovirus 31 infection, had only extensive pneumonias.[367,439] Willems and colleagues[440] described an infant with echovirus 11 infection who had pneumonia, persistent pulmonary hypertension, and purpura fulminans.

PARECHOVIRUSES

Neonatal parechovirus type 3 infections often involve the CNS, and extensive white matter injury has been repeatedly noted.[441-443]

Clinical Manifestations

In this section, we present clinical manifestations by the specific viral agents and also by serotypes of the specific viruses. However, in recent years, a large number of enteroviral and parechoviral infections are now diagnosed by PCR assay, and serotype information is not always available. Because of this, much of the specific information in this section was determined more than 2 decades ago. In recent years, phenotypic presentations have been altered by recombination between different enteroviruses, and therefore clinical characteristics of specific enteroviral types today may be different from the findings identified 4 and 5 decades ago.

ABORTION

Polioviruses

Poliomyelitis is associated with an increased incidence of abortion. Horn[201] reported 43 abortions in 325 pregnancies complicated by maternal poliomyelitis. Abortion was directly related to the severity of the maternal illness, including the degree of fever during the acute phase of illness. However, abortion also was associated with mild, nonparalytic poliomyelitis. Schaeffer and colleagues[216] studied the placenta and abortus 12 days after the onset of illness in a mother. Poliovirus type 1 was isolated from the placenta and the fetal tissues.

Other investigators[439,444-447] have reported an increased incidence of abortions in cases of maternal poliomyelitis. Siegel and Greenberg[220] noticed that fetal death occurred in 14 (46.7%) of 30 instances of maternal poliomyelitis during the first trimester. Kaye and colleagues[448] reviewed the literature in 1953 and found 19 abortions in 101 cases of poliomyelitis in pregnancy. In a small study in Evanston Hospital in Illinois, the abortion rate associated with maternal poliomyelitis was little different from the expected rate.[446] In a study of 310 pregnant women who received trivalent OPV, there was no increase in abortions above the expected rate.[226] In a later study in Finland that involved about 9000 pregnant women immunized with OPV, there was no evidence of an increase in stillbirths.[449]

Coxsackieviruses

Although in the late 1950s and early 1960s there were extensive outbreaks of illness caused by coxsackievirus A16, there was no evidence of adverse outcomes of pregnancy related to this virus. Because infections with other coxsackieviruses rarely involve large segments of the population, rate studies have not been performed.

Frisk and Diderholm[450] found that 33% of women with abortions had IgM antibody to coxsackieviruses B, whereas only 8% of controls had similar antibody. In a second, larger study, the same research group confirmed their original findings.[451]

Echoviruses

There is no available evidence suggesting that echovirus infections during pregnancy are a cause of spontaneous abortion. Landsman and associates[266] studied 2631 pregnancies during an epidemic of echovirus 9 and could find no difference in antibody to echovirus 9 between mothers who aborted and those who delivered term infants. A similar study in Finland revealed no increase in the abortion rate among mothers infected in early pregnancy with echovirus 9.[267]

Parechoviruses

Ljungan virus (a parechovirus) is endemic in some rodent populations, and it can cause fetal death in these animals.[452-454] It has been suggested that this virus may be the cause of some intrauterine deaths in humans. In one study, both PCR assay and immunohistochemical staining identified Ljungan virus in specimens from five human intrauterine fetal deaths.[454]

PREMATURITY AND STILLBIRTHS

Polioviruses

In the study by Horn[201] of 325 pregnancies, 9 infants died in utero. In each instance, the mother was critically ill with poliomyelitis. Horn[201] also observed that 45 infants weighed less than 6 pounds, and 17 of these had a birth weight of less than 5 pounds. These low-birth-weight infants were born predominantly to mothers who had had poliomyelitis early in pregnancy. A similar finding was reported by Aycock.[204,455] In New York City, Siegel and Greenberg[220] also documented an increase in prematurity after maternal poliomyelitis infection. This was specifically related to maternal paralytic poliomyelitis. There has been no observation of stillbirth or prematurity in relation to vaccine administration.[449]

Coxsackieviruses

Bates[251] reported a fetus of 8 months of gestational age who was stillborn and had calcific pancarditis and hydrops fetalis at autopsy. Fluorescent antibody study revealed coxsackievirus B3 antigen in the myocardium. Burch and colleagues[261] described three stillborn infants who had fluorescent antibody evidence of coxsackievirus B myocarditis, one each with coxsackieviruses B2, B3, or B4. They also reported a premature boy who had histologic and immunofluorescent evidence of cardiac infection with coxsackieviruses B2 through B4; he lived only 24 hours. A macerated stillborn girl was delivered 2 weeks after the occurrence of aseptic meningitis caused by coxsackievirus A9 in a 27-year-old woman.[385] Virus was recovered from the placenta but not from the infant. Coxsackievirus B6 has been recovered from the brain, liver, and placenta of a stillborn infant.[250] A baby of 26 weeks of gestation with nonimmune hydrops fetalis with an intrauterine infection with coxsackievirus B3 was reported by Ouellet and coworkers.[456]

Echoviruses and Numbered Enteroviruses

Freedman[457] reported the occurrence of a full-term, fresh stillbirth in a woman infected with echovirus 11. Because the infant had no pathologic or virologic evidence of infection, he attributed the event to a secondary consequence of maternal infection from fever and dehydration rather than primary transplacental infection. Echovirus 27 has been associated with intrauterine death on two occasions.[250,274]

In an extensive study of neonatal enteroviral infections in Milwaukee in 1979, Piraino and associates[273] found that 12 of 19 stillbirths occurred from July through October, coincident with a major outbreak of enterovirus disease. Echovirus 11 was the main agent isolated during this period. A 1300-g fetus, stillborn after 26 weeks of gestation, had hydrocephalus, fibrotic peritonitis, and hepatosplenomegaly and was found to have an enterovirus 71 infection by PCR assay and immunohistochemical study.[281]

CONGENITAL MALFORMATIONS

Polioviruses

The congenital malformation rate associated with poliovirus infection, as determined in the National Institutes of Health (NIH)-sponsored Collaborative Perinatal Research Project of 45,000 pregnancies, was 4.1%.[458] Although isolated instances of congenital malformation and maternal poliomyelitis have been reported, there is little statistical evidence demonstrating that polioviruses are teratogens. In their review of the literature, Kaye and colleagues[448] identified six anomalies in 101 infants born to mothers with poliomyelitis during pregnancy. In the reviews of Horn,[201] Bates,[207] and Siegel and Greenberg,[220] there was no evidence of maternal poliovirus infection–induced anomalies.

The possibility of congenital anomalies associated with attenuated OPV has also been studied.[225,226,448,458-460] Pearson and coworkers[225] studied the fetal malformation rate in a community in which a large vaccine field trial had been carried out; although it is probable that pregnant women became infected with vaccine virus by secondary spread, there was no community increase in fetal malformations. Prem and associates[226] studied the infants of 69 women who received attenuated vaccine before 20 weeks of gestation and found that none had anomalies. In contrast, the rate of congenital defects in Blackburn, England, increased coincident with mass vaccination with trivalent poliomyelitis vaccine.[459] However, there is no evidence of cause and effect related to this observation. Connelly and colleagues[460] commented on a child with a unique renal disease acquired in utero. The child's mother had received OPV during the second month of pregnancy.

In February 1985, a mass vaccination program with live OPV was carried out in Finland.[461] Although pregnant women received vaccine, there was no evidence that vaccine virus had a harmful effect on developing fetuses.

Coxsackieviruses

In a large prospective study, Brown,[462-464] Evans and Brown,[465] Brown and Evans,[466] and Brown and Karunas[467] made a serologic search for selected maternal enteroviral infections in association with congenital malformations. In one study,[467] serum samples from 22,935 women had been collected. From this group, serum samples from 630 mothers of infants with anomalies and from 1164 mothers of children without defects were carefully studied. Specifically, serologic evidence was sought for infection during the first trimester and last 6 months of pregnancy with coxsackieviruses B1 through B5 and A9 and with echoviruses 6 and 9. In this study, infants were examined for 113 specific abnormalities; these anomalies were grouped into 12 categories for analysis. The investigators demonstrated a positive correlation between maternal infection and infant anomaly with coxsackieviruses B2 through B4 and A9. The overall first-trimester infection rate with coxsackievirus B4 was significantly higher in patients with anomalies than that in control subjects. Maternal coxsackievirus B2 infection throughout pregnancy, coxsackievirus B4 infections during the first trimester of pregnancy, and infection with at least one of the five coxsackieviruses B during pregnancy were all associated with urogenital anomalies. Coxsackievirus A9 infection was associated with digestive anomalies, and coxsackieviruses B3 and B4 were associated with cardiovascular defects. When coxsackieviruses B were analyzed as a group (B1-B5), there was an overall association with congenital heart disease; the likelihood of cardiovascular anomalies was increased when maternal infection with two or more coxsackieviruses B occurred. In this study, the mothers had been instructed to keep illness diary sheets. There was no correlation between reported maternal clinical illnesses and serologic evidence of infection with the selected enteroviruses. This suggests that many infections that may have been causally related to the anomalies were asymptomatic. A disturbing finding in this study was the lack of seasonal occurrence of the births of children with specific defects. Because enteroviral transmission is most common in the summer and fall, the birth rate of children with malformations should have been greatest in the spring and summer if coxsackieviruses were a major cause of malformation.

In the NIH-sponsored Collaborative Perinatal Research Project, Elizan and coworkers[468] were unable to find any relationships between maternal infections with coxsackieviruses B and congenital CNS malformations. Scattered case reports in the literature describe congenital anomalies associated with maternal coxsackievirus infections. Makower and colleagues[256] reported a child with congenital malformations who was born at 32 weeks of gestation and from whom a coxsackievirus A4 strain was recovered from the meconium. The child's mother had been well throughout pregnancy, except for a febrile illness during the first month. The relationship of the viral infection to the congenital malformations or to the prematurity is uncertain.

Gauntt and associates[469] studied the ventricular fluids from 28 newborn infants with severe congenital anatomic defects of the CNS. In four infants (two with hydranencephaly, one with an occipital meningocele, and one with aqueductal stenosis), neutralizing antibody to one or more coxsackievirus B types was found in the fluid. In one case, IgM-neutralizing antibody to coxsackievirus B6 was found. The investigators concluded that their data suggested the possibility of an association between congenital infections with coxsackieviruses B and severe CNS defects.

Echoviruses

In the large prospective study of Brown and Karunas,[467] the possible association of maternal infections with echoviruses 6 and 9 and congenital malformations was examined. Maternal infection with these selected echoviruses apparently was not associated with any anomaly. In three other studies,[265-267] no association was found between maternal echovirus 9 infection and congenital malformation.

Parechoviruses

Niklasson and associates[453] studied CNS malformations in terminated pregnancies. Ljungan virus, generally considered a parechovirus of rodents, was identified in 9 of 10 cases of hydrocephalus and in 5 of 9 cases of anencephaly, whereas this virus was found in only one of 18 trisomy 21 control subjects.

NEONATAL INFECTION

Nonpolio Enteroviruses and Parechoviruses

Illnesses caused by nonpolio enteroviruses and parechoviruses are discussed by clinical classification (Table 25-5) in the following sections.

Inapparent Infection. Inapparent infections in neonates occasionally occur with many different enteroviruses and parechoviruses. Infections without evidence of illness have occurred with coxsackieviruses A9, B1, B4, and B5 and with echoviruses 3, 5, 9, 11, 13, 14, 20, 30, and 31.[†a] The incidence of such cases is unclear. Cherry and coworkers[254] studied 590 normal newborns during a 6-month period and found only one infection without clinical signs of illness, a child infected in utero or immediately thereafter with coxsackievirus B2. The mother had an upper respiratory illness 10 days before delivery. In a similar but more comprehensive study, Jenista and associates[294] failed to isolate any enteroviruses from cultures from 666 newborns on the first postpartum day. However, during weekly cultures during the month after birth, 75 enteroviruses were isolated. Symptomatic enteroviral disease occurred in 21% (16 of 75).

During a survey of perinatal virus infections, 44 infants were found to be infected with parechovirus 1 during the study period from May to December 1966.[363] The virus prevalence and the incidence of new infections during this period were fairly uniform. No illness was attributed to parechovirus 1 infection, and the virus disappeared from the nursery in mid-December 1966. Inapparent infections with parechovirus 1 have been reported on two other occasions.[352,373] In the present molecular virologic era, data suggest that subclinical human parechoviral infections are common in infants.[115] However, specific neonatal data are lacking in this regard.

Mild, Nonspecific Febrile Illness. In a review of 338 enteroviral infections in early infancy, 9% were classified as nonspecific febrile illnesses.[472] Illness may be sporadic in nature or part of an outbreak with a specific viral type. In the latter situation, clinical manifestations vary depending on the viral type; some infants have aseptic meningitis and other signs and symptoms, and some have only nonspecific fever. Coxsackievirus B5 and echovirus types 5, 11, and 33 have been those found most commonly in nonspecific fevers; other agents identified have included coxsackieviruses A9, A16, and B1 through B4; echoviruses 4, 7, 9, and 17; and human parechovirus types 1, 3, and 4.[‡a] A 6-day-old infant with parechovirus 4 and fever and poor feeding has been described.[476]

Mild, nonspecific febrile illness occurs most commonly in full-term infants after uneventful pregnancies and deliveries without complications. Illness can occur at any time during the first month of life. When the onset occurs after the infant is 7 days old, a careful history frequently reveals a trivial illness in a family member. The onset of illness is characterized by mild irritability and fever, which is usually in the range of 38° to 39° C, but higher temperatures occasionally occur. Poor feeding is frequently observed. One or two episodes of vomiting or diarrhea, or both, may occur in some infants. The usual duration of illness is 2 to 4 days.

Routine laboratory study is not helpful, but cerebrospinal fluid (CSF) examination may reveal an increased protein concentration and leukocyte count indicative of aseptic meningitis. Although, by definition, illness in this category is mild, the degree of viral infection may be extensive. When looked for, virus may be isolated from the blood, urine, and spinal fluid of infants with mild illnesses.[327,470]

Sepsis-like Illness. The major diagnostic problem in neonatal enteroviral and human parechovirus infections is differentiation of bacterial from viral disease. Even in the infant with mild, nonspecific fever, bacterial disease must be strongly considered. The sepsis-like illness described here is always alarming. This illness is characterized by fever, poor feeding, abdominal distention, irritability, rash, lethargy, and hypotonia.[433,477-479] Other findings include diarrhea, vomiting, seizures, shock, disseminated intravascular coagulation, thrombocytopenia, hepatomegaly, jaundice, and apnea. The onset of illness is introduced by irritability, poor feeding, and fever and followed within 24 hours by other manifestations. In a group of 27 neonates, Lake and associates[433] observed that 54% had temperatures of 39° C or higher. The duration of fever varies from 1 to 8 days, most commonly 3 to 4 days. Barre and colleagues[480] reported a 3-day-old boy with an enterovirus-associated hemophagocytic syndrome. This neonate presented with a typical sepsis-like picture with fever, hepatosplenomegaly, coagulopathy, thrombocytopenia, and anemia. This child recovered and had no hemophagocytic relapses.

Sepsis-like illness is common. Morens[472] described its occurrence in one fifth of 338 enteroviral infections in infants.

[†a] References 279, 280, 294, 326, 367, 372, 430, 457, 470-472.

[‡a] References 28, 254, 273, 294, 311, 327, 334, 340, 343, 351, 355, 359, 360, 364, 369, 372, 380, 470, 473-475.

Table 25-5 Major Manifestations of Neonatal Nonpolio Enteroviral and Parechoviral Infections

Specific Involvement	Common	Rare
Inapparent infection	Parechovirus 1	Coxsackievirus A9, B1, B2, B4, B5
		Echovirus 3, 5, 9, 11, 13, 14, 20, 30, 31
Mild, nonspecific, febrile illness	Coxsackievirus B5	Coxsackievirus B1, B2, B3, B4, A9, A16
	Echovirus 5, 11, 33	Echovirus 4, 7, 9, 17, 30
		Parechovirus 1, 3, 4
Sepsis-like illness	Coxsackievirus B2, B3, B4, B5	Coxsackievirus B1, A9
	Echovirus 5, 11, 15	Echovirus 2, 3, 4, 6, 9, 14, 19, 21
	Parechovirus 3	Parechovirus 1, 2
Respiratory illness (general)	Echovirus 11	Coxsackievirus B1, B4, B5, A9
	Parechovirus 1, 3	Echovirus 9, 17
Herpangina		Coxsackievirus A5
Coryza		Coxsackievirus A9
		Echovirus 11, 17, 19
		Parechovirus 1
Pharyngitis		Coxsackievirus B4
		Echovirus 11, 17, 18
Laryngotracheitis or bronchitis		Coxsackievirus B1, B4
		Echovirus 11
Pneumonia		Coxsackievirus B4, A9
		Echovirus 6, 9, 11, 17, 31
		Parechovirus 1
Cloud baby		Echovirus 20
Gastrointestinal		
Vomiting or diarrhea	Echovirus 5, 17, 18	Coxsackievirus B1, B2, B5
		Echovirus 4, 6, 8, 9, 11, 16, 19, 21
		Parechovirus 1
		Enterovirus 71
Hepatitis	Echovirus 11, 19	Coxsackievirus B1, B3, B4, A9
		Echovirus 5, 6, 7, 9, 14, 20, 21
		Parechoviruses
Pancreatitis		Coxsackievirus B3, B4, B5
Necrotizing enterocolitis		Coxsackievirus B2, B3
		Parechovirus 1
Cardiovascular		
Myocarditis and pericarditis	Coxsackievirus B1, B2, B3, B4	Coxsackievirus B5, A9
		Echovirus 11, 19
Skin	Coxsackievirus B5	Coxsackievirus B1
	Echovirus 5, 17	Echovirus 4, 7, 9, 11, 18
	Parechovirus 1, 3	Enterovirus 71
Neurologic		
Aseptic meningitis	Coxsackievirus B2, B3, B4, B5	Coxsackievirus B1, A9, A14
	Echovirus 3, 9, 11, 17	Echovirus 1, 5, 13, 14, 21, 30
		Enterovirus 71
		Parechovirus 3
Encephalitis	Coxsackievirus B1, B2, B3, B4	Coxsackievirus B5
	Parechovirus 3	Echovirus 6, 9, 23
		Parechovirus 2
		Enterovirus 71
Paralysis		Coxsackievirus B2
Sudden infant death		Coxsackievirus B1, B3, B4, A4, A5, A8
		Parechovirus 1, 3

Data from Cherry JD, Krogstad P: Enteroviruses, parechoviruses, and saffold viruses. In Cherry JD, Harrison GJ, Kaplan SL, Steinback WJ, Hotez PT, editors: *Textbook of pediatric infectious diseases*, ed 7, Philadelphia, 2014, Saunders.

In an attempt to differentiate bacterial from viral disease, Lake and coworkers[433] studied 27 infants with enteroviral infections. White blood cell counts were not helpful because the total count, the number of neutrophils, and the number of band-form neutrophils were elevated in most instances. Of most importance were historical data. Most mothers had evidence of a recent febrile, viral-like illness. Other factors often associated with bacterial sepsis, such as prolonged rupture of membranes, prematurity, and low Apgar scores, were unusual in the enteroviral infection group.

Historically, sepsis-like illness has been identified most often with coxsackieviruses B2 through B5, echovirus types 5, 11, and 16 and parechovirus 3; other viruses detected include coxsackieviruses A9 and B1; echoviruses 2, 3, 4, 6, 9, 14, 19, 21, and 30; and parechovirus 1.[§a] Since the early 1980s, echovirus 11 has been associated most frequently with fatal septic events, with hepatic necrosis, and disseminated intravascular coagulation.[31,271-273,368,415-419,504]

In recent years, the use of human parechovirus–specific PCR assay has led to the realization that human parechovirus type 3 is a relatively common cause of sepsis-like illness in neonates. These human parechovirus type 3 illnesses often have exanthema and abdominal distention.[‖a] Yuzurihara and associates[503] have reported nine parechovirus type 3–infected neonates who presented with hemophagocytic lymphohistiocytosis.

Respiratory Illness. Respiratory complaints are generally overshadowed by other manifestations of neonatal enteroviral and parechoviral diseases. Only 7% of 338 enteroviral infections in early infancy were classified as respiratory illness.[472] Except for echoviruses 11 and parechovirus 1, respiratory illness associated with enteroviruses has been sporadic.[352,362]

Hercík and coworkers[362] reported an epidemic of respiratory illness in 22 newborns associated with echovirus 11 infection. All of these infants had rhinitis and pharyngitis, 50% had laryngitis, and 32% had interstitial pneumonitis. Berkovich and Pangan[352] studied respiratory illnesses in premature infants and reported 64 with illness, 18 of whom had virologic or serologic evidence of parechovirus 1 infection. Many had high but constant levels of serum antibody to parechovirus 1. Some of the 18 infants were probably also infected with parechovirus 1. The children with proven parechovirus 1 infections could not be clinically differentiated from those without evidence of parechovirus 1 infection. Ninety percent of the infants had coryza, and 39% had radiographic evidence of pneumonia. Respiratory tract symptoms were noted in about one half of the neonates in two parechovirus studies in the Netherlands.[408,482] In an outbreak of parechovirus type 1 infection in a nursery in Croatia, all 7 patients had respiratory symptoms.[283] These symptoms were apnea, rhinitis, retractions, and tachypnea.

Herpangina. Chawareewong and associates[505] described several infants with herpangina and coxsackievirus A5 infection. A vesicular lesion on an erythematous base on a tonsillar pillar in a 6-day-old infant with coxsackievirus B2 meningitis has also been reported.[506] Two 1-month-old infants were described in an outbreak of herpangina caused by coxsackievirus B3 in a welfare home in Japan.[507]

Coryza. Several agents have been associated with coryza: coxsackievirus A9; and echoviruses 11, 17, and 19; and parechoviruses 1 and 3.[282,283,362,373,376,480]

Pharyngitis. Pharyngitis is uncommon in neonatal enteroviral infections. In more than 50 infants with enteroviral infections studied by Linnemann and colleagues[487] and Lake and associates,[433] pharyngitis did not occur. Suzuki and coworkers[508] observed pharyngitis in 3 of 42 neonates with echovirus 11 infections. In contrast, in the same study, 67% of children 1 month to 4 years of age had pharyngitis. Pharyngitis has been associated with coxsackievirus B4 and with echoviruses 11, 17, and 18.[340,362,366,485,488]

Laryngotracheobronchitis or Bronchitis. A few enteroviruses have been identified in cases of laryngotracheobronchitis or bronchitis: coxsackieviruses B1 and B4 and echovirus 11.[362,509] Specific clinical descriptions of laryngotracheobronchitis or bronchitis associated with enteroviral infections are scanty. Hercík and coworkers[362] observed laryngitis in 11 and croup in 4 of 22 neonates during an echovirus 11 outbreak. All of the affected infants had upper respiratory tract findings, vomiting, and lethargy. Many were also cyanotic and had hepatosplenomegaly.

Pneumonia. Pneumonia as the main manifestation of neonatal enteroviral and parechoviral infections is rare. Morens[472] documented only seven instances of pneumonia in 338 neonatal enteroviral infections. Outbreaks of pneumonia in neonates have been reported with echovirus 11 and parechovirus 1.[352,362] During a nursery echovirus 11 outbreak, 7 of 22 neonates had pneumonia.[362] All infants had signs of upper respiratory infection and general signs of sepsis-like illness. In infants with pneumonia associated with parechovirus 1 nursery epidemic, coryza, cough, and dyspnea were early signs.[352] The illnesses tended to be protracted, with radiographic changes persisting for 10 to 100 days. Pneumonia resulting from other enteroviruses is a sporadic event and has been reported for coxsackieviruses A9 and B4 and echoviruses 9, 17, and 31.

Cloud Baby. Eichenwald and associates[357] recovered echovirus 20 from four full-term infants younger than 8 days. Although these infants apparently were well, it was found that they were extensively colonized with staphylococci and that they disseminated these organisms into the air around them. Because of this ability to disseminate staphylococci, they were called cloud babies. The investigators believed that these cloud babies contributed to the epidemic spread of staphylococci in the nursery. Because active staphylococcal dissemination occurred only during the time that echovirus 20 could be recovered from the nasopharynx, it was theorized that viral-bacterial synergism occurred.

Gastrointestinal Manifestations

Vomiting or Diarrhea. Vomiting and diarrhea are common but usually just part of the overall illness complex and not the major manifestations. In 1958, Eichenwald and colleagues[356] described epidemic diarrhea associated with echovirus 18 infections.

In 22 infants with epidemic respiratory disease caused by echovirus 11, all had vomiting as a manifestation of the

[§a] References 28, 30, 31, 37, 38, 249, 259, 260, 268, 269, 271-273, 276, 283-285, 333, 350, 354, 355, 358, 368, 372, 376, 381, 415, 416, 418, 420, 429, 432, 433, 435, 436, 438, 441-443, 475, 477, 481-503.

[‖a] References 37, 38, 443, 475, 491, 492, 494-496, 498, 500, 501, 503.

illness.[362] Linnemann and colleagues[487] reported vomiting in 36% and diarrhea in 7% of neonates with echoviral infections. In another study, Lake and associates[433] found diarrhea in 81% and vomiting in 33% of neonates with nonpolio enteroviral infections. Vomiting and diarrhea in neonates have been associated with coxsackieviruses B1, B2, and B5; echoviruses 4 through 6, 8, 9, 11, 16, 17, 18, 19, and 21; parechovirus 1 and 3; and enterovirus 71.[¶a]

Abdominal Distention. Abdominal distention may be a prominent feature of parechovirus infections; it was noted in 5 of 8 infants in one report, and occurred in association with seizures and irritability.[#a]

Hepatitis. Morens[472] observed that 2% of neonates with clinically severe enteroviral disease had hepatitis. Lake and colleagues[433] found that 37% of neonates with enteroviral infections had hepatomegaly, and hepatosplenomegaly was observed by Hercík and associates[362] in 12 of 22 newborns with echovirus 11 respiratory illnesses.

Severe hepatitis, frequently with hepatic necrosis, has been associated with echoviruses 5, 6, 7, 9, 11, 14, 19, 20, 21 and 30.[*b] In 1980, Modlin[370] reported four fatal echovirus 11 illnesses in premature infants. All had hepatitis, disseminated intravascular coagulation, thrombocytopenia, lethargy, poor feeding, and jaundice. Since 1980, there have been many reports of sepsis-like illness with fatal hepatitis related to echovirus 11.[†b]

Coxsackieviruses B1, B3, B4, and other B types have been associated with neonatal hepatitis.[‡b] Abzug[514] reviewed medical records of 16 neonates with hepatitis and coagulopathy and found a case-fatality rate of 31%. All of the five patients who died had myocarditis, and three had encephalitis. Although sepsis-like illness frequently occurs in parechoviral infections, hepatitis is relatively uncommon.[37,38,476] Verboon-Maciolek and colleagues[37] noted two neonates with hepatitis and thrombocytopenia in association with parechovirus infection.

Pancreatitis. Pancreatitis was recognized in three of four newborns with coxsackievirus B5 meningitis[331] and in coxsackievirus B3 and B4 infections at autopsy.[347] In other fatal coxsackievirus B infections, pancreatic involvement has been identified, but clinical manifestations have rarely been observed.

Necrotizing Enterocolitis. Lake and associates[433] described three infants with necrotizing enterocolitis. Coxsackievirus B3 was recovered from two of these infants and coxsackievirus B2 from the third. Parechovirus 1 has been associated with a necrotizing enterocolitis outbreak.[515]

Cardiovascular Manifestations. In contrast with enteroviral cardiac disease in children and adults, in which pericarditis is common, neonatal disease virtually always involves the myocardium.[§b] Most cases of neonatal myocarditis are related to coxsackievirus B infections, and nursery outbreaks have occurred on several occasions. In 1961, Kibrick[29] reviewed the clinical findings in 45 cases of neonatal myocarditis; his findings are summarized in Table 25-6. Many of the early experiences, particularly in South Africa, involved catastrophic nursery epidemics. Since the observation in 1972 of five newborns with echovirus 11 infections and myocarditis, there have been no further reports of nursery epidemics.[518]

Table 25-6 Findings in Neonatal Coxsackievirus B Myocarditis

Finding	Frequency (%)
Feeding difficulty	84
Listlessness	81
Cardiac signs	81
Respiratory distress	75
Cyanosis	72
Fever	70
Pharyngitis	64
Hepatosplenomegaly	53
Biphasic course	35
Central nervous system signs	27
Hemorrhage	13
Jaundice	13
Diarrhea	8

Modified from Kibrick S: Viral infections of the fetus and newborn, *Perspect Virol* 2:140, 1961.

The illness as described by Kibrick[29] most commonly had an abrupt onset and was characterized by listlessness, anorexia, and fever. A biphasic pattern was observed in about one third of the patients. Progression was rapid, and signs of circulatory failure appeared within 2 days. If death did not occur, recovery was occasionally rapid but usually occurred gradually during an extended period. Most patients had cardiac findings, such as tachycardia, cardiomegaly, electrocardiographic changes, and transitory systolic murmurs. Many patients showed signs of respiratory distress and cyanosis. About one third of the infants had signs suggesting neurologic involvement. Of the 45 patients analyzed by Kibrick, only 12 survived.

In the echovirus 11 nursery outbreak reported by Drew,[519] 5 of 10 infants had tachycardia out of proportion to their fevers. Three of these infants had electrocardiograms; supraventricular tachycardia occurred in all, and ST segment depression was observed in two of the records. Supraventricular tachycardia has also been seen in patients with coxsackievirus B infections.[326] Echovirus 19 has been associated with myocarditis.[524]

Until recently, neonatal myocarditis related to enteroviruses was less common than it was 5 decades ago. In his review in 1978, Morens[472] reported only two instances among 248 severe neonatal enteroviral illnesses. In 2007 severe neonatal disease associated with coxsackievirus B1 infection was noted in several areas of the United States.[172,259,260] In Los Angeles County, California, 12 neonates had myocarditis. Similarly in Chicago, Illinois, 11 neonates aged from younger than 1 day to 12 days had myocarditis. Other cases with coxsackievirus B1 myocarditis occurred in Alaska and Colorado.

¶a References 280, 283, 327, 333, 350, 351, 356, 358, 359, 362, 369, 376, 477, 487, 510-512.

#a References 443, 475, 491, 496, 498, 500, 501, 503.

*b References 268, 276, 278, 285, 375, 417-420, 432, 434, 437, 483, 486, 490.

†b References 31, 271, 273, 368, 415, 417, 418, 436.

‡b References 12, 28, 289, 323, 349, 431, 505, 506, 513.

§b References 12, 15, 28, 30, 37, 38, 246, 251, 252, 257, 261, 271, 273, 309, 310, 313, 316, 317, 319, 321-323, 326, 330, 334, 335, 338, 339, 341-346, 348, 416, 418, 431, 482, 486, 490, 513, 516-523.

Exanthem. Exanthem as a manifestation of neonatal enteroviral and parechoviral infections has occurred with coxsackieviruses B1, B3, and B5; echoviruses 4, 5, 7, 9, 11, 16, 17, 18, and 21; and parechoviruses 1 and 3.[‖b] In most instances, rash is just a minor manifestation of moderate-to-severe neonatal disease. Of 27 infants studied by Lake and colleagues, 41% had exanthem.[433] Similarly, Linnemann and coworkers[487] reported exanthem in 4 of 14 neonates with echoviral infections.

Cutaneous manifestations usually have their onset between the third and fifth day of illness. The rash is usually macular or maculopapular, and petechial lesions occasionally are seen. Surprisingly, vesicular lesions have been reported only once with coxsackievirus B3 infection and once with enterovirus 71 infection in neonates. Theodoridou and associates[525] described a full-term newborn boy with vesicular lesions at birth. PCR assay revealed coxsackievirus B3. A 1-month-old infant with enterovirus 71 infection and hand-foot-and-mouth syndrome has been reported.[526] Hall and associates[477] reported two neonates with echovirus 16 infections in which the illnesses were similar to roseola. The patients had fevers for 2 and 3 days, defervescence, and then the appearance of maculopapular rashes.

Recent studies suggest that exanthem is a common manifestation in neonatal parechovirus type 3 infections.[¶b] In one study, 15 of 15 young infants had a rash.[501] The rash had its onset on the third day (range, 1-5 days) and lasted 3 days (range, 2-7 days). The rash was erythematous only in 87% of the patients, and in 13%, it was erythematous and maculopapular. In 80% of the infants, it was palmar/plantar in location, and in some, it involved the trunk and extremities.

Neurologic Manifestations

Meningitis and Meningoencephalitis. As shown in Table 25-5, meningitis and meningoencephalitis have been associated with coxsackieviruses B1 through B5, many echoviruses, and with parechoviruses.[#b] In most instances, the differentiation of meningitis from meningoencephalitis is difficult in neonates. Meningoencephalitis is common in infants with sepsis-like illness, and autopsy studies reveal many infants with disseminated viral disease (e.g., heart, liver, adrenals) in addition to CNS involvement. In the review of Morens,[472] 50% of the neonates with enteroviral infections had encephalitis or meningitis.

The initial clinical findings in neonatal meningitis or meningoencephalitis are similar to those in nonspecific febrile illness or sepsis-like illness. Most often, the child is quite normal and then becomes febrile, anorectic, and lethargic. Jaundice frequently affects newborns, and vomiting occurs in neonates of all ages. Less common findings include apnea, tremulousness, and general increased tonicity. Seizures occasionally occur.

CSF examination reveals considerable variation in protein, glucose, and cellular values. In 7 newborns with meningitis related to coxsackievirus B5 as studied by Swender and associates,[350] the mean CSF protein value was 244mg/dL, and the highest value was 480 mg/dL. The mean CSF glucose value was 57mg/dL, and one of the 7 had pronounced hypoglycorrhachia (12mg/dL). The mean CSF leukocyte count for the 7 infants was 1069cells/mm^3, with 67% polymorphonuclear cells. The highest cell count was 4526cells/mm^3, with 85% polymorphonuclear cells. In another study involving 28 infants younger than 2 months in whom coxsackievirus B5 was the implicated pathogen, 36% of the infants had CSF leukocyte counts of 500 cells/mm^3 or more.[488] In this same study, only 13% of the infants had CSF protein values of 120mg/dL or more; 12% of the infants had glucose values of less than 40 mg/dL.

The CSF findings in cases of neonatal nonpolio enteroviral and parechoviral infections are frequently similar to those in bacterial disease. In particular, the most consistent finding in bacterial disease, hypoglycorrhachia, affects about 10% of newborns with enteroviral meningitis.[350,430,510,512,547]

Of particular note in neonatal parechovirus type 3 infections is the occurrence of extensive white matter injury.[441-443] Also of note in parechovirus type 3 neonatal CNS infections is the general lack of pleocytosis, even with the presence of virus in the CSF.[499,502]

Paralysis. Johnson and associates[540] reported a 1-month-old boy with a right facial paralysis and loss of abdominal reflexes. The facial paralysis persisted through convalescence; the reflexes returned to normal within 2 weeks. The boy was infected with coxsackievirus B2. A 1-month-old boy with hand-foot-and-mouth syndrome and bilateral lower limb weakness caused by enterovirus 71 infection has been described.[526]

Sudden Infant Death. Balduzzi and Greendyke[427] recovered coxsackievirus A5 from the stool of a 1-month-old child after sudden infant death. In a similar investigation of sudden infant death, Gold and coworkers[428] recovered coxsackievirus A4 from the brains of three infants. Coxsackievirus A8 was recovered from the stool of a child in whom anorexia was diagnosed on the day before death. Coxsackievirus B3 was recovered at autopsy from an infant who died suddenly on the eighth day of life.[427] Morens and associates[15] reported eight cases of sudden infant death associated with enteroviral infection; parechovirus 1 was found on two occasions. In five instances of cot death in one study, echovirus 11 was isolated from the lungs in two children, from the myocardium in one, and from the nose or feces in the other two.[415]

Grangeot-Keros and coworkers[548] looked for evidence of enteroviral infections using PCR assay and an IgM immunoassay in cases of sudden and unexplained infant deaths. They divided their infant death population into two groups. One group had clinical, biologic, or histologic signs of viral infection, and the other group had no indicators of an antecedent infection. Fifty-four percent of infants with evidence of a preceding infection had PCR assay evidence of an enterovirus in samples from the respiratory tract or lung, or both, whereas none of those without evidence of a prior infection had similar positive PCR findings. Their IgM antibody studies supported their PCR findings. Sedmak

‖b References 28, 30, 37, 38, 257, 269, 273, 282, 312, 314, 336, 354, 359, 369, 376, 382, 383, 414, 443, 475, 477-479, 486, 487, 496, 498, 500, 501, 503, 518, 524, 525.

¶b References 443, 475, 491, 496, 498, 500, 501, 503.

#b References 28, 30, 31, 37, 38, 172, 179, 261, 273, 280, 284, 317, 336, 351, 354, 358, 368, 369, 377, 418, 422, 429, 430, 441-443, 471, 478, 479, 482, 488, 489, 492, 493, 495, 496, 499, 502, 506, 510, 511, 513, 517, 518, 526-546.

and associates[549] noted a 4-week-old and a 4-month-old infant who had sudden infant death and were found to have parechovirus type 3 infections of the respiratory tract.

Manifestations of Polioviruses

General Considerations. Polioviral infection in children classically results in a spectrum of clinical illness. As described by Paul[550] and accepted by others, 90% to 95% of infections in nonneonatal children are inapparent, 4% to 8% are abortive, and 1% to 2% are frank cases of poliomyelitis. Whether neonatal polioviral infection is acquired in utero, during birth, or after birth, it appears that the more severe manifestations of clinical illness are similar to those of older children. However, the available reports in the literature suggest that the frequencies of occurrence of inapparent, abortive, and frank cases are quite different from those in older children. Most reports describe severely affected infants.[203,205-217,219-221,223,224] Asymptomatic infection does occur, however.[204,218]

In the excellent review by Bates[207] in 1955, 58 cases of clinically overt poliomyelitis in infants younger than 1 month were described. Although complete data were not available on many of the cases, 51 had paralysis or died from their disease, or both. Of the total number of infants for whom there were clinical data, only one had nonparalytic disease. Because follow-up observation was recorded for only a short time in many infants, the evaluation of residual paralysis (presence or absence) may not be reliable. Pertinent clinical data from the study by Bates are presented in Table 25-7, and these data show that more than one half of the cases resulted from maternal disease. Because others have identified congenital infection without symptomatic maternal infection, it is probable that infection in the mothers was the source for an even greater percentage of the neonatal illnesses. Because the incubation period of neonatal poliomyelitis has not been determined, it is difficult to know how many infants were infected in utero. Most illnesses occurring within the first 5 days of life probably were congenital. Most neonates had symptoms of fever, anorexia or dysphagia, and listlessness. Almost one half the infants described in this review died, and of those surviving, 48% had residual paralysis.

Table 25-7 Clinical Findings in 58 Cases of Neonatal Poliomyelitis

Finding	No. of Cases With a Particular Finding/No. of Cases Evaluated (%)
TIME OF ONSET AFTER BIRTH	
≤5 days	13/55 (24)
6-14 days	25/55 (45)
≥15 days	17/55 (31)
INFECTION SOURCE FOR SYMPTOMATIC ILLNESS	
Mother	22/42 (52)
Other contact	6/42 (14)
Unknown	14/42 (34)
ACUTE ILLNESS	
Fever	17/29 (59)
Anorexia or dysphagia	16/24 (67)
Listlessness	24/33 (73)
Irritability	3/33 (9)
Diarrhea	2/11 (18)
Paralysis	43/44 (98)
OUTCOME	
Death	21/44 (48)
Residual paralysis	12/44 (27)
Recovery without paralysis	11/44 (25)

Modified from Bates T: Poliomyelitis in pregnancy, fetus, and newborn, *Am J Dis Child* 90:189, 1955.

Inapparent Infection. Shelokov and Habel[218] followed a virologically proven infected newborn without signs of illness. The infant was normal when 1 year of age. Wingate and coworkers[222] studied an infant delivered by cesarean section from a woman with poliomyelitis who died 1 hour after delivery. Her infant was treated with gamma globulin intramuscularly at the postnatal age of 21 hours. He remained asymptomatic; poliovirus 1 was recovered from a stool specimen on the fifth day of life.

Infection Acquired In Utero. Elliott and colleagues[210] described an infant girl in whom "complete flaccidity" was observed at birth. This child's mother had had mild paralytic poliomyelitis, with the onset of minor illness occurring 19 days before the infant's birth. Fetal movements had ceased 6 days before delivery, suggesting that paralysis had occurred at this time. On examination, the infant was severely atonic; when supported under the back, she was passively opisthotonic. Respiratory efforts were abortive and confined to accessory muscles, and laryngoscopy revealed complete flaccidity in the larynx.

Johnson and Stimson[212] reported a case in which the mother's probable abortive infection occurred 6 weeks before the birth of the infant. The newborn was initially thought to be normal but apparently had no medical examination until the fourth day of life. At that time, the physician diagnosed a right hemiplegia. On the next day, a more complete examination revealed a lateral bulging of the right abdomen accompanied by crying and the maintenance of the lower extremities in a frog-leg position. Adduction and flexion at the hips were weak, and the knee and ankle jerks were absent. Laboratory studies were unremarkable except for the examination of the CSF, which revealed 20 lymphocytes/mm^3 and a protein concentration of 169 mg/dL. During a 6-month period, this child's paralysis gradually improved and resulted in only residual weakness of the left lower extremity.

Paresis of the left arm occurred in another child with apparent transplacentally acquired poliomyelitis shortly after birth.[215] The 2-day-old infant was quadriplegic, but patellar reflexes were present, and there were no respiratory or swallowing difficulties. This child had pneumonia when 3 weeks of age, but general neurologic improvement occurred. Examination when the infant was 8 weeks of age revealed bilateral atrophy of the shoulder girdle muscles. The CSF in this case revealed 63 leukocytes/mm^3, with 29% of them polymorphonuclear cells, and a protein value of 128mg/dL.

All three of the infants previously discussed were apparently infected in utero several days before birth. Their symptoms were exclusively neurologic; fever, irritability, and vomiting did not occur.

Postnatally Acquired Infection. In contrast to infections acquired in utero, those acquired postnatally are more typical of classic poliomyelitis. Shelokov and Weinstein[219] described a child who was asymptomatic at birth. Onset of minor symptoms in the mother occurred 3 weeks before delivery, and major symptoms occurred 1 day before delivery. On the sixth day of life, the infant became suddenly ill with watery diarrhea. He looked grayish and pale. On the next day, he was irritable, lethargic, and limp and had a temperature of 38° C. Mild opisthotonos and weakness of both lower extremities developed. He was responsive to sound, light, and touch. The CSF had an elevated protein level and an increased number of leukocytes. His condition worsened during a total period of 3 days, and then gradual improvement began. At 1 year of age, he had severe residual paralysis of the right leg and moderate weakness in the left leg.

Baskin and associates[206] described two infants with neonatal poliomyelitis. The first child, whose mother had severe poliomyelitis at the time of delivery, was well for 3 days and then developed a temperature of 38.3° C. On the fifth day of life, the boy became listless and cyanotic. CSF examination revealed a protein level of 300mg/dL and 108 leukocytes/mm^3. His condition worsened, and extreme flaccidity, irregular respiration, and progressive cyanosis developed; he died on the seventh day of life. The second infant was a boy who was well until he was 8 days of age, but he then became listless and developed a temperature of 38.3° C. During the next 5 days, he developed flaccid quadriplegia; irregular, rapid, and shallow respirations; and an inability to swallow. The child died on the 14th day of life. His mother had developed acute poliomyelitis 6 days before the onset of his symptoms.

Abramson and colleagues[203] reported four children with neonatal poliomyelitis, two of whom died. In three of the children, the illnesses were typical of acute poliomyelitis seen in older children; they were similar to the cases of Baskin and associates[206] described previously. The fourth child died at 13 days of age with generalized paralysis. The onset of his illness was difficult to define, and he was never febrile. Swarts and Kercher[221] also described a child whose illness had an insidious onset. When 10 days of age, the child gradually became lethargic and anorectic and regurgitated formula through his nose. On the next day, flaccid quadriplegia developed. Winsser and associates[223] and Bates[207] reported infants with acute poliomyelitis with clinical illnesses similar to those that occur in older individuals.

Vaccine Viral Infections. Administration of oral polio vaccines to newborns has been carried out in numerous studies.[226,295-307] Vaccine viral infection occurs in newborns with all three types of poliovirus, although the rate of infection is less than that for immunized older children. This rate is governed by the dose of virus, transplacentally acquired maternal antibody, and antibody acquired from colostrum and breast milk. Although clinical illness rarely has resulted from attenuated polioviral infections in older children and adults, there is only one specific report of paralytic poliomyelitis in a newborn associated with infection with a vaccine viral strain.[308] In that case, the possible source for the infection was the recently vaccinated child of the babysitter. In a review of 118 cases of vaccine-associated paralytic poliomyelitis in the United States between 1980 and 1992, the age of patients ranged from 1 month to 69 years, but details about neonates were not presented.[551]

Manifestations of Specific Nonpolio Enteroviruses

Coxsackieviruses

COXSACKIEVIRUS A. There have been few reports of neonatal coxsackievirus A infections. Baker and Phillips[426] reported a small-for-gestational-age infant with pneumonia and a sepsis-like illness with disseminated intravascular coagulation. This newborn died on the second day of life, and when cultured, the CSF grew coxsackievirus A3. Balduzzi and Greendyke[427] recovered a coxsackievirus A5 from the stool of a 1-month-old child with sudden infant death. In a similar investigation of sudden infant death, Gold and coworkers[428] recovered coxsackievirus A4 from the brains of three infants. Coxsackievirus A8 was also recovered from the stool of a child in whom anorexia was observed on the day before death. Berkovich and Kibrick[351] reported a 3-day-old neonate with nonspecific febrile illness (38.3° C) who was infected with coxsackievirus A9. Coxsackievirus A9 was also recovered from an 11-day-old infant with rhinitis, lethargy, anorexia, and fever.[376] This illness lasted 3 days. Jack and associates[363] described a 3-day-old newborn with fever, cyanosis, and respiratory distress who died on the seventh day of life; an autopsy revealed bronchopneumonia. Coxsackievirus A9 was isolated from the feces on the fourth and sixth days of life.

Lake and associates[433] reported two neonates with coxsackievirus A9 infections, but no clinical details were presented. Jenista and coworkers[294] recovered coxsackievirus A9 strains from seven nonhospitalized neonates who were thought to be well. In the Netherlands, a neonate with coxsackievirus A9 illness had pericarditis, meningitis, pneumonitis, and hepatitis; he recovered completely.[523] Krajden and Middleton[30] described a neonate with a sepsis-like illness who died. Coxsackievirus A9 was recovered from the liver and lung. Morens[472] also reported a death associated with this same virus type. Eisenhut and colleagues[429] reported an outbreak that included four neonates with coxsackievirus A9 infections. One infant who had meningitis, myocarditis, and disseminated intravascular coagulation died. A second neonate had vomiting, rhinitis, and abdominal distention, and two neonates had asymptomatic infections. Forty-eight of 598 neonates admitted to a regular nursery in Bangkok, Thailand, in the spring of 1977 had herpangina.[429] Coxsackievirus A5 was isolated from nine specimens from the afflicted infants, and a rise in the serum antibody titer was identified in 10 instances. Helin and colleagues[540] described 16 newborns with aseptic meningitis caused by coxsackievirus A14. During a 2.5-year follow-up period, they all developed normally, and no sequelae were identified. Coxsackievirus A16 was recovered from one newborn with nonspecific illness; his mother had had hand-foot-and-mouth syndrome 4 days previously.[539]

COXSACKIEVIRUS B1. Until recently, coxsackievirus B1 has only occasionally been recovered from newborns (Table 25-8). Eckert and coworkers[510] recovered a coxsackievirus B1 strain from the stool of a 1-month-old boy with bronchitis. Jahn and Cherry[327] described a 4-day-old infant who became febrile and lethargic. This illness persisted for 5 days without other signs or symptoms. An

Table 25-8 Clinical and Pathologic Findings in Coxsackievirus B Infection of Newborns

	REFERENCES FOR COXSACKIEVIRUS				
Finding	**B1**	**B2**	**B3**	**B4**	**B5**
Exanthem	314, 487		252		257, 312, 336, 534
Nonspecific febrile illness		258	343	334, 340	473
Sepsis-like illness	28, 325, 338, 487, 491, 514	28	30, 325	271, 426	28
Paralysis	491	541			
Diarrhea		513			
Sudden infant death	549		427, 549	549	
Pneumothorax					363
Aseptic meningitis, meningoencephalitis, encephalomyelitis	172, 327, 333, 349, 514, 533	261, 318, 324, 339, 426, 430, 474, 507, 528, 543	28, 30, 246, 255, 335, 336, 341, 456	28, 312, 316, 319, 323, 336, 430	30, 247, 257, 261, 326, 331, 332, 337, 342, 350, 471, 489, 521, 537, 553
Myocarditis	172, 259, 260, 320, 325, 333, 346, 349, 432, 487, 491	28, 261, 315, 318, 321, 326, 339, 426, 474, 529	28, 30, 109, 246, 252, 313, 324, 338, 340, 358, 376, 455, 523	30, 261, 273, 312, 316, 319, 323, 330, 334, 344, 426, 517, 518, 529	30, 257, 342, 471, 537
Hepatitis	172, 325, 349, 432, 487, 506		289, 325	323, 330	
Pancreatitis				347	331
Adrenocortical necrosis			335		
Bronchitis				510	

examination of the CSF showed a slight increase in the number of leukocytes, and most were mononuclear cells. Coxsackievirus B1 was recovered from the throat, stool, urine, and serum.

Wright and colleagues[349] reported an infant fatality associated with coxsackievirus B1 infection. This premature boy was well until he was 4 days of age, when he had two episodes of cyanosis and apnea. After this, he became anorexic and listless and lost the Moro reflex. On the ninth day of life, he had shallow respirations, hepatomegaly, jaundice, petechiae, and thrombocytopenia. He was edematous and lethargic, and he had a temperature of 34.5°C, a pulse rate of 130 beats per minute, and a respiratory rate of 20 breaths per minute. He became weaker, unresponsive, and apneic and died. Positive laboratory findings included the following values: less than 10,000 platelets/mm^3,[349] 283 mg of CSF protein/dL, 20.5 mg of serum bilirubin/dL, and 100 units of serum aspartate aminotransferase. Autopsy revealed hepatic necrosis, meningoencephalitis, and myocarditis. Coxsackievirus B1 was recovered from the throat, urine, liver, lung, kidney, and brain.

Twin boys with a sepsis-like illness with hepatitis and disseminated intravascular coagulation have been reported.[28] The first twin died on the 16th day of life, and the second twin survived. Another set of twins had coxsackievirus B1 infections shortly after birth; one twin had myocarditis, and the other had hepatitis with subsequent progressive liver calcifications.[432] A third set of twins had coxsackievirus B1 infections with illness that began when they were 5 days old.[513] One twin had disseminated intravascular coagulation, and the other had meningitis. Three other newborns with fatal sepsis-like illnesses with hepatitis have been described.[486,490]

Isacsohn[325] described four severe cases of neonatal illnesses caused by coxsackievirus B1; three of the four neonates died. Of the three fatalities, one was caused by myocarditis and the other two resulted from multiorgan dysfunction. The surviving infant had hepatitis, congestive heart failure, thrombocytopenia, and residual neurologic damage.

McLean and colleagues[333] described a male newborn who had a temperature of 39° C, vomiting, and diarrhea on the fourth day of life. When 6 days of age, he appeared gray and mottled and developed shallow respirations. He died on the seventh day of life after increased respiratory distress (90 breaths per minute), hepatomegaly, generalized edema, and cardiac enlargement. Coxsackievirus B1 was recovered from the heart and brain.

Gear[320] studied an extensive epidemic of Bornholm disease related to coxsackievirus B1 in Johannesburg in the summers of 1960 to 1961. After the first coxsackievirus B1 isolations, the medical officers of the area were on the alert for nursery infections and the prevention of nursery epidemics. Despite careful isolation procedures, Gear[320] reported that infection "was introduced into all the large maternity homes in Johannesburg." About 20 cases of neonatal myocarditis were documented, as were three deaths. The isolation procedures apparently prevented secondary nursery cases.

Volakova and Jandasek[346] reported epidemic myocarditis related to coxsackievirus B1. Cherry and Jahn[314] described a child with a mild febrile exanthematous illness, which had its onset within 10 minutes of birth. In 2007, coxsackievirus B1 was the predominant enterovirus in the United States.[172] Associated with this was the finding of an increased detection of severe neonatal disease due to this virus. Five fatal cases were noted. Manifestations included myocarditis, meningitis/meningoencephalitis, sepsis-like illness, hepatitis, and coagulopathy.

Coxsackievirus B2. The reported instances of coxsackievirus B2 infections in neonates are provided Table 25-8. In most instances, the infants had myocarditis or neurologic manifestations. Eleven of 12 of the infants with myocarditis died. The one child with myocarditis who survived was reexamined when 2 years of age and was found to be normal.[315] This child's mother became ill with sore throat, coryza, and malaise on the day after delivery. When 3 days of age, the child became febrile (38.9° C) and had periods of apnea and cardiac irregularities. The cry was "pained." The electrocardiogram showed a left-sided heart pattern in the V leads and T wave abnormalities. The child's symptoms lasted less than 48 hours. Coxsackievirus B2 was isolated from the nose, urine, throat, and CSF of the child and from the mother's stool. The mother breastfed the infant (while she wore a mask) during her illness. A later specimen of breast milk was cultured for virus without successful recovery of an agent.

Puschak[258] reported a child who became febrile (39.5° C) 8 hours after birth. During the next 9 days, the infant's temperature fluctuated between 36.7° and 38.9° C. The patient had no other symptoms. Serologic evidence of coxsackievirus B2 infection was found.

Johnson and associates[540] described a 1-month-old infant with aseptic meningitis who developed a persistent right facial paralysis. In a study of undifferentiated diarrheal syndromes, Ramos-Alvarez[512] observed a child with coxsackievirus B2 infection. Eilard and associates[474] reported a nursery outbreak in which 12 infants were infected. All had aseptic meningitis, and 2 also had myocarditis. One of the two infants died on the 13th day of life. One child with thrombocytopenia and respiratory failure died.[433]

Coxsackievirus B3. Neonatal infections with coxsackievirus B3 are summarized in Table 25-8. Most reported cases have been severe illnesses with myocarditis or meningoencephalitis, or both. One case involved sudden infant death[427] in which coxsackievirus B3 was recovered from a pool of organs from an infant who died on the eighth day of life.

Tuuteri and coworkers[343] studied a nursery outbreak of coxsackievirus B3 infection. Seven children had mild disease characterized by anorexia, listlessness, and fever, and two infants had fatal myocarditis. Of the 57 reported neonatal infections with coxsackievirus B3, 30 deaths occurred, and most were associated with myocarditis and sepsis-like illness. Three infants had febrile illnesses with meningitis and were reported to have suffered no residual effects; long-term follow-up is not available, however.[255,336]

Isacsohn and colleagues[325] reported two neonates with multiorgan dysfunction who survived. A full-term boy delivered by caesarean section had scattered vesicular lesions at birth.[525] New lesions appeared over a 5-day period, and the rash lasted for 10 days. The child had no other symptoms, and the mother had no febrile illness during pregnancy.

Chesney and associates[534] studied a 3-week-old girl with meningoencephalitis. This child had hypoglycorrhachia; the CSF glucose value on the sixth day of illness was 23mg/dL, with a corresponding blood glucose level of 78mg/dL. As described in another review,[433] two infants who died had thrombocytopenia and respiratory failure; a clinical picture suggestive of necrotizing enterocolitis also was observed.

During a 5-year period in Toronto, Krajden and Middleton[30] assessed 24 neonates with enteroviral infections who were admitted to the Hospital for Sick Children. Nine children were infected with coxsackievirus B3; of these, 2 infants had meningitis, 3 had myocarditis, and 4 had a sepsis-like illness. Of this group, 1 infant with meningitis, 1 with myocarditis, and all with sepsis-like illness died. All the neonates with sepsis-like illness had clinical evidence of multiorgan involvement; they had respiratory distress, hepatomegaly, hemorrhagic manifestations, and congestive heart failure. Two neonates with herpangina and coxsackievirus B3 infections were described in an outbreak involving 25 infants.[507] Fatal myocarditis has been noted recently in two cases.[109,522] In one case, the infecting virus was found to be a recombinant human enterovirus-B variant.[109] The genomic chimera arose from recombination between coxsackievirus B3 and enteroviruses B86 and B97.

Coxsackievirus B4. Table 25-8 summarizes coxsackievirus B4 neonatal infections. Most were severe and frequently were fatal illnesses with neurologic and cardiac involvement. An infant with less severe disease was described by Sieber and associates.[340] This child was well until 6 days after delivery, when he developed pharyngitis, diarrhea, and gradually increasing lethargy. This was followed by fever for 36 hours. No other signs or symptoms were observed, and the child was well when 11 days of age. He had virologic and serologic evidence of coxsackievirus B4 infection.

Winsser and Altieri[347] studied an infant who suddenly became cyanotic and convulsed and died at 2 days of age. At autopsy, the only findings were bronchopneumonia, congestive splenomegaly, and chronic interstitial pancreatitis. Coxsackievirus B4 was isolated from the spleen.

Barson and associates[516] reported the survival of an infant with myocarditis. Cardiac calcification was revealed on radiographs when the child was 4 weeks of age, and the electrocardiogram revealed a left bundle branch block. When the child was 7 months of age, the conduction defect remained, but the myocardial calcification had resolved.

Coxsackievirus B5. The spectrum of neonatal infection with coxsackievirus B5 is greater than that with the other coxsackieviruses B. Studies are summarized in Table 25-8. Meningitis and encephalitis are common neonatal manifestations of coxsackievirus B5 infection.[*c] Nursery epidemics have been observed. Rantakallio and associates[337] studied 17 infants in one nursery with aseptic meningitis. None of the infants was severely ill. All had fever, with a temperature of 38° to 40° C. Eleven of the 17 neonates were boys. Signs included irritability, nuchal rigidity, increased tone, anorexia, opisthotonos, whimpering, loose stools, and diminution of alertness. In another nursery outbreak, Farmer and Patten[471] found 28 infected infants. Of the group of 28, 15 had aseptic meningitis, 4 had diarrhea, and 9 had no signs of illness. Six years later, the 15 children who had had meningitis were studied. Thirteen were found to be physically normal and to have normal intelligence. Two children had intelligence levels below the mean for the group and had residual spasticity. At the time of the initial illness, these two infants and one additional child were twitching, irritable, or jittery.

Swender and associates[350] studied seven cases of aseptic meningitis in an intensive care nursery during a 6-week period during the summer of 1972. Two of the infants had apnea. One of the infants had a CSF glucose level of 12mg/dL. During a community outbreak

---

[*c]References 30, 247, 257, 261, 331, 332, 337, 342, 350, 471, 488, 536.

of coxsackievirus B5 infections, Marier and colleagues[489] studied 32 infants with aseptic meningitis. In this group, 36% had CSF leukocyte counts of 500 cells/mm^3 or higher,[488] and in 19%, neutrophils accounted for 50% or more of the count. In 12% of patients, the CSF glucose level was less than 40 mg/dL. Thirty-eight percent of the infants had blood leukocyte counts of 15,000 cells/mm^3 or higher values.

Of particular interest is the observation of exanthem in four reports. Cherry and coworkers[533] described a 3-week-old boy with fever, a maculopapular rash, and enlarged cervical and postauricular lymph nodes. Examination of the CSF revealed 141 leukocytes/mm^3, of which 84% were lymphocytes, and a protein value of 100 mg/dL. An electrocardiogram was normal. In this child, the rash appeared before the fever. Coxsackievirus B5 was isolated from the pharynx and the CSF. Nogen and Lepow[336] reported an infant with a similar illness. This child had a nonspecific erythematous papular rash on the face and scalp. One week later, he became febrile and irritable. The CSF contained 440 white blood cells/mm^3, and 96% of them were mononuclear. Virus was isolated from the feces, throat, and CSF.

Artenstein and associates[312] reported a 23-day-old girl with a fever and an erythematous macular rash that spread from the scalp to the entire body, except the palms and soles, and lasted 4 days. Coxsackievirus B5 was recovered from the stool, but no evidence of serum antibody to this virus was found. McLean and coworkers[257] also described a child with a papular rash on the trunk and limbs that was present at birth. On the fourth day of life, the rash had disappeared, but the patient then developed a temperature of 39.4° C. Irritability, twitching, and fullness of the anterior fontanelle were observed, and CSF examination showed meningitis. During an 8-day period, the child had repeated episodes of vomiting and diarrhea. On the 11th day of life, the infant had hyperpnea, tachycardia, and an enlarging liver. The child died on the 13th day of life. Autopsy revealed extensive encephalitis and focal myocardial necrosis. Virus was recovered from the brain, heart, lungs, and liver.

It appears that neonatal infection with coxsackievirus B5 is less likely to be fatal than infection with the other coxsackieviruses B. Only 6 of 36 infants described in Table 25-8 died. In contrast to coxsackieviruses B2, B3, and B4, coxsackievirus B5 appears to be more neurotropic than cardiotropic.

Echoviruses

ECHOVIRUS 1. Dömök and Molnár[317] described aseptic meningitis related to echovirus 1.

ECHOVIRUS 2. Krajden and Middleton[30] described three infants with echovirus 2 infections. Two of the neonates had meningitis and recovered. The third child, who died, had a sepsis-like illness. Virus was isolated from the CSF, lung, liver, and urine. One other neonate with echovirus 2 infection has been observed, but no details are available.[433]

ECHOVIRUS 3. In the summer of 1970, Haynes and coworkers[537] studied an epidemic of infection caused by echovirus 3. Three infected neonates were observed, all of whom had meningitis. One child, a full-term girl, developed tonic seizures and an inability to suck on the third day of life. The serum bilirubin level was 28 mg/dL. Shortly thereafter, the child became cyanotic, flaccid, and apneic and developed a bulging anterior fontanelle; she was in shock. She received assisted ventilation with a respirator for 3 days. When the child was 1 month of age, severe neurologic damage with developing hydrocephalus was obvious. Echovirus 3 was recovered from the CSF, and the CSF protein level was 880 mg/dL on the sixth day of life.

The other two infants in this study apparently had uncomplicated aseptic meningitis. The CSF findings in one child revealed 1826 white blood cells/mm^3, and 91% of them were polymorphonuclear cells. The other child had 320 cells/mm^3, 98% of which were polymorphonuclear cells.

A 4-day-old infant from whom echovirus 3 was recovered from the CSF has been reported.[30] This child had fewer than 3 white blood cells/mm^3 in the CSF. Other neonates with echovirus 3 infection have been observed, but no details are available.[294,433]

ECHOVIRUS 4. Linnemann and associates[487] studied 11 infants with echovirus 4 infections. All infants had fevers, and most were irritable. Four infants had a fine maculopapular rash, which was located on the face or abdomen, or both. In two children, the extremities were also involved. Other neonates with echovirus 4 infections have been reported, but details of their illness are not available.[294,433]

ECHOVIRUS 5. There have been six reports of neonatal illnesses associated with echovirus 5 infections.[417,430,472,525] In one nursery epidemic, six infants were involved.[360] All infants had fever (38.3° C to 39.7° C) that lasted 4 to 8 days. Two neonates had tachycardia that was disproportionately rapid when compared with the degree of fever, but in neither was there evidence of myocarditis. Four infants had splenomegaly and enlarged lymph nodes; these findings persisted for several weeks.

In 1966 (July to October), an epidemic of echovirus 5 infection involved 23% of the infants in the maternity unit at the Royal Air Force Hospital in Chargi, Singapore.[359] Fifty-six infants were symptomatically infected, and 10 were asymptomatically infected. Those who were ill were 2 to 12 days of age at the onset of disease. All 56 symptomatic infants had fever; 87% of them had a temperature of 38.3° C or greater. The mean duration of fever was 3.5 days, with a range of 2 to 7 days. Twenty infants had a faint erythematous macular rash that was most prominent on the limbs and buttocks but also occurred on the trunk and face. The rash, which began 24 to 36 hours after the beginning of fever, lasted 48 hours. Diarrhea occurred in 17 infants, 4 of whom passed blood and mucus. Vomiting was observed in about one half the neonates. All infants apparently recovered completely.

One newborn girl had a nonspecific, biphasic febrile illness.[406] Echovirus 5 was recovered from the CSF, but the cell count, protein level, and glucose value were normal.

Another study included a 9-day-old infant with aseptic meningitis.[552] During an epidemiologic investigation in Rochester, New York, 13 of 75 enteroviral isolates were echovirus 5.[294] Six of the infants were asymptomatic; no clinical details of the other seven patients were presented. A neonate with sepsis-like illness and hepatic failure died 9 days after birth.[420]

ECHOVIRUS 6. Sanders and Cramblett[376] reported a boy who was well until 9 days of age, when he developed a fever (38° C), severe diarrhea, and dehydration. His white blood cell count was 27,900 cells/mm^3, and virologic and serologic evidence of echovirus 6 infection was found. Treatment consisted of intravenous hydration, to which there was a good response. Krous and colleagues[419] described an infant who died on the ninth day of life with a sepsis-like illness. The child had meningitis, disseminated intravascular coagulation, hepatic necrosis, and adrenal and renal hemorrhage. Ventura and associates[437] reported the death of a full-term neonate with sepsis-like syndrome who at postmortem examination had massive hepatic necrosis, adrenal hemorrhagic necrosis, renal medullary hemorrhage, hemorrhagic noninflammatory pneumonia, and severe encephalomalacia. Yen and coworkers[276] reported a premature boy who developed a sepsis-like illness on the fifth day of life. This infant had hepatic failure and was treated with intravenous immune globulin. He recovered gradually, but on the 62nd day of life, he died of a nosocomial *Enterobacter cloacae* infection. Echovirus type 6 has been associated with neonatal illness on two other occasions, but no clinical details are available.[433,487] A premature boy with a birth weight of 2460 g was lethargic at birth. At 5 days of age, he had a sepsis-like illness with hepatitis and disseminated intravascular coagulation.[276] This child was treated with intravenous immune globulin (IVIG) but later died of nosocomial sepsis caused by *Enterobacter cloacae.*

ECHOVIRUS **7.** Piraino and colleagues[273] reported three infants with echovirus 7 infections. All three had fever, one had respiratory distress and exanthem, and one had irritability and loose stools. Two neonates with fatal sepsis-like illnesses with massive disseminated intravascular coagulation have been reported.[379,438] One neonate with severe hepatitis was treated with pleconaril and survived.[553] Daboval and colleagues[382] described an outbreak of echovirus 7 infection in 6 newborns over a 12-day period. The index case was the mother of one of the infants. The baby of the index case developed fever on day 6 of life. The subsequent five babies all had illnesses suggestive of sepsis. Five of the babies had macular rashes. All six of the babies had high C-reactive protein levels, but none had evidence of bacterial infection.

ECHOVIRUS **8.** In a search for etiologic associations in infantile diarrhea, Ramos-Alvarez[512] identified one neonate from whom echovirus 8 was recovered from the stool. The antibody titer to this virus rose fourfold.

ECHOVIRUS **9.** Echovirus 9 is the most prevalent of all the enteroviruses (see Table 25-4). From 1955 to 1958, epidemic waves of infection spread throughout the world.[554] Since that time, echovirus 9 has been a common cause of human illness. Despite its prevalence and its frequent association with epidemic disease, descriptions of neonatal illness are uncommon. Unlike experiences with several other enteroviruses, newborn nursery epidemics caused by echovirus 9 have not often been described.

Neonatal echovirus 9 experiences are provided in Table 25-9. Moscovici and Maisel[279] described an asymptomatic infant with echovirus 9 infection. When echovirus 9 was prevalent in Erie County, New York, during the summer of 1971, seven neonatal cases were observed.[511] Four children had aseptic meningitis, but only moderate elevations of CSF protein values and white blood cells were observed. One child, a 15-day-old infant, had radiologic evidence of bronchopneumonia, and two infants had gastroenteritis. Rawls and coworkers[436] described an infant who was well until the seventh day of life, when progressive lethargy, anorexia, and irritability developed. The child became moribund, and jaundice, scattered petechiae, and hypothermia were observed. The pulse rate was 90 beats per minute, the respiratory rate was 40 breaths per minute, and the liver was enlarged. The infant died 3 days after the onset of symptoms. Echovirus 9 was recovered from the lung, brain, and CSF. Cho and colleagues[484] described a similar severe neonatal illness in a child from whom echovirus 9 was recovered from the CSF. This child was hypothermic and hypotonic on the third day of life. He had bilateral pneumonia and leukopenia. After a stormy course, which included an exchange transfusion for suspected sepsis and mechanical ventilation for apnea, he eventually recovered.

Table 25-9 Neonatal Infection With Echovirus 9

Study	Finding
Moscovici and Maisel[279]	Asymptomatic infection
Mirani et al[511]	Meningitis (4 cases)
	Gastroenteritis (2 cases)
	Pneumonia (1 case)
Rawls et al[436]	Hepatic necrosis
Cho et al[484]	Severe, generalized disease
Jahn and Cherry[327]	Mild febrile illness
Eichenwald and Kostevalov[280]	Aseptic meningitis
	Gastroenteritis (2 cases)
Haynes et al[538]	Meningoencephalitis
Cheeseman et al[269]	Fatal interstitial pneumonia
Krajden and Middleton[30]	Meningitis

A child who became febrile (38.3° C), irritable, and anorectic on the sixth day of life was described by Jahn and Cherry.[327] This child became asymptomatic within 2 days; echovirus 9 was recovered from the throat, feces, serum, and CSF. Eichenwald and Kostevalov[280] reported two children with mild irritability, fever, and diarrhea and a third child with diarrhea and convulsions in whom laboratory findings showed aseptic meningitis. Haynes and colleagues[538] studied a large outbreak of meningoencephalitis caused by echovirus 9 and described nine children who were 2 weeks to 2 months of age. Cheeseman and associates[269] studied a neonate with fatal interstitial pneumonia, and Krajden and Middleton[30] reported a 4-day-old infant from whom echovirus 9 was recovered from the CSF. This child had fewer than 3 white blood cells/mm^3 in the CSF.

ECHOVIRUS **11.** A wide array of neonatal illnesses have been associated with echovirus 11 infection. Reported cases are listed in Table 25-10. Eleven of the reports involved nursery outbreaks, and, in five reports, the neonatal cases were part of a larger community epidemic. Miller and associates[369] studied an epidemic of aseptic meningitis and other acute febrile illnesses in New Haven, Connecticut, in the summer of 1965. This epidemic was unique in that one half of the patients with meningitis from whom virus was isolated were younger than 6 months. The echovirus 11 in this epidemic was a prime strain. Three neonatal illnesses were reported. One of the patients, a 1-month-old infant, was initially irritable and feverish and had diarrhea. Chest radiographs revealed bilateral pneumonitis. A generalized,

Table 25-10 Neonatal Infection With Echovirus 11

Study	Finding
Miller et al[369]	Exanthem and pneumonia (1 case)
	Nonspecific febrile illness (1 case)
	Aseptic meningitis (1 case)
Sanders and Cramblett[376]	Gastroenteritis (2 cases)
Berkovich and Kibrick[351]	Gastroenteritis (1 case)
	Meningitis (1 case)
Cramblett et al[354]	Meningitis (3 cases, 1 with rash)
	Severe, nonspecific febrile illness (1 case)
Hercík et al[362]	Respiratory illness (22 cases)
Hasegawa [361]	Fever (31 cases)
	Stomatitis (4 cases)
	Fever and stomatitis (6 cases)
Davies et al[355]	Encephalopathy (1 case)
	Nonspecific febrile illness (1 case)
	Sepsis-like illness with cardiac failure (1 death)
	Lower respiratory infection (1 case)
Jones et al[270]	Sepsis-like illness with hepatitis and rash (1 case)
Lapinleimu and Hakulinen [366]	Aseptic meningitis (4 cases)
	Gastroenteritis and/or respiratory distress (3 cases)
Nagington et al[372]	Sepsis-like illness with shock, diffuse bleeding, and renal hemorrhage (3 deaths)
Suzuki et al[508]	Fever (100%); pharyngitis (7%) (42 cases)
Krous et al[419]	Sepsis-like illness with disseminated intravascular coagulation, hepatic necrosis (1 death)
Modlin[370]	Sepsis-like illness with apnea, lethargy, poor feeding, jaundice, hepatitis, disseminated intravascular coagulation (4 deaths)
Drew[519]	Myocarditis (5 cases)
Piraino et al[273]	Meningitis and rash (2 cases)
	Meningitis (4 cases)
	Fatal case with cardiac failure, interstitial pneumonia, and interventricular cerebral hemorrhage
Krajden and Middleton[30]	Meningitis
Mertens et al[368]	Fever (2 cases)
	Meningitis (4 cases)
Reyes et al[272]	Fatal sepsis-like illness
Berry and Nagington[415]	Sepsis-like illness (11 deaths)
	Sudden death
Mostoufizadeh et al[416]	Sepsis-like illness (5 deaths)
Bose et al[271]	Sepsis-like illness (1 death, 1 survived)
Bowen et al[531]	Meningitis (34 infants ≤4 months of age)
Halfon and Spector[418]	Sepsis-like illness (2 deaths)
Steinmann and Albrecht[377]	Sepsis-like illness with meningitis and apnea (5 cases)
	Meningitis (4 cases)
	Gastroenteritis (3 cases)
Gitlin et al[417]	Sepsis-like illness with hepatic necrosis (4 deaths)
Kinney et al[365]	Meningitis (8 cases with 1 death)
	Mild illness (4 cases)
	Inapparent infection (2 cases)
Rabkin et al[375]	Sepsis-like illness (9 cases: 5 with meningitis)
	Inapparent infection (1 case)
Isaacs et al[608]	Meningitis (2 cases: 1 with myocarditis)
	Pneumonia (1 case)
	Inapparent infection (7 cases)
	Apnea (1 case)
Wang et al[420]	Sepsis-like illness with hepatic failure
Tarcan et al[555]	Bone marrow failure
Bina Rai et al[380]	11 cases: 11 fever, 5 diarrhea, 3 coryza, 2 breathing difficulty, 1 jaundice
Tang et al[489]	Mother had pleurodynia and newborn aseptic meningitis
Chen et al[381]	Fever 10 babies; 3 asymptomatic fatal cases with sepsis-like illness and pulmonary hemorrhage
	Sepsis-like illness with hepatitis
Willems et al[440]	Fatal sepsis-like illness with pulmonary hypertension

discrete maculopapular rash, which lasted 24 hours, was seen on the third day of illness. Fever persisted for 6 days. A 12-day-old girl had fever (39.4° C) lasting 1 day but no other findings. Echovirus 11 was recovered from her throat. Another 1-month-old infant had aseptic meningitis.

Sanders and Cramblett[376] described two infants with diarrhea. Both infants were acutely ill; one was jaundiced and irritable and had feeding difficulty. In another study, two infants with echovirus 11 infections had diarrhea.[351] One infant had a temperature of 39.3° C and a "stuffy nose," and the other had a temperature of 39.8° C and aseptic meningitis. Cramblett and coworkers[354] observed an outbreak of nosocomial infections caused by echovirus 11 in a neonatal ICU. In a 1-month-old, premature infant with frequent apneic episodes, the CSF contained 2200 white blood cells/mm^3, 89% of them polymorphonuclear cells, and the protein level was 280 mg/dL. The infant made a gradual recovery. Echovirus 11 was isolated from the CSF and stool. In another premature infant, apneic episodes and bradycardia suddenly began on the 20th day of life. Fever developed, the apneic spells continued, and digitalis therapy was necessary because of congestive heart failure. Examination of the CSF revealed aseptic meningitis, and echovirus 11 was recovered from the CSF, throat, and stool. A third child with aseptic meningitis had an exanthem. The disease began suddenly, and the child had shallow respirations and poor skin color. On the next day, generalized seizures occurred, and a maculopapular rash developed on the trunk, extremities, and face. The patient made a gradual recovery. A fourth child had a severe, nonspecific febrile illness.

A particularly noteworthy finding in neonatal echovirus 11 infection has been severe sepsis-like illness with hepatitis or hepatic necrosis, disseminated intravascular coagulation, and extensive hemorrhagic manifestations.[†c] During the past 15 years, more than 40 such cases have been described, and most of the illnesses have been fatal.

Hercík and coworkers[362] reported an epidemic of respiratory illness in 22 newborns. Six of the infants were severely ill, and one subsequently died. The incubation period varied from 17 hours to 9 days, with an average of 3 days. Seven infants had an interstitial pneumonia, and all had rhinitis, pharyngitis, and vomiting. Toce and Keenan[275] reported two newborns with respiratory distress and pneumonia at birth. Both infants died of their echovirus 11 infections. Tarcan and colleagues[555] described a 5-day-old boy who developed fever and diarrhea. He developed a maculopapular rash on the face, generalized petechiae and hemorrhagic bullae, and pancytopenia caused by bone marrow failure. This infant was treated with IVIG and recovered.

An outbreak of echovirus 11 infections in neonates in a confinement home in Penang, Malaysia, was noted in September and October 2004.[380] Of the two primary cases from a hospital nursery, one went to the confinement home and there became symptomatic. Eleven of the 13 babies in the confinement home developed febrile illnesses. In addition, 5 had diarrhea, 3 coryza, 2 difficulty breathing, and 1 jaundice.

Three days after birth, a baby in a neonatal unit in London, England developed lethargy and fed poorly.[489] The neonate had temperature fluctuations and recurrent hypoglycemia and aseptic meningitis. The mother of the baby had pleurodynia at the time of delivery. An echovirus 11 outbreak occurred in a nursery in Taipei, Taiwan, in November 2003.[556] Twelve neonates had symptomatic illness, and there were 3 asymptomatically infected babies. One of the infants developed respiratory failure, hypotonia, disseminated intravascular coagulopathy and bacterial grade IV intraventricular hemorrhage and died at a referral center from extensive pulmonary hemorrhage 6 days after admission. A second baby had fulminant hepatitis, anemia, aseptic meningitis, and disseminated intravascular coagulopathy but survived after a lengthy hospital stay. The other 10 infants who were referred because of fever all recovered without sequelae. The source of infection in the index patient was the mother.

Echovirus 13. Before 2000, infection with echovirus 13 was rare in neonates. The virus was isolated from one asymptomatic infant in a neonatal surveillance study.[294] In 2001 in the United States, echovirus 13 was the leading cause of aseptic meningitis, and during 2001 and 2002, aseptic meningitis outbreaks with this agent occurred in a number of countries.[422,536,539,557] A substantial number of cases were infants who were 3 months of age or younger.[558] A 28-day-old boy in Tennessee had aseptic meningitis and hepatitis.[559] Neonatal cases were reported in Israel and Spain, but details were not presented.[560,561]

Echovirus 14. Hughes and colleagues[278] reported an infant boy who became febrile (38° C) and had cyanotic episodes on the third day of life. When 4 days of age, his temperature was 38.9° C, and he experienced recurrent apneic spells. Liver enlargement, hypothermia, bradycardia, periodic breathing, and spontaneous ecchymoses developed, and the infant died on the seventh day of life. Laboratory studies revealed the presence of leukopenia and thrombocytopenia, and autopsy showed severe hepatic necrosis. Drouhet[562] described a child with aseptic meningitis and echovirus 14 infection, and Hinuma and associates[563] reported four newborns with apparent asymptomatic echovirus 14 infections.

Echovirus 16. In 1974, Hall and colleagues[477] studied five neonates with echovirus 16 infections. All five infants were admitted to the hospital because sepsis was suspected. Four of five were febrile, all were lethargic and irritable, and two had abdominal distention. Three of the neonates had erythematous maculopapular exanthems, and in two, the rash appeared after or with defervescence. Leukocyte counts in four infants revealed an increased percentage of band form neutrophils. Two neonates had aseptic meningitis. Lake and associates[433] observed three infants with echovirus 16 infections. In their study, clinical findings were not itemized by virus type, but it is inferred that sepsis-like illnesses occurred.

Echovirus 17. Neonatal infection with echovirus 17 has been observed by three investigators. Cherry and coworkers[254] reported two ill infants. A 19-day-old infant developed otitis media 5 days after his mother had a flu-like illness. Echovirus 17 was isolated from his feces, and serologic evidence of echovirus 17 infection was found in the infant and the mother. The second child had a nonspecific febrile illness at the age of 4 weeks, which was severe enough to require hospitalization. Virus was isolated from the infant's throat, feces, and serum.

[†c]References 270-272, 355, 370, 372, 415-419, 432, 436.

Sanders and Cramblett[376] described two neonates with exanthem associated with echovirus 17. The first child, a 3-week-old girl, became drowsy, anorectic, and febrile. She had a fine maculopapular rash on the trunk, a slightly injected pharynx, and a few petechiae on the soft palate. She remained febrile for 5 days. Echovirus 17 was recovered from the CSF and the feces. The second infant became ill when 3 weeks old. His symptoms were mild rhinitis and cough, followed by lethargy and refusal to eat. Four days after the onset of symptoms, his temperature was 39° C, and his respiratory rate was 60 breaths per minute. A fine maculopapular rash appeared on the trunk, and radiographs revealed an infiltrate in the right lung. The patient's course was uneventful, and he was much improved 12 days after the onset of symptoms.

Faulkner and van Rooyen[358] described an outbreak of echovirus 17 infection with illness in a nursery in mid-August of 1971. Seven infants were involved, including one with aseptic meningitis who was 7 weeks of age. All the infants had fever, four had CNS signs, three had abdominal distention, four had diarrhea, and three had a rash. One other infant from another community was also studied by the investigators. This child had a febrile pneumonitis when 3.5 weeks old. The findings abated in 5 days, but the child suddenly died 6 days later. Autopsy revealed interstitial pneumonitis with extensive edema and scattered petechial hemorrhages of the viscera. Echovirus 17 was isolated from the liver, lung, spleen, and kidney.

Echovirus 18. In 1958, Eichenwald and colleagues[356] described epidemic diarrhea associated with echovirus 18 infections. In a nursery unit of premature infants, 12 of 21 were mildly ill. Neither temperature elevation nor hypothermia occurred. Six infants were lethargic and listless, and two developed moderate abdominal distention. The diarrhea lasted 1 to 5 days; there were five or six watery, greenish stools per day, occasionally expelled explosively. In two infants, a small amount of blood was seen in the stools, but there were no mucus or pus cells. Five other infants in another nursery had similar diarrheal illness. Echovirus 18 was recovered from all ill infants.

Medearis and coworkers[564] reported a 3-week-old girl with fever, irritability, lethargy, pharyngitis, and postnasal drainage. Admitted to the hospital because of apneic spells, she developed a generalized erythematous blotchy macular rash and had frequent stools. The illness lasted about 7 days. Echovirus 18 was recovered from the blood, throat, and feces. Berkovich and Kibrick[351] found echovirus 18 in the stool of a 12-day-old twin infant with fever and a red throat. The relationship of echovirus 18 to the illness is uncertain because the patient's twin was infected with echovirus 11, and the patient also had serologic evidence of echovirus 11 infection. The fever and red throat may have been caused by echovirus 11 rather than echovirus 18 infection. Wilfert and associates[557] observed a 9-day-old infant with aseptic meningitis.

Kusuhara and coworkers[383] described an outbreak of echovirus 18 infection in a neonatal intensive care unit involving 20 patients. This outbreak occurred between November 3 and November 24, 2003, and involved patients aged 1 week to 6 months. Eight of the infants had acute exanthematous diseases, 1 had transient fever, and the other 11 patients were asymptomatic.

Echovirus 19. Cramblett and coworkers[524] described two neonates with echovirus 19 infections. One child had an upper respiratory infection, cough, and paroxysmal atrial tachycardia. The other child also had an upper respiratory infection, but in addition to echovirus 19 infection, coxsackievirus B4 was recovered from the throat of this infant. Butterfield and associates[353] isolated echovirus 19 postmortem from the brain, lung, heart, liver, spleen, lymph nodes, and intestine of a premature infant who had cystic emphysema. The relationship between the generalized viral infection and the pulmonary disease is not understood.

Philip and Larson[268] reported three catastrophic neonatal echovirus 19 infections, which resulted in hepatic necrosis and massive terminal hemorrhage. One infant, infected in utero, was symptomatic at birth. The Apgar score was 3, and multiple petechiae were observed. The infant had generalized ecchymoses and apneic episodes and died when 3.5 hours of age. Thrombocytopenia was identified, and echovirus 19 was isolated from the brain, liver, spleen, and lymph nodes. The other two infants who died of echovirus 19 infection were twins. They were normal during the first 3 days of life but then became mildly cyanotic and lethargic. Shortly thereafter, apneic episodes occurred, and jaundice and petechiae developed. Both twins became oliguric, and they died on the eighth and ninth days of life with severe gastrointestinal bleeding. Both twins were thrombocytopenic, and virus was recovered from systemic sites in both. Two similar catastrophic cases have been described.[547]

Purdham and associates[374] reported an outbreak of echovirus 19 in a neonatal unit in which 12 infants were affected. Eleven infants were febrile, 10 were irritable, 7 had marked abdominal distention with decreased bowel sounds, and 5 had apneic episodes. Bacon and Sims[481] described two neonates with sepsis-like illness. The infants were cyanotic with peripheral circulatory failure. In another study involving the same echovirus 19 epidemic, five infants younger than 3 months were reported.[485] All had sepsis-like illness with hypotonia and peripheral circulatory failure. Two infants had aseptic meningitis, and two others had diarrhea.

Echovirus 20. Eichenwald and Kostevalov[280] recovered echovirus 20 from four asymptomatic infants younger than 8 days (see "Cloud Baby"). Five neonates with severe illness caused by echovirus 20 have also been described.[434,504] All had hepatitis, and two died.

Echovirus 21. Jack and coworkers[363] recovered echovirus 21 from the feces of a 7-day-old infant with jaundice and diarrhea. No other details of the child's illness are available. Chonmaitree and associates[518] studied a 19-day-old infant with aseptic meningitis and rash, and Georgieff and colleagues[435] reported a newborn with fulminant hepatitis. Lake and colleagues[433] also mentioned one infected infant but presented no specific details.

Echovirus 25. Linnemann and colleagues[487] reported one neonate with echovirus 25 infection. They gave no virus-specific details, except that fever and irritability occurred.

Echovirus 30. Matsumoto and associates[541] described a nursery outbreak involving 11 infants during a 2-week period. All the neonates had aseptic meningitis, and all recovered. Two symptomatic and six asymptomatic neonates were reported in the Rochester, New York, surveillance study.[294] Chen and associates[483] described twin neonates who had fever, followed by thrombocytopenia, coagulopathy, and hepatic failure. One of the neonates died and the other survived and had no obvious sequelae at 1 year of age. In another study, twins had a sepsis-like illness with hepatitis.[482] These twins survived and had normal development and normal liver function at 1 year of age.

ECHOVIRUS 31. McDonald and associates[367] described three neonates in an intensive care nursery with echovirus 31 infections. One infant had a fatal encephalitis-like illness, with hypertonicity, hyperreflexia, and apneic spells. The other two infants also experienced apneic spells, and in addition, one had pneumonia and meningitis.

ECHOVIRUS 33. In a study of epidemic illness related to echovirus 33 disease in the Netherlands, Kapsenberg[364] stated that 7- to 8-day-old neonates in a maternity ward had a febrile illness. No further data were presented.

Enterovirus 71. Schmidt and colleagues[422] mentioned one 3-week-old infant with meningitis and enterovirus 71 infection. Chonmaitree and colleagues[510] described one 9-day-old neonate with aseptic meningitis and one 14-day-old infant with gastroenteritis from enterovirus 71. Chen and associates[526] reported a child with bilateral lower limbs weakness in association with the hand-foot-and-mouth syndrome.

Parechoviruses

PARECHOVIRUS 1. Parechovirus 1 has been associated with three epidemics of nursery infections. During a survey of perinatal virus infections by Jack and associates,[363] 44 infants were found to be infected with parechovirus 1 during a study period from May to December 1966. The virus prevalence and the incidence of new infections during this period were fairly uniform. No illness was attributed to parechovirus 1 infection, and the virus disappeared from the nursery in mid-December of 1966. Berkovich and Pangan[352] studied respiratory illnesses in premature infants and reported 64 infants with illness, 18 of whom had virologic or serologic evidence of parechovirus 1 infection. Many had high but constant levels of serum antibody to parechovirus 1. Some of these infants were probably also infected with parechovirus 1. The children with proven parechovirus 1 infections could not be clinically differentiated from those without evidence of parechovirus 1 infection. Of 18 infants with documented parechovirus 1 infections, 90% had coryza, 39% had pneumonia, and 11% had morbilliform rash or conjunctivitis, or both. In contrast to the studies of Jack and coworkers,[363] only 3 of 35 asymptomatic infants were found to be infected with parechovirus 1. Nakao and associates[373] recovered parechovirus 1 from 29 premature infants. Many of the infected infants were asymptomatic, and those who were ill had only mild symptoms of coryza, cough, and diarrhea. Jenista and colleagues[294] described 17 parechovirus 1 infections in nonhospitalized neonates. Clinical details were not presented, but it appears that all of these infants were asymptomatic. Parechovirus 1 infection was associated with a nosocomial necrotizing enterocolitis outbreak.[530]

In a study of Dutch children, Benschop and colleagues[482] compared the clinical findings in 27 children with parechovirus 1 with those of 10 children with parechovirus 3. Unfortunately, they only identified the median ages of the children, so we do not know the number of neonates with illnesses. They found that sepsis-like illness and CNS symptoms were more common in the parechovirus 3 cases compared with the parechovirus 1 cases.

In 2009 in a neonatal unit in Zagreb, Croatia, an outbreak involving seven infants with parechovirus type 1 was noted.[283] The characteristics of infection in these infants were apnea, rhinitis, tachypnea and retractions. In addition, four of the infants had mild gastrointestinal symptoms manifested by diarrhea, abdominal distention, and poor feeding.

PARECHOVIRUS 2. Ehrnst and Eriksson[535] reported a 1-month-old girl with encephalopathy resulting from a nosocomial parechovirus 2 infection. No further details of this case were provided.

PARECHOVIRUS 3. A number of recent studies of illness with parechovirus 3 infections in neonates and young infants have been presented.[‡c] Four studies occurred in the Netherlands. In one study of 10 neonates and young infants, 90% had fever, 70% had sepsis-like illness, 70% had gastrointestinal tract symptoms, 50% had CNS symptoms, and 30% had respiratory tract symptoms.[482] In a subsequent study of 29 young children (median age, 1.2 months) by members of the same group, the following findings were noted: fever, 97%; irritability, 86%; sepsis-like illness, 75%; meningitis, 12%; seizures, 7%; encephalitis, 4%; paralysis, 4%; rash, 17%; gastrointestinal tract symptoms, 39%; and respiratory tract symptoms, 36%.

Boivin and associates[475] in Quebec, Canada reported 3 neonates with high fever, erythematous rash, and tachypnea. Verboon-Maciolak and coworkers[37]compared neonatal illness with parechovirus 3 with illness caused by enteroviruses, and the only differences noted were that gastrointestinal tract symptoms were more common in the parechovirus 3 group and that the C-reactive protein and the CSF protein were higher in the enterovirus group.[443] Members of the same group carefully studied encephalitis in 10 neonates. All had white matter injury. Six of the 10 were normal at later follow-up; of the 4 others, 1 child had cerebral palsy with epilepsy, 1 child had learning disabilities, 1 child had epilepsy but normal cognitive outcome at 3 years of age, and 1 child had mild distal hypertonia at 18 months of age.

In contrast with enterovirus infections in neonates, exanthem is common in parechovirus type 3 infections.[§c] It is most often erythematous and macular and most often involves the hands and feet.

PARECHOVIRUS 4. A neonate with fever and poor feeding was found to be infected with parechovirus 4.[476]

Diagnosis and Differential Diagnosis

CLINICAL DIAGNOSIS

The clinical differentiation of neonatal infectious diseases frequently seems to be an impossible task. Although it is true that treatable bacterial and viral illnesses should always be considered and treated first, it is also true that when all the circumstances of a particular neonatal illness are

‡c References 37, 38, 441-443, 475, 482, 492-496, 498, 500-502.

§c References 475, 491, 492, 494, 496, 500, 501.

considered, enterovirus and parechovirus diseases can be suspected on clinical grounds. The most important factors in clinical diagnosis are season of the year, geographic location, exposure, incubation period, and clinical symptoms.

In temperate climates, enteroviral and parechovirus prevalence is distinctly seasonal, and disease is usually seen in the summer and fall. Neonatal enterovirus disease is less likely in the winter. In the tropics, enteroviruses are prevalent throughout the year, and the season therefore is not helpful diagnostically.

As with all infectious illnesses, knowledge of exposure and incubation time is important. A careful history of maternal illness is vital, particularly the symptoms of maternal illness. For example, nonspecific mild febrile illness in the mother that occurs in the summer and fall should warn of the possibility of more severe neonatal illness. More specific findings in the mother (e.g., aseptic meningitis, pleurodynia, herpangina, pericarditis, myocarditis) should alert the clinician to look for more specific enteroviral illnesses. Minor illness in nursery personnel during enteroviral seasons and the short incubation period of enteroviral and parechovirus infections should be taken into consideration. Manifestations of neonatal nonpolio enteroviral and parechoviral infections are given in Table 25-5.

LABORATORY DIAGNOSIS

Virus Isolation

Most viral diagnostic laboratories have facilities for the recovery of most enteroviruses and parechoviruses that cause congenital and neonatal illness. Three tissue culture systems—primary rhesus, cynomolgus, or African green monkey kidney tissue culture; a diploid, human embryonic lung fibroblast cell strain; and the RD cell line—allow the isolation of all polioviruses, coxsackieviruses B, echoviruses, newer enteroviruses, parechoviruses, and many coxsackieviruses A. In a 1988 study in which Buffalo green monkey kidney cells and subpassages of primary human embryonic kidney cells were used in addition to primary monkey kidney and human diploid fibroblast (MRC-5) cells, the enterovirus recovery rate was increased by 11%.[565] Also useful for parechovirus isolation are HT 29 (primary colorectal adenocarcinoma) cells and A549 (human lung carcinoma) cells.[132] For a complete diagnostic isolation spectrum, suckling mouse inoculation should also be performed. Optimally, at least one blind passage should be carried out in each of the culture systems.

Proper selection and handling of specimens are most important in the isolation of viruses from ill neonates. Because infection in neonates tends to be generalized, collection of material from multiple sites is important. Specimens should be taken from any or all of the following: nasopharynx, throat, stool, blood, urine, CSF, and any other body fluids that are available. Swabs from the nose, throat, and rectum should be placed in a transport medium.

Transport medium provides a protective protein, neutral pH, and antibiotics for control of microbial contamination and, most importantly, prevents desiccation. Many viral transport and storage media are commercially available or are prepared readily in the laboratory; their utility has been reviewed elsewhere.[566] Convenient and practical collection devices, such as the Culturette (Becton-Dickinson, Cockeysville, Md) or Virocult (Medical Wire and Equipment Co., Victory Gardens, NY), consist of a swab, usually Dacron or rayon, on a plastic or aluminum shaft, accompanied by a self-contained transport medium (Stuart or Amies), and are routinely available in most hospitals for bacteriologic culture. Calcium alginate swabs, which are toxic to herpes simplex virus, and wooden shafts, which may be toxic for viruses and the cell culture system itself, should not be used. Saline or holding media that contain serum also should be avoided. Useful liquid transport media (2-mL aliquots in screw-capped vials) consist of tryptose phosphate broth with 0.5% bovine albumin; Hanks balanced salt solution with 5% gelatin or 10% bovine albumin; or buffered sucrose phosphate (0.2M, 2-SP medium),[566,567] which has been used as a combined transport for viral, chlamydial, and mycoplasmal culture requests and is appropriate for long-term frozen storage of specimens and isolates.[568]

Fluid specimens should be collected in sterile vials. Specimens of autopsy material are best collected in vials that contain transport medium. In general, specimens should be refrigerated immediately after collection and during transportation to the laboratory. Specimens should not be exposed to sunlight during transportation. If an extended period is likely to elapse before a specimen can be processed in the laboratory, it is advisable to ship and store it frozen.

Contrary to popular belief, evidence of enteroviral growth from tissue cultures takes only a few days in many cases and less than a week in most.[131] The use of the spin amplification, shell vial technique, and monoclonal antibodies has significantly reduced the time for detection of enteroviral cultures.[75,569] After isolation of an enterovirus, identification of its type has historically done by neutralization, which is unfortunately an expensive and lengthy process. "Molecular serotyping," by determining the sequence of the VP1 coding domain of the viral genome, is increasingly being used for epidemiologic purposes.[97,99,103,104]

Rapid Virus Identification

Because of the number of different serotypes of enteroviruses and parechoviruses, the use of immunofluorescence, agglutination, counterimmunoelectrophoresis, and ELISA techniques for the direct detection of antigen in suspected enteroviral infections has not been useful. Nucleic acid techniques with complementary DNA and RNA probes have been useful for the direct identification of enteroviruses.[90,551,559-561] Of most importance has been the development of numerous PCR techniques. Since 1990, innumerable reports have described enteroviral and, more recently, parechovirus PCR methods and their use in identifying enterovirus and parechovirus RNA in clinical specimens.[‖c] PCR assay has proved most useful for the direct identification of enteroviruses and parechoviruses in the CSF of patients with meningitis. Compared with culture of CSF specimens, PCR assay is more rapid and sensitive, and the specificity is equal.

PCR assay also has proved useful in the identification of enteroviruses and parechoviruses in blood, urine, and throat specimens.[¶c] Particularly impressive are the findings of Byington and associates.[22] Using the PCR on specimens

‖c References 71-73, 75-78, 81-87, 115, 131, 132, 554, 562, 565-570.
¶c References 22, 71, 78, 84, 115, 565, 566, 571, 573.

of blood and CSF, they found that more than 25% of infants admitted to the hospital for suspected sepsis in 1997 had nonpolio enterovirus infections. Based on this study and a subsequent study in Utah and the work of Andréoletti and coworkers,[72,73] we believe the general workup for febrile neonates hospitalized for possible sepsis should include PCR for enteroviruses in blood and CSF. This is most important during enterovirus and parechovirus season (summer and fall in temperate climates), but because enteroviral circulation continues all year, it is reasonable to also perform PCR in the off seasons. Although the PCR detects enterovirus RNA, the specific enteroviral type is not identified. Because of this shortcoming, we recommend that conventional culture should be performed along with PCR assay. It should be noted that parechoviruses will not be identified using the PCR designed to amplify enterovirus nucleotide sequences. Therefore neonatal parechovirus cases will be missed unless specific PCR assay for parechovirus is also performed.

PCR assay has also identified enteroviruses in frozen and formalin-fixed biopsy and autopsy specimens of myocardium.[71,78,84,565,566] In one study, enteroviruses were identified in myocardial tissue from four neonates who died of myocarditis.[573] In one case, the specimen was obtained during life by a right ventricular endomyocardial biopsy, and in the other three, frozen or formalin-fixed autopsy samples were used. Most PCR methods can detect one tissue culture infective dose of enterovirus in CSF, stool, or throat specimen.[574] Polioviruses can be separated from other enteroviruses, and poliovirus vaccine strains can be rapidly identified by PCR assay.[131,567-570,575]

Enteroviral RNA has been identified in numerous tissue specimens from patients with chronic medical conditions, such as idiopathic dilated cardiomyopathy. However, the possibility of lack of specificity is a concern; false-positive results could be due to technical factors (e.g., PCR contamination) or due to persistence of viral RNA in tissue.

Serology

Except in special circumstances, the use of serologic techniques in the primary diagnosis of suspected neonatal enterovirus infections is impractical. Standard serologic study depends on the demonstration of an antibody titer rise to a specific virus as an indication of infection with that agent. Although hemagglutination inhibition, ELISA, and complement fixation tests take only a short time to perform, these tests can be done only after the collection of a second, convalescent-phase blood specimen. These tests are also impractical in searching for the cause of a specific illness in a child because there are so many antigenically different enteroviruses. As discussed in "Antigenic Characteristics," group antigens can be produced that allow serologic diagnosis by IgM EIA and complement fixation, but these tests lack specificity.[133,134,576]

In the evaluation of an infant with a suspected enterovirus infection, serum should be collected as soon as possible after the onset of illness and then again 2 to 4 weeks later. This serum should be stored frozen. In most clinical situations, it is not necessary to carry out serologic tests on the collected serum because demonstration of an antibody titer rise in the serum of an infant from whom a specific virus has been isolated from a body fluid is obviously superfluous. However, collected serum can be useful diagnostically if the prevalence of specific enteroviruses or parechoviruses in a community is known. In this situation, it is relatively easy to look for antibody titer changes to a selected number of viral types. More rapid diagnosis using a single serum sample is possible if a search for specific IgM enteroviral antibody is made.[340,571,573,574,577-582]

Unfortunately, enterovirus IgM antibody tests are not commercially available. Commercial laboratories do offer enteroviral complement fixation antibody panels. However, these tests are expensive, and their results in the clinical setting are almost always meaningless unless acute- and convalescent-phase sera are analyzed.

Histology

There are no specific histologic findings in enteroviral infections, such as those seen in cytomegalovirus or herpes simplex viral infections. However, tissues can be examined for specific enteroviral antigens by immunofluorescent study and by PCR assay.[261,554,583,584]

Differential Diagnosis

The differential diagnosis of congenital and neonatal enterovirus infections depends on the clinical manifestations. In general, the most important illness categories are generalized bacterial sepsis or meningitis, congenital heart disease, and congenital and neonatal infections with other viruses.

Hypothermia and hyperthermia associated with nonspecific signs such as lethargy and poor appetite are common in neonatal enteroviral infections; they are also the presenting manifestations in bacterial sepsis. Proper bacterial cultures are essential. Differentiation between congenital heart disease and neonatal myocarditis is frequently difficult. However, the occurrence of fever or hypothermia, generalized lethargy and weakness, and characteristic electrocardiographic changes should suggest a viral cause.

Congenital infections with rubella virus, cytomegalovirus, *Toxoplasma gondii*, or *Treponema pallidum* are frequently associated with intrauterine growth retardation; this is not usual with enterovirus infections. Generalized herpes simplex infections are clinically similar to severe infections with several enteroviruses; in herpes infections, skin lesions are common, and a scraping of a lesion and a culture should allow a rapid diagnosis. In infants with signs of CNS involvement, it is particularly important to consider herpes simplex virus infection as a possible cause because infection with this agent is treatable and early treatment is essential. In infants with meningitis, proper cultures and PCR testing are essential because the CSF findings in bacterial and viral illnesses are frequently similar.

Prognosis

POLIOVIRUSES

As substantiated in the review by Bates[207] and the summary in Table 25-7, poliovirus infections in neonates are generally severe. Of the 44 cases with available follow-up data, there were 21 deaths; of the survivors, 12 had residual paralyses. Because infant survivors of poliomyelitis are susceptible to infection by the other two types of poliovirus, they should receive polio vaccine.

NONPOLIO ENTEROVIRUSES AND PARECHOVIRUSES

It is apparent that the immediate prognosis for patients with coxsackievirus and echovirus infections is related to the specific manifestations. Mortality rates are highest for infants with myocarditis, encephalitis, or sepsis-like illness with liver involvement. Differences in the severity of illness depend on viral type and strain variations. In general, infections with coxsackieviruses B1 to B4 and with echovirus 11 appear to carry the most ominous initial prognoses. Also of concern are CNS infections with parechovirus 3.

There is a surprising dearth of information related to long-term sequelae of neonatal coxsackievirus and echovirus infections. Gear,[322] in a 4-year follow-up study, found no evidence of permanent cardiac damage in several children who had coxsackievirus B myocarditis. For children with aseptic meningitis, there is little available evidence of neurologic damage. One of five infants studied by Nogen and Lepow,[336] from whom virus was recovered from the CSF, was suspected of having brain damage. Cho and colleagues[484] reported that a child who had had severe neonatal echovirus 9 disease was developing normally at 1 year of age. Tuuteri and associates[343] reported that 2 children who had had clinically mild neonatal coxsackievirus B3 infections were thriving when seen at 1 year of age. After an epidemic of mild febrile disease related to echovirus 5, 51 children were examined at 1 year of age and found to be normal.[359]

Farmer and colleagues[536] did a careful follow-up study of 15 children who had meningoencephalitis related to coxsackievirus B5 during the neonatal period. When 6 years of age, 2 of the children were found to have developed spasticity, and their intelligence was below the mean for the study group as a whole and below the mean of a carefully selected control group. Three children who had myocarditis and meningoencephalitis had no cardiac sequelae at 6 years of age. Sells and associates[543] described neurologic impairment at later follow-up study of some children who had CNS enteroviral infections during the first year of life.

In a study in which 9 children with enteroviral meningitis during the first 3 months of life were compared with nine matched control children, Wilfert and associates[552] found that the receptive language functioning of patients was significantly less than that of the control children. Head circumference, hearing, and intellectual function were similar for patients and control children. Bergman and colleagues[528] reported an extensive study in which 33 survivors of enteroviral meningitis during infancy were compared with their siblings. In this comprehensive study, none of the survivors had major neurologic sequelae, and they performed as well as their siblings on a large number of cognitive, achievement, perceptual-motor skills, and language tests. Rantakallio and coworkers[520] found that 16 of 17 patients with neonatal meningitis related to coxsackievirus B5 had normal neurologic development on follow-up. The one exception was a child with suspected intrauterine myocarditis. In another study, 16 newborns with meningitis related to coxsackievirus A14 were normal 2.5 years later.

The most alarming report is that of Eichenwald,[356] who gave details of a 5-year follow-up study of infants who had had neonatal diarrhea associated with echovirus 18 infection. Thirteen of 16 infants who had had an echovirus 18 infection during the neonatal period showed neurologic damage; these children had an IQ of less than 70, spasticity, deafness, blindness, or a combination of these effects.

In most instances, the antibody response of neonates after enterovirus infection is good. It is therefore to be expected that one attack of infection with a particular viral type provides immunity to the specific agent in the future. From the evidence derived from polio vaccine studies, it is probable that reinfection with all enteroviruses is common but that after an initial antibody response, a secondary inapparent infection occurs and is confined to the gastrointestinal tract.

Therapy

SPECIFIC THERAPY

No specific therapy for any enterovirus infection is approved for use in the United States. In severe, catastrophic, and generalized neonatal infection, it is likely that the infant received no specific antibody for the particular virus from the mother. In this situation, it is probably advisable to administer human immune serum globulin to the infant. Dagan and associates[586] examined three lots of human serum globulin and found the presence of neutralizing antibodies to several commonly circulating and infrequently circulating enteroviruses. Although there is no evidence that this therapy is beneficial in treating acute neonatal infections, there is evidence of some success in the treatment of chronic enteroviral infections in agammaglobulinemic patients.[587] Because it was found by Hammond and coworkers[588] that a single dose of intramuscular immunoglobulin resulted in little change in circulating neutralizing antibodies to coxsackievirus B4 and echovirus 11 in seven infants, it seems advisable, when therapy is decided on, to use high-dose IVIG. One neonate with disseminated echovirus 11 infection with hepatitis, pneumonitis, meningitis, disseminated intravascular coagulation, decreased renal function, and anemia survived after receiving a large dose of IVIG and supportive care.[589]

Abzug and colleagues[590] performed a small but controlled study of nine enterovirus-infected neonates who received IVIG and seven similarly infected infants who received supportive care. In this study, there was no significant difference in clinical scores, antibody values, or magnitude of viremia and viruria in those treated compared with the control infants. However, five infants received IVIG with a high neutralizing antibody titer (≥1:800) to their individual viral isolates, and they had a more rapid cessation of viremia and viruria.

Jantausch and associates[591] reported an infant with a disseminated echovirus 11 infection who survived after maternal plasma transfusions. The role, if any, of these transfusions in the infant's recovery is unknown, and this form of therapy cannot be recommended.

Many antipicornavirus drugs and biologicals have been studied during the past 30 years.[67,68,592] The antiviral drug pleconaril offers promise for the treatment of enteroviral infections.[#c] This drug is a novel compound that integrates into the capsid of enteroviruses. It prevents the virus from

[#c] References 67, 70, 490, 506, 586, 587, 593, 594.

attaching to cellular receptors and therefore prevents uncoating and subsequent release of viral RNA into the host cell. In a double-blinded, placebo-controlled study of 39 patients with enteroviral meningitis, a statistically significant shortening of the disease duration was noted, from 9.5 days in control subjects to 4.0 days in drug recipients.[67] Pleconaril was also used on a compassionate-release basis in the treatment of patients with life-threatening infection.[594] Several categories of enteroviral illnesses were treated: chronic meningoencephalitis in patients with agammaglobulinemia or hypogammaglobulinemia, neonatal sepsis, myocarditis, poliomyelitis (wild type or vaccine associated), encephalitis, and bone marrow transplant patients. Favorable clinical responses were observed in 22 of 36 treated patients, including 12 of 18 patients with chronic meningoencephalitis. After a study of its effectiveness in treatment of the common cold in adults,[595,596] the United States Food and Drug Administration rejected pleconaril, citing concerns about both safety and efficacy that may not be germane to its use in infants with life-threatening enterovirus infections. A double-blind, placebo-controlled efficacy trial of pleconaril (vs. placebo) in neonates with enteroviral sepsis was completed in 2012 and is currently undergoing data analysis. Pleconaril is not currently available in the United States, even for compassionate use.

In severe illnesses, such as neonatal myocarditis or encephalitis, it is frequently tempting to administer corticosteroids. Although some investigators thought this approach was beneficial in treating coxsackievirus myocarditis, we believe that corticosteroids should not be given during acute enterovirus infections. The deleterious effects of these agents in coxsackievirus infections of mice[597] are particularly persuasive. Immunosuppressive therapy for myocarditis of unknown origin with prednisone and cyclosporine or azathioprine was evaluated in a controlled trial of 111 adults, and no beneficial effect was observed.[598]

Because the possibility of bacterial sepsis cannot initially be excluded in most instances of neonatal enteroviral infections, antibiotics should be administered for the most likely potential pathogens. Care in antibiotic selection and administration is urged so that drug toxicity is not added to the problems of the patient. In neonates with meningitis or meningoencephalitis and in some infants with sepsis-like illnesses, the possibility of herpes simplex virus infections should be strongly considered, and empirical treatment with intravenous acyclovir should be instituted after obtaining appropriate herpesvirus studies.

NONSPECIFIC THERAPY

Mild, Nonspecific Febrile Illness

In infants in whom fever is the only symptom, careful observation is most important. Many infants who eventually become severely ill have 2 to 3 days of fever initially without other localized findings. Care should be taken to administer adequate fluids to febrile infants, and excessive elevation of temperature should be prevented, if possible.

Sepsis-like Illness

In infants with severe sepsis-like illness, the major problems are shock, hepatitis and hepatic necrosis, and disseminated intravascular coagulation. For shock, attention should be directed toward treating hypotension and acidosis and ensuring adequate oxygenation.

Myocarditis and Severe Hepatitis

There is no specific therapy for myocarditis. However, congestive heart failure and arrhythmias should be treated by the usual methods. In administering digitalis preparations to infants with enteroviral myocarditis, careful attention to the initial dosage is most important because the heart is often extremely sensitive; frequently, only small amounts of digoxin are necessary.

In cases of severe hepatitis with hyperammonemia, administration of neomycin and rifaximin or other nonabsorbable antibiotics, alone or with lactulose, is used to suppress the bacterial intestinal microbiome. Coagulopathy is corrected with infusions of fresh-frozen plasma or other blood products.

Several infants with echovirus-induced liver failure and who survived after undergoing orthotopic liver transplantation have been reported.[293,599,600] Similarly, three infants have been described who underwent successful heart transplantation after neonatal enterovirus myocarditis at 11 days to 8 weeks of life.[259,521,601] It is worth noting that in several of these cases, transplantation and the use of immunosuppression occurred in the first month of life, yet recrudescent infection and dysfunction of the grafts did not occur.

Meningoencephalitis

In patients with meningoencephalitis, convulsions, cerebral edema, and disturbances of fluid and electrolyte balance occur frequently and respond to treatment. Seizures are best treated with phenobarbital, phenytoin, or lorazepam. Cerebral edema can be treated with urea, mannitol, or large doses of corticosteroids. However, it seems unwise to use corticosteroids in active enterovirus infections because the potential benefits may be outweighed by deleterious effects. Fluid status should be monitored closely, and frequent determinations of serum electrolyte levels should be made because inappropriate antidiuretic hormone secretion may occur.

Paralytic Poliomyelitis

Infants should be observed carefully for evidence of respiratory paralysis. If respiratory failure occurs, the early use of a positive-pressure ventilator is essential. In newborns, this is better performed without tracheotomy. Careful attention to pooling of secretions is important. Blood gas levels should be monitored frequently. Passive exercises of all involved extremities should be started if the infant has been afebrile for 3 days.

Prevention

IMMUNIZATION

Congenital and neonatal poliomyelitis should be illnesses of historical interest only. However, because segments of populations in a few regions of the world have not been adequately immunized with polioviral vaccines, clinical poliomyelitis will continue to occur. In adequately immunized populations, congenital and neonatal poliomyelitis has been eliminated.

Attenuated or inactivated viral vaccines for other enteroviruses are not currently available, although vaccines for enterovirus 71 are being been developed.[602,603] In one recent study, an inactivated EV71 vaccine was given to children 6 to 35 months of age and demonstrated 90% efficacy in the prevention of hand-foot-and-mouth disease and 80% against any serious EV71-related disease; this study demonstrates that the approaches used to produce inactivated poliovirus vaccine can be used to induce protective immunity to nonpoliovirus vaccine.[603]

Passive protection with intramuscular immune globulin (0.15-0.5 mL/kg) or perhaps IVIG can be useful in preventing disease.[590,591,604,605] In practice, however, this approach seems to be worthwhile only in sudden and virulent nursery outbreaks. For example, if several cases of myocarditis occurred in a nursery, it would seem wise to administer immune globulin to all infants in the nursery. Pooled human immune globulin in most instances can be expected to contain antibodies against coxsackievirus types B1 through B5 and echovirus 11. This procedure could offer protection to infants without transplacentally acquired specific antibody who had not yet become infected.

OTHER MEASURES

Breastfeeding should be encouraged in all newborns. Sadeharju and associates[606] found that infants exclusively breastfed for greater than 2 weeks had fewer enteroviral infections by the age of 1 year compared with those exclusively breastfed for less than or equal to 2 weeks.

Careful attention to routine nursery infection control procedures is important in preventing and controlling epidemics of enteroviral diseases. Nursery personnel should exercise strict care in washing their hands after handling each infant. It is also important to restrict the nursery area to personnel who are free of even minor illnesses.

Nursery infection, when it occurs, is best controlled in units that follow a cohort system. When illness occurs, the infant in question should be immediately isolated, and the nursery should be closed to all new admissions.

References

1. Pallansch MA, Roos RP: *Enteroviruses: polioviruses, coxsackieviruses, echoviruses, and newer enteroviruses*, Philadelphia, 2001, Lippincott Williams & Wilkins.
2. Racaniello VR: *Picornaviridae: the viruses and their replication*, Philadelphia, 2001, Lippincott Williams & Wilkins.
3. Stanway G, Hyypia T: Parechoviruses, *J Virol* 73:5249, 1999.
4. Stanway G, Joki-Korpela P, Hyypiä T: Human parechoviruses—biology and clinical significance, *Rev Med Virol* 10:57, 2000.
5. Zoll J, Erkens Hulshof S, Lanke K, et al: Saffold virus, a human Theiler's-like cardiovirus, is ubiquitous and causes infection early in life, *PLoS Pathog* 5: e1000416, 2009.
6. Bodian D, Horstmann DM: *Polioviruses*, Philadelphia, 1965, JB Lippincott.
7. Cherry JD, Nelson DB: Enterovirus infections: their epidemiology and pathogenesis, *Clin Pediatr* 5:659, 1966.
8. Dalldorf G, Melnick JL: *Coxsackie viruses*, Philadelphia, 1965, JB Lippincott.
9. Kibrick S: Current status of coxsackie and ECHO viruses in human disease, *Prog Med Virol* 6:27, 1964.
10. Melnick JL: *Echoviruses*, Philadelphia, 1965, JB Lippincott.
11. Cherry JD, Krogstad P: Enteroviruses, parechoviruses, and saffold viruses. In Cherry JD, Harrison GJ, Kaplan SL, Steinback WJ, Hotez PT, editors: *Textbook of pediatric infectious diseases*, ed 7, Philadelphia, 2014, Saunders.
12. Gear JHS, Measroch V: Coxsackievirus infections of the newborn, *Prog Med Virol* 15:42, 1973.
13. Grist NR, Bell EJ, Assaad F: Enteroviruses in human disease, *Prog Med Virol* 24:114, 1978.
14. Melnick JL: *Enteroviruses*, New York, 1989, Plenum Publishing.
15. Morens DM, Zweighaft RM, Bryan JM: Nonpolio enterovirus disease in the United States, 1971-1975, *Int J Epidemiol* 8:49, 1979.
16. Scott TFM: Clinical syndromes associated with entero virus and REO virus infections, *Adv Virus Res* 8:165, 1961.
17. Wenner HA, Behbehani AM: *Echoviruses*, New York, 1968, Springer-Verlag.
18. Blinkova O, Kapoor A, Victoria J, et al: Cardioviruses are genetically diverse and cause common enteric infections in South Asian children, *J Virol* 83:4631, 2009.
19. Itagaki T, Abiko C, Aoki Y, et al: Saffold cardiovirus infection in children associated with respiratory disease and its similarity to coxsackievirus infection, *Pediatr Infect Dis J* 30:680, 2011.
20. Nielsen AC, Bottiger B, Banner J, et al: Serious invasive Saffold virus infections in children, 2009, *Emerg Infect Dis* 18:7, 2012.
21. Blattner RJ, Heys FM: Role of viruses in the etiology of congenital malformations, *Prog Med Virol* 3:311, 1961.
22. Byington CL, Taggart W, Carroll KC, et al: A polymerase chain reaction-based epidemiologic investigation of the incidence of nonpolio enteroviral infections in febrile and afebrile infants 90 days and younger, *Pediatrics* 103:E27, 1999.
23. Eichenwald HF, McCracken GH, Kindberg SJ: Virus infections of the newborn, *Prog Med Virol* 9:35, 1967.
24. Hanshaw JB, Dudgeon JA: *Viral diseases of the fetus and newborn*, Philadelphia, 1978, WB Saunders.
25. Hardy JB: Viral infection in pregnancy: a review, *Am J Obstet Gynecol* 93:1052, 1965.
26. Hardy JB: Viruses and the fetus, *Postgrad Med* 43:156, 1968.
27. Horstmann DM: Viral infections in pregnancy, *Yale J Biol Med* 42:99, 1969.
28. Kaplan MH, Klein SW, McPhee J, et al: Group B coxsackievirus infections in infants younger than three months of age: a serious childhood illness, *Rev Infect Dis* 5:1019, 1983.
29. Kibrick S: Viral infections of the fetus and newborn, *Perspect Virol* 2:140, 1961.
30. Krajden S, Middleton PJ: Enterovirus infections in the neonate, *Clin Pediatr* 22:87, 1983.
31. Modlin JF: Perinatal echovirus infection: insights from a literature review of 61 cases of serious infection and 16 outbreaks in nurseries, *Rev Infect Dis* 8:918, 1986.
32. Monif GRG: *Viral infections of the human fetus*, Toronto, 1969, Macmillan.
33. Overall JC Jr, Glasgow LA: Virus infections of the fetus and newborn infant, *J Pediatr* 77:315, 1970.
34. Plotz EJ: Virus disease in pregnancy, *N Y J Med* 65:1239, 1965.
35. Wang SM, Liu CC, Yang YJ, et al: Fatal coxsackievirus B infection in early infancy characterized by fulminant hepatitis, *J Infect* 37:270, 1998.
36. Khetsuriani N, Lamonte A, Oberste MS, et al: Neonatal enterovirus infections reported to the national enterovirus surveillance system in the United States, 1983-2003, *Pediatr Infect Dis J* 25:889, 2006.
37. Verboon-Maciolek MA, Krediet TG, Gerards LJ, et al: Severe neonatal parechovirus infection and similarity with enterovirus infection, *Pediatr Infect Dis J* 27:241, 2008.
38. Wolthers KC, Benschop KS, Schinkel J, et al: Human parechoviruses as an important viral cause of sepsislike illness and meningitis in young children, *Clin Infect Dis* 47:358, 2008.
39. Paul JR: *A history of poliomyelitis*, New Haven, Conn, 1971, Yale University Press.
40. Horstmann DM: The poliomyelitis story: a scientific hegira, *Yale J Biol Med* 58:79, 1985.
41. Melnick JL: Portraits of viruses: the picornaviruses, *Intervirology* 20:61, 1983.
42. Underwood M: *A treatise on the diseases of children*, ed 2, London, 1789, J Mathews.
43. Wickman I: On the epidemiology of Heine-Medin's disease, *Rev Infect Dis* 2:319, 1980.
44. Landsteiner K, Popper E: Übertragung der Poliomyelitis acuta auf Affen, *Z Immun Forsch* 2:377, 1909.
45. Enders JF, Weller TH, Robbins FC: Cultivation of the Lansing strain of poliomyelitis virus in cultures of various human embryonic tissues, *Science* 109:85, 1949.
46. Hannaeus G. Dissertation, Copenhagen. 1735.

47. Dalldorf G, Sickles GM: An unidentified, filtrable agent isolated from the feces of children with paralysis, *Science* 108:61, 1948.
48. Melnick JL, Dalldorf G, Enders JF, et al: The enteroviruses, *Am J Public Health* 47:1556, 1957.
49. Jones MS, Lukashov VV, Ganac RD, Schnurr DP: Discovery of a novel human picornavirus in a stool sample from a pediatric patient presenting with fever of unknown origin, *J Clin Microbiol* 45:2144, 2007.
50. Abed Y, Boivin G: New Saffold cardioviruses in 3 children, Canada, *Emerg Infect Dis* 14:834, 2008.
51. Chiu CY, Greninger AL, Kanada K, et al: Identification of cardioviruses related to Theiler's murine encephalomyelitis virus in human infections, *Proc Natl Acad Sci U S A* 105:14124, 2008.
52. Harada S, Okada M, Yahiro S, et al: Surveillance of pathogens in outpatients with gastroenteritis and characterization of sapovirus strains between 2002 and 2007 in Kumamoto Prefecture, Japan, *J Med Virol* 81:1117, 2009.
53. Itagaki T, Abiko C, Ikeda T, et al: Sequence and phylogenetic analyses of Saffold cardiovirus from children with exudative tonsillitis in Yamagata, Japan, *Scand J Infect Dis* 42:950, 2010.
54. Khamrin P, Chaimongkol N, Nantachit N, et al: Saffold cardioviruses in children with diarrhea, Thailand, *Emerg Infect Dis* 17:1150, 2011.
55. Ren L, Gonzalez R, Xiao Y, et al: Saffold cardiovirus in children with acute gastroenteritis, Beijing, China, *Emerg Infect Dis* 15:1509, 2009.
56. Ren L, Gonzalez R, Xie Z, et al: Saffold cardioviruses of 3 lineages in children with respiratory tract infections, Beijing, China, *Emerg Infect Dis* 16:1158, 2010.
57. Tsukagoshi H, Masuda Y, Mizutani T, et al: Sequencing and phylogenetic analyses of Saffold cardiovirus (SAFV) genotype 3 isolates from children with upper respiratory infection in Gunma, Japan, *Jpn J Infect Dis* 63:378, 2010.
58. Xu ZQ, Cheng WX, Qi HM, et al: New Saffold cardiovirus in children, China, *Emerg Infect Dis* 15:993, 2009.
59. Tsukagoshi H, Mizuta K, Abiko C, et al: The impact of Saffold cardiovirus in patients with acute respiratory infections in Yamagata, Japan, *Scand J Infect Dis* 43:669, 2011.
60. Centers for Disease Control and Prevention: Progress toward global poliomyelitis eradication, 1985-1994, *MMWR Morb Mortal Wkly Rep* 44:273, 1995.
61. World Health Organization. Poliomyelitis. Fact sheet no. 114 [last revised 2003]. Available at http://www.who.int/mediacentre/factsheets/fs114/en/print.html. Accessed September 11, 2014.
62. Centers for Disease Control and Prevention: Progress toward global eradication of poliomyelitis, 2002, *MMWR Morb Mort Wkly Rep* 52:366, 2003.
63. Cochi SL, Hull HF, Sutter RW, et al: Commentary: the unfolding story of global poliomyelitis eradication, *J Infect Dis* 175: S1, 1997.
64. Hull HF, Ward NA, Hull BP, et al: Paralytic poliomyelitis: seasoned strategies, disappearing disease, *Lancet* 343:1331, 1994.
65. Robbins FC, de Quadros CA: Certification of the eradication of indigenous transmission of wild poliovirus in the Americas, *J Infect Dis* 175: S281, 1997.
66. Cochi SL, Linkins RW: The final phase of polio eradication: new vaccines and complex choices, *J Infect Dis* 205:169-171, 2012.
67. Rotbart HA, O'Connel JF, McKinlay MA: Treatment of human enterovirus infections, *Antiviral Res* 38:1, 1998.
68. Diana GD, Pevear DC: Antipicornavirus drugs: current status, *Antivir Chem Chemother* 8:401, 1997.
69. Rotbart HA, Webster AD: Treatment of potentially life-threatening enterovirus infections with pleconaril, *Clin Infect Dis* 32:228, 2001.
70. Desmond RA, Accortt NA, Talley L, et al: Enteroviral meningitis: natural history and outcome of pleconaril therapy, *Antimicrob Agents Chemother* 50:2409, 2006.
71. Abzug MJ, Loeffelholz M, Rotbart HA: Clinical and laboratory observations, *J Pediatr* 126:447, 1995.
72. Andréoletti L, Blassel-Damman N, Dewilde A, et al: Comparison of use of cerebrospinal fluid, serum, and throat swab specimens in the diagnosis of enteroviral acute neurological infection by a rapid RNA detection PCR assay, *J Clin Microbiol* 36:589, 1998.
73. Andréoletti L, Hober D, Belaich S, et al: Rapid detection of enterovirus in clinical specimens using PCR and microwell capture hybridization assay, *J Virol Methods* 62:1, 1996.
74. Ishiko H, Shimada Y, Yonaha M, et al: Molecular diagnosis of human enteroviruses by phylogeny-based classification by use of the VP4 sequence, *J Infect Dis* 185:744, 2002.
75. Klespies SL, Cebula DE, Kelley CL, et al: Detection of enterovirus from clinical specimens by spin amplification shell vial culture and monoclonal antibody assay, *J Clin Microbiol* 34:1465, 1996.
76. Lina B, Pozzetto B, Andréoletti L, et al: Multicenter evaluation of a commercially available PCR assay for diagnosing enterovirus infection in a panel of cerebrospinal fluid specimens, *J Clin Microbiol* 34:3002, 1996.
77. Marshall GS, Hauck MA, Buck G, et al: Potential cost savings through rapid diagnosis of enteroviral meningitis, *Pediatr Infect Dis J* 16:1086, 1997.
78. Nielsen LP, Modlin JF, Rotbart HA: Detection of enteroviruses by polymerase chain reaction in urine samples of patients with aseptic meningitis, *Pediatr Infect Dis J* 15:125, 1996.
79. Oberste MS, Nix WA, Maher K, et al: Improved molecular identification of enteroviruses by RT-PCR and amplicon sequencing, *J Clin Virol* 26:375, 2003.
80. Romero JR, Rotbart HA: Sequence diversity among echoviruses with different neurovirulence phenotypes, *Pediatr Res* 33:181A, 1993.
81. Rotbart HA: Reproducibility of AMPLICOR enterovirus PCR test results, *J Clin Microbiol* 35:3301, 1997.
82. Sawyer MH, Holland D, Aintablian N, et al: Diagnosis of enteroviral central nervous system infection by polymerase chain reaction during a large community outbreak, *Pediatr Infect Dis J* 13:177, 1994.
83. Schlesinger Y, Sawyer MH, Storch GA: Enteroviral meningitis in infancy: potential role for polymerase chain reaction in patient management, *Pediatrics* 94:157, 1994.
84. Sharland M, Hodgson J, Davies EG, et al: Enteroviral pharyngitis diagnosed by reverse transcriptase-polymerase chain reaction, *Arch Dis Child* 74:462, 1996.
85. Tanel RE, Kao S, Niemiec TM, et al: Prospective comparison of culture vs genome detection for diagnosis of enteroviral meningitis in childhood, *Arch Pediatr Adolesc Med* 150:919, 1996.
86. Uchio E, Yamazaki K, Aoki K, et al: Detection of enterovirus 70 by polymerase chain reaction in acute hemorrhagic conjunctivitis, *Am J Ophthalmol* 122:273, 1996.
87. Yerly S, Gervaix A, Simonet V, et al: Rapid and sensitive detection of enteroviruses in specimens from patients with aseptic meningitis, *J Clin Microbiol* 34:199, 1996.
88. Diedrich S, Driesel G, Schreier E: Sequence comparison of echovirus type 30 isolates to other enteroviruses in the 5′ noncoding region, *J Med Virol* 46:148, 1995.
89. Fenner F: Classification and nomenclature of viruses: second report of the International Committee on Taxonomy of Viruses, *Intervirology* 7:1, 1976.
90. Hyypiä T, Hovi T, Knowles NJ, et al: Classification of enteroviruses based on molecular and biological properties, *J Gen Virol* 78:1, 1997.
91. Kew OM, Mulders MN, Lipskaya GY, et al: Molecular epidemiology of polioviruses, *Virology* 6:401, 1995.
92. Kubo H, Iritani N, Seto Y: Molecular classification of enteroviruses not identified by neutralization tests, *Emerg Infect Dis* 8:298, 2002.
93. Melnick JL: Enteroviruses: polioviruses, coxsackieviruses, echoviruses and newer enteroviruses. In Fields BN, Knipe DM, editors: *Virology*, ed 2, New York, 1990, Raven Press. p 549.
94. Melnick JL: My role in the discovery and classification of the enteroviruses, *Annu Rev Microbiol* 50:1, 1996.
95. Melnick JL, Cockburn WC, Dalldorf G, et al: Picornavirus group, *Virology* 19:114, 1963.
96. Melnick JL, Wenner HA: *Enteroviruses*, New York, 1969, American Public Health Association.
97. Norder H, Bjerregaard L, Magnius L, et al: Sequencing of 'untypable' enteroviruses reveals two new types, EV-77 and EV-78, within human enterovirus type B and substitutions in the BC loop of the VP1 protein for known types, *J Gen Virol* 84:827, 2003.
98. Pöyry T, Hyypiä T, Horsnell C, et al: Molecular analysis of coxsackievirus A16 reveals a new genetic group of enteroviruses, *Virology* 202:962, 1994.
99. Pöyry T, Kinnunen L, Hyypiä T, et al: Genetic and phylogenetic clustering of enteroviruses, *J Gen Virol* 77:1699, 1996.
100. Pulli T, Koskimies P, Hyypiä T: Molecular comparison of coxsackie A virus serotypes, *Virology* 212:30, 1995.
101. Rueckert RR: *Picornaviridae and their replication*, New York, 1990, Raven Press.
102. Stanway G, Brown F, Christian P, et al: Family Picornaviridae. In Fauquet CM, Mayo MA, Maniloff J, Desselberger U, Ball LA, editors: *Virus taxonomy eighth report of the International Committee on Taxonomy of Viruses*, London, 2005, Elsevier/Academic Press, p 757.

103. Knowles N, Hovi T, Hyypiä T, et al: Picornaviridae. In King A, Adams M, Carstens E, Lefkowitz E, editors: *Virus taxonomy: classification and nomenclature of viruses: ninth report of the International Committee on Taxonomy of Viruses*, San Diego, 2012, Elsevier, p 855.
104. Oberste MS, Maher K, Kilpatrick DR, et al: Typing of human enteroviruses by partial sequencing of VP1, *J Clin Microbiol* 37:1288, 1999.
105. Oberste MS, Maher K, Nix WA, et al: Molecular identification of 13 new enterovirus types, EV79-88, EV97, and EV100-101, members of the species human enterovirus B, *Virus Res* 128:34, 2007.
106. Benschop KS, Williams CH, Wolthers KC, et al: Widespread recombination within human parechoviruses: analysis of temporal dynamics and constraints, *J Gen Virol* 89:1030, 2008.
107. Chan YF, AbuBakar S: Recombinant human enterovirus 71 in hand, foot and mouth disease patients, *Emerg Infect Dis* 10:1468, 2004.
108. Chevaliez S, Szendroi A, Caro V, et al: Molecular comparison of echovirus 11 strains circulating in Europe during an epidemic of multisystem hemorrhagic disease of infants indicates that evolution generally occurs by recombination, *Virology* 325:56, 2004.
109. Krogstad P, Hammon R, Halnon N, et al: Fatal neonatal myocarditis caused by a recombinant human enterovirus-B variant, *Pediatr Infect Dis J* 27:668, 2008.
110. Lukashev AN: Role of recombination in evolution of enteroviruses, *Rev Med Virol* 15:157, 2005.
111. Lukashev AN, Lashkevich VA, Ivanova OE, et al: Recombination in circulating enteroviruses, *J Virol* 77:10423, 2003.
112. Lukashev AN, Lashkevich VA, Ivanova OE, et al: Recombination in circulating human enterovirus B: independent evolution of structural and non-structural genome regions, *J Gen Virol* 86:3281, 2005.
113. Oberste MS, Maher K, Pallansch MA: Evidence for frequent recombination within species human enterovirus B based on complete genomic sequences of all thirty-seven serotypes, *J Virol* 78:855, 2004.
114. Oberste MS, Penaranda S, Pallansch MA: RNA recombination plays a major role in genomic change during circulation of coxsackie B viruses, *J Virol* 78:2948, 2004.
115. Romero JR, Selvarangan R: The human parechoviruses: an overview, *Adv Pediatr* 58:65, 2011.
116. Benschop KS, de Vries M, Minnaar RP, et al: Comprehensive full-length sequence analyses of human parechoviruses: diversity and recombination, *J Gen Virol* 91:145, 2010.
117. Calvert J, Chieochansin T, Benschop KS, et al: Recombination dynamics of human parechoviruses: investigation of type-specific differences in frequency and epidemiological correlates, *J Gen Virol* 91:1229, 2010.
118. Badorff C, Lee GH, Lamphear BJ, et al: Enteroviral protease 2A cleaves dystrophin: evidence of cytoskeletal disruption in an acquired cardiomyopathy, *Nat Med* 5:320, 1999.
119. Doedens JR, Kirkegaard K: Inhibition of cellular protein secretion by poliovirus proteins 2B and 3A, *EMBO J* 14:894, 1995.
120. Krogerus C, Egger D, Samuilova O, et al: Replication complex of human parechovirus 1, *J Virol* 77:8512, 2003.
121. Triantafilou K, Triantafilou M, Takada Y, et al: Human parechovirus 1 utilizes integrins alphavbeta3 and alphavbeta1 as receptors, *J Virol* 74:5856, 2000.
122. Samuilova O, Krogerus C, Poyry T, et al: Specific interaction between human parechovirus nonstructural 2A protein and viral RNA, *J Biol Chem* 279:37822, 2004.
123. Himeda T, Ohara Y: Saffold virus, a novel human cardiovirus with unknown pathogenicity, *J Virol* 86:1292, 2012.
124. Noordhoek GT, Weel JF, Poelstra E, et al: Clinical validation of a new real-time PCR assay for detection of enteroviruses and parechoviruses, and implications for diagnostic procedures, *J Clin Virol* 41:75, 2008.
125. Romero JR: Enteroviruses and parechoviruses. In Murray PR, Baron EJ, Jorgensen JH, Landry ML, Pfaller MA, editors: *Manual of clinical microbiology*, ed 9, Washington, DC, 2007, American Society for Microbiology Press, p 1392.
126. Bryden AS: Isolation of enteroviruses and adenoviruses in continuous simian cell lines, *Med Lab Sci* 49:60, 1992.
127. Cherry JD, Bobinski JE, Horvath FL, et al: Acute hemangiomalike lesions associated with ECHO viral infections, *Pediatrics* 44:498, 1969.
128. Hatch MH, Marchetti GE: Isolation of echoviruses with human embryonic lung fibroblast cells, *Appl Microbiol* 22:736, 1971.
129. Kelen AE, Lesiak JM, Labzoffsky NA: An outbreak of aseptic meningitis due to ECHO 25 virus, *Can Med Assoc J* 90:1349, 1964.
130. Bell EJ, Cosgrove BP: Routine enterovirus diagnosis in a human rhabdomyosarcoma cell line, *Bull World Health Organ* 58:423, 1980.
131. Herrmann EC Jr: Experience in providing a viral diagnostic laboratory compatible with medical practice, *Mayo Clin Proc* 42:112, 1967.
132. Westerhuis BM, Jonker SC, Mattao S, et al: Growth characteristics of human parechovirus 1 to 6 on different cell lines and cross-neutralization of human parechovirus antibodies: a comparison of the cytopathic effect and real time PCR, *Virol J* 10:146, 2013.
133. Terletskaia-Ladwig E, Metzger C, Schalasta G, et al: Evaluation of enterovirus serological tests IgM-EIA and complement fixation in patients with meningitis, confirmed by detection of enteroviral RNA by RT-PCR in cerebrospinal fluid, *J Med Virol* 61:221, 2000.
134. Terletskaia-Ladwig E, Metzger C, Schalasta G, et al: A new enzyme immunoassay for the detection of enteroviruses in faecal specimens, *J Med Virol* 60:439, 2000.
135. Gelfand HM: The occurrence in nature of the coxsackie and ECHO viruses, *Prog Med Virol* 3:193, 1961.
136. Melnick JL, Emmons J, Coffey JH, et al: Seasonal distribution of coxsackie viruses in urban sewage and flies, *Am J Hyg* 59:164, 1954.
137. Downey TW: Polioviruses and flies: studies on the epidemiology of enteroviruses in an urban area, *Yale J Biol Med* 35:341, 1963.
138. Melnick JL, Dow RP: Poliomyelitis in Hidalgo County, Texas 1948: poliomyelitis and coxsackie viruses from flies, *Am J Hyg* 58:288, 1953.
139. Verlinde JD, Versteeg J, Beeuwkes H: Mogelijkheid van een besmetting van de mens door varkens lijdende aan een Coxsackievirus pneumonie, *Ned Tijdschr Geneeskd* 102:1445, 1958.
140. Moscovici C, Ginevri A, Felici A, et al: Virus 1956, *Rend 1st Sup Sanit* 20:1137, 1957.
141. Lundgren DL, Clapper WE, Sanchez A: Isolation of human enteroviruses from beagle dogs, *Proc Soc Exp Biol Med* 128:463, 1968.
142. Lundgren DL, Sanchez A, Magnuson MG, et al: A survey for human enteroviruses in dogs and man, *Arch Gesamte Virusforsch* 32:229, 1970.
143. Koprowski H: Counterparts of human viral disease in animals, *Ann N Y Acad Sci* 70:369, 1958.
144. Sommerville RG: Type I poliovirus isolated from a budgerigar, *Lancet* 1:495, 1959.
145. Makower H, Skurska Z: Badania nad wirusami Coxsackie. Doniesienie III. Izolacja wirusa Coxsackie z mózgu lisa, *Arch Immunol Ter Dosw* 5:219, 1957.
146. Bendinelli M, Ruschi A: Isolation of human enterovirus from mussels, *Appl Microbiol* 18:531, 1969.
147. Chang PW, Liu OC, Miller LT, et al: Multiplication of human enteroviruses in northern quahogs, *Proc Soc Exp Biol Med* 136:1380, 1971.
148. Metcalf TG, Stiles WC: Enterovirus within an estuarine environment, *Am J Epidemiol* 88:379, 1968.
149. Horstmann DM, Manuelidis EE: Russian Coxsackie A-7 virus ("AB IV" strain)—neuropathogenicity and comparison with poliovirus, *J Immunol* 81:32, 1958.
150. Harvala H, McIntyre CL, Imai N, et al: High seroprevalence of enterovirus infections in apes and old world monkeys, *Emerg Infect Dis* 18:283, 2012.
151. Bartell P, Klein M: Neutralizing antibody to viruses of poliomyelitis in sera of domestic animals, *Proc Soc Exp Biol Med* 90:597, 1955.
152. Morris JA, O'Connor JR: Neutralization of the viruses of the Coxsackie group by sera of wild rabbits, *Cornell Vet* 42:56, 1952.
153. Metcalf TG, Stiles WC: Accumulation of enteric viruses by the oyster, Crassostrea virginica, *J Infect Dis* 115:68, 1965.
154. Atwood RP, Cherry JD, Klein JO: Clams and viruses, *Hepat Surveill Rep* 20:26, 1964.
155. Duff MF: The uptake of enteroviruses by the New Zealand marine blue mussel Mytilus edulis aoteanus, *Am J Epidemiol* 85:486, 1967.
156. Liu OC, Seraichekas HR, Murphy BL: Viral depuration of the Northern quahaug, *Appl Microbiol* 15:307, 1967.
157. Lynt RK: Survival and recovery of enterovirus from foods, *Appl Microbiol* 14:218, 1966.
158. Keswick BH, Gerba CP, Goyal SM: Occurrence of enteroviruses in community swimming pools, *Am J Public Health* 71:1026, 1981.
159. Johnson I, Hammond GW, Verma MR: Nosocomial coxsackie B4 virus infections in two chronic-care pediatric neurological wards, *J Infect Dis* 151:1153, 1985.

160. Maus MV, Posencheg MA, Geddes K, et al: Detection of echovirus 18 in human breast milk, *J Clin Microbiol* 46:1137, 2008.
161. Chang ML, Tsao KC, Huang CC, et al: Coxsackievirus B3 in human milk, *Pediatr Infect Dis J* 25:955, 2006.
162. Kalter SS: A serological survey of antibodies to selected enteroviruses, *Bull World Health Organ* 26:759, 1962.
163. van der Sanden S, de Bruin E, Vennema H, et al: Prevalence of human parechovirus in the Netherlands in 2000 to 2007, *J Clin Microbiol* 46:2884, 2008.
163a. Fox JP: Epidemiological aspects of coxsackie and ECHO virus infections in tropical areas, *Am J Public Health* 54:1134, 1964.
164. Centers for Disease Control and Prevention. Enterovirus surveillance: report 1970-1979, Issued November 1981.
165. Bodian D, Horstmann DM: *Poliomyelitis*, Philadelphia, 1965, JB Lippincott.
166. Assaad F, Ljungars-Esteves K: World overview of poliomyelitis: regional patterns and trends, *Rev Infect Dis* 6: S302, 1984.
167. Phillips CA, Aronson MD, Tomkow J, et al: Enteroviruses in Vermont, 1969-1978: an important cause of illness throughout the year, *J Infect Dis* 141:162, 1980.
168. Drebit MA, Nguan CY, Campbell JJ, et al: Molecular epidemiology of enterovirus outbreaks in Canada during 1991-1992: identification of echovirus 30 and coxsackievirus B1 strains by amplicon sequencing, *J Med Virol* 44:340, 1994.
169. Ishiko H, Takeda N, Miyanura K, et al: Phylogenetic analysis of a coxsackievirus A24 variant: the most recent worldwide pandemic was caused by progenies of a virus prevalent around 1981, *Virology* 187:748, 1992.
170. Lin KH, Wang HL, Sheu MM, et al: Molecular epidemiology of a variant of coxsackievirus A24 in Taiwan: two epidemics caused by phylogenetically distinct viruses from 1985 to 1989, *J Clin Microbiol* 31:1160, 1993.
171. Mulders MN, Lipskaya GY, van der Avoort H, et al: Molecular epidemiology of wild poliovirus type 1 in Europe, the Middle East, and the Indian subcontinent, *J Infect Dis* 171:1399, 1995.
172. Centers for Disease Control and Prevention: Increased detections and severe neonatal disease associated with coxsackievirus B1 infection—United States, 2007, *MMWR Morb Mortal Wkly Rep* 57:553, 2008.
173. Centers for Disease Control and Prevention: Nonpolio enterovirus and human parechovirus surveillance—United States, 2006-2008, *MMWR Morb Mortal Wkly Rep* 59:1577, 2010.
174. Centers for Disease Control and Prevention: Enterovirus surveillance—United States, 1985, *MMWR Morb Mortal Wkly Rep* 34:494, 1985.
175. Centers for Disease Control and Prevention: Nonpolio enterovirus surveillance—United States, 1993-1996, *JAMA* 278:975, 1997.
176. Centers for Disease Control and Prevention: Enterovirus surveillance—United States, 1997-1999, *MMWR Morb Mortal Wkly Rep* 49:913, 2000.
177. Centers for Disease Control and Prevention: Enterovirus surveillance—United States, 2000-2001, *MMWR Morb Mortal Wkly Rep* 51:1047, 2002.
178. Centers for Disease Control and Prevention: Enterovirus surveillance—United States, 2002-2004, *MMWR Morb Mortal Wkly Rep* 55:153, 2006.
179. Alexander JP, Anderson LJ: (Respiratory and Enterovirus Branch, Centers for Disease Control), Personal communication, 1990.
180. Gary H: (Respiratory and Enteric Viruses Branch, Centers for Disease Control and Prevention), Personal communication, 1996.
181. Strikas RA, Anderson LJ, Parker RA: Temporal and geographic patterns of isolates of nonpolio enterovirus in the United States, 1970-1983, *J Infect Dis* 153:346, 1986.
182. Druyts-Voets E: Epidemiological features of entero non-poliovirus isolations in Belgium 1980-94, *Epidemiol Infect* 119:71, 1997.
183. Trallero G, Casas I, Tenorio A, et al: Enteroviruses in Spain: virological and epidemiological studies over 10 years (1988-97), *Epidemiol Infect* 124:497, 2000.
184. Brown BA, Oberste MS, Alexander JP Jr, et al: Molecular epidemiology and evolution of enterovirus 71 strains isolated from 1970 to 1998, *J Virol* 73:9969, 1999.
185. Chan LG, Parashar UD, Lye MS, et al: Deaths of children during an outbreak of hand, foot, and mouth disease in Sarawak, Malaysia: clinical and pathological characteristics of the disease, *Clin Infect Dis* 31:678, 2000.
186. Ho M, Chen ER, Hsu KH, et al: An epidemic of enterovirus 71 infection in Taiwan, *N Engl J Med* 341:929, 1999.
187. Komatsu H, Shimizu Y, Takeuchi Y, et al: Outbreak of severe neurologic involvement associated with enterovirus 71 infection, *Pediatr Neurol* 20:17, 1999.
188. Cardosa MJ, Perera D, Brown BA, et al: Molecular epidemiology of human enterovirus 71 strains and recent outbreaks in the Asia-Pacific region: comparative analysis of the VP1 and VP4 genes, *Emerg Infect Dis* 9:461, 2003.
189. Chan KP, Goh KT, Chong CY, et al: Epidemic hand, foot and mouth disease caused by human enterovirus 71, Singapore, *Emerg Infect Dis* 9:78, 2003.
190. Chan LG, Parashar UD, Lye MS, et al: Deaths of children during an outbreak of hand, foot, and mouth disease in Sarawak, Malaysia: clinical and pathological characteristics of the disease. For the Outbreak Study Group, *Clin Infect Dis* 31:678, 2000.
191. Chang LY, Tsao KC, Hsia SH, et al: Transmission and clinical features of enterovirus 71 infections in household contacts in Taiwan, *JAMA* 291:222, 2004.
192. Chong CY, Chan KP, Shah VA, et al: Hand, foot and mouth disease in Singapore: a comparison of fatal and non-fatal cases, *Acta Paediatr* 92:1163, 2003.
193. Hosoya M, Kawasaki Y, Sato M, et al: Genetic diversity of enterovirus 71 associated with hand, foot and mouth disease epidemics in Japan from 1983 to 2003, *Pediatr Infect Dis J* 25:691, 2006.
194. Li CC, Yang MY, Chen RF, et al: Clinical manifestations and laboratory assessment in an enterovirus 71 outbreak in southern Taiwan, *Scand J Infect Dis* 34:104, 2002.
195. Lu CY, Lee CY, Kao CL, et al: Incidence and case-fatality rates resulting from the 1998 enterovirus 71 outbreak in Taiwan, *J Med Virol* 67:217, 2002.
196. McMinn P, Stratov I, Nagarajan L, et al: Neurological manifestations of enterovirus 71 infection in children during an outbreak of hand, foot, and mouth disease in Western Australia, *Clin Infect Dis* 32:236, 2001.
197. McMinn PC: An overview of the evolution of enterovirus 71 and its clinical and public health significance, *FEMS Microbiol Rev* 26:91, 2002.
198. Centers for Disease Control and Prevention: Neurotropic diseases surveillance, No. 3, annual summary, Washington, DC, 1970, Department of Health, Education, and Welfare.
199. Communicable Disease Center: Poliomyelitis surveillance, No. 274, Washington, DC, 1963, U.S. Department of Health, Education, and Welfare.
200. Horstmann DB, Emmons J, Gimpel L, et al: Enterovirus surveillance following a community-wide oral poliovirus vaccination program: a seven-year study, *Am J Epidemiol* 97:173, 1973.
201. Horn P: Poliomyelitis in pregnancy: a twenty-year report from Los Angeles County, California, *Obstet Gynecol* 6:121, 1955.
202. Gresser I, Chany C, Enders JF: Persistent polioviral infection of intact human amniotic membrane without apparent cytopathic effect, *J Bacteriol* 89:470, 1965.
203. Abramson H, Greenberg M, Magee MC: Poliomyelitis in the newborn infant, *J Pediatr* 43:167, 1953.
204. Aycock WL: The frequency of poliomyelitis in pregnancy, *N Engl J Med* 225:405, 1941.
205. Barsky P, Beale AJ: The transplacental transmission of poliomyelitis, *J Pediatr* 51:207, 1957.
206. Baskin JL, Soule EH, Mills SD: Poliomyelitis of the newborn: pathologic changes in two cases, *Am J Dis Child* 80:10, 1950.
207. Bates T: Poliomyelitis in pregnancy, fetus, and newborn, *Am J Dis Child* 90:189, 1955.
208. Blattner RJ: Intrauterine infection with poliovirus, type I, *J Pediatr* 62:625, 1963.
209. Carter HM: Congenital poliomyelitis, *Obstet Gynecol* 8:373, 1956.
210. Elliott GB, McAllister JE, Alberta C: Fetal poliomyelitis, *Am J Obstet Gynecol* 72:896, 1956.
211. Jackson AL, Louw JX: Poliomyelitis at birth due to transplacental infection, *S Afr Med J* 33:357, 1959.
212. Johnson JF, Stimson PM: Clinical poliomyelitis in the early neonatal period, *J Pediatr* 40:733, 1956.
213. Kreibich H, Wold W: Ueber einen Fall von diaplazenter poliomyelitis Infektion des Feten in 9 Schwangerschaftsmonat, *Zentralbl Gynaekol* 72:694, 1950.
214. Lance M: Paralysis infantile (poliomyelité) constatée des la naissance, *Bull Soc Pediatr (Paris)* 31:2297, 1933.

215. Lycke E, Nilsson LR: Poliomyelitis in a newborn due to intrauterine infection, *Acta Paediatr* 51:661, 1962.
216. Schaeffer M, Fox MJ, Li CP: Intrauterine poliomyelitis infection, *JAMA* 155:248, 1954.
217. Severin G: Case of poliomyelitis in newborn, *Nord Med* 1:55, 1939.
218. Shelokov A, Habel K: Subclinical poliomyelitis in a newborn infant due to intrauterine infection, *JAMA* 160:465, 1956.
219. Shelokov A, Weinstein L: Poliomyelitis in the early neonatal period: report of a case of possible intrauterine infection, *J Pediatr* 38:80, 1951.
220. Siegel M, Greenberg M: Poliomyelitis in pregnancy: effect on fetus and newborn infant, *J Pediatr* 49:280, 1956.
221. Swarts CL, Kercher EF: A fatal case of poliomyelitis in a newborn infant delivered by cesarean section following maternal death due to poliomyelitis, *Pediatrics* 14:235, 1954.
222. Wingate MB, Meller HK, Ormiston G: Acute bulbar poliomyelitis in late pregnancy, *Br Med J* 1:407, 1961.
223. Winsser J, Pfaff ML, Seanor HE: Poliomyelitis viremia in a newborn infant, *Pediatrics* 20:458, 1957.
224. Wyatt HV: Poliomyelitis in the fetus and the newborn: a comment on the new understanding of the pathogenesis, *Clin Pediatr* 18:33, 1979.
225. Pearson RJC, Miller DG, Palmier ML: Reactions to the oral vaccine, *Yale J Biol Med* 34:498, 1962.
226. Prem KA, Fergus JW, Mathers JE, et al: Vaccination of pregnant women and young infants with trivalent oral attenuated live poliomyelitis vaccine, Washington, DC, 1960, Pan American Sanitary Bureau.
227. Prem KA, McKelvey JL: Immunologic response of pregnant women to oral trivalent poliomyelitis vaccine, Washington, DC, 1959, Pan American Sanitary Bureau.
228. Cabasso VJ, Jungherr EL, Moyer AW, et al: Oral poliomyelitis vaccine, Lederle: thirteen years of laboratory and field investigation, *N Engl J Med* 263:1321, 1960.
229. Horstmann DM: Epidemiology of poliomyelitis and allied diseases—1963, *Yale J Biol Med* 36:5, 1963.
230. Horstmann DM, Opton EM, Klemperer R, et al: Viremia in infants vaccinated with oral poliovirus vaccine (Sabin), *Am J Hyg* 79:47, 1964.
231. Katz SL: Efficacy, potential and hazards of vaccines, *N Engl J Med* 270:884, 1964.
232. McKay HW, Fodor AR, Kokko UP: Viremia following the administration of live poliovirus vaccines, *Am J Public Health* 53:274, 1963.
233. Melnick JL, Proctor RO, Ocampo AR, et al: Free and bound virus in serum after administration of oral poliovirus vaccine, *Am J Epidemiol* 84:329, 1966.
234. Payne AMM: Summary of the conference, Washington, DC, 1960, Pan American Sanitary Bureau.
235. White LR: Comment. Viral etiology of congenital malformations, May 19-20, 1967, Washington, DC, U.S. Government Printing Office; 1968.
236. Dalldorf G, Gifford R: Susceptibility of gravid mice to coxsackie virus infection, *J Exp Med* 99:21, 1954.
237. Berger E, Roulet F: Beitrage zur Ausscheidung und Tierpathogenitüt des Coxsackie-virus, *Schweiz Z Allg Pathol* 15:462, 1952.
238. Selzer G: Transplacental infection of the mouse fetus by Coxsackie viruses, *Israel J Med Sci* 5:125, 1969.
239. Soike K: Coxsackie B-3 virus infection in the pregnant mouse, *J Infect Dis* 117:203, 1967.
240. Modlin JF, Crumpacker CS: Coxsackievirus B infection in pregnant mice and transplacental infection of the fetus, *Infect Immun* 37:222, 1982.
241. Flamm H: Some considerations concerning the pathogenesis of prenatal infections, Washington, DC, 1966, U.S. Government Printing Office.
242. Flamm H: Untersuchungen über die diaplazentare Übertragung des Coxsackievirus, *Schweiz Z Allg Pathol* 18:16, 1955.
243. Palmer AL, Rotbart HA, Tyson RW, et al: Adverse effects of maternal enterovirus infection on the fetus and placenta, *J Infect Dis* 176:1437, 1997.
244. Abzug MJ: Maternal factors affecting the integrity of the late gestation placental barrier to murine enterovirus infection, *J Infect Dis* 176:41, 1997.
245. Benirschke K: Viral infection of the placenta, Washington, DC, 1968, U.S. Government Printing Office.
246. Kibrick S, Benirschke K: Acute aseptic myocarditis and meningoencephalitis in the newborn child infected with Coxsackie virus group B, type 3, *N Engl J Med* 255:883, 1956.
247. Brightman VJ, Scott TFM, Westphal M, et al: An outbreak of coxsackie B-5 virus infection in a newborn nursery, *J Pediatr* 69:179, 1966.
248. Konstantinidou A, Anninos H, Spanakis N, et al: Transplacental infection of Coxsackievirus B3 pathological findings in the fetus, *J Med Virol* 79:754, 2007.
249. Euscher E, Davis J, Holzman I, et al: Coxsackie virus infection of the placenta associated with neurodevelopmental delays in the newborn, *Obstet Gynecol* 98:1019, 2001.
250. Basso NGS, Fonseca MEF, Garcia AGP, et al: Enterovirus isolation from foetal and placental tissues, *Acta Virol* 34:49, 1990.
251. Bates HR: Coxsackie virus B3 calcific pancarditis and hydrops fetalis, *Am J Obstet Gynecol* 106:629, 1970.
252. Bendig J, Franklin O, Hebden A, et al: Coxsackievirus B3 sequences in the blood of a neonate with congenital myocarditis, plus serological evidence of maternal infection, *J Med Virol* 70:606, 2003.
253. Benirschke K, Pendleton ME: Coxsackie virus infection: an important complication of pregnancy, *Obstet Gynecol* 12:305, 1958.
254. Cherry JD, Soriano F, Jahn CL: Search for perinatal viral infection: a prospective, clinical, virologic and serologic study, *Am J Dis Child* 116:245, 1968.
255. Hanson L, Lundgren S, Lycke E, et al: Clinical and serological observations in cases of Coxsackie B3 infections in early infancy, *Acta Paediatr Scand* 55:577, 1966.
256. Makower H, Skurska Z, Halazinska L: On transplacental infection with Coxsackie virus, *Texas Rep Biol Med* 16:346, 1958.
257. McLean DM, Donohue WL, Snelling CE, et al: Coxsackie B5 virus as a cause of neonatal encephalitis and myocarditis, *Can Med Assoc J* 85:1046, 1961.
258. Puschak RB: Coxsackie virus infection in the newborn with case report, Harrisburg Polyclinic Hosp, 1962.
259. Verma NA, Zheng XT, Harris MU, et al: Outbreak of life-threatening coxsackievirus B1 myocarditis in neonates, *Clin Infect Dis* 49: 759, 2009.
260. Wikswo ME, Khetsuriani N, Fowlkes AL, et al: Increased activity of Coxsackievirus B1 strains associated with severe disease among young infants in the United States, 2007-2008, *Clin Infect Dis* 49: e44, 2009.
261. Burch GE, Sun SC, Chu KC, et al: Interstitial and coxsackievirus B myocarditis in infants and children, *JAMA* 203:1, 1968.
262. Plager H, Beeve R, Miller JK: Coxsackie B-5 pericarditis in pregnancy, *Arch Intern Med* 110:735, 1962.
263. Euscher E, Davis J, Holzman I, et al: Coxsackievirus virus infection of the placenta associated with neurodevelopmental delays in the newborn, *Obstet Gynecol* 98:1019, 2001.
264. Yoshioka I, Horstmann DM: Viremia in infection due to ECHO virus type 9, *N Engl J Med* 262:224, 1960.
265. Kleinman H, Prince JT, Mathey WE, et al: ECHO 9 virus infection and congenital abnormalities: a negative report, *Pediatrics* 29:261, 1962.
266. Landsman JB, Grist NR, Ross CAC: Echo 9 virus infection and congenital malformations, *Br J Prev Soc Med* 18:152, 1964.
267. Rantasalo I, Penttinen K, Saxen L, et al: ECHO 9 virus antibody status after an epidemic period and the possible teratogenic effect of the infection, *Ann Paediatr Fenn* 6:175, 1960.
268. Philip AGS, Larson EJ: Overwhelming neonatal infection with ECHO 19 virus, *J Pediatr* 82:391, 1973.
269. Cheeseman SH, Hirsch MS, Keller EW, et al: Fatal neonatal pneumonia caused by echovirus type 9, *Am J Dis Child* 131:1169, 1977.
270. Jones MJ, Kolb M, Votava HJ, et al: Intrauterine echovirus type 11 infection, *Mayo Clin Proc* 55:509, 1980.
271. Bose CL, Gooch WM 3rd, Sanders GO, et al: Dissimilar manifestations of intrauterine infection with echovirus 11 in premature twins, *Arch Pathol Lab Med* 107:361, 1983.
272. Reyes MP, Ostrea EM Jr, Roskamp J, et al: Disseminated neonatal echovirus 11 disease following antenatal maternal infection with a virus-positive cervix and virus-negative gastrointestinal tract, *J Med Virol* 12:155, 1983.
273. Piraino FF, Sedmak G, Raab K: Echovirus 11 infections of newborns with mortality during the 1979 enterovirus season in Milwaukee, Wisc, *Public Health Rep* 97:346, 1982.
274. Nielsen JL, Berryman GK, Hankins GD: Intrauterine fetal death and the isolation of echovirus 27 from amniotic fluid, *J Infect Dis* 158:501, 1988.

275. Toce SS, Keenan WJ: Congenital echovirus 11 pneumonia in association with pulmonary hypertension, *Pediatr Infect Dis J* 7:360, 1988.
276. Yen H, Lien R, Fu R, et al: Hepatic failure in a newborn with maternal peripartum exposure to echovirus 6 and enterovirus 71, *Eur J Pediatr* 162:648, 2003.
277. Otonkoski T, Roivainen M, Vaarala O, et al: Neonatal type I diabetes associated with maternal echovirus 6 infection: a case report, *Diabetologia* 43:1235, 2000.
278. Hughes JR, Wilfert CM, Moore M, et al: Echovirus 14 infection associated with fatal neonatal hepatic necrosis, *Am J Dis Child* 123:61, 1972.
279. Moscovici C, Maisel J: Intestinal viruses of newborn and older prematures, *Am J Dis Child* 101:771, 1961.
280. Eichenwald HF, Kostevalov O: Immunologic responses of premature and full-term infants to infection with certain viruses, *Pediatrics* 25:829, 1960.
281. Chow K, Lee C, Lin T, et al: Congenital enterovirus 71 infection: a case study with virology and immunochemistry, *Clin Infect Dis* 31:509, 2000.
282. Berkovich S, Smithwick EM: Transplacental infection due to ECHO virus type 22, *J Pediatr* 72:94, 1968.
283. Ljubin-Sternak S, Juretic E, Santak M, et al: Clinical and molecular characterization of a parechovirus type 1 outbreak in neonates in Croatia, *J Med Virol* 83:137, 2011.
284. Zhong H, Lin Y, Su L, et al: Prevalence of human parechoviruses in central nervous system infections in children: a retrospective study in Shanghai, China, *J Med Virol* 85:320, 2013.
285. Pino-Ramirez RM, Pertierra-Cortada A, Iriondo-Sanz M, et al: Neonatal echovirus 30 infection associated with severe hepatitis in twin neonates, *Pediatr Infect Dis J* 27:88, 2008.
286. Kleger B, Prier JE, Rosato DJ, et al: Herpes simplex infection of the female genital tract. I. Incidence of infection, *Am J Obstet Gynecol* 102:745, 1968.
287. Montgomery R, Youngblood L, Medearis DN Jr: Recovery of cytomegalovirus from the cervix in pregnancy, *Pediatrics* 49:524, 1972.
288. Reyes MP, Zalenski D, Smith F, et al: Coxsackievirus-positive cervices in women with febrile illnesses during the third trimester in pregnancy, *Am J Obstet Gynecol* 155:159, 1986.
289. Cheng LL, Ng PC, Chan PK, et al: Probable intrafamilial transmission of coxsackievirus b3 with vertical transmission, severe early-onset neonatal hepatitis, and prolonged viral RNA shedding, *Pediatrics* 118: e929, 2006.
290. Cole RM, Bell JA, Beeman EA, et al: Studies of Coxsackie viruses: observations on epidemiologic aspects of group A viruses, *Am J Public Health* 41:1342, 1951.
291. Ramos-Alvarez M, Sabin AB: Intestinal viral flora of healthy children demonstrable by monkey kidney tissue culture, *Am J Public Health* 46:295, 1956.
292. Vandeputte M: L'endémicité des virus entériques à Léopoldville, *Congo Bull WHO/OMS* 22:313, 1960.
293. Katz SL: Case records of the Massachusetts General Hospital. Case 20-1965, *N Engl J Med* 272:907, 1965.
294. Jenista JA, Powell KR, Menegus MA: Epidemiology of neonatal enterovirus infection, *J Pediatr* 104:685, 1984.
295. Földes P, Bános A, Bános Z, et al: Vaccination of newborn children with live poliovirus vaccine, *Acta Microbiol Acad Sci Hung* 9:305, 1962.
296. Katz M, Plotkin SA: Oral polio immunization of the newborn infant: a possible method of overcoming interference by ingested antibodies, *J Pediatr* 73:267, 1968.
297. Keller R, Dwyer JE, Oh W, et al: Intestinal IgA neutralizing antibodies in newborn infants following poliovirus immunization, *Pediatrics* 43:330, 1969.
298. Lepow ML, Warren RJ, Gray N, et al: Effect of Sabin type 1 poliomyelitis vaccine administered by mouth to newborn infants, *N Engl J Med* 264:1071, 1961.
299. Lepow ML, Warren RJ, Ingram VG, et al: Sabin type 1 (LSc2ab) oral poliomyelitis vaccine, *Am J Dis Child* 104:67, 1962.
300. Murphy W: Response of infants to trivalent poliovirus vaccine (Sabin strains), *Pediatrics* 40:980, 1967.
301. Pagano JS, Plotkin SA, Cornely D: The response of premature infants to infection with type 3 attenuated poliovirus, *J Pediatr* 65:165, 1964.
302. Pagano JS, Plotkin SA, Cornely D, et al: The response of premature infants to infection with attenuated poliovirus, *Pediatrics* 29:794, 1962.
303. Pagano JS, Plotkin SA, Koprowski H: Variations in the response of infants to living attenuated poliovirus vaccines, *N Engl J Med* 264:155, 1961.
304. Plotkin SA, Katz M, Brown RE, et al: Oral poliovirus vaccination in newborn African infants, *Am J Dis Child* 111:27, 1966.
305. Sabin AB, Michaels RH, Krugman S, et al: Effect of oral poliovirus vaccine in newborn children. I. Excretion of virus after ingestion of large doses of type 1 or of mixture of all three types, in relation to level of placentally transmitted antibody, *Pediatrics* 31:623, 1963.
306. Sabin AB, Michaels RH, Ziring P, et al: Effect of oral poliovirus vaccine in newborn children. II. Intestinal resistance and antibody response at 6 months in children fed type 1 vaccine at birth, *Pediatrics* 31:641, 1963.
307. Warren RJ, Lepow ML, Bartsch GE, et al: The relationship of maternal antibody, breast feeding, and age to the susceptibility of newborn infants to infection with attenuated polioviruses, *Pediatrics* 34:4, 1964.
308. Bergeisen GH, Bauman RJ, Gilmore RL: Neonatal paralytic poliomyelitis: a case report, *Arch Neurol* 43:192, 1986.
309. Javett SN, Heymann S, Mundel B, et al: Myocarditis in the newborn infant, *J Pediatr* 48:1, 1956.
310. Kipps A, Naudé WDT, Don P, et al: Coxsackie virus myocarditis of the newborn, *Med Proc* 4:401, 1958.
311. Archibald E, Purdham DR: Coxsackievirus type A16 infection in a neonate, *Arch Dis Child* 54:649, 1979.
312. Artenstein MS, Cadigan FC, Buescher EL: Epidemic coxsackie virus infection with mixed clinical manifestations, *Ann Intern Med* 60:196, 1964.
313. Butler N, Skelton MO, Hodges GM, et al: Fatal Coxsackie B3 myocarditis in a newborn infant, *BMJ* 1:1251, 1962.
314. Cherry JD, Jahn CL: Virologic studies of exanthems, *J Pediatr* 68:204, 1966.
315. Cherry JD, Lerner AM, Klein J, et al: Unpublished data, 1962.
316. Delaney TB, Fakunaga FH: Myocarditis in a newborn with encephalomeningitis due to Coxsackie virus group B, type 5, *N Engl J Med* 259:234, 1958.
317. Dömök I, Molnár E: An outbreak of meningoencephalomyocarditis among newborn infants during the epidemic of Bornholm disease of 1958 in Hungary. II. Aetiological findings, *Ann Pediatr* 194:102, 1960.
318. Farber S, Vawter GF: Clinical pathological conference, *J Pediatr* 62:786, 1963.
319. Fechner RE, Smith MG, Middelkamp JN: Coxsackie B virus infection of the newborn, *Am J Pathol* 42:493, 1963.
320. Gear J: Coxsackie virus infections in Southern Africa, *Yale J Biol Med* 34:289, 1961.
321. Gear J, Measroch V, Prinsloo FR: The medical and public health importance of the coxsackie viruses, *S Afr Med J* 30:806, 1956.
322. Gear JHS: Coxsackie virus infection of the newborn, *Prog Med Virol* 1:106, 1958.
323. Hosier DM, Newton WA: Serious Coxsackie infection in infants and children, *Am J Dis Child* 96:251, 1958.
324. Hurley R, Norman AP, Pryse-Davies J: Massive pulmonary hemorrhage in the newborn associated with coxsackie B virus infection, *BMJ* 3:636, 1969.
325. Isacsohn M, Eidelman AI, Kaplan M, et al: Neonatal coxsackievirus group B infections: experience of a single department of neonatology, *Israel J Med Sci* 30:371, 1994.
326. Jack I, Townley RRW: Acute myocarditis of newborn infants, due to Coxsackie viruses, *Med J Aust* 2:265, 1961.
327. Jahn CL, Cherry JD: Mild neonatal illness associated with heavy enterovirus infection, *N Engl J Med* 274:394, 1966.
328. Jennings RC: Coxsackie group B fatal neonatal myocarditis associated with cardiomegaly, *J Clin Pathol* 19:325, 1966.
329. Johnson WR: Manifestations of Coxsackie group B infections in children, *Del Med J* 32:72, 1960.
330. Kibrick S, Benirschke K: Severe generalized disease (encephalohepatomyocarditis) occurring in the newborn period and due to infection with Coxsackie virus, group B, *Pediatrics* 22:857, 1958.
331. Koch VF, Enders-Ruckle G, Wokittel E: Coxsackie B5-Infektionen mit signifikanter Antikörperentwicklung bei Neugeborenen, *Arch Kinderheilkd* 165:245, 1962.
332. Lapinleimu K, Kaski U: An outbreak caused by coxsackievirus B5 among newborn infants, *Scand J Infect Dis* 4:27, 1972.
333. McLean DM, Coleman MA, Larke RPB, et al: Viral infections of Toronto children during 1965. I. Enteroviral disease, *Can Med Assoc J* 94:839, 1966.

334. Montgomery J, Gear J, Prinsloo FR, et al: Myocarditis of the newborn: an outbreak in a maternity home in Southern Rhodesia associated with Coxsackie group-B virus infection, *S Afr Med J* 29:608, 1955.
335. Moossy J, Geer JC: Encephalomyelitis, myocarditis and adrenal cortical necrosis in coxsackie B3 virus infection, *Arch Pathol* 70:614, 1960.
336. Nogen AG, Lepow ML: Enteroviral meningitis in very young infants, *Pediatrics* 40:617, 1967.
337. Rantakallio P, Lapinleimu K, Mäntyjärvi R: Coxsackie B5 outbreak in a newborn nursery with 17 cases of serious meningitis, *Scand J Infect Dis* 2:17, 1970.
338. Rapmund G, Gauld JR, Rogers NG, et al: Neonatal myocarditis and meningoencephalitis due to Coxsackie virus group B, type 4: virologic study of a fatal case with simultaneous aseptic meningitis in the mother, *N Engl J Med* 260:819, 1959.
339. Robino G, Perlman A, Togo Y, et al: Fatal neonatal infection due to Coxsackie B2 virus, *J Pediatr* 61:911, 1962.
340. Sieber OF, Kilgus AH, Fulginiti VA, et al: Immunological response of the newborn infant to Coxsackie B-4 infection, *Pediatrics* 40:444, 1967.
341. Suckling PV, Vogelpoel L: Coxsackie myocarditis of the newborn, *Med Proc* 4:372, 1958.
342. Sussman ML, Strauss L, Hodes HL: Fatal Coxsackie group B infection in the newborn, *Am J Dis Child* 97:483, 1959.
343. Tuuteri L, Lapinleimu K, Meurman L: Fatal myocarditis associated with coxsackie B3 infection in the newborn, *Ann Paediatr Fenn* 9:56, 1963.
344. Van Creveld S, De Jager H: Myocarditis in newborns, caused by Coxsackie virus: clinical and pathological data, *Ann Pediatr* 187:100, 1956.
345. Verlinde JD, Van Tongeren HAE, Kret A: Myocarditis in newborns due to group B Coxsackie virus: virus studies, *Ann Pediatr* 187:113, 1956.
346. Volakova N, Jandasek L: Epidemic of myocarditis in newborn infants caused by Coxsackie B1 virus, *Cesk Epidemiol* 13:88, 1963.
347. Winsser J, Altieri RH: A three-year study of coxsackie virus, group B, infection in Nassau County, *Am J Med Sci* 247:269, 1964.
348. Woodward TE, McCrumb FR Jr, Carey TN, et al: Viral and rickettsial causes of cardiac disease, including the Coxsackie virus etiology of pericarditis and myocarditis, *Ann Intern Med* 53:1130, 1960.
349. Wright HT Jr, Okuyama K, McAllister RM: An infant fatality associated with Coxsackie B1 virus, *J Pediatr* 63:428, 1963.
350. Swender PT, Shott RJ, Williams ML: A community and intensive care nursery outbreak of coxsackievirus B5 meningitis, *Am J Dis Child* 127:42, 1974.
351. Berkovich S, Kibrick S: ECHO 11 outbreak in newborn infants and mothers, *Pediatrics* 33:534, 1964.
352. Berkovich S, Pangan J: Recoveries of virus from premature infants during outbreaks of respiratory disease: the relation of ECHO virus type 22 to disease of the upper and lower respiratory tract in the premature infant, *Bull N Y Acad Med* 44:377, 1968.
353. Butterfield J, Moscovici C, Berry C, et al: Cystic emphysema in premature infants: a report of an outbreak with the isolation of type 19 ECHO virus in one case, *N Engl J Med* 268:18, 1963.
354. Cramblett HG, Haynes RE, Azimi PH, et al: Nosocomial infection with echovirus type 11 in handicapped and premature infants, *Pediatrics* 51:603, 1973.
355. Davies DP, Hughes CA, MacVicar J, et al: Echovirus-11 infection in a special-care baby unit, *Lancet* 1:96, 1979.
356. Eichenwald HF, Ababio A, Arky AM, et al: Epidemic diarrhea in premature and older infants caused by ECHO virus type 18, *JAMA* 166:1563, 1958.
357. Eichenwald HF, Kostevalov O, Fasso LA: The "cloud baby": an example of bacterial-viral interaction, *Am J Dis Child* 100:161, 1960.
358. Faulkner RS, van Rooyen CE: Echovirus type 17 in the neonate, *Can Med Assoc J* 108:878, 1973.
359. German LJ, McCracken AW, Wilkie KM: Outbreak of febrile illness associated with ECHO virus type 5 in a maternity unit in Singapore, *BMJ* 1:742, 1968.
360. Hart EW, Brunton GB, Taylor CED, et al: Infection of newborn babies with ECHO virus type 5, *Lancet* 2:402, 1962.
361. Hasegawa A: Virologic and serologic studies on an outbreak of echovirus type 11 infection in a hospital maternity unit, *Jpn J Med Sci Biol* 28:179, 1975.
362. Hercík L, Huml M, Mimra J, et al: Epidemien der Respirationstrakterkrankunger bei Neugeborenen durch ECHO 11-Virus, *Zentrabl Bakteriol* 213:18, 1970.
363. Jack I, Grutzner J, Gray N, et al: A survey of prenatal virus disease in Melbourne, Personal communication, July 21, 1967.
364. Kapsenberg JG: ECHO virus type 33 as a cause of meningitis, *Arch Gesamte Virusforschl* 23:144, 1968.
365. Kinney JS, McCray E, Kaplan JE, et al: Risk factors associated with echovirus 11 infection in a hospital nursery, *Pediatr Infect Dis* 5:192, 1986.
366. Lapinleimu K, Hakulinen A: A hospital outbreak caused by ECHO virus type 11 among newborn infants, *Ann Clin Res* 4:183, 1972.
367. McDonald LL, St. Geme JW, Arnold BH: Nosocomial infection with ECHO virus type 31 in a neonatal intensive care unit, *Pediatrics* 47:995, 1971.
368. Mertens T, Hager H, Eggers HJ: Epidemiology of an outbreak in a maternity unit of infections with an antigenic variant of echovirus 11, *J Med Virol* 9:81, 1982.
369. Miller DG, Gabrielson MO, Bart KJ, et al: An epidemic of aseptic meningitis, primarily among infants, caused by echovirus 11-prime, *Pediatrics* 41:77, 1968.
370. Modlin JF: Fatal echovirus 11 disease in premature neonates, *Pediatrics* 66:775, 1980.
371. Modlin JF: Echovirus infections of newborn infants, *Pediatr Infect Dis* 7:311, 1988.
372. Nagington J, Wreghitt TG, Gandy G, et al: Fatal echovirus 11 infections in outbreak in special-care baby unit, *Lancet* 2:725, 1978.
373. Nakao T, Miura R, Sato M: ECHO virus type 22 in a premature infant, *Tohoku J Exp Med* 102:61, 1970.
374. Purdham DR, Purdham PA, Wood BSB, et al: Severe ECHO 19 virus infection in a neonatal unit, *Arch Dis Child* 51:634, 1976.
375. Rabkin CS, Telzak EE, Ho MS, et al: Outbreak of echovirus 11 infection in hospitalized neonates, *Pediatr Infect Dis J* 7:186, 1988.
376. Sanders DY, Cramblett HG: Viral infections in hospitalized neonates, *Am J Dis Child* 116:251, 1968.
377. Steinmann J, Albrecht K: Echovirus 11 epidemic among premature newborns in a neonatal intensive care unit, *Zentralbl Bakteriol Mikrobiol Hyg* 259:284, 1985.
378. Wilson CW, Stevenson DK, Arvin AM: A concurrent epidemic of respiratory syncytial virus and echovirus 7 infections in an intensive care nursery, *Pediatr Infect Dis J* 8:24, 1989.
379. Wreghitt TG, Sutehall GM, King A, et al: Fatal echovirus 7 infection during an outbreak in a special care baby unit, *J Infect* 19:229, 1989.
380. Bina Rai S, Wan Mansor H, Vasantha T, et al: An outbreak of echovirus 11 amongst neonates in a confinement home in Penang, Malaysia, *Med J Malaysia* 62:223, 2007.
381. Chen JH, Chiu NC, Chang JH, et al: A neonatal echovirus 11 outbreak in an obstetric clinic, *J Microbiol Immunol Infect* 38:332, 2005.
382. Daboval T, Ferretti E, Duperval R: High C-reactive protein levels during a benign neonatal outbreak of echovirus type 7, *Am J Perinatol* 23:299, 2006.
383. Kusuhara K, Saito M, Sasaki Y, et al: An echovirus type 18 outbreak in a neonatal intensive care unit, *Eur J Pediatr* 167:587, 2008.
384. Sato K, Yamashita T, Sakae K, et al: A new-born baby outbreak of echovirus type 33 infection, *J Infect* 37:123, 1998.
385. Batcup G, Holt P, Hambling MH, et al: Placental and fetal pathology in coxsackie virus A9 infection: a case report, *Histopathology* 9:1227, 1985.
386. Ramsingh AI, Collins DN: A point mutation in the VP4 coding sequence of coxsackievirus B4 influences virulence, *J Virol* 69:7278, 1995.
387. Rinehart JE, Gomez RM, Roos RP: Molecular determinants for virulence in coxsackievirus B1 infection, *J Virol* 71:3986, 1997.
388. Heineberg H, Gold E, Robbins FC: Differences in interferon content in tissues of mice of various ages infected with coxsackie B1 virus, *Proc Soc Exp Biol Med* 115:947, 1964.
389. Levy O: Innate immunity of the newborn: basic mechanisms and clinical correlates, *Nat Rev Immunol* 7:379, 2007.
390. Behbehani AM, Sulkin SE, Wallis C: Factors influencing susceptibility of mice to coxsackie virus infection, *J Infect Dis* 110:147, 1962.
391. Boring WD, Angevine DM, Walker DL: Factors influencing host-virus interactions. I. A comparison of viral multiplication and histopathology in infant, adult, and cortisone-treated adult mice infected with the Conn-5 strain of coxsackie virus, *J Exp Med* 102:753, 1955.
392. Kunin CM: Cellular susceptibility to enteroviruses, *Bacteriol Rev* 28:382, 1964.
393. Kunin CM: Virus-tissue union and the pathogenesis of enterovirus infections, *J Immunol* 88:556, 1962.

394. Ito M, Kodama M, Masuko M, et al: Expression of coxsackievirus and adenovirus receptor in hearts of rats with experimental autoimmune myocarditis, *Circ Res* 86:275, 2000.
395. Teisner B, Haahr S: Poikilothermia and susceptibility of suckling mice to coxsackie B1 virus, *Nature* 247:568, 1974.
396. Arola A, Kalimo H, Ruuskanen O, et al: Experimental myocarditis induced by two different coxsackievirus B3 variants: aspects of pathogenesis and comparison of diagnostic methods, *J Med Virol* 47:251, 1995.
397. Gauntt CJ, Arizpe HM, Higdon AL, et al: Molecular mimicry, anti-coxsackievirus B3 neutralizing monoclonal antibodies, and myocarditis, *J Immunol* 154:2983, 1995.
398. Gauntt CJ, Higdon AL, Arizpe HM, et al: Epitopes shared between coxsackievirus B3 (CVB3) and normal heart tissue contribute to CVB3-induced murine myocarditis, *Clin Immunol Immunopathol* 68:129, 1993.
399. Henke A, Huber S, Stelzner A, et al: The role of CD8+ T lymphocytes in coxsackievirus B3-induced myocarditis, *J Virol* 69:6720, 1995.
400. Hosier DM, Newton WA Jr: Serious coxsackie infection in infants and children: myocarditis, meningoencephalitis, and hepatitis, *Am J Dis Child* 96:251, 1958.
401. Pague RE: Role of anti-idiotypic antibodies in induction, regulation, and expression of coxsackievirus-induced myocarditis, *Prog Med Virol* 39:204, 1992.
402. Rabausch-Starz I, Scwaiger A, Grünewald K, et al: Persistence of virus and viral genome in myocardium after coxsackievirus B3-induced murine myocarditis, *Clin Exp Immunol* 96:69, 1994.
403. Seko Y, Yoshifumi E, Yagita H, et al: Restricted usage of T-cell receptor Va genes in infiltrating cells in murine hearts with acute myocarditis caused by coxsackie virus B3, *J Pathol* 178:330, 1996.
404. Neu N, Beisel KW, Traystman MD, et al: Autoantibodies specific for the cardiac myosin isoform are found in mice susceptible to coxsackievirus B3-induced myocarditis, *J Immunol* 183:2488, 1987.
405. Herskowitz A, Beisel KW, Wolfgram LJ, et al: Coxsackievirus B3 murine myocarditis: wide pathologic spectrum in genetically defined inbred strains, *Hum Pathol* 16:671, 1985.
406. Wolfgram LJ, Rose NR: Coxsackievirus infection as a trigger of cardiac autoimmunity, *Immunol Res* 8:61, 1989.
407. Chehadeh W, Weill J, Vantyghem MC, et al: Increased level of interferon-alpha in blood of patients with insulin-dependent diabetes mellitus: relationship with coxsackievirus B infection, *J Infect Dis* 181:1929, 2000.
408. Hober D, Andréoletti L, Shen L, et al: Coxsackievirus B3-induced chronic myocarditis in mouse: use of whole blood culture to study the activation of TNF alpha-producing cells, *Microbiol Immunol* 40:837, 1996.
409. Juhela S, Hyöty H, Roivainen M, et al: T-cell responses to enterovirus antigens in children with type 1 diabetes, *Diabetes* 49:1308, 2000.
410. Lane JR, Neumann DA, Lafond-Walker A, et al: Role of IL-1 and tumor necrosis factor in coxsackie virus-induced autoimmune myocarditis, *J Immunol* 151:1682, 1993.
411. Roivainen M, Knip M, Hyöty H, et al: Several different enterovirus serotypes can be associated with prediabetic autoimmune episodes and onset of overt IDDM. Childhood Diabetes in Finland (DiMe) Study Group, *J Med Virol* 56:74, 1998.
412. McManus BM, Chow LH, Wilson JE, et al: Direct myocardial injury by enterovirus: a central role in the evolution of murine myocarditis, *Clin Immunol Immunopathol* 68:159, 1993.
413. Philipson L: Association between a recently isolated virus and an epidemic of upper respiratory disease in a day nursery, *Arch Gesamte Virusforsch* 8:204, 1958.
414. Cherry JD, Lerner AM, Klein JO, et al: Echo 11 virus infections associated with exanthems, *Pediatrics* 32:509, 1963.
415. Berry PJ, Nagington J: Fatal infection with echovirus 11, *Arch Dis Child* 57:22, 1982.
416. Mostoufizadeh M, Lack EE, Gang DL, et al: Postmortem manifestations of echovirus 11 sepsis in five newborn infants, *Hum Pathol* 14:818, 1983.
417. Gitlin N, Visveshwara N, Kassel SH, et al: Fulminant neonatal hepatic necrosis associated with echovirus type 11 infection, *West J Med* 138:260, 1983.
418. Halfon N, Spector SA: Fatal echovirus type 11 infections, *Am J Dis Child* 135:1017, 1981.
419. Krous HF, Dietzman D, Ray CG: Fatal infections with echovirus types 6 and 11 in early infancy, *Am J Dis Child* 126:842, 1973.
420. Wang J, Atchinson R, Walpusk J, et al: Echovirus hepatic failure in infancy: report of four cases with speculation on the pathogenesis, *Pediatr Dev Pathol* 4:454, 2001.
421. Kennett ML, Birch CJ, Lewis FA, et al: Enterovirus type 71 infection in Melbourne, *Bull World Health Organ* 51:609, 1974.
422. Schmidt NJ, Lennette EH, Ho HH: An apparently new enterovirus isolated from patients with disease of the central nervous system, *J Infect Dis* 129:304, 1974.
423. Kew O, Morris-Glasgow V, Landaverde M, et al: Outbreak of poliomyelitis in Hispaniola associated with circulating type 1 vaccine-derived poliovirus, *Science* 296:356, 2002.
424. Santti J, Hyypia T, Kinnunen L, Salminen M: Evidence of recombination among enteroviruses, *J Virol* 73:8741, 1999.
425. Simmonds P, Welch J: Frequency and dynamics of recombination within different species of human enteroviruses, *J Virol* 80:483, 2006.
426. Baker DA, Phillips CA: Maternal and neonatal infection with coxsackievirus, *Obstet Gynecol* 55:12S, 1980.
427. Balduzzi PC, Greendyke RM: Sudden unexpected death in infancy and viral infection, *Pediatrics* 38:201, 1966.
428. Gold E, Carver DH, Heineberg H, et al: Viral infection: a possible cause of sudden, unexpected death in infants, *N Engl J Med* 264:53, 1961.
429. Eisenhut M, Algawi G, Wreghitt T, et al: Fatal coxsackie A9 virus infection during an outbreak in a neonatal unit, *J Infect* 40:297, 2000.
430. Estes ML, Rorke LB: Liquefactive necrosis in coxsackie B encephalitis, *Arch Pathol Lab Med* 110:1090, 1986.
431. Iwasaki T, Monma N, Satodate R, et al: An immunofluorescent study of generalized coxsackie virus B3 infection in a newborn infant, *Acta Pathol Jpn* 35:741, 1985.
432. Konen O, Rathaus V, Bauer S, et al: Progressive liver calcifications in neonatal coxsackievirus infection, *Pediatr Radiol* 30:343, 2000.
433. Lake AM, Lauer BA, Clark JC, et al: Enterovirus infections in neonates, *J Pediatr* 89:787, 1976.
434. Chambon M, Delage C, Bailly J, et al: Fatal hepatitis necrosis in a neonate with echovirus 20 infection: use of the polymerase chain reaction to detect enterovirus in the liver tissue, *Clin Infect Dis* 24:523, 1997.
435. Georgieff MK, Johnson DE, Thompson TR, et al: Fulminant hepatic necrosis in an infant with perinatally acquired echovirus 21 infection, *Pediatr Infect Dis* 6:71, 1987.
436. Rawls WE, Shorter RG, Herrmann EC Jr: Fatal neonatal illness associated with ECHO 9 (coxsackie A-23) virus, *Pediatrics* 33:278, 1964.
437. Ventura K, Hawkins H, Smith M, et al: Fatal neonatal echovirus 6 infection: autopsy case report and review of the literature, *Mod Pathol* 14:85, 2001.
438. Wreghitt TG, Gandy GM, King A, et al: Fatal neonatal echo 7 virus infection, *Lancet* 2:465, 1984.
439. Boyd MT, Jordan SW, Davis LE: Fatal pneumonitis from congenital echovirus type 6 infection, *Pediatr Infect Dis J* 6:1138, 1987.
440. Willems A, Benne CA, Timmer A, et al: Fatal illness associated with pulmonary hypertension in a neonate caused by intrauterine echovirus 11 infection, *Am J Perinatol* 23:59, 2006.
441. Gupta S, Fernandez D, Siddiqui A, et al: Extensive white matter abnormalities associated with neonatal parechovirus (HPeV) infection, *Eur J Paediatr Neurol* 14:531, 2010.
442. Renna S, Bergamino L, Pirlo D, et al: A case of neonatal human parechovirus encephalitis with a favourable outcome, *Brain Dev* 36:70, 2014.
443. Verboon-Maciolek MA, Groenendaal F, Hahn CD, et al: Human parechovirus causes encephalitis with white matter injury in neonates, *Ann Neurol* 64:266, 2008.
444. Anderson GW, Anderson G, Skaar A, et al: Poliomyelitis in pregnancy, *Am J Hyg* 55:127, 1952.
445. Aycock WL, Ingalls TH: Maternal disease as a principle in the epidemiology of congenital anomalies, *Am J Med Sci* 212:366, 1946.
446. Bowers VM Jr, Danforth DN: The significance of poliomyelitis during pregnancy—an analysis of the literature and presentation of twenty-four new cases, *Am J Obstet Gynecol* 65:34, 1953.
447. Schaefer J, Shaw EB: Poliomyelitis in pregnancy, *Calif Med* 70:16, 1949.
448. Kaye BM, Rosner DC, Stein I: Viral diseases in pregnancy and their effect upon the embryo and fetus, *Am J Obstet Gynecol* 65:109, 1953.
449. Harjulehto-Mervaala T, Aro T, Hiilesmaa VK, et al: Oral polio vaccination during pregnancy: lack of impact on fetal development and perinatal outcome, *Clin Infect Dis* 18:414, 1994.

450. Frisk G, Diderholm H: Increased frequency of coxsackie B virus IgM in women with spontaneous abortion, *J Infect* 24:141, 1992.
451. Axelsson C, Bondestam K, Frisk G, et al: Coxsackie B virus infections in women with miscarriage, *J Med Virol* 39:282, 1993.
452. Krous HF, Langlois NE: Ljungan virus: a commentary on its association with fetal and infant morbidity and mortality in animals and humans, *Birth Defects Res A Clin Mol Teratol* 88:947, 2010.
453. Niklasson B, Samsioe A, Papadogiannakis N, et al: Zoonotic Ljungan virus associated with central nervous system malformations in terminated pregnancy, *Birth Defects Res A Clin Mol Teratol* 85:542, 2009.
454. Samsioe A, Papadogiannakis N, Hultman T, et al: Ljungan virus present in intrauterine fetal death diagnosed by both immunohistochemistry and PCR, *Birth Defects Res A Clin Mol Teratol* 85:227, 2009.
455. Aycock WL: Acute poliomyelitis in pregnancy: its occurrence according to month of pregnancy and sex of fetus, *N Engl J Med* 235:160, 1946.
456. Ouellet A, Sherlock R, Toye B, et al: Antenatal diagnosis of intrauterine infection with coxsackievirus B3 associated with live birth, *Infect Dis Obstet Gynecol* 12:23, 2004.
457. Freedman PS: Echovirus 11 infection and intrauterine death, *Lancet* 1:96, 1979.
458. Berendes HW, Weiss W: The NIH collaborative study. A progress report. In Fraser FC, McKusick VA, editors: *Congenital malformations. Proceedings of the Third International Conference on Congenital Malformations, The Hague, Netherlands, September 7-13, 1969*, Amsterdam, 1970, Exerpta Medica International Congress. (Series no. 204, p 293).
459. News and notes. Polio vaccine and congenital defects, *BMJ* 1:510, 1967.
460. Connelly JP, Reynolds S, Crawford JD, et al: Viral and drug hazards in pregnancy, *Clin Pediatr* 3:587, 1964.
461. Harjulehto T, Hovi T, Aro T, et al: Congenital malformations and oral poliovirus vaccination during pregnancy, *Lancet* 1:771, 1989.
462. Brown GC: Maternal virus infection and congenital anomalies, *Arch Environ Health* 21:362, 1970.
463. Brown GC: Recent advances in the viral aetiology of congenital anomalies, *Adv Teratol* 1:55, 1966.
464. Brown GC: Coxsackie virus infections and heart disease, *Am Heart J* 75:145, 1968.
465. Evans TN, Brown GC: Congenital anomalies and virus infections, *Am J Obstet Gynecol* 87:749, 1963.
466. Brown GC, Evans TN: Serologic evidence of coxsackievirus etiology of congenital heart disease, *JAMA* 199:183, 1967.
467. Brown GC, Karunas RS: Relationship of congenital anomalies and maternal infection with selected enteroviruses, *Am J Epidemiol* 95:207, 1972.
468. Elizan TS, Ajero-Froehlich L, Fabiyi A, et al: Viral infection in pregnancy and congenital CNS malformations in man, *Arch Neurol* 20:115, 1969.
469. Gauntt CJ, Gudvangen RJ, Brans YW, et al: Coxsackievirus group B antibodies in the ventricular fluid of infants with severe anatomic defects in the central nervous system, *Pediatrics* 76:64, 1985.
470. Barton LL: Febrile neonatal illness associated with echo virus type 5 in the cerebrospinal fluid, *Clin Pediatr* 16:383, 1977.
471. Farmer K, Patten PT: An outbreak of coxsackie B5 infection in a special care unit for newborn infants, *N Z Med J* 68:86, 1968.
472. Morens DM: Enteroviral disease in early infancy, *J Pediatr* 92:374, 1978.
473. News and notes: Coxsackie B virus infections in 1971, *BMJ* 1:453, 1972.
474. Eilard T, Kyllerman M, Wennerblom I, et al: An outbreak of coxsackie virus type B2 among neonates in an obstetrical ward, *Acta Paediatr Scand* 63:103, 1974.
475. Boivin G, Abed Y, Boucher FD: Human parechovirus 3 and neonatal infections, *Emerg Infect Dis* 11:103, 2005.
476. Benschop KS, Schinkel J, Luken ME, et al: Fourth human parechovirus serotype, *Emerg Infect Dis* 12:1572, 2006.
477. Hall CB, Cherry JD, Hatch MH, et al: The return of Boston exanthem, *Am J Dis Child* 131:323, 1977.
478. Abzug MJ, Levin MJ, Rotbart HA: Profile of enterovirus disease in the first two weeks of life, *Pediatr Infect Dis J* 12:820, 1993.
479. Haddad J, Gut JP, Wendling MJ, et al: Enterovirus infections in neonates: a retrospective study of 21 cases, *Eur J Med* 2:209, 1993.
480. Barre V, Marret S, Mendel I, et al: Enterovirus-associated haemophagocytic syndrome in a neonate, *Acta Paediatr* 87:467, 1998.
481. Bacon CJ, Sims DG: Echovirus 19 infection in infants under six months, *Arch Dis Child* 51:631, 1976.
482. Benschop KS, Schinkel J, Minnaar RP, et al: Human parechovirus infections in Dutch children and the association between serotype and disease severity, *Clin Infect Dis* 42:204, 2006.
483. Chen CA, Tsao PN, Chou HC, et al: Severe echovirus 30 infection in twin neonates, *J Formos Med Assoc* 102:59, 2003.
484. Cho CT, Janelle JG, Behbehani A: Severe neonatal illness associated with ECHO 9 virus infection, *Clin Pediatr* 12:304, 1973.
485. Codd AA, Hale JH, Bell TM, et al: Epidemic of echovirus 19 in the northeast of England, *J Hyg (Lond)* 76:307, 1976.
486. Grossman M, Azimi P: Fever, hepatitis and coagulopathy in a newborn infant, *Pediatr Infect Dis J* 11:1069, 1992.
487. Linnemann CC Jr, Steichen J, Sherman WG, et al: Febrile illness in early infancy associated with ECHO virus infection, *J Pediatr* 84:49, 1974.
488. Marier R, Rodriguez W, Chloupek RJ, et al: Coxsackievirus B5 infection and aseptic meningitis in neonates and children, *Am J Dis Child* 129:321, 1975.
489. Tang JW, Bendig JW, Ossuetta I: Vertical transmission of human echovirus 11 at the time of Bornholm disease in late pregnancy, *Pediatr Infect Dis J* 24:88, 2005.
490. Wong SN, Tam AYC, Ng THK, et al: Fatal coxsackie B1 virus infection in neonates, *Pediatr Infect Dis J* 8:638, 1989.
491. Bangalore H, Ahmed J, Bible J, et al: Abdominal distension: an important feature in human parechovirus infection, *Pediatr Infect Dis J* 30:260, 2011.
492. Eis-Hubinger AM, Eckerle I, Helmer A, et al: Two cases of sepsis-like illness in infants caused by human parechovirus traced back to elder siblings with mild gastroenteritis and respiratory symptoms, *J Clin Microbiol* 51:715, 2013.
493. Escuret A, Mirand A, Dommergues MA, et al: [Epidemiology of parechovirus infections of the central nervous system in a French pediatric unit], *Arch Pediatr* 20:470, 2013.
494. Eyssette-Guerreau S, Boize P, Thibault M, et al: [Neonatal parechovirus infection, fever, irritability and myositis.], *Arch Pediatr* 20:772, 2013.
495. Harvala H, Robertson I, Chieochansin T, et al: Specific association of human parechovirus type 3 with sepsis and fever in young infants, as identified by direct typing of cerebrospinal fluid samples, *J Infect Dis* 199:1753, 2009.
496. Pineiro L, Vicente D, Montes M, et al: Human parechoviruses in infants with systemic infection, *J Med Virol* 82:1790, 2010.
497. Schuffenecker I, Javouhey E, Gillet Y, et al: Human parechovirus infections, Lyon, France, 2008-10: evidence for severe cases, *J Clin Virol* 54:337, 2012.
498. Selvarangan R, Nzabi M, Selvaraju SB, et al: Human parechovirus 3 causing sepsis-like illness in children from midwestern United States, *Pediatr Infect Dis J* 30:238, 2011.
499. Sharp J, Harrison CJ, Puckett K, et al: Characteristics of young infants in whom human parechovirus, enterovirus or neither were detected in cerebrospinal fluid during sepsis evaluations, *Pediatr Infect Dis J* 32:213, 2013.
500. Shoji K, Komuro H, Kobayashi Y, et al: An infant with human parechovirus type 3 infection with a distinctive rash on the extremities, *Pediatr Dermatol* 31:258, 2014.
501. Shoji K, Komuro H, Miyata I, et al: Dermatologic manifestations of human parechovirus type 3 infection in neonates and infants, *Pediatr Infect Dis J* 32:233, 2013.
502. Walters B, Penaranda S, Nix WA, et al: Detection of human parechovirus (HPeV)-3 in spinal fluid specimens from pediatric patients in the Chicago area, *J Clin Virol* 52:187, 2011.
503. Yuzurihara SS, Ao K, Hara T, et al: Human parechovirus-3 infection in nine neonates and infants presenting symptoms of hemophagocytic lymphohistiocytosis, *J Infect Chemother* 19:144, 2013.
504. Verboon-Maciolek MA, Swanink CM, Krediet TG, et al: Severe neonatal echovirus 20 infection characterized by hepatic failure, *Pediatr Infect Dis J* 16:524, 1997.
505. Chawareewong S, Kiangsiri S, Lokaphadhana K, et al: Neonatal herpangina caused by coxsackie A-5 virus, *J Pediatr* 93:492, 1978.
506. Murray D, Altschul M, Dyke J: Aseptic meningitis in a neonate with an oral vesicular lesion, *Diagn Microbiol Infect Dis* 3:77, 1985.
507. Nakayama T, Urano T, Osano M, et al: Outbreak of herpangina associated with coxsackievirus B3 infection, *Pediatr Infect Dis J* 8:495, 1989.

508. Suzuki N, Ishikawa K, Horiuchi T, et al: Age-related symptomatology of ECHO 11 virus infection in children, *Pediatrics* 65:284, 1980.
509. Eckert HL, Portnoy B, Salvatore MA, et al: Group B Coxsackie virus infection in infants with acute lower respiratory disease, *Pediatrics* 39:526, 1967.
510. Chonmaitree T, Menegus MA, Schervish-Swierkosz EM, et al: Enterovirus 71 infection: report of an outbreak with two cases of paralysis and a review of the literature, *Pediatrics* 67:489, 1981.
511. Mirani M, Ogra PL, Barron A: Epidemic of echovirus type 9 infection: certain clinical and epidemiologic features, *N Y J Med* 73:403, 1973.
512. Ramos-Alvarez M: Cytopathogenic enteric viruses associated with undifferentiated diarrheal syndromes in early childhood, *Ann N Y Acad Sci* 67:326, 1957.
513. Bauer S, Gottesman G, Sirota L, et al: Severe coxsackie virus B infection in preterm newborns treated with pleconaril, *Eur J Pediatr* 161:491, 2002.
514. Abzug MJ: Prognosis for neonates with enterovirus hepatitis and coagulopathy, *Pediatr Infect Dis J* 20:758, 2001.
515. Birenbaum E, Handsher R, Kuint J, et al: Echovirus type 22 outbreak associated with gastro-intestinal disease in a neonatal intensive care unit, *Am J Perinatol* 14:469, 1997.
516. Barson WJ, Craenen J, Hosier DM, et al: Survival following myocarditis and myocardial calcification associated with infection by coxsackie virus B4, *Pediatrics* 68:79, 1981.
517. Chan SH, Lun KS: Ventricular aneurysm complicating neonatal coxsackie B4 myocarditis, *Pediatr Cardiol* 22:247, 2001.
518. Chonmaitree T, Menegus MA, Powell KR: The clinical relevance of "CSF viral culture." A two-year experience with aseptic meningitis in Rochester, NY, *JAMA* 247:1843, 1982.
519. Drew JH: ECHO 11 virus outbreak in a nursery associated with myocarditis, *Aust Paediatr J* 9:90, 1973.
520. Rantakallio P, Saukkonen AL, Krause U, et al: Follow-up study of 17 cases of neonatal coxsackie B5 meningitis and one with suspected myocarditis, *Scand J Infect Dis* 2:25, 1970.
521. Simmonds J, Cubitt D, Ashworth M, Burch M: Successful heart transplantation following neonatal necrotic enterovirus myocarditis, *Pediatr Cardiol* 29:834, 2008.
522. Smets K, Keymeulen A, Wollants E, et al: Detection of enteroviral RNA on Guthrie card dried blood of a neonate with fatal Coxsackie B3 myocarditis on day 17, *J Clin Virol* 42:207, 2008.
523. Talsma M, Vegting M, Hess J: Generalised coxsackie A9 infection in a neonate presenting with pericarditis, *Br Heart J* 52:683, 1984.
524. Cramblett HG, Moffet HL, Middleton GK Jr, et al: ECHO 19 virus infections, *Arch Intern Med* 110:574, 1962.
525. Theodoridou M, Kakourou T, Laina I, et al: Vesiculopapular rash as a single presentation in intrauterine coxsackie virus infection, *Eur J Pediatr* 161:412, 2002.
526. Chen CY, Chang YC, Huang CC, et al: Acute flaccid paralysis in infants and young children with enterovirus 71 infection: MR imaging findings and clinical correlates, *Am J Neuroradiol* 22:200, 2001.
527. Barson WJ, Reiner CB: Coxsackievirus B2 infection in a neonate with incontinentia pigmenti, *Pediatrics* 77:897, 1986.
528. Bergman I, Painter MJ, Wald ER, et al: Outcome in children with enteroviral meningitis during the first year of life, *J Pediatr* 110:705, 1987.
529. Blokziji ML, Koskiniemi M: Echovirus 6 encephalitis in a preterm baby, *Lancet* 2:164, 1989.
530. Boccia D, Stolfi I, Lana S, et al: Nosocomial necrotising enterocolitis outbreaks: epidemiology and control measures, *Eur J Pediatr* 160:385, 2001.
531. Bowen GS, Fisher MC, Deforest A, et al: Epidemic of meningitis and febrile illness in neonates caused by echo type 11 virus in Philadelphia, *Pediatr Infect Dis* 2:359, 1983.
532. Callen J, Paes BA: A case report of a premature infant with coxsackie B1 meningitis, *Adv Neonatal Care* 7:238, 2007.
533. Cherry JD, Lerner AM, Klein JO, et al: Coxsackie B5 infections with exanthems, *Pediatrics* 31:445, 1963.
534. Chesney PJ, Quennec P, Clark C: Hypoglycorrhachia and coxsackie B3 meningoencephalitis, *Am J Clin Pathol* 70:947, 1978.
535. Ehrnst A, Eriksson M: Echovirus type 23 observed as a nosocomial infection in infants, *Scand J Dis* 28:205, 1996.
536. Farmer K, MacArthur BA, Clay MM: A follow-up study of 15 cases of neonatal meningoencephalitis due to coxsackie virus B5, *J Pediatr* 87:568, 1975.
537. Haynes RE, Cramblett HG, Hilty MD, et al: ECHO virus type 3 infections in children: clinical and laboratory studies, *J Pediatr* 80:589, 1972.
538. Haynes RE, Cramblett HG, Kronfol HJ: Echovirus 9 meningoencephalitis in infants and children, *JAMA* 208:1657, 1969.
539. Helin I, Widell A, Borulf S, et al: Outbreak of coxsackievirus A-14 meningitis among newborns in a maternity hospital ward, *Acta Paediatr Scand* 76:234, 1987.
540. Johnson RT, Shuey HE, Buescher EL: Epidemic central nervous system disease of mixed enterovirus etiology. I. Clinical and epidemiologic description, *Am J Hyg* 71:321, 1960.
541. Matsumoto K, Yokochi T, Matsuda S, et al: Characterization of an echovirus type 30 variant isolated from patients with aseptic meningitis, *Microbiol Immunol* 30:333, 1986.
542. Schurmann W, Statz A, Mertens T, et al: Two cases of coxsackie B2 infection in neonates: clinical, virological, and epidemiological aspects, *Eur J Pediatr* 140:59, 1983.
543. Sells CJ, Carpenter RL, Ray CG: Sequelae of central-nervous-system enterovirus infections, *N Engl J Med* 293:1, 1975.
544. Sumaya CV, Corman LI: Enteroviral meningitis in early infancy: significance in community outbreaks, *Pediatr Infect Dis* 1:151, 1982.
545. King RL, Lorch SA, Cohen DM, et al: Routine cerebrospinal fluid enterovirus polymerase chain reaction testing reduces hospitalization and antibiotic use for infants 90 days of age or younger, *Pediatrics* 120:489, 2007.
546. Tavakoli NP, Wang H, Nattanmai S, et al: Detection and typing of enteroviruses from CSF specimens from patients diagnosed with meningitis/encephalitis, *J Clin Virol* 43:207, 2008.
547. Arnon R, Naor N, Davidson S, et al: Fatal outcome of neonatal echovirus 19 infection, *Pediatr Infect Dis J* 10:788, 1991.
548. Grangeot-Keros L, Broyer M, Briand E, et al: Enterovirus in sudden unexpected deaths in infants, *Pediatr Infect Dis J* 15:123, 1996.
549. Sedmak G, Nix WA, Jentzen J, et al: Infant deaths associated with human parechovirus infection in Wisconsin, *Clin Infect Dis* 50:357, 2010.
550. Paul JR: Epidemiology of poliomyelitis, *Monogr Ser World Health Organ* 26:9, 1955.
551. Weibel RE, Benor DE: Reporting vaccine-associated paralytic poliomyelitis: concordance between the CDC and the National Vaccine Injury Compensation Program, *Am J Public Health* 86:734, 1996.
552. Wilfert CM, Thompson RJ Jr, Sunder TR, et al: Longitudinal assessment of children with enteroviral meningitis during the first three months of life, *Pediatrics* 67:811, 1981.
553. Aradottir E, Alonso E, Shulman S: Severe neonatal enteroviral hepatitis treated with pleconaril, *Pediatr Infect Dis J* 20: e457, 2001.
554. Sabin AB, Krumbiegel ER, Wigand R: ECHO type 9 virus disease, *Am J Dis Child* 96:197, 1958.
555. Tarcan A, Özbek N, Gürakan B: Bone marrow failure with concurrent enteroviral infection in a newborn, *Pediatr Infect Dis J* 20: e719, 2001.
556. Chen KT, Chang HL, Wang ST, et al: Epidemiologic features of hand-foot-mouth disease and herpangina caused by enterovirus 71 in Taiwan, 1998-2005, *Pediatrics* 120: e244, 2007.
557. Wilfert CM, Lauer BA, Cohen M, et al: An epidemic of echovirus 18 meningitis, *J Infect Dis* 131:75, 1975.
558. Mullins JA, Khetsuriani N, Nix WA, et al: Emergence of echovirus type 13 as a prominent enterovirus, *Clin Infect Dis* 38:70, 2004.
559. Kirschke DL, Jones TF, Buckingham SC, et al: Outbreak of aseptic meningitis associated with echovirus 13, *Pediatr Infect Dis J* 21:1034, 2002.
560. Somekh E, Cesar K, Handsher R, et al: An outbreak of echovirus 13 meningitis in central Israel, *Epidemiol Infect* 130:257, 2003.
561. Trallero G, Casas I, Avellón CA, et al: First epidemic of aseptic meningitis due to echovirus type 13 among Spanish children, *Epidemiol Infect* 130:251, 2003.
562. Drouhet V: Enterovirus infection and associated clinical symptoms in children, *Ann Inst Pasteur* 98:562, 1960.
563. Hinuma Y, Murai Y, Nakao T: Two outbreaks of echovirus 14 infection: a possible interference with oral poliovirus vaccine and a probable association with aseptic meningitis, *J Hyg (Lond)* 63:277, 1965.
564. Medearis DN Jr, Kramer RA: Exanthem associated with ECHO virus type 18 viremia, *J Pediatr* 55:367, 1959.
565. Chonmaitree T, Ford C, Sanders C, et al: Comparison of cell cultures for rapid isolation of enteroviruses, *J Clin Microbiol* 26:2576, 1988.

566. Johnson FB: Transport of viral specimens, *Clin Microbiol Rev* 3:120, 1990.
567. Howell CL, Miller MJ: Effect of sucrose phosphate and sorbitol on infectivity of enveloped viruses during storage, *J Clin Microbiol* 18:658, 1983.
568. August MJ, Warford A: Evaluation of a commercial monoclonal antibody for detection of adenovirus antigen, *J Clin Microbiol* 25:2233, 1987.
569. Trabelsi A, Grattard F, Nejmeddine M, et al: Evaluation of an enterovirus group-specific anti-VPI monoclonal antibody, 5-D8/1, in comparison with neutralization and PCR for rapid identification of enteroviruses in cell culture, *J Clin Microbiol* 33:2454, 1995.
570. Carstens JM, Tracy S, Chapman NM, et al: Detection of enteroviruses in cell cultures by using in situ transcription, *J Clin Microbiol* 30:25, 1992.
571. Abraham R, Chonmaitree T, McCombs J, et al: Rapid detection of poliovirus by reverse transcription and polymerase chain amplification: application for the differentiation between poliovirus and nonpoliovirus enteroviruses, *J Clin Microbiol* 31:295, 1993.
572. Rittichier KR, Bryan PA, Bassett KE, et al: Diagnosis and outcomes of enterovirus infections in young infants, *Pediatr Infect Dis J* 24:546, 2005.
573. Martin AB, Webber S, Fricker FJ, et al: Acute myocarditis: rapid diagnosis by PCR in children, *Circulation* 90:330, 1994.
574. Muir P, Ras A, Klapper PE, et al: Multicenter quality assessment of PCR methods for detection of enteroviruses, *J Clin Microbiol* 37:1409, 1999.
575. De L, Nottay B, Yang CF, et al: Identification of vaccine-related polioviruses by hybridization with specific RNA probes, *J Clin Microbiol* 33:562, 1995.
576. Rotbart HA: Nucleic acid detection systems for enteroviruses, *Clin Microbiol Rev* 4:156, 1991.
577. Chezzi C: Rapid diagnosis of poliovirus infection by PCR amplification, *J Clin Microbiol* 34:1722, 1996.
578. Egger D, Pasamontes L, Ostermayer M, et al: Reverse transcription multiplex PCR for differentiation between polio and enteroviruses from clinical and environmental samples, *J Clin Microbiol* 33:1442, 1995.
579. Gorgievski-Hrisoho M, Schumacher JD, Vilimomovic N, et al: Detection by PCR of enteroviruses in cerebrospinal fluid during a summer outbreak of aseptic meningitis in Switzerland, *J Clin Microbiol* 36:2408, 1998.
580. Muir P, Nicholson F, Jhetam M, et al: Rapid diagnosis of enterovirus infection by magnetic bead extraction and polymerase chain reaction detection of enterovirus RNA in clinical specimens, *J Clin Microbiol* 31:31, 1993.
581. Petitjean J, Freymuth F, Kopecka H, et al: Detection of enteroviruses in cerebrospinal fluids: enzymatic amplification and hybridization with a biotinylated riboprobe, *Mol Cell Probes* 8:15B22, 1994.
582. Redline RW, Genest DR, Tycko B: Detection of enteroviral infection in paraffin-embedded tissue by the RNA polymerase chain reaction technique, *Am J Clin Pathol* 96:568, 1991.
583. Ramers C, Billman G, Hartin M, et al: Impact of a diagnostic cerebrospinal fluid enterovirus polymerase chain reaction test on patient management, *JAMA* 283:2680, 2000.
584. Yang CF, De L, Holloway BP, et al: Detection and identification of vaccine-related polioviruses by the polymerase chain reaction, *Viral Res* 20:159, 1991.
585. Dagan R, Prather SL, Powell KR, et al: Neutralizing antibodies to non-polio enteroviruses in human immune serum globulin, *Pediatr Infect Dis* 2:454, 1983.
586. McKinney RE Jr, Katz SL, Wilfert CM: Chronic enteroviral meningoencephalitis in agammaglobulinemic patients, *Rev Infect Dis* 9:334, 1987.
587. Hammond GW, Lukes H, Wells B, et al: Maternal and neonatal neutralizing antibody titers to selected enteroviruses, *Pediatr Infect Dis* 4:32, 1985.
588. Johnston JM, Overall JC Jr: Intravenous immunoglobulin in disseminated neonatal echovirus 11 infection, *Pediatr Infect Dis J* 8:254, 1989.
589. Abzug MJ, Keyerling HL, Lee ML, et al: Neonatal enterovirus infection: virology, serology, and effects of intravenous immune globulin, *Clin Infect Dis* 20:1201, 1995.
590. Jantausch BA, Luban NLC, Duffy L, et al: Maternal plasma transfusion in the treatment of disseminated neonatal echovirus 11 infection, *Pediatr Infect Dis J* 14:154, 1995.
591. Thibaut HJ, De Palma AM, Neyts J: Combating enterovirus replication: state-of-the-art on antiviral research, *Biochem Pharmacol* 83:185, 2012.
592. United States Public Health Service: The prevention of mental retardation through control of infectious diseases, Washington, DC, 1966, U.S. Government Printing Office.
593. Bryant PA, Tingay D, Dargaville PA, et al: Neonatal coxsackie B virus infection—a treatable disease? *Eur J Pediatr* 163:223, 2004.
594. Rotbart HA, Abzug MJ, Levin MJ: Development and application of RNA probes for the study of picornaviruses, *Mol Cell Probes* 2:65, 1988.
595. Hayden FG, Herrington DT, Coats TL, et al: Efficacy and safety of oral pleconaril for treatment of colds due to picornaviruses in adults: results of 2 double-blind, randomized, placebo-controlled trials, *Clin Infect Dis* 36:1523, 2003.
596. Fleischer R, Laessig K: Safety and efficacy evaluation of pleconaril for treatment of the common cold, *Clin Infect Dis* 37:1722, 2003.
597. Kilbourne ED, Wilson CB, Perrier D: The induction of gross myocardial lesions by a Coxsackie (pleurodynia) virus and cortisone, *J Clin Invest* 35:367, 1956.
598. Mason JW, O'Connell JB, Herskowitz A, et al: A clinical trial of immunosuppressive therapy for myocarditis, *N Engl J Med* 333:269, 1995.
599. Grabhorn E, Richter A, Fischer L, et al: Emergency liver transplantation in neonates with acute liver failure: long-term follow-up, *Transplantation* 86:932, 2008.
600. Colombani PM, Cigarroa FG, Schwarz K, et al: Liver transplantation in infants younger than 1 year of age, *Ann Surg* 223:658, 1996. discussion 662.
601. Ramachandra G, Shields L, Brown K, Ramnarayan P: The challenges of prompt identification and resuscitation in children with acute fulminant myocarditis: case series and review of the literature, *J Paediatr Child Health* 46:579, 2010.
602. Liang ZL, Mao QY, Wang YP, et al: Progress on the research and development of inactivated EV71 whole-virus vaccines, *Hum Vaccin Immunother*, 9:1701, 2013.
603. Zhu FC, Meng FY, Li JX, et al: Efficacy, safety, and immunology of an inactivated alum-adjuvant enterovirus 71 vaccine in children in China: a multicentre, randomised, double-blind, placebo-controlled, phase 3 trial, *Lancet* 381:2024, 2013.
604. Bell EJ, McCartney RA, Basquill D, et al: Mu-antibody capture ELISA for the rapid diagnosis of enterovirus infections in patients with aseptic meningitis, *J Med Virol* 19:213, 1986.
605. Chuang E, Maller ES, Hoffman MA, et al: Successful treatment of fulminant echovirus 11 infection in a neonate by orthotopic liver transplantation, *J Pediatr Gastroenterol Nutr* 17:211, 1993.
606. Sadeharju K, Knip M, Virtanen SM, et al: Maternal antibodies in breast milk protect the child from enterovirus infections, *Pediatrics* 119:941, 2007.
607. Cherry JD: Enteroviruses: Polioviruses (poliomyelitis), coxsackieviruses, echoviruses, and enteroviruses. In Feigin RD, Cherry JD, editors: *Textbook of pediatric infectious diseases*, ed 2, Philadelphia, 1987, WB Saunders, p 1729.
608. Isaacs D, Wilkinson AR, Eglin R, et al: Conservative management of an echovirus 11 outbreak in a neonatal unit, *Lancet* 1:543, 1989.

26 Hepatitis

WIKROM KARNSAKUL and KATHLEEN B. SCHWARZ

CHAPTER OUTLINE

Knowledge about the hepatotropic viruses has grown dramatically in the past century, with contributions from clinicians, molecular virologists, immunologists, and pharmacologists.

Hepatotropic viruses (hepatitis A through G viruses and torque teno virus [TTV]) are not a common cause of neonatal morbidity and mortality in the developed world. When hepatitis E virus (HEV) is contracted during the second or third trimester, pregnant women are at risk of developing fulminant fatal hepatitis.[1] In pregnant mothers with a high viral load and positive hepatitis B early antigen (HBeAg) status, transmission from mother to newborn may occur in 5% to 10% of pregnancies,[2] even with the use of appropriate prophylaxis with hepatitis B virus (HBV) immunoglobulin and active HBV vaccination. The prevention of perinatal transmission is still a high priority in the attempt to reduce the global burden of chronic HBV.

During pregnancy, a significant shift in the maternal T-helper type 1 (Th1)–T-helper type 2-(Th2) cell paradigm, with a definite skew toward Th2 cells, causes a reduction of most cytokines during the first 20 weeks of pregnancy, to sustain the fetal life.[3] Whether or not this suppresses the maternal immune system may increase the risk of infections during pregnancy and requires further study. Because pregnancy involves two genetically distinct individuals (a pregnant mother and fetus), a pregnant woman infected with any hepatitis virus cannot be simply considered as an infected adult alone when planning the antiviral treatment. The treatment during the entire pregnancy should be judiciously considered to balance the maternal benefits with the exposure of the fetus to potentially toxic drugs during its entire prenatal life.

This chapter reviews up-to-date information on the hepatotropic viruses (hepatitis A through G viruses and TTV), with a particular focus on pregnant women, the fetus, and newborn infants, as well as breakthroughs in vaccine development and global preventive measures (Table 25-1).

Hepatitis A Virus

Hepatitis A virus (HAV) is one of the most common communicable diseases and has a worldwide distribution, with estimated recognized cases of 1.5 million annually.[4] This virus accounts for 20% to 40% of cases of adult viral hepatitis in the Western world.[5] The rate of HAV in the United States has significantly declined since hepatitis A vaccine was first available in 1995.[6] In May 2006, the Advisory Committee on Immunization Practices recommended routine HAV vaccination for all children, beginning at 12 months of age.[7] The same year, the lowest incidence of HAV ever was recorded at 1.2 per 100,000.[8] Routine HAV immunization is close to cost-neutral on a cost-per-quality–adjusted-life-year basis.[9]

EPIDEMIOLOGY AND TRANSMISSION

Hepatitis A virus infection is one of the most common causes of acute viral hepatitis in the general population; however, it

Table 25-1 Hepatitis Viruses and Primary Route of Transmission

Viruses	Virus Structure	Primary Route of Neonatal/Fetal Infection	Transmission in Children and Adults
HAV (picornavirus)	SS RNA, nonenveloped	Perinatal	Fecal-oral
HBV (hepadnavirus)	DS circular DNA, enveloped	Perinatal	Bloodborne
HCV (flavivirus)	SS RNA, enveloped	Perinatal	Bloodborne
HDV (deltavirus)	SS, circular RNA (HBV envelope)	Not reported	Bloodborne
HEV (calicivirus)	SS RNA, nonenveloped	In utero, perinatal	Fecal-oral
HGV (flavivirus)	SS RNA, nonenveloped	In utero, perinatal	Bloodborne, sexual
TTV (circovirus)	SS, circular DNA, nonenveloped	Perinatal	Fecal-oral, bloodborne, sexual contact

DS, Double-stranded; *HAV*, hepatitis A virus; *HBV*, hepatitis B virus; *HCV*, hepatitis C virus; *HDV*, hepatitis D virus; *HEV*, hepatitis E virus; *HGV*, hepatitis G virus (GB virus type C); *SS*, single-stranded; *TTV*, torque teno virus.

has been infrequently reported among pregnant females.[10-13] In a study from Ireland,[10] in which 13,181 consecutive deliveries were retrospectively reviewed, only 2% developed HAV during pregnancy. Of 127 consecutive pregnant patients in an Indian series, no cases of acute or fulminant hepatitis from HAV were identified.[11] No cases of HAV infection were identified among the 76-patient prospective 3-year study of pregnant women with acute hepatitis.[12] In other retrospective patient series, the incidence of HAV infection during pregnancy was also extremely low.[13] In a U.S. study of 313 patients affected by the urban HAV epidemic in Tennessee, 4 individuals were pregnant and 2 in their third trimester of pregnancy experienced premature delivery with subsequent full recovery of mothers and children.[14]

In the United States, person-to-person transmission through the fecal-oral route is probably the primary mode of HAV transmission in all subjects, including pregnant women.[15] Infections usually result from a contact from a family member or a sex partner. In most infected individuals, the stool contains a higher concentration of virus and is likely highly contagious during the 1 to 2 weeks before the illness compared with later in the course.[6] The risk of transmission subsequently diminishes by 1 week after onset of jaundice.[16] HAV can be detected in stool for longer periods, however, especially in neonates and young children.[17] The majority of index cases, who are usually unaware of this risk, are international travelers to developing countries, regardless of travel budget, who account for 11% of documented cases of infection without a known source.[18]

HAV is not commonly associated with a severe outcome or complications during pregnancy. Mother-to-child HAV transmission seems to be very rare.[19-22] In four cases, infections occurred after maternal symptomatic hepatitis A in both second and third trimesters. Nosocomial transmission is unusual, but outbreaks caused by transmission from hospitalized patients to health care staff have been reported.[17,23] In addition, outbreaks have occurred in neonatal intensive care units from neonates receiving infected transfused blood and subsequently transmitting HAV to other neonates and health care staff.[17,23]

MICROBIOLOGY AND PATHOGENESIS

Hepatitis A virus is a single-stranded RNA virus classified as a member of the picornavirus group. Most human strains belong to genotype I or III.[16] The three major proteins of viral capsid—VP1, VP2, and VP3 (structural proteins)—are encoded by P1 region on viral genome. The structural arrangement of capsid proteins VP1 and VP3 forms a single, dominant, serologic epitope on the virus capsid and accounts for a neutralizing antibody response. The virus can be stable in the environment for several months. HAV can live outside the body for months, which is likely explained by the slow translation rate, depending on the environmental conditions.[24]

HAV crosses through the gastrointestinal tract by an uncharacterized mechanism to the liver, where it solely replicates in hepatocytes.[25] The pathogenetic mechanism leading to liver tissue injury by HAV is not a viral cytopathogenic effect. Rather, it is suggested to be an immunopathologic reaction of sensitized cytotoxic T lymphocytes against infected hepatocytes, where these T lymphocytes are present as an antiviral reaction similar to that directed against HBV.[16,26] A low translation rate and RNA replication rate may play a role in escaping host cell defenses.[19] Almost all individuals infected with HAV develop immunoglobulin G (IgG) and IgM antibodies to VP1.[16]

PATHOLOGY

After the availability of serology to confirm HAV, a liver histopathology study was performed in patients with acute viral hepatitis caused by HAV or HBV. The liver parenchymal changes in patients with HAV, including focal necrosis, hepatocellular ballooning, and acidophilic degeneration, were milder than changes seen in patients with HBV, but the degree of portal inflammation seemed similar in these two groups.[27]

CLINICAL MANIFESTATIONS

In pregnant women, HAV typically is an acute, self-limited illness associated with fever, malaise, jaundice, anorexia, nausea, and abdominal discomfort after an incubation period of approximately 28 days (range, 15-50 days).[6] A significant number (69%) of pregnant women with acute HAV infection during the second and third trimesters of pregnancy have gestational complications leading to preterm labor, including premature contractions, placental separation, and premature rupture of membranes.[28,29] Fulminant hepatitis from HAV was reported in one mother who received a liver transplant at the second trimester and lost her fetus after her transplant period.[30]

Although uncommon, neonatal cholestasis resulting from maternal-to-fetal transmission has been reported.[31,32] Four cases of intrauterine infection have been reported. Two mothers had symptomatic HAV at 20 and 13 weeks of gestation. The fetuses developed ascites, meconium peritonitis, and perforation of the distal ileum in utero, requiring surgery after birth. The newborn infants subsequently recovered. In two other mothers with HAV at 20 days before delivery, infants developed neonatal icteric hepatitis A on day 3 of life and had a full recovery.[32,33] Mild acute hepatitis in newborn infants followed the onset of hepatitis in their mothers, developing in late third trimester (gestational week >33), probably resulting from a perinatal contact with infected blood or feces.[19-22] Although typically self-limited, HAV can be potentially life threatening, with an estimated fatality rate of 0.3% to 0.6%, reaching 1.8% among adults older than 50 years.[15] Fulminant hepatitis is rare, but is more common in people with underlying liver disease.[34] Chronic infection does not occur with HAV.[35] Rare extrahepatic manifestations include pancreatitis, renal failure, arthritis, vasculitis, thrombocytopenia, aplastic anemia, red blood cell aplasia, transverse myelitis, and toxic epidermal necrolysis.[8] The appearance of jaundice usually leads to further investigation and the diagnosis of HAV; however, 70% of infected children younger than 6 years are anicteric or have a mild flulike illness. Jaundice is observed in only 7% of children younger than 4 years, including newborns.[35] Symptoms usually last less than 2 months, although 10% to 15% of individuals with HAV have prolonged or relapsing hepatitis for up to 6 months.

DIAGNOSIS

Serologic tests for HAV-specific total and IgM antibody are available commercially.[1] Serum IgM is present at the onset of illness and usually disappears within 4 months but may persist for 6 months or longer.[6] The presence of serum IgM may indicate current infection, recent infection, or HAV vaccination, although false-positive results can occur. Anti-HAV IgG is detectable shortly after the appearance of IgM. The presence of anti-HAV IgG alone indicates past infection and immunity.

TREATMENT

Treatment generally is supportive. In addition to standard precautions, contact precautions are recommended for diapered and incontinent patients for at least 1 week after the onset of symptoms.[6] One of the most important aspects of management of infected individuals is active and passive immunization of close contacts (see "Prevention," next). Some patients with cholestasis may not tolerate a fatty diet. In individuals with fulminant hepatitis or liver failure, specific management is determined by the complications, and evaluation for liver transplant may be required.[16]

PREVENTION

Acute HAV infection during pregnancy and perinatal transmission seem to be rare, especially at the time of delivery. There have been no data to suggest cesarean section as a mode of delivery for HAV-infected pregnant women; infants born via vaginal delivery to mothers with acute HAV infection have a favorable outcome.[28] No data exist about administration of the hepatitis A vaccine to pregnant women. Because the vaccine does not contain a live virus, the risk to mother and fetus should be extremely low to nonexistent.[36,37] The prevalence of HAV infection in young children seems to be decreasing in countries that are moving from high-to-intermediate endemic areas. It is expected that an increased number of adolescents and adults susceptible to HAV may be associated with greater morbidity, mortality, and treatment costs.[38] On the other hand, in areas of low endemicity for HAV, outbreaks of HAV infection could put individuals, including pregnant women who are not immune to HAV, at risk. Although rare, acute HAV infection during pregnancy is associated with a high risk of maternal complications and preterm labor; HAV serology and maternal immunization during prenatal or pre-pregnancy evaluation could be considered in areas in which adult populations are susceptible to HAV.

The infant usually has exposure to HAV before the diagnosis is made in the mother. HAV has been detected in breast milk, but only one newborn case of HAV transmission in breast milk has been reported.[19] Although the efficacy has not yet been established, immunoglobulin (0.02 mL/kg) is advised to be administered to the infant if the mother's symptoms of HAV began between 2 weeks before and 1 week after delivery.[6] To prevent nosocomial transmission, particularly in the neonatal intensive care unit or newborn nursery, the infected mother and the neonate should be isolated, and careful hygiene practices should be emphasized.[39]

The presence of passive maternal HAV antibody during the first 6 to 12 months of life would interfere with vaccine immunogenicity.[40-44] HAV vaccination is recommended and licensed in the United States for all children 1 to 18 years of age; for adults who are at increased risk for infection; for adults who are at increased risk for complications from HAV, such as persons with underlying liver disease; and for any person wishing to obtain immunity to HAV. HAV vaccines are given intramuscularly in a two-dose schedule with a 6- to 12-month interval.[6] Doses and schedules for HAV vaccines and formulations produced by different manufacturers are recommended by American Academy of Pediatrics (AAP).[6] Current HAV vaccines have been shown to be safe, to be highly immunogenic, and to confer long-lasting protection. Vaccine-induced antibodies persist for longer than 12 years in vaccinated adults, and mathematical modeling predicts antibody persistence for longer than 25 years in greater than 95% of vaccine recipients.[38] Intramuscular immunoglobulin is more than 85% effective in preventing symptomatic infection when given within 2 weeks after the most recent exposure to HAV in a household or sexual contact.[6]

Hepatitis B Virus and Hepatitis D Virus

Hepatitis B virus (HBV) is believed to have infected 2 billion persons worldwide; more than 350 million individuals are currently infected.[45] The maternal-to-fetal route of transmission is responsible for most infections. Past efforts to prevent this route of transmission resulted in the strategy of providing a combination of passive and active immunization within 24 hours of birth. Although this strategy is 90% to 95% effective when properly administered, remaining areas of concern are the need to disseminate this practice for all high-risk infants and to achieve universal vaccination of all infants, as recommended by the World Health Organization. In addition, there is a need to develop effective measures to prevent transmission in 100% of newborns born to infected mothers. Such measures would be highly cost-effective, given the ongoing morbidity and mortality from HBV, which accounts for 500,000 to 1 million deaths from cirrhosis, liver failure, and hepatocellular carcinoma worldwide per year.[46] The delta virus or hepatitis D virus [HDV] is always linked to HBV because it requires the surface coat of HBV for replication. Little information exists regarding perinatal transmission of HDV; even in highly endemic areas, infection with HDV is infrequent in infants and is mainly acquired during the second and third decades of life, suggesting a horizontal rather than vertical transmission of the virus.[47]

EPIDEMIOLOGY AND TRANSMISSION

Acute HBV infection does not appear to increase mortality during pregnancy or to have teratogenic effects. However, a higher incidence of low birth weight and prematurity has been reported.[48] In addition, acute HBV early in pregnancy is associated with a 10% perinatal transmission rate, and the rate increases substantially with HBV infection in the third trimester.[1] The effects of chronic HBV infection on pregnancy outcomes have not been clearly defined. In a study of pregnancy outcome comparing hepatitis B surface antigen (HBsAg)-positive and HBsAg-negative women, there were no differences in gestational age at delivery, birth weight, incidence of prematurity, neonatal jaundice, congenital anomalies, or perinatal mortality.[1] In general, women with chronic hepatitis B do well during pregnancy. Although the infection is usually well tolerated, cases of exacerbation of hepatitis[49] and even fulminant hepatic failure[50] have been described in the peripartum period. The strategy to control HBV viremia during pregnancy is prudent.

Before the development of the combination vaccination strategy (hepatitis B immunoglobulin [HBIG] plus vaccine) for high-risk neonates, most neonates born to HBV-infected mothers were infected with HBV. Chen and colleagues[51] reported that the presence of HBsAg in gastric aspirates of newborns was strongly associated with the acquisition of HBsAg by the infants; there was no correlation between the rate of infant antigenemia and the duration of the first stage of labor, and cesarean section did not decrease the rate of vertical HBV transmission.

The prevalence of chronic HBV infection in pregnant women in urban areas of the United States varies by race and ethnicity,[52] the highest rate being in Asian women (6%); the rates in black, white, and Hispanic women are 1.0, 0.6, and 0.14%, respectively. European studies show similar data, with highest rates among immigrants and low immunization-induced protection rates.[53,54] In areas of high endemicity, such as China, other Far East countries, and Africa, rates of chronic HBV infection are higher. According to recent data from the Centers for Disease Control and Prevention (CDC), prenatal screening for HBsAg in the United States showed that 97% of pregnant women undergo screening before delivery.[55] Among infants at risk of acquiring HBV infection, 92% completed the three-dose vaccination by the time they are 3 years of age. Outside the United States, however, many high-prevalence countries lack immunization coverage, and perinatal transmission is common. In 87 countries with a prevalence of HBV infection that exceeds 8%, the infant immunization coverage was only 36%.[56]

Perinatal transmission occurs at or near the time of birth because of exposure to cervical secretions and maternal blood. To a minor degree, transplacental transmission presumably is responsible for perinatal infections, depending on risk factors: maternal HBeAg positivity, HBsAg titer, and HBV DNA level.[57] Despite the use of effective active and passive immunoprophylaxis, perinatal transmission might still occur.[1] Mothers positive for HBeAg and mothers with very high serum DNA levels (e.g., 10^9 copies/mL) have the greatest risk of transmitting HBV to their offspring, despite adherence to the recommended combination of active and passive immunization of newborns within 24 hours of birth.[58] In one Chinese study, 7.4% of infants born to HBV-infected mothers were infected with HBV during the first year of life, despite receiving passive and active immunoprophylaxis in the immediate newborn period.[58] Mode of delivery does not influence the likelihood of HBV transmission. Wang and colleagues[49] compared outcomes among three groups of 144 infants born by spontaneous vaginal delivery, 40 by forceps or vacuum extraction, and 117 by cesarean section. All infants received HBIG and HBV vaccine at the recommended schedule. Chronic HBV infection was detected at the rates of 7.3, 7.7, and 6.8%, respectively, and response rates to immunization were the same in all groups.[49]

Sexual intercourse in the second trimester of pregnancy has also been implicated in HBV intrauterine transmission.[59] Although the prevalence is low, another risk of HBV transmission is amniocentesis in HBsAg-positive mothers. In one series of 21 mothers with positive HBsAg who underwent amniocentesis for accepted indications at a mean of 19.5 weeks of gestation, none of the infants who received the HBIG and HBV vaccine as recommended was HBsAg positive at 1 or 12 months of age.[50] In a study of 47 HBsAg positive women who presented for amniocentesis, 32% of the amniotic-fluid samples were HBsAg positive, but HBV DNA was undetectable in all. Although cord blood from 27% of the infants contained HBsAg, none contained HBV DNA.[60] Although HBsAg can be detected in the breast milk of HBV-infected mothers, several studies have shown there is no additional risk of transmission of HBV to breast-fed infants of infected mothers, provided that proper active and passive immunoprophylaxis is carried out.[61]

MICROBIOLOGY AND PATHOGENESIS

Hepatitis B virus is a well-characterized, partially double-stranded DNA virus. HBsAg is the hallmark of chronic infection. This marker is the first to appear in acute infection. The presence of HBsAg for 6 months or more connotes chronic infection. HBeAg is associated with infectivity and indicates active replication of HBV. More recent reports have described "occult HBV," as defined by the presence of HBV DNA in serum or tissue in the absence of other markers. Several HBV genotypes are now recognized, and knowledge is emerging regarding their clinical significance. It is recognized that HBV genotype C is associated with an increased risk of development of hepatocellular carcinoma, as are the basal core promoter mutant and the pre-S deletion mutant.[62] Whether or not there is a role for quantification of HBV antigens or intrahepatic HBV covalently closed circular DNA, or both, is currently under investigation.

HBV is thought to cause liver injury in immunocompetent subjects via cytotoxic T cells directed to the infected hepatocyte. Functionally impaired dendritic cells may play a role in viral persistence,[63] and B and T cells are involved in viral clearance. In immunocompromised subjects, such as individuals who have undergone liver transplantation, the virus itself may be hepatotoxic because HBV recurrence in the allograft is associated with poor patient and graft survival. The HB-X protein is a transcriptional activator of cellular genes and may play a role in the hepatocarcinogenesis of HBV via effects on apoptosis, DNA repair, mitogen-activated protein kinase, and Janus kinase (JAK)/signal transducer and activator of transcription (STAT) pathways.[64]

PATHOLOGY

There are few reports of HBV hepatic histopathology in young infants, although hepatocellular carcinoma has been reported at 8 months of age.[65] In case series of children with active HBV hepatitis enrolled in antiviral trials, liver biopsy specimens generally show mild-to-moderate inflammation and mild-to-moderate fibrosis.[66]

CLINICAL MANIFESTATIONS

The clinical manifestations of HBV infection depend on the age of acquisition. Neonates have a greater than 90% risk of chronic infection, and children and adolescents have a 25% to 50% risk; chronic infection is observed in only 5% of adults exposed to HBV.[67] Most newborns who acquire HBV remain in the immunotolerant stage for 1 or 2 decades. This stage is characterized by HBsAg and HBeAg antigenemia, high levels of HBV DNA, normal or minimally elevated serum aminotransferases, and minimal inflammation in the liver biopsy specimen. Approximately 6% of infants born to mothers who are positive for anti–hepatitis B early antibody develop acute hepatitis at 2 months of age.[68] Infants are ill with fever, jaundice, and hepatic tenderness. Serum aminotransferases are elevated, and there is active inflammation in the liver biopsy specimen. About one third of older children and adolescents with acute HBV develop these classic symptoms.[69] Most infants, children, and adolescents have chronic infection (lasting >6 months) of the asymptomatic immunotolerant type. In infants who are perinatally infected, the estimated spontaneous clearance of HBV is 0.6% per year over the first decade of life, but in subjects infected as adolescents and adults, the rate of clearance is 1.8% per year.[70] A few young subjects have active hepatitis with elevation of serum aminotransferases and active inflammation in the liver biopsy specimen. These subjects are most likely to respond to antiviral treatment. Inactive carriers are characterized by HBsAg positivity, seroconversion of HBeAg to anti–hepatitis B early antibody, undetectable HBV DNA, and normal serum aminotransferases. Individuals with active hepatitis are at greatest risk for developing cirrhosis and hepatocellular carcinoma, but there is a growing concern that persistently high levels of HBV DNA for decades, even in immunotolerant subjects, are associated with an increased risk of hepatocellular carcinoma.[71] In one Chinese study, HBV infection in pregnancy was associated with high rates of complications (abortion, 16.7%; preterm births, 43%; neonatal asphyxia, 15.6%; and fetal death, 4.5%).[72]

DIAGNOSIS

The diagnosis of HBV is most commonly made by the presence of HBsAg in the circulation. Other studies commonly performed include HBeAg, HBV DNA, and anti–core antibody. IgM anti–core antibody is indicative of recent exposure to HBV, whereas IgG core antibody is positive in individuals with chronic infection and in individuals who have cleared infection. Subjects who have been successfully immunized with HBV vaccine exhibit anti-HBsAg positivity. If a liver biopsy specimen is obtained, immunohistochemistry can be performed using an antibody against the surface antigen. Screening has been recommended for all pregnant women and for newly arrived immigrants to the United States from countries where HBV prevalence rate is 2% or greater.[73] Whether or not there should be screening of pregnant women living in areas of high HBV endemicity for occult HBV infection by using sensitive assays for HBV DNA is a matter of current study.

TREATMENT

There are currently two treatments for chronic HBV infection approved by the U.S. Food and Drug Administration (FDA) for children 2 to 18 years of age: standard interferon (IFN), which is given parenterally three times per week for 16 to 24 weeks, and lamivudine, which is given via the oral route. IFN therapy should not be given to infants younger than 1 year because of the risk of spastic diplegia; in older children, side effects are common and are usually flulike in nature. Drug resistance has not been a problem. When IFN is administered to children with active hepatitis B, 20% to 58% show undetectable HBV DNA or HBeAg, or both, in serum.[74] Lamivudine is much better tolerated by children than IFN, but drug resistance is common—approximately 20% per year of administration. Currently, complete and ongoing pediatric trials of more potent nucleoside/nucleotide analogues include adefovir dipivoxil and entecavir.[75] Adefovir dipivoxil was recently approved for children aged 12 years and older; entecavir is approved for children aged 16 years and older.

PREVENTION

Immunoprophylaxis with HBIG and hepatitis B vaccine is known to be safe and effective but is applied variably in different geographic regions. Compliance issues have been reported even in countries such as Canada, where the government mandates screening of all pregnant women for HBV and provides prophylaxis to infants born to HBV-infected women. Less than 85% completed prophylaxis, suggesting that there is a need for public health programs with more effective universal neonatal immunization for infants at highest risk of HBV acquisition.[76] Even with proper vaccination, 5% to 10% of infants of HBeAg-positive women become infected, so there is opportunity for improvement in prevention strategies.[1] Different doses and routes of HBIG administration during pregnancy have been studied in an attempt to reduce the rate of perinatal transmission with varying efficacy.[77-79] Shi and colleagues[80] reported a meta-analysis of 37 randomized controlled trials (RCTs) that investigated the efficacy of administration of HBIG to the mother to prevent transmission to the offspring. A group of 5900 newborns of asymptomatic HBsAg-seropositive mothers received HBIG injection to prevent transmission from mother to newborn. Newborns in the HBIG group had a higher protection rate compared with the control group. Although HBIG appears to be safe, a few RCTs have reported adverse events.[80]

Another strategy to interrupt this process is maternal treatment with a nucleoside analogue late in pregnancy. In the largest randomized, double-blind, placebo-controlled trial of 114 highly viremic women, viral load reduction to less than 1000 mEq/mL was achieved in 98% of the lamivudine-treated mothers and 31% of control subjects.[81] At 1 year of age, 18% of infants of lamivudine-treated mothers were HBsAg positive versus 39% in placebo group, even though all infants received HBIG and vaccine in the standard regimen. No adverse effects of lamivudine were noted in either the mothers or their infants.[82] Although there is no consensus regarding using HBIG or a nucleoside analogue in pregnant women to prevent perinatal transmission, telbivudine or tenofovir should be selected when the treatment of chronic hepatitis B infection is necessary because these drugs have been classified as FDA pregnancy risk category B and because they are more effective against HBV than lamivudine, as well as being associated with much lower drug-resistance rates than lamivudine. Seven clinical trials involving 644 pregnant women were included in the meta-analysis study by Liu and colleagues.[83] Telbivudine resulted in lower HBsAg rates and HBV DNA values in newborns and infants.[83]

Detailed HBV vaccine schedules are available from the AAP *Red Book*.[67] Schedules are provided for the various pediatric age groups, for vaccination of preterm infants, and for newborns, depending on maternal HBsAg status (Table 25-2). Systematic HBV vaccination has markedly decreased the incidence of new HBV infections in the pediatric age group over the last 2 decades. Although much less is known about the impact of HBV vaccine programs on HDV incidence, one Italian study showed the incidence decreased from 1.7 to 0.5 cases per 1 million population after introduction of a universal anti-HBV campaign.[84] Efforts have been made to assess the impact of maternal HBV screening on perinatal HBV vaccination. In a U.S. study, to assess the completeness of maternal screening for newborn prophylaxis, the mother's HBsAg status was known within 12 hours of delivery for 84% of mothers screened; however, of the infants whose mothers' HBsAg status was unknown, only 28% were vaccinated the first day of life.[85]

Guo and colleagues[86] studied 1133 HBsAg-positive mothers and their babies in China. A total of 101 neonates had positive HBsAg and/or HBV DNA; thus the intrauterine transmission rate was 8.9%. Maternal vaginal bleeding and severe nausea during the first trimester were associated with an increased risk of intrauterine transmission, whereas

Table 25-2 Hepatitis B Neonatal Intervention Strategies Based on Maternal Hepatitis B Virus Screening Status

Maternal HBV Status	Interpretation on Maternal History	Laboratory Evaluation at Birth and During Infancy	Neonatal and Infant Intervention
HBsAg positive	Mother is infectious; significant risk of neonatal infection	HBsAg on peripheral venous blood sampling to diagnose intrauterine infection; check infant after age 9 mo for anti-HBs and HBsAg	All infants: HBIG 0.5 mL ≤12 hr after birth; in addition, 12 hr after birth, second and third doses of vaccine for infants with birth weight <2000 g, as for HBsAg-negative status Preterm infants < 2000 g birth weight: Initial birth dose should not be counted as one of immunizing series because of immature response to vaccine; subsequent three immunizations in primary immunizing series for these infants should start at age 1-2 mo
HBsAg status unknown	Mother's infectious status should be determined by HBsAg testing as soon as possible	None required at birth; in infants whose mothers are subsequently found to be HBsAg-positive, check infant after age 9 mo for anti-HBs and HBsAg	Full-term infants: Give first dose of hepatitis B vaccine ≤12 hr of birth; if maternal HBsAg is positive, give HBIG 0.5 mL as soon as possible, ≤7 days of age; if maternal HBsAg is negative, HBIG is not needed; subsequent doses, as for HBsAg-negative status Preterm infants <2000 g birth weight: If maternal HBsAg status cannot be determined ≤12 hr of birth, give HBIG in addition to hepatitis vaccine ≤12 hr of birth; provide subsequent three hepatitis B immunizations for primary series, starting at 1 mo of age, as above for preterm infants
HBsAg negative	Mother is not considered infectious; no risk to neonate	None required	All newborn infants: Standard three-dose immunization regimen with hepatitis B vaccine recommended: Dose 1 given soon after birth before discharge, dose 2 given at age 1-2 mo at least 4 wk after dose 1; dose 3 given at age 6-18 mo, at least 16 wk after dose 1, and at least 8 wk after dose 2, with last dose not before 24 wk of age

This table recommends only single-antigen vaccine to be given between birth and 6 weeks of age. Single-antigen or combination vaccine may be used to complete the series; four doses of vaccine may be administered if a birth dose is given, and a combination vaccine containing a hepatitis B component is used to complete the series. Refer to American Academy of Pediatrics: Hepatitis B. In Pickering LK, Baker CJ, Kimberlin DW, Long SS, editors: *Red book: 2012 report of the Committee on Infectious Diseases,* ed 29, Elk Grove Village, Ill, 2012, American Academy of Pediatrics, pp 369-390.
HBIG, Hepatitis B immunoglobulin; *HBsAg,* hepatitis B surface antigen; *HBV,* hepatitis B virus.

cesarean delivery (odds ratio, 0.32; 95% confidence interval, 0.20 to 0.51) was associated with a decreased risk after adjusting for potential confounders. Maternal HBeAg positivity was a strong independent predictor for intrauterine transmission. A positive association between maternal HBV DNA levels and intrauterine transmission was suggested. Neither maternal treatment with HBIG nor a family history of HBV infection nor premature rupture of membranes was associated with the risk of intrauterine transmission.[86] HBV DNA virus levels increase during the last trimester of pregnancy and early in the postpartum period; the value of assessing these levels to modify immunoprophylaxis of the newborn is a matter of current study.[87] Although serum alanine aminotransferase levels are often used as surrogate markers of HBV DNA in HBeAg-negative pregnant women, they do not seem to correlate well with these levels.[88] Because of possible in utero HBV transmission among pregnant women with high HBV DNA titers, studies have been done regarding the possible added efficacy of using HBIG during the third trimester of pregnancy to prevent maternal-to-fetal transmission of HBV; results to date have been conflicting. One study reported that protective anti-HBsAg rates at 6 months were higher in infants born to either HBeAg-positive or HBeAg-negative mothers who had received three doses of HBIG in late pregnancy, along with infant passive and active immunization.[89] Another study showed no difference in the protective efficacy rates assessed at 12 months of age in infants of mothers receiving HBIG or not receiving HBIG.[90]

The benefits of detection of infected pregnant women include the identification not only of infants who require prophylaxis but also of women who might need treatment, and of sexual and household contacts who will benefit from testing, counseling, vaccination, or therapy if indicated.

The AAP states that HBV infection should not be considered a contraindication to breastfeeding of infants who receive the HBIG and HBV vaccine as advised.[91] Breastfeeding does not interfere with the immune response to the HBV vaccine.

Although the high efficacy of neonatal HBV vaccination suggests that most cases are transmitted perinatally, some neonates who have failed vaccine have been found to be positive for HBsAg or HBeAg at birth, suggestive of intrauterine transmission.[92] There is a need to elucidate the role of nucleoside nucleotide agents in treating chronic HBV in the last part of pregnancy in women with high HBV DNA levels who are positive for HBeAg and who are most likely to infect their newborns.[93,94]

Hepatitis C Virus

Since the discovery of hepatitis C virus (HCV) in 1989, HCV has become a global public health problem, infecting approximately 170 million individuals. Although transfusion-transmitted HCV was the major form of HCV in the pediatric age group when the virus was first described,[95] since 1992, when most blood units transfused have been free of HCV, the maternal-to-fetal route of transmission of this virus has become the dominant route for new cases of HCV. Jhaveri and colleagues[96] estimated the direct medical costs related to HCV in childhood projected for the next decade. Expressed as U.S. dollars, these include $26 million for screening, $117 to $206 million for monitoring, and $56 to $104 million for treatment costs. There are currently two FDA-approved treatments for HCV in children starting at age 3 years.[74] No strategy to date has been shown to be effective in interrupting maternal-to-fetal transmission, so this is a major research goal in the future.

EPIDEMIOLOGY AND TRANSMISSION

Maternal-to-fetal transmission has been studied extensively. The prevalence of anti-HCV antibody in pregnant women is 0.1% to 2.4%, and 60% to 70% are viremic. Transmission rates are 4% to 7% when the mother is viremic, and mothers with HCV RNA greater than 10^6 copies/mL are more likely to transmit the infection to the fetus compared with mothers with lower levels of viremia.[97] Coinfection with human immunodeficiency virus (HIV) increases the risk of transmission fourfold to fivefold, but highly active retroviral therapy may significantly decrease this risk.[98] In the setting of coinfection with HCV and HIV, there is no evidence that HCV neutralizing antibodies are associated with the prevention of maternal-to-fetal transmission of HCV.[99] Female infants are more likely than male infants to acquire HCV from their mothers.[100] One Japanese study, which reported higher maternal-to-fetal transmission rates than most (14.2%), found positive associations between transmission rate and maternal viral load, liver dysfunction, and blood loss of greater than 500 mL at delivery.[101] Although it is unknown when during pregnancy and delivery HCV transmission occurs, one study suggested that one third to one half of infants acquiring HCV from their mothers were infected in utero.[102]

Amniocentesis has been considered a risk factor for maternal fetal transmission. HCV RNA in amniotic fluid is rarely positive. In one case report in which amniotic fluid HCV RNA was positive, the anterior position of the placenta suggested that the amniotic fluid could have been contaminated by placental blood during the transplacental procedure.[103]

MICROBIOLOGY AND PATHOGENESIS

HCV is a well-characterized, single-stranded enveloped RNA virus, 10 kb in length and 30 to 60 nm in diameter. It contains a single open reading frame that encodes a polyprotein of approximately 3000 amino acids. There are three structural proteins (one core and two envelope [E1 and E2])—and five nonstructural proteins (NS2, NS3, NS4A, NSB, and NS5B). The related genes encode the NS2-3 protease, the NS3/NS4A serine protease, and the NS5B RNA-dependent RNA polymerase.[104] The polyprotein undergoes cleavage by cellular and viral proteases to yield functional proteins. Tissue culture studies in the past had used replicon systems that produced viral proteins but not infectious virions. In 2005, Kato and Wakita[104a] reported a major breakthrough when they were able to culture the JFH-1 HCV virus in human hepatoma (HuH)-7 cells to produce infectious virions. There are at least six genotypes of HCV and more than 50 subtypes; genotypes differ at 31% to 34% of nucleotide positions on pairwise comparisons of complete sequences, and there is a similar difference between encoded polyproteins. The major utility of the genotypes so far has been to characterize differential susceptibility to antiviral treatments, with genotypes I and IV being most resistant to IFN-based therapies.

HCV is not considered a cytopathic virus. Viral clearance and hepatic injury are related to the immune response to the virus. The antigen nonspecific arm is the first line of defense and consists of natural killer cells, neutrophils, and macrophages. Dendritic cells assume the role of professional antigen-presenting cells; these induce the virus-specific immune response from CD4 T-helper cells, B cells, and CD8 cytotoxic T cells. The liver is the only known site of viral replication because negative RNA is detected only in the liver. The immunopathogenesis of HCV liver disease is still being elaborated, but cytokines and Fas ligand–induced apoptosis of hepatocytes probably play major roles.[105] Extrahepatic manifestations of HCV include mixed cryoglobulinemia, membranoproliferative glomerulonephritis, diabetes mellitus, retinopathy, peripheral neuropathy, and lymphoma; pathogenesis of these entities is under current investigation.[106]

PATHOLOGY

Several histologic features are characteristic of HCV, including bile duct damage, steatosis, and lymphoid follicles.[107] In a multicenter antiviral trial of children 5 to 18 years of age, 121 liver biopsy specimens were reviewed at entry. Inflammation in the biopsy specimen was minimal in 42%, mild in 17%, moderate in 38%, and severe in only 3%. Five specimens had bridging fibrosis, and two had cirrhosis.[108]

CLINICAL MANIFESTATIONS

Pergam and coworkers[109] reported that infants of HCV-positive mothers were more likely to have low birth weight, to be small for gestational age, to need assisted ventilation, and to require admission to a neonatal intensive care unit. HCV-positive mothers with excess weight gain also had a greater risk of gestational diabetes.[109] Cholestasis of pregnancy is increased in HCV-infected mothers.[110] The European Paediatric Hepatitis C Virus Network reported the natural history of 266 children with vertical HCV infection; approximately 20% seemed to clear the infection, 50% had evidence of chronic asymptomatic infection, and 30% had evidence of chronic active infection.[111] Infants and children with HCV are usually asymptomatic, and liver disease generally develops slowly, with spontaneous clearance of HCV occurring more often in children than in adults.[112,113] Children with transfusion-acquired HCV also tend to have mild asymptomatic infection, although rarely, infection may proceed to decompensated liver disease and liver transplantation.[114] In another large pediatric natural history study, 1.8% of children progressed to decompensated cirrhosis (mean age, 9.6 years). These children were mostly perinatally infected with genotype 1a, and most of the mothers were intravenous drug users.[115]

DIAGNOSIS

The acute stage of HCV infection is usually asymptomatic. In most instances, HCV infection remains undetected until a chronic stage and is discovered during the course of testing for an unrelated condition or during blood donation.[116]

Universal screening in pregnancy is not yet recommended in most countries. Therefore routine testing for HCV is not recommended for pregnant women because treatments or modes of delivery do not appear to modify the risk of transmission and because the timing, mode, and risk factors for transmission remain unclear. Diagnosis in pregnant mothers is usually made by screening of high-risk cases with an anti-HCV antibody.

The AAP recommends that infants born to HCV-infected mothers be screened by anti-HCV at 18 months postpartum because passively acquired maternal antibody can persist for 18 months.[117] Infants born to HCV-positive mothers using illicit drugs are often in foster homes. During a decision for adopting those infants who have positive anti-HCV antibody, physicians are frequently asked to perform a test for a definite diagnosis of HCV infection. If requested by the family, the serum HCV RNA can be tested before 18 months of age. The infants should be at least 2 months of age.[117] If serum HCV RNA is positive in early infancy, HCV RNA should be rechecked after 12 months of age to determine presence of chronic hepatitis C (CHC).[117] HCV infection is confirmed by HCV RNA by a polymerase chain reaction (PCR) assay in older children. Cost effectiveness should be considered in such an investigation.

TREATMENT

There is no known treatment to prevent perinatal transmission and none for infants younger than 3 years.[118,119] Parents should be counseled regarding certain mechanisms in infants that may explain low rates of mother-to-infant HCV transmission. Infants with human leukocyte antigen (HLA) DR13 are less likely to develop CHC after mother-to-infant transmission.[120] However, other HLA loci may also influence disease transmission.[119,121] Infants with the Rs12979860 CC genotype for the IL28B polymorphism are likely to have spontaneous clearance of the virus after the vertical HCV infection.[122] Nevertheless, it is encouraging that the development of antiviral therapy for HCV infection has progressed rapidly in the last few years. Therapy should not be given to pregnant patients with chronic hepatitis C because all current therapies are contraindicated in this population. In terms of fetal risk, IFN is classified as category C by the FDA. Studies have shown that the drug exerts teratogenic or embryocidal effects in animals. Ribavirin is contraindicated in pregnancy (FDA pregnancy category X) and in men whose partners may become pregnant. After approximately 5 years of operation, the Ribavirin Pregnancy Registry enrolled 49 live births with direct exposure and 69 live births after indirect exposure. Six outcomes (three each from direct and indirect exposures), with birth defects have been reported in all live-born infants: torticollis (three), hypospadias (one), polydactyly and a neonatal tooth (one), glucose-6-phosphate dehydrogenase deficiency (one), ventricular septal defect and cyst of fourth ventricle of the brain (one).[123]

There are currently two FDA-approved antiviral therapies for children: pegylated IFN-α2b plus ribavirin, which is indicated for children 3 to 18 years old with HCV infection, and pegylated IFN-α2a plus ribavirin, which is indicated for children 5 to 18 years of age; both regimens are given for 48 weeks for children with genotypes 1 and 4. Children with genotypes 2 and 3 may require only 24 weeks of therapy, similar to adults, but this has not been well studied. Many small-molecule inhibitors of HCV replication, such as inhibitors of the NS3 serine protease and the RNA polymerase, are being studied in adults with positive preliminary results, although none have been approved by the FDA as yet. IFN-free regimes are currently under development. Such therapies will be tested in children after safety and efficacy are well established in adults.

PREVENTION

At present, there is no effective way to interrupt transmission of HCV from mother to infant. At present, neither elective cesarean section nor avoidance of breastfeeding should be recommended to HCV-infected women,[124] although scattered reports do show a higher risk of HCV transmission for infants whose mothers have HCV RNA in breast milk.[125] In one report, membrane rupture lasting 6 or more hours and internal fetal monitoring were associated with increased rates of transmission of HCV from mother to infant, suggesting there may be obstetric practices that can reduce transmission.[45] Others have reported an association of higher transmission rates with intrapartum exposure to virus-contaminated maternal blood secondary to a perineal or vaginal laceration,[126] HCV RNA is detectable in maternal colostrum. HCV transmission via breastfeeding has not been well documented, however. Inactivation of the virus by gastric acid and very low levels of virus in breast milk may explain this potential protective mechanism. The AAP and the American College of Obstetricians and Gynecologists support breastfeeding by mothers with HCV infection.[127] There is definitely a role for public education about risk avoidance for high-risk children and adolescents. Steininger and colleagues[126] reported that 19% of homeless caregivers were anti–HCV-positive, although no cases of HCV infection were found in their children, suggesting the importance of directing preventive education to the young.

Hepatitis E Virus

Hepatitis E virus is endemic in many developing countries, where it is responsible for more than 50% of cases of acute viral hepatitis.[127] Recent data have shown that HEV is more common worldwide than HAV.[128] HEV is an important public health concern as a major cause of enterically transmitted hepatitis worldwide. Cases of sporadic HEV in people with no history of recent travel (autochthonous infection) in developed countries are far more common than previously thought.[129] HEV is frequently misdiagnosed as drug-induced liver injury or hepatitis of unknown etiology. HEV has a poor prognosis in patients with preexisting chronic liver disease and pregnant women in their third trimester. Patients with unexplained hepatitis should be tested for HEV, regardless of their age, demographics, or travel history.

EPIDEMIOLOGY AND TRANSMISSION

Hepatitis E virus is spread through food or water contaminated by feces from an infected individual. Transmission of HEV is by the fecal-oral route. Waterborne outbreaks have often been reported in developing countries.[129] The outbreaks of HEV are large, affecting 1% to 15% of individuals exposed (3%-30% in adults to 0.2%-10% in children).[128,130,131] In contrast to the other agents of viral hepatitis, HEV commonly is found in wild and domestic animals, which may provide an important source of infections in humans.[128] Person-to-person transmission seems to be much less efficient than with HAV. HEV has occasionally been linked to nosocomial spread.[132] It is infrequently transmitted by transfusion of blood or blood products.[133,134] HEV transmission is highly endemic in Asia, the Middle East, and Africa. Sporadic HEV infection has been reported in developing countries, particularly on the Indian subcontinent, where some studies have shown HEV to be the most common etiology of acute viral hepatitis.[130]

Pregnant women are at a high risk of developing acute liver failure from HEV. This association was first reported during outbreaks,[135,136] but has been found in sporadic cases in endemic areas such as in Indian subcontinent and Africa.[137-139] HEV infection has both a high incidence and a severe course in pregnant women in some geographic regions of HEV-endemic countries, such as Northern India and Africa,[140] whereas in other HEV-endemic countries, such as Egypt, a benign course is observed with little or no morbidity.[141] In a large prospective study from Northern India on the maternal and fetal outcomes of HEV infection, nearly 60% of viral hepatitis in pregnant women was attributed to HEV. Fulminant hepatic failure (FHF) was more common among HEV-infected women (55%), who were at a 2.7-times higher risk than non–HEV-infected women (20%). Maternal mortality was also higher secondarily to FHF in the HEV-infected group (41%) versus 7% in the non-HEV group.[1] In pregnant women with HEV infection, FHF was significantly higher than other causes of acute viral hepatitis (69.2 vs. 10%; $P = .001$). The prevalence and severity of HEV infection in pregnant women did not differ significantly in various gestational stages.[1] However, this more severe pathogenesis in pregnant women is not seen in all populations with HEV infection. By contrast, in Egypt, where the anti-HEV prevalence was 84.3% in one study of 2428 pregnant women, no patients with acute viral hepatitis were reported.[141] Infected pregnant women in Egypt and South India experienced lower case fatality rates (0%-3.4%) in some studies.[142] The reasons for this discrepancy in clinical presentation are not understood. Different subtypes causing infection, differential exposures in early childhood, or prevalence of micronutrient deficiencies may play a role in pathogenesis.[143]

In the United Arab Emirates, the risk of vertical transmission of HEV infection is up to 100% in maternal-fetal pairs studied. Twenty-six HEV RNA–positive mothers who developed acute/ongoing clinical infection transmitted the infection to all 26 infants.[144] This high transmission rate is not the only important factor for neonatal outcome. Nevertheless, HEV infection transmitted from mother-to-fetus results in high neonatal mortality. HEV infection in surviving newborn infants is self-limiting, with short-lasting viremia.[96] In the United States, HEV infection is more recognized in individuals not only returning from countries with high endemicity but having autochthonous infection. Autochthonous infection is an infection that has originated in a location where individuals have lived. This type of HEV infection has been reported in developed regions, such as North America, Europe, Japan, New Zealand, and Australia, and a porcine zoonosis has been suggested as the mode of transmission.[114,145] Compared with HEV infections in the developing world, in developed countries, most autochthonous HEV infections are reported in middle-aged and elderly men.[141]

Studies in endemic regions show high seroprevalence rates of HEV, ranging from 15% to 60%.[146-148] The anti-HEV seroprevalence rate reaches more than 95% by the age of 10 years in children living in endemic areas. Anti-HEV antibodies are rarely detected in children living in developed countries. Anti-HEV seroprevalence increases to 40% in young adults, without substantial increases later in life.[146]

Maternal-to-fetal transmission of HEV ranges from 50% to 100%, depending on endemicity and geography.[144,149] Acute HEV infection is severe for the mother during the third trimester of pregnancy, resulting in a mortality rate of 15% to 25%.[150]

MICROBIOLOGY AND PATHOGENESIS

Hepatitis E virus causing epidemic non-A, non-B hepatitis was identified in 1983 from a human challenge experiment and subsequently cloned in 1990. HEV is a spherical, nonenveloped, positive-strand RNA virus, classified as a member of the Caliciviridae family, that is approximately 32 to 34 nm in diameter.[151] Two major species of the virus are recognized: mammalian HEV, a virus that causes acute hepatitis in humans and has a reservoir in pigs and possibly a range of other mammals, and avian HEV. Four major genotypes of mammalian HEV have been reported. Genotype 1 HEV is the main cause of sporadic and epidemic HEV in developing regions of Asia, Africa, and South America. Genotype 2 has so far been identified in patients in Mexico, Chad, and Nigeria.[152-154] Genotype 3 HEV has been found in patients with autochthonous HEV in many developed regions and in pig populations worldwide.[155] Genotype 4 has been found in developed countries such as Japan, China, and Taiwan and in pig populations in those countries and India.[156,157]

Peak viremia occurs during the incubation period and the early acute phase of disease. Immediately before the onset of clinical symptoms, HEV RNA can be detected in the blood and stool. The concentration of serum liver enzymes increases, with a marked elevation of aminotransferases peaking at about 6 weeks after exposure coincident with anti-HEV in serum and decreasing HEV antigen in hepatocytes. Although the mechanism of liver injury in HEV is unclear, it is postulated that the severe pathogenesis in pregnant women may be immune mediated.[143] Infiltrating lymphocytes in the liver have been found to be a cytotoxic/suppressor immunophenotype, and this supports the role of an immune-mediated response in the pathogenesis of liver injury.[158] A few days to weeks after the onset of clinical symptoms, HEV RNA is cleared from the blood; however, the virus continues to be shed in stool for another 2 weeks.[159] Researchers have been unable to explain the high HEV morbidity in pregnancy, why it is different from other hepatitis viruses such as HAV with similar epidemiologic features, and the difference in HEV morbidity in pregnant women in different geographic regions. Most of the studies have shown that pregnant women have a differential immune response that triggers FHF. The increased pathogenicity in pregnant women could be explained by viral mutations. In experiments involving culture of HEV isolated from two chronically infected patients in a hepatic cell line containing a human genome sequence encoding for a ribosomal protein, this insertion seemed to promote viral growth and enable the virus to better adapt to the cell culture.[160] A study in India comparing the genome of genotype 1 strains from FHF cases with acute viral hepatitis cases showed that the viruses that caused FHF had many more nucleotide substitutions compared with the strains that caused acute hepatitis only. Six substitutions that were significantly associated with FHF, including one nonsynonymous mutation, suggest that mutations may play a role in determining outcome of HEV infection.[161]

PATHOLOGY

In general, individuals with HEV who travel from developing countries are diagnosed with serology without a liver biopsy. Few patients with autochthonous HEV require a liver biopsy because they have a self-limiting illness. In a few patients with more severe hepatitis, a liver biopsy may be required. The few data on hepatic histopathology of acute autochthonous HEV are limited to patients with severe disease. Liver histology in noncirrhotic liver is similar to that seen in other cases of acute viral hepatitis, with lobular disarray with reticulin framework distortion, portal tract expansion with severe mixed polymorphonuclear and lymphocytic inflammatory infiltrates, moderate-to-severe interface hepatitis, and cholangiolitis.[162,163] In patients with HEV who have underlying cirrhosis, the liver histology is nonspecific.[164] In the few transplant patients receiving immunosuppression who have developed chronic HEV infection, liver histology shows progressive fibrosis, portal hepatitis with lymphocytic infiltration, and piecemeal necrosis with progression to cirrhosis.[165,166]

CLINICAL MANIFESTATIONS

In most previously healthy individuals, HEV manifests as a self-limiting, acute, icteric hepatitis with symptoms including jaundice, malaise, anorexia, fever, abdominal pain, and arthralgia. Clinical disease is more common among adults than among children. Mortality rates associated with HEV are low and are thought to be about 1% in the general population.[167] HEV is more severe in pregnant women, however, in whom mortality rates vary between 30% to 100%.[143,168,169] The incubation period ranges from 2 to 9 weeks. Populations endemic for genotype 1 HEV show a high disease attack rate among pregnant women, leading to a more severe pathogenesis and increased fatality rates. HEV infection may lead to FHF, hepatic encephalopathy, disseminated intravascular coagulation, fetal distress, premature deliveries, and death of both the mother and fetus.[2] The risks of these adverse events escalate with trimester of pregnancy.[143]

The presentation of HEV in individuals infected in developed countries seems to be similar to individuals from endemic regions; however, the mortality rate is higher, ranging from 8% to 11%. Most autochthonous HEV infections are self-limiting[129]; 8% to 11% of infected individuals develop fulminant hepatitis and liver failure. Individuals with underlying chronic liver disease can have a poor outcome, with mortality approaching 70%.[170,171] A study from India showed that patients with chronic liver disease and HEV superinfection have a 1-year mortality rate of 70%.[172] Chronic HEV infection has been documented in patients receiving immunosuppressive therapy after organ transplantation.[165]

DIAGNOSIS

The antibody response to HEV infection follows a conventional course, with specific IgM usually detectable at the onset of symptoms or deranged liver function, followed shortly by HEV-specific IgG.[173] Most primary serologic tests are enzyme immunoassays that use recombinant antigens derived from different strains of HEV. Conventional and real-time reverse-transcriptase PCR assays have been used to detect HEV RNA in clinical specimens (mainly blood). Although reverse-transcriptase PCR seems to be more sensitive than serology for HEV diagnosis,[174-176] the window of detectable HEV viremia is narrow.[177] Because patients might not present until sometime after the onset of illness, a negative result does not exclude infection.

TREATMENT

Hepatitis E virus illness usually is self-limiting over several weeks to months, and treatment is usually supportive in healthy individuals. Patients with preexisting chronic liver disease who develop FHF as a result of HEV infection should be considered for liver transplantation because such patients have a poor outcome. Administration of immunoglobulin has not been helpful in preventing the disease in HEV-endemic areas.[158,178]

There is no consensus as to how to treat patients with HEV infection in pregnancy. In pregnant women with a near-term fetus, it is logical that early delivery of the viable fetus could be suggested to prevent maternal mortality. Therapeutic termination of pregnancy has not been reported in mothers with HEV infection as a beneficial therapy, as in pregnancy-related disorders such as HELLP (hemolysis, elevated liver enzymes, and low platelet count) syndrome and acute fatty liver of pregnancy.[179]

PREVENTION

The only way to prevent HEV disease is to reduce the risk of exposure to the virus. The risk for HEV transmission in infants born to asymptomatic anti–HEV-positive mothers seems to be low. No data suggest cesarean section prevents HEV transmission.[180] Given the low amount of HEV in colostrum (low infectivity), breastfeeding, an important nutritional source in endemic areas, should not be discouraged.[180] Mothers with symptomatic HEV with high viral loads should be advised not to breastfeed, however, because of potential risk of transmission.[180] Although there is no FDA-approved vaccine for HEV, several vaccines are under development, including a completed phase II, randomized, placebo-controlled trial in Nepal of a vaccine with efficacy of 95.5%.[181] At 2 years of follow-up, only 56% of vaccinated individuals had detectable anti-HEV. The most important issue is the safety and efficacy of the vaccine in women because mortality is high in pregnant women and individuals with chronic liver disease infected with HEV. Other issues include the durability of vaccine-induced immunity and its cost-effectiveness. A new vaccine has just completed a large, phase III trial with promising results[182] and is now licensed for use in China. Because women of childbearing age are the target for prevention of the disease during pregnancy, the issues of vaccine effectiveness in genotype 1–predominant populations and the safety and efficacy are important.

Other Hepatotropic Viruses

Some cases of viral hepatitis cannot be attributed to the hepatitis A, B, C, D, or E viruses or even less common viruses that can infect the liver, such as cytomegalovirus, Epstein-Barr virus, herpesvirus, parvovirus, and adenovirus. These cases are called non–A-E hepatitis. Scientists continue to study the causes of non–A-E hepatitis. GB virus type C/hepatitis G virus (GBV-C/HGV)[183-187] and TTV[188-197]) and its species variants, such as SEN virus (SEN-V) have been a health care concern and received extensive investigation as possible agents of acute non–A-E hepatitis. Although they do not seem to be responsible for most sporadic acute non–A-E hepatitis cases, more research is needed.

Conclusion

Translational research has made many contributions to knowledge about the hepatotropic viruses, but knowledge gaps remain. The incidence and health care costs related to HAV should decrease dramatically with the use of the highly effective hepatitis A vaccine for all subjects 1 to 18 years of age; universal vaccination for all adults, as well, may be a more practical strategy, rather than targeted immunization in high-risk groups. More effective strategies are needed to prevent maternal-to-fetal transmission of HBV because vaccine failures still occur in at least 10% of mother-infant pairs. New data have emerged in recent years on the natural history and treatment of chronic HBV infection in children, but antiviral resistance remains a main concern during long-term treatment of chronic HBV. For the last decade, several government and nongovernment organizations have held consensus conferences on the management of acute and chronic viral hepatitis to update previous management recommendations, in particular against HCV infection. Advances have been made in treatment of HCV in children, and promising results are seen with specifically targeted antiviral therapies. A novel hepatitis E vaccine was shown to be efficacious; however, more investigations to improve immunogenicity and safety are needed, especially for pregnant women, in whom morbidity and mortality are high. More attention should be paid to disease burden associated with HEV, an emergent pathogen, especially in developing countries with low- and middle-incomes. Close observations of HGV and TTV are needed to see if these viruses are truly of clinical significance.

References

1. Patra S, Kumar A, Trivedi SS, et al: Maternal and fetal outcomes in pregnant women with acute hepatitis E virus infection, *Ann Intern Med* 147:28-33, 2007.
2. Fiore S, Savasi V: Treatment of viral hepatitis in pregnancy, *Expert Opin Pharmacother* 10:2801-2809, 2009.
3. Fiore S, Newell ML, Trabattoni D, et al: Antiretroviral therapy-associated modulation of Th1 and Th2 immune responses in HIV-infected pregnant women, *J Reprod Immunol* 70:143-150, 2006.
4. Berge JJ, Drennan DP, Jacobs RJ, et al: The cost of hepatitis A infections in American adolescents and adults in 1997, *Hepatology* 31:469-473, 2000.
5. Shapiro CN, Coleman PJ, McQuillan GM, et al: Epidemiology of hepatitis A: seroepidemiology and risk groups in the USA, *Vaccine* 10:S59-S62, 1992.
6. American Academy of Pediatrics: Hepatitis A. In Pickering LK, Baker CJ, Kimberlin DW, Long SS, editors: *Red book: 2012 report of the Committee on Infectious Diseases*, ed 29, Elk Grove Village, Ill, 2012, American Academy of Pediatrics, pp 361-369.
7. Advisory Committee on Immunization Practices (ACIP): Fiore AE, Wasley A, Bell BP: Prevention of hepatitis A through active or passive immunization: recommendations of the Advisory Committee on Immunization Practices (ACIP), *MMWR Recomm Rep* 55(RR-7): 1-23, 2006.
8. Koslap-Petraco MB, Shub M, Judelsohn R: Hepatitis A: disease burden and current childhood vaccination strategies in the United States, *J Pediatr Health Care* 22:3-11, 2008.
9. Armstrong GL, Billah K, Rein DB, et al: The economics of routine childhood hepatitis A immunization in the United States: the impact of herd immunity, *Pediatrics* 119:e22-e29, 2007.
10. O'Donoghue K, Byrne BM: Antenatal detection of abnormal liver function tests—a marker for poor perinatal outcome, *J Obstet Gynaecol* 20:475-478, 2000.
11. Jaiswal SP, Jain AK, Naik G, et al: Viral hepatitis during pregnancy, *Int J Gynaecol Obstet* 72:103-108, 2001.
12. Khuroo MS, Kamili S: Aetiology, clinical course and outcome of sporadic acute viral hepatitis in pregnancy, *J Viral Hepat* 10:61-69, 2003.
13. Nayak NC, Panda SK, Datta R, et al: Aetiology and outcome of acute viral hepatitis in pregnancy, *J Gastroenterol Hepatol* 4:345-352, 1989.
14. Willner IR, Uhl MD, Howard SC, et al: Serious hepatitis A: an analysis of patients hospitalized during an urban epidemic in the United States, *Ann Intern Med* 128:111-114, 1998.
15. Wheeler C, Vogt TM, Armstrong GL, et al: An outbreak of hepatitis A associated with green onions, *N Engl J Med* 353:890-897, 2005.
16. Cuthbert JA, Hepatitis A: old and new, *Clin Microbiol Rev* 14:38-58, 2001.
17. Rosenblum LS, Villarino ME, Nainan OV, et al: Hepatitis A outbreak in a neonatal intensive care unit: risk factors for transmission and evidence of prolonged viral excretion among preterm infants, *J Infect Dis* 164:476-482, 1991.
18. Hamer DH, Connor BA: Travel health knowledge, attitudes and practices among United States travelers, *J Travel Med* 11:23-26, 2004.
19. Watson JC, Fleming DW, Borella AJ, et al: Vertical transmission of hepatitis A resulting in an outbreak in a neonatal intensive care unit, *J Infect Dis* 167:567-571, 1993.
20. Tanaka I, Shima M, Kubota Y, et al: Vertical transmission of hepatitis A virus, *Lancet* 345:397, 1995.
21. Erkan T, Kutlu T, Cullu F, Tümay GT: A case of vertical transmission of hepatitis A virus infection, *Acta Paediatr* 87:1008-1009, 1998.
22. Urganci N, Arapoglu M, Akyildiz B, et al: Neonatal cholestasis resulting from vertical transmission of hepatitis A infection, *Pediatr Infect Dis J* 22:381-382, 2003.
23. Noble RC, Kane MA, Reeves SA, et al: Posttransfusion hepatitis A in a neonatal intensive care unit, *JAMA* 252:2711-2715, 1984.
24. Pinto RM, Aragonès L, Costafreda MI, et al: Codon usage and replicative strategies of hepatitis A virus, *Virus Res* 127:158-163, 2007.
25. Stapleton JT: Host immune response to hepatitis A virus, *J Infect Dis* 171(Suppl 1):S9-S14, 1995.
26. Fleischer B, Vallbracht A: Demonstration of virus-specific cytotoxic T lymphocytes in liver tissue in hepatitis A—a model for immunopathological reactions, *Behring Inst Mitt* 89:226-230, 1991.
27. Kryger P, Christoffersen P: Liver histopathology of the hepatitis A virus infection: a comparison with hepatitis type B and non-A, non-B, *J Clin Pathol* 36:650-654, 1983.
28. Elinav E, Ben-Dov IZ, Shapira Y, et al: Acute hepatitis A infection in pregnancy is associated with high rates of gestational complications and preterm labor, *Gastroenterology* 130:1129-1134, 2006.
29. Gall SA: Expanding the use of hepatitis vaccines in obstetrics and gynecology, *Am J Med* 118(Suppl 10A):96S-99S, 2005.
30. Simsek Y, Isik B, Karaer A, et al: Fulminant hepatitis A infection in second trimester of pregnancy requiring living-donor liver transplantation, *J Obstet Gynaecol Res* 38:745-748, 2012.
31. Renge RL, Dani VS, Chitambar SD, et al: Vertical transmission of hepatitis A, *Indian J Pediatr* 69:535-536, 2002.
32. Leikin E, Lysikiewicz A, Garry D, Tejani N: Intrauterine transmission of hepatitis A virus, *Obstet Gynecol* 88:690-691, 1996.
33. McDuffie RS Jr, Bader T: Fetal meconium peritonitis after maternal hepatitis A, *Am J Obstet Gynecol* 180:1031-1032, 1999.
34. Vento S, Garofano T, Renzini C, et al: Fulminant hepatitis associated with hepatitis A virus superinfection in patients with chronic hepatitis C, *N Engl J Med* 338:286-290, 1998.
35. Armstrong GL, Bell BP: Hepatitis A virus infections in the United States: model-based estimates and implications for childhood immunization, *Pediatrics* 109:839-845, 2002.
36. American Academy of Pediatrics Committee on Infectious Diseases: Hepatitis A vaccine recommendations, *Pediatrics* 120:189-199, 2007.
37. Sharapov UM, Bulkow LR, Negus SE, et al: Passively transferred maternal antibodies to hepatitis A virus (maternal anti-HAV) may reduce the infant's immune response to the routine immunization in infancy, *Hepatology* 56:516-522, 2012.
38. Nothdurft HD: Hepatitis A vaccines, *Expert Rev Vaccines* 7:535-545, 2008.
39. Crowcroft NS, Walsh B, Davison KL, et al: PHLS Advisory Committee on Vaccination and Immunisation: guidelines for the control of hepatitis A virus infection, *Commun Dis Public Health* 4:213-227, 2001.
40. Lieberman JM, Chang SJ, Partridge S, et al: Kinetics of maternal hepatitis a antibody decay in infants: implications for vaccine use, *Pediatr Infect Dis J* 21:347-348, 2002.
41. Dagan R, Amir J, Mijalovsky A, et al: Immunization against hepatitis A in the first year of life:priming despite the presence of maternal antibody, *Pediatr Infect Dis J* 19:1045-1052, 2000.
42. Letson GW, Shapiro CN, Kuehn D, et al: Effect of maternal antibody on immunogenicity of hepatitis A vaccine in infants, *J Pediatr* 144:327-332, 2004.
43. Bell BP, Negus S, Fiore AE, et al: Immunogenicity of an inactivated hepatitis A vaccine in infants and young children, *Pediatr Infect Dis J* 26:116-122, 2007.
44. Stojanov S, Liese JG, Belohradsky BH, et al: Administration of hepatitis A vaccine at 6 and 12 months of age concomitantly with hexavalent (DTaP-IPV-PRP approximately T-HBs) combination vaccine, *Vaccine* 25:7549-7558, 2007.
45. Mast EE, Alter MJ, Margolis HS: Strategies to prevent and control hepatitis B and C virus infections: a global perspective, *Vaccine* 17:1730-1733, 1999.
46. Lee WM: Hepatitis B virus infection, *N Engl J Med* 337:1733-1745, 1997.
47. Ramia S, Bahakim H: Perinatal transmission of hepatitis B virus-associated hepatitis D virus, *Ann Inst Pasteur Virol* 139:285-290, 1988.
48. Shepard TH: *Catalog of teratogenic agents*, ed 9, Baltimore, 1998, Johns Hopkins University Press, p 1309.
49. Wang J, Zhu Q, Zhang X: Effect of delivery mode on maternal–infant transmission of hepatitis B virus by immunoprophylaxis, *Chin Med J* 115:1510-1512, 2002.
50. Alexander JM, Ramus R, Jackson G, et al: Risk of hepatitis B transmission after amniocentesis in chronic hepatitis B carriers, *Infect Dis Obstet Gynecol* 7:283-286, 1999.
51. Chen WH, Yin CS, Chang YK, et al: Neonatal gastric aspirates as a predictor of perinatal hepatitis B virus infections, *Int J Gynaecol Obstet* 60:15-21, 1998.
52. Euler GL, Wooten KG, Baughman AL, et al: Hepatitis B surface antigen prevalence among pregnant women in urban areas: implications for testing, reporting, and preventing perinatal transmission, *Pediatrics* 111:1192-1197, 2003.
53. Hahne S, Ramsay M, Balogun K, et al: Incidence and routes of transmission of hepatitis B virus in England and Wales, 1995–2000: implications for immunisation policy, *J Clin Virol* 29:211-220, 2004.

54. Elefsiniotis IS, Glynou I, Zorou I, et al: Surveillance for hepatitis B virus infection in pregnant women in Greece shows high rates of chronic infection among immigrants and low vaccination-induced protection rates: preliminary results of a single center study, *Euro Surveill* 14:5-7, 2009.
55. Schrag SJ, Arnold KE, Mohle-Boetani JC, et al: Prenatal screening for infectious diseases and opportunities for prevention, *Obstet Gynecol* 102:753-760, 2003.
56. Centers for Disease Control and Prevention (CDC): Implementation of newborn hepatitis B vaccination—worldwide, 2006, *MMWR Morb Mortal Wkly Rep* 57:1249-1252, 2008.
57. Xu DZ, Yan YP, Choi BC, et al: Risk factors and mechanism of transplacental transmission of hepatitis B virus: a case-control study, *J Med Virol* 67:20-26, 2002.
58. Soderstrom A, Norkrans G, Lindh M: Hepatitis B virus DNA during pregnancy and post partum: aspects on vertical transmission, *Scand J Infect Dis* 35:814-819, 2003.
59. Shao ZJ, Xu DZ, Xu JQ, et al: Maternal hepatitis B virus (HBV) DNA positivity and sexual intercourse are associated with HBV intrauterine transmission in China: a prospective case-control study, *J Gastroenterol Hepatol* 22:165-170, 2007.
60. Towers CV, Asrat T, Rumney P: The presence of hepatitis B surface antigen and deoxyribonucleic acid in amniotic fluid and cord blood, *Am J Obstet Gynecol* 184:1514-1518, 2001; discussion 1518–1520.
61. Hill JB, Sheffield JS, Kim MJ, et al: Risk of hepatitis B transmission in breast-fed infants of chronic hepatitis B carriers, *Obstet Gynecol* 99:1049-1052, 2002.
62. Kao JH: Diagnosis of hepatitis B virus infection through serological and virological markers, *Expert Rev Gastroenterol Hepatol* 2:553-562, 2008.
63. Zhang Z, Zou ZS, Fu JL, et al: Severe dendritic cell perturbation is actively involved in the pathogenesis of acute-on-chronic hepatitis B liver failure, *J Hepatol* 49:396-406, 2008.
64. Arbuthnot P, Capovilla A, Kew M: Putative role of hepatitis B virus X protein in hepatocarcinogenesis: effects on apoptosis, DNA repair, mitogen-activated protein kinase and JAK/STAT pathways, *J Gastroenterol Hepatol* 15:357-368, 2000.
65. Wu TC, Tong MJ, Hwang B, et al: Primary hepatocellular carcinoma and hepatitis B infection during childhood, *Hepatology* 7:46-48, 1987.
66. Woynarowski M, Cielecka-Kuszyk J, Kałuzyński A, et al: Inter-observer variability in histopathological assessment of liver biopsies taken in a pediatric open label therapeutic program for chronic HBV infection treatment, *World J Gastroenterol* 12:1713-1717, 2006.
67. American Academy of Pediatrics: Hepatitis B. In Pickering LK, Baker CJ, Kimberlin DW, Long SS, editors: *Red book: 2012 report of the Committee on Infectious Diseases*, ed 29, Elk Grove Village, Ill, 2012, American Academy of Pediatrics, pp 369-390.
68. Shiraki K, Yoshihara N, Sakurai M, et al: Acute hepatitis B in infants born to carrier mother with the antibody to hepatitis B e antigen, *J Pediatr* 97:768-770, 1980.
69. Bortolotti F, Iorio R, Resti M, et al: An epidemiological survey of hepatitis C virus infection in Italian children in the decade 1990–1999, *J Pediatr Gastroenterol Nutr* 32:562-566, 2001.
70. Huo TI, Wu JC, Lee PC, et al: Sero-clearance of hepatitis B surface antigen in chronic carriers does not necessarily imply a good prognosis, *Hepatology* 28:231-236, 1998.
71. Lok AS, McMahon BJ: Chronic hepatitis B, *Hepatology* 45:507-539, 2007.
72. Su GG, Pan KH, Zhao NF, et al: Efficacy and safety of lamivudine treatment for chronic hepatitis B in pregnancy, *World J Gastroenterol* 10:910-912, 2004.
73. Belongia EA, Costa J, Gareen IF, et al: NIH consensus development statement on management of hepatitis b: draft, *NIH Consens State Sci Statements* 25:1-29, 2008.
74. Hsu EK, Murray KF: Hepatitis B and C in children, *Nat Clin Pract Gastroenterol Hepatol* 5:311-320, 2008.
75. Jonas MM, Kelly D, Pollack H, et al: Safety, efficacy, and pharmacokinetics of adefovir dipivoxil in children and adolescents (age 2 to <18 years) with chronic hepatitis B, *Hepatology* 47:1863-1871, 2008.
76. Plitt SS, Somily AM, Singh AE: Outcomes from a Canadian public health prenatal screening program for hepatitis B: 1997–2004, *Can J Public Health* 98:194-197, 2007.
77. Xiao XM, Li AZ, Chen X, et al: Prevention of vertical hepatitis B transmission by hepatitis B immunoglobulin in the third trimester of pregnancy, *Int J Gynecol Obstet* 96:167-170, 2007.
78. Yuan J, Lin J, Xu A, et al: Antepartum immunoprophylaxis of three doses of hepatitis B immunoglobulin is not effective: a single-centre randomized study, *J Virol Hepatol* 13:597-604, 2006.
79. Xu Q, Xiao L, Lu XB, et al: A randomized controlled clinical trial: interruption of intrauterine transmission of hepatitis B, *World J Gastroenterol* 12:3434-3437, 2006.
80. Shi Z, Li X, Ma L, Yang Y: Hepatitis B immunoglobulin injection in pregnancy to interrupt hepatitis B virus mother-to-child transmission-a meta-analysis, *Int J Infect Dis* 14:e622-e634, 2010.
81. Xu WM, Cui YT, Wang L, et al: Lamivudine in late pregnancy to prevent perinatal transmission of hepatitis B virus infection: a multicentre, randomized, double-blind, placebo-controlled Study, *J Viral Hep* 16:94-103, 2009.
82. Köse S, Türken M, Devrim I, Taner C: Efficacy and safety of lamivudine treatment in late pregnancy with high HBV DNA: a perspective for mother and infants, *J Infect Dev Ctries* 26:303-306, 2011.
83. Liu MH, Sheng YJ, Liu JY, et al: Efficacy of telbivudine on interruption of hepatitis B virus vertical transmission: a meta-analysis, *Ann Saudi Med* 33:169-176, 2013.
84. Mele A, Mariano A, Tosti ME, et al: Acute hepatitis delta virus infection in Italy: incidence and risk factors after the introduction of the universal anti-hepatitis B vaccination campaign, *Clin Infect Dis* 44:e17-e24, 2007.
85. Gonzalez-Quintero VH, Katz D, Pandya-Smith I, et al: Assessing perinatal hepatitis B screening and neonatal prophylaxis in a large, multiethnic county, *J Reprod Med* 51:101-108, 2006.
86. Guo ZZ, Shi XH, Feng YL, et al: Risk factors of HBV intrauterine transmission among HBsAg-positive pregnant women, *J Viral Hepat* 20:317-321, 2013.
87. Soderstrom A, Norkrans G, Lindh M: Hepatitis B virus DNA during pregnancy and post partum: aspects on vertical transmission, *Scand J Infect Dis* 35:814-819, 2003.
88. Sangfelt P, Von Sydow M, Uhnoo I, et al: Serum ALT levels as a surrogate marker for serum HBV DNA levels in HBeAg-negative pregnant women, *Scand J Infect Dis* 36:182-185, 2004.
89. Xiao XM, Li AZ, Chen X, et al: Prevention of vertical hepatitis B transmission by hepatitis B immunoglobulin in the third trimester of pregnancy, *Int J Gynaecol Obstet* 96:167-170, 2007.
90. Yuan J, Lin J, Xu A, et al: Antepartum immunoprophylaxis of three doses of hepatitis B immunoglobulin is not effective: a single-centre randomized study, *J Viral Hepat* 13:597-604, 2006.
91. Gartner LM, Morton J, Lawrence RA, et al: Breastfeeding and the use of human milk, *Pediatrics* 115:496-506, 2005.
92. Vranckx R, Alisjahbana A, Meheus A: Hepatitis B virus vaccination and antenatal transmission of HBV markers to neonates, *J Viral Hepat* 6:135-139, 1999.
93. Bacq Y: Hepatitis B and pregnancy, *Gastroenterol Clin Biol* 32: S12-S19, 2008.
94. Gambarin-Gelwan M: Hepatitis B in pregnancy, *Clin Liver Dis* 11:945-963, 2007.
95. Luban NL, Colvin CA, Mohan P, et al: The epidemiology of transfusion-associated hepatitis C in a children's hospital, *Transfusion* 47:615-620, 2007.
96. Jhaveri R, Grant W, Kauf TL, McHutchison J: The burden of hepatitis C virus infection in children: estimated direct medical costs over a 10-year period, *J Pediatr* 148:353-358, 2006.
97. Roberts EA, Yeung L: Maternal-infant transmission of hepatitis C virus infection, *Hepatology* 36:S106-S113, 2002.
98. Airoldi J, Berghella V: Hepatitis C and pregnancy, *Obstet Gynecol Surv* 61:666-672, 2006.
99. Dowd KA, Hershow RC, Yawetz S, et al: Maternal neutralizing antibody and transmission of hepatitis C virus to infants, *J Infect Dis* 198:1651-1655, 2008.
100. Bortolotti F, Iorio R, Resti M, et al: Epidemiological profile of 806 Italian children with hepatitis C virus infection over a 15-year period, *J Hepatol* 46:783-790, 2007.
101. Hayashida A, Inaba N, Oshima K, et al: Re-evaluation of the true rate of hepatitis C virus mother-to-child transmission and its novel risk factors based on our two prospective studies, *J Obstet Gynaecol Res* 33:417-422, 2007.
102. Mok J, Pembrey L, Tovo PA, et al: European Paediatric Hepatitis C Virus Network. When does mother to child transmission of hepatitis C virus occur, *Arch Dis Child Fetal Neonatal* 90:F156-F160, 2005.
103. Delamare C, Carbonne B, Heim N, et al: Detection of hepatitis C virus RNA (HCV RNA) in amniotic fluid: a prospective study, *J Hepatol* 31:416-420, 1999.

104. Thomson M, Liang TJ: Molecular biology of hepatitis C virus in hepatitis C: biomedical research reports. In Liang TJ, Hoofnagle JH, editors: *Hepatitis C*, San Diego, 2000, Academic Press, pp 1-24.
104a. Wakita T, Pietschmann T, Kato T, et al: Production of infectious hepatitis C virus in tissue culture from a cloned viral genome. *Nat Med* 11:791-796, 2005.
105. Zaki MS, Auf FA, Ghawalby NA, et al: Clinical significance of serum soluble Fas, Fas ligand and fas as in intrahepatic lymphocytes in chronic hepatitis C, *Immunol Invest* 37:163-170, 2008.
106. Himoto T, Masaki T: Extrahepatic manifestations and autoantibodies in patients with hepatitis C virus infection, *Clin Dev Immunol* 871401:2012, 2012.
107. Bach N, Thung SN, Schaffner F: The histological features of chronic hepatitis C and autoimmune chronic hepatitis: a comparative analysis, *Hepatology* 15:572-577, 1992.
108. Goodman ZD, Makhlouf HR, Liu L, et al: Pathology of chronic hepatitis C in children: liver biopsy findings in the Peds-C Trial, *Hepatology* 47:836-843, 2008.
109. Pergam SA, Wang CC, Gardella CM, et al: Pregnancy complications associated with hepatitis C: data from a 2003–2005 Washington State birth cohort, *Am J Obstet Gynecol* 199:38, e1–38.e9, 2008.
110. Berkley EM, Leslie KK, Arora S, et al: Chronic hepatitis C in pregnancy, *Obstet Gynecol* 112:304-310, 2008.
111. European Paediatric Hepatitis C Virus Network: Three broad modalities in the natural history of vertically acquired hepatitis C virus infection, *Clin Infect Dis* 41:45-51, 2005.
112. Slowik MK, Jhaveri R: Hepatitis B and C viruses in infants and young children, *Semin Pediatr Infect Dis* 16:296-305, 2005.
113. England K, Thorne C, Pembrey L, et al: Policies and practices for the clinical management of HIV/HCV coinfected children in Europe: an epidemiological survey, *Eur J Pediatr* 168:915-917, 2009.
114. Mohan P, Colvin C, Glymph C, et al: Clinical spectrum and histopathologic features of chronic hepatitis C infection in children, *J Pediatr* 150:168, e1–174.e1, 2007.
115. Bortolotti F, Verucchi G, Cammà C, et al: Long-term course of chronic hepatitis C in children: from viral clearance to end-stage liver disease, *Gastroenterology* 134:1900-1907, 2008.
116. Alter MJ, Seeff LB, Bacon BR, et al: Testing for hepatitis C virus infection should be routine for persons at increased risk for infection, *Ann Intern Med* 9:715-717, 2004.
117. Mack CL, Gonzalez-Peralta RP, Gupta N, et al: NASPGHAN practice guidelines: diagnosis and management of hepatitis C infection in infants, children, and adolescents, *J Pediatr Gastroenterol Nutr* 54:838-855, 2012.
118. Zanetti AR, Tanzi E, Newell ML: Mother-to-infant transmission of hepatitis C virus, *J Hepatol* 31:96-100, 1999.
119. Bevilacqua E, Fabris A, Floreano P, et al: Genetic factors in mother-to-child transmission of HCV infection, *Virology* 390:64-70, 2009.
120. Bosi I, Ancora G, Mantovani W, et al: HLA DR13 and HCV vertical infection, *Pediatr Res* 51:746-749, 2002.
121. Martinetti M, Pacati I, Cuccia M, et al: Hierarchy of baby-linked immunogenetic risk factors in the vertical transmission of hepatitis C virus, *Int J Immunopathol Pharmacol* 19:369-378, 2006.
122. Ruiz-Extremera A, Muñoz-Gámez JA, Salmerón-Ruiz MA, et al: Genetic variation in interleukin 28B with respect to vertical transmission of hepatitis C virus and spontaneous clearance in HCV-infected children, *Hepatology* 53:1830-1838, 2011.
123. Roberts SS, Miller RK, Jones JK, et al: The Ribavirin Pregnancy Registry: Findings after 5 years of enrollment, 2003-2009, *Birth Defects Res A Clin Mol Teratol* 88:551-559, 2010.
124. Pembrey L, Newell ML, Tovo PA, EPHN Collaborators: The management of HCV infected pregnant women and their children; European paediatric HCV network, *J Hepatol* 43:515-525, 2005.
125. Ruiz-Extremera A, Salmerón J, Torres C, et al: Follow-up of transmission of hepatitis C to babies of human immunodeficiency virus-negative women: the role of breastfeeding in transmission, *Pediatr Infect Dis J* 19:511-516, 2000.
126. Steininger C, Kundi M, Jatzko G, et al: Increased risk of mother-to-infant transmission of hepatitis C virus by intrapartum infantile exposure to maternal blood, *J Infect Dis* 187:345-351, 2003.
127. Schwarz KB, Garrett B, Alter MJ, et al: Seroprevalence of HCV infection in homeless Baltimore families, *J Health Care Poor Underserved* 19:580-587, 2008.
128. Tsega E, Hansson BG, Krawczynski K, et al: Acute sporadic viral hepatitis in Ethiopia: causes, risk factors, and effects on pregnancy, *Clin Infect Dis* 14:961-965, 1992.
129. Aggarwal R, Naik SR: Epidemiology of hepatitis E: past, present and future, *Trop Gastroenterol* 18:49-56, 1997.
130. Dalton HR, Bendall R, Ijaz S, et al: Hepatitis E: an emerging infection in developed countries, *Lancet Infect Dis* 8:698-709, 2008.
131. Kane MA, Bradley DW, Shrestha SM, et al: Epidemic non-A, non-B hepatitis in Nepal: recovery of a possible etiologic agent and transmission studies in marmosets, *JAMA* 252:3140-3145, 1984.
132. Robson SC, Adams S, Brink N, et al: Hospital outbreak of hepatitis E, *Lancet* 339:1424-1425, 1992.
133. Psichogiou M, Tzala E, Boletis J, et al: Hepatitis E virus infection in individuals at high risk of transmission of non-A, non-B hepatitis and sexually transmitted diseases, *Scand J Infect Dis* 28:443-445, 1996.
134. Brazilai A, Schulman S, Karetnyi YV, et al: Hepatitis E virus infection in hemophiliacs, *J Med Virol* 46:153-156, 1995.
135. Viswanathan R: Epidemiology, *Indian J Med Res* 45(Suppl):1-29, 1957.
136. Khuroo MS: Study of an epidemic of non-A, non-B hepatitis. Possibility of another human hepatitis virus distinct from post-transfusion non-A, non-B type, *Am J Med* 68:818-824, 1980.
137. Khuroo MS, Duermeyer W, Zargar SA, et al: Acute sporadic non-A, non-B hepatitis in India, *Am J Epidemiol* 118:360-364, 1983.
138. Strand RT, Franque-Ranque M, Bergström S, Weiland O: Infectious aetiology of jaundice among pregnant women in Angola, *Scand J Infect Dis* 35:401-403, 2003.
139. Guthmann JP, Klovstad H, Boccia D, et al: A large outbreak of hepatitis E among a displaced population in Darfur, Sudan, 2004: the role of water treatment methods, *Clin Infect Dis* 42:1685-1691, 2006.
140. Kumar A, Beniwal M, Kar P, et al: Hepatitis E in pregnancy, *Int J Gynaecol Obstet* 85:240-244, 2004.
141. Stoszek SK, Abdel-Hamid M, Saleh DA, et al: High prevalence of hepatitis E antibodies in pregnant Egyptian women, *Trans R Soc Trop Med Hyg* 100:95-101, 2006.
142. Rasheeda CA, Navaneethan U, Jayanthi V: Liver disease in pregnancy and its influence on maternal and fetal mortality: a prospective study from Chennai, Southern India, *Eur J Gastroenterol Hepatol* 20:362-364, 2008.
143. Navaneethan U, Al Mohajer M, Shata MT: Hepatitis E and pregnancy: understanding the pathogenesis, *Liver Int* 28:1190-1199, 2008.
144. Kumar RM, Uduman S, Rana S, et al: Sero-prevalence and mother-to-infant transmission of hepatitis E virus among pregnant women in the United Arab Emirates, *Eur J Obstet Gynecol Reprod Biol* 100:9-15, 2001.
145. Purcell RH, Emerson SU: Hepatitis E: an emerging awareness of an old disease, *J Hepatol* 48:494-503, 2008.
146. Arankalle VA, Tsarev SA, Chadha MS, et al: Age-specific prevalence of antibodies to hepatitis A and E viruses in Pune, India, 1982 and 1992, *J Infect Dis* 171:447-450, 1995.
147. Clayson ET, Shrestha MP, Vaughn DW, et al: Rates of hepatitis E virus infection and disease among adolescents and adults in Kathmandu, Nepal, *J Infect Dis* 176:763-766, 1997.
148. Tran HT, Ushijima H, Quang VX, et al: Prevalence of hepatitis virus types B through E and genotypic distribution of HBV and HCV in Ho Chi Minh City, Vietnam, *Hepatol Res* 26:275-280, 2003.
149. Singh S, Mohanty A, Joshi YK, et al: Mother-to-child transmission of hepatitis E virus infection, *Indian J Pediatr* 70:37-39, 2003.
150. Ranger-Rogez S, Alain S, Denis F: Hepatitis viruses: mother to child transmission, *Pathol Biol (Paris)* 50:568-575, 2002.
151. Hyams KC: New perspectives on hepatitis E, *Curr Gastroenterol Rep* 4:302-307, 2002.
152. Buisson Y, Grandadam M, Nicand E, et al: Identification of a novel hepatitis E virus in Nigeria, *J Gen Virol* 81:903-909, 2000.
153. van Cuyck-Gandre H, Zhang HY, Tsarev SA, et al: Characterization of hepatitis E virus (HEV) from Algeria and Chad by partial genome sequence, *J Med Virol* 53:340-347, 1997.
154. Tam AW, Smith MM, Guerra ME, et al: Hepatitis E virus (HEV): molecular cloning and sequencing of the full-length viral genome, *Virology* 185:120-131, 1991.
155. Banks M, Heath GS, Grierson SS, et al: Evidence for the presence of hepatitis E virus in pigs in the United Kingdom, *Vet Rec* 154: 223-227, 2004.
156. Lu L, Li C, Hagedorn CH: Phylogenetic analysis of global hepatitis E virus sequences: genetic diversity, subtypes and zoonosis, *Rev Med Virol* 16:5-36, 2006.
157. Wang YC, Zhang HY, Xia NS, et al: Prevalence, isolation, and partial sequence analysis of hepatitis E virus from domestic animals in China, *J Med Virol* 67:516-521, 2002.

158. Aggarwal R, Krawczynski K: Hepatitis E: an overview and recent advances in clinical and laboratory research, *J Gastroenterol Hepatol* 15:9-20, 2000.
159. Clayson ET, Myint KS, Snitbhan R, et al: Viremia, fecal shedding, and IgM and IgG responses in patients with hepatitis E, *J Infect Dis* 172:927-933, 1995.
160. Nguyen HT, Torian U, Faulk K, et al: A naturally occurring human/hepatitis E recombinant virus predominates in serum but not in faeces of a chronic hepatitis E patient and has a growth advantage in cell culture, *J Gen Virol* 93:526-530, 2012.
161. Mishra N, Walimbe AM, Arankalle VA: Hepatitis E virus from India exhibits significant amino acid mutations in fulminant hepatic failure patients, *Virus Genes* 46:47-53, 2013.
162. Peron JM, Danjoux M, Kamar N, et al: Liver histology in patients with sporadic acute hepatitis E: a study of 11 patients from South-West France, *Virchows Arch* 450:405-410, 2007.
163. Malcolm P, Dalton H, Hussaini HS, et al: The histology of acute autochthonous hepatitis E virus infection, *Histopathology* 51: 190-194, 2007.
164. Lockwood GL, Fernandez-Barredo S, Bendall R, et al: Hepatitis E autochthonous infection in chronic liver disease, *Eur J Gastroenterol Hepatol* 20:800-803, 2008.
165. Haagsma EB, van den Berg AP, Porte RJ, et al: Chronic hepatitis E virus infection in liver transplant recipients, *Liver Transpl* 14: 547-553, 2008.
166. Kamar N, Selves J, Mansuy JM, et al: Hepatitis E virus and chronic hepatitis in organ-transplant recipients, *N Engl J Med* 358 :811-817, 2008.
167. Mast EE, Krawczynski K: Hepatitis E: an overview, *Annu Rev Med* 47:257-266, 1996.
168. Khuroo MS, Teli MR, Skidmore S, et al: Incidence and severity of viral hepatitis in pregnancy, *Am J Med* 70:252-255, 1981.
169. Khuroo MS, Kamili S: Aetiology and prognostic factors in acute liver failure in India, *J Viral Hepat* 10:224-231, 2003.
170. Dalton HR, Hazeldine S, Banks M, et al: Locally acquired hepatitis E in chronic liver disease, *Lancet* 369:1260, 2007.
171. Peron JM, Bureau C, Poirson H, et al: Fulminant liver failure from acute autochthonous hepatitis E in France: description of seven patients with acute hepatitis E and encephalopathy, *J Viral Hepat* 14:298-303, 2007.
172. Kumar Acharya S, Kumar Sharma P, Singh R, et al: Hepatitis E virus (HEV) infection in patients with cirrhosis is associated with rapid decompensation and death, *J Hepatol* 46:387-394, 2007.
173. Bendall R, Ellis V, Ijaz S, et al: Serological response to hepatitis E virus genotype 3 infection: IgG quantitation, avidity, and IgM response, *J Med Virol* 80:95-101, 2008.
174. Lin CC, Wu JC, Chang TT, et al: Diagnostic value of immunoglobulin G (IgG) and IgM antihepatitis E virus (HEV) tests based on HEV RNA in an area where hepatitis E is not endemic, *J Clin Microbiol* 38: 3915-3918, 2000.
175. El-Sayed Zaki M, El-Deen Zaghloul MH, El Sayed O: Acute sporadic hepatitis E in children: diagnostic relevance of specific immunoglobulin M and immunoglobulin G compared with nested reverse transcriptase PCR, *FEMS Immunol Med Microbiol* 48:16-20, 2006.
176. Jothikumar N, Cromeans TL, Robertson BH, et al: A broadly reactive one-step real-time RT-PCR assay for rapid and sensitive detection of hepatitis E virus, *J Virol Methods* 131:65-71, 2006.
177. Takahashi M, Tanaka T, Azuma M, et al: Prolonged fecal shedding of hepatitis E virus (HEV) during sporadic acute hepatitis E: evaluation of infectivity of HEV in fecal specimens in a cell culture system, *J Clin Microbiol* 45:3671-3679, 2007.
178. Khuroo MS, Dar MY: Hepatitis E: evidence for person-to-person transmission and inability of low dose immune serum globulin from an Indian source to prevent it, *Indian J Gastroenterol* 11:113-116, 1992.
179. Mjahed K, Charra B, Hamoudi D, et al: Acute fatty liver of pregnancy, *Arch Gynecol Obstet* 274:349-353, 2006.
180. Chibber RM, Usmani MA, Al-Sibai MH: Should HEV infected mothers breast feed? *Arch Gynecol Obstet* 270:15-20, 2004.
181. Shrestha MP, Scott RM, Joshi DM, et al: Safety and efficacy of a recombinant hepatitis E vaccine, *N Engl J Med* 356:895-903, 2007.
182. Zhu FC, Zhang J, Zhang XF, et al: Efficacy and safety of a recombinant hepatitis E vaccine in healthy adults: a large-scale, randomised, double-blind placebo-controlled, phase 3 trial, *Lancet* 376:895-902, 2010.
183. Ohto H, Ujiie N, Sato A, et al: Mother-to-infant transmission of GB virus type C/HGV, *Transfusion* 40:725-730, 2000.
184. Reshetnyak VI, Karlovich TI, Ilchenko LU: Hepatitis G virus, *World J Gastroenterol* 14:4725-4734, 2008.
185. Pawlotsky JM, Dhumeaux D: The G virus: the orphan virus, *Presse Med* 28:1882-1883, 1999.
186. Dal Molin G, D'Agaro P, Biagi C, et al: Vertical transmission of HGV and outcome of the infected babies, *Ann Ig* 16:109-114, 2004.
187. Woelfle J, Berg T, Keller KM, et al: Persistent hepatitis G virus infection after neonatal transfusion, *J Pediatr Gastroenterol Nutr* 26: 402-407, 1998.
188. Mutlu D, Abacioglu H, Altunyurt S: Investigation of transplacental transmission of TT virus in mother-newborn pairs, *Mikrobiyol Bul* 41:71-77, 2007.
189. Gerner P, Oettinger R, Gerner W, et al: Mother-to-infant transmission of TT virus: prevalence, extent and mechanism of vertical transmission, *Pediatr Infect Dis J* 19:1074-1077, 2000.
190. Davidson F, MacDonald D, Mokili JL, et al: Early acquisition of TT virus (TTV) in an area endemic for TTV infection, *J Infect Dis* 179:1070-1076, 1999.
191. Iso K, Suzuki Y, Takayama M: Mother-to-infant transmission of TT virus in Japan, *Int J Gynaecol Obstet* 75:11-19, 2001.
192. Inaba N, Oshima K, Okajima Y, et al: TTV materno-infantile infection—a study on the TTV frequency in Japanese pregnant women and the natural history of TTV mother-to-infant infection, *Nippon Rinsho* 57:1406-1409, 1999.
193. Hino S, Miyata H: Torque teno virus (TTV): current status, *Rev Med Virol* 17:45-57, 2007.
194. Hu ZJ, Lang ZW, Zhou YS, et al: Clinicopathological study on TTV infection in hepatitis of unknown etiology, *World J Gastroenterol* 8:288-293, 2002.
195. Zaki M, el-Hady NA: Molecular detection of transfusion transmitted virus coinfection with some hepatotropic viruses, *Arch Pathol Lab Med* 130:1680-1683, 2006.
196. Garbuglia AR, Grasso F, Donà MG, et al: TT virus infection: role of interferons, interleukin-28 and 29, cytokines and antiviral proteins, *Int J Immunopathol Pharmacol* 20:249-258, 2007.
197. Moreno J, Moraleda G, Barcena R, et al: Response of TT virus to IFN plus ribavirin treatment in patients with chronic hepatitis C, *World J Gastroenterol* 10:143-146, 2004.

27 Herpes Simplex Virus Infections

DAVID W. KIMBERLIN and KATHLEEN M. GUTIERREZ

CHAPTER OUTLINE

Neonatal herpes simplex virus infection (HSV) was identified as a distinct disease in the 1930s. The first written descriptions of neonatal HSV were attributed to Hass, who described the histopathologic findings of a fatal case, and to Batignani, who described a newborn child with HSV keratitis.[1,2] During the initial decades that followed, our understanding of neonatal HSV infections was based on histopathologic descriptions of the disease, which indicated a broad spectrum of organ involvement in infants.

An important scientific breakthrough occurred in the mid-1960s, when Nahmias and Dowdle[3] demonstrated two antigenic types of HSV. The development of viral typing methods provided the tools required to clarify the epidemiology of these infections. HSV infection "above the belt," primarily of the lip and oropharynx, was found in most cases to be caused by HSV type 1 (HSV-1). Infections "below the belt," particularly genital infections, were usually caused by HSV type 2 (HSV-2). The finding in the 1960s and 1970s that genital HSV infections and neonatal HSV infections were most often caused by HSV-2 suggested a cause and effect relationship between these two entities. This causal relationship was strengthened by detection of the virus in the maternal genital tract at the time of delivery, indicating that acquisition of the virus occurs by contact with infected genital secretions during birth.

Knowledge of HSV structure and function, epidemiology, and natural history, and of the pathogenesis of neonatal HSV infection, has increased during the past 5 decades.[4] The development of antiviral therapy represented a significant advance in the management of infected children and has substantially decreased the morbidity and mortality associated with neonatal HSV infections. Neonatal HSV infection is more amenable to prevention and treatment than many other viral and bacterial diseases affecting neonates because it is acquired most often at birth rather than in utero. Postnatal acquisition of HSV-1 has been documented from nonmaternal sources, and more cases of genital herpes caused by HSV-1 have been identified more recently, including HSV-1 in the maternal genital tract from changes in sexual practices that result in increased likelihood of oral-genital contact. This evolving natural history of genital herpetic infection has the potential to impact the incidence and outcomes of neonatal HSV infections. Perspectives on the changing presentations of neonatal HSV infection, the obstacles to diagnosis, and the value of antiviral therapy are addressed in this chapter.

Herpes Simplex Virus

STRUCTURE

Herpes simplex virus types 1 and 2 are members of the large family of herpesviruses.[4] Other human herpesviruses include cytomegalovirus, varicella-zoster virus, Epstein-Barr virus, and human herpesviruses 6 (including variants

6A and 6B), 7, and 8. Structurally, these viruses are virtually indistinguishable. The viral DNA genome is packaged inside an icosahedral capsid that is surrounded by a layer of proteins called the tegument. A lipid envelope that contains viral glycoproteins surrounds the capsid and tegument. These glycoproteins mediate virion attachment and entry into cells.

The HSV-1 and HSV-2 genomes consist of approximately 150,000 base pairs and encode more than 100 proteins.[4] The viral genomes consist of two components, L (long) and S (short), each of which contains unique sequences that can invert, generating four isomers. Viral genomic DNA extracted from virions or infected cells consists of four equal populations that differ in the relative orientation of these two unique components. Although the two viruses diverged millions of years ago, the order of genes in the HSV-1 and HSV-2 genomes follows the same linear pattern, and most genes have counterparts in both viruses. The nucleotide sequence of related genes and the amino acid residues of the proteins they encode often differ significantly, however.[5,6] The two viral types can be distinguished by using restriction enzyme analysis of genomic DNA or, more recently, by sequencing of selected genes or regions of the genome, which allows precise epidemiologic investigation of virus transmission.

REPLICATION

Herpes simplex virus replication is characterized by the transcription of three gene classes—α, β, and γ—that encode viral proteins made at immediate-early, early, and late times after virus entry into the cell.[4] Many of these genes can be removed from the viral genome without blocking the capacity of the virus to replicate in cultured cells, but most have important functions during infection of the host. The HSV genome can also be manipulated to insert foreign genes without inhibiting viral replication. Mutations that modify the virulence of HSV-1 and HSV-2 may provide an opportunity to design genetically engineered herpesviruses for use as vaccines for genital herpes or as therapeutic agents in the treatment of brain tumors.[7]

HSV α genes are expressed at immediate-early times after infection and are responsible for the initiation of replication. These genes are transcribed in infected cells in the absence of viral protein synthesis. Products of the β genes, or early genes, include the enzymes necessary for viral replication, such as HSV thymidine kinase, which is targeted by acyclovir and related antiviral drugs, and other regulatory proteins. β genes require functional α gene products for expression. The onset of expression of β genes coincides with a decline in the rate of expression of α genes and an irreversible shutoff of host cellular macromolecular protein synthesis. Structural proteins, such as proteins that form the viral capsid, are usually of the γ, or late, gene. The γ genes are heterogeneous and are differentiated from β genes by their requirement for viral DNA synthesis for maximal expression. Most glycoproteins are expressed predominantly as late genes. In addition to its regulatory and structural genes, the virus encodes genes that allow initial evasion of the innate host cell response, including gene products that block the interferon (IFN) pathway. HSV-1 and HSV-2 also express proteins that interfere with adaptive immunity, as exemplified by an immediate-early protein, ICP47, that mediates the downregulation of major histocompatibility complex class I molecules, which are required for recognition of HSV-infected cells by HSV-specific CD8+ T cells.[8,9] Replication of viral DNA occurs in the nucleus of the cell. Assembly of the virus begins with formation of nucleocapsids in the nucleus, followed by egress across the nuclear membrane and envelopment at cytoplasmic locations. Virus particles are transported to the plasma membrane, where progeny virions are released. HSV glycoproteins have been designated as glycoproteins B, C, D, E, G, H, I, L, and M.[4,5] Glycoproteins B, D, and H (gB, gD, and gH) are required for infectivity and are targets of neutralizing antibodies against HSV, glycoprotein C (gC) binds to the C3b component of complement, and the glycoprotein E (gE) and glycoprotein I (gI) complex binds to the Fc portion of immunoglobulin G (IgG). The amino acid sequences of glycoprotein G (gG) produced by HSV-1 and HSV-2 are sufficiently different to elicit antibody responses that are specific for each virus type. The fact that the antibody response to the two G molecules exhibits minimal cross-reactivity has provided the basis for type-specific serologic methods that can be used to detect recent or past HSV-1 and HSV-2 infections.[10-13] The close antigenic relatedness between HSV-1 and HSV-2 interferes with the serologic diagnosis of these infections when using standard, type-common serologic assays, which do not distinguish between individuals who have had past infection with HSV-1 only, infection with HSV-2 only, or dual infection. Commercial type-specific tests based on gG must be used for diagnosis of HSV-2 infection (Table 27-1).[12,14] Clinicians should be knowledgeable regarding the type of testing performed by the laboratory to interpret results correctly.

LATENCY AND REACTIVATION

A common characteristic of all members of the human herpesvirus family is the ability to establish latency, to persist in this latent state for various intervals of time, and to reactivate and cause active infection (with or without disease) and viral transmission at mucosal or other sites. After primary infection, the HSV genome persists in sensory ganglion neurons for the lifetime of the individual. The biologic phenomenon of latency was first described at the beginning of the 20th century, when Cushing[15] observed in 1905 that patients treated for trigeminal neuralgia by sectioning a branch of the trigeminal nerve developed herpetic lesions in areas innervated by the sectioned branch. This specific association of HSV with the trigeminal ganglion was suggested by Goodpasture.[16] Past observations have shown that microvascular surgery of the trigeminal nerve tract to alleviate pain associated with tic douloureux resulted in recurrent lesions in greater than 90% of seropositive individuals.[17,18]

Accumulated experience in animal models and from clinical observations suggests that inoculation of virus at the portal of entry, usually oral or genital mucosal tissue, results in infection of sensory nerve endings at that site, with subsequent transport of the virus to the dorsal root ganglia.[19] Replication at the site of inoculation enhances access of the virus to ganglia but usually does not produce

Table 27-1 Quick Reference Guide for Blood Tests to Accurately Detect Type-Specific HSV Antibodies

	Biokit HSV-2 Rapid Test (Also Sold as SureVue HSV-2 Rapid Test by Fisher HealthCare)	BioPlex HSV	Captia ELISA	Euroimmun Anti-HSV-1 and Anti–HSV-2 ELISA	HerpeSelect HSV-1 ELISA and HerpeSelect HSV-2 ELISA	HerpeSelect 1 and 2 Differentiation Immunoblot	Liaison HSV-2	AtheNA MultiLyte
Supplier	Biokit USA	Bio-Rad Laboratories	Trinity Biotech USA	Euroimmun US LLC	Focus Diagnostics	Focus Diagnostics	DiaSorin	Inverness Medical
FDA approved	1999	2009	2004	2007	2000/2002	2000	2008	2008
Antibodies detected	HSV-2 only	HSV-1 or HSV-2 or both	HSV-1 or HSV-2 or both	HSV-1 or HSV-2	HSV-1 or HSV-2 or both	HSV-1 and/or HSV-2	HSV-1 or HSV-2	HSV-1 and/or HSV-2
Best use of test	POC test to screen or test individuals > 3 months post-exposure	Screening or testing (high volume)	Screening or testing pregnant women or STD clinic patients (moderate volume)	Moderate volume	Screening or testing STD patients or pregnant women (moderate volume)	Low volume	High volume	Screening or testing (moderate-to-high volume)
Collection method	Finger stick, whole blood or serum in clinic	Blood draw (sent to laboratory)	Blood draw (sent to laboratory)	Blood draw (sent to laboratory)	Blood draw (sent to laboratory)	Blood draw (sent to laboratory)	Blood draw (sent to laboratory)	Blood draw (sent to laboratory)
Test time	10 minutes	45 minutes	≈2 hours	≈2 hours	≈2 hours	≈2 hours	35 minutes	≈2 hours
FDA approved for use during pregnancy		Yes	Yes		Yes	Yes		
Test availability	Limited	Limited	Widely available		Widely available			
Website	www.biokitusa.com	www.bio-rad.com	www.trinitybiotech.com	www.euroimmunus.com	www.herpeselect.com	www.herpeselect.com	www.diasorin.com	www.invernessmedicalpd.com
For more information	800-926-3353	800-224-6723	800-325-3424	800-913-2022			800-328-5669	877-546-8633

From Kimberlin DW, Baley J: Guidance on management of asymptomatic neonates born to women with active genital herpes lesions, *Pediatrics* 131:e635-e646, 2013.
ELISA, Enzyme-linked immunosorbent assay; *HSV*, herpes simplex virus; *POC*, point of care; *STD*, sexually transmitted disease.

signs of mucocutaneous disease; only a fraction of new infections with HSV-1 and HSV-2 cause clinically recognizable disease. When viral reactivation occurs at oral or genital sites, virus then is transported back down axons to mucocutaneous sites, where viral replication and shedding of infectious HSV then occurs.

Recognizing that excretion of infectious virus during reactivation is not usually associated with clinical signs of recurrent herpes lesions is essential for understanding the transmission of HSV to newborns. Clinically, silent viral reactivations are much more common than recurrent lesions that are clinically apparent. This distinction between asymptomatic infection and symptomatic disease underlies much of the challenge in neonatal HSV prevention because only those relatively fewer situations where there are clinically apparent lesions can be expected to initiate a response from treating physicians. Reactivation with or without symptoms occurs in the healthy host in the presence of HSV-specific humoral and cell-mediated immunity. Reactivation seems to be spontaneous, although symptomatic recurrences have been associated with physical or emotional stress, exposure to ultraviolet light, or tissue damage; immunosuppression is associated with an increased predilection for symptomatic HSV disease when reactivation occurs. Persistence of viral DNA has been documented in neuronal tissue of animal models and humans.[4,20-22] Because the latent virus does not multiply, it is not susceptible during latency to drugs such as acyclovir, which affect DNA synthesis, and cannot be eradicated from the infected host. Understanding of the mechanisms by which HSV establishes a latent state and persists in this form remains limited.

Epidemiology and Transmission

Transmission of HSV most often occurs as a consequence of intimate person-to-person contact. Virus must come in contact with mucosal surfaces or abraded skin for infection to be initiated.

The usual mode of HSV-1 transmission is through direct contact of a susceptible individual with infected secretions, although transfer in respiratory droplets is possible. Acquisition often occurs during childhood. Primary HSV-1 infection in a young child usually is asymptomatic, but clinical illness is associated with HSV gingivostomatitis. Primary infection in young adults has been associated with pharyngitis only or with a mononucleosis-like syndrome. Seroprevalence studies have shown that acquisition of HSV-1 infection, similar to that of other herpesvirus infections, is related to socioeconomic factors.[23,24] Antibodies, indicative of past infection, are found early in life more often among individuals of lower socioeconomic groups, presumably reflecting the crowded living conditions that provide a greater opportunity for direct contact with infected individuals. By the end of the first decade of life, 75% to 90% of individuals from lower socioeconomic populations develop antibodies to HSV-1.[25-27] In middle and upper-middle socioeconomic groups, 30% to 40% of individuals are seropositive by the middle of the second decade of life.

A change in seroprevalence rates of HSV-1 has been recognized in the past few decades, which reflects a delay in acquisition of infection until later in life. Data from the National Health and Nutrition Examination Surveys (NHANES) recently have revealed that in 2005 to 2010 the seroprevalence of HSV-1 was 53.9%.[28] From 1999 to 2004 and 2005 to 2010, HSV-1 seroprevalence declined by nearly 7% ($P < .01$), with the largest decline being observed among 14- to 19-year-olds, among whom seroprevalence declined by nearly 23%, from 39.0% to 30.1% ($P < .01$). In this age group, HSV-1 seroprevalence declined more than 29% from 1976 to 1980 and 2005 to 2010 ($P < .01$).[28] As a result, an increasing number of adolescents lack HSV-1 antibodies at sexual debut. This is occurring at a time when almost half of teenagers 15 to 19 years of age and more than four fifths of young adults 20 to 24 years of age have engaged in oral sex.[29] Increasing rates of genital HSV-1 infection already are being seen in several studies published over the past decade, with 60% to 80% of cases of genital herpes now being attributed to this virus type.[30-32]

Because infection with HSV-2 is usually acquired through sexual contact, antibodies to this virus are rarely found until the age of onset of sexual activity.[26] A progressive increase in infection rates with HSV-2 in all populations begins in adolescence. In earlier studies, the precise seroprevalence of antibodies to HSV-2 had been difficult to determine because of cross-reactivity with HSV-1 antigens. During the late 1980s, seroepidemiologic studies performed using type-specific antigen for HSV-2 (glycoprotein G-2) identified this virus in approximately 25% to 35% of middle-class women in several geographic areas of the United States.[11,33-35] Based on national health surveys, the seroprevalence of HSV-2 in the United States from 1988 to 1994 was 21.9% for individuals 12 years and older, representing a 30% increase compared with data collected from 1976 to 1980.[35] Among individuals with serologic evidence of infection, less than 10% had a history of genital herpes symptoms. A statistically significant decline in HSV-2 seroprevalence was observed from 1988 to 1994 and 1999 to 2004, but since that time findings suggest seroprevalence has plateaued.[36] HSV-2 seroprevalence was 15.7% in 2005 to 2010, which was not significantly different from the estimate in 1999 to 2004.[28] Overall, HSV-2 seroprevalence has increased significantly since 1976 to 1980, primarily because of the large increase from 1976-1980 to 1988-1994.[35] HSV-2 seroprevalence is highly variable and depends on geographic region, sex, age, race, and high-risk behaviors.[37] The molecular epidemiology of HSV infections can be determined by restriction enzyme analysis of viral DNA or polymerase chain reaction (PCR) assay and sequencing of regions of the HSV genome obtained from infected individuals. Viruses have essentially identical genetic profiles when they are from the same host or are epidemiologically related.[38] In a few circumstances, it has been shown, however, that superinfection or exogenous reinfection with a new strain of HSV is possible. Such occurrences are uncommon in a nonimmunocompromised host with recurrent genital HSV infection.[38-40] Differences in the genetic sequence of viral DNAs indicating exogenous infections are more common in immunocompromised individuals who are exposed to different HSVs, such as patients with acquired immunodeficiency syndrome.

MATERNAL INFECTION

Infection with HSV-2, which reactivates and is shed at genital sites, is common in pregnant women. Using assays to detect type-specific antibodies to HSV-2, seroepidemiologic investigations have shown that approximately one in five pregnant women has had HSV-2 infection.[24,34,41-45] Given the capacity of HSV to establish latency, the presence of antibodies is a marker of persistent infection of the host with the virus. The incidence of infection in women of upper socioeconomic class was 30% or greater in three large studies.[43,45,46] These investigations have shown that most women with serologic evidence of HSV-2 infection have no history of symptomatic primary or recurrent disease. New HSV-2 infections are acquired during pregnancy with a frequency that is comparable to seroconversion rates among nonpregnant women, and these infections also usually occur without clinical signs or symptoms.[42-46] Even so, most genital HSV shedding occurs from reactivation of viral infection, rather than from primary HSV disease.[47-49]

HSV-1 is less likely than HSV-2 to reactivate in the genital tract of nonpregnant women, especially after the first year after infection.[50] HSV-1 reactivations may occur after mid-pregnancy, however, when women are relatively immunosuppressed.[51] In contrast, genital HSV-2 continues to recur, often frequently, for many years.[52]

Evaluation of pregnant women and their partners has shown that women can remain susceptible to HSV-2 despite prolonged sexual contact with a partner who has known genital herpes.[44] In this study, 1 in 10 women were found to be at unsuspected risk for acquiring HSV-2 infection during pregnancy as a result of contact with a partner whose HSV-2 infection was asymptomatic. Most maternal infections are clinically silent during gestation. However, infection during gestation may manifest in several clinical syndromes, the most severe of which is widely disseminated disease. As first reported by Flewett and coworkers[53] in 1969 and by others[54,55] subsequently, disseminated infection during pregnancy has been documented to involve multiple visceral sites in addition to cutaneous ones. In a few cases, dissemination after primary oropharyngeal or genital infection has led to severe manifestations of disease, including necrotizing hepatitis with or without thrombocytopenia, leukopenia, disseminated intravascular coagulopathy, and encephalitis. Although rare, the mortality rate for these pregnant women is greater than 50%. Fetal deaths occur in greater than 50% of cases, although neonatal mortality does not correlate with the death of the mother. Surviving fetuses have been delivered by cesarean section during the acute illness or at term, and may not have evidence of neonatal HSV infection.

Earlier studies described an association of maternal primary infection before 20 weeks of gestation,[56] with spontaneous abortion in some women. Although the original incidence of spontaneous abortion after a symptomatic primary infection during gestation was thought to be 25%, this estimate was not substantiated by prospective studies and was erroneous because of the small number of women followed. More precise data obtained from a prospective analysis of susceptible women showed that 2% or greater acquired infection, but acquisition of infection was not associated with a risk of spontaneous abortion.[57] With the exception of rare case reports, primary infection that develops later in gestation is not generally associated with premature rupture of membranes or premature termination of pregnancy.[58]

Localized genital infection, whether it is associated with lesions or remains asymptomatic, is the most common form of HSV infection during pregnancy. Overall, prospective investigations using cytologic and virologic screening indicate that genital herpes occurs with a frequency of about 1% in women tested at any time during gestation.[43,57] Most maternal genital infections are due to recurrent HSV-2 infections when characterized virologically and serologically.[49] This potentially could change as the incidence of HSV-1 genital infection, which is more likely to be primary than recurrent, increases in the population.[29] Because HSV infection of the infant is usually the consequence of contact with infected maternal genital secretions at the time of delivery, the incidence of viral excretion at this time point has been of particular interest. The reported incidence of viral excretion at delivery is 0.01% to 0.39% for all women, regardless of their history of genital herpes.[43,46]

Several prospective studies have evaluated the frequency and nature of viral shedding in pregnant women with a known history of genital herpes. These women represent a subset of the population of women with HSV-2 infection because they had a characteristic genital lesion from which virus was isolated. In a predominantly white, middle-class population, symptomatic recurrent infection occurred during pregnancy in 84% of pregnant women with a history of symptomatic disease.[59] Viral shedding from the cervix occurred in only 0.56% of symptomatic infections and 0.66% of asymptomatic infections. These data are similar to data obtained from other populations.[33] The incidence of cervical shedding in asymptomatic pregnant women has been reported to range from 0.2% to 7.4%, depending on the numbers of cultures that were obtained between symptomatic episodes. Overall, these data indicate that the frequency of cervical shedding is low, which may reduce the risk of transmission of virus to the infant when the maternal infection is recurrent. The frequency of maternal genital shedding does not seem to vary by trimester during gestation.

Most infants who develop neonatal disease are born to women who are completely asymptomatic for genital HSV infection during the pregnancy and at the time of delivery. These women usually have neither a past history of genital herpes nor a sexual partner reporting a genital vesicular rash and account for 60% to 80% of all women whose infants become infected.[60, 61]

FACTORS INFLUENCING TRANSMISSION OF INFECTION TO THE FETUS

The development of serologic assays that distinguish HSV-1–specific antibodies from HSV-2–specific antibodies allowed an accurate analysis of risks related to perinatal transmission of HSV.[10-13] The category of maternal genital infection at the time of delivery influences the frequency of neonatal acquisition of infection. Maternal infections are classified as caused by HSV-1 or HSV-2 and as newly acquired or recurrent.[62] These categories of maternal infection status are based on virologic and serologic laboratory criteria and are independent of clinical signs.

Women with recurrent infections are those who have preexisting antibodies to the virus type that is isolated from the genital tract, which, until recently, has usually been HSV-2.

Most women classified as having recurrent infection have no history of symptomatic genital herpes. Infections that are newly acquired, which have been referred to as first-episode infections, are categorized further as either primary or nonprimary based on type-specific serologic testing. This differentiation is made whether clinical signs are present or not. First-episode primary infections are infections in which the mother is experiencing a new infection with HSV-1 or HSV-2 and has not already been infected with the other virus type. These mothers are seronegative for any HSV antibodies (i.e., negative for both HSV-1 and HSV-2 antibodies) at the onset of infection. First-episode nonprimary infections are infections in which the mother has a new infection with one virus type, usually HSV-2, but has antibodies to the other virus type, usually HSV-1, because of an infection that was acquired previously.

Because transmission has been studied using type-specific serologic methods, it has become apparent that attempts to distinguish primary and recurrent disease by clinical criteria are unreliable. Use of both serologic and virologic data to classify the category of maternal infection is an important advance because many "new" genital herpes infections in pregnancy are actually recurrent infections and represent the first symptomatic episode of a genital HSV infection acquired at some time in the past. In one study designed to evaluate acyclovir therapy, pregnant women who were thought to have recent acquisition of HSV-2 based on symptoms all had been infected previously. These women were experiencing genital symptoms, caused by reactivation of latent virus, for the first time.[55]

A hierarchy of risk of transmission has emerged using virologic and serologic laboratory tools to classify maternal infection. Infants born to mothers who have a first-episode primary infection at the time of delivery are at highest risk, with transmission rates approaching 60%.[49,57,60] Infants born to mothers with first-episode nonprimary infections are at lower risk, with transmission rates of approximately 25%.[49] The lowest risk of neonatal acquisition occurs with recurrent infection, when the mother has active infection caused by shedding of virus that she acquired before the pregnancy or earlier in gestation; the estimated attack rate for neonatal herpes among these infants is approximately 2%.[49] This estimate is reliable because it is based on the cumulative experience from large, prospective studies of pregnant women in which viral shedding was evaluated at delivery, regardless of the mother's history of genital herpes or contact with a partner with suspected or documented genital herpes.

The higher risk of transmission to the infant when the mother has a new infection can be attributed to differences in the quantity and duration of viral shedding in the mother and in the transfer of passive antibodies from the mother to the infant before delivery. Primary infection is associated with larger quantities of virus replication in the genital tract (>10^6 viral particles/0.2 mL of inoculum) and a period of viral excretion that may persist for an average of 3 weeks.[63] Many women with new infections have no symptoms but shed virus in high titers. In some mothers, these infections cause signs of systemic illness, including fever, malaise, myalgias, dysuria, and headache. Viremia during primary HSV infection in women is common and is associated with systemic maternal symptoms.[64] In a small percentage of cases, significant complications, such as urinary retention and aseptic meningitis, occur in the mother.

In contrast, virus is shed for an average of only 2 to 5 days and at lower concentrations (approximately 10^2-10^3 viral particles/0.2 mL of inoculum) in women with symptomatic recurrent genital infections. Asymptomatic reactivation is also associated with short periods of viral replication, often less than 24 to 48 hours. One of the most important observations about HSV infections that has emerged from the evaluation of pregnant women is that new HSV-1 and HSV-2 infections often occur without any of the manifestations that were originally described as the classic findings in primary and recurrent genital herpes.

In parallel with the classification of maternal infection, the mother's antibody status to HSV at delivery is an additional factor that influences the likelihood of transmission and probably affects the clinical course of neonatal herpes. Transplacental maternal neutralizing antibodies have a protective, or at least an ameliorative, effect on acquisition of infection for infants inadvertently exposed to virus.[65] Maternal first-episode primary or nonprimary infection late in gestation may not result in significant passage of maternal antibodies across the placenta to the fetus. Based on available evidence, the highest risk of transmission from mothers with newly acquired genital herpes is observed when the infant is born before the transfer of passive antibodies to HSV-1 or HSV-2, when the infant is exposed at delivery, or within the first few days of life.[57,66]

The duration of ruptured membranes has also been described as an indicator of risk for acquisition of neonatal infection. Observations in the early 1970s of a small cohort of women (n = 22) with symptomatic genital herpes indicated that prolonged rupture of membranes (>6 hours) increased the risk of acquisition of virus, perhaps as a consequence of ascending infection from the cervix.[56] This small case series resulted in the recommendation that women with active genital lesions at the time of onset of labor be delivered by cesarean section.[67] It was not until 2003, however, that it was proven in a large, landmark study that cesarean delivery protects against neonatal HSV infection in infants born to women from whom HSV was isolated at the time of delivery (1.2% vs. 7.7%; P = .047).[49] In the single baby in this trial to develop neonatal HSV disease after cesarean delivery, membranes were ruptured in the mother for 19 hours. It is important to note, however, that infection of the newborn with HSV-2 has occurred despite delivery by cesarean section.[61,68]

Certain forms of medical intervention during labor and delivery may increase the risk of neonatal herpes if the mother has active shedding of the virus, although in most instances, viral shedding is not suspected clinically. Fetal scalp monitors can be a site of viral entry through disrupted skin.[49,69,70] The benefits and risks of these devices should be considered for women with a history of recurrent genital HSV infections. Because most women with genital infections caused by HSV are asymptomatic during labor and have no history of genital herpes, it is usually impossible to make this assessment.

INCIDENCE OF NEWBORN INFECTION

Estimates of the incidence of neonatal herpes have varied from 1 in 3000 to 1 in 20,000 live births.[71] Although fluctuations in the incidence of neonatal HSV disease have been observed,[46,71] the current estimated rate of occurrence is approximately 1 in 3200 deliveries.[49] Although a progressive increase in the number of cases of neonatal HSV infection has been noted in some areas of the country,[72] neonatal HSV infections still occur far less frequently than do genital HSV infections in the adult childbearing population. Overall, the United States, with approximately 4.0 million deliveries per year, has an estimated 1500 cases of neonatal HSV infection annually.

In studies where maternal serologic status during pregnancy and virologic status at the time of delivery are evaluated prospectively, the rate of transmission leading to neonatal HSV infection ranges from 12 to 54 newborn infections per 100,000 births (1/8300 and 1/1850 births, respectively). Higher rates of transmission are seen in infants born to seronegative mothers and mothers infected with HSV-1.[49] Based on seroprevalence studies, the highest risk of HSV transmission would be expected to occur in infants born to non-Hispanic white mothers, whose HSV seroprevalence is the lowest.[24] Some countries do not report a significant number of cases of neonatal HSV infection despite a similar high prevalence of antibodies to HSV-2 in women. In the United Kingdom, genital herpes infection is relatively common, but very few cases of neonatal HSV infection are recognized. Neonatal HSV infection in the Netherlands occurs in only 2.4 of 100,000 newborns.[73] Although underreporting of cases may explain some differences between countries, unidentified factors may account for these differences. The interpretation of incidence data must also include the potential for postnatal acquisition of HSV infection. Not all cases of neonatal infection are the consequence of intrapartum contact with infected maternal genital secretions, which alters the overall estimate of delivery-associated infection. The prevalence of neonatal HSV infection relative to serious bacterial infections in hospitalized neonates was evaluated more recently in a retrospective study and found to be 0.2% compared with 0.4% and 4.5% for infants with bacterial meningitis and serious bacterial infections, respectively.[74]

TIMES OF TRANSMISSION OF INFECTION

Herpes simplex virus infection of the newborn can be acquired in utero, intrapartum, or postnatally. The mother is the source of infection for the first two of these three routes of transmission of infection. With regard to postnatal acquisition of HSV infection, the mother can be a source of infection from a nongenital site, or other contacts or environmental sources of virus can lead to infection of the infant. A maternal source is suspected when maternal herpetic lesions are discovered during or shortly after the birth of the infant, or when the infant's illness is caused by HSV-2. Although intrapartum transmission accounts for approximately 85% of cases of neonatal HSV, in utero and postnatal infection must be recognized for public health and prognostic purposes.

In utero transmission is very rare, causing approximately 5% of all cases of neonatal HSV disease.[75-78] Although it was originally presumed that in utero acquisition of infection resulted in a totally normal infant or premature termination of gestation,[56] it has become apparent that intrauterine acquisition of infection can lead to severe clinical disease and sequelae. When using stringent diagnostic criteria, more than 70 infants with symptomatic congenital disease have been described in the literature.[75] These criteria include identification of infected infants with lesions present at birth or within the first 24 hours of life; virologic confirmation of HSV at that time; and exclusion of other infectious agents whose pathogenesis mimics the clinical findings of HSV infections, such as congenital cytomegalovirus infection, rubella, syphilis, or toxoplasmosis. Virologic diagnosis is a necessary criterion because no standard method for reliable detection of IgM antibodies is available, and infected infants often fail to produce IgM antibodies detectable by research methods.[66,79] Intrauterine HSV disease occurs in approximately 1 in 300,000 deliveries.[75] Although rare, in utero disease is unlikely to be missed due to the extent of involvement of affected babies. Infants acquiring HSV in utero typically have a triad of clinical findings consisting of cutaneous manifestations (scarring, active lesions, hypopigmentation and hyperpigmentation, aplasia cutis, and/or an erythematous macular exanthem), ophthalmologic findings (microopthalmia, retinal dysplasia, optic atrophy, and/or chorioretinitis), and neurologic involvement (microcephaly, encephalomalacia, hydranencephaly, and/or intracranial calcification).[76,77,80,81]

In utero infection can result from transplacental or ascending infection. The placenta can show evidence of necrosis and inclusions in the trophoblasts, which suggests a transplacental route of infection.[82] The situation can result in an infant who has hydranencephaly at the time of birth, or it may be associated with spontaneous abortion and intrauterine HSV viremia. Virus has been isolated from the products of conception under such circumstances. Histopathologic evidence of chorioamnionitis suggests ascending infection as an alternative route for in utero infection.[83] Risk factors associated with intrauterine transmission are unknown. Primary and recurrent maternal infections can result in infection of the fetus in utero. HSV DNA has been detected in the amniotic fluid of two women experiencing a first-episode nonprimary infection and in one woman during a symptomatic recurrent infection. All three infants were healthy at birth and showed no clinical or serologic evidence of HSV infection during follow-up.[84]

The second and most common route of infection is intrapartum contact of the fetus with infected maternal genital secretions. Intrapartum transmission can occur when a baby passes through a birth canal when HSV is present. Approximately 85% of cases of neonatal HSV are acquired in the intrapartum period. Intrapartum transmission is more likely to occur when the neonate is being delivered to a mother with newly acquired infection (25%-60% likelihood of transmission if virus is present in the genital tract) but can also occur with recurrent maternal infection (approximately a 2% likelihood of transmission if virus is present in the genital tract).

Postnatal acquisition is the third route of transmission, accounting for approximately 10% of cases of neonatal HSV disease. Postnatal acquisition of neonatal HSV is virtually always due to HSV-1 because the source of transmission is nongenital. However, with the increasing incidence of genital HSV-1 disease in sexually active adults, simply detecting HSV-1 in a neonate does not define the timing of transmission as postnatal. The most recent data on the proportion of neonatal HSV that is caused by HSV-1 are from the 1980s, when the National Institute of Allergy and Infectious Diseases (NIAID) Collaborative Antiviral Study Group (CASG) reported that approximately 25% to 35% of cases of neonatal herpes are caused by this virus type.[61,85]

The documentation of postnatal transmission of HSV-1 has focused attention on nongenital sources of virus.[86-90] Postpartum transmission from mother to child has been reported as a consequence of nursing on an infected breast.[91] Transmission from fathers and grandparents has also been documented.[90] When the infant's mother has not had HSV infection, the infant may be inoculated with the virus from a nonmaternal contact in the absence of any possible protection from maternally derived passive antibodies. Because of the high prevalence of HSV-1 infection in the general population, many individuals have intermittent episodes of asymptomatic excretion of the virus from the oropharynx and can provide a source of infection for the newborn. The occurrence of herpes labialis, commonly referred to as fever blisters or cold sores, has ranged from 16% to 46% in various groups of adults.[92]

Population studies conducted in two hospitals indicated that 15% to 34% of hospital personnel had a history of nongenital herpetic lesions.[92,93] In both hospitals surveyed, at least 1 in 100 individuals documented a recurrent cold sore each week. As is true of genital herpes, many individuals have HSV-1 infection with no clinical symptoms at the time of acquisition or during episodes of reactivation and shedding of infectious virus in oropharyngeal secretions. Prospective virologic monitoring of hospital staff increased the frequency with which infection was detected by twofold; however, no cases of neonatal HSV infection were documented in these nurseries.

The risk of nosocomial infection in the hospital environment is a concern. Identification by restriction endonuclease or sequence analysis of virus recovered from an index case and a nursery contact leaves little doubt about the possibility of spread of virus in a high-risk nursery population.[87,89] The possible vectors for nosocomial transmission have not been defined. The risk of transmission to infants by health care professionals who have herpes labialis or who are asymptomatic oral shedders of virus is low. Compromising patient care by excluding health care professionals with cold sores who are essential for the operation of the hospital nursery must be weighed against the potential risk of newborn infants becoming infected. Health care professionals with cold sores who have contact with infants should cover and not touch their lesions and should comply with hand hygiene policies. Transmission of HSV infection from health care professionals with genital lesions is not likely as long as they comply with hand hygiene policies. Health care professionals with an active herpetic whitlow should not have responsibility for direct care of neonates or immunocompromised patients and should wear gloves and use hand hygiene during direct care of other patients.

Because most mothers have antibodies to HSV, and these antibodies are transferred to their infants, postnatal exposures to the virus in the neonatal period usually do not result in neonatal disease. If the mother is seronegative, nosocomial exposure may pose a more significant risk to the neonate, however.

Immunologic Response

The neonatal host response to HSV is impaired compared with older children and adults.[66,79,94-98] There is no evidence for differences in virulence of particular HSV strains. The severity of the manifestations of HSV-1 and HSV-2 infections in the newborn can be attributed to immunologic factors. Relevant issues are protection by transplacental antibodies, the innate immune response of the exposed infant, and the acquisition of adaptive immunity by the infected newborn.

Passive antibodies to HSV influence the acquisition of infection and its severity and clinical signs.[45,60,66,79] Transplacentally acquired antibodies from the mother are not totally protective against neonatal infection, but transplacentally acquired neutralizing antibodies correlate with a lower attack rate in exposed newborns.[60,65,66] Although the absence of any detectable antibodies has been associated with dissemination and systemic disease in the neonate, the presence of antibodies at the time that clinical signs appear does not predict the subsequent outcome.[61,79]

Most infected newborns eventually produce HSV IgM antibodies, but the interval to detection is prolonged, requiring at least 2 to 4 weeks.[66] These antibodies increase rapidly during the first 2 to 3 months but may be detectable for 1 year after infection. The quantity of neutralizing antibodies and antibodies that mediate antibody-dependent cellular cytotoxicity in infants with disseminated disease is lower than in infants with more limited disease.[66,97] Humoral antibody responses to specific viral proteins, especially glycoproteins, have been evaluated by assays for antibodies to gG and by immunoblot.[10,79] Immunoblot studies indicate that the severity of infection correlates directly with the number of antibody bands to defined polypeptides. Children with a more limited infection, such as infection of the skin, eye, or mouth (SEM disease), have fewer antibody bands compared with children with disseminated disease.

A vigorous antibody response to the ICP4 α gene product, which is responsible for initiating viral replication, has been correlated with poor long-term neurologic outcome, suggesting that these antibodies reflect the extent of viral replication. A regression analysis that compared neurologic impairment with the quantity of antibodies to ICP4 identified the child at risk for severe neurologic impairment.[79]

Adaptive cellular immunity is a crucial component of the host response to primary herpetic infection. Newborns with HSV infections have a delayed T-lymphocyte proliferative response compared with older individuals.[66,94,95] Most infants have no detectable T-lymphocyte responses to HSV when evaluated 2 to 4 weeks after the onset of clinical symptoms.[66] The delayed T-lymphocyte response to viral antigens in infants whose initial disease is localized to the SEM may be an important determinant of the frequent progression to more severe disease in infants.[66,94] The importance of IFN-γ may be related to its effect on the induction of innate immune mechanisms, such as natural killer–cell responses.[96] Other mechanisms of the innate immune system of the newborn that may be deficient in controlling HSV include other nonspecific cytokine responses and complement-mediated effects. T lymphocytes from infected infants have decreased IFN-γ production during the first month of life. This defect can be predicted to limit the clonal expansion of helper and cytotoxic T lymphocytes specific for herpes viral antigens, allowing more extensive and prolonged viral replication. Antibody-dependent cell-mediated cytotoxicity has been shown to be an important component of adaptive immunity to viral infection.[97] Lymphocytes, monocytes, macrophages, or polymorphonuclear leukocytes and antibodies and complement lyse HSV-infected cells in vitro.[99] However, newborns appear to have fewer effector lymphocytes than older individuals do. The immaturity of neonatal monocytes and macrophage function against HSV infection has been demonstrated in vitro and in animal models.[100,101] Additional information regarding the immune response to HSV is provided in Chapter 4.

Neonatal Infection

PATHOGENESIS AND PATHOLOGY

After direct exposure, replication of HSV is presumed to occur at the portal of entry, which is probably the mucous membranes of the mouth or eye, or at sites where the skin integrity has been compromised. Factors that determine whether the infection causes symptoms at the site of inoculation or disseminates to other organs are poorly understood. Sites of replication during the incubation period have not been well defined, but the virus evades the host response during this early stage, probably by mechanisms such as interfering with expression of the IFN response genes and blocking cell-mediated immune recognition of viral peptides by preventing major histocompatibility complex class I molecules from reaching the surface of infected cells.

Intraneuronal transmission of viral particles may provide a privileged site that is relatively inaccessible to circulating humoral and cell-mediated defense mechanisms, facilitating the pathogenesis of encephalitis. Transplacental maternal antibodies may be less effective under such circumstances. Disseminated infection seems to be the consequence of viremia. HSV DNA has been detected in peripheral blood mononuclear cells, even in infants who have localized infection.[102] Extensive cell-to-cell spread could help explain primary HSV pneumonia after aspiration of infected secretions.

After the virus has adsorbed to cell membranes and penetration has occurred, viral replication proceeds, leading to release of progeny virus and cell death. The synthesis of cellular DNA and protein ceases as large quantities of HSV are produced. Many infants with disseminated HSV infection have high viral loads and higher concentrations of inflammatory cytokines compared with infants with central nervous system (CNS) infection alone or SEM disease.[103] Uncontrolled host immune responses may contribute to the development of multiorgan dysfunction. Cell death in critical organs of the newborn, such as the brain, results in devastating consequences, as reflected by the long-term morbidity of herpes encephalitis. Cellular swelling, hemorrhagic necrosis, development of intranuclear inclusions, and cytolysis all result from the replication process and ensuing inflammatory response. Small, punctate, yellow-to-gray areas of focal necrosis are the most prominent gross lesions in infected organs. When infected tissue is examined by microscopy, there is extensive evidence of hemorrhagic necrosis, clumping of nuclear chromatin, dissolution of the nucleolus, cell fusion with formation of multinucleate giant cells, and, ultimately, a lymphocytic inflammatory response.[104] Irreversible organ damage results from ischemia and direct viral destruction of cells. A major advance in our understanding of the pathogenesis of sequelae of neonatal HSV CNS disease is the finding that subclinical reactivation of virus within the CNS occurs after successful treatment of the acute disease and that this contributes to the long-term neurologic sequelae of this manifestation of neonatal HSV disease.[105]

CLINICAL MANIFESTATIONS

Pediatricians should consider the diagnosis of neonatal herpes in infants who have clinical signs consistent with the disease, regardless of the maternal history of genital herpes. Only a minority (20%-40%) of mothers whose infants develop neonatal herpes have had symptomatic genital herpes or sexual contact with a partner who has recognized HSV infection during or before the pregnancy.

The clinical presentation of infants with neonatal HSV infection depends on the initial site of infection and the extent of viral replication. In contrast to human cytomegalovirus, neonatal infections caused by HSV-1 and HSV-2 are almost invariably symptomatic. Case reports of asymptomatic infection in the newborn exist but are uncommon, and long-term follow-up of these children to document absence of subtle disease or sequelae is not sufficient to determine if neonatal infection actually occurred.

Classification of newborns with HSV infection is used for prognostic and therapeutic considerations.[106] Historically, infants with neonatal HSV infection were classified as having localized or disseminated disease, with the former group being subdivided into infants with SEM disease versus infants with CNS infection. This classification system understated the significant differences in outcome within each category, however.[107] In a revised classification scheme, infants who are infected intrapartum or postnatally are divided into three groups: disease localized to the skin, eyes, or mouth (SEM disease); encephalitis, with or without SEM involvement (CNS disease); and disseminated infection that involves multiple organs, including the CNS, lung, liver, adrenals, and SEM (disseminated disease). This classification system is predictive of both morbidity and mortality.[85,106,108-110] Patients with disseminated or SEM disease generally present to medical attention at 10 to 12 days of life, whereas patients with CNS disease on average present somewhat later at 16 to 19 days of life.[85]

Knowledge of the patterns of clinical disease caused by HSV-1 and HSV-2 in the newborn is based on prospectively acquired data obtained through the NIAID CASG. These analyses have used uniform case record forms from one study interval to the next. Approximately 25% of babies with neonatal HSV infection are classified as having disseminated disease, whereas 30% have CNS disease and 45% have SEM disease.[61,111]

Intrauterine Infection

Intrauterine infection is very rare, constituting only about 5% of cases of neonatal HSV infection.[75] When infection occurs in utero, severe disease follows acquisition of infection at virtually any time during gestation. In the most severely affected group of infants, evidence of infection is apparent at birth or within the first 24 hours of life and is characterized by a triad of findings: skin vesicles or scarring, eye damage, and severe manifestations of microcephaly or hydranencephaly. CNS damage is caused by intrauterine encephalitis. Infants do not have evidence of embryopathy, such as cardiac malformations. Often, chorioretinitis combined with other eye findings, such as keratoconjunctivitis or microphthalmia, is a component of the clinical presentation.

Serial ultrasound examination of the mothers of infants infected in utero has demonstrated the presence of hydranencephaly, but cases are seldom diagnosed before delivery. Chorioretinitis alone should alert the pediatrician to the possibility of this diagnosis, although it is a sign for other, more commonly encountered congenital infections as well. A few infants have been described who have signs of HSV infection at birth after prolonged rupture of membranes. These infants may have no other findings of invasive multiorgan involvement—no chorioretinitis, encephalitis, or evidence of other diseased organs—and can be expected to respond to antiviral therapy. Antiviral therapy cannot be expected to improve long-term outcomes for infants who are born with very severe CNS involvement or hydranencephaly. Intrauterine HSV infection has been reported as a cause of hydrops fetalis.[112]

Disseminated Disease

Infants with disseminated neonatal HSV disease have the highest mortality rate of the three intrapartum and postnatal disease classifications. Many of these infants are born to mothers who are experiencing a first-episode primary or nonprimary HSV-1 or HSV-2 infection and may lack any passively acquired antibodies against the infecting virus type.[10,60,113] Patients with disseminated disease generally present to medical attention at 10 to 12 days of life.[85] The short incubation period of disseminated herpes reflects an acute viremia, which allows transport of the virus to all organs; the principal organs involved are the adrenals and the liver, resulting in fulminant hepatitis in some cases.[106,114-117] Viremia is associated with infection of circulating mononuclear cells in these infants.[102,114,116,118,119]

Disseminated infection can affect multiple organs, including the CNS, larynx, trachea, lungs, esophagus, stomach, lower gastrointestinal tract, spleen, kidneys, pancreas, and heart. Initial signs and symptoms are irritability, seizures, respiratory distress, jaundice, coagulopathy, and shock. The characteristic vesicular exanthem oftentimes is not present when the symptoms begin. Untreated infants may develop cutaneous lesions resulting from viremia, but greater than 40% of children with disseminated infection do not develop skin vesicles during the course of their illness.[61,85,114] Disseminated infections caused by HSV-1 and HSV-2 are indistinguishable by clinical criteria.

The diagnosis of disseminated neonatal herpes is exceedingly difficult because the clinical signs are often vague and nonspecific, mimicking signs of neonatal bacterial sepsis (e.g., group B streptococcal or *Escherichia coli* sepsis) or neonatal enteroviral sepsis syndrome.

Evaluation of the extent of dissemination is imperative to provide appropriate supportive interventions early in the clinical course. Infants should be assessed for hypoxemia, acidosis, hyponatremia, transaminitis, direct hyperbilirubinemia, neutropenia, thrombocytopenia, and bleeding diathesis. Chest radiographs also should be obtained. Depending on signs and whether the infant is stable enough, abdominal radiography, electroencephalography, and computed tomography (CT) or magnetic resonance imaging (MRI) of the head should be obtained to determine further the extent of disease. The radiographic picture of HSV lung disease is characterized by a diffuse, interstitial pattern, which progresses to a hemorrhagic pneumonitis and, rarely, a significant pleural effusion.[120] Frequently, necrotizing enterocolitis with pneumatosis intestinalis can be detected when gastrointestinal disease is present. Meningoencephalitis seems to be a common component of disseminated infection, occurring in about 60% to 75% of children. Usual examinations of cerebrospinal fluid (CSF), including PCR for HSV DNA and viral culture, should be performed along with noninvasive neurodiagnostic tests to assess the extent of brain disease.

The mortality rate for disseminated HSV in the absence of therapy exceeds 80%, and many survivors are impaired. The most common causes of death of infants with disseminated disease are intravascular coagulopathy or HSV pneumonitis. Premature infants seem to be at particularly high risk for disseminated disease with pneumonitis and have a high mortality rate, even with appropriate antiviral therapy.[121]

Central Nervous System Disease

Almost one third of all infants with neonatal HSV infection have only encephalitis as the initial manifestation of disease.[122,123] These infants have clinical manifestations distinct from infants who have CNS infection associated with disseminated HSV, and the pathogenesis of these two forms of brain infection is probably different. The virus is likely to reach brain parenchyma by a hematogenous route in infants with disseminated infection, resulting in multiple areas of cortical hemorrhagic necrosis. In contrast, neonates who present with only CNS disease are likely to develop brain infection because of retrograde axonal transport of the virus to the CNS. Patients with CNS disease on average present at 16 to 19 days of life.[85] Clinical manifestations of encephalitis include seizures (focal or generalized), fever, lethargy, irritability, tremors, poor feeding, temperature instability, bulging fontanelle, and pyramidal tract signs. Similar signs are observed when disseminated herpesvirus is associated with encephalitis. Approximately one third of infants with CNS disease do not have skin vesicles when signs of illness begin. Some infants have a history or residual signs of lesions of the SEM that were not recognized as herpetic.

Anticipated findings on CSF examination include a mononuclear cell pleocytosis, moderately low glucose concentrations, and elevated protein. A few infants with CNS infection, proven by brain biopsy done immediately after the onset of seizures, have no abnormalities of CSF, but most infants have some degree of pleocytosis and mild reduction of the glucose level. The hemorrhagic nature of the encephalitis may result in an apparent "bloody tap," although this is seen less frequently in the current era compared with the 1970s, when awareness of neonatal HSV infection was lower and earlier assessment less likely to occur. Although initial protein concentrations may be normal or only slightly elevated, infants with localized brain disease usually show progressive increases in protein. The importance of CSF examination in all infants is underscored by the finding that even subtle abnormalities have been associated with significant developmental sequelae.[106]

Electroencephalography and MRI or CT can be very useful in defining the presence and extent of CNS abnormalities and should be obtained before discharge of all infants with this diagnosis.[124,125] Abnormalities may also be detected by ultrasound examination.[125] Typical abnormalities seen by neuroimaging include localized or multifocal areas of abnormal parenchymal attenuation, atrophy, edema, and hemorrhage involving the temporal, frontal, parietal, and subcortical regions of the brain (Fig. 27-1).[126] Predominant brainstem involvement is rare but reported.[127]

Localized CNS disease is fatal in approximately 50% of infants who are not treated. With rare exceptions, survivors who are not treated are left with neurologic impairment.[106] With parenteral antiviral therapy, mortality is decreased to approximately 5%,[108] and 30% of survivors who also receive 6 months of oral acyclovir suppressive therapy have some degree of neurologic impairment,[105] often in association with microcephaly, hydranencephaly, porencephalic cysts, spasticity, blindness, chorioretinitis, or learning disabilities. Quantitative PCR methods show a greater amount of HSV-2 DNA in CSF from patients with more extensive neurologic impairment.[128] Although many infants have obvious severe sequelae within a few weeks after onset of HSV encephalitis,[109,129] recent data document that without follow-up suppressive oral therapy progressive, subclinical neurologic damage occurs after parenteral treatment of the acute infection.[105]

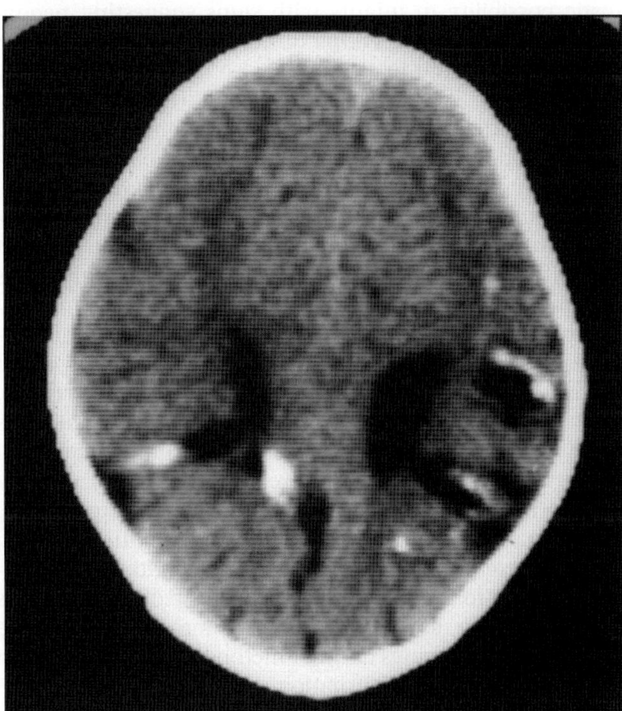

Figure 27-1 Herpes simplex encephalitis. Computed tomography scan of an infant with herpes simplex virus type 2 infection and severe sequelae.

Despite the presumed differences in pathogenesis, neurologic manifestations of disease in children with CNS disease are virtually identical to the findings for brain infection in disseminated disease. For infants with CNS disease, approximately two thirds develop evidence of a vesicular rash characteristic of HSV infection. A newborn with pleocytosis and elevated protein in the CSF but without the characteristic rash of neonatal HSV can easily be misdiagnosed as having another viral or bacterial infection unless HSV infection is considered.

Skin, Eye, or Mouth Disease

Infection localized to the SEM or some combination of these sites seems benign at the onset but is associated with a high risk of progression to serious disease. When infection is localized to the skin, the presence of discrete vesicles remains the hallmark of disease (Fig. 27-2). Vesicles occur in greater than 80% of children with SEM disease. The skin vesicles usually erupt from an erythematous base and typically are 1 to 2 mm in diameter. The formation of new lesions adjacent to the original vesicles is typical, creating a cluster that may coalesce into larger, irregular vesicles. In some cases, the lesions progress to bullae larger than 1 cm in diameter. Clusters of vesicles may appear initially on the presenting part of the body, presumably because of prolonged contact with infectious secretions during birth, or at sites of trauma (e.g., scalp monitor sites). However, it also is common for the first herpetic lesions in infants with localized cutaneous disease to be on the trunk, extremities, and other sites.

Patients with SEM disease generally present to medical attention at 10 to 12 days of life.[85] Although discrete vesicles are usually encountered, crops and clusters of vesicles have been described, particularly before antiviral treatment was available or when the cause of the first lesions was not recognized. In these cases, the rash can progress to involve other cutaneous sites, presumably by viremia and hematogenous spread. The scattered vesicles can resemble varicella. Although progression is expected without treatment, a few infants have had infection of the skin limited to one or two vesicles, with no further evidence of cutaneous disease. These infants may be identified after the newborn period and should have a careful evaluation because many are likely to have had neurologic disease that was not detected. A zosteriform eruption is another manifestation of herpetic skin disease reported in infants.[130]

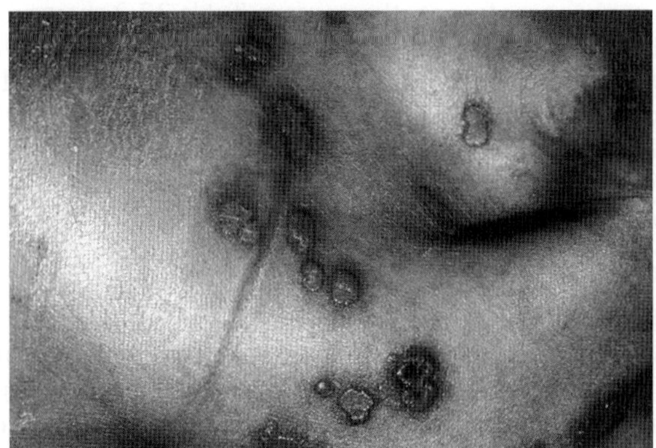

Figure 27-2 Cutaneous herpes simplex virus infection. Initial vesicular lesion in a premature infant with herpes simplex type 2 infection.

Table 27-2 Morbidity and Mortality Among Patients After 12 Months by Viral Type, 1981-1997

	DISEASE CLASSIFICATION					
	SEM		CNS		DISSEMINATED	
Outcome	**HSV-1**	**HSV-2**	**HSV-1**	**HSV-2**	**HSV-1**	**HSV-2**
Normal	24 (100%)	19 (95%)	4 (57%)	7 (17.5%)	3 (23%)	14 (41%)
Mild impairment	0 (0%)	0 (0%)	0 (0%)	7 (17.5%)	0 (0%)	1 (3%)
Moderate impairment	0 (0%)	1 (5%)	1 (14%)	7 (17.5%)	0 (0%)	0 (0%)
Severe impairment	0 (0%)	0 (0%)	2 (29%)	13 (32.5%)	1 (8%)	3 (9%)
Death	0 (0%)	0 (0%)	0 (0%)	6 (15%)	9 (69%)	16 (47%)
Unknown	Total of 20		Total of 16		Total of 12	

Data from Douglas J, Schmidt O, Corey L: Acquisition of neonatal HSV-1 infection from a paternal source contact, *J Pediatr* 103:908-910, 1983.
CNS, Central nervous system; *SEM,* skin, eyes, or mouth.

Infections involving the eye may manifest as keratoconjunctivitis. Ocular infection may be the only site of involvement in a newborn. When localized eye infection is observed in infants who also have microphthalmos and retinal dysplasia, intrauterine acquisition should be suspected, and a thorough neurologic evaluation should be done. Before antiviral therapy was available, persistent ocular disease resulted in chorioretinitis caused by HSV-1 or HSV-2.[131] Keratoconjunctivitis can progress to chorioretinitis, cataracts, and retinal detachment despite therapy. Cataracts have been detected as a long-term consequence in infants with HSV infections acquired intrapartum.

Localized infection of the oropharynx involving the mouth or tongue occurs, but newborns do not develop the classic herpetic gingivostomatitis caused by primary HSV-1 infection in older children. Overall, approximately 10% of patients have evidence of HSV infection of the oropharynx by viral culture. Many of these children did not undergo a thorough oral examination to determine whether the detection of infectious virus in oropharyngeal secretions was associated with lesions.

Long-term neurologic impairment has been encountered in children whose disease seemed to be localized to the SEM during the newborn period.[61,106,109] Significant findings included spastic quadriplegia, microcephaly, and blindness. However, these outcomes were described before routine use of CSF PCR analysis for HSV DNA and likely occurred in babies who were PCR positive and now would be classified as having CNS disease.[132]

Most newborns who have skin lesions experience cutaneous recurrences for months or years. Table 27-2 shows morbidity and mortality 12 months after infection by HSV viral type and disease classification in patients enrolled in two studies conducted by the NIAID CASG from 1981 to 1997. Although HSV-2 outcomes appear to be more severe than HSV-1 outcomes, the differences between viral types do not reach statistical significance in regression analysis ($P = .10$).[85]

Subclinical Infection

A few cases of apparent subclinical infection with HSV proven by culture isolation of virus in the absence of symptoms have been described.[133] It has been difficult to document such cases in the course of prospective evaluations of several hundred infants from many centers around the United States. Conversely, infants who were exposed to active maternal infection at the time of delivery and who did not develop symptoms have been followed for the first year of life and did not have immunologic evidence of subclinical infection.[60] HSV-1 or HSV-2 may be recovered from the infant's oropharyngeal secretions transiently, without representing true infection. Because of the propensity of the newborn to develop severe or life-threatening disease, laboratory evidence of neonatal HSV infection requires careful follow-up for clinical signs and administration of antiviral therapy.

Diagnosis

CLINICAL EVALUATION

The clinical diagnosis of neonatal HSV infection is difficult because the appearance of skin vesicles cannot be relied on as an initial component of disease presentation. Neonatal enteroviral sepsis syndrome is a major differential diagnostic possibility in infants with signs suggesting neonatal HSV. Bacterial infections of newborns, such as group B streptococcal and *E. coli* sepsis, also can mimic neonatal HSV infection. Skin lesions may resemble lesions seen with bullous or crusted impetigo. Some infants infected by HSV have been described who had concomitant bacterial infections, including group B streptococci, *Staphylococcus aureus*, *Listeria monocytogenes*, and gram-negative bacteria. A positive culture for one of these pathogens does not rule out HSV infection if the clinical suspicion for neonatal herpes infection is present.

Many other disorders of the newborn can be indistinguishable from neonatal HSV infections, including acute respiratory distress syndrome, intraventricular hemorrhage, necrotizing enterocolitis, and various ocular or cutaneous diseases. When vesicles are present, alternative causes of neonatal exanthems should be excluded (Box 27-1). Cutaneous disorders such as erythema toxicum, neonatal melanosis, acrodermatitis enteropathica, and incontinentia pigmenti often confuse physicians who suspect neonatal HSV infections. HSV lesions can be distinguished rapidly from lesions caused by these diseases using direct immunofluorescence stain of lesion scrapings or other methods for rapid detection of viral proteins and confirmation by viral culture.

Neonatal HSV CNS disease is a difficult clinical diagnosis to make, particularly because many such neonates do not have a vesicular rash at the time of clinical presentation. Infection of the CNS is suspected in a child who has evidence

Box 27-1 Differential Diagnosis for Vesicular Eruptions in the Neonate

Infectious Etiologies

HSV
Staphylococcus aureus
Pseudomonas
Haemophilus influenzae type b
Treponema pallidum
Candida
Aspergillus
VZV
CMV
Listeria monocytogenes
Group B streptococci

Noninfectious Conditions

Erythema toxicum
Pustular melanosis
Miliaria
Letterer-Siwe disease
Urticaria pigmentosa
Bullous mastocytosis
Pemphigus vulgaris
Dermatitis herpetiformis
Herpes gestationis
Incontinentia pigmenti
Neonatal lupus
Epidermolysis bullosa
Epidermolytic hyperkeratosis
Acropustulosis
Neonatal bullous dermatitis
Langerhans cell histiocytosis
Bednar aphthae

Modified from Kohl S: Neonatal herpes simplex virus infection, Clin Perinatol *24:129-150, 1997.*

of acute neurologic deterioration, often but not always associated with the onset of seizure, and in the absence of intraventricular hemorrhage and metabolic causes. Using PCR assay to detect viral DNA in CSF has become the gold standard diagnostic methodology for confirming neonatal HSV CNS involvement, replacing the need for diagnosis by brain biopsy.[134] Infants with localized CNS disease usually have increases in CSF cell counts and protein concentrations and negative bacterial cultures of CSF. Noninvasive neurodiagnostic studies such as MRI and CT can be used to define sites of involvement.

LABORATORY ASSESSMENT

The appropriate use of laboratory methods is essential if a timely diagnosis of HSV infection is to be achieved. Virus isolation remains the gold standard diagnostic method from non-CNS sites. HSV grows readily in cell culture. Special transport media are available that allow transport to local or regional laboratories for culture. Cytopathogenic effects typical of HSV infection usually are observed 1 to 3 days after inoculation. Methods of culture confirmation include fluorescent antibody staining, enzyme immunoassays, and monolayer culture with typing. Cultures that remain negative by day 5 likely will continue to remain negative.

Of the sites routinely cultured for HSV during a recent study,[85] skin or eye/conjunctival cultures consistently provided the greatest yields regardless of disease classification, with greater than or equal to 90% of cultures being positive. Overall, 58 (94%) of 62 patients had a positive skin or eye culture, 33 (48%) of 69 patients had a positive mouth/oropharyngeal culture, and 17 (40%) of 42 patients with CNS involvement (CNS disease or disseminated disease with CNS involvement) had a positive CSF or brain biopsy culture.[85]

Viral DNA detection by PCR assay is the gold standard diagnostic method for CNS involvement.[132,134-136] PCR was used in the retrospective analysis of materials collected from 24 infants enrolled in the NIAID CASG antiviral studies.[132] HSV was detected by PCR assay of CSF in 71% of infants before antiviral therapy was initiated. At least one specimen was positive in 76% of infants, and all samples that were positive by viral culture were positive by PCR. Similar findings were reported by Swedish investigators when stored CSF specimens obtained from infants with neonatal HSV infection were tested for HSV by PCR. HSV DNA was detected from CSF in the acute phase of illness from 78% of patients with CNS disease.[137] Older patients with herpes simplex encephalitis can have initial HSV PCR results that are negative early in the course of illness; CSF obtained 4 to 7 days after the initial CSF samples was subsequently positive for HSV DNA in a few patients.[138] Most studies of PCR for the diagnosis of HSV CNS infections indicate the test is sensitive in approximately 75% to 100% of cases in small cohorts of infants.[132,135-137] Specificity of the test ranges from 71% to 100%. The broad range of values for sensitivity and specificity of HSV PCR probably results from different study methods and disease classifications.[111] In difficult cases in which repeated CSF PCRs are negative, histologic examination and viral culture of a brain tissue biopsy specimen is the most definitive method of confirming the diagnosis of HSV CNS disease. Viral cultures of CSF from a patient with neonatal HSV CNS disease are positive in 25% to 40% of cases.

Application of PCR testing to blood specimens from infants with suspected HSV disease appears promising.* Data are insufficient at the current time to allow use of serial blood PCR measurements to establish response to antiviral therapy or guide decisions about the duration of therapy.

Cytologic methods, such as Papanicolaou, Giemsa, or Tzanck staining, have a sensitivity of only approximately 60% to 70%. A negative result must not be interpreted as excluding the diagnosis of HSV, and a positive result should not be the sole diagnostic determinant of HSV infection in the newborn. Intranuclear inclusions and multinucleated giant cells may be consistent with, but not diagnostic of, HSV infection.

For diagnosis of neonatal HSV infection, the following specimens should be obtained[141]: (1) swab specimens from the mouth, nasopharynx, conjunctivae, and anus ("surface cultures") for HSV culture and, if desired, for HSV PCR assay (all surface swab specimens can be obtained with a single swab, ending with the anal swab, and placed in one viral transport media tube); (2) specimens of skin vesicles and CSF for HSV culture and PCR assay; (3) whole-blood sample for HSV PCR assay; and (4) whole-blood sample for measuring alanine aminotransferase. The performance of PCR assay on skin and mucosal specimens from neonates has not

*References 102, 128, 135, 137, 139, 140.

been studied; if used, surface PCR assay should be performed in addition to, and not instead of, the gold standard surface culture. Positive cultures obtained from any of the surface sites more than 12 to 24 hours after birth indicate viral replication and therefore are suggestive of infant infection rather than merely contamination after intrapartum exposure. As with any PCR assay, false-negative and false-positive results can occur. Whole-blood PCR assay may be of benefit in diagnosis of neonatal HSV disease, but its use should not supplant the standard workup of such patients, which includes surface cultures and CSF PCR assay; no data exist to support use of serial blood PCR assay to monitor response to therapy. Rapid diagnostic techniques also are available, such as direct fluorescent antibody staining of vesicle scrapings or enzyme immunoassay detection of HSV antigens. These techniques are as specific but slightly less sensitive than culture. Typing HSV strains differentiates between HSV-1 and HSV-2 isolates. Histologic examination of lesions for presence of multinucleated giant cells and eosinophilic intranuclear inclusions typical of HSV (e.g., with Tzanck test) has low sensitivity and should not be performed.

Interpretation of negative or positive HSV cultures and PCR results must depend on clinical findings. A negative PCR result for HSV in CSF in the setting of clinical, laboratory, or radiologic findings consistent with CNS infection does not rule out HSV infection. It is important to continue to use standard clinical and laboratory diagnostic methods for the evaluation of infants with possible neonatal HSV.

In contrast to some other neonatal infections, serologic diagnosis of HSV infection has little clinical value. The interpretation of serologic assays is complicated by the fact that transplacentally acquired maternal IgG cannot be differentiated from endogenously produced antibodies, making it difficult to assess the neonate's antibody status during acute infection. Serial type-specific antibody testing may be useful for retrospective diagnosis if a mother without a prior history of HSV infection has a primary infection late in gestation and transfers little or no antibody to the fetus. However, therapeutic decisions cannot await a diagnostic approach based on comparing acute-phase and convalescent-phase antibody titers. IgM production is delayed or does not occur in infected infants because of inherent immaturity in the immune response to systemic viral infections in the newborn, and commercially available assays for IgM antibodies to HSV have limited reliability. The results of specific laboratory tests for HSV should be used in conjunction with clinical findings and general laboratory tests, such as platelet counts, CSF analysis, and liver function tests, to establish a disease classification.

Treatment

BACKGROUND

The cumulative experience of the past 4 decades shows that intrapartum-acquired HSV infections are amenable to treatment with antiviral agents, with parenteral acyclovir being the standard of care.[122] Because most infants acquire infection at the time of delivery or shortly thereafter, antiviral therapy has the potential to decrease mortality and improve long-term outcome. The benefits that antiviral therapy can provide are influenced substantially by earlier diagnosis, when possible. Without treatment, approximately 70% of infants presenting with disease localized to the SEM develop involvement of the CNS or disseminated infection. Treatment initiated after disease progression is not optimal because many of these children die or are left with significant neurologic impairment.

ANTIVIRAL DRUGS

Historically, four nucleoside analogues have been used to treat neonatal herpes: idoxuridine, cytosine arabinoside, vidarabine, and acyclovir. Of these, the first three are nonspecific inhibitors of cellular and viral replication. The fourth, acyclovir, is monophosphorylated by HSV-specific thymidine kinases and then converted to its diphosphate and triphosphate forms by cellular enzymes. Acyclovir acts as a competitive inhibitor of HSV DNA polymerase and terminates DNA chain elongation.[142] Idoxuridine and cytosine arabinoside have no value as systemic therapy for any viral infection because of toxicity and equivocal efficacy. Vidarabine was the first drug shown to be efficacious, with decreased mortality and improved morbidity in neonatal HSV infections.[110]

In the preantiviral era, 85% of patients with disseminated neonatal HSV disease died by 1 year of age, as did 50% of patients with CNS neonatal HSV disease (Table 27-3).[110] Evaluations of two different doses of vidarabine and of a lower dose of acyclovir (30 mg/kg/day for 10 days) documented that both of these antiviral drugs reduce mortality to comparable degrees,[109,110,143] with mortality rates at 1 year from disseminated disease decreasing to 54% and from CNS disease decreasing to 14% (see Table 27-3).[109] Despite its lack of therapeutic superiority, the lower dose of acyclovir quickly supplanted vidarabine as the treatment of choice for neonatal HSV disease because of its favorable safety profile and its ease of administration. Unlike acyclovir, vidarabine had to be administered over prolonged infusion times and in large volumes of fluid. With use of a higher dose of acyclovir (60 mg/kg/day for 21 days), 12-month mortality is further reduced to 29% for disseminated neonatal HSV disease and to 4% for CNS HSV disease (Fig. 27-3A and B, respectively).[108] Differences in mortality at 24 months among patients treated with the higher dose of acyclovir and the lower dose of acyclovir are statistically significant after stratification for disease category (CNS vs. disseminated) (P = .0035; odds ratio, 3.3 with 95% confidence interval of 1.5 to 7.3).[108] Lethargy and severe hepatitis are associated with mortality among patients with disseminated disease, as are prematurity and seizures in patients with CNS disease.[85]

Improvements in morbidity rates with antiviral therapies have not been as dramatic as with mortality. In the preantiviral era, 50% of survivors of disseminated neonatal HSV infections were developing normally at 12 months of age (see Table 27-3).[110] With use of the higher dose of acyclovir for 21 days, this percentage has increased to 83% (Fig. 27-4).[108] In the case of CNS neonatal HSV disease, 33% of patients in the preantiviral era were developing normally at 12 months of age (see Table 27-3), whereas 31% of higher-dose acyclovir recipients develop normally at 12 months today (see Fig. 27-4).[108,110] Seizures at or before the time of initiation of antiviral therapy are associated with increased

Table 27-3 Mortality and Morbidity Outcomes Among 295 Infants With Neonatal HSV Infection, Evaluated by the National Institute of Allergy and Infectious Diseases Collaborative Antiviral Study Group Between 1974 and 1997

EXTENT OF DISEASE	TREATMENT			
	Placebo[110]	**Vidarabine[109]**	**Acyclovir[109] 30 mg/kg/day**	**Acyclovir[108] 60 mg/kg/day**
DISSEMINATED DISEASE	*n* = 13	*n* = 28	*n* = 18	*n* = 34
Dead	11 (85%)	14 (50%)	11 (61%)	10 (29%)
Alive	2 (15%)	14 (50%)	7 (39%)	24 (71%)
Normal	1 (50%)	7 (50%)	3 (43%)	15 (63%)
Abnormal	1 (50%)	5 (36%)	2 (29%)	3 (13%)
Unknown	0 (0%)	2 (14%)	2 (29%)	6 (25%)
CENTRAL NERVOUS SYSTEM INFECTION	*n* = 6	*n* = 36	*n* = 35	*n* = 23
Dead	3 (50%)	5 (14%)	5 (14%)	1 (4%)
Alive	3 (50%)	31 (86%)	30 (86%)	22 (96%)
Normal	1 (33%)	13 (42%)	8 (27%)	4 (18%)
Abnormal	2 (67%)	17 (55%)	20 (67%)	9 (41%)
Unknown	0 (0%)	1 (3%)	2 (7%)	9 (41%)
SKIN, EYE, OR MOUTH INFECTION	*n* = 8	*n* = 31	*n* = 54	*n* = 9
Dead	0 (0%)	0 (0%)	0 (0%)	0 (0%)
Alive	8 (100%)	31 (100%)	54 (100%)	9 (100%)
Normal	5 (62%)	22 (71%)	45 (83%)	2 (22%)
Abnormal	3 (38%)	3 (10%)	1 (2%)	0 (0%)
Unknown	0 (0%)	6 (19%)	8 (15%)	7 (78%)

Modified from Kimberlin DW: Advances in the treatment of neonatal herpes simplex infections, *Rev Med Virol* 11:157-163, 2001.
HSV, Herpes simplex virus.

risk of morbidity, both in patients with CNS disease and in patients with disseminated infection.[85] Unlike disseminated or CNS neonatal HSV disease, morbidity after SEM disease has dramatically improved during the antiviral era. Before use of antiviral therapies, 38% of SEM patients experienced developmental difficulties at 12 months of age (see Table 27-3).[110] With vidarabine and lower-dose acyclovir, these percentages were reduced to 12% and 2%, respectively.[109] In the high-dose acyclovir study, no SEM patients developed neurologic sequelae at 12 months of life (see Fig. 27-4).[108]

The improvements in mortality and morbidity achieved with use of higher-dose acyclovir support use of acyclovir at 60 mg/kg/day delivered intravenously in three divided daily doses, as is currently recommended.[108,141] The dosing interval of intravenous acyclovir may need to be increased in premature infants, based upon their creatinine clearance.[144] Duration of therapy is 21 days for patients with disseminated or CNS neonatal HSV disease and 14 days for patients with HSV infection limited to the SEM.[145] All patients with CNS HSV involvement should have a repeat lumbar puncture at the end of intravenous acyclovir therapy to determine that the specimen is PCR negative in a reliable laboratory and to document the end-of-therapy CSF indices.[85] Those persons who remain PCR positive should continue to receive intravenous antiviral therapy until PCR negativity is achieved.[85,132]

The primary apparent toxicity associated with the use of intravenous acyclovir administered at 60 mg/kg/day is neutropenia, with approximately one fifth of patients developing an absolute neutrophil count (ANC) of less than or equal to 1000/μL.[108] Although the neutropenia resolves either during continuation of intravenous acyclovir or after its cessation, it is prudent to monitor neutrophil counts at least twice weekly throughout the course of intravenous acyclovir therapy, with consideration being given to decreasing the dose of acyclovir or administering granulocyte colony-stimulating factor (G-CSF) if the ANC remains less than 500/μL for a prolonged period of time.[108]

Determining which infants admitted to the hospital with presumed sepsis should be treated empirically with acyclovir remains a topic of debate.[146,147] In all cases of presumptive therapy, specimens should be obtained before initiation of antiviral treatment for laboratory testing to guide the decision of whether to continue treatment. During the course of therapy, careful monitoring is important to assess the therapeutic response. Even in the absence of clinical evidence of encephalitis, evaluation of the CNS should be done for prognostic purposes when starting antiviral therapy. Serial evaluations of hepatic and hematologic parameters may indicate changes caused by the viral infection or by drug toxicity. Intravenous acyclovir is tolerated well by infants. Adequate hydration is necessary to minimize the risk of nephrotoxicity, and dosage adjustments are necessary if renal clearance is impaired. As for all drugs, the possibility of acute toxicity should be considered in any child receiving parenteral antiviral therapy and should be assessed by serially evaluating bone marrow, renal, and hepatic functions.

Acyclovir resistance has been reported in neonatal HSV disease, but only rarely and in the form of case reports. One infant with acute HSV infection of the larynx in the newborn period developed antiviral resistance during the course of therapy; in this case, the initial isolate was not inhibited by acyclovir, although the source of this infection could not be explained.[148] Acyclovir resistance has also been reported in a premature infant with cutaneous and CNS disease caused by an initially acyclovir-susceptible

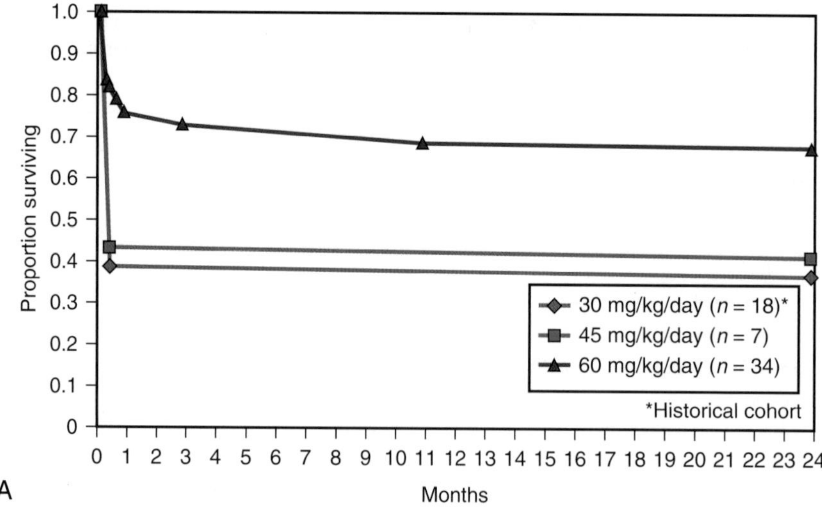

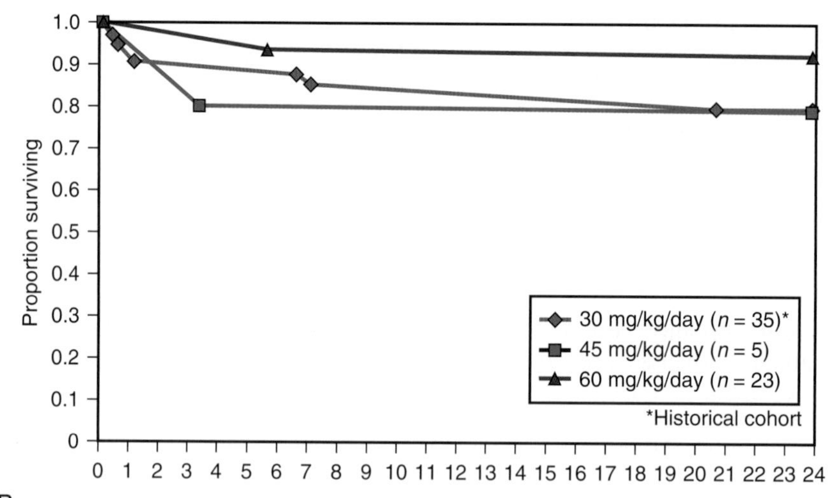

Figure 27-3 Mortality rates for patients with disseminated disease **(A)** and central nervous system disease **(B)** depending on dose of acyclovir. (Data from Kimberlin DW, Lin CY, Jacobs RF, et al: Safety and efficacy of high-dose intravenous acyclovir in the management of neonatal herpes simplex virus infections, *Pediatrics* 108:230-238, 2001.)

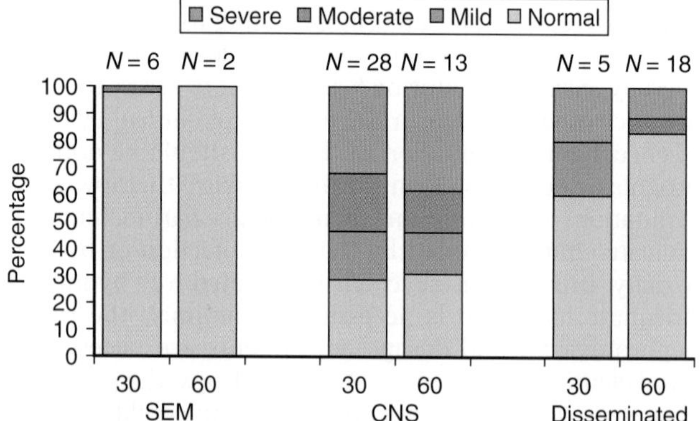

Figure 27-4 Morbidity among patients with known outcomes after 12 months of life. *CNS,* Central nervous system; *SEM,* skin, eyes, or mouth. (Modified from Kimberlin DW, Lin CY, Jacobs RF, et al: Safety and efficacy of high-dose intravenous acyclovir in the management of neonatal herpes simplex virus infections, *Pediatrics* 108:230-238, 2001.)

HSV. The infant developed recurrent disseminated HSV infection 8 days after a 21-day course of acyclovir. The virus isolated at the onset of recurrent symptoms was found to lack thymidine kinase activity on the basis of a frameshift mutation in the thymidine kinase gene.[149] Another infant born to a mother with severe systemic primary HSV-2 infection developed an acyclovir-resistant mutant during acyclovir therapy for disseminated HSV infection and eventually died. The use of steroids to treat blood pressure instability may have hampered this infant's immune response to infection further.[150] Emergence of viral resistance to acyclovir also has been described in patients requiring prolonged or repeated treatment with this drug. One infant who was given long-term oral acyclovir for suppression of recurrences during the first 6 months of life had a resistant HSV isolated from a lesion after therapy was discontinued, but subsequent isolates were susceptible.[151] However, isolates of HSV recovered from infants who received intravenous acyclovir for cutaneous disease in the newborn period and had subsequent recurrent cutaneous lesions typically remain sensitive to acyclovir,[152] and antiviral resistance generally does not explain the failure of infants with the disseminated or CNS form of the disease to respond well to antiviral therapy. Rather, clinical deterioration despite appropriate therapy and supportive care can almost always be attributed to virus-induced destruction of cells compromising infected organs, such as liver or brain, or irreversible changes, such as disseminated intravascular coagulopathy.

The NIAID CASG recently completed a multicenter, randomized, placebo-controlled, double-blind study of 6 months of oral acyclovir suppressive therapy after parenteral treatment of acute disease.[105] Subjects were stratified by CNS versus SEM disease and were randomized to either oral acyclovir at 300 mg/m^2/dose administered three times per day or to a matching placebo. If a subject had two cutaneous recurrences, the blinded suppression drug was stopped and open-label suppression was provided. Subjects randomized to receive acyclovir had significantly higher (better) mean Bayley Mental Scores at 1 year (88.24 vs. 68.12; $P = .046$). Distribution of neurologic outcomes was: 69% normal, 6% mild impairment, 6% moderate impairment, and 19% severe impairment for subjects randomized to acyclovir suppression versus 33%, 8%, 25%, and 33%, respectively, for subjects randomized to placebo. Of note, this distribution of outcomes was virtually identical to that from a small uncontrolled case series ($N = 16$) of oral acyclovir suppression after neonatal HSV CNS disease in which patients received five times the dose for four times the duration (69% having normal outcomes in both studies).[153] In the CASG study, the 12-month Bayley Mental Scores were incrementally higher because subjects were on active suppression for longer periods of time. For subjects in the SEM study, no differences in Bayley Mental Scores were noted. Combining the 74 subjects with either CNS or SEM disease, time to a second cutaneous HSV recurrence was statistically significantly longer for the group randomized to acyclovir suppression. Time to first ANC less than or equal to 500 cells/mm^3 was not statistically different for those subjects randomized to acyclovir versus placebo, although a trend for neutropenia in those who received acyclovir was noted ($P = .09$). In total, 25% and 20% of subjects on the CNS study and SEM study, respectively, who were randomized to acyclovir developed an ANC of less than or equal to 500 cells/mm^3, compared with 5% and 7% of placebo recipients in the respective trials. Neutropenia resolved in all affected subjects both with and without cessation of suppressive therapy, and none had associated complications.[105] These results have led to routine use of oral acyclovir suppressive therapy for the 6 months after treatment of acute neonatal HSV disease to improve neurodevelopmental outcomes in infants with HSV CNS disease and to prevent skin recurrences in infants with any disease classification of neonatal HSV.[141]

OTHER ISSUES IN ACUTE MANAGEMENT

Neonates with HSV infection should be hospitalized and managed with contact precautions if mucocutaneous lesions are present. Many infants with this infection have life threatening problems, including disseminated intravascular coagulation, shock, and respiratory failure, and they require supportive care that is available only at tertiary medical centers.

There is no indication that administration of immunoglobulin or hyperimmunoglobulin is of value for the treatment of neonatal HSV infection. Although a series of studies have suggested that the quantity of transplacental neutralizing antibodies affects the attack rate among exposed infants and may influence the initial disease manifestations, the presence of antibodies may or may not influence the subsequent course of infection.[60,61,65,66,97] The administration of standard preparations of intravenous immunoglobulin does not enhance the titers of functional antibodies against HSV in infants with low birth weight.[154]

No other forms of adjunctive therapy are useful for treating neonatal HSV infections. Various experimental modalities, including interferon, immunomodulators, and immunization, have been attempted, but none has produced demonstrable effects.

LONG-TERM MANAGEMENT OF INFECTED INFANTS

With the advent of antiviral therapy, an increasing number of newborns with HSV infection are surviving and require careful long-term follow-up. The most common complications of neonatal HSV infection include neurologic and ocular sequelae that may be detected only on long-term follow-up. It is necessary that these children receive serial long-term evaluation from qualified pediatric specialists in these areas, which should include neurodevelopmental, ophthalmologic, and hearing assessments.

Recurrent skin vesicles are present in many children, including children who did not have obvious mucocutaneous disease during the acute phase of the clinical illness. Skin vesicles provide a potential source for transmission of infection to other children or adults who have direct contact with these infants. The increasing use of daycare for children, including children surviving neonatal HSV infections, stimulates many questions from daycare providers about these children. There is some risk that children with recurrent HSV skin lesions would transmit the virus to other children in this environment. The most reasonable recommendation in this situation is to cover the lesions to prevent direct contact. HSV-1 is much more likely to be present in the daycare environment in the form of asymptomatic infection or gingivostomatitis. In both cases, virus is present in the mouth and pharynx, and the frequent exchange of saliva and other respiratory droplets that occurs among children in this setting makes this route of transmission more likely. Education of daycare workers and the general public about herpesvirus infections, their implications, and the frequency with which they occur in the population as a whole can calm fears and correct common misconceptions.

Parents of children with neonatal HSV infection often have significant feelings of guilt. Parents often require support from psychologists, psychiatrists, or counselors. The family physician or pediatrician can provide a valuable supportive role to the family in this situation. Most parents and many physicians are unaware of the high prevalence of HSV-2 infection and the increasing incidence of HSV-1 genital infection in the United States and of the lifelong persistence and subclinical nature of these infections. Concern about the risk of fetal and neonatal infection during subsequent pregnancies is often a major issue that can be addressed effectively based on the low risks as proven from large, prospective studies.

Prevention

BACKGROUND

Despite the progress that has been made in antiviral treatment of neonatal HSV infection, the ideal approach is to prevent the exposure of infants to active maternal infection at the time of delivery. Genital infections caused by HSV often are clinically silent when they are acquired as new infections

Table 27-4 Projected Risk of Transmission of Herpes Simplex Virus Type 2 (HSV-2) From Mothers to Infants at Delivery in a Cohort of 100,000 Pregnant Women

25% with past HSV-2 infection	75% susceptible to HSV-2 infection
25,000 women	75,000 women
1.5% reactivation at delivery	0.02% seroconversion/week
375 women with reactivation	30 women with infection <2 weeks before delivery
<5% risk of transmission	50% risk of transmission
19 infected infants	15 infected infants

Data from Arvin AM: The epidemiology of perinatal herpes simplex infections. In Stanberry L, editor: *Genital and neonatal herpes,* New York, 1996, John Wiley & Sons, pp 179-192.

and when the virus reactivates. With the high prevalence of HSV-2 infection in the U.S. population and the increasing practice of oral-genital sexual contact, women are at risk for acquiring new genital infections during pregnancy. The problem of asymptomatic genital HSV infection means that the transmission of HSV from mothers to infants cannot be eliminated even with the best obstetric management.

Sequential genital cultures during the last weeks of gestation in women with a history of genital herpes do not predict the infant's risk of exposure at delivery[59] because of the usually brief duration of asymptomatic shedding and the time required for the culture to become positive. Because of the attention of the lay press to the devastating outcome of neonatal HSV infections, many women who know that they have genital herpes experience severe anxiety about the potential risks to the fetus and the newborn. As a consequence, these women may have an unnecessarily high frequency of cesarean deliveries. The risk of neonatal HSV infection in the newborn is approximately equivalent for women who have no prior history of genital herpes or a partner with known infection (Table 27-4).

Although development of a vaccine has received substantial industry and government support, a recent large clinical trial of the vaccine product that was farthest along in development failed to show protection.[31] Although development efforts continue, it will be many years, if ever, before a vaccine for genital herpes is available.

MANAGEMENT OF PREGNANT WOMEN WITH KNOWN GENITAL HERPES

Women who have a history of recurrent genital herpes should be reassured that the risk of fetal or neonatal infection is very low. Intrauterine HSV infections are very rare, with an estimated overall risk of 1 in 300,000 pregnancies.[77] Information about the risk of exposure to asymptomatic viral reactivation at delivery derived from six large-scale prospective studies is sufficient to conclude that the incidence of asymptomatic reactivation in these women is about 2% and that the attack rate for their exposed infants is approximately 2% or less. Because laboratory methods cannot be used to detect asymptomatic infection in a timely manner, the current approach to management is to perform a careful vaginal examination at presentation and to elect cesarean delivery if the mother has signs or symptoms of recurrent genital herpes at the onset of labor. Given the low probability of neonatal infection, it is appropriate to deliver infants of women who have a history of recurrent genital herpes but who have no active clinical disease at delivery by the vaginal route.[67] An analysis of the occurrence of HSV infections in infants in California showed no change from 1985 to 1995, despite a documented decrease in deliveries by cesarean section and an increase in the proportion of women with a previous diagnosis of genital herpes whose infants were delivered vaginally.[155]

A culture for HSV obtained at the time of delivery may be useful in establishing whether the virus was present at delivery to facilitate recognition of neonatal infection if it occurs. The value of this approach has not been established, however. Alternative diagnostic approaches, such as those based on PCR assay to detect virus, may ultimately expedite identification of women at risk for delivering infected infants.[156,157] Evidence indicates that detection of viral presence in genital samples by PCR assay is more sensitive than culture methods. The significance of a positive PCR result in predicting risk of transmission of HSV to the infant is unknown, however.[158] Viral DNA can persist for a longer interval than infectious virus.

The utility of suppressive therapy of genital herpes in women with a known history of recurrent infection remains a question for clinical investigation because of risk-benefit considerations. Some studies indicate that prophylactic acyclovir (400 mg three times daily) reduces the number of genital lesions from HSV. Despite prophylaxis, a few women continue to have virus detectable by PCR assay.[158] Use of prophylactic valacyclovir also reduced clinical HSV recurrences but did not decrease shedding of HSV within 7 days of delivery compared with placebo.[159] Even with suppressive therapy, the potential for neonatal HSV infection is not eliminated entirely, and cases of neonatal HSV after delivery to women on antiviral suppression have been reported.[160] Based on limited scientific evidence, the American College of Obstetricians and Gynecologists recommends that women with active recurrent genital herpes should be offered suppressive viral therapy at or beyond 36 weeks of gestation until delivery.[67] Universal antenatal type-specific HSV screening to prevent neonatal HSV is not recommended.[161]

MANAGEMENT OF INFANTS OF MOTHERS WITH GENITAL HERPES

Infants of mothers with histories of genital herpes delivered vaginally or by cesarean section and whose mothers have no evidence of active genital herpetic infection are at low risk for acquiring neonatal HSV infection. These infants need no special evaluation during the newborn period.

Infants delivered to women with clinically apparent genital herpetic lesions are at known risk for acquisition of neonatal HSV. However, the magnitude of the risk is influenced by the category of maternal infection, with women with first episode primary or nonprimary genital infection being at 30 to 50 times the likelihood of having their babies acquire neonatal HSV than women with recurrent genital infection. The American Academy of Pediatrics (AAP) recently released a clinical report that seeks to provide guidance on the management of these babies, using serologic and virologic testing to ascertain the level of risk and then providing recommendations on management of the infants accordingly.[14] The algorithms from this clinical report are reproduced in Figures 27-5 and 27-6.

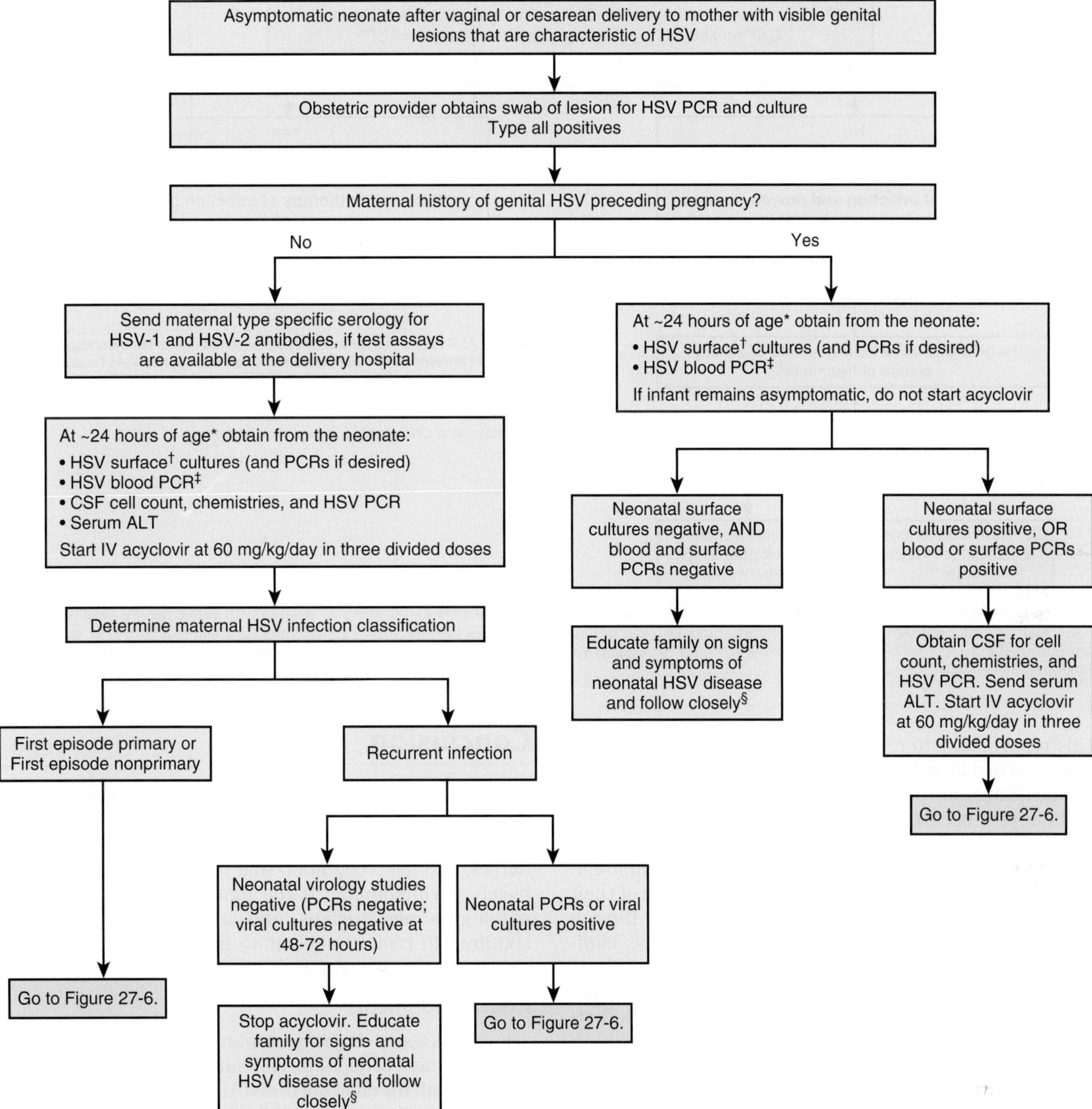

This algorithm should be applied only in facilities where access to PCR and type-specific serologic testing is readily available and turnaround time for test results is appropriately short. In situations where this is not possible, the approach detailed in the algorithm will have limited, and perhaps no, applicability.

**Evaluation and treatment is indicated before 24 hours of age if the infant develops signs and symptoms of neonatal HSV disease. In addition, immediate evaluation and treatment may be considered if:*

- *There is prolonged rupture of membranes (>4-6 hours)*
- *The infant is premature (≤37 weeks' gestation)*

†Conjunctivae, mouth, nasopharynx, and rectum, and scalp electrode site, if present

‡HSV blood PCR is not used for assignment of disease classification

§Discharge after 48 hours of negative HSV cultures (and negative PCRs) is acceptable if other discharge criteria have been met, there is ready access to medical care, and a person who is able to comply fully with instructions for home observation will be present. If any of these conditions is not met, the infant should be observed in the hospital until HSV cultures are finalized as negative or are negative for 96 hours after being set up in cell culture, whichever is shorter.

Figure 27-5 Algorithm for the evaluation of asymptomatic neonates after vaginal or cesarean delivery to women with active genital herpes lesions. *ALT,* Alanine aminotransferase; *CSF,* cerebrospinal fluid; *HSV,* herpes simplex virus; *IV,* intravenous; *PCR,* polymerase chain reaction. (Modified from Kimberlin DW, Baley J: Guidance on management of asymptomatic neonates born to women with active genital herpes lesions, *Pediatrics* 131:e635-e646, 2013.)

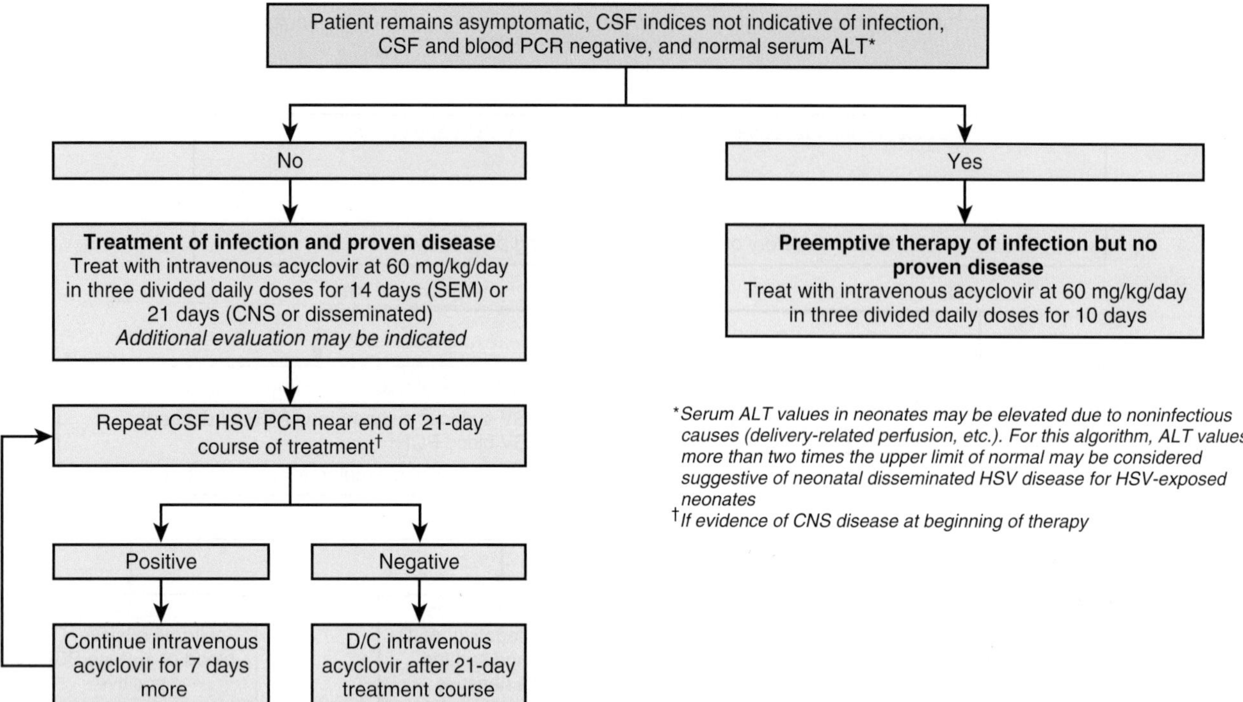

Figure 27-6 Algorithm for the treatment of asymptomatic neonates after vaginal or cesarean delivery to women with active genital herpes lesions. *ALT,* Alanine aminotransferase; *CSF,* cerebrospinal fluid; D/C, discontinue; *HSV,* herpes simplex virus; *PCR,* polymerase chain reaction; *SEM,* skin, eyes, or mouth. (Modified from Kimberlin DW, Baley J: Guidance on management of asymptomatic neonates born to women with active genital herpes lesions, *Pediatrics* 131:e635-e646, 2013.)

This report seeks to move beyond the recommendations that preceded its publication in 2013 that "some experts" do one thing and "other experts" do something else. Parts of the report use expert consensus in some of its recommendations, such as preemptive therapy with parenteral acyclovir in neonates delivered to women with first-episode primary and nonprimary infections because of their substantial risk of neonatal HSV disease, even though such an approach has not been, and never will be, clinically investigated. However, these expert consensus recommendations are grounded in the risk assessments derived from categorizing the mother's infection as first-episode primary, first-episode nonprimary, and recurrent. The clinical report was written by the AAP Committee on Infectious Diseases and Committee on Fetus and Newborn and was supported by the American College of Obstetricians and Gynecologists.

An issue of frequent concern is whether the mother with an active genital HSV infection at delivery should be isolated from her infant after delivery. Women with recurrent orolabial HSV infection and cutaneous HSV infections at other sites (e.g., breast lesions) are at similar risk for transmission of virus to their newborns. Because transmission occurs by direct contact with the virus, appropriate precautions by the mother, including careful hand washing before touching the infant, should prevent any need to separate mother and child. In some cases, it is possible to have the exposed infant room-in with the mother as a means of isolating the infant from other newborns. Breastfeeding is contraindicated if the mother has vesicular lesions involving the breast.

Conclusion

Neonatal HSV infection is a life-threatening disease in the newborn. With an increasing prevalence of HSV-1 genital herpes, a continuing high prevalence of HSV-2 genital herpes, and the recognition that many infections are completely asymptomatic in the mother, pediatricians, neonatologists, obstetricians, and family practitioners must continue to remain vigilant to infants whose symptoms may be compatible with HSV infections.

Acknowledgments

The databases on clinical presentations, diagnosis, and antiviral treatment of neonatal HSV infections have been generated through the efforts of the NIAID Collaborative Antiviral Study Group for more than 35 years, with support from the National Institute of Allergy and Infectious Diseases. The Institute also has supported prognostic studies of HSV infection in pregnancy and newborns in the United States.

References

1. Hass M: Hepatoadrenal necrosis with intranuclear inclusion bodies: report of a case, *Am J Pathol* 11:127, 1935.
2. Batignani A: Conjunctivite da virus erpetico in neonato, *Boll Ocul* 13:1217, 1934.
3. Nahmias AJ, Dowdle WR: Antigenic and biologic differences in herpesvirus hominis, *Prog Med Virol* 10:110-159, 1968.
4. Roizman B, Knipe DM, Whitley RJ: Herpes simplex viruses. In Knipe DM, Howley PM, editors: *Fields virology*, ed 5, vol 2, Philadelphia, 2007, Lippincott Williams & Wilkins, pp 2501-2601.
5. Spear PG: Membrane fusion induced by herpes simplex virus. In Bentz J, editor: *Viral fusion mechanisms*. Boca Raton, Fla, 1993, CRC Press, pp 201-232.

6. Roizman B, Norrild B, Chan C, et al: Identification and preliminary mapping with monoclonal antibodies of a herpes simplex virus 2 glycoprotein lacking a known type 1 counterpart, *Virology* 133: 242-247, 1984.
7. Markert JM, Gillespie GY, Weichselbaum RR, et al: Genetically engineered HSV in the treatment of glioma: a review, *Rev Med Virol* 10:17-30, 2000.
8. York IA, Roop C, Andrews DW, et al: A cytosolic herpes simplex virus protein inhibits antigen presentation to CD8+ T lymphocytes, *Cell* 77:525-535, 1994.
9. Jugovic P, Hill AM, Tomazin R, et al: Inhibition of major histocompatibility complex class I antigen presentation in pig and primate cells by herpes simplex virus type 1 and 2 ICP47, *J Virol* 72: 5076-5084, 1998.
10. Sullender WM, Yasukawa LL, Schwartz M, et al: Type-specific antibodies to herpes simplex virus type 2 (HSV-2) glycoprotein G in pregnant women, infants exposed to maternal HSV-2 infection at delivery, and infants with neonatal herpes, *J Infect Dis* 157:164-171, 1988.
11. Coleman RM, Pereira L, Bailey PD, et al: Determination of herpes simplex virus type-specific antibodies by enzyme-linked immunosorbent assay, *J Clin Microbiol* 18:287-291, 1983.
12. Wald A, Ashley-Morrow R: Serological testing for herpes simplex virus (HSV)-1 and HSV-2 infection, *Clin Infect Dis* 35:S173-S182, 2002.
13. Ashley RL, Wu L, Pickering JW, et al: Premarket evaluation of a commercial glycoprotein G-based enzyme immunoassay for herpes simplex virus type-specific antibodies, *J Clin Microbiol* 36:294-295, 1998.
14. Kimberlin DW, Baley J: Guidance on management of asymptomatic neonates born to women with active genital herpes lesions, *Pediatrics* 131:e635-e646, 2013.
15. Cushing H: Surgical aspects of major neuralgia of trigeminal nerve: report of 20 cases of operation upon the gasserian ganglion with anatomic and physiologic notes on the consequence of its removal, *JAMA* 44:1002-1009, 1905.
16. Goodpasture EW: Herpetic infection, with especial reference to involvement of the nervous system 1929, *Medicine (Baltimore)* 72:125-132, 1993; discussion 133–135.
17. Carton CA, Kilbourne ED: Activation of latent herpes simplex by trigeminal sensory-root section, *N Engl J Med* 246:172-176, 1952.
18. Pazin GJ, Armstrong JA, Lam MT, et al: Prevention of reactivated herpes simplex infection by human leukocyte interferon after operation on the trigeminal root, *N Engl J Med* 301:225-230, 1979.
19. Cunningham AL, Diefenbach RJ, Miranda-Saksena M, et al: The cycle of human herpes simplex virus infection: virus transport and immune control, *J Infect Dis* 194(Suppl 1):S11-S18, 2006.
20. Stevens JG, Cook ML: Latent herpes simplex virus in spinal ganglia of mice, *Science* 173:843-845, 1971.
21. Rock DL, Fraser NW: Detection of HSV-1 genome in central nervous system of latently infected mice, *Nature* 302:523-525, 1983.
22. Baringer JR: Recovery of herpes simplex virus from human sacral ganglions, *N Engl J Med* 291:828-830, 1974.
23. Xu F, Lee FK, Morrow RA, et al: Seroprevalence of herpes simplex virus type 1 in children in the United States, *J Pediatr* 151:374-377, 2007.
24. Xu F, Markowitz LE, Gottlieb SL, et al: Seroprevalence of herpes simplex virus types 1 and 2 in pregnant women in the United States, *Am J Obstet Gynecol* 196:43.e1-43.e6, 2007.
25. Wentworth BB, Alexander ER: Seroepidemiology of infections due to members of the herpesvirus group, *Am J Epidemiol* 94:496-507, 1971.
26. Arvin AM: The epidemiology of perinatal herpes simplex infections. In Stanberry L, editor: *Genital and neonatal herpes*, New York, 1996, John Wiley and Sons, pp 179-192.
27. Nahmias AJ, Josey WE, Naib ZM, et al: Antibodies to *Herpesvirus hominis* types 1 and 2 in humans. I. Patients with genital herpetic infections, *Am J Epidemiol* 91:539-546, 1970.
28. Bradley H, Markowitz LE, Gibson T, et al: Seroprevalence of herpes simplex virus types 1 and 2—United States, 1999-2010, *J Infect Dis* 209:325-333, 2013.
29. Kimberlin DW: The scarlet H, *J Infect Dis* 209:315-317, 2013.
30. Roberts CM, Pfister JR, Spear SJ: Increasing proportion of herpes simplex virus type 1 as a cause of genital herpes infection in college students, *Sex Transm Dis* 30:797-800, 2003.
31. Belshe RB, Leone PA, Bernstein DI, et al: Efficacy results of a trial of a herpes simplex vaccine, *N Engl J Med* 366:34-43, 2012.
32. Bernstein DI, Bellamy AR, Hook EW 3rd, et al: Epidemiology, clinical presentation, and antibody response to primary infection with herpes simplex virus type 1 and type 2 in young women, *Clin Infect Dis* 56:344-351, 2013.
33. Wald A, Zeh J, Selke S, et al: Virologic characteristics of subclinical and symptomatic genital herpes infections, *N Engl J Med* 333: 770-775, 1995.
34. Frenkel LM, Garratty EM, Shen JP, et al: Clinical reactivation of herpes simplex virus type 2 infection in seropositive pregnant women with no history of genital herpes, *Ann Intern Med* 118:414-418, 1993.
35. Fleming DT, McQuillan GM, Johnson RE, et al: Herpes simplex virus type 2 in the United States, 1976 to 1994, *N Engl J Med* 337: 1105-1111, 1997.
36. Xu F, Sternberg MR, Kottiri BJ, et al: Trends in herpes simplex virus type 1 and type 2 seroprevalence in the United States, *JAMA* 296:964-973, 2006.
37. Smith JS, Robinson NJ: Age-specific prevalence of infection with herpes simplex virus types 2 and 1: a global review, *J Infect Dis* 186: S3-S28, 2002.
38. Buchman TG, Roizman B, Nahmias AJ: Demonstration of exogenous genital reinfection with herpes simplex virus type 2 by restriction endonuclease fingerprinting of viral DNA, *J Infect Dis* 140:295-304, 1979.
39. Schmidt OW, Fife KH, Corey L: Reinfection is an uncommon occurrence in patients with symptomatic recurrent genital herpes, *J Infect Dis* 149:645-646, 1984.
40. Lakeman AD, Nahmias AJ, Whitley RJ: Analysis of DNA from recurrent genital herpes simplex virus isolates by restriction endonuclease digestion, *Sex Transm Dis* 13:61-66, 1986.
41. Boucher FD, Yasukawa LL, Bronzan RN, et al: A prospective evaluation of primary genital herpes simplex virus type 2 infections acquired during pregnancy, *Pediatr Infect Dis J* 9:499-504, 1990.
42. Brown ZA, Vontver LA, Benedetti J, et al: Genital herpes in pregnancy: risk factors associated with recurrences and asymptomatic viral shedding, *Am J Obstet Gynecol* 153:24-30, 1985.
43. Prober CG, Hensleigh PA, Boucher FD, et al: Use of routine viral cultures at delivery to identify neonates exposed to herpes simplex virus, *N Engl J Med* 318:887-891, 1988.
44. Kulhanjian JA, Soroush V, Au DS, et al: Identification of women at unsuspected risk of primary infection with herpes simplex virus type 2 during pregnancy, *N Engl J Med* 326:916-920, 1992.
45. Brown ZA, Vontver LA, Benedetti J, et al: Effects on infants of a first episode of genital herpes during pregnancy, *N Engl J Med* 317:1246-1251, 1987.
46. Brown ZA, Benedetti J, Ashley R, et al: Neonatal herpes simplex virus infection in relation to asymptomatic maternal infection at the time of labor, *N Engl J Med* 324:1247-1252, 1991.
47. Wald A, Zeh J, Selke S, et al: Reactivation of genital herpes simplex virus type 2 infection in asymptomatic seropositive persons, *N Engl J Med* 342:844-850, 2000.
48. Tronstein E, Johnston C, Huang ML, et al: Genital shedding of herpes simplex virus among symptomatic and asymptomatic persons with HSV-2 infection, *JAMA* 305:1441-1449, 2011.
49. Brown ZA, Wald A, Morrow RA, et al: Effect of serologic status and cesarean delivery on transmission rates of herpes simplex virus from mother to infant, *JAMA* 289:203-209, 2003.
50. Engelberg R, Carrell D, Krantz E, et al: Natural history of genital herpes simplex virus type 1 infection, *Sex Transm Dis* 30:174-177, 2003.
51. Gardella C, Brown ZA: Managing genital herpes infections in pregnancy, *Cleve Clin J Med* 74:217-224, 2007.
52. Wald A, Corey L, Cone R, et al: Frequent genital herpes simplex virus 2 shedding in immunocompetent women. Effect of acyclovir treatment, *J Clin Invest* 99:1092-1097, 1997.
53. Flewett TH, Parker RG, Philip WM: Acute hepatitis due to herpes simplex virus in an adult, *J Clin Pathol* 22:60-66, 1969.
54. Young EJ, Killam AP, Greene JF Jr: Disseminated herpesvirus infection. Association with primary genital herpes in pregnancy, *JAMA* 235:2731-2733, 1976.
55. Hensleigh PA, Andrews WW, Brown Z, et al: Genital herpes during pregnancy: inability to distinguish primary and recurrent infections clinically, *Obstet Gynecol* 89:891-895, 1997.
56. Nahmias AJ, Josey WE, Naib ZM, et al: Perinatal risk associated with maternal genital herpes simplex virus infection, *Am J Obstet Gynecol* 110:825-837, 1971.

57. Brown ZA, Selke S, Zeh J, et al: The acquisition of herpes simplex virus during pregnancy, *N Engl J Med* 337:509-515, 1997.
58. Dietrich YM, Napolitano PG: Acyclovir treatment of primary herpes in pregnancy complicated by second trimester preterm premature rupture of membranes with term delivery: case report, *Am J Perinatol* 19:235-238, 2002.
59. Arvin AM, Hensleigh PA, Prober CG, et al: Failure of antepartum maternal cultures to predict the infant's risk of exposure to herpes simplex virus at delivery, *N Engl J Med* 315:796-800, 1986.
60. Prober CG, Sullender WM, Yasukawa LL, et al: Low risk of herpes simplex virus infections in neonates exposed to the virus at the time of vaginal delivery to mothers with recurrent genital herpes simplex virus infections, *N Engl J Med* 316:240-244, 1987.
61. Whitley RJ, Corey L, Arvin A, et al: Changing presentation of herpes simplex virus infection in neonates, *J Infect Dis* 158:109-116, 1988.
62. Kimberlin DW, Rouse DJ: Genital herpes, *N Engl J Med* 350:1970-1977, 2004.
63. Corey L, Adams HG, Brown ZA, et al: Genital herpes simplex virus infections: clinical manifestations, course, and complications, *Ann Internl Med* 98:958-972, 1983.
64. Johnston C, Magaret A, Selke S, et al: Herpes simplex virus viremia during primary genital infection, *J Infect Dis* 198:31-34, 2008.
65. Yeager AS, Arvin AM, Urbani LJ, et al: Relationship of antibody to outcome in neonatal herpes simplex virus infections, *Infect Immun* 29:532-538, 1980.
66. Sullender WM, Miller JL, Yasukawa LL, et al: Humoral and cell-mediated immunity in neonates with herpes simplex virus infection, *J Infect Dis* 155:28-37, 1987.
67. ACOG Committee on Practice Bulletins: ACOG Practice Bulletin: Management of herpes in pregnancy. No. 82 June 2007. Clinical management guidelines for obstetrician-gynecologists, *Obstet Gynecol* 109:1489-1498, 2007.
68. Stone KM, Brooks CA, Guinan ME, et al: National surveillance for neonatal herpes simplex virus infections, *Sex Transm Dis* 16: 152-156, 1989.
69. Kaye EM, Dooling EC: Neonatal herpes simplex meningoencephalitis associated with fetal monitor scalp electrodes, *Neurology* 31: 1045-1047, 1981.
70. Parvey LS, Ch'ien LT: Neonatal herpes simplex virus infection introduced by fetal-monitor scalp electrodes, *Pediatrics* 65:1150-1153, 1980.
71. Nahmias AJ, Keyserling HL, Kerrick GM: Herpes simplex. In Remington JS, Klein JO, editors: *Infectious diseases of the fetus and newborn infants*, ed 2, Philadelphia, 1983, Saunders, pp 636-678.
72. Sullivan-Bolyai J, Hull HF, Wilson C, et al: Neonatal herpes simplex virus infection in King County, Washington. Increasing incidence and epidemiologic correlates, *JAMA* 250:3059-3062, 1983.
73. Gaytant MA, Steegers EA, van Cromvoirt PL, et al: Incidence of herpes neonatorum in Netherlands, *Ned Tijdschr Geneeskd* 144: 1832-1836, 2000.
74. Caviness AC, Demmler GJ, Almendarez Y, et al: The prevalence of neonatal herpes simplex virus infection compared with serious bacterial illness in hospitalized neonates, *J Pediatr* 153:164-169, 2008.
75. Baldwin S, Whitley RJ: Intrauterine herpes simplex virus infection, *Teratology* 39:1-10, 1989.
76. Florman AL, Gershon AA, Blackett PR, et al: Intrauterine infection with herpes simplex virus. Resultant congenital malformations, *JAMA* 225:129-132, 1973.
77. Hutto C, Arvin A, Jacobs R, et al: Intrauterine herpes simplex virus infections, *J Pediatr* 110:97-101, 1987.
78. South MA, Tompkins WA, Morris CR, et al: Congenital malformation of the central nervous system associated with genital type (type 2) herpesvirus, *J Pediatr* 75:13-18, 1969.
79. Kahlon J, Whitley RJ: Antibody response of the newborn after herpes simplex virus infection, *J Infect Dis* 158:925-933, 1988.
80. Karesh JW, Kapur S, MacDonald M: Herpes simplex virus and congenital malformations, *South Med J* 76:1561-1563, 1983.
81. Monif GR, Kellner KR, Donnelly WH Jr: Congenital herpes simplex type II infection, *Am J Obstet Gynecol* 152:1000-1002, 1985.
82. Garcia AG: Maternal herpes-simplex infection causing abortion. Histopathologic study of the placenta, *Hospital (Rio J)* 78:1267-1274, 1970.
83. Arvin AM: Fetal and neonatal infections. In Nathanson N, Murphy F, editors: *Viral pathogenesis*, New York, 1996, Lippincott-Raven, pp 801-814.
84. Alanen A, Hukkanen V: Herpes simplex virus DNA in amniotic fluid without neonatal infection, *Clin Infect Dis* 30:363-367, 2000.
85. Kimberlin DW, Lin CY, Jacobs RF, et al: Natural history of neonatal herpes simplex virus infections in the acyclovir era, *Pediatrics* 108:223-229, 2001.
86. Douglas J, Schmidt O, Corey L: Acquisition of neonatal HSV-1 infection from a paternal source contact, *J Pediatr* 103:908-910, 1983.
87. Hammerberg O, Watts J, Chernesky M, et al: An outbreak of herpes simplex virus type 1 in an intensive care nursery, *Pediatr Infect Dis* 2:290-294, 1983.
88. Light IJ: Postnatal acquisition of herpes simplex virus by the newborn infant: a review of the literature, *Pediatrics* 63:480-482, 1979.
89. Linnemann CC Jr, Buchman TG, Light IJ, et al: Transmission of herpes-simplex virus type 1 in a nursery for the newborn. Identification of viral isolates by D.N.A. "fingerprinting", *Lancet* 1:964-966, 1978.
90. Yeager AS, Ashley RL, Corey L: Transmission of herpes simplex virus from father to neonate, *J Pediatr* 103:905-907, 1983.
91. Sullivan-Bolyai JZ, Fife KH, Jacobs RF, et al: Disseminated neonatal herpes simplex virus type 1 from a maternal breast lesion, *Pediatrics* 71:455-457, 1983.
92. Hatherley LI, Hayes K, Jack I: Herpes virus in an obstetric hospital. II: Asymptomatic virus excretion in staff members, *Med J Aust* 2: 273-275, 1980.
93. Hatherley LI, Hayes K, Jack I: Herpes virus in an obstetric hospital. III: Prevalence of antibodies in patients and staff, *Med J Aust* 2: 325-329, 1980.
94. Burchett SK, Corey L, Mohan KM, et al: Diminished interferon-gamma and lymphocyte proliferation in neonatal and postpartum primary herpes simplex virus infection, *J Infect Dis* 165:813-818, 1992.
95. Chilmonczyk BA, Levin MJ, McDuffy R, et al: Characterization of the human newborn response to herpesvirus antigen, *J Immunol* 134:4184-4188, 1985.
96. Kohl S, Harmon MW: Human neonatal leukocyte interferon production and natural killer cytotoxicity in response to herpes simplex virus, *J Interferon Res* 3:461-463, 1983.
97. Kohl S, West MS, Prober CG, et al: Neonatal antibody-dependent cellular cytotoxic antibody levels are associated with the clinical presentation of neonatal herpes simplex virus infection, *J Infect Dis* 160:770-776, 1989.
98. Pass RF, Dworsky ME, Whitley RJ, et al: Specific lymphocyte blastogenic responses in children with cytomegalovirus and herpes simplex virus infections acquired early in infancy, *Infect Immun* 34:166-170, 1981.
99. Kohl S: Neonatal herpes simplex virus infection, *Clin Perinatol* 24:129-150, 1997.
100. Mintz L, Drew WL, Hoo R, et al: Age-dependent resistance of human alveolar macrophages to herpes simplex virus, *Infect Immun* 28: 417-420, 1980.
101. Hirsch MS, Zisman B, Allison AC: Macrophages and age-dependent resistance to Herpes simplex virus in mice, *J Immunol* 104:1160-1165, 1970.
102. Diamond C, Mohan K, Hobson A, et al: Viremia in neonatal herpes simplex virus infections, *Pediatr Infect Dis J* 18:487-489, 1999.
103. Kawada J, Kimura H, Ito Y, et al: Evaluation of systemic inflammatory responses in neonates with herpes simplex virus infection, *J Infect Dis* 190:494-498, 2004.
104. Singer DB: Pathology of neonatal herpes simplex virus infection, *Perspect Pediatr Pathol* 6:243-278, 1981.
105. Kimberlin DW, Whitley RJ, Wan W, et al: Oral acyclovir suppression and neurodevelopment after neonatal herpes, *N Engl J Med* 365:1284-1292, 2011.
106. Whitley R, Arvin A, Prober C, et al: Predictors of morbidity and mortality in neonates with herpes simplex virus infections, *N Engl J Med* 324:450-454, 1991.
107. Nahmias AJ, Alford CA, Korones SB: Infection of the newborn with herpesvirus hominis, *Adv Pediatr* 17:185-226, 1970.
108. Kimberlin DW, Lin CY, Jacobs RF, et al: Safety and efficacy of high-dose intravenous acyclovir in the management of neonatal herpes simplex virus infections, *Pediatrics* 108:230-238, 2001.
109. Whitley R, Arvin A, Prober C, et al: A controlled trial comparing vidarabine with acyclovir in neonatal herpes simplex virus infection, *N Engl J Med* 324:444-449, 1991.

110. Whitley RJ, Nahmias AJ, Soong SJ, et al: Vidarabine therapy of neonatal herpes simplex virus infection, *Pediatrics* 66:495-501, 1980.
111. Kimberlin DW: Neonatal herpes simplex infection, *Clin Microbiol Rev* 17:1-13, 2004.
112. Anderson MS, Abzug MJ: Hydrops fetalis: an unusual presentation of intrauterine herpes simplex virus infection, *Pediatr Infect Dis J* 18:837-839, 1999.
113. Malm G, Berg U, Forsgren M: Neonatal herpes simplex: clinical findings and outcome in relation to type of maternal infection, *Acta Paediatr* 84:256-260, 1995.
114. Arvin AM, Yeager AS, Bruhn FW, et al: Neonatal herpes simplex infection in the absence of mucocutaneous lesions, *J Pediatr* 100:715-721, 1982.
115. Greenes DS, Rowitch D, Thorne GM, et al: Neonatal herpes simplex virus infection presenting as fulminant liver failure, *Pediatr Infect Dis J* 14:242-244, 1995.
116. Lee WS, Kelly DA, Tanner MS, et al: Neonatal liver transplantation for fulminant hepatitis caused by herpes simplex virus type 2, *J Pediatr Gastroenterol Nutr* 35:220-223, 2002.
117. Ford A, Swing DC Jr, Tobin JR, et al: A 10-day-old neonate with fulminant hepatitis, *J Paediatr Child Health* 44:471-472, 2008.
118. Golden SE: Neonatal herpes simplex viremia, *Pediatr Infect Dis J* 7:425-427, 1988.
119. Gressens P, Martin JR: HSV-2 DNA persistence in astrocytes of the trigeminal root entry zone: double labeling by in situ PCR and immunohistochemistry, *J Neuropathol Exp Neurol* 53:127-135, 1994.
120. Langlet C, Gaugler C, Castaing M, et al: An uncommon case of disseminated neonatal herpes simplex infection presenting with pneumonia and pleural effusions, *Eur J Pediatr* 162:532-533, 2003.
121. O'Riordan DP, Golden WC, Aucott SW: Herpes simplex virus infections in preterm infants, *Pediatrics* 118:e1612-e1620, 2006.
122. Whitley RJ, Kimberlin DW: Treatment of viral infections during pregnancy and the neonatal period, *Clin Perinatol* 24:267-283, 1997.
123. Kimberlin DW: Herpes simplex virus infections of the central nervous system, *Semin Pediatr Infect Dis* 14:83-89, 2003.
124. Mizrahi EM, Tharp BR: A characteristic EEG pattern in neonatal herpes simplex encephalitis, *Neurology* 32:1215-1220, 1982.
125. O'Reilly MA, O'Reilly PM, de Bruyn R: Neonatal herpes simplex type 2 encephalitis: its appearances on ultrasound and CT, *Pediatr Radiol* 25:68-69, 1995.
126. Toth C, Harder S, Yager J: Neonatal herpes encephalitis: a case series and review of clinical presentation, *Can J Neurol Sci* 30:36-40, 2003.
127. Pelligra G, Lynch N, Miller SP, et al: Brainstem involvement in neonatal herpes simplex virus type 2 encephalitis, *Pediatrics* 120: e442-e446, 2007.
128. Kimura H, Ito Y, Futamura M, et al: Quantitation of viral load in neonatal herpes simplex virus infection and comparison between type 1 and type 2, *J Med Virol* 67:349-353, 2002.
129. Gutman LT, Wilfert CM, Eppes S: Herpes simplex virus encephalitis in children: analysis of cerebrospinal fluid and progressive neurodevelopmental deterioration, *J Infect Dis* 154:415-421, 1986.
130. Music SI, Fine EM, Togo Y: Zoster-like disease in the newborn due to herpes-simplex virus, *N Engl J Med* 284:24-26, 1971.
131. Nahmias AJ, Hagler WS: Ocular manifestation of herpes simplex in the newborn (neonatal ocular herpes), *Int Ophthalmol Clin* 12: 191-213, 1972.
132. Kimberlin DW, Lakeman FD, Arvin AM, et al: Application of the polymerase chain reaction to the diagnosis and management of neonatal herpes simplex virus disease, *J Infect Dis* 174:1162-1167, 1996.
133. Cherry JD, Soriano F, Jahn CL: Search for perinatal viral infection. A prospective, clinical, virologic, and serologic study, *Am J Dis Child* 116:245-250, 1968.
134. Whitley RJ, Lakeman F: Herpes simplex virus infections of the central nervous system: therapeutic and diagnostic considerations, *Clin Infect Dis* 20:414-420, 1995.
135. Kimura H, Futamura M, Kito H, et al: Detection of viral DNA in neonatal herpes simplex virus infections: frequent and prolonged presence in serum and cerebrospinal fluid, *J Infect Dis* 164:289-293, 1991.
136. Troendle-Atkins J, Demmler GJ, Buffone GJ: Rapid diagnosis of herpes simplex virus encephalitis by using the polymerase chain reaction, *J Pediatr* 123:376-380, 1993.
137. Malm G, Forsgren M: Neonatal herpes simplex virus infections: HSV DNA in cerebrospinal fluid and serum, *Arch Dis Child Fetal Neonatal Ed* 81:F24-F29, 1999.
138. Weil AA, Glaser CA, Amad Z, et al: Patients with suspected herpes simplex encephalitis: rethinking an initial negative polymerase chain reaction result, *Clin Infect Dis* 34:1154-1157, 2002.
139. Barbi M, Binda S, Primache V, et al: Use of Guthrie cards for the early diagnosis of neonatal herpes simplex virus disease, *Pediatr Infect Dis J* 17:251-252, 1998.
140. Lewensohn-Fuchs I, Osterwall P, Forsgren M, et al: Detection of herpes simplex virus DNA in dried blood spots making a retrospective diagnosis possible, *J Clin Virol* 26:39-48, 2003.
141. American Academy of Pediatrics: Herpes simplex. In Pickering LK, Baker CJ, Kimberlin DW, Long SS, editors: *Red book: 2012 report of the Committee on Infectious Diseases*, ed 29, Elk Grove Village, Ill, 2012, American Academy of Pediatrics, pp 398-408.
142. Elion GB, Furman PA, Fyfe JA, et al: Selectivity of action of an antiherpetic agent, 9-(2-hydroxyethoxymethyl) guanine, *Proc Natl Acad Sci U S A* 74:5716-5720, 1977.
143. Whitley RJ, Yeager A, Kartus P, et al: Neonatal herpes simplex virus infection: follow-up evaluation of vidarabine therapy, *Pediatrics* 72:778-785, 1983.
144. Englund JA, Fletcher CV, Balfour HH Jr: Acyclovir therapy in neonates, *J Pediatr* 119:129-135, 1991.
145. American Academy of Pediatrics: Herpes simplex. In Pickering LK, editor: *Red book: 2000 report of the Committee on Infectious Diseases*, ed 25, Elk Grove Village, Ill, 2000, American Academy of Pediatrics, pp 309-318.
146. Long SS: In defense of empiric acyclovir therapy in certain neonates, *J Pediatr* 153:157-158, 2008.
147. Kimberlin DW: When should you initiate acyclovir therapy in a neonate? *J Pediatr* 153:155-156, 2008.
148. Nyquist AC, Rotbart HA, Cotton M, et al: Acyclovir-resistant neonatal herpes simplex virus infection of the larynx, *J Pediatr* 124: 967-971, 1994.
149. Oram RJ, Marcellino D, Strauss D, et al: Characterization of an acyclovir-resistant herpes simplex virus type 2 strain isolated from a premature neonate, *J Infect Dis* 181:1458-1461, 2000.
150. Levin MJ, Weinberg A, Leary JJ, et al: Development of acyclovir-resistant herpes simplex virus early during the treatment of herpes neonatorum, *Pediatr Infect Dis J* 20:1094-1097, 2001.
151. Kimberlin D, Powell D, Gruber W, et al: Administration of oral acyclovir suppressive therapy after neonatal herpes simplex virus disease limited to the skin, eyes and mouth: results of a phase I/II trial, *Pediatr Infect Dis J* 15:247-254, 1996.
152. Rabalais GP, Nusinoff-Lehrman S, Arvin AM, et al: Antiviral susceptibilities of herpes simplex virus isolates from infants with recurrent mucocutaneous lesions after neonatal infection, *Pediatr Infect Dis J* 8:221-223, 1989.
153. Tiffany KF, Benjamin DK Jr, Palasanthiran P, et al: Improved neurodevelopmental outcomes following long-term high-dose oral acyclovir therapy in infants with central nervous system and disseminated herpes simplex disease, *J Perinatol* 25:156-161, 2005.
154. Kohl S, Loo LS, Rench MA, et al: Effect of intravenously administered immune globulin on functional antibody to herpes simplex virus in low birth weight neonates, *J Pediatr* 115:135-139, 1989.
155. Gutierrez KM, Falkovitz Halpern MS, Maldonado Y, et al: The epidemiology of neonatal herpes simplex virus infections in California from 1985 to 1995, *J Infect Dis* 180:199-202, 1999.
156. Cone RW, Hobson AC, Brown Z, et al: Frequent detection of genital herpes simplex virus DNA by polymerase chain reaction among pregnant women, *JAMA* 272:792-796, 1994.
157. Hardy DA, Arvin AM, Yasukawa LL, et al: Use of polymerase chain reaction for successful identification of asymptomatic genital infection with herpes simplex virus in pregnant women at delivery, *J Infect Dis* 162:1031-1035, 1990.
158. Watts DH, Brown ZA, Money D, et al: A double-blind, randomized, placebo-controlled trial of acyclovir in late pregnancy for the reduction of herpes simplex virus shedding and cesarean delivery, *Am J Obstet Gynecol* 188:836-843, 2003.
159. Andrews WW, Kimberlin DF, Whitley R, et al: Valacyclovir therapy to reduce recurrent genital herpes in pregnant women, *Am J Obstet Gynecol* 194:774-781, 2006.
160. Pinninti SG, Angara R, Feja KN, et al: Neonatal herpes disease following maternal antenatal antiviral suppressive therapy: a multicenter case series, *J Pediatr* 161:134-138.e1-e3, 2012.
161. Tita AT, Grobman WA, Rouse DJ: Antenatal herpes serologic screening: an appraisal of the evidence, *Obstet Gynecol* 108:1247-1253, 2006.

28 Human Parvovirus

STUART P. ADLER and WILLIAM C. KOCH

CHAPTER OUTLINE

The parvoviruses are a family of single-stranded DNA viruses that have a wide cellular tropism and broad host range, causing infection in invertebrate species and vertebrates, from insects to mammals. Although many parvoviruses are important veterinary pathogens, there are only two human pathogens in the family: human parvovirus B19 and the more recently described human bocavirus.[1,2] Human bocavirus seems to be primarily a respiratory pathogen of young children and is not discussed further here. Human parvovirus B19 is most commonly referred to as parvovirus B19 or simply B19. B19 is the prototype of the genus *Erythrovirus* in the Parvoviridae family, and a new genus and name have been proposed for this virus, *Erythrovirus* B19,[3] based on its cellular tropism for erythroid lineage cells and to distinguish it from the other mammalian parvoviruses. Compared with most other common human viruses, B19 is a relatively new pathogen, but since its initial description, B19 has come to be associated with a variety of seemingly diverse clinical syndromes in many different patient populations (Table 28-1). Although

Table 28-1 Clinical Manifestations Associated With Parvovirus B19 Infection

Diseases	Primary Patient Groups
DISEASES ASSOCIATED WITH ACUTE INFECTION	
Erythema infectiosum (fifth disease)	Normal children
Polyarthropathy	Normal adolescents and adults
Transient aplastic crisis	Patients with hemolytic anemia or accelerated erythropoiesis or both
Papular-purpuric "gloves and socks" syndrome	Normal adolescents and adults
DISEASES ASSOCIATED WITH CHRONIC INFECTION	
Persistent anemia (red blood cell aplasia)	Immunodeficient or immunocompromised children and adults
Nonimmune fetal hydrops	Intrauterine infection
Congenital anemia	Intrauterine infection
Chronic arthropathy	Rare patients with parvovirus B19–induced joint disease
Infection-associated hemophagocytosis	Normal or immunocompromised patients
Vasculitis or purpura	Normal adults and children
Myocarditis	Intrauterine infection, normal infants and children, immunocompromised patients

Modified from Young NS, Brown KE: Parvovirus B19, *N Engl J Med* 350:586-597, 2004.

the list of clinical manifestations caused by B19 infection is probably not yet complete, some proposed relationships, such as to rheumatologic disease and neurologic disorders, remain controversial.[4,5]

Parvovirus B19 was accidentally discovered by Cossart and associates[6] in 1975 as an anomalous band of precipitation while screening blood donor serum for hepatitis B antigen by counterimmunoelectrophoresis. The name *B19* refers to the donor unit from which it was originally isolated. Initial analysis of the new virus revealed it had physical features characteristic of the known parvoviruses,[7] allowing classification in this family. Because the donors from whom it was originally isolated were asymptomatic, B19 infection was not initially associated with any illness, and for the next several years after its description, it was a virus in search of a disease.

In 1981, Pattison and colleagues[8] noted a high prevalence of antibodies to this virus in the serum of children hospitalized with transient aplastic crisis of sickle cell disease and proposed B19 as the viral cause of this clinically well-described event. Serjeant and colleagues[9] later confirmed this association in population studies of sickle cell patients in Jamaica. In 1983, 8 years after its initial description, Anderson and coworkers[10] proposed B19 as the cause of the common childhood exanthem erythema infectiosum (EI), or fifth disease. The name *fifth disease* derives from the 19th century practice of numbering the common exanthems of childhood—EI was the fifth rash designated in this scheme, and it is the only one for which this numeric designation has persisted in clinical practice.[11] The others in the series included measles, scarlet fever, rubella, and Filatov-Dukes disease (a mild variant of scarlet fever that is no longer recognized).

The possibility of fetal disease associated with EI was considered long before the viral etiology was known primarily because of comparison with rubella and the incidence of congenital rubella syndrome after community epidemics.[12-14] Advances in knowledge of the virology of other animal parvoviruses and their known propensity to cause disease in the fetus and newborn animal further fueled this concern.[15] This suspicion was confirmed in 1984 when two reports of B19 infection in pregnant women associated with adverse fetal outcomes appeared[16,17] and were later followed by a larger report of a series of cases of nonimmune hydrops fetalis caused by intrauterine infections with B19.[18] Over the ensuing decade, various clinical manifestations associated with acute and chronic infection have since been attributed to this virus in different patient groups (see Table 28-1).

Since the initial reports of fetal infection, knowledge of the epidemiology, pathophysiology, and short-term outcome of fetal and neonatal infection with B19 has increased immensely based on numerous large population-based studies.[19-23] B19 infection during pregnancy has probably been the subject of more such studies than any of the other manifestations with the possible exception of transient aplastic crisis of sickle cell disease. There is still much to be learned, however, regarding the long-term outcome of fetal infection, the clinical spectrum of infection in neonates, and the immunologic response to infection. Last, the potential for prevention through vaccine development is a topic of current interest and ongoing research.

Microbiology

Similar to other members of the family Parvoviridae, parvovirus B19 is a small, nonenveloped, single-stranded DNA virus. The taxonomy for this family has been revised to include two subfamilies, the Densovirinae, which are insect viruses, and the Parvovirinae, which infect vertebrates.[24,25] The Parvovirinae subfamily is composed of five genera, four of which are capable of infecting humans: *Dependovirus*, *Parvovirus*, *Erythrovirus*, and *Bocavirus*. The dependoviruses require coinfection with another unrelated helper virus (adenovirus or herpesvirus) to complete their life cycle. Some *Dependovirus* strains infect humans (e.g., adeno-associated viruses), but the infection is asymptomatic and without clinical consequence. In contrast to *Dependovirus* strains, members of the genera *Parvovirus*, *Erythrovirus*, and *Bocavirus* are able to replicate autonomously. Previously included in the genus *Parvovirus*, B19 is now classified as an *Erythrovirus*. At present, the genus *Erythrovirus* consists of only two members: B19 and a simian parvovirus that has a genomic organization similar to B19 and several related viruses identified in cynomolgus monkeys and macaques that have a similar genomic organization and a similar tropism for erythroid cells.[26] Although many parvoviruses are pathogenic to other mammals (e.g., canine parvovirus, feline panleukopenia virus), B19 and human bocavirus are the only parvoviruses proven to cause disease in humans. A fourth human parvovirus, termed Parv4, has been recently described.[27] Originally isolated from the blood of an intravenous drug abuser with hepatitis C, it has subsequently been found in plasma pools and asymptomatic blood donors.

To date, no disease has been associated with Parv4 infection, and its classification into a parvovirus genus awaits further evaluation of its genomic organization.[24]

There is only one recognized serotype of B19. Minor variations in the nucleotide sequence occur among different B19 viral isolates from different geographic areas, but these have not been definitely shown to affect clinical patterns of infection or pathogenicity.[28-29] Two isolates of human parvovirus, V9 and V6, whose nucleotide sequence differs significantly (>10%) from B19, have been described.[30,31] Both were isolated from patients with transient red blood cell aplasia indistinguishable clinically from typical B19-induced aplastic crisis. The clinical significance of these variants and whether they represent different genotypes or merely geographic variants of B19 remain topics of debate.[29,32]

The B19 genome is very small (approximately 5.6 kb) and contained within an icosahedral protein capsid. The capsid structure and lack of an envelope make the virus very resistant to heat and detergent inactivation, features that seem to be important in transmission. The genome seems to encode only three proteins. Two are capsid proteins, designated VP1 and VP2. VP2 is smaller but more abundant and makes up approximately 96% of the capsid protein. VP1 is larger and makes up about 4% of the capsid but contains a unique region that extends out from the capsid surface and serves as the attachment site for the cellular receptor.[4] VP2 has the unique ability to self-assemble into capsids that are morphologically and antigenically similar to B19 viruses when expressed in cell culture systems in vitro.[33,34] When present with VP1, the capsids incorporate proteins, but VP1 alone does not self-assemble.[33]

The third gene product is a nonstructural protein designated NS1. The function of this protein is unclear, but it has been shown to be involved in regulation of the viral promoter and seems to have a role in DNA replication.[25] Studies of NS1 have been hampered by the observation that it seems to be toxic to cells by an unknown mechanism.[35] More recent studies have further suggested that production of NS1 can lead to programmed cell death (apoptosis) mediated by stimulation of cytokine production.[36,37]

Because of its limited genomic complement, B19 requires a mitotically active host cell for replication. It can replicate only in certain erythroid lineage cells stimulated by erythropoietin, such as erythroid precursors found in bone marrow, fetal liver, umbilical cord blood, and a few erythroleukemic cell lines.[25,38-42] B19 cannot be propagated in standard cell cultures,[43] a fact that had previously limited the availability of viral products for development of diagnostic assays. Much of this limitation has been overcome by the development of molecular methods for the detection of viral nucleic acid and commercial assays for detection of both antibodies and viral DNA are available.

The cellular receptor for the virus has been identified as globoside, a neutral glycosphingolipid that is present on erythrocytes, where it represents the P blood group antigen.[44] The presence of this lipid is necessary for viral infection to occur, and individuals who lack this antigen (p phenotype) are naturally immune to B19 infection.[45] The P antigen is also present on other cells, such as endothelial cells, fetal myocardial cells, placenta, and megakaryocytes.[44] The tissue distribution of this receptor may explain some of the clinical manifestations of infection with this virus (see "Clinical Manifestations Other Than Intrauterine Infection").

Although the P antigen is necessary for B19 viral infection, it is insufficient because some cells, particularly nonerythroid tissues, that express the receptor are incapable of productive viral infection.[46] More recently, a co-receptor has been described on human cells that are permissive for B19 infection.[47] The hypothesis is that the globoside is necessary for viral attachment, but the co-receptors somehow allow viral entry into the cell where viral replication can occur. If confirmed, this hypothesis may provide an alternative explanation of the pathogenesis of infection in nonerythroid tissues that express globoside without a co-receptor.

General Aspects of Pathogenesis

Parvovirus B19 requires a mitotically active host cell to complete its full replicative life cycle. The primary target for B19 infection seems to be erythroid progenitor cells that are near the pronormoblast stage of development. The virus can be propagated only in human erythroid progenitor cells from bone marrow, umbilical cord blood, fetal liver, peripheral blood, and a few erythroid leukemic cell lines.[48] B19 lytically infects these cells with progressive loss of targeted cells as infection proceeds. In vitro hematopoietic assays show that B19 suppresses formation of erythroid colony-forming units, and this effect can be reversed by addition of serum containing anti-B19 immunoglobulin G (IgG) antibodies.[49]

The virus has little to no effect on the myeloid cell line in vitro but causes inhibition of megakaryocytopoiesis in vitro without viral replication or cell lysis.[50] Clinically, this is best illustrated in transient aplastic crisis of sickle cell disease. Patients have fever, weakness, and pallor on presentation, with a sudden and severe decrease in their reticulocyte count. This cessation of red blood cell production coupled with the shortened red blood cell survival because of chronic hemolysis produces a profound anemia. Examination of the bone marrow typically reveals hypoplasia of the erythroid cell line and a maturational arrest; giant pronormoblasts are often seen with intranuclear viral inclusions.[49] With development of specific antibodies, viral infection is controlled, and reticulocyte counts begin to increase.

Evaluation of infection in normal volunteers has shown similar hematologic changes, but because of the longer life of red blood cells, these changes are clinically insignificant.[51] Adult volunteers inoculated intranasally with B19 developed viremia after 5 to 6 days with a mild illness. Their reticulocyte counts decreased to undetectable levels, and this was accompanied by a modest decline in hemoglobin and hematocrit. Platelets and granulocyte counts also declined. Specific antibody production with IgM followed by IgG developed, and viremia was cleared rapidly. A second phase of illness developed at 17 to 18 days, with rash and arthralgias but without fever, and hematologic indices had returned to normal.

The tissue distribution of the cellular receptor for the virus (P antigen) may explain the predominance of hematologic findings associated with B19 infection. Its presence on other tissues may help to explain other clinical manifestations, such as myocardial disease, congenital infection, and vasculitis syndromes. Although the cellular receptor is present and the virus can attach, in contrast to the erythroid cell, these cells are nonpermissive for viral replication; that is, the virus is unable to undergo a complete life cycle with the resultant lysis of the host cells, as described previously. Instead, interaction in these tissues leads to accumulation of the nonstructural protein NS1. This protein is essential for viral replication and has various proposed functions,[25] but it seems to be toxic to most mammalian cell lines when present in excess.[35] NS1 has been associated with apoptosis and programmed cell death.[37,42] NS1 has also been linked to production of tumor necrosis factor-α and interleukin-6, a potent proinflammatory cytokine.[36,42,52] Cellular injury may occur through cytokine pathways and provide another mechanism aside from lytic infection for some of the clinical manifestations.

Chronic infections in immunocompromised patients develop when patients are unable to mount an adequate neutralizing antibody response. These infections are characterized by viral persistence in serum or bone marrow and lack of detectable circulating antibody. Clinical manifestations include chronic anemia or red blood cell aplasia and may include granulocytopenia and thrombocytopenia. The mechanism for leukopenia and thrombocytopenia is unknown, although it has been shown that B19 causes disturbances in megakaryocytic replication when infected in vitro.[50]

Epidemiology and Transmission

OVERVIEW

Parvovirus B19 is a highly contagious and common infection worldwide. In the United States, 60% or greater of white adults are seropositive (have IgG antibodies to B19 in their sera). This seropositivity indicates a previous infection usually acquired in childhood. Among African Americans, the rate of seropositivity is about 30%.[21] Transmission of B19 from person to person is probably by droplets from oral or nasal secretions. This mode of transmission is suggested by the rapid transmission among individuals in close physical contact, such as schoolmates or family members, and from a study of healthy adult volunteers experimentally infected with B19, in whom virus was found in blood and nasopharyngeal secretions for several days beginning 1 or 2 days before symptoms appeared.[51] In the volunteer study, no virus was detected in urine or stool.

Given the highly contagious nature of B19 infections, it is not surprising that most outbreaks occur in elementary schools and occasionally child care centers. Susceptible seronegative adult school personnel are at high risk for acquiring the infection from students.[21,53] Some outbreaks in schools may be seasonal, often late winter and spring, and epidemic, with many children and staff acquiring the infection and developing symptoms of EI. At other times, the infection is endemic, with transmission occurring slowly and with only a few manifesting symptoms.

GLOBAL DISTRIBUTION

Parvovirus B19 infections occur worldwide. Serologic evidence of B19 infection has been found everywhere studied, including developed countries, undeveloped countries, urban and rural areas, and isolated island populations.[54-59] The diseases and associated signs and symptoms are the same worldwide. No clinically or epidemiologically important strain or antigenic differences have been detected, and serologic assays are independent of the source or location of patient serum. Disease resulting from B19 seems to be unrelated to specific viral genotypes, although analysis of the antigenic variation or nucleotide sequences of widely dispersed B19 isolates shows some heterogeneity of unknown significance.[27,28,60-65]

SEASONALITY AND PERIODICITY

Transmission of parvovirus B19 continues throughout the year; however, there are seasonal variations in transmission rates. Outbreaks of EI most often occur in winter and spring in temperate climates and less frequently in fall and summer.[66-68] In schools or daycare centers, outbreaks of EI may persist for months, usually starting in late winter or early spring and ending with summer vacation. Figure 28-1 highlights multiyear outbreaks of B19 exposure among pregnant women and the associated seasonal variation in Pittsburgh, Pennsylvania. Yearly, most cases occurred in late spring and summer.

In the island nation of Jamaica, careful studies of people with sickle cell disease showed that epidemics of transient aplastic crises occurred about every 5 years, with little disease inside this interval.[69] Epidemics of B19 infections at 5-year intervals were also observed in Rio de Janeiro, Brazil.[70] In Japan, age-related serologic evaluation of stored serum samples showed no evidence for B19 epidemics over a 10-year period.[71] The prevalence of IgG antibodies to B19 among three tribes of Amerindians living in remote regions of Brazil was very low (<11%), and in one tribe, it was zero for people younger than 30 years.[57] School nursing records in Iowa over 14 years identified cases of EI in all but one year.[72]

SEROPREVALENCE BY AGE

In numerous studies of parvovirus B19 infection based on serologic testing, the seroprevalence of B19 infection increases with age.[6,69,73-78] Figure 28-2 shows the age-dependent increase in seroprevalence from Richmond, Virginia.[79] Transplacentally acquired maternal antibodies are undetectable by 1 year of age. In children younger than 5 years, the prevalence of IgG antibodies to B19 is usually less than 5%. The greatest increase in seroprevalence and B19 infection occurs between 5 and 20 years of age. By age 20 years, the seroprevalence of B19 infection increases from about 5% at 5 years of age to nearly 40%. Afterward, without regard to risk factors, B19 seroprevalence increases slowly. In adult blood donors, the seroprevalence of IgG antibodies to B19 ranges from 29% to 79% (median, 45%).[76-82] By age 50 years, the seroprevalence may be greater than 75%. Similar results on age-related seroprevalence of B19 infections were observed in India.[80-86]

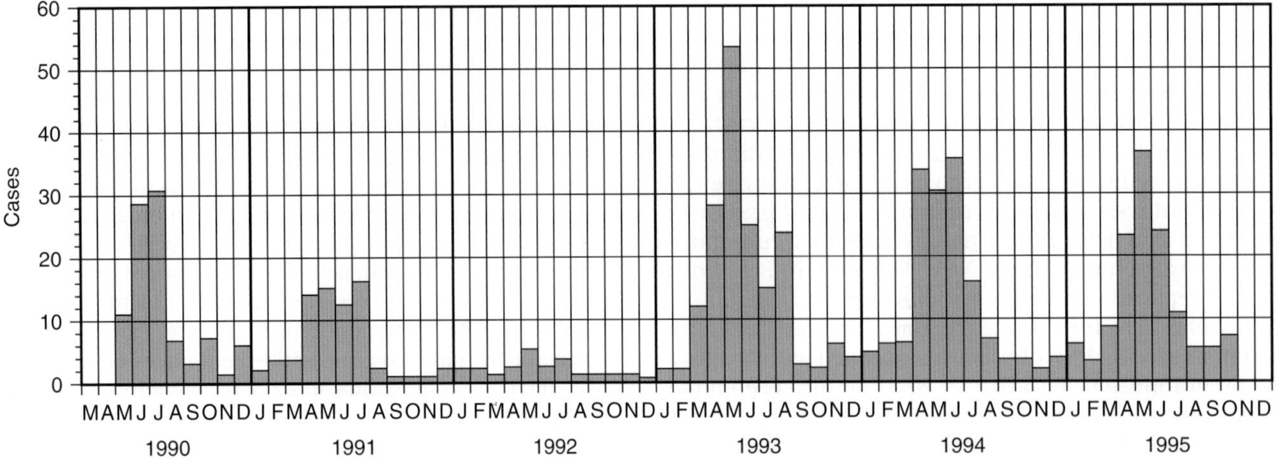

Figure 28-1 Seasonal variation in reported parvovirus B19 exposures in pregnant women. Each month is indicated by its first letter. (Data from Harger J, Koch W, Harger GF: Prospective evaluation of 618 pregnant women exposed to parvovirus B19: risks and symptoms, *Obstet Gynecol* 91:413-420, 1998.)

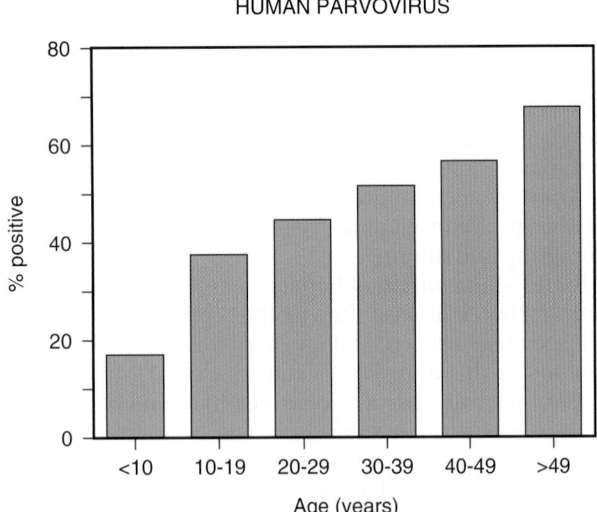

Figure 28-2 Percentage of family subjects positive for IgG antibody to parvovirus B19 by age. The sample includes 283 subjects from 111 families. Subjects were one twin of each twin pair, nontwin parents, and the oldest child of each family. (Data from Adler SP, Koch W: Human parvovirus B19 infections in women of childbearing age and within families, *J Pediatr Infect Dis* 8:83-87, 1989.)

SEROPREVALENCE BY GENDER

In most studies, the prevalence of antibodies to parvovirus B19 in sera obtained from men and women is similar.[59,74] At least six studies have reported that women have a higher rate of B19 infection than men, however.*

In one study of adult blood donors, the proportion of women who were seropositive, 47.5%, was 1.5 times higher than in men. The prevalence of IgG antibodies averaged 51% for women of all ages compared with 38% for men in one of two family studies in Richmond, Virginia, and 64% for women and 50% for men in the other study.[21,79] In Taiwan, the prevalence of IgG antibodies to B19 among women was significantly higher than among men (36.4% vs. 29.4%; $P < .001$).[89] The most likely explanation for the higher rates of B19 infection among women compared with men is that women are likely to have more frequent contact with children, especially school-age children who, because of school attendance, are the major sources of B19 transmission. For adults, contact with school-age children is the major risk factor for B19 infection.[21]

*References 21, 59, 79, 81, 87, 88.

SEROPREVALENCE BY RACE

In the United States, there are significant differences in the seroprevalence to parvovirus B19 between African Americans and whites. In Richmond, Virginia, approximately 60% of whites are seropositive compared with 45% of African Americans.[21] The reasons for the lower rate of infection among African Americans are unknown but likely reflect the racial segregation of children in schools.

INCIDENCE

In tests of serum from random blood donors for evidence of a recent parvovirus B19 infection, the rate of infection using antigen detection is 0 to 2.6 per 10,000 individuals tested, with a median of 1 per 10,000, whereas using DNA detection, the rate is 0 to 14.5 per 10,000, with a median of 2 per 10,000.[90-95] By contrast, when IgM antibodies to B19 were used to detect recent infection, the rate was zero, but all studies included fewer than 1000 patients.[80,96,97] As for seroprevalence, women may have a greater risk for infection during outbreaks of EI. During an epidemic of EI in Port Angeles, Washington, the attack rate for women was 15.6%, more than twice the rate of 7.4% for men.[12]

In Spain and Chile, children have the highest rates of B19 infection, which is true for children ages 0 to 4 years and 5 to 9 years.[98,99] A study of 633 children with sickle cell disease, followed at Children's Hospital in Philadelphia from 1996 to 2001, found that 70% were seronegative (susceptible), and during this period, 110 of these patients developed B19 infections, for an incidence of 11.3 per 100 patients per year.[100] Of the 110 patients infected, there were 68 episodes of transient aplastic crisis, characterized not only by an acute exacerbation of anemia but also by acute chest syndrome, pain, and fever. The high incidence of disease among children with sickle cell disease emphasizes the need for a vaccine against B19.

RISK FACTORS FOR ACQUISITION

Parvovirus B19 is efficiently transmitted among persons residing in the same home, with attack rates, based on the development of signs and symptoms of EI, of 17% to 30%.[12,101] Using serologic testing to identify asymptomatic infection and to exclude immune individuals, the secondary attack rate for susceptible household contacts is 50%. Most secondary cases of EI or aplastic crisis in the home occur 6 to 12 days after symptoms develop in the index case.[10,12,101-104] A serologic study of pregnant Danish women indicated that seropositivity was significantly correlated with increasing number of siblings, having a sibling of the same age, number of own children, and occupational exposure to children.[105]

During epidemics, B19 transmission is widespread among school-age children. Studies of school or classroom outbreaks of EI with at least one serologically confirmed case of acute B19 infection revealed student infection rates of 1% to 62% based on the occurrence of a rash illness. The median infection rate for all studies was 23%.[106-113] Because asymptomatic infections are common, and other signs and symptoms of EI may be mild and overlooked, these studies undoubtedly underestimate the true incidence of infection. Studies of students using serologic assays to identify B19 infection during outbreaks report infection rates of 34% to 72%, with most not associated with a rash illness.[107,112,113] Higher rates of infection occur in elementary schools and daycare centers compared with secondary schools, and in students in boarding schools compared with students who live at home.[12,75,111-113]

During school epidemics, employees in contact with children have the highest rates of infection compared with community control subjects. The attack rate based on detection of rash illness or arthropathy may be relatively low—12% to 25%.[107,111] The seroprevalence of B19 IgG antibodies to B19 in school employees is greater than in adult community control subjects, however—50% to 75%.[21,113,114] When serologic testing is used to identify employees with asymptomatic infection and to exclude immune employees, the attack rate among the susceptible individuals is usually very high. In four school outbreaks where serologic testing was used, the attack rate among teachers ranged from 19% to 84%, and the frequency of asymptomatic infection was greater than 50% in all but one outbreak.[107,110,113,114] The highest infection rates occurred among susceptible elementary school teachers compared with middle and high school teachers; this may reflect either exposure to more infected children or a greater likelihood of contact with respiratory secretions in younger children.[113,114] During a community-wide outbreak of EI in Connecticut in 1988, the infection rate among susceptible women was 16% for school teachers, 9% for daycare workers and homemakers, but only 4% for other women working outside the home.[113]

The risk of infection may be increased for school employees even in the absence of recognized epidemics of EI. In a study of 927 susceptible school employees conducted during a 3.5-year period when no community outbreaks were detected, the annual incidence of specific IgG seroconversion was 2.9% compared with 0.4% for a control population of 198 hospital employees.[21] The rate was higher, 3.4%, for school employees with jobs involving direct contact with children compared with only 0.6% observed for persons with jobs that did not involve contact with children.[21] Most (>50%) of the individuals who seroconverted did not recall an illness characterized by rash or arthropathy.

Salivary antibodies can be used to detect IgG and IgM antibodies to B19 because serum antibodies passively diffuse into saliva. Testing saliva for antibodies to B19 was useful in documenting outbreaks in schools and households. In an outbreak in England, school attack rates ranged from 8% to 50%, including an attack rate of 45% among the teaching staff.[115] The household transmission attack rate was 45% for 11 susceptible individuals. These rates are similar to what has been previously observed.[115] Crowding and low socioeconomic status are not proven risk factors for B19 infection. These risk factors are suggested, however, by the observation that in Rio de Janeiro, the seroprevalence of IgG antibodies to B19 is 35% in children aged 5 years or younger, and in Niger, it was 90% by 2 years of age.[56,74]

HOSPITAL TRANSMISSION

Parvovirus B19 can be transmitted from infected patients to hospital workers.[111] Most, but not all, investigations reveal that hospital transmission of B19 to laboratory personnel is common and includes direct patient-to-patient transmission and indirect transmission from materials or specimens known to contain B19.[116-119] One patient with sickle cell anemia became ill with aplastic crisis 9 to 11 days after contact in the hospital with a patient with hereditary spherocytosis hospitalized for aplastic crisis; B19 infection was confirmed in both patients.[120] An outbreak of EI occurred on a pediatric ward where 13 (26%) of 50 children developed a rash illness.[121] B19 seroconversion occurred in 5 (71%) of 7 children with rash illness and in 9 (35%) of 26 children who were asymptomatic.

Transmission from patient to health care worker occurred twice in one hospital after admission of patients with aplastic crisis.[116] In the first case, 4 (36%) of 11 susceptible employees with close contact had IgM antibodies to B19, indicating recent infection; in the second case, 10 (48%) of 21 employees either had specific IgM antibodies to B19 or seroconverted from IgG negative to positive. Eleven (79%) of 14 employees were symptomatic with rash or arthropathy. Another study of an outbreak of EI among health care workers on a pediatric ward found that 10 (33%) of 30 susceptible health care workers had serologic evidence of acute B19 infection, along with 2 (17%) of 12 immunocompromised patients being cared for on the ward.[117,122] The two infected patients were not symptomatic, but analysis of preexisting sera showed they acquired B19 while hospitalized. Onset of symptoms among the employees was temporally clustered, indicating a chronic source, such as an immunocompromised patient or person-to-person transmission.

Studies in Hong Kong identified three immunocompromised patients who seemed to transmit genetically identical strains of B19 from patient to patient.[123] At least one of these three patients seemed to be able to transmit the virus over many months. Immunocompromised patients often have chronic infections and may be infectious for long periods. DNA sequence analysis was also used in Japan to document B19 transmission between hospital staff members, including nursing staff, office workers, and a physiotherapist.[124]

Other investigations have observed little, if any, risk for hospital transmission. No evidence of patient-to-employee transmission was found among 10 susceptible health care workers with frequent contact with a chronically infected patient hospitalized for 24 days before institution of isolation precautions.[125] Transmission to hospital employees did not occur after exposure to a B19-infected mother, her infected stillborn fetus, and contaminated objects in the hospital room.[126] During a community outbreak of B19, none of 17 susceptible pregnant health care workers with possible exposure had serologic evidence (IgM antibodies to B19) of a recent infection.[127] In a case-control study of hospital transmission, serologic testing was used to determine the infection rates among personnel exposed to patients with sickle cell disease and transient aplastic crisis before the patients were placed in isolation.[128] Only 1 of 32 susceptible exposed hospital workers acquired a B19 infection compared with 3 of 37 susceptible workers not exposed. This study suggested that hospital workers who cared for patients with aplastic crisis were not at an increased risk for B19 acquisition.

Two prospective studies from one institution determined the incidence of infection in health care workers during endemic (nonepidemic) periods. The first study found the annual seroconversion rate to be 1.4% for 124 susceptible female health care workers followed for an average of 1.7 years. In a subsequent study of 198 susceptible hospital employees, the annual rate was 0.4% compared with 2.9% for school employees.[21] Taken as a whole, the evidence indicates that one must assume that B19 may be highly contagious in the hospital, although perhaps not in every circumstance. Many potential variables may affect rates of transmission from patients to staff, including the type of patient, immunocompromised status or nonimmunocompromised status, the duration of B19 infection at the time of hospitalization, and potentially the viral load of the infected patient. Patients with erythrocyte aplasia or others with suspected EI or B19 infection should be presumed to have a B19 infection until proven otherwise. These patients should receive respiratory and contact isolation while hospitalized.

ROUTES OF VIRAL SPREAD

Person-to-person spread of parvovirus B19 probably occurs through contact with respiratory secretions. Viral DNA is present in saliva[51,112,128,129] at levels similar to those in blood, and in a volunteer study infection was initiated by intranasal inoculation of B19.[51,130] B19 cannot be detected in columnar epithelial cells of the large airways.[131] Indirect evidence suggests B19 is not transmitted by aerosols. Viruses transmitted by aerosols, such as measles and influenza, are rapidly spread during outbreaks, but new cases of EI are spread out over many months during school outbreaks, suggesting that B19 transmission is inefficient. B19 DNA may be found in the urine, but it is unlikely that this is associated with infectious virus.

The only well-documented route of spread for B19 is vertically from mother to fetus and from parenteral transfusion with contaminated blood products or needles. Vertical transmission is discussed later. Although transmission of B19 by transfusion occurs, it is rare because of the low prevalence of B19 viremia among donors of blood and blood products; however, the risk increases for pooled blood products.[130-135] B19 DNA is frequently found in clotting factor concentrates, including products treated with solvents and detergents, steam, or monoclonal antibodies, and even treated products may be infectious.[95,133,135-138] Seroprevalence of IgG antibodies to B19 is high among hemophiliacs compared with age-matched controls and is higher for individuals who received frequent infusions of clotting factors prepared from large donor pools, compared with infusions prepared from small donor pools.[134]

Parvoviruses are resistant to chemical inactivation. In one hospital, B19 transmission occurred without recognized direct patient contact, suggesting possible transmission via fomites or environmental contamination.[116] That B19 is transmitted by fomites has not been directly established, but, considering the stability of related animal parvoviruses, this possibility exists. B19 DNA, not infectious virus, was found in a study of a suspected nosocomial outbreak in a maternity ward.[127] B19 DNA was detected by polymerase chain reaction (PCR) assay on the hands of the mother of a stillborn fetus infected with B19 and on the sink handles in her hospital room. Samples from countertops, an intravenous pump, and telephone were also positive by a sensitive nested PCR DNA technique. PCR assay is so sensitive that minute quantities of DNA can be detected via this technique, and the presence of B19 DNA on surfaces does not imply that these surfaces are sources of infection. Infected fetal tissues and placental or amniotic fluids are more likely sources of infection for health care workers than fomites.

RISK OF PARVOVIRUS B19 ACQUISITION FOR WOMEN OF CHILDBEARING AGE

We completed a large epidemiologic study to determine the relative risk of parvovirus B19 acquisition for women of childbearing age in daily contact with children, including nurses, daycare employees, and teachers at all levels.[21] We identified risk factors for B19 infections for hospital and school employees during an endemic period. Serologic testing was used to monitor 2730 employees of 135 schools in three school systems and 751 employees of a hospital, all in Richmond, Virginia. Of participants, 60% were initially seropositive. After adjusting for age, race, and gender, risk factors for seropositivity were contact with children 5 to 18 years of age at home or at work and employment in elementary schools. Over 42 months, only 1 of 198 susceptible hospital employees seroconverted (0.42% annual rate), compared with 62 of 927 (2.93% annual rate) school employees (relative risk, 6.9). Four factors associated with seroconversion were employment at elementary schools, contact with children 5 to 11 years of age at home, contact with children 5 to 18 years of age at work, and age younger than 30 years. Women in daily contact with school-age children had a fivefold increased annual occupational risk for B19 infection.[21]

Several observations indicate that B19 infections were endemic but not epidemic or pandemic in the Richmond area during the 42-month prospective evaluation.[21] First, few cases of B19 infection were reported by the school nurses, and no cluster of cases was observed at any single school or group of schools. Second, the seroconversion rates during each of three consecutive study periods were the same for all groups or subgroups. Third, for employees, B19 infections were not clustered at individual schools or groups of schools. Fourth, the infection rates that we observed in employees, even for elementary school teachers, were less than those observed for the 1988 Connecticut epidemic, where 46 infections occurred among 236 susceptible individuals exposed in the schools, for a minimum annual infection rate of 19%.[113] Also, in a study of secondary B19 infections among exposed household members, rates ranged from 30% to 50%.[102]

B19 infections are often asymptomatic or without a rash, and low-level endemics go unnoticed. We observed that 28 of 60 infected employees were asymptomatic, and only 20 knew of a specific exposure. In a study of 52 household contacts of patients with B19 infections during an Ohio epidemic, infections without a rash occurred in 15 of 16 (94%) African Americans and 17 of 35 (47%) whites, and completely asymptomatic infections occurred in 11 of 16 (69%) African Americans and 6 of 30 (20%) whites.[102] During the Connecticut outbreak, 5 of 65 (8%) teachers who were never exposed to a child with a rash became infected.[113] The observations of high secondary attack rates during epidemics and the high rates of infections without a rash or asymptomatic infections provide strong evidence that even during periods when EI is inapparent in the community, school or hospital personnel in contact with children have a significant occupational risk for B19 infections.

Contact with elementary school–age children, whether at home or at work, may be the most important risk factor for B19 acquisition. When seropositivity for persons with children at home was stratified by the child's age, the association between seropositivity and children at home was significant ($P < .05$) when all children 5 to 18 years of age were included; for seroconversion, the significant association was with elementary school–age children at home.[21] The low seroprevalence and seroconversion rate among hospital employees without known contact with children indicates that this group has a low occupational risk for acquiring B19 infections. We and others have not observed an increased rate of seroprevalence among daycare workers, but this has been observed in other studies.[139,140]

The major conclusions from these studies were that when EI is inapparent in the community, school or hospital personnel in contact with children still have a significant occupational risk for B19 infections and that school employees have an approximately twofold greater risk of acquiring B19 from children at work than from elementary school–age children at home. We also found that hospital employees without contact with children have a low risk for acquiring B19.

Using the Richmond data and assuming that on average 50% of pregnant women are immune, we estimate that, in endemic periods, 1% to 4% of susceptible women become infected during pregnancy. If the rate of fetal death after maternal infection is 5% to 10% (see "Intrauterine Transmission Rates, Clinical Manifestations, and Fetal Outcomes"), the occupational risk of fetal death for a pregnant woman with unknown serologic status is between 1 in 500 and 1 in 4000. These rates are so low that during endemic periods, they do not justify intervention, such as serologic testing for pregnant women or furloughing or temporary transfer of pregnant seronegative employees to administrative or other positions without child contact (see "Prevention").

Knowing B19 infection rates during endemic periods may be more important than knowing rates during epidemic periods. In the United States, B19 infections are endemic most of the time. Because greater than 75% of B19 infections are inapparent, most women who acquire B19 infection during pregnancy do so during endemic periods, not during epidemics. For establishing public health policy and assessing the potential importance of immunizing against B19, knowing that for seronegative women the endemic infection rate is 1% to 4% is more important than knowing epidemic rates, which vary widely depending on the frequency of susceptible individuals in a given population at a particular time.

Clinical Manifestations (Other Than Intrauterine Infection)

ERYTHEMA INFECTIOSUM

The most common clinical manifestation of infection with parvovirus B19 is EI, or fifth disease, a well-known rash illness of children. EI begins with a mild prodromal illness consisting of low-grade fever, headache, malaise, and upper respiratory tract symptoms. This prodrome may be so mild as to go unnoticed. The hallmark of the illness is the characteristic exanthem. The rash usually occurs in three phases, but these are not always distinguishable.[12,106] The initial stage consists of an erythematous facial flushing described as a "slapped-cheek" appearance. In the second stage, the rash spreads quickly to the trunk and proximal extremities as a diffuse macular erythema. The third stage is central clearing of macular lesions, which occurs promptly, giving the rash a lacy, reticulated appearance. Palms and soles are usually spared, and the rash tends to be more prominent on the extensor surfaces. Affected children at this point are afebrile and feel well. Adolescents and adults often complain of pruritus or arthralgias concurrent with the rash. The rash resolves spontaneously but typically may recur over 1 to 3 weeks in response to various environmental stimuli, such as sunlight, heat, exercise, and stress.

Lymphadenopathy is not a consistent feature but has been reported in association with EI[101] and as a sole manifestation of infection.[141-143] A mononucleosis-like illness associated with confirmed B19 infections has occasionally been reported, but B19 does not typically cause a mononucleosis-like illness. Atypical rashes not recognizable as classic EI have also been associated with acute B19 infections; these include morbilliform, vesiculopustular, desquamative, petechial, and purpuric rashes.[4]

Asymptomatic infection with B19 also occurs commonly in children and adults. In studies of large outbreaks, asymptomatic infection is reported in approximately 20% to 30% of serologically proven cases.[101,102]

TRANSIENT APLASTIC CRISIS

As noted earlier, transient aplastic crisis was the first clinical illness to be definitively linked to infection with parvovirus B19. An infectious etiology had been suspected for this condition because it usually occurred only once in a given patient, had a well-defined course and duration of illness, and tended to occur in clusters within families and communities. Attempts to link it to infection with any particular agent had repeatedly failed until 1981, when Pattison and colleagues[8] reported six positive tests for B19 (seroconversion or antigenemia) among 600 admissions to a London hospital; all six positive tests were in children with sickle cell anemia admitted with aplastic crisis. This association was confirmed by studies of an outbreak of aplastic crisis in the population with sickle cell disease in Jamaica.[9]

Although such transient aplastic crises are most commonly associated with sickle cell anemia, any patient with a condition of increased red blood cell turnover and accelerated erythropoiesis can experience a similar transient red blood cell aplasia with B19 infection. B19-induced aplastic crises have been described in many hematologic disorders, including other hemoglobinopathies (e.g., thalassemia, sickle-C hemoglobin), red blood cell membrane defects (e.g., hereditary spherocytosis, stomatocytosis), enzyme deficiencies (e.g., pyruvate kinase deficiency, glucose-6-phosphate dehydrogenase deficiency), antibody-mediated red blood cell destruction (autoimmune hemolytic anemia), and decreased red blood cell production (e.g., iron deficiency, blood loss).[49,144] B19 is not a significant cause of transient erythroblastopenia of childhood, another condition of transient red blood cell hypoplasia that usually occurs in younger, hematologically normal children and follows a more indolent course.[4]

In contrast to EI, patients with a transient aplastic crisis are ill at presentation with fever, malaise, and signs and symptoms of profound anemia (e.g., pallor, tachypnea, tachycardia). Rash is rarely present in these patients.[104,144] The acute infection causes a transient arrest of erythropoiesis (see "General Aspects of Pathogenesis") with a profound reticulocytopenia. Given the short half-life of red blood cells in these patients and their dependence on active erythropoiesis to counterbalance their increased red blood cell turnover, this arrest of erythropoiesis leads to a sudden and potentially life-threatening decrease in serum hemoglobin. Children with sickle hemoglobinopathies may also develop a concurrent vasoocclusive pain crisis, which may complicate the clinical picture further.

Leukopenia and thrombocytopenia may also occur during a transient aplastic crisis, but the incidence varies with the underlying condition. In a French study of 24 episodes of aplastic crisis (mostly in individuals with hereditary spherocytosis), 35% to 40% of patients were either leukopenic or thrombocytopenic, compared with 10% to 15% reported in a large U.S. study of mostly sickle cell patients.[104,145] These transient declines in leukocyte count or platelets follow a time course similar to reticulocytopenia, although they are not as severe, and recovery occurs without clinical sequelae. The relative preservation of leukocyte and platelet counts in sickle cell anemia, compared with other hereditary hemolytic anemias, is presumably due to the functional asplenia associated with sickle cell disease.[49]

As noted in experimental infection in human volunteers, B19 infection in normal subjects results in a decrease in the reticulocyte count, but because of the normal red blood cell half-life, this is not clinically significant or noticeable. Varying degrees of leukopenia and thrombocytopenia also occur after natural B19 infection in hematologically normal patients.[51] Some cases of idiopathic thrombocytopenic purpura and cases of childhood neutropenia have been reported in association with acute B19 infection.[146,147] Aside from these few anecdotal reports, larger studies have not confirmed B19 as a common cause of either idiopathic thrombocytopenic purpura or chronic neutropenia in children.[48]

ARTHROPATHY

Joint symptoms are reported by 80% of adolescents and adults with parvovirus B19 infection, whereas joint symptoms are uncommon in children.[12,106] Arthritis or arthralgia may occur in association with the symptoms of typical EI or may be the only manifestation of infection. Women are more frequently affected with joint symptoms than men.[12,106]

The joint symptoms of B19 infection usually manifest as the sudden onset of a symmetrical peripheral polyarthropathy.[148] The joints most often affected are the hands, wrists, knees, and ankles, but the larger joints can also be involved.[110,149] The joint symptoms have a wide range of severity, from mild morning stiffness to frank arthritis with the classic combination of erythema, warmth, tenderness, and swelling. Similar to the rash of EI, the arthropathy has been presumed to be immunologically mediated because the onset of joint symptoms occurs after the peak of viremia and coincides with the development of specific IgM and IgG antibodies.[51] Rheumatoid factor may also be transiently positive, leading to some diagnostic confusion with rheumatoid arthritis in adult patients.[150] There is no joint destruction, and, in most patients, joint symptoms resolve within 2 to 4 weeks. For some patients, joint discomfort may last for months or, in rare individuals, years. The role of B19 in these more chronic arthropathies is unclear.

The arthritis associated with B19 infection may persist long enough to satisfy clinical diagnostic criteria for rheumatoid arthritis or juvenile idiopathic (formerly juvenile) arthritis.[89,97,149,151,152] This finding has led some authors to suggest that B19 may be the etiologic agent of these conditions.[5] This speculation has been supported by the detection of B19 DNA in synovial tissue from patients with rheumatoid arthritis and reports of increased seropositivity among patients with these conditions.[98,153-155] The more recent findings of DNA from other viruses, in addition to B19 in synovial tissue from patients with arthritis and B19 DNA in synovium from persons without arthritis, suggest that this may be a nonspecific effect of inflammation.[156,157] A review of the accumulated evidence on this topic has concluded that B19 is unlikely to be a primary etiology in these rheumatic diseases, but it may be one of several viral triggers capable of initiating joint disease in genetically predisposed individuals.[158]

INFECTION IN IMMUNOCOMPROMISED HOSTS

Patients with impaired humoral immunity are at risk for developing chronic and recurrent infections with parvovirus B19. Persistent anemia, sometimes profound, with reticulocytopenia is the most common manifestation of such infections, which may also be accompanied by neutropenia, thrombocytopenia, or complete marrow suppression. Chronic infections with B19 occur in children with cancer who receive cytotoxic chemotherapy,[159,160] children with congenital immunodeficiency states,[161] children and adults with acquired immunodeficiency syndrome (AIDS),[162] and transplant recipients.[163] Chronic infections may even occur in patients with more subtle defects in immunoglobulin production, who are able to produce measurable antibodies to B19 but are unable to generate adequate neutralizing antibodies.[164]

B19 has also been linked to viral-associated hemophagocytic syndrome,[159,160] more generally referred to as infection-associated hemophagocytic syndrome. This condition of histiocytic infiltration of bone marrow and associated cytopenias usually occurs in immunocompromised patients. B19 is only one of several viruses that have been implicated as causing viral-associated hemophagocytic syndrome. Infection-associated hemophagocytic syndrome is generally considered to be a nonspecific response to various viral and bacterial insults, rather than a specific manifestation of a single pathogen.

Infections in immunocompromised hosts can lead to chronic infection; this is most often manifested as chronic anemia (red blood cell aplasia), but varying degrees of cytopenia have been described, ranging from thrombocytopenia or neutropenia to complete bone marrow failure.[144] Patients with an inability to produce neutralizing antibodies are at greatest risk, and this complication of B19 infection has been described in children with congenital immunodeficiency syndromes, patients receiving cytoreductive chemotherapy, transplant patients receiving immunosuppressive therapy, and adults and children with AIDS.[144] Increased recognition of B19 infection in solid-organ transplant patients has led to many more recent reports.[165-167] Although most such infections are manifested as the typical persistent anemia, an association of B19 viremia with acute graft rejection has been described.[168]

OTHER DERMATOLOGIC SYNDROMES

Vasculitis and Purpura

Various atypical skin eruptions have been described in association with parvovirus B19 infections. Most of these are petechial or purpuric in nature, often with evidence of vasculitis in descriptions of eruptions that report skin biopsy results, and may resemble the rash of other connective tissue diseases.[4,169] There are reports of confirmed acute B19 infections associated with nonthrombocytopenic purpura and vasculitis, including several cases clinically diagnosed as Henoch-Schönlein purpura,[90,170] an acute leukocytoclastic vasculitis of unknown etiology in children. Chronic B19 infection has also been associated with a necrotizing vasculitis, including cases of polyarteritis nodosa and Wegener granulomatosis.[171] These patients had no underlying hematologic disorder and were generally not anemic at diagnosis. The pathogenesis is unknown but could suggest an endothelial cell infection as occurs with some other viruses such as rubella.

Data from skin biopsy of rashes temporally associated with B19 infection are limited, although several reports have been published. B19 capsid antigens and DNA were found in a skin biopsy specimen from a patient with EI, and this observation lends support to a role for B19 in these vascular disorders.[172] Rashes resembling those of systemic lupus erythematosus, Henoch-Schönlein purpura, and other connective tissue disorders have been described.[169,173] In a controlled study of 27 children with Henoch-Schönlein purpura, B19 was not a common cause.[174] Only 3 of 27 children had detectable B19 IgM antibodies, indicating a recent infection. The role of B19 in these conditions remains speculative.

Papular-Purpuric "Gloves and Socks" Syndrome

Papular-purpuric "gloves and socks" syndrome (PPGSS) is a distinctive, self-limited dermatosis first described in the dermatologic literature in 1990.[175] PPGSS is characterized by fever, pruritus, and painful edema and erythema localized to the distal extremities in a distinct glove-and-sock distribution. The distal erythema is usually followed by petechiae or papules or purpura, and oral lesions often develop as well. Resolution of all symptoms usually occurs in 1 to 2 weeks. A search for serologic evidence of viral infection led to the discovery of an association with acute parvovirus B19 infection in many of these patients, based on demonstration of specific IgM or seroconversion. This association has been confirmed further with subsequent reports and demonstration of B19 DNA in skin biopsy samples and sera from these patients.[175,176] Initially described in adults, numerous children have now been described with this condition.[177] There seems to be sufficient evidence to suggest that PPGSS is a rare but distinctive manifestation of primary, acute infection with B19, occurring mainly in young adults but also affecting children.

CENTRAL NERVOUS SYSTEM INFECTION AND NEUROLOGIC DISORDERS

Although various neurologic symptoms and disorders have been described in patients clinically diagnosed as having EI or laboratory-confirmed parvovirus B19 infection,[4] the issue of whether B19 causes central nervous system (CNS) infection or is etiologic for other neurologic conditions remains unresolved. Cases of meningitis,[178,179] encephalitis,[180] and encephalopathy[181] secondary to B19 infection all have been reported. Many of these cases were reported during outbreaks of EI from older reports based on clinical diagnosis only, before reliable laboratory tests for B19 were available. In one study, headache was reported in 32% of children with rash illness.[178]

There are no controlled comparative studies to evaluate the frequency of signs or symptoms suggestive of meningeal inflammation or CNS infection in B19 infection. Cerebrospinal fluid (CSF) abnormalities, such as pleocytosis and increased levels of CSF protein, have been reported in some, but not all, patients with meningismus or altered level of consciousness associated with EI.[5] B19 DNA has been detected in CSF using PCR assay in several cases of serologically confirmed acute B19 infection with meningoencephalitis or encephalopathy.[182-184] Most of these reported patients were also viremic at the time, however, so the possibility that CSF PCR was positive secondary to contamination from blood could not be completely excluded.

B19 infection has been associated with vasculitis and histopathologic changes in the CNS that potentially may lead to stroke.[185] Most cases of stroke in association with documented B19 infection have been reported in children; some of these children have had other concurrent medical conditions that could contribute to stroke, particularly sickle cell disease.[186-188] At least two cases of neonatal stroke have been reported in association with B19 infection: one related to maternal infection during gestation and the other associated with infection of the newborn infant.[189,190]

Disorders of the peripheral nervous system have also been described, including brachial plexus neuropathy,[191] carpal tunnel syndrome,[192] extremity paresthesias and dysesthesias,[193] and myasthenia-like weakness.[194] The onset of most of these peripheral nerve symptoms has been coincident with the onset of rash or joint pain, or both, at a time when the patient should have a brisk immune response, suggesting that the neurologic abnormalities could be immunologically mediated.[5] In the course of one well-described outbreak of EI among intensive care nurses, numbness and tingling of the fingers was reported in 54% of the 13 nurses infected with B19.[193] The neurologic symptoms persisted for more than 1 year in three of the nurses, and one had low levels of B19 DNA in serum for more than 3 years in association with recurrent episodes of paresthesias. She was never anemic and had no demonstrable immunodeficiency.[195] Although these cases are suggestive, the role of B19 in neurologic disease, stroke, and CNS infection remains unresolved until the pathogenesis of the viral infection in these conditions can be elucidated.[5,196]

RENAL DISEASE

Reports of renal disease after parvovirus B19 infection, previously rare, have increased.[197-199] Most have been case reports of glomerulonephritis or focal glomerulosclerosis temporally related to an acute B19 infection. Immune complex deposition has been shown in renal tissue, and B19 DNA can occasionally be found in renal tissue by PCR assay as well.[200] Renal failure is rarely reported. The virus is not known to infect kidney cells in vitro, and its presence in renal tissue could be secondary to filtration from the viremia of acute infection. B19 DNA has been detected in urine in studies of infants with evidence of intrauterine infections. It is possible that B19 antigens could trigger an immune complex–mediated nephritis, but this may be a nonspecific effect, and further study is necessary to define the relationship between B19 infection and the potential for renal disease.

MYOCARDIAL DISEASE

Parvovirus B19 is now a well-established, although infrequent, cause of myocarditis in children and adults. B19 DNA is often present within the myocardium of patients with myocarditis and idiopathic left ventricular failure.[201-206] B19 infection has also been associated with acute dilated cardiopathy, but the etiologic significance of B19 in the myocardium is unclear.[207] Myocarditis resulting from B19 infection usually resolves over several weeks but is occasionally fatal.[208-210]

General Aspects of Diagnosis

The diagnosis of EI (fifth disease) is usually based on the clinical recognition of the typical exanthem, benign course, and exclusion of other similar conditions. Laboratory confirmation is rarely necessary. A presumptive diagnosis of a parvovirus B19–induced transient aplastic crisis in a patient with known sickle cell disease (or other condition associated with chronic hemolysis) is based on an acute febrile illness, a sudden and severe decline in serum hemoglobin, and an absolute reticulocytopenia. Likewise, a clinical diagnosis of PPGSS can be based on the characteristic skin eruption in the distinct acral distribution.

LABORATORY DIAGNOSTIC METHODS

Specific laboratory diagnosis depends on identification of parvovirus B19 antibodies, viral antigens, or viral DNA. In an immunologically normal patient, determination of anti-B19 IgM is the best marker of recent or acute infection on a single serum sample. IgM antibodies develop rapidly after infection and are detectable for 6 to 8 weeks.[211] Specific IgG antibodies become detectable a few days after IgM and persist for years and probably for life. Seroconversion from IgG-negative to IgG-positive on paired acute and convalescent sera confirms a recent infection. Anti-B19 IgG primarily serves as a marker of past infection or immunity, however. Patients with EI or acute B19 arthropathy are almost always IgM-positive, so a diagnosis can generally be made from a single serum sample. Patients with B19-induced aplastic crisis may present before antibodies are detectable; however, IgM is detectable within 1 to 2 days of presentation, and detection of IgG follows within days.[104]

The availability of serologic assays for B19 had previously been limited by the lack of a reliable and renewable source of antigen for diagnostic studies. The development of recombinant cell lines that express B19 capsid proteins has provided more reliable sources of antigen suitable for use in commercial test kits.[212,213] Several commercial kits are currently available for detection of B19 antibodies, but they use a variety of different antigens (e.g., recombinant capsid proteins, fusion proteins, synthetic peptides), and their performance in large studies has varied.[212] Based on studies of the humoral immune response to the various B19 viral antigens, it seems to be important to have serologic assays based on intact capsids that provide conformational epitopes. Antibody responses to these antigens are more reliable and longer lasting than the responses to linear epitopes used in some assays.[214]

At present, only one commercial assay based on such capsids has received approval from the U.S. Food and Drug Administration (FDA); other commercial assays for this purpose are considered research tests.[215] Until serologic tests are more standardized and results are more consistent, some knowledge of the assay and antigens used is necessary for proper interpretation of B19 antibody test results.

In immunocompromised or immunodeficient patients, serologic diagnosis is unreliable because humoral responses are impaired, so methods to detect viral particles or viral DNA are necessary to make the diagnosis of a B19 infection. As noted, the virus cannot be isolated on routine cell cultures, so viral culture is not useful. Detection of viral DNA by DNA hybridization techniques[216] or by PCR assay[217,218] is useful in these patients. Both techniques can be applied to various clinical specimens, including serum, amniotic fluid, fresh tissues, bone marrow, and paraffin-embedded tissues.[148] Histologic examination is also helpful in diagnosing B19 infection in certain situations. Examination of bone marrow aspirates in anemic patients typically reveals giant pronormoblasts or "lantern cells" against a background of general erythroid hypoplasia. The absence of such cells does not exclude B19 infection, however.[219,220] Electron microscopy has proven useful and may reveal viral particles in serum of some infected patients and in cord blood or tissues of hydropic infants (see "Pathogenesis of Infection in the Fetus").

Epidemiology of Parvovirus B19 Infections and Risk of Acquisition in Pregnant Women

PREVALENCE AND INCIDENCE IN THE UNITED STATES

We completed three studies using complementary strategies to determine the incidence of parvovirus B19 infection during pregnancy. First, using the data from a study of school personnel, we estimated the average B19 infection rate among pregnant school personnel.[21] Of the 60 individuals who seroconverted in that study, 8 (13%) were pregnant. Not all pregnant women in the school system participated in the study. Although we had data on the pregnancy rates for the female school personnel who participated, these volunteers may have been biased toward younger women, raising the possibility that their pregnancy rates may not have been representative of all school employees. Of approximately 11,637 total school employees in Richmond, Virginia, we enrolled 2730 (24%) in our study. To determine if the sample enrolled was representative, we performed a random survey of 733 school employees at the schools studied. The results provided strong evidence that the seroprevalence and annual infection rates observed among study subjects were representative and applicable to the entire school employee population.[21] Assuming no seasonality to B19 infections, because none was observed, and that pregnancy does not affect susceptibility, we predicted that without regard to risk factors, seronegative pregnant personnel have an average annual infection rate of 3%, for a rate of 2.25% per pregnancy.[21]

Second, in Richmond, Virginia, from 1989 to 1991, we collected sera from 1650 pregnant women from a lower socioeconomic group, who attended a high-risk pregnancy clinic for patients without medical insurance. This group was 80% African American, with an average maternal age of 24 years. We randomly selected a subset of 395 women for serologic testing and monitoring, 35% of whom were seropositive. Of the 256 seronegative women, 2 (0.8%) seroconverted, for an annual rate of 1.7%. This rate was similar to the rate observed among low-risk African-American school personnel in Richmond.[21]

Finally, we also obtained serial sera from a large group of private practice obstetric patients from Birmingham, Alabama.[221] From this serum bank, we randomly selected 200 patients per year over 4 years, 1987 to 1990. No significant differences in seroprevalence were observed by year among the 800 patients (average age, 27 years, and 88% white), and 46% were seropositive overall. Of 413 seronegative women serially tested over the 4 years, 5 seroconverted. Overall, the annual seroconversion rate was 2%. Combining data from the studies of pregnant women done in Richmond and Birmingham, we observed that 7 of 669 seronegative women seroconverted in pregnancy for a rate of 1% per pregnancy with a 95% confidence interval of 0.3% to 21%.

PREVALENCE AND INCIDENCE IN OTHER COUNTRIES

In numerous studies conducted worldwide, including pregnant women and women of reproductive age, the seroprevalence of IgG antibodies to parvovirus B19 has ranged from 16% to 81%, with most estimates between 35% and 55%.[73,78,79,88,222-225] In Denmark, a serologic survey of 31,000 pregnant Danish women found 65% had evidence of past infection.[105] The seroprevalence of IgG antibody among 1610 pregnant women in Barcelona was 35.03%.[22] Of pregnant Swedish women, 81% had parvovirus antibodies.[226] In Japan, the seroprevalence of IgG antibodies to B19 was 26% for women 21 to 30 years of age and 44% for women 31 to 40 years of age.[78] In Germany, 62.9% of 40,517 pregnant women had IgG antibodies to B19.[217] The prevalence of IgG antibodies to B19 in cord blood from normal newborns also provides estimates of maternal immunity of 50% to 75%.[19,227,228]

Without regard to maternal age or other potential risk factors, a South African study found that 64 (3.3%) of 1967 pregnant women acquired B19 infection during pregnancy, and another study in Barcelona found that 60 (3.7%) of 1610 pregnant women became infected with B19 during pregnancy.[22,229] Seroconversion rates among susceptible pregnant Danish women during endemic and epidemic periods were 1.5% and 13%. In Denmark, risk of infection increased with the number of children in the household, and having children ages 6 to 7 years resulted in the highest rate of seroconversion. Nursery school teachers had a threefold increased risk of acute infection.[105] Extrapolating to a 40-week period would place the infection rate during pregnancy among susceptible women at approximately 1.1%, with a range of 1% to 4% depending on risk factors. The Danish and Barcelona data are similar to data obtained in Richmond, Virginia.[21]

A prospective study conducted from 1998 to 2000 of 2567 pregnant women found that 70% had IgG antibodies to B19 at the beginning of pregnancy, and of those seronegative, 2.4% acquired B19 during pregnancy.[222] A similar study of 13,449 women conducted in five European countries found that the risk of a seronegative woman acquiring B19 during pregnancy ranged from 0.61% in Belgium to 1.58% in Poland.[223]

A few studies have tried to estimate the infection rate based on the prevalence of IgM antibodies to B19 in pregnancy or in women of reproductive age. Although B19-specific IgM is an accurate diagnostic test for recent infection, it is a poor test for epidemiology studies. B19 IgM persists for only a few months and underestimates the maternal infection rate because women who have had a B19 infection 6 to 9 months before testing would not be detected by this assay. Another problem with IgM surveys is that most studies have surveyed high-risk populations, such as women with rash illness, possible exposure to cases of EI, or recent diagnosis of adverse reproductive outcomes. Sampling high-risk populations biases the results toward rates higher than would be observed in population-based studies. A few studies have used B19-specific IgM to test pregnant women or women of reproductive age who did not have risk factors for infection. The observed range in these studies was 0% to 2.6%.[19,227,230] For susceptible women of reproductive age in populations known to be at increased risk for infection, the prevalence of IgM has ranged from 0% and 12.5%.[19,78,128,231,232]

In countries other than the United States, the prevalence of IgG antibodies to B19 among pregnant women and women of reproductive age varies widely and is likely to reflect exposure during prior epidemics. Studies on infections during pregnancy are fraught with potentially confounding variables, such as use of IgM testing, which lacks sensitivity, and selection bias introduced by selection criteria for the population studied. Despite these problems, it is likely the risk for B19 infection during pregnancy in other countries is similar to that observed in the United States.

Clinical Manifestations of Parvovirus B19 Infections in Pregnant Women

The symptoms reported by pregnant women with a proven recent parvovirus B19 infection are usually vague and nonspecific, so serologic confirmation is essential to establish the diagnosis. The signs and symptoms of classic EI in children are significantly different in adults; the sunburned or slapped-cheek facial rash common in children rarely occurs in adults. Malaise is a common feature of B19 infection in children and in adults but is nonspecific. In pregnant women and adolescents, the most characteristic symptom is symmetrical arthralgias, occasionally with signs of arthritis, and usually involving the small distal joints of hands, wrists, and feet.

The proportion of pregnant women with serologically proven B19 infection who are asymptomatic varies with the inclusion criteria in the few studies that address symptoms. In a cohort of 1610 pregnant women studied in Barcelona, the sera of 30 women had IgM antibodies to B19 at the first prenatal visit, and another 30 seroconverted during pregnancy.[22] Of these 60 women, only 18 (30%) reported any combination of fever, rash, and arthralgias; 70% were asymptomatic. The authors did not report when questions about symptoms were asked in relation to the serologic results, and no comment was made about the distribution of symptoms or about which joints were affected by the arthralgias.[22] Similarly, during an epidemic of EI in Connecticut, 69% of nonpregnant adults with serologically proven B19 infection were asymptomatic. In this study, symptoms were assessed by mailed questionnaires after the women were provided their serologic results.[113,127] In a British multicenter study, only 6 (3%) of 184 patients were asymptomatic, but the population was ascertained largely by recruiting women with typical symptoms, so this study is not comparable to the others.[20]

We studied 618 pregnant women in Pittsburgh, Pennsylvania, with known exposure to someone with a rash illness highly suggestive of EI. Each exposed patient was questioned about symptoms before serologic testing. Only 33% of the 52 women with serologically proven B19 infection reported no symptoms, whereas the remaining 67% reported rash, fever, arthralgias, coryza, or malaise.[233] Malaise, although a very vague and nonspecific finding, was reported by 27 (52%) of the 52 infected women.[233] In contrast, only 5.5% of 307 exposed, but not susceptible (IgG seropositive, IgM seronegative), women reported this symptom. After malaise, symmetrical arthralgias were the second most common symptom reported. Of the 618 pregnant women with known exposures, 24 (46%) of the 52 infected pregnant women reported arthralgias, compared with 11 (3.6%) of 307 immune women and 12 (4.6%) of 259 susceptible but uninfected women ($P < .0001$).[233] Of the 24 women with arthralgias in this study, 23 also reported malaise, 16 reported rash, 7 reported coryza, and 7 reported fever. Among the 24 IgM-positive women with arthralgias, the symmetrical joints most commonly affected by pain, swelling, and erythema were the knees (75%), followed by wrists (71%), fingers (63%), ankles (42%), feet (29%), elbows (29%), shoulders (17%), hips (13%), and back and neck (8%). Only 2 of the 24 women had only one set of joints involved, and very few other women reported monarticular pain or swelling. In most women, the arthralgias were easily controlled by antiinflammatory drugs and lasted only 1 to 5 days. Arthralgias occasionally lasted 10 to 14 days, however, and in some women were so painful that they were incapacitated for 2 to 3 days.

The high frequency of arthralgia in pregnant women with B19 infection is consistent with reports that distal arthralgias and arthritis are the most frequent finding in adults with EI. The frequency of arthralgias among nonpregnant adults with proven B19 infection in the Torrington, Connecticut, epidemic was 24% (11 of 46 adults) compared with 12% (61 of 512 adults) in adults without B19 infection ($P < .05$).[113] In another study in Connecticut, arthralgias occurred significantly more often (26%) in 19 adults with IgM antibodies to B19 than in 460 adults (7%) who lacked IgM antibodies to B19 ($P < .01$).[127] Arthralgias were even more common during outbreaks in Ireland, occurring in 79% of 47 recently infected women and men. Of patients with arthralgias, 93% reported that their knees were involved.[234]

Rash is less frequent in pregnant women than in children with EI, and the rash in pregnant women is not characteristic. In one report of the Connecticut epidemic, rashes occurred in 6 (13%) of 46 infected adults compared with 49 (10%) of 512 individuals who were uninfected. In another report, rashes occurred in 3 (16%) of 19 infected adults compared with 33 (7%) of 460 uninfected individuals. This difference was not significant ($P = .16$) and may represent random variation.[113] In contrast to the classic "curtain lace" rash in children, pregnant women (80%) often have a maculopapular rash that rarely involves the face and may be urticarial or morbilliform. In adults, these rashes are rarely pruritic and usually resolve within 1 to 5 days. A Japanese study reported that of 100 pregnant women with a confirmed B19 infection during pregnancy, 51 had a facial, body, or limb rash, and 49 were without symptoms.[235] In the Pittsburgh series, coryza was reported by 23% of the 52 B19-infected pregnant women but was reported in only 6.8% of the 307 previously infected women and 5.8% of the 259 seronegative women.[233] This difference was significant ($P < .0001$), but the nonspecific nature of coryza in pregnant women means this symptom alone is not diagnostically helpful.

In the Pittsburgh series, a temperature 38° C or greater occurred in 19% of 52 IgM-seropositive B19-infected women compared with 2.6% of 307 previously infected patients and 3.1% of 259 susceptible, noninfected patients ($P < .0001$).[226] In 9 of 10 women with fever, at least one other symptom was present. No woman's temperature exceeded 38.9° C. In 16 uninfected women with fever, all had at least one other symptom, and temperatures ranged up to 40° C, suggesting that a temperature greater than 39° C in a pregnant woman indicates infections other than B19. In a London outbreak of B19 infection, 7 of the 10 infected adults had an elevated temperature.[117] In the Connecticut epidemic, fever was reported in 15% of the 46 infected individuals but also in 16% of the 512 uninfected individuals.[113] On occasion, pregnant women infected with B19 develop rapidly increasing fundal height, preterm labor, or preeclampsia. Such symptoms are nonspecific and rarely indicate B19 infection.

Intrauterine Transmission Rates, Clinical Manifestations, and Fetal Outcomes

OVERVIEW

Primary maternal infection with parvovirus B19 during gestation has been associated with adverse outcomes, such as nonimmune hydrops fetalis, intrauterine fetal death, and asymptomatic neonatal infection, but also with normal delivery at term.[16,17] Initial reports of fetal hydrops related to maternal B19 infection were anecdotal and retrospective, suggesting rates of adverse outcomes of 26% and generating concern that B19 might be more fetotropic than rubella or CMV.[236,237] Subsequent reports of normal births after documented maternal B19 infection made clear the need for better estimates of the rate of intrauterine transmission and the risk of adverse outcomes.[238,239]

FETAL DEATH

Parvovirus B19 was first linked to fetal death in 1984.[17] As anticipated based on the epidemiology of B19 transmission, the percentage of all fetal deaths attributable to B19 varies, probably depending on the frequency of B19 infections in the population being studied. Overall, the contribution of B19 infection to fetal death is variable.

Prospective studies report rates of intrauterine viral transmission ranging from 25% to 50%.[20,240,241] Initial studies indicated that the risk of an adverse fetal outcome after a recent maternal infection is less than 10% and probably much less, with greatest risk in the first 20 weeks of pregnancy.[148] A large British prospective study identified 186 pregnant women with confirmed B19 infections during an epidemic and followed these women to term.[20] There were 30 (16%) fetal deaths in all, with 17 (9%) estimated to be due to B19 on the basis of DNA studies of a sample of the abortuses. Most of the fetal deaths occurred in the first 20 weeks of gestation, with an excess fetal loss in the second trimester.[20,242-244] The intrauterine transmission rate was estimated at 33%, based on analysis of the abortuses, fetal IgM in cord blood, and persistence of B19 IgG at 1-year follow-up of the infants. A smaller study of 39 pregnancies complicated by maternal B19 infection and followed to term found two fetal deaths (fetal loss rate of 5%), one (3%) of which was attributable to B19 and occurred at 10 weeks of gestation.[240]

A prospective study conducted by the Centers for Disease Control and Prevention (CDC) identified 187 pregnant women with B19 infection and compared their outcomes with 753 matched control women.[241] The overall fetal loss rate in the infected group was 5.9%, with 10 of 11 occurring before the 18th week of gestation, compared with 3.5% fetal loss rate in the control group, suggesting a fetal loss rate of 2.5% attributable to B19. In a prospective Spanish study during an endemic period, 1610 pregnant women were screened for B19 infection, and 60 (3.7%) were identified.[22] There were five abortions among this group, but only one (1.7%) was caused by B19, based on histologic and virologic analysis of fetal samples. The incidence of vertical transmission was estimated at 25%, based on serologic evaluation of the infants at delivery and at 1 year of age. In a similar prospective study of an obstetric population, 1967 pregnant women were screened, and 64 (3.3%) were identified as recently infected.[229] Among this group, no adverse effects were seen by serial ultrasound examinations, and no fetal hydrops was noted; one abortion occurred, but the fetus was not examined for evidence of B19 infection (maximal fetal loss attributable, 1.6%).

In a Japanese study of 100 women with a confirmed B19 infection during pregnancy, the fetal loss rate, including hydrops and fetal death, was 7%, with all maternal infections occurring before the 20th week of gestation.[235] These results are similar to results from a larger study from Germany, where 1018 pregnant women with a confirmed B19 infection during pregnancy were studied.[245] The overall fetal death rate was 6.3%, with the highest death rate (11%) occurring among women infected before 20 weeks of gestation. The overall rate of hydrops was 3.9%.[235] In a case-control study of 192 women with fetal deaths, half occurring before 20 weeks of gestation and half after, there was serologic evidence of acute B19 infection in 1% of case and control groups.[19] The prevalence of IgG antibodies was also similar. In this study, the percentage of fetal deaths attributed to B19 infection was unlikely to exceed 3% in cases not selected for parvovirus exposure.

In another study, 5 (6.3%) of 80 women with spontaneous abortions between 4 and 17 weeks of gestation had IgM antibodies to B19 compared with 2 (2%) of 100 control women, but this difference was not statistically significant.[232] In addition, these investigators studied the aborted fetuses from the five seropositive cases and found B19 DNA in only two.

In a prospective study of 39 pregnant women infected with B19 during a community-wide outbreak in Connecticut, there were two fetal deaths, and only one (3%) was attributable to B19 infection.[240] Among women followed prospectively and who acquired B19 infection during pregnancy, there was no evidence of fetal damage in 43 in Richmond, Virginia, 52 in Pittsburgh, Pennsylvania, and one fetal loss among 56 pregnancies in women from Barcelona.[22,23,233]

Two Chinese studies found fetal B19 infection frequently associated with fetal death.[246,247] The first study in China found that of 116 spontaneously aborted fetuses tested for B19 DNA, 27.3% were positive for parvovirus B19, but only 4% (1/25) of nonaborted fetal tissues in the control group tested positive.[246] This difference was significant. It was unknown when these samples were collected or whether B19 was endemic or epidemic in the community. The second Chinese study examined 175 biopsy tissues from spontaneous abortions from 1994 to 1995 and found that 25% were positive for B19 DNA in the fetal tissues.[247] A control group of 20 fetal tissues came from induced abortions, and only 2 (5%) were positive. This difference was not statistically significant but did support the observation that in China, B19 may be an important cause of fetal death, especially if B19 is epidemic in the community.

In contrast to the Chinese studies, a study from the Netherlands of fetal and placental tissue from 273 cases of first-trimester and second-trimester fetal loss tested the tissues for serologic or virologic evidence of B19 infection.[248] Of the 273 cases, 149 were from seronegative women, and the fetal deaths for these women were considered unrelated to B19. The mothers had IgM antibodies to B19 at the time of abortion in only 2 of the remaining 124 cases (0.7% for all 273 cases). This study indicates that B19 infection was a rare cause of fetal loss during the first and second trimesters. No congenital anomalies were observed among the fetal tissues examined.

In a study of 1047 pregnant women in Kuwait, maternal blood samples were obtained in the first, second, and third trimesters and tested for serologic evidence of recent B19 infection.[249] Of the mothers, 47% were seronegative, and in these women, the incidence of seroconversion was 16.5%. Among the women who seroconverted to B19, the rate of fetal loss was 5.4%. All the fetal deaths occurred in the first two trimesters, suggesting that fetal death after maternal B19 infection is common, particularly during the first and second trimesters.

A report from Toledo, Ohio, described five unexpected fetal deaths that occurred in the second trimester.[250] Only one of the fetuses was hydropic, but all five contained viral inclusions in the liver, and all five women were seropositive to B19.

Fetal deaths in the third trimester have also been reported (Table 28-2). A Swedish study of fetal deaths among 33,759 pregnancies found 93 cases of third-trimester fetal deaths, and of these, 7 (7.5%) had detectable B19 DNA in frozen placental tissue.[251] None of the seven fetuses was hydropic. The authors suggested B19 occasionally caused fetal death in the third trimester.

Table 28-2 Fetal Deaths From Parvovirus B19 Infection

Infection-to-Death Interval (wk)	Gestational Age at Death (wk)	Fetal Weight at Death (g)	Reference
1	39	3840	17
10	25	NR	316
13	22	409	18
4	20	161	18
4	24	420	317
4	26	695	315
9	24	580	315
7	18	300	318
8	19	236	277
1	4	NR	319
3	NR	NR	319
6	17	NR	319
10-19	23	NR	320
5	15	NR	320
(10)*	(11)†	Hydrops fetalis	291
(4)	(25)	Hydrops, 3320	321
(11)	(21)	Hydrops, 3111	322
(7)	(13)	Hydrops fetalis	277
(4)	(24)	Hydrops, 1495	277
(3)	(30)	Hydrops, 3550	320
(8)	(25)	Hydrops fetalis	144

NR, not reported.
*Numbers in parentheses in this column refer to intervals between exposure or onset of symptoms and diagnosis of hydrops fetalis.
†Numbers in parentheses in this column refer to gestational age at time of diagnosis of hydrops fetalis.

A study of 13 pregnant women who acquired B19 infection during pregnancy and in whom the time of acquisition was known was completed in Japan.[252] Nonimmune hydrops occurred in three fetuses whose mothers acquired B19 infection in the first half of pregnancy. Spontaneous abortion without hydrops and intrauterine growth restriction occurred in two fetuses whose mothers also developed B19 infection during the first half of pregnancy. The remaining eight fetuses, whose mothers acquired infection in the first and second half of pregnancy, were asymptomatic, although B19 DNA was detected in the immune serum of all of the infants. These results suggest that B19 transmission to the fetus is frequent, and fetal death may occur in almost half of the fetuses of infected mothers.

A Swedish study of 92 pregnancies with unexpected fetal death occurring after 22 weeks of gestation found B19 DNA in 13 (14%) of the 92 fetuses.[253] Only 2 of the 13 were hydropic. The Swedish study again suggests that B19 infection may infect the fetus in the third trimester and result in fetal death or hydrops. This observation was confirmed in a larger study also from Sweden, where 47 cases of fetal deaths occurring after 22 weeks of gestation were identified and compared with 53 normal pregnancies.[254] Seven of the 43 intrauterine fetal deaths were positive for parvovirus B19 DNA, whereas B19 DNA was not detected in any of the normal pregnancies. Finally, a large Danish study of 2918 pregnancies with fetal loss and more than 8000 control pregnancies estimated that during an endemic period the overall rate of fetal loss attributable to B19 was 0.1%, which could rise to 1% during epidemics.[255]

Dichorionic twin pregnancies affected by maternal B19 infections have also been reported.[256,257] These reports indicate that one or both fetuses may be infected, and only one fetus may be symptomatic even if both are infected.

In two studies, the presence of IgM to B19 or B19 DNA or both in maternal sera of pregnant women with a history of unexplained recurrent abortions was significantly higher than in pregnant women without a history of recurrent abortion, suggesting that women who are prone to recurrent abortion may be more likely to abort after a B19 infection than others.[258,259]

B19 is a likely cause of fetal death in the first, second, and third trimesters, and most infected infants are not hydropic. The estimates of fetal deaths attributable to B19 range from 0% to 27%, making it difficult to assess the precise increase in fetal mortality attributable to B19.

ASYMPTOMATIC FETAL INFECTION

Although published prospective studies of parvovirus B19 infection in pregnancy have varied in their estimates of adverse fetal outcome and rates of vertical transmission, most women infected during pregnancy deliver normal-appearing infants at term. Among these infants, some have asymptomatic infection.[260] A prospective study that combined serologic with virologic markers of infection suggested that intrauterine transmission is very high.[23] In this study, 43 pregnant women with a confirmed B19 infection were followed to delivery. The infants were tested at birth and at intervals throughout the first year of life for IgM and IgG to B19 and by PCR for viral DNA in serum, urine, or saliva. No fetal losses or cases of fetal hydrops were observed in this study; however, the rate of intrauterine viral transmission was 51%.[23]

BIRTH DEFECTS

There is circumstantial evidence that intrauterine parvovirus B19 infection may occasionally cause birth defects. The first case was reported in 1987.[261] An aborted fetus at 11 weeks of gestation was described with striking ocular abnormalities, including microphthalmia; aphakia; and dysplastic changes of the cornea, sclera, and choroid of one eye and retinal folds and degeneration of the lens in the other eye.[262,263] The mother had a history of a rash illness with arthropathy at 6 weeks that was serologically confirmed as B19 infection. There have been few additional reports of malformations or developmental abnormalities in aborted fetuses or live-born infants after intrauterine infection, and the few cases that have been described could not be unequivocally attributed to infection with B19.

There are no other data suggesting that B19 is an important cause of birth defects in live-born infants. In an uncontrolled study of 243 infants with birth defects and younger than 4 months, none had IgM antibodies to B19 detected.[227] In a controlled study of 57 infants with structural abnormalities or stigmata of congenital infection, specific B19 IgM was not detected in cord blood of any of the affected infants or of the matched normal newborn controls.[19] There are also no data suggesting that structural defects are common in newborns after maternal B19 infection. After a large community-wide outbreak of EI, there was no increase in congenital malformations compared with the preepidemic and postepidemic periods.[264] In the British study of maternal infections during pregnancy, outcomes were available for 186 patients; anencephaly was reported in 1 of the 30 fatal cases but was not attributed to B19 infection, and hypospadias was present in 2 of the 156 live-born infants.[20] No new anomalies or serious neurodevelopmental problems were detected in the 114 infants followed clinically for at least 1 year.[264] In another prospective but uncontrolled study of 39 pregnancies with maternal B19 infection, hypospadias was reported in 1 of the 37 live-born infants, and no abnormalities were reported in the one fatal case for which tissues were available.[240]

OTHER FETAL MANIFESTATIONS

Meconium ileus and peritonitis has been associated with maternal parvovirus B19 infection in a few reports.[144] Three infants with congenital anemia after maternal infection and intrauterine hydrops have also been reported.[16] All three infants had abnormalities on bone marrow examination and B19 DNA detected in bone marrow by PCR assay. Hyperechogenic bowel, common in fetuses infected with cytomegalovirus, has also been observed in a fetus with intrauterine B19 infection.[265]

FETAL HYDROPS

Although parvovirus B19 infection in utero may cause nonimmune hydrops fetalis, it is one of many causes of this syndrome and probably accounts for only 10% to 15% of fetal hydrops.[144] Hydrops fetalis is rare, occurring in only 1 in 3000 births; in 50% of cases, the etiology is unknown. In a study of 50 cases, B19 DNA was detected by in situ hybridization in the tissues of 4 fetuses; most of the cases were due to chromosomal or cardiovascular abnormalities.[266] In another study, B19 DNA was shown in 4 of 42 cases of nonimmune hydrops fetalis.[267]

B19 infection is frequently associated with nonimmune fetal hydrops during local epidemics of EI. In a hospital series from England, 10 cases of B19-associated hydrops, representing 8% of all cases of nonimmune hydrops and 27% of anatomically normal cases of nonimmune hydrops, occurred over 17 years.[268] In a consecutive series of 72 patients with nonimmune hydrops from Germany, 3 (4.2%) had B19 infection.[269] In a series of 673 fetal and neonatal autopsies conducted over 6 years in Rhode Island, 32 (0.7%) cases of hydrops were identified, and 5 (16%) of these had histologic and laboratory evidence of B19 infection.[270,271] In the British study, 1 of the 156 live-born infants had been diagnosed with intrauterine hydrops and recovered after intrauterine transfusion; of the six fatal cases that were positive for B19 DNA, hydrops was present in one of three fatal cases with laboratory-confirmed intrauterine infection.[20,268] Postmortem examination may be unable to identify hydrops in fetal death occurring in early pregnancy. Published reports suggest that nonimmune hydrops is an uncommon manifestation of fetal infection with B19.

FETAL OUTCOME IN RELATION TO MATERNAL MANIFESTATIONS

No data suggest that the clinical manifestation of parvovirus B19 infection in the mother influences the pregnancy outcome. There is evidence for an association between a B19-affected fetus and maternal hypertension. Pregnancy-induced hypertension, preeclampsia, and eclampsia have been reported in some women with B19-associated fetal hydrops, and there is a record of improvement with spontaneous resolution of hydrops in one case.[18,268,269] Hypertension of pregnancy may be caused by poor fetal-placental perfusion, and there is an increased risk in pregnancies complicated by hydrops. It is unknown if there is an increased frequency of hypertensive disorders in B19-infected women compared with uninfected women, or if more careful monitoring of B19-infected women to detect findings of preeclampsia would be useful in identifying women at increased risk of B19-associated fetal hydrops.

LONG-TERM OUTCOMES

The long-term outcomes of live-born infants infected in utero with parvovirus B19 are discussed in "Prognosis."

Pathogenesis of Infection in the Fetus

FETAL IMMUNE RESPONSES TO PARVOVIRUS B19

In studies in which serologic and virologic markers of infection have been examined, fetal immune responses to parvovirus B19 are variable.[23,148,272] B19-specific IgM in cord blood is a recognized marker of fetal infection, but sensitivity can be increased by adding other markers, such as IgA, PCR positivity, and persistence of B19 IgG at 1 year of age.[23,148,272] Infants exposed to B19 earlier in gestation may be less likely to show a positive IgM response because of immaturity of the fetal immune system; for infants exposed later in gestation, the IgM response may be delayed because of interference by passively acquired maternal antibodies. In one study of pregnancies complicate by B19 infection and where fetal blood was sampled, B19 DNA was detected in 100%, but B19 IgM and IgG were only detected one quarter of the cases.[273] IgG in fetal blood was associated with lower levels of IgG.[273] In another study, only two of nine infected infants whose exposure occurred in the first 14 weeks of pregnancy were positive for B19 IgM at delivery, whereas all four infected infants exposed in the last trimester had B19-specific IgM in cord blood.[23] Serum IgA, similar to IgM, does not cross the placenta, so for some other congenital viral infections (e.g., rubella and human immunodeficiency virus), viral-specific IgA responses in cord blood have been used to provide evidence of intrauterine infection. In the only study of B19 in which this response was examined, B19 IgA in cord blood was associated with maternal infection with B19, and for a few infants, this was the only marker of intrauterine infection.[23]

The fetal immune response to B19 may be important for preventing B19-induced red blood cell aplasia in the fetus and is suggested by the observed decreased rates of fetal death after 20 weeks of gestation. Viral clearance by the fetus may be prolonged. IgM specific to B19 may be detected at 18 weeks of gestation.[274] Fetal serum collected at 21 weeks of gestation neutralizes B19 virus in vitro.[275]

PATHOGENESIS OF PARVOVIRUS B19 HYDROPS

Nonimmune hydrops is the best-characterized complication of fetal parvovirus B19 infection. Several mechanisms have been proposed, and more than one may contribute to hydrops.[269] Severe fetal anemia and thrombocytopenia are present in most cases.[276] Hemoglobin levels less than 2 g/dL are detected by cordocentesis of hydropic fetuses.[277,278] Hypoxic injury to tissues may result in increased capillary permeability. Severe anemia may also increase cardiac output, as evidenced by increases in umbilical venous pressure, and subsequently result in high-output heart failure.[279] Alternatively, myocarditis may precipitate heart failure. Reduced fetal myocardial function, as shown by echocardiography, occurs in some cases of fetal hydrops. Regardless of the etiology, congestive heart failure could cause an increase in capillary hydrostatic pressure. Decreased venous return caused by massive ascites or organomegaly may lead to further cardiac decompensation. Hepatic function may be compromised by the extreme levels of extramedullary hematopoiesis, and lysis of B19-infected erythrocytes in the liver may cause hemosiderin deposition, fibrosis, and esophageal varices. Impaired production of albumin could lead to a decrease in colloid osmotic pressure with transfer of fluid to the extravascular compartment. Placental hydrops may compromise further oxygen delivery to the fetus.

Finally, there is considerable evidence that fetal tissues other than erythroid cells may be susceptible to B19 infection. Virus has been shown in fetal myocytes, including cardiac myocytes, along with inflammatory changes; fetal myocarditis associated with B19 infection is well documented.[131,280] Histologic studies show vascular damage and perivascular infiltrates in other fetal tissues; it is unknown if this is due to B19 infection in endothelial cells or a nonspecific effect related to hypoxic damage.

Pathology in the Fetus

ANATOMIC AND HISTOLOGIC FEATURES

The hallmarks of fetal infection with parvovirus B19 are edema, anemia, and myocarditis, and these are reflected in the pathologic findings at autopsy, but otherwise, postmortem reports of gross and histopathologic pathology reveal few features specific for intrauterine B19 infection.[18,268,270]

At postmortem, B19-infected fetuses are often described as pale with subcutaneous edema. Rashes are almost always absent; however, a "blueberry muffin" rash caused by extramedullary hematopoiesis in the skin may occur.[281]

Fetal anemia is common in fetal deaths caused by B19 but does not occur in all cases.[277,278]

The histologic findings suggestive of B19 infection include erythroid hypoplasia or occasionally hyperplasia characteristic of recovery. Extramedullary hematopoiesis is common in many organs, especially the liver and spleen.

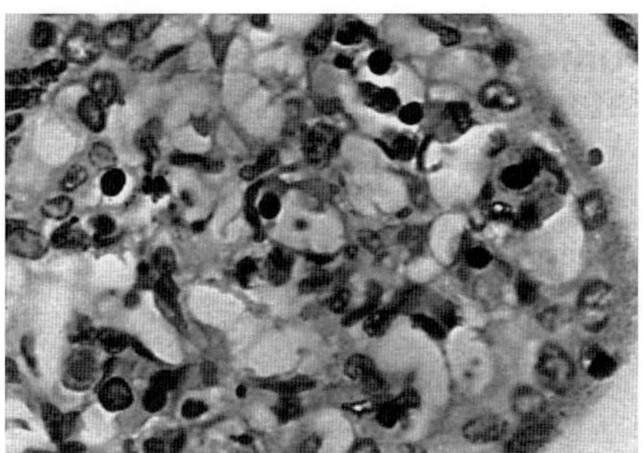

Figure 28-3 Placenta from a case of parvovirus B19–associated nonimmune hydrops shows fetal capillaries filled with erythroblasts, most with marginated chromatin and typical amphophilic intranuclear inclusions [hematoxylin and eosin stain].

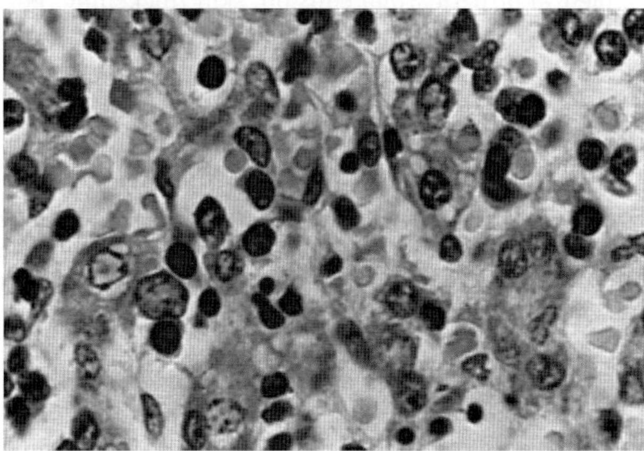

Figure 28-4 Fetal liver from a case of parvovirus B19–associated nonimmune hydrops shows extramedullary hematopoiesis, intranuclear inclusions in erythroblasts, and focal areas with hemosiderin and fibrosis [hematoxylin and eosin stain].

Nucleated red blood cells with amphophilic intranuclear inclusions (Figs. 28-3 and 28-4) are highly suggestive of B19 infection. These nucleated red blood cells are often found in the lumens of vessels and at sites of extramedullary hematopoiesis.[131] When stained with hematoxylin and eosin, the nuclei have an irregular band of dark chromatin. The center of the nucleus is lighter with a smooth texture. The specificity of intranuclear inclusions for fetal B19 infection is unknown, but it is probably high when associated with anemia and hydrops. Viral DNA or inclusions may also be present in macrophages and myocytes.[131,280] PCR assay to detect B19 DNA is the best method to diagnose B19 infection in a postmortem fetus. In one study, 6 of 34 cases of idiopathic nonimmune hydrops contained B19 DNA in either fetal or placental tissues compared with no positive PCR results among 23 cases of hydrops that were noninfectious.[282] Histologic examination of these cases found no nucleated red blood cells with intranuclear inclusions.

PLACENTA

Parvovirus B19 infection of the placenta probably precedes fetal infection. The placenta is usually abnormal when associated with fetal death resulting from B19. Grossly, the placenta is often enlarged and edematous. Histologically, the placenta also contains nucleated red blood cells with typical intranuclear inclusions (see Fig. 28-4). Foci of red blood cell production also occur in the placenta, as does vascular inflammation.[268,280] In one study, vasculitis of villous capillaries or stem arteries occurred in 9 of 10 placentas.[268] There was swelling of endothelial cells, fragmentation of endothelial cell nuclei, and fibrin thrombi. B19 DNA occurs in endothelial cells of patients with myocarditis and in patients with cutaneous lesions but has not been sought in placental endothelial cells.

The human placenta contains a B19 receptor, the neutral glycosphingolipid globoside, on the villous trophoblast layer of the placenta; the concentration of the globoside decreases with advancing pregnancy.[283] The highest concentration occurs in the first trimester with diminished reactivity in the second trimester. The presence of this globoside in the placenta provides a mechanism by which the virus infects the placenta and fetus. It also may explain why there is a difference in fetal outcome associated with gestational age. Maternal infections in late pregnancy have a better prognosis than infections occurring early in pregnancy. In addition to B19 receptors, there is also a B19-induced inflammatory response in the placenta, characterized by a significant number of $CD3^+$ T cells and the inflammatory cytokine interleukin-2.[284]

HEART

The anemia associated with parvovirus B19 infection is due to a specific viral tropism for progenitor erythroid cells, specifically P antigen, which is found on these cells.[285] Clinical and laboratory evidence suggests, however, that B19 has a wider tropism than only erythroblasts.[286] Fetal myocardial cells contain P antigen.[287] Direct infection of myocardial cells after fetal B19 infection of extramedullary erythroid progenitor cells has been shown by in situ DNA hybridization or electron microscopy.[60,72,131] B19 myocarditis is also associated with acute lymphocytic infiltration. Case reports have described at least eight fetuses, five children, and four adults with myocarditis associated with a concurrent B19 infection.[288-290] B19 causes acute and chronic myocarditis in infants. This myocarditis and the cardiac enlargement present in some B19-infected fetuses with hydrops suggest that B19 is pathogenic for the myocardium.[†]

In infected fetuses, the heart may be normal or symmetrically enlarged, suggesting congestive heart failure. Pericardial effusions are common. Myocytes with intranuclear inclusions occur infrequently. Mononuclear cell infiltrates occur occasionally, and B19 DNA, not associated with cells, can be found in the lumens of large vessels. As a response to injury, focal areas with dystrophic calcification or fibroelastosis have been reported.

One case-control study examined the relationship between congenital heart disease and B19 infection.[292] Five of 29 cases of congenital heart disease had B19 DNA detected in cardiac tissue by using PCR assay compared with none of 30 matched case control subjects. This difference was significant ($P < .02$). Other infections, including

---

[†]References 131, 268, 270, 274, 280, 288, 291.

herpes simplex virus, cytomegalovirus, rubella, and toxoplasmosis, were excluded. Additional studies testing for B19 infection of congenital heart disease are appropriate.

OTHER ORGANS

Numerous other anatomic abnormalities have been described in association with parvovirus B19 infection of the fetus. The occurrence of these abnormalities is so infrequent, however, that it is unlikely that any are related to B19. These associated abnormalities include dystrophic calcification of the brain and adrenal glands, anencephaly and ventriculomegaly, pulmonary hypoplasia, hypospadias, cleft lip, meconium peritonitis, corneal opacification and angioedema, and thymic abnormalities.

Diagnostic Evaluation and Management of the Woman and Fetus Exposed to or Infected by Parvovirus B19 During Pregnancy

OVERVIEW

Management of a pregnant woman exposed to parvovirus B19 requires knowledge of the prevailing status of EI in the community, a detailed history of the exposure, knowledge of characteristic symptoms and signs of maternal EI and B19 infection in the fetus, appropriate laboratory tests needed to confirm maternal and fetal infection, knowledge of the methods for monitoring the fetus at risk for nonimmune hydrops, knowledge of therapeutic approaches for treating the hydropic fetus, and information about the prognosis of maternal and fetal infection and the expected outcomes for the therapeutic intervention.

PREVALENCE OF ERYTHEMA INFECTIOSUM

The community health or school health departments may know if EI is endemic or epidemic in the community, increasing the probability of primary infection in susceptible pregnant women.

HISTORY OF EXPOSURE

Pregnant women who are potentially exposed to a person with EI should be asked about the type of exposure, including duration and location, brief or prolonged, household or workplace, indoor or outdoor, and contact with respiratory secretions. Exposure to a child within the household constitutes the highest risk.

Did the contact have symptoms typical of EI, including a low-grade fever and a typical slapped-cheek rash that soon spread to the trunk or limbs in a lacy pattern? Did the rash disappear and then reappear when the child was warm from exercise or bathing? Had the child been exposed to any known source of EI, such as an outbreak in school, preschool, or daycare center; a family gathering; a play group; or church nursery? Was the child evaluated by a physician familiar with viral exanthems?

CLINICAL FEATURES SUGGESTING SIGNS AND SYMPTOMS OF PARVOVIRUS B19 INFECTION IN THE PREGNANT WOMAN

It should be determined if the mother's signs and symptoms are compatible with parvovirus B19 infection in adults, including at least one or more of the following: malaise, arthralgia, rash, coryza, or fever ($\geq 38°$ C). Pregnant women with such symptoms, especially malaise with symmetric arthralgias in the hands, wrists, knees, or feet, should be considered at high risk and tested for a recent B19 infection. In Barcelona, Gratacos and coworkers[22] found that only 30% of 60 IgM-positive women recalled any such symptoms. Pregnant women without such systemic symptoms but with a rapidly enlarging uterus (fundal height exceeding dates by >3 cm), an elevated serum α-fetoprotein, preterm labor, or decreased fetal movement should be asked about B19 exposure. If ultrasonography reveals evidence of hydrops fetalis or the fetus has ascites, pleural or pericardial effusion, skin thickening, polyhydramnios, or placentomegaly, maternal B19 testing is appropriate.

LABORATORY DIAGNOSIS IN THE PREGNANT WOMAN

With evidence of maternal parvovirus B19 exposure or maternal disease, maternal serum should be tested for IgG and IgM antibodies to B19. If there is probable or possible exposure, the first serum should be drawn at least 10 days after the exposure. Fetal morbidity is unlikely to occur within 2 weeks of exposure, so immediate serologic testing is appropriate for a woman or fetus with symptoms or signs of B19 infection.

If an initial serum sample is IgG-positive but IgM-negative, this indicates a previous maternal infection, and additional testing is usually unnecessary. The IgM assay is sensitive, with few false-negative reactions. If an initial serum sample is negative for IgM and IgG, this indicates no previous maternal infection, and B19 is not responsible for maternal symptoms and signs or for hydrops fetalis.

If the IgM result is positive, a recent B19 infection is established regardless of the IgG titer. A concomitant negative IgG titer indicates an early B19 infection without time for IgG to be detectable. If PCR is available, detection of maternal and fetal viremia by PCR for B19 DNA is also diagnostic of B19 infection. Viremia may precede the development of IgM antibodies by 7 to 14 days and may persist for several months after a primary infection.

A useful adjunct to IgM testing is measurement of IgG avidity to the VP1 capsid protein.[286,293] After a primary infection, initial IgG antibodies have low avidity for binding to the VP1 capsid. This avidity increases slowly over several weeks or months, and avidity can be used as a confirmatory test for the occasional patient for whom the diagnosis is initially unclear.

With a positive maternal IgM, the fetus must be examined for signs of hydrops fetalis by ultrasonography within 24 to 48 hours. If the gestational age is less than 18 weeks, the absence of hydrops may not be reassuring because hydrops could appear later. Several cases of severe hydrops fetalis spontaneously reverting to normal over 3 to 6 weeks have been reported, so advice about pregnancy termination is difficult.[272]

Detection of maternal and fetal levels of B19 DNA (viral load) is a highly sensitive test for identifying B19 infection.[286,294-296] Peak maternal viral loads occur about 1 week after maternal infection, and fetal viral loads, approximately equal to maternal levels, occur 1 to 3 weeks after maternal infection. The prolonged persistence of B19 DNA in the blood means additional testing is required to establish the time of maternal infection. Viral loads are not predictive of the severity of fetal infection. Among 72 pregnancies complicated by B19 infections, IgM assay correctly diagnosed 94% of maternal infections, and PCR assay for B19 DNA diagnosed 96%, with combination of the two tests yielding maximal sensitivity.[244]

FETAL MONITORING

For a fetal gestational age of greater than 20 weeks, an initial negative ultrasound scan should be repeated weekly to detect hydrops. The number of weekly ultrasound scans that should be performed is controversial: Rodis and colleagues[298] originally suggested continuing weekly scans for 6 to 8 weeks after exposure. They reported a fetal death at 23 weeks after maternal fever and arthralgias in the first trimester. The interval between maternal B19 infection and fetal morbidity is uncertain. Based on this report, other authors recommended weekly ultrasound scans for 14 weeks after maternal B19 infection.[297] This monitoring often appeals to pregnant women fearful of fetal death, but it is time-consuming and expensive.

The duration of monitoring for hydrops fetalis might be best determined by examination of the interval between maternal exposure or symptoms of B19 infection and the appearance of hydrops fetalis or fetal death. Table 28-2 summarizes reports with adequate information to evaluate the interval, which include 14 intervals between maternal B19 exposure or infection and fetal death and 7 intervals between maternal exposure or infection and the first diagnosis of hydrops fetalis. The intervals range from 1 to 19 weeks (median, 6 weeks). Between 3 and 11 weeks, 17 of 21 (81%) cases of hydrops fetalis developed. Because 11 of the 21 cases developed 4 to 8 weeks after maternal exposure or infection, this is the most common interval between infection and the detection of fetal hydrops.

Based on these observations, weekly ultrasound monitoring of the fetus for 12 weeks after maternal exposure is optimal but does not detect all delayed cases and may be expensive. Such frequent scanning may not be considered cost-effective because the incidence of hydrops after maternal B19 infection is low in many studies. In our study, none of the 52 fetuses born to pregnant women positive for B19 IgM developed hydrops fetalis; however, the 95% confidence interval, based on our sample size, ranged from 0% to 8.6% risk for hydrops fetalis.[233] Using maternal symptoms as criteria for maternal B19 infection, other studies have suggested a 9% incidence of fetal death because of B19 in women positive for B19 IgM.[20]

The fetus in a B19-infected woman may be monitored with serial maternal serum α-fetoprotein (MSAFP) measurements.[299] One report found elevated MSAFP in five B19 IgM–positive pregnancies associated with fetal death but no fetal deaths in 11 IgM-positive women with B19 infection although having normal MSAFP values.[277] A case of B19-associated fetal death discovered because of elevated MSAFP at 16 weeks in a routine test in an asymptomatic woman has also been described.[18] In adding a seventh case of fetal death associated with elevated MSAFP among women positive for B19 IgM, Bernstein and Capeless[299] suggested using MSAFP values to indicate a good fetal prognosis.

A German study found, however, that neither MSAFP nor human gonadotropin was a marker of B19-infected pregnancies, although both were frequently elevated when complications occurred.[300] The study included 35 pregnant women with fetal complications associated with B19; significant elevations of MSAFP occurred in 13 of 35 women, and elevations of human gonadotropin occurred in 25 of 35 women. The investigators tested 137 serum samples from 65 pregnant women without acute B19 infection and no fetal complications. Of the 30 women without fetal complications, there were significant elevations of MSAFP in only 2 women, and elevations of human gonadotropin occurred in only 5 women. Neither MSAFP nor human gonadotropin was a marker for a poor pregnancy outcome early on, but these proteins were frequently elevated when complications developed. Despite this study, there is insufficient experience using MSAFP, and MSAFP measurements at any gestational age are relatively nonspecific indicators of fetal well-being.

Electronic fetal monitoring is ineffective in detecting hydrops fetalis and predicting the outcome of pregnancy in women positive for B19 IgM. Contraction stress tests and nonstress tests are not accurate predictors of fetal well-being in cases of fetal anemia and hydrops fetalis. Similarly, fetal assessment with estriol measurements or other biochemical markers have no documented role in cases of hydrops fetalis.

Because fetal ultrasonography is readily available and provides rapid specific information about hydrops fetalis, it is the best method to monitor the fetus after maternal B19 infection. Doppler ultrasonography of the middle cerebral artery may also be used to reveal increased peak systolic velocity suggestive of fetal anemia.[301]

FETAL THERAPY

If hydrops fetalis is detected before 18 weeks of gestation, there is no effective intervention. Other causes of hydrops, such as chromosomal disorders or anatomic abnormalities, should be assessed. If the fetus is still viable, as determined by ultrasonography, at 18 weeks of gestation, percutaneous umbilical blood sampling, or cordocentesis, can be considered. At 18 weeks of gestation, the umbilical vein diameter is about 4 mm, the minimum size required for successful percutaneous umbilical blood sampling. Fetal blood should be obtained for hematocrit, reticulocyte count, platelet count, leukocyte count, anti–B19 IgM, karyotype, and tests for B19 DNA by PCR assay. The hematocrit must be determined immediately, and if fetal anemia is present, an intrauterine intravascular fetal transfusion is performed with the same needle puncture.

If the fetus is between 18 and 32 weeks of gestation when hydrops fetalis is detected, fetal transfusion should be considered. There are many successful reported cases of fetal transfusion for B19-induced hydrops fetalis, and some have long-term follow-up data, but the success rate of the procedure remains unknown.[291] Two or three separate transfusions are usually required before resolution of the fetal anemia and hydrops fetalis, increasing the 1% to 2% risk of each single percutaneous umbilical blood sampling procedure. Resolution of the hydrops usually occurs 3 to 6 weeks after the first transfusion. Although spontaneous resolution has been reported, it seems appropriate not to risk an uncertain outcome because the longer the fetal transfusion is delayed, the less likely it is to be successful, and the worse the potential harm to the fetus caused by continued fetal hypoxia.[291,294]

Thrombocytopenia is also common and, if severe, may require intrauterine platelet transfusion.[276] There is also one report of a hydropic infant successfully treated with intraperitoneal gamma globulin high in titer to B19.[302] For fetuses at 32 weeks of gestation or greater when hydrops is discovered, immediate delivery with neonatal exchange transfusion, thoracentesis, and paracentesis as indicated is usually the safest management.[303]

Differential Diagnosis

Recalling that the hallmarks of fetal infection with parvovirus B19 are anemia, hydrops, and myocarditis helps in compiling a differential diagnosis. For infants with anemia, the differential diagnosis includes all the known causes of fetal anemia, such as fetal-maternal transfusion, intracranial bleeding, blood group incompatibilities, congenital anemias such as Diamond-Blackfan syndrome, nutritional deficiencies, and inborn metabolic errors. Fetal hydrops and fetal and placental edema may be associated with other congenital infections, particularly congenital syphilis, chromosomal abnormalities, immune hydrops associated with blood group incompatibilities, hypothyroidism, and heart and renal failure.

Prognosis

Pregnant women can be reassured about the relatively low risk of fetal morbidity resulting from exposure to parvovirus B19. About half of women are already seropositive, and the seronegative maternal B19 infection rate ranges from about 29% for exposures by the woman's own children to 10% to 18% for other exposures. The expected fetal morbidity and mortality risk is about 2% ($\frac{1}{50}$). The overall risk of fetal death ranges from 0.3% ($\frac{1}{2} \times \frac{3}{10} \times \frac{1}{50} = \frac{3}{1000}$) to a mere 0.1% ($\frac{1}{2} \times \frac{1}{10} \times \frac{1}{50} = \frac{1}{1000}$).[233] Live-born infants infected in utero may die shortly after birth. There is one report of two infants born prematurely at 24 weeks and 35 weeks of gestational age, respectively, who developed an illness characteristic of congenital viral infection, including placentomegaly, petechial rash, edema, hepatomegaly, anemia, thrombocytopenia, and respiratory insufficiency; both died postnatally.[304] Both infants had nuclear inclusions in erythroid precursor cells, and PCR assay confirmed the presence of B19 DNA in one of the infants.

There is one report describing three live-born infants with severe CNS abnormalities after serologically confirmed maternal B19 infection.[305] Subsequent case reports have also identified CNS manifestations, including mild-to-moderate hydrocephalus, with CNS scarring associated with fetal B19 infection.[306] These reports suggest possible long-term neurologic sequelae in surviving infants that may not be apparent at birth.

Data regarding the long-term outcomes of live-born children infected in utero or born of mothers infected during pregnancy are very limited. In one study, 113 pregnant women with B19 infection during pregnancy and a control group of immune women were questioned about the health and development of their children when the median age of the children was 4 years for both groups.[264] The incidence of development delays in speech, language, information processing, and attention was similar in the study and control groups (7.3% vs. 7.5%, respectively). Two cases of cerebral palsy were found in the study group compared with none in the control group. Although not statistically significant, this 2% incidence of cerebral palsy in the infected group is 10-fold higher than the reported national incidence.[264]

In a British study of 427 pregnant women with B19 infection and 367 of their surviving infants, 129 surviving infants were followed up at 7 to 10 years of age.[307] The follow-up included questionnaires to obstetricians and general practitioners on outcome of pregnancy and health of surviving infants. Maternal infection was confirmed by B19-specific IgM assay or IgG seroconversion, or both. An excess rate of fetal loss was confined to the first 20 weeks of gestation and averaged 9%. There were seven cases of fetal hydrops with maternal infections between 9 and 20 weeks of gestation. There were no abnormalities attributable to B19 infection found at birth in surviving infants. There were no late effects observed between 7 and 10 years of age. The conclusions of this study were as follows: (1) Approximately 1 in 10 women infected before 20 weeks of gestation have a fetal loss resulting from B19; (2) the risk of an adverse outcome of pregnancy beyond this stage is unlikely; and (3) infected women can be reassured that the risk of congenital abnormality resulting from B19 is less than 1%, and long-term development will be normal.

One study used IQ testing and standard neurodevelopmental tests to assess 20 children who had B19-induced fetal hydrops and intrauterine transfusion of packed red blood cells.[308] IQ testing of the 20 children between 13 months and 9 years of age revealed that all of the children ranged within 2 standard deviations of a population norm. There was no significant developmental delay. This study concluded that children who survived successful intrauterine transfusion from B19 anemia and hydrops had a good neurodevelopmental prognosis.

Another study came to an opposite conclusion.[309] That study used Bayley scales of infant development to assess 16 transfused B19 hydropic fetuses who were live-born and survived. Assessments were done between 6 months and 8 years of age. Postnatal growth and health status were reported to be normal. Mild-to-severe developmental delay was observed in 5 of the children, suggesting that B19 infection may induce brain damage.[309] A Dutch study reported severe neurodevelopmental impairment in 3 of 28 infants infected in utero and treated with intrauterine transfusion, including an infant with cerebral palsy.[310]

In summary, most infants infected in utero with B19 survive and develop normally, but it is unlikely that all infected infants, whether because of direct viral infection of the brain or as a consequence of intrauterine hypoxia, will develop normally.

Prevention

GENERAL MEASURES

Because parvovirus B19 is usually endemic in most communities, what is the appropriate management for pregnant women with daily contact with children? The prevalence of seropositivity (immunity) to B19 among pregnant women varies according to geographic location, sex, age, and race. Assuming that on average 50% of pregnant women are immune, that during endemic periods between 1% and 4% of susceptible women become infected during pregnancy, and that the rate of fetal death after maternal infection is 2%, the occupational risk of fetal death for a pregnant woman with unknown serologic status would be between 1 in 1000 and 1 in 2500. These rates are so low that they would not justify intervention, such as serologic testing for pregnant women or furloughing or temporarily transferring pregnant seronegative employees to administrative or other positions without child contact. A detailed cost-benefit analysis for Germany reached the same conclusion.[311] During epidemic periods in specific schools, when the infection rates may be 5-fold to 20-fold higher, serologic testing or temporary transfer of pregnant employees may occasionally be appropriate, and some anxious women may choose to leave the workplace.

Given the low risk for individual pregnant women, seronegative women should not send their own children away. Schools and daycare centers cannot stop B19 outbreaks by excluding children with rash illnesses because B19 is transmissible before the rash appears. Whether B19 can be transmitted via breastfeeding is unknown.

VACCINE DEVELOPMENT

For most women, fetal B19 infections during pregnancy do not occur from occupational exposure, but rather from exposure to school-age children at home. Given this factor, the highly communicable and endemic nature of the infection, the broad spectrum of illness that B19 causes, and the large portion of the population (30%-50%) who are susceptible, an effective B19 vaccine, preferably administered in infancy, is appropriate, and at least one vaccine has been developed.[312] This vaccine comprises the major B19 capsid proteins VP1 and VP2 and is administered with a squalene adjuvant, MF59. After testing in a limited number of subjects, this vaccine seems safe and induces neutralizing antibodies but was reactogenic.[313,314] Studies using volunteers challenged with wild-type B19 should be able to assess efficacy. A vaccine that induces sustained neutralizing antibody IgG levels to B19 should be effective given that prior immunity to natural B19 infection protects against reinfection.

References

1. Allander T, Tammi MT, Eriksson M, et al: Cloning of a human parvovirus by molecular screening of respiratory tract samples, *Proc Natl Acad Sci U S A* 102:12891-12896, 2005.
2. Kesebir D, Vazquez M, Weibel C, et al: Human bocavirus infection in young children in the United States: molecular epidemiological profile and clinical characteristics of a newly emerging respiratory virus, *J Infect Dis* 194:1276-1282, 2006.
3. Tattersall P, Bergoin M, Bloom ME, et al: Parvoviridae. In Fauquet CM, Mayo MA, Maniloff J, Desselberger U, Ball LA, editors: *Virus taxonomy: classification and nomenclature of viruses: eighth report of the International Committee on Taxonomy of Viruses*, New York, 2005, Elsevier Academic Press, pp 353-369.
4. Young NS, Brown KE: Parvovirus B19, *N Engl J Med* 350:586-597, 2004.
5. Koch WC: Fifth (human parvovirus B19) and sixth (herpesvirus 6) diseases, *Curr Opin Infect Dis* 14:343-356, 2001.
6. Cossart YE, Field AM, Cant B, et al: Parvovirus-like particles in human sera, *Lancet* 1:72-73, 1975.
7. Summers J, Jones SE, Anderson MJ: Characterization of the genome of the agent of erythrocyte aplasia permits its classification as a human parvovirus, *J Gen Virol* 64:2527-2532, 1983.
8. Pattison JR, Jones SE, Hodgson J: Parvovirus infections and hypoplastic crisis in sickle-cell anemia, *Lancet* 1:664-665, 1981.
9. Serjeant GR, Topley JM, Mason K, et al: Outbreak of aplastic crises in sickle cell anemia associated with parvovirus-like agent, *Lancet* 2:595-597, 1981.
10. Anderson MJ, Jones SE, Fisher-Hoch SP, et al: Human parvovirus, the cause of erythema infectiosum (fifth disease)? *Lancet* 1:1378, 1983.
11. Thurn J: Human parvovirus B19: historical and clinical review, *Rev Infect Dis* 10:1005-1011, 1988.
12. Ager EA, Chin TDY, Poland JD: Epidemic erythema infectiosum, *N Engl J Med* 275:1326-1331, 1966.
13. Cramp JE, Armstrong BD: Erythema infectiosum: no evidence of teratogenicity, *Br Med J* 2:1031, 1977.
14. Pattison JR: B19 virus infections in pregnancy. In Pattison JR, editor: *Parvoviruses and human disease*, Boca Raton, Fla, 1988, CRC Press.
15. Siegel G: Patterns of parvovirus disease in animals. In Pattison JR, editor: *Parvoviruses and human disease*, Boca Raton, Fla, 1988, CRC Press.
16. Brown T, Anand A, Ritchie LD, et al: Intrauterine parvovirus infection associated with hydrops fetalis, *Lancet* 2:1033-1034, 1984.
17. Knott PD, Welply GA, Anderson MJ: 1984 Serologically proved intrauterine infection with parvovirus, *Br Med J (Clin Res Ed)* 289 (6459):1660, 1960.
18. Anand A, Gray ES, Brown T, et al: Human parvovirus infection in pregnancy and hydrops fetalis, *N Engl J Med* 316:183-186, 1987.
19. Kinney JS, Anderson LJ, Farrar J, et al: Risk of adverse outcomes of pregnancy after human parvovirus B19 infection, *J Infect Dis* 157:663-667, 1988.
20. Hall SM: Public Health Laboratory Service Working Party on Fifth Disease. Prospective study of human parvovirus (B19) infection in pregnancy, *BMJ* 300:1166-1170, 1990.
21. Adler SP, Manganello AM, Koch WC, et al: Risk of human parvovirus B19 infections among school and hospital employees during endemic periods, *J Infect Dis* 168:361-368, 1993.
22. Gratacos E, Torres PJ, Vidal J, et al: The incidence of human parvovirus B19 infection during pregnancy and its impact on perinatal outcome, *J Infect Dis* 171:1360-1363, 1995.
23. Koch WC, Harger JH, Barnstein B, et al: Serologic and virologic evidence for frequent intrauterine transmission of human parvovirus B10 with a primary maternal infection during pregnancy, *Pediatr Infect Dis J* 17:489-494, 1998.
24. Brown KE: The expanding range of parvoviruses which infect humans, *Rev Med Virol* 20:231-244, 2010.
25. Astell CR, Luo W, Brunstein J, et al: B19 parvovirus: biochemical and molecular features. In Anderson LJ, Young NS, editors: *Human parvovirus B19. Monographs in virology*, vol 20, Basel, 1997, Karger.
26. O'Sullivan MG, Anderson DC, Fikes JD, et al: Identification of a novel simian parvovirus from cynomolgus monkey with severe anemia: a paradigm for human B19 parvovirus infection, *J Clin Invest* 93:1571-1576, 1994.

27. Jones MS, Kapoor A, Lukashov VV, et al: New DNA viruses identified in patient with acute viral infection syndrome, *J Virol* 79:8230-8236, 2005.
28. Umene K, Nunoue T: Genetic diversity of human parvovirus B19 determined using a set of restriction endonucleases recognizing four or five base pairs and partial nucleotide sequencing: use of sequence variability in virus classification, *J Gen Virol* 72:1997-2001, 1991.
29. Gallinella G, Venturoli S, Manaresi E, et al: B19 virus genome diversity: epidemiological and clinical correlations, *J Clin Virol* 76:9124-9134, 2003.
30. Nguyen QT, Sifer C, Schneider V, et al: Novel human erythrovirus associated with transient aplastic crisis, *J Clin Microbiol* 37:2483-2487, 1999.
31. Nguyen QT, Wong S, Heegaard ED, et al: Identification and characterization of a second human erythrovirus variant, A6, *Virology* 30:374-380, 2002.
32. Servant A, Laperche S, Lallemand F, et al: Genetic diversity within human erythroviruses: identification of three genotypes, *J Virol* 76:9124-9134, 2002.
33. Brown CS, Van Lent JW, Vlak JM, et al: Assembly of empty capsids by using baculovirus recombinants expressing human parvovirus B19 structural proteins, *J Virol* 65:2702-2706, 1991.
34. Kajigay S, Fujii H, Field A, et al: Self-assembled B19 parvovirus capsids, produced in a baculovirus system, are antigenically and immunogenically similar to native virions, *Proc Natl Acad Sci U S A* 88:4646-4650, 1991.
35. Ozawa K, Ayub J, Kajigaya S, et al: The gene encoding the nonstructural protein of B19 (human) parvovirus may be lethal in transfected cells, *J Virol* 62:2884-2889, 1988.
36. Moffat S, Yaegashi N, Tada K, et al: Human parvovirus B19 nonstructural protein NS1 induces apoptosis in erythroid lineage cells, *J Virol* 72:3018-3028, 1998.
37. Sol N, Le Junter J, Vassias I, et al: Possible interactions between the NS-1 protein and tumor necrosis factor alpha pathways in erythroid cell apoptosis induced by parvovirus B19, *J Virol* 73:8762-8770, 1999.
38. Ozawa K, Kurtzman G, Young N: Replication of the B19 parvovirus in human bone marrow cell cultures, *Science* 233:883-886, 1986.
39. Srivastava A, Lu L: Replication of B19 parvovirus in highly enriched hematopoietic progenitor cells form normal human bone marrow, *J Virol* 62:3059-3063, 1988.
40. Yaegashi N, Shiraishi H, Takeshita T, et al: Propagation of human parvovirus B19 in primary culture of erythroid lineage cells derived from fetal liver, *J Virol* 63:2422-2426, 1989.
41. Takahashi T, Ozawa K, Mitani K, et al: B19 parvovirus replicates in erythroid leukemic cells in vitro, *J Infect Dis* 160:548-549, 1989.
42. Miyagawa E, Yoshida T, Takahashi H, et al: Infection of the erythroid cell line KU812Ep6 with human parvovirus B19 and its application to titration of B19 infectivity, *J Virol Methods* 83:45-54, 1999.
43. Brown KE, Young NS, Liu JM: Molecular, cellular and clinical aspects of parvovirus B19 infection, *Crit Rev Oncol Hematol* 16:1-31, 1994.
44. Brown KE, Anderson SM, Young NS: Erythrocyte P antigen: cellular receptor for B19 parvovirus, *Science* 262:114-117, 1993.
45. Brown KE, Hibbs JR, Gallinella G, et al: Resistance to parvovirus B19 infection due to a lack of virus receptor (erythrocyte P antigen), *N Engl J Med* 330:1192-1196, 1994.
46. Weigel-Kelley KA, Yoder MC, Srivastava A: Recombinant human parvovirus B19 vectors: erythrocyte P antigen is necessary but not sufficient for successful transduction of human hematopoietic cells, *J Virol* 75:4110-4116, 2001.
47. Weigel-Kelley KA, Yoder MC, Srivastava A: Alpha5 beta 1 integrin as a cellular coreceptor for human parvovirus B19: requirement of functional activation of beta 1 integrin for viral entry, *Blood* 102:3927-3933, 2003.
48. Brown KE, Young NS: Parvovirus B19 infection and hematopoiesis, *Blood Rev* 9:176-182, 1995.
49. Young N: Hematologic and hematopoietic consequences of B19 infection, *Semin Hematol* 25:159-172, 1988.
50. Srivastava A, Bruno E, Briddell R, et al: Parvovirus B19-induced perturbation of human megakaryocytopoiesis in vitro, *Blood* 76:1997-2004, 1990.
51. Anderson MJ, Higgins PG, Davis LR, et al: Experimental parvovirus infection in humans, *J Infect Dis* 152:257-265, 1985.
52. Moffat S, Tanaka N, Tada K, et al: A cytotoxic nonstructural protein, NS1, of human parvovirus B19 induces activation of interleukin-6 gene expression, *J Virol* 70:8485-8491, 1996.
53. Gilbert NL, Gyorkos TW, Béliveau C, et al: Seroprevalence of parvovirus B19 infection in daycare educators, *Epidemiol Infect* 133:299-304, 2005.
54. Teuscher T, Baillod B, Holzer BR: Prevalence of human parvovirus B19 in sickle cell disease and healthy controls, *Trop Geogr Med* 43:108-110, 1991.
55. Schwarz TF, Gürtler LG, Zoulek G, et al: Seroprevalence of human parvovirus B19 infection in São Tomé and Principe, Malawi and Mascarene Islands, *Int J Med Microbiol* 271:231-236, 1989.
56. Jones PH, Pickett LC, Anderson MJ, et al: Human parvovirus infection in children and severe anaemia seen in an area endemic for malaria, *J Trop Med Hyg* 93:67, 1990.
57. de Freitas RB, Wong D, Boswell F, et al: Prevalence of human parvovirus (B19) and rubellavirus infections in urban and remote rural areas in northern Brazil, *J Med Virol* 32:203-208, 1990.
58. Gaggero A, Rivera J, Calquín E, et al: Seroprevalence of IgG antibodies against parvovirus B19 among blood donors from Santiago, Chile, *Rev Med Chil* 135:443-448, 2007.
59. Rohrer C, Gärtner B, Sauerbrei A, et al: Seroprevalence of parvovirus B19 in the German population, *Epidemiol Infect* 16:1-12, 2008.
60. Brown CS, Jensen T, Meloen RH, et al: Localization of an immunodominant domain on baculovirus-produced parvovirus B19 capsids: correlation to a major surface region on the native virus particle, *J Virol* 66:69-89, 1992.
61. Morey AL, O'Neill HJ, Coyle PV, et al: Immunohistological detection of human parvovirus B19 in formalin-fixed, paraffin-embedded tissues, *J Pathol* 166:105-108, 1992.
62. Loughrey AC, O'Neill HJ, Coyle PV, et al: Identification and use of a neutralizing epitope of parvovirus B19 for the rapid detection of virus infection, *J Med Virol* 39:97-100, 1993.
63. Morinet F, Tratschin JD, Perol Y, et al: Comparison of 17 isolates of the human parvovirus B19 by restriction enzyme analysis, *Arch Virol* 90:165-172, 1986.
64. Umene K, Nunoue T: The genome type of human parvovirus B19 strains isolated in Japan during 1981 differs from types detected in 1986 to 1987: a correlation between genome type and prevalence, *J Gen Virol* 71:983-986, 1990.
65. Umene K, Nunoue T: Partial nucleotide sequencing and characterization of human parvovirus B19 genome DNAs from damaged human fetuses and from patients with leukemia, *J Med Virol* 39:333, 1993.
66. Lawton AL, Smith RE: Erythema infectiosum: a clinical study of an epidemic in Branford, Connecticut, *Arch Intern Med* 47:28-41, 1931.
67. Chargin L, Sobel N, Goldstein H: Erythema infectiosum: report of an extensive epidemic, *Arch Dermatol Syphilol* 47:467, 1943.
68. Galvon FAC: An outbreak of erythema infectiosum—Nova Scotia, *Can Dis Wkly Rep* 9:69, 1983.
69. Serjeant GR, Serjeant BE, Thomas PW, et al: Human parvovirus infection in homozygous sickle cell disease, *Lancet* 341:1237-1240, 1993.
70. Oliveira SA, Camacho LA, Pereira AC, et al: Clinical and epidemiological aspects of human parvovirus B19 infection in an urban area in Brazil (Niteroi city area, State of Rio de Janeiro, Brazil), *Mem Inst Oswaldo Cruz* 97:965-970, 2002.
71. Yamashita K, Matsunaga Y, Taylor-Wiedeman J, et al: A significant age shift of the human parvovirus B19 antibody prevalence among young adults in Japan observed in a decade, *Jpn J Med Sci Biol* 45: 49-58, 1992.
72. Naides SJ: Erythema infectiosum (fifth disease) occurrence in Iowa, *Am J Public Health* 78:1230-1231, 1988.
73. Cohen BJ, Buckley MM: The prevalence of antibody to human parvovirus B19 in England and Wales, *J Med Microbiol* 25:151-153, 1988.
74. Nascimento JP, Buckley MM, Brown KE, et al: The prevalence of antibody to human parvovirus B19 in Rio de Janeiro, Brazil, *Rev Inst Med Trop São Paulo* 32:41-45, 1990.
75. Edelson RN, Altman RA: Erythema infectiosum: a statewide outbreak, *J Med Soc N J* 67:805-809, 1970.
76. Werner GH, Brachman PS, Ketler A, et al: A new viral agent associated with erythema infectiosum, *Ann N Y Acad Sci* 67:338-345, 1957.
77. Greenwald P, Bashe WJ Jr: An epidemic of erythema infectiosum, *Am J Dis Child* 107:30-34, 1964.
78. Yaegashi N, Okamura K, Hamazaki Y, et al: Prevalence of antihuman parvovirus antibody in pregnant women, *Nippon Sanka Fujinka Gakkai Zasshi* 42:162-166, 1990.

79. Koch WC, Adler SP: Human parvovirus B19 infections in women of childbearing age and within families, *Pediatr Infect Dis J* 8:83-87, 1989.
80. Cohen BJ, Mortimer PP, Pereira MS: Diagnostic assays with monoclonal antibodies for the human serum parvovirus-like virus (SPLV), *J Hyg (Lond)* 91:113-130, 1983.
81. Schwarz TF, Roggendorf M, Deinhardt F: Häufigkeit der parovirus-B19-infektionen. Seroepidemiologishe untersuchungen, *Dtsch Med Wochenschr* 112:1526-1531, 1987.
82. Bartolomei Corsi O, Azzi A, Morfini M, et al: Human parvovirus infection in haemophiliacs first infused with treated clotting factor concentrates, *J Med Virol* 25:165-170, 1988.
83. Eiffert H, Köchel HG, Heuer M, et al: Expression of an antigenic polypeptide of the human parvovirus B19, *Med Microbiol Immunol* 179:169-175, 1990.
84. Brown CS, van Bussel MJ, Wassenaar AL, et al: An immunofluorescence assay for the detection of parvovirus B19 IgG and IgM antibodies based on recombinant viral antigen, *J Virol Methods* 29:53-62, 1990.
85. Rollag H, Patou G, Pattison JR, et al: Prevalence of antibodies against parvovirus B19 in Norwegians with congenital coagulation factor defects treated with plasma products from small donor pools, *Scand J Infect Dis* 23:675-679, 1991.
86. Salimans MM, van Bussel MJ, Brown CS, et al: Recombinant parvovirus B19 capsids as a new substrate for detection of B19-specific IgG and IgM antibodies by an enzyme-linked immunosorbent assay, *J Virol Methods* 39:247-258, 1992.
87. Schwarz TF, Hottenträger B, Roggendorf M: Prevalence of antibodies to parvovirus B19 in selected groups of patients and healthy individuals, *Int J Med Microbiol Virol Parasitol Infect Dis* 276:437-442, 1992.
88. Vyse AJ, Andrews NJ, Hesketh LM: The burden of parvovirus B19 infection in women of childbearing age in England and Wales. *Epidemiol Infect* 135:1354-1362, 2007.
89. Lin KH, You SL, Chen CJ, et al: Seroepidemiology of human parvovirus B19 in Taiwan, *J Med Virol* 57:169-173, 1999.
90. Courouсé AM, Ferchal F, Morinet F, et al: Parvovirus (SPLV) et antigène Aurillac, *Rev Fr Transfus Immunohematol* 27:5-19, 1984.
91. Cossart Y: Parvovirus B19 finds a disease, *Lancet* 2:988-989, 1981.
92. O'Neill HJ, Coyle PV: Two anti-parvovirus B19 IgM capture assays incorporating a mouse monoclonal antibody specific for B19 viral capsid proteins VP1 and VP2, *Arch Virol* 123:125-134, 1992.
93. Cohen BJ, Field AM, Gudnadottir S, et al: Blood donor screening for parvovirus B19, *J Virol Methods* 30:233-238, 1990.
94. da Silva Cruz A, Serpa MJ, Barth OM, et al: Detection of the human parvovirus B19 in a blood donor plasma in Rio de Janeiro, *Mem Inst Oswaldo Cruz* 84:279-280, 1989.
95. McOmish F, Yap PL, Jordan A, et al: Detection of parvovirus B19 in donated blood: a model system for screening by polymerase chain reaction, *J Clin Microbiol* 31:323-328, 1993.
96. Yaegashi N, Shiraishi H, Tada K, et al: Enzyme-linked immunosorbent assay for IgG and IgM antibodies against human parvovirus B19: use of monoclonal antibodies and viral antigen propagated in vitro, *J Virol Methods* 26:171-181, 1989.
97. Naides SJ, Scharosch LL, Foto F, et al: Rheumatologic manifestations of human parvovirus B19 infection in adults, *Arthritis Rheum* 33:1297-1309, 1990.
98. Martinez-Campillo F, López J, Verdú M, et al: Parvovirus B19 outbreak in a rural community in Alicante, *Enferm Infecc Microbiol Clin* 20:376-379, 2002.
99. Abarca K, Cohen BJ, Vial PA: Seroprevalence of parvovirus B19 in urban Chilean children and young adults, 1990 and 1996, *Epidemiol Infect* 128:59-62, 2002.
100. Smith-Whitley K, Zhao H, Hodinka RL, et al: The epidemiology of human parvovirus B19 in children with sickle cell disease, *Blood* 103:422-427, 2003.
101. Plummer FA, Hammond GW, Forward K, et al: An erythema infectiosum-like illness caused by human parvovirus infection, *N Engl J Med* 313:74-79, 1985.
102. Chorba T, Coccia P, Holman RC, et al: The role of parvovirus B19 in aplastic crisis and erythema infectiosum (fifth disease), *J Infect Dis* 154:383-393, 1986.
103. Mortimer PP: Hypothesis: the aplastic crisis of hereditary spherocytosis is due to a single transmissible agent, *J Clin Pathol* 36:445-448, 1983.
104. Saarinen UA, Chorba TL, Tattersall P, et al: Human parvovirus B19 induced epidemic red-cell aplasia in patients with hereditary hemolytic anemia, *Blood* 67:1411-1417, 1986.
105. Valeur-Jensen A, Pedersen CB, Westergaard T, et al: Risk factors for parvovirus B19 infection in pregnancy, *JAMA* 281:1099-1105, 1999.
106. Anderson MJ, Lewis E, Kidd IM, et al: An outbreak of erythema infectiosum associated with human parvovirus infection, *J Hyg (Lond)* 93:85-93, 1984.
107. Tuckerman JG, Brown T, Cohen BJ: Erythema infectiosum in a village primary school: clinical and virological studies, *J R Coll Gen Pract* 36:267-270, 1986.
108. Morgan-Capner P, Wright J, Longley JP, et al: Sex ratio in outbreaks of parvovirus B19 infection, *Lancet* 2:98, 1987.
109. Mansfield F: Erythema infectiosum: slapped face disease, *Aust Fam Physician* 17:737-738, 1988.
110. Woolf AD, Campion GV, Chishick A, et al: Clinical manifestations of human parvovirus B19 in adults, *Arch Intern Med* 149:1153-1156, 1989.
111. Turner A, Olojugba O: Erythema infectiosum in a primary school: investigation of an outbreak in Bury, *Public Health* 103:391-393, 1989.
112. Grilli EA, Anderson MJ, Hoskins TW: Concurrent outbreaks of influenza and parvovirus B19 in a boys' boarding school, *Epidemiol Infect* 103:359-369, 1989.
113. Gillespie SM, Cartter ML, Asch S, et al: Occupational risk of human parvovirus B19 infection for school and day-care personnel during an outbreak of erythema infectiosum, *JAMA* 263:2061-2065, 1990.
114. Anderson LJ, Gillespie SM, Török TJ, et al: Risk of infection following exposures to human parvovirus B19, *Behring Inst Mitt* 85:60-63, 1990.
115. Rice PS, Cohen BJ: A school outbreak of parvovirus B19 infection investigated using salivary antibody assays, *Epidemiol Infect* 6:331-338, 1996.
116. Bell LM, Naides SJ, Stoffman P, et al: Human parvovirus B19 infection among hospital staff members after contact with infected patients, *N Engl J Med* 321:485-491, 1989.
117. Pillay D, Patou G, Hurt S, et al: Parvovirus B19 outbreak in a children's ward, *Lancet* 339:107-109, 1992.
118. Cohen BJ, Courouсé AM, Schwarz TF, et al: Laboratory infection with parvovirus B19, *J Clin Pathol* 41:1027-1028, 1988.
119. Shiraishi H, Sasaki T, Nakamura M, et al: Laboratory infection with human parvovirus B19, *J Infect* 22:308-310, 1991.
120. Evans JP, Rossiter MA, Kumaran TO, et al: Human parvovirus aplasia: case due to cross infection in a ward, *Br Med J (Clin Res Ed)* 288:681, 1984.
121. Ueda K, Akeda H, Tokugawa K, et al: Human parvovirus infection, *N Engl J Med* 314:645-647, 1986.
122. Pillay D, Patou G, Griffiths PD, et al: Secondary parvovirus B19 infection in an immunocompromised child, *Pediatr Infect Dis J* 10:623-624, 1991.
123. Lui SL, Luk WK, Cheung CY, et al: Nosocomial outbreak of parvovirus B19 infection in a renal transplant unit, *Transplantation* 71:59-64, 2001.
124. Miyamoto K, Ogami M, Takahashi Y, et al: Outbreak of human parvovirus B19 in hospital workers, *J Hosp Infect* 45:238-241, 2000.
125. Koziol DE, Kurtzman G, Ayub J, et al: Nosocomial human parvovirus B19 infection: lack of transmission from a chronically infected patient to hospital staff, *Infect Control Hosp Epidemiol* 13:343-348, 1992.
126. Dowell SF, Török TJ, Thorp JA, et al: Parvovirus B19 infection in hospital workers. Community or hospital acquisition, *J Infect Dis* 172:1076-1079, 1995.
127. Carter ML, Farley TA, Rosengren S, et al: Occupational risk factors for infection with parvovirus B19 among pregnant women, *J Infect Dis* 163:282-285, 1991.
128. Ray SM, Erdman DD, Berschling JD, et al: Nosocomial exposure to parvovirus B19: low risk of transmission to healthcare workers, *Infect Control Hosp Epidemiol* 18:109-114, 1997.
129. Patou G, Pillay D, Myint S, et al: Characterization of a nested polymerase chain reaction assay for detection of parvovirus B19, *J Clin Microbiol* 31:540-546, 1993.
130. Potter CG, Potter AC, Hatton CS, et al: Variation of erythroid and myeloid precursors in the marrow of volunteer subjects infected with human parvovirus (B19), *J Clin Invest* 79:1486-1492, 1987.

131. Morey AL, Porter HJ, Keeling JW, et al: Non-isotopic in situ hybridisation and immunophenotyping of infected cells in investigation of human fetal parvovirus infection, *J Clin Pathol* 45:673-678, 1992.
132. Mortimer PP, Luban NL, Kelleher JF, et al: Transmission of serum parvovirus-like virus by clotting-factor concentrates, *Lancet* 2:482-484, 1983.
133. Lyon DJ, Chapman CS, Martin C, et al: Symptomatic parvovirus B19 infection and heat-treated factor IX concentrate, *Lancet* 1:1085, 1989.
134. Williams MD, Cohen BJ, Beddall AC, et al: Transmission of human parvovirus B19 by coagulation factor concentrates, *Vox Sang* 58:177-181, 1990.
135. Morfini M, Longo G, Rossi Ferrini P, et al: Hypoplastic anemia in a hemophiliac first infused with a solvent/detergent treated factor VIII concentrate: the role of human B19 parvovirus, *Am J Hematol* 39:149-150, 1992.
136. Zakrzewska K, Azzi A, Patou G, et al: Human parvovirus B19 in clotting factor concentrates: B19 DNA detection by the nested polymerase chain reaction, *Br J Haematol* 81:407-412, 1992.
137. Schwarz TF, Roggendorf M, Hottenträger B, et al: Removal of parvovirus B19 from contaminated factor VIII during fractionation, *J Med Virol* 35:28-31, 1991.
138. Azzi A, Ciappi S, Zakrzewska K, et al: Human parvovirus B19 infection in hemophiliacs infused with two high purity, virally attenuated factor VIII concentrates, *Am J Hematol* 39:228-230, 1992.
139. Stelma FF, Smismans A, Goossens VJ, et al: Occupational risk of human cytomegalovirus and parvovirus B19 infection in female day care personnel in the Netherlands; a study based on seroprevalence, *Eur J Clin Microbiol Infect Dis* 28:393-397, 2009.
140. van Rijckevorsel GG, Bovée LP, Damen M, et al: Increased seroprevalence of IgG-class antibodies against cytomegalovirus, parvovirus B19, and varicella-zoster virus in women working in child day care, *BMC Public Health* 12:475, 2012.
141. Garcia-Tapia AM, Fernandez-Gutiérrez del Alamo C, Girón JA, et al: Spectrum of parvovirus B19 infection: analysis of an outbreak of 43 cases in Cadiz, Spain, *Clin Infect Dis* 21:424-430, 1995.
142. Zerbini M, Musiani M, Venturoli S, et al: Different syndromes associated with B19 parvovirus viraemia in paediatric patients: report of four cases, *Eur J Pediatr* 151:815-817, 1992.
143. Tsuda H, Maeda Y, Nakagawa K: Parvovirus B19-related lymphadenopathy, *Br J Haematol* 85:631-632, 1993.
144. Brown KE: Human parvovirus B19 epidemiology and clinical manifestations. In Anderson LJ, Young NS, editors: *Human parvovirus B19. Monographs in virology*, vol 20, Basel, 1997, Karger, pp 42-60.
145. Lefrere JJ, Courouce AM, Soulier JP, et al: Henoch-Schönlein purpura and human parvovirus infection, *Pediatrics* 78:183-184, 1986.
146. Saunders PW, Reid MM, Cohen BJ: Human parvovirus induced cytopenias: a report of five cases, *Br J Haematol* 63:407-410, 1986.
147. Lefrere JJ, Couroucé AM, Kaplan C: Parvovirus and idiopathic thrombocytopenic purpura, *Lancet* 1:279, 1989.
148. Török TJ: Parvovirus B19 and human disease, *Adv Int Med* 37:431-455, 1992.
149. White DG, Woolf AD, Mortimer PP, et al: Human parvovirus arthropathy, *Lancet* 1:419-421, 1985.
150. Naides SJ, Field EH: Transient rheumatoid factor positivity in acute human parvovirus B19 infection, *Arch Intern Med* 148:2587-2589, 1988.
151. Reid DM, Reid TM, Brown T, et al: Human parvovirus-associated with arthritis: a clinical and laboratory description, *Lancet* 1:422-425, 1985.
152. Nocton JJ, Miller LC, Tucker LB, et al: Human parvovirus B19-associated arthritis in children, *J Pediatr* 122:186-190, 1993.
153. Dijkmans BA, van Elsacker-Niele AM, Salimans MM, et al: Human parvovirus B19 DNA in synovial fluid, *Arthritis Rheum* 31:279-281, 1998.
154. Saal JG, Steidle M, Einsele H, et al: Persistence of B19 parvovirus in synovial membranes of patients with rheumatoid arthritis, *Rheumatology* 12:147-151, 1992.
155. Mimori A, Misaki Y, Hachiya T, et al: Prevalence of antihuman parvovirus B19 IgG antibodies in patients with refractory rheumatoid arthritis and polyarticular juvenile rheumatoid arthritis, *Rheumatol Int* 14:87-90, 1994.
156. Soderlund M, von Essen R, Haapasaari J, et al: Persistence of parvovirus B19 DNA in synovial membranes of young patients with and without chronic arthropathy, *Lancet* 349:1063-1065, 1997.
157. Stahl HD, Hubner B, Seidl B, et al: Detection of multiple viral DNA species in synovial tissue and fluid of patients with early arthritis, *Ann Rheum Dis* 59:342-346, 2000.
158. Kerr JR: Pathogenesis of human parvovirus B19 in rheumatic disease, *Ann Rheum Dis* 59:672-683, 2000.
159. Koch WC, Massey G, Russell CE, et al: Manifestations and treatment of human parvovirus B19 infection in immunocompromised patients, *J Pediatr* 116:355-359, 1990.
160. Van Horn DK, Mortimer PP, Young N, et al: Human parvovirus-associated red cell aplasia in the absence of hemolytic anemia, *Am J Pediatr Hematol-Oncol* 8:235-239, 1986.
161. Kurtzman GJ, Ozawa K, Cohen B, et al: Chronic bone marrow failure due to persistent B19 parvovirus infection, *N Engl J Med* 317: 287-294, 1987.
162. Frickhofen N, Abkowitz JL, Safford M, et al: Persistent B19 parvovirus infection in patients infected with human immunodeficiency virus type 1 (HIV-1): a treatable cause of anemia in AIDS, *Ann Intern Med* 113:926-933, 1990.
163. Weiland HT, Salimans MM, Fibbe WE, et al: Prolonged parvovirus B19 infection with severe anaemia in a bone marrow transplant recipient, *Br J Haematol* 71:300, 1989.
164. Kurtzman G, Frickhofen N, Kimball J, et al: Pure red-cell aplasia of ten years' duration due to persistent parvovirus B19 infection and its cure with immunoglobulin therapy, *N Engl J Med* 321:519-523, 1989.
165. Wong TY, Chan PK, Leung CB, et al: Parvovirus B19 infection causing red cell aplasia in renal transplantation on tacrolimus, *Am J Kidney Dis* 34:1119-1123, 1999.
166. Geetha D, Zachary JB, Baldado HM, et al: Pure red cell aplasia caused by parvovirus B19 infection in solid organ transplant recipients: a case report and review of the literature, *Clin Transplant* 14:586-591, 2000.
167. Pamidi S, Friedman K, Kampalath B, et al: Human parvovirus infection presenting as persistent anemia in renal transplant recipients, *Transplantation* 69:2666-2669, 2000.
168. Zolnourian ZR, Curran MD, Rima BK, et al: Parvovirus B19 in kidney transplant patients, *Transplantation* 69:2198-2202, 2000.
169. Seishima M, Kanoh H, Izumi T: The spectrum of cutaneous eruptions in 22 patients with isolated serological evidence of infection by parvovirus B19, *Arch Dermatol* 135:1556-1557, 1999.
170. Lefrere JJ, Couroucé AM, Bertrand Y, et al: Human parvovirus and aplastic crisis in chronic hemolytic anemias: a study of 24 observations, *Am J Hematol* 23:271-275, 1986.
171. Finkel TH, Török TJ, Ferguson PJ, et al: Chronic parvovirus B19 infection and systemic necrotising vasculitis. Opportunistic infection or aetiological agent, *Lancet* 343:1255-1258, 1994.
172. Schwarz TF, Wiersbitzky S, Pambor M: Case report: detection of parvovirus B19 in skin biopsy of a patient with erythema infectiosum, *J Med Virol* 43:171-174, 1994.
173. Magro CM, Dawood MR, Crowson AN: The cutaneous manifestations of human parvovirus B19 infection, *Hum Pathol* 31:488-497, 2000.
174. Ferguson PJ, Saulsbury FT, Dowell SF, et al: Prevalence of human parvovirus B19 infection in children with Henoch-Schonlein purpura, *Arthritis Rheum* 39:880-881, 1996.
175. Smith PT, Landry ML, Carey H, et al: Papular-purpuric gloves and socks syndrome associated with acute parvovirus B19 infection: case report and review, *Clin Infect Dis* 27:164-168, 1997.
176. Grilli R, Izquierdo MJ, Fariña MC, et al: Papular-purpuric "gloves and socks" syndrome: polymerase chain reaction demonstration of parvovirus B19 DNA in cutaneous lesions and sera, *J Am Acad Dermatol* 41:793-796, 1999.
177. Saulsbury FT: Petechial gloves and socks syndrome caused by parvovirus B19, *Pediatr Dermatol* 15:35-37, 1998.
178. Brass C, Elliott LM, Stevens DA: Academy rash: a probable epidemic of erythema infectiosum ("fifth disease"), *JAMA* 248:568-572, 1982.
179. Tsuji A, Uchida N, Asamura S, et al: Aseptic meningitis with erythema infectiosum, *Eur J Pediatr* 149:449-450, 1990.
180. Balfour HH Jr, Schiff GM, Bloom JE: Encephalitis associated with erythema infectiosum, *JAMA* 77:133-136, 1970.
181. Hall CB, Horner FA: Encephalopathy with erythema infectiosum, *Am J Dis Child* 131:65-67, 1977.
182. Okumura A, Ichikawa T: Aseptic meningitis caused by human parvovirus B19, *Arch Dis Child* 68:784-785, 1993.

183. Cassinotti P, Schultze D, Schlageter P, et al: Persistent human parvovirus B19 infection following an acute infection with meningitis in an immunocompetent patient, *Eur J Clin Microbiol Infect Dis* 12: 701-704, 1993.
184. Watanabe T, Satoh M, Oda Y: Human parvovirus B19 encephalopathy, *Arch Dis Child* 70:71, 1994.
185. Magro CM, Crowson AN, Dawood M, et al: Parvoviral infection of endothelial cells and its possible role in vasculitis and autoimmune diseases, *J Rheumatol* 29:1227-1235, 2002.
186. Douvoyiannis M, Litman N, Goldman L: Neurologic manifestations associated with parvovirus B19 infection, *Clin Infect Dis* 48:1713-1723, 2009.
187. Guidi B, Bergonzini P, Crisi G, et al: Case of stroke in a 7-year-old male after parvovirus B19 infection, *Pediatr Neurol* 28:69-71, 2003.
188. Wierenga KJ, Serjeant BE, Serjeant GR: Cerebrovascular complications and parvovirus infection in homozygous sickle cell disease, *J Pediatr* 139:438-442, 2001.
189. Craze JL, Salisbury AJ, Pike MG: Prenatal stroke associated with maternal parvovirus infection, *Dev Med Child Neurol* 38:84-85, 1996.
190. De Haan TR, Van Wezel-Meijler G, Beersma MF, et al: Fetal stroke and congenital parvovirus B19 infection complicated by activated protein C resistance, *Acta Paediatr* 95:863-867, 2006.
191. Walsh KJ, Armstrong RD, Turner AM: Brachial plexus neuropathy associated with human parvovirus infection, *Br Med J (Clin Res Ed)* 296:896, 1988.
192. Samii K, Cassinotti P, de Freudenreich J, et al: Acute bilateral carpal tunnel syndrome associated with human parvovirus B19 infection, *Clin Infect Dis* 22:162-164, 1996.
193. Faden H, Gary GW Jr, Korman M: Numbness and tingling of fingers associated with parvovirus B19 infection, *J Infect Dis* 161:354-355, 1990.
194. Dereure O, Montes B, Guilhou JJ: Acute generalized livedo reticularis with myasthenia-like syndrome revealing parvovirus B19 primary infection, *Arch Dermatol* 131:744-745, 1995.
195. Faden H, Gary GW Jr, Anderson LJ: Chronic parvovirus infection in a presumably immunologically healthy woman, *Clin Infect Dis* 15:595-597, 1992.
196. Barah F, Vallely PJ, Cleator GM, et al: Neurological manifestations of human parvovirus B19 infection, *Rev Med Virol* 13:185-199, 2003.
197. Nakazawa T, Tomosugi N, Sakamoto K, et al: Acute glomerulonephritis after human parvovirus B19 infection, *Am J Kidney Dis* 35:E31, 2000.
198. Komatsuda A, Ohtani H, Nimura T, et al: Endocapillary proliferative glomerulonephritis in a patient with parvovirus B19 infection, *Am J Kidney Dis* 36:851-854, 2000.
199. Diaz F, Collazos J: Glomerulonephritis and Henoch-Schoenlein purpura associated with acute parvovirus B19 infection, *Clin Nephrol* 53:237-238, 2000.
200. Tanawattanacharoen S, Falk RJ, Jennette JC, et al: Parvovirus B19 DNA in kidney tissue of patients with focal segmental glomerulosclerosis, *Am J Kidney Dis* 35:1166-1174, 2000.
201. Klein RM, Jiang H, Niederacher D, et al: Frequency and quantity of the parvovirus B19 genome in endomyocardial biopsies from patients with suspected myocarditis or idiopathic left ventricular dysfunction, *Z Kardiol* 93:300-309, 2004.
202. Munro K, Croxson MC, Thomas S, et al: Three cases of myocarditis in childhood associated with human parvovirus (B19 virus), *Pediatr Cardiol* 24:473-475, 2003.
203. Lamparter S, Schoppet M, Pankuweit S, et al: Acute parvovirus B19 infection associated with myocarditis in an immunocompetent adult, *Hum Pathol* 34:725-728, 2003.
204. Wang X, Zhang G, Liu F, et al: Prevalence of human parvovirus B19 DNA in cardiac tissues of patients with congenital heart diseases indicated by nested PCR and in situ hybridization, *J Clin Virol* 31: 20-24, 2004.
205. Bultmann BD, Klingel K, Näbauer M, et al: High prevalence of viral genomes and inflammation in peripartum cardiomyopathy, *Am J Obstet Gynecol* 195:330-331, 2006.
206. Kuhl U, Pauschinger M, Seeberg B, et al: Viral persistence in the myocardium is associated with progressive cardiac dysfunction, *Circulation* 112:1965-1970, 2005.
207. Kuethe F, Sigusch HH, Hilbig K, et al: Detection of viral genome in the myocardium: lack of prognostic and functional relevance in patients with acute dilated cardiomyopathy, *Am Heart J* 153: 850-858, 2007.
208. Tavora F, Gonzalez-Cuyar LF, Dalal JS, et al: Fatal parvoviral myocarditis: a case report and review of literature, *Diagn Pathol* 3:21, 2008.
209. Marton T, Martin WL, Whittle MJ: Hydrops fetalis and neonatal death from human parvovirus B19: an unusual complication, *Prenat Diagn* 7:543-545, 2005.
210. Nyman M, Skjoldebrand-Sparre L, Broliden K: Non-hydropic intrauterine fetal death more than 5 months after primary parvovirus B19 infection, *J Perinat Med* 33:176-178, 2005.
211. Anderson LJ, Tsou C, Parker RA, et al: Detection of antibodies and antigens of human parvovirus B19 by enzyme-linked immunosorbent assay, *J Clin Microbiol* 24:522-526, 1986.
212. Cohen BJ, Bates CM: Evaluation of 4 commercial test kits for parvovirus B19-specific IgM, *J Virol Methods* 55:11-25, 1995.
213. Koch WC: A synthetic parvovirus B19 capsid protein can replace viral antigen in antibody-capture enzyme immunoassays, *J Virol Methods* 55:67-82, 1995.
214. Jordan JA: Comparison of a baculovirus-based VP2 enzyme immunoassay (EIA) to an *Escherichia coli*-based VP1 EIA for detection of human parvovirus B19 immunoglobulin M and immunoglobulin G in sera of pregnant women, *J Clin Microbiol* 38:1472-1475, 2000.
215. Doyle S: The detection of parvoviruses, *Methods Mol Biol* 665:213-231, 2011.
216. Clewly JP: Detection of human parvovirus using a molecularly cloned probe, *J Med Virol* 15:383-393, 1985.
217. Clewly JP: Polymerase chain reaction assay of parvovirus B19 DNA in clinical specimens, *J Clin Microbiol* 27:2647-2651, 1989.
218. Koch WC, Adler SP: Detection of human parvovirus B19 DNA by using the polymerase chain reaction, *J Clin Microbiol* 28:65-69, 1990.
219. Heegard ED, Hasle H, Clausen N, et al: Parvovirus B19 infection and Diamond-Blackfan anemia, *Acta Pediatr* 85:299-302, 1996.
220. Crook TW, Rogers BB, McFarland RD, et al: Unusual bone marrow manifestations of parvovirus B19 infection in immunocompromised patients, *Hum Pathol* 31:161-168, 2000.
221. Adler SP, Harger JH, Koch WC: Infections due to human parvovirus B19 during pregnancy. In Martens M, Faro S, Soper D, editors: *Infectious diseases in women*, Philadelphia, 2001, Saunders.
222. van Gessel PH, Gaytant MA, Vossen AC, et al: Incidence of parvovirus B19 infection among an unselected population of pregnant women in the Netherlands: a prospective study, *Eur J Obstet Gynecol Reprod Biol* 128:46-49, 2006.
223. Mossong J, Hens N, Friederichs V, et al: Parvovirus B19 infection in five European countries: seroepidemiology, force of infection and maternal risk of infection, *Epidemiol Infect* 24:1-10, 2007.
224. Enders M, Weidner A, Enders G: Current epidemiological aspects of human parvovirus B19 infection during pregnancy and childhood in the western part of Germany, *Epidemiol Infect* 135:563-569, 2007.
225. Candotti D, Danso K, Parsyan A, et al: Maternal-fetal transmission of human parvovirus B19 genotype 3, *J Infect Dis* 194:608-611, 2006.
226. Skjoldebrand-Sparre L, Fridell E, Nyman M, et al: A prospective study of antibodies against parvovirus B19 in pregnancy, *Acta Obstet Gynecol Scand* 75:336-339, 1996.
227. Mortimer PP, Cohen BJ, Buckley MM, et al: Human parvovirus and the fetus, *Lancet* 2:1012, 1985.
228. Wiersbitzky VS, Schwarz TF, Bruns R, et al: Seroprävalenz von Antikörpern gegen das humane parvovirus B19 (Ringelröteln/erythema infectiosum) in der DDR-Bevölkerung, *Kinderärztl Prax* 58:185-189, 1990.
229. Schoub BD, Blackburn NK, Johnson S, et al: Primary and secondary infection with human parvovirus B19 in pregnant women in South Africa, *S Afr Med J* 83:505-506, 1993.
230. Barros De Freitas R, Buarque De Gusmão SR, Durigon EL, et al: Survey of parvovirus B19 infection in a cohort of pregnant women in Belem, Brazil, *Braz J Infect Dis* 3:6-14, 1999.
231. Enders G, Biber M: Parvovirus B19 infections in pregnancy, *Behring Inst Mitt* 85:74-78, 1990.
232. Rogers BB, Singer DB, Mak SK, et al: Detection of human parvovirus B19 in early spontaneous abortuses using serology, histology, electron microscopy, in situ hybridization, and the polymerase chain reaction, *Obstet Gynecol* 81:402-408, 1993.
233. Harger JH, Adler SP, Koch WC, et al: Prospective evaluation of 618 pregnant women exposed to parvovirus B19: risks and symptoms, *Obstet Gynecol* 91:413-420, 1998.

234. Kerr JR, Curran MD, Moore JE: Parvovirus B19 infection—persistence and genetic variation, *Scand J Infect Dis* 27:551-557, 1995.
235. Chisaka H, Ito K, Niikura H, et al: Clinical manifestations and outcomes of parvovirus B19 infection during pregnancy in Japan, *Tohoku J Exp Med* 209:277-283, 2006.
236. Schwarz TF, Roggendorf M, Hottenträger B, et al: Human parvovirus B19 infection in pregnancy, *Lancet* 2:566-567, 1988.
237. Gray ES, Anand A, Brown T: Parvovirus infections in pregnancy, *Lancet* 1:208, 1986.
238. Brown T, Ritchie LD: Infection with parvovirus during pregnancy, *BMJ* 290:559-560, 1985.
239. Kinney JS, Anderson LJ, Farrar J, et al: Risk of adverse outcomes of pregnancy after human parvovirus B19 infection, *J Infect Dis* 157:663-667, 1988.
240. Rodis JF, Quinn DL, Gary GW Jr, et al: Management and outcomes of pregnancies complicated by human B19 parvovirus infection: a prospective study, *Am J Obstet Gynecol* 163:1168-1171, 1990.
241. Török TJ, Anderson U, Gary GW, et al: Reproductive outcomes following human parvovirus B19 infection in pregnancy (abstract 1374). In *Program and abstracts of 31st Interscience Conference on Antimicrobial Agents and Chemotherapy, Chicago*, Washington, DC, 1991, American Society for Microbiology.
242. Simms RA, Liebling RE, Patel RR, et al: Management and outcome of pregnancies with parvovirus B19 infection over seven years in a tertiary fetal medicine unit, *Fetal Diagn Ther* 25:373-378, 2009.
243. Enders M, Klingel K, Weidner A, et al: Risk of fetal hydrops and non-hydropic late intrauterine fetal death after gestational parvovirus B19 infection, *J Clin Virol* 49:163-168, 2010.
244. Bonvicini F, Puccetti C, Salfi NC, et al: Gestational and fetal outcomes in B19 maternal infection: a problem of diagnosis, *J Clin Microbiol* 49:3514-3518, 2011.
245. Enders M, Weidner A, Zoellner I, et al: Fetal morbidity and mortality after acute human parvovirus B19 infection in pregnancy: prospective evaluation of 1018 cases, *Prenat Diagn* 24:513-518, 2004.
246. Xu D, Zhang G, Wang R: The study on detection of human parvovirus B19 DNA in spontaneous abortion tissues, *Zhonghua Shi Yan He Lin Chuang Bing Du Xue Za Zhi* 12:158-160, 1998.
247. Wang R, Chen X, Han M: Relationship between human parvovirus B19 infection and spontaneous abortion, *Zhonghua Fu Chan Ke Za Zhi* 32:541-543, 1997.
248. De Krijger RR, van Elsacker-Niele AM, Mulder-Stapel A, et al: Detection of parvovirus B19 infection in first and second trimester fetal loss, *Pediatr Pathol Lab Med* 18:23-34, 1998.
249. Makhseed M, Pacsa A, Ahmed MA, et al: Pattern of parvovirus B19 infection during different trimesters of pregnancy in Kuwait, *Infect Dis Obstet Gynecol* 7:287-292, 1997.
250. Lowden E, Weinstein L: Unexpected second trimester pregnancy loss due to maternal parvovirus B19 infection, *South Med J* 90: 702-704, 1997.
251. Skjoldebrand-Sparre L, Tolfvenstam T, Papadogiannakis N, et al: Parvovirus B19 infection: association with third-trimester intrauterine fetal death, *Br J Obstet Gynaecol* 107:476-480, 2000.
252. Nunoue T, Kusuhara K, Hara T: Human fetal infection with parvovirus B19: maternal infection time in gestation, viral persistence and fetal prognosis, *Pediatr Infect Dis J* 21:1133-1136, 2002.
253. Norbeck O, Papadogiannakis N, Petersson K, et al: Revised clinical presentation of parvovirus B19-associated intrauterine fetal death, *Clin Infect Dis* 35:1032-1038, 2002.
254. Tolfvenstam T, Papadogiannakis N, Norbeck O, et al: Frequency of human parvovirus B19 infection in intrauterine fetal death, *Lancet* 357:1494-1497, 2001.
255. Lassen J, Jensen AK, Bager P, et al: Parvovirus B19 infection in the first trimester of pregnancy and risk of fetal loss: a population-based case-control study, *Am J Epidemiol* 176:803-807, 2012.
256. Leung TN, Leung TY, Chan PK, et al: Fetal parvovirus B19 infection in a twin pregnancy with 1 twin presenting with hydrops fetalis and the other asymptomatic: a case report, *J Reprod Med* 5:419-421, 2007.
257. Dickinson JE, Keil AD, Charles AK: Discordant fetal infection for parvovirus B19 in a dichorionic twin pregnancy, *Twin Res Hum Genet* 9:456-459, 2006.
258. el-Sayed Zaki M, Goda H: Relevance of parvovirus B19, herpes simplex virus 2, and cytomegalovirus virologic markers in maternal serum for diagnosis of unexplained recurrent abortions, *Arch Pathol Lab Med* 131:956-960, 2007.
259. Kishore J, Gupta I: Serological study of parvovirus B19 infection in women with recurrent spontaneous abortions, *Indian J Pathol Microbiol* 49:548-550, 2006.
260. Koch WC, Adler SP, Harger J: Intrauterine parvovirus B19 infection may cause an asymptomatic or recurrent postnatal infection, *Pediatr Infect Dis J* 12:747-750, 1993.
261. Weiland HT, Vermey-Keers C, Salimans MM, et al: Parvovirus B19 associated with fetal abnormality, *Lancet* 1:682-683, 1987.
262. Hartwig NG, Vermeij-Keers C, Van Elsacker-Niele AM, et al: Embryonic malformations in a case of intrauterine parvovirus B19 infection, *Teratology* 39:295-302, 1989.
263. Hartwig NG, Vermeij-Keers C, Versteeg J: The anterior eye segment in virus induced primary congenital aphakia, *Acta Morphol Neerl Scand* 26:283-292, 1988-1989.
264. Rodis JF, Rodner C, Hansen AA, et al: Long-term outcome of children following maternal human parvovirus B19 infection, *Obstet Gynecol* 91:125-128, 1998.
265. Jouannic JM, Gavard L, Créquat J, et al: Isolated fetal hyperechogenic bowel associated with intrauterine parvovirus B19 infection, *Fetal Diagn Ther* 20:498-500, 2005.
266. Porter HJ, Khong TY, Evans MF, et al: Parvovirus as a cause of hydrops fetalis: detection by in situ DNA hybridisation, *J Clin Pathol* 41:381-383, 1988.
267. Yaegashi N, Okamura K, Yajima A, et al: The frequency of human parvovirus B19 infection in nonimmune hydrops fetalis, *J Perinat Med* 22:159-163, 1994.
268. Morey AL, Keeling JW, Porter HJ, et al: Clinical and histopathological features of parvovirus B19 infection in the human fetus, *Br J Obstet Gynaecol* 99:566-574, 1992.
269. Gloning KP, Schramm T, Brusis E, et al: Successful intrauterine treatment of fetal hydrops caused by parvovirus B19 infection, *Behring Inst Mitt* 85:79-85, 1990.
270. Rogers BB, Mark Y, Oyer CE: Diagnosis and incidence of fetal parvovirus infection in an autopsy series, I. Histology, *Pediatr Pathol* 13:371-379, 1993.
271. Mark Y, Rogers BB, Oyer CE: Diagnosis and incidence of fetal parvovirus infection in an autopsy series. II. DNA amplification, *Pediatr Pathol* 13:381-386, 1993.
272. Zerbini M, Musiani M, Gentilomi G, et al: Comparative evaluation of virological and serological methods in prenatal diagnosis of parvovirus B19 fetal hydrops, *J Clin Microbiol* 34:603-608, 1996.
273. Weiffenbach J, Bald R, Gloning KP, et al: Serological and virological analysis of maternal and fetal blood samples in prenatal human parvovirus B19 infection, *J Infect Dis* 205:782-788, 2012.
274. Török TJ, Wang QY, Gary GW Jr, et al: Prenatal diagnosis of intrauterine infection with parvovirus B19 by the polymerase chain reaction technique, *Clin Infect Dis* 14:149-155, 1992.
275. Morey AL, Patou G, Myint S, et al: In vitro culture for the detection of infectious human parvovirus B19 and B19-specific antibodies using foetal haematopoietic precursor cells, *J Gen Virol* 73:3313-3317, 1992.
276. de Haan TR, van den Akker ES, Porcelijn L, et al: Thrombocytopenia in hydropic fetuses with parvovirus B19 infection: incidence, treatment and correlation with fetal B19 viral load, *Br J Obstet Gynaecol* 115:76-81, 2008.
277. Carrington D, Gilmore DH, Whittle MJ, et al: Maternal serum alpha-fetoprotein-a marker of fetal aplastic crisis during intrauterine human parvovirus infection, *Lancet* 1:433-435, 1987.
278. Anderson MJ, Khousam MN, Maxwell DJ, et al: Human parvovirus B19 and hydrops fetalis, *Lancet* 1:535, 1988.
279. Sahakian V, Weiner CP, Naides SJ, et al: Intrauterine transfusion treatment of nonimmune hydrops fetalis secondary to human parvovirus B19 infection, *Am J Obstet Gynecol* 164:1090-1091, 1991.
280. Porter HJ, Quantrill AM, Fleming KA: B19 parvovirus infection of myocardial cells, *Lancet* 1:535-536, 1988.
281. Glaser C, Tannenbaum J: Newborn with hydrops and a rash, *Pediatr Infect Dis J* 11:980-984, 1992.
282. Jordan JA: Identification of human parvovirus B19 infection in idiopathic nonimmune hydrops fetalis, *Am J Obstet Gynecol* 174:37-42, 1996.
283. Jordan JA, DeLoia JA: Globoside expression within the human placenta, *Placenta* 20:103-108, 1999.
284. Jordan JA, Huff D, DeLoia JA: Placental cellular immune response in women infected with human parvovirus B19 during pregnancy, *Clin Diagn Lab Immunol* 8:288-292, 2001.

285. Brown KE: Human parvovirus B19 infections in infants and children, *Adv Pediatr Infect Dis* 13:101-126, 1998.
286. Enders M, Weidner A, Rosenthal T, et al: Improved diagnosis of gestational parvovirus B19 infection at the time of nonimmune fetal hydrops, *J Infect Dis* 197:58-62, 2008.
287. Heegaard ED, Hornsleth A: Parvovirus: the expanding spectrum of disease, *Acta Paediatr* 84:109-117, 1995.
288. Nigro G, Bastianon V, Colloridi V, et al: Acute and chronic lymphocytic myocarditis in infancy is associated with parvovirus B19 infection and high cytokine levels, *Clin Infect Dis* 31:65-69, 2000.
289. Heegaard ED, Eiskjaer H, Baandrup U, et al: Parvovirus B19 infection associated with myocarditis following adult cardiac transplantation, *Scand J Infect Dis* 30:607-610, 1998.
290. Papadogiannakis N, Tolfvenstam T, Fischler B, et al: Active, fulminant, lethal myocarditis associated with parvovirus B19 infection in an infant, *Clin Infect Dis* 35:1027-1031, 2002.
291. Kovacs BW, Carlson DE, Shahbahrami B, et al: Prenatal diagnosis of human parvovirus B19 in nonimmune hydrops fetalis by polymerase chain reaction, *Am J Obstet Gynecol* 167:461-466, 1992.
292. Wang X, Zhang G, Han M, et al: Investigation of parvovirus B19 in cardiac tissue from patients with congenital heart disease, *Chin Med J (Engl)* 112:995-997, 1999.
293. Enders M, Schalasta G, Baisch C, et al: Human parvovirus B19 infection during pregnancy—value of modern molecular and serological diagnostics, *J Clin Virol* 35:400-406, 2006.
294. de Haan TR, Beersma MF, Claas EC, et al: Parvovirus B19 infection in pregnancy studies by maternal viral load and immune responses, *Fetal Diagn Ther* 22:55-62, 2007.
295. de Haan TR, Beersma MF, Oepkes D, et al: Parvovirus B19 infection in pregnancy: maternal and fetal viral load measurements related to clinical parameters, *Prenat Diagn* 27:46-50, 2007.
296. Dobec M, Juchler A, Flaviano A: Prolonged parvovirus B19 viremia in spite of neutralizing antibodies after erythema infectiosum in pregnancy, *Gynecol Obstet Invest* 63:53-54, 2007.
297. Sheikh AU, Ernest JM, O'Shea M: Long-term outcome in fetal hydrops from parvovirus B19 infection, *Am J Obstet Gynecol* 167:337-341, 1992.
298. Rodis JF, Hovick TJ Jr, Quinn DL, et al: Human parvovirus infection in pregnancy, *Obstet Gynecol* 72:733-738, 1988.
299. Bernstein IA, Capeless EL: Elevated maternal serum alpha-fetoprotein and hydrops fetalis in association with fetal parvovirus B19 infection, *Obstet Gynecol* 774:456-457, 1989.
300. Komischke K, Searle K, Enders G: Maternal serum alpha-fetoprotein and human chorionic gonadotropin in pregnant women with acute parvovirus B19 infection with and without fetal complications, *Prenat Diagn* 17:1039-1046, 1997.
301. Kempe A, Rösing B, Berg C, et al: First-trimester treatment of fetal anemia secondary to parvovirus B19 infection, *Ultrasound Obstet Gynecol* 29:226-228, 2007.
302. Matsuda H, Sakaguchi K, Shibasaki T, et al: Intrauterine therapy for parvovirus B19 infected symptomatic fetus using B19 IgG-rich high titer gammaglobulin, *J Perinat Med* 33:561-563, 2005.
303. Chauvet A, Dewilde A, Thomas D, et al: Ultrasound diagnosis, management and prognosis in a consecutive series of 27 cases of fetal hydrops following maternal parvovirus B19 infection, *Fetal Diagn Ther* 30:41-47, 2011.
304. Vogel H, Kornman M, Ledet SC, et al: Congenital parvovirus infection, *Pediatr Pathol Lab Med* 17:903-912, 1997.
305. Török TJ: Human parvovirus B19. In Remington JS, Klein JO, editors: *Infectious diseases of the fetus and newborn infant*, ed 5, Philadelphia, 2001, Saunders.
306. Katz VL, McCoy MC, Kuller JA, et al: An association between fetal parvovirus B19 infection and fetal anomalies: a report of two cases, *Am J Perinatol* 13:43-45, 1996.
307. Miller E, Fairley CK, Cohen BJ, et al: Immediate and long term outcome of human parvovirus B19 infection in pregnancy, *Br J Obstet Gynaecol* 105:14-18, 1998.
308. Dembinski J, Haverkamp F, Maara H, et al: Neurodevelopmental outcome after intrauterine red cell transfusion for parvovirus B19-induced fetal hydrops, *Br J Obstet Gynaecol* 109:1232-1234, 2002.
309. Nagel HT, de Haan TR, Vandenbussche FP, et al: Long-term outcome after fetal transfusion for hydrops associated with parvovirus B19 infection, *Obstet Gynecol* 109:42-47, 2007.
310. De Jong EP, Lindenburg IT, van Klink JM, et al: Intrauterine transfusion for parvovirus B19 infection: long-term neurodevelopmental outcome, *Am J Obstet Gynecol* 204:e1-e5, 2012.
311. Gärtner B, Enders M, Luft-Duchow C, et al: Parvovirus B19 infections in pregnant women in day care facilities: health economic analysis of prohibition to employ seronegative women, *Bundesgesundheitsblatt Gesundheitsforschung Gesundheitsschutz* 50:1369-1378, 2007.
312. Ballou WR, Reed JL, Noble W, et al: Safety and immunogenicity of a recombinant parvovirus B19 vaccine formulated with MF59C.1, *J Infect Dis* 187:675-678, 2003.
313. Bernstein DI, El Sahly HM, Keitel WA, et al: Safety and immunogenicity of a candidate parvovirus B19 vaccine, *Vaccine* 29:7357-7363, 2011.
314. Chandramouli S, Medina-Selby A, Coit D, et al: Generation of a parvovirus B19 vaccine candidate, *Vaccine* 31:3872-3878, 2013.
315. Maeda H, Shimokawa H, Satoh S, et al: Nonimmunologic hydrops fetalis resulting from intrauterine human parvovirus B19 infection: report of 2 cases, *Obstet Gynecol* 71:482-485, 1988.
316. Bond PR, Caul EO, Usher J, et al: Intrauterine infection with human parvovirus, *Lancet* 1:448-449, 1986.
317. Woernle CH, Anderson LJ, Tattersall P, et al: Human parvovirus B19 infection during pregnancy, *J Infect Dis* 156:17-26, 1987.
318. Samra JS, Obhrai MS, Constantine G: Parvovirus infection in pregnancy, *Obstet Gynecol* 73:832-834, 1989.
319. Mortimer PP, Cohen BJ, Buckley MM, et al: Human parvovirus and the fetus, *Lancet* 2:1012, 1985.
320. Weiner CP, Naides SJ: Fetal survival after human parvovirus B19 infection: spectrum of intrauterine response in a twin gestation, *Am J Perinatol* 9:66-68, 1992.
321. Humphrey W, Magoon M, O'Shaughnessy R: Severe nonimmune hydrops secondary to parvovirus B-19 infection: spontaneous reversal in utero and survival of a term infant, *Obstet Gynecol* 78: 900-902, 1991.
322. Morey AL, Nicolini U, Welch CR, et al: Parvovirus B19 infection and transient fetal ascites, *Lancet* 337:496, 1991.

29 Rubella

SUSAN E. REEF and STANLEY A. PLOTKIN*

CHAPTER OUTLINE

The impact of rubella virus infection and the progress made toward controlling congenital rubella infection have been well chronicled.[1-9] Rubella was first recognized in the mid-18th century as a clinical entity by German researchers, who called it *Rötheln*. They considered it to be a modified form of measles or scarlet fever.[1] Manton[10] first described it as a separate disease in the English literature in 1815. In 1866, Veale[11] gave it a "short and euphonious" name—*rubella*. The disease was considered mild and self-limited.

Rubella became a focus of major interest in 1941, after Gregg,[12] an Australian ophthalmologist, associated intrauterine acquisition of infection with production of cataracts and heart disease. Although his findings were initially doubted, numerous reports of infants with congenital defects after maternal rubella infection soon appeared in the literature.[1] Subsequent investigations showed that the major defects associated with congenital rubella infection included congenital heart disease, cataracts, and deafness. Mental retardation and many defects involving almost every organ have also been reported.[2-4,7,13,14] Before the availability of specific viral diagnostic studies, the frequency of fetal damage after maternal infection in the first trimester was estimated to be greater than 20%, a figure now known to be much too low.

Recognition of the teratogenic potential of rubella infection led to increased efforts to isolate the etiologic agent. The viral cause of rubella was suggested by experimental infections in humans and monkeys in 1938 but was not confirmed until the isolation of the viral agent in cell cultures was reported independently in 1962 by Weller and Neva at Harvard University School of Public Health and by Parkman, Buescher, and Artenstein at Walter Reed Army Institute for Research.[15-20] This accomplishment paved the way for the development of serologic tests and a vaccine.[2-4,21-23] Efforts to develop a vaccine were hastened by events associated with a worldwide rubella pandemic in 1962 to 1964, which in the United States resulted in approximately 12.5 million cases of clinically acquired rubella, 11,000 fetal deaths, and 20,000 infants born with defects collectively referred to as congenital rubella syndrome (CRS); 2100 infants with CRS died in the neonatal period.[24] The estimated cost to the U.S. economy was approximately $2 billion. Routine use of rubella vaccine, in a two-dose schedule as measles-mumps-rubella vaccine (MMR), has not prevented importation-related infection, but it has eliminated endemic rubella in the United States.[25] CRS remains a problem in many countries, however, with current estimates of more than 100,000 new cases annually in developing countries.[26]

In 1969, three strains of live-attenuated rubella vaccine were licensed in various countries: HPV-77 (high-passage virus, 77 times), grown in duck embryo for five passages

*Drs. Louis Cooper and Charles Alford, Jr., previously contributed to this chapter.

(DE-5) or dog kidney cell culture for 12 passages (DK-12); Cendehill, grown in primary rabbit cells; and RA 27/3 (rubella abortus, 27th specimen, third explant), grown in human diploid fibroblast culture.[27-29] The RA 27/3 vaccine has been used exclusively in the United States since 1979 and is now the only strain in global use outside of Japan and China.[2-4,7,30,31]

In addition to providing the impetus for vaccine research and development, the rubella pandemic provided the scientific community with a unique opportunity to gain knowledge about the nature of intrauterine and extrauterine infections and the immunity stimulated by both. The quest for more knowledge using the tools of molecular biology has continued since vaccine licensure and serves as a tribute to Gregg's historic contribution to our understanding of intrauterine infection.

Much interest has focused on the epidemiology of rubella and CRS in countries with immunization programs, the desirability of introducing vaccine in countries without a program, and the optimal strategy to control congenital rubella (i.e., universal immunization vs. selective immunization of females vs. combined strategy of universal vaccination and selective immunization).[3,5-7,32-38] Vaccination of all children and of susceptible adolescents and young adults, particularly women, has had such a dramatic impact on the occurrence of rubella and congenital rubella in the United States that it has resulted in the elimination of endemic rubella and CRS from the United States.[5,24,33,39,40] Given the magnitude of international travel, the goal of eradication of rubella will remain elusive until similar goals are adopted by other countries. In 2003, the Pan American Health Organization (PAHO) adopted a resolution calling on all countries of the Western Hemisphere to eliminate rubella by 2010, a goal that appears to have now been achieved.[41] Among developing countries, rubella immunization has not yet been given priority, however.

Duration and quality of vaccine-induced immunity[5,8,42-61] and adverse events associated with immunization, particularly arthritis and the risk of the vaccine to the fetus,[5,8,62-69] have been a concern, but the vaccine continues to confer long-lasting immunity, while placing the vaccinated person at minimal risk of adverse events. Success in eliminating endemic disease in the United States and the absence of teratogenicity observed after massive immunization programs (2001-2002) in Latin America offer considerable assurance about the long-term efficacy and safety of rubella vaccine. In Brazil, 28 million women were immunized in mass campaigns, and in Costa Rica, more than 2400 susceptible pregnant women were immunized. Although infants were infected, none had evidence of CRS.

Research on the characteristics of the rubella virus, its effect on the developing fetus, the host's immune response, and diagnostic methodology has yielded new information about the structural proteins of the virus and about the difference in the immune response to these proteins after congenital and acquired infections.[70-90] Differences in antibody profile may be useful in diagnosing congenital infection retrospectively and may provide further information on the pathogenesis of congenital infection.[68,89,91] Techniques that detect rubella-specific antibodies within minutes have been developed by using latex agglutination and passive hemagglutination.[92-98] Studies to examine the subclass distribution of IgG and the kinetics of rubella-specific immunoglobulins (including immunoglobulin A [IgA], IgD, and IgE) after acquired rubella, congenital infection, and vaccination may eventually lead to the development of additional diagnostic tools.[99-103] In particular, rubella IgG avidity testing can be helpful in distinguishing between recently acquired and remote infection.[104-106]

Improved laboratory methods defined the risk of fetal infection and congenital damage in all stages of pregnancy.[107-114] The risk of fetal infection after first-trimester maternal infection and subsequent congenital anomalies after fetal infection may be higher than previously reported (81% and 85%, respectively, in one study).[109] The fetus may be at risk of infection throughout pregnancy, even near term, although the occurrence of defects after infection beyond 16 to 18 weeks of gestation is small. Sensitive laboratory assays have shown that subclinical reinfection after previous natural infection, as after vaccination, may be accompanied by an IgM response, making differentiation between subclinical reinfection and asymptomatic primary infection difficult sometimes.[45,55,57,59] IgG avidity testing may be helpful in this situation. Although reinfection usually poses no threat to the fetus, rare instances of congenital infection after maternal reinfection have been reported.*

Follow-up of patients with congenital rubella has provided information about the pathogenesis, immune status, interplay between congenital infection and human leukocyte antigen (HLA) haplotypes, and long-term outcome associated with congenital infection.[121-138] These studies have documented that congenital infection is persistent, that virtually every organ may be affected, and that autoimmunity and immune complex formation are probably involved in many of the disease processes, particularly in the delayed and persistent clinical manifestations. They also confirm earlier studies, noting an increased risk of diabetes mellitus and other endocrinopathies in patients with CRS compared with rates for the general population.

Virus

MORPHOLOGY AND PHYSICAL AND CHEMICAL COMPOSITION

Rubella virus is a generally spherical particle, 50 to 70 nm in diameter, with a dense central nucleoid measuring 30 nm in diameter. The central nucleoid is surrounded by a 10-nm thick, single-layered envelope acquired during budding of the virus into cytoplasmic vesicles or through the plasma membrane.[139-153] Surface projections or spikes with knobbed ends that are 5 to 6 nm long have been reported. The specific gravity of the complete viral particle is 1.184 ± 0.004 g/mL, corresponding to a sedimentation constant of 360 ± 50 Svedberg units.[139]

The wild-type virus contains within its core infectious positive-strand RNA (molecular weight of $3\text{-}4 \times 10^6$) containing 9800 nucleotides.[124] Full-length and subgenomic RNA are produced, and it is from the latter that viral structural proteins are translated. The rubella virus envelope contains lipids that differ quantitatively from lipids of the plasma

*References 45, 47, 49, 51, 55-57, 59, 115-120.

membrane and are essential for infectivity.[154,155] Rubella virus is heat labile and has a half-life of 1 hour at 57° C.[156] In the presence of protein (e.g., 2% serum albumin), infectivity is maintained for 1 week or more at 4° C, however, and indefinitely at −60° C. Storage at freezer temperatures of −10° to −20° C should be avoided because infectivity is rapidly lost.[156,157] Rubella virus can also be stabilized against heat inactivation by the addition of magnesium sulfate to virus suspensions.[158] Specimens for virologic examination should be transported to distant laboratories packed in ice rather than frozen, with the addition of stabilizer if possible. Infectivity is rapidly lost at pH levels less than 6.8 or greater than 8.1 and exhausted in the presence of ultraviolet light; lipid-active solvents; or other chemicals, such as formalin, ethylene oxide, and β-propiolactone.[156,159-161] Infectivity of rubella in cell culture is inhibited by amantadine, but this drug seems to have no therapeutic effect.[162-165]

Several laboratories have described the structural proteins of rubella virus and determined the nucleotide sequence of the genes coding for these proteins.[70,85,139,166-169] Originally, three structural proteins were identified and designated as VP-1, VP-2, and VP-3.[166] These three major structural proteins now are designated E1, E2, and C, respectively, with relative molecular weights of 58,000, 42,000 to 47,000, and 33,000 Da, respectively.[71-73] E1 and E2 are envelope glycoproteins and make up the characteristic spikelike projections that are located on the viral membrane. Structural protein C, which is not glycosylated, is associated with the infectious 40S genomic RNA to form the nucleocapsid.[75] The E2 glycopeptide has been shown on polyacrylamide gels to be heterogeneous with two bands, which are designated E2a (relative molecular weight of 42,000 Da) and E2b (relative molecular weight of 47,000 Da).[71]

Monoclonal antibody studies have begun to delineate the functional activities of these structural proteins. E1 seems to be the viral hemagglutinin and binds hemagglutination-inhibiting and hemolysis-inhibiting antibody; E2 does not seem to be involved in hemagglutination.[70,72,74,76-79] Monoclonal antibodies specific for E1 and E2 have neutralizing activity because both proteins are involved in cell entry.[†]

Studies also indicate that there are multiple epitopes on the structural proteins that are involved in hemagglutination inhibition (HI) and neutralizing activities.[79,82] Molecular analyses of rubella viruses isolated during 1961 to 1997 from specimens obtained in North America, Europe, and Asia have documented the remarkable antigenic stability of the E1 envelope glycoprotein.[84] E1 amino acid sequences have differed by no more than 3%, indicating no major antigenic variation over the 36-year period that spanned the major worldwide pandemic of 1962 to 1964 and the 30 years since introduction of rubella vaccine. Two clades, 12 genotypes, and one provisional genotype are now recognized: 1A-1J and 2A-2C.[172,173] Genotype I was isolated before 1970 and grouped into a single diffuse clade, indicating intercontinental circulation, whereas most of the post-1975 viruses segregated into geographic clades from each continent, indicating evolution in response to vaccination programs. Clade 2 seems to be Asian in origin.[174]

Figure 29-1 shows the geographic distribution of the genotypes.[175] The availability of molecular analysis and the minor variations in amino acid sequences have provided an additional tool for monitoring the sources of infection in areas where indigenous rubella has been greatly reduced by high levels of immunization. As discussed in more detail later, the complexity of the antigenic nature of the rubella virion affects the ability of the host to respond to the full complement of antigens and affects the various antibody assays required to detect all the corresponding antibody responses (see "Natural History").

CLASSIFICATION

Rubella has been classified as a member of the Togaviridae family (from the Latin word *toga,* meaning "cloak"), genus

[†]References 74, 80, 89, 90, 170, 171.

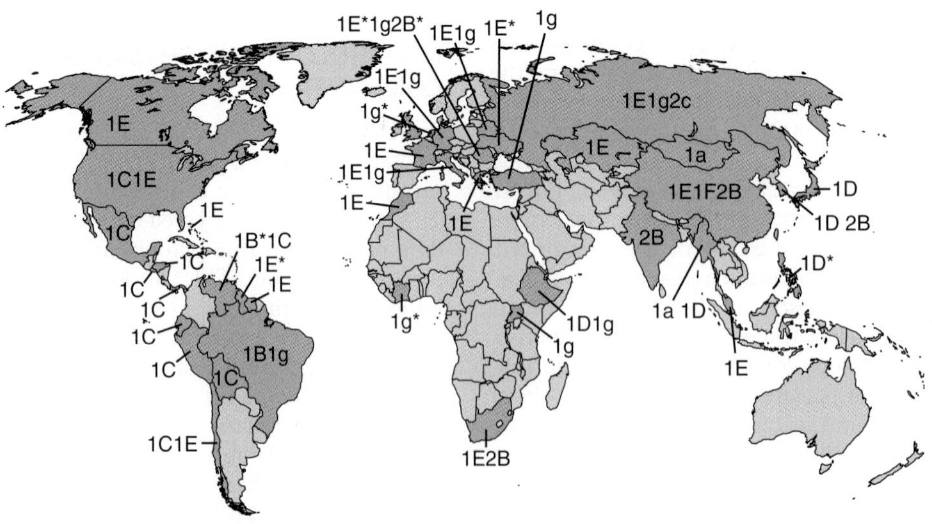

Figure 29-1 Global distribution of indigenous rubella viruses, 1995-2006. Data summarize information available as of the end of November 2006. *Beige shading* indicates countries where circulating rubella viruses have been identified. During this period, some countries reduced indigenous rubella transmission to low levels (e.g., Canada, United Kingdom, and United States).

Rubivirus.[176,177] No serologic relationship exists between rubella and other known viruses. Minor biologic differences identified in different passaged strains of rubella virus are not reflected in the antigenic differences assessed by comparing protein composition or serologic reactions.[139,169,178,179] Differences in the immune response after immunization with the various vaccines now in use are not caused by inherent differences in the viral strain, but rather by modification of the viruses during their attenuation in cell culture.[30] The reported variation in the virulence of rubella epidemics does not seem to be explained by the molecular analyses described earlier, but it may result from differences in population susceptibility and underreporting of cases of congenital rubella.[180-187]

ANTIGEN AND SEROLOGIC TESTING

Rubella virus may be isolated in cell culture from nasopharynx, serum, urine, cataracts, placenta, amniotic fluid, and fetal tissues. The nasopharynx is the best source because excretion is more persistent there. RK-13 and Vero cells are the best substrates. Virus isolation takes many days to become positive and confirmed by neutralization, however. During pregnancy, it is important to attempt more rapid diagnosis through the use of reverse-transcriptase polymerase chain reaction (RT-PCR).[188] Amniotic fluid is the best source, although chorionic villi and placenta may be positive. Primers come from nucleotides located between 731 and 854 of the *E1* gene.[189,190]

Purified rubella virus has many antigenic components associated with the viral envelope and the ribonucleoprotein core.[161,167] These antigens and the ability of specific antiserum to neutralize virus form the basis for the wide variety of serologic methods available to measure humoral immunity after natural and vaccine-induced infection.

The ability of antibodies against E1 and E2 proteins to inhibit agglutination of erythrocytes by the surface hemagglutinin (HA antigen) forms the basis for the HI test, which previously was the most popular rubella serologic test. The HA antigen was originally prepared from BHK tissue culture fluids and then from alkaline extracts of infected BHK-21 cells.[23,191] This antigen can agglutinate various red blood cells, including newborn chick, adult goose, pigeon, and human group O erythrocytes.[192] Rubella hemagglutinin is unique in its dependency on calcium ions to attach to red blood cell receptors.[192,193] After extraction from infected cells, rubella hemagglutinin is stable for months at −20° C, several weeks at 4° C, and overnight at 37° C, but is destroyed within minutes after heating to 56° C.[191,193] The HA antigen can be protected from ether inactivation by pretreatment with polysorbate 80 (Tween 80).

Cells and serum contain heat-stable β-lipoproteins that can inhibit rubella hemagglutination and give rise to false-positive results.[23,161] Although it has been reported that nonspecific inhibitors do not interfere in the HI test if the HA antigen and erythrocytes are mixed before addition of serum, the recommended method is to pretreat the sera to remove these inhibitors.[161,194] Earlier test procedures used kaolin adsorption for removal of these nonspecific inhibitors; however, many faster and more specific methods are now used, such as treatment with heparin–manganese chloride or dextran sulfate–calcium chloride.[195,196]

Cell-associated complement fixation antigen was first derived from infected rabbit kidney (RK-13) and African green monkey kidney cell cultures and later prepared from alkaline extracts of infected BHK-21 cells.[22,197] There are two complement fixation antigens: One is similar in size and weight to the hemagglutinin and infectious virus, and the other is smaller and "soluble."[170,198,199] The antibody response as measured by the soluble antigen develops more slowly than the response to the larger antigen, which parallels the HI response. In contrast to the HA antigen, complement fixation antigens do not lose their antigenicity after either treatment.[197,199]

Various precipitin antigens have been shown serologically; two of these, the theta and iota antigens, are associated with the viral envelope and core.[200-202] The antibody response to these two antigens is of interest. Antibodies to the theta antigen rise promptly and persist. Antibodies to the iota antigen are detectable later and for a shorter time.[203] The RA 27/3 vaccine seems to be unique among vaccine strains in its ability to elicit a response to the iota antigen, making its immune response more similar to natural infection. The significance of this observation is unclear.[204]

Rubella virus antigen-antibody complexes (involving the envelope and the core antigens) cause aggregation of platelets.[205,206] The main platelet aggregation activity seems to reside with the viral envelope, however.

Antibody directed against the rubella virus can also be measured by virus neutralization in tissue culture.[2-4,21,207-209] Although the presence of neutralizing antibodies correlates best with protective immunity, neutralization assays are time-consuming, expensive, and relatively difficult to perform. Laboratories have traditionally performed the complement fixation and HI tests. Because the complement fixation test is insensitive for screening purposes and cannot detect an early rise in antibody in acute acquired infection, the HI test was been the most widely used assay.[‡]

Numerous more rapid, easily performed, reliable, and sensitive tests have replaced the HI test for routine use,[92,211,212] including passive (or indirect) hemagglutination; single radial hemolysis (also known as hemolysis in gel), which is used widely abroad; radioimmunoassay; immunofluorescence; and enzyme immunoassay tests, also referred to as enzyme-linked immunosorbent assays.[207,210-241] Rapid latex agglutination and passive hemagglutination assays can provide results in minutes for screening and diagnostic purposes.[92-98] The numerous assays now available, and their greater sensitivity compared with the HI test have led to some confusion about the level of antibody that should be considered indicative of immunity (see "Update on Vaccine Characteristics").[48,58,61,211,239] The HI test remains the reference test against which other assays are compared, however.

Immunoglobulin class-specific antibody can be measured in most of the serologic systems.[§] This most frequently involves detection of IgM in whole or fractionated sera. Numerous techniques are used to fractionate and then test the serum. An important consideration in any IgM assay is the possibility of false-positive results because of the presence of rheumatoid factor. Solid-phase IgM capture assays seem to be unaffected, however, by rheumatoid factor.[104-107,222,237,248]

[‡]References 2-4, 161, 203, 207, 210, 211.

[§]References 161, 218-222, 225, 227, 236-239, 242-250.

GROWTH IN CELL CULTURE

Rubella replicates in a wide variety of cell culture systems, primary cell strains, and cell lines.[157,161,251] The time required for virus recovery varies markedly, depending partly on the culture system being used.

In general, rubella growing in primary cell cultures (i.e., human, simian, bovine, rabbit, canine, or duck) produces interference to superinfection by a wide variety of viruses (especially enteroviruses, but also myxoviruses, papovaviruses, arboviruses, and, to some extent, herpesviruses) but no cytopathic effect.[19,20,156] In contrast, a cytopathic effect of widely varying natures results from infection of continuous cell lines (i.e., hamster, rabbit, simian, and human). In general, primary cells, especially African green monkey kidney, have proved superior for isolation of virus from human material by the interference technique. The continuous RK-13 and Vero (vervet monkey kidney) cell lines are also used, however, because cytopathic effect is produced, and there is no problem with adventitious simian agents.[157] Continuous cell lines, such as BHK-21 and Vero, are best suited for antigen production because of the higher levels of virus produced.

All cell lines support chronic infection with serial propagation, but some are limited by the occurrence of cytopathic effect. These cells grow slowly and can be subcultivated fewer times than when not infected.[157] The mechanisms of rubella-induced interference and persistent infection in cell cultures are not completely understood. Although interferon (IFN) production has been described after rubella infection of cell cultures, interference seems to be an intrinsic phenomenon.[157,161,252–254] As with other viruses, generation of defective interfering particles can be found in tissue culture.[255] These particles are thought to be nonessential for persistence, however.

Rubella virus can be plaqued in RK-13, BHK-21, SIRC (i.e., rabbit cornea), and Vero cells.[161] Plaquing forms the basis of neutralization assays, and differences in plaquing characteristics can be used as markers to differentiate strains.[21,161,179,207-209]

PATHOGENICITY FOR ANIMALS

Rubella virus grows in primates and in various small laboratory animals. The acquired or congenital disease has not been completely reproduced in any animal, however.

Vervet and particularly rhesus monkeys are susceptible to infection by the intranasal, intravenous, or intramuscular routes.[256–258] Although no rash develops, there is nasopharyngeal excretion of virus in all of the inoculated monkeys and demonstrable viremia in 50%. Attempts to produce transplacental infection in pregnant monkeys have been partially successful. Rubella virus has been recovered from the amnion and the placenta, but the embryo itself has not been shown to be consistently infected.[259,260]

The ferret is the most useful of the small laboratory animals in rubella studies. Ferret kits are highly sensitive to subcutaneous and particularly to intracerebral inoculations. Virus has been recovered from the heart, liver, spleen, lung, brain, eye, blood, and urine for 1 month or longer after inoculation, and neutralizing and complement fixation antibodies have developed.[261] Ferret kits inoculated at birth develop corneal clouding. Virus appears in fetal ferrets after inoculation of pregnant animals.[262]

Rabbits, hamsters, guinea pigs, rats, and suckling mice all have been infected with rubella virus, but none has proved to be a consistent and reliable animal model system for study of rubella infection.[180,181,263-266] Studies indicating that Japanese strains of rubella virus were less teratogenic to offspring of infected rabbits than U.S. strains have not been confirmed.[180,181] These experiments were conducted to examine further the hypothesis referred to earlier that there is a difference in the virulence among rubella virus strains circulating in Japan and other parts of the world,[178,180-184,186] which appears to be untrue.

Epidemiology

Humans are the only known host for rubella virus. Continuous cycling in humans is the only apparent means for the virus to be maintained in nature. Because rubella is predominantly a self-limited infection seen in late winter and spring, questions have arisen about how the virus persists throughout the remainder of the year. Person-to-person transmission probably occurs at very low levels in the general population throughout summer and winter and probably at much higher levels in closed populations of susceptible individuals.[267-288] Congenitally infected infants can shed virus from multiple sites and can serve as reservoirs of virus during periods of low transmission.[165,289-294] This is of particular concern in the hospital setting.[165,286] Efficiency of transmission may also vary among individuals, with some being better "spreaders" than others. This phenomenon may contribute to continued circulation of the virus.[295]

Rubella has a worldwide distribution.[296-302] The virus circulates almost continually, at least in continental populations. In the continental temperate zones of the Northern Hemisphere, rubella is consistently more prevalent in the spring, with peak attack rates in March, April, and May; infection is much less prevalent during the remainder of the year, increasing or decreasing during the 2 months before or after the peak period.[299,301] Before widespread rubella immunization, sizable epidemics occurred every 5 to 9 years in temperate climates; however, the periodicity of rubella epidemics was highly variable in developed and developing countries, with major epidemics occurring at intervals ranging from 10 to 30 years. Epidemics usually built up and receded gradually over a 3- to 4-year interval, peaking at the midpoint.[9,296,299,301]

The apparent increased infectivity and virulence of rubella, as exemplified in the major epidemics, have been the subject of considerable speculation. One popular thesis has been the unproven emergence of a more virulent strain of virus at widely separated intervals.[178,180-184,186] No convincing evidence exists concerning clinically different strains of rubella, however, and molecular analysis of the E1 envelope glycoprotein does not support the hypothesis of an epidemic versus endemic strain difference.[84] The apparent severity of the epidemic seems to be related to the number of susceptible adults, especially pregnant women, in any given population at the outset of an epidemic.[185,187,301,303] Host factors, such as the differences in the ability to transmit rubella, and still unknown factors may also be involved.[295,303]

Attack rates in open populations have not been defined precisely for many reasons. Because rubella is such a mild disease, it is underreported, even in areas where reporting has been mandatory for years. Mandatory reporting did not begin in the United States until 1966 (Fig. 29-2).[299,304] The high and variable rate of inapparent infection poses a major problem when attempting to interpret the recorded data, which are based usually on clinical findings.[272,305-310]

In childhood, the most common time of infection, 50% or more of serologically confirmed infections result in inapparent illness. The ratio may be 6:1 or 7:1 in adults, perhaps as a result of silent reinfection in naturally immune individuals who have lost detectable antibody.[272,308] The frequent occurrence of infections that clinically mimic rubella makes it even more difficult to determine attack rates in open populations.[311] Attack rates undoubtedly depend on the number of susceptible individuals, which varies widely in different locations.

Serologic assessments of rubella attack rates have been performed in closed populations, such as military recruits, isolated island groups with small populations, boarding home residents, and household members.[272-274,295,307,310-318] In such situations, individual exposure to the virus is more intense than encountered in open populations. Under these circumstances, 90% to 100% of children and adults who are susceptible may become infected. Attack rates in susceptible persons on college and university campuses and in other community settings range from 50% to 90%.[9,303] Similar to primary infection, reinfection probably is increased as exposure becomes more intense.[272,308,316,317]

In most of the world, including the United States before the introduction of mass immunization of children in 1969, rubella was typically a childhood disease that was most prevalent in the 5- to 14-year-old age group.[2,3,7,297-304] It was rare in infants younger than 1 year. The incidence increased slowly for the first 4 years of age, increased steeply between 5 and 14 years of age, peaked around 20 to 24 years of age, and then leveled off. In developed countries before mass immunization, the incidence of infection did not reach 100% before the ages of 35 to 40 years; 5% to 20% of women of childbearing age remained susceptible to infection.

In the era before a rubella vaccine, in isolated or island populations, such as in Trinidad, some areas of Japan, Panama, rural Peru, and Hawaii, a relatively high rate of susceptibility was found among young adults[297,298,300,301,314]; 26% to 70% of women of childbearing age remained susceptible. This situation existed even though rubella was endemic with ample opportunity for multiple introductions of virus from the outside. Low population density, tropical climate, low concentration of effective spreaders, and genetic factors all have been invoked to explain these low attack rates, but none can adequately account for this peculiar epidemiologic phenomenon by itself.[295,300,301,303] Later studies from 45 developing nations where rubella immunization efforts have been minimal have revealed a wide range of susceptibility (≤10% to approximately 25%).[315]

In other areas, particularly in South America, infections begin earlier in life, and peak incidence occurs before puberty.[300] Infection rates in most South American countries reach a plateau at approximately the same level as seen in Europe and North America, however, leaving 10% or more of young women who are susceptible, based on serologic tests. Chile seemed to be an exception, with almost all persons being infected before puberty.[300] The impact of major immunization programs in the PAHO countries to reach a goal of eliminating rubella by 2010 appears to have eliminated new infections to date (http://new.paho.org/).

Recently, some information has become available from other parts of the world. In Vietnam, 29% of mothers were shown to be seronegative,[319] and in Africa rubella infection was shown to be widespread.[320] The incidence of CRS in Vietnam was estimated to be 234 per 100,000 live births, caused by serotype 2B.[319,321] Japan has had a recent major outbreak of rubella with thousands of cases, because of insufficient immunization of women of childbearing

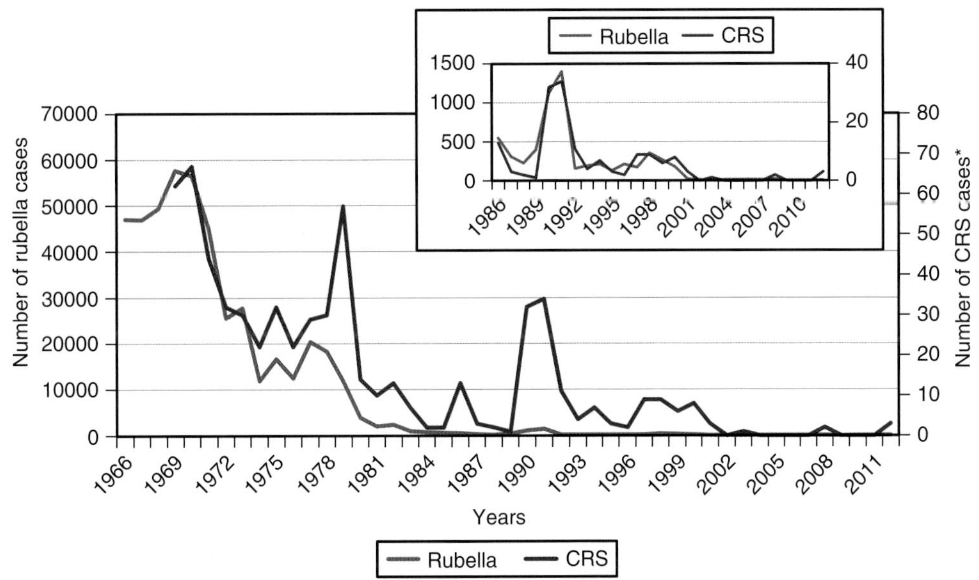

Figure 29-2 Reported rubella and congenital rubella syndrome—United States, 1966-2012. *Year of birth.

age.[322,323] At least 30 CRS cases have been reported. Surveillance in India is insufficient to give an accurate picture, but many women are susceptible to rubella, and CRS is frequently reported.[324,325] Overall, CRS is reported in significant numbers throughout the world except for the Americas.[326]

Initial mass vaccination of children with distribution of more than 29 million doses over the first year after licensure, followed by routine vaccination of 1-year-old children and vaccination of susceptible adolescents and adults, has been extremely successful in controlling rubella and CRS in the United States.[‖] The characteristic 6- to 9-year epidemic cycle has been interrupted, and the reported incidence of rubella that ranged from approximately 200 to 400 cases annually during the period 1992 to 2000 decreased to less than 25 since 2001. For comparison, there were approximately 58,000 cases reported in 1969, the year of vaccine licensure in the United States (see Fig. 29-2).

Age-specific declines in the occurrence of rubella have been greatest in children, who, because they were the major reservoir of the virus, have been the primary target of the U.S. immunization program. The risk of rubella decreased by 99% in all age groups, however, after efforts to increase vaccination levels in older, susceptible persons, especially women of childbearing age (see "Prevention of Congenital Rubella").[267,269] Until the late 1990s, serologic surveys documented susceptibility of 20% in this adult population; however, the National Health and Nutrition Examination Survey (1999-2004) documented susceptibility of less than 11%.[328-331]

Adolescents and young adults now account for most reported cases, with more cases reported among individuals older than 15 years than in children. Although there are fewer and smaller outbreaks since elimination was achieved, outbreaks are still reported in colleges, cruise ships, and other settings in which people live or work in proximity.[278-280,283-288] Outbreaks no longer occur among military recruits because they receive rubella vaccine as soon as they arrive for basic training.[275]

Although the reported incidence of cases of CRS has decreased dramatically, the number of cases of rubella and congenital rubella reported in the United States increased in 1989 to 1991, documenting that the potential for cases will continue as long as immunization of children and women of childbearing age is not close to 100%.[39] The outbreak of rubella and subsequent clusters of congenital rubella among the Amish in Pennsylvania in 1991 and 1992 provided a reminder that there are still pockets of susceptible individuals in the United States.[282] The epidemiology of rubella is closely linked with the epidemiology of CRS. From 1997 to 1999, more than 90% of the mothers of infants with CRS were born outside the United States. Since 2000, the incidence of CRS has been the lowest reported at a rate of less than 1 per 1 million live births and with most of the mothers of these infants born outside the United States and presumably unimmunized.[332] In 2012, three cases of CRS were reported in the United States, but all three mothers were infected in Africa.

‖References 5, 24, 33, 39, 270, 304, 327.

Transmission In Utero

In pregnant women with clinical or inapparent primary rubella, the virus infects the placenta during the period of viremia and subsequently infects the fetus.[2,6,296,311,333-348] Intrauterine transmission of virus associated with maternal reinfection is rare. It is presumed that this difference is a reflection that viremia is absent or greatly reduced because of immunity induced by the primary infection (natural or vaccine induced).[¶]

Maternal infection may result in no infection of the conceptus, resorption of the embryo (seen only with infections occurring in the earliest stages of gestation), spontaneous abortion, stillbirth, infection of the placenta without fetal involvement, or infection of the placenta and fetus.[6] Infected infants can have obvious multiorgan system involvement or, as is frequently observed, no immediately evident disease.[6,13,111,349-356] After long-term follow-up, many of these seemingly unaffected infants have evidence of hearing loss or central nervous system (CNS) or other defects.[#]

Gestational age at the time of maternal infection is the most important determinant of intrauterine transmission and fetal damage.[2-4,6,296,311,336] The risk of fetal infection and congenital anomalies decreases with increasing gestational age. Fetal damage is rare much beyond the first trimester of pregnancy, as was shown in large British and American studies (Table 29-1).

Availability of more sensitive antibody assays has led to refinement of understanding of the risk of fetal infection and subsequent congenital defects throughout all stages of pregnancy.[107,114] Although the risk of defects does decrease with increasing gestational age, fetal infection can occur at any time during pregnancy. Data on the risk of fetal infection are inconsistent when maternal rubella infection occurs before conception.[1,12,112,114,357-360] If some risk exists, it is small.

¶References 5, 6, 44, 46, 49, 51, 55-57, 59, 115, 120, 340-378.
#References 6, 13, 14, 116, 135, 136, 349, 350, 352-355.

Table 29-1 Fetal Abnormality Induced by Confirmed Rubella at Various Stages of Pregnancy

Stage of Pregnancy (wk)	United Kingdom Study (% Defective)*	United States Study (% Defective)†
≤4	—	70
5-8	—	40
≤10	90	—
11-12	33	—
9-12	—	25
13-14	11	—
15-16	24	—
13-16	—	40
≥17	—	8

From Plotkin SA, Orenstein WA, Offit PA, editors: *Vaccines*, ed 5, Philadelphia, 2008, Saunders.
*Data from Miller E, Cradock-Watson JE, Pollock TM: Consequences of confirmed maternal rubella at successive stage of pregnancy, *Lancet* 2:781, 1982.
†Data from South MA, Stever JL: Teratogen update: the congenital rubella syndrome, *Teratology* 31:297, 1985.

RISK OF FETAL INFECTION

Early attempts to define the risk of fetal infection relied on isolation of virus from products of conception.[333-339] Of products of conception obtained from women with clinical rubella during the first trimester, 40% to 90% were found to be infected. The higher rates were observed in serologically confirmed cases of maternal rubella and when improved isolation techniques were employed.[338,339] Attempts were made to refine the risk estimates by evaluating placental and fetal tissue separately. In some of these studies, equal rates of persistent placental and fetal infection were observed, ranging from 80% to 90%.[338,339]

In other studies, persistent placental infection was found to be twice as frequent as fetal infection: 50% to 70% versus 20% to 30%.[333,336] High rates of fetal infection accompanied placental infection, however, when specimens obtained during the first 8 weeks of gestation were examined. Of 14 cases in which virus was cultured from placental tissue, six of seven fetuses were culture-positive when maternal rubella occurred during the first 8 weeks of pregnancy. In contrast, only one of seven fetal specimens was positive when infection occurred between 9 and 14 weeks of gestation.[333] In another similar study, fetal infection rates decreased sharply after the 8th week of gestation; placental infection rates decreased, but less rapidly.[336] After the 8th week, placental infection occurred in 36% (8/22), and fetal infection occurred in 10% (2/20) of cases. Although fetal infection was not documented beyond the 10th week of gestation, placental infections were identified up to the 16th week.

Further data on the risk of fetal infection have been obtained from studies using sensitive laboratory tests to detect congenital infection in children born to mothers with serologically confirmed rubella.[107,114] Because congenital rubella is often subclinical in infants and young children, use of such tests is necessary to assess accurately the risk of congenital infection.[6,107-112,350,352-355] In investigations in which this approach was used, with detection of rubella-specific IgM antibody in sera to document congenital infection, the discrepancy between rates of placental and fetal infection seen in viral isolation studies is less apparent. These studies have provided new information on the events after maternal infection in the second and third trimesters.

In a study involving 273 children (269 of whom had IgM antibody assessment), Miller and colleagues[109] reported that fetal infection after serologically documented symptomatic maternal rubella in the first trimester was, as expected, quite high: 81% (13/16), with rates of 90% for fetuses exposed before 11 weeks of gestation and 67% for fetuses exposed at 11 to 12 weeks of gestation (Table 29-2). Of greater interest is that the infection rate was 39% (70/178) after exposure in the second trimester (decreasing steadily from 67% at 13-14 weeks to 25% at 23-26 weeks) but increased to 53% (34/64) with third-trimester infection (with infection rates of 35%, 60%, and 100%, respectively, during the last 3 months of pregnancy).

In another investigation of fetal infection after first-trimester maternal rubella infection based on IgM determination, Cradock-Watson and associates[107] found that 32% of 166 children were infected after exposure in the second trimester and that a comparable proportion (24% of 100) were infected after exposure in the third trimester. The rate of infection increased during the latter stages of gestation after initially decreasing to a low of 12% by the 28th week and was 58% (11/19) when maternal infection occurred near term. Even higher rates were observed when persistence of IgG antibody was used as the criterion for congenital infection. The true fetal infection rate probably lies between the rates calculated by using the IgM and persistent IgG data.

In both studies, the fetal infection rate declined between 12 and 28 weeks of gestation, suggesting that the placenta may prevent transfer of virus, although not completely.[107] Some of the infections recorded during the last weeks of pregnancy could have been perinatally or postnatally acquired (e.g., by means of exposure to virus in the birth canal or from breast milk), but the available evidence

Table 29-2 Risk of Serologically Confirmed Congenital Rubella Infection and Associated Defects in Children Exposed to Symptomatic Maternal Rubella Infection, by Weeks of Gestation

	INFECTION		DEFECTS*		
Weeks of Gestation	**No. Tested**	**Rate (%)**	**No. Followed**	**Rate (%)**	**Overall Risk of Defects (%)†**
<11	10	90 (9)‡	9	100	90
11-12	6	67 (4)	4	50	33
13-14	18	67 (12)	12	17	11
15-16	36	47 (17)	14	50	24
17-18	33	39 (13)	10		
19-22	59	34 (20)			
23-26	32	25 (8)			
27-30	31	35 (11)	53		
31-36	25	60 (15)			
>36	8	100 (8)			
Total	258§	45 (117)	102	20	

Modified from Miller E, Cradock-Watson JE, Pollock TM: Consequences of confirmed maternal rubella at successive stages of pregnancy, *Lancet* 2:781, 1982.
*Defects in seropositive patients only.
†Overall risk of defects = rate of infection × rate of defects.
‡Numbers in parentheses are number of children infected.
§None of 11 infants whose mothers had subclinical rubella were infected.

indicates that the placental barrier to infection may be relatively ineffective during the last month, perhaps to the same degree as that seen during the first trimester, and that the fetus is susceptible to infection throughout pregnancy, albeit to various degrees.[361-363]

RISK OF CONGENITAL DEFECTS

Estimates of the risk of congenital anomalies in live-born infants after fetal infection have been affected by numerous factors. Early retrospective and hospital-based studies led to overestimates of the risk of congenital defects after first-trimester infection (up to 90%).[6,111,303] The risk of abnormalities as determined by prospective studies relying on a clinical diagnosis of maternal rubella varied considerably (10%-54% overall, with a 10%-20% risk for major defects recognizable in children ≤3 years of age) and tended to underestimate the risk because serologic evaluation of infants was not performed.[111,357,364-368] The proportion of pregnancies electively terminated can affect observed malformation rates. The fact that fetal infection can occur during all stages of pregnancy also influences assessments of the risk of congenital defects.

Because most infants born with congenital rubella who were exposed after the 12th week of gestation do not have grossly apparent defects, long-term follow-up is necessary to detect subtle, late-appearing abnormalities, such as deafness and mental impairment.[*a] This is especially true for infants infected beyond the 16th to 29th week of gestation, who seem to be at little, if any, risk of congenital anomalies.[107,113] Studies by Peckham[111,354] showed that estimates of the risk of defects are affected by the serologic status and age at evaluation of the child. The overall incidence of defects in 218 children studied when they were about 2 years of age was 23%; it was 52% if maternal infection occurred before 8 weeks of gestation, 36% at 9 to 12 weeks, and 10% at 13 to 20 weeks. No defects were observed when maternal infection occurred after 20 weeks of gestation. When considering only seropositive children, the overall risk of defects increased to 38%, with increased risks of 75%, 52%, and 18%, respectively, for the three gestational periods previously cited. At follow-up, when the children were 6 to 8 years of age, the overall risk of abnormalities in infected children who were seropositive when 2 years of age increased from 38% to 59%; the risk after first-trimester infection increased from 58% to 82%.

Miller and colleagues[109] observed higher rates of defects in infected children observed for only 2 years (see Table 29-2). Defects were seen in 9 of 9 seropositive children exposed during the first 11 weeks of gestation, 2 of 4 children exposed at 11 to 12 weeks, 2 of 12 children exposed at 13 to 14 weeks, and 7 of 14 children exposed at 15 to 16 weeks. Congenital heart disease and deafness were observed after infection before the 11th week; deafness was the sole defect identified after infection at 11 to 16 weeks of gestation. No defects were observed in 63 children infected after 16 weeks of gestation. Some children infected in the third trimester had growth restriction, however.

Although the number of subjects is small, results of the study of Miller and colleagues[109] indicate that the risk of damage is 85% in infants who were infected as fetuses during the first trimester and 35% after infection during weeks 13 to 16 of gestation. These rates of defects are higher than previously reported, but they may be an accurate reflection of intrauterine events because all maternal cases were serologically confirmed, and sensitive antibody assays were used to detect congenital infection. With further follow-up, higher rates of defects may be observed.

*a References 6, 13, 14, 116, 135, 136, 349, 350, 352-355.

These rates pertain to offspring known to be infected and are useful in evaluating the risk of defects given fetal infection. For counseling purposes, it is essential to know the risk of congenital defects after confirmed maternal infection. This risk can be derived by multiplying the rates of defects in infected fetuses by the rates of fetal infection. Based on the reported experience of Miller and colleagues,[109] the risks are 90% for maternal infection before the 11th week of gestation, 33% for infection during weeks 11 to 12, 11% for weeks 13 to 14, and 24% for weeks 15 to 16 (see Table 29-2). The overall risk after maternal infection in the first trimester was 69%.

Natural History

POSTNATAL INFECTION

Virologic Findings

The pertinent virologic findings of postnatal infection are depicted in Figure 29-3. The portal of entry for rubella virus is believed to be the upper respiratory tract. Virus spreads through the lymphatic system or by a transient viremia to regional lymph nodes, where replication first occurs. Virus is released into the blood 7 to 9 days after exposure and may seed multiple tissues, including the placenta. By the 9th to 11th day, viral excretion begins from the nasopharynx, kidneys, cervix, gastrointestinal tract, and various other sites.[†a]

The viremia peaks at 10 to 17 days, just before rash onset, which usually occurs 16 to 18 days after exposure. Virus disappears from the serum in the next few days, as antibody becomes detectable.[290,306,321,369] Infection may persist, however, in peripheral blood lymphocytes and monocytes for 1 to 4 weeks.[63,68,370,371] Virus is excreted in high titers from nasopharyngeal secretions. Nasopharyngeal shedding

†a References 9, 290, 314, 321, 361-363, 369.

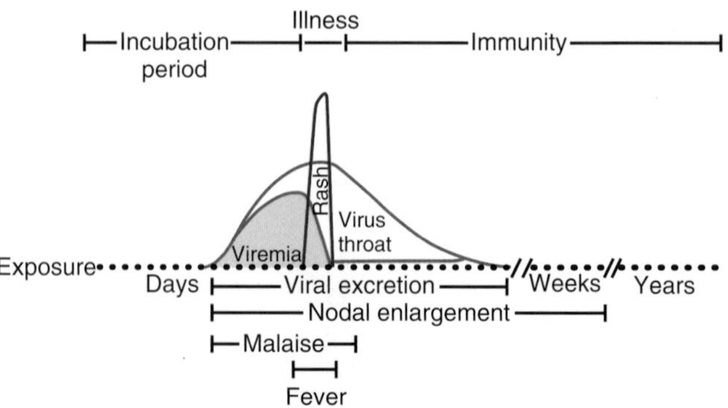

Figure 29-3 **Relationship of viral excretion and clinical findings in postnatally acquired rubella.** (Data from Alford CA: Chronic congenital and perinatal infections. In Avery GB, editors: *Neonatology*, Philadelphia, 1987, Lippincott.)

rarely may be detected for 3 to 5 weeks. Although virus can usually be cultured from the nasopharynx from 7 days before to 14 days after rash onset, the highest risk of virus transmission is believed to be from 5 days before to 6 days after the appearance of rash. Viral shedding from other sites is not as consistent, intense, or prolonged.[306,369] Rubella virus has been cultured from skin at sites where rash was present and where it was absent.[372,373]

Humoral Immune Response

In challenge studies conducted in the early 1960s, Green and coworkers[306] showed that neutralizing antibody was first detected in serum 14 to 18 days after exposure (usually 2-3 days after rash onset), peaked within 1 month, and persisted for the duration of the follow-up period of 6 to 12 months. The HI test soon became the standard method for detecting rubella antibodies after acute postnatal rubella infection because of its reliability and ease compared with the neutralization test. Several other methods for measuring rubella antibody responses have supplanted the HI test in popularity (see "Virus").[92,211,212] Figure 29-4 depicts the kinetics of the immune response to acute infection detected by these various serologic assays, which have been exhaustively compared with the HI technique.[‡a]

There are generally three distinct patterns of antibody kinetics. Antibodies of the IgG class measured by HI, latex agglutination, neutralization, immunofluorescence, single radial hemolysis (or hemolysis in gel) (not shown in Fig. 29-5), radioimmunoassay, and enzyme-linked immunoassay theta precipitation (not shown) follow the first pattern. These IgG antibodies usually become detectable 5 to 15 days after rash onset, although they may appear earlier and may even be detected 1 or 2 days before the rash appears. The antibody titers rapidly increase to reach peak values at 15 to 30 days and then gradually decline over years to a constant titer that varies from person to person. In some patients with low levels of residual antibody, a second exposure to rubella virus may lead to low-grade reinfection of the pharynx. A booster antibody response can be detected with any of the assays. This antibody response rapidly terminates the new infection, which is most often subclinical, and little or no viremia occurs.[§a]

A second pattern of immune response to rubella infection is seen when IgG antibodies are measured by passive hemagglutination. The peak titer of these antibodies is similar to that measured by HI, but the passive hemagglutination antibodies are relatively delayed in appearance, and levels increase only slowly to their maximal titers. They first become detectable 15 to 50 days after the onset of the rash and often take 200 days to reach peak titers. The antibodies probably persist for life. Booster responses may be seen with reinfections.

Studies indicate that the predominant IgG subclass detected by all these various assays is probably IgG1.[99,101] Failure to detect IgG3 may be indicative of reinfection.[102] A third distinct pattern of antibody production is represented in Figure 29-4 by the IgM antibody–class immune response. Rubella-specific IgM antibody can be measured by HI, immunofluorescence, radioimmunoassay, or enzyme immunoassay.[‖a]

IgM antibodies are most consistently detectable 5 to 10 days after the onset of the rash, increase rapidly to peak values at around 20 days, and then decline so rapidly that they usually disappear by 50 to 70 days. In a few patients, low levels may persist for 1 year.[374-376] The booster IgG antibody response to reinfection described earlier does not usually involve the IgM class of antibody, and the presence of high-titer IgM antibodies usually indicates recent primary infection with rubella. More sensitive techniques, such as radioimmunoassay or enzyme immunoassay, may occasionally detect low levels of specific IgM antibodies in some

‡a References 92-96, 203, 207-217, 219, 226-236, 238, 241.

§a References 42, 48, 51, 54, 58, 60, 280, 325, 348.

‖a References 103, 161, 218-222, 225, 227, 236, 237.

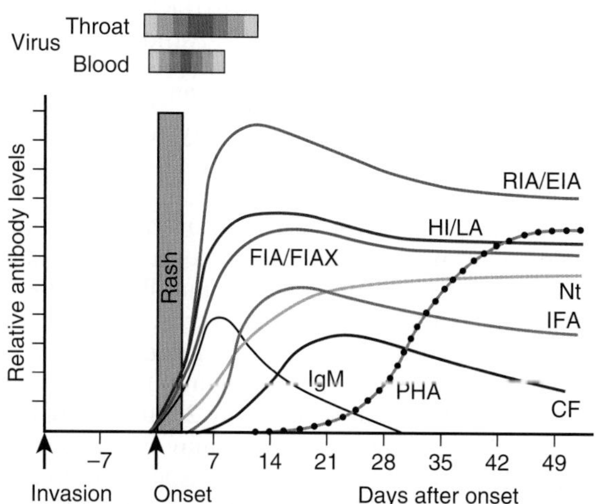

Figure 29-4 Diagram of immune response in acute rubella infection. *CF*, Complement fixation; *EIA*, enzyme immunoassay; *FIA*, fluorescence immunoassay; *FIAX*, commercial solid-phase indirect fluorescence immunoassay (Bioproducts, Walkersville, Md); *IFA*, immunofluorescence assays; *IgM*, immunoglobulin M; *HI*, hemagglutination inhibition; *LA*, latex agglutination; *Nt*, neutralization; *PHA*, passive agglutination; *RIA*, radioimmunoassay. (Data from Herrmann KL: Rubella virus. In Lennette EH, Schmidt NJ, editors: *Diagnostic procedures for viral, rickettsial and chlamydial infections*, Washington, DC, 1979, American Public Health Association, p 725; and Herrmann KL: Available rubella serologic tests, *Rev Infect Dis* 7[Suppl 1]:S108, 1985.)

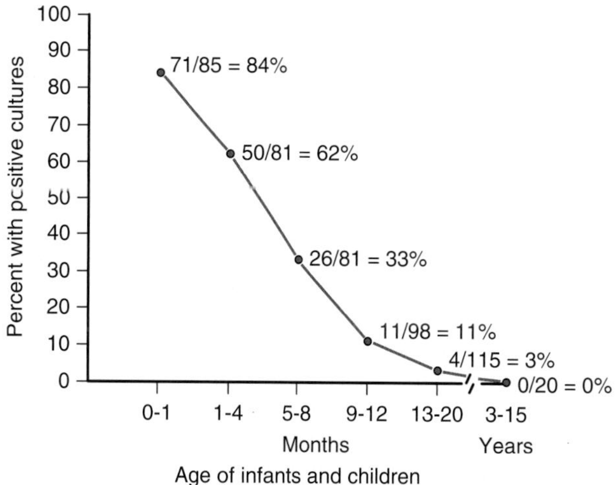

Figure 29-5 Rate of virus excretion by age in infants and children with congenital rubella infection. (Data from Cooper LZ, Krugman S: Clinical manifestations of postnatal and congenital rubella, *Arch Ophthalmol* 77:434, 1967.)

patients with reinfections, which may cause some difficulty in differentiating subclinical reinfection, which is almost always of no consequence, from acute primary subclinical infection.[45,55,57,59] Determination of avidity of rubella-specific IgG may help resolve this problem.[377-379] Primary infection seems to be associated with low-avidity IgG, and reinfection seems to be associated with high-avidity IgG.

The kinetics of the immune response to rubella infection detected by other serologic assays is not as distinct as the three patterns just described, and marked variability among patients has been observed. Complement fixation antibodies or iota precipitins (not shown in Fig. 29-5) are lacking in the first 10 days after the rash and increase slowly to peak at 30 to 90 days.[203] These antibodies persist for several years in one third of patients and may reappear during reinfections. Iota precipitins do not persist for more than a few months and do not usually reappear with reinfections.

Antibodies of the IgA class appear within 10 days, but may disappear within another 20 days or persist for several years.[100,103,218,243] IgD and IgE antibodies appear rapidly (6-9 days) after infection, remain high for at least 2 months, and then decline slightly at 6 months.[100] IgE antibodies reach an early peak similar to that seen for IgM and IgA. In contrast, the IgD response is delayed, similar to that of IgG.

The antibody response after infection is generally considered to confer complete and permanent immunity. Clinical reinfection is rare, and reinfections usually pose little risk to the fetus because placental exposure to the virus is minimal.[¶a] Some rare instances of fetal infection after maternal reinfection may be caused by an incomplete immune response to the various antigenic domains on each structural protein of the virus (see "Virus").[78-80,115,119,340,345-349] Three cases after natural infection have been reported involving women who had positive HI results but who had no detectable levels of neutralizing antibody.[340,345,347] The sensitivity of the neutralizing assay itself is an important determinant in interpreting these results.[115,208] This phenomenon also may account for the four reported cases of congenital infection that followed reinfection of women who had presumably been immunized previously.[46,49,56,120] Some reported instances of maternal reinfection probably (and in at least one case definitely) represent cases of primary acute infection.[5,6,117,342-344]

Cellular Immune Response

Cellular immunity to rubella virus has been measured by lymphocyte transformation response, secretion of IFN, secretion of macrophage migration-inhibitory factor, induction of delayed hypersensitivity to skin testing, and release of lymphokines by cultured lymphocytes.[380-391] Peripheral blood lymphocytes from seropositive individuals respond better in each of these tests than do lymphocytes from uninfected persons, suggesting that these assays measure parameters of the cellular immune response to rubella virus. The results from other studies in which chromium-51 microcytotoxicity assays have been used are difficult to interpret because syngeneic cell lines have not been used to control for HLA-restricted responses.[381,384]

In the first weeks after natural rubella infection, some degree of transient lymphocyte suppression may occur.[385,387] In general, cell-mediated immune responses precede the appearance of humoral immunity by 1 week, reach a peak value at the same time as the antibody response, and subsequently persist for many years, probably for life.[350] Acute infection may suppress skin reactivity to tuberculin testing for approximately 30 days.[392]

Local Immune Response

The local antibody response at the portal of entry in the nasopharynx is essentially IgA in character, although IgG antibody from serum may diffuse into nasopharyngeal secretions. The nasopharyngeal IgA antibody persists at detectable levels for at least 1 year after infection. Its persistence apparently minimizes the tendency for reinfection after natural rubella infection. The lack of local IgA nasopharyngeal response after parenteral administration of live rubella vaccines (less so with the RA 27/3 strain than with other strains) probably plays a key role in the increased incidence of subclinical reinfection after vaccination.[#a] Local antibody levels tend to be higher in individuals resistant to challenge with live virus, but no specific titer of antibody has been associated with complete protection.

A cell-mediated immune response in tonsillar cells has been detected by lymphocyte transformation and secretion of migration-inhibitory factor after natural rubella and after intranasal challenge with live RA 27/3 vaccine.[397] In guinea pigs, the response first becomes detectable 1 to 2 weeks after intranasal vaccination, peaks at 4 weeks, and disappears at about 6 weeks.[398]

CONGENITAL INFECTION

Virologic Findings

An important feature that distinguishes congenital infection from postnatal infection is that the former is chronic.[*b] During the period of maternal viremia, the placenta may become infected and transmit virus to the fetus (see "Transmission In Utero").[2,6,296,311,333-339] Although virus may persist for months in the placenta, recovery of virus from the placenta at birth occurs infrequently.[401] In contrast, after the fetus is infected, the virus persists typically throughout gestation and for months postnatally. It can infect many fetal organs or only a few.[336]

In infected infants, virus can be recovered from multiple sites (e.g., pharyngeal secretions, urine, conjunctival fluid, feces) and is detectable in cerebrospinal fluid (CSF), bone marrow, and circulating white blood cells.[†b]

Pharyngeal shedding of virus is more common, prolonged, and intense during the early months after delivery (see Fig. 29-5). By 1 year of age, only 2% to 20% of infants shed virus.[289-291] Rarely, shedding may continue beyond the age of 2 years.[292-294] Virus can be isolated from the eye and CSF, particularly when disease is evident in the corresponding organs and can persist for more than 1 year in the eye and CNS.[402-405] Virus has been isolated from the brain of a 12-year-old boy with later-appearing subacute panencephalitis occurring after congenital rubella infection.[405-407]

¶a References 42, 45, 48, 51, 54, 55, 57-60, 348.

#a References 42, 44, 48, 54, 58, 60, 393-396.

*b References 2, 13, 296, 336, 399, 400.

†b References 2, 13, 165, 289-294, 296, 333, 334, 336, 338, 399-402, 403.

Humoral Immune Response

Studies have shown that placental infection does not prevent passive transfer of maternal antibody and that the infected fetus can mount an immune response.[296,333-339,408-410] Although the development and function of the other components of the immune response of the fetus may be important, critical factors that allow fetal infection to occur in the presence of antibody may be the timing when antibody is present in the fetal circulation, the quality of the antibody that the fetus produces, or both.

Although placental transfer of antibody occurs despite persistent infection, levels of antibody in fetal blood during the first half of gestation are only 5% to 10% of levels in maternal serum.[411,412] As the placental transfer mechanisms mature by midgestation (16-20 weeks), increasing levels of maternal IgG antibody are transferred to the fetus (Fig. 29-6).[413,414]

The development of the fetal humoral immune system apparently is too late to limit the effects of the virus. Cells with membrane-bound immunoglobulins of all three major classes—IgM, IgG, and IgA—appear in the fetus by 9 to 11 weeks of gestation.[412] Circulating fetal antibody levels remain low until midgestation, however, despite the presence of high titers of virus and the development of antigen receptors on the cell surface (Fig. 29-7). At this time, levels of fetal antibody increase, with IgM antibody predominating.[408,415-419] Fetal IgA, IgD, and IgG also are made, although in lesser amounts.[100,416,419] As in the case with other chronic intrauterine infections, congenital rubella infection may lead to an increase in total IgM antibody levels.[408,410,414,419] Total IgA levels are also occasionally increased, but IgG levels seldom exceed levels of uninfected infants.[408,419-421] At the time of delivery of infected infants, levels of IgG rubella antibodies in cord sera are equal to or greater than levels in maternal sera, even if the infant is born prematurely.[408] IgG is the dominant antibody present at delivery in rubella-infected infants and is mainly maternal in origin. In contrast, the IgM levels are lower but are totally fetus derived.

In the first 3 to 5 months after birth, the levels of maternally derived IgG decrease as maternal antibody is catabolized (see Fig. 29-7).[408] In contrast, IgM antibodies increase in titer and can predominate. Later, as viral excretion wanes and disappears, the IgM antibody levels diminish, and IgG becomes the dominant and persistent antibody type. Cradock-Watson and colleagues[419] found that total IgM was elevated in nearly all sera obtained from infected infants during the first 3 months of life and in half of sera from infected infants 3 to 6 months of age. Rubella-specific IgM has been shown consistently to persist for 6 months, frequently for 1 year, and rarely longer when assayed by sensitive serologic procedures, such as radioimmunoassay and immunofluorescence.[224,419] Cradock-Watson and colleagues[419] also reported that IgM was detectable in 48 (96%) of 50 serum samples during the first 6 months of life and in 11 (29%) of 38 serum samples from children 6.5 months to 2 years of age. The total level of antibody, as measured by various serologic tests, remains virtually unchanged throughout the first year of life, despite the fluctuations in immunoglobulin composition.[408,419]

High levels of IgG antibody are usually maintained for several years after detectable virus excretion ends, suggesting that there may be continued antigenic stimulation. During the first few years of life, some patients have a relative hypergammaglobulinemia, particularly of the IgM and IgG classes of antibody, which results from the increased antigenic stimulus accompanying the chronic infection.[414,419] With increasing time, antibody levels may decrease and even become undetectable in 10% to 20% of patients.[354,422-424] Cooper and coworkers[424] found that

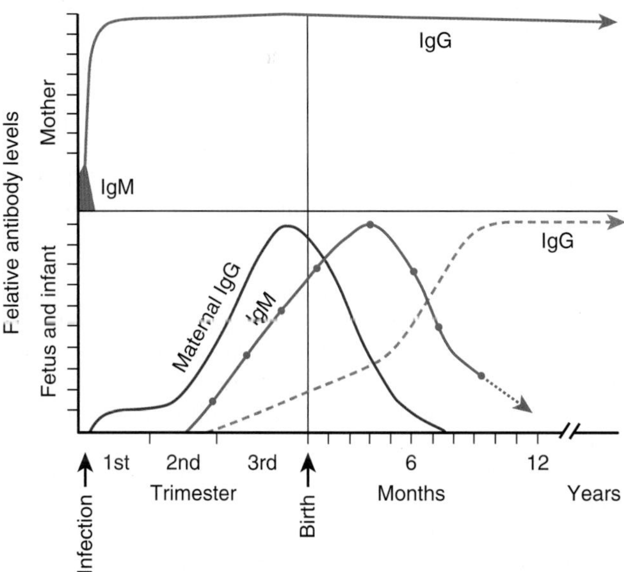

Figure 29-6 Diagram of immune response in the mother, fetus, and infant after maternal and fetal rubella infections in the first trimester of pregnancy. *IgG, IgM,* Immunoglobulins G and M, respectively. (Data from Alford CA: Immunology of rubella. In Friedman H, Prier JE, editors: *Rubella,* Springfield, Ill, 1972, Charles C Thomas.)

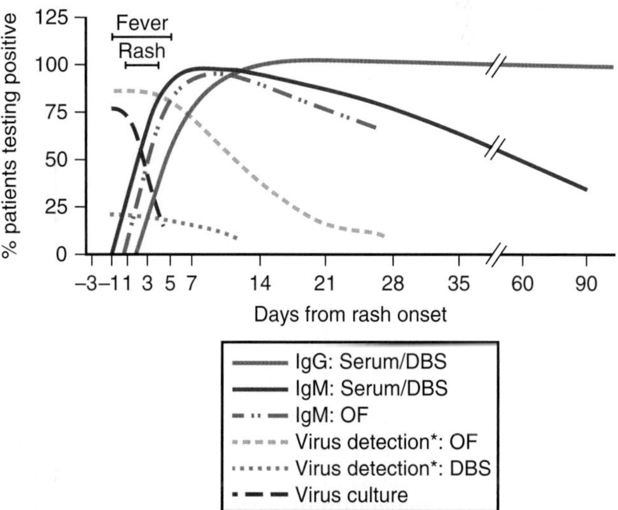

Figure 29-7 Pattern of test results among patients with mild rubella virus infection, by day from rash onset and type of sampling method used. Incubation period: 14-17 days. *DBS,* Dried blood spots; *IgG, IgM,* immunoglobulins G and M, respectively; *OF,* oral fluid. *Virus RNA detection by conventional, nested, or real-time reverse-transcription polymerase chain reaction. (Based on data presented at the Measles and Rubella Alternative Sampling Techniques Review Meeting, convened in Geneva in June 2007. World Health Organization Measles and Rubella Laboratory Network.)

the geometric mean HI titer decreased by a factor of 16 by age 5 years in 223 children with CRS. No HI antibodies were detected in 8 of 29 5-year-old children. In a study from Japan, only 3% of 381 children with congenital infection observed for more than 17 years had undetectable HI titers.[425] There was an initial rapid decline from a geometric mean titer of 1:416 ($2^{8.7}$) to 1:84 ($2^{6.4}$) over the first 2 years of follow-up. After this, there was a modest continuing decline, and the final geometric mean titer was 1:42 ($2^{5.4}$).

Cooper and coworkers[424] reported that congenitally infected children who have lost detectable rubella-specific antibody did not develop a boost in antibody titer after rubella vaccination. This finding may reflect some sort of immunologic tolerance that follows intrauterine exposure to rubella virus. None of the children with congenital rubella in Japan had evidence of significant boosts in antibody or a history of clinical disease when exposed during recent outbreaks of rubella.[425,426] RA 27/3 vaccine virus administered intranasally succeeded in inducing an immune response, however, so the problem may be less tolerance than low systemic levels of humoral or cellular immunity.[424]

Hypogammaglobulinemia with low levels of all three major classes of immunoglobulins has been reported in a few instances of congenital rubella.[137,165,427,428] Usually, only IgA is affected; there may also be instances when IgG levels are low, whereas levels of IgM are two or three times the upper limit of normal for adults. These IgG and IgM abnormalities may occur with or without IgA abnormalities.[427] Over time, immunoglobulin development may become normal, and this can occur despite continued viral excretion but is more likely if viral titers are decreasing.[292]

In addition to defects in the immunoglobulin levels, defects in specific antibody production have been observed. One such defect is a complete lack of antibody response to any antigen, including the rubella virus itself. Response only to the virus, in the absence of a response to most other antigens, has also been reported.[292] This state of immunologic unresponsiveness resolves in many patients. Antibody production becomes normal as the patient's general condition improves and as immunoglobulin levels normalize.

Immunoprecipitation studies of sera from patients with CRS provide further information on defective antibody production. The studies indicate that the antibody profile to the three structural proteins of the rubella virus is qualitatively different from that observed in sera from persons with postnatally acquired infection (see "Virus").[88,89,91] Little or no antibody to the core structural protein (C) is found, and the absolute and relative amounts of antibody to structural proteins E1 and E2 seem to vary with age.[88,89] These findings further suggest that the immune response of the infected fetus may be incomplete and may explain why detectable antibodies are not present in some serum samples.[91,354,422-425] If a serum sample contains relatively little antibody to structural protein E1 (i.e., hemagglutinin), assays that detect antibody to the whole virion are more likely to be positive than assays that detect antibody only to E1 (e.g., HI assay). It is unclear whether these abnormal antibody patterns persist for life.

Cellular Immune Response

Similar to the cells responsible for the humoral immune response (i.e., B cells), the cells involved in cellular immunity (i.e., T cells and macrophages) develop some of their functions early in gestation.[429-431] Little is known about their response in utero, however, because appropriate specimens have not been obtainable for study. The cellular immune response of the infected fetus has been inferred from studies of infected infants and children. Available evidence indicates that some infants with congenital rubella have impaired cellular immune responses.

Retarded development of the thymus and lymphocyte depletion have been reported, but these abnormalities may result from the stress of infection, rather than the virus itself.[432] Abnormal delayed hypersensitivity skin reactions to numerous antigens (e.g., diphtheria toxoid, *Candida*, dinitrofluorobenzene) have also been reported.[292,433] This defect has been associated with abnormalities in the humoral system and resolves as antibody production returns to normal.

Results of studies of in vitro lymphocyte blastogenesis in congenitally infected infants and children have been confusing. Early studies showed a poor response to phytohemagglutinin, vaccinia, and diphtheria toxoid.[433-436] Because rubella virus can depress the lymphocyte blastogenic response and the virus can be isolated from lymphocytes of chronically infected infants, the abnormality may be a result of viral infection of the circulating blood cells, rather than an inherent defect in cell-mediated immunity.[434,435,437,438] This diminished cellular response may normalize over time because elevated lymphocyte responses have been detected in some older infected children.[429,439]

Buimovici-Klein and colleagues[391,440] showed that lymphocytes from older children and adolescents with congenital rubella had no or very poor lymphocyte proliferative responses to rubella virus antigens and had markedly reduced IFN and migration-inhibition factor production. These studies indicated that these defects were greater in children exposed early in gestation than those exposed later, with the greatest degree of abnormality in children whose mothers had been infected during the first 8 weeks of pregnancy. The studies also pointed out that these defects could persist long after viral excretion had ceased. It remains unclear if these cellular immune defects are responsible for viral persistence or are yet another manifestation of intrauterine infection.[440]

Other investigators have confirmed that patients with congenital rubella have defects in cell-mediated immunity.[124,137,138] Verder and colleagues[138] reported a decreased proportion of suppressor or cytotoxic ($CD8^+$) T cells in an infant with congenital rubella. Rabinowe and coworkers[137] documented persistent T-cell abnormalities in patients with congenital infection who were 9 to 21 years of age. Compared with normal subjects, congenitally infected patients had depressed ratios of $CD4^+$ T cells (helper or inducer) to $CD8^+$ T cells (from a decreased proportion of $CD4^+$ T cells and an increased percentage of $CD8^+$ T cells). Such findings persist for only 1 month after acute postnatal rubella infection.[441]

Lymphocytes of infected children were unable to kill rubella-infected cells in a cytotoxicity assay.[442] These results were questioned because syngeneic target cells were not used, and these responses are known to be HLA restricted. Similar results have been reported by Verder and associates,[138] however, who observed abnormal killer and natural killer cell activities.

Morag and associates[398] detected cytotoxic T lymphocytes in tonsillar lymphocytes after intranasal administration of

RA 27/3 vaccine but not after subcutaneous administration of another attenuated strain. Elevation of cytokines interleukin-4, interleukin-10, and tumor necrosis factor-α after vaccination has also been observed.[443]

Interferon Response

It has long been suggested that the fetus has a deficient IFN response to viral infections, including rubella, but this evidence has been derived from indirect studies with in vitro cell systems or animal models.[182,183,338,444,445] Technical difficulties have hampered direct studies of humans. IFN that seemed to be specifically stimulated by the presence of rubella virus in rubella-infected human embryos has been shown, however.[446] The IFN was found at 7 weeks of gestation and persisted 12 weeks after symptoms ceased in the mothers. Direct study of fetal blood and amniotic fluid has also shown that the fetus can produce IFN in response to the virus.[447]

Children with congenital infection have the capacity to make IFN on challenge. Desmyter and coworkers[448] reported that IFN could not be detected from the serum or urine of nine children 11 to 18 months of age who were excreting virus. After vaccination with live measles vaccine (i.e., Edmonston B or Schwarz strains), all the children seroconverted, however, and produced detectable levels of IFN.

Pathogenesis

POSTNATAL INFECTION

The events leading to acute postnatal infection are relatively well known and have been discussed in detail in "Natural History." Available information indicates that viral replication and postinfection immune phenomena are involved in the clinical manifestations of the illness.

Viremia may lead to seeding of multiple organs, but few are clinically affected.[6] Speculation that the rash may be an immune phenomenon caused by circulating immune complexes has not been documented. Few persons with uncomplicated illness have immune complexes containing rubella virus, and virus has been isolated from involved and uninvolved skin.[127,132,372,373] Virus has been isolated from lymph nodes and conjunctiva, accounting for the lymph node enlargement and conjunctivitis observed in many patients.[369,449] Virus has been isolated from synovial fluid, but immune mechanisms may play a role in some cases of arthralgia and arthritis, particularly if symptoms are persistent.[127,449-453] Encephalitis is probably a manifestation of the immune response, but direct viral invasion may be involved, particularly in the rare case of progressive panencephalitis that has been reported to follow postnatal infection.[125,454-456] It has been suggested that pregnant women are at increased risk of serious complications because of the impaired immune response associated with pregnancy, but there are few data to support this claim.[456-458] There has also been interest, especially in Japan, in the influence of HLA type and other genetic factors on the incidence and severity of postnatal infection. [‡b] No consistent pattern has been reported.

‡b References 122, 123, 126, 128, 131, 459.

CONGENITAL INFECTION

The outcome of maternal rubella infection follows a logical sequence of events, beginning with maternal infection, followed by viremia, placental seeding, and dissemination of infection to the fetus (see "Transmission In Utero" and "Natural History").[2,6,296,311,333-339] The fetus may escape infection entirely, die in utero, be born with multiple obvious defects, or seem to be normal at birth only to develop abnormalities later in life.[6,13,111,290,349-356] The variability in outcome is highlighted by the observation that one identical twin may be infected and the other spared.[6,460,461]

The most important determinant of fetal outcome is gestational age at the time of infection.[§b] The disease is more severe and has a greater tendency to involve multiple organs when acquired during the first 8 weeks of gestation. The factors that govern the influence of gestation are unknown. It is possible that immature cells are more easily infected and support the growth of virus better than older, more differentiated cells. It is also possible that the placenta becomes increasingly resistant to infection (or at least more able to limit infection) as it rapidly matures during the first trimester. A third possibility is that maturing fetal defense mechanisms become capable of confining and clearing the infection. This last explanation is probably important after 18 or 20 weeks of gestation but seems unlikely in the latter half of the first trimester, when attenuation of fetal infection begins. It is likely that a combination of these and other factors are responsible for the decrease in virulence of fetal infection with increasing gestational age.

The hallmark of fetal infection is its chronicity, with the tendency for virus to persist throughout fetal life and after birth.[‖b] The fact that virus can be isolated long after birth also raises the possibility of reactivation, at least in brain tissue.[407] It is unclear why the virus has these properties because the fetus is not truly immunologically tolerant and seems to be able to produce IFN.[¶b] In any case, chronic or reactivated infection can lead to ongoing pathologic processes.[#b]

The causes of cellular and tissue damage from congenital rubella infection are poorly defined.[444,445] Only a variable, small number of cells are infected (1/1000-250,000).[339] In tissue culture, infection with rubella virus has diverse effects, ranging from no obvious effect to cell destruction (see "Virus"); this is also likely to be the case in vivo,[161] but cytolysis is uncommon (see "Pathology").[2,3,6,9,462-466] Inflammation is minimal and consists mainly of infiltration of small lymphocytes. Polymorphonuclear leukocytes and plasma cells are lacking, particularly compared with other viral infections of the human fetus, in which inflammation and general necrosis are quite extensive. In contrast, vascular insufficiency seems to be more important than cell destruction or secondary inflammatory damage in the genesis of congenital defects.[2,3,6,9,462-466] This suggestion is supported by the observation that rubella virus has low destructive potential for cells growing in vitro, including those of human origin. Numerous investigators have maintained multiple types of rubella-infected human fetal cells

§b References 2, 3, 6, 107, 114, 296, 311, 333, 336.
‖b References 2, 13, 165, 289-294, 296, 311, 333-339, 391-407.
¶b References 224, 296, 342, 400, 401, 411, 444-448.
#b References 6, 13, 14, 111, 135, 136, 349, 350, 352-355.

in culture for years without loss of viability or evidence of cytopathic effect.[467-469]

Other defects have been reported in chronically infected cells that might help explain the mechanism of congenital defects. These include chromosomal breaks, increased cellular multiplication time, and increased production of a protein inhibitor that causes mitotic arrest of certain cell types.[399,467,470-475] The mitotic arrest is presumably responsible for the reduced replication of infected cells.

A report by Bowden and associates[476] indicates that rubella virus may interfere with mitosis by having an adverse effect on actin microfilaments. Observations of Yoneda and coworkers[477] show that rubella virus may alter cell receptors to specific growth factors. All of these abnormalities, if occurring in vivo, may result in decreased cell multiplication because of slow growth rates and limited doubling potential during the period of embryogenesis, when cell division and turnover are normally very rapid. Naeye and Blanc[478] found histopathologic evidence for mitotic arrest and reduced cell numbers in infants who died of CRS. These observations have been offered to explain the increased incidence of intrauterine growth restriction seen in infants with congenital rubella, but this explanation probably represents an oversimplification of the actual mechanisms involved.

More recently, it has been shown that rubella virus capsid protein interacts with host cell proteins to inhibit translation.[479] Although infection of adult human cells often results in apoptosis, infection of fetal cells does not.[480] The reduction of apoptosis would favor the chronic infection that is the hallmark of congenital rubella. Excess cytokine stimulation from persistent infection may also play a role.

Immunologic responses also have been proposed as causes of cellular damage. Although cellular immune defects may be a result of chronic infection, it is possible that these defects contribute to ongoing tissue damage.[391,436,440] Excessive serum immunoglobulin development, persistent antibody production in the face of viral replication for prolonged periods, and production of rheumatoid factor, all indicative of overstimulation of the immune system, also may have a role in the pathogenesis of CRS.[481,482] The presence of immune complexes and autoantibodies and the influence of certain HLA types may contribute to the delayed expression of some signs of congenital rubella, such as pneumonitis, diabetes mellitus, thyroid dysfunction, and progressive rubella panencephalitis (see "Clinical Manifestations").[*c] Some of these immunologic events may be directly involved in tissue damage (e.g., immune complexes, autoantibodies), whereas others may allow the virus to persist or reactivate.

Pathology

POSTNATAL INFECTION

Little is known about the pathology of postnatally acquired rubella because patients seldom die of this mild disease. As observed by Cherry,[9] the histologic findings of tissues that have been examined (i.e., lymph nodes and autopsy specimens from patients dying with encephalitis) are unremarkable. Changes in lymphoreticular tissue have been limited-to-mild edema, nonspecific follicular hyperplasia, and some loss of normal follicular morphology. Examination of brain tissue has revealed diffuse swelling, nonspecific degeneration, and little meningeal and perivascular infiltrate.

CONGENITAL INFECTION

In contrast to the situation with postnatal rubella, much is known about the pathology of congenital rubella infection.[†c] In general, small foci of infected cells are seen in apparently normal tissue. Cellular necrosis and secondary inflammation are seldom obvious, although a generalized vasculitis predominates (see "Pathogenesis").

The pathologic findings of the placenta include hypoplasia, inflammatory foci in chorionic villi, granulomatous changes, mild edema, focal hyalinization, and necrosis.[462,463,483,484] Disease usually causes extensive damage to the endothelium of the capillaries and smaller blood vessels of the chorion. The vessel lesions consist mainly of endothelial necrosis, with fragmentation of intraluminal blood cells. Töndury and Smith[462] postulated that emboli of infected endothelial cells originating from the chorion might seed target organs in the fetus. These emboli may also contribute to organ damage by obstructing the fetal blood supply. Petechiae and the presence of hemosiderin-laden phagocytes in surrounding tissue are evidence of functional vascular damage.[463]

Although not nearly as common as vascular lesions, specific cytolysis, presumably caused by direct viral effect on the cell, is also present in the placenta. This condition is characterized by cytoplasmic eosinophilia, nuclear pyknosis or karyorrhexis, and cellular necrosis. Specific nuclear and cytoplasmic cellular inclusion bodies are rare but have been observed.[484] Although placentitis would be expected to be present in all affected placentas, regardless of when fetal infection occurred, Garcia and colleagues[484] found that placental lesions seemed to be more intense when infection occurred in the last trimester of pregnancy. This finding is consistent with the observation that the placenta is not a barrier to fetal infection in the latter stages of pregnancy.[107,113,352,354]

Autopsies show that virtually every organ may be involved, with hypoplasia being a common finding. The necrotizing angiopathy of small blood vessels seen in the placenta is the most characteristic lesion in fetal organs. Cytolysis with tissue necrosis and accompanying inflammatory changes is also far less common but has been found in the myocardium, brain, spinal cord, skeletal muscle, viscera, and epithelial cells of the developing lens, inner ear (organ of Corti), and teeth.

The overall pathologic process of congenital rubella, in keeping with its chronic nature, is progressive. Healing and new lesions can be found in specimens obtained in the later stages of gestation.[462,463] The pathologic changes vary among embryos in quantity and in organ distribution, and the location and nature of organ lesions depend on the gestational age at the time of infection.[462] The pathologic findings parallel the enormous variability of the clinical disease seen in infected newborns.

[*c]References 13, 14, 121, 124, 125, 127, 129, 130, 133-138, 407, 420.

[†c]References 2, 3, 6, 9, 462-466, 481.

Clinical Manifestations

POSTNATAL INFECTION

Rubella is usually a mild disease with few complications. Clinical illness may be more severe in adults.[‡c] Measles, varicella, and some enteroviruses acquired close to delivery may be associated with serious illness in the newborn, probably because of fetal exposure to transplacental viremia in the absence of protective levels of maternal antibody. One case report suggests that the same may be true in rubella. Sheinis and associates[486] reported the death of a neonate with rash onset when 12 days of age; the mother developed rash on the day of delivery. This single observation needs to be confirmed. There are no conclusive data to indicate that infection in the immunocompromised host is associated with an increased risk of complications.

The first symptoms of rubella occur after an incubation period of 16 to 18 days (range, 14-21 days). In a child, rash is often the first sign detected. In adolescents and adults, the eruption is commonly preceded by a 1- to 5-day prodromal period characterized by low-grade fever, headache, malaise, anorexia, mild conjunctivitis, coryza, sore throat, cough, and lymphadenopathy usually involving suboccipital, postauricular, and cervical nodes.

The constitutional symptoms often subside rapidly with the appearance of the rash. The rash can last 1 to 5 days or longer and can be pruritic in adults. Infection without a rash is quite common. The ratio of subclinical to clinical infections has varied from 1:9 to 7:1.[272,308] Subclinical infection can lead to fetal infection, although it is unclear whether the risk is as great as that associated with clinically apparent infection.[§c]

Arthralgia and frank arthritis with recrudescence of low-grade fever and other constitutional symptoms may appear after the rash fades. Joint involvement typically lasts 5 to 10 days, but may be more persistent. The frequency of these symptoms is variable, but they are more common in adults, particularly women.[9] In some studies of adult patients, the frequency has been 70%.[487] Thrombocytopenia (occurring in ≈1/3000 patients) and acute postinfection encephalitis (occurring in 1/5000-6000 patients) are rare complications that usually occur 2 to 4 days after rash onset[9] but may be more frequent.[488] Rare complications associated with postnatal rubella include myocarditis, Guillain-Barré syndrome, relapsing encephalitis, optic neuritis, and bone marrow aplasia.[9,489-493] In a rubella outbreak in the Tongan islands, encephalitis was particularly frequent.[494] Two cases of a progressive panencephalitis, similar to measles-associated subacute sclerosing panencephalitis, have been reported.[454,455] This CNS disturbance is more likely to manifest in patients with CRS, although it still occurs infrequently.[407,495,496] Testalgia has also been reported in patients with rubella, but this may have been a coincidental finding.[497,498]

An ophthalmic disease called Fuchs heterochromic cyclitis, a form of uveitis, has been associated more recently with rubella virus infection.[499-503] The disease usually affects only one eye, with manifestations of chronic, low-grade anterior uveitis that may lead to cataract, glaucoma, vitreous opacities, and change of iris color. This condition is painless. All patients are seropositive for rubella, and intraocular antibody production of rubella (but not other pathogens) has been shown in adults and in a 13-year-old unvaccinated child.[501,504] Fuchs uveitis occurred in one patient with CRS who had persistent intraocular rubella virus.[505]

CONGENITAL INFECTION

Gregg's original report[12] in 1941 defined CRS as a constellation of defects, usually involving some combination of congenital heart, eye, and hearing abnormalities, with or without mental retardation and microcephaly. After the extensive studies in the mid-1960s, in which virologic and serologic methods of assessment were used, the pathologic potential associated with intrauterine rubella infection had to be greatly expanded.[2,3] The recognition of various new defects associated with congenital rubella infection led to speculation that they had not existed before the 1962 to 1964 pandemic. A review of the abnormalities in infants born during previous nonepidemic periods indicated, however, that they were not new but had not been appreciated previously because of the small number of affected infants studied.[506]

The virus can infect one or virtually all fetal organs and, when established, can persist for long periods (see "Transmission In Utero," "Natural History," "Pathogenesis," and "Pathology").[‖c] Congenital rubella, a chronic infection, may kill the fetus in utero, causing miscarriage or stillbirth. At the other extreme, the infection may have no apparent effect clinically detectable at the delivery of a normal-appearing infant. Alternatively, severe multiple birth defects may be obvious in the newborn period. The wide spectrum of disease is discussed later and summarized in Tables 29-3 and 29-4.

Silent infections in the infant are much more common than symptomatic ones. Schiff and colleagues[353] prospectively examined 4005 infants born after the 1964 rubella epidemic. Based on virologic and serologic techniques to detect infection in the newborns, the overall rate of congenital rubella was greater than 2% compared with only approximately 0.1% in endemic years.[353,360] Of the infected newborns, 68% had subclinical infection during the neonatal period. Among infants who were followed, 71% developed manifestations of infection at various times in the first 5 years of life. Many important rubella defects can be undetectable or overlooked in the early months of life. Existing manifestations of infection can progress, and new manifestations may appear throughout life.[¶c] Some abnormalities of CRS usually are not detected until the second year of life or later (see Table 29-3). The silent and progressive nature of congenital rubella infection has important implications for accurate, timely diagnosis and appropriate short-term and long-term management.

It is useful to group the clinical features of congenital rubella into three categories: transient manifestations in newborns and infants; permanent manifestations, which may be present at birth or become apparent during the first year of life; and developmental and late-onset manifestations,

[‡c] References 6, 9, 302, 305, 370, 485.

[§c] References 2, 3, 6, 109, 112, 354, 360.

[‖c] References 6, 13, 14, 111, 135, 136, 165, 289-294, 296, 311, 333-339, 349-356, 399-407, 420.

[¶c] References 6, 13, 14, 111, 135, 136, 349-356.

which usually appear and progress during childhood, adolescence, and early adult life.[13,461,507] These groupings overlap.

Transient Manifestations

Transient manifestations seem to reflect ongoing heavy viral infection, perhaps abetted by the newborn's emerging, often abnormal immune function.[6,124,138] Examples of these manifestations include hepatosplenomegaly, hepatitis, jaundice, thrombocytopenia with petechiae and purpura, discrete bluish red ("blueberry muffin") lesions of dermal erythropoiesis, hemolytic anemia, chronic rash, adenopathy, meningoencephalitis (in some cases), large anterior fontanelle, interstitial pneumonia, myositis, myocarditis, diarrhea, cloudy cornea, and disturbances in bone growth that appear as striated radiolucencies in the long bones. More than 50% of infants with these transient findings usually have evidence of intrauterine growth restriction and may continue to fail to thrive during infancy.[290] These transient abnormalities were referred to as the *expanded rubella syndrome* when widely reported after the pandemic of 1962 to 1964. Careful review of early observations during the 1940s and 1950s revealed that these were not new manifestations of congenital rubella.

Table 29-3 Abnormalities of Congenital Rubella Usually Not Detected Until Second Year or Later

Defects	References
Hearing	
Peripheral	13, 342, 347, 528-531
Central	
Language	13, 523, 531, 532
Developmental	
Motor	13, 533, 534
Intellectual	13, 509, 533
Behavioral	13, 533
Psychiatric	13, 533
Autism	13, 455
Endocrine	
Diabetes	13, 116, 124, 129, 130
Precocious puberty	13, 14
Hypothyroidism	536-540
Thyroiditis	537-539
Hyperthyroidism	116, 541
Growth hormone deficiency	544, 545, 569
Addison disease	14
Visual	
Glaucoma (later onset)	546
Subretinal neovascularization	547, 548
Keratic precipitates	546
Keratoconus	549
Corneal hydrops	549
Lens absorption	550
Dental	524, 561
Progressive panencephalitis	401, 487, 489
Educational difficulties	13
Hypertension	562

These conditions usually are self-limiting and clear spontaneously over days or weeks.[2] These lesions are important from a diagnostic and prognostic standpoint. They may be associated with other, more severe defects; this applies especially to thrombocytopenia and bone lesions.[13,507] The mortality rate was approximately 35% in one group of infants who presented with neonatal thrombocytopenia. Extreme prematurity, gross cardiac lesions or myocarditis with early heart failure, rapidly progressive hepatitis, extensive meningoencephalitis, and fulminant interstitial pneumonitis contributed to the mortality during infancy.[461]

Permanent Manifestations

Permanent manifestations include heart and other blood vessel defects, eye lesions, CNS abnormalities, deafness, and various other congenital anomalies. These structural defects result from defective organogenesis (i.e., some cardiac, eye, and other organ defects) and from tissue destruction and scarring (i.e., hearing loss, brain damage, cataracts, chorioretinopathy, and vascular stenosis). Relatively few defects result from gross anatomic abnormalities. It is uncertain that all of the malformations listed in Table 29-5 are associated with congenital rubella.[13,334,400,474,506-534] Because many of them occur in the absence of intrauterine rubella infection, their presence in affected infants may be coincidental.[9]

Congenital heart disease is present in more than half of children infected during the first 2 months of gestation. The most common lesions, in descending order, are patent ductus arteriosus, pulmonary artery stenosis, and pulmonary valvular stenosis. Aortic valvular stenosis and tetralogy of Fallot have also been recorded. A patent ductus arteriosus occurs alone in approximately one third of cases; otherwise, it is frequently associated with pulmonary artery or valvular stenosis.[13,507,519] Stenosis of other vessels plays

Table 29-4 Maximal Theoretical Risks of Congenital Rubella Syndrome (CRS) after Rubella Vaccination by Vaccine Strain, United States, 1971-1988*

			RISK OF CRS	
Vaccine Strain	**Susceptible Vaccinated Subjects**	**Normal Live Births**	**Observed**	**Theoretical**
RA 27/3	226	229†	0	0-1.8
Cendehill or HPV-77	94	94	—	0-3.8
Unknown	1	1	0	—
Total	321	324	0	0-1.2

*No women entered in the register after 1980 were vaccinated with Cendehill or HPV-77 vaccine.
†Includes three twin births.

an important role in the spectrum of CRS.[465,528,529] These lesions may be related to coronary, cerebral, renal, and peripheral vascular disease seen in adults.[135,535]

A "salt and pepper" retinopathy caused by disturbed growth of the pigmentary layer of the retina is the most common ocular finding.[6,13,461,507] Cataracts, often accompanied by microphthalmia, occur in approximately one third of all cases of congenital rubella. Bilateral cataracts are found in half of affected children. Primary glaucoma is uncommon; it does not affect a cataractous eye. Cataracts and infantile glaucoma may not be present or detectable at birth, but usually become apparent during the early weeks of life. Other ocular abnormalities occur later in life (see "Developmental and Late-Onset Manifestations").

Table 29-5 Clinical Findings and Their Estimated Frequency of Occurrence in Young Symptomatic Infants With Congenitally Acquired Rubella

Clinical Findings	Frequency*	References
Adenopathies	++	492, 493
Anemia	+	493, 495
Bone		
Micrognathia	+	491
Extremities	+	491
Bony radiolucencies	++	492, 496-498, 506
Brain		
Encephalitis (active)	++	507, 508
Microcephaly	+	507, 508, 645
Brain calcification	Rare	508, 510, 511
Bulging fontanelle	+	393, 492
Cardiovascular system		
Pulmonary arterial hypoplasia	++	512
Patent ductus arteriosus	++	512
Coarctation of aortic isthmus	+	512
Interventricular septal defect	Rare	
Interauricular septal defect	Rare	
Others	Rare	13
Chromosomal abnormalities	?	467
Dermal erythropoiesis (blueberry muffin syndrome)	+	513, 514
Dermatoglyphic abnormalities	+	515, 516
Ear		
Hearing defects (severe)	+++	492
Peripheral	+++	492
Central	+	
Eye	++	492, 517-519
Retinopathy	+++	13
Cataracts	++	393, 491-493, 507, 517, 520, 645
Cloudy cornea	Rare	492
Glaucoma	Rare	493, 507, 517
Microphthalmos	+	492, 517
Genitourinary tract	+	492
Undescended testicle	+	492, 524
Polycystic kidney†	Rare	522
Bilobed kidney with reduplicated ureter†	Rare	522
Hypospadias	Rare	14, 523
Unilateral agenesis†	Rare	522
Renal artery stenosis with hypertension†	Rare	523
Hydroureter and hydronephrosis†	Rare	508
Growth restriction		
Intrauterine	+++	393, 491-493, 507, 520, 645
Extrauterine	+++	524, 645
Hepatitis	Rare	491, 492, 507, 525
Hepatosplenomegaly	+++	393, 491, 493, 507, 520, 645
Immunologic dyscrasias	Rare	526
Interstitial pneumonitis (acute, subacute, chronic)	++	125, 492, 507, 527
Jaundice (regurgitative)	+	507, 520
Leukopenia	+	495
Myocardial necrosis	Rare	507, 508, 518, 525
Neurologic deficit	++	
Prematurity	+	393, 491-493, 507, 520, 525, 645
Thrombocytopenia with or without purpura	++	491-493, 507, 520, 645
Others†	Rare	
Esophageal atresia		645
Tracheoesophageal fistula		520
Anencephaly		520
Encephalocele		491, 520
Meningomyelocele		509
Cleft palate		520, 645
Inguinal hernia		
Asplenia		
Nephritis (vascular)		508
Clubfoot		520
High palate		524
Talipes equinovarus		524
Depressed sternum		524
Pes cavus		524
Clinodactyly		524
Brachydactyly		524
Syndactyly		524
Elfin facies		524

*Frequency of occurrence is classified as follows: +, <20%; ++, 20%-50%; +++, 50%-75%.

†Rarely associated with rubella syndrome (whether caused by infection is unknown). Incidence is seemingly increased in infants with congenital rubella.

Children with CRS exhibit numerous CNS abnormalities that follow widespread insult to the brain. Microcephaly can be a feature of this syndrome. Mental retardation and motor retardation are common and are directly related to the acute meningoencephalitis in 10% to 20% of affected children at birth.[9] Behavioral and psychiatric disorders have been confirmed in many patients.[13,461] Of particular interest is autism, which has been reported to occur with a frequency of approximately 6%.[461] Chronic encephalitis has been reported in young children.[6] Late-onset progressive panencephalitis may occur in the second decade of life.[407,494,495] This condition is discussed later with other developmental manifestations.

The incidence of deafness has been underestimated because many cases had been missed in infancy and early childhood. Follow-up studies showed that deafness was the most common manifestation of congenital rubella, however, occurring in 80% or more of children infected.[#c] In contrast to other serious defects, hearing impairment often is the only significant consequence of congenital rubella. Rubella-related defects of organogenesis (i.e., cataracts and some heart lesions) are uncommon after infection beyond 8 weeks of gestation. The organ of Corti is vulnerable to the effects of the virus up to the first 16 weeks of gestation, however, and perhaps up to the first 18 to 20 weeks of gestation. Deafness, ranging from mild to profound and from unilateral or bilateral, is usually peripheral (sensorineural) and is more commonly bilateral. Central auditory impairment and language delay may lead to a misdiagnosis of mental retardation.[13,536-540]

Developmental and Late-Onset Manifestations

Developmental and late-onset manifestations have been reviewed by Sever and Shaver and their colleagues.[135,136] These manifestations include endocrinopathies, deafness, ocular damage, vascular effects, and progression of CNS disease (see Table 29-3).[*d] Numerous mechanisms may be responsible for the continuing disease process that leads to these abnormalities, including persistent viral infection, viral reactivation, vascular insufficiency, and immunologic insult. The last problem may be mediated by circulating immune complexes and autoantibodies. Hyper-IgM syndrome with combined immunodeficiency and autoimmunity has been reported.[560] Abnormalities in cellular immunity and genetic factors have also been studied.

Insulin-dependent diabetes mellitus is the most frequent of all these manifestations, occurring in approximately 20% of patients by adulthood.[13,121,129,134-136,541] This reported prevalence is 100 to 200 times that observed for the general population. A Japanese study of CRS patients with 40 years of follow-up reported only 1.1% diabetics, however.[542] Studies of HLA type indicate that CRS patients with diabetes have the same frequencies of selected HLA haplotypes as diabetic patients without CRS (e.g., increased HLA-DR3 and decreased HLA-DR2). The presence of pancreatic islet cell and cytotoxic surface antibodies in children with CRS does not seem to be related to any specific HLA type. It has been postulated that congenital infection increases the penetrance of a preexisting susceptibility to diabetes in these patients.[134] Rabinowe and coworkers[137] also reported an elevation in the number of Ia-positive ("activated") T cells in patients with CRS. They suggested that this T-cell abnormality may be related in these patients to the increased incidence of diabetes mellitus and other diseases associated with autoantibodies.

Thyroid dysfunction affects about 5% of patients and manifests as hyperthyroidism, hypothyroidism, and thyroiditis.[121,133,543-548] Autoimmune mechanisms seem to be responsible for these abnormalities. Clarke and colleagues[133] reported that 23% of 201 deaf teenagers with congenital infection had autoantibodies to the microsomal or globulin fraction, or both fractions, of the thyroid and that 20% of those with autoantibodies had thyroid gland dysfunction. Coexistence of diabetes and thyroid dysfunction has been reported, but the significance of the association is unknown.[121,137]

Two cases of growth hormone deficiency have been reported.[549] The defect seems to be hypothalamic in origin. Among eight growth-restricted older children with CRS, Oberfield and associates[550] found no evidence, however, of functional abnormality in the hypothalamic-pituitary axis and normal or elevated levels of somatomedin C. Growth patterns in 105 subjects in late adolescence revealed three patterns: growth consistently below the fifth percentile; growth in the normal range, but early cessation of growth, usually with a final height below the fifth percentile; and normal growth. The magnitude of the cognitive deficits was closely correlated with growth failure.[561] Ziring[14] commented on a case with Addison disease, and precocious puberty has been observed.[13,14]

The delayed diagnosis of preexisting deafness has already been mentioned. The hearing deficit can increase over time, however, and sudden onset of sensorineural deafness may occur after years of normal auditory acuity.[365,551,562] As reported by Sever and coworkers,[135] the latter has been observed in a 10-year-old child.

Many late-onset ocular defects can occur. Glaucoma has been reported in patients 3 to 22 years of age who did not previously have the congenital or infantile variety of glaucoma associated with CRS.[552] Other reported manifestations are keratic precipitates, keratoconus, corneal hydrops, and spontaneous lens absorption.[553]

The retinopathy of congenital rubella, which was previously believed to be completely benign, has more recently been associated with the delayed occurrence of visual difficulties caused by subretinal neovascularization.[554-556] Another delayed manifestation associated with vascular changes is hypertension resulting from renal artery and aortic stenosis.[535]

Mental retardation, autism, and other behavioral problems may be delayed in appearance and can be progressive.[13,461] The most serious delayed CNS manifestation is the occurrence of a progressive and fatal panencephalitis resembling subacute sclerosing panencephalitis, which manifests during the second decade of life. The first cases were reported by Weil and Townsend and their coworkers.[407,495] At the time of their review, Waxham and Wolinsky[496] found that 10 cases of progressive rubella panencephalitis had been identified among patients with CRS. Two cases have been reported after postnatally acquired rubella.[454,455] Patients with this condition present with increasing loss of mental function, seizures, and ataxia. These symptoms continue

[#c] References 6, 9, 13, 14, 111, 135, 136, 349, 350, 352-355.

[*d] References 13, 14, 121, 129, 134, 135, 137, 349, 354, 420, 496, 497, 516, 529, 535-559.

to progress until the patient is in a vegetative state and ultimately dies. Rubella virus has been recovered from the brain of one congenitally infected patient.[407] Elevated serum and CSF antibodies and increased amounts of CSF protein and gamma globulin have been detected. Virus has also been isolated from lymphocytes, and rubella-specific immune complexes have been identified.[125,557] Although rare, this syndrome focuses attention on the ability of the virus to persist and to become reactivated after years of latency.

Long-Term Prognosis

Investigators examined 50 survivors of the congenital rubella epidemic of 1939 to 1943 in Australia at age 25 years of age, and their status was reviewed again in 1991.[563] Seven subjects had died in the interval: 3 with malignancies, 3 with cardiovascular disease, and 1 with acquired immunodeficiency syndrome. Among the survivors in 1991, 5 were diabetic, all 40 examined were deaf, 23 had eye defects, and 16 had cardiovascular defects. Despite these conditions, the group was characterized by remarkably good social adjustment. Most (29) were married, and they had 51 children—only 1 with a congenital defect (deafness presumed to be hereditary from his deaf father, who did not have congenital rubella). Most survivors were of normal stature, although 6 of the 40 were less than the third percentile for height.

The group of survivors from Australia is quite different from the approximately 300 survivors followed in New York since the rubella epidemic of 1963 to 1965.[39] In their late 20s, approximately one third of these survivors were leading relatively normal lives in the community, one third were living with their parents with "noncompetitive" employment, and one third were residing in facilities with 24-hour care. Neither the Australian nor the New York group is a representative sample of all survivors of maternal rubella infection, but these groups do offer insight on long-term prognosis. The differences in outcome between the Australian group (survivors of Gregg's original patients) and the New York group probably reflect the different methods by which the groups were collected and the significant differences in the medical technology of the 1940s compared with the 1960s.

Laboratory Diagnosis

Timely, accurate diagnosis of acute primary rubella infection in a pregnant woman and congenital rubella infection in an infant is imperative if appropriate management is to be undertaken (see "Management Issues"). The diagnosis must be confirmed serologically or virologically because clinical diagnosis of postnatal and congenital rubella is unreliable. In any suspected exposure of a pregnant woman, every effort should be made to confirm rubella infection so that accurate counseling can be offered about the risks to the fetus. Laboratory proof of congenital infection facilitates proper treatment, follow-up, and long-term management.

MATERNAL INFECTION

All women of childbearing age should have been vaccinated against rubella as children or in gynecologic care before conception. In addition, they should be screened for rubella IgG antibodies at the first obstetric visit and tested further for IgM antibodies (see later in this section) if they give a history of rash or exposure to rash illness earlier in pregnancy. Most experts accept an enzyme-linked immunosorbent assay titer of 10 IU or greater as an indication of immunity; however, some experts accept greater than 15 IU.[564,565] Women who are IgG antibody negative at the first visit should be retested 2 to 3 weeks later if the fetus is less than 16 weeks of gestational age, to exclude intercurrent infection. All seronegative women should be vaccinated postpartum.[566]

Because of inapparent infection, the variable clinical manifestations of rubella, and the mimicking of rubella by other viral exanthems, laboratory diagnosis is essential in managing potential rubella infection during pregnancy (see "Natural History" and "Clinical Manifestations").[161,211,238,239,567] Although virus can be cultured from the nose and throat, isolation techniques are slow and labor-intensive. RT-PCR offers another reliable tool for confirming the diagnosis during acute rubella, but laboratory confirmation of acquired infection in nonpregnant persons is usually limited to serologic testing (see "Virus").

Acute primary infection can usually be documented by showing a significant increase in rubella IgG antibody level between acute and convalescent sera or the presence of rubella-specific IgM antibody. Appropriate timing of specimen collection with regard to rash onset (or exposure in the case of subclinical infection) is crucial for accurate interpretation of results. Diagnosis is greatly facilitated if the immune status is known before disease onset or exposure.[271] Women with laboratory evidence of immunity are not considered to be at risk. From a practical point of view, women with a history of vaccination on or after the first birthday should also be considered immune.[268,269] Because seroconversion is not 100% (see "Prevention of Congenital Rubella"), serologic testing may be indicated on an individual basis in vaccinated women who have a known exposure or a rash and illness consistent with rubella to rule out acute primary infection or reinfection.

Traditionally, a fourfold or greater increase in antibody titer (i.e., HI, complement fixation, or latex agglutination tests) has been considered a significant increase in antibody. With the advent of enzyme immunoassay, the diagnosis may be based on significant changes in optical density expressed as an index rather than a titer. The acute phase specimen should be obtained as soon as possible after onset of the rash, ideally within 7 days. If a positive titer is obtained for a specimen taken on the day of rash onset or 1 to 2 days later, the risk of acute infection is low but cannot be excluded. The convalescent-phase serum sample should be taken 10 to 14 days later. If the first serum sample is obtained more than 7 days after rash onset, some assays (e.g., HI) may be unable to detect a significant antibody increase because titers may have already peaked. In this situation, measurement of antibodies that appear later in the course of infection may be useful. A significant increase in complement fixation titer or a high HI, latex agglutination, or enzyme immunoassay titer and little or no antibody as measured by passive hemagglutination suggests recent infection.

When multiple serum samples are obtained in the course of the diagnostic workup, all should be tested simultaneously in the same laboratory to avoid misinterpretation of laboratory-related variations in titer. Although a single high titer is consistent with recent infection, it is not specific enough to conclude that recent infection has occurred.[271]

Detection of rubella-specific IgM is a very useful method for confirming acute recent infection. Although rubella-specific IgM testing is valuable, numerous factors can affect test results. Results must be interpreted with careful attention to the timing of the specimens. Samples obtained within the first several days after onset of rash may have low or undetectable levels of rubella-specific IgM, but a specimen obtained 7 to 14 days later invariably shows higher titers of antibody. The levels of rubella-specific IgM may decline promptly thereafter. Many of the methods previously described for detecting IgM have some limitations (see "Virus"). IgM antibody testing may involve pretreatment of the serum by various techniques to separate IgM from IgG, such as column chromatography, sucrose gradient centrifugation, or adsorption of IgG with staphylococcal protein A.

The serum IgM fraction can be assayed by HI, immunofluorescence, radioimmunoassay, or enzyme immunoassay.[†d] A false-positive result may occur if the serum was pretreated with protein A because about 5% of IgG is not removed. The radioimmunoassay and enzyme immunoassay techniques can detect specific IgM antibodies directly in unfractionated sera, but false-positive results may be produced by the presence of rheumatoid factor.[161,219,221] A solid-phase, immunosorbent (i.e., capture) technique seems to be unaffected by rheumatoid factor.[104,222,237,248]

Although high or moderate titers provide very good evidence of recent infection, low rubella-specific IgM titers detected by sensitive assays must be interpreted cautiously. Low titers have been shown to persist for many months in a few patients after natural infection and can be detected in some immune patients with subclinical reinfection.[45,55,57,59,366-371] Diagnosis of subclinical infection is straightforward if the woman is known to be susceptible, the exposure is recognized, and a serum sample is obtained approximately 28 days after exposure.

The diagnosis of subclinical infection is more difficult if the immune status of the woman is unknown. It can be facilitated, however, if the acute-phase serum specimen is obtained as soon as possible after a recognized exposure that did not occur more than 5 weeks earlier.[271] The convalescent serum sample, if necessary, should be obtained approximately 3 weeks later. If the first specimen lacks detectable antibody, continued close clinical observance and serologic follow-up are necessary. If the first specimen has detectable antibody and was obtained within 7 to 10 days of exposure, there is no risk of infection, and further evaluation is unnecessary. A positive titer in a specimen obtained after this period indicates a need for further serologic investigation. If test results of paired serum specimens are inconclusive, rubella-specific IgM testing may be helpful, but a negative test result may be difficult to interpret. Dried blood spots have been useful in the detection of IgM antibodies because they show concordance with serum determinations.[568,569]

More significant diagnostic difficulties arise when women of unknown immune status are exposed at an unknown time, were exposed more than 5 weeks earlier, or had rash onset more than 3 weeks earlier.[271] In these situations, expert consultation may be necessary if positive titers are obtained. Where available, avidity testing of rubella IgG may be used to help clarify the timing of infection. Recent rubella infection is characterized by antibody of low avidity. When such low-avidity antibody is found in the presence of rubella-specific IgM, it supports a diagnosis of recent rubella infection.[377-379] Avidity results, which relate to the binding of antibody to the E1 protein, can be crucial in distinguishing recent from past infection.[570,571]

Table 29-6 Percentage of Patients Testing Positive for Wild Measles and Rubella Virus Infection, by Time of Specimen Collection, Type of Specimen, and Type of Sampling Method Used—World Health Organization (WHO) Measles and Rubella Laboratory Network

Time of Collection	Serum (%)	Dried Blood Spots (%)	Oral Fluid (%)
IMMUNOGLOBULIN M			
Early (day 0-3)	50	50	40
Intermediate (day 4-14)	60-90	60-90	50-90
Late (day 15-28)	100	100	100
VIRUS DETECTION (RT-PCR)			
Early (day 0-3)	—	20	60-70
Intermediate (day 4-14)	—	—	50
Late (day 15-28)	—	—	—

RT-PCR, Reverse-transcriptase polymerase chain reaction.

Table 29-6 gives information on the prevalence of IgM antibodies and positive RT-PCR results in acquired infection according to time since onset of rash.[572] Figure 29-7 shows the pattern of test results according to the stage of infection.[25]

Conclusive information about the timing of past infection and risk to the fetus is often unavailable, even when a combination of antibody assays is used. These situations can be minimized if prenatal rubella testing is done routinely. Laboratories performing prenatal screening should store these specimens until delivery in case retesting is necessary.[268,567]

CONGENITAL INFECTION

A presumptive diagnosis of congenital rubella infection should be considered for any infant born to a mother who had documented or suspected rubella infection at any time during pregnancy (see "Transmission In Utero").[107,113] The diagnosis should also be considered in any infant with evidence of stigmata consistent with congenital infection, regardless of maternal history (see "Clinical Manifestations"). Although such findings are sensitive for clinically apparent disease, they are nonspecific because many of them can be associated with other intrauterine infections, such as cytomegalovirus infection, syphilis, and toxoplasmosis. Many affected infants are asymptomatic. As with maternal rubella, congenital infection must be confirmed by laboratory tests.

In contrast to maternal rubella, attempting to isolate rubella virus in tissue culture is a valuable tool for diagnosing congenital rubella in newborns. The virus is most

†d References 161, 218-222, 225, 227, 236-240, 242-250.

readily isolated from the posterior pharynx and less consistently from the conjunctivae, CSF, or urine.[‡d] Virus isolation should be attempted as soon as congenital rubella is suspected clinically because viral excretion wanes during infancy (see Fig. 29-6). In older children in whom virus shedding has ceased from other sites, virus may be isolated from cataractous lens tissue.[404] In children with encephalitis, virus may persist in the CSF for several years.[379-381,526]

There are two approaches for serologic diagnosis. First, cord serum can be assayed for the presence of rubella-specific IgM antibody.[408,410,419,420] Detectable IgM antibody is a reliable indicator of congenital infection because IgM is fetally derived. False-positive results may occur, however, because of rheumatoid factor or incomplete removal of IgG (largely maternal), depending on the techniques used. A few newborns with stigmata of congenital rubella may not have detectable levels of rubella-specific IgM in sera taken during the first days of life, and some infections may go undiagnosed if infection occurred late in pregnancy because it is theoretically possible that there was inadequate time for the fetus to produce detectable levels of specific IgM antibodies by the time of delivery.[13,107,113]

A second approach is to monitor IgG levels in the infant over time to see if they persist. Maternally derived antibodies have a half-life of approximately 30 days.[408,410,420] As measured by the HI test, they usually decline at a rate of one twofold dilution per month and would be expected to disappear by 6 to 12 months of age (see Fig. 29-4). Persistence of IgG antibody at this age, especially in high titer, is presumptive evidence of intrauterine infection with rubella virus. Sera should be drawn when the infant is 3 months and then 5 to 6 months of age, with a repeat specimen at 12 months of age if necessary. All serum samples should be tested in parallel.

Important limitations of this method are the delay in diagnosis and the fact that rubella infections occurring after birth may be mistaken for congenital infections.[107,573] The latter is usually more of a problem when attempting to diagnose congenital infection retrospectively in patients beyond infancy, especially if the incidence of rubella in childhood is high or vaccine has already been administered. A third limitation is that some infants and children with CRS (particularly older children) may lack antibody as measured by HI.[354,422-424] If the diagnosis is still suspected and the HI, IgM, and culture results are negative, retesting with an assay that detects antibody to all components of the virion, such as some enzyme immunoassays, is advised.[91] Some cases with undetectable HI antibody may be from an incomplete immune response to all the structural proteins of the virus, including the hemagglutinin (see "Virus").[86,87]

Other diagnostic methods, such as measurement of cellular immunity and response to vaccine (i.e., a failure to boost antibody titer), may also be helpful in this situation, but a definitive retrospective diagnosis often cannot be made.[391,440,574,575] CSF may also be examined for the presence of rubella-specific IgM.[576] As in the case for acquired infection, determination of avidity of IgG may be useful.[377,379,577]

The availability of sensitive and specific tests for prenatal diagnosis of fetal infection after suspected or documented maternal rubella can greatly facilitate counseling. Although positive diagnoses were reported from examination of amniotic fluid, fetal blood, and chorionic villus sampling for virus isolation, rubella-specific IgM and antigens, IFN, and RNA,[103,447,578–584] the low sensitivity of these assays added little to the counseling process. Reverse-transcriptase nested PCR has been reported to offer a far more reliable and rapid tool and, where available, a valuable aid to counseling.[189,585,586] Timing of the specimen collection related to the timing of maternal infection may influence sensitivity, which reached 100% (eight of eight specimens) for amniotic fluid in one study and 83% (five of six specimens) for chorionic villus sampling in another study. Repeat testing may increase the yield of positive specimens.[189,578]

Postnatal diagnosis of congenital rubella infection is based on one or more of the following tests: isolation of virus or positive RT-PCR from fetal tissues or postnatal respiratory secretions, the demonstration of rubella-specific IgM antibodies in cord blood or neonatal serum, and persistence of rubella IgG antibodies beyond the 3 to 6 months required for elimination of maternally transmitted antibodies.[187] Figure 29-8 is an algorithm for diagnosis of maternal and congenital rubella proposed by Mendelson and colleagues.[187]

Management Issues

The major management issues associated with postnatal infection arise when a pregnant woman is at risk of acquiring infection. Confirming the diagnosis, counseling about the risks of infection of and damage to the fetus, and discussing courses of action, including the use of immunoglobulin and consideration of termination of pregnancy, require a thorough understanding of the natural history and consequences of rubella in pregnancy. In the case of congenital infection, the emphasis is on diagnosis and acute and long-term management. Isolation may be important to reduce spread of infection.

USE OF IMMUNOGLOBULIN

The role of passive immunization with immunoglobulin after exposure to rubella is controversial.[§d] Brody and coworkers[588] reported that large doses of immunoglobulin may have some efficacy, but immunoglobulin generally proved to be more useful when given prophylactically than when administered after exposure. This finding is not surprising because extensive viral replication is demonstrable 1 week or more before symptoms appear, with initial replication probably beginning even earlier. The amount of antirubella antibody in commercial immunoglobulin preparations is variable and unpredictable; specific hyperimmunoglobulin preparations are unavailable.[590,591]

In theory, the role of circulating antibodies in rubella is mainly to limit the viremia and possibly to prevent replication at the portal of entry; antibody is less valuable after infection has begun. Fetal infection occurred when immunoglobulin was administered to the mother in what seemed to be adequate amounts soon after exposure. Another disadvantage of immunoglobulin is that it may eliminate or

[‡d] References 2, 13, 165, 289-294, 296, 333, 334, 336, 338, 402, 405.

[§d] References 2, 6, 9, 314, 320, 351, 354, 587-590.

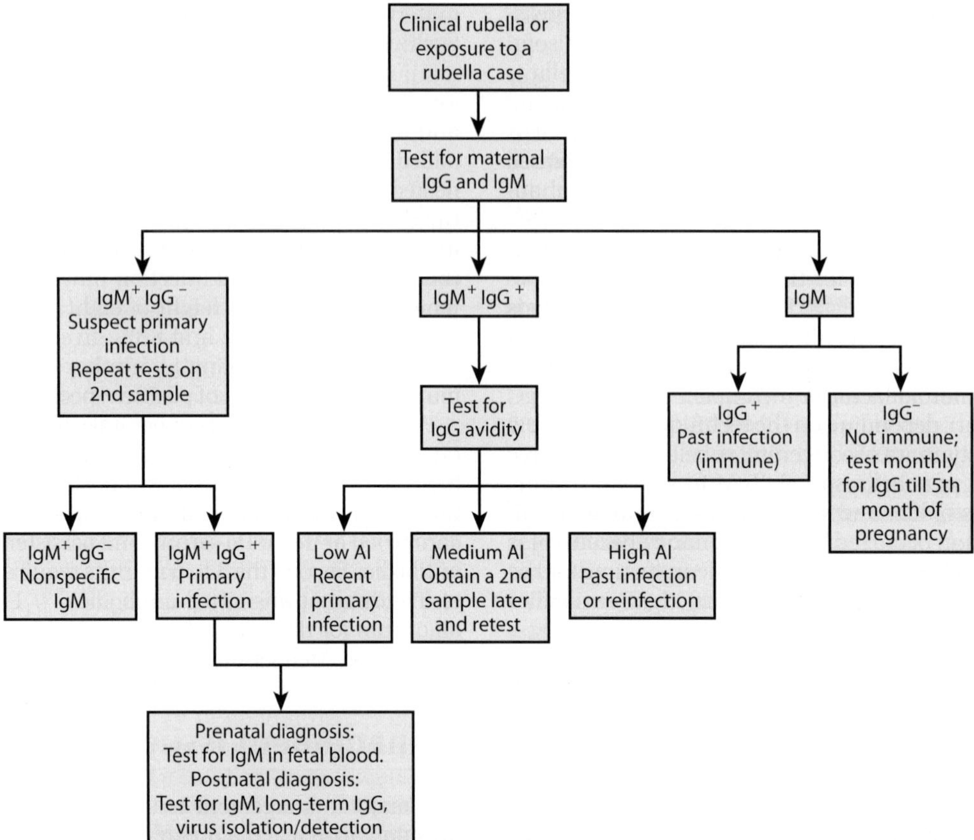

Figure 29-8 Algorithm for assessment of rubella infection in pregnancy shows a stepwise procedure, beginning with testing of maternal blood for immunoglobulin M (IgM) and IgG. If maternal blood is negative for IgM (IgM⁻), the IgG results determine if the woman is seropositive (immune) or seronegative (not immune). If not immune, the woman should be retested monthly for seroconversion until the end of the fifth month of pregnancy. If the maternal blood is positive for IgM (IgM⁺) and IgG (IgG⁺), the next step would be an IgG avidity assay on the same blood sample to estimate the time of infection. Low avidity index (AI) indicates recent infection, whereas high AI indicates past positive and IgG negative (IgG⁻); recent primary infection is suspected, and the same tests should be repeated on a second blood sample obtained 2 to 3 weeks later. If the results remain the same (IgM⁺ IgG⁻), the IgM result is considered nonspecific, indicating that the woman has not been infected; however, she is seronegative and should be followed until the end of the 5th month. If the woman has seroconverted (IgM⁺ IgG⁺), recent primary infection is confirmed, and a prenatal diagnosis should be made if the woman wishes to continue her pregnancy. Determination of IgM in cord blood is the preferred diagnostic method with the highest prognostic value. Postnatal diagnosis is based on the newborn's serology (IgM for 6-12 months and IgG for >6 months) and on virus isolation from the newborn's respiratory secretions. (Modified from Mendelson E, Aboudy Y, Smetana Z, et al: Laboratory assessment and diagnosis of congenital viral infections: rubella, cytomegalovirus [CMV], varicella-zoster virus [VZV], herpes simplex virus [HSV], parvovirus B19 and human immunodeficiency virus [HIV], *Reprod Toxicol* 21:350, 2006.)

reduce clinical findings without affecting viral replication. Clinical clues of maternal infection would be masked without adequate protection of the fetus, resulting in a false sense of security.

It is recommended that use of immunoglobulin be confined to rubella-susceptible women known to have been exposed and who do not wish to interrupt their pregnancy under any circumstances.[267,269] In this situation, large doses (20 mL in adults) should be administered. The patient should be advised that protection from fetal infection cannot be guaranteed.

TERMINATION OF PREGNANCY

A discussion of the complex issues involved in the decision about termination of pregnancy for maternal rubella is beyond the scope of this chapter. The decision must be carefully weighed by the physician and the prospective parents. The physician must have a thorough understanding of the known facts about the pathogenesis and diagnosis of congenital rubella and the risks to the fetus, depending on the timing of maternal infection. Where available, analysis of amniotic fluid, fetal blood, or chorionic villus sampling by reverse-transcriptase nested PCR may assist in antenatal diagnosis of infection.[189,585,586] Expert consultation is desirable to ensure that the most current information is used in the decision-making process.

CLINICAL MANAGEMENT

Acute rubella infection usually requires little clinical management. A patient with congenital infection may require medical, surgical, educational, and rehabilitative management, however. Many lesions are not apparent at birth because they have not yet appeared or cannot be detected. In keeping with its chronicity, congenital rubella must be managed as a dynamic rather than a static disease state. A continuing effort on the part of the physician must be made to define initially the extent of the problem and to detect evidence of progressive disease or emergence of new problems over time. Because of the broad range of problems, a multidisciplinary team approach to care is essential.

Complete pediatric, neurologic, cardiac, ophthalmologic, and audiologic examinations should be complemented by complete blood cell count, radiologic bone surveys, and often evaluation of CSF for all newborns in whom the diagnosis is suspected, whether the infant is symptomatic or not. Some defects, such as interstitial pneumonitis, can be slowly progressive and apparently cause major functional difficulties months after birth. Infected infants require scrutiny during the first 6 months of life. Serial assessment for immunologic dyscrasias is necessary during this period because the humoral defects may be masked by the presence of maternal immunoglobulin.

Hearing defects and psychomotor difficulties are the most important problems because of their high incidence. Both often occur in infants who are initially asymptomatic. The new techniques for detection of hearing impairment in newborns and the state-mandated universal newborn hearing screening testing requirements have been initiated too recently to determine their utility in detection of unsuspected congenital rubella. Delay in diagnosis and therapeutic intervention has a profound impact on language development and skills acquisition and can magnify psychosocial adjustment problems within the entire family constellation.

Because many children with congenital rubella have multiple handicaps, early interdisciplinary treatment is warranted. Appropriate hearing aids; visual aids, including contact lenses; speech, language, occupational, and physical therapy; and special educational programs are frequently required for such children. Serial psychological and perceptual testing may be very helpful for ongoing management, particularly when performed by individuals experienced in assessing children with multiple handicaps who are sensorially deprived. In many cases, repeated testing is important because the problems seem to be progressive and require continuing assessment of the therapeutic approach. In the United States, most infants suspected to have congenital rubella are eligible for early intervention and habilitation services authorized by the Individuals with Disabilities Education Act. These programs offer services to affected children beginning in infancy, a critical time for children who may be hearing impaired. The impact of universal newborn hearing screening programs as another tool for early detection of congenital rubella and of cochlear implants for children with severe rubella deafness remains to be determined.

CHEMOTHERAPY

Because postnatal rubella is usually mild, there has been little need to pursue chemotherapeutic regimens, and the literature on this subject is sparse. IFN has been used to treat chronic arthritis, and inosine pranobex (Isoprinosine) has been administered to a patient with postnatally acquired progressive rubella panencephalitis.[455,557,592] Chance temporal association between IFN administration and reported improvement in joint symptoms cannot be differentiated from potential therapeutic benefits of the IFN. In the trial of inosine pranobex, no improvement was observed.

Reports regarding treatment of infants with congenital rubella are limited. The course of congenital infection does not seem to be altered by any available chemotherapeutic agent. Because amantadine reduces the replication of rubella virus in vitro, it has theoretical possibilities as a chemotherapeutic agent.[162-164] Its use has been confined, however, to a 5-month-old infant with congenital infection.[165] Neither virus excretion nor clinical status was affected. IFN has also been administered to a few infants with CRS. Arvin and associates[593] reported that nasopharyngeal excretion in three infants (3-5 months of age) persisted throughout IFN administration, although at reduced titers compared with baseline. There was, however, no clinical effect. Larsson and coworkers[594] administered IFN to a 14-month-old child and reported regression of a cutaneous eruption resulting from vasculitis and disappearance of viremia. Viruria and other signs of viral persistence (e.g., rubella-specific IgM in the CSF) were unaffected. It is also uncertain whether improvement in the rash was from IFN administration or was coincidental. A 10-month-old infant treated by Verder and coworkers[138] may have benefited from IFN, but improvement was also seen after exchange transfusions that preceded the IFN treatment. Inosine pranobex has been administered to some patients with progressive rubella panencephalitis.[557,595] As for postnatally acquired disease, the results in this case have been disappointing.

ISOLATION

Patients with rubella are considered infectious from the 7th day before to the 5th to 7th day after the onset of the rash and should be placed in contact isolation.[596,597] Exposed rubella-susceptible patients confined to the hospital should be placed in contact isolation from the 7th through 21st day after exposure and tested appropriately to rule out asymptomatic infection.[598] Infectious patients with congenital rubella should also be in contact isolation.[596] Isolation precautions should be instituted as soon as rubella or congenital rubella is suspected. Only persons known to be immune (i.e., persons with serologic evidence of immunity or documentation of vaccination on or after the first birthday) should care for infectious or potentially infectious patients.[267,269]

Children with CRS should be considered infectious for the first year of life unless repeated pharyngeal and urine culture results are negative.[269,596] Culture results are unlikely to become negative until the child is 3 to 6 months of age (see Fig. 29-4). From a practical point of view, children older than 1 year are unlikely to be a significant source of infection. In the home situation, susceptible pregnant visitors should be informed of the potential risk of exposure.

Prevention of Congenital Rubella

RUBELLA VACCINE AND IMMUNIZATION STRATEGIES

Active immunization is the only practical means to prevent congenital rubella because passive immunization provides unreliable, transient protection (see "Management Issues"). There has been considerable debate, however, about the best way to use the vaccine.[3,5-7,32,37,599] Because rubella vaccination is not aimed primarily at protecting the individual, but rather the unborn fetus, (although as mentioned above, acquired rubella may have serious sequelae) two basic strategies have been proposed: universal childhood immunization and selective vaccination of susceptible girls and women of childbearing age. The former approach is designed to interrupt transmission of virus by vaccinating the reservoir of infection; reduce the overall risk of infection in the general population; and provide indirect protection of unvaccinated, postpubertal women. The latter approach directly protects women at risk of being infected when pregnant, limits overall vaccine use, and allows virus to circulate and boost vaccine-induced immunity in the population. Experience gained during the past 30 years indicates that integration of both approaches is necessary to achieve maximal control in the shortest possible time.[5,32,35,37]

At the time of licensure in 1969, available information indicated that the live-attenuated rubella vaccines were safe, noncommunicable, and highly effective.[3,4,27-29] Although information on the duration of vaccine-induced immunity was limited, public health policy makers in the United States believed that vaccination of all children would provide protection into the childbearing years. The duration and quality of the immunity would have to be monitored continually. Because vaccine virus could cross the placenta and infect the fetus, cautious recommendations for vaccination of susceptible women of childbearing age were also proposed.[352,600,601] Vaccine was to be administered in this population only after susceptibility had been documented by serologic testing. Vaccinated women were also advised to avoid conception for 2 months after vaccination. After Fleet and colleagues[602] isolated virus from the fetus of a woman who had conceived 7 weeks before vaccination, this time interval was increased to 3 months as an extra precaution.[267,269]

In some areas of the world, mass vaccination was considered undesirable because of concerns about the duration of vaccine-induced immunity.[5-7,34,111] Instead, vaccine was targeted for all girls 11 to 14 years of age and postpubertal women known to be seronegative. As with the U.S. program, pregnancy was to be avoided for 3 months after immunization. The goal was to immunize at least 90% of the women immediately at risk and simultaneously to provide a higher level of immunity throughout the group of women of childbearing age. It was recognized that this approach would take many years to have a significant effect on the incidence of congenital infection.

The U.S. strategy prevented epidemic disease, but initially had little effect on the occurrence of infection in young adults, particularly women of childbearing age (see "Epidemiology").[ld] There was no evidence that infection was occurring in individuals who had been vaccinated years earlier (see "Update on Vaccine Characteristics"). Childhood vaccination decreased the overall risk of infection, but virus could still circulate in the community, especially wherever unvaccinated adolescents and adults congregated.[272-280,283-288] Although CRS could eventually be eliminated as vaccinated cohorts of children entered the childbearing years, this process would take many years, and potentially preventable cases of congenital infection would continue to occur.[280] Specific recommendations were made to increase vaccination levels in older individuals, particularly women of childbearing age (see "Vaccination Recommendations").[267,269]

Selective vaccination programs have not been successful because of the inability to immunize a sufficient proportion of the female population.[7,35,36] With this immunization approach, large-scale epidemics continue to occur, and the incidence of congenital rubella has not declined significantly since the introduction of vaccines. Because of these problems, in 1988, the United Kingdom implemented a program of MMR vaccination for all children in the second year of life and initial catch-up in 2- to 4-year-olds. In 1994, a mass measles-rubella vaccine program for 5- to 16-year-old recipients was conducted to avert a measles epidemic. A preschool MMR booster was added in 1996.[35,37,603]

As highlighted earlier, the U.S. and U.K. programs adopted a combined approach to rubella control and elimination by the universal vaccination of children and selective vaccination of women of childbearing age. In 1997, as part of a regional initiative for rubella control and CRS prevention, PAHO developed a rubella and CRS control strategy that included introduction of a rubella-containing vaccine into routine childhood immunization programs, ensuring rubella vaccination of women of childbearing age to reduce the number of susceptible women and to develop specific vaccination strategies for accelerated rubella control and CRS prevention. Two strategies for accelerated rubella control and CRS prevention were provided: Countries wishing to prevent and control CRS promptly were advised to conduct a one-time mass campaign to vaccinate all females 5 to 39 years of age with measles and rubella–containing vaccine, and countries wishing to prevent and control rubella and CRS promptly were advised to carry out a one-time mass campaign to vaccinate males and females 5 to 39 years of age with measles and rubella–containing vaccine.[604]

In 2011, the World Health Organization (WHO) rubella vaccine recommendations were updated.[605] WHO recommends that countries that have not introduced rubella vaccination take the opportunity offered by accelerated measles control and elimination to introduce rubella vaccine. The measles vaccine strategy platform provides the opportunity to use combined vaccines and an integrated measles-rubella surveillance system. The preferred strategy for introduction of rubella vaccination is to begin with MR/MMR vaccine in a campaign targeting a wide range of ages, together with immediate introduction of MR/MMR vaccine into the routine program for infants. Figure 29-9 shows the state of rubella vaccination throughout the world.

These strategies have been highly successful in North and South America, with elimination having been achieved.[606] Australia has also successfully eliminated rubella, and modeling confirmed that immunization of young girls gave an immediate reduction of CRS, whereas immunization of infants sharply reduced viral circulation.[607] Certainly, rubella vaccination is cost-effective in high- and middle-income countries.[608] Of interest, it has been estimated that more than 1200 cases of autism were prevented between 2001 and 2010 in the United States because of rubella vaccination.[609]

Update on Vaccine Characteristics

Approximately 200 million doses of vaccine have been administered in the United States since rubella vaccines were licensed in 1969. The RA 27/3 strain of vaccine was licensed for use in Europe in 1971 and in the United States

[ld] References 5, 24, 33, 39, 270, 304.

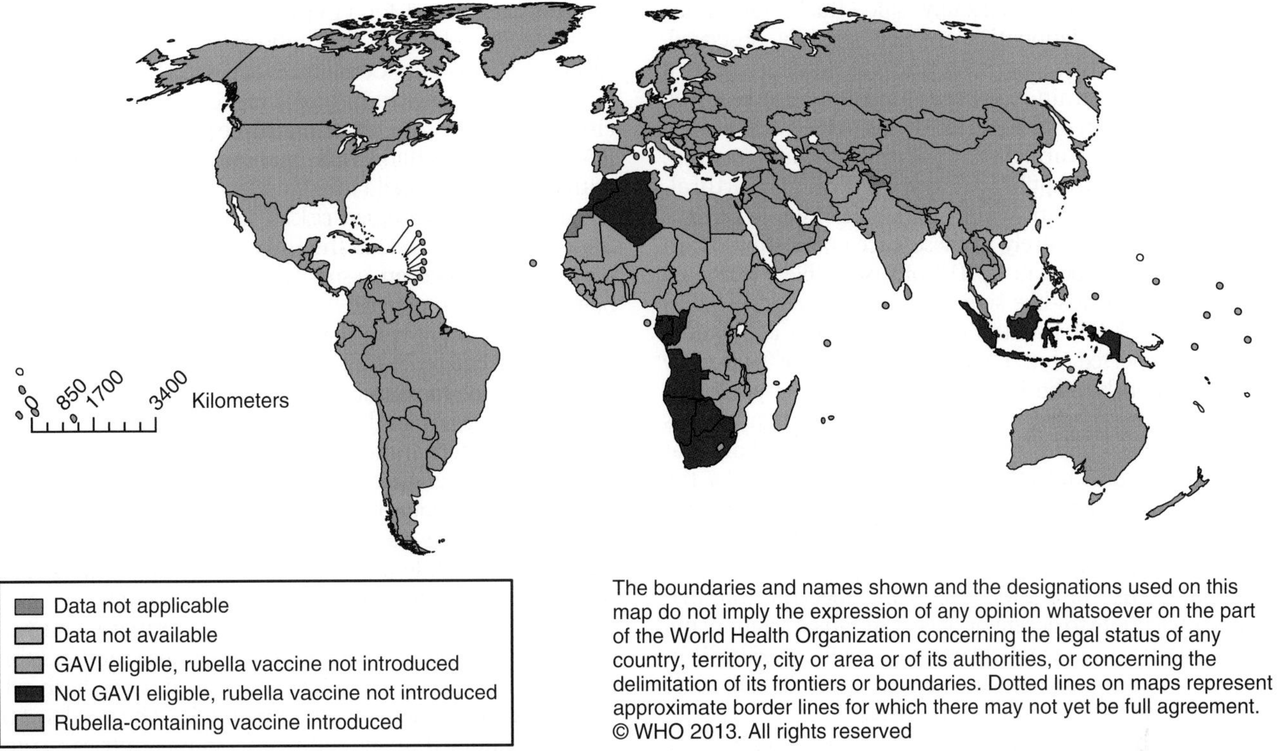

Figure 29-9 Status of rubella vaccination throughout the world in 2013. *GAVI,* Global Alliance for Vaccines and Immunizations. (From World Health Organization/Immunization Vaccines and Biologicals database, as of November 5, 2013.)

in 1979 and is now the only vaccine available. It was attenuated by serial passage in the WI-38 fetal human diploid cell strain with adaptation to growth at 30° C and is manufactured in the MRC-5 human diploid cell strain.[398,602,610] Although it has been used successfully by the intranasal and aerosol routes,[611,612] it is licensed only for subcutaneous administration, usually as part of a combination with measles and mumps vaccines.[613] Compared with the Cendehill or HPV-77 strains of vaccines, the RA 27/3 vaccine elicits an immune response that more closely resembles the response occurring after natural infection.[31,204,395,396] There are no data to indicate the need for revaccination of persons who had previously received vaccine strains other than the RA 27/3.

Appropriate administration of the RA 27/3 vaccine induces an antibody response in 95% or greater of persons 12 months or older when vaccinated. Antibody is induced to the three major rubella virus structural proteins.[86] Vaccine efficacy and challenge studies indicate that greater than 90% to 95% of vaccinated persons are protected against clinical illness or asymptomatic viremia. Although vaccine-induced titers are lower than titers after natural infection and are more likely to increase after reexposure, protection after a single dose of vaccine lasts for at least 18 years, if not for life.[¶d]

Detectable HI antibodies persist in almost all vaccinated subjects who initially seroconvert.[#d] In current practice, most children receive two doses of a rubella-containing vaccine, however, which does seem to improve seropositivity.[624,625] A survey of U.S. military recruits showed that 93% were seropositive for rubella.[626] Long-term studies of vaccinated persons who initially seroconverted and then lost detectable HI antibodies indicate that most of these individuals are also immune because they have detectable antibodies as measured by other, more sensitive assays or have a booster immune response (i.e., absence of IgM antibody and a rapid increase and decrease in IgG antibody) after revaccination.[47,53,627] A study done in Taiwan followed women for up to 22 years postvaccination and did not show an increase in seronegativity with time.[628] Measurements of memory B cells indicate higher numbers after rubella vaccination than after measles or mumps vaccination.[629]

Viremia and reinfection have been documented in some vaccinated persons and some naturally immune individuals who had very low titers of antibody.[42,44,48,54,60] It is unknown how often this phenomenon occurs or places the fetus at risk, but the incidence of both events is believed to be low.[8] There are rare case reports of congenital infection after reinfection of mothers who had been previously infected or vaccinated (see "Virus" and "Natural History").[*e]

The lack of an international standard level of antibody considered to be protective frequently complicates the interpretation of serologic data when antibodies are detected only by tests more sensitive than the HI test. Cutoff levels ranging from 5 to 15 IU have been used.[†e] Available information indicates that any appropriately measured level of detectable antibody should be considered presumptive evidence of past infection and immunity.[267,269] This applies to naturally acquired and vaccine-induced immunity.

[¶d] References 42-44, 47, 48, 50, 52-54, 58, 60, 61, 272, 317, 614-617.
[#d] References 43, 47, 50, 52, 58, 61, 331, 618-623.

[*e] References 47, 49, 56, 115, 120, 340, 345-347.
[†e] References 58, 61, 211, 239, 614, 627.

Rubella vaccine is remarkably safe. Rash, low-grade fever, and lymphadenopathy are occasionally observed. The polyneuropathies, myositis, and vasculitis associated with the HPV-77 strain of vaccine have not been reported after administration of the RA 27/3 strain.[9,615]

Vaccine-related arthralgia and arthritis remain a concern, particularly for susceptible women.[‡e] Although arthralgia has been reported in 3% of susceptible children, arthritis has been reported rarely in these vaccinated subjects. In contrast, joint pain occurs in 40% of susceptible vaccinated women, with arthritis-like signs and symptoms reported in 10% to 20%.[5,68] Persistent and recurring joint complaints have been reported, but most studies indicate that they occur infrequently. The high frequency (5%) of persistent joint symptoms reported by one group of investigators has not been confirmed.[8,68] This rate is still far less than that (30%) after natural infection, however, as reported by the same group of researchers.[68] Permanent disability and joint destruction have also been reported, but only rarely.[65,68] In the 2011 report reviewing adverse events associated with vaccines, the Institute of Medicine concluded that the evidence is inadequate to accept or reject the causal relationship between MMR vaccine and chronic arthralgia or arthritis in women.[630] Vaccination of patients with juvenile idiopathic arthritis with MMR did not worsen disease.[631]

Most published data indicate that these and other adverse events associated with rubella vaccine occur only in susceptible vaccinated persons.[5,8] There is no conclusive evidence that there is an increased risk of reactions in persons who are already immune at the time of vaccination.[8,68,127] Vaccination programs of adults have not led to significant rates of absenteeism or disruption in everyday, work-related activities.[8,283,285-288] Single cases of rash and lymphadenopathy, anterior uveitis and cataract, and encephalitis have been reported in which the vaccine virus has been isolated.[632-634]

Although some vaccinated persons intermittently shed virus in low titers from the pharynx 7 to 28 days after vaccination, there is no evidence that vaccine virus is spread to susceptible contacts.[5,494] Vaccine virus can be recovered from breast milk, however, and may be transmitted to the breastfed neonate.[65,362,616,617] The vaccine virus may elicit an immune response in some exposed neonates. There is no evidence of a significant alteration in the immune response or increased risk of reactions after vaccination at a later date.[66,68] Although a mild clinical infection from transmitted vaccine virus has been reported, infection with wild-type virus might have occurred.[635]

The fetotropic and teratogenic potential of rubella vaccine virus has greatly influenced vaccination practices in the United States and worldwide. With the increased emphasis on vaccinating susceptible, postpubertal women in the United States, especially recent immigrants, the need to have accurate information on the risks of the vaccine virus on the fetus became even more important.

From 1971 to 1988, the Centers for Disease Control and Prevention followed to term prospectively 321 pregnant women known to be susceptible to rubella by serologic testing and who were vaccinated in the period from 3 months before to 3 months after conception (see Table 29-4).[69,267] Approximately one third received vaccine during the highest risk period for viremia and fetal defects (1 week before to 4 weeks after conception).[62,69] Of the women, 94 received HPV-77 or Cendehill vaccines, 1 received a vaccine of unknown strain, and 226 received RA 27/3 vaccine. None of the 229 offspring (three mothers who received RA 27/3 vaccine had twins) had malformations consistent with congenital rubella infection.

Although the observed risk of congenital defects is zero, from the data obtained in the United Kingdom, United States, Germany, and Sweden, a small theoretical risk of 0.5% (upper bound of 95% confidence limit, 0.05%) cannot be ruled out. Limiting the analysis to the 293 infants born to susceptible mothers vaccinated 1 to 2 weeks before to 4 to 6 weeks after conception, the maximum theoretical risk is 1.3%. This risk is substantially less than the greater than 20% risk for CRS associated with maternal infection during the first 20 weeks of pregnancy and is no greater than the 2% to 3% rate of major birth defects in the absence of exposure to rubella vaccine.[69,109,572]

These favorable data are consistent with the experience reported with Cendehill and RA 27/3 vaccines in the Federal Republic of Germany and the United Kingdom.[64,67] None of 98 infants in the Federal Republic of Germany and none of 21 infants in the United Kingdom, whose mothers were known to be susceptible when vaccinated, were born with congenital anomalies consistent with CRS. The results of the studies conducted in six Latin American countries (Argentina, Brazil, Costa Rica, Ecuador, El Salvador, and Paraguay) provide the largest collection of new evidence to support existing documentation of a negligible or absent risk for CRS after administration of rubella vaccine shortly before or during pregnancy. Of the 1980 susceptible pregnant women followed, 70 (3.5%) of the infants had congenital rubella infection, but none had congenital defects associated with CRS.[630] In the Brazilian study, one rubella IgM antibody–positive infant had clinical features of CRS but had wild-type rubella virus identified by molecular genotyping of viral culture.[636-638] Similar negative data were reported from Costa Rica.[639] Although fetal infection occurs, if rubella vaccine has any teratogenic potential, it must be rare.

Vaccination Recommendations

The control of rubella and congenital rubella in the United States has been predicated on universal immunization of children, with a single dose of vaccine given after the first birthday, and selective immunization of postpubertal and susceptible postpartum women. This approach remains the basis for current recommendations of the Advisory Committee on Immunization Practices (ACIP) of the Public Health Service and the American Academy of Pediatrics (AAP).[267,269] Part of this success in control of rubella and congenital rubella has come from the recommended use of rubella vaccine as a component of the combined MMR vaccine, which in the United States is given routinely to 15-month-old children. As concerns arose about measles in adolescents and adults, attributed to the existence of a cohort of young adults representing the 2% to 10% failure rate for a single dose of measles vaccine and the theoretical possibility of waning immunity after successful immunization in early childhood, the ACIP and AAP added a second dose to the measles immunization schedule in 1989. The specific recommendation was that the second dose be given just before school entry or in the prepubertal period and that the vaccine be given as the MMR vaccine.[267,269]

‡e References 5, 8, 63, 65, 66, 68.

Rubella immunization (as MMR vaccine) should be offered to all women of childbearing age who do not have acceptable evidence of rubella immunity. Given the current data, routine screening of postpubertal women for susceptibility before rubella vaccination is no longer recommended. Women should understand the theoretical risk of fetal infection, however, and be advised not to become pregnant for at least 28 days after vaccination.[277] Known pregnancy is still considered a contraindication.

Missed opportunities should not be confused with bona fide contraindications for rubella immunization. These include the following:

1. Severe febrile illness
2. Altered immunity from congenital immunodeficiency; from acquired diseases such as leukemia, lymphoma, and generalized malignancy; and from therapy with radiation, corticosteroids, alkylating drugs, and antimetabolites
3. History of an anaphylactic reaction to neomycin (the vaccine does not contain penicillin)
4. Pregnancy, albeit because of theoretical concerns

Because vaccine virus is not transmitted through the nasopharynx, the presence of a susceptible pregnant woman in a household is not a contraindication for vaccination of other household members. Vaccine virus is present in breast milk and can infect the neonate, but breastfeeding also is not a contraindication to vaccination. Although vaccination is usually deferred for 8 to 12 weeks after receipt of immunoglobulin, receipt of anti-Rho (D) immunoglobulin (human) or blood products does not generally interfere with seroconversion and is not a contraindication to postpartum vaccination.[640-643] In this situation, 6- to 8-week postvaccination serologic testing should be performed, however, to ensure that seroconversion has occurred.[642] This is the only situation in which postvaccination testing is recommended as routine.

OUTBREAK CONTROL

Although outbreak control is an after-the-fact method of prevention, rapid, aggressive responses to outbreaks are necessary to limit the spread of infection and can serve as a catalyst to increase immunization levels. Although there is no conclusive evidence that vaccination after exposure prevents rubella, there are also no data to suggest that vaccinating an individual incubating rubella is harmful. Vaccination programs initiated in the middle of an outbreak serve to protect persons not adequately exposed in the current outbreak from future exposures.

Although laboratory confirmation of cases is important, control measures, including isolation of suspected cases or susceptible exposed persons, vaccination or exclusion of susceptible persons, and confirmation of the immune status of exposed pregnant women, should be implemented as soon as a suspected case has been identified (see "Management Issues"). Ideally, mandatory exclusion and vaccination of susceptible individuals should be practiced to ensure high rates of vaccination in the shortest possible period, particularly in the medical setting. Vaccination during an outbreak has not been associated with significant absenteeism in the workplace.[8,283,285-288] Vaccination before the occurrence of an outbreak is preferable, however, because vaccination causes far less disruption of routine work activities and schedules than rubella infection.

SURVEILLANCE

Surveillance of rubella and CRS is necessary for rubella prevention because the information can be used to evaluate the progress of the immunization program; to identify high-risk groups that would benefit from specific interventions; and to monitor the safety, efficacy, and durability of the vaccine. Surveillance can also draw attention to small numbers of cases before they develop into sizable outbreaks. Because rubella and CRS are reportable diseases, all suspected cases should be reported to local health officials.

STRATEGIES FOR ELIMINATION OF RUBELLA AND CONGENITAL RUBELLA SYNDROME

Elimination of rubella and CRS has been achieved in many countries and WHO regions have established elimination goals. As part of the strategy, integration with the measles elimination goal is critical. For all strategies for elimination, universal childhood vaccination is crucial with maintenance of high coverage. Although various elimination strategies have been used, the strategy that PAHO has recommended includes introduction of rubella-containing vaccines into routine vaccination programs for children 12 months of age and conducting a one-time mass campaign in adolescents and adults and periodic follow-up campaigns in children younger than 5 years. In the PAHO experience, it is necessary to vaccinate both males and females.[25]

Given the frequency of international travel, all countries will remain at risk of imported disease during the foreseeable future. Maintaining high levels of immunization, ongoing surveillance (recognizing that the sporadic nature of new cases likely will add to delay in diagnosis), and prompt outbreak control measures remain critical for achieving and maintaining elimination of rubella. The efforts under way in the Western Hemisphere can be a global model that eventually will make rubella and CRS matters of historic interest.[644]

References

1. Wesselhoff C: Rubella (German measles), *N Engl J Med* 236:943, 1947.
2. Krugman S: Rubella symposium, *Am J Dis Child* 110:345, 1965.
3. Krugman S: Proceedings of the International Conference on Rubella Immunization, *Am J Dis Child* 118:2, 1969.
4. Regamy RH: International Symposium on Rubella Vaccines, *Symp Ser Immunobiol Stand* 11:1, 1969.
5. Preblud SR, Serdula MK, Frank JA Jr, et al: Rubella vaccination in the United States: a ten-year review, *Epidemiol Rev* 2:171, 1980.
6. Hanshaw JB, Dudgeon JA, Marshall WC, editors: *Viral diseases of the fetus and newborn*, ed 2, Philadelphia, 1985, Saunders.
7. Krugman S: International Symposium on Prevention of Congenital Rubella Infection, *Rev Infect Dis* 7(Suppl 1):S1, 1985.
8. Preblud SR: Some current issues relating to rubella vaccine, *JAMA* 254:253, 1985.
9. Cherry JD: Rubella. In Feigin RD, Cherry JD, editors: *Textbook of pediatric infectious diseases*, ed 3, Philadelphia, 1992, Saunders.
10. Manton WG: Some accounts of rash liable to be mistaken for scarlatina, *Med Trans R Coll Physicians (Lond)* 5:149, 1815.
11. Veale H: History of epidemic Roetheln, with observations on its pathology, *Edinb Med J* 12:404, 1866.

12. Gregg NM: Congenital cataract following German measles in the mother, *Trans Ophthalmol Soc Aust* 3:35, 1941.
13. Cooper LZ: Congenital rubella in the United States. In Krugman S, Gershon AA, editors: *Infections of the fetus and the newborn infant*, New York, 1975, Alan R Liss.
14. Ziring PR: Congenital rubella: the teenage years, *Pediatr Ann* 6:762, 1977.
15. Hiro Y, Tasaka S: Die Rötheln sind eine Viruskrankheit, *Monatsschr Kinderheilkd* 76:328, 1938.
16. Habel K: Transmission of rubella to *Macaca mulatta* monkeys, *Public Health Rep* 57:1126, 1942.
17. Anderson SB: Experimental rubella in human volunteers, *J Immunol* 62:29, 1949.
18. Krugman S, Ward R, Jacobs KG, Lazar M: Studies on rubella immunization. I. Demonstration of rubella without rash, *JAMA* 151:285, 1953.
19. Weller TH, Neva FA: Propagation in tissue culture of cytopathic agents from patients with rubella-like illness, *Proc Soc Exp Biol Med* 111:215, 1962.
20. Parkman PD, Buescher EL, Artenstein MS: Recovery of rubella virus from army recruits, *Proc Soc Exp Biol Med* 111:225, 1962.
21. Parkman PD, Mundon FK, McCown JM, Buescher EL: Studies of rubella. II. Neutralization of the virus, *J Immunol* 93:608, 1964.
22. Sever JL, Huebner RJ, Castellano GA, et al: Rubella complement fixation test, *Science* 148:385, 1965.
23. Stewart GL, Parkman PD, Hopps HE, et al: Rubella-virus hemagglutination-inhibition test, *N Engl J Med* 276:554, 1967.
24. Orenstein WA, Bart KJ, Hinman AR, et al: The opportunity and obligation to eliminate measles from the United States, *JAMA* 251:1988, 1984.
25. Centers for Disease Control and Prevention: Progress toward elimination of rubella and congenital rubella syndrome—the Americas, 2003-2008, *MMWR Morb Mortal Wkly Rep* 57:1176, 2008.
26. Cutts FT, Vynnycky E: Modelling the incidence of congenital rubella syndrome in developing countries, *Int J Epidemiol* 28:1176, 1999.
27. Meyer HM Jr, Parkman PD, Panos TC: Attenuated rubella virus. II. Production of an experimental live-virus vaccine and clinical trial, *N Engl J Med* 275:575, 1966.
28. Prinzie A, Huygelen C, Gold J, et al: Experimental live attenuated rubella virus vaccine: clinical evaluation of Cendehill strain, *Am J Dis Child* 118:172, 1969.
29. Plotkin JA, Farquhar JD, Katz M: Attenuation of RA 27/3 rubella virus in WI-38 human diploid cells, *Am J Dis Child* 118:178, 1969.
30. Perkins FT: Licensed vaccines, *Rev Infect Dis* 7(Suppl 1):S73, 1985.
31. Plotkin SA, Orenstein WA, Offit PA, editors: *Vaccines*, ed 5, Philadelphia, 2008, Saunders.
32. Hinman AR, Bart KJ, Orenstein WA, Preblud SR: Rational strategy for rubella vaccination, *Lancet* 1:39, 1983.
33. Bart KJ, Orenstein WA, Preblud SR, Hinman AR: Universal immunization to interrupt rubella, *Rev Infect Dis* 7(Suppl 1):S177, 1985.
34. Dudgeon JA: Selective immunization: protection of the individual, *Rev Infect Dis* 7(Suppl 1):S185, 1985.
35. Walker D, Carter H, Jones IJ: Measles, mumps, and rubella: the need for a change in immunisation policy, *Br Med J (Clin Res Ed)* 292:1501, 1986.
36. Best JM, Welch JM, Baker DA, Banatvala JE: Maternal rubella at St. Thomas' Hospital in 1978 and 1986: support for augmenting the rubella vaccination programme, *Lancet* 2:88, 1987.
37. Badenoch J: Big bang for vaccination: eliminating measles, mumps, and rubella, *BMJ* 297:750, 1988.
38. Centers for Disease Control and Prevention: Recommendations from an ad hoc Meeting of the WHO Measles and Rubella Laboratory Network (LabNet) on use of alternative diagnostic samples for measles and rubella surveillance, *MMWR Morb Mortal Wkly Rep* 57:657, 2008.
39. Centers for Disease Control and Prevention: Increase in rubella and congenital rubella in the United States, 1988-1990, *MMWR Morb Mortal Wkly Rep* 40:93, 1991.
40. Centers for Disease Control and Prevention: Elimination of rubella and congenital rubella syndrome—United States, 1969-2004, *MMWR Morb Mortal Wkly Rep* 54:279, 2005.
41. Castillo-Solorzano C, Marsigli C, Bravo-Alcantara P, et al: Elimination of rubella and congenital rubella syndrome in the Americas, *J Infect Dis* 204(Suppl 2):S571, 2011.
42. Harcourt GC, Best JM, Banatvala JE: Rubella-specific serum and nasopharyngeal antibodies in volunteers with naturally acquired and vaccine-induced immunity after intranasal challenge, *J Infect Dis* 142:145, 1980.
43. Weibel RE, Buynak EB, McLean AA, et al: Persistence of antibody in human subjects 7 to 10 years following administration of combined live attenuated measles, mumps, and rubella virus vaccines, *Proc Soc Exp Biol Med* 165:260, 1980.
44. Balfour HH, Groth KE, Edelman CK, et al: Rubella viraemia and antibody responses after rubella vaccination and reimmunisation, *Lancet* 1:1078, 1981.
45. Cradock-Watson JE, Ridehalgh MK, Anderson MJ, Pattison JR: Outcome of asymptomatic infection with rubella virus during pregnancy, *J Hyg (Lond)* 87:147, 1981.
46. Bott LM, Eizenberg DH: Congenital rubella after successful vaccination, *Med J Aust* 1:514, 1982.
47. Herrmann KL, Halstead SB, Wiebenga NH: Rubella antibody persistence after immunization, *JAMA* 247:193, 1982.
48. O'Shea S, Best JM, Banatvala JE: Viremia, virus excretion, and antibody responses after challenge in volunteers with low levels of antibody to rubella virus, *J Infect Dis* 148:639, 1983.
49. Enders G, Calm A, Schaub J: Rubella embryopathy after previous maternal rubella vaccination, *Infection* 12:96, 1984.
50. Hillary IB, Griffith AH: Persistence of rubella antibodies 15 years after subcutaneous administration of Wistar 27/3 strain live attenuated rubella virus vaccine, *Vaccine* 2:274, 1984.
51. Morgan-Capner R, Hodgson J, Sellwood J, Tippett J: Clinically apparent rubella reinfection, *J Infect* 9:97, 1984.
52. O'Shea S, Best JM, Banatvala JE, et al: Persistence of rubella antibody 8-18 years after vaccination, *Br Med J (Clin Res Ed)* 288:1043, 1984.
53. Serdula MK, Halstead SB, Wiebenga NH, Herrmann KL: Serological response to rubella revaccination, *JAMA* 251:1974, 1984.
54. Banatvala JE, Best JM, O'Shea S, Dudgeon JA: Persistence of rubella antibodies after vaccination: detection after experimental challenge, *Rev Infect Dis* 7(Suppl 1):S86, 1985.
55. Cradock-Watson M, Ridehalgh KS, Anderson MJ, et al: Rubella reinfection and the fetus, *Lancet* 325:1039, 1985.
56. Forsgren M, Soren L: Subclinical rubella reinfection in vaccinated women with rubella-specific IgM response during pregnancy and transmission of virus to the fetus, *Scand J Infect Dis* 17:337, 1985.
57. Grangeot-Keros L, Nicolas JC, Bricout F, Pillot J: Rubella reinfection and the fetus, *N Engl J Med* 313:1547, 1985.
58. Horstmann DM, Schluederberg A, Emmons JE, et al: Persistence of vaccine-induced immune responses to rubella: comparison with natural infection, *Rev Infect Dis* 7(Suppl 1):S80, 1985.
59. Morgan-Capner P, Hodgson J, Hambling MH, et al: Detection of rubella-specific IgM in subclinical rubella reinfection in pregnancy, *Lancet* 1:244, 1985.
60. Schiff GM, Young BC, Stefanovic GM, et al: Challenge with rubella virus after loss of detectable vaccine-induced antibody, *Rev Infect Dis* 7(Suppl 1):S157, 1985.
61. Chu SY, Bernier RH, Stewart JA, et al: Rubella antibody persistence after immunization: sixteen-year follow-up in the Hawaiian Islands, *JAMA* 259:3133, 1988.
62. Bart SW, Stetler HC, Preblud SR, et al: Fetal risk associated with rubella vaccine: an update, *Rev Infect Dis* 7(Suppl 1):S95, 1985.
63. Chantler JK, Tingle AJ, Perry RE: Persistent rubella virus infection associated with chronic arthritis in children, *N Engl J Med* 313:1117, 1985.
64. Enders G: Rubella antibody titers in vaccinated and nonvaccinated women and results of vaccination during pregnancy, *Rev Infect Dis* 7(Suppl 1):S103, 1985.
65. Tingle AJ, Chantler JK, Pot KH, et al: Postpartum rubella immunization: association with development of prolonged arthritis, neurological sequelae, and chronic rubella viremia, *J Infect Dis* 152:606, 1985.
66. Preblud PR, Orenstein WA, Lopez C, Herrmann KL, Hinman AR: Postpartum rubella immunization, *J Infect Dis* 154:367, 1986.
67. Sheppard S, Smithells RW, Dickson A, Holzel H: Rubella vaccination and pregnancy: preliminary report of a national survey, *Br Med J (Clin Res Ed)* 292:727, 1986.
68. Tingle AJ: Postpartum rubella immunization (reply), *J Infect Dis* 154:368, 1986.
69. Centers for Disease Control and Prevention: Rubella vaccination during pregnancy—United States, 1971-1988, *MMWR Morb Mortal Wkly Rep* 38:290, 1989.
70. Ho-Terry L, Cohen A: Degradation of rubella virus envelope components, *Arch Virol* 65:1, 1980.
71. Oker-Blom C, Kalkkinen N, Kääriäinen L, Pettersson RF: Rubella virus contains one capsid protein and three envelope glycoproteins, E1, E2a, and E2b, *J Virol* 46:964, 1983.

72. Waxham MN, Wolinsky JS: Immunochemical identification of rubella virus hemagglutinin, *Virology* 126:194, 1983.
73. Bowden DS, Westway EG: Rubella virus: structural and non-structural proteins, *J Gen Virol* 65:933, 1984.
74. Ho-Terry L, Cohen A, Tedder RS: Immunologic characterisation of rubella virion polypeptides, *J Med Microbiol* 17:105, 1984.
75. Oker-Blom C, Ulmanen I, Kääriäinen L, Pettersson RF: Rubella virus 40S genome RNA specifies a 24S subgenomic mRNA that codes for a precursor to structural proteins, *J Virol* 49:403, 1984.
76. Dorsett PH, Miller DC, Green KY, Byrd FI: Structure and function of the rubella virus proteins, *Rev Infect Dis* 7(Suppl 1):S150, 1985.
77. Pettersson RF, Oker-Blom C, Kalkkinen N, et al: Molecular and antigenic characteristics and synthesis of rubella virus structural proteins, *Rev Infect Dis* 7(Suppl 1):S140, 1985.
78. Waxham MN, Wolinsky JS: A model of the structural organization of rubella virions, *Rev Infect Dis* 7(Suppl 1):S133, 1985.
79. Waxham MN, Wolinsky JS: Detailed immunologic analysis of the structural polypeptides of rubella virus using monoclonal antibodies, *Virology* 143:153, 1985.
80. Green KY, Dorsett PH: Rubella virus antigens: localization of epitopes involved in hemagglutination and neutralization by using monoclonal antibodies, *J Virol* 57:893, 1986.
81. Vidgren G, Takkinen K, Kalkkinen N, et al: Nucleotide sequence of the genes coding for the membrane glycoproteins E1 and E2 of rubella virus, *J Gen Virol* 68:2347, 1987.
82. Terry GM, Ho-Terry L, Londesborough P, Rees KR: Localization of the rubella E1 epitopes, *Arch Virol* 98:189, 1988.
83. Clarke DM, Loo TW, McDonald H, Gillam S: Expression of rubella virus cDNA coding for the structural proteins, *Gene* 65:23, 1988.
84. Frey TK, Marr LD: Sequence of the region coding for virion proteins C and E2 and the carboxy terminus of the nonstructural proteins of rubella virus: comparison with alphaviruses, *Gene* 62:85, 1988.
85. Takkinen K, Vidgren G, Ekstrand J, et al: Nucleotide sequence of the rubella virus capsid protein gene reveals an unusually high G/C content, *J Gen Virol* 69:603, 1988.
86. Cusi MG, Rossolini GM, Cellesi C, Valensin PE: Antibody response to wild rubella virus structural proteins following immunization with RA 27/3 live attenuated vaccine, *Arch Virol* 101:25, 1988.
87. Frey TK, Abernathy ES, Bosma TJ, et al: Molecular analysis of rubella virus epidemiology across three continents, North America, Europe and Asia, 1961-1997, *J Infect Dis* 178:642, 1998.
88. Katow S, Sugiura A: Antibody response to the individual rubella virus proteins in congenital and other rubella virus infections, *J Clin Microbiol* 21:449, 1985.
89. de Mazancourt A, Waxham MN, Nicolas JC, Wolinsky JS: Antibody response to the rubella virus structural proteins in infants with the congenital rubella syndrome, *J Med Virol* 19:111, 1986.
90. Chaye H, Chong P, Tripet B, et al: Localization of the virus neutralizing and hemagglutinin epitopes of E1 glycoprotein of rubella virus, *Virology* 189:483, 1992.
91. Hancock EJ, Pot K, Puterman ML, Tingle AJ: Lack of association between titers of HAI antibody and whole-virus ELISA values for patients with congenital rubella syndrome, *J Infect Dis* 154:1031, 1986.
92. Castellano GA, Madden DL, Hazzard GT, et al: Evaluation of commercially available diagnostic kits for rubella, *J Infect Dis* 143:578, 1981.
93. Storch GA, Myers N: Latex-agglutination test for rubella antibody: validity of positive results assessed by response to immunization and comparison with other tests, *J Infect Dis* 149:459, 1984.
94. Safford JW, Abbott GG, Diemier CM: Evaluation of a rapid passive hemagglutination assay for anti-rubella antibody: comparison to hemagglutination inhibition and a vaccine challenge study, *J Med Virol* 17:229, 1985.
95. Skendzel LP, Edson DC: Latex agglutination test for rubella antibodies: report based on data from the College of American Pathologists surveys, 1983 to 1985, *J Clin Microbiol* 24:333, 1986.
96. Vaananen P, Häivä VM, Koskela P, Meurman O: Comparison of a simple latex agglutination test with hemolysis-in-gel, hemagglutination inhibition, and radioimmunoassay for detection of rubella virus antibodies, *J Clin Microbiol* 21:973, 1985.
97. Chernesky MA, DeLong DJ, Mahony JB, Castriciano S: Differences in antibody responses with rapid agglutination tests for the detection of rubella antibodies, *J Clin Microbiol* 23:772, 1986.
98. Pruneda RC, Dover JC: A comparison of two passive agglutination procedures with enzyme-linked immunosorbent assay for rubella antibody status, *Am J Clin Pathol* 86:768, 1986.
99. Linde GA: Subclass distribution of rubella virus-specific immunoglobulin G, *J Clin Microbiol* 21:117, 1985.
100. Salonen EM, Hovi T, Meurman O, et al: Kinetics of specific IgA, IgD, IgE, IgG, and IgM antibody responses in rubella, *J Med Virol* 16:1, 1985.
101. Stokes A, Mims A, Grahame R: Subclass distribution of IgG and IgA responses to rubella virus in man, *J Med Microbiol* 21:283, 1986.
102. Thomas HIJ, Morgan-Capner P: Specific IgG subclass antibody in rubella virus infections, *Epidemiol Infect* 100:443, 1988.
103. Grangeot-Keros L, Pillot J, Daffos F, Forestier F: Prenatal and postnatal production of IgM and IgA antibodies to rubella virus studied by antibody capture immunoassay, *J Infect Dis* 158:138, 1988.
104. Nedeljkovic J, Jovanovic T, Oker-Blom C: Maturation of IgG avidity to individual rubella virus structural proteins, *J Clin Virol* 22:47, 2001.
105. Mehta NM, Thomas RM: Antenatal screening for rubella infection or immunity? *BMJ* 325:90, 2002.
106. Best JM, O'Shea S, Tipples G, et al: Interpretation of rubella serology in pregnancy—pitfalls and problems, *BMJ* 325:147, 2002.
107. Cradock-Watson JE, Ridehalgh MK, Anderson MJ, et al: Fetal infection resulting from maternal rubella after the first trimester of pregnancy, *J Hyg (Lond.)* 85:381, 1980.
108. Vejtorp M, Mansa B: Rubella IgM antibodies in sera from infants born after maternal rubella later than the twelfth week of pregnancy, *Scand J Infect Dis* 12:1, 1980.
109. Miller E, Cradock-Watson JE, Pollock TM: Consequences of confirmed maternal rubella at successive stages of pregnancy, *Lancet* 2:781, 1982.
110. Grillner L, Forsgren M, Barr B, et al: Outcome of rubella during pregnancy with special reference to the 17th-24th weeks of gestation, *Scand J Infect Dis* 15:321, 1983.
111. Peckham C: Congenital rubella in the United Kingdom before 1970: the prevaccine era, *Rev Infect Dis* 7(Suppl 1):S11, 1985.
112. Bitsch M: Rubella in pregnant Danish women 1975-1984, *Dan Med Bull* 34:46, 1987.
113. Munro ND, Sheppard S, Smithells RW, et al: Temporal relations between maternal rubella and congenital defects, *Lancet* 2:201, 1987.
114. Enders G, Nickerl-Pacher U, Miller E, et al: Outcome of confirmed periconceptional maternal rubella, *Lancet* 1:1445, 1988.
115. Partridge JW, Flewett TH, Whitehead JEM: Congenital rubella affecting an infant whose mother had rubella antibodies before conception, *Br Med J (Clin Res Ed)* 282:187, 1981.
116. Best JM, Harcourt GC, Banatvala JE, et al: Congenital rubella affecting an infant whose mother had rubella antibodies before conception, *Br Med J (Clin Res Ed)* 282:1235, 1981.
117. Levine JB, Berkowitz CD, St. Geme JW: Rubella virus reinfection during pregnancy leading to late-onset congenital rubella syndrome, *J Pediatr* 100:589, 1982.
118. Sibille G, Sarda P, Jalaguier J, et al: [Reinfection after rubella and congenital polymalformation syndrome], *J Genet Hum* 34:305, 1986.
119. Hornstein L, Levy U, Fogel A: Clinical rubella with virus transmission to the fetus in a pregnant woman considered to be immune, *N Engl J Med* 319:1415, 1988.
120. Saule H, Enders G, Zeller J, Bernsau U: Congenital rubella infection after previous immunity of the mother, *Eur J Pediatr* 147:195, 1988.
121. Floret D, Rosenberg D, Hage GN, Monnet P: Hyperthyroidism, diabetes mellitus and the congenital rubella syndrome, *Acta Paediatr Scand* 69:259, 1980.
122. Hansen HE, Larsen SO, Leerhoy J: Lack of correlation between the incidence of rubella antibody and the distribution of HLA antigens in a Danish population, *Tissue Antigens* 15:325, 1980.
123. Kato S, Kimura M, Takakura I, et al: HLA-linked genetic control in natural rubella infection, *Tissue Antigens* 15:86, 1980.
124. Tardieu M, Grospierre B, Durandy A, Gariscelli C: Circulating immune complexes containing rubella antigens in late-onset rubella syndrome, *J Pediatr* 97:370, 1980.
125. Coyle PK, Wolinsky JS: Characterization of immune complexes in progressive rubella panencephalitis, *Ann Neurol* 9:557, 1981.
126. Ishii K, Nakazono N, Sawada H, et al: Host factors and susceptibility to rubella virus infection: the association of HLA antigens, *J Med Virol* 7:287, 1981.
127. Coyle PK, Wolinsky JS, Buimovici-Klein E, et al: Rubella-specific immune complexes after congenital infection and vaccination, *Infect Immun* 36:498, 1982.
128. Kato S, Muranaka S, Takakura I, et al: HLA-DR antigens and the rubella-specific immune response in man, *Tissue Antigens* 19:140, 1982.

129. Rubinstein P, Walker ME, Fedun B, et al: The HLA system in congenital rubella patients with and without diabetes, *Diabetes* 31:1088, 1982.
130. Boner A, Wilmott RW, Dinwiddie R, et al: Desquamative interstitial pneumonia and antigen-antibody complexes in two infants with congenital rubella, *Pediatrics* 72:835, 1983.
131. Ilonen J, Anttila AC, Lehtinen M, et al: HLA antigens in rubella seronegative young adults, *Tissue Antigens* 22:379, 1983.
132. Ziola B, Lund G, Meurman O, Salmi A: Circulating immune complexes in patients with acute measles and rubella virus infections, *Infect Immun* 41:578, 1983.
133. Clarke WL, Shaver KA, Bright GM, et al: Autoimmunity in congenital rubella syndrome, *J Pediatr* 104:370, 1984.
134. Ginsberg-Fellner F, Witt ME, Fedun B, et al: Diabetes mellitus and autoimmunity in patients with congenital rubella syndrome, *Rev Infect Dis* 7(Suppl 1):S170, 1985.
135. Sever JL, South MA, Shaver KA: Delayed manifestations of congenital rubella, *Rev Infect Dis* 7(Suppl 1):S164, 1985.
136. Shaver KA, Boughman JA, Nance WE: Congenital rubella syndrome and diabetes: a review of epidemiologic, genetic, and immunologic factors, *Am Ann Deaf* 130:526, 1985.
137. Rabinowe SL, George KL, Loughlin R, et al: Congenital rubella: monoclonal antibody-defined T cell abnormalities in young adults, *Am J Med* 81:779, 1986.
138. Verder H, Dickmeiss E, Haahr S, et al: Late-onset rubella syndrome: coexistence of immune complex disease and defective cytotoxic effector cell function, *Clin Exp Immunol* 63:367, 1986.
139. Bardeletti G, Kessler N, Aymard-Henry M: Morphology, biochemical analysis and neuraminidase activity of rubella virus, *Arch Virol* 49:175, 1975.
140. Best JM, Banatvala JE, Almeida JD, Waterson AP: Morphological characteristics of rubella virus, *Lancet* 2:237, 1967.
141. Murphy FA, Halonen PE, Harrison AK: Electron microscopy of the development of rubella virus in BHK-21 cells, *J Virol* 2:1223, 1968.
142. Oshiro LS, Schmidt NJ, Lennette EH: Electron microscopic studies of rubella virus, *J Gen Virol* 5:205, 1969.
143. Bardeletti G, Tektoff J, Gautheron D: Rubella virus maturation and production in two host cell systems, *Intervirology* 11:97, 1979.
144. Holmes IH, Wark MC, Warburton MF: Is rubella an arbovirus? II. Ultrastructural morphology and development, *Virology* 37:15, 1969.
145. Maes R, Vaheri A, Sedwick D, Plotkin S: Synthesis of virus and macromolecules by rubella-infected cells, *Nature* 210:384, 1966.
146. Nakhasi HL, Zheng DX, Hewlett IK, Liu TY: Rubella virus replication: effect of interferons and actinomycin D., *Virus Res.* 10:1, 1988.
147. Sato M, Yamada T, Yamamoto K, Yamamoto N: Evidence for hybrid formation between rubella virus and a latent virus of BHK21/WI-2 cells, *Virology* 69:691, 1976.
148. Sato M, Tanaka H, Yamada T, Yamamoto N: Persistent infection of BHK21/WI-2 cells with rubella virus and characterization of rubella variants, *Arch Virol* 54:333, 1977.
149. Sato M, Urade M, Maeda N, et al: Isolation and characterization of a new rubella variant with DNA polymerase activity, *Arch Virol* 56:89, 1978.
150. Sato M, Maeda N, Urade M, et al: Persistent infection of primary human cell cultures with rubella variant carrying DNA polymerase activity, *Arch Virol* 56:181, 1978.
151. Sato M, Maeda N, Shirasuna K, et al: Presence of DNA in rubella variant with DNA polymerase activity, *Arch Virol* 61:251, 1979.
152. Mifune K, Matsuo S: Some properties of temperature-sensitive mutant of rubella virus defective in the induction of interference to Newcastle disease virus, *Virology* 63:278, 1975.
153. Norval M: Mechanism of persistence of rubella virus in LLC-MK2 cells, *J Gen Virol* 43:289, 1979.
154. Bardeletti G, Gautheron DC: Phospholipid and cholesterol composition of rubella virus and its host cell BHK21 grown in suspension cultures, *Arch Virol* 52:19, 1978.
155. Voiland A, Bardeletti G: Fatty acid composition of rubella virus and BHK21/13S infected cells, *Arch Virol* 64:319, 1980.
156. Parkman PD, Buescher EL, Artenstein MS, et al: Studies of rubella. I. Properties of the virus, *J Immunol* 93:595, 1964.
157. McCarthy K, Taylor-Robinson CH: Rubella, *Br Med Bull* 23:185, 1967.
158. Wallis C, Melnick JL, Rapp F: Different effects of MgCl2 and MgSO4 on the thermostability of viruses, *Virology* 26:694, 1965.
159. Chagnon A, Laflamme P: Effect of acidity on rubella virus, *Can J Microbiol* 10:501, 1964.
160. Fabiyi A, Sever JL, Ratner N, Caplan B: Rubella virus: growth characteristics and stability of infectious virus and complement-fixing antigen, *Proc Soc Exp Biol Med* 122:392, 1966.
161. Herrmann KL: Rubella virus. In Lennette EH, Schmidt NJ, editors: *Diagnostic procedures for viral, rickettsial, and chlamydial infections*, Washington, DC, 1979, American Public Health Association.
162. Cochran KW, Maassab HF: Inhibition of rubella virus by 1-adamantanamine hydrochloride, *Fed Proc* 23:387, 1964.
163. Plotkin SA: Inhibition of rubella virus by amantadine, *Arch Gesamte Virusforsch* 16:438, 1965.
164. Oxford JS, Schild GC: In vitro inhibition of rubella virus by 1-adamantanamine hydrochloride, *Arch Gesamte Virusforsch* 17:313, 1965.
165. Plotkin SA, Klaus RM, Whitely JA: Hypogammaglobulinemia in an infant with congenital rubella syndrome: failure of 1-adamantanamine to stop virus excretion, *J Pediatr* 69:1085, 1966.
166. Vaheri A, Hovi T: Structural proteins and subunits of rubella virus, *J Virol* 9:10, 1972.
167. Vesikari T: Immune response in rubella infection, *Scand J Infect Dis* 4:1, 1972.
168. Liebhaber H, Gross PA: The structural proteins of rubella virus, *Virology* 47:684, 1972.
169. Chantler JK: Rubella virus: intracellular polypeptide synthesis, *Virology* 98:275, 1979.
170. Ho-Terry L, Londesborough P, Cohen A: Analysis of rubella virus complement-fixing antigens by polyacrylamide gel electrophoresis, *Arch Virol* 87:219, 1986.
171. Claus A, Hofmann J, Uberla K, Liebert UG: Rubella virus pseudotypes and a cell-cell fusion assay as tools for functional analysis of the rubella virus E2 and E1 envelope glycoproteins, *J Gen Virol* 87:3029, 2006.
172. Zhou Y, Ushijima H, Frey TK: Genomic analysis of diverse rubella virus genotypes, *J Gen Virol* 88:932, 2007.
173. Rubella virus nomenclature update, 2013, *Wkly Epidemiol Rec* 88:337, 2013.
174. Katow S: Molecular epidemiology of rubella virus in Asia: utility for reduction in the burden of diseases due to congenital rubella syndrome, *Pediatr Int* 46:207, 2004.
175. Global distribution of measles and rubella genotypes—update, *Wkly Epidemiol Rec* 81:474, 2006.
176. Fenner F: The classification and nomenclature of viruses, *Intervirology* 6:1, 1975.
177. Melnick JL: Taxonomy of viruses, *Prog Med Virol* 22:211, 1976.
178. Best JM, Banatvala JE: Studies on rubella virus strain variation by kinetic hemagglutination-inhibition tests, *J Gen Virol* 9:215, 1970.
179. Fogel A, Plotkin SA: Markers of rubella virus strains in RK13 culture, *J Virol* 3:157, 1969.
180. Kono R: Antigenic structures of American and Japanese rubella virus strains and experimental vertical transmission of rubella virus in rabbits, *Symp Ser Immunobiol Stand* 11:195, 1969.
181. Kono R, Hayakawa Y, Hibi M, Ishii K: Experimental vertical transmission of rubella virus in rabbits, *Lancet* 1:343, 1969.
182. Banatvala JE, Best JM: Cross-serological testing of rubella virus strains, *Lancet* 1:695, 1969.
183. Potter JE, Banatvala JE, Best JM: Interferon studies with Japanese and U.S. rubella virus, *Br Med J* 1:197, 1973.
184. Banatvala JE, Potter JE, Webster MJ: Foetal interferon responses induced by rubella virus, *Ciba Found New Ser* 10:77, 1973.
185. Ueda K, Nishida Y, Oshima K, et al: An explanation for the high incidence of congenital rubella syndrome in Ryukyu, *Am J Epidemiol* 107:344, 1978.
186. Kono R, Hirayama M, Sugishita C, Miyamura K: Epidemiology of rubella and congenital rubella infection in Japan, *Rev Infect Dis* 7(Suppl 1):S56, 1985.
187. Ueda K, Tokugawa K, Nishida Y, Kimura M: Incidence of congenital rubella syndrome in Japan (1965-1985): a nationwide survey of the number of deaf children with history of maternal rubella attending special schools for the deaf in Japan, *Am J Epidemiol* 124:807, 1986.
188. Mendelson E, Aboudy Y, Smetana Z, et al: Laboratory assessment and diagnosis of congenital viral infections: rubella, cytomegalovirus (CMV), varicella-zoster virus (VZV), herpes simplex virus (HSV), parvovirus B19 and human immunodeficiency virus (HIV), *Reprod Toxicol* 21:350, 2006.
189. Frey TK, Marr LD, Hemphill ML, Dominguez G: Molecular cloning and sequencing of the region of the rubella virus genome coding for glycoprotein E1, *Virology* 154:228, 1986.

190. Revello MG, Baldanti F, Sarasini A, et al: Prenatal diagnosis of rubella virus infection by direct detection and semiquantitation of viral RNA in clinical samples by reverse transcription-PCR, *J Clin Microbiol* 35:708, 1997.
191. Halonen PE, Ryan JM, Stewart JA: Rubella hemagglutinin prepared with alkaline extraction of virus grown in suspension culture of BHK-21 cells, *Proc Soc Exp Biol Med* 125:162, 1967.
192. Schmidt NJ, Dennis J, Lennette EH: Rubella virus hemagglutination with a wide variety of erythrocyte species, *Appl Microbiol* 22:469, 1971.
193. Furukawa T, Plotkin SA, Sedwick WD, et al: Studies on hemagglutination by rubella virus, *Proc Soc Exp Biol Med* 126:745, 1967.
194. Haukenes G: Simplified rubella haemagglutination inhibition test not requiring removal of nonspecific inhibitors, *Lancet* 2:196, 1979.
195. Liebhaber H: Measurement of rubella antibody by hemagglutination inhibition. I. Variables affecting rubella hemagglutination, *J Immunol* 104:818, 1970.
196. Liebhaber H: Measurement of rubella antibody by hemagglutination inhibition. II. Characteristics of an improved test employing a new method for the removal of non-immunoglobulin HA inhibitors from serum, *J Immunol* 104:826, 1970.
197. Schmidt NJ, Lennette EH: Rubella complement-fixing antigens derived from the fluid and cellular phases of infected BHK-21 cells: extraction of cell-associated antigen with alkaline buffers, *J Immunol* 97:815, 1966.
198. Schmidt NJ, Lennette EH, Gee PS: Demonstration of rubella complement-fixing antigens of two distinct particle sizes by gel filtration on Sephadex G-200, *Proc Soc Exp Biol Med* 123:758, 1966.
199. Schmidt NJ, Lennette EH: Antigens of rubella virus, *Am J Dis Child* 118:89, 1969.
200. Schmidt NJ, Styk B: Immunodiffusion reactions with rubella antigens, *J Immunol* 101:210, 1968.
201. Salmi AA: Gel precipitation reactions between alkaline extracted rubella antigens and human sera, *Acta Pathol Microbiol Scand* 76:271, 1969.
202. LeBouvier GL: Precipitinogens of rubella virus infected cells, *Proc Soc Exp Biol Med* 130:51, 1969.
203. Cappel R, Schluederberg A, Horstmann DM: Large-scale production of rubella precipitinogens and their use in the diagnostic laboratory, *J Clin Microbiol* 1:201, 1975.
204. LeBouvier GL, Plotkin SA: Precipitin responses to rubella vaccine RA27/3, *J Infect Dis* 123:220, 1971.
205. Vaheri A, Vesikari T: Small size rubella virus antigens and soluble immune complexes, analysis by the platelet aggregation technique, *Arch Gesamte Virusforsch* 35:10, 1971.
206. Penttinen K, Myllyla G: Interaction of human blood platelets, viruses, and antibodies. I. Platelet aggregation test with microequipment, *Ann Med Exp Biol Fenn* 46:188, 1968.
207. Lennette EH, Schmidt NJ: Neutralization, fluorescent antibody and complement fixation tests for rubella. In Friedman H, Prier JE, editors: *Rubella*, Springfield, Ill, 1973, Charles C Thomas.
208. Schluederberg A, Horstmann DM, Andiman WA, Randolph MF: Neutralizing and hemagglutination-inhibition antibodies to rubella virus as indicators of protective immunity in vaccinees and naturally immune individuals, *J Infect Dis* 138:877, 1978.
209. Sato H, Albrecht P, Krugman S, Ennis FA: Sensitive neutralization test for rubella antibody, *J Clin Microbiol* 9:259, 1979.
210. Meurman OH: Antibody responses in patients with rubella infection determined by passive hemagglutination, hemagglutination inhibition, complement fixation, and solid-phase radioimmunoassay tests, *Infect Immun* 19:369, 1978.
211. Herrmann KL: Available rubella serologic tests, *Rev Infect Dis* 7(Suppl 1):S108, 1985.
212. Skendzel LP, Wilcox KR, Edson DC: Evaluation of assays for the detection of antibodies to rubella: a report based on data from the College of American Pathologists surveys of 1982, *Am J Clin Pathol* 80(Suppl 4):594, 1983.
213. Hauknes G: Experience with an indirect (passive) hemagglutination test for the demonstration of rubella virus antibody, *Acta Pathol Microbiol Scand* 88:85, 1980.
214. Kilgore JM: Further evaluation of a rubella passive hemagglutination test, *J Med Virol* 5:131, 1980.
215. Inouye S, Satoh K, Tajima T: Single-serum diagnosis of rubella by combined use of the hemagglutination inhibition and passive hemagglutination tests, *J Clin Microbiol* 23:388, 1986.
216. Harnett GB, Palmer CA, Mackay-Scollay EM: Single-radial-hemolysis test for the assay of rubella antibody in antenatal, vaccinated, and rubella virus-infected patients, *J Infect Dis* 140:937, 1979.
217. Nommensen FE: Accuracy of single radial hemolysis test for rubella immunity when internal reference standards are used to estimate antibody levels, *J Clin Microbiol* 25:22, 1987.
218. Halonen P, Meurman O, Matikainen MT, et al: IgA antibody response in acute rubella determined by solid-phase radioimmunoassay, *J Hyg (Lond)* 83:69, 1979.
219. Kangro HO, Pattison JR, Heath RB: The detection of rubella-specific IgM antibodies by radioimmunoassay, *Br J Exp Pathol* 59:577, 1978.
220. Meurman OH, Viljanen MK, Granfors K: Solid-phase radioimmunoassay of rubella virus immunoglobulin M antibodies: comparison with sucrose density gradient centrifugation test, *J Clin Microbiol* 5:257, 1977.
221. Meurman OH, Ziola BR: IgM-class rheumatoid factor interference in the solid-phase radioimmunoassay of rubella-specific IgM antibodies, *J Clin Pathol* 31:483, 1978.
222. Mortimer PP, Tedder RS, Hamblig MH, et al: Antibody capture radioimmunoassay for anti-rubella IgM, *J Hyg (Lond)* 86:139, 1981.
223. Brown GC, Maassab HF, Veronelli JA, Francis TJ Jr: Rubella antibodies in human serum: detection by the indirect fluorescent-antibody technic, *Science* 145:943, 1964.
224. Cradock-Watson JE, Ridehalgh MK, Pattison JR, et al: Comparison of immunofluorescence and radioimmunoassay for detecting IgM antibody in infants with the congenital rubella syndrome, *J Hyg (Lond.)* 83:413, 1979.
225. Leinikki PO, Shekarchi I, Dorsett P, Sever JL: Determination of virus-specific IgM antibodies by using ELISA: elimination of false-positive results with protein A-Sepharose absorption and subsequent IgM antibody assay, *J Lab Clin Med* 92:849, 1978.
226. Vejtorp M: Enzyme-linked immunosorbent assay for determination of rubella IgG antibodies, *Acta Pathol Microbiol Scand* 86:387, 1978.
227. Vejtorp M, Fanoe E, Leerhoy J: Diagnosis of postnatal rubella by the enzyme-linked immunosorbent assay for rubella IgM and IgG antibodies, *Acta Pathol Microbiol Scand* 87:155, 1979.
228. Bidwell D, Chantler SM, Morgan-Capner P, Pattison JR: Further investigation of the specificity and sensitivity of ELISA for rubella antibody screening, *J Clin Pathol* 33:200, 1980.
229. Skendzel LP, Edson DC: Evaluation of enzyme immunosorbent rubella assays, *Arch Pathol Lab Med* 109:391, 1985.
230. Morgan-Capner P, Pullen HJ, Pattison JR, et al: A comparison of three tests for rubella antibody screening, *J Clin Pathol* 32:542, 1979.
231. Champsaur H, Dussaix E, Tournier P: Hemagglutination inhibition, single radial hemolysis, and ELISA tests for the detection of IgG and IgM to rubella virus, *J Med Virol* 5:273, 1980.
232. Deibel R, D'Arcangelis D, Ducharme CP, Schryver GD: Assay of rubella antibody by passive hemagglutination and by a modified indirect immunofluorescence test, *Infection* 8(Suppl 3):S255, 1980.
233. Zartarian MV, Friedly G, Peterson EM, de la Maza LM: Detection of rubella antibodies by hemagglutination inhibition, indirect fluorescent-antibody test, and enzyme-linked immunosorbent assay, *J Clin Microbiol* 14:640, 1981.
234. Weissfeld AS, Gehle WD, Sonnenworth AC: Comparison of several test systems used for the determination of rubella immune status, *J Clin Microbiol* 16:82, 1982.
235. Truant AL, Barksdale BL, Huber TW, Elliott LB: Comparison of an enzyme-linked immunosorbent assay with indirect hemagglutination inhibition for determination of rubella virus antibody: evaluation of immune status with commercial reagents in a clinical laboratory, *J Clin Microbiol* 17:106, 1983.
236. Field PR, Gong CM: Diagnosis of postnatally acquired rubella by use of three enzyme-linked immunosorbent assays for specific immunoglobulins G and M and single radial hemolysis for specific immunoglobulin G, *J Clin Microbiol* 20:951, 1984.
237. Cubie H, Edmond E: Comparison of five different methods of rubella IgM antibody testing, *J Clin Pathol* 38:203, 1985.
238. Enders G: Serologic test combinations for safe detection of rubella infections, *Rev Infect Dis* 7(Suppl 1):S113, 1985.
239. Forsgren M: Standardization of techniques and reagents for the study of rubella antibody, *Rev Infect Dis* 7(Suppl 1):S129, 1985.
240. Grillner L, Forsgren M, Nordenfelt E: Comparison between a commercial ELISA, Rubazyme, and hemolysis-in-gel test for determination of rubella antibodies, *J Virol Methods* 10:111, 1985.
241. Chernesky MA, Smaill F, Mahony JB, Castriciano S: Combined testing for antibodies to rubella non-structural and envelope proteins sentinels infections in two outbreaks, *Diagn Microbiol Infect Dis* 8:173, 1987.

242. Ankerst J, Christensen P, Kjellén L, Kronvall G: A routine diagnostic test for IgA and IgM antibodies to rubella virus: absorption of IgG with *Staphylococcus aureus*, *J Infect Dis* 130:268, 1974.
243. Pattison JR, Mace JE: Elution patterns of rubella IgM, IgA, and IgG antibodies from a dextran and an agarose gel, *J Clin Pathol* 28:670, 1975.
244. Pattison JR, Mace JE, Dane DS: The detection and avoidance of false-positive reactions in tests for rubella-specific IgM, *J Med Microbiol* 9:355, 1975.
245. Pattison JR, Mace JE: The detection of specific IgM antibodies following infection with rubella virus, *J Clin Pathol* 28:377, 1975.
246. Pattison JR, Jackson CM, Hiscock JA, et al: Comparison of methods for detecting specific IgM antibody in infants with congenital rubella, *J Med Microbiol* 11:411, 1978.
247. Caul EO, Hobbs SJ, Roberts PC, Clarke SK: Evaluation of a simplified sucrose gradient method for the detection of rubella-specific IgM in routine diagnostic practice, *J Med Virol* 2:153, 1978.
248. Krech U, Wilhelm JA: A solid-phase immunosorbent technique for the rapid detection of rubella IgM by haemagglutination inhibition, *J Gen Virol* 44:281, 1979.
249. Morgan-Capner P, Davies E, Pattison JR: Rubella-specific IgM detection using Sephacryl S-300 gel filtration, *J Clin Pathol* 33:1072, 1980.
250. Kobayashi N, Suzuki M, Nakagawa T, Matumoto M: Separation of hemagglutination-inhibiting immunoglobulin M antibody to rubella virus in human serum by high-performance liquid chromatography, *J Clin Microbiol* 23:1143, 1986.
251. Cunningham AL, Fraser JRE: Persistent rubella virus infection of human synovial cells cultured in vitro, *J Infect Dis* 151:638, 1985.
252. Parkman PD, Meyer HM Jr, Kirschstein RL, Hopps HE: Attenuated rubella virus. I. Development and laboratory characterization, *N Engl J Med* 275:569, 1966.
253. Desmyter J, De Somer P, Rawls WE, Melnick JL: The mechanism of rubella virus interference, *Symp Ser Immunobiol Stand* 11:139, 1969.
254. Kleiman MB, Carver DH: Failure of the RA 27/3 strain of rubella virus to induce intrinsic interference, *J Gen Virol* 36:335, 1977.
255. Frey TK, Hemphill ML: Generation of defective-interfering particles by rubella virus in Vero cells, *Virology* 164:22, 1988.
256. Sigurdardottir B, Givan KF, Rozee KR, Rhodes AJ: Association of virus with cases of rubella studied in Toronto: propagation of the agent and transmission to monkeys, *Can Med Assoc J* 88:128, 1963.
257. Heggie AD, Robbins FC: Rubella in naval recruits: a virologic study, *N Engl J Med* 271:231, 1964.
258. Parkman PD, Phillips PE, Kirschstein RL, Meyer Jr HM: Experimental rubella virus infection in the rhesus monkey, *J Immunol* 95:743, 1965.
259. Parkman PD, Phillips PE, Meyer HM: Experimental rubella virus infection in pregnant monkeys, *Am J Dis Child* 110:390, 1965.
260. Sever JL, Meier GW, Windle WF, et al: Experimental rubella in pregnant rhesus monkeys, *J Infect Dis* 116:21, 1966.
261. Fabiyi A, Gitnick GL, Sever JL: Chronic rubella virus infection in the ferret *(Mustela putorius fero)* puppy, *Proc Soc Exp Biol Med* 125:766, 1967.
262. Barbosa L, Warren J: Studies on the detection of rubella virus and its immunogenicity for animals and man, Semi-annual contract progress report to the National Institute for Neurological Diseases and Blindness, September 1, 1966 to March 1, 1967.
263. Belcourt RJ, Wong FC, Walcroft MJ: Growth of rubella virus in rabbit foetal tissues and cell cultures, *Can J Public Health* 56:253, 1965.
264. Oxford JS: The growth of rubella virus in small laboratory animals, *J Immunol* 98:697, 1967.
265. Cotlier E, Fox J, Bohigian G, et al: Pathogenic effects of rubella virus on embryos and newborn rats, *Nature* 217:38, 1968.
266. Carver DH, Seto DS, Marcus PI, Rodrigues L: Rubella virus replication in the brains of suckling mice, *J Virol* 1:1089, 1967.
267. Centers for Disease Control and Prevention: Recommendation of the Immunization Practices Advisory Committee (ACIP). Rubella prevention, *MMWR Morb Mortal Wkly Rep* 39:1, 1990.
268. Centers for Disease Control and Prevention: Revised ACIP recommendation for avoiding pregnancy after receiving a rubella containing vaccine, *MMWR Morb Mortal Wkly Rep* 50:1117, 2001.
269. American Academy of Pediatrics Committee on Infectious Diseases: Rubella. In Peter G, editor: *Report of the Committee on Infectious Diseases*, ed 22, Elk Grove Village, Ill, 1991, American Academy of Pediatrics.
270. Bart KJ, Orenstein WA, Preblud SR, et al: Elimination of rubella and congenital rubella from the United States, *Pediatr Infect Dis* 4:14, 1985.
271. Mann JM, Preblud SR, Hoffman RE, et al: Assessing risks of rubella infection during pregnancy: a standardized approach, *JAMA* 245:1647, 1981.
272. Horstmann DM, Liebhaber H, Le Bouvier GL, et al: Rubella: reinfection of vaccinated and naturally immune persons exposed in an epidemic, *N Engl J Med* 283:771, 1970.
273. Lehane DE, Newberg NR, Beam WE Jr: Evaluation of rubella herd immunity during an epidemic, *JAMA* 213:2236, 1970.
274. Pollard RB, Edwards EA: Epidemic survey of rubella in a military recruit population, *Am J Epidemiol* 101:435, 1975.
275. Crawford GE, Gremellion DH: Epidemic measles and rubella in Air Force recruits: impact of immunization, *J Infect Dis* 144:403, 1981.
276. Blouse LE, Lathrop GD, Dupuy HJ, Ball RJ: Rubella screening and vaccination program for US Air Force trainees: an analysis of findings, *Am J Public Health* 72:280, 1982.
277. Chretien JH, Esswein JG, McGarvey MA, deStwolinski A: Rubella: pattern of outbreak in a university, *South Med J* 69:1042, 1976.
278. Centers for Disease Control: Rubella in colleges—United States, 1983-1984, *MMWR Morb Mortal Wkly Rep* 34:228, 1985.
279. Centers for Disease Control: Rubella outbreaks in prisons—New York City, West Virginia, California, *MMWR Morb Mortal Wkly Rep* 34:615, 1985.
280. Centers for Disease Control: Rubella and congenital rubella syndrome—New York City, *MMWR Morb Mortal Wkly Rep* 35:770, 1986.
281. Centers for Disease Control and Prevention: Increase in rubella and congenital rubella syndrome in the United States, *MMWR Morb Mortal Wkly Rep* 40:93, 1991.
282. Centers for Disease Control: Congenital rubella syndrome among the Amish—Pennsylvania, 1991-1992, *MMWR Morb Mortal Wkly Rep* 41:468, 1992.
283. Goodman AK, Friedman SM, Beatrice ST, Bart SW: Rubella in the workplace: the need for employee immunization, *Am J Public Health* 77:725, 1987.
284. McLaughlin MC, Gold LH: The New York rubella incident: a case for changing hospital policy regarding rubella testing and immunization, *Am J Public Health* 79:287, 1979.
285. Polk BF, White JA, DeGirolami PC, Modlin JF: An outbreak of rubella among hospital personnel, *N Engl J Med* 303:541, 1980.
286. Greaves WL, Orenstein WA, Stetler HC, et al: Prevention of rubella transmission in medical facilities, *JAMA* 248:861, 1982.
287. Strassburg MA, Stephenson TG, Habel LA, Fannin SL: Rubella in hospital employees, *Infect Control* 5:123, 1984.
288. Storch GA, Gruber C, Benz B, et al: A rubella outbreak among dental students: description of the outbreak and analysis of control measures, *Infect Control* 6:150, 1985.
289. Sever JL, Monif G: Limited persistence of virus in congenital rubella, *Am J Dis Child* 110:452, 1965.
290. Cooper LZ, Krugman S: Clinical manifestations of postnatal and congenital rubella, *Arch Ophthalmol* 77:434, 1967.
291. Rawls WE, Phillips A, Melnick JL, Desmond MM: Persistent virus infection in congenital rubella, *Arch Ophthalmol* 77:430, 1967.
292. Michaels RH: Immunologic aspects of congenital rubella, *Pediatrics* 43:339, 1969.
293. Menser MA, Slinn RF, Forrest JM, et al: Rubella viruria in a 29-year-old woman with congenital rubella, *Lancet* 2:797, 1971.
294. Shewmon DA, Cherry JD, Kirby SE: Shedding of rubella virus in a 4½-year-old boy with congenital rubella, *Pediatr Infect Dis* 1:342, 1982.
295. Hattis RP, Halstead SB, Herrmann KL, Witte JJ: Rubella in an immunized island population, *JAMA* 223:1019, 1973.
296. Weller TH, Alford CA Jr, Neva FA: Changing epidemiologic concepts of rubella, with particular reference to unique characteristics of the congenital infection, *Yale J Biol Med* 37:455, 1965.
297. Rawls WE, Melnick JL, Bradstreet CM, et al: WHO collaborative study on the seroepidemiology of rubella, *Bull World Health Organ* 37:79, 1967.
298. Cockburn WC: World aspects of the epidemiology of rubella, *Am J Dis Child* 118:112, 1969.
299. Witte JJ, Karchmer AW, Case G, et al: Epidemiology of rubella, *Am J Dis Child* 118:107, 1969.
300. Dowdle WR, Ferrera W, De Salles Gomes LF, et al: WHO collaborative study on the seroepidemiology of rubella in Caribbean and Middle and South American populations in 1968, *Bull World Health Organ* 42:419, 1970.

301. Horstmann DM: Rubella: the challenge of its control, *J Infect Dis* 123:640, 1971.
302. Assad R, Ljungars-Esteves K: Rubella—world impact, *Rev Infect Dis* 7(Suppl 1):S29, 1985.
303. Horstmann DM: Rubella. In Evans AS, editor: *Viral infections of humans: epidemiology and control*, ed 2, New York, 1985, Plenum Publishing.
304. Reef SE, Frey TK, Theall K, et al: The changing epidemiology of rubella in the 1990s: on the verge of elimination and new challenges for control and prevention, *JAMA* 287:464, 2002.
305. Buescher EL: Behavior of rubella virus in adult populations, *Arch Gesamte Virusforsch* 16:470, 1965.
306. Green RH, Balsamo MR, Giles JP, et al: Studies of the natural history and prevention of rubella, *Am J Dis Child* 110:348, 1965.
307. Horstmann DM, Riordan JT, Ohtawara M, Niederman JC: A natural epidemic of rubella in a closed population, *Arch Gesamte Virusforsch* 16:483, 1965.
308. Brody JA: The infectiousness of rubella and the possibility of reinfection, *Am J Public Health* 56:1082, 1966.
309. Bisno AL, Spence LP, Stewart JA, Casey HL: Rubella in Trinidad: seroepidemiologic studies of an institutional outbreak, *Am J Epidemiol* 89:74, 1969.
310. Gale JL, Detels R, Kim KS, et al: The epidemiology of rubella on Taiwan. III. Family studies in cities of high and low attack rates, *Int J Epidemiol* 1:261, 1972.
311. Neva FA, Alford CA Jr, Weller TH: Emerging perspective of rubella, *Bacteriol Rev* 28:444, 1964.
312. Brody JA, Sever JL, McAlister R, et al: Rubella epidemic on St. Paul Island in the Pribilofs, 1963. I. Epidemiologic, clinical, and serologic findings, *JAMA* 191:619, 1965.
313. Sever JL, Brody JA, Schiff GM, et al: Rubella epidemic on St. Paul Island in the Pribilofs, 1963. II. Clinical and laboratory findings for the intensive study population, *JAMA* 191:624, 1965.
314. Halstead SB, Diwan AR, Oda AI: Susceptibility to rubella among adolescents and adults in Hawaii, *JAMA* 210:1881, 1969.
315. Hinman AR, Irons B, Lewis M, Kandola K: Economic analyses of rubella and rubella vaccines: a global review, *Bull World Health Organ* 80:264, 2003.
316. Wilkins J, Leedom JM, Portnoy B, Salvatore MA: Reinfection with rubella virus despite live vaccine-induced immunity, *Am J Dis Child* 118:275, 1969.
317. Chang TW, DesRosiers S, Weinstein L: Clinical and serologic studies of an outbreak of rubella in a vaccinated population, *N Engl J Med* 283:246, 1970.
318. Gross PA, Portnoy B, Mathies AW Jr, et al: A rubella outbreak among adolescent boys, *Am J Dis Child* 119:326, 1970.
319. Miyakawa M, Yoshino H, Yoshida LM, et al: Seroprevalence of rubella in the cord blood of pregnant women and congenital rubella incidence in Nha Trang, Vietnam, *Vaccine* 32:1192, 2014.
320. Goodson JL, Masresha B, Dosseh A, et al: Rubella epidemiology in Africa in the prevaccine era, 2002-2009, *J Infect Dis* 204(Suppl 1): S215, 2011.
321. Pham VH, Nguyen TV, Nguyen TT, et al: Rubella epidemic in Vietnam: characteristic of rubella virus genes from pregnant women and their fetuses/newborns with congenital rubella syndrome, *J Clin Virol* 57:152, 2013.
322. Minakami H, Kubo T, Unno N: Causes of a nationwide rubella outbreak in Japan, 2012-2013, *J Infect* 68:99, 2014.
323. Yamada T, Kubo T, Mochizuki J, et al: Immune status among Japanese during nationwide rubella outbreak in Japan 2012-2013, *J Infect* 68:300, 2014.
324. Chandy S, Abraham AM, Jana AK, et al: Congenital rubella syndrome and rubella in Vellore, South India, *Epidemiol Infect* 139:962, 2011.
325. Dewan P, Gupta P: Burden of congenital rubella syndrome (CRS) in India: a systematic review, *Indian Pediatr* 49:377, 2012.
326. Centers for Disease Control and Prevention: Rubella and congenital rubella syndrome control and elimination—global progress, 2000-2012, *MMWR Morb Mortal Wkly Rep* 62:983, 2013.
327. Bloom S, Smith P, Stanwyck C, Stokley S: Has the United States population been adequately vaccinated to achieve rubella elimination? *Clin Infect Dis* 43(Suppl 3):S141, 2006.
328. Miller KA: Rubella susceptibility in an adolescent female population, *Mayo Clin Proc* 59:31, 1984.
329. Allen S: Rubella susceptibility in young adults, *J Fam Pract* 21:271, 1985.
330. Dykewicz CA, Kruszon-Moran D, McQuillan GM, et al: Rubella seropositivity in the United States, 1988-1994, *Clin Infect Dis* 33:1279, 2001.
331. Hyde TB, Kruszon-Moran D, McQuillan GM, et al: Rubella immunity levels in the United States population: has the threshold of viral elimination been reached? *Clin Infect Dis* 43(Suppl 3):S146, 2006.
332. Reef SE, Redd SB, Abernathy E, et al: The epidemiological profile of rubella and congenital rubella syndrome in the United States, 1998-2004: the evidence for absence of endemic transmission, *Clin Infect Dis* 43(Suppl 3):S126, 2006.
333. Alford CA, Neva FA, Weller TH: Virologic and serologic studies on human products of conception after maternal rubella, *N Engl J Med* 271:1275, 1964.
334. Horstmann DJ, Banatvala JE, Riordan JT, et al: Maternal rubella and the rubella syndrome in infants, *Am J Dis Child* 110:408, 1965.
335. Monif GRG, Sever JL, Schiff GM, Traub RG: Isolation of rubella virus from products of conception, *Am J Obstet Gynecol* 91:1143, 1965.
336. Alford CA Jr: Congenital rubella: a review of the virologic and serologic phenomena occurring after maternal rubella in the first trimester, *South Med J* 59:745, 1966.
337. Heggie AD: Intrauterine infection in maternal rubella, *J Pediatr* 71:777, 1967.
338. Rawls WE, Desmyter J, Melnick JL: Serologic diagnosis and fetal involvement in maternal rubella, *JAMA* 203:627, 1968.
339. Thompson KM, Tobin JO: Isolation of rubella virus from abortion material, *Br Med J* 2:264, 1970.
340. Strannegard O, Holm SE, Hermodsson S, et al: Case of apparent reinfection with rubella, *Lancet* 1:240, 1970.
341. Boué A, Nicholas A, Montagnon B: Reinfection with rubella in pregnant women, *Lancet* 2:1251, 1971.
342. Haukenes G, Haram KO: Clinical rubella after reinfection, *N Engl J Med* 287:1204, 1972.
343. Northrop RL, Gardner WM, Geittman WF: Rubella reinfection during early pregnancy, *Obstet Gynecol* 39:524, 1972.
344. Northrop RL, Gardner WM, Geittman WF: Low-level immunity to rubella, *N Engl J Med* 287:615, 1972.
345. Eilard T, Strannegard O: Rubella reinfection in pregnancy followed by transmission to the fetus, *J Infect Dis* 129:594, 1974.
346. Snijder JAM, Schroder FP, Hoekstra JH: Importance of IgM determination in cord blood in cases of suspected rubella infection, *Br Med J* 1:23, 1977.
347. Forsgren M, Carlstrom G, Strangert K: Congenital rubella after maternal reinfection, *Scand J Infect Dis* 11:81, 1979.
348. Fogel A, Handsher R, Barnea B: Subclinical rubella in pregnancy—occurrence and outcome, *Isr J Med Sci* 21:133, 1985.
349. Sheridan MD: Final report of a prospective study of children whose mothers had rubella in early pregnancy, *Br Med J* 2:536, 1964.
350. Butler NR, Dudgeon JA, Hayes K, et al: Persistence of rubella antibody with and without embryopathy: a follow-up study of children exposed to maternal rubella, *Br Med J* 2:1027, 1965.
351. Phillips GA, Melnick JL, Yow MD, et al: Persistence of virus in infants with congenital rubella and in normal infants with a history of maternal rubella, *JAMA* 193:1027, 1965.
352. Hardy JB, McCracken GH Jr, Gilkeson MR, Sever JL: Adverse fetal outcome following maternal rubella after the first trimester of pregnancy, *JAMA* 207:2414, 1969.
353. Schiff GM, Sutherland J, Light I: Congenital rubella. In Thalhammer O, editor: *Prenatal infections, International Symposium of Vienna*, Stuttgart, September 2-3, 1970, 1971, Georg Thieme Verlag.
354. Peckham GS: Clinical and laboratory study of children exposed in utero to maternal rubella, *Arch Dis Child* 47:571, 1972.
355. Menser MA, Forrest JM: Rubella—high incidence of defects in children considered normal at birth, *Med J Aust* 1:123, 1974.
356. Dudgeon JA: Infective causes of human malformations, *Br Med Bull* 32:77, 1976.
357. Lundstrom R: Rubella during pregnancy: a follow-up study of children born after an epidemic of rubella in Sweden, 1951, with additional investigations on prophylaxis and treatment of maternal rubella, *Acta Paediatr Suppl* 133:1, 1962.
358. Whitehouse WL: Rubella before conception as a cause of foetal abnormality, *Lancet* 1:139, 1963.
359. Monif GRG, Hardy JB, Sever JL: Studies in congenital rubella, Baltimore 1964-65. I. Epidemiologic and virologic, *Bull Johns Hopkins Hosp* 118:85, 1966.

360. Sever JL, Hardy JB, Nelson KB, Gilkeson MR: Rubella in the Collaborative Perinatal Research Study. II. Clinical and laboratory findings in children through 3 years of age, *Am J Dis Child* 118:123, 1969.
361. Seppala M, Vaheri A: Natural rubella infection of the female genital tract, *Lancet* 1:46, 1974.
362. Buimovici-Klein E, Hite RL, Byrne T, Cooper LZ: Isolation of rubella virus in milk after postpartum immunization, *J Pediatr* 91:939, 1977.
363. Klein EB, Bryne T, Cooper LZ: Neonatal rubella in a breast-fed infant after postpartum maternal infection, *J Pediatr* 97:774, 1980.
364. Manson MM, Logan WPD, Loy RM: *Rubella and other virus infections during pregnancy*, Reports on Public Health and Medical Subjects, No. 101. London, 1960, Her Majesty's Stationery Office.
365. Siegel M, Greenberg M: Fetal death, malformation and prematurity after maternal rubella: results of prospective study, 1949-1958, *N Engl J Med* 262:389, 1960.
366. Liggins GC, Phillips LI: Rubella embryopathy: an interim report on a New Zealand epidemic, *Br Med J* 1:711, 1963.
367. Pitt D, Keir EH: Results of rubella in pregnancy, III, *Med J Aust* 2:737, 1965.
368. Sallomi SJ: Rubella in pregnancy: a review of prospective studies from the literature, *Obstet Gynecol* 27:252, 1966.
369. Heggie AD, Robbins FC: Natural rubella acquired after birth: clinical features and complications, *Am J Dis Child* 118:12, 1969.
370. Chantler JK, Tingle AJ: Isolation of rubella virus from human lymphocytes after acute infection, *J Infect Dis* 145:673, 1982.
371. O'Shea S, Mutton D, Best JM: In vivo expression of rubella antigens on human leucocytes: detection by flow cytometry, *J Med Virol* 25:297, 1988.
372. Heggie AD: Pathogenesis of the rubella exanthem: isolation of rubella virus from the skin, *N Engl J Med* 285:664, 1971.
373. Heggie AD: Pathogenesis of the rubella exanthem: distribution of rubella virus in the skin during rubella with and without rash, *J Infect Dis* 137:74, 1978.
374. Al-Nakib W, Best JM, Banatvala JE: Rubella-specific serum and nasopharyngeal immunoglobulin responses following naturally acquired and vaccine-induced infection: prolonged persistence of virus-specific IgM, *Lancet* 1:182, 1975.
375. Pattison JR, Dane DS, Mace JE: The persistence of specific IgM after natural infection with rubella virus, *Lancet* 1:185, 1975.
376. Meurman OH: Persistence of immunoglobulin G and immunoglobulin M antibodies after postnatal rubella infection determined by solid-phase radioimmunoassay, *J Clin Microbiol* 7:34, 1978.
377. Rousseau S, Hedman K: Rubella infection and reinfection distinguished by avidity of IgG, *Lancet* 1:1108, 1988.
378. Hedman K, Seppala I: Recent rubella virus infection indicated by a low avidity of specific IgG, *J Clin Immunol* 8:214, 1988.
379. Morgan-Capner P, Thomas HIJ: Serological distinction between primary rubella and reinfection, *Lancet* 1:1397, 1988.
380. Smith KA, Chess L, Mardiney MR Jr: The relationship between rubella hemagglutination inhibition antibody (HIA) and rubella induced in vitro lymphocyte tritiated thymidine incorporation, *Cell Immunol* 8:321, 1973.
381. Steele RW, Hensen SA, Vincent MM, et al: A 52Cr microassay technique for cell-mediated immunity to viruses, *J Immunol* 110:1502, 1973.
382. Honeyman MC, Forrest JM, Dorman DC: Cell-mediated immune response following natural rubella and rubella vaccination, *Clin Exp Immunol* 17:665, 1974.
383. McMorrow L, Vesikari T, Wolman SR, et al: Suppression of the response of lymphocytes to phytohemagglutinin in rubella, *J Infect Dis* 130:464, 1974.
384. Steele RW, Hensen SA, Vincent MM, et al: Development of specific cellular and humoral immune responses in children immunized with liver rubella virus vaccine, *J Infect Dis* 130:449, 1974.
385. Kanra GY, Vesikari T: Cytotoxic activity against rubella-infected cells in the supernatants of human lymphocyte cultures stimulated by rubella virus, *Clin Exp Immunol* 19:17, 1975.
386. Vesikari T, Kanra GY, Buimovici-Klein E, Cooper LZ: Cell-mediated immunity in rubella assayed by cytotoxicity of supernatants from rubella virus-stimulated human lymphocyte cultures, *Clin Exp Immunol* 19:33, 1975.
387. Ganguly R, Cusumano CL, Waldman RH: Suppression of cell-mediated immunity after infection with attenuated rubella virus, *Infect Immun* 13:464, 1976.
388. Buimovici-Klein E, Weiss KE, Cooper LZ: Interferon production in lymphocyte cultures after rubella infection in humans, *J Infect Dis* 135:380, 1977.
389. Rossier E, Phipps PH, Polley JR, Webb T: Absence of cell-mediated immunity to rubella virus 5 years after rubella vaccination, *Can Med Assoc J* 116:481, 1977.
390. Rossier E, Phipps PH, Weber JM, Meurman OH: Persistence of humoral and cell-mediated immunity to rubella virus in cloistered nuns and in schoolteachers, *J Infect Dis* 144:137, 1981.
391. Buimovici-Klein E, Cooper LZ: Cell-mediated immune response to rubella infections, *Rev Infect Dis* 7(Suppl 1):S123, 1985.
392. Mori T, Shiozawa K: Suppression of tuberculin hypersensitivity caused by rubella infection, *Am Rev Respir Dis* 131:886, 1985.
393. Ogra PL, Kerr-Grant D, Umana G, et al: Antibody response in serum and nasopharynx after naturally acquired and vaccine-induced infection with rubella virus, *N Engl J Med* 285:1333, 1971.
394. Al-Nakib W, Best JM, Banatvala JE: Detection of rubella-specific serum IgG and IgA and nasopharyngeal IgA responses using a radioactive single radial immunodiffusion technique, *Clin Exp Immunol* 22:293, 1975.
395. Plotkin SA, Farquhar JD: Immunity to rubella: comparison between naturally and artificially induced resistance, *Postgrad Med J* 48(Suppl 3):47, 1972.
396. Plotkin SA, Farquhar JD, Ogra PL: Immunologic properties of RA 27/3 rubella virus vaccine: a comparison with strains presently licensed in the United States, *JAMA* 225:585, 1973.
397. Morag A, Beutner KR, Morag B, Ogra PL: Development and characteristics of in vitro correlates of cellular immunity to rubella virus in the systemic and mucosal sites in guinea pigs, *J Immunol* 113:1703, 1974.
398. Morag A, Morag B, Bernstein JM, et al: In vitro correlates of cell-mediated immunity in human tonsils after natural or induced rubella virus infection, *J Infect Dis* 131:409, 1975.
399. Selzer G: Virus isolation, inclusion bodies, and chromosomes in a rubella-infected human embryo, *Lancet* 2:336, 1963.
400. Rudolph AJ, Yow MD, Phillips A, et al: Transplacental rubella infection in newly born infants, *JAMA* 191:843, 1965.
401. Catalano LW Jr, Fuccillo DA, Traub RG, Sever JL: Isolation of rubella virus from placentas and throat cultures of infants: a prospective study after the 1964-65 epidemic, *Obstet Gynecol* 38:6, 1971.
402. Monif GRG, Sever JL: Chronic infection of the central nervous system with rubella virus, *Neurology* 16:111, 1966.
403. Plotkin SA, Cochran W, Lindquist JM, et al: Congenital rubella syndrome in late infancy, *JAMA* 200:435, 1967.
404. Desmond MM, Wilson GS, Melnick JL, et al: Congenital rubella encephalitis, *J Pediatr* 71:311, 1967.
405. Menser MA, Harley JD, Hertzberg R, et al: Persistence of virus in lens for three years after prenatal rubella, *Lancet* 2:387, 1967.
406. Cremer NE, Oshiro LS, Weil ML, et al: Isolation of rubella virus from brain in chronic progressive panencephalitis, *J Gen Virol* 29:143, 1975.
407. Weil ML, Itabashi H, Cremer NE, et al: Chronic progressive panencephalitis due to rubella virus simulating subacute sclerosing panencephalitis, *N Engl J Med* 292:994, 1975.
408. Alford CA Jr: Studies on antibody in congenital rubella infections. I. Physicochemical and immunologic investigations of rubella-neutralizing antibody, *Am J Dis Child* 110:455, 1965.
409. Weller TH, Alford CA Jr, Neva FA: Retrospective diagnosis by serologic means of congenitally acquired rubella infections, *N Engl J Med* 270:1039, 1964.
410. Alford CA Jr, Blankenship WJ, Straumfjord JV, et al: The diagnostic significance of IgM-globulin elevations in newborn infants with chronic intrauterine infections. In Bergsma D, editor: *Birth defects original article series*, vol. 4, New York, 1968, National Foundation–March of Dimes.
411. Gitlin D: The differentiation and maturation of specific immune mechanisms, *Acta Paediatr Scand Suppl* 172:60, 1967.
412. Lawton AR, Self KS, Royal SA, Cooper MD: Ontogeny of lymphocytes in the human fetus, *Clin Immunol Immunopathol* 1:104, 1972.
413. Gitlin D, Biasucci A: Development of gamma G, gamma A, beta IC-beta IA, CI esterase inhibitor, ceruloplasmin, transferrin, hemopexin, haptoglobin, fibrinogen, plasminogen, alpha 1-antitrypsin, orosomucoid, beta-lipoprotein, alpha 2-macroglobulin, and prealbumin in the human conceptus, *J Clin Invest* 48:1433, 1969.
414. Alford CA Jr: Fetal antibody in the diagnosis of chronic intrauterine infections. In Thalhammer O, editor: *Prenatal infections, International Symposium of Vienna*, Stuttgart, 1971, Georg Thieme Verlag, p 1971.

415. Bellanti JA, Artenstein MS, Olson LC, et al: Congenital rubella: clinicopathologic, virologic, and immunologic studies, *Am J Dis Child* 110:464, 1965.
416. Baublis JV, Brown GC: Specific response of the immunoglobulins to rubella infection, *Proc Soc Exp Biol Med* 128:206, 1968.
417. Cohen SM, Ducharme CP, Carpenter CA, Deibel R: Rubella antibody in IgG and IgM immunoglobulins detected by immunofluorescence, *J Lab Clin Med* 72:760, 1968.
418. Vesikari T, Vaheri A, Pettay O, Kunnas M: Congenital rubella: immune response of the neonate and diagnosis by demonstration of specific IgM antibodies, *J Pediatr* 75:658, 1969.
419. Cradock-Watson JE, Ridehalgh MKS, Chantler S: Specific immunoglobulins in infants with the congenital rubella syndrome, *J Hyg (Lond.)* 76:109, 1976.
420. Alford CA Jr: Immunoglobulin determinations in the diagnosis of fetal infection, *Pediatr Clin North Am* 18:99, 1971.
421. McCracken GH Jr, Hardy JB, Chen TC, et al: Serum immunoglobulin levels in newborn infants. II. Survey of cord and follow-up sera from 123 infants with congenital rubella, *J Pediatr* 74:383, 1969.
422. Kenrick KG, Slinn RF, Dorman DC, Menser MA: Immunoglobulins and rubella-virus antibodies in adults with congenital rubella, *Lancet* 1:548, 1968.
423. Hardy JB, Sever JL, Gilkeson MR: Declining antibody titers in children with congenital rubella, *J Pediatr* 75:213, 1969.
424. Cooper LZ, Florman AL, Ziring PR, Krugman S: Loss of rubella hemagglutination-inhibition antibody in congenital rubella, *Am J Dis Child* 122:397, 1971.
425. Ueda K, Tokugawa K, Fukushige J, et al: Hemagglutination inhibition antibodies in congenital rubella: a 17-year follow-up in the Ryukyu Islands, *Am J Dis Child* 141:211, 1987.
426. Ueda K, Tokugawa K, Fukushige J, et al: Continuing problem in congenital rubella syndrome in southern Japan: its outbreak in Fukuoka and the surrounding areas after the 1965-1969 and 1975-1977 rubella epidemics, *Fukuoka Acta Med* 77:309, 1986.
427. Soothill JF, Hayes K, Dudgeon JA: The immunoglobulins in congenital rubella, *Lancet* 1:1385, 1966.
428. Hancock MP, Huntley CC, Sever JL: Congenital rubella syndrome with immunoglobulin disorder, *J Pediatr* 72:636, 1968.
429. Hayward AR, Ezer G: Development of lymphocyte populations in the human foetal thymus and spleen, *Clin Exp Immunol* 17:169, 1974.
430. Cooper MD, Dayton DH, editors: *Development of host defenses*, New York, 1977, Raven Press.
431. Miller ME, editor: *Host defenses in the human neonate*, New York, 1978, Grune & Stratton.
432. Berry CL, Thompson EN: Clinicopathological study of thymic dysplasia, *Arch Dis Child* 43:579, 1968.
433. White LR, Leikin S, Villavicencio O, et al: Immune competence in congenital rubella: lymphocyte transformation, delayed hypersensitivity and response to vaccination, *J Pediatr* 73:229, 1968.
434. Montgomery JR, South MA, Rawls WE, et al: Viral inhibition of lymphocyte response to phytohemagglutinin, *Science* 157:1068, 1967.
435. Olson GB, South MA, Good RA: Phytohemagglutinin unresponsiveness of lymphocytes from babies with congenital rubella, *Nature* 214:695, 1967.
436. Dent PB, Olson GB, Good RA, et al: Rubella-virus/leukocyte interaction and its role in the pathogenesis of the congenital rubella syndrome, *Lancet* 1:291, 1968.
437. Olson GB, Dent PB, Rawls WE, et al: Abnormalities of in vitro lymphocyte responses during rubella virus infections, *J Exp Med* 128:47, 1968.
438. Simmons JJ, Fitzgerald MG: Rubella virus and human lymphocytes in culture, *Lancet* 2:937, 1968.
439. Marshall WC, Cope WA, Soothill JF, Dudgeon JA: In vitro lymphocyte response in some immunity deficiency diseases and in intrauterine virus infections, *Proc R Soc Med* 63:351, 1970.
440. Buimovici-Klein E, Lang PB, Ziring PR, Cooper LZ: Impaired cell-mediated immune response in patients with congenital rubella: correlation with gestational age at time of infection, *Pediatrics* 64: 620, 1979.
441. Hyypiä T, Eskola J, Laine M, Meurman O: B-cell function in vitro during rubella infection, *Infect Immun* 43:589, 1984.
442. Fuccillo DA, Steele RW, Hensen SA, et al: Impaired cellular immunity to rubella virus in congenital rubella, *Infect Immun* 9:81, 1974.
443. Pukhalsky AL, Shmarina GV, Bliacher MS, et al: Cytokine profile after rubella vaccine inoculation: evidence of the immunosuppressive effect of vaccination, *Mediators Inflamm* 12:203, 2003.
444. Mims CA: Pathogenesis of viral infections in the fetus, *Prog Med Virol* 10:194, 1968.
445. Rawls WE: Congenital rubella: the significance of virus persistence, *Prog Med Virol* 10:238, 1968.
446. Alford CA Jr: Production of interferon-like substance by the rubella-infected human conceptus, Program and abstracts of the American Pediatric Society and Society of Pediatric Research Meeting, Atlantic City, NJ, April 29-May 2, 1970.
447. Lebon P, Daffos F, Checoury A, et al: Presence of an acid-labile alpha-interferon in sera from fetuses and children with congenital rubella, *J Clin Microbiol* 21:755, 1985.
448. Desmyter J, Rawls WE, Melnick JL, et al: Interferon in congenital rubella: response to live attenuated measles vaccine, *J Immunol* 99:771, 1967.
449. McCarthy K, Taylor-Robinson CH, Pillinger SE: Isolation of rubella virus from cases in Britain, *Lancet* 2:593, 1963.
450. Hildebrandt HM, Maassab HF: Rubella synovitis in a 1-year-old patient, *N Engl J Med* 274:1428, 1966.
451. Yanez JE, Thompson GR, Mikkelsen WM, Bartholomew LE: Rubella arthritis, *Ann Intern Med* 64:772, 1966.
452. McCormick JN, Duthie JJ, Gerber H, et al: Rheumatoid polyarthritis after rubella, *Ann Rheum Dis* 37:266, 1978.
453. Graham R, Armstrong R, Simmons NA, et al: Isolation of rubella virus from synovial fluid in five cases of seronegative arthritis, *Lancet* 2:649, 1981.
454. Lebon P, Lyon G: Noncongenital rubella encephalitis, *Lancet* 2:468, 1974.
455. Wolinsky JS, Berg BO, Maitland CJ: Progressive rubella panencephalitis, *Arch Neurol* 33:722, 1976.
456. Squadrini F, Taparelli F, De Rienzo B, et al: Rubella virus isolation from cerebrospinal fluid in postnatal rubella encephalitis, *Br Med J* 2:1329, 1977.
457. Thong YH, Steele RW, Vincent MM, et al: Impaired in vitro cell-mediated immunity to rubella virus during pregnancy, *N Engl J Med* 289:604, 1973.
458. Weinberg ED: Pregnancy-associated depression of cell-mediated immunity, *Rev Infect Dis* 6:814, 1984.
459. Honeyman MC, Dorman DC, Menser MA, et al: HL-A antigens in congenital rubella and the role of antigens 1 and 8 in the epidemiology of natural rubella, *Tissue Antigens* 5:12, 1975.
460. Forrester RM, Lees VT, Watson GH: Rubella syndrome: escape of a twin, *Br Med J* 1:1403, 1966.
461. Cooper LZ: The history and medical consequences of rubella, *Rev Infect Dis* 7(Suppl 1):S1, 1985.
462. Töndury G, Smith DW: Fetal rubella pathology, *J Pediatr* 68:867, 1966.
463. Driscoll SG: Histopathology of gestational rubella, *Am J Dis Child* 118:49, 1969.
464. Dudgeon JA: Teratogenic effect of rubella virus, *Proc R Soc Med* 63:1254, 1970.
465. Menser MA, Reye RDK: The pathology of congenital rubella: a review written by request, *Pathology* 6:215, 1974.
466. Esterly JR, Oppenheimer EH: Intrauterine rubella infection. In Rosenberg HS, Bolande RP, editors: *Perspectives in pediatric pathology*, vol. 1, Chicago, 1973, Year Book Medical Publishers.
467. Boué A, Boué JG: Effects of rubella virus infection on the division of human cells, *Am J Dis Child* 118:45, 1969.
468. Smith JL, Early EM, London WT, et al: Persistent rubella virus production in embryonic rabbit chondrocyte cell cultures (37465), *Proc Soc Exp Biol Med* 143:1037, 1973.
469. Heggie AD: Growth inhibition of human embryonic and fetal rat bones in organ culture by rubella virus, *Teratology* 15:47, 1977.
470. Rawls WE, Melnick JL, Rosenberg HS, Bayatpour M: Spontaneous virus carrier cultures and postmortem isolation of virus from infants with congenital rubella, *Proc Soc Exp Biol Med* 120:623, 1965.
471. Boué A, Plotkin SA, Boué JG: Action du virus de la rubéole sur différents systemes de cultures de cellules embryonnaires humaines, *Arch Gesamte Virusforsch* 16:443, 1965.
472. Plotkin SA, Boué A, Boué JG: The in vitro growth of rubella virus in human embryo cells, *Am J Epidemiol* 81:71, 1965.
473. Chang TH, Moorhead PS, Boué JG, et al: Chromosome studies of human cells infected in utero and in vitro with rubella virus, *Proc Soc Exp Biol Med* 122:236, 1966.
474. Nusbacher J, Hirschhorn K, Cooper LZ: Chromosomal studies on congenital rubella, *N Engl J Med* 276:1409, 1967.

475. Plotkin SA, Vaheri A: Human fibroblasts infected with rubella virus produce a growth inhibitor, *Science* 156:659, 1967.
476. Bowden DS, Pedersen JS, Toh BH, Westaway EG: Distribution by immunofluorescence of viral products and actin-containing cytoskeleton filaments in rubella virus-infected cells, *Arch Virol* 92:211, 1987.
477. Yoneda T, Urade M, Sakuda M, Miyazaki T: Altered growth, differentiation, and responsiveness to epidermal growth factor of human embryonic mesenchymal cells of palate by persistent rubella virus infection, *J Clin Invest* 77:1613, 1986.
478. Naeye RL, Blanc W: Pathogenesis of congenital rubella, *JAMA* 194:1277, 1965.
479. Ilkow CS, Mancinelli V, Beatch MD, Hobman TC: Rubella virus capsidprotein interacts with poly(a)-binding protein and inhibits translation, *J Virol* 82:4284, 2008.
480. Adamo MP, Zapeta M, Frey TK: Analysis of gene expression in fetal and adult cells infected with rubella virus, *Virology* 370:1, 2007.
481. Reimer CB, Black CM, Phillips DJ, et al: The specificity of fetal IgM. Antibody or anti-antibody, *Ann N Y Acad Sci* 254:77, 1975.
482. Robertson PW, Kertesz V, Cloonan MJ: Elimination of false-positive cytomegalovirus immunoglobulin M-fluorescent-antibody reactions with immunoglobulin M serum fractions, *J Clin Microbiol* 6:174, 1977.
483. Altshuler G: Placentitis with a new light on an old TORCH, *Obstet Gynecol Ann* 6:197, 1977.
484. Garcia AGP, Marques RL, Lobato YY, et al: Placental pathology in congenital rubella, *Placenta* 6:281, 1985.
485. Krugman S: Rubella. In Krugman S, editor: *Infectious diseases of children*, St. Louis, 1985, Mosby.
486. Sheinis M, Sarov I, Maor E, Gorodischer R: Severe neonatal rubella following maternal infection, *Pediatr Infect Dis* 4:202, 1985.
487. Judelsohn RG, Wyll SA: Rubella in Bermuda: termination of an epidemic by mass vaccination, *JAMA* 223:401, 1973.
488. Ben AN, Benrhouma H, Rouissi A, et al: [Epidemic of rubella encephalitis], *Arch Pediatr* 20:858, 2013.
489. Fujimoto T, Katoh C, Hayakawa H, et al: Two cases of rubella infection with cardiac involvement, *Jpn Heart J* 20:227, 1979.
490. Saeed AA, Lange LS: Guillain-Barré syndrome after rubella, *Postgrad Med J* 54:333, 1978.
491. Callaghan N, Feely M, Walsh B: Relapsing neurological disorder associated with rubella virus infection in two sisters, *J Neurol Neurosurg Psychiatry* 40:1117, 1977.
492. Connolly JH, Hutchinson WM, Allen IV, et al: Carotid artery thrombosis, encephalitis, myelitis and optic neuritis associated with rubella virus infections, *Brain* 98:583, 1975.
493. Choutet P, Binet CH, Goudeau A, et al: Bone-marrow aplasia and primary rubella infection, *Lancet* 2:966, 1979.
494. Plotkin SA: Rubella vaccine. In Plotkin SA, Orenstein WA, Offit PA, editors: *Vaccines*, ed 5, Philadelphia, 2008, Saunders.
495. Townsend JJ, Baringer JR, Wolinsky JS, et al: Progressive rubella panencephalitis: late onset after congenital rubella, *N Engl J Med* 292:990, 1975.
496. Waxham MN, Wolinsky JS: Rubella virus and its effect on the nervous system, *Neurol Clin* 2:267, 1984.
497. Schlossberg D, Topolosky MR: Military rubella, *JAMA* 238:1273, 1974.
498. Preblud SR, Dobbs HI, Sedmak GV, et al: Testalgia associated with rubella infection, *South Med J* 73:594, 1980.
499. Quentin CD, Reiber H: Fuchs heterochromic cyclitis: rubella virus antibodies and genome in aqueous humor, *Am J Ophthalmol* 138:46, 2004.
500. Gordon L: Fuch's heterochromic cyclitis: new clues regarding pathogenesis, *Am J Ophthalmol* 138:133, 2004.
501. de Groot-Mijnes JD, de Visser L, Rothova A, et al: Rubella virus is associated with Fuchs heterochromic iridocyclitis, *Am J Ophthalmol* 141:212, 2006.
502. Rothova A: The riddle of Fuchs heterochromic uveitis, *Am J Ophthalmol* 144:447, 2007.
503. Van Gelder RN: Idiopathic no more: clues to the pathogenesis of Fuchs heterochromic iridocyclitis and glaucomatocyclitic crisis, *Am J Ophthalmol* 145:769, 2008.
504. Siemerink MJ, Sijssens KM, de Groot-Mijnes JD, de Boer JH: Rubella virus-associated uveitis in a nonvaccinated child, *Am J Ophthalmol* 143:899, 2007.
505. Winchester SA, Varga Z, Parmar D, Brown KE: Persistent intraocular rubella infection in a patient with Fuchs' uveitis and congenital rubella syndrome, *J Clin Microbiol* 51:1622, 2013.
506. White LR, Sever JL, Alepa FP: Maternal and congenital rubella before 1964: frequency, clinical features, and search for isoimmune phenomena, *Pediatrics* 74:198, 1969.
507. Cooper LZ: Rubella: a preventable cause of birth defects. In Bergsma D, editor: *Birth defects original article series*, vol. 4 no. 5, New York, 1968, National Foundation–March of Dimes, p 1968.
508. Cooper LZ, Green RH, Krugman S, et al: Neonatal thrombocytopenic purpura and other manifestations of rubella contracted in utero, *Am J Dis Child* 110:416, 1965.
509. Zinkham WH, Medearis DN, Osborn JE: Blood and bone marrow findings in congenital rubella, *J Pediatr* 71:512, 1967.
510. Rudolph AJ, Singleton EB, Rosenberg HS, et al: Osseous manifestations of the congenital rubella syndrome, *Am J Dis Child* 110:428, 1965.
511. Rabinowitz JG, Wolf BS, Greenberg EI, Rausen AR: Osseous changes in rubella embryopathy, *Radiology* 85:494, 1965.
512. Wall WL, Altman DH, Gair DR, Litt RE: Roentgenological findings in congenital rubella, *Clin Pediatr* 4:704, 1965.
513. Reed GB Jr: Rubella bone lesions, *J Pediatr* 74:208, 1969.
514. Korones SB, Ainger LE, Monif GR, et al: Congenital rubella syndrome: study of 22 infants, *Am J Dis Child* 110:434, 1965.
515. Rorke LB, Spiro AJ: Cerebral lesions in congenital rubella syndrome, *J Pediatr* 70:243, 1967.
516. Streissguth AP, Vanderveer BB, Shepard TH: Mental development of children with congenital rubella syndrome: a preliminary report, *Am J Obstet Gynecol* 108:391, 1970.
517. Rowen M, Singer MI, Moran ET: Intracranial calcification in the congenital rubella syndrome, *AJR Am J Roentgenol* 115:86, 1972.
518. Peters ER, Davis RL: Congenital rubella syndrome: cerebral mineralizations and subperiosteal new bone formation as expressions of this disorder, *Clin Pediatr (Phila)* 5:743, 1966.
519. Hastreiter AR, Joorabchi B, Pujatti G, et al: Cardiovascular lesions associated with congenital rubella, *J Pediatr* 71:59, 1967.
520. Klein HZ, Markarian M: Dermal erythropoiesis in congenital rubella: description of an infected newborn who had purpura associated with marked extramedullary erythropoieses in the skin and elsewhere, *Clin Pediatr (Phila)* 8:604, 1969.
521. Brough AJ, Jones D, Page RH, Mizukami I: Dermal erythropoieses in neonatal infants, *Pediatrics* 40:627, 1967.
522. Achs R, Harper KG, Siegal M: Unusual dermatoglyphic findings associated with the rubella embryopathy, *N Engl J Med* 274:148, 1966.
523. Purvis-Smith SG, Howard PR, Menser MA: Dermatoglyphic defects and rubella teratogenesis, *JAMA* 209:1865, 1969.
524. Murphy AM, Reid RR, Pollard I, et al: Rubella cataracts: further clinical and virologic observations, *Am J Ophthalmol* 64:1109, 1967.
525. Collis WJ, Cohen DN: Rubella retinopathy: a progressive disorder, *Arch Ophthalmol* 84:33, 1970.
526. Kresky B, Nauheim JS: Rubella retinitis, *Am J Dis Child* 113:305, 1967.
527. Schiff GM, Sutherland JM, Light IJ, Bloom JE: Studies on congenital rubella, *Am J Dis Child* 110:441, 1965.
528. Menser MA, Dorman DC, Reye RD, Reid RR: Renal artery stenosis in the rubella syndrome, *Lancet* 1:790, 1966.
529. Menser MA, Robertson SE, Dorman DC, et al: Renal lesions in congenital rubella, *Pediatrics* 40:901, 1967.
530. Kaplan GW, McLaughlin AP 3rd: Urogenital anomalies and congenital rubella syndrome, *Urology* 2:148, 1973.
531. Forrest JM, Menser MA: Congenital rubella in schoolchildren and adolescents, *Arch Dis Child* 45:63, 1970.
532. Korones SB, Ainger Lorin E, Monif Gilles RG, et al: Congenital rubella syndrome: new clinical aspects with recovery of virus from affected infants, *J Pediatr* 67:166, 1965.
533. South MA, Alford CA Jr: The immunology of chronic intrauterine infections. In Stiehm ER, Fulginiti VA, editors: *Immunologic disorders in infants and children*, Philadelphia, 1973, Saunders.
534. Phelan P, Campbell P: Pulmonary complications of rubella embryopathy, *J Pediatr* 75:202, 1969.
535. Fortuin NJ, Morrow AG, Roberts WC: Late vascular manifestations of the rubella syndrome: a roentgenographic-pathologic study, *Am J Med* 51:134, 1971.
536. Karmody GS: Subclinical maternal rubella and congenital deafness. *N Engl J Med* 278:809, 1968.
537. Ames MD, Plotkin SA, Winchester RA, Atkins TE: Central auditory imperception: a significant factor in congenital rubella deafness, *JAMA* 213:419, 1970.

538. Peckham CS, Martin JA, Marshall WC, Dudgeon JA: Congenital rubella deafness: a preventable disease, *Lancet* 1:258, 1979.
539. Rossi M, Ferlito A, Polidoro F: Maternal rubella and hearing impairment in children, *J Laryngol Otol* 94:281, 1980.
540. Weinberger MM, Masland MW, Asbed RA, Sever JL: Congenital rubella presenting as retarded language development, *Am J Dis Child* 120:125, 1970.
541. Menser MA, Forrest JM, Bransby RD: Rubella infection and diabetes mellitus, *Lancet* 1:57, 1978.
542. Takasu N, Ikema T, Komiya I, Mimura G: Forty-year observation of 280 Japanese patients with congenital rubella syndrome, *Diabetes Care* 28:2331, 2005.
543. Hanid TK: Hypothyroidism in congenital rubella, *Lancet* 2:854, 1976.
544. Nieberg PI, Gardner LI: Thyroiditis and congenital rubella syndrome, *J Pediatr* 89:156, 1976.
545. Perez Comas A: Congenital rubella and acquired hypothyroidism secondary to Hashimoto thyroiditis, *J Pediatr* 88:1065, 1976.
546. Ziring PR, Gallo G, Finegold M, Buimovici-Klein E, Ogra P: Chronic lymphocytic thyroiditis: identification of rubella virus antigen in the thyroid of a child with congenital rubella, *J Pediatr* 90:419, 1977.
547. AvRuskin TW, Brakin M, Juan C: Congenital rubella and myxedema, *Pediatrics* 69:495, 1982.
548. Ziring PR, Fedun BA, Cooper LZ: Thyrotoxicosis in congenital rubella, *J Pediatr* 87:1002, 1975.
549. Preece MA, Kearney PJ, Marshall WC: Growth hormone deficiency in congenital rubella, *Lancet* 2:842, 1977.
550. Oberfield SE, Casullo AM, Chiriboga-Klein S, et al: Growth hormone dynamics in congenital rubella syndrome, *Brain Dysfunct* 1:303, 1988.
551. Anderson H, Barr B, Wedenberg E: Genetic disposition—a prerequisite for maternal rubella deafness, *Arch Otolaryngol* 91:141, 1970.
552. Boger WP 3rd: Late ocular complications in congenital rubella syndrome, *Ophthalmology* 87:1244, 1980.
553. Boger WP 3rd, Petersen RA, Robb RM: Spontaneous absorption of the lens in the congenital rubella syndrome, *Arch Ophthalmol* 99:433, 1981.
554. Deutman AF, Grizzard WS: Rubella retinopathy and subretinal neovascularization, *Am J Ophthalmol* 85:82, 1978.
555. Frank KE, Purnell EW: Subretinal neovascularization following rubella retinopathy, *Am J Ophthalmol* 86:462, 1978.
556. Orth DH, Fishman GA, Segall M, et al: Rubella maculopathy, *Br J Ophthalmol* 64:201, 1980.
557. Wolinsky JS, Dau PC, Buimovici-Klein E, et al: Progressive rubella panencephalitis: immunovirological studies and results of isoprinosine therapy, *Clin Exp Immunol* 35:397, 1979.
558. Schiff GM, Dine MS: Transmission of rubella from newborns: a controlled study among young adult women and report of an unusual case, *Am J Dis Child* 110:447, 1965.
559. Boger WP 3rd, Petersen RA, Robb RM: Keratoconus and acute hydrops in mentally retarded patients with congenital rubella syndrome, *Am J Ophthalmol* 91:231, 1981.
560. Palacin PS, Castilla Y, Garzón P, et al: Congenital rubella syndrome, hyper-IgM syndrome and autoimmunity in an 18-year-old girl, *J Paediatr Child Health* 43:716, 2007.
561. Chiriboga-Klein S, Oberfield SE, Casullo AM, et al: Growth in congenital rubella syndrome and correlation with clinical manifestations, *J Pediatr* 115:251, 1989.
562. Desmond MM, Fisher ES, Vorderman AL, et al: The longitudinal course of congenital rubella encephalitis in nonretarded children, *J Pediatr* 93:584, 1978.
563. McIntosh ED, Menser MA: A fifty-year follow-up of congenital rubella, *Lancet* 340:414, 1992.
564. Robinson JL, Lee BE, Preiksaitis JK, et al: Prevention of congenital rubella syndrome—what makes sense in 2006? *Epidemiol Rev* 28:81, 2006.
565. Skendzel LP: Rubella immunity. Defining the level of protective antibody, *Am J Clin Pathol* 106:170, 1996.
566. Dontigny L, Arsenault MY, Martel MJ, et al: Rubella in pregnancy, *J Obstet Gynaecol Can* 30:152, 2008.
567. Preblud SR, Kushubar R, Friedman HM: Rubella hemagglutination inhibition titers, *JAMA* 247:1181, 1982.
568. Helfand RF, Cabezas C, Abernathy E, et al: Dried blood spots versus sera for detection of rubella virus-specific immunoglobulin M (IgM) and IgG in samples collected during a rubella outbreak in Peru, *Clin Vaccine Immunol* 14:1522, 2007.
569. Hardelid P, Williams D, Dezateux C, et al: Agreement of rubella IgG antibody measured in serum and dried blood spots using two commercial enzyme-linked immunosorbent assays, *J Med Virol* 80:360, 2008.
570. Wilson KM, Di Camillo C, Doughty L, Dax EM: Humoral immune response to primary rubella virus infection, *Clin Vaccine Immunol* 13:380, 2006.
571. Vauloup-Fellous C, Grangeot-Keros L: Humoral immune response after primary rubella virus infection and after vaccination, *Clin Vaccine Immunol* 14:644, 2007.
572. Centers for Disease Control and Prevention: Revised ACIP recommendation for avoiding pregnancy after receiving a rubella-containing vaccine, *MMWR Morb Mortal Wkly Rep* 50:1117, 2001.
573. Munro ND, Wild NJ, Sheppard S, et al: Fall and rise of immunity to rubella, *Br Med J (Clin Res Ed)* 294:481, 1987.
574. Hoskins CS, Pyman C, Wilkins B: The nerve deaf child—intrauterine rubella or not? *Arch Dis Child* 58:327, 1983.
575. Iurio JL, Hoskins CS, Pyman C: Retrospective diagnosis of congenital rubella, *Br Med J (Clin Res Ed)* 289:1566, 1984.
576. Vesikari T, Meurman OH, Maki R: Persistent rubella-specific IgM-antibody in the cerebrospinal fluid of a child with congenital rubella, *Arch Dis Child* 55:46, 1980.
577. Fitzgerald MG, Pullen GR, Hosking CS: Low affinity antibody to rubella antigen in patients after rubella infection in utero, *Pediatrics* 81:812, 1988.
578. Alestig K, Bartsch FK, Nilsson LA, Strannegard O: Studies of amniotic fluid in women infected with rubella, *J Infect Dis* 129:79, 1974.
579. Levine MJ, Oxman MN, Moore MG, et al: Diagnosis of congenital rubella in utero, *N Engl J Med* 290:1187, 1974.
580. Cederqvist LL, Zervoudakis IA, Ewool LC, et al: Prenatal diagnosis of congenital rubella, *Br Med J* 276:615, 1977.
581. Daffos F, Forestier F, Grangeot-Keros L, et al: Prenatal diagnosis of congenital rubella, *Lancet* 2:1, 1984.
582. Terry GM, Ho-Terry L, Warren RC, et al: First trimester prenatal diagnosis of congenital rubella: a laboratory investigation, *Br Med J (Clin Res Ed)* 292:930, 1986.
583. Enders G, Jonatha W: Prenatal diagnosis of intrauterine rubella, *Infection* 15:162, 1987.
584. Ho-Terry L, Terry GM, Londesborough P, et al: Diagnosis of fetal rubella infection by nucleic acid hybridization, *J Med Virol* 24:175, 1988.
585. Bosma TJ, Corbett KM, O'Shea S, et al: PCR for detection of rubella virus RNA in clinical samples, *J Clin Microbiol* 33:1075, 1995.
586. Tanemura M, Suzumori K, Yagami Y, Katow S: Diagnosis of fetal rubella infection with reverse transcription and nested polymerase chain reaction: a study of 34 cases diagnosed in fetuses, *Am J Obstet. Gynecol* 174:578, 1996.
587. McDonald JC: Gamma-globulin for prevention of rubella in pregnancy, *Br Med J* 2:416, 1963.
588. Brody JA, Sever JL, Schiff GM: Prevention of rubella by gamma globulin during an epidemic in Barrow, Alaska, in 1964, *N Engl J Med* 272:127, 1965.
589. McCallin PF, Fuccillo DA, Ley AC, et al: Gammaglobulin as prophylaxis against rubella-induced congenital anomalies, *Obstet Gynecol* 39:185, 1972.
590. Urquhart GED, Crawford RJ, Wallace J: Trial of high-titre human rubella immunoglobulin, *Br Med J* 2:1331, 1978.
591. Schiff GM, Sever JL, Huebner RJ: Rubella virus: neutralizing antibody in commercial gamma globulin, *Science* 142:58, 1963.
592. Armstrong RD, Sinclair A, O'Keeffe G, Grahame R: Interferon treatment of chronic rubella associated arthritis, *Clin Exp Rheumatol* 3:93, 1985.
593. Arvin AM, Schmidt NJ, Cantell K, Merigan TC: Alpha interferon administration to infants with congenital rubella, *Antimicrob Agents Chemother* 21:259, 1982.
594. Larsson A, Forsgren M, Hård AF, Segerstad S, et al: Administration of interferon to an infant with congenital rubella syndrome involving persistent viremia and cutaneous vasculitis, *Acta Paediatr Scand* 65:105, 1976.
595. Jan JE, Tingle AJ, Donald G, et al: Progressive rubella panencephalitis: clinical course and response to "Isoprinosine", *Dev Med Child Neurol* 21:648, 1979.
596. Garner JS, Simmons BP: CDC guidelines for isolation precautions in hospitals, *Infect Control* 4:245, 1983.
597. Reef SE, Reed S: *Manual for the surveillance of vaccine-preventable diseases*, Atlanta, 2008, Centers for Disease Control and Prevention.

598. Williams WW: CDC guidelines for infection control in hospital personnel, *Infect Control* 4:326, 1983.
599. Schoenbaum SC, Hyde JN Jr, Bartoshesky L, Crampton K: Benefit-cost analysis of rubella vaccination policy, *N Engl J Med* 294:306, 1976.
600. Furukawa T, Miyata T, Kondo K, et al: Clinical trials of RA 27/3 (Wistar) rubella vaccine in Japan, *Am J Dis Child.* 118:262, 1969.
601. Vaheri A, Vesikari T, Oker-Blom N, et al: Transmission of attenuated rubella vaccines to the human fetus: a preliminary report, *Am J Dis Child* 118:243, 1969.
602. Fleet WF Jr, Benz EW Jr, Karzon DT, et al: Fetal consequences of maternal rubella immunization, *JAMA* 227:621, 1974.
603. Vyse AJ, Gay NJ, White JM, et al: Evolution of surveillance of measles, mumps, and rubella in England and Wales: providing the platform for evidence-based vaccination policy, *Epidemiol Rev* 24:125, 2002.
604. Castillo-Solorzano C, Carrasco P, Tambini G, et al: New horizons in the control of rubella and prevention of congenital rubella syndrome in the Americas, *J Infect Dis* 187(Suppl 1):S146, 2003.
605. Rubella vaccines: WHO position paper, *Wkly Epidemiol Rec* 86:301, 2011.
606. Andrus JK, de Quadros CA, Solorzano CC, Periago MR, Henderson DA: Measles and rubella eradication in the Americas, *Vaccine* 29(Suppl 4):D91, 2004.
607. Gao Z, Wood JG, Burgess MA, et al: Models of strategies for control of rubella and congenital rubella syndrome—a 40 year experience from Australia, *Vaccine* 3:691, 2004.
608. Babigumira JB, Morgan I, Levin A: Health economics of rubella: a systematic review to assess the value of rubella vaccination, *BMC Public Health* 13:406, 2013.
609. Berger BE, Navar-Boggan AM, Omer SB: Congenital rubella syndrome and autism spectrum disorder prevented by rubella vaccination United States, 2001-2010, *BMC Public Health* 11:340, 2011.
610. Plotkin SA, Cornfeld D, Ingalls TH: Studies of immunization with living rubella virus: trials in children with a strain cultured from an aborted fetus, *Am J Dis Child* 110:381, 1965.
611. Freestone DS: Clinical trials carried out to assess non-parenteral routes for administration of Wistar RA 27/3 strain live attenuated rubella vaccine, *Dev Biol Stand* 33:237, 1976.
612. Ganguly R, Ogra PL, Regas S, Waldman RH: Rubella immunization of volunteers via the respiratory tract, *Infect Immun* 8:497, 1973.
613. Weibel RE, Carlson AJ Jr, Villarejos VM, et al: Clinical and laboratory studies of combined live measles, mumps, and rubella vaccines using the RA 27/3 rubella virus, *Proc Soc Exp Biol Med* 165:323, 1980.
614. Orenstein WA, Herrmann KL, Holmgreen P, et al: Prevalence of rubella antibodies in Massachusetts schoolchildren, *Am J Epidemiol* 124:290, 1986.
615. Rutledge SL, Snead OC 3rd: Neurologic complications of immunizations, *J Pediatr* 109:917, 1986.
616. Losonsky GA, Fishaut JM, Strussenberg J, Ogra PL: Effect of immunization against rubella on lactation products. I. Development and characterization of specific immunologic reactivity in breast milk, *J Infect Dis* 145:654, 1982.
617. Losonsky GA, Fishaut JM, Strussenberg J, Ogra PL: Effect of immunization against rubella on lactation products. II. Maternal-neonatal interactions, *J Infect Dis* 145:661, 1982.
618. de Haas R, van den Hof S, Berbers GA, et al: Prevalence of antibodies against rubella virus in The Netherlands 9 years after changing from selective to mass vaccination, *Epidemiol Infect* 123:263, 1999.
619. Mossong J, Putz L, Schneider F: Seroprevalence of measles, mumps and rubella antibodies in Luxembourg: results from a national cross-sectional study, *Epidemiol Infect* 132:11, 2004.
620. Al Mazrou YY, Khalil MK, Tischer A, et al: Serosurvey of measles, mumps and rubella antibodies in Saudi children, *Saudi Med J* 26:1551, 2005.
621. Zanetta DM, Cabrera EM, Azevedo RS, et al: Seroprevalence of rubella antibodies in the State of São Paulo, Brazil, 8 years after the introduction of vaccine, *Vaccine* 21:25, 2003.
622. Kremer JR, Schneider F, Muller CP: Waning antibodies to measles and rubella vaccinees—a longitudinal study, *Vaccine* 24:2594, 2006.
623. Best JM: Rubella vaccines: past, present and future, *Epidemiol Infect* 107:17, 1999.
624. Vandermeulen C, Mathieu R, Geert LR, et al: Long-term persistence of antibodies after one or two doses of MMR-vaccine, *Vaccine* 25:6672, 2007.
625. Davidkin I, Jokinen S, Broman M, et al: Persistence of measles, mumps, and rubella antibodies in an MMR-vaccinated cohort: a 20-year follow-up, *J Infect Dis* 197:950, 2008.
626. Eick AA, Hu Z, Wang Z, Nevin RL: Incidence of mumps and immunity to measles, mumps and rubella among US military recruits, 2000-2004, *Vaccine* 26:494, 2008.
627. Mortimer PP, Edwards JM, Porter AD, et al: Are many women immunized against rubella unnecessarily? *J Hyg (Lond.)* 87:131, 1981.
628. Lin CC, Yang CY, Shih YL, et al: Persistence and titer changes of rubella virus antibodies in primiparous women who had been vaccinated with strain RA 27/3 in junior high school, *Clin Vaccine Immunol* 19:1, 2012.
629. Latner DR, McGrew M, Williams N, et al: Enzyme-linked immunospot assay detection of mumps-specific antibody-secreting B cells as an alternative method of laboratory diagnosis, *Clin Vaccine Immunol* 18:35, 2011.
630. Institute of Medicine: *Adverse effects of vaccines: evidence and causality*, Washington, DC, 2011, National Academies Press.
631. Heijstek MW, Kamphuis S, Armbrust W, et al: Effects of the live attenuated measles-mumps-rubella booster vaccination on disease activity in patients with juvenile idiopathic arthritis: a randomized trial, *JAMA* 309:2449, 2013.
632. Gualberto FA, Curti SP, de Oliveira MI, Moraes-Vasconcelos D, Figueiredo CA: Intermittent rash, lymph node swelling, arthralgia and vaccinal viral detection after rubella immunization, *J Clin Virol* 56:93, 2013.
633. Ferrini W, Aubert V, Balmer A, Munier FL, Abouzeid H: Anterior uveitis and cataract after rubella vaccination: a case report of a 12-month-old girl, *Pediatrics* 132:e1035, 2013.
634. Gualberto FA, de Oliveira MI, Alves VA, et al: Fulminant encephalitis associated with a vaccine strain of rubella virus, *J Clin Virol* 58:737, 2013.
635. Landes RD, Bass JW, Millunchick EW, Oetgen WJ: Neonatal rubella following maternal immunization, *J Pediatr* 97:465, 1980.
636. da Silva GR, Camacho LA, Siqueira MM: Seroepidemiological profile of pregnant women after inadvertent rubella vaccination in the state of Rio de Janeiro, Brazil, 2001-2002, *Rev Panam Salud Publica* 19:371, 2006.
637. Minussi L, Mohrdieck R, Bercini M, et al: Prospective evaluation of pregnant women vaccinated against rubella in southern Brazil, *Reprod Toxicol* 25:120, 2008.
638. Soares RC, Siqueira MM, Toscano CM, et al: Follow-up study of unknowingly pregnant women vaccinated against rubella in Brazil, 2001-2002, *J Infect Dis* 204(Suppl 2):S729, 2011.
639. Badilla X, Morice A, Avila-Aguero ML, et al: Fetal risk associated with rubella vaccination during pregnancy, *Pediatr Infect Dis J* 26:830, 2007.
640. Centers for Disease Control and Prevention: Immunization practices in colleges—United States, *MMWR Morb Mortal Wkly Rep* 36:209, 1987.
641. Edgar WM, Hambling MH: Rubella vaccination and anti-D immunoglobulin administration in the puerperium, *Br J Obstet Gynaecol* 84:754, 1977.
642. Watt RW, McGucken RB: Failure of rubella immunization after blood transfusion: birth of congenitally infected infant, *Br Med J* 281:977, 1980.
643. Black NA, Parsons A, Kurtz JB, et al: Post-pubertal rubella immunisation: a controlled trial of two vaccines, *Lancet* 2:990, 1983.
644. Bloom S, Rguig A, Berraho A, et al: Congenital rubella syndrome burden in Morocco: a rapid retrospective assessment, *Lancet* 365:135, 2005.
645. Preblud PR, Gross F, Halsey NA, et al: Assessment of susceptibility to measles and rubella, *JAMA* 247:1134, 1982.

30 Less Common Viral Infections

JULIA A. MCMILLAN and YVONNE A. MALDONADO

CHAPTER OUTLINE

Human Papillomavirus

Human papillomaviruses (HPV) are the most common cause of sexually transmitted infection in the United States, with approximately 14 million new infections annually, according to the Centers for Disease Control and Prevention (CDC).[1] These DNA viruses are the cause of condyloma acuminata (i.e., genital warts), cervical condylomata, and cervical cancer, but most infections are asymptomatic and resolve spontaneously within 2 years.[2,3] More than 40 human HPV serotypes have been found to infect the anogenital tract, and at least 12 serotypes are regarded as carcinogenic. Of these, serotypes 16 and 18 account for greater than 70% of cervical cancer worldwide, and serotypes 6 and 11 account for greater than 90% of anogenital warts (condylomata acuminata).[4,5] The 2011 National Health and Nutrition Study found that greater than 40% of women in the United States were infected with at least one serotype of HPV, and that women in the 20- to 25-year age group were most likely to be infected.[6]

The infant born to a mother with HPV infection is at risk for development of juvenile laryngeal papillomatosis and/or of anogenital warts, primarily because of HPV serotypes 6 and 11.[7] Hajek[8] associated the presence of condyloma acuminatum in a mother at the time of delivery with the subsequent development of laryngeal papilloma in her infant (Table 30-1). Cook and colleagues[9] described a similar association in nine children with laryngeal papilloma. Five of the children who developed laryngeal papilloma when younger than 6 months of age were born to mothers who had condylomata acuminata at the time of delivery, and the mothers of two of the other four had genital warts but did not have them at the time of delivery. Seven (78%) of the nine children with laryngeal papilloma had mothers with condylomata acuminata. Six of the nine children also had skin warts. The expected incidence of condylomata acuminata in women in the population studied by Cook and colleagues[9] was 1.5%. Quick and coworkers[10] also described a strong association between laryngeal papilloma in young children and maternal condylomata. Twenty-one (68%) of the 31 patients with laryngeal papilloma they studied had been born to mothers who had had condylomata.

HPV cannot be isolated by tissue culture, but HPV DNA sequences can be detected in cervical cells. HPV can be detected in epithelial cells that have a normal histologic appearance and from tissue samples of patients whose papillomatous lesions are in remission.[11] The frequency of HPV detection has ranged from 5% to 20% in studies of women of childbearing age, with the highest incidence occurring among younger women.[12,13] It has been estimated that greater than 70% of sexually active women will contract HPV during their lifetime, and that the frequency of infection is correlated with the number of sexual partners.[14] Pregnancy has not been associated with a higher rate of infection. Most pregnant women with HPV infection do not have a history of genital warts.

Results of studies investigating the frequency of subclinical transmission from mothers to infants vary widely. The results are likely confounded by the method and site of attempted detection, the quantity of maternal virus, the HPV strain(s) with which the mother is infected, and the duration of infant follow-up. Recent studies using nucleic acid techniques to detect virus have found that 20% to 30% of infants born to HPV-infected mothers are HPV positive early in life, but the strains detected in those infants during the first few weeks of life are generally no longer detected by 6 to 12 months.[15,16,17] Perinatal transmission through exposure to the virus at delivery has been proposed as the means of transmission, but HPV DNA has also been found in cord blood, placenta, and breast milk of mothers whose infants were positive for the same genotype, and papillomatosis has been described in infants delivered by cesarean section.[18]

Despite the prevalence of genital HPV infection, juvenile laryngeal papillomatosis remains a rare disease. The

Table 30-1 Effects of Other Viral Infections of the Fetus and Newborn

Infectious Agent	Increased Incidence of Abortion	Increased Risk of Prematurity	Major Clinical Manifestations in Infants
Human papillomavirus	No	No	Laryngeal papilloma, anogenital warts
Epstein-Barr virus	Possibly	Possibly	?
Human herpes-virus 6	No	No	Febrile illness in postnatal period
Influenza viruses	No	No	Respiratory illness during neonatal period
Respiratory syncytial virus	No	No	Pneumonia, bronchiolitis, in postnatal period
Lymphocytic choriomeningitis virus	Yes	No	Hydrocephalus, chorioretinitis, viral meningitis, jaundice, thrombocytopenia (?)
Molluscum contagiosum virus	No	No	Rash
Rabies	No	No	None known
West Nile Virus	No	No	Meningitis, rash
Smallpox	Yes	Yes	Rash, variable illness
Dengue	Unknown	Possibly	Fever, thrombocytopenia, hepatomegaly, rash, hemorrhage
Chikungunya	Possibly	No	Fever, pain, poor feeding, and rash

incidence of recurrent respiratory papillomatosis is variable, depending upon the epidemiology of HPV infection among women of childbearing age in the population. A national surveillance study in Canada determined that between 1994 and 2007 the incidence was 0.24 per 100,000 children.[19] Others have estimated that the incidence is 7 of every 1000 children born to mothers with vaginal condyloma.[20] Because of the high prevalence of asymptomatic HPV infection, the feasibility of preventing the rare cases of laryngeal papillomatosis by considering maternal condyloma acuminatum as an indication for cesarean delivery is questionable.

Treatment of anogenital warts is not optimal, but podophyllum resin or podofilox is often used in older children and adults. Neither has been tested for safety or efficacy in children, and both are contraindicated for use in pregnancy. Laryngeal papillomas recur even after repeated surgical removal. Interferon has been used with some success for treatment of laryngeal papillomas.[21,22] Although the mainstay of surgical management has traditionally been the carbon dioxide laser,[23] newer surgical techniques have demonstrated efficacy in the management of pediatric patients, including powered instrumentation and the pulse-dye laser. Adjuvant medical therapies used for pediatric recurrent respiratory papillomatosis include topical interferon-α2a, retinoic acid, and indol-3-carbinol diindolylmethane (I3C/DIM). Topical cidofovir has not demonstrated efficacy compared with placebo.[24]

Two HPV vaccines are available for the prevention, but not therapy, of HPV infection. One vaccine is protective against the two most common serotypes associated with cervical cancer (HPV serotypes 16 and 18) as well as the two most common serotypes associated with anogenital warts (HPV serotypes 6 and 11); this vaccine is licensed in the United States for use in females and males 9 to 26 years of age. A second vaccine protects only against HPV serotypes 16 and 18 associated with cervical cancer and is licensed only for females 10 to 25 years of age. Although two approaches, preventive and therapeutic, have been pursued for HPV vaccines, to date only preventive vaccines, which evoke a robust neutralizing antibody response to selected HPV serotype, have been successful. There is evidence from recent epidemiologic studies that implementation of HPV vaccine recommendations have reduced the prevalence of HPV infection.[24,25] Further research to develop therapeutic vaccines that generate cytotoxic T lymphocytes and destroy HPV-infected neoplastic cells is underway.[26]

Epstein-Barr Virus

Epstein-Barr virus (EBV) is a human herpesvirus that is most familiar as the cause of infectious mononucleosis; however, most women of childbearing age have been infected asymptomatically in childhood. Because EBV cannot be isolated directly in tissue culture, serologic tests are used to detect recent primary or past infection.

Persons infected with EBV form immunoglobulin G (IgG) and IgM antibodies to viral capsid antigens (VCAs) soon after infection.[27] About 80% form antibodies to early antigens (EAs), which usually fall to undetectable levels 6 months after infection. The presence of antibodies to EAs at later times after acute infection may indicate viral reactivation.[28] Antibodies to EBV-associated nuclear antigen (EBNA) develop weeks to months after primary infection in most people and probably persist for life, as do IgG antibodies to VCAs.

Prospective studies using antibodies to EAs as a marker of recent maternal EBV infection have yielded conflicting results. In a group of 719 women evaluated by Icart and Didier,[29] pregnancies resulting in early fetal death, birth of infants with a congenital abnormality, prematurity or intrauterine growth retardation, and deaths or illnesses during the first week of life were more common in women who were EA antibody positive during the first 3 months of pregnancy than in those who were not. Whether these women had a recent primary EBV infection or reactivation of an infection cannot be determined. In contrast, Fleisher and Bolognese[30] found that the frequency of antibodies to EA in pregnant women was 55%, compared with 22% to 32% among nonpregnant adults, but the incidence of low birth weight, neonatal jaundice, or congenital anomalies was not increased among infants of women with anti-EA antibodies. Esklid and colleagues[31] found no association between EBV reactivation after the first trimester of pregnancy and the likelihood of fetal death in a large Norwegian cohort, but in their study, pregnancy was shorter and birth weight was lower for infants born to mothers found to have high levels of IgM antibody against EA during pregnancy.

The rate of congenital anomalies was not determined. Avgil and colleagues[32] found no difference in pregnancy outcome, including miscarriage, prematurity, birth weight, or congenital anomalies for 126 women who had serologic evidence of primary or reactivated EBV infection during pregnancy, compared with 1434 control women. Primary EBV infection during pregnancy is unusual[33] because only 3.0% to 3.4% of pregnant women are susceptible.[31,34] Recent primary EBV infection is diagnosed by the presence of VCA IgG and IgM antibodies in the absence of antibodies to EBV-associated nuclear antigen.[35] Among six women who had primary EBV infections during pregnancy, as established by the presence of IgM antibody to VCA and the absence of antibody to EBNA in their sera, only one had symptoms compatible with mononucleosis during pregnancy; she gave birth to a normal infant.[36] Four of the remaining five pregnancies terminated abnormally. One woman had a spontaneous abortion, and the other three were delivered of premature infants. All three of the premature infants were abnormal. One was stillborn, one had multiple congenital anomalies, and one was small for gestational age. The products of abortion and the premature infants were not studied for evidence of an EBV infection. The abnormal infants in this study did not have a characteristic syndrome but instead had a variety of abnormalities.

Fleisher and Bolognese[37] identified three infants born to women who had had silent EBV seroconversion during the first trimester. Two infants were normal; one infant had tricuspid atresia. EBV IgM was not detected in cord blood serum, and EBV was not recovered from the cord blood lymphocytes. Three infants of mothers with a primary EBV infection and infectious mononucleosis were normal at birth and had no serologic or virologic evidence of intrauterine infection.[38]

Early reports implicated EBV as a cause of congenital anomalies, particularly congenital heart disease; however, Tallqvist and colleagues[39] were unable to detect an increase in incidence of antibodies to EBV in 6- to 23-month-old children with congenital heart disease compared with normal, age-matched controls. EBV may cause congenital heart disease in an individual case, but this study suggests that it is not a common cause of cardiac defects. Goldberg and associates[40] described an infant born with hypotonia, micrognathia, bilateral cataracts, metaphyseal lucencies, and thrombocytopenia. Immunologic evidence suggesting possible EBV infection included an elevated total IgM level, the presence of IgM anti-VCA antibody at 22 days of age, and a delay in development of anti-EBNA antibody until 42 days of age. Weaver and coworkers[41] described an infant with extrahepatic bile duct atresia and evidence of intrauterine EBV infection; EBV IgM was identified in serum obtained when the infant was 3 and 6 weeks of age, and persistent EBV IgG was seen at 1 year.

Although EBV cannot be recovered by standard tissue culture methods, the virus can be detected by its capacity to transform B lymphocytes into persistent lymphoblastoid cell lines. In studies conducted to identify cases of intrauterine EBV infection, Visintine and colleagues[42] and Chang and Blankenship[43] observed spontaneous transformation of lymphocytes obtained from cord blood, but EBV could not be associated. EBV-transformed cells were not found in any samples of cord blood from 2000 newborns studied by Chang and Seto[44] or from the 25 newborns tested by Joncas and associates.[45,46] One study used nested polymerase chain reaction (PCR) methods for amplifying EBV DNA regions in circulating lymphocytes from 67 mother-infant pairs within 1 week of birth.[47] Approximately 50% of the women and two of the neonates were EBV PCR positive. Visintine and colleagues[42] studied 82 normal-term infants, 28 infants with congenital anomalies, and 29 infants suspected of having congenital infections; they were unable to isolate EBV from any of these infants. Two infants have been described in whom there was evidence of infection with EBV at birth.[46,48] A congenital cytomegalovirus (CMV) infection coexisted in both. Most of the clinical findings in the infants were compatible with those typical of congenital CMV infections and included microcephaly, periventricular calcifications, hepatosplenomegaly, and inclusions characteristic of CMV in sections of tissues or cells in urinary sediments. One infant had deformities of the hands similar to those seen in arthrogryposis. Neither CMV nor EBV was isolated from the saliva or secretions of these infants. In the first infant, IgM antibody to EBV was present at birth and EBNA-positive permanent lymphoblastoid cell lines were established on five occasions between 3 and 30 months of age. In the second infant, permanent lymphoblastoid cell lines were established from the peripheral blood at birth and from postmortem heart blood at 3 days of age. EBNA and EBV RNA were identified in these cells, and CMV DNA was identified in the cells from the liver of the same infant.

Attempts to isolate EBV from secretions obtained from the maternal cervix have been unsuccessful,[42,44] but the virus can be detected at this site by DNA hybridization.[49] There is little evidence suggesting that natal transmission of EBV occurs. However, EBV was recovered from genital ulcers in a young woman with infectious mononucleosis.[50] Fatal EBV infection was diagnosed by DNA hybridization of lymph node tissue from one infant who presented with failure to thrive, emesis, diarrhea, and a macular rash at 14 days of age, but this infection might have been acquired in utero.[51]

EBV can be transmitted to newborns in the perinatal period by blood transfusion.[42,45] Permanent lymphoblastoid lines that contained EBV antigens were established by Joncas and coworkers[45] from the blood of two infants who had been transfused. One of these infants did not develop permanent antibodies to EBV.

There is no convincing evidence at present that EBV causes congenital anomalies. Because the early and the late serologic responses of young infants to a primary EBV infection differ from those found when a primary infection occurs at an older age,[28,45,52] it will be difficult to screen large numbers of newborns for serologic evidence of an EBV infection sustained in utero.

Human Herpesvirus 6

Human herpesvirus 6 (HHV-6) is a member of the Betaherpesvirinae subfamily of herpesviruses; HHV-6 has been identified as a cause of exanthema subitum (i.e., roseola).[53-55] The virus exhibits tropism for T lymphocytes and is most closely related to human CMV by genetic analysis.[56]

Seroepidemiologic studies have shown that HHV-6 is ubiquitous in the human population, regardless of geographic area, and that it infects greater than 90% of infants during the first year of life.[57-59] IgG antibodies to HHV-6 are detected in almost all infants at birth, with a subsequent decline in seropositivity rates by 4 to 6 months of age as transplacentally acquired antibody is lost. The highest rate of acquisition of HHV-6 infection appears to occur during the first 6 months to 1 year of life as maternal antibodies wane.

The seroepidemiologic evidence and restriction enzyme analysis of paired virus isolates from mothers and their infants suggest that the usual route of transmission is perinatal or postnatal.[60] HHV-6 is present in the cord bloods of approximately 1% of newborns[61,62], and HHV-6 genome was found in the amniotic fluid of a similar proportion (7/729) of pregnancies.[63] Hall and colleagues[64] have demonstrated that the majority of congenitally acquired infection is transmitted as chromosomally integrated HHV-6 transmitted from a parent, and in those cases, HHV-6 DNA can be demonstrated in all tissues tested. Among 43 infants with congenital infection, they found evidence of chromosomal integration in 86%, whereas the remaining 14% had acquired their infection transplacentally. Cord blood anti–HHV-6 antibodies were similar whether the infection was chromosomally integrated or transplacentally acquired.

Primary HHV-6 infection should be rare during pregnancy because almost all adult women have been infected in childhood. One case of a spontaneous abortion has been described in a woman who was seronegative to HHV-6 at the beginning of pregnancy and had developed anti-HHV-6 antibody by the time of the pregnancy loss. HHV-6 was detected by PCR assay in fetal tissues, the placenta, umbilical cord blood, and maternal serum.[65] Symptoms attributable to congenital HHV-6 infection have been only rarely described in live-born infants. Lanari and colleagues[66] described a term newborn who developed seizures during the first few hours of life and was found to have HHV-6 DNA in the cerebrospinal fluid (CSF) on day 2. The infant developed evidence of neurologic compromise with developmental delay. Evidence of reinfection after presumed congenital HHV-6 infection also has been demonstrated.[67]

In addition to the roseola syndrome, HHV-6 has been detected by PCR in peripheral blood lymphocytes obtained from infants younger than 3 months who had acute, nonspecific, febrile illnesses.[68,69] Two neonates who had fulminant hepatitis associated with HHV-6 infection have been described.[70,71] Other associations found among infants include a mononucleosis-like syndrome,[72] pneumonitis,[73,74] and one case report of possible immunodeficiency and pneumonitis associated with HHV-6 infection.[74] However, all clinical associations between disease in infants and HHV-6 infection must be evaluated with care because of the evidence that most infants become infected with this virus within a few months after birth and that the virus persists after primary infection, as is characteristic of herpesviruses. In an attempt to identify clinical symptoms related to HHV-6 infection, Rentz and colleagues[75] tested infants hospitalized in their neonatal intensive care unit for HHV-6 and compared clinical findings in 12 infants whose plasma was positive for HHV-6 DNA with 144 HHV-6–negative infants. In this small study, no significant differences were found in clinical characteristics of the two groups.

Human Herpesvirus 7

Human herpesvirus 7 (HHV-7) was discovered in the peripheral blood lymphocytes of a healthy adult in 1990.[76] Like HHV-6, HHV-7 belongs to the *Roseolovirus* genus within the Betaherpesvirinae subfamily, along with HHV-6 and CMV. Like HHV-6, it causes primary infection in most individuals during childhood. However, clinically symptomatic infection with HHV-7 appears to be significantly less common and occurs later in life than HHV-6.[77-79]

The average age at infection is about 2 years, and 75% of children are seropositive by 5 years of age. The primary mechanism of transmission is from contact with saliva of infected individuals. Because HHV-7 DNA has been detected in breast milk, breastfeeding may be another source of infection.[80] However, antibodies to HHV-7 in breast milk may protect against infection, and in one study, breastfeeding was associated with a lower risk of early acquisition of HHV-7 infection.[81] HHV-7 DNA has been detected in 2.7% of cervical swabs obtained from women in their third trimester of pregnancy but from none of the swabs of control women, suggesting that pregnancy may be associated with reactivation of HHV-7.[82] However, perinatal transmission from contact with infected maternal secretions is unknown, and neonatal infections with HHV-7 have not been reported.[83] Clinical symptoms are rarely associated with HHV-7 infection but include nonspecific fever, with or without rash, which resembles exanthema subitum.[84-89] Clinically apparent HHV-7 infections appear to have a high rate of central nervous system (CNS) involvement.[90]

Influenza A and B

Early investigations of the teratogenic potential of influenza virus were epidemiologic studies in which the diagnosis of influenza was not confirmed serologically.[91] Some of those studies suggested that infants born to mothers who experienced clinical influenza infection during pregnancy were more likely to be born with congenital anomalies, particularly CNS anomalies, including anencephaly.[92,93] Record[94] and Leck[95] analyzed previously collected data and were unable to find an association between influenza and malformations of the CNS. An increase in congenital defects in infants of mothers who had influenza-like symptoms at 5 to 11 weeks of gestation was reported by Hakosalo and Saxen.[93] Most of these anomalies involved the CNS, but there was no increase in incidence of anencephaly in infants of women who had symptoms compatible with influenza compared with those who remained asymptomatic.

All of these studies were undertaken during influenza epidemics. It was assumed that, under these circumstances, there would be a high correlation between a history of influenza, as elicited from the patient, and infection with influenza virus. MacKenzie and Houghton[96] summarized the reports implicating influenza virus as a cause of maternal morbidity and congenital anomalies and came to the conclusion that probably no association exists between maternal influenza infection and subsequent congenital malformations or neoplasms in childhood.

Several studies have been performed in which influenza infection during pregnancy has been serologically confirmed. Hardy and coworkers[97] reported that the incidence of stillbirths was higher in 332 symptomatic pregnant women with serologically confirmed influenza infections than in 206 women with serologically confirmed infections who had remained asymptomatic or in 73 uninfected women. The control group of uninfected women was smaller than expected because the attack rate during the period of the study was very high. Major congenital anomalies occurred in 5.3% of women whose infections occurred during the first trimester compared with 2.1% of 183 women infected during the second trimester and 1.1% of 275 women infected during the third trimester. Supernumerary digits, syndactyly, and skin anomalies were excluded from these figures. Among infants of mothers infected during the first trimester, cardiac anomalies were the most common type of abnormality; none of these infants had anencephaly. Griffiths and associates[98] observed a slight increase in congenital anomalies in infants born to women who had had serologically confirmed influenza during pregnancy compared with infants of women who had not; however, all of the infants with congenital anomalies were born to women who had had influenza in the second or third trimester, suggesting that congenital infection was an unlikely cause.

Influenza infections during pregnancy are more likely to result in hospitalization for respiratory symptoms in the pregnant woman than in nonpregnant adults. Hartert and associates[99] conducted a matched cohort study of pregnant women to determine pregnancy outcomes associated with respiratory hospitalizations during influenza seasons from 1985 to 1993. During those influenza seasons, 293 pregnant women were hospitalized for respiratory symptoms at a rate of 5.1 per 1000 pregnant women. The prevalence of prematurity and low birth weight was not higher than a matched cohort of pregnant women hospitalized with nonrespiratory diagnoses. However, pregnant women with asthma had higher rates of respiratory hospitalizations than those without asthma, and all of three fetal deaths in this cohort were singleton, late third-trimester, intrauterine fetal deaths in mothers who had asthma and were current smokers. During the 2009 H1N1 influenza pandemic, the CDC requested state and local health departments to report all pregnant women hospitalized with influenza. Over an 8.5-month period in 2009, the CDC received reports of 347 severely ill women, 272 of whom were admitted to intensive care units but survived, and 75 of whom died. Preterm delivery was more common for the women who were severely ill and delivered during their hospitalization, compared with the general population, and infants delivered following their mother's hospitalization for influenza infection were more likely to be born small for gestational age.[100] In this group of very sick women, antiviral therapy was provided earlier for the women who survived. A report from Great Britain of 256 pregnant women hospitalized during the 2009 pandemic described an increase in perinatal mortality compared with the general population, primarily because of an increase in stillbirths.[101]

It can be said with certainty that intrauterine exposure to influenza virus does not cause a consistent syndrome. If there is a cause-and-effect association between influenza virus infections during pregnancy and congenital anomalies, the latter occur with low frequency. Hakosalo and Saxen[93] have documented an increase in the use of nonprescription drugs during influenza outbreaks and have suggested that drugs rather than infection with influenza virus may exert an erratic teratogenic influence. A number of studies have investigated the possible association between influenza infection in pregnant women and subsequent development of bipolar affective disorders or schizophrenia among their offspring, with mixed results.[102-104]

Viremia is rare during influenza infections, but it does occur. Few attempts have been made to demonstrate transplacental passage of the virus to the fetus. Ruben and colleagues[105] tested the cord sera of infants born to 22 mothers who had been pregnant during an influenza A/England/42/72 outbreak and had serologic evidence of infection. All seven infants with evidence of antigenic recognition of influenza virus at birth had uncomplicated deliveries and remained healthy. Influenza A/Bangkok was isolated from the amniotic fluid of a mother with amnionitis and acute influenza infection at 36 weeks of gestation; the infant who was born at 39 weeks of gestation had serologic evidence of infection but was asymptomatic.[106]

Yawn and associates[107] studied a woman who developed influenza in the third trimester and died of pulmonary edema. A virus similar to the prototype strain A_2/Hong Kong/8/68 was isolated from the lung, hilar nodes, heart, spleen, liver, kidney, brain, and spinal cord of the mother and from the amniotic fluid and myocardium of the fetus, which did not survive. Ramphal and colleagues[108] studied another woman who died of complications of an influenza infection at term. A virus similar to strain A/Texas/77 was isolated from maternal tissues, but influenza virus was not isolated from any of the fetal tissues tested.

In contrast to intrauterine infections with influenza virus, which are rare, infections acquired by infants in the neonatal period are common. Passively transferred antibody to influenza virus may prevent symptomatic infections during the first few months of life if it is present in sufficient quantity.[109,110] Outbreaks of influenza virus infection have occurred in neonatal intensive care units. Although some newborns found to be infected during outbreaks remain asymptomatic, others have a variety of respiratory symptoms, including pneumonia.[111,112] Influenza virus infection may be fatal in the neonatal period.[113] In December 2012, the U.S. Food and Drug Administration (FDA) approved the use of oseltamivir for treatment of infants as young as 2 weeks of age. Safety of this drug during the neonatal period had been demonstrated in studies performed during the 2009 H1N1 influenza pandemic.[111,114] Oseltamivir is the only antiviral agent approved for use in newborns, and it is not approved for prophylactic use.

Infants younger than 6 months cannot be protected by influenza vaccine. All health care professionals should receive influenza vaccine annually in the fall. Several studies have demonstrated that immunization of pregnant women provides protection for their newborns exposed to influenza.[115-117] Since 2004, the CDC has recommended that all pregnant women receive influenza vaccine during pregnancy, regardless of the trimester in which it is available.[118]

Respiratory Syncytial Virus

Although respiratory syncytial virus (RSV) is a common cause of upper respiratory tract infection in children and adults, there is no evidence that the virus causes intrauterine infection. Maternal infection has no known adverse effect on the fetus.

RSV infections are frequently acquired by infants during the first few weeks of life and are associated with a high mortality rate, particularly in infants born prematurely.[119] Immaturity of the immune system in premature and very young infants and the small caliber of their airways are both thought to contribute to their susceptibility to severe disease. It is known that passively transmitted maternal antibody plays a role in protecting newborns from infection.[120,121] Two thirds of all infants become infected with RSV in the first year of life, and one third of those will develop lower respiratory tract symptoms, 2.5% will be hospitalized, and 1 in 1000 infants will die as a result of RSV infection. Breastfeeding can be demonstrated to protect against severe RSV infection in developing countries.[122] Because breastfeeding and crowded living conditions affect the incidence of RSV infection in infants, it has been difficult to define effects attributable solely to breastfeeding in the United States. Passive smoke exposure, daycare attendance, presence of older siblings in the household, and lower socioeconomic status have all been found to increase the likelihood of lower respiratory tract infection and hospitalization resulting from RSV infection.[119] Infection with RSV in infants who are younger than 4 weeks may be asymptomatic, consist of an afebrile upper respiratory syndrome, or be accompanied by fever, bronchiolitis or pneumonia, and apnea.[123]

RSV accounted for 55% of cases of viral pneumonia in infants younger than 1 month in one study that evaluated hospitalized infants over a 5-year period.[124] Most infants who died had underlying medical conditions that involved the heart or lungs. Premature infants who have had respiratory distress syndrome and who have bronchopulmonary dysplasia are especially likely to develop severe infections, but it has been reported that morbidity and mortality have also increased among late preterm infants.[125] Infants with underlying neuromuscular difficulties are also thought to be at increased risk.[126] The A subtype of RSV may have the potential to cause more severe disease than the B subtype.[127] There is some evidence that infants born with low cord blood concentrations of vitamin D are at increased risk of developing RSV lower respiratory tract infection.[128]

Nosocomial RSV outbreaks that have occurred in nurseries caring for premature and ill term infants have varied in severity.[129-131] Symptoms, when they occur, can include fever alone, rhinorrhea, apnea, and evidence of lower respiratory tract involvement. Infants who are younger than 1 month have a higher mean maximal titer of virus in their secretions than those who are older.[129] Ninety-six percent of the infected infants studied by Hall and coworkers[129] shed virus for 9 days. Objects contaminated with secretions from infected infants may be important sources of infection in nursery personnel. RSV in infected secretions is viable for up to 6 hours on countertops, for up to 45 minutes on cloth gowns and paper tissues, and for up to 20 minutes on skin.[132,133] Evidence suggests that personnel are at least as important in spreading the infection to infants as are other infected infants housed in the same area and that infection control measures can reduce the risk of transmission.[132,133]

Any hospitalized infant with rhinorrhea, nasal congestion, or unexplained apnea should be segregated and investigated for RSV infection or other pathogens that may produce similar signs and symptoms. Personnel should be made aware that RSV, which causes only mild colds in adults, can cause fatal illnesses in infants. Strict hand hygiene, cohorting of infected infants, requiring gowns, gloves, and masks when entering the room of an infected patient, limiting visitors, and cohorting staff have all been recommended to halt nosocomial spread.[134] Palivizumab, which is recommended for certain high-risk infants to prevent serious RSV lower respiratory tract infection (see later), has been used in some neonatal intensive care unit RSV outbreaks[134,135] and has seemed to halt the spread of infection. There has been no randomized, controlled trial that confirms its effectiveness in this regard, however.

Infants with RSV infection should be supported to ensure adequate hydration and oxygenation. Some infants with RSV-induced bronchiolitis will benefit from inhaled bronchodilator therapy, but bronchodilators are not generally recommended. Similarly, use of corticosteroid therapy for wheezing infants with RSV infection has not been shown to be of benefit and is not recommended for routine use in these patients.[136] Ribavirin, a guanosine analogue that acts by interfering with RSV replication, has been used in an aerosol form to treat infants with severe RSV lower respiratory tract infection, but consistent benefit has not been demonstrated, and its use is limited by the difficulty of administration, concerns about secondary exposure of medical staff, and cost. Therefore ribavirin aerosol therapy is not routinely recommended for RSV infection.[136,137]

There is clear evidence for the benefit of prophylaxis against severe RSV lower respiratory tract infection in infants at high risk for complications by using palivizumab, a humanized anti-RSV monoclonal antibody preparation. Palivizumab administered monthly during the annual RSV season has been shown to reduce the risk of hospitalization related to RSV infection by 39% to 82% in high-risk infants. It is recommended for use during the RSV season for infants born less than 29 weeks of gestation, premature infants with chronic lung disease, some forms of congenital heart disease, congenital airway abnormalities, and some neuromuscular conditions.[137]

Improved survival of infants with RSV infection and underlying cardiopulmonary disease has been reported with advances in intensive care management.[138,139] Nevertheless, families of infants with medical conditions that predispose to severe RSV disease should be advised to avoid the higher risk of exposure associated with group daycare and tobacco smoke.[137] Neonatal RSV infection is known to predispose to subsequent episodes of recurrent wheezing.[140,141] Administration of palivizumab to prevent severe lower respiratory tract RSV infection during the first year of life appears to significantly reduce subsequent episodes of wheezing, even after therapy has ended and after the RSV season has ended.[142]

Table 30-2 Sources of Maternal or Neonatal Infection

Infectious Agent	Other Affected Populations	Vector
Human papillomavirus	Yes	No
Epstein-Barr virus	Yes	No
Human herpesvirus 6	Yes	No
Influenza viruses	Yes	No
Respiratory syncytial virus	Yes	No
Lymphocytic choriomeningitis virus	No	House mice, pet Syrian hamsters, laboratory rats, rabbits
Molluscum contagiosum virus	Yes	No
Rabies	?	Yes
West Nile Virus	No	Yes
Smallpox	Yes	No
Dengue	No	Yes
Chikungunya	No	Yes

Lymphocytic Choriomeningitis Virus

Lymphocytic choriomeningitis virus (LCV) is spread from animals, primarily rodents, to humans. Person-to-person spread has not been described (Table 30-2).[143] Mice and hamsters have most often been implicated as the source of human infections. Mice and hamsters acquire LCV transplacentally or as newborns but remain asymptomatic; however, they shed the virus in large quantities in urine, saliva, feces, and nasal secretions for months.[144,145]

Beyond the neonatal period, human infection with LCV is acquired through contaminated fomites or through inhalation of aerosolized virus. The illness typically is biphasic. Symptoms in the first phase include fever, headache, nausea, vomiting, malaise, and myalgia, lasting as long as a week. After a brief asymptomatic period, many infected individuals will then develop CNS illness ranging from meningitis to severe encephalitis. Unusual manifestations have included orchitis, pneumonitis, parotitis, and pharyngitis. Children and adults generally recover without sequelae after 1 to 3 weeks. Infection is asymptomatic in as many as 30% of infected individuals.[146]

LCV infection during pregnancy may result in spontaneous abortion or congenital infection. Infants who survive in utero infection are at risk to develop chorioretinitis and severe brain injury resulting in hydrocephalus and failure of brain growth.[147-150] Periventricular calcifications can be seen.[151,152] Effects on the brain can include periventricular cysts, porencephalic cysts, encephalomalacia, and neuronal migration disturbances. Clinically, congenital infection can result in intellectual disability, epilepsy, cerebral palsy, and blindness. Less severe consequences of congenital infection have been described, and the variability of damage is thought to be related to the gestational age of the fetus at the time of infection.[153] Unlike other forms of congenital infection, LCV generally does not cause organ-system damage other than to the CNS, birth weight is generally appropriate for gestational age, and rash is uncommon.

The incidence of LCV infection during pregnancy is unknown, as is the frequency of asymptomatic or only mildly symptomatic infection of the fetus. The prevalence of mice in the homes of humans suggests that infection likely occurs more frequently than is appreciated. Epidemiologic studies in Baltimore, Maryland, and Birmingham, Alabama, have found that approximately 5% of healthy adults are seropositive, suggesting past infection.[154,155]

The diagnosis of infection with LCV can be made by isolation of the virus or by serology, but because the virus may not be viable by the time an infant is born, congenital infection is best diagnosed using serology. The immunofluorescent antibody test detects both IgM and IgG and is commercially available for testing CSF and/or serum.[156] The enzyme-linked immunosorbent assay is a more sensitive test but is available only from the CDC. PCR has also been used to identify virus in CSF. LCV infections during pregnancy may be underdiagnosed as causes of congenital infections.[157-160] Ocular and CNS findings may overlap with those of congenital cytomegalovirus and *Toxoplasma* infection. Absence of organomegaly, jaundice, rash, intrauterine growth restriction, and thrombocytopenia can help distinguish congenital LCV from congenital CMV infection. Intracranial calcifications, if they are present, are generally parenchymal in patients with congenital toxoplasmosis, whereas they are typically periventricular in LCV infection, but definitively distinguishing LCV from other causes of congenital infection requires laboratory diagnostic testing. Because apparently healthy mice and hamsters may shed LCV chronically, pregnant women should avoid direct contact with these animals and with their aerosolized excreta. Unless appropriate measures have been taken to ensure that laboratory animals are free of LCV, these precautions should apply to laboratory as well as domestic rodents. Although the total number of intrauterine and perinatal infections from LCV is not large, the incidence of serious sequelae in the infant appears to be high. No treatment is available.

Molluscum Contagiosum

Molluscum contagiosum is a papular rash consisting of multiple discrete lesions that are acanthomas by histologic examination. The skin lesions are caused by a poxlike virus that has been difficult to study because it cannot be propagated in tissue culture. Epidemiologically, molluscum contagiosum is a disease of children and young adults. The virus can be transmitted by sexual conduct, and the incidence increases among adolescents and young adults.

Five women who delivered infants at a time when they had the lesions of molluscum contagiosum in the genital area have been described by Wilkin.[161] None of the infants developed molluscum contagiosum. Mandel and Lewis[162] reported an infant who developed two papules on the thigh when 1 week of age. These enlarged and were excised when the child was 1 year of age. The results of histologic examination and the findings on electron microscopy were compatible with molluscum contagiosum. Another report describes an infant born to a mother with molluscum lesions on her labia majora and inner thighs in the third trimester of pregnancy. Her child, who was born at term and otherwise healthy, was found to have developed more than 50 pearly papules on her face, chest, back, and inner thigh at 9 months of age. The child was treated successfully with topical cantharidin.[163]

The mode of transmission of molluscum contagiosum is not known, but it is thought to occur as an ascending infection after rupture of membranes or through transmission of virus during passage through the birth canal.

Rabies Virus

Transplacental transmission of rabies virus to the human fetus has been described only once,[164] although it is known that transplacental transmission occurs in experimental infections in many species.[165] Several instances of maternal rabies have been reported, and despite the inevitable demise of the mother, infants, other than the one noted by Sipahioglu and Alpaut,[164] have been healthy after receiving rabies immune globulin or vaccine or both.[166-170]

Administration of human rabies immune globulin and rabies vaccine as prophylaxis against rabies in pregnant women appears to be safe for both the mother and the fetus.[171,172] No serious reactions have been reported after administration of this vaccine, and it is possible to achieve titers that are about 10-fold higher than those found after administration of the previously used duck embryo vaccine.

Because of the high likelihood of fatal disease after the bite of a rabid animal, postexposure prophylaxis should always be given. Pregnancy is not a contraindication. When it is necessary to administer prophylaxis to a pregnant woman, human rabies immune globulin and human diploid cell vaccine should be used to minimize potential adverse effects on the pregnancy. After reviewing the available data, the Advisory Committee on Immunization Practices of the CDC has recommended human diploid cell vaccine to rabies virus as a preexposure immunization that is safe for use in pregnant women who will likely be exposed to wild rabies virus before completion of pregnancy.[173]

West Nile Virus

West Nile virus (WNV) is a mosquito-borne flavivirus that has caused epidemic infections in the United States since its introduction in 1999.[174] In 2002, a previously healthy woman at 27 weeks of gestation developed a febrile illness, followed by lower extremity paresis and meningoencephalitis. At 38 weeks of gestation, she delivered an infant with bilateral chorioretinitis and severe, bilateral white matter loss in the temporal and occipital lobes. Maternal, cord, and infant blood samples at birth were positive for WNV-specific IgM and neutralizing antibodies; CSF from the infant was WNV IgM positive; and the placenta was WNV PCR positive.[175,176] In 2003, the CDC established a surveillance registry with state health departments to investigate and assess birth outcomes for infants born to mothers who develop WNV infection during pregnancy. The results of 77 such pregnancies were reported by O'Leary and colleagues.[177] The frequency of preterm delivery, spontaneous abortion, or low birth weight was no higher than expected among infants born to infected mothers. Of 77 infants whose mothers had clinical illness caused by WNV, outcome was reported for 72. Birth defects noted in 10% of the 72 infants included coarctation of the aorta, cleft palate, Down syndrome, polydactyly, and microcephaly; however, none of those conditions could be linked to WNV through serologic testing or the fetal developmental stage at the time of maternal infection. Three of the infants developed WNV infection within a month of birth; in each case, their mothers had become infected near the time of delivery. One of the three, whose mother became ill 6 days before delivery, developed WNV meningitis at 10 days of life but recovered with normal growth and development at 12-months follow-up. Infection postdelivery could not be excluded for this breastfed infant. A second breastfed infant, whose mother had WNV fever at delivery, developed a transient rash. A third infant, whose mother was febrile 3 weeks before delivery, developed seizures at 7 days of life and was found to have WNV encephalitis. Evaluation also revealed lissencephaly, and the infant died at 7 weeks of life.

Since 2003, the CDC has also collected information regarding breastfeeding for mothers experiencing WNV infection during pregnancy or the breastfeeding period.[178] In addition to the two breastfed infants whose mothers experienced WNV infection near delivery (see earlier), six infants who were breastfed by mothers with WNV fever have been reported. Of these six, five remained well and had no serologic evidence of infection, and one, who had no serologic testing performed, developed a transient rash but was otherwise well. Two additional infants developed symptomatic WNV infection while breastfeeding, but in neither case was preceding maternal infection documented. The frequency and concentration of WNV shed in breast milk is not known. Forty-five samples of breast milk and colostrum were tested from women enrolled in the CDC's registry, and only two, collected 50 and 70 days after the onset of illness, were found to have low levels of WNV RNA by PCR. Neither of the infants of these mothers developed infection. WNV IgM was found in 11 colostrum and 3 breast-milk samples.

No specific therapy is available for WNV infection, and the CDC does not recommend WNV screening of asymptomatic pregnant women. Pregnant women who have meningitis, encephalitis, acute flaccid paralysis, or unexplained fever in an area of ongoing WNV transmission should have serum and CSF, if clinically indicated, tested for antibody to WNV. If WNV illness is diagnosed in the pregnant woman, ultrasound examination of the fetus should be considered no sooner than 2 to 4 weeks after maternal onset of illness, and fetal or amniotic fluid testing can be considered. Infants born to women with known or suspected WNV infection during pregnancy should be evaluated for congenital WNV infection. Prevention of WNV infection should include application of insect repellent to skin and clothes when exposed to mosquitoes and avoidance of peak mosquito feeding times at dawn and dusk.[179]

Smallpox

Smallpox is a severe exanthemous clinical disease caused by the variola virus. Variola is a member of the genus *Orthopoxvirus* in the Poxviridae family, a genus that also includes monkeypox, cowpox, and rabbitpox, as well as vaccinia. Variola infection occurs only in humans, a fact that allowed eradication of this infection in the latter part of the 20th century. The global smallpox eradication program used vaccine derived from the relatively benign vaccinia virus. The last case of smallpox in the United States occurred in 1949. In 1980, the world was declared free of smallpox by the World Health Organization (WHO). All variola isolates, except stocks to be maintained in WHO-designated laboratories in the United States and the Soviet Union, were destroyed in 1986.

In 2002, the U.S. Department of Defense initiated a pre-event vaccination program to protect its personnel from possible smallpox exposures, and in 2003, the U.S. Public Health Service began vaccinating health care and public health workers who might be involved in caring for patients with smallpox or investigating circumstances surrounding the use of smallpox as an agent of bioterrorism. It is in this context that discussion of smallpox and vaccinia virus and their potential effects on the mother and fetus have again become a matter of potential concern.

VARIOLA IN PREGNANCY

The mortality rate caused by smallpox among pregnant women was high. The more lethal hemorrhagic form of smallpox was more likely to occur in pregnant women.

Past recorded experience regarding the frequency of transmission of variola from mother to fetus must be considered against the backdrop of near-universal childhood vaccination. Infection during the first half of gestation resulted in an increased likelihood of fetal death or prematurity. Overall, the rate of fetal loss or death after premature delivery ranged from 57% to 81%.[180,181] There are some documented cases of live-born infants infected in utero near term. In those instances, the likelihood of congenital or neonatal infection was greatest when the mother became ill during the period 4 days before delivery through the 9 days after delivery.[182,183] It is thought that transplacental transmission of variola can occur at any time during gestation.

The pattern of rash and the characteristics of individual pox lesions should help distinguish it from other conditions, such as rubella, measles, meningococcemia, rickettsial diseases, rat-bite fever, and enteroviral infections. The rash of smallpox begins as papules, progressing to fluid-filled vesicles, and then to firm, tense pustules that scab after 10 days to 2 weeks. The lesions are distributed over the entire body but predominate on the face and extremities, including palms and soles.

Today, suspicion that a patient may have smallpox would imply introduction of the disease through bioterrorism, and great care should be taken to prevent spread of the infection and to confirm the diagnosis in the laboratory. Local and state health authorities should be contacted immediately.

If maternal smallpox is suspected, contact and airborne isolation precautions, in addition to universal precautions, should be instituted immediately, and if possible, the patient should be cared for in a negative-pressure room. Family and community contacts, emergency medical personnel, and health care workers who might have been exposed to the patient should be identified and immunized as soon as possible. Immunization within 4 days can ameliorate illness and, in some cases, prevent infection completely.

VACCINIA

Vaccinia virus transmission to the fetus after vaccination of pregnant women has been documented,[184-186] although the frequency with which it occurs and the severity of resulting disease are difficult to determine from published studies.[187,188] Levine and coworkers[189] reviewed 20 cases of fetal vaccinia reported between 1932 and 1972. At least 13 of the 20 women involved had received their first smallpox vaccination during that pregnancy. Ten infected infants were born alive, and three survived. Other studies have failed to find an increased risk of fetal death, miscarriage, or fetal malformations.[189,190] Primary vaccination during pregnancy in the years in which these studies were conducted was unusual, however, and the potential impact on the fetus after vaccination of nonimmune pregnant women cannot be extrapolated accurately.

Congenital vaccinia among live-born infants is rare, and inadvertent vaccination during pregnancy should not be a reason to recommend termination of pregnancy. In utero vaccinia infection has not been associated with serious birth defects or with other long-term adverse events in surviving infants. Vaccinia immune globulin (VIG) has been used to treat some complications associated with smallpox vaccination, and it may be used for those same reasons during pregnancy, but VIG is not recommended as prophylaxis against congenital vaccinia. Cidofovir is available for treatment of complications of smallpox vaccination only under the investigational new drug protocol administered by the CDC. It will be released only as secondary treatment for complications that do not respond to treatment with VIG.

In early 2003, the National Smallpox Vaccine in Pregnancy Registry was established by the U.S. Department of Defense and the CDC to enroll and prospectively follow women who had been inadvertently vaccinated while pregnant or within 4 weeks of conception as a part of the military or civilian public health preparedness effort.[191] As of September 2006, 376 women had enrolled in the registry, 354 (94.1%) of whom had never received smallpox vaccine in the past. The majority of the women in the registry (76.9%) were vaccinated during the first 4 weeks of their pregnancies. There have been no cases of fetal vaccinia and no increase in fetal loss, prematurity, low birth weight, or major anomalies compared with the expected rates in the U.S. population.

Although these recent studies offer reassurance that smallpox vaccination during pregnancy does not have adverse consequences for the fetus, caution must be used in extrapolating these results to a larger population whose overall health may be more variable.

In September 2007, ACAM2000 replaced Dryvax as the only smallpox vaccine licensed by the FDA. Like Dryvax, which was initially approved in 1931, ACAM2000 is a live vaccinia virus vaccine; unlike Dryvax, ACAM2000 is produced in cell culture, allowing more rapid and uniform large-scale production.

Dengue

Dengue is a febrile illness caused by four closely related flaviviruses: DENV-1, DENV-2, DENV-3, and DENV-4. Dengue is transmitted to humans by mosquitoes, primarily *Aedes aegypti*, in tropical and subtropical areas of the world. Approximately 40% of the world's human population lives in areas where DENV is transmitted, and dengue is the most frequent cause of febrile illness among travelers returning from tropical areas. Infection with one of the four DENV types conveys immunity only to that type, so that individuals in endemic areas are at risk for multiple episodes of dengue illness.

Pregnant women living or traveling in dengue-endemic regions are at risk of infection, and case reports and case series of DENV infection during pregnancy have been published.[192-197] DENV infection is asymptomatic in as many as 75% of infected individuals, but the proportion of asymptomatic infection during pregnancy is not known. As is the case with nonpregnant individuals, symptoms of DENV in pregnancy include fever and myalgia, but severe dengue, with thrombocytopenia, hemorrhage, and hemorrhagic shock have been described. In one study reported from the Sudan, greater than 20% of infected pregnant women died as a result of dengue complicated by multiorgan failure and hemorrhage.[193] Pouliot and colleagues[194] reviewed 30 published reports (19 case reports, 9 case series, and 2 comparison studies) of dengue during pregnancy and concluded that, although premature birth, low birth weight, and fetal death occurred in association with maternal dengue, the limited number of comparative studies precludes the conclusion that the risk of these outcomes is greater than for infants of noninfected mothers. Individuals who are seropositive for one DENV strain are thought to suffer more severe disease when infected by a second strain, but the limited available evidence does not indicate that pregnant women with second infections with a distinct serotype have an increased risk of complications of pregnancy or delivery.[195]

Viremia during DENV infection persists for approximately 7 days; transmission of infection from pregnant woman to the fetus has been reported, but the frequency and relationship to the stage of pregnancy is not known. Among the 30 reports summarized by Pouliot and colleagues,[194] 5 of 34 infected infants were asymptomatic; among symptomatic infants, clinical findings included fever, thrombycytopenia, hepatomegaly, hemorrhage, pleural effusion, and rash. The average time between maternal fever and neonatal symptoms for 19 mother-infant pairs was 7 days (range, 5-13 days). Evidence suggests that both in utero and peripartum transmission occurs. There is no evidence that vertical transmission of DENV leads to fetal anomalies.

Diagnosis of DENV infection can be confirmed by testing for anti-DENV IgM antibodies, which can be detected approximately 4 to 5 days after illness onset, in sera or CSF. DENV RNA can be detected during the febrile phase of illness. No specific antiviral agent is available for treatment of dengue. Supportive care involves hydration, avoidance of aspirin and other nonsteroidal antiinflammatory medications, and provision of intensive supportive care if signs of shock or bleeding occur. There is currently no vaccine for prevention of dengue, but candidate vaccines are in development.

Chikungunya

Chikungunya is a mosquito-borne RNA alphavirus spread by bites of various strains of *Aedes* mosquitoes found until recently only in eastern Africa, Southeast Asia, India, and the western Pacific. In late 2013 chikungunya virus was first found in the Caribbean, and in 2014 it was diagnosed in hundreds of travellers returning to the U.S. from Caribbean islands. As of September, 2014, seven cases of locally transmitted chikungunya had been identified in Florida. Symptoms include high fever and musculoskeletal pain. Nausea, vomiting, headache, photophobia, and rash may occur. Some patients experience hemorrhagic symptoms, such as bleeding from mouth or gums. The febrile illness is self-resolving in approximately a week, but associated joint pain and swelling may persist for weeks and may be migratory. Mortality is unusual.

Chikungunya virus was first identified in 1952 in Tanzania, and epidemics have been described in various parts of the endemic region since then. Perhaps the most extensively studied outbreak occurred in 2005 to 2006 on Reunion Island, a French territory in the Indian Ocean east of Madagascar. Mother-to-child transmission of chikungunya had not been reported before the Reunion Island epidemic. Ramful and colleagues[198] identified 38 newborn infants with chikungunya diagnosed by reverse-transcriptase PCR detection of the virus in CSF or serum or by virus-specific IgM during the first week of life during the Reunion Island epidemic. Gerardin and colleagues[199] prospectively screened the 7504 women who delivered at one hospital for evidence of infection during or immediately after delivery. In both studies, maternal symptoms began during the week before delivery or within 2 days postdelivery. Onset of symptoms in newborns ranged from day 3 to 7 of life and included fever, pain, poor feeding, and rash. The rash described by Ramful and colleagues[198] began as generalized erythroderma, followed by brownish discoloration of the skin, particularly of the limbs and face. Gerardin and colleagues[199] describe the rashes they observed as polymorphous and "rubella-like" or "roseola-like." Peripheral edema was common. Complications included diarrhea, gastrointestinal and intracerebral hemorrhage, hypotonia, seizures, coma, and hemorrhagic conjunctivitis. Laboratory abnormalities included thrombocytopenia (severe in some), lymphopenia, elevated liver enzymes, and hypoprothrombinemia. Magnetic resonance imaging was performed in infants with CNS symptoms, and scattered white matter lesions and intraparenchymal hemorrhage were seen in some. Cardiac abnormalities included coronary artery dilatation, ventricular dysfunction, pericarditis, and heart failure. Mechanical ventilation was required for infants with severe neurologic abnormalities or multiorgan failure. One infant died because of necrotizing enterocolitis, gastrointestinal hemorrhage, and *Klebsiella pneumoniae* sepsis. Among the 9 patients with encephalopathy reported by Gerardin and colleagues,[199] 4 developed persistent neurologic and developmental abnormalities, which has also been reported in other patients with perinatally transmitted chikungunya who developed encephalopathy.

In their prospective study during the Reunion Island epidemic, which compared the outcome of pregnancies for 705 pregnant women who developed chikungunya infection during pregnancy to 668 who did not, Fritel and colleagues[200] found no difference in risk for stillbirth, preterm delivery, low birth weight, or admission to a neonatal intensive care unit. Congenital anomalies were more frequent in infants born to women who experienced infection during pregnancy than those born to uninfected women (19 vs. 15), but the difference was not statistically significant. The number of women who experienced infection in the first trimester was too small to reach a definitive conclusion about risks associated with maternal infection early in pregnancy. Early fetal death was reported due to maternal chikungunya infection in three cases during the Reunion Island epidemic.[201]

Diagnosis of chikungunya virus infection can be made using enzyme immunoassay to detect IgM or with PCR detection of viral RNA. There are no antiviral agents available for treatment, and no vaccine has been developed. Treatment of infected infants involves supportive care and management of hemorrhagic, neurologic, and cardiac complications.

References

1. Centers for Disease Control and Prevention: *Incidence, prevalence, and cost of sexually transmitted infections in the United States.* Available at http://www.cdc.gov/std/stats/STI-Estimates-Fact-Sheet-Feb-2013.pdf. Accessed October 7, 2013.
2. Richardson H, Kelsall G, Tellier P, et al: The natural history of type-specific human papillomavirus infections in female university students, *Cancer Epidemiol Biomarkers Prev* 12:485-490, 2003.
3. Ho GY, Bierman R, Beardsley L, et al: Natural history of cervicovaginal papillomavirus infection in young women, *N Engl J Med* 338:423-428, 1998.
4. Muñoz N, Bosch FX, de Sanjosé S, et al: Epidemiologic classification of human papillomavirus types associated with cervical cancer, *N Engl J Med* 348:518-527, 2003.
5. Clifford GM, Smith JS, Aguado T, et al: Comparison of HPV type distribution in high-grade cervical lesions and cervical cancer: a meta-analysis, *Br J Cancer* 89:101-105, 2003.
6. Hariri S, Unger ER, Sternberg M, et al: Prevalence of genital human papillomavirus among females in the United States, The National Health And Nutrition Examination Survey, 2003-2006, *J Infect Dis* 204:66-73, 2011.
7. Allen AL, Seigfried EC: The natural history of condyloma in children, *J Am Acad Dermatol* 39:951-955, 1998.
8. Hajek EF: Contribution to the etiology of laryngeal papilloma in children, *J Laryngol* 70:166-168, 1956.
9. Cook TA, Brunschwig JP, Butel JS, et al: Laryngeal papilloma: etiologic and therapeutic considerations, *Ann Otol* 82:649-655, 1973.
10. Quick CA, Watts SL, Krzyzek RA, et al: Relationship between condylomata and laryngeal papillomata, *Ann Otol* 89:467-471, 1980.
11. Steinberg BM, Topp WC, Schneider PS, et al: Laryngeal papillomavirus infection during clinical remission, *N Engl J Med* 308: 1261-1264, 1983.
12. Hording U, Iversen AK, Sebbelov A, et al: Prevalence of human papillomavirus types 11, 16 and 18 in cervical swabs: a study of 1362 pregnant women, *Eur J Obstet Gynecol Reprod Biol* 35:191-198, 1990.
13. Trottier H, Burchell AN: Epidemiology of mucosal human papillomavirus infection and associated diseases, *Public Health Genomics* 12:291-307, 2009.
14. Baseman JG, Koutsky LA: The epidemiology of human papillomavirus infections, *J Clin Virol* 32(Suppl 1):S16-S24, 2005.
15. Rombaldi RL, Serafini EP, Mandelli J, et al: Transmission of human papillomavirus, *Virol J* 5:106, 2008.
16. Rombaldi RL, Serafini EP, Mandelli J, et al: Perinatal transmission of human papillomavirus DNA, *Virol J* 6:83, 2009.
17. Smith EM, Parker MA, Rubenstein LM, et al: Evidence for vertical transmission of HPV from mothers to infants, *Infect Dis Obstet Gynecol* 326369:2010, 2010.
18. Koskimaa HM, Waterboer T, Pawlita M, et al: Human papillomavirus genotypes present in the oral mucosa of newborns and their concordance with maternal cervical human papillomavirus genotypes, *J Pediatr* 260:837-843, 2012.
19. Campisi P, Hawkes M, Simpson K: Canadian Juvenile Onset Recurrent Respiratory Papillomatosis Working Group: the epidemiology of juvenile onset recurrent respiratory papillomatosis derived from a population level national database, *Laryngoscope* 120:1233-1245, 2010.
20. Silverberg MJ, Thorsen P, Lindeberg H, et al: Condyloma in pregnancy is strongly predictive of juvenile-onset recurrent respiratory papillomatosis, *Obstet Gynecol* 101:645-652, 2003.
21. Avidano MA, Singleton GT: Adjuvant drug strategies in the treatment of recurrent respiratory papillomatosis, *Otolaryngol Head Neck Surg* 112:197-202, 1995.
22. Sjogren PP, Sidman JD: Use of the carbon dioxide laser for tracheobronchial lesions in children, *JAMA Otolaryngol Head Neck Surg* 139:231-235, 2013.
23. Chadha NK, James A: Adjuvant antiviral therapy for recurrent respiratory papillomatosis, *Cochrane Database Syst Rev* 12:CD005053, 2012.
24. Ali H, Donovan B, Wand H, et al: Genital warts in young Australians five years into national human papillomavirus vaccination programme: national surveillance data, *BMJ* 346:12032-12041, 2013.
25. Leval A, Herweijer E, Arnheim-Dahlström L, et al: Incidence of genital warts in Sweden before and after quadrivalent human papillomavirus vaccine availability, *J Infect Dis* 206:860-866, 2012.
26. Roden R, Wu TC: Preventative and therapeutic vaccines for cervical cancer, *Expert Rev Vaccines* 2:495-516, 2003.
27. Henle W, Henle G, Horwitz CA: Epstein-Barr virus-specific diagnostic tests in infectious mononucleosis, *Hum Pathol* 5:551-565, 1974.
28. Fleisher G, Henle W, Henle G, et al: Primary Epstein-Barr virus infection in infants in the United States: clinical and serological observations, *J Infect Dis* 139:553-558, 1979.
29. Icart J, Didier J: Infections due to Epstein-Barr virus during pregnancy, *J Infect Dis* 143:499, 1981.
30. Fleisher G, Bolognese R: Persistent Epstein-Barr virus infection and pregnancy, *J Infect Dis* 147:982-986, 1983.
31. Eskild A, Bruu AL, Stray-Pedersen B, et al: Epstein-Barr virus infection during pregnancy and risk of adverse pregnancy outcome, *BJOG* 112:1620-1624, 2005.
32. Avgil M, Diav-Citrin O, Shechtman S, et al: Epstein-Barr virus infection in pregnancy–a prospective, controlled study, *Reproduct Toxicol* 25:468-471, 2008.
33. Le CT, Chang S, Lipson MH: Epstein-Barr virus infections during pregnancy, *Am J Dis Child* 137:466-468, 1983.
34. Gervais F, Joncas JH: Seroepidemiology in various population groups of the greater Montreal area, *Comp Immunol Microbiol Infect Dis* 2:207-212, 1979.
35. Horowitz CA, Henle W, Henle G, et al: Long-term serologic follow-up of patients for Epstein-Barr virus after recovery from infectious mononucleosis, *J Infect Dis* 151:1150-1153, 1985.
36. Icart J, Enjalbert L, Didier J, et al: Étude prospective de l'infection à virus Epstein-Barr (EBV) au cours de la grossesse, *Biomedicine* 34:160, 1981.
37. Fleisher G, Bolognese R: Epstein-Barr virus infections in pregnancy: a prospective study, *J Pediatr* 104:374-379, 1984.
38. Fleisher G, Bolognese R: Infectious mononucleosis during gestation: report of three women and their infants studied prospectively, *Pediatr Infect Dis* 3:308-311, 1984.
39. Tallqvist H, Henle W, Klemola E, et al: Antibodies to Epstein-Barr virus at the ages of 6 to 23 months in children with congenital heart disease, *Scand J Infect Dis* 5:159-161, 1973.
40. Goldberg GN, Fulginiti VA, Ray CG, et al: In utero Epstein-Barr virus (infectious mononucleosis) infection, *JAMA* 246:1579-1581, 1981.
41. Weaver LT, Nelson R, Bell TM: The association of extrahepatic bile duct atresia and neonatal Epstein-Barr virus infection, *Acta Paediatr Scand* 73:155-157, 1984.
42. Visintine AJ, Gerber P, Nahmias AJ: Leukocyte transforming agent (Epstein-Barr virus) in newborn infants and older individuals, *J Pediatr* 89:571-575, 1976.
43. Chang RS, Blankenship W: Spontaneous in vitro transformation of leukocytes from a neonate, *Proc Soc Exp Biol Med* 144:337-339, 1973.
44. Chang RS, Seto DY: Perinatal infection by Epstein-Barr virus, *Lancet* 2:201, 1979.
45. Joncas J, Boucher J, Granger-Julien M, et al: Epstein-Barr virus in the neonatal period and in childhood, *Can Med Assoc J* 140:33-37, 1974.
46. Joncas JH, Wills A, McLaughlin B: Congenital infection with cytomegalovirus and Epstein-Barr virus, *Can Med Assoc J* 117:1417-1418, 1977.
47. Meyohas MC, Maréchal V, Desire N, et al: Study of mother-to-child Epstein-Barr virus transmission by means of nested PCRs, *J Virol* 70:6816-6819, 1996.
48. Joncas J, Alfieri C, Leyritz-Wills M, et al: Dual congenital infection with the Epstein-Barr virus (EBV) and the cytomegalovirus (CMV), *N Engl J Med* 304:1399-1403, 1981.

49. Sixbey JW, Lemon SM, Pagano JS: A second site for Epstein-Barr virus shedding: the uterine cervix, *Lancet* 2:1122-1124, 1986.
50. Portnoy J, Ahronheim GA, Ghibu F, et al: Recovery of Epstein-Barr virus from genital ulcers, *N Engl J Med* 311:966-968, 1984.
51. Horwitz CA, McClain K, Henle W, et al: Fatal illness in a 2 week old infant: diagnosis by detection of Epstein-Barr virus genomes from a lymph node biopsy, *J Pediatr* 103:752-755, 1983.
52. Gervais F, Joncas JH: Correspondence-an unusual antibody response to Epstein-Barr virus during infancy, *J Infect Dis* 140:273-275, 1979.
53. Salahuddin SZ, Ablashi DV, Markham PD, et al: Isolation of a new virus, HBLV, in patients with lymphoproliferative disorders, *Science* 234:596-601, 1986.
54. Lopez C, Pellett P, Stewart J, et al: Characteristics of human herpesvirus-6, *J Infect Dis* 157:1271-1273, 1988.
55. Leach CT, Sumaya CV, Brown NA: Human herpesvirus-6: clinical implications of a recently discovered, ubiquitous agent, *J Pediatr* 1231:173-181, 1992.
56. Lawrence GL, Chee M, Craxton MA, et al: Human herpes virus 6 is closely related to human cytomegalovirus, *J Virol* 64:287-299, 1990.
57. Baillargeon J, Piper J, Leach CT: Epidemiology of human herpesvirus 6 (HHV-6) infection in pregnant and non-pregnant women, *J Clin Virol* 16:149-157, 2000.
58. Dahl H, Fjaertoft G, Norsted T, et al: Reactivation of human herpesvirus 6 during pregnancy, *J Infect Dis* 180:2035-2038, 1999.
59. Adams O, Krempe C, Kögler G, et al: Congenital infections with human herpesvirus 6, *J Infect Dis* 178:544-546, 1998.
60. Okada K, Ueda K, Kusuhara K, et al: Exanthem subitum and human herpes virus 6, *Pediatr Infect Dis J* 12:204-208, 1993.
61. Caserta MT, Hall CB, Schnabel K, et al: Human herpesvirus (HHV)-6 and HHV-7 infections in pregnant women, *J Infect Dis* 196: 1296-1303, 2007.
62. Hall CB, Caserta MT, Schnabel KC, et al: Congenital infections with human herpesvirus 6 (HHV6) and human herpesvirus 7 (HHV7), *J Pediatr* 145:472-477, 2004.
63. Gervasi MT: Viral invasion of the amniotic cavity (VIAC) in the midtrimester of pregnancy, *J Matern Fetal Neonatal Med* 25:2002-2013, 2012.
64. Hall CB, Caserta MT, Schnabel K, et al: Chromosomal integration of human herpesvirus 6 is the major mode of congenital human herpesvirus 6 infection, *Pediatrics* 122:513-522, 2008.
65. Revest M, Minjolle S, Veyer D, et al: Detection of HHV6 in over a thousand samples: new types of infection revealed by analysis of positive results, *J Clin Virol* 51:20-24, 2011.
66. Lanari M: Congenital infection with human herpesvirus 6 variant B associated with neonatal seizures and poor neurological outcome, *J Med Virol* 70:628-632, 2003.
67. van Loon NM, Gummuluru S, Sherwood DJ, et al: Direct sequence analysis of human herpesvirus 6 (HHV-6) sequences from infants and comparison of HHV-6 from mother/infant pairs, *Clin Infect Dis* 21:1017-1019, 1995.
68. Pruksananonda P, Hall CB, Insel RA, et al: Primary human herpes virus 6 infection in young children, *N Engl J Med* 122:1445-1450, 1992.
69. Kawaguchi S, Suga S, Kozawa T, et al: Primary human herpesvirus 6 infection (exanthem subitum) in the newborn, *Pediatrics* 90:628-630, 1992.
70. Tajiri H, Nose O, Baba K, et al: Human herpesvirus-6 infection with liver injury in neonatal hepatitis, *Lancet* 335:863, 1990.
71. Asano Y, Yoshikawa T, Suga S, et al: Fatal fulminant hepatitis in an infant with human herpesvirus-6 infection, *Lancet* 335:862-863, 1990.
72. Kanegane C, Katayama K, Kyoutani S, et al: Mononucleosis-like illness in an infant associated with human herpesvirus 6 infection, *Acta Paediatr Jpn* 37:227-229, 1995.
73. Hammerling JA, Lambrecht RS, Kehl KS, et al: Prevalence of human herpesvirus 6 in lung tissue from children with pneumonitis, *J Clin Pathol* 49:802-814, 1996.
74. Knox KK, Pietryga D, Harrington DJ, et al: Progressive immunodeficiency and fatal pneumonitis associated with human herpesvirus 6 infection in an infant, *Clin Infect Dis* 20:406-413, 1995.
75. Rentz AC, Stevenson J, Hymas W, et al: Human herpesvirus 6 in the newborn intensive care unit, *Eur J Clin Microbiol Infect Dis* 26: 297-299, 2007.
76. Black JB, Pellett PE: Human herpesvirus 7, *Rev Med Virol* 3:217-223, 1993.
77. Frenkel N, Schirmer EC, Wyatt LS, et al: Isolation of a new herpesvirus from human CD4+ T cells, *Proc Natl Acad Sci U S A* 87:748-752, 1990.
78. Krueger GR, Koch B, Leyssens N, et al: Comparison of seroprevalences of human herpesvirus-6 and -7 in healthy blood donors from nine countries, *Vox Sang* 75:193-197, 1998.
79. Clark DA, Freeland ML, Mackie LK, et al: Prevalence of antibody to human herpesvirus 7 by age, *J Infect Dis* 168:251-252, 1993.
80. Fujisaki H, Tanaka-Taya K, Tanabe H, et al: Detection of human herpesvirus 7 (HHV-7) DNA in breast milk by polymerase chain reaction and prevalence of HHV-7 antibody in breast-fed and bottle-fed children, *J Med Virol* 56:275-279, 1998.
81. Lanphear BP, Hall CB, Black J, et al: Risk factors for the early acquisition of human herpesvirus 6 and human herpesvirus 7 infections in children, *Pediatr Infect Dis J* 17:792-795, 1998.
82. Okuno T, Oishi H, Hayashi K, et al: Human herpesviruses 6 and 7 in cervixes of pregnant women, *J Clin Microbiol* 133:1968-1970, 1995.
83. Boutolleau D, Cointe D, Gautheret-Dejean A, et al: No evidence for a major risk of roseolovirus vertical transmission during pregnancy, *Clin Infect Dis* 36:1634-1635, 2003.
84. Torigoe S, Kumamoto T, Koide W, et al: Clinical manifestations associated with human herpesvirus 7 infection, *Arch Dis Child* 72:518-519, 1995.
85. Clark DA, Kidd IM, Collingham KE, et al: Diagnosis of primary human herpesvirus 6 and 7 infections in febrile infants by polymerase chain reaction, *Arch Dis Child* 77:42-45, 1997.
86. Portolani M, Cermelli C, Mirandola P, et al: Isolation of human herpesvirus 7 from an infant with febrile syndrome, *J Med Virol* 45:282-283, 1995.
87. Torigoe S, Kumamoto T, Koide W, et al: Clinical manifestations associated with human herpesvirus 7 infection, *Arch Dis Child* 72:518-519, 1995.
88. Clark DA, Kidd IM, Collingham KE, et al: Diagnosis of primary human herpesvirus 6 and 7 infections in febrile infants by polymerase chain reaction, *Arch Dis Child* 77:42-45, 1997.
89. Portolani M, Cermelli C, Mirandola P, et al: Isolation of human herpesvirus 7 from an infant with febrile syndrome, *J Med Virol* 45: 282-283, 1995.
90. Torigoe S, Koide W, Yamada M, et al: Human herpesvirus 7 infection associated with central nervous system manifestations, *J Pediatr* 129:301-305, 1996.
91. Coffey VP, Jessup WJE: Maternal influenza and congenital deformities, *Lancet* 2:935-938, 1959.
92. Doll R, Hill AB: Asian influenza in pregnancy and congenital defects, *Br J Prev Soc Med* 14:167-172, 1960.
93. Hakosalo J, Saxen L: Influenza epidemic and congenital defects, *Lancet* 2:1346-1347, 1971.
94. Record RG: Anencephalus in Scotland, *Br J Prev Soc Med* 15:93-105, 1961.
95. Leck I: Incidence of malformations following influenza epidemics, *Br J Prev Soc Med* 17:70-80, 1963.
96. MacKenzie JS, Houghton M: Influenza infections during pregnancy: association with congenital malformations and with subsequent neoplasms in children, and potential hazards of live virus vaccines, *Bacteriol Rev* 38:356-370, 1974.
97. Hardy JMB, Azarowicz EN, Mannini A, et al: The effect of Asian influenza on the outcome of pregnancy. Baltimore 1957-1958, *Am J Public Health* 51:1182-1188, 1961.
98. Griffiths PD, Ronalds CJ, Heath RB: A prospective study of influenza infections during pregnancy, *J Epidemiol Community Health* 34: 124-128, 1980.
99. Hartert TV, Neuzil KM, Shintani AK, et al: Maternal morbidity and perinatal outcomes among pregnant women with respiratory hospitalizations during influenza season, *Am J Obstet Gynecol* 189: 1705-1712, 2003.
100. Centers for Disease Control and Prevention: Maternal and infant outcomes among severely ill pregnant and postpartum women with 2009 pandemic influenza A (H1N1)— United States, April 2009–August 2010, *MMWR Morb Mortal Wkly Rep* 60:1193-1196, 2011.
101. Pierce M, Kurinczuk JJ, Spark P, et al: Perinatal outcomes after maternal 2009/H1N1 infection: national cohort study, *BMJ* 342:d3214, 2011.

102. Mortensen PB, Pedersen CB, Melbye M, et al: Individual and familial risk factors for bipolar affective disorders in Denmark, *Arch Gen Psychiatry* 60:1209-1215, 2003.
103. Limosin F, Rouillon F, Payan C, et al: Prenatal exposure to influenza as a risk factor for adult schizophrenia, *Acta Psychiatr Scand* 107:331-335, 2003.
104. Brown AS, Susser ES: In utero infection and adult schizophrenia, *Ment Retard Dev Disabil Res Rev* 8:51-57, 2002.
105. Ruben FL, Winkelstein A, Sabbagha RE: In utero sensitization with influenza virus in man, *Proc Soc Exp Biol Med* 149:881-883, 1975.
106. McGregor JA, Burns JC, Levin MJ, et al: Transplacental passage of influenza A/Bangkok (H3N2) mimicking amniotic fluid infection syndrome, *Am J Obstet Gynecol* 149:856-859, 1984.
107. Yawn DH, Pyeatte JC, Joseph JM, et al: Transplacental transfer of influenza virus, *JAMA* 216:1022-1023, 1971.
108. Ramphal R, Donnelly WH, Small PA: Fatal influenzal pneumonia in pregnancy: failure to demonstrate transplacental transmissions of influenza virus, *Am J Obstet Gynecol* 138:347-348, 1980.
109. Puck JM, Glezen WP, Frank AL, et al: Protection of infants from infection with influenza A virus by transplacentally acquired antibody, *J Infect Dis* 142:844-849, 1980.
110. Reuman PD, Ayoub EM, Small PA: Effect of passive maternal antibody on influenza illness in children: a prospective study of influenza A in mother-infant pairs, *Pediatr Infect Dis J* 6:398-403, 1987.
111. Pannaraj PS, Tam B, Akan D: Oseltamivir treatment and prophylaxis in a neonatal intensive care unit during a 2009 H1N1 influenza outbreak, *J Perinatol* 31:487-493, 2011.
112. Tsagris V, Nika A, Kyriakou D, et al: Influenza A/H1N1/2009 outbreak in a neonatal intensive care unit, *J Hosp Infect* 81:36-40, 2012.
113. Joshi VV, Escobar MR, Stewart L, et al: Fatal influenza A2 viral pneumonia in a newborn infant, *Am J Dis Child* 126:839-840, 1973.
114. Standing JF, Nika A, Tsagris V, et al: Oseltamivir pharmcokinetics and clinical experience in neonates and infants during an outbreak of H1N1 influenza A virus infection in a neonatal intensive care unit, *Antimicrob. Agents Chemother.* 56:3833-3840, 2012.
115. Zaman K, Roy E, Arifeen SE, et al: Effectiveness of maternal influenza immunization in mothers and infants, *N Engl J Med* 359:1555-1564, 2008.
116. Eick AA, Uyeki TM, Klimov A, et al: Maternal influenza vaccination and effect on influenza virus infection in young infants, *Arch Pediatr Adolesc Med* 165:104-111, 2011.
117. Benowitz I, Esposito DB, Gracey KD, et al: Influenza vaccine given to pregnant women reduces hospitalization due to influenza in their infants, *Clin Infect Dis* 51:1355-1361, 2010.
118. Centers for Disease Control and Prevention: Prevention and control of influenza with vaccines: recommendations of the Advisory Committee on Immunization Practices (ACIP), *MMWR Recomm Rep* 59(RR-8):1-62, 2010. 2010.
119. Simoes EAF: Environmental and demographic risk factors for respiratory syncytial virus lower respiratory tract disease, *J Pediatr* 143:S118-S126, 2003.
120. Lamprecht CL, Krause HE, Mufson MA: Role of maternal antibody in pneumonia and bronchiolitis due to respiratory syncytial virus, *J Infect Dis* 134:211-217, 1976.
121. Glezen WP, Paredes A, Allison JE, et al: Risk of respiratory syncytial virus infection for infants from low-income families in relationship to age, sex, ethnic group, and maternal antibody level, *J Pediatr* 98:708-715, 1981.
122. Lopez-Alarcon M, Villalpando S, Fajardo A: Breastfeeding lowers the frequency and duration of acute respiratory infection and diarrhea in infants under six months of age, *J Nutr* 127:436-443, 1997.
123. Bruhn FW, Mokrohisky ST, McIntosh K: Apnea associated with respiratory syncytial virus infection in young infants, *J Pediatr* 90:382-386, 1977.
124. Abzug MJ, Beam AC, Gyorkos EA, et al: Viral pneumonia in the first month of life, *Pediatr Infect Dis J* 9:881-885, 1990.
125. Resch B, Paes B: Are late preterm infants as susceptible to RSV infection as full term infants? *Early Human Dev* 87S:S47-S49, 2011.
126. Resch B, Manzoni P, Lanari M: Severe respiratory syncytial virus (RSV) infection in infants with neuromuscular diseases and immune deficiency syndromes, *Paediatric Resp Rev* 10:148-153, 2009.
127. McConnochie KM, Hall CB, Walsh EE, et al: Variation in severity of respiratory syncytial virus infections with subtype, *J Pediatr* 117:52-62, 1990.
128. Belderbos ME, Houben ML, Wilbrink B, et al: Cord blood vitamin D deficiency is associated with respiratory syncytial virus bronchiolitis, *Pediatr* 127:e1513-e1520, 2011.
129. Hall CB, Kopelman AE, Douglas RG Jr, et al: Neonatal respiratory syncytial virus infection, *N Engl J Med* 300:393-396, 1979.
130. Wilson CW, Stevenson DK, Arvin AM: A concurrent epidemic of respiratory syncytial virus and echovirus 7 infections in an intensive care nursery, *Pediatr Infect Dis J* 8:24-29, 1989.
131. Unger A, Tapia L, Minnich LL, et al: Atypical neonatal respiratory syncytial virus infection, *J Pediatr* 100:762-764, 1982.
132. Hall CB, Douglas RG Jr, Geiman JM: Respiratory syncytial virus infections in infants: quantitation and duration of shedding, *J Pediatr* 89:11-15, 1976.
133. Hall CB, Douglas RG Jr, Geiman JM: Possible transmission by fomites or respiratory syncytial virus, *J Infect Dis* 41:98-102, 1980.
134. Snydman DR, Greer C, Meissner HC, et al: Prevention of nosocomial transmission of respiratory syncytial virus in a newborn nursery, *Infect Control Hosp Epidemiol* 9:105-108, 1988.
135. Groothuis J, Bauman J, Malinoski F, et al: Strategies for prevention of RSV nosocomial infection, *J Perinatol* 28:319-323, 2008.
136. American Academy of Pediatrics Subcommittee on Diagnosis and Management of Bronchiolitis: Diagnosis and management of bronchiolitis, *Pediatrics* 118:1774-1793, 2006.
137. Committee on Infectious Diseases and Bronchiolitis Guidelines Committee: Prophylaxis among infants and young children at increased risk of respiratory syncytial virus infection, *Pediatr* 134:415-420, 2014.
138. Moler FW, Khan AS, Meliones JN, et al: Respiratory syncytial virus morbidity and mortality estimates in congenital heart disease patients: a recent experience, *Crit Care Med* 20:1406-1413, 1992.
139. Navas L, Wang E, de Carvalho V, et al: Improved outcome of respiratory syncytial virus infection in a high-risk hospitalized population of Canadian children, *J Pediatr* 121:348-354, 1992.
140. Escobar GJ, Ragins A, Li SX, et al: Recurrent wheezing in the third year of life among children born at 32 weeks gestation or later: relationship to laboratory-confirmed, medically attended infection with respiratory syncytial virus during the first year of life, *Arch Pediatr Adolesc Med* 164:915-922, 2010.
141. You D: Exposure of neonates to respiratory syncytial virus is critical in determining subsequent airway response in adults, *Respir Res* 7:107-116, 2006.
142. Blanken MO, Rovers MM, Molenaar JM, et al: Respiratory syncytial virus and recurrent wheeze in healthy preterm infants, *N Engl J Med* 368:1791-1799, 2013.
143. Diebel R, Woodall JP, Decher WJ, et al: Lymphocytic choriomeningitis virus in man: serologic evidence of association with pet hamster, *JAMA* 232:501-504, 1975.
144. Smadel JE, Wall MJ: Lymphocytic choriomeningitis in the Syrian hamster, *J Exp Med* 75:581-591, 1942.
145. Traub E: Persistence of lymphochoriomeningitis virus in immune animals and its relation to immunity, *J Exp Med* 63:847-861, 1936.
146. Jahrling PB, Peters CJ: Lymphocytic choriomeningitis virus: a neglected pathogen of man, *Arch Pathol Lab Med* 116:486-488, 1992.
147. Bonthius DJ: Lymphocytic choriomeningitis virus: a prenatal and postnatal threat, *Advances in Pediatr* 56:75-86, 2009.
148. Komrower GM, Williams BL, Stones PB: Lymphocytic choriomeningitis in the newborn, *Lancet* 1:697-698, 1955.
149. Biggar RJ, Woodall JP, Walter PD, et al: Lymphocytic choriomeningitis outbreak associated with pet hamsters: fifty-seven cases from New York state, *JAMA* 232:494-500, 1975.
150. Barton LL, Peters CJ, Ksiazek TG: Lymphocytic choriomeningitis virus: an unrecognized teratogenic pathogen, *Emerg Infect Dis* 1:152-153, 1995.
151. Wright R, Johnson D, Neumann M, et al: Congenital lymphocytic choriomeningitis virus syndrome: a disease that mimics congenital toxoplasmosis or cytomegalovirus infection, *Pediatrics* 100:1-6, 1997.
152. Bonthius DJ, Wright R, Tseng B, et al: Congenital lymphocytic choriomeningitis virus infection: spectrum of disease, *Ann Neurol* 62:347-355, 2007.
153. Bonthius DJ, Nichols B, Harb H, et al: Lymphocytic choriomeningitis virus infection of the developing brain: critical role of host age, *Ann Neurol* 62:356-374, 2007.

154. Childs JE, Glass GE, Korch GW, et al: Lymphocytic choriomeningitis virus infection and house mouse *(Mus musculus)* distribution in urban Baltimore, *Am J Trop Med Hyg* 47:27-34, 1992.
155. Stephensen CB, Blount SR, Lanford RE, et al: Prevalence of serum antibodies against lymphocytic choriomeningitis virus in selected populations from two U.S. cities, *J Med Virol* 38:27-31, 1992.
156. Lehmann-Grube F, Kallay M, Ibscher B, et al: Serologic diagnosis of human infections with lymphocytic choriomeningitis virus: comparative evaluation of seven methods, *J Med Virol* 4:25-36, 1979.
157. Wright R, Johnson D, Neumann M, et al: Congenital lymphocytic choriomeningitis virus syndrome: a disease that mimics congenital toxoplasmosis or cytomegalovirus infection, *Pediatrics* 100:e9, 1997.
158. Bale JF, Murph JR: Congenital infections and the nervous system, *Pediatr Clin North Am* 39:669-690, 1992.
159. Ackermann R, Körver G, Turss R, et al: Pränatale Infektion mit dem Virus der lymphozytären Choriomeningitis, *Dtsch Med Wochenschr* 99:629-632, 1974.
160. Mets MB, Barton LL, Khan AS, et al: Lymphocytic choriomeningitis virus: an underdiagnosed cause of congenital chorioretinitis, *Am J Ophthalmol* 130:209-215, 2000.
161. Wilkin JK: Molluscum contagiosum venereum in a women's outpatient clinic: a venereally transmitted disease, *Am J Obstet Gynecol* 128:531-535, 1977.
162. Mandel MJ, Lewis RJ: Molluscum contagiosum of the newborn, *Br J Dermatol* 84:370-372, 1970.
163. Luke JD, Silverberg NB: Vertically transmitted molluscum contagiosum infection, *Pediatr* 125:e423-e425, 2010.
164. Sipahioglu U, Alpaut S: Transplacental rabies in humans, *Mikrobiyol Bul* 19:95-99, 1985.
165. Martell MA, Montes FC, Alcocer RB: Transplacental transmission of bovine rabies after natural infection, *J Infect Dis* 127:291-293, 1973.
166. Cates W Jr: Treatment of rabies exposure during pregnancy, *Obstet Gynecol* 44:893-896, 1974.
167. Geneverlay J, Dodero J: Note sur un enfant né d'une mere en etat du rage, *Ann Inst Pasteur Paris* 55:124, 1935.
168. Spence MR, Davidson DE, Dill Jr GS, et al: Rabies exposure during pregnancy, *Am J Obstet Gynecol* 123:655-656, 1975.
169. Lumbiganon P, Wasi C: Survival after rabies immunisation in newborn infant of infected mother, *Lancet* 336:319-320, 1990.
170. Iehle C, Dacheux L, Ralandison S, et al: Delivery and follow-up of a healthy newborn from a mother with clinical rabies, *J Clin Virol* 42:82-85, 2008.
171. Chabala S: Confirmed rabies exposure during pregnancy: treatment with human rabies immune globulin and human diploid cell vaccine, *Am J Med* 91:423-424, 1991.
172. Chutivongse S, Wilde H, Benjavongkulchai M: Postexposure rabies vaccination during pregnancy: effect on 202 women and their infants, *Clin Infect Dis* 20:818-820, 1995.
173. Rupprecht CE, Briggs D, Brown CM: Centers for Disease Control and Prevention: Use of a reduced 4-dose schedule for postexposure prophylaxis to prevent human rabies: recommendations of the Advisory Committee on Immunization Practices, *MMWR Recomm Rep* 59(RR-2):1-9, 2010.
174. Nash D, Mostashari F, Fine A, et al: The outbreak of West Nile infection in the New York City area in 1999, *N Engl J Med* 344:1807-1814, 2001.
175. Centers for Disease Control and Prevention: Intrauterine West Nile virus infection—New York, 2002, *MMWR Morb Mortal Wkly Rep* 51:1135-1136, 2002.
176. Alpert SG, Fergerson J, Noel LP: Intrauterine West Nile virus: ocular and systemic findings, *Am J Ophthalmol* 136:733-735, 2003.
177. O'Leary DR, Kuhn S, Kniss KL, et al: Birth outcomes following West Nile virus infection of pregnant women in the United States: 2003-2004, *Pediatrics* 117:e537-e545, 2006.
178. Hinckley AF, O'Leary DR, Hayes EB: Transmission of West Nile virus through human milk seems to be rare, *Pediatrics* 119:e666-e671, 2007.
179. Centers for Disease Control and Prevention: Interim guidelines for the evaluation of infants born to mothers infected with West Nile virus during pregnancy, *MMWR Morb Mortal Wkly Rep* 53:154-157, 2004.
180. Lynch FW: Dermatologic conditions of the fetus with particular reference to variola and vaccinia, *Arch Dermatol Syphilis Chic* 26:997-1019, 1932.
181. Rao AR, Prahlad I, Swaminathan M, et al: Pregnancy and smallpox, *J Indian Med Assoc* 40:353-363, 1963.
182. Marsden JP, Greenfield CRM: Inherited smallpox, *Arch Dis Child* 9:309-314, 1934.
183. Sharma R, Jagdev DK: Congenital smallpox, *Scand J Infect Dis* 3: 245-247, 1971.
184. MacArthur P: Congenital vaccinia and vaccinia gravidarum, *Lancet* 2:1104-1106, 1952.
185. Bourke GJ, Whitty RJ: Smallpox vaccination in pregnancy: a prospective study, *Br Med J* 1:1544-1546, 1964.
186. Green DM, Reid SM, Rhaney K: Generalized vaccinia in the human foetus, *Lancet* 1:1296-1298, 1966.
187. Lane JM, Ruben FL, Neff JM, et al: Complications of smallpox vaccination, 1968: results of ten statewide surveys, *J Infect Dis* 122:303-309, 1970.
188. Lane JM, Ruben FL, Neff JM, et al: Complications of smallpox vaccination, 1968: national surveillance in the United States, *N Engl J Med* 281:1201-1208, 1969.
189. Levine MM, Edsall G, Bruce-Chwatt LJ: Live-virus vaccines in pregnancy: risks and recommendations, *Lancet* 2:34-38, 1974.
190. Greenberg M, Yankauer A Jr, Krugman S, et al: The effect of smallpox vaccination during pregnancy on the incidence of congenital malformations, *Pediatrics* 3:456-467, 1949.
191. Ryan MAK, Seward JF: Pregnancy, birth, and infant health outcomes from the national smallpox vaccine in pregnancy registry, 2003-2006, *Clin Infect Dis* 46(Suppl 3):S221, 2008.
192. Chitra TV, Panicker S: Maternal and fetal outcome of dengue fever in pregnancy, *J Vector Borne Dis* 48:210-213, 2011.
193. Ishag A, Jumaa AM, Elbashir HM, et al: Maternal and perinatal outcomes of dengue on Port Sudan, Eastern Sudan, *Virolog J* 7:153-157, 2010.
194. Pouliot SH, Xiong X, Harville E, et al: Maternal dengue and pregnancy outcomes: a systematic review, *Obstet Gynecol Surv* 65:107-118, 2010.
195. Tan P, Rajasingam G, Devi S, et al: Dengue infection in pregnancy, *Obstet Gynecol* 111:1111-1117, 2008.
196. Phongsamart W, Yoksan S, Vanaprapa N, et al: Dengue virus infection in late pregnancy and transmission to the infants, *Pediatr Infect Dis J* 27:500-504, 2008.
197. Kariyawasam S, Senanayake H: Dengue infections during pregnancy: case series from a tertiary care hospital in Sri Lanka, *J Infect Dev Ctries* 4:767-775, 2010.
198. Ramful D, Carbonnier M, Pasquet M, et al: Mother-to-child transmission of chikungunya virus infection, *Pediatr Infect Dis J* 26: 811-815, 2007.
199. Gerardin P, Barau G, Michault A, et al: Multidisciplinary prospective study of mother-to-child chikungunya virus infection on the island of La Reunion, *PLoS Med* 5:e260, 2008.
200. Fritel X, Rollot O, Gerardin P, et al: Chikungunya virus infection during pregnancy, Reunion, France, 2006, *Emerg Infect Dis* 16:419-425, 2010.
201. Touret Y, Randrianaivo H, Michault A, et al: Early maternal-fetal transmission of the chikungunya virus [in French], *Presse Med* 35:1656-1658, 2006.

SECTION **IV**

PROTOZOAN, HELMINTH, AND FUNGAL INFECTIONS

SECTION OUTLINE

31 Toxoplasmosis

FRANÇOIS PEYRON, MARTINE WALLON, FRANÇOIS KIEFFER, and JUSTUS GARWEG

CHAPTER OUTLINE

Infectious diseases will never disappear. New ones will forever come to light; some may dissipate slowly; those that remain will no longer keep the form that we recognize today.

CHARLES NICOLLE, *The Fate of Infectious Diseases*

Toxoplasma gondii is a worldwide, intracellular protozoan parasite that can infect humans and almost all warm-blooded animals. Among the fetal and neonatal pathogens, *T. gondii* is certainly one of the most:

- Widespread, because it affects one third of the world's human population,[1] although a wide discrepancy is observed between countries (range, 10%-80%), its prevalence is continually evolving, and it is related to regional socioeconomic parameters and population habits[2]
- Heterogeneous, in terms of its clinical presentation, because the spectrum of the disease ranges from asymptomatic to devastating[3]

- Unpredictable, in terms of evolution because ocular lesions can emerge or relapse during childhood and adolescence or even later in life[4]
- Perplexing, because although *T. gondii* has elicited a huge body of scientific evidence in different fields,[5] no consensus has been reached regarding systematic screening for this infection in pregnant women, data on the efficacy of prenatal and postnatal treatment are contradictory, and little is known about the burden of disease in different countries[6,7]
- Challenging to prevent, because of multiple routes of infection

Biology of the Parasite

HISTORY

Toxoplasma gondii was first described in a rodent (*Ctenodactylus gondii*) by Nicolle in Tunisia in 1908[8] and simultaneously by Splendore[9] in rabbits in Brazil. Initially, toxoplasmosis was thought to be an animal disease, but since its discovery, our awareness of its clinical importance in humans has increased tremendously, and it is now known to have diverse manifestations requiring oversight by a wide range of medical specialties.

- In 1923, Janku,[10] a Czech ophthalmologist, described the first human case of toxoplasmosis and demonstrated the presence of the parasite in the retina of an 11-month-old boy.
- In 1938, Wolf and colleagues[11,12] in the United States reported the first case of congenital toxoplasmosis in a girl who developed seizures 3 days after birth and presented with macular lesion in both eyes. She died at 1 month of age, and free parasites were found in her brain and eyes. When inoculated intracerebrally into mice and rabbits, these parasites induced encephalitis.
- In 1970, the full life cycle of the parasite and the role of cats as its definitive host were described by Frenkel and colleagues.[13]
- In 1983, necrotizing encephalitis was reported in 10 patients by Luft and colleagues,[14] and the necessity of including toxoplasmosis in the differential diagnosis of encephalitis of unknown etiology was highlighted.
- In 1984, toxoplasmic encephalitis was reported in 70 patients with acquired immune deficiency syndrome (AIDS),[15] and *T. gondii* was included in the list of opportunistic pathogens. Since that time, the rate of life-threatening toxoplasmic infections in human immunodeficiency virus (HIV)-positive patients has decreased,[16] but they are still reported regularly in transplant patients.[17,18]
- In 1994, an important outbreak of human toxoplasmic infections was associated with the presence of *T. gondii* in the water system in Vancouver, Canada.[19] Waterborne transmission of the disease therefore appeared to be more common than had previously been estimated.[20]
- In 1988, Dardé and coworkers[21] described three isoenzyme pattern groups, launching the era of strain typing for strains of *T. gondii*. In 1998, atypical strains that were highly virulent for immunocompetent humans were reported in French Guiana.[22] Since then, many publications have reported on this issue, giving a better understanding of the worldwide parasite population structure, identifying virulent atypical strains from South America, and determining their clinical importance.

STAGES AND LIFE CYCLE

Toxoplasma gondii has *three* infective stages: tachyzoites, bradyzoites, and oocysts. The first determines the proliferative phase of the parasite, and the other two play an important role in the epidemiology of disease and its transmission. Only the first two stages are encountered in humans.

Tachyzoites

These represent a rapidly dividing stage (from the Greek word *tachos*, which means speed); they invade nucleated cells, where they multiply. Tachyzoites appear as crescent-shaped structures of 2 by 6 μm with a pointed apical and round posterior end (Fig. 31-1). They are limited by a membrane called the pellicle. At the apical end, tachyzoites display a structure called the apical complex, which plays a vital role in cell invasion and is composed of different elements: two polar rings that encircle the conoid, a truncated cone made of six to eight microtubular elements that are wound like a compressed spring (Fig. 31-2).[23] Other structures include rhoptries, which comprise 8 to 10 club-shaped organelles[24] that have a secretory function associated with cell invasion and virulence; micronemes, which are rodlike structures located on the anterior part of the parasite; and dense granules, which are also secretory structures involved in the development of a microtubule within the parasitophorous vacuole (PV)[25] (see "Host Cell Penetration"). The nucleus is centrally located, and other organs, such as the Golgi complex, endoplasmic reticulum, and mitochondrion, are also present.[23] More recently, a vestigial plasmid was described in the apical region. This body, which is apparently an ancestor of algae present in most apicomplexan species, was named an "apicoplast" and appears to play a role in some metabolic pathways (Fig. 31-3).[26] Tachyzoites multiply within host cells by endodyogeny, an asexual method of replication in which two progeny form within the parent tachyzoite. They can invade all nucleated cells, where they multiply within a specific vacuole (see "Host Cell Penetration"). Tachyzoites are sensitive to acid pepsin digestion and gastric juice.[27]

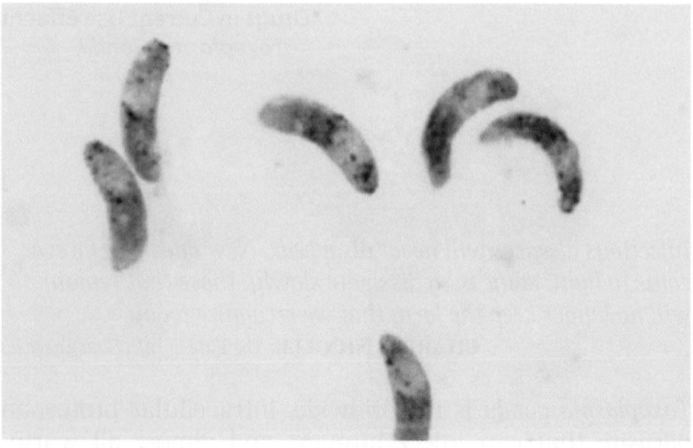

Figure 31-1 Tachyzoites of *Toxoplasma gondii*. Staining: May-Grünwald–Giemsa.

They are killed by the combined action of immunoglobulin and complement[28] and do not appear to be able to survive extracellularly in the bloodstream.[29]

Bradyzoites and Cysts

The bradyzoite stage results from the conversion of tachyzoites into slowly multiplying organisms that replicate by endodyogeny within a PV (see "Host Cell Penetration") and form cysts in tissues throughout the body.[30] Its structure differs slightly from that of the tachyzoite. The nucleus is located in the posterior part, and the shape of the rhoptries differs in that some can be looped back on themselves (Fig. 31-4). Intracellular cysts vary in size (range, 5 μm-100 μm) and can contain from two to thousands of packed bradyzoites (Fig. 31-5). Their form varies according to their location: In the brain, they are spheroidal, and their diameter is less than 70 μm, whereas in muscles, they are elongated and may be 100 μm in length (Fig. 31-6).

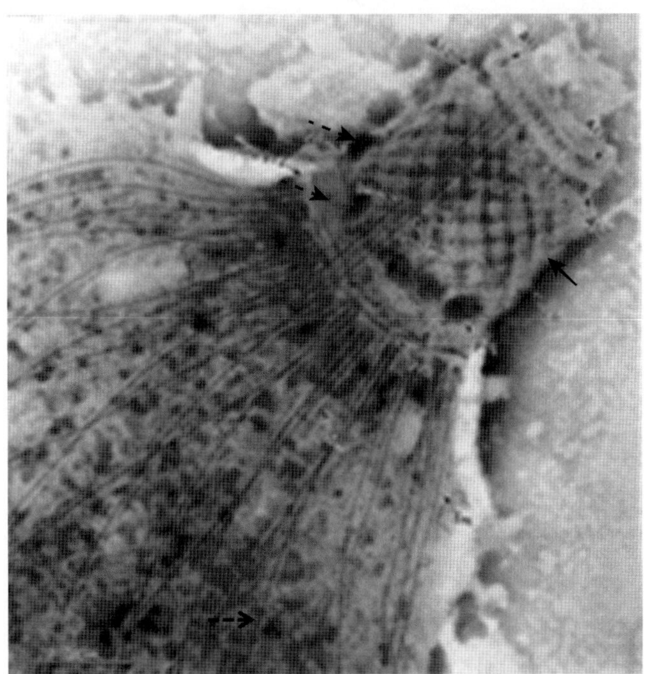

Figure 31-2 Apical complex. Polar ring *(arrow)*. Microtubular element of conoid *(dotted arrows)*. (From Morrissette NS, Murray JM, Roos DS: Subpellicular microtubules associate with an intramembranous particle lattice in the protozoan parasite *Toxoplasma gondii*, *J Cell Sci* 110[Pt 1]:35-42, 1997; with permission.)

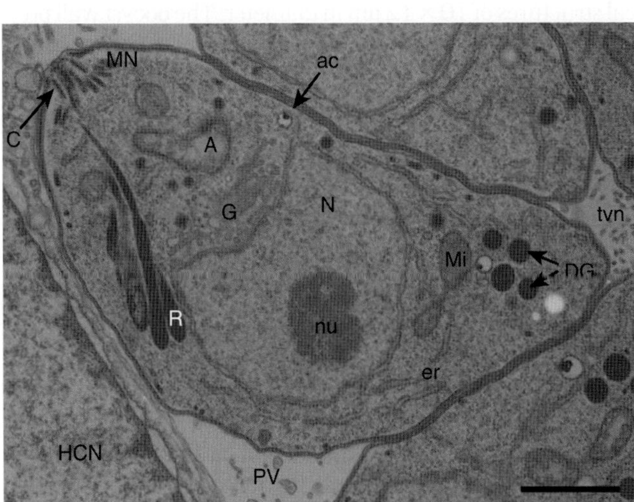

Figure 31-3 Sagittal section of an intravacuolar tachyzoite. *A*, Apicoplast; ac, acidocalcisomes; *C*, conoid; *DG*, dense granule; *er*, endoplasmic reticulum; *G*, Golgi body; *HCN*, host cell nucleus; *MN*, micronemes; *Mi*, mitochondria; *N*, nucleus; *nu*, nucleolus; *PV*, parasitophorous vacuole; *R*, rhoptry; *tvn*, tubovesicular network. Bar = 1 mm. (From Ferguson DJP, Dubremetz D: The ultrastructure of *Toxoplasma gondii*. In Weiss LM, Kim K, editors: *Toxoplasma gondii*, ed 2, [Figure 2.1A], London, 2014, Academic Press.)

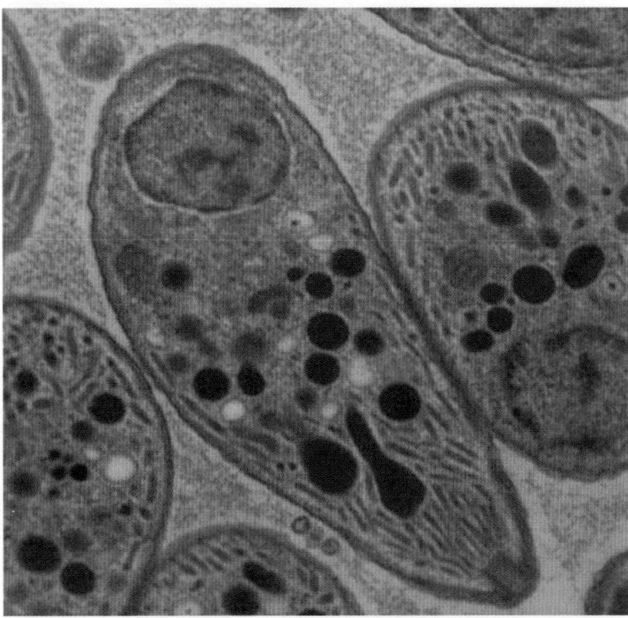

Figure 31-4 Bradyzoite of *Toxoplasma gondii*. (Courtesy M.L. Dardé, Limoges, France.)

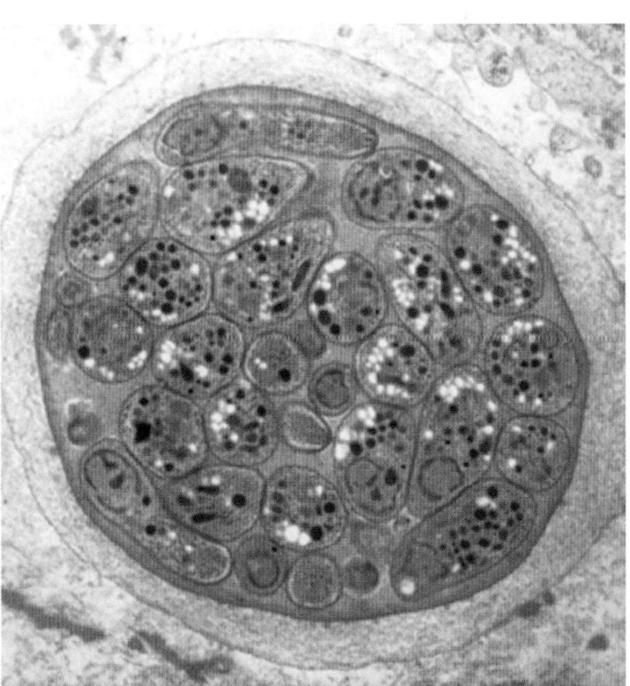

Figure 31-5 Cyst containing bradyzoites. (Courtesy M.L. Dardé, Limoges, France.)

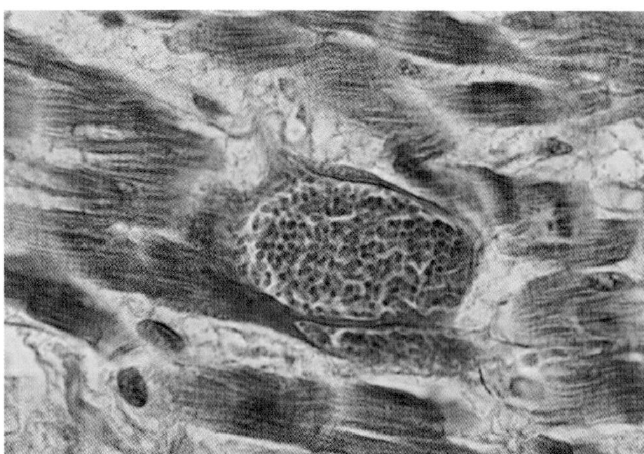

Figure 31-6 Cyst in human myocardium. Invasive toxoplasmosis after heart transplantation.

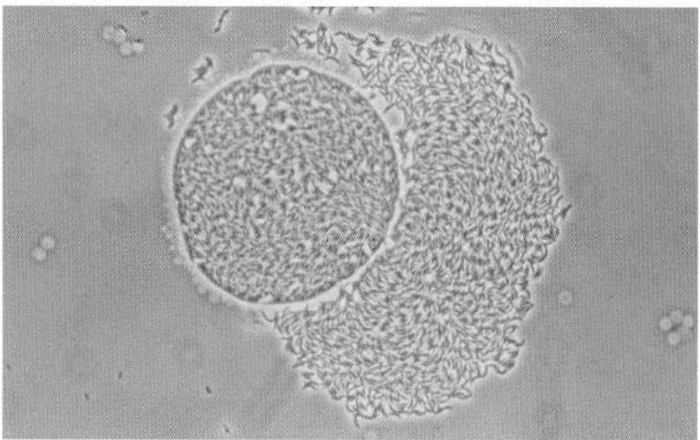

Figure 31-7 Cyst releasing bradyzoites after trypsin digestion. (Courtesy M.L. Dardé, Limoges, France.)

The cyst wall is less than 0.5 μm thick and is composed of host cell and parasitic antigens.[31]

Cysts are distributed in different organs, depending on the host. In rats, they are more abundant in neural tissue, whereas in cattle, they are more abundant in muscles. It is tempting to speculate that this distribution of cysts is the result of a very powerful adaption of the parasite to create a successful life cycle. Indeed, prey with preferential parasitic load in the muscle are more liable to be infectious when eaten by cats or other intermediate hosts. The presence of cysts in the muscles of pigs and cattle is also of the utmost importance with respect to transmission to humans through the consumption of meat.[32] Intact cysts can last for the entire life of the host and probably do not cause harm, provided that the immune system is intact and efficient.[27] They are not static structures because they can break down (Fig. 31-7), releasing parasites, which can re-invade other cells.[33]

Whether the presence of cysts can alter host behavior is certainly one of the most intriguing questions in the field of clinical toxoplasmosis. Rats that have cysts in their brain approach cat odors that they usually avoid; this change in behavior of the intermediate host increases its chances of capture by and infection of the definitive host[34] (see "Management of Children, Long-Term Outcome").

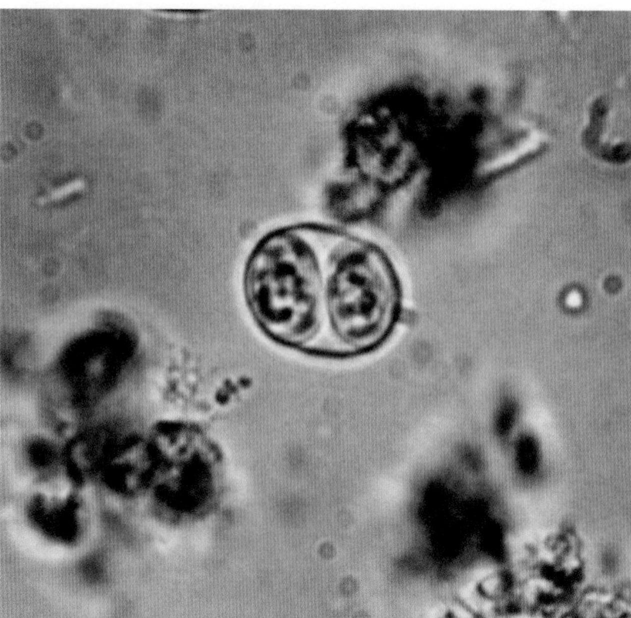

Figure 31-8 Sporulated oocyst of *Toxoplasma gondii.* (Courtesy M.L. Dardé, Limoges, France.)

Bradyzoites contained within the cyst display a latent metabolism and are less susceptible than tachyzoites to proteolytic enzymes, which allows their transmission through ingestion.[35] They are also resistant to low temperatures (refrigeration) but are killed after 3 days at −12° C.[23] Conversely, heating to 67° C kills cysts but, for meat to be safe, this temperature should be reached at its center.

Sporozoites and Oocysts

Sporozoites are derived from the sexual replication of *T. gondii,* which occurs in the intestine of cats and other felids. They are contained within mature oocysts, which are initially shed unsporulated in cat feces. Unsporulated oocysts are subspherical structures of 10 × 12 μm in diameter. The oocyst wall presents a strong five-layered structure that enables the parasite to survive once shed into the environment.[36] Sporulation begins within 1 to 5 days after excretion, depending on environmental conditions. Before the start of sporulation, oocysts are not infective. The nucleus of the unsporulated oocyst divides twice, a second limiting membrane is formed, then the cytoplasm divides and two sporocysts of 6 by 8 μm are formed (Fig. 31-8). At the end of the maturation process, each sporocyst contains four sporozoites. Oocysts can survive for up to 548 days in native feces and for 54 months in cold water. They are resistant to freezing and to water treatment such as chlorination, ozonation, and ultraviolet light.[37]

Life Cycle of *Toxoplasma gondii*

The life cycle of *T. gondii* operates in a prey-predator system[38] that alternates between the definitive host (in which sexual replication occurs), which includes cats and other felids, and the intermediate host (in which asexual replication occurs), mainly mammals, including humans, although birds can also be involved. Moreover, the life cycle can occur not only between the definitive and intermediate host but also between carnivorous intermediate hosts or between definitive hosts.

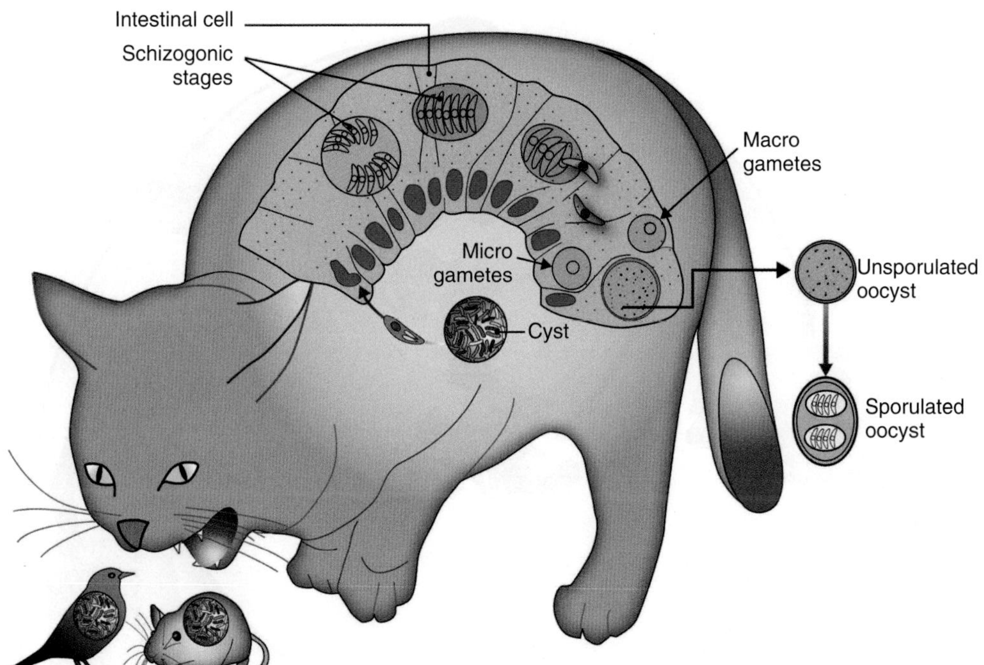

Figure 31-9 Sexual reproduction of *Toxoplasma gondii* in cats. (Courtesy Université Claude Bernard Lyon 1. Illustration by Monique Billaud, Service ICAP.)

Sexual Cycle. Cats (and other felids) are infected by the ingestion of cysts present within the tissues of their prey or by ingestion of oocysts. The cyst wall is dissolved by gastric enzymes, and released bradyzoites penetrate the epithelial cells of the small intestine and undergo asexual multiplication, resulting in merozoites being released from schizonts. The sexual cycle then starts 2 days after the tissue cysts have been ingested,[27] producing male and female gametes[39] within the intestinal cells. Male microgametes use their flagella to penetrate and fertilize female macrogametes to form oocysts. Cells bearing parasites rupture and release immature oocysts ((Fig. 31-9); see earlier). Under certain conditions, for instance, after feeding on one infected mouse, domestic cats can shed millions of oocysts,[32] indicating the high reproductive potential of this parasite.

Oocysts are shed mostly for 1 week (generally < 3 weeks) after feline infection, but prepatent periods depend on the infective stages: 3 to 10 days after ingesting tissue cysts, more than 18 days after ingesting oocysts.[27] Cats usually shed oocysts only after primary infection, but exceptions have been reported[32]; concomitant infection, malnutrition, and immunodepression can induce the reshedding of oocysts.[32]

Asexual Cycle. Intermediate hosts are infected either by ingestion of cysts present in meat or oocysts that are present in food or water. In the intestinal tract, oocysts liberate sporozoites that penetrate the intestinal epithelium, where they differentiate into tachyzoites. When ingested by the intermediate host via raw or undercooked meat, cysts rupture in the digestive tract and invade the epithelial cells of the intestine before spreading within the new host. Little information is available on how tachyzoites invade and spread in the intestinal cells. In orally infected mice, an overrepresentation of neutrophils among infected leucocytes in the small intestine has been reported.[40] These infected cells migrate across the epithelium to the lumen, suggesting a possible transmission of parasites from one villus to another and an increase in the number of infection entry sites.[40] The other fate of tachyzoites after replicating in intestinal cells is dissemination throughout the body (Fig. 31-10).

If it is accepted that the transmission of *T. gondii* from the mother to the fetus reflects parasitemia, this stage is the key point for the understanding of congenital toxoplasmosis. Infected mothers have a temporary parasitemia,[41] but the delay between maternal infection and the occurrence and duration of parasitemia is not known. Polymerase chain reactions (PCRs) performed on the blood of pregnant women, sequentially sampled after seroconversion, have given inconsistent results (Peyron and colleagues' unpublished data).

Dissemination can also reach the lymphoid organs during the acute phase of infection.[42] In a mouse model, infected subpopulations of dendritic cells have been reported to shuttle tachyzoites from the gut to the brain.[43] Tachyzoites can exist as free extracellular parasites but do not contribute to any great extent to the dissemination of parasites.[29] The infection of organs occurs when infected leukocytes migrate into the parenchyma as "Trojan horses," but tachyzoites can also egress the leukocyte and invade the parenchyma, crossing the vascular endothelium in a short-lived extracellular form.[29] How the parasite survives in these cells with microbicidal properties is not fully understood, but it is clear that the parasite has to subvert the host immune response (see "Parasite-Host Interaction in the Brain and the Eye").

Tachyzoites can enter almost all nucleated cells. After cell invasion, they convert to bradyzoites, and tissue cysts are formed. Tissue cysts persist for several months and perhaps for life, depending on the host and the strains.[27] The ingestion of tissue cysts by cats will "close" the cycle.

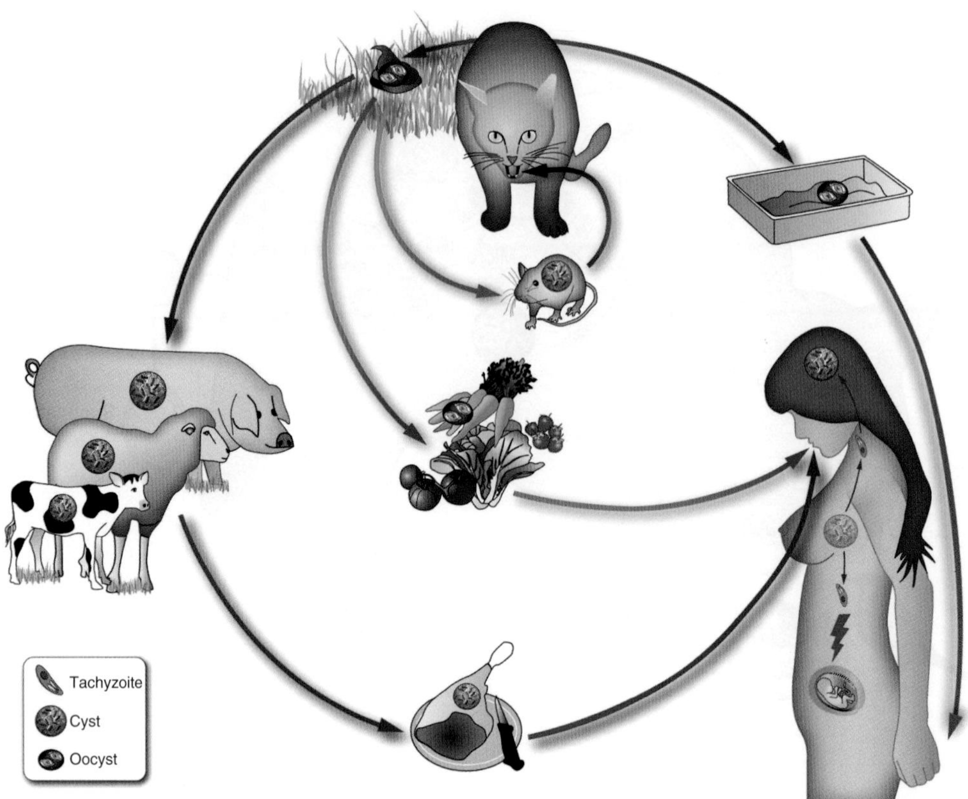

Figure 31-10 Asexual cycle of *Toxoplasma gondii.* (Courtesy Université Claude Bernard Lyon 1. Illustration by Monique Billaud, Service ICAP.)

Host Cell Penetration. Parasites invade cells by a self-driven multistep process that differs from endocytosis because of the rapid nature of the phenomenon (≈30 seconds).[44] The first step entails attachment to the host cell membrane and involves the surface antigen proteins (SAGs) of the parasite. This interaction is reversible and allows the parasite to disengage when the host cells are suboptimal.[45] Otherwise, the process continues, and the parasite glides along the cell membrane (Fig. 31-11).

T. gondii expresses a wide range of adhesive proteins, one of which allows it to select a given host cell.[45] Among these, micronemal proteins (MICs) that are released from the apical end of the parasite through a calcium-dependent mechanism bind to the host cell membrane. The parasite then initiates the penetration process through adhesion to the host cell membrane by extruding its conoid. Another micronemal protein, known as apical membrane antigen 1 (AMA1), forms a stable complex with other proteins secreted by "the neck" region of the rhoptries (termed RON proteins) and cooperates to form a ringlike structure called the moving junction (MJ).[46] The parasite jumps through this loop[45] and invades the cell. The MJ does not move but may rather provide a point of traction through which the parasites glide.[46]

The parasite migrates from the apical end to the posterior end, leading to its internalization into the PV. During this process, AMA1 is distributed on the parasite surface, and rhoptry-secreted proteins, as well as dense granule proteins, participate in the formation of PV membranes (PVM). The MJ appears to act as a sieve to remove host and parasite proteins, thus modifying the biochemical structure of the PVM and preventing its fusion with lysosomes.

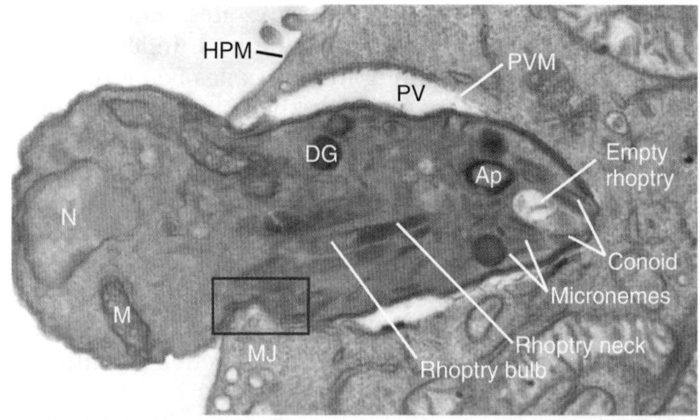

Figure 31-11 Tachyzoite penetrating a cell. Parasite's internal structures: *Ap,* Apicoplast; *DG,* dense granules; *M,* mitochondrion; *N,* nucleus. Structures associated with parasite: *HPM,* Host cell plasma membrane; *MJ,* moving junction; *PVM,* parasitophorous vacuole membranes. (From Lebrun M, Carruthers VB, Cesbron-Delauw M : *Toxoplasma* secretory proteins and their roles in cell invasion and intracellular survival. In Weiss LM, Kim K, editors: *Toxoplasma gondii,* ed 2, [Figure 2.1A], London, 2014, Academic Press.)

Repressor of primer (ROP) proteins are involved in the formation of PVM. Among them, ROP18, a member of ROP2 family proteins, possesses a protein kinase activity and plays an important role in parasitic growth. Overexpression of ROP18 in transgenic parasites causes a dramatic increase in intravacuolar parasite multiplication rate.[47] When the MJ has reached the posterior end of the parasite, the PV is closed by pinching off and separating the PVM from the host plasma membrane.

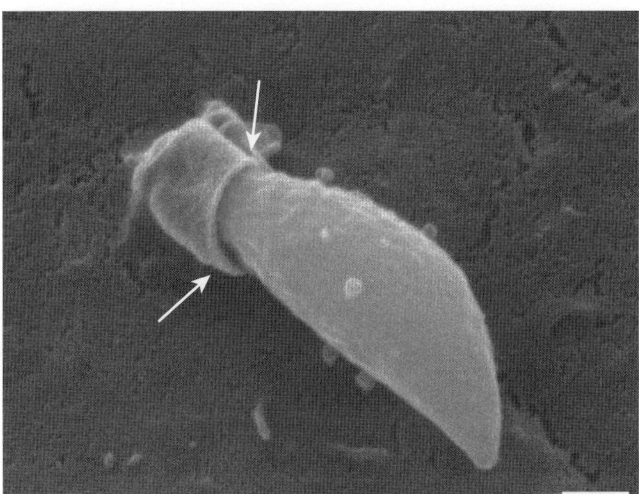

Figure 31-12 Formation of a collar-like structure *(arrows)* during invasion of the host cell by *Toxoplasma gondii*. Scanning electron micrograph; bar = 1 μm. (From Meissner M, Ferguson DJ, Frischknecht F: Invasion factors of apicomplexan parasites: essential or redundant? *Curr Opin Microbiol* 16:438-444, 2013; Figure 2A.)

Dense granule proteins participate in the development of a tubulovesicular membranous network that appears within the PV just after penetration (see Fig. 31-3). This network is assumed to play a role in exchanges between the parasite and the host cell. Protected by the PV, tachyzoites divide by endodyogeny and exit the cell when their numbers have reached 64 to 128 parasites.[48] Alternatively, the tachyzoites remain within the cell and differentiate into bradyzoites.

Cell invasion is thought to be driven by the parasite through an actin/myosin interaction.[45] However, some studies suggest that the host cell may play an active role in parasite penetration in that host cell actin and tubulin are recruited at the attachment site and involved in parasitic invasion.[49] Moreover, the host cell plasmalemma develops a collar-like structure around the invading *T. gondii* (Fig. 31-12).[44]

Tachyzoite to Bradyzoite Interconversion. This process is central to the pathogenesis and longevity of infection.[30] As described above, cysts that harbor bradyzoites persist for a long time in various tissues of the intermediate host. They are assumed to induce a protective, but not sterilizing, immune response. Initially, it was proposed that the host immune response triggered the differentiation of tachyzoites to bradyzoites.[50] This view was supported by the fact that, in immunocompromised patients, bradyzoites can transform back into fast-replicating tachyzoites, resulting in life-threatening lesions.[1] In vitro, stress conditions in culture, such as alkaline pH, proinflammatory cytokines, heat shock proteins, deprivation of nutriment, and drug pressure, have been shown to induce bradyzoite differentiation, demonstrating that these stages are the result of an adaptation to a hostile environment.[50] However, spontaneous bradyzoite development has also been observed in culture in the absence of immune response or stress conditions, suggesting that spontaneous transformation can occur in vivo.[50] Whether this phenomenon depends on cell type remains to be elucidated. Of interest, bradyzoites appear spontaneously in rat central nervous system (CNS) cells,[51] and in cultures of primary skeletal muscle cells, high levels of spontaneous bradyzoite transformation have been observed.[50]

GENETIC DIVERSITY

Population Structure

The nuclear genome of *T. gondii* comprises 14 chromosomes that range in size from 2 to 7 mega–base pairs.[52] The first studies on *T. gondii* strain genotyping began in the early 1990s. Despite worldwide distribution and sexual reproduction, the results, mainly from France and the United States, initially described a clonal population structure with three main lineages, designated as types I, II, and III.[53] The limited diversity within these three lineages strongly suggested that they have expanded relatively recently (10,000 years ago) from a common ancestor.[54] Further studies using new PCR–restriction fragment length polymorphism (RFLP) markers and microsatellite analysis allowed more precise investigations and reported a more heterogeneous structure of parasite populations than that described previously. Currently, the majority of isolates from South America, Africa, and Asia do not correspond to one of the three major lineages.

In Europe, the population is highly clonal, and type II is largely predominant. In France, this type represents 90% of strains isolated in animals and humans,[55,56] even in immunocompromised patients with severe clinical expression of the disease[57] or in ocular toxoplasmosis.[58] Type III is occasionally isolated, perhaps more frequently in southern Europe.[59] Type I is only observed as an exception.[38] Atypical strains isolated in Europe originated from the consumption of imported meat or were contracted during oversea journeys.[57]

In the United States, type II is predominant.[53] Recently, a completely new lineage, closely related to type II and named haplogroup 12, has been found in wild animals and occasionally in humans, and appears to be highly prevalent.[60] Other isolates that differ from existing lineages through a minor mutational drift have also been reported.[61]

In South America, studies from Brazil have revealed parasites with high genetic diversity, many isolates of which are virulent for mice,[62] although type II is very rare. Clonal lineages designated as Br I, Br II, Br III, and Br IV have been observed in domestic animals in Brazil,[63] but 88 atypical genotypes have been reported, and new genotypes have regularly been identified.[38] The Amazonian area displays a greater genetic diversity than that usually observed for *T. gondii* isolates. In French Guiana, two populations of "wild" and "anthropized" were differentiated genetically, and anthropization of the environment appears to be accompanied by a decrease in the diversity of *T. gondii*.[38] Interpenetration and genetic exchanges lead to hybridization between these two environmental populations, which may present a risk for human health because "wild" genotypes have been reported to be more pathogenic.[64] This difference between the strains that circulate in South America and Europe was confirmed by serotyping methods.[65,66]

In Asia, the population structure revealed limited diversity compared with South America with some shared genotypes.[38] In China, a recent study investigating 23 isolates from humans and animals revealed five genotypes, three of which were atypical. Genotype Chinese 1 is predominant and widespread in mainland China.[67] Types I and II are rarely observed, and atypical genotypes have intermediate or high virulence in mice.[67]

In Africa, information is scarce but the population structure appears to be more clonal than that in South America. In a study conducted on animal isolates in Gabon, the majority of strains belonged to the ubiquitous type III. The remaining strains were distributed into two haplogroups (Africa 1 and 3).[68]

See the next section for discussion of genotype and virulence.

Pathogenesis of Congenital Toxoplasmosis

FACTORS ASSOCIATED WITH PATHOGENICITY

Parasitic Factors

For clinicians, the link between strain genotype and pathogenicity is an important issue but is still controversial. It has to be borne in mind that virulence, from a clinical point of view, is a multifactorial phenomenon that results from a combination of host factors, such as genetic susceptibility[69,70] and immune status, and parasitic factors, such as genetic diversity.[71] Moreover, pathogenicity is usually determined in animal models, but the range of intermediate host susceptibility is highly variable. Regarding mouse virulence, among the three archetypal groups observed in Europe, type I is highly virulent in mice, for which an inoculum of less than 10 tachyzoites is lethal within 10 days. Types II and III are considered to be less virulent, and mice can survive after inoculation of more than 10^3 tachyzoites. Type II, which is largely dominant in North America and Europe, where the majority of acquired infections are subclinical, can induce deleterious lesions in immunocompromised patients[57] or in congenital toxoplasmosis acquired early in pregnancy. Crosses between strains allowed the identification of polymorphic genes coding for secreted factors associated with virulence in mice: Deletion of the ROP5 cluster in a highly pathogenic strain resulted in the complete loss of virulence,[72] and crosses between type II and III strains identified kinases (ROP18 and ROP16, respectively) as the key molecules for virulence.[73] These kinases, which are secreted into the host cell, exert a kinase activity that appears to be crucial to the host-pathogen interaction.

In humans, several studies in Europe, North America, and South America have argued that the clinical manifestations and severity of human toxoplasmosis are determined in part by parasite genotype. In French Guiana, infection of immunocompetent patients by atypical strains led to severe multiorgan infections.[74] In France, an atypical genotype that is uncommon in Europe but has already been described in South America was observed in a case of congenital toxoplasmosis that was unusually severe for European cases but not for cases typical of Brazil.[75] Atypical strains have also been isolated in a case of severe pulmonary toxoplasmosis in an immunocompetent patient.[76]

A prospective cohort study revealed more severe ocular lesions in congenital toxoplasmosis in Brazil, where atypical strains are common, than those observed in Europe, where the parasitic population is highly clonal.[77] Higher virulence of atypical strains has also been confirmed by severe cases of congenital toxoplasmosis after the mothers consumed imported horse meat from South America.[78] Genetic diversity also questions the dogma of immunoprotection provided by prior infection. In a pregnant woman who was immune before conception, immunity acquired against European *Toxoplasma* strains appeared not to protect against reinfection by atypical strains acquired outside Europe or through eating imported meat.[79]

Host Factors

After parasite virulence and genetics, there are two well-established factors associated with outcome: gestational age at the time when primary maternal infection is acquired and the parasite load in amniotic fluid. If a pregnant woman becomes infected with *Toxoplasma* during the first weeks of gestation, the likelihood of vertical transmission to her offspring is low. Nevertheless, if it does occur, the embryo may incur severe damage. The transmission probability increases in parallel with gestation time and rises to a value of 80% by the end of pregnancy, whereas the risk of organ damage decreases[80] (see "Exploring Cellular Immunity"). Evaluation of *T. gondii* concentration in amniotic fluid by quantitative PCR assay is also a good indicator of risk of severe fetal outcome in humans.[81]

Genetic factors may also contribute to risk. Several genes involved in host innate and adaptive immune response are induced during active infection in the pregnant woman to control the rapidly replicating tachyzoites. Transgenic murine models have been useful in illuminating genes and pathways that control the innate immune response.[82-85] However, the data gleaned from these studies have not been of great value in helping to identify factors that determine human susceptibility.

In humans, an association between the human leukocyte antigen (HLA) class II gene *DQ3* and hydrocephalus has been reported in cases of congenital toxoplasmosis, as well as in AIDS patients with *Toxoplasma* encephalitis. This finding is supported by data gleaned from a study with transgenic mice carrying the HLA class II *DQ3* locus. In these mice, the CNS load of *Toxoplasma* was higher than in those carrying the *DQ1* locus.[69] Other genetic associations with disease susceptibility and disease severity include mutations in the collagen gene *COL2A* and the lipid transporter gene *ABC4r*, as well as alleles of the genes encoding the Toll-like receptor 9 (TLR9), the purinergic receptor P2X7R, and the endoplasmic reticulum aminopeptidase associated with antigen processing (ERAAP2).[70,86,87] Finally, in children with congenital toxoplasmosis who have undergone treatment, the female gender has been reported to predominate; the basis for this difference remains speculative, but hormonal differences are not likely to be involved at the young ages studied.[88]

Cellular Immunity and Immunopathology of Toxoplasmosis

Innate immune mechanisms,[89] including natural killer cells, help to control acute infection with *Toxoplasma*, but resolution of active infection is dependent on adaptive, T-cell–mediated immunity. T-helper 1 (Th1)-cell responses, with appropriate regulation of this response by interleukin-10 (IL-10), regulatory T cells, and Th2-cell responses to protect against untoward tissue injury, are known to be important in the control of infections with intracellular pathogens generally and with *T. gondii* in mouse models.[82,90] In principle, during pregnancy, such a balanced response would help to control primary infection with *Toxoplasma*, while maintaining placental-fetal integrity.[91] However, little is known concerning the degree to which balanced regulation of the Th1-cell microenvironment influences vertical transmission during the early stages of pregnancy. By contrast, and not surprisingly, a Th2-cell environment has been found to favor the transplacental dissemination of *Toxoplasma* and fetal infection in a mouse model.[85]

In the context of placental infection, HLA class II antigens are expressed at the trophoblast interface, which is not the case in the absence of infection.[91,92] Hence the almost threefold increase in the risk of abortion among women with pregnancy-associated primary infection can be readily explained.[93] The expression of HLA class II antigens is mediated by interferon-γ (IFN-γ). The IFN-γ–mediated response, produced both by $CD4^+$ and $CD8^+$ T cells, is essential for controlling tachyzoite proliferation during both acute acquired infection and reactivation of infection. Some data suggest, however, that IFN-γ may enhance, directly or indirectly, the transplacental transmission of *T. gondii*.[94] In experimental animals, IFN-γ has been shown to play a pivotal role in the upregulation of the intracellular adhesion molecule 1 (ICAM-1) during the process of congenital transmission.[95,96] IFN-γ also seems to have a crucial role in the recruitment of T cells into the brain after infection by inducing expression of the adhesion molecule vascular cell adhesion molecule 1 (VCAM-1) on cerebrovascular endothelial cells, and several chemokines, including CXCL10.[97] Whether similar mechanisms facilitate transplacental passage of the parasite is unknown.

The increase in the rate of vertical transmission with increased gestational age could be due, at least in part, to immunologic factors. In human placental explants, the expression levels of macrophage-migration inhibitory factor (MIF) increases in parallel with gestational age, and this response correlates with the susceptibility of the placenta to *Toxoplasma* infection.[98]

Whether, when, and in which aspects antigen-specific T-cell responses are impaired in congenital *Toxoplasma* infection compared with those with acquired infection is debated. T-cell hyporesponsiveness to parasite antigens in congenitally infected infants has been observed, followed by resolution later during childhood.[99,100] One group reported that the degree of impairment was greater in young children with significant organ damage and required years to reach the strength of responses observed in infected adults.[101] Another group found that although impaired in young infants with congenital infection, T-cell responses to the granule antigen 1 (GRA1) of *Toxoplasma* matured during childhood such that in older children with congenital infection, the strength, epitope specificity, and cytokine responses were comparable to those of immunocompetent adults with asymptomatically acquired *T. gondii* infection.[100] This maturation was unrelated to the presence or severity of disease manifestations. A more recent study found that nearly all congenitally infected neonates, such as older *Toxoplasma* immune individuals, had responses to soluble *Toxoplasma* antigens measured as antigen-stimulated induction of IL-2 receptor-α (CD25).[102]

During chronic infection, control of *T. gondii* infection is, at least in the mouse, kept latent through Th1-type T cells and the cytokines they produce, including IFN-γ and CXCL10.[103] Waning of this response over time may contribute to the development of recurrent eye disease. In line with this speculation, 41% of the new ocular lesions in congenital toxoplasmosis are observed in individuals older than 10 years.[103] By contrast, in patients with ocular toxoplasmosis not known to be associated with congenital infection, the risk of a recurrence seems to decrease with time after the last outbreak.[104,105]

REINFECTION OR REACTIVATION?

Fifty years ago, we learned that if mice survive the acute stage of an initial infection with *T. gondii*, they become resistant to reinfection.[106] More than a decade later, this belief was revised by the finding that reinfection in mice was feasible under experimental conditions,[107,108] but vertical transmission after reinfection during pregnancy did not occur in mice or rabbits.[109]

In humans, the first clinical cases of reinfection were reported for three Brazilian brothers, who in parallel exhibited both clinical and serologic signs of acute toxoplasmosis. Reactivation of a latent disease in all three was deemed unlikely.[110] Ten years later, a spontaneous abortion in a pregnant woman was suspected to have resulted from reinfection.[111] Also, in the first reported human case of vertical transmission by an immunocompetent woman who was shown to be immune before conception, serologic signs of active infection were observed; it was not clear whether this case resulted from reactivation or from reinfection acquired through known contact with kittens.[112]

Since the field became aware of the importance of strain and virulence in toxoplasmosis, the issue of reinfection has been addressed in model systems. In one study, cerebral reinvasion with parasites and cyst formation was reported to occur in the face of prior immunity after challenge with a strain of heterologous genotype. This finding indicates that immunity to a particular strain does not necessarily protect the host against infection with *T. gondii* of a different genotype.[113,114]

Moreover, whereas it was previously thought that all cases of congenital infection resulted from primary infection of the mother during pregnancy, in recent years, a few cases of congenital *Toxoplasma* infection have been reported in the offspring of immunocompetent mothers who were confirmed to be *Toxoplasma* immune before pregnancy.[79,115-117] In these rare cases, congenital toxoplasmosis may result either from reinfection, which has been confirmed in one instance only, or from reactivation; band patterns in comparative immunoblot analyses of sera can help to clarify whether disease recurrence results from reactivation or reinfection.[118] Reactivation might be triggered by pregnancy-associated modulation of T-cell immunity[119,120]; consistent with this possibility, susceptibility to reinfection in a murine model of toxoplasmosis is related to the balance between protective Th1-type cytokines and modulatory cytokines, such as IL-10.[121]

WHAT IS THE DRIVING FORCE BEHIND A RECURRENCE?

A prerequisite for the virtually lifelong persistence of the parasite is its ability to undergo conversion from the proliferative stage (tachyzoite) to a latent tissue cyst (bradyzoite). Reactivation represents a switch back to the proliferative trophozoite stage. The driving force behind a recurrence in immunocompetent individuals is unknown.[122] Recurrences can be triggered by senescent changes in tissue cysts, which are accompanied by the release of parasites or antigens, by hormonal fluctuations, and by transient changes in humoral or cellular immune responses,[123] as well as by pregnancy[124,125] and by surgical trauma, such as that induced by the extraction of a cataract.[126] Better understanding of the mechanisms whereby these factors lead to reprogramming of gene expression in *Toxoplasma* that is required for bradyzoite conversion could open up the way to the development of new drug targets for eradication of the parasite before the attainment of this chronic stage.[127]

In animal models of toxoplasmosis, parasitemia regularly occurs in the absence of overt disease.[128] Likewise in humans, circulating parasites have been observed in the absence of disease activity.[129] This circumstance would account for the well-documented occurrence of fluctuations in serum antibody titers and could contribute mechanistically to the development of recurrences.[129-133] Low-level, periodic parasitemia could thus be a normal physiologic state in chronic infection, which leads only randomly to clinically manifested disease activity at immunoprivileged sites.[129]

After follow-up times of 5 to 6 years, recurrence rates for ocular toxoplasmosis of 50% and 80 % have been reported.[105,134,135] Although greater than 30% of treated as well as untreated individuals with congenital toxoplasmosis manifest ocular lesions by the age of 10 years, new ones also occur later in life.[136-138] The risk of a recurrence is highest immediately and up to 2 years after the last outbreak, and it decreases with an increase in the disease-free interval. The age of the patient impacts risk of a recurrence with younger individuals being at higher risk.[104,105]

Modulation of the Host Environment by *Toxoplasma* and Host Immune Countermeasures

Toxoplasma gondii has the capacity to infect virtually all warm-blooded animals, which it does by active invasion of the host's nucleated cells, where it replicates within the cytosol (see "Host Cell Penetration"). The range of hosts that can be infected with the parasite is extraordinarily high because of the facility with which it can invade cells, its ability to modulate their gene expression, and its successful evasion of the immune response. Consistent with data derived from PCR analyses, the parasite's dissemination throughout the body is mediated largely by intracellular tachyzoites, which escape immune surveillance[29,139]; comparable to many other apicomplexans, tachyzoites of *Toxoplasma* survive for only a short period of time within an extracellular environment.

Infection with the parasite is usually asymptomatic; only rarely does it elicit a serious clinical condition. Indeed, the host's survival and the asymptomatic persistence of the parasite for the lifetime of that host probably contribute to the unique evolutionary success of *Toxoplasma*.[140] Already at the time of its entry into a host's cell, *T. gondii* secretes effector proteins into the cytosol. These virulence factors interfere with the innate immune response and promote the parasite's survival.[141] Once within a cell, the parasite envelops itself within a vacuole that protects it from surveillance and destruction by macrophages.[142,143] In an attempt to eliminate the parasite and in response to protective cytokines, such as IFN-γ, macrophages upregulate a family of immunity-related p47–guanosine triphosphatases (IRGs), which aim to modify the membrane of the vacuole to promote phagosome-lysosome fusion and digestion of the enclosed parasite. However, the parasite can escape this lysosomal attack of the host's immune system by a unique maneuver, which involves coating the external surface of the vacuole in which it is contained with a secretory enzyme, the serine/threonine kinase ROP18. Together with pseudokinase ROP5, an essential cofactor, ROP18 phosphorylates and inactivates IRGs on the surface of the vacuole, thereby protecting the parasite from destruction.[144-146]

Host resistance also may be mediated in part by CD40-induced autophagy. Engagement of CD40 on infected macrophages by CD40 ligand expressed on activated $CD4^+$ T cells stimulates the formation of autophagosomes around the PV, particularly in neural tissues. By this means, lysosomal degradation of the parasite is facilitated.[147-149] It is conceivable that this mechanism could be used to help eliminate cysts through the use of therapeutic anti-CD40 antibodies, a form of intervention that is currently being tested in the context of antitumor immunotherapy and prevention of allograft rejection.[150-152] Given the theoretical risk for the development of cerebral and ocular recurrences in *Toxoplasma*-seropositive individuals, such intervention might be considered only if the risk profile was sufficiently favorable.

The virulence of *T. gondii* and the resistance of a host to the parasite depend also on other factors, including the innate immune response. However, our knowledge of innate immunity to *Toxoplasma* is still incomplete, and that knowledge is essentially confined to the murine model; little is known about these aspects of the infection in humans. Experiments with mice have revealed TLR/myeloid differentiation primary response 88 protein (MyD88) signaling to be important in recognition of the pathogen by the innate immune system. The various points at which the parasite impacts TLR/MyD88 signaling could serve as candidate targets for pharmacologic intervention.[153]

The host proinflammatory response to *Toxoplasma* is counteracted by the parasite's secretion of specific effector proteins, various combinations of which help to maintain an optimal parasite burden for forward transmission in different hosts.[154] These effector proteins are secreted by the parasite upon penetration of the targeted cell, with a view to manipulating or disarming the host's innate immunity and thereby promoting its own survival.[141]

Understanding the regulatory mechanisms during *Toxoplasma* infection that limit excessive inflammation and tissue injury, which could result if protective Th1-type immunity[155] was not modulated, and of the events that lead to the development of immunopathology are also incomplete.[156] Together, this modulation of cytokine secretion to limit tissue injury, parasite-mediated inhibition of signal transduction within host cells and parasite adaptation to the host immune response may facilitate the establishment of latency and chronic, lifelong infection.[157] Thereafter, waning of protective Th1-type immunity over time may contribute to reactivation. Such waning may be due in part to T-cell exhaustion, as observed in certain persistent viral infections,[119,120,158] and to inhibition of antigen presentation on host HLA (i.e., HLA/major histocompatibility complex [MHC]) molecules, thereby averting T-cell–mediated recognition.[159,160]

Parasite-Host Interaction in Brain and Eye

A hallmark of *T. gondii*–induced infection is the ability of the parasite to cross normally nonpermissive biologic barriers, namely, the intestine, the blood-brain barrier, the blood-retina barrier, and the placenta, and consequently to spread to organs with restricted access. *T. gondii* migrates through the body within host leukocytes, using them as "Trojan horses" and hijacking their ICAM-1–dependent cell trafficking pathways to facilitate its own dissemination and to escape the immune attacks of the host.[161,162]

Parasite-Host Interaction in Brain and Eye

Typical examples of immunoprivileged tissue compartments that are accessible to *T. gondii* include the CNS and the eye. Primary invasion of the CNS is the consequence of an interaction between *T. gondii* and vascular endothelial cells that constitute the blood-brain barrier.[163] In addition to the ICAM-1–dependent trafficking within host leukocytes noted above, the parasite may gain access by direct transmigration through either retinal or choroidal vascular endothelial cells.[164] In humans, accumulation of bradyzoites and clinical manifestations of infection are encountered more frequently within ocular and neuronal tissues than within any other organs. This observation probably reflects the fact that in humans, vascular endothelial cells of the retina are more susceptible than those of other tissues to infection with *T. gondii*, which leads to a higher tachyzoite invasion efficiency and to the attainment of higher parasitic loads in this compartment than elsewhere in the body.[165]

After the primary invasion of neuronal cells by the parasites and their conversion into bradyzoites, the infection commonly persists in a chronically latent form without reactivation until the end of the host's life, if the individual remains immunocompetent. Small vessels in the vicinity of intact bradyzoites are occasionally subject to infiltration with inflammatory cells, and lymphocytes may be observed to adhere to the vascular endothelium and to perivascular tissues but not to neurons.[166] The adhering lymphocytes have been identified as locally resident, antigen-specific host CD8$^+$ T cells, which survey latent forms of the parasite but ignore intact bradyzoites. In the CNS, production of IFN-γ by T cells plays a key role in the control and clearance of parasites during the acute phase of infection and to prevent or control reactivation. It mediates the control of parasitic proliferation by the activation of microglia, astrocytes, and macrophages, as well as by the local recruitment of T cells.[97] If bradyzoites lodged within the CNS rupture and early recognition by CD8$^+$ T cells does not occur, which would be the case in immunocompromised individuals or in instances of primary congenital infection, severe tissue damage may ensue.[167]

Ocular lesions are the most typical clinical manifestation of congenital as well as of acquired toxoplasmosis. Ocular lesions represent a local manifestation of systemic infection that has spread to the eye by parasite transit through the blood-retina barrier. Reactivation of a latent retinal infection is presumed to follow the rupturing of bradyzoites in the vicinity of preexisting scars and may secondarily involve the choroid, thereby leading to retinochoroiditis. Because toxoplasmic retinochoroiditis is deemed to be a local event, it does not usually evoke a systemic immune response.[168] Replication of the parasite within the retina is followed by a breakdown of the blood-retina barrier. Invasion of the retinal compartment ensues and leads to local tissue damage.[156,169]

Recurrences

Clinically manifest recurrences can occur even in immunocompetent individuals, even after several decades of quiescence, and in the absence of previous signs of active disease. These delayed manifestations have been attributed to the local rupture of cysts within the specific immunoprivileged environment of the eye and brain. In animal models, a positive effect of treatment on the number of tissue cysts in the brain has been reported.[170,171] This finding has been used to argue in favor of therapeutic intervention to limit tachyzoites and thereby lower the tissue cyst burden, which, even though this would not reduce the rate of vertical transmission, could reduce the risk of clinical disease later in life. However, there is at present no direct evidence that risk is correlated with the number of cysts in the affected tissue compartment. Rupturing of cysts may, however, not represent the sole mechanism underlying recurrences.[172] In the brains of chronically infected mice, large and small cysts are often encountered close to one another. This finding might imply that leakage, rather than rupturing of cysts, may lead to the formation of smaller satellite cysts.[31,173,174] In any case, bradyzoite-containing cysts serve as an important source of the parasite in the brain and probably contribute greatly to the successful maintenance of the microbe and to its wide, almost ubiquitous distribution in warm-blooded animals.[175]

Special Problems Relating to Brain and Eyes

Histopathologic studies in murine models of congenital toxoplasmosis have revealed great variability in the degree of tissue destruction, both in the eye and in the brain. *Toxoplasma*-containing cysts are encountered within the retina and the optic nerve, irrespective of whether the disease is severe or mild, but less frequently in the latter case. Mild forms of the disease are characterized by low-grade uveitis and by lymphatic perivasculitis. In more severely affected eyes, the retinal destruction may be focal, affect only certain sectors, or be complete. Inflammatory destruction of the outer retina is also sometimes evident and is associated with death of cells or infiltration of lymphocytes and plasma cells; granulomatous reactions are rare. In very severe cases, the retina may be subject to complete necrosis and calcification.[176] The formation of cataracts and a selective destruction of the photoreceptor cell layers appear to occur specifically in congenitally infected mice. In the adult murine brain, subacute inflammatory tissue changes are manifested in the vicinity of intact bradyzoites in chronic infection.[177,178]

The eye is generally considered to be an immunologically privileged organ because of the existence of a tight blood-vascular barrier, the absence of a lymphatic drainage system, and the paucity of classic antigen-presenting cells. However, this dogma is now being challenged in the face of evidence for active interaction between the immune system and the eye and for an ocular presentation of exogenous and endogenous antigens. According to current knowledge, cell-mediated immune responses and noninflammatory humoral ones are regulated in the eye by cytokine-mediated, active immunosuppressive mechanisms, which include the apoptosis of alloreactive lymphocytes to curb the tissue-destructive effects of inflammatory reactions, both locally and in the brain.[179-181]

The structure of the retina is complex, both architecturally and antigenically. Because it develops as an extension of the neural tube, it shares in common with the brain several membranous and cytoplasmic antigens, which include those of the neural and glial filaments. Several antigens that are specific to the nervous system are also abundant in the retina. Antigens that are specific to the eye include those of the retinal pigmented epithelium, retinal ganglion cells, and astrocytes. The outer segments of the photoreceptor cells contain soluble antigens which, when injected into rats, rabbits, guinea-pigs, or monkeys, evoke varying degrees of intraocular inflammation. The inflammatory response can lead to uveitis, to retinal detachment, to degeneration of the photoreceptor cells and occasionally to retinovasculitis.

Both cell-mediated and humoral immunity to photoreceptor cell–specific antigens have been demonstrated in various types of uveitis, including those associated with ocular toxoplasmosis and sarcoidosis. Autoimmunity that is specific to the retina can develop upon its detachment and in conjunction with diabetic retinopathy; in the latter case, particularly after photocoagulation with argon laser light. In patients with systemic immune disorders, such as lupus erythematosus, antibodies against retinal antigens have been detected even in the absence of ocular involvement. Hence the precise pathogenetic role of retinal autoimmunity in ocular diseases, including *Toxoplasma*-related ocular disease, is not known with certainty. It may represent no more than an epiphenomenon that develops after physically, immunologically, or microbially induced retinal damage. On the other hand, although retinal autoimmunity alone may fail to evoke ocular inflammation, it could perpetuate and sustain the level of a preexisting inflammatory state, thereby leading to further destruction of ocular tissues.[182]

Support for this latter contention has been furnished by Muiño and colleagues: Fivefold to 10-fold higher concentrations of immunoglobulin E (IgE) and two- to threefold higher concentrations of the soluble CD23 (sCD23) B-cell marker were detected in patients with either autoimmune uveitis or ocular toxoplasmosis than in healthy control subjects.[183] Immunoglobulins specific to the retinal S-antigen were detected in greater than 80% of the cases, and those of the IgE class accounted for nearly 70% of these immune responses. Specific IgE was detected in two thirds of the patients with autoimmune uveitis but not in the control group or in individuals with bacterial uveitis. Elevated levels of total IgE and of sCD23 and the presence of antibodies against S-antigen reflect an activation of Th2 cells. In patients with ocular toxoplasmosis, a strong antiretinal signal in the photoreceptor cell layers was reported to occur in greater than 90% of the individuals, whereas in healthy control subjects and in subjects with retinovasculitis, a lower level of reactivity was detected at the same site in only 40% of cases. Antibodies against the retinal S-antigen were detected in 75% of the patients suffering from either ocular toxoplasmosis or retinovasculitis but also in greater than 60% of the healthy control subjects. Hence antiretinal reactivity in patients with ocular toxoplasmosis seems not to be specific and cannot be accounted for solely by the presence of anti–S-antigen.

The prevalence of antiphotoreceptor antibodies indicates that they occur naturally, although the higher degree of reactivity in those with ocular toxoplasmosis suggest that such antibodies could play a contributory role in disease pathogenesis.[181,183,184] More recently, mononuclear cells derived from the peripheral blood of patients suffering from mild ocular toxoplasmosis were reported to respond more frequently to one or several retinal antigens than did those stemming from either healthy subjects or individuals with severe ocular toxoplasmosis. The production of cytokines by the proliferating mononuclear cells did not follow a specific pattern, but a trend was observed toward greater production of IL-4 and IL-5, which are Th2-type cytokines, than in healthy subjects, suggesting that this response to self-antigens might help to curb, rather than exacerbate, acute inflammation-related injury.[185] However, at least in animal models, this temporally limited response may be directed solely against the retinal and cerebral antigens that are liberated by disturbance of the blood-brain barrier in the context of infection-associated tissue destruction.[186,187]

Pathology in Congenital Toxoplasmosis*

In reviewing the literature on the pathology of congenital toxoplasmosis, it is immediately apparent that the genesis of the natural infection in the fetus is entirely comparable with that observed in experimental toxoplasmosis in animals. The position of necrotic foci and lesions in general suggests that the organisms reach the brain and all other organs through the bloodstream. Noteworthy is the remarkable variability in distribution of lesions and parasites among the different reported cases.[188-191] Age at the time of autopsy is a major modifying factor, but others include the virulence of the strain of *T. gondii*, the number of organisms actually transmitted from the mother to the fetus, the time during pregnancy when the infection occurred, the developmental maturity of the infant's immune system, and the number of organs and tissues carefully examined. After the appearance of early reports of cases of congenital toxoplasmosis, the prevailing impression was that the infection manifested itself in infants mainly as an encephalomyelitis and that visceral lesions were uncommon and insignificant. This view reflected the observation of a marked degree of damage

*In the absence of relevant new data, this portion of the chapter has remained unchanged from the 7th edition Chapter 31, by Jack S. Remington, Rima McLeod, Christopher B. Wilson, and George Desmonts, with permission of the authors. The list of references, however, has been updated.

to the CNS without a comparable degree of extraneural involvement in these infants. In some cases, however, extraneural lesions are severe and may even predominate.[191-193] Thus at autopsy, in some cases, only the CNS and eyes may be involved, whereas in others, wide dissemination of lesions and parasites may be noted. Between these two extremes are wide variations in the degree of organ and tissue involvement, but the CNS is never spared. The clinical importance of lesions in the CNS and eye is magnified by the limited ability of these tissues to regenerate, compared with the remarkable regenerative capacity of other tissues in the body. Active regeneration of extraneural tissues may be observed even in the most acute stages of infection in the infant.[194] Thus in extraneural organs, residual lesions may be so slight and insignificant that they are easily overlooked. In the CNS and eye, on the other hand, the lesser ability of nerve cells to regenerate leads to more severe permanent damage.[194-196] The presence of *T. gondii* in the cells lining alveoli and in the endothelium of pulmonary vessels led Callahan and coworkers[188] to suggest that aspiration of infected amniotic fluid in the lungs may be a route of entry of the organism into the fetus. That infection by this route may occur cannot be disputed. The diffuse character of the lung changes contrasts with the more focal lesions found in other organs and tissues. Zuelzer[197] pointed out that this difference may be due to the position of the lungs in the route of circulation. Before dissemination to other tissues of the body all blood with parasites entering the venous circulation must first pass through the alveolar capillaries. Thus the lungs are exposed to more parasites than any other single organ.

PLACENTA

The first description of *T. gondii* in placental tissues was by Neghme and coworkers.[198] Subsequently, a number of similar observations have been made.[199-203] Evidence for the likelihood of the hematogenous route of spread of *T. gondii* to the placenta is supplied by the fact that groups of tachyzoites can be found widely dispersed in the chorionic plate, decidua, and amnion, and organisms have been observed in the placental villi and umbilical cord without associated significant lesions (Fig. 31-13).[198,199,203-206] The first description of the histopathologic features of a *T. gondii*–infected placenta of a woman with AIDS was by Piche and colleagues[207] in 1997. The woman experienced a spontaneous abortion associated with fever and *T. gondii* pneumonia. In five cases studied by Benirschke and Driscoll,[203] the most consistent findings in the placentas were chronic inflammatory reactions in the decidua capsularis and focal reactions in the villi. The lesions appeared to be more severe in infants who died soon after birth. Villous lesions develop at random throughout the placenta. Single or multiple neighboring villi with low-grade chronic inflammation, activation of Hofbauer cells, necrobiosis of component cells, and proliferative fibrosis may be seen. Although villous lesions frequently are observed in placental toxoplasmosis, histologic examination of these foci does not reveal parasites; they occur in free villi and in villi attached to the decidua. Lymphocytes and other mononuclear cells, but rarely plasma cells, make up the intravillous and perivillous infiltrates. The decidual infiltrate consists primarily of lymphocytes. Inflammation of

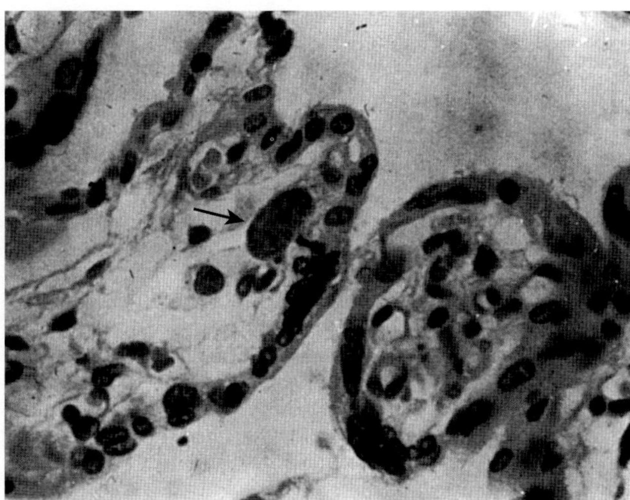

Figure 31-13 *Toxoplasma* cyst in the placenta of an infected fetus *(arrow).*

the umbilical cord is uncommon. When fetal hydrops is present, the placenta also is hydropic.[208] The organism is seen mainly in the tissue cyst form and may be present in the connective tissues of the amnionic and chorionic membranes, Wharton jelly, and in the decidua. Mellgren and coworkers,[201] Benirschke and Driscoll,[203] and Nowakowska and coworkers[209] observed one specimen from which the parasite was isolated, in which contiguous decidua capsularis, chorion, and amnion contained organisms. In a retrospective histologic examination of 13 placentas of newborns with serologic test results suggestive of congenital *T. gondii* infection, Garcia and associates[210] observed organisms that had the morphology of *T. gondii* tachyzoites in 4 cases. Of interest is that in 10 of their cases, on gross examination, the placenta was found to be abnormal, suggesting the diagnosis of prolonged fetal distress, hematogenous infection, or both. In some cases, the diagnosis was made initially from examination of the placenta.[205,211,212] Altshuler[211] made a premortem diagnosis by noting cysts in connective tissue beneath the amnion in a very hydropic placenta. The fetal villi showed hydrops, an abundance of Hofbauer cells, and vascular proliferation. Numerous erythroblasts were present within the vessels of the terminal villi. Elliott[202] described lesions in a placenta after a third-month spontaneous abortion of a macerated fetus. The placenta showed nodular accumulations of histiocytes beneath the syncytial layer. In villi that had pronounced histiocytic infiltrates, the syncytial layer was raised away from the villous stroma, and the infiltrate had spilled into the intervillous space. Disruption of the syncytium was associated with coagulation necrosis of the villous stroma and fibrinous exudate. Both encysted and free forms of *T. gondii* were present in the areas of histiocytic inflammation, in the zones of coagulation necrosis, and in the villi without either necrotizing inflammation or syncytial loss. The location of the organisms varied, but they seemed to be concentrated at the interface between the stroma and the trophoblast. This aggregation of histiocytes and organisms at the stroma-trophoblast interface suggested to Elliott that this is a favored site of growth for the parasite.

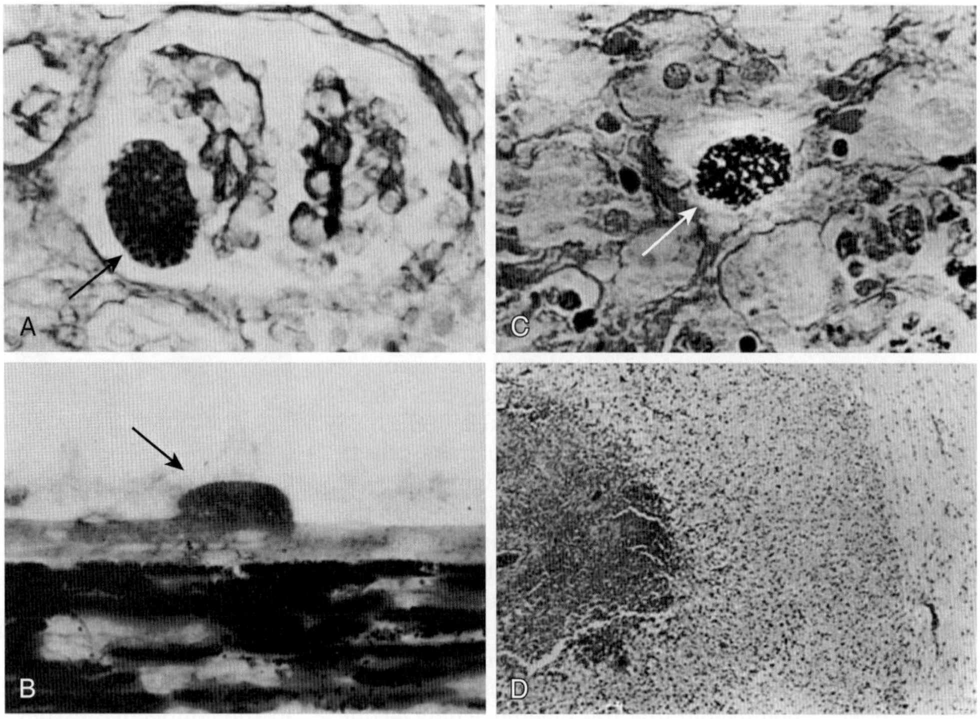

Figure 31-14 A, Large cyst *(arrow)* in glomerular space. **B,** *Toxoplasma* cyst *(arrow)* in the retina. Note incomplete pigmentation of the choroid. **C,** *Toxoplasma* cyst *(arrow)* in the cortex of the fetal adrenal gland. **D,** Section of brain showing abscess *(left),* normal brain *(right),* and area of gliosis *(middle).* Encysted parasites were abundant at the periphery of these areas. (From Miller MJ, Seaman E, Remington JS: The clinical spectrum of congenital toxoplasmosis: problems in recognition, *J Pediatr* 70:714-723, 1967.)

CENTRAL NERVOUS SYSTEM

In infants who die in the newborn period, the severity of the cellular reaction in the leptomeninges of both brain and spinal cord reflects the amount of damage done to underlying tissue. The pia-arachnoid overlying destructive cortical or spinal cord lesions shows congestion of the vessels and infiltration of large numbers of lymphocytes, plasma cells, macrophages, and eosinophils. This type of change is particularly noticeable around small arterioles, venules, and capillaries. Complete obliteration of the gyri and sulci may be noted; the line of demarcation between the pia-arachnoid and brain substance is obscured. Parasites frequently are found within intimal cells of the arterioles, venules, and capillaries.[188,213-216] Only recently, it has been recognized that continued parasite proliferation and tissue destruction can occur within the fetal brain despite sufficient maternal immune response.[217] This strongly argues for a treatment of recently acquired congenital infection to control proliferating parasites in immunologically protected sites, such as the fetal brain.

In the cerebral hemispheres, brainstem, and cerebellum, extensive diffuse and focal alterations of the parenchymal architecture are seen (Figs. 31-14 and 31-15).[188,192,197,218-220] The most characteristic change is the extensive necrosis of the brain parenchyma resulting from vascular involvement by lesions (Fig. 31-16). The lesions are most intense in the cortex and basal ganglia and at times in the periventricular areas (Fig. 31-17). They are marked by the formation of glial nodules,[218] which Wolf and coworkers[220] referred to as characteristic miliary granulomas. Necrosis may progress to actual formation of cystic areas, which have a homogeneous eosinophilic material at the center of the cyst cavity. At the periphery of these cystic areas, focal calcification of necrotic, individual nerve cells may be evident (Fig. 31-18). Calcification within zones of necrosis may be extensive, with the formation of broad bands of calcific material involving most of the cortical layers, or it may be scattered diffusely throughout the foci of necrosis. Calcium salts are deposited in coarse granules or in finely divided particles, which give the appearance of "calcium dust." Many cells become completely calcified, whereas others contain only a few particles of finely divided calcium. Some pathologists have suggested that the *T. gondii* organisms themselves become encrusted with calcium salts.[197,221] Cells containing fine particles of calcium also are observed in cytomegalovirus infection and ischemic brain damage of the fetus or newborn and may be mistakenly construed as evidence of *T. gondii*.[222-224] The extent of calcification appears to depend on the severity of the reaction and the duration of the infection.[189] *T. gondii* tachyzoites and cysts are seen in and adjacent to the necrotic foci, near or in the glial nodules, in perivascular regions, and in cerebral tissue uninvolved by inflammatory change (see Figs. 31-14D and 31-15D).[219,225] Hervas and colleagues[226] described an infant who developed progressive drowsiness, a weak cry, and grunting in the newborn period. Computed tomography (CT) revealed cerebral calcifications, multiple ring-enhancing lesions mimicking brain abscesses, and moderate ventricular enlargement. At autopsy, *T. gondii* organisms were seen in the ventricular cerebrospinal fluid (CSF). Widespread necrosis and granulomatous lesions with mononuclear infiltrates also were noted. The degree of change in the spinal cord is extremely variable. It may consist of local infiltration of lymphocytes and plasma cells or, on the other hand, almost complete disruption of the normal architecture, caused by the transformation of the gray and white matter into a mass of necrotic granulation tissue, may be seen. *T. gondii* cysts, which can be identified in the white matter, usually are unassociated with inflammatory reaction.[227-229] Periaqueductal and periventricular vasculitis with necrosis

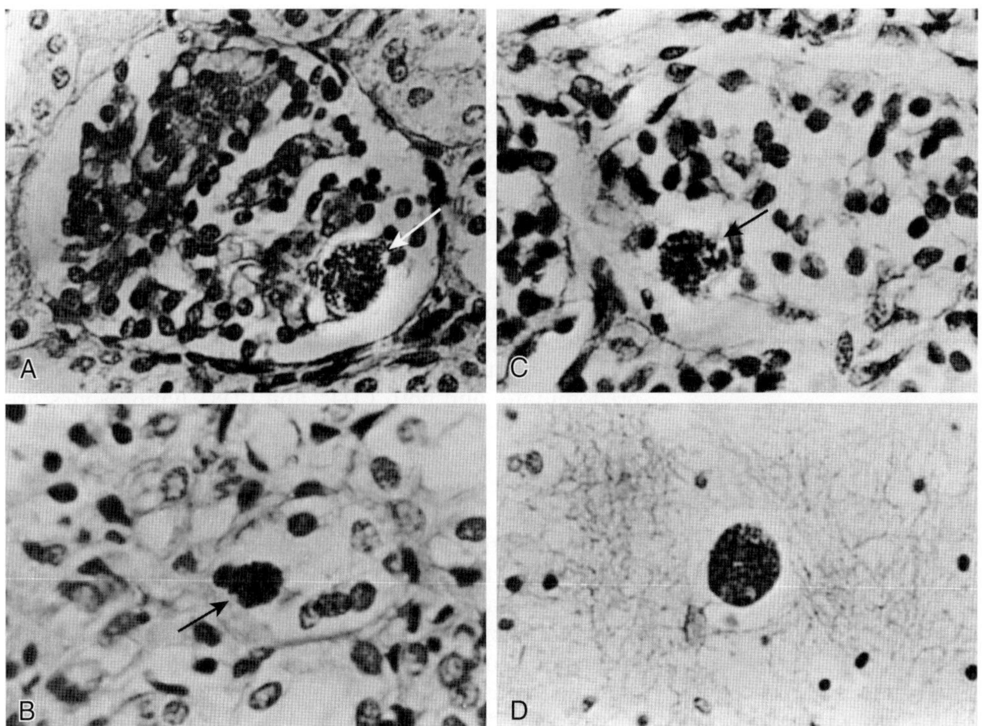

Figure 31-15 A, *Toxoplasma* cyst *(arrow)* within a glomerulus. Similar cysts were identified in endothelial cells of the glomeruli and free in the glomerular spaces. **B,** Encysted parasites *(arrow)* in a renal tubule cell. Other cysts were present within lumina of several tubules. **C,** *Toxoplasma* cyst *(arrow)* in immature testicular tissue. **D,** *Toxoplasma* cyst in cerebral cortex. Note lack of inflammatory response. (From Miller MJ, Seaman E, Remington JS: The clinical spectrum of congenital toxoplasmosis: problems in recognition, *J Pediatr* 70:714-723, 1967.)

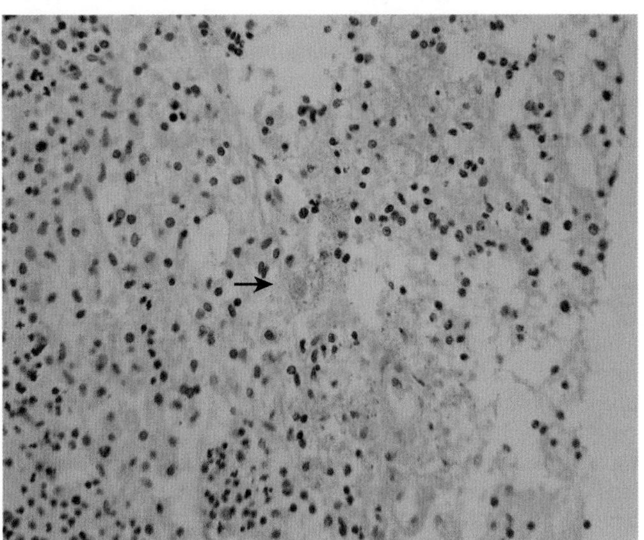

Figure 31-16 Brain of an infected fetus: cyst *(arrow)* in a necrotic area. (Courtesy F. Arbez-Gindre, Besançon, France.)

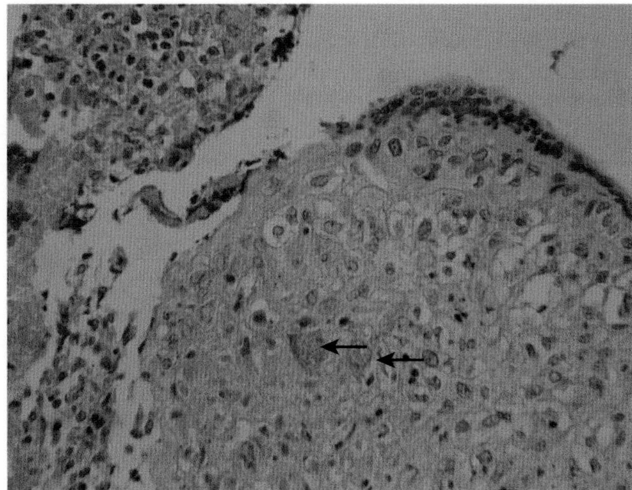

Figure 31-17 Cysts *(arrows)* in the subependymal areas with moderate inflammatory reaction. (Courtesy F. Arbez-Gindre, Besançon, France.)

is a lesion that occurs only in toxoplasmosis.[218,230] The large areas of necrosis have been attributed to vascular thrombosis. The necrotic brain tissue autolyzes and gradually sloughs into the ventricles. The protein content of such ventricular fluid may be in the range of grams per deciliter, and the fluid has been shown to contain significant amounts of *T. gondii* antigens.[196] If the cerebral aqueduct of Sylvius becomes obstructed by the ependymitis, the lateral and third ventricles begin to resemble an abscess cavity containing accumulations of *T. gondii* and inflammatory cells.[231] Hydrocephalus develops in such children, and the necrotic brain tissue may calcify and become visible on radiographs. The fourth ventricle may show ulcers and ependymal nodules but is free from periventricular vasculitis and necrosis, apparently as a consequence of adequate drainage of its fluid through the foramina of Luschka and Magendie. The CSF that communicates with the fourth ventricle often contains several hundred milligrams per deciliter of protein and fewer inflammatory cells than are seen in the lateral ventricle fluid.[231] Frequently, inflammation and necrosis are seen to involve the hypothalamus surrounding the third ventricle. Wolf and coworkers[220] suggested that such lesions in the floor of the third ventricle probably cause the temperature lability observed in infants with congenital toxoplasmosis. Destruction of brain tissue, especially intense periventricular necrosis, rather than obstruction of ventricular passages, appears to account for the development of hydrocephalus in some cases.[197,220]

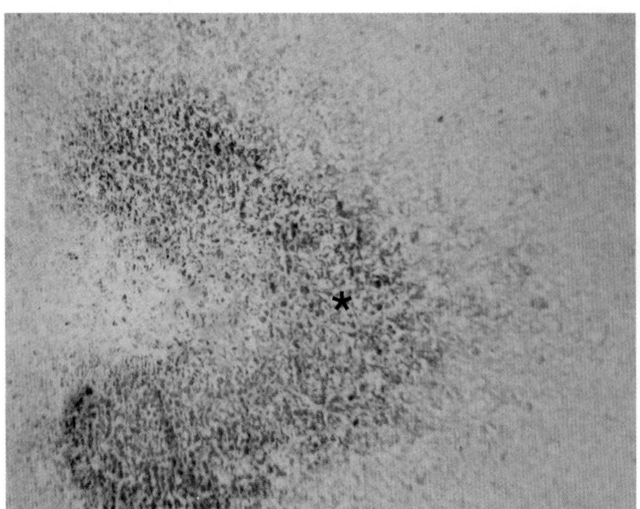

Figure 31-18 Cerebral necrosis punctuated with dystrophic calcifications. (Courtesy F. Arbez-Gindre, Besançon, France.)

EYES

The histopathologic features of the ocular lesions depend on their stage of development at the time of the examination; a number of studies describing lesions in the earliest-recognized cases have been published,[194,232-236] and were reviewed by Hogan[237] in his classic thesis. The description that follows is based on Hogan's summary of his and other cases. The primary and principal lesions are found in the retina and choroid; secondary changes, such as iridocyclitis and cataracts,[236] that occur in other portions of the eye are considered to represent complications of the chorioretinitis. Intraocular inflammation may cause microphthalmia resulting from arrest in development of the eye, or a secondary atrophy may result in shrinkage of the globe. The frequently reported failure of regression of the fetal pupillary vessels may indicate that an arrest in development occurred. The inflammation commences in the retina (see Fig. 31-14B), and a copious exudate in the vitreous produces a marked haze. Secondary involvement of the choroid causes marked elevation; small satellite foci are common. After healing, the lesions are atrophic and pale, with a variable amount of pigmentation at the margins.[238] The organisms first lodge in the capillaries of the inner layers of the retina, invade the endothelium, and extend into adjacent tissues. An intense focal inflammatory reaction results, with edema and infiltration of polymorphonuclear leukocytes, lymphocytes, plasma cells, mononuclear cells, and, in some cases, eosinophils. The reaction results in disruption and disorganization of the retinal layers. Cells are dislocated from the nuclear layers into the adjacent fiber layers. The external limiting membrane may be ruptured, displacing retinal cells into the subretinal space. The inner limiting membrane may also be interrupted, and cells from the inner nuclear layers are then displaced into the adjacent vitreous. Glial tissue, vascular connective tissue, and inflammatory exudate also extend through the interruptions in the inner and outer limiting membranes. In the zones of most acute inflammation, all retinal supporting and neural tissues are completely destroyed. The pigmentary epithelium shows extensive destruction. The retina may detach.[237,239] In the healing process, proliferation of the retinal pigment epithelial cells bordering the inflammatory foci occurs. Large lesions cause considerable necrosis and destruction, resulting in marked central atrophy of the retina and choroid. Disorganization of retinal cells has occurred.[240] Inflammation in the choroid is most acute beneath the retinal foci and is rather well demarcated. The Bruch membrane frequently is destroyed, and proliferation of connective tissue into the subretinal space may be seen. Retina and choroid thereby become fixed to each other by a scar. The choroidal vessels usually are engorged and show perivascular infiltration of lymphocytes, plasma cells, mononuclear cells, and eosinophils. Lymphocytes predominate, and both $CD4^+$ and $CD8^+$ lymphocytes are present.[240-242]

Organisms are present in the retinal lesions and, in general, are most numerous where the lesions are most severe (see Fig. 31-14B). Occasional parasites without an accompanying reaction are observed in relatively normal portions of the retina near the margins of inflammatory foci. The organisms may occur singly or in clusters, free or intracellularly, or in cysts. They are rarely seen in the choroid. They also have been found in the tissues of the optic papilla and in optic nerves associated with inflammatory cells in congenital cases.[190,240]

Serofibrinous exudate and inflammatory cells extend into the vitreous through dehiscences in the inner limiting membrane of the retina. The exudate may be accompanied by masses of budding capillaries, and the vitreous becomes infiltrated with granulation tissue.[243,244] The optic disc may show papillitis, sometimes associated with optic neuritis and sometimes secondary to inflammation in the adjacent retina, or papilledema caused by the hydrocephalus.[240,245] Leptomeningeal inflammation may be present around the optic nerve.

EARS

The presence of the parasite in the mastoid and inner ear and the accompanying inflammatory and pathologic changes have been considered to be causes of deafness in congenital toxoplasmosis.[188,246,247] This may be related to ossal damage or neural damage resulting from ongoing active tachyzoite proliferation after birth,[248] which strongly argues for neonatal treatment as soon as the diagnosis is made.[217] Also, brainstem involvement affecting auditory nuclei can lead to inability to process auditory input.

LUNG AND HEART

The alveolar septa may be widened, edematous, and infiltrated with mononuclear cells, occasional plasma cells, and rare eosinophils. The walls of small blood vessels may be infiltrated with lymphocytes and mononuclear cells, and parasites may be found in endothelial cells.[188] In many cases, some degree of bronchopneumonia, often caused by suprainfection with other agents, is present. *T. gondii* has been identified in the epithelial cells lining alveoli and within the endothelium of small blood vessels in such cases; in some affected patients, the pneumonic process was considered to be a prominent part of the general disease.[188] Single organisms have been found free in alveoli in the cases described by Zuelzer[197] and Paige and coworkers.[232] Of interest, their pathologic findings are identical to those described for adults in whom the lungs were particularly involved.[233] For a review of this subject in congenital and acquired cases, the reader is referred to the publications by Couvreur[249,250] and Pomeroy and Filice.[251] *T. gondii* is almost always found in the heart in the form of cysts in myocardial fibers, accompanied by pathologic changes in the heart muscle. A focal infiltration with lymphocytes, plasma cells, mononuclear cells, and occasional eosinophils is seen. These foci usually do not contain organisms. In the focal areas of infiltration, the myocardial cells may undergo hyaline necrosis and fragmentation. Parasites are found in myocardial fibers in large aggregates and in cysts without any accompanying inflammatory reaction (see Fig. 31-6).[252-254] Single parasites often may be present in areas of beginning necrosis and peripherally in larger areas of necrosis.[188,197,219] Extensive calcification of the heart, involving primarily the right ventricle and intraventricular septum, was observed in a 3-hour-old infant and was attributed to congenital toxoplasmosis.[188] Involvement of the heart has been demonstrated in a congenitally infected infant with AIDS who died of *Pneumocystis* pneumonia and toxoplasmosis.[255-258] Cardiac biopsy may reveal marked autolytic changes without evidence of inflammatory reaction or fibrosis. *T. gondii* organisms were identified in the muscle fibers.[255]

SPLEEN, LIVER, ASCITES, AND KIDNEYS

Marked engorgement of the splenic pulp may be noted, along with erythropoiesis. In general, no significant pathologic changes that could be attributed to direct destruction by the parasite have been noted in the spleen. In some cases, an eosinophilic leukocytic infiltration has been described.[197,232] Organisms are rarely seen in the spleen. In most cases, parasites are not identified in the liver, and neither necrosis nor inflammatory cell infiltrations are present. In some instances, in areas of marked hepatocellular degenerative changes are observed, but without associated cellular infiltration.[197,232] The periportal spaces may be infiltrated with mononuclear cells, neutrophils, and eosinophils. Enlargement of the liver frequently is pronounced and is accompanied by erythropoiesis, as occurs also in the spleen. In a few cases, hepatic cirrhosis has been observed as a sequel to congenital toxoplasmosis.[259] Caldera and coworkers[260] have described calcification in the liver seen both radiologically and at autopsy. Congenital toxoplasmosis was diagnosed by exfoliative cytologic examination of ascitic fluid in a 7-week-old infant born at 38 weeks of gestation. Hepatomegaly and anemia developed shortly after birth, and liver failure and ascites during the first week of life. Because an extensive workup failed to reveal a cause, a paracentesis was performed, which revealed tachyzoites both in Wright-stained smear preparations and in electron microscopy sections. This case is reminiscent of that of an adult patient with AIDS in whom the diagnosis of toxoplasmosis was first established on examination of Wright-Giemsa–stained smears of ascitic fluid obtained because of suspected bacterial peritonitis.[261]

Numerous foci of hematopoiesis may be seen in the kidney. Focal glomerulitis often has been observed; in such cases, a majority of glomeruli remain intact.[188,197] In fully developed lesions, glomerular tufts undergo massive necrosis, and necrosis of adjacent tubules may be seen. In the earlier stages of the glomerular lesion, some capillary loops are still intact; in others, necrotic areas are observed in the basement membrane and epithelium, and the lumina are occluded by fibrin thrombi. In some of these partly preserved glomeruli, single parasites have been found in cells of the exudate within the capsular space or embedded in the necrotic remains of the capillary loop.[197] *T. gondii* cysts have been found in glomeruli and renal tubules of kidneys, in which there were no other associated lesions (see Figs. 31-14A and 31-15A and B).[262-264] In severely affected kidneys, focal areas of necrosis also are found in the collecting tubules in the medulla. The inflammatory infiltrations are predominantly mononuclear, although in some cases, numerous eosinophil cells also are seen scattered throughout. In 1966, Fediushina and Sherstennikova[265] reported the pathologic findings in the kidneys in nine cases of congenital toxoplasmosis. In three of these cases, distinct changes in the glomeruli were noted, and, as described by these investigators, many of the changes appear to resemble those observed in glomerulonephritis from other causes, including streptococcal infection. In 1972, Wickbom and Winberg[266] reported a case of a 10-week-old boy with congenital toxoplasmosis who developed severe nephritis with the nephrotic syndrome. In that same year, Shahin and associates[267] reported a case of nephrotic syndrome in a 4-month-old infant with congenital toxoplasmosis. Granular and pseudolinear glomerular deposits of IgM, fibrinogen, and *T. gondii* antigen and antibody were demonstrated in the glomeruli of the initial biopsy of renal tissue. After approximately 7 months of treatment, a second renal biopsy showed no evidence of the *T. gondii* antigen-antibody complexes previously noted, but IgM, fibrinogen, and the fourth component of complement (C4) were present. IgG and C3 were not demonstrable in the glomeruli in either biopsy specimen. Light microscopy of the first renal biopsy revealed glomeruli with a diffuse mild increase in mesangial cells and matrix. One glomerulus contained a segmented area of sclerosis that adhered to the Bowman capsule. Other findings included rare foci of tubular atrophy and associated interstitial fibrosis, occasional hyaline casts, focal tubular and interstitial calcification, and prominent tubular hyaline droplets. The second renal biopsy specimen, obtained after treatment with prednisone for 7 months and with pyrimethamine and sulfadiazine for 3 weeks, revealed glomeruli with varying degrees of damage, ranging from total hyalinization to partial collapse and segmental sclerosis. The tubulointerstitial changes were not significantly different from those observed in the first biopsy specimen. The results of electron microscopy also were reported.

ENDOCRINE ORGANS

Parasites and numerous foci of necrosis have been identified in the adrenal cortex (see Fig. 31-14C). Similar areas of necrosis have been found in the pancreas.[188,193,197,232] Parasites, usually without associated inflammation, have been found in the pituitary.[188,193] Large clusters of organisms, without accompanying inflammation or necrosis, have been found in the acini of the thyroid gland.[232] In the testes and ovaries, acute interstitial inflammation with focal areas of necrosis is frequently observed.[188,193,197,218,232] Necrosis of the seminiferous tubules with preservation of adjacent units is common, with infiltration with plasma cells, lymphocytes, mononuclear cells, and eosinophils. Parasites often are observed in the spermatogonia of intact tubules (see Fig. 31-15C). Focal hematopoiesis has been observed in the interstitia of these organs.

SKELETAL MUSCLE

Involvement varies, ranging in degree from parasitized fibers without pathologic changes to focal areas of infiltration or widespread myositis with necrosis. The organisms in parasitized fibers are found beneath the sarcolemmal sheaths. Hundreds of organisms may be present in a single long tubular space in a fiber, and *T. gondii* cysts frequently are seen in muscle fibers. The affected fibers are swollen and lose their striations, but as a rule, no inflammatory reactions are noted. By contrast, focal areas of inflammation and necrosis may be present in areas where only a few parasites or none can be identified. The cellular infiltrate consists mainly of mononuclear cells, but lymphocytes, plasma cells, and eosinophils also are present. In rare instances, focal inflammatory lesions may be found adjacent to heavily parasitized but unbroken muscle fibers.[197] Noteworthy is the description of severe involvement of the extraocular muscles in the case described by Rodney and coworkers.[219]

THYMUS

Sarrut observed a hypoplastic thymus in an infant who died of congenital toxoplasmosis at the age of 1 month (personal communication to G. Desmonts, 1980). The disease was not diagnosed before autopsy. *T. gondii* organisms were isolated from the brain and heart. The histologic picture in this case was quite different from that described in experimental infection in newborn mice[268] because in the former, hypoplasia involved both lymphocytes and Hassall corpuscles. Newborn thymic hypoplasia in congenital toxoplasmosis can be differentiated from that following advanced congenital HIV infection.[269]

SKIN

Torres found *T. gondii* tachyzoites without formation of lesions in the subcutaneous tissue of one infant.[270] In one case ("case 5") reported by Paige and associates,[232] *T. gondii* organisms were present in the subcutaneous tissue, again with no associated inflammatory lesion or necrosis. No rash was noted in the infant. Clinically, these changes may present with blister formation and scarring similar to that seen in aplasia cutis congenita.[271]

BONE

Milgram[193] described osseous changes in a fatal case of congenital toxoplasmosis. The infant died on day 17, and at autopsy, widespread active infection was discovered. The parasite was found in almost all tissues of the body. Large numbers of inflammatory cells were found in the bone marrow, with deficient osteogenesis and remodeling in the primary spongiosa. Intracellular aggregates of *T. gondii* were present in macrophages in the bone marrow.

IMMUNOGLOBULIN ABNORMALITIES

Subtle abnormalities have been noted in the development of immunoglobulins in infants with subclinical congenital toxoplasmosis.[272,273] In several infants, retarded development of IgA for the first 3 years of life and excessive development of IgG and IgM were noted. The latter abnormality also is seen in congenital rubella, cytomegalic inclusion disease, and syphilis. In *T. gondii*–infected children, the degree of increase in IgG and IgM appears to be directly related to the severity of the infection.[274]

Oxelius[275] described monoclonal (M) immunoglobulins of the IgG class in the serum and CSF of three newborns with severe clinical signs of congenital toxoplasmosis. Because these M proteins were found in the sera of newborns but not in the sera of their mothers, Oxelius concluded that the M immunoglobulins were either selectively transferred or synthesized by the newborn. Reports by Van Camp and associates[276] and Griscelli and colleagues[277] suggest that the observation by Oxelius may not be uncommon. Griscelli and colleagues performed a survey of 27 newborns and older infants who had the severe form of congenital toxoplasmosis. In 11 of the infants, IgG components of M proteins were noted. These authors concluded that these components were synthesized by the fetus because they could be detected up to 75 days postpartum and were absent in maternal serum. They were unable to define any anti–*T. gondii* antibody in isolated IgG components of M proteins. Absorption of the hypergammaglobulinemic sera with antigens of *T. gondii* resulted in almost complete loss of anti-*Toxoplasma* antibodies detected by using the Sabin-Feldman dye test but did not affect the presence of the M component or significantly reduce the immunoglobulin levels. Similar results have been reported in *T. gondii*–infected mice; hypergammaglobulinemia and a condition that appeared to be a monoclonal spike were observed.[278] The underlying mechanism or the cause of the appearance of M components in infants with congenital toxoplasmosis is unknown. M components have also been described in congenital syphilis.[279]

TOXOPLASMA GONDII–CYTOMEGALOVIRUS INFECTION

A number of reports of dual infection with *T. gondii*–cytomegalovirus have appeared.[280-284] In systematically searching for cytomegalovirus infection among nine autopsies in cases of congenital toxoplasmosis, Vinh and coworkers[282] found these two diseases coexisting in two instances. Sotelo-Avila and associates[283] described a case of coexisting congenital toxoplasmosis and cytomegalovirus infection in a microcephalic infant who died at the age of 15 days. Microscopically, numerous areas of calcification and necrosis and large cells with the characteristic nuclear inclusions of cytomegalovirus were seen. Aggregates of *T. gondii* were found in the cytoplasm of many of the cytomegalic inclusion cells in the CNS, lungs, retina, kidneys, and liver. Maszkiewicz and colleagues[281] described a case of cytomegalic inclusion disease with toxoplasmosis in a premature infant.

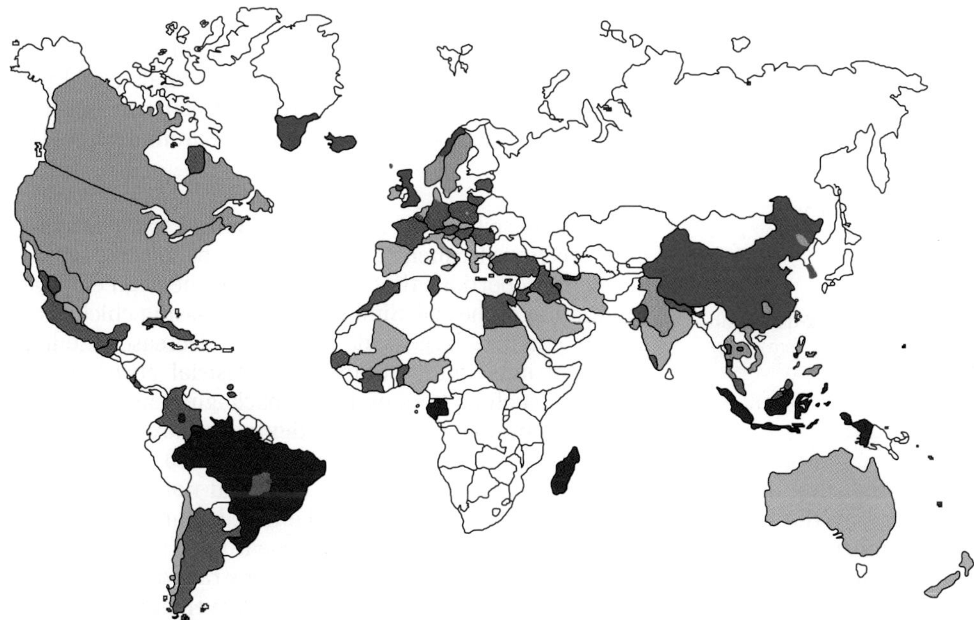

Figure 31-19 Global status of *Toxoplasma gondii* seroprevalence. Dark red equals prevalence greater than 60%, light red equals 40% to 60%, yellow equals 20% to 40%, blue equals 10% to 20%, and green equals prevalence <10%. White equals absence of data. (Modified from Pappas G, Roussos N, Falagas ME: Toxoplasmosis snapshots: global status of *Toxoplasma gondii* seroprevalence and implications for pregnancy and congenital toxoplasmosis, *Int J Parasitol* 39:1385-1394, 2009; with permission.)

Epidemiology

SEROPREVALENCE IN THE GENERAL POPULATION

Toxoplasma gondii is prevalent worldwide (Fig. 31-19). As reviewed in several publications,[2,285,286] recent seropositivity rates show extreme geographic variations, ranging from less than 1%[287] to greater than 95%.[288] The highest overall rates are found in Latin American countries (mostly in Brazil), sub-Saharan Africa, the Middle East, and some parts of Asia. The lowest rates are reported in Southeast Asia. Estimates for North America are less than 25%, and those for Europe are mostly less than 36%, except for subclasses of non-American or non-European immigrants, who tend to have higher rates. Significant differences are found between countries within the same continent, as well as between areas or ethnic groups within the same country (see "Epidemiology and Diagnosis of Infections in the Mother and the Unborn Child"). Local rates of seropositivity depend on many factors, and climate plays an important role by influencing the sporulation and survival of oocysts. Prevalence rates are usually higher in areas where the climate is humid and warm than in dryer and colder climates and at high altitude. The prevalence of domestic and stray cats also influences the burden of oocysts in the environment.[286] Direct contacts with cats or their litter are not thought to be major risk factors, but concordant evidence shows that contact with oocyst-contaminated soil is a source of infection. This can occur in the context of poor housing conditions,[289-291] through occupational activities or gardening, and, indirectly, by eating unwashed vegetables. Present or past residence in rural areas and having lived on a farm have been factors associated with a greater likelihood of infection.

High seroprevalence rates in younger age groups, as reported, for example, in surveys in Brazil,[292] São Tomé and Principe,[293] and Ethiopia,[294] are good indicators of this risk of environmental exposure. Waterborne transmission through ingestion of oocysts in the drinking water is also supported by epidemiologic data.[20] It was hypothesized that Jains are primarily infected through drinking contaminated water because their lifestyle excludes most other routes of infection.[295] Infection is also thought to be possible through inadvertent swallowing of water from ponds, lakes, and streams during recreational activities.[20,296] The distribution of oocysts in the environment also influences the risk of infection in meat animals that are raised outdoors and consequently affects the risk for humans to ingest viable tissue cysts when eating undercooked meat from these animals. This risk is also highly dependent on farming conditions and local culinary habits. Seropositivity rates were found to be lower for vegetarians,[297,298] and in countries where most meat is eaten well cooked compared with areas where traditional dishes are based on raw/undercooked meat. A low level of education, which is often linked to low socioeconomic status and is likely to be predictive of low awareness of toxoplasmosis and an increased risk for exposure, was commonly found to be associated with higher seroprevalence, which tends to increase with age.

A comparison of rates over the last few decades has indicated a significant decrease in most countries.[2,299] Industrialized, high-density animal husbandry, more frequent use of frozen meat, and urbanization have been suggested as possible explanations. However, stable or increasing seroprevalence has also been reported.[300-303] The higher rates of infection in Korea are thought to be due to an increased consumption of imported pork meat[301,302] and/or a greater prevalence of cats, although the increased sensitivity of more recent serologic tests may also have contributed to the findings.

ORAL ROUTES OF INFECTION

The Role of Meat

The association between eating raw or undercooked meat and acute *Toxoplasma* infection in humans has been a consistent finding in many epidemiologic studies. The distribution

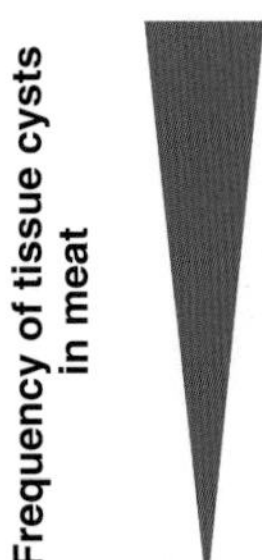

Figure 31-20 Relative importance of meat-producing and game animals in the transmission of *Toxoplasma gondii* to humans. (From Tenter AM, Heckeroth AR, Weiss LM: *Toxoplasma gondii*: from animals to humans, *Int J Parasitol* 30:1217-1258, 2000; with permission.)

of *T. gondii* in a large variety of meat-producing animals is widespread. This diversity is illustrated by the various types of meat potentially involved in a number of outbreaks recorded over the last few decades: seal and caribou meat in Canada,[304] kangaroo and lamb in Australia,[305] raw pig liver in Korea,[306] grilled lamb in Great Britain,[307] and raw mutton in Brazil.[285,308]

The risk of infection is influenced by many factors that have been discussed in several reviews.[285,309-312] The first is the type of meat and the susceptibility of animals to *Toxoplasma* infection (Fig. 31-20). The conditions of production and the amount of time mainly spent outdoors are other major factors. Animals that are raised indoors are more likely to be protected from exposure to oocysts than those that are reared outdoors. An equally important factor is age, which increases the risk of animals becoming infected. The risk also varies with the parts of animals that are eaten because some tissues harbor more cysts than others and are therefore more infective. In addition, postslaughter treatments, including heating and freezing, play an important role. Cooking meat to at least 67° C kills the parasite. Freezing at −12° C for 24 hours is also considered to improve the safety of the meat. Findings on the isolation of parasites from various food animals in the United States were reviewed by Hill and Dubey.[309]

Pigs have traditionally been considered to be a major source of *Toxoplasma* infection in humans.[285,311] Ingestion of uncooked pork meat was identified as a significant factor for acute infection in several seroprevalence or case-control studies in Europe in the 1990s[313-316] and in America.[317] However, the risks of infection have decreased in many parts of the world through modern farming practices that enclose animals in environmentally regulated buildings, which have reduced infection rates sharply in the United States[318] and Europe.[312]

Nevertheless, pork meat could reemerge as a significant risk factor as a consequence of the increasing trend in animal-friendlier production methods that have been demanded by consumers.[309,319] A survey carried out in 2004 in the Netherlands found that the prevalence of *Toxoplasma* was almost 0.38% in pigs raised using modern high-production farming practices but was 2.9% in organically-raised pigs and close to 6% in free-range animals.[319] Infection rates remain high in unconfined or poorly confined animals, and prevalence rates as high as 68% have been recorded in the United States.[318] Because the prevalence of infection increases with age, meat products that are traditionally generated from older animals could represent a higher risk. Feral pigs are also frequently infected, and eating undercooked meat from these animals should be avoided.[309]

Poultry. Despite being resistant to clinical toxoplasmosis, chickens have frequently been found to be infected with *T. gondii* in proportions that correlate with the degree of contamination of the soil. Similarly to pigs, raising chickens in strictly confined large-scale operations decreases the likelihood of infection.[309] Common industrial postslaughter methods, such as freezing before packaging, also decrease the risk of human infection by killing the parasites. Analysis of 2094 chicken meat samples obtained from grocery stores in the United States in 2005 did not find any viable cysts. However, it should be noted that antibodies to *T. gondii* were found in 1.4% of meat juice samples.[320] In contrast to confined animals, chickens raised in backyards are commonly infected, especially in developing countries, and could represent an important source of infection.[309] Eating chicken meat more than twice a week was found to be independently associated with past infection in pregnant women interviewed in 2005 in Fortaleza (Brazil).[321] This is concordant with the high rates of infection found in chickens in Brazil.[322-324] Infection is also common in commercial free-range chickens. Edelhofer and Prossinger[325] reported mean seroprevalence rates of 36% (up to 98%) in the hearts of chickens slaughtered after 1 year spent on organic farms in Austria. The risk of acquiring infection from commercial free-range broilers is considered to be low because of their very short life span.[312,326] However, a small series of young commercial free-range chickens in Australia showed high rates of infection, as measured by serologic tests and DNA detection.[327]

Viable cysts were isolated from experimentally infected turkeys,[328] ducks,[329,330] and geese,[331] and seroprevalence was 20% in domestic turkeys raised on turkey farms in Germany.[332] A survey of pregnant women in Mexico found a strong association between the consumption of turkey meat and the presence of *T. gondii* antibodies.[333] Seroprevalence in naturally exposed domestic ducks varied from 6% in Germany[334] to 16% in China[335] and 55% in Egypt.[336] In domestic geese, infection rates were 25% in Germany[334] and 14% to 17% in China.[337] In the German study, rates were lower in farms that kept ducks and geese indoors.

Beef. Cattle are considered to be a poor host for *T. gondii*, and viable cysts have rarely been isolated from edible beef parts despite high seroprevalence rates that exceeded 40%[338,339] and even 90% in some studies.[285] Eating undercooked beef was nonetheless identified as a significant risk factor in several studies in Europe[316,340] and North America.[341] This significant association has been thought to be due to cross-contamination or the adulteration of beef products with other types of meat, such as lamb, which is a common practice.[312]

Sheep. Sheep are highly susceptible to *Toxoplasma* infection and, being free-range grazing animals, are widely exposed to infection.[309] Dubey reported worldwide infection rates between 3% and 96%[342]; rates recorded in Europe ranged from 4% to 92% in farmed sheep. Analysis of the hearts from 383 lambs that were raised in the United States and butchered in commercial abattoirs for human consumption found that greater than 27% were seropositive, and viable cysts were isolated from 78% of the positive animals.[343] The risk of infection increases with age, but lamb meat is more frequently eaten raw than is mutton and therefore is probably more dangerous. The consumption of undercooked mutton or lamb was found to be associated with acute infection in pregnant European women: in France,[340] where it is traditionally considered to be an important source of infection, but also in Norway,[315] in a study in five European countries,[316] and it was also involved in several outbreaks.[307,308,344]

Goats. *Toxoplasma gondii* infection is also common in goats, and prevalence rates reached 75% in some surveys.[285,325] Dubey and colleagues[345] reported a prevalence of 53% in 234 goats originating from American farms, and bioassays isolated parasites in 29 of 122 goat hearts. Unpasteurized goat's milk has also been implicated in human infections.[298,346-348]

Horses. The seroprevalence of *T. gondii* in horses varies worldwide.[349] Most estimates reviewed by Tenter and colleagues[285] or published since[350-354] were less than 20%, but higher rates have also been reported, mainly in China (25%-31%)[355,356] and the Middle East (25%-71%).[357-359] In some European countries and Japan, the consumption of raw or undercooked horse meat is a common practice,[360,361] and severe cases of human toxoplasmosis have been reported in France after the consumption of horse meat originating from Brazil and Canada.[78]

Rabbits. Viable cysts of *T. gondii* have been isolated from farmed domestic rabbits.[362] However, only a few seroprevalence rates are available, and they vary from 6% to 53%.[285,336,362-364]

Game. Humans can also be infected by the ingestion of cysts of *T. gondii* found in the tissues of venison and other wild animals, such as wild boars, hares, and pheasants. These animals are good indicators of environmental contamination with *T. gondii*, and seroprevalence can be high, especially in older animals. High rates were reported in the United States for white-tailed deer (30%-65%), wild boars (up to 37%), and bears (75%-85%).[318] Eating undercooked venison or wildlife meat was found in several surveys to be associated with acute infection or seropositivity,[304,317,365,366] and kangaroo meat was implicated in one outbreak in Australia.[305] Marsupials are highly susceptible to infection; they have high prevalence rates, and viable tissue cysts have been isolated from their meat.[285]

Handling infected meat may generate a risk of infection, and skinning animals for fur was one of the factors implicated in the infection of pregnant women in a small outbreak in an Inuit population in the North of Canada.[304] Professional contact with meat was found to be associated with a higher risk of *Toxoplasma* infection in the United States[341] and Poland.[313] Conversely, workers occupationally exposed to raw meat in Mexico were not found to have higher infection rates.[367]

The Role of Milk and Eggs

The milk of several intermediary hosts, including sheep, goats, and cows, has been found to contain tachyzoites of *T. gondii*, and infected milk has been reported to transmit infection to animals.[285] The consumption of milk and milk products was not thought to represent a significant risk for humans because of the widespread practice of pasteurizing milk. Also, gastric juices are expected to inactivate tachyzoites in raw milk. Cases of infection have been reported, however, that brought to light the possibility of acquiring infection through the consumption of nonpasteurized goat's milk. These were reported in newborns[347] and adolescents,[348] as well as in adults.[298,346] Drinking goat's milk was also identified as a significant factor for acute infection in adults in the United States[341] and for past infection in pregnant women in Brazil.[368] A case of acute toxoplasmosis has also been reported in a breastfed infant.[369] The lower concentration of proteolytic enzymes in the intestinal tract of children and the penetration of tachyzoites through the oropharyngeal mucosa[285] may contribute to the ability of low numbers of parasites in milk to be transmitted to infants.

Raw eggs from hens raised in contemporary high-density production facilities are unlikely to transmit *Toxoplasma* infection,[326] but caution is probably warranted for eggs from free-range hens, although any cooking will kill the parasite.[285]

The Role of Oocysts

Humans can also be infected through the ingestion of environmentally stable oocysts. Epidemiologic studies have provided indirect evidence that this route contributes to a large proportion of human infections in South America and Africa and, to a lesser extent, in Asia. Recent findings suggested that it may also play a predominant role in developed countries. A new test has been developed that enables the recognition in serum samples of antibody responses to an 11-kDa sporozoite protein, which indicate that infection was acquired by the ingestion of oocysts within the previous 6 to 8 months.[370] Analysis of sera collected in the United States and Canada in the context of maternal and congenital infections found that the ingestion of oocysts was the predominant cause of infection in 78% of cases.[296]

Oocysts can only be shed by felids, which are the definitive hosts of *T. gondii*. Cats usually become infected soon after they begin to hunt and ingest contaminated prey, and oocysts in their environment are less pathogenic than viable cysts in infected prey.[371] Indoor cats can also be contaminated if fed raw meat. Shedding of oocysts in the feces begins on average 3 to 5 days after initial infection and lasts for up to 21 days, with a median of 8 days.[32,286] Up to 55 million oocysts are deposited daily in soil, grass, water, and in the cat litter of indoor cats. After this short period, cats are unlikely to shed oocysts again in their lifetime.[32,286] Reinfection with *T. gondii* is unlikely to lead to renewed shedding of oocysts unless the cat is exposed more than 6 years after the initial ingestion, is given high doses of corticosteroids, is undernourished, or is infected with other coccidian parasites.[286]

Because of the short duration of shedding, owning a cat or having contact with a cat is not thought to be a major risk factor for humans, and it is estimated that only 1% of cats shed oocysts at any given time.[318] Kittens are likely to represent a higher risk than adult cats, and having three kittens or more was associated with acute infection in a case-control study in the United States.[341] Keeping an adult cat at home is unlikely to represent any risk; should the cat still be shedding oocysts, changing the soiled litter on a daily basis (before oocysts become infective, which occurs 1-5 days after elimination[20]) would further decrease the risk of infection. Given their grooming habits, adult cats do not carry oocysts in their fur,[32] and cat bites or scratches are not considered to be risk factors for *Toxoplasma* infection.

Of five European case-control studies that investigated a possible association between cat ownership and acute infections in pregnancy, only one identified cleaning the litter box as a significant risk factor,[315] although an association between cat ownership and past *Toxoplasm*a infection was found in several seroprevalence surveys. The significance of these findings is difficult to determine because, in most studies, other factors were also detected that indirectly result from the presence of cats at or close to the home, such as contact with the soil, which might be the true risk factor.

Contact with oocysts contained in soil and water, rather than contact with cats, is thought to be a source of infection in humans, including non–pet owners. The burden of oocysts has been demonstrated to be very high[20,286,318] as a consequence of two factors. The first is the remarkable stability of oocysts, which may remain viable for more than 1 year in the soil, especially when they are deposited at moist, temperate, and shady locations.[372,373] The second is the high and globally increasing number of domestic and feral cats.

In a review, Jones and Dubey[20] found that the seroprevalence in domestics cats worldwide varied from 2% in China to 89% in South America. Variations exist within countries and within cities because of the influences of lifestyle and age. It has been estimated that 32% of domestic cats in the United States have *T. gondii* antibodies[374]; higher rates were reported in feral cats[318] (>90% in several studies[375]). Oocysts were found to be widely distributed in rural[376] as well as residential urban[377,378] areas. High densities were reported around elementary schools,[379] sandpits, and playgrounds,[380] which are favorite defecation sites for cats.[286] Occupation as a farmer or an agricultural worker, or gardening or having contact with the soil has been found in many epidemiologic surveys to be associated with an increased likelihood of infection.[316,333,381-392] Eating unwashed vegetables was also reported to be an independent risk factor.[315,321] In a French rural population, of whom 97% had a garden and 90% grew vegetables, seroprevalence was higher than the average national level.[393] PCR analysis of 216 samples of fruit and vegetables failed to identify *Toxoplasma* DNA on the 41 samples that were bought in supermarkets, but DNA was detected on 8% (14/175) of the vegetables bought from local stores and bazaars and in 17% of those grown in home gardens. Higher detection rates were observed for carrots and lettuce.[380]

Oocysts can also be washed from the soil into water bodies and persist for several years in cold water.[20] They can therefore be found in drinking water that has not been adequately filtered, boiled, or treated. Standard municipal systems in developed countries should be able to filter oocysts, but small or malfunctioning systems could fail to do so. Contaminated drinking water has been implicated in several outbreaks,[20] and consistent evidence from several epidemiologic surveys has shown that contaminated drinking water also causes endemic *Toxoplasma* infection.[313,394-397] It has also been suggested that infection can be acquired through the inadvertent swallowing of contaminated water from rivers, lakes, and ponds. Drinking untreated lake and river water was identified as a risk factor in a survey that compared seropositivity rates among military personnel involved in jungle operations and urban soldiers in Colombia.[366] Drinking creek water was also suspected to have caused infection in British soldiers in Panama.[398]

NON-ORAL ROUTES OF INFECTION

Human infection can also be acquired through transplantation, blood transfusion, and laboratory accidents.[399] Of these routes, transmission by transplantation is the most important.[18] Toxoplasmosis can affect recipients of solid-organ and hematopoietic stem cell transplants. In solid-organ transplantations, infection results from the transmission of the parasite via the transplanted organ from an infected donor to an uninfected recipient. This risk is highest for heart transplants and is significantly lower for other solid organs. In hematopoietic stem cell transplants, complications result mainly from the reactivation of a preexisting latent infection under intense suppressive therapy. Allogeneic hematopoietic stem cell transplant recipients are exposed to a much higher risk than those receiving autologous hematopoietic stem cell transplants.

Tachyzoites have also been transmitted via blood products, in particular those containing the white cell fraction, and by accidental injection in the laboratory.[285,399,400] Acquiring infection from a blood transfusion is thought to be rare because of the limited duration of parasitemia after an acute infection.[41]

In addition to milk and blood, tachyzoites have also been detected in tears, saliva, sputum, urine, and semen.[285] It has been hypothesized that sheep[401] and dogs[402] inseminated with *T. gondii*–contaminated semen could develop toxoplasmosis, but no evidence is currently available that any of these routes could cause horizontal transmission in humans.

Drugs Active Against *Toxoplasma gondii*

GENERAL CONSIDERATIONS

The strain of the parasite and its genetic characteristics, as well as the immunologic status of the host, are important determinants of the clinical outcome.[403] Current clinical studies frequently draw on archival control data, which may not be compatible with the current situation because of the lower sensitivity of the diagnostic techniques applied at these earlier times than now and because of the greater severity of disease.[404] Because none of the currently available antiparasitic drugs are effective against bradyzoites, treatment regimens do not produce sterilizing cure, and long-term clinical monitoring is advisable.

The optimal duration of treatment has not been clearly established. Results from one retrospective study involving patient cohorts in France supported the notion that treatment of congenitally infected infants should be continued for 12 or more months to avert late clinical manifestations of disease and recurrences, although changes in specific antibody titers did not differ, depending on duration of treatment.[405] Data from a prospective, randomized clinical trial, likewise involving patient cohorts in France, will soon be published.[406]

HISTORICAL EVOLUTION OF THERAPEUTIC STRATEGIES

The first drugs that were established to be effective against *Toxoplasma* were sulfonamides,[407] and their combination with pyrimethamine dates back to 1953.[408,409] Five years later, in 1958, spiramycin was demonstrated to be effective in the treatment of *Toxoplasma*-induced uveitis[410] as well as in the inhibition of vertical transmission.[411] Subsequently, atovaquone was shown to be effective in the treatment of AIDS patients suffering from ocular toxoplasmosis.[412-415] The combined use of trimethoprim (TMP) and sulfamethoxazole (SMZ) has found wide acceptance in the treatment of acute forms of toxoplasmosis in older individuals because of the ease with which the two drugs can be applied, their low toxicity, and the satisfying clinical results; however, in experimental murine models of the disease, this combination has not met with success in the handling of recurrences.[416-419] By contrast to the results in mice, in AIDS patients suffering from encephalic and ocular toxoplasmosis, TMP/SMZ has been successful in reducing symptoms[420-424] and is frequently used clinically as a prophylactic measure against recurrences.[425-427] The combination of pyrimethamine plus sulfadoxine (Fansidar), which is marketed for the prophylactic treatment of malaria, has been used increasingly for the treatment of toxoplasmosis in some regions but is not used for this purpose in the United States because of, in part, concerns regarding risk for severe adverse events, for instance, Stevens-Johnson syndrome and the long duration of action of sulfadoxine.[405,428-432]

DRUGS IN CURRENT USE EFFECTIVE AGAINST *TOXOPLASMA GONDII*

Pyrimethamine and Sulfonamides

Pyrimethamine (Daraprim) has a long plasma half-life (approximately 100 hours) in adults,[433,434] which is attributable to its high binding affinity (94%) for proteins in serum.[435] In children younger than 1.5 years, the serum half-life of pyrimethamine is approximately 60 hours. Pyrimethamine dosages of 1 mg/kg of body weight/day yield serum drug levels of approximately 1000 to 2000 ng/mL 4 hours after the administration of the drug. When the same dose is administered on alternate days three times per week, serum levels of approximately 500 ng/mL are attained

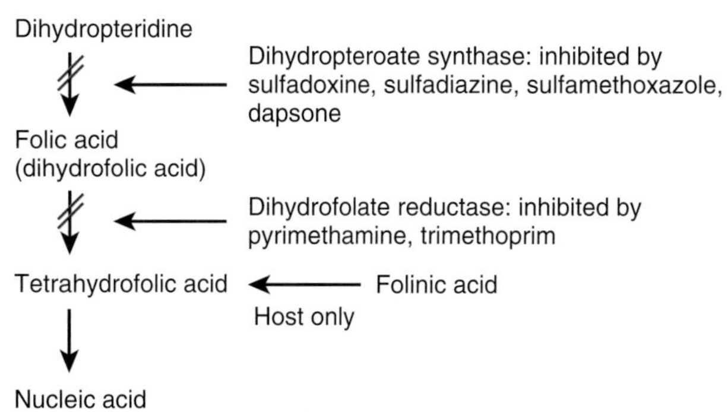

Figure 31-21 Mechanism of action of inhibitors of folate biosynthesis.

4 hours after the each dose. The corresponding levels in the CSF are 10% to 25% of those in the serum.[436]

Pyrimethamine is typically used in combination with sulfadiazine or another sulfonamide. This combination acts to inhibit two enzymes that are essential for parasite nucleic acid synthesis, namely dihydropteroate synthase and dihydrofolate reductase, as illustrated in Figure 31-21.

The inhibitory and the parasiticidal concentrations of these drugs depend upon the nature of the assay and the calibration systems, as well as upon the strain of the parasite.[436] In one study that was conducted using a cell culture system, pyrimethamine alone was reported to have an IC_{50} (the concentration at which 50% inhibition of growth was observed) of 0.48 μM and to be cidal at 11.2 μM.[437] In another in vitro study, the levels of pyrimethamine and sulfadiazine that were required to inhibit the growth of the type-I RH strain of *T. gondii* were determined. Twenty-four hours after monotherapy with each drug, the IC_{50} for pyrimethamine was 100 ng/mL, and the IC_{90} for sulfadiazine was 6.25 μg/mL, whereas when the two agents were administered together, the corresponding values were 25 ng/mL and 6.25 μg/mL, respectively.[436] The actual concentrations of the drugs that are required in a combined approach to prevent disease activity and recurrences in children have not been established.[429]

Because the synergistic effect of combined therapy with pyrimethamine and sulfadiazine was first recognized in the treatment of toxoplasmosis,[408,438-441] numerous investigations have been undertaken to identify other useful drug combinations that would be more efficacious in averting vertical transmission, combating chronic infection, and/or eliciting less severe side effects.[170,405,442-454] However, none of the tested combinations have been significantly superior in these regards than pyrimethamine/sulfadiazine. Although several triple therapies have been shown to afford some benefits, they are not generally advocated for routine clinical use because the number of tablets that would need to be swallowed would be increased to an unpalatable level (7-8 times per day). To date, pyrimethamine/sulfadiazine is the most widely applied therapy and is generally well tolerated, whereas the combination of pyrimethamine/sulfadoxine is also used outside of the United States. Compared with sulfadiazine or sulfadoxine, other tested sulfonamides, namely, sulfapyrazine, sulfamethazine, sulfamerazine, sulfathiazole, sulfapyridine, sulfadimidine, and sulfisoxazole, have not been found to confer any benefits and are, moreover, not so universally available.

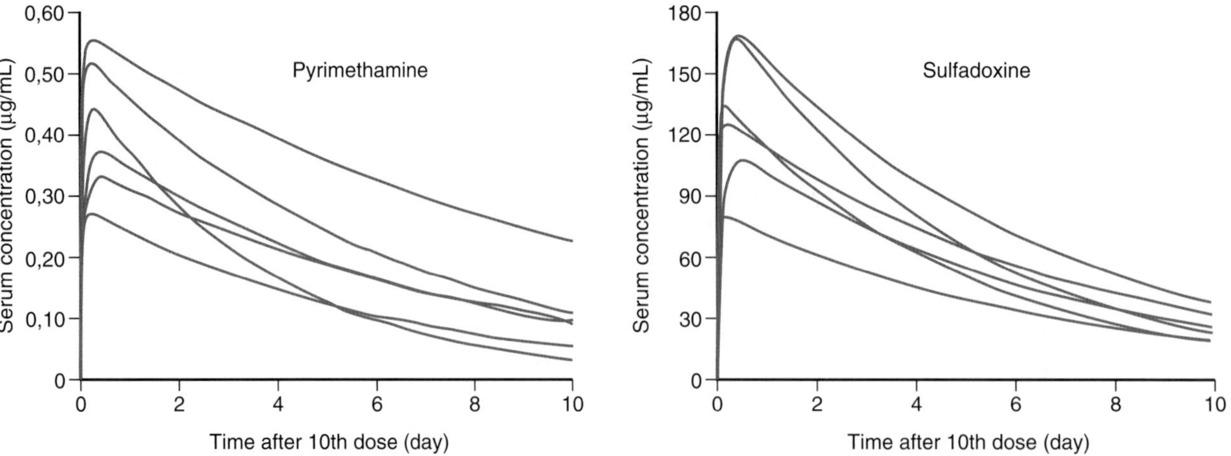

Figure 31-22 Simulated concentration: time curves for pyrimethamine and sulfadoxine in six infants after the 10th dose. (Modified from Corvaisier S, Charpiat B, Mounier C, et al: Population pharmacokinetics of pyrimethamine and sulfadoxine in children treated for congenital toxoplasmosis, *Antimicrob Agents Chemother* 48:3794-3800, 2004.)

The serum concentrations of pyrimethamine and sulfonamides are unpredictable, even when the dose is adjusted according to body weight (Fig. 31-22). Of note, levels of pyrimethamine achieved in infants being treated for overt congenital toxoplasmosis can vary by factors of 8- to 25-fold, and those of sulfonamides between 4- and 5-fold.[429,430,436,445,455] The variability is probably accounted for in part by the use of different assays and by the mode of their calibration, as well as biologic variability and other factors. The latter includes cotreatment with barbiturates[436]; the administration of certain anti-HIV drugs, such as zidovudine[456]; delayed dose adjustment in response to weight gain; differences in the dosing intervals; dietary factors; and parental compliance.[430] Because of this variability, dosage recommendations in individual cases need to be considered with care. The lack of commercially available suspensions of pyrimethamine and sulfonamide, specifically for pediatric use, exacerbates the problem of defining suitable doses for infants.[457]

The combination of pyrimethamine/sulfadiazine (plus folinic acid) has been standard therapy for the treatment of infants with congenital toxoplasmosis for more than 50 years and is the regimen recommended for use in the United States; this combination is also used for treatment in utero of the fetus with proven infection (see "Treatment in the Mother and Unborn Child"). A regimen of pyrimethamine, sulfadiazine, and spiramycin was used in the past but is not currently used extensively in France.

An alternative regimen of pyrimethamine in combination with sulfadoxine, marketed commercially as Fansidar, is used by some groups outside of the United States. Because sulfadoxine has a much longer half-life than sulfadiazine, this combination is typically administered orally every 10 days for 1 year at doses of 1.25 mg/kg of body weight and 25 mg/kg of body weight for pyrimethamine and sulfadoxine, respectively, with dose adjustments for changes in body weight every 3 months thereafter. Outside of the United States, Fansidar is available as syrup, which simplifies administration. In our experience, this regimen is well tolerated and seldom leads to relevant neutropenia[405]; regular hematologic testing is nevertheless needed as with the standard pyrimethamine/sulfadiazine treatment regimen (see later).[436] Over the past 20 years, this strategy has been used in several large cohort studies.[405,428-432] After the administration of 1.25 mg of Fansidar every 14 days to infants, the serum levels of pyrimethamine may attain peak levels of 350 ng/mL and trough levels of 25 ng/mL.[458] Because concentrations of pyrimethamine in the CSF are 10% to 25% of those in the serum,[436] with this dosing regimen, the levels of pyrimethamine in the CSF exceed the IC_{50} for only a fraction of the dosing interval. However, in the cerebral tissue of rhesus monkeys, the concentrations of pyrimethamine have been reported to be three- to fourfold higher than those in the serum,[459,460] which might compensate therapeutically for the lower levels in the CSF.

In a small cohort study, Fansidar has also been used to treat pregnant women in whom fetal infection was confirmed using a dosage of 25 mg of pyrimethamine and 500 mg of sulfadoxine per 20 kg of body weight and 50 mg of folinic acid on a twice-monthly basis. Under steady-state conditions, the ratio of fetal-to-maternal drug concentrations in umbilical vein blood at the time of delivery ranged from 0.43 to 1.03 (mean ± SD, 0.66 ± 0.22) for pyrimethamine and from 0.65 to 1.16 (mean ± SD, 0.97 ± 0.14) for sulfadoxine. After birth, the combination was continued, with the dose adjusted to the weight of the infant.[430] Children who were treated in utero and during infancy with this regimen and evaluated after a median follow-up of more than 10 years had an apparently favorable clinical course compared with expectations based on historical experience,[136,405,428,461-463] with severe manifestations seen in less than 30%.[463] However, in utero treatment with pyrimethamine and sulfadoxine failed to reduce the risk of developing ocular lesions and intracerebral calcifications. Whether this reflects the lower in vitro activity of sulfadoxine compared with sulfadiazine,[436,464] lower concentrations of pyrimethamine in the CSF than in the plasma,[436] or other contributing factors, such as a delay in the instigation of treatment because of a deferred confirmation of fetal infection by screening,[4,88,465] is unclear.

In any case, and despite the lack of evidence from randomized controlled trials, the body of evidence from large nonrandomized case series indicates that the combination of pyrimethamine with sulfadiazine or sulfadoxine is beneficial, based on differences in the incidences of sequelae between treated and untreated individuals.[465,466] Moreover, three recent autopsy reports on aborted fetuses with untreated congenital toxoplasmosis revealed the presence of numerous tissue cysts but few or no tachyzoites in the placenta, adrenal gland, and heart, but large numbers of actively dividing, tissue-destructive tachyzoites were noted in the brain.[217,248,467] These cases further suggest that treatment helps to control active replication and reduce tissue destruction in the brain, although it has little impact on parasite burden in the placenta.

Adverse Effects of Pyrimethamine and Sulfonamides. Because pyrimethamine inhibits the activity of dihydrofolate reductase, a precursor of folic acid, it induces, as expected, a reversible and usually gradual suppression of hematopoiesis. Neutropenia is the most severe and common side effect of treatment with pyrimethamine, although reduced platelet counts and anemia are not uncommon.[468] Other, less serious side effects include gastrointestinal distress, headaches, and a disagreeable taste in the mouth. When the drugs are administered at the recommended doses, their plasma concentrations usually fall within the expected therapeutic limits, and the intervention is generally well tolerated (in 86% of cases).[445] However, if the recommended dosage of pyrimethamine is exceeded by 10-fold for several days, its plasma concentrations may rise to more than 6000 ng/mL; this has been associated with seizures.[469] Accidental overdosing of infants can induce vomiting, tremor, convulsions, and depressed bone marrow activity.[470-473] In all patients undergoing treatment with pyrimethamine-containing regimens, it is essential to monitor the peripheral blood leukocyte and platelet counts twice weekly until a steady-state condition is attained, and thereafter once per week. Available data afford no evidence of teratogenicity when administered in the recommended dosage,[474,475] but pyrimethamine/sulfonamides should not be given in the first 14 weeks of gestation in any case.

Because the toxic effects of pyrimethamine on hematopoiesis are a consequence of the induced deficiency in folic acid, which is required for cell division, this problem can be ameliorated by the co-administration of folinic acid (leucovorin). Folinic acid is metabolized by mammalian cells but not by the parasite[476]; by contrast, folic acid can be used by the parasite and should NOT be used (see Fig. 31-21). Leucovorin calcium is usually administered three times per week at a dose of 5 to 20 mg, with which regimen the inhibitory action of pyrimethamine on the proliferation of *T. gondii* is not markedly impacted.[436]

At 20-fold higher levels than the clinically applied doses, pyrimethamine retards fetal growth (resulting in reduced body weight) and may be associated with microcephaly and malformations of the limbs, for instance, micromelia, brachydactyly, and adactyly.[477] Because the damage to the fetal DNA is partially attributable to folate deficiency,[478] these adverse effects can be attenuated by co-administration of folinic acid.[479] Treatment of pregnant rats with doses of pyrimethamine that are comparable to those administered in human patients leads to fetal resorption but not to teratogenic effects.[480] However, because tremendous species differences are observed in the responses of rodent offspring to pyrimethamine, the potentially harmful effects in humans cannot be realistically assessed from these animal experiments.[481]

The major side effects of treatment with sulfonamides include changes in the pH of the urine, which leads to the deposition of crystals in the upper urinary tract and skin allergies. In rare cases, the latter can lead to severe or even fatal allergic dermatitis (Stevens-Johnson and Luell syndromes).[431]

Spiramycin

Because of the known and undesired side effects of treatment with pyrimethamine, spiramycin is usually administered instead during the first trimester of pregnancy. During this phase, spiramycin can clear the parasite from the blood and reduce the frequency of placental infection. The infectious load of the placenta is also reduced, although, to attain this effect, a longer treatment duration is necessary than is required with a pyrimethamine/sulfonamide regimen.[460,482]

The in vitro experimental and clinical activities of spiramycin against *T. gondii* are comparable to those reported for other macrolide antibiotics. Under in vivo and in vitro conditions, spiramycin exerts an antitoxoplasmic effect, which appears to be clinically useful in preventing congenital infection with *T. gondii* during pregnancy. However, because spiramycin is not parasiticidal, its use is not recommended for the treatment of fetal toxoplasmosis.[483,484]

Spiramycin is commercially available in many countries, but not in the United States, as a syrup or as capsules. The usual dose in adults is 1 g three times per day. The serum levels of this drug can vary greatly. However, inhibitory concentrations are barely attained in fetal tissues and not at all in the brain.[485,486]

In pregnant women who are undergoing therapy with spiramycin at a daily dose of 1 g given 3 times daily, the levels of the drug in the maternal serum, the umbilical cord serum, and the placental serum have been reported to be 1.7 μg/mL (range, 1-4 μg/mL), 0.8 μg/mL (range, 0.75-2.0 μg/mL) and 6.2 μg/mL (range, 3.25-10 μg/mL), respectively.[487] However, in other studies, the levels were found to be lower by half in each case.[488] The levels of spiramycin in umbilical cord serum are generally 50% lower, and those in placental serum are three- to fivefold higher than the concentrations in maternal serum; however, the levels of spiramycin in umbilical cord serum do not correlate closely with those in maternal serum.[488-490]

Data pertaining to the consequences of maternal spiramycin treatment on the clinical manifestations of toxoplasmosis in newborn infants are scarce. No carefully designed prospective studies have been undertaken. There exists no evidence that prenatal treatment with spiramycin reduces the risk of developing clinical manifestations in infants who become infected despite treatment of the mother.[451,491] Nonetheless, if treatment with spiramycin is begun early during the first trimester of pregnancy, it reduces the incidence of placental infection from 89% to 90% to 75%.[461,488] Compared with untreated historical controls, long-term outcomes in terms of severity of manifestations are favorable.[457,461] If treatment is continued until the time of birth, even when a PCR analysis of the amniotic fluid yields negative results, the risk of late transmission of a placental infection to the fetus may be reduced to 17%, with only 25% of treated cases presenting with overt clinical manifestations.[461]

If fetal infection is confirmed, because of limited transplacental passage of spiramycin and insufficient levels of the drug in the fetal brain,[492] a switch to pyrimethamine/sulfonamide treatment regimen is recommended.[447,493] Similarly, this drug is no longer recommended for treating congenitally infected newborn infants, who should be treated with a pyrimethamine/sulfonamide regimen (see "Postnatal Treatment").

Although spiramycin is generally well tolerated, overdosage of newborn infants can induce potentially severe side effects. Doses greater than 35 mg/kg of body weight can provoke local vasospasm, changes in taste perception, vertigo, dizziness, flushing of the face, tearing of the eyes, nausea, vomiting, diarrhea, and anorexia.[494] In neonates, spiramycin doses of 300,000 IU/kg of body weight/day can induce reversible prolongation of the Q-T interval and life-threatening arrhythmias (including cardiac arrest).

Other Drugs

For the drugs described in the following sections, no clinical data are available that would support their being recommended for use in the treatment of the immunocompetent pregnant woman, the fetus, or the newborn infant. Further evaluations in both animal models and human patients are required. To date, no randomized controlled clinical trials have been conducted.[495]

The treatment of immunocompromised individuals with a combination of *TMP* and *SMZ* (cotrimoxazole) has proved to be efficacious in the prophylaxis and treatment of toxoplasmic encephalitis, and this drug combination is well tolerated.[496] Treatment with cotrimoxazole has also been shown to reduce the risk of recurrences in individuals with ocular toxoplasmosis who are particularly prone to these intermittent flare-ups.[427] In murine models of toxoplasmosis, treatment with cotrimoxazole alone proved to be more efficacious than that with spiramycin alone.[497]

No clinical experience has been gained relating to the use of cotrimoxazole in the prevention of congenital toxoplasmosis. Although cotrimoxazole has been used in combination with spiramycin to treat pregnancy-associated toxoplasmosis and was well tolerated by the patients, this agent cannot be recommended on the basis of the available data.[422]

Clindamycin has been shown to be effective in the treatment of murine toxoplasmosis. In this model, the drug averted the fatal consequences of acute infection in, and eradicated the parasite from, the livers, spleens, and brains of approximately 30% to 50% of acutely surviving animals. During the acute phase of infection in mice, clindamycin effectively inhibited the vertical transmission of the parasite from the mother to the fetus.[498-500]

More recently, treatment of ocular toxoplasmosis with intravitreal clindamycin has attracted attention. A weekly intravitreal injection of this drug, together with dexamethasone, over a 4-week period, proved to be as effective as the recommended oral therapy with pyrimethamine and sulfadiazine in terms of the primary outcome and the prevention of recurrences over a 2-year follow-up course.[424,501-504] However, available data afford no evidence that clindamycin, either alone or together with other drugs, is equally or more efficacious than established systemic combination therapies for the treatment of congenital infection in either pregnant women or their newborn offspring.

Atovaquone has been shown to potently inhibit the replication of both tachyzoites and bradyzoites in vitro and to reduce the fatality rate in a murine model of toxoplasmosis in a strain-dependent manner.[412,505] Although this drug has been reported to suppress the tissue-destructive activity of bradyzoites in a murine model of toxoplasmosis,[170,506] in AIDS patients, it prevented the recurrence of toxoplasmic encephalitis in no more than 50% of the individuals.[507,508] The effect of atovaquone on bradyzoites may be both strain- and time-dependent and enhanced by combining it with either pyrimethamine or clindamycin.[171,442]

DRUGS UNDER CONSIDERATION AND NOVEL DRUG TARGETS

Recently, *artemisinin* has gained interest for the treatment of toxoplasmosis. In one in vitro study, the effects of artesunate, a derivative of artemisinin, on the intracellular replication of tachyzoites were compared with those of cotrimoxazole, pentamidine, pyrimethamine, quinine, or TMP. The IC_{50} for artesunate-induced tachyzoitic toxicity was, at 0.075 μM, 25-fold lower than that for host cell cytotoxicity (2.0 μM). The corresponding values for pyrimethamine were 0.48 μM and 11.2 μM, respectively. Trimethoprim and cotrimoxazole were also effective against the parasite but at higher concentrations than those observed for artesunate and pyrimethamine. If a similar effect of artesunate could be demonstrated in vivo, without eliciting deleterious side effects, this agent could find a role in the treatment of toxoplasmosis.[437]

Artemisinin-based combination therapies are currently recommended by the World Health Organization for the treatment of uncomplicated cases of malaria caused by *Plasmodium falciparum*. In contrast to sulfonamides, artemisinin and its semisynthetic derivatives artesunate, artemether, and dihydroartemisinin, are short-acting antimalarial agents that destroy the parasites more rapidly than conventional ones.[509] A 1:1 combination of artesunate and its metabolite dihydroartemisinin has experimentally been shown to have some effect but does not eradicate cerebral bradyzoites of *T. gondii* at concentrations of 0.1 to 0.5 μg/mL.[510]

Other drugs, which have been used to treat toxoplasmic patients with complications, include rifampin, tetracyclines, fluoroquinolones, and macrolides—roxithromycin, clarithromycin, and azithromycin. However, none of these agents have been clinically tested in the context of congenital toxoplasmosis, nor, indeed, even been investigated in a murine model of toxoplasmosis.[7,511-515]

In *Plasmodium*, genetic mutations, as well as overexpression of genes encoding drug targets and adenosine triphosphate (ATP)-binding cassette (ABC) transporters, have led to the development of resistance. As yet, genetic resistance has not been observed with drugs used to treat infection with *T. gondii*. Although three sulfadiazine-resistant strains of *T. gondii* have been recently isolated, the resistance does not appear to have a genetic background. Consequently, these variants do not pose a clinically relevant problem.[516]

Recently, protein kinases have been shown to play crucial roles in the proliferation, differentiation, and pathogenesis of *T. gondii*. Two are involved in motility and host cell invasion (the calcium-dependent protein kinase 1 and the cyclic guanosine monophosphate–dependent protein kinase), two in stage interconversion (the mitogen-activated protein kinase 1 and the cyclic adenosine monophosphate–dependent protein kinase), and two in cell-cycle control (the casein kinase 1 and the cdc2 cyclin-dependent kinase) cell.[517,518] Moreover, the rhoptry kinases, which are specific to *T. gondii*, combat the parasite's intracellular digestion by manipulating the host cell's enzymes. Because the rhoptry kinases differ greatly from mammalian protein kinase in structure and function, they would be ideal drug targets.

A plant-type redox apparatus, consisting of ferredoxin–nicotinamide adenine dinucleotide phosphate$^+$ reductase and its redox partner ferredoxin, as well as lipoic acid synthase and enzymes of the isoprenoid biosynthetic pathway, could also serve as drug targets because both systems are implicated in metabolic processes that are vital for the parasite.[519]

The biosynthesis of type II fatty acids has likewise been shown to be a promising target for drug intervention in toxoplasmosis. Analogues of 8-thiolactomycin act selectively against *T. gondii* by interfering with its membrane-bound organelles and its division, thereby influencing the development of the parasite and its survival, as demonstrated in vitro.[520]

In conclusion, many antibiotics have been shown to be highly efficacious against both active and chronic forms of infection with *T. gondii*, and several potentially new drug targets have been identified. However, as yet, studies with these drugs have been conducted exclusively under experimental conditions and have not been pursued to the stage of preclinical development and clinical evaluation.

Epidemiology and Diagnosis of Infections in the Mother and the Unborn Child

EPIDEMIOLOGY OF MATERNAL INFECTION

Seroprevalence of Infection with *Toxoplasma gondii* and Related Risk Factors

Detailed knowledge of the proportion of susceptible pregnant women in any given area is important to determine the best strategy for the local prevention of congenital toxoplasmosis. Because the rates of seropositivity decline to the same extent in pregnant women and in the general population, recent data are required to avoid an underestimation of the proportion of susceptible pregnant women. Accurate knowledge of the manner in which pregnant women acquire infection in a given location is also a prerequisite for the development of appropriate education campaigns.

Pappas and colleagues[2] provided a worldwide overview for the period 1999 to 2008, and Roberts and colleagues[521] reviewed seroprevalence in the developing world between 1950 and 2010. Risk factors for seropositivity or for acute infection have also been discussed in several reviews.[522-524] Analysis of the data published since 2000 for America, Europe, Africa, and Asia demonstrates wide variations in transmission patterns.

North America. Only a few studies have been published on the seroprevalence of *T. gondii* infection in the United States. The most recent figures were estimated from a nationwide survey of subjects sampled between 1999 and 2004 and indicated that the overall age-adjusted seroprevalence of *T. gondii* for persons aged 6 to 49 years was 10.8% (95% confidence limits [CL], 9.6% to 11.9%) and that for U.S.-born women aged 15 to 44 years was 11.0% (95% CL, 9.5% to 12.4%). Among persons born in the United States aged 12 to 49 years, seroprevalence declined from 14.1% to 9.0% ($P < .001$) in the period between the National Health and Nutrition Examination Survey (NHANES) III (1988-1994) and NHANES IV (1999-2004). The prevalence of *T. gondii* infection was higher in Mexican Americans than in non-Hispanic white subjects. Seroprevalence was also found to increase significantly with age group and poverty.[299]

Risk factors for *Toxoplasma* infection were investigated in a case-control study of recently infected adults.[341] Case patients were 148 adults, including 76 pregnant women, who were diagnosed with a profile of recent (<6 months) infection at the Palo Alto Medical Foundation *Toxoplasma* Serology Laboratory between 2002 and 2007. Control patients (two or three control patients for every infected case patient) were 413 persons, including 301 pregnant women, randomly selected among those who tested negative within the year before each case was diagnosed and lived in the same state or geographic region. Multivariate analysis was performed for the whole study population, for women and pregnant women only, and for a subset of responders who were also questioned about raw seafood consumption. In all four models, a number of risk factors were found to increase the risk of infection (Table 31-1) and were related to exposure to oocysts (owning three kittens or more) and to consumption of meat (eating rare lamb, raw ground beef, and/or locally produced cured, dried, or smoked meat). Eating previously frozen ground pork was an additional risk factor in pregnant women. Cooking meat in a microwave oven was consistently found to decrease the risk of infection. Drinking unpasteurized goat's milk increased the risk of infection, except in the model that identified the consumption of raw oysters, mussels, and clams as a significant risk factor. The risk of infection was higher in persons living in the Northeast vs. the West, or in the Midwest vs. the West.[341] A previous study also reported higher prevalence rates in persons living in the Northeast compared with those in the West, the Midwest, and the South.[525]

Potential predictors of infection were also assessed in 131 mothers of infants with congenital *Toxoplasma* infection who were questioned by Boyer and colleagues[526] in Chicago. Thirty-one percent of these women reported having eaten undercooked meat during pregnancy, and 27% had potential exposure to oocysts through gardening or contacts with a sandbox. The proportion of African-American women in this group was lower than that in the general population, but women from Asia or the Pacific Islands were overrepresented.[526] Similar findings on geographic origins were reported among mothers of congenitally

Table 31-1 Adjusted Odds Ratios (aORs) Based on Four Multivariate Models Comparing Case and Control Patients

Model, Associated Factor	aOR (95% CLs)	AR (95% CLs),* %
Model 1[†]	All persons responding to the questions in the model ($n = 473$)	
Age		
≥50 vs. 18-29 years	3.21 (1.01, 10.19)	8 (0, 11)
30-49 vs. 18-29 years	1.13 (0.64, 1.97)	—
Sex, male vs. female	5.13 (2.10, 12.58)	12 (8, 14)
Region		
Midwest vs. West	3.67 (1.53, 8.79)	43 (26, 53)
Northeast vs. West	3.43 (1.66, 7.09)	—
South vs. West	1.50 (0.65, 3.47)	—
Work with meat; yes vs. no	3.15 (1.09, 9.10)	5 (2, 7)
Have kittens		
≥ 3 vs. 0	27.89 (5.72, 135.86)	10 (9, 13)
1-2 vs. 0	0.64 (0.26, 1.56)	
Eat locally produced cured, dried, or smoked meat; yes vs. no	1.97 (1.18, 3.28)	22 (7, 32)
Eat rare lamb; yes vs. no	8.39 (3.68, 19.16)	20 (17, 21)
Eat raw ground beef; yes vs. no	6.67 (2.09, 21.24)	7 (5, 8)
Microwave meat; yes vs. no	0.44 (0.24, 0.81)	22 (8, 46)[‡]
Drink unpasteurized goat's milk; yes vs. no	5.09 (1.45, 17.80)	4 (1, 5)
Drink untreated water from a stream, lake, or pond; yes vs. no	3.11 (0.92, 10.51)	—
Model 2[§]	Persons receiving amended questionnaire (including oyster, mussel, and clam consumption) and responding to the questions in the model ($n = 380$)	
Age		
≥50 vs. 18-29 years	2.50 (0.54, 11.56)	
30-49 vs. 18-29 years	0.72 (0.38, 1.38)	—
Sex, male vs. female	7.30 (2.34, 22.82)	13 (8, 14)
Region		
Midwest vs. West	3.32 (1.23, 8.91)	39 (13, 54)
Northeast vs. West	2.67 (1.15, 6.16)	—
South vs. West	1.60 (0.61, 4.20)	—
Work with meat; yes vs. no	2.75 (0.83, 9.15)	—
Have kittens		
≥ 3 vs. 0	35.36 (4.00, 312.94)	10 (8, 13)
1-2 vs. 0	0.62 (0.23, 1.70)	—
Eat locally produced cured, dried, or smoked meat; yes vs. no	2.10 (1.16, 3.82)	23 (7, 33)
Eat rare lamb; yes vs. no	9.26 (3.79, 22.63)	20 (17, 22)
Eat raw ground beef; yes vs. no	7.55 (1.75, 32.65)	7 (4, 8)
Microwave meat; yes vs. no	0.42 (0.21, 0.83)	23 (7, 50)[‡]
Eat any raw oysters, clams, or mussels; yes vs. no	2.22 (1.07, 4.61)	16 (4, 24)
Model 3[‖]	All women responding to the questions in the model ($n = 446$)	
Age		
≥50 vs. 18-29 years	3.42 (0.84, 13.96)	
30-49 vs. 18-29 years	1.14 (0.63, 2.07)	—
Region		
Midwest vs. West	4.92 (1.96, 12.34)	47 (28, 57)
Northeast vs. West	3.48 (1.60, 7.58)	—
South vs. West	1.42 (0.56, 3.60)	—
Have kittens		
≥ 3 vs. 0	72.74 (8.78, 602.80)	11 (10, 14)
1-2 vs. 0	0.63 (0.25, 1.60)	—
Eat locally produced cured, dried, or smoked meat; yes vs. no	2.48 (1.45, 4.26)	28 (15, 36)
Eat sausage; yes vs. no	1.72 (0.94, 3.16)	—
Eat rare lamb; yes vs. no	10.27 (4.40, 24.01)	20 (17, 21)
Eat raw ground beef; yes vs. no	5.78 (1.78, 18.71)	7 (4, 9)
Microwave meat; yes vs. no	0.41 (0.22, 0.79)	24 (7, 49)[‡]

Table 31-1 Adjusted Odds Ratios (aORs) Based on Four Multivariate Models Comparing Case and Control Patients—cont'd

Model, Associated Factor	aOR (95% CLs)	AR (95% CLs),* %
Drink unpasteurized goat's milk; yes vs. no	5.92 (1.59, 22.09)	4 (1, 5)
Model 4¶	All pregnant women responding to the questions in the model (n = 300)	
Region		
Midwest vs. West	4.57 (1.29, 16.17)	58 (30, 71)
Northeast vs. West	4.65 (1.58, 13.67)	—
South vs. West	1.37 (0.37, 5.11)	—
Have kittens		
≥ 3 vs. 0	76.15 (8.27, 701.12)	13 (12, 19)
1-2 vs. 0	1.10 (0.37, 3.26)	—
Eat previously frozen ground pork; often/sometimes vs. never	2.30 (1.12, 4.74)	22 (6, 33)
Eat rare lamb; yes vs. no	5.20 (1.58, 17.09)	13 (6, 16)
Eat raw ground beef; yes vs. no	5.39 (1.38, 21.01)	9 (3, 11)
Microwave meat; yes vs. no	0.33 (0.12, 0.87)	26 (5, 73) ‡
Drink unpasteurized goat's milk; yes vs. no	7.12 (1.56, 32.44)	6 (2, 7)
Wash hands after handling raw meat; always/sometimes vs. never	0.32 (0.09, 1.10)	—

From Jones JL, Dargelas V, Roberts J, et al: *Toxoplasma gondii* case-control study, United States, August 2002 through May 2007, *Clin Infect Dis* 49:878-884, 2009.
AR, Attributable risk; *CLs,* confidence limits.
*Denoted for aORs significant at $P < .05$ only. Data are ARs unless otherwise indicated.
†Summary AR, 78% (95% CLs, 69%, 83%); summary AR excluding region, sex, and age: 52% (95% CLs, 40%, 58%).
‡Prevented fraction.
§Summary AR, 77% (95% CLs, 63%, 83%); summary AR excluding region and sex: 57% (95% CLs, 42%, 63%).
‖Summary AR, 75% (95% CLs, 64%, 81%); summary AR excluding region: 54% (95% CLs, 41%, 59%).
¶Summary AR, 79% (95% CLs, 59%-86%); summary AR excluding region: 50% (95% CLs, 30%, 56%).

infected children identified by the screening of newborns in Massachusetts.[527] Women who were born in Vietnam, Laos, and Cambodia were 8.9 times more likely to give birth to an infected child than those born in the United States. Higher gravidity (three or more) and education (college graduate or higher) were also independent risk factors for congenital infection.

Few epidemiologic data are available for pregnant or women of childbearing age in Canada. A survey of providers for young children in the Toronto area reported seropositivity rates as low as 4.6% in Canadian-born women aged 30 years or younger, whereas those born outside of Canada had rates of 23.1%.[528] Similarly low rates (5%) were found in two Cree communities.[528a] In contrast, much higher rates (59.8%) were reported in a cross-sectional survey of Inuit communities in Nunavik.[529] Independent risk factors for past infection were being a woman, having a low level of education, being in the older age group, drinking municipal or natural water, infrequently cleaning the domestic water tank, and frequently eating birds and seal meat.[529] In a previous study in Inuit women, the consumption of raw seal and caribou meat and skinning animals for fur were suspected to be responsible for clusters of cases of acute infection in pregnancy.[304]

South America. Most estimates have been calculated from studies in Brazil, where the seropositivity rates in pregnant women are highest, as described in a recent review.[530] Except for one study in Brasilia, quoted by Pappas and coworkers,[2] which reported a seroprevalence of only 7.3%, estimates in the most recent studies ranged between 49% and 75%.[321,382,391,392,531-534] Limited information is available for other countries. The rates reported over the last decade ranged between 18%[535] and 49%[536] in Argentina, and they were 33% in Venezuela[537] and 46% in Colombia.[300] In Mexico, the rates of seroprevalence were less than 10%[333,538] in the Durango state but were estimated to be 16% in a meta-analysis of national data.[539] Seroprevalence generally increased with age and decreased with calendar time, except in Cali, Colombia, where no decline was observed.[300]

Information on risk factors for seropositivity was provided by nine surveys in Brazil and one in Mexico. Nine reported at least one factor that involved exposure to oocysts: having contact with soil and sand,[382,392,540] not wearing gloves when working in the yard,[391] living in a house with a soil floor[333,538] or without garbage collection[382] or sewage,[368] eating raw vegetables[534] or vegetables that were washed with untreated water,[321] drinking water that did not come from the public water supply[540] or eating homemade water ice,[321] and having contact with or owning cats and/or dogs.[321,382,391,531,534] Geophagia was listed in one survey. Current or previous residence in a rural area was also reported to be associated with past infection.[333,368,540] Only four studies found the consumption of meat to be a significant factor: poultry meat was involved in two (eating turkey[333] or eating chicken more than twice a day[321]), whereas the other two mentioned eating undercooked meat with no further specification.[368,382] The consumption of unpasteurized goat's milk[368] or raw/undercooked eggs[368] was rarely found to be associated with past infection. Women who were less well educated† and/or had the lowest per-capita income‡ were often found to be more likely to have been in contact with the parasite. Pregnancy was found to be the main risk factor for infection in one Brazilian study.[368]

†References 368, 391, 392, 532, 534, 540.
‡References 321, 368, 391, 392, 534, 540.

Risk factors for acute infections were investigated in Colombia in a case-control study of 14 pregnant women who had a serologic profile of acute infection and 34 seronegative pregnant control subjects.[395] Consumption of undercooked meat and contact with kittens aged less than 6 months accounted for 42% of all infections. Drinking beverages prepared with water that had not been boiled was a third, significant risk factor.

Africa. Recent information on the seroprevalence in pregnant women or women of childbearing age in Africa is limited but suggests high variations between, and probably within, countries. The highest estimates (>50%) were found in five countries located in North, West, Central and East Africa: Morocco (51%),[541] Ivory Coast (60%),[303] Gabon(56%),[542] São Tomé and Principe (75% or greater),[543] and Ethiopia (81%).[544,545] The lowest seroprevalence was found in South Africa, where only 6% of the pregnant women who were surveyed had a positive test for anti–*T. gondii* IgG.[546] In all other surveys, the reported overall seroprevalence rates were moderate, ranging from19% to 41% (49% in Tunisia,[547] 20% to 31% in Burkina Faso,[548-551] 27% in Mali,[552] 34.5% to 40% in Senegal,[553-555] 29% to 41% in Nigeria,[556,557] 19% in Mozambique,[558] 31% in Tanzania,[559] and 34% in Sudan[560]). In contrast to the overall decreasing trend over the past decades, prevalence was found to be stable in Côte d'Ivoire[303] and increasing in Ethiopia.[545]

The risk factors for *T. gondii* infection were only assessed through seroprevalence surveys. Similarly to South America, exposure to oocysts (through contact with soil[541,555] or cats/pets,[303,542,543,545] or the consumption of treated/not boiled water[543,556] or raw/unwashed vegetables[543,544]) was more frequently reported than the consumption of undercooked meat[555,560] or tasting meat during the cooking process.[556] No information was provided on the implication of hand and kitchen hygiene. A low level of education was less frequently reported to be a significant risk factor than in South America. Seroprevalence increased with age. A comparison between HIV-positive and HIV-negative pregnant women in Burkina Faso[548,549] and Mozambique[558] indicated higher rates of infection in the HIV-positive group.

Europe. The majority of rates of seropositivity for *T. gondii* infection in pregnant women or women of child-bearing age in Europe published since 2000 ranged from 20% to 37%.[2,561-573] Lower rates were found in northern Europe[574-577] but also in Spain[578-581] and Italy.[582] This suggests the absence of a significant gradient according to latitude across countries, which was also confirmed among pregnant women of diverse ethnic origins in London.[577] Seroprevalences of 50% or higher were still observed in two studies conducted in Albania[583] and Switzerland.[584] In pregnant French women, seroprevalence decreased from 44% in 2003 to 37% in 2010,[585] and a similar trend was observed throughout Europe. Seropositivity for *T. gondii* was also found to increase with age and to be generally higher in rural than in metropolitan areas. Several studies have indicated differences between native and immigrant pregnant women.[568,577,579-581,586] In most cases, immigrant pregnant women had higher rates of infection, except when they originated from Asia.

The findings of three case-control studies carried out on European women with infection in and around the time of pregnancy are summarized in Table 31-2. Information on risk factors for *T. gondii* infection was also collected in

Table 31-2 Risk Factors for Incident *Toxoplasma* Infection in Pregnant Women in Europe: Selection of Case-Control Studies

Location and Period of Study, Study Reference	Study Population	Factors Related to Exposure to Tissue Cysts	Factors Related to Exposure to Oocysts*	Other Factors
Six European centers: Brussels, Copenhagen, Lausanne, Milan, Naples, and Oslo 1994-1995[316]	252 pregnant women with a proven seroconversion or a profile of recent infection vs. 858 seronegative pregnant control women (3 per case in the same laboratory minus 150 exclusions)	Eating undercooked meat: Lamb: OR, 3.13; 95% CI, 1.4 to 7.2 Beef: OR, 1.73; 95% CI, 1.1 to 7.2 Other meat: OR, 4.12; 95% CI, 1.1 to 10.9 Note: Undercooked pork: OR, 1.40; 95% CI, 0.7 to 2.8	Contact with soil: OR, 1.81; 95% CI, 1.2 to 2.7	Travel outside Europe, United States, or Canada: OR, 2.33; 95% CI, 1.3 to 4.1
France 1995[340]	80 pregnant women with seroconversion vs. 80 seronegative control subjects (same physician as cases) matched by gestational age, and geographic area	Eating undercooked meat: Beef: OR, 5.5; 95% CI, 1.1 to 27, Lamb: OR, 3.1; 95% CI, 0.85 to 14.	Poor hand hygiene: OR, 9.9; 95% CI, 0.8 to 125 Having a pet cat: OR, 4.5; 95% CI, 1.0 to 19.9 Frequent consumption of raw vegetables outside the home: OR, 3.1; 95% CI, 1.2 to 7.7	
Norway 1992-1994[315]	63 pregnant women with a serologic profile of acute infection vs. 128 seronegative pregnant control subjects matched by age, gestational age, and geographic area	Eating undercooked meat: Minced meat products: OR,4.1; $P = .007$ (AF, 0.288) Mutton: OR, 11.4; $P = .005$ (AF, 0.221) Pork: OR, 3.4; $P = .03$ (AF, 0.179) Infrequently washing kitchen knives after preparation of raw meat: OR, 7.3; $P = .04$ (AF, 0.111) No increased risk with consumption of beef and poultry	Eating unwashed raw vegetables or fruits: OR, 2.4; $P = .03$ (AF, 0.278) Cleaning the cat litter box: OR, 5.5; $P = .02$ (AF, 0.155)	

AF, Attributable fraction; *CI*, confidence interval; *OR*, odds ratio.

seroprevalence surveys. All but one[577] of the studies identified in the same population risk factors that were related to oocysts and tissue cysts. Exposure to oocysts involved contact with soil[314,316,383,569] or consumption of fruits and vegetables[315,340,569] more frequently than pet ownership.[315,340] Consumption of undercooked meat was regularly reported,[314-316,340,569,577] and rare mutton or lamb was listed in three case-control studies.[383,587] Undercooked beef or processed pork products were also commonly implicated.[314-316,340,569] Other factors included feeding dogs pieces of raw meat,[575] not washing kitchen utensils[315] or hands[340] adequately, and traveling outside Europe and North America.[315]

Asia. The lowest seroprevalence rates for *T. gondii* infection in Asia were found in pregnant women and women of childbearing age who were surveyed in Korea (<4%),[287,396] Vietnam (11%),[588] Thailand (3%-28%),[589,590] and in Japan[361] and China[591,592] (≈10%). Rates reported in surveys from Bahrain (22%)[593] and Palestine (8%-28%)[594, 595] were moderate and were much higher in other Middle Eastern countries: Iran and Turkey (the majority reported ranged from 30% to 65%[397,596-604]), Saudi Arabia (35%-51%),[605-607] Egypt (45%-70%),[608,609] Jordan (30%-90%),[387,610,611] Kuwait (53%),[612] and Beirut (62%).[613] A high proportion (70%) of pregnant women surveyed in Jakarta had anti-*Toxoplasma* antibodies[614]; variations from 9% to 45% were found in India[615-619]; and seroprevalence in pregnant women was reported to be 30% in Taiwan[616] and 39% in Malaysia.[620]

In several studies, participants were questioned on exposure to risk factors, but only a few items related to food and hygiene reached significance and involved either consumption of raw meat[361,600,605] or ingestion of oocysts,[397,589,597,609] and, more rarely, both routes of infection in the same population.[387,396,591,616] A number of sociodemographic characteristics were associated with past infection, including residence in more rural[§] or remote areas,[589] older age,[‖] low level of education[591,600] or low family income,[605] unemployment[595,598] or occupation as an agricultural worker,[615] belonging to an ethnic group in Malaysia,[620] or being indigenous versus being an immigrant in Taiwan.[616]

The prevalence of *T. gondii* antibodies was 33% in pregnant women in Auckland, New Zealand.[621]

Incidence of *Toxoplasma* Infections During Pregnancy

Precise information on how many women seroconvert during pregnancy in any given setting is important because it contributes to decisions on which preventive interventions are the most appropriate and to an assessment of their impact. The direct observation of cases is complex because acute infections are relatively rare events, and retesting during pregnancy is required on a large sample of pregnant women who were found to be susceptible at the time of an early prenatal test. Cross-sectional surveys are widely used as alternatives but are prone to errors because of the absence of reliable markers for acute infection in a single test. Including serologic profiles that only suggest the possibility of infection (i.e., detection of IgM antibody and IgG antibodies of low avidity) as criteria for proven infection will overestimate the cumulative incidence.

§References 387, 591, 595, 601, 604, 605.

‖References 397, 589, 595, 598, 600, 605.

Modeling age- and time-specific seroprevalence data has been demonstrated to afford a valuable substitute,[585,622,623] provided that the information available is satisfactory. Incidence is expressed as the number of primary infections per 1000 susceptible pregnant women per year.

Published data are rather limited and have mostly originated from Europe. The incidence of primary infection during pregnancy varied between 0.5 and 3 per 1000 susceptible pregnant women in most European countries, including Sweden (0.5/1000),[624] Belgium (0.9/1000),[625] Spain (1/1000),[626] Austria (1.7/1000),[563] France (2.1/ 1000),[585] Denmark (2.1/1000),[627] and Finland (2.4/1000),[628] but higher estimates were also found in Italy (7.7/1000),[629] Greece (8/1000),[561] and in Hungary (17/1000).[630] The incidence was estimated to be between 2 and 10 per 1000 in the United States,[631,631a,631b] and two Brazilian surveys[632,633] reported a cumulative incidence of 4.8 per 1000 and 5.7 per1000, respectively. The analysis of data collected in France suggested that the incidence of primary *Toxoplasma* infection among women aged 15 to 45 years decreased by 70% over the last 30 years.[585]

Incidence of Congenital Infections

The incidence of congenital infection depends on the proportion of susceptible pregnant women and on the incidence of primary infection acquired during or immediately preceding pregnancy. Information can be obtained from prenatal and postnatal screening for *Toxoplasma* infection and also by testing dried blood spots from newborn screening. The quality of estimates varies according to the methods used, and those obtained in the context of neonatal screening need to be corrected for the less-than-perfect sensitivity of tests for IgM antibodies at birth.

The incidence of congenital infection was estimated to be 0.8 per 10,000 live births by Guerina and coworkers[631] and 1 to 20 per 10,000 by Remington and coworkers.[634] The incidence varied from 3 to 9 per 10,000 in Brazil[632,633,635-639] (except in one study that reported a record incidence of 50/10,000[640]) and from 39 to 62 per 10,000 in Colombia.[641,642] In Europe, the estimates ranged from 0.5 to 1.6 per 10,000,[624,627,643-645] except for two surveys in Spain[626] and the Netherlands[646] that reported estimates of 3 per 10,000 and 20 per 10,000, respectively. The lowest incidence was found in Greece (0.1/10,000), based on reporting by physicians.[647] Togerson and Mastroiacovo assessed the global burden of congenital toxoplasmosis in a systematic review of the available data and estimated that congenital toxoplasmosis causes 190,000 cases annually (95% confidence interval: 179,300-206,300), equivalent to a burden of 1.20 million DALYs (95% confidence interval: 0.76-1.90) per year. Table 31-3 summarizes the global incidence and burden of congenital toxoplasmosis by region of the World Health Organization, further subdivided into subregions based on mortality strata. As expected, incidence of congenital toxoplasmosis was the highest in South America.

CLINICAL SIGNS OF MATERNAL INFECTION

The clinical diagnosis of maternal *Toxoplasma* infection is complex because most pregnant women who acquire infection during pregnancy show no or only benign symptoms that are often unrecognized or not reported and are not specific.

Table 31-3 Global incidence and Burden of Congenital Toxoplasmosis, by Region of the World Health Organization

Region	Incident Cases (95% CI)	Incidence* (95% CI)	DALYs (95% CI)	DALYs* (95% CI)
AFR D	26,500 (24,300-30,100)	2.0 (1.8-2.3)	171,500 (92,300-294,500)	13 (6.9-22)
AFR E	37,000 (33,900-41,000)	2.4 (2.2-2.5)	235,900 (129,600-379,000)	15 (8.3-24)
AMR A	2,940 (2360-3540)	0.6 (0.5-0.8)	19,700 (14,100-26,700)	4.2 (3.0-5.7)
AMR B	15,300 (13,100-17,800)	1.8 (1.5-2.0)	105,300 (82,500-127,500)	12 (9.4-15)
AMR C	5077 (4225-6792)	3.4 (2.5-4.1)	35,000 (24,400-41,200)	19 (13-22)
EMR B	8450 (6950-9530)	2.5 (2.1-2.9)	53,900 (27,800-84,800)	17 (8.5-26)
EMR D	26,300 (21,200-31,200)	2.2 (1.7-2.6)	164,900 (84,600-277,800)	14 (6.9-23)
EUR A	2170 (1900-2896)	0.5 (0.4-0.6)	13,600 (7,508-23,400)	2.8 (1.3-4.3)
EUR B	5200 (4500-6090)	1.5 (1.3-1.7)	32,200 (17,500-54,700)	9.2 (5.0-16)
EUR C	4200 (3700-4800)	1.6 (1.4-1.8)	26,400 (14,400-42,700)	10 (5.4-16)
SEAR B	6430 (4240-8600)	1.3 (0.9-1.7)	40,300 (18,700-71,800)	8.1 (3.8-14)
SEAR D	25,400 (20,700-30,700)	0.8 (0.7-1.0)	158,300 (85,900-275,400)	5.1 (2.8-8.9)
WPR A	960 (720-1200)	0.6 (0.9-1.3)	5950 (2900-10,100)	3.9 (1.9-6.6)
WPR B	24,200 (20,500-28,100)	1.1 (0.9-1.3)	154,700 (81,200-253,000)	7.1 (3.7-12)
Total	190,100 (179,300-206,300)	1.5 (1.4-1.6)	1,200,000 (760,000-1,900,000)	9.6 (5.8-15)

From Torgerson PR, Mastroiacovo P: The global burden of congenital toxoplasmosis: a systematic review, *Bull World Health Organ* 91:501-508, 2013.
AFR, African Region; *AMR,* Region of the Americas; *CI,* confidence interval; *DALY,* disability-adjusted life year; *EMR,* Eastern Mediterranean Region; *EUR,* European Region; *SEAR,* Southeast Asia Region; *WPR,* Western Pacific Region.
*Per 1000 live births.

In immunocompetent pregnant women, lymphadenopathy and fatigue are the most common manifestations and appear, on average, 1 week after infection is acquired, although the incubation period can be longer. Cervical nodes are most frequently involved, the most typical manifestation being enlarged posterior cervical nodes.[648] Adenopathy can also be multiple and involve other groups of nodes (axillary, supraclavicular, inguinal, retroperitoneal, or mesenteric). Lymph nodes may or not be tender and are usually firm, discreet, smooth, and mobile, with no tendency toward suppuration. Fatigue is also commonly reported and can be associated with low-grade fever, headaches, malaise, pharyngitis, and myalgia, mimicking infectious mononucleosis. Splenomegaly, hepatomegaly, and erythematous exanthem are rarer.[648]

The clinical course is usually self-limited, and symptoms resolve within a few weeks or months. However, fatigue can occasionally persist for several months after the regression of lymph nodes. The frequency and severity of symptoms have been reported to be greater after the ingestion of oocysts than after that of tissue cysts.[649] Retinochoroiditis is thought to affect no more than 2% of healthy infected patients in the United States.[650] However, lesions that were consistent with, or reminiscent of, ocular toxoplasmosis were found in 7.7% of 130 mothers of children who had congenital toxoplasmosis.[651]

Immunodepression during pregnancy could explain why the frequency is higher than that in the nonpregnant population. Higher rates of 11%[652] and 18%,[653] respectively, were reported in Brazil in two studies of immunocompetent nonpregnant patients who had an acute acquired *Toxoplasma* infection. Pregnant women with HIV infection and acquired immunodeficiency syndrome also run a higher risk of severe symptoms that take the form of encephalitis. Direct inoculation of the parasite during laboratory accidents can also lead to severe forms.[654]

Clinical signs were reported by 5% of patients in the context of the French screening program.[80] Higher rates were reported in the United States by Boyer and colleagues[526] in mothers who gave birth to a child with congenital toxoplasmosis. Of 131 respondents, 48% could recall having had clinical signs compatible with toxoplasmosis during their pregnancy, including lymphadenopathy in 23%. Awareness of the clinical signs that are compatible with a *Toxoplasma* infection in pregnant women offers the chance for a prompt diagnosis and treatment of the maternal and fetal infections. Retrospective enquiries about clinical signs can also help estimate the timing of an acute infection detected through serologic screening.

DIAGNOSIS OF MATERNAL INFECTION

Circumstances

Two main circumstances can lead to the detection of a *Toxoplasma* infection in a pregnant woman. The first occurs within the context of a prenatal retesting programs, whether organized, as in France and in Austria, or performed at the initiative of a clinician or at the request of the patient in the majority of countries, including the United States, where screening is not organized. Recognition of an acute infection is usually less of a challenge in this context than in the second one, which arises when clinical signs suggestive of acute *Toxoplasma* infection (see earlier) are recognized in a pregnant woman. In both situations, laboratory tests are required to establish whether or not the patient has preexisting immunity or has acquired the infection postconception and, if so, to establish when it occurred.

Available Tests

Serologic tests are the most useful, in part because the prompt formation of tissue cysts after an acute infection limits the possibilities of direct detection of the parasite or its nucleic acids. Those for the detection of specific anti-*Toxoplasma* IgG and IgM antibodies are the most widely used.[648,655] Tests for the exploration of cellular immunity are only available in a few centers, and their utility and performance characteristics are less established than for serologic tests.

Table 31-4 Serologic Tests for the Diagnosis of *Toxoplasma* Infection in Pregnancy

Technique	Principles and Main Advantages
TECHNIQUES THAT USE WHOLE TACHYZOITES	
Sabin-Feldman dye test (SFDT)	Live virulent tachyzoites are used as antigens and incubated with a dilution of the serum and complement accessory factor. The test is based on the ability of live parasites to take up methylene blue in the presence of serum that does not contain any antibodies (staining = negative test), but not when specific anti-*Toxoplasma* antibodies are present, and cause complement-mediated cytolysis of the parasites (no staining = positive test). This reference test has the highest sensitivity and specificity for the early and late detection of total specific immunoglobulins, mostly IgG, including low titers. Comparison with a standard reference serum allows results to be expressed in IU/mL.
Indirect fluorescent antibody test (IFAT)	Less demanding than SFDT because it uses slide preparations of fixed tachyzoites that are washed with dilutions of the test serum. IgG or IgM are revealed by specific fluorescent-labeled conjugates. Its sensitivity is lower than that of SFDT but still satisfactory, and its specificity is excellent. Comparison with a standard reference serum allows results to be expressed in IU/mL.
Direct agglutination test: modified agglutination test (MAT)	Formalin-treated tachyzoites are exposed to serum. The presence of IgG antibodies will cause the parasite to agglutinate and form a precipitate that can be detected visually. Treatment with 2-mercaptoethanol can be used to eliminate IgM and detect IgG only (MAT). A kit is commercially available; interpreting the test is not automated but is done by direct visualization, and accuracy requires operator proficiency.
Differential agglutination test	Chemical modification of the outer membrane of tachyzoites allows differential agglutination (HS/AC test) to differentiate between recent and chronic infection
Immunosorbent agglutination assay (ISAGA)	ISAGA plates are coated with an anti-IgM monoclonal antibody to capture serum IgM. After addition of a suspension of formalin-treated *T. gondii,* a positive test result is associated with agglutination of the parasite, whereas a negative reaction results in sedimentation of parasites forming a compact button. Results are expressed as an ISAGA index. There is high sensitivity but low specificity for diagnosing the acute phase of the disease because of long-lasting specific IgM. The technique can be adapted for detection of IgA or IgE by changing the monoclonal antibody.
TECHNIQUES THAT USE SOLUBLE ANTIGENS	
Agglutination	Different agglutination methods can be used. Red blood cells (hemagglutination) or latex particles coated with *Toxoplasma* antigens agglutinate in the presence of specific anti-*Toxoplasma* antibodies. The test detects IgG and IgM (the contribution of IgM can be eliminated by addition of 2- mercaptoethanol). Results are expressed as an index.
Enzyme-linked immunosorbent assays (ELISA)	ELISA is the most widely used technique. Plates are coated with soluble antigens of *T. gondii.* Specific immunoglobulins are revealed by enzyme-labeled anti–human globulins; numerous commercial kits are available. Results depend on the nature of the antigens used, which are usually a mixture of membrane and cytoplasmic antigens. Coating plates with recombinant antigens increases the standardization. This technique can be used to demonstrate IgG, IgM, and IgA. Its scoring depends on the nature of the antigen. Results are expressed in IU/mL.
IgG avidity	IgG avidity is determined by an adaptation of commercial ELISA kits that incorporates a hydrogen bond–disrupting agent (most commonly urea), which dissociates low-affinity antigen/antibody complexes. Results are expressed as an avidity index, that is, the percentage of antibodies that resist elution.
Western blot	Preferentially for diagnosing congenital infection in newborn infants (see "Infection in the Newborn," under Laboratory Diagnosis). *Toxoplasma* antigens are first separated by electrophoresis, according to their molecular weight, before being transferred to a nitrocellulose membrane. Serum is incubated with this membrane, and antibodies are revealed by an enzymatic tracer. The technique has high sensitivity but is not automated; interpretation is sometimes difficult.

IgA, IgE, IgG, and IgM, Immunoglobulins A, E, G, and M, respectively.

A large number of kits are commercially available that are very useful for routine frontline screening tests. However, they vary in characteristics and quality and have certain limitations in terms of performance; it is also sometimes necessary to send the serum samples to a reference laboratory, where more highly specialized tests are available to confirm atypical findings and to help establish the timing of an infection (Table 31-4). Biologists and clinicians should also be aware of another limitation, which is the impossibility of comparing the findings obtained with different kits or performed by different laboratories because of large intertest variations in the principles and mixtures of antigens used, which influence the kinetics and performance.

Detection of Immunoglobulin G. IgG anti-*Toxoplasma* antibodies are detectable 2 to 4 weeks after infection (Fig. 31-23), depending on the tests and the individual responses of patients. Upon reaching a peak after 2 or 3 months, IgG titers stabilize at a plateau phase for several months before declining progressively and can decrease to very low levels with time but persist throughout life. This persistence of IgG provides a reliable means to recognize which pregnant women or women of childbearing age are immune because of a past infection and who are seronegative and therefore susceptible to infection. A positive test for IgG before pregnancy indicates that the fetus is not at risk, with the possible caveat that rare cases of congenital toxoplasmosis have been reported in children born to mothers who were immune before conception; these rare cases involved specific medical conditions in the mother that were likely to weaken her immunity and thereby to foster recrudescent infection or reinfection with a different strain.[79,111,112,656-667] These rare cases do not warrant

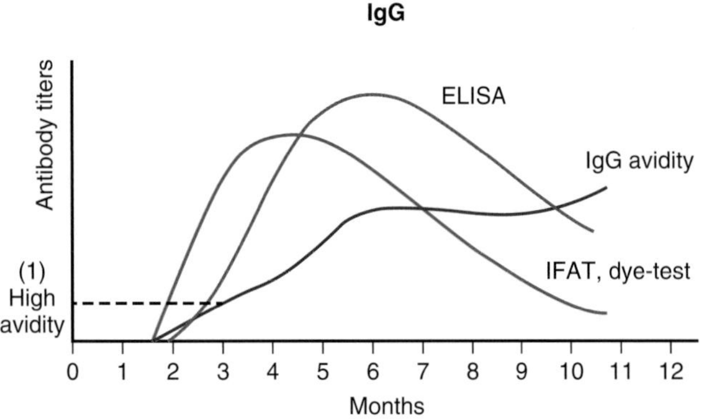

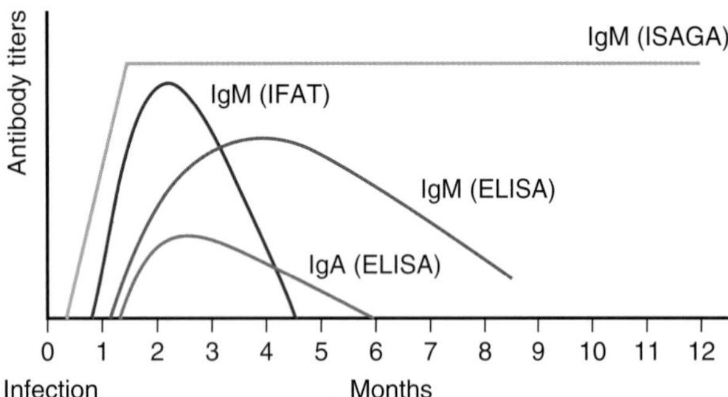

Figure 31-23 Kinetics of antibody response. Trends in kinetics according to different isotypes and techniques are represented here. The use of techniques with different immunoglobulin kinetics allows a retrospective estimate of the date of infection that can, however, be hampered by interindividual variation. (1) Cutoff of the high-avidity IgG index and its interpretation depend on the test used. Here, an avidity index above the cutoff demonstrates a previous infection of greater than 3 months. Because of delayed maturation of avidity, a low-avidity index does not demonstrate an acute infection. *ELISA,* Enzyme-linked immunosorbent assay; *IFAT,* indirect fluorescent antibody test; *IgA, IgG,* and *IgM,* immunoglobulins A, G, and M, respectively; *ISAGA,* immunosorbent agglutination assay.

a change to the general rule that women who have proven immunity before conception do not need to be treated or to be tested for antibodies during pregnancy.

Detection of Immunoglobulin M. Anti-*Toxoplasma* IgM is traditionally tested in parallel to IgG and is useful for two reasons. First, in a susceptible patient, IgM alerts the physician to a possible acute infection before IgG antibodies are detected because IgM antibodies are the first to appear in the context of acute infection (1 or 2 weeks before IgG). They can even be detected within 1 week of infection with hypersensitive immunocapture tests, such as the immunosorbent agglutination assay (ISAGA) or newer commercialized enzyme-linked immunosorbent assay (ELISA) kits (see Fig. 31-23). After increasing for 1 month, IgM antibodies persist for a period that varies between patients. The main advantage of testing for IgM is therefore that its absence when IgG antibodies are detected helps to exclude a recent infection. This is even truer with very sensitive assays such as ISAGA.[668]

The interpretation of a positive test result for IgM antibodies requires great caution for several reasons, mainly because IgM can remain positive for months and even years, especially with hypersensitive techniques. In a large study based on 446 women who acquired *Toxoplasma* infection during pregnancy, the persistence of IgM was longest when tested with ISAGA, which still yielded positive results in 27% of patients 2 years after infection, compared with 9% when using the indirect fluorescent antibody test.[668] Positive IgM should therefore never be used alone as a sign of acute infection. The difficulty of interpreting positive IgM tests in the presence of IgG antibodies is even greater when the IgM tests used only provide qualitative results and cannot distinguish between low-to-moderate levels versus high levels that are more likely to indicate a recent infection. False-positive test results for IgM and the possibility for natural IgM (see "Natural Immunoglobulin M") represent a further challenge for the interpretation of test results.

Measurement of Immunoglobulin G Avidity. Because the level of specific IgG in a single test does not provide a reliable indication of the acuteness of infection, and IgM can still be detected many years after infection, the measurement of IgG avidity is often useful in pregnant women who present with antibodies in their first sample.[669] IgG avidity measures the strength of the antigen-antibody binding, which increases with the time elapsed since infection.

IgG antibodies produced during the first month after primary infection are of low avidity, whereas those produced several months or a year past infection exhibit high avidity. IgG avidity is assessed by using ELISA assays that incorporate a washing step, using a protein denaturing agent (urea classically), that will dissociate the low-avidity antibodies from the antigens but not the high-avidity ones. An avidity index is then computed by using the ratio of the IgG titers obtained with and without the dissociating treatment.

Several commercial assays are available that rely on different principles to denature proteins and compute the IgG avidity results and, as a consequence, often differ in terms of performance. The majority have a very high predictive value for ruling out a recent infection. According to the test, high avidity allows the exclusion of an infection acquired in the last 12 to 20 weeks (see Fig. 31-23). However, it is important to note that the converse is not true. A delay in maturation and a lack of maturation are indeed not uncommon, and low avidity or doubtful results can still be found more than 1 year after an infection.[670-672] A later stage of gestation at the time of infection and anti-*Toxoplasma* treatment may contribute to delayed maturation.[672,673]

From a clinical point of view, a low IgG avidity index offers no significant informative value because it does not rule in nor exclude recent infection. Conversely, a high-avidity index is very useful because it indicates with a high degree of confidence that infection did not occur in the preceding 3 to 4 months. Provided that the test was performed in the first trimester, a high-avidity index will exclude that infection took place during pregnancy. The clinical benefits of using avidity testing in early pregnancy were analyzed in several studies. It was estimated in a U.S. study to have contributed to ruling out infection acquired during or immediately before pregnancy in 56% of patients who exhibited a positive IgM, thus avoiding a large number of unnecessary abortions.[674]

Detection of Specific Immunoglobulin A and Immunoglobulin E. Specific anti-IgA antibodies can be measured using commercial ISAGA or ELISA assays. Their appearance is somewhat delayed compared with IgM, with a peak around the second or third month after infection.[675] They usually disappear earlier than IgM but can also persist for a long time after infection. Their appearance is also inconstant, which further limits their ability to accurately establish the acuteness of infection in a pregnant woman.[675-677] In contrast, the measurement of IgA plays an important role in the diagnosis of congenital infection in newborns (see "Infection in the Newborn")

Specific IgE can also be detected using ISAGA or ELISA assays, which are not commercially available. The presence of specific IgE in a pregnant woman points toward an acute infection because they appear at an early stage (similar to IgA and IgM) but disappear earlier than IgM.[678,679] However, their presence is inconstant,[680,681] and their detection is performed in only a few reference centers.

Immunoblot. Qualitative tests based on immunoblotting, which detect anti–*T. gondii*–specific IgG, are also now available and can be used to confirm serologic test results for low titers of IgG antibodies.[682] They are useful in the context of prenatal screening to determine whether a pregnant woman can be considered to be immune or whether she should be retested.

Exploring Cellular Immunity. It has been shown that specific cellular immunity can be detected in patients infected with *Toxoplasma*, including pregnant women.[683,684] An IFN-γ–based test is available, but not commercialized, and can recognize an IFN-γ response after stimulation of whole blood with a crude toxoplasmic antigen with a high level of accuracy (97% sensitivity and 97% specificity).[685] It can be used to ascertain previous contact with the parasite in women who have doubtful IgG titers or to recognize acute infection in a patient who presents with IgM but not IgG antibodies. It is also useful for the diagnosis of congenital infection (see "Infection in the Newborn")

Interpretation of Serologic Tests Based on the Results for Immunoglobulin M and Immunoglobulin G Antibodies

This section along with Table 31-5 and Figure 31-24 provide guidelines for the interpretation of IgM and IgG tests for *Toxoplasma* antibodies in the pregnant woman. Reflexive testing that should be performed based on these results is also described. The subsequent section describes pitfalls that may confound test interpretation.

Negative Immunoglobulin G and Negative Immunoglobulin M. This profile indicates the absence of previous contact with the parasite and the need to take specific measures to avoid infection during pregnancy. If the pregnant

Table 31-5 Most Frequent Serologic Profiles for *Toxoplasma gondii* in Pregnancy: Interpretations and Actions to Be Taken

	TESTS RESULTS INTERPRETATION	ACTIONS TO BE TAKEN	
		First Test During the First 12 Weeks of Gestation	**First Test After 12 Weeks of Gestation**
1	*Negative IgM and negative IgG:* No infection	Give advice on how to avoid infection. Follow local instructions for prenatal screening.	
2	*Equivocal IgG ("gray zone") and negative IgM:* Suggests past infection Note: If IgM is positive, see situation 4	Perform additional tests to confirm that the patient is immune. If results are not available or are inconclusive, consider that the patient is not immune. Follow local policies regarding prenatal screening.	
3	*Positive IgG and negative IgM:* Past infection	Retest 4 weeks later at the same laboratory. If stable, infection occurred at least 3 months earlier. Stop testing.	Supplementary tests, including avidity, required to estimate whether infection postconception can be excluded. If uncertainty remains, perform fetal ultrasound evaluation, check for the absence of specific IgM and IgA at day 3 after birth and monitor the clearance of IgG over the first year of life.
4	*Positive IgG and positive IgM:* Recent infection or persistent IgM	Measure IgG avidity and/or retest 2 and 4 weeks later at the same laboratory. If IgG avidity is high and IgG titers are stable, infection occurred at least 3 months earlier. Stop testing. A rise in IgG could indicate a recent infection: see situation 6.	Measure IgG avidity and/or retest 2 and 4 weeks later at the same laboratory. If IgG avidity is high and IgG titers are stable, infection occurred at least 3 months earlier. If an infection postconception cannot be excluded because of a late first sample, benefit and risk of amniocentesis should be discussed with an expert. Check for the absence of specific IgM and IgA at day 3 after birth and monitor the clearance of IgG over the first year of life. A rise in IgG could indicate a recent infection: see situation 6.
5	*Negative IgG and positive IgM:* Early seroconversion, or natural or false-positive IgM	Confirm with another test. Retest for IgG and IgM at 7- to 10-day intervals at the same laboratory for 2 months to monitor the appearance of IgG, which would confirm seroconversion; if not, conclude that the IgM is nonspecific. Note: IgG avidity is not helpful in this context.	
6	*Change from negative to positive IgG or rise in IgG with high IgM:* Seroconversion	Refer the patient to a reference center to estimate the stage of gestation at the time of maternal infection and to decide on treatment and evaluation.	

IgA, IgG, and IgM, Immunoglobulins A, G, and M, respectively.

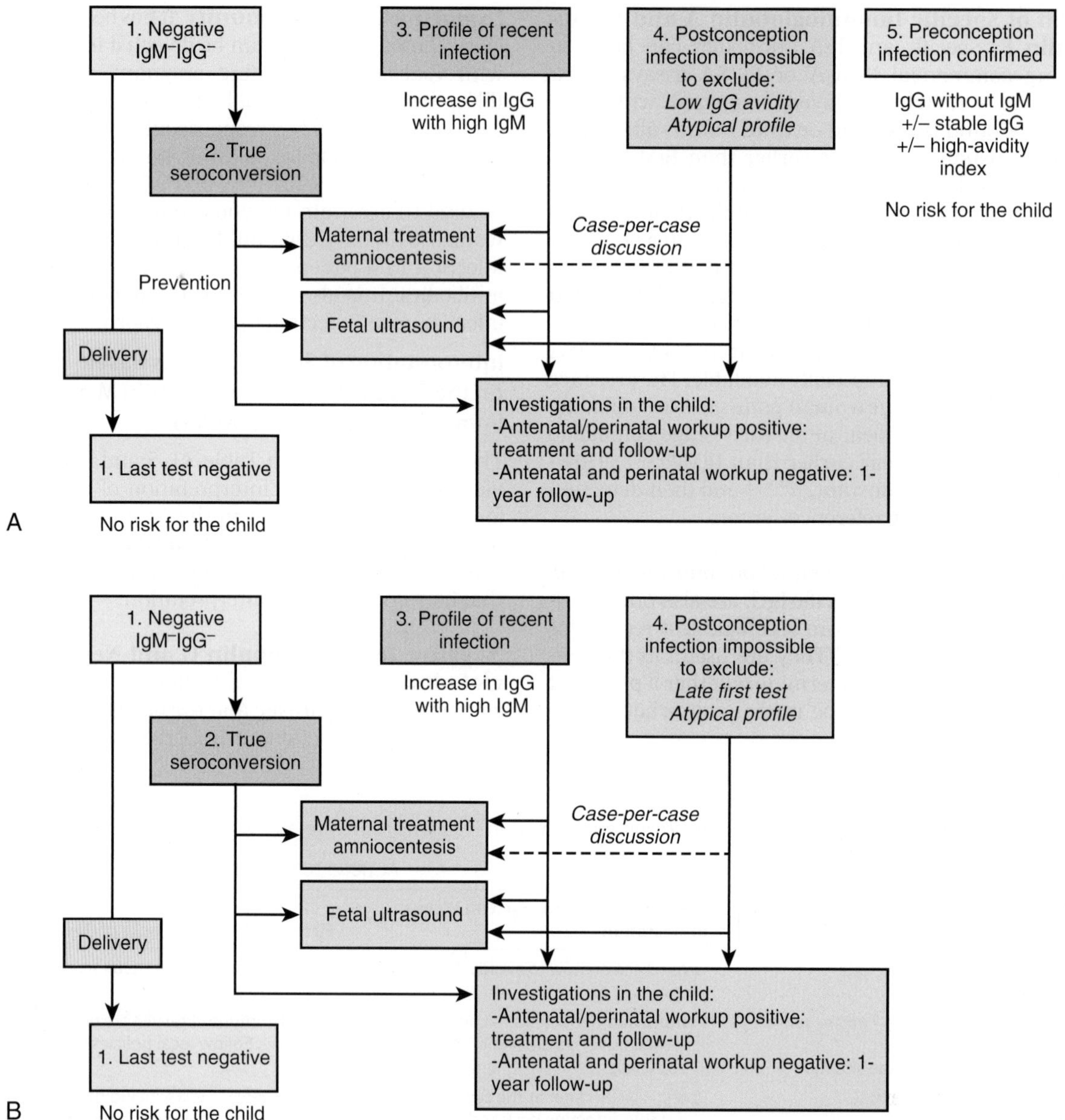

Figure 31-24 Actions to be taken according to serologic findings in pregnancy. **A,** First prenatal test before 12 weeks of pregnancy: the different possible situations. **B,** First prenatal test after 12 weeks of pregnancy: the different possible situations. *IgG* and *IgM*, immunoglobulins G and M, respectively.

patient takes part in follow-up testing program, the subsequent tests should be scheduled according to local recommendations. The last test to check for the absence of late infection should be performed on maternal blood rather than cord blood at delivery. This avoids missing late infections that would only be recognized by the detection of IgM antibodies in maternal blood because a test on cord blood would still be negative at that time.[686] If the test is performed in the context of very recent clinical signs or shortly after a potential risk of exposure, an additional test performed 7 to 10 days later may be useful to definitively exclude a recent infection.

Positive Immunoglobulin G and Negative Immunoglobulin M. The detection of IgG without IgM indicates that the patient is immune as a consequence of an infection acquired at least 3 to 4 months previously (or up to 6 months earlier if hypersensitive immunocapture tests are used). If the patient is less than 12 weeks pregnant, no supplementary tests are needed after the initial test. Some centers recommend testing a second sample taken 4 weeks later, using the same kit as an additional guarantee that IgG titers have remained stable and that infection is not recent. The patient can then be reassured with regard to the absence of risk and should be given a copy of her results to keep so that she may present this as evidence of prior infection should caregivers in the future be concerned about the possibility of recent infection.

If the pregnancy is more advanced and no earlier samples are available, supplementary tests based on different kinetics and principles should be performed. These will establish whether the time elapsed since infection is sufficient to exclude infection postconception or at least narrow down the "uncertainty window"—during which infection is impossible to exclude—to the beginning of pregnancy. If uncertainty remains about infection postconception, a recommendation should be given as a precautionary measure to check for the absence of specific IgM and IgA antibodies in the child at birth and even to monitor the clearance of maternal antibodies during his/her first year of life.

Equivocal Immunoglobulin G and Negative Immunoglobulin M. Equivocal IgG, in the "gray" zone, as defined by the manufacturer of the test, without IgM favors a past infection. Ideally, additional tests based on other principles should be performed to confirm that the patient is immune and that her unborn child is not at risk. Hypersensitive tests for IgG and immunoblotting are useful under these circumstances. If uncertainty remains, the patient should preferably be considered as not being immune. The situation should be explained to the patient to avoid confusion if subsequent tests are performed with kits that have different cutoffs. It is also important not to label the results as "negative" on the laboratory report or in the patient's file but to mention the details of the low titers and the decision to consider them as nonprotective.

Negative Immunoglobulin G and Positive Immunoglobulin M. Isolated IgM without IgG can be an early marker of an acute infection, but, on a first serum specimen, false-positive IgM results or natural IgM cannot be excluded (see "Possible Pitfalls"). Confirmation of the presence of IgM through a second test is therefore recommended. Repeated tests at 7- to 10-day intervals will confirm an acute infection when IgG antibodies are detected or rule it out when IgG antibodies are not detected over a 2-month interval.

When IgM antibodies are confirmed, treatment should be offered without delay to increase the possibility of preventing fetal infection if acute maternal infection is indeed present. Starting treatment within 21 days of infection has been found in several studies[4,88,491,687] to be associated with a lower risk of maternal-fetal transmission. Treatment can eventually be stopped if subsequent tests are not confirmatory. Those who perform the follow-up serology tests must be informed of this treatment because it might delay or attenuate the IgG response.[688]

A search for clinical signs in the patient and her relatives or for significant risk factors could increase the pretest likelihood of an acute infection and be informative regarding the date of its occurrence. Conversely, knowledge of earlier IgM antibody detection during the current or previous pregnancies would make the possibility of natural IgM antibodies, which are not indicative of acute infection (see "Natural Immunoglobulin M"), more likely.

Positive Immunoglobulin G and Positive Immunoglobulin M. The detection of IgG and IgM antibodies in the first prenatal test requires differentiating between two options: a long-standing latent infection with long-lasting IgM, which is the most frequent situation in any given laboratory, or a recent primary infection, which is uncommon. Discounting the possibility of persistent IgM antibodies can cause much undue anxiety and lead to many unjustified abortions.[689]

The levels of IgM antibodies tend to favor a chronic infection when they are low and point toward a possible recent infection when they are higher. However, additional tests are required to estimate the acuteness of infection more accurately. High IgG avidity and stable IgG titers over a 4-week interval confirm that the infection is not acute and took place at least 3 to 4 months earlier. Further actions will depend on the trimester of pregnancy at the time of sampling and on whether the estimated time elapsed since infection is or is not sufficient to exclude infection postconception. No additional tests are required if the first test was performed during the first trimester. When initial maternal testing was later than 12 weeks of gestation, a limited evaluation is recommended, which should include fetal ultrasonography, tests for IgM and IgA antibodies at birth, and serologic follow-up until the first birthday. Significant increases in IgG indicate an acute infection. Estimating the stage of gestation at the time of infection is important toward making informed decisions on treatment, amniocentesis, and ultrasound surveillance.

Diagnostic Criteria for a Recent Infection

No assay exists that can determine precisely when the initial *Toxoplasma* infection occurred. The best indicator of a recent infection is true seroconversion, with a change from a negative to a positive result for IgG. Recognizing seroconversion in a patient who is known to have had a negative IgG test at the beginning of pregnancy is usually not a problem. The appearance of IgM antibodies acts as an alert for probable acute infection, but the diagnosis can only be confirmed by the appearance of IgG antibodies. In such cases, no subsequent test, such as the measurement of avidity, is needed. The second best indicator is a significant increase in IgG in a patient who presents with high IgM titers. As previously stated, the detection of IgM alone or low avidity alone are not sufficient to conclude a recent infection.

Possible Pitfalls

Natural Immunoglobulin M. As mentioned earlier, pregnant women can present with IgM antibodies that are not followed by the appearance of specific IgG, even with very sensitive tests such as the Sabin-Feldman test, that do not reflect an acute infection. The mechanism that underlies their production is not well known but could involve nonspecific reactions to glycolipids.[690] They are more frequently detected after 20 weeks of pregnancy and up to delivery but can also occur earlier and persist for only a couple of months. They have been detected at similar stages of gestation in successive pregnancies (M. Wallon, personal communication). Confirmation that the IgM antibodies are natural can be provided by follow-up tests showing no appearance of IgG, even when using highly sensitive tests. A 2-month observation period is recommended, especially when anti-*Toxoplasma* therapy has been prescribed that might delay the IgG response. Because natural IgA antibodies do not exist, positive IgA antibody test results favor the diagnosis of incident infection.[678] A positive cellular immunity test also favors an early infection. Natural IgG antibodies are less frequent and more difficult to identify. Comparing the kinetics between tests and exploring cellular immunity helps in their recognition.

Intravenous Injection of Immunoglobulins. Intravenous injection of immunoglobulins during pregnancy, to prevent fetal alloimmunization or for any other indication, can complicate the interpretation of serologic tests for toxoplasmosis.[691] Because they are obtained from a large number of donors, these blood products contain anti-*Toxoplasma* IgG and can lead to the erroneous conclusion that a patient is immune if no results from previous tests during pregnancy are available. In the context of screening, one risk would be to mistake this sudden appearance of IgG as a sign of acute infection. However, an atypical serologic profile, presenting low and stable IgG titers, the absence of IgM and high-avidity titers, and a progressive and rapid clearance of IgG would draw the attention to their exogenous origin. Passively transmitted IgG antibodies do not protect against *T. gondii*, and patients should be advised to continue taking all necessary precautions.

Atypical Seroconversion with Transient or No Immunoglobulin M. Some patients exhibit very atypical seroconversion profiles in the course of their pregnancy, such as a switch from a negative IgG test to IgG titers that remain low. Seroconversions with only transient or barely detectable IgM have also been described.[692] These atypical profiles need to be confirmed by a reference laboratory. When a clear distinction between natural or false-positive IgG or seroconversion cannot be established, it is safer to consider these situations as atypical seroconversions and to ensure that the child has no clinical and biologic signs of infection at birth and during the first year of life.

Importance of Estimating the Stage of Gestation at the Time of Maternal Infection

The risk of giving birth to an infected child and that of the child having lesions vary greatly with the stage of gestation at the time of maternal infection. Based on a French cohort study, the risk that the parasite will cross the placenta rises steadily with each week, from less than 5% to 70% during the last weeks of pregnancy.[80] Congenital infection of the fetus in women infected just before conception is extremely rare. The clinical consequences of congenital infection vary inversely: The risk of severe malformations decreases with each additional week of pregnancy. Estimates based on the European study group are summarized in Figures 31-25 and 31-26A and B. The probability that an infected child will have some clinical signs at the age of 3 years was found to be approximately 50% when maternal infection was acquired during the first 4 months of pregnancy and to decrease to less than 10% when this occurred during the last month. The risk of giving birth to a child who had a congenital infection with clinical signs at the age of 3 years was highest for maternal infections that occurred between 20 and 27 weeks of gestation (Table 31-6).

The ability to estimate when infection occurred, as precisely as possible, is important in order to answer parents' questions and to make decisions on treatment and surveillance. The trimester of pregnancy also influences the performance of tests to detect fetal infection. This has been shown for PCR assay of amniotic fluid, the sensitivity of which was maximal for infections during the second trimester,[693] and for tests for IgM and IgA antibodies at birth.[694]

Referral to an Expert Laboratory. The serologic diagnosis of toxoplasmosis during pregnancy presents several

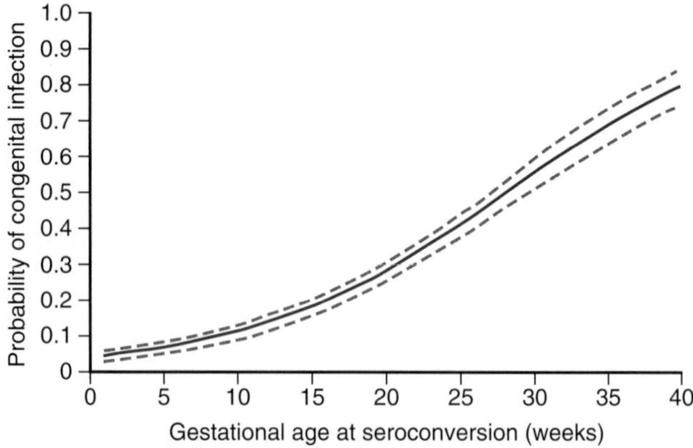

Figure 31-25 Risk of mother-to-child transmission of *Toxoplasma gondii* by gestational age at maternal seroconversion (n = 1721). *Dotted lines* are bounds of 95% confidence interval. (Modified from SYROCOT (Systematic Review on Congenital Toxoplasmosis) Study Group; Thiébaut R, Leproust S, Chêne G, Gilbert R: Effectiveness of prenatal treatment for congenital toxoplasmosis: a meta-analysis of individual patients' data, *Lancet* 369:115-122, 2007; with permission.)

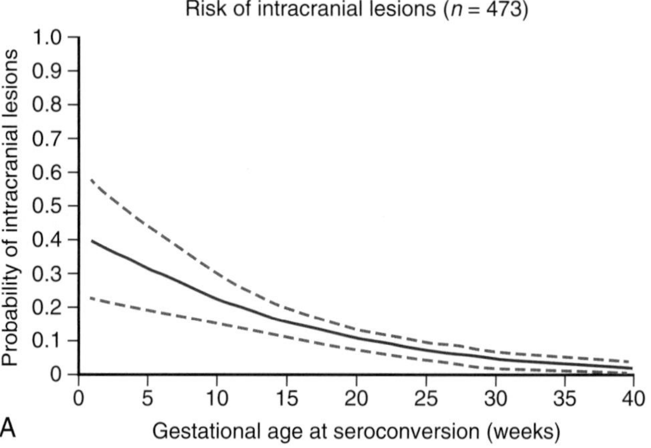

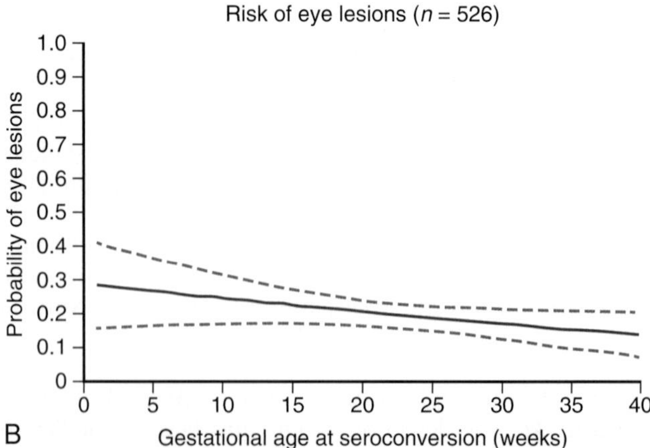

Figure 31-26 A, Risk of clinical manifestation in children infected by *Toxoplasma gondii* gestational age at maternal seroconversion: intracranial lesions. *Dotted lines* are bounds of 95% confidence interval. **B,** Risk of clinical manifestation in children infected *by T. gondii* gestational age at maternal seroconversion: risk of eye lesions. *Dotted lines* are bounds of 95% confidence interval. (Modified from SYROCOT (Systematic Review on Congenital Toxoplasmosis) Study Group; Thiébaut R, Leproust S, Chêne G, Gilbert R: Effectiveness of prenatal treatment for congenital toxoplasmosis: a meta-analysis of individual patients' data, *Lancet* 369:115-122, 2007; with permission.)

Table 31-6 Lyon Cohort (Antenatal and Postnatal Treatment): Risk Estimate by Gestational Age at the Time of Maternal Infection for the Risk of Congenital Infection*

				RISK OF CLINICAL SIGNS† AT 3 YEARS OF AGE (PER 100 CHILDREN)					
	CHILDREN (388 CONGENITAL INFECTION/1624)			ALL LIVE-BORN CHILDREN (*n* = 1150)			INFECTED LIVE-BORN CHILDREN (*n* = 207)		
Weeks of Gestation	**%**	**(95% CI)**	**No.‡**	**%**	**(95% CI)**	**No.‡**	**%**	**(95% CI)**	**No.‡**
0	6.4	(1.7-21.8)	26	0	(.0-§)	143	48.2	(2.8-96.8)	1
1	3.7	(1.7-8.2)	25						
2	2.8	(1.4-5.6)	78						
3	2.6	(1.3-5.2)	61						
4	2.8	(1.4-5.5)	63	1.3	(.3-4.9)	161	57.0	(22.5-85.8)	2
5	3.4	(1.9-6.0)	55						
6	4.3	(2.7-6.8)	53						
7	5.5	(3.6-8.2)	50						
8	6.6	(4.5-9.8)	57	3.0	(1.2-6.9)	147	59.5	(33.0-81.5)	7
9	7.7	(5.2-11.3)	48						
10	8.7	(6.0-12.4)	57						
11	9.5	(6.8-13.1)	49						
12	10.2	(7.6-13.7)	62	3.7	(2.0-6.5)	141	56.1	(36.8-73.6)	11
13	10.9	(8.3-14.2)	41						
14	11.7	(9.0-15.0)	41						
15	12.6	(9.7-16.1)	41						
16	13.7	(10.5-17.8)	52	5.0	(2.9-8.6)	130	46.3	(29.6-63.8)	13
17	15.4	(11.8-19.7)	48						
18	17.4	(13.6-22.1)	52						
19	20.0	(16.0-24.8)	37						
20	23.1	(19.0-27.9)	44	7.0	(4.4-10.9)	98	31.1	(19.2-46.2)	26
21	26.7	(22.3-31.5)	32						
22	30.6	(26.0-35.6)	31						
23	34.7	(29.6-40.2)	31						
24	38.9	(33.3-44.9)	47	7.8	(4.7-12.7)	117	17.3	(8.8-31.3)	41
25	42.9	(69.9-49.2)	34						
26	46.6	(40.4-52.8)	40						
27	49.7	(43.8-55.6)	44						
28	52.3	(46.7-57.8)	35	6.2	(3.6-10.5)	97	14.3	(6.9-27.2)	48
29	54.4	(48.9-59.9)	34						
30	56.2	(50.3-61.9)	49						
31	57.7	(51.3-63.9)	33						
32	59.1	(52.1-65.7)	26	4.8	(2.2-10.1)	82	10.8	(4.1-25.5)	37
33	60.3	(53.0-67.1)	35						
34	61.5	(54.2-68.3)	34						
35	62.8	(55.2-69.8)	28						
36	64.2	(55.2-72.3)	18	6.0	(1.6-20.30)	34	9.5	(2.4-31.1)	21
37	65.8	(53.2-76.5)	24						
38	67.6	(49.0-82.0)	6						
39	69.8	(42.6-87.7)	3						

From Wallon M, Peyron F, Cornu C, et al: Congenital *Toxoplasma* infection: monthly prenatal screening decreases transmission rate and improves clinical outcome at age 3 years, *Clin Infect Dis* 56:1223-1231, 2013; with permission.

CI, Confidence interval.

*Based on 1624 maternal infections diagnosed since mid-1992 and on clinical signs at 3 years of age, based on 1150 maternal infections diagnosed after 1995.

†Systematic, neurologic, and ophthalmic signs.

‡Number of patients per week or per 4-week interval.

§No upper limit.

characteristics that often complicate the interpretation of test results. These include persistent, natural or false-positive IgM titers, long-lasting low-avidity IgG, uneven performance of frontline tests, and the need to estimate precisely the stage of gestation at the time of maternal infection to enable appropriate counseling. It is therefore often necessary to refer samples for additional testing to an expert laboratory that will be able to confirm findings and estimate the risks for the unborn child. Relevant information on the due date, the dates of potential exposure to risk factors, clinical history, previous test results, and dates of treatment should also be provided. These centers will also help to make decisions on amniocentesis, prenatal and postnatal treatment, and surveillance.

INFECTION IN THE UNBORN CHILD

Risk and Severity

Fetal infection results from hematogenous transmission of the parasite across the placenta. In almost all cases, it is secondary to primary infection of the mother during pregnancy. Rare cases of congenital toxoplasmosis have been described after maternal primary infection in immunocompetent women during the 3 months immediately preceding conception. In most of these cases, the maternal primary infection was symptomatic, with posterior cervical nodes.[695-697] Current evidence suggests that when primary infection predates conception by greater than 6 months, and perhaps by greater than 3 months, there is little or no risk to the fetus.[697] However, some exceptional cases of acquired congenital toxoplasmosis in immunocompetent women with preexisting immunity to *Toxoplasma* have also been reported.[698,699] The mechanisms for such cases remain speculative (reinfection with a particularly virulent strain?). Finally, vertical transmission after reactivation of infection has also been described in severely immunocompromised women infected with HIV,[700] although the risk of such infections is low.[701]

After maternal primary infection during pregnancy, the overall risk of transmission is about 30%. However, this risk increases considerably with the term at which maternal infection is acquired: from 15% at 13 weeks to 44% at 26 weeks and 71% at 36 weeks (see Fig. 31-25).[702] Conversely, when the child is infected, the risk of clinical symptoms at birth or during the first 3 years of life decreases with increasing gestational age at the time of maternal primary infection (57% between 4 and 7 weeks, 31% between 20 and 23 weeks, and 9.5% after 36 weeks) (see Table 31-6).[703] This effect of gestational age on the symptomatic/asymptomatic nature of the congenital infection has been consistently demonstrated over several decades.[704-706] However, the two most common clinical manifestations of congenital toxoplasmosis—neurologic and ophthalmologic problems—were always considered together until the middle of the 2000s. Their analysis as separate entities led to the demonstration that the incidence of neurologic problems was, effectively, inversely correlated with the term at which maternal infection occurred, whereas the risk of ophthalmologic problems was not greatly affected by gestational age at the time of maternal infection (see Fig. 31-26A and B).[702,707,708] For 1.4%[709] and 2.5%[703,710] of infected fetuses, the pregnancy ends in miscarriage or fetal death in utero, respectively. These events follow infections acquired during the first 3 months of pregnancy or at the start of the second trimester.

Fetal brain damage takes the form of focal necrotic lesions, mostly in the periventricular and/or cortical parenchyma of the brain (see Fig. 31-18). These lesions are often few in number—between 1 and about 12 lesions—and may display secondary calcification. Obstruction of the cerebral aqueduct rapidly leads to hydrocephalus (within 1-2 weeks),[703,710] which has been reported in 1.3% to 1.8% of published series.[703,709]

Most of the fetal ocular damage takes the form of chorioretinitis (see "Infection in the Newborn") that cannot currently be diagnosed prenatally. Nevertheless, the presence of other clinical signs of congenital toxoplasmosis is associated with a 2.6- to 4.3-times higher risk of chorioretinitis, depending on the study.[707,708] The incidence of ophthalmologic lesions at birth is about 3% in European children[708,711] and close to 50% in Brazil. The apparent virulence of *T. gondii* strains is much higher in South America than in Europe, but some of this difference is due to differences in the method of diagnosis (prenatal screening vs. neonatal diagnosis on the basis of clinical signs) and the type of treatment prescribed (prenatal and postnatal vs. postnatal only). Signs of disseminated disease in the fetus (hepatomegaly, splenomegaly, ascites, pericardial, or pleural effusion) may also be observed, together with thickening of the placenta.

Based on these signs, infected fetuses are classically categorized as having asymptomatic, benign, or severe forms. The definitions of benign and severe congenital toxoplasmosis differ between authors. All agree that the severe forms should include hydrocephalus and that the presence of fewer than three cerebral calcifications[457] and/or peripheral chorioretinitis is associated with benign forms. By contrast, macular chorioretinitis and multiple calcifications are sometimes classified as benign, sometimes as severe, and even sometimes not classified.

Antenatal Diagnosis

The prenatal diagnosis of fetal infection is based on ultrasound scans and PCR testing of amniotic fluid. In countries in which prenatal screening to detect maternal seroconversion for toxoplasmosis is not performed, the diagnosis may be suggested by detection of signs compatible with fetal infection on routine ultrasound examination. In such cases, further evaluations using serologic testing and, when indicated, amniotic fluid assessment should be carried out to determine if the abnormalities are related to *Toxoplasma* infection.

Ultrasound Evaluation. In cases in which maternal seroconversion occurs during the pregnancy, ultrasound scans should be carried out monthly or every 2 weeks. The most characteristic ultrasound signs concern the brain: hyperechogenic lesions several millimeters in diameter in the parenchyma or in a periventricular position (Fig. 31-27). These lesions may be associated with ventricular dilatation, which is generally symmetrical, and rapid progression, which is associated with a poor long-term prognosis (Fig. 31-28).[710] In addition to these images, Malinger and colleagues,[712] in 2011, described cysts similar to those observed in congenital cytomegalovirus infections. Despite being a classic symptom of toxoplasmosis, microcephaly is not observed in utero (head circumference is normal or larger than normal, in cases of hydrocephalus).[713] Other ultrasound signs are less specific

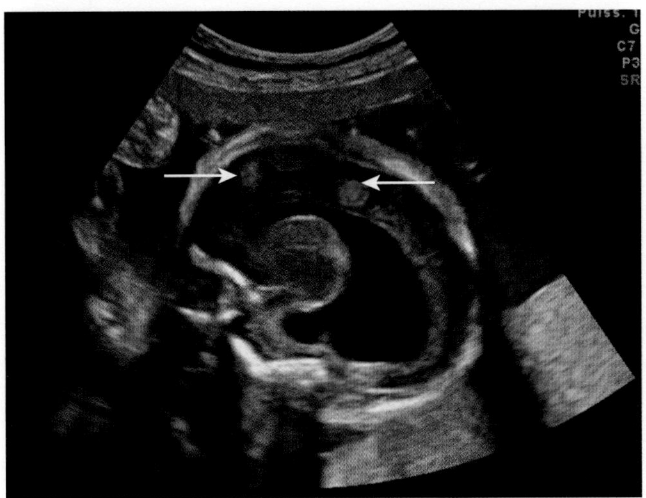

Figure 31-27 Fetal rounded hyperechogenic brain lesions *(arrows)* and ventricular dilatation on prenatal ultrasound scan (sagittal section). (Courtesy R. Levy, Paris.)

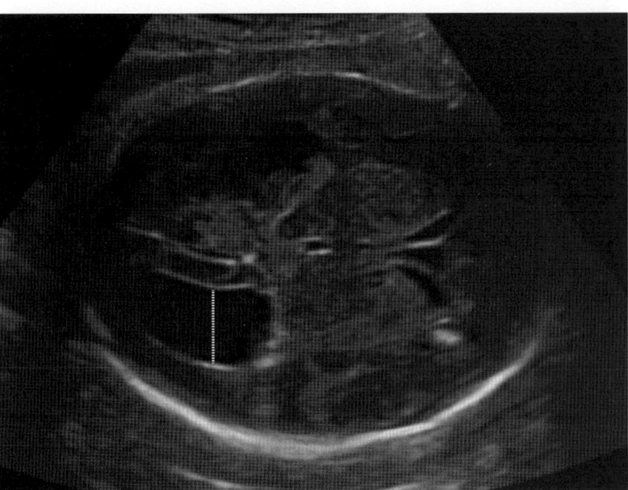

Figure 31-28 Prenatal ultrasound scan calcification and ventricular dilatation *(dotted line)*. (Courtesy F. Jacquemard, Paris.)

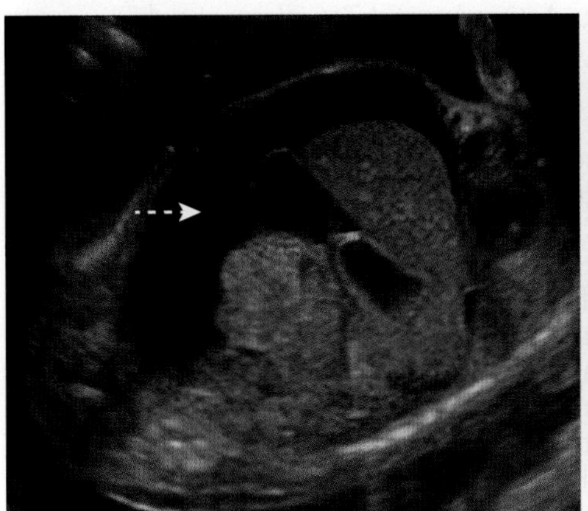

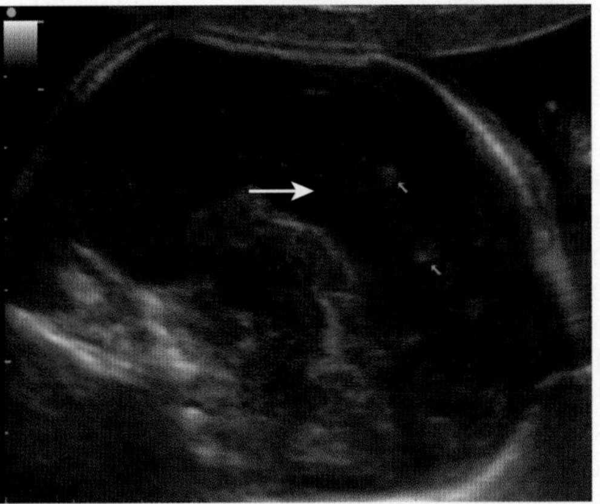

Figure 31-29 Maternal seroconversion between 19 and 23 weeks of gestation; at 23 weeks of gestation, ultrasound normal, spiramycin started; at 26 weeks of gestation, fetal ascites *(dotted arrow)* associated with enlarged ventricles *(arrow)* and intracerebral densities *(small green arrows)*. (Courtesy L. Mandelbrot, Paris.)

and may be observed in most infectious diseases of the fetus: hyperechogenic intestine, hepatomegaly, ascites (Fig. 31-29), pleural effusion, or increase in the size of the placenta.[710]

Fetal magnetic resonance imaging (MRI) shows the same cerebral lesions: focal necrosis and ventricular dilatation[714] (Fig. 31-30). The correlation observed with ultrasound scans obtained with high-frequency probes is excellent, rendering MRI less relevant,[712] although MRI may provide additional information, in some cases, concerning the occurrence of partial cerebellar hypoplasia, for example.[715] Confirmed first trimester fetal infections can now be considered an indication for antenatal MRI.

Amniocentesis and Direct Detection of the Parasite. Prenatal biologic diagnosis should be offered to pregnant women who seroconvert for toxoplasmosis during pregnancy or whose fetuses display ultrasound signs suggestive of fetal disease caused by *T. gondii*. The reference technique is PCR testing of amniotic fluid. This technique was developed in the 1990s and initially made use of conventional PCR amplification of the *B1* gene of the parasite, which is used as a target. The specificity of this technique was 100%, but its overall sensitivity was only 65%.[716] From 2000 onward, quantitative real-time PCR techniques were developed, allowing a prognostic marker to be included in the testing procedure: Maternal infections acquired before 20 weeks of gestation with a parasite load in amniotic fluid of more than 100 parasites/mL are associated with a very high risk (odds ratio [OR], 15.4; 95% CI, 2.45 to 98) of severe fetal infection (fetal death, anasarca, hydrocephalus).[717] The target gene was changed to a 529-bp DNA fragment present at much higher copy number in the genome of the parasite (200-300 copies) than the *B1* gene (35 copies).[718] The new technique had a better sensitivity at 92% (95% CI, 81 to 95), while retaining a specificity and a positive predictive value of 100%.[719]

It is recommended to carry out amniocentesis after 18 weeks of gestation and at least 4 weeks after the estimated date of maternal infection, to minimize the risk of a false-negative result because of the late passage of the parasite across the placenta into the fetus.[720] The performance of PCR tests with amniotic fluid is impressive but must be balanced against the risk of inducing a miscarriage by amniocentesis, which is estimated to be 0.3% to 0.6%. This point is of particular importance in cases of maternal periconceptional seroconversion, for which the rate of parasite transmission is less than 2%. The benefit-to-risk ratio of amniocentesis must be clearly explained to all future parents. The psychological issues, with considerable parental anxiety linked to the announcement of the diagnosis and/or to the amniocentesis procedure itself, have also been highlighted.[721] These negative psychological

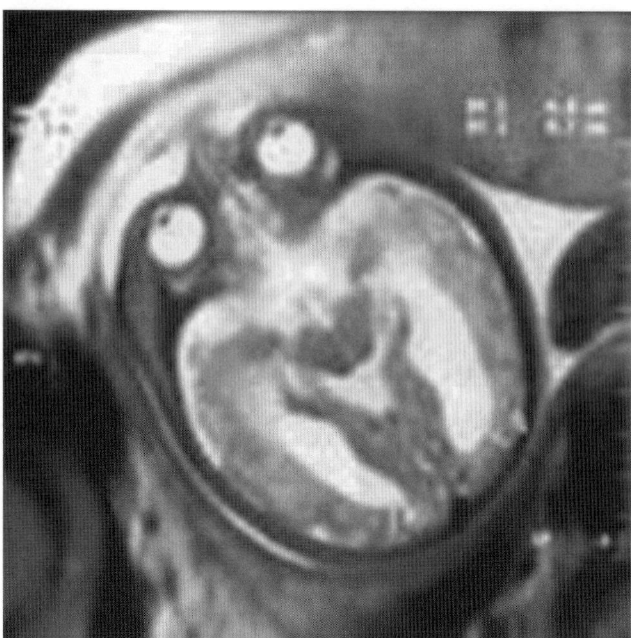

Figure 31-30 Magnetic resonance image of fetal brain: bilateral ventricular dilatation.

effects have to be balanced with the expected benefits: In first trimester infection, a negative result is associated with a 99% probability that the child is not infected.[722]

Inoculation of mice has also been used to detect parasites. The amniotic fluid is injected intraperitoneally into nonimmune mice, which are killed 3 to 6 weeks later and examined for brain cysts. The specificity of this approach is 100%, and its sensitivity is between 42% and 64%.[720,723] The better performance of PCR testing, contrasting with the poor sensitivity and the longer time required to obtain results by inoculating mice, has led to this technique being gradually abandoned.

Fetal Blood Sampling. Fetal blood sampling for the detection of nonspecific biologic signs (hypereosinophilia, high total IgM levels, thrombocytopenia) or specific biologic signs (IgM or IgA against *Toxoplasma*, inoculation of mice with fetal blood) is not very sensitive[720] and is accompanied by a high risk of fetal loss (2%-6%). It is no longer used for the routine diagnosis of congenital toxoplasmosis.

Treatment and Prevention of Infections in the Mother and the Unborn Child

TREATMENT IN THE MOTHER AND UNBORN CHILD

Indications

Acute maternal infection is usually benign and does not require any treatment per se. The infection is self-limited, and symptoms disappear within a few weeks or months. Drug treatment has been recommended for the lymphadenopathy or to reduce the duration of fatigue, but data demonstrating benefit is limited.[724,725] However, treatment is recommended in pregnant women to reduce the risks and severity of fetal infection. It should also be considered when infection occurred during the 3 months before pregnancy, especially when clinical signs were reported during this period, and in cases where periconception or postconception infection is suspected or cannot be excluded. Treatment of maternal infection is a key issue in countries where monthly or trimonthly retesting is performed during pregnancy but is also important in cases where infection was diagnosed as the consequence of individual testing or of clinical signs.

Early treatment of fetal infection is expected to reduce the short- and long-term severity of congenital infection. This is the rationale for identifying maternal infection through organized or individual retesting programs.

Drugs Available

Drug regimens used routinely for treatment of the mother rely primarily on spiramycin and a pyrimethamine/sulfonamide combination. Other drugs, such as azithromycin, atovaquone, clindamycin, and clarithromicin, are potential candidates but have not been validated for use in this context (see "Drugs Active Against *Toxoplasma gondii*").

Strategies for First-Line Treatment of Maternal Infections

There have been no randomized controlled trials of treatment for *Toxoplasma* infection during pregnancy.[491] In the absence of such data and in the face of other evidence suggesting the benefit of treatment, the strategies for using these drugs differ widely by country.

In France, in the framework of the monthly prenatal serologic testing program, the prevention of fetal infection relies mainly on treatment with spiramycin, which is started as soon as maternal infection is suspected in an attempt to prevent transplacental transmission. If maternal infection is confirmed or cannot be excluded, it is prescribed until delivery (Table 31-7), unless an analysis of amniotic fluid confirms the presence of fetal infection (see "Amniocentesis"). In such cases, treatment with spiramycin is stopped and is switched to the combination of pyrimethamine and sulfadiazine. An alternative regimen that is widely used in France, but not in the United States, is Fansidar, which is a fixed-dose combination of pyrimethamine plus sulfadoxine (see "Drugs Active Against *Toxoplasma gondii*"). Either regimen is given continuously until delivery. In our view, indications for presumptive treatment with pyrimethamine/sulfonamides in the absence of confirmed fetal infection are limited to situations in which the risk is estimated to be high because maternal infection occurred in the last 2 months of pregnancy and when amniocentesis cannot be performed. Two advantages of basing the decision to administer pyrimethamine/sulfonamides on the amniotic fluid analysis are (1) to avoid subjecting many uninfected fetuses to drugs that have potential hematologic toxicity and (2) to encourage the prenatal identification of infected children, which greatly simplifies the decisions to be made at birth regarding treatment and follow-up evaluation.

A similar approach to management and treatment of the pregnant woman is recommended by expert groups in the United States. The drug regimens recommended in pregnancy by the *Toxoplasma* Serology Laboratory at the Palo Alto Medical Foundation for the prevention and the treatment of congenital toxoplasmosis are summarized in Table 31-8.

Table 31-7 Antenatal Treatment: Guidelines of the Study Group on Congenital Toxoplasmosis: Croix Rousse Hospital (Lyon, France), Timone Hospital (Marseille, France), Trousseau Hospital (Paris, France)

These guidelines apply to maternal infections that were confirmed by a reference laboratory that could estimate the gestational age at maternal infection. Management varies according to the gestational age at the time of the infection.

1. Maternal infection before 33 weeks

- Spiramycin should be started immediately (or as soon as it can be obtained in the United States and other countries where it is not widely available; see Table 31-8): 3 g (9 million IU)/day in three divided daily doses.
- Amniocentesis should be done on or after the 18th week and at least 4 weeks after the date of the estimated maternal infection. Send 20 mL of amniotic fluid to the laboratory for PCR assay.
- Monthly fetal ultrasound follow-up.

According to the results of the amniocentesis and ultrasound examinations:

A. No ultrasound abnormalities and negative PCR on amniotic fluid: Spiramycin and monthly ultrasound monitoring should be continued until delivery.

B. No or minor ultrasound abnormalities and positive PCR on amniotic fluid: Stop spiramycin and treat continuously until delivery, according to one of the two following regimens:

Pyrimethamine	50 mg/day
Sulfadiazine	1.5 g twice daily
Folinic acid	25 mg twice weekly
Or	
Pyrimethamine 50 mg and sulfadoxine 1 g (Fansidar)*	Every 10 days
Folinic acid	50 mg every week

Warning: Rare but severe cutaneous side effects such as Lyell syndrome or DRESS syndrome are possible with both treatments.

Monitoring: Check blood cell counts before the first dose and every 15 days thereafter. Pyrimethamine and sulfonamide should be withheld and folinic acid continued when neutropenia <1500/mm^3 occurs; check blood cell counts 15 days later, and resume treatment if absolute neutrophil count returns to >1500/mm^3.

Patients treated with pyrimethamine and sulfadiazine should be advised to take abundant fluids regularly.

Continue ultrasound monitoring every 2 to 4 weeks.

C. Severe cerebral involvement: It is our practice to discuss prognostic implications of this finding with the parent(s), so that they may make an informed decision regarding treatment or pregnancy termination. If the pregnancy is continued, treat according to one of the two previous regimens.

2. Maternal infection beyond 33 weeks

- Until delivery, give one of the above-mentioned treatments.
- Monitoring as described above.
- Discuss amniocentesis (a PCR-positive result on amniotic fluid will inform appropriate treatment for the newborn immediately after birth, without waiting for postnatal serologic findings).
- Schedule follow-up ultrasound monitoring

DRESS, Drug reaction with eosinophilia and systemic symptoms; *PCR*, polymerase chain reaction.
*In the United States, Fansidar is not used; see Table 31-8 for regimens recommended for use by U.S. authorities.

Table 31-8 Guidelines for Treatment of *Toxoplasma gondii* Infection in the Pregnant Woman and Congenital *Toxoplasma* Infection in the Fetus in the United States*

Medication	Dosage	Indication for Therapy	Duration of Therapy
Spiramycin†	1 g every 8 hr without food	Primary maternal *Toxoplasma* infection without evidence of fetal infection	Until term or until fetal infection is documented
Pyrimethamine‡ *plus*	Loading dose: 50 mg every 12 hr for 2 days; then beginning on day 3, 50 mg/day	When fetal infection is documented (after 12 or 18 weeks of gestation)	Until term§
Sulfadiazine *plus*	Loading dose: 75 mg/kg; then 50 mg/kg every 12 hr (maximum, 4 g/day)		Until term§
Leucovorin (folinic acid) †	10 20 mg daily		During and for 1 wk after pyrimethamine therapy

*Regimen recommended in pregnancy by the Palo Alto Medical Foundation *Toxoplasma* Serology Laboratory [PAMF-TSL]; phone: 650-853-4828; http://www.pamf.org/serology/; email: toxolab@pamf.org.

†Available only on request from the U.S. Food and Drug Administration (phone: 301-796-1600; fax: 301-796-9881) and after consultation with PAMF-TSL.

‡Adjusted for megaloblastic anemia, granulocytopenia, or thrombocytopenia; blood cell counts, including platelets, should be monitored as described in text.

§Subsequent treatment of the infant is the same as that described under treatment of congenital infection. When the diagnosis of infection in the fetus is established earlier, we suggest that sulfadiazine be used alone until after the first trimester, at which time pyrimethamine should be added to the regimen. The decision about when to begin pyrimethamine/sulfadiazine/leucovorin for the pregnant woman is based on an assessment of the risk of fetal infection, incidence of false-positive and false-negative results of amniocentesis with polymerase chain reaction (PCR) assay, and risks associated with medicines. Although reliability of PCR assay results is laboratory dependent, results from the best reference laboratories have a sensitivity of 92% for detection of the *T. gondii* 300-copy 529-bp DNA using the amniotic fluid PCR assay (see text). Thus PCR assay results reasonably determine therapeutic approach. (Data from Wallon M, Franck J, Thulliez P, et al: Accuracy of real-time polymerase chain reaction for *Toxoplasma gondii* in amniotic fluid, *Obstet Gynecol* 115:727-733, 2010). With maternal acquisition of infection after 31 weeks of gestation, incidence of transmission exceeds 60%, and manifestations of infection are in general less severe. When infection is acquired between 21 and 29 weeks of gestation, management varies. After 24 weeks of gestation, we recommend that amniocentesis be performed and that pyrimethamine/leucovorin/sulfadiazine be used instead of spiramycin. Consultation with the reference laboratory is advised. Amniocentesis is not performed before 17 to 18 weeks of gestation.

In other countries, including Austria, Germany, and Italy, the practice regarding the use of amniocentesis and PCR assay to guide the use of pyrimethamine/sulfonamides may differ. When maternal infection is documented, treatment with pyrimethamine/sulfonamide may be recommended beginning at 14, 16,[567] or 18[726] weeks of pregnancy in the absence of an amniocentesis for a period of 4 or 6 weeks or until amniocentesis is performed, depending on the center. If amniocentesis is performed and yields positive results, this combination is continued, given continuously until delivery,[726] or alternating with spiramycin,[567] according to the protocols of the centers. When *Toxoplasma* is not detected in the amniotic fluid and fetal ultrasound does not show any abnormality, pyrimethamine/sulfonamide treatment is either stopped[726] or replaced with spiramycin as a precautionary approach.[726]

No controlled data are currently available that compare the benefits of treatment with pyrimethamine/sulfonamide only after PCR confirmation of fetal infection versus presumptive treatment before or in the absence of such confirmation. Our concern about exposing a large number of noninfected fetuses for several weeks or months to pyrimethamine/sulfonamide treatment has led us to restrict the administration of these drugs to fetuses identified as infected on the basis of a positive PCR assay of amniotic fluid. We also offer these drugs, presumptively, in cases of maternal infections occurring in the last 2 months of pregnancy, which are associated with a risk of fetal infection of 60% to 70%.[4] Any evidence from the ongoing TOXOGEST randomized trial,[511] or any other trial investigating the impact of pyrimethamine and sulfonamides on preventing maternal to fetal transmission, would, of course, lead us to review and possibly update our strategy. The efficacy of maternal treatment is discussed in a specific chapter on the effectiveness of all possible interventions (see "Treatment Efficacy").

In Utero Treatment of Proven Fetal Infection

If PCR testing of the amniotic fluid is positive but ultrasound scans are normal, a combination of pyrimethamine/sulfonamide should be substituted for spiramycin or continued if presumptively given to the mother before amniotic fluid testing. Pyrimethamine and sulfonamides cross the placenta and reach therapeutic concentrations in the fetus (see "Drugs Active Against *Toxoplasma gondii*"). This treatment is continued until delivery, with regular monitoring of blood cell counts (see Table 31-7).

If PCR testing of the amniotic fluid is positive and ultrasound scans are abnormal, prenatal treatment with pyrimethamine and sulfonamide should be identical to that in the preceding situation. Such treatment is practiced both in countries with ultrasound monitoring of known maternal seroconversion and in countries in which there is no program of screening for maternal seroconversion, with infected fetuses diagnosed on the basis of ultrasound abnormalities. With prenatal treatment, the abnormalities observed on ultrasound scans may regress,[727] stabilize, or become accentuated. Repeated evaluation of the severity of the fetal condition is required, and abortion for medical reasons may be considered in the most serious forms (hydrocephalus) (see Fig. 31-28 and 31-30). In our experience, when antenatal treatment is introduced soon after maternal infection is acquired, severe disease is observed in less than 1% of cases (Lyon cohort unpublished data).

Particular Cases. Abortion was frequently proposed in confirmed first-trimester fetal infections until the 1980s. The more general use of prenatal treatment with pyrimethamine/sulfonamide and improvements in the quality of ultrasound surveillance raised questions about this practice.[728] Subsequent studies with long-term follow-up of children infected during the first trimester and treated both in utero and postnatally confirmed that systematically proposing abortion was no longer justified because these children had a good prognosis in the absence of antenatal ultrasound abnormalities.[729]

Maternal seroconversion during the last 2 months of pregnancy is a particular problem in that only a limited time period is available for the confirmation of maternal seroconversion at a time when the risk of maternal-fetal transmission is maximal (60%-70%) and the risks of amniocentesis are high.[730] Presumptive prenatal treatment with pyrimethamine/sulfonamide without amniocentesis is recommended in cases where amniocentesis is contraindicated for obstetric reasons.[731] Neonatal diagnosis may be more difficult or delayed by this approach.[732]

In conclusion, when maternal infection (at least infection by type II strains) is treated early in pregnancy, fetal infection is rarely severe and should never automatically lead to pregnancy termination. Fetal ultrasonography should be carried out regularly, and amniocentesis should be performed when possible because of the excellent performance of PCR tests for the detection of fetal infection.

Other molecules, such as cotrimoxazole, have been suggested for both the prevention of maternal-fetal transmission and for the treatment of fetal disease caused by *Toxoplasma*, but experience with this approach remains theoretical or limited.[733,734]

PREVENTION OF *TOXOPLASMA* INFECTION DURING PREGNANCY

The prevention of maternal infection is certainly the most satisfying strategy to reduce the number of infected children due to our limited ability to prevent or reduce the severity of congenital infection. The prevention of maternal infection also saves much stress and anxiety in parents[735] and reduces the costs involved in the management of maternal and congenital infections.

Primary Prevention in the Individual

In the absence of an effective vaccine for humans[736] and of possibilities for readily marketing *Toxoplasma*-free food,[310] the education of women regarding the avoidance of risk behavior is the best means of preventing prenatal infections.

Rationale. Educating pregnant women on the avoidance of *Toxoplasma* infection has the advantage of reducing both the human and financial costs involved in the prevention and management of congenital infection before and after birth and is less costly than other secondary or tertiary prevention approaches. Costs can be further reduced by combining this advice with that on other preventive measures directed at pregnant women, using the same channels to deliver the information. The promotion of improved hand and food hygiene and recommendations not to eat undercooked meat would also help to preclude contact with other pathogens. A review of eight medical economics studies on the prevention of congenital toxoplasmosis found that health education was always cost-effective compared with no intervention, regardless of the underlying hypotheses. Patient education was estimated to be more cost-effective than screening in all studies but one.[737]

Prerequisites. Several prerequisites are essential for the effective education of pregnant women at risk. First, up-to-date information on the routes by which pregnant women at any given location acquire *Toxoplasma* infection is vital and requires that case-control studies of patients with a proven postgestational infection be carried out. Participants should ideally be representative of all social classes and cultural backgrounds and live in both rural and urban areas. These studies should be performed under the guidance of epidemiologists to guarantee that appropriate methods are used to select patients and to collect and analyze data.

Second, the efficient communication of how to avoid these risk factors during pregnancy requires the establishment of means and opportunities to provide information that is comprehensible for all women at risk. The help of health educators and parasitologists should be sought to produce attractive material that delivers clear and accurate information that is accessible to the largest possible audience, including women born in other countries and those with little knowledge of health hygiene. This material should include some information on *Toxoplasma* infection but should mainly provide advice on the adoption of risk-free behaviors.

Third, face-to-face counseling is important to provide tailored guidance and encouragement and requires that health professionals have up-to-date knowledge of the main risk factors and of those that are free of risk. The diffusion of identical information to all professionals in charge of patient education is important to avoid the dissemination of prejudicial, conflicting advice.[738]

Limited data are available on the manner in which patient education on *T. gondii* infection is provided and on its efficacy worldwide, but they suggest that all of these steps need to be strengthened.

KNOWLEDGE OF RISK FACTORS FOR *TOXOPLASMA* INFECTION IN PREGNANCY. Prevention relies on a set of recommendations based on the life cycle of the parasite and on factors that are traditionally associated with human infections. Because many sources of infection are involved, the establishment of specific modes of transmission for a pregnant woman at a given location is imperative so that recommendations can be ranked accordingly. Risk assessment should include the type and amount of meat eaten and how it is produced and traditionally prepared.

The large majority of recent data on risk factors was collected from seroprevalence surveys (see "Epidemiology of Maternal Infection") and may therefore not reflect adequately the risk of acquiring infection during pregnancy. The quality of the surveys was also often hampered by their small sample size and the lack of adjustment for confounders and of attributable risk computations. Only a few case-control studies have been performed in pregnant women with incident infections, and most were carried out in developed countries and date back 1 decade or longer. Even those that were well designed could not explain all infections. A case-control study in the United States could not account for 48% of infections,[341] and a multicenter study in Europe was unable to explain 14% to 49% of the risk for *T. gondii* infection, depending on the center.[316] This suggests that we probably do not yet know all of the factors involved in human infections. Well-designed, large-scale, case-control studies are needed to provide up-to-date information on the role played by known factors and to explore the contribution of others, especially those associated with the consumption of seafood and waterborne transmission.

KNOWLEDGE, ATTITUDES, AND PRACTICES OF OBSTETRICIANS AND MIDWIVES REGARDING THE PREVENTION OF *TOXOPLASMA GONDII* INFECTION. Perinatal health professionals play a major role in the prevention of prenatal infections, including *Toxoplasma*. Only a few surveys have assessed their knowledge of the risk factors involved and the manner in which they counsel pregnant women on how to avoid such infections. Table 31-9 summarizes the findings from five surveys, four of which were performed in the United States with obstetricians,[739-741] internists, and family practitioners,[742] and the fifth included French midwives.[743] Although the questionnaires differed widely between studies, the participants' answers shared many similarities.

Knowledge was assessed in four surveys.[739,740,742,743] A high proportion (90%-100%) of obstetricians in three studies correctly identified eating raw or undercooked meat as a main source of infection. Of interest, many (79%-99.9%) also perceived handling cat litter as a risky procedure that required the use of gloves. In the fourth study, when surveying obstetricians, changing cat litter was also listed as the primary factor, to the same extent as eating raw meat, or to a much larger extent for the internists and family practitioners.[742] Overall, the participants in all studies were less knowledgeable about the other risk factors.

Almost all (96%-100%) clinicians and midwives were reported to have mentioned cats in their recommendations. In two studies, not eating raw or undercooked meat was only mentioned by 77.6%[741] and 82%[739] of respective responders. A discrepancy between knowledge and frequency of counseling was a general finding and was especially striking among midwives surveyed in France, almost 50% of whom would not recommend washing hands before meals, and more than 65% of whom would not warn against gardening without gloves or manipulating unwashed vegetables grown in a domestic garden, although almost 90% of responders were knowledgeable of the potential risks involved.[743]

Undergraduate and postgraduate teaching and continuous medical education should include information on the prevention of *Toxoplasma* infection. A clear message should be conveyed that priority should be given to other factors than those that directly involve cat litter. As discussed in the section "Epidemiology and Diagnosis of Infections in the Mother and the Unborn Child," it is important that cat owners be well informed about the risks involved, but these explanations should principally be aimed at reassuring

Table 31-9 Knowledge, Attitudes, and Practice of Obstetricians and Midwives Regarding *Toxoplasma gondii* Prevention

		KNOWLEDGE OF RISK FACTORS		COUNSELING	
Authors (Year of Publication), Country, Year of Survey	**Study population**	**Item Investigated**	**% of Answers**	**Items Investigated**	**% of Answers**
Jones et al (2001), United States, 1999[740]	Random sample of 2% (*n* = 786) of ACOG members and 224 of CARN/ACOG members; questionnaires available for 364/768 (47%): CARN group: 147; random sample: 217	"In order to prevent toxoplasmosis, it is helpful for women to":		"Your counseling includes information about":	
		Keep cat completely outdoors	52.5	Eating undercooked food	83.3
		Wear gloves when changing litter	78.7	Handling raw food	76.5
		Wear gloves when gardening	76.8	Handling cat litter	100
		Cover sand boxes	72.3	Inadvertent contact with cat feces	96.5
		Wash hands after handling raw meat	86.2	Gardening	67.6
		Eat only well-cooked meat	89.8		
		Not consume unpasteurized foods	64.2		
Jones et al (2010), United States, 2006[741]	Random sample of 1200 ACOG fellows; questionnaires available for 502 (42%)	—		"Which issues would you include in counseling?"	
		-		Eating undercooked meat	77.6
		-		Handling raw meat	67.4
		-		Handling cat litter	99.6
		-		Inadvertent contact with cat feces	98.0
		-		Gardening	65.4
		-		Washing fruit and vegetables	34.2
Kravetz and Federman (2005), United States, [742]	Random sample (*n* = 339) of obstetricians (OB), internists (IM) and family practitioners (FP); questionnaires available for 102 (30%): 49 OB, 40 IM, 13 FP	Most likely mode for transmission?	Overall OB IM/FP	Advice given	OB IM-FP
		Changing cat litter	58 43 72	Avoid changing cat litter $P = .15$	98 88
		Eating undercooked meat	28 42 15	Avoid raw meat $P < = .001$	98 65
		Gardening without gloves	8	Garden only with gloves $P = .026$	73 46
		Living with cats	4	Avoid contact with cats $P = .82$	26 31
		Eating unwashed vegetables/fruit	1	Avoid unwashed vegetables $P = .15$	61 41
Ross et al (2009), United States, 2007[739]	Random sample of 787 CARN members equivalent to 2% of ACOG members and matched for demographic characteristics; questionnaires available for 305/606 (50%)	Knowledge*		Recommendations given*	
		On avoiding cat litter	98.1	On avoiding cat litter	97.7
		On cooking meat until well done	92.0	On cooking meat until well done	82.2
Sellier et al (2012) France, 2011[743]	Random sample (*n* = 139) of midwives involved in prenatal education in 8 areas of the Rhône-Alpes region; answers available for 102 (73.4%)	"Can infection be acquired from: ?"		"Do you warn against: ?"	
		Eating raw meat	100	Eating raw meat	99.0
		Eating unwashed vegetable from garden	100	Eating unwashed vegetables from garden	90.2
		Handling the cat litter	99.0	Handling cat litter	96.1
		Not washing hands before eating	95.1	Not washing hands before eating	51.0
		Gardening "without precautions"	89.2	Gardening "without precautions"	32.4
		Handling unwashed vegetables from the garden	88.2	Handling unwashed vegetables from garden	35.3
		Handling raw meat	76.5	Handling raw meat	81.3

ACOG, American College of Obstetricians and Gynecologists; *CARN*, Collaborative Ambulatory Research Network of ACOG.
*Questions on *Toxoplasma* infection were included among questions on other perinatal infections.

Table 31-10 Frequency of Counseling on *Toxoplasma* Infection Among Obstetricians in Two Surveys Performed in 1999 and 2006 in the United States

	Jones et al (2001)[740]	Jones et al (2010)[741]
Frequencies	%	%
At the initial visit	65.5	53.4
At every visit	1.4	0.2
If the patient has asked questions	42.6	20.2
If the patient mentioned she was ill	7.6	4.7
If the patient is considered at high risk	37.0	18.2
Never	3.1	3.3

them and dissuading them from getting rid of their cats under pressure from their family and friends. A pamphlet for cat owners can be downloaded from the Centers for Disease Control and Prevention (CDC) website.[744]

Ideally, information on the avoidance of toxoplasmosis should be provided before conception[745,746] to allow the implementation of preventive behaviors early in pregnancy. Information at the first prenatal visit is also widely recommended. In two of the studies mentioned above, only 53% and 65% of obstetricians,[740,741] respectively, reported the systematic provision of information on prevention at this early visit (Table 31-10). Also of concern is the lack of adaptation to their patients' profile, which was reported by the French midwives. Time, rather than a lack of conviction or motivation, was listed as the main barrier to providing or repeating information.[739,743] A majority of the obstetricians surveyed by Ross and colleagues[739] indicated that other persons in their department would help to educate patients, including staff, midwives, and nurses. Recommendations also need to be distributed to these professionals on giving priority to the promotion of healthy behaviors not directly related to cat ownership.

PATIENT EDUCATION HANDOUTS. Providing physicians with prepared material would be useful to help them counsel their patients. It would also solve the problem of forgetting important recommendations. The vast majority of the French midwives (84%) expressed the wish to have access to such material, for their own education and to help counsel their patients. The majority of obstetricians surveyed by Ross and colleagues[739] indicated that they would find handouts, office posters, or downloadable web-based material useful.

This material should meet a number of standards listed by Newton and Hall.[747] It should best be designed with the help of experts on *Toxoplasma* infection to guarantee complete and accurate information. Collaboration with health education specialists is also important to ensure easy readability and attractiveness.

Newton and Hall[747] reviewed 18 leaflets or booklets on *Toxoplasma* infection that were produced in Great Britain, by local districts or nationally, for the education of patients (n = 14) or professionals (n = 4). None were found to meet the standards for preventive advice set by the Department of Health. All but two mentioned avoiding eating undercooked meat, but eight did not advise that hands be washed after handling raw meat. Twelve advised wearing gloves while gardening, but only four mentioned washing hands afterward. The clinical and epidemiologic information that was provided was also considered to be incomplete, irrelevant, or too vague.

ASSESSMENT OF KNOWLEDGE AND PRACTICE OF PREGNANT WOMEN REGARDING THE PREVENTION OF *TOXOPLASMA* INFECTION. Information on what knowledge pregnant women have about the possibility of preventing *Toxoplasma* infection and on the precautions they actually take is limited. Several studies have provided evidence of a low level of knowledge of risk factors, which was clearly the case for the majority of women who participated as control subjects in a case-control study carried out by Cook and coworkers[316] in six European centers. Overall, only 6% mentioned contact with soil as a risk factor, and 58% only identified eating raw meat as a source of infection. A lack of awareness of *Toxoplasma* infection was also reported in a small cohort of 15 women who were diagnosed with acute pregnancy-associated infection in Ireland.[748] However, three surveys performed in the United States and the Netherlands suggested that knowledge of preventive measures might not be a reliable indicator of preventive behavior. Of 403 pregnant women surveyed by Jones and colleagues[749] in 2002, only 48% had heard of or seen information about toxoplasmosis; only 40% knew that it was an infection; less than 30% were aware that it could be acquired by eating undercooked meat, by handling raw venison, or by gardening without gloves; and many could not provide exact answers on ways to avoid toxoplasmosis. However, the preventive behaviors reported by responders were quite satisfactory.[749] (Table 31-11).

Ogunmodede and colleagues[750] observed the same contrast between knowledge and behavior in a sample of 322 pregnant women in Minnesota, of whom only about a fourth knew that the parasite could be found in raw or undercooked meat (26%) and that infection could be acquired from eating undercooked pork (24%) or gardening without gloves (26%); however, their reported hand-washing practice was satisfactory.[750] In both surveys, knowledge increased with level of education. Similar findings were found among 1097 pregnant women included in the DELIVER study in the Netherlands.[751] Their knowledge of the possibilities of preventing *Toxoplasma* infection was imperfect (see Table 31-11), but their reported preventive behavior was in general correct, although it was more heavily influenced by the patient's profile (having a higher education, being of Dutch nationality, and having worked at a daycare center) than by knowledge of the disease. This led the authors to suggest that pregnant women receive such a large amount of information during their prenatal visits that they convert it into practical cognitive shortcuts, allowing them to take preventive steps without exactly knowing or remembering why they do it. Another explanation (not discussed by the authors) could be that social desirability led responders to overrate their preventive behaviors.

Less satisfactory findings were reported by Costa and coworkers,[752] who analyzed the preventive behavior of 320 pregnant adolescents aged 12 to 19 years who attended a prenatal care facility in Brazil. Only 50 (16.3%) reported having taken preventive measures that were based on the recommendations established by the CDC[753] and are listed in Box 31-1. The most frequent failings involved not

Table 31-11 Findings From a Selection of Surveys on the Knowledge and Practice of Pregnant Women Regarding the Prevention of *Toxoplasma* Infection

Authors (Year of Publication), Country, Year of Survey	Study Population	Knowledge of Preventive Practice	% of Correct Answers	Question on Preventive Behaviors	% of Affirmative Answers
Jones et al (2003), United States, 2002[749]	403 pregnant women recruited by 225 CARN physician members	Letting someone else change the cat's litter box	65	Since becoming pregnant, do you	
		Cleaning all cutting boards and utensils thoroughly after each use	49	Routinely wash your hands after handling raw meat?	96
		Cooking meat well	48	Routinely wash your hands after gardening?	93
		Avoiding stray cats	47	Routinely wash your hands after changing cat litter?	80
		Making sure the cat's litter box is changed daily	45	Eat rare meat?	6
		Washing and/or peeling fruits and vegetables before eating them	39		
		Feeding cat dry or commercial cat food and not letting it kill and eat rodents	29		
Pereboom et al (2013), Netherlands, 2010[751]	1977 pregnant women included in the DELIVER study. Questionnaire available for 1097(66%)	Letting someone else change the cat's litter box	77.9	Let someone else change the cat litter box	95.6
		Gardening with gloves	74.3	Eat well cooked meat	91.7
		Washing and/or peeling fruits and vegetables before eating them	48.2	Eat washed raw vegetables or fruits	53.3
		Cooking meat well	48.1	Garden with gloves	78.6
Costa et al (2012), Brazil, 2009-2010[753]	341 pregnant adolescents provided prenatal assistance in the public health care system in Fortaleza Questionnaire available for 320			Drinking water from the public water supply	92.2
				Not handling sand	93.5
				Not eating undercooked or partially cooked meat weekly	82.4
				Not having kittens as pets	78.2
				Wearing gloves when cleaning the kittens' litter box	25.0
				Washing fruits and vegetables before eating them	15.1
				Cleaning kitchen utensils and washing hands with warm water and soap after handling raw meat and unwashed fruits and vegetables	9.4
Ogunmodede (2005), United States, 2003[750]	Representative sample of pregnant women in Minnesota. Questionnaires available for 322 patients	Cooking meat thoroughly	30	Hand washing after changing cat litter	72
				Hand washing after gardening	81
				Hand washing after handling raw meat	93

CARN, Collaborative Ambulatory Research Network of the American College of Obstetricians and Gynecologists.

washing hands and vegetables, eating raw vegetables, and not wearing gloves when cleaning litter boxes. The responders who were aged 12 to 14 years and had attended two prenatal visits were more likely to report better behavior.[752]

In summary, patient education remains an important issue, especially for those who are less well educated. The key message should focus on the required achievements, in terms of behaviors and healthy lifestyle, rather than on a perfect knowledge of *Toxoplasma* infection.[751] Understanding the rationale for changing behaviors may still be critical for some patients. Negative attitudes and misconceptions about the disease, its prevention, and treatment are not uncommon and might explain why an understanding of risk factors does not always lead to the avoidance of risk. These obstacles could best be identified and overcome by face-to-face counseling with perinatal health professionals or health educators.

Recommendations

UNIVERSAL RECOMMENDATIONS. A large number of recommendations have been circulated, not all of which are supported by solid evidence. These messages may mislead and

Box 31-1 General Measures to Prevent *Toxoplasma* Infection During Pregnancy

To Minimize Exposure to Tissue Cysts

- Do not eat raw or uncooked meat of any animal, especially lamb, pork, and venison/game. Meat should be cooked to at least 67° C (153° F) or frozen for at least 3 days at −12° C.
- Do not taste meat while it is cooking.
- Do not handle raw meat (especially lamb, pork and venison), or use thorough hand-washing techniques afterwards.
- Wash cutting boards, dishes, countertops and utensils with hot soapy water after contact with raw meat. Use separate cutting boards for meat and vegetables.

To Minimize Exposure to Oocysts

- Avoid contact with potentially contaminated soil, sand, or cat litter, or wear gloves and wash hands carefully afterward.
- Peel or thoroughly wash fruits and vegetable before eating them raw.
- Wash cutting boards, dishes, countertops, utensils, and hands after contact with unwashed fruits and vegetables.
- Do not drink water from sources that are not filtered or treated sufficiently to remove parasites (see text for details).

confuse patients and diminish the emphasis on the principles of risk factors. Health education should primarily target the two main risk factors, which are the consumption of undercooked meat and contact with soil (see Box 31-1).

The first important message is not to eat undercooked meat or meat products. The risk exists for all types of meat, but special attention should be given to lamb, pork, and chicken (especially when raised outdoors or organically) and venison. All types of meat should be cooked until an internal temperature of 67° C (153° F) is reached, including meat cooked in conventional and microwave ovens or on charcoal/wood grills.[754,755] Temperature is best checked by using a thermometer or by verifying that the meat has turned uniformly dark brown both inside and outside. Freezing the meat for at least 3 days at a minimum of −12° C before consumption is also considered to kill the parasite.[756] Industrially frozen meat offers the highest guarantee because household freezers do not always sustain temperature at or below −12° C. Tasting meat while it is cooking should also be avoided. Pregnant women should be specially warned about traditional dishes based on raw or undercooked meat[757] or against consuming certain types of meat that are supposed to be healthy for pregnancy when eaten raw.[758]

To avoid accidental ingestion of tissue cysts, it is also important not to handle raw meat and to wash the hands thoroughly after such exposure. Hands should also be kept away from the mouth and eyes while handling raw meat. To prevent cross-contamination, cutting boards, dishes, counter tops, and utensils should be washed with soapy water after contact with raw meat.

To minimize exposure to oocysts, pregnant women at risk should have no contact with potentially contaminated soil or sand because oocysts can remain infectious in soil and sand for more than 1 year.[373] They are therefore advised not to garden or have contact with sand, even in the absence of evidence of recent cat feces, or to wear gloves and to wash their hands carefully afterward, even when gloves are worn. Vegetables and fruit that are potentially soiled need to be peeled or washed thoroughly before being eaten raw. Washing the hands, cutting boards, dishes, counter tops, and utensils after contact with unwashed fruit and vegetables is also advisable.

It has been demonstrated that oocysts can survive in oysters,[759] but additional studies are needed to quantify the risk of infection in humans through seafood consumption. Consumption of raw fish is not a risk factor for *Toxoplasma* infection.

Pregnant women should avoid drinking untreated or inadequately treated water. This is especially important for those who live in locations where untreated surface water is the main source of drinking water, and for travelers, who should be aware that, in some areas, municipal water may not be adequately treated or filtered.[20] The possibility was also raised recently that infection could be acquired via the inadvertent swallowing of oocysts contained in recreational water, such as lakes, ponds, and streams.[20]

Traveling outside of Europe, the United States, and Canada was found to be a significant risk factor for seroconversion during pregnancy in a multicenter study of European women,[316] probably because of the difficulties in controlling food, water, and hand hygiene. The risk of acquiring a *Toxoplasma* infection has been documented in travelers returning from countries where the incidence of infection is high[760] and underlines the importance of adapting preventive behaviors to changes in the environment.

Because of the growing tendency for consumers to experiment with new types of food, pregnant women should be discouraged from consuming new, exotic types of meat, such as kangaroo, that are often eaten raw and could represent a significant new source of infection in pregnancy.[305,758]

Consumption of raw cow's milk is not thought to be a significant risk factor for *Toxoplasma* infection. However, because raw cow's milk may be contaminated with other pathogens that pose serious risks for pregnant women and their fetuses, raw cow's milk should not be consumed by pregnant women. Any other type of raw milk or milk products, especially goat's milk, should only be consumed if pasteurized, sterilized, or ultra–heat-treated.

RECOMMENDATIONS FOR CAT OWNERS. Despite a large body of concordant evidence to the contrary,[286,524,761] many people are under the misconception that owning a cat or having contact with a cat is a major risk of infection. This causes unnecessary suspicion and alarm in pregnant cat owners and could also lead pregnant women who do not own a cat to feel falsely less exposed to the risk of acquiring a *Toxoplasma* infection.

It is important for cat owners to be reassured that they do not need to abandon their animals. Concordant messages from clinicians and veterinarians are important to avoid confusion. A few simple recommendations will contribute to reassure pregnant women fully and prevent them from incriminating their pets should infection acquired after conception be diagnosed as a consequence of other sources of infection.

Litter box hygiene is the first precaution. Because oocysts are not infectious until 24 hours after shedding, the soiled litter should be changed daily and the litter disposed of in the garbage. The litter box or tray should be washed regularly with boiling water and kept outside of the kitchen or dining room area. Pregnant women should preferably not handle the litter and the box themselves but ask someone else to take care of them or wear gloves and wash their hands thoroughly afterward. Keeping cats indoors and not feeding them uncooked meat is also important to prevent them from becoming infected. Cats that are only fed commercially prepared food do not represent a risk of infection. Pregnant women should not acquire a new cat, and especially not a kitten, which is more likely to eliminate oocysts than older cats.[762] Cat bites and scratches do not represent a significant risk for *Toxoplasma* infection.

RECOMMENDATIONS REGARDING WORK-RELATED RISKS. Pregnant women who are exposed to specific risks in the course of their work, such as animal caretakers, including veterinarians, farmers, gardeners, workers in the food industry, or laboratory technicians, should receive appropriate advice. The recommendations issued by the Canadian Center for Occupational Health and Safety can be useful for this purpose (Box 31-2).[763]

Collective Efforts

Public health strategies to reduce the transmission of *T. gondii* to animals and humans have been detailed in several publications.[20,286,310,764,765]

The first strategy entails the control of cat populations, with the objective of reducing the burden of oocysts in the environment and the contamination of soil and water. Veterinarians should educate cat owners on the importance of spaying or neutering their cats. Attempts should also be made to reduce the number of feral cats[286] through trap-neuter-return programs, adoption, or other options discussed in expert reports.[766] Domestic cats should be kept indoors if at all possible to prevent them from hunting and depositing cat feces outside, and they should not be fed raw meat. Soiled litter should be safely deposited in garbage destined for landfills designed to prevent waste material from leaking into groundwater.[286] The cat feces should not be flushed into the municipal sanitation systems in developing countries.[20] Access of cats should be limited in areas around drinking-water tanks and reservoirs and close to recreational waters,[20] and in areas where wildlife that could be susceptible to cat predation can be found,[286] as well as close to children's playgrounds and sandboxes.

The second series of measures aim to prevent infection in farm animals. These preharvest strategies require the identification and elimination of a number of sources of infections. Keeping animals strictly indoors decreases the risk of infection by avoiding contact with oocysts present in the environment and preventing omnivorous animals from feeding on infected prey. However, this is insufficient, and other precautions should also be taken that include using sterilized feed and bedding, providing animals with clean drinking water, and avoiding the access of cats, rodents, and birds to stables. Rodent controls have been proven to be effective in maintaining organically raised pigs free of *Toxoplasma* infection[312] (Fig. 31-31).

Were an effective vaccine available, vaccination of farm animals would offer the double advantage of reducing infection in animals and production losses and of limiting the

Box 31-2 Precautions to Avoid Infection in Pregnant Women Involved in Specific Risk Activities

Animal Care Workers and Zoo Attendants

Remove all feline feces daily. Dried litter should be disposed of without shaking. Flush feces down the toilet, carefully bag them for disposal, burn them, or bury them deeply. Disinfect litter pans daily by treating with near-boiling water.

Wear disposable gloves when handling litter boxes or working in soil or sand that is possibly contaminated with cat feces. Wash hands after removing gloves. House all members of the cat family in a separate room or building to prevent infecting other animals. Autoclave or heat to 70° C (for at least 10 minutes) any brooms, shovels, and other equipment that have been used to clean cat cages or enclosures.

Do not feed cats raw meat. If this is not possible, feed meat that has previously been frozen because it is less likely to be infectious than fresh meat. Where practical, use and store equipment and tools for cleaning up cat feces in the area where cats are housed.

Slaughterhouse Workers, Meat Inspectors, Line Processors, Butchers, Cooks, and Others in Contact With Raw Meat

Where appropriate, wear gloves when in contact with raw meat. Wash hands thoroughly with soap and water.

Do not touch mouth and eyes while handling raw meat. Wash all cutting boards, knives, sink tops, and other materials that come into contact with raw meat with soap and water. Control cockroaches or other insects that can come into contact with food or areas where food is prepared. They may transfer oocysts to uncovered food.

Agricultural Workers

Soil can be a source of transmission, particularly if it is used by cats. Wash hands after working in the soil or after contact with animals. Confirm the cause of abortion in animals. Send the placenta, fetus, and blood samples to a laboratory to confirm the presence of *Toxoplasma gondii*. Do not handle fetal membranes and dead fetuses with bare hands. Fetal material that is not sent to the laboratory should be buried or incinerated. Remove placentas and aborted material from access by cats or rodents as a potential source of further infection. Do not allow cats access to stored feed.

Remove all cat feces from feed. Keep only adult barn cats by spaying females and driving new cats away. Adult cats are likely to have acquired resistance and are thus unlikely to shed oocysts in their feces.

Landscapers and Gardeners

Wear gloves to avoid exposure to *Toxoplasma gondii* when in contact with soil contaminated with infected cat feces. Wash hands after removing gloves.

Laboratory Workers

Pregnant women should be discouraged from working with *Toxoplasma* spp. Protective clothing should be worn by workers exposed to contaminated materials. Contaminated clothing should be labeled with a biohazard warning and washed using laundry procedures for disinfection. Pregnant women should avoid handling contaminated needles. Production and exposure to aerosols from animal tissues should be minimized. Acceptable laboratory techniques, as outlined in "Laboratory Biosafety Guidelines," should be used.

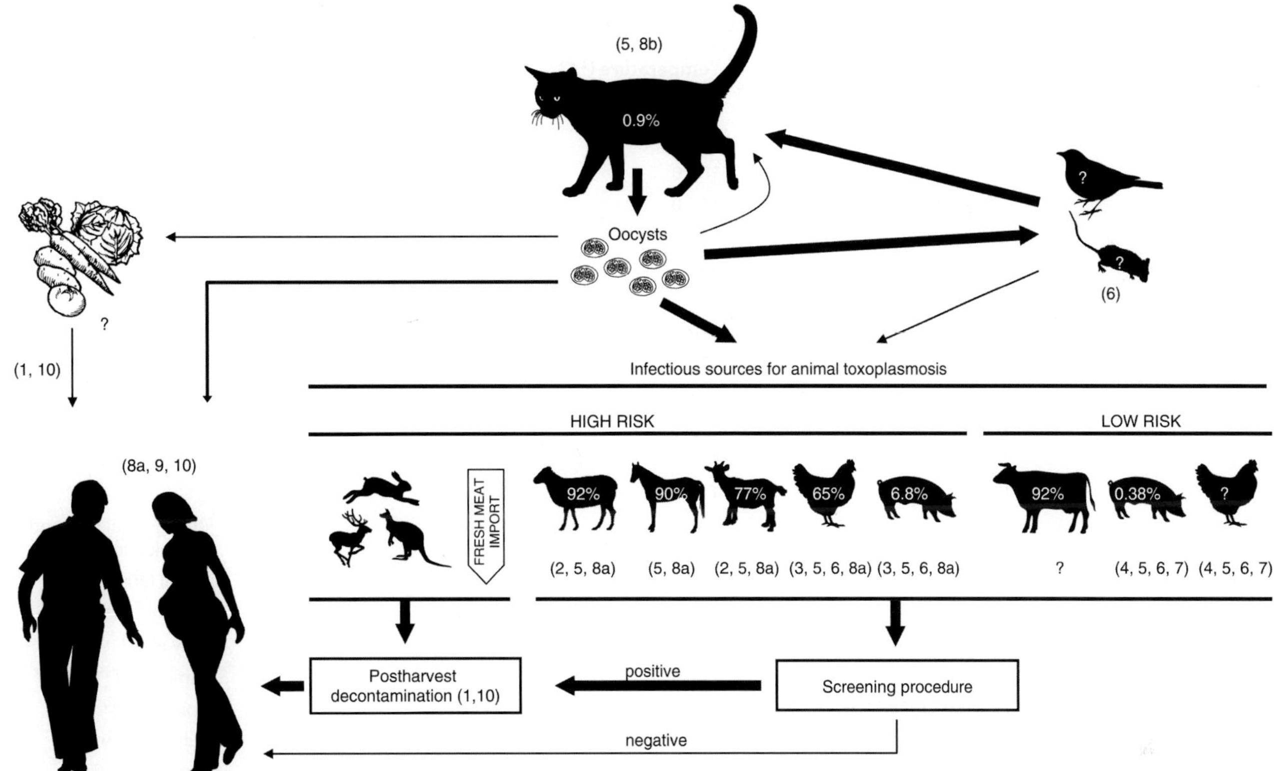

Figure 31-31 Preharvest and postharvest risk management for the control of infectious sources of animal and human toxoplasmosis. *(1)* Freezing and/or heating, *(2)* heating of milk products, *(3)* animal-friendly production system, *(4)* indoor production system, *(5)* cat control, *(6)* rodent control, *(7)* animal feed and bedding decontamination by heating, *(8)* vaccination against tissue cyst formation *(a)* or oocyst shedding *(b)*, *(9)* serologic monitoring of people at risk, *(10)* consumer education on food hygiene and decontamination procedures. Percentages indicate highest observed seroprevalence per species. Thickness of arrows represents the likeliness of transmission without risk management procedure. Percentages indicate the highest observed seroprevalence per animal species or the percentage of cats actively shedding oocysts. (From Kijlstra A, Jongert E: Control of the risk of human toxoplasmosis transmitted by meat, *Int J Parasitol* 38:1359-1370, 2008; with permission.)

presence of viable cysts in meat and thus the risk of infection to humans (see later).

The final option to reduce infection in humans is by killing *T. gondii* in infected meat. Several processes that can be used are listed in Table 31-12 and include cooking meat above 66° C, freezing until −12° C for 3 days, curing with greater than 2% salt or greater than 1.4% lactate salts for at least 1 day,[767] and using gamma irradiation and high hydrostatic pressure.

Outlook for Vaccines

Immunization against toxoplasmosis is awaited with impatience. The natural course of infection in humans that confers protective, but nonsterile immunity indicates that it is possible to create an effective vaccine. Currently, despite a huge body of research,[736] no vaccine has been licensed for human use. These circumstances apply to all parasitic infections and, in particular, to malaria. The reasons for this situation are complex, and the most important include the antigenic diversity of parasites and their ability to evade the immune system.[768]

Research on vaccines has taken into account the progress made in all scientific fields, and numerous trials on immunization have been performed with a range of attenuated strains, crude parasitic extracts, and, more recently, recombinant peptides and DNA vaccines by using different vectors or adjuvants. To date, no long-lasting protective immunity has been achieved.[736] Because infection occurs through the ingestion of either cysts or oocytes, a vaccine would not only target humans but also food animals (to prevent cyst formation in meat) and cats (to reduce the shedding of oocytes). In addition to reducing human infection, such vaccines would also lower the economic impact of abortion in cattle.

Vaccination to Prevent Abortion in Sheep. The only commercial vaccine licensed solely for veterinary use is the live-attenuated tachyzoite of strain S48 (Toxovax).[769] This strain was originally isolated from an aborted lamb and has been passaged 3000 times in mice and has lost its ability to form cysts in tissues. Subcutaneous Toxovax immunization protected sheep against abortion for 18 months[769] but did not completely eradicate the parasite. Immunization with a MIC1 and MIC3 knockout RH strain mutant was as effective as Toxovax in protecting ewes against abortion.[770]

Perspectives for a Vaccine in Humans. Studies in experimental mouse models reported that immunization against different antigens of *T. gondii* did not induce safe, long-lasting protective immunity.[771] Live-attenuated vaccines can induce an efficient $CD8^+$ T-cell response, but they are not practical in humans because they can revert to pathogenic strains.[771] Inactivated, killed, and crude antigen vaccines do not appear to be sufficiently effective.[772] Epitope vaccines

Table 31-12 Effect of Salting, Freezing, and Heating on Viability of *Toxoplasma gondii* Tissue Cysts

Sample	Salt	Temperature (° C)	Time	Efficacy*	Reference
Tissue cysts from infected rat brain	0.85%	4	0-24 days	–	Jacobs et al (1960)[35]
	0.1%	18-20	12 hr	+	
	0%	18-20	30 min	+	
	0.1%-2.1%	18-20	24 hr	+	
	0.85%	50	1 hr	+	
	0.85%	56	10 min	+	
	0.85%	50	15 min	+	
Tissue cysts from infected mouse brain	6%	Various		+	Dubey et al (1997)[33]
	0.85%		56 days	–	
	2%		49 days	–	
	3.3%		21 days	–	
	2%	4	7 days	+	Hill et al (2004)[767]
	1%	4	45 days	–	
		−20	3 days	+	Djurkovic-Djakovic and Milenkovic (2000)[862]
Pork meat spiked with *Toxoplasma* cysts	2%	4	7 days	+	Hill et al (2004)[767]
	1%	4	45 days	–	
		67	Immediate	+	Dubey et al (1990)[956]
		−20	2 days	+	Sommer et al (1965)[957]
	15% $NaNO_3$/NaCl	5	4-21 days	+†	Scupin (1968)[958]
		−12		+	Kotula et al (1991)[959]
	Various enhancing solutions	4	8 hr	+	Hill et al (2006)[960]
Meat from experimentally infected pigs		−25	6-35 days	+‡	Grossklaus and Baumgarten (1968)[961]
	Various enhancing solutions	4	8 hr	+	Hill et al (2006)[960]
		−7 to −12		–	Kuticic and Wikerhauser (1996)[962]
Meat from infected sheep	Salt and sugar	4	64 hr	+	Lunden and Uggla (1992)[755]
	Smoking	<50	24-48 hr	+	

From Kijlstra A, Jongert E: Control of the risk of human toxoplasmosis transmitted by meat, *Int J Parasitol* 38:1359-1370, 2008; with permission.
NaCl, Sodium chloride; *NaNO₃*, sodium nitrate.
*Efficacy was scored as +/–; indicates that the procedure did not kill all parasites and "+" indicates a 100% killing effect of the procedure on the parasite, unless stated otherwise. Parasite viability was evaluated by mice or cat bioassay.
†*Toxoplasma gondii* cysts could be isolated up to 13 days after preparation of smoked hams.
‡One of 54 deep-frozen samples was still positive in a mouse bioassay after storage at 25° C for 35 days.

have been tested, either individually or in the form of multiple antigenic peptides (MAP). A tri-epitope MAP construct, including one B-cell and two T-cell epitopes derived from *T. gondii* antigens (SAG1, GRA4, and GRA1) in Freund adjuvant, induced both humoral and cellular immune responses in mice, leading to increased survival time compared with unvaccinated control mice after a lethal challenge.[773] Recombinant protein vaccines and, more recently, DNA vaccines have been widely evaluated.[771] DNA vaccines appear to be very promising because they are safe, but their efficacy needs to be improved, for example, by using a live-vector vaccine that induces humoral and cellular immune responses.

Despite these research activities in animal models, no human vaccine against toxoplasmosis will be available in the foreseeable future. Moreover, the extent to which findings of increased survival or decreased tissue cysts burden in rodent models can be translated into a vaccine that protects the childbearing-age woman and her fetus is not known. A better understanding of the mechanism of cell invasion, the subversion of the immune system and the pathogenicity of *T. gondii* is a prerequisite for a safe and effective vaccine. Antigenic combinations that cover different parasitic stages should, in theory, be more effective than a single-antigen vaccine, but the criteria by which to select among the candidate antigens must be established. As pointed out by some authors,[774] the identification of the antigen relies on empirical testing rather than a prediction of its efficacy. $CD8^+$ T cells are considered to be the main protective response to clear intracellular parasites through the MHC class I response. The development of a predictive binding algorithm for MHC-I peptides in humans could be used to predict the protective epitope among all of the *T. gondii* vaccine candidates.[774] Completion of the genome for different strains has facilitated proteomic studies,[775] which will allow a more accurate selection of candidate proteins, especially antigens recognized by T lymphocytes. Concomitant use of animal vaccines may lead to a reduction in parasitic biomass and have a positive impact on human health.

Infection in the Newborn

CLINICAL EVALUATION

Clinical Presentation

Clinical examination is most often normal, with 80% to 90% of children with congenital toxoplasmosis having no symptoms at birth.[776,777] The complete classic triad of hydrocephalus, intracerebral calcifications, and retinochoroiditis, as described by Wolf and colleagues,[778] is observed in only a small proportion of infected newborn infants. The clinical signs, if present, may be nonspecific signs of progressive generalized fetal disease: hepatomegaly, splenomegaly (Fig. 31-32), jaundice, skin rash (Fig. 31-33), myocarditis, thrombopenic purpura, anemia, myocarditis, respiratory distress (Fig. 31-34), or CNS sequelae (microcephaly, hydrocephalus (Fig. 31-35), convulsions.[779,780] Congenital toxoplasmosis is not associated with intrauterine growth retardation[781] but has been associated with prematurity when maternal seroconversion has occurred before 20 weeks of gestation (OR, 4.71; 95% CI, 2.03 to 10.9)[781] and with infection caused by non–type II serotypes.[782]

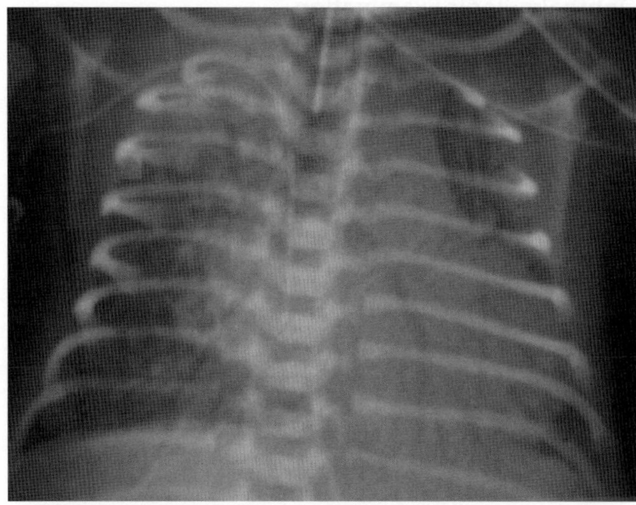

Figure 31-34 Disseminated congenital *Toxoplasma* infection: chest radiograph showing nonconfluent mottled opacities.

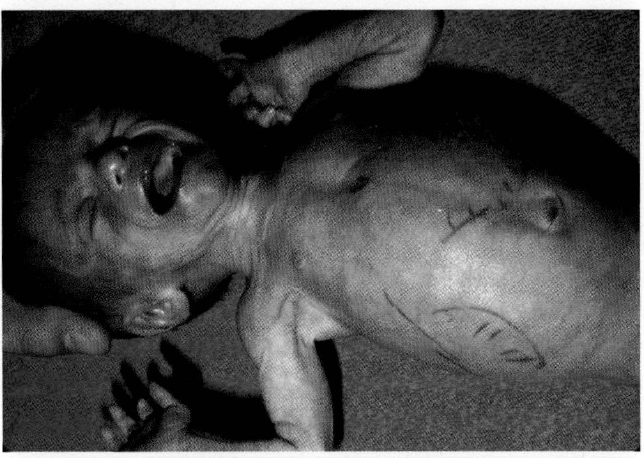

Figure 31-32 Hepatosplenomegaly.

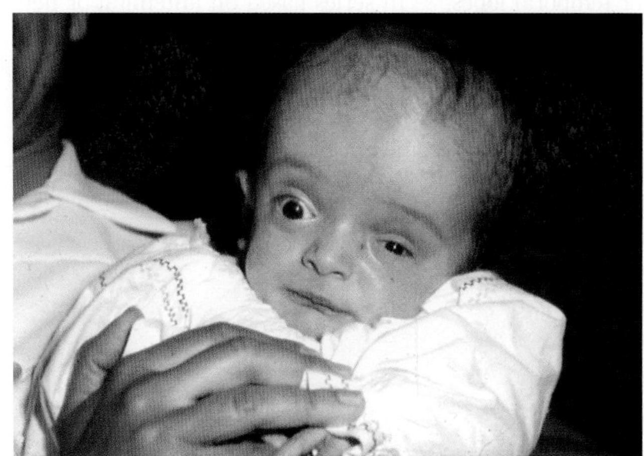

Figure 31-35 Hydrocephalus and left microphthalmia.

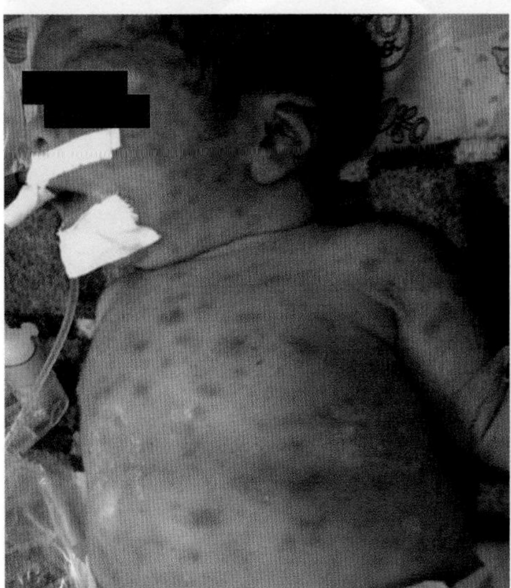

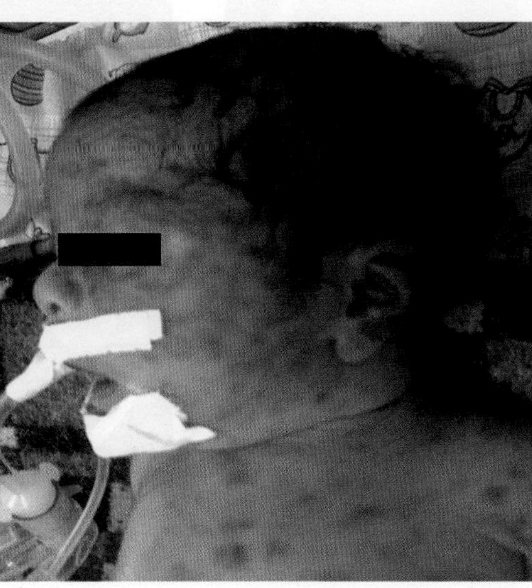

Figure 31-33 Petechiae, ecchymoses and "blueberry muffin rash": a diffuse blue maculopapular rash. (Courtesy J. Gomez-Marin, Armenia, Colombia.)

Ophthalmologic Examination

Ophthalmologic examination is best carried out by indirect ophthalmoscopy, with the results reported on a standardized chart. The ophthalmologic lesion most characteristic of toxoplasmosis is focal chorioretinitis, the size of which is expressed relative to the diameter of the optical disc, varying from between less than one half to four diameters. The active or healed nature of the lesions and their macular, juxtamacular, or peripheral location should be determined. At birth, 3% to 5% of children with congenital toxoplasmosis have one or several chorioretinitis lesions.[707,708,783] Other associated ophthalmologic abnormalities (cataracts, microphthalmia, etc.) are very rare (<1% in Kodjikian's series).[783]

Neonatal Neuroimaging

As in prenatal examination, the aim of neonatal brain imaging is to detect symmetrical ventricular dilatation after stenosis of the cerebral aqueduct, possibly progressing to moderate ventriculomegaly and marked hydrocephalus (Fig. 31-36). Small (1-3 mm) round calcifications are the most specific finding. They may occur singly (Fig. 31-37) or in larger numbers (Fig. 31-38). They predominate in the periventricular regions of the parietal-occipital or temporal lobes.[784] In series based on antenatal or neonatal screening, the incidence of calcification and/or brain dilatation at birth is between 6.5% and 18% of children with congenital toxoplasmosis.[702,708,777,785,786] Other less specific aspects have been described: curvilinear calcifications, a hyperechogenic appearance of the thalamostriatal vessels known as the "candlestick" sign, and subependymal cysts.[784] Cerebral atrophy, with porencephalic cavities or even brain destruction and microcephaly, may be observed in cases of severe congenital toxoplasmosis.[780] Neuroimaging is most commonly performed with ultrasound scans in Europe[702,708,786,787] and with CT scans in the United States.[788,789] Those favoring ultrasonography highlight the high sensitivity of current probes, the widespread availability of machines, and the absence of irradiation.[790] Supporters of CT scans stress the higher sensitivity of this technique for the detection of calcifications.[791] These arguments are based on old studies, and the correlation between the results obtained in these two examinations has been shown to be excellent in recent studies, such as that carried out by Lago and coworkers.[792] MRI may be used in addition to ultrasonography or CT scans to search for parenchymatous or cortical abnormalities, but it makes only a minor contribution.[784]

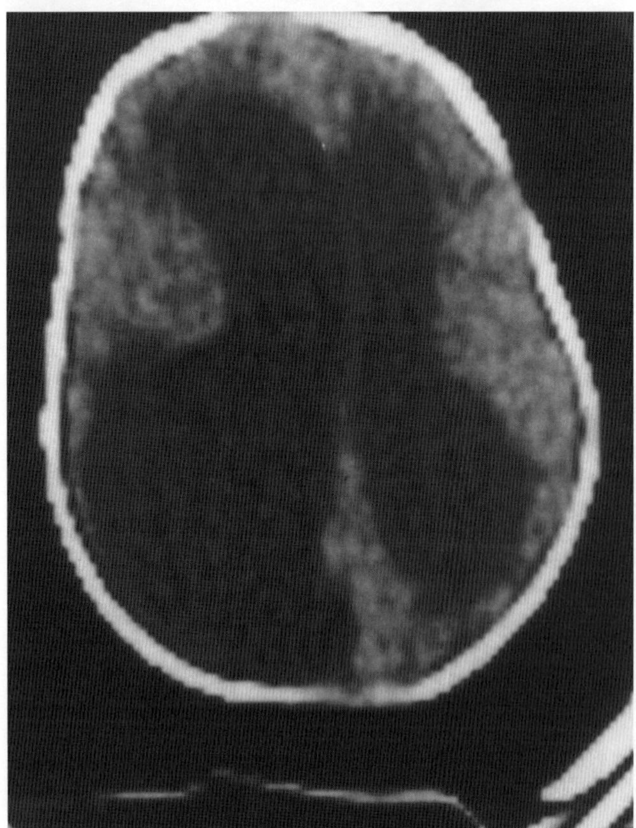

Figure 31-36 Computed tomography scan: major asymmetrical hydrocephalus.

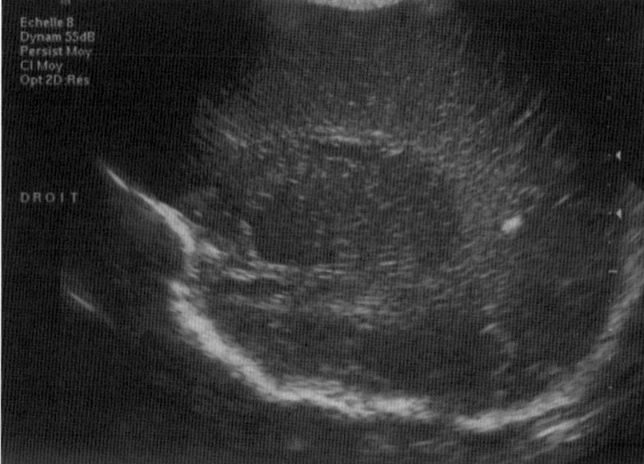

Figure 31-37 Sagittal section on a brain ultrasonography: a single parietal-occipital calcification.

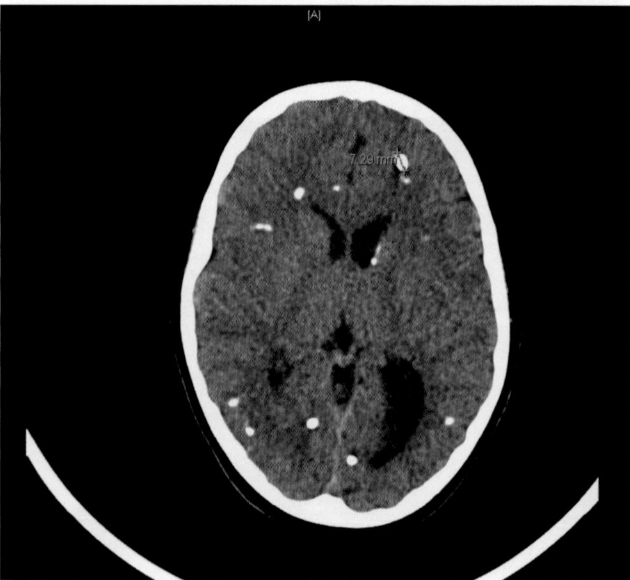

Figure 31-38 Computed tomography scan: numerous intracranial calcifications and moderate ventricular dilatation.

Differential Diagnosis

Infection with one of two viruses most closely mimics congenital *Toxoplasma* infection.

Cytomegalovirus (CMV) infection (see Chapter 24) is the most frequent congenital infection, with a prevalence at birth of 3 to 6 per thousand.[793] Symptomatic congenital infections are frequently associated with small brain calcifications, predominantly in the periventricular area and the central gray matter nuclei. Candlestick images are more frequently observed than for congenital toxoplasmosis. These images are rarely isolated, and the presence of intrauterine growth restriction, microcephaly, abnormalities of the cerebral cortical gyri, and hepatosplenomegaly suggest congenital CMV infection rather than toxoplasmosis. Chorioretinitis is much rarer (<1%) in the context of CMV infection than in that of toxoplasmosis.[794,795]

Lymphocytic choriomeningitis virus (LCMV) is an arenavirus (see Chapter 30). Rodents serve as the reservoir of this virus, and human infections occur through contact with infected rodents (mice, hamsters, laboratory animals). Congenital infections are acquired after primary maternal infection during pregnancy. In greater than 90% of cases, chorioretinitis similar to that observed in the context of toxoplasmosis develops.[796] Diffuse cerebral calcifications (Fig. 31-39) and hydrocephalus were described for greater than 80% of the published cases.[797,798] Diagnosis is serologic, and the incidence of this infection is probably underestimated.[799] There is no treatment.

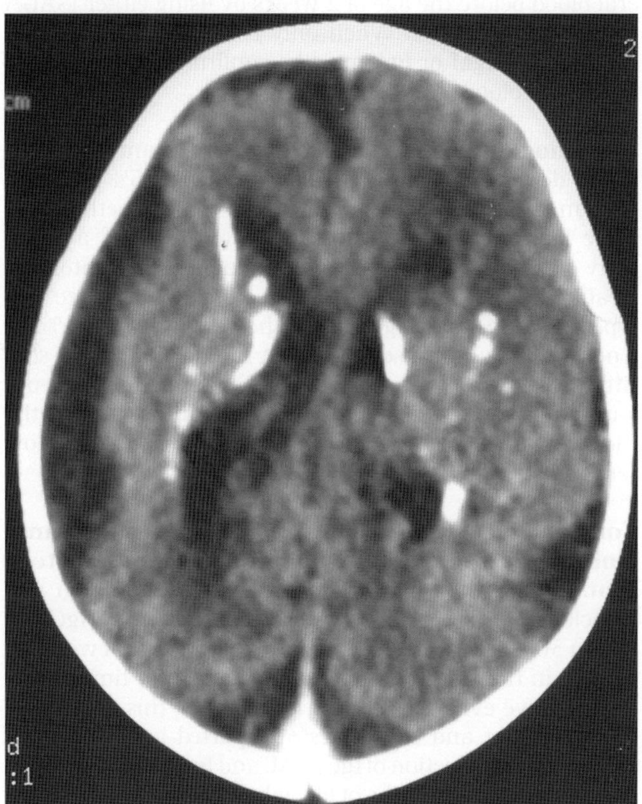

Figure 31-39 Lymphocytic choriomeningitis congenital infection: ventricular dilatation and diffuse brain calcifications predominantly in the periventricular area.

Particular Situations: Twin Pregnancy, Human Immunodeficiency Virus–Infected Mothers

Twin Pregnancies. Congenital *T. gondii* infections in twins have been reported as clinical cases or small series.[800,801] In monozygotic twin pregnancies, the infectious status of the two fetuses has been concordant, with one exception,[802] and the severity is often similar in cases of congenital infection.[800] In dizygotic twin pregnancies, the situation is less uniform because cases in which one of the twins was infected, whereas the other was not, have regularly been reported.[800,803,804] This heterogeneity is also evident in the clinical data. In more than half of the cases of dizygotic twin infection, one of the children was asymptomatic, and the other had severe infection.[800,805] Prenatal diagnosis is carried out as in singleton pregnancies, by sampling amniotic fluid from each of the amniotic sacs.

Human Immunodeficiency Virus–Infected Mothers. In HIV-infected pregnant women, the reactivation of latent toxoplasmosis may lead to maternal-fetal transmission. The risk of vertical transmission is unclear: One small European study described a risk of 0%,[806] and one small series reported a risk of 3.7% (95% CI, 0.09 to 18.9) (one child with congenital toxoplasmosis among 27 children born to pregnant women seropositive for both HIV and *Toxoplasma*[807]). Severe maternal immunodepression with low CD4 lymphocyte counts (<200/μL) during pregnancy has been reported in almost all the cases described to date.[700,806-808]

LABORATORY DIAGNOSIS

The laboratory plays a key role in the workup of congenital toxoplasmosis at birth. Both indirect (detection of antibodies) and direct (detection of parasites or parasitic DNA in body fluids) are used. Laboratory evaluation should be undertaken whenever either of two situations arises:

1. Maternal infection during pregnancy has been documented (see "Epidemiology and Diagnosis of Infections in the Mother and the Unborn Child") or is suspected; because congenital infection is often subclinical, a complete checkup should be performed systematically, regardless of the results of the antenatal diagnosis (when undertaken) and postnatal presentation.[41]
2. The newborn presents clinical manifestations that resemble those of congenital toxoplasmosis, and the mother has not been followed up serologically for toxoplasmosis during pregnancy; because none of the signs are pathognomonic for toxoplasmosis and can be mimicked by other pathogens, such as cytomegalovirus, herpes, rubella, and syphilis,[1] a full evaluation should be made.

Indirect Diagnosis by Detection of Antibodies

Immunoglobulin G. Immunoglobulin G antibodies cross the placenta but are not a reliable marker of congenital infection in newborns because they will inevitably be observed in all babies born to mothers who have positive IgG antibody titers and, in some cases, are found at higher levels in newborns than in mothers. This phenomenon has also been observed in other clinical settings[809] and has no value with respect to diagnosis because it only reflects the dynamics of the placental transfer of IgG, which increases with gestation and peaks during the last weeks of pregnancy.[810] However, maternal serology is a valuable tool for later comparisons with newborn IgG (see later).

Numerous methods are available for the detection of IgG antibodies (see "Available Tests"). The dye test described by Sabin and Feldman is the most sensitive but does not detect IgG alone. It requires living parasites, is not automated, and is used only in some reference laboratories. The indirect fluorescent antibody test, which has been widely used until recently, is a sensitive, nonautomated test that is now frequently replaced by ELISA tests. Numerous commercial kits are available, but it is essential that, for all specific isotypes assayed, the kit has been validated for newborns and infants before use. IgG subclasses that react with recombinant antigens have been reported to be good markers for neurologic and ocular lesions,[811] and these findings deserve further investigation.

Immunoglobulin M and Immunoglobulin A. Neither IgM nor IgA cross the placenta; therefore their presence in newborn blood demonstrates congenital infection. Several studies have addressed the performance of the detection of IgM and IgA in the neonatal diagnosis of congenital toxoplasmosis. The sensitivity of these tests ranges from 54%[812] to 76.5%[813] for IgM, from 53%[814] to 70.6%[813] for IgA. Combination of IgM and IgA on peripheral blood scored a sensitivity of 71.4% versus 69.5% in cord blood.[813]

The most convenient sample to use for testing newborns is cord blood, but this can be contaminated by maternal blood.[726] Moreover, tests for IgM and IgA antibodies appeared to be significantly less specific in cord blood than in peripheral blood in some studies,[694,813,815,816] although other studies confirmed greater specificity in peripheral blood for IgM only[817] and did not find significantly better specificity for IgM and IgA in samples of cord blood.[818] Nevertheless, it is advisable, when testing for specific IgM or IgA in cord blood, to confirm the results by testing samples of peripheral blood.

The results from different studies are often difficult to compare because many factors that were not always evaluated can affect test performance (gestational age at maternal infection, the type of sample and the techniques used, and antenatal treatment). Gestational age at which maternal infection is acquired appears to affect the performance of these tests. In a multicenter study, Gilbert and colleagues[818] found that tests for IgM or IgA detected only 52% to 55% of infected infants and that sensitivity for IgM was lowest when maternal infection occurred during the first or second trimester, whereas the sensitivity of IgA was not affected. Wallon and colleagues[816] confirmed that the date of maternal infection should be taken into account when interpreting such results because IgA sensitivity was slightly higher, whereas IgM sensitivity was substantially higher, for infections that occurred during the third trimester compared with those during the second trimester. False-negative serologic tests in the newborn infant can be observed when mothers seroconvert shortly before delivery and transmission of antibodies from the mother to the fetus has not yet occurred. Tests for IgM and IgA antibodies should be performed as soon as possible after delivery because it has been reported that better scores are achieved when they are performed before 2 weeks of age and that sensitivity declines thereafter.[818]

Some studies have reported satisfactory results of screening performed on eluates from blood specimens collected on filter paper.[819] The detection of IgM and IgA showed a sensitivity of 72% in a retrospective study, in which no cases were diagnosed solely by the detection of IgA.[820] The techniques used are also of key importance: The ISAGA gave reliable results for both isotypes, whereas ELISA scored better for detecting IgA than IgM,[818] and the immunofluorescence assay was found to be less sensitive (10%) for the detection of IgM.[818]

Whether or not antenatal treatment has an impact on serologic workup at birth is difficult to assess. Several parameters that are not always addressed in studies, such as the components of the treatment (spiramycin or pyrimethamine/sulfonamide), compliance with treatment, or the stage of pregnancy at the onset of treatment, could bias the results. Some authors have reported that antenatal treatment, especially with a combination of pyrimethamine/sulfadoxine can induce false-negative serologic test results at birth.[821] However, Gilbert and colleagues[818] did not report any significant reduction in IgM or IgA sensitivity after antenatal treatment with pyrimethamine/sulfonamide in agreement with other authors.[815] The components of the treatment may be an important factor because spiramycin was reported to induce fewer false-negative test results than pyrimethamine/sulfadoxine.[822]

Taken together, these results indicate that good practice should include tests to detect both IgM and IgA in peripheral blood before the age of 2 weeks by using either ISAGA or ELISA techniques. When only cord blood is available, positivity for IgM or IgA must be confirmed on samples of peripheral blood.

Immunoglobulin E. The sensitivity of IgE antibody testing to detect congenital toxoplasmosis was 25% using an immunocapture method.[823] With an ELISA method, the same team achieved a sensitivity of 59.5% and a specificity of 91%; results were not influenced by antenatal treatment.[678] Combining the detection of the three isotypes (IgM, IgA, and IgE) raised the sensitivity to 81%.[678] Another study that used an ELISA method showed a sensitivity of 40.2% and reported that IgE antibodies were not found in infected infants older than 5 months.[3] Currently, the detection of IgE is not commonly used because of its low sensitivity.

Comparative Analysis of Mother/Newborn Immunoglobulin G and Immunoglobulin M Using Western Blot. This method was first described by Remington and associates,[824] who reported specific band patterns of IgG and IgM in 50% of congenitally infected newborns that were not present in their respective mothers. Since that time, many studies have evaluated the performance of this technique. Tissot Dupont and colleagues[825] reported a sensitivity of 82.6% for the detection of IgG, IgM, and IgA by Western blot within the first 3 months of life, whereas at birth, the same combination had a sensitivity of 65.2%.[825] IgA detection was the least sensitive, whereas the combination of IgG and IgM yielded the best score.[825] The combination of Western

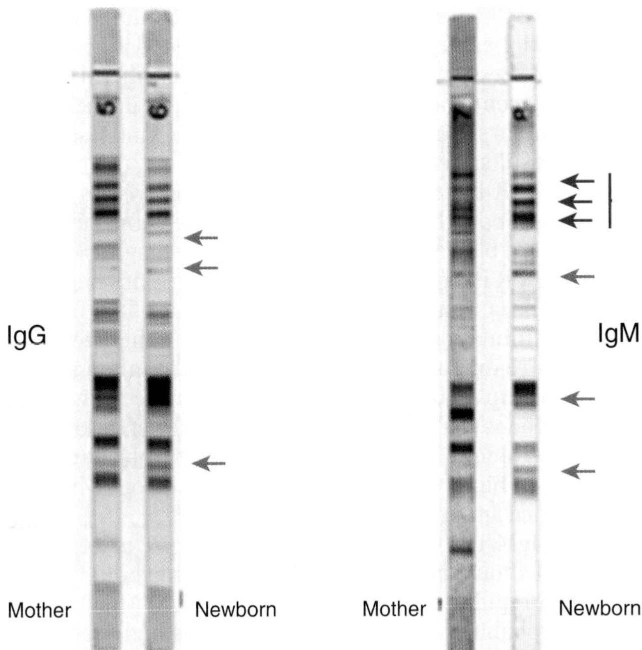

Figure 31-40 Comparison of mother/newborn Western blots. *Arrows* indicate neosynthesized immunoglobulin. *Red arrows* indicate the immunoglobulin M triplet bands of 75 to 100 kDa. Diagnosis kit commercialized by Ldbio Diagnostics, Lyon, France.

blot and conventional serologic analysis increased the sensitivity at birth to 78%, and within the first 3 months of life to 85%.[826] Simultaneous detection of IgG, IgM, and IgA by Western blot achieved a sensitivity of 91% and a specificity of 100%.[827] The sensitivity of IgM has been improved by a new interpretation standard: The presence of three IgM-reactive bands at 75, 90, and 100 kDa increased the sensitivity to 95.8%, in combination with prenatal and other neonatal tests (Fig. 31-40).[828] Comparative Western blot testing nevertheless presents some drawbacks: Readings can be complicated because of the presence of novel bands, and band intensity must also be taken into account; scanning the bands could improve interpretation by eliminating reader variability. Because the Western blot test is not automated and is expensive, in our opinion, it should not be performed systematically but, rather, used only in cases for which the results of other tests are doubtful or negative in situations in which the likelihood of congenital toxoplasmosis is high (i.e., in the case of late maternal infection or a positive antenatal diagnosis) and should be delegated to reference laboratories.

Direct Detection of the Parasite

Toxoplasma gondii can be detected at birth in the placenta, blood, CSF, or urine by either PCR assay or mouse inoculation. The former is the simplest, fastest, and therefore the most commonly used method.

The sensitivity of PCR on the placenta varied from 60%[452] to 79.5%,[829] and its specificity ranged from 92%[829] to 97%.[830] Of interest, parasites were detected more often when maternal infection occurred during the third trimester of pregnancy, regardless of the type of treatment.[830] In the same study, out of 74 uninfected infants, 2 (3%) displayed false-positive results not confirmed by mouse inoculation, which may have been caused by persistent DNA from nonviable parasites. In both cases, the high cycle threshold (Ct) value (>36) confirmed the low amount of parasitic DNA. The PCR target was either the highly repetitive REP-529 sequence (Genbank AF487550) or gene *B1* (Genbank AB703302), and one study reported better scores for REP-529.[831]

Intraperitoneal mouse inoculation of placental fragments and cord blood displayed a sensitivity of 42% and inoculation of placenta alone 21%.[452] Other studies reported a sensitivity of 50%[832] or 67%,[830] with a specificity of 100%.[830] Mouse inoculation has been used for many years, and when combined with PCR, increases the sensitivity of the detection of parasites in the placenta.[832] Nevertheless, it is time consuming and requires digestion for 2 hours with trypsin of a 100-g tissue sample that has been shipped under appropriate conditions (see the protocol in reference 634). Moreover, it requires animal facilities, and the results are not obtained until 4 and 6 weeks after inoculation: First serology is performed on the mice, and when serology on the mice is positive, cysts must also be detected in their brains. Robert-Gangneux and colleagues[830] suggested that the combination of PCR and mouse inoculation has the advantage of early diagnosis, along with the specificity of parasite isolation, but mouse inoculation is restricted to specialized laboratories. When the volume of amniotic fluid is limited, the priority in any case should be given to PCR testing.[831] Placental samples have been inoculated into cell cultures, but this method is no longer recommended because of its low sensitivity (29.6 %).[833]

Cord blood is often processed together with the placenta. Using cord blood and a PCR targeting gene *B1* yielded a sensitivity of 21.2%, with a specificity of 100%.[829] Using mouse inoculation, parasites were isolated from cord blood in 43% of cases.[452]

PCR has also been used on a limited number of samples of neonatal amniotic fluid with promising results.[831] In our experience, this type of sampling is limited by difficulties in the appropriate collection of neonatal amniotic fluid during labor.

Parasites have been detected in the CSF of 46% of infected infants[3]; however, this invasive method of diagnosis should be reserved solely for newborns with neurologic signs, for whom the diagnosis of toxoplasmosis is not certain. The quality of the results depends on the purity of the CSF, which is often contaminated by blood that hampers the performance of the serologic test and the detection of biochemical markers, such as an increased concentration of protein in the CSF.[834]

PCR on urine is a noninvasive, simple method to detect the presence of parasites, but few data are available on this approach. Olariu and colleagues[3] reported a sensitivity of 50% in a cohort of 10 infected infants, and another study reported positive results for urinary PCR in 4 infants who displayed hydrocephalus or cerebral calcification.[835]

Cellular Immunity

Few studies have investigated the importance of assays based on the detection of *Toxoplasma* antigen-stimulated cellular immune responses in the diagnosis of congenital toxoplasmosis during the perinatal period. Moreover, reports have been contradictory, with some finding a lack of response[99] or age-related impairment.[100] Others, including one in which antigen-stimulated expression of CD25 (IL-2 receptor) was determined by flow cytometry, detected a cellular immune response in most congenitally infected infants or newborns.[102,836] An in vitro IFN-γ release assay has also been evaluated using blood collected from infants for serologic purposes. Plasma was kept for the serologic investigation, cell pellets were re-suspended in culture medium, stimulated for 24 hours with crude parasitic antigen, and the IFN-γ released into the medium was assayed by ELISA. In a cohort of 62 infants younger than 1 year who received antenatal treatment, the sensitivity and specificity of the assay were 94% and 98%, respectively.[685] This test, which does not require additional sample collection from the infants, appears to be very promising. However, one drawback is that it has to be performed on freshly withdrawn blood.

INTERPRETATION OF TEST RESULTS TO MAKE AN INFORMED DECISION REGARDING TREATMENT

The diagnosis of congenital toxoplasmosis often relies on a wide range of tests that do not always give consistent results. Anecdotal reports abound that present cases in which only one test gave positive results. Doctors are therefore tempted to prescribe all possible tests and disregard the cost-benefit aspect. It must be borne in mind that, when one test is positive, this might be due to its high sensitivity but also to a lack of specificity. Various factors can have an impact on test performance, including the stage of pregnancy at maternal infection; others, such as antenatal treatment, are more questionable but have to be considered in the final interpretation. Some tests do not carry the same weight in the decision to treat a patient, which complicates the task of care providers. Therefore two different situations have to be considered:

1. *Information on infection during pregnancy is available: The pretest probability of congenital infection is known* (Table 31-13).

Table 31-13 Probability of Congenital Toxoplasmosis According to the Gestational Age at Infection of the Mother and Antenatal Diagnosis (PCR on Amniotic Fluid): Majority of Mothers Received Treatment

	GESTATIONAL AGE AT INFECTION OF THE MOTHER		
	6 weeks	**18 weeks**	**30 weeks**
Pretest probability %	2.2	23.0	56.0
Probability with a positive antenatal diagnosis % (95% CI)	64.0 (39-100)	95.4 (91-100)	98.2 (69.2-100)
Probability with a negative antenatal diagnosis % (95% CI)	1.0 (0.2-1.7)	10.0 (7-12.5)	22.6 (13.2-31.4)

Modified from Rabilloud M, Wallon M, Peyron F: In utero and at birth diagnosis of congenital toxoplasmosis: use of likelihood ratios for clinical management, *Pediatr Infect Dis J* 29:421-425, 2010; with permission.
CI, Confidence interval; *PCR*, polymerase chain reaction.

Tests for the presence of IgM and IgA should be carried out on peripheral blood. When only cord blood is available, all positive tests must be confirmed on peripheral blood. PCR on placenta (and cord blood, particularly if placenta is not available) should also be performed. When all tests yield positive results, treatment should be given.

When PCR is negative but IgM or IgA is present in the peripheral blood, the infant should be treated and comparative Western blot carried out to confirm the diagnosis.

When PCR is positive but tests for IgM/IgA are negative, additional tests, such as comparative Western blot or lymphocyte stimulation should be undertaken. If these tests are negative, treatment may be withheld, but the infant should be followed up regularly until the disappearance of IgG (see "Management of Congenitally Infected Children and Long-Term Outcome"); if the pretest probability of congenital infection is high, serologic investigations should be performed once again by 2 weeks of age.

When IgM/IgA are not detected and PCR is negative, treatment should be withheld, but the infant should be followed up regularly until the disappearance of IgG; if the pretest probability of congenital infection is high, serologic investigations should be repeated by 2 weeks of age. If these tests are also negative, the infant should be followed up until the disappearance of IgG.

2. *No information on infection during pregnancy is available.*

A specific workup is required when the clinical presentation resembles congenital toxoplasmosis or on the basis of neonatal screening (as is performed in Massachusetts and New Hampshire). Because none of the clinical signs are pathognomonic,[1] laboratory investigation plays a pivotal role in diagnostic evaluation.

First, maternal serology must be checked (see "Diagnosis of Maternal Infection"). If the results are negative or do not favor recent infection (low IgG titers and negative IgM), congenital toxoplasmosis is very improbable. When the results are positive, the entire workup must be undertaken and treatment decisions based on the results obtained.

In conclusion, the diagnosis of congenital toxoplasmosis at birth is often a complicated task, and interpretation can be difficult when heterogeneous results are found for subclinical infections. The decision to treat with potentially toxic compounds relies entirely on laboratory findings; it is therefore advisable to refer samples to specialized laboratories and consult with experts in the management of this condition.

POSTNATAL TREATMENT

Anti-*Toxoplasma* Therapy (See "Drugs Active Against *Toxoplasma gondii*")

There are no universal guidelines for postnatal treatment, and practices vary between centers. Spiramycin is no longer used for the postnatal treatment of congenital toxoplasmosis because of the lack of diffusion of this molecule into the brain parenchyma. This lack of diffusion has been known since the 1990s because of the occurrence of *Toxoplasma* encephalitis in subjects with AIDS taking spiramycin[837] and thanks to modeling studies on rhesus monkeys.[838]

Current treatment regimens are based on the continuous use of pyrimethamine and a sulfonamide.[779,839] We recommend that severe forms of congenital toxoplasmosis be treated with pyrimethamine and sulfadiazine for 1 year (Table 31-14). The dosage of pyrimethamine is 1 mg/kg/day for the first 6 months and then 0.5 mg/kg/day for the following months; folinic acid should be given as well to diminish bone marrow suppression (either 10 mg three times per week or 25 mg twice per week). For subclinical or milder forms, different regimens can be used (see Table 31-14). One such alternative regimen, particularly for treatment beyond the first 2 months of age and in countries other than the United States, where it is not used, is the combination of pyrimethamine and sulfadoxine (Fansidar): 1.25 mg/kg and 25 mg/kg, respectively, given every 10 days.[840]

In newborns, pyrimethamine has a half-life of 64 ± 12 hours; its concentration in the CSF is 10% to 25% of that in serum, but its concentration in the brain parenchyma is three to four times higher than that in serum.[841,842] In children, sulfadiazine has a half-life of 21.3 hours,[843] and its concentration in the CSF is 10% to 80% of that in serum.[844] The half-life of sulfadoxine is 6.6 days[845,846] but varies from 1.5 to 22.4 days[845]; the concentration of this drug in the CSF has not been studied other than in the context of meningitis. For pyrimethamine, as for sulfadiazine and sulfadoxine, all the pharmacokinetic studies carried out to date indicate considerable interindividual variability. The pharmacologic and clinical data for other antiparasitic drugs, such as azithromycin, clindamycin, and atovaquone, are too fragmentary for these drugs to be used in newborns or infants.[847]

Table 31-14 Postnatal Treatment for Infants With Congenital Toxoplasmosis

FOR SEVERE FORMS OF CONGENITAL TOXOPLASMOSIS (HYDROCEPHALUS, >3 CEREBRAL CALCIFICATIONS, MACULAR CHORIORETINITIS)*

Pyrimethamine	1 mg/kg/day for 6 months, then 0.5 mg/kg/day for 6 months
Sulfadiazine	100 mg/kg/day in two daily divided doses, 1 year
Folinic acid	10 mg 3× weekly or 25 mg 2× weekly, 1 year

FOR SUBCLINICAL AND MILDER FORMS OF CONGENITAL TOXOPLASMOSIS:

Two possible protocols:

Protocol A†

Primary regimen:

Pyrimethamine	1 mg/kg/day for 2 months, then 0.5 mg/kg/day for 10 months
Sulfadiazine	100 mg/kg/day in two daily divided doses, 1 year
Folinic acid	10 mg 3× weekly or 25 mg 2× weekly, 1 year

Alternative regimen: May be used for subclinical/mild forms, and/or for difficulties in compliance, and/or frequent hematologic adverse effects

Pyrimethamine and sulfadoxine (Fansidar)	1.25 mg/kg every 10 days 25 mg/kg every 10 days, 1 year
Folinic acid	10 mg 3× weekly or 25 mg 2× weekly, 1 year

The authors recommend starting with the primary regimen of pyrimethamine plus sulfadiazine for the first 2 months then continuing treatment with pyrimethamine plus sulfadoxine, which has a longer half-life and is more convenient as it is administered every 10 days.

With either regimen, leukocyte counts should be checked at day 0 and 15 and monthly thereafter. Therapy should be discontinued (but folinic acid continued) whenever neutrophils decrease below 750/mm^3. Monthly tests for proteinuria are recommended in children treated with pyrimethamine and sulfadiazine.

Protocol B‡

Postnatal treatment of the infant and child

Medication	Dosage Therapy	Indication for Therapy	Duration of Therapy
Pyrimethamine	Loading dose: 1 mg/kg every 12 hours for 2 days; then beginning on day 3, 1 mg/kg per day for 2 or 6 months; then this dose every Monday, Wednesday, and Friday	When congenital toxoplasmosis diagnosed in infant	1 year
Sulfadiazine *plus*	50 mg/kg every 12 hours		1 year
Folinic acid (Leucovorin)	10 mg 3×/week		1 year
Corticosteroids§ (prednisone)	0.5 mg/kg every 12 hours	When CSF protein is ≥1 g/dL or when active chorioretinitis threatens vision	During and for 1 week after

CI, Confidence interval; *CSF,* cerebrospinal fluid.

*Authors' recommendations, which are modified from McAuley J, Boyer KM, Patel D, et al: Early and longitudinal evaluations of treated infants and children and untreated historical patients with congenital toxoplasmosis: the Chicago Collaborative Treatment Trial, *Clin Infect Dis* 18:38-72, 1994.

†Modified from: Guidelines of the work group on congenital toxoplasmosis: Croix Rousse hospital (Lyon, France), Timone hospital (Marseille, France), Trousseau hospital (Paris, France).

‡Recommendations from the *Toxoplasma* Serology Laboratory at the Palo Alto Medical Foundation [PAMF-TSL], Palo Alto, Calif ; phone: 650-853-4828; http://www.pamf.org/serology/; email: toxolab@pamf.org.

§Corticosteroids should be used only in conjunction with pyrimethamine, sulfadiazine, and folinic acid treatment and should be continued until signs of inflammation (high CSF protein, ≥1 g/dL) or active chorioretinitis that threatens vision have subsided; dosage can then be tapered and the steroids discontinued.

The optimal duration of postnatal treatment is unknown. Treatment for 1 month does not seem to improve the neurologic or ophthalmologic prognosis of children versus children receiving no treatment.[779,848] Most current treatment regimens are given for 1 year.[462,779,785,849] Treatment durations of between 3 months in Denmark,[787] and 2 years in France have also been used,[839] resulting in apparently similar long-term results. A prospective randomized study is currently underway comparing 3 and 12 months of postnatal treatment for nonsevere forms of congenital toxoplasmosis (ClinicalTrials.gov; identifier: NCT01202500).

Treatment monitoring and adverse effects: Hematologic toxicity is the principal adverse effect of pyrimethamine. Blood cell counts should be performed at weekly to monthly intervals, depending on initial tolerance and the dose schedule used for pyrimethamine. Anemia and thrombopenia occur, but both are rare.[785,850] By contrast, neutropenia ($<1000/mm^3$) is observed in more than half the children treated with pyrimethamine and sulfadiazine[779,785] but more rarely in children treated with pyrimethamine and sulfadoxine.[839] The addition of folinic acid (leucovorin) to the drug combination reduces the risk of neutropenia. Folinic acid is thus administered throughout treatment.[785,850,851] If severe neutropenia (<750 mm^3) is observed, the pyrimethamine and sulfonamide treatment should be stopped and the dose of folinic acid increased to 75 mg to 100 mg/week.[851] Treatment can generally be restarted 1 to 2 weeks later, once the neutropenia has resolved. Convulsions have been reported in cases of pyrimethamine overdose resulting from the lack of a pediatric formulation, but the convulsions have resolved without sequelae.[852,853]

Depending on the ethnicity of the patient, it may be necessary to check levels of erythrocyte glucose-6-phosphate dehydrogenase activity before initiating sulfonamide treatment, to avoid the risk of hemolysis. The use of other sulfonamides or sulfonamide-containing combinations such as cotrimoxazole during the treatment phase is contraindicated because of the possibility of aggravating hematologic toxicity.

Skin allergies resulting from the use of sulfonamides occur at a frequency of 1% to 2% in treated children; they are manifested in the form of a skin rash or urticaria during initial treatment.[839,849] Rare, severe, generalized allergic reactions, such as drug reaction with eosinophilia and systemic symptoms (DRESS) syndrome, have been described after the reintroduction of treatment for late ophthalmologic events.[854] A few reports of Stevens-Johnson syndrome and toxic epidermal necrolysis have been published related to the use of sulfadiazine for AIDS patients.[855,856] Digestive problems (abdominal pain, nausea) are frequent at the start of treatment and gradually resolve over the course of a few weeks.

Children should receive all routine immunisations,[857] although if severe neutropenia has occurred (<500-600 per mm^3) as a result of therapy, immunization may be delayed until it has resolved.

Adjunctive Therapy

Corticosteroid treatment (1 mg/kg/day prednisone equivalent) should be administered in association with antiparasitic treatment in cases of inflammatory chorioretinitis or active damage to the CNS, with CSF protein concentrations exceeding 1 g/dL.[851] In cases of obstructive hydrocephalus, a CSF shunt may be required.[848] If antiepileptic treatments are given, the clinician should be aware that doing so can complicate treatment because phenobarbital decreases the half-life of pyrimethamine[841] and carbamazepine frequently causes neutropenia.[851]

BREASTFEEDING

Breastfeeding is not contraindicated for infants born from mothers who experienced primary infection with *Toxoplasma gondii* during pregnancy. Only one published case report suggested possible transmission of toxoplasmosis through breastfeeding.[858] Moreover, extensive experience by numerous teams involved in the care for children with congenital toxoplasmosis has found that breastfeeding is not associated with untoward effects.

Management of Congenitally Infected Children and Long-Term Outcome

SEROLOGIC FOLLOW-UP

In Treated Infants

When congenital toxoplasmosis is confirmed, the newborn is treated immediately. However, no consensus has been reached on the frequency of follow-up serologic testing. In our setting, to alleviate any constraints on parents and infants, serologic tests are performed at 1 month of age and then every 3 months, when ophthalmologic and clinical follow-up are also performed.

Typical patterns of serologic evolution reflect the combined effects of elimination of passively acquired maternal IgG and active production of IgG by the infant. Reductions in IgG titers, in some instances transiently declining to undetectable, are observed during treatment, followed by a rebound when treatment is discontinued (Fig. 31-41); this is true even when the Sabin-Feldman dye test is used.[405,859]

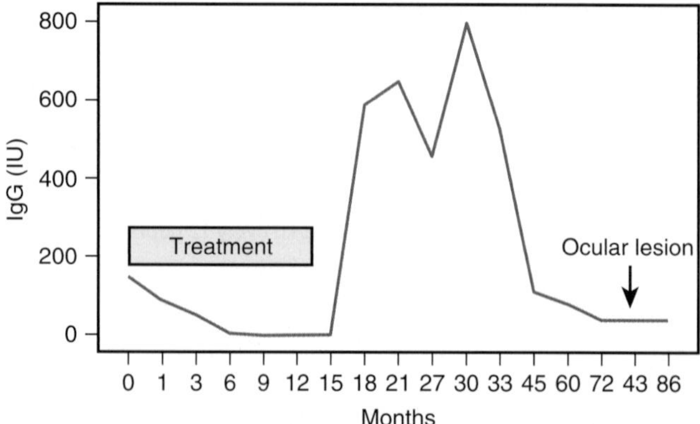

Figure 31-41 Evolution of immunoglobulin G (IgG) in an infant treated for congenital toxoplasmosis. Note transient negativity of IgG under treatment, followed by a rebound with high titers lasting for 27 months. Funduscopy was normal up to the age of 43 months, when the infant presented with chorioretinitis (inactive lesion). Serology remained unchanged at low levels.

This transient phenomenon has been observed more frequently when maternal infection occurred during the first two trimesters of pregnancy.[859] Because wide interindividual variations in the pharmacokinetics of the combination of pyrimethamine and sulfadoxine have been observed even when dosage is adjusted for body weight,[429] one hypothesis is that high concentrations of antiparasitic drugs alter the production of IgG directly or by acting on the multiplication of parasites. Of interest, the same pattern has been observed with in vitro antigen-stimulated IFN-γ release assays, in that the responses in these assays paralleled the fluctuations in IgG titers in treated infants.[685] Therefore it is crucial not to question the initial diagnosis of congenital toxoplasmosis based on transient changes in IgG antibody titers but rather to continue regular, routine monitoring to determine whether these changes are transient or sustained, with only sustained loss indicating the absence of infection. Although rare, four cases of congenital infection in which IgG antibodies were never detected were reported by McAuley and colleagues.[457]

Serologic rebound occurs very frequently (58%-98%) when treatment is discontinued.[457,860-862] Although not observed by other authors in this context,[861] Djurkovic-Djakovic and colleagues[862] found an atypical pattern during rebound in which the differential agglutination (AC/HS) test and IgG avidity were suggestive of chronic disease despite a high rate of detection of IgA and IgM. Some authors have suggested that rebounds are due to the reactivation of parasites,[457] because rebound is common after discontinuation and rare during treatment. Perhaps consistent with this hypothesis, in children experiencing a rebound, increased numbers of circulating specific IgG antibody–secreting cells,[863] a switch toward the Th2 immune response,[864] and the presence of IgE antibodies in 50% of the cases have been reported.[405,864] In contrast, although polyclonal activation of antibody production can be ruled out because of stable overall IgG concentrations, nonspecific oligoclonal activation cannot be excluded because 15% of children who exhibited a rebound displayed the same kinetic profile for rubella IgG.[861] In monozygotic twins, we observed a similar diphasic pattern in each child.[800]

Intracranial calcifications are associated with risk of rebound, whereas antenatal treatment was not found to influence its occurrence.[861] These authors did not find any benefit in prescribing additional treatment, which did not reduce risk of rebound or ocular lesions. Moreover, serologic rebounds, although frequent, are not associated with unfavorable ocular outcomes. Nevertheless, we believe it prudent to perform regular follow-up evaluations of such infants, especially follow-up ophthalmologic examinations[41]; we suggest that funduscopy be performed every 3 months while the IgG titers remain elevated. It also important that parents and care providers be informed of the likelihood of the occurrence of rebounds and their good prognosis before treatment is stopped.

As illustrated in Figure 31-41, the development of ocular lesions may not be associated with a change in antibody titers. In the case shown, an ocular lesion was diagnosed at the age of 3.5 years, whereas all previous funduscopy examinations performed by a trained ophthalmologist had been normal. Thus serology is not a useful way to monitor ocular status, for which regular funduscopy is essential.

In Untreated Infants

A negative workup at birth cannot exclude congenital toxoplasmosis. Presentation of the disease is frequently subclinical,[136] and the results of serologic tests in early infancy may not be definitive (see "Clinical Investigation" and "Laboratory Diagnosis"), necessitating regular serologic follow-up to provide clarity. The unanimously accepted criterion to rule out congenital infection is the complete, sustained loss of specific IgG antibodies, which occurs within the first year of life in an untreated infant, demonstrating that the fetus has eliminated maternally transmitted IgG and has not synthesized his or her own.[865] The half-life of IgG is approximately 30 days; therefore the decline in IgG antibodies in infant sera is expected to be approximately 50% per month (Fig. 31-42). This follow-up, which requires regular sampling in a healthy looking infant, may not be easily accepted by parents, to whom the importance of ruling out congenital toxoplasmosis, with its attendant risk of ocular lesions later in life, should be explained. To alleviate the burden of the follow-up, we have implemented a noninvasive salivary sampling test to monitor the decrease in IgG (E. Chapey and associates; to be published). The saliva is collected using two microsponges (Beaver Visitec, Waltham, Mass) (Fig. 31-43) placed between the lower gum and the cheek for at least 2 minutes. The microsponges are then placed in a swab

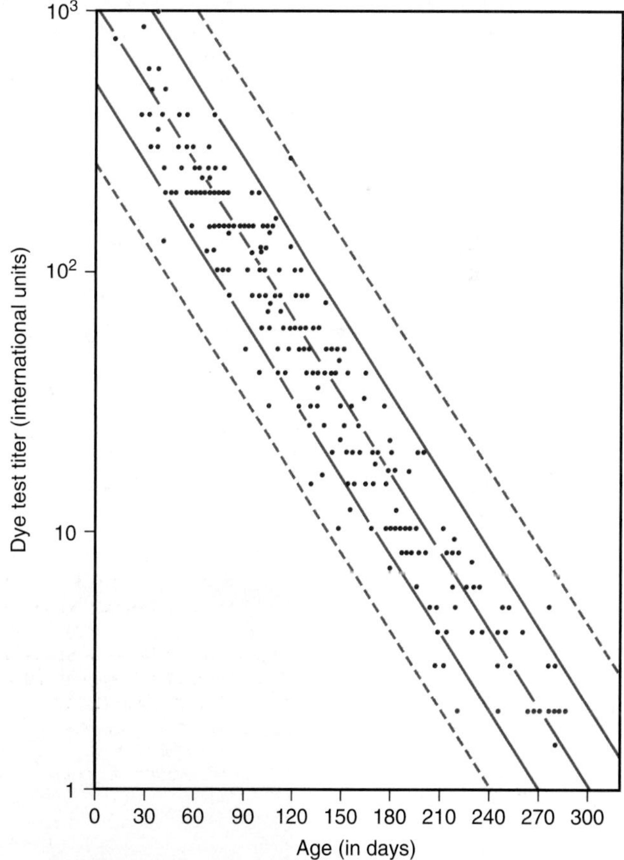

Figure 31-42 Decrease in maternally transmitted *Toxoplasma* antibodies (dye test) in uninfected infants. The two parallel lines indicate one-half and twice the titer, plus or minus one twofold dilution. The result in one serum sample of each pair is on the theoretical line and is not represented by a dot. The result in the other serum sample of each pair is represented by a dot.

storage tube (Salimetrics, State College, Pa) and kept at 4° C. The saliva is recovered by centrifugation at 3000 g for 15 minutes at 4° C and stored at −20° C until use in a routine ELISA. Figure 31-44 shows the parallel between IgG patterns obtained from blood and saliva in noninfected infants.

LONG-TERM OUTCOME

Congenital toxoplasmosis is essentially a neurologic and ophthalmologic chronic disease because recurrences and relapses of ocular lesions can occur throughout life. Therefore the outcome of the disease and the evaluation of its burden are dependent on the duration of follow-up.

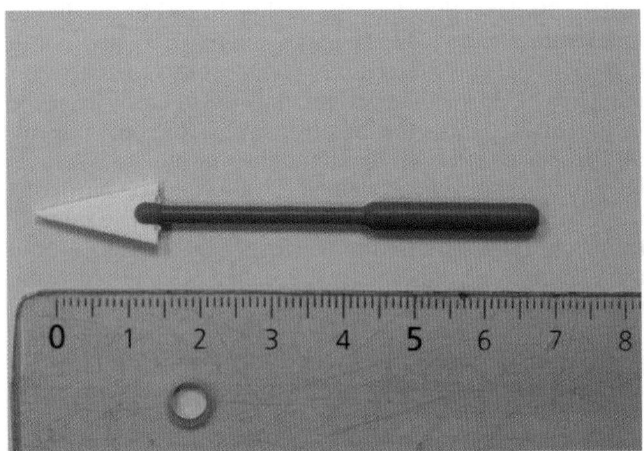

Figure 31-43 Microsponges (Beaver Visitec, Waltham, Mass) used for saliva tests.

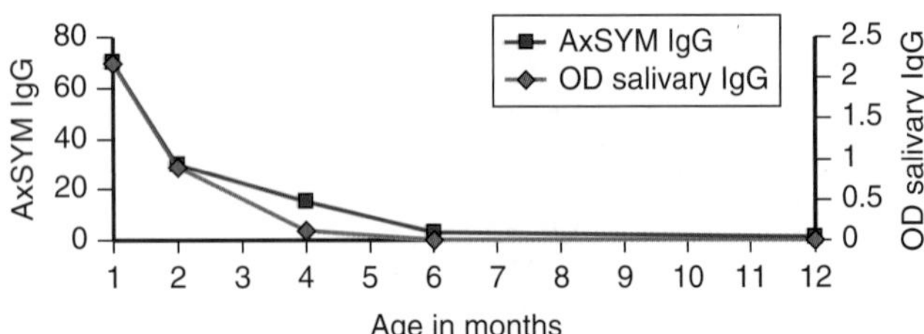

Figure 31-44 Similar pattern of immunoglobulin G disappearance in blood (ELISA AxSYM, Abbott Diagnostics, Abbott Park, Ill) and optical density (OD) in saliva in an uninfected infant. *IgG*, Immunoglobulin G.

Ophthalmologic Evolution

General Considerations. From the clinical picture of an ocular lesion, be it active or healed, it is virtually impossible to differentiate lesions resulting from congenital or postnatal infection.[866] Patients with active ocular disease resulting from congenital toxoplasmosis tend to be younger at the time of diagnosis of their ocular manifestation (9.1 ± 8.8 compared with 21.7 ± 12.6 years)[867] and to present more frequently with bilateral disease (44%- 64% vs. 2%-4%) and macular involvement (49% vs. 25%) (Fig. 31-45).[867-869] Moreover, long-term secondary eye pathologies, such as strabismus, cataracts, and microphthalmia are more prevalent after congenital than acquired infection.[870] Certain manifestations are more commonly associated with acquired disease, for example, atypical large retinochoroidal lesions in the periphery in the absence of a scar in an elderly person.[242,871] In either situation, specific IgM is not usually found because active ocular disease usually arises long after primary parasitemia and specific IgM have disappeared.[181,867,872] Thus, in practice, the ophthalmologist is usually not able to differentiate between congenital and acquired disease.[866,873] Herein, any information pertaining to the management and long-term outcome of ocular lesions in congenital toxoplasmosis has been derived from cases in which the congenital route of acquisition was confirmed in advance. Nonetheless, it is worth noting that the possibility that an active lesion in an individual with documented congenital infection occurred as a result of superinfection rather than reactivation cannot be excluded.

Evolution of Ocular Disease in Children. Unbiased data derived from untreated cohorts are not available for European patients,[874,875] and reports from American referral centers are alarming.[3] In children treated in utero and throughout infancy, in contrast, the severity of disease in general and specifically of ocular lesions may be remarkably less severe.[466]

The frequency of ocular lesions in treated children increases with the length of follow-up. Lesions are first detected in many instances before the age of 5 years (Table 31-15)[461,876] but may arise more than 12 years after birth[428,463] (Figs. 31-46 and 31-47). Lesions are present in 17% after follow-up over 3 years[877] and in 24% after 6 years.[136]

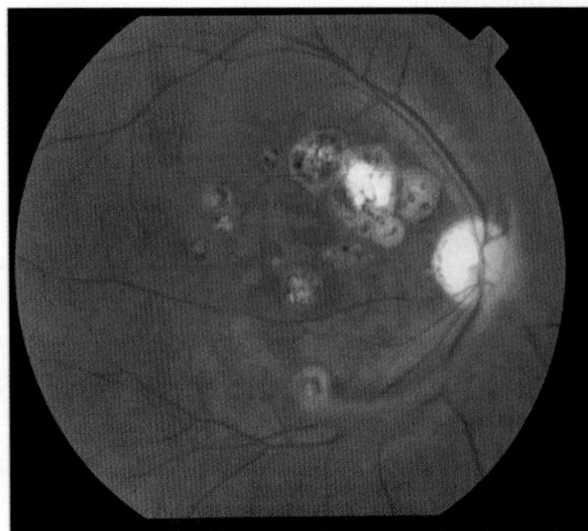

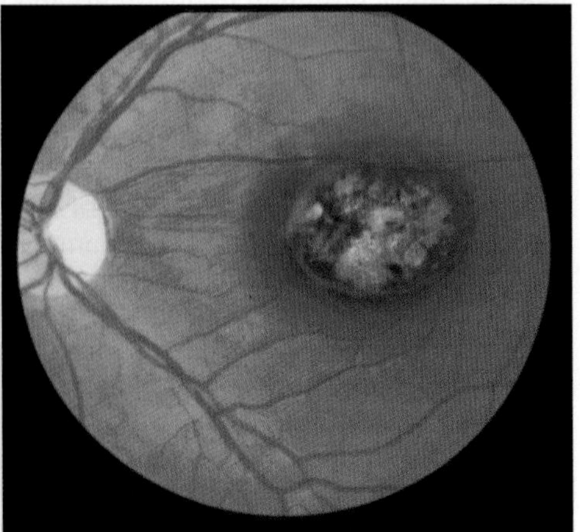

Figure 31-45 Typical appearance of bilateral, inactive, scarred ocular lesions in a 20-year-old male with congenital toxoplasmosis who had previously experienced recurrent ocular disease. Note the multiple small scars in the right eye *(left image)*, each resulting from disease reactivation over an interval of 12 years, and the large colobomatous macular scar *(right image)* typical of congenital infection and probably present since birth.

Expanding the follow-up to more 10.5 years, Wallon and colleagues[136,461,877] reported ocular lesions in 29.8%, which were unilateral in 69.0% and did not cause vision loss in 80.6%. Bilateral visual impairment is fortunately rare, and two thirds may present with normal vision in either eye. Recurrences or new ocular lesions may occur up to 12 years after birth[463] and sometimes even later (Fig. 31-48). Only every sixth case (17%) has active ocular disease at diagnosis. In treated children, secondary ocular pathologies resulting from the inflammatory tissue damage of ocular toxoplasmosis were reported in 19%, with squinting in 16%, microphthalmia in 5%, and unilateral cataract formation in 3%, as the three most frequently encountered pathologies.[870] This is below expectations from other series, suggesting that the underlying treatment was able to ameliorate the severity of ocular disease.[457,878]

Evolution of Disease in Congenital Toxoplasmosis in Europe and the Americas. Despite central localization of the lesion in up to 65% of instances, the overall functional prognosis of congenital toxoplasmosis in Europe is better than would be expected on the basis of literature findings, with less than 2% to 9% suffering bilateral visual impairment[870,877] Although the consequences of congenital toxoplasmosis are rarely severe in European children treated in utero and until the end of their first year of life, annual postnatal monitoring may be justified because of the persisting risk of ocular disease.[137,463,876] Indeed, regular follow-up until adulthood was performed in the great majority of affected individuals (98%) and, in most instances (92%), was reported to be reassuring. Nevertheless, 11% found the follow-ups frightening; these were predominantly patients with low visual acuity and visual function scores.[879]

By contrast to European patients, in North American patients, macular involvement was reported in 54% and bilateral involvement in 41% of those with postnatally treated congenital ocular toxoplasmosis.[138] There exists some evidence that severity of clinical manifestations is related to delayed onset and shorter duration of therapy.[457] In one Dutch study, the risk for recurrences was estimated at 0.2 episodes per year after a follow-up of up to 41 years, and a decreased risk was associated with the duration of the recurrence-free interval and increasing age at first clinical episode.[104] In South America, in contrast, the burden of disease,[636,641,869] and, in particular, the incidence and severity of ocular manifestations and their impact on visual function, are much more severe, with 60% to 80% of affected individuals presenting ocular lesions.[77,530,869,878,880]

Recurrences are observed in more than 50% of Colombian patients during childhood and may thus be more frequent than in Europe (34%),[137,463] whereas the recurrence rate, in contrast, does not differ.[881] In Brazilian patients, ocular involvement is already observed in up to 70% shortly after

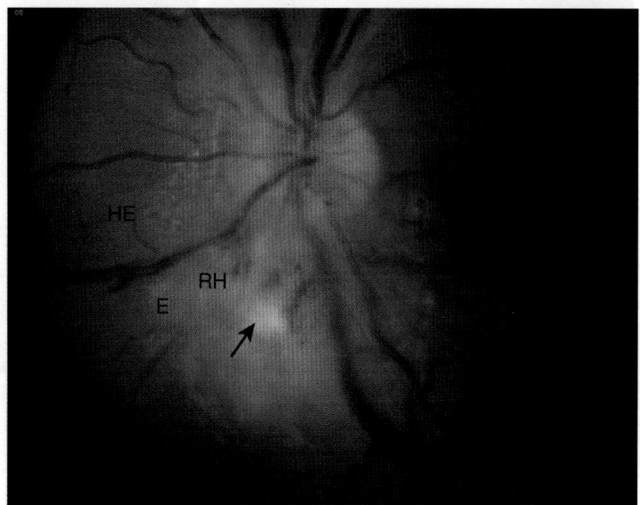

Figure 31-46 Young male with confirmed congenital toxoplasmosis who developed a first ocular lesion at the age of 17 years close to the optic nerve head (arrow). Note the surrounding edema *(E)*, hard exudates *(HE)* and retinal hemorrhage *(RH)*, together with the hyperemic vessels indicative of vasculitis, which contrasts with discrete (here not visible) areas of vitreal infiltration.

Table 31-15 Ocular Disease in Congenital Toxoplasmosis in Different Areas of the World: France, Europe, Denmark, United States, and Brazil

Author	Reference	Follow-up (years)	Treatment	*n* (CT)*	*n* (OD)†	% (OD)†	% Present at Birth	% With New Lesions‡	% With Bilateral Disease
Wallon (F), 2014	935	10.5	Yes	477	142	29.8	5.6	94.4	31
Faucher (F), 2012	428	>10	Yes	127	24	18.9	8.7	12.6	
Berrébi (F), 2010	461	>10	Yes	107	28	26			
Tan (EU), 2007	877	4.8	NA	281	49	17			
Schmidt (DK), 2006	786	3	Yes	47	9	19.2	14.9	6.4	4.3
Phan (US), 2008	137	10.8	Yes	108	34	31	25	14	12
Vasconcelos-Santos (BR), 2009	869	0.3	No	178	142	79.8	79.8		63.5
Melamed (BR), 2010	880	0.4	No	44	29	65.9	84.3	15.7	71

BR, Brazil; *CT*, congenital toxoplasmosis; *DK*, Denmark; *EU*, Europe; *F*, France; *NA*, not available; *US*, United States.
*Number of cases of congenital toxoplasmosis evaluated.
†Number and percent of cases with ocular disease (OD) resulting from congenital toxoplasmosis.
‡New lesions detected after birth.

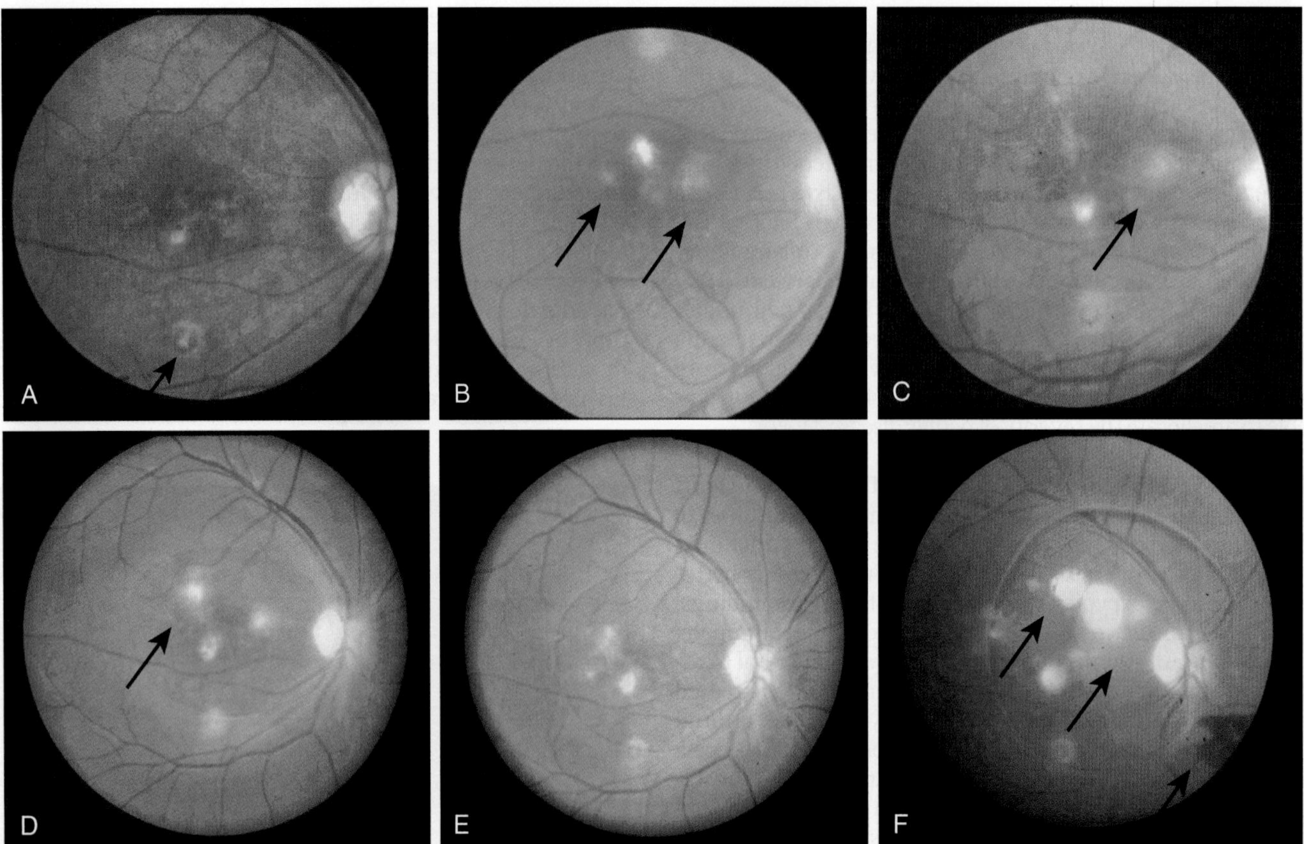

Figure 31-47 Same patient as in Figure 31-45. Although the large old lesion in his left eye remained stable over a period of 14 years, his right eye went through several recurrences. The six images represent, in chronologic order, the evolution of his disease before reaching the quiescent state represented in Figure 31-45. The left eye had a visual acuity of 20/400 but never developed recurrences. By contrast, he experienced several recurrences of active disease in his right eye between 8 and 20 years of age, which, although still having a normal visual acuity, is at lifelong risk of severe permanent vision loss because of the proximity of lesions to the macula. This patient had first presented at the age of 6 years at the Department of Ophthalmology, University of Bern when he was sent with suspected squinting by his school physician. The small lesion on the first image (**A,** *arrow*) outside the vascular arcades and the macular scar in his left eye (Fig. 31-45) had been noted shortly after birth. The remaining central lesions in his right eye had developed asymptomatically. At the age of 8 years, he reported visual irritation, and two new active lesions (**B,** *arrows*) were discovered. Eighteen months later, a discrete reactivation was found during routine screening (**C,** *arrow*), whereas the next recurrence at the age of 12 years was symptomatic **(D).** The retinal lesions remained quiet **(E)** until the age of 16 years, when he developed two new foveal lesions (**F,** *upper two arrows*) with progressive loss of vision and secondary vitreal detachment, which was associated with a preretinal hemorrhage (**F,** *bottom arrow*) and adding to the discrete preretinal ring structure, best detectable superior to the optic nerve head.

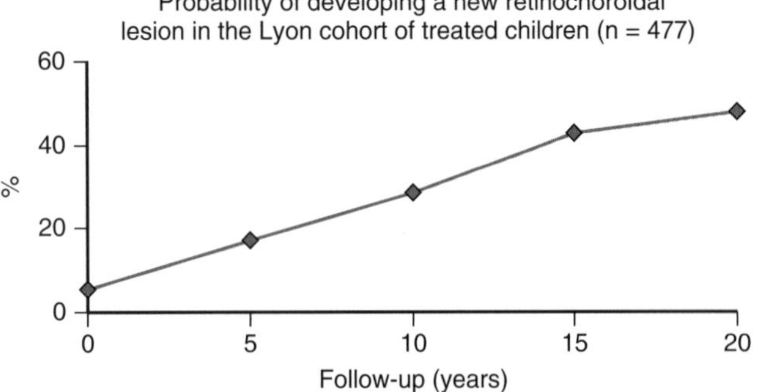

Figure 31-48 Probability of developing a new retinochoroidal lesion in the Lyon cohort of treated children (n = 477.) Among the children, 5.6% had a first lesion detected shortly after birth, as had nearly half (48.1%) of the patients followed up for 20 years. (Modified from Wallon M, Peyron F, Cornu C, et al: Congenital *Toxoplasma* infection: monthly prenatal screening decreases transmission and improves clinical outcome at age 3 years, *Clin Infect Dis* 56:1223-1231, 2013.)

birth, the central retina is involved in the majority, and in two thirds (65.9%), disease is already bilateral. Secondary eye lesions are identified in 50%, with cataract, microphthalmia, and strabismus being the most prevalent.[880]

Macular lesions and bilateral involvement are more frequently reported in congenital than in postnatally-acquired disease in European cohorts. Moreover, congenital infection seems to be a risk factor for vision loss.[428,449] From cohorts of European individuals with ocular toxoplasmosis in whom congenital and acquired infection are not differentiated, it is known that visual function is generally good. Ocular lesions are found in the visual field in 94% of eyes, whereas visual acuity is normal in 59% and nearly normal (>20/40) in 13.5%, which is consistent with the observation that chorioretinal damage is greater in the peripheral than central retina.[882,883] Moderate-to-severe functional impairment may be evident in 65.2% as visual field reduction and in 27.5% as reduced visual acuity.[883] Of interest, visual field defects are compensated by neural mechanisms of filling-in at the blind spot and thus not recognized as scotoma by the patient.[884]

Table 31-16 Diagnostic and Therapeutic Follow-up for Children With Ocular Disease Caused by Congenital Toxoplasmosis: Protocol of the Interdisciplinary Group of the University of Bern

Age (months)	Therapy	Serology IgG, IgA, IgM	Skull Sonography	Psychomotoric Evaluations*	Ophthalmologic Examinations†
0	+*	+	+		+
3	+		+		+
6	+	+	+	+†	
12	Stop	+		+†	+
15-18		+		+†	+
2 years				+†	+‡
4 years				+†	+‡
10 years				+†	+‡

IgA, IgG, and IgM, Immunoglobulins A, G, and M, respectively.
*See text and Table 31-14 for recommendations regarding treatment regimens.
†Together with routine pediatric examinations and, if pathologic manifestations are detected, referral to a neuropediatric center.
‡Annual examination of the eyes until the age of 10 years. Thereafter follow-up evaluations are not routinely performed in the absence of symptoms and recurrences. In case of disease reactivation, the intervals should be shortened to 6 months for 2 years.

Therapy and Follow-up of Ocular Disease in Congenital Toxoplasmosis. Any newly detected ocular lesion may be congenital or acquired in origin. In cases with confirmed congenital toxoplasmosis, the first detected lesion confirms the presence of ocular involvement and sets the stage for possible recurrences. Therefore treatment and regular follow-up may be prudent. Based on published evidence and clinical experience, the interdisciplinary consensus group in the University of Bern has proposed systematic follow-up as presented in Table 31-16.

There is no generally accepted therapeutic strategy for ocular recurrences of congenital toxoplasmosis after 1 year of age. No treatment kills bradyzoites, and available treatments have not been clearly demonstrated to affect visual outcomes and recurrence rates. Nevertheless, there exists general agreement that any lesion in an immunocompromised person needs to be treated. Because of the differences in parasite virulence, different treatment considerations are necessary for Europe and South America, with virulence in North America ranging in between. In South American patients, antiparasitic treatment should be considered for virtually any active ocular lesion because of the destructive potency of parasites, to ameliorate the inflammatory tissue response, and possibly reduce the risk for recurrences.[424] In European patients, the treatment strategy respects the localization and size of a lesion and the secondary tissue response.[885] It is widely accepted that (1) a lesion located in the retinal periphery does not benefit from treatment, and (2) an active lesion in the foveal region or close to the fovea or optic nerve head should be treated to minimize the risk of permanent vision loss[873] (Fig. 31-49).

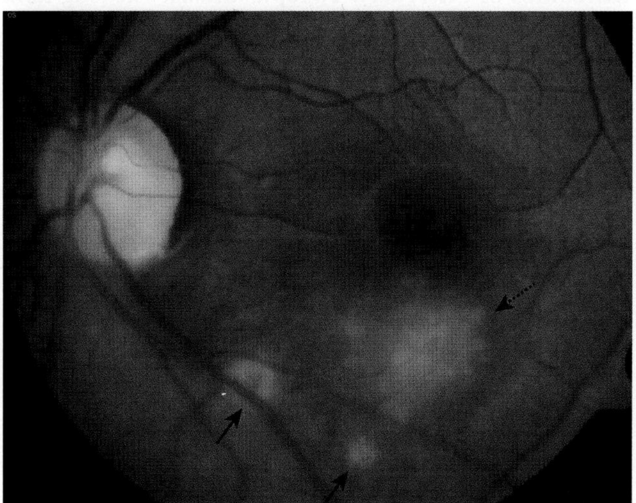

Figure 31-49 Typical fundus image of a 23-year-old male patient with known congenital toxoplasmosis, demonstrating two scars at the inferior vessel arcade of his left eye *(solid-line arrows)* and full vision before noticing a central shadow and loss of vision resulting from a new lesion developing right next to the fovea *(dashed-line arrow)*. The patient qualified for antiparasitic treatment to protect his fovea and maintain good vision.

Most established is therapy with pyrimethamine and sulfadiazine given over 4 to 8 weeks; the risk of bone marrow suppression with this combination[886] necessitates regular hematologic testing.[887] Although less effective in vitro and in animal models (see "Drugs Active Against *Toxoplasma gondii*"), the use of cotrimoxazole (a fixed combination of TMP and SMZ) for the treatment of ocular disease beyond infancy is increasing since the publication of a prospective clinical trial showing identical outcome in those receiving cotrimoxazole or the combination of pyrimethamine-sulfonamide.[423,424,888] Intravitreal administration of clindamycin in isolated ocular disease is also used by some.[424,501-504] However, it has to be borne in mind that congenital toxoplasmosis is not a local ocular disease; parasite DNA has sporadically been detected in the blood in ocular toxoplasmosis, more frequently so in South American cases.[129,131,133] Local treatment with clindamycin might thus be considered in adults with recurrent nonaggressive disease. If local or systemic steroids are used, they should only be used as an adjunct in combination with antiparasite therapy—corticosteroid use without antiparasitic coverage is contraindicated.[885] Anti-*Toxoplasma* prophylaxis may reduce the recurrence rate in endemic areas and in patients with severe immune defect and might be considered in individuals with more than one to two recurrences per year.[427,885]

Based on growing prospective clinical and experimental evidence,[4] it is the strong conviction of the authors, although the incidence of congenital toxoplasmosis is declining in European countries, that screening is the only effective way to diagnose and treat affected individuals at the earliest possible time, to promote the best achievable outcomes. The burden of disease is even higher in South American countries, particularly in Brazil; thus frequent and regular prenatal screening and earliest possible fetal and postnatal therapy is strongly recommended in this region. Moreover, based on the evidence from all large prospective cohort studies conducted worldwide, we recommend that all affected individuals should have regular ophthalmologic follow-up evaluations in early childhood, until they are able to report visual symptoms, then minimally thereafter until the age of 10 to 12 years of life. The aim of regular follow-up evaluation is the prevention of unnecessary loss of visual function; such follow-up is in our experience not only accepted, but appreciated by the affected patients.[879]

Neurologic Outcome

Outcomes of Untreated Toxoplasmosis. The long-term neurologic outcome for untreated children has been studied in several series, the most recent of which are those of Saxon, Wilson, and Koppe.[889-891] Saxon found that mean IQ was significantly lower in children who were asymptomatic at birth and not treated than in matched control subjects without congenital toxoplasmosis (93.2 vs. 109.8; $P = .016$). There was no difference in mean IQ between treated infected children and their matched control group (121 vs. 116).[890] Wilson studied 24 children allocated to two groups. Group I contained 13 infected asymptomatic children diagnosed at birth, and group II contained 11 symptomatic children (Table 31-17). Six of the children in group I and nine of those in group II had not been treated or were treated for less than 2 weeks, and those who had been treated had been so for only a short period ("at least 3 weeks").[891] With 8 to 10 years of follow-up, 3 of the children had severe neurologic sequelae, and the mean IQ was 85.3 for group I and 88.6 for group II. In the Dutch study of Koppe,[889] 7 subclinical congenitally infected children were untreated. After 20 years of follow-up, their school performance did not differ from a group of infected children born to mothers who had a seroconversion during pregnancy. These results are not in accordance with those of Saxon and Wilson, but the number of followed children (7) was very small.

The geographic origin of the studies (the United States vs. Europe) with different strains may also explain these conflicting results. These studies were not controlled and have methodologic limitations necessitating caution in their interpretation. Furthermore, they were carried out some time ago, and epidemiologic changes in toxoplasmosis suggest that the virulence of current strains and the parasite load during primary infection have substantially decreased over the last few decades, at least in Europe and North America. Because it is no longer possible to carry out prospective follow-up in the absence of postnatal treatment in children with congenital toxoplasmosis, this question will remain unanswered. Nevertheless, recent clinical data for children born in the United States with untreated toxoplasmosis diagnosed during the first 6 months of life are consistent with older data (brain calcification in 79.6% of cases, hydrocephalus in 67.7% of cases).[780]

Table 31-17 Adverse Sequelae in Children With Subclinical Congenital *Toxoplasma* Infection at Birth

Neurologic and Ophthalmologic Findings	Group I (Subclinical Infection at Birth, $n = 13$)	Group II (Symptomatic Infection at Birth, $n = 11$)
Untreated / treated	6 (46.2%) / 7 (53.8%)	9 (71.8%) / 2 (18.2%)
Mean age at last examination (years)	7.4	10.2
Hydrocephalus/microcephalus	1 (7.7%)	2 (18.2%)
Seizures	1 (7.7%)	3 (27.3%)
Severe psychomotor retardation	1 (7.7%)	2 (18.2%)
Transiently delayed psychomotor development	2 (15.4%)	2 (18.2%)
IQ (mean)	88.6	85.3
Bilateral blindness	0	5 (45.5%)
Unilateral blindness	3 (23.1%)	3 (27.3%)

Modified from Wilson CB, Remington JS, Stagno S, Reynolds DW: Development of adverse sequelae in children born with subclinical congenital *Toxoplasma* infection, *Pediatrics* 66:767-774, 1980; with permission.
IQ, Intelligence quotient.

Outcomes of Treated Congenital Toxoplasmosis. When present, systemic signs of active infection have regressed over a few weeks after the initiation of treatment.[779] Long-term neurologic fate has been assessed in only few studies with prospective follow-up of cohorts of children, principally in the United States and Europe. These studies recruited children with congenital toxoplasmosis diagnosed by prenatal or neonatal screening in Europe, or postnatal diagnosis on the basis of clinical signs for studies in the United States. The children in the European cohorts had few symptoms during the neonatal period. In each series, 10% to 20% had intracranial lesions detectable by imaging, less than 2% had hydrocephalus, and 2% to 3% had clinical neurologic signs (abnormalities of motor tone, seizures). In the North American cohorts, 20% to 87% displayed intracranial calcifications, and 2% to 50% displayed hydrocephalus. The duration of postnatal treatment was between 3 months[786] and 2 years,[461,776,839] follow-up lasted from a little more than 1 year[786] until adolescence,[462,788] and the methods used to assess neurologic development were diverse: questionnaires for the parents,[892] general pediatric neurologic evaluation,[461,776,849,893] and standardized neuropsychological tests[788,839] with[892] or without[¶] a control group. These studies are summarized in Table 31-18. Despite this heterogeneity, the following points emerge:

- Whatever the durations of treatment and follow-up, the children in European cohorts who had normal or only slightly abnormal (e.g., a few intracranial calcifications) brain imaging results had normal neurologic development. The children with sequelae (epilepsy, delayed language acquisition, abnormalities of motor tone) had pathologic neuroimaging findings, generally including ventricular dilatation.[776,786,839]

¶References 461, 711, 776, 786, 788, 839, 849, 893.

- The progression of severe forms of treated congenital toxoplasmosis has been extensively described by the team in Chicago.[779,788,848,851] Severe forms were defined as congenital toxoplasmosis at birth, with at least three cerebral calcifications or white matter density abnormalities, seizures, hydrocephalus, microcephaly, motor tone abnormalities, macular lesions, microphthalmia, optic atrophy, or high protein concentrations in the CSF. After postnatal treatment for 1 year, with a mean follow-up that now extends over more than 10 years, 48 of the 66 children (72.7%) have an IQ of at least 70, and 44 of 55 (80%) have no abnormalities of motor tone.
- These results are consistent with the regression or disappearance of intracranial lesions observed in children treated for congenital toxoplasmosis[789] and are clearly better than those reported in previous decades for untreated children.[788]

Analysis, in future studies, of factors such as strain virulence[719,894] or genetic and epigenetic factors[895,896] may make it possible to refine evaluations of the prognosis of treated children. There is, however, still no explanation of the substantial contrast between the improvements in clinical neurologic and radiologic symptoms over time in treated children[789,792] and the increase in the incidence of ophthalmologic lesions over the same period.

Association of congenital toxoplasmosis with sensorineural hearing loss is controversial. As in older studies, Wilson

Table 31-18 Long-Term Outcome of Prospective Cohorts of Congenital Toxoplasmosis in Children Receiving Postnatal Treatment

Author/ Year of Publication	Country	*n*	Main Clinical Signs	Postnatal Treatment Duration	Follow-up	Evaluation	Main Results
Guerina/1994[849]	United States	*n* = 49	Neonatal screening Intracranial calcifications at birth: 19.6% Hydrocephalus: 2%	1 year	1-4 years	Pediatric examination	4 (8.2%) children with transiently abnormal motor tone 1 (2%) child with hemiplegia
Villena/1998[839]	France	*n* = 78	Prenatal screening Intracranial calcifications at birth: 5.1% Hydrocephalus: 3.8%	12-24 months	1-18 years	Standardized neuropsychological tests	1 (1.3%) epileptic child
Sáfadi/2003[893]	Brazil	*n* = 43	Postnatal diagnosis (clinical signs) Intracranial calcifications at birth: 65.1% Hydrocephalus: 30.2%	1 year	≥5 years	Standardized scale	Frequency of 54% for neurologic sequelae if intracranial calcifications present, 47% if not
Wallon/2004[711]	France	*n* = 327	Prenatal screening Intracranial calcifications at birth: 9% Hydrocephalus: 2% Microcephalus: 0.3%	12 months	Median, 6 years (range, 6 months-14 years)	General pediatric examination	Seizures: 2 (0.6%)
Freeman/2005[892]	Europe	*n* = 178	Prenatal or neonatal screening Intracranial lesions at birth: 8.4%	12-24 months	3-4 years	Parental questionnaire Control group: children without congenital toxoplasmosis born to mothers displaying seroconversion during pregnancy	Development and behavior similar in infected and uninfected children. Greater parental anxiety among the parents of infected children
Schmidt/2006[786]	Netherlands	*n* = 5 5	Neonatal screening Intracranial calcifications at birth: 19.1% Hydrocephalus: 2.1%	3 months	1-3 years	Pediatric examination	Severe neurologic signs: 1 child (1.8%)
McLeod/2006[788]	United States	*n* = 120	Postnatal diagnosis (clinical signs) Intracranial calcifications at birth: 87% Hydrocephalus: 50%	1 year	10.5 ± 4.8 years	Standardized neuropsychological tests	Asymptomatic or moderate forms: IQ < 70: 0 Motor tone abnormalities: 0 Severe forms: IQ < 70: 27.3% Motor tone abnormalities: 20%
Berrébi/2010[776]	France	*n* = 107	Prenatal screening Intracranial calcifications at birth: ? Hydrocephalus: 3.7%	2 years	Median, 7.8 years (range, 1-20)	Pediatric examination	Epilepsy: 1 (0.9%) Psychomotor retardation + epilepsy: 1 (0.9%)

IQ, Intelligence quotient.

found an increased incidence (5/19 children, 26.3%) of mild-to-moderate hearing loss.[891] These findings were not confirmed by the longitudinal follow-up of the Chicago group: 0 of 30 with sensorineural hearing loss, with a median age of 22 months in the study of McGee,[897] and 0 of 68, with a mean age at evaluation greater than or equal to 5 years.[788] The most plausible explanation is a more intensive treatment (1 year) for the children followed by the Chicago team than those studied by Wilson (0-1 month). Nevertheless, a recent histopathologic study found tachyzoites in the internal auditory canal, the spiral ligament, and saccular macula of the temporal bone in 3 of 9 (33%) of children with congenital toxoplasmosis.[898]

A Brazilian study evaluated hearing of children with congenital toxoplasmosis detected by newborn screening. Seventy-five percent were asymptomatic at birth, and they were treated for 12 months. At a median age of 2 years at the last evaluation, 21.1% (4/19) of the children had mild-to-profound sensorineural impairment.[899] Further studies are mandatory to identify risk factors for hearing loss (such as the influence of strains) with congenital toxoplasmosis.

CONGENITAL TOXOPLASMOSIS IN ADULTS

Quality of Life and Visual Function in Adult Patients

Bilateral macular involvement has been associated with reduced cognitive functional scores. Although children with bilateral visual impairment may compensate with higher verbal skills, their verbal scores are still less than those of children with normal vision, indicating that their intellectual performance is generally reduced.[900] This indicates a substantial impact of congenital toxoplasmosis on the quality of life of affected individuals. Of interest, this has received little attention in the literature.

By contrast, one French study addressed this topic and found a surprisingly low long-term impact of treated congenital toxoplasmosis on quality of life and visual performance in patients treated during pregnancy and until the end of the first year of life. Of the 102 patients, 12% presented with neurologic manifestations and 59% with ocular manifestations: 13% had reduced visual function in one eye. Nevertheless, the overall global quality-of-life score (74.7 ± 14.2) was close to the expected normal range for the general population (73.7 ± 15.3), and visual function was only slightly impaired (mean compound score, 97.3; 95% CI, 95.8 to 98.8). Neurologic abnormalities, reduced visual acuity, foveal location of the retinal lesion, and squinting contributed to decreased visual function at follow-up. Thus, in European cohorts who are diagnosed and treated early, congenital toxoplasmosis appears to have little effect on the quality of life and visual function of the affected individuals.[901]

This may not be generalized to other parts of the world. Although prospective data from South America are lacking, it is not surprising that quality of life seems to be much more compromised in less early diagnosed, less well-treated, and more severely affected individuals, as is the rule in South America.[902] This has been confirmed in a small study from Colombia, where a group of 29 cases with ocular toxoplasmosis was found to have significantly lower visual performance scores than control subjects, except for color vision, with a significantly reduced compound score of 79 (range, 35-99) compared with the control subject score of 95 (range, 72-98), especially if they have bilateral lesions and more recurrences.[903]

Behavioral Abnormalities

Many studies have reported behavioral changes in infected rodents that increase their chance of being eaten by cats because they become less afraid of cat odors and, specifically, the smell of cat urine.[904,905] From an evolutionary point of view, these behavioral changes may promote the completion of the life cycle of the parasite by an as yet unknown mechanism. Increased levels of dopamine in the brain of infected mice have been reported.[906] This neurotransmitter is produced by some brain cells in response to IL-2, which is produced by leukocytes at the site of inflammation.[907] In addition, it has been demonstrated that the genome of *T. gondii* possesses two genes for key enzymes that are involved in the synthesis of dopamine,[908] and cysts release dopamine in surrounding tissues.[909] Taken together, these data support an adaptive manipulation of the intermediate host by *T. gondii* that has also been observed in many other parasitic diseases.[910]

This theory is not universally accepted. Worth and coworkers[911] argued that the experimental evidence was not convincing because the findings were not consistent across all studies. They stated that these behavioral changes may be coincidental; mice infected by *Eimeria vermiformis*, a parasite that does not require predation, presented the same attraction to cat odor, but, when eaten by a cat, both the mouse and the parasite will die.[911] Another study reported transient behavioral changes, possibly induced as a byproduct of the immune response of the host rather than as a direct effect of *T. gondii*.[912]

In humans, many studies have suggested a link between *Toxoplasma* infection (based on positive serology) and numerous psychiatric disorders or behavioral changes, including schizophrenia,[913,914] bipolar disorders,[915,916] obsessive compulsive disorders,[917] Parkinson disease,[918] recurrent migraines,[919] epilepsy,[920] suicide,[921,922] and traffic accidents.[923] The mechanism underlying such disorders has not been explained, nor has a causal role for *Toxoplasma* infection been established. A questionnaire study found that infection appeared to induce opposite shifts in personality factors in men and women; the scoring for relationships was lower in infected than in uninfected men, whereas the scoring in women was not affected by infection,[924] which they proposed might be explained by different levels of testosterone, which are increased in men after infection.[907] Other neurotransmitters could in theory also be affected by toxoplasmic infection, such as serotonin, which is synthesized from tryptophan and can be decreased by infection (tryptophan is an essential amino acid for *Toxoplasma*, and its catabolism by host cells is induced by IFN-γ; see "Factors Associated with Pathogenicity"). Low levels of serotonin could hypothetically explain depression and irritability that some have observed in infected subjects.[925]

Among this large body of literature, no study to date has specifically addressed mental disorders or behavioral changes in congenital toxoplasmosis or the underlying biologic or psychosocial mechanisms. Also largely unexplored are the potential impact of congenital toxoplasmosis on mother/infant relationships and infant psychological development or maternal anxiety, especially when a termination of pregnancy has been considered during a moment of despair, and the impact of maternal feelings of guilt for having transmitted the disease to the fetus on its anxiety. To address these gaps, we conducted a questionnaire study with 102 congenitally infected adults, 11.8% of whom presented with neurologic effects, and 58.8% presented with ocular lesions. The outcome used was the Psychological General Well-Being Index, which measures quality of life and has been specifically designed to assess psychological distress.[926] The overall scores did not differ from those observed in a control population. Anxiety, positive well-being, vitality, and depressed mood scores were similar to those observed in the age-matched general population.[901]

In summary, several observational epidemiologic studies have been carried out in humans, but little evidence has been found for a causal link between *T. gondii* infection and psychiatric disorders. Nevertheless, because of the huge amount of indirect evidence that has been published in recent years and the striking findings in animal models, this issue deserves further investigation because its impact on public health could be considerable.

Effectiveness of Current Approaches to Prevent Congenital Toxoplasmosis and Its Sequelae and Proposal for Improvement

EFFICACY OF PATIENT EDUCATION IN THE PRIMARY PREVENTION OF MATERNAL INFECTION

The goal of patient education is to reduce exposure to oocysts and tissue cysts to such an extent that maternal infection in pregnancy is avoided. Thus the optimal outcome to assess the impact of preventive intervention is the incidence of maternal infection, which should decrease among patients who participated in the intervention compared with those who did not. This was attempted in one prevention trial performed in France in the 1990s, but seroconversion rates were lower than those anticipated in both groups, and no conclusion could be reached.[927] To guarantee sufficient power in such a randomized trial, Di Mario and colleagues[928] estimated that each arm should include 102,000 women in a low-incidence country in the Western world and 6300 in higher-incidence areas such as Brazil.

Several different approaches were used in the few other studies carried out on this topic, which were analyzed as part of the Eurotoxo project[927] and in a Cochrane Review.[928] In one study conducted by Breugelmans and colleagues[625] in Brussels, Belgium, incidence rates were monitored at three time points that coincided with educational interventions carried out over a 22-year period (1979-2001). Incidence rates were found to have declined from 1.43% during the first period to 0.58% during the second and to 0.09% during the last. However, in the absence of a control group, it is not possible to exclude the possibility that some epidemiologic changes contributed to this decline. Pawlowski and colleagues[929] analyzed the impact of a large range of educational activities implemented between 1991 and 1997 that were targeted toward obstetricians, midwives, nurses, students, and pregnant women and included oral information given at school, at medical conferences, and during prenatal classes, as well as the distribution of flyers and brochures. The proportion of pregnant women who knew the correct preventive measures increased from 24.3%, in 1991 to 1992, to 45.3%, in 1997,[929] but because follow-up ended in 1997, this study was not able to determine the impact of this increased knowledge on risk of infection.

A randomized trial was carried out in Canada[930] in the late 1980s to assess the impact of a 10-minute educational program on pet, food, and personal hygiene. This program was presented to 26 randomly selected early prenatal classes, whereas the matched control group of 26 other classes did not receive any specific information. The outcome was measured through self-administered questionnaires, which were completed before and after the intervention. After the intervention, the reported behavior for pet hygiene and for cooking beef and hamburgers had improved in the intervention group compared with the control group. However, the sample size was too small to assess the impact on the risk of infection of these improved behaviors, but it would probably have been low because of the minor role played by the two risk factors involved.

An intervention trial was initiated in the French Rhône-Alpes region in 1994.[927] Pregnant women, who were seronegative for *T. gondii*, were enrolled by physicians during the first trimester of gestation and were randomly allocated to two groups, according to the city of the medical practice. Physicians in the intervention cities were asked to give their patients a booklet and an audiotape including advice on how to avoid toxoplasmosis, together with global information regarding pregnancy. Physicians in the control cities were instructed not to change anything in their usual practice. Knowledge of and risk behavior relating to toxoplasmosis and other topics related to pregnancy were measured through two questionnaires at inclusion and at delivery. Analysis was limited to 2790 women (56%) for whom both questionnaires were available. No difference was found between the arms of the study at baseline regarding knowledge of toxoplasmosis or risk-preventing behavior. Greater than 80% of study participants provided correct answers on the risk of infection through the consumption of raw meat (92%) or unwashed salad (90%) and through handling cat litter (80%), but only 55% were aware that infection could be prevented by washing hands after handling raw meat. A high proportion reported washing their hands after handling unwashed fruit and vegetables, but more than half of the participants acknowledged having eaten uncooked meat in the last 2 months preceding inclusion. At delivery, knowledge in the intervention group had improved on all main aspects (the consequences of infection and the routes of infection involving food and hygiene) compared with that at baseline. Participants in the control group also had a better knowledge of factors linked to food and hygiene but to a lesser extent than the intervention group. In both groups, the change was highest for items related to hygiene.

Better habits were also reported but were not associated with assignment to the intervention group.[927]

As pointed out in a recent update of a Cochrane review on this topic,[928] evidence for the true benefits of education is still lacking. A priority would be to implement systems for monitoring the incidence of maternal and congenital infections, which are necessary for measuring the impact of any educational intervention. Because these parameters are also influenced by epidemiologic factors and by prenatal screening, the evidence regarding prenatal effectiveness should best be collected through randomized trials. As recommended by Di Mario and colleagues,[928] the adoption of a cluster-trial design would help to enroll the very large number of participants required.[928]

EFFICACY OF SECONDARY PREVENTION THROUGH TREATMENT OF INFECTION

Efficacy of Antenatal Treatment

The efficacy of antenatal treatment to prevent and reduce the severity of congenital *T. gondii* infection is a central question that remains unanswered, despite numerous studies that have been performed over the past 4 decades and reviewed in several publications.[491,931-933] As discussed by Gilbert,[934] congenital *Toxoplasma* infection poses several challenges that might explain why so little is known about the efficacy of treatment. First, maternal infections are often asymptomatic, and their incidence is low—less than 1% in the majority of studies (see "Infection in Pregnant Women"). As a consequence, the effectiveness of antenatal treatment on transmission can only be assessed in the context of mass screening involving a large number of patients. Second, proving the absence of infection in all uninfected children and detecting 100% of infected children requires a 1-year postnatal follow-up to monitor the clearance or persistence of IgG antibodies, and the organization of such a follow-up for a large group of newborns requires substantial effort and resources. Third, the risk of transmission is relatively low during the first and second trimesters when the incidence of fetal lesions, which are of interest for the reduction of severity, is highest. Fourth, measuring the impact of treatment on the onset of sequelae later in life requires the extension of clinical follow-up far beyond birth for all infected children. In a cohort of 477 French children who were followed up for a median of 10.5 years, 25% of first lesions were detected after 8 years of age.[935] The occurrence of new lesions during adolescence was also reported in the United States.[137,936] Postnatal treatment is given to most neonates who are diagnosed with congenital toxoplasmosis. Therefore, the fifth challenge for assessing the efficacy of prenatal treatment is to take postnatal interventions into account, although they might not be as effective as prenatal interventions.[934] Sixth, gestational stage at the time of maternal infection is a strong determinant of the risks of infection and of intracerebral lesions and also determines the timing and duration of prenatal treatment. It is important to control for this variable to avoid confounding,[513] which is best achieved with a randomized, controlled study design. Estimating gestational stage at the time of maternal infection as precisely as possible is also important to determine the time interval between infection and onset of treatment, which plays an important role in its efficacy. Seventh, the extrapolation of findings from one setting to another may be difficult because of differences in virulence of the local parasite strains (see "Biology of the Parasite"). Similarly, differences in host susceptibility may also interfere with the response to treatment.

Reduction of Mother-to-Child Transmission. Prenatal screening was implemented in France and in Austria based on the belief that prompt treatment could reduce mother-to-child transmission of *T. gondii* by at least 50%.[937] This belief was based on results from in vivo studies in mice[483] and a foundational study by Desmonts and colleagues.[411] However, this notion has not been tested in a randomized controlled study. Rather, the studies that have been carried out in the context of prenatal screening programs were designed to provide information on the prognosis or on diagnostic performance, rather than to address the efficacy of treatment. In these studies, nearly all pregnant women were treated, except those who were diagnosed late in pregnancy; given the absence of an adequate untreated control group, the potential benefit of treatment could not be directly determined.

This conclusion was supported by the findings of a systematic review (search dates, 1966-1997) published in 1999.[931] Of the 2591 reports identified, only 9 small cohort studies met the inclusion criteria. In these studies, pregnant women were treated with spiramycin alone, pyrimethamine/sulfonamide, or with a combination of both, and the rate of infection in the fetus was assessed; however, gestational stage was not adequately controlled, treatment was not randomized, and the untreated controls were generally not directly comparable to the treatment groups. In addition, congenital infection was common in the treated groups. Five of these studies reported significantly lower transmission rates in children born to treated mothers, and four reported no reduction in fetal infection. An additional study was included in an updated version of the review, but the overall level of evidence in favor of treatment remained low.[938]

Several other approaches have been used to investigate the potential impact of treatment. In 2000, a study was carried out that compared mother-to-child transmission of *T. gondii* in four cohorts of pregnant women managed according to different strategies, including intensive treatment after monthly (France) or every3-months (Austria) prenatal screening, short-term treatment in Dutch women, and no treatment in Denmark. This comparison failed to find that more intensive treatment was more effective in terms of risk prevention than no or shorter treatment. The relative risk for mother-to-child transmission, compared with Lyon, was 1.24 (95% CI, 0.88 to 1.59) in Austria, 0.59 (95% CI, 0.41 to 0.81) in Denmark, and 0.65 (95% CI, 0.37 to 1.01) in the Netherlands.[939]

To determine whether early treatment was more effective than later treatment, the Systematic Review on Congenital Toxoplasmosis (SYROCOT) meta-analysis analyzed the interval between the estimated time of infection and the administration of treatment in 1438 patients from 26 observational cohorts and found that the introduction of treatment within 3 versus 8 weeks reduced transmission by half (OR, 0.48; 95% CI, 0.28 to 0.80).[491] The importance of prompt maternal treatment was indirectly confirmed by findings from the French Lyon cohort, which were based on a comparison of transmission rates for maternal infections diagnosed over two periods: between 1988 and 1992, when no specific follow-up testing schedule was recommended, and after 1992, when monthly follow-up testing became mandatory. This change in screening was associated with a significantly faster initiation of antenatal treatment after mid-1992 ($P < .001$). The median delay until treatment was reduced by 4 days (33 vs. 37 days; 95% CI, 0.6 to 8.6; $P = .0007$) in the first trimester, by 6 days (33 vs. 27 days; 95% CI, 2.1 to 9.9; $P = .0004$) in the second trimester, and by 8 days (28 vs. 20 days; 95% CI, 3.2 to 12.8; $P = .0001$) in the third trimester. As shown in Figure 31-50, the apparent reduction in maternal transmission and in clinical signs at 3 years of age was greatest for third-trimester infections, for which treatment was begun on average within 20 days after infection,[4] which is concordant with the conclusions of the SYROCOT meta-analysis. These findings provide indirect evidence that early treatment can reduce transmission (Table 31-19) but do not indicate to what extent, compared with no treatment. Therefore they do not replace the need for randomized controlled studies to evaluate the efficacy of existing regimens or to compare the efficacy of new with that of existing treatments.[932,934,940] If placebo-controlled trials are considered to be unethical by the relevant local authorities, randomized trials could still provide valuable indirect information by comparing different treatment strategies and protocols. Priority should be given to carrying out these trials in settings where infections are most severe because of virulent strains and/or increased host susceptibility.

Evidence is lacking for several specific points. First is the ability to generalize conclusions from the findings in Europe to other settings. These conclusions could probably be extrapolated to North America, as discussed in several publications.[4,631a,782,941] However, caution should be exercised in their extrapolation to other epidemiologic contexts, especially South America, although to date no evidence has shown a reduced sensitivity of *T. gondii* from South America or Africa to antifolates or other drugs.[125,782,942] Second is whether the benefit of prompt treatment would be greater with pyrimethamine/sulfonamides as the frontline treatment instead of spiramycin. In the SYROCOT study and in several reports from the European Multicentre Study on Congenital Toxoplasmosis (EMSCOT) study, the type of treatment (spiramycin or pyrimethamine and sulfonamides) did not seem to have a significant effect.[491] The overall transmission rate was low (4.5%) in a German study that included patients who were systematically treated with pyrimethamine/sulfonamides at 16 weeks of pregnancy. However, because follow-up testing was rarely performed, a majority of infections were diagnosed at the first test during the first trimester. This overrepresentation of early infections and the impossibility of excluding that some were acquired before pregnancy prevented a fair comparison with the higher rate found in France in the context of the monthly follow-up testing program.[943] The third interesting question is whether improved compliance with screening at monthly intervals, and thereby an increase in the number of mothers treated within 3 weeks after infection, would further prevent congenital infection. A survey performed on 34,000 pregnant women in France suggested that as many as 80% were not consistently

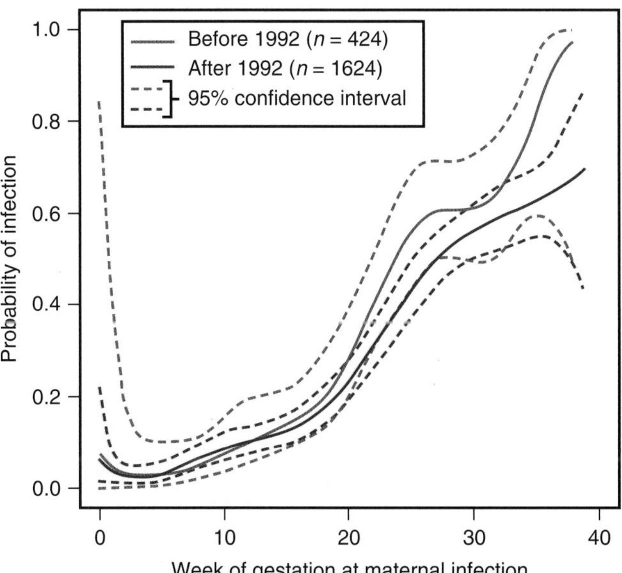

Figure 31-50 Probability of fetal infection according to gestational age at maternal infection before and after 1992 in the Lyon cohort. (Modified from Wallon M, Peyron F, Cornu C, et al: Congenital *Toxoplasma* infection: monthly prenatal screening decreases transmission and improves clinical outcome at age 3 years, *Clin Infect Dis* 56:1223-1231, 2013; with permission.)

Table 31-19 Reduction in the Risk of Infection and of Clinical Signs After Changes in the Retesting Policy (1992) and in Antenatal Diagnosis and Treatment Procedure (1995)

Risk and Clinical Signs	1987-1991	1992-1995	1996-2008	P Value
RISK OF INFECTION				
Retesting policy for women identified as susceptible at the first prenatal test implemented in 1985	Recommended without specified frequency	Mandatory and monthly		
Infected children/mothers	125/424	366/1624		$P < .018$
RISK OF CLINICAL SIGNS AT AGE 3 YEARS				
PCR availability on amniotic fluid	No		Yes	
PS antenatal treatment	Alternating with spiramycine for 3-week periods		Continuous	
Clinical signs/infected children	87/794		46/1150	$P < 10^{-4}$

From Wallon M, Peyron F, Cornu C, et al: *Toxoplasma* infection: monthly prenatal screening decreases transmission and improves clinical outcome at age 3 years, *Clin Infect Dis* 56:1223-1231, 2013; with permission.
PCR, Polymerase chain reaction; *PS*, pyrimethamine and sulfadiazine.

retested on a monthly schedule.[944] Finally, treatment is often continued until delivery despite a negative amniocentesis and the absence of fetal ultrasound abnormalities. If it was determined that such treatment was not beneficial, cessation of this practice could alleviate human and financial costs.

Reduction of the Severity of Congenital Toxoplasmosis. The early treatment of an infected fetus is expected to reduce the risks of immediate and long-term lesions of toxoplasmosis. In the absence of data from controlled trials, the available evidence is derived from observational studies, which were not designed to address the efficacy of treatment. In the absence of comparable control groups, it was impossible to attribute any observed benefits solely to the administration of prenatal treatment in the vast majority of these studies. Further confounding interpretation, the few untreated mothers in such studies were also the least likely to give birth to a child with an overt infection because they acquired infections in the last trimester of pregnancy, and the risk for neurologic signs was typically predicted by gestational stage at the time of maternal infection, rather than by the absence of treatment. Some reports also provided information on the postnatal outcome, but, except for a few cohorts, the median length of follow-up did not extend beyond early childhood.

In several noncontrolled studies, a different approach, based on the association between treatment delay and risk of infection, provided indirect evidence suggesting that prenatal treatment reduces the risk of lesions in utero or during the first 3 years of life.

Cortina-Borja and colleagues[687] analyzed the data collected from 293 cases of congenital infection diagnosed by prenatal or postnatal screening as part of the EMSCOT study and demonstrated that prenatal treatment reduced the risk of severe neurologic sequelae or death, with an OR, adjusted for gestational stage at the time of maternal infection, of 0.24 (95% Bayesian credible intervals, 0.07-0.71). This risk was not found to be reduced by treatment with pyrimethamine/sulfonamide compared with spiramycin alone or increased by a delay in the administration of treatment, but the power to detect both associations was limited.[687]

Another report that was based on the EMSCOT study concluded that treatment initiated within 4 weeks after infection significantly reduced the risk of intracranial calcifications (OR, 0.28; 95% CI, 0.08 to 0.75) compared with a treatment initiated later. The effect of pyrimethamine and sulfonamide alone or after spiramycin was similar to that of spiramycin alone. The risk of ocular lesions at 12 months of age was not found to be increased when prenatal treatment was delayed by more than 4 weeks after the estimated gestational stage at the time of maternal infection.[945]

Conversely, Kieffer and colleagues[88] analyzed a cohort of 300 children with congenital *Toxoplasma* infection and found that a shorter delay between maternal infection and the start of treatment (spiramycin or pyrimethamine and sulfonamide) reduced the risk of ocular lesions at 2 years of age (hazard ratio: 2.54; 95% confidence interval: 1.14-4.01).

The fourth indication of a positive effect on short-term lesions was seen in the French Lyon cohort through the analysis of the risk of clinical lesions both before 1995 and after that time, when PCR assay of amniotic fluid had become routinely available. The risk of clinical signs at 3 years of age was found to be reduced after PCR assay became available in 1995, presumably as a consequence of earlier treatment of infected children with pyrimethamine and sulfadiazine. The proportion of live-born infected children who had been diagnosed as being infected antenatally was greater after 1995 (87/272, 32.0%) than before 1995 (46/213, 21.6%; $P = .011$). In addition, the probabilities of clinical signs developing in live-born children (either uninfected or, when infected, followed for 3 years) were significantly lower in infected children born to mothers who were diagnosed after 1995 than those who were diagnosed before 1995 (46/1150 vs. 87/794; OR, 0.59; 95% CI, 0.40 to 0.89; $P = .012$) (see Table 31-19).[4]

Efficacy of Postnatal Treatment

The evidence for the efficacy of postnatal treatment is limited and relies solely on observational studies that can be divided into two groups, according to the severity of infection at the time of treatment. Those carried out in the United States on newborns, whose infections were detected because of an overt infection and not through an organized screening program, provided the greatest amount of information. In this context, postnatal treatment was primarily aimed at reducing neurologic impairment and attempting to prevent new retinochoroidal lesions. Despite the absence of concurrent comparative studies, these provided indirect evidence of a positive effect of a 12-month treatment with pyrimethamine and sulfadiazine on neurologic prognosis[457,466,946] (see "Management of Congenitally Infected Children and Long-Term Outcome"). Two cohort studies published in 2008 suggested that postnatal treatment might also have an impact on the risk of long-term ocular lesions. The first included 108 patients who had received 12 months of treatment with pyrimethamine and sulfadiazine after birth,[936] whereas the second included 25 patients who were not treated in their first year of life despite probable congenital infection.[137] At a mean age of 10.8 and 10.9 years, respectively, 31% of patients in the first cohort, compared with 72% in the second, had new lesions, which were central in 14% of those who had been treated versus 52% of those who had not.

Little evidence is available on the impact of postnatal treatment as a prophylactic measure to prevent long-term lesions in children who show no or only benign lesions at birth and who were diagnosed with congenital infection by prenatal or neonatal screening. Neonatal screening was implemented in Denmark in 1999, then discontinued in 2007 after follow-up evaluation of the 100 patients identified with congenital infection demonstrated that the 3-month postnatal treatment regimen provided no benefit.[643] Table 31-20 summarizes the findings reported by three French cohort studies,[136,428,461] which included 107 to 327 newborns diagnosed by prenatal screening, treated for 12 months after birth, and followed up for a median of 4 to 10 years. New lesions or relapses were not rare in these children but seldom caused significant impairment. The advantages of such long-term postnatal treatment in newborns

Table 31-20 Long-Term Outcomes From Three Cohort Studies of Children With Congenital *Toxoplasma* Infection, Detected Through the French Prenatal Screening Program and Treated for 1 Year After Birth

	Berrébi et al[461]	Faucher et al[428]	Wallon et al[136]
Study period and location	1985-2005, Toulouse	1995-2010, Marseille	1988-2001, Lyon
Number of patients	107	127	327
Median length of follow-up (years)	8 (1-20)	4	6 (interquartile range, 3-10)
Asymptomatic infection at the last examination	79 (74%)	96 (76%)	232 (71%)
Non-ocular lesions	6 (5%)	11 (9%)	35 (11%)
Retinal lesions			
At the last examination	28 (26%) Unilateral visual impairment: 6 (21%) No bilateral impairment	24 (19%) Unilateral visual impairment: 7 Bilateral visual impairment: 1	79 (24%) Unilateral visual impairment: 24 (30%) No bilateral impairment
Time of detection of first lesions	Birth: 11 (39%) <5 years: 24 (55%) <10 years: 27 (96%)	Birth: 11 <2 years: 18 (75%) <5 years: 22 (92%)	First month: 9 (11%) <1 year: 38 (48%) <2 years: 46 (58%) <5 years: 60 (76%) <10 years: 75 (95%)

with subclinical lesions need to be evaluated through carefully randomized studies. In the meantime, consideration must be given to reducing the constraints of and any harm that may be caused from such treatment by reducing its length in these nonseverely infected children. This is the objective of the TOSCANE trial, which is currently in progress in France (ClinicalTrials.gov; NCT01202500)[406] and compares the effects of two durations of treatment—3 months and 12 months—in children with nonsevere congenital *T. gondii* infection. Outcome variables are the age at which new retinochoroidal lesions occur, neurologic developments, the anxiety levels of parents, and the quality of life of parents and children.

SCREENING

Screening for *Toxoplasma* infection includes different types of intervention that vary in terms of advantages, limitations, constraints, and costs. These various aspects of screening have been analyzed and discussed extensively.[#]

Option 1

A single test, before pregnancy or during the first trimester of pregnancy in women who are not known to be immune, is useful in terms of primary prevention because it discerns those who are susceptible to infection and need to be educated on its avoidance. It also promotes the collection of relevant epidemiologic data, such as time and geographic trends in the prevalence of *Toxoplasma* infection among pregnant women in different age groups, and the investigation of factors involved in past infection in women of different socioeconomic and cultural backgrounds. Constraints include the timing of the test, which should be performed as early as possible in pregnancy—or ideally before pregnancy—to allow the timely adoption of healthy, risk-free behaviors. When the result is positive, an early test also facilitates the exclusion of a perigravidic infection. Requirements for testing include the availability of high-performance tests that can determine precisely the immune status of patients and the training for laboratory biologists and clinicians on the interpretation of test results and on explaining their implications to patients, respectively. Their attention should be drawn to the risk of false-positive test results and to the danger of misinterpreting residual IgM or low-avidity antibodies as signs of acute infection (see "Diagnosis of Maternal Infection"). Reference centers or groups should be available and their expertise requested to assess the risks for the fetus whenever atypical findings or a suspicion of infection are detected. Costs for follow-up testing should also be included in planning, as part of this option. Sufficient funding should also be available for educational material and campaigns and for the training of perinatal care providers, who should be able to give accurate advice on how a pregnant woman with a negative test can avoid infection, according to her level of risk and sociocultural profile. An inability to provide clear answers to their questions on risky or risk-free behaviors may be a source of stress in pregnant women who have been identified as susceptible.

Option 2

The provision of a second test during the third trimester of pregnancy, or at delivery, for women who tested negative at the first test allows the identification of those who seroconverted during pregnancy, and the detection of *Toxoplasma* infection in their children. However, it also increases the technical constraints, in terms of test performance and the interpretation of their results in pregnant women and newborns, and the need for reliable reference centers or groups to be available to counsel obstetricians and pediatricians, who should be provided with criteria and guidelines for treatment, despite the uncertainty regarding the impact of postnatal treatment on the reduction of long-term ocular lesions.

Option 3

Any additional testing during pregnancy offers the opportunity to detect incident maternal infections and to attempt to prevent transmission to the fetus by antenatal treatment.

[#]References 735, 737, 745, 933, 937, 941, 942, 945, 948.

Additional benefits are the possibility of performing an amniocentesis and intensifying fetal ultrasound surveillance when fetal infection is diagnosed. Retesting is performed at 3-monthly or monthly intervals according to the clinical settings. More frequent testing increases the costs of screening but might also increase its efficacy by expanding the opportunities of implementing prenatal treatment within 21 days of infection and thus reducing the risks[4,491] and the severity[88,687] of a congenital infection. However, any economic assessment of such procedures is limited by the lack of knowledge on the extent to which treatment reduces the proportion of disease compared with no treatment.

Decision analysis is an ideal tool that takes into account the magnitude of disease in a local population and can hypothesize the proportion that can be prevented. A decision tree was designed by Binquet in 2003 to compare antenatal and neonatal screening by using a cost-effectiveness approach.[948] It was updated in 2010 to incorporate the 20% reduction in seroprevalence and the incidence of seroconversion in France, the knowledge gained on long-term outcomes, and updated costs used by the French Health Insurance System. This decision analysis confirmed that the risk of an event was reduced by antenatal screening, regardless of whether the outcome considered was congenital toxoplasmosis, fetal loss and termination, or long-term sequelae. The cost-effectiveness ratios were almost 8000 euros for each additional event that was avoided by antenatal screening compared with neonatal screening with regard to congenital toxoplasmosis, fetal loss, and termination, and more than 15,500 euros with regard to long-term sequelae. A cost-utility analysis is under consideration to include the quality of life of the patients. To determine whether the French approach might be cost saving in the United States, Stillwaggon and coworkers[631a] used a decision-analytic and a cost-minimization model to compare universal monthly maternal serologic screening (including prenatal and postnatal treatment and follow-up) versus no systematic screening or perinatal treatment. The probabilities were estimated from published results and clinical practices in the United States and France, and costs were based on current diagnostic and treatment costs and on published estimates of lifetime societal costs for disabilities. Universal monthly maternal screening was found to lead to savings of $620 per child screened and to be cost saving for rates of congenital infection greater than 1 per 10,000 live births, taking the cost of a maternal screening test as $12.[631a]

Instead of universal screening, some countries recommend a selective approach, which is restricted to pregnant women who are estimated to be at risk for infection because of a known or suspected exposure, and this approach was adopted in some states in the United States[631b,739] and Canada.[949]

Option 4

Neonatal screening permits the diagnosis of a larger number of congenitally infected children than would have been detected based on clinical signs alone and to organize their treatment and surveillance. It was found to be very appropriate in Colombia, where a high proportion of pregnant women do not attend prenatal care clinics despite the high risks of congenital infection.[642] Other advantages of neonatal screening are the avoidance of anxiety in pregnant women and the approximately 10-fold lower cost compared with prenatal screening.[950] The detection of infection relies on tests for specific IgM that can be performed on blood taken for other neonatal screening tests and stored on filter papers. The main limitations are the inability to detect greater than 50% to 70% of infected newborns and the uncertainty of the efficacy of postnatal treatment.

The choices made between these options vary largely between countries or even within a given country, as illustrated by the diversity of screening programs found in Brazil. Screening relies on a single test in Mato Grosso do Sul and Gioia, on two tests (early and late) in Belo Horizonte, State of Minas Gerais, and on 3-monthly follow-up testing in Porto Alegre and Curitiba.[951] The situation is also very heterogeneous in Europe.[952] The French and Austrian universal retesting programs are the longest standing. Several other programs have been implemented since, but some countries, including the United Kingdom,[953] have also taken a firm position against any type of screening. Universal screening is not organized in the United States, but a large proportion of obstetricians were reported to screen patients who are considered at high risk, ask for it, or show symptoms.[740]

PROPOSAL FOR IMPROVEMENT

How Can You Counsel When You Do Not Know?

One of the numerous unanswered questions concerning congenital toxoplasmosis is for how long and according to what schedule should these patients be followed after treatment has been stopped. Infants with neurologic lesions are likely to present severe sequelae, and some of them need to be placed in institutions. For others, congenital toxoplasmosis, especially when treated before delivery, is subclinical at birth.[4] Because of the unpredictable risk of the occurrence or relapse of ocular lesions, even many years after birth, congenital toxoplasmosis can be viewed as a chronic ophthalmologic disease. Because there is no consensus concerning the necessity of ophthalmologic follow-up, pediatricians must decide how the disease should be monitored and provide explanations to the parents. It has been proposed that regular funduscopy be performed until the age of 4 years, after which children are able to communicate verbally regarding visual disturbances.[954] This option, although acceptable from a medical point of view, prevents the creation of population-based prospective cohort studies that are irreplaceable because they obtain information on long-term outcomes, providing they have a sufficiently long follow-up to cover the occurrence of ocular lesions.[4] Moreover, addressing key issues, such as the efficacy of antenatal or postnatal treatment, is difficult without properly designed randomized controlled trials. Such studies are difficult to organize, and none have been conducted to date.

Population-based prospective cohort studies are a good proxy, in the context where randomized trials have not been conducted, for investigating the effect of treatment, providing they are not based on referred cases. In our setting, we are following a cohort of 700 cases of congenital toxoplasmosis. Their ages range from 3 weeks to 37 years. Each patient undergoes a yearly follow-up, including funduscopy and clinical evaluation. When they reach the age of reason, the importance for the community of a regular follow-up is explained to them. Thanks to the existence of this cohort, it has been possible to obtain a clear picture of the evolution of the disease and to investigate the risk of ocular recurrences during pregnancy, the possibility of vertical transmission,[124] and the quality of life and visual function in infected adults.[901] Our results are tremendously helpful for counseling parents. It has to be remembered that our results are specific for a particular setting: type II strains and infants who received antenatal and postnatal treatment and are monitored in one center; these results cannot be extrapolated to other centers.[902] Findings could be totally different in other settings where, such as in the United States, infants are not given antenatal treatment, or in South America, where strain virulence is completely different.

In some parts of the world, similar studies have delineated the local burden of disease, which has allowed the approach to be tailored appropriately for those settings.[902] We advocate long-term follow-up because this is the only way that a clear understanding of the evolution of the disease in specific contexts can be defined. One can argue that such a follow-up will result in overcrowded ophthalmologic consultations, be costly, and be frightening for the patients. The two first arguments are admissible, but, if accepted, will leave doctors alone to answer the questions of parents and make decisions. Regarding the third argument, we asked 102 adults who have congenital toxoplasmosis and have been followed regularly since birth how they perceived this monitoring: 98% of them stated that follow-up was useful, and 92% found it reassuring. The majority wanted to continue and, among the reasons for doing so, 65% said it was to improve knowledge of the disease.[879,955]

Conclusion

Since its discovery, the significance of *T. gondii* has changed dramatically: From its determination as a rodent pathogen, it has been acknowledged to cause subclinical or devastating fetal infections and life-threatening manifestations in immunocompromised patients. For scientists, *T. gondii* offers an attractive model for scientific exploration. Over the last 2 decades, many studies have generated an abundance of information concerning its life cycle, genetics, and immunology. In the future, breakthroughs in the area of vaccines and treatments with novel compounds, especially those that target protein kinases, may be enabled through the application of new technologies.

For clinicians, congenital toxoplasmosis presents pathologic difficulties, and for parents and children, it can be a tragedy. Tremendous progress has been made in the field of diagnosis through IgG avidity, recombinant antigens, and fully automated tests that allow rapid accurate detection at a reasonable cost. The most important breakthrough concerns antenatal diagnosis, for which amniocentesis with PCR detection of the parasite and ultrasonography allow the determination of fetal infection and an accurate monitoring of the evolution of the disease in the infected fetus, respectively. Nevertheless, the lack of guidelines on screening and contradictory information on the efficacy of treatment and outcomes cast doubts that prevent the communication of reliable information and might lead to inappropriate advice such as unjustified terminations of pregnancy.

Failure to respond to the anxieties of pregnant women is totally unacceptable. There is no universal solution because the prevalence and burden of the disease varies among countries. Each country should evaluate the national dimensions of the disease and rank congenital toxoplasmosis among its public health priorities. For some, congenital toxoplasmosis is not a public health concern, except for its severity in vulnerable groups. In others, such as Brazil, where in some areas 17.7% of the adult population has ocular toxoplasmosis, the disease cannot be disregarded.

Precise information on the prevalence of toxoplasmosis and its routes of infection, which are sometimes linked to culinary or cultural habits, are prerequisites to launch a campaign for information and primary prevention. Awareness of the disease needs to be increased among care providers and health educators through workshops or continuing medical education, which will target updated information and basic rules for the interpretation of serologic tests. The main question is the cost-benefit aspect of mass screening of pregnant women, such as that performed in France and Austria. The advocates will put forward evidence for the efficacy of antenatal treatment in reducing fetal transmission or abating sequelae and for the importance of an information campaign. The opponents will underline the lack of randomized controlled trials that demonstrate the efficacy of treatment and the cost-benefit aspects of such programs, especially in countries such as the United States, where seroprevalence of the disease is low among pregnant women.

Another option would entail implementing neonatal screening, such as the screening that has been initiated for phenylketonuria. In Massachusetts and New Hampshire, unlike other states in the United States, all newborns are tested for toxoplasmosis. Such screening detects approximately 75% of cases but allows a rapid onset of postnatal treatment, even for children who present with subclinical congenital toxoplasmosis. In the light of recent literature, randomized controlled studies that address the efficacy of antenatal or postnatal treatment are both impractical and unfeasible because of ethical limitations, and population-based prospective cohort studies should be undertaken instead. Associated with epidemiologic investigations, they appear to be the only means to gather information in precise clinical settings and enable doctors to provide parents-to-be with unbiased information and help policy makers to take the appropriate decisions.

In the meantime, working groups should issue standardized guidelines on which doctors can rely for counselling pregnant women, initiate information campaigns for both the public and doctors, and implement networks with referral laboratories and referral physicians, who would be available for face-to-face interviews with patients whenever requested.

Acknowledgments

The authors are grateful to Marie Laure Dardé, Valeria Meroni, and Eskild Petersen for their advice and help. They also thank Jane Mitchell and Monique Billaud for providing technical assistance, Jack Remington for his helpful suggestions, and Christopher Wilson for assistance in editing the manuscript. This chapter is dedicated to Professor J.P. Garin, who passed away in October 2014. Dr. Garin founded the toxoplasmosis center in Lyon, France.

References

1. Montoya JG, Liesenfeld O: Toxoplasmosis, *Lancet* 363:1965-1976, 2004.
2. Pappas G, Roussos N, Falagas ME: Toxoplasmosis snapshots: global status of *Toxoplasma gondii* seroprevalence and implications for pregnancy and congenital toxoplasmosis, *Int J Parasitol* 39:1385-1394, 2009.
3. Olariu TR, Remington JS, McLeod R, et al: Severe congenital toxoplasmosis in the United States: clinical and serologic findings in untreated infants, *Pediatr Infect Dis J* 30:1056-1061, 2011.
4. Wallon M, Peyron F, Cornu C, et al: Congenital Toxoplasma infection: monthly prenatal screening decreases transmission rate and improves clinical outcome at age 3 years, *Clin Infect Dis* 56:1223-1231, 2013.
5. Boothroyd JC: *Toxoplasma gondii*: 25 years and 25 major advances for the field, *Int J Parasitol* 39:935-946, 2009.
6. Kirby T: Calls for more detailed studies on toxoplasmosis, *Lancet Infect Dis* 12:912-913, 2012.
7. Peyron F: When are we going to celebrate the centenary of the discovery of efficient treatment for congenital toxoplasmosis? *Mem Inst Oswaldo Cruz* 104:316-319, 2009.
8. Nicolle C, Manceaux L: Sur un protozoaire nouveau du gondi, *Arch Inst Pasteur Tunis* 2:97-107, 1909.
9. Splendore A: Un nuovo parassita deconigli incontrato nelle lesioni anatomiche d'une malattia che ricorda in molti punti il Kala-azar dell' uomo. Nota preliminar, *Rev Soc Sci São Paulo* 3:109-112, 1908.
10. Janku J: Pathogenesa a pathologicka anatomie tak nazvaneho vrozeneho kolobomu zlute skvrny v oku normalne velikem a mikrophtalmickem s nalezem parasitu v sitnicio, *Cas Lek Cesk* 62:1021-1027, 1923.
11. Wolf A, Cowen D, Paige B: Human toxoplasmosis: occurrence in infants as an encephalomyelitis verification by transmission to animals, *Science* 89:226-227, 1939.
12. Wolf A, Cowen D, Paige B: Toxoplasmic encephalomyelitis: III. A new case of granulomatous encephalomyelitis due to a protozoon, *Am J Pathol* 15:657-694, 1939.
13. Frenkel JK, Dubey JP, Miller NL: *Toxoplasma gondii* in cats: fecal stages identified as coccidian oocysts, *Science* 167:893-896, 1970.
14. Luft BJ, Conley F, Remington JS, et al: Outbreak of central-nervous-system toxoplasmosis in western Europe and North America, *Lancet* 1:781-784, 1983.
15. Luft BJ, Brooks RG, Conley FK, et al: Toxoplasmic encephalitis in patients with acquired immune deficiency syndrome, *JAMA* 252:913-917, 1984.
16. Jones JL, Roberts JM: Toxoplasmosis hospitalizations in the United States, 2008, and trends, 1993-2008, *Clin Infect Dis* 54:e58-e61, 2012.
17. Bautista G, Ramos A, Fores R, et al: Toxoplasmosis in cord blood transplantation recipients, *Transpl Infect Dis* 14:496-501, 2002.
18. Derouin F, Pelloux H: Prevention of toxoplasmosis in transplant patients, *Clin Microbiol Infect* 14:1089-1101, 2008.
19. Bowie WR, King AS, Werker DH, et al: Outbreak of toxoplasmosis associated with municipal drinking water. The BC *Toxoplasma* Investigation Team, *Lancet* 350:173-177, 1997.
20. Jones JL, Dubey JP: Waterborne toxoplasmosis—recent developments, *Exp Parasitol* 124:10-25, 2010.
21. Dardé ML, Bouteille B, Pestre-Alexandre M: Isoenzymic characterization of seven strains of *Toxoplasma gondii* by isoelectrofocusing in polyacrylamide gels, *Am J Trop Med Hyg* 39:551-558, 1988.
22. Dardé ML, Villena I, Pinon JM, et al: Severe toxoplasmosis caused by a *Toxoplasma gondii* strain with a new isoenzyme type acquired in French Guyana, *J Clin Microbiol* 36:324, 1998.
23. Dubey JP: Advances in the life cycle of *Toxoplasma gondii*, *Int J Parasitol* 28:1019-1024, 1998.
24. Sulzer AJ, Strobel PL, Springer EL, et al: A comparative electron microscopic study of the morphology of *Toxoplasma gondii* by freeze-etch replication and thin sectioning technic, *J Protozool* 21:710-714, 1974.
25. Mercier C, Adjogble KD, Daubener W, et al: Dense granules: are they key organelles to help understand the parasitophorous vacuole of all apicomplexa parasites? *Int J Parasitol* 35:829-849, 2005.
26. Fichera ME, Roos DS: A plastid organelle as a drug target in apicomplexan parasites, *Nature* 390:407-409, 1997.
27. Dubey JP, Lindsay DS, Speer CA: Structures of *Toxoplasma gondii* tachyzoites, bradyzoites, and sporozoites and biology and development of tissue cysts, *Clin Microbiol Rev* 11:267-299, 1998.
28. Kaneko Y, Takashima Y, Xuaun X, et al: Natural IgM antibodies in sera from various animals but not the cat kill *Toxoplasma gondii* by activating the classical complement pathway, *Parasitology* 128(Pt 2): 123-129, 2004.
29. Unno A, Suzuki K, Xuan X, et al: Dissemination of extracellular and intracellular *Toxoplasma gondii* tachyzoites in the blood flow, *Parasitol Int* 57:515-518, 2008.
30. Lyons RE, McLeod R, Roberts CW: *Toxoplasma gondii* tachyzoite-bradyzoite interconversion, *Trends Parasitol* 18:198-201, 2002.
31. Sims TA, Hay J, Talbot IC: Host-parasite relationship in the brains of mice with congenital toxoplasmosis, *J Pathol* 156:255-261, 1988.
32. Dubey JP: Duration of immunity to shedding of *Toxoplasma gondii* oocysts by cats, *J Parasitol* 81:410-415, 1995.
33. Dubey JP, Speer CA, Shen SK, et al: Oocyst-induced murine toxoplasmosis: life cycle, pathogenicity, and stage conversion in mice fed *Toxoplasma gondii* oocysts, *J Parasitol* 83:870-882, 1997.
34. House PK, Vyas A, Sapolsky R: Predator cat odors activate sexual arousal pathways in brains of *Toxoplasma gondii* infected rats, *PLoS One* 6:e23277, 2011.
35. Jacobs L, Remington JS, Melton ML: The resistance of the encysted form of *Toxoplasma gondii*, *J Parasitol* 46:11-21, 1960.
36. Mai K, Sharman PA, Walker RA, et al: Oocyst wall formation and composition in coccidian parasites, *Mem Inst Oswaldo Cruz* 104:281-289, 2009.
37. Dubey JP: *Toxoplasma gondii* oocyst survival under defined temperatures, *J Parasitol* 84:862-865, 1998.
38. Robert-Gangneux F, Dardé ML: Epidemiology of and diagnostic strategies for toxoplasmosis, *Clin Microbiol Rev* 25:264-296, 2012.
39. Ferguson DJ: *Toxoplasma gondii* and sex: essential or optional extra? *Trends Parasitol* 18:355-359, 2002.
40. Coombes JL, Charsar BA, Han SJ, et al: Motile invaded neutrophils in the small intestine of *Toxoplasma gondii*-infected mice reveal a potential mechanism for parasite spread, *Proc Natl Acad Sci U S A* 110:E1913-E1922, 2013.
41. Hill DE, Chirukandoth S, Dubey JP: Biology and epidemiology of *Toxoplasma gondii* in man and animals, *Anim Health Res Rev* 6:41-61, 2005.
42. Sumyuen MH, Garin YJ, Derouin F: Early kinetics of *Toxoplasma gondii* infection in mice infected orally with cysts of an avirulent strain, *J Parasitol* 81:327-329, 1995.
43. Courret N, Darche S, Sonigo P, et al: CD11c- and CD11b-expressing mouse leukocytes transport single *Toxoplasma gondii* tachyzoites to the brain, *Blood* 107:309-316, 2006.
44. Meissner M, Ferguson DJ, Frischknecht F: Invasion factors of apicomplexan parasites: essential or redundant? *Curr Opin Microbiol* 16:438-444, 2013.
45. Carruthers V, Boothroyd JC: Pulling together: an integrated model of Toxoplasma cell invasion, *Curr Opin Microbiol* 10:83-89, 2007.
46. Shen B, Sibley LD: The moving junction, a key portal to host cell invasion by apicomplexan parasites, *Curr Opin Microbiol* 15:449-455, 2012.
47. El Hajj H, Lebrun M, Arold ST, et al: ROP18 is a rhoptry kinase controlling the intracellular proliferation of *Toxoplasma gondii*, *PLoS Pathog* 3:e14, 2007.
48. Black MW, Boothroyd JC: Lytic cycle of *Toxoplasma gondii*, *Microbiol Mol Biol Rev* 64:607-623, 2000.
49. Sweeney KR, Morrissette NS, LaChapelle S, et al: Host cell invasion by *Toxoplasma gondii* is temporally regulated by the host microtubule cytoskeleton, *Eukaryot Cell* 9:1680-1689, 2010.
50. Ferreira da Silva Mda F, Barbosa HS, Gross U, et al: Stress-related and spontaneous stage differentiation of *Toxoplasma gondii*, *Mol Biosyst* 4:824-834, 2008.
51. Luder CG, Giraldo-Velasquez M, Sendtner M, et al: *Toxoplasma gondii* in primary rat CNS cells: differential contribution of neurons, astrocytes, and microglial cells for the intracerebral development and stage differentiation, *Exp Parasitol* 93:23-32, 1999.
52. Sibley LD, Boothroyd JC: Construction of a molecular karyotype for *Toxoplasma gondii*, *Mol Biochem Parasitol* 51:291-300, 1992.
53. Howe DK, Sibley LD: *Toxoplasma gondii* comprises three clonal lineages: correlation of parasite genotype with human disease, *J Infect Dis* 172:1561-1566, 1995.
54. Dardé ML: *Toxoplasma gondii*, "new" genotypes and virulence, *Parasite* 15:366-371, 2008.
55. Ajzenberg D, Cogne N, Paris L, et al: Genotype of 86 *Toxoplasma gondii* isolates associated with human congenital toxoplasmosis, and correlation with clinical findings, *J Infect Dis* 186:684-689, 2002.

56. Aubert D, Ajzenberg D, Richomme C, et al: Molecular and biological characteristics of *Toxoplasma gondii* isolates from wildlife in France, *Vet Parasitol* 171:346-349, 2010.
57. Ajzenberg D, Yera H, Marty P, et al: Genotype of 88 *Toxoplasma gondii* isolates associated with toxoplasmosis in immunocompromised patients and correlation with clinical findings, *J Infect Dis* 199:1155-1167, 2009.
58. Fekkar A, Ajzenberg D, Bodaghi B, et al: Direct genotyping of *Toxoplasma gondii* in ocular fluid samples from 20 patients with ocular toxoplasmosis: predominance of type II in France, *J Clin Microbiol* 49:1513-1517, 2011.
59. de Sousa S, Ajzenberg D, Canada N, et al: Biologic and molecular characterization of *Toxoplasma gondii* isolates from pigs from Portugal, *Vet Parasitol* 135:133-136, 2006.
60. Dubey JP, Velmurugan GV, Rajendran C, et al: Genetic characterisation of *Toxoplasma gondii* in wildlife from North America revealed widespread and high prevalence of the fourth clonal type, *Int J Parasitol* 41:1139-1147, 2011.
61. Khan A, Dubey JP, Su C, et al: Genetic analyses of atypical *Toxoplasma gondii* strains reveal a fourth clonal lineage in North America, *Int J Parasitol* 41:645-655, 2011.
62. Carneiro AC, Andrade GM, Costa JG, et al: Genetic characterization of *Toxoplasma gondii* revealed highly diverse genotypes for isolates from newborns with congenital toxoplasmosis in southeastern Brazil, *J Clin Microbiol* 51:901-907, 2013.
63. Pena HF, Gennari SM, Dubey JP, et al: Population structure and mouse-virulence of *Toxoplasma gondii* in Brazil, *Int J Parasitol* 38:561-569, 2008.
64. Mercier A, Ajzenberg D, Devillard S, et al: Human impact on genetic diversity of *Toxoplasma gondii*: example of the anthropized environment from French Guiana, *Infect Genet Evol* 11:1378-1387, 2011.
65. Peyron F, Lobry JR, Musset K, et al: Serotyping of *Toxoplasma gondii* in chronically infected pregnant women: predominance of type II in Europe and types I and III in Colombia (South America), *Microbes Infect* 8:2333-2340, 2006.
66. Morisset S, Peyron F, Lobry JR, et al: Serotyping of *Toxoplasma gondii*: striking homogeneous pattern between symptomatic and asymptomatic infections within Europe and South America, *Microbes Infect* 10:742-747, 2008.
67. Wang L, Chen H, Liu D, et al: Genotypes and mouse virulence of *Toxoplasma gondii* isolates from animals and humans in China, *PLoS One* 8:e53483, 2013.
68. Mercier A, Devillard S, Ngoubangoye B, et al: Additional haplogroups of *Toxoplasma gondii* out of Africa: population structure and mouse-virulence of strains from Gabon, *PLoS Negl Trop Dis* 4: e876, 2010.
69. Mack DG, Johnson JJ, Roberts F, et al: HLA-class II genes modify outcome of *Toxoplasma gondii* infection, *Int J Parasitol* 29:1351-1358, 1999.
70. Jamieson SE, de Roubaix LA, Cortina-Borja M, et al: Genetic and epigenetic factors at COL2A1 and ABCA4 influence clinical outcome in congenital toxoplasmosis, *PLoS One* 3: e2285, 2008.
71. Dubremetz JF, Lebrun M: Virulence factors of *Toxoplasma gondii*, *Microbes Infect* 14:1403-1410, 2012.
72. Reese ML, Zeiner GM, Saeij JP, et al: Polymorphic family of injected pseudokinases is paramount in Toxoplasma virulence, *Proc Natl Acad Sci U S A* 108:9625-9630, 2011.
73. Saeij JP, Boyle JP, Coller S, et al: Polymorphic secreted kinases are key virulence factors in toxoplasmosis, *Science* 314:1780-1783, 2006.
74. Carme B, Demar M, Ajzenberg D, et al: Severe acquired toxoplasmosis caused by wild cycle of *Toxoplasma gondii*, French Guiana, *Emerg Infect Dis* 15:656-658, 2009.
75. Delhaes L, Ajzenberg D, Sicot B, et al: Severe congenital toxoplasmosis due to a *Toxoplasma gondii* strain with an atypical genotype: case report and review, *Prenat Diagn* 30:902-905, 2010.
76. Sobanski V, Ajzenberg D, Delhaes L, et al: Severe toxoplasmosis in immunocompetent hosts: be aware of atypical strains, *Am J Respir Crit Care Med* 187:1143-1145, 2013.
77. Gilbert RE, Freeman K, Lago EG, et al: Ocular sequelae of congenital toxoplasmosis in Brazil compared with Europe, *PLoS Negl Trop Dis* 2:e277, 2008.
78. Pomares C, Ajzenberg D, Bornard L, et al: Toxoplasmosis and horse meat, France, *Emerg Infect Dis* 17:1327-1328, 2011.
79. Elbez-Rubinstein A, Ajzenberg D, Dardé ML, et al: Congenital toxoplasmosis and reinfection during pregnancy: case report, strain characterization, experimental model of reinfection, and review, *J Infect Dis* 199:280-285, 2009.
80. Dunn D, Wallon M, Peyron F, et al: Mother-to-child transmission of toxoplasmosis: risk estimates for clinical counselling, *Lancet* 353:1829-1833, 1999.
81. Romand S, Chosson M, Franck J, et al: Usefulness of quantitative polymerase chain reaction in amniotic fluid as early prognostic marker of fetal infection with *Toxoplasma gondii*, *Am J Obstet Gynecol* 190:797-802, 2004.
82. Ortiz-Alegria LB, Caballero-Ortega H, Canedo-Solares I, et al: Congenital toxoplasmosis: candidate host immune genes relevant for vertical transmission and pathogenesis, *Genes Immun* 11: 363-373, 2010.
83. Bela SR, Dutra MS, Mui E, et al: Impaired innate immunity in mice deficient in interleukin-1 receptor-associated kinase 4 leads to defective type 1 T cell responses, B cell expansion, and enhanced susceptibility to infection with *Toxoplasma gondii*, *Infect Immun* 80:4298-4308, 2012.
84. Shiono Y, Mun HS, He N, et al: Maternal-fetal transmission of *Toxoplasma gondii* in interferon-gamma deficient pregnant mice, *Parasitol Int* 56:141-148, 2007.
85. Thouvenin M, Candolfi E, Villard O, et al: Immune response in a murine model of congenital toxoplasmosis: increased susceptibility of pregnant mice and transplacental passage of *Toxoplasma gondii* are type 2-dependent, *Parassitologia* 39:279-283, 1997.
86. Lees MP, Fuller SJ, McLeod R, et al: P2X7 receptor-mediated killing of an intracellular parasite, *Toxoplasma gondii*, by human and murine macrophages, *J Immunol* 184:7040-7046, 2010.
87. Peixoto-Rangel AL, Miller EN, Castellucci L, et al: Candidate gene analysis of ocular toxoplasmosis in Brazil: evidence for a role for toll-like receptor 9 (TLR9), *Mem Inst Oswaldo Cruz* 104:1187-1190, 2009.
88. Kieffer F, Wallon M, Garcia P, et al: Risk factors for retinochoroiditis during the first 2 years of life in infants with treated congenital toxoplasmosis, *Pediatr Infect Dis J* 27:27-32, 2008.
89. Mason NJ, Artis D, Hunter CA: New lessons from old pathogens: what parasitic infections have taught us about the role of nuclear factor-kappaB in the regulation of immunity, *Immunol Rev* 201: 48-56, 2004.
90. Jamieson SE, Cordell H, Petersen E, et al: Host genetic and epigenetic factors in toxoplasmosis, *Mem Inst Oswaldo Cruz* 104:162-169, 2009.
91. Coutinho LB, Gomes AO, Araujo EC, et al: The impaired pregnancy outcome in murine congenital toxoplasmosis is associated with a pro-inflammatory immune response, but not correlated with decidual inducible nitric oxide synthase expression, *Int J Parasitol* 42:341-352, 2012.
92. Biedermann K, Flepp M, Fierz W, et al: Pregnancy, immunosuppression and reactivation of latent toxoplasmosis, *J Perinat Med* 23:191-203, 1995.
93. Vado-Solis IA, Suarez-Solis V, Jimenez-Delgadillo B, et al: *Toxoplasma gondii* presence in women with spontaneous abortion in Yucatan, Mexico, *J Parasitol* 99:383-385, 2013.
94. Abou-Bacar A, Pfaff AW, Georges S, et al: Role of NK cells and gamma interferon in transplacental passage of *Toxoplasma gondii* in a mouse model of primary infection, *Infect Immun* 72:1397-1401, 2004.
95. Pfaff AW, Georges S, Abou-Bacar A, et al: *Toxoplasma gondii* regulates ICAM-1 mediated monocyte adhesion to trophoblasts, *Immunol Cell Biol* 83:183-189, 2005.
96. Senegas A, Villard O, Neuville A, et al: *Toxoplasma gondii*-induced foetal resorption in mice involves interferon-gamma-induced apoptosis and spiral artery dilation at the maternofoetal interface, *Int J Parasitol* 39:481-487, 2009.
97. Suzuki Y, Sa Q, Gehman M, et al: Interferon-gamma- and perforin-mediated immune responses for resistance against *Toxoplasma gondii* in the brain, *Expert Rev Mol Med* 13:e31, 2011.
98. de Oliveira Gomes A, de Oliveira Silva DA, Silva NM, et al: Effect of macrophage migration inhibitory factor (MIF) in human placental explants infected with *Toxoplasma gondii* depends on gestational age, *Am J Pathol* 178:2792-2801, 2011.
99. McLeod R, Beem MO, Estes RG: Lymphocyte anergy specific to *Toxoplasma gondii* antigens in a baby with congenital toxoplasmosis, *J Clin Lab Immunol* 17:149-153, 1985.
100. Guglietta S, Beghetto E, Spadoni A, et al: Age-dependent impairment of functional helper T cell responses to immunodominant epitopes of *Toxoplasma gondii* antigens in congenitally infected individuals, *Microbes Infect* 9:127-133, 2007.

101. McLeod R, Mack DG, Boyer K, et al: Phenotypes and functions of lymphocytes in congenital toxoplasmosis, *J Lab Clin Med* 116: 623-635, 1990.
102. Fatoohi AF, Cozon GJ, Wallon M, et al: Cellular immunity to *Toxoplasma gondii* in congenitally infected newborns and immunocompetent infected hosts, *Eur J Clin Microbiol Infect Dis* 22:181-184, 2003.
103. Norose K, Kikumura A, Luster AD, et al: CXCL10 is required to maintain T-cell populations and to control parasite replication during chronic ocular toxoplasmosis, *Invest Ophthalmol Vis Sci* 52:389-398, 2011.
104. Holland GN, Crespi CM, ten Dam-van Loon N, et al: Analysis of recurrence patterns associated with toxoplasmic retinochoroiditis, *Am J Ophthalmol* 145:1007-1013, 2008.
105. Garweg JG, Scherrer JN, Halberstadt M: Recurrence characteristics in European patients with ocular toxoplasmosis, *Br J Ophthalmol* 92:1253-1256, 2008.
106. De Lalla F, Sampieri L, Bechelli G, et al: [Relations between the resistance to reinfection and serum antibodies in mice used in isolation tests of human Toxoplasma], *Boll Soc Ital Biol Sper* 40:297-298, 1964.
107. Werner H: [The effect of Toxoplasma antibodies after reinfection with *T. gondii*. II. Communication: investigations over the incidence of Toxoplasma in peripheral blood after primary and secondary infection] (author's transl), *Zentralbl Bakteriol Orig A* 238:122-127, 1977.
108. Werner H, Egger I: [Protective effect of Toxoplasma antibody against re-infection] (author's transl), *Z Tropenmed Parasitol* 24:174-180, 1973.
109. Werner H, Janitschke K, Masihi M, et al: The effect of Toxoplasma antibodies after reinfection with *T. gondii*. III. Communication: investigations on the question of placental transmission of Toxoplasma in immunised pregnant animals (author's transl), *Zentralbl Bakteriol Orig A* 238:128-142, 1977.
110. Coutinho SG, Leite MA, Amendoeira MR, et al: Concomitant cases of acquired toxoplasmosis in children of a single family: evidence of reinfection, *J Infect Dis* 146:30-33, 1982.
111. Fortier B, Aissi E, Ajana F, et al: Spontaneous abortion and reinfection by *Toxoplasma gondii*, *Lancet* 338:444, 1991.
112. Gavinet MF, Robert F, Firtion G, et al: Congenital toxoplasmosis due to maternal reinfection during pregnancy, *J Clin Microbiol* 35:1276-1277, 1997.
113. Araujo F, Slifer T, Kim S: Chronic infection with *Toxoplasma gondii* does not prevent acute disease or colonization of the brain with tissue cysts following reinfection with different strains of the parasite, *J Parasitol* 83:521-522, 1997.
114. Dao A, Fortier B, Soete M, et al: Successful reinfection of chronically infected mice by a different *Toxoplasma gondii* genotype, *Int J Parasitol* 31:63-65, 2001.
115. Ladas ID, Rallatos CL, Kanaki CS, et al: Presumed congenital ocular toxoplasmosis in two successive siblings, *Ophthalmologica* 213:320-322, 1999.
116. Kodjikian L, Hoigne I, Adam O, et al: Vertical transmission of toxoplasmosis from a chronically infected immunocompetent woman, *Pediatr Infect Dis J* 23:272-274, 2004.
117. Valdes V, Legagneur H, Watrin V, et al: Congenital toxoplasmosis due to maternal reinfection during pregnancy, *Arch Pediatr* 18: 761-763, 2011.
118. Dzitko K, Staczek P, Gatkowska J, et al: *Toxoplasma gondii*: serological recognition of reinfection, *Exp Parasitol* 112:134-137, 2006.
119. Gigley JP, Bhadra R, Khan IA: CD8 T Cells and *Toxoplasma gondii*: a new paradigm, *J Parasitol Res* 2011:243796, 2011.
120. Gigley JP, Bhadra R, Moretto MM, et al: T cell exhaustion in protozoan disease, *Trends Parasitol* 28:377-384, 2012.
121. Brandao GP, Melo MN, Gazzinelli RT, et al: Experimental reinfection of BALB/c mice with different recombinant type I/III strains of *Toxoplasma gondii*: involvement of IFN-gamma and IL-10, *Mem Inst Oswaldo Cruz* 104:241-245, 2009.
122. Bodaghi B, Touitou V, Fardeau C, et al: Toxoplasmosis: new challenges for an old disease, *Eye (Lond)* 26:241-244, 2012.
123. Holland GN: Ocular toxoplasmosis: new directions for clinical investigation, *Ocul Immunol Inflamm* 8:1-7, 2000.
124. Garweg JG, Scherrer J, Wallon M, et al: Reactivation of ocular toxoplasmosis during pregnancy, *BJOG* 112:241-242, 2005.
125. Andrade GM, Vasconcelos-Santos DV, Carellos EV, et al: Congenital toxoplasmosis from a chronically infected woman with reactivation of retinochoroiditis during pregnancy, *J Pediatr (Rio J)* 86:85-88, 2010.
126. Bosch-Driessen LH, Plaisier MB, Stilma JS, et al: Reactivations of ocular toxoplasmosis after cataract extraction, *Ophthalmology* 109: 41-45, 2002.
127. Sullivan WJ Jr, Jeffers V: Mechanisms of *Toxoplasma gondii* persistence and latency, *FEMS Microbiol Rev* 36:717-733, 2012.
128. Remington JS, Melton ML, Jacobs L: Induced and spontaneous recurrent parasitemia in chronic infections with avirulent strains of *Toxoplasma gondii*, *J Immunol* 87:578-581, 1961.
129. Silveira C, Vallochi AL, Rodrigues da Silva U, et al: *Toxoplasma gondii* in the peripheral blood of patients with acute and chronic toxoplasmosis, *Br J Ophthalmol* 95:396-400, 2011.
130. Siegel SE, Lunde MN, Gelderman AH, et al: Transmission of toxoplasmosis by leukocyte transfusion, *Blood* 37:388-394, 1971.
131. Garweg J, Boehnke M, Koerner F: Restricted applicability of the polymerase chain reaction for the diagnosis of ocular toxoplasmosis, *Ger J Ophthalmol* 5:104-108, 1996.
132. Lee SE, Hong SH, Lee SH, et al: Detection of ocular *Toxoplasma gondii* infection in chronic irregular recurrent uveitis by PCR, *Korean J Parasitol* 50:229-231, 2012.
133. Kompalic-Cristo A, Frotta C, Suarez-Mutis M, et al: Evaluation of a real-time PCR assay based on the repetitive B1 gene for the detection of *Toxoplasma gondii* in human peripheral blood, *Parasitol Res* 101:619-625, 2007.
134. Accorinti M, Bruscolini A, Pirraglia MP, et al: Toxoplasmic retinochoroiditis in an Italian referral center, *Eur J Ophthalmol* 19: 824-830, 2009.
135. Bosch-Driessen LE, Berendschot TT, Ongkosuwito JV, et al: Ocular toxoplasmosis: clinical features and prognosis of 154 patients, *Ophthalmology* 109:869-878, 2002.
136. Wallon M, Kodjikian L, Binquet C, et al: Long-term ocular prognosis in 327 children with congenital toxoplasmosis, *Pediatrics* 113: 1567-1572, 2004.
137. Phan L, Kasza K, Jalbrzikowski J, et al: Longitudinal study of new eye lesions in children with toxoplasmosis who were not treated during the first year of life, *Am J Ophthalmol* 146:375-384, 2008.
138. Mets MB, Holfels E, Boyer KM, et al: Eye manifestations of congenital toxoplasmosis, *Am J Ophthalmol* 122:309-324, 1996.
139. Meganathan P, Singh S, Ling LY, et al: Detection of *Toxoplasma gondii* DNA by PCR following microwave treatment of serum and whole blood, *Southeast Asian J Trop Med Public Health* 41:265-273, 2010.
140. Boothroyd JC: Expansion of host range as a driving force in the evolution of Toxoplasma, *Mem Inst Oswaldo Cruz* 104:179-184, 2009.
141. Hunter CA, Sibley LD: Modulation of innate immunity by *Toxoplasma gondii* virulence effectors, *Nat Rev Microbiol* 10:766-778, 2012.
142. Molestina RE, El-Guendy N, Sinai AP: Infection with *Toxoplasma gondii* results in dysregulation of the host cell cycle, *Cell Microbiol* 10:1153-1165, 2008.
143. Sinai AP: Biogenesis of and activities at the *Toxoplasma gondii* parasitophorous vacuole membrane, *Subcell Biochem* 47:155-164, 2008.
144. Fentress SJ, Sibley LD: The secreted kinase ROP18 defends Toxoplasma's border, *Bioessays* 33:693-700, 2011.
145. Fleckenstein MC, Reese ML, Konen-Waisman S, et al: *Toxoplasma gondii* pseudokinase inhibits host IRG resistance proteins, *PLoS Biol* 10: e1001358, 2012.
146. Zhao YO, Rohde C, Lilue JT, et al: *Toxoplasma gondii* and the immunity-related GTPase (IRG) resistance system in mice: a review, *Mem Inst Oswaldo Cruz* 104:234-240, 2009.
147. Portillo JA, Okenka G, Reed E, et al: The CD40-autophagy pathway is needed for host protection despite IFN-Gamma-dependent immunity and CD40 induces autophagy via control of P21 levels, *PLoS One* 5: e14472, 2010.
148. Subauste CS: Autophagy in immunity against *Toxoplasma gondii*, *Curr Top Microbiol Immunol* 335:251-265, 2009.
149. Van Grol J, Muniz-Feliciano L, Portillo JA, et al: CD40 induces anti-*Toxoplasma gondii* activity in nonhematopoietic cells dependent on autophagy proteins, *Infect Immun* 81:2002-2011, 2013.
150. Khong A, Nelson DJ, Nowak AK, et al: The use of agonistic anti-CD40 therapy in treatments for cancer, *Int Rev Immunol* 31: 246-266, 2012.
151. Kornbluth RS, Stempniak M, Stone GW: Design of CD40 agonists and their use in growing B cells for cancer immunotherapy, *Int Rev Immunol* 31:279-288, 2012.
152. Webber A, Hirose R, Vincenti F: Novel strategies in immunosuppression: issues in perspective, *Transplantation* 91:1057-1064, 2011.

153. Egan CE, Sukhumavasi W, Butcher BA, et al: Functional aspects of Toll-like receptor/MyD88 signalling during protozoan infection: focus on *Toxoplasma gondii*, *Clin Exp Immunol* 156:17-24, 2009.
154. Melo MB, Jensen KD, Saeij JP: *Toxoplasma gondii* effectors are master regulators of the inflammatory response, *Trends Parasitol* 27:487-495, 2011.
155. Dzierszinski FS, Hunter CA: Advances in the use of genetically engineered parasites to study immunity to *Toxoplasma gondii*, *Parasite Immunol* 30:235-244, 2008.
156. Dupont CD, Christian DA, Hunter CA: Immune response and immunopathology during toxoplasmosis, *Semin Immunopathol* 34:793-813, 2012.
157. Leng J, Butcher BA, Denkers EY: Dysregulation of macrophage signal transduction by *Toxoplasma gondii*: past progress and recent advances, *Parasite Immunol* 31:717-728, 2009.
158. Bhadra R, Gigley JP, Weiss LM, et al: Control of Toxoplasma reactivation by rescue of dysfunctional CD8+ T-cell response via PD-1-PDL-1 blockade, *Proc Natl Acad Sci U S A* 108:9196-9201, 2011.
159. Luder CG, Campos-Salinas J, Gonzalez-Rey E, et al: Impact of protozoan cell death on parasite-host interactions and pathogenesis, *Parasit Vectors* 3:116, 2010.
160. Luder CG, Stanway RR, Chaussepied M, et al: Intracellular survival of apicomplexan parasites and host cell modification, *Int J Parasitol* 39:163-173, 2009.
161. Barragan A, Hitziger N: Transepithelial migration by Toxoplasma, *Subcell Biochem* 47:198-207, 2008.
162. Barragan A, Sibley LD: Migration of *Toxoplasma gondii* across biological barriers, *Trends Microbiol* 11:426-430, 2003.
163. Feustel SM, Meissner M, Liesenfeld O: *Toxoplasma gondii* and the blood-brain barrier, *Virulence* 3:182-192, 2012.
164. Furtado JM, Bharadwaj AS, Chipps TJ, et al: *Toxoplasma gondii* tachyzoites cross retinal endothelium assisted by intercellular adhesion molecule-1 in vitro, *Immunol Cell Biol* 90:912-915, 2012.
165. Zamora DO, Rosenbaum JT, Smith JR: Invasion of human retinal vascular endothelial cells by *Toxoplasma gondii* tachyzoites, *Br J Ophthalmol* 92:852-855, 2008.
166. Sims TA, Hay J: Host-parasite relationship between congenital Toxoplasma infection and mouse brain: role of small vessels, *Parasitology* 110(Pt 2):123-127, 1995.
167. Schaeffer M, Han SJ, Chtanova T, et al: Dynamic imaging of T cell-parasite interactions in the brains of mice chronically infected with *Toxoplasma gondii*, *J Immunol* 182:6379-6393, 2009.
168. Garweg JG: Determinants of immunodiagnostic success in human ocular toxoplasmosis, *Parasite Immunol* 27:61-68, 2005.
169. Dutton GN: The causes of tissue damage in toxoplasmic retinochoroiditis, *Trans Ophthalmol Soc U K* 105(Pt 4):404-412, 1986.
170. Gormley PD, Pavesio CE, Minnasian D, et al: Effects of drug therapy on Toxoplasma cysts in an animal model of acute and chronic disease, *Invest Ophthalmol Vis Sci* 39:1171-1175, 1998.
171. Djurkovic-Djakovic O, Milenkovic V, Nikolic A, et al: Efficacy of atovaquone combined with clindamycin against murine infection with a cystogenic (Me49) strain of *Toxoplasma gondii*, *J Antimicrob Chemother* 50:981-987, 2002.
172. Reiter-Owona I, Seitz H, Gross U, et al: Is stage conversion the initiating event for reactivation of *Toxoplasma gondii* in brain tissue of AIDS patients? *J Parasitol* 86:531-536, 2000.
173. Ferguson DJ, Huskinson-Mark J, Araujo FG, et al: A morphological study of chronic cerebral toxoplasmosis in mice: comparison of four different strains of *Toxoplasma gondii*, *Parasitol Res* 80:493-501, 1994.
174. Ferguson DJ, Hutchison WM: The host-parasite relationship of *Toxoplasma gondii* in the brains of chronically infected mice, *Virchows Arch A Pathol Anat Histopathol* 411:39-43, 1987.
175. Afonso C, Paixao VB, Costa RM: Chronic Toxoplasma infection modifies the structure and the risk of host behavior, *PLoS One* 7, 2012. e32489.
176. Lee WR, Hay J, Hutchison WM, et al: A murine model of congenital toxoplasmic retinochoroiditis, *Acta Ophthalmol (Copenh)* 61:818-830, 1983.
177. Graham DI, Hay J, Hutchison WM, et al: Encephalitis in mice with congenital ocular toxoplasmosis, *J Pathol* 142:265-277, 1984.
178. Hutchison WM, Hay J, Lee WR, et al: A study of cataract in murine congenital toxoplasmosis, *Ann Trop Med Parasitol* 76:53-70, 1982.
179. Esterre P: Immune reactions in the brain, *Arch Inst Pasteur Madagascar* 63:24-30, 1996.
180. Caspi RR: Ocular autoimmunity: the price of privilege? *Immunol Rev* 213:23-35, 2006.
181. Garweg JG, Peyron F: Clinical and laboratory diagnosis of ocular toxoplasmosis, *Expert Rev Ophthalmol* 3:333-346, 2008.
182. Rahi AH, Addison DJ: Autoimmunity and the outer retina, *Trans Ophthalmol Soc U K* 103(Pt 4):428-437, 1983.
183. Muiño JC, Juarez CP, Luna JD, et al: The importance of specific IgG and IgE autoantibodies to retinal S antigen, total serum IgE, and sCD23 levels in autoimmune and infectious uveitis, *J Clin Immunol* 19:215-222, 1999.
184. Whittle RM, Wallace GR, Whiston RA, et al: Human antiretinal antibodies in Toxoplasma retinochoroiditis, *Br J Ophthalmol* 82:1017-1021, 1998.
185. Vallochi AL, da Silva Rios L, Nakamura MV, et al: The involvement of autoimmunity against retinal antigens in determining disease severity in toxoplasmosis, *J Autoimmun* 24:25-32, 2005.
186. Garweg JG, de Kozak Y, Goldenberg B, et al: Anti-retinal autoantibodies in experimental ocular and systemic toxoplasmosis, *Graefes Arch Clin Exp Ophthalmol* 248:573-584, 2010.
187. Garweg JG, Candolfi E: Immunopathology in ocular toxoplasmosis: facts and clues, *Mem Inst Oswaldo Cruz* 104:211-220, 2009.
188. Callahan WP Jr, Russell WO, Smith MG: Human toxoplasmosis; a clinicopathologic study with presentation of five cases and review of the literature, *Medicine* 25:343-397, 1946.
189. Hayes K, Billson FA, Jack I, et al: Cell culture isolation of *Toxoplasma gondii* from an infant with unusual ocular features, *Med J Aust* 1:1297-1299, 1973.
190. Manschot WA, Daamen CB: Connatal ocular toxoplasmosis, *Arch Ophthalmol* 74:48-54, 1965.
191. Pratt-Thomas HR, Cannon WM: Systemic infantile toxoplasmosis, *Am J Pathol* 22:779-795, 1946.
192. Wolf A, Cowen D, Paige BH: Fetal encephalomyelitis: prenatal inception of infantile toxoplasmosis, *Science* 93:548-549, 1941.
193. Milgram JW: Osseous changes in congenital toxoplasmosis, *Arch Pathol* 97:150-151, 1974.
194. Heath P, Zuelzer WW: Toxoplasmosis (report of eye findings in infant twins), *Trans Am Ophthalmol Soc* 42:119-132, 1944.
195. Dunn D, Weisberg LA: Serial changes in a patient with congenital CNS toxoplasmosis as observed with CT, *Comput Radiol* 8:133-139, 1984.
196. Frenkel JK: Pathology and pathogenesis of congenital toxoplasmosis, *Bull N Y Acad Med* 50:182-191, 1974.
197. Zuelzer WW: Infantile toxoplasmosis, with a report of three cases, including two in which the patients were identical twins, *Arch Pathol* 38:1-19, 1944.
198. Neghme A, Thiermann E, Pino F, et al: Toxoplasmosis in Chile; preliminary communication, *Bol Inf Parasit Chil* 7:6-8, 1952.
199. Beckett RS, Flynn FJ Jr: Toxoplasmosis; report of two new cases, with a classification and with a demonstration of the organisms in the human placenta, *N Engl J Med* 249:345-350, 1953.
200. Sarrut S: Histological study of the placenta in congenital toxoplasmosis, *Ann Pediatr (Paris)* 14:2429-2435, 1967.
201. Mellgren J, Alm L, Kjessler A: The isolation of Toxoplasma from the human placenta and uterus, *Acta Pathol Microbiol Scand* 30:59-67, 1952.
202. Elliott WG: Placental toxoplasmosis. Report of a case, *Am J Clin Pathol* 53:413-417, 1970.
203. Benirschke K, Driscoll SG. *The pathology of the human placenta*, New York, 1967, Springer-Verlag.
204. Farber S, Craig JM: Clinical Pathological Conference (Children's Medical Center, Boston, Mass), *J Pediatr* 49:752-764, 1956.
205. Glasser L, Delta BG: Congenital toxoplasmosis with placental infection in monozygotic twins, *Pediatrics* 35:276-283, 1965.
206. Cardoso RA, Guimaraes FN, Garcia AP: Congenital toxoplasmosis, *Mem Inst Oswaldo Cruz* 54:571-597, 1956.
207. Piche M, Battaglione V, Monticelli I, et al: Placenta toxoplasmosis in the course of AIDS. Immunohistochemical and ultrastructural study of a case, *Ann Pathol* 17:337-339, 1997.
208. Altshuler G: Placentitis, with a new light on an old ToRCH, *Obstet Gynecol Annu* 6:197-221, 1977.
209. Nowakowska D, Golab E, Czichos E, et al: Detection of *Toxoplasma gondii* in human placenta by PCR and placental histologic findings, *Wiad Parazytol* 48:301-309, 2002.
210. Garcia AG, Coutinho SG, Amendoeira MR, et al: Placental morphology of newborns at risk for congenital toxoplasmosis, *J Trop Pediatr* 29:95-103, 1983.

211. Altshuler G: Toxoplasmosis as a cause of hydranencephaly, *Am J Dis Child* 125:251-252, 1973.
212. Volchenko KL: Case of congenital generalized toxoplasmosis with specific changes in the placenta and reactive myeloerythroblastosis, *Arkh Patol* 29:66-68, 1967.
213. Dos Santos Neto JG: Toxoplasmosis. Historical review, direct diagnostic microscopy, and report of a case, *Am J Clin Pathol* 63:909-915, 1975.
214. Gordon N: Toxoplasmosis: a preventable cause of brain damage, *Dev Med Child Neurol* 35:567-573, 1993.
215. Jacquemard F: Ultrasonographic signs of congenital toxoplasmosis, *Arch Pediatr* 10(Suppl 1):35-38, 2003.
216. Weber F: The cerebral lesions in congenital toxoplasmosis. Study of 9 personal cases and 61 cases in the literature, *Helv Paediatr Acta Suppl* 48:1-51, 1983.
217. Ferguson DJ, Bowker C, Jeffery KJ, et al: Congenital toxoplasmosis: continued parasite proliferation in the fetal brain despite maternal immunological control in other tissues, *Clin Infect Dis* 56:204-208, 2013.
218. Frenkel JK, Friedlander S: *Toxoplasmosis: pathology of neonatal disease*, Washington, DC, 1952, US Government Printing Office.
219. Rodney MB, Mitchell N, Redner B, et al: Infantile toxoplasmosis: report of a case with autopsy, *Pediatrics* 5:649-663, 1950.
220. Wolf A, Cowen D, Paige BH: Toxoplasmic encephalomyelitis. VI. Clinical diagnosis of infantile or congenital toxoplasmosis; survival beyond infancy, *Arch Neurol Psychiatry* 48:689-739, 1942.
221. Wolf A, Cowen D, Paige B: Toxoplasmic encephalomyelitis, *Trans Am Neurol Assoc* 65:76-79, 1939.
222. Ansari MQ, Chincanchan CA, Armstrong DL: Brain calcification in hypoxic-ischemic lesions: an autopsy review, *Pediatr Neurol* 6:94-101, 1990.
223. Kulkarni AM, Baskar S, Kulkarni ML, et al: Fetal intracranial calcification: pseudo-TORCH phenotype and discussion of related phenotypes, *Am J Med Genet A* 152A:930-937, 2010.
224. Eyaid W, Al-Tassan RS, Al-Nouri DM: Intracranial calcifications, microcephaly, and seizure. If not congenital infection, what could it be? *Neurosciences (Riyadh)* 17:248-252, 2012.
225. Taccone A, Fondelli MP, Ferrea G, et al: An unusual CT presentation of congenital cerebral toxoplasmosis in an 8-month-old boy with AIDS, *Pediatr Radiol* 22:68-69, 1992.
226. Hervas JA, Fiol M, Caimari M, et al: Central nervous system congenital toxoplasmosis mimicking brain abscesses, *Pediatr Infect Dis J* 6:491-492, 1987.
227. Mehren M, Burns PJ, Mamani F, et al: Toxoplasmic myelitis mimicking intramedullary spinal cord tumor, *Neurology* 38:1648-1650, 1988.
228. Wende-Fischer R, Ehrenheim C, Heyer R, et al: In spinal symptoms remember toxoplasmosis, *Monatsschr Kinderheilkd* 141:789-791, 1993.
229. al Shahwan S, Rossi ML, al Thagafi MA: Ascending paralysis due to myelitis in a newborn with congenital toxoplasmosis, *J Neurol Sci* 139:156-159, 1996.
230. Shefer-Kaufman N, Mimouni FB, Stavorovsky Z, et al: Incidence and clinical significance of echogenic vasculature in the basal ganglia of newborns, *Am J Perinatol* 16:315-319, 1999.
231. Frenkel JK: Toxoplasmosis. Mechanisms of infection, laboratory diagnosis and management, *Curr Top Pathol* 54:27-75, 1971.
232. Paige BH, Cowen D, Wolf A: Toxoplasmic encephalomyelitis. V. Further observations of infantile toxoplasmosis; intrauterine inception of the disease; visceral manifestations, *Am J Dis Child* 63: 474-514, 1942.
233. Pinkerton H, Henderson RG: Adult toxoplasmosis, *JAMA* 116: 807-814, 1941.
234. Bamatter F, Bamatter F: La choriorétinite toxoplasmique, *Ophthalmologica* 114:340-358, 1947.
235. Binkhorst CD: Toxoplasmosis; report of four cases, with demonstration of parasites in one case, *Ophthalmologica* 115:65-77, 1948.
236. Koch FL: Toxoplasmic encephalomyelitis. VII. Significance of ocular lesions in the diagnosis of infantile or congenital toxoplasmosis, *Arch Ophthalmol* 29:1-25, 1943.
237. Hogan MJ: *Ocular toxoplasmosis*, New York, 1951, Columbia University Press.
238. Wilder HC: Toxoplasma chorioretinitis in adults, *AMA Arch Ophthalmol* 48:127-136, 1952.
239. Butler NJ, Furtado JM, Winthrop KL, et al: Ocular toxoplasmosis II: clinical features, pathology and management, *Clin Experiment Ophthalmol* 41:95-108, 2013.
240. Roberts F, Mets MB, Ferguson DJ, et al: Histopathological features of ocular toxoplasmosis in the fetus and infant, *Arch Ophthalmol* 119:51-58, 2001.
241. Tetz M, Holz FG, Gallasch G, et al: Segmental retinal arteritis and retinochorioiditis, *Ophthalmologe* 89:71-76, 1992.
242. Smith JR, Cunningham ET Jr: Atypical presentations of ocular toxoplasmosis, *Curr Opin Ophthalmol* 13:387-392, 2002.
243. Dutton GN, McMenamin PG, Hay J, et al: The ultrastructural pathology of congenital murine toxoplasmic retinochoroiditis. Part II: the morphology of the inflammatory changes, *Exp Eye Res* 43:545-560, 1986.
244. Furtado JM, Ashander LM, Mohs K, et al: *Toxoplasma gondii* migration within and infection of human retina, *PLoS One* 8:e54358, 2013.
245. Meenken C, Assies J, van Nieuwenhuizen O, et al: Long term ocular and neurological involvement in severe congenital toxoplasmosis, *Br J Ophthalmol* 79:581-584, 1995.
246. Kelemen G: Toxoplasmosis and congenital deafness, *AMA Arch Otolaryngol* 68:547-561, 1958.
247. Wright I: Congenital toxoplasmosis and deafness. An investigation, *Pract Otorhinolaryngol (Basel)* 33:377-387, 1971.
248. Salviz M, Montoya JG, Nadol JB, et al: Otopathology in congenital toxoplasmosis, *Otol Neurotol* 34:1165-1169, 2013.
249. Couvreur J, Desmonts G: Congenital and maternal toxoplasmosis. A review of 300 congenital cases, *Dev Med Child Neurol* 4:519-530, 1962.
250. Couvreur J: The lungs in toxoplasmosis, *Rev Mal Respir* 3:525-532, 1975.
251. Pomeroy C, Filice GA: Pulmonary toxoplasmosis: a review, *Clin Infect Dis* 14:863-870, 1992.
252. Theologides A, Kennedy BJ: Toxoplasmic myocarditis and pericarditis, *Am J Med* 47:169-174, 1969.
253. van der Horst R, Klenerman P, Schonland M, et al: Fatal myocardial necrosis probably due to Toxoplasma myocarditis, *S Afr Med J* 46:951-952, 1972.
254. Rosenberg HS: Cardiovascular effects of congenital infections, *Am J Cardiovasc Pathol* 1:147-156, 1987.
255. Medlock MD, Tilleli JT, Pearl GS: Congenital cardiac toxoplasmosis in a newborn with acquired immunodeficiency syndrome, *Pediatr Infect Dis J* 9:129-132, 1990.
256. Mitchell CD, Erlich SS, Mastrucci MT, et al: Congenital toxoplasmosis occurring in infants perinatally infected with human immunodeficiency virus 1, *Pediatr Infect Dis J* 9:512-518, 1990.
257. Escribano Subias J, Bilbao Sustacha J, Balaguer Santamaria A, Bofarull Bosch JM: Congenital toxoplasmosis in a newborn infant with AIDS, *An Esp Pediatr* 39:349-350, 1993.
258. Schweickert B, Bollmann R, Loui A, et al: Fatal disseminated toxoplasmosis with congenital transmission in an African migrant, *AIDS* 22:1523-1525, 2008.
259. Lelong M, Lepage F, Alison F, et al: Alagille: Toxoplasmosis of the newborn with icterus and liver cirrhosis, *Arch Fr Pediatr* 10: 530-536, 1953.
260. Caldera R, Sarrut S, Rossier A: Hepatic calcifications associated with congenital toxoplasmosis, *Arch Fr Pediatr* 19:1087-1093, 1962.
261. Israelski DM, Skowron G, Leventhal JP, et al: Toxoplasma peritonitis in a patient with acquired immunodeficiency syndrome, *Arch Intern Med* 148:1655-1657, 1988.
262. Roussel B, Pinon JM, Birembaut P, et al: Congenital nephrotic syndrome associated with congenital toxoplasmosis, *Arch Fr Pediatr* 44:795-797, 1987.
263. Kean BH, Grocott RG: Sarcosporidiosis or toxoplasmosis in man and guinea-pig, *Am J Pathol* 21:467-483, 1945.
264. Miller MJ, Seaman E, Remington JS: The clinical spectrum of congenital toxoplasmosis. Problems in recognition, *J Pediatr* 70:714-723, 1967.
265. Fediushina NA, Sherstennikova GE: Damage of the kidneys in congenital toxoplasmosis, *Vrach Delo* 4:121-122, 1966.
266. Wickbom B, Winberg J: Coincidence of congenital toxoplasmosis and acute nephritis with nephrotic syndrome, *Acta Paediatr Scand* 61:470-472, 1972.
267. Shahin B, Papadopoulou ZL, Jenis EH: Congenital nephrotic syndrome associated with congenital toxoplasmosis, *J Pediatr* 85:366-370, 1974.
268. Huldt G, Gard S, Olovson SG: Effect of *Toxoplasma gondii* on the thymus, *Nature* 244:301-303, 1973.
269. Cohen-Addad NE, Joshi VV, Sharer LR, et al: Congenital acquired immunodeficiency syndrome and congenital toxoplasmosis: pathologic support for a chronology of events, *J Perinatol* 8:328-331, 1988.

270. Torres CM: Affinité de l'encephalitozoon chagasi agent étiologique d'une méningoencephalomyélitis congénitale avec myocardité et myosité chez l'homme, *C R Soc Biol* 86:1797-1799, 1927.
271. McCrossin DB, Roberton NR: Congenital skin defects, twins and toxoplasmosis, *J R Soc Med* 82:108-109, 1989.
272. Arnaud JP, Griscelli C, Couvreur J, et al: Hematological and immunological abnormalities in congenital toxoplamosis, *Nouv Rev Fr Hematol* 15:496-505, 1975.
273. Alford CA Jr, Stagno S, Reynolds DW: Congenital toxoplasmosis: clinical, laboratory, and therapeutic considerations, with special reference to subclinical disease, *Bull N Y Acad Med* 50:160-181, 1974.
274. Wilson CB: Immunologic basis for increased susceptibility of the neonate to infection, *J Pediatr* 108:1-12, 1986.
275. Oxelius VA: Monoclonal immunoglobulins in congenital toxoplasmosis, *Clin Exp Immunol* 11:367-380, 1972.
276. Van Camp B, Reynaert P, Van Beers D: Congenital toxoplasmosis associated with transient monoclonal IgGl-lambda gammopathy, *Rev Infect Dis* 4:173-178, 1982.
277. Griscelli C, Desmonts G, Gny B, et al: Congenital toxoplasmosis. Fetal synthesis of oligoclonal immunoglobulin G in intrauterine infection, *J Pediatr* 83:20-26, 1973.
278. Remington JS, Hackman R: Changes in mouse serum proteins during acute and chronic infection with an intracellular parasite (*Toxoplasma gondii*), *J Immunol* 95:1023-1033, 1965.
279. Koch F, Schlagetter K, Schultze HE, et al: Symptomatic macroglobulinemia in congenital lues, *Z Kinderheilkd* 78:283-300, 1956.
280. de Zegher F, Sluiters JF, Stuurman PM, et al: Concomitant cytomegalovirus infection and congenital toxoplasmosis in a newborn, *Eur J Pediatr* 147:424-425, 1988.
281. Maszkiewicz W, Wojnar A, Sujakowa A, et al: Coexistence of cytomegalic inclusion disease, toxoplasmosis and in a premature infant, *Pediatr Pol* 57:821-826, 1982.
282. Le Tan V, Tran Van D, Aicardi J, et al: Association of congenital toxoplasmosis and cytomegaly in infants. Study of 2 anatomoclinical cases, *Arch Fr Pediatr* 27:511-521, 1970.
283. Sotelo-Avila C, Perry CM, Parvey LS, et al: Clinicopathologic conference: coexistent congenital cytomegalovirus and toxoplasmosis in a newborn infant, *J Tenn Med Assoc* 67:588-592, 1974.
284. Demian SD, Donnelly Jr WH, Monif GR: Coexistent congenital cytomegalovirus and toxoplasmosis in a stillborn, *Am J Dis Child* 125:420-421, 1973.
285. Tenter AM, Heckeroth AR, Weiss LM: *Toxoplasma gondii*: from animals to humans, *Int J Parasitol* 30:1217-1258, 2000.
286. Dabritz HA, Conrad PA: Cats and Toxoplasma: implications for public health, *Zoonoses Public Health* 57:34-52, 2010.
287. Song KJ, Shin JC, Shin HJ, et al: Seroprevalence of toxoplasmosis in Korean pregnant women, *Korean J Parasitol* 43:69-71, 2005.
288. Boia MN, Carvalho-Costa FA, Sodre FC, et al: Seroprevalence of *Toxoplasma gondii* infection among indian people living in Iauarete, São Gabriel da Cachoeira, Amazonas, Brazil, *Rev Inst Med Trop São Paulo* 50:17-20, 2008.
289. Alvarado-Esquivel C, Estrada-Martinez S, Liesenfeld O: *Toxoplasma gondii* infection in workers occupationally exposed to unwashed raw fruits and vegetables: a case control seroprevalence study, *Parasit Vectors* 4:235, 2011.
290. Dattoli VC, Veiga RV, Cunha SS, et al: Oocyst ingestion as an important transmission route of *Toxoplasma gondii* in Brazilian urban children, *J Parasitol* 97:1080-1084, 2011.
291. Minbaeva G, Schweiger A, Bodosheva A, et al: *Toxoplasma gondii* infection in Kyrgyzstan: seroprevalence, risk factor analysis, and estimate of congenital and AIDS-related toxoplasmosis, *PLoS Negl Trop Dis* 7:e2043, 2013.
292. Ferreira MU, Hiramoto RM, Aureliano DP, et al: A community-based survey of human toxoplasmosis in rural Amazonia: seroprevalence, seroconversion rate, and associated risk factors, *Am J Trop Med Hyg* 81:171-176, 2009.
293. Fan CK, Lee LW, Liao CW, et al: *Toxoplasma gondii* infection: relationship between seroprevalence and risk factors among primary schoolchildren in the capital areas of Democratic Republic of São Tomé and Príncipe, West Africa, *Parasit Vectors* 5:141, 2012.
294. Dubey JP, Tiao N, Gebreyes WA, et al: A review of toxoplasmosis in humans and animals in Ethiopia, *Epidemiol Infect* 140:1935-1938, 2012.
295. Hall SM, Pandit A, Golwilkar A, et al: How do Jains get Toxoplasma infection? *Lancet* 354:486-487, 1999.
296. Boyer K, Hill D, Mui E, et al: Unrecognized ingestion of *Toxoplasma gondii* oocysts leads to congenital toxoplasmosis and causes epidemics in North America, *Clin Infect Dis* 53:1081-1089, 2011.
297. Roghmann MC, Faulkner CT, Lefkowitz A, et al: Decreased seroprevalence for *Toxoplasma gondii* in Seventh Day Adventists in Maryland, *Am J Trop Med Hyg* 60:790-792, 1999.
298. Proctor EM, Banerjee SN: The seroepidemiology of toxoplasmosis in the lower Fraser Valley of British Columbia, *Can J Infect Dis* 5:218-223, 1994.
299. Jones JL, Kruszon-Moran D, Sanders-Lewis K, et al: *Toxoplasma gondii* infection in the United States, 1999-2004, decline from the prior decade, *Am J Trop Med Hyg* 77:405-410, 2007.
300. Rosso F, Les JT, Agudelo A, et al: Prevalence of infection with *Toxoplasma gondii* among pregnant women in Cali, Colombia, South America, *Am J Trop Med Hyg* 78:504-508, 2008.
301. Yang Z, Cho PY, Ahn SK, et al: A surge in the seroprevalence of toxoplasmosis among the residents of islands in Gangwha-gun, Incheon, Korea, *Korean J Parasitol* 50:191-197, 2012.
302. Lim H, Lee SE, Jung BK, et al: Serologic survey of toxoplasmosis in Seoul and Jeju-do, and a brief review of its seroprevalence in Korea, *Korean J Parasitol* 50:287-293, 2012.
303. Adou-Bryn KD, Ouhon J, Nemer J, et al: Serological survey of acquired toxoplasmosis in women of child-bearing age in Yopougon (Abidjan, Côte d'Ivoire), *Bull Soc Pathol Exot* 97:345-348, 2004.
304. McDonald JC, Gyorkos TW, Alberton B, et al: An outbreak of toxoplasmosis in pregnant women in northern Quebec, *J Infect Dis* 161:769-774, 1990.
305. Robson J, Sullivan J, Nicolaides N, et al: A probable foodborne outbreak of toxoplasmosis, *Commun Dis Intell* 19:517-522, 1995.
306. Choi WY, Nam HW, Kwak NH, et al: Foodborne outbreaks of human toxoplasmosis, *J Infect Dis* 175:1280-1282, 1997.
307. Fertig A, Selwyn S, Tibble MJ: Tetracycline treatment in a food-borne outbreak of toxoplasmosis, *Br Med J* 1:1064, 1977.
308. Bonametti AM, Passos Jdo N, da Silva EM, Bortoliero AL: Outbreak of acute toxoplasmosis transmitted thru the ingestion of ovine raw meat, *Rev Soc Bras Med Trop* 30:21-25, 1996.
309. Hill DE, Dubey JP: *Toxoplasma gondii* prevalence in farm animals in the United States, *Int J Parasitol* 43:107-113, 2013.
310. Kijlstra A, Jongert E: Toxoplasma-safe meat: close to reality? *Trends Parasitol* 25:18-22, 2009.
311. European Food Safety Authority: Surveillance and monitoring of Toxoplasma in humans, food and animals. Scientific opinion of the Panel on Biological Hazards, *EFSA J* 583:1-64, 2007.
312. Kijlstra A, Jongert E: Control of the risk of human toxoplasmosis transmitted by meat, *Int J Parasitol* 38:1359-1370, 2008.
313. Paul M: Potential risk factors for *Toxoplasma gondii* infection in cases with recently acquired toxoplasmosis, *Przegl Epidemiol* 52:447-454, 1998.
314. Buffolano W, Gilbert RE, Holland FJ, et al: Risk factors for recent Toxoplasma infection in pregnant women in Naples, *Epidemiol Infect* 116:347-351, 1996.
315. Kapperud G, Jenum PA, Stray-Pedersen B, et al: Risk factors for *Toxoplasma gondii* infection in pregnancy. Results of a prospective case-control study in Norway, *Am J Epidemiol* 144:405-412, 1996.
316. Cook AJ, Gilbert RE, Buffolano W, et al: Sources of Toxoplasma infection in pregnant women: European multicentre case-control study, European Research Network on Congenital Toxoplasmosis, *BMJ* 321:142-147, 2000.
317. Jimenez-Coello M, Guzman-Marin E, Ortega-Pacheco A, et al: Immunological status against *Toxoplasma gondii* in non-cat owners from an endemic region of Mexico, *Vector Borne Zoonotic Dis* 11:1057-1061, 2011.
318. Dubey JP, Jones JL: *Toxoplasma gondii* infection in humans and animals in the United States, *Int J Parasitol* 38:1257-1278, 2008.
319. van der Giessen J, Fonville M, Bouwknegt M, et al: Seroprevalence of Trichinella spiralis and *Toxoplasma gondii* in pigs from different housing systems in The Netherlands, *Vet Parasitol* 148:371-374, 2007.
320. Dubey JP, Hill DE, Jones JL, et al: Prevalence of viable *Toxoplasma gondii* in beef, chicken, and pork from retail meat stores in the United States: risk assessment to consumers, *J Parasitol* 91:1082-1093, 2005.
321. Sroka S, Bartelheimer N, Winter A, et al: Prevalence and risk factors of toxoplasmosis among pregnant women in Fortaleza, Northeastern Brazil, *Am J Trop Med Hyg* 83:528-533, 2010.

322. Beltrame MA, Pena HF, Ton NC, et al: Seroprevalence and isolation of *Toxoplasma gondii* from free-range chickens from Espirito Santo state, southeastern Brazil, *Vet Parasitol* 188:225-230, 2012.
323. Costa DG, Marvulo MF, Silva JS, et al: Seroprevalence of *Toxoplasma gondii* in domestic and wild animals from the Fernando de Noronha, Brazil, *J Parasitol* 98:679-680, 2012.
324. de Oliveira LN, Costa LM Jr, de Melo CF, et al: *Toxoplasma gondii* isolates from free-range chickens from the northeast region of Brazil, *J Parasitol* 95:235-237, 2009.
325. Edelhofer R, Prossinger H: Infection with *Toxoplasma gondii* during pregnancy: seroepidemiological studies in Austria, *Zoonoses Public Health* 57:18-26, 2010.
326. Dubey JP: *Toxoplasma gondii* infections in chickens *(Gallus domesticus)*: prevalence, clinical disease, diagnosis and public health significance, *Zoonoses Public Health* 57:60-73, 2010.
327. Chumpolbanchorn K, Lymbery AJ, Pallant LJ, et al: A high prevalence of Toxoplasma in Australian chickens, *Vet Parasitol* 196:209-211, 2013.
328. Dubey JP, Camargo ME, Ruff MD, et al: Experimental toxoplasmosis in turkeys, *J Parasitol* 79:949-952, 1993.
329. Dubey JP, Graham DH, Dahl E, et al: Isolation and molecular characterization of *Toxoplasma gondii* from chickens and ducks from Egypt, *Vet Parasitol* 114:89-95, 2003.
330. Bartova E, Dvorakova H, Barta J, et al: Susceptibility of the domestic duck *(Anas platyrhynchos)* to experimental infection with *Toxoplasma gondii* oocysts, *Avian Pathol* 33:153-157, 2004.
331. Dubey JP, Webb DM, Sundar N, et al: Endemic avian toxoplasmosis on a farm in Illinois: clinical disease, diagnosis, biologic and genetic characteristics of *Toxoplasma gondii* isolates from chickens *(Gallus domesticus)*, and a goose *(Anser anser)*, *Vet Parasitol* 148:207-212, 2007.
332. Koethe M, Pott S, Ludewig M, et al: Prevalence of specific IgG-antibodies against *Toxoplasma gondii* in domestic turkeys determined by kinetic ELISA based on recombinant GRA7 and GRA8, *Vet Parasitol* 180:179-190, 2011.
333. Alvarado-Esquivel C, Sifuentes-Alvarez A, Narro-Duarte SG, et al: Seroepidemiology of *Toxoplasma gondii* infection in pregnant women in a public hospital in northern Mexico, *BMC Infect Dis* 6:113, 2006.
334. Maksimov P, Buschtons S, Herrmann DC, et al: Serological survey and risk factors for *Toxoplasma gondii* in domestic ducks and geese in Lower Saxony, Germany, *Vet Parasitol* 182:140-149, 2011.
335. Yan C, Yue CL, Yuan ZG, et al: *Toxoplasma gondii* infection in domestic ducks, free-range and caged chickens in southern China, *Vet Parasitol* 165:337-340, 2009.
336. Harfoush M, Tahoon Ael N: Seroprevalence of *Toxoplasma gondii* antibodies in domestic ducks, free-range chickens, turkeys and rabbits in Kafr El-Sheikh Governorate Egypt, *J Egypt Soc Parasitol* 40:295-302, 2010.
337. Yan C, Yue CL, Zhang H, et al: Serological survey of *Toxoplasma gondii* infection in the domestic goose *(Anser domestica)* in southern China, *Zoonoses Public Health* 58:299-302, 2011.
338. Berger-Schoch AE, Bernet D, Doherr MG, et al: *Toxoplasma gondii* in Switzerland: a serosurvey based on meat juice analysis of slaughtered pigs, wild boar, sheep and cattle, *Zoonoses Public Health* 58:472-478, 2011.
339. Frazao-Teixeira E, de Oliveira FC: Anti-*Toxoplasma gondii* antibodies in cattle and pigs in a highly endemic area for human toxoplasmosis in Brazil, *J Parasitol* 97:44-47, 2011.
340. Baril L, Ancelle T, Goulet V, et al: Risk factors for Toxoplasma infection in pregnancy: a case-control study in France, *Scand J Infect Dis* 31:305-309, 1999.
341. Jones JL, Dargelas V, Roberts J, et al: Risk factors for *Toxoplasma gondii* infection in the United States, *Clin Infect Dis* 49:878-884, 2009.
342. Dubey JP: Toxoplasmosis in sheep—the last 20 years, *Vet Parasitol* 163:1-14, 2009.
343. Dubey JP, Sundar N, Hill D, et al: High prevalence and abundant atypical genotypes of *Toxoplasma gondii* isolated from lambs destined for human consumption in the USA, *Int J Parasitol* 38:999-1006, 2008.
344. Masur H, Jones TC, Lempert JA, et al: Outbreak of toxoplasmosis in a family and documentation of acquired retinochoroiditis, *Am J Med* 64:396-402, 1978.
345. Dubey JP, Rajendran C, Ferreira LR, et al: High prevalence and genotypes of *Toxoplasma gondii* isolated from goats, from a retail meat store, destined for human consumption in the USA, *Int J Parasitol* 41:827-833, 2011.
346. Sacks JJ, Roberto RR, Brooks NF: Toxoplasmosis infection associated with raw goat's milk, *JAMA* 248:1728-1732, 1982.
347. Riemann HP, Meyer ME, Theis JH, et al: Toxoplasmosis in an infant fed unpasteurized goat milk, *J Pediatr* 87:573-576, 1975.
348. Skinner LJ, Timperley AC, Wightman D, et al: Simultaneous diagnosis of toxoplasmosis in goats and goat owner's family, *Scand J Infect Dis* 22:359-361, 1990.
349. Tassi P: *Toxoplasma gondii* infection in horses. A review, *Parassitologia* 49:7-15, 2007.
350. Evers F, Garcia JL, Navarro IT, et al: Diagnosis and isolation of *Toxoplasma gondii* in horses from Brazilian slaughterhouses, *Rev Bras Parasitol Vet* 22:58-63, 2013.
351. Karatepe B, Babur C, Karatepe M, et al: Seroprevalence of toxoplasmosis in horses in Nigde Province of Turkey, *Trop Anim Health Prod* 42:385-389, 2010.
352. Jakubek EB, Lunden A, Uggla A: Seroprevalences of *Toxoplasma gondii* and Neospora sp. infections in Swedish horses, *Vet Parasitol* 138:194-199, 2006.
353. Gupta GD, Lakritz J, Kim JH, et al: Seroprevalence of Neospora, *Toxoplasma gondii* and Sarcocystis neurona antibodies in horses from Jeju island, South Korea, *Vet Parasitol* 106:193-201, 2002.
354. Alvarado-Esquivel C, Rodriguez-Pena S, Villena I, et al: Seroprevalence of *Toxoplasma gondii* infection in domestic horses in Durango State, Mexico, *J Parasitol* 98:944-945, 2012.
355. Miao Q, Wang X, She LN, et al: Seroprevalence of *Toxoplasma gondii* in horses and donkeys in Yunnan Province, Southwestern China, *Parasit Vectors* 6:168, 2013.
356. Yang N, Mu MY, Yuan GM, et al: Seroprevalence of *Toxoplasma gondii* in slaughtered horses and donkeys in Liaoning province, northeastern China, *Parasit Vectors* 6:140, 2013.
357. Haridy FM, Shoukry NM, Hassan AA, et al: ELISA-seroprevalence of *Toxoplasma gondii* in draught horses in Greater Cairo, Egypt, *J Egypt Soc Parasitol* 39:821-826, 2009.
358. Hajialilo E, Ziaali N, Harandi MF, et al: Prevalence of anti-*Toxoplasma gondii* antibodies in sport horses from Qazvin, Iran, *Trop Anim Health Prod* 42:1321-1322, 2010.
359. Alanazi AD, Alyousif MS: Prevalence of antibodies to *Toxoplasma gondii* in horses in Riyadh Province, Saudi Arabia, *J Parasitol* 97:943-945, 2011.
360. Gill CO: Safety and storage stability of horse meat for human consumption, *Meat Sci* 71:506-513, 2005.
361. Sakikawa M, Noda S, Hanaoka M, et al: Anti-Toxoplasma antibody prevalence, primary infection rate, and risk factors in a study of toxoplasmosis in 4,466 pregnant women in Japan, *Clin Vaccine Immunol* 19:365-367, 2012.
362. Shin HG, Lee SE, Hong SH, et al: Prevalence of *Toxoplasma gondii* infection in rabbits of Korea by serological tests and nested polymerase chain reaction, *J Vet Med Sci* 75: 1609-1613, 2013.
363. Alvarado-Esquivel C, Alvarado-Esquivel D, Villena I, et al: Seroprevalence of *Toxoplasma gondii* infection in domestic rabbits in Durango State, Mexico, *Prev Vet Med* 111:325-328, 2013.
364. Ashmawy KI, Abuakkada SS, Awad AM: Seroprevalence of antibodies to Encephalitozoon cuniculi and *Toxoplasma gondii* in farmed domestic rabbits in Egypt, *Zoonoses Public Health* 58:357-364, 2011.
365. Sacks JJ, Delgado DG, Lobel HO, et al: Toxoplasmosis infection associated with eating undercooked venison, *Am J Epidemiol* 118:832-838, 1983.
366. Gomez-Marin JE, de-la-Torre A, Barrios P, et al: Toxoplasmosis in military personnel involved in jungle operations, *Acta Trop* 122:46-51, 2012.
367. Alvarado-Esquivel C, Liesenfeld O, Estrada-Martinez S, et al: *Toxoplasma gondii* infection in workers occupationally exposed to raw meat, *Occup Med (Lond)* 61:265-269, 2011.
368. Avelino MM, Campos D Jr, Parada JB, et al: Risk factors for *Toxoplasma gondii* infection in women of childbearing age, *Braz J Infect Dis* 8:164-174, 2004.
369. Bonametti AM, Passos JN: Koga da Silva EM, Macedo ZS: Probable transmission of acute toxoplasmosis through breast feeding, *J Trop Pediatr* 43:116, 1997.
370. Hill D, Coss C, Dubey JP, et al: Identification of a sporozoite-specific antigen from *Toxoplasma gondii*, *J Parasitol* 97:328-337, 2011.
371. Dubey JP: Infectivity and pathogenicity of *Toxoplasma gondii* oocysts for cats, *J Parasitol* 82:957-961, 1996.
372. Yilmaz SM, Hopkins SH: Effects of different conditions on duration of infectivity of *Toxoplasma gondii* oocysts, *J Parasitol* 58:938-939, 1972.

373. Frenkel JK, Ruiz A, Chinchilla M: Soil survival of Toxoplasma oocysts in Kansas and Costa Rica, *Am J Trop Med Hyg* 24:439-443, 1975.
374. Vollaire MR, Radecki SV, Lappin MR: Seroprevalence of *Toxoplasma gondii* antibodies in clinically ill cats in the United States, *Am J Vet Res* 66:874-877, 2005.
375. Al-Kappany YM, Rajendran C, Ferreira LR, et al: High prevalence of toxoplasmosis in cats from Egypt: isolation of viable *Toxoplasma gondii*, tissue distribution, and isolate designation, *J Parasitol* 96:1115-1118, 2010.
376. Afonso E, Thulliez P, Gilot-Fromont E: Local meteorological conditions, dynamics of seroconversion to *Toxoplasma gondii* in cats (Felis catus) and oocyst burden in a rural environment, *Epidemiol Infect* 138:1105-1113, 2010.
377. Dabritz HA, Miller MA, Atwill ER, et al: Detection of *Toxoplasma gondii*-like oocysts in cat feces and estimates of the environmental oocyst burden, *J Am Vet Med Assoc* 231:1676-1684, 2007.
378. Afonso E, Thulliez P, Gilot-Fromont E: Transmission of *Toxoplasma gondii* in an urban population of domestic cats *(Felis catus)*, *Int J Parasitol* 36:1373-1382, 2006.
379. dos Santos TR, Nunes CM, Luvizotto MC, et al: Detection of *Toxoplasma gondii* oocysts in environmental samples from public schools, *Vet Parasitol* 171:53-57, 2010.
380. Lass A, Pietkiewicz H, Modzelewska E, et al: Detection of *Toxoplasma gondii* oocysts in environmental soil samples using molecular methods, *Eur J Clin Microbiol Infect Dis* 28:599-605, 2009.
381. Jones JL, Muccioli C, Belfort R Jr, et al: Recently acquired *Toxoplasma gondii* infection, Brazil, *Emerg Infect Dis* 12:582-587, 2006.
382. Spalding SM, Amendoeira MR, Klein CH, et al: Serological screening and toxoplasmosis exposure factors among pregnant women in South of Brazil, *Rev Soc Bras Med Trop* 38:173-177, 2005.
383. Bobic B, Jevremovic I, Marinkovic J, et al: Risk factors for Toxoplasma infection in a reproductive age female population in the area of Belgrade, Yugoslavia, *Eur J Epidemiol* 14:605-610, 1998.
384. Ferreira EC, Marchioro AA, Guedes TA, et al: Association between seropositivity for *Toxoplasma gondii*, scholastic development of children and risk factors for T. gondii infection, *Trans R Soc Trop Med Hyg* 107:390-396, 2013.
385. Uneke CJ, Duhlinska DD, Ngwu BA, et al: Seroprevalence of *Toxoplasma gondii* infection in Kwal, a rural district of Plateau-Nigeria, *Afr J Med Med Sci* 36:109-113, 2007.
386. Jafari R, Sadaghian M, Safari M: Seroprevalence of *Toxoplasma gondii* infection and related risk factors in Tabriz City, Iran, 2008, *J Res Health Sci* 12:119-121, 2012.
387. Jumaian NF: Seroprevalence and risk factors for Toxoplasma infection in pregnant women in Jordan, *East Mediterr Health J* 11:45-51, 2005.
388. Kortbeek LM, De Melker HE, Veldhuijzen IK, Conyn-Van Spaendonck MA: Population-based Toxoplasma seroprevalence study in The Netherlands, *Epidemiol Infect* 132:839-845, 2004.
389. Rahman H, Murugkar HV, Kumar A, et al: Seroprevalence of toxoplasmosis in a district of Assam, India, *Indian J Public Health* 52: 48-49, 2008.
390. Weigel RM, Dubey JP, Dyer D, et al: Risk factors for infection with *Toxoplasma gondii* for residents and workers on swine farms in Illinois, *Am J Trop Med Hyg* 60:793-798, 1999.
391. Barbosa IR, de Carvalho Xavier Holanda CM, de Andrade-Neto VF: Toxoplasmosis screening and risk factors amongst pregnant females in Natal, northeastern Brazil, *Trans R Soc Trop Med Hyg* 103: 377-382, 2009.
392. Lopes-Mori FM, Mitsuka-Bregano R, Bittencourt LH, et al: Gestational toxoplasmosis in Paraná State, Brazil: prevalence of IgG antibodies and associated risk factors, *Braz J Infect Dis* 17:405-409, 2013.
393. Fromont EG, Riche B, Rabilloud M: Toxoplasma seroprevalence in a rural population in France: detection of a household effect, *BMC Infect Dis* 9:76, 2009.
394. Sroka J, Wojcik-Fatla A, Dutkiewicz J: Occurrence of *Toxoplasma gondii* in water from wells located on farms, *Ann Agric Environ Med* 13:169-175, 2006.
395. Lopez-Castillo CA, Diaz-Ramirez J, Gomez-Marin JE: [Risk factors for *Toxoplasma gondii* infection in pregnant women in Armenia, Colombia], *Rev Salud Publica (Bogota)* 7:180-190, 2005.
396. Han K, Shin DW, Lee TY, et al: Seroprevalence of *Toxoplasma gondii* infection and risk factors associated with seropositivity of pregnant women in Korea, *J Parasitol* 94:963-965, 2008.
397. Ertug S, Okyay P, Turkmen M, et al: Seroprevalence and risk factors for Toxoplasma infection among pregnant women in Aydin province, Turkey, *BMC Public Health* 5:66, 2005.
398. Benenson MW, Takafuji ET, Lemon SM, et al: Oocyst-transmitted toxoplasmosis associated with ingestion of contaminated water, *N Engl J Med* 307:666-669, 1982.
399. Herwaldt BL: Laboratory-acquired parasitic infections from accidental exposures, *Clin Microbiol Rev* 14:659-688, 2001.
400. Field PR, Moyle GG, Parnell PM: The accidental infection of a laboratory worker with *Toxoplasma gondii*, *Med J Aust* 2:196-198, 1972.
401. Lopes WD, Rodriguez JD, Souza FA, et al: Sexual transmission of *Toxoplasma gondii* in sheep, *Vet Parasitol* 195:47-56, 2013.
402. Arantes TP, Lopes WD, Ferreira RM, et al: *Toxoplasma gondii*: evidence for the transmission by semen in dogs, *Exp Parasitol* 123: 190-194, 2009.
403. McLeod R, Boyer KM, Lee D: Prematurity and severity are associated with *Toxoplasma gondii* alleles (NCCCTS, 1981-2009), *Clin Infect Dis* 54:1595-1605, 2012.
404. Petersen E: Prevention and treatment of congenital toxoplasmosis, *Expert Rev Anti Infect Ther* 5:285-293, 2007.
405. Villena I, Aubert D, Leroux B, et al: Pyrimethamine-sulfadoxine treatment of congenital toxoplasmosis: follow-up of 78 cases between 1980 and 1997. Reims Toxoplasmosis Group, *Scand J Infect Dis* 30:295-300, 1998.
406. Wallon M, Kieffer F, Binquet C, et al: Congenital toxoplasmosis: randomised comparison of strategies for retinochoroiditis prevention, *Therapie* 66:473-480, 2011.
407. Sabin AB, Warren J: Therapeutic effect of the sulfonamides on the infection with intracellular protozoa (Toxoplasma), *J Bacteriol* 41:80-86, 1941.
408. Eyles DE, Coleman N: Synergistic effect of sulfadiazine and daraprim against toxoplasmosis in mice, *Antibiot Chemother* 3:483-490, 1953.
409. Beverley JK, Fry BA: Sulphadimidine, pyrimethamine and dapsone in the treatment of toxoplasmosis in mice, *Br J Pharmacol Chemother* 12:189-193, 1957.
410. Beverley JK: A rational approach to the treatment of toxoplasmic uveitis, *Trans Opthal Soc U K* 78:109-121, 1958.
411. Desmonts G, Couvreur J: Congenital toxoplasmosis. A prospective study of 378 pregnancies, *N Engl J Med* 290:1110-1116, 1974.
412. Araujo FG, Huskinson J, Remington JS: Remarkable in vitro and in vivo activities of the hydroxynaphthoquinone 566C80 against tachyzoites and tissue cysts of *Toxoplasma gondii*, *Antimicrob Agents Chemother* 35:293-299, 1991.
413. Araujo FG, Huskinson-Mark J, Gutteridge WE, et al: In vitro and in vivo activities of the hydroxynaphthoquinone 566C80 against the cyst form of *Toxoplasma gondii*, *Antimicrob Agents Chemother* 36:326-330, 1992.
414. Kovacs JA: Efficacy of atovaquone in treatment of toxoplasmosis in patients with AIDS. The NIAID-Clinical Center Intramural AIDS Program, *Lancet* 340:637-638, 1992.
415. Romand S, Pudney M, Derouin F: In vitro and in vivo activities of the hydroxynaphthoquinone atovaquone alone or combined with pyrimethamine, sulfadiazine, clarithromycin, or minocycline against *Toxoplasma gondii*, *Antimicrob Agents Chemother* 37:2371-2378, 1993.
416. Sander J, Midtvedt T: The effect of trimethoprim on acute experimental toxoplasmosis in mice, *Acta Pathol Microbiol Scand B Microbiol Immunol* 78:664-668, 1970.
417. Terragna A, Cellesi C, Barberi A: Activity of the trimethoprim-sulfamethoxazole association in experimental toxoplasmosis in mice. Histological and immuno histological study, *Boll Ist Sieroter Milan* 52:60-69, 1973.
418. Stadtsbaeder S, Calvin-Preval MC: The trimethoprim-sulfamethoxazole association in experimental toxoplasmosis in mice, *Acta Clin Belg* 28:34-39, 1973.
419. Dumas JL, Pizzolato G, Pechere JC: Evaluation of trimethoprim and sulphamethoxazole as monotherapy or in combination in the management of toxoplasmosis in murine models, *Int J Antimicrob Agents* 13:35-39, 1999.
420. Norrby R, Eilard T, Svedhem A, et al: Treatment of toxoplasmosis with trimethoprim-sulphamethoxazole, *Scand J Infect Dis* 7:72-75, 1975.
421. Derouin F, Jacqz-Aigrain E, Thulliez P, et al: Cotrimoxazole for prenatal treatment of congenital toxoplasmosis? *Parasitol Today* 16:254-256, 2000.
422. Valentini P, Annunziata ML, Angelone DF, et al: Role of spiramycin/cotrimoxazole association in the mother-to-child transmission of toxoplasmosis infection in pregnancy, *Eur J Clin Microbiol Infect Dis* 28:297-300, 2009.

423. Soheilian M, Sadoughi MM, Ghajarnia M, et al: Prospective randomized trial of trimethoprim/sulfamethoxazole versus pyrimethamine and sulfadiazine in the treatment of ocular toxoplasmosis, *Ophthalmology* 112:1876-1882, 2005.
424. de-la-Torre A, Stanford M, Curi A, et al: Therapy for ocular toxoplasmosis, *Ocul Immunol Inflamm* 19:314-320, 2011.
425. O'Farrell N, Bradbeer C, Fitt S, et al: Cerebral toxoplasmosis and co-trimoxazole prophylaxis, *Lancet* 337:986, 1991.
426. Lee YH, Lee DY, Shin DW: Prophylactic effects of trimethoprim-sulfamethoxazole in *Toxoplasma*-infected mice, *Korean J Parasitol* 31:363-370, 1993.
427. Silveira C, Belfort R Jr, Muccioli C, et al: The effect of long-term intermittent trimethoprim/sulfamethoxazole treatment on recurrences of toxoplasmic retinochoroiditis, *Am J Ophthalmol* 134:41-46, 2002.
428. Faucher B, Garcia-Meric P, Franck J, et al: Long-term ocular outcome in congenital toxoplasmosis: a prospective cohort of treated children, *J Infect* 64:104-109, 2012.
429. Corvaisier S, Charpiat B, Mounier C, et al: Population pharmacokinetics of pyrimethamine and sulfadoxine in children treated for congenital toxoplasmosis, *Antimicrob Agents Chemother* 48:3794-3800, 2004.
430. Trenque T, Simon N, Villena I, et al: Population pharmacokinetics of pyrimethamine and sulfadoxine in children with congenital toxoplasmosis, *Br J Clin Pharmacol* 57:735-741, 2004.
431. Dorangeon PH, Marx-Chemla C, Quereux C, et al: The risks of pyrimethamine-sulfadoxine combination in the prenatal treatment of toxoplasmosis, *J Gynecol Obstet Biol Reprod (Paris)* 21:549-556, 1992.
432. Maisonneuve H, Faber C, Piens MA, et al: [Congenital toxoplasmosis. Tolerability of the sulfadoxine-pyrimethamine combination. 24 cases], *Presse Med* 13:859-862, 1984.
433. Ahmad RA, Rogers HJ: Pharmacokinetics and protein binding interactions of dapsone and pyrimethamine, *Br J Clin Pharmacol* 10: 519-524, 1980.
434. Coleman MD, Mihaly GW, Edwards G, et al: Pyrimethamine pharmacokinetics and its tissue localization in mice: effect of dose size, *J Pharm Pharmacol* 37:170-174, 1985.
435. Rudy AC, Poynor WJ: Binding of pyrimethamine to human plasma proteins and erythrocytes, *Pharm Res* 7:1055-1060, 1990.
436. McLeod R, Mack D, Foss R, et al: Levels of pyrimethamine in sera and cerebrospinal and ventricular fluids from infants treated for congenital toxoplasmosis. Toxoplasmosis Study Group, *Antimicrob Agents Chemother* 36:1040-1048, 1992.
437. Gomes TC, de Andrade Junior HF, Lescano SA, Amato-Neto V: In vitro action of antiparasitic drugs, especially artesunate, against *Toxoplasma gondii*, *Rev Soc Bras Med Trop* 45:485-490, 2012.
438. Eyles DE, Coleman N: An evaluation of the curative effects of pyrimethamine and sulfadiazine, alone and in combination, on experimental mouse toxoplasmosis, *Antibiot Chemother* 5:529-539, 1955.
439. Sheffield HG, Melton ML: Effect of pyrimethamine and sulfadiazine on the fine structure and multiplication of *Toxoplasma gondii* in cell cultures, *J Parasitol* 61:704-712, 1975.
440. Schoondermark-van de Ven E, Vree T, Melchers W, et al: In vitro effects of sulfadiazine and its metabolites alone and in combination with pyrimethamine on *Toxoplasma gondii*, *Antimicrob Agents Chemother* 39:763-765, 1995.
441. van der Ven AJ, Schoondermark-van de Ven EM, Camps W, et al: Anti-Toxoplasma effect of pyrimethamine, trimethoprim and sulphonamides alone and in combination: implications for therapy, *J Antimicrob Chemother* 38:75-80, 1996.
442. Araujo FG, Lin T, Remington JS: The activity of atovaquone (566C80) in murine toxoplasmosis is markedly augmented when used in combination with pyrimethamine or sulfadiazine, *J Infect Dis* 167:494-497, 1993.
443. Martins-Duarte ES, de Souza W, Vommaro RC: *Toxoplasma gondii*: the effect of fluconazole combined with sulfadiazine and pyrimethamine against acute toxoplasmosis in murine model, *Exp Parasitol* 133:294-299, 2013.
444. Lopes CD, Silva NM, Ferro EA, et al: Azithromycin reduces ocular infection during congenital transmission of toxoplasmosis in the Calomys callosus model, *J Parasitol* 95:1005-1010, 2009.
445. Schmidt DR, Hogh B, Andersen O, et al: Treatment of infants with congenital toxoplasmosis: tolerability and plasma concentrations of sulfadiazine and pyrimethamine, *Eur J Pediatr* 165:19-25, 2006.
446. Lescano SA, Amato Neto V, Chieffi PP, et al: Evaluation of the efficacy of azithromycin and pyrimethamine, for treatment of experimental infection of mice with *Toxoplasma gondii* cystogenic strain, *Rev Soc Bras Med Trop* 37:460-462, 2004.
447. Gilbert R, Gras L: Effect of timing and type of treatment on the risk of mother to child transmission of *Toxoplasma gondii*, *BJOG* 110: 112-120, 2003.
448. Mahmoud MS: Effect of deferoxamine alone and combined with pyrimethamine on acute toxoplasmosis in mice, *J Egypt Soc Parasitol* 29:791-803, 1999.
449. Bosch-Driessen LH, Verbraak FD, Suttorp-Schulten MS, et al: A prospective, randomized trial of pyrimethamine and azithromycin vs pyrimethamine and sulfadiazine for the treatment of ocular toxoplasmosis, *Am J Ophthalmol* 134:34-40, 2002.
450. Kieffer F, Thulliez P, Brezin A, et al: Treatment of subclinical congenital toxoplasmosis by sulfadiazine and pyrimethamine continuously during 1 year: apropos of 46 cases, *Arch Pediatr* 9:7-13, 2002.
451. Gras L, Gilbert RE, Ades AE, et al: Effect of prenatal treatment on the risk of intracranial and ocular lesions in children with congenital toxoplasmosis, *Int J Epidemiol* 30:1309-1313, 2001.
452. Bessières MH, Berrébi A, Rolland M, et al: Neonatal screening for congenital toxoplasmosis in a cohort of 165 women infected during pregnancy and influence of in utero treatment on the results of neonatal tests, *Eur J Obstet Gynecol Reprod Biol* 94:37-45, 2001.
453. Khan AA, Slifer TR, Araujo FG, et al: Activity of gatifloxacin alone or in combination with pyrimethamine or gamma interferon against *Toxoplasma gondii*, *Antimicrob Agents Chemother* 45:48-51, 2001.
454. Braz LM, Di Pietro AO, Amato Neto V, et al: The evaluation of the efficacy of azithromycin and pyrimethamine used alone or in combination in the treatment of an experimental infection in mice by *Toxoplasma gondii*, *Rev Soc Bras Med Trop* 32:401-403, 1999.
455. Lipka B, Milewska-Bobula B, Filipek M: Monitoring of plasma concentration of pyrimethamine (PYR) in infants with congenital *Toxoplasma gondii* infection—own observations, *Wiad Parazytol* 57:87-92, 2011.
456. Israelski DM, Tom C, Remington JS: Zidovudine antagonizes the action of pyrimethamine in experimental infection with *Toxoplasma gondii*, *Antimicrob Agents Chemother* 33:30-34, 1989.
457. McAuley J, Boyer KM, Patel D, et al: Early and longitudinal evaluations of treated infants and children and untreated historical patients with congenital toxoplasmosis: the Chicago Collaborative Treatment Trial, *Clin Infect Dis* 18:38-72, 1994.
458. Dorangeon P, Fay R, Marx-Chemla C, et al: Transplacental passage of the pyrimethamine-sulfadoxine combination in the prenatal treatment of congenital toxoplasmosis, *Presse Med* 19:2036, 1990.
459. Schoondermark-van de Ven E, Galama J, Vree T, et al: Study of treatment of congenital *Toxoplasma gondii* infection in rhesus monkeys with pyrimethamine and sulfadiazine, *Antimicrob Agents Chemother* 39:137-144, 1995.
460. Schoondermark-van de Ven EM, Melchers WJ, Galama JM, et al: Prenatal diagnosis and treatment of congenital *Toxoplasma gondii* infections: an experimental study in rhesus monkeys, *Eur J Obstet Gynecol Reprod Biol* 74:183-188, 1997.
461. Berrébi A, Assouline C, Bessières MH, et al: Long-term outcome of children with congenital toxoplasmosis, *Am J Obstet Gynecol* 203:552, 2010. e551–e556.
462. Peyron F, Wallon M, Bernardoux C: Long-term follow-up of patients with congenital ocular toxoplasmosis, *N Engl J Med* 334:993-994, 1996.
463. Wallon M, Garweg JG, Abrahamowicz M, et al: Ophthalmic outcomes of congenital toxoplasmosis followed until adolescence, *Pediatrics* 133:e601-e608, 2014.
464. Mack DG, McLeod R: New micromethod to study the effect of antimicrobial agents on *Toxoplasma gondii*: comparison of sulfadoxine and sulfadiazine individually and in combination with pyrimethamine and study of clindamycin, metronidazole, and cyclosporin A, *Antimicrob Agents Chemother* 26:26-30, 1984.
465. Foulon W, Villena I, Stray-Pedersen B, et al: Treatment of toxoplasmosis during pregnancy: a multicenter study of impact on fetal transmission and children's sequelae at age 1 year, *Am J Obstet Gynecol* 180(2 Pt 1):410-415, 1999.
466. McLeod R, Boyer K, Karrison T, et al: Outcome of treatment for congenital toxoplasmosis, 1981-2004: the National Collaborative Chicago-Based, Congenital Toxoplasmosis Study, *Clin Infect Dis* 42:1383-1394, 2006.
467. Gupta K, Vasishta RK, Bansal A, et al: Cortical cysts with hydrocephalus and ventriculitis: an unusual presentation of congenital toxoplasmosis at autopsy, *J Clin Pathol* 64:272-274, 2011.
468. Perkins ES, Schofield PB, Smith CH: Treatment of uveitis with pyrimethamine (daraprim), *Br J Ophthalmol* 40:577-586, 1956.

469. Tracqui A, Mikail I, Kintz P, et al: Nonfatal prolonged overdosage of pyrimethamine in an infant: measurement of plasma and urine levels using HPLC with diode-array detection, *J Anal Toxicol* 17:248-250, 1993.
470. Genuini M, Freihuber C, Girard I, et al: [Neonatal intoxication with pyrimethamine: risk due to the absence of pediatric formulation]? *Arch Pediatr* 18:1084-1086, 2011.
471. Aguemon AR, Atchade D, Houngbe F, et al: [A case of acute pyrimethamine poisoning], *Bull Soc Pathol Exot* 90:117-119, 1997.
472. Nano HD, Plaza A: [Intoxication with pyrimethamine (Daraprim)], *Arch Oftalmol B Aires* 42:224-229, 1967.
473. Elmalem J, Poulet B, Garnier R, et al: [Severe complications arising from the prescription of pyrimethamine for infants being treated for toxoplasmosis], *Therapie* 40:357-359, 1985.
474. Phillips-Howard PA, Wood D: The safety of antimalarial drugs in pregnancy, *Drug Saf* 14:131-145, 1996.
475. Peters PJ, Thigpen MC, Parise ME, et al: Safety and toxicity of sulfadoxine/pyrimethamine: implications for malaria prevention in pregnancy using intermittent preventive treatment, *Drug Saf* 30:481-501, 2007.
476. Frenkel JK, Hitchings GH: Relative reversal by vitamins (*p*-aminobenzoic, folic and folinic acids) of the effects of sulfadiazine and pyrimethamine on Toxoplasma, mouse and man, *Antibiot Chemother* 7:630-638, 1957.
477. Klementiev B, Bichevaja N, Novikova T, et al: A peptide agonist of the neural cell adhesion molecule (NCAM), C3, protects against developmental defects induced by a teratogen pyrimethamine, *Int J Dev Neurosci* 20:527-536, 2002.
478. Tsuda S, Kosaka Y, Matsusaka N, et al: Detection of pyrimethamine-induced DNA damage in mouse embryo and maternal organs by the modified alkaline single cell gel electrophoresis assay, *Mutat Res* 415:69-77, 1998.
479. Horvath C, Compagnon A, Petter C: Teratogenic effect of pyrimethamine in the rat. In vivo prevention by calcium folinate, *C R Seances Soc Biol Fil* 182:158-166, 1988.
480. Krahe M: Studies on the teratogenic effect of drugs in the treatment of toxoplasmosis during pregnancy, *Arch Gynakol* 202:104-109, 1965.
481. Sullivan GE, Takacs E: Comparative teratogenicity of pyrimethamine in rats and hamsters, *Teratology* 4:205-210, 1971.
482. Schoondermark-Van de Ven E, Melchers W, Camps W, et al: Effectiveness of spiramycin for treatment of congenital *Toxoplasma gondii* infection in rhesus monkeys, *Antimicrob Agents Chemother* 38:1930-1936, 1994.
483. Garin JP, Paillard B: Experimental toxoplasmosis in mice. Comparative activity of clindamycin, midecamycin, josamycin, spiramycin, pyrimethamine-sulfadoxine, and trimethoprim-sulfamethoxazole, *Ann Pediatr (Paris)* 31:841-845, 1984.
484. Chang HR, Pechere JC: Activity of spiramycin against *Toxoplasma gondii* in vitro, in experimental infections and in human infection, *J Antimicrob Chemother* 22(Suppl B):87-92, 1988.
485. Gratzl R, Sodeck G, Platzer P, et al: Treatment of toxoplasmosis in pregnancy: concentrations of spiramycin and neospiramycin in maternal serum and amniotic fluid, *Eur J Clin Microbiol Infect Dis* 21:12-16, 2002.
486. Schoondermark-Van de Ven E, Galama J, Camps W, et al: Pharmacokinetics of spiramycin in the rhesus monkey: transplacental passage and distribution in tissue in the fetus, *Antimicrob Agents Chemother* 38:1922-1929, 1994.
487. Garin JP, Pellerat J, Maillard, et al: Theoretical bases of the prevention by spiramycin of congenital toxoplasmosis in pregnant women, *Presse Med* 76:2266, 1968.
488. Couvreur J, Desmonts G, Thulliez P: Prophylaxis of congenital toxoplasmosis. Effects of spiramycin on placental infection, *J Antimicrob Chemother* 22(Suppl B):193-200, 1988.
489. Hudson DG, Yoshihara GM, Kirby WM: Spiramycin; clinical and laboratory studies, *AMA Arch Intern Med* 97:57-61, 1956.
490. Forestier F, Daffos F, Rainaut M, et al: Fetomaternal therapeutic follow-up of spiramycin during pregnancy, *Arch Fr Pediatr* 44: 539-544, 1987.
491. Thiebaut R, Leproust S, Chene G, et al: Effectiveness of prenatal treatment for congenital toxoplasmosis: a meta-analysis of individual patients' data, *Lancet* 369:115-122, 2007.
492. Beverley JK, Henry L: Histopathological changes caused by congenital toxoplasmosis in mice, *Lyon Med* 225:883-887, 1971.
493. Thulliez P: Commentary: efficacy of prenatal treatment for toxoplasmosis: a possibility that cannot be ruled out, *Int J Epidemiol* 30:1315-1316, 2001.
494. Back N, Ambrus JL, Velasco H, et al: Clinical and experimental pharmacology of parenteral spiramycin, *Clin Pharmacol Ther* 3:305-313, 1962.
495. Petersen E, Schmidt DR: Sulfadiazine and pyrimethamine in the postnatal treatment of congenital toxoplasmosis: what are the options? *Expert Rev Anti Infect Ther* 1:175-182, 2003.
496. Beraud G, Pierre-Francois S, Foltzer A, et al: Cotrimoxazole for treatment of cerebral toxoplasmosis: an observational cohort study during 1994-2006, *Am J Trop Med Hyg* 80:583-587, 2009.
497. Nguyen BT, Stadtsbaeder S: Comparative effects of cotrimoxazole (trimethoprim-sulphamethoxazole) and spiramycin in pregnant mice infected with *Toxoplasma gondii* (Beverley strain), *Br J Pharmacol* 85:713-716, 1985.
498. Araujo FG, Remington JS: Effect of clindamycin on acute and chronic toxoplasmosis in mice, *Antimicrob Agents Chemother* 5:647-651, 1974.
499. Tabbara KF, Nozik RA, O'Connor GR: Clindamycin effects on experimental ocular toxoplasmosis in the rabbit, *Arch Ophthalmol* 92: 244-247, 1974.
500. Garweg JG, Kuenzli H, Boehnke M: Experimental ocular toxoplasmosis in naive and primed rabbits, *Ophthalmologica* 212:136-141, 1998.
501. Soheilian M, Ramezani A, Azimzadeh A, et al: Randomized trial of intravitreal clindamycin and dexamethasone versus pyrimethamine, sulfadiazine, and prednisolone in treatment of ocular toxoplasmosis, *Ophthalmology* 118:134-141, 2011.
502. Baharivand N, Mahdavifard A, Fouladi RF: Intravitreal clindamycin plus dexamethasone versus classic oral therapy in toxoplasmic retinochoroiditis: a prospective randomized clinical trial, *Int Ophthalmol* 33:39-46, 2013.
503. Sobrin L, Kump LI, Foster CS: Intravitreal clindamycin for toxoplasmic retinochoroiditis, *Retina* 27:952-957, 2007.
504. Lasave AF, Diaz-Llopis M, Muccioli C, et al: Intravitreal clindamycin and dexamethasone for zone 1 toxoplasmic retinochoroiditis at twenty-four months, *Ophthalmology* 117:1831-1838, 2010.
505. Huskinson-Mark J, Araujo FG, Remington JS: Evaluation of the effect of drugs on the cyst form of *Toxoplasma gondii*, *J Infect Dis* 164:170-171, 1991.
506. Ferguson DJ, Huskinson-Mark J, Araujo FG, et al: An ultrastructural study of the effect of treatment with atovaquone in brains of mice chronically infected with the ME49 strain of *Toxoplasma gondii*, *Int J Exp Pathol* 75:111-116, 1994.
507. Morlat P, Leport C: Prevention of toxoplasmosis in immunocompromised patients, *Ann Med Interne (Paris)* 148:235-239, 1997.
508. Torres RA, Weinberg W, Stansell J, et al: Atovaquone for salvage treatment and suppression of toxoplasmic encephalitis in patients with AIDS. Atovaquone/Toxoplasmic Encephalitis Study Group, *Clin Infect Dis* 24:422-429, 1997.
509. German PI, Aweeka FT: Clinical pharmacology of artemisinin-based combination therapies, *Clin Pharmacokinet* 47:91-102, 2008.
510. Sarciron ME, Saccharin C, Petavy AF, et al: Effects of artesunate, dihydroartemisinin, and an artesunate-dihydroartemisinin combination against *Toxoplasma gondii*, *Am J Trop Med Hyg* 62:73-76, 2000.
511. Mandelbrot L: Prevention of mother-to-child transmission of toxoplasmosis: perspectives, *Gynecol Obstet Fertil* 40:591-598, 2012.
512. Peyron F, Wallon M: Options for the pharmacotherapy of toxoplasmosis during pregnancy, *Expert Opin Pharmacother* 2:1269-1274, 2001.
513. Thiebaut R, Leroy V, Alioum A, et al: Biases in observational studies of the effect of prenatal treatment for congenital toxoplasmosis, *Eur J Obstet Gynecol Reprod Biol* 124:3-9, 2006.
514. Peyron F, Wallon M, Liou C, et al: Treatments for toxoplasmosis in pregnancy, *Cochrane Database Syst Rev*: CD001684, 2000.
515. Franco PS, Gomes AO, Barbosa BF, et al: Azithromycin and spiramycin induce anti-inflammatory response in human trophoblastic (BeWo) cells infected by *Toxoplasma gondii* but are able to control infection, *Placenta* 32:838-844, 2011.
516. Doliwa C, Escotte-Binet S, Aubert D, et al: Sulfadiazine resistance in *Toxoplasma gondii*: no involvement of overexpression or polymorphisms in genes of therapeutic targets and ABC transporters, *Parasite* 20:19, 2013.
517. Jacot D, Soldati-Favre D: Does protein phosphorylation govern host cell entry and egress by the Apicomplexa? *Int J Med Microbiol* 302:195-202, 2012.
518. Wei F, Wang W, Liu Q: Protein kinases of *Toxoplasma gondii*: functions and drug targets, *Parasitol Res* 112:2121-2129, 2013.

519. Seeber F, Aliverti A, Zanetti G: The plant-type ferredoxin-NADP+ reductase/ferredoxin redox system as a possible drug target against apicomplexan human parasites, *Curr Pharm Des* 11:3159-3172, 2005.
520. Martins-Duarte ES, Lemgruber L, Lorente SO, et al: Evaluation of three novel azasterols against *Toxoplasma gondii*, *Vet Parasitol* 177:157-161, 2011.
521. Roberts T, Gravett CA, Velu PP, et al: Epidemiology and aetiology of maternal parasitic infections in low- and middle-income countries, *J Glob Health* 1:189-200, 2011.
522. Elsheikha HM: Congenital toxoplasmosis: priorities for further health promotion action, *Public Health* 122:335-353, 2008.
523. Petersen E, Vesco G, Villari S, et al: What do we know about risk factors for infection in humans with *Toxoplasma gondii* and how can we prevent infections? *Zoonoses Public Health* 57:8-17, 2010.
524. Kravetz JD, Federman DG: Toxoplasmosis in pregnancy, *Am J Med* 118:212-216, 2005.
525. Jones JL, Kruszon-Moran D, Wilson M, et al: *Toxoplasma gondii* infection in the United States: seroprevalence and risk factors, *Am J Epidemiol* 154:357-365, 2001.
526. Boyer KM, Holfels E, Roizen N, et al: Risk factors for *Toxoplasma gondii* infection in mothers of infants with congenital toxoplasmosis: implications for prenatal management and screening, *Am J Obstet Gynecol* 192:564-571, 2005.
527. Jara M, Hsu HW, Eaton RB, et al: Epidemiology of congenital toxoplasmosis identified by population-based newborn screening in Massachusetts, *Pediatr Infect Dis J* 20:1132-1135, 2001.
528. Ford-Jones E, Kitai I, Corey M, et al: Seroprevalence of Toxoplasma antibody in a Toronto population, *Can J Infect Dis* 7:326-328, 1996.
528a. Campagna S, Lévesque B, Anassour-Laouan-Sid E, et al: Seroprevalence of 10 zoonotic infection in two Canadian Cree communities, *Diagn Microbiol Infect Dis* 70:191-199, 2011.
529. Messier V, Levesque B, Proulx JF, et al: Seroprevalence of *Toxoplasma gondii* among Nunavik Inuit (Canada), *Zoonoses Public Health* 56:188-197, 2009.
530. Dubey JP, Lago EG, Gennari SM, et al: Toxoplasmosis in humans and animals in Brazil: high prevalence, high burden of disease, and epidemiology, *Parasitology* 139:1375-1424, 2012.
531. Fonseca AL, Silva RA, Fux B, et al: Epidemiologic aspects of toxoplasmosis and evaluation of its seroprevalence in pregnant women, *Rev Soc Bras Med Trop* 45:357-364, 2012.
532. Bittencourt LH, Lopes-Mori FM, Mitsuka-Bregano R, et al: Seroepidemiology of toxoplasmosis in pregnant women since the implementation of the Surveillance Program of Toxoplasmosis Acquired in Pregnancy and Congenital in the western region of Paraná, Brazil, *Rev Bras Ginecol Obstet* 34:63-68, 2012.
533. Reboucas EC, Dos Santos EL, Do Carmo ML, Cavalcante Z, Favali C: Seroprevalence of Toxoplasma infection among pregnant women in Bahia, Brazil, *Trans R Soc Trop Med Hyg* 105:670-671, 2011.
534. Lopes FM, Mitsuka-Bregano R, Goncalves DD, et al: Factors associated with seropositivity for anti-*Toxoplasma gondii* antibodies in pregnant women of Londrina, Paraná, *Brazil. Mem Inst Oswaldo Cruz* 104:378-382, 2009.
535. Carral L, Kaufer F, Olejnik P, et al: Prevention of congenital toxoplasmosis in a Buenos Aires hospital, *Medicina (B Aires)* 73:238-242, 2013.
536. Marquez M, Etcheverry I: Seroprevalence of toxoplasmosis in pregnant women in La Plata area, *Acta Bioquím Clín Latinoam* 37:413-415, 2003.
537. Diaz-Suarez O, Estevez J: Seroepidemiology of toxoplasmosis in women of childbearing age from a marginal community of Maracaibo, Venezuela, *Rev Inst Med Trop São Paulo* 51:13-17, 2009.
538. Alvarado-Esquivel C, Torres-Castorena A, Liesenfeld O, et al: Seroepidemiology of *Toxoplasma gondii* infection in pregnant women in rural Durango, Mexico, *J Parasitol* 95:271-274, 2009.
539. Galvan-Ramirez Mde L, Troyo R, Roman S, et al: A systematic review and meta-analysis of *Toxoplasma gondii* infection among the Mexican population, *Parasit Vectors* 5:271, 2012.
540. Dias RC, Lopes-Mori FM, Mitsuka-Bregano R, et al: Factors associated to infection by *Toxoplasma gondii* in pregnant women attended in Basic Health Units in the city of Rolandia, Paraná, Brazil, *Rev Inst Med Trop São Paulo* 53:185-191, 2011.
541. El Mansouri B, Rhajaoui M, Sebti F, et al: Seroprevalence of toxoplasmosis in pregnant women in Rabat, Morocco, *Bull Soc Pathol Exot* 100:289-290, 2007.
542. Mpiga Mickoto R, Akue JP, Bisvigou U, et al: Serological study on toxoplasmosis among pregnant women from Franceville, Gabon, *Bull Soc Pathol Exot* 103:41-43, 2010.
543. Hung CC, Fan CK, Su KE, et al: Serological screening and toxoplasmosis exposure factors among pregnant women in the Democratic Republic of São Tomé and Principe, *Trans R Soc Trop Med Hyg* 101:134-139, 2007.
544. Gebremedhin EZ, Abebe AH, Tessema TS, et al: Seroepidemiology of *Toxoplasma gondii* infection in women of child-bearing age in central Ethiopia, *BMC Infect Dis* 13:101, 2013.
545. Zemene E, Yewhalaw D, Abera S, et al: Seroprevalence of *Toxoplasma gondii* and associated risk factors among pregnant women in Jimma town, Southwestern Ethiopia, *BMC Infect Dis* 12:337, 2012.
546. Kistiah K, Frean J, Winiecka-Krusnell J, et al: Unexpectedly low seroprevalence of toxoplasmosis in South Africa, *Onderstepoort J Vet Res* 79:E1, 2012.
547. Sellami H, Amri H, Cheikhrouhou F, et al: Toxoplasmosis in Sfax, Tunisia, *Bull Soc Pathol Exot* 103:37-40, 2010.
548. Simpore J, Savadogo A, Ilboudo D, et al: *Toxoplasma gondii*, HCV, and HBV seroprevalence and co-infection among HIV-positive and -negative pregnant women in Burkina Faso, *J Med Virol* 78:730-733, 2006.
549. Ouermi D, Simpore J, Belem AM, et al: Co-infection of *Toxoplasma gondii* with HBV in HIV-infected and uninfected pregnant women in Burkina Faso, *Pak J Biol Sci* 12:1188-1193, 2009.
550. Bamba S, Some DA, Chemla C, et al: Serological analysis of toxoplasmosis during pregnancy: risk assessment and perspectives of prenatal screening at the University Hospital of Bobo Dioulasso in Burkina Faso, *Pan Afr Med J* 12:43, 2012.
551. Linguissi LS, Nagalo BM, Bisseye C, et al: Seroprevalence of toxoplasmosis and rubella in pregnant women attending antenatal private clinic at Ouagadougou, Burkina Faso, *Asian Pac J Trop Med* 5:810-813, 2012.
552. Ouologuem DT, Djimde AA, Diallo N, et al: *Toxoplasma gondii* seroprevalence in Mali, *J Parasitol* 99:371-374, 2013.
553. Diallo S, Ndir O, Dieng Y, et al: Seroprevalence of toxoplasmosis in Dakar (Senegal) in 1993: study of women in their reproductive years, *Sante* 6:102-106, 1996.
554. Ndiaye D, Ndiaye A, Sene PD, et al: Evaluation of serological tests of toxoplasmosis in pregnant women realized at the Laboratory of Parasitology and Mycology of Le Dantec Teaching Hospital in 2002, *Dakar Med* 52:58-61, 2007.
555. Ndir I, Gaye A, Faye B, et al: Seroprevalence of toxoplasmosis among women having spontaneous abortion and pregnant women following in a center of health up-town in Dakar, *Dakar Med* 49:5-9, 2004.
556. Ishaku B, Ajogi I, Umoh J, et al: Seroprevalence and risk factors for *Toxoplasma gondii* infection among antenatal women in Zaria, Nigeria, *Res J Med Sci* 4:483-488, 2009.
557. Akinbami AA, Adewunmi AA, Rabiu KA, et al: Seroprevalence of *Toxoplasma gondii* antibodies amongst pregnant women at the Lagos State University Teaching Hospital, Nigeria, *Niger Postgrad Med J* 17:164-167, 2010.
558. Sitoe SP, Rafael B, Meireles LR, et al: Preliminary report of HIV and *Toxoplasma gondii* occurrence in pregnant women from Mozambique, *Rev Inst Med Trop São Paulo* 52:291-295, 2010.
559. Mwambe B, Mshana SE, Kidenya BR, et al: Sero-prevalence and factors associated with *Toxoplasma gondii* infection among pregnant women attending antenatal care in Mwanza, Tanzania, *Parasit Vectors* 6:222, 2013.
560. Elnahas A, Gerais AS, Elbashir MI, et al: Toxoplasmosis in pregnant Sudanese women, *Saudi Med J* 24:868-870, 2003.
561. Diza E, Frantzidou F, Souliou E, et al: Seroprevalence of *Toxoplasma gondii* in northern Greece during the last 20 years, *Clin Microbiol Infect* 11:719-723, 2005.
562. Bobic B, Nikolic A, Klun I, et al: Kinetics of Toxoplasma infection in the Balkans, *Wien Klin Wochenschr* 123(Suppl 1):2-6, 2011.
563. Sagel U, Kramer A, Mikolajczyk RT: Incidence of maternal Toxoplasma infections in pregnancy in Upper Austria, 2000-2007, *BMC Infect Dis* 11:348, 2011.
564. Mosti M, Pinto B, Giromella A, et al: A 4-year evaluation of toxoplasmosis seroprevalence in the general population and in women of reproductive age in central Italy, *Epidemiol Infect* 11:1-4, 2012.
565. Stricker R, Sitavanc R, Liassine N, et al: Toxoplasmosis during pregnancy and infancy, *Swiss Med Wkly* 139:643-644, 2009. author reply 643–644.
566. Dentico P, Volpe A, Putoto G, et al: Toxoplasmosis in Kosovo pregnant women, *New Microbiol* 34:203-207, 2011.

567. Prusa AR, Kasper DC, Olischar M, et al: Evaluation of serological prenatal screening to detect *Toxoplasma gondii* infections in Austria, *Neonatology* 103:27-34, 2013.
568. Tomasoni LR, Sosta E, Beltrame A, et al: Antenatal screening for mother to child infections in immigrants and residents: the case of toxoplasmosis in northern Italy, *J Immigr Minor Health* 12:834-840, 2010.
569. Lopes AP, Dubey JP, Moutinho O, et al: Seroepidemiology of *Toxoplasma gondii* infection in women from the north of Portugal in their childbearing years, *Epidemiol Infect* 140:872-877, 2012.
570. Ricci M, Pentimalli H, Thaller R, et al: Screening and prevention of congenital toxoplasmosis: an effectiveness study in a population with a high infection rate, *J Matern Fetal Neonatal Med* 14:398-403, 2003.
571. Vilibic-Cavlek T, Ljubin-Sternak S, Ban M, et al: Seroprevalence of TORCH infections in women of childbearing age in Croatia, *J Matern Fetal Neonatal Med* 24:280-283, 2011.
572. Ferguson W, Mayne PD, Lennon B, et al: Susceptibility of pregnant women to Toxoplasma infection—potential benefits for newborn screening, *Ir Med J* 101:220-221, 2008.
573. Cvetkovic D, Bobic B, Jankovska G, et al: Risk factors for Toxoplasma infection in pregnant women in FYR of Macedonia, *Parasite* 17: 183-186, 2010.
574. Hofhuis A, van Pelt W, van Duynhoven YT, et al: Decreased prevalence and age-specific risk factors for *Toxoplasma gondii* IgG antibodies in The Netherlands between 1995/1996 and 2006/2007, *Epidemiol Infect* 139:530-538, 2011.
575. Nash JQ, Chissel S, Jones J, et al: Risk factors for toxoplasmosis in pregnant women in Kent, United Kingdom, *Epidemiol Infect* 133:475-483, 2005.
576. Birgisdottir A, Asbjornsdottir H, Cook E, et al: Seroprevalence of *Toxoplasma gondii* in Sweden, Estonia and Iceland, *Scand J Infect Dis* 38:625-631, 2006.
577. Flatt A, Shetty N: Seroprevalence and risk factors for toxoplasmosis among antenatal women in London: a re-examination of risk in an ethnically diverse population, *Eur J Public Health* 23:648-652, 2013.
578. Gutiérrez-Zufiaurre N, Sánchez-Hernández J, Muñoz S, et al: Seroprevalence of antibodies against Treponema pallidum, *Toxoplasma gondii*, rubella virus, hepatitis B and C virus, and HIV in pregnant women, *Enferm Infecc Microbiol Clin* 22:512-516, 2004.
579. Ramos JM, Milla A, Rodriguez JC, et al: Seroprevalence of *Toxoplasma gondii* infection among immigrant and native pregnant women in Eastern Spain, *Parasitol Res* 109:1447-1452, 2011.
580. Bartolome Alvarez J, Martinez Serrano M, Moreno Parrado L, et al: Prevalence and incidence in Albacete, Spain, of *Toxoplasma gondii* infection in women of childbearing age: differences between immigrant and non-immigrant (2001-2007), *Rev Esp Salud Publica* 82:333-342, 2008.
581. Sampedro A, Mazuelas P, Rodriguez-Granger J, et al: Serological markers in immigrant and Spanish pregnant women in Granada, *Enferm Infecc Microbiol Clin* 28:694-697, 2010.
582. Pinto B, Castagna B, Mattei R, et al: Seroprevalence for toxoplasmosis in individuals living in north west Tuscany: access to Toxo-test in central Italy, *Eur J Clin Microbiol Infect Dis* 31:1151-1156, 2012.
583. Maggi P, Volpe A, Carito V, et al: Surveillance of toxoplasmosis in pregnant women in Albania, *New Microbiol* 32:89-92, 2009.
584. Frischknecht F, Sell W, Trummer I, et al: Serological testing for infectious diseases in pregnant women: are the guidelines followed? *Swiss Med Wkly* 140:w13138, 2011.
585. Nogareda F, Le Strat Y, Villena I, et al: Incidence and prevalence of *Toxoplasma gondii* infection among women in France, 1980-2020: model-based estimation, *Epidemiol Infect* 142:1661-1670, 2014.
586. Bjerke SE, Vangen S, Holter E, et al: Infectious immune status in an obstetric population of Pakistani immigrants in Norway, *Scand J Public Health* 39:464-470, 2011.
587. Bobic B, Nikolic A, Klun I, et al: Undercooked meat consumption remains the major risk factor for Toxoplasma infection in Serbia, *Parassitologia* 49:227-230, 2007.
588. Buchy P, Follezou JY, Lien TX, et al: Serological study of toxoplasmosis in Vietnam in a population of drug users (Ho Chi Minh city) and pregnant women (Nha Trang), *Bull Soc Pathol Exot* 96:46-47, 2003.
589. Nissapatorn V, Suwanrath C, Sawangjaroen N, et al: Toxoplasmosis-serological evidence and associated risk factors among pregnant women in southern Thailand, *Am J Trop Med Hyg* 85:243-247, 2011.
590. Sakae C, Natphopsuk S, Settheetham-Ishida W, et al: Low prevalence of *Toxoplasma gondii* infection among women in northeastern Thailand, *J Parasitol* 99:172-173, 2013.
591. Liu Q, Wei F, Gao S, et al: *Toxoplasma gondii* infection in pregnant women in China, *Trans R Soc Trop Med Hyg* 103:162-166, 2009.
592. Xiao Y, Yin J, Jiang N, et al: Seroepidemiology of human *Toxoplasma gondii* infection in China, *BMC Infect Dis* 10:4, 2010.
593. Tabbara KS, Saleh F: Serodiagnosis of toxoplasmosis in Bahrain, *Saudi Med J* 26:1383-1387, 2005.
594. Al-Hindi A, Al-Helou T, Al-Helou Y: Seroprevalence of *Toxoplasma gondii*, cytomegalovirus, rubella virus and *Chlamydia trachomatis* among infertile women attending in vitro fertilization center, Gaza strip, Palestine, *J Egypt Soc Parasitol* 40:451-458, 2010.
595. Nijem KI, Al-Amleh S: Seroprevalence and associated risk factors of toxoplasmosis in pregnant women in Hebron district, Palestine, *East Mediterr Health J* 15:1278-1284, 2009.
596. Koksaldi-Motor V, Evirgen O, Azaroglu I, et al: Prevalence of toxoplasmosis, cytomegalovirus and rubella IgG antibodies in Hatay women and children, *West Indian Med J* 61:154-157, 2012.
597. Saeedi M, Veghari GR, Marjani A: Seroepidemiologic evaluation of anti-Toxoplasma antibodies among women in north of Iran, *Pak J Biol Sci* 10:2359-2362, 2007.
598. Hashemi HJ, Saraei M: Seroprevalence of *Toxoplasma gondii* in unmarried women in Qazvin, Islamic Republic of Iran, *East Mediterr Health J* 16:24-28, 2010.
599. Tamer GS, Dundar D, Caliskan E: Seroprevalence of *Toxoplasma gondii*, rubella and cytomegalovirus among pregnant women in western region of Turkey, *Clin Invest Med* 32:E43-E47, 2009.
600. Fallah M, Rabiee S, Matini M, et al: Seroepidemiology of toxoplasmosis in primigravida women in Hamadan, Islamic Republic of Iran, 2004, *East Mediterr Health J* 14:163-171, 2008.
601. Youssefi MR, Sefidgar AA, Mostafazadeh A, et al: Serologic evaluation of toxoplasmosis in matrimonial women in Babol, Iran, *Pak J Biol Sci* 10:1550-1552, 2007.
602. Ocak S, Zeteroglu S, Ozer C, et al: Seroprevalence of *Toxoplasma gondii*, rubella and cytomegalovirus among pregnant women in southern Turkey, *Scand J Infect Dis* 39:231-234, 2007.
603. Mostafavi N, Ataei B, Nokhodian Z, et al: *Toxoplasma gondii* infection in women of childbearing age of Isfahan, Iran: a population-based study, *Adv Biomed Res* 1:60, 2012.
604. Hajsoleimani F, Ataeian A, Nourian A, et al: Seroprevalence of *Toxoplasma gondii* in pregnant women and bioassay of IgM positive cases in Zanjan, Northwest of Iran, *Iran J Parasitol* 7:82-86, 2012.
605. Al-Mohammad HI, Amin TT, Balaha MH, et al: Toxoplasmosis among the pregnant women attending a Saudi maternity hospital: seroprevalence and possible risk factors, *Ann Trop Med Parasitol* 104:493-504, 2010.
606. Almogren A: Antenatal screening for *Toxoplasma gondii* infection at a tertiary care hospital in Riyadh, Saudi Arabia, *Ann Saudi Med* 31:569-572, 2011.
607. Ghazi HO, Telmesani AM, Mahomed MF: TORCH agents in pregnant Saudi women, *Med Princ Pract* 11:180-182, 2002.
608. El-Gozamy BR, Mohamed SA, Mansour HA: Toxoplasmosis among pregnant women in Qualyobia Governorate, Egypt, *J Egypt Soc Parasitol* 39:389-401, 2009.
609. El Deeb HK, Salah-Eldin H, Khodeer S, et al: Prevalence of *Toxoplasma gondii* infection in antenatal population in Menoufia governorate, Egypt, *Acta Trop* 124:185-191, 2012.
610. Nimri L, Pelloux H, Elkhatib L: Detection of *Toxoplasma gondii* DNA and specific antibodies in high-risk pregnant women, *Am J Trop Med Hyg* 71:831-835, 2004.
611. Singh S, Pandit AJ: Incidence and prevalence of toxoplasmosis in Indian pregnant women: a prospective study, *Am J Reprod Immunol* 52:276-283, 2004.
612. Iqbal J, Khalid N: Detection of acute *Toxoplasma gondii* infection in early pregnancy by IgG avidity and PCR analysis, *J Med Microbiol* 56(Pt 11):1495-1499, 2007.
613. Bouhamdan SF, Bitar LK, Saghir HJ, et al: Seroprevalence of Toxoplasma antibodies among individuals tested at hospitals and private laboratories in Beirut, *J Med Liban* 58:8-11, 2010.
614. Terazawa A, Muljono R, Susanto L, et al: High Toxoplasma antibody prevalence among inhabitants in Jakarta, Indonesia, *Jpn J Infect Dis* 56:107-109, 2003.
615. Hu IJ, Chen PC, Su FC, et al: Perinatal toxoplasmosis, northern Taiwan, *Emerg Infect Dis* 12:1460-1461, 2006.

616. Lin YL, Liao YS, Liao LR, et al: Seroprevalence and sources of Toxoplasma infection among indigenous and immigrant pregnant women in Taiwan, *Parasitol Res* 103:67-74, 2008.
617. Khurana S, Bagga R, Aggarwal A, et al: Serological screening for antenatal Toxoplasma infection in India, *Indian J Med Microbiol* 28:143-146, 2010.
618. Sarkar MD, Anuradha B, Sharma N, et al: Seropositivity of toxoplasmosis in antenatal women with bad obstetric history in a tertiary-care hospital of Andhra Pradesh, India, *J Health Popul Nutr* 30:87-92, 2012.
619. Borkakoty BJ, Borthakur AK, Gohain M: Prevalence of *Toxoplasma gondii* infection amongst pregnant women in Assam, India, *Indian J Med Microbiol* 25:431-432, 2007.
620. Nissapatorn V, Noor Azmi MA, Cho SM, et al: Toxoplasmosis: prevalence and risk factors, *J Obstet Gynaecol* 23:618-624, 2003.
621. Morris A, Croxson M: Serological evidence of *Toxoplasma gondii* infection among pregnant women in Auckland, *N Z Med J* 117:U770, 2004.
622. Ades AE, Nokes DJ: Modeling age- and time-specific incidence from seroprevalence: toxoplasmosis, *Am J Epidemiol* 137:1022-1034, 1993.
623. Naoi K, Yano A: A theoretical analysis of the relations between the risk of congenital toxoplasmosis and the annual infection rates with a convincing argument for better public intervention, *Parasitol Int* 51:187-194, 2002.
624. Evengard B, Petersson K, Engman ML, et al: Low incidence of Toxoplasma infection during pregnancy and in newborns in Sweden, *Epidemiol Infect* 127:121-127, 2001.
625. Breugelmans M, Naessens A, Foulon W: Prevention of toxoplasmosis during pregnancy—an epidemiologic survey over 22 consecutive years, *J Perinat Med* 32:211-214, 2004.
626. Muñoz Batet C, Guardià Llobet C, Juncosa Morros T, et al: [Toxoplasmosis and pregnancy. Multicenter study of 16,362 pregnant women in Barcelona], *Med Clin (Barc)* 123:12-16, 2004.
627. Lebech M, Andersen O, Christensen NC, et al: Feasibility of neonatal screening for Toxoplasma infection in the absence of prenatal treatment. Danish Congenital Toxoplasmosis Study Group, *Lancet* 353:1834-1837, 1999.
628. Lappalainen M, Koskela P, Hedman K, et al: Incidence of primary Toxoplasma infections during pregnancy in southern Finland: a prospective cohort study, *Scand J Infect Dis* 24:97-104, 1992.
629. Capretti MG, De Angelis M, Tridapalli E, et al: Toxoplasmosis in pregnancy in an area with low seroprevalence: is prenatal screening still worthwhile? *Pediatr Infect Dis J* 33:5-10, 2014.
630. Szenasi Z, Ozsvar Z, Nagy E, et al: Prevention of congenital toxoplasmosis in Szeged, Hungary, *Int J Epidemiol* 26:428-435, 1997.
631. Guerina NG, Hsu HW, Meissner HC, et al: Neonatal serologic screening and early treatment for congenital *Toxoplasma gondii* infection. The New England Regional Toxoplasma Working Group, *N Engl J Med* 330:1858-1863, 1994.
631a. Stillwaggon E, Carrier CS, Sautter M, et al: Maternal serologic screening to prevent congenital toxoplasmosis: a decision-analytic economic model, *PLoS Negl Trop Dis* 5:e1333. 2011.
631b. Lopez A, Dietz VJ, Wilson M, et al: Preventing congenital toxoplasmosis, *MMWR Recomm Rep* 49:59-68, 2000.
632. Varella IS, Canti IC, Santos BR, et al: Prevalence of acute toxoplasmosis infection among 41,112 pregnant women and the mother-to-child transmission rate in a public hospital in South Brazil, *Mem Inst Oswaldo Cruz* 104:383-388, 2009.
633. Nobrega OT, Karnikowski MG: An estimation of the frequency of gestational toxoplasmosis in the Brazilian Federal District, *Rev Soc Bras Med Trop* 38:358-360, 2005.
634. Remington J, Klein J, editors: *Infectious diseases of the fetus and the newborn infant*, ed 7, Philadelphia, 2011, Saunders.
635. Lago EG, Neto EC, Melamed J, et al: Congenital toxoplasmosis: late pregnancy infections detected by neonatal screening and maternal serological testing at delivery, *Paediatr Perinat Epidemiol* 21:525-531, 2007.
636. de Melo Inagaki AD, Carvalheiro CG, Cipolotti R, et al: Birth prevalence and characteristics of congenital toxoplasmosis in Sergipe, North-east Brazil, *Trop Med Int Health* 17:1349-1355, 2012.
637. Mozzatto L, Procianoy RS: Incidence of congenital toxoplasmosis in southern Brazil: a prospective study, *Rev Inst Med Trop São Paulo* 45:147-151, 2003.
638. Carvalheiro CG, Mussi-Pinhata MM, Yamamoto AY, et al: Incidence of congenital toxoplasmosis estimated by neonatal screening: relevance of diagnostic confirmation in asymptomatic newborn infants, *Epidemiol Infect* 133:485-491, 2005.
639. Segundo GR, Silva DA, Mineo JR, et al: Congenital toxoplasmosis in Uberlandia, MG, Brazil, *J Trop Pediatr* 50:50-53, 2004.
640. Segundo GR, Silva DA, Mineo JR, et al: A comparative study of congenital toxoplasmosis between public and private hospitals from Uberlandia, MG, Brazil, *Mem Inst Oswaldo Cruz* 99:13-17, 2004.
641. Gomez-Marin JE, de-la-Torre A, Angel-Muller E, et al: First Colombian multicentric newborn screening for congenital toxoplasmosis, *PLoS Negl Trop Dis* 5:e1195, 2011.
642. Gomez-Marin JE, Gonzalez MM, Montoya MT, et al: A newborn screening programme for congenital toxoplasmosis in the setting of a country with less income, *Arch Dis Child* 92:88, 2007.
643. Roser D, Nielsen HV, Petersen E, et al: Congenital toxoplasmosis—a report on the Danish neonatal screening programme 1999-2007, *J Inherit Metab Dis* 33(Suppl 2):S241-S247, 2010.
644. Gilbert RE, Stanford MR, Jackson H, et al: Incidence of acute symptomatic Toxoplasma retinochoroiditis in south London according to country of birth, *BMJ* 310:1037-1040, 1995.
645. Signorell LM, Seitz D, Merkel S, et al: Cord blood screening for congenital toxoplasmosis in northwestern Switzerland, 1982-1999, *Pediatr Infect Dis J* 25:123-128, 2006.
646. Kortbeek LM, Hofhuis A, Nijhuis CD, et al: Congenital toxoplasmosis and DALYs in the Netherlands, *Mem Inst Oswaldo Cruz* 104:370-373, 2009.
647. Aptouramani M, Theodoridou M, Syrogiannopoulos G, et al: A dedicated surveillance network for congenital toxoplasmosis in Greece, 2006-2009: assessment of the results, *BMC Public Health* 12:1019, 2012.
648. Durlach RA, Kaufer F, Carral L, et al: Toxoplasmic lymphadenitis—clinical and serologic profile, *Clin Microbiol Infect* 9:625-631, 2003.
649. Burnett AJ, Shortt SG, Isaac-Renton J, et al: Multiple cases of acquired toxoplasmosis retinitis presenting in an outbreak, *Ophthalmology* 105:1032-1037, 1998.
650. Holland GN: Ocular toxoplasmosis: a global reassessment. Part I: epidemiology and course of disease, *Am J Ophthalmol* 136:973-988, 2003.
651. Noble AG, Latkany P, Kusmierczyk J, et al: Chorioretinal lesions in mothers of children with congenital toxoplasmosis in the National Collaborative Chicago-based, Congenital Toxoplasmosis Study, *Sci Med (Porto Alegre)* 20:20-26, 2010.
652. Neves ES, Bicudo LN, Curi AL, et al: Acute acquired toxoplasmosis: clinical-laboratorial aspects and ophthalmologic evaluation in a cohort of immunocompetent patients, *Mem Inst Oswaldo Cruz* 104: 393-396, 2009.
653. Glasner PD, Silveira C, Kruszon-Moran D, et al: An unusually high prevalence of ocular toxoplasmosis in southern Brazil, *Am J Ophthalmol* 114:136-144, 1992.
654. Abboud P, Harika G, Saniez D, et al: Ultrasonic signs of fetal toxoplasmosis. Review of the literature, *J Gynecol Obstet Biol Reprod (Paris)* 24:733-738, 1995.
655. Montoya JG, Remington JS: Studies on the serodiagnosis of toxoplasmic lymphadenitis, *Clin Infect Dis* 20:781-789, 1995.
656. Vogel N, Kirisits M, Michael E, et al: Congenital toxoplasmosis transmitted from an immunologically competent mother infected before conception, *Clin Infect Dis* 23:1055-1060, 1996.
657. Hennequin C, Dureau P, N'Guyen L, et al: Congenital toxoplasmosis acquired from an immune woman, *Pediatr Infect Dis J* 16:75-77, 1997.
658. Dollfus H, Dureau P, Hennequin C, et al: Congenital Toxoplasma chorioretinitis transmitted by preconceptionally immune women, *Br J Ophthalmol* 82:1444-1445, 1998.
659. Pons JC, Sigrand C, Grangeot-Keros L, et al: Congenital toxoplasmosis: transmission to the fetus of a pre-pregnancy maternal infection, *Presse Med* 24:179-182, 1995.
660. Boumahni B, Randrianivo H, Flodrops H, et al: [Maternal toxoplasmosis before conception and chorioretinitis in twin sisters], *J Gynecol Obstet Biol Reprod (Paris)* 33:248-250, 2004.
661. Lebas F, Ducrocq S, Mucignat V, et al: [Congenital toxoplasmosis: a new case of infection during pregnancy in an previously immunized and immunocompetent woman], *Arch Pediatr* 11:926-928, 2004.
662. D'Ercole C, Boubli L, Franck J, et al: Recurrent congenital toxoplasmosis in a woman with lupus erythematosus, *Prenat Diagn* 15: 1171-1175, 1995.
663. Villena I, Chemla C, Quereux C, et al: Prenatal diagnosis of congenital toxoplasmosis transmitted by an immunocompetent woman infected before conception. Reims Toxoplasmosis Group, *Prenat Diagn* 18:1079-1081, 1998.
664. Desmonts G, Couvreur J, Thulliez P: Congenital toxoplasmosis. 5 cases of mother-to-child transmission of pre-pregnancy infection, *Presse Med* 19:1445-1449, 1990.

665. Silveira C, Ferreira R, Muccioli C, et al: Toxoplasmosis transmitted to a newborn from the mother infected 20 years earlier, *Am J Ophthalmol* 136:370-371, 2003.
666. Bachmeyer C, Mouchnino G, Thulliez P, et al: Congenital toxoplasmosis from an HIV-infected woman as a result of reactivation, *J Infect* 52:e55-e57, 2006.
667. Robert-Gangneux F, Yera H, D'Herve D, et al: Congenital toxoplasmosis after a preconceptional or periconceptional maternal infection, *Pediatr Infect Dis J* 28:660-661, 2009.
668. Gras L, Gilbert RE, Wallon M, et al: Duration of the IgM response in women acquiring *Toxoplasma gondii* during pregnancy: implications for clinical practice and cross-sectional incidence studies, *Epidemiol Infect* 132:541-548, 2004.
669. Lappalainen M, Hedman K: Serodiagnosis of toxoplasmosis. The impact of measurement of IgG avidity, *Ann Ist Super Sanita* 40:81-88, 2004.
670. Remington JS, Thulliez P, Montoya JG: Recent developments for diagnosis of toxoplasmosis, *J Clin Microbiol* 42:941-945, 2004.
671. Lefevre-Pettazzoni M, Le Cam S, Wallon M, et al: Delayed maturation of immunoglobulin G avidity: implication for the diagnosis of toxoplasmosis in pregnant women, *Eur J Clin Microbiol Infect Dis* 25:687-693, 2006.
672. Lefevre-Pettazzoni M, Bissery A, Wallon M, et al: Impact of spiramycin treatment and gestational age on maturation of *Toxoplasma gondii* immunoglobulin G avidity in pregnant women, *Clin Vaccine Immunol* 14:239-243, 2007.
673. Sensini A, Pascoli S, Marchetti D, et al: IgG avidity in the serodiagnosis of acute *Toxoplasma gondii* infection: a multicenter study, *Clin Microbiol Infect* 2:25-29, 1996.
674. Liesenfeld O, Montoya JG, Kinney S, et al: Effect of testing for IgG avidity in the diagnosis of *Toxoplasma gondii* infection in pregnant women: experience in a US reference laboratory, *J Infect Dis* 183:1248-1253, 2001.
675. Bessières MH, Roques C, Berrébi A, et al: IgA antibody response during acquired and congenital toxoplasmosis, *J Clin Pathol* 45:605-608, 1992.
676. Jenum PA, Stray-Pedersen B: Development of specific immunoglobulins G, M, and A following primary *Toxoplasma gondii* infection in pregnant women, *J Clin Microbiol* 36:2907-2913, 1998.
677. Nascimento FS, Suzuki LA, Rossi CL: Assessment of the value of detecting specific IgA antibodies for the diagnosis of a recently acquired primary Toxoplasma infection, *Prenat Diagn* 28:749-752, 2008.
678. Foudrinier F, Villena I, Jaussaud R, et al: Clinical value of specific immunoglobulin E detection by enzyme-linked immunosorbent assay in cases of acquired and congenital toxoplasmosis, *J Clin Microbiol* 41:1681-1686, 2003.
679. Wong SY, Hajdu MP, Ramirez R, et al: Role of specific immunoglobulin E in diagnosis of acute Toxoplasma infection and toxoplasmosis, *J Clin Microbiol* 31:2952-2959, 1993.
680. Gross U, Keksel O, Dardé ML: Value of detecting immunoglobulin E antibodies for the serological diagnosis of *Toxoplasma gondii* infection, *Clin Diagn Lab Immunol* 4:247-251, 1997.
681. Ashburn D, Joss AW, Pennington TH, et al: Do IgA, IgE, and IgG avidity tests have any value in the diagnosis of Toxoplasma infection in pregnancy? *J Clin Pathol* 51:312-315, 1998.
682. Franck J, Garin YJ, Dumon H: LDBio-Toxo II immunoglobulin G Western blot confirmatory test for anti-Toxoplasma antibody detection, *J Clin Microbiol* 46:2334-2338, 2008.
683. Kahi S, Cozon GJ, Greenland T, et al: A rapid flow cytometric method to explore cellular immunity against *Toxoplasma gondii* in humans, *Clin Diagn Lab Immunol* 5:745-748, 1998.
684. Fatoohi AF, Cozon GJ, Greenland T, et al: Cellular immune responses to recombinant antigens in pregnant women chronically infected with *Toxoplasma gondii*, *Clin Diagn Lab Immunol* 9:704-707, 2002.
685. Chapey E, Wallon M, Debize G, et al: Diagnosis of congenital toxoplasmosis by using a whole-blood gamma interferon release assay, *J Clin Microbiol* 48:41-45, 2010.
686. Wallon M, Franck J, Romand S, et al: Value of Toxoplasma serology at delivery in women seronegative during pregnancy, *J Gynecol Obstet Biol Reprod (Paris)* 30(7 Pt 1):697-699, 2001.
687. Cortina-Borja M, Tan HK, Wallon M, et al: Prenatal treatment for serious neurological sequelae of congenital toxoplasmosis: an observational prospective cohort study, *PLoS Med* 7(10):2010. doi: 10.1371/journal.pmed.1000351. pii: e1000351.
688. Sensini A: *Toxoplasma gondii* infection in pregnancy: opportunities and pitfalls of serological diagnosis, *Clin Microbiol Infect* 12:504-512, 2006.
689. Liesenfeld O, Montoya JG, Tathineni NJ, et al: Confirmatory serologic testing for acute toxoplasmosis and rate of induced abortions among women reported to have positive Toxoplasma immunoglobulin M antibody titers, *Am J Obstet Gynecol* 184:140-145, 2001.
690. Dao A, Azzouz N, Eloundou Nga C, et al: Unspecific reactivity of IgM directed against the low-molecular-weight antigen of *Toxoplasma gondii*, *Eur J Clin Microbiol Infect Dis* 22:418-421, 2003.
691. Pelloux H, Fricker-Hidalgo H, Brochier G, et al: Intravenous immunoglobulin therapy: confounding effects on serological screening for toxoplasmosis during pregnancy, *J Clin Microbiol* 37:3423-3424, 1999.
692. Fricker-Hidalgo H, Cimon B, Chemla C, et al: Toxoplasma seroconversion with negative or transient immunoglobulin M in pregnant women: myth or reality? A French multicenter retrospective study, *J Clin Microbiol* 51:2103-2111, 2013.
693. Wallon M, Franck J, Thulliez P, et al: Accuracy of real-time polymerase chain reaction for *Toxoplasma gondii* in amniotic fluid, *Obstet Gynecol* 115:727-733, 2010.
694. Rabilloud M, Wallon M, Peyron F: In utero and at birth diagnosis of congenital toxoplasmosis: use of likelihood ratios for clinical management, *Pediatr Infect Dis J* 29:421-425, 2010.
695. Pons J, Sigrand C, Grangeot-Keros L, et al: Congenital toxoplasmosis: transmission to the fetus of a pre-pregnancy maternal infection, *Presse Med* 24:179-182, 1995.
696. Villena I, Chemla C, Quereux C, et al: Prenatal diagnosis of congenital toxoplasmosis transmitted by an immunocompetent woman infected before conception, *Prenat Diagn* 18:1079-1081, 1998.
697. Vogel N, Kirisits M, Michael E, et al: Congenital toxoplasmosis transmitted from an immunologically competent mother infected before conception, *Clin Infect Dis* 23:1055-1060, 1996.
698. Hennequin C, Dureau P, N'Guyen L, et al: Congenital toxoplasmosis acquired from an immune woman, *Pediatr Infect Dis J* 16:75-77, 1997.
699. Lebas F, Ducrocq S, Mucignat V, et al: Congenital toxoplasmosis: a new case of infection during pregnancy in a previously immunized and immunocompetent woman], *Arch Pediatr* 11:926-928, 2004.
700. Fernandes R, Vasconcellos VP, Araújo LC, et al: Vertical transmission of HIV and Toxoplasma by reactivation in a chronically infected woman, *Braz J Infect Dis* 13:70-71, 2009.
701. Lago E, Conrado GS, Piccoli CS, et al: *Toxoplasma gondii* antibody profile in HIV-infected pregnant women and the risk of congenital toxoplasmosis, *Eur J Clin Microbiol Infect Dis* 28:345-351, 2009.
702. SYROCOT (Systematic Review on Congenital Toxoplasmosis) Study Group, Thiébaut R, Leproust S, et al: Effectiveness of prenatal treatment for congenital toxoplasmosis: a meta-analysis of individual patients' data, *Lancet* 369:115-122, 2007.
703. Wallon M, Peyron F, Cornu C, et al: Congenital Toxoplasma infection: monthly prenatal screening decreases transmission rate and improves clinical outcome at age 3 years, *Clin Infect Dis* 56: 1223-1231, 2013.
704. Daffos F, Forestier F, Capella-Pavlovsky M, et al: Prenatal management of 746 pregnancies at risk for congenital toxoplasmosis, *N Engl J Med* 318:271-275, 1988.
705. Desmonts G, Couvreur J: Congenital toxoplasmosis. A prospective study of 378 pregnancies, *N Engl J Med* 290:1110-1116, 1974.
706. Dunn D, Wallon M, Peyron F, et al: Mother-to-child transmission of toxoplasmosis: risk estimates for clinical counselling, *Lancet* 353:1829-1833, 1999.
707. Binquet C, Wallon M, Quantin C, et al: Prognostic factors for the long-term development of ocular lesions in 327 children with congenital toxoplasmosis, *Epidemiol Infect* 131:1157-1168, 2003.
708. Kieffer F, Wallon M, Garcia P, et al: Risk factors for retinochoroiditis during the first 2 years of life in infants with treated congenital toxoplasmosis, *Pediatr Infect Dis J* 27:27-32, 2008.
709. Villena I, Ancelle T, Delmas C, et al: Congenital toxoplasmosis in France in 2007: first results from a national surveillance system, *Euro Surveill* 15:19600, 2010.
710. Jacquemard F: Clinical aspects of infection during pregnancy. In Ambroise-Thomas P, Petersen E, editors: *Congenital toxoplasmosis: scientific background, clinical management and control*, Paris, 2000, Springer-Verlag, pp 111-120.
711. Wallon M, Kodjikian L, Binquet C, et al: Long-term ocular prognosis in 327 children with congenital toxoplasmosis, *Pediatrics* 113: 1567-1572, 2004.

712. Malinger G, Werner H, Rodriguez Leonel JC, et al: Prenatal brain imaging in congenital toxoplasmosis, *Prenat Diagn* 31:881-886, 2011.
713. Abboud P, Harika G, Saniez D, et al: Ultrasonic signs of fetal toxoplasmosis. Review of the literature, *J Gynecol Obstet Biol Reprod (Paris)* 24:733-738, 1995.
714. Barkovich A, Girard N: Fetal brain infections, *Childs Nerv Syst* 19:501-507, 2003.
715. Cuillier F, Avignon M: Case of the week #168, *The Fetusnet*, 2012.
716. Romand S, Wallon M, Franck J, et al: Prenatal diagnosis using polymerase chain reaction on amniotic fluid for congenital toxoplasmosis, *Obstet Gynecol* 97:296-300, 2001.
717. Romand S, Chosson M, Franck J, et al: Usefulness of quantitative polymerase chain reaction in amniotic fluid as early prognostic marker of fetal infection with *Toxoplasma gondii*, *Am J Obstet Gynecol* 190:797-802, 2004.
718. Homan W, Vercammen M, De Braekeleer J, et al: Identification of a 200- to 300-fold repetitive 529 bp DNA fragment in *Toxoplasma gondii*, and its use for diagnostic and quantitative PCR, *Int J Parasitol* 30:69-75, 2000.
719. Delhaes L, Yera H, Ache S, et al: Contribution of molecular diagnosis to congenital toxoplasmosis, *Diagn Microbiol Infect Dis* 76:244-247, 2013.
720. Hohlfeld P, Daffos F, Costa JM, et al: Prenatal diagnosis of congenital toxoplasmosis with a polymerase-chain-reaction test on amniotic fluid, *N Engl J Med* 331:695-699, 1994.
721. Khoshnood B, De Vigan C, Goffinet F, et al: Prenatal screening and diagnosis of congenital toxoplasmosis: a review of safety issues and psychological consequences for women who undergo screening, *Prenat Diagn* 27:395-403, 2007.
722. Chapey E, Wallon M, Debize G, et al: Diagnosis of congenital toxoplasmosis by using a whole-blood gamma interferon release assay, *J Clin Microbiol* 48:41-45, 2010.
723. Sterkers Y, Pratlong F, Albaba S, et al: Novel interpretation of molecular diagnosis of congenital toxoplasmosis according to gestational age at the time of maternal infection, *J Clin Microbiol* 50:3944-3951, 2012.
724. Rajapakse S, Chrishan Shivanthan M, Samaranayake N, et al: Antibiotics for human toxoplasmosis: a systematic review of randomized trials, *Pathog Glob Health* 107:162-169, 2013.
725. Alavi SM, Alavi L: Treatment of toxoplasmic lymphadenitis with co-trimoxazole: double-blind, randomized clinical trial, *Int J Infect Dis* 14(Suppl 3):e67-e69, 2010.
726. Moncada PA, Montoya JG: Toxoplasmosis in the fetus and newborn: an update on prevalence, diagnosis and treatment, *Expert Rev Anti Infect Ther* 10:815-828, 2012.
727. Friedman S, Ford-Jones LE, Toi A, et al: Congenital toxoplasmosis: prenatal diagnosis, treatment and postnatal outcome, *Prenat Diagn* 19:330-333, 1999.
728. Berrébi A, Kobuch WE, Bessières MH, et al: Termination of pregnancy for maternal toxoplasmosis, *Lancet* 344:36-39, 1994.
729. Berrébi A, Bardou M, Bessières MH, et al: Outcome for children infected with congenital toxoplasmosis in the first trimester and with normal ultrasound findings: a study of 36 cases, *Eur J Obstet Gynecol Reprod Biol* 135:53-57, 2007.
730. Zalud I, Janas S: Risks of third-trimester amniocentesis, *J Reprod Med* 53:45-48, 2008.
731. Garcia-Méric P, Franck J, Dumon H, et al: Management of congenital toxoplasmosis in France: current data, *Presse Med* 39:530-538, 2010.
732. Wallon M, Franck J, Thulliez P, et al: Accuracy of real-time polymerase chain reaction for *Toxoplasma gondii* in amniotic fluid, *Obstet Gynecol* 115:727-733, 2010.
733. Derouin F, Jacqz-Aigrain E, Thulliez P, et al: Cotrimoxazole for prenatal treatment of congenital toxoplasmosis? *Parasitol Today* 16:254-256, 2000.
734. Valentini P, Annunziata ML, Angelone DF, et al: Role of spiramycin/cotrimoxazole association in the mother-to-child transmission of toxoplasmosis infection in pregnancy, *Eur J Clin Microbiol Infect Dis* 28:297-300, 2009.
735. Khoshnood B, De Vigan C, Goffinet F, et al: Prenatal screening and diagnosis of congenital toxoplasmosis: a review of safety issues and psychological consequences for women who undergo screening, *Prenat Diagn* 27:395-403, 2007.
736. Jongert E, Roberts CW, Gargano N, et al: Vaccines against *Toxoplasma gondii*: challenges and opportunities, *Mem Inst Oswaldo Cruz* 104:252-266, 2009.
737. Binquet C, Wallon M, Quantin C, et al: Evaluation of prevention strategies for congenital toxoplasmosis: a critical review of medico-economic studies, *Rev Epidemiol Sante Publique* 50:475-487, 2002.
738. Mulder E, Davis A, Gawley L, et al: Negative impact of non-evidence-based information received by women taking antidepressants during pregnancy from health care providers and others, *J Obstet Gynaecol Can* 34:66-71, 2012.
739. Ross DS, Rasmussen SA, Cannon MJ, et al: Obstetrician/gynecologists' knowledge, attitudes, and practices regarding prevention of infections in pregnancy, *J Womens Health (Larchmt)* 18:1187-1193, 2009.
740. Jones JL, Dietz VJ, Power M, et al: Survey of obstetrician-gynecologists in the United States about toxoplasmosis, *Infect Dis Obstet Gynecol* 9:23-31, 2001.
741. Jones JL, Krueger A, Schulkin J, et al: Toxoplasmosis prevention and testing in pregnancy, survey of obstetrician-gynaecologists, *Zoonoses Public Health* 57:27-33, 2010.
742. Kravetz JD, Federman DG: Prevention of toxoplasmosis in pregnancy: knowledge of risk factors, *Infect Dis Obstet Gynecol* 13:161-165, 2005.
743. Sellier Y, Dupont C, Peyron F, et al: Prévention de la toxoplasmose maternelle en cours de grossesse: connaissances et pratiques de sages-femmes de la région Rhône-Alpes (France), *Rev Med Perinat* 4:9-16, 2012.
744. Centers for Disease Control and Prevention: Toxoplasmosis: an important message for cat owners. Available at http://www.cdc.gov/parasites/toxoplasmosis/resources/printresources/catowners.pdf. Accessed April 2, 2014.
745. Haute Autorité de Santé: Surveillance sérologique et prévention de la toxoplasmose et de la rubéole au cours de la grossesse et dépistage prénatal de l'hépatite B : pertinence des modalités de réalisation, Paris, 2009, Haute Autorité de Santé.
746. Coonrod DV, Jack BW, Stubblefield PG, et al: The clinical content of preconception care: infectious diseases in preconception care, *Am J Obstet Gynecol* 199(6 Suppl 2):S296-S309, 2008.
747. Newton LH, Hall SM: A survey of health education material for the primary prevention of congenital toxoplasmosis, *Commun Dis Rep CDR Rev* 5:R21-R27, 1995.
748. Ferguson W, Mayne PD, Cafferkey M, et al: Lack of awareness of risk factors for primary toxoplasmosis in pregnancy, *Ir J Med Sci* 180:807-811, 2011.
749. Jones JL, Ogunmodede F, Scheftel J, et al: Toxoplasmosis-related knowledge and practices among pregnant women in the United States, *Infect Dis Obstet Gynecol* 11:139-145, 2003.
750. Ogunmodede F, Scheftel J, Jones JL, et al: Toxoplasmosis prevention knowledge among pregnant women in Minnesota, *Minn Med* 88: 32-34, 2005.
751. Pereboom MT, Mannien J, Spelten ER, et al: Observational study to assess pregnant women's knowledge and behaviour to prevent toxoplasmosis, listeriosis and cytomegalovirus, *BMC Pregnancy Childbirth* 13:98, 2013.
752. Costa FF, Gondim AP, de Lima MB, et al: Preventive behavior for toxoplasmosis in pregnant adolescents in the state of Ceara, Brazil, *BMC Public Health* 12:73, 2012.
753. Centers for Disease Control and Prevention: Parasites: toxoplasmosis (Toxoplasma infection) and pregnant women. Available at http://www.cdc.gov/parasites/toxoplasmosis/gen_info/pregnant.html. Accessed April 2, 2014.
754. El-Nawawi FA, Tawfik MA, Shaapan RM: Methods for inactivation of *Toxoplasma gondii* cysts in meat and tissues of experimentally infected sheep, *Foodborne Pathog Dis* 5:687-690, 2008.
755. Lunden A, Uggla A: Infectivity of *Toxoplasma gondii* in mutton following curing, smoking, freezing or microwave cooking, *Int J Food Microbiol* 15:357-363, 1992.
756. Dubey JP: Long-term persistence of *Toxoplasma gondii* in tissues of pigs inoculated with *T. gondii oocysts* and effect of freezing on viability of tissue cysts in pork, *Am J Vet Res* 49:910-913, 1988.
757. Vitale M, Di Marco Lo Presti V: Food safety or typical dishes?: *Toxoplasma gondii* and educational preventive campaign, *Foodborne Pathog Dis* 10:196, 2013.
758. Tenter AM: *Toxoplasma gondii* in animals used for human consumption, *Mem Inst Oswaldo Cruz* 104:364-369, 2009.
759. Lindsay DS, Collins MV, Mitchell SM, et al: Survival of *Toxoplasma gondii* oocysts in Eastern oysters (Crassostrea virginica), *J Parasitol* 90:1054-1057, 2004.

760. Anand R, Jones CW, Ricks JH, et al: Acute primary toxoplasmosis in travelers returning from endemic countries, *J Travel Med* 19:57-60, 2012.
761. Elmore SA, Jones JL, Conrad PA, et al: *Toxoplasma gondii*: epidemiology, feline clinical aspects, and prevention, *Trends Parasitol* 26: 190-196, 2010.
762. Kramer L: Human toxoplasmosis and the role of veterinary clinicians, *Int J Med Sci* 6:133-134, 2009.
763. Canadian Centre for Occupational and Health Safety: Toxoplasmosis. Available at http://www.ccohs.ca/oshanswers/diseases/toxoplasmosis.html. Accessed October 9, 2014.
764. Dubey JP: Strategies to reduce transmission of *Toxoplasma gondii* to animals and humans, *Vet Parasitol* 64:65-70, 1996.
765. Jones JL, Dubey JP: Foodborne toxoplasmosis, *Clin Infect Dis* 55: 845-851, 2012.
766. American Veterinary Medical Association Collections: Feral cats. Available at https://www.avma.org/News/Journals/Collections/Pages/AVMA-Collections-Feral-cats.aspx. Accessed October 9, 2014.
767. Hill DE, Sreekumar C, Gamble HR, et al: Effect of commonly used enhancement solutions on the viability of *Toxoplasma gondii* tissue cysts in pork loin, *J Food Prot* 67:2230-2233, 2004.
768. Mutapi F, Billingsley PF, Secor WE: Infection and treatment immunizations for successful parasite vaccines, *Trends Parasitol* 29:135-141, 2013.
769. Buxton D, Thomson KM, Maley S, et al: Experimental challenge of sheep 18 months after vaccination with a live (S48) *Toxoplasma gondii* vaccine, *Vet Rec* 133:310-312, 1993.
770. Mevelec MN, Ducournau C, Bassuny Ismael A, et al: Mic1-3 Knockout *Toxoplasma gondii* is a good candidate for a vaccine against *T. gondii*-induced abortion in sheep, *Vet Res* 41:49, 2010.
771. Kur J, Holec-Gasior L, Hiszczynska-Sawicka E: Current status of toxoplasmosis vaccine development, *Expert Rev Vaccines* 8:791-808, 2009.
772. Liu Q, Singla LD, Zhou H: Vaccines against *Toxoplasma gondii*: status, challenges and future directions, *Hum Vaccin Immunother* 8:1305-1308, 2012.
773. Wang Y, Wang M, Wang G, et al: Increased survival time in mice vaccinated with a branched lysine multiple antigenic peptide containing B- and T-cell epitopes from *T. gondii* antigens, *Vaccine* 29:8619-8623, 2011.
774. Henriquez FL, Woods S, Cong H, et al: Immunogenetics of *Toxoplasma gondii* informs vaccine design, *Trends Parasitol* 26:550-555, 2010.
775. Weiss LM, Fiser A, Angeletti RH, et al: *Toxoplasma gondii* proteomics, *Expert Rev Proteomics* 6:303-313, 2009.
776. Berrébi A, Assouline C, Bessières MH, et al: Long-term outcome of children with congenital toxoplasmosis, *Am J Obstet Gynecol* 203:552, 2010.
777. Gras L, Wallon M, Pollak A, et al: Association between prenatal treatment and clinical manifestations of congenital toxoplasmosis in infancy: a cohort study in 13 European centres, *Acta Paediatr* 94:1721-1731, 2005.
778. Wolf A, Cowen D, Paige B: Toxoplasmic encephalomyelitis: a new case of granulomatous encephalomyelitis due to a protozoan, *Am J Pathol* 15:657-694, 1939.
779. McAuley J, Boyer KM, Patel D, et al: Early and longitudinal evaluations of treated infants and children and untreated historical patients with congenital toxoplasmosis: the Chicago Collaborative Treatment Trial, *Clin Infect Dis* 18:38-72, 1994.
780. Olariu T, Remington JS, McLeod R, et al: Severe congenital toxoplasmosis in the United States: clinical and serologic findings in untreated infants, *Pediatr Infect Dis J* 30:1056-1061, 2011.
781. Freeman K, Oakley L, Pollak A, et al: Association between congenital toxoplasmosis and preterm birth, low birthweight and small for gestational age birth, *BJOG* 112:31-37, 2005.
782. McLeod R, Boyer KM, Lee D, et al: Prematurity and severity are associated with *Toxoplasma gondii* alleles (NCCCTS, 1981–2009), *Clin Infect Dis* 54:1595-1605, 2012.
783. Kodjikian L, Wallon M, Fleury J, et al: Ocular manifestations in congenital toxoplasmosis, *Arch Clin Exp Ophthalmol* 244:14-21, 2006.
784. Virkola K, Lappalainen M, Valanne L, et al: Radiological signs in newborns exposed to primary Toxoplasma infection in utero, *Pediatr Radiol* 27:133-138, 1997.
785. Kieffer F, Thulliez P, Brézin A, et al: Treatment of subclinical congenital toxoplasmosis by sulfadiazine and pyrimethamine continuously during 1 year: apropos of 46 cases, *Arch Pediatr* 9:7-13, 2002.
786. Schmidt D, Hogh B, Andersen O, et al: The national neonatal screening programme for congenital toxoplasmosis in Denmark: results from the initial four years, *Arch Dis Child* 91:661-665, 2006.
787. Lebech M, Andersen O, Christensen NC, et al: Feasibility of neonatal screening for Toxoplasma infection in the absence of prenatal treatment. Danish Congenital Toxoplasmosis Study Group, *Lancet* 353:1834-1837, 1999.
788. McLeod R, Boyer K, Karrison T, et al: Outcome of treatment for congenital toxoplasmosis, 1981-2004: the National Collaborative Chicago-Based, Congenital Toxoplasmosis Study, *Clin Infect Dis* 42:1383-1394, 2006.
789. Patel D, Holfels EM, Vogel NP, et al: Resolution of intracranial calcifications in infants with treated congenital toxoplasmosis, *Radiology* 199:433-440, 1996.
790. Brenner D, Elliston C, Hall E, et al: Estimated risks of radiation-induced fatal cancer from pediatric CT, *Am J Roentgenol* 176: 289-296, 2001.
791. Grant E, Williams AL, Schellinger D, et al: Intracranial calcification in the infant and neonate: evaluation by sonography and CT, *Radiology* 157:63-68, 1985.
792. Lago E, Baldisserotto M, Hoefel Filho JR, et al: Agreement between ultrasonography and computed tomography in detecting intracranial calcifications in congenital toxoplasmosis, *Clin Radiol* 62:1004-1011, 2007.
793. Townsend C, Forsgren M, Ahlfors K, et al: Long-term outcomes of congenital cytomegalovirus infection in Sweden and the United Kingdom, *Clin Infect Dis* 56:1232-1239, 2013.
794. Fink K, Thapa MM, Ishak GE, et al: Neuroimaging of pediatric central nervous system cytomegalovirus infection, *Radiographics* 30: 1779-1796, 2010.
795. Townsend C, Peckham CS, Tookey PA: Surveillance of congenital cytomegalovirus in the UK and Ireland, *Arch Dis Child Fetal Neonatal Ed* 96:F398-F403, 2011.
796. Barton L, Mets B: Congenital lymphocytic choriomeningitis virus infection: decade of rediscovery, *Clin Infect Dis* 33:370-374, 2001.
797. Enders G, Varho-Göbel M, Löhler J, et al: Congenital lymphocytic choriomeningitis virus infection: an underdiagnosed disease, *Pediatr Infect Dis J* 18:652-655, 1999.
798. Wright R, Johnson D, Neumann M, et al: Congenital lymphocytic choriomeningitis virus syndrome: a disease that mimics congenital toxoplasmosis or cytomegalovirus infection, *Pediatrics* 100:E9, 1997.
799. Anderson J, Levy PT, Leonard KB, et al: Congenital lymphocytic choriomeningitis virus: when to consider the diagnosis, *J Child Neurol* 29:837-842, 2013.
800. Peyron F, Ateba AB, Wallon M, et al: Congenital toxoplasmosis in twins: a report of fourteen consecutive cases and a comparison with published data, *Pediatr Infect Dis J* 22:695-701, 2003.
801. Lipka B, Milewska-Bobula B, Dunin-Wasowicz D, et al: Congenital toxoplasmosis in twins in own material, *Wiad Parazytol* 50: 187-191, 2004.
802. Couveur J, Thulliez T, Daffos F, et al: 6 cases of toxoplasmosis in twins, *Ann Pediatr (Paris)* 38:63-68, 1991.
803. Thapa R, Banerjee P, Akhtar N, et al: Discordance for congenital toxoplasmosis in twins, *Indian J Pediatr* 76:1069-1070, 2009.
804. Tjalma W, Vanderheyden T, Naessens A, et al: Discordant prenatal diagnosis of congenital toxoplasmosis in a dizygotic pregnancy, *Eur J Obstet Gynecol Reprod Biol* 79:107-108, 1998.
805. Falavigna D, Roncada EV, Nakazora D, et al: Congenital toxoplasmosis in dizygotic twins, Paraná, Brazil, *Rev Inst Med Trop São Paulo* 49:117-118, 2007.
806. Low incidence of congenital toxoplasmosis in children born to women infected with human immunodeficiency virus. European Collaborative Study and Research Network on Congenital Toxoplasmosis, *Eur J Obstet Gynecol Reprod Biol* 68:93-96, 1996.
807. Minkoff H, Remington JS, Holman S, et al: Vertical transmission of Toxoplasma by human immunodeficiency virus-infected women, *Am J Obstet Gynecol* 176:555-559, 1997.
808. Bachmeyer C, Mouchnino G, Thulliez P, et al: Congenital toxoplasmosis from an HIV-infected woman as a result of reactivation, *J Infect* 52:e55-e57, 2006.
809. Argolo AF, Feres VC, Silveira LA, et al: Prevalence and incidence of dengue virus and antibody placental transfer during late pregnancy in central Brazil, *BMC Infect Dis* 13:254, 2013.

810. Palmeira P, Quinello C, Silveira-Lessa AL, et al: IgG placental transfer in healthy and pathological pregnancies, *Clin Dev Immunol* 2012: 985646, 2012.
811. de Souza-e-Silva CH, Vasconcelos-Santos DV, de Andrade GQ, et al: Association between IgG subclasses against *Toxoplasma gondii* and clinical signs in newborns with congenital toxoplasmosis, *Pediatr Infect Dis J* 32:13-16, 2013.
812. Fricker-Hidalgo H, Pelloux H, Racinet C, et al: Congenital toxoplasmosis: specific IgM in fetal blood, cord blood and in the newborn, *Ann Biol Clin (Paris)* 54:165-168, 1996.
813. Robert-Gangneux F, Commerce V, Tourte-Schaefer C, et al: Performance of a Western blot assay to compare mother and newborn anti-Toxoplasma antibodies for the early neonatal diagnosis of congenital toxoplasmosis, *Eur J Clin Microbiol Infect Dis* 18:648-654, 1999.
814. Bessières MH, Berrébi A, Cassaing S, et al: Diagnosis of congenital toxoplasmosis: prenatal and neonatal evaluation of methods used in Toulouse University Hospital and incidence of congenital toxoplasmosis, *Mem Inst Oswaldo Cruz* 104:389-392, 2009.
815. Naessens A, Jenum PA, Pollak A, et al: Diagnosis of congenital toxoplasmosis in the neonatal period: a multicenter evaluation, *J Pediatr* 135:714-719, 1999.
816. Wallon M, Dunn D, Slimani D, et al: Diagnosis of congenital toxoplasmosis at birth: what is the value of testing for IgM and IgA? *Eur J Pediatr* 158:645-649, 1999.
817. Prusa AR, Hayde M, Pollak A, et al: Evaluation of the liaison automated testing system for diagnosis of congenital toxoplasmosis, *Clin Vaccine Immunol* 19:1859-1863, 2012.
818. Gilbert RE, Thalib L, Tan HK, et al: Screening for congenital toxoplasmosis: accuracy of immunoglobulin M and immunoglobulin A tests after birth, *J Med Screen* 14:8-13, 2007.
819. Patel B, Holliman RE: Antibodies to *Toxoplasma gondii* in eluates from filter paper blood specimens, *Br J Biomed Sci* 51:104-108, 1994.
820. Sorensen T, Spenter J, Jaliashvili I, et al: Automated time-resolved immunofluorometric assay for *Toxoplasma gondii*-specific IgM and IgA antibodies: study of more than 130,000 filter-paper blood-spot samples from newborns, *Clin Chem* 48:1981-1986, 2002.
821. Villena I, Quereux C, Pinon JM: Congenital toxoplasmosis: value of prenatal treatment with pyrimethamine-sulfadoxine combination, *Prenat Diagn* 18:754-756, 1998.
822. Couvreur J, Thulliez P, Daffos F, et al: In utero treatment of toxoplasmic fetopathy with the combination pyrimethamine-sulfadiazine, *Fetal Diagn Ther* 8:45-50, 1993.
823. Villena I, Aubert D, Brodard V, et al: Detection of specific immunoglobulin E during maternal, fetal, and congenital toxoplasmosis, *J Clin Microbiol* 37:3487-3490, 1999.
824. Remington JS, Araujo FG, Desmonts G: Recognition of different Toxoplasma antigens by IgM and IgG antibodies in mothers and their congenitally infected newborns, *J Infect Dis* 152:1020-1024, 1985.
825. Tissot Dupont D, Fricker-Hidalgo H, Brenier-Pinchart MP, et al: Usefulness of Western blot in serological follow-up of newborns suspected of congenital toxoplasmosis, *Eur J Clin Microbiol Infect Dis* 22:122-125, 2003.
826. Rilling V, Dietz K, Krczal D, et al: Evaluation of a commercial IgG/IgM Western blot assay for early postnatal diagnosis of congenital toxoplasmosis, *Eur J Clin Microbiol Infect Dis* 22:174-180, 2003.
827. Gallego-Marin C, Henao AC, Gomez-Marin JE: Clinical validation of a western blot assay for congenital toxoplasmosis and newborn screening in a hospital in Armenia (Quindio) Colombia, *J Trop Pediatr* 52:107-112, 2006.
828. L'Ollivier C, Wallon M, Faucher B, et al: Comparison of mother and child antibodies that target high-molecular-mass *Toxoplasma gondii* antigens by immunoblotting improves neonatal diagnosis of congenital toxoplasmosis, *Clin Vaccine Immunol* 19:1326-1328, 2012.
829. Sterkers Y, Pratlong F, Albaba S, et al: Novel interpretation of molecular diagnosis of congenital toxoplasmosis according to gestational age at the time of maternal infection, *J Clin Microbiol* 50:3944-3951, 2012.
830. Robert-Gangneux F, Dupretz P, Yvenou C, et al: Clinical relevance of placenta examination for the diagnosis of congenital toxoplasmosis, *Pediatr Infect Dis J* 29:33-38, 2010.
831. Delhaes L, Yera H, Ache S, et al: Contribution of molecular diagnosis to congenital toxoplasmosis, *Diagn Microbiol Infect Dis* 76:244-247, 2013.
832. Robert-Gangneux F, Gavinet MF, Ancelle T, et al: Value of prenatal diagnosis and early postnatal diagnosis of congenital toxoplasmosis: retrospective study of 110 cases, *J Clin Microbiol* 37:2893-2898, 1999.
833. Fricker-Hidalgo H, Pelloux H, Racinet C, et al: Detection of *Toxoplasma gondii* in 94 placentae from infected women by polymerase chain reaction, in vivo, and in vitro cultures, *Placenta* 19:545-549, 1998.
834. Wallon M, Caudie C, Rubio S, et al: Value of cerebrospinal fluid cytochemical examination for the diagnosis of congenital toxoplasmosis at birth in France, *Pediatr Infect Dis J* 17:705-710, 1998.
835. Fuentes I, Rodriguez M, Domingo CJ, et al: Urine sample used for congenital toxoplasmosis diagnosis by PCR, *J Clin Microbiol* 34:2368-2371, 1996.
836. Ciardelli L, Meroni V, Avanzini MA, et al: Early and accurate diagnosis of congenital toxoplasmosis, *Pediatr Infect Dis J* 27:125-129, 2008.
837. Leport C, Vilde JL, Katlama C, et al: Failure of spiramycin to prevent neurotoxoplasmosis in immunosuppressed patients, *JAMA* 255:2290, 1986.
838. Schoondermark-Van de Ven E, Melchers W, Camps W, et al: Effectiveness of spiramycin for treatment of congenital *Toxoplasma gondii* infection in rhesus monkeys, *Antimicrob Agents Chemother* 38:1930-1936, 1994.
839. Villena I, Aubert D, Leroux B, et al: Pyrimethamine-sulfadoxine treatment of congenital toxoplasmosis: follow-up of 78 cases between 1980 and 1997. Reims Toxoplasmosis Group, *Scand J Infect Dis* 30:295-300, 1998.
840. Wallon M, Cozon G, Ecochard R, et al: Serological rebound in congenital toxoplasmosis: long-term follow-up of 133 children, *Eur J Pediatr* 160:534-540, 2001.
841. McLeod R, Mack D, Foss R, et al: Levels of pyrimethamine in sera and cerebrospinal and ventricular fluids from infants treated for congenital toxoplasmosis. Toxoplasmosis Study Group, *Antimicrob Agents Chemother* 36:1040-1048, 1992.
842. Schoondermark-Van de Ven E, Galama J, Vree T, et al: Study of treatment of congenital *Toxoplasma gondii* infection in rhesus monkeys with pyrimethamine and sulfadiazine, *Antimicrob Agents Chemother* 39:137-144, 1995.
843. Mehta S, Nain CK, Sharma B, et al: Metabolism of sulfadiazine in children with protein calorie malnutrition, *Pharmacology* 21: 369-374, 1980.
844. Berman J, Fleckenstein L: Pharmacokinetic justification of antiprotozoal therapy. A US perspective, *Clin Pharmacokinet* 21:479-493, 1991.
845. Corvaisier S, Charpiat B, Mounier C, et al: Population pharmacokinetics of pyrimethamine and sulfadoxine in children treated for congenital toxoplasmosis, *Antimicrob Agents Chemother* 48:3794-3800, 2004.
846. Trenque T, Simon N, Villena I, et al: Population pharmacokinetics of pyrimethamine and sulfadoxine in children with congenital toxoplasmosis, *Br J Clin Pharmacol* 57:735-741, 2004.
847. Petersen E, Schmidt D: Sulfadiazine and pyrimethamine in the postnatal treatment of congenital toxoplasmosis: what are the options? *Expert Rev Anti Infect Ther* 1:175-182, 2003.
848. Roizen N, Swisher CN, Stein MA, et al: Neurologic and developmental outcome in treated congenital toxoplasmosis, *Pediatrics* 95:11-20, 1995.
849. Guerina N, Hsu HW, Meissner HC, et al: Neonatal serologic screening and early treatment for congenital *Toxoplasma gondii* infection. The New England Regional Toxoplasma Working Group, *N Engl J Med* 330:1858-1863, 1994.
850. Schmidt D, Hogh B, Andersen O, et al: Treatment of infants with congenital toxoplasmosis: tolerability and plasma concentrations of sulfadiazine and pyrimethamine, *Eur J Pediatr* 165:19-25, 2006.
851. McLeod R, Boyer K: Toxoplasmosis Study Group and Collaborators: Management of and outcome for the newborn infant with congenital toxoplasmosis. In Ambroise-Thomas P, Petersen E, editors: *Congenital toxoplasmosis: scientific background, clinical management and control*, Paris, 2000, Springer-Verlag, pp 189-213.
852. Duveau E, Chomienne F, Seguin G: Convulsions associated with pyrimethamine overdose, *Arch Pediatr* 3:286-287, 1996.
853. Genuini M, Freihuber C, Girard I, et al: Neonatal intoxication with pyrimethamine: risk due to the absence of pediatric formulation? *Arch Pediatr* 18:1034-1036, 2011.
854. McLeod R, Khan AR, Noble GA, et al: Severe sulfadiazine hypersensitivity in a child with reactivated congenital toxoplasmic chorioretinitis, *Pediatr Infect Dis J* 25:270-272, 2006.
855. Carrión-Carrión C, Morales-Suárez-Varela M, Llopis-González A: Fatal Stevens-Johnson syndrome in an AIDS patient treated with sulfadiazine, *Ann Pharmacother* 33:379-380, 1999.
856. Caumes E, Bocquet H, Guermonprez G, et al: Adverse cutaneous reactions to pyrimethamine/sulfadiazine and pyrimethamine/clindamycin in patients with AIDS and toxoplasmic encephalitis, *Clin Infect Dis* 21:656-658, 1995.

857. Lakshman R, Finn A: Neutrophil disorders and their management, *J Clin Pathol* 54:7-19, 2001.
858. Bonametti A, Passos JN, Koga da Silva EM, et al: Probable transmission of acute toxoplasmosis through breast feeding, *J Trop Pediatr* 43:116, 1997.
859. Jaisson-Hot I, Wallon M, al Kurdi M, et al: Congenital toxoplasmosis. Transitory negative serology, *Presse Med* 30:1001-1004, 2001.
860. Fortier B, Coignard-Chatain C, Dao A, et al: Study of developing clinical outbreak and serological rebounds in children with congenital toxoplasmosis and follow-up during the first 2 years of life, *Arch Pediatr* 4:940-946, 1997.
861. Wallon M, Cozon G, Ecochard R, et al: Serological rebound in congenital toxoplasmosis: long-term follow-up of 133 children, *Eur J Pediatr* 160:534-540, 2001.
862. Djurkovic-Djakovic O, Romand S, Nobre R, et al: Serologic rebounds after one-year-long treatment for congenital toxoplasmosis, *Pediatr Infect Dis J* 19:81-83, 2000.
863. Kahi S, Cozon GJ, Greenland T, et al: Circulating *Toxoplasma gondii*-specific antibody-secreting cells in patients with congenital toxoplasmosis, *Clin Immunol Immunopathol* 89:23-27, 1998.
864. Kahi S, Cozon GJ, Pinon JM, et al: A switch towards Th2 during serological rebound in children with congenital toxoplasmosis, *Clin Exp Immunol* 117:524-528, 1999.
865. Lebech M, Joynson DH, Seitz HM, et al: Classification system and case definitions of *Toxoplasma gondii* infection in immunocompetent pregnant women and their congenitally infected offspring. European Research Network on Congenital Toxoplasmosis, *Eur J Clin Microbiol Infect Dis* 15:799-805, 1996.
866. Stanford MR, Tan HK, Gilbert RE: Toxoplasmic retinochoroiditis presenting in childhood: clinical findings in a UK survey, *Br J Ophthalmol* 90:1464-1467, 2006.
867. Delair E, Monnet D, Grabar S, et al: Respective roles of acquired and congenital infections in presumed ocular toxoplasmosis, *Am J Ophthalmol* 146:851-855, 2008.
868. Balasundaram MB, Andavar R, Palaniswamy M, et al: Outbreak of acquired ocular toxoplasmosis involving 248 patients, *Arch Ophthalmol* 128:28-32, 2010.
869. Vasconcelos-Santos DV, Machado Azevedo DO, Campos WR, et al: Congenital toxoplasmosis in southeastern Brazil: results of early ophthalmologic examination of a large cohort of neonates, *Ophthalmology* 116:2199-2205, 2009.
870. Kodjikian L, Wallon M, Fleury J, et al: Ocular manifestations in congenital toxoplasmosis, *Graefes Arch Clin Exp Ophthalmol* 244:14-21, 2006.
871. Labalette P, Delhaes L, Margaron F, et al: Ocular toxoplasmosis after the fifth decade, *Am J Ophthalmol* 133:506-515, 2002.
872. Garweg JG, de Groot-Mijnes JD, Montoya JG: Diagnostic approach to ocular toxoplasmosis, *Ocul Immunol Inflamm* 19:255-261, 2011.
873. Wakefield D, Cunningham ET Jr, Pavesio C, et al: Controversies in ocular toxoplasmosis, *Ocul Immunol Inflamm* 19:2-9, 2011.
874. Koppe JG, Loewer-Sieger DH, de Roever-Bonnet H: Results of 20-year follow-up of congenital toxoplasmosis, *Lancet* 1:254-256, 1986.
875. Koppe JG, Kloosterman GJ: Congenital toxoplasmosis: long-term follow-up, *Padiatr Padol* 17:171-179, 1982.
876. Garweg JG, Kodjikian L, Peyron F, et al: [Congenital ocular toxoplasmosis–ocular manifestations and prognosis after early diagnosis of infection], *Klin Monbl Augenheilkd* 222:721-727, 2005.
877. Tan HK, Schmidt D, Stanford M, et al: Risk of visual impairment in children with congenital toxoplasmic retinochoroiditis, *Am J Ophthalmol* 144:648-653, 2007.
878. Delair E, Latkany P, Noble AG, et al: Clinical manifestations of ocular toxoplasmosis, *Ocul Immunol Inflamm* 19:91-102, 2011.
879. Beraud L, Rabilloud M, Fleury J, et al: Congenital toxoplasmosis: long-term ophthalmologic follow-up praised by patients, *J Fr Ophtalmol* 36:494-498, 2013.
880. Melamed J, Eckert GU, Spadoni VS, et al: Ocular manifestations of congenital toxoplasmosis, *Eye (Lond)* 24:528-534, 2010.
881. de-la-Torre A, Rios-Cadavid AC, Cardozo-Garcia CM, et al: Frequency and factors associated with recurrences of ocular toxoplasmosis in a referral centre in Colombia, *Br J Ophthalmol* 93:1001-1004, 2009.
882. Stanford MR, Tomlin EA, Comyn O, et al: The visual field in toxoplasmic retinochoroiditis, *Br J Ophthalmol* 89:812-814, 2005.
883. Scherrer J, Iliev ME, Halberstadt M, et al: Visual function in human ocular toxoplasmosis, *Br J Ophthalmol* 91:233-236, 2007.
884. Alvarenga DP, Couto MF, Pessoa VF: Perceptual visual filling-in of toxoplasmic retinochoroiditis scotomas, *Neuroreport* 18: 1679-1681, 2007.
885. Garweg JG, Stanford MR: Therapy for ocular toxoplasmosis - the future, *Ocul Immunol Inflamm* 21:300-305, 2013.
886. Iaccheri B, Fiore T, Papadaki T, et al: Adverse drug reactions to treatments for ocular toxoplasmosis: a retrospective chart review, *Clin Ther* 30:2069-2074, 2008.
887. Kim SJ, Scott IU, Brown GC, et al: Interventions for Toxoplasma retinochoroiditis: a report by the American Academy of Ophthalmology, *Ophthalmology* 120:371-378, 2013.
888. Yazici A, Ozdal PC, Taskintuna I, et al: Trimethoprim/sulfamethoxazole and azithromycin combination therapy for ocular toxoplasmosis, *Ocul Immunol Inflamm* 17:289-291, 2009.
889. Koppe J, Loewer-Sieger D, de Roever-Bonnet H: Results of 20-year follow-up of congenital toxoplasmosis, *Lancet* 1:254-256, 1986.
890. Saxon S, Knight W, Reynolds DW, et al: Intellectual deficits in children born with subclinical congenital toxoplasmosis: a preliminary report, *J Pediatr* 82:792-797, 1973.
891. Wilson C, Remington JS, Stagno S, et al: Development of adverse sequelae in children born with subclinical congenital Toxoplasma infection, *Pediatrics* 66:767-774, 1980.
892. Freeman K, Salt A, Prusa A, et al: Association between congenital toxoplasmosis and parent-reported developmental outcomes, concerns, and impairments, in 3 year old children, *BMC Pediatr* 13:23, 2005.
893. Sáfadi M, et al: Clinical presentation and follow up of children with congenital toxoplasmosis in Brazil, *Braz J Infect Dis* 7:325-331, 2003.
894. Kieffer F, et al: Disseminated congenital Toxoplasma infection with a type II strain, *Pediatr Infect Dis J* 30:813-815, 2011.
895. Jamieson S, de Roubaix LA, Cortina-Borja M, et al: Genetic and epigenetic factors at COL2A1 and ABCA4 influence clinical outcome in congenital toxoplasmosis, *PLoS One* 3:e2285, 2008.
896. Lees M, Fuller SJ, McLeod R, et al: P2X7 receptor-mediated killing of an intracellular parasite, *Toxoplasma gondii*, by human and murine macrophages, *J Immunol* 184:7040-7046, 2010.
897. McGee T, Wolters C, Stein L, et al: Absence of sensorineural hearing loss in treated infants and children with congenital toxoplasmosis, *Otolaryngol Head Neck Surg* 106:75-80, 1992.
898. Salviz M, Montoya JG, Nadol JB, et al: Otopathology in congenital toxoplasmosis, *Otol Neurotol* 34:1165-1169, 2013.
899. Andrade G, Resende LM, Goulart EM, et al: Hearing loss in congenital toxoplasmosis detected by newborn screening, *Braz J Otorhinolaryngol* 74:21-28, 2008.
900. Roizen N, Kasza K, Karrison T, et al: Impact of visual impairment on measures of cognitive function for children with congenital toxoplasmosis: implications for compensatory intervention strategies, *Pediatrics* 118:e379-e390, 2006.
901. Peyron F, Garweg JG, Wallon M, et al: Long-term impact of treated congenital toxoplasmosis on quality of life and visual performance, *Pediatr Infect Dis J* 30:597-600, 2011.
902. Vasconcelos-Santos, DVQueiroz Andrade GM: Geographic difference in outcomes of congenital toxoplasmosis, *Pediatr Infect Dis J* 30:816-817, 2011. author reply 817.
903. de-la-Torre A, Gonzalez-Lopez G, Montoya-Gutierrez JM, et al: Quality of life assessment in ocular toxoplasmosis in a Colombian population, *Ocul Immunol Inflamm* 19:262-266, 2011.
904. Vyas A, Kim SK, Giacomini N, et al: Behavioral changes induced by Toxoplasma infection of rodents are highly specific to aversion of cat odors, *Proc Natl Acad Sci U S A* 104:6442-6447, 2007.
905. Berdoy M, Webster JP, Macdonald DW: Fatal attraction in rats infected with *Toxoplasma gondii*, *Proc Biol Sci* 267:1591-1594, 2000.
906. Stibbs HH: Changes in brain concentrations of catecholamines and indoleamines in *Toxoplasma gondii* infected mice, *Ann Trop Med Parasitol* 79:153-157, 1985.
907. Flegr J: How and why Toxoplasma makes us crazy, *Trends Parasitol* 29:156-163, 2013.
908. Gaskell EA, Smith JE, Pinney JW, et al: A unique dual activity amino acid hydroxylase in *Toxoplasma gondii*, *PLoS One* 4:e4801, 2009.
909. Prandovszky E, Gaskell E, Martin H, et al: The neurotropic parasite *Toxoplasma gondii* increases dopamine metabolism, *PLoS One* 6:e23866, 2011.
910. Moore J: An overview of parasite-induced behavioral alterations - and some lessons from bats, *J Exp Biol* 216(Pt 1):11-17, 2013.

911. Worth AR, Lymbery AJ, Thompson RC: Adaptive host manipulation by *Toxoplasma gondii*: fact or fiction? *Trends Parasitol* 29:150-155, 2013.
912. Hrda S, Votypka J, Kodym P, et al: Transient nature of *Toxoplasma gondii*-induced behavioral changes in mice, *J Parasitol* 86:657-663, 2000.
913. Torrey EF, Bartko JJ, Lun ZR, et al: Antibodies to *Toxoplasma gondii* in patients with schizophrenia: a meta-analysis, *Schizophr Bull* 33:729-736, 2007.
914. Pedersen MG, Stevens H, Pedersen CB, et al: Toxoplasma infection and later development of schizophrenia in mothers, *Am J Psychiatry* 168:814-821, 2011.
915. Hinze-Selch D, Daubener W, Erdag S, et al: The diagnosis of a personality disorder increases the likelihood for seropositivity to *Toxoplasma gondii* in psychiatric patients, *Folia Parasitol (Praha)* 57:129-135, 2010.
916. Hamdani N, Daban-Huard C, Lajnef M, et al: Relationship between *Toxoplasma gondii* infection and bipolar disorder in a French sample, *J Affect Disord* 148:444-448, 2013.
917. Miman O, Mutlu EA, Ozcan O, et al: Is there any role of *Toxoplasma gondii* in the etiology of obsessive-compulsive disorder? *Psychiatry Res* 177:263-265, 2010.
918. Miman O, Kusbeci OY, Aktepe OC, et al: The probable relation between *Toxoplasma gondii* and Parkinson's disease, *Neurosci Lett* 475:129-131, 2010.
919. Koseoglu E, Yazar S, Koc I: Is *Toxoplasma gondii* a causal agent in migraine? *Am J Med Sci* 338:120-122, 2009.
920. Yazar S, Arman F, Yalcin S, et al: Investigation of probable relationship between *Toxoplasma gondii* and cryptogenic epilepsy, *Seizure* 12:107-109, 2003.
921. Yagmur F, Yazar S, Temel HO, et al: May *Toxoplasma gondii* increase suicide attempt-preliminary results in Turkish subjects? *Forensic Sci Int* 199:15-17, 2010.
922. Pedersen MG, Mortensen PB, Norgaard-Pedersen B, et al: *Toxoplasma gondii* infection and self-directed violence in mothers, *Arch Gen Psychiatry* 69:1123-1130, 2012.
923. Flegr J, Klose J, Novotna M, et al: Increased incidence of traffic accidents in Toxoplasma-infected military drivers and protective effect RhD molecule revealed by a large-scale prospective cohort study, *BMC Infect Dis* 9:72, 2009.
924. Lindova J, Novotna M, Havlicek J, et al: Gender differences in behavioural changes induced by latent toxoplasmosis, *Int J Parasitol* 36:1485-1492, 2006.
925. Russo S, Kema IP, Haagsma EB, et al: Irritability rather than depression during interferon treatment is linked to increased tryptophan catabolism, *Psychosom Med* 67:773-777, 2005.
926. Gaston JE, Vogl L: Psychometric properties of the general well-being index, *Qual Life Res* 14:71-75, 2005.
927. Gollub EL, Leroy V, Gilbert R, et al: Effectiveness of health education on Toxoplasma-related knowledge, behaviour, and risk of seroconversion in pregnancy, *Eur J Obstet Gynecol Reprod Biol* 136:137-145, 2008.
928. Di Mario S, Basevi V, Gagliotti C, et al: Prenatal education for congenital toxoplasmosis, *Cochrane Database Syst Rev*, CD006171. 2013.
929. Pawlowski ZS, Gromadecka-Sutkiewicz M, Skommer J, et al: Impact of health education on knowledge and prevention behavior for congenital toxoplasmosis: the experience in Poznan, Poland, *Health Educ Res* 16:493-502, 2001.
930. Carter AO, Gelmon SB, Wells GA, et al: The effectiveness of a prenatal education programme for the prevention of congenital toxoplasmosis, *Epidemiol Infect* 103:539-545, 1989.
931. Wallon M, Liou C, Garner P, et al: Congenital toxoplasmosis: systematic review of evidence of efficacy of treatment in pregnancy, *BMJ* 318:1511-1514, 1999.
932. Kravetz J: Congenital toxoplasmosis, *Clin Evid (Online)*, 2013. pii:0906
933. Eskild A, Oxman A, Magnus P, et al: Screening for toxoplasmosis in pregnancy: what is the evidence of reducing a health problem? *J Med Screen* 3:188-194, 1996.
934. Gilbert R: Treatment for congenital toxoplasmosis: finding out what works, *Mem Inst Oswaldo Cruz* 104:305-311, 2009.
935. Wallon M, Garweg J, Abrahamowicz M, et al: Ophthalmic outcomes of congenital toxoplasmosis followed until adolescence, *Pediatrics* 133:e601-e608, 2014.
936. Phan L, Kasza K, Jalbrzikowski J, et al: Longitudinal study of new eye lesions in treated congenital toxoplasmosis, *Ophthalmology* 115:553-559, 2008.
937. Chevallier M: Etude coût-avantage d'un système de prévention de la toxoplasmose congénitale, *Bull Stat Santé-Securité Sociale* 3:71-84, 1974.
938. Peyron F, Wallon M, Liou C, et al: Treatments for toxoplasmosis in pregnancy, *Cochrane Database System Rev*: CD001684, 2010.
939. Gilbert R, Dunn D, Wallon M, et al: Ecological comparison of the risks of mother-to-child transmission and clinical manifestations of congenital toxoplasmosis according to prenatal treatment protocol, *Epidemiol Infect* 127:113-120, 2001.
940. Chêne G, Thiébaut R: Options for clinical trials of pre and post-natal treatments for congenital toxoplasmosis, *Mem Inst Oswaldo Cruz* 104:299-304, 2009.
941. McLeod R, Kieffer F, Sautter M, et al: Why prevent, diagnose and treat congenital toxoplasmosis? *Mem Inst Oswaldo Cruz* 104:320-344, 2009.
942. Mui EJ, Schiehser GA, Milhous WK, et al: Novel triazine JPC-2067-B inhibits *Toxoplasma gondii* in vitro and in vivo, *PLoS Negl Trop Dis* 2:e190, 2008.
943. Hotop A, Hlobil H, Gross U: Efficacy of rapid treatment initiation following primary *Toxoplasma gondii* infection during pregnancy, *Clin Infect Dis* 54:1545-1552, 2012.
944. Cornu C, Bissery A, Malbos C, et al: Factors affecting the adherence to an antenatal screening programme: an experience with toxoplasmosis screening in France, *Euro Surveill* 14:21-25, 2009.
945. Gras L, Wallon M, Pollak A, et al: Association between prenatal treatment and clinical manifestations of congenital toxoplasmosis in infancy: a cohort study in 13 European centres, *Acta Paediatr* 94:1721-1731, 2005.
946. Roizen N, Swisher CN, Stein MA, et al: Neurologic and developmental outcome in treated congenital toxoplasmosis, *Pediatrics* 95:11-20, 1995.
947. Abdel-Fattah SA, Bhat A, Illanes S, et al: TORCH test for fetal medicine indications: only CMV is necessary in the United Kingdom, *Prenat Diagn* 25:1028-1031, 2005.
948. Binquet C: *Evaluation des stratégies de dépistage et de prise en charge de la toxoplasmose congénitale*, Thèse d'Université, Dijon, France, 2003, Université de Bourgogne.
949. Paquet C, Yudin MH: Toxoplasmosis in pregnancy: prevention, screening, and treatment, *J Obstet Gynaecol Can* 35:78-79, 2013.
950. Gilbert R, Dezateux C: Newborn screening for congenital toxoplasmosis: feasible, but benefits are not established, *Arch Dis Child* 91:629-631, 2006.
951. Lopes-Mori FM, Mitsuka-Bregano R, Capobiango JD, et al: Programs for control of congenital toxoplasmosis, *Rev Assoc Med Bras* 57: 594-599, 2011.
952. Leroy V, Raeber P, Petersen E, et al: National public health policies and routines programs to prevent congenital toxoplasmosis, Europe, 2005 (unpublished report), Bordeaux, France, 2005, Eurotoxo Groupe, p 19.
953. Gilbert RE, Peckham CS: Congenital toxoplasmosis in the United Kingdom: to screen or not to screen? *J Med Screen* 9:135-141, 2002.
954. Sauer A, de la Torre A, Gomez-Marin J, et al: Prevention of retinochoroiditis in congenital toxoplasmosis: Europe versus South America, *Pediatr Infect Dis J* 30:601-603, 2011.
955. Beraud L, Rabilloud M, Fleury J, et al: Congenital toxoplasmosis: long-term ophthalmologic follow-up praised by patients, *J Fr Ophtalmol* 36:494-498, 2013.
956. Dubey JP, Kotula AW, Sharar A, Andrews CD, Lindsay DS: Effect of high-temperature on infectivity of *Toxoplasma gondii* tissue cysts in pork, *J Parasitol* 76:201-204, 1990.
957. Sommer R, Rommel M, Levetzov R: Die überlebensdauer von toxoplasmazysten in fleisch und fleischzubereitungen, *Fleischwirtsch* 45:454-457, 1965.
958. Scupin E: Weitere untersuchungen der überlebensmöglichkeiten von toxoplasma in schinken, *Archiv für Lebensmittelhygiene* 12:11-13, 1968.
959. Kotula AW, Dubey JP, Sharar AK, et al: Effect of freezing on infectivity of *Toxoplasma gondii* tissue cysts in pork, *J Food Prot* 54:687-690, 1991.
960. Hill AE, Benedetto SMC, Coss C, et al: Effects of time and temperature on the viability of *Toxoplasma gondii* tissue cysts in enhanced pork loin, *J Food Prot* 69:1961-1965, 2006.
961. Grossklaus D, Baumgarten H-J: Die überlebensdauer von *Toxoplasma*-cysten in schweinefleisch I. Mitteilung: ergebnisse von lagerungsversuchen bei verschiedenen temperature, *Fleischwirtschaft* 48:930-932, 1968.
962. Kuticic V, Wikerhauser T: Studies of the effect of various treatments on the viability of *Toxoplasma gondii* tissue cysts and oocysts, *Toxoplasma gondii*, *Curr Top Microbiol Immunol* 219:261-265, 1996.

32 Malaria and Less Common Protozoan and Helminth Infections

YVONNE A. MALDONADO

CHAPTER OUTLINE

Parasitic infections are highly prevalent in many developing areas of the world and are common among pregnant women in developed countries. They may exacerbate maternal and fetal anemia, and contribute to low birth weight and poor infant survival. The placenta serves as an effective barrier, even in infections such as malaria and schistosomiasis in which systemic involvement and hematogenous spread are common. Although transplacental infections of the fetus are uncommon, the prevalence of parasitic infections among infants younger than 1 month is high in developing countries, and infections occur primarily through transmission during or shortly after birth.

In a study conducted in Guatemala, Kotcher and colleagues[1] found that 30% of newborns had acquired a protozoal infection by 2 weeks of age. Although these infants were infected with *Entamoeba histolytica*, *Entamoeba coli*, *Endolimax nana*, and *Iodamoeba buetschlii*, they remained asymptomatic. *Giardia lamblia* was found by the fifth week of life and *Trichuris trichiura* by the 16th week of life. A study conducted in a regional hospital in Togo revealed that 55% of infants and children from birth to 16 years of age demonstrated evidence of parasitic infections in stool or urine, with obvious neonatal infections occurring as well.[2]

Soil-transmitted helminths (STHs), primarily *Ascaris*, *Trichuris*, and hookworm, through gastrointestinal infection and chronic blood loss, can result in or exacerbate iron deficiency anemia and nutritional deficits. Worldwide, it is estimated that more than 1 billion people are infected with at least one STH, including at least 44 million pregnant women infected with hookworm alone. Although few random controlled trials have failed to demonstrate a beneficial impact of anthelmintics in pregnancy, results from observational studies suggest a potential benefit on maternal anemia, birth weight, and infant mortality, and further studies are needed.[3]

Pneumocystis jirovecii (previously classified as *Pneumocystis carinii*) is considered in Chapter 34.[4]

Ascaris

Ascaris lumbricoides is the most prevalent parasitic infection worldwide, affecting up to 1 billion people. In humans, *Ascaris* eggs are ingested through fecal-oral contamination, hatch in the small intestine, and then penetrate the intestinal lumen to migrate extensively through blood and lymphatics. Larvae eventually reach the pulmonary circulation, where they migrate into the alveolar sacs, through the respiratory tree to the esophagus, and into the small intestine. Because *Ascaris* may migrate to many organs, worms are occasionally found in the uterus and the fallopian tubes.[5]

Human fetuses apparently can mount an immune response to maternal *Ascaris* infection, and congenital infections are rare. Sanjeevi and associates[6] studied the immunoglobulin G (IgG) and IgM responses to *Ascaris* antigens from matched maternal and cord bloods in south India and found evidence of fetal IgM directed against *Ascaris* antigens in 12 of 28 samples. Clinical status of the infants was not reported. Chu and coworkers,[7] however, described an infant whose delivery was complicated by the simultaneous delivery of 12 adult *A. lumbricoides* worms. During preparations for a cesarean section, which was being undertaken because of prolonged premature labor and fetal distress, one worm passed from the vagina, and another was found in the vagina. When the placenta was removed, 10 worms were found on the maternal side of the placenta. The infant was delivered in good condition. The infant passed two female worms, which were 28 and 30 cm long, on the second and sixth days of life. He was treated with piperazine citrate, but no other worms were passed, and no eggs were seen after the 11th day of life. Fertilized ova of *A. lumbricoides* were found in the amniotic fluid and in the newborn's feces. An adhesion connected the mother's intestine and uterus, but it is uncertain whether the worms passed directly from the mother's intestine to the placenta and amniotic fluid, and were swallowed by the fetus; whether larvae passed hematogeneously from the mother's lung to the placenta and thereby reached the fetal circulation, lung, and gastrointestinal tract; or whether female worms in the placenta produced fertile eggs that reached the amniotic fluid and were swallowed by the fetus. Other investigators have reported fetal evidence of *Ascaris* infection in infants as young as 1 to 2 weeks of age and in one infant with failure to thrive and bloody diarrhea at 3 weeks who responded to levamisole therapy.[8]

Giardiasis

Giardia lamblia causes a localized intestinal infection, with no systemic involvement, and *G. lamblia* infection in pregnancy has not been associated with fetal infection. Severe maternal infection that compromises nutrition can affect fetal growth, but such a severe illness is rare.[9] Neonatal *G. lamblia* infection can result from fecal contamination at birth. Infected infants are usually asymptomatic.[10] Treatment of pregnant women with giardiasis is generally deferred until after the first trimester unless symptoms are severe. There is some evidence that maternal antibody may be protective against neonatal giardiasis.[11]

American Trypanosomiasis: Chagas Disease

Millions of people in Central and South America are infected by *Trypanosoma cruzi* and related protozoa. Because of the chronicity of these infections, they have a significant impact on public health. One estimate suggests that approximately 40,000 women and 2000 newborns may be infected on an annual basis in North America, primarily in Mexico, although up to 3780 infected pregnant women and 189 congenitally infected infants could be born among Hispanic populations in the United States.[12]

THE ORGANISM

The form of the organism that circulates in human blood is the trypomastigote. Cell division does not occur in the bloodstream. In tissue, the flagellum and undulating membrane are lost, and the organism differentiates into a leishmanial form, the amastigote.[13,14] Amastigotes multiply by binary fission, and masses of amastigotes are grouped into pseudocysts. The amastigotes in pseudocysts may evolve into trypanomastigotes and, on rupture of the pseudocyst, can gain access to the bloodstream or to new cells. Two strains of *T. cruzi* that cause human infections have been identified by biochemical differences among nine enzymes produced by the parasite.[15]

EPIDEMIOLOGY AND TRANSMISSION

T. cruzi infects primates, marsupials, armadillos, bats, and many rodents, including guinea pigs, opossums, and raccoons; birds are not infected.[16] Infection of insects and mammals with *T. cruzi* is most common between the latitudes 398N (i.e., northern California and Maryland) and 438S (i.e., southern Argentina and Chile) and on the islands of Aruba and Trinidad.[1] The usual vectors are in the family Reduviidae, subfamily Triatominae. The main vector in Venezuela is *Rhodnius prolixus*; in Brazil, *Panstrongylus megistus*; and in Argentina, *Triatoma infestans* (cone-nosed bug).[16] These species are well adapted to human dwellings. Triatominae are hematophagous insects. They acquire and transmit the infection by biting infected vertebrates, including humans. The life span of the insect is not shortened by infection with *T. cruzi*; infected insects live up to a year after the onset of infection. In North America, the sylvatic habitat of the vector and the low virulence of the strains of *Trypanosoma* are responsible for the relative rarity of the disease. Colloquial terms used for the usual vector include the kissing or assassin bug in the southwestern United States; pito, hito, or vinchuca in Spanish America; and barbeiro in Portuguese America.[17]

The vector is most commonly found in huts of mud and sticks and in other housing containing cracks. In vectors infected with *T. cruzi*, metacyclic trypomastigotes congregate in the rectum. Bites become contaminated when defecation occurs. The infective form reaches the bloodstream through the site of the bite or by penetrating mucous membranes, conjunctivae, or abraded skin.[13] *Trypanosoma rangeli* is spread by a few species of the triatomid bug. These metacyclic trypanosomes develop, divide, and multiply in the salivary gland. They are injected directly into the site of the bite.

Infections can also be acquired by blood transfusion[18] and transplacentally. The isoenzyme patterns of *T. cruzi* recovered from congenitally infected infants and their mothers are identical, but transplacental transmission may not always follow maternal infection with enzymatically similar strains.[19]

PATHOLOGY

Placenta

The placenta is a relatively effective barrier to the spread of infection to the fetus.[14] The organism reaches the placenta by the hematogenous route and traverses the placental villi to the trophoblasts. After differentiation into amastigotes, the organism remains within Hofbauer (phagocytic) cells of the placenta until it is liberated into the fetal circulation.[20-22]

Maternal parasitemia is greatest in the acute phase of infection; however, the period of intense parasitemia is short. Of the reported cases of congenital Chagas disease, only four have originated during the acute phase of infection.[14] Most congenital infections occur in infants born to women with the chronic form of the disease.

Infected placentas are pale, yellow, and bulky. They have an appearance similar to the placentas of infants with erythroblastosis fetalis. Infection of the placenta is much more common than infection of the fetus.

BIOPSY AND AUTOPSY STUDIES

Two histologic types of lesions are recognized: those that contain parasites and those that do not.[14] In tissue sections, the parasite assumes the morphology of *Leishmania* bodies, which are round and contain an ovoid nucleus and a rodlike blepharoplast. Inflammation usually does not occur unless a pseudocyst ruptures. Tissue reactions induced by an antibody are believed to be responsible for lesions in which the parasite cannot be demonstrated. After infection, an antibody that cross reacts with the endocardium, the interstitium, and the blood vessels of the heart is formed and is referred to as an endocardial-vascular-interstitial antibody.[23-25] This antibody has an affinity for the plasma membranes of the endocardium, endothelial cell, and striated muscle, and for *T. cruzi*. Endocardial-vascular-interstitial antibody is present in 95% of persons with Chagas heart disease and in 45% of asymptomatic patients with serologic evidence of having had Chagas disease.[25]

Tissue replication of the organism causes damage to the ganglia of the autonomic nervous system and to muscle.[16] Injury to the Auerbach plexus results in megaesophagus, megacolon, and dilatation of other parts of the gastrointestinal tract and gallbladder. Similarly, the conducting system of the heart and the myocardium may be infected. Sudden death from arrhythmias can occur.

CLINICAL MANIFESTATIONS

In the mother, urticaria is often present at the site of the bite, regardless of whether the insect was infected.[13] The favored site for the bite is the face, presumably because this is the part of the body that is most often exposed during sleep. In acute infections, an inflammatory nodule, referred to as a chagoma, may develop at the site of the bite. If the bite is on the face, it is often associated with a unilateral, nonpurulent edema of the palpebral folds and an ipsilateral regional lymphadenopathy (i.e., Romaña sign). Between 2 and 3 weeks after the bite, parasitemia, fever, and a moderate local and general lymphadenopathy develop. The infection can extend and involve the myocardium, resulting in tachycardia, arrhythmia, hypotension, distant heart sounds, cardiomegaly, and congestive heart failure. The latter feature is more severe in pregnant and postpartum women than in nonpregnant women. Hepatosplenomegaly and encephalitis also occur. The mortality rate during the acute phase is 10% to 20%. Death is usually attributed to cardiac dysfunction. Many survivors have abnormal electrocardiograms.

In the chronic phase, the placenta and fetus may be infected despite the fact that the mother is asymptomatic.[13] Chronic Chagas disease often comes to medical attention because of the occurrence of an arrhythmia. These patients often do not have signs or symptoms of congestive heart failure.[16] Of 503 patients with myocardiopathy of chronic Chagas disease studied by Vasquez,[26] 19.8% died during an observation period of 6 years—37.5% suddenly and 55.2% with congestive heart failure.

ABORTIONS AND STILLBIRTHS

Of 300 abortions in Argentina, 3 (1%) were performed because of Chagas disease.[27] In Chile and Brazil, 10% of all abortions are attributed to Chagas disease.[13] When the fetus is aborted, massive infection of the placenta is usually found.

CONGENITAL INFECTIONS

Bittencourt and coworkers[28] found *T. cruzi* antibodies in 226 of 2651 pregnant women; 28.3% of seropositive mothers had parasitemia. Nevertheless, the risk of transmission to the fetus is low, and live births of infants congenitally infected with *T. cruzi* are rare.[29] It is postulated that upregulation of fetal or neonatal immunity might be important in preventing vertical infection.[30,31] Congenital infections occur in 1% to 5% of women with serologic evidence of having had Chagas disease.* Among infants with a birth weight of 2500 g or more, congenital infections are rare.[20,34-37] Among low-birth-weight infants, congenitally infected infants can be premature or small for gestational age, or both. Congenital infections were found in 10 (2.3%) of 425 infants by Saleme and associates[27] in Argentina, in 10 (2%) of 500 infants weighing less than 2000 g by Bittencourt and coworkers[28] in Brazil, and in 3 (1.6%) of 186 infants with birth weights of more than 2000 g and in 1 (0.5%) of 200 premature infants with birth weights of 2000 g or less by Howard in Chile.[38,39]

Congenitally infected infants may develop symptoms at birth or during the first few weeks of life. Early-onset jaundice, anemia, and petechiae are common. These symptoms are similar to those associated with erythroblastosis fetalis.[14] As occurs in older patients, congenitally infected infants may have hepatosplenomegaly, cardiomegaly, and congestive heart failure and have involvement of the esophagus leading to dysphagia, regurgitation, and megaesophagus.[25,40] Some infants have myxedematous edema. Pneumonitis has been associated with infection of the amnionic epithelium.[41] Congenitally infected infants can be born with encephalitis or can develop it postnatally. It is generally associated with hypotonia, a poor suck, and seizures.[13] The cerebrospinal fluid shows mild pleocytosis, which consists primarily of lymphocytes. Cataracts and opacification of the media of the eye have also been observed.[32] Both twins may be congenitally infected, or one may escape infection.[42]

Of 64 congenitally infected infants for whom follow-up results were known, Bittencourt[14] reported that 7.8% died the first day, 35.9% died when younger than 4 months, 9.3% died between the ages of 4 and 24 months, and 42.2% survived for more than 24 months. Of those who survived for 2 years or longer, 74% had no serious clinical symptoms

*References 1, 13, 14, 22, 32, 33.

despite continued parasitemia. However, subclinical abnormalities might have been found if electrocardiography or radiography had been performed.

As with other congenital infections, the immune system of the fetus is stimulated. IgM antibody to *T. cruzi* and endocardial-vascular-interstitial antibody are formed.[14,25]

DIAGNOSIS

The diagnosis should be suspected at the time of abortions and stillbirths, and in infants who develop symptoms compatible with congenital infection. An easy, but often omitted, means of making a diagnosis of congenital infection is to examine the placenta for the amastigote of *T. cruzi*. The gross appearance of the placenta is similar to that seen in erythroblastosis fetalis. It appears that examination of infected amniotic fluid by polymerase chain reaction is not useful in diagnosing congenital infection.[43]

Motile trypomastigotes can also be demonstrated by examining blood under a coverslip.[14] The number of parasites is low initially but increases subsequently. Thin and thick smears can be examined after being stained with Giemsa stain. Microhematocrit concentration and examination of the buffy coat enhance the detection of parasites in congenital Chagas disease.[44] If more than 10 parasites/mm^3 are found, the infant generally dies.[27]

Xenodiagnosis is performed by allowing laboratory-bred uninfected insects to feed and ingest the patient's blood. The fecal contents of the insects are examined for trypomastigotes 30 to 60 days later. Blood may also be injected into mice. In mothers with acute Chagas disease, the parasites are found in blood smears beginning 3 weeks after onset of the infection, and they persist for several months. Parasites can be demonstrated for years by xenodiagnosis.

In the chronic stages of the disease, the diagnosis can be made histologically by sampling skeletal muscle. The histologic appearance of the parasite in tissue sections is similar to that of toxoplasmosis. However, the amastigotes in Chagas disease contain a blepharoplast that is lacking in toxoplasmosis.

Several tests for antibody are available. Complement-fixing antibody crosses the placenta from mother to infant. This test, referred to as the Machado-Guerreiro reaction, demonstrates antibodies that exhibit a cross-reaction with *Leishmania donovani* and with sera from patients with lepromatous leprosy. In uninfected infants, complement-fixing antibodies are no longer demonstrable after the 40th day of life; in infected infants, these antibodies persist.[14]

Agglutinating antibodies may also be demonstrable. Uninfected infants with titers of agglutinating antibody of 1:512 or less at birth have negative titers by 2 months of age.[32] The titer of agglutinating antibody in uninfected infants with initial titers of 1:1024 or higher becomes negative by 6 months of age. IgM fluorescent antibodies can be demonstrated in some infants, but infected infants do not always have a positive test result.[25,42] Data suggest that fetal IgG to specific acute-phase antigens may be useful in the diagnosis of congenital Chagas disease, but maternal and neonatal serologic tests using the microhematocrit, direct parasitologic visualization, and indirect hemagglutination or enzyme-linked immunosorbent assay have proved to be reliable.[45,46]

PROGNOSIS FOR RECURRENCE

Congenital infections can recur during subsequent pregnancies.[47] The same mother, however, often has healthy children before and after the affected one.[25]

THERAPY

In the past, various drugs, including nitrofurans, 8-aminoquinolines, and metronidazole, were thought to have some effect on the bloodborne form of the parasite. They were ineffective in eliminating the tissue form, the amastigote. There is no therapy available for prevention of congenital infection, but early detection of neonatal infection and treatment with nifurtimox has resulted in cure rates of up to 90%.[48] Information regarding treatment can be obtained from the Parasitic Disease Drug Service, Centers for Disease Control and Prevention (CDC), Atlanta, Georgia.

PREVENTION

The main means of prevention is to improve housing so that the vector cannot reach the inhabitants, especially during sleep. In endemic areas, potential blood donors should be tested, and only those who lack serologic evidence of having had Chagas disease should be permitted to donate blood. The addition of gentian violet (1:4000 solution) to blood has been useful as a means of preventing transmission of the infection to the recipient of the blood.[16]

African Trypanosomiasis: African Sleeping Sickness

Whereas few cases of congenital disease have been reported, infection with *Trypanosoma brucei gambiense* and *T. brucei rhodesiense* in adults is severe and often fatal, and congenital infection is most likely underreported. Humans are infected by the bite of an infected male or female tsetse fly, which injects trypomastigotes into the host. Humans are the primary reservoir for *T. gambiense* and large, wild game the hosts for *T. rhodesiense*. Once injected, the organism disseminates throughout the bloodstream. Signs and symptoms of infection appear after 2 to 4 weeks, and a chronic infection develops 6 months to 1 to 2 years later. The chronic stage includes a progressive meningoencephalitis, which is often fatal if left untreated. Infection with *T. gambiense* is associated with lymphadenopathy and is slowly progressive, whereas infection with *T. rhodesiense* is rapidly progressive.

The parasite can be transmitted transplacentally, but few cases have been reported.[49,50] Transplacental infection can cause prematurity, abortion, and stillbirth. Transplacental infection has been proved in infants who were born in nonendemic areas to infected mothers or if the parasite was identified in the peripheral blood in the first 5 days of life. Central nervous system involvement is common in congenital infection and, in some infants, may be slowly progressive.

The diagnosis should be suspected in an infant with unexplained fever, anemia, hepatosplenomegaly, or progressive neurologic symptoms whose mother is from an endemic area. The parasite can be identified in thick smears from peripheral blood or in the cerebrospinal fluid. In infants, treatment with suramin or melarsoprol has been reported with good results; however, in a case report of congenital trypanosomiasis,[49] severe neurologic symptoms persisted after delayed diagnosis and treatment when the child was 22 months of age.

Entamoeba Histolytica

There is some evidence that amebiasis during pregnancy may be more severe and have a higher fatality rate than that expected in nonpregnant women of the same age.[51,52] Abioye[52] found that 68% of fatal cases of amebiasis in females 15 to 34 years of age occurred in pregnant women, whereas only 17.1% and 12.5% of fatal cases of typhoid or other causes of enterocolitis, respectively, in women in this age group occurred during pregnancy. Czeizel and coworkers[53] found a significantly higher incidence of positive stool cultures for *E. histolytica* among women who had spontaneous abortions than among those who gave birth to living infants at term.

Amebiasis has been reported in infants as young as 3 to 6 weeks of age.[54-56] In most instances, person-to-person transmission was considered likely, and the mother was the probable source of the infant's infection.[54] In one fatal case, the father had cysts of *E. histolytica* in his stool, whereas no evidence of infection with *E. histolytica* was found in the mother.[55] Perinatal infections have occurred in countries such as the United States in which the disease is rare.

Most infants reported with amebiasis in the perinatal period had illnesses with sudden, dramatic onset and were seriously ill. Bloody diarrhea was followed by development of hepatomegaly and hepatic abscess, rectal abscess, and gangrene of the appendix and colon with perforation and peritonitis. Persistent bloody diarrhea that is complicated by the development of a mass in or around the liver should lead to a thorough investigation about whether infection with *E. histolytica* could be the cause. Maternal amebiasis has also been associated with low birth weight.[57]

Routine stool examinations for ova and parasites may be negative. Despite this, trophozoites of *E. histolytica* can usually be found in biopsy specimens of gastrointestinal ulcers and of the wall of the liver abscesses. The organisms cannot always be demonstrated in pus aspirated from the center of the abscess. An elevated indirect hemagglutination titer to *E. histolytica* can be helpful in diagnosing extraintestinal amebiasis. However, high titers are not usually seen until 2 weeks or more after onset of the infection in older patients and are not always present in neonates with severe extraintestinal infections.[54] Infants have been successfully treated with oral metronidazole.[56] Critically ill children should receive intravenous therapy with dehydroemetine or metronidazole.

Malaria

The risk of malaria exists for about half of the world's population, including approximately 125 million pregnant women who live in malaria-endemic regions annually.[58,59] Eighty percent of overall malaria cases and 90% of deaths occur in sub-Saharan Africa.[60] Approximately 627,000 malaria deaths occurred in 2012, 77% of these among children younger than 5 years.[61]

THE ORGANISMS

In addition to the four known species of malaria, *Plasmodium knowlesi* is a nonhuman primate species that can also infect humans. *Plasmodium vivax* has the widest distribution, but *Plasmodium falciparum* tends to predominate in tropical areas. *Plasmodium malariae* distribution overlaps considerably but is less prevalent, and *Plasmodium ovale* is found primarily in sub-Saharan Africa. Malaria is spread to humans by the bite of anopheline mosquitoes. Of the many species of anopheline mosquito capable of becoming infected with malarial parasites, those that enter houses are more important than those preferring an outdoor habitat.[62] Mosquitoes that feed at night on human blood while the victim is asleep are the most important vectors.

After the bite of the mosquito, sporozoites are injected into the bloodstream but are cleared within one-half hour. The parasites mature in the parenchymal cells of the liver and form a mature schizont, which contains 7500 to 40,000 merozoites, depending on the species. The release of the merozoites results in the appearance of the ring stage in erythrocytes in the peripheral blood. Within hours, the parasite assumes an ameboid form and is referred to as a trophozoite. The sexual form is called a gametocyte. In infections with *P. vivax*, *P. malariae*, and *P. ovale*, all forms are seen in the peripheral blood from early ring forms through mature schizonts and gametocytes. In infections with *P. falciparum*, usually only rings and gametocytes are found in the peripheral blood.

EPIDEMIOLOGY AND TRANSMISSION

In addition to transmission by the bite of mosquitoes, malaria can be transmitted by transfusion of blood products. In infants, this has occurred after simple transfusion and after exchange transfusion.[63-66] The onset of symptoms in neonates infected by blood products has varied from 13 to 21 days.

Malaria parasites survive in blood for weeks. Relapses can occur from *P. vivax* for up to 2 years and rarely for up to 4 years. Relapses from *P. malariae* have occasionally occurred 5 years or more after infection, but low-grade chronic parasitemia that is unassociated with symptoms is more common.

Malaria may be transmitted by reuse of syringes and needles and has spread by this route among heroin addicts. Infection in heroin addicts who become pregnant can result in congenital infections.[67]

PATHOLOGY

Effect of Pregnancy on Malaria

The density and the prevalence of parasitemia are increased in pregnant women compared with women who are not pregnant but who reside in the same geographic area.[68-72] For *P. falciparum*, Campbell and colleagues[73] found a parasite density of 6896/mm^3 in pregnant women and 3808/mm^3

in nonpregnant women; for *P. vivax*, the parasite density was 3564/mm^3 for pregnant women and 1949/mm^3 for nonpregnant women. The prevalence and the density of the parasitemia decrease with increasing parity. Reinhardt and associates[69] found that the placenta was infected in 45% of primiparous women compared with 19% of women with a parity of five. This trend toward an increase in resistance to malaria with parity has been attributed by some to the increase in immunity that would be expected with an increase in age. However, the prevalence and the density of parasitemia are increased in pregnant women of all parities compared with those in nonpregnant women of the same parity.[68-70] This suggests that pregnancy, as well as age, is an important factor in determining susceptibility to malaria.[68]

Infection of the Placenta

The intervillous spaces of infected placentas are packed with lymphoid macrophages, which contain phagocytosed pigment in large granules. Lymphocytes and immature polymorphonuclear leukocytes are also present in large numbers. Numerous young and mature schizonts are present. Trophozoites and gametocytes are uncommon.[74,75] Jelliffe[76] has suggested that the intensity of the infection in the placenta is related to the severity of the effect on the fetus. In general, the inflammatory response in placentas infected with *P. falciparum* is more intense than that in those infected with *P. malariae*.

Effect of Malaria on Fetal Survival and Birth Weight

Up to 40% of the world's pregnant women are exposed to malaria infection during pregnancy. In those with little or no preexisting immunity, malaria may be associated with a high risk for maternal and perinatal mortality. Fetal and perinatal loss may be as high as 60% to 70% in nonimmune women with malaria.[77] In 1941, Torpin[78] reviewed 27 cases of malaria that had occurred in pregnant women during the preceding 20 years in a city in the United States. The maternal mortality rate was 4%, and the fetal mortality rate was 60%. In 1951, in Vietnam, Hung[79] found a fetal death rate of 14% among women who had infected placentas. Many of these women had had severe attacks of malaria during the first trimester and had sustained spontaneous abortions at that time.

Low birth weight is more common when the placenta is infected by parasites than when the mother is infected, but the placenta is not.[69,70,76,80,81] The mean birth weight is lower if the placenta is infected with *P. falciparum* than if it is infected with *P. malariae*. Maternal anemia and placental insufficiency probably affect the fetus. It has been postulated that heavy infiltrations of parasites, lymphocytes, and macrophages interfere with the circulation of maternal blood through the placenta and result in diminished transport of oxygen and nutrients to the fetus.[70] The transport through the placenta of antibody to malaria may also be decreased when placental inflammation is severe.[68]

Bruce-Chwatt[74] found that when the placenta was infected, infant weight at birth was an average of 145 g less than the weight of infants born to women with uninfected placentas. Similarly, Archibald[82] found infant weight at birth to be 170 g less, and Jelliffe[76,81] found it to be 263 g less in infants of women with infected placentas than in infants of women with uninfected placentas. In the studies performed by Bruce-Chwatt[67] and Jelliffe,[76,81] 20% of the infants born to mothers with infected placentas weighed 2500 g or less, whereas 10% and 11%, respectively, of those born to mothers with uninfected placentas weighed 2500 g or less. Cannon[70] found that 37% of women who had infected placentas gave birth to infants weighing 2500 g or less compared with 12% of those who had uninfected placentas. For primiparous women, 44% of those with infected placentas and 27% of those with uninfected placentas gave birth to infants weighing 2500 g or less.[83] Infants who have parasites demonstrable in their cord blood appear to be more severely affected than those who do not have parasitemia at the time of delivery; the mean weight gain of the mothers of these infants and the head and chest circumferences of the infants at birth are lower than expected.[69] Larkin[84] studied the prevalence of *P. falciparum* infection among 63 pregnant women and their newborns in southern Zambia and found peripheral parasitemia in 63% (40/63) of mothers and 29% (19/65) of newborns. Infected newborns had a mean average birth weight 469 g lower than uninfected newborns but did not have a higher incidence of preterm delivery.

Using the method developed by Dubowitz and associates[85] for scoring gestational age, Reinhardt and colleagues[69] found no evidence that the incidence of infants who were small for gestational age was increased when the placenta was infected. This finding suggested that low birth weight resulted from prematurity of infants born to women with malaria.

Jelliffe[76] observed that because malaria influences birth weight, it has an important effect on infant survival in countries in which it is endemic. In 1925, Blacklock and Gordon[86] found that 35% of infants born to mothers with infected placentas died within the first 7 days of life, whereas only 5% of those born to mothers with uninfected placentas died during this period. In 1958, Cannon[70] found that the mortality rate among infants 7 days of age or younger was 6.9% for those whose mothers' placentas were infected compared with 3.4% for those whose mothers' placentas were uninfected.

The data suggesting that malaria has an important influence on birth weight and therefore on infant survival have been given further credence by the demonstration by MacGregor and Avery[83] that control of malaria in a region is followed by an increase in mean birth weight of infants born there. After dichlorodiphenyltrichloroethane (DDT) spraying on the island of Malaita in the British Solomon Islands, the mean birth weight for infants of mothers of all parities increased by 165 g. For infants of primiparous women, the mean birth weight increased by 252 g.[83] There was a concomitant decrease in the number of infants with birth weights of 2500 g or less; the incidence of births in this weight range fell by 8% for all births and by 20% for infants of primiparous women.[83]

Steketee and colleagues[87] reviewed studies between 1985 and 2000 and summarized the population attributable risk of malaria on anemia, low birth weight, and infant mortality in malaria endemic areas. Approximately 3% to 15% of anemia, 8% to 14% of low birth weight, 8% to 36% of preterm low birth weight, 13% to 70% of intrauterine growth retardation and low birth weight, and 3% to 8% of infant mortality were attributable to malaria. Maternal anemia was associated with low birth weight, and fetal anemia was associated with increased infant mortality. It was estimated that 75,000 to 200,000 annual infant deaths are associated with malaria infection in pregnancy.[87] Recently, it was also demonstrated that maternal malaria in the first half of pregnancy may result in delayed decreases in fetal growth as late as the third trimester, emphasizing the importance of early maternal infection on later fetal and neonatal growth.[88] Malaria therefore contributes to fetal loss, stillbirth, prematurity, low birth weight, and neonatal death.[81,89]

Influence of Maternal Antibody on Risk of Infection

Antimalarial antibodies are transferred from the mother to the infant. The prevalence of precipitating antibody to *P. falciparum* within 24 hours of birth in The Gambia was 87% in newborns and 87.5% in their mothers.[90] The prevalence of antibody in these newborns reflected the extent to which malaria had been controlled in the area in which their mothers lived. In infants born in the provinces with more malaria, 97% had antibodies to malaria, whereas 75.8% of infants born in an urban area had antibodies to malaria.

Antibodies to malaria can be detected by complement fixation, indirect hemagglutination, and indirect fluorescence. Agglutinating and precipitating antibodies are also formed.[91] Levels of precipitating antibodies and antibodies detected by indirect hemagglutination decrease from birth to 25 weeks of age.[92,93] Subsequently, as a result of postnatal acquisition of infection, endogenous antibody synthesis begins and antibody levels rise.

Bray and Anderson[68] have suggested that the amount of IgG transferred to the fetus is decreased when the placenta is heavily infested with parasites. They found that women who were pregnant during the wet season in The Gambia had higher mean antibody titers to *P. falciparum* than those who were pregnant during the dry season. This pattern reflected the mothers' serologic responses to the increase in exposure to malaria during the wet season. The antibody titers of the infants born to women who were pregnant during the wet season were not higher than those of infants born to women who had been pregnant during the dry season. The infants born to women who had been pregnant during the wet season had lower mean titers of antibody to malaria at birth than infants born during other seasons. In infants 2 to 3 months of age, parasitemia was found in 32% born during the wet season but in only 3% to 15% born in other seasons.

Other Factors Influencing Risk of Infection

Infants younger than 3 months have a lower than expected incidence of clinical disease, death from malaria, and parasitemia.[90,92] This has been attributed to a variety of factors, including the possibility that infants of this age are less exposed to and therefore less often bitten by mosquitoes. However, the two most important causes are probably the fact that the level of serologic immunity is high at this age and that fetal hemoglobin is present in the circulating red blood cells. Sehgal and associates[94] studied the role of humoral immunity in acquired malaria infection among newborns in Papua New Guinea. Among 104 newborns, there was a 3.8% incidence of congenital malaria and a cumulative incidence of acquired malaria of 3% at 12 weeks, 16% by 24 weeks, 24% by 36 weeks, and 38% by 48 weeks of age. Ninety-six percent of infants lost maternal antibody between 4 and 7 months of age, and most cases of asymptomatic malaria occurred among infants with detectable malaria antibody.

Although there were seasonal fluctuations in the overall incidence of parasitemia, Gilles[95] showed that the corrected rates were always lower for infants from birth to 2 months of age than for infants 3 to 4 or 5 to 6 months of age. He did not find differences in sleeping habits or in the amount of exposure to mosquitoes among infants in these age groups. In June to October, parasitemia was found in 10% of those from birth to 2 months of age, 42% of those 3 to 4 months of age, and 53% of those 5 to 6 months of age; in May, parasitemia was found in 0% of infants from birth to 2 months of age, 11% of those 3 to 4 months of age, and 16% of those 5 to 6 months of age. The rise in prevalence of parasitemia corresponded with a fall in the amount of fetal hemoglobin in the red blood cells.[95] The fact that cells containing fetal hemoglobin are poor hosts for the malarial parasite had been previously suggested by Allison[96,97] as one of the reasons for the selective advantage of sickle cell anemia and sickle cell trait in areas in which malaria is endemic. Although antibody is undoubtedly important in protecting newborns from malaria, Campbell and coworkers[7] and Reinhardt and associates[73] pointed out that antibody levels in infants from birth to 2 months of age might be low or absent even when the mother has had parasitemia and placental infection. The presence of fetal hemoglobin in the red cells may serve as a source of protection for infants who do not derive high levels of antibody from their mothers.

Placental infection as a risk for congenital malaria was studied in 197 infants in Cameroon. Infants born to placenta-infected mothers were more likely to develop malaria than infants born to women without placental infection.[98] Rates of infant infection and parasitemia were not related to maternally derived malaria antibodies.

CONGENITAL MALARIA

Occurrence

There has been no consistently accepted definition of congenital malaria. Some have taken the position that parasites must be demonstrable in the peripheral blood of the infant during the first day of life; others have accepted cases that were confirmed within the first 7 days of life.[89] In areas in which malaria is endemic, infants are exposed to mosquitoes and may become infected by this route at a very young age. It may be difficult to distinguish congenital cases from acquired cases. However, a sufficient number of cases of congenital malaria have been reported from countries that are free of malaria, thereby eliminating the possibility of postnatal transmission, to establish the fact that the clinical onset of disease in a congenitally infected infant can be delayed for weeks and rarely even for months.[66,67,99,100] The prevalence of parasitemia in infants younger than 3 months was 0.7% among those born during the dry season in the rural part of The Gambia compared with 11.4%

among those born during the wet season, which suggests that postnatal infection is a more common event than congenital malaria.[65] It is probable that IgG antibody transmitted from the mother to the infant is an important factor in determining whether parasites that reach the fetal circulation establish an infection. The presence of passively transferred antibody in the neonate may lengthen the incubation period beyond that which would be expected in the nonimmune host.

The frequency of placental infection varies according to the prevalence of malaria in the population, the vigor of measures of control, and the availability of nonprescription antimalarial drugs. However, among Nigerian women who did not receive antimalarial agents, three studies suggested that the frequency of infection of the placenta remained relatively stable over a 30-year period. In 1948 through 1950, Bruce-Chwatt[74] found that 20% of the placentas from 228 pregnancies were infected. One (0.4%) of the 235 neonates had the trophozoites of *P. falciparum* in a peripheral smear obtained on the fifth day of life. In 1958, Cannon[70] found that 26% of the placentas were infected; in 1970, Williams and McFarlane[101] found that 37% of the placentas were infected. None of the cord blood samples of the infants in these latter studies contained parasites. In 1964 through 1965 in Uganda, Jelliffe[76] found that 16% of the 570 placentas were infected, but only one (0.18%) infant was infected at birth.

The studies of Kortmann,[102] Reinhardt and colleagues,[69] and Schwetz and Peel[103] suggest that parasitemia in cord blood may be more common than had been previously believed and that the presence of parasites does not necessarily indicate that the infant will become infected. Reinhardt and colleagues[69] found 33% of 198 placentas to be infected. Thick smears of the cord blood were positive for 21.7% of the 198 infants and 55% of the infants of mothers who had had parasitemia during the pregnancy. Thin smears were negative for all 198 infants. Kortmann[102] was able to demonstrate parasites in 19.7% of the placentas of 1009 women but in only 3.8% of cord blood from their infants. Eleven infants who had parasites in their cord blood also had peripheral smears performed; parasites were demonstrable in the peripheral blood of only 2 (18%). Lehner and Andrews[104] found a 14.6% incidence of cord parasitemia and a 7.7% incidence of peripheral parasitemia among 48 newborns in Papua New Guinea. Whereas all maternal and cord samples had malaria antibodies, low levels of cord malaria antibody were found to correlate with cord parasitemia. Schwetz and Peel[103] demonstrated parasites in 6% of cord blood samples and 3.6% of peripheral blood samples of infants born to mothers in Central Africa. Because the rate of infection of the placenta was 74%, this study demonstrates that the placenta, although frequently infected, serves as a relatively effective barrier and that parasites infrequently reach the fetus. The relative importance of transplacental infection or transmission by transfer from mother to infant during labor as mechanisms by which the infant acquires malaria remains uncertain.[103]

Despite massive involvement of the placenta, it is generally agreed that clinically apparent congenital infections are rare in areas in which malaria is endemic and levels of maternal immunity are high. Covell[90] reviewed cases of congenital malaria that had been reported up to 1950 and estimated the incidence at 16 (0.3%) infections per 5324 live births. This rate pertained to areas of the world in which malaria was endemic. For women having an overt attack of malaria during pregnancy, the rate of congenital infection was higher and was estimated to be 1% to 4%.[90] Congenital malaria is more common among infants of women who have clinical attacks of malaria during pregnancy than in those with chronic subclinical infections; however, congenital malaria may occur in infants of mothers who are asymptomatic throughout their pregnancies.[89,100,105] Often, parasitemia is not demonstrable in the mother; splenomegaly occurs frequently.[79] Congenital malaria is more common in infants of women who have immigrated to areas in which malaria is endemic than in women who have been raised to maturity in such areas because their levels of immunity are lower than those of the native population. Conversely, congenital malaria is also more common among women who emigrate from areas in which malaria is endemic to areas that are free of malaria. Loss of immunity results from lack of frequent exposure. Although rare, congenital malaria may also occur as a result of maternal infection by chloroquine-resistant *P. falciparum*. A number of reported cases of chloroquine-resistant congenital malaria in Africa and Indonesia responded to treatment with intravenous quinine.[106-108]

Clinical Presentation

Cases of congenital malaria have been identified in countries in which malaria is endemic and in countries in which it is not, including Great Britain and the United States. Most infants with congenital malaria have had the onset of the first sign or symptom when 10 to 28 days of age.[66,109,110] However, onsets occurring as early as 8 hours and as late as 8 weeks of age have been reported.[89,99,107,111-114] Keitel and coworkers[67] described a case of malaria in a 15-month-old child who had been separated from her mother when 6 weeks of age but who was breastfed during this 6-week period. The infection was caused by *P. malariae*. The source of the mother's infection was probably contaminated needles and syringes used to inject heroin. The infant must have derived the infection from her mother because she had always lived in an area that was free of malaria. Hulbert[110] reviewed the 49 cases of congenital malaria reported in the United States since 1950 and found that the mean age at onset of symptoms was 5.5 weeks (range, 0 to 60 weeks) and that 96% of these children had signs or symptoms when 2 to 8 weeks of age. There was no association found between age of symptom onset and *Plasmodium* species.

Most cases of congenital infection have occurred in infants of mothers who had overt attacks of malaria during pregnancy. However, Harvey and associates[100] and McQuay and colleagues[112] reported cases of congenital infection with *P. malariae* in which the mother had lived in an area that was free of malaria for 3 years or more. In these cases, it is likely that the mothers had had onset of their infection many years before their move from an endemic area.

The most common clinical findings in cases of congenital malaria are fever, anemia, and splenomegaly, which occur in greater than 80% of cases.[66,115] The anemia, which may be accompanied by pallor, is associated with a reticulocytosis in about one half of the cases. Jaundice and hyperbilirubinemia are found in about one third of the cases. The direct or the indirect bilirubin level may be elevated, depending on whether liver dysfunction or hemolysis is the most important process in an individual case.[66] Hepatomegaly may occur but is less common than splenomegaly. Nonspecific findings include failure to thrive, poor feeding, regurgitation, and loose stools. In developing countries, when malaria occurs during the first few months of life, it is frequently complicated by other illness, such as pneumonia, septicemia, and diarrhea.[113]

Of the 107 cases of congenital malaria summarized by Covell,[90] 40% were caused by *P. falciparum*, 32% were caused by *P. vivax*, and 1.9% were caused by *P. malariae*. The clinical findings of congenital malaria are not distinguishable from the signs and symptoms of malaria that has been acquired by the bite of a mosquito. IgM antibody to *P. falciparum* was found in the cord blood of one infant.[111] The mother had probably had her first attack of malaria during that pregnancy and had high fever and parasitemia at delivery. Reinhardt and colleagues[69] found that the total IgM levels in the cord blood of infants of infected mothers were similar to those of infants of uninfected mothers. Although fever and parasitemia may occur within 24 hours of birth, hepatosplenomegaly and anemia at birth as a result of a chronic intrauterine infection have not been described. Normal red blood cells can cross from the maternal to the fetal circulation.[69] If parasitized cells cross, however, they must usually be destroyed by the immune defenses of the fetus and by the maternal antimalarial antibodies that have passed transplacentally.

Treatment

Chloroquine is the drug of choice for sensitive strains of *P. falciparum* and for *P. malariae*. For these infections, chloroquine phosphate should be administered orally in an initial dose of 10 mg/kg of chloroquine base (maximum, 600 mg of base), followed in 6 hours by a dose of 5 mg/kg of chloroquine base (maximum, 300 mg of base). Subsequent doses of 5 mg/kg of chloroquine base should be given 24 and 48 hours after the first dose (maximum, 300 mg of base). Parenteral therapy consists of quinidine gluconate at a dose of 10 mg/kg as a loading dose (maximum, 600 mg) in normal saline given over 1 to 2 hours and then 0.02 mg/kg per minute until oral therapy can be given. Infections with *P. vivax* may be treated with chloroquine alone because sporozoite forms are not transmitted, and there is no exoerythrocytic phase in congenital infections; administration of primaquine is unnecessary. The treatment of transfusion-acquired infections is the same as that for congenital infections because there is no exoerythrocytic phase in these infections.

Recommended therapy for *P. falciparum* infection in areas with known chloroquine resistance is variable, depending on ability to appropriately diagnose resistant *P. falciparum*, the percentage of parasitemia, signs of organ involvement (especially of the central nervous system), and other systemic manifestations of malaria. Severe malaria may require intensive care, and exchange transfusion may be necessary if the degree of parasitemia is greater than 10%. Sequential smears should be monitored to ensure adequacy of therapy. For serious infections in those who may have been exposed to chloroquine-resistant strains of *P. falciparum*, intravenous quinidine plus doxycycline, tetracycline, or clindamycin are recommended by the CDC.[116] Intravenous quinidine in combination with exchange transfusion has been used in a severe case of maternal *P. falciparum* malaria.[117] Intravenous artesunate is available through a CDC investigational new drug protocol for patients with severe malaria in the United States who do not tolerate or cannot easily access quinidine.

Recommended, up-to-date treatment regimens can be found at the CDC Malaria website (http://www.cdc.gov/malaria/resources/pdf/treatmenttable.pdf). Additional current recommendations regarding treatment can also be obtained from the Malaria Branch, CDC, Atlanta, Georgia.†

Globally, the World Health Organization (WHO) recommends artemisinin-based combination therapies (ACTs) for the treatment of uncomplicated malaria caused by *P. falciparum*. The choice of ACT should be based on the results of therapeutic efficacy studies against local strains of *P. falciparum* malaria. Artemisinin and its derivatives must not be used as oral monotherapy because this promotes the development of artemisinin resistance. Fixed-dose formulations are recommended over loose tablet combinations because they facilitate adherence to treatment and reduce the potential use of the individual components as monotherapy.[118] In the United States, the combination of artemether (20 mg) and lumefantrine (120 mg) was approved for therapy of *P. falciparum* malaria in 2009. The recommended dose for adults is 4 tablets twice daily for 3 days (6 doses). Artesunate (Adamsunate) is also available on a named-patient basis from the CDC Malaria Hotline.†

Prevention

Because malaria chemoprophylaxis may not be 100% effective, decreasing or eliminating exposure to mosquitoes is an important strategy for preventing malaria during pregnancy. Exposure to mosquitoes should be avoided by use of mosquito netting around beds, wire mesh screening on windows, insecticides, and mosquito repellents.

Pregnant women living in malaria-endemic countries must have access to prompt, safe, and effective treatment for malaria. In these settings, the WHO recommends that in addition to antenatal care, these women receive a dose of intermittent preventive treatment (IPT) (e.g., with sulfadoxine-pyrimethamine) at each antenatal care visit during the second and third trimester, as well as use of insecticide-treated bed nets during pregnancy through the postpartum period, effective case management of malaria, and screening and treatment of anemia frequently resulting from malaria infection.[119-121] Although the possible toxicity of administering prophylactic antimalarial agents to women during pregnancy has been much discussed, controlled trials have shown that there is little risk and much to gain from such a practice. Recent studies have demonstrated that IPT is associated with reduced maternal disease, including anemia and placental infection, birth weight, risk of preterm delivery, and neonatal mortality.[122] In contrast, treatment only for identified cases of maternal malaria, rather than the administration of malaria prophylaxis,

†CDC Malaria Hotline: 770-488-7788 or 855-856-4713, toll-free Monday through Friday 9 AM to 5 PM EST; 770-488-7100 after hours, weekends, and holidays

failed to reduce the incidence of malaria-related low birth weight because only 12 of 65 women who had plasmodial pigmentation of the placenta had symptoms leading to an antenatal diagnosis of malaria.[106-108,123] Morley and associates[124] showed that administration of a prophylactic monthly dose of 50 mg of pyrimethamine during pregnancy resulted in improved maternal weight gain and in an increase in the mean birth weight of 157 g compared with administration of antimalarial drugs only for febrile episodes. Pyrimethamine prophylaxis had been avoided in pregnant women because of concern that this dihydrofolate reductase inhibitor may cause abnormalities by interference with folic acid metabolism. Congenital defects have occurred in the offspring of animals ingesting pyrimethamine during pregnancy.[125] Evidence of embryo resorption has been documented in pregnant Wistar rats given sulfadoxine-pyrimethamine.[126] However, more recent literature has demonstrated the overall strong safety profile of intermittent administration of pyrimethamine in combination with sulfadoxine to pregnant women.[127] Sulfadoxine/pyrimethamine administered in two to four treatment doses over 6 months has been well tolerated in multiple IPT trials but should not be administered concurrently with cotrimoxazole because of the potential for synergistic worsening of adverse drug reactions. Therefore HIV-infected pregnant women in malaria endemic areas who are already receiving cotrimoxazole prophylaxis should not also receive IPT. Large case-control studies have demonstrated that sulfadoxine/pyrimethamine administered as IPT in the second and third trimesters does not result in an increased risk of teratogenesis. Folic acid supplementation is recommended for all pregnant women to reduce the rate of congenital anomalies at a standard dose of 0.4 mg/day; higher doses might affect antimalarial efficacy. No clinical association between sulfadoxine/pyrimethamine use and kernicterus has been reported.

Chloroquine prophylaxis is recommended for pregnant women traveling to areas with chloroquine-sensitive *P. falciparum*. There have been no safety concerns for the fetus when used in the recommended doses for malaria prophylaxis. Chloroquine and the other 4-aminoquinolines, such as amodiaquine and hydroxychloroquine, have similar activities and toxicities. The usual recommendation for prophylaxis is 300 mg of chloroquine base once each week. Hart and Naunton[128] attributed the abnormal outcome of four pregnancies in a single patient to the administration of chloroquine during the pregnancies. This patient, who had systemic lupus erythematosus (SLE), took 150 to 300 mg chloroquine base daily. Two of the children who had had intrauterine exposures to chloroquine had severe cochleovestibular paresis and posterior column defects. Another had a Wilms tumor and hemihypertrophy. The fourth pregnancy ended in a spontaneous abortion at 12 weeks of gestation. The dose given to this pregnant patient was three to seven times higher than the dose recommended for prophylaxis against malaria. Two other studies reported pregnancy outcomes after exposure to antimalarials. Parke[129] described 14 pregnancies among 8 patients with SLE who took chloroquine or hydroxychloroquine during pregnancy. Three pregnancies ended in spontaneous abortion or neonatal death during periods of increased SLE activity; of the remaining 11 pregnancies, 6 were normal full-term deliveries, 1 ended in stillbirth, and 4 ended in spontaneous abortion. No congenital deformities occurred. Levy and coworkers[130] reviewed the cases of 24 women who took chloroquine or hydroxychloroquine during a total of 27 pregnancies. Eleven women had SLE, 3 had rheumatoid arthritis, and 4 were taking malaria prophylaxis. There were 14 normal deliveries, 6 abortions attributed to severe underlying disease or social conditions, 3 stillbirths, and 4 spontaneous abortions. No congenital abnormalities were identified. The risk of poor outcome was higher among women with connective tissue disease, for which chloroquine and hydroxychloroquine doses are much higher than for malaria prophylaxis. Despite widespread use of weekly doses of chloroquine in pregnant women, teratogenic effects have not been confirmed in controlled trials.[131]

Mefloquine is the only medication recommended for malaria chemoprophylaxis during pregnancy in areas with chloroquine-resistant *P. falciparum*. In 2011, the U.S. Food and Drug Administration reclassified mefloquine from category C (animal reproduction studies have shown an adverse effect on the fetus, and there are no adequate and well-controlled studies in humans, but potential benefits may warrant use of the drug in pregnant women despite potential risks) to category B (animal reproduction studies have failed to demonstrate a risk to the fetus, and there are no adequate and well-controlled studies in pregnant women). A retrospective review of 1627 reports of women exposed to mefloquine before or during pregnancy revealed a 4% prevalence of congenital malformations among infants of these women, reportedly similar to that observed in the general population.[132] A second report demonstrated a high rate of spontaneous abortions, but not congenital malformations, among 72 female U.S. soldiers who inadvertently received mefloquine during pregnancy.[133,134]

Atovaquone-proguanil, doxycycline, and primaquine are not recommended as malaria prophylaxis in pregnant women. There is insufficient data regarding use of atovaquone-proguanil in pregnancy; doxycycline is contraindicated during pregnancy because of the fetal adverse effects associated with tetracycline, a related drug, including discoloration and dysplasia of the teeth and inhibition of bone growth. Primaquine may be passed transplacentally to a glucose-6-phosphate dehydrogenase (G6PD)-deficient fetus and causes hemolytic anemia in utero.

Concerns regarding breastfeeding in infants who require chemoprophylaxis are minimal. These infants are not protected against malaria by antimalarials excreted in breast milk and should therefore receive their own chemoprophylaxis as indicated. The possibility of adverse events in infants of lactating women on doxycycline is considered to be unlikely. Both lactating mothers and their infants should be tested for G6PD before administering primaquine to the mother because of the possible risk of hemolytic anemia.

The safety of atovaquone-proguanil prophylaxis in infants weighing less than 5 kg is unknown and is not recommended for those infants nor for women breastfeeding infants weighing less than 5 kg, except when the potential benefit outweighs the potential risk to the infant (e.g., treatment of maternal *P. falciparum* malaria in an area of multidrug-resistant strains in those who cannot tolerate other treatment options). Depending on geographic resistance patterns, chloroquine and mefloquine may be used as chemoprophylaxis in infants and children. Primaquine can be used for children who are not G6PD-deficient as part of a chemoprophylactic regimen against *P. vivax*. Doxycycline may be used for children who are aged greater than or equal to 8 years. Atovaquone-proguanil may be used for prophylaxis for infants and children weighing greater than or equal to 5 kg but is off-label use in the United States for children weighing less than 11 kg.[135]

The consequences of an attack of malaria during pregnancy are serious. Hindi and Azimi[99] described a woman who became pregnant while living in Nigeria but who stopped taking prophylactic doses of pyrimethamine at the onset of pregnancy. At 6 months of gestation, she had a febrile illness and was treated with chloroquine for 2 weeks. At 8 months of gestation, she had a second attack of malaria and was delivered of an infant who was 4 weeks premature and small for gestational age. The infant developed malaria during the first few weeks of life and was treated with chloroquine. The total exposure of this infant to chloroquine would have been less if the mother had been taking it weekly in prophylactic doses.

Women living in or returning from areas in which malaria is endemic should continue to take prophylactic antimalarial agents. Although primaquine is not known to have teratogenic effects, experience with its use during pregnancy is limited; it is therefore recommended that treatment with primaquine to eradicate the exoerythrocytic phase in *P. vivax* infections be deferred until after delivery.[136]

Some investigators think the widespread use of prophylaxis may lower the level of maternal immunity and increase the severity of cases of malaria seen in children who are younger than 1 year. There is no evidence that administration of antimalarial drugs prophylactically to pregnant women has changed the expected incidence of infection during the first few months of life.

Because of the tremendous global burden of disease imposed by malaria infections, a key initiative in the prevention of malaria is the emphasis on development of malaria vaccines. The cloning of the *P. falciparum* receptor protein, which allows red blood cell attachment, should facilitate the development of a malarial vaccine.[137,138] Vaccine candidates are in development, but no effective vaccine will be immediately available.[139-141] Development of animal models for malaria infection in which to test vaccines and antimalarial drugs would be ideal. A rhesus monkey model mimicking human infection after exposure to *Plasmodium coatneyi* has been tested with potential for use in animal studies.[142] Clinical development of the malaria vaccine candidate RTS,S/AS01 is the most advanced and expected to gain licensure in 2015.[143] This vaccine targets the pre-erythrocytic stages in the life cycle of the parasite and has shown modest efficacy of 31.3% (95% confidence interval [CI], 23.6 to 38.3) against prevention of malaria in African infants and against severe malaria (36.6% [95% CI, 4.6 to 57.7]).[144]

There is an increased risk of maternal and placental malaria among human immunodeficiency virus (HIV)-infected pregnant women, although the influence of malaria on the clinical course of maternal HIV infection and maternal-to-child transmission of HIV remains unclear.[145-149] IPT with sulfadoxine-pyrimethamine is contraindicated among pregnant women already receiving cotrimoxazole prophylaxis because of added toxicity, emphasizing the need for research to identify additional antimalarial treatment, especially in this population. Furthermore, interactions between antimalarial and antiretroviral drugs are poorly understood.[148] There remains a need for effective, practical, and well-tolerated strategies to prevent and treat malaria in women with HIV.

Schistosomiasis

Schistosomiasis (i.e., bilharziasis) contributes to infertility by causing sclerosis of the fallopian tubes or cervix.[150] It is estimated that 9 to 13 million women may be afflicted by genital schistosomiasis in Africa alone.[151] The placenta usually does not become infected until the third month of pregnancy or thereafter.[152] Although the frequency of placental infection is as high as 25% in endemic areas, the infestations are light and cause little histologic reaction.[152,153] In their study of the impact of placental infection on the outcome of pregnancy, Renaud and coworkers[152] concluded that there was little evidence that the size or weight of the infant was affected and that placental bilharziasis was not an important cause of intrauterine growth retardation or prematurity.

Trichomonas Vaginalis

Infection of the vagina of the pregnant woman with *Trichomonas vaginalis* is not uncommon, but no adverse effect on the fetus has been documented.[154-156] There are six reports in the literature of *T. vaginalis* recovered from a respiratory source among neonates, all with respiratory illness whose viral and bacterial cultures revealed no other pathogens, but a causal relationship was not certain.[157,158] During the first 2 weeks of life, female newborns may be particularly susceptible to infection because of the influence of maternal estrogens on the vaginal epithelium. By 3 to 6 weeks of age, the vaginal pH is no longer acid.[159] *T. vaginalis* has been found in 0% to 4.8% of sequentially studied female newborns.[159-161] Among infants younger than 3 weeks who had vaginal discharges, *T. vaginalis* was the probable cause of the discharge in 17.2%.[162] In addition to causing a vaginal discharge,[163] infection of the newborn with *T. vaginalis* may aggravate candidal infections and may be associated with urinary tract infections.[159] In most infants, the white blood cells found in the urine originate from the vagina rather than from the bladder.[164] However, several reports suggest that a bacterial urinary tract infection can be present concomitantly.[165,166] In symptomatic cases, metronidazole has been used at a dosage of 500 mg twice daily or 15 mg/kg/day divided in three doses for 5 to 7 days.[159,164,167]

Trichinosis

Prenatal transmission of trichinosis from mother to infant is rare. Four larvae, however, were found in the diaphragm of a fetus by Kuitunen-Ekbaum.[168] No evidence of infection with trichinosis was found in 25 newborns studied by McNaught and Anderson.[169] Despite this, *Trichinella spiralis* has been found in the placenta, in the milk of nursing women, and in the tissue from the mammary gland.[170] In 1939, Hood and Olson[171] found *T. spiralis* in pressed muscle preparations from 4 (8.3%) of 48 infants from birth to 12 months of age. Although transplacental transmission is rare, *T. spiralis* is present in the placenta of women with acute trichinosis and can be passed to the infant by means of breast milk.

Babesiosis

Babesia microti is a tick-borne protozoan that infects erythrocytes and causes a malaria-like illness. Most cases in the United States have occurred in the Northeast. Raucher and colleagues[172] described a *B. microti* infection in a pregnant woman that began in the 19th week of gestation; the infant was born at term without evidence of infection. Ten neonatal cases have been reported in the literature. Of those, seven were transfusion-related, two were congenital, and one was secondary to tick transmission.[173]

Pneumocystis Jirovecii

P. jirovecii is an infectious agent with a history. In 1988, DNA analysis demonstrated that *Pneumocystis* was not a protozoan but a fungus.[174,175] Subsequent DNA analysis has led to the change in nomenclature of *P. carinii* to *P. jirovecii*, a name chosen in honor of the parasitologist Otto Jirovec, who is credited by some with the original description of this organism.[174,175] *P. carinii* as a fungus has been defined based on molecular analysis.[176,177] Previous controversy over the classification *Pneumocystis* existed because of the difficulty in cultivating and further characterizing the biochemical nature of the organism. Questions remained until polymerase chain reaction techniques established that *P. jirovecii* was not found in lung samples from any other mammals.[178] However, genetic analysis clearly demonstrated differences between human and nonhuman *Pneumocystis* isolates.[179] This organism is covered in detail in Chapter 34: "*Pneumocystis* and Other Less Common Fungal Infections."

References

1. Kotcher E, et al: Acquisition of intestinal parasites in newborn infants, *Fed Proc* 24:442, 1965.
2. Agbere AD, Atakouma DY, Balaka B, et al: Gastrointestinal and urinary parasitic infection in children at a regional hospital center in Togo: some epidemiological aspects, *Med Trop* 55:65, 1995.
3. Imhoff-Kunsch B, Briggs V: Antihelminthics in pregnancy and maternal, newborn, and child health, *Paediatr Perinat Epidemiol* 26(Suppl 1):223, 2012.
4. Stringer JR, Beard CB, Miller RF, et al: A new name *(Pneumocystis jiroveci)* for *Pneumocystis* from humans, *Emerg Infect Dis* 8:891, 2002.
5. Sterling R, Guay AJL: Invasion of the female generative tract by *Ascaris lumbricoides*, *JAMA* 107:2046, 1936.
6. Sanjeevi CB, Vivekanandan S, Narayanan PR: Fetal response to maternal ascariasis as evidenced by anti-*Ascaris lumbricoides* IgM antibodies in the cord blood, *Acta Paediatr Scand* 80:1134, 1991.
7. Chu W, Chen PM, Huang CC, et al: Neonatal ascariasis, *J Pediatr* 81:783, 1972.
8. Costa-Macedo LM, Rey L: *Ascaris lumbricoides* in neonate: evidence of congenital transmission of intestinal nematodes, *Rev Soc Bras Med Trop* 33:371, 1991.
9. Roberts NS, Copel JA, Bhutani V, et al: Intestinal parasites and other infections during pregnancy in Southeast Asian refugees, *J Reprod Med* 30:720, 1985.
10. Kreutner AK, Del Bene VE, Amstey MS: Giardiasis in pregnancy, *Am J Obstet Gynecol* 140:895, 1981.
11. Tellez A, Winiecka-Krusnell J, Paniagua M, et al: Antibodies in mother's milk protect children against giardiasis, *Scand J Infect Dis* 35:322, 2003.
12. Buekens P, Almendares O, Carlier Y, et al: Mother-to-child transmission of Chagas' disease in North America: why don't we do more? *Matern Child Health J* 12:283, 2008.
13. Edgcomb JH, Johnson CM: American trypanosomiasis (Chagas' disease). In Binford CH, Connor OH, editors: *Pathology of tropical and extraordinary disease*, vol. 1, Washington, DC, 1976, Armed Forces Institute of Pathology, p 244.
14. Bittencourt A: Congenital Chagas' disease, *Am J Dis Child* 130:97, 1976.
15. Miles MA: The epidemiology of South American trypanosomiasis—biochemical and immunological approaches and their relevance to control, *Trans R Soc Trop Med Hyg* 77:5, 1983.
16. Marsden PD: South American trypanosomiasis (Chagas' disease), *Int Rev Trop Med* 4:97, 1981.
17. Santos-Buch CA: American trypanosomiasis: Chagas' disease, *Int Rev Exp Pathol* 19:63, 1979.
18. Amato Neto V, Doles J, Rassi A, et al: Relato de novos casos de transmissão da doença de Chagas por transfusão de sangue, *Rev Inst Med Trop São Paulo* 10:46, 1968.
19. Bittencourt AL, Mota E: Isoenzyme characterization of *Trypanosoma cruzi* from congenital cases of Chagas' disease, *Ann Trop Med Parasitol* 4:393, 1985.
20. Bittencourt AL, Sadigursky M, Barbosa HA: Doença de Chagas congenita: estudo de 29 caspiatos, *Rev Inst Med Trop São Paulo* 17:146, 1975.
21. Rassi A, Borges C, Koeberle F, et al: Sobre a transmissão congenita da doença de Chagas, *Rev Goiana Med* 4:319, 1958.
22. Delgado MA, Santos Buch CA: Transplacental transmission and fetal parasitosis of *Trypanosoma cruzi* in outbred white Swiss mice, *Am J Trop Med Hyg* 27:1108, 1978.
23. Cossio PM, Diez C, Szarfman A, et al: Chagasic cardiopathy: demonstration of a serum gamma globulin factor which reacts with endocardium and vascular structures, *Circulation* 49:13, 1974.
24. Cossio PM, Laguens RP, Diez C, et al: Antibodies reacting with plasma membrane of striated muscle and endothelial cells, *Circulation* 50:1252, 1974.
25. Szarfman A, Cossio PM, Arana RM, et al: Immunologic and immunopathologic studies in congenital Chagas' disease, *Clin Immunol Immunopathol* 4:489, 1975.
26. Vasquez AD: Doctoral thesis, Universidad del los Andes, Venezuela, 1959.
27. Saleme A, Yanicelli GL, Iñigo LA, et al: Enfermedad de Chagas-Mazza congenita en Tucuman, *Arch Argent Pediatr* 59:162, 1971.
28. Bittencourt AL, Mota E, Ribeiro Filho R, et al: Incidence of congenital Chagas' disease in Bahia, Brazil, *J Trop Pediatr* 31:242, 1985.
29. De Rissio AM, Riarte AR, Garcia MM, et al: Congenital *Trypanosoma cruzi* infection. Efficacy of its monitoring in an urban reference health center in a non-endemic area of Argentina, *Am J Trop Med Hyg* 82:838, 2010.
30. Bekemans J, Truyens C, Torrico F, et al: Maternal *Trypanosoma cruzi* infection upregulated capacity of uninfected neonate cells to produce pro- and anti-inflammatory cytokines, *Infect Immun* 68:5430, 2000.
31. Cuna WR, Choque AG, Passera R, et al: Pro-inflammatory cytokine production in chagasic mothers and their uninfected newborns, *J Parasitol* 95:891, 2009.
32. Barousse AP, Eposto MO, Mandel S, et al: Enfermedad de Chagas congenita en area no endemica, *Medicina (B Aires)* 38:611, 1978.
33. Blanco SB, Segura EL, Gurtler RE: Control of congenital transmission of *Trypanosoma cruzi* in Argentina, *Medicina (B Aires)* 59(Suppl 2):138, 1999.
34. Stagno S, Hurtado R: Enfermedad de Chagas congenita: studio immunologico y diagnostico mediante immunofluorescencia con anti IgM, *Bol Chil Parasitol* 26:20, 1971.
35. Bittencourt AL, Barbosa HS, Santos I, et al: Incidencia da transmissão congenita da doença de Chagas em partos a termo, *Rev Inst Med Trop São Paulo* 16:197, 1974.

36. Rubio M, Howard BJ: Enfermedad de Chagas congenita. II. Halazgo anatomopatologico en 9 casos, *Bol Chil Parasitol* 23:113, 1968.
37. Azogue E, LaFuente C, Darras C: Congenital Chagas' disease in Bolivia: epidemiological aspects and pathological findings, *Trans R Soc Trop Med Hyg* 79:176, 1985.
38. Yadon ZE, Schmunis GA: Congenital Chagas disease: estimating the potential risk in the United States, *Am J Trop Med Hyg* 81:927, 2010.
39. Howard JE: *La enfermedad de Chagas congenita [thesis]*, Santiago, Chile, 1962, Universidad de Chile.
40. Bittencourt AL, Vieira GO, Tavares HC, et al: Esophageal involvement in congenital Chagas' disease, *Am J Trop Med Hyg* 33:30, 1984.
41. Bittencourt AL, Rodrigues de Freitas LA, Galvão de Araujo MO, et al: Pneumonitis in congenital Chagas' disease: a study of ten cases, *Am J Trop Med Hyg* 30:38, 1981.
42. Hoff R, Mott KE, Milanesi ML: Congenital Chagas' disease in an urban population: investigation of infected twins, *Trans R Soc Trop Med Hyg* 72:247, 1978.
43. Virreira M, Martinez S, Alonso-Vega C, et al: Amniotic fluid is not useful for diagnosis of congenital *Trypanosoma cruzi* infection, *Am J Trop Med Hyg* 75:1082, 2006.
44. Feilij H, Muller L, Gonzalez Cappa SM: Direct micromethod for diagnosis of acute and congenital Chagas' disease, *J Clin Microbiol* 18:327, 1983.
45. Reyes MB, Lorca M, Muñoz P, et al: Fetal IgG specificities against *Trypanosoma cruzi* antigens in infected newborns, *Proc Natl Acad Sci U S A* 87:2846, 1990.
46. Blanco SB, Segura EL, Cura EN, et al: Congenital transmission of *Trypanosoma cruzi*: an operational outline for detecting and treating infected infants in north-western Argentina, *Trop Med Int Health* 5:293, 2000.
47. Bittencourt AL, Gomes MC: Gestacoes sucessivas de uma paciente chagasica com ocorrencia de casos de transmissao congenital da doença, *Rev Med Bahia* 67:166, 1967.
48. Moya PR, Paolasso RD, Blanco S, et al: Tratamiento de la enfermedad de Chagas con Nifurtimox durante los primeros meses de vida, *Medicina (B Aires)* 45:553, 1985.
49. Lingam S, Marshall WC, Wilson J, et al: Congenital trypanosomiasis in a child born in London, *Dev Med Child Neurol* 27:664, 1985.
50. Reinhardt MC, Macleod CL: *Parasitic infections in pregnancy and the newborn*, New York, 1988, Oxford University Press.
51. Armon PJ: Amoebiasis in pregnancy and the puerperium, *Br J Obstet Gynaecol* 85:264, 1978.
52. Abioye AA: Fatal amoebic colitis in pregnancy and puerperium: a new clinico-pathological entity, *J Trop Med Hyg* 76:97, 1973.
53. Czeizel E, Hancsók M, Palkovich I, et al: Possible relation between fetal death and *E. histolytica* infection of the mother, *Am J Obstet Gynecol* 96:264, 1966.
54. Dykes AC, Ruebush TK 2nd, Gorelkin L, et al: Extraintestinal amebiasis in infancy: report of three patients and epidemiologic investigations of their families, *Pediatrics* 65:799, 1980.
55. Botman T, Ruys PJ: Amoebic appendicitis in a newborn infant, *Trop Geogr Med* 15:221, 1963.
56. Axton JHM: Amoebic proctocolitis and liver abscess in a neonate, *S Afr Med J* 46:258, 1972.
57. Dreyfuss ML, Msamanga GI, Spiegelman D, et al: Determinants of low birth weight among HIV-infected pregnant women in Tanzania, *Am J Clin Nutr* 74:814, 2001.
58. Millner DA Jr, Montgomery J, Seydel KB, et al: Severe malaria in children and pregnancy: an update and perspective, *Trends Parasitol* 24:590, 2008.
59. Conroy AL, McDonald CR, Kain KC: Malaria in pregnancy: diagnosing infection and identifying fetal risk, *Expert Rev Anti Infect Ther* 10:1331, 2012.
60. World Health Organization: *WHO Global Malaria Programme*, World Malaria Report 2008. Geneva, 2008, World Health Organization.
61. World Health Organization: *World malaria report*, Geneva, 2013, World Health Organization. Available at http://www.who.int/malaria/publications/world_malaria_report_2013/wmr2013_no_profiles.pdf?ua=1. Accessed October 13, 2014.
62. Young MD: Malaria. In Hunter GW 3rd, Schwartzwelder JC, Clyde F, editors: *Tropical medicine*, Philadelphia, 1976, WB Saunders, p 353.
63. Shulman IA, Saxena S, Nelson JM, et al: Neonatal exchange transfusions complicated by transfusion-induced malaria, *Pediatrics* 73:330, 1984.
64. Piccoli DA, Perlman S, Ephros M: Transfusion-acquired *Plasmodium malariae* infection in two premature infants, *Pediatrics* 72:560, 1983.
65. Sinclair S, Mittal SK, Singh M: Neonatal transfusion malaria, *Indian Pediatr* 8:219, 1971.
66. Ghosh S, Patwari A, Mohan M, et al: Clinical and hematologic peculiarities of malaria in infancy, *Clin Pediatr (Phila)* 17:369, 1978.
67. Keitel HG, Goodman HC, Havel RJ, et al: Nephrotic syndrome in congenital quartan malaria, *JAMA* 161:521, 1956.
68. Bray RS, Anderson MJ: Falciparum malaria and pregnancy, *Trans R Soc Trop Med Hyg* 73:427, 1979.
69. Reinhardt MC, Ambroise-Thomas P, Cavallo-Serra R, et al: Malaria at delivery in Abidjan, *Helv Paediatr Acta* 33(Supp. 41):65, 1978.
70. Cannon DSH: Malaria and prematurity in the western region of Nigeria, *Br Med J* 2:877, 1958.
71. Gilles HM, Lawson JB, Sibelas M, et al: Malaria, anaemia and pregnancy, *Ann Trop Med Parasitol* 63:245, 1969.
72. McGregor I: Epidemiology, malaria and pregnancy, *Am J Trop Med Hyg* 33:517, 1984.
73. Campbell CC, Martinez JM, Collins WE: Seroepidemiological studies of malaria in pregnant women and newborns from coastal El Salvador, *Am J Trop Med Hyg* 29:151, 1980.
74. Bruce-Chwatt LJ: Malaria in African infants and children in southern Nigeria, *Ann Trop Med Parasitol* 46:173, 1952.
75. Taufa T: Malaria and pregnancy, *P N G Med J* 21:197, 1978.
76. Jelliffe EFP: Low birth-weight and malarial infection of the placenta, *Bull World Health Organ* 38:69, 1968.
77. Shulman CE, Dorman EK: Importance and prevention of malaria in pregnancy, *Trans R Soc Trop Med Hyg* 97:30, 2003.
78. Torpin R: Malaria complicating pregnancy with a report of 27 cases, *Am J Obstet Gynecol* 41:882, 1941.
79. Hung LV: [Malaria and pregnancy in Saigon], *Rev Palud Med Trop* 83:75, 1951.
80. Spita AJ: Malaria infection of the placenta and its influence on the incidence of prematurity in eastern Nigeria, *Bull World Health Organ* 21:242, 1959.
81. Jelliffe EFP: *1967 Placental malaria and foetal growth. Nutrition and infection*, London, 1967, CIBA Foundation Study Group No. 31, J&A Churchill, p 18.
82. Archibald HM: The influence of malarial infection of the placenta on the incidence of prematurity, *Bull World Health Organ* 15:842, 1956.
83. MacGregor JD, Avery JG: Malaria transmission and fetal growth, *Br Med J* 3:433, 1974.
84. Larkin GL, Thuma PE: Congenital malaria in a hyperendemic area, *Am J Trop Med Hyg* 45:587, 1991.
85. Dubowitz LMS, Dubowitz V, Goldberg G: Clinical assessment of gestational age in the newborn infant, *J Pediatr* 77:1, 1970.
86. Blacklock DB, Gordon RM: Malaria parasites in the placental blood, *Ann Trop Med Parasitol* 19:37, 1925.
87. Steketee RW, Nahlen BL, Parise ME, et al: The burden of malaria in pregnancy in malaria-endemic areas, *Am J Trop Med Hyg* 64(Suppl 1-2):28, 2001.
88. Schmiegelow C, Minja D, Oesterholt M, et al: Malaria and fetal growth alterations in the 3rd trimester of pregnancy: a longitudinal ultrasound study, *PLoS One* 8:e53794, 2013.
89. Meno R: Pregnancy and malaria, *Med J Malaysia* 27:115, 1972.
90. Covell G: Congenital malaria, *Trop Dis Bull* 47:1147, 1950.
91. McGregor IA: Immunity to plasmodial infections; consideration of factors relevant to malaria in man, *Int Rev Trop Med* 4:1, 1971.
92. Molineaux L, Cornille-Brögger R, Mathews HM, et al: Longitudinal serological study of malaria in infants in the West African savanna, *Bull World Health Organ* 56:573, 1978.
93. Mathews HM, Lobel HO, Breman JG: Malarial antibodies measured by the indirect hemagglutination test in West African children, *Am J Trop Med Hyg* 25:217, 1976.
94. Sehgal VM, Siddiqui WA, Alpers MP: A seroepidemiological study to evaluate the role of passive maternal immunity to malaria in infants, *Trans R Soc Trop Med Hyg* 83:105, 1989.
95. Gilles HM: The development of malarial infection in breast-fed Gambian infants, *Ann Trop Med Parasitol* 51:58, 1957.
96. Allison AC: Genetic factors in resistance to malaria, *Ann N Y Acad Sci* 91:710, 1961.
97. Allison AC: Malaria in carriers of the sickle cell trait and in newborn children, *Exp Parasitol* 6:418, 1957.

98. Le Hesran JY, Cot M, Personne P, et al: Maternal placental infection with *Plasmodium falciparum* and malaria morbidity during the first two years of life, *Am J Epidemiol* 146:826, 1997.
99. Hindi RD, Azimi PH: Congenital malaria due to *Plasmodium falciparum*, *Pediatrics* 66:977, 1980.
100. Harvey B, Remington JS, Sulzer AJ: IgM malaria antibodies in a case of congenital malaria in the United States, *Lancet* 1:333, 1969.
101. Williams AIO, McFarlane H: Immunoglobulin levels, malarial antibody titres and placental parasitaemia in Nigerian mothers and neonates, *Afr J Med Sci* 1:369, 1970.
102. Kortmann HF: *Malaria and pregnancy [thesis]*, Utrecht, Netherlands, 1972, Manuel Drukkrig Elinkwijk.
103. Schwetz J, Peel M: Congenital malaria and placental infections amongst the Negroes of Central Africa, *Trans R Soc Trop Med Hyg* 28:167, 1934.
104. Lehner PJ, Andrews CJ: Congenital malaria in Papua New Guinea, *Trans R Soc Trop Med Hyg* 82:822, 1988.
105. Davies HD, Keystone J, Lester ML, et al: Congenital malaria in infants of asymptomatic women, *Can Med Assoc J* 146:1755, 1992.
106. Dianto RTH: Congenital falciparum malaria with chloroquine resistance type II, *Paediatr Indones* 29:237, 1989.
107. Chabasse D, De Gentile L, Ligny C, et al: Chloroquine-resistant *Plasmodium falciparum* in Mali revealed by congenital malaria, *Trans R Soc Trop Med Hyg* 82:547, 1988.
108. Airede AI: Congenital malaria with chloroquine resistance, *Ann Trop Paediatr* 11:267, 1991.
109. Centers for Disease Control and Prevention: Congenital malaria infection in an infant born to a Kampuchean refugee, *MMWR Morb Mortal Wkly Rep* 29:3, 1980.
110. Hulbert TV: Congenital malaria in the United States: report of a case and review, *Clin Infect Dis* 14:922, 1992.
111. Thomas V, Wing Chit C: A case of congenital malaria in Malaysia with IgM malaria antibodies, *Trans R Soc Trop Med Hyg* 74:73, 1980.
112. McQuay RM, Silberman S, Mudrik P, et al: Congenital malaria in Chicago: a case report and a review of published reports (U.S.A.), *Am J Trop Med* 16:258, 1967.
113. Dhatt PS, Singh H, Singhal SC, et al: A clinicopathological study of malaria in early infancy, *Indian Pediatr* 26:331, 1979.
114. Olowu WA, Torimiro SE: Congenital malaria in 8 hours old newborn: case report, *Niger J Med* 11:81, 2002.
115. Subramanian D, Moise KJ, White AC: Imported malaria in pregnancy: report of four cases and review of management, *Clin Infect Dis* 15:408, 1992.
116. Centers for Disease Control and Prevention: Guidelines for treatment of malaria in the United States. Available at http://www.cdc.gov/malaria/resources/pdf/treatmenttable.pdf. Accessed February 2, 2014.
117. Malaria LH: In Hoeprich PD, editor: *Infectious diseases: a modern treatise of infectious processes*, ed 2, Hagerstown, Md, 1977, Harper & Row, p 1075.
118. World Health Organization: Overview of malaria treatment. Available at http://www.who.int/malaria/areas/treatment/overview/en/index.html. Accessed February 2, 2014.
119. Brabin BJ, Warsame M, Uddenfeldt-Wort U, et al: Monitoring and evaluation of malaria in pregnancy—developing a rational basis for control, *Malar J* 7(Suppl 1):S6, 2008.
120. World Health Organization/Regional Office for Africa: A strategic framework for malaria prevention and control during pregnancy in the African region, Brazzaville, 2004, Republic of the Congo, World Health Organization/Regional Office for Africa.
121. World Health Organization (WHO) Global Malaria Programme, WHO Department of Reproductive Health and Research, WHO Department of Maternal, Newborn, Child and Adolescent Health: WHO policy brief for the implementation of intermittent preventive treatment of malaria in pregnancy using sulfadoxine-pyrimethamine (IPTpSP). Available at http://www.who.int/malaria/publications/atoz/Policy_brief_IPTp-SP_implementation_11april2013.pdf. Accessed February 2, 2014.
122 Garner P, Gulmezoglu AM: Drugs for preventing malaria in pregnant women, *Cochrane Database Syst Rev* (4):CD000169, 2006.
123. Quinn TC, Jacobs RF, Mertz GJ, et al: Congenital malaria: a report of four cases and a review, *J Pediatr* 101:229, 1982.
124. Watkinson M, Rushton DI: Plasmodial pigmentation of placenta and outcome of pregnancy in West African mothers, *Br Med J (Clin Res Ed)* 287:251, 1983.
125. Morley D, Woodland M, Cuthbertson WFJ: Controlled trial of pyrimethamine in pregnant women in an African village, *Br Med J* 1:667, 1964.
126. Harpy JP, Darbois Y, Lefebvre G: Teratogenicity of pyrimethamine, *Lancet* 2:399, 1983.
127. Peters PJ, Thigpen MC, Parise ME, et al: Safety and toxicity of sulfadoxine/pyrimethamine: implications for malaria prevention in pregnancy using intermittent preventive treatment, *Drug Safety* 30:481, 2007.
128. Hart CW, Naunton RF: The ototoxicity of chloroquine phosphate, *Arch Otolaryngol* 80:407, 1964.
129. Parke A: Antimalarial drugs and pregnancy, *Am J Med* 85(Suppl 4A):30, 1988.
130. Levy M, Buskila D, Gladman DD, et al: Pregnancy outcome following first trimester exposure to chloroquine, *Am J Perinatol* 8:174, 1991.
131. Wolfe MS, Cordero JF: Safety of chloroquine in chemosuppression of malaria during pregnancy, *Br Med J (Clin Res Ed)* 290:1466, 1985.
132. Uche-Nwachi EO: Effect of intramuscular sulfadoxine-pyrimethamine on pregnant Wistar rats, *Anat Rec* 250:426, 1998.
133. Vanhauwere B, Maradi H, Kerr L: Post-marketing surveillance of prophylactic mefloquine (Lariam) use in pregnancy, *Am J Trop Med Hyg* 58:17, 1998.
134. Smoak BL, Writer JV, Keep LW, et al: The effects of inadvertent exposure of mefloquine chemoprophylaxis on pregnancy outcomes and infants of US Army servicewomen, *J Infect Dis* 176:831, 1997.
135. Centers for Disease Control and Prevention: *Malaria*. Available at http://wwwnc.cdc.gov/travel/yellowbook/2014/chapter-3-infectious-diseases-related-to-travel/malaria. Accessed February 2, 2014.
136. Katz M: Treatment of protozoan infections: malaria, *Pediatr Infect Dis* 2:475, 1983.
137. Dame JB, Williams JL, McCutchan TF, et al: Structure of the gene and coding the immunodominant surface antigen of the sporozoite of the human malarial parasite, *Science* 225:593, 1984.
138. Enea V, Ellis J, Zavala F, et al: DNA cloning of *Plasmodium falciparum* circumsporozoite gene: amino acid sequence of repetitive epitope, *Science* 225:628, 1984.
139. Soares IS, Rodrigues MM: Malaria vaccine: roadblocks and possible solutions, *Braz J Med Biol Res* 31:317, 1998.
140. Graves PM: Comparison of the cost-effectiveness of vaccines and insecticide impregnation of mosquito nets for the prevention of malaria, *Ann Trop Med Parasitol* 92:399, 1996.
141. Moorthy VS, Good MF, Hill AV: Malaria vaccine developments, *Lancet* 363:150, 2004.
142. Davison BB, Cogswell FB, Baskin GB, et al: *Plasmodium coatneyi* in the rhesus monkey *(Macaca mulatta)* as a model of malaria in pregnancy, *Am J Trop Med Hyg* 59:189, 1998.
143. von Seidlein L, Bejon P: Malaria vaccines: past, present and future, *Arch Dis Child* 98:981, 2013.
144. RTS,S Clinical Trials Partnership, Agnandji ST Lell B, et al: A phase 3 trial of RTS,S/AS01 malaria vaccine in African infants, *N Engl J Med* 367:2284, 2012.
145. Brahmbhatt H, Kigozi G, Wabwire-Mangen F, et al: The effects of placental malaria on mother-to-child HIV transmission in Rakai Uganda, *AIDS* 17:2539, 2003.
146. Ladner J, Leroy V, Karita E, et al: Malaria, HIV and pregnancy, *AIDS* 17:275, 2003.
147. van Eijk AM, Ayisi JG, ter Kuile FO, et al: HIV increases the risk of malaria in women of all gravidities in Kisumu, Kenya, *AIDS* 17:595, 2003.
148. Briand V, Badaut C, Cot M: Placental malaria, maternal HIV infection and infant morbidity, *Ann Trop Paediatr* 29:71, 2009.
149. Ticconi C, Mapfumo M, Dorrucci M, et al: Effect of maternal HIV and malaria infection on pregnancy and perinatal outcome in Zimbabwe, *J Acquir Immune Defic Syndr* 34:289, 2003.
150. Bullough CHW: Infertility and bilharziasis of the female genital tract, *Br J Obstet Gynaecol* 83:819, 1976.
151. Poggensee G, Kiwelu I, Saria M, et al: Schistosomiasis of the lower reproductive tract without egg excretion in urine, *Am J Trop Med Hyg* 59:782, 1998.
152. Renaud R, Carrie J, Brettes JP, et al: Placental bilharziasis, *Int J Gynaecol Obstet* 10:25, 1972.

153. Bittencourt AL, Cardoso de Almeida MA, Iunes MA, et al: Placental involvement in schistosomiasis mansoni, *Am J Trop Med Hyg* 29:571, 1980.
154. Ross SM, Van Middelkoop A: *Trichomonas* infection in pregnancy—does it affect perinatal outcome? *S Afr Med J* 63:566, 1983.
155. Franjola RT, Añazco R, Puente R, et al: *Trichomonas vaginalis* en embarazadas y en recien nacidos, *Rev Med Chil* 117:142, 1989.
156. Carter JE, Whithaus KC: Neonatal respiratory tract involvement by *Trichomonas vaginalis*: a case report and review of the literature, *Am J Trop Med Hyg* 78:17, 2008.
157. McLaren LC, Davis LE, Healy GR, et al: Isolation of *Trichomonas vaginalis* from the respiratory tract of infants with respiratory disease, *Pediatrics* 71:888, 1983.
158. Hiemstra I, Van Bel F, Berger HM: Can *Trichomonas vaginalis* cause pneumonia in newborn babies? *Br Med J (Clin Res Ed)* 289:355, 1984.
159. Al-Salihi FL, Curran JP, Wang JS: Neonatal *Trichomonas vaginalis*: report of three cases and review of the literature, *Pediatrics* 53:196, 1974.
160. Feo LG: The incidence of *Trichomonas vaginalis* in the various age groups, *Am J Trop Med* 5:786, 1956.
161. Trussell RE, Wilson Mary E: Vaginal trichomoniasis: complement fixation, puerperal morbidity and early infection of newborn infants, *Am J Obstet Gynecol* 44:292, 1942.
162. Komorowska A, Kurnatowska A, Liniecka J: Occurrence of *Trichomonas vaginalis* (Donne) in girls in relation to hygiene conditions, *Wiad Parazytol* 8:247, 1962.
163. Danesh IS, Stephen JM, Gorbach J: Neonatal *Trichomonas vaginalis* infection, *J Emerg Med* 13:1, 1995.
164. Littlewood JM, Kohler HG: Urinary tract infection by *Trichomonas vaginalis* in a newborn baby, *Arch Dis Child* 41:693, 1966.
165. Postlethwaite RJ: *Trichomonas vaginitis* and *Escherichia coli* urinary infection in a newborn infant, *Clin Pediatr (Phila)* 14:866, 1975.
166. Dagenais-Perusse P, Baril E, Ouadahi S, et al: Vaginite á trichomonas du nourrison, *Union Med Can* 93:1228, 1964.
167. Crowther IA: *Trichomonas* vaginitis in infancy, *Lancet* 1:1074, 1962.
168. Kuitunen-Ekbaum E: The incidence of trichinosis in humans in Toronto: findings in 420 autopsies, *Can Public Health J* 32:569, 1941.
169. McNaught JB, Anderson EV: The incidence of trichinosis in San Francisco, *JAMA* 107:1446, 1936.
170. Salzer BF: A study of an epidemic of 14 cases of trichinosis with cures by serum therapy, *JAMA* 67:579, 1916.
171. Hood M, Olson SW: Trichinosis in the Chicago area, *Am J Hyg* 29:51, 1939.
172. Raucher HS, Jaffin H, Glass JL: Babesiosis in pregnancy, *Obstet Gynecol* 63:75, 1984.
173. Fox LM, Wingerter S, Ahmed A, et al: Neonatal babesiosis: case report and review of the literature, *Pediatr Infect Dis J* 25:169, 2006.
174. Hughes WT: *Pneumocystis carinii* vs. *Pneumocystis jiroveci*: another misnomer (response to Stringer et al), *Emerg Infect Dis* 9:276, 2003.
175. Wakefield AE, Banerji S, Pixley FJ, et al: Molecular probes for the detection of *Pneumocystis carinii*, *Trans R Soc Trop Med Hyg* 84(Suppl 1):17, 1990.
176. Li J, Edlind T: Phylogeny of *Pneumocystis carinii* based on β-tubulin sequence, *J Eukaryotic Microbiol* 41:97S, 1994.
177. Mazars E, Odberg-Ferragut C, Dei-Cas E: Polymorphism of the thymidylate synthase gene of *Pneumocystis carinii* from different host species, *J Eukaryot Microbiol* 42:26, 1995.
178. Ma L, Kovacs JA: Expression and characterization of recombinant human-derived *Pneumocystis carinii* dihydrofolate reductase, *Antimicrob Agents Chemother* 44:3092, 2000.
179. Banerji S, Lugli EB, Miller RF, et al: Analysis of genetic diversity at the arom locus in isolates of *Pneumocystis carinii*, *J Eukaryot Microbiol* 42:675, 1995.

33 Candidiasis

CATHERINE M. BENDEL

CHAPTER OUTLINE

Candida species are important pathogens in the neonate. After a significant increase in the incidence of systemic candidiasis in neonatal intensive care (NICU) patients in the late 1990s, since 2000 the incidence has remained stable or even decreased slightly.[1-4] However, this has clearly become a disease of the extremely-low-birth-weight (ELBW; birth weight ≤ 1000 g) or medically complex larger infant.[5-8] Infections range from superficial colonization to widely disseminated, life-threatening disease. Unfortunately, the most dramatic rise has been in the incidence of invasive or systemic candidiasis. With improvements in technology, more aggressive approaches to the treatment of very-low-birth-weight (VLBW; ≤1500 g) infants have become the standard of care. Concomitantly, there has been an increase in risk factors for neonates to develop candidemia, most notably the prolonged use of indwelling intravascular catheters and multiple courses of broad-spectrum antimicrobial agents.[6,9]

Candida albicans remains the most frequently isolated yeast species among infected neonates; however, the incidence of infection with other species, particularly *Candida parapsilosis* and *Candida glabrata*, has increased exponentially over the past 10 years.[4,10,11] The importance of *Candida* as a pathogen in VLBW infants is reflected by a mortality rate approaching 30% in this fragile group of immunocompromised patients, even among those who receive appropriate antifungal therapy, and a significant accompanying morbidity among survivors.[11-13]

Epidemiology and Transmission

Infections with *Candida* spp. afflict neonates, immunocompromised hosts, diabetics, trauma patients, postoperative patients (particularly after gastrointestinal procedures), and are most often nosocomially acquired.[1,7,13,14] The SENTRY Antimicrobial Surveillance Program, monitoring bloodstream infections caused by both *Candida* spp. and bacteria among all patients in participating hospitals, reports *Candida* spp. as the fourth most common nosocomial bloodstream infection overall, with *C. albicans* the most common single pathogen.[13,15] In neonates, the numbers are equally striking. Approximately 1% of early-onset neonatal infections result from *Candida* spp.; for late-onset sepsis, center-specific incidence reports vary from 2% to 28%, with combined study averages of 5% to 10% among the VLBW infants and 8% to 15% for the ELBW infants .[7,9,16-19] Among hospitals participating in the Neonatal Institute of Child Health and Human Development (NICHD) National Research Network, *C. albicans* was the third most frequent single organism isolated among all pathogens responsible for late-onset sepsis.[5]

Although *C. albicans* remains the leading cause of disseminated fungal infection among hospitalized patients, the isolation of other yeast species, including *C. glabrata*, *C. parapsilosis*, *Candida tropicalis*, *Candida krusei*, *Candida lusitaniae*, *Candida dubliniensis*, and even *Saccharomyces cerevisiae*, is occurring more frequently.[3,4,11,15,20] Table 33-1 displays the relative distribution of *Candida* spp. recovered from the bloodstream of all NICU patients in the National Nosocomial Infection Surveillance (NNIS) system compared with the overall population reported in the SENTRY program.[4,15] Among neonates, *C. albicans* and *C. parapsilosis* remain the predominant species compared with adults, in whom the predominant species isolated is *C. albicans*—responsible for approximately 50% of infections—followed by *C. parapsilosis* and *C. glabrata*, each of which accounts for approximately 15% of yeast infections.[11,15] Historically, *C. albicans* has been considered the most virulent species. A retrospective study of neonatal candidiasis before 2000 revealed a 24% mortality rate among infants infected with *C. albicans* but no deaths among those infected with *C. parapsilosis*.[21] However, more recent reports dispute this assumption: Overall, mortality rates have increased to 25% to 40% with *C. albicans* infections, and there has been an overall increase in infections with non–*Candida albicans Candida* (NCAC) spp., with mortality for neonates infected with *C. glabrata* and *C. parapsilosis* equivalent to that for *C. albicans* infections.[7,11,22,23] Although

Table 33-1 Frequency of Isolation of *Candida* Species Causing Candidemia Sepsis

	PERCENT OF BLOOD CULTURE ISOLATES	
***Candida* Species**	**Neonates***	**All Patients†**
C. albicans	58	50
C. parapsilosis	34	15
C. glabrata	2	18
C. tropicalis	4	10
Other species	2	7

*Data from Fridkin SK, Kaufman D, Edwards JR, et al: Changing incidence of *Candida* bloodstream infections among NICU patients in the United States: 1995-2004, *Pediatrics* 117:1680-1687, 2006.

†Data from Pfaller MA, Messer SA, Moet GJ, et al: *Candida* bloodstream infections: comparison of species distribution and resistance to echinocandin and azole antifungal agents in intensive care unit (ICU) and non-ICU settings in the SENTRY Antimicrobial Surveillance Program (2008-2009), *Int J Antimicrob Agents* 38:65-69, 2011.

C. albicans may be responsible for more infections than NCAC species, almost all *Candida* spp. have been implicated in disease, and any candidal infection in the neonate can be life threatening.

Candida spp. are commensal organisms, colonizing the human skin, gastrointestinal tract, and female genitourinary tract.[15,24,25] Studies evaluating gastrointestinal tract colonization document approximately 5% of neonates are colonized with *Candida* on admission to the NICU; up to 50% are colonized by the end of the first week and almost three fourths by the end of the first month of life.[26,27] A variety of *Candida* spp. colonize the human gastrointestinal tract, including *C. albicans, C. tropicalis, C. glabrata,* and *C. parapsilosis* in neonates.[27,28] More than one species may be recovered from a single host, but there is usually a predominant colonizing species.[29] The *Candida* strain colonizing the infant most often is acquired by vertical transmission from the maternal vaginal mucosa after passage through the birth canal.[29-31] Using molecular typing techniques, vertical transmission of *C. albicans, C. parapsilosis,* and *C. glabrata* has been documented in term and preterm infants.[29,30] Heavy maternal colonization or maternal *Candida* vaginitis is an important risk factor for efficient transmission, resulting in increased neonatal colonization and the potential for disease.[30-33] Intrauterine fetal infections occur rarely, but they have been attributed to ascending infection from the vagina of the mother and transplacental transmission.[34] Breastfeeding can result in transmission of yeast present on the maternal skin to the infant's oral mucosa, and *Candida* spp. have been recovered from expressed breast milk, although lactoferrin present in human milk can inhibit the growth of *C. albicans.*[35] Candidal mastitis increases the risk of transmission. Perinatal transmission can result in colonization, congenital candidiasis, or mucocutaneous infections in the term infant, whereas the result can be disseminated or systemic candidiasis in the preterm infant.[36]

Although maternal vertical transmission is more common, acquisition of *Candida* from care providers may occur and historically was considered the primary mode of transmission for *C. parapsilosis.*[26,29,30] In one study evaluating 19 mother-infant pairs, no maternal reservoir could be demonstrated among infants colonized with *C. parapsilosis.*[29] More recent studies have demonstrated maternal gastrointestinal colonization, highlighting the changing epidemiology as colonization rates alter with antimicrobial pressure.[33,37] After birth, NICU personnel, rather than the mother, may have the greatest contact with the preterm or sick infant. Because *C. parapsilosis* is the most common *Candida* spp. recovered from the hands of health care providers, transmission can be expected and may be a contributing factor to the increased incidence of *C. parapsilosis* catheter-associated infections in high-risk neonates.[38-41]

Colonization is important in the development of disease because the *Candida* strain recovered in infection usually is identical to the colonizing strain.[42,43] Disseminated infections result from translocation across the gastrointestinal tract epithelium of commensal *Candida* spp.[14,18,42] However, colonization does not inevitably lead to disease, and infection does occur in the absence of apparent colonization.[44] Direct transmission of *Candida* to NICU infants has been documented from exogenous yeast carried by hands of hospital personnel or found on equipment.[41,45,46] This emphasizes the need for proper hand hygiene among health care workers in the NICU. It is primarily the mechanical action of hand washing that decreases the burden of *Candida* spp. present because most of the antimicrobial soaps available are not fungicidal.[47] Vaudry and colleagues[48] described an outbreak of candidemia in seven infants without central intravascular catheters, and molecular typing of the *C. albicans* strains grouped the isolates into two cohorts corresponding with the timing of infections and the geographic location of babies in the nursery. The use of intravascular pressure-monitoring devices has been associated with *C. parapsilosis* fungemia in a NICU.[49] *Candida* infections have resulted from retrograde administration of medications by multiple-use syringes in infants receiving total parenteral nutrition; in these cases, the responsible organisms, *C. albicans, C. tropicalis,* and *C. parapsilosis,* were isolated from the blood of the infants and the medication syringe.[41] The outbreak subsided with a change to single-use syringes. A nursery outbreak of *Candida guilliermondii,* a typically nonpathogenic NCAC, was traced to contaminated heparin vials used for flushing needles for blood drawing.[49] All of these examples point to the ubiquitous nature of *Candida* spp. and the need for stringent infection control practices on the NICU to decrease the acquisition of nosocomial infections.[50,51]

Microbiology

The name *Candida* comes from the Latin term *candidus,* meaning "glowing white," which refers to the smooth, glistening white colonies formed by these yeasts when grown on culture media. The taxonomy of the genus *Candida* is somewhat challenging and incomplete because of the reclassification of certain species (e.g., *Torulopsis glabrata* has been correctly identified as *C. glabrata*) and the discovery of new species, such as *C. dubliniensis, Candida orthopsilosis,* and *Candida metapsilosis* (the last two previously classified as part of the *C. parapsilosis* complex).[52-54] Previously used terms, such as Fungi Imperfecti, *Oidium,* and *Monilia,* are no longer used in classifying the genus *Candida.* Fungi Imperfecti, or Deuteromycetes, refers to the class of fungi that reproduce asexually. This was the prevailing theory regarding *Candida*; however, a teleomorph, or sexual stage, has been described for certain *Candida* spp. (e.g., *C. krusei*, *C. guilliermondii*), eliminating this characteristic as a useful tool in classification.[55] *Oidium* and *Monilia* were 19th century terms that are no longer used to refer to the genus *Candida*, although the term monilial is still commonly used to describe the characteristic rash observed in cutaneous *Candida* infections.[55,56]

Although more than 150 species of *Candida* have been described, relatively few species infect humans. Most exist as environmental saprophytes, and more than one half the *Candida* spp. described cannot even grow at 37° C, making them unlikely candidates to be successful human pathogens.[55,56] *C. albicans* is the most prevalent species causing human disease, but other pathogenic species include *C. parapsilosis*, *C. glabrata*, *C. tropicalis*, *Candida pseudotropicalis*, *Candida paratropicalis*, *C. krusei*, *Candida lusitaniae*, *C. guilliermondii*, *C. dubliniensis*, and *C. orthopsilosis*. The primary pathogens among neonates are *C. albicans* and *C. parapsilosis* (see Table 33-1).

Members of the genus *Candida* are ubiquitous and form a heterogeneous group of eukaryotic, dimorphic, or polymorphic organisms. All *Candida* spp. grow as yeast cells or blastoconidia under general culture conditions between 25° C and 35° C, and growth is augmented by increased sugar or fat content in the media. Yeast cells are approximately 2 to 10 μm in the largest dimension, round to oval, and reproduce by budding. *C. albicans* is among the larger yeast at 4 to 6 × 6 to 10 μm, whereas *C. glabrata* and *C. parapsilosis* are among the smallest at 1 to 4 μm × 2 to 9 μm and 2 to 4 × 2 to 9 μm, respectively.[55] Figure 33-1A shows *C. albicans* single blastoconidia and budding yeast cells. Most members of the genus also produce a filamentous form: pseudohyphae (Fig. 33-1B) or true hyphae (Fig. 33-1C). *C. glabrata* is the only pathogenic species that does not produce filamentous forms, existing exclusively as blastoconidia.[55] *C. parapsilosis* forms pseudohyphae but not true hyphae. Only *C. dubliniensis* and *C. albicans* form true hyphae (see Fig. 33-1C), distinguishing these two species as polymorphic rather than dimorphic. Formation of a germ tube precedes the development of true hyphae, and this change in morphology can be induced by growth in serum or other specialized media or by incubation at 37° C. The clinical diagnostic microbiology laboratory has exploited this distinction by use of the germ tube formation test to rapidly identify *C. albicans* or *C. dubliniensis* over other *Candida* spp.[57]

The ability to form true hyphae is considered one of the prime virulence factors for *C. albicans*.[58] Microscopic examination of infected human and animal tissue usually demonstrates the presence of *C. albicans* hyphae.[59-62] Conversely, nonfilamentous yeast, such as *S. cerevisiae*, rarely cause human disease, and genetically altered strains of *C. albicans*, which cannot filament normally, are generally less virulent in animal models of fungemia.[63-65] Other commonly recognized virulence factors for *C. albicans* include the production of proteinases and phospholipases, hydrophobicity, the presence of various surface molecules (e.g., receptors, adhesions), and the production of biofilm, which may be particularly important in catheter-associated infections.[59,62,64,66,67]

A variety of surface molecules of *C. albicans* are responsible for modulating epithelial adhesion by interacting with host ligands on the epithelial or endothelial surface.[63,66]

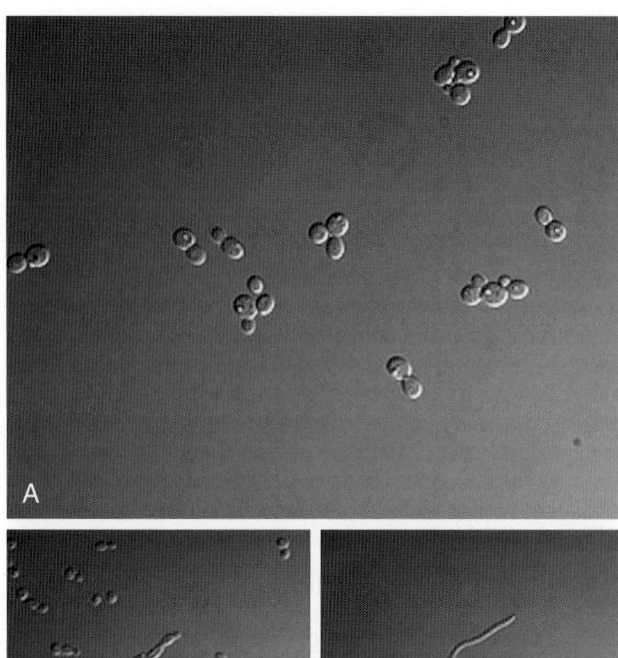

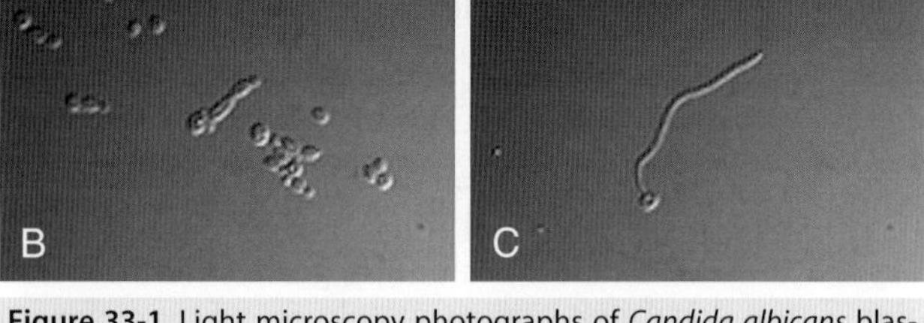

Figure 33-1 Light microscopy photographs of *Candida albicans* blastoconidia or yeast cells **(A)**, pseudohyphae **(B)**, and true hyphae **(C)**. (Courtesy Cheryl A. Gale, MD, University of Minnesota Medical School, Minneapolis.)

Ligands include sugar residues on human buccal epithelial cells and a wide variety of extracellular matrix proteins, such as fibronectin, fibrinogen, types I and IV collagen, laminin, and the complement components iC3b and C3d.[68] Reciprocally, human cells recognize yeast cell ligands via pattern recognition receptors, such as Toll-like receptors (TLR) or the β-glucan receptor (βGR) dectin-1.[69] In tissue culture assays, *C. albicans* is more adherent than other *Candida* spp. to every form of human epithelium and endothelium available, including cultured buccal epithelium, enterocytes (adult and fetal), cervical epithelium, and human umbilical vein endothelial cells.[32,70-72] The adhesive molecules responsible for epithelial and endothelial adhesion may also facilitate binding between individual *Candida* cells and the subsequent development of "fungus balls" found in infected organs.[68] No single adhesin molecule is completely responsible for the adherence of *C. albicans* to human epithelium, and multiple methods of interacting with the host surface are postulated for this commensal organism.[68] *C. albicans* and *C. parapsilosis* both adhere well to the surface of catheters and, in the process, form a biofilm, although the biofilms formed by *C. albicans* are more dense and complex than those formed by other *Candida* spp.[73,74] The biofilm microenvironment promotes fungal growth with hyphal transformation and may confer relative drug resistance because of poor penetration of antimicrobial agents into this mass of extracellular matrix, yeast cells, and hyphae.[67,73,75] In vitro studies of *C. albicans* biofilms document the development of fluconazole resistance within 6 hours of formation.[73] Biofilm formation is associated with persistent fungemia and with coinfection by nosocomial bacterial pathogens, such as *Staphylococcus* spp.[73,76,77] *Candida* spp. induce a strong TLR-mediated proinflammatory response in cultured oral epithelial cells, resulting in profound interleukin-8 secretion.[78,79] In addition, the βGR dectin-1 and Toll-like receptors TLR2 and TLR4 (thought to be the main receptors for the innate immune system recognition of *C. albicans*) appear to work synergistically, with dectin-1 amplifying tumor necrosis factor-α (TNF-α) production via the TLR pathway.[69] The ability to adhere to human epithelium and endothelium (and to itself and catheters), resulting in microenvironmental changes, is a significant virulence factor setting *C. albicans* apart from other *Candida* spp. and may be a prominent reason for the increased frequency with which *C. albicans* is found colonizing the host and causing disease at epithelial and endothelial sites.

Virulence factors of other *Candida* spp. have not been well studied. A fibronectin receptor that facilitates epithelial adhesion has been described in *C. tropicalis*.[66,80] *C. glabrata* colonizes the gastrointestinal tract, and this nonfilamentous *Candida* spp. can form biofilms.[75] *C. parapsilosis* has been recovered from the alimentary tract of neonates, but no work has been done to implicate or exclude the gastrointestinal tract as a possible source of infection among neonates, and no specific virulence factors have been identified in this *Candida* spp.[23,29,74] *C. glabrata* and *C. parapsilosis* produce biofilms; however, this area has not been well investigated for either of these pathogenic NCAC species.[67,74,81] Overall, *Candida* spp. exhibit relatively low-level virulence factors compared with organisms that typically cause disease in an immunocompetent host. Candidal virulence factors serve to differentiate the more virulent from the less virulent *Candida* spp., rather than to distinguish *Candida* from other more pathogenic microbes.

Pathogenesis

The pathogenesis of invasive candidiasis involves a common sequence of events in all at-risk hosts: colonization, resulting from adhesion of the yeast to the skin or mucosal epithelium (particularly the gastrointestinal tract); penetration of the epithelial barriers; and locally invasive or widely disseminated disease. Dissemination to deep visceral organs results from hematogenous spread.[14] However, not every colonized patient develops a *Candida* infection. The unique combination of host factors and yeast virulence mechanisms results in the persistence of benign colonization or the progression to infection among high-risk neonatal patients, as outlined in Figure 33-2. Yeast virulence factors were described in the preceding section. Host risk factors, listed in Box 33-1, are potentially more important in the development of neonatal candidal infections.[6,51,82] Limitation of exposure to all predisposing conditions for candidal infection is highly desirable but rarely feasible, especially in the VLBW infant. However, we should consider limiting any of these risk factors, if possible, in the ELBW infant. Benjamin and colleagues[7] have reported that the most significant "potentially modifiable" risk factors for invasive candidiasis are broad-spectrum antibiotic exposure (adjusted odds ratio [aOR], 1.98), central catheter in place (aOR, 1.94), intravenous lipid emulsion (aOR, 1.66), endotracheal tube in place (aOR, 1.58), and exposure to antenatal antibiotics (aOR, 1.40)]. They also reported the following "predictors" of invasive candidiasis: *Candida*-like dermatitis (aOR, 3.22), central catheter in place (aOR, 1.85), vaginal versus cesarean delivery (aOR, 1.84), enteral feeding (aOR, 1.52), lower gestational age (aOR, 1.29), hyperglycemia (aOR, 1.22), thrombocytopenia (aOR, 1.17), and antibiotic exposure in the week before infection (aOR, 1.13).[7]

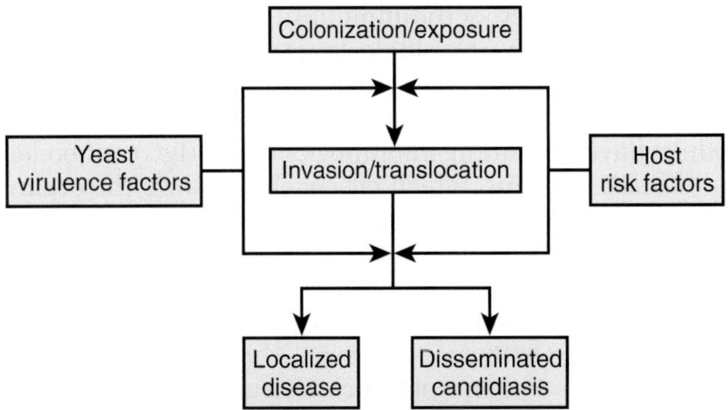

Figure 33-2 The pathogenesis of neonatal candidiasis follows a pathway from colonization to infection, modified by multiple host factors and yeast virulence factors.

Box 33-1 Host Factors Enhancing Risk for Candidiasis in Neonates

High burden of colonization with *Candida* species
Prematurity, especially gestational age < 28 weeks
Very low birth weight (<1500 g)
Apgar score < 5 at 5 minutes
Prolonged broad-spectrum antimicrobial therapy
Third-generation cephalosporin exposure
Indwelling catheters, especially central intravascular catheters
Total parenteral hyperalimentation > 5 days
Intravenous lipid emulsion > 7 days
Intubation
Exposure to an H2 blocker
Abdominal surgery
Necrotizing enterocolitis
Spontaneous intestinal perforation
Cardiac surgery
Prolonged hospitalization > 7 days
Steroid therapy
Neutropenia
Hyperglycemia

Indiscriminate, frequent, or prolonged use of broad-spectrum antimicrobial agents, resulting in alterations of the normal skin and intestinal microbial flora, allows overgrowth of the colonizing strain of *Candida* and a concomitant increased risk for translocation and hematogenous spread.[18] The greater the density of organisms in the neonatal gastrointestinal tract, the greater is the chance of dissemination.[83] High levels of *Candida* colonization found in certain nurseries are linked to patterns of antibiotic usage, including a particularly strong association with third-generation cephalosporin use.[26,43,84]

The immunocompromised state predisposes an infant to candidal infection, whether caused by the developmentally immature immune system of the newborn, a congenital immunodeficiency, or the immunosuppression accompanying steroid therapy. No single defect in the immune system appears to be solely responsible for an increased susceptibility of premature neonates to candidal infections. Healthy adults have circulating immunoglobulin G (IgG) antibodies to *Candida* antigens, which effectively opsonize the organism and activate the alternative complement pathway.[85] Neonatal IgG levels depend on maternal exposure to the yeast, accompanied by transplacental transmission of candidal antibodies, and the ability for the infant to respond to a new challenge with a *Candida* spp., which may be slow and inadequate.[86] Polymorphonuclear leukocytes ingest and kill *Candida*; therefore neutropenia is an important risk factor.[6,18] Disseminated candidiasis in neonates is associated with the intravenous administration of dexamethasone and hydrocortisone.[87,88] Steroid therapy results in immunosuppression and may have direct effects on colonization and translocation from the gastrointestinal tract. In vitro studies have shown that *C. albicans* is more adherent to monolayers of cultured enterocytes treated with dexamethasone than to untreated control monolayers, whereas mice injected with dexamethasone demonstrate higher levels of gastrointestinal tract colonization with *C. albicans* and increased rates of dissemination to the kidney.[61] Steroids may have a direct effect on the yeast by regulation of gene expression, including multidrug-resistance genes and other modulators of virulence.[89] The presence of indwelling catheters is a significant predisposing risk factor for neonatal candidiasis. Endotracheal tubes, urinary catheters, peritoneal catheters, chest tubes, mediastinal tubes, and ventriculoperitoneal shunts can all become infected, but the greatest risk lies with intravascular catheters, particularly central venous catheters (CVCs).[7,51,82] All catheters in the vascular space for more than a day begin to develop a thrombin sheath with a matrix-like substance providing an optimal site for accumulation of microorganisms.[73] *Candida* spp. adhere extremely well to the inert surface of the catheter, and electron microscopy studies have shown that *Candida* spp. are able to burrow into the catheter and form a surrounding biofilm.[73,90] This sequence results in a unique microenvironment, providing a barrier to host defenses and offering optimal conditions for growth and proliferation of the *Candida* organism, often resulting in the development of an infected mural thrombus extending from the tip of the catheter.[91-93] The "fungal mass" adherent to the catheter can then serve as a source for persistent fungemia or embolic spread of *Candida* spp. to distant organs.[1,18] The original source of the yeast that "sticks" to the line may be from hematogenous spread of endogenous gastrointestinal tract *Candida* strains or from nosocomial transmission through placement or handling of the catheter itself.[41,48] Use of the catheter for hyperalimentation is an additional risk, especially with the infusion of high-dextrose–containing total parenteral solutions and intralipids.[6,7,18] Any compromise of epithelial barriers can predispose the neonate to candidal infections. Abdominal surgery and cardiac surgery are associated with an increased risk for disseminated candidiasis, especially among term infants.[18,76] Necrotizing enterocolitis (NEC) is strongly associated with *Candida* fungemia.[6,7,14] The loss of mucosal integrity after mesenteric ischemia and NEC provides a portal of entry for the dissemination of endogenous gastrointestinal flora.[14] Spontaneous intestinal perforation, occurring most often in the extremely preterm infant, is highly associated with candidemia.[19,94] As with any nosocomially acquired organism, prolonged hospitalization is a significant risk factor for the development of candidiasis.[6,7,14,18]

Prematurity is a key risk factor for candidiasis, especially infants born at less than 28 weeks of gestation or VLBW neonates.[3,7,18] With improvements in technology, the current standard of care in the NICU includes an aggressive approach to the treatment of VLBW infants such that life for an extremely premature infant combines nearly all the risk factors for candidiasis in one patient.[7,18] The premature infant is born with immature epithelial barriers and an immature immune system. The skin and mucosal epithelium of these very tiny infants are minimally protective, readily breaking down with exposure to air and routine nursing procedures.[19,95,96] Preterm infants have the lowest levels of circulating maternal IgG of all neonates, having lost the opportunity for transplacental transfer that occurs during the third trimester of pregnancy.[97] Even if specific anti-*Candida* IgG is present, opsonization and complement activation are diminished.[85] Complement levels are low in preterm infants (see Chapter 4), with biochemical abnormalities of C3 resulting in inadequate activation of this pathway for fighting infections.[98] Neutropenia is common among infants born at less than 28 weeks of gestation.[99,100] Virtually every premature infant begins life with a course of empirical broad-spectrum antibiotics, leading to an interruption in the process of establishing the normal gastrointestinal microflora and the potential for unchecked proliferation of *Candida*.[36,100] Endotracheal and intravascular catheters are true lifelines for the VLBW premature infant needing respiratory, inotropic agent, and nutritional support. Because venous access is often difficult to obtain and maintain in these infants, intravascular access lines are not automatically rotated and frequently remain in place for weeks. Even the fairly healthy VLBW infant often displays feeding intolerance that can require prolonged central total parenteral nutrition (TPN) rather than enteral feeds.[6,7] As reported by the NICHD Neonatal Research Network, the aOR for any episode of late-onset sepsis is 3.1 in VLBW infants receiving TPN for 8 to14 days, rising to 4.0 for an infant receiving TPN for more than 22 days.[5] Saiman and colleagues[18] reported odds ratios for developing candidemia of 2.93 for infants less than 1000 g receiving TPN for more than 5 days and 2.91 for intravenous (IV) intralipid use for more than 7 days. Unfortunately, NEC may also accompany feeding intolerance, leading to an additional risk for disseminated candidiasis.[101,102] Corticosteroid use is also common in these patients.[87,88] Multiple reviews report that almost one half of the infants with a birth weight of less than 750 g are postnatally exposed to corticosteroids: hydrocortisone used to treat hypotension; dexamethasone, methylprednisolone, or hydrocortisone used for severe lung disease.[87,88,102] Hyperglycemia and hyperlipidemia are common in these immature patients receiving TPN, steroids, or both.[88] Prolonged length of stay is the rule rather than the exception for the NICU infant, with or without a nosocomially acquired infection. The average corrected gestational age at discharge from the NICU is between 35 and 37 weeks, and the average NICU hospitalization is approximately 62 days; however, the length of stay to achieve 36 weeks of gestational age is even longer for the infant born at less than 28 weeks of gestation.[5,18] Each of these factors, especially in combination, makes the VLBW preterm infant an extremely high-risk candidate for the development of candidiasis.

Pathology

The tissue pathology observed in *Candida* spp. infections depends on the site of involvement and the extent of invasion or dissemination. Histologic evaluation of mucosal or epithelial lesions reveals superficial ulcerations with the presence of yeast and filamentous forms of *Candida* spp., including a prominent polymorphonuclear (PMN) leukocyte infiltration.[96] ELBW infants can develop invasive fungal dermatitis with erosive lesions; biopsy of these lesions reveals invasion of fungal elements through the epidermis into the dermis.[19,96] In disseminated neonatal infections, *Candida* spp. can invade virtually any tissue. Microabscesses are commonly found in the kidney, retina, and brain, but they also have been described in the liver, spleen, peritoneum, heart, lungs, and joints.[96,103-105] When *C. albicans* is the infecting organism, abscesses contain a predominance of hyphal elements with a significant accompanying infiltration of PMNs and prominent tissue necrosis, especially in the kidney.[59,91,104] Mycelia are frequently found invading the walls of blood vessels within infected tissues.[13,60,104] Retinal lesions, vitreal fungal lesions, and even lens abscesses with cataract formation have been described in neonates.[106,107] Evaluation of brain material shows significant inflammation with seeding of the meninges and may include parenchymal lesions, ventriculitis, perivasculitis, and ependymal inflammation.[105,108-110] Macroscopic fungus balls can form in fluid-filled spaces lined with epithelial or endothelial cells, such as the urinary tract, the central nervous system (CNS), and the intravascular space (particularly the right atrium).[92,111] Fungus balls are large collections of intertwined hyphae, pseudohyphae, and yeast cells that presumably grow from *Candida* spp. initially adherent to the epithelial or endothelial surface of the involved organ.[104,112,113] Foreign bodies present in these fluid-filled spaces, such as urinary catheters, ventricular shunts, or CVCs, can also serve as the nidus for infection and precipitate the formation of a fungus ball.[92,103,104,112,113]

In intrauterine candidal infections, macroscopic chorioamnionitis is evident, and histologic examination of the fetal membranes and the chorionic plate often reveals fungal elements with an extensive PMN infiltration.[114] Along with diffuse placental inflammation, focal granulomatous lesions can be present in the chorioamniotic membranes and umbilical cord.[114-116] The detection of placental pathology consistent with candidal chorioamnionitis can lead to the early detection of congenital candidiasis in the infant.[114]

Clinical Manifestations

Candida spp. are responsible for a variety of infections in neonates with a broad spectrum of clinical presentations, ranging from mild, irritating thrush and diaper dermatitis in the healthy term infant to life-threatening systemic disease in the extremely premature infant. The primary forms of candidiasis among infants are mucocutaneous infections, congenital candidiasis, catheter-related candidemia, and systemic or disseminated candidiasis. Individual organ system involvement (e.g., urinary tract infection, isolated meningitis, endophthalmitis) can occur, but infection occurs much more often as a component of disseminated infection, especially in the premature infant. Table 33-2 lists features of the various presentations of neonatal candidiasis.

OROPHARYNGEAL CANDIDIASIS

Oropharyngeal candidiasis (i.e., thrush) can occur at any time during infancy. Among hospitalized infants, the overall incidence is reported as 3%, with a median age of onset of 9 to 10 days in NICU patients.[19,117,118] Specific risk factors include vaginal delivery, maternal vaginal *Candida* spp. infection, and birth asphyxia.[118,119] In a study of more than 500 mother-infant pairs, an eightfold increase was observed in the incidence of thrush among infants born to mothers with symptomatic candidal vaginitis compared with infants born to asymptomatic mothers.[119] A multivariate analysis of factors among NICU infants reported that birth asphyxia was the only event significantly associated with the development of thrush.[118] Although *Candida* spp. can be transmitted from mother to infant during breastfeeding, thrush occurs more often among formula-fed infants.[120] *C. albicans* is the most common species isolated from infants with thrush, but other NCAC species, such as *C. parapsilosis* and *C. glabrata*, increasingly are found as commensals and infecting agents.[120,121]

Thrush manifests as irregular white plaques on the oral mucosa, including the buccal and lingual surfaces and the palate. The underlying mucosa may appear normal or erythematous and may have an ulcerative base to the white lesion. Physical removal of the plaques usually is difficult and often results in mucosal damage. Infected infants can be healthy or quite irritable, with disinterest in oral feedings and obvious discomfort with any care involving contact with the oral lesions.

DIAPER DERMATITIS

Diaper dermatitis can occur any time during infancy, with a peak incidence at age 7 to 9 months in term infants (10% incidence) and approximately 10 to 11 weeks among VLBW infants (28% incidence).[28,36,122] Most infants with candidal diaper dermatitis have gastrointestinal colonization, with stool cultures positive for a *Candida* spp.[122] Some infants also have oropharyngeal candidiasis. *C. albicans* is the most common species isolated, but there has been an increase in the recovery of other NCAC species, particularly *C. glabrata* and *C. parapsilosis*, when cultures are obtained.[19]

The characteristic rash of candidal diaper dermatitis is confluent and intensely erythematous with satellite lesions and pustules.[19,122] As with oral thrush, the lesions can be very irritating to the infant, especially during normal perineal care. In the term infant, the rash resolves rapidly after treatment with an appropriate topical antifungal agent.[120]

Table 33-2 Features of Neonatal Candidiasis

Clinical Syndrome	Age at Onset	Host Risk Factors*	Presentation	Diagnosis	Treatment	Multiorgan Involvement	Prognosis
MUCOCUTANEOUS INFECTIONS							
Thrush	Throughout infancy	Birth asphyxia	White plaques on oral mucosa	Physical examination	Topical or oral antifungal therapy	None	Excellent
Diaper dermatitis	Throughout infancy; peak at 7-9 mo (term) and 10-11 wk (preterm)	Gastrointestinal colonization	Intense erythema of perineal area with satellite lesions	Physical examination	Topical antifungal therapy	None in term infants	Excellent
Congenital candidiasis	Birth	Premature rupture of membranes or uterine foreign body	Widespread erythematous maculopapular rash ± vesicles Pneumonia in preterm infants	Physical examination Culture of lesions for *Candida* spp.	Topical antifungal therapy Systemic antifungal therapy for pneumonia	Uncommon Dissemination can occur in preterm infants	Excellent in term infants; excellent in preterm infants without dissemination
Invasive fungal dermatitis	<2 weeks	<1000 g Vaginal delivery Postnatal steroids—hyperglycemia	Erosive, crusting lesions in dependent areas	Physical examination Biopsy and culture of lesions	Systemic antifungal therapy	Common	Good if localized without dissemination
SYSTEMIC INFECTIONS							
Catheter-related infections	>7 days	Intravascular catheters	Sepsis	Blood culture by catheter grows *Candida* spp. but peripheral blood cultures sterile	Catheter removal and systemic antifungal therapy	Rare endocarditis or right atrial mass or thrombus	Good without dissemination or complication
Candidemia	>7 days		Sepsis	Only blood cultures grow *Candida* spp.	Systemic antifungal therapy	Common in VLBW infants	Good to fair Risk of ROP in VLBW infants
Disseminated candidiasis	>7 days		Severe sepsis Multiorgan involvement	Blood and urine, CSF or other sites grow *Candida* spp. Clinical and/or radiographic evidence for multiorgan involvement	Systemic antifungal therapy	Always (sites most often involved are kidneys, CNS, eyes, heart)	Fair to poor
Renal candidiasis	>7 days	Congenital urinary tract anomalies Neurogenic bladder	Sepsis Urinary tract obstruction	Urine culture grows *Candida* spp. Ultrasound evidence of renal fungal lesions	Systemic antifungal therapy	Uncommon with isolated UTI	Good
CNS candidiasis	>7 days	Neural tube defects	Indwelling CSF shunt or catheter Sepsis None to focal neurologic signs	CSF culture grows *Candida* spp. CSF culture grows *Candida* spp. ± signs of inflammation; lesions by cranial imaging	Systemic antifungal therapy	Common	Poor

CNS, Central nervous system; *CSF*, cerebrospinal fluid; *ROP*, retinopathy of prematurity; *UTI*, urinary tract infection; *VLBW*, very low birth weight.
*Factors, in addition to those listed in Box 33-1, pertaining to the specific clinical syndrome listed.

The preterm infant has a greater risk for spread beyond the diaper area. In a prospective study, Faix and colleagues[117] found mucocutaneous disease in 7.8% of all preterm infants, and most had diaper dermatitis. Among preterm infants with dermatitis and an associated change in clinical status, 32% developed systemic disease compared with 2.1% of healthy preterm infants without dermatitis.[117] Therefore it is prudent to monitor the preterm infants with candidal diaper dermatitis for signs of systemic infection.

CONGENITAL CANDIDIASIS

Congenital candidiasis typically presents at birth or within the first 24 hours of life, resulting from a maternal intrauterine infection or from massive exposure to maternal vaginal colonization with *Candida* during labor and delivery.[114,115] *Candida* chorioamnionitis has been associated with intrauterine fetal death and preterm delivery.[115,123] Hematogenous dissemination from mother to fetus, direct invasion of intact membranes, and ascending infection after ruptured membranes have been postulated as mechanisms for intrauterine infection.[19,123] Recognized risk factors for congenital candidiasis differ from those associated with postnatal infection and include prolonged rupture of membranes and the presence of an intrauterine foreign body, most commonly a cerclage suture.[123,124] Infants with the latter risk factor are more likely to be born prematurely and to have more severe skin involvement with disseminated disease.[115,123] Although *C. albicans* is the predominant species responsible for congenital candidiasis, cases of congenital infections with *C. glabrata* and *C. parapsilosis* have been described.[19,124,125]

Although there are rare case reports of infants with congenital candidiasis without skin involvement, the classic presentation is one of diffuse cutaneous disease.[34,126] Dermatologic findings include a widespread erythematous maculopapular rash, often with well-demarcated borders, that evolves into vesicles or pustules with eventual desquamation.[124,126] Any part of the skin may be involved, including the palms and soles, but the lesions typically are more prominent in the skin folds or intertriginous areas.[19,127] Preterm infants can have a diffuse, widespread, intensely erythematous dermatitis that resembles a mild burn or the early stages of staphylococcal scalded skin syndrome.[19,96] This form of congenital candidiasis often leads to massive desquamation, often accompanied by a prominent leukocytosis.[34] Extensive desquamation can lead to severe fluid and electrolyte imbalances in the extremely premature infant.[34]

In term infants, clinical findings usually are limited to the skin, and recovery is uneventful after topical antifungal therapy. However, meningitis has been reported in the term infant with congenital candidiasis, and some infants may have nonspecific clinical signs of sepsis, such as poor perfusion, hypotonia, and temperature instability, suggesting systemic disease.[126,128] In preterm infants, cutaneous findings can be coupled with pulmonary invasion and early respiratory distress. In this circumstance, the chest radiograph is atypical for surfactant deficiency, and the expected ground-glass appearance is replaced by a nodular or alveolar infiltrate.[127] Hematogenous dissemination is uncommon, but it can occur more frequently among preterm neonates and infants with widespread cutaneous involvement, pulmonary disease, and central intravascular catheters.[124,126] Every attempt should be made to avoid placing central intravascular catheters through the infected skin of patients with congenital cutaneous candidiasis.

INVASIVE FUNGAL DERMATITIS

Invasive fungal dermatitis is a unique clinical entity described in the ELBW infant occurring during the first 2 weeks of life.[96,129] *Candida* spp. are frequently isolated, but infection with other filamentous non-*Candida* fungi, including species of *Aspergillus, Trichosporon, Curvularia*, and *Bipolaris*, can result in this clinical presentation.[96,130,131] Specific risk factors for invasive fungal dermatitis include a gestational age less than 26 weeks, vaginal birth, postnatal steroid administration, and hyperglycemia.[96] The immature skin of the extremely preterm infant is not an efficient barrier to the external invasion of *Candida*, making these neonates more susceptible to invasive cutaneous disease. The stratum corneum of the preterm infant is extremely thin, and keratinization with maturation of the barrier properties typically occurs beyond the second week of life.[124]

Neonates with invasive fungal dermatitis have characteristic skin lesions with severe erosions, serous drainage, and crusting, often occurring on dependent surfaces such as the back or abdomen.[96] Biopsy of the affected area shows invasion of fungal elements through the epidermis into the dermis.[96] Without prompt and appropriate therapy, dissemination with resulting widespread systemic disease is a frequent complication. As with congenital candidiasis, infants with extensive erosive lesions are at risk for the development of fluid and electrolyte abnormalities and secondary infections with other skin microorganisms.

CATHETER-RELATED CANDIDAL INFECTIONS

Catheter-related candidal infections are disease processes of the sick, hospitalized preterm or term infant requiring prolonged use of intravascular catheters or other invasive means of support.[7,18,51] Almost any type of indwelling foreign body can become infected, but vascular catheter-related candidemia is the most frequent and serious infection. The incidence increases after a central vascular catheter has been in place for more than 7 days. These infections have been associated with umbilical venous and arterial catheters and with percutaneously placed arterial or CVCs (i.e., femoral venous, subclavian, Broviac, or Silastic lines).[6,50] Peripheral venous catheters have the same potential for fungemia in the premature infant, especially when used for the delivery of hyperalimentation fluid, and have been associated with the development of skin abscesses at the insertion site.[132,133] Catheter-related *Candida* infection can occur in the absence of cutaneous infection in neonates with one or more of the predisposing conditions listed in Box 33-1, and the infection can arise from endogenous gastrointestinal organisms or from nosocomial transmission. Infected neonates exhibit nonspecific signs of sepsis, including feeding intolerance, apnea, hyperglycemia, and temperature instability, but no evidence of multiorgan involvement. Preterm infants also may exhibit hemodynamic instability or respiratory distress. Thrombocytopenia is a common presenting feature.[3,134] The vascular catheter tip provides an excellent nidus for growth of *Candida* and affords a source of ongoing fungemia. An infected thrombus or fungus ball can form on the catheter tip, serving as a source of platelet consumption or embolic dissemination.[104] By definition, catheter-related candidemia is infection of the catheter only; there is no dissemination or multiorgan involvement. Prompt catheter removal at the earliest sign of infection, although often impractical in the management of many of the highest-risk neonates, is necessary to contain the infection and prevent persistent candidemia with the attendant risk of developing disseminated infection or other complications.[135,136] Candidal infections of right atrial catheters are associated with endocarditis and intracardiac fungal masses; the latter may result in cardiac dysfunction because of the enlarging right atrial mass.[92,137]

Although infected intravascular catheters provide the greatest concern for dissemination, infection can occur with almost any type of catheter used in the treatment of the VLBW infant. Prolonged endotracheal intubation for mechanical ventilation can be required in the extremely premature infant with respiratory distress and in the sick term infant after cardiac or other extensive surgery. The concurrent ongoing presence of the endotracheal tube can lead to candidal colonization with the potential for development of pneumonia, although invasive lung infection is uncommon.[7,9,76] Candidal cystitis can accompany the prolonged use of indwelling bladder catheters by facilitating ascending infection, and cystic fungal masses can form, resulting in urethral obstruction.[50,51,111-113,138] Infants with vesicoureteral reflux and a candidal bladder infection are at increased risk for renal parenchymal infection.[112,138] Candidal peritonitis can develop with the prolonged use of peritoneal catheters placed intraoperatively for drainage or, more often, placed for peritoneal dialysis.[103] Peritoneal dialysis catheters are at extremely high risk for infection because of the frequent handling required and the high dextrose concentration of the indwelling dialysis fluid.[103] *Candida* spp. have been recovered from the pleural fluid draining from thoracic tubes and from the fluid draining through surgically placed mediastinal tubes.[127] With cystitis, dissemination and widespread disease can be complications, but *Candida* peritonitis or pleuritis rarely leads to fungemia.[112,138]

Candidemia and Disseminated Candidiasis

Candidemia and disseminated or systemic candidiasis usually are associated with multiple invasive infection enhancing factors and are infections of the sick preterm or term infant who is in the NICU more than 7 days.[7,8,104] However, most cases occur among ELBW infants, who have an incidence of candidemia ranging from 5.5% to 20%.[7,18,51] The source of the infecting *Candida* spp. can be the infant's endogenous flora or from nosocomial transmission, and all the *Candida* spp. listed in Table 33-1 have been implicated in systemic disease.[5,18] Although candidemia without organ involvement can occur, *Candida* spp. have such high affinity for certain organs (e.g., kidney, eye, heart, CNS) that dissemination appears to be the rule rather than the exception, particularly in the neonate with persistent fungemia.[2,51,104,105] The clinical presentation of the infant with candidemia can vary greatly depending upon the extent of systemic disease. The most common presentation is one with clinical features typical of generalized sepsis, including lethargy, feeding intolerance, hyperbilirubinemia, apnea, cardiovascular instability, and the development or worsening of respiratory distress. The preterm infant can become critically ill, requiring a significant escalation in cardiorespiratory support. Fever rarely occurs, even with widespread disease. New-onset glucose intolerance and thrombocytopenia are common presenting findings that can persist until adequate therapy has been instituted and the infection contained.[18,50,88,134] This association is so strong that the presence of persistent hyperglycemia with thrombocytopenia in a neonate cared for in the NICU is almost diagnostic for untreated candidemia.[134] Leukocytosis with either a neutrophil predominance or neutropenia can be seen.[100] Neutropenia is more often associated with overwhelming systemic disease. Skin abscesses have been described with systemic disease and are attributed to the deposition of septic emboli in end vessels of the skin.[139] Infants also can have specific organ involvement, such as renal insufficiency, meningitis, endophthalmitis, endocarditis, or osteomyelitis, confirming dissemination. Complex multiorgan involvement is the hallmark of disseminated candidiasis, especially among VLBW premature infants, and results from diffuse hematogenous spread.[50,140] The suspicion or diagnosis of candidemia or the diagnosis of candidal infection of any single organ system should prompt a thorough examination and survey of the infant for additional organ involvement.[2,50,140] Almost any organ can become infected, but the most common sites for candidal dissemination are the urinary tract, the CNS, and the eye.[2,50,140] The specific clinical presentation for each of these systems is described separately in the following sections. For the infant with disseminated candidiasis, complications can be extensive, multiorgan system failure common, and the need for escalated intensive support frequent and prolonged.[50,104]

Renal Candidiasis

Renal involvement occurs in most infants with candidemia because each of the risk factors that predispose to disseminated disease specifically increases the risk for renal disease.[112,138] Every infant with candidemia should have an evaluation of the urinary tract for candidal infection. Infants with congenital urinary tract anomalies and those requiring frequent catheterization for neurologic reasons are at increased risk for an isolated *Candida* spp. urinary tract infection (UTI).[111,112] Congenital urinary tract anomalies, such as cloacal exstrophy, can provide a portal of entry for *Candida* spp. present on the skin. Urinary stasis, whether caused by a congenital anatomic obstruction or a functional obstruction (e.g., in the neurogenic bladder with myelomeningocele), increases the risk of candidal bladder infections.[112] Regardless of the underlying cause, candidal UTIs generally manifest with the same nonspecific systemic signs as with candidemia, whereas specific renal findings can be silent or manifest as urinary tract obstruction, hypertension, or renal failure.[111,112,141-144] Acute renal insufficiency or failure is a common clinical presentation and may be nonoliguric, oliguric, or anuric. In the nonoliguric form, urine output remains normal or near normal, but elevation of the serum creatinine level may be quite dramatic.[111] Renal ultrasonography often reveals parenchymal abnormalities suggestive of single or multiple abscesses; however, lesions may not be obvious at initial presentation, becoming evident only later in the disease process.[112,141] With oliguria, obstruction of the urinary tract by a discrete fungus ball or balls must be considered.[142] These fungal masses commonly are found in the ureteropelvic junction and usually are diagnosed by ultrasonography but are found rarely by physical examination as a palpable flank mass.[59,144] Hypertension may be the only initial clinical feature in neonatal renal candidiasis.[143]

Central Nervous System Candidiasis

Central nervous system candidiasis most often accompanies disseminated candidiasis, with up to 50% of VLBW infants having some form of CNS infection.[6,18,50,145] Neonates with neural tube defects and those requiring indwelling cerebrospinal fluid (CSF) shunts are at increased risk for isolated candidal infections of the CNS. Meningitis is the most frequently reported form of CNS infection, but parenchymal abscesses, ventriculitis, vasculitis and perivasculitis, ependymal inflammation, osteomyelitis of the skull or vertebral bodies, and even fungus balls within the subarachnoid space have been described, although rarely.[2,105,113,141,146] The specific clinical presentation is extremely variable but typically occurs when infants are older than 1 week.[6,147] The initial presentation is similar to that of disseminated candidiasis, subtle or quite severe, with cardiorespiratory instability and rapid overall deterioration.[105] Less frequently, an infant may have only neurologic signs, such as seizures, focal neurologic changes, an increase in head circumference, or a change in fontanelle quality.[105,145,147] Because clinical findings may be limited or nonexistent, the possibility of CNS involvement with *Candida* must always be considered in neonates with candidemia or evidence for invasive candidal disease at other sites. A high index of suspicion is required; in one reported series, blood cultures were negative in up to half the ELBW infants with *Candida* meningitis.[6]

Candidal Ophthalmologic Infections

Endophthalmitis results from hematogenous spread of *Candida* spp. to the eye of the infant and is a diagnosed complication in approximately 6% of infants with systemic candidiasis.[106] Overall risk factors for ophthalmologic infection are the same as factors predisposing to disseminated disease. Infants with prolonged candidemia (i.e., blood cultures positive for more than 4 days) are significantly more likely to develop end-organ involvement of the eye, kidney, or heart.[140] Ophthalmic infections have been reported with all *Candida* spp. listed in Table 33-1.[106,140] Because the clinical presentation of candidal chorioretinitis is frequently silent, an indirect ophthalmoscopic examination should be performed on all infants diagnosed with or suspected of having candidemia or systemic candidiasis. Lesions can be unilateral or bilateral, and these appear as individual yellow-white, elevated lesions with indistinct borders in the posterior fundus.[106] Vitreous lesions occasionally occur, and some infants show vitreal inflammation or a nonspecific choroidal lesion with hemorrhage or Roth spots in the posterior retina.[50,108] Infection of the lens occurs rarely; five case reports of lens abscesses in preterm infants exist, and each infant presented with a unilateral cataract.[108,148-150]

In addition to the ophthalmologic infections caused by *Candida* spp., an association between candidemia and retinopathy of prematurity (ROP) has been described in neonates with no previous evidence for chorioretinitis or endophthalmitis.[151-156] Early reports suggested a significant increase in the incidence of any stage ROP among infants with *Candida* sepsis compared with those without candidiasis (95% vs. 69%) and an increased probability of severe ROP requiring laser surgery (41% vs. 9%).[151] Subsequent retrospective studies have demonstrated a greater incidence of threshold ROP and need for laser surgery among infants with *Candida* sepsis but no greater overall incidence of ROP of any severity.[153,155,156] Data are inconclusive as to cause and effect, but an association clearly is documented.[151,155] Premature infants of any gestational age who develop candidal sepsis should be followed closely by an ophthalmologist for the late development of severe ROP.

Spontaneous Intestinal Perforation

Invasive disseminated candidiasis is associated with the occurrence of spontaneous intestinal perforation in preterm infants.[96,103,157,158] This syndrome is distinct from NEC, occurring predominantly during the first 2 to 3 weeks of life among the smallest, most premature infants on the NICU (median gestational age, 24 weeks; median birth weight, 634 g).[94] Specific predisposing factors identified for spontaneous intestinal perforation include umbilical arterial catheterization, hypothermia, indomethacin therapy (prophylactic or treatment), and cyanotic congenital heart disease.[96,103,159] Neonates typically have bluish discoloration of the abdomen and a gasless pattern on abdominal radiographs, without pneumatosis intestinalis, often accompanied by systemic signs such as hypotension.[94] Disseminated candidiasis frequently is diagnosed in association with this syndrome; one series reported up to 33% of affected infants with cultures of blood, peritoneal fluid, CSF, or urine positive for *Candida* spp.[94] Pathologic examination of the involved intestinal area demonstrates mucosal invasion by yeast and filamentous forms of *Candida* spp.[96,157,159] It is not clear from these specimens, nor from the clinical picture, whether the perforation is a result of primary candidal invasion of the intestinal mucosa or the colonizing *Candida* strain merely invades bowel damaged by another insult. Whatever the cause, the association exists, suggesting that clinicians should consider extensive evaluation for disseminated candidiasis with the diagnosis of a spontaneous intestinal perforation in the extremely premature infant.

Diagnosis

The diagnosis of most mucocutaneous disease is based on the characteristic clinical findings described earlier. Culture of the lesions of oral thrush or diaper dermatitis usually is not indicated. However, in an infant refractory to therapy, culture with susceptibility determination of the recovered organism may identify a NCAC species with a susceptibility pattern requiring modification of specific therapy.[121,124] In congenital candidiasis, a presumptive diagnosis can be made by Gram stain of vesicular contents of an individual lesion or by potassium hydroxide preparations of skin scrapings, with confirmation by culture of discrete lesions or swabs of skin folds or intertriginous areas. Cultures of blood, urine, and CSF are indicated for term infants with systemic signs of infection and for all affected preterm infants, healthy or ill appearing.[34] In the infant with change in respiratory or radiographic status, endotracheal aspirate cultures that grow *Candida* spp. are difficult to interpret because most often this represents colonization rather than pulmonary invasion.[24] The characteristic skin lesions of invasive fungal dermatitis often are diagnostic, but a skin biopsy provides a definitive diagnosis and tissue for culture and species determination. Biopsy is more sensitive than skin swabs in identifying other non-*Candida* filamentous fungi included in the differential diagnosis for this disease process.[96]

Given the increasing incidence of invasive candidiasis among premature infants, clinicians caring for these infants must be alert to the possibility of *Candida* in any infant who develops signs of systemic infection, especially neonates with predisposing conditions (see Box 33-1). The differential diagnosis includes primarily other microorganisms responsible for nosocomial sepsis.[5,6] At a minimum, any infant with systemic signs of infection should have blood cultures obtained from a peripheral venipuncture and from all indwelling intravascular catheters. Most *Candida* spp. are identified by growth on standard bacteriologic culture media with aerobic processing, and requesting separate fungal cultures does not increase the yield of *Candida* spp.[57] Previous recommendations were to monitor such cultures for up to 10 days to ensure adequate growth of the slower-growing *Candida* spp.[57,127] However, in one report, 90% of cultures for *Candida* spp. were positive by 72 hours, before and immediately after the initiation of antifungal therapy.[160] Multiple or repeat blood cultures increase the likelihood of obtaining a positive result.[161,162] For infants with an indwelling intravascular catheter or catheters, samples obtained through each catheter and from a peripheral vessel are recommended for culture. Recovery of a *Candida* spp. from the culture sample obtained from an intravascular catheter and not from the peripheral blood supports the diagnosis of catheter-related candidemia without dissemination. However, caution should be used in making this distinction in neonates. First, the sensitivity of a single blood culture in diagnosing candidiasis is low; a single sterile peripheral blood culture does not exclude disseminated candidiasis.[51,161] Second, by the time the culture results are known (usually 24-48 hours after collection), dissemination might have occurred, especially in the preterm infant. Disparate results do indicate that the catheter tip is infected, and prompt removal of the catheter is indicated to prevent dissemination and other complications.

If disseminated candidiasis is suspected based on the clinical picture or a positive blood culture is obtained from a peripheral vessel, additional studies are indicated. Even after the initiation of appropriate antifungal therapy, daily blood samples should be collected until culture results are negative because the risk for multiorgan involvement increases the longer fungemia persists.[140] Because renal and CNS candidiasis can be clinically silent at presentation, urine and CSF should be obtained for analyses and culture. The presence of budding yeast or filamentous fungal forms by microscopic examination of the urine or CSF suggests invasive disease. Because *Candida* spp. are frequent contaminants of nonsterilely collected urine samples, urine should be obtained by sterile urethral catheterization or suprapubic aspiration.[51,112] In clinical practice, suprapubic aspiration is infrequently performed in many NICUs, and sterile urethral catheterization is reported to be an efficient method for obtaining urine cultures from infants younger than 6 months.[163] The current consensus is that a *Candida* spp. UTI in neonates be defined as 10^4 or more colony-forming units of *Candida* spp. per milliliter in a culture obtained by sterile urethral catheterization.[112] Cultures of the CSF are more likely to be positive if the volume of CSF obtained is at least 1 mL.[105] Even when an optimal volume of CSF is cultured, a negative result does not eliminate the possibility of CNS disease because infection can occur in areas of the brain not in communication with the CSF.[105,110] Analysis of the CSF for abnormalities suggestive of inflammation, including an elevated white blood cell count or protein level or a decreased glucose level, suggests meningitis, but normal values do not exclude CNS infection.[147,164] Interpretation of CSF values can be complicated by the presence of blood resulting from a traumatic lumbar puncture or preexisting intracranial hemorrhage in the preterm infant. Cultures of other clinically suspicious sites, such as peritoneal fluid or a skin abscess or vesicle, can help to confirm the diagnosis in an ill infant. However, cultures of healthy-appearing skin and mucous membranes or cultures of endotracheal secretions without the presence of pulmonary symptoms are not helpful in diagnosing systemic infections. Endotracheal tube secretion cultures may not be helpful in the infant with respiratory symptoms because *Candida* pneumonia is more often a result of hematogenous spread.[26,50,82] If any other catheters are present, such as chest or mediastinal tubes, cultures of the fluid drainage also should be obtained.

A culture from a usually sterile body site that grows *Candida* spp. confirms the diagnosis of candidiasis. Determination of the *Candida* spp. involved is equally important. Historically, because most infections were caused by *C. albicans*, many laboratories did not go beyond the initial identification of a yeast in culture as *Candida*.[13,57,165] Today, the incidence of infections with the NCAC species has increased dramatically, and identification of the species involved is important for epidemiologic and therapeutic reasons.[127,166,167] Knowledge of the infecting *Candida* spp. can help to determine whether the source of the infection is endogenous or from nosocomial transmission. This can be especially important in determining whether an apparent outbreak of candidiasis in a particular NICU is a coincidence or caused by a common source.[45,48,49,165,167] From the therapeutic perspective, when comparing the various pathogenic *Candida* spp., variations exist in susceptibility to the common antifungal agents (Table 33-3), and defining the infecting *Candida* spp. is important in determining appropriate antifungal therapy.[51,82]

To determine the extent and severity of candidiasis, additional laboratory tests are indicated when evaluating the infant with suspected disseminated candidiasis, including a complete blood count with differential and platelet counts and determinations of the levels of serum glucose, creatinine, blood urea nitrogen, bilirubin, liver aminotransferases, and C-reactive protein. The white blood cell count may be normal, high, or low; however, in the neonate, neutropenia may suggest a severe, overwhelming infection.[99] Thrombocytopenia is strongly associated with systemic candidiasis and may be an early indicator of this disease.[125,134] Elevations in the blood urea nitrogen and serum creatinine levels may indicate renal infection. Mild elevations in the serum bilirubin levels may be a part of the sepsis syndrome, but

Table 33-3 General Patterns of Susceptibility of *Candida* Species to Antifungal Agents

Candida Species	Amphotericin B	Fluconazole	Voriconazole	Echinocandins
C. albicans	S	S	S	S
C. parapsilosis	S	S	S	S to I*
C. glabrata	S to I†	I to R‡	S to I§	S
C. tropicalis	S	S	S	S
C. krusei	S to I†	R‖	S	S
C. lusitaniae	I to R	S	S	S

Data from references 18, 135, 176-178, 187, 216, and 220.
I, Intermediately resistant; *R*, resistant; *S*, susceptible.
*Isolates of *C. parapsilosis* have slightly higher minimal inhibitory concentrations.
†A significant proportion of clinical isolates of *C. glabrata* and *C. krusei* have reduced susceptibility to amphotericin B.
‡Between 30% and 65% of clinical isolates of *C. glabrata* are resistant to fluconazole.
§Susceptibility is dose dependent.
‖*C. krusei* is intrinsically resistant to fluconazole.

marked elevations in the serum bilirubin concentration or liver enzymes indicate extensive liver involvement.[6] Elevation of the C-reactive protein level is a nonspecific indicator of systemic infection.[50,51] Unfortunately, obtaining normal values for any or all of these ancillary laboratory tests does not completely exclude the possibility of candidiasis, especially CNS disease, in the high-risk neonate.[105]

Because of the predilection of *Candida* for certain organs, specific imaging studies are indicated to diagnose the extent of dissemination. Renal ultrasonography, echocardiography, and cranial imaging are recommended for all infants with candidemia or systemic candidiasis.[140] Renal and bladder ultrasonography are extremely sensitive, but nonspecific, in their ability to define abnormalities resulting from *Candida* infections. The ultrasonographic appearance of a nonshadowing echogenic focus strongly suggests a renal fungus ball, particularly when the infant has a urine culture that grows *Candida*.[168] However, blood clots, fibrinous deposits, and nephrocalcinosis may have the same ultrasound appearance, confounding interpretation.[168] Another common ultrasonographic finding is renal parenchymal infiltration characterized by enlarged kidneys with diffusely increased echogenicity. In any given infant with renal candidiasis, one or both of these ultrasound findings can be seen. Limited information exists about the accuracy of computed tomography (CT) or magnetic resonance imaging (MRI) in diagnosing renal candidiasis.[168,169] Echocardiography is useful in neonates with CVCs when the primary concern is for endocarditis with an infected thrombus at the catheter tip site or a right atrial mass.[92,137] Cranial ultrasonography easily can reveal enlarged ventricles, calcifications, cystic changes, and intraventricular fungus balls in infants with CNS candidiasis.[109,141] Ventriculitis can be diagnosed by the appearance of intraventricular septations or debris.[105] Interpretation of the cranial ultrasonography can be difficult in the preterm neonate who has experienced an intraventricular hemorrhage in the past or has developed periventricular leukomalacia. Cranial CT and MRI offer certain advantages over ultrasonography, including superior imaging of the posterior fossa and infratentorial and nonmidline structures.[169] Calcifications are seen best with CT, and the addition of intravenous contrast can aid in the identification of intracranial abscesses. However, as a practical matter, cranial ultrasonography is more frequently used because it can be performed at the bedside of a critically ill infant. In addition to these imaging studies, all neonates with confirmed or suspected candidemia should have a dilated ophthalmologic examination, preferably by a pediatric ophthalmologist.[106] The infant who has characteristic lesions of *Candida* endophthalmitis has a confirmed diagnosis of disseminated disease.

Despite heightened awareness of the more subtle presentations of disseminated candidiasis and improvements in the ancillary and imaging studies available to clinicians, an accurate and timely diagnosis of candidal infections in the neonate remains a challenge. This largely reflects continued reliance on a positive culture for *Candida* spp. from a normally sterile body fluid (e.g., blood, urine, CSF, peritoneal fluid) or a potentially infected site to confirm the diagnosis and guide therapy. Autopsy studies suggest that the specificity of blood cultures for candidiasis approaches 100%; however, the sensitivity in the diagnosis of disseminated candidiasis is low, ranging from 30% with single-organ involvement up to 80% with four or more organs involved.[161] The situation in the neonate is further complicated by the fact that fluid volumes as low as 1 mL may be obtained for culture, additionally diminishing the sensitivity, especially if the total burden of organisms in the fluid is low.[161] The development of techniques for more sensitive, reliable, and rapid diagnosis of candidal infections is a priority and is an active area of investigation.[161,170] A number of molecular diagnostic assays that exploit recognition of small amounts of *Candida* spp. proteins or DNA, including the β-glucan antigen assay, scanning electron microscopy of fluid containing yeast, and polymerase chain reaction (PCR) testing, are being evaluated in adults and older children.[170-172] None of these assays has been rigorously evaluated in a population of neonates.[173-176] β-1,3-D-Glucan is a major component of the fungal cell wall found in all clinically relevant *Candida* spp. Various assays are reported to have 85% sensitivity and 95% specificity for candidemia by detecting very small amounts of this fungal cell wall antigen.[173] PCR amplification of an area of the genome common to *C. albicans* and other pathogenic *Candida* spp. can be successfully performed, again using very small volumes of blood, urine, or CSF; this assay appears to be the best hope for rapid diagnosis.[171] Extensive use of PCR assays has previously been limited by unacceptably high rates of fungal

Table 33-4 Systemic Antifungal Agents for the Treatment of Invasive Candidiasis in Neonates

Drug	Dose	Interval	Route	Indications	Toxicities	Toxicity Monitoring	Comments
Amphotericin B	0.5-1.0 mg/kg/day	q24h	IV	Candidemia, invasive candidiasis	Renal, hematologic, hepatic	Urine output, creatinine, potassium, magnesium, liver enzymes	Not indicated to treat *C. lusitaniae* Dose adjustments may be required for renal failure
Lipid-associated amphotericin B preparations	1-5 mg/kg/day	q24h	IV	Invasive candidiasis with severe preexisting renal insufficiencies	Similar to amphotericin B; decreased renal toxicities	Urine output, creatinine, potassium, magnesium, liver enzymes	May be indicated in patients failing therapy or requiring higher doses
Fluconazole	6-12 mg/kg/day (consideration may be given to 25 mg/kg loading dose)	≤14 days,* q72h; 15-27 days, q48h; ≥28 days, q24h	PO, IV	Alternative therapy to amphotericin B for localized urinary tract infection, mucocutaneous disease	Hepatic, gastrointestinal	Liver enzymes	Excellent CSF penetration; oral formulation well absorbed; not indicated to treat *Candida krusei* or *Candida glabrata*
Micafungin†	4-10 mg/kg/day (as high as 15 mg/kg/day has been well tolerated and may be indicated for CNS disease)	q24h	IV	Severe and/or refractory systemic infections; hepatic and renal infections	Minimal, potential	Creatinine, urine output, liver enzymes	CSF penetration variable

Data from references 82, 135, 176, 179, 186, 187, and 210.

CNS, Central nervous system; *CSF*, cerebrospinal fluid; *IV*, intravenous; *PO*, oral.

*Age in days.

†Published reports on echinocandin use in neonates include small studies of patients with caspofungin and micafungin, neither of which is currently licensed for use in neonates. However, the data suggest safety and efficacy (see text for further details). We recommend verifying dosage and indications based on most current publications.

Note: Recommendations are not included for the use of 5-fluorocytosine because of potential toxicities, nor voriconazole and caspofungin because of potential toxicities and lack of adequate published data in neonates (see text for further details and Chapter 37).

contamination resulting in false-positive tests, but newer assays are more specific and sensitive.[171,174,175] Each of these assays holds promise for the rapid detection of fungus in small volumes of body fluids and does not require the presence of live *Candida* spp. One major drawback to many early PCR assays, compared with culture, was the lack of differentiation between pathogenic *Candida* spp.; the diagnosis they provided was simply candidiasis. However, newer PCR assays are able to distinguish between various yeast species.[175] With specific culture or PCR results, the clinician knows which *Candida* spp. is causing the infection and can tailor the therapeutic plan accordingly. Without specific results, more generic management plans must be used. However, because the institution of therapy often is delayed because of the lack of a positive culture when clinical deterioration begins, which may lead to systemic complications from persistent fungemia, knowing the neonate has a *Candida* spp. may lead to improved therapeutic management.

Treatment

Therapy and management of candidiasis in the neonate require an effective antifungal agent coupled with appropriate supportive care and measures to eliminate factors favoring ongoing infection. In the NICU, the first two objectives are easier to achieve than the last. Multiple antifungal therapies are available, but few have been studied for determination of appropriate dose and interval, safety, and efficacy in neonates, especially VLBW infants. Amphotericin B has been the mainstay of antifungal therapy for more than 40 years, but newer agents may be indicated in certain settings.[82,135,136,176-179] Table 33-3 summarizes the antimicrobial susceptibility pattern of pathogenic *Candida* spp. to the most common antifungal agents, and Table 33-4 and the following discussion outline important features regarding use of each agent in the neonate with candidiasis. Because candidiasis often is a nosocomially acquired infection, most infected infants are already in the NICU, where appropriate intensive care to support these critically ill infants is readily available. If the hospital nursery is unable to address the needs of a critically ill neonate, transfer to a higher-level NICU should be considered. Unfortunately, the elimination of all risk factors for ongoing candidemia often is an unattainable goal, and the clinician frequently must settle for a less than optimal reduction of risk factors (see Table 33-2 and preceding section on pathogenesis regarding reduction of risk factors).[7]

With the diagnosis of candidemia or disseminated candidiasis, immediate consideration should be given to the removal of all potentially contaminated medical hardware, especially central intravascular catheters.[180] For ongoing fungemia, successful medical treatment of *Candida* spp. infections while the catheters remain in place is rare.[51,82,91,104] The risk of dissemination also increases with every day the infant remains fungemic, as does the rate of infection of previously uninfected intravascular lines.[104,181] The clinician must face the reality that most preterm infants with systemic candidiasis require central access because of the clinical instability directly attributable to the ongoing candidemia, which in large part is caused by the ongoing presence of the infected catheter. If all lines cannot be removed, removal of a potentially infected catheter with insertion of a new line at a different site or a sequential reduction in the number of catheters is preferable to inaction. Infants with more than one catheter may not have all lines infected at the time of diagnosis, and removal of the catheter known or most likely to be infected may resolve the problem and allow continued therapy through the remaining line.[93] Antifungal therapy should be administered through the remaining central catheter to maximize drug delivery to a potential site of ongoing infection. Daily blood cultures to determine whether fungemia is persistent and whether additional infected catheters should be removed are necessary. Consideration should be given to surgical resection of infected tissue if antifungal therapy does not achieve sterilization (e.g., urine) or if mechanical complications caused by the presence of a fungus ball arise (e.g., right atrial mass). Although successful medical therapy for endocarditis caused by *Candida* spp. can often be achieved, large right atrial masses are almost impossible to sterilize and may also compromise hemodynamic function, necessitating surgical removal.[92,93,137,169,182] Surgical removal of an enlarging right atrial candidal mass in the face of ongoing fungemia and hemodynamic instability may be lifesaving for the premature infant.[137] Most renal fungal balls can be treated medically because of the high levels of most antifungal agents attained in the urine.[112,138] However, in an infant with complete obstruction of urinary flow caused by the presence of one or more fungal balls, surgical removal is indicated.[142,143] Hyperglycemia can be avoided by judicious administration of dextrose and insulin therapy if glucose intolerance persists. Corticosteroid therapy should be avoided or tapered as tolerated.

ANTIFUNGAL AGENTS

Topical Antifungal Therapy

Topical antifungal agents are indicated for thrush, diaper dermatitis, and uncomplicated congenital candidiasis in the term infant.[19] Nystatin, the most commonly used topical therapy, is a polyene drug that is not absorbed by the gastrointestinal tract, making it a topical agent in any of the three common formulations: oral suspension, ointment, or powder. The oral suspension is indicated for the treatment of thrush in patients of all ages. However, because of the high osmolality of the oral suspension (caused by the added sucrose excipient), care should be taken and use limited in the very premature infant or the neonate with compromise of the gastrointestinal tract.[120] Reports of clinical cure vary widely, from as low as 30% to as high as 85%.[120,121] Nystatin should be applied directly to the lesions of oral thrush. If swallowed rapidly, there is minimal contact with the lesions and little efficacy. Nystatin ointment or powder, when applied to diaper dermatitis, has an 85% cure rate.[120] Because thrush often accompanies diaper dermatitis, many clinicians add oral Nystatin when prescribing perineal therapy, even if no oral lesions exist. Data suggest no added efficacy with this practice, which should be discouraged.[120,183] If oral lesions are present, treatment is indicated. However, if oral lesions are not present, the source of the *Candida* spp. probably is the lower gastrointestinal tract, in which Nystatin is not an optimal agent.

Miconazole gel is a nonabsorbable formulation of this azole, developed particularly for treatment of thrush, which is not available in the United States.[120,184] The gel formulation is said to offer more prolonged contact with the oral lesions and has a reported efficacy of greater than 90%.[120] Side effects predominantly are gastrointestinal, similar to Nystatin, but use of this agent has been evaluated only in a limited number of preterm infants.[154] Miconazole creams and ointments and other topical azole formulations frequently are prescribed for diaper dermatitis with excellent results.[120,185]

Gentian violet, the first topical therapy for oral thrush, has become the treatment of last resort. Although effective, the liquid treatment must be applied directly to the lesions, and it causes unsightly dark purple stains on the infant's mouth, clothes, bedclothes, and often on the hands and clothes of the care provider. Complications include local irritation and ulceration from the direct application of the treatment to adjacent normal mucosa.[120] Given these inconveniences, most clinicians avoid gentian violet in favor of administering systemic therapy when topical treatments fail.[121]

Systemic Antifungal Therapy

For all the drugs discussed in this section, see Chapter 37 for complete details on antimicrobial activity, pharmacokinetics, safety, and alternative dosing.

Amphotericin B. Amphotericin B deoxycholate is an antifungal agent available since 1958. The American Academy of Pediatrics Committee on Infectious Diseases, the Pediatric Infectious Disease Society, and the Infectious Disease Society of America (IDSA) recommend amphotericin B as the primary antifungal agent for the treatment of candidemia, disseminated candidiasis, and any form of invasive candidiasis in the neonate.* Most pathogenic *Candida* spp. are susceptible to amphotericin B (see Table 33-3). However, reports suggest a proportion of *C. glabrata* and *C. krusei* isolates have a somewhat reduced susceptibility to amphotericin B, which can be overcome by using higher-dose therapy, and resistance has been described for isolates of *C. lusitaniae*.[15,177-179,188] Very occasional resistance with *C. parapsilosis* has been reported.[189]

Toxicities reported in neonates receiving amphotericin B include renal insufficiency with occasional renal failure, hypokalemia, and hypomagnesemia caused by excessive renal losses; bone marrow suppression with anemia and thrombocytopenia; and abnormalities in hepatic enzymes.[82,164] Most toxicities are dose dependent and reversible on cessation of therapy.[82] Nephrotoxicity is the most common and worrisome toxic effect. A substantial rise in creatinine and decrease in urine output can be

*References 82, 135, 136, 179, 186, 187.

observed; however, it is frequently difficult to differentiate between renal insufficiency caused by inadequately treated systemic renal candidiasis and that caused by amphotericin B. Although there is a potential for renal failure, most infants display no or mild nephrotoxicity that resolves with decreasing the dose of amphotericin B or after completion of therapy. A common and very uncomfortable side effect in adults and older children receiving amphotericin B is an infusion-related reaction consisting of fever, chills, nausea, headache, and occasionally hypotension.[190] No such toxicity has been described in neonates, and test doses are not indicated.[190] The risk for dissemination is so high among infants that no delay should occur in delivering treatment doses. Any neonate receiving amphotericin B should have serial monitoring of serum potassium and magnesium levels and of renal, liver, and bone marrow function.

The recommended treatment dose is 1 mg/kg given every 24 hours, intravenously.[82] Reports suggest variable CSF concentrations, ranging from 40% to 90% of plasma levels in one study of preterm infants.[191] CSF and brain tissue penetration is generally better in neonates than adults, so a change in dosing is not necessarily indicated with concerns for CNS disease.[82] Successful treatment of CNS disease with amphotericin monotherapy has been reported.[82,164]

Amphotericin B Lipid Formulations. As an alternative to standard amphotericin B, three lipid-associated formulations are approved for use in adults: liposomal amphotericin B (L-amphotericin B), amphotericin B lipid complex (ABLC), and amphotericin B cholesterol sulfate complex (ABCD). Fungal susceptibility patterns for these lipid-associated formulations are the same as for conventional amphotericin B deoxycholate.[192,193] Each is significantly more expensive than conventional amphotericin B.[176] The main purported advantage to these amphotericin B preparations is the ability to deliver a higher dose of medication with lower levels of toxicity. In adults and older children receiving a lipid-formulation of amphotericin B, significantly lower rates of infusion-related reactions and serum creatinine elevations are reported, compared with conventional amphotericin B.[194] Several case reports of successful use of these preparations in neonates have been published, demonstrating no major adverse events, diminished toxicities associated with conventional amphotericin (i.e., hypokalemia and hyperbilirubinemia), and treatment success rates of 70% to 100%, but no controlled trials have been performed.[82,193,195] Studies of ABLC in pediatric patients have included small numbers of neonates and demonstrated efficacy rates of 75% to 85%, with no significant toxicities.[82,193] Renal penetration of the lipid-associated formulations is poor compared with conventional amphotericin, and treatment failure at this site of infection has been reported.[194]

Although randomized, controlled trials of the lipid-associated preparations in neonates are lacking, available information suggests that they may be safe and effective, although not superior to conventional amphotericin B. Treatment with amphotericin B deoxycholate remains the most appropriate therapy for infants with invasive infections with *Candida* spp., especially for those with renal infection.[82,135,136,179] The amphotericin B lipid formulations may have a role in the treatment of invasive candidiasis in neonates with preexisting severe renal disease or in infants who fail to respond to conventional amphotericin B after removal of all intravascular catheters, but more data are needed. Current dosing recommendations suggest 1-5 mg/kg/day.[82,135]

5-Fluorocytosine. 5-Fluorocytosine (5-FC) is a fluorinated analogue of cytosine. All pathogenic *Candida* spp. are susceptible to this agent, but resistance develops rapidly when used as monotherapy (see Table 33-3).[177] 5-FC has excellent CNS penetration and historically was used in combination with amphotericin B in the treatment of neonatal CNS candidiasis because early studies demonstrated synergy with these two agents.[177,196] However, more recent reports suggest no added therapeutic benefit when 5-FC is combined with amphotericin B.[6,179] The potential benefit of 5-FC added to amphotericin B must be carefully weighed against common significant toxicities, including azotemia, renal tubular acidosis, and myelosuppression.[82] Serum levels must be followed closely.[82] 5-Fluorocytosine is available only in an enteral preparation, significantly limiting its use in most critically ill neonates with systemic candidiasis, who are also at risk for necrotizing enterocolitis.

Azoles. The azoles are a class of synthetic fungistatic agents that inhibit fungal growth. The most common side effects are alterations in the pharmacokinetics of concomitant medications the infant is receiving and mild hepatotoxicity.[197] Clinically significant hepatotoxicity is rare with use of the newer azoles, such as fluconazole and voriconazole, in adults and older children, and their overall safety profile is favorable.[198] However, monitoring of aminotransferases and serum bilirubin levels in neonates receiving azoles is recommended.[198] In addition, not all *Candida* spp. are sensitive to all members of this class of antifungal agents (see Table 33-3), limiting use in empirical therapy.[13,15]

Fluconazole, the azole used most frequently in neonates, is water soluble, available in oral or intravenous preparations, and highly bioavailable in the neonate.[198,199] Fluconazole has a long plasma half-life, with excellent levels achieved in the blood, CSF, brain, liver, spleen, and especially the kidneys, where it is excreted unchanged in the urine.[176,179,199] The pharmacokinetics of fluconazole in neonates change dramatically over the first weeks of life, presumably because of increased renal clearance with maturity; therefore the dosing interval is based on both postnatal and postconceptual age (see Table 33-4 and Chapter 37).[82,199] Transient thrombocytopenia, elevations in creatinine, mild hyperbilirubinemia, and transient increases in liver aminotransferases have been documented in neonates.[28,176,179,200]

Several studies have shown fluconazole to be efficacious in the treatment of invasive candidiasis in the neonate. In one prospective, randomized trial versus amphotericin B, rates of survival and clearance of the organism were equivalent for both treatment groups.[201] Infants treated with fluconazole had less renal and hepatic toxicity and had a shorter time to the complete removal of central intravascular catheters, which was attributed to the ability to convert to oral therapy for completion of the treatment course.[201]

Although these features make the use of fluconazole appear quite attractive, the primary concern with fluconazole is fungal resistance, limiting its use as a first-line therapeutic medication.[13,15,202] Although most pathogenic *Candida* spp. are susceptible to fluconazole, *C. krusei* is intrinsically resistant to this azole, as are up to 65% of *C. glabrata* isolates (see Table 33-3).[176-178] Both of these NCAC species can cause neonatal disease; therefore the use of fluconazole as empirical single therapy is not recommended. The IDSA guidelines recommend the administration of fluconazole as an alternative therapy to amphotericin B for disseminated, invasive neonatal candidiasis or congenital candidiasis with systemic signs after the pathogenic *Candida* spp. is identified and susceptibility determination completed.[135] Because of its unaltered renal clearance, fluconazole is an excellent choice for the treatment of isolated urinary tract infections resulting from susceptible *Candida* spp., and oral fluconazole is an alternative therapy in refractory mucocutaneous disease.[121,199] Combination therapy with amphotericin B was evaluated in a multicellular trial of nonneutropenic adults with candidemia with excellent results.[181]

Voriconazole is a second-generation azole, derived from fluconazole, with increased potency and a broader spectrum of activity (see Table 33-3 and Chapter 37).[203,204] Voriconazole is active in vitro against all clinically relevant *Candida* spp., including *C. krusei* and *C. glabrata*, and no resistance by fluconazole-resistant strains has been reported.[176,179,203] Voriconazole is metabolized by the liver, and the only clinically significant adverse event reported in adults is the occurrence of visual disturbances.[203] For this reason, concerns have been raised about the possibility of unknown interactions with the developing retina, discouraging therapeutic trials in neonates.[186] The neonatal literature is limited, but one case report does describe successful combination therapy with voriconazole and liposomal amphotericin B in a premature infant with disseminated fluconazole-resistant *C. albicans* infection.[205] A more recent report showed safety and efficacy in a very small group of neonates treated with voriconazole.[206] Although this agent appears to be safe and effective in children, further trials in neonates are indicated before a routine recommendation can be established.[207] There is genetic variation in the metabolism of voriconazole, and slow metabolizers may accumulate concentrations up to four times greater than others, which along with the paucity of data regarding pharmacokinetics in neonates suggest caution in the use of this agent at this age and, if used, that drug concentrations be monitored (see Chapter 37).

Echinocandins. Echinocandins are a novel class of antifungal drugs that act by a unique and completely fungal-specific mechanism—inhibition of the synthesis of β-1,3-D-glucan, an essential component of the fungal cell wall.[207] Because there is no mammalian equivalent to the fungal cell wall, the safety profile for the echinocandins, in adults and older children, is excellent and significantly better than the polyenes or azoles.[207] Three drugs in this class—anidulafungin, caspofungin, and micafungin—are currently licensed for use in the United States for adults; use in neonates is considered off-label by the U.S. Food and Drug Administration,[176,179,186] whereas micafungin is approved for use in neonates by the European Medicines Agency. Echinocandins are fungicidal against all pathogenic *Candida* spp.[203,208] Because the mechanism of action is completely different from the other antifungal agents currently in use, the echinocandins are excellent candidates for use in combined therapy, especially for refractory infections. Pharmacokinetic studies in the neonatal population are limited, but those completed show caspofungin and micafungin are well tolerated but have a shorter serum half-life and more rapid clearance, emphasizing the importance of evaluating the neonatal population separate from older children and adults.[179,186,209] Recommendations for optimal dosage in the neonate, especially a preterm one, for either of these agents remain unclear (see Chapter 37).[82,179] Multiple case reports suggest safety and efficacy.[179,186,210] The most current guidelines from the IDSA recommend caspofungin as a second-line agent for neonatal candidemia without dissemination.[135] Development of this novel class of truly fungicidal agents against *Candida* spp. has greatly expanded our options for treating invasive candidiasis in adults. If the echinocandins prove to be as safe and effective for neonates, clinicians could have the ability to combine antifungal agents with different general mechanisms of action (i.e., amphotericin B plus an echinocandin, or an azole plus an echinocandin) to optimize therapeutic efficacy.

Length of Therapy

No matter which antifungal therapy is chosen, the length of therapy to adequately treat invasive neonatal candidiasis is prolonged (see Table 33-2). There are no controlled clinical trials to provide the optimal length of therapy for any of the antifungal agents and no consensus among neonatologists and pediatric infectious disease specialists.[50,82,176,179] The IDSA recommends a minimum of 14 to 21 days of systemic therapy after negative blood, urine, and CSF culture results have been obtained, along with the resolution of clinical findings.[135] Therapy for endocarditis typically lasts 6 weeks.[135,136] In neonates with isolated *Candida* cystitis, treatment for 7 days appears to be adequate. Therapy must be administered intravenously initially, but in an infant who responds to fluconazole, completion of the course with oral therapy is acceptable.[112,199] Infants with fungal abscesses, renal lesions, intracranial lesions, or right atrial fungal masses should have sonographic or radiographic evidence of resolution before completing therapy.[51,111] Close monitoring for relapse after the cessation of therapy is necessary given the high rate of recurrence, especially in infants with CNS disease.[2,105,148]

Prognosis

Despite the current advances in neonatal care and antifungal therapy, the prognosis for the infant who develops an invasive fungal infection is still quite variable but generally poor. Mortality rates range from 20% to 50%, with significant accompanying morbidity and length of stay on the NICU.[6,51,117,211] Factors determining the final prognosis include the degree of prematurity, extent of dissemination, severity of illness, and the rapidity of institution of appropriate antifungal and supportive therapy.[7,211,212] Infants with isolated catheter-related candidal infections, uncomplicated urinary tract infections, or candidemia without dissemination tend to have a good outcome with the potential for complete recovery without sequelae. Infants with extreme prematurity, widely disseminated disease, multiorgan involvement, renal or hepatic failure, and ophthalmologic or CNS infection have a much worse prognosis. In studies of VLBW infants surviving candidemia, disseminated candidiasis, or candidal meningitis, candidiasis survivors were significantly more likely to have a major neurologic abnormality (40%-60% vs. 11%-25%) and a subnormal (<70) Mental Developmental Index (40% vs. 14%) than noninfected infants of the same gestational age and birth weight.[108,211] In a series of ELBW neonates with disseminated candidiasis, including meningitis, Friedman and colleagues[212] found a higher incidence of chronic lung disease (100% vs. 33%), periventricular leukomalacia (26% vs. 12%), severe ROP (22% vs. 9%), and adverse neurologic outcomes at 2 years of corrected age (60% vs. 35%) for infected infants than for gestational age- and birth weight–matched, noninfected controls. Among the infected neonates with adverse neurologic outcomes, 41% had severe disabilities compared with 12% of the control infants, and all infants with parenchymal brain lesions diagnosed by cranial ultrasonography at the time of candidiasis had poor neurologic outcomes.[11,50] The visual outcome after endophthalmitis is generally good after provision of appropriate systemic antifungal therapy. Only a small percentage of infants have significant visual impairment, although most have some decrease in visual acuity.[106] Severe ROP has developed in preterm infants who recovered from candidiasis but never had endophthalmitis.[152,154] These infants may require laser surgery and may be at significant risk for vision loss.[154] Great strides have been made in our ability to diagnose and treat invasive candidiasis, but we must strive to continue to improve therapeutic management and address the issues of morbidity.

Prevention

The old adage that "an ounce of prevention is worth a pound of cure" could never be truer than when considering neonatal candidiasis. Treatment is difficult, prolonged, and prevents mortality and morbidity little more than one half of the time. In addition, as outlined in the preceding section on prognosis, neonatal systemic candidal infections lead to an increase in both risk of neurodevelopmental impairment and length of stay.[211] The development of strategies to prevent neonatal candidal infections should be a priority on the NICU. Many of the factors listed in Box 33-1 that enhance the risk for candidiasis are unavoidable, such as prematurity and low birth weight, but every attempt should be made to address conditions that can be reduced, starting with exposure to the yeast itself (see Table 33-2 and preceding section on pathogenesis regarding reduction of host risk factors).[7] Appropriate diagnosis and treatment of maternal candidal vaginosis and urinary tract infections during pregnancy may decrease vertical transmission.[135] Prevention of horizontal transmission from caregivers by the use of good hand hygiene and gloves should always be encouraged but has resulted in limited success.[44,45,180] In studies of health care workers, appropriate hand hygiene is helpful in reducing superficial and transient flora, and the mechanical action of scrubbing does reduce the fungal burden on the hands of providers.[47] However, antimicrobial or alcohol washes do not alter the deep or permanent yeast flora, with no significant reduction in the recovery of *C. albicans* detected on the hands of providers.[47,213] Elimination of artificial fingernails among care providers has been shown to drastically reduce exposure and transmission.[45] The meticulous care of long-term indwelling catheters is recommended, including standard procedures for insertion and maintenance, especially if used to administer hyperalimentation[136] The use of topical petrolatum ointment in skin care of the ELBW infant is associated with a significantly increased incidence of invasive candidal infections.[214] Although attempts at providing good skin care to prevent epidermal breakdown in the ELBW infant are laudable, the use of petrolatum ointment does not appear to be the best choice, and the increased risk of infection appears to outweigh any potential benefits.

Reduction in exposures to medications associated with neonatal candidiasis is likely the most important part of prevention. Broad-spectrum antibiotic therapy (especially third-generation cephalosporins) and the postnatal use of H2 antagonists, hydrocortisone, and dexamethasone are each associated with a higher incidence of fungal sepsis.[18,87,61,151,180] These medications alter the enteric microenvironment, favoring increased candidal colonization and potential dissemination. Reviews of these risk factors suggest that judicious use of antimicrobial agents may be the most important step in preventing systemic candidiasis.[7,10] Optimization of all the strategies described above should precede implementation of any protocol for widespread chemoprophylaxis.

FLUCONAZOLE PROPHYLAXIS

Chemoprophylaxis with antifungal agents such as oral Nystatin and especially fluconazole has been a major area for investigation in recent years, with the goal of reducing candidal colonization and the accompanying potential for invasive disseminated disease. The cardinal rule of antimicrobial prophylaxis is to use one agent with minimal toxicities for prophylaxis and others for therapy. The use of oral Nystatin to prevent systemic candidiasis has been practiced in many NICUs for decades, is tolerated well by neonates, with no fungal resistance documented, but efficacy in preventing invasive infection is not consistently achieved.[132,215,216] Based on studies demonstrating safety and efficacy, fluconazole is currently recommended for targeted anticandidal prophylaxis among ELBW infants in NICUs with moderate (5%-10%) or high (>10%) rates of invasive candidiasis.[47,216,217] The recommended regimen is to provide 3 mg/kg/dose, twice weekly, starting at 48 to 72 hours and continuing for 4 to 6 weeks or until IV access is no longer present.[47,216,218] No increase in fungal resistance to fluconazole has been noted.[216,219] Efficacy is less conclusive among NICUs with low rates of systemic infection (<5%), and there is no consensus as to the appropriate recommendation for these patients.[82,220,221]

Although multiple randomized controlled trials have suggested that fluconazole prophylaxis will reduce invasive candidiasis in ELBW infants in high-risk NICUs, none has looked at the combined outcome of infection or death.[82] A meta-analysis of prophylactic fluconazole versus death before discharge showed no difference between the groups.[22] In addition, little is known about long-term outcomes and potential effects of early fluconazole exposure in ELBW infants. One study of 38 ELBW infants suggested no differences in neurodevelopmental outcomes at 8 to 10 years of age, comparing those who received fluconazole prophylaxis versus placebo.[222] This small study suggests no adverse neurodevelopmental outcomes after early exposure to fluconazole on a prophylaxis regimen, but as we have learned over time in neonatology, caution must be exercised until more information is known. Additional studies are indicated to look at the long-term outcomes of additional ELBW infants, as well as to explore the use of additional novel therapies for the prevention of *Candida* spp. colonization and systemic disease. Vigilance in our monitoring and adherence to the reduction of all risk factors for invasive candidiasis in the care of the ELBW infant is still the best approach and may preclude the need for chemoprophylaxis in a low-incidence NICU.

Thus the role for fluconazole prophylaxis, targeted or not, requires further clarification.

References

1. Pfaller MA: Nosocomial candidiasis: emerging species, reservoirs, and modes of transmission, *Clin Infect Dis* 22:S89-S94, 1996.
2. Chapman RL, Faix RG: Invasive neonatal candidiasis: an overview, *Semin Perinatol* 27:352-356, 2003.
3. Rangel-Frausto MS, Wiblin T, Blumberg HM, et al: National epidemiology of mycoses survey (NEMIS): variations in rates of bloodstream infections due to *Candida* species in seven surgical intensive care units and six neonatal intensive care units, *Clin Infect Dis* 29:253-258, 1999.
4. Fridkin SK, Kaufman D, Edwards JR, et al: Changing incidence of *Candida* bloodstream infections among NICU patients in the United States: 1995–2004, *Pediatrics* 117:1680-1687, 2006.
5. Stoll BJ, Hansen N: Infections in VLBW infants: studies from the NICHD Neonatal Research Network. *Semin Perinatol* 27:293-301, 2003.
6. Benjamin DK, Stoll BJ, Fanaroff AA, et al: Neonatal candidiasis among extremely low birth weight infants: risk factors, mortality rates, and neurodevelopmental outcomes at 18 to 22 months, *Pediatrics* 117:84-92, 2006.
7. Benjamin DK, Stoll BJ, Gantz MG, et al: Neonatal candidiasis: epidemiology, risk factors, and clinical judgement, *Pediatrics* 126:e865-e873, 2010.
8. Brissard O, Tandonnet O, Guichoux J: Invasive candidiasis in neonatal intensive care units, *Arch Pediatr* 18(Suppl 1):S22-S32, 2011.
9. Chapman RL: Prevention and treatment of *Candida* infections in neonates, *Semin Perinatol* 31:39-46, 2007.
10. Lin MY, Carmeli Y, Zumsteg J, et al: Prior antimicrobial therapy and risk for hospital-acquired *Candida glabrata* and *Candida krusei* fungemia: a case-case-control study, *Antimicrob Agents Chemother* 49:4555-4560, 2005.
11. Pammi M, Holland L, Butler G, et al: *Candida parapsilosis* is a significant neonatal pathogen: a systemic review and meta-analysis, *Pediatric Infect Dis J* 32:e206-e216, 2013.
12. Smith PB, Morgan J, Benjamin JD, et al: Excess costs of hospital care associated with neonatal candidemia, *Pediatr Infect Dis J* 26:197-200, 2007.
13. Pfaller MA, Diekema DJ, Jones RN, et al: International surveillance of bloodstream infections due to *Candida* species: frequency of occurrence and in vitro susceptibilities to fluconazole, ravuconazole, and voriconazole of isolates collected from 1997 through 1999 in the SENTRY antimicrobial surveillance program, *J Clin Microbiol* 39:3254-3259, 2001.
14. Cole GT, Halawa AA, Anaissie EJ: The role of the gastrointestinal tract in hematogenous candidiasis: from the laboratory to the bedside, *Clin Infect Dis* 22:S73-S88, 1996.
15. Pfaller MA, Messer SA, Moet GJ, et al: *Candida* bloodstream infections: comparison of species distribution and resistance to echinocandin and azole antifungal agents in intensive care unit (ICU) and non-ICU settings in the SENTRY Antimicrobial Surveillance Program (2008-2009), *Int J Antimicrob Agents* 38:65-69, 2011.
16. Stoll BJ, Hansen N, Fanaroff AA, et al: Changes in pathogens causing early-onset sepsis in very-low-birth-weight infants, *N Engl J Med* 347:240-247, 2002.
17. Stoll BJ, Hansen NI, Sánchez PJ, et al: Early onset neonatal sepsis: the burden of group B streptococal and *E. coli* disease continues, *Pediatrics* 127:817-826, 2011.
18. Saiman L, Ludington E, Pfaller M, et al: Risk factors for candidemia in neonatal intensive care unit patients. The National Epidemiology of Mycosis Survey study group, *Pediatr Infect Dis J* 19:319-324, 2000.
19. Rowen JL: Mucocutaneous candidiasis, *Semin Perinatol* 27:406-413, 2003.
20. Baradkar VP, Mathur M, Kumar S: Neonatal septicaemia in a premature infant due to *Candida dubliniensis*, *Indian J Med Microbiol* 26:382-389, 2008.
21. Faix RG: Invasive neonatal candidiasis: comparison of albicans and parapsilosis infection, *Pediatr Infect Dis J* 11:88-93, 1992.
22. Clerihew L, Austin N, McGuire W: Systemic antifungal prophylaxis for very low birthweight infants: a systematic review, *Arch Dis Child Fetal Neonatal Ed* 93:F198-F200, 2008.
23. Trofa D, Gacser A, Nosanchuk JD: *Candida parapsilosis*, an emerging fungal pathogen, *Clin Microbiol Rev* 21:606-625, 2008.
24. Farmaki E, Evdoridou J, Pouliou T, et al: Fungal colonization in the neonatal intensive care unit: risk factors, drug susceptibility, and association with invasive fungal infections, *Am J Perinatol* 24:127-135, 2007.
25. Kai-Larsen Y, Bergsson G, Gudmundsson GH, et al: Antimicrobial components of the neonatal gut affected upon colonization, *Pediatr Res* 61:530-536, 2007.
26. Kaufman D, Gurka MJ, Hazen KC, et al: Patterns of fungal colonization in preterm infants weighing less than 1000 grams at birth, *Pediatr Infect Dis J* 25:733-737, 2006.
27. Vendettuoli V, Tana M, Tirone C, et al: The role of *Candida* surveillance cultures for identification of a preterm subpopulation at highest risk for invasive fungal infection, *Pediatr Infect Dis J* 27:1114-1118, 2008.
28. Kaufman D, Boyle R, Hazen KC: Fluconazole prophylaxis against fungal colonization and infection in preterm infants, *N Engl J Med* 345:1660-1666, 2001.
29. Waggoner-Fountain LA, Walker MW, Hollis RJ, et al: Vertical and horizontal transmission of unique *Candida* species to premature newborns, *Clin Infect Dis* 22:803-808, 1996.
30. Bliss JM, Basavegowda KP, Watson WJ, et al: Vertical and horizontal transmission of *Candida albicans* in very low birth weight infants using DNA fingerprinting techniques, *Pediatr Infect Dis J* 27:231-235, 2008.
31. She XD, Wang XJ, Fu MH, et al: Genotype comparisons of strains of *Candida albicans* from patients with cutaneous candidiasis and vaginal candidiasis, *Chin Med J* 121:1450-1455, 2008.
32. Bendel CM: Colonization and epithelial adhesion in the pathogenesis of neonatal candidiasis, *Semin Perinatol* 27:357-364, 2003.
33. Ali GY, Algohary EH, Rashed KA, et al: Prevalence of *Candida* colonization in preterm newborns VLBW in neonatal intensive care unit: role of maternal colonization as a risk factor in transmission of disease, *J Matern Fetal Neonatal Med* 25:789-795, 2012.
34. Johnson DE, Thompson TR, Ferrieri P: Congenital candidiasis, *Am J Dis Child* 135:273-275, 1981.
35. Morrill JF, Pappagianis D, Heinig MJ, et al: Detecting *Candida albicans* in human milk, *J Clin Microbiol* 41:475-478, 2003.
36. Manzoni P, Farina D, Galletto P, et al: Type and number of sites colonized by fungi and risk of progression to invasive fungal infection in preterm neonates in neonatal intensive care unit, *J Perinat Med* 35:220-226, 2007.
37. Hedderwick SA, Lyons MJ, Liu M, et al: Epidemiology of yeast colonization in the intensive care unit, *Eur J Clin Microbiol Infect Dis* 19:663-670, 2000.
38. Bonassoli LA, Bertoli M, Svidzinski TI, et al: High frequency of *Candida parapsilosis* on the hands of healthy hosts, *J Hosp Infect* 59:159-162, 2005.
39. vanAsbeck EC, Huang YC, Markham AN, et al: *Candida parapsilosis* fungemia in neonates: genotyping results suggest heathcare workers hands as source, and review of published articles, *Mycopathologia* 164:287-293, 2007.
40. Hernandez-Castro R, Arroyo-Escalante S, Carrillo-Casas EM, et al: Outbreak of *Candida parapsilosis* in a neonatal intensive care unit: a health care workers source, *Eur J Pediatr* 169:763-787, 2010.

41. Sheretz RJ, Gledhill KS, Hampton KD, et al: Outbreak of *Candida* blood stream infections associated with retrograde medication administration in a neonatal intensive care unit, *J Pediatr* 120:455-461, 1992.
42. Fox BC, Mobley HL, Wade JC: The use of a DNA probe for epidemiological studies of candidiasis in immunocompromised hosts, *J Infect Dis* 159:488-494, 1989.
43. White MH: Epidemiology of invasive candidiasis: recent progress and current controversies, *Int J Infect Dis* 1:S7-S10, 1997.
44. Huang YC, Lin TY, Peng HL, et al: Outbreak of *Candida albicans* fungaemia in a neonatal intensive care unit, *Scand J Infect Dis* 30:137-142, 1998.
45. Reef SE, Lasker BA, Butcher DS, et al: Nonperinatal nosocomial transmission of *Candida albicans* in a neonatal intensive care unit: prospective study, *J Clin Microbiol* 36:1255-1259, 1998.
46. Asmundsdóttir LR, Erlendsdóttir H, Haraldsson G, et al: Molecular epidemiology of candidemia: evidence of clusters of smoldering nosocomial infections, *Clin Infect Dis* 47:E17-E24, 2008.
47. Boyce JM, Pittet D: Guideline for hand hygiene in health-care settings: recommendations of the healthcare infection control practices advisory committee and the HICPAC/SHEA/APIC/IDSA hand hygiene task force, *Infect Control Hosp Epidemiol* 23:S3-S40, 2002.
48. Vaudry WL, Tierney AJ, Wenman WM: Investigation of a cluster of systemic *Candida albicans* infections in a neonatal intensive care unit, *J Infect Dis* 158:1375-1379, 1988.
49. Solomon SL, Alexander H, Eley JW, et al: Nosocomial fungemia in neonates associated with intravascular pressure-monitoring devices, *Pediatr Infect Dis J* 5:680-685, 1986.
50. Kaufman DA: Neonatal candidiasis: clinical manifestations, management and prevention strategies, *J Pediatr* 156:S53-S67, 2010.
51. Kaufman DA: Challenging issues in neonatal candidiasis, *Curr Med Res Opin* 26:1769-1778, 2010.
52. St-Germain G, Laverdière M: Torulopsis Candida, a new opportunistic pathogen, *J Clin Microbiol* 24:884-885, 1986.
53. Lockhart SR, Messer SA, Pfaller MA, et al: Geographic distribution and antifungal susceptibility of the newly described species *Candida orthopsilosis* and *Candida metapsilosis* in comparison to the closely related species *Candida parapsilosis*, *J Clin Microbiol* 46:2659-2664, 2008.
54. Sullivan D, Coleman D: *Candida dubliniensis*: characteristics and identification, *J Clin Microbiol* 36:329-334, 1998.
55. Calderone RA, Clancy CJ: Candida *and candidiasis*, ed 2, Washington, DC, 2012, American Society for Microbiology Press.
56. Moran GP, Sullivan DJ, Colema DC: *Emergence of non-*Candida albicans Candida *species as pathogens*, Washington, DC, 2002, American Society for Microbiology Press.
57. Emori TG, Gaynes RP: An overview of nosocomial infections, including the role of the microbiology laboratory, *Clin Microbiol Rev* 6:428-442, 1993.
58. San-Blas G, Travassos LR, Fries BC, et al: Fungal morphogenesis and virulence, *Med Mycol* 38:79-86, 2000.
59. Bendel CM, Hess DJ, Garni RM, et al: Comparative virulence of *Candida albicans* yeast and filamentous forms in orally and intravenously inoculated mice, *Crit Care Med* 31:501-507, 2003.
60. Bendel CM, Kinneberg KM, Jechorek RP, et al: Systemic infection following intravenous inoculation of mice with *Candida albicans* int1 mutant strains, *Mol Genet Metab* 67:343-351, 1999.
61. Bendel CM, Wiesner SM, Garni RM, et al: Cecal colonization and systemic spread of *Candida albicans* in mice treated with antibiotics and dexamethasone, *Pediatr Res* 51:290-295, 2002.
62. Calderone RA: In vitro and ex vivo assays of virulence in *Candida albicans*, *Methods Mol Biol* 56:85-93, 2009.
63. Gale CA, Bendel CM, McClellan M, et al: Linkage of adhesion, filamentous growth, and virulence in *Candida albicans* to a single gene, INT1, *Science* 279:1355-1358, 1998.
64. Lo HJ, Köhler JR, DiDomenico B, et al: Nonfilamentous *C. albicans* mutants are avirulent, *Cell* 90:939-949, 1997.
65. Hoyer LL: The ALS gene family of *Candida albicans*, *Trends Microbiol* 9:176-180, 2001.
66. Mayer FL, Wilson D, Hube B, et al: *Candida albicans* pathogenicity mechanisms, *Virulence* 4:119-128, 2013.
67. Seneviratne CJ, Jin L, Samaranayake LP: Biofilm lifestyle of *Candida*: a mini review, *Oral Dis* 14:582-590, 2008.
68. Hostetter MK: New insights into candidal infections, *Adv Pediatr* 43:209-230, 1996.
69. Ferwerda G, Meyer-Wentrup F, Kullberg BJ, et al: Dectin-1 synergizes with TLR2 and TLR4 for cytokine production in human primary monocytes and macrophages, *Cell Microbiol* 10:2058-2066, 2008.
70. Bendel CM, St Sauver J, Carlson S, et al: Epithelial adhesion in yeast species: correlation with surface expression of the integrin analog, *J Infect Dis* 171:1660-1663, 1995.
71. Wiesner SM, Bendel CM, Hess DJ, et al: Adherence of yeast and filamentous forms of *Candida albicans* to cultured enterocytes, *Crit Care Med* 30:677-683, 2002.
72. Gustafson KS, Vercellotti GM, Bendel CM, et al: Molecular mimicry in *Candida albicans*-role of an integrin analog in adhesion of the yeast to human endothelium, *J Clin Invest* 87:1896-1902, 1991.
73. Bonhomme J, d'Enfert C: *Candida albicans* biofilms: building a heterogeneous, drug-tolerant environment, *Curr Opin Microbiol* 16:1-6, 2013.
74. Rossignol T, Ding C, Guida A, et al: Correlation between biofilm formation and the hypoxic response in *Candida parapsilosis*, *Eukaryot Cell* 8:550-559, 2009.
75. Douglas LJ: Penetration of antifungal agents through *Candida* biofilms, *Methods Mol Biol* 499:37-44, 2009.
76. Eubanks PJ, de Virgilio C, Klein S, et al: *Candida* sepsis in surgical patients, *Am J Surg* 166:617-620, 1993.
77. Faix RG, Kovarik SM: Polymicrobial sepsis among intensive care nursery infants, *J Perinatol* 9:131-136, 1989.
78. Li L, Dongari-Bagtzoglou A: Oral epithelium–*Candida glabrata* interactions in vitro, *Oral Microbiol Immunol* 22:182-187, 2007.
79. Falgier C, Kegley S, Podgorski H, et al: *Candida* species differ in their interactions with immature human gastrointestinal epithelial cells, *Pediatr Res* 69:384-389, 2011.
80. Bendel CM, Hostetter MK, McClellan M: Distinct mechanisms of epithelial adhesion for *Candida albicans* and *Candida tropicalis* identification of the participating ligands and development of inhibitory peptides, *J Clin Invest* 92:1840-1849, 1993.
81. Cuellar-Cuz M, López-Romero E, Villagómez-Castro JC, et al: *Candida* species: new insights into biofilm formation, *Future Microbiol* 7:755-771, 2012.
82. Tripathi N, Watt K, Benjamin DK: Treatment and prophylaxis of invasive candidiasis, *Semin Perinatol* 36:416-423, 2012.
83. Pappu-Katikaneni LD, Rao KPP, Banister E: Gastrointestinal colonization with yeast and *Candida* septicemia in very low birth weight infants, *Mycoses* 33:20-23, 1999.
84. Cotton MS, McDonald S, Stoll B, et al: The association of third-generation cephalosporin use and invasive candidiasis in extremely low birth-weight infants, *Pediatrics* 118:717-722, 2006.
85. Gordon DL, Johnson GM, Hostetter MK: Characteristics of iC3b binding to human polymorphonuclear leucocytes, *Immunology* 60:553-558, 1987.
86. Stanley VC, Carroll CJ, Hurley R: Distribution and significance of *Candida* precipitins in sera from pregnant women, *J Med Microbiol* 5:313-320, 1972.
87. Botas CM, Kurlat I, Young SM, et al: Disseminated candidal infections and intravenous hydrocortisone in preterm infants, *Pediatrics* 95:883-887, 1995.
88. Stark AR, Carlo WA, Tyson JE, et al: Adverse effects of early dexamethasone in extremely-low-birth-weight infants, National Institute of Child Health and Human Development Neonatal Research Network, *N Engl J Med* 344:95-101, 2001.
89. Banerjee D, Martin N, Nandi S, et al: A genome-wide steroid response study of the major human fungal pathogen *Candida albicans*, *Mycopathologia* 164:1-17, 2007.
90. Andes D, Nett J, Oschel P, et al: Development and characterization of an in vivo central venous catheter *Candida albicans* biofilm model, *Infect Immun* 72:6023-6031, 2004.
91. Chapman RL, Faix RG: Persistently positive cultures and outcome in invasive neonatal candidiasis, *Pediatr Infect Dis J* 19:822-827, 2000.
92. Johnson DE, Base JL, Thompson TR, et al: *Candida* septicemia and right atrial mass secondary to umbilical vein catheterization, *Am J Dis Child* 135:275-277, 1981.
93. Faix RG: Nonsurgical treatment of *Candida* endocarditis, *J Pediatr* 120:665-666, 1992.
94. Adderson EE, Pappin A, Pavia AT: Spontaneous intestinal perforation in premature infants: a distinct clinical entity associated with systemic candidiasis, *J Pediatr Surg* 33:1463-1467, 1998.

95. Darmstadt GL, Dinulos JG: Neonatal skin care, *Pediatr Clin North Am* 47:757-782, 2000.
96. Rowen JL, Atkins JT, Levy ML, et al: Invasive fungal dermatitis in the less-than-or-equal-to 1000 gram neonate, *Pediatrics* 95:682-687, 1995.
97. Ballow M, Cates KL, Rowe JC, et al: Development of the immune system in very low birth weight (less than 1500 g) premature infants: concentrations of plasma immunoglobulins and patterns of infections, *Pediatr Res* 20:899-904, 1986.
98. Zach TL, Hostetter MK: Biochemical abnormalities of the third component of complement in neonates, *Pediatr Res* 26:116-120, 1989.
99. al-Mulla ZS, Christensen RD: Neutropenia in the neonate, *Clin Perinatol* 22:711-739, 1995.
100. Manzoni P, Farina D, Monetti C, et al: Early-onset neutropenia is a risk factor for *Candida* colonization in very low-birth-weight neonates, *Diagn Microbiol Infect Dis* 57:77-83, 2007.
101. Parra-Herran CE, Pelaez L, Sola JE, et al: Intestinal Candidiasis: an uncommon cause of necrotizing enterocolitis (NEC) in neonates, *Fetal Pediatr Pathol* 29:172-180, 2010.
102. Fanaroff AA, Hack M, Walsh MC: The NICHD Neonatal Research Network: changes in practice and outcomes during the first 15 years, *Semin Perinatol* 27:281-287, 2003.
103. Johnson DE, Conroy MM, Foker JE, et al: *Candida* peritonitis in the newborn infant, *J Pediatr* 97:298-300, 1980.
104. Benjamin DK, Poole C, Steinbach WJ, et al: Neonatal candidemia and end-organ damage: a critical appraisal of the literature using meta-analytic techniques, *Pediatrics* 112:634-640, 2003.
105. Faix RG, Chapman RL: Central nervous system candidiasis in the high-risk neonate, *Semin Perinatol* 27:384-392, 2003.
106. Baley JE, Ellis F: Neonatal candidiasis: ophthalmologic infection, *Semin Perinatol* 27:401-405, 2003.
107. Drohan L, Colby CE, Brindle ME, et al: *Candida* (amphotericin-sensitive) lens abscess associated with decreasing arterial blood flow in a very low birth weight preterm infant, *Pediatrics* 110:e65, 2002.
108. Doctor BA, Newman N, Minich NM, et al: Clinical outcomes of neonatal meningitis in very-low-birth-weight infants, *Clin Pediatr* 40:473-480, 2001.
109. Marcinkowski M, Bauer K, Stoltenburg-Didinger G, et al: Fungal brain abscesses in neonates: sonographic appearances and corresponding histopathologic findings, *J Clin Ultrasound* 29:417-421, 2001.
110. Carter JE, Laurini JA, Evans TN, et al: Neonatal *Candida parapsilosis* meningitis and empyema related to epidural migration of a central venous catheter, *Clin Neurol Neurosurg* 110:614-618, 2008.
111. Benjamin DK, Fisher RG, McKinney RE: Candidal mycetoma in the neonatal kidney, *Pediatrics* 104:1126-1129, 1999.
112. Karlowicz MG: Candidal renal and urinary tract infections in neonates, *Semin Perinatol* 27:393-400, 2003.
113. Winters WD, Shaw DWW, Weinberger E: *Candida* fungus balls presenting as intraventricular masses in cranial sonography, *J Clin Ultrasound* 23:266-270, 1995.
114. Schwartz DA, Reef S: *Candida albicans* placentitis and funisitis-early diagnosis of congenital candidemia by histopathologic examination of umbilical cord vessels, *Pediatr Infect Dis J* 9:661-665, 1990.
115. Ito F, Okubo T, Yasuo T, et al: Premature delivery due to intrauterine *Candida* infection that caused neonatal congenital cutaneous candidiasis: a case report, *J Obstet Gynaecol Res* 39:341-343, 2013.
116. Smolinski KN, Shah SS, Honig PJ, et al: Neonatal cutaneous fungal infections, *Curr Opin Pediatr* 17:486-493, 2005.
117. Faix RG, Kovarik SM, Shaw TR, et al: Mucocutaneous and invasive candidiasis among very low birth weight (less than 1,500 grams) infants in intensive care nurseries: a prospective study, *Pediatrics* 83:101-107, 1989.
118. Gupta P, Faridi MM, Rawat S, et al: Clinical profile and risk factors for oral candidosis in sick newborns, *Indian Pediatr* 33:299-303, 1996.
119. Daftary SS, Desai SV, Shah MV, et al: Oral thrush in the new-born, *Indian Pediatr* 17:287-288, 1980.
120. Hoppe JE: Treatment of oropharyngeal candidiasis and candidal diaper dermatitis in neonates and infants: review and reappraisal, *Pediatr Infect Dis J* 16:885-894, 1997.
121. Goins RA, Ascher D, Waecker N, et al: Comparison of fluconazole and nystatin oral suspensions for treatment of oral candidiasis in infants, *Pediatr Infect Dis J* 21:1165-1167, 2002.
122. Leyden JJ: Diaper dermatitis, *Dermatol Clin* 4:23-28, 1986.
123. Roque H, Abdelhak Y, Young BK: Intra amniotic candidiasis. Case report and meta-analysis cases, *J Perinat Med* 27:253-262, 1999.
124. Darmstadt GL, Dinulos JG, Miller Z: Congenital cutaneous candidiasis: clinical presentation, pathogenesis, and management guidelines, *Pediatrics* 105:438-444, 2000.
125. Fairchild KD, Tomkoria S, Sharp EC, et al: Neonatal *Candida glabrata* sepsis: clinical and laboratory features compared with other *Candida* species, *Pediatr Infect Dis J* 21:39-43, 2002.
126. Wang SM, Hsu CH, Chang JH: Congenital candidiasis, *Pediatr Neonatol* 3:94-96, 2008.
127. Bendel CM, Hostetter MK: Systemic candidiasis and other fungal infections in the newborn, *Semin Pediatr Infect Dis* 5:35-41, 1994.
128. Barone SR, Krilov LR: Neonatal candidal meningitis in a full-term infant with congenital cutaneous candidiasis, *Clin Pediatr (Phila)* 34:217-219, 1995.
129. Melville C, Kempley S, Graham J, et al: Early onset systemic *Candida* infection in extremely preterm neonates, *Eur J Pediatr* 155:904-906, 1996.
130. Fernandez M, Noyola DE, Rossmann SN, et al: Cutaneous phaeohyphomycosis caused by *Curvularia lunata* and a review of *Curvularia* infections in pediatrics, *Pediatr Infect Dis J* 18:727-731, 1999.
131. Bryan MG, Elston DM, Hivnor C, et al: Phaeohyphomycosis in a premature infant, *Cutis* 65:137-140, 2000.
132. Leibovitz E, Iuster-Reicher A, Amitai M, et al: Systemic candidal infections associated with use of peripheral venous catheters in neonates: a 9-year experience, *Clin Infect Dis* 14:485-491, 1992.
133. Hensey OJ, Hart CA, Cooke RWI: *Candida albicans* skin abscesses, *Arch Dis Child* 59:479-480, 1984.
134. Dyke MP, Ott K: Severe thrombocytopenia in extremely low birth weight infants with systemic candidiasis, *J Paediatr Child Health* 29:298-301, 1993.
135. Pappas PG, Kauffman CA, Andes D, et al: Clinical practice guidelines for the management of candidiasis: 2009 update by the Infectious Diseases Society of America, *Clin Infect Dis* 48:503-535, 2009.
136. Pickering LK: Candidiasis. In Pickering LK, Baker CJ, Kimberlin DW, Long SS, editors: *Red book, 2012 report of the Committee on Infectious Diseases*, ed 29, Elk Grove Village, Ill, 2012, American Academy of Pediatrics.
137. Foker JE, Bass JL, Thompson T, et al: Management of intracardiac fungal masses in premature infants, *J Thorac Cardiovasc Surg* 87:244-250, 1984.
138. Robinson JL, Davies HD, Barton M, et al: Characteristics and outcomes of infants with candiduria in neonatal intensive care: a Paediatric Investigators Collaborative Network on Infections in Canada (PICNIC) study, *BMC Infect Dis* 9:183-192, 2009.
139. Bodey GP, Luna M: Skin lesions associated with disseminated candidiasis, *JAMA* 229:1466-1468, 1974.
140. Noyola DE, Fernandez M, Moylett EH, et al: Ophthalmologic, visceral, and cardiac involvement in neonates with candidemia, *Clin Infect Dis* 32:1018-1023, 2001.
141. Tung KT, MacDonald LM, Smith JC: Neonatal systemic candidiasis diagnosed by ultrasound, *Acta Radiol* 31:293-295, 1990.
142. Khan MY: Anuria from *Candida* pyelonephritis and obstructing fungal balls, *Urology* 21:421-423, 1983.
143. Sirinelli D, Biriotti V, Schmit P, et al: Urinoma and arterial hypertension complicating neonatal renal candidiasis, *Pediatr Radiol* 17:156-158, 1987.
144. McDonnell M, Lam AH, Isaacs D: Nonsurgical management of neonatal obstructive uropathy due to *Candida albicans*, *Clin Infect Dis* 21:1349-1350, 1995.
145. Faix RG: Systemic *Candida* infections in infants in intensive care nurseries-high incidence of central nervous system involvement, *J Pediatr* 105:616-622, 1984.
146. Goldsmith LS, Rubenstein SD, Wolfson BJ, et al: Cerebral calcifications in a neonate with candidiasis, *Pediatr Infect Dis J* 9:451-453, 1990.
147. Cohen-Wolkowiez M, Smith PB, Mangum B, et al: Neonatal *Candida* meningitis: significance of cerebrospinal fluid parameters and blood cultures, *J Perinatol* 27:97-100, 2007.
148. Stern JH, Calvano C, Simon JW: Recurrent endogenous candidal endophthalmitis in a premature infant, *J AAPOS* 5:50-51, 2001.
149. Todd Johnston W, Cogen MS: Systemic candidiasis with cataract formation in a premature infant, *J AAPOS* 4:386-388, 2000.
150. Shah GK, Vander J, Eagle RC: Intralenticular *Candida* species abscess in a premature infant, *Am J Ophthalmol* 129:390-391, 2000.

151. Mittal M, Dhanireddy R, Higgins RD: *Candida* sepsis and association with retinopathy of prematurity, *Pediatrics* 101:654-657, 1998.
152. Noyola DE, Bohra L, Paysse EA, et al: Association of candidemia and retinopathy of prematurity in very low birthweight infants, *Ophthalmology* 109:80-84, 2002.
153. Karlowicz MG, Giannone PJ, Pestian J, et al: Does candidemia predict threshold retinopathy of prematurity in extremely low birth weight (</= 1000 g) neonates? *Pediatrics* 105:1036-1040, 2000.
154. Haroon Parupia MF, Dhanireddy R: Association of postnatal dexamethasone use and fungal sepsis in the development of severe retinopathy of prematurity and progression to laser therapy in extremely low-birth-weight infants, *J Perinatol* 21:242-247, 2001.
155. Tadesse M, Dhanireddy R, Mittal M, et al: Race, *Candida* sepsis, and retinopathy of prematurity, *Biol Neonate* 81:86-90, 2002.
156. Manzoni P, Maestri A, Leonessa M, et al: Fungal and bacterial sepsis and threshold ROP in preterm very low birth weight neonates, *J Perinatol* 26:23-30, 2006.
157. Robertson NJ, Kuna J, Cox PM, et al: Spontaneous intestinal perforation and *Candida* peritonitis presenting as extensive necrotizing enterocolitis, *Acta Paediatr* 92:258-261, 2003.
158. Bond S, Stewart DL, Bendon RW: Invasive *Candida* enteritis of the newborn, *J Pediatr Surg* 35:1496-1498, 2000.
159. Kaplan M, Eidelman AI, Dollberg L, et al: Necrotizing bowel disease with *Candida* peritonitis following severe neonatal hypothermia, *Acta Paediatr Scand* 79:876-879, 1990.
160. Schelonka RL, Moser SA: Time to positive culture results in neonatal *Candida* septicemia, *J Pediatr* 142:564-565, 2003.
161. Ellepola AN: Laboratory diagnosis of invasive candidiasis, *J Microbiol* 43:65-84, 2005.
162. Schelonka RL, Chai MK, Yoder BA, et al: Volume of blood required to detect common neonatal pathogens, *J Pediatr* 129:275-278, 1996.
163. Pollack CV Jr, Pollack ES, Andrew ME: Suprapubic bladder aspiration versus urethral catheterization in ill infants: success, efficiency and complication rates, *Ann Emerg Med* 23:225-230, 1994.
164. Fernandez M, Moylett EH, Noyola DE, et al: Candidal meningitis in neonates: a 10-year review, *Clin Infect Dis* 31:458-463, 2000.
165. Villari P, Iacuzio L, Torre I, et al: Molecular epidemiology as an effective tool in the surveillance of infections in the neonatal intensive care unit, *J Infect* 37:274-281, 1998.
166. Pfaller MA: Epidemiology of nosocomial candidiasis: the importance of molecular typing, *Braz J Infect Dis* 4:161-167, 2000.
167. Reiss E, Lasker BA, Lott TJ, et al: Genotyping of *Candida parapsilosis* from three neonatal intensive care units (NICUs) using a panel of five multilocus microsatellite markers: broad genetic diversity and a cluster of related strains in one NICU, *Infect Genet Evol* 12:1654-1660, 2012.
168. Erden A, Fitoz S, Karagülle T, et al: Radiological findings in the diagnosis of genitourinary candidiasis, *Pediatr Radiol* 30:875-877, 2000.
169. Huang CC, Chen CY, Yang HB, et al: Central nervous system candidiasis in very low-birth-weight premature neonates and infants: US characteristics and histopathologic and MR imaging correlates in five patients, *Radiology* 209:49-56, 1998.
170. Lain A, Elguezabal N, Brena S, et al: Diagnosis of invasive candidiasis by enzyme-linked immunosorbent assay using the N-terminal fragment of *Candida albicans* hyphal wall protein I, *BMC Microbiol* 7:35, 2007.
171. Metwally L, Fairley DJ, Coyle PV, et al: Improving molecular detection of *Candida* DNA in whole blood: comparison of seven fungal DNA extraction protocols using real-time PCR, *J Med Microbiol* 57:296-303, 2008.
172. Naja G, Hrapovic S, Male K, et al: Rapid detection of microorganisms with nanoparticles and electron microscopy, *Microsc Res Tech* 71:742-748, 2008.
173. Kedzierska A, Kochan P, Pietrzyk A, et al: Current status of fungal cell wall components in the immunodiagnostics of invasive fungal infections in humans: galactomannan, mannan and (1→3)-beta-d-glucan antigens, *Eur J Clin Microbiol Infect Dis* 26:755-766, 2007.
174. Gebert S, Siegel D, Wellinghausen N: Rapid detection of pathogens in blood culture bottles by real-time PCR in conjunction with the pre-analytic tool MolYsis, *J Infect* 57:307-316, 2008.
175. Lau A, Sorrell TC, Chen S, et al: Multiplex tandem PCR: a novel platform for rapid detection and identification of fungal pathogens from blood culture specimens, *J Clin Microbiol* 46:3021-3027, 2008.
176. Wiley JM: Fungal infections in pediatric immunocompromised patients: epidemiology, principles of treatment and promising antifungal agents, *J Pediatr* 156:S74-S82, 2010.
177. Pfaller MA, Messer SA, Boyken L, et al: In vitro activities of 5-fluorocytosine against 8,803 clinical isolates of *Candida* spp.: global assessment of primary resistance using national committee for clinical laboratory standards susceptibility testing methods, *Antimicrob Agents Chemother* 46:3518-3521, 2002.
178. Hajjeh RA, Sofair AN, Harrison LH, et al: Incidence of bloodstream infections due to *Candida* species and in vitro susceptibilities of isolates collected from 1998-2000 in a population-based active surveillance program, *J Clin Microbiol* 42:1519-1527, 2004.
179. Lestner JM, Smith PB, Cohen-Wolkowiez M, et al: Antifungal agents and therapy for infants and children with invasive fungal infections; a pharmacological perspective, *Br J Clin Pharmacol* 75:1381-1395, 2012.
180. Karlowicz MG, Hashimoto LN, Kelly RE Jr, et al: Should central venous catheters be removed as soon as candidemia is detected in neonates? *Pediatrics* 106:e63, 2000.
181. Rex JH, Pappas PG, Karchmer AW: A randomized and blinded multicenter trial of high-dose fluconazole plus placebo versus fluconazole plus amphotericin B as therapy for candidemia and its consequences in nonneutropenic subjects, *Clin Infect Dis* 36:1221-1228, 2003.
182. Faix RG, Feick HJ, Frommelt P, et al: Successful medical treatment of *Candida parapsilosis* endocarditis in a premature infant, *Am J Perinatol* 7:272-275, 1990.
183. Munz D, Powell KR, Pai CH: Treatment of candidal diaper dermatitis: a double-blind placebo-controlled comparison of topical nystatin with topical plus oral nystatin, *J Pediatr* 101:1022-1025, 1982.
184. Wainer S, Cooper PA, Funk E, et al: Prophylactic oral gel for the prevention of neonatal fungal rectal colonization and systemic infection, *Pediatr Infect Dis J* 11:713-716, 1992.
185. Concannon P, Gisoldi E, Phillips S, et al: Diaper dermatitis: a therapeutic dilemma. Results of a double-blind placebo controlled trial of miconazole nitrate 0.25%, *Pediatr Dermatol* 18:149-155, 2001.
186. Almirante B, Rodriguez D: Antifungal agents in neonates: issues and recommendations, *Pediatr Drugs* 9:311-321, 2007.
187. Zaoutis T, Walsh TJ: Antifungal therapy for neonatal candidiasis, *Curr Opin Infect Dis* 6:592-597, 2007.
188. McClenny NB, Fei H, Baron EJ, et al: Change in colony morphology of *Candida lusitaniae* in association with development of amphotericin B resistance, *Antimicrob Agents Chemother* 46:1325-1328, 2002.
189. Linder N, Klinger G, Shalit I: Treatment of candidaemia in premature infants: comparison of three amphotericin B preparations, *J Antimicrob Chemother* 52:663-667, 2003.
190. Kingo AR, Smyth JA, Waisman D: Lack of evidence of amphotericin B toxicity in very low birth weight infants treated for systemic candidiasis, *Pediatr Infect Dis J* 16:1002-1003, 1997.
191. Baley JE, Meyers C, Kliegman RM, et al: Pharmacokinetics, outcome of treatment, and toxic effects of amphotericin B and 5-fluorocytosine in neonates, *J Pediatr* 116:791-797, 1990.
192. Juster-Reicher A, Leibovitz E, Linder N, et al: Liposomal amphotericin B (AmBisome) in the treatment of neonatal candidiasis in very low birth weight infants, *Infection* 28:223-226, 2000.
193. Adler-Shohet F, Waskin H, Lieberman JM: Amphotericin B lipid complex for neonatal invasive candidiasis, *Arch Dis Child Fetal Neonatal Ed* 84:F131-F133, 2001.
194. Dupont B: Overview of the lipid formulations of amphotericin B, *J Antimicrob Chemother* 49:31-36, 2002.
195. Ferrari P, Chiarolanza J, Capriotti T, et al: Favorable course of cerebral candidiasis in a low-birth weight newborn treated with liposomal amphotericin B, *Pediatr Med Chir* 23:197-199, 2001.
196. Chesney PJ, Justman RA, Bogdanowicz WM: *Candida* meningitis in newborn infants-review and report of combined amphotericin B flucytosine therapy, *Johns Hopkins Med J* 142:155-160, 1978.
197. Johnson EM, Richardson MD, Warnock DW: In vitro resistance to imidazole antifungals in *Candida albicans*, *J Antimicrob Chemother* 13:547-558, 1984.
198. Novelli V, Holzel H: Safety and tolerability of fluconazole in children, *Antimicrob Agents Chemother* 43:1955-1960, 1999.
199. Triolo V, Gari-Toussaint M, Casagrande F, et al: Fluconazole therapy for *Candida albicans* urinary tract infections in infants, *Pediatr Nephrol* 17:550-553, 2002.

200. Kicklighter SD, Springer SC, Cox T, et al: Fluconazole for prophylaxis against candidal rectal colonization in the very low birth weight infant, *Pediatrics* 107:293-298, 2001.
201. Driessen M, Ellis JB, Cooper PA, et al: Fluconazole vs. amphotericin B for the treatment of neonatal fungal septicemia: a prospective randomized trial, *Pediatr Infect Dis J* 15:1107-1112, 1996.
202. Manzoni P, Leonessa M, Galletto P, et al: Routine use of fluconazole prophylaxis in a neonatal intensive care unit does not select natively fluconazole-resistant *Candida* subspecies, *Pediatr Infect Dis J* 27:731-737, 2008.
203. Sabo JA, Abdel-Rahman SM: Voriconazole: a new triazole antifungal, *Ann Pharmacother* 34:1032-1043, 2000.
204. Walsh TJ, Driscoll T: Pharmacokinetics and safety of intravenous voriconazole in children after single- or multiple-dose administration, *Antimicrob Agents Chemother* 48:2166-2172, 2004.
205. Muldrew KM, Maples HD, Stowe CD: Intravenous voriconazole therapy in a preterm infant, *Pharmacotherapy* 25:893-898, 2005.
206. Kohli V, Taneja V, Sachdev P, et al: Voriconazole in newborns, *Indian Pediatr* 45:236-238, 2008.
207. Stone EA, Fung HB, Kirschenbaum HL: Caspofungin: an echinocandin antifungal agent, *Clin Ther* 24:351-377, 2002.
208. Roling EE, Klepser ME, Wasson A, et al: Antifungal activities of fluconazole, caspofungin (MK0991), and anidulafungin (LY 303366) alone and in combination against *Candida* spp. and *Cryptococcus neoformans* via time-kill methods, *Diagn Microbiol Infect Dis* 43:13-17, 2002.
209. Saez-Llorens X, Macias M, Maiya P, et al: Pharmacokinetics and safety of caspofungin in neonates and infants less than 3 months of age, *Antimicrob Agents Chemother* 53:869-875, 2008.
210. Heresi GP, Gerstmann DR, Reed MD: The pharmacokinetics and safety of micafungin, a novel echinocandin, in premature infants, *Pediatr Infect Dis J* 25:1110-1115, 2006.
211. Adams-Chapman I, Bann CM, Das A, et al: Neurodevelopmental outcome of extremely low birth weight infants with *Candida* infection, *J Pediatr* 162:1047-1053, 2013.
212. Friedman S, Richardson SE, O'Brien K: Systemic *Candida* infection in extremely low birth weight infants: short term morbidity and long term neurodevelopmental outcome, *Pediatr Infect Dis J* 19:499-504, 2000.
213. Larson E, Silberger M, Jakob K, et al: Assessment of alternative hand hygiene regimens to improve skin health among neonatal intensive care unit nurses, *Heart Lung* 29:136-142, 2000.
214. Campbell JR, Zaccaria E, Baker CJ: Systemic candidiasis in extremely low birth weight infants receiving topical petrolatum ointment for skin care: a case-control study, *Pediatrics* 105:1041-1045, 2000.
215. Isaacs D: Fungal prophylaxis in very low birth weight neonates: nystatin, fluconazole or nothing? *Curr Opin Infect Dis* 3:246-250, 2008.
216. Kaufman DA: Aiming for zero: preventing invasive *Candida* infections in extremely preterm infants, *Neoreviews* 12:e381-e392, 2011.
217. Healy CM, Baker CJ: Fluconazole prophylaxis in the neonatal intensive care unit, *Pediatr Infect Dis J* 28:49-52, 2009.
218. Manzoni P, Stolfi I, Pugni L, et al: A multicenter, randomized trial of prophylactic fluconazole in preterm neonates, *N Engl J Med* 356:2483-2495, 2007.
219. Rex JH, Rinaldi MG, Pfaller MA: Resistance of *Candida* species to fluconazole, *Antimicrob Agents Chemother* 39:1-8, 1995.
220. Weitkamp JH, Ozdas A, LaFleur B, et al: Fluconazole prophylaxis for prevention of invasive fungal infections in targeted highest risk preterm infants limits drug exposure, *J Perinatol* 28:405-411, 2008.
221. Martin A, Pappas A, Lulic-Botica M, et al: Impact of "targeted" fluconazole prophylaxis for preterm neonates: efficacy of a highly selective approach? *J Perinatol* 32:21-26, 2012.
222. Kaufman DA, Cuff AL, Wamstad JB, et al: Fluconazole prophylaxis in extremely low birth weight infants and neurodevelopmental outcomes at 8 to 10 years of age, *J Pediatric* 158:759-765, 2011.

34 *Pneumocystis* and Other Less Common Fungal Infections

FRANCIS GIGLIOTTI, TERRY W. WRIGHT, and DAMIAN J. KRYSAN

CHAPTER OUTLINE

Fungal infections, other than those caused by *Candida* spp., rarely are considered in the differential diagnosis for an acutely ill newborn infant because disorders of bacterial and viral etiology are vastly more common. Nevertheless, fungal infections do occur in neonates, especially in premature infants and those of very low birth weight (less than 1500 g), and can cause serious and frequently fatal disease. As with any other infectious disease, the risk of fungal infection depends on the host and risk of exposure. The neonate has some risk of exposure to either *Malassezia furfur* or *Pneumocystis jirovecii* (previously *Pneumocystis carinii*), has a limited risk of exposure to *Aspergillus* spp., and has an extremely low risk of exposure to other fungi, especially in the neonatal intensive care unit (NICU) setting. Therefore it is not surprising that the most common fungal infection in neonates is candidiasis.

Although much has been learned regarding the pathogenesis, immune response, and treatment of fungal infections in older children and adults, studies to determine the cause of increased susceptibility or resistance to infection with fungi, especially in neonates, are incomplete. The intent of this chapter is to review current knowledge regarding fungal diseases, other than those caused by *Candida*, in the neonate and infant. Infections caused by *Candida* are reviewed in Chapter 33.

Pneumocystis jirovecii (Formerly Known as *Pneumocystis carinii*) Infection

P. jirovecii, a fungus with a history of unsettled taxonomy, was discovered in the lungs of small mammals and humans in Brazil more than 100 years ago. Today it is a cause of often fatal pneumonia in patients with primary immunodeficiencies or secondary immunodeficiencies, such as those resulting from the treatment of hematologic malignancies, collagen-vascular disorders, or organ allografts, and in those who receive corticosteroids and immunosuppressive drug therapy. Although congenital infection with *Pneumocystis* is unproven, it does occur in infants younger than 1 year in two well-defined epidemiologic settings: (1) in epidemics in nurseries located in impoverished areas of the world and (2) in isolated cases in which the infected child has an underlying primary immunodeficiency disease or acquired immunodeficiency syndrome (AIDS).

This section of the chapter reviews the problem of *Pneumocystis* infection in the newborn. Much of our knowledge of the epidemiologic, pathologic, and clinical features of pneumocystosis, however, is drawn from observations of the infection in older children and adults, as well as from animal models. As a result, we have elected to include data derived from such observations to present a more complete picture of the infectious process caused by this unique organism.

HISTORY

In 1909 in Brazil, Chagas[1] first described the morphologic forms of *Pneumocystis* in the lungs of guinea pigs infected with *Trypanosoma cruzi*. He believed the forms to represent a sexual stage in the life cycle of the trypanosome and not a different organism. Carini,[2] an Italian working in Brazil, saw the same organism-like cysts in the lungs of rats experimentally infected with *Trypanosoma lewisi*. His slide material subsequently was reviewed by P. and M. Delanoë and their colleagues[3] at the Pasteur Institute in Paris. They recognized that these alveolar cysts were present in the lungs of local Parisian sewer rats and thereby established that the "organisms" were independent of trypanosomes. They proposed the name *Pneumocystis carinii* for the new species.

At about this time, Chagas may have unwittingly described the first human case of pneumocystosis when he reported the presence of similar organisms in the lungs of a patient with interstitial pneumonia who had died of American trypanosomiasis.[4] Nevertheless, no definite etiologic connection was made between *P. carinii* and human pneumonic disease for another 30 years. The reason for this delay was the belief during this period that infantile syphilis was responsible for virtually all instances of interstitial plasma cell pneumonia. In 1938, Benecke[5] and Ammich[6] identified a histologically similar pneumonic illness in nonsyphilitic children that was characterized by a peculiar honeycombed exudate in alveoli. Subsequent scrutiny of photomicrographs in their reports revealed the presence of *Pneumocystis* organisms,[7] but it was not until 1942 that Van der Meer and Brug,[8] in the Netherlands, unequivocally recognized the organism in lungs from two infants and one adult. The first epidemics of interstitial plasma cell pneumonia were reported shortly thereafter among premature debilitated babies in nurseries and foundling homes in central Europe. In 1952, Vanek and Jirovec[7] in Czechoslovakia provided the most convincing demonstration of the etiologic relationship of *Pneumocystis* to this disease in an autopsy study of 16 cases.

Pneumocystosis was first brought to the attention of pediatricians in the United States in 1953 by Deamer and Zollinger,[9] who reviewed the pathologic and epidemiologic features of the European disease. In 1957, Gajdusek[10] presented an in-depth perspective on the history of the infection that included an extensive bibliography. This review was particularly timely because the next decade was to see the disturbing emergence of *P. carinii* pneumonia in the Western world—even while the epidemic disease in central Europe was waning—to the degree that it would become preeminent among the so-called opportunistic pulmonary infections in the immunosuppressed host. In 1988, DNA analysis demonstrated that *Pneumocystis* was not a protozoan but a fungus.[11] Most recently, a change in nomenclature from *P. carinii* to *P. jirovecii*, a name chosen in honor of the parasitologist Otto Jirovec, who now is credited by some with the original description of this organism, has been put forth.[12] The rationale for this change is the unique antigenic, genetic, and restricted infectivity profile of the *Pneumocystis* organisms associated with each mammalian species.[12-15]

THE ORGANISM

The taxonomic status of *P. jirovecii* as a fungus has been defined on the basis of molecular analysis.[11,12] Because the organism cannot be adequately propagated in vitro, efforts to classify it and to elucidate its structure and life cycle have been based exclusively on morphologic observations of infected lungs from animals and humans. The earliest of these investigations was performed by parasitologists; in accordance, the terminology applied to the forms of *Pneumocystis* seen in diseased tissue has been that reserved for protozoal organisms.

Three developmental forms of this presumably unicellular microbe have been described: a thick-walled cyst, an intracystic sporozoite (intracystic body), and a thin-walled trophozoite (trophic form).[4] The form of *Pneumocystis* that assists with diagnosis is the cyst, which may contain up to eight sporozoites. Each sporozoite is round to crescent shaped, measures 1 to 2 μm in diameter, and contains an eccentric nucleus. This cystic unit with its intracystic bodies is seen well in Giemsa-stained imprint smears of infected fresh lung.[10,16] Giemsa stain, however, results in staining of background alveoli and host cell fragments and does not stain empty cysts. Gomori methenamine silver stain (GMS), which highlights only the cyst wall of *Pneumocystis*, is preferable to Giemsa stain when tissues must be screened for the presence of organisms.[17] The cysts stained with silver have a black cell wall and appear round, crescentic, or disk shaped. Cysts measure 4 to 6 μm in diameter and must be distinguished from erythrocytes. The cysts often occur in clusters within an alveolus.

The typical honeycombed intraalveolar exudate of *Pneumocystis* pneumonia is a result of negative staining of clumps of cysts held together by proteinaceous debris. The internal structure of the silver-stained cyst is variable. In the lighter-staining round cysts, there are sometimes visible thickenings in the cell wall that are circular or comma shaped (Fig. 34-1).[18] The significance of these cell wall variations is unknown, but they are helpful in confirming the identification of *Pneumocystis*.

Staining procedures, other than those using Giemsa and methenamine silver, have been used less frequently to delineate the cyst form of the organism. The cyst wall stains red with periodic acid–Schiff (PAS) stain.[19] A modified Gram-Weigert method stains both the cyst wall and the intracystic sporozoites.[20] Gridley fungus stain may identify cyst outlines. More reliable stains for this purpose are the modified toluidine blue stain of Chalvardjian and Grawe[21] and the crystal violet stain,[22] which color the cyst wall purple. Electron microscopy has been an invaluable tool in morphologic studies of *P. jirovecii*.[23-26] It has helped to confirm that the structures regarded as *Pneumocystis* under light microscopy are, in fact, typical microorganisms and not just degradation products of host cells.

The trophozoite is thin walled and measures between 1.5 and 2.0 μm in diameter. It has numerous evaginations or pseudopodia-like projections that appear to interdigitate with those of other organisms in the alveolar space.[25,26] The projections have been postulated to allow for attachment of *Pneumocystis*, but the prevailing opinion, however, is that no specialized organelle of attachment exists. Rather, the surfaces of *P. jirovecii* and alveolar cells (specifically, type I pneumonocytes) are closely opposed, without fusion of cell membranes.[27] This adherence of *P. jirovecii* to alveolar lining cells may explain why organisms are not commonly found in expectorated mucus or tracheal secretions.[25]

The intracystic bodies (sporozoites) measure 1.0 to 1.7 μm across and bear a marked similarity to small trophozoites.[26] In addition, thick-walled cysts rich in glycogen particles but without intracystic bodies ("precysts"), partly empty cysts, and collapsed cystic structures have been identified. The collapsed cysts are crescentic and presumably are the same crescentic forms seen frequently in silver-stained specimens under light microscopy.

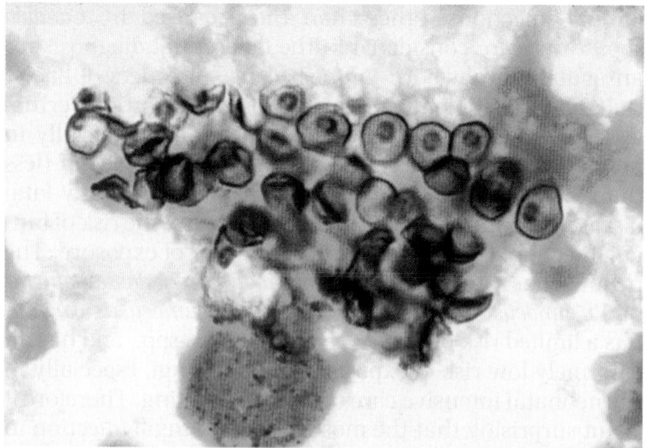

Figure 34-1 Cysts of *Pneumocystis jirovecii* in a smear from bronchoalveolar lavage. (Gomori methenamine silver stain, ×400.) (Courtesy Dr. Russell K. Brynes, Centers for Disease Control and Prevention Public Health Image Library.)

Life cycles for *P. jirovecii* have been proposed. They have been based on the variant forms of the fungus detected by light[18,28,29] and electron microscopy.[26,30] One scheme suggests that the thick-walled round cyst undergoes dissolution or "cracking," whereupon the intracystic bodies pass through tears in the wall (Fig. 34-2).[26] It is not known whether the bodies escape from the cyst by active motility or whether they are extruded passively as a consequence of cyst collapse. At this stage, the intracystic bodies resemble free thin-walled trophozoites. The small trophozoites evolve to larger forms, their walls thicken, and a precyst develops that is devoid of intracystic bodies. The cyclic process is completed when formation of the mature cyst, containing eight daughter cysts, is achieved.

Classification of *Pneumocystis* as a protozoan or as a fungus was complicated by the inability to maintain the organism in culture to further characterize the biochemical nature of the organism. Arguments in favor of a protozoan taxonomy were based mainly on the resemblance of its structural features to those of other protozoa. The organism has cystic and trophozoite stages, pseudopodia in cell walls, and pellicles around intracystic sporozoites. In addition, the disease caused by *Pneumocystis* responds to antiprotozoal medications, such as pentamidine, atovaquone, fansidar, trimethoprim-sulfamethoxazole (TMP-SMX), while not responding to many antifungal drugs, namely, amphotericin, azoles, 5-flucytosine, and Nystatin. On the other hand, like fungi, *P. jirovecii* contains a paucity of cellular organelles, its nucleus is not visibly prominent, and its cell membrane is layered throughout an entire life cycle. Finally, there is a high degree of homology between "housekeeping" genes of *Pneumocystis* and other fungi.[11,31,32]

The question of host species specificity of *Pneumocystis* remained similarly unanswered until the development of highly specific monoclonal antibodies provided the tools to demonstrate the uniqueness of *Pneumocystis* isolated from

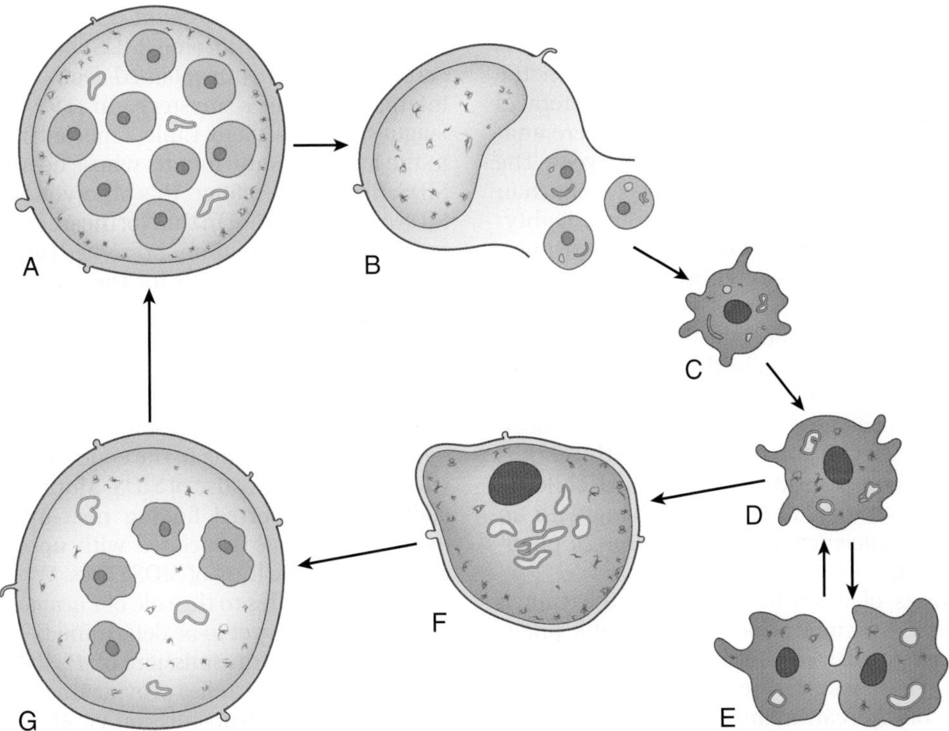

Figure 34-2 Probable life cycle of *Pneumocystis* within pulmonary alveoli. **A,** Mature cyst with intracystic bodies. **B,** Empty cyst and recently escaped intracystic body. **C,** Small trophozoite. **D,** Larger trophozoite. **E,** Possible budding or conjugating form. **F,** Large trophozoite undergoing thickening of pellicle. **G,** Precyst.

different mammalian hosts.[13,33,34] Subsequent genetic analyses confirmed the host species specificity of *Pneumocystis*.[15,35-39] The initial demonstration that *Pneumocystis* could not be transmitted between different host species provided biologic confirmation for the observed host-defined phenotypic and genotypic differences among *Pneumocystis*.

EPIDEMIOLOGY AND TRANSMISSION

The distribution of human infection is worldwide, and a wide variety of wild and domestic animal species has been demonstrated to be infected by *Pneumocystis*. The natural habitat of *P. jirovecii* is unknown, but what is known of the biology of *Pneumocystis* strongly supports the idea that it is maintained in the population through subclinical or mild infection of immunologically normal persons, especially infants.[40] The prevalence of infection with *Pneumocystis* remains to be determined because studies to detect latent carriage of the organism in large populations have not been performed. Serologic surveys, however, indicate that infection is widespread and acquired in early life. Meuwissen and colleagues,[41] in the Netherlands, noted that antibodies to *P. jirovecii* are first detectable in healthy children at 6 months of age, and by age 4 years, nearly all children are seropositive. Pifer and associates,[42] in the United States, found significant titers of antibody to *Pneumocystis* in healthy 7-month-old infants and in two thirds of normal children by age 4 years. Gerrard and coworkers,[43] in England, detected *P. jirovecii* antibodies in serum from 48% of 94 young healthy children. Pifer[44] also found that serologic evidence of *Pneumocystis* infection is present before immunosuppressive therapy with corticosteroids and that *Pneumocystis* elicits pneumonia in healthy rats. A prospective, longitudinal study of infants bled every 2 months from birth to 2 years demonstrated 85% of the infants seroconverted by 20 months of age.[45] Authors of a number of autopsy reviews have attempted to determine the incidence of *Pneumocystis* infection, but the results have been divergent, because of the heterogeneity of the populations studied.[46-52] Those studies conducted in central Europe after World War II[47] or in cancer referral centers in the United States[52] have yielded higher rates of infection.

Few published reports have been devoted exclusively to the descriptive epidemiology of *Pneumocystis* pneumonia in the United States. In a literature review of the subject, Le Clair[53] accumulated 107 accounts of the disease recorded from 1955 through 1967. The male-to-female ratio of infected persons was in excess of 2:1, but ethnic distribution was even. The disease was reported from diverse geographic locales (21 of the 50 states). The largest number of cases[33] occurred in infants younger than 1 year. Proved or presumptive congenital immunodeficiencies were identifiable in virtually all of the children in this group. In patients 1 to 10 years of age, who constituted the next largest group,[26] only six had a primary immune deficit, whereas most of the other children had an underlying hematologic malignancy. The remaining patients, ranging in age from 10 to 81 years, were persons with assorted malignancies or renal allografts, who almost always had had prior exposure to corticosteroids, radiation, or cytotoxic drugs. The mortality rate for the entire group of patients was 95%.

The Centers for Disease Control and Prevention (CDC) updated Le Clair's study by investigating the epidemiologic, clinical, and diagnostic aspects of all confirmed cases of pneumocystosis reported to its Parasitic Disease Drug Service between 1967 and 1970.[54,55] The first of these reports has particular relevance because it focused only on the infectious episodes in infants and young children. A total of 194 documented cases of *P. jirovecii* pneumonia were analyzed, and 29 occurred in infants younger than 1 year. The attack rate for this group (8.4 per million) was more than five times higher than that for other age groups. Eighty-three percent of these infants had an underlying primary immunodeficiency disease. Moreover, because the inheritance of the primary immunodeficiency state often was sex linked, the preponderance of infection (88%) occurred in males. The mean age at diagnosis in the immunodeficient infants was 7.5 months, whereas the epidemic form of the infection in European and Asian infants was associated with peak morbidity in the third and fourth months of life.[10,16] Twenty-four percent of the infected children with immunodeficiencies had at least one sibling with an identifiable immune deficiency in whom *P. jirovecii* pneumonia also developed.

After this analysis of cases indigenous to the United States was complete, it became evident that infantile pneumocystosis could be introduced into the United States from epidemics abroad. The first such case was reported in 1966, when a 3-month-old Korean infant died of *Pneumocystis* infection after being brought to the United States from an orphanage in Korea.[56] The potential for imported pneumocystosis received renewed publicity with the cessation of the war in Vietnam. Surveillance for *Pneumocystis* infection in American-adopted Vietnamese orphans was urged when it was recognized that large numbers of infants exposed to the hardships of war and malnutrition in Indochina had experienced fulminant *Pneumocystis* pneumonia.[57,58] In quick succession, multiple cases of *Pneumocystis* infection among these refugee Vietnamese were reported.[59] Most of the affected infants were approximately 3 months of age; this was exactly the age at which pneumocystosis had emerged in the marasmic children infected during the earlier nursery epidemics in central Europe and Asia.

The epidemiology of *P. jirovecii* infection has changed as cases of human immunodeficiency virus (HIV) infection have occurred in infants.[60] As is true in adults with acquired AIDS, infants with AIDS are at high risk for this opportunistic infection. Among children with perinatally acquired HIV infection, *P. jirovecii* pneumonitis occurs most often among infants 3 to 6 months of age.[61] Another important change in the epidemiology of *Pneumocystis* pneumonia relates to the use of more potent immunosuppressive therapies, which places new patient groups at risk for *Pneumocystis* pneumonia. For example, it is now suggested that patients with inflammatory bowel disease who are receiving anti–tumor necrosis factor (TNF) treatment should be considered for *Pneumocystis* pneumonia prophylaxis because of the recognized risk of *Pneumocystis* infection in these patients.[62]

It has been suggested[63-67] that *P. jirovecii* may be an important cause of pneumonitis in immunologically intact infants. As noted above, primary infection with *Pneumocystis* occurs in most healthy infants by 2 years of age.[45] However, seroconversion occurred for the most part without a recognizeable clinical illness. More cases need to be confirmed histologically before it is established that *Pneumocystis* infection produces morbidity in previously healthy infants.

A role for *Pneumocystis* in the pathogenesis of the sudden infant death syndrome (SIDS) has been postulated. The cause of SIDS, the unexplained death of previously healthy infants, remains a mystery. In 1999, Vargas and colleagues,[68] in Santiago, Chile, reported finding *Pneumocystis* in the lungs of many infants whose death was diagnosed as SIDS. Shortly thereafter, this observation was confirmed in SIDS cases occurring in the Northeast United States.[69] Interpreting these observations presented two problems: defining appropriate case controls for the presence of *Pneumocystis* in infants without SIDS and explaining the mechanism of death, given the light infections and lack of demonstrable pathology in these infants. After a series of investigations, which included control infants, Vargas and colleagues[70] clearly established the presence of *Pneumocystis* in infants dying of SIDS but came to the conclusion that *Pneumocystis* was not likely the cause of SIDS. More recently, Vargas and colleagues[71] reported finding near-universal focal *Pneumocystis* that was associated with upregulation of mucus expression in the lung of SIDS cases. Whether and how this observation relates to the role of *Pneumocystis* in the pathogenesis of SIDS is yet to be determined.

The mode of transmission of *P. jirovecii* is difficult to prove, but animal studies provide unequivocal evidence for animal-to-animal transmission via the airborne route.[72-74] Epidemiologic studies support a similar mode of transmission among humans. For example, *Pneumocystis* infections among transplant patients have been shown to increase as their exposure to patients with or at risk for *Pneumocystis* pneumonia increases.[75-79] Furthermore, using molecular probes, it is possible to demonstrate that clusters of *Pneumocystis* pneumonia appear to be caused by the same organism.[75,77,78] Occurrence of pneumocystosis among family members also has been reported with pneumonia developing in three family members in a strikingly related time sequence.[64] More commonly, cases within a family emerge over a period of several years, and affected members almost always are infant siblings with either proven or suspected underlying immunodeficiencies. In at least three family studies, no fewer than three siblings succumbed to the infection.[80-83] It is unlikely, however, that direct patient-to-patient transfer of the organism occurred in any of these settings because, in almost all instances, development of disease in the sibling occurred months or years later. Contagion could still be implicated in the family milieu if a reservoir of asymptomatic infection with *P. jirovecii* existed among healthy family members. Supporting evidence suggests that infants may serve in the role of reservoir.[40,45] Maternal transfer of *Pneumocystis* to infants from colostrum or from the genital tract at parturition also might maintain *Pneumocystis* within a family, but it is difficult to test this hypothesis. The paucity of documented cases of overt *Pneumocystis* pneumonia in stillborn infants or in the early neonatal period, however, argues against frequent intrauterine passage of the organism. Congenital infection has been suggested based on very few case reports, but the data presented is inconclusive.[84-86]

The possibility that *Pneumocystis* pneumonia is a zoonotic disease and that infestation of rodents or even domesticated pets could provide a sizable reservoir for human infection has been postulated based on the frequent finding of *Pneumocystis* in animals. For example, abundant infection of rodents with *Pneumocystis* was discovered in patients' homes in many of the index cases in ward epidemics in Czechoslovakia.[87] However, with only microscopy, it is not possible to distinguish animal from human *Pneumocystis.* The development of reagents that could distinguish *Pneumocystis* from one host species from that infecting a different host allowed for definitive experiments to address host species specificity. Controlled experiments demonstrated that *Pneumocystis* from ferrets could not infect severe combined immunodeficient (SCID) mice.[14] These results were quickly confirmed using *Pneumocystis* from different hosts, including *P. jirovecii* from humans.[88-90] Thus the concept of *Pneumocystis* pneumonia as a zoonosis is not tenable.

PATHOLOGY

The gross and microscopic pathologic features of *P. jirovecii* pneumonia have been elucidated in a number of excellent reviews.[9,10,16,20,91-93] At autopsy in typically advanced infection, both lungs are heavy and diffusely affected. The most extensive involvement often is seen in posterior or dependent areas. At the lung margins anteriorly, a few remaining air-filled alveoli may constitute the only portion of functioning lung at the time of death.[9] Subpleural air blebs not infrequently are seen in these anterior marginal areas. On occasion, prominent mediastinal emphysema or frank pneumothorax can be noted. The color of the lungs is variously described as dark bluish purple, yellow-pink, or pale gray-brown. The pleural surfaces are smooth and glistening, with little inflammatory reaction. Hilar adenopathy is uncommon. Necrosis of tissue is not a feature of the disease.

Although these gross features of widespread infection are strikingly characteristic, focal or subclinical pneumocystosis presents a less recognizable picture. In this condition, the lung has tiny 3- to 5-mm reddish brown retracted areas contained within peribronchial and subpleural lobules, where hypostasis is greatest.[16,19] Even these features, however, may be absent because of variable involvement of adjacent lung tissue by concomitant pathologic processes.

The microscopic appearance of both the contents and the septal walls of pulmonary alveoli in *Pneumocystis* pneumonia are virtually pathognomonic of the infection. The outstanding histologic finding with hematoxylin and eosin stain is an intensely eosinophilic, foamy, or honeycomb-like material uniformly filling the alveolar sacs (Fig. 34-3). This intraalveolar material is composed largely of *Pneumocystis*, host cells, immunoglobulin, and proteinaceous debris.[94,95] Typical cyst forms of the organism within alveoli are visible only after application of special stains such as methenamine silver.

The type and degree of cellular inflammatory responses provoked by the intraalveolar cluster of *Pneumocystis* organisms vary based on host response (see "Pathogenesis"). The descriptive histologic term for pneumocystosis—interstitial plasma cell pneumonia—is derived from the pronounced plasma cellular infiltration of the interalveolar septa observed almost exclusively in newborns in European nursery epidemics. Distention of alveolar walls to 5 to 10 times the normal thickness, with resultant compression of alveolar spaces and capillary lumens, typically is noted in this form of the disease. Hyaline membranes develop

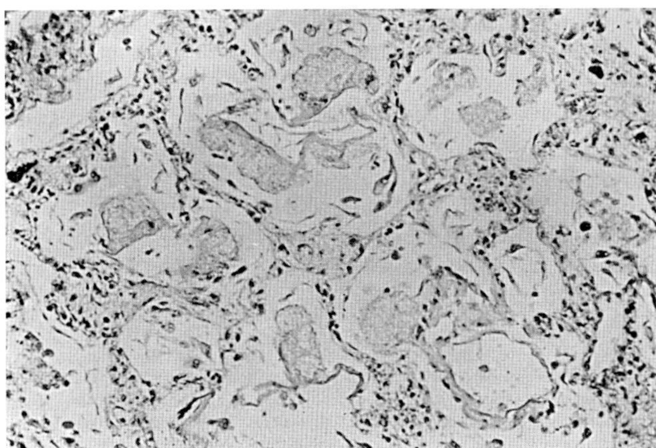

Figure 34-3 Section of lung tissue obtained at autopsy showing the amorphous, proteinaceous intraalveolar infiltrate characteristic of pneumonitis caused by *Pneumocystis jirovecii*. Hematoxylin and eosin stain, ×160. (From Remington JS: The compromised host, *Hosp Practice* 7:59-70, 1972.)

occasionally.[9] Septal cell hyperplasia, a nonspecific reaction of lung tissue to injury induced by infections of diverse etiology, is also seen.[96]

Hughes and colleagues[97] studied the histologic progression of typical *Pneumocystis* pneumonia based on the number and location of organisms and the cellular response in pulmonary tissue. The lung samples were from children with underlying malignancy who had received intensive chemotherapy. The authors categorized three sequential stages in the course of the disease. In the first stage, no septal inflammatory or cellular response is seen, and only a few free cyst forms are present in the alveolar lumen; the remainder are isolated on the alveolar septal wall. The second stage is characterized by an increase in the number of organisms within macrophages fixed to the alveolar wall and desquamation of these cells into the alveolar space; again, only minimal septal inflammatory response is seen at this time. Finally, a third stage is identified, in which extensive reactive and desquamative alveolitis can be seen. Such diffuse alveolar damage may be the major pathologic feature in certain cases.[98] Variable numbers of cysts of the organism, presumably undergoing dissolution, are present within the alveolar macrophages. These findings underscore the thought that the so-called foamy exudate within alveoli is neither foamy edema fluid nor the product of an exudative inflammatory reaction but largely a collection of coalesced alveolar cells and macrophages that contain sizable digestive vacuoles and remnant organisms.

The mechanism of spread of *Pneumocystis* throughout pulmonary tissue is not completely understood. Direct invasion by the organism through septal walls into the interstitium or the lymphatic or blood vascular spaces of the lung is considered unlikely,[19,97] except in rare instances when systemic dissemination of the organism occurs.

Interstitial fibrosis is a distinct but infrequently reported complication of *Pneumocystis* pneumonia in older children and adults but has been reported in infants only rarely.[92,93,99-101] Nowak,[100] in Europe, first emphasized that fibrosis was not unusual in the lungs of infants at autopsy who had especially protracted infection with *P. jirovecii*. *Pneumocystis*-infected lungs sometimes demonstrate, in addition to fibrosis, other pathologic features compatible with a more chronic destructive inflammatory process. Multinucleate alveolar giant cells occasionally accompany alveolar cell proliferation.[16,19,93] Whether presence of these cells is more often a response to undetected concomitant viral infection is unknown. Typical granulomatous reactions with organisms visible in the granulomas also have been described.[93,102,103] Extensive calcification of *Pneumocystis* exudate and adjacent lung tissue may ultimately develop.[93]

PATHOGENESIS

The clinical conditions that predispose patients to the development of *Pneumocystis* pneumonia are associated with impaired immune responses, leading to the presumption that *Pneumocystis* causes disease, not because it is intrinsically virulent but because the host's immune mechanisms fail to contain it. The severity of *P. jirovecii* pneumonia in infants with AIDS illustrates this phenomenon dramatically. The primary role of immunocompromise also would explain, in part, why *Pneumocystis* pneumonia did not emerge as a serious health problem until more than 30 years after the disease was first recognized. European epidemics of *Pneumocystis* arose out of the devastation of World War II and widespread use of antibacterial drugs. Each of these two seemingly unrelated events served ultimately to disrupt the normal host-organism immunologic interaction in favor of the organism. The war resulted in institutionalization of inordinate numbers of orphans under conditions of overcrowding and malnutrition. At the same time, antibacterial therapy dramatically enhanced survival rates of these institutionalized infants, who would otherwise have succumbed to bacterial sepsis during the first days or weeks of life. In addition, it was realized that *Pneumocystis* infection appeared in these marasmic children at an age when their immunoglobulin G (IgG) levels reached a physiologic nadir. By 1960, the orphanage epidemics had abated in Europe as environmental conditions improved, but they persisted in Asia, where poverty and overcrowding continued.[84,104] Subsidence of the epidemic disease and more widespread antibacterial drug therapy, as well as sophisticated immunosuppressive drug treatment, contributed thereafter to awareness in Europe and North America of isolated instances of *Pneumocystis* infection among children suffering from a variety of identifiable immunodeficiencies.

Weller,[105,106] in Europe, was among the first to experimentally induce *Pneumocystis* pneumonia in animals. His crucial observation relative to pathogenesis of the infection was that in rats pretreated with cortisone (and penicillin) and exposed to suspensions of *Pneumocystis*-containing lung tissue, *Pneumocystis* pneumonia develops with the same frequency and severity as in corticoid-treated animals that were not subsequently inoculated with organisms. The intensity of such artificially induced animal infection also was noted to be less marked than that in spontaneous human pneumocystosis of the epidemic variety. Comparable observations in the rabbit model were made by Sheldon[107] in the United States. He showed that cortisone and antimicrobial agents were sufficient to induce *Pneumocystis* infection without direct exposure of animals to an exogenous source of organisms. The inescapable conclusion of these carefully designed studies was that *Pneumocystis* infection is latent in rats and rabbits and becomes clinically manifest only when host resistance is altered or that *Pneumocystis* is ubiquitous in the environment and capable of infecting a susceptible host.

The issue of latency is an important one in defining the pathogenesis of *Pneumocystis* pneumonia. To determine whether *Pneumocystis* establishes latency after infection, SCID mice, which resolve naturally acquired *Pneumocystis carinii* pneumonia (PCP) after reconstitution with immunocompetent spleen cells, were observed for evidence of a latent *Pneumocystis* infection.[108] Neither *P. carinii* nor amplified *P. carinii* DNA was detected in the lungs of SCID mice killed 21 days after spleen cell reconstitution. Furthermore, SCID mice that recovered from *P. carinii* infection failed to reactivate the infection after they were either depleted of $CD4^+$ cells for up to 84 days or depleted of $CD4^+$ cells and treated with corticosteroid for 35 days. These results indicate that an immune response to *P. carinii* can completely clear the organism from the host. This supports the hypothesis that *P. carinii* pneumonia that develops in immunocompromised patients is due to exposure to an exogenous source of *P. carinii* rather than reactivation of latent infection. Experiments using the steroid-treated rat model of *Pneumocystis* infection demonstrated similar findings.[109]

In 1966, Frenkel and colleagues[110] published a hallmark study of rat pneumocystosis. They showed that clinical and histopathologically significant involvement with *Pneumocystis* is regularly inducible in rats by "conditioning" them with parenteral cortisone over a period of 1 to 2 months. Premature death from complicating bacterial infection was prevented by simultaneous administration of antibacterial agents. Of interest is their finding that regression of established interstitial pneumonitis occurs if cortisone conditioning is stopped early enough; on the other hand, rats continuing to receive cortisone die of coalescent alveolar *Pneumocystis* infiltration, and the infiltrate is almost devoid of inflammatory cells. These histologic changes are, in fact, an exact replica of those observed in sporadic cases of human *Pneumocystis* infection developing in congenitally immunodeficient and exogenously immunosuppressed patients. Attempts to precipitate clinical pneumocystosis with a variety of immunosuppressants other than cortisone were also explored. Of eight cytotoxic agents and antimetabolites tested, only cyclophosphamide was shown to make the rats susceptible to infection by *Pneumocystis*. Total-body irradiation and lymphoid tissue ablation (splenectomy, thymectomy) by themselves were incapable of inducing overt *Pneumocystis* pneumonia.

The clinical association between pneumocystosis and protein-calorie malnutrition also has been reproduced in a rat model.[111] Healthy rats given either a regular or a low-protein diet gain weight and exhibit little to no evidence of pneumocystosis postmortem. By contrast, in rats fed a protein-free diet, which produces weight loss and hypoalbuminemia, fatal infection regularly developed; administration of corticosteroid only foreshortened their median survival time.[102]

None of the experimental models described thus far permit a precise appraisal of the relative importance of the cellular and humoral components of host defense against *Pneumocystis*. Although corticosteroids, cytotoxic drugs, and starvation interfere primarily with cell-mediated immunity, they do not always induce purely functional cellular defects. Rather, the immunosuppressive effects of chemotherapeutic agents or of malnutrition are far more complex, and ultimately both cellular and humoral arms of the immune system may be impaired by them.

The production of pneumocystosis in the nude mouse without the use of exogenous immunosuppressants implies that susceptibility to the infection relates most to a defect in thymic-dependent lymphocytes.[112] The role of antibody deficiency is less clear. A role for antibody in control of infection with the organism has been shown in vitro by demonstrating that *Pneumocystis* organisms adherent to rat alveolar macrophages become interiorized only after anti-*Pneumocystis* serum is added to the culture system.[113]

That primary humoral immune deficits could predispose to sporadic pneumocystosis was first reported, unwittingly, by Hutchison[114] in England in 1955. He described male siblings with congenital agammaglobulinemia who died of pneumonia of "similar and unusual" histology. *P. jirovecii* was implicated as the etiologic agent of these fatal infections only when the pathologic sections were reviewed by Baar.[115] Burke and colleagues[116] stressed what was to be regarded as a typical histologic finding in *Pneumocystis*-infected agammaglobulinemic children, namely, the absence or gross deficiency of plasma cells in pulmonary lesions (and in hematopoietic tissues). This deficiency contrasted sharply with the extensive plasmacytosis seen in epidemic infections.

Pneumocystis been reported in association with a pure T-cell deficiency, namely, in DiGeorge syndrome.[117] That the integrity of the cellular immune system is critical for resistance to *Pneumocystis* may be inferred from the steroid-induced and congenitally athymic animal models of pneumocystosis described earlier. Most *Pneumocystis* infections occurred in infants with SCID, a state characterized by profound depression of both cellular and humoral immunity.

For many years it had not been possible to study in vitro the cellular immune response to *P. jirovecii* because of the impurity of available antigens. Preliminary experiments with an antigen derived from a cell culture suggested that specific cell-mediated immunity may be depressed in children with active *Pneumocystis* pneumonia. Lymphocytes from two such children failed to transform in the presence of the antigen,[118] whereas lymphocytes from healthy, seropositive adults were, in most cases, stimulated specifically to undergo blastogenesis.[118,119]

Although PCP was clearly defined as an opportunistic pathogen causing clinical disease in patients suffering from primary or, more commonly, secondary immunodeficiencies, for many years the pathogenic mechanisms by which *Pneumocystis* caused lung injury and respiratory impairment remained mostly undefined. Histologic observations of infected lung tissue demonstrated that *Pneumocystis* attaches to alveolar epithelial cells in the distal lung and that these cells are preferentially damaged during severe PCP. However, the nature of the injury was unclear, and progress in understanding this organism and identifying potential toxins or virulence factors was hampered by the lack of an axenic culture system. Clinical observations offered some insight into the nature of PCP-associated lung injury. A positive correlation between the degree of pulmonary inflammation and the severity of PCP was noted and suggested that the host response to infection affects the clinical manifestation of PCP.[120,121] Before the AIDS epidemic, the majority of PCP cases occurred in patients with hematologic malignancies, and often it was noted that the onset of PCP coincided with cessation of corticosteroid treatment. Similarly, the onset of PCP in bone marrow transplant recipients often coincided with engraftment. In both examples, *Pneumocystis* infection likely occurred during the period of immunosuppression, but the clinical manifestation was not evident until a degree of immune function was restored, suggesting that the host-driven pulmonary immune response contributed to the disease process. The onset of the AIDS epidemic offered a distinct subset of PCP patients who suffered from profound immunosuppression. Comparison of patients with AIDS-related PCP to patients with non-AIDS PCP revealed that AIDS patients had a more subtle onset of symptoms with better pulmonary function and better prognosis, despite harboring higher lung fungal burdens. Furthermore, the severity and prognosis for PCP patients was found to correlate with the degree of pulmonary inflammation but not with organism burden. Together, these findings suggest that the host response to *Pneumocystis* infection contributes to lung injury and respiratory impairment during PCP.

The development of animal models of *Pneumocystis* infection has proved invaluable for elucidating the immunopathogenesis of PCP.[122-126] SCID mice lack functional lymphocytes and are highly susceptible to *Pneumocystis* infection. An early study found that when *Pneumocystis*-infected (SCID) mice were immune reconstituted by the adoptive transfer of functional lymphocytes, the mice suffered from rapid deterioration and high mortality rates. Subsequent studies found that immune reconstitution of *Pneumocystis*-infected SCID mice induced a rapid increase in the pulmonary expression of proinflammatory cytokines and chemokines and the recruitment of cellular infiltrates into the lungs. Although immune reconstitution provided the benefit of restoring an effective $CD4^+$ T-cell–dependent immune response against *Pneumocystis* infection, it also had profound effects on physiology, including severe weight loss, tachypnea, hypoxia, and decreased lung compliance. Of importance, nonreconstituted SCID mice with similar fungal burdens appeared physiologically normal and showed little evidence of PCP-related disease, suggesting that *Pneumocystis* itself is not the direct cause of pulmonary damage, at least early in the evolution of the disease process. The immune-reconstituted SCID mouse model of PCP is similar to the clinical syndrome termed immune reconstitution inflammatory syndrome (IRIS), which has been reported in AIDS patients after institution of combined antiretroviral therapy. The rapid recovery of $CD4^+$ T lymphocytes causes an intense pathologic pulmonary immune response to preexisting pulmonary infections, including *Pneumocystis*. Patients with PCP-related IRIS suffer severe pulmonary decompensation and have poorer survival rates than patients with a classic AIDS-related presentation of PCP. These observations highlight the contribution of the immune response to PCP pathogenesis.

Classic AIDS-related PCP has also been effectively modeled in mice. Continual administration of anti-CD4 monoclonal antibody maintains mice in a chronic $CD4^+$

T-cell–depleted state. CD4-depleted mice are susceptible to *Pneumocystis* infection and develop a clinical syndrome very similar to AIDS-related PCP in humans. Several studies have demonstrated that in the absence of $CD4^+$ lymphocytes, large numbers of $CD8^+$ T cells are recruited to the lung in response to *Pneumocystis* infection.[122-124] These lymphocytes are unable to control *Pneumocystis* infection but directly contribute to lung injury and PCP-related pathogenesis. Mice depleted of both $CD4^+$ and $CD8^+$ lymphocytes are much healthier compared with mice depleted of only $CD4^+$ lymphocytes. Together, these findings support the immunopathogenic features of PCP. Although infection is necessary to cause pneumonia, certain aspects of the immune response cause disease symptoms. Differences in the degree of immunosuppression among PCP patients likely affect their ability to produce an immunopathogenic response to infection and may account for variability in the severity of PCP between different patient groups.

The mechanisms of PCP-related immunopathogenesis are not clearly defined. Although both $CD4^+$ and $CD8^+$ lymphocyte-driven events have been implicated in immunopathogenesis, the specific mechanisms have not been elucidated. The appearance of neutrophils and neutrophil chemotactic factors in the lung correlate with a poorer prognosis for PCP patients.[120,121] However, these cells do not appear to directly contribute to either host defense against *Pneumocystis* infection or to PCP-related immunopathogenesis.[126] The proinflammatory cytokine TNF appears to be required for successful host defense against *Pneumocystis* infection, and signaling through TNF receptors is also a major contributor to immunopathogenesis.[127] A possible physiologic consequence of PCP-driven inflammation is pulmonary surfactant dysfunction.[128,129] Surfactant is critical to normal gas exchange and proper lung function. Pulmonary inflammation elicited during *Pneumocystis* infection was found to directly disrupt surfactant function, contributing to PCP-related respiratory impairment. Although the specific mechanisms of immunopathogenesis are not defined, the contribution of inflammation and the immune response to this disease process is recognized, and standard treatment of moderate-to-severe PCP typically includes corticosteroids as adjunctive therapy to dampen inflammation.

CLINICAL MANIFESTATIONS

General Considerations

With the exception of hypoxia, no clinical features are pathognomonic for *P. jirovecii* infection. As discussed earlier, the clinical presentation of PCP is influenced by the patient's residual capacity to mount an immune response. For example, severely immunosuppressed AIDS patients often have a very subacute onset of PCP with a lower mortality than a patient being treated for a hematologic malignancy who develops PCP while receiving maintenance chemotherapy. Clinical syndromes ascribable to *Pneumocystis* may be simulated by other infections (cytomegalovirus[10]), or by inflammatory processes (drug-induced pulmonary toxicity,[130] radiation fibrosis[131]) and neoplasia (pulmonary leukemia[132]) capable of producing interstitial pulmonary infiltrates in older children and adults. Thus recognition of pneumocystosis on clinical grounds requires, above all, a high index of suspicion whenever interstitial pneumonia occurs in settings known to predispose to infection with the organism. It may be inferred from these observations that pneumocystosis is not merely an end-stage infection in a host with a preterminal illness but, on the contrary, often represents a potentially treatable cause of death in patients whose primary immunodeficiency or malignancy is being controlled.

Symptoms and Signs

Epidemic Infection in Infants. The onset of epidemic-type infection, essentially nonexistent in developed countries, in infants is reported to be slow and insidious. Initially, nonspecific signs of restlessness or languor, poor feeding, and diarrhea are common. Tachypnea and periorbital cyanosis gradually develop. Cough productive of sticky mucus, although not prominent, may appear later.[10,19] Respiratory insufficiency progresses over 1 to 4 weeks, and patients exhibit increasingly severe tachypnea, dyspnea, intercostal retractions, and flaring of the nasal alae. Fever is absent or of low grade.[133] Physical findings are strikingly minimal and consist primarily of fine crepitant rales with deep inspiration. Chest radiographs, however, typically demonstrate pulmonary infiltrates early in the illness. The duration of untreated disease is 4 to 6 weeks, but it often is difficult to determine an exact date of onset of illness. Before the introduction of pentamidine therapy, the mortality rate for such epidemic infant infection is estimated to have been between 20% and 50%.[134]

Sporadic Infection in Infants. The typical clinical syndrome is less evident in sporadic cases of pneumocystosis occurring in infants with acquired or congenital immunodeficiency and in older children with acquired immunodeficiency. In infants with primary immunodeficiency diseases, the onset of clinical infection can be insidious, and illness can extend over weeks or possibly months,[135] a course not unlike that seen in epidemic pneumocystosis. By contrast, in most infants with congenital immunodeficiency or AIDS and in older children with acquired immune deficits, *Pneumocystis* pneumonia manifests abruptly and is a more symptomatic, short-lived disease.[50,55,97,135] Among infants with HIV infection, the median age at onset is 4 to 5 months, and the mortality rate is between 39% and 59%.[136] High fever and nonproductive cough are initial findings, followed by tachypnea, coryza, and, later, cyanosis. Death may supervene within a week or so. If no treatment is given, essentially all patients with this form of pneumocystosis die.

Radiologic Findings

Because the extent of pulmonary involvement in *P. jirovecii* pneumonia rarely is detectable by physical examination, a chest radiograph showing diffuse infiltrative disease is the most useful indicator of infection in a susceptible host.[137] Although certain characteristic patterns of radiographic involvement have been ascribed to *Pneumocystis* pneumonitis, it is worth emphasizing that the findings may vary depending on the presence of coincident pulmonary infection as well as on the nature of the underlying disease state.

The radiographic findings of mild ("focal") *Pneumocystis* pneumonia described by Vessal and associates[138] in infants from an Iranian orphanage included hilar interstitial infiltrate, thymic atrophy, pulmonary hyperaeration, and scattered lobular atelectasis. Although none of these signs is specific for *Pneumocystis* infection, they persist longer (3 weeks-2 months) in serologically proven cases. Indeed, surviving infants may exhibit focal interstitial infiltrates after organisms are cleared from the lung and for as long as 1 year.[133,139]

In infants, especially those with immunodeficiency syndromes, the initial radiograph often shows haziness spreading from the hilar regions to the periphery, which assumes a finely granular, interstitial pattern. An antecedent gross alveolar infiltrate usually is not seen. The peripheral granularity may progress to coalescent nodules. These changes resemble the "atelectatic" radiographic abnormalities of hyaline membrane disease. In both conditions, aeration is absent peripherally. Pneumothorax with subcutaneous and interstitial emphysema and pneumomediastinum are not uncommon and are associated with a poor prognosis.[140] Even with therapy, radiographic clearing can lag far behind clinical improvement.

As experience with *Pneumocystis* has broadened, especially in older children and adults, a number of atypical radiographic abnormalities have been described.[141] These atypical findings include hilar and mediastinal adenopathy, pleural effusions, parenchymal cavitation, pneumatoceles, nodular densities, and unilateral or lobar distribution of infiltrates. By contrast, the chest radiographic appearance can remain essentially normal well after the onset of fever, dyspnea, and hypoxemia. The presence of such radiographically silent lung disease can be visualized as abnormal findings by pulmonary computed tomography.

Laboratory Studies

Routine laboratory studies yield little diagnostic information in *Pneumocystis* infection. Abnormalities in hemoglobin concentration or white blood cell count are more likely to result from an underlying disease of the hematopoietic system or cytotoxic drug effect. Neither laboratory value is consistently altered by secondary pneumocystosis. Nevertheless, a subgroup of infants with primary immunodeficiency disease and infection caused by *P. jirovecii* can exhibit significant eosinophilia.[19,83,134,135] Jose and associates [83] first emphasized the association of peripheral blood eosinophilia and pneumocystosis in a report describing three infected male siblings with infantile agammaglobulinemia. In one of the infants, eosinophilia developed very early in the course of the illness, and the differential eosinophil count peaked at 42% as the respiratory disease worsened. In accordance, it has been suggested that the combination of cough, tachypnea, diffuse haziness on chest radiographs, and eosinophilia in an infant with immunodeficiency can be indicative of *Pneumocystis* pneumonia. A constant pathophysiologic finding in pneumocystosis, as well as in other interstitial pulmonary diseases, is that of ventilation and perfusion defects most compatible with an "alveolar-capillary block" syndrome.[135,142] Arterial blood gas determinations in infected patients show severe hypoxemia and hypocapnia, often before profound subjective respiratory insufficiency or even radiologic abnormalities supervene. Less commonly, modest hypercapnia with respiratory acidosis is recorded. This respiratory pathophysiology correlates well with the anatomic pulmonary lesion in *Pneumocystis* pneumonia. Concentration of organisms within alveoli and inflammation of the surrounding alveolar septa not unexpectedly lead to interference in gas transfer, whereas persistence of areas of normal lung parenchyma and lack of significant airway obstruction account for the usual absence of carbon dioxide retention.

Concurrent Infection

The clinical presentation of pneumocystosis may be altered by simultaneous infection with other organisms. Certainly, infection with a variety of opportunistic pathogens is not surprising in patients with broadly compromised immunologic defense mechanisms. Infection with one or more organisms was found in 56% of *Pneumocystis*-infected infants and children with primary immunodeficiency disease reported to the CDC.[54] Comparable rates of multiple infections also have been noted in several large series of patients with acquired immune defects and pneumocystosis.[96,135,143]

Infection with cytomegalovirus appears to be the most common "unusual" infection associated with pneumocystosis. Indeed, in his 1957 review, Gajdusek[10] already was able to cite numerous published studies referring to the "unexpectedly high frequency of association" of the two infections. He conceded that one infection most probably predisposed the affected patient to the other. On the basis of electron micrographic observations of cytomegalovirus-like particles within pneumocysts, histopathologic examination of lung biopsy specimens from infants with AIDS often demonstrates concomitant cytomegalovirus and *P. jirovecii* infections.[144,145]

DIAGNOSIS

The diagnosis of *Pneumocystis* pneumonia remains difficult. The organism must be visualized in the respiratory tract of ill persons, and often this can be accomplished only by bronchoalveolar lavage (BAL) or, in infants, a lung biopsy. Recently, polymerase chain reaction (PCR) assay has been used for diagnosis in fluid specimens obtained by BAL. Nevertheless, this technique is still not generally available for routine clinical use. Attempts to isolate *Pneumocystis* from clinical specimens on synthetic media or in tissue culture have not been successful, and serologic techniques to detect active infection have been too insensitive.

Examination of Pulmonary Secretions

Diagnosis of sporadic cases of pneumocystosis by examination of sputum or tracheal and gastric aspirates has never been rewarding. The rate of recovery of *Pneumocystis* from upper airway secretions in the cases compiled by the CDC was estimated to be only about 6%.[55] Japanese investigators have described a method of concentrating sputum samples with acetyl-L-cysteine in 0.2 N sodium hydroxide solution, which permits filtration and centrifugation of a pellet of *Pneumocystis*.[146] Ognibene and associates[147] reported the use of induced sputa in the diagnosis of pneumonia in 18 children with HIV infection or malignancy. Nine sputum samples were positive for *P. jirovecii* by immunofluorescent antibody testing. Four of the patients with negative findings by examination of sputum samples subsequently underwent BAL; BAL fluid was negative for *P. jirovecii* in all four. The remaining five patients received treatment for bacterial pneumonia and responded to therapy. This technique required ultrasonic nebulization in the children, and the youngest patient in this report was 2 years of age.

Percutaneous Lung Aspiration

The need to obtain lung tissue for a more accurate assessment of the presence of *Pneumocystis* pneumonia has been appreciated for some time. Percutaneous needle aspiration of the lung was successfully used in infected infants and children with underlying primary and acquired immunodeficiencies.[148,149] The procedure is performed without general anesthesia so that the child's respiratory function is not further compromised. Under fluoroscopy, a 20-gauge spinal needle with syringe in place is guided into the midportion of the lung. The resultant aspirate (usually < 0.1 mL) may be transferred directly to slides, allowed to air dry, and then stained with Gram, GMS, and toluidine blue O stains. Children with platelet counts of less than 60,000/mm^3 receive fresh whole-blood or platelet transfusions before the procedure. Pneumothorax appears to be the major complication encountered. In one series, it occurred in 37% of the patients, and evacuation of air by thoracotomy tube was required in 14%.[149]

Lung Biopsy

It has been argued that aspiration is inferior to biopsy in that the former does not permit histologic examination of lung tissue. Open lung biopsy has been proposed as the most reliable method for identifying and estimating the extent of *Pneumocystis* infection, as well as for demonstrating the presence of complicating pathologic conditions, such as coexistent infection, malignancy, or interstitial fibrosis.[150-152] It may be hazardous, however, to perform a thoracotomy using general anesthesia in patients with marginal pulmonary reserve. Although the procedure has been associated with an acceptably low incidence of serious complications in critically ill children,[153-156] determination of its risk-to-benefit ratio based on the infant's underlying disease, expected life span, and clinical condition is appropriate in individual cases. Unfortunately, these analyses have not yet been applied rigorously to infants and young children with suspected pneumocystosis. Technical modification in the performance of open biopsy that would avoid general anesthesia and endotracheal intubation (e.g., using thoracoscopy) may be particularly advantageous for diagnosis of *Pneumocystis* pneumonia in small children.[157]

Once obtained, there are a variety of acceptable staining techniques that can be used to identify *Pneumocystis*. The most commonly used staining methods include methenamine silver, toluidine blue O, Diff-Quick, calcofluor white, and immunofluorescence.[158,159]

Serologic Tests

It is clear that sensitive and specific serologic methods are desirable to detect active *Pneumocystis* infection. It is disappointing that despite extensive investigation, no method has been proved to be entirely satisfactory.

Serodiagnosis of *P. jirovecii* infection in infants by detection of immunofluorescent antibodies was first reported in 1964 in Europe.[160] It was found that IgM and IgG anti-*Pneumocystis* immunofluorescent antibodies appear sequentially in sera during the course of clinical infection. Both classes of antibodies are present in sera of diseased infants during the first weeks of pneumonia, but only IgG antibodies persist during convalescent periods or in cases of protracted infection.[161]

The worth of immunofluorescent antibody tests in the diagnosis of sporadic pneumocystosis was examined subsequently in the United States by Norman and Kagan[162] at the CDC. They observed low rates of serologic reactivity among patients with suspected and confirmed cases, positive results in sera from patients who seemed to have only cytomegalovirus and other fungal infections, and negative results in sera from six infants with primary immunodeficiency diseases and documented pneumocystosis. Although it is possible to increase the specificity and sensitivity of these tests for *Pneumocystis*,[163,164] such tests detect background levels of *Pneumocystis* antibody in clinically healthy persons and, as a result, fail to discriminate between patients with active disease and those with past unrecognized infection.

To avoid the problem posed by the insensitivity of antibody determinations per se in pneumocystosis, Perera and colleagues[52] developed a counterimmunoelectrophoretic assay for detecting circulating *Pneumocystis* antigen in suspected cases. In an initial evaluation of the test, antigenemia was demonstrated in up to 95% of children with *Pneumocystis* pneumonia and was absent in normal control children. Antigen also was found in the sera of 15% of oncology patients who did not have pneumonia, however. Unfortunately, this ability to detect circulating antigens has not been duplicated by other laboratories and as a result detection of antigenemia is not used to diagnose PCP.

TREATMENT

Specific Therapy

Hughes and coworkers,[165] in 1974, first demonstrated that the combination of TMP-SMX was effective in treatment of cortisone-induced rat pneumocystosis. This combination was shown to be as efficacious as pentamidine in children infected with *Pneumocystis* who also had underlying malignancy.[166] Several uncontrolled trials of TMP-SMX in congenitally immunodeficient infants and in older immunosuppressed children and adults confirmed the efficacy and low toxicity of this combination agent.[167,168] The dosage used was 20 mg of TMP and 100 mg of SMX/kg body weight/day, given orally in four divided doses for 14 days. This daily dose was two to three times that used in treatment of bacterial infections. The equivalent efficacy of TMP-SMX and of pentamidine has been confirmed in pediatric cancer patients with *P. jirovecii* pneumonia.[169]

TMP-SMX is the drug of choice for treatment of *P. jirovecii* pneumonia in infants and children. The oral route of administration can be used in mild cases, for which the recommended dosage is 20 mg TMP plus 100 mg SMX/kg/day in divided doses every 6 to 8 hours apart. Infants with moderate or severe disease require treatment by the intravenous route, with 15 to 20 mg TMP plus 75 to 100 mg SMX/kg/day in divided doses 6 to 8 hours apart. In general, treatment is given for 3 weeks. Adverse reactions to TMP-SMX will develop in approximately 5% of infants and children without HIV infection and 40% of children with HIV infection; most commonly seen is a maculopapular rash that clears after discontinuation of the drug. Other adverse reactions are uncommon and include neutropenia, anemia, renal dysfunction, and gastrointestinal symptoms or signs.

In infants who do not respond to TMP-SMX or in whom serious adverse reactions develop, pentamidine isethionate in a single daily dose of 4 mg/kg given intravenously may be used. Other drugs have been tested in limited studies in infants and young children with HIV infection and *P. jirovecii* pneumonia, including atovaquone, trimetrexate-leucovorin, oral TMP-dapsone, pyrimethamine-sulfadoxine, clindamycin plus primaquine, and aerosolized pentamidine.

The ease with which TMP-SMX can be administered and its lack of adverse side effects make it an attractive combination for empirical therapy for suspected pneumocystosis. Such treatment is reasonable in infants who are gravely ill and whose outlook for recovery from underlying disease is bleak. Several objections to the universal adoption of this approach have been raised. In at least half of the immunosuppressed children with typical clinical and radiographic features of *Pneumocystis* pneumonia, the illness is in fact not related to infection with *P. jirovecii*.[170] Identification of the etiologic agent and proper management of the disorder can be accomplished only by first performing appropriate diagnostic procedures.

Until 1958, no therapy specific for *P. jirovecii* infection was available. In that year, Ivady and Paldy[171] in Hungary recorded the first successful use of several aromatic diamidines, including pentamidine isethionate, in 16 of 19 infected infants. By 1962, the Hungarian investigators had used pentamidine therapy in 212 patients with epidemic *Pneumocystis* pneumonia.[172] During the next several years, favorable responses to this drug were observed in infants and children with both the epidemic and the sporadic forms of the infection.[97,135] Treatment effected a dramatic reduction in the mortality rate for the epidemic disease from 50% to less than 4%.[169,173] In the cases of sporadic infection reported to the CDC,[55,174,175] survival rates ranged from 42% to 63% for those patients who received the drug for 9 or more days. In cases confined largely to young children and managed at a single institution, cure rates were noted to be as high as 68% to 75%.[97,166] Because spontaneous recovery from *Pneumocystis* pneumonia in immunodepressed persons is rare, it is clear that pentamidine therapy reduced the mortality rate in such patients to nearly 25%.

The recommended dose of the drug is 4 mg/kg intravenously once daily for 14 days. Clinical improvement becomes evident 4 to 6 days after initiation of therapy, but radiographic improvement may be delayed for several weeks.

Pentamidine toxicity from intravenous and intramuscular use has been reported. Although toxicity from pentamidine apparently was not a significant problem in the marasmic infants with *Pneumocystis* infection treated during the European epidemics,[176] the CDC determined that 189 (47%) of 404 children and adults given the drug for confirmed or suspected *Pneumocystis* infection suffered one or more adverse effects.[55] Immediate systemic reactions, such as hypotension, tachycardia, nausea, vomiting, facial flushing, pruritus, and subjective experience of unpleasant taste in the mouth, were noted particularly after intravenous administration of the drug. Herxheimer reactions occurred rarely.[177] Local reactions at injection sites, namely, pain, erythema, and frank abscess formation, developed in 10% to 20% of patients.[55,175] Elevation in serum glutamic-oxaloacetic aminotransferase levels was frequently recorded and may have resulted partly from this local trauma. Hypoglycemia ensued not uncommonly after the fifth day of pentamidine therapy but often was asymptomatic.[174] Hypoglycemia also was observed in pediatric patients with AIDS who were given pentamidine for treatment of *P. jirovecii* pneumonia.[178] Pentamidine-associated pancreatitis also has been reported in children and adults with HIV infection.[179-181] Although overt anemia was rare, megaloblastic bone marrow changes or depressed serum folate levels were noted.[174]

Supportive Care

A critical component in the management of *Pneumocystis* pneumonia is oxygen therapy. Because hypoxemia can be profound, the fraction of inspired oxygen should be adjusted to maintain the arterial oxygen tension at 70 mm Hg or greater. The inspired oxygen concentration should not exceed 50%, to avoid oxygen toxicity. Assisted or controlled ventilation may be required.

The use of early adjunctive corticosteroid therapy in the treatment of *P. jirovecii* pneumonia in adults with AIDS can increase survival and reduce the risk of respiratory failure.[182,183] A national consensus panel has recommended the use of corticosteroids in adults and adolescents with HIV infection and documented or suspected *P. jirovecii* pneumonia.[184] Two studies have supported the use of corticosteroids in decreasing the morbidity and mortality associated with *P. jirovecii* pneumonia.[185,186]

PROGNOSIS

Chronic Sequelae

Little is known about the residual effects of successfully treated *Pneumocystis* pneumonia on pulmonary function. Patients may suffer additional "pulmonary" morbidity from other opportunistic infections or from noninfectious complications of underlying disease or its therapy. Hughes and coworkers[97] evaluated 18 children with underlying malignancies over periods of 1 to 4 years after surviving *Pneumocystis* infection. Although pulmonary function tests were not performed, none of the subjects demonstrated clinical or radiographic evidence of residual pulmonary disease. In a subsequent study from the same institution, pulmonary function was assessed serially in surviving children.[187] Significant improvement in function was noted within 1 month of the infection, and all abnormalities resolved by 6 months.

It seems inevitable that respiratory dysfunction can result from severe episodes of *Pneumocystis* pneumonia that provoke interstitial fibrosis or extensive calcification (as discussed earlier under "Pathology"). Cor pulmonale has been observed in infants with such protracted infection.[135] In one notably well-studied patient, an adult with biopsy-proven fibrosis that appeared 4 months after curative pentamidine therapy, serial tests of pulmonary function revealed persistent ventilatory defects of the restrictive type and impairment of carbon monoxide–diffusing capacity.[101] Although a possible link between pentamidine therapy per se and lung fibrosis was suggested by earlier observations in rat pneumocystosis,[110,188] healthy animals given the drug exhibit no histologic abnormalities.[97] Moreover, pulmonary fibrosis has been described after *Pneumocystis* pneumonia in patients who received treatment with pyrimethamine and sulfonamide[189] and TMP-SMX.[190]

Recurrent Infection

Recurrence of *Pneumocystis* pneumonia after apparently curative courses of therapy has been documented in infants and children with underlying congenital immunodeficiency or malignancy. As early as 1966, Patterson[191] reported the case of an infant with probable SCID who experienced one presumptive and two substantiated bouts of pneumocystosis at approximately 5-month intervals; treatment with pentamidine resulted in "cure" on each occasion, although radiographic abnormalities persisted. A few years later, Richman and associates[192] and then Saulsbury and colleagues[193] described recurrent pneumocystosis in two children with hypogammaglobulinemia. In the first case, three proven attacks responded to pentamidine, and in the second child, two separate episodes of infection were treated successfully with TMP-SMX. At St. Jude Children's Research Hospital, a study of 28 children with malignancy whose pneumocystosis was treated with pentamidine revealed that 4 (14%) suffered a second infection.[97,194] The clinical manifestations, radiographic findings, and response to therapy were similar for each child in both infectious episodes. In addition, no differences in host factors were discernible in those patients who had recurrent infection and those who did not. Other examples of recurrent pneumocystosis emerging rather soon after clinical recovery have been observed in patients given either pentamidine or TMP-SMX.[195] Whether recurrences of *Pneumocystis* pneumonia result from reinfection or from relapse of previously treated infection is not known.

Clinical and morphologic studies provide conflicting views on the completeness of *Pneumocystis* killing by specific drugs. The Hungarian workers, who first used pentamidine in epidemic pneumocystosis among infants, witnessed progressive degeneration of *P. jirovecii* in tracheal mucus from the sixth day of therapy; by the tenth day, the organisms had almost entirely disintegrated.[172] In their review of sporadic pneumocystosis in the United States, Western and associates[174] similarly concluded that pentamidine probably eliminates organisms from the lung. In two patients, no microscopically visible *P. jirovecii* organisms were present at 5 and 14 days, respectively, after initiation of therapy. Also, none of 11 patients who died more than 20 days after receiving pentamidine had demonstrable organisms in their lungs, even though they survived an average of 189.5 days after administration of the drug. In ultrastructural studies, Campbell[26] detected what he believed to be the destructive effects of pentamidine on the organisms. In a lung biopsy specimen obtained surgically 16 hours after onset of therapy, structurally normal trophozoites or mature cysts with intracystic bodies were absent. A few apparent "ghosts" of trophozoites were noted within phagosomes of intraalveolar macrophages.

By contrast, pentamidine does not promptly eradicate potentially viable forms of the organism. Hughes and coworkers[97] identified intact *P. jirovecii* in lung aspirates (or autopsy material) 10 to 20 days after institution of drug treatment. Richman and associates[192] demonstrated normal-appearing *Pneumocystis* organisms in a lung aspirate from a clinically cured patient 3 days after completion of his 14-day course of pentamidine. Similarly, Fortuny and colleagues[196] recovered organisms from induced sputa on each of 11 days of pentamidine injections.

TMP-SMX appears to have only a limited and nonlethal effect on organisms. Experiments have shown that short-term treatment with the drug combination ultimately fails to prevent emergence of recrudescent *Pneumocystis* infection. In one study, a therapeutic dosage of TMP-SMX was given prophylactically to children with acute lymphocytic leukemia for a 2-week period beginning 28 days after initiation of antineoplastic treatment.[197] Although the incidence of *Pneumocystis* infection in these children after TMP-SMX was discontinued was not different from that observed in persons who did not receive the drug, the time interval to development of infection was lengthened. Reinfection rather than relapse may have accounted for the late infections, but relapse seems more likely in view of the following results in experimental animals.[198] Immunocompetent rats were given TMP-SMX for as long as 6 weeks and then placed in individual isolator cages to exclude the possibility of acquisition of new organisms from the environmental air. After 12 weeks of immunosuppressive therapy with prednisone, *P. jirovecii* was still found in the lungs of at least 90% of both the animals given TMP-SMX and the control animals (given no treatment). These human and animal data are particularly relevant to the design of prophylactic regimens to prevent *Pneumocystis* infection in humans. They provide a compelling argument for the need to continue prophylaxis for as long as host defenses are considered to be too compromised to keep patients protected from *Pneumocystis* infection. Survival and permanent immunity to reinfection relate not to chemotherapy but to specific anti-*Pneumocystis* immunity in the affected infants. Unfortunately, the congenitally immunodeficient or exogenously immunosuppressed child does not possess such normal immune responsiveness and thus is subject to recurrent infection.

PREVENTION

The first successful attempts to prevent pneumocystosis with drugs were reported in infants with the epidemic form of the infection. In a controlled trial conducted in an Iranian orphanage where the infection was endemic (attack rate of 28%), the biweekly administration of a pyrimethamine and sulfadoxine combination to marasmic infants before the second month of life entirely eradicated *Pneumocystis* pneumonia from the institution.[16] In a children's hospital in Budapest, Hungary, pentamidine given every other day for a total of seven doses to premature infants from the second week of life provided equally effective prophylaxis. During the 6 years of the study, *Pneumocystis* infection did not develop among 536 premature babies who received this treatment, whereas 62 fatal cases were recorded elsewhere in the city.[199]

On the basis of promising results in a rat model of infection, TMP-SMX was evaluated in a randomized, double-blind, controlled trial in children with cancer who were at extremely high risk for *Pneumocystis* pneumonitis.[200] The daily dosage for prophylaxis was 5 mg of TMP plus 20 mg of SMX/kg body weight, administered orally in two divided doses. Seventeen (21%) of 80 children receiving placebo acquired pneumocystosis, whereas the infection developed in none of 80 patients given TMP-SMX. No adverse effects of TMP-SMX administration were observed, although oral candidiasis was more prevalent among the patients in the treatment group than among the control patients. In a subsequent uncontrolled trial, the prophylactic efficacy of TMP-SMX was confirmed; cases of infection developed only in those children in whom the TMP-SMX was discontinued while they were still receiving anticancer chemotherapy.[201] More recently, a regimen of TMP-SMX prophylaxis given 3 days per week was shown to be as effective as daily administration.[202]

The gratifying success of TMP-SMX prophylaxis in prevention of *Pneumocystis* infection has been duplicated in other medical centers caring for children with underlying malignancy.[203] Administration of the drug for the duration of antineoplastic therapy has become standard practice. Congenitally immunodeficient children and infants with AIDS who have had a prior episode of *Pneumocystis* pneumonia would appear to be prime candidates for preventive therapy. The CDC issues a set of guidelines for chemoprophylaxis against *P. jirovecii* pneumonia in children with HIV infection.[204] These guidelines recommend promptly identifying infants and children born to HIV-infected women, initiating prophylaxis at 4 to 6 weeks of age for all of these children, and continuing prophylaxis through 12 months of age for HIV-infected children and offer new algorithms based on clinical and immunologic status to continue prophylaxis beyond 12 months of age. Although no chemoprophylactic regimens for *P. jirovecii* pneumonia among HIV-infected children have been approved as labeling indications by the U.S. Food and Drug Administration (FDA), TMP-SMX currently is recommended as the drug of choice in children with HIV infection. This recommendation is based on the known safety profile of TMP-SMX and its efficacy in adults with HIV infection and in children with malignancies. Alternative regimens recommended for HIV-infected children who cannot tolerate TMP-SMX include aerosolized pentamidine in children older than 5 years of age, oral dapsone, and oral atovaquone. One study suggests that TMP-SMX use is associated with a decreased incidence of *P. jirovecii* pneumonitis and an increased incidence of HIV encephalopathy, both as initial AIDS-defining conditions in infants and children.[205] Most likely this was related to an "unmasking" of progressive encephalopathy among infants who otherwise would have died earlier because of *P. jirovecii* pneumonia.

Aspergillosis

Aspergillosis is the most common cause of human mold infections, and the most common species isolated from patients is *Aspergillus fumigatus*. Invasive infections are extremely rare in preterm and term infants and are much less common than in older patients with compromised immunity.[206] Immunocompromised older children and adults typically present with pulmonary aspergillosis and, although pulmonary aspergillosis occurs in term and preterm infants, primary cutaneous aspergillosis (PCA) comprises a much larger proportion of aspergillosis in this age group compared with older children and adults.[207] For example, a large case series of invasive aspergillosis in children younger than 3 months (44 cases) reported by Groll and coworkers[208] found that the number of children with pulmonary aspergillosis (10) was nearly identical to those with PCA.[11] The most common underlying condition associated with invasive aspergillosis in this series was prematurity (43% of patients), followed by chronic granulomatous disease (14%). Of interest, whereas 10 of 11 patients with PCA were preterm, only 2 of 10 patients with pulmonary aspergillosis were preterm; 5 of 10 term infants with pulmonary aspergillosis were later diagnosed with chronic granulomatous disease, indicating that it would be reasonable to evaluate infants who develop pulmonary aspergillosis for chronic granulomatous disease.

Aspergillus spp. are ubiquitous environmental molds and are an opportunistic pathogen in that the vast majority of exposed people do not develop disease. In the hospital setting, there have been numerous reports of outbreaks or clusters of aspergillosis within specific units or in groups of at-risk patients. For example, a number of outbreaks in NICUs have been associated with construction or renovation projects at the hospitals housing these units.[209] Presumably, the disruption of dirt and soil caused by these projects increases the burden of exposure and, correspondingly, the likelihood of disease in high-risk patients. However, it is important to note that clusters of cases in preterm infants have also been linked to contaminated equipment within the units themselves. For example, Etienne and associates[210] described a cluster of invasive aspergillosis in a NICU that was ultimately linked to contaminated humidity chambers. Invasive aspergillosis is sufficiently rare in term and preterm infants that any cases within a unit should prompt a careful consideration of possible sources of environmental contamination as a means to avoid larger outbreaks.

THE ORGANISM

The genus *Aspergillus* is within the family Moniliaceae and is classified as an ascomycetous, saprophytic mold. The species that cause disease most commonly are *Aspergillus fumigatus*, which causes at least 90% of all disease, followed by *Aspergillus flavus*, *Aspergillus niger*, and *Aspergillus terreus*.[206] However, as the number of people living with profound immunosuppression has increased, the number of *Aspergillus* spp. that have been reported to cause invasive disease has increased; the list contains at least 20 different species. Almost all cases of neonatal aspergillosis have been caused by *A. fumigatus*.[208] A distinguishing feature of pathogenic species is their ability to grow at human body temperature (37° C); *A. fumigatus*, for example, can grow at temperatures as high as 50° C, and this characteristic can be used to identify this specific species. Microscopically, *Aspergillus* is a hyaline, septate, monomorphic mold that shows dichotomous branching. The species are differentiated using a variety of distinguishing morphologic, mycologic, and biochemical characteristics. It is important to note that it can be difficult to differentiate *Aspergillus* spp.

from other types of molds during the initial evaluation of clinical samples.

EPIDEMIOLOGY AND TRANSMISSION

Aspergillosis is a rare infection in neonates and infants, and the literature of such infections is limited to case reports and case series. Consequently, it is not possible to estimate an incidence rate. In general, the two primary modes of transmission are inhalation of airborne conidia or through direct, localized inoculation of damaged or compromised tissues. Person-to-person transmission has not been documented, whereas the clustering of multiple cases has been linked to exposure to a common environmental source, such as humidifying units.[210] Thus isolating affected patients is unlikely to prevent additional cases within a closed unit. The identification and control of possible sources of environmental contamination is more likely to lead to the prevention of additional cases.

For preterm infants in the NICU setting, PCA is the most common manifestation of aspergillosis, as illustrated by the large case series reported by Groll and associates.[208] As discussed in depth by Walsh,[211] it is likely that the well-characterized fragility of the skin of preterm infants is the primary reason for the disproportionate rate of PCA relative to pulmonary aspergillosis. A large multicenter retrospective analysis of 139 cases of invasive aspergillosis in children of all ages found that cutaneous aspergillosis was more common in children than adults; however, this study did not correlate age with incidence of PCA.[212] In other populations, a primary risk factor acquiring invasive aspergillosis is decreased levels or function of peripheral neutrophils. Although neutropenia is not generally a complication of prematurity, there are numerous studies indicating that premature infants have defects in specific neutrophil functions, including migration, phagocytosis, and microbial killing.[213] No specific studies have examined the ability of neutrophils from premature infants to respond to *Aspergillus*, but it is certainly possible that an inability of premature neutrophils to make an effective response to microbial pathogens contributes to their risk for aspergillosis. The study of Groll and associates[208] underscores this possibility in that it found that a significant portion of term infants who developed pulmonary aspergillosis also had chronic granulomatous disease. Chronic granulomatous disease is genetic disease caused by mutation of the *phox* gene, leading to decreased respiratory burst in phagocytes, and is characterized by increased susceptibility to aspergillosis as well as other pathogens.[214] The findings of Groll suggest that infants who develop pulmonary aspergillosis be evaluated for defects in neutrophil function, including chronic granulomatous disease.[208]

PATHOGENESIS

Consistent with their opportunistic nature, *Aspergillus* spp. do not display virulence factors in the traditional microbiologic sense (e.g., cholera toxin). To replicate and cause disease, the fungus must be able to withstand the host environment, and the thermotolerant nature of *Aspergillus* spp. that cause disease is an important trait required for virulence. For example, mutants of specific genes (e.g., *crgA*[215]) that lead to decreased growth at 37° C are attenuated for virulence in animal models of aspergillosis. Other genes that have been associated with decreased virulence in animal models include amino acid metabolism and iron acquisition, as well as others.[215] Once the fungus has breached the pulmonary epithelium or epidermis, it is well known to invade tissue and blood vessels. Consistent with its saprophytic nature, it is well adapted to growth along environmental gradients, which is thought to contribute to its characteristic angiotropism. Invasion of blood vessels has two consequences. First, it leads to additional tissue damage and necrosis by destroying the blood vessel and depriving the local tissue of oxygen and nutrients. Second, angioinvasion facilitates dissemination to other organ systems within the host. The latter characteristic is particularly relevant to neonatal aspergillosis because many cases of PCA ultimately lead to disseminated disease accompanied by sepsis and multiorgan system involvement.[208,211] A commonly encountered target organ of *Aspergillus* is the central nervous system (CNS), and its angiotropism appears to also allow it to readily penetrate the blood-brain barrier.[216] As one might expect, CNS involvement is a complication of aspergillosis that is associated with a very poor prognosis.

PATHOLOGY

Because PCA is one of the primary manifestations of aspergillosis in neonates, the histopathologic analysis of biopsy specimens of infected tissue and skin is an important mode of diagnosis.[208] *Aspergillus* is readily demonstrated in tissue using standard GMS or PAS stains. The hyphae are septate and hyaline and, classically, display dichotomous branches that emerge at an acute angle to the primary filament (<90 degrees). Although these features can allow one to distinguish *Aspergillus* from Zygomycetes (aseptate, right-angle branching), the histopathologic characteristics of *Aspergillus* are similar to a wide range of other pathogenic molds, including *Fusarium* and *Scedosporium*. However, because these molds are exceedingly rare in infants and are generally treated with the same agents, this ambiguity rarely has clinical significance. Because of its angiotropic nature and destructive effect on blood vessels, hemorrhagic necrosis is typical of infected tissue and is consistent with the necrotic skin lesions that are part and parcel of PCA in neonates.[207-210]

CLINICAL MANIFESTATIONS

The most distinctive manifestation of aspergillosis in neonates and infants is the high percentage of PCA. The characteristic clinical feature of PCA is the appearance of skin lesions. Initially, these lesions can be nonspecific raised erythematous plaques and pustules.[207-210] However, they generally progress to macerated, ulcerated lesions with a punched out appearance. In almost all cases, the lesions form necrotic eschars. Although these lesions are almost characteristic of PCA, it is important to note that their appearance is not pathognomonic of PCA, and they cannot be distinguished from skin lesions resulting from the systemic dissemination of other microbial pathogens such as *Pseudomonas aeruginosa* or *Staphylococcus aureus*. Similarly, as a number of authors have noted, pulmonary aspergillosis does not have distinctive clinical characteristics that allow it to be readily identified.[207-210]

Regardless of the initial site of infection, many neonates develop disseminated disease with a sepsis-like syndrome and multiorgan system involvement. Symptoms accompanying dissemination include hypotension, coagulopathy, and hepatosplenomegaly. Although almost any organ can be involved after dissemination, CNS disease is a frequent complication. Because aspergillosis is difficult to diagnose, it is not surprising that CNS symptoms or findings may be the initial clue to the diagnosis, as for the patient described by Fuchs and coworkers.[216] In the series of children younger than 3 months reported by Groll and coworkers,[208] four patients with CNS disease as the only manifestation were identified.

DIAGNOSIS/DIFFERENTIAL DIAGNOSIS

The diagnosis of aspergillosis in the neonate and infant is extremely difficult for a wide variety of reasons, including its rarity and the fact that its clinical manifestations overlap with other, much more commonly encountered pathogens. The most important method of diagnosing invasive infections in any patient population is the blood culture. Unfortunately, blood cultures are almost invariably negative in the setting of invasive aspergillosis, a fact that is somewhat counterintuitive, given its angiotropism.[206,212] In older patients, radiographic characteristics of pulmonary aspergillosis, such as the halo sign, can be suggestive of the diagnosis in an at-risk patient population.[212] However, no such characteristics have been identified in neonates or infants. The skin lesions characteristic of PCA provide the most direct opportunity for diagnosis through biopsy, stains, and culture. In contrast to blood cultures, tissue culture yields reasonable results; however, histologic identification of hyphal elements in a biopsy specimen in the absence of culture results should prompt immediate treatment and is certainly sufficient for a presumptive diagnosis. It is also important to consider other potential diagnoses that are associated with a critically ill infant displaying ulcerative or necrotic skin lesions; these include other fungal infections such as invasive candidiasis, bacterial infections such as *P. aeruginosa*, and disseminated viral infections such as congenital herpes or enterovirus.

Non–culture-based methods for the diagnosis of aspergillosis have been the subject of intensive interest.[206,212] The most widely used and best characterized of these tests is the serum galactomannan assay. The assay uses an enzyme-linked immunosorbent assay (ELISA)–based technology to detect the presence of galactomannan in serum and, less commonly, other fluids such as BAL samples. Galactomannan is a component of the *Aspergillus* cell wall but is absent from *Candida* spp. The assay has been widely adopted to monitor for and diagnose aspergillosis in adult patients. Initial, small studies of the assay in children found that neonates had a significantly higher rate of false-positive tests. Subsequent studies indicate that this high false-positive rate may be due to the high levels of *Bifidobacterium* in the gut of neonates[217]; the lipoteichoic acid from this organism cross-reacts with the galactomannan ELISA. The galactomannan assay has been studied in older children and seems to perform similarly to adult patients.[218] However, no prospective studies have evaluated its use in neonates and infants, and thus its value for this patient population remains unknown and may be complicated by false-positive results. Other tests that have been developed for aspergillosis, including serum 1,3-β-glucan and PCR-based methods, remain experimental or have not been sufficiently studied in this population to warrant routine use.

THERAPY

All three classes of antifungal agents used as monotherapy (polyenes, azoles, and echinocandins) have specific agents with activity against *Aspergillus*. Of these, amphotericin B, either as the deoxycholate or as a lipid-based formulation, is the recommended therapy for neonatal aspergillosis. The recommended dose of amphotericin B deoxycholate is 1 mg/kg day for infants and neonates.[219] Three lipid formulations of amphotericin B are available: L-amB (AmBisome), amphotericin B lipid complex (ABLC, or Abelcet), and ABCD (Amphotec). The pharmacokinetics and pharmacodynamics of the lipid-based amphotericin B preparations have not been studied extensively in neonates or infants, but doses of 3 to 5 mg/kg/day are typically used.[219] Amphotericin B deoxycholate appears to be tolerated better in neonates than in older patients,[220] and a small study comparing amphotericin B with liposomal amphotericin and amphotericin B colloidal dispersion found no difference in efficacy or adverse events.[221] In adult patients, liposomal preparations generally are associated with less renal toxicity and would be reasonable to use for a neonate with decreased renal function. However, it is important to note that the lipid preparations do not penetrate renal tissue well.

In adult patients with aspergillosis, voriconazole, an azole antifungal, was found to be superior to amphotericin B.[222] Two case reports have been published describing the use of voriconazole, either alone or in combination with amphotericin B and micafungin, to treat infants with PCA.[223,224] In both case reports, the infants had not responded to treatment with amphotericin B–based agents. Although Santos and coworkers[224] measured a variety of pharmacokinetic data for voriconazole, the routine use of voriconazole in infants and neonates awaits studies designed to establish effective dosing in this age group. This is particularly important for voriconazole because studies in older children have revealed significant age-based variations in pharmacokinetics and pharmacodynamics. Of the other azole agents available, itraconazole and posaconazole also have activity against *Aspergillus*. However, neither agent has been studied in neonates and, in general, should not be considered as a first-line treatment option. It is extremely important to note that fluconazole, the most widely used antifungal in NICUs, has no activity toward *Aspergillus*. If the diagnosis of aspergillosis is being considered and the patient is being treated empirically with fluconazole, then the antifungal agent should be changed to a mold-active drug.

The echinocandins have been approved for salvage treatment of aspergillosis in adults. In contrast to voriconazole, a reasonable amount of data is available to guide dosing of this class of agents in neonates and infants.[219] Currently, three echinocandins are available: caspofungin, micafungin, and anidulafungin. The recommended doses for these agents vary with age and agent: caspofungin (25 mg/m^2/day for neonates younger than 30 days, 50 mg/m²/day for infants 31 days-2 years of age), micafungin (10 mg/kg/day for infants and neonates up to 2 years of age), and anidulafungin (3 mg/kg/loading dose, followed by 1.5 mg/kg/day for infants and neonates up to 2 years of age). The echinocandins are only available as intravenous preparations. In addition, they have an excellent safety profile and few drug-drug interactions. Echinocandins are primarily used in the NICU to treat invasive candidiasis caused by *Candida* spp. with reduced susceptibility to fluconazole, for instance, *Candida glabrata* and *Candida krusei.* Thus it seems reasonable to consider the echinocandins as a logical choice as second-line or salvage therapy for aspergillosis in a neonate or infant who is either intolerant of, or not a candidate for, amphotericin B–based treatment.

PROGNOSIS

In general, invasive aspergillosis carries a very poor prognosis, regardless of underlying conditions. Because most of the information regarding neonatal and infant aspergillosis is based on relatively small case series and case reports, it is subject to significant ascertainment bias as well as other confounding factors. The large case series by Groll and coworkers[208] suggests that neonates and infants with PCA that does not disseminate respond to therapy much more frequently than those with secondary dissemination. In that study, 73% of patients with limited PCA were cured with either medical or a combination of medical surgical therapy, whereas all patients with disseminated disease died. However, because a significant number of cases of PCA are complicated by dissemination, the serious nature of this infection cannot be underestimated and, as with other fungal infection, early recognition and institution of appropriate therapy is crucial.

PREVENTION

Outbreaks of aspergillosis in the health care setting have been linked to environmental contamination related to construction at the health care sites as well as to contaminated equipment within NICUs per se.[209,210] Therefore adherence to standard maintenance and practices with respect to humidifiers and other equipment that could harbor extensive contamination of mold is important. Because this is a rare disease, it would seem prudent to strongly consider investigating any case of aspergillosis within a NICU for a potential environmental source.

Blastomycosis

Blastomycosis is an endemic mycosis caused by *Blastomyces dermatitides*, a dimorphic environmental fungus. In general, it is thought that the majority of *B. dermatitides* infections lead to a subclinical or nonspecific illness that is followed by resolution and the development of protective immunity.[225] Outside of epidemic outbreaks, children rarely present with clinically apparent disease.[226] In addition, immunocompromise does not appear to predispose a patient to blastomycosis, but such patients may develop more severe disease.[225] A number of cases of pregnant women with blastomycosis have been described in the literature.[227-229] Of importance, transplacental transmission to the fetus appears to occur only rarely. For example, Lemos and coworkers[228] reviewed the literature reports of pregnancies complicated by blastomycosis and found that the fetus was infected in 2 of 20 cases (10%). Both of the infected infants, however, died of blastomycosis.[228,229]

THE ORGANISM

B. dermatitidis is a dimorphic fungus that grows naturally in the environment. At ambient temperature in the soil, it exists as a mycelial form. The conidia are the infectious form of the organism, which, upon entrance into a mammalian host, rapidly germinate into the yeast form; a process that can be triggered in vitro by cultivation at 37° C. The yeast form has a thick cell wall and forms a characteristically wide bud-neck with daughter cells.

EPIDEMIOLOGY AND TRANSMISSION

B. dermatitidis is endemic to specific regions of North America.[225] Most cases occur in states that are located along the Mississippi and Ohio Rivers of the Midwest. In addition, cases have been reported in states and Canadian provinces that border the Great Lakes and the St. Lawrence River. Within these regions are areas of hyperendemicity as well as isolated epidemics. Although sporadic cases of blastomycosis have been reported outside of the traditional range, many appear to be due to exposures within an endemic region, followed by travel.

B. dermatitidis infects a mammalian host when the spores are inhaled.[225] Once inside the host, the organism germinates to the yeast form, which replicates. The organism is not generally considered as being transmitted from person to person, although there are reports of transmission via the bite of an infected dog.[230]

PATHOGENESIS

Once the conidial form enters the pulmonary system, it rapidly germinates to the yeast form. This transition appears to be required for pathogenesis. The conidia are more susceptible to killing by phagocytes, such as alveolar macrophages, than the yeast form.[231] The surviving yeast forms are then thought to replicate within the lung and spread to other body sites via the bloodstream. Infected tissues are subject to an acute inflammatory response involving both neutrophils and macrophages; ultimately, cellular immunity to *Blastomyces* develops.[232]

PATHOLOGY

Infected tissues are characterized by a pyogranulomatous response involving neutrophils, followed by macrophages. The granulomas are generally not caseating, in distinction from mycobacterial infections.

CLINICAL MANIFESTATIONS

The most common symptoms associated with blastomycosis are nonspecific, including fever, malaise, and weight loss.[225] Pulmonary symptoms include cough and pleuritic chest pain. Disseminated disease can involve skin, bones, CNS, and deep organs. Skin is the most common extrapulmonary site of infection. There have not been sufficient cases in neonates or infants to formulate a typical set of presenting findings.

DIAGNOSIS

As with the clinical manifestations, radiographic findings associated with blastomycosis are not specific. The diagnosis is most commonly made by microscopic or histologic identification within infected tissue or fluid samples. It is cultivable in the laboratory and can be isolated from blood, lavage fluid, and tissue. Non–culture-based methods, such as serologic and skin testing, are not helpful clinically, and none have been studied in the setting of neonates and/or infants.

THERAPY

Because there are very few cases of blastomycosis in neonates and because amphotericin B–based therapy has been used in adults for serious infections, it would seem most prudent to use this agent.[225] Fluconazole has been used in mild-to-moderate disease in older children and adults and could be regarded as an alternative. Again, there is almost no experience available, and any treatment plan must be devised on a case-by-case basis by analogy to those used in adults and older children.

PROGNOSIS

All reported cases of blastomycosis in neonates have been fatal. On a more encouraging note, very few infants appear to be born to pregnant women with disseminated disease.

PREVENTION

Because many of the pregnant women with blastomycosis were treated, it is possible that treatment could play a role in preventing transmission to the fetus.

Histoplasmosis

Histoplasmosis is an endemic mycosis caused by the dimorphic fungus, *Histoplasma capsulatum*. Histoplasmosis is the most common endemic mycosis in the United States.[233] However, like blastomycosis, very few cases of histoplasmosis have been reported in neonates and young infants. A relatively large case series of histoplasmosis in older infants has been reported, with the youngest patient being 6 weeks of age.[234] There have been two cases of congenital transmission of histoplasmosis in the literature, including one patient with congenital HIV infection.[235,236] In contrast to the neonates who contracted blastomycosis, both infants with histoplasmosis responded well to antifungal therapy and survived.

THE ORGANISM

H. capsulatum is a dimorphic, environmental fungus that appears to thrive in soil containing the droppings of birds or bats.[233] In its environmental niche, *H. capsulatum* exists in a mycelial form and, like *B. dermatitidis*, transitions to the yeast form upon infection of a mammalian host or incubation at 37° C. The conidia of *H. capsulatum* are of two types: macroconidia with thick walls that contain projections and microconidia with smooth walls. The budding yeast forms are frequently seen with macrophages in histologic samples.

EPIDEMIOLOGY AND TRANSMISSION

H. capsulatum is distributed worldwide but has a well-characterized endemic region within the United States that includes the Mississippi and Ohio River Valleys of the Midwest and Southeastern regions of the country.[233] The microconidia of *H. capsulatum* in its mycelial phase are small (2-4 μm), readily aerosolized, and pass into the alveoli when inhaled. The vast majority of histoplasmosis is subclinical or results in a self-limited nonspecific illness.[225,233] Almost all cases are due to sporadic, local exposure, but two large outbreaks have been associated with urban construction projects in Indianapolis.[237] Before the advent of highly active antiretroviral therapy for HIV/AIDS, attack rates were much higher for persons living with HIV/AIDS in *Histoplasma*-endemic areas.[238]

PATHOGENESIS

The inhaled conidia undergo morphogenesis to the yeast form. Alveolar macrophages phagocytose both conidia and yeast cells, but the yeast cells are able to survive within the phagolysosome and replicate. Within the macrophages, the organisms traffic to hilar and mediastinal lymph nodes from which they disseminate to other sites of the reticuloendothelial system. The crucial factor for containment of the infection is the development of T-cell immunity.[233] The sensitized T cells activate macrophages which, in turn, are able to kill the organism and clear the infection. As discussed by Kauffman,[233] the severity of disease is also dependent on the size of the infecting inoculum. An immunocompetent person, for example, can develop severe disease if they are exposed to a large amount of conidia. Thus the nature of the clinical outcome of histoplasmosis is a function of both the nature of the patient's exposure and the immune response that the patient mounts to the pathogen. With that said, the majority of patients who develop severe disease also have deficiencies in cell-mediated immunity.

PATHOLOGY

Tissue biopsy, from lymph nodes most commonly, will demonstrate yeast cells either within macrophages or free in the tissue upon staining with GMS or periodic acid–Schiff. BAL samples rarely are positive unless there is a very large organism burden; in such cases, it can also be possible to identify organisms within neutrophils from smears of peripheral blood. Infected lymph nodes also typically demonstrate caseating granulomas.

CLINICAL MANIFESTATIONS

Histoplasmosis is generally asymptomatic or leads to an illness that is nonspecific, mild, and self-limited. The most common clinically apparent manifestation of histoplasmosis is acute pulmonary disease; most of these cases resolve without the need for antifungal therapy, whereas severe and chronic cases require antifungal therapy.[233] As noted earlier, dissemination of histoplasmosis throughout the reticular-endothelial system occurs in almost all cases. However, clinical disease accompanies this dissemination only in immunosuppressed patients. Based on the case series reported by Odio and coworkers,[234] dissemination also occurs in otherwise normal infants.[234] Of interest, many of these infants have T-cell abnormalities at the time of infection that resolve with treatment of the histoplasmosis. Both children who were reported to have contracted histoplasmosis congenitally presented with disseminated disease[235,236] and, for one case, yeast forms were demonstrated within placental villi.[235] The CNS can also be infected either as part of disseminated histoplasmosis or in isolation. In accordance, cultures of the cerebrospinal fluid (CSF) of both infants with congenital histoplasmosis were positive, indicating CNS involvement.[235,236]

DIAGNOSIS

H. capsulatum is cultivatable from tissue, blood, bone marrow, BAL, as well as other patient samples. In addition, it is readily identified in biopsy samples by standard histopathologic techniques. An antigen assay that detects a polysaccharide in serum or urine is also available. It is most sensitive in the setting of disseminated disease and severe pulmonary disease (75%-90%) but is much less so in the setting of mild or chronic disease (10%-20%). The urine antigen assay was positive in one of the congenitally infected infants. A complement fixation test is also available and can be used to aid diagnosis, particularly in the setting of disseminated or chronic pulmonary disease. Like many serologic tests, it can be falsely negative in immunocompromised patients who are unable to generate a normal humoral response. However, Odio and coworkers[234] found that 93% of infants with disseminated histoplasmosis were positive by complement fixation at the time of diagnosis, indicating that the test should be useful in this age group.

TREATMENT

The recommended treatment of histoplasmosis is dependent on the severity of disease[233]; mild-to-moderate infections are treated with itraconazole, and severe infections are treated with amphotericin B–based drugs. In the two reported congenital infections,[235,236] the children were treated with amphotericin B and a combination of amphotericin B and itraconazole. The infants described in the series reported by Odio and coworkers[234] were treated with amphotericin B for 40 days, followed by ketoconazole for a total of 3 months.

PROGNOSIS

Both congenitally infected infants responded to treatment and were cured.[235,236] The cure rate for the series of infants with disseminated disease was similarly good, with 88% of patients cured; four died and one had recurrent disease. The child with relapse was cured after a second treatment course.[234]

Coccidiodomycosis

Coccidioides immitis is a dimorphic fungus that is found in the soil of the Western Hemisphere. *C. immitis* is geographically restricted to area between 40°N and 40°S and, in the United States, is found in the southwestern states, including California, Nevada, Utah, Arizona, New Mexico, and Texas.[239] *C. immitis* is the etiologic agent of so-called valley fever, which refers to its endemicity within the San Joaquin Valley in central California. Like other endemic fungi, *C. immitis* is a mold in the soil that then undergoes morphogenesis to a spherule form within the host. Also similar to other endemic dimorphs, the majority of *C. immitis* infections are asymptomatic, and most symptomatic infections are self-limited. Severe pulmonary disease and dissemination occur in a minority of cases, and people with deficits in cell-mediated immunity are at higher risk for these complications. Pregnant women are at increased risk for severe primary and disseminated coccidioidomycosis during the second and third trimester.[240,241] Based on the fact that there have been many cases of coccidioidomycosis in pregnant women and relatively few cases of neonatal infections, it appears that vertical transmission of *C. immitis* is relatively rare. However, there have been 15 cases of neonatal coccidioidomycosis described in the literature.[242,243] The majority of neonates infected with *C. immitis* have developed disseminated disease, with many resulting in the death of the infant.

THE ORGANISM

C. immitis is classified as an ascomycete, and ribosomal DNA analysis indicates that *C. immitis* is related to the endemic dimorphic fungi *H. capsulatum* and *B. dermatitidis*.[241] In the soil, *C. immitis* forms septate hyphae that fragment into barrel-shaped arthroconidia that are thought to be the infectious particle. Within the host, the organism undergoes morphogenesis to a large (120 μm) compartmented, multinucleate structure called a spherule. The internal structures within the spherule are referred to as endospores.[241]

EPIDEMIOLOGY AND TRANSMISSION

Within endemic regions, seropositivity of residents has been reported to be quite high, particularly based on older studies. A seroprevalence study performed in Arizona in 1985 indicated that 30% of those tested were seropositive.[244] A study comparing the incidence from 1937 to 1939 to that in 1995 within the San Joaquin Valley indicated that it had decreased from 10% per year to 2% per year, respectively.[245] Outbreaks of coccidioidomycosis have been associated with strong wind storms or earthquakes that generated large dust clouds.[246] Transmission is primarily through inhalation of dust containing aerosolized arthroconidia. However, direct inoculation of skin through traumatic wounds contaminated with soil has also been reported.[247] Direct person-to-person transmission of pulmonary coccidioidomycosis has not been reported. Contact with infected fomites in the health care setting has been documented.[239] Some controversy exists in the literature as to whether neonatal cases result from intrauterine transmission or from contact with infected body fluids within the birth canal.[241]

PATHOGENESIS

The inhaled arthrocondia of *C. immitis* undergo germination, followed by isotropic growth that ultimately results in the formation of large spherules.[239] The cycle of pathogenesis has been characterized as a parasitic life cycle. In this model, the initial arthroconidia lead to spherule formation that contains a large number of small endospores. The spherule then releases the endospores, which undergo dispersion and additional rounds of growth, spherule formation, and endospore release. The spherules are too large to be effectively phagocytosed by macrophages, whereas there is also evidence that the endospores are relatively resistant to phagocyte-mediated killing. Ultimately, an effective cell-mediated immune response appears to be required to contain the infection. For example, people who have mild, self-limited infections develop delayed-type hypersensitivity to *C. immitis*, whereas failure to mount this response is associated with more severe or disseminated disease.[248]

PATHOLOGY

Pathologic specimens of tissue infected with *C. immitis* show necrotizing granulomas, classically. In addition, the spherules can be seen by histopathology and are diagnostic of coccidioidomycosis. Histopathology studies of the placenta from pregnant women with disseminated disease have shown the presence of *C. immitis* spherules.[249]

CLINICAL MANIFESTATIONS

Many infections with *C. immitis* are asymptomatic or lead to mild, nonspecific symptoms, such as fever, cough, and headache.[239] Primary pulmonary disease is characterized by an atypical pneumonia with radiographic findings that are indistinguishable from other types of pneumonia. Coccidiodomycosis is associated with a pruritic skin rash as well as the development of erythema nodosum or erythema multiforme in up to 25% of patients. Symptoms generally manifest 1 to 4 weeks after infection and resolve without treatment over weeks to months. Disseminated disease is associated with a poor cellular immune response[248] and has been estimated to occur in less than 1% of patients. Dissemination frequently involves the skin, bones, and joints. Meningitis can also develop. The majority of neonatal coccidioidomycosis reported in the literature have been cases of disseminated disease involving CNS as well as deep organs.[242,243]

DIAGNOSIS

C. immitis can be cultured in the laboratory from infected tissues.[239] The yields are highest in respiratory secretions; for example, *C. immitis* was cultured from deep tracheal aspirate from two of the neonatal cases.[242,243] It is important to note that *C. immitis* presents a risk to laboratory workers and requires special precautions in the laboratory. Therefore the laboratory should be notified when samples from a patient suspected of being infected with *C. immitis* are submitted for processing. The diagnosis of coccidioidomycosis can also be established by histopathologic identification of the characteristic spherules within biopsy or other clinical samples. The organisms are readily stained with GMS and PAS procedures. Finally, serologic assays are available. The IgM and IgG responses can both be determined using a variety of methods. Neonates infected with *C. immitis* appear to generate antibodies reactive in these assays.[242,243]

TREATMENT

Similar to the approaches used for other pathogenic dimorphic fungi, amphotericin B is the drug of choice for severe or disseminated disease. Azoles (fluconazole, itraconazole, and ketoconazole) also have activity against *C. immitis* and have been used as well. Sequential treatment with an initial course of amphotericin B, followed by oral fluconazole, has also been used. For example, the neonate described in the report by Charlton and coworkers[243] was successfully treated with a three-week course of amphotericin B, followed by oral fluconazole. In adult patients, the relapse rate is between 15% and 30% after discontinuation of azole therapy.

PROGNOSIS

The outcome of disseminated disease in neonates and infants based on the available case reports is grim, with the majority of patients succumbing to infection. The infant described by Charlton and coworkers[243] responded to therapy and was well after a 6-month follow-up.

Cryptococcosis

Cryptococcosis is caused by *Cryptococcus* species and primarily manifests as meningoencephalitis and pneumonia in immunocompromised persons.[250] It is a global health problem primarily because people living with HIV/AIDS are at increased risk, and it is one of the most common life-threatening, opportunistic infections within that patient population.[251] Otherwise healthy pregnant women also appear to be at increased risk of cryptococcosis.[252] However, even in the setting of infants born to HIV-positive mothers with cryptococcosis, vertical transmission of *Cryptococcus* seems to be a rare event.[253] With that said, a dozen cases of congenital and presumed congenital infection in neonates have been reported. The majority of these involved CNS and pulmonary manifestations.[253]

THE ORGANISM

Cryptococcosis is caused by three varieties of the *Cryptococcus neoformans:* var. neoformans; var. grubii; and var. gattii.[250] *C. neoformans* is a basidiomycetous budding yeast that has a polysaccharide capsule. Five serotypes (A, B, C, D, and A/D) have been identified based on the antigenic properties of the capsule. The capsule plays an important role in pathogenesis. *C. neoformans* is an environmental organism associated with bird droppings, particularly pigeon, as well as eucalyptus trees. The organism can undergo mating, which results in the formation of mycelia and basidiospores. However, mating has not been observed outside of the laboratory.

EPIDEMIOLOGY AND TRANSMISSION

Park and coworkers[251] have estimated that approximately 1 million new cases of cryptococcosis occur each year worldwide. The majority of these cases occur in regions with high rates of HIV; in sub-Saharan Africa, more people die each year from cryptococcal meningitis than from tuberculosis. The majority of these cases are caused by *C. neoformans* var. grubii and affect immunocompromised individuals. In the Pacific Northwest region of North America, *C. neoformans* var. gattii is causing an ongoing outbreak that has mainly involved people without apparent deficits in immunity.[254] Transmission is thought to occur via inhalation of the organism; however, it is unclear as to whether the yeast form or the basidiospore is the infectious form.[250] There are rare reports of local inoculation leading to skin infection. Person-to-person transmission through an aerosol route has not been reported. Vertical transmission to newborns has been documented.[253] The mechanism of vertical transmission appears to involve both intrauterine and extrauterine exposure, with the latter thought to be more common. A study of the seroprevalence of response to *C. neoformans* antigens indicates that exposure before the age of 2 years is rare, but common in children older than 2 years.[255]

PATHOGENESIS

The pathogenesis of *C. neoformans* has been the subject of intensive study.[250,254,256] The inhaled organism enters into the bronchioles, where it establishes an initial infection. The alveolar macrophage appears to be the first line of host defense and is involved in containing the infection; however, the interaction between macrophages and *C. neoformans* is complex. The polysaccharide capsule of *C. neoformans* is an important virulence factor and is antiphagocytic as well as immunomodulatory.[256] Once inside the macrophage, *C. neoformans* is also able to replicate within the phagolysosome and lyse macrophages.[256,257] The ability of *C. neoformans* to survive within the hostile environment of the phagolysosome is partly dependent upon its ability to produce the antioxidant melanin. Ultimately, a cell-mediated immune response is required to clear the infection; although it is clear that cell-mediated immunity is critical, there are also data to suggest that humoral immunity contributes to the host response to *C. neoformans.*[256] In the absence of this response, *C. neoformans* disseminates to the CNS and causes a meningoencephalitis.[250] The mechanistic details of dissemination are not understood completely. In addition to hematogenous spread and direct transmigration across the blood-brain barrier, a "Trojan horse–type" mechanism, where *C. neoformans* enters the CNS within macrophages, may also play a role.[257] Once CNS infection is established, it is generally fatal in the absence of effective treatment.

PATHOLOGY

C. neoformans is detectable in infected tissue using standard GMS and PAS stains but is generally hard to identify in hematoxylin and eosin–stained samples. *C. neoformans* has been identified within placental tissue by histopathology and involved both villi and intravillous space.

CLINICAL MANIFESTATIONS

The pulmonary disease caused by *C. neoformans* in older children and adults does not have a specific presentation.[250] Immunocompetent people are generally asymptomatic or have very mild disease, and constitutional symptoms are uncommon even in the setting of confirmed pulmonary infection. Pulmonary disease in an immunocompromised patient, however, is frequently accompanied by extrapulmonary disease, including subclinical meningoencephalitis[258]; therefore such patients require a full evaluation for CNS and extrapulmonary disease. The meningoencephalitis caused by *C. neoformans* is notable for its general lack of meningismus and wide range of severity, from asymptomatic disease to fulminant symptoms.[250] Cranial nerve deficits are common, as is evidence of elevated intracranial pressure. Seizures can occur and are frequently related to cryptococcomas within the brain parenchyma. Skin lesions occur frequently (≈15%) and also range widely in appearance from pustules and papules to frank ulcers and abscesses. It is also important to note that disseminated disease can involve almost any organ. The majority of cases in neonates have had evidence of CNS involvement, and many cases involved sepsis-like presentations. Finally, a number of cases of cryptococcosis in pregnant mothers without vertical transmission have been reported, including cases in which placental infection was documented.[259]

DIAGNOSIS

The clinical symptoms of cryptococcosis are not sufficiently specific to directly suggest the diagnosis, but in the context of high-risk patients with pulmonary or CNS symptoms, cryptococcosis should be part of the differential diagnosis.[250] The diagnosis of cryptococcosis is most readily established in the setting of CNS disease. Lumbar puncture will generally show elevated opening pressure, lymphocytic pleocytosis, decreased glucose, and increased protein. However, the CSF parameters can also be near normal, particularly in HIV-positive patients. Culture of CSF is positive in 89% to 95% of patients with cryptococcal meningitis, and blood cultures are positive in 55% of patients.[260] Cryptococcal polysaccharide antigen is readily detectable in CSF, serum, and urine by using a latex-agglutination test. The sensitivity is highest for meningitis in HIV-infected patients (90%-95%) and much lower for pulmonary disease in HIV-uninfected patients. Classically, India ink preparations can be used to demonstrate the presence of *C. neoformans* in clinical samples, but testing for the presence of antigen is more widely used. Culture and antigen testing have been positive in cases of neonatal cryptococcosis.[253]

TREATMENT

The gold standard therapy for cryptocococcal meningoencephalitis is amphotericin B combined with 5-flucytosine. A randomized clinical trial demonstrated the superiority of the combination relative to amphotericin B alone for cryptococcal meningitis.[261] Fluconazole and other azoles have activity against *C. neoformans* but are less effective compared with amphotericin B–based therapy because of the fact that azoles are fungistatic, and early fungicidal activity is correlated with better outcome.[262] Current recommendations for treatment of adults are to treat with an amphotericin B–based preparation in combination with 5-flucytosine for at least 2 weeks, followed by a maintenance treatment of oral fluconazole for at least 10 weeks.[263]

PROGNOSIS

The outcome of treatment varies significantly, based on the immune status of the patient, access to amphotericin B, and geoeconomic factors. As summarized by Patel and coworkers,[253] the mortality rate for neonatal cases reported in the literature has been quite high (60%).

Malassezia

Malassezia spp. are among the most commonly isolated organisms colonizing human skin.[264] In older children and adults, these organisms are associated with tinea versicolor, seborrheic dermatitis, and dandruff; in neonates and infants, *Malassezia* spp. cause catheter-related bloodstream infections in patients receiving intralipid infusions and have been associated with neonatal cephalic pustulosis.[263] The causal nature of the latter association has, however, not been established.[265]

THE ORGANISM

Malassezia spp. are dimorphic fungi and thus are isolated as both yeast and filamentous forms. Fourteen species of *Malassezia* are recognized, with *M. furfur* being the most widely reported in the setting of invasive infections in preterm infants.[266] Sequencing studies of organisms isolated from the skin of adult humans have shown that *Malessezia* spp. are the predominant microorganism (fungi or bacteria) inhabiting this medically important niche.[264] With the exception of *M. pachydermatis, Malassezia* spp. are characterized as obligate lipophilic organisms.[265] Consequently, the recommended culture conditions for the isolation of *Malassezia* spp. include incubation on Sabouraud medium supplemented with olive oil.[267] This feature of their biology provides a reasonable explanation for the association of bloodstream infections with the administration of concentrated lipid.

EPIDEMIOLOGY AND TRANSMISSION

Malassezia spp. have been shown to rapidly colonize the skin of newborn infants and remain an important component of the human microbiome throughout life.[264,268] This fungus is associated with a variety of dermatoses and invasive disease in a small set of immunocompromised patients. The latter infections are associated with colonization of intravascular catheters and the administration of lipid-containing parenteral nutrition.[265,269] Given the near-universal colonization of health care workers and patients, it is important to recognize that the rate of invasive disease is quite low.

PATHOGENESIS

The pathogenesis of diseases caused by *Malassezia* is poorly understood at the microbiologic and molecular level.[270] With respect to invasive disease associated with intravascular catheters and intralipid infusions, it appears most plausible that the skin is first colonized as part of the normal establishment of the human microbiome. The high concentration of lipid within the catheter could then allow the lipid-dependent organism to establish colonization, leading to systemic infection.

CLINICAL MANIFESTATIONS

Malassezia have been linked to a variety of skin diseases, such as neonatal pustulosis, tinea versicolor, seborrheic dermatitis, and eczema.[265] A prospective study of newborns, however, showed that infants without pustulosis were as likely to be colonized with *Malassezia* as children without pustulosis.[266] The symptoms associated with *Malassezia* fungemia are nonspecific and similar to those associated with other infections, including poor feeding, temperature instability, lethargy, and respiratory distress.

DIAGNOSIS

Malassezia spp. infection is diagnosed by culture of the organism, and because the optimal growth of the organism requires special media (supplementation with oil), it is crucial to notify the clinical microbiology laboratory when the diagnosis is suspected.[267]

TREATMENT

The treatment of *Malessezia* fungemia is prompt removal of the infected catheter, which eliminates the colonization site from the bloodstream and the source of highly concentrated lipid. Although dissemination is rare, systemic therapy with amphotericin B has also been administered after removal of catheter to ensure clearance. No treatment is required for neonatal pustulosis.

PROGNOSIS

In general, the outcome for invasive disease in neonates is excellent, although some deaths in extremely-low-birth-weight infants have been reported.

PREVENTION

The prevention of *Malassezia* infections in neonates has not been studied. The judicious use of intralipids may significantly limit the risk. In patients in whom intralipid therapy cannot be avoided, this fungal infection should be suspected if the central venous catheter malfunctions or if mild, nonspecific signs of infection are noted.

Zygomycosis

Zygomycosis refers to mold infections caused by organisms of the class Zygomycetes and order Mucorales.[271,272] In previous editions of this book, these infections were termed phycomycosis, which was the name of this class of organisms. This name is no longer used, and to maintain consistency with other references, we will use zygomycosis to refer to infections caused by molds of the genera *Mucor, Rhizopus,* and *Rhizomucor.*[272] Zygomycosis is a rare infection within neonates and infants, with approximately fewer than 80 cases reported in the literature.[273] Zygomycosis is increasing in incidence among older children and adults with compromised immunity.[271] Classically, major risk factors for zygomycosis are diabetic ketoacidosis, iron chelation therapy, malignancy, steroids, and other immunosuppressive factors or conditions.[271,272] A review of the published cases of neonatal zygomycosis reported before, and including, 2007 found that most occurred in premature infants independent of other risk factors, with the gastrointestinal tract and skin being the most commonly affected organs.[273] Consistent with other uncommon invasive mold infections in premature infants, the fatality rate in this case series was very high (64%). It is difficult to ascertain whether the incidence of zygomycosis is increasing in neonates and infants because no prospective data are available, but the number of reported cases has increased since 1990.[273]

THE ORGANISM

Zygomycetes is a class of molds that includes the orders Mucorales and Entomophthorales.[272] The majority of invasive infections are due to genera within Mucorales, including *Rhizopus, Mucor,* and *Rhizomucor.*[271] Classically, the morphology of these molds includes ribbon-like aseptate hyphae that display right-angle branching. Zygomycetes can be difficult to distinguish from other molds, such as *Aspergillus* spp., on biopsy, but the latter organisms typically have acute-angle branching and visible septa.[272] The Zygomycetes are ubiquitous environmental organisms found within the soil and in association with decaying matter. They are spore forming, and the airborne spores are likely to play a role in pathogenesis. Based on the review of reported cases published by Roilides and coworkers,[273] the most common species affecting neonates are *Rhizopus* spp. (72% of reported cases).

EPIDEMIOLOGY AND TRANSMISSION

The incidence of zygomycosis appears to be increasing in populations of immunocompromised adult patients.[271] Part of that increase may be due to the fact that the agents used for prophylaxis against candidiasis and aspergillosis are not active against Zygomycetes.[271] As noted above, the number of neonatal cases reported in the literature has increased in recent years; however, it is not possible to firmly determine if this represents a true increase in incidence. The two primary modes of transmission of zygomycosis are inhalation of spores and direct inoculation of damaged skin.

PATHOGENESIS

The pathogenesis of zygomycosis has not been as extensively studied as other organisms.[274] Animal models have confirmed the importance of phagocytes in the host response. For example, immunocompetent mice do not develop zygomycosis after inhalation of spores, whereas those treated with steroids or with diabetes develop disseminated infection.[275] The alveolar macrophages harvested from immunocompetent mice ingest the spores and prevent germination, whereas those from immunocompromised mice are unable to prevent germination.[275] Iron levels and receipt of iron chelation therapy appear to contribute to susceptibility of patients to zygomycosis.[274] It is thought that the iron chelators may act as siderophores, providing essential iron to the organism.

PATHOLOGY

Histopathologic evidence of tissue damage, along with the presence of hyphal elements of the characteristic morphology, is part and parcel of the diagnosis of zygomycosis.

CLINICAL MANIFESTATIONS

In neonates, the most common sites of infection are the gastrointestinal tract and skin.[273,276] Of interest, pulmonary and rhinocerebral disease has been reported in only 10% of cases. Of importance, a number of neonates have presented with signs and symptoms similar to necrotizing enterocolitis, albeit without pneumatosis intestinalis.[273] In these cases, the diagnosis was made based on cultures or histopathologic analysis of surgical specimens. Approximately half of the cases of neonatal zygomycosis progressed to disseminated disease, whereas dissemination was much less common in infants older than 1 month.[273]

TREATMENT

The treatment of zygomycosis should involve a consideration of both surgical and medical approaches. Amphotericin B is the drug of choice for neonatal zygomycosis. Echinocandins have no activity against Zygomycetes. Itraconazole and posaconazole are the two azoles with in vitro activity against Zygomycetes. Posaconazole has been used to treat zygomycosis in adult patients, but this agent is limited to an oral formulation, and no dosing data are available for neonates. According to the review by Roilides and coworkers,[273] neonates who were treated with a combination of surgery and amphotericin B had better outcomes than patients treated with amphotericin B alone.

PROGNOSIS

Neonatal zygomycosis is associated with high mortality (64%) and high rates of disseminated disease.

Dermatophytoses

The dermatophytoses are caused by three genera of fungi that infect the keratinized regions of the skin: *Microsporum, Trichophyton,* and *Epidermophyton.*[277,278] Collectively, these organisms cause tinea, which is then further modified by a description of the affected region of the body, that is, tinea capitis.[278] Despite the fact that young children are frequently affected by the various tineas, neonates and young infants only rarely develop dermatophytoses.[279] Because these dermatophytoses are thought to result from contact with persons or animals harboring the causative organisms, the low incidence in neonates and young infants is most likely due to the fact that the pathogenic cycle of exposure, establishment of infection, and development of symptoms are rarely completed within the first few weeks of life. However, as with other less common fungal infections of this age group, a number of cases of neonatal dermatophytosis have been reported over the years.[279] Consistent with tinea in other age groups, the most common organisms isolated from neonatal cases have been *Trichophyton rubrum* and *Microsporum canis.* Nosocomial outbreaks of *M. canis* have been reported in a number of newborn nurseries.[280,281]

THE ORGANISM

Dermatophytoses are caused by organisms of the genera *Microsporum, Trichophyton,* and *Epidermophyton.* All form septate hyphae as well as a wide range of morphologic types of macroconidia, microconidia, and arthoconidia.[277,278]

EPIDEMIOLOGY AND TRANSMISSION

The etiologic organisms for the dermatophytoses vary according to the affected body site and the geographic location of the patient. The most common cause of tinea corpis is *T. rubrum,* whereas *M. canis* is the typical agent responsible for tinea capitis.[277,278] Of the neonatal dermatophytosis cases reported in the literature, *M. canis* and *T. rubrum* have been the organisms most commonly isolated.[279] Transmission is person to person or through contact with infected animals. The nosocomial outbreaks of neonatal dermatophytosis reported in the literature have been due to *M. canis.*[280,281]

PATHOGENESIS

Our understanding of pathogenesis and virulence mechanisms of dermatophytes is quite rudimentary relative to other fungal pathogens.[282] Proteases that digest keratin have been thought to play a role and, consistent with this notion, genome sequencing has shown that genes encoding these enzymes are increased in dermatophytes when compared with closely related fungi.[283]

PATHOLOGY

Histopathologic sections show yeast and hyphae within the stratum corneum. A very brisk inflammatory response within affected areas is part and parcel of many dermatophytoses, although chronic, less inflammatory presentations can also be seen.[268,278]

CLINICAL MANIFESTATIONS

Tinea corporis and tinea capitis are the two most commonly reported manifestations of dermatophyte infections in the neonate. Presentations of tinea corporis vary widely and include relatively noninflammatory scaly plaques to highly inflammatory pustules. The classic plaque of ringworm (annular plaque with raised, erythematous border) has been reported.[284]

DIAGNOSIS

Classically, the diagnosis of dermatophytes is made by microscopic examination of potassium hydroxide preparations of skin scrapings.[277,278] Potassium hydroxide digests the epithelial cells and leaves the fungal elements intact. Culture of the specimens will then confirm the diagnosis and identify the organism. Typically, selective medium supplemented with antibiotics is used to suppress the growth of bacteria, and cycloheximide is used to prevent the growth of other molds. No molecular or serologic tests are available.

TREATMENT

The majority of neonates were treated with topical agents, such as clotrimazole, econazole, ketoconazole, or miconazole.[279-281,284] For older children, griseofulvin has been the gold standard therapy for years and has been used as systemic therapy as has itraconazole.

PROGNOSIS

All cases of neonatal dermatophytoses have responded well to topical, systemic, or combination therapy.

PREVENTION

Because a number of outbreaks of nosocomial dermatophytoses have occurred within nurseries, it seems prudent that health care workers with symptoms of dermatophyte infection identify themselves to their institution's infection control group, to institute effective precautions to prevent transmission to neonates in the unit.

References

1. Chagas C: Nova trypanomiazaea humana, *Mem Inst Oswaldo Cruz* 1:159-218, 1909.
2. Carini A: Formas de eschizogonia do *Trypanosoma lewisii*, Soc Med Cir São Paulo 16 Aoakut, *Bull Inst Pasteur* 9:937-939, 1911.
3. Delanoë P, Delanoë M: Sur les rapports des kystes de carini du poumon des rats avec le *Trypanosoma lewisii*, Presenté par M. Laveran. Note de Delanoë et Delanoë, *C R Acad Sci* 155:658-661, 1912.
4. Chagas C: Nova entidade morbida do homen; rezumo geral de estudos etiologicos e clinicos, *Mem Inst Oswaldo Cruz* 3:219-275, 1911.
5. Benecke E: Eigenartige Bronchiolenerkrankung im ersten Lebensjahr, *Verh Dtsch Pathol Ges* 31:402-406, 1938.
6. Ammich O: Über die nichtsyphilitische interstitielle Pneumonie des ersten Kindesalters, *Virchows Arch Pathol Anat* 302:539-554, 1938.
7. Vanek J, Jirovec O: Parasitäre Pneumonie. "Interstitielle" plasmazellen Pneumonie der Frühgeborenen, verursacht durch *Pneumocystis carinii*, *Zentralbl Bakteriol (Orig)* 158:120-127, 1952.
8. Van der Meer G, Brug SL: Infection par *Pneumocystis* chez l'homme et chez les animaux, *Ann Soc Belge Med Trop* 22:301-309, 1942.
9. Deamer WC, Zollinger HU: Interstitial "plasma cell" pneumonia of premature and young infants, *Pediatrics* 12:11-22, 1953.
10. Gajdusek DC: *Pneumocystis carinii*—etiologic agent of interstitial plasma cell pneumonia of premature and young infants, *Pediatrics* 19:543-565, 1957.
11. Edman JC, Kovacs JA, Masur H, et al: Ribosomal RNA sequence shows *Pneumocystis carinii* to be a member of the fungi, *Nature* 334:519-522, 1988.
12. Stringer JR, Beard CB, Miller RF, et al: A new name (*Pneumocystis jiroveci*) for *Pneumocystis* from humans, *Emerg Infect Dis* 8:891-896, 2002.

13. Gigliotti F, Haidaris CG: Antigenic characterization of *Pneumocystis carinii*, *Semin Respir Infect* 13:313-322, 1998.
14. Gigliotti F, Harmsen AG, Haidaris CG, et al: *Pneumocystis carinii* is not universally transmissible between mammalian species, *Infect Immun* 61:2886-2890, 1993.
15. Gigliotti F, Haidaris PJ, Haidaris CG, et al: Further evidence of host species-specific variation in antigens of *Pneumocystis carinii* using the polymerase chain reaction, *J Infect Dis* 168:191-194, 1993.
16. Dutz W: *Pneumocystis carinii* pneumonia, *Pathol Annu* 5:309-341, 1970.
17. Esterly JA, Warner NE: *Pneumocystis carinii* pneumonia, *Arch Pathol* 80:433-441, 1965.
18. Kim HK, Hughes WT, Feldman S: Studies of morphology and immunofluorescence of *Pneumocystis carinii*, *Proc Soc Exp Biol Med* 141:304-309, 1972.
19. Sheldon WH: Pulmonary *Pneumocystis carinii* infection, *J Pediatr* 61:780-791, 1962.
20. Le TV, Cochard AM, Vu-Trieu-Dong, Solonar W: Diagnostic "in vivo" de la pneumonie á *"Pneumocystis," Arch Fr Pediatr* 20:773-792, 1963.
21. Chalvardjian AM, Grawe LA: A new procedure for the identification of *Pneumocystis carinii* cysts in tissue sections and smears, *J Clin Pathol* 16:383-384, 1963.
22. Bowling MC, Smith IM, Wescott SL: A rapid staining procedure for *Pneumocystis carinii*, *Am J Med Tech* 39:267-268, 1973.
23. Bommer W: *Pneumocystis carinii* from human lungs under electron microscope, *Am J Dis Child* 104:657-661, 1962.
24. Barton EG Jr, Campbell WG Jr: Further observations on the ultrastructure of *Pneumocystis*, *Arch Pathol* 83:527-534, 1967.
25. Huang SN, Marshall KG: *Pneumocystis carinii* infection: a cytologic, histologic and electron microscopic study of the organism, *Am Rev Respir Dis* 102:623-635, 1970.
26. Campbell WG Jr: Ultrastructure of *Pneumocystis* in human lung: life cycle in human pneumocystosis, *Arch Pathol* 93:312-329, 1972.
27. Yoneda K, Walzer PD: Attachment of *Pneumocystis carinii* to type I alveolar cells studied by freeze-fracture electron microscopy, *Infect Immun* 40:812-815, 1983.
28. Kucera K: *On the morphology and developmental cycle of Pneumocystis carinii of human and rat origin*, Prague, August 22-31, 1961, Proceedings of the First International Conference on Protozoology, pp 482–484.
29. Kucera K, Valousek T: The direct proof of *Pneumocystis carinii* in alive nurslings and a new evolutive stage of *Pneumocystis*, *Folia Parasitol* 13:113, 1966.
30. Vossen M, Beckers PJ, Meuwissen JH, et al: Developmental biology of *Pneumocystis carinii*, an alternative view on the life cycle of the parasite, *Z Paracitesmnkd* 55:101-118, 1978.
31. Pixley FJ, Wakefield AE, Banerji S, et al: Mitochondrial gene sequences show fungal homology for *Pneumocystis carinii*, *Mol Microbiol* 5:1347-1351, 1991.
32. Wakefield AE, Peters SE, Banerji S, et al: *Pneumocystis carinii* shows DNA homology with the ustomycetous red yeast fungi, *Mol Microbiol* 6:1903-1911, 1992.
33. Gigliotti F, Stokes DC, Cheatham AB, et al: Development of murine monoclonal antibodies to *Pneumocystis carinii*, *J Infect Dis* 152:315-322, 1986.
34. Gigliotti F: Host species-specific antigenic variation of a mannosylated surface blycoprotein of *Pneumocystis carinii*, *J Infect Dis* 165:329-336, 1992.
35. Wakefield AE, Banerji S, Pixley FJ, et al: Molecular probes for the detection of *Pneumocystis carinii*, *Trans R Soc Trop Med Hyg* 84(Suppl 1): 17-18, 1990.
36. Li J, Edlind T: Phylogeny of *Pneumocystis carinii* based on β-tubulin sequence, *J Eukaryot Microbiol* 41:97S, 1994.
37. Mazars E, Odberg-Ferragut C, Dei-Cas E, et al: Polymorphism of the thymidylate synthase gene of *Pneumocystis carinii* from different host species, *J Eukaryot Microbiol* 42:26-32, 1995.
38. Ma L, Kovacs JA: Expression and characterization of recombinant human-derived *Pneumocystis carinii* dihydrofolate reductase, *Antimicrob Agents Chemother* 44:3092-3096, 2000.
39. Banerji S, Lugli EB, Miller RF, et al: Analysis of genetic diversity at the arom locus in isolates of *Pneumocystis carinii*, *J Eukaryot Microbiol* 42:675-679, 1995.
40. Gigliotti F, Wright TW: Pneumocystis: where does it live? *PLoS Pathog* 8:e1003025, 2012.
41. Meuwissen J, Tauber I, Leeuwenberg AD, et al: Parasitological and serologic observations of infection with *Pneumocystis* in humans, *J Infect Dis* 136:43-48, 1977.
42. Pifer LL, Hughes WT, Stagno S, et al: *Pneumocystis carinii* infection: evidence for high prevalence in normal and immunosuppressed children, *Pediatrics* 61:35-41, 1978.
43. Gerrard MP, Eden OB, Jameson B, et al: Serological study of *Pneumocystis carinii* infection in the absence of immunosuppression, *Arch Dis Child* 62:177-179, 1987.
44. Pifer L: Serodiagnosis of *Pneumocystis carinii*, *Chest* 87:698-699, 1985.
45. Vargas SL, Hughes WT, Santolaya ME, et al: Search for primary infection by *Pneumocystis carinii* in a cohort of normal, healthy infants, *Clin Infect Dis* 15:855-861, 2001.
46. Robinson JJ: Two cases of pneumocystosis: observation in 203 adult autopsies, *Arch Pathol* 71:156-159, 1961.
47. Weisse K, Wedler E: Über das Vorkommen der sogenannten *"Pneumocystis carinii," Klin Wochenschr* 32:270-271, 1954.
48. Hamlin WB: Pneumocystis carinii, *JAMA* 204:173-174, 1968.
49. Esterly JA: *Pneumocystis carinii* in lungs of adults at autopsy, *Am Rev Respir Dis* 97:935-937, 1968.
50. Vogel CL, Cohen MH, Powell RD Jr, et al: *Pneumocystis carinii* pneumonia, *Ann Intern Med* 68:97-108, 1968.
51. Sedaghatian MR, Singer DB: *Pneumocystis carinii* in children with malignant disease, *Cancer* 29:772-777, 1972.
52. Perera DR, Western KA, Johnson HD, et al: *Pneumocystis carinii* pneumonia in a hospital for children: epidemiologic aspects, *JAMA* 214:1074-1078, 1970.
53. Le Clair RA: Descriptive epidemiology of interstitial pneumocystic pneumonia, *Am Rev Respir Dis* 99:542-547, 1969.
54. Walzer PD, Schultz MG, Western KA, et al: *Pneumocystis carinii* pneumonia and primary immune deficiency diseases of infancy and childhood, *J Pediatr* 92:416-422, 1973.
55. Walzer PD, Perl DP, Krogstad DJ, et al: *Pneumocystis carinii* pneumonia in the United States: epidemiologic, diagnostic and clinical features, *Ann Intern Med* 80:83-93, 1974.
56. Hyun BH, Varga CF, Thalheimer LJ: *Pneumocystis carinii* pneumonitis occurring in an adopted Korean infant, *JAMA* 195:784-786, 1966.
57. Editorial: a call to recognize *Pneumocystis carinii* pneumonia, Danilevicius Z, editor: *JAMA* 231:1168-1169, 1975.
58. Eidelman A, Nkongo A, Morecki R: *Pneumocystis carinii* pneumonitis in Vietnamese infant in U.S., *Pediatr Res* 8:424, 1974.
59. Eidelman AI, Giebink GS, Stracener CE: *Pneumocystis carinii* pneumonia in Vietnamese orphans, *MMWR Morb Mortal Wkly Rep* 25:15, 1976.
60. Centers for Disease Control and Prevention: Update: acquired immunodeficiency syndrome—United States, *MMWR Morb Mortal Wkly Rep* 35:757-760, 1986.
61. Simonds RJ, Oxtoby MJ, Caldwell MB, et al: *Pneumocystis carinii* pneumonia among U.S. children with perinatally acquired HIV infection, *JAMA* 270:470-473, 1993.
62. Poppers DM, Scherl EJ: Prophylaxis against *Pneumocystis* pneumonia in patients with inflammatory bowel disease: toward a standard of care, *Inflamm Bowel Dis* 14:106-113, 2008.
63. Lyons HA, Vinijchaikul K, Hennigar GR: *Pneumocystis carinii* pneumonia unassociated with other disease, *Arch Intern Med* 108:929-936, 1961.
64. Watanabe JM, Chinchinian H, Weitz C, et al: *Pneumocystis carinii* pneumonia in a family, *JAMA* 193:685-686, 1965.
65. Weinberg AG, McCracken Jr GH, LoSpalluto J, et al: Monoclonal macroglobulinemia and cytomegalic inclusion disease, *Pediatrics* 51:518-524, 1973.
66. Rao M, Steiner P, Victoria MS, et al: *Pneumocystis carinii* pneumonia: occurrence in a healthy American infant, *JAMA* 238:2301, 1977.
67. Heresi GP, Caceres E, Atkins JT, et al: *Pneumocystis carinii* pneumonia in infants who were exposed to human immunodeficiency virus but were not infected: an exception to the AIDS surveillance case definition, *Clin Infect Dis* 25:739-740, 1977.
68. Vargas SL, Ponce CA, Hughes WT, et al: Association of primary *Pneumocystis carinii* infection and sudden infant death syndrome, *Clin Infect Dis* 29:1489-1493, 1999.
69. Morgan D, Vargas SL, Reyes-Mugica M, et al: Identification of *Pneumocystis carinii* in the lungs of infants dying of sudden infant death syndrome, *Pediatr Infect Dis J* 20:306-309, 2001.
70. Vargas SL, Ponce CA, Gálvez P, et al: *Pneumocystis* is not a direct cause of sudden infant death syndrome, *Pediatr Infect Dis J* 26:81-83, 2007.

71. Vargas SL, Ponce CA, Gallo M, et al: Near-universal prevalence of *Pneumocystis* and associated increase in mucus in the lungs of infants with sudden unexpected death, *Clin Infect Dis* 56:171-179, 2013.
72. Hendley JO, Weller TH: Activation and transmission in rats of infection with *Pneumocystis*, *Proc Soc Exp Biol Med* 137:1401-1404, 1971.
73. Hughes WT: Natural mode of acquisition for de novo infection with *Pneumocystis carinii*, *J Infect Dis* 145:842-848, 1982.
74. Gigliotti F, Harmsen AG, Wright TW: Characterization of transmission of *Pneumocystis carinii* f. sp. muris through immunocompetent BALB/c mice, *Infect Immun* 71:3852-3856, 2003.
75. Le Gal S, Damiani C, Rouillé A, et al: A cluster of *Pneumocystis* infections among renal transplant recipients: molecular evidence of colonized patients as potential infectious sources of *Pneumocystis jirovecii*, *Clin Infect Dis* 54:e62-e71, 2012.
76. Brunot V, Pernin V, Chartier C, et al: An epidemic of *Pneumocystis jiroveci* pneumonia in a renal transplantation center: role of T-cell lymphopenia, *Transplant Proc* 44:2818-2820, 2012.
77. Rabodonirina M, Vanhems P, Couray-Targe S, et al: Molecular evidence of interhuman transmission of *Pneumocystis* pneumonia among renal transplant recipents hospitalized with HIV-infected patients, *Emerg Infect Dis* 10:1766-1773, 2004.
78. Sassi M, Ripamonti C, Mueller NJ, et al: Outbreaks of *Pneumocystis* pneumonia in 2 renal transplant centers linked to a single strain of *Pneumocystis*: implications for transmission and virulence, *Clin Infect Dis* 54:1437-1444, 2012.
79. Brazinsky JH, Phillips JE: *Pneumocystis* pneumonia transmission between patients with lymphoma, *JAMA* 209:1527-1529, 1969.
80. Robbins JD, Fodor T: *Pneumocystis carinii* pneumonia, *MMWR Morb Mortal Wkly Rep* 17:51-55, 1968.
81. Gentry LO, Remington JS: *Pneumocystis carinii* pneumonia in siblings, *J Pediatr* 76:769-772, 1970.
82. Bazaz GR, Manfredi OL, Howard RG, et al: *Pneumocystis carinii* pneumonia in three full-term siblings, *J Pediatr* 76:767-773, 1970.
83. Jose DG, Gatti RA, Good RA: Eosinophilia with *Pneumocystis carinii* pneumonia and immune deficiency syndromes, *J Pediatr* 79:748-754, 1971.
84. Post C, Dutz W, Nasarian I: Endemic *Pneumocystis carinii* pneumonia in South Iran, *Arch Dis Child* 39:35-40, 1964.
85. Brock P, Ninane J, Cornu G, et al: AIDS in two African infants born in Belgium, *Acta Paediatr Scand* 76:175-178, 1987.
86. Beach RS, Garcia ER, Sosa R, et al: *Pneumocystis carinii* pneumonia in a human immunodeficiency virus 1-infected neonate with meconium aspiration. *Pediatr Infect Dis J* 10:953-955, 1991.
87. Kucera K: Some new views on the epidemiology of infections caused by *Pneumocystis carinii*. In Corradetti A, editor: *Proceedings of the First International Congress of Parasitology*, Oxford, 1964, Pergamon Press, p 452.
88. Furuta T, Fujita M, Mukai R, et al: Severe pulmonary pneumocystosis in simian acquired immunodeficiency syndrome induced by simian immunodeficiency virus: its characterization by the polymerase-chain-reaction method and failure of experimental transmission to immunodeficient animals, *Parasitol Res* 78:624-628, 1993.
89. Aliouat EM, Mazars E, Dei-Cas E, et al: *Pneumocystis* cross inection experiments using SCID mice and nuderats as recipient host, showed strong host-species specificity, *J Eukaryot Microbiol* 41:71S, 1994.
90. Durand-Joy I, Aliouat el M, Recourt C, et al: *Pneumocystis carinii* f. sp. hominis is not infectious for SCID mice, *J Clin Micro* 40:1862-1865, 2002.
91. Price RA, Hughes WT: Histopathology of *Pneumocystis carinii* infestation and infection in malignant disease in childhood, *Hum Pathol* 5:737-752, 1974.
92. Rosen P, Armstrong D, Ramos C: *Pneumocystis carinii* pneumonia: a clinicopathologic study of 20 patients with neoplastic diseases, *Am J Med* 53:428-436, 1972.
93. Weber WR, Askin FB, Dehner LP: Lung biopsy in *Pneumocystis carinii* pneumonia: a histopathologic study of typical and atypical features, *Am J Clin Pathol* 67:11-19, 1977.
94. Merlier JF, Valade SP, Mayaud CM, et al: Immunohistological localization of immunoglobulins in pneumocystosis of adults, *Bull Eur Physiopathol Respir* 23:43-49, 1987.
95. Durand-Joly I, Wakefield AE, Palmer RJ, et al: Ultrastructural and molecular characterization of *Pneumocystis carinii* isolated from a rhesus monkey *(Macaca mulatta)*, *Med Mycol* 38:61-72, 2000.
96. Rifkind D, Faris TD, Hill RB: *Pneumocystis carinii* pneumonia: studies on the diagnosis and treatment, *Ann Intern Med* 65:943-956, 1966.
97. Hughes WT, Price RA, Kim HK, et al: *Pneumocystis carinii* pneumonitis in children with malignancies, *J Pediatr* 82:404-415, 1973.
98. Askin FB, Katzenstein AA: *Pneumocystis* infection masquerading as diffuse alveolar damage: a potential source of diagnostic error, *Chest* 79:420-422, 1981.
99. Nicastri AD, Hutter RVP, Collins HS: *Pneumocystis carinii* pneumonia in an adult: emphasis on antemortem morphologic diagnosis, *N Y State J Med* 65:2149-2154, 1965.
100. Nowak J: Late pulmonary changes in the course of infection with *Pneumocystis carinii*, *Acta Med Pol* 7:23-41, 1966.
101. Whitcomb ME, Schwarz MI, Charles MA, et al: Interstitial fibrosis after *Pneumocystis carinii* pneumonia, *Ann Intern Med* 73:761-765, 1970.
102. Schmid KO: Studien zur *Pneumocystis*-erkrankung des Menschen: I. Mitteilung, das wechselnde Erscheinungsbild der *Pneumocystis* Pneumonie beim Säugling: konkordante und discordante Form, Pneumocystosis granulomatose, *Frankfurt Z Pathol* 74:121-145, 1964.
103. Cruickshank B: Pulmonary granulomatous pneumocystosis following renal transplantation: report of a case, *Am J Clin Pathol* 63:384-390, 1975.
104. Dutz W, Jennings-Khodadad E, Post C, et al: Marasmus and *Pneumocystis carinii* pneumonia in institutionalized infants: observations during an endemic, *Z Kinderheilkd* 117:241-258, 1974.
105. Weller R: Zur Erzeugung der Pneumocystosen im Tierver-such, *Z Kinderheilkd* 76:366, 1955.
106. Weller R: Weitere Untersuchungen über experimentele Rattenpneumocystose in Hinblick auf die interstitielle Pneumonie der Frühgeborenen, *Z Kinderheilkd* 78:166-176, 1956.
107. Sheldon WH: Experimental pulmonary *Pneumocystis carinii* infection in rabbits, *J Exp Med* 110:147-160, 1959.
108. Chen W, Gigliotti F, Harmsen AG: Latency is not an inevitable outcome of infection with *Pneumocystis carinii*, *Infect Immun* 61:5406-5409, 1993.
109. Vargas SL, Hughes WT, Wakefield AE, et al: Limited persistence in and subsequent elimination of *Pneumocystis carinii* from the lungs after *P. carinii* pneumonia, *J Infect Dis* 172:506-510, 1995.
110. Frenkel JK, Good JT, Shultz JA: Latent *Pneumocystis* infection of rats, relapse and chemotherapy, *Lab Invest* 15:1559-1577, 1966.
111. Hughes WT, Price RA, Sisko F, et al: Protein-calorie malnutrition: a host determinant for *Pneumocystis carinii* infection, *Am J Dis Child* 128:44-52, 1974.
112. Walzer PD, Schnelle V, Armstrong D, et al: Nude mouse: a new experimental model for *Pneumocystis carinii* infection, *Science* 197:177-179, 1977.
113. Walzer PD, Rutledge ME: Humoral immune responses in experimental *Pneumocystis carinii* pneumonia, *Clin Res* 28:381, 1980.
114. Hutchison JH: Congenital agammaglobulinemia, *Lancet* 266:844-847, 1955.
115. Baar HS, cited in Hutchison JH: Congenital agammaglobulinemia, *Lancet* 266:1196, 1955.
116. Burke BA, Krovetz LJ, Good RA: Occurrence of *Pneumocystis carinii* pneumonia in children with agammaglobulinemia, *Pediatrics* 28:196-205, 1961.
117. DiGeorge AM: Congenital absence of the thymus and its immunologic consequences: occurrence with congenital hypoparathyroidism. In Bergsma D, Good RA, editors: *Immunological deficiency diseases in man*, New York, 1968, National Foundation Press.
118. Quittell LM, Fisher M, Foley CM: *Pneumocystis carinii* pneumonia in infants given adrenocorticotropic hormone for infantile spasms, *J Pediatr* 110:901-903, 1987.
119. Herrod HG, Valenski WR, Woods DR, et al: The in vitro response of human lymphocytes to *Pneumocystis carinii*, *Clin Res* 27:811, 1979.
120. Limper AH, Offord KP, Smith TF, et al: *Pneumocystis carinii* pneumonia. Differences in lung parasite number and inflammation in patients with and without AIDS, *Am Rev Respir Dis* 140:1204-1209, 1989.
121. Benfield TL, Vestbo J, Junge J, et al: Prognostic value of interleukin-8 in AIDS-associated *Pneumocystis carinii* pneumonia, *Am J Respir Crit Care Med* 151:1058-1062, 1995.
122. Wright TW, Gigliotti F, Finkelstein JN, et al: Immune-mediated inflammation directly impairs pulmonary function, contributing to the pathogenesis of *Pneumocystis carinii* pneumonia, *J Clin Invest* 104:1307-1317, 1999.

123. Bhagwat SP, Gigliotti F, Xu H, et al: Contribution of T cell sumsets to the pathophysiology of *Pneumocystis*-related immunorestitution disease, *Am J Physiol Lung Cell Mol Physiol* 291:L1256-L1266, 2006.
124. Gigliotti F, Crow EL, Bhagwat SP, et al: Sensitized CD8+ T cells fail to control organism burden but accelerate the onset of lung injury during *Pneumocystis carinii* pneumonia, *Infect Immun* 74:6310-6316, 2006.
125. Roths JB, Sidman CL: Both immunity and hyperresponsiveness to *Pneumocystis carinii* result from transfer of CD4+ but not CD8+ T cells into severe combined immunodeficiency, *J Clin Invest* 90:673-678, 1992.
126. Swain SD, Wright TW, Degel PM, et al: Neither neutrophils nor reactive oxygen species contribute to tissue damage during *Pneumocystis* pneumonia in mice, *Infect Immun* 72:5722-5732, 2004.
127. Wright TW, Pryhuber GS, Chess PR, et al: TNF receptor signaling contributes to chemokine secretion, inflammation, and respiratory deficits during *Pneumocystis* pneumonia, *J Immunol* 172:2511-2521, 2004.
128. Sheehan PM, Stokes DC, Yeh YY, et al: Surfactant phospholipids and lavage phospholipase A2 in experimental *Pneumocystis carinii* pneumonia, *Am Rev Respir Dis* 134:526-531, 1986.
129. Wright TW, Notter RH, Wang Z, et al: Pulmonary inflammation distrupts surfactant function during *Pneumocystis carinii* pneumonia, *Infect Immun* 69:758-764, 2001.
130. Weiss RB, Muggia FM: Cytotoxic drug-induced pulmonary disease: update 1980, *Am J Med* 68:259-266, 1980.
131. Richards MJS, Wara WM: Radiation pneumonitis complicated by *Pneumocystis carinii*, *Int J Radiat Oncol Biol Phys* 4:287-291, 1978.
132. Wells RJ, Weetman RM, Ballantine TV, et al: Pulmonary leukemia in children presenting as diffuse interstitial pneumonia, *J Pediatr* 96:262-264, 1980.
133. Thomas SF, Dutz W, Khodadad EJ: *Pneumocystis carinii* pneumonia (plasma cell pneumonia): roentgenographic, pathologic and clinical correlations, *AJR Am J Roentgenol* 98:318-322, 1966.
134. Ahvenainen EK: Interstitial plasma cell pneumonia, *Pediatr Clin North Am* 4:203-214, 1957.
135. Burke BA, Good RA: *Pneumocystis carinii* infection, *Medicine* 52:23-51, 1973.
136. Hauger SB: Approach to the pediatric patient with HIV infection and pulmonary symptoms, *J Pediatr* 119:S25-33, 1991.
137. Ruskin J, Remington JS: The compromised host and infection: I. *Pneumocystis carinii* pneumonia, *JAMA* 202:1070-1074, 1967.
138. Vessal K, Post C, Dutz W, et al: Roentgenologic changes in infantile *Pneumocystis carinii* pneumonia, *AJR Am J Roentgenol* 120:254-260, 1974.
139. Falkenbach KH, Bachmann KD, O'Laughlin BJ: *Pneumocystis carinii* pneumonia, *AJR Am J Roentgenol* 85:706-713, 1961.
140. Robillard G, Bertrand R, Gregoire H, et al: Plasma cell pneumonia in infants: review of 51 cases, *J Can Assoc Radiol* 16:161-168, 1965.
141. Pitcher RD, Zar HJ: Radiographic features of paediatric pneumocystis pneumonia—a historical perspective, *Clin Radiol* 63:666-672, 2008.
142. Hughes WT, Sanyal SK, Price RA: Signs, symptoms, and pathophysiology of *Pneumocystis carinii* pneumonitis, *Natl Cancer Inst Monogr* 43:77-88, 1976.
143. Gentry LO, Ruskin J, Remington JS: *Pneumocystis carinii* pneumonia: problems in diagnosis and therapy in 24 cases, *Calif Med* 116:6-14, 1972.
144. Rubenstein A, Morecki R, Silverman B, et al: Pulmonary disease in children with acquired immunodeficiency syndrome and AIDS-related complex, *J Pediatr* 108:498-503, 1986.
145. Joshi VV, Oleske JM, Saad S, et al: Pathology of opportunistic infections in children with acquired immunodeficiency syndrome, *Pediatr Pathol* 6:145-150, 1986.
146. Yoshida Y, Ikai T, Ogino K, et al: Studies of *Pneumocystis carinii* and *Pneumocystis carinii* pneumonia: V. Diagnosis by cyst concentration from sputum, *Jpn J Parasitol* 27:473, 1978.
147. Ognibene FP, Gill VJ, Pizzo PA, et al: Induced sputum to diagnose *Pneumocystis carinii* pneumonia in immunosuppressed pediatric patients, *J Pediatr* 115:430-433, 1989.
148. Johnson HD, Johnson WW: *Pneumocystis carinii* pneumonia in children with cancer: diagnosis and treatment, *JAMA* 214:1067-1073, 1970.
149. Chaudhary S, Hughes WT, Feldman S, et al: Percutaneous transthoracic needle aspiration of the lung: diagnosing *Pneumocystis carinii* pneumonitis, *Am J Dis Child* 131:902-907, 1977.
150. Rosen PP, Martini N, Armstrong D: *Pneumocystis carinii* pneumonia: diagnosis by lung biopsy, *Am J Med* 58:794-802, 1975.
151. Tyras DH, Campbell W, Corley C, et al: The role of early open lung biopsy in the diagnosis and treatment of *Pneumocystis carinii* pneumonia, *Ann Thorac Surg* 18:571-577, 1974.
152. Michaelis LL, Leight GS, Pouell Jr RD, et al: *Pneumocystis* pneumonia: the importance of early open lung biopsy, *Ann Surg* 183:301-306, 1976.
153. Roback SA, Weintraub WH, Nesbit M, et al: Diagnostic open lung biopsy in the critically ill child, *Pediatrics* 52:605-608, 1973.
154. Wolff LJ, Bartlett MS, Baehner RL, et al: The causes of interstitial pneumonitis in immunocompromised children: an aggressive systematic approach to diagnosis, *Pediatrics* 41:41-45, 1977.
155. Ballantine TVN, Grosfeld JL, Knapek RM, et al: Interstitial pneumonitis in the immunologically suppressed child: an urgent surgical condition, *J Pediatr Surg* 12:504-508, 1977.
156. Mason WH, Siegel SE, Tucker BL: Diagnostic open lung biopsy in immunosuppressed pediatric patients, *Clin Res* 27:114, 1979.
157. Rodgers BM, Moazam F, Talbert JL: Thoracoscopy: early diagnosis of interstitial pneumonitis in the immunologically suppressed child, *Chest* 75:126-130, 1979.
158. Elvin K: Laboratory diagnosis and occurrence of *Pneumocystis carinii*, *Scand J Infect Dis Suppl* 94:1-34, 1994.
159. Procop GW, Haddad S, Quinn J, et al: Detection of *Pneumocystis jiroveci* in respiratory specimens by four staining methods, *J Clin Microbiol* 42:3333-3335, 2004.
160. Nowoslawski A, Brzosko WJ: Indirect immunofluorescent test for serodiagnosis of *Pneumocystis carinii* infection, *Bull Acad Pol Sci* 12:143-147, 1964.
161. Brzosko W, Madalinski K, Nowoslawski A: Fluorescent antibody and immuno-electrophoretic evaluation of the immune reaction in children with pneumonia induced by *Pneumocystis carinii*, *Exp Med Microbiol* 19:397-405, 1967.
162. Norman L, Kagan IG: A preliminary report of an indirect fluorescent antibody test for detecting antibodies to cysts of *Pneumocystis carinii* in human sera, *Am J Clin Pathol* 58:170-176, 1972.
163. Lau WK, Young LS: Immunofluorescent antibodies against *Pneumocystis carinii* in patients with and without pulmonary infiltrates, *Clin Res* 25:379, 1977.
164. Shepherd V, Jameson B, Knowles GK: *Pneumocystis carinii* pneumonitis: a serological study, *J Clin Pathol* 32:773-777, 1979.
165. Hughes WT, McNabb PC, Makres TD, et al: Efficacy of trimethoprim and sulfamethoxazole in the prevention and treatment of *Pneumocystis carinii* pneumonitis, *Antimicrob Agents Chemother* 5:289-293, 1974.
166. Hughes WT, Feldman S, Chaudhary SC, et al: Comparison of pentamidine isethionate and trimethoprim-sulfamethoxazole in the treatment of *Pneumocystis carinii* pneumonia, *J Pediatr* 92:28-291, 1978.
167. Lipson A, Marshall WC, Hayward AR: Treatment of *Pneumocystis carinii* pneumonia in children, *Arch Dis Child* 52:314-319, 1977.
168. Larter WE, John TJ, Sieber Jr OF, et al: Trimethoprim-sulfamethoxazole treatment of *Pneumocystis carinii* pneumonitis, *J Pediatr* 92:826-828, 1978.
169. Seigel SE, Wolff LJ, Baehner RL, et al: Treatment of *Pneumocystis carinii* pneumonitis: a comparative trial of sulfamethoxazole-trimethoprim vs pentamidine in pediatric patients with cancer: report from the Children's Cancer Study Group, *Am J Dis Child* 138:1051-1054, 1984.
170. Overturf GD: Use of trimethoprim-sulfamethoxazole in pediatric infections: relative merits of intravenous administration, *Rev Infect Dis* 9(Suppl 2):168-176, 1987.
171. Ivady G, Paldy L: Ein neues Behandlungsverfahren der interstitiellen plasmazelligen Pneumonie Frühgeborener mit fünfwertigen Stibium und aromatischen Diamidinen, *Monatsschr Kinderheilkd* 106:10-14, 1958.
172. Ivady G, Paldy L, Koltay M, et al: *Pneumocystis carinii* pneumonia, *Lancet* 1:616-617, 1967.
173. Lörinczi K, Mérth J, Perényi K: Pentamidinnel szerzett tapasztalatink az interstitialis plasmasejtes pneumonia kezelésében, *Gyermekgyogyaszat* 15:207-212, 1964.
174. Western KA, Perera DR, Schultz MG: Pentamidine isethionate in the treatment of *Pneumocystis carinii* pneumonia, *Ann Intern Med* 73:695-702, 1970.
175. Parasitic Disease Drug Service: Pentamidine releases for *Pneumocystis* pneumonia, *MMWR Morb Mortal Wkly Rep* 25:365-366, 1976.
176. Ivady G, Paldy L: Treatment of *Pneumocystis carinii* pneumonia in infancy, *Natl Cancer Inst Monogr* 43:201-209, 1976.
177. Stark FR, Crast F, Clemmer T, et al: Fatal Herxheimer reaction after pentamidine in *Pneumocystis* pneumonia, *Lancet* 1:1193-1194, 1976.

178. Stahl-Bayliss CM, Kalman CM, Laskin OL: Pentamidine-induced hypoglycemia in patients with the acquired immune deficiency syndrome, *Clin Pharmacol Ther* 39:271, 1986.
179. Pauwels A, Eliaszewicz M, Larrey D, et al: Pentamidine-induced acute pancreatitis in a patient with AIDS, *J Clin Gastroenterol* 12:457-459, 1990.
180. Wood G, Wetzig N, Hogan P, et al: Survival from pentamidine induced pancreatitis and diabetes mellitus, *N Z J Med* 21:341-342, 1991.
181. Miller TL, Winter HS, Luginbuhl LM, et al: Pancreatitis in pediatric human immunodeficiency virus infection, *J Pediatr* 120:223-227, 1992.
182. Gagnon S, Boota AM, Fischl MA, et al: Corticosteroids as adjunctive therapy for severe *Pneumocystis carinii* pneumonia in the acquired immunodeficiency syndrome, *N Engl J Med* 323:1444-1450, 1990.
183. Bozzette SA, Sattler FR, Chiu J, et al: A controlled trial of early adjunctive treatment with corticosteroids for *Pneumocystis carinii* pneumonia in the acquired immunodeficiency syndrome. *N Engl J Med* 323:1451-1457, 1990.
184. Consensus statement on the use of corticosteroids as adjunctive therapy for pneumocystis pneumonia in the acquired immunodeficiency syndrome: NIH-University of California Expert Panel for Corticosteroids as Adjunctive Therapy for *Pneumocystis* Pneumonia, *N Engl J Med* 323:1500-1504, 1990.
185. McLaughlin GE, Virdee SS, Schleien CL, et al: Effect of corticosteroids on survival of children with acquired immunodeficiency syndrome and *Pneumocystis carinii*-related respiratory failure, *J Pediatr* 126:821-824, 1995.
186. Bye MR, Cairns-Bazarian AM, Ewig JM: Markedly reduced mortality associated with corticosteroid therapy of *Pneumocystis carinii* pneumonia in children with acquired immunodeficiency syndrome, *Arch Pediatr Adolesc Med* 148:638-641, 1994.
187. Sanyal SK, Mariencheck WC, Hughes WT, et al: Course of pulmonary dysfunction in children surviving *Pneumocystis carinii* pneumonitis, *Am Rev Respir Dis* 124:161-166, 1981.
188. Kluge RM, Spaulding DM, Spain AJ: Combination of pentamidine and trimethoprim-sulfamethoxazole in the therapy of *Pneumocystis carinii* pneumonia in rats, *Antimicrob Agents Chemother* 13:975-978, 1978.
189. Kirby HB, Kenamore B, Guckian JC: *Pneumocystis carinii* pneumonia treated with pyrimethamine and sulfadiazine, *Ann Intern Med* 75:505-509, 1971.
190. Ruskin J: Parasitic diseases in the immunocompromised host. In Rubin RH, Young LS, editors: *Clinical approach to infection in the compromised host*, New York, 1981, Plenum Publishing.
191. Patterson JH: *Pneumocystis carinii* pneumonia; pentamidine therapy, *Pediatrics* 38:926-927, 1966.
192. Richman DD, Zamvil L, Remington JS: Recurrent *Pneumocystis carinii* pneumonia in a child with hypogammaglobulinemia, *Am J Dis Child* 125:102-103, 1973.
193. Saulsbury FT, Bernstein MT, Winkelstein JA: *Pneumocystis carinii* pneumonia as the presenting infection in congenital hypogammaglobulinemia, *J Pediatr* 95:559-560, 1979.
194. Hughes WT, Johnson WW: Recurrent *Pneumocystis carinii* pneumonia following apparent recovery, *J Pediatr* 79:755-759, 1971.
195. Ross L, et al: Recurrent *Pneumocystis carinii* pneumonia, *Clin Res* 25:183, 1977.
196. Fortuny IE, Tempero KF, Amsden TW: *Pneumocystis carinii* pneumonia diagnosed from sputum and successfully treated with pentamidine isethionate, *Cancer* 26:911-913, 1970.
197. Wolff LJ, Baehner RL: Delayed development of *Pneumocystis* pneumonia following administration of short-term high-dose trimethoprim-sulfamethoxazole, *Am J Dis Child* 132:525-526, 1978.
198. Hughes WT: Limited effect of trimethoprim-sulfamethoxazole prophylaxis on *Pneumocystis carinii*, *Antimicrob Agents Chemother* 16:333-335, 1979.
199. Post C, Fakouhi T, Dutz W, et al: Prophylaxis of epidemic infantile pneumocystosis with a 20:1 sulfadoxine and pyrimethamine combination, *Curr Ther Res* 13:273-279, 1971.
200. Hughes WT, Kuhn S, Chaudhary S, et al: Successful chemoprophylaxis for *Pneumocystis carinii* pneumonitis, *N Engl J Med* 297:1419-1426, 1977.
201. Wilber RB, Feldman S, Malone WJ, et al: Chemoprophylaxis for *Pneumocystis carinii* pneumonitis: outcome of unstructured delivery, *Am J Dis Child* 134:643-648, 1980.
202. Hughes WT, Rivera GK, Schell MJ, et al: Successful intermittent chemoprophylaxis for *Pneumocystis carinii* pneumonitis, *N Engl J Med* 316:1627-1632, 1987.
203. Harris RE, McCallister JA, Allen SA, et al: Prevention of *Pneumocystis* pneumonia: use of continuous sulfamethoxazole-trimethoprim therapy, *Am J Dis Child* 134:35-38, 1980.
204. Siberry GK, Abzug MJ, Nachman S, et al, for the Department of Health and Human Services: Guidelines for the prevention and treatment of opportunistic infections in HIV-exposed and HIV-infected children. Available at http://aidsinfo.nih.gov/contentfiles/lvguidelines/oi_guidelines_pediatrics.pdf Accessed September 23, 2014.
205. Maldonado YA, Araneta RG, Hersh A: *Pneumocystis carinii* pneumonia prophylaxis and early clinical manifestations of severe perinatal human immunodeficiency virus type 1 infection. Northern California Pediatric HIV Consortium, *Pediatr Infect Dis J* 17:398-402, 1998.
206. Steinbach WJ: Invasive aspergillosis in pediatric patients, *Curr Med Res Opin* 26:1779-1787, 2010.
207. Langan EW, Agarwal RP, Subudhi CP, et al: *Aspergillus* fumigatus: a potentially lethal ubiquitous fungus in extremely low birthweight neonates, *Pediatr Dermatol* 27:403-404, 2010.
208. Groll AH, Jaeger G, Allendorf A, et al: Invasive pulmonary aspergillosis in a critically ill neonate: case report and review of the literature, *Clin Infect Dis* 27:437-452, 1988.
209. Horii KA, Nopper AJ: Emerging cutaneous infection in the premature neonate, *Adv Dermatol* 23:177-195, 2007.
210. Etienne KA, Subudhi CP, Chadwick PR, et al: Investigation of a cluster of aspergillosis in a neonatal intensive care unit, *J Hosp Infect* 79:344-348, 2011.
211. Editorial response: primary cutaneous aspergillosis: an emerging infection among immmunocompromised patients, Walsh TJ, editor, *Clin Infect Dis* 27:452-457, 1998.
212. Burgos A, Zaoutis TE, Dvorak CC, et al: Pediatric invasive aspergillosis: a multicenter retrospective analysis of 139 contemporary cases, *Pediatrics* 121:e1286-e1294, 2008.
213. Melville JM, Moss TJ: The immune consequences of preterm birth, *Front Neurosci* 7:1-9, 2013.
214. Henriet S, Verweij PE, Holland SM, et al: Invasive fungal infections in patients with chronic granulomatous disease, *Adv Exp Med Biol* 764:27-55, 2013.
215. McCormick A, Loeffler J, Ebel F: *Aspergillus* fumigatus: contours of an opportunistic human pathogen, *Cell Microbiol* 12:1535-1543, 2010.
216. Fuchs H, von Baum H, Meth M, et al: CNS-manifestation of aspergillosis in an extremely low-birth-weight infant, *Eur J Pediatr* 165: 476-480, 2006.
217. Mennink-Kersten MA, Ruegebrink D, Klont RR, et al: Bifidobacterial lipoglycan as a new cause for false-positive platelia *Aspergillus* enzyme-linked immunosorbent assay reactivity, *J Clin Microbiol* 43:3925-3931, 2005.
218. Steinbach WJ, Addison RM, McLaughlin L, et al: Prospective *Aspergillus* galatomannan antigen testing in pediatric hematopoietic stem cell transplant recipients, *Pediatr Infect Dis J* 26:558-564, 2007.
219. Testoni D, Smith PB, Benjamin Jr DK: The use of antifungal therapy in neonatal intensive care, *Clin Perinatol* 39:83-98, 2012.
220. Fisher BT, Zaoutis TE: Treatment of invasive candidiasis in immunocompromised pediatric patients, *Paediatr Drugs* 10:281-298, 2008.
221. Linder N, Klinger G, Shalit I, et al: Treatment of candidaemia in premature infants: comparison of three amphotericin B preparations, *J Antimicrob Chemother* 52:663-667, 2003.
222. Herbrecht R, Denning DW, Patterson TF, et al: Voriconazole versus amphotericin B for primary therapy of invasive aspergillosis, *N Engl J Med* 347:408-415, 2002.
223. Frankenbusch K, Eifinger F, Kribs A, et al: Severe primary cutaneous aspergillosis refractory to amphotericin B and the successful treatment with systemic voriconazole in two premature infants with extremely low birth weight, *J Perinatol* 26:511-514, 2006.
224. Santos RP, Sánchez PJ, Mejias A, et al: Successful medical treatment of cutaneous aspergillosis in a premature infant using liposomal amphotericin B, voriconazole, and micafungin, *Pediatr Infect Dis J* 26:364-366, 2007.
225. Kauffman CA: Endemic mycoses: blastomycosis, histoplasmosis, and sporotrichosis, *Infect Dis Clin N Am* 20:645-662, 2006.
226. Steele RW, Abernathy RS: Systemic blastomycosis in children, *Pediatr Infect Dis* 2:304-307, 1983.
227. Youseff D, Raval B, El-Abbassi A, et al: Pulmonary blastomycosis during pregnancy: case report and review of the literature, *Tenn Med* 106:37-39, 2013.

228. Lemos L, Soofi M, Amir E: Blastomycosis and pregnancy, *Ann Diagn Path* 6:211-215, 2002.
229. Maxson S, Miller SF, Tryka AF, et al: Perinatal blastomycosis: a review, *Pediatr Infect Dis J* 11:760-763, 1992.
230. Gnann JW, Bressler GS, Bodet CA 3rd, et al: Human blastomycosis after a dog bite, *Ann Int Med* 98:48-49, 1983.
231. Sugar AM, Picard M: Macrophage-and oxidant-mediated inhibition of the ability of live *Blastomyces dermatitides* conidia to transform to pathogenic yeast phase, *J Infect Dis* 163:371-375, 1991.
232. Klein BS, Bradsher RW, Vergeront JM, et al: Development of long-term specific cellular immunity after acute *Blastomyces dermatitidis* infection: assessments following a large point-source outbreak in Wisconsin, *J Infect Dis* 161:1310-1316, 1990.
233. Kauffman CA: Histoplasmosis, *Clin Chest Med* 30:217-225, 2009.
234. Odio CM, Navarrete M, Carrillo JM, et al: Disseminated histoplasmosis in infants, *Pediatr Infect Dis J* 18:1065-1068, 1999.
235. Whitt SP, Koch GA, Fender B, et al: Histoplasmosis in pregnancy, *Arch Intern Med* 164:454-458, 2004.
236. Alverson B, Alexander N, LeGolvan MP, et al: A human immunodeficiency virus-positive infant with probable congenital histoplasmosis in a nonendemic area, *Pediatr Infect Dis J* 29:1055-1057, 2010.
237. Wheat LJ, Wass J, Norton J, et al: Cavitary histoplasmosis occurring during two large urban outbreaks: analysis of clinical epidemiologic, roentgenographic, and laboratory features, *Medicine (Baltimore)* 63:201-209, 1984.
238. Dupont B, Crewe Brown HH, Westermann K, et al: Mycoses in AIDS, *Med Mycol* 38(Suppl 1):259-267, 2000.
239. Ampel NM: Coccidioidomycosis. In Dismukes WE, Pappas PG, Sobel JD, editors: *Clinical mycology*, Oxford, UK, 2003, Oxford University Press, pp 311-327.
240. Caldwell JW, Arsura EL, Kilgore WB, et al: Coccidioidomycosis in pregnancy during an epidemic in California, *Obstet Gynecol* 95:236-239, 2000.
241. Bercovitch RS, Catanzaro A, Schwartz BS, et al: Coccidioidomycosis during pregnancy: a review and recommendations for management, *Clin Infect Dis* 53:363-368, 2011.
242. Linsangan LS, Ross L: *Coccidioides immitis* infection of the neonate: two routes of infection, *Pediatr Infect Dis J* 18:171-173, 1999.
243. Charlton V, Ramsdell K, Sehring S: Intrauterine transmission of coccidioidomycosis, *Pediatr Infect Dis J* 18:561-563, 1999.
244. Dodge RR, Lebowitz MD, Barbee R, et al: Estimates of *C. immitis* infection by skin test reactivity in an endemic community, *Am J Public Health* 75:863-865, 1985.
245. Larwood TR: Coccidioidin skin testing in Kern County, California: decrease in infection rate over 58 years, *Clin Infect Dis* 30:612-613, 2000.
246. Schneider E: A coccidioidomycosis outbreak following the Northridge, Calif earthquake, *JAMA* 277:904-908, 1997.
247. O'Brien J, Gilsdorf JR: Primary cutaneous coccidioidomycosis in childhood, *Pediatr Infect Dis* 5:485-486, 1986.
248. Drutz DJ, Cantanzaro A: Coccidioidomycosis. Part I, *Am Rev Respir Dis* 117:559-585, 1978.
249. Spark RP: Does transplacental spread of coccidioidomycosis occur? Report of a neonatal fatality and review of the literature, *Arch Pathol Lab Med* 105:347-350, 1981.
250. Chayakulkeeree M, Perfect JR: Cryptococcosis, *Infect Dis Clin North Am* 20:507-544, 2006.
251. Park BJ, Wannemuehler KA, Marston BJ, et al: Estimation of the current global burden of cryptococcal meningitis among persons living with HIV/AIDS, *AIDS* 23:525-530, 2009.
252. Ely EW, Peacock Jr JE, Haponik EF, et al: Cryptococcal pneumonia complicating pregnancy, *Medicine (Baltimore)* 77:153-167, 1998.
253. Patel M, Beckerman KP, Reznik S, et al: Transplacental transmission of *Cryptococcus neoformans* to an HIV-exposed premature infant, *J Perinatol* 32:235-237, 2012.
254. Kronstad JW, Attarian R, Cadieux B, et al: Expanding fungal pathogenesis: *Cryptococcus* breaks out of the opportunistic box, *Nat Rev Microbiol* 9:193-203, 2011.
255. Goldman DL, Khine H, Abadi J, et al: Serologic evidence for *Cryptococcus neoformans* infection in early childhood, *Pediatrics* 107:e66, 2001.
256. Voelz K, May RC: Cryptococcal interactions with the host immune system, *Eukaryot Cell* 9:835-846, 2010.
257. Casadevall A: *Cryptococcus* at the gate: break and enter or use a Trojan horse? *J Clin Invest* 120:1389-1392, 2010.
258. Cameron ML, Bartlett JA, Gallis HA, et al: Manifestations of pulmonary cryptococcosis in patients with acquired immunodeficiency syndrome, *Rev Infect Dis* 13:64-67, 1991.
259. Darko AD, Dim DC, Taylor G, et al: Placental *Cryptococcus neoformans* infection without neonatal disease: case report and review of the literature, *Pediatr Dev Pathol* 12:249-252, 2009.
260. Baddley JW, Dismukes WE: Cryptococcosis. In Dismukes WE, Pappas PG, Sobel JD, editors: *Clinical mycology*, Oxford, UK, 2003, Oxford University Press, pp 194-195.
261. Day JN, Chau TT, Wolbers M, et al: Combination therapy for cryptococcal meningitis, *N Engl J Med* 368:1291-1302, 2013.
262. Bicanic T, Muzoora C, Brouwer AE, et al: Independent association of clearance of infection and clinical outcome of HIV-associated cryptococcal meningitis: analysis of combined cohort of 262 patients, *Clin Infect Dis* 49:702-709, 2009.
263. Perfect JR, Dismukes WE, Dromer F, et al: Clinical practice guidelines for the management of cryptococcal disease: 2010 update by the Infectious Diseases Society of America, *Clin Infect Dis* 50:291-322, 2010.
264. Findley K, Oh J, Yang J, et al: Topographic diversity of fungal and bacterial communities in human skin, *Nature* 498:367-370, 2013.
265. Gaitanis G, Magiatis P, Hantschke M, et al: The *Malassezia* genus in skin and systemic disease, *Clin Microbiol Rev* 25:106-141, 2012.
266. Ayhan M, Sancak B, Karaduman A, et al: Colonization of neonate skin by *Malassezia* species: relationship with neonatal cephalic pustulosis, *J Am Acad Dermatol* 57:1012-1018, 2007.
267. Weeks J, Moser SA, Elewski BE: Superficial cutaneous fungal infections. In Dismukes WE, Pappas PG, Sobel JD, editors: *Clinical mycology*, Oxford, UK, 2003, Oxford University Press, pp 367-368.
268. Lemming JP, Sutton TM, Fleming PJ: Neonatal skin as a reservoir of *Malassezia* species, *Pediatr Infect Dis J* 14:719-720, 1995.
269. Danker WH, Spector SA, Fierer J, et al: *Malassezia* fungemia in neonates and adults: complication of hyperalimentation, *Rev Infect Dis* 9:743-753, 1987.
270. Saunders CW, Scheynius A, Heitman J: *Malassezia* fungi are specialized to live on skin and associated with dandruff, eczema, and other skin diseases, *PLoS Pathog* 8:e1002701, 2012.
271. Petrikkos G, Skiada A, Lortholary O, et al: Epidemiology and clinical manifestations of mucormycosis, *Clin Infect Dis* 54:S23-34, 2012.
272. Ibrahim AS, Edwards Jr JE, Filler SG: Zygomycosis. In Dismukes WE, Pappas PG, Sobel JD, editors: *Clinical mycology*, Oxford, UK, 2003, Oxford University Press.
273. Roilides E, Zaoutis TE, Katragkou A, et al: Zygomycosis in neonates: an uncommon but life-threatening infection, *Am J Perinatol* 26:565-573, 2009.
274. Ibrahim AS, Spellberg B, Walsh TJ, et al: Pathogenesis of mucormycosis, *Clin Infect Dis* 54:S16-S22, 2012.
275. Waldorf AR, Ruderman N, Diamond RD: Specific susceptibility to mucormycosis in murine diabetes and bronchoalveolar macrophage defense against *Rhizopus*, *J Clin Invest* 74:150-160, 1984.
276. Inoue S, Odaka A, Hashimoto D, et al: Rare case of disseminated neonatal zygomycosis mimicking necrotizing enterocolitis with necrotizing fascititis, *J Pediatr Surg* 46:E29-E32, 2011.
277. Weitzman I, Summerbell RC: The dermatophytes, *Clin Microbiol Rev* 8:240-259, 1995.
278. Weeks J, Moser SA, Elewski BE: Superficial cutaneous fungal infections. In Dismukes WE, Pappas PG, Sobel JD, editors: *Clinical mycology*, Oxford, UK, 2003, Oxford University Press.
279. Atanasovski M, El Tal AK, Hamzavi F, et al: Neonatal dermatophytosis: report of a case and review of the literature, *Pediatr Dermatol* 28:185-188, 2011.
280. Snider R, Landers S, Levy ML: The ringworm riddle: an outbreak of *Microsporum canis* in the nursery, *Pediatr Infect Dis J* 12:145-148, 1993.
281. Drusin LM, Ross BG, Rhodes KH, et al: Nosocomial ringworm in a neonatal intensive care unit: a nurse and her cat, *Infect Control Hosp Epidemiol* 21:605-607, 2000.
282. Achterman RR, White TC: A foot in the door for dermatophyte research, *PLoS Pathog* 8:e1002564, 2012.
283. Burmester A, Shelest E, Glöckner G, et al: Comparative and functional genomics provide insight into the pathogenicity of dermatophytic fungi, *Genome Biol* 12:R7, 2011.
284. Sproul AV, Whitehall J, Engler C: *Trichophyton tonsurans*: ringworm in the NICU, *Neonatal Netw* 28:305-308, 2009.

SECTION V

DIAGNOSIS AND MANAGEMENT

SECTION OUTLINE

35 Health Care–Associated Infections in the Nursery

JULIA S. SAMMONS and SUSAN E. COFFIN

CHAPTER OUTLINE

Neonates, especially premature neonates who require intensive medical care, are among the patients at highest risk for nosocomial or health care–associated infections (HAIs). Although the rate of HAIs varies with the specific patient population and institution, many institutions have achieved impressive reductions in the incidence of HAI over the past decade. For example, some reports from the early 2000s found that greater than 20% of critically ill neonates who survived more than 48 hours acquired a nosocomial infection.[1-3] In contrast, a report from the Vermont Oxford Network found that rates of HAI among very-low-birth-weight (VLBW) infants ranged from 9% to 16% in 2009.[4] The overall rate of late bacterial or fungal infections (presumed HAI) among surviving infants weighing 501 to 1500 g also dropped from 20% in 2000 to 15% in 2009.[5] Neonatal HAIs are associated with significant morbidity, mortality, and excessive direct health care costs.[3] Prevention of these infections should be a major priority in all neonatal intensive care units (NICUs) and nurseries. The most important risk factors for HAIs in neonates, gestational age and birth weight, cannot be modified. However, consistent use of evidence-based clinical practices and scrupulous attention to the patient care environment have been shown to minimize the risk of infections. This chapter reviews the epidemiology, microbiology, pathogenesis, and prevention of neonatal HAIs.

Special Issues for Neonates

The innate and adaptive arms of the neonatal immune system are functionally less mature than that of older infants, children, and adults (see Chapter 4). Compared with term infants, preterm infants have less developed specific components of the innate immune system, particularly factors that maintain physiologic barriers. Immature and easily damaged skin is a major factor in the relative immunocompromised state of preterm infants. Iatrogenic breaches in skin integrity, such as those caused by percutaneous medical devices and surgical wounds, also increase the risk for HAI.

Although the cellular precursors of the human immune system are present around the beginning of the second trimester, T cells, neutrophils, monocytes, and the complement pathways are functionally impaired at this time. Neonatal neutrophils show decreased chemotaxis, diminished adherence to the endothelium, and impaired phagocytosis (see Chapter 4); neonatal complement levels and opsonic capacity are also reduced, particularly in premature neonates. In addition, immature T-cell function results in diminished production of cytokines, T-cell killing of virally infected cells, and B-cell differentiation and maturation.[6,7]

Passively acquired maternal immunoglobulin G (IgG) is the sole source of neonatal IgG. Because transplacental transfer of maternal IgG occurs primarily in the third trimester, the serum IgG levels of many preterm neonates are very low. Soon after birth, maternal IgG levels begin to decline, and neonatal production of antigen-specific immunoglobulins begins. Serum IgG concentrations reach about 60% of adult levels by 1 year of age in term neonates (see Chapter 4). Given the incomplete transfer of maternal IgG and an impaired ability to produce antigen-specific immunoglobulins, premature infants typically have significantly lower levels of serum IgG than their term counterparts, a difference that can persist throughout the first year of life. Developmental issues of other organ systems can also affect the risk of HAIs. The immature gastrointestinal tract, characterized by reduced acidification of gastric contents and the fragile integrity of the intestinal epithelium, provides another potential portal of entry for pathogens.

Colonization resistance, the incomplete passive protection associated with colonization of skin and mucous membranes with "normal flora," also provides protection from invasive infections caused by pathogenic or commensal bacteria. The in utero environment is sterile; however, colonization begins within the first few days of life. The colonizing flora of a hospitalized newborn varies markedly from that of a healthy infant. Environmental exposures, including the presence of pathogenic bacteria in the hospital environment and on the hands of health care workers, the frequent use of antimicrobial agents, and exposure to invasive procedures, appear to influence the infant microbiome to a much greater extent than do genetic factors.[8,9] As a result, the microbiota of infants in the NICU can be markedly different from healthy term infants. Multidrug-resistant coagulase-negative staphylococci (CoNS) and gram-negative species colonize the skin and respiratory and gastrointestinal tracts of a high proportion of NICU neonates by the second week of hospitalization.[10] By the fourth week of life, more than half of all organisms isolated from the intestinal tract of VLBW infants are gram-negative organisms.[11] In addition, hospitalized neonates can become colonized with *Candida* and other yeasts.[12,13]

Epidemiology

INCIDENCE

The incidence of HAIs varies markedly by birth weight, gestational age, underlying conditions, and exposure to medical devices.[14,15] Reported rates of specific infections in similar patient populations differ dramatically by institution. In the past, much of this variation likely arose from differences in patient populations and clinical practices. As noted above, however, the patient safety movement has resulted in marked reductions in the rates of many specific HAIs in numerous NICU settings.

In 1999, a nationwide multicenter surveillance study, the Pediatric Prevention Network (PPN) Point-Prevalence Survey, was undertaken to determine the point prevalence of and to define risk factors associated with nosocomial infections in NICU patients.[16] This study included data from 29 NICUs and found that 11.4% of infants had an active nosocomial infection on the day of the survey. Bacteremia was the most common infection (53%). Lower respiratory tract infections; ear, nose, or throat infections; and urinary tract infections accounted for 13%, 9%, and 9% of infections, respectively. A more recent nationwide point-prevalence survey conducted in Canada in 2009 found that the overall rate of HAI in NICUs was 6.6% (95% confidence interval (CI), 4.68 to 9.19) and that bacteremia accounted for 60% of all infections.[17]

In contrast to the NICU setting, the frequency of nosocomial infection in well-infant nurseries has been estimated to be 0.3% to 1.7%.[18-20] In general, non–life-threatening infections such as conjunctivitis account for most infections in the well-infant population. The remainder of this chapter focuses on nosocomial infections in NICUs.

MATERNALLY ACQUIRED INFECTIONS

Differentiating maternally acquired and hospital-acquired infections can be difficult. Surveillance definitions typically describe nosocomial infections as infections that arise 2 or more days after initial admission to a nursery or NICU. No precise time point or definition perfectly discriminates infections that clinically were likely attributable to vertical transmission from infections transmitted within the NICU. Approximately 90% of hospitalized neonates with an infection presumed to be of maternal origin had onset of symptoms within 48 hours of birth. Maternally acquired bloodstream infections were more likely to be caused by group B streptococci, other streptococci, and *Escherichia coli* and were rarely caused by CoNS.[21,22]

NONMATERNAL ROUTES OF TRANSMISSION

Nonmaternal routes of transmission generally can be divided into three categories: contact (from either direct or indirect contact from an infected person or a contaminated source), droplet (from large respiratory droplets that fall out of the air at a maximum distance of 3 feet), and airborne (from microscopic droplet nuclei, which can remain suspended in air for long periods and as a result travel longer distances). Specific microorganisms can be spread by more than one mechanism; however, in most instances, a single mode of spread predominates. The U.S. Centers for Disease Control and Prevention (CDC) has developed a system of precautions to prevent the spread of HAIs that is based on these modes of transmission.[23]

Most neonatal HAIs are caused by the infant's own flora. The "abnormal flora" of the neonate residing in the NICU is determined at least in part by the NICU environment and the hands of health care workers. Contact transmission of bacteria, viruses, and fungi on the hands of health care workers is arguably the most important, yet seemingly preventable, mechanism by which potentially pathogenic organisms are spread. Poor compliance with hand hygiene has been repeatedly shown as a cause of outbreaks and transmission of resistant microorganisms.[24-27] In a study of infants with CoNS bloodstream infections, investigators used pulsed-field gel electrophoresis to demonstrate a high rate of concordance between the isolates that caused invasive infection in hospitalized neonates and those carried on the hands of nurses who cared for them.[28] In contrast, gram-negative organisms isolated from neonatal bloodstream infections differed from those cultured from the clean hands of their nurses.[29]

Transmission via contaminated inanimate objects also occurs and has been described as a potential mechanism of spread of pathogens in multiple NICU outbreaks.[27,30-32] Implicated items have included linens, medical devices, soap dispensers, and breast pumps. These observations highlight the need for careful attention to disinfecting items shared among infants.

Spread of infection through large respiratory droplets is an important mode of transmission for pertussis and certain respiratory viruses. The early identification and appropriate use of precautions for suspected cases are particularly important for nurseries that admit infants from the community. Recent reports of NICU-based outbreaks of pertussis have highlighted both the morbidity and cost associated with these outbreaks.[33,34] Parents and health care workers with unrecognized infection have been found to be the source of NICU-based pertussis outbreaks. Measles, varicella, and pulmonary tuberculosis are usually spread via the airborne route by means of microscopic droplet nuclei but are not typical risks in a nursery or NICU.

Other sources of HAIs include contaminated infusions, medications, and feeding powders or solutions, which can be either intrinsically or extrinsically contaminated, and have been reported as the source of outbreaks caused by a variety of different pathogens. It is important, when possible, to mix infusions in a controlled environment (usually the pharmacy), to avoid multiuse sources of medication, and to use bottled or sterilized feeding solutions when breast milk is unavailable.

RISK FACTORS FOR HEALTH CARE–ASSOCIATED INFECTIONS

Patient-Related Factors

As discussed earlier, infants in NICUs have intrinsic factors that predispose them to infection, such as an immature immune system and compromised skin or mucous membranes. In addition, multiple extrinsic factors play important roles in the development of infection, such as the presence of indwelling catheters, performance of invasive procedures, and administration of certain medications, such as steroids and antimicrobial agents.

Although the relationship between birth weight and HAIs is likely confounded by multiple other unmeasured factors, such as immune system immaturity, birth weight remains one of the strongest risk factors for HAIs. Data from the CDC and other investigators have consistently demonstrated an inverse association between birth weight and the risk of developing either bloodstream infections or ventilator-associated pneumonia (VAP).[15,21,35] Similarly, in the PPN Point-Prevalence Survey, infants weighing 1500 g or less at birth were 2.69 times (95% CI, 1.75 to 4.14; $P < .001$) more likely to have an infection than infants weighing more than 1500 g.[16]

Severity-of-illness scores have been developed to derive risk-adjusted rates of morbidity and mortality in NICU patients. Stratification by birth weight is the most common strategy used to risk adjust NICU infection data. Other scores used by some institutions include the Score for Neonatal Acute Physiology (SNAP) and the Clinical Risk Index for Babies (CRIB).[36] Risk adjustment using these scores can provide more accurate predictions of neonatal mortality and nosocomial infections, although they are not universally used, even within narrow birth-weight strata.

Medical Devices

The presence of indwelling intravascular or transmucosal medical devices has been identified repeatedly as one of the greatest risk factors for HAIs in neonates. Of importance, these associations persist after adjustment for birth weight.[16] The epidemiology of HAIs related to medical devices is discussed in more detail later in this chapter.

Therapeutic Agents

Numerous medications and other therapeutic agents crucial to the survival of infants in the NICU increase risk of infection. The widespread use of broad-spectrum antimicrobial agents has been associated with fundamental alterations in the neonatal microbiome[8,9] and increased colonization with resistant organisms.[14,37] In addition to increasing colonization, use of antimicrobial agents increases the risk of invasive infection with resistant bacteria[38] and fungal pathogens.[12] Other medications can also be associated with the development of HAIs. Infants who receive corticosteroids after delivery are at approximately 1.3 to 1.6 times higher risk for nosocomial bacteremia in the subsequent 2 to 6 weeks than infants who do not receive this intervention.[39,40] In addition, colonization and infection with bacterial and fungal pathogens have been shown to increase with the use of H2 blockers.[12,41,42]

Parenteral alimentation and intravenous fat emulsion have been shown in some studies to increase risk of bloodstream infection in premature infants even after adjustment for other covariables, such as birth weight and central venous catheter (CVC) use; the pathogenesis of this possible association remains unclear.[43,44] Investigators have suggested that fat emulsions could have a direct effect on the immune system.[45] Alternatively, as with any intravenous fluids, parenteral alimentation has the potential for intrinsic and extrinsic contamination, and fat emulsion especially may serve as a growth medium for certain bacteria and fungi. Finally, total parenteral alimentation and intravenous administration of fats likely delay the normal development of gastrointestinal mucosa because of lack of enteral feeding, encouraging translocation of pathogens across the gastrointestinal mucosa. Other risk factors related to infection include poor hand hygiene and environmental issues, such as understaffing and overcrowding.[4,46-48]

Etiologic Agents

The microbiology of neonatal HAIs is diverse (Table 35-1). Detailed discussions of the microbiology of sepsis and meningitis and of specific organisms can be found in other chapters.

COAGULASE-NEGATIVE STAPHYLOCOCCI

Since the early 1980s, CoNS have been the most common cause of HAIs, particularly bloodstream infections, in the NICU.[15,47] Data from 2006 to 2008, reported to the National Healthcare Safety Network (NHSN), estimate that

Table 35-1 Most Common Nosocomial Pathogens in Neonatal Intensive Care Unit Patients: Distribution by Site

	NO. INFECTIONS (%)				
Pathogen	**Bloodstream**	**EENT**	**GI**	**Pneumonia**	**Surgical Site**
CoNS	3833 (51)	787 (29.3)	102 (9.6)	434 (16.5)	119 (19.2)
Staphylococcus aureus	561 (7.5)	413 (15.4)	—	440 (16.7)	138 (22.3)
Group B streptococci	597 (7.9)	—	—	150 (5.7)	—
Enterococcus	467 (6.2)	92 (3.4)	—	120 (4.6)	55 (8.9)
Candida	518 (6.9)	—	—	—	—
Escherichia coli	326 (4.3)	163 (6.1)	147 (13.9)	152 (5.8)	74 (12)
Other streptococci	205 (2.7)	199 (7.4)	—	86 (3.3)	—
Enterobacter	219 (2.9)	120 (4.5)	58 (5.5)	215 (8.2)	47 (7.6)
Klebsiella pneumoniae	188 (2.5)	76 (2.8)	104 (9.8)	152 (5.8)	39 (6.3)
Pseudomonas aeruginosa	—	178 (6.6)	—	308 (11.7)	—
Haemophilus influenzae	—	72 (2.7)	—	38 (1.4)	—
Viruses	—	136 (5.1)	317 (30*)	—	—
Gram-positive anaerobes	—	—	99 (9.4)	—	—
Other enteric bacilli	—	—	8 (0.8)	—	—
Miscellaneous organisms	607 (8.1)	449 (26.7)	223 (21)	570 (21.7)	147 (23.7)
Total	*7521 (100)*	*2685 (100)*	*1058 (100)*	*2665 (100)*	*619 (100)*

Modified from Gaynes RP: Nosocomial infections among neonates in high-risk nurseries in the United States. National Nosocomial Infections Surveillance System, *Pediatrics* 98:357-361, 1996.
CoNS, Coagulase-negative staphylococci; *EENT,* eye, ear, nose, or throat; *GI,* gastrointestinal.
*Rotavirus constituted 96.4% of viruses isolated from gastrointestinal infections.

28% of bloodstream infections are caused by these organisms.[15] Although an infrequent cause of fatal infection, bacteremia caused by CoNS has been associated with prolonged NICU stay and increased hospital charges, even after adjustment for birth weight and severity of illness on admission.[49] Molecular techniques suggest that infections caused by *Staphylococcus epidermidis* can result from clonal dissemination and that there is often concordance between the strains infecting infants and strains carried on the hands of health care workers.[28,50,51] Several studies have demonstrated that a small number of CoNS clones accounted for the isolates from both infected infants and the health care workers that cared for them.[28,50] These findings suggest that a significant proportion of CoNS infections may be preventable by strict adherence to appropriate hand hygiene practices.[52]

OTHER GRAM-POSITIVE BACTERIA

Enterococcus accounts for approximately 10% of all neonatal HAIs, 6% to 15% of bloodstream infections, 0% to 5% of cases of pneumonia, 17% of urinary tract infections, and 9% of surgical site infections.[15,16,21] Sepsis and meningitis are common manifestations of enterococcal infection during NICU outbreaks.[52-54] The presence of a nonumbilical CVC, prolonged presence of a CVC, and bowel resection all have been identified as independent risk factors for enterococcal infections in NICU patients,[54] whereas prolonged antibiotic exposure and low birth weight (LBW) were found to be risk factors for colonization with vancomycin-resistant enterococci.[55] Because *Enterococcus* colonizes the gastrointestinal tract and can survive for long periods on inanimate surfaces, the patient's environment may become contaminated and, along with the infant, serve as a reservoir for ongoing spread of the organism.

Historically, before the recognized importance of hand hygiene and the availability of antimicrobial agents, group A streptococci were a major cause of puerperal sepsis and fatal neonatal sepsis. Although less common now, group A streptococci remain a cause of outbreaks in nurseries and NICUs.[56-59] Early-onset infections caused by group A streptococci are often characterized by severe sepsis and respiratory distress, whereas clinical manifestations of late-onset infections typically include meningitis and soft tissue infections.[60] Molecular techniques have enhanced the ability to define outbreaks, and use of these techniques has suggested that transmission can occur between mother and infant, between health care worker and infant, and between infants—probably indirectly via the hands of health care workers.[57,58] In one recurring outbreak, inadequate laundry practices seemed to have been a contributing factor.[61]

Data from the CDC and the Neonatal Research Network have shown that group B streptococcal infections account for less than 2% of non–maternally acquired nosocomial bloodstream infections and pneumonia.[21,62] Numerous studies from the 1970s and 1980s showed nosocomial colonization of infants born to women negative for group B streptococci.[63-67] These studies suggested a rate of transmission to infants born to seronegative mothers of 12% to 27%.[64,65] A case-control study evaluating risk factors for late-onset infection caused by group B streptococci showed that premature birth was a strong predictor.[68] In that study, 50% of the infants with late-onset infection caused by group B streptococci were born at less than 37 weeks of gestation compared with 15% of control subjects, and only 38% of the mothers of these infants were colonized with group B streptococci, suggesting possible nosocomial transmission of group B streptococci during the NICU stay.

GRAM-NEGATIVE BACTERIA

Organisms from the Enterobacteriaceae family have long been recognized as an important cause of HAIs, including sepsis, pneumonia, urinary tract infections, and soft tissue infections; morbidity and mortality rates are frequently high.[62,69] *Enterobacter* species, *Klebsiella pneumoniae,* and *E. coli* are the members of the Enterobacteriaceae family that are most commonly encountered in the NICU. Many outbreaks caused by gram-negative bacteria have been reported. Underlying causes of these outbreaks include contaminated equipment,[32,70-73] formula or breast milk,[73-78] and intravenous fluids,[79-81] understaffing, overcrowding, and poor hand hygiene practices.[82-85] Risk factors for endemic bloodstream infections caused by gram-negative organisms include LBW, gastrointestinal tract pathology, and proton-pump inhibitors.[86] The origins of these organisms are often unclear, although many authors hypothesize that at least some episodes of gram-negative bacteremia are a consequence of intestinal translocation. This hypothesis is consistent with the observation that enteric feedings have been associated with a reduced risk of gram-negative infections[87] but awaits future studies for confirmation.

Pseudomonas aeruginosa, an opportunistic pathogen that can persist in relatively harsh environments, has frequently been associated with HAIs and outbreaks in NICUs. Nosocomial *P. aeruginosa* infections vary in their clinical presentation, but the most common manifestations are respiratory; ear, nose, or throat; and bloodstream infections.[16] *P. aeruginosa* infections, particularly bloodstream infections, have been associated with a very high mortality rate.[62,88] Risk factors for infection include feeding intolerance, prolonged parenteral alimentation, and long-term intravenous antimicrobial therapy.[88] Outbreaks caused by *P. aeruginosa* have been linked to contaminated hand lotion,[89] respiratory therapy solutions,[90] a water bath used to thaw fresh-frozen plasma,[91] a blood gas analyzer,[92] and bathing equipment.[93]

Health care workers and their contaminated hands have also been linked with *Pseudomonas* infections in the NICU. In a study of a New York outbreak, recovery of *Pseudomonas* species from the hands of health care workers was associated with older age and history of use of artificial nails.[94] This and other studies suggest that the risk of transmission of *Pseudomonas* to patients is higher among health care workers with onychomycosis or who wear long artificial or long natural nails.[94,95] As a result of these and other findings, the CDC revised its 2002 hand hygiene recommendations to include a recommendation against the presence of health care workers with artificial fingernails in intensive care units.[96]

MULTIDRUG-RESISTANT ORGANISMS

Staphylococcus aureus has frequently been identified as a cause of nosocomial infection and outbreaks in well-infant nurseries and NICUs. Methicillin-resistant *S. aureus* (MRSA) has become a serious nosocomial pathogen, and outbreaks have been reported in many areas of hospitals, including nurseries.[97-99] Recent data from the NHSN demonstrated that approximately one third of NICU infections caused by *S. aureus* were due to MRSA.[15] With the emergence of community strains of MRSA, nosocomial transmission of MRSA with the molecular phenotype of either community-associated or hospital-associated strains has been shown.[12,100,101] In addition to the usual manifestations of neonatal nosocomial infection, *S. aureus* HAIs (caused by methicillin-sensitive strains or MRSA strains) can manifest as skin infections,[102] bone and joint infections,[103] parotitis,[104] staphylococcal scalded skin syndrome,[105,106] toxic shock syndrome,[97] and disseminated sepsis. No significant differences in clinical manifestations have been noted between infections caused by methicillin-sensitive *S. aureus* compared with MRSA.[107]

Direct contact is the presumed mechanism of most instances of *S. aureus* transmission. Several distinct reservoirs of MRSA have been identified and associated with MRSA outbreaks, including parents, visitors, and health care workers.[98,105,108,109] Understaffing and overcrowding have been associated with *S. aureus* outbreaks in NICUs.[98,110] The potential for airborne transmission has been suggested by "cloud babies," described by Eichenwald and colleagues,[111] in which the respiratory secretions or desquamated skin from a colonized infant carry *S. aureus* over relatively long distances. "Cloud" health care workers also have been described; in such cases, the point source of an outbreak was determined to be a colonized health care worker with a viral respiratory infection.[102,112] Parents can also transmit MRSA to their newborn infants on passage through a colonized birth canal or postpartum handling.[113,114]

The emergence of vancomycin-resistant enterococci (VRE) is a concern in all hospital settings, and several VRE outbreaks have been reported in NICUs.[115,116] In neonates, VRE seem to cause clinical syndromes indistinguishable from syndromes caused by susceptible enterococci.[54] Vancomycin use, which is especially prevalent in the NICU, has increased markedly and has probably contributed to the growing prevalence of resistant gram-positive organisms in neonatal patients.[117] More recent observations suggest that clinical infections caused by VRE may signal the presence of a larger reservoir of VRE among asymptomatic colonized infants,[55] and some authors have suggested that active surveillance may be required to interrupt ongoing transmission.[118,119]

Over the past decade, the array and prevalence of resistant gram-negative organisms have expanded rapidly. Extended-spectrum β-lactamases (ESBLs) are plasmid-mediated resistance factors produced by members of the Enterobacteriaceae family. ESBLs inactivate third-generation cephalosporins and aztreonam. *K. pneumoniae* and *E. coli* are the organisms most commonly recognized as ESBL-producing organisms, but other ESBL-producing gram-negative bacilli are being increasingly reported in both NICU outbreaks as well as endemic infections in NICUs in some settings.[120-122] Transfer of ESBL-carrying plasmids to other Enterobacteriaceae organisms has been shown in several NICU outbreaks.[123,124] Two mechanisms of acquisition of resistant gram-negative organisms have been shown through molecular epidemiologic investigations: patient-to-patient transfer (presumably via contaminated health care worker hands or medical equipment) and de novo emergence as a consequence of antibiotic exposure.[12,125]

FUNGI

Candida species are the third most common pathogen identified in patients with late-onset sepsis and are associated with morbidity and mortality rates similar to those observed with sepsis from gram-negative bacteria.[74] More recent reports have also linked neonatal candidiasis to increased neurodevelopmental impairment in infancy,[126] retinopathy of prematurity,[127] and death.[128] In addition, investigators have quantified the cost of an episode of candidemia in the NICU to be $28,000 to $39,000.[129,130]

Chitnis and colleagues[131] reported on data from the National Nosocomial Infections Surveillance (NNIS) network, including 128 NICUs covering 130,523 patients over a 10-year period ending in 2004. Of 1997 cases of candidemia in these patients, 57.9% were *Candida albicans*, 33.7% were *Candida parapsilosis*, 3.8% were *Candida tropicalis*, 2% were *Candida glabrata*, and 0.2% were *Candida krusei*. Over time, there was an overall decrease in candidemia in neonates weighing less than 1000 g, but there was variability in the incidence of candidemia in different NICUs, ranging from 2.4% to 20.4%. During this time period, there was no change in the distribution of *Candida* species. The combined mortality rate for neonates with candidemia was 13%, which did not significantly differ among infecting species.

A retrospective cohort study of neonatal candidiasis using the 2003 Kids Inpatient Database reported the incidence of candidiasis at 15 per 10,000 NICU admissions.[130] Two thirds of the cases occurred in neonates with a birth weight of less than 1000 g. Of these patients, neonates with extremely LBW were twice as likely to die as propensity-matched neonates with extremely LBW without candidiasis. The overall mortality attributable to candidiasis in neonates with extremely LBW was 11.9%.

Many risk factors have been associated with neonatal candidemia. Colonization likely precedes infection, and this can occur either vertically (via the maternal genitourinary tract) or horizontally (nosocomial spread). The relative roles of gastrointestinal tract colonization and enteric translocation versus skin surface colonization and catheter-related infection are unclear and not mutually exclusive.[132] Studies have identified gestational age 32 weeks or younger, APGAR score less than 5, shock, disseminated intravascular coagulation, delayed enteral feeding, intralipid use, parenteral nutrition, CVCs, H2 blockers, intubation, and prolonged length of stay as risk factors for neonatal candidemia.[133-135] Use of broad-spectrum antibiotics has also been associated with an increased risk of candidemia.[134,136,137]

Fluconazole prophylaxis at dosage of 3 mg/kg or 6 mg/kg twice weekly reduces rates of candidemia in premature neonates in NICUs that have a high incidence of candidemia.[138,139] Recent data suggest the risk of invasive candidiasis in infants is decreasing.[131] At present, fluconazole prophylaxis is only recommended for infants with extremely LBWs in nurseries that have a moderate (5%-10%) or high (>10%) incidence of invasive candidiasis.[140] A long-term follow-up study of surviving infants who had participated in a randomized controlled trial of fluconazole prophylaxis revealed no difference in neurodevelopmental outcomes at 8 to 10 years of life.[141]

Malassezia species, which are lipophilic yeasts, frequently colonize NICU patients. In one French study, 30 of 54 preterm neonates (56%) became colonized with *Malassezia furfur*.[142] *Malassezia pachydermatis*, a zoonotic organism present on the skin and in the ear canals of healthy dogs and cats, has also been associated with nosocomial outbreaks in NICUs.[142,143] In one report, the outbreak seemed to be linked to colonization of health care workers' pet dogs.[142]

Invasive mold infections are a rare cause of nosocomial infection in neonates, but when they occur, they are associated with a high mortality rate. *Aspergillus* infections may manifest as pulmonary, central nervous system, gastrointestinal, or disseminated disease. A cutaneous presentation, with or without subsequent dissemination, seems to be the most common presentation for hospitalized premature infants without underlying immunodeficiency.[144,145] Often, skin maceration is the presumed portal of entry. In a series of four patients who died of disseminated *Aspergillus* infection that started cutaneously, a contaminated device used to collect urine from the male infants was implicated.[145] Investigation of a recent cluster of *Aspergillus* infections implicated contaminated humidity chambers of incubators as a source.[146] Contaminated wooden tongue depressors, used as splints for intravenous and arterial cannulation sites, were associated with cutaneous infection caused by *Rhizopus microsporus* in four premature infants.[147] In addition to preterm birth, use of broad-spectrum antimicrobial agents, steroid therapy, and hyperglycemia are thought to be risk factors for mold infection.

VIRAL PATHOGENS

Nosocomial viral infections can be a significant problem for neonates.[148] Introduction of common viral pathogens into the NICU can be associated with (1) admission of infants from the community, (2) health care workers who work while ill or infectious, and (3) visitors.

Enteric Viruses

Although many pathogens can cause nosocomial gastroenteritis, rotavirus has been reported to be responsible for up to 95% or greater of viral infections in high-risk nurseries, including the NICU,[21,149] although adoption of rotavirus immunization is likely to reduce both the incidence of community-onset and health care–associated rotavirus.[150] The clinical picture of rotavirus infections in newborns can vary markedly; there are many reports of asymptomatic rotavirus infection in nurseries.[151] In addition, rotavirus can manifest as frequent and watery stools in term infants and as abdominal distention and bloody, mucoid stools in preterm neonates.[149,152,153] A high titer of virus is excreted in stool of infected persons, and the organism is viable on hands and in the environment for relatively prolonged periods.[154,155] Attention to hand hygiene and disinfection of potential fomites are crucial in preventing spread of infection. Rotavirus outbreaks in NICUs have been associated with poor hand hygiene, ill health care workers, and ill visitors.[154,155] A large outbreak in a Spanish neonatal unit identified four risk factors for nosocomial rotavirus: premature birth, infections other than rotavirus, congenital anomalies, and jaundice.[156] In addition, rotaviruses[156] and other enteric viruses, including norovirus,[157,158] astrovirus,[159] and toroviruses[160] have been associated with necrotizing enterocolitis.

Respiratory Viruses

Using prospective active surveillance data from eight NICUs, the Canadian Nosocomial Infection Surveillance Program estimated the incidence of health care–associated febrile respiratory tract infections in NICUs to be 0.25 infections per 1000 patient days.[161] Virtually all respiratory viruses, including influenza A virus, parainfluenza virus, coronavirus, respiratory syncytial virus, and adenovirus, have been reported to cause nosocomial infections in NICU patients.[162-166] Associated clinical findings include rhinorrhea, tachypnea, retractions, nasal flaring, rales, and wheezing, but illness can also be manifested as apnea, sepsis-like illness, and gastrointestinal symptoms.[155,165,167,168] Investigators at two New York NICUs conducted active surveillance for occult respiratory infections over a 12-month period. They found that more than half of premature infants (26/50) were positive for one or more respiratory viruses during their hospital stay.[169] Identified risk factors for acquisition vary from study to study but have included LBW, low gestational age, twin pregnancy, mechanical ventilation, and high CRIB score.[163-165,167] Contact and droplet transmission are the most common modes of spread of infection, highlighting the importance of scrupulous hand hygiene and adherence to transmission-based precautions (see later for a more detailed discussion of these measures). Additional measures, such as rapid diagnosis and cohorting of infected patients and assigned staff, have also been recognized as important adjuncts for prevention.[170]

Enteroviruses

Numerous nursery and NICU outbreaks of enteroviral infection have been reported.[171-173] In neonates with enteroviral infection, clinical manifestations can range from mild gastroenteritis to a severe and fulminant sepsis-like syndrome or meningitis and encephalitis. The latter presentation can be associated with a high mortality rate.[172] Several outbreak investigations have shown the introduction of enterovirus into a nursery via vertical transmission to an index case, with subsequent horizontal spread.[172,174] Enteroviruses are typically shed in the stool of infected neonates for long periods, providing a reservoir of organisms that can be transmitted when breaches of infection control practices occur.

Cytomegalovirus

Congenital cytomegalovirus (CMV) infection can be asymptomatic or fulminant. Postnatally acquired CMV infections almost always follow a benign course in healthy term infants. Postnatal CMV infection in premature infants can be severe, particularly when associated with transfusion of CMV-positive blood in VLBW infants. Signs and symptoms may include hepatitis, bone marrow suppression, or pneumonitis.[175-177] The incidence of postnatal CMV infections in preterm infants has decreased significantly with the routine use of CMV-seronegative blood products. At present, most postnatal CMV infections are acquired through breast milk.[93] Approximately one third of infants who are breastfed by mothers with CMV detected in breast milk can develop infection.[93] In one study, approximately 50% of these infants had clinical features of infection, and 12% presented with a sepsis-like syndrome. At present, no proven, highly effective method is available for removing CMV from breast milk without destroying its beneficial components. Some data suggest, however, that freezing breast milk before use may decrease the CMV titer, limiting subsequent transmission.[178] Person-to-person transmission within the NICU has also been documented,[179,180] but the extent to which this occurs is controversial.[181] More detailed information on the clinical features and management of CMV is presented in Chapter 24.

Herpes Simplex Virus

Most neonates with herpes simplex virus (HSV) acquire the infection from their mother, although nursery transmission of HSV infection has been described.[182-184] Although the precise mechanism of transmission remains unclear in some cases, contact transmission has been commonly implicated. Presumed patient-to-patient transmission, apparently via the hands of health care workers, has been described.[184] In addition, HSV can frequently be recovered from the hands of parents and health care workers with herpes labialis.[185] Strict attention to hand hygiene is critical to prevent nursery spread of HSV. Health care workers with herpetic whitlow are typically restricted from patient contact until the lesion is healed. An in-depth discussion of the clinical features and management of HSV is provided in Chapter 27.

Varicella-Zoster Virus

With the adoption of varicella vaccine and health care worker screening for varicella immunity, nosocomial transmission of varicella-zoster virus has become rare.[186] Infants at greatest risk are premature infants born at less than 28 weeks of gestation who did not receive transplacental maternal antibodies. Transmission is most likely to occur from an adult with early, unrecognized symptoms of varicella because the virus is excreted in respiratory secretions 24 to 48 hours before onset of the characteristic rash. Management of neonates exposed to and infected with varicella-zoster virus is discussed in Chapter 23.

Hepatitis A

Neonatal intensive care unit outbreaks of hepatitis A have been reported and have typically been recognized after diagnosis of a symptomatic adult.[187-189] Transmission has been documented via blood transfusion from a donor with acute infection.[189] In addition, indirect patient-to-patient transmission through fomites or health care worker hands can occur when there are subclinical cases (as is typical in neonatal hepatitis A infection) and lapses in the adherence to standard precautions. Neonatal hepatitis is discussed in depth in Chapter 26.

Device-Related Infections

CATHETER-ASSOCIATED BLOODSTREAM INFECTIONS

Epidemiology and Pathogenesis

Bloodstream infections account for a significant proportion of all HAIs in NICU patients,[16,190] and most are related to the use of an intravascular catheter.[191,192] Peripheral intravenous catheters are the most frequently used devices for neonatal patients. When a longer duration of access is necessary, nontunneled CVCs, such as umbilical catheters or peripherally inserted central catheters (PICCs), are commonly used.[193]

The CDC has monitored rates of HAIs for many years, originally in the NNIS system and more recently in the NHSN. Using standardized definitions, NHSN reported rates of device-associated HAIs among 413 participating level III NICUs during 2011.[194] Pooled mean rates for catheter-associated bloodstream infections among neonates were inversely proportional to birth weight (Table 35-2). The mean rate of infections for infants with birth weights less than 750 g was higher than that for patients in both pediatric and adult medical and medical/surgical ICUs.[194] The most recent data regarding pathogen frequencies in NICU patients with catheter-associated bloodstream infections is available from NHSN during 2006 to 2008: Among bloodstream infection isolates, CoNS was most common (28%), followed by *S. aureus* (19%) and *Candida* species (13%).[15]

Most catheter-associated bloodstream infections result from two primary mechanisms: migration of microorganisms colonizing the skin at the insertion site along the external catheter surface and into the blood vessel (extraluminal contamination) and contamination of the catheter or catheter hub during catheter maintenance (intraluminal contamination).[195] Extraluminal contamination predominates in the first 10 days after catheter insertion (likely related to contamination during insertion), whereas the potential for intraluminal contamination increases with prolonged catheterization.[195] Molecular analysis has shown that most CoNS isolated from neonates with catheter-associated bloodstream infections are concordant with isolates recovered from lumens of catheter hubs, suggesting that many of these episodes of infection may be a consequence of intraluminal contamination.[196] Hematogenous seeding from another focus of infection and infusion of contaminated fluids, medications, or blood products are other potential mechanisms of infection but are less common.

Prevention and Control

Several advisory groups, including the CDC, the Vermont Oxford Network, and the Infectious Diseases Society of America (IDSA), have published detailed recommendations of strategies to reduce the incidence of catheter-associated bloodstream infections that strike a balance between patient safety and cost-effectiveness.[191,197,198] A compendium of strategies to prevent specific HAIs has been endorsed by the Society of Healthcare Epidemiologists of America (SHEA) and the IDSA and includes detailed information on strategies to prevent catheter-associated bloodstream infections during insertion and maintenance (Box 35-1).[198] An update to the compendium is currently in progress.

A key strategy to minimize the risk of catheter-associated bloodstream infections is the prompt removal of indwelling catheters when no longer medically necessary. A recent study evaluating risk of catheter-associated bloodstream infection in neonates with PICCs found that catheter duration significantly increased risk of infection, particularly after 35 days.[199] Practices such as early enteral feeding and rapid conversion to oral medications whenever possible can shorten the length of time a patient requires a catheter. In addition, participation in quality improvement activities focused on improved hand hygiene and better adherence to best practices for catheter placement and maintenance has been shown to reduce the rate of catheter-associated bloodstream infections in NICUs.[200-202] Other specific preventive measures are discussed later.

Careful skin antisepsis before inserting an intravascular catheter is crucial to the prevention of intravascular device–related bacteremia. The CDC recommends chlorhexidine-based preparations because these products have been found to be superior to povidone-iodine in reducing the risk of catheter colonization (a recognized surrogate marker of catheter-associated bloodstream infections). Chlorhexidine use in neonates has been limited due to concerns regarding the potential for local skin irritation and even burns, particularly in premature infants; however, off-label use of this product has been reported[203,204] and the U.S. Food and

Table 35-2 Rates of Device-Associated Infections for Level III NICUs, by Birth Weight Category*

Birth Weight Category	Pooled Mean CLABSI Rate†	Pooled Mean VAP Rate‡
≤750 g	2.5	1.6
751-1000 g	2.0	1.4
1001-1500 g	1.3	1.0
1501-2500 g	0.9	0.5
>2500 g	0.9	0.2

Modified from Dudeck MA, Horan TC, Peterson KD, et al: National Healthcare Safety Network (NHSN) report, data summary for 2011, device-associated module, *Am J Infect Control* 41:286-300, 2013.

CLABSI, Central line–associated bloodstream infection; *NICUs*, neonatal intensive care units; *VAP*, ventilator-associated pneumonia.

*Neonatal intensive care unit component of reported data, 2011.

†Number central catheter–associated bloodstream infections × 1000/number central catheter days.

‡Number ventilator-associated pneumonia cases × 1000/number ventilator days.

Box 35-1 Evidence-Based Strategies to Prevent Catheter-Associated Bloodstream Infections

Conduct surveillance for catheter-associated bloodstream infections (B-II).

Educate health care workers who insert and maintain catheters (A-II).

Use checklist to ensure adherence to proper practices during insertion (B-II).

Perform hand hygiene before catheter insertion (B-II).

Use a catheter cart or kit that contains all necessary materials for catheter insertion (B-II).

Adhere to maximal sterile barrier precautions during catheter insertion (A-I).

Disinfect skin with appropriate antiseptic before catheter insertion and during dressing changes (A-I).

Disinfect catheter hubs and needleless connectors before accessing catheter (B-II).

Remove nonessential catheters promptly (A-II).

Perform dressing changes every 7 days, or more frequently, if dressing is loose or soiled (A-I).

Modified from Marschall J, Mermel LA, Classen D, et al: Strategies to prevent central line-associated bloodstream infections in acute care hospitals, Infect Control Hosp Epidemiol *29(Suppl 1):S22-S30, 2008.*

Drug Administration (FDA) modified its drug safety label for chlorhexidine in May 2012 from a restriction to infants older than 2 months to a statement advising that clinicians "use with care in premature infants or infants under 2 months of age." Daily bathing with 2% chlorhexidine wash has also been shown to decrease rates of bloodstream infection in adult and pediatric ICU patients,[205-209] and its use is recommended in current guidelines, but dedicated studies on skin cleansing with chlorhexidine in neonatal populations are limited.[210-212]

Catheter insertion site has been identified as a factor influencing infection risk in adults, and evidence-based guidelines recommend avoiding catheter placement in the lower extremity in adult patients, likely because of a higher density of local skin microorganisms in the groin.[191] However, studies in pediatric populations have not shown an increased risk of infection associated with femoral catheters in neonates and children,[213-215] and current guidelines recommend catheter placement in either the upper or lower extremity in pediatric patients.[191] Umbilical vessels provide a catheter insertion site unique to neonates, allowing easy collection of blood specimens and hemodynamic measurements. However, the umbilicus becomes heavily colonized with skin flora and other microorganisms soon after birth. Still, rates of catheter colonization and catheter-associated bloodstream infections attributable to umbilical catheters are similar to rates associated with other catheter types.[191] Current guidelines recommend that umbilical venous catheters be removed as soon as no longer clinically necessary but that they may remain in place up to 14 days if aseptically maintained.[191]

The use of antibiotic or antiseptic solutions "locked" into a catheter lumen has also been evaluated as a strategy to prevent catheter-associated bloodstream infections. In pediatric patients, a meta-analysis found that the use of ethanol locks reduced catheter-associated bloodstream infections among children with chronic parenteral nutrition dependence.[216] Only a few studies have evaluated lock therapy in infants. In a randomized study comparing lock therapy with vancomycin-heparin solution versus heparin alone among high-risk infants (VLBW or critical illnesses) in a community level III nursery, the investigators noted a significant reduction in the incidence of catheter-related bloodstream infections among infants receiving lock therapy with the vancomycin-containing solution.[217] Similarly, a single-center randomized clinical trial found a significant reduction in the incidence of catheter-associated bloodstream infections among infants receiving lock therapy with fusidic acid–heparin solutions, but the high rate of infections in the control group suggests that this intervention may not be beneficial in settings with already low infection rates.[218] Because many NICUs achieve substantial reductions in catheter-associated bloodstream infections through other evidence-based practices, the role of antiseptic lock solutions needs further investigation.

Routine use of systemic prophylactic antibiotics is not recommended as a strategy to prevent catheter-associated bloodstream infections in any patient population.[191] A dedicated 2008 Cochrane review identified only three small studies evaluating whether prophylactic systemic antibiotics prevented neonatal infection or death. Although the use of prophylactic antibiotics was associated with a decreased risk of bloodstream infections in these studies, there was no significant difference in overall mortality, and there were significant safety concerns related to the potential selection of resistant organisms.[219]

Other strategies that are commonly used by clinicians caring for adult patients are not commonly used to prevent catheter-associated bloodstream infections in NICU patients. Antiseptic-impregnated catheters are recommended for short-term catheters when infection rates remain elevated despite the reliable implementation of bundle measures[191]; however, these catheters are not available in sizes small enough for neonates. In addition, although the replacement of peripheral intravenous catheters to prevent infection remains an unresolved issue in adults, data suggest that leaving peripheral intravenous catheters in place in pediatric patients does not increase the risk of complications,[220] and current guidelines recommend that peripheral catheters be removed in children only when clinically indicated.[191]

VENTILATOR-ASSOCIATED PNEUMONIA

Epidemiology and Pathogenesis

Health care–associated pneumonia is the second most common HAI in NICU patients; most of these cases are VAP. Neonatal VAP has been associated with increased direct costs and prolonged hospitalization.[221] Rates of neonatal VAP reported by level III NICUs to the CDC's NHSN are available from 2011 (see Table 35-2).[194] Similar to catheter-associated bloodstream infections, rates of neonatal VAP are inversely proportional to birth weight. Gram-negative organisms are the most commonly recovered pathogens from tracheal specimens of patients with VAP.[221] Among NICUs contributing data on pathogen distribution for neonatal VAP to NHSN from 2006 to 2008, *Pseudomonas* species were identified most often (19%), followed by *Klebsiella* species (15%), *Enterobacter* species (12%), and *S. aureus* (12%).[15]

The pathogenesis of VAP is most commonly attributed to one of three different mechanisms: aspiration of secretions, colonization of the aerodigestive tract, or use of contaminated equipment.[222] Specific risk factors for VAP are associated with these basic pathogenic mechanisms and include host characteristics (prematurity, LBW, sedation, or use of paralytic agents), exposure to medical devices (endotracheal intubation, mechanical ventilation, orogastric or nasogastric tube placement), and factors that increase bacterial colonization of the aerodigestive tract (broad-spectrum antimicrobial agents, antacids, or H2 blockers).[223-226]

Prevention and Control

Few studies have assessed the effectiveness of VAP prevention strategies in children; thus most commonly used VAP prevention strategies in NICU patients are based on adult studies. In 2008, infectious disease experts and hospital epidemiologists published a broad compendium of VAP prevention strategies; this document should continue to serve as a guideline for NICUs working to reduce VAP in their patients (Box 35-2).[222] The core recommendations are designed to interrupt the three most common mechanisms by which VAP typically develops. An obvious but key component of VAP prevention is to minimize use of invasive mechanical

Box 35-2 Evidence-Based Strategies to Prevent Ventilator-Associated Pneumonia

- Conduct surveillance for ventilator-associated pneumonia (A-II).
- Educate health care workers who care for ventilated patients (A-II).
- Implement practices for disinfection, sterilization, and maintenance of respiratory equipment (A-II).
- Perform regular oral care (A-I).
- Ensure patients are maintained in semirecumbent position, unless medical contraindication exists (B-II).
- Promote use of noninvasive ventilation when possible (B-III).

Modified from Coffin SE, Klompas M, Classen D, et al: Strategies to prevent ventilator-associated pneumonia in acute care hospitals, Infect Control Hosp Epidemiol *29(Suppl 1):S31-S40, 2008.*

ventilation. This can be accomplished through weaning protocols, daily sedation vacations to assess readiness to wean, and increased use of noninvasive ventilation.[227,228]

Practices designed to minimize aspiration of pathogenic organisms are central to VAP prevention efforts. Patient positioning in a semirecumbent angle is a key strategy. A single-center study involving 60 intubated infants found that lateral positioning delayed onset of tracheal colonization; however, no studies have shown a clear reduction in neonatal VAP associated with strict adherence to this practice.[229] Appropriate placement of enteral feeding tubes should be verified before their use.[230,231] To prevent regurgitation and potential aspiration of stomach contents by a sedated patient, overdistention of the stomach should be avoided by regular monitoring of intestinal motility, serial measurement of residual gastric volume or abdominal girth, reducing the use of narcotics and anticholinergic agents, and adjusting the rate and volume of enteral feedings.[230, 231] Other strategies to minimize aspiration include avoiding unplanned extubations.

Decreasing oropharyngeal colonization through oral decontamination has been shown to reduce the incidence of VAP in adults,[232-234] and many NICUs have adopted regular oral care as a component of their VAP prevention activities. Avoidance of gastric acid suppression in patients without a high risk of stress gastritis may also reduce the risk of VAP by minimizing bacterial colonization of the stomach.[235] Two small studies in pediatric patients failed to show a significant benefit; however, the authors stressed that additional studies with larger sample sizes are needed to confirm these findings.[236,237] Further studies are needed to define the most important VAP prevention strategies for young infants and to determine the relative contribution of each of these strategies in neonates.

Careful attention to the appropriate disinfection and reprocessing of reusable components of respiratory care equipment is also important.[238] Circuits should be monitored for the accumulation of condensate and drained periodically, with care taken to prevent the condensate, a potential reservoir for pathogens, to drain toward the patient.[231] Other basic infection control measures, such as hand hygiene and standard precautions, can also reduce the risk of VAP and other types of nosocomial pneumonia and are generally recommended for all ventilated patients.[222]

CATHETER-ASSOCIATED URINARY TRACT INFECTIONS

Urinary tract infections are recognized as the most common cause of HAIs in adults worldwide.[229,239] However, catheter-associated urinary tract infections comprise a much smaller proportion of device-related HAIs among hospitalized children (≈14%),[194] largely related to differences in frequency of urinary tract catheterization between children and adults. Still, pooled means of catheter-associated urinary tract infections are similar between adult and pediatric units reporting to the CDC's NHSN in 2011,[194] suggesting that the infectious risk associated with urinary catheter use is the same. Data on catheter-associated urinary tract infections in NICUs are not currently collected by NHSN.

Duration of catheterization is the most important risk factor for development of catheter-associated urinary tract infections.[239] Young age has been identified as an additional risk factor among children.[240,241] Gram-negative organisms, yeast, and enterococci are the most frequently isolated pathogens;[239,240,242] however, CoNS have been reported in excess of 30% of catheter-associated urinary tract infections in NICU patients.[243,244] Although few studies have prospectively evaluated strategies to prevent catheter-associated urinary tract infections in neonates, implementation of the strategies outlined in current practice guidelines is recommended.[239,245]

VENTRICULAR SHUNT–ASSOCIATED INFECTIONS

Premature infants are at significant risk of intraventricular hemorrhage and may require temporary or permanent diversion of cerebrospinal fluid (CSF) to manage obstructive hydrocephalus. Placement of CSF shunts is associated with a significant risk of postoperative infections, either ventriculitis or more superficial surgical site infections. Premature births, myelomeningocele, prior shunt placement, shunt revisions, breaches in aseptic technique during shunt placement, presence of a perioperative CSF leak, and use of a neuroendoscope have each been identified as risk factors for shunt infections.[246-250] In general, appropriate skin antisepsis, adherence to hand hygiene, proper sterile technique, and appropriate use of perioperative antibiotic prophylaxis are all strategies to reduce the risk of infection at the surgical site.[251] Use of antimicrobial-impregnated suture material and shunt catheters are additional strategies that may reduce the risk of these infections, but their evaluation in children is limited.[251-254]

Preventing Transmission of Health Care–Associated Infections

An effective infection prevention and control program can decrease the incidence of HAIs by focusing on reducing risk on a prospective basis.[74,255] The principal function of such a program is to protect the infant and the health care worker from risk of HAI in a cost-effective manner. Activities crucial to achieving and maintaining this goal include collection and management of critical data relating to surveillance for nosocomial infections and direct intervention to interrupt the transmission of infectious diseases.[256]

SURVEILLANCE

Surveillance is an essential component of any infection prevention program. The definitions provided by the CDC's NHSN have been widely adopted and provide specific definitions and data collection for the NICU population.[257] The application of these surveillance definitions can be challenging within a neonatal population. In particular, these definitions do not distinguish late-onset infections caused by transplacentally acquired organisms or organisms acquired via passage through the maternal genital tract (e.g., group B streptococcal infections) from more typical nosocomial infections.[257] The distinction between maternal and hospital sources of infection is important, although difficult at times, because control measures designed to prevent acquisition from hospital sources would be ineffective in preventing perinatal transmission. Infections can also develop after discharge, particularly in healthy newborns with short lengths of stay, which are more difficult to capture. Methods for postdischarge surveillance have been developed, but because most neonatal infections occurring after discharge are noninvasive,[258] such surveillance has not been widely implemented because of concerns regarding the cost-effectiveness of these labor-intensive processes.

Surveillance data must be analyzed and presented in a way that facilitates interpretation, comparison of data both internally and with comparable external benchmarks, and dissemination within the organization. Quality improvement tools (e.g., control and run charts) can be useful for these purposes. Statistical tools should be used to determine the significance of findings, although statistical significance should always be balanced with the evaluation of clinical significance.[259] External benchmarking through interhospital comparison is a valuable tool for improving quality of care but should be performed only when surveillance methodologies (e.g., case definitions, case finding, data collection methods, intensity of surveillance) can be assumed to be reasonably consistent between facilities.[256]

Infection data must be shared with personnel who can effect change and implement infection prevention interventions. Written reports summarizing the data and appropriate control charts should be provided to the facility's infection prevention and control committee, unit leaders, and members of the hospital administration on an ongoing basis. The interval between reports is determined by the needs of the institution. In addition to formal written reports, face-to-face discussion of data is appropriate in the event of identification of a serious problem or an outbreak. Infection preventionists can serve as consultants to assist NICU or neonatology service leaders in addressing infection rate increases or outbreak management.

More recently, controversy has emerged over the use of active surveillance cultures to identify infants colonized with multidrug-resistant organisms. Although many adult ICUs now screen all patients routinely on admission for carriage of various multidrug-resistant organisms, this practice has not yet been consistently adopted by NICUs. Factors such as the perceived low rate of carriage of resistant organisms by infants have undoubtedly led some neonatologists to question the need for universal screening on NICU admission. Data have shown, however, that a significant reservoir of resistant organisms can exist in hospitalized neonates. After two patients developed clinical infections caused by VRE, surveillance cultures revealed that greater than 15% of other patients in the same unit had unsuspected VRE colonization.[118,119] In addition, current data suggest that greater than 25% of all *S. aureus* infections in NICUs are due to methicillin-resistant strains.[260] Some units have adopted regularly scheduled point-prevalence surveys as an alternative strategy to universal surveillance. Point-prevalence surveys are most useful in units with a known low prevalence of multidrug-resistant organisms and can be used for early detection of increasing rates of carriage of multidrug-resistant organisms. Other NICUs have used active surveillance for carriage of multidrug-resistant organisms to guide programs that have led to the successful eradication of MRSA.[261,262]

STANDARD AND TRANSMISSION-BASED PRECAUTIONS IN THE NURSERY

The most widely accepted guideline for preventing transmission of infections in hospitals was developed by the CDC's Healthcare Infection Control Practices Advisory Committee (HICPAC).[23] Updated in 2007, the guideline recommends using two tiers of precautions. The first and most important, standard precautions, was designed for the management of all hospitalized patients regardless of diagnosis or presumed infection status. The second, transmission-based precaution, is intended for patients documented or suspected to be infected or colonized with highly transmissible or epidemiologically important pathogens for which additional precautions are needed to interrupt transmission.

Standard Precautions

Standard precautions are designed to reduce the risk of transmission of microorganisms from recognized and unrecognized sources and are to be applied during the care of all patients, including neonates. They apply to blood; all body fluids, secretions, and excretions except sweat; nonintact skin; and mucous membranes. Components of standard precautions include hand hygiene and the use of gloves, gowns, masks, and other forms of eye protection.

Hand Hygiene. Hand hygiene plays a critical role in the prevention of HAIs.[26,42,263] In 2009, the World Health Organization (WHO) published updated guidelines for hand hygiene, including recommendations for successful implementation.[264] Hand hygiene should be performed before and after touching a patient; before handling an invasive device, regardless of whether gloves are worn; after contact with body fluids or excretions, mucous membranes, nonintact skin, or wound dressings; in moving from a contaminated to a clean body site during patient care; after contact with inanimate objects in the immediate vicinity of the patient; and after removing sterile or nonsterile gloves.[96,264] Specific activities that have been independently associated with increased density of pathogens on health care worker hands include skin contact, respiratory care, and diaper changes; of note, investigators have shown that the use of gloves during these activities does not fully protect health care workers' hands from bacterial contamination, thus underscoring the need for appropriate hand hygiene after glove removal.[265]

Soap and water should be used for hand hygiene when hands are visibly soiled; contaminated with proteinaceous materials, blood, or body fluids; and after using the restroom. When hands are not visibly soiled, alcohol-based hand rubs, foams, or gels are recommended by both the CDC and the WHO for all clinical settings.[96,264] Compared with washing with soap and water, use of the alcohol-based products is at least as effective against a variety of pathogens, requires less time, and is less damaging to skin.[266]

It is common practice among health care workers providing care to neonates to wash hands and forearms to the elbows upon arrival in the nursery. Consensus on the optimal duration of initial hand washing is lacking but should be long enough to ensure thorough washing and rinsing of all parts of the hands and forearms. Routine hand washing throughout care delivery should consist of wetting the hands, applying product, rubbing all surfaces of the hands and fingers vigorously for at least 15 seconds, rinsing, and patting dry with disposable towels.[96] Wearing hand jewelry has been associated with increased microbial load on hands; whether this results in increased transmission of pathogens is unknown.[264] Current CDC and WHO guidelines state that staff with direct patient care should not wear artificial fingernails or nail extenders.[96,264] Only natural nails kept less than ¼-inch long should be allowed; at least one outbreak in a NICU was associated with a health care worker who wore artificial nails.[267]

Programs that have been successful in improving hand hygiene and decreasing nosocomial infection have used multidisciplinary teams to develop interventions focusing on the use of alcohol rubs in the setting of institutional commitment and support for the initiative.[26,264,268,269] Monitoring health care workers' adherence to hand hygiene practices and providing feedback is an important component of hand hygiene promotion.[264]

Gloves. It should be emphasized that wearing gloves does not replace the need for hand hygiene. Clean, nonsterile gloves are to be worn whenever contact with blood or other potentially infectious materials, mucous membranes, or nonintact skin is anticipated. Health care workers should change gloves when moving from dirty to clean tasks performed on the same patient, such as after changing a diaper and before suctioning a patient, and whenever they are soiled. Because hands may become contaminated during glove removal, and because gloves may have tiny, unnoticeable defects, hand hygiene must be performed immediately after glove removal.[264,270]

Gowns. The use of cover gowns during all routine patient care has been a common historical practice by personnel in nurseries and NICUs. However, this practice has not been found to reduce infection or colonization in neonates and is unnecessary.[23,271-273] Instead, CDC guidelines recommend nonsterile, fluid-resistant gowns to be worn as barrier protection when soiling of clothing is anticipated and in performing procedures likely to result in splashing or spraying of body substances.[23] Possible examples of such procedures in the NICU include placement of an arterial line and irrigating a wound.

Face Protection. Nonsterile masks, face shields, goggles, and other eye protectors are worn in various combinations to provide barrier protection and should be used during procedures and patient care activities that are likely to generate splashes or sprays of body substances and fluids.[23]

Other Standard Precautions. Standard precautions also require that reusable patient care equipment be cleaned and appropriately reprocessed between patients; that soiled linen be handled carefully to prevent contamination of skin, clothing, or the environment; that sharps (i.e., needles, scalpels) be handled carefully to prevent exposure to bloodborne pathogens; and that mouthpieces and other resuscitation devices be used rather than mouth-to-mouth methods of resuscitation.[23,270]

Transmission-Based Precautions

In addition to standard precautions, which must be used for every patient, the CDC recommends use of transmission-based precautions when providing care to patients known or suspected to be infected or colonized with epidemiologically important or highly transmissible organisms. Always used in addition to standard precautions, transmission-based precautions comprise three categories: contact precautions, droplet precautions, and airborne precautions.

Contact Precautions. Contact precautions involve the use of barriers to prevent transmission of organisms by direct or indirect contact with the patient or contaminated objects in the patient's immediate environment.[23] Sources of indirect contact transmission in nurseries include monitor leads, thermometers, isolettes, breast pumps,[274] toys, and contaminated hands.[275]

Ideally, a patient requiring contact precautions should be placed in a private room. However, many nurseries have few, if any, isolation rooms available. Cohorting of patients infected with the same microorganism can be a safe and effective alternative and should be discussed with infection control personnel.[23] The American Academy of Pediatrics states that infected neonates requiring contact precautions can be safely cared for without an isolation room if staffing is adequate to allow appropriate hand hygiene, a 4- to 6-foot-wide space can be provided between care stations, adequate hand hygiene facilities are available, and staff members are well trained regarding infection transmission modes.[276]

Health care workers should wear clean, nonsterile gloves and don a cover gown upon entering the room or space of a patient requiring contact precautions to address unintentional contact with contaminated surfaces.[23] Infant care equipment should be dedicated to the patient if possible so that it is not shared with others. Examples of conditions in the neonate that require contact precautions include neonatal mucocutaneous HSV infection, respiratory syncytial virus infection, varicella (also see airborne precautions), and infection or colonization with a multidrug resistant organism such as MRSA.

Droplet Precautions. Droplet precautions are intended to reduce the risk of transmission during care of patients known or suspected to be infected with microorganisms that are transmitted via large-particle droplets. Large droplets may be generated when infected persons cough, sneeze, or talk, or during procedures such as suctioning. These relatively large droplets travel only short distances and do not remain suspended in the air but can be deposited on the conjunctiva, nasal mucosa, or mouth of persons working within 3 feet of the infected patient.[23] Patients requiring droplet precautions should be placed in private rooms (see earlier discussion of isolation rooms in nurseries in "Contact Precautions"), and staff should wear masks when working within 3 feet of the patient.[23] Examples of conditions in the neonate requiring droplet precautions include pertussis and invasive *Neisseria meningitidis* infection.

Airborne Precautions. Airborne precautions are designed to reduce the risk of airborne transmission of infectious agents.[23] Because of their small size, airborne droplet nuclei and dust particles containing infectious agents or spores can be widely spread on air currents or through ventilation systems and inhaled by or deposited on susceptible hosts. Special air-handling systems and ventilation are required to prevent transmission. Patients requiring airborne precautions should be placed in private rooms in negative air-pressure ventilation with 6 to 12 air changes per hour. Air should be externally exhausted or subjected to high-efficiency particulate air (HEPA) filtration if it is recirculated.[23]

Examples of conditions in neonates for which airborne precautions are required are varicella-zoster virus infections and measles. Whenever possible, susceptible health care workers should not enter the rooms of patients with these viral infections.[23] If such assignments cannot be avoided, susceptible staff members should wear masks to deliver care. Persons with proven immunity to these viruses need not wear a mask. Airborne precautions are also required for active pulmonary tuberculosis, and although neonates are rarely contagious, the CDC recommends isolating patients while they are being evaluated.[23] A more important consideration is the need to isolate the family of a suspected tuberculosis patient until an evaluation for pulmonary tuberculosis has been completed, as the source of tuberculosis is often a member of the child's family.[277,278]

Other Related Issues

HEALTH CARE WORKERS

Health care workers caring for neonates have the potential to transmit and acquire infections while providing care to infant patients. Health care workers are at high risk of acquiring infections such as pertussis and respiratory syncytial virus when caring for infected children and can subsequently spread infection to other patients.[279-282] In general, health care workers with respiratory, cutaneous, mucocutaneous, or gastrointestinal infections should not deliver direct patient care to neonates. In addition, nonimmune staff members exposed to highly communicable diseases, such as varicella and measles, should not care for infected patients during the contagious portion of the incubation period.[23,283] In contrast, staff members with HSV infection have rarely been implicated in transmission of HSV to infants and do not need to be routinely excluded from direct patient care. Lesions should be covered, and health care workers should be instructed not to touch their lesions and to practice excellent hand hygiene.

Acquisition of CMV is often a concern of pregnant health care workers because of the potential effect on the fetus. The prevalence of asymptomatic CMV secretion is approximately 1% among infants in most nurseries.[275] Because the risk of acquiring CMV infection is the same for health care workers compared with the general population, pregnant caregivers can safely provide care to neonates who are shedding CMV with the use of standard precautions.

Nurse-to-patient ratios have been inversely correlated with the rates of nosocomial infections and mortality.[4,46,284,285] Although optimal staffing ratios have not been established for NICUs and vary according to characteristics of individual units and patients, one study showed that the incidence of clustered *S. aureus* infections was 16 times higher after periods when the infant-to-nurse ratio exceeded 7:1. Decreased compliance with hand hygiene during a period of understaffing has been associated with increased rates of nosocomial infection.[82]

FAMILY-CENTERED CARE

Family-centered care has emerged as a guiding principle of pediatric health care. In many NICUs, parents are encouraged to become actively involved in the nonmedical aspects of their infant's care. Principles of family-centered care also include liberal visitation for relatives, siblings, and family friends and the involvement of parents in the development of nursery policies and programs promoting parenting skills.[286] The benefits of family-centered care can be undermined by an increased risk of infection for neonatal patients. Mothers can transmit infections to neonates postpartum, although separation of mother and newborn is rarely indicated. To ensure the risk of postpartum transmission is minimal, all mothers should wash their hands before handling their infants. For mothers with postpartum fever, care should be taken to ensure that the infant does not have contact with contaminated dressings, linens, or pads.[276]

Mothers with other infections can also safely visit their infants. Mothers with active herpes labialis should not kiss or nuzzle their infants until lesions have cleared; lesions should be covered, and a surgical mask may be worn until the lesions are crusted and dry. The importance of hand hygiene should also be emphasized. Mothers with viral respiratory infections should be educated about how to interrupt transmission of these pathogens. Strategies such as covering a cough, prompt disposal of used tissues, and scrupulous hand hygiene should be taught before visiting. In addition, masks can be worn to reduce the risk of droplet transmission.[276,287]

As previously mentioned, a few infections do require brief separations of mother and infant. Women with untreated active pulmonary tuberculosis should be separated from their infants until they are no longer contagious. Mothers with group A streptococcal infections, especially with draining wounds, should also be isolated from their infants until they are no longer contagious.

BREASTFEEDING

Numerous studies support the value of human milk for infants (see Chapter 5). Breast milk provides optimal nutritional content for infants, and breastfed infants experience fewer episodes of infection (including respiratory tract infections and otitis media) during the first year of life.[288] In addition, preterm infants who are breastfed experience fewer episodes of sepsis and necrotizing enterocolitis.[288] There are, however, several infectious contraindications to breastfeeding: mothers who have active untreated tuberculosis, breast abscesses (as opposed to simple mastitis that is being treated with antimicrobial therapy), or HSV lesions around the nipples should not breastfeed; however, expressed breast milk can be used because there is no concern about these organisms passing though milk.[288] Human immunodeficiency virus (HIV) infection is also a contraindication to breastfeeding (except in countries where the risk of not breastfeeding outweighs the potential risk of HIV transmission [see Chapters 5 and 22]). In contrast, mothers who are positive for hepatitis B surface antigen may safely breastfeed their infants because ingestion of infected milk has not been shown to increase the risk of transmission to an infant who has received hepatitis B virus immunoglobulin and vaccine immediately after birth.[288]

Transmission of CMV has been observed in preterm infants who receive breast milk of CMV-seropositive mothers, presumably because of the infant's low titers of anti-CMV antibody. Decisions regarding breastfeeding should weigh the benefits of human milk against the risk of CMV transmission. Freezing breast milk has been shown to decrease viral titers but does not eliminate CMV; pasteurization of human milk can inactivate CMV but also affects the nutritional content (see Chapter 24). Either method may be considered in attempts to decrease risk of transmission for breastfeeding NICU neonates; however, mother's own fresh milk is generally preferred for routine feeding of preterm infants.[288]

Neonates in the NICU are frequently incapable of breastfeeding because of maternal separation, unstable respiratory status, and immaturity of the sucking reflex. For these reasons, mothers of such infants must use a breast pump to collect milk for administration through a feeding tube. Pumping, collection, and storage of breast milk create opportunities for contamination of the milk and for cross-infection if equipment is shared between mothers. Several studies have shown contamination of breast pumps, contamination of expressed milk that had been frozen and thawed, and higher levels of stool colonization with aerobic bacteria in infants fed precollected breast milk.[272,289-291] Mothers who are able to pump or express their breast milk should be taught optimal collection, storage, and administration techniques. Cleaning and disinfection of breast pumps should be included in educational material provided to nursing mothers. In addition, mothers should be instructed to perform hand hygiene and cleanse nipples with cotton and plain water before expressing milk in sterile containers.

Proper storage and handling of expressed breast milk is essential. Newer data suggest that expressed breast milk can be safely refrigerated for up to 96 hours[292] and may be safely frozen (−20° C ± 2° C [−4° F ± 3.6° F]) for up to 6 months. Vessels containing frozen breast milk can be thawed quickly under warm running water (avoiding contamination with tap water) or gradually in a refrigerator.[288] Exposure to high temperatures, as in a microwave, can destroy valuable components of the milk and should be avoided.[288] Thawed breast milk can be stored in the refrigerator for 24 hours before it must be discarded. To avoid proliferation of microorganisms, milk administered through a feeding tube by continuous infusion should hang no longer than 4 to 6 hours before replacement of the milk, container, and tubing.[276]

VISITORS

The principles of family-centered care encourage liberal visitation policies in the well-infant nursery (or rooming-in scenario) and in the NICU. Parents, including fathers, should be allowed unlimited visitation to their newborns, and siblings should be allowed liberal visitation. Still, expanding the number of visitors to neonates may increase the risk of disease exposure if education and screening for symptoms of infection are not implemented. Written policies should be in place to guide sibling visits, and parents should be encouraged to share the responsibility of protecting their newborn from contagious illnesses.

Adult visitors to neonates, including parents, have been implicated in outbreaks of infections including *P. aeruginosa* infection, pertussis, and *Salmonella* infection.[68,284,293] The principles for sibling visitation should be applied to adult visitors as well. Visitors should be screened for symptoms of contagious illness, should be instructed to perform hand hygiene before entering the NICU and before and after touching the neonate, and should interact only with the family member they came to the hospital to visit. Families of neonates who have prolonged NICU stays may come to know each other well and serve as sources of emotional support to one another. Nevertheless, they should be educated about the potential of transmitting microorganisms and infections between families if standard precautions and physical separation are not maintained, even though they may be sharing an inpatient space.

SKIN AND CORD CARE

Bathing the newborn is standard practice in nurseries, but very little standardization in frequency or cleansing product exists. If not performed carefully, bathing can be detrimental to the infant, resulting in hypothermia and increased crying, with resulting increases in oxygen consumption, respiratory distress, and instability of vital signs.[203] Although the initial bath or cleansing should be delayed until the neonate's temperature has been stable for several hours, removing blood and drying the skin immediately after delivery may remove potentially infectious microorganisms such as hepatitis B virus, HSV, and HIV, minimizing risk to the neonate from maternal infection.[276] When the newborn requires an intramuscular injection in the delivery room, injection sites should be cleansed with alcohol to prevent transmission of organisms that may be present in maternal blood and body fluids.[193] For routine bathing in the first few weeks of life, plain warm water should be used. This is especially important for preterm infants and full-term infants with barrier compromise, such as abrasions or dermatitis. If soap is necessary for heavily soiled areas, a mild pH-neutral product without additives should be used, and duration of soaping should be restricted to less than 5 minutes no more than three times per week.[203]

Few randomized studies comparing cord care regimens and infection rates have been performed, and consensus has not been reached on best practice regarding care of the umbilical cord stump. A review published in 2003 described care regimens used for more than 2 decades, including combinations of triple dye, chlorhexidine, 70% alcohol, bacitracin, hexachlorophene, povidone-iodine, and "dry care" (soap and water cleansing of soiled periumbilical skin), and found variable impact on colonization of the stump.[294] The study authors suggested that dry cord care alone may be insufficient and that chlorhexidine seemed to be a favorable antiseptic choice for cord care because of its activity against gram-positive and gram-negative bacteria, but went on to stress that large, well-designed studies were required before firm conclusions could be drawn. A more recent Cochrane review of 34 randomized and quasi-randomized trials found that there is significant evidence to suggest that topical chlorhexidine reduces neonatal mortality and omphalitis in developing countries but that the evidence is insufficient to support the use of an antiseptic versus dry care of the umbilical cord in hospital settings in developed countries.[295]

References

1. Zafar N, Wallace CM, Kieffer P, et al: Improving survival of vulnerable infants increases neonatal intensive care unit nosocomial infection rate, *Arch Pediatr Adolesc Med* 155:1098-1104, 2001.
2. Nagata E, Brito AS, Matsuo TL: Nosocomial infections in a neonatal intensive care unit: incidence and risk factors, *Am J Infect Control* 30:26-31, 2002.
3. Payne NR, Carpenter JH, Badger GJ, et al: Marginal increase in cost and excess length of stay associated with nosocomial bloodstream infections in surviving very low birth weight infants, *Pediatrics* 114:348-355, 2004.
4. Rogowski JA, Staiger D, Patrick T, et al: Nurse staffing and NICU infection rates, *JAMA Pediatr* 167:444-450, 2013.
5. Horbar JD, Carpenter JH, Badger GJ, et al: Mortality and neonatal morbidity among infants 501 to 1500 grams from 2000 to 2009, *Pediatrics* 129:1019-1026, 2012.
6. Sharma AA, Jen R, Butler A, et al: The developing human preterm neonatal immune system: a case for more research in this area, *Clin Immunol* 145:61-68, 2012.
7. Ygberg S, Nilsson A: The developing immune system—from foetus to toddler, *Acta Paediatr* 101:120-127, 2012.
8. Johnson CL, Versalovic J: The human microbiome and its potential importance to pediatrics, *Pediatrics* 129:950-960, 2012.
9. Madan JC, Farzan SF, Hibberd PL, et al: Normal neonatal microbiome variation in relation to environmental factors, infection and allergy, *Curr Opin Pediatr* 24:753-759, 2012.
10. Pessoa-Silva CL, Meurer Moreira B, Camara Almeida V, et al: Extended-spectrum beta-lactamase-producing *Klebsiella pneumoniae* in a neonatal intensive care unit: risk factors for infection and colonization, *J Hosp Infect* 53:198-206, 2003.
11. Milisavljevic V, Garg M, Vuletic I, et al: Prospective assessment of the gastroesophageal microbiome in VLBW neonates, *BMC Pediatr* 13:49, 2013.
12. Carey AJ, Della-Latta P, Huard R, et al: Changes in the molecular epidemiological characteristics of methicillin-resistant *Staphylococcus aureus* in a neonatal intensive care unit, *Infect Control Hosp Epidemiol* 31:613-619, 2010.
13. Parm U, Metsvaht T, Sepp E, et al: Risk factors associated with gut and nasopharyngeal colonization by common gram-negative species and yeasts in neonatal intensive care units patients, *Early Hum Dev* 87:391-399, 2011.
14. Baltimore RS: Neonatal nosocomial infections, *Semin Perinatol* 22:25-32, 1998.
15. Hocevar SN, Edwards JR, Horan TC, et al: Device-associated infections among neonatal intensive care unit patients: incidence and associated pathogens reported to the National Healthcare Safety Network, 2006-2008, *Infect Control Hosp Epidemiol* 33:1200-1206, 2012.
16. Sohn AH, Garrett DO, Sinkowitz-Cochran RL, et al: Prevalence of nosocomial infections in neonatal intensive care unit patients: results from the first national point-prevalence survey, *J Pediatr* 139:821-827, 2001.
17. Rutledge-Taylor K, Matlow A, Gravel D, et al: A point prevalence survey of health care-associated infections in Canadian pediatric inpatients, *Am J Infect Control* 40:491-496, 2012.
18. Scheckler WE, Brimhall D, Buck AS, et al: Requirements for infrastructure and essential activities of infection control and epidemiology in hospitals: a consensus panel report. Society for Health Care Epidemiology of America, *Am J Infect Control* 26:47-60, 1998.
19. Neumann PW, O'Shaughnessy M, Garnett M: Laboratory evidence of human immunodeficiency virus infection in Canada in 1986, *Can Med Assoc J* 137:823, 1987.
20. Bureau of Communicable Disease Epidemiology, Laboratory Centre for Disease Control, Health and Welfare, Canada: Canadian nosocomial infection surveillance program: annual summary, June 1984-May 1985, *Can Dis Wkly Rep* 12:S1, 1986.
21. Gaynes RP, Edwards JR, Jarvis WR, et al: Nosocomial infections among neonates in high-risk nurseries in the United States. National Nosocomial Infections Surveillance System, *Pediatrics* 98:357-361, 1996.
22. Stoll BJ, Hansen NI, Sanchez PJ, et al: Early onset neonatal sepsis: the burden of group B streptococcal and *E. coli* disease continues, *Pediatrics* 127:817-826, 2011.
23. Siegel JD, Rhinehart E, Jackson M, et al: 2007 Guideline for isolation precautions: preventing transmission of infectious agents in health care settings, *Am J Infect Control* 35:S65-S164, 2007.
24. Pittet D, Dharan S, Touveneau S, et al: Bacterial contamination of the hands of hospital staff during routine patient care, *Arch Intern Med* 159:821-826, 1999.
25. Larson EL, Bryan JL, Adler LM, et al: A multifaceted approach to changing handwashing behavior, *Am J Infect Control* 25:3-10, 1997.
26. Pittet D, Hugonnet S, Harbarth S, et al: Effectiveness of a hospital-wide programme to improve compliance with hand hygiene. Infection Control Programme, *Lancet* 356:1307-1312, 2000.
27. Nguyen DM, Bancroft E, Mascola L, et al: Risk factors for neonatal methicillin-resistant *Staphylococcus aureus* infection in a well-infant nursery, *Infect Control Hosp Epidemiol* 28:406-411, 2007.
28. Milisavljevic V, Wu F, Cimmotti J, et al: Genetic relatedness of *Staphylococcus epidermidis* from infected infants and staff in the neonatal intensive care unit, *Am J Infect Control* 33:341-347, 2005.
29. Larson EL, Cimiotti JP, Haas J, et al: Gram-negative bacilli associated with catheter-associated and non-catheter-associated bloodstream infections and hand carriage by healthcare workers in neonatal intensive care units, *Pediatr Crit Care Med* 6:457-461, 2005.
30. Zafar AB, Sylvester LK, Beidas SO: *Pseudomonas aeruginosa* infections in a neonatal intensive care unit, *Am J Infect Control* 30:425-429, 2002.
31. Rabier V, Bataillon S, Jolivet-Gougeon A, et al: Hand washing soap as a source of neonatal *Serratia marcescens* outbreak, *Acta Paediatr* 97:1381-1385, 2008.
32. Jhung MA, Sunenshine RH, Noble-Wang J, et al: A national outbreak of *Ralstonia mannitolilytica* associated with use of a contaminated oxygen-delivery device among pediatric patients, *Pediatrics* 119:1061-1068, 2007.
33. Baggett HC, Duchin JS, Shelton W, et al: Two nosocomial pertussis outbreaks and their associated costs—King County, Washington, 2004, *Infect Control Hosp Epidemiol* 28:537-543, 2007.
34. Yasmin E, Balen AH, Barth JH: The association of body mass index and biochemical hyperandrogenaemia in women with and without polycystic ovary syndrome, *Eur J Obstet Gynecol Reprod Biol* 166:173-177, 2013.
35. Perlman SE, Saiman L, Larson EL: Risk factors for late-onset health care-associated bloodstream infections in patients in neonatal intensive care units, *Am J Infect Control* 35:177-182, 2007.
36. Richardson DK, Gray JE, McCormick MC, et al: Score for Neonatal Acute Physiology: a physiologic severity index for neonatal intensive care, *Pediatrics* 91:617-623, 1993.
37. Sprunt K: Practical use of surveillance for prevention of nosocomial infection, *Semin Perinatol* 9:47-50, 1985.
38. Sirot D: Extended-spectrum plasmid-mediated beta-lactamases, *J Antimicrob Chemother* 36(Suppl A):19-34, 1995.
39. Stoll BJ, Temprosa M, Tyson JE, et al: Dexamethasone therapy increases infection in very low birth weight infants, *Pediatrics* 104: e63, 1999.

40. Papile LA, Tyson JE, Stoll BJ, et al: A multicenter trial of two dexamethasone regimens in ventilator-dependent premature infants, *N Engl J Med* 16:1112-1118, 1998.
41. Beck-Sague CM, Azimi P, Fonseca SN, et al: Bloodstream infections in neonatal intensive care unit patients: results of a multicenter study, *Pediatr Infect Dis J* 13:1110-1116, 1994.
42. Graham PL 3rd, Begg MD, Larson E, et al: Risk factors for late onset gram-negative sepsis in low birth weight infants hospitalized in the neonatal intensive care unit, *Pediatr Infect Dis J* 25:113-117, 2006.
43. Brodie SB, Sands KE, Gray JE, et al: Occurrence of nosocomial bloodstream infections in six neonatal intensive care units, *Pediatr Infect Dis J* 19:56-65, 2000.
44. Holmes A, Dore CJ, Saraswatula A, et al: Risk factors and recommendations for rate stratification for surveillance of neonatal healthcare-associated bloodstream infection, *J Hosp Infect* 68:66-72, 2008.
45. Sirota L, Straussberg R, Notti I, et al: Effect of lipid emulsion on IL-2 production by mononuclear cells of newborn infants and adults, *Acta Paediatr* 86:410-413, 1997.
46. Tucker J: Patient volume, staffing, and workload in relation to risk-adjusted outcomes in a random stratified sample of UK neonatal intensive care units: a prospective evaluation, *Lancet* 359:99-107, 2002.
47. Goldmann DA, Durbin WA Jr, Freeman J: Nosocomial infections in a neonatal intensive care unit, *J Infect Dis* 144:449-459, 1981.
48. Cimiotti JP, Haas J, Saiman L, et al: Impact of staffing on bloodstream infections in the neonatal intensive care unit, *Arch Pediatr Adolesc Med* 160:832-836, 2006.
49. Gray JE, Richardson DK, McCormick MC, et al: Coagulase-negative staphylococcal bacteremia among very low birth weight infants: relation to admission illness severity, resource use, and outcome, *Pediatrics* 95:225-230, 1995.
50. Villari P, Sarnataro C, Iacuzio L: Molecular epidemiology of *Staphylococcus epidermidis* in a neonatal intensive care unit over a three-year period, *J Clin Microbiol* 38:1740-1746, 2000.
51. Carlos CC, Ringertz S, Rylander M, et al: Nosocomial *Staphylococcus epidermidis* septicaemia among very low birth weight neonates in an intensive care unit, *J Hosp Infect* 19:201-207, 1991.
52. Sharek PJ, Benitz WE, Abel NJ, et al: Effect of an evidence-based hand washing policy on hand washing rates and false-positive coagulase negative *Staphylococcus* blood and cerebrospinal fluid culture rates in a level III NICU, *J Perinatol* 22:137-143, 2002.
53. Coudron PE, Mayhall CG, Facklam RR, et al: *Streptococcus faecium* outbreak in a neonatal intensive care unit, *J Clin Microbiol* 20: 1044-1048, 1984.
54. Luginbuhl LM, Rotbart HA, Facklam RR, et al: Neonatal enterococcal sepsis: case-control study and description of an outbreak, *Pediatr Infect Dis J* 6:1022-1026, 1987.
55. Malik RK, Montecalvo MA, Reale MR, et al: Epidemiology and control of vancomycin-resistant enterococci in a regional neonatal intensive care unit, *Pediatr Infect Dis J* 18:352-356, 1999.
56. Geil CC, Castle WK, Mortimer EA Jr: Group A streptococcal infections in newborn nurseries, *Pediatrics* 46:849-854, 1970.
57. Campbell JR, Arango CA, Garcia-Prats JA, et al: An outbreak of M serotype 1 group A *Streptococcus* in a neonatal intensive care unit, *J Pediatr* 129:396-402, 1996.
58. Bingen E, Denamur E, Lambert-Zechovsky N, et al: Mother-to-infant vertical transmission and cross-colonization of *Streptococcus pyogenes* confirmed by DNA restriction fragment length polymorphism analysis, *J Infect Dis* 165:147-150, 1992.
59. Isenberg HD, Tucci V, Lipsitz P, et al: Clinical laboratory and epidemiological investigations of a *Streptococcus pyogenes* cluster epidemic in a newborn nursery, *J Clin Microbiol* 19:366-370, 1984.
60. Miyairi I, Berlingieri D, Protic J, et al: Neonatal invasive group A streptococcal disease: case report and review of the literature, *Pediatr Infect Dis J* 23:161-165, 2004.
61. Brunton WA: Infection and hospital laundry, *Lancet* 345:1574-1575, 1995.
62. Stoll BJ, Hansen N, Fanaroff AA, et al: Late-onset sepsis in very low birth weight neonates: the experience of the NICHD Neonatal Research Network, *Pediatrics* 110:285-291, 2002.
63. Paredes A, Wong P, Mason EO Jr, et al: Nosocomial transmission of group B streptococci in a newborn nursery, *Pediatrics* 59:679-682, 1977.
64. Aber RC, Allen N, Howell JT, et al: Nosocomial transmission of group B streptococci, *Pediatrics* 58:346-353, 1976.
65. Anthony BF, Okada DM, Hobel CJ: Epidemiology of the group B *Streptococcus*: maternal and nosocomial sources for infant acquisitions, *J Pediatr* 95:431-436, 1979.
66. Easmon CS, Hastings MJ, Clare AJ, et al: Nosocomial transmission of group B streptococci, *Br Med J* 283:459-461, 1981.
67. Noya FJ, Rench MA, Metzger TG, et al: Unusual occurrence of an epidemic of type Ib/c group B streptococcal sepsis in a neonatal intensive care unit, *J Infect Dis* 155:1135-1144, 1987.
68. Cartolano GL, Moulies ME, Seguier JC, et al: A parent as a vector of *Salmonella brandenburg* nosocomial infection in a neonatal intensive care unit, *Clin Microbiol Infect* 9:560-562, 2003.
69. Ayan M, Kuzucu C, Durmaz R, et al: Analysis of three outbreaks due to *Klebsiella* species in a neonatal intensive care unit, *Infect Control Hosp Epidemiol* 24:495-500, 2003.
70. van den Berg RW, Claahsen HL, Niessen M, et al: *Enterobacter cloacae* outbreak in the NICU related to disinfected thermometers, *J Hosp Infect* 45:29-34, 2000.
71. Jeong SH, Kim WM, Chang CL, et al: Neonatal intensive care unit outbreak caused by a strain of *Klebsiella oxytoca* resistant to aztreonam due to overproduction of chromosomal beta-lactamase, *J Hosp Infect* 48:281-288, 2001.
72. Macrae MB, Shannon KP, Rayner DM, et al: A simultaneous outbreak on a neonatal unit of two strains of multiply antibiotic resistant *Klebsiella pneumoniae* controllable only by ward closure, *J Hosp Infect* 49:183-192, 2001.
73. Berthelot P, Grattard F, Amerger C, et al: Investigation of a nosocomial outbreak due to *Serratia marcescens* in a maternity hospital, *Infect Control Hosp Epidemiol* 20:233-236, 1999.
74. Adams-Chapman I, Stoll BJ: Prevention of nosocomial infections in the neonatal intensive care unit, *Curr Opin Pediatr* 14:157-164, 2002.
75. Donowitz LG, Marsik FJ, Fisher KA, et al: Contaminated breast milk: a source of *Klebsiella* bacteremia in a newborn intensive care unit, *Rev Infect Dis* 3:716-720, 1981.
76. Fleisch F, Zimmermann-Baer U, Zbinden R, et al: Three consecutive outbreaks of *Serratia marcescens* in a neonatal intensive care unit, *Clin Infect Dis* 34:767-773, 2002.
77. Gransden WR, Webster M, French GL, et al: An outbreak of *Serratia marcescens* transmitted by contaminated breast pumps in a special care baby unit, *J Hosp Infect* 7:149-154, 1986.
78. Moloney AC, Quoraishi AH, Parry P, et al: A bacteriological examination of breast pumps, *J Hosp Infect* 9:169-174, 1987.
79. Archibald LK, Ramos M, Arduino MJ, et al: *Enterobacter cloacae* and *Pseudomonas aeruginosa* polymicrobial bloodstream infections traced to extrinsic contamination of a dextrose multidose vial, *J Pediatr* 133:640-644, 1998.
80. Matsaniotis NS, Syriopoulou VP, Theodoridou MC, et al: *Enterobacter* sepsis in infants and children due to contaminated intravenous fluids, *Infect Control* 5:471-477, 1984.
81. Lalitha MK, Kenneth J, Jana AK, et al: Identification of an IV-dextrose solution as the source of an outbreak of *Klebsiella pneumoniae* sepsis in a newborn nursery, *J Hosp Infect* 43:70-73, 1999.
82. Harbarth S, Sudre P, Dharan S, et al: Outbreak of *Enterobacter cloacae* related to understaffing, overcrowding, and poor hygiene practices, *Infect Control Hosp Epidemiol* 20:598-603, 1999.
83. Wang H, Song W, Huang G, et al: *Candida albicans* Zcf37, a zinc finger protein, is required for stabilization of the white state, *FEBS Lett* 585:797-802, 2011.
84. Archibald LK, Corl A, Shah B, et al: *Serratia marcescens* outbreak associated with extrinsic contamination of 1% chlorxylenol soap, *Infect Control Hosp Epidemiol* 18:704-709, 1997.
85. van Ogtrop ML, van Zoeren-Grobben D, Verbakel-Salomons EM, et al: *Serratia marcescens* infections in neonatal departments: description of an outbreak and review of the literature, *J Hosp Infect* 36:95-103, 1997.
86. Patel S, Saiman L: Antibiotic resistance in neonatal intensive care unit pathogens: mechanisms, clinical impact, and prevention including antibiotic stewardship, *Clin Perinatol* 37:547-563, 2010.
87. Dalben M, Varkulja G, Basso M, et al: Investigation of an outbreak of *Enterobacter cloacae* in a neonatal unit and review of the literature, *J Hosp Infect* 70:7-14, 2008.
88. Leigh L, Stoll BJ, Rahman M, et al: *Pseudomonas aeruginosa* infection in very low birth weight infants: a case-control study, *Pediatr Infect Dis J* 14:367-371, 1995.
89. Becks VE, Lorenzoni NM: *Pseudomonas aeruginosa* outbreak in a neonatal intensive care unit: a possible link to contaminated hand lotion, *Am J Infect Control* 23:396-398, 1995.

90. McNeil MM, Solomon SL, Anderson RL, et al: Nosocomial *Pseudomonas pickettii* colonization associated with a contaminated respiratory therapy solution in a special care nursery, *J Clin Microbiol* 22:903-907, 1985.
91. Muyldermans G, de Smet F, Pierard D, et al: Neonatal infections with *Pseudomonas aeruginosa* associated with a water-bath used to thaw fresh frozen plasma, *J Hosp Infect* 39:309-314, 1998.
92. Garland SM, Mackay S, Tabrizi S, et al: *Pseudomonas aeruginosa* outbreak associated with a contaminated blood-gas analyser in a neonatal intensive care unit, *J Hosp Infect* 33:145-151, 1996.
93. Hamprecht K, Maschmann J, Vochem M, et al: Epidemiology of transmission of cytomegalovirus from mother to preterm infant by breastfeeding, *Lancet* 357:513-518, 2001.
94. Foca M, Jakob K, Whittier S, et al: Endemic *Pseudomonas aeruginosa* infection in a neonatal intensive care unit, *N Engl J Med* 343:695-700, 2000.
95. Moolenaar RL, Crutcher JM, San Joaquin VH, et al: A prolonged outbreak of *Pseudomonas aeruginosa* in a neonatal intensive care unit: did staff fingernails play a role in disease transmission? *Infect Control Hosp Epidemiol* 21:80-85, 2000.
96. Boyce JM, Pittet D: Guideline for hand hygiene in healthcare settings. Recommendations of the Health Care Infection Control Practices Advisory Committee and the HICPAC/SHEA/APIC/IDSA Hand Hygiene Task Force. Society for Health Care Epidemiology of America/Association for Professionals in Infection Control/Infectious Diseases Society of America, *MMWR Recomm Rep* 51(RR-16):1-45, 2002.
97. Nakano M, Miyazawa H, Kawano Y, et al: An outbreak of neonatal toxic shock syndrome-like exanthematous disease (NTED) caused by methicillin-resistant *Staphylococcus aureus* (MRSA) in a neonatal intensive care unit, *Microbiol Immunol* 46:277-284, 2002.
98. Andersen BM, Lindemann R, Bergh K, et al: Spread of methicillin-resistant *Staphylococcus aureus* in a neonatal intensive unit associated with understaffing, overcrowding and mixing of patients, *J Hosp Infect* 50:18-24, 2002.
99. Saito Y, Seki K, Ohara T, et al: Epidemiologic typing of methicillin-resistant *Staphylococcus aureus* in neonate intensive care units using pulsed-field gel electrophoresis, *Microbiol Immunol* 42:723-729, 1998.
100. Eckhardt C, Halvosa JS, Ray SM, et al: Transmission of methicillin-resistant *Staphylococcus aureus* in the neonatal intensive care unit from a patient with community-acquired disease, *Infect Control Hosp Epidemiol* 24:460-461, 2003.
101. Seybold U, Halvosa JS, White N, et al: Emergence of and risk factors for methicillin-resistant *Staphylococcus aureus* of community origin in intensive care nurseries, *Pediatrics* 122:1039-1046, 2008.
102. Belani A, Sherertz RJ, Sullivan ML, et al: Outbreak of staphylococcal infection in two hospital nurseries traced to a single nasal carrier, *Infect Control* 7:487-490, 1986.
103. Ish-Horowicz MR, McIntyre P, Nade S: Bone and joint infections caused by multiply resistant *Staphylococcus aureus* in a neonatal intensive care unit, *Pediatr Infect Dis J* 11:82-87, 1992.
104. Sabatino G, Verrotti A, de Martino M, et al: Neonatal suppurative parotitis: a study of five cases, *Eur J Pediatr* 158:312-314, 1999.
105. Saiman L, Jakob K, Holmes KW, et al: Molecular epidemiology of staphylococcal scalded skin syndrome in premature infants, *Pediatr Infect Dis J* 17:329-334, 1998.
106. Dave J, Reith S, Nash JQ, et al: A double outbreak of exfoliative toxin-producing strains of *Staphylococcus aureus* in a maternity unit, *Epidemiol Infect* 112:103-114, 1994.
107. Carey AJ, Duchon J, Della-Latta P, et al: The epidemiology of methicillin-susceptible and methicillin-resistant *Staphylococcus aureus* in a neonatal intensive care unit, 2000-2007, *J Perinatol* 30:135-139, 2010.
108. Otter JA, Klein JL, Watts TL, et al: Identification and control of an outbreak of ciprofloxacin-susceptible EMRSA-15 on a neonatal unit, *J Hosp Infect* 67:232-239, 2007.
109. James L, Gorwitz RJ, Jones RC, et al: Methicillin-resistant *Staphylococcus aureus* infections among healthy full-term newborns, *Arch Dis Child Fetal Neonatal Ed* 93:F40-F44, 2008.
110. Haley RW, Bregman DA: The role of understaffing and overcrowding in recurrent outbreaks of staphylococcal infection in a neonatal special-care unit, *J Infect Dis* 145:875-885, 1982.
111. Eichenwald HF, Kotsevalov O, Fasso LA: The "cloud baby": an example of bacterial-viral interaction, *Am J Dis Child* 100:161-173, 1960.
112. Sheretz RJ, Reagan DR, Hampton KD, et al: A cloud adult: the *Staphylococcus aureus*-virus interaction revisited, *Ann Intern Med* 124:539-547, 1996.
113. Morel AS, Wu F, Della-Latta P, et al: Nosocomial transmission of methicillin-resistant *Staphylococcus aureus* from a mother to her preterm quadruplet infants, *Am J Infect Control* 30:170-173, 2002.
114. Reusch M, Ghosh P, Ham C, et al: Prevalence of MRSA colonization in peripartum mothers and their newborn infants, *Scand J Infect Dis* 40:667-671, 2008.
115. McNeeley DF, Saint-Louis F, Noel GJ: Neonatal enterococcal bacteremia: an increasingly frequent event with potentially untreatable pathogens, *Pediatr Infect Dis J* 15:800-805, 1996.
116. Golan Y, Doron S, Sullivan B, et al: Transmission of vancomycin-resistant enterococcus in a neonatal intensive care unit, *Pediatr Infect Dis J* 24:566-567, 2005.
117. Arnold C, Clark R, Bosco J, et al: Variability in vancomycin use in newborn intensive care units determined from data in an electronic medical record, *Infect Control Hosp Epidemiol* 29:667-670, 2008.
118. Singh AE, Guenette T, Gratrix J, et al: Seroreversion of treponemal tests in infants meeting Canadian surveillance criteria for confirmed early congenital syphilis, *Pediatr Infect Dis J* 32:199-202, 2013.
119. Duchon J, Graham P 3rd, Della-Latta P, et al: Epidemiology of enterococci in a neonatal intensive care unit, *Infect Control Hosp Epidemiol* 29:374-376, 2008.
120. Maltezou HC, Kontopidou F, Katerelos P, et al: Infections caused by carbapenem-resistant gram-negative pathogens in hospitalized children, *Pediatr Infect Dis J* 32:e151-e154, 2013.
121. Tamma PD, Savard P, Pal T, et al: An outbreak of extended-spectrum beta-lactamase-producing *Klebsiella pneumoniae* in a neonatal intensive care unit, *Infect Control Hosp Epidemiol* 33:631-634, 2012.
122. Wojkowska-Mach J, Chmielarczyk A, Borszewska-Kornacka M, et al: Enterobacteriaceae infections of very low birth weight infants in Polish neonatal intensive care units: resistance and cross-transmission, *Pediatr Infect Dis J* 32:594-598, 2013.
123. Venezia RA, Scarano FJ, Preston KE, et al: Molecular epidemiology of an SHV-5 extended-spectrum beta-lactamase in enterobacteriaceae isolated from infants in a neonatal intensive care unit, *Clin Infect Dis* 21:915-923, 1995.
124. Shannon K, Fung K, Stapleton P, et al: A hospital outbreak of extended-spectrum beta-lactamase-producing *Klebsiella pneumoniae* investigated by RAPD typing and analysis of the genetics and mechanisms of resistance, *J Hosp Infect* 39:291-300, 1998.
125. Anderson B, Nicholas S, Sprague B, et al: Molecular and descriptive epidemiology of multidrug-resistant Enterobacteriaceae in hospitalized infants, *Infect Control Hosp Epidemiol* 29:250-255, 2008.
126. Anaissie EJ, Segal BH, Graybill JR, et al: Clinical research in the lay press: irresponsible journalism raises a huge dose of doubt, *Clin Infect Dis* 43:1031-1039, 2006.
127. Manzoni P, Maestri A, Leonessa M, et al: Fungal and bacterial sepsis and threshold ROP in preterm very low birth weight neonates, *J Perinatol* 26:23-30, 2006.
128. Zaoutis TE, Prasad PA, Localio AR, et al: Risk factors and predictors for candidemia in pediatric intensive care unit patients: implications for prevention, *Clin Infect Dis* 51:e38-e45, 2010.
129. Lee JH, Hornik CP, Benjamin DK Jr, et al: Risk factors for invasive candidiasis in infants >1500 g birth weight, *Pediatr Infect Dis J* 32:222-226, 2013.
130. Gerber JS, Coffin SE, Smathers SA, et al: Trends in the incidence of methicillin-resistant *Staphylococcus aureus* infection in children's hospitals in the United States, *Clin Infect Dis* 49:65-71, 2009.
131. Chitnis AS, Magill SS, Edwards JR, et al: Trends in *Candida* central line-associated bloodstream infections among NICUs, 1999-2009, *Pediatrics* 130:e46-e52, 2012.
132. Fridkin SK, Kaufman D, Edwards JR, et al: Changing incidence of *Candida* bloodstream infections among NICU patients in the United States: 1995-2004, *Pediatrics* 117:1680-1687, 2006.
133. Saiman L, Ludington E, Pfaller M, et al: Risk factors for candidemia in neonatal intensive care unit patients. The National Epidemiology of Mycosis Survey study group, *Pediatr Infect Dis J* 19:319-324, 2000.
134. Cotten CM, McDonald S, Stoll B, et al: The association of third-generation cephalosporin use and invasive candidiasis in extremely low birth-weight infants, *Pediatrics* 118:717-722, 2006.
135. Dotis J, Prasad PA, Zaoutis T, et al: Epidemiology, risk factors and outcome of *Candida parapsilosis* bloodstream infection in children, *Pediatr Infect Dis J* 31:557-560, 2012.

136. Benjamin DK Jr, Stoll BJ, Fanaroff AA, et al: Neonatal candidiasis among extremely low birth weight infants: risk factors, mortality rates, and neurodevelopmental outcomes at 18 to 22 months, *Pediatrics* 117:84-92, 2006.
137. Lee WI, Huang JL, Yeh KW, et al: Clinical features and genetic analysis of Taiwanese patients with the hyper IgM syndrome phenotype, *Pediatr Infect Dis J* 32:1010-1016, 2013.
138. Feja KN, Wu F, Roberts K, et al: Risk factors for candidemia in critically ill infants: a matched case-control study, *J Pediatr* 147:156-161, 2005.
139. Manzoni P, Stolfi I, Pugni L, et al: A multicenter, randomized trial of prophylactic fluconazole in preterm neonates, *N Engl J Med* 356:2483-2495, 2007.
140. Pappas PG, Kauffman CA, Andes D, et al: Clinical practice guidelines for the management of candidiasis: 2009 update by the Infectious Diseases Society of America, *Clin Infect Dis* 48:503-535, 2009.
141. Kaufman DA, Cuff AL, Wamstad JB, et al: Fluconazole prophylaxis in extremely low birth weight infants and neurodevelopmental outcomes and quality of life at 8 to 10 years of age, *J Pediatr* 158:759-765, 2011.
142. Chryssanthou E, Broberger U, Petrini B: *Malassezia pachydermatis* fungaemia in a neonatal intensive care unit, *Acta Paediatr* 90:323-327, 2001.
143. Chang HJ, Miller HL, Watkins N, et al: An epidemic of *Malassezia pachydermatis* in an intensive care nursery associated with colonization of health care workers' pet dogs, *N Engl J Med* 338:706-711, 1998.
144. Groll AH, Jaeger G, Allendorf A, et al: Invasive pulmonary aspergillosis in a critically ill neonate: case report and review of invasive aspergillosis during the first 3 months of life, *Clin Infect Dis* 27:437-452, 1998.
145. Singer S, Singer D, Ruchel R, et al: Outbreak of systemic aspergillosis in a neonatal intensive care unit, *Mycoses* 41:223-227, 1998.
146. Etienne KA, Subudhi CP, Chadwick PR, et al: Investigation of a cluster of cutaneous aspergillosis in a neonatal intensive care unit, *J Hosp Infect* 79:344-348, 2011.
147. Mitchell SJ, Gray J, Morgan ME, et al: Nosocomial infection with *Rhizopus microsporus* in preterm infants: association with wooden tongue depressors, *Lancet* 348:441-443, 1996.
148. Gelber SE, Ratner AJ: Hospital-acquired viral pathogens in the neonatal intensive care unit, *Semin Perinatol* 26:346-356, 2002.
149. Sharma R, Hudak ML, Premachandra BR, et al: Clinical manifestations of rotavirus infection in the neonatal intensive care unit, *Pediatr Infect Dis J* 21:1099-1105, 2002.
150. Anderson EJ, Rupp A, Shulman ST, et al: Impact of rotavirus vaccination on hospital-acquired rotavirus gastroenteritis in children, *Pediatrics* 127:e264-e270, 2011.
151. Flores J, White L, Blanco M, et al: Serological response to rotavirus infection in newborn infants, *J Med Virol* 42:97-102, 1994.
152. Lee CN, Lin CC, Kao CL, et al: Genetic characterization of the rotaviruses associated with a nursery outbreak, *J Med Virol* 63:311-320, 2001.
153. Verhagen P, Moore D, Manges A, et al: Nosocomial rotavirus gastroenteritis in a Canadian paediatric hospital: incidence, disease burden and patients affected, *J Hosp Infect* 79:59-63, 2011.
154. Sattar SA, Jacobsen H, Rahman H, et al: Interruption of rotavirus spread through chemical disinfection, *Infect Control Hosp Epidemiol* 15:751-756, 1994.
155. Widdowson MA, van Doornum GJ, van der Poel WH, et al: An outbreak of diarrhea in a neonatal medium care unit caused by a novel strain of rotavirus: investigation using both epidemiologic and microbiological methods, *Infect Control Hosp Epidemiol* 23:665-670, 2002.
156. Herruzo R, Omenaca F, Garcia S, et al: Identification of risk factors associated with nosocomial infection by rotavirus P4G2 in a neonatal unit of a tertiary-care hospital, *Clin Microbiol Infect* 15:280-285, 2009.
157. Turcios-Ruiz RM, Axelrod P, St John K, et al: Outbreak of necrotizing enterocolitis caused by norovirus in a neonatal intensive care unit, *J Pediatr* 153:339-344, 2008.
158. Stuart RL, Tan K, Mahar JE, et al: An outbreak of necrotizing enterocolitis associated with norovirus genotype GII.3, *Pediatr Infect Dis J* 29:644-647, 2010.
159. Bagci S, Eis-Hubinger AM, Franz AR, et al: Detection of astrovirus in premature infants with necrotizing enterocolitis, *Pediatr Infect Dis J* 27:347-350, 2008.
160. Lodha A, de Silva N, Petric M, et al: Human torovirus: a new virus associated with neonatal necrotizing enterocolitis, *Acta Paediatr* 94:1085-1088, 2005.
161. Vayalumkal JV, Gravel D, Moore D, et al: Surveillance for healthcare–acquired febrile respiratory infection in pediatric hospitals participating in the Canadian Nosocomial Infection Surveillance Program, *Infect Control Hosp Epidemiol* 30:652-658, 2009.
162. Birenbaum E, Linder N, Varsano N, et al: Adenovirus type 8 conjunctivitis outbreak in a neonatal intensive care unit, *Arch Dis Child* 68:610-611, 1993.
163. Sizun J, Soupre D, Legrand MC, et al: Neonatal nosocomial respiratory infection with coronavirus: a prospective study in a neonatal intensive care unit, *Acta Paediatr* 84:617-620, 1995.
164. Cunney RJ, Bialachowski A, Thornley D, et al: An outbreak of influenza A in a neonatal intensive care unit, *Infect Control Hosp Epidemiol* 21:449-554, 2000.
165. Moisiuk SE, Robson D, Klass L, et al: Outbreak of parainfluenza virus type 3 in an intermediate care neonatal nursery, *Pediatr Infect Dis J* 17:49-53, 1998.
166. Kurz H, Herbich K, Janata O, et al: Experience with the use of palivizumab together with infection control measures to prevent respiratory syncytial virus outbreaks in neonatal intensive care units, *J Hosp Infect* 70:246-252, 2008.
167. Sagrera X, Ginovart G, Raspall F, et al: Outbreaks of influenza A virus infection in neonatal intensive care units, *Pediatr Infect Dis J* 21: 196-200, 2002.
168. Halasa NB, Williams JV, Wilson GJ, et al: Medical and economic impact of a respiratory syncytial virus outbreak in a neonatal intensive care unit, *Pediatr Infect Dis J* 24:1040-1044, 2005.
169. Bennett NJ, Tabarani CM, Bartholoma NM, et al: Unrecognized viral respiratory tract infections in premature infants during their birth hospitalization: a prospective surveillance study in two neonatal intensive care units, *J Pediatr* 161:814-818, 2012.
170. Groothuis JT, van Kuppevelt DH: Postpartum spinal cord injury in a woman with HELLP syndrome, *J Spinal Cord Med* 31:309-311, 2008.
171. Syriopoulou VP, Hadjichristodoulou C, Daikos GL, et al: Clinical and epidemiological aspects of an enterovirus outbreak in a neonatal unit, *J Hosp Infect* 51:275-280, 2002.
172. Jankovic B, Pasic S, Kanjuh B, et al: Severe neonatal echovirus 17 infection during a nursery outbreak, *Pediatr Infect Dis J* 18:393-394, 1999.
173. Kusuhara K, Saito M, Sasaki Y, et al: An echovirus type 18 outbreak in a neonatal intensive care unit, *Eur J Pediatr* 167:587-589, 2008.
174. Chambon M, Bailly JL, Beguet A, et al: An outbreak due to echovirus type 30 in a neonatal unit in France in 1997: usefulness of PCR diagnosis, *J Hosp Infect* 43:63-68, 1999.
175. Griffin MP, O'Shea M, Brazy JE, et al: Cytomegalovirus infection in a neonatal intensive care unit. Subsequent morbidity and mortality of seropositive infants, *J Perinatol* 10:43-45, 1990.
176. Vochem M, Hamprecht K, Jahn G, et al: Transmission of cytomegalovirus to preterm infants through breast milk, *Pediatr Infect Dis J* 17:53-58, 1998.
177. Sawyer MH, Edwards DK, Spector SA: Cytomegalovirus infection and bronchopulmonary dysplasia in premature infants, *Am J Dis Child* 141:303-305, 1987.
178. Sharland M, Khare M, Bedford-Russell A: Prevention of postnatal cytomegalovirus infection in preterm infants, *Arch Dis Child Fetal Neonatal Ed* 86:F140, 2002.
179. Aitken C, Booth J, Booth M, et al: Molecular epidemiology and significance of a cluster of cases of CMV infection occurring on a special care baby unit, *J Hosp Infect* 34:183-189, 1996.
180. Spector SA: Transmission of cytomegalovirus among infants in hospital documented by restriction-endonuclease-digestion analyses, *Lancet* 1:378-381, 1983.
181. Demmler GJ, Yow MD, Spector SA, et al: Nosocomial cytomegalovirus infections within two hospitals caring for infants and children, *J Infect Dis* 156:9-16, 1987.
182. Linnemann CC Jr, Buchman TG, Light IJ, et al: Transmission of herpes-simplex virus type 1 in a nursery for the newborn. Identification of viral isolates by D.N.A. "fingerprinting", *Lancet* 1:964-966, 1978.
183. Hammerberg O, Watts J, Chernesky M, et al: An outbreak of herpes simplex virus type 1 in an intensive care nursery, *Pediatr Infect Dis* 2:290-294, 1983.
184. Sakaoka H, Saheki Y, Uzuki K, et al: Two outbreaks of herpes simplex virus type 1 nosocomial infection among newborns, *J Clin Microbiol* 24:36-40, 1986.

185. Turner R, Shehab Z, Osborne K, et al: Shedding and survival of herpes simplex virus from 'fever blisters', *Pediatrics* 70:547-549, 1982.
186. Hayakawa M, Kimura H, Ohshiro M, et al: Varicella exposure in a neonatal medical centre: successful prophylaxis with oral acyclovir, *J Hosp Infect* 54:212-215, 2003.
187. Klein BS, Michaels JA, Rytel MW, et al: Nosocomial hepatitis A. A multinursery outbreak in Wisconsin, *JAMA* 252:2716-2721, 1984.
188. Watson JC, Fleming DW, Borella AJ, et al: Vertical transmission of hepatitis A resulting in an outbreak in a neonatal intensive care unit, *J Infect Dis* 167:567-571, 1993.
189. Rosenblum LS, Villarino ME, Nainan OV, et al: Hepatitis A outbreak in a neonatal intensive care unit: risk factors for transmission and evidence of prolonged viral excretion among preterm infants, *J Infect Dis* 164:476-482, 1991.
190. Klevens RM, Edwards JR, Richards CL Jr, et al: Estimating health care-associated infections and deaths in U.S. hospitals, 2002, *Public Health Rep* 122:160-166, 2007.
191. O'Grady NP, Alexander M, Burns LA, et al: Guidelines for the prevention of intravascular catheter-related infections, *Clin Infect Dis* 52:e162-e193, 2011.
192. Glumac N, Hocevar M, Zadnik V, et al: Inguinal or inguino-iliac/obturator lymph node dissection after positive inguinal sentinel lymph node in patients with cutaneous melanoma, *Radiol Oncol* 46:258-264, 2012.
193. Siegel JD: *The newborn nursery*, Philadelphia, 1998, Lippincott-Raven.
194. Dudeck MA, Horan TC, Peterson KD, et al: National Healthcare Safety Network report, data summary for 2011, device-associated module, *Am J Infect Control* 41:286-300, 2013.
195. Raad I, Costerton W, Sabharwal U, et al: Ultrastructural analysis of indwelling vascular catheters: a quantitative relationship between luminal colonization and duration of placement, *J Infect Dis* 168:400-407, 1993.
196. Garland JS, Alex CP, Sevallius JM, et al: Cohort study of the pathogenesis and molecular epidemiology of catheter-related bloodstream infection in neonates with peripherally inserted central venous catheters, *Infect Control Hosp Epidemiol* 29:243-249, 2008.
197. Horbar JD, Rogowski J, Plsek PE, et al: Collaborative quality improvement for neonatal intensive care. NIC/Q Project Investigators of the Vermont Oxford Network, *Pediatrics* 107:14-22, 2001.
198. Marschall J, Mermel LA, Classen D, et al: Strategies to prevent central line-associated bloodstream infections in acute care hospitals, *Infect Control Hosp Epidemiol* 29(Suppl 1):S22-S30, 2008.
199. Sengupta A, Lehmann C, Diener-West M, et al: Catheter duration and risk of CLA-BSI in neonates with PICCs, *Pediatrics* 125:648-653, 2010.
200. Capretti MG, Sandri F, Tridapalli E, et al: Impact of a standardized hand hygiene program on the incidence of nosocomial infection in very low birth weight infants, *Am J Infect Control* 36:430-435, 2008.
201. Kaplan HC, Lannon C, Walsh MC, et al: Ohio statewide quality-improvement collaborative to reduce late-onset sepsis in preterm infants, *Pediatrics* 127:427-435, 2011.
202. Wirtschafter DD, Powers RJ, Pettit JS, et al: Nosocomial infection reduction in VLBW infants with a statewide quality-improvement model, *Pediatrics* 127:419-426, 2011.
203. Darmstadt GL, Dinulos JG: Neonatal skin care, *Pediatr Clin North Am* 47:757-782, 2000.
204. Tamma PD, Aucott SW, Milstone AM: Chlorhexidine use in the neonatal intensive care unit: results from a national survey, *Infect Control Hosp Epidemiol* 31:846-849, 2010.
205. Karki S, Cheng AC: Impact of non-rinse skin cleansing with chlorhexidine gluconate on prevention of healthcare-associated infections and colonization with multi-resistant organisms: a systematic review, *J Hosp Infect* 82:71-84, 2012.
206. Milstone AM, Elward A, Song X, et al: Daily chlorhexidine bathing to reduce bacteraemia in critically ill children: a multicentre, cluster-randomised, crossover trial, *Lancet* 381:1099-1106, 2013.
207. Climo MW, Yokoe DS, Warren DK, et al: Effect of daily chlorhexidine bathing on hospital-acquired infection, *N Engl J Med* 368:533-542, 2013.
208. O'Horo JC, Silva GL, Munoz-Price LS, et al: The efficacy of daily bathing with chlorhexidine for reducing healthcare-associated bloodstream infections: a meta-analysis, *Infect Control Hosp Epidemiol* 33:257-267, 2012.
209. Huang SS, Septimus E, Kleinman K, et al: Targeted versus universal decolonization to prevent ICU infection, *N Engl J Med* 368:2255-2265, 2013.
210. Garland JS, Alex CP, Uhing MR, et al: Pilot trial to compare tolerance of chlorhexidine gluconate to povidone-iodine antisepsis for central venous catheter placement in neonates, *J Perinatol* 29:808-813, 2009.
211. Milstone AM, Budd A, Shepard JW, et al: Role of decolonization in a comprehensive strategy to reduce methicillin-resistant Staphylococcus aureus infections in the neonatal intensive care unit: an observational cohort study, *Infect Control Hosp Epidemiol* 31:558-560, 2010.
212. Tielsch JM, Darmstadt GL, Mullany LC, et al: Impact of newborn skin-cleansing with chlorhexidine on neonatal mortality in southern Nepal: a community-based, cluster-randomized trial, *Pediatrics* 119:e330-e340, 2007.
213. Hoang V, Sills J, Chandler M, et al: Percutaneously inserted central catheter for total parenteral nutrition in neonates: complication rates related to upper versus lower extremity insertion, *Pediatrics* 121:e1152-e1159, 2008.
214. Niedner MF, Huskins WC, Colantuoni E, et al: Epidemiology of central line-associated bloodstream infections in the pediatric intensive care unit, *Infect Control Hosp Epidemiol* 32:1200-1208, 2011.
215. Reyes JA, Habash ML, Taylor RP: Femoral central venous catheters are not associated with higher rates of infection in the pediatric critical care population, *Am J Infect Control* 40:43-47, 2012.
216. Oliveira C, Nasr A, Brindle M, et al: Ethanol locks to prevent catheter-related bloodstream infections in parenteral nutrition: a meta-analysis, *Pediatrics* 129:318-329, 2012.
217. Garland JS, Alex CP, Henrickson KJ, et al: A vancomycin-heparin lock solution for prevention of nosocomial bloodstream infection in critically ill neonates with peripherally inserted central venous catheters: a prospective, randomized trial, *Pediatrics* 116:e198-e205, 2005.
218. Filippi L, Pezzati M, Di Amario S, et al: Fusidic acid and heparin lock solution for the prevention of catheter-related bloodstream infections in critically ill neonates: a retrospective study and a prospective, randomized trial, *Pediatr Crit Care Med* 8:556-562, 2007.
219. Jardine LA, Inglis GD, Davies MW: Prophylactic systemic antibiotics to reduce morbidity and mortality in neonates with central venous catheters, *Cochrane Database Syst Rev* (1): CD006179, 2008.
220. Garland JS, Dunne WM Jr, Havens P, et al: Peripheral intravenous catheter complications in critically ill children: a prospective study, *Pediatrics* 89:1145-1150, 1992.
221. Yuan TM, Chen LH, Yu HM: Risk factors and outcomes for ventilator-associated pneumonia in neonatal intensive care unit patients, *J Perinat Med* 35:334-338, 2007.
222. Coffin SE, Klompas M, Classen D, et al: Strategies to prevent ventilator-associated pneumonia in acute care hospitals, *Infect Control Hosp Epidemiol* 29(Suppl 1):S31-S40, 2008.
223. Kawagoe JY, Segre CA, Pereira CR, et al: Risk factors for nosocomial infections in critically ill newborns: a 5-year prospective cohort study, *Am J Infect Control* 29:109-114, 2001.
224. Petdachai W: Nosocomial pneumonia in a newborn intensive care unit, *J Med Assoc Thai* 83:392-397, 2000.
225. O'Grady NP, Murray PR, Ames N: Preventing ventilator-associated pneumonia: does the evidence support the practice? *JAMA* 307:2534-2539, 2012.
226. Pepe R: *Nosocomial pneumonia*, Washington, DC, 2002, Association for Professionals in Infection Control and Epidemiology.
227. Lesiuk W, Lesiuk L, Maliczowska M, et al: [Non-invasive mandatory ventilation in extremely low birth weight and very low birth weight newborns with failed respiration], *Przegl Lek* 59(Suppl 1):57-59, 2002.
228. Fernandez-Jurado MI, Fernandez-Baena M: Use of laryngeal mask airway for prolonged ventilatory support in a preterm newborn, *Paediatr Anaesth* 12:369-370, 2002.
229. Aly H, Badawy M, El-Kholy A, et al: Randomized, controlled trial on tracheal colonization of ventilated infants: can gravity prevent ventilator-associated pneumonia? *Pediatrics* 122:770-774, 2008.
230. Centers for Disease Control and Prevention: Guidelines for prevention of nosocomial pneumonia, *MMWR Recomm Rep* 46(RR-1):1-79, 1997.
231. Kollef MH: The prevention of ventilator-associated pneumonia, *N Engl J Med* 340:627-634, 1999.
232. Bergmans DC, Bonten MJ, Gaillard CA, et al: Prevention of ventilator-associated pneumonia by oral decontamination: a prospective, randomized, double-blind, placebo-controlled study, *Am J Respir Crit Care Med* 164:382-388, 2001.

233. Labeau SO, Van de Vyver K, Brusselaers N, et al: Prevention of ventilator-associated pneumonia with oral antiseptics: a systematic review and meta-analysis, *Lancet Infect Dis* 11:845-854, 2011.
234. Pugin J, Auckenthaler R, Lew DP, et al: Oropharyngeal decontamination decreases incidence of ventilator-associated pneumonia. A randomized, placebo-controlled, double-blind clinical trial, *JAMA* 265:2704-2710, 1991.
235. Cook DJ, Reeve BK, Guyatt GH, et al: Stress ulcer prophylaxis in critically ill patients. Resolving discordant meta-analyses, *JAMA* 275:308-314, 1996.
236. Ildizdas K, Yapicioglu H, Yilmaz H: Occurrence of ventilator-associated pneumonia in mechanically ventilated pediatric intensive care patients during stress ulcer prophylaxis with sucralfate, ranitidine, and omeprazole, *J Crit Care* 17:240-245, 2002.
237. Lopriore E, Markhorst DG, Gemke RJ: Ventilator-associated pneumonia and upper airway colonisation with gram negative bacilli: the role of stress ulcer prophylaxis in children, *Intensive Care Med* 28:763-767, 2002.
238. Tablan OC, Anderson LJ, Besser R, et al: Guidelines for preventing health-care–associated pneumonia, 2003: recommendations of CDC and the Healthcare Infection Control Practices Advisory Committee, *MMWR Recomm Rep* 53(RR-3):1-36, 2004.
239. Hooton TM, Bradley SF, Cardenas DD, et al: Diagnosis, prevention, and treatment of catheter-associated urinary tract infection in adults: 2009 International Clinical Practice Guidelines from the Infectious Diseases Society of America, *Clin Infect Dis* 50:625-663, 2010.
240. Langley JM, Hanakowski M, Leblanc JC: Unique epidemiology of nosocomial urinary tract infection in children, *Am J Infect Control* 29:94-98, 2001.
241. Lohr JA, Downs SM, Dudley S, et al: Hospital-acquired urinary tract infections in the pediatric patient: a prospective study, *Pediatr Infect Dis J* 13:8-12, 1994.
242. Aziz M, Patel AL, Losavio J, et al: Efficacy of fluconazole prophylaxis for prevention of invasive fungal infection in extremely low birth weight infants, *Pediatr Infect Dis J* 29:352-356, 2010.
243. Lohr JA, Donowitz LG, Sadler JE 3rd: Hospital-acquired urinary tract infection, *Pediatrics* 83:193-199, 1989.
244. Davies HD, Jones EL, Sheng RY, et al: Nosocomial urinary tract infections at a pediatric hospital, *Pediatr Infect Dis J* 11:349-354, 1992.
245. Lo E, Nicolle L, Classen D, et al: Strategies to prevent catheter-associated urinary tract infections in acute care hospitals, *Infect Control Hosp Epidemiol* 29(Suppl 1):S41-S50, 2008.
246. Kulkarni AV, Drake JM, Lamberti-Pasculli M: Cerebrospinal fluid shunt infection: a prospective study of risk factors, *J Neurosurg* 94:195-201, 2001.
247. McGirt MJ, Zaas A, Fuchs HE, et al: Risk factors for pediatric ventriculoperitoneal shunt infection and predictors of infectious pathogens, *Clin Infect Dis* 36:858-862, 2003.
248. Odio C, McCracken GH Jr, Nelson JD: CSF shunt infections in pediatrics. A seven-year experience, *Am J Dis Child* 138:1103-1108, 1984.
249. Jeelani NU, Kulkarni AV, Desilva P, et al: Postoperative cerebrospinal fluid wound leakage as a predictor of shunt infection: a prospective analysis of 205 cases. Clinical article, *J Neurosurg Pediatr* 4:166-169, 2009.
250. Simon TD, Whitlock KB, Riva-Cambrin J, et al: Revision surgeries are associated with significant increased risk of subsequent cerebrospinal fluid shunt infection, *Pediatr Infect Dis J* 31:551-556, 2012.
251. Alexander JW, Solomkin JS, Edwards MJ: Updated recommendations for control of surgical site infections, *Ann Surg* 253:1082-1093, 2011.
252. Eymann R, Chehab S, Strowitzki M, et al: Clinical and economic consequences of antibiotic-impregnated cerebrospinal fluid shunt catheters, *J Neurosurg Pediatrics* 1:444-450, 2008.
253. Rozzelle CJ, Leonardo J, Li V: Antimicrobial suture wound closure for cerebrospinal fluid shunt surgery: a prospective, double-blinded, randomized controlled trial, *J Neurosurg Pediatrics* 2:111-117, 2008.
254. Pattavilakom A, Xenos C, Bradfield O, et al: Reduction in shunt infection using antibiotic impregnated CSF shunt catheters: an Australian prospective study, *J Clin Neurosci* 14:526-531, 2007.
255. Haley RW, Culver DH, White JW, et al: The efficacy of infection surveillance and control programs in preventing nosocomial infections in US hospitals, *Am J Epidemiol* 121:182-205, 1985.
256. Lee TB, Montgomery OG, Marx J, et al: Recommended practices for surveillance: Association for Professionals in Infection Control and Epidemiology (APIC), Inc, *Am J Infect Control* 35:427-440, 2007.
257. Horan TC, Andrus M, Dudeck MA: CDC/NHSN surveillance definition of health care-associated infection and criteria for specific types of infections in the acute care setting, *Am J Infect Control* 36: 309-332, 2008.
258. Sinha A, Yokow D, Platt R: Epidemiology of neonatal infections: experience during and after hospitalization, *Pediatr Infect Dis J* 22:244-250, 2003.
259. Lee T, Baker-Montgomery O: *Surveillance*, Washington, DC, 2002, Association for Professionals in Infection Control and Epidemiology.
260. Lessa FC, Edwards JR, Fridkin SK, et al: Trends in incidence of late-onset methicillin-resistant *Staphylococcus aureus* infection in neonatal intensive care units: data from the National Nosocomial Infections Surveillance System, 1995-2004, *Pediatr Infect Dis J* 28:577-581, 2009.
261. Khoury J, Jones M, Grim A, et al: Eradication of methicillin-resistant *Staphylococcus aureus* from a neonatal intensive care unit by active surveillance and aggressive infection control measures, *Infect Control Hosp Epidemiol* 26:616-621, 2005.
262. Axelrod FB, Rolnitzky L, Gold von Simson G, et al: A rating scale for the functional assessment of patients with familial dysautonomia (Riley Day syndrome), *J Pediatr* 161:1160-1165, 2012.
263. Pessoa-Silva CL, Hugonnet S, Pfister R, et al: Reduction of health care associated infection risk in neonates by successful hand hygiene promotion, *Pediatrics* 120:e382-e390, 2007.
264. Pittet DAB, Allegranzi B, Boyce J: World Health Organization World Alliance for Patient Safety First Global Patient Safety Challenge Core Group of Experts: the World Health Organization Guidelines on Hand Hygiene in Health Care and their consensus recommmendations, *Infect Control Hosp Epidemiol* 30:611-622, 2009.
265. Pessoa-Silva CL, Dharan S, Hugonnet S, et al: Dynamics of bacterial hand contamination during routine neonatal care, *Infect Control Hosp Epidemiol* 25:192-197, 2004.
266. Larson EL, Cimiotti J, Haas J, et al: Effect of antiseptic handwashing vs alcohol sanitizer on health care-associated infections in neonatal intensive care units, *Arch Pediatr Adolesc Med* 159:377-383, 2005.
267. Gupta A, Della-Latta P, Todd B, et al: Outbreak of extended-spectrum beta-lactamase-producing *Klebsiella pneumoniae* in a neonatal intensive care unit linked to artificial nails, *Infect Control Hosp Epidemiol* 25:210-215, 2004.
268. Pittet D: Improving adherence to hand hygiene practice: a multidisciplinary approach, *Emerg Infect Dis* 7:234-240, 2001.
269. Won SP, Chou HC, Hsieh WS, et al: Handwashing program for the prevention of nosocomial infections in a neonatal intensive care unit, *Infect Control Hosp Epidemiol* 25:742-746, 2004.
270. Garner JS: Guideline for isolation precautions in hospitals. The Hospital Infection Control Practices Advisory Committee, *Infect Control Hosp Epidemiol* 17:53-80, 1996.
271. Pelke S, Ching D, Easa D, et al: Gowning does not affect colonization or infection rates in a neonatal intensive care unit, *Arch Pediatr Adolesc Med* 148:1016-1020, 1994.
272. Birenbaum HJ, Glorioso L, Rosenberger C, et al: Gowning on a postpartum ward fails to decrease colonization in the newborn infant, *Am J Dis Child* 144:1031-1033, 1990.
273. Webster J, Pritchard MA: Gowning by attendants and visitors in newborn nurseries for prevention of neonatal morbidity and mortality, *Cochrane Database Syst Rev* (3): CD003670, 2003.
274. Lee TB, Baker OG, Lee JT, et al: Recommended practices for surveillance. Association for Professionals in Infection Control and Epidemiology, Inc. Surveillance Initiative working group, *Am J Infect Control* 26:277-288, 1998.
275. Centers for Disease Control and Prevention: Division of Health Care Quality Promotion: National Nosocomial Infections Surveillance (NNIS) System Report, data summary from January 1992 through June 2003, issued August 2003, *Am J Infect Control* 30:481-498, 2003.
276. American Academy of Pediatrics, American College of Obstetricians and Gynecologists: Infection control. In *Guidelines for perinatal care*, ed 6, Washington, DC, 2007, AAP//ACOG, pp 349-370.
277. Bozzi D, Burwen D, Dooley S, et al: Guideline for preventing the transmission of Mycobacterium tuberculosis in health care facilities, *MMWR Morb Mortal Wkly Rep* 43:1-132, 1994.
278. Munoz FM, Ong LT, Seavy D, et al: Tuberculosis among adult visitors of children with suspected tuberculosis and employees at a children's hospital, *Infect Control Hosp Epidemiol* 23:568-572, 2002.

279. De Serres G, Shadmani R, Duval B, et al: Morbidity of pertussis in adolescents and adults, *J Infect Dis* 182:174-179, 2000.
280. Hall CB, Douglas RG Jr, Geiman JM, et al: Nosocomial respiratory syncytial virus infections, *N Engl J Med* 293:1343-1346, 1975.
281. Hall CB, Geiman JM, Douglas RG Jr, et al: Control of nosocomial respiratory syncytial viral infections, *Pediatrics* 62:728-732, 1978.
282. Hall CB, Kopelman AE, Douglas RG Jr, et al: Neonatal respiratory syncytial virus infection, *N Engl J Med* 300:393-396, 1979.
283. Bolyard EA, Tablan OC, Williams WW, et al: Guideline for infection control in healthcare personnel, 1998. Hospital Infection Control Practices Advisory Committee, *Infect Control Hosp Epidemiol* 19: 407-463, 1998.
284. Spearing NM, Horvath RL, McCormack JG: Pertussis: adults as a source in healthcare settings, *Med J Aust* 177:568-569, 2002.
285. Fridkin SK, Pear SM, Williamson TH, et al: The role of understaffing in central venous catheter-associated bloodstream infections, *Infect Control Hosp Epidemiol* 17:150-158, 1996.
286. Harrison H: The principles for family-centered neonatal care, *Pediatrics* 92:643-650, 1993.
287. Moore D: *Newborn nursery and neonatal intensive care unit*, Washington, DC, 2002, Association for Professionals in Infection Control and Epidemiology.
288. Section on Breastfeeding, Johnston M, Landers S, et al: Breastfeeding and the use of human milk, *Pediatrics* 129:e827-e841, 2012.
289. el-Mohandes AE, Picard MB, Simmens SJ, et al: Use of human milk in the intensive care nursery decreases the incidence of nosocomial sepsis, *J Perinatol* 17:130-134, 1997.
290. el-Mohandes AE, Schatz V, Keiser JF, et al: Bacterial contaminants of collected and frozen human milk used in an intensive care nursery, *Am J Infect Control* 21:226-230, 1993.
291. D'Amico CJ, DiNardo CA, Krystofiak S: Preventing contamination of breast pump kit attachments in the NICU, *J Perinat Neonatal Nurs* 17:150-157, 2003.
292. Slutzah M, Codipilly CN, Potak D, et al: Refrigerator storage of expressed human milk in the neonatal intensive care unit, *J Pediatr* 156:26-28, 2010.
293. Wittrock B, Lavin MA, Pierry D, et al: Parents as a vector for nosocomial infection in the neonatal intensive care unit, *Infect Control Hosp Epidemiol* 22:472, 2001.
294. Mullany LC, Darmstadt GL, Tielsch JM: Role of antimicrobial applications to the umbilical cord in neonates to prevent bacterial colonization and infection: a review of the evidence, *Pediatr Infect Dis J* 22:996-1002, 2003.
295. Imdad A, Bautista RM, Senen KA, et al: Umbilical cord antiseptics for preventing sepsis and death among newborns, *Cochrane Database Syst Rev* (5): CD008635, 2013.

36 Laboratory Aids for Diagnosis of Neonatal Sepsis

GEOFFREY A. WEINBERG and CARL T. D'ANGIO

CHAPTER OUTLINE

For years, investigators have sought a test or panel of tests able to diagnose neonatal sepsis accurately and more rapidly than is possible with the recovery of microorganisms from specimens of sterile body fluids or tissues. Although results of some studies have been encouraging, microbial isolation from blood, cerebrospinal fluid (CSF), urine, other body fluids (peritoneal, pleural, joint, middle ear), or tissues (bone marrow, liver, spleen) remains the most valid method of diagnosing bacterial sepsis. Many advances in non–culture-based methods, which may nevertheless remain microorganism specific, such as tests using polymerase chain reaction (PCR) amplification technology, are promising for more rapid diagnosis of infection. This chapter discusses nonspecific laboratory aids for the diagnosis of invasive bacterial infections. Specific microbiologic techniques are discussed in Chapter 6 and in chapters addressing specific pathogens.

Diagnostic Utility of Laboratory Tests

In establishing the usefulness of any laboratory determination, a balance must be reached between sensitivity and specificity.[1] For a clinician needing to decide whether to institute or withhold therapy on the basis of a test result, the predictive values (and perhaps likelihood ratios [LRs])[2] of that test are also important. In relation to neonatal infection, these terms can be defined as follows (Fig. 36-1):

Sensitivity: If infection is present, how often is the test result abnormal?

Specificity: If infection is absent, how often is the test result normal?

Positive predictive value: If the test result is abnormal, how often is infection present?

Negative predictive value: If the test result is normal, how often is infection absent?

LR, positive test result: If the test result is abnormal, how much does that result increase the pretest probability of disease?

LR, negative test result: If the test result is normal, how much does that result decrease the pretest probability of disease?

In attempting to discover the presence of a serious illness such as neonatal bacteremia, which is life-threatening yet treatable, diagnostic tests with maximal (100%) sensitivity and negative predictive value are desirable. In other words, if infection were present, the result would always be abnormal; if the result were normal, infection would always be absent. The reduced specificity and positive predictive value that this combination may engender usually are acceptable because overtreatment with antibiotics on the basis of a false-positive result is likely to be of limited harm compared with withholding therapy on the basis of

		Bacterial infection present: Yes	Bacterial infection present: No	
Laboratory test result	Positive	True positives (a)	False positives (b)	***Positive predictive value*** *(a)/(a+b)*
	Negative	False negatives (c)	True negatives (d)	***Negative predictive value*** *(d)/(c+d)*
		Sensitivity *(a)/(a+c)*	***Specificity*** *(d)/(b+d)*	

Likelihood ratio, positive
Sensitivity/(1-specificity)

Likelihood ratio, negative
(1-sensitivity)/specificity

Prevalence
(a+c)/(a+b+c+d)

Figure 36-1 Diagnostic test characteristics. Sensitivity, specificity, positive predictive value, and negative predictive value are commonly expressed as percentages; likelihood ratios represent x-fold increases or y-fold decreases in probability. (From Feinstein AR: Clinical biostatistics: XXXI. On the sensitivity, specificity, and discrimination of diagnostic tests, *Clin Pharmacol Ther* 17:104-116, 1975; Jaeschke R, Guyatt GH, Sackett DL: Users' guides to the medical literature. III. How to use an article about a diagnostic test. B. What are the results and will they help me in caring for my patients? *JAMA* 271:703-707, 1994; and Radetsky M: The laboratory evaluation of newborn sepsis, *Curr Opin Infect Dis* 8:191-199, 1995.)

a false-negative result. Some authorities prefer the use of LRs because predictive values vary with the prevalence of a disease, whereas LRs relate only to the test performance (sensitivity, specificity).[3,4] Large LRs (>10) imply that a test result would conclusively increase the probability of the disease being present, whereas small LRs (<0.1) minimize the probability of the disease being present.

In reviewing a report of a new laboratory aid for the diagnosis of neonatal sepsis, the first consideration is to determine what reference standard was used to evaluate the new test (i.e., what was the gold standard applied). In one study of infants who died with unequivocal evidence of infection at autopsy, bacteria were grown from 32 of 39 antemortem blood cultures (sensitivity of only 82%).[5] Among 50 infants without pathologic findings of infection at autopsy, 48 had negative blood culture results (specificity of 96%). A positive blood or CSF culture result had a 94% chance of being associated with serious neonatal infection (positive predictive value of 94%), whereas a negative blood culture result indicated absence of serious infection only 87% of the time (negative predictive value of 87%). It is likely that the predictive values cited in this study already are different from the values that may be observed in practice because of the high prevalence (44%) of positive bacterial culture results in the autopsy cases reviewed.[5] High prevalence inflates the positive predictive value and depresses the negative predictive value; low prevalence depresses the positive predictive value and inflates the negative predictive value.

The lack of perfection of the generally accepted gold standard of bacterial culture complicates the search for new laboratory aids in the diagnosis of neonatal sepsis; it may be unclear whether a new test is truly functioning better than culture, which itself may not be "perfect." Interpretation of bacterial culture results may become even more complicated as intrapartum antibiotic prophylaxis to prevent early-onset group B streptococcal sepsis becomes more common.[6-9] Yet, it may not be clinically necessary to require detection of only *bacterial* sepsis. Tests that yield results considered "falsely positive" in the absence of bacterial disease may still be clinically useful in assigning normal versus abnormal status if the results register positive because of *serious viral disease* that may require antiviral therapy (e.g., neonatal enterovirus or herpes simplex infections).

In addition, even the most useful test serving as a gold standard may function well in one population of infants, for example, very low birth weight with a greater prevalence of sepsis, and yet may function quite poorly in another population—that of older infants with larger birth weights who are growing normally and have a lesser prevalence of sepsis. Each report of a new test claiming superiority to current tests (e.g., bacterial culture) must be critically evaluated in the extended clinical setting, including target populations, with standardization within clinical laboratories and among institutions.

In Search of the Ideal Laboratory Test

Because the body's response to an infection necessarily begins after the invasion of a pathogen, it may never be possible to diagnose an infection immediately: There may always be a lag in the physiologic response on which the diagnostic test is based. Even bacterial blood cultures performed with modern, continuously computer-monitored detection technology do not reach 100% sensitivity for the diagnosis of neonatal infection. Incubation of bacteria may take several days, and genuine bacteremia may be missed because of the small volume of blood taken from infants with very low birth weight. A set of properties of the ideal or perfect diagnostic test has been proposed.[10,11] These characteristics should be kept in mind as the different laboratory tests for neonatal infection are discussed in this chapter.

First, the laboratory analyte would be biochemically stable (to ease transport requirements), easy to analyze (quick laboratory turnaround time), and obtainable from a small volume of blood. Second, the analyte would have clear diagnostic cutoffs between normal and abnormal, across various gestational ages, and across birth weights. Third,

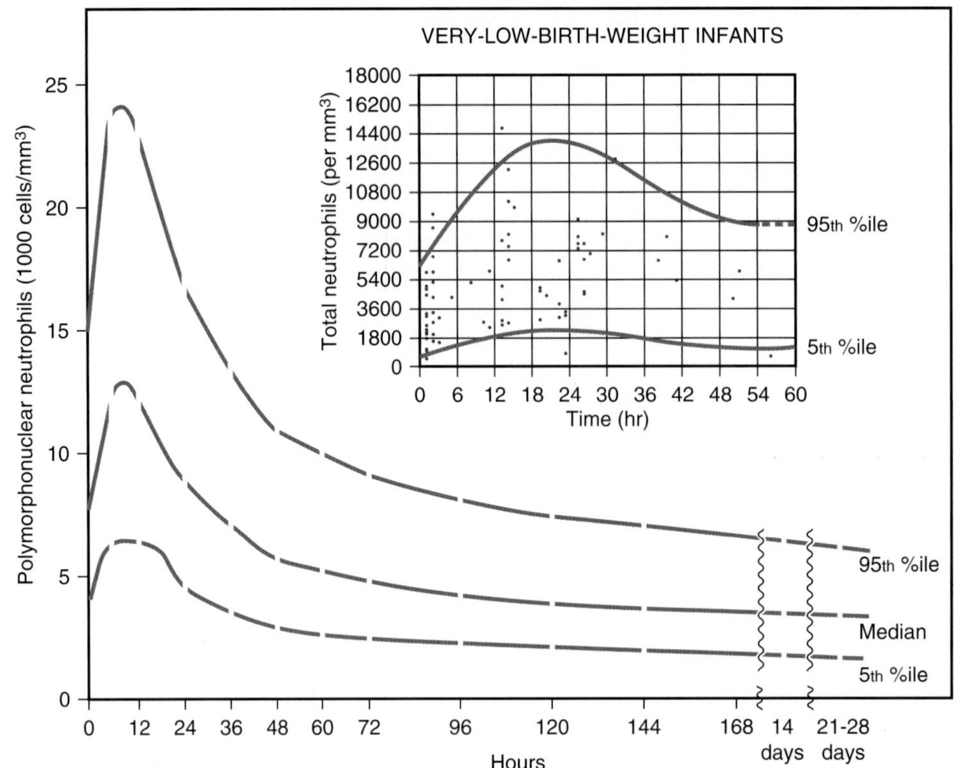

Figure 36-2 Total neutrophil counts in normal term infants and in very-low-birth-weight infants *(inset)*. (The data are for term infants[25] and align well with those from most[14,24,27] but not all[21] other sources. The data for the inset are from Mouzinho and colleagues[26] and align well with other studies.)

the test would be inexpensive and comparable among different laboratories so that it could be widely applied.

In addition, the ideal laboratory test for the diagnosis of neonatal infection would be maximally sensitive (no false-negative results) and highly specific (few false-positive results) and have a physiologic window of opportunity for sampling. More precisely, the test would become abnormal just as infection was present and remain abnormal for some time, to allow clinicians to use it as a diagnostic aid even if the clinical symptoms of infection were initially missed.

Finally, the ideal marker would correlate well with progress of infection, perhaps even predicting outcome.[10,11] As we review each test in this chapter, it will become apparent that none of the currently available laboratory aids for the diagnosis of infection fulfills these ideal properties. Although new tests are continually being studied, it is uncertain whether any will ever achieve perfection. For a more extensive review of the older literature on laboratory aids for the diagnosis of neonatal sepsis, the reader is referred to the previous edition of this text.[12]

Blood Cell Counts, Ratios, and Flow Cytometric Markers

TOTAL LEUKOCYTE COUNT, DIFFERENTIAL LEUKOCYTE COUNT, AND MORPHOLOGY

Total leukocyte counts (white blood cell [WBC] counts) are of limited value in the diagnosis of septicemia in newborns.[13] Total leukocyte counts are particularly unreliable indicators of infection during the first several hours of early-onset sepsis because they are normal at the time of initial evaluation in more than one half of infants with proven bacteremia.[13-18] Optimal interpretation of the WBC count also requires examination of the newborn's age in hours.[14]

Differential leukocyte counts also have not functioned well as markers for infectious disease in the newborn period. Increased percentages of lymphocytes have been described in association with pertussis and congenital syphilis, and increased monocyte counts with congenital syphilis, and perinatal listeriosis; however, either or both may also be affected by ABO incompatibility and recovery from sepsis.[12,17] Eosinophilia, a common finding in premature infants, has been related to numerous factors, including low birth weight, immaturity, establishment of positive nitrogen balance, improved nutritional status, and use of total parenteral nutrition or blood transfusions, in addition to sepsis.[12,19,20] Basophil counts tend to follow the fluctuations in eosinophil numbers in ill or healthy newborns.[12]

Several investigators have shown that significant changes in neutrophil morphology occur in association with serious bacterial infection, with the appearance of toxic granules, Döhle bodies, and vacuolization.[12,20-22] These features are of limited value in establishing a diagnosis; their presence has, at best, a positive predictive value for sepsis of only slightly more than 50%[5,12,21,22] and, at worst, a positive predictive value of 33% to 37%.[12,23]

ABSOLUTE NEUTROPHIL COUNT

Recognizing the low predictive value of total leukocyte counts in serious neonatal bacterial disease, several investigators have studied the dynamics of neutrophil counts during the first month of life.[12,20,21,24-27] These researchers and others uncovered patterns of change sufficiently constant to establish limits of normal variation (Fig. 36-2) and

Table 36-1 Clinical Factors Affecting Neutrophil Counts in Newborn Infants

	NEUTROPHIL COUNTS*				
Factor	**Decrease**	**Increase**	**Total Immature Increase**	**Increased I:T Ratio†**	**Approximate Duration (hr)**
Maternal hypertension	++++	0	+	+	72
Maternal fever, neonate healthy	0	++	+++	++++	24
≥6 hours intrapartum oxytocin administration	0	++	++	++++	120
Asphyxia (5-min Apgar score ≤ 5)	+	++	++	+++	24-60
Meconium aspiration syndrome	0	++++	+++	++	72
Pneumothorax with uncomplicated hyaline membrane disease	0	++++	++++	++++	24
Seizures: No hypoglycemia, asphyxia, or central nervous system hemorrhage	0	+++	+++	++++	24
Prolonged (≥4 min) crying	0	++++	++++	++++	1
Asymptomatic blood glucose ≤ 30 mg/dL	0	+++	+++	+++	24
Hemolytic disease	++	++	+++	++	7-28 days
Surgery	0	++++	++++	+++	24
High altitude	0	++++	++++	0	6

Data from Weinberg GA, D'Angio CT: Laboratory aids for diagnosis of neonatal sepsis. In Remington JS, Klein JO, Wilson CB, et al, editors: *Infectious diseases of the fetus and newborn infant*, ed 7, Philadelphia, 2011, Saunders, pp 1144-1160; Xanthou M: Leucocyte blood picture in ill newborn babies, *Arch Dis Child* 47:741-746, 1972; Manroe BL, Weinberg AG, Rosenfeld CR, et al: The neonatal blood count in health and disease. I. Reference values for neutrophilic cells, *J Pediatr* 95:89-98, 1979; Gregory J, Hey E: Blood neutrophil response to bacterial infection in the first month of life, *Arch Dis Child* 47:747-753, 1972; and Rodwell RL, Tudehope DI, Gray PH: Hematologic scoring system in early diagnosis of sepsis in neutropenic newborns, *Pediatr Infect Dis* 12:372-376, 1993.

*+, <25% of neonates affected; ++, 25%-50%; +++, 50%-75%; ++++, 75%-100%.

†Ratio of immature forms to total neutrophils.

Box 36-1 **Clinical Factors With No Effect on Neutrophil Counts in Newborn Infants**

- Race
- Gender
- Maternal diabetes
- Fetal bradycardia
- Mode of delivery*
- Premature rupture of membranes, mother afebrile
- Meconium staining, no lung disease
- Uncomplicated hyaline membrane disease
- Uncomplicated transient tachypnea of the newborn
- Hyperbilirubinemia, physiologic, unexplained
- Phototherapy
- Diurnal variation

Data from Weinberg GA, D'Angio CT: Laboratory aids for diagnosis of neonatal sepsis. In Remington JS, Klein JO, Wilson CB, et al, editors: Infectious diseases of the fetus and newborn infant, *ed 7, Philadelphia, 2011, Saunders, pp 1144-1160; Manroe BL, Weinberg AG, Rosenfeld CR, et al: The neonatal blood count in health and disease. I. Reference values for neutrophilic cells,* J Pediatr *95:89-98, 1979; Xanthou M: Leucocyte blood picture in healthy full-term and premature babies during neonatal period,* Arch Dis Child *45:242-249, 1970; and Gregory J, Hey E: Blood neutrophil response to bacterial infection in the first month of life,* Arch Dis Child *47:747-753, 1972.*

*Total neutrophil counts in cord blood of infants delivered vaginally or by cesarean section after labor (2-14 hr) are twice those of infants delivered by cesarean section without labor.

defined noninfectious conditions involving the mother or the infant that might have significant effects on neutrophil values (Table 36-1 and Box 36-1). Largely on the basis of these data, it was suggested that calculation of the absolute number of circulating neutrophils (polymorphonuclear plus immature forms) might provide a useful index of neonatal infection. Clinical experience has only partly supported this premise.

Most series of consecutive cases of neonatal sepsis have shown abnormal neutrophil counts at the *time of onset of symptoms* in only about two thirds of infants.* In some series, 80% to 90% of infected infants have had abnormal values,[23,25,29] whereas in other series, initial neutrophil counts were reduced or elevated in only one fourth to one third of infants with bacteremia, particularly when counts were determined early in the course of illness.[12,14,24,30]

However, the absolute neutrophil count (ANC) may be of value in specific clinical situations. The association of neutropenia, respiratory distress, and early-onset (<48 hours) sepsis caused by group B streptococci is well documented,[12,14,31] although the recognition that a similar association exists for early sepsis caused by other microorganisms (e.g., *Haemophilus influenzae*,[32] pneumococci,[33] and *Escherichia coli*[12,14]) has not been adequately emphasized. Because all infants were noted to be ill at birth or shortly thereafter, when neutrophil counts normally are increasing, a low count (0-4000 cells/mm^3) in this clinical setting is a highly significant finding, often reflecting a depletion of bone marrow granulocyte reserves[34] and indicating a poor prognosis.[5,12,16,20,35]

TOTAL NONSEGMENTED NEUTROPHIL (BAND) COUNT

The blood smear and differential cell count during the newborn period are strikingly different from values seen at any other time of life. Immature forms are present in relatively large numbers, particularly among premature infants and during the first few days of life.[21,22,24] The number of immature neutrophils, mostly nonsegmented (band, stab) forms, increases from a maximum normal value of 1100 cells/

*References 5, 12, 13, 16, 21, 22, 28.

mm³ in cord blood to 1500 cells/mm³ at 12 hours of life and gradually decreases to 600 cells/mm³ by 60 hours of life. Between 60 and 120 hours, the maximum count decreases from 600 to 500 cells/mm³ and remains unchanged through the first month of life.[21] Metamyelocytes and myelocytes also are often present in significant numbers during the first 72 hours after delivery but disappear almost entirely toward the end of the first week of life.[24] Even occasional promyelocytes and blast cells may be seen during the early days of life in healthy infants.[24]

As neutrophils are released from the bone marrow in response to infection, an increasing number of immature cells enter the bloodstream, producing a differential cell count with a "shift to the left" even greater than that normally present in the neonate.[29] This response is so inconstant, however, that, with few exceptions,[12] the absolute band or immature (bands, metamyelocytes) neutrophil count has been found to be of little diagnostic value.[5,12,16,23,31] In many infants with infection, despite an increased proportion of immature cell types in the differential leukocyte count, exhaustion of the bone marrow reserves prevents an increase in the absolute number of band neutrophils in the circulation.[34,36] This is particularly common in more seriously ill patients, in whom early diagnosis is most critical.[5,29,34]

Despite its relative insensitivity, the immature neutrophil count has been found to have good positive predictive value in some,[5,22,29,31] although not all,[23] studies. In infants with clinical evidence of sepsis and high band counts in whom culture results remain negative, follow-up cultures and investigation for a history of perinatal events that might explain the discrepancy (see Table 36-1) or for the possibility of infection related to other causes, such as enteroviruses, are indicated.

NEUTROPHIL RATIOS

The unreliability of absolute band counts led to the investigation of neutrophil ratios as an index of neonatal infection. Determinations have included the ratio of either bands or all immature neutrophils (e.g., bands, metamyelocytes, and myelocytes) to either segmented neutrophils (the immature-to-mature neutrophil ratio [I:M ratio]) or to all neutrophils (the immature-to-total neutrophil ratio [I:T ratio]). Despite the early enthusiasm of researchers, the clinical studies that include these determinations have failed to show a consistent correlation with the presence of serious bacterial disease. As might be expected, low band counts caused by exhaustion of marrow can produce misleadingly low ratios in the presence of serious or overwhelming infection.[†]

The I:T ratio is the best studied of the ratios.[14,28,37] Inclusion in the numerator of all immature forms, rather than just band cells, heightens accuracy by accounting for the increase in metamyelocytes that is sometimes seen with accelerated release from the neutrophil storage pool.[29] Use of total rather than segmented neutrophils in the denominator has the advantage of always yielding a value between 0 and 1 inclusive. The upper limit of normal for the first 24 hours is variably reported as between approximately 0.2 to 0.4.[14,21] It gradually declines to about 0.12 by 60 hours of age and remains unchanged for the remainder of the first month.[21] A normal value up to 0.2, with age unspecified, has been found in some laboratories.[15] I:T ratios during the first 5 days of life are less than 0.2 in 96% of healthy premature infants with a gestational age of 32 weeks or less.[12]

However, numerous clinical studies of the I:T ratio have found it too unreliable to achieve more than limited usefulness by itself, with diagnostic sensitivity of at most 60% to 90% and specificity of only 50% to 75%.[‡] Perhaps the greatest value of the I:T ratio lies in its good negative predictive value: If the I:T ratio is normal, the likelihood that infection is absent is very high.[3,12,15,23,31]

PLATELET COUNT

Several extensive studies have established that the normal platelet count in newborns, regardless of birth weight, is rarely less than 100,000/mm³ during the first 10 days of life or less than 150,000/mm³ during the next 3 weeks.[12,40,41] Although it would behoove the clinician to perform a workup for sepsis in any infant with unexplained thrombocytopenia,[41] a reduction in the number of circulating platelets has been shown to be an insensitive, nonspecific, and relatively late indicator of serious bacterial infection during the neonatal period. Automated measurements of mean platelet volume have added little to the platelet count as a diagnostic aid.[42] Thrombocytopenia accompanying bacterial infection is thought to be caused by a direct effect of bacteria or bacterial products on platelets and vascular endothelium, leading to increased aggregation and adhesion, or by increased platelet destruction caused by immune mechanisms.[12,22] However, thrombocytopenia is not specific for bacterial sepsis; it also may accompany intrauterine syphilis, toxoplasmosis, rubella, cytomegalovirus, enterovirus, and herpes simplex virus infections, as well as complications associated with umbilical catheter placement, birth asphyxia, mechanical ventilation, meconium aspiration, multiple exchange transfusions, and necrotizing enterocolitis.[12]

NEUTROPHIL AND LYMPHOCYTE FLOW CYTOMETRIC MARKERS

Neutrophil and lymphocyte surface markers and receptors are modified during the inflammatory response to infection, and such changes are readily detected by flow cytometry. However, flow cytometry analyses are not able to be determined in a timely fashion in many hospitals and may require several milliliters of whole blood, depending upon the equipment at hand. The surface expression of the neutrophil surface marker CD11b yielded good sensitivity, specificity, and predictive values in diagnosing neonatal bacterial and fungal infection in several studies.[43,44] The expression of CD11b and other markers, such as soluble CD40 ligand, may be affected by duration of labor and chronologic age; further studies are required to define normal ranges and clinical utility.[43,45] Expression of another neutrophil surface marker, CD64, has been found to correlate with early-onset and late-onset nosocomial newborn sepsis in some studies.[46-48] Automated hematology analyzers can evaluate neutrophil volume, scatter, and distribution width (similar to what is done for erythrocytes and platelets); modest sensitivity and specificity for detection of

†References 15, 16, 22, 28, 29, 31, 34.

‡References 12, 14, 21, 23, 31, 38, 39.

bacterial sepsis has been reported.[49] Activation of T lymphocytes after infection results in upregulation of the lymphocyte surface marker CD45RO isoform, coupled to loss of the CD45RA isoform. Sequential analysis of the distribution of early CD45RA-CD45RO dual expression and later CD45RO expression alone discriminated bacterial (and viral) infection from respiratory distress or erythrocyte incompatibility in a few infants.[50]

Acute-Phase Reactants

In the presence of inflammation caused by infection, trauma, or other cellular destruction, the liver, under the influence of proinflammatory cytokines interleukin-1β (IL-1β), IL-6, and tumor necrosis factor-α (TNF-α), rapidly synthesizes large amounts of certain proteins collectively known as *acute-phase reactants*.[51-53] Serum levels of these proteins usually increase together, and generally the degree of change in one is proportional to the degree of change in the others; two important exceptions are albumin and transferrin, which decrease together (Fig. 36-3). Acute-phase reactants are produced very early in fetal life, beginning in the fourth to fifth week of gestation.[54] Their exact role in the inflammatory process is not completely defined, but many components appear to be part of a primitive nonspecific (innate) defense mechanism. Several acute-phase reactants have been extensively evaluated in neonatal sepsis, including C-reactive protein (CRP), procalcitonin, and proteins such as fibrinogen, which influence the erythrocyte sedimentation rate (ESR); haptoglobin; and α1-acid glycoprotein (orosomucoid).

Most of the acute-phase reactants, including the ESR, have not been found to be sufficiently sensitive or specific for the diagnosis of neonatal sepsis. Two major exceptions, CRP and procalcitonin, are further discussed later in this chapter.

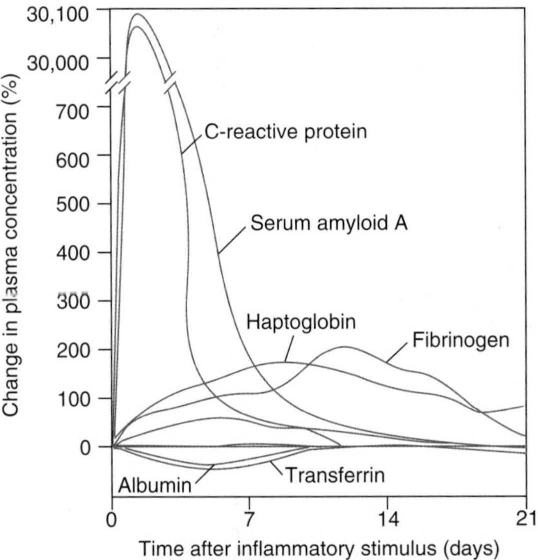

Figure 36-3 Acute-phase reactants in patients with inflammatory illnesses. The response of C-reactive protein is greater than that of all other acute phase proteins except serum amyloid A. Levels of certain plasma proteins decrease during the acute-phase response. (Data from Gabay C, Kushner I: Acute-phase proteins and other systemic responses to inflammation, *N Engl J Med* 340:448-454, 1999.)

ERYTHROCYTE SEDIMENTATION RATE AND MISCELLANEOUS ACUTE-PHASE REACTANTS

The development more than 50 years ago of an *ESR* technique, by use of a microhematocrit tube and a few drops of capillary blood, permitted the application of this test in very small infants.[55,56] Attempts at standardization have shown that the ESR increases slowly during the first weeks of life, perhaps as a result of increasing fibrinogen and decreasing hematocrit levels. Maximal normal rates have varied so widely, however, that any laboratory attempting to use this test in neonates must establish its own normal values.[12,57] Sedimentation rates do not vary significantly with gestational age, birth weight, or gender but are related inversely to the hematocrit level, particularly in infants with hematocrit readings of less than 0.40.[12,57] The ESR generally is normal or only mildly elevated in noninfectious conditions, such as respiratory distress syndrome, aspiration pneumonia, and asphyxia, and in superficial infections.[12,57] Significant elevations are unusual in healthy infants but can occur in the presence of Coombs-positive hemolytic disease and physiologic hyperbilirubinemia.[12,57] Although extensive clinical experience has shown that the ESR eventually becomes elevated in most infants with systemic bacterial infections, this increase may not have occurred at the time of the initial evaluation in 30% to 70% of infants with proven sepsis, particularly when disseminated intravascular coagulopathy is present.[12,35,57]

The increase in plasma *fibrinogen* level associated with infection has been recognized for many years through its effects on the erythrocyte sedimentation rate. Clinical experience with the use of fibrinogen levels is limited but generally disappointing. Median fibrinogen concentrations in infected infants overlapped to a great extent with levels obtained from normal infants, and low values despite severe infection also have been reported.[58] Concentrations may be affected by birth weight and test methodology and decrease dramatically in the presence of disseminated intravascular coagulopathy (which is, of course, associated with sepsis). *Haptoglobin* is an α2-glycoprotein that reacts with free hemoglobin to form a complex that is removed by the reticuloendothelial system. Gestational age, neonatal asphyxia, gender, and hemolytic ABO/Rh disease have no significant influence on haptoglobin levels in cord blood or during the postnatal period; however, elevated levels usually persist for several days after exchange transfusion, probably as a result of passive transfer of blood with adult concentrations of the protein. Inaccuracies related to phenotypic variants of haptoglobin, although seen when levels are measured by radial immunodiffusion, have not presented a problem when concentrations are determined by laser nephelometry. More important, clinical studies have raised serious doubts about the reliability of haptoglobin concentrations in the prediction of neonatal sepsis.[15,59-61] *α1-Acid glycoprotein* is produced by lymphocytes, monocytes, neutrophils, and hepatocytes. It exists as an integral membrane protein of leukocytes and is liberated into the plasma as the cells disintegrate. The function of α1-acid glycoprotein is unknown, but it may have a role in forming collagen, binding steroid hormones, and modifying lymphocyte responsiveness.[62] Although early studies suggested that α1-acid glycoprotein might be a specific and sensitive indicator of neonatal bacterial infection, subsequent surveys have been unable to confirm this favorable experience.[15,59,62-64] Other acute-phase proteins evaluated for the early diagnosis of neonatal sepsis include *serum amyloid protein,*[65,66] *α1-proteinase inhibitor* (α1-antitrypsin),[64] the complex of elastase and α1-proteinase inhibitor,[65] *α1-antichymotrypsin,* [64] *inter-α-inhibitor proteins,*[67] *ceruloplasmin,*[68] *hepcidin,*[69] and *secretory phospholipase A2.*[70] No definitive clinical studies suggest that any of these reactants are helpful for diagnosis or management in the neonate suspected to have a bacterial infection.

C-REACTIVE PROTEIN

Serum CRP is one of the most useful of the acute-phase reactants for assisting in the diagnosis of neonatal sepsis. CRP is a pathogen-associated molecular pattern recognition protein of the pentraxin family, so named because it forms a precipitate when combined with the C-polysaccharide of *Streptococcus pneumoniae.*[52,53] CRP not only recognizes microbial polysaccharides but also necrotic cells, chromatin subunits, and small nuclear riboproteins. CRP and other pentraxins (e.g., serum amyloid protein, pentraxin 3) have long been known to activate the classical complement pathway and were recently found to bind cellular immunoglobulin Fc receptors as well. This has led to the recognition that CRP participates both in opsonization of pathogens and apoptotic cells to stimulate their complement-mediated destruction, and also the promotion of phagocytosis and release of cellular inflammatory mediators.[52] Thus it is not surprising that CRP is elevated as part of the acute-phase response to inflammation or infection. In fact, CRP and other pentraxins are ancient immune mediators present in invertebrates, amphibians, and mammals; they may be viewed as a nonspecific, rapid, first line of immune defense.[52]

Differences in laboratory techniques and in the interpretation of what constitutes a positive result for CRP assay have been partly responsible for conflicting opinions about the reliability of this test during the neonatal period.[28,53,71] Early clinical laboratory techniques (capillary tube precipitation and gel immunodiffusion) were less sensitive and specific than more modern immunochemical methods.[28,71] Newer rapid, reliable, and quantitative monoclonal antibody-based turbidimetric and nephelometric methods have been developed, providing results in 30 to 60 minutes, whereas enzyme immunoassays, such as the enzyme-multiplied immunoassay technique, can give results in less than 10 minutes.[71]

Analysis of paired serum specimens obtained from mothers and their infants (fetuses, premature infants, and full-term neonates) has shown that CRP crosses the placenta either only in very low concentrations or not at all.[53] Determination of CRP levels in neonatal serum by numerous authors using several modern assay techniques has shown the upper limit of normal to be approximately 10 mg/L (1 mg/dL) during the neonatal period.[53,59,72] CRP normal ranges do vary slightly with gestational and postnatal age over the first 48 hours of life, however, with 95th percentile values of 0.6, 6, 10, and 12 mg/L at 0, 12, 24, and 48 hours of age, respectively, for term neonates and 0.6, 5, 10, and 9 mg/L, respectively, for preterm neonates (Fig. 36-4).[53,71-73]

Most surveys in sera of neonates with systemic bacterial infections have shown significant elevations of CRP levels *at the time of onset of signs* (i.e., diagnostic test sensitivity) in 50% to 90% of cases.[12,28,53,73-78] A poor response is particularly frequent among infants whose infection occurs during the first 12 to 24 hours of life and among infants with infection caused by gram-positive bacteria, including group B streptococci.[38,75] Although the intensity of the response does not always reflect the severity of the infection, the relationship between formation of CRP and the degree of tissue injury indicates that infants who show a positive response usually have systemic infections or inflammation.[12]

Yet measurement of CRP levels is not completely specific; diagnostic specificity has been reported to be 85% to 95%.[12,38,74,75,79] The response of CRP to nonbacterial infections is variable, and increased serum levels have been found in infants born to women with chorioamnionitis, as well as those with viral infections, fetal asphyxia, respiratory distress syndrome, intracerebral hemorrhage, and meconium aspiration pneumonitis.[12,59,75]

It is clear from the foregoing discussion that despite new technology permitting more rapid and precise measurement, reliance on *single* CRP levels *alone* as an early indicator of neonatal bacterial infection cannot be recommended. Although CRP levels possibly are helpful in combination with other tests as part of a sepsis screening panel (see later discussion), when a single CRP assay is used alone as an initial test for infection, even if the most favorable results are assumed, approximately 10% of cases would be missed, and 5% of uninfected infants would be incorrectly diagnosed as having infection.

Nevertheless, determination of *serial* CRP levels does seem to be of some value in excluding serious infection.[28,53,77,79] Although assay results in a few infants are normal at the onset of invasive bacterial disease, CRP levels increase rapidly and usually are abnormal within 1 day (CRP doubling time is 8 hours). CRP levels peak at 2 to 3 days and remain elevated until infection is controlled and resolution of the inflammatory process begins.[12,38,53,80] Thereafter, by virtue of a relatively short serum half-life of about 19 hours, CRP levels decline promptly and return to normal within 5 to 10 days in most infants who have a favorable outcome.[12,79]

Serial measurements of CRP levels over 1 to 3 days after onset of possible neonatal bacterial infection may help determine the duration of antibiotic therapy and identify the occurrence of relapse or complications during or after treatment of known infection. Several studies document that serial determination of CRP levels in this fashion yields diagnostic sensitivity of 75% to 98%, specificity of 90%, and, perhaps most notably, negative predictive value of 99%.[62,75-81] These studies suggest that although the relatively low sensitivity of initial CRP determination precludes the firm diagnosis of bacterial infection, the very high negative predictive value of several normal CRP determinations in combination allows the early cessation of empirical 7- to 10-day courses of intravenous antibiotics. It is less likely, however, that serial CRP determinations would allow cessation of empirical 2- to 3-day courses of antibiotics. Also, the kinetics of increase and decrease of elevated CRP levels does not differ sufficiently to allow distinction between newborns with positive bacterial blood cultures and newborns with negative bacterial blood cultures.[80]

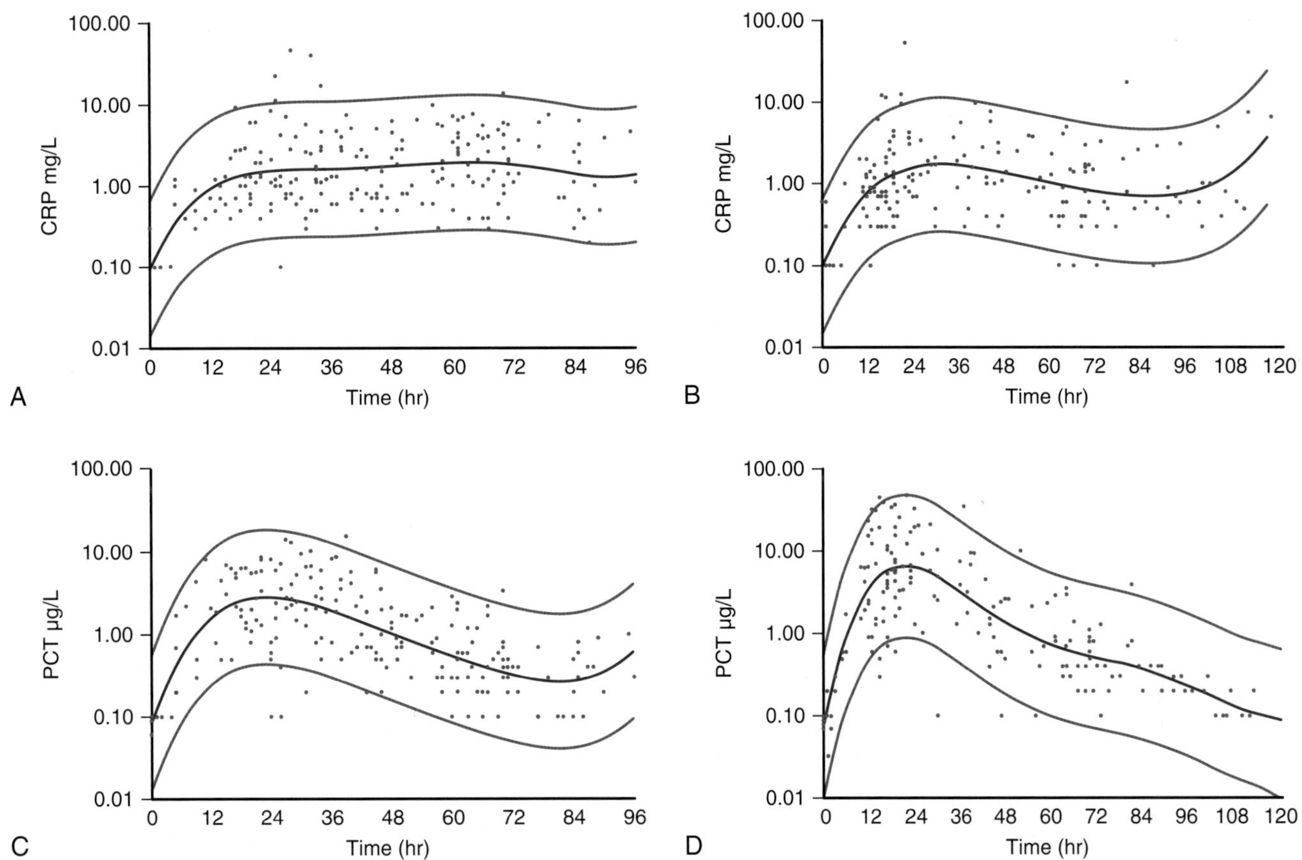

Figure 36-4 Age-specific 95% reference intervals for C-reactive protein (CRP) and procalcitonin (PCT) in otherwise healthy term and preterm neonates. Circles represent single values; the black line represents the geometric means and the blue lines the 95% reference limits. Note that the vertical axis is logarithmic. **A,** CRP, term infants. **B,** CRP, preterm infants. **C,** PCT, term infants. **D,** PCT, preterm infants. (Modified from Chiesa C, Natale F, Pascone R, et al: C-reactive protein and procalcitonin: reference intervals for preterm and term newborns during the early neonatal period, *Clin Chim Acta* 412:1053-1059, 2011.)

PROCALCITONIN

Serum procalcitonin (PCT) is a useful aid for the diagnosis of bacterial sepsis in older children and adults. Several authors also have described an early and specific elevation in serum levels of PCT in infants with invasive bacterial disease.[82-84] Procalcitonin concentrations naturally fluctuate during the first 48 hours of life, however, mandating careful (perhaps hourly) adjustments in the normal reference ranges and complicating use of PCT relative to CRP as a diagnostic aid (see Fig. 36-4).[71,73,85-87] In addition, the normal reference ranges for PCT require adjustment for the estimated gestational age of the premature newborn (see Fig. 36-4).[71,88] In early studies, elevation of PCT levels was only modestly reliable (75%-80% sensitivity and specificity) even for the diagnosis of late-onset sepsis in older neonates in whom the fluctuations after birth had resolved.[89] In a more recent meta-analysis of 16 studies involving nearly 2000 neonates, the pooled sensitivity and specificity of PCT for culture-proven or clinically diagnosed probable sepsis were 81% and 79%, respectively.[90] Marked heterogeneity among studies was present, however, likely due in part to variability of the gestational and chronologic age range of newborns studied and the diagnostic cutoff points for elevated PCT.[90,91] Thus PCT is likely less useful in the diagnosis of neonatal sepsis than it is in the diagnosis of bacterial infections in older children and adults.

Other Biomarkers of Host Inflammation

CYTOKINES AND CHEMOKINES

Cytokines such as IL-1β, IL-6, IL-10, and TNF-α and chemokines such as IL-8 and others are endogenous mediators of the innate immune response to inflammation, including, but not limited to, inflammation caused by bacterial infections. Cord and postnatal blood cytokine concentrations may vary as a result of clinical complications during the perinatal period. IL-1β is elevated in cord plasma specimens from infants born after induced vaginal or urgent cesarean delivery, whereas IL-6 is elevated in the presence of chorioamnionitis and delivery room intubation, yet depressed in the presence of pregnancy-induced hypertension.[74,92,93] Because of the confounding effects of maternal complications, differences in chronologic age from the first hours to days of life, and illness severity, the reported performance of various cytokine markers must be viewed with some caution.[4,71,74] Also, the first reported available laboratory method of measuring a cytokine may not be the most appropriate one. For example, the sensitivity and specificity of IL-8 assays were improved markedly by newer assays of detergent-lysed whole-blood samples, rather than those using plasma samples as reported in earlier studies, because it was found that the majority of IL-8 in blood is not free but is bound to cells via high-affinity receptors and must be released by detergent lysis.[94]

Nevertheless, several studies suggest that elevated levels of IL-6 detected after birth may provide an early and sensitive parameter for the diagnosis of neonatal bacterial infection.[59,73,74,93-96] Similarly, levels of IL-8 were found to be elevated in cord blood from infants in whom histologic evidence of chorioamnionitis was noted and in infants with sepsis.[12,95] Because of variations in study design and methodology, estimates of diagnostic sensitivity and specificity for IL-6 and IL-8 levels range from 60% to greater than 95% for each interleukin.[12,97-99] Both plasma and tracheal aspirate IL-8 and IL-10 levels correlate with bacterial sepsis but are nonspecific in neonates with necrotizing enterocolitis.[100]

ADHESION MOLECULES AND CELLULAR RECEPTORS

Upregulation of adhesion molecules, such as E-selectin, L-selectin, and intercellular adhesion molecule-1, has been suggested as a discriminating feature of bacterial sepsis.[43,76,101] Genetic polymorphisms in mannose-binding lectins seem to underlie susceptibility to infection in some premature neonates; it is unknown whether this analyte could be used for diagnostic purposes.[102] Cytokine receptors and receptor antagonists, such as soluble TNF-α, IL-2 receptors, and an IL-1 receptor antagonist, have been explored as potential aids in the laboratory diagnosis of neonatal sepsis.[96,97,103,104] Further clinical data are needed to determine whether measurement of these analytes is truly useful for the diagnosis and follow-up evaluation of neonatal sepsis.

MISCELLANEOUS ANALYTES

Fibronectin is an adhesive, high-molecular-weight glycoprotein of 450,000 kDa that has been identified on cell surfaces and in extracellular fluids. It is thought that fibronectin acts both as an intercellular cement to maintain microvascular integrity and as an opsonin to aid in WBC phagocytosis.[52,105] In general, the concentration of fibronectin in fetal plasma increases with gestational age to concentrations at term of approximately half the concentrations found in healthy adults.[105] Plasma concentrations usually decrease significantly during the course of neonatal sepsis, and the rate of recovery of fibronectin concentrations as infection resolves is relatively rapid, occurring over 5 to 7 days.[105] However, attempts to characterize a decrease in fibronectin concentrations as a specific marker for sepsis have been disappointing.[12]

Demonstration of increased amounts of *total serum IgM* in umbilical cord blood previously was thought to be helpful in identifying infants with infections acquired in the intrauterine environment, particularly infections caused by rubella virus, cytomegalovirus, *Treponema pallidum*, and *Toxoplasma gondii*.[106] On the basis of this experience, several studies, mainly in the late 1960s and early 1970s, attempted to use serially determined IgM concentrations in the evaluation of infants suspected to have acute postnatal bacterial infections. The sensitivity and specificity of IgM concentrations in infants with bacterial sepsis, meningitis, pneumonia, or urinary tract infection were too low for general use.[12,106] Other analytes proposed, but not found to be adequately sensitive, specific, or standardized enough for general use, include *neutrophil reduction of nitroblue tetrazolium (NBT)*, changes in *leukocyte lactate dehydrogenase* or *alkaline phosphatase*, and changes in *host glucose regulation*.[12,107-110]

An exciting discovery in the field of immunology is that multicellular organisms share many evolutionarily conserved aspects of their innate immune systems. Innate immunity depends on molecules such as specialized cellular receptors and binding proteins (e.g., *Toll-like receptors* and *mannose-binding proteins*), serum complement proteins, and several substances produced and released at the site of infection by neutrophils.[111,112] This last group includes the antimicrobial peptides of the defensin and cathelicidin classes, bactericidal/permeability-increasing protein, lysozyme, and lactoferrin.[111-113] Some of these substances are found in vernix caseosa, the lipid-rich substance covering the skin of the fetus and newborn infant.[114] Further studies on the kinetics of these molecules in health and disease may lead to diagnostic aids for newborn sepsis.[113-115]

A novel proteomic approach to identify host biomarkers for the diagnosis of neonatal late-onset sepsis and necrotizing enterocolitis identified prophospholipoprotein CII and a desarginine variant of serum amyloid A as valid predictors, especially when combined into a transformed "*ApoSAA score*."[116] The laboratory turnaround time was fast (<4 hr), and the analytical volume of plasma required was minimal (<50 μL). The apparent diagnostic utility of the ApoSAA score requires confirmation in multicenter trials, but the proteomic approach to finding improved methods of diagnosis of neonatal sepsis may turn out to be important.[116]

Finally, sepsis or, more properly, the systemic inflammatory response to sepsis causes hemodynamic changes in regional blood flow. Early in sepsis, peripheral vasoconstriction is seen, whereas in advanced sepsis, generalized vasodilation and shock occur. An interesting concept in diagnostic techniques for neonatal sepsis is to attempt to measure noninvasively deviations in peripheral vascular reactivity or heart rate characteristics. In one small study, newborns with early-onset sepsis (clinical or bacteriologic) had lower degrees of mean peripheral skin perfusion and a higher amount of postocclusion reactive hyperemia as measured by a laser-Doppler instrument; the sensitivity and specificity for the measurement of reactive hyperemia were equivalent to or greater than those for measurement of IL-6, IL-8, and TNF-α.[95] A number of studies have described a commercially available system for the continuous monitoring of neonatal heart rate characteristics (reductions in heart rate variability and transient decelerations in heart rate; HeRO system[117]). Using this device in combination with a clinical scoring system, including factors such as severe apnea, feeding intolerance, increases in level of ventilator support, I:T ratio, and so forth, predicted sepsis with high levels of sensitivity and specificity.[117] A bedside risk assessment tool using the HeRO monitor, along with the clinical scoring system, led to reduction in mortality in a two-group, randomized multicenter clinical trial in nine neonatal intensive care units (NICUs) (reduction in mortality from 10.2%-8.1%; hazard ratio, 0.78 [95% confidence interval, 0.61 to 0.99]).[118]

Improvements in Pathogen Detection

Microscopic examination of tissues or body fluids is a time-honored but insensitive and nonspecific aid in the diagnosis of neonatal sepsis. An association of neonatal sepsis with pathologic changes in the placenta and umbilical cord was suggested more than 40 years ago.[119,120] Neonatal infection acquired at or about the time of birth often is associated with chorioamnionitis or funisitis.[12,121] Histologic sections of the placenta may show acute inflammatory changes, with infiltration of the umbilical vein by neutrophils and gross or microscopic evidence of chorioamnionitis. However, some inflammatory changes are apparent in the placenta and its membranes or the umbilical cord in 30% of live-born infants, and the presence of chorioamnionitis and placentitis does not automatically imply significant neonatal infection.[12] The stomach of the newborn contains fluid swallowed before and during delivery, and the ear canal may also be filled with amniotic fluid. The presence of neutrophils and bacteria in a stained smear of the gastric or ear canal aspirate indicates inflammation of the amniotic fluid, placenta, and other tissues of the birth canal.[12,122,123] The presence of these maternal leukocytes indicates exposure to possible infection and does not identify an infectious disease in the newborn. Pathogens frequently are isolated when daily tracheal aspirates for intubated infants are cultured. Because many, if not all, intubated newborns eventually become colonized with potentially pathogenic microbes, however, the positive predictive value of this test is less than 30%.[124] Similar to gastric aspirates or external ear canal fluid, tracheal aspirates reflect environmental influences but do not imply sepsis.

Molecular detection tests for bacteria or bacterial products have been applied to amniotic fluid and neonatal blood. The limulus lysate assay for the detection of endotoxin did not prove to be clinically useful.[12] PCR amplification of bacterial DNA from blood seems promising but is not ready for general clinical use.[125,126] A recent systematic review and meta-analysis of molecular nucleic acid amplification assays for pathogens in blood found a pooled sensitivity and specificity of 90% and 96%, respectively, when measured against the gold standard of microbial blood culture.[126] Although amplification methodology changes over time, variability of gestational age, and type of sepsis likely contributed to some study heterogeneity, the analysis used clinically relevant diagnostic criteria and was methodologically sound. Nucleic acid amplification tests such as PCR are likely to be improved over time and perhaps someday will become the new gold standard for the diagnosis of neonatal sepsis.

Combination Diagnostic Screening Panels

As we have seen by this point, no single laboratory test—even nucleic acid amplification assays of blood—provides a rapid, reliable, and early identification of neonates with bacterial sepsis. This has led to efforts to devise a panel of screening tests, combining data from several different determinations, as a means of increasing the joint predictive value of the tests.[57,71,76,127] The results generally have shown disappointingly little increase in positive predictive value (if a test result is abnormal, disease is present) compared with most individual screening tests, although their negative predictive value (if a result is normal, disease is absent) has been remarkably good, approaching 100% in some studies. Performance characteristics of some screening panel tests are summarized in Table 36-2 and compared with single tests.

One attempt to diagnose neonatal sepsis through multiple, simple, standard laboratory determinations involved more than 500 infants younger than 7 days studied by Philip and colleagues.[15,128] The authors devised a "sepsis screen" for use with infants believed to be at risk for, or showing clinical evidence of, serious bacterial infection. In addition to the standard procedures (blood, CSF, urine cultures, and chest radiographs), the evaluation included a screening panel consisting of total leukocyte count, determination of the I:M ratio, CRP and haptoglobin assays, and microerythrocyte sedimentation rate. An abnormality in any two or more of these items was considered to reflect a "positive sepsis screen," and no abnormality or an abnormality in one item reflected a "negative sepsis screen"; the test turnaround time was 1 hour.

Analysis of the results[12,15,128] showed a 39% probability that serious bacterial infection was present if two or more test results were positive (positive predictive value) and a 99% probability that infection was not present if only one or no result was positive (negative predictive value). In actual numbers, as a result of the sepsis screen, 60 of 524 infants with clinically suspected sepsis received unnecessary treatment with antimicrobial agents (false positives; specificity of 88%), and 3 with subsequently proven bacterial infection were missed (false negatives; sensitivity of 93%). Comparable results have been reported by others who used only hematologic or clinical indices.[12,13,21,30] Panels of screening tests have not always functioned better than relying solely on the I:T neutrophil ratio, however, particularly in the first week of life.[12,15,23,30,31]

By virtue of its high negative predictive value, one of the screening panels described above resulted in a significant decrease in the use of antimicrobial agents in a NICU in which it was applied.[128] Not only did fewer neonates receive antimicrobial agents, but also treatment could be discontinued earlier with greater confidence in the infants who were being administered these agents. As with serial CRP testing, the ability to safely discontinue antibiotics once started has value in today's modern NICU. Similarly, a screening panel combining clinical evaluation and IL-8 and CRP assays led to fewer antibiotic courses being administered compared with neonates treated with standard clinical diagnosis.[127] However, neither the IL-8 nor the CRP assays detected all bacteremic neonates at the time of the first evaluation.[127] As noted above, the combination of continuous monitoring of heart rate characteristics and clinical factors together may form a type of screening panel that has value in predicting onset of sepsis and in decreasing mortality.[117,118]

An increasingly important area in which a screening test panel might be useful is in the evaluation of asymptomatic infants whose mothers have been given intrapartum antibiotics to decrease the risk of early-onset neonatal group B

Table 36-2 Performance Characteristics of Tests and Screening Panels for Early-Onset Neonatal Bacteremia: Selected Reports

Source, Test (Test Cutoff*)	No. Evaluated	Prevalence of Bacterial Sepsis (%)	Sens. (%)	Spec. (%)	PPV (%)	NPV (%)	LR+	LR−
Philip[15]								
Any ≥2 abnormalities in I:T ratio, total WBC, CRP, ESR, haptoglobin	376	8	93	88	39	99	7.8	0.08
Chiesa[73]	134	8						
CRP: At birth (4 mg/L)			73	83	28	97	4.3	0.33
CRP: At 24 hr of age (10 mg/L)			91	87	38	99	7	0.10
IL-6: At birth (200 ng/L)			73	89	36	97	6.6	0.30
IL-6: At 24 hr of age (30 ng/L)			64	71	16	96	2.2	0.50
PCT: At birth (1 μg/L)			82	95	60	98	16.4	0.19
PCT: At 24 hr of age (100 μg/L)			100	96	69	100	2.5	≈0
Døllner[74]	166	14.5						
CRP (10 mg/L)			63	89	48	93	5.7	0.42
IL-6 (20 ng/L)			78	64	27	95	2.2	0.34
CRP, IL-6, or both			96	58	28	99	3.7	0.07
Franz[127]	1291	1	80	87	68	93	6.2	0.23
Clinical signs, plus CRP (10 mg/L), IL-8 (70 ng/L), or both								
Benitz[77]	999	1.5	89	70	5	99	3	0.16
Serial CRP levels: Any of 3 tests performed over 48 hr (10 mg/L)								
Auriti[91]	762	N/A	77	69	19	97	2.5	0.3
PCT: At >48 hr of age (1 μg/L)								
Vouloumanou[90]	1959	N/A	81	79	N/A	N/A	3.9	0.24
PCT: Meta-analysis (varied, 0.5-5 μg/L)								
Pammi[126]	5670	8%	90	96	N/A	N/A	22.5	0.1
Molecular amplification of blood cultures, meta-analysis (positive/negative)								

CRP, C-reactive protein; *ESR*, erythrocyte sedimentation rate; *IL-6*, interleukin-6; *IL-8*, interleukin-8; *I:T*, immature-to-total neutrophil ratio; *LR+*, positive likelihood ratio; *LR−*, negative likelihood ratio; *N/A*, not available from data cited; *NPV*, negative predictive value; *PCT*, procalcitonin; *PPV*, positive predictive value; *Sens.*, sensitivity; *Spec.*, specificity; *WBC*, white blood cell count.

*Test cutoff refers to the value above which the test result is considered abnormal.

streptococcal sepsis.[6,8] The American Academy of Pediatrics and the U.S. Centers for Disease Control and Prevention recommend that a "limited evaluation," consisting of complete blood cell count and a blood culture, be performed in infants whose mothers met the criteria for intrapartum antibiotic prophylaxis but who did not receive a complete course of prophylactic treatment. The goal is to identify infants with sepsis, including infants whose blood cultures may have been sterilized temporarily by maternal antibiotic prophylaxis.[129]

Ottolini and colleagues[18] tested the utility of a complete blood count screening panel in 1665 initially asymptomatic infants whose mothers met the criteria for intrapartum antibiotic prophylaxis but did not receive a full course of treatment. The diagnostic test sensitivity and specificity of an abnormal white blood cell count (i.e., total white blood cell count of ≤5000/mm^3 or ≥30,000/mm^3, ANC of <1500/mm^3, or I:M ratio of >0.2) were 41% and 73%, respectively.[18] Because of the low incidence of true sepsis, even after only partial maternal antibiotic prophylaxis, the positive predictive value of the complete blood count panel was only 1.5% and the positive LR only 1.5. A positive test result was not indicative of newborn sepsis. The negative predictive value of the screen was 99%, implying that a normal test result would at least reassure the clinician that sepsis was not present. However, the negative predictive value of an infant appearing asymptomatic also was 99%; the complete blood count panel did not add any diagnostic information beyond that gained simply by obtaining a careful history and physical examination of the infant. Similar conclusions were reached by Escobar and colleagues[130]; in their study of nearly 3000 neonates evaluated for sepsis, clinical signs were essentially equivalent to low ANC or I:T ratios in predicting sepsis. The ineffectiveness of the screening panel in these studies may have been due to the low rates of culture-proven sepsis, especially among asymptomatic infants, but many U.S. centers where group B streptococcal sepsis prophylaxis is used now do have such low (or even lower) rates of sepsis.[6,8]

Perspectives and Conclusions

WHY HAVE WE NOT YET IDENTIFIED A "BEST TEST"?

As discussed previously, on examining all of the data published to date, it is difficult to choose one cytokine, acute-phase reactant, or screening panel for current use as the "best" test (see Table 36-2).[71,97,98,127] Why is this still the case in the 21st century, after so many advances in medical science and biotechnology and with the plethora of studies of newborn sepsis? Why has the "ideal test" not been discovered[10,11]? Besides the difficulties in constructing a quick, easy-to-analyze, stable, analytic test with clear diagnostic cutoffs across gestational ages, birth weights, and optimal sensitivity and specificity,[10,11] there are further epidemiologic and clinical constraints in study design that are limiting.

Recall that the meta-analysis of nucleic acid amplification assays of blood cultures found a pooled sensitivity and specificity of 90% and 96%, respectively.[126] The authors correctly note that even with their best-case scenario of a diagnostic test with 90% sensitivity and 96% specificity (a positive LR of 22.5 and negative LR of 0.1) in a modern NICU with a 2% prevalence of early-onset sepsis, two cases of sepsis would be missed among 1000 newborns tested, and 39 would be overtreated with antibiotics.[126] To not miss any neonate with early-onset sepsis in this idealized setting, a test with greater than or equal to 98% sensitivity would be required, a rate not yet achievable with any of the molecular methods surveyed.[126]

Second, while designing studies of new diagnostic tests, some authors do not differentiate between perinatal (early-onset) and postnatal (late-onset) sepsis. This omission can lead to bias because different neonatal pathogens cause early-onset and late-onset disease, and the sepsis rate differs among these two populations. In addition, the normal ranges of the test analytes vary across gestational and chronologic age, again confounding the results or, at least, reducing their clinical validity.[71-73]

Third, not all reports of neonatal sepsis diagnostic tests include healthy control subjects, and consequently, construction of the normal range of results for an analytic test poses difficulties. Another problem is the lack of universal agreement on the definition of newborn sepsis or systemic inflammatory response syndrome. Some studies restrict the analyses to culture-proven sepsis, although false-negative cultures resulting from low blood sample volume or maternal antibiotic therapy may lead to bias. Other studies analyze clinical septicemia, although no universal definition of this entity exists, which also may lead to diagnostic bias; very few studies separately analyze data using proven and clinically diagnosed sepsis as different gold standards for the practitioner to review.[74] A fifth problem is that the current neonatal illness severity scores (e.g., Score for Neonatal Acute Physiology [SNAP], SNAP-Perinatal Extension [SNAP-PE], Clinical Risk Index for Babies [CRIB]), which theoretically could lead to better stratification of patients and more accurate interstudy comparisons, are cumbersome to use.[71]

Finally, as noted by Chiesa and colleagues,[71] "the usefulness of a test will depend, above all, on the clinical condition of the baby. If the baby is really very sick, the test will not give very much additional information...if the baby is evidently well...a positive test result [will] not dramatically increase the probability that the baby is infected...." In other words, it is essential for the clinician to heed Bayesian statistical theory: One must consider the pretest (prior) probability (essentially, the disease prevalence) of infection and the test characteristics (sensitivity, specificity) to interpret and apply diagnostic test results properly.[131] Intuitively, one would expect that a group of tests, each with at least a modestly high positive LR value (or reasonably low negative LR value) could be combined to form a panel with a summary positive LR value great enough to diagnose sepsis (or a summary negative LR low enough to exclude it). However, depending on the pretest (prior) probability of sepsis in any one neonate, such a panel still may not be informative, even though on average it would be for a NICU population as a whole.

Many of the confounding effects just discussed are evident in the data of Table 36-2, in which various studies have used different populations of infants, definitions of sepsis, and laboratory cutoff points, leading to different estimates of the utility of any one laboratory test.

WHAT MUST WE DO WITHOUT AN IDENTIFIED "BEST TEST"?

Faced with the imperfection of currently available laboratory aids for the diagnosis of neonatal sepsis, what is today's practitioner to do? History, physical examination, and clinical impression still constitute a large part of clinical medicine, even in the era of molecular diagnostics and therapeutics. A single normal laboratory test should not sway a clinician against empirical therapy for a newborn if it seems to be clinically indicated, and an isolated abnormal test result should not be enough for the clinician to demand therapy. This concept may be restated in diagnostic test statistical terminology as follows: At present, there is no one test or test panel with a high enough positive LR or a low enough negative LR to recommend it uniquely over all others. The negative predictive values of available tests are not yet high enough, when results are normal, to lead to the withholding of therapy for an uncommon but possibly life-threatening disease (neonatal sepsis). Conversely, the positive predictive values of available tests are not yet high enough when results are abnormal to lead to routine institution of antimicrobial therapy.

When laboratory testing is combined with clinical impression, and perhaps serial laboratory monitoring, predictive values may increase enough to help the clinician make decisions. When the risk of an uncommon disease with a poor outcome is high, however, and the risk of antimicrobial therapy is low, it may be difficult ever to find a test with predictive values high enough to "rule in" or "rule out" disease with complete confidence.

Clinical judgment, using standardized definitions of historical risk factors, signs, and symptoms, may sometimes perform as well as laboratory screening panels.[18,130] This point may be especially important to remember in resource-poor settings in developing countries.[132] Much future work is needed in the area of rapid diagnosis of neonatal sepsis to move beyond the current best menu of simple, rapid, and inexpensive (albeit imperfect) tests, such as total neutrophil counts, total leukocyte counts, I:T ratios, and CRP assay.[116,133] Continued improvements in pathogen detection techniques are decreasing the time to positivity of neonatal blood cultures or molecular assays, which may at least speed up bacteriologic confirmation of septicemia.[126,133]

References

1. Feinstein AR: Clinical biostatistics: XXXI. On the sensitivity, specificity, and discrimination of diagnostic tests, *Clin Pharmacol Ther* 17:104-116, 1975.
2. Jaeschke R, Guyatt GH, Sackett DL: Users' guides to the medical literature. III. How to use an article about a diagnostic test. B. What are the results and will they help me in caring for my patients? *JAMA* 271:703-707, 1994.
3. Radetsky M: The laboratory evaluation of newborn sepsis, *Curr Opin Infect Dis* 8:191-199, 1995.

4. Escobar GJ: Effect of the systemic inflammatory response on biochemical markers of neonatal bacterial infection: a fresh look at old confounders, *Clin Chem* 49:21-22, 2003.
5. Squire E, Favara B, Todd J: Diagnosis of neonatal bacterial infection: hematologic and pathologic findings in fatal and nonfatal cases, *Pediatrics* 64:60-64, 1979.
6. Stoll BJ, Hansen N, Fanaroff AA, et al: Changes in pathogens causing early-onset sepsis in very-low-birth-weight infants, *N Engl J Med* 347:240-247, 2002.
7. Stoll BJ, Hansen N, Fanaroff AA, et al: Late-onset sepsis in very low birth weight neonates: the experience of the NICHD Neonatal Research Network, *Pediatrics* 110:285-291, 2002.
8. Stoll BJ, Hansen NI, Sánchez PJ, et al: Early onset neonatal sepsis: the burden of group B streptococcal and *E. coli* disease continues, *Pediatrics* 127:817-826, 2011.
9. Boghossian NS, Page GP, Bell EF, et al: Late-onset sepsis in very low birth weight infants from singleton and multiple-gestation births, *J Pediatr* 162:1120-1124, 2013.
10. Ng PC, Lam HS: Diagnostic markers for neonatal sepsis, *Curr Opin Pediatr* 18:125-131, 2006.
11. Lam HS, Ng PC: Biochemical markers of neonatal sepsis, *Pathology* 40:141-148, 2008.
12. Weinberg GA, D'Angio CT: Laboratory aids for diagnosis of neonatal sepsis. In Remington JS, Klein JO, Wilson CB, et al: *Infectious diseases of the fetus and newborn infant*, ed 7, Philadelphia, 2011, Saunders, pp 1144-1160.
13. Spector SA, Ticknor W, Grossman M: Study of the usefulness of clinical and hematologic findings in the diagnosis of neonatal bacterial infections, *Clin Pediatr* 20:385-392, 1981.
14. Newman TB, Puopolo KM, Wi S, et al: Interpreting complete blood counts soon after birth in newborns at risk for sepsis, *Pediatrics* 126:903-909, 2010.
15. Philip AGS, Hewitt JR: Early diagnosis of neonatal sepsis, *Pediatrics* 65:1036-1041, 1980.
16. Jahnke S, Bartiromo G, Maisels MJ: The peripheral white blood cell count in the diagnosis of neonatal infection, *J Perinatol* 5:50-56, 1985.
17. Rozycki HJ, Stahl GE, Baumgart S: Impaired sensitivity of a single early leukocyte count in screening for neonatal sepsis, *Pediatr Infect Dis J* 6:440-442, 1987.
18. Ottolini MC, Lundgren K, Mirkinson LJ, et al: Utility of complete blood count and blood culture screening to diagnose neonatal sepsis in the asymptomatic at risk newborn, *Pediatr Infect Dis J* 22:430-434, 2003.
19. Weinberg AG, Rosenfeld CR, Manroe BL, et al: Neonatal blood cell count in health and disease. II. Values for lymphocytes, monocytes, and eosinophils, *J Pediatr* 106:462-466, 1985.
20. Xanthou M: Leucocyte blood picture in ill newborn babies, *Arch Dis Child* 47:741-746, 1972.
21. Manroe BL, Weinberg AG, Rosenfeld CR, et al: The neonatal blood count in health and disease. I. Reference values for neutrophilic cells, *J Pediatr* 95:89-98, 1979.
22. Zipursky A, Palko J, Milner R, et al: The hematology of bacterial infections in premature infants, *Pediatrics* 57:839-853, 1976.
23. Rodwell RL, Leslie AL, Tudehope DI: Early diagnosis of neonatal sepsis using a hematologic scoring system, *J Pediatr* 112:761-767, 1988.
24. Xanthou M: Leucocyte blood picture in healthy full-term and premature babies during neonatal period, *Arch Dis Child* 45:242-249, 1970.
25. Gregory J, Hey E: Blood neutrophil response to bacterial infection in the first month of life, *Arch Dis Child* 47:747-753, 1972.
26. Mouzinho A, Rosenfeld CR, Sánchez PJ, et al: Revised reference ranges for circulating neutrophils in very-low-birth-weight neonates, *Pediatrics* 94:76-82, 1999.
27. Schelonka RL, Yoder BA, desJardins SE, et al: Peripheral leukocyte count and leukocyte indexes in healthy newborn term infants, *J Pediatr* 125:603-606, 1994.
28. Da Silva O, Ohlsson A, Kenyon C: Accuracy of leukocyte indices and C-reactive protein for diagnosis of neonatal sepsis: a critical review, *Pediatr Infect Dis J* 14:363-366, 1995.
29. Christensen RD, Bradley PP, Rothstein G: The leukocyte left shift in clinical and experimental neonatal sepsis, *J Pediatr* 98:101-105, 1981.
30. Rodwell RL, Tudehope DI, Gray PH: Hematologic scoring system in early diagnosis of sepsis in neutropenic newborns, *Pediatr Infect Dis* 12:372-376, 1993.
31. Manroe BL, Rosenfeld CR, Weinberg AG, et al: The differential leukocyte count in the assessment and outcome of early-onset neonatal group B streptococcal disease, *J Pediatr* 91:632-637, 1977.
32. Courtney SE, Hall RT: *Haemophilus influenzae* sepsis in the premature infant, *Am J Dis Child* 132:1039-1040, 1978.
33. Bortolussi R, Thompson TR, Ferrieri P: Early-onset pneumococcal sepsis in newborn infants, *Pediatrics* 60:352-355, 1977.
34. Christensen RD, Rothstein G: Exhaustion of mature marrow neutrophils in neonates with sepsis, *J Pediatr* 96:316-318, 1980.
35. Boyle RJ, Chandler BD, Stonestreet BS, et al: Early identification of sepsis in infants with respiratory distress, *Pediatrics* 62:744-750, 1978.
36. Wheeler JG, Chauvenet AR, Johnson CA, et al: Neutrophil storage pool depletion in septic, neutropenic neonates, *Pediatr Infect Dis* 3:407-409, 1984.
37. Gerdes JS: Clinicopathologic approach to the diagnosis of neonatal sepsis, *Clin Perinatol* 18:361-381, 1991.
38. Mathers NJ, Pohlandt F: Diagnostic audit of C-reactive protein in neonatal infection, *Eur J Pediatr* 146:147-151, 1987.
39. Kite P, Millar MR, Gorham P, et al: Comparison of five tests used in diagnosis of neonatal bacteraemia, *Arch Dis Child* 63:639-643, 1988.
40. Aballi AJ, Puapondh Y, Desposito F: Platelet counts in thriving premature infants, *Pediatrics* 42:685-689, 1968.
41. Andrew M, Kelton J: Neonatal thrombocytopenia, *Clin Perinatol* 11:359-390, 1984.
42. Guida JD, Kunig AM, Leef KH, et al: Platelet count and sepsis in very low birth weight neonates. Is there an organism-specific response, *Pediatrics* 111:1411-1415, 2003.
43. Kim SK, Keeney SE, Alpard SK, et al: Comparison of L-selectin and CD11b on neutrophils of adults and neonates during the first month of life, *Pediatr Res* 53:132-136, 2003.
44. Turunen R, Andersson S, Nupponen I, et al: Increased CD11b-density on circulating phagocytes as an early sign of late-onset sepsis in extremely low-birth-weight infants, *Pediatr Res* 57:270-275, 2005.
45. Cholette JM, Blumberg N, Phipps RP, et al: Developmental changes in soluble CD40 ligand, *J Pediatr* 152:50-54, 2008.
46. Ng PC, Li K, Wong RP, et al: Neutrophil CD64 expression: a sensitive diagnostic marker for late-onset nosocomial infection in very low birthweight infants, *Pediatr Res* 51:296-303, 2002.
47. Ng PC, Li G, Chui KM, et al: Neutrophil CD64 is a sensitive diagnostic marker for early-onset neonatal infection, *Pediatr Res* 56:796-803, 2004.
48. Bhandari V, Wang C, Rinder C, et al: Hematologic profile of sepsis in neonates: neutrophil CD64 as a diagnostic marker, *Pediatrics* 121:129-134, 2008.
49. Celik IH, Demirel G, Aksoy HT, et al: Automated determination of neutrophil VCS parameters in diagnosis and treatment efficacy of neonatal sepsis, *Pediatr Res* 71:121-125, 2012.
50. Hodge S, Hodge G, Flower R, et al: Surface activation markers of T lymphocytes: role in the detection of infection in neonates, *Clin Exp Immunol* 113:33-38, 1998.
51. Gabay C, Kushner I: Acute-phase proteins and other systemic responses to inflammation, *N Engl J Med* 340:448-454, 1999.
52. Lu J, Marjon KD, Mold C, et al: Pentraxins and Fc receptors, *Immunol Rev* 250:230-238, 2012.
53. Jaye DL, Waites KB: Clinical applications of C-reactive protein in pediatrics, *Pediatr Infect Dis J* 16:735-747, 1997.
54. Gitlin D, Biasucci A: Development of IgG, IgA, IgM, β1C/β1A, Cv'1 esterase inhibitor, ceruloplasmin, transferrin, hemopexin, haptoglobin, fibrinogen, plasminogen, α1-antitrypsin, orosomucoid, β-lipoprotein, α2-macroglobulin, and prealbumin in the human conceptus, *J Clin Invest* 48:1433-1446, 1969.
55. Barratt BA, Hill PI: A micromethod for the erythrocyte sedimentation rate suitable for use on venous or capillary blood, *J Clin Pathol* 33:1118, 1980.
56. Lascari AD: The erythrocyte sedimentation rate, *Pediatr Clin North Am* 19:1113-1121, 1972.
57. Adler SM, Denton RL: The erythrocyte sedimentation rate in the newborn period, *J Pediatr* 86:942-948, 1975.
58. Jensen AH, Josso F, Zamet P, et al: Evolution of blood clotting factor levels in premature infants during the first 10 days of life: a study of 96 cases with comparison between clinical status and blood clotting factor levels, *Pediatr Res* 7:638-644, 1973.

59. Pourcyrous M, Bada HS, Korones SB, et al: Acute phase reactants in neonatal bacterial infection, *J Perinatol* 11:319-325, 1991.
60. Salmi TT: Haptoglobin levels in the plasma of newborn infants with special reference to infections, *Acta Paediatr Scand* 241:7-55, 1973.
61. Kanakoudi F, Drossou V, Tzimouli V, et al: Serum concentrations of 10 acute-phase proteins in healthy term and preterm infants from birth to age 6 months, *Clin Chem* 41:605-608, 1995.
62. Philip AGS: Acute-phase proteins in neonatal infection, *J Pediatr* 105:940-942, 1984.
63. Philip AGS, Hewitt JR: α1β-Acid glycoprotein in the neonate with and without infection, *Biol Neonate* 43:118-124, 1983.
64. Gutteberg TJ, Haneberg B, Jergensen T: Lactoferrin in relation to acute phase proteins in sera from newborn infants with severe infections, *Eur J Pediatr* 142:37-39, 1984.
65. Rodwell RL, Taylor KM, Tudehope DI, et al: Capillary plasma elastase alpha-1-proteinase inhibitor in infected and non-infected neonates, *Arch Dis Child* 67:436-439, 1992.
66. Arnon S, Litmanovitz I, Regev RH, et al: Serum amyloid A: an early and accurate marker of neonatal early-onset sepsis, *J Perinatol* 27:297-302, 2007.
67. Baek YW, Brokat S, Padbury JF, et al: Inter-alpha inhibitor proteins in infants and decreased levels in neonatal sepsis, *J Pediatr* 143:11-15, 2003.
68. Suri M, Sharma VK, Thirupuram S: Evaluation of ceruloplasmin in neonatal septicemia, *Indian Pediatr* 28:489-493, 1991.
69. Wu TW, Tabangin M, Kusano R, et al: The utility of serum hepcidin as a biomarker for late-onset neonatal sepsis, *J Pediatr* 162:67-71, 2013.
70. Schrama AJJ, de Beaufort AJ, Poorthuis BJ, et al: Secretory phospholipase A2 in newborn infants with sepsis, *J Perinatol* 28:291-296, 2008.
71. Chiesa C, Panero A, Osborn JF, et al: Diagnosis of neonatal sepsis: a clinical and laboratory challenge, *Clin Chem* 50:279-287, 2004.
72. Chiesa C, Natale F, Pascone R, et al: C-reactive protein and procalcitonin: reference intervals for preterm and term newborns during the early neonatal period, *Clin Chim Acta* 412:1053-1059, 2011.
73. Chiesa C, Pellegrini G, Panero A, et al: C-reactive protein, interleukin-6, and procalcitonin in the immediate postnatal period: influence of illness severity, risk status, antenatal and perinatal complications, and infection, *Clin Chem* 49:60-68, 2003.
74. Døllner H, Vatten L, Austgulen R: Early diagnostic markers for neonatal sepsis: comparing C-reactive protein, interleukin-6, soluble tumour necrosis factor receptors and soluble adhesion molecules, *J Clin Epidemiol* 54:1251-1257, 2001.
75. Pourcyrous M, Bada HS, Korones SB, et al: Significance of serial C-reactive protein responses in neonatal infection and other disorders, *Pediatrics* 92:431-435, 1993.
76. Ng PC, Cheng SH, Chui KM, et al: Diagnosis of late onset neonatal sepsis with cytokines, adhesion molecule, and C-reactive protein in preterm very low birthweight infants, *Arch Dis Child* 77:F221-F227, 1997.
77. Benitz WE, Han MY, Madan A, et al: Serial C-reactive protein levels in the diagnosis of neonatal infection, *Pediatrics* 102:e41, 1998.
78. Ehl S, Gering B, Bartmann P, et al: C-reactive protein is a useful marker for guiding duration of antibiotic therapy in suspected neonatal bacterial infection, *Pediatrics* 99:216-221, 1997.
79. Bomela HN, Ballot DE, Cory BJ, et al: Use of C-reactive protein to guide duration of empiric antibiotic therapy in suspected early neonatal sepsis, *Pediatr Infect Dis J* 19:531-535, 2000.
80. Ehl S, Gehring B, Pohlandt F: A detailed analysis of changes in serum C-reactive protein levels in neonates treated for bacterial infection, *Eur J Pediatr* 158:238-242, 1999.
81. Franz AR, Steinbach G, Kron M, et al: Reduction of unnecessary antibiotic therapy in newborn infants using interleukin-8 and C-reactive protein as markers of bacterial infections, *Pediatrics* 104:447-453, 1999.
82. Assicot M, Gendrel D, Carsin H, et al: High serum procalcitonin concentrations in patients with sepsis and infection, *Lancet* 1:515-518, 1993.
83. Gendrel D, Assicot M, Raymond J, et al: Procalcitonin as a marker for the early diagnosis of neonatal infection, *J Pediatr* 128:570-573, 1996.
84. Gendrel D, Bohuon C: Procalcitonin as a marker of bacterial infection, *Pediatr Infect Dis J* 19:679-687, 2000.
85. Van Rossum AMC, Wulkan RW, Oudesluys-Murphy AM: Procalcitonin as an early marker of infection in neonates and children, *Lancet Infect Dis* 4:620-630, 2004.
86. Chiesa C, Panero A, Rossi N, et al: Reliability of procalcitonin concentrations for the diagnosis of sepsis in critically ill neonates, *Clin Infect Dis* 26:664-672, 1998.
87. Lapillone A, Basson E, Monneret G, et al: Lack of specificity of procalcitonin for sepsis diagnosis in premature infants, *Lancet* 351: 1211-1212, 1998.
88. Turner D, Hammerman C, Rudensky B, et al: Procalcitonin in preterm infants during the first few days of life: introducing an age related nomogram, *Arch Dis Child Fetal Neonatal Ed* 91:F283-F286, 2006.
89. López Sastre JB, Pérez Solís D, Roqués Serradilla V, et al: Procalcitonin is not sufficiently reliable to be the sole marker of neonatal sepsis of nosocomial origin, *BMC Pediatr* 6:16, 2006.
90. Vouloumanou EK, Plessa E, Karageorgopoulos DE, et al: Serum procalcitonin as a diagnostic marker for neonatal sepsis: a systematic review and meta-analysis, *Intensive Care Med* 37:747-762, 2011.
91. Auriti C, Fiscarelli E, Ronchetti MP, et al: Procalcitonin in detecting neonatal nosocomial sepsis, *Arch Dis Child Fetal Neonatal Ed* 97: F368-F370, 2012.
92. Miller LC, Isa S, LoPreste G, et al: Neonatal interleukin-1α, interleukin-6, and tumor necrosis factor: cord blood levels and cellular production, *J Pediatr* 117:961-965, 1990.
93. Kashlan F, Smulian J, Shen-Schwarz S, et al: Umbilical vein interleukin 6 and tumor necrosis factor alpha plasma concentrations in the very preterm infant, *Pediatr Infect Dis J* 19:238-243, 2000.
94. Orlikowsky TW, Neunhoeffer F, Goelz R, et al: Evaluation of IL-8 concentrations in plasma and lysed EDTA-blood in healthy neonates and those with suspected early onset bacterial infection, *Pediatr Res* 56:804-809, 2004.
95. Martin H, Olander B, Norman M: Reactive hyperemia and interleukin 6, interleukin 8, and tumor necrosis factor-α in the diagnosis of early-onset neonatal sepsis, *Pediatrics* 108:e61, 2001.
96. Messer J, Eyer D, Donato L, et al: Evaluation of interleukin-6 and soluble receptors of tumor necrosis factor for early diagnosis of neonatal infection, *J Pediatr* 129:574-580, 1996.
97. Malik A, Hui CP, Pennie RA, et al: Beyond the complete blood cell count and C-reactive protein: a systematic review of modern diagnostic tests for neonatal sepsis, *Arch Pediatr Adolesc Med* 157: 511-516, 2003.
98. Mehr S, Doyle LW: Cytokines as markers of bacterial sepsis in newborn infants: a review, *Pediatr Infect Dis J* 19:879-887, 2000.
99. Verboon-Maciolek MA, Thijsen SF, Hemels MA, et al: Inflammatory mediators for the diagnosis and treatment of sepsis in early infancy, *Pediatr Res* 59:457-461, 2006.
100. Harris MC, D'Angio CT, Gallagher PR, et al: Cytokine elaboration in critically ill infants with bacterial sepsis, necrotizing enterocolitis, or sepsis syndrome: correlation with clinical parameters of inflammation and mortality, *J Pediatr* 147:462-468, 2005.
101. Figueras-Aloy J, Gómez-López L, Rodríguez-Miguélez JM, et al: Serum soluble ICAM-1, VCAM-1, L-selectin, and P-selectin levels as markers of infection and their relation to clinical severity in neonatal sepsis, *Am J Perinatol* 24:331-338, 2007.
102. Israëls J, Frakking FN, Kremer LC, et al: Mannose-binding lectin and infection risk in newborns: a systematic review, *Arch Dis Child Fetal Neonatal Ed* 95:F452-F461, 2010.
103. De Bont E, de Leij LH, Okken A: Increased plasma concentrations of interleukin-1 receptor antagonist in neonatal sepsis, *Pediatr Res* 37:626-629, 1995.
104. Spear ML, Stefano JL, Fawcett P, et al: Soluble interleukin-2 receptor as a predictor of neonatal sepsis, *J Pediatr* 126:982-985, 1995.
105. Yang KD, Bohnsack JF, Hill HR: Fibronectin in host defense: implications in the diagnosis, prophylaxis and therapy of infectious diseases, *Pediatr Infect Dis* 12:234-239, 1993.
106. Alford CS Jr: Immunoglobulin determinations in the diagnosis of fetal infection, *Pediatr Clin North Am* 18:99-113, 1971.
107. Baehner RL: Use of the nitroblue tetrazolium test in clinical pediatrics, *Am J Dis Child* 128:449-451, 1974.
108. Powers DW, Ayoub EM: Leukocyte lactate dehydrogenase in bacterial meningitis, *Pediatrics* 54:27-33, 1974.
109. Donato H, Gebara E, de Cosen RH, et al: Leukocyte alkaline phosphatase activity in the diagnosis of neonatal bacterial infections, *J Pediatr* 94:242-244, 1979.
110. Leake RD, Fiser RH Jr, Oh W: Rapid glucose disappearance in infants with infection, *Clin Pediatr* 20:397-401, 1981.
111. Zasloff M: Vernix, the newborn, and innate defense, *Pediatr Res* 53:203-204, 2003.

112. Levy O: Impaired innate immunity at birth: deficiency of bactericidal/permeability-increasing protein (BPI) in the neutrophils of newborns, *Pediatr Res* 51:667-669, 2002.
113. Thomas NJ, Carcillo JA, Doughty LA, et al: Plasma concentrations of defensins and lactoferrin in children with severe sepsis, *Pediatr Infect Dis J* 21:34-38, 2002.
114. Yoshio H, Tollin M, Gudmundsson GH: Antimicrobial polypeptides of human vernix caseosa and amniotic fluid: implications for newborn innate defense, *Pediatr Res* 53:211-216, 2003.
115. Nupponen I, Turunen R, Nevalainen T, et al: Extracellular release of bactericidal/permeability-increasing protein in newborn infants, *Pediatr Res* 51:670-674, 2002.
116. Ng PC, Ang IL, Chiu RW, et al: Host-response biomarkers for diagnosis of late-onset septicemia and necrotizing enterocolitis in preterm infants, *J Clin Invest* 120:2989-3000, 2010.
117. Fairchild KD, O'Shea TM: Heart rate characteristics: physiomarkers for detection of late-onset neonatal sepsis, *Clin Perinatol* 37:581-598, 2010.
118. Moorman JR, Carlo WA, Kattwinkel J, et al: Mortality reduction by heart rate characteristic monitoring in very low birth weight neonates: a randomized trial, *J Pediatr* 159:900-906, 2011.
119. Benirschke K: Routes and types of infection in the fetus and the newborn, *Am J Dis Child* 99:714-721, 1960.
120. Blanc WA: Pathways of fetal and early neonatal infection: viral placentitis, bacterial and fungal chorioamnionitis, *J Pediatr* 59:473-496, 1961.
121. Overbach M, Daniel SJ, Cassady G: The value of umbilical cord histology in the management of potential perinatal infection, *J Pediatr* 76:22-31, 1970.
122. Vasan U, Lim DM, Greenstein RM, et al: Origin of gastric polymorphonuclear leukocytes in infants born after prolonged rupture of membranes, *J Pediatr* 91:69-72, 1977.
123. Scanlon J: The early detection of neonatal sepsis by examination of liquid obtained from the external ear canal, *J Pediatr* 79:247-249, 1971.
124. Lau YL, Hey E: Sensitivity and specificity of daily tracheal aspirate cultures in predicting organisms causing bacteremia in ventilated neonates, *Pediatr Infect Dis J* 10:290-294, 1991.
125. Jordan JA, Durso MB: Comparison of 16S rRNA gene PCR and BACTEC 9240 for detection of neonatal bacteremia, *J Clin Microbiol* 38:2574-2578, 2000.
126. Pammi M, Flores A, Leeflang M, et al: Molecular assays in the diagnosis of neonatal sepsis: a systematic review and meta-analysis, *Pediatrics* 128:e973-e985, 2011.
127. Franz AR, Bauer K, Schalk A, et al: Measurement of interleukin 8 in combination with C-reactive protein reduced unnecessary antibiotic therapy in newborn infants: a multicenter, randomized, controlled trial, *Pediatrics* 114:1-8, 2004.
128. Philip AGS: Decreased use of antibiotics using a neonatal sepsis screening technique, *J Pediatr* 98:795-799, 1981.
129. American Academy of Pediatrics: 2012 Group B streptococcal infections. In Pickering LK, Baker CJ, Kimberlin. DW, Long SS, editors: *Red book: report of the Committee on Infectious Diseases*, ed 29, Elk Grove Village, Ill, 2012, American Academy of Pediatrics.
130. Escobar GJ, Li DK, Armstrong MA, et al: Neonatal sepsis workups in infants >2000 grams at birth: a population-based study, *Pediatrics* 106:256-263, 2000.
131. Gill CJ, Sabin L, Schmid CH: Why clinicians are natural Bayesians, *BMJ* 330:1080-1083, 2005. [Erratum in *BMJ* 330:1369, 2005].
132. Weber MW, Carlin JB, Gatchalian S, et al: Predictors of neonatal sepsis in developing countries, *Pediatr Infect Dis J* 22:711-717, 2003.
133. Srinivasan L, Harris MC: New technologies for the rapid diagnosis of neonatal sepsis, *Curr Opin Pediatr* 24:165-171, 2012.

37 Clinical Pharmacology of Antiinfective Drugs

KELLY C. WADE and DANIEL K. BENJAMIN, JR.

CHAPTER OUTLINE

Effective antimicrobial treatment typically begins with empirical therapy at a dose that is most likely to cure the infection with the minimal risk of toxic effects. To select the correct dosage, clinicians need to understand and apply the principles of pharmacokinetics (PK) and pharmacodynamics (PD). This chapter will focus on basic pharmacology and the application of PK and PD principles to the most commonly used antiinfective drugs, to guide optimal therapy of common infections in the newborn and young infant.

Since the seventh edition of this book, progress has been made in understanding the PK and PD of many antimicrobial drugs in preterm and term neonates. We have added relevant new information for several drugs and added metronidazole to the list of drugs reviewed. To focus the reader's attention on the most relevant and available literature we have trimmed the reference list. Information on antimicrobial drugs that are no longer used or rarely used have been omitted to make room for new information.

The clinical pharmacology, indication, dosing, and toxicity of licensed drugs from well-controlled studies submitted to and approved by the U.S. Food and Drug Administration (FDA) are included in the product label and available at www.daily.med.nlm.nih.gov or on the FDA general website at www.accessdata.fda.gov.[1] However, the use of many drugs remains off-label in term and premature neonates because of inadequate PK, safety, and efficacy studies. We have organized drugs into the following five categories: (1) gram-positive infections, including methicillin-resistant *Staphylococcus aureus* (MRSA); (2) gram-negative infections; (3) polymicrobial or complicated serious infections; (4) viral infections; and (5) fungal infections. The pharmacology of drugs in neonates is unique and should not be extrapolated from data derived from studies in older patients, whenever possible. Few drugs have been adequately studied in the extremely preterm infant, so many of the dosing guidelines in this high-risk patient group remain empirical. In such cases, we will review the mechanism of action and dosing relative to known PK-PD properties and safety. The National Institute of Child Health and Development (NICHD)-sponsored Pediatric Trials Network (www.pediatrictrialsnetwork.org) is conducting several antimicrobial trials in neonates with the goal of improved dosing and label guidance.

A few antimicrobial drugs have been associated with serious toxicity (Table 37-1), and therefore their use in neonates is discouraged in developed countries. The most notable on this list is chloramphenicol. Chloramphenicol has been associated with circulatory collapse, otherwise known as "gray baby syndrome," and death in infants resulting from drug accumulation after excessive dosages. This complication can be traced to immaturity of the glucuronyl transferase activity in the fetus and young newborn infants, coupled with diminished renal function.[2] Chloramphenicol toxicity appears to be related to impaired mitochondrial protein synthesis, as well as to direct inhibition of myocardial contractile activity. Because this toxicity results from free-drug accumulation, multiple exchange transfusions or charcoal hemoperfusion may reverse the clinical syndrome by removing the free drug from the blood.[3] Anemia resulting from dose-related marrow suppression is the most common untoward reaction to chloramphenicol; however, severe idiosyncratic bone marrow aplasia occurs in approximately 1 in 40,000 patients of all ages receiving the antibiotic.[4]

Table 37-1 Drugs Not Routinely Used in Neonates*

Drug	Potential Adverse Effect
Tetracycline	Depressed bone growth and teeth abnormalities
Chloramphenicol	Circulatory collapse, impaired mitochondrial protein synthesis, bone marrow aplasia; gray baby syndrome
Sulfonamide	Bilirubin displacement with rare but possible kernicterus; increased risk of hemolysis in G6PD-deficient infants
Trimethoprim-sulfamethoxazole	Bilirubin displacement with rare but possible kernicteru; increased risk of hemolysis in G6PD-deficient infants. Possible bone marrow suppression
Ceftriaxone	Highly protein bound, potential to displace bilirubin; cannot be co-administered with calcium-containing fluids because of risk of precipitation of ceftriaxone-calcium salts and serious cardiovascular adverse events

G6PD, Glucose-6-phosphate dehydrogenase.
*Information from References 2, 3, and 4.

Basic Principles of Clinical Pharmacology

The rapidly changing physiologic processes characteristic of fetal and neonatal development profoundly affect the PK properties of antibiotics.[5,6] Maturation affects total body water, drug metabolism, and drug elimination. Gastric absorption is highly variable. These changes can result either in subtherapeutic drug concentrations, thereby delaying bacterial eradication, or in toxic drug concentrations that cause morbidity. Common PK terms and abbreviations are defined in Table 37-2.

The PK of a drug describes the relationship between drug dose and subsequent concentration in the blood over time. Four basic components explain the PK of a drug: absorption, distribution, metabolism, and excretion. Absorption of drugs administered at extravascular sites typically occurs by passive diffusion across biologic membranes. This process is affected by chemical properties of the drug, such as its molecular weight, ionization, and lipid solubility, as well as by physiologic factors, such as local pH and blood flow, which undergo developmental changes as the newborn matures. The severity of infections and the inconsistent absorption after extravascular administration warrant that most antimicrobial therapies be delivered by the intravenous (IV) route in developed countries.

Oral absorption of antimicrobial agents is difficult to predict and can only be determined by carefully executed experiments. Bioavailability describes the fraction of an administered dose of a drug that reaches the systemic circulation. By definition, IV medications have 100% bioavailability. However, oral medications have decreased bioavailability because of incomplete absorption and first-pass hepatic metabolism. Unique neonatal features that impact absorption change with gestational and chronologic age include the alkaline gastric pH, slow gastric emptying, high gastrointestinal-to-whole body surface area ratio, increased permeability of bowel mucosa, irregular peristalsis, prolonged intestinal transit time, differences in first-pass

Table 37-2 Common Pharmacokinetic and Neonatal Terminology

Term	Abbreviation	Definition	Units
PHARMACOKINETIC TERMS			
Maximum concentrations	C_{max}	Maximum drug concentration at end of infusion. Alternatively, for drugs that are rapidly distributed (α-phase), the peak concentrations may be evaluated 30 minutes after end of infusion to give the concentration after the initial rapid phase of distribution	μg/mL
Minimum concentrations	C_{min}	Minimum drug concentration just before subsequent dose	μg/mL
Clearance	CL	The amount of blood from which all drug is removed per unit time through both renal and nonrenal mechanisms	mL/min/kg L/hr/kg
Volume of distribution	Vd	Hypothetical volume of fluid through which a drug is dispersed	L/kg
Elimination rate constant	k_e k_e = Vd/CL	For drugs with first-order kinetics, the ratio of clearance to volume of distribution (CL/Vd)	L/hr
Half-life	$t_{½}$ of β-phase = (0.693)/k_e	Time it takes to clear half of the drug from plasma. It is directly proportional to the Vd and inversely proportional to CL	hours
Bioavailability	F	The fraction of the administered dose that reaches the systemic circulation. F = 1 for intravenous administration. After oral administration, F is reduced by incomplete absorption, first-pass metabolism, and distribution into other tissue	%
Area under the concentration-time curve	AUC	Measure of total drug exposure, typically over 24-hour period	mg*hr/L
NEONATAL TERMS			
Gestational age	GA	Gestational age at birth, typically rounded down to completed weeks	weeks
Postnatal age	PNA	Chronologic age of infant, i.e., day of life	days
Postmenstrual age	PMA	Corrected GA on day of study, GA + PNA	weeks

hepatic metabolism, and the deconjugational activity of the intestinal enzyme β-glucuronidase.

Intramuscular (IM) absorption of antimicrobial agents is generally comparable to IV administration; however, substantial differences can exist because IM antibiotic absorption is dependent upon regional blood flow. IM absorption can be profoundly reduced in infants with hypoxia, hypotension, or poor tissue perfusion.

After drug absorption into the bloodstream, the dose of a drug is distributed into all of the body compartments and tissues that the product is physically able to penetrate, including water compartments and adipose tissue. This distributive phase is typically rapid, and the drug is said to distribute into its volume of distribution, or Vd. This volume is considered hypothetical because it is based on sampling drug concentrations in serum or plasma after dosing. Interpretation of these samples requires the assumption that the drug is uniformly distributed throughout the body. However, drugs do not distribute in a uniform fashion. Drugs that are water soluble or highly bound to plasma proteins have a high plasma concentration and a low Vd because the drug tends to remain in the blood. Drugs that are lipid soluble or bind extensively to tissue are present in the plasma in low concentrations and therefore have large Vds. Vd in the neonate is usually larger than in children (and premature infants larger than term infants) because of the larger extracellular water compartment in neonates.

The extracellular fluid volume in newborns is considerably greater than that in children and adults. In the first 3 months of life, it decreases substantially and then remains nearly constant throughout infancy and early childhood. Extracellular fluid volume is also increased with prematurity so that peak serum concentrations are lower in preterm infants compared to term infants after similar dosages. Expanded extracellular volumes prolong drug elimination and lead to longer half-lives. The clinical application of these concepts is particularly relevant to aminoglycosides because the efficacy is associated with the peak concentration, whereas toxicity is associated with trough concentrations.

Protein binding can also impact drug distribution and elimination. Quantitative and qualitative differences exist between the serum proteins of newborns and those of older infants. These differences affect the degree to which antimicrobial agents are protein bound. Variables that impact protein binding include concentrations of plasma proteins (such as albumin), concentration of drug, drug affinity for protein binding sites, presence of competing substances for protein binding sites (e.g., furosemide, bilirubin), and plasma pH. Protein-bound drug has negligible antibacterial activity and remains in the intravascular space with limited distribution into tissue and limited excretion. Because only free drug is active and available for elimination, changes in protein binding can dramatically affect exposure and efficacy. Protein binding for some antibiotics is lower in neonates than in adults, so extrapolation is not advised, and the PK of the free drug needs to be determined.

Some antibacterial agents are capable of displacing bilirubin from albumin-binding sites, including the sulfonamides and ceftriaxone. Theoretically, jaundiced neonates receiving these antibiotics are at increased risk of developing kernicterus. This complication, however, has been documented only for sulfonamides.[7] Most antimicrobial drugs do not displace bilirubin because most have a much lower binding affinity for albumin than bilirubin, and thus the extent of protein binding by an antibiotic does not necessarily correlate with bilirubin displacement.[8]

Drugs start to be eliminated from the body as soon as they are delivered. If doses are given at a rate that balances the drug clearance (CL) rate, then target steady-state drug concentrations can be maintained. Drug CL represents the volume of blood, serum, or plasma completely cleared of drug per unit of time and has the units of volume/time, for example, L/hr or mL/min, or L/hr/kg for weight normalized CL. Clearance is not only related to infant size (L/hr/kg) but also to clinical characteristics, such as renal disease, hepatic disease, and drug interactions. Clearance of water-soluble drugs usually occurs via excretion into the urine, whereas lipid-soluble drugs are often metabolized to water-soluble metabolites by the liver before they can be excreted.

Drug elimination occurs through hepatic metabolism, renal excretion, or both, and is affected by physiologic maturation.[6] Hepatic metabolism involves chemical transformation of the drug into a form that is more fat soluble for elimination in the bile and feces or a form more water soluble for elimination by the kidneys. The ontogeny of the cytochrome P-450–metabolizing enzymes in newborn development has been evaluated and reviewed.[9] Newborns are at risk for toxicity from drug accumulation because of deficiencies in hepatic glucuronyl transferase or hepatic esterases. Drugs can also induce P-450 enzyme production, leading to drug interaction. Phenobarbital stimulates hepatic enzyme production, thereby increasing the CL and lowering serum concentrations of some drugs, including anticoagulants, corticosteroids, phenytoin, metronidazole, and theophylline.

Renal elimination of active drug or metabolites occurs via glomerular filtration and/or tubular secretion. Some drugs are reabsorbed in renal tubules, thus further altering their elimination rate. Renal function varies with gestational age (GA), postnatal age (PNA), and postmenstrual age (PMA) (neonatal abbreviations are reviewed in Table 37-2). The constant state of renal function fluctuation has a profound impact on antibiotic PK. In newborns, the glomerular filtration rate is 30% to 60% of adult levels. A remarkable increase in renal function occurs over the first 2 weeks of life.[5,10] As a result, sustained serum concentrations and prolonged half-life values of many drugs eliminated through the kidneys are observed in the first days of life. After birth, renal function improves more slowly in premature infants, leading to prolonged drug elimination over the first few weeks of life. Drug elimination is also reduced in sick infants because of decreased renal blood flow resulting from respiratory insufficiency, hypotension, or dehydration. For example, hypoxemic infants have a prolonged serum half-life ($t_{½}$) of aminoglycosides. Therapeutic hypothermia is associated with reduced hepatic CL of morphine. Because renal function is constantly changing in the first month of life and with advancing GA, a PK profile needs to be determined on multiple occasions during this period to define the proper dosage and frequency of administration of an antibiotic.

Most drugs are cleared through first-order elimination. This means that a constant proportion of drug is cleared per unit of time. Initially, there is a steep fall in concentration, after which the decline becomes shallower as the amount of drug remaining decreases. When the concentration-time profile is plotted on a log-linear scale, the decline is linear because the shape of the relationship between concentration and time is described by an exponential function. The elimination rate constant (k_e) is the ratio of CL to Vd and is usually expressed in units of L/hr.

Each patient has their own unique elimination rate constant (k_e) that reflects the CL and Vd of the drug. The elimination rate constant can be converted into the clinically meaningful concept of drug half-life, the time it takes for the concentration of a drug to fall to half (see Table 37-2). Half-life estimates are patient specific. For drugs eliminated by first-order kinetics, the elimination rate constant represents the ratio of drug CL and Vd. For patients with renal insufficiency, delayed renal CL of gentamicin will result in a half-life that can be three times as long as patients with normal renal function. Patients with fluid overload have a large Vd and a longer half-life and therefore may need to receive a higher dose of medication less frequently.

OPTIMIZING ANTIMICROBIAL THERAPY USING PK-PD PRINCIPLES

Optimizing antimicrobial therapy in neonates requires a thorough understanding of the relationship between dose and exposure (PK) and between exposure and optimal response to therapy (PD).[11,12] Our goal is to provide an integrative approach using knowledge from microbiology (minimal inhibitory concentration [MIC], minimal bactericidal concentration [MBC]), PK, and PD such that we can have a high probability that a specific dose of an antibiotic can cure a particular infection in a defined population of infants. Carefully designed clinical trials can then be performed to confirm the results of such an integrative modeling and simulation approach.

Minimal Inhibitory Concentration

The in vitro drug susceptibilities of commonly encountered bacterial pathogens allow comparison of potencies for eradication. Ideally, both the MIC and the MBC should be determined. To account for the great variation in pathogens and susceptibilities in different nurseries and geographic regions, this knowledge can be generated for each specific newborn unit. The higher the MIC, the more difficult it is to eradicate a pathogen with that drug, even if the MIC falls within the established sensitivity range.

Pharmacokinetic Data

New analytic techniques and the computer algorithms for population PK model analysis have made PK evaluation of drugs in infants more feasible. PK explains the relationship between drug dose and the concentration of drug in the plasma or serum over time. PK studies are performed after a single dose and after multiple doses to determine concentrations at steady state. Drug levels can now be measured using mass spectroscopy in as little as 0.1 mL obtained by heel stick. For drugs that exhibit protein binding, it is important to measure the quantity of total and non–protein-bound drug. Subsequently, multiple serum samples are obtained to determine concentrations of the drug at a given time after the dose. The serum half-life ($t_{½}$) and Vd are calculated by plotting the serum concentration-time curves and calculating the CL, a measure of the disappearance of drug from serum.[13] Population PK analysis allows investigators to study a medication in a diverse group of preterm and term infants of different ages so that changes in drug CL and Vd can be explained by maturational covariates (GA at birth, PNA, PMA reviewed in Table 37-2), weight, or renal function in a mathematical model. Monte Carlo simulation using these models of drug CL and Vd is used to predict and compare drug exposure from different dosing regimens to provide dose adjustments for maturational changes in an infant.

It is clinically important to determine the active drug concentrations in the cerebrospinal fluid (CSF).[14] Central nervous system (CNS) penetration of drugs is usually expressed as the fraction of CSF drug concentrations divided by the plasma or serum concentrations because most studies link a single CSF sample with a simultaneous blood sample. In the 1980s, new antibiotics were tested in a rabbit model of meningitis before use in infants to determine the CSF penetration and bactericidal activity of the drug against commonly encountered meningeal pathogens.[15] More data are needed to understand the CSF penetration of antimicrobial drugs in the presence or absence of meningitis in neonates. Some current antimicrobial trials are attempting to collect CSF from standard-of-care sampling to measure drug levels in CSF.

Although CSF concentrations represent the closest approximation of drug concentration in the CNS, they only represent one compartment and can underrepresent drug exposure in brain parenchymal tissue.[16,17] Amphotericin and echinocandins have been used successfully to eradicate CNS fungal infections, yet they are detected at very low levels in the CSF. Drugs cross the blood-brain and blood-CSF barrier through diffusion and transport systems.[16,17] Efflux channels can remove drugs from the CSF. CNS infection also tends to cause an increase in permeability of the blood-brain and blood-CSF barriers. In addition to CSF evaluation, it remains important to consider the physiochemical properties of the drug, including molecular size, lipophilicity, plasma protein binding, and active transport mechanisms. Higher serum exposures are often warranted when treating CNS infections to allow for drug entry into both the parenchymal tissue and the CSF. Intraventricular therapy is traditionally avoided if systemic therapy is available because studies of intraventricular aminoglycosides administration show an association with threefold increase in mortality compared with standard treatment with IV antibiotics alone.[18,19]

Pharmacodynamics

Pharmacodynamics equations describe the relationships between the drug concentration-time profile and the ability to eradicate the organism, prevent emerging resistance, and minimize adverse effects. Dose and dosing interval determine the minimum concentration, maximum concentration, and overall drug exposure per 24-hour interval (24-hour area under the concentration-time curve = AUC_{24}) (Figure 37-1). Bacterial eradication is typically evaluated in relation to the maximal drug concentration, the AUC, or the percentage of dosing interval time that the drug concentration is above a minimum threshold, as determined by the MIC of the target organism (see Figure 37-1).

Pharmacokinetic-Pharmacodynamic Approach

To achieve the best therapeutic response, drug dose should be related to antimicrobial effect through an integrated PK-PD approach, in which a dose is chosen to target a therapeutic drug concentration relative to the MIC of the offending

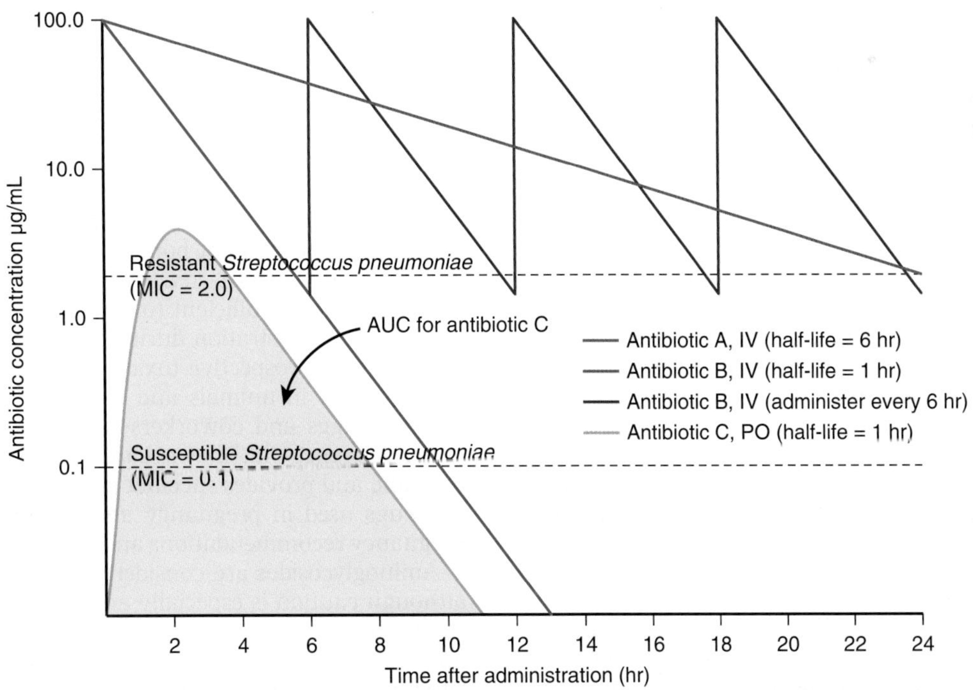

Figure 37-1 Effects of dose (mg/kg), dosing interval and route of administration on total drug exposure, as defined by the AUC and its relationship to the minimal inhibitory concentration (MIC) of the pathogen being treated. Antibiotics administered intravenously with a long serum half-life of 6 hours (antibiotic A) achieve a relatively large area under the curve (AUC) compared with antibiotics with a shorter half-life of 1 hour (antibiotic B), which require more frequent dosing (every 6 hours in this example) to achieve similar drug exposure to the pathogen. Orally administered antibiotics (antibiotic C) generally produce a much lower AUC than those administered intravenously. The MICs for penicillin-susceptible and -resistant *Streptococcus pneumoniae* are superimposed on the graph. (From Bradley JS, Dudley MN, Drusano GL: Predicting efficacy of antiinfectives with pharmacodynamics and Monte Carlo simulation, *Pediatr Infect Dis J* 22:982-992, 2003; Figure 2.)

Table 37-3 PK-PD Relationships for Optimal Antimicrobial Treatment

Antimicrobial Activity	PK-PD Parameter and Goal of Therapy	Definition	Drug Class	Dosing Goal
Concentration-dependent killing with postantibiotic effect	C_{max}/MIC	Bacterial killing is proportional to maximal concentration achieved relative to MIC of offending organism	Aminoglycosides Fluoroquinolones Daptomycin	Enhance peak concentration
Time-dependent killing	T > MIC	Bacterial killing is proportional to the amount of time the drug concentration is maintained greater than the MIC of offending organism	β-Lactams: Penicillins Cephalosporins Carbapenems	Enhance duration of exposure by short dosing intervals
Time-dependent killing with postantibiotic effect	AUC/MIC	Bacterial killing is proportional to the amount of total drug exposure relative to MIC of offending organism	Vancomycin Clindamycin Linezolid Azoles	Enhance amount of drug using both dose and interval

AUC, Area under the concentration-time curve; C_{max}, maximum drug concentration; *MIC*, minimal inhibitory concentration; *PD*, pharmacodynamic; *PK*, pharmacokinetic; *T*, time.

organism.[12] Three important PK parameters are the peak serum level (C_{max}), the trough level (C_{min}), and the AUC (see Tables 37-2 and 37-3; see Figure 37-1). These PK-PD parameters are used to quantify the activity of an antibiotic. Antimicrobial agents are typically associated with one of three patterns of activity (see Table 37-3 and Figure 37-1)[11,20]: (1) those that exhibit concentration-dependent killing and prolonged persistent postantibiotic effects (PAEs) and thus achieve optimal killing when the maximum concentration exceeds a threshold peak/MIC ratio, (2) agents that exhibit time-dependent killing patterns and therefore achieve optimal killing when the duration of drug exposure above a MIC exceeds a percentage of time (T) greater than the MIC, and (3) agents that are most effective when the maximal total drug exposure exceeds a threshold AUC/MIC ratio. Threshold PK-PD therapeutic exposure targets are determined through in vitro experiments, animal models, and human studies that relate drug exposure to MIC and efficacy.

Placental Transport of Antimicrobial Drugs

Antimicrobial agents are prescribed for approximately 20% of pregnant women,[21] and many of these drugs are given at the end of pregnancy for amnionitis or intrauterine bacterial infections. Understanding placental transport is therefore an important component of antimicrobial therapy in the neonate.

Drugs may be transported across the placenta either passively, by simple diffusion, or actively through energy-dependent processes.[22,23] Factors influencing transplacental passage include lipid solubility, degree of ionization, molecular weight, protein-binding affinity, surface area of the fetal-maternal interface, placental blood flow, stage of pregnancy, and placental metabolism. Drug transport across the placenta changes greatly with advancing GA because of the thickness of barrier and also differential expression of drug transporters. Placental drug biotransformation ensues by oxidation, reduction, hydrolysis, or conjugation with endogenous chemicals. In addition, antibiotics can concentrate to various degrees in fetal tissues, depending on lipid solubility, specific binding to biologic constituents, changes in fetal circulation, and GA.

Many antimicrobial drugs rapidly cross the placenta (Table 37-4). Maternal serum concentrations are usually lower than those reported in nonpregnant women because of larger plasma Vd and an increased renal CL during pregnancy. As a result of differences in maternal dosage, route of administration, GA, timing of sample collection, and methods of measuring antimicrobial activity, a wide range of serum values for pregnant women and infants and of percentages of transplacental penetration is obtained for most drugs. Most penicillins and cephalosporins are considered compatible with pregnancy, typically cross the placenta rapidly, and quickly achieve fetal levels that approach or even exceed those in maternal serum. The high and rapidly attainable fetal penicillin serum concentrations explain, in part, the benefit of intrapartum administration of penicillins to pregnant women colonized with group B streptococci in reducing early-onset neonatal sepsis. Antibiotics with lower transplacental penetration with fetal to maternal ratios of 10% to 50% include dicloxacillin, erythromycin, nafcillin, and aminoglycosides.

Serious adverse fetal and maternal events have been associated with antibiotic use in pregnancy. Examples include kernicterus (sulfonamides), ototoxicity (streptomycin), inhibition of infant bone growth (tetracyclines), and discoloration of teeth (tetracyclines). Anecdotal clinical experience is not sufficient to assess properly the safety of antibiotic administration during pregnancy. Rather, carefully planned prospective toxicity studies in the fetus and neonate, first in animals and then in humans, are warranted. Briggs and coworkers[24] published an up-to-date online reference that allows searching for a drug of interest by name and provides succinct summaries of the research on drugs used in pregnancy and lactation and provides pregnancy recommendations and fetal risk summaries.

Aminoglycosides are considered low risk in pregnancy, although caution is especially advised for kanamycin and streptomycin.[24] Aminoglycosides rapidly cross the placenta into the fetal circulation. Eighth nerve toxicity in the human fetus has been reported after exposure to kanamycin and streptomycin but not other aminoglycosides.[24] Although possible, ototoxicity has not been directly reported after fetal exposure to tobramycin, amikacin, and gentamicin.

Carbapenems are considered low risk in pregnancy based on animal data and sparse human data. Imipenem-cilastatin crosses the placenta and achieves fetal levels of about 30% of

Table 37-4 Transplacental Passage of Antimicrobial Agents*

Antimicrobial Agent	Trimester	Serum Infant-to-Maternal Ratio(s) (%)	Potential Adverse Effects on Fetus or Infant
Ampicillin	1, 2	50-250	None
	3	20-200	
Penicillin G	1, 2	26-70	None
Cefazolin	1, 2	2-27	None
	3	36-69	
Cefotaxime	2	80-150	None
Ceftriaxone	3	9-120	None
Cefuroxime	3	18-108	None
Cephalexin	3	33	None
Clindamycin	2	10-25	None
	3	30-50	
Gentamicin	2, 3	21-44	Very rare association with ototoxicity; potentiation of $MgSO_4$-induced neuromuscular weakness
Tobramycin	1, 2	20	Ototoxicity
Amikacin	1, 2	8-16	Ototoxicity
	3	30-50	
Imipenem	3	14-52	Seizure activity
Nitrofurantoin	3	38-92	Hemolysis in G6PD deficiency
Chloramphenicol	3	30-106	Circulatory collapse
Sulfonamides	3	13-275	Hemolysis in G6PD deficiency; jaundice and potential kernicterus
Tetracyclines	3	10-90	Depressed bone growth; abnormal teeth; possible inguinal hernia
Trimethoprim	1, 2	27-131	Teratogenic in animals

G6PD, Glucose-6-phosphate dehydrogenase; *$MgSO_4$,* magnesium sulfate.
*As reviewed in References 21, 24, and 440.

that seen in maternal circulation.[24] No significant fetal toxicity has been observed in different animal models. Placental transfer of meropenem has apparently not been studied; however, the molecular properties of the drug suggest placental transfer will occur with subsequent distribution into the fetus.[24]

MEDICATIONS CONTRAINDICATED OR CONSIDERED TO BE HIGH RISK IN PREGNANCY

Sulfonamides should be avoided in the third trimester, particularly if close to delivery.[24] Sulfonamides cross the placenta and the fetal levels are 70% to 90% of maternal levels after 2 to 3 hours. Significant fetal levels can persist for several days after birth. Fetal toxicities include jaundice, hemolytic anemia, and, theoretically, kernicterus.

Tetracyclines are associated with both maternal and fetal risk and are therefore contraindicated in pregnancy, particularly in the second and third trimester.[24] Tetracycline-induced hepatotoxicity is a rare, although serious, adverse event that does not spontaneously resolve after delivery of infant. Tetracyclines readily cross the placental barrier and concentrate in many tissues of the developing fetus. Of particular interest is the deposition of tetracycline in fetal bones and deciduous teeth.[25] Calcification of deciduous teeth begins during the fourth month of gestation, and crown formation of the anterior teeth is almost complete at term. Tetracycline administered during this gestational period produces yellow discoloration, enamel hypoplasia, and abnormal development of those teeth. These effects have been documented for tetracycline, oxytetracycline, and demethylchlortetracycline.

Chloramphenicol crosses the placenta and achieves fetal levels 30% to 100% of maternal levels.[24] Chloramphenicol use in pregnancy has not been associated with major or minor fetal anomalies. However, chloramphenicol is not recommended in newborns because it has been associated with circulatory collapse (gray baby syndrome) and death.[26] Therefore many suggest that chloramphenicol should only be administered to pregnant women near term with caution and if alternative medicines are not available.

The use of metronidazole in pregnancy is controversial because the drug is mutagenic in bacteria and carcinogenic in rodents.[24,27] However, these properties have not been shown in humans. Most published evidence suggests that metronidazole does not pose significant risk; however, carcinogenic potential cannot be excluded. The use of metronidazole for trichomoniases or vaginosis during the second and third trimester is acceptable. For other indications, alternative drugs with acceptable profiles would be preferred.

ANTIVIRAL AND ANTIFUNGAL MEDICATIONS IN PREGNANCY

Many antiviral medications can be administered to pregnant women, particularly when the maternal benefit outweighs the potential for fetal risk. Valacyclovir and acyclovir are the most common antiviral medications used in pregnancy, often administered to women for treatment or prophylaxis of genital herpes infections. No increase in fetal abnormalities has been ascribed to acyclovir.[23,24] Because valacyclovir is quickly converted to acyclovir, the placenta and fetus are most exposed to acyclovir. Acyclovir readily crosses the placenta and achieves a cord blood–to-maternal ratio of approximately 1.3.[23,24]

Pregnancy is also a risk factor for morbidity and mortality caused by severe influenza infections. Oseltamivir is recommended in pregnant women with influenza to decrease mortality and hospital intensive care unit (ICU) admission.[23,24] Oseltamivir exhibits low transplacental permeability to the fetus, with fetal concentrations predicted to be less than 20%, with even lower concentrations of the active drug oseltamivir carboxylase. Drug transporters may be important in the apparent restrictive placental transfer of oseltamivir and its metabolites.[23] Case series and a review of the Roche Company safety database suggest that oseltamivir is unlikely to cause adverse pregnancy or fetal outcomes, but available data are limited.[24]

Ganciclovir is rarely indicated in pregnancy, and its use is restricted to pregnant women with severe cytomegalovirus (CMV) infections, typically in immunocompromised pregnant women.[23,24] Both ganciclovir and valganciclovir are associated with concerns for bone marrow toxicity and animal reports of mutagenesis. Very rare cases of ganciclovir use during pregnancy of women with a history of organ transplant have described healthy infant outcomes.

Most antifungal medications must be used with caution in pregnant women. Amphotericin B is the only antifungal agent thought to be compatible with pregnancy.[24] Amphotericin does cross the placenta with cord blood–to-maternal serum ratios ranging from 40% to 100%. No evidence of adverse fetal effects has been reported.

Alternatively, fluconazole at doses greater than or equal to 400 mg/day in the first trimester is associated with teratogenicity in human and animal models, similar to the skeletal anomalies seen in Antley-Bixler syndrome.[24] Exposure to short-course, low-dose fluconazole has not been associated with increased congenital anomalies. Fluconazole is a small enough molecule that placental transfer is expected; however, placental transfer across the human placenta has not been evaluated.

The echinocandin class of antifungal medications has not been adequately studied in pregnancy. Animal data suggest moderate risk for embryotoxicity and teratogenicity.[24] The physical/chemical properties of caspofungin and micafungin, specifically their relatively large size, low lipid solubility, and high protein binding, may limit placental transfer. However, given the absence of human data and suggestion of risk in animal models, most clinicians would attempt to avoid echinocandins, specifically in the first trimester if alternative agents are available.[24]

Excretion of Antibiotics in Human Milk

Postpartum women are often prescribed an antibiotic. However, the concentration of antimicrobial agents in breast milk is typically so low that neither therapeutic nor harmful effects are likely to occur. The amount of drug could be significant if the drug accumulates in breast milk, the infant ingests a large volume of milk, infant feeding times correlate with maximal maternal plasma concentrations, or the drug has reasonable bioavailability in the infant.[28] Assessment of the safety of antibiotics in milk has relied primarily on anecdotal clinical experience, rather than on carefully controlled long-term studies. Two important, updated and referenced sources of information to aid clinicians about medications in breastfeeding mothers are LactMed from the National Library of Medicine (http://toxnet.nlm.nih.gov/cgi-bin/sis/htmlgen?LACT) and Dr. Thomas Hale's *Medications and Mother's Milk* (http://www.medsmilk.com/).

Most drugs are transferred into breast milk by passive diffusion, exocytosis, or reverse pinocytosis. Factors influencing the transfer of antibiotics from plasma to milk include maternal serum concentration of unbound drug and the physiochemical properties of the drug, for instance, molecular weight, lipid solubility, degree of ionization, and protein-binding capability.[28] Small, lipid-soluble, non-ionized drugs traverse the lipid bilayers into milk more readily than larger, ionized, water-soluble drugs. Although drugs with high lipid solubility tend to accumulate in milk, the extent varies with the fat content of the milk. The ionization power of drugs depends on the pH of the milk and the drug dissociation constant (pKa). Weak bases become more ionized with decreasing pH. Early postpartum human milk has a pH of 7.0 to 7.1, whereas mature milk after 2 weeks has a pH of approximately 7.3 to 7.4, each compared with the normal serum pH of 7.35 to 7.45. Therefore drugs that are weak bases (pKa > pH), such as erythromycin, isoniazid, metronidazole, and tetracyclines, would be expected to ionize and accumulate in the lower pH environment of colostrum. Weak acids, such as ampicillin, are more likely to be ionized in maternal serum and therefore not transferred at high levels into breast milk. Drugs that are highly serum-protein bound, such as ceftriaxone, tend to remain in the intravascular space in the maternal circulation. Data pertaining to antibiotic concentrations in the colostrum are not available. Because blood flow and permeability are increased during the colostral phase, it is possible that these drugs are present in concentrations equal to or greater than those found in mature milk.

The maternal serum and breast milk concentrations of commonly used antimicrobial agents have been reviewed.[28,29] Milk-to-plasma ratios show considerable variability because of the extremely small number of women studied and the differences in age, gestation, dosing regimen, and underlying pathophysiology. In general, the concentrations of metronidazole, sulfonamides, and trimethoprim in breast milk are similar to those in maternal serum (milk-to-serum ratio of 1.0), whereas those of chloramphenicol, erythromycin, and tetracycline are approximately 50% of maternal serum values. The concentrations of penicillin, oxacillin, various cephalosporins, and aminoglycosides in milk are low.

Although the milk-to-plasma ratio is frequently quoted to predict drug distribution into breast milk, its utility for those drugs with higher milk-to-serum ratios is suspect. The milk-to-plasma ratio is typically obtained at a single point in time; however, the concentration of drug in breast milk and plasma is not constant, and the ratio of milk-to-plasma concentrations varies greatly over time. Most studies are not performed at steady state. Furthermore, most studies usually do not expose the infant to the breast milk and cannot comment on infant systemic exposure. Instead, Chung and coworkers[28] recommend that the milk-to-plasma ratio be used as a qualitative estimate of the possible magnitude of infant drug exposure. By taking the peak breast-milk concentration and an assumed ingestion of breast-milk intake (150 mL/kg/day), they have derived an estimated potential infant dose correlated with predicted infant exposure (Table 37-5).[28] In addition, infant maturity, developmental characteristics of drug disposition, and tolerance of drug when given directly to the infant, and the possible extent to which the drug may modify the infant's intestinal gut flora need to be taken into consideration.

Most drugs are predicted to yield limited exposure to newborns (see Table 37-5). Penicillin, amoxicillin, ampicillin, ticarcillin, cephalosporins, and aminoglycosides are detected in very low concentrations in breast milk.[28,29] Clavulanic acid was not detected in breast milk. One study observed higher-than-expected concentrations of ceftazidime in breast milk from women receiving a high-dose regimen at steady state.[30] The predicted infant ceftazidime exposure remains limited, especially given the poor

Table 37-5 Summary of Reported Breast Milk Concentrations of Selected Antibiotic and Estimated Maximal Potential Infant Daily Dose for Medications That Distribute Into Breast Milk*

Drug	Maternal Dose Regimen†	Peak Milk (μg/mL)‡	Corresponding Potential Infant Dose§ (mg/kg/day)	Infant Clinical Dose (mg/kg/day)	Theoretical Safety Concerns
DRUGS FOR WHICH THE EFFECT ON NURSING INFANTS IS UNKNOWN BUT MAY BE OF CONCERN; CONSIDER DISCARDING MILK IN SOME CASES OF REPEATED DOSING					
Metronidazole	2 g once	45.8	6.87	7.5-30	In vitro mutagen
Metronidazole	400 mg tid for 3-4 days	15.5	2.44	7.5-30	
Chloramphenicol	250 mg q6h for 7-10 days	2.8	0.43	50-75	Idiosyncratic bone marrow suppression; extremely unlikely to achieve levels to cause gray baby syndrome
Chloramphenicol	500 mg q6h for 7-10 days	6.1	0.92	50-75	
MATERNAL MEDICATION USUALLY COMPATIBLE WITH BREASTFEEDING WITH ONGOING OBSERVATION OF INFANT					
Erythromycin	2 g/day	3.2	0.48	15-50	GI distress Pyloric stenosis
Azithromycin	1 g then 500 mg/day for 3 days	2.8	0.42	5-10	GI distress
Clindamycin	600 mg q6h	3.8	0.57	25-40	*Clostridium difficile* colitis
Clindamycin	150 mg tid for at least 7 days	3.1	0.47	25-40	*C. difficile* colitis
Co-trimoxazole (trimethoprim/ sulfamethoxazole 80/400)	3 tablets bid for 5 days	2.0 (trim) 5.3 (sulf)	0.3 (trim) 0.8 (sulf)	6-10 (trim) 75-150 (sulf)	Hemolytic anemia with sulfa drugs in infants with G6PD deficiency
Nitrofurantoin	100 mg tid for 4 doses	2.2	0.33	5-7	Hemolytic anemia in infants with G6PD deficiency
Tetracycline	2 g /day	0.4-2	0.3	25-50	Teeth staining
Ciprofloxacin	750 mg q12h for 3 doses	8.2	1.23	100-150	Arthropathy, none reported
Ofloxacin	400 mg q12h for 3 doses	2.4	0.36	none	Arthropathy, none reported

BID, Twice daily; *GI*, gastrointestinal; *G6PD*, glucose-6-phospate dehydrogenase; *qxh*, every x hours; *sulf*, sulfamethoxazole; *tid*, three times daily; *trim*, trimethoprim.

*As described and referenced in Chung AM, Reed MD, Blumer JL: Antibiotics and breast-feeding: a critical review of the literature, *Paediatr Drugs* 4:817-837, 2002; Hale TW: *Medications and mothers' milk online,* Amarillo, Tex, 2012, Hale Publishing; and Academy of Pediatrics Committee on Drugs: Transfer of drugs and other chemicals into human milk, *Pediatrics* 108:776-789, 2001.

†Highest possible concentration was used.

‡Assuming infant consumes approximately 150 mL/kg/day of breast milk.

§Varies with detail given in citation.

bioavailability of ceftazidime. The overall tolerability profile of penicillin and cephalosporins, along with the low concentration of these drugs in breast milk, support their use in breastfeeding infants.[29,31] The rare possibility of hypersensitivity reactions or altered intestinal flora–associated diarrhea in breastfeeding infants remains a theoretical concern.

Broad-acting agents should be reserved for the most serious infections. A recent review of antibiotics in breastfeeding[28] reported personal communication with Merck of limited data on detectable low levels of imipenem in breast milk of women; typically 0.2 to 0.5 μg/mL. Cilastatin was not detected. Despite this low exposure in breast milk, infant exposure would be further limited by poor bioavailability and drug inactivation at alkaline or acidic pH. Meropenem is also detected at very low levels in breast milk, with a maximal infant exposure reported to be less than 1%.[32] The physiochemical properties of aztreonam suggest limited transfer into breast milk because it is inactivated in acidic solutions and exhibits moderate protein binding and low lipid solubility. Single-dose PK studies confirmed a minimal amount of aztreonam in breast milk of women.[33]

The physiochemical properties of fluoroquinolones (weak acid, low molecular weight, high lipid solubility, low protein binding, and good bioavailability) suggest that fluoroquinolones can accumulate in breast milk[34]; however, the predicted infant dose exposure is limited to 2% to 6% (see Table 37-5). A case report of one infant revealed negligible ciprofloxacin infant serum concentrations (<0.03 μg/mL) despite accumulation in breast milk after 10 days of maternal exposure (maternal serum, 0.21 mg/mL; breast milk, 0.98 μg/mL).[35] This report highlighted the difficulty of predicting infant exposure from maternal plasma and milk concentrations. The risk of fluoroquinolone induced arthropathies or cartilage erosion in neonates has not been explored. The predicted fluoroquinolone exposure to an infant is predicted to be negligible and the American Academy of Pediatrics (AAP) and Hale's *Medications in Mother's Milk* have determined that the medication is usually compatible with breastfeeding and moderately safe.[29,31]

Sulfonamides and tetracycline both distribute relatively poorly into breast milk yet have theoretical concerns for associated adverse events in neonates. The amount of sulfamethoxazole and tetracyclines in breast milk is low and of unclear clinical significance. One breastfed infant with glucose-6-phosphate dehydrogenase (G6PD) deficiency experienced hemolytic anemia while the mother was receiving sulfamethoxypyridazine.[36] The adverse effects of tetracyclines on developing teeth and bones are well documented when the drug is given directly to infants and children; however, the limited exposure in breast milk has not been directly associated with abnormalities.[24,29] The AAP and Hale agree that most sulfamethoxazole (with trimethoprim) and tetracyclines are usually compatible with breastfeeding and moderately safe.[24,29,31] Caution is advised for infants with jaundice, G6PD deficiency, severe illness, or significant prematurity.[31]

Macrolides, including azithromycin, and clindamycin distribute into breast milk. However, the actual amount the infant would receive from breastfeeding remains very small (see Table 37-5). Neonatal exposure may be further limited by bioavailability. One case report of erythromycin-induced pyloric stenosis during breastfeeding exposure in a 3-week-old infant has been reported.[29] One report incriminated the administration of clindamycin to a mother in the development of antibiotic-induced colitis in her breastfed infant. The AAP has described erythromycin and clindamycin as usually compatible with breastfeeding and moderately safe.[29,31] Azithromycin is likely to be compatible with breastfeeding as well.[28]

Metronidazole effectively distributes into breast milk and achieves infant plasma concentrations approximately one fifth of the exposure observed in the mother's plasma.[37] The relative infant dose is estimated to be 13% of maternal dose, and metronidazole has been detected in infant plasma. Given the mutagenesis and carcinogenicity in animal models, its use in lactation is controversial. Breastfed infants whose mothers were administered metronidazole therapy had no difference in adverse events compared with infants whose mothers received ampicillin or no antibiotics. The AAP considers metronidazole to have an unknown effect on nursing infants but may be of concern.[31] Hale, on the other hand, reports metronidazole as "safer" and thus usually compatible with breastfeeding.[29]

The decision to allow or stop breastfeeding is based on the likelihood that high milk concentrations are attained for a particular antibiotic, whether the drug is expected to be absorbed into neonatal plasma, and whether significant adverse events are commonly associated with this agent. Online resources are now available to rapidly review the most up-to-date knowledge about specific drugs and their use in lactating mothers.[29] In general, the severity of the woman's infection, rather than the drug that she is receiving, most often is the more important contraindication to breastfeeding.

Penicillin

Penicillin has been used for treatment of neonatal bacterial infections for more than 3 decades. It is safe and well tolerated. However, its efficacy is limited by the development of resistance. Many species of streptococci, *Listeria monocytogenes*, meningococci, and *Treponema pallidum* remain susceptible to penicillin, whereas most species of staphylococci, pneumococci, and gonococci have become resistant.

MICROBIOLOGIC ACTIVITY

Penicillin and other β-lactam derivatives interfere with bacterial cell wall synthesis by reacting with one or more penicillin-binding proteins (PBPs) to inhibit transpeptidation.[38] The transpeptidase activity of PBPs is essential for cross-linking adjacent peptides and for incorporating newly formed peptidoglycan into an already existing strand. Subsequently, this event promotes bacterial cell lysis.

Several mechanisms of bacterial resistance to penicillin and other β-lactams have been identified. The most important is by inactivation through enzymatic hydrolysis of the β-lactam ring by β-lactamases.[39] These enzymes are produced by most staphylococci and enteric gram-negative bacilli and by many *Neisseria gonorrhoeae* strains. Another mechanism of resistance involves decreased permeability of the outer membrane of gram-negative bacteria, which can prevent this drug from reaching its target site.[40] In addition, by poorly defined mechanisms, some group B streptococci are inhibited but not killed by penicillin, a phenomenon termed tolerance.[41] The first group B streptococci isolates with elevated MIC to β-lactamase antibiotics by a mutation in the PBP have recently been described.[42] Usual MICs of penicillin against streptococci are between 0.005 and 0.1 μg/mL. For *T. pallidum*, the corresponding concentration ranges are between 0.02 and 0.2 μg/mL. Many pneumococcal strains isolated around the world are considered to be relatively (MICs of 0.1-1 μg/mL) or highly (MICs of 2 μg/mL or greater) resistant to multiple antibiotics, including penicillins, macrolides, and third-generation cephalosporins.[43]

PHARMACOKINETIC DATA

Most of the penicillin dose is excreted in the urine in unchanged form. Tubular secretion accounts for approximately 90% of urinary penicillin, whereas glomerular filtration contributes the remaining 10%. Biliary excretion also occurs, and this may be an important route of elimination in newborns with renal failure. A review of the clinical PK of penicillin in neonates has recently been published and serves to reference historical publications.[44]

Aqueous Penicillin G

A mean peak serum concentration of 24 μg/mL (range, 8-41 μg/mL) is observed after a dose of 25,000 units/kg of penicillin G is given intramuscularly to infants with birth weights of less than 2000 g.[45] The peak values do not change appreciably with increasing birth weight or chronologic age up to 14 days. After a dose of 50,000 units/kg, peak serum values of 35 to 40 μg/mL were detected in neonates of different ages. The concentrations at 4 and 8 hours after the dose were not substantially different from those after a dose of 25,000 units/kg. The half-life of penicillin in serum becomes longer in smaller and younger infants. Half-life values of 1.5 to 10 hours are observed in the first week of life, with the longer half-lives being in the smallest infants, having birth weights less than 1500 g. A shorter half-life of 1.5 to 4 hours was observed after 7 days of age. The half-life of penicillin also decreases as creatinine clearance improves.

Procaine Penicillin G

In the first week after birth, a 50,000 units/kg IM dose of procaine penicillin G produces mean serum values of 7 to 9 μg/mL for up to 12 hours and a 24-hour trough concentration of 1.5 μg/mL.[45] Older neonates have lower 24-hour trough concentrations (0.4 μg/mL) because of their increased clearance and shorter half-lives. These serum values are approximately twice those obtained in the original study (22,000 units/kg) and suggest a linear relationship between dose and serum concentration. No accumulation of penicillin in serum is observed after 7 to 10 days of daily doses of procaine penicillin G. The drug was well tolerated, without evidence of local reaction at the site of injection.

Benzathine Penicillin G

Penicillin can be detected in serum and urine for up to 12 days after a single IM injection of 50,000 units/kg of benzathine penicillin G in newborns. Peak serum concentrations of 0.4 to 2.5 μg/mL (mean, 1.2 μg/mL) are observed 12 to 24 hours after administration, and levels of 0.07 to 0.09 μg/mL are present at 12 days.[46,47] This preparation has been well tolerated by infants. Muscle damage from IM injection as judged from creatinine values does not appear to be appreciably different from that after IM administration of procaine penicillin.

Cerebrospinal Fluid Penetration

Penicillin does not penetrate CSF well, even when meninges are inflamed. Peak concentrations of 1 to 2 μg/mL occur after an IV dose of 40,000 units/kg of penicillin G is given to infants and children with bacterial meningitis.[48] Although these values are 2% to 5% of concomitant serum concentrations, the concentrations exceed the MIC values for streptococci and susceptible pneumococci by 50- to 100-fold. CSF concentrations of penicillin are not optimal to treat neonatal meningitis caused by penicillin-resistant pneumococci. CSF concentrations decrease as meningeal inflammation is reduced. Concentrations of penicillin in CSF during the first several days of therapy are maintained in the range of 0.5 to 1 μg/mL; thereafter the values are 0.1 μg/mL or less by 4 hours after the dose.

Procaine penicillin G administered by IM injection in newborns provides sufficient CSF exposure for the treatment of congenital neurosyphilis. Procaine penicillin G administered intramuscularly at a dose of 50,000 units/kg provides mean CSF concentrations ranging from 0.12 to 0.7 μg/mL between 4 and 24 hours after a dose.[49,50] These CSF values are at least severalfold greater than the required minimal spirocheticidal concentration.[51] Benzathine penicillin G does not provide adequate CSF exposure and is not recommended for the treatment of congenital neurosyphilis.

SAFETY

All forms of penicillin are typically well tolerated in newborns. Cutaneous allergic manifestations to penicillin are rare in the newborn and young infant.

PK-PD AND CLINICAL IMPLICATIONS FOR DOSING

Penicillin remains effective for therapy for infections caused by group B streptococci and *T. pallidum*. The dosage recommended for neonatal sepsis or pneumonia is 50,000 to 100,000 units/kg/day administered in two to four divided doses, whereas that for meningitis is 250,000 to 450,000 units/kg/day in two to four divided doses, depending on birth weight and chronologic age.[52] The PD target for β-lactam antibiotics is the T greater than MIC.[11] The trough penicillin levels ideally will remain above the MIC for streptococci.

Penicillin remains effective therapy for congenital syphilis. However, because CNS involvement in congenital syphilis is difficult to exclude with certainty, benzathine penicillin G is not routinely used for therapy. Benzathine penicillin G is reserved for asymptomatic infants with normal findings on CSF examination and radiographic studies and who have positive results on treponemal serologic studies (presumably from maternal origin), and only if follow-up can be ensured.[52] For symptomatic infants and for asymptomatic infants with laboratory or radiologic evidence suggestive of congenital syphilis, the recommended regimen is either aqueous crystalline penicillin G, 100,000 to 150,000 units/kg/day (divided every 12 hours for first 7 days and then every 8 hours thereafter) and administered IV for 10 to 14 days. Alternatively, procaine penicillin G, 50,000 units/kg/day, can be administered intramuscularly for at least 10 days.[52]

Ampicillin

ANTIMICROBIAL ACTIVITY

Ampicillin remains the preferred penicillin for initial empirical therapy for neonatal septicemia and meningitis because it provides broader antimicrobial activity without sacrificing safety. Ampicillin is commonly used in combination with aminoglycosides. Compared with penicillin G, ampicillin has increased in vitro efficacy against most strains of enterococci and *L. monocytogenes*, as well as against some gram-negative pathogens, such as *Haemophilus influenzae, Escherichia coli, Proteus mirabilis,* and *Salmonella* spp. It is only rarely active against *S. aureus*. Approximately 90% of group B streptococci and *L. monocytogenes* organisms are inhibited by 0.06 μg/mL or less of ampicillin. Almost two thirds of the gram-negative enteric bacilli isolated from CSF cultures of infants enrolled in the Second Neonatal Meningitis Cooperative Study (1976-1978) were inhibited by 10 μg/mL or less of ampicillin.[19] However, an increased rate of ampicillin-resistant gram-negative bacilli has been reported.

PHARMACOKINETIC DATA

Ampicillin, similar to many β-lactam antibiotics, is cleared by renal elimination. Therefore drug CL and half-life are dependent on renal maturation. Plasma drug CL increases (and half-life decreases) with increasing birth weight, GA, and chronologic age. Despite its frequent use, the PK of ampicillin in extremely-low-birth-weight (ELBW) infants remains sparse.

Serum ampicillin concentration-time curves have been determined after IM doses in newborns.[44] The mean peak serum concentrations 0.5 to 1 hour after 5-, 10-, 20-, and 25-mg/kg doses were 16, 25, 54, and 57 μg/mL, respectively, whereas the values at 12 hours were from 1 to 15 μg/mL (mean, 5 μg/mL). After 50-mg/kg doses, the mean peak values were higher in LBW infants (100-130 μg/mL) compared with larger-term infants (80-85 μg/mL). Peak serum concentrations as high as 300 μg/mL (mean values,

180-216 μg/mL) are observed 1 to 2 hours after a 100-mg/kg dose. These latter values exceed the MIC_{90} values of group B streptococci by at least 3000-fold. Half-life decreases with advancing age from 3 to 6 hours in the first week of life to 2 to 3.5 hours thereafter.

Serum ampicillin concentration-time curves after IV doses have been characterized for preterm and term infants. After a 100-mg/kg IV dose, premature infants of 26 to 33 weeks of gestation had a lower mean peak serum concentration (135 μg/mL) compared with more mature 34- to 40-week infants (153 μg/mL).[53] When the loading dose was followed by maintenance ampicillin doses of 50 mg/kg IV at 12- to 18-hour intervals, the mean peak and trough serum concentrations in steady-state conditions were 113 and 30 μg/mL, respectively, for premature neonates, and 140 and 37 μg/mL, respectively, for full-term neonates. Despite the lower peak concentration in premature infants, the trough value was maintained, likely given the longer half-life in premature newborn (9.5 hours) compared with full-term newborns (7 hours). Trough values of 30 μg/mL exceed the MIC_{90} value for group B streptococci by 300-fold.

CEREBROSPINAL FLUID PENETRATION

Concentrations of ampicillin in CSF vary greatly. The largest concentrations (3-18 μg/mL) occur approximately 2 hours after a 50-mg/kg IV dose and exceed the MIC_{90} values for group B streptococci and *L. monocytogenes* by 50- to 300-fold.[54] By contrast, these peak concentrations equal or exceed the MIC values against many *E. coli* strains by only severalfold. The values in CSF are lower later in the course of meningitis, when meningeal inflammation subsides.

SAFETY

Ampicillin is well tolerated when administered parenterally to newborns. Nonspecific rashes and urticaria are rarely observed, and diarrhea is uncommon. In older children and adults, very large doses can result in CNS excitation or seizures.[55] Moderately prolonged bleeding times have been reported with repeated doses. Elevations of serum glutamic-oxaloacetic aminotransferase and creatinine values frequently are detected in neonates and probably represent local tissue destruction at the site of IM injection. Mild eosinophilia may be noted in newborns and young infants. Alteration of the microbial flora of the bowel may occur after parenteral administration of ampicillin, but overgrowth of resistant gram-negative organisms and *Candida albicans* occurs more frequently after oral administration. Diarrhea usually subsides on discontinuation of therapy.

PK-PD AND CLINICAL IMPLICATIONS FOR DOSING

Vast clinical experience has demonstrated that ampicillin is a safe and effective drug for therapy for neonatal bacterial infections caused by susceptible organisms. Combined ampicillin and aminoglycoside therapy is appropriate initial empirical management of suspected bacterial infections of neonates because it provides broad antimicrobial activity and potential synergism against many strains of group B streptococci, *L. monocytogenes*, and enterococci. β-Lactam antibiotics exhibit time-dependent killing; therefore the PK-PD target is T greater than MIC.[11] Frequent dosing intervals are used to maintain drug exposure over the dosing interval. For systemic bacterial infections other than meningitis, a dosage of 25 to 50 mg/kg per dose given two to three times per day in the first week of life, and then three to four times per day thereafter, is recommended.[52,55] For therapy of bacterial meningitis, we recommend a dosage of at least 200 mg/kg/day, although some consultants use dosages as high as 300 mg/kg/day. Premature infants may continue to receive ampicillin 2 to 3 times per day for up to 4 weeks, depending on GA, chronologic age, and renal function (Table 37-6).

Antistaphylococcal Treatment

S. aureus infections occur in nurseries either as sporadic cases or in the form of disease outbreaks. In recent years, multiply-resistant strains, especially MRSA and coagulase-negative staphylococcal species, such as methicillin-resistant *Staphylococcus epidermidis* (MRSE), have been responsible for an increasing number of nosocomially-acquired staphylococcal infections in many neonatal care units.

ANTISTAPHLOCOCCAL PENICILLINS (TABLE 37-7)

Antimicrobial Activity

Nafcillin and oxacillin are the mainstays of methicillin-sensitive staphylococcal therapy. These semisynthetic agents are engineered to be resistant to hydrolysis by most staphylococcal β-lactamases by virtue of a substituted side chain that acts by steric hindrance at the site of enzyme attachment. Most penicillinase-producing staphylococci are inhibited by less than 0.5 μg/mL of nafcillin and oxacillin.[56]

Pharmacokinetic Data (See Table 37-7)

Nafcillin. Unlike other penicillins, nafcillin exhibits primarily *hepatic* CL rather than renal CL. The administration of 5-, 10-, 15-, and 20-mg/kg IM doses of nafcillin to full-term newborns in the first 4 days of life produces mean peak serum concentrations 1 hour later of 10, 25, 30, and 37 μg/mL, respectively.[57,58] These concentrations are significantly higher than those obtained in older children receiving comparable amounts of this drug.[58] Preterm infants weighing less than 2000 g had higher steady-state peak concentrations—100 to 160 μg/mL after receiving 33- to 50-mg/kg IV doses.[59] In these preterm infants, the half-life ranged from 2.2 to 5.5 hours.

Oxacillin. Oxacillin exhibits primarily renal CL. Despite this difference in clearance mechanism, the PK of oxacillin in neonates is similar to that of nafcillin. Mean peak serum concentrations of approximately 50 and 100 μg/mL are produced by 20- and 50-mg/kg IM doses, respectively.[60,61] The serum half-life of oxacillin in premature infants is about 3 hours in the first week of life and 1.5 hours thereafter.

Safety

The antistaphylococcal penicillins are well tolerated in newborn and young infants. Repeated IM injections can result in muscle damage, sterile muscle abscess, and elevation of creatinine concentrations. Nephrotoxicity

Table 37-6 Suggested Dosage Schedules for Systemic Antibiotics Used in Newborns*

		DOSAGE (mg/kg) AND INTERVAL OF ADMINISTRATION BY WEIGHT				
	WEIGHT	<1200 G*	1200-2000 G		>2000 G	
Antibiotics	**Route**	**Age 0 to 28 Days**	**Age 0 to 7-14 Days**	**Age >7 to 14 Days**	**Age 0 to 7 Days**	**Age >7 Days**
Amikacin† (ODD)	IV, IM	15-18 q36-48h	18 q36-48h	15 q24-36h	15 q24h	15 q12-24h
Ampicillin	IV, IM					
Meningitis		100 q12h	100 q12h	75-100 q8h	100 q8-12h	75 q6h
Other infections		50 q12h	50 q12h	50 q8h	50 q12h	50 q8h
Aztreonam	IV, IM	30 q12h	30 q12h	30 q8h	30 q8-12h	30 q8h
Cefazolin	IV, IM	25 q12h	25 q8h	25 q8h	25 q12h	25 q8h
Cefepime	IV, IM	30-50 q12h	30-50 q12h	30-50 q8h	30-50 q12h	30-50 q8h
Cefotaxime	IV, IM	50 q12h	50 q12h	50 q8h	50 q12h	50 q8h
Clindamycin	IV, IM	5 q12h	5 q12h	5 q8h	5 q12h	5 q8h
Gentamicin† (ODD)	IV, IM	4-5 q48h	4-5 q36-48h	4 q24h	4 q24h	4 q24h
Linezolid	IV	10 q8-12h	10 q12h	10 q8h	10 q8h	10 q8h
Metronidazole‡	IV	7.5 q24h	7.5 q12h	7.5 q12h	7.5 q12h	7.5 q8h
Meropenem	IV, IM	20 q12h	20 q12h	20 q8h	20 q8h	20-30 q8h
Nafcillin	IV	25 q12h	25 q12h	25 q8h	25 q8h	25-50 q6-8h
Oxacillin	IV, IM	25 q12h	25 q12h	25 q8h	25 q8h	25-50 q6-8h
Penicillin G (units)	IV					
Meningitis		50,000 q12h	50,000 q12h	50,000 q8h	50,000 q8h	50,000 q6h
Other infections		25,000 q12h	25,000 q12h	25,000 q8h	25,000 q8h	25,000 q6h
Piperacillin-tazobactam	IV, IM	50-100 q12	100 q12h	100 q8h	100 q12h	100 q8h
Rifampin	IV	5-10 q12	5-10 q12h	5-10 q12h	5-10 q12h	5-10 q12h
Ticarcillin-clavulanate	IV	75 q12h	75 q12h	75 q8h	75 q8-12h	75 q6-8h
Tobramycin† (ODD)	IV, IM	4-5 q36-48h	4-5 q36h	4 q24h	4 q24h	4 q24h
Vancomycin†	IV	15 q18-24h	15 q12h	15 q8-12h	15 q12h	15 q8h

IM, Intramuscular; *IV*, intravenous; *ODD*, once-daily dosing.
*Based upon anecdotal clinical experience, neonatal and hospital formularies,[52,55] and notable references cited in text. Dosing for infants < 1200 g or often infants with gestational age < 29 weeks is typically based upon limited pharmacokinetic (PK) information and many prefer to use postmenstrual age–based dosing for these infants. Use of most of these drugs remains off-label in neonates because of the need for more pharmacokinetic and safety information. Higher dosing may be indicated for treatment of meningitis or microorganisms with higher minimal inhibitory concentration, such as *Pseudomonas*. In the absence of complete pharmacokinetic information across gestation age and postnatal ages, interhospital variability in dosing guidance is expected. National Institute of Child Health and Development–sponsored Pediatric Trials Network (https://pediatrictrials.org/) has several ongoing PK studies to evaluate dosing of antimicrobial drugs in neonates to improve labeling of drugs by the U.S. Food and Drug Administration.
†Adjustments of further dosing intervals should be based on therapeutic drug monitoring.
‡Consider loading dose, given long half-life.

(interstitial nephritis or cystitis) is rare in newborns but occurs in 3% to 5% of children who receive large doses of methicillin and possibly the other antistaphylococcal penicillins, with the exception of nafcillin.[62] Reversible hematologic abnormalities, such as neutropenia or eosinophilia, commonly are observed in children undergoing treatment with these drugs, but their incidence in newborns is unknown.[63] Because nafcillin has a predominant biliary excretion, accumulation of this drug in serum can occur in jaundiced neonates, and potential adverse effects can develop. Extravasation of nafcillin at the injection site can result in necrosis of local tissue.

PK-PD and Clinical Implications for Dosing (See Tables 37-6 and 37-7)

Nafcillin and oxacillin are the antistaphylococcal drugs most often used for treatment of methicillin-sensitive staphylococcal infections in neonates. Like other β-lactam antibiotics, it is important to maintain the drug concentrations over the dosing interval (T > MIC). Therefore, as infants mature, drug CL improves and dosing intervals shorten. The dosage of oxacillin is 25 to 50 mg/kg every 12 hours (50-150 mg/kg/day) in the first week of life and every 6 to 8 hours (75-200 mg/kg/day) thereafter. The larger dosage is indicated for infants with disseminated staphylococcal disease or meningitis. For nafcillin, the dosage is 25 mg/kg (50 mg/kg for meningitis) per dose given every 12 hours in the first week of life and every 6 to 8 hours thereafter. Depending on GA at birth and chronologic age, extremely preterm infants may have delayed clearance and therefore should continue twice daily dosing for 2 to 4 weeks (see Table 37-6). If an infant does not respond to antimicrobial therapy as anticipated, one should consider an occult site of staphylococcal disease (e.g., abscess, osteomyelitis, endocarditis), pathogen resistance, or the need to shorten the dosing interval to maintain the drug concentration above the MIC throughout the dosing interval. Appropriate drainage of purulent foci, addition of an aminoglycoside or rifampin to the regimen, and use of vancomycin are among several options to consider in management of unresponsive infections.

Table 37-7 Drugs Used in Treatment of *Staphylococcus aureus*

Drug	Route Elimination	Peak (µg/mL)	Half-Life (hr)	CLSI Sensitivity Breakpoint MIC*	PK-PD Target[11,12,82,441]	CSF Penetration[16]	Safety and Clinical Pearls
MRSA							
Vancomycin 15 mg/kg	Renal	25-30	PNA<7d 6.7 (<2 kg) 5.9 (>2 kg) 4 at ≈90 days	≤2	AUC/MIC > 400 Trough 10 (15 if MRSA pneumonia) Keep level > the MIC	30%-50% inflamed[442] 0%-20% noninflamed	Check levels in renal insufficiency or change renal function. Steady state before fourth to fifth dose 10%-20% penetration epithelial lung fluid Consider increased trough target (15-20) with difficult-to-treat infection Limited protein binding Very high variability
Clindamycin 5-6.5 mg/kg	Hepatic	10	8.7 (preterm) 3.6 (term)	≤0.5	AUC/MIC	Poor	Good bone penetration, often effective against MSSA (check D-test)
Linezolid 10 mg/kg	Renal 30% Nonrenal 65% Metabolites renally excreted	12	5.6 (PNA<7d, GA <34wk GA) 2.8 (PNA<80d, 25-40wk GA)	≤4	AUC/MIC > 80	27%-100%	Monitor blood counts to evaluate for rare thrombocytopenia and anemia if used > 14 days. Enhanced lung penetration with accumulation in epithelial lung lining fluid CSF penetration unreliable; case report of linezolid efficacy in treatment of ventriculostomy related CSF infection in preterm infants[443]
Rifampin 10 mg/kg/day	Hepatic	4	Not defined	≤1	Not defined	5%-20%	Light sensitive Use in combination therapy due to induction of resistance
Daptomycin 6 mg/kg	Hepatic	25	6.2 (range, 3.7-9.0)	≤1	C_{max}/MIC AUC/MIC	Low	Myopathy, elevated CPK Sparse PK, safety evaluation No lung penetration
MSSA							
Oxacillin 50 mg/kg	Renal	100	3 (day 0-7 PNA<7d) 1.5 (day > 7 PNA>7d)	≤2	T > MIC > 50%	Low	Bone marrow suppression Monitor CBC

Dose, peak, and half-life as reported in references 60, 61, 64, 95, 115, 128, and 142.

AUC, Area under the concentration-time curve; *CBC,* complete blood count; *CPK,* creatine phosphokinase; *CSF,* cerebrospinal fluid; *CLSI,* Clinical and Laboratory Standards Institute; C_{max}, maximum drug concentration; *MIC,* minimum inhibitory concentration; *MRSA,* methicillin-resistant *Staphylococcus aureus; MSSA,* methicillin-sensitive *S. aureus; PD,* pharmacodynamic; *PK,* pharmacokinetic; *T,* time.

*CLSA. Performance Standard for Antimicrobial Susceptibility Testing; Twenty-Fourth Informational Supplement. CLSI document M100-S24. Wayne, Pa: Clinical and Laboratory Standards Institute; 2014. Bacteria with intermediate sensitivities have higher MIC.

METHICILLIN-RESISTANT STAPHYLOCOCCAL INFECTIONS (MRSE AND MRSA) (SEE TABLE 37-7)

MRSA now constitutes a relatively common cause of infection outbreaks in some nurseries, and MRSE strains are an important cause of catheter-associated disease, particularly among LBW premature infants. Glycopeptide antibiotics such as vancomycin or teicoplanin (in Europe) are the drugs of choice for infections caused by these resistant strains. Infections may be treated with combination therapy: a glycopeptide with an aminoglycoside or rifampin. More recently, the use of linezolid, clindamycin, and daptomycin have been explored for the treatment of MRSA infections.

VANCOMYCIN (SEE TABLE 37-7)

Antimicrobial Activity

Vancomycin is bactericidal against most aerobic and anaerobic gram-positive cocci and bacilli. The drug interferes with the phospholipid cycle of cell wall synthesis, alters plasma membrane function, and inhibits RNA synthesis.[1,64] There is no cross-resistance between vancomycin and other antibiotics. Synergistic bacterial killing has been demonstrated for vancomycin with aminoglycosides.

Pharmacokinetic Data (See Table 37-7)

Vancomycin is not metabolized by the body and is excreted unchanged in the urine primarily by glomerular filtration.[64] Vancomycin CL reflects renal maturation and increases with GA and chronologic age. Vancomycin is approximately 55% protein bound.

Neonates have increased extracellular fluid volume and limited renal elimination capacity and therefore are expected to have lower C_{max} and delayed clearance of vancomycin. The PK of vancomycin in preterm and term infants has been thoroughly reviewed by Pacifici and Allegaert.[64] Clearance estimates are lowest in the most preterm neonates (≈0.9 mL/min/kg), with a two- to threefold increase in clearance within the neonatal age range, reflecting renal maturation and improvement in renal function, with clinical stability over time. Serum creatinine (SCr) remains an important predictor of renal clearance, even after accounting for GA and postchronologic age. The use of neonatal creatinine is controversial, however, because it is affected by maternal creatinine load, the natural decline with PNA, analytic variation in creatinine measurement, and concomitant diseases and medications. Currently, creatinine remains the best clinically available estimate of renal function despite these limitations. Vancomycin CL is also reduced in growth restriction and in the setting of indomethacin exposure for patent ductus arteriosus (PDA). Infants on extracorporeal membrane oxygenation (ECMO) have delayed CL and increased Vd.

In the first week after birth, peak concentrations of 17 to 30 μg/mL are produced at the end of a 30-minute infusion of a 15-mg/kg dose given to neonates weighing less than 2000 g. Slightly higher values are observed in larger infants. In infants up to 12 months of age, doses of 10 mg/kg produce similar peak serum concentrations.

Population PK studies have attempted to explain the observed variability of vancomycin with chronologic age, maturity, and renal function. In a large population PK study of 1103 vancomycin concentrations from 374 newborns and infants less than 2 years of age, creatinine levels were strongly correlated with vancomycin elimination, whereas chronologic age and prematurity (<28 weeks) were significant but less important predictors of vancomycin CL.[65] Vancomycin CL for a typical 27-day-old, 1.8-kg, ex–33-week-GA infant with creatinine at 0.6 mg/dL is estimated to be 0.10 to 0.12 L/hr.[65-67] The Vd (0.5- 0.8 L/kg) varies with weight and is larger than that reported in older children.

Traditional and population PK studies consistently report improved clearance and shorter half-lives with advancing GA and chronologic age. However, PK studies in preterm infants still show remarkable variability. Vancomycin half-life is prolonged in the first week of life, ranging from 6 to 10 depending on prematurity and renal function. The half-life then decreases to 4 to 7 hours in the first 1 to 2 months, then eventually to 2 to 2.5 hours in childhood.

Neonates undergoing ECMO receiving vancomycin have a larger Vd, lower CL, and longer half-life.[68] However, because infants on ECMO typically have renal insufficiency, some of the delayed vancomycin CL may be explained by elevated SCr.[65]

Vancomycin does not readily penetrate the CSF unless the meninges are inflamed. The CSF concentrations of vancomycin are 10% to 15% of the concomitant serum concentrations in infants with minimal meningeal inflammation.[69] In premature infants born at 26 to 31 weeks of GA, dosages of 20 mg/kg every 18 to 24 hours were associated with CSF vancomycin concentrations of 2.2 to 5.6 μg/mL, 26% to 68% of their corresponding serum values.[70]

Safety

Initial experience with vancomycin in the 1950s suggested a moderate incidence of ototoxicity and nephrotoxicity. These adverse effects were presumably related to the impurities found in early preparations of the drug. Further studies have indicated that vancomycin is well tolerated and safe when administered intravenously, particularly in newborns and young infants.[71] Rare cases of ototoxicity and nephrotoxicity typically involved excessive doses, underlying hearing loss or renal disease, and concomitant therapy with other ototoxic or nephrotoxic agents. To minimize risk of nephrotoxicity or ototoxicity, vancomycin trough levels are monitored in patients with underlying renal dysfunction or those receiving concomitant therapy with aminoglycoside. There is also no proven association between therapeutic drug monitoring and the prevention of ototoxicity. Renal function should be monitored during vancomycin therapy.

In adults, the most important risk factors for developing nephrotoxicity include trough concentrations greater than 10 μg/mL, concomitant treatment with aminoglycosides, and/or prolonged therapy greater than 21 days.[72] Other risk factors include extremely high peak concentrations greater than 60, high total dose, preexisting renal failure, and concurrent treatment with amphotericin and/or furosemide. Nephrotoxicity is not well characterized in pediatrics but appears to be less common in neonates and young infants.[73-76] After rapid administration, some older patients develop a histamine reaction characterized by an erythematous pruritic rash that can persist for several hours but tends to resolve with antihistamine medications. Use of a slower infusion rate (i.e., >45-60 minutes) usually avoids this adverse event. Vancomycin is irritating to tissue and is thus always administered through the IV route. In neonates, an association between vancomycin exposure and ototoxicity or renal toxicity has not been described.

PK-PD and Clinical Implications for Dosing (See Tables 37-6 and 37-7)

The primary indication for vancomycin therapy in newborns is for infections caused by MRSA and by ampicillin-resistant enterococci. Vancomycin is the initial drug of choice for documented infections caused by *S. epidermidis* because most strains are resistant to penicillin, methicillin, cephalosporins, and aminoglycosides. Of interest, *Staphylococcus warneri* has a somewhat reduced glycopeptide susceptibility (MIC > 2 μg/mL) compared with *S. epidermidis* (MIC < 2 μg/mL). The rate of killing of staphylococci is slow for vancomycin compared with β-lactams. If susceptibility data for staphylococcal infections reveals methicillin sensitivity, then the antibiotic regimen should be adjusted. For β-lactam–sensitive staphylococci and enterococci, vancomycin was inferior to nafcillin and ampicillin when comparing bactericidal rate and rapidity of blood sterility.[77,78]

Vancomycin is a concentration-independent, time-dependent antibiotic with moderate PAE.[79] The continued suppression of bacterial growth against gram-positive bacteria can persist for several hours, depending on the organism and initial antibiotic concentration, typically ranging from 0.6 to 2 hours for *S. aureus* and 4 to 6 hours for *S. epidermidis*.[80] Both increased AUC/MIC (>400) and increased T greater than MIC have been shown to promote bacterial clearance.[81,82] MRSA and *S. epidermidis* are typically sensitive to vancomycin, with MIC less than 2 μg/mL. Serum bactericidal titers of 1:8 (approximate serum concentrations of 12 μg/mL) have been associated with clinical cures in children.[83] Bactericidal activity appears to be maintained if the vancomycin concentrations exceed the MIC for 100% of the dosing interval,[84] or if the vancomycin trough concentration is greater than 10 μg/mL.[85]

Therapeutic drug monitoring focused on trough serum concentrations can be used to optimize PK-PD efficacy targets. Trough values of at least 10 ensure that the non–protein-bound vancomycin concentration will typically remain above the MIC of the offending organism and should achieve an $AUC_{0\text{-}24}$/MIC greater than 400 if the MIC is less than 1 mg/dL. In adults, higher trough concentrations, that is, 15 to 20 μg/mL, are indicated when treating serious MRSA infections, deep-seated infections, or those caused by organisms with a MIC greater than 1 μg/mL.[86] Peak levels are no longer recommended. The safety of these higher exposures has not been evaluated in neonates and children. Extremely preterm infants, infants with renal insufficiency or variable renal function, and infants on ECMO are likely to need more therapeutic drug monitoring.

The timing of trough monitoring is critical. Trough values near steady state are typically drawn around the fourth dose. Trough values evaluated before steady state may need to be repeated after subsequent dosing to evaluate probable drug accumulation until steady state is reached and also with any change in renal function or with prolonged treatment regimens.

Several vancomycin dosing regimens have been proposed.[65,87] The traditional dosage schedule for vancomycin in neonates is typically 10 to 15 mg/kg every 12 hours (20-30 mg/kg/day) in the first week of life and every 8 hours (30-45 mg/kg/day) thereafter. Extremely premature infants have unique dosing requirements to account for changes in body water composition and postnatal maturation in renal function. It is also reasonable to consider SCr and/or changes in SCr in setting of infection when determining vancomycin dosage.[65] The larger dosage (15 mg/kg) is used for treatment of CSF infection or pneumonia. Extremely preterm infants, infants with renal insufficiency or variable renal function, and infants on ECMO are likely to need more frequent drug monitoring.

Prospective evaluation of these dosing regimens continues to demonstrate the large degree of variability in exposure, consistent with variability seen in PK studies.[64,88] Until prospectively validated dosing guidelines are available, individual units should consider monitoring the frequency of vancomycin trough concentrations outside of the target range and the MIC of their local organisms to evaluate the appropriateness of their current dosing guidance in their specific population.[64,88,89]

To maintain an AUC/MIC PD target and maintain vancomycin concentration above a given threshold, some clinicians have considered dosing by continuous infusion. One study in 145 preterm neonates showed that continuous infusions of either 15 to 25 mg/kg/day or 20 to 30 mg/kg/day both resulted in therapeutic vancomycin exposures.[90] In another study, one group of 27- to 41-week PMA infants received vancomycin 10 to 30 mg/kg/day continuous infusion, whereas a second group of 28- to 51-week PMA infants received a loading dose of 7 mg/kg, followed by a continuous infusion of 10 to 40 mg/kg/day, according to PMA.[91] Both groups had therapeutic vancomycin concentrations at steady state. Group 1 steady-state vancomycin concentration was 11 μg/mL, and group 2 steady-state vancomycin concentration after loading dose was 15 μg/mL. These continuous infusions appear to have been well tolerated; however, the infusions would likely require a dedicated IV line.

The dramatic increase in worldwide prevalence of vancomycin-resistant enterococci (VRE) and the serious threat posed by the spread of vancomycin-resistant staphylococci has discouraged the use of vancomycin for antimicrobial prophylaxis or empirical therapy.

LINEZOLID (SEE TABLE 37-7)

Antimicrobial Activity

Linezolid is a synthetic oxazolidinone antibiotic that inhibits bacterial protein synthesis in a broad range of gram-positive organisms.[92,93] In kill-curve experiments, linezolid is bacteriostatic against staphylococci and enterococci but can be bactericidal against streptococci.[94] Linezolid has a unique mechanism of action and therefore does not exhibit cross-resistance with antistaphylococcal penicillins or vancomycin. It is FDA approved for treatment of infections caused by glycopeptide-resistant strains of *Enterococcus faecium*, *S. aureus*, and *Streptococcus pneumoniae* in neonates.[1]

Pharmacokinetic Data (See Table 37-7)

Linezolid is known for its rapid and nearly complete absorption after oral dosing.[92] Bioavailability is approximately 100% in adults but has not been well characterized in neonates. Only 30% of linezolid is eliminated via the kidneys as active drug in the urine. Nonrenal pathways account for approximately 65% of total body clearance for linezolid. Linezolid is oxidized on the morpholine ring, resulting in two inactive metabolites that are then excreted in the urine. The specific biotransformation pathways in children have not been defined. Linezolid is not a cytochrome P-450 substrate. Single-dose PK for IV linezolid has been assessed in 42 neonates (25-40 weeks of gestation) in the first 80 days of life.[10,95,96] Linezolid CL increases rapidly in the first week of life and is relatively constant from day 8 to 79 after birth. The increases in clearance are likely related to the development of biotransformation pathways after birth- and age-associated increases in glomerular filtration for the residual renal elimination of the drug. Linezolid Vd varies inversely with GA. In the first week of life, preterm infants have a slower CL and longer half-life (2.0 mL/kg*min and 5.6 hours, respectively) compared with more mature infants (3.8 mL/kg*min and 3 hours, respectively). Beyond the first week of life, CL and half-life estimates are similar (5.1 mL/kg*min and 1.5 hours, respectively) in preterm and term infants up to 90 days of age. Linezolid trough concentrations at 11 hours are 0 to 4 µg/mL. Infants receiving a 10-mg/kg dose are predicted to have a mean AUC of 54.9 mg*hr/L. Infants have faster CLs and shorter half-lives than older infants such that infants (>7 days of age) dosed every 8 hours achieve AUCs similar to older children. Linezolid rapidly penetrates the CSF in children; however, CSF concentrations are inconsistent; children with ventricular peritoneal shunts receiving the drug did not consistently achieve or maintain therapeutic concentrations in the CSF.[97] In adults, moderate hepatic or renal insufficiency does alter the PK of linezolid. The drug's metabolites accumulate in adults with renal insufficiency; however, the clinical significance of these metabolites is unknown.

Safety

Linezolid has been well tolerated in the small number of infants and children in PK and efficacy trials. In pediatric comparator trials, the most common drug-related adverse events in children treated with linezolid were diarrhea, nausea, vomiting, anemia, and thrombocytopenia.[98-100] Drug-related adverse events rarely led to discontinuation of therapy. Linezolid is a reversible, nonselective inhibitor of monoamine oxidase[1,101]; therefore it has the potential for interaction with adrenergic and serotonergic agents. Patients receiving linezolid may have an enhanced pressor response to sympathomimetic agents, including dopamine. Myelosuppression has been reported, and therefore complete blood counts should be monitored weekly in patients on linezolid therapy, particularly for therapy beyond 2 weeks.[101] One noncomparative study found good therapeutic outcomes, but a high rate of adverse reactions, in adults with serious gram-positive infections treated with linezolid for a mean of 28 days.[102]

PK-PD and Clinical Implications for Dosing (See Tables 37-6 and 37-7)

Linezolid is indicated for the treatment of vancomycin-resistant *E. faecium* (VRE) infections; pneumonia caused by MRSA or *S. pneumoniae*; and severe, complicated skin infections caused by susceptible organisms. Linezolid penetrates respiratory secretions and epithelial lining fluid better than vancomycin.[103] Linezolid exhibits time-dependent killing with moderate-to-prolonged persistent antimicrobial effects.[94] The primary PD determinant associated with efficacy in the neutropenic thigh-infection model for *S. pneumoniae* and *S. aureus* is an AUC/MIC ratio of 50 and 80, respectively.[104] Susceptible strains of *Enterococcus* and *Streptococcus* spp. have MICs less than or equal to 2 µg/mL, whereas the susceptible strains of staphylococci have a MIC less than or equal to 4 µg/mL. In adults with MRSA or VRE, favorable outcomes were experienced in 97% of those who achieved a linezolid AUC/MIC ratio of greater than 95 compared with 75% of those who had lower AUC/MIC ratios.[105] Administration of continuous linezolid infusions, such that drug concentrations are maintained above the MIC for entire dosing interval, has been associated with bactericidal activity.[106,107] For adults with MRSA infections, there appears to be no significant difference in clinical cure or microbiologic cure between linezolid and vancomycin.[108] However, linezolid was superior to vancomycin in one adult comparator trial of complicated skin and soft tissue infections.[109]

Linezolid clinical trials have been performed in hospitalized young infants and children with documented gram-positive infections.[99,110,111] Linezolid was well tolerated at a dosage of 10 mg/kg every 8 hours and as effective as vancomycin for treatment of resistant gram-positive infections. Infants require dosing every 8 hours to maintain AUCs similar to those achieved in adolescents and adults dosed every 12 hours.[101] An AUC of 100 would achieve AUC/MIC ratios of greater or equal to 50 if the MIC of the organism was less than or equal to 2, as would be expected for most enterococcal or streptococcal infections. Higher doses may be needed to achieve this AUC/MIC target in infants with faster CL or infants with MRSA infections, where the MIC may be between 2 to 4 µg/mL; PD targets have not been confirmed in clinical trials. In the first few days of life, infants may accumulate linezolid as CL is rapidly changing. For extremely preterm infants younger than 7 days of chronologic age, we would consider a dose of 10 mg/kg every 12 hours.[55] The risk of drug accumulation is balanced with the need to rapidly achieve and maintain adequate plasma and tissue concentrations of drug during a developmental period of rapidly improving CL. The potential for line zolid resistance has been documented; further emergence and spread of such resistance may depend on its prudent use.

A new oxazolidinone antibiotic, tedizolid (marketed as Sivextro), was approved by the FDA in 2014 for once-daily dosing against acute gram-positive bacterial infections, including MRSA; information on its potential use and safety in pregnancy and infants is not yet available.

CLINDAMYCIN (SEE TABLE 37-7)

Antimicrobial Activity

Clindamycin replaced its parent compound lincomycin because it is more completely absorbed from the gut, has fewer adverse effects, and has greater antibacterial activity in vitro.[112,113] Clindamycin is primarily a bacteriostatic agent that acts by inhibiting protein synthesis through reversible binding to bacterial ribosomes, thus inhibiting bacterial protein synthesis. Clindamycin is active against gram-positive cocci such as *S. aureus*, *S. pneumoniae* (including many multidrug-resistant strains), and *S. pyogenes*. It also maintains notable activity against anaerobic bacteria, especially members of the *Bacteroides* group. Aerobic gram-negative bacteria are not usually susceptible to this antibiotic. Resistance to clindamycin is related to alterations of its target site and not to reduced uptake or to breakdown of the drug by the resistant bacteria.

Pharmacokinetic Data

Clindamycin pharmacology has been recently reviewed; however, there is a paucity of information in neonates.[112,113] Clindamycin exhibits significant (94%) protein binding. The drug is eliminated primarily through the liver, with only about 10% excreted in unchanged form in the urine. Clindamycin is reported to be a cytochrome P-450 substrate that may increase the neuromuscular blocking action of tubocurarine and pancuronium. Clindamycin has been shown to accumulate in patients with hepatic dysfunction. It is widely distributed throughout the body, including pleural fluid, ascites, bone, and bile. However, no significant levels (≈20%) are seen in the CSF, even in the setting of meningitis. Experimental meningitis animal models have demonstrated CSF penetration after parenteral administration.[114] In adults, clindamycin exhibits excellent bioavailability after oral administration.

When IV clindamycin was administered to infants in the first 4 weeks after birth, in a dosage schedule of 6.5 mg/kg every 8 hours (preterm) or 5 mg/kg every 6 hours (term), the mean peak serum concentration was 10 μg/mL, and trough values ranged from 2.8 to 5.5 μg/mL.[115] The serum elimination half-life was inversely related to GA and birth weight. Premature neonates demonstrated a mean serum half-life of 8.7 hours, compared with 3.6 hours for term newborns.[115] Another study of 12 neonates demonstrated a serum elimination half-life of 3.5 to 9.8 hours (mean, 6.3 hours).[116] Neonates have longer elimination half-lives for clindamycin than the 3-hour half-life observed in infants aged 1 month to 1 year of age.

Safety

Adverse effects of clindamycin include diarrhea, rashes, elevated levels of hepatic enzymes, granulocytopenia, thrombocytopenia, and, rarely, Stevens-Johnson syndrome. The most serious potential complication to consider is pseudomembranous colitis. Many asymptomatic neonates are colonized with *Clostridium difficile*, the presumed etiologic agent of pseudomembranous colitis.[117] However, evidence for an association of *C. difficile* colonization with colitis in newborns is lacking, and pseudomembranous colitis is rare in both newborns and young infants. This adverse effect also is observed with the use of β-lactam and other antimicrobial agents.

PK-PD and Clinical Implications for Dosing (See Tables 37-6 and 37-7)

Clinical information suggests that clindamycin can be effectively used to treat MRSA infections.[118] Caution is advised, however, because resistance to clindamycin can be induced after selective antimicrobial pressure, particularly in MRSA organisms that initially are clindamycin susceptible and erythromycin resistant. Use of clindamycin in selected MRSA-infected newborn patients can obviate the need for vancomycin therapy. For treatment of the rare *Bacteroides fragilis* infections in newborns, especially those involving the CSF, metronidazole or clindamycin have been used. Clindamycin is said to have poor penetration into the CSF[119] albeit good penetration into brain tissue.[120]

Considerable debate exists regarding the optimal dose of clindamycin. Antibacterial activity is concentration independent and time dependent, with considerable PAE.[121] Clindamycin has antibacterial activity that appears to be maximized as drug concentrations approach one to four times the MIC and also has a considerable PAE (4-6 hours).[122] In the murine thigh infection model, clindamycin has been effective against clindamycin-susceptible (and noninducible) MRSA.[123] One proposed PK-PD target is to maintain the clindamycin concentration above the MIC for greater than or equal to 50% of the dosing interval. Most staphylococcal species have a low MIC (<1 μg/mL) for the drug. Much lower dosing than is currently used in adults was shown to achieve equivalent killing and maintain the clindamycin concentration above the MIC for 100% of the dosing interval.[122] Empirical dosing information based upon the limited PK information available is 5 mg/kg/dose administered every 12 hours in the first week of life and every 6 to 8 hours thereafter. Preterm infants may have decreased CL of clindamycin; therefore dosing interval is typically maintained at 8 to 12 hours for the first 2 weeks after birth. These doses are less than recommended in infants and young children (25-40 mg/kg/day divided every 6-8 hours). More neonatal PK data is needed, especially in ELBW infants with serious bacterial infections in the first 90 days after birth. Because clindamycin is highly protein bound, assays need to clearly quantify the molecularly active non–protein-bound exposure to clindamycin.

RIFAMPIN

In selected neonates with persistent, systemic staphylococcal infections, rifampin has been used to provide a synergistic effect when given with other antistaphylococcal drugs.[124,125] Resistance rapidly emerges with rifampin monotherapy. In adults, rifampin is widely distributed throughout the body, including the CSF.[126] Rifampin is 80% protein bound and is eliminated in bile after progressive deacetylation to metabolites that remain microbiologically active. No dose adjustment is needed for renal insufficiency. Rifampin is bactericidal through the inhibition of bacterial-specific DNA-dependent RNA polymerase activity. It is active against most strains of *Neisseria meningitidis*, *Mycobacterium tuberculosis*, and aerobic gram-positive bacteria, including methicillin-sensitive *S. aureus* (MSSA), MRSA, and *S. epidermidis*. Safety concerns regarding rifampin are focused on thrombocytopenia, liver dysfunction and jaundice; liver function and blood count monitoring is recommended. Rifampin has been found to compete with bilirubin for biliary excretion, and increased bilirubin has been observed. Rifampin is also known to induce cytochrome P-450 enzymes, and therefore drug interactions are possible.[127] Rifampin has been shown to accelerate elimination of drugs that are used in the neonatal population, including phenytoin, azole antifungal agents, narcotic analgesics, diazepam, and corticosteroids.

Neonatal PK information for IV rifampin is sparse, and dosing remains empirical.[124,128] In one small study, infants (mean age, 23 days) received rifampin 10 mg/kg/day and had a mean peak concentration of 4.02 μg/mL and a mean 12-hour trough concentration of 1.11 μg/mL.[128] In children, rifampin CL is induced after 8 days of therapy. As rifampin CL increases and half-life decreases, the dosing interval may need to be shortened to accommodate induced clearance in prolonged therapy.[129] Uncontrolled clinical case series suggest that rifampin used as an adjunct to vancomycin therapy can provide prompt clearance of persistent staphylococcal bacteremia or ventriculitis in high-risk neonates.[124,125,128]

TEICOPLANIN

Teicoplanin is a glycopeptide antibiotic that is almost identical to vancomycin with regard to its antibacterial spectrum of activity. It is used frequently in Europe, where it is approved for the treatment of gram-positive infections[130,131]; however, it is not approved for use in the United States. Teicoplanin may have some advantages over vancomycin in terms of tolerability, with a lower propensity to cause nephrotoxicity and histaminic-type reactions. Teicoplanin also has a longer elimination half-life, allowing for longer dosing intervals. It rapidly penetrates into tissue and reaches high concentrations in the kidney, trachea, lungs, and adrenals but does not penetrate well into the CSF. It is excreted unchanged in the urine after a prolonged elimination phase.

Despite these potential advantages, teicoplanin PK data adequate to formulate dosage regimens in neonates are lacking. In one study, four neonates received a single dose of 6 mg/kg, and the mean peak serum teicoplanin concentration was 19.6 μg/mL, with a mean half-life of 30 hours.[132] In several noncomparative trials, the clinical and bacteriologic response rates ranged between 80% and 100% in 173 infected neonates given IV teicoplanin 8 to 10 mg/kg once daily after a loading dose of 10 to 20 mg/kg.[133] A recent study of 37 episodes of staphylococcal bacteremia in neonates treated with a loading dose of 16 mg/kg teicoplanin, followed by a maintenance dose of 8 mg/kg/day, achieved bacterial eradication in 89% and survival of 94% with no documented drug-related adverse events.[134] One neonate was reported to have tolerated teicoplanin overdose (20 mg/kg/day for 5 days).[135]

DAPTOMYCIN

Daptomycin is the first-in-class member of the cyclic lipopeptide family.[1,136,137] Lipopeptides have a unique mechanism of action. They insert into bacteria membranes and cause a rapid membrane depolarization, leading to inhibition of protein, DNA and RNA synthesis, cell leakage, and ultimately cell death. Daptomycin exhibits rapid, concentration-dependent, bactericidal activity against MRSA, MRSE, vancomycin-resistant *S. aureus*, and VRE. The product is approved in the United States for the treatment of complicated skin and skin structure infections, and *S. aureus* bacteremia.[1,136] Daptomycin is not indicated for the treatment of pneumonia because of its inactivation by surfactant.[138] Daptomycin exhibits a high degree of protein binding and is primarily excreted unchanged by the kidney. In clinical trials, a few adults receiving daptomycin had elevated creatine phosphokinase (CPK) enzyme and, rarely, myopathy.[1,136,139] The manufacturer recommends monitoring CPK weekly while on therapy and discontinuing therapy for myopathy, myalgia, or CPK greater than 1000 mg/dL.[136]

Daptomycin is not approved for use in children or neonates. One single-dose PK study of 25 children with suspected or proven gram-positive infections revealed more rapid CL in younger children.[140] Two infants with complicated MRSA infections who received 6 mg/kg dose every 12 hours had peak and trough concentrations that were consistent with concentrations observed in adults treated with a 4-mg/kg daily dose.[141] These infants achieved microbiologic and clinical cure; however, their exposure was less than that achieved in adults receiving daptomycin at the approved dose of 6 mg/kg per day for treatment of MRSA bacteremia.

A single-dose PK study, after giving 6 mg/kg daptomycin IV, was carried out on 20 neonates at risk for infection, having a median gestation age at birth of 32 weeks (range, 23-40 weeks) and median PNA of 3 days (range, 1-85 days).[142] The median AUC at 24 hours, Vd, total-body clearance, and half-life of daptomycin were 262.4 mg*hr/L (range, 166.7-340.2), 0.21 L/kg (range, 0.11-0.34), 0.021 L/hr/kg (range, 0.016-0.034), and 6.2 hours (3.7-9.0), respectively. CPK concentrations were not elevated. No adverse events related to daptomycin were observed. Daptomycin concentrations were lower than that achieved in adults receiving similar doses. Clearance in young infants was similar to that in children 2 to 6 years of age and higher than that observed in adolescents and adults. Young infants are likely to need higher doses of daptomycin to achieve adult efficacy targets. Additional studies, including multiple-dose PK and safety studies, are needed to derive appropriate PK-PD dosing guidance.[142]

Aminoglycosides (Table 37-8)

HISTORY

For more than 3 decades, the aminoglycosides have been relied upon for therapy for neonatal sepsis because of their broad-spectrum antibacterial activity against gram-negative bacilli. However, their use in some centers is decreasing because of the emergence of resistant strains. Currently, gentamicin, tobramycin, and amikacin are the aminoglycosides of choice in most nurseries. Because amikacin is resistant to degradation by most of the plasmid-mediated bacterial enzymes that inactivate gentamicin and tobramycin, some centers have held amikacin in reserve for treatment of nosocomially acquired infections caused by multidrug-resistant gram-negative organisms. Gentamicin resistance occurs frequently enough in some European, Latin American, and U.S. centers to warrant use of amikacin as a first-line drug

Table 37-8 Aminoglycosides and Aztreonam for the Treatment of Gram-Negative Infections in the First Week After Birth

Drug	Route Elimination	Peak μg/mL	Half-Life (hr)	PK-PD Target[11,12]	Protein Binding %	CSF Penetration[16]	CLSI Sensitivity Breakpoint MIC* *Enterobacteriaceae*	CLSI Sensitivity Breakpoint MIC* *Pseudomonas aeruginosa*	Safety and Clinical Pearls
Gentamicin 2.5 mg/kg q12h 4 mg/kg q24h 5 mg/kg q24h	Renal	 3-6 7-8 8-12	 8-12 (<2000 g) 5 (>2000 g) 3-5 (PNA > 7 days)	Peak/MIC > 8-10 TDM goal Peak 6-12 Trough <2	0%-30%	5%	≤4	≤4	Extended-interval dosing more likely to achieves PK-PK target but requires dosing every 36 or 48 hours in premature infants TDM especially if premature or if treatment > 48 hr Follow urine output, creatinine Consider hearing screen
Amikacin 7.5 mg/kg q12 15 mg/kg q24h	Renal	 15 25	6-9 (<2000 g) 5-6 (>2000 g) 4-5 (PNA >7 days)	Peak/MIC Peak 20-30 Trough < 5	0%-10%	20%-34%	≤16	≤16	
Tobramycin 2-4 mg/kg	Renal	 3-8	 8-12 (<2500 g) 3-5 (>2500 g)	Peak/MIC Peak 6-12 Trough < 2		0	≤4	≤4	
Aztreonam 30 mg/kg	Renal	 80 (<2500g) 100 (>2500g)	 5-8 (<2500g) 2-3 (>2500g)	Peak/MIC	56%	17%-33%	≤4	≤8	Measure glucose 1 hr after dose Rare AE: rash, diarrhea Monitor CBC, LFT

Dose, peak, and half-life as reported in References 143, 149, 199, 200, and 201.

AE, Antibiotic effects; *CBC,* complete blood count; *CLSI,* Clinical and Laboratory Standards Institute; *CSF,* cerebrospinal fluid; *LFT,* liver function tests; *MIC,* minimal inhibitory concentration; *PD,* pharmacodynamic; *PK,* pharmacokinetic; *PNA,* postnatal age; *TDM,* therapeutic drug monitoring.

*CLSA. Performance Standard for Antimicrobial Susceptibility Testing; Twenty-Fourth Informational Supplement. CLSI document M100-S24. Wayne, Pa: Clinical and Laboratory Standards Institute; 2014. Bacteria with intermediate sensitivities have higher MIC.

for therapy of life-threatening gram-negative infections. Thus far, its routine use has not resulted in emergence of resistant strains.

The history of aminoglycoside usage in the late 1950s and 1960s is an excellent example of the inherent problems of adapting dosages derived from studies in adults to newborns. Irreversible ototoxicity in neonates was caused by excessive doses of streptomycin or kanamycin. By contrast, the PK of gentamicin, tobramycin, amikacin, and netilmicin were carefully defined in the neonate before routine use of these drugs; appropriate studies thus provided a scientific basis for safe and effective dosage regimens. The risk of aminoglycoside toxicity is minimal when these agents are administered to infants in the proper dosage and when serum concentrations are closely monitored and kept within the recommended therapeutic range.

The evolution of gentamicin dosing over recent years is also an excellent example of dosing modifications that target PD to achieve optimal therapeutic exposure. Aminoglycoside administration using extended-dosing intervals appears to be at least as safe and effective as giving these drugs in two or three divided doses. The extended-dosing interval schedule provides a higher peak concentration to maximize the concentration-dependent bacterial killing and take advantage of the prolonged PAE of the aminoglycosides.[143,144]

ANTIMICROBIAL ACTIVITY

Aminoglycosides act on microbial ribosomes to irreversibly inhibit protein synthesis. In general, gentamicin, tobramycin, and amikacin have good antibacterial activity against most gram-negative strains. Tobramycin has the greatest antipseudomonal activity, whereas amikacin is the only drug of this class that reliably provides activity against *Serratia* spp. and other coliforms with nosocomially acquired resistance. Although staphylococci are susceptible in vitro to aminoglycosides, infections caused by these pathogens usually do not respond satisfactorily to aminoglycoside therapy alone. Synergistic bactericidal activity between aminoglycosides and the penicillins has been demonstrated in vitro and in animals against *S. aureus*, group B streptococci, *L. monocytogenes*, and enterococci, despite low-level resistance of each microorganism to the aminoglycoside alone.

Possible mechanisms of bacterial resistance to these drugs include alteration of the ribosomal binding site, changes in the cell surface proteins to prevent entrance of drug into the cell, and induction of aminoglycoside-inactivating enzymes. Antibiotic resistance in clinical situations is most often a result of extrachromosomally controlled (R-factor) enzymes. Phosphorylation, adenylation, and acetylation are the three most common enzymatic mechanisms encountered.[145] High concentrations of aminoglycosides may reduce the emergence of resistance by targeting resistant subpopulations.

Some gram-negative organisms, notably *Pseudomonas aeruginosa* and *Enterobacter* spp., demonstrate reduced uptake of aminoglycosides after initial exposure.[146] Such reduced uptake can decrease bacterial killing and is referred to as adaptive resistance; it may last for several hours after initial antibiotic exposure but appears to be reversible after a duration of low plasma aminoglycoside concentrations.

PHARMACOKINETIC DATA

Gentamicin (See Table 37-8)

Gentamicin is the most methodically studied aminoglycoside in newborns; however, there is considerable interpatient variability in gentamicin concentrations achieved in neonates. This variability is typically due to changes in renal function and body-water composition with advancing GA, chronologic age, and creatinine clearance as well as differences in clinical disease state of the infant and concomitant medications.

Gentamicin is administered via IM or IV injection. Studies of gentamicin concentrations demonstrate that IM and IV administration of gentamicin provide similar exposure.[147,148] Aminoglycosides such as gentamicin cannot be administered orally for treatment of systemic infection because they are not absorbed from the intact gastrointestinal tract.

Neonates have reduced gentamicin CL, longer half-life, and increased Vd compared with older patients. Neonatal population PK studies of gentamicin have attempted to explain the variability of gentamicin disposition with demographic and clinical variables.[143,149] Vd is consistently associated with infant weight and ranges from 0.45 to 0.69 L/kg. The mean relative clearance is 0.04 to 0.06 L/hr/kg, typically depending on how many premature infants were included in the model and their chronologic age. Clearance improves with advancing GA, chronologic age, PMA, and creatinine clearance as expected for improved renal maturation. Half-life of gentamicin is longer in younger, smaller, more immature infants, and those with reduced creatinine clearance. During the first week of life, premature (<30 weeks) infants have delayed CL (≈0.03 L/kg/hr) and long half-life (10-14 hours), compared with moderately preterm infants (30-34 weeks) who have delayed CL (≈0.04 L/kg/hr) and modest half-life (8-10 hours).[143] Late preterm and term infants have a much shorter half-life of 4 to 5 hours, given their faster CL of approximately 0.05 L/kg/hr.[143] Perinatal asphyxia, PDA (or its treatment), and unrepaired congenital heart disease are associated with prolonged serum gentamicin half-life, likely resulting from decreased renal clearance.[150,151]

CSF concentrations of gentamicin in infants with meningitis are from 0.3 to 3.7 μg/mL (mean, 1.6 μg/mL) 1 to 6 hours after a 2.5-mg/kg dose.[19] Peak values are observed 4 to 6 hours after the dose and are correlated with the degree of meningeal inflammation and dosage. During the 1970s, the Neonatal Meningitis Cooperative Study Group evaluated lumbar intrathecal and intraventricular gentamicin administration in comparative studies with systemic antibiotic therapy alone.[19] Despite higher CSF and intraventricular fluid concentrations, neither route of administration of therapy was associated with a better outcome in infants with meningitis caused by gram-negative enteric organisms. In fact, case-fatality rates were significantly greater in intraventricular gentamicin recipients. Poor outcomes may in part be explained by the rapid lysis of gram-negative bacteria associated with high ventricular fluid gentamicin concentrations, the subsequent release of significantly larger amounts of endotoxin into the ventricular fluid, and greater meningeal inflammation.[152]

Serum gentamicin concentrations are altered by exchange transfusion and ECMO; after a two–volume exchange transfusion, serum aminoglycoside concentrations are reduced by 19% to 62%.[153,154] Whenever possible, such procedures are best timed to precede the next scheduled dose of gentamicin. Therapeutic drug monitoring is needed to guide dosing for infants on ECMO because gentamicin, and probably other aminoglycosides, exhibits a higher Vd, a lower clearance, and a longer half-life.[155]

Tobramycin (See Table 37-8)

Tobramycin offers two theoretical advantages over gentamicin for therapy for neonatal infections: increased in vitro activity against *P. aeruginosa* and decreased nephrotoxicity. The lower incidence of nephrotoxicity for tobramycin has been documented in laboratory animals and human adults but not in neonates.[156] Neonates appear to be less sensitive to aminoglycoside nephrotoxicity; therefore this advantage is uncertain in young infants.

Neonatal PK of tobramycin data are not as well defined as gentamicin. After a 2-mg/kg dose of tobramycin, mean peak serum concentrations of 4 to 6 µg/mL are observed at 30 to 60 minutes.[157] Predose trough concentrations are higher in smaller and more premature infants. The serum tobramycin half-life is also prolonged in smaller, younger, and more premature infants and in those infants with delayed creatinine clearance. In the first week after birth, very-low-birth-weight (VLBW) infants (<1500 g) have half-life values as long as 9 to 17 hours, compared with values of 3 to 4.5 hours for larger infants (>2500g) and older infants who are 1 to 4 weeks of age. Premature infants born at less than 30 weeks of gestation often require dosage intervals of 18 to 24 hours.[158]

More recently, population PK models of tobramycin CL and Vd have been developed using retrospective, existing datasets of peak and trough concentrations obtained in clinical care.[149,159,160] In the largest study, in 470 neonates with suspected septicemia in the first week of life, tobramycin CL was delayed in prematurity (0.04 L/hr/kg in ≤36-week infants and 0.05-0.06 L/hr/kg in >36-week infants), and Vd varied with weight but was somewhat higher in premature infants (0.07 L/kg in ≤36-week infants compared with 0.54 L/kg in >36-week infants). Tobramycin half–life ranged from 7 hours in mature infants to 11 hours in premature infants. Infants received tobramycin 3.5 mg/kg every 24 hours (<28 weeks), 2.5 mg/kg every 12 hours (28-36 weeks), or 2.5 mg/kg every 12 hours (>36 weeks). Target trough levels (<2 µg/mL) and peak levels (5-10 µg/mL) occurred in 67% and 21% of samples respectively. Nearly half of the significant preterm infants less than 28 weeks of gestation had aberrant trough levels. Population PK models determined that dosing of 4 mg/kg is needed to achieve desired peak concentration. Dosing intervals to achieve trough concentrations less than 2 µg/mL varied with degree of prematurity: 24 hours for term, 36 hours for 32- to 37-week infants, and every 48 hours for infants less than 32 weeks of gestation. Using this dosing scheme, simulated peak and trough targeted concentrations were predicted to be achieved in greater than 90% of infants. Therapeutic drug monitoring and individualization of the dosage schedule are often needed to provide the optimal therapy for VBLW infants.

Amikacin (See Table 37-8)

Neonatal amikacin PK data are limited. Historically, infants receiving 7.5-mg/kg doses of amikacin achieved mean peak and 12-hour trough serum concentrations of 15 to 25 µg/mL and 3 to 6 µg/mL, respectively.[161] Serum half-life of amikacin is longer in younger and more premature infants. LBW infants exhibit a half-life of 7 to 8 hours at 1 to 3 days of age compared with the much shorter half-life of 4 to 5 hours in term infants who are older than 1 week. The serum half-life is also prolonged in hypoxemic newborns.

Neonatal population PK studies of amikacin have explored the wide variability of disposition.[162-166] Amikacin CL increased with GA, weight, and PNA, whereas Vd varied with body weight. In the largest dataset created from 874 neonates (GA, 24-43 weeks; PNA, 1 to 30 days; and birth weight, 385-4650 g), amikacin CL varied most with PMA; however, the combination of both birth weight and PNA was somewhat superior.[164] Concomitant administration of ibuprofen also was associated with reduced clearance, and many datasets include a high percentage of preterm infants who were receiving ibuprofen. Body weight was the most important covariate for Vd. In the final PK model, CL was 0.05 L/hr and Vd was 0.82 L.[164] De Cock and colleagues[164] concluded that amikacin CL reflects the glomerular filtration rate in neonates and can therefore be predicted by the birth weight representing the antenatal state of renal maturation, the PNA representing postnatal maturation, and co-administration of ibuprofen representing affects of renal perfusion. At birth, clearance varied fourfold from preterm 1-kg infants (CL ≈0.026 L/hr) to term 3-kg infants (CL ≈0.112 L/hr). Even though clearance improves with PNA, premature infants still exhibit delay of clearance at 28 days when compared with larger-term infants. Ibuprofen reduced clearance by 16%. Wide patient variability was also observed.

Reports of CSF concentrations of amikacin are scarce.[167] In the presence of uninflamed meninges in 1-day-old infants, CSF values ranged from 0.2 to 2.7 µg/mL when measured at 1 to 4 hours after a single 10-mg/kg dose administered by slow IV infusion.[168] Simultaneous concentrations in serum ranged from 15 to 29 µg/mL. The highest CSF concentration reported has been 9.2 µg/mL after a 7.5-mg/kg dose was administered intramuscularly to an infant with meningitis.[161] Amikacin concentration in ventricular fluid 12 hours after 1- or 2-mg intraventricular doses and 2 to 8 hours after IM doses varies, ranging from 4.5 to 11.6 µg/mL (mean, 7.3 µg/mL). In the largest and most recent study of 43 preterm and term infants (mean PMA, 36 weeks; range, 26-41 weeks), the median amikacin CSF concentration was 1.09 µg/mL (range, 0.34-2.65 µg/mL), and the mean peak and trough serum concentration were 35.7 µg/mL and 3.8 µg/mL, respectively.[167] Concentrations in CSF were low, likely because the CSF sampling occurred at a median of 25 hours after amikacin administration; no correlation between CSF white blood cell count and CSF amikacin levels was identified.

SAFETY

The major adverse effects of aminoglycoside antibiotics are renal toxicity, ototoxicity, and, rarely, neuromuscular blockade. Aminoglycosides are eliminated through glomerular filtration, but some drug is reabsorbed in the proximal tubule. Aminoglycosides may accumulate in renal tubular cells, where they fuse with cytoplasmic lysosomes and inhibit phospholipases, with the resultant accumulation of phospholipid aggregates and release of lysosomal contents within the renal tubular cells. The potential for nephrotoxicity varies among the aminoglycosides because of differences in the rate of uptake and amount of drug accumulation in the renal cortex. This renal cortical uptake is saturable in rats.[169] Human nephrectomy studies have also demonstrated saturable uptake: higher renal cortical aminoglycoside (amikacin and gentamicin but not tobramycin) concentrations when doses were administered by continuous infusion or twice daily compared with once daily.[170,171] Toxicity is correlated with elevated drug trough concentrations and prolonged therapy but not with high peak concentrations. Extended aminoglycoside dosing intervals produce longer periods at low drug concentrations, thereby lessening the potential for renal drug accumulation and toxicity.

Meta-analysis of adult trials of extended-interval aminoglycoside administration compared with conventional multidose daily administration showed that the rate of nephrotoxicity with extended-interval dosing was less than or equal to that observed with traditional regimens.[172] In addition to drug dose and administration regimen, the risk factors for nephrotoxicity also include the concomitant medications and the patient's clinical condition.

The reported incidence of aminoglycoside nephrotoxicity ranges from 5% to 25% and is thought to be lower in children than adults.[173] It has been suggested that the immature kidney of the neonate may be protected from major toxic effects of aminoglycosides. Transient cylindruria and proteinuria may occur after prolonged administration of any of these drugs, but significant elevations in blood urea nitrogen and creatinine values are rarely observed.[174,175]

In a meta-analysis of neonatal comparative trials of once-daily extended-interval dosing, compared with multidose standard dosing of aminoglycosides, nephrotoxicity was rare, and there was no significant difference noted between the two dosing administration groups.[144] Because renal excretion accounts for the elimination of approximately 80% of an aminoglycoside dose, the risk of toxicity is greatest when drug elimination is impaired by reduction in renal function for any reason. Therapeutic drug monitoring is often helpful in neonates receiving greater than 48 hours of therapy.

Therapeutic drug monitoring, however, has not been shown to prevent renal or ototoxicity in neonates but rather serves as a guide to provide individual dosing, given large interpatient variability in kinetics, especially in premature infants or infants who are expected to receive aminoglycosides for greater than 48 hours. Other factors that may be associated with increased risk for aminoglycoside nephrotoxicity include acidosis, hypovolemia, hypoalbuminemia, sodium depletion, duration of therapy, increased total aminoglycoside dose, and frequency of administration and co-administration of furosemide, vancomycin, or prostaglandin synthesis inhibitors such as indomethacin.

Neomycin, streptomycin, kanamycin, and gentamicin each have been implicated as a cause of sensorineural hearing loss in infants and children. Gentamicin and streptomycin also have been associated with vestibular impairment. However, it is difficult to incriminate the aminoglycosides as the single causative agent of hearing loss in most studies because of the high-risk conditions present in affected patients, such as asphyxia, hyperbilirubinemia, and incubator/ventilator noise exposure, that have been independently associated with ototoxicity.[176] In a prospective evaluation of long-term toxicity of kanamycin and gentamicin, neither was incriminated as the sole agent responsible for hearing impairment.[177] Historically, ototoxicity has been related primarily to very high total aminoglycoside dosages: High-frequency sensorineural hearing loss in infants with normal renal function is more likely if the total dosage exceeds 500 mg/kg.[177] Data from the first Neonatal Meningitis Cooperative Study[19] indicated that profound deafness, potentially related to gentamicin exposure, developed in only 1 (1.3%) of 79 infants who received a minimum of 5 to 7.5 mg/kg per day of the drug for 3 weeks or longer. Auditory toxicity was reported in a very small number of infants in the largest meta-analysis to date of once-daily gentamicin compared with standard-interval dose regimen.[144] Vestibular toxicity is difficult to assess in neonates and has not been evaluated.

The precise mechanism involved in ototoxicity is unknown. Some evidence suggests that point mutations in mitochondrial DNA are relevant to explain hearing loss in selected persons after aminoglycoside treatment.[178] Mutations in 12S ribosomal RNA (rRNA) gene have also been associated with aminoglycoside-induced ototoxicity. However, in a recent study of 436 neonates, mutations in 12S rRNA occurred in only 0.9%.[179] In this cohort, 39 (9%) infants failed initial hearing assessment, but only 1 of these infants had a 12S rRNA mutation. Low birth weight remained the largest risk factor for failed hearing screen. Even for the rare hospitalized infant with ototoxicity after receiving concurrent dosages of aminoglycosides, it is difficult to establish a direct causal relationship in many of the published studies because of their complicated clinical histories.

Aminoglycoside-associated neuromuscular blockade has been reported only rarely.[180] The underlying mechanism appears to be inhibition of acetylcholine release at the neuromuscular junction by these drugs.[181] The aminoglycoside may act alone or synergistically with other neuromuscular blocking agents. Hypermagnesemia in newborns, often resulting from antenatal exposure to maternal magnesium administered for preeclampsia, may potentiate the neuromuscular blocking effects of aminoglycosides. Diagnosis is made by nerve conduction studies, which reveal a progressive fatigue and posttetanic facilitation characteristic of a nondepolarizing, curare-like neuromuscular block. Reversal of this block is achieved by neostigmine or calcium (or both). Potentiation of neuromuscular blockade can be observed in infant botulism when aminoglycosides are administered to treat suspected sepsis.[182] Prophylactic treatment with calcium is not indicated because this cation may interfere with the antimicrobial activity of aminoglycosides against certain organisms.

PK-PD AND CLINICAL IMPLICATIONS FOR DOSING (SEE TABLES 37-6, 37-8, AND 37-9)

The aminoglycosides still remain effective for the initial empirical therapy in newborns with suspected early onset sepsis. The choice of aminoglycoside to be routinely used

Table 37-9 Serum Peak and Trough Concentrations of Gentamicin in Preterm and Term Neonate*

		ODD REGIMEN				SDD REGIMEN				
Study	**GA (wk)**	**N**	**Daily Dose (mg/kg)**	**Peak (μg/mL)**	**Trough (μg/mL)**	**N**	**Daily Dose (mg/kg)**	**Peak (μg/mL)**	**Trough (μg/mL)**	**Reference**
GENTAMICIN										
Skopnik	≥38	10	4	10.9	0.8 ± 0.2	10	4	7.4	1.0 ± 0.4	178
Hayani	≥34	11	5	10.7 ± 2.1	1.7 ± 0.4	15	5	6.6 ±1.3	1.7 ± 0.5	444
de Alba-Romero	≥38	13	5	9.2 ± 1.5	1.1 ± 0.4	15	5	5.7 ± 1.3	1.5 ± 0.6	445
de Alba-Romero	29-37	20	5	9.7 ± 1.8	1.6 ± 0.8	17	5	7.1 ± 1.7	2.7 ± 0.9	445
Skopnik	32-38	28	4	7.9 ± 1.6	1.0 ± 0.5	27	5	6.1 ± 1.1	2.0 ± 1.1	446
Miron	32-37	17	5	9.9 ± 4.6	1.5 ± 0.5	18	5	5.9 ± 1.7	2.4 ± 0.9	447
Agrawal	≥2500 g	20	4	8.2 ± 1.7	0.9 ± 0.4	21	5	6.2 ± 1.5	1.9 ± 0.5	448
Chotigeat	≥34	27	4-5	8.9 ± 1.6	0.9 ± 0.4	27	4-5	5.9 ± 1.6	1.4 ± 0.5	449
Kosalaraksa	≥2000 g	33	5	10 ± 3.0	1.6 ± 1.1	31	5	7.8 ± 2.0	2.6 ± 1.2	450
Krishnan	32-36	9	4	5.9 ± 1.1	1.96 ± 0.6	9	5	3.9 ± 0.8	2.8 ± 0.7	451
Solomon	32-36	13	4	7.4 ± 2.3	1.8 ± 0.9	12	5	6.7 ± 2.4	2.0 ±1.1	452
Solomon	≥37	24	4	7.1 ± 2.6	1.3 ± 1.0	24	5	7.0 ± 2.8	1.5 ± 1.0	452
Thureen	≥34	27	4	7.9 ± 0.2	1.0 ± 0.5	28	5	6.7 ± 0.3	2.1 ± 1.1	453
Rastogi	<33	30	5 (q48h)	8.2 ± 1.3	1.7 ± 0.6	18	2.5 (q18h)	6.0 ± 2.2	1.2 ± 0.4	191
Mercado (concentration range)	<33		5 (q48h)	5-12	0.4-1.6		2.5 (q18h)	2-9	0.3-2.1	454
AMIKACIN										
Langhendries	>34	10	15	23.6 ± 3.3	2.7 ± 1.2	12	15	13.6 ± 3.3	3.5 ± 1.4	455
Kotze	≥38	20	15	30.6 ± 2.8	1.7 ± 0.8	20	15	18.5 ± 4.0	3.5 ± 2.4	196

GA, Gestational age; *ODD*, once-daily dosing; *SDD*, standard daily dosing.

*Neonates who received standard daily dosing q12h (SDD) or once-daily dosing q24h (ODD) in several randomized comparison trials included in 2011 Cochrane review[144] with the addition of data from Skopnik and Heimann[446] (1995); Rastogi, Agarwal, Pyati, et al[191] (2002); Mercado, Brodsky, McGuire, et al[454] (2004); Langhendries, Battisti, Bertrand, et al[455] (1993); and Kotze[196] (1999).

is mainly dependent on the patterns of microbial resistance within a nursery. Amikacin remains one option for empirical treatment when multidrug-resistant coliforms are frequently isolated within an individual neonatal unit. The aminoglycosides are usually safe to use in the newborn when administered according to the recommended dosage schedules. Therapeutic drug monitoring is helpful, particularly in premature infants and infants with hypoxemia, renal dysfunction, or critical illness. Therapeutic drug monitoring is needed to guide dosing in infants on ECMO.

Systemic aminoglycoside therapy remains an acceptable initial empirical treatment choice when meningitis is present because, in combination with ampicillin, this agent offers potential synergistic activity against group B streptococci and *L. monocytogenes*. Aminoglycosides have been demonstrated to be effective for therapy for meningitis caused by susceptible gram-negative bacteria. However, if gram-negative bacilli are seen on CSF smears or later isolated as the causative agent of meningitis, third-generation cephalosporins or carbapenems should be considered. Combined therapy with a cephalosporin and an aminoglycoside is often used for the first 7 to 10 days of therapy for possible synergistic bacterial killing and to prevent emergence of bacterial resistance during the treatment, especially for meningitis caused by *Serratia*, *Pseudomonas*, *Acinetobacter*, *Citrobacter*, and *Enterobacter* spp.

Aminoglycosides demonstrate concentration-dependent bactericidal activity (see Table 37-8).[11] In vitro time-kill curves and animal studies both demonstrate increased rate and extent of killing with increasing concentration of aminoglycosides. Early studies in gram-negative infections showed clinical response was associated with peak serum concentrations of greater than 7 μg/mL for gentamicin and tobramycin and 28 μg/mL for amikacin.[183,184] Subsequently, adult studies demonstrated effective response to therapy near 90% for a peak/MIC ratio of greater than 8:1 for *E. coli* bacteremia[185] or greater than or equal to 10:1 for gram-negative pneumonia.[186] The PD of aminoglycosides in the treatment of gram-negative infections has not been evaluated in infants.

In addition to therapeutic killing, high concentrations of aminoglycosides also provide a PAE, that is, the sustained suppression of bacterial growth even after the antibiotic concentration is below the MIC of the target organism.[187] In vitro, aminoglycosides demonstrate a PAE of 1 to 3 hours against *P. aeruginosa* and 1 to 2 hours against *Enterobacteriaceae*.[188] Animal models suggest an even longer period of PAE: 2 to 7.5 hours.[188,189] The PAE is prolonged by increasing aminoglycoside concentration and in the presence of neutrophils.[190] PAE has not been demonstrated in clinical trials, given ethical restraints of such studies. The duration of PAE is unknown in neonates, but given the immature immunity of neonates, it may be less than calculated in animal models.

Ideally, dosing regimens for aminoglycosides would attempt to maximize killing, take advantage of the PAE, minimize adaptive resistance, reduce emergence of resistance, and diminish the potential for toxicity. Therapeutic drug monitoring is used to individualize dosage regimens. To achieve this PD target, peak serum concentrations should be maintained at 8 to 12 μg/mL for gentamicin and tobramycin, and at 20 to 30 μg/mL for amikacin, in other words, a peak (C_{max})/MIC ratio of greater than 8 to 10. To potentially minimize the rare risk of toxicity, trough values are typically kept below 2 μg/mL for the former drugs and below 5 μg/mL for amikacin. To determine peak serum concentrations, blood samples are obtained 30 minutes after completion of the IV infusion or 45 to 60 minutes after an IM administration. Trough serum concentrations are measured just before the next dose of the aminoglycoside.

USE OF EXTENDED-DOSING INTERVALS TO ACHIEVE PHARMACODYNAMIC EXPOSURE TARGETS (SEE TABLES 37-6 AND 37-9)

Analysis of peak and trough concentrations reveals significant interpatient variability within and between studies. Clinical trials have compared gentamicin concentrations using traditional and extended-interval dosing regimens in primarily term and near-term neonates in the first week after birth. A Cochrane review meta-analysis concludes that once-daily extended-interval dosing was associated with fewer failures to attain a peak level of at least 5 μg/mL and fewer failures to achieve trough levels of less than or equal to 2 μg/mL compared with multiple-doses-per-day regimens.[144] Ototoxicity and nephrotoxicity were not noted with either treatment regimen. Both regimens showed adequate clearance of sepsis; however, the studies may have been underpowered to show a difference in efficacy with true bacteremia.

The rationale for use of extended-dosing intervals is based on several PK, PD, and microbiologic principles of aminoglycosides.[144] (1) Aminoglycosides exhibit concentration-dependent bacterial killing in which higher peak/MIC ratios are associated with improved bactericidal response; C_{max}/MIC ratios greater than 8 to 10 have been linked to superior efficacy of aminoglycosides against gram-negative bacteria. (2) Aminoglycosides exhibit a PAE in which bacterial growth is suppressed despite serum concentrations below the MIC; drug concentrations, therefore, can remain below the pathogen's MIC for a period without compromising efficacy. (3) Nephrotoxicity is associated with aminoglycoside uptake into renal cells and possibly into the cochlea and vestibular membrane, but cellular uptake is more efficicent with low sustained concentrations, and (in animals) uptake is a saturable process so that transient high peak levels do not lead to excessive drug accumulation. (4) Gram-negative bacteria have been shown to exhibit adaptive resistance after continuous exposure to aminoglycosides, a property that may be minimized by providing high bactericidal exposures minimizing time for bacterial growth in presence of antibiotic. (5) The lower glomerular filtration rate in neonates, especially the first few days of life, and preterm infants suggests that more time for clearance may be needed to avoid toxic accumulation of aminoglycosides. (6) Finally, once-daily dosing is associated with lower hospital costs. Although increased peak concentrations lengthen the duration of PAE, the pharmacodynamics of this phenomenon in neonates has not been defined.

Considerable evidence generated in adults with extended-dosing intervals of aminoglycoside administration prompted studies in the pediatric and neonatal populations. A meta-analysis of the comparison trials has been conducted in neonates to evaluate peak and trough gentamicin, tobramycin, or amikacin concentrations after administration of standard dosing and once-daily-dosing regimens (see Table 37-9).[144] Mean peak concentrations in each study were higher in the once-daily regimen than in the twice-daily group, and mean trough concentrations were lower in the daily group than in the standard group. Dose adjustment was indicated more often in the standard-dosing groups. One study compared 2.5- to 3-mg/kg dosing every 24 hours with 4.5- to 5-mg/kg dosing every 48 hours in 58 VLBW infants (600-1500g).[191] The 48-hour dosing schedule achieved therapeutic serum concentrations and higher peak/MIC ratios for infecting microorganisms. Nearly one third of these infants, however, had extremely low serum gentamicin concentrations before the next dose, suggesting that a 36-hour interval might be more appropriate for VLBW infants. Another study evaluated single doses of 5 mg/kg of tobramycin and gentamicin administered at extended intervals and found that only 1.3% of these infants had subtherapeutic concentrations compared with 26.8% of those given the traditional 2.5-mg/kg doses.[192]

Once-daily interval dosing was also explored for amikacin (see Table 37-9).[164-166,193-196] In term infants, 15 mg/kg daily amikacin therapy in the first 3 days of life leads to significantly increased peak levels that are more likely to achieve the PD target compared with multiple-doses-per-day traditional regimens. Both regimens yield trough levels less than 5 μg/mL. Preterm infants required higher doses and longer dosing intervals to achieve desired targets, depending on GA group. It was also proposed that dosage interval be extended for infants with a history of hypoxia or who were receiving concurrent indomethacin therapy. Amikacin-associated nephrotoxicity was not observed, and results of auditory evaluation were similar in study participants and nonstudy control subjects.

However, when amikacin dosing guidance was prospectively evaluated, patient variability was notable. De Cock and colleagues[164] reviewed amikacin concentrations in 874 neonates (24-43 weeks GA) and determined that when routine dosing strategies are used, 20% of infants did not achieve targeted exposure resulting from the inherent inter-individual variability in kinetics of drug CL in preterm and term infants, typically because of slightly higher peak and trough concentrations. They then created a population PK model from these amikacin concentrations and used simulated exposure profiles to explore dosing strategies for more consistent exposures. Their very detailed dosing algorithm (10 strata) recommends dose (12-20 mg/kg) and interval (20-48 hours) adjustment based upon current body weight (<800 g, 800-1200 g, 122-2000 g, 2000-2800 g, and >2800 g) and PNA (<14 days of age, ≥14 days of age).[164] Even using the most elaborate dosing guidance that takes into account weight, PNA, and GA, therapeutic drug monitoring will likely remain necessary for preterm neonates and those receiving greater than 48 hours of amikacin.

In summary, a Cochrane review meta-analysis concludes that once-daily or extended-interval gentamicin dosing was associated with fewer failures to attain a peak level of at least 5 μg/mL and fewer failures to achieve trough levels of less than or equal to 2 μg/mL compared with multiple-doses-per-day regimens. Analysis of peak and trough concentrations reveals significant interpatient variability within and between studies. Many recommend using population PK–derived dosing for first dose, then therapeutic drug monitoring 24 hours after the first dose to determine the individual patient's kinetics, and then modifying dosing and interval on an individual basis.[149] Ototoxicity and nephrotoxicity were not noted with either treatment regimen. Both regimens showed adequate clearance of sepsis; however, the studies may have been underpowered to show a difference in efficacy with true bacteremia. They conclude that based on PK properties and PD targets, the once-per-day regimen may be superior in treating sepsis in neonates greater than 32 weeks of gestation.

Aztreonam

Aztreonam is the first synthetic monocyclic β-lactam (monobactam) antibiotic approved for use in clinical medicine. Its aminoglycoside-like activity, good CSF penetration, and absence of nephrotoxic or ototoxic side effects make aztreonam potentially useful when combined with ampicillin for initial empirical therapy in newborns with severe, suspected sepsis.

ANTIMICROBIAL ACTIVITY

Aztreonam has good activity against a broad spectrum of aerobic gram-negative bacteria, but its activity against gram-positive or anaerobic organisms is poor.[197,198] Most *E. coli, Klebsiella pneumoniae,* and *Citrobacter* spp. are inhibited by less than 1 μg/mL of aztreonam. *Serratia* and *Enterobacter* are less susceptible (MIC_{90}, 1-4 μg/mL), whereas *H. influenzae* and *N. gonorrhoeae* are more susceptible (MIC_{90}, 0.2 μg/mL or less). Higher concentrations of aztreonam are needed to inhibit growth of *P. aeruginosa* (MIC, 8-12 μg/mL).[198,199] Like other β-lactams, aztreonam exerts its antimicrobial activity by interfering with bacterial cell wall synthesis by binding to PBPs, especially PBP-3 of aerobic gram-negative bacteria. This drug is stable to hydrolysis by chromosome- or plasmid-mediated β-lactamases of the Enterobacteriaceae and does not induce chromosomal β-lactamase production.

PHARMACOKINETIC DATA

The PK of IV aztreonam (20-30 mg/kg/dose of body weight) has been evaluated in a limited number of neonates.[200] Serum concentrations and half-life decreased with chronologic age. The mean serum aztreonam concentration was 54 μg/mL in first week of life and 45 μg/mL in infants 2 to 22 days of age. The half-life decreased from 3.5 to 6.6 hours in 0-3 day-old neonates to 2.0 to 4.0 hours thereafter. Small premature infants weighing less than 1500 g have longer half-lives compared with larger preterm infants: 5.3 versus 4.1 hours respectively.[201] A larger 30-mg/kg IV dose of aztreonam administered to infants weighing less than 2000 g during their first week of life resulted in peak serum concentrations from 65 to 79 μg/mL after the first dose and 77 to 83 μg/mL after 3 to 6 days of therapy.[199] Trough values were highly variable and ranged between 8.2 and 70.7 μg/mL. The half-life decreased from 7.6 to 5.5 hours after 3 to 6 doses. Older infants and young children have a shorter mean half-life of 1.7 hours.[202]

Aztreonam has good penetration into the CSF of newborns with bacterial meningitis.[203] In a 7-day-old infant with newly diagnosed bacterial meningitis, a CSF concentration of 13.3 μg/mL was obtained 1.3 hours after an aztreonam dose, representing 18.8% of a simultaneously measured serum concentration. Pediatric patients with acute bacterial meningitis have concentrations of aztreonam in CSF that are 17% to 33% of serum values.[204]

SAFETY

Aztreonam appears to be well tolerated with no apparent side effects when given intravenously to newborns in PK studies. Adverse reactions described in adults include rashes, nausea, diarrhea, and eosinophilia, but their incidence is low.[197,198] Aztreonam effects on bowel flora are limited to a reduction in coliforms without significant changes in anaerobic bacteria. Colonization by resistant bacteria resulting from aztreonam therapy does not appear to be as much of a problem as that encountered with the use of the third-generation cephalosporins. Because aztreonam contains 780 mg arginine/g of antibiotic, concern has been raised regarding possible arginine-induced hypoglycemia.[205] Arginine is rapidly metabolized and can be transformed to glucose, leading to transient hyperglycemia. As a result of this transient hyperglycemia, insulin concentrations can immediately rise, with the subsequent induction of hypoglycemia. These fluctuations in blood glucose and subsequent variation in insulin concentration can be potentially important in premature infants exposed to a metabolic stress. A study addressing this safety issue indicated that aztreonam was well tolerated and safe in premature infants when a glucose solution was concomitantly infused (at a glucose infusion rate greater than 5 mg/kg/min).[206]

PK-PD AND CLINICAL IMPLICATIONS FOR DOSING

Aztreonam remains off-label for neonates and infants younger than 3 months. Data from a prospective, randomized study of 58 neonates with infections caused by gram-negative bacilli, including *P. aeruginosa*, suggest that the use of aztreonam in combination with ampicillin is as effective as treatment with ampicillin and amikacin.[205] Individual aztreonam doses of 30 mg/kg given two to four times daily can achieve median peak serum bactericidal titers of about 1:16 and can maintain trough serum concentrations that exceed the MIC_{90} for most gram-negative bacteria.

Cephalosporins

Cephalosporins are semisynthetic derivatives of a 7-aminocephalosporanic acid nucleus.[207,208] Individual derivatives differ chemically by the addition of various side chains. The cephalosporins exert their antibacterial action in a manner similar to that described earlier for penicillin. It has become customary to group cephalosporins into generations of agents on the basis of their antibacterial spectrum of activity. In the following section, we have focused on the most-well-studied cephalosporins in neonates.

ANTIMICROBIAL ACTIVITY

The *first-generation* cephalosporins have good activity against gram-positive organisms but limited activity against gram-negative bacteria. First-generation cephalosporins include cefazolin, cephalothin, cephalexin, and cefadroxil. Susceptible pathogens include streptococci, penicillin-susceptible and penicillin-resistant staphylococci, and penicillin-susceptible pneumococci. Although typically the activity against coliforms is good, other antibiotics are often preferred for treatment of infections caused by these organisms. *P. aeruginosa*, *Serratia marcescens*, *Enterococci*, MRSA, *L. monocytogenes*, *Enterobacter* spp., indole-positive *Proteus* spp., and *B. fragilis* all are resistant to these antibacterial agents.

Compared with first-generation cephalosporins, *second-generation* agents have improved stability to hydrolysis by β-lactamases and therefore have increased activity against many gram-negative bacteria. Second-generation agents include cefaclor, cefprozil, cefamandole, cefuroxime, and loracarbef. Cefuroxime is more active than cephalothin against group B streptococci, pneumococci, and gram-negative enteric bacilli and also is active against *H. influenzae*, meningococci, gonococci, and staphylococci. The second-generation agents have very poor activity against *P. aeruginosa*, enterococci, and *L. monocytogenes*.

The *third-generation* cephalosporins have excellent in vitro activity against *H. influenzae*, gonococci, meningococci, and many gram-negative enteric bacilli. Third-generation agents include cefoperazone, cefotaxime, ceftizoxime, ceftriaxone, and ceftazidime. Ceftazidime and cefoperazone, however, are the only ones with adequate anti-*Pseudomonas* activity. *L. monocytogenes* and enterococci are uniformly resistant to these agents. Resistance has emerged as a problem with ceftazidime. Susceptibility of gram-positive organisms to these agents is variable but generally is lower than first- or second- generation cephalosporins.

The *fourth-generation* cephalosporins, notably cefepime, demonstrate activity against gram-positive and gram-negative bacterial pathogens, including *P. aeruginosa*. Cefepime has been shown to be effective for therapy for meningitis in children and is useful for treatment of multidrug-resistant gram-negative bacillary infections in pediatric patients. Some isolates of ceftazidime- and cefotaxime-resistant *Enterobacter* spp. are susceptible to cefepime. Resistant organisms include enterococci, *L. monocytogenes*, MRSA, MRSE, and anaerobes.

Cephalosporins interfere with bacterial cell wall synthesis, thus lysing bacteria. Cephalosporins must pass through the bacterial cell membrane and bind the PBPs that cross-link peptidoglycan polymers. *Enterococcus* is resistant to cephalosporins because their PBPs do not bind cephalosporins.

Resistance to the cephalosporins develops through several mechanisms.[209] Cephalothin and cefazolin can be inactivated by β-lactamases. Exposure of some gram-negative bacteria, such as *P. aeruginosa* or *Enterobacter cloacae*, to second- or third-generation agents can induce the production of chromosomally mediated potent β-lactamases by these bacteria, which can hydrolyze even the β-lactamase–stable cephalosporins. Several plasmid-mediated β-lactamases have been shown to play a role in the resistance of certain gram-negative enteric bacilli to third-generation cephalosporins. Other mechanisms of resistance include alterations in the permeability of the outer membranes of gram-negative bacteria to these drugs that limit their ability to reach the PBP target sites. Mutations leading to functional or quantitative changes in PBPs constitute an additional means by which bacteria can resist the antimicrobial action of these drugs.

PHARMACOKINETIC DATA

Cefazolin (Table 37-10)

The IM administration of 25-mg/kg doses of cefazolin produces peak serum concentrations of 55 to 65 μg/mL 1 hour after the dose. The concentrations at 12 hours drop to 13 to 18 μg/mL.[210] IV doses of 25 mg/kg administered to 6 premature infants 2 to 12 days of age resulted in mean serum concentrations of 92, 79, 48, and 12 μg/mL at 0.5, 1, 4, and 12 hours, respectively, after the end of the infusion.[211] In a study of 11 late preterm infants (mean, 35 weeks; mean PNA, 9 days), cefazolin CL was estimated to be 0.048 L/hr/kg, and Vd was 0.28 L/kg.[209] The drug is excreted in the urine in unchanged form. The serum half-life of cefazolin decreases from 4.5 to 5 hours in the first week of life to approximately 3 hours by 3 to 4 weeks of age. Cefazolin often exhibits significant protein binding (range, 20%-80%). CSF penetration of cefazolin is poor.

Cefuroxime (See Table 37-10)

Intramuscular doses of 25 mg/kg given to neonates weighing less than 2.5 kg during their first week of life produce mean serum concentrations of 49, 30, and 15 μg/mL at 2, 4, and 8 hours after the injection, respectively.[212] For larger newborns, the corresponding values were lower (34, 21, and 9 μg/mL, respectively). A study of preterm and term infants receiving cefuroxime 25 mg/kg every 12 hours resulted in median steady-state serum concentrations of 45, 26, and 11 μg/mL after 0.5, 5, and 12 hours, respectively.[213] Repeated administration of the drug did not result in serum accumulation. About 70% of the daily cefuroxime dose could be recovered in the urine in a 24-hour period. Half-life times have been reported to range from 2 to 11 hours (mean, 6 hours). CSF cefuroxime concentrations of 2.3 to 5.3 μg/mL were measured in three newborns with meningitis.[214] These values represented 12% to 25% of the corresponding serum concentrations. In three other neonates without meningeal inflammation, concentrations were lower and ranged from 0.4 to 1.5 μg/mL.

Cefotaxime (See Table 37-10)

About 80% of the cefotaxime dose is excreted in the urine; however, only a third of the drug is eliminated in unchanged form. Cefotaxime is rapidly metabolized in the body to desacetylcefotaxime through the action of esterases found in the liver, erythrocytes, and other tissues.[209] This metabolite is biologically active, but its antibacterial activity is generally lower than that of cefotaxime. Synergistic interactions against many organisms can be demonstrated when these two compounds are combined in vitro. Desacetylcefotaxime accounts for 15% to 45% of the peak and 45% to 70% of the trough concentrations of total cefotaxime.[215]

Several investigators have evaluated the PK properties of cefotaxime in newborns.[209] A 25-mg/kg IV dose produces concentrations of 60 to 80 μg/mL immediately after the

Table 37-10 Pharmacology of Cephalosporins

Drug Dose	Route of Elimination	Infant Characteristics	Peak (μg/mL)	Half-Life (hr)	PK-PD Target[11,12]	Protein Binding	CSF Penetration[16]	CLSI Sensitivity Breakpoint MIC* *Enterobacteriaceae*	CLSI Sensitivity Breakpoint MIC* *Pseudomonas aeruginosa*	Clinical Pearls†
Cefazolin 25 mg/kg	Renal	PNA < 14 days	55-80	4-5 PNA <7 days 3 PNA > 14 days	T > MIC >60%-70%	80%	Poor	≤2	Resistant	Perioperative prophylaxis
Cefotaxime 50 mg/kg	Liver/RBC esterase Renal 30%	0-7 days <2000 g >2000 g	 116 ±38 132 ±38	 4.6 ± 1.1 3.5 ± 0.9 2 if term, >7 days	T > MIC >60%-70%	30%	45 ± 12%	≤1	Resistant	Does not cover *P. aeruginosa* Metabolites maintain some antimicrobial activity
Cefepime 50 mg/kg	Renal	PNA 0-14 days PNA > 14 days	90-120	4.5 PNA < 14 days 1.8 PNA > 14 days	T > MIC >60%-70%	18%	25 ± 30%	≤2	≤8	Covers *P. aeruginosa*

Dose, peak, and half-life as reviewed in Pacifici GM: Pharmacokinetics of cephalosporins in the neonate: a review, *Clinics (São Paulo)* 66:1267-1274, 2011.

CLSI, Clinical and Laboratory Standards Institute; C_{max}, maximum concentration; *CSF*, cerebrospinal fluid; *MIC*, minimal inhibitory concentration; *PD*, pharmacodynamic; *PK*, pharmacokinetic; *PNA*, postnatal age; *RBC*, red blood cell; *T*, time.

*CLSA. Performance Standard for Antimicrobial Susceptibility Testing; Twenty-Fourth Informational Supplement. CLSI document M100-S24. Wayne, Pa: Clinical and Laboratory Standards Institute; 2014. Bacteria with intermediate sensitivities have higher MIC.

†Safety considerations for cephalosporins: hypersensitivity, diarrhea, eosinophilia, bone marrow suppression, risk factor for candidiasis in extremely preterm infants, seizures related to massive exposure.

end of drug infusion, which decreases to 35 to 50 μg/mL 30 minutes later. Serum cefotaxime concentrations are higher in premature newborns and in those younger than 1 week. The administration of a 50-mg/kg IV dose during the first week of life results in peak serum concentrations of 116 μg/mL (range, 46-186 μg/mL) in LBW infants compared with 133 μg/mL (range, 76-208 μg/mL) in term neonates.[215] Values decline thereafter to approximately 34 to 38 μg/mL 6 hours after the dose. The mean half-life is 4.6 hours for LBW neonates and 3.4 hours for larger newborns.[215]

Both cefotaxime and its metabolite penetrate well into the CSF of infants with meningitis.[209] Concentrations of 7.1 to 30 μg/mL are detected 1 to 2 hours after a 50-mg/kg IV dose and represented 27% to 63%, respectively, of simultaneously measured serum values. CSF concentrations as high as 20 μg/mL in neonates with or without meningitis have been reported.[216]

The PK of cefotaxime and its metabolite desacetylcefotaxime was recently described for infants during ECMO.[217] Plasma samples from 37 neonates on ECMO were evaluated. Infants received cefotaxime 50 mg/kg every 12 hours (PNA < 1 week), every 8 hours (PNA of 1-4 weeks), or 37.5 mg/kg every 6 hours for infants older than 4 weeks. Cefotaxime CL was 0.36 L/hr, with wide variability of 0.19 to 0.75 L/hr. The Vd was 1.82 L and ranged from 0.73 to 3.02 L. Vd for desacetylcefotaxime was very large, 11 L (range, 2-28 L). Elimination half-life for cefotaxime and desacetylcefotaxime were 3.5 and 5.4 hours, respectively. Cefotaxime concentrations were well above the MIC of 8 μg/mL for the entire dosing interval. Desacetylcefotaxime concentrations were variable, with a median concentration of 10 μg/mL in the first 12 hours postdose. For infants on ECMO, the cefotaxime standard-dosing regimen seemed to provide for cefotaxime concentrations to remain above the MIC of typical organisms for the dosing intervals.[217]

Cefepime (See Table 37-10)

Cefepime is eliminated through the kidney, mainly unchanged in the urine. PK studies in neonates given a 50-mg/kg IV dose every 12 hours have shown a mean C_{max} of 89 to 121 μg/mL, half-life of 4.3 to 4.9 hours, and CL of 1.2 mL/min/kg.[218,219] Premature infants have delayed clearance and prolonged half–life because of immature renal function and increased Vd resulting from increased total body-water composition. SCr is negatively associated with cefepime CL. Penetration into CSF appears to be good, with CSF concentrations averaging 3.3 to 5.7 μg/mL at 0.5 and 8 hours, respectively, after drug administration.[220] Clearance increases twofold in older infants, leading to a much shorter half- life and drug administration at shorter intervals.[221]

SAFETY

In general, cephalosporins are well tolerated by neonates. Adverse reactions that have been observed, mostly in older patients, include hypersensitivity reactions, diarrhea, thrombophlebitis, pain on IM injection, eosinophilia, leukopenia, granulocytopenia, and seizures related to the administration of massive doses of these drugs.[208,222] Falsely elevated SCr concentrations have been observed in patients who received cefoxitin or cephalothin. Alterations of the bowel bacterial flora are most pronounced with the third-generation agents, especially ceftriaxone and cefoperazone, and can lead to intestinal colonization by resistant organisms, such as *Candida, Pseudomonas, Enterobacter,* or *Enterococcus* spp. Subsequent superinfections by these drug-resistant pathogens have been described in neonates.[208,223] Another potential adverse effect related to disruption of bacterial intestinal flora by potent cephalosporins is the induction of antibiotic-associated colitis, presumably caused by overgrowth of toxin-producing *C. difficile.*

Bleeding disorders occurring with the use of cephalosporins have been well documented, mostly in adults. Hemostatic abnormalities associated with the use of cephalosporins can be mediated by several mechanisms. Immune-mediated platelet destruction with resultant thrombocytopenia is very rare but has been associated with cephalosporin exposure in older patients.[224] A second rare mechanism involves the development of antibodies, usually immunoglobulin G, against certain clotting factors, such as factor V or VIII. Platelet dysfunction can be observed after several days of therapy with any of the cephalosporins. These drugs may inhibit adenosine diphosphate–induced platelet aggregation, with resultant prolongation of the bleeding time. The effect is slowly reversible after discontinuation of the drug.[225] Another mechanism is defective fibrinogen-to-fibrin conversion, which has been observed with drugs such as cefazolin and cefamandole, particularly in patients with renal failure, who have very high serum antibiotic concentrations.[225]

The most important mechanism of hemostatic abnormalities involves interference with the production of vitamin K–dependent clotting factors (II, VII, IX, and X), with resultant hypoprothrombinemia.[225] This effect, observed most commonly with moxalactam and cefamandole therapy and rarely with cefotaxime and ceftriaxone therapy, may be related to, but not necessarily caused by, the presence of the *N*-methylthiotetrazole side chain in moxalactam, cefamandole, and cefoperazone. In patients with inadequate dietary intake, inhibition of colonic bacteria such as *E. coli* or *Bacteroides,* which are capable of vitamin K production, may lead to hypoprothrombinemia secondary to vitamin K deficiency. This side effect usually is avoidable or reversible by the administration of supplemental vitamin K.

Ceftriaxone is not generally recommended in neonates. Fatal outcomes have occurred in neonates who received ceftriaxone and calcium-containing products and had calcium-ceftriaxone precipitates discovered in their lungs and kidneys.[226,227] In addition, because ceftriaxone has a high avidity for protein binding, a theoretical concern is that its use in the neonatal period can be associated with a significant displacement of bilirubin from albumin-binding sites, thereby inducing a hyperbilirubinemia. Ceftriaxone, when given to neonates in the first days of life, has been associated with an immediate and prolonged decrease in the reserve albumin concentration, which could predispose a vulnerable infant to bilirubin encephalopathy. In older children and adults, an immune-mediated severe hemolytic reaction to ceftriaxone has been described in children and adults.

PK-PD AND CLINICAL IMPLICATIONS FOR DOSING

Cephalosporins, like other β-lactams, have time-dependent bacterial killing properties.[11] Therefore the PD target associated with bacterial killing is T greater than MIC. For most of these drugs, clearance occurs through renal elimination. As neonatal kidneys mature, dosing intervals need to decrease to provide therapeutic drug concentrations above the MIC of target organisms.

The usefulness of first-generation cephalosporins for therapy for neonatal bacterial infections is restricted. Their activity against gram-negative bacteria is limited and unpredictable, and their penetration into the CSF is relatively poor; thus these drugs are not typically indicated for initial therapy for suspected neonatal bacterial infections. Cefazolin dosing is typically 25 mg/kg given intravenously every 12 hours for newborns weighing less than 2000 g in the first 2 weeks of life and every 8 hours for older infants. Extremely preterm infants may continue twice-per-day dosing for up to 28 days of life. For infants weighing greater than 2000 g, the dose is given every 8 to 12 hours in first week of life and every 8 hours thereafter. Use in neonates is generally limited to prophylaxis of perioperative infections and treatment of urinary tract and soft tissue infections caused by susceptible organisms.

Although second-generation cephalosporins have been successfully used to treat neonatal infections caused by susceptible bacteria, these antibiotics are not typically recommended for routine use because of limited experience in newborns and because of their inferior activity to that of third-generation agents against gram-negative bacteria.

As a group, third- and fourth-generation cephalosporins are useful agents for the treatment of suspected or proven bacterial infections in newborns. Their advantages include excellent in vitro activity against the major pathogens for newborns, including aminoglycoside-resistant gram-negative bacilli, adequate CSF penetration with resultant high bactericidal activity in CSF of infants with meningitis, and a proven record of safety and tolerability. Indications for use of individual agents vary in accordance with their pharmacologic properties.

The clinical efficacy and safety of cefotaxime in the treatment of neonatal infections have been well documented in several studies.[228] Cefotaxime is typically not used alone for initial therapy in suspected sepsis because of its poor activity against *L. monocytogenes* and enterococci. The addition of ampicillin provides antibacterial coverage against these organisms. One potential problem associated with the routine use of this drug is the possible emergence of cefotaxime-resistant gram-negative bacteria in the nursery. Cefotaxime reaches CSF concentrations that are 50 to several hundred times greater than the MIC_{90} of susceptible gram-negative enteric bacilli or group B streptococci isolated from newborns with meningitis and has therefore been shown to be effective for the treatment of neonatal meningitis caused by susceptible bacteria.[229] The dosage of cefotaxime in newborns is 50 mg/kg every 12 hours during the first week of life and every 8 hours thereafter. In full-term infants older than 3 weeks, a 6-hour regimen can be used for treatment of meningitis.[230]

We do not recommend using ceftazidime alone for initial therapy for suspected neonatal sepsis because this antibiotic is not active against enterococci and *L. monocytogenes* and because of the possibility for emergence of cephalosporin-resistant gram-negative organisms. Treatment failures have occurred when the offending organism proved to be a gram-positive bacterium. Increased colonization and superinfection by resistant organisms, such as enterococci and *C. albicans*, are additional concerns. Other drugs such as piperacillin/tazobactam, cefepime, or carbapenems are preferred for the treatment of *P. aeruginosa*.

Cefepime has been evaluated in young children with serious bacterial infections, including meningitis, and has been comparable in safety and efficacy to third-generation cephalosporins.[231] PK information supports the typical dosing regimen: 30 mg/kg every 12 hours during first 2 to 4 weeks of life and 50 mg/kg every 12 hours thereafter. Meningitis or severe infections caused by *Pseudomonas* or *Enterobacter* spp. may require dosing every 8 hours or prolonged infusion times (4 hours) to maintain the concentrations above the MIC of offending organism. Although data on the use of cefepime in the neonatal period are sparse, because of its extended activity and stability against β-lactamase–producing bacteria, cefepime can be used for treatment of multidrug-resistant gram-negative infections. In a small randomized trial of 90 infants, cefepime was safe and therapeutically equivalent to cefotaxime for treatment of bacterial meningitis in infants and children.[232]

Broad-Acting Agents With Activity Against *Pseudomonas* or Anaerobes (See Table 37-10)

β-LACTAM/β-LACTAMASE INHIBITOR ANTIBIOTICS

Antimicrobial Activity

Combination β-lactam and β-lactamase inhibitor antibiotics (piperacillin-tazobactam, ticarcillin-clavulanate) offer broad-spectrum activity and have reemerged as an alternative to extended-spectrum cephalosporins, particularly given the development of resistant pathogens.[233] These drugs are bactericidal against many organisms, with the exception of methicillin-resistant *Staphylococcus* and *Enterococcus* (ticarcillin-clavulanate). Recently, the use of β-lactam/β-lactamase combination antibiotics have become appealing in neonates because of their safety profiles and their decreased likelihood to propagate bacterial resistance compared with extended-spectrum cephalosporins. However, more PK and PD knowledge in neonates is needed to optimize dosing guidelines. These agents are not typically recommended for treatment of CSF infections because penetration of β-lactamase inhibitors has not been well defined.

PIPERACILLIN-TAZOBACTAM

Antimicrobial Activity

Piperacillin-tazobactam is not approved by the FDA for use in infants younger than 2 months. However, it has been considered for neonates with proven bacterial infections, particularly those infected with difficult-to-treat polymicrobial sepsis or infections caused by *P. aeruginosa, K. pneumoniae*, or necrotizing enterocolitis. Piperacillin is formulated with the β-lactamase inhibitor tazobactam in an 8:1 ratio for IV preparation.[234] Piperacillin is an acylampicillin, a semisynthetic penicillin that is a piperazine derivative of ampicillin. Piperacillin is active against a broad range of gram-positive and gram-negative bacteria, including *S. aureus*, streptococci, *H. influenzae*, *N. meningitidis*, *L. monocytogenes*, *K. pneumoniae*, *P. mirabilis*, *S. marcescens*, and many anaerobes. In contrast to ticarcillin, piperacillin has better activity against enterococci and *P. aeruginosa*. In vitro synergistic activity with gentamicin has been demonstrated against *P. aeruginosa*, coliforms, and susceptible *S. aureus* strains. Synergy and antagonism has been demonstrated with cephalosporins, perhaps because of the ability of some cephalosporins to induce β-lactamase production.

Pharmacokinetic Data (See Table 37-10)

Piperacillin and tazobactam are widely distributed into tissue and body fluids, including the intestinal mucosa and biliary system; however, distribution into CSF is low in adults with noninflamed meninges, as with most penicillins.[234,235] Protein binding is estimated to be 30% for both piperacillin and tazobactam. Each drug is eliminated primarily through the kidneys via glomerular filtration and tubular secretion, with approximately 70% excreted as unchanged, active drug in the urine in children and adults. The primary nonrenal route of elimination is biliary excretion. The piperacillin metabolite desethyl-piperacillin maintains some microbiologic activity, whereas the single metabolite of tazobactam does not.

Piperacillin-tazobactam elimination is dependent on renal function and therefore improves with age until adult clearance is achieved at about 2 years of age. Children receiving piperacillin-tazobactam have somewhat reduced piperacillin elimination and prolonged half-life (0.7 vs. 0.5 hours, respectively) compared with piperacillin alone, likely the result of competitive antagonism for renal tubular secretion.[236,237]

The PK of piperacillin as a solo agent has been evaluated in 98 neonates (29-40 weeks of gestation) in the first 2 weeks of life.[238,239] Preterm neonates have lower peak piperacillin concentrations because of their higher Vd. In the first week after birth, the mean peak serum concentration after an IV 75-mg/kg dose is 180 μg/mL, 233 μg/mL, and 207 μg/mL for infants 29 to 31 weeks, 33 to 35 weeks, or 38 to 40 weeks of gestation, respectively. Immature renal function leads to prolonged half-life and delayed CL, thus allowing preterm infants to maintain concentrations over the dosing interval. The mean 12-hour trough concentrations decreased from 20 μg/mL in 29- to 31-week GA infants to 5 μg/mL in term infants.[239] In the second week of life, 8-hour trough concentrations decreased from 19 μg/mL for less than 33-week GA infants to 6 μg/mL for term infants.[239] Piperacillin half-life similarly decreases with advanced GA, chronologic age, and birth weight consistent with renal maturation. The prolonged half-life in neonates decreases from 6 hours in the first 2 days after birth, to 4 hours in the first week, and to 2 hours by the second week.[238,239] Infants with septic shock and significant renal insufficiency have prolonged half-life up to 14 hours. In older infants, the reported half-life of piperacillin is 0.75 hours in 1- to 6-month-old infants.[240]

The PK of piperacillin after administration of piperacillin-tazobactam combination has recently been explored.[241] Piperacillin concentrations were evaluated from 32 young infants younger than 61 days , with a median GA at birth of 32 weeks (range, 23-40 weeks), who received open-label piperacillin-tazobactam at a dose of 80 to 100 mg/kg every 8 hours based on GA and PNA.[241] Population PK models determined that CL improved with PMA, and Vd varied with weight. CL estimates were 0.08 L/hr/kg (95% confidence interval [CI], 0.068 to 0.93), and Vd was 0.42 L/kg). The estimated half-life of 4 to 6 hours in neonates is longer than the half-life of 1.4 hours reported in older infants aged 2 to 6 months.[236]

CSF piperacillin concentrations of 2.6 to 6 μg/mL were measured in three neonates without meningitis within 7 hours of the IV administration of a 100-mg/kg dose.[238,242,243] In one infant with *Pseudomonas* meningitis, piperacillin reached a concentration of 19 μg/mL in the CSF 2.5 hours after administration of a 200-mg/kg IV dose.[238,242,243] Human and animal models suggest that modest CSF penetration is expected for β-lactamase inhibitors.[244]

Safety

In a prospective, randomized, comparative, open-label trial of children with severe intraabdominal infections, patients receiving piperacillin-tazobactam had a similar rate of adverse reactions when compared with those receiving cefotaxime and metronidazole.[242,243] Adverse events were reported in greater than 1% of children in this study, including diarrhea, fever, vomiting, local reaction, abscess, sepsis, abdominal pain, infection, bloody diarrhea, pharyngitis, constipation and elevated liver enzyme. These adverse events were infrequent compared with transient complications encountered in adult trials. Bleeding manifestations, neuromuscular excitability, and seizures have occurred in patients receiving β-lactam antibiotics, including piperacillin. Impaired hemostasis secondary to platelet dysfunction occurs less frequently than with carbenicillin and ticarcillin.[225] The sodium content in piperacillin is less than half that in ticarcillin, which may be important in some newborns with cardiac or renal disease.

PK-PD and Clinical Implications for Dosing

Piperacillin-tazobactam, either alone or combined with aminoglycosides, has been used successfully for the treatment of bacteriologically proven neonatal infections.[233] Neonatal PK knowledge and clinical experience are limited, and dosing recommendations remain empirical. Piperacillin and tazobactam are both mainly eliminated through the kidney by glomerular filtration and tubular secretion. Therefore dosing adjustment with PMA is rational. In a recent review, the most common indications in piperacillin-tazobactam use in pediatric patients were nosocomial infections caused by resistant gram-negative bacteria, exacerbation of pulmonary colonization with *P. aeruginosa* in patients with cystic fibrosis, intraabdominal infections, and fever and neutropenia in pediatric cancer patients.[235]

The PD of efficacy for β-lactam antibiotics depends on the time that the drug concentration exceeds the MIC for the pathogen. To maintain piperacillin concentrations above the MIC, the dosing interval may need to be shortened or infusion time extended when treating susceptible pathogens with MICs greater than 4 to 8 μg/mL, such as can be seen for *Pseudomonas*, *Enterobacter*, or *Klebsiella*.[236,245] Given the modest CSF penetration, higher dosages may be considered for meningitis.

Dosing recommendations are variable and hindered by the paucity of PK data. Recent piperacillin-tazobactam population PK study,[241] with modeling and simulation of piperacillin dose-exposure relationship, suggested that a dose of 80 to 100 mg/kg every 4 to 8 hours, depending on PMA, could allow for greater than 90% of infants to maintain piperacillin concentrations above the MIC (32) for at least 75% of dosing interval. Specifically, infants with PMA less than 30 weeks receive 100 mg/kg every 8 hours, infants with PMA 30 to 35 weeks receive 80 mg/kg every 8 hours, and infants with PMA 35 to 49 weeks receive 80 mg/kg every 4 hours. This target MIC of 32 is the upper breakpoint for susceptibility for very-difficult-to-treat pseudomonal infections. This dosing is consistent with previous recommendations, with more specific PMA adjustments now offered.[238,239] Dosing guidance in NeoFax (50- to 100-mg/kg dose every 8-12 hours, based on PMA and PNA) would maintain exposure for at least 75% of dosing interval only if MIC was less than 8 μg/mL.[55,241] Evaluation of neonatal trough concentrations at 8 hours would help ensure that levels can be maintained above the MIC for at least 50% to 75% of the dosing interval.

Ticarcillin-Clavulanate (See Table 37-10)

Ticarcillin is a semisynthetic penicillin with pharmacologic and toxic properties virtually identical to those of other semisynthetic penicillin. The co-administration of clavulanic acid with ticarcillin significantly enhances the antibacterial activity of the latter drug against several organisms, including some ticarcillin-resistant strains of *E. coli, K. pneumoniae, P. mirabilis*, and staphylococci. *Enterococcus* spp. are resistant to ticarcillin. Clavulanate is a β-lactam with weak antibacterial activity, but it has the property of being a potent irreversible inhibitor of several β-lactamases produced by gram-positive and gram-negative bacteria. Current ticarcillin-clavulanate combination formulation (Timentin R) is approved for children older than 3 months for the treatment of bacterial sepsis, respiratory infections, urinary tract infections, and intraabdominal infections.[1] Information regarding the use of this compound in newborns is limited. Ticarcillin activity against *P. aeruginosa* and its formulation with the β-lactamase inhibitor clavulanate make it attractive for serious bacterial disease of neonates. Synergy with aminoglycosides has been demonstrated for the treatment of some strains of *Pseudomonas*.

PHARMACOKINETIC DATA

Ticarcillin-clavulanate is available for IV administration in a 30:1 ticarcillin:clavulanate ratio. Like piperacillin, ticarcillin is eliminated via glomerular filtration and renal tubular secretion. Approximately 60% to 70% of ticarcillin is excreted unchanged in urine during the first 6 hours after administration. However, only 30% to 40% of clavulanic acid is excreted unchanged in the urine, whereas the remainder undergoes nonrenal metabolism. Ticarcillin is approximately 45% protein bound, whereas clavulanic acid is approximately 25% protein bound. Ticarcillin penetrates well into bile and pleural fluid.

PK data for ticarcillin-clavulanic acid has been assessed in a limited number of preterm and term neonates; however, the ratio of ticarcillin:clavulanate was not consistent between reports. In a study of 24 newborns (25-39 weeks of gestation) who received 80 mg/kg ticarcillin and 3.5 mg/kg clavulanate, the ticarcillin peak serum concentrations (mean, 183 μg/mL; range, 100-400 μg/mL) and half-life (mean, 4.5 hours; range, 1.2-9.5) are similar to those observed after administration of ticarcillin alone.[246] The ticarcillin and clavulanate half-lives were shorter in term infants (ticarcillin, 2.7 hours; clavulanate, 1.4 hours) than preterm infants (ticarcillin, 4.2 hours; clavulanate, 2.6 hours).[247] Similar results were reported for the one PK study that evaluated the commercially available product with a 30:1 ratio of ticarcillin:clavulanate.[248]

Ticarcillin and clavulanate have different PK profiles. Ticarcillin is renally eliminated, and clearance improves with renal maturation and chronologic age. Alternatively, clavulanate is eliminated through nonrenal mechanisms, and clearance is more rapid. Ticarcillin accumulates in young neonates because of renal immaturity; however, clavulanate does not, and therefore the ticarcillin:clavulanate ratio observed in older patients is not likely to be maintained in neonates. Simulation of ticarcillin and clavulanate exposure using a population PK model[248] suggested that a lower dose (50 mg/kg ticarcillin) administered more frequently, that is, every 6 hours, was needed to maintain both ticarcillin and clavulanate levels. The significance of altered ticarcillin:clavulanate ratios is unclear,[249] because we do not know the optimal duration or concentration for serum clavulanate.

SAFETY

Ticarcillin-clavulanate possesses the characteristic safety profile of other penicillin antibiotics. Adverse reactions include anaphylaxis, bleeding disorders, seizures, headache, gastrointestinal disturbances, transient elevation hepatic enzymes, hypernatremia, and hypokalemia. Ticarcillin-clavulanate has been studied in 296 children (>3 months of age) in controlled trials and another 408 children in uncontrolled clinical trials.[1] Clinical trials in neonates are lacking. Anecdotal reports and small case series suggest that ticarcillin-clavulanate is well tolerated in neonates.

PK-PD AND CLINICAL IMPLICATIONS FOR DOSING

Ticarcillin-clavulanate is typically used along with an aminoglycoside for infants with severe gram-negative enteric infections or *Pseudomonas* sepsis and anecdotally with satisfactory safety and effectiveness. The most consistent dosing recommendation for neonates is 50 mg/kg every 6 hours, the same dose as recommended in infants older than 3 months with moderate infections. Frequent dosing is needed to maintain clavulanic acid levels because clavulanic acid clearance is more rapid than ticarcillin in infants. Clavulanic acid CSF penetration is only modest and is inconsistent in adult and animal models; therefore its use in treatment of CNS infections is discouraged. Ticarcillin-clavulanate should not be mixed in the same container or administered simultaneously with an aminoglycoside because of the physical and chemical incompatibilities between these two drug classes.

Carbapenems (See Table 37-10)

Carbapenems are β-lactam antibiotics known for their exceptionally broad activity and activity against extended-spectrum β-lactamase (ESBL)-producing gram-negative organisms.[250] *Imipenem* was the first drug in this new class. However, imipenem is susceptible to degradation by the enzyme dehydropeptidase-1 in the kidney, and therefore imipenem is now formulated with cilastatin, a dehydropeptidase inhibitor. The co-administration of both imipenem-cilastatin (1:1 ratio) increases the urinary concentration of imipenem, prolongs the imipenem serum half-life, and appears to prevent the nephrotoxicity induced by high doses of imipenem. Cilastatin itself has no intrinsic antimicrobial activity.

Meropenem is a newer carbapenem that is not susceptible to dehydropeptidase degradation. Meropenem is structurally different from imipenem in two ways: The carbapenem ring structure of meropenem includes an additional β-methyl group in the C-1 position, providing stability against the human renal tubular enzyme dehydropeptidase, and a long, substituted pyrrolidine side chain present in the C-2 position allows greater activity against intracellular target sites in organisms such as *P. aeruginosa*.[251] Meropenem was approved by the FDA for use in children older than 3 months on the basis of extensive pediatric investigations across a wide range of infections, including meningitis and complicated abdominal infections.[252] Meropenem is being increasingly studied in neonates for the treatment of complicated intraabdominal infections and infections caused by *Pseudomonas* or ESBL-producing bacterial infections. The newest carbapenems, ertapenem and doripenem, have yet to be studied in young infants.

ANTIMICROBIAL ACTIVITY

Imipenem and meropenem have an exceptionally broad spectrum of activity. The bacterial species considered resistant to these drugs are MRSA, methicillin-resistant *S. epidermidis*, *Stenotrophomonas maltophilia*, *Burkholderia cepacia*, and *Enterococcus faecium*.[250] These drugs maintain activity against ESBL-producing organisms. Carbapenems produce in vitro MIC_{90} values of less than or equal to 1 μg against the most commonly isolated species of gram-positive and enteric gram-negative aerobic bacteria, including group B streptococci, penicillin-susceptible and penicillin-resistant *S. pneumoniae*, MSSA, *L. monocytogenes*, *Citrobacter freundii*, *E. coli*, *H. influenzae*, *Klebsiella*, *Proteus*, *Serratia*, *and Acinetobacter* spp. The MIC_{90} values are typically less than 2 μg/mL for anaerobic bacteria.[250] *P. aeruginosa* has an MIC_{50} and MIC_{90} of 1 and greater than 8 for imipenem-cilastatin and of 0.5 and 16 for meropenem, respectively. Meropenem is consistently more active against *P. aeruginosa* than imipenem. Synergistic interactions between carbapenems and aminoglycosides can be demonstrated in vitro against *P. aeruginosa* and *S. aureus* isolates. Antagonistic interactions have been observed when imipenem is combined with other β-lactams, probably as a result of chromosomal β-lactamase induction by imipenem.[253]

Carbapenem's unusually broad antibacterial spectrum is related to its ability to penetrate efficiently the outer membrane of gram-negative bacteria, its high binding affinity for PBP-2, and its resistance to hydrolysis by both plasmid- and chromosomally mediated β-lactamases.[250] Some β-lactamases produced by *Stenotrophomonas maltophilia*, *Aeromonas hydrophila*, and *B. fragilis*, however, are capable of hydrolyzing imipenem and meropenem. Emergence of carbapenem-resistant strains during therapy with this drug is rare, except in the case of *P. aeruginosa*, in which resistance occurs in as many as 17% of isolates.

PHARMACOKINETIC DATA

Imipenem-Cilastatin (Table 37-11)

For both imipenem and cilastatin, serum concentration is directly proportional to the administered dose. Higher serum concentrations are achieved with cilastatin than with identical doses of imipenem. Imipenem, when co-administered with cilastatin, is eliminated as active drug through the kidneys. Cilastatin is excreted primarily unchanged in the urine, but about 12% of the drug appears as the metabolite *N*-acetylcilastatin.

In neonatal studies, the IV administration of 10-, 15-, 20-, and 25-mg/kg doses of both drugs results in mean peak imipenem concentrations of 11, 21, 30, and 55 μg/mL, respectively, compared with mean peak cilastatin values of 28, 37, 57, and 69 μg/mL, respectively.[254,255] After 3 to 4 days of treatment with 20-mg/kg IV doses of imipenem-cilastatin every 12 hours, peak serum concentrations are 35 and 86 μg/mL for imipenem and cilastatin, respectively. The mean serum half-life of imipenem is about 2 hours, whereas that of cilastatin is 5 to 6.4 hours.[254] The half-life for both drugs is inversely related to birth weight and GA and is considerably longer than the 1-hour half-life reported for both drugs in older infants and in healthy adult volunteers.[254,255] During the neonatal period, plasma clearance of cilastatin is only about 25% of that of imipenem.[254]

Although both imipenem and cilastatin penetrate well into the CSF in the presence of meningeal inflammation,[16] data derived from neonatal studies are scant. In one newborn who received a 15-mg/kg IV dose, concentrations of 1.1 and 0.8μg/mL were noted for imipenem and cilastatin, respectively, at 1.5 hours after injection. In a second neonate who received a 25-mg/kg dose, CSF values of 5.6 and 1.8 μg/mL were found for imipenem and cilastatin, respectively.[255]

Meropenem (See Table 37-11)

Meropenem was approved by the FDA for use in children older than 3 months on the basis of extensive pediatric investigations across a wide range of infections, including meningitis and complicated abdominal infections.[1,256] Meropenem exhibits dose-proportional linear PK properties with dosages of meropenem from 10 to 40 mg/kg. A large PK and safety study of meropenem in 200 infants with a mean GA of 28 weeks (range, 23-40 weeks) and a mean of 21 days of age (range, 1-92 days) confirmed prior associations of meropenem clearance with SCr and PMA.[251,257-259] Half-life becomes shorter with advancing GA and PNA, whereas the Vd remains relatively constant. In the first 2 weeks of life, the PK of meropenem was consistent with smaller meropenem PK studies: Preterm (<32-weeks GA) infants had a longer half-life of 3.8 hours, larger Vd

Table 37-11 Broad-Acting Agents With Activity Against *Pseudomonas*

Drug	Infant Characteristics	Peak µg/mL	Half-Life (hr)	Elimination	Protein Binding	PK/PD Target[11,12]	CSF Penetration[16]	ESBL	CLSI MIC* *Enterobacteriaceae*	CLSI MIC* *Pseudomonas aeruginosa*	Clinical Pearls†
Piperacillin-tazobactam (PK pip only) 75 mg/kg	<14 days 29-31 wk 33-40 wk	 180 230	6 at 2 days 4 at 7 days 2 at 14 days	Renal Biliary	30%	T/MIC > 50%	5%-30% (pip)	No	≤16	≤16	2.8 mEq Na/g Superior to tic for *Pseudomonas* and anaerobes
Ticarcillin-clavulanate 75 mg/kg tic	<2200 g ≤34 wk ≤19 days old	≈200	5 at 4 days 4 at 9 days 3 at 18 days 2 at >30 days	Renal: tic Non renal: C	45%	T/MIC > 50%	40% (tic)	No	≤16	<16	5 mEq Na/g Resistant to enterococci, *Klebsiella*
Imipenem-cilastatin 25 mg/kg	Preterm (mean, 29 wk) Full term	75 97	2.5 1.9 (cilastatin = 5 hr)	Renal metabolism (inhibited by cilastatin)	20%	T/MIC > 50%-75%	15%-27% (imip)	Yes	≤1	≤2	Rare incidence seizures in pt with CNS disease
Meropenem 20 mg/kg	<32 wk, <14 days <32 wk, ≥14 days ≥32 wk, <14 days ≥32 wk, ≥14 days	44 46 45 61	3.8 2.7 2.7 1.6	Renal	2%	T/MIC > 50%-75%	10%-70%	Yes	≤1	≤2	Possibly lower-risk seizures PK safety study in 200 infants

Dose, peak, and half life as reported in References 241, 248, 254, 255, and 257. CSF penetration reviewed in Nau R, Sorgel F, Eiffert H: Penetration of drugs through the blood-cerebrospinal fluid/blood-brain barrier for treatment of central nervous system infections, *Clin Microbiol Rev* 23:858-883, 2010. CSF penetration relates only to piperacillin, ticarcillin, and imipenem components.

C, Clavulanate; *CLSI,* Clinical Laboratory Standards Institute; *CNS,* central nervous system; *CSF,* cerebrospinal fluid; *ESBL,* extended-spectrum β-lactamase–producing organism; *imip,* imipenem; *MIC,* minimal inhibitory concentration; *Na,* sodium; *PD,* pharmacodynamic target for efficacy; *pip,* piperacillin; *PK* pip, pharmacokinetics derived from piperacillin alone; *T,* time; *tic,* ticarcillin; *wk,* weeks gestational age.

A neonatal PD has not been performed. Neonates may need longer T > MIC to account for immunodeficiencies.

*CLSA. Performance Standard for Antimicrobial Susceptibility Testing; Twenty-Fourth Informational Supplement. CLSI document M100-S24. Wayne, Pa: Clinical and Laboratory Standards Institute; 2014. Bacteria with intermediate sensitivities have higher MIC.

†Safety considerations similar to β-lactams: hypersensitivity, diarrhea, seizures (notably in patients with CNS disease and imipenem), rare risk of bleeding.

(0.49-0.74 L/kg), and slower CL (0.089 L/hr/kg) compared with more mature (≥32-weeks GA) infants who had a half-life of 2.7 hours, Vd of 0.46 L/kg, and CL of 0.135 L/hr/kg.[257] Beyond the first 2 weeks of life, the more premature infants (<32 weeks GA) show improved CL and shorter half-life, but they continued to differ from the more mature (≥32 week GA) infants: CL of 0.122 compared with 0.202 L/hr/kg and half-life of 2.68 hours compared with 1.58 hours.[257] The half-life decreases to 1.6 hours at 2 to 5 months of age as renal maturation occurs.

SAFETY

Both imipenem-cilastatin and meropenem appear to be well tolerated when administered intravenously to newborns. In a review of studies conducted worldwide, including thousands of patients, most of whom were adults, it was observed that the nature and frequency of side effects were similar to those of other β-lactam antibiotics; these adverse effects consisted mainly of nausea, vomiting, diarrhea, thrombophlebitis, thrombocytosis, eosinophilia, and elevation of hepatic enzyme concentrations.[260] Colonization by *Candida* or imipenem-resistant bacteria occurred in about 16% of patients, and secondary superinfection was noted in about 6%.[260] Alterations of bowel flora in children given imipenem-cilastatin have been minimal in the few patients studied in detail.[261]

A worrisome report suggests that imipenem treatment in infants with bacterial meningitis was possibly associated with drug-related seizure activity.[262] In infants with bacterial meningitis, seizures developed in 7 of 21 infants (33%), aged 3 to 48 months, after imipenem therapy. In this study,[262] CSF imipenem and cilastatin peak concentrations ranged from 1.4 to 10 μg/mL and 0.8 to 7.2 μg/mL, respectively. It is believed that interference of β-lactam antibiotics with the inhibitory effects of the neurotransmitter γ-aminobutyric acid (GABA) can result in epileptiform bursts. In mice, imipenem has been shown to induce seizure activity at serum concentrations two to three times lower than those of penicillin and cefotaxime.[263]

Meropenem has less affinity than imipenem for the GABA receptor and consequently has demonstrated a lower propensity to cause seizures in animal models.[264] In infants and children with meningitis, treatment with meropenem was well tolerated, and no drug-related seizure activity was observed.[256] In a 200-patient PK trial of preterm and term infants younger than 3 months, meropenem was well tolerated, with no adverse events that were probably or definitely attributed to meropenem.[265,266] The most commonly reported adverse events were sepsis (6%), seizures (5%), elevated conjugated bilirubin (5%), and hypokalemia (5%).

Adverse events associated with carbapenem exposure were recently evaluated in a retrospective study of 5566 hospitalized infants with a mean GA of 29 weeks exposed to meropenem (58.5%), imipenem-cilastatin (37.5%), or both (4%).[267] Infants exposed to meropenem had fewer seizures and death but a higher incidence of laboratory adverse events (elevated creatinine or liver enzymes) compared with infants exposed to imipenem-cilastatin. This retrospective study was not able to control for carbapenem indication or severity of illness. Although this association does not confer causality, laboratory monitoring is reasonable during exposure to carbapenems.

PK-PD AND CLINICAL IMPLICATIONS FOR DOSING (SEE TABLE 37-11)

Imipenem-cilastatin and meropenem are not recommended for routine use in the treatment of suspected or proven neonatal infections, with rare exceptions. Both agents should be primarily reserved to treat infections caused by multidrug-resistant microorganisms or serious abdominal infections. Data in 25 neonates with proven bacterial infections suggest that single-drug therapy with imipenem-cilastatin, using a 25-mg/kg dose given two to four times daily, is both efficacious and safe.[268] Because newborns have lower renal clearance capability and somewhat greater blood-brain permeability than those in older infants and children, high concentrations of imipenem-cilastatin could be achieved in the CSF of neonates, especially those with bacterial meningitis, potentially resulting in drug-related seizure activity.

Meropenem also appears to be safe and effective for treatment of neonatal infections.[265,266] Because meropenem is more active against *P. aeruginosa*, not metabolized in the kidney, and has not been linked to the potential induction of seizures, we believe that if a carbapenem is selected for therapy in a newborn, meropenem should be the agent of choice.

Meropenem, like other β-lactam antibiotics, exhibits time-dependent killing, so the goal of therapy is to keep meropenem serum concentrations above the MIC for at least 40% of the dosing interval for immunocompetent patients.[269] Some authors have recommended higher T-greater-than-MIC intervals in immunocompromised patients and particularly those with *Pseudomonas* infections, resulting from the higher MIC_{50} of 4 and MIC_{90} of 32. The meropenem dose-exposure relationship has been evaluated using Monte Carlo simulation and population PK models.[257,258,270-272] Monte Carlo simulation of PK-PD relationships using the population PK model derived from the largest dataset determined the following dosing scheme: (1) 20 mg/kg every 12 hours if less than 32-weeks GA, PNA less than 14 days; (2) 20 mg/kg every 8 hours if less than 32-weeks GA, PNA greater than or equal to 14 days; (3) 20 mg/kg every 8 hours if greater than or equal to 32-weeks GA, PNA less than 14 days; and (4) 30 mg/kg every 8 hours if greater than or equal to 32-weeks GA, PNA greater than or equal to 14 days.[257] Using these dosing guidelines, greater than 90% of infants will have simulated meropenem concentrations greater than 4 μg/mL for 50% of the dosing interval and greater than 2 μg/mL for 75% of the dosing interval. Neonatal intensive care unit (NICU)-specific sensitivities for nosocomial pathogens must be taken into account when considering appropriate exposure. Higher dosage and longer infusion times may need to be considered for the treatment of meningitis and more resistant organisms, such as *P. aeruginosa* with MIC 4 to 8 μg/mL.

Metronidazole

Metronidazole is a synthetic, trichomonacidal and bactericidal agent, 1-(β-hydroxyethyl)-2-methyl-5-nitroimidazole that is produced in an oral and IV formulation. Metronidazole is approved by the FDA for the treatment of adults with serious infections caused by susceptible anaerobic bacteria but is not approved for use in children.[1] In young infants, the IV formulation is used off-label to treat complicated intraabdominal infections, such as necrotizing enterocolitis and, in rare cases, anaerobic bacteremia. Clinical pharmacology of metronidazole is not well characterized in either premature or term neonates or young infants. Metronidazole distributes in total body water, to the CSF, saliva, and into erythrocytes and is minimally protein bound (20%). Metronidazole is extensively metabolized by the liver, yet the specific biotransformation pathways, particularly in neonates, are not well described.[273] Metronidazole and metabolites are primarily eliminated in urine. In adults, single-dose PK plasma clearance is reduced in patients with liver dysfunction but not renal dysfunction. Hepatic transformation seems to be reduced in neonates; therefore the kidneys may be responsible for elimination of higher fraction of unchanged metronidazole.

PHARMACOKINETICS

Limited PK data of metronidazole in neonates have led to highly variable dosing recommendations. Recently, three population PK studies of metronidazole in a total of 88, mostly preterm, less than 32-week GA infants consistently demonstrate that clearance improves with advancing PNA and PMA, whereas Vd is primarily affected by weight. Only 2 infants (2%) were 32 to 37 weeks GA at birth. Infants enrolled in these three PK studies shared many characteristics, including a median GA of 25 to 27 weeks and PMA of 30 to 32 weeks. They differed in the median PNA of infants, ranging from 12 days[274] to 27 days[275] to 41 days.[276] Metronidazole dosing varied; two studies had infants treated with standard of care, and one study had protocol-derived dosing adjusted for PMA and PNA. All studies developed one-compartment population PK models, with clearance associated with weight and PMA and volume associated with weight. Bayesian estimates were similar between studies: CL estimates for a 30-week PMA infant were 0.029, 0.025, and 0.038 L/hr/kg, respectively, whereas Vd estimates were 0.71, 0.735, and 0.93 L/kg, respectively.[274-276] Suyagh and coworkers[274] predicted a fivefold increase in CL from a PMA of 25 to 32 weeks and a concomitant twofold reduction in half-life (40-19 hours). Clearance also improves with PNA, from an estimate of 0.027 L/hr/kg at less than 14 days of age to 0.042 L/hr/kg at greater than or equal to 14 days of age, whereas the half-life shortens from 24 hours (<14 days of age) to 15 hours beyond 14 days of age.[275] The most recent study showed somewhat larger Vd and CL, potentially resulting from slightly lower median GA, older PNA, relatively small sample size in all studies, and variation in concomitant medications, pathophysiology, and drug metabolizing enzymes.[275]

SAFETY

The safety and efficacy of metronidazole in pediatrics has not been clearly established, especially in the treatment of complicated intraabdominal infections. It has been well tolerated in small PK studies. Metronidazole has been shown to be carcinogenic in mice and rats; therefore unnecessary use of the drug should be avoided. Its use should be reserved for the serious conditions caused by organisms known to be susceptible. Carcinogenic risk has not been established in humans.[277] Adult patients taking metronidazole have experienced seizures and peripheral neuropathy; therefore it is used very cautiously in patients with CNS disease.[1] Metronidazole can have significant drug interactions with concomitant medications that affect the P-450 cytochrome oxidase systems, such as phenobarbital, phenytoin, and warfarin.[1] Additional adverse reactions typically refer to the gastrointestinal systems, particularly nausea and reversible neutropenia, and rarely thrombocytopenia. Dose adjustments are indicated in adults with severe hepatic dysfunction.

PK-PD AND CLINICAL IMPLICATIONS FOR DOSING

In the absence of well-defined PD targets, recent studies have aimed to have the trough (C_{min}) at steady state exceed the MIC (6-8 μg/mL) of the organisms responsible for intraabdominal infections.[274-276] The Clinical and Laboratory Standards Institute recommended that the MIC susceptibility breakpoint of metronidazole for anaerobic organisms is 8 μg/mL; however, most anaerobic bacteria have a MIC of less than 2 μg/mL. Loading doses are indicated, given the long half-life and wide distribution.

Metronidazole PMA-based dosing that accounts for apparent developmental differences in CL is required to achieve the surrogate PD target of C_{min} greater than MIC of either 6 μg/mL[274] or 8 μg/mL[275,276] and is superior to commonly used dosing references in clinical pediatrics. Dosing recommendations based on these population PK models and simulation to target C_{min} greater than MIC all indicate a loading dose of 15 mg/kg, followed by variable maintenance dosing based on PMA as follows: dosing regimen 1[275]—for infants 7.5 mg/kg: every 12 hours for PMA less than 34 weeks, every 8 hours for PMA 34 to 40 weeks, every 6 hours for PMA greater than 40 weeks, and consider every 24 hours if within the first 14 days of life; or dosing regimen 2[274]—compared with 7.5 mg/kg: every 24 hours for PMA 24 to 25 weeks, 10 mg/kg every 24 hours for PMA 26 to 27 weeks, 7.5 mg/kg every 12 hours for PMA 28 to 33 weeks, and 10 mg/kg every 12 hours for PMA 24 to 27 weeks. Because the surrogate PD target is to maintain the C_{min} greater than MIC, we prefer more frequent interval dosing with advancing PMA. More prospective evaluations of dose-exposure relationships, safety, and efficacy are needed.

Antiviral Medications

Viral infections in the neonate are fortunately rare yet associated with significant morbidity and mortality. Viral therapy is available for the treatment of human immunodeficiency virus (HIV), herpes simplex virus (HSV), CMV, and varicella zoster virus (VZV). The pharmacology of medications used to treat or prevent HIV infections is discussed in Chapter 22. The pharmacology of acyclovir, ganciclovir, valganciclovir, and oseltamivir will be reviewed here.

ACYCLOVIR FOR THE TREATMENT OF HERPES SIMPLEX VIRUS

Acyclovir is a nucleoside analogue used with HSV and VSV. It is the most common antiviral drug used for the management of HSV.

Pharmacokinetics

The PK of acyclovir in neonates is limited. In a very small PK study of three infants (<60 days of age) receiving oral acyclovir (300 mg/m^2) for three doses showed that the maximum concentration (1.88 µg/mL) was higher than observed in adults receiving a larger dose (400 mg/m^2) and suggests adequate bioavailability.[278] The elimination half-life in infants was longer than adults. IV doses of 2.5 to 15 mg/kg are associated with steady-state acyclovir concentrations that range from 6.7 to 20.6 µg/mL.[279] Acyclovir is widely distributed and achieves high concentrations in the kidneys, lung, liver, heart, and skin vesicles. CSF concentrations are about 50% of those in the plasma.[280] Most of the drug is excreted unchanged in the urine through glomerular filtration and tubular secretion. Acyclovir has a 2- to 3-hour half-life in children and adults. Neonates with normal creatinine clearance have a prolonged half-life of 3 to 4 hours in small studies that do not include the GA of infants and up to 5 hours in a small study that included premature infants but had a median GA of 38 weeks.[279-283] Elimination is prolonged in patients with renal dysfunction. The PK of the currently recommended neonatal dosing schedule (20 mg/kg/dose every 8 hours) has not been described.

Prematurity is a risk factor for mortality in infants with HSV infections. Recently, the PK of acyclovir has been described in 28 preterm and term infants (median [range], 31 (23-40) weeks GA and 3.5 [0-30 days] PNA).[284] The acyclovir population PK model predicted a greater than fivefold increase in clearance from 23 to 40 weeks GA. Clearance was associated with PMA. Vd was larger (3 L/kg) than previously described in infants and adults, likely relating to the increased extracellular water in preterm and very young infants.

Safety

Acyclovir is generally a well-tolerated and safe drug. High doses of IV acyclovir, as is used in neonates, have been associated with neutropenia. Less common adverse effects include rash, nausea, headache, hematuria, and hypotension. Renal dysfunction can result from obstructive nephropathy caused by the formation of acyclovir crystals precipitating in renal tubules. Neurotoxicity has been reported in subjects with compromised renal function who attain high acyclovir serum concentrations. In the most recent PK trial of 28 neonates (23-41 weeks of GA), acyclovir was well tolerated, with only one adverse event attributed to acyclovir (worsening SCr), and no episodes of neutropenia were reported. The study of oral acyclovir suppressive therapy, 300 mg/m^2/dose bovine serum albumin (BSA), found neutropenia in 20% to 25% of infants compared with 5% to 7% in the placebo arm. These episodes of neutropenia resolved and were not associated with complications.

PK-PD and Clinical Implications for Dosing

Mortality was reduced in infants with neonatal HSV disease who received a high dose (60 mg/kg/day) compared with infants receiving 45 mg/kg/day (given every 8 hours) for 21 days.[285,286] The survival rate was similar for infants with CNS disease. Neutropenia was the most significant adverse event reported; however, there were no reported adverse sequelae, and the neutropenia was transient. The dosing interval may need to be increased in premature infants who are expected to have decreased creatinine clearance.[281] HSV isolates typically have an acyclovir half-maximal inhibitory concentration (IC_{50}) of less than 1 µg/mL.[287] It is reasonable to dose acyclovir to maintain acyclovir concentrations greater than 1 µg/mL and greater than 3 µg/mL if attempting to exceed 1 µg/mL in the CSF. In infants with disseminated or CNS infections, acyclovir should be administered for 21 days and until CSF testing for HSV is negative.[52,288]

Most formularies recommend 20-mg/kg dosing every 8 hours, which results in improved survival in efficacy trials. The population PK model of acyclovir in very young preterm and term infants was used to derive PMA-based dosing to achieve the theoretical PD target of steady-state concentration exceeding 3 µg/mL for at least 50% of dosing interval.[284] According to simulated dose-related exposures, the most premature infants with PMA less than 30 weeks should receive 20 mg/kg every 12 hours, whereas the more mature 30- to 36-week PMA infants can receive acyclovir 20 mg/kg every 8 hours, and the most mature infants with a PMA of 36 to 41 weeks should receive acyclovir 20 mg/kg every 6 hours.[284]

Infants with recurrent skin lesions are at higher risk of neurodevelopmental sequelae. Oral acyclovir has recently been shown to reduce the recurrence risk and improve neurodevelopmental outcomes.[289,290] Randomized, controlled trials show long-term benefit after 6 months of suppressive therapy (300 mg/m^2/dose BSA three times per day).[289] Another, uncontrolled study of 16 infants also showed improved neurodevelopmental outcomes after 2 years of treatment with higher-dose oral acyclovir suppression.[290] In this study, dosing began at 400 mg twice per day (≈1200-1600 mg/m^2 BSA) and then was adjusted based on acyclovir concentrations to maintain a minimum concentration greater than 3 µg/mL. Approximate doses for term infants by age were 400 mg for age 1 to 5 months, 600 mg for age 5 to 9 months, 800 mg for age 9 to 15 months, and 1000 mg for age 15 to 24 months (maximum dosage, 1200 mg). Acyclovir was also well tolerated in both studies; however, there was a trend toward more neutropenia in the acyclovir-treated infants compared with infants receiving placebo.[289]

GANCICLOVIR AND VALGANCICLOVIR FOR TREATMENT OF CONGENITAL CYTOMEGALOVIRUS WITH CENTRAL NERVOUS SYSTEM SEQUELAE

Antimicrobial Activity

Ganciclovir is approved for the prevention or treatment of CMV virus in adults.[1] Ganciclovir is a synthetic guanine derivative that specifically inhibits viral DNA synthesis by inhibiting viral DNA polymerase, resulting in termination of viral DNA elongation.[291] Ganciclovir is active against CMV and, to a lesser extent, HSV.

Pharmacokinetic Data

Ganciclovir is phosphorylated by viral protein kinases to ganciclovir triphosphate, the active metabolite that persists for days in CMV-infected cells.[291] To a lesser degree, normal, uninfected cells can generate monophosphorylated ganciclovir, thus possibly explaining its cytotoxic side effects.[292] Ganciclovir exhibits low protein binding. CSF penetration is 24% to 70% of the respective plasma concentrations. Renal excretion of unchanged drug occurs by glomerular filtration and active tubular secretion. The half-life in adults is 3.5 hours. Dose adjustment is advised in renal insufficiency. Ganciclovir exhibits linear kinetics with dose escalation.

Single-dose, IV ganciclovir PK has been evaluated in 27 neonates younger than 50 days. After a 4- or 6-mg/kg IV dose, the peak concentration was 5.5 and 7.0 μg/mL, respectively; systemic CL was 3.14 and 3.56 mL/kg/min, respectively, and the half-life was 2.4 hours for both doses.[293] Clearance was less than reported in children, but the half-life was similar; neonates had high interpatient variability. Population PK analysis of these newborns showed that ganciclovir CL was associated with body weight and creatinine CL.[294] The mean population CL was 0.4 L/hr, and the Vd was 1.73 L. A recent population PK analysis in young infants receiving IV ganciclovir or oral valganciclovir showed similar results, namely, a mean CL of 0.32 L/hr and Vd of 1.78 L.[295] Because ganciclovir is eliminated through the kidney, ganciclovir CL accelerates with PNA such that the AUC at the end of 6 weeks of therapy is expected to be less than the AUC during the first week. Extremely preterm infants with decreased renal elimination pathways would be expected to have delayed CL.

Valganciclovir is the oral prodrug of ganciclovir. Valganciclovir is rapidly hydrolyzed to ganciclovir and has similar indications to ganciclovir when oral therapy is acceptable. The bioavailability of valganciclovir exceeds 60% and is enhanced by concomitant administration of food. Typically, the AUC of ganciclovir after oral administration of valganciclovir is 33% to 50% of that which would have been achieved with IV ganciclovir. Dosing is modified for age and renal function. PK studies of valganciclovir show adequate bioavailability.[295-299] A recent study of 24 neonates reported that 16-mg/kg/dose oral valganciclovir administered twice daily achieves similar exposure as the 6-mg/kg/dose IV ganciclovir regimen and the target AUC_{0-12} of 27 mg*hr/L.[299] The median bioavailability was 41%. Ganciclovir CL doubled over the 6 weeks of therapy in young infants. However, infants receiving valganciclovir had more consistent AUC over 6 weeks of therapy compared with those receiving IV ganciclovir, likely because the valganciclovir bioavailability increased by 32% over the course of treatment. This dose was consistent with the 15-mg/kg dose recommended in smaller studies.[298] Viral load decreased in all infants (median, 0.7-log viral DNA copies/mL); however, this decrease in viral load was not associated with C_{max} or AUC. Neutropenia remained the most significant adverse effect.

Safety

Ganciclovir label contains a black-box warning for risk of granulocytopenia, anemia, and thrombocytopenia, and the drug should be avoided in patients with cytopenia or history of cytopenia. Dose reduction is also indicated in renal impairment. Dose-related neutropenia is the most common hematologic abnormality with both ganciclovir and valganciclovir and occurs in approximately 40% of patients and is reversible. Less frequent reported adverse events include fever, anorexia, vomiting, rash, elevated hepatic enzymes, and seizures. Ganciclovir has important drug interactions; it should not be combined with imipenem-cilastatin because of concern for seizures, and caution is required when combined with other nucleoside analogues, cyclosporine, and amphotericin B because of potential additive toxicity.

In a placebo-controlled trial of ganciclovir in infants, neutropenia occurred in 63% of infants receiving ganciclovir compared with 21% in the control infants.[300] Adverse events in infants participating in a phase II study of 8 versus 12 mg/kg/day included retinal detachment, neutropenia, and a moderate increase in creatinine and liver enzymes.[301] It remains unclear if these adverse events were attributed to either progression of CMV disease, adverse drug effect, or both. In valganciclovir trial for congenital CMV, neutropenia remained the most significant adverse effect, and grade 3 to 4 neutropenia occurred in 38% of infants and was correlated with a higher C_{max} and a higher AUC.[298] Periodic monitoring of blood counts, SCr, and liver function is recommended. Hematologic manifestations are typically transient.

PK-PD and Clinical Indication

Ganciclovir is licensed outside the newborn period for the treatment of CMV retinitis in immunocompromised patients and the prevention of CMV disease in transplant recipients. The relationship between ganciclovir exposure and clinical response has not been established. In vitro studies have shown that median inhibitory concentrations ranged from 0.02 to 3.48 μg/mL. A placebo-controlled trial in neonates with CSF manifestations of CMV demonstrated a reduction of hearing deterioration in infants receiving IV ganciclovir 12 mg/kg/day (6 mg/kg/dose administered every 12 hours) for 6 weeks.[300] Safety and efficacy of ganciclovir have not been established for congenital CMV disease without CNS manifestations. However, there was a high incidence of neutropenia in infants receiving ganciclovir compared with placebo, and dose modification was common. Controversy exists regarding the potential benefits of prolonged ganciclovir therapy to neonates, given the prolonged duration of IV access required and risk of adverse drug events.[302] Oral valganciclovir, an oral prodrug of ganciclovir, has been shown to have adequate bioavailability in neonates to achieve therapeutic ganciclovir plasma concentrations.

OSELTAMIVIR FOR THE TREATMENT OF INFLUENZA

The Centers for Disease Control and Prevention (CDC) estimates that each year more than 200,000 hospitalizations and 36,000 deaths are attributable to influenza in the United States.[303,304] In the 2003 to 2004 influenza seasons, the CDC reported 153 influenza-related deaths in children with a median age of 3 years. The highest mortality rate in children was among children younger than 6 months. In addition to mortality, children are known to have high rates of hospitalization and can suffer chronic neurologic or neuromuscular conditions.[52] Neonates and young infants are particularly vulnerable because vaccination is ineffective and antiviral treatment was previously not recommended in infancy. Immunization of pregnant mothers and all adults who contact infants is the best means of preventing influenza infection in infants. Neuraminidase inhibitors are effective in the treatment of sensitive influenza species in infants older than 1 year if initiated within 48 hours of symptoms.

Antimicrobial Activity

Neuraminidase inhibitors inhibit influenza virus type A and type B by binding to a highly conserved region of the neuraminidase protein on the viral surface, to inhibit viral penetration, replication, and disease.[305] The only neuraminidase inhibitor available for oral treatment in children younger than 6 years is oseltamivir. Oseltamivir has been shown to be safe and effective at reducing both the duration and severity of influenza symptoms in adult and pediatric patients older than 1 year.[1] However, neuraminidase inhibitor resistance among circulating influenza strains is increasing.

Pharmacokinetic Data

Oseltamivir PK has been established in adults and children older than 1 year.[306,307] Oseltamivir has excellent bioavailability after oral dosing and is extensively converted by hepatic esterase to oseltamivir carboxylate. In adults, at least 75% of an oral dose reaches the systemic circulation as the active form oseltamivir carboxylate. This active form is then renally excreted. Oseltamivir carboxylate is not a substrate for, nor an inhibitor of, cytochrome P-450 enzymes. PK analysis in children revealed that younger patients cleared both the prodrug and the active metabolite faster than adult patients, resulting in a lower exposure for a given mg/kg dose. In animals, oseltamivir carboxylate accumulates in the lung, middle ear, and nasal mucosa at concentrations exceeding those measured in the blood.[306]

The PK of oseltamivir in young infants has only recently been reported. Neonates are expected to have unique and variable PK properties because they typically exhibit altered renal clearances of drug and metabolite, variation in oral bioavailability, and large variability in the expression of human carboxylesterase. As infants mature, human carboxylesterase 1 increases expression and exhibits decreased intersubject variability. What is most striking in these studies is the large variation in oseltamivir and oseltamivir carboxylate exposure. Fortunately, preterm and term neonates are able to generate active oseltamivir carboxylate at plasma concentrations that are associated with antiviral efficacy. This extreme variation in exposures likely reflects differences in bioavailability, carboxylesterase expression, efflux of drug out of the liver and renal elimination, disease state, and enteral feeding frequency.

The first PK reports described preterm and term infants in the NICU who were treated with oseltamivir for postexposure prophylaxis, or a few were treated for influenza infections.[308-310] These studies all show large between-subject variability, delayed gastric absorption, effective albeit slower conversion to oseltamivir carboxylate (slower metabolite appearance), and accumulation of oseltamivir carboxylate over time. However, the observed oseltamivir concentrations reported as AUC_{0-12} are relatively consistent (2900-6700 μg*hr/L) for preterm neonates with PMA of less than 37 weeks receiving 1 mg/kg twice daily and in older subjects receiving 2 to 3 mg/kg twice daily.

A larger PK of oseltamivir in 87 infants younger than 2 years was recently published.[311] This study is unique in that all infants had confirmed influenza and that the investigators set the desired oseltamivir carboxylate AUC_{0-12} target to be 3800 ng*hr/mL (acceptable range, 2660 ng*hr/mL-7700 ng*hr/mL). This target was based on effective adult AUC targets, and the lower limit was set to minimize the development of antiviral resistance previously observed in 1- to 2-year-old infants who received 2-mg/kg dosing and had an AUC_{0-12} of 2880 ng*hr/mL. Dose adjustment in study protocol occurred if the first 9 subjects did not achieve this target. Infants 0 to 8 months of age receiving twice-daily dosing of 3 mg/kg had drug exposures within the target range. Older 9- to 11-month-old infants needed a higher dose of 3.5 mg/kg to produce adequate drug-exposure targets. For 11- to 24-month-old infants, standard non–weight-based 30-mg dosing, as recommended in clinical guidance, did not consistently produce target drug exposures, but the increased weight-based dosing of 3.5 mg/kg was able to achieve the target. The youngest infants (<3 months of age) showed the highest degree of variation. They had a delay in the formation of the metabolite; however, the overall oseltamivir carboxylate exposures were similar.

Safety

Oseltamivir has been well tolerated in adult and pediatric clinical trials.[1] The most common reported adverse events are related to gastrointestinal disturbances, particularly nausea and vomiting. Initially, there was concern about the safety of oseltamivir in infants younger than 1 year. Roche Laboratory issued an alert in 2003 that oseltamivir should not be used in infants younger than 1 year because an animal study revealed CNS toxicity and death in some very young rats who were exposed to excessively high doses of oseltamivir (500-1000 mg/kg).[312] There was great uncertainty in extrapolating juvenile animal data to human infants. Early retrospective case series in more than 300 oseltamivir-exposed infants revealed no serious complications or neurotoxicity.[313-315]

In response to the 2009 H1N1 flu pandemic, the FDA issued an emergency use authorization for oseltamivir in young infants. Subsequently, safety data have been collected in hospitalized neonates and young infants who were receiving oseltamivir for treatment or prophylaxis.[308-310,316-318] Oseltamivir was well tolerated in young infants, with rare association with gastrointestinal symptoms and no reports of encephalopathy. In one retrospective study of infants with confirmed influenza, vomiting was noted to be present upon admission before receiving oseltamivir and improved with treatment.[317] In one study, 3 infants presented with seizures as a symptom of illness before the receipt of oseltamivir, and seizures did not recur on therapy. No neurologic side effects were seen. A few infants exhibited gastrointestinal symptoms (vomiting and diarrhea) during their course of treatment, and causality to oseltamivir was unclear because symptoms were also attributed to concomitant antibiotics or associated viral gastroenteritis infections. Oseltamivir was well tolerated in the largest published study of oseltamivir in 87 infants younger than 2 years with confirmed influenza.[311] No unexpected adverse drug events were reported, no infants had the drug discontinued because of tolerability issues, and no seizures were reported. Expected adverse events considered related to oseltamivir were rare and included emesis ($N = 5$, 6%) and skin rash ($N = 2$, 2.5%). One infant had a serious adverse event (cutaneous hypersensitivity reaction) that was considered related to oseltamivir.

PK-PD and Clinical Implications for Dosing

Infants are at high risk for influenza-associated morbidity and mortality. In infants hospitalized with influenza, the possible benefit of therapy likely outweighs the risks. More PK studies are needed to better define the dose-exposure relationship in young infants. PK-PD studies are needed in young infants to best define exposure targets based on infant outcomes. At this time, twice-daily dosing recommendations based on the most thorough PK study are stratified by age[311]: 1 mg/kg in preterm infants with PMA less than 37 weeks, 3-mg/kg dose in 0- to 8-month-old infants, 3.5-mg/kg dose in 9- to 11-month-old infants, and 3.5-mg/kg dose in 12- to 24-month-old infants. Some clinicians recommend 30-mg flat dosing for 12- to 24-month-old infants. A lower dose of 2 mg/kg has been advocated for young, term infants with severe preexisting medical problems, prolonged newborn ICU hospitalizations, or infants on parenteral nutrition instead of enteral nutrition.

Antifungal Therapy

In the extremely premature infant, invasive candidiasis is common, often fatal, and frequently results in severe neurodevelopmental impairment. The therapeutic agents of choice in the nursery have been fluconazole and amphotericin products. Echinocandins are emerging as first-line therapy in older patients, and their PK, safety, and efficacy are under investigation in young infants.

A hallmark of neonatal candidiasis is CNS infection.[319] The incidence of CNS involvement is higher in the young infant than older patients, and invasive candidiasis (isolation of *Candida* from normally sterile body fluids) from any source has been associated with neurodevelopmental impairment. The diagnosis of CNS disease is very difficult, thus CNS involvement should be presumed in the young, premature infant.

MENINGOENCEPHALITIS

Central nervous system infection is not limited to meningitis; CNS infection with *Candida* is more accurately described as meningoencephalitis. Because the infection is based in brain tissue, it is likely that brain tissue penetration of antifungal drugs is more important to management of CNS infection with *Candida* rather than a strict assessment of penetration into the CSF.[17] CSF concentrations do not reliably predict outcome. This helps explain why amphotericin B deoxycholate and the echinocandins are likely to be effective in treating invasive candidiasis in young infants, provided that the levels of these products in the blood are sufficiently high to drive the product into the brain.

AMPHOTERICIN B

Amphotericin B (approved in 1958) is so named because it is amphoteric, forming soluble salts in both acidic and basic environments.[320] However, because of its insolubility in water, amphotericin B for clinical use is actually amphotericin B mixed with the detergent deoxycholate in a 3:7 mixture.[320,321]

Antimicrobial Activity

Amphotericin products bind to ergosterol, the major sterol found in fungal cytoplasmic membranes.[322] The lipophilic amphotericin B acts by preferential binding to fungal membrane ergosterols, creating transmembrane channels, which result in an increased permeability to monovalent cations. The fungicidal activity is believed to be due to a damaged barrier and subsequent cell death through leakage of essential nutrients from the fungal cell. Amphotericin B also has oxidant activity, which disrupts cellular metabolism, inhibits proton adenosine triphosphatase pumps, depletes cellular energy reserves, and promotes lipid peroxidation to result in an increase in membrane fragility and ionized calcium leakage.[322]

Pharmacokinetic Data

Amphotericin B is released from its carrier and is distributed very efficiently (>90%) with lipoproteins. The antifungal drug is taken up preferentially by organs of the reticuloendothelial system and follows a three-compartment distribution model. There is an initial 24- to 48-hour half-life, reflecting uptake by host lipids, very slow release and excretion into urine and bile, and a subsequent terminal half-life of up to 15 days.[323] In a small series ($n = 13$) evaluating the PK of amphotericin B among premature infants (27.4 ± 5 weeks), nine subjects showed elimination of amphotericin B at steady state, with an estimated elimination half-life of 14.8 hours. The rest of the infants, however, showed minimal drug elimination during the dosing interval, suggesting substantial drug accumulation and interindividual variability[324] in a small series of premature infants born at 27.4 ± 5) weeks GA ($n = 5$). In one study of five premature infants and five older children, the Vd was smaller and the elimination clearance more rapid than previously reported in adults. Serum levels were approximately half of those in adults with comparable doses, and interpatient variability was marked in the premature infants.[325]

Safety

Tolerance to amphotericin B deoxycholate is limited by its acute and chronic toxicities, particularly in children and adults. In addition to fungal ergosterol, the drug also interacts with cholesterol in human cell membranes; this likely accounts for its toxicity.[326] Amphotericin B also has a constrictive effect on renal arterioles, leading to a reduction in the glomerular filtration rate.[327] Up to 80% of older patients receiving amphotericin B develop either infusion-related toxicity or nephrotoxicity[320]; however, the product is likely better tolerated in young infants. Renal function usually returns to normal after cessation of amphotericin B, although permanent renal impairment is common after larger doses in older patients.[328]

PK-PD and Clinical Implication

Experimental in vitro and in vivo studies support concentration-dependent killing with a prolonged postantifungal effect, suggesting large daily doses will be most effective and that achieving optimal peak concentrations is important.[329] Peak levels are achieved 1 hour after a 4-hour infusion and reach a plateau at the third consecutive day of a constant dose. There is a relationship between total dose administered and tissue concentrations, suggesting a progressive accumulation with continued drug administration.[330] However, there is no evidence of a clinical dose effect to support higher doses (>1 mg/kg/day) of amphotericin B.[331] CSF values are only 2% to 4% of serum concentrations and sometimes difficult to detect,[332] yet a small case series completed in young infants suggests that the penetration of the product may be greater in this population.[324] As the drug penetrates well into brain tissue, 1-mg/kg dosing should be sufficient for CNS infections (see "Meningoencephalitis").

AMPHOTERICIN B LIPID-ASSOCIATED FORMULATIONS

In addition to conventional amphotericin B deoxycholate, three fundamentally different lipid-associated formulations have been developed that offer the advantage of an increased daily dose of the parent drug, better delivery to the primary reticuloendothelial organs (lungs, liver, spleen), and reduced toxicity: amphotericin B lipid complex (ABLC), amphotericin B colloidal dispersion (ABCD), and liposomal amphotericin B (L-amphotericin B).[322,333]

ABLC is a tightly packed, ribbon-like structure of a bilayered membrane formed by combining dimyristoyl phosphatidylcholine, dimyristoyl phosphatidylglycerol, and amphotericin B in a ratio of 7:3:3. ABCD is composed of disklike structures of cholesteryl sulfate complexed with amphotericin B in an equimolar ratio. L-Amphotericin B consists of small, uniformly sized unilamellar vesicles of a lipid bilayer of hydrogenated soy phosphatidylcholine–distearoyl phosphatidylglycerol–cholesterol–amphotericin B in the ratio 2:0.8:1:0.4.

Pharmacokinetic Data

Lipid formulations of amphotericin B generally have a slower onset of action and are less active than amphotericin B alone in time-kill studies, presumably because of the required disassociation of free amphotericin B from the lipid vehicle.[334] It is postulated that activated monocytes/macrophages take up drug-laden lipid formulations and transport them to the site of infection, where phospholipases release the free drug.[335] The different PK and toxicities of the lipid formulations are reflected in the dosing recommendations: ABLC is recommended at 5 mg/kg/day, ABCD at 3 to 5 mg/kg/day, and L-amphotericin B at 1 to 5 mg/kg/day. However, most clinical data have been obtained with the use of these preparations at 5 mg/kg/day.

The dosage of 5 mg/kg/day is especially pertinent to the young infant, given the frequency of CNS disease (see "Meningoencephalitis"). Animal studies suggest that on a similar dosing schedule, the lipid products are almost always not as potent as amphotericin B but that the ability to safely administer higher daily doses of the parent drug improves their efficacy[332] such that they compare favorably with the amphotericin B deoxycholate preparation with less toxicity. A multicenter maximum-tolerated-dose study of L-amphotericin B, using doses from 7.5 to 15 mg/kg/day, found a nonlinear plasma PK profile with a maximum concentration at 10 mg/kg/day and no demonstrable dose-limiting nephrotoxicity or infusion-related toxicity.[336]

Lipid formulations have the added benefit of increased tissue concentration compared with conventional amphotericin B, specifically in the liver, lungs, and spleen. However, it is not entirely clear whether these higher concentrations in tissue are truly available to the microfoci of infection. L-Amphotericin B has a comparatively higher peak plasma level and prolonged circulation in plasma,[337] whereas ABCD has a lower plasma level than amphotericin B after infusion but a longer half-life and larger Vd.[338]

The PK of amphotericin B lipid complex (ABLC) has been investigated in 28 neonates (median GA, 27 weeks; weight, 1 kg with range 0.48-4.9 kg) with invasive candidiasis.[339] Infants received IV ABLC at 2.5 (n = 15) or 5 (n = 13) mg/kg/day for a median of 21 days. Weight was the only factor that influenced clearance. The terminal half-life was estimated to be 395 hours. CSF concentrations in a limited number of samples were very low or undetectable. Dosing is therefore recommended at 2.5 and 5.0 mg/kg/day for treatment of invasive *Candida* infections in neonates, with higher dosing for any infant with suspected CNS involvement. High doses (5-7 mg/kg/day) and early treatment have been associated with improved outcomes.[340]

Safety Data

Lipid formulations appear to stabilize amphotericin B in a self-associated state so that it is not available to interact with the cholesterol of human cellular membranes.[337,341] Another theory for the decreased nephrotoxicity of lipid formulations is the preferential binding of its amphotericin B to serum high-density lipoproteins compared with amphotericin B's binding to low-density lipoproteins.[342] The high-density lipoprotein-bound amphotericin B appears to be released to the kidney more slowly, or to a lesser degree. For infusion-related toxicity, there is a general agreement that L-amphotericin B has less toxicity than ABLC, whereas ABCD appears closer in toxicity to conventional amphotericin B.[343,344] Liposomal amphotericin is generally well tolerated in VLBW neonates. In a recent cohort of 71 infants, nephrotoxicity, defined as a hypokalemia, elevated creatinine levels, or decrease urine output, occurred in 2.8% of infants who were receiving 3 to 5 mg/kg/day for an average of 14 days.[345] A small case control study of ABLC in 35 VLBW infants also concluded that treatment with ABLC for 2 weeks did not increase blood urea nitrogen or SCr, nor decrease sodium or potassium.[346]

PK-PD and Clinical Implications for Dosing

Antifungal efficacy is dependent on the $AUC_{0\text{-}24}$. The key target organ is the brain, even if the lumbar puncture is normal. Killing of the organism in the brain depends not only on $AUC_{0\text{-}24}$ but also total AUC exposure during therapy. That is, CNS disease usually requires extended therapy.[347] The typical duration of therapy is at least 21 days.[348] We acknowledge that the optimal length of therapy is not known as of this writing.

There are no data or consensus opinions among authorities indicating improved efficacy of any new amphotericin B lipid formulation over conventional amphotericin B, especially in neonates where renal toxicity is uncommon.[348,349] The clearest indication for a lipid formulation over amphotericin B is to reduce nephrotoxicity; however, nephrotoxicity in the young infant is thought to be uncommon. In neonates, early administration of high-dose (5-7 mg/kg/day) liposomal amphotericin has been associated with improved outcomes in retrospective analysis.[340]

PYRIMIDINE ANALOGUES: 5-FLUOROCYTOSINE

5-Fluorocytosine (5-FC) is a fluorinated analogue of cytosine synthesized as a potential antitumor agent and initially approved for use in 1972. Unfortunately, most reports detail clinical failure with monotherapy for yeast infections. The antimycotic activity of the drug results from the rapid conversion of 5-FC into 5-fluorouracil (5-FU) within susceptible fungal cells.[350] The two mechanisms of action of 5-FU are incorporation into fungal RNA in place of uridylic acid to inhibit fungal protein synthesis, and inhibition of thymidylate synthetase to inhibit fungal DNA synthesis.[350] The latter appears to be the dominant mechanism. Clinical and microbiologic antifungal resistance to 5-FC monotherapy appears to develop quickly.

Pharmacokinetic Data

Fungistatic 5-FC is thought to enhance the antifungal activity of amphotericin B, especially in anatomic sites where amphotericin B penetration is often suboptimal, such as the CSF, heart valves, and the vitreal body.[351] 5-FC penetrates well into most body sites because it is small, highly water soluble, and not bound by serum proteins to any great extent.[350] In a study involving 33 neonates in the United Kingdom treated with IV or oral 5-FC who underwent therapeutic drug monitoring, drug concentrations were low (trough, <20 μg/mL or peak, <50 μg/mL) in 40.5%; undetectable in 5.1%; high (trough level >40 μg/mL or peak > 80 μg/mL) in 38.9%; and potentially toxic (>100 μg/mL) in 9.9%.[352]

Safety

The mechanism of toxicity for 5-FC is unknown; but toxicity is common and substantial. 5-FC may exacerbate myelosuppression; toxic levels may develop when in combination with amphotericin B because of the nephrotoxicity of the amphotericin B and the decreased renal clearance of 5-FC.[353] If 5-FC is used, routine serum level monitoring is warranted because peak serum concentrations of 100 μg/mL or greater are associated with bone marrow aplasia. Approximately 50% of patients who receive the product experience substantial toxicity, including azotemia, renal tubular acidosis, and myelosuppression.[354] The product is also known to cause gastrointestinal complications, and in the premature infant at risk for necrotizing enterocolitis, its use should be undertaken with extreme caution. Given the narrow therapeutic range and need for therapeutic drug monitoring and the need for oral administration in the United States, this drug is seldom used in neonates.

Clinical Implications

Nearly all clinical studies involving 5-FC are combination antifungal protocols for cryptococcal meningitis because of the inherently rather weak antifungal activity of 5-FC monotherapy. The use of 5-FC in premature neonates is discouraged. A study evaluating risk factors and mortality rates of neonatal candidiasis among extremely premature infants showed that infants with *Candida* meningitis who received amphotericin B in combination with 5-FC experience a prolonged time to sterilization of the CSF compared with those receiving amphotericin B monotherapy (median of 17.5 vs. 6 days, respectively).[319]

AZOLES: FLUCONAZOLE AND VORICONAZOLE

The azoles are subdivided into imidazoles and triazoles on the basis of the number of nitrogens in the azole ring.[322,333] The structural differences result in different binding affinities for the cytochrome P-450 (CYP) enzyme system. The triazoles are the products used in young infants and will be covered here. Fluconazole is effective against most *Candida* spp., but it is unreliable for the treatment of *Candida glabrata*, and it is ineffective against the very rare cases of neonatal *Aspergillus* infections. Newer, second-generation triazoles (voriconazole, posaconazole, and ravuconazole) are modifications of prior triazoles with an expanded antifungal spectrum of activity and generally lower MIC values than the older compounds.[355] Only voriconazole has been investigated in children younger than 12 years.

Antimicrobial Activity

The azole antifungals are heterocyclic synthetic compounds that inhibit the fungal cytochrome P-450_{14DM} (also known as lanosterol 14α-demethylase), which catalyzes a late step in ergosterol biosynthesis.[333] The drugs bind to the heme group in the target protein and block demethylation of the C-14 of lanosterol, leading to substitution of methylated sterols in the membrane and depletion of ergosterol. The result is an accumulation of precursors with abnormalities in fungal membrane permeability, membrane-bound enzyme activity, and lack of coordination of chitin synthesis.[356,357]

FLUCONAZOLE

Fluconazole (Diflucan; Pfizer, New York) is a bis-triazole approved by the FDA for use in treating cryptococcosis and *Candida* infections in 1990. An in vitro time-kill study showed that the rate of fluconazole fungistatic activity was not influenced by concentration once the maximal fungistatic concentration was surpassed, which is in contrast to the concentration-dependent fungicidal activity of amphotericin B[358] or caspofungin.[359] Fluconazole is well-absorbed from the gastrointestinal tract and is cleared predominantly by the renal route as unchanged drug, whereas metabolism accounts for only a minor proportion of fluconazole CL.[360] Binding to plasma proteins is low (12%).[361] Gastric absorption of oral fluconazole is virtually unaffected by pH or the presence of food in the stomach.

Fluconazole is available as either an oral or an IV form. Oral fluconazole has a high bioavailability of approximately 90% relative to its IV administration. Fluconazole passes into tissues and fluids very rapidly, probably because of its relatively low lipophilicity and limited degree of binding to plasma proteins. Concentrations of fluconazole are 10- to 20-fold higher in urine than in blood, and drug concentrations in the CSF and vitreous humor of the eye are approximately 80% of those found simultaneously in blood.[361] The concentrations of fluconazole in body fluids, such as vaginal secretions, breast milk, saliva, and sputum, are also similar to those in blood, and the fluid-to-blood ratio remains stable after multiple doses. There is a linear plasma concentration-dose relationship.

Simple conversion of the corresponding adult dosage of fluconazole on a weight basis is inappropriate for young infants. A population PK study in premature infants showed that Vd varies with weight, and CL varies with renal maturation. Maintenance fluconazole doses of 12 mg/kg/day are necessary to achieve exposures similar to older children and adults.[362] In addition, a loading dose of 25 mg/kg is necessary to achieve therapeutic concentrations after the first dose.[363]

Candida infections are a leading cause of infectious disease-related death in infants supported with ECMO. The PK of fluconazole in 10 infants supported by ECMO demonstrated that infants on ECMO had higher Vd but similar CL.[364] Oxygenator extraction was minimal. A fluconazole dose of 25 mg/kg once per week was able to provide adequate exposure for prophylaxis; however, higher doses would be indicated for treatment of invasive *Candida* infection.

Safety

Side effects of fluconazole are uncommon. In one study of 24 immunocompromised children, elevated aminotransferases were observed in only 2 cases.[365] A large review of 78 reports of fluconazole use in a total of 726 children younger than 1 year showed it was generally well tolerated.[366] Another review of 562 children from 12 clinical studies confirmed that pediatric results mirror the excellent safety profile seen in adults. The most common side effects were gastrointestinal upset (7.7%; vomiting, diarrhea, nausea) and a skin rash (1.2%).[367] Fluconazole affects the metabolism of cyclosporine, leading to its increased concentration when they are used together.[368]

PK-PD and Clinical Implications for Dosing

Fluconazole may be used as monotherapy for treatment of candidiasis in the nursery. It should be given 12 mg/kg daily. There does not appear to be antagonism if the product is used with amphotericin B. In a multicenter trial of 236 patients with invasive candidiasis, those treated with fluconazole plus amphotericin B versus fluconazole alone trended toward better success and more rapid resolution of *Candida* fungemia with the combination.[369] Fluconazole is particularly appropriate for urinary tract infections because of its concentrating effect in the bladder. Fluconazole is also effective for superficial skin infections because the stratum corneum-to-serum ratio is high.[370]

Some centers use fluconazole for prophylaxis; however, this is not yet considered standard of care. In a single-center blind trial over a 30-month period of 100 infants with birth weights less than 1000 g, those infants who received fluconazole for 6 weeks had a decrease in the development of invasive fungal infection compared with placebo (0% vs. 20%).[371] A larger prospective, randomized double-blind, controlled trial conducted in eight NICUs in Italy among 322 infants with birth weights less than1500 g showed that a fluconazole prophylaxis regimen of 3 to 6 mg/kg several times per week for 4 to 6 weeks reduced the incidence of *Candida* colonization (9.8% in the 6-mg group, 7.7% in the 3-mg group, and 29.2% in the placebo group [$P <$ .001]) and invasive fungal infections (2.7% in the 6-mg group [$P = .005$], 3.8% in the 3-mg group [$P = .02$], and 13.2% in the placebo group).[372] A retrospective study evaluating the incidence of invasive candidiasis and *Candida*-related mortality among infants with birth weights less than1000 g who received fluconazole prophylaxis (3 mg/kg several times per week) for 6 weeks showed that the incidence of invasive candidiasis and *Candida*-associated mortality decreased. In the group receiving fluconazole, no increase in fluconazole-resistant *Candida* strains was observed.[373] Similarly, another report demonstrated that the use of fluconazole prophylaxis for 4 to 6 weeks in infants with birth weights less than 1500 g did not increase the incidence of fungal colonization and infections caused by natively fluconazole-resistant *Candida* spp.[374]

Results of fluconazole prophylaxis studies in premature infants are encouraging; however, the universal implementation of such strategy across nurseries has not been recommended because (1) the rate of *Candida* infections varies greatly among centers[375] and (2) there are insufficient neurodevelopmental follow-up data in these infants to justify prophylaxis.[376] A multicenter international trial is underway to answer questions regarding the need of prophylaxis based on rates of systemic *Candida* infections in individual nurseries.

VORICONAZOLE

Voriconazole (VFend; Pfizer) is a second-generation triazole and a synthetic derivative of fluconazole. Voriconazole has activity against most *Candida* spp. and against *Aspergillus*.[377,378] It is not well studied in neonates and young infants, and therapeutic drug monitoring is advised.

Pharmacokinetic Data

Voriconazole is extensively metabolized by the liver, and its bioavailability in adults is approximately 90%. It appears that CYP2C19 plays a major role in the metabolism of voriconazole, and this enzyme exhibits genetic polymorphism, dividing the population into poor and extensive metabolizers as a result of a point mutation in the gene encoding the protein CYP2C19.[379] About 5% to 7% of the white population has a deficiency in expressing this enzyme, so genotype plays a key role in the PK of voriconazole.[380] As many as 20% of non-Indian Asians have low CYP2C19 activity and can achieve voriconazole levels as much as fourfold greater than those homozygous subjects who metabolize the drug more extensively.[377]

Voriconazole is 44% to 67% plasma bound with nonlinear PK; has a variable half-life of approximately 6 hours,[381] with large interpatient variation in blood levels[382]; and good CSF penetration.[356,383,384] Time-kill studies against *Candida* spp. and *Cryptococcus neoformans* revealed in vitro non–concentration-dependent fungistatic activity, similar to that of fluconazole.[358]

Oral absorption is nonlinear and rapid, with an approximately fivefold accumulation over 14 days in one study of hematologic malignancy patients.[385] In a study assessing voriconazole levels after IV-to-oral switching, mean voriconazole levels did fall after oral administration compared with IV administration, but most subjects achieved steady state 4 days after dosing began. Maximal plasma voriconazole levels occurred at the end of the 1-hour IV infusion and between 1.4 and 1.8 hours after oral administration.[377] A PK study in six cirrhosis patients demonstrated hepatic-impaired patients should receive the same oral loading dose but half the maintenance dose.[386]

In contrast to adults, elimination of voriconazole can follow linear kinetics in children, although large interpatient and intrapatient variation remains. They have a higher elimination capacity and therefore require a larger (4 mg/kg twice daily vs. 3 mg/kg twice daily) maintenance dose after a 6-mg/kg load for two doses the first day of therapy.[387,388] The kinetics of the product in young infants are not known. One case series describes the therapeutic drug monitoring of voriconazole in 10 young infants and toddlers (aged 2 weeks-35 months).[389] These young children received doses of 3.4 to 14.7 mg/kg/dose administered every 12 hours. Trough concentrations ranged from 0.1 to 3.2 μg/mL. Only three trough values met the PD target of greater than or equal to 1 μg/mL. Most patients experienced dose increases after therapeutic drug monitoring to meet this metric. Trough levels were difficult to predict based on weight-based dosing. Variation in young children may be exacerbated by developmental changes in CYP2C19 expression, differences in protein binding, drug interaction, and underlying disease states.

Safety

Voriconazole's main side effects include reversible dose-dependent visual disturbances (increased brightness, blurred vision)[385,390] in as many as one third of treated patients, elevated hepatic aminotransferases with increasing doses,[390] and occasional skin reactions likely resulting from photosensitization.[391] The visual side effects have resulted in great caution in the use of the product in premature infants because of the concern of the developing retina as a target organ for toxicity. No such long-term effects have been observed nor studied in the young infant; however, most clinicians reserve this product for the occasional case of aspergillosis[392] and as a third-line agent for candidiasis. Trough values exceeding 5 to 6 μg/mL have been associated with increased risk of adverse events.[393,394]

PK-PD and Clinical Implications

Voriconazole is recommended for the treatment of invasive aspergillosis.[395] There are insufficient data to guide dosing in neonates and infants. Very high variation of voriconazole levels makes therapeutic drug monitoring imperative.[396] Voriconazole therapeutic drug monitoring may improve efficacy and safety.[393,394,397] Trough levels greater than or equal to 1 μg/mL are associated with improved response, and trough levels exceeding 5 to 6 μg/mL are associated with adverse events.

A multicenter trial of voriconazole versus fluconazole in treating esophageal candidiasis in 391 immunocompromised patients showed similar success rates with voriconazole (98.3%) and fluconazole (95.1%).[398] Overall, safety and tolerability of both antifungals was acceptable. In an open-label evaluation of 58 children with a proven or probable invasive fungal infection (most had aspergillosis), 45% of children had a complete or partial response, and only 7% were discontinued from voriconazole because of intolerance. The most commonly reported adverse events in these children included elevation in hepatic aminotransferases, skin rash and photosensitivity reaction, and abnormal vision. Intravenously administered voriconazole has been used successfully in VLBW preterm infants with primary cutaneous aspergillosis.[389,399]

ECHINOCANDINS

Antimicrobial Activity

A relatively new class of antifungals, the echinocandins and the amino-containing pneumocandin analogues, are cyclic hexapeptide agents that interfere with cell wall biosynthesis by noncompetitive inhibition of 1,3-β-D-glucan synthase, an enzyme present in fungi but absent in mammalian cells.[355,356] This 1,3-β-D-glucan, an essential cell wall polysaccharide, forms a fibril of three helically entwined linear polysaccharides and provides structural integrity for the fungal cell wall.[400] Their use is increasing in NICUs, yet PK, safety, and efficacy data are limited.[401] All of these agents remain off-label by the FDA for neonates.

Echinocandins prevent cell division by *Candida*, inhibit germination, and interfere with hyphal tip growth, thus converting the mycelium into small clumps of cells.[402] Therefore the echinocandin activity end point is morphologic change, not in vitro medium clearing. Echinocandins are generally fungicidal in vitro against *Candida* spp., although not as rapidly as amphotericin B,[329,355] but appear to be fungistatic against *Aspergillus*.[403] As a class, these agents are not metabolized through the CYP enzyme system but through a presumed *O*-methyltransferase, lessening some of the drug interactions and side effects seen with the azole class. The echinocandins appear to have a prolonged and dose-dependent fungicidal antifungal effect on *C. albicans* compared with the fungistatic fluconazole.[404]

Three compounds in this class (caspofungin, micafungin, and anidulafungin) are FDA approved for use in adults. Recently, more studies have evaluated the use of echinocandins in children; most constitute early phase I/II safety and PK studies. Micafungin is the only well-studied echinocandin in neonates and young infants. Because neonates with candidemia often suffer from disseminated disease in the CSF, which is associated with neurodevelopmental impairment, dosing of antifungal agents in this population should target the CNS. Echinocandins are relatively large-molecular-weight compounds; therefore large doses are likely required to penetrate the CNS.

MICAFUNGIN

Pharmacokinetic Data

Micafungin (Fujisawa Healthcare, Deerfield, Ill) is the only echinocandin lipopeptide compound authorized for neonatal use in Europe, but it is not approved for use in neonates by the FDA.[405] It exhibits linear PK, with the highest drug concentrations detected in the lung, followed by the liver, spleen, and kidney, and does not require dose adjustment for patients with renal disease.[406] Micafungin (like the other echinocandins) does not penetrate the CSF,[407] but levels were detected in the brain tissue, choroidal layer, meninges, and cerebellum in an experimental rabbit animal model.[347] Therefore the product can be considered in premature and young infants (see "Meningoencephalitis"). A time-kill study of micafungin against *Candida* spp. demonstrated potent fungicidal activity against most isolates, including a concentration-dependent postantifungal effect.[408]

The PK of micafungin has been well studied in young infants, perhaps more thoroughly than any other antifungal agent as of this writing. Of interest, micafungin CL in premature infants weighing greater than 1000 g is 1.7 times greater than children 2 to 8 years of age and 2.6 times greater than adults and older children. This higher clearance may be attributed to differences in micafungin plasma protein binding in neonates. A phase I, sequential and single-dose (0.75, 1.5, and 3.0 mg/kg) study of IV micafungin in 18 premature infants (mean GA, 26.4 ± 2.4 weeks) weighing greater than 1000 g showed that micafungin PK in preterm infants were linear; premature infants displayed a shorter half-life (8 hours) and a more rapid rate of clearance (≈39 mL/hr/kg) compared with older children and adults.[409] In this study, an additional 4 infants weighing less than 1000 g received 0.75 mg/kg/day of micafungin and demonstrated shorter mean half-life (5.5 hours) and more rapid mean clearance per body weight (79.3 ± 12.5 mL/hr/kg) when compared with the heavier infants.[409] These results suggest that young infants may require higher micafungin doses when compared with older children and adults. Data from 12 premature infants (mean birth weight and GA, 851 g and 27 weeks, respectively) suggests that a micafungin dose of 15 mg/kg/day achieves similar exposures (mean AUC, 437.5 ± 99.4 mg*hr/L) to adults receiving 5 mg/kg/day.[410] Micafungin doses of 7 mg/kg/day (infants > 1000 g) and 10 mg/kg/day (infants < 1000 g) administered to 13 premature infants (mean birth weight and GA, 1449 ± 1211 g and 27.3 ± 4.68 weeks, respectively) provided adequate exposures (median AUC of 258.1 and 291.2 mg/hr/L, respectively) to treat CSF candidiasis (as determined in animal models).[411]

PK of micafungin in the first 48 hours of life has been evaluated in one small ($n = 25$) PK study in VLBW (<1500 g) infants that evaluated exposure after low-dose (1 mg/kg/day) micafungin was administered on the day of birth and continued for an average of 13 days (range, 4-32 days) for prophylaxis.[412] The Vd and CL were larger and the half-life shorter than previously reported in older neonates and young infants. These differences likely result from dynamic changes in extracellular fluid volume, particularly in preterm infants shortly after birth. The average micafungin concentrations after the first dose were peak (2 hours) of 1.3 μg/mL (range, 0.39-3.1 μg/mL) and 24-hour trough of 0.2 μg/mL (range, 0.076-0.62μg/mL). Micafungin accumulation over time was minimal, with last-dose trough values of 0.26 μg/mL (range, 0.1-0.73 μg/mL).[412]

Safety

The safety profile of micafungin is optimal when compared with other antifungal agents in adults and children.[401,413,414] In clinical trials of micafungin, patients have demonstrated fewer adverse events compared with liposomal amphotericin B and fluconazole. No dose-limiting toxicities have been described. The most common adverse events include liver function test abnormalities, headache, diarrhea, vomiting, arthralgias, hypophosphatemia, insomnia, and rash. Hypersensitivity reactions associated with micafungin have been reported, and 5% of patients receiving the product may develop liver enzyme elevation. Hyperbilirubinemia, renal impairment, and hemolytic anemia related to micafungin use have also been identified in postmarketing surveillance of the drug. One 44-day-old premature infant developed hepatitis after micafungin (8 mg/kg/day) was added to an ongoing regimen of amphotericin for the treatment of protracted candidemia.[415] The most common adverse events in a phase I micafungin study of 77 children (2-17 years of age) with fever and neutropenia were diarrhea (19.5%), epistaxis (18.2%), abdominal pain (16.9%), and headache (16.9%).[416] Micafungin has very few drug interactions; however, when administered simultaneously, it increases overall exposure (AUC) of sirolimus (21%), nifedipine (18%), and itraconazole (22%).

Higher doses of 10 to 15 mg/kg/day have been well tolerated in small PK studies in neonates and young infants, and rare adverse events included elevated liver function tests, hypokalemia, and elevated temperature.[410,411] In a pooled analysis of pediatric trials, 2% of children stopped treatment because of adverse events that were possibly drug related because of neutropenia, jaw and joint pain, rash, and abnormal liver function tests, with two serious adverse events reported to be hyperbilirubinemia and increased SCr.[414]

PK-PD and Clinical Implications

Clinical studies in adults suggest that micafungin dosed at 100 to 150 mg/day provides a similar clinical response compared with caspofungin (70-mg load, followed by 50 mg/day). However, given infants' predilection for disseminated candidiasis with CNS involvement, higher doses are necessary. A micafungin AUC_{0-24} of 166.5 mg*hr/L in a rabbit model of hematogenous *Candida* meningoencephalitis has been associated with reduction in CNS fungal burden. Dosages of at least 10 mg/kg/day are required to achieve this PD target. Higher dosages in infants likely reflect increased rates of clearance and also increase the need to penetrate the CNS.

A pediatric substudy ($n = 106$, ages 0-16 years, including 14 neonates) was conducted between 2003 and 2005 as part of a double-blind, randomized, multinational trial comparing micafungin (2 mg/kg/day) with liposomal amphotericin B (3 mg/kg/day) as first-line treatment for invasive candidiasis.[417] Treatment success was defined as clinical and mycologic response at the end of therapy. The median duration of study drug administration was 15 days for micafungin (range, 3-42 days) and 14.5 days for liposomal amphotericin B (range, 2-34 days). In a modified intent-to-treat analysis the rate of overall treatment success was similar for micafungin (72.9%, 35/48) when compared with liposomal amphotericin B (76.0%, 38/50), with an adjusted difference between treatment groups of −2.4 (95% CI,15.3 to 20.1) when stratified by neutropenic status. However, when stratified by age group, liposomal amphotericin B out-performed micafungin in all age groups except for the neonatal group.[417] This observation could be related to the low micafungin dose used in this trial. In general, micafungin was better tolerated than liposomal amphotericin B, as evidenced by the fewer adverse events that led to discontinuation of therapy.[417]

Dosing has been recently derived from population PK analysis using data from 47 infants with proven or presumptive disseminated candidiasis previously enrolled in three clinical trials. Infants received a daily micafungin dose of 0.75 to 15 mg/kg and had serum concentrations evaluated after the first dose and at steady state. In the final population PK model, weight-based estimates of CL and Vd approximated those previously described for adults.[418] Monte Carlo simulation of dose-exposure relationships in young infants suggested that 82.6% of infants receiving a dosage of 10 mg/kg/day would have an AUC greater than or equal to 166.5 mg*hr/L. The PD target was associated with near-maximal decline in fungal burden in a rabbit model of *Candida* meningoencephalitis. All neonates also achieved an AUC/MIC ratio of at least 1332 for MICs of 0.007 to 0.0625 μg/mL.

CASPOFUNGIN

Pharmacokinetic Data

Caspofungin (Cancidas; Merck, Whitehouse Station, NJ) is a fungicidal, water-soluble, semisynthetic derivative of the natural product pneumocandin B_0. It has linear PK,[419] is hepatically excreted with a β-phase half-life of 9 to 10 hours in adults,[420] and has uncommon adverse effects.[421] Parenteral administration is preferred due to the low bioavailability when administered orally. It is not metabolized by the CYP isozyme system. The rate of killing for caspofungin in time-kill studies is greater than that of amphotericin B.

There is no known maximal tolerated dose and no toxicity-determined maximal length of therapy in adults. The usual course is to begin with a "load," followed by a lesser daily dose. PK appears slightly different in children compared with adults; smaller children exhibit lower levels and shorter half-lives.[422] PK projections suggest that dosing at 50 mg/m^2 appears to be more appropriate in children, rather than using 1 mg/kg/day.[423] The PK in young infants are highly variable and not well described, especially at dosages that should be used to clear CSF infections. Peak and trough levels were evaluated in 18 infants (GA, 24-41 weeks), with a PNA of 1 to 11 weeks, who received caspofungin at a daily dose of 25 mg/m^2. Caspofungin given 25 mg/m^2 is thought to provide similar exposure to adults receiving caspofungin at 50 mg/day for the treatment of esophageal and or oropharyngeal candidiasis; however, this exposure is unlikely to clear CNS infections in young infants.[424] Thus a recommended dosage cannot be provided from these data. Caspofungin exhibits reduced clearance in neonates and young infants relative to older children. Clearance appears to be primarily determined by the rate of distribution from plasma to hepatocytes and possibly other tissue. Differences in clearance could be due to difference in hepatic uptake transporters, organ size, or blood flow velocity.[424]

Safety

1,3-β-D-Glucan is a selective target present only in fungal cell walls and not in mammalian cells; therefore the echinocandins are rarely toxic in humans.[400] There appears to be no apparent myelotoxicity or nephrotoxicity with the agent.[333] Adverse events reported in a small retrospective study of caspofungin-exposed neonates included thrombophlebitis, hypokalemia, and elevated liver enzymes.[425]

PK-PD and Clinical Implications

Caspofungin was approved by the FDA in February 2001 for refractory aspergillosis or intolerance to other therapies, and in January 2003, it was approved for candidemia and various other sites of invasive *Candida* infections in adults. In a multicenter trial of 239 patients with invasive candidiasis, 73.4% of patients who received caspofungin had a favorable response at the end of therapy compared with 61.7% in the amphotericin B group.[426] Mortality was similar in both groups, and the proportion of patients with drug-related adverse events was higher in the amphotericin B group.

Caspofungin in newborns has been used off-label as single or adjuvant therapy for refractory cases of disseminated candidiasis. A study from Costa Rica reported the use of caspofungin (0.5-1 mg/kg/day for the first 2-3 days and 1-2 mg/kg/day for the remainder of the course) among 10 neonates (mean GA, 33.5 ± 1.77) with refractory disseminated candidiasis; all patients had a sterile blood culture within 3 to 7 days of starting caspofungin, and the drug was well tolerated.[427] Through a retrospective chart review, another center identified 13 cases of neonates with a median GA of 27 weeks (range, 24-28 weeks) who were treated with caspofungin (1-1.5 mg/kg/day) for refractory disseminated candidiasis; 11 of the infants achieved blood sterilization within a median of 3 days (range, 1-21 days). However, all but 3 patients had their intravascular lines removed before the onset of caspofungin therapy.[425]

Additional studies of caspofungin in the neonatal and young infant population are necessary to assess its safety and efficacy. In addition, PK studies in neonates, to determine optimal dose, are needed before the widespread use of this antifungal agent in the nursery.

ANIDULAFUNGIN

Pharmacokinetic Data

Anidulafungin (Eraxis, Pfizer) is a semisynthetic terphenyl-substituted antifungal derived from echinocandin B, a lipopeptide fungal product.[428] It has linear PK, with the longest half-life of all the echinocandins (≈18 hours)[429] and has shown fungistatic or fungicidal activity in different settings.[430] Analysis in healthy rabbits revealed linear PK with dose-proportional increases in AUC.[431] Anidulafungin lacks significant hepatic metabolism and is not renally excreted. Therefore neither end-stage renal impairment, dialysis, nor mild-to-moderate hepatic failure changes the PK of anidulafungin in adults.[432]

Tissue concentrations after multiple dosing were highest in the lung and liver, followed by the spleen and kidney, with measurable concentrations in brain tissue. The PK showed approximately sixfold lower mean peak concentrations in plasma and twofold lower AUC values compared with values with similar doses of caspofungin and micafungin.

PK data of anidulafungin in children and young infants are sparse.[433,434] Two commercially available anidulafungin formulations exist. One requires reconstitution with 20% dehydrated alcohol and therefore is not appropriate for young infants. One PK study in 15 young infants and neonates used a newer formulation that is alcohol free.[434] Young infants and neonates received a loading dose of

3 mg/kg, followed by maintenance dosing of 1.5 mg/kg/day, and PK samples were collected after the first dose and at steady state around dose 3 to 5. The concentration-time profiles and steady-state AUC estimates in these young infants and neonates (median AUC was 75 μg*hr/mL in neonates and 98 μg*hr/mL in infants) were similar to the AUC of 100 μg*hr/mL seen in older children receiving the same weight-based dosing and adults receiving 100 mg/day. Neonates had a faster median steady-state CL of 0.02 L/kg/hr compared with young infants' CL of 0.015 L/kg/hr. Because anidulafungin undergoes nonenzymatic degradation in blood and is not renally cleared nor metabolized in the liver, consistency across patient age populations is not too surprising.

Safety

Anidulafungin has an excellent safety profile and appears to be well tolerated.[435] A phase I study reported anidulafungin to be well tolerated in 29 healthy volunteers, with the highest-dose cohort experiencing transient liver function test elevations that exceeded twice the upper limit of normal.[436] In a separate study, 12 subjects with mild or moderate hepatic impairment did not show clinically significant changes in the PK parameters of anidulafungin.[437] However, in patients with severe hepatic impairment, the plasma concentrations of anidulafungin are decreased and plasma clearance increased.[438] In a study of 25 neutropenic children receiving anidulafungin as empirical therapy, rare adverse events included facial erythema and rash, elevation in serum blood urea nitrogen, fever, and hypotension.[433] Anidulafungin was well tolerated, with few adverse events in a small PK study in neonates and young infants. Two infants had worsening in elevated bilirubin levels; however, these biliary effects were not attributed to study drug because these infants had preexisting hyperbilirubinemia.[434] Larger pediatric trials are warranted to evaluate a possible association with hepatobiliary side effects.

PK-PD and Clinical Implications

Clinical trials with anidulafungin are ongoing. A phase III, randomized, double-blind study of adult patients with invasive candidiasis showed that anidulafungin was not inferior to fluconazole in the treatment of invasive candidiasis.[439] The frequency and types of adverse events were similar in the two groups.[439] Neonatal and pediatric studies are needed. The dose and drug exposure necessary to treat *Candida* meningoencephalitis is unknown.

Conclusions

Effective dosing of antimicrobial therapy for neonates must be based on rigorous PK studies performed in premature and term neonates. We remain grateful to the exhaustive efforts of Dr. George McCracken, a previous author of this chapter for many editions and author of more than 500 publications, many relating to the pharmacology of antimicrobial drugs and the treatment of neonatal infections. Advances in tandem mass spectroscopy are now allowing drug concentrations to be measured in very small blood samples and even dried blood spots. Population PK trials allow sparse sampling that accommodates standard-of-care blood-drawing times. Research networks have emerged that support collaborative efforts designed to perform rigorous studies that will lead to approved drug labels for neonates. We anticipate continued improvements in our understanding of the PK-PD of antimicrobial drugs in neonates and thus improved dosing guidance.

References

1. Federal Drug Administration: Drug labels, Available at http://www.daily.med.nlm.nih.gov or http://www.accessdata.fda.gov. Accessed April 1, 2013.
2. Weiss CF, Glazko AJ, Weston JK: Chloramphenicol in the newborn infant. A physiologic explanation of its toxicity when given in excessive doses, *N Engl J Med* 262:787-794, 1960.
3. Chavers B, Kjellstrand CM, Mauer SM: Exchange transfusion in acute chloramphenicol toxicity, *J Pediatr* 101:652, 1982.
4. Mulhall A, de Louvois J, Hurley R: Chloramphenicol toxicity in neonates: its incidence and prevention, *Br Med J (Clin Res Ed)* 287:1424-1427, 1983.
5. Allegaert K, Verbesselt R, Naulaers G, et al: Developmental pharmacology: neonates are not just small adults, *Acta Clin Belg* 63:16-24, 2008.
6. Kearns GL, Abdel-Rahman SM, Alander SW, et al: Developmental pharmacology—drug disposition, action, and therapy in infants and children, *N Engl J Med* 349:1157-1167, 2003.
7. Silverman WA, Andersen DH, Blanc WA, et al: A difference in mortality rate and incidence of kernicterus among premature infants allotted to two prophylactic antibacterial regimens, *Pediatrics* 18:614-625, 1956.
8. Robertson A, Karp W, Brodersen R: Bilirubin displacing effect of drugs used in neonatology, *Acta Paediatr Scand* 80:1119-1127, 1991.
9. Blake MJ, Castro L, Leeder JS, et al: Ontogeny of drug metabolizing enzymes in the neonate, *Semin Fetal Neonatal Med* 10:123-138, 2005.
10. Kearns GL, Jungbluth GL, Abdel-Rahman SM, et al: Impact of ontogeny on linezolid disposition in neonates and infants, *Clin Pharmacol Ther* 74:413-422, 2003.
11. Drusano GL: Pharmacokinetics and pharmacodynamics of antimicrobials, *Clin Infect Dis* 45(Suppl 1):S89-S95, 2007.
12. Lodise TP, Drusano GL: Pharmacokinetics and pharmacodynamics: optimal antimicrobial therapy in the intensive care unit, *Crit Care Clin* 27:1-18, 2011.
13. Winter ME: *Basic clinical pharmacokinetics*, ed 4, Philadelphia, 2004, Lippincott Williams & Wilkins.
14. Andes DR, Craig WA: Pharmacokinetics and pharmacodynamics of antibiotics in meningitis, *Infect Dis Clin North Am* 13:595-618, 1999.
15. McCracken GH Jr, Sakata Y, Olsen KD: Aztreonam therapy in experimental meningitis due to *Haemophilus influenzae* type b and *Escherichia coli* K1, *Antimicrob Agents Chemother* 27:655-656, 1985.
16. Nau R, Sorgel F, Eiffert H: Penetration of drugs through the blood-cerebrospinal fluid/blood-brain barrier for treatment of central nervous system infections, *Clin Microbiol Rev* 23:858-883, 2010.
17. Kethireddy S, Andes D: CNS pharmacokinetics of antifungal agents, *Expert Opin Drug Metab Toxicol* 3:573-581, 2007.
18. Shah S, Ohlsson A, Shah V: Intraventricular antibiotics for bacterial meningitis in neonates, *Cochrane Database Syst Rev* (4):CD004496, 2004.
19. McCracken GH Jr, Mize SG, Threlkeld N: Intraventricular gentamicin therapy in gram-negative bacillary meningitis of infancy. Report of the Second Neonatal Meningitis Cooperative Study Group, *Lancet* 1:787-791, 1980.
20. Bradley JS, Dudley MN, Drusano GL: Predicting efficacy of antiinfectives with pharmacodynamics and Monte Carlo simulation, *Pediatr Infect Dis J* 22:982-992, quiz 93–95, 2003.
21. Niebyl JR: Antibiotics and other antiinfective agents in pregnancy and lactation, *Am J Perinatol* 20:405-414, 2003.
22. Syme MR, Paxton JW, Keelan JA: Drug transfer and metabolism by the human placenta, *Clin Pharmacokinet* 43:487-514, 2004.
23. Tomi M, Nishimura T, Nakashima E: Mother-to-fetus transfer of antiviral drugs and the involvement of transporters at the placental barrier, *J Pharm Sci* 100:3708-3718, 2011.

24. Briggs GG, Freeman CD, Roger K, et al: *Drugs in pregnancy and lactation: a reference guide to fetal and neonatal risk*, ed 9, Philadelphia, 2011, Lippincott Williams & Wilkins.
25. Grossman ER: Tetracycline and staining of the teeth, *JAMA* 255:2442-2443, 1986.
26. Krasinski K, Perkin R, Rutledge J: Gray baby syndrome revisited, *Clin Pediatr (Phila)* 21:571-572, 1982.
27. Koss CA, Baras DC, Lane SD, et al: Investigation of metronidazole use during pregnancy and adverse birth outcomes, *Antimicrob Agents Chemother* 56:4800-4805, 2012.
28. Chung AM, Reed MD, Blumer JL: Antibiotics and breast-feeding: a critical review of the literature, *Paediatr Drugs* 4:817-837, 2002.
29. Hale TW: *Medications and mothers' milk online*, Amarillo, Tex, 2012, Hale Publishing.
30. Blanco JD, Jorgensen JH, Castaneda YS, et al: Ceftazidime levels in human breast milk, *Antimicrob Agents Chemother* 23:479-480, 1983.
31. Academy of Pediatrics Committee on Drugs: Transfer of drugs and other chemicals into human milk, *Pediatrics* 108:776-789, 2001.
32. Sauberan JB, Bradley JS, Blumer J, et al: Transmission of meropenem in breast milk, *Pediatr Infect Dis J* 31:832-834, 2012.
33. Fleiss PM, Richwald GA, Gordon J, et al: Aztreonam in human serum and breast milk, *Br J Clin Pharmacol* 19:509-511, 1985.
34. Giamarellou H, Kolokythas E, Petrikkos G, et al: Pharmacokinetics of three newer quinolones in pregnant and lactating women, *Am J Med* 87:49S-51S, 1989.
35. Gardner DK, Gabbe SG, Harter C: Simultaneous concentrations of ciprofloxacin in breast milk and in serum in mother and breast-fed infant, *Clin Pharm* 11:352-354, 1992.
36. Atkinson HC, Begg EJ, Darlow BA: Drugs in human milk. Clinical pharmacokinetic considerations, *Clin Pharmacokinet* 14:217-240, 1988.
37. Heisterberg L, Branebjerg PE: Blood and milk concentrations of metronidazole in mothers and infants, *J Perinat Med* 11:114-120, 1983.
38. Neu HC: Penicillin-binding proteins and beta-lactamases: their effects on the use of cephalosporins and other new beta-lactams, *Curr Clin Top Infect Dis* 8:37-61, 1987.
39. Neu HC: Contribution of beta-lactamases to bacterial resistance and mechanisms to inhibit beta-lactamases, *Am J Med* 79:2-12, 1985.
40. Nayler JH: Resistance to beta-lactams in gram-negative bacteria: relative contributions of beta-lactamase and permeability limitations, *J Antimicrob Chemother* 19:713-732, 1987.
41. Tuomanen E, Durack DT, Tomasz A: Antibiotic tolerance among clinical isolates of bacteria, *Antimicrob Agents Chemother* 30:521-527, 1986.
42. Dahesh S, Hensler ME, Van Sorge NM, et al: Point mutation in the group B streptococcal *pbp2x* gene conferring decreased susceptibility to beta-lactam antibiotics, *Antimicrob Agents Chemother* 52: 2915-2918, 2008.
43. Van Bambeke F, Reinert RR, Appelbaum PC, et al: Multidrug-resistant *Streptococcus pneumoniae* infections: current and future therapeutic options, *Drugs* 67:2355-2382, 2007.
44. Pacifici GM, Labatia J, Mulla H, et al: Clinical pharmacokinetics of penicillins in the neonate: a review of the literature, *Eur J Clin Pharmacol* 65:191-198, 2009.
45. McCracken GH Jr, Ginsberg C, Chrane DF, et al: Clinical pharmacology of penicillin in newborn infants, *J Pediatr* 82:692-698, 1973.
46. Kaplan JM, McCracken GH: Clinical pharmacology of benzathine penicillin G in neonates with regard to its recommended use in congenital syphilis, *J Pediatr* 82:1069-1072, 1973.
47. Klein JO, Schaberg MJ, Buntin M, et al: Levels of penicillin in serum of newborn infants after single intramuscular doses of benzathine penicillin G, *J Pediatr* 82:1065-1068, 1973.
48. Hieber JP, Nelson JD: A pharmacologic evaluation of penicillin in children with purulent meningitis, *N Engl J Med* 297:410-413, 1977.
49. McCracken GH Jr, Kaplan JM: Penicillin treatment for congenital syphilis. A critical reappraisal, *JAMA* 228:855-858, 1974.
50. Speer ME, Taber LH, Clark DB, et al: Cerebrospinal fluid levels of benzathine penicillin G in the neonate, *J Pediatr* 91:996-997, 1977.
51. Speer ME, Mason EO, Scharnberg JT: Cerebrospinal fluid concentrations of aqueous procaine penicillin G in the neonate, *Pediatrics* 67:387-388, 1981.
52. Pickering LK: *Red book: report of the Committee on Infectious Diseases*, Elk Grove Village, Ill, 2012, American Academy of Pediatrics.
53. Dahl LB, Melby K, Gutteberg TJ, et al: Serum levels of ampicillin and gentamycin in neonates of varying gestational age, *Eur J Pediatr* 145:218-221, 1986.
54. Kaplan JM, McCracken GH Jr, Horton LJ, et al: Pharmacologic studies in neonates given large dosages of ampicillin, *J Pediatr* 84:571-577, 1974.
55. Thomson Reuters Clinical Editorial Staff: *NeoFax Mobile*, ed 24, New York, 2011, Thomson Reuters via Skyscape.
56. Neu HC: Antistaphylococcal penicillins, *Med Clin North Am* 66: 51-60, 1982.
57. Grossman M, Ticknor W: Serum levels of ampicillin, cephalothin, cloxacillin, and nafcillin in the newborn infant, *Antimicrob Agents Chemother* 5:214-219, 1965.
58. O'Connor WJ, Warren GH, Mandala PS, et al: Serum concentration of nafcillin in newborn infants and children, *Antimicrob Agents Chemother* 10:188-191, 1964.
59. Banner W Jr, Gooch WM 3rd, Burckart G, et al: Pharmacokinetics of nafcillin in infants with low birth weights, *Antimicrob Agents Chemother* 17:691-694, 1980.
60. Axline SG, Yaffe SJ, Simon HJ: Clinical pharmacology of antimicrobials in premature infants. II. Ampicillin, methicillin, oxacillin, neomycin, and colistin, *Pediatrics* 39:97-107, 1967.
61. Burns LE, Hodgman JE, Wehrle PF: Treatment of premature infants with oxacillin, *Antimicrob Agents Chemother* 10:192-199, 1964.
62. Kitzing W, Nelson JD, Mohs E: Comparative toxicities of methicillin and nafcillin, *Am J Dis Child* 135:52-55, 1981.
63. Nahata MC, DeBolt SL, Powell DA: Adverse effects of methicillin, nafcillin and oxacillin in pediatric patients, *Dev Pharmacol Ther* 4:117-123, 1982.
64. Pacifici GM, Allegaert K: Clinical pharmacokinetics of vancomycin in the neonate: a review, *Clinics (São Paulo)* 67:831-837, 2012.
65. Capparelli EV, Lane JR, Romanowski GL, et al: The influences of renal function and maturation on vancomycin elimination in newborns and infants, *J Clin Pharmacol* 41:927-934, 2001.
66. de Hoog M, Schoemaker RC, Mouton JW, et al: Vancomycin population pharmacokinetics in neonates, *Clin Pharmacol Ther* 67:360-367, 2000.
67. Seay RE, Brundage RC, Jensen PD, et al: Population pharmacokinetics of vancomycin in neonates, *Clin Pharmacol Ther* 56:169-175, 1994.
68. Mulla H, Pooboni S: Population pharmacokinetics of vancomycin in patients receiving extracorporeal membrane oxygenation, *Br J Clin Pharmacol* 60:265-275, 2005.
69. Schaad UB, McCracken GH Jr, Nelson JD: Clinical pharmacology and efficacy of vancomycin in pediatric patients, *J Pediatr* 96:119-126, 1980.
70. Reiter PD, Doron MW: Vancomycin cerebrospinal fluid concentrations after intravenous administration in premature infants, *J Perinatol* 16:331-335, 1996.
71. de Hoog M, van Zanten BA, Hop WC, et al: Newborn hearing screening: tobramycin and vancomycin are not risk factors for hearing loss, *J Pediatr* 142:41-46, 2003.
72. Elyasi S, Khalili H, Dashti-Khavidaki S, et al: Vancomycin-induced nephrotoxicity: mechanism, incidence, risk factors and special populations. A literature review, *Eur J Clin Pharmacol* 68:1243-1255, 2012.
73. Bhatt-Mehta V, Schumacher RE, Faix RG, et al: Lack of vancomycin-associated nephrotoxicity in newborn infants: a case-control study, *Pediatrics* 103:e48, 1999.
74. Timpe EM: Nephrotoxicity with combination vancomycin-aminoglycoside therapy, *J Pediatr Pharmacol Ther* 10:174-182, 2005.
75. McKamy S, Hernandez E, Jahng M, et al: Incidence and risk factors influencing the development of vancomycin nephrotoxicity in children, *J Pediatr* 158:422-426, 2011.
76. Moffett BS, Kim S, Edwards M: Vancomycin nephrotoxicity may be overstated, *J Pediatr* 158:865-866, author reply 866, 2011.
77. Chambers HF, Miller RT, Newman MD: Right-sided *Staphylococcus aureus* endocarditis in intravenous drug abusers: two-week combination therapy, *Ann Intern Med* 109:619-624, 1988.
78. Small PM, Chambers HF: Vancomycin for *Staphylococcus aureus* endocarditis in intravenous drug users, *Antimicrob Agents Chemother* 34:1227-1231, 1990.
79. Nightengale CH, Ambrose PG, Drusano GL, Murakawa T, editors: *Antimicrobial pharmacodynamics in theory and clinical practice*, ed 2, New York, 2007, Informa Healthcare.

80. Lowdin E, Odenholt I, Cars O: In vitro studies of pharmacodynamic properties of vancomycin against *Staphylococcus aureus* and *Staphylococcus epidermidis*, *Antimicrob Agents Chemother* 42:2739-2744, 1998.
81. Moise-Broder PA, Forrest A, Birmingham MC, et al: Pharmacodynamics of vancomycin and other antimicrobials in patients with *Staphylococcus aureus* lower respiratory tract infections, *Clin Pharmacokinet* 43:925-942, 2004.
82. Rybak MJ: The pharmacokinetic and pharmacodynamic properties of vancomycin, *Clin Infect Dis* 42(Suppl 1):S35-S39, 2006.
83. Schaad UB, McCracken GH Jr, Loock CA, et al: Pharmacokinetics and bacteriological efficacy of moxalactam (LY127935), netilmicin, and ampicillin in experimental gram-negative enteric bacillary meningitis, *Antimicrob Agents Chemother* 17:406-411, 1980.
84. Lacy MK, Tessier PR, Nicolau DP, et al: Comparison of vancomycin pharmacodynamics (1 g every 12 or 24 h) against methicillin-resistant staphylococci, *Int J Antimicrob Agents* 15:25-30, 2000.
85. Klepser ME, Patel KB, Nicolau DP, et al: Comparison of bactericidal activities of intermittent and continuous infusion dosing of vancomycin against methicillin-resistant *Staphylococcus aureus* and *Enterococcus faecalis*, *Pharmacotherapy* 18:1069-1074, 1998.
86. Liu C, Bayer A, Cosgrove SE, et al: Clinical practice guidelines by the Infectious Diseases Society of America for the treatment of methicillin-resistant *Staphylococcus aureus* infections in adults and children, *Clin Infect Dis* 52:e18-e55, 2011.
87. de Hoog M, Mouton JW, van den Anker JN: Vancomycin: pharmacokinetics and administration regimens in neonates, *Clin Pharmacokinet* 43:417-440, 2004.
88. Mehrotra N, Tang L, Phelps SJ, et al: Evaluation of vancomycin dosing regimens in preterm and term neonates using Monte Carlo simulations, *Pharmacotherapy* 32:408-419, 2012.
89. van den Anker JN: Getting the dose of vancomycin right in the neonate, *Int J Clin Pharmacol Ther* 49:247-249, 2011.
90. Plan O, Cambonie G, Barbotte E, et al: Continuous-infusion vancomycin therapy for preterm neonates with suspected or documented gram-positive infections: a new dosage schedule, *Arch Dis Child Fetal Neonatal Ed* 93:F418-F421, 2008.
91. Pawlotsky F, Thomas A, Kergueris MF, et al: Constant rate infusion of vancomycin in premature neonates: a new dosage schedule, *Br J Clin Pharmacol* 46:163-167, 1998.
92. Simon A, Mullenborn E, Prelog M, et al: Use of linezolid in neonatal and pediatric inpatient facilities—results of a retrospective multicenter survey, *Eur J Clin Microbiol Infect Dis* 31:1435-1442, 2012.
93. Stevens DL, Dotter B, Madaras-Kelly K: A review of linezolid: the first oxazolidinone antibiotic, *Expert Rev Anti Infect Ther* 2:51-59, 2004.
94. Craig WA: Basic pharmacodynamics of antibacterials with clinical applications to the use of beta-lactams, glycopeptides, and linezolid, *Infect Dis Clin North Am* 17:479-501, 2003.
95. Jungbluth GL, Welshman IR, Hopkins NK: Linezolid pharmacokinetics in pediatric patients: an overview, *Pediatr Infect Dis J* 22: S153-S157, 2003.
96. Kearns GL, Abdel-Rahman SM, Blumer JL, et al: Single dose pharmacokinetics of linezolid in infants and children, *Pediatr Infect Dis J* 19:1178-1184, 2000.
97. Yogev R, Damle B, Levy G, et al: Pharmacokinetics and distribution of linezolid in cerebrospinal fluid in children and adolescents, *Pediatr Infect Dis J* 29:827-830, 2010.
98. Jantausch BA, Deville J, Adler S, et al: Linezolid for the treatment of children with bacteremia or nosocomial pneumonia caused by resistant gram-positive bacterial pathogens, *Pediatr Infect Dis J* 22: S164-S171, 2003.
99. Kaplan SL, Deville JG, Yogev R, et al: Linezolid versus vancomycin for treatment of resistant gram-positive infections in children, *Pediatr Infect Dis J* 22:677-686, 2003.
100. Kaplan SL, Patterson L, Edwards KM, et al: Linezolid for the treatment of community-acquired pneumonia in hospitalized children. Linezolid Pediatric Pneumonia Study Group, *Pediatr Infect Dis J* 20: 488-494, 2001.
101. Pharmacia & Upjohn Company. Zyvox: Linezolid injection, linezolid tablets, linezolid for oral suspension package insert, *Kalamazoo (MI)*, 2002.
102. Bishop E, Melvani S, Howden BP, et al: Good clinical outcomes but high rates of adverse reactions during linezolid therapy for serious infections: a proposed protocol for monitoring therapy in complex patients, *Antimicrob Agents Chemother* 50:1599-1602, 2006.
103. Conte JE Jr, Golden JA, Kipps J, et al: Intrapulmonary pharmacokinetics of linezolid, *Antimicrob Agents Chemother* 46:1475-1480, 2002.
104. Andes D, van Ogtrop ML, Peng J, et al: In vivo pharmacodynamics of a new oxazolidinone (linezolid), *Antimicrob Agents Chemother* 46:3484-3489, 2002.
105. Rayner CR, Forrest A, Meagher AK, et al: Clinical pharmacodynamics of linezolid in seriously ill patients treated in a compassionate use programme, *Clin Pharmacokinet* 42:1411-1423, 2003.
106. Adembri C, Fallani S, Cassetta MI, et al: Linezolid pharmacokinetic/pharmacodynamic profile in critically ill septic patients: intermittent versus continuous infusion, *Int J Antimicrob Agents* 31:122-129, 2008.
107. Jacqueline C, Batard E, Perez L, et al: In vivo efficacy of continuous infusion versus intermittent dosing of linezolid compared to vancomycin in a methicillin-resistant *Staphylococcus aureus* rabbit endocarditis model, *Antimicrob Agents Chemother* 46:3706-3711, 2002.
108. Stevens DL, Herr D, Lampiris H, et al: Linezolid versus vancomycin for the treatment of methicillin-resistant *Staphylococcus aureus* infections, *Clin Infect Dis* 34:1481-1490, 2002.
109. Weigelt J, Itani K, Stevens D, et al: Linezolid versus vancomycin in treatment of complicated skin and soft tissue infections, *Antimicrob Agents Chemother* 49:2260-2266, 2005.
110. Deville JG, Adler S, Azimi PH, et al: Linezolid versus vancomycin in the treatment of known or suspected resistant gram-positive infections in neonates, *Pediatr Infect Dis J* 22:S158-S163, 2003.
111. Lyseng-Williamson KA, Goa KL: Linezolid: in infants and children with severe gram-positive infections, *Paediatric Drugs* 5:419-429, discussion 30–1, 2003.
112. Guay D: Update on clindamycin in the management of bacterial, fungal and protozoal infections, *Expert Opin Pharmacother* 8:2401-2444, 2007.
113. Spizek J, Novotna J, Rezanka T: Lincosamides: chemical structure, biosynthesis, mechanism of action, resistance, and applications, *Adv Appl Microbiol* 56:121-154, 2004.
114. Paris MM, Shelton S, Trujillo M, et al: Clindamycin therapy of experimental meningitis caused by penicillin- and cephalosporin-resistant *Streptococcus pneumoniae*, *Antimicrob Agents Chemother* 40:122-126, 1996.
115. Bell MJ, Shackelford P, Smith R, et al: Pharmacokinetics of clindamycin phosphate in the first year of life, *J Pediatr* 105: 482-486, 1984.
116. Koren G, Zarfin Y, Maresky D, et al: Pharmacokinetics of intravenous clindamycin in newborn infants, *Pediatr Pharmacol* 5:287-292, 1986.
117. Donta ST, Myers MG: *Clostridium difficile* toxin in asymptomatic neonates, *J Pediatr* 100:431-434, 1982.
118. Newland JG, Kearns GL: Treatment strategies for methicillin-resistant *Staphylococcus aureus* infections in pediatrics, *Paediatr Drugs* 10: 367-378, 2008.
119. Feldman WE: *Bacteroides fragilis* ventriculitis and meningitis. Report of two cases, *Am J Dis Child* 130:880-883, 1976.
120. de Louvois J: Bacteriological examination of pus from abscesses of the central nervous system, *J Clin Pathol* 33:66-71, 1980.
121. Ambrose PG, Bhavnani SM, Rubino CM, et al: Pharmacokinetics-pharmacodynamics of antimicrobial therapy: it's not just for mice anymore, *Clin Infect Dis* 44:79-86, 2007.
122. Lewis RE, Klepser ME, Ernst EJ, et al: Evaluation of low-dose, extended-interval clindamycin regimens against *Staphylococcus aureus* and *Streptococcus pneumoniae* using a dynamic in vitro model of infection, *Antimicrob Agents Chemother* 43:2005-2009, 1999.
123. LaPlante KL, Leonard SN, Andes DR, et al: Activities of clindamycin, daptomycin, doxycycline, linezolid, trimethoprim-sulfamethoxazole, and vancomycin against community-associated methicillin-resistant *Staphylococcus aureus* with inducible clindamycin resistance in murine thigh infection and in vitro pharmacodynamic models, *Antimicrob Agents Chemother* 52:2156-2162, 2008.
124. Shama A, Patole SK, Whitehall JS: Intravenous rifampicin in neonates with persistent staphylococcal bacteraemia, *Acta Paediatr* 91:670-673, 2002.
125. Yee-Guardino S, Kumar D, Abughali N, et al: Recognition and treatment of neonatal community-associated MRSA pneumonia and bacteremia, *Pediatr Pulmonol* 43:203-205, 2008.
126. Bedford Laboratories: Bedford, Ohio: Rifampin, for injection only: product label. Available at http://www.fda.gov/cder/foi/anda/99/64-217_Rifampin_prntlbl.pdf, 1997. Accessed April 1, 2013.

127. Niemi M, Backman JT, Fromm MF, et al: Pharmacokinetic interactions with rifampicin: clinical relevance, *Clin Pharmacokinet* 42: 819-850, 2003.
128. Tan TQ, Mason EO Jr, Ou CN, et al: Use of intravenous rifampin in neonates with persistent staphylococcal bacteremia, *Antimicrobial Agents Chemother* 37:2401-2406, 1993.
129. Koup JR, Williams-Warren J, Weber A, et al: Pharmacokinetics of rifampin in children. I. Multiple dose intravenous infusion, *Ther Drug Monit* 8:11-16, 1986.
130. Sanofi-Aventis: Teicoplanin drug label. Available at http://www.sanofi-aventiscouk/products/Targocid_SPCpdf. Accessed April 1, 2013.
131. Pryka RD, Rodvold KA, Rotschafer JC: Teicoplanin: an investigational glycopeptide antibiotic, *Clin Pharm* 7:647-658, 1988.
132. Tarral E, Jehl F, Tarral A, et al: Pharmacokinetics of teicoplanin in children, *J Antimicrob Chemother* 21(Suppl A):47-51, 1988.
133. Fanos V, Kacet N, Mosconi G: A review of teicoplanin in the treatment of serious neonatal infections, *Eur J Pediatr* 156:423-427, 1997.
134. Yalaz M, Cetin H, Akisu M, et al: Experience with teicoplanin in the treatment of neonatal staphylococcal sepsis, *J Int Med Res* 32: 540-548, 2004.
135. Fanos V, Mussap M, Khoory BJ, et al: Renal tolerability of teicoplanin in a case of neonatal overdose, *J Chemother* 10:381-384, 1998.
136. Cubicin, daptomycin for injection. Full prescribing information, Lexington, Mass, 2006, Cubist Pharmaceuticals.
137. Weis F, Beiras-Fernandez A, Schelling G: Daptomycin, a lipopeptide antibiotic in clinical practice, *Curr Opin Investig Drugs* 9:879-884, 2008.
138. Silverman JA, Mortin LI, Vanpraagh AD, et al: Inhibition of daptomycin by pulmonary surfactant: in vitro modeling and clinical impact, *J Infect Dis* 191:2149-2152, 2005.
139. Dvorchik BH, Brazier D, DeBruin MF, et al: Daptomycin pharmacokinetics and safety following administration of escalating doses once daily to healthy subjects, *Antimicrob Agents Chemother* 47:1318-1323, 2003.
140. Abdel-Rahman SM, Benziger DP, Jacobs RF, et al: Single-dose pharmacokinetics of daptomycin in children with suspected or proved gram-positive infections, *Pediatr Infect Dis J* 27:330-334, 2008.
141. Cohen-Wolkowiez M, Smith PB, Benjamin DK Jr, et al: Daptomycin use in infants: report of two cases with peak and trough drug concentrations, *J Perinatol* 28:233-234, 2008.
142. Cohen-Wolkowiez M, Watt KM, Hornik CP, et al: Pharmacokinetics and tolerability of single-dose daptomycin in young infants, *Pediatr Infect Dis J* 31:935-937, 2012.
143. Touw DJ, Westerman EM, Sprij AJ: Therapeutic drug monitoring of aminoglycosides in neonates, *Clin Pharmacokinet* 48:71-88, 2009.
144. Rao SC, Srinivasjois R, Hagan R, et al: One dose per day compared to multiple doses per day of gentamicin for treatment of suspected or proven sepsis in neonates, *Cochrane Database Syst Rev* (11)CD005091, 2011.
145. Shakil S, Khan R, Zarrilli R, et al: Aminoglycosides versus bacteria—a description of the action, resistance mechanism, and nosocomial battleground, *J Biomed Sci* 15:5-14, 2008.
146. Daikos GL, Lolans VT, Jackson GG: First-exposure adaptive resistance to aminoglycoside antibiotics in vivo with meaning for optimal clinical use, *Antimicrob Agents Chemother* 35:117-123, 1991.
147. Lian WB, Yeo CL, Ho LY: Once-daily-dosing intramuscular gentamicin in neonates, *Ann Acad Med Singapore* 41:227-229, 2012.
148. McCracken GH Jr, Threlkeld N, Thomas ML: Intravenous administration of kanamycin and gentamicin in newborn infants, *Pediatrics* 60:463-466, 1977.
149. Pacifici GM: Clinical pharmacokinetics of aminoglycosides in the neonate: a review, *Eur J Clin Pharmacol* 65:419-427, 2009.
150. Friedman CA, Parks BR, Rawson JE: Gentamicin disposition in asphyxiated newborns: relationship to mean arterial blood pressure and urine output, *Pediatr Pharmacol (New York)* 2:189-197, 1982.
151. Watterberg KL, Kelly HW, Johnson JD, et al: Effect of patent ductus arteriosus on gentamicin pharmacokinetics in very low birth weight (less than 1,500 g) babies, *Dev Pharmacol Ther* 10:107-117, 1987.
152. Mustafa MM, Mertsola J, Ramilo O, et al: Increased endotoxin and interleukin-1 beta concentrations in cerebrospinal fluid of infants with coliform meningitis and ventriculitis associated with intraventricular gentamicin therapy, *J Infect Dis* 160:891-895, 1989.
153. Kliegman RM, Bertino JS Jr, Fanaroff AA, et al: Pharmacokinetics of gentamicin during exchange transfusions in neonates, *J Pediatr* 96:927-930, 1980.
154. Bertino JS Jr, Kliegman RM, Myers CM, et al: Alterations in gentamicin pharmacokinetics during neonatal exchange transfusion, *Dev Pharmacol Ther* 4:205-215, 1982.
155. Cohen P, Collart L, Prober CG, et al: Gentamicin pharmacokinetics in neonates undergoing extracorporal membrane oxygenation, *Pediatr Infect Dis J* 9:562-566, 1990.
156. Itsarayoungyuen S, Riff L, Schauf V, et al: Tobramycin and gentamicin are equally safe for neonates: results of a double-blind randomized trial with quantitative assessment of renal function, *Pediatr Pharmacol (New York)* 2:143-155, 1982.
157. Kaplan JM, McCracken GH Jr, Thomas ML, et al: Clinical pharmacology of tobramycin in newborns, *Am J Dis Child* 125:656-660, 1973.
158. Nahata MC, Powell DA, Durrell DE, et al: Tobramycin pharmacokinetics in very low birth weight infants, *Br J Clin Pharmacol* 21:325-327, 1986.
159. Falcao AC, Buelga DS, Mendez ME, et al: Population kinetics of tobramycin in neonates, *Ther Drug Monit* 23:202-208, 2001.
160. de Hoog M, Schoemaker RC, Mouton JW, et al: Tobramycin population pharmacokinetics in neonates, *Clin Pharmacol Ther* 62:392-399, 1997.
161. Howard JB, McCraken GH Jr, Trujillo H, et al: Amikacin in newborn infants: comparative pharmacology with kanamycin and clinical efficacy in 45 neonates with bacterial diseases, *Antimicrob Agents Chemother* 10:205-210, 1976.
162. Bleyzac N, Varnier V, Labaune JM, et al: Population pharmacokinetics of amikacin at birth and interindividual variability in renal maturation, *Eur J Clin Pharmacol* 57:499-504, 2001.
163. Botha JH, du Preez MJ, Miller R, et al: Determination of population pharmacokinetic parameters for amikacin in neonates using mixed-effect models, *Eur J Clin Pharmacol* 53:337-341, 1998.
164. De Cock RF, Allegaert K, Schreuder MF, et al: Maturation of the glomerular filtration rate in neonates, as reflected by amikacin clearance, *Clin Pharmacokinet* 51:105-117, 2012.
165. Schreuder MF, Wilhelm AJ, Bokenkamp A, et al: Impact of gestational age and birth weight on amikacin clearance on day 1 of life, *Clin J Am Soc Nephrol* 4:1774-1778, 2009.
166. Sherwin CM, Svahn S, Van der Linden A, et al: Individualised dosing of amikacin in neonates: a pharmacokinetic/pharmacodynamic analysis, *Eur J Clin Pharmacol* 65:705-713, 2009.
167. Allegaert K, Scheers I, Adams E, et al: Cerebrospinal fluid compartmental pharmacokinetics of amikacin in neonates, *Antimicrob Agents Chemother* 52:1934-1939, 2008.
168. Yow MD: An overview of pediatric experience with amikacin, *Am J Med* 62:954-958, 1977.
169. Giuliano RA, Verpooten GA, Verbist L, et al: In vivo uptake kinetics of aminoglycosides in the kidney cortex of rats, *J Pharmacol Exp Ther* 236:470-475, 1986.
170. Verpooten GA, Giuliano RA, Verbist L, et al: Once-daily dosing decreases renal accumulation of gentamicin and netilmicin, *Clin Pharmacol Ther* 45:22-27, 1989.
171. De Broe ME, Verbist L, Verpooten GA: Influence of dosage schedule on renal cortical accumulation of amikacin and tobramycin in man, *J Antimicrob Chemother* 27(Suppl C):41-47, 1991.
172. Smyth AR, Bhatt J: Once-daily versus multiple-daily dosing with intravenous aminoglycosides for cystic fibrosis, *Cochrane Database Syst Rev* (2):CD002009, 2012.
173. Swan SK: Aminoglycoside nephrotoxicity, *Semin Nephrol* 17:27-33, 1997.
174. Gouyon JB, Aujard Y, Abisror A, et al: Urinary excretion of N-acetylglucosaminidase and beta-2-microglobulin as early markers of gentamicin nephrotoxicity in neonates, *Dev Pharmacol Ther* 10:145-152, 1987.
175. Tessin I, Trollfors B, Bergmark J, et al: Enzymuria in neonates during treatment with gentamicin or tobramycin, *Pediatr Infect Dis J* 6: 870-871, 1987.
176. Winkel S, Bonding P, Larsen PK, et al: Possible effects of kanamycin and incubation in newborn children with low birth weight, *Acta Paediatr Scand* 67:709-715, 1978.
177. Finitzo-Hieber T, McCracken GH Jr, Roeser RJ, et al: Ototoxicity in neonates treated with gentamicin and kanamycin: results of a four-year controlled follow-up study, *Pediatrics* 63:443-450, 1979.
178. Skopnik H, Wallraf R, Nies B, et al: Pharmacokinetics and antibacterial activity of daily gentamicin, *Arch Dis Child* 67:57-61, 1992.
179. Johnson RF, Cohen AP, Guo Y, et al: Genetic mutations and aminoglycoside-induced ototoxicity in neonates, *Otolaryngol Head Neck Surg* 142:704-707, 2010.

180. Warner WA, Sanders E: Neuromuscular blockade associated with gentamicin therapy, *JAMA* 215:1153-1154, 1971.
181. Yamada S, Kuno Y, Iwanaga H: Effects of aminoglycoside antibiotics on the neuromuscular junction: part I, *Int J Clin Pharmacol Ther Toxicol* 24:130-138, 1986.
182. Santos JI, Swensen P, Glasgow LA: Potentiation of *Clostridium botulinum* toxin aminoglycoside antibiotics: clinical and laboratory observations, *Pediatrics* 68:50-54, 1981.
183. Moore RD, Smith CR, Lietman PS: Association of aminoglycoside plasma levels with therapeutic outcome in gram-negative pneumonia, *Am J Med* 77:657-662, 1984.
184. Moore RD, Smith CR, Lietman PS: The association of aminoglycoside plasma levels with mortality in patients with gram-negative bacteremia, *J Infect Dis* 149:443-448, 1984.
185. Moore RD, Lietman PS, Smith CR: Clinical response to aminoglycoside therapy: importance of the ratio of peak concentration to minimal inhibitory concentration, *J Infect Dis* 155:93-99, 1987.
186. Kashuba AD, Nafziger AN, Drusano GL, et al: Optimizing aminoglycoside therapy for nosocomial pneumonia caused by gram-negative bacteria, *Antimicrob Agents Chemother* 43:623-629, 1999.
187. Craig WA: Post-antibiotic effects in experimental infection models: relationship to in-vitro phenomena and to treatment of infections in man, *J Antimicrob Chemother* 31(Suppl D):149-158, 1993.
188. Fantin B, Ebert S, Leggett J, et al: Factors affecting duration of in-vivo postantibiotic effect for aminoglycosides against gram-negative bacilli, *J Antimicrob Chemother* 27:829-836, 1991.
189. Vogelman B, Gudmundsson S, Turnidge J, et al: In vivo postantibiotic effect in a thigh infection in neutropenic mice, *J Infect Dis* 157: 287-298, 1988.
190. Kapusnik JE, Hackbarth CJ, Chambers HF, et al: Single, large, daily dosing versus intermittent dosing of tobramycin for treating experimental *Pseudomonas* pneumonia, *J Infect Dis* 158:7-12, 1988.
191. Rastogi A, Agarwal G, Pyati S, et al: Comparison of two gentamicin dosing schedules in very low birth weight infants, *Pediatr Infect Dis J* 21:234-240, 2002.
192. Avent ML, Kinney JS, Istre GR, et al: Gentamicin and tobramycin in neonates: comparison of a new extended dosing interval regimen with a traditional multiple daily dosing regimen, *Am J Perinatol* 19:413-420, 2002.
193. Abdel-Hady E, El Hamamsy M, Hedaya M, et al: The efficacy and toxicity of two dosing-regimens of amikacin in neonates with sepsis, *J Clin Pharm Ther* 36:45-52, 2011.
194. Siddiqi A, Khan DA, Khan FA, et al: Therapeutic drug monitoring of amikacin in preterm and term infants, *Singapore Med J* 50:486-489, 2009.
195. Langhendries JP, Battisti O, Bertrand JM, et al: Adaptation in neonatology of the once-daily concept of aminoglycoside administration: evaluation of a dosing chart for amikacin in an intensive care unit, *Biol Neonate* 74:351-362, 1998.
196. Kotze A, Bartel PR, Sommers DK: Once versus twice daily amikacin in neonates: prospective study on toxicity, *J Paediatr Child Health* 35:283-286, 1999.
197. Lebel MH, McCracken GH Jr: Aztreonam: review of the clinical experience and potential uses in pediatrics, *Pediatr Infect Dis J* 7:331-339, 1988.
198. Tunkel AR, Scheld WM: Aztreonam, *Infect Control Hosp Epidemiol* 11:486-494, 1990.
199. Likitnukul S, McCracken GH Jr, Threlkeld N, et al: Pharmacokinetics and plasma bactericidal activity of aztreonam in low birth weight infants, *Antimicrob Agents Chemother* 31:81-83, 1987.
200. Stutman HR: Clinical experience with aztreonam for treatment of infections in children, *Rev Infect Dis* 13(Suppl 7):S582-S585, 1991.
201. Cuzzolin L, Fanos V, Zambreri D, et al: Pharmacokinetics and renal tolerance of aztreonam in premature infants, *Antimicrob Agents Chemother* 35:1726-1728, 1991.
202. Millar MR, Gorham P, Baxter H, et al: Pharmacokinetics of aztreonam in very low birthweight neonates, *Eur J Clin Microbiol* 6:691-692, 1987.
203. Greenman RL, Arcey SM, Dickinson GM, et al: Penetration of aztreonam into human cerebrospinal fluid in the presence of meningeal inflammation, *J Antimicrob Chemother* 15:637-640, 1985.
204. Stutman HR, Marks MI, Swabb EA: Single-dose pharmacokinetics of aztreonam in pediatric patients, *Antimicrob Agents Chemother* 26:196-199, 1984.
205. Umana MA, Odio CM, Castro E, et al: Evaluation of aztreonam and ampicillin vs. amikacin and ampicillin for treatment of neonatal bacterial infections, *Pediatr Infect Dis J* 9:175-180, 1990.
206. Uauy R, Mize C, Argyle C, et al: Metabolic tolerance to arginine: implications for the safe use of arginine salt-aztreonam combination in the neonatal period, *J Pediatr* 118:965-970, 1991.
207. Elks J: Structural formulae and nomenclature of the cephalosporin antibiotics, *Drugs* 34(Suppl 2):240-246, 1987.
208. Schaad UB: The cephalosporin compounds in severe neonatal infection, *Eur J Pediatr* 141:143-146, 1984.
209. Pacifici GM: Pharmacokinetics of cephalosporins in the neonate: a review, *Clinics (São Paulo)* 66:1267-1274, 2011.
210. Chang N, Ito T, Saito H, et al: *Studies on cefazolin in obstetrics and gynecology with special reference to its clinical pharmacology in the neonate*, Baltimore, 1972, University Park Press.
211. Sakata Y: The pharmacokinetic studies of cephalothin, cefazolin and cefmetazole in the neonates and the premature babies, *Kurume Med J* 27:275-298, 1980.
212. Dash CH, Kennedy MR, Ng SH, editors: *Cefuroxime in the first week of life*, Washington, DC, 1980, American Society for Microbiology.
213. de Louvois J, Mulhall A, Hurley R: Cefuroxime in the treatment of neonates, *Arch Dis Child* 57:59-62, 1982.
214. Renlund M, Pettay O: Pharmacokinetics and clinical efficacy of cefuroxime in the newborn period, *Proc R Soc Med* 70(Suppl 9):183, 1977.
215. McCracken GH Jr, Threlkeld NE, Thomas ML: Pharmacokinetics of cefotaxime in newborn infants, *Antimicrob Agents Chemother* 21: 683-684, 1982.
216. von Loewenich V, Miething R, Uihlein M, et al: Cefotaxime and desacetylcefotaxime in cerebrospinal fluid of newborn and premature infants, *Padiatr Padol* 18:361-366, 1983.
217. Ahsman MJ, Wildschut ED, Tibboel D, et al: Pharmacokinetics of cefotaxime and desacetylcefotaxime in infants during extracorporeal membrane oxygenation, *Antimicrob Agents Chemother* 54:1734-1741, 2010.
218. Capparelli E, Hochwald C, Rasmussen M, et al: Population pharmacokinetics of cefepime in the neonate, *Antimicrob Agents Chemother* 49:2760-2766, 2005.
219. Lima-Rogel V, Medina-Rojas EL, Del Carmen Milan-Segovia R, et al: Population pharmacokinetics of cefepime in neonates with severe nosocomial infections, *J Clin Pharm Ther* 33:295-306, 2008.
220. Blumer JL, Reed MD, Knupp C: Review of the pharmacokinetics of cefepime in children, *Pediatr Infect Dis J* 20:337-342, 2001.
221. Reed MD, Yamashita TS, Knupp CK, et al: Pharmacokinetics of intravenously and intramuscularly administered cefepime in infants and children, *Antimicrob Agents Chemother* 41:1783-1787, 1997.
222. Roos R, editor: *New beta-lactams*, Amsterdam, 1986, Elsevier.
223. Bryan CS, John JF Jr, Pai MS, et al: Gentamicin vs cefotaxime for therapy of neonatal sepsis. Relationship to drug resistance, *Am J Dis Child* 139:1086-1089, 1985.
224. Bang NU, Kammer RB: Hematologic complications assoicated with β-lactam antibiotics, *Rev Infec Dis* 5:S380-S393, 1983.
225. Johnson GJ, editor: *Antibiotic-induced hemostatic abnormalities*, Amsterdam, 1986, Elsevier.
226. Bradley JS, Wassel RT, Lee L, et al: Intravenous ceftriaxone and calcium in the neonate: assessing the risk for cardiopulmonary adverse events, *Pediatrics* 123:e609-e613, 2009.
227. Steadman E, Raisch DW, Bennett CL, et al: Evaluation of a potential clinical interaction between ceftriaxone and calcium, *Antimicrob Agents Chemother* 54:1534-1540, 2010.
228. McCracken GH Jr: Use of third-generation cephalosporins for treatment of neonatal infections, *Am J Dis Child* 139:1079-1080, 1985.
229. Hoogkamp-Korstanje JA: Activity of cefotaxime and ceftriaxone alone and in combination with penicillin, ampicillin and piperacillin against neonatal meningitis pathogens, *J Antimicrob Chemother* 16:327-334, 1985.
230. Hall MA, Ducker DA, Lowes JA, et al: A randomised prospective comparison of cefotaxime versus netilmicin/penicillin for treatment of suspected neonatal sepsis, *Drugs* 35(Suppl 2):169-177, 1988.
231. Saez-Llorens X, O'Ryan M: Cefepime in the empiric treatment of meningitis in children, *Pediatr Infect Dis J* 20:356-361, 2001.
232. Saez-Llorens X, Castano E, Garcia R, et al: Prospective randomized comparison of cefepime and cefotaxime for treatment of bacterial meningitis in infants and children, *Antimicrob Agents Chemother* 39:937-940, 1995.
233. Rubino CM, Gal P, Ransom JL: A review of the pharmacokinetic and pharmacodynamic characteristics of beta-lactam/beta-lactamase inhibitor combination antibiotics in premature infants, *Pediatr Infect Dis J* 17:1200-1210, 1998.

234. Gin A, Dilay L, Karlowsky JA, et al: Piperacillin-tazobactam: a beta-lactam/beta-lactamase inhibitor combination, *Expert Rev Anti Infect Ther* 5:365-383, 2007.
235. Wolf MF, Simon A: The use of piperacillin-tazobactam in neonatal and paediatric patients, *Expert Opin Drug Metab Toxicol* 5:57-69, 2009.
236. Reed MD, Goldfarb J, Yamashita TS, et al: Single-dose pharmacokinetics of piperacillin and tazobactam in infants and children, *Antimicrob Agents Chemother* 38:2817-2826, 1994.
237. Wise R, Logan M, Cooper M, et al: Pharmacokinetics and tissue penetration of tazobactam administered alone and with piperacillin, *Antimicrob Agents Chemother* 35:1081-1084, 1991.
238. Placzek M, Whitelaw A, Want S, et al: Piperacillin in early neonatal infection, *Arch Dis Child* 58:1006-1009, 1983.
239. Kacet N, Roussel-Delvallez M, Gremillet C, et al: Pharmacokinetic study of piperacillin in newborns relating to gestational and postnatal age, *Pediatr Infect Dis J* 11:365-369, 1992.
240. Thirumoorthi MC, Asmar BI, Buckley JA, et al: Pharmacokinetics of intravenously administered piperacillin in preadolescent children, *J Pediatr* 102:941-946, 1983.
241. Cohen-Wolkowiez M, Watt KM, Zhou C, et al: Population pharmacokinetics of piperacillin and tazobactam in infants. In *Proceedings of Pediatric Academic Society Annual Meeting*, Washington, DC, May 4-7, 2013.
242. Arguedas A, Sifuentes-Osornio J, Loaiza C, et al: An open, multicenter clinical trial of piperacillin/tazobactam in the treatment of pediatric patients with intra-abdominal infections, *J Chemother* 8:130-136, 1996.
243. Maltezou HC, Nikolaidis P, Lebesii E, et al: Piperacillin/tazobactam versus cefotaxime plus metronidazole for treatment of children with intra-abdominal infections requiring surgery, *Eur J Clin Microbiol Infect Dis* 20:643-646, 2001.
244. Kern W, Kennedy SL, Sachdeva M, et al: Evaluation of piperacillin-tazobactam in experimental meningitis caused by a beta-lactamase-producing strain of K1-positive *Escherichia coli*, *Antimicrob Agents Chemother* 34:697-701, 1990.
245. Nichols KR, Knoderer CA, Cox EG, et al: System-wide implementation of the use of an extended-infusion piperacillin/tazobactam dosing strategy: feasibility of utilization from a children's hospital perspective, *Clin Ther* 34:1459-1465, 2012.
246. Fayed SB, Sutton AM, Turner TL, et al: The prophylactic use of ticarcillin/clavulanate in the neonate, *J Antimicrob Chemother* 19:113-118, 1987.
247. Fricke G, Doerck M, Hafner D, et al: The pharmacokinetics of ticarcillin/clavulanate acid in neonates, *J Antimicrob Chemother* 24(Suppl B): 111-120, 1989.
248. Burstein AH, Wyble LE, Gal P, et al: Ticarcillin-clavulanic acid pharmacokinetics in preterm neonates with presumed sepsis, *Antimicrob Agents Chemother* 38:2024-2028, 1994.
249. Abdel-Rahman SM, Kearns GL: The beta-lactamase inhibitors: clinical pharmacology and rational application to combination antibiotic therapy, *Pediatr Infect Dis J* 17:1185-1194, 1998.
250. Zhanel GG, Wiebe R, Dilay L, et al: Comparative review of the carbapenems, *Drugs* 67:1027-1052, 2007.
251. Blumer JL: Pharmacokinetic determinants of carbapenem therapy in neonates and children, *Pediatr Infect Dis J* 15:733-737, 1996.
252. Bradley JS, Garau J, Lode H, et al: Carbapenems in clinical practice: a guide to their use in serious infection, *Int J Antimicrob Agents* 11:93-100, 1999.
253. Clissold SP, Todd PA, Campoli-Richards DM: Imipenem/cilastatin. A review of its antibacterial activity, pharmacokinetic properties and therapeutic efficacy, *Drugs* 33:183-241, 1987.
254. Freij BJ, McCracken GH Jr, Olsen KD, et al: Pharmacokinetics of imipenem-cilastatin in neonates, *Antimicrob Agents Chemother* 27: 431-435, 1985.
255. Gruber WC, Rench MA, Garcia-Prats JA, et al: Single-dose pharmacokinetics of imipenem-cilastatin in neonates, *Antimicrob Agents Chemother* 27:511-514, 1985.
256. Bradley JS: Meropenem: a new, extremely broad spectrum beta-lactam antibiotic for serious infections in pediatrics, *Pediatr Infect Dis J* 16:263-268, 1997.
257. Smith PB, Cohen-Wolkowiez M, Castro LM, et al: Population pharmacokinetics of meropenem in plasma and cerebrospinal fluid of infants with suspected or complicated intra-abdominal infections, *Pediatr Infect Dis J* 30:844-849, 2011.
258. Bradley JS, Sauberan JB, Ambrose PG, et al: Meropenem pharmacokinetics, pharmacodynamics, and Monte Carlo simulation in the neonate, *Pediatr Infect Dis J* 27:794-799, 2008.
259. van Enk JG, Touw DJ, Lafeber HN: Pharmacokinetics of meropenem in preterm neonates, *Ther Drug Monit* 23:198-201, 2001.
260. Calandra GB, Brown KR, Grad LC, et al: Review of adverse experiences and tolerability in the first 2,516 patients treated with imipenem/cilastatin, *Am J Med* 78:73-78, 1985.
261. Modai J, Vittecoq D, Decazes JM, et al: Penetration of imipenem and cilastatin into cerebrospinal fluid of patients with bacterial meningitis, *J Antimicrob Chemother* 16:751-755, 1985.
262. Wong VK, Wright HT Jr, Ross LA, et al: Imipenem/cilastatin treatment of bacterial meningitis in children, *Pediatr Infect Dis J* 10:122-125, 1991.
263. Eng RH, Munsif AN, Yangco BG, et al: Seizure propensity with imipenem, *Arch Intern Med* 149:1881-1883, 1989.
264. Day IP, Goudie J, Nishiki K, et al: Correlation between in vitro and in vivo models of proconvulsive activity with the carbapenem antibiotics, biapenem, imipenem/cilastatin and meropenem, *Toxicol Lett* 76:239-243, 1995.
265. Cohen-Wolkowiez M, Poindexter B, Bidegain M, et al: Safety and effectiveness of meropenem in infants with suspected or complicated intra-abdominal infections, *Clin Infect Dis* 55:1495-1502, 2012.
266. Smith PB, Cohen-Wolkowiez M, Castro LM , et al: Population pharmacokinetics of meropenem in plasma and cerebrospinal fluid of infants with suspected or complicated intra-abdominal infections. *Pediatr Infect Dis J* 30:844-849, 2011.
267. Hornik CP, Herring AH, Benjamin DK Jr, et al: Adverse events associated with meropenem versus imipenem/cilastatin therapy in a large retrospective cohort of hospitalized infants, *Pediatr Infect Dis J* 32:748-753, 2013.
268. Collins MA, Tolpin M, Group atcI-Cs: *Clinical evaluation of imipenem-cilastatin as a single agent therapy for sepsis neonatorum. Program and abstracts of the 27th Interscience Conference on Antimicrobial Agents and Chemotherapy*, October 4-7. Washington, DC, 1987, American Society for Microbiology, abstract 188.
269. Drusano GL: Antimicrobial pharmacodynamics: critical interactions of 'bug and drug', *Nat Rev Microbiol* 2:289-300, 2004.
270. Ohata Y, Tomita Y, Nakayama M, et al: Optimal dosage regimen of meropenem for pediatric patients based on pharmacokinetic/pharmacodynamic considerations, *Drug Metab Pharmacokinet* 26:523-531, 2011.
271. Padari H, Metsvaht T, Korgvee LT, et al: Short versus long infusion of meropenem in very-low-birth-weight neonates, *Antimicrob Agents Chemother* 56:4760-4764, 2012.
272. van den Anker JN, Pokorna P, Kinzig-Schippers M, et al: Meropenem pharmacokinetics in the newborn, *Antimicrob Agents Chemother* 53:3871-3879, 2009.
273. Houghton GW, Smith J, Thorne PS, et al: The pharmacokinetics of oral and intravenous metronidazole in man, *J Antimicrob Chemother* 5:621-623, 1979.
274. Suyagh M, Collier PS, Millership JS, et al: Metronidazole population pharmacokinetics in preterm neonates using dried blood-spot sampling, *Pediatrics* 127:e367-e374, 2011.
275. Cohen-Wolkowiez M, Sampson M, Bloom BT, et al: Determining population and developmental pharmacokinetics of metronidazole using plasma and dried blood spot samples from premature infants, *Pediatr Infect Dis J* 32:956-961, 2013.
276. Cohen-Wolkowiez M, Ouellet D, Smith PB, et al: Population pharmacokinetics of metronidazole evaluated using scavenged samples from preterm infants, *Antimicrob Agents Chemother* 56:1828-1837, 2012.
277. Beard CM, Noller KL, O'Fallon WM, et al: Lack of evidence for cancer due to use of metronidazole, *N Engl J Med* 301:519-522, 1979.
278. Sullender WM, Arvin AM, Diaz PS, et al: Pharmacokinetics of acyclovir suspension in infants and children, *Antimicrob Agents Chemother* 31:1722-1726, 1987.
279. Whitley RJ: The use of antiviral drugs during the neonatal period, *Clin Perinatol* 39:69-81, 2012.
280. Blum MR, Liao SH, de Miranda P: Overview of acyclovir pharmacokinetic disposition in adults and children, *Am J Med* 73:186-192, 1982.
281. Englund JA, Fletcher CV, Balfour HH Jr: Acyclovir therapy in neonates, *J Pediatr* 119:129-135, 1991.
282. Hintz M, Connor JD, Spector SA, et al: Neonatal acyclovir pharmacokinetics in patients with herpes virus infections, *Am J Med* 73: 210-214, 1982.

283. Whitley RJ, Blum MR, Barton N, et al: Pharmacokinetics of acyclovir in humans following intravenous administration. A model for the development of parenteral antivirals, *Am J Med* 73:165-171, 1982.
284. Sampson M, Bloom B, Anand R, et al: Population pharmacokinetics of acyclovir in preterm and term infants. In *Proceedings of Pediatric Academic Society Annual Meeting* Washington, DC, May 4-7, 2013.
285. Kimberlin DW: Management of HSV encephalitis in adults and neonates: diagnosis, prognosis and treatment, *Herpes* 14:11-16, 2007.
286. Kimberlin DW, Lin CY, Jacobs RF, et al: Safety and efficacy of high-dose intravenous acyclovir in the management of neonatal herpes simplex virus infections, *Pediatrics* 108:230-238, 2001.
287. Rabalais GP, Nusinoff-Lehrman S, Arvin AM, et al: Antiviral susceptibilities of herpes simplex virus isolates from infants with recurrent mucocutaneous lesions after neonatal infection, *Pediatr Infect Dis J* 8:221-223, 1989.
288. Kimberlin DW, Baley J: Guidance on management of asymptomatic neonates born to women with active genital herpes lesions, *Pediatrics* 131:383-386, 2013.
289. Kimberlin DW, Whitley RJ, Wan W, et al: Oral acyclovir suppression and neurodevelopment after neonatal herpes, *N Engl J Med* 365:1284-1292, 2011.
290. Tiffany KF, Benjamin DK Jr, Palasanthiran P, et al: Improved neurodevelopmental outcomes following long-term high-dose oral acyclovir therapy in infants with central nervous system and disseminated herpes simplex disease, *J Perinatol* 25:156-161, 2005.
291. McGavin JK, Goa KL: Ganciclovir: an update of its use in the prevention of cytomegalovirus infection and disease in transplant recipients, *Drugs* 61:1153-1183, 2001.
292. Wutzler P, Thust R: Genetic risks of antiviral nucleoside analogues—a survey, *Antiviral Res* 49:55-74, 2001.
293. Trang JM, Kidd L, Gruber W, et al: Linear single-dose pharmacokinetics of ganciclovir in newborns with congenital cytomegalovirus infections. NIAID Collaborative Antiviral Study Group, *Clin Pharmacol Ther* 53:15-21, 1993.
294. Zhou XJ, Gruber W, Demmler G, et al: Population pharmacokinetics of ganciclovir in newborns with congenital cytomegalovirus infections. NIAID Collaborative Antiviral Study Group, *Antimicrob Agents Chemother* 40:2202-2205, 1996.
295. Acosta EP, Brundage RC, King JR, et al: Ganciclovir population pharmacokinetics in neonates following intravenous administration of ganciclovir and oral administration of a liquid valganciclovir formulation, *Clin Pharmacol Ther* 81:867-872, 2007.
296. Meine Jansen CF, Toet MC, Rademaker CM, et al: Treatment of symptomatic congenital cytomegalovirus infection with valganciclovir, *J Perinat Med* 33:364-366, 2005.
297. Schulzke S, Buhrer C: Valganciclovir for treatment of congenital cytomegalovirus infection, *Eur J Pediatr* 165:575-576, 2006.
298. Galli L, Novelli A, Chiappini E, et al: Valganciclovir for congenital CMV infection: a pilot study on plasma concentration in newborns and infants, *Pediatr Infect Dis J* 26:451-453, 2007.
299. Kimberlin DW, Acosta EP, Sanchez PJ, et al: Pharmacokinetic and pharmacodynamic assessment of oral valganciclovir in the treatment of symptomatic congenital cytomegalovirus disease, *J Infect Dis* 197:836-845, 2008.
300. Kimberlin DW, Lin CY, Sanchez PJ, et al: Effect of ganciclovir therapy on hearing in symptomatic congenital cytomegalovirus disease involving the central nervous system: a randomized, controlled trial, *J Pediatr* 143:16-25, 2003.
301. Whitley RJ, Cloud G, Gruber W, et al: Ganciclovir treatment of symptomatic congenital cytomegalovirus infection: results of a phase II study. National Institute of Allergy and Infectious Diseases Collaborative Antiviral Study Group, *J Infect Dis* 175:1080-1086, 1997.
302. Smets K, De Coen K, Dhooge I, et al: Selecting neonates with congenital cytomegalovirus infection for ganciclovir therapy, *Eur J Pediatr* 165:885-890, 2006.
303. Thompson WW, Shay DK, Weintraub E, et al: Influenza-associated hospitalizations in the United States, *JAMA* 292:1333-1340, 2004.
304. Thompson WW, Shay DK, Weintraub E, et al: Mortality associated with influenza and respiratory syncytial virus in the United States, *JAMA* 289:179-186, 2003.
305. Noyola DE: Neuraminidase inhibitors in pediatric patients: potential place in influenza therapy, *Paediatr Drugs* 5:125-131, 2003.
306. He G, Massarella J, Ward P: Clinical pharmacokinetics of the prodrug oseltamivir and its active metabolite Ro 64-0802, *Clin Pharmacokinet* 37:471-484, 1999.
307. Oo C, Hill G, Dorr A, et al: Pharmacokinetics of anti-influenza prodrug oseltamivir in children aged 1-5 years, *Eur J Clin Pharmacol* 59:411-415, 2003.
308. Standing JF, Nika A, Tsagris V, et al: Oseltamivir pharmacokinetics and clinical experience in neonates and infants during an outbreak of H1N1 influenza A virus infection in a neonatal intensive care unit, *Antimicrob Agents Chemother* 56:3833-3840, 2012.
309. Maltezou HC, Drakoulis N, Siahanidou T, et al: Safety and pharmacokinetics of oseltamivir for prophylaxis of neonates exposed to influenza H1N1, *Pediatr Infect Dis J* 31:527-529, 2012.
310. Acosta EP, Jester P, Gal P, et al: Oseltamivir dosing for influenza infection in premature neonates, *J Infect Dis* 202:563-566, 2010.
311. Kimberlin DW, Acosta EP, Prichard MN, et al: Oseltamivir pharmacokinetics, dosing, and resistance among children aged <2 years with influenza, *J Infect Dis* 207:709-720, 2013.
312. Hoffmann-La Roche: "Dear healthcare professional letter,"2003, Available at http://www.fda.gov/medwatch/SAFETY/2003/tamiflu_deardoc.pdf. Accessed April 1, 2013.
313. Tamura D, Miura T, Kikuchi Y: Oseltamivir phosphate in infants under 1 year of age with influenza infection, *Pediatr Int* 47:484, 2005.
314. Okamoto S, Kamiya I, Kishida K, et al: Experience with oseltamivir for infants younger than 1 year old in Japan, *Pediatr Infect Dis J* 24:575-576, 2005.
315. Kimberlin DW, Shalabi M, Abzug MJ, et al: Safety of oseltamivir compared with the adamantanes in children less than 12 months of age, *Pediatr Infect Dis J* 29:195-198, 2010.
316. Morioka I, Nonoyama S, Tanaka-Taya K, et al: Survey of Japanese infants younger than 3 months who were treated with oseltamivir for influenza: safety of oseltamivir treatment, *Scand J Infect Dis* 44:605-609, 2012.
317. Khandaker G, Zurynski Y, Lester-Smith D, et al: Clinical features, oseltamivir treatment and outcome in infants aged <12 months with laboratory-confirmed influenza A in 2009, *Antivir Ther* 16: 1005-1010, 2011.
318. Siedler K, Skopnik H: Oseltamivir for treatment of influenza in infants less than one year: a retrospective analysis, *Pediatr Infect Dis J* 29:495-498, 2010.
319. Benjamin DK Jr, Stoll BJ, Fanaroff AA, et al: Neonatal candidiasis among extremely low birth weight infants: risk factors, mortality rates, and neurodevelopmental outcomes at 18 to 22 months, *Pediatrics* 117:84-92, 2006.
320. Gallis HA, Drew RH, Pickard WW, et al: 30 years of clinical experience, *Rev Infect Dis* 12:308-329, 1990.
321. Latge JP: *Aspergillus fumigatus* and aspergillosis, *Clin Microbiol Rev* 12:310-350, 1999.
322. Meis JF, Verweij PE: Current management of fungal infections, *Drugs* 61(Suppl 1):13-25, 2001.
323. Atkinson AJ Jr, Bennett JE: Amphotericin B pharmacokinetics in humans, *Antimicrob Agents Chemother* 13:271-276, 1978.
324. Baley JE, Meyers C, Kliegman RM, et al: Pharmacokinetics, outcome of treatment, and toxic effects of amphotericin B and 5-fluorocytosine in neonates, *J Pediatr* 116:791-797, 1990.
325. Starke JR, Mason EO Jr, Kramer WG, et al: Pharmacokinetics of amphotericin B in infants and children, *J Infect Dis* 155:766-774, 1987.
326. De Pauw BE: New antifungal agents and preparations, *Int J Antimicrob Agents* 16:147-150, 2000.
327. Albengres E, Le Louet H, Tillement JP: Systemic antifungal agents. Drug interactions of clinical significance, *Drug Saf* 18:83-97, 1998.
328. Kullberg BJ, de Pauw BE: Therapy of invasive fungal infections, *Neth J Med* 55:118-127, 1999.
329. Groll AH, Piscitelli SC, Walsh TJ: Antifungal pharmacodynamics: concentration-effect relationships in vitro and in vivo, *Pharmacotherapy* 21:133S-148S, 2001.
330. Christiansen KJ, Bernard EM, Gold JW, et al: Distribution and activity of amphotericin B in humans, *J Infect Dis* 152:1037-1043, 1985.
331. Ellis M: Amphotericin B preparations: a maximum tolerated dose in severe invasive fungal infections? *Transpl Infect Dis* 2:51-61, 2000.
332. Luna B, Drew RH, Perfect JR: Agents for treatment of invasive fungal infections, *Otolaryngol Clin North Am* 33:277-299, 2000.
333. Frattarelli DA, Reed MD, Giacoia GP, et al: Antifungals in systemic neonatal candidiasis, *Drugs* 64:949-968, 2004.
334. Ralph ED, Khazindar AM, Barber KR, et al: Comparative in vitro effects of liposomal amphotericin B, amphotericin B-deoxycholate, and free amphotericin B against fungal strains determined by using MIC and minimal lethal concentration susceptibility studies and time-kill curves, *Antimicrob Agents Chemother* 35:188-191, 1991.

335. Wong-Beringer A, Jacobs RA, Guglielmo BJ: Lipid formulations of amphotericin B: clinical efficacy and toxicities, *Clin Infect Dis* 27:603-618, 1998.
336. Walsh TJ, Goodman JL, Pappas P, et al: Safety, tolerance, and pharmacokinetics of high-dose liposomal amphotericin B (AmBisome) in patients infected with *Aspergillus* species and other filamentous fungi: maximum tolerated dose study, *Antimicrob Agents Chemother* 45:3487-3496, 2001.
337. Hiemenz JW, Walsh TJ: Lipid formulations of amphotericin B: recent progress and future directions, *Clin Infect Dis* 22(Suppl 2)S133-S144, 1996.
338. Fielding RM, Smith PC, Wang LH, et al: Comparative pharmacokinetics of amphotericin B after administration of a novel colloidal delivery system, ABCD, and a conventional formulation to rats, *Antimicrob Agents Chemother* 35:1208-1213, 1991.
339. Wurthwein G, Groll AH, Hempel G, et al: Population pharmacokinetics of amphotericin B lipid complex in neonates, *Antimicrob Agents Chemother* 49:5092-5098, 2005.
340. Juster-Reicher A, Flidel-Rimon O, Amitay M, et al: High-dose liposomal amphotericin B in the therapy of systemic candidiasis in neonates, *Eur J Clin Microbiol Infect Dis* 22:603-607, 2003.
341. Schmitt HJ: New methods of delivery of amphotericin B, *Clin Infect Dis* 17(Suppl 2):S501-S506, 1993.
342. Wasan KM, Rosenblum MG, Cheung L, et al: Influence of lipoproteins on renal cytotoxicity and antifungal activity of amphotericin B, *Antimicrob Agents Chemother* 38:223-227, 1994.
343. Graybill JR, Tollemar J, Torres-Rodriguez JM, et al: Antifungal compounds: controversies, queries and conclusions, *Med Mycol* 38(Suppl 1):323-333, 2000.
344. Ringden O, Jonsson V, Hansen M, et al: Severe and common side-effects of amphotericin B lipid complex (Abelcet), *Bone Marrow Transplant* 22:733-734, 1998.
345. Manzoni P, Galletto P, Rizzollo S, et al: Liposomal amphotericin B does not induce nephrotoxicity or renal function impairment in premature neonates, *Early Hum Dev* 88(Suppl 2):S86-S91, 2012.
346. Auron A, Auron-Gomez M, Raina R, et al: Effect of amphotericin B lipid complex (ABLC) in very low birth weight infants, *Pediatr Nephrol (Berlin)* 24:295-299, 2009.
347. Hope WW, Mickiene D, Petraitis V, et al: The pharmacokinetics and pharmacodynamics of micafungin in experimental hematogenous *Candida* meningoencephalitis: implications for echinocandin therapy in neonates, *J Infect Dis* 197:163-171, 2008.
348. Pappas PG, Kauffman CA, Andes D, et al: Clinical practice guidelines for the management of candidiasis: 2009 update by the Infectious Diseases Society of America, *Clin Infect Dis* 48:503-535, 2009.
349. Turkova A, Roilides E, Sharland M: Amphotericin B in neonates: deoxycholate or lipid formulation as first-line therapy—is there a 'right' choice? *Curr Opin Infect Dis* 24:163-171, 2011.
350. Vermes A, Guchelaar HJ, Dankert J: Flucytosine: a review of its pharmacology, clinical indications, pharmacokinetics, toxicity and drug interactions, *J Antimicrob Chemother* 46:171-179, 2000.
351. Denning DW, Stevens DA: Antifungal and surgical treatment of invasive aspergillosis: review of 2,121 published cases, *Rev Infect Dis* 12:1147-1201, 1990.
352. Pasqualotto AC, Howard SJ, Moore CB, et al: Flucytosine therapeutic monitoring: 15 years experience from the UK, *J Antimicrob Chemother* 59:791-793, 2007.
353. Stevens DA, Kan VL, Judson MA, et al: Practice guidelines for diseases caused by *Aspergillus*. Infectious Diseases Society of America, *Clin Infect Dis* 30:696-709, 2000.
354. Stamm AM, Diasio RB, Dismukes WE, et al: Toxicity of amphotericin B plus flucytosine in 194 patients with cryptococcal meningitis, *Am J Med* 83:236-242, 1987.
355. Ernst EJ: Investigational antifungal agents, *Pharmacotherapy* 21:165S-174S, 2001.
356. Walsh TJ, Viviani MA, Arathoon E, et al: New targets and delivery systems for antifungal therapy, *Med Mycol* 38(Suppl 1):335-347, 2000.
357. De Beule K, Van Gestel J: Pharmacology of itraconazole, *Drugs* 61(Suppl 1):27-37, 2001.
358. Klepser ME, Malone D, Lewis RE, et al: Evaluation of voriconazole pharmacodynamics using time-kill methodology, *Antimicrob Agents Chemother* 44:1917-1920, 2000.
359. Ernst EJ, Klepser ME, Ernst ME, et al: In vitro pharmacodynamic properties of MK-0991 determined by time-kill methods, *Diagn Microbiol Infect Dis* 33:75-80, 1999.
360. Brammer KW, Coates PE: Pharmacokinetics of fluconazole in pediatric patients, *Eur J Clin Microbiol Infect Dis* 13:325-329, 1994.
361. Wildfeuer A, Laufen H, Schmalreck AF, et al: Fluconazole: comparison of pharmacokinetics, therapy and in vitro susceptibility, *Mycoses* 40:259-265, 1997.
362. Wade KC, Wu D, Kaufman DA, et al: Population pharmacokinetics of fluconazole in young infants, *Antimicrob Agents Chemother* 52:4043-4049, 2008.
363. Piper L, Smith PB, Hornik CP, et al: Fluconazole loading dose pharmacokinetics and safety in infants, *Pediatr Infect Dis J* 30:375-378, 2011.
364. Watt KM, Benjamin DK Jr, Cheifetz IM, et al: Pharmacokinetics and safety of fluconazole in young infants supported with extracorporeal membrane oxygenation, *Pediatr Infect Dis J* 31:1042-1047, 2012.
365. Viscoli C, Castagnola E, Fioredda F, et al: Fluconazole in the treatment of candidiasis in immunocompromised children, *Antimicrob Agents Chemother* 35:365-367, 1991.
366. Schwarze R, Penk A, Pittrow L: Administration of fluconazole in children below 1 year of age, *Mycoses* 42:3-16, 1999.
367. Novelli V, Holzel H: Safety and tolerability of fluconazole in children, *Antimicrobial Agents Chemother* 43:1955-1960, 1999.
368. Debruyne D: Clinical pharmacokinetics of fluconazole in superficial and systemic mycoses, *Clin Pharmacokinet* 33:52-77, 1997.
369. Rex JH, Pappas PG, Karchmer AW, et al: A randomized and blinded multicenter trial of high-dose fluconazole plus placebo versus fluconazole plus amphotericin B as therapy for candidemia and its consequences in nonneutropenic subjects, *Clin Infect Dis* 36:1221-1228, 2003.
370. Faergemann J, Laufen H: Levels of fluconazole in serum, stratum corneum, epidermis-dermis (without stratum corneum) and eccrine sweat, *Clin Exp Dermatol* 18:102-106, 1993.
371. Kaufman D, Boyle R, Hazen KC, et al: Fluconazole prophylaxis against fungal colonization and infection in preterm infants [see comment], *N Engl J Med* 345:1660-1666, 2001.
372. Manzoni P, Stolfi I, Pugni L, et al: A multicenter, randomized trial of prophylactic fluconazole in preterm neonates [see comment], *N Engl J Med* 356:2483-2495, 2007.
373. Healy CM, Campbell JR, Zaccaria E, et al: Fluconazole prophylaxis in extremely low birth weight neonates reduces invasive candidiasis mortality rates without emergence of fluconazole-resistant *Candida* species, *Pediatrics* 121:703-710, 2008.
374. Manzoni P, Leonessa M, Galletto P, et al: Routine use of fluconazole prophylaxis in a neonatal intensive care unit does not select natively fluconazole-resistant *Candida* subspecies, *Pediatr Infect Dis J* 27:731-737, 2008.
375. Cotten CM, McDonald S, Stoll B, et al: The association of third-generation cephalosporin use and invasive candidiasis in extremely low birth-weight infants, *Pediatrics* 118:717-722, 2006.
376. Benjamin DK Jr: First, do no harm, *Pediatrics* 121:831-832, 2008.
377. Johnson LB, Kauffman CA: Voriconazole: a new triazole antifungal agent, *Clin Infect Dis* 36:630-637, 2003.
378. Johnson E, Espinel-Ingroff A, Szekely A, et al: Activity of voriconazole, itraconazole, fluconazole and amphotericin B in vitro against 1763 yeasts from 472 patients in the voriconazole phase III clinical studies, *Int J Antimicrob Agents* 32:511-514, 2008.
379. Goldstein JA, de Morais SM: Biochemistry and molecular biology of the human CYP2C subfamily, *Pharmacogenetics* 4:285-299, 1994.
380. Purkins L, Wood N, Ghahramani P, et al: Pharmacokinetics and safety of voriconazole following intravenous- to oral-dose escalation regimens, *Antimicrob Agents Chemother* 46:2546-2553, 2002.
381. Ghannoum MA, Kuhn DM: Voriconazole: better chances for patients with invasive mycoses, *Eur J Med Res* 7:242-256, 2002.
382. Denning DW, Ribaud P, Milpied N, et al: Efficacy and safety of voriconazole in the treatment of acute invasive aspergillosis, *Clin Infect Dis* 34:563-571, 2002.
383. Sheehan DJ, Hitchcock CA, Sibley CM: Current and emerging azole antifungal agents, *Clin Microbiol Rev* 12:40-79, 1999.
384. Groll AH, Lehrnbecher T: New antifungal drugs and the pediatric cancer patient: current status of clinical development, *Klin Padiatr* 217:158-168, 2005.
385. Lazarus HM, Blumer JL, Yanovich S, et al: Safety and pharmacokinetics of oral voriconazole in patients at risk of fungal infection: a dose escalation study, *J Clin Pharmacol* 42:395-402, 2002.
386. Tan KKC, Wood N, Weil A: Multi-dose pharmacokinetics of voriconazole in chronic hepatic impairment. Program and abstracts of the 41st Interscience Conference on Antimicrobial Agents and Chemotherapy, December 16-19, 2001. Chicago abstract A-16.

387. Walsh TJ, Karlsson MO, Driscoll T, et al: Pharmacokinetics and safety of intravenous voriconazole in children after single- or multiple-dose administration, *Antimicrob Agents Chemother* 48:2166-2172, 2004.
388. Walsh TJ, Lutsar I, Driscoll T, et al: Voriconazole in the treatment of aspergillosis, scedosporiosis and other invasive fungal infections in children, *Pediatr Infect Dis J* 21:240-248, 2002.
389. Doby EH, Benjamin DK Jr, Blaschke AJ, et al: Therapeutic monitoring of voriconazole in children less than three years of age: a case report and summary of voriconazole concentrations for ten children, *Pediatr Infect Dis J* 31:632-635, 2012.
390. Tan K, Brayshaw N, Tomaszewski K, et al: Investigation of the potential relationships between plasma voriconazole concentrations and visual adverse events or liver function test abnormalities, *J Clin Pharmacol* 46:235-243, 2006.
391. Bernhard S, Kernland Lang K, Ammann RA, et al: Voriconazole-induced phototoxicity in children, *Pediatr Infect Dis J* 31:769-771, 2012.
392. Santos RP, Sanchez PJ, Mejias A, et al: Successful medical treatment of cutaneous aspergillosis in a premature infant using liposomal amphotericin B, voriconazole and micafungin, *Pediatr Infect Dis J* 26:364-366, 2007.
393. Neely M, Rushing T, Kovacs A, et al: Voriconazole pharmacokinetics and pharmacodynamics in children, *Clin Infect Dis* 50:27-36, 2009.
394. Pascual A, Calandra T, Bolay S, et al: Voriconazole therapeutic drug monitoring in patients with invasive mycoses improves efficacy and safety outcomes, *Clin Infect Dis* 46:201-211, 2008.
395. Walsh TJ, Anaissie EJ, Denning DW, et al: Treatment of aspergillosis: clinical practice guidelines of the Infectious Diseases Society of America, *Clin Infect Dis* 46:327-360, 2008.
396. Spriet I, Cosaert K, Renard M, et al: Voriconazole plasma levels in children are highly variable, *Eur J Clin Microbiol Infect Dis* 30: 283-287, 2011.
397. Pieper S, Kolve H, Gumbinger HG, et al: Monitoring of voriconazole plasma concentrations in immunocompromised paediatric patients, *J Antimicrob Chemother* 67:2717-2724, 2012.
398. Ally R, Schurmann D, Kreisel W, et al: A randomized, double-blind, double-dummy, multicenter trial of voriconazole and fluconazole in the treatment of esophageal candidiasis in immunocompromised patients, *Clin Infect Dis* 33:1447-1454, 2001.
399. Frankenbusch K, Eifinger F, Kribs A, et al: Severe primary cutaneous aspergillosis refractory to amphotericin B and the successful treatment with systemic voriconazole in two premature infants with extremely low birth weight, *J Perinatol* 26:511-514, 2006.
400. Bartizal K, Gill CJ, Abruzzo GK, et al: In vitro preclinical evaluation studies with the echinocandin antifungal MK-0991 (L-743,872), *Antimicrob Agents Chemother* 41:2326-2332, 1997.
401. Caudle KE, Inger AG, Butler DR, et al: Echinocandin use in the neonatal intensive care unit, *Ann Pharmacother* 46:108-116, 2012.
402. Graybill JR: The echinocandins, first novel class of antifungals in two decades: will they live up to their promise? *Int J Clin Pract* 55:633-638, 2001.
403. Kontoyiannis DP: A clinical perspective for the management of invasive fungal infections: focus on IDSA guidelines. Infectious Diseases Society of America, *Pharmacotherapy* 21:175S-187S, 2001.
404. Ernst EJ, Klepser ME, Pfaller MA: Postantifungal effects of echinocandin, azole, and polyene antifungal agents against *Candida albicans* and *Cryptococcus neoformans*, *Antimicrob Agents Chemother* 44: 1108-1111, 2000.
405. Manzoni P, Benjamin DK, Hope W, et al: The management of *Candida* infections in preterm neonates and the role of micafungin, *J Matern Fetal Neonatal Med* 24(Suppl 2):24-27, 2011.
406. Groll AH, Stergiopoulou T, Roilides E, et al: Micafungin: pharmacology, experimental therapeutics and clinical applications, *Expert Opin Investig Drugs* 14:489-509, 2005.
407. Okugawa S, Ota Y, Tatsuno K, et al: A case of invasive central nervous system aspergillosis treated with micafungin with monitoring of micafungin concentrations in the cerebrospinal fluid, *Scand J Infect Dis* 39:344-346, 2007.
408. Ernst EJ, Roling EE, Petzold CR, et al: In vitro activity of micafungin (FK-463) against *Candida* spp.: microdilution, time-kill, and postantifungal-effect studies, *Antimicrob Agents Chemother* 46:3846-3853, 2002.
409. Heresi GP, Gerstmann DR, Reed MD, et al: The pharmacokinetics and safety of micafungin, a novel echinocandin, in premature infants, *Pediatr Infect Dis J* 25:1110-1115, 2006.
410. Smith PB, Walsh TJ, Hope W, et al: Pharmacokinetics of an elevated dosage of micafungin in premature neonates, *Pediatr Infect Dis J* 28:412-415, 2009.
411. Benjamin DK Jr, Smith PB, Arrieta A, et al: Safety and pharmacokinetics of repeat-dose micafungin in young infants, *Clin Pharmacol Ther* 87:93-99, 2010.
412. Kawada M, Fukuoka N, Kondo M, et al: Pharmacokinetics of prophylactic micafungin in very-low-birth-weight infants, *Pediatr Infect Dis J* 28:840-842, 2009.
413. Arrieta AC, Maddison P, Groll AH: Safety of micafungin in pediatric clinical trials, *Pediatr Infect Dis J* 30:e97-e102, 2011.
414. Ascher S, Smith PB, Benjamin DK Jr: Safety of micafungin in infants: insights into optimal dosing, *Expert Opin Drug Saf* 10:281-286, 2011.
415. King KY, Edwards MS, Word BM: Hepatitis associated with micafungin use in a preterm infant, *J Perinatol* 29:320-322, 2009.
416. Seibel NL, Schwartz C, Arrieta A, et al: Safety, tolerability, and pharmacokinetics of Micafungin (FK463) in febrile neutropenic pediatric patients, *Antimicrob Agents Chemother* 49:3317-3324, 2005.
417. Queiroz-Telles F, Berezin E, Leverger G, et al: Micafungin versus liposomal amphotericin B for pediatric patients with invasive candidiasis: substudy of a randomized double-blind trial, *Pediatr Infect Dis J* 27:820-826, 2008.
418. Hope WW, Smith PB, Arrieta A, et al: Population pharmacokinetics of micafungin in neonates and young infants, *Antimicrob Agents Chemother* 54:2633-2637, 2010.
419. Groll AH, Walsh TJ: Caspofungin: pharmacology, safety and therapeutic potential in superficial and invasive fungal infections, *Expert Opin Investig Drugs* 10:1545-1558, 2001.
420. Stone JA, Holland SD, Wickersham PJ, et al: Single- and multiple-dose pharmacokinetics of caspofungin in healthy men, *Antimicrob Agents Chemother* 46:739-745, 2002.
421. Chiou CC, Groll AH, Walsh TJ: New drugs and novel targets for treatment of invasive fungal infections in patients with cancer, *Oncologist* 5:120-135, 2000.
422. Lehrnbecher T, Groll AH: Experiences with the use of caspofungin in paediatric patients, *Mycoses* 51(Suppl 1):58-64, 2008.
423. Walsh TJ, Adamson PC, Seibel NL, et al: Pharmacokinetics, safety, and tolerability of caspofungin in children and adolescents, *Antimicrob Agents Chemother* 49:4536-4545, 2005.
424. Saez-Llorens X, Macias M, Maiya P, et al: Pharmacokinetics and safety of caspofungin in neonates and infants less than 3 months of age, *Antimicrob Agents Chemother* 53:869-875, 2009.
425. Natarajan G, Lulic-Botica M, Rongkavilit C, et al: Experience with caspofungin in the treatment of persistent fungemia in neonates, *J Perinatol* 25:770-777, 2005.
426. Mora-Duarte J, Betts R, Rotstein C, et al: Comparison of caspofungin and amphotericin B for invasive candidiasis, *N Engl J Med* 347:2020-2029, 2002.
427. Odio CM, Araya R, Pinto LE, et al: Caspofungin therapy of neonates with invasive candidiasis, *Pediatr Infect Dis J* 23:1093-1097, 2004.
428. Joseph JM, Kim R, Reboli AC: Anidulafungin: a drug evaluation of a new echinocandin, *Expert Opin Pharmacother* 9:2339-2348, 2008.
429. Lucas R, De Sante K, Hatcher B, et al: LY303366 single dose pharmacokinetics and safety in healthy volunteers (abstract F50). Abstracts of the 36th Annual Interscience Conference on Antimicrobial Agents and Chemotherapy (September 15-18, 1996, New Orleans), Washington, DC, 1996, American Society for Microbiology, p 108.
430. Petraitis V, Petraitiene R, Groll AH, et al: Antifungal efficacy, safety, and single-dose pharmokinetics of LY303366, a novel echinocandin B, in experimental pulmonary aspergillosis in persistently neutropenic rabbits, *Antimicrob Agents Chemother* 42:2898-2905, 1998.
431. Groll AH, Mickiene D, Petraitiene R, et al: Pharmacokinetic and pharmacodynamic modeling of anidulafungin (LY303366): reappraisal of its efficacy in neutropenic animal models of opportunistic mycoses using optimal plasma sampling, *Antimicrob Agents Chemother* 45:2845-2855, 2001.
432. Dowell JA, Stogniew M, Krause D, et al: Anidulafungin does not require dosage adjustment in subjects with varying degrees of hepatic or renal impairment, *J Clin Pharmacol* 47:461-470, 2007.
433. Benjamin DK Jr, Driscoll T, Seibel NL, et al: Safety and pharmacokinetics of intravenous anidulafungin in children with neutropenia at high risk for invasive fungal infections, *Antimicrob Agents Chemother* 50:632-638, 2006.
434. Cohen-Wolkowiez M, Benjamin DK Jr, Piper L, et al: Safety and pharmacokinetics of multiple-dose anidulafungin in infants and neonates, *Clin Pharmacol Ther* 89:702-707, 2011.

435. Vazquez JA: The safety of anidulafungin, *Expert Opin Drug Saf* 5: 751-758, 2006.
436. Thye D, Shepherd B, White RJ, et al: Anidulafungin: a phase 1 study to identify the maximum tolerated dose in healthy volunteers (abstract A-36). Abstracts of the 41st Annual Interscience Conference on Antimicrobial Agents and Chemotherapy (December 16-19, 2001, Chicago), Washington, DC, 2001, American Society for Microbiology.
437. Thye D, Kilfoil T, White RJ, et al: Anidulafungin: pharmacokinetics in subjects with mild and moderate hepatic impairment. Abstracts of the 41st Annual Interscience Conference on Antimicrobial Agents and Chemotherapy (December 16-19, 2001, Chicago), Washington, DC, 2001, American Society for Microbiology.
438. Thye D, Kilfoil T, Kilfoil G, et al: Anidulafungin: pharmacokinetics in subjects with severe hepatic impairment. Abstracts of the 42nd Annual Interscience Conference on Antimicrobial Agents and Chemotherapy (San Diego), Washington, DC, 2002, American Society for Microbiology.
439. Reboli AC, Rotstein C, Pappas PG, et al: Anidulafungin versus fluconazole for invasive candidiasis, *N Engl J Med* 356:2472-2482, 2007.
440. Amann U, Egen-Lappe V, Strunz-Lehner C, et al: Antibiotics in pregnancy: analysis of potential risks and determinants in a large German statutory sickness fund population, *Pharmacoepidemiol Drug Saf* 15: 327-337, 2006.
441. Rybak MJ: Therapeutic options for gram-positive infections, *J Hosp Infect* 49(Suppl A):S25-S32, 2001.
442. Albanese J, Leone M, Bruguerolle B, et al: Cerebrospinal fluid penetration and pharmacokinetics of vancomycin administered by continuous infusion to mechanically ventilated patients in an intensive care unit, *Antimicrob Agents Chemother* 44:1356-1358, 2000.
443. Langgartner M, Mutenthaler A, Haiden N, et al: Linezolid for treatment of catheter-related cerebrospinal fluid infections in preterm infants, *Arch Dis Child Fetal Neonatal Ed* 93:F397, 2008.
444. Hayani KC, Hatzopoulos FK, Frank AL, et al: Pharmacokinetics of once-daily dosing of gentamicin in neonates, *J Pediatr* 131:76-80, 1997.
445. de Alba Romero C, Gomez Castillo E, Manzanares Secades C, et al: Once daily gentamicin dosing in neonates, *Pediatr Infect Dis J* 17:1169-1171, 1998.
446. Skopnik H, Heimann G: Once daily aminoglycoside dosing in full term neonates, *Pediatr Infect Dis J* 14:71-72, 1995.
447. Miron D, Steinfeld M, Hasanein J, et al: Tolerability of once-daily-dosing of intravenous gentamicin in preterm neonates born at 32-37 weeks of gestation, *Harefuah* 142:413-415, 2003.
448. Agarwal G, Rastogi A, Pyati S, et al: Comparison of once-daily versus twice-daily gentamicin dosing regimens in infants > or = 2500 g, *J Perinatol* 22:268-274, 2002.
449. Chotigeat U, Narongsanti A, Ayudhya DP: Gentamicin in neonatal infection: once versus twice daily dosage, *J Med Assoc Thai* 84: 1109-1115, 2001.
450. Kosalaraksa P, Janthep P, Jirapradittha J, et al: Once versus twice daily dose of gentamicin therapy in Thai neonates, *J Med Assoc Thai* 87:372-376, 2004.
451. Krishnan L, George SA: Gentamicin therapy in preterms: a comparison of two dosage regimens, *Indian Pediatr* 34:1075-1080, 1997.
452. Solomon R, Kuruvilla KA, Job V, et al: Randomized controlled trial of once vs. twice daily gentamicin therapy in newborn, *Indian Pediatr* 36:133-137, 1999.
453. Thureen PJ, Reiter PD, Gresores A, et al: Once- versus twice-daily gentamicin dosing in neonates >/=34 weeks' gestation: cost-effectiveness analyses, *Pediatrics* 103:594-598, 1999.
454. Mercado MC, Brodsky NL, McGuire MK, et al: Extended interval dosing of gentamicin in preterm infants, *Am J Perinatol* 21:73-77, 2004.
455. Langhendries JP, Battisti O, Bertrand JM, et al: Once-a-day administration of amikacin in neonates: assessment of nephrotoxicity and ototoxicity, *Dev Pharmacol Ther* 20:220-230, 1993.

38 Prevention of Fetal and Early Life Infections Through Maternal–Neonatal Immunization

JAMES E. CROWE, JR.

CHAPTER OUTLINE

Overall Principles

Vaccination has been the most effective medical intervention in the modern era. Historically, the focus on vaccine development and implementation programs has been on preventing infectious diseases during infancy and early childhood. The current vaccine schedule for early childhood is replete with dozens of inoculations with an array of safe and effective vaccines that have dramatically reduced the incidence of many previously formidable childhood infectious diseases. Close review of the schedule, however, reveals that most vaccines are clustered in the 2- to 15-months age group, whereas there is a paucity of approved vaccines for the neonatal period (Fig. 38-1). Safe and effective vaccination of pregnant women and neonates is difficult to achieve but clearly is now an important target of development. Some of the major pathogens that cause disease in the neonatal period, such as group B streptococcal sepsis, meningitis, respiratory syncytial virus (RSV) bronchiolitis, and pneumonia, remain neonatal plagues that can only be addressed by new strategies.

A number of fundamental general principles have been defined through our experience in childhood vaccination programs. First, the usual goal of vaccination is to prevent disease, rather than to induce sterilizing protection against infection. In fact, most licensed vaccines do not completely prevent infection. Eradication of microorganisms in the population is a very difficult goal, whereas excellent protection against severe disease is often achievable. Second, whereas vaccines generally benefit the individual being immunized, additional public health benefits are often observed when herd immunity is induced in a previously susceptible population. This principle is especially important for protecting neonates because there often is insufficient time to induce an adequate immune response for protection in the early weeks of life, and vaccines may not be safe, tested, or immunogenic in this age group. Protecting all of the household contacts and caregivers against infection is currently the most feasible approach for protection of neonates against many diseases. Third, the mechanism by which many vaccines induce protection is poorly understood. In general, current vaccine development programs are accomplished using correlates of protection rather than definitive knowledge of protective immune mechanisms. A correlate of protection is typically a serologic test with an estimated cutoff of protection that allows comparison of the relatively common data on immunogenicity for different vaccines or vaccine preparations, in contrast to efficacy data, which are difficult to achieve without large numbers of subjects. Examples of correlates of protection that have been established by historical practice are summarized in Table 38-1. Finally, there is significant variation in response to vaccines among individuals that is poorly understood. Responses are affected by many factors, such as age, immune status, nutritional status, genetic polymorphisms, and environmental exposures.

Disclosure: This chapter is meant to review the principles of vaccination, and many specific indications, practices, and recommendations are discussed later that were current at the time of writing. Vaccine practice is, however, a constantly changing enterprise. Practitioners should consult the vaccine package inserts for U.S. Food and Drug Administration (FDA)-approved uses and the relevant current documents of the regulatory and advisory bodies for up-to-date information. The recommendations and guidelines of the Advisory Committee on Immunization Practices (ACIP) of the Centers for Disease Control and Prevention (CDC) are regularly updated on the website www.cdc.gov. The ACIP is the only entity in the federal government that makes such recommendations. The American Academy of Pediatrics (AAP) also issues guidelines, as published in notices in the

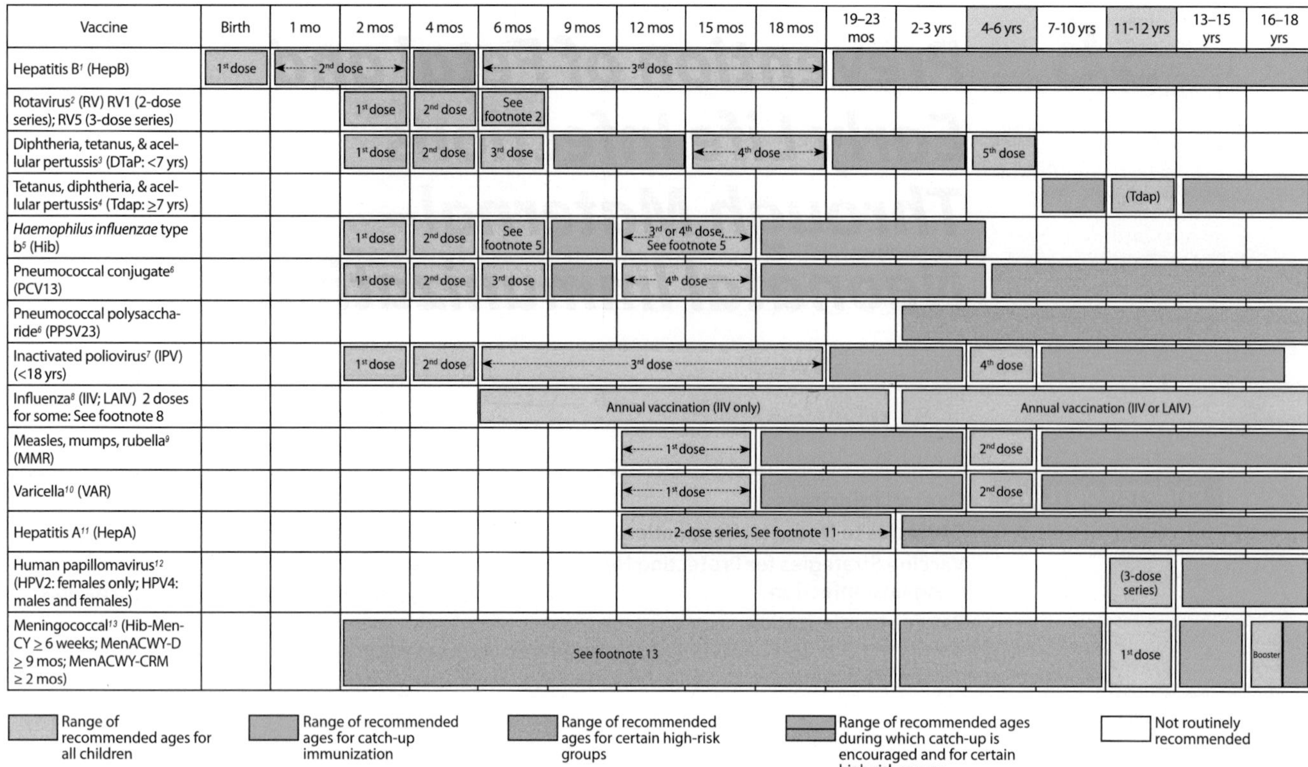

Vaccine	Birth	1 mo	2 mos	4 mos	6 mos	9 mos	12 mos	15 mos	18 mos	19–23 mos	2-3 yrs	4-6 yrs	7-10 yrs	11-12 yrs	13–15 yrs	16–18 yrs
Hepatitis B[1] (HepB)	1st dose	←2nd dose→			←3rd dose→											
Rotavirus[2] (RV) RV1 (2-dose series); RV5 (3-dose series)			1st dose	2nd dose	See footnote 2											
Diphtheria, tetanus, & acellular pertussis[3] (DTaP: <7 yrs)			1st dose	2nd dose	3rd dose			←4th dose→				5th dose				
Tetanus, diphtheria, & acellular pertussis[4] (Tdap: ≥7 yrs)														(Tdap)		
Haemophilus influenzae type b[5] (Hib)			1st dose	2nd dose	See footnote 5		←3rd or 4th dose, See footnote 5→									
Pneumococcal conjugate[6] (PCV13)			1st dose	2nd dose	3rd dose		←4th dose→									
Pneumococcal polysaccharide[6] (PPSV23)																
Inactivated poliovirus[7] (IPV) (<18 yrs)			1st dose	2nd dose	←3rd dose→							4th dose				
Influenza[8] (IIV; LAIV) 2 doses for some: See footnote 8					Annual vaccination (IIV only)						Annual vaccination (IIV or LAIV)					
Measles, mumps, rubella[9] (MMR)							←1st dose→					2nd dose				
Varicella[10] (VAR)							←1st dose→					2nd dose				
Hepatitis A[11] (HepA)							←2-dose series, See footnote 11→									
Human papillomavirus[12] (HPV2: females only; HPV4: males and females)														(3-dose series)		
Meningococcal[13] (Hib-MenCY ≥ 6 weeks; MenACWY-D ≥ 9 mos; MenACWY-CRM ≥ 2 mos)			See footnote 13											1st dose		Booster

Range of recommended ages for all children | Range of recommended ages for catch-up immunization | Range of recommended ages for certain high-risk groups | Range of recommended ages during which catch-up is encouraged and for certain high-risk groups | Not routinely recommended

Figure 38-1 Recommended immunization schedule for persons aged 0 through 18 years—United States, 2014. These recommendations must be read with the footnotes that follow. For those who fall behind or start late, provide catch-up vaccination at the earliest opportunity as indicated by the green bars. To determine minimum intervals between doses, see the catch-up schedule (http://www.cdc.gov/vaccines/schedules/downloads/child/catchup-schedule-pr.pdf). School entry and adolescent vaccine age groups are shaded in grey. This schedule includes recommendations in effect as of January 1, 2014. Any dose not administered at the recommended age should be administered at a subsequent visit, when indicated and feasible. The use of a combination vaccine generally is preferred over separate injections of its equivalent component vaccines. Vaccination providers should consult the relevant Advisory Committee on Immunization Practices (ACIP) statement for detailed recommendations, available online at http://www.cdc.gov/vaccines/hcp/acip-recs/index.html. Clinically significant adverse events that follow vaccination should be reported to the Vaccine Adverse Event Reporting System (VAERS) online (http://www.vaers.hhs.gov) or by telephone (800-822-7967). Suspected cases of vaccine-preventable diseases should be reported to the state or local health department. Additional information, including precautions and contraindications for vaccination, is available from CDC online (http://www.cdc.gov/vaccines/recs/vac-admin/contraindications.htm) or by telephone (800-CDC-INFO [800-232-4636]). This schedule is approved by the Advisory Committee on Immunization Practices (http://www.cdc.gov/vaccines/acip), the American Academy of Pediatrics (http://www.aap.org), the American Academy of Family Physicians (http://www.aafp.org), and the American College of Obstetricians and Gynecologists (http://www.acog.org). (From Centers for Disease Control and Prevention: Recommended immunization schedule for persons aged 0 through 18 years—United States, 2014. Available at http://www.cdc.gov/vaccines/schedules/downloads/child/0-18yrs-schedule.pdf. Accessed March 20, 2014.)

Additional information

- For contraindications and precautions to use of a vaccine and for additional information regarding that vaccine, vaccination providers should consult the relevant ACIP statement available online at http://www.cdc.gov/vaccines/hcp/acip-recs/index.html.
- For purposes of calculating intervals between doses, 4 weeks = 28 days. Intervals of 4 months or greater are determined by calendar months.
- Vaccine doses administered 4 days or less before the minimum interval are considered valid. Doses of any vaccine administered ≥5 days earlier than the minimum interval or minimum age should not be counted as valid doses and should be repeated as age appropriate. The repeat dose should be spaced after the invalid dose by the recommended minimum interval. For further details, see General recommendations on immunization and reports, *MMWR* 60(2):2011; Table 1. Recommended and minimum ages and intervals between vaccine doses available online at http://www.cdc.gov/mmwr/pdf/rr/rr6002.pdf.
- Information on travel vaccine requirements and recommendations is available at http://wwwnc.cdc.gov/travel/destinations/list.
- For vaccination of persons with primary and secondary immunodeficiencies, see Table 13, "Vaccination of persons with primary and secondary immunodeficiencies," in General Recommendations on Immunization (ACIP), available at http://www.cdc.gov/mmwr/pdf/rr/rr6002.pdf; and American Academy of Pediatrics: Immunization in special clinical circumstances. In Pickering LK, Baker CJ, Kimberlin DW, Long SS, editors: *Red book: 2012 report of the Committee on Infectious Diseases,* ed 29, Elk Grove Village, Ill, 2012, American Academy of Pediatrics.

1. **Hepatitis B (HepB) vaccine. (Minimum age: birth)**
   Routine vaccination:
   At birth:
   - Administer monovalent HepB vaccine to all newborns before hospital discharge.
   - For infants born to hepatitis B surface antigen (HBsAg)-positive mothers, administer HepB vaccine and 0.5 mL of hepatitis B immune globulin (HBIG) within 12 hours of birth. These infants should be tested for HBsAg and antibody to HBsAg (anti-HBs) 1 to 2 months after completion of the HepB series, at age 9 through 18 months (preferably at the next well-child visit).
   - If mother's HBsAg status is unknown, within 12 hours of birth administer HepB vaccine regardless of birth weight. For infants weighing less than 2000 g, administer HBIG in addition to HepB vaccine within 12 hours of birth. Determine mother's HBsAg status as soon as possible and, if mother is HBsAg positive, also administer HBIG for infants weighing 2000 g or more as soon as possible, but no later than age 7 days.

   Doses following the birth dose:
   - The second dose should be administered at age 1 or 2 months. Monovalent HepB vaccine should be used for doses administered before age 6 weeks.
   - Infants who did not receive a birth dose should receive 3 doses of a HepB-containing vaccine on a schedule of 0, 1 to 2 months, and 6 months starting as soon as feasible. See the catch-up schedule.

- Administer the second dose 1 to 2 months after the first dose (minimum interval of 4 weeks), administer the third dose at least 8 weeks after the second dose AND at least 16 weeks after the first dose. The final (third or fourth) dose in the HepB vaccine series should be administered no earlier than age 24 weeks.
- Administration of a total of 4 doses of HepB vaccine is permitted when a combination vaccine containing HepB is administered after the birth dose.

Catch-up vaccination:

- Unvaccinated persons should complete a 3-dose series.
- A 2-dose series (doses separated by at least 4 months) of adult formulation Recombivax HB is licensed for use in children aged 11 through 15 years.
- For other catch-up guidance, see the catch-up schedule.

2. **Rotavirus (RV) vaccines. (Minimum age: 6 weeks for both RV1 [Rotarix] and RV5 [RotaTeq])**

Routine vaccination:

- Administer a series of RV vaccine to all infants as follows:
  If Rotarix is used, administer a 2-dose series at 2 and 4 months of age.
  If RotaTeq is used, administer a 3-dose series at ages 2, 4, and 6 months.
  If any dose in the series was RotaTeq or vaccine product is unknown for any dose in the series, a total of 3 doses of RV vaccine should be administered.

Catch-up vaccination:

- The maximum age for the first dose in the series is 14 weeks, 6 days; vaccination should not be initiated for infants aged 15 weeks, 0 days, or older.
- The maximum age for the final dose in the series is 8 months, 0 days.
- For other catch-up guidance, see the catch-up schedule.

3. **Diphtheria and tetanus toxoids and acellular pertussis (DTaP) vaccine. (Minimum age: 6 weeks. Exception: DTaP-IPV [Kinrix]: 4 years)**

Routine vaccination:

- Administer a 5-dose series of DTaP vaccine at ages 2, 4, 6, 15 through 18 months, and 4 through 6 years. The fourth dose may be administered as early as age 12 months, provided at least 6 months have elapsed since the third dose.

Catch-up vaccination:

- The fifth dose of DTaP vaccine is not necessary if the fourth dose was administered at age 4 years or older.
- For other catch-up guidance, see the catch-up schedule.

4. **Tetanus and diphtheria toxoids and acellular pertussis (Tdap) vaccine. (Minimum age: 10 years for Boostrix, 11 years for Adacel)**

Routine vaccination:

- Administer 1 dose of Tdap vaccine to all adolescents aged 11 through 12 years.
- Tdap may be administered regardless of the interval since the last tetanus and diphtheria toxoid–containing vaccine.
- Administer 1 dose of Tdap vaccine to pregnant adolescents during each pregnancy (preferred during 27 through 36 weeks gestation) regardless of time since prior Td or Tdap vaccination.

Catch-up vaccination:

- Persons aged 7 years and older who are not fully immunized with DTaP vaccine should receive Tdap vaccine as 1 (preferably the first) dose in the catch-up series; if additional doses are needed, use Td vaccine. For children 7 through 10 years who receive a dose of Tdap as part of the catch-up series, an adolescent Tdap vaccine dose at age 11 through 12 years should NOT be administered. Td should be administered instead 10 years after the Tdap dose.
- Persons aged 11 through 18 years who have not received Tdap vaccine should receive a dose followed by tetanus and diphtheria toxoids (Td) booster doses every 10 years thereafter.
- Inadvertent doses of DTaP vaccine:
  - If administered inadvertently to a child aged 7 through 10 years may count as part of the catch-up series. This dose may count as the adolescent Tdap dose, or the child can later receive a Tdap booster dose at age 11 through 12 years.
  - If administered inadvertently to an adolescent aged 11 through 18 years, the dose should be counted as the adolescent Tdap booster.
- For other catch-up guidance, see the catch-up schedule.

5. ***Haemophilus influenzae* type b (Hib) conjugate vaccine. (Minimum age: 6 weeks for PRP-T [ActHIB, DTaP-IPV/Hib (Pentacel) and Hib-MenCY (MenHibrix)], PRP-OMP [PedvaxHIB or COMVAX], 12 months for PRP-T [Hiberix])**

Routine vaccination:

- Administer a 2- or 3-dose Hib vaccine primary series and a booster dose (dose 3 or 4 depending on vaccine used in primary series) at age 12 through 15 months to complete a full Hib vaccine series.
- The primary series with ActHIB, MenHibrix, or Pentacel consists of 3 doses and should be administered at 2, 4, and 6 months of age. The primary series with PedvaxHIB or COMVAX consists of 2 doses and should be administered at 2 and 4 months of age; a dose at age 6 months is not indicated.
- One booster dose (dose 3 or 4 depending on vaccine used in primary series) of any Hib vaccine should be administered at age 12 through 15 months. An exception is Hiberix vaccine. Hiberix should only be used for the booster (final) dose in children aged 12 months through 4 years who have received at least 1 prior dose of Hib-containing vaccine.
- For recommendations on the use of MenHibrix in patients at increased risk for meningococcal disease, please refer to the meningococcal vaccine footnotes and also to *MMWR* 62(RR-02):1-22, 2013; available at http://www.cdc.gov/mmwr/pdf/rr/rr6202.pdf.

Catch-up vaccination:

- If dose 1 was administered at ages 12 through 14 months, administer a second (final) dose at least 8 weeks after dose 1, regardless of Hib vaccine used in the primary series.
- If the first 2 doses were PRP-OMP (PedvaxHIB or COMVAX), and were administered at age 11 months or younger, the third (and final) dose should be administered at age 12 through 15 months and at least 8 weeks after the second dose.
- If the first dose was administered at age 7 through 11 months, administer the second dose at least 4 weeks later and a third (and final) dose at age 12 through 15 months or 8 weeks after second dose, whichever is later, regardless of Hib vaccine used for first dose.
- If first dose is administered at younger than 12 months of age and second dose is given between 12 through 14 months of age, a third (and final) dose should be given 8 weeks later.
- For unvaccinated children aged 15 months or older, administer only 1 dose.
- For other catch-up guidance, see the catch-up schedule. For catch-up guidance related to MenHibrix, please see the meningococcal vaccine footnotes and also *MMWR* 62(RR-02):1-22, 2013; available at http://www.cdc.gov/mmwr/pdf/rr/rr6202.pdf.

Vaccination of persons with high-risk conditions:

- Children aged 12 through 59 months who are at increased risk for Hib disease, including chemotherapy recipients and those with anatomic or functional asplenia (including sickle cell disease), human immunodeficiency virus (HIV) infection, immunoglobulin deficiency, or early component complement deficiency, who have received either no doses or only 1 dose of Hib vaccine before 12 months of age, should receive 2 additional doses of Hib vaccine 8 weeks apart; children who received 2 or more doses of Hib vaccine before 12 months of age should receive 1 additional dose.

Continued

- For patients younger than 5 years of age undergoing chemotherapy or radiation treatment who received a Hib vaccine dose(s) within 14 days of starting therapy or during therapy, repeat the dose(s) at least 3 months following therapy completion.
- Recipients of hematopoietic stem cell transplant (HSCT) should be revaccinated with a 3-dose regimen of Hib vaccine starting 6 to 12 months after successful transplant, regardless of vaccination history; doses should be administered at least 4 weeks apart.
- A single dose of any Hib-containing vaccine should be administered to unimmunized children and adolescents 15 months of age and older undergoing an elective splenectomy; if possible, vaccine should be administered at least 14 days before procedure.
- Hib vaccine is not routinely recommended for patients 5 years or older. However, 1 dose of Hib vaccine should be administered to unimmunized persons aged 5 years or older who have anatomic or functional asplenia (including sickle cell disease) and unvaccinated persons 5 through 18 years of age with human immunodeficiency virus (HIV) infection.
- Patients who have not received a primary series and booster dose or at least 1 dose of Hib vaccine after 14 months of age are considered unimmunized.

6. **Pneumococcal vaccines. (Minimum age: 6 weeks for PCV13, 2 years for PPSV23)**
   Routine vaccination with PCV13:
   - Administer a 4-dose series of PCV13 vaccine at ages 2, 4, and 6 months and at age 12 through 15 months.
   - For children aged 14 through 59 months who have received an age-appropriate series of 7-valent PCV (PCV7), administer a single supplemental dose of 13-valent PCV (PCV13).

   Catch-up vaccination with PCV13:
   - Administer 1 dose of PCV13 to all healthy children aged 24 through 59 months who are not completely vaccinated for their age.
   - For other catch-up guidance, see the catch-up schedule.

   Vaccination of persons with high-risk conditions with PCV13 and PPSV23:
   - All recommended PCV13 doses should be administered prior to PPSV23 vaccination if possible.
   - For children 2 through 5 years of age with any of the following conditions: chronic heart disease (particularly cyanotic congenital heart disease and cardiac failure); chronic lung disease (including asthma if treated with high-dose oral corticosteroid therapy); diabetes mellitus; cerebrospinal fluid leak; cochlear implant; sickle cell disease and other hemoglobinopathies; anatomic or functional asplenia; HIV infection; chronic renal failure; nephrotic syndrome; diseases associated with treatment with immunosuppressive drugs or radiation therapy, including malignant neoplasms, leukemias, lymphomas, and Hodgkin disease; solid organ transplantation; or congenital immunodeficiency:
     - Administer 1 dose of PCV13 if 3 doses of PCV (PCV7 and/or PCV13) were received previously.
     - Administer 2 doses of PCV13 at least 8 weeks apart if fewer than 3 doses of PCV (PCV7 and/or PCV13) were received previously.
     - Administer 1 supplemental dose of PCV13 if 4 doses of PCV7 or other age-appropriate complete PCV7 series was received previously.
     - The minimum interval between doses of PCV (PCV7 or PCV13) is 8 weeks.
     - For children with no history of PPSV23 vaccination, administer PPSV23 at least 8 weeks after the most recent dose of PCV13.
   - For children aged 6 through 18 years who have cerebrospinal fluid leak; cochlear implant; sickle cell disease and other hemoglobinopathies; anatomic or functional asplenia; congenital or acquired immunodeficiencies; HIV infection; chronic renal failure; nephrotic syndrome; diseases associated with treatment with immunosuppressive drugs or radiation therapy, including malignant neoplasms, leukemias, lymphomas, and Hodgkin disease; generalized malignancy; solid organ transplantation; or multiple myeloma:
     - If neither PCV13 nor PPSV23 has been received previously, administer 1 dose of PCV13 now and 1 dose of PPSV23 at least 8 weeks later.
     - If PCV13 has been received previously but PPSV23 has not, administer 1 dose of PPSV23 at least 8 weeks after the most recent dose of PCV13.
     - If PPSV23 has been received but PCV13 has not, administer 1 dose of PCV13 at least 8 weeks after the most recent dose of PPSV23.
   - For children aged 6 through 18 years with chronic heart disease (particularly cyanotic congenital heart disease and cardiac failure), chronic lung disease (including asthma if treated with high-dose oral corticosteroid therapy), diabetes mellitus, alcoholism, or chronic liver disease, who have not received PPSV23, administer 1 dose of PPSV23. If PCV13 has been received previously, then PPSV23 should be administered at least 8 weeks after any prior PCV13 dose.
   - A single revaccination with PPSV23 should be administered 5 years after the first dose to children with sickle cell disease or other hemoglobinopathies; anatomic or functional asplenia; congenital or acquired immunodeficiencies; HIV infection; chronic renal failure; nephrotic syndrome; diseases associated with treatment with immunosuppressive drugs or radiation therapy, including malignant neoplasms, leukemias, lymphomas, and Hodgkin disease; generalized malignancy; solid organ transplantation; or multiple myeloma.

7. **Inactivated poliovirus vaccine (IPV). (Minimum age: 6 weeks)**
   Routine vaccination:
   - Administer a 4-dose series of IPV at ages 2, 4, 6 through 18 months, and 4 through 6 years. The final dose in the series should be administered on or after the fourth birthday and at least 6 months after the previous dose.

   Catch-up vaccination:
   - In the first 6 months of life, minimum age and minimum intervals are only recommended if the person is at risk for imminent exposure to circulating poliovirus (i.e., travel to a polio-endemic region or during an outbreak).
   - If 4 or more doses are administered before age 4 years, an additional dose should be administered at age 4 through 6 years and at least 6 months after the previous dose.
   - A fourth dose is not necessary if the third dose was administered at age 4 years or older and at least 6 months after the previous dose.
   - If both OPV and IPV were administered as part of a series, a total of 4 doses should be administered, regardless of the child's current age. IPV is not routinely recommended for U.S. residents aged 18 years or older.
   - For other catch-up guidance, see the catch-up schedule.

8. **Influenza vaccines. (Minimum age: 6 months for inactivated influenza vaccine [IIV], 2 years for live, attenuated influenza vaccine [LAIV])**
   Routine vaccination:
   - Administer influenza vaccine annually to all children beginning at age 6 months. For most healthy, nonpregnant persons aged 2 through 49 years, either LAIV or IIV may be used. However, LAIV should NOT be administered to some persons, including (1) those with asthma, (2) children 2 through 4 years who had wheezing in the past 12 months, or (3) those who have any other underlying medical conditions that predispose them to influenza complications. For all other contraindications to use of LAIV, see *MMWR* 62(RR-7):1-43, 2013; available at http://www.cdc.gov/mmwr/pdf/rr/rr6207.pdf.

   For children aged 6 months through 8 years:
   - For the 2013-2014 season, administer 2 doses (separated by at least 4 weeks) to children who are receiving influenza vaccine for the first time. Some children in this age group who have been vaccinated previously will also need 2 doses. For additional guidance, follow dosing guidelines in the 2013-2014 ACIP influenza vaccine recommendations, *MMWR* 62(RR-7):1-43, 2013; available at http://www.cdc.gov/mmwr/pdf/rr/rr6207.pdf.
   - For the 2014-2015 season, follow dosing guidelines in the 2014 ACIP influenza vaccine recommendations.

   For persons aged 9 years and older:
   - Administer 1 dose.

9. **Measles, mumps, and rubella (MMR) vaccine. (Minimum age: 12 months for routine vaccination)**
   Routine vaccination:
   - Administer a 2-dose series of MMR vaccine at ages 12 through 15 months and 4 through 6 years. The second dose may be administered before age 4 years, provided at least 4 weeks have elapsed since the first dose.

- Administer 1 dose of MMR vaccine to infants aged 6 through 11 months before departure from the United States for international travel. These children should be revaccinated with 2 doses of MMR vaccine, the first at age 12 through 15 months (12 months if the child remains in an area where disease risk is high), and the second dose at least 4 weeks later.
- Administer 2 doses of MMR vaccine to children aged 12 months and older before departure from the United States for international travel. The first dose should be administered on or after age 12 months and the second dose at least 4 weeks later.

Catch-up vaccination:

- Ensure that all school-aged children and adolescents have had 2 doses of MMR vaccine; the minimum interval between the 2 doses is 4 weeks.

10. Varicella (VAR) vaccine. (Minimum age: 12 months)

Routine vaccination:

- Administer a 2-dose series of VAR vaccine at ages 12 through 15 months and 4 through 6 years. The second dose may be administered before age 4 years, provided at least 3 months have elapsed since the first dose. If the second dose was administered at least 4 weeks after the first dose, it can be accepted as valid.

Catch-up vaccination:

- Ensure that all persons aged 7 through 18 years without evidence of immunity (see *MMWR* 56[RR-4]:1-40, 2007; available at http://www.cdc.gov/mmwr/pdf/rr/rr5604.pdf) have 2 doses of varicella vaccine. For children aged 7 through 12 years, the recommended minimum interval between doses is 3 months (if the second dose was administered at least 4 weeks after the first dose, it can be accepted as valid); for persons aged 13 years and older, the minimum interval between doses is 4 weeks.

11. Hepatitis A (HepA) vaccine. (Minimum age: 12 months)

Routine vaccination:

- Initiate the 2-dose HepA vaccine series at 12 through 23 months; separate the 2 doses by 6 to 18 months.
- Children who have received 1 dose of HepA vaccine before age 24 months should receive a second dose 6 to 18 months after the first dose.
- For any person aged 2 years and older who has not already received the HepA vaccine series, 2 doses of HepA vaccine separated by 6 to 18 months may be administered if immunity against hepatitis A virus infection is desired.

Catch-up vaccination:

- The minimum interval between the two doses is 6 months.

Special populations:

- Administer 2 doses of HepA vaccine at least 6 months apart to previously unvaccinated persons who live in areas where vaccination programs target older children, or who are at increased risk for infection. This includes persons traveling to or working in countries that have high or intermediate endemicity of infection; men having sex with men; users of injection and non-injection illicit drugs; persons who work with hepatitis A virus (HAV)-infected primates or with HAV in a research laboratory; persons with clotting-factor disorders; persons with chronic liver disease; and persons who anticipate close, personal contact (e.g., household or regular babysitting) with an international adoptee during the first 60 days after arrival in the United States from a country with high or intermediate endemicity. The first dose should be administered as soon as the adoption is planned, ideally 2 or more weeks before the arrival of the adoptee.

12. Human papillomavirus (HPV) vaccines. (Minimum age: 9 years for HPV2 [Cervarix] and HPV4 [Gardasil])

Routine vaccination:

- Administer a 3-dose series of HPV vaccine on a schedule of 0, 1-2, and 6 months to all adolescents aged 11 through 12 years. Either HPV4 or HPV2 may be used for females, and only HPV4 may be used for males.
- The vaccine series may be started at age 9 years.
- Administer the second dose 1 to 2 months after the first dose (minimum interval of 4 weeks); administer the third dose 24 weeks after the first dose and 16 weeks after the second dose (minimum interval of 12 weeks).

Catch-up vaccination:

- Administer the vaccine series to females (either HPV2 or HPV4) and males (HPV4) at age 13 through 18 years if not previously vaccinated.
- Use recommended routine dosing intervals (see above) for vaccine series catch-up.

13. Meningococcal conjugate vaccines. (Minimum age: 6 weeks for Hib-MenCY [MenHibrix], 9 months for MenACWY-D [Menactra], 2 months for MenACWY-CRM [Menveo])

Routine vaccination:

- Administer a single dose of Menactra or Menveo vaccine at age 11 through 12 years, with a booster dose at age 16 years.
- Adolescents aged 11 through 18 years with human immunodeficiency virus (HIV) infection should receive a 2-dose primary series of Menactra or Menveo with at least 8 weeks between doses.
- For children aged 2 months through 18 years with high-risk conditions, see below.

Catch-up vaccination:

- Administer Menactra or Menveo vaccine at age 13 through 18 years if not previously vaccinated.
- If the first dose is administered at age 13 through 15 years, a booster dose should be administered at age 16 through 18 years with a minimum interval of at least 8 weeks between doses.
- If the first dose is administered at age 16 years or older, a booster dose is not needed.
- For other catch-up guidance, see the catch-up schedule.

Vaccination of persons with high-risk conditions and other persons at increased risk of disease:

- Children with anatomic or functional asplenia (including sickle cell disease):
  - For children younger than 19 months of age, administer a 4-dose infant series of MenHibrix or Menveo at 2, 4, 6, and 12 through 15 months of age.
  - For children aged 19 through 23 months who have not completed a series of MenHibrix or Menveo, administer 2 primary doses of Menveo at least 3 months apart.
  - For children aged 24 months and older who have not received a complete series of MenHibrix or Menveo or Menactra, administer 2 primary doses of either Menactra or Menveo at least 2 months apart. If Menactra is administered to a child with asplenia (including sickle cell disease), do not administer Menactra until 2 years of age and at least 4 weeks after the completion of all PCV13 doses.
- Children with persistent complement component deficiency:
  - For children younger than 19 months of age, administer a 4-dose infant series of either MenHibrix or Menveo at 2, 4, 6, and 12 through 15 months of age.
  - For children 7 through 23 months who have not initiated vaccination, two options exist depending on age and vaccine brand:
    a. For children who initiate vaccination with Menveo at 7 months through 23 months of age, a 2-dose series should be administered with the second dose after 12 months of age and at least 3 months after the first dose.
    b. For children who initiate vaccination with Menactra at 9 months through 23 months of age, a 2-dose series of Menactra should be administered at least 3 months apart.
    c. For children aged 24 months and older who have not received a complete series of MenHibrix, Menveo, or Menactra, administer 2 primary doses of either Menactra or Menveo at least 2 months apart.

Continued

- For children who travel to or reside in countries in which meningococcal disease is hyperendemic or epidemic, including countries in the African meningitis belt or the Hajj, administer an age appropriate formulation and series of Menactra or Menveo for protection against serogroups A and W meningococcal disease. Prior receipt of MenHibrix is not sufficient for children traveling to the meningitis belt or the Hajj because it does not contain serogroups A or W.
- For children at risk during a community outbreak attributable to a vaccine serogroup, administer or complete an age- and formulation-appropriate series of MenHibrix, Menactra, or Menveo.
- For booster doses among persons with high-risk conditions, refer to *MMWR* 62(RR-02):1-22, 2013; available at http://www.cdc.gov/mmwr/preview/mmwrhtml/rr6202a1.htm.

  Catch-up recommendations for persons with high-risk conditions:
  - If MenHibrix is administered to achieve protection against meningococcal disease, a complete age-appropriate series of MenHibrix should be administered.
  - If the first dose of MenHibrix is given at or after 12 months of age, a total of 2 doses should be given at least 8 weeks apart to ensure protection against serogroups C and Y meningococcal disease.
  - For children who initiate vaccination with Menveo at 7 months through 9 months of age, a 2-dose series should be administered with the second dose after 12 months of age and at least 3 months after the first dose.
  - For other catch-up recommendations for these persons, refer to *MMWR* 62(RR02):1-22, 2013; available at http://www.cdc.gov/mmwr/preview/mmwrhtml/rr6202a1.htm.

    For complete information on use of meningococcal vaccines, including guidance related to vaccination of persons at increased risk of infection, see *MMWR* 62(RR-02):1-22, 2013; available at http://www.cdc.gov/mmwr/pdf/rr/rr6202.pdf.

Table 38-1 Selected Correlates of Protection for Common Childhood Vaccines

Vaccine	Type of Test	Correlate of Protection	Reference(s)
Diphtheria	Toxin neutralization	0.01-0.1 international units (IU)/mL	129-131
Hepatitis A virus	Enzyme-linked immunosorbent assay (ELISA)	10 mIU/mL	132, 133
Hepatitis B virus	ELISA	10 mIU/mL	134
Haemophilus influenzae type b polysaccharides	ELISA	1 μg/mL	135, 136
H. influenzae type b conjugate	ELISA	0.15 μg/mL	137, 138
Influenza virus	Hemagglutination inhibition	1:40 dilution	139
Measles virus	Microneutralization	120 mIU/mL	140, 141
Pneumococcus	ELISA; opsonophagocytosis	0.20-0.35 μg/mL (for children); 1:8 dilution	142-144
Polioviruses	Serum neutralizing	1:4 to 1:8 dilution	145-147
Rotavirus	Serum immunoglobulin A	Not determined	148-152
Rubella virus	Immunoprecipitation	10-15 mIU/mL	153-155
Tetanus	Toxin neutralization	0.1 IU/mL	156
Varicella virus	Serum neutralizing; ELISA	1:64 dilution; 5 IU/mL	157, 158

Modified from Table 2 in Plotkin SA: Correlates of protection induced by vaccination. *Clin Vaccine Immunol* 17:1055-1065, 2010.

Academy's journal *Pediatrics* and in the periodic handbook called the *Red Book*.

OBSTACLES TO NEONATAL VACCINATION

To date, there are many vaccines for infancy and early childhood; however, very few vaccines have been implemented successfully in the neonatal period. A large number of obstacles make it difficult to establish a safe and effective neonatal vaccination program (Box 38-1).

Box 38-1 Obstacles to Safe and Effective Vaccination of Neonates and Young Infants

Safety Concerns

Occult or late presentation of congenital immunodeficiency
Occurrence of sudden infant death syndrome during this period
Presentation of developmental delay and neurologic syndromes during this period
Increased risk of intussusception with gut inflammation at young age
Increased risk of wheezing with provocation due to high-resistance airways
Need for medical workup for sepsis/meningitis when neonates present with fever without localizing symptoms

Immunologic Immaturity

Antibody genes lacking somatic mutations
Poor magnitude of antibody immune responses
Poor quality of antibody immune responses
Poor durability of antibody responses
Cytokine bias in response to infection (low Th1/Th2 ratio)
Low levels of complement
Inability to respond to polysaccharides
Concern for inducing tolerance
Antibody-mediated suppression of humoral responses caused by transplacentally-acquired maternal antibodies
Interference by concomitant exposure to antigens from other infections, environmental antigens, or vaccine antigens

Safety Concerns

The Hippocratic principle *primum non nocere*, first do no harm, is the supreme driving principle in all vaccination programs, but even more so in the development of neonatal vaccines. Many events and factors that occur during the neonatal period can complicate the interpretation of vaccine safety at this age. The population at risk for birth defects is estimated to be about 3% or 4%, and not all of these defects are fully apparent at the time of birth. Many neonates in the United States are discharged from hospitals and birthing centers before 24 hours of age. If a defect was present at birth but not detected until later, it might be falsely linked to a vaccine given to the neonate. Many, if not most, congenital immunodeficiencies do not declare themselves this early in life. In some areas of the world, a high percentage of infants are infected with human immunodeficiency virus (HIV), but this status is not known at the time of birth. Live-virus vaccines and the live *Mycobacterium* bacillus Calmette-Guérin (BCG), although generally effective, are usually contraindicated in immunodeficient individuals. Other types of congenital defects first become apparent during early infancy, a time in which many vaccinations are given. For instance, many neurologic disorders, including seizure disorders and neurodegenerative diseases, manifest in the first few months of life. Many cardiopulmonary disorders, for instance, cyanotic heart disease or cystic fibrosis, do not cause symptoms in the neonatal period. Sudden infant death syndrome (SIDS) also occurs early in life during the target period of vaccination. The cause of this fatal disorder is not well understood; therefore it is very difficult to assess the risk of exacerbation of SIDS by infection or vaccination. A large number of physiologic changes occur during the first few months of life. Young infants possess airways with very small diameters, which exhibit high resistance, especially during airway inflammation. Therefore young infants are prone to wheezing with relatively minor provocation. Infants are obligate nose breathers. Therefore a vaccine that has the potential to cause an increase in nasal secretions leading to nasal obstruction, such as live-attenuated respiratory virus vaccines, can interfere with feeding, which is a significant problem at this age. Also, infants are susceptible to intestinal intussusception during inflammation of the gastrointestinal tract, which complicates approaches such as live-attenuated rotavirus vaccines. However, careful epidemiology studies and experimental trial designs can overcome these obstacles.

There are also medical factors that complicate the evaluation of vaccines in this age group. Infants in the first 2 months of life who exhibit fever without localizing symptoms generally undergo a complete medical workup for sepsis and meningitis. A vaccine that causes even a low rate of fever in this age group will be associated with a large number of expensive and unnecessary medical workups.

Immunologic Immaturity

Neonates are clearly in transition in their immunologic development as they move from a sterile environment enveloped in the placenta, through the birth canal, into a world with vast numbers of environmental and microbial exposures. In general, it is thought that fetal immune systems are regulated in utero to avoid robust innate and adaptive immune responses to self-antigens or to maternal antigens that cross the placenta. Mouse models suggest that fetuses can be tolerized to antigens after in utero exposure, whereas human studies are more limited. Suppressive T-regulatory (Treg) cells in the fetus are generated against noninherited maternal antigens, and these cells establish functional tolerance to foreign antigens present during development in utero. For instance, one study observed Treg cells in the lymph nodes of fetal products of conception at 18 to 22 weeks of gestation that promoted maternal microchimerism (presence of maternal cells in the fetus) in 15 of 18 lymph node samples.[1] Foreign antigens clearly do cross the placenta.[2,3] Some human studies suggest that fetal adaptive immune responses to non–self-antigens are relatively intact.[4-7] Overall, the evidence suggests that the fetal immune system promotes a relatively high level of tolerance, but it is not devoid of functional activity.

After parturition, a rapid transition must be made to deal with new antigens from food, the environment, and commensal bacteria, and to differentiate them from harmful microorganisms. It is likely that this transition takes time and that human neonates still exhibit some features of predisposition to tolerance, associated with persistence of long-lived Treg cells[1] and significant evidence of B-cell tolerance.[8] Theoretical concerns are sometimes raised that exposure to antigens early in life during a phase when the immune milieu exhibits a residual tolerogenic status might result in the infant becoming *less* well able to respond to the antigen rather than achieving immunologic priming for memory.

Neonates tend to make poor immune responses after infection or vaccination in terms of quantity, quality, and durability. The magnitude of antibody responses, as measured by serology, is reduced. The time to peak titer of serum antibodies is often delayed by a month or more compared with the response of older children. The level of function of neonatal antibodies often is low, for example, the neutralizing activity of antiviral antibody responses, suggesting that neonates secrete antibodies that bind but do not kill viruses. The durability of the antibody response to particular microbes made early in life also is poor. Young infants who are demonstrated to be infected with a virus early in life, as evidenced by disease and virus shedding, may seroconvert in the months after infection but then appear to be seronegative the following year. It is likely that this observation suggests a neonatal B-cell response characterized by differentiation of naïve antigen-specific cells to antibody-secreting plasma cells without induction of long-lived plasma cells or significant numbers of memory B cells. The B cells of neonates are markedly predisposed to apoptosis after stimulation, compared with adult cells, because of reduced expression of interleukin-4 (IL-4) receptor and higher levels of gene expression related to pro-apoptotic programs.[9]

Neonatal mice exhibit skewed antibody gene-segment usage compared with adult mice; however, most evidence in human infants suggests that the antibody variable gene repertoire is very similar to that of adults, including microbial-specific B-cell repertoires. The antibody sequences of B cells of infants exhibit mature levels of junctional diversity, including nontemplated and palindromic types of additions at the V-D and D-J gene-segment junctions and the lengths of the antibody variable loops (complementarity-determining regions) are similar to those of adults.[10] The distinguishing molecular difference between adult and infant antibodies is the striking lack of somatic mutations in infant antibody sequences.[10] The use of germline sequences to encode antibodies to microorganisms early in life leads to the generation of low-affinity antibodies.[11] Somatic mutations, which occur in the germinal center during antigen exposure, are the driving molecular force behind antibody affinity maturation and increases in antibody function. It is not clear currently whether the lack of mutations stems from the fact that neonatal B cells are encountering antigen for the first time (as opposed to the secondary responses made by older previously exposed individuals) or whether there are intrinsic B-cell defects in affinity maturation. After stimulation with the CD40 ligand and cytokines (mimicking helper T-cell interaction), human cord blood B cells do upregulate the transcription of genes involved in somatic hypermutation, including activation-induced cytidine deaminase and error-prone DNA polymerases.[12]

There are also factors extrinsic to B cells that affect antibody responses early in life. T-cell responses, although perhaps more robust than B-cell responses early in life, exhibit some altered features compared with adult T cells. In particular, neonatal responses generally appear to be reduced in the magnitude of T-helper 1 (Th1)-type cytokines, with relatively preserved levels of Th2 cytokines, leading to an overall Th2-biased response. The model of Th1 versus Th2 biases in this age group is an oversimplification of very complex and highly regulated responses that are skewed early in life in various ways. Studies in recent years of Th-cell differentiation have revealed further complexity in Th-cell subsets, such as Th17, Th9, and Th22 cells. In the presence of IL-1 and IL-23 in humans, the naïve Th cell expresses retinoic acid–related orphan receptor (ROR)γt and differentiates into a Th17 cell that produces a host of cytokines, including IL-17. These cells appear to contribute protection against extracellular bacteria and fungi, but they also may have potential for autoimmune effects. In the presence of IL-4 and transforming growth factor-β, the Th2 cell can further differentiate into Th9 cells, which produce IL-9 and IL-10. In the presence of tumor necrosis factor-α and IL-6, naïve Th cells can differentiate into Th22 cells that express the aryl hydrocarbon receptor and secrete IL-22. The level of maturity of regulation of such subsets of Th cells in neonates is poorly understood. Recent work suggests that fetal T cells arise from different populations of hematopoietic cells than adult T cells and that the fetal T-cell lineage is biased toward immune tolerance.[13] In addition, professional antigen-presenting cells, such as dendritic cells and macrophages, may exhibit developmental programs that affect the outcome of humoral responses.

The basis for the profile of the neonatal response likely stems not only from relative deficiencies, compared with adults, but also from active suppression or regulation of immune responses. For example, neonates exhibit high numbers of circulating $CD71^+$ red blood cells, which express the enzyme arginase-2, whose activity mediates immunosuppressive properties.[14] These cells appear to afford some cell-mediated protection against unwanted immune cell activation in the intestine during transition to postnatal life but also inhibit active responses to pathogens such as *Listeria monocytogenes*.

There are also extrinsic factors that affect the function of antibody proteins. For instance, complement protein levels are low in neonates, especially terminal elements of the complement cascade. Even if complement-fixing antimicrobial antibodies are induced, they may not be able to induce effective formation of membrane attack complexes in neonates when terminal complement components are in short supply. Complement also is necessary for optimal antigen presentation in many cases.

Infants exhibit a particular deficiency in responding to capsular polysaccharides, such as those of pathogenic bacteria, including *Neisseria meningitidis*, *Haemophilus influenzae*, *Streptococcus pneumoniae*, and others. A functional response to the small repeating units of these carbohydrates is usually not observed until the age of 2 years, although this deficiency has been overcome with conjugate vaccines, discussed later. For a more detailed discussion of fetal and neonatal immunity, see Chapter 4.

Maternal Antibodies

Antibodies from the mother cross the placenta into the fetus, beginning at about 32 weeks, and increasing until term. The transfer is an active process, mediated by a receptor (FcRn) that specifically transports immunoglobulin G (IgG), especially IgG1, but not other immunoglobulin isotypes. In many cases, the IgG titer of antibodies to particular pathogens at birth exceeds those of the mother. If the mother has malaria or HIV infection, the transplacental transfer of specific IgG often is reduced, likely resulting from placental dysfunction. Transfer of IgG is beneficial because the infant effectively becomes passively immunized against all of the pathogens to which the mother had mounted an effective response. Acquisition of these antibodies affords protection against severe disease in many cases, but the antibodies are lost over time. The specific half-life of transferred IgG in older subjects is typically about 3 weeks, but some reports in neonates suggest that maternal antibodies may possess a longer half-life in infants. Passively acquired maternal antibodies may, however, interfere with the response of neonates to infection or immunization, a phenomenon termed antibody-mediated immune suppression.

Interference

In some cases, the suboptimal responses exhibited by neonates may be due to interference caused when multiple exposures, infections, or immunizations occur simultaneously. Combination vaccines have been carefully developed, with an eye toward adding new vaccine antigens in such a way as to maintain effective responses to existing vaccines. However, in some cases, investigators have observed that addition of new antigens can affect the quantitative response to other components of the vaccine. Forcing multiple exposures early in life could lead to interference.[15] It should be remembered that vaccines are not the only exposures because neonates are also exposed to a myriad of naturally acquired infections, food and environmental antigens, and allergens. Vaccine antigens, in fact, represent a very small component of the antigen exposures early in life.

Logistics of Immunization Programs

Immunization programs have to be implemented in the context of an overall public health approach. In many areas of the world, children have the highest rate of access to medical interventions in the newborn period. Investigators interested in global health have often dreamed of a single efficacious vaccination given at birth for all major childhood infections because access to children is highest at birth. However, this goal is not really realistic, given the obstacles outlined earlier. Therefore each country has to develop an approach to vaccinating infants that achieves the highest feasible coverage based on local resources, infrastructure, financial commitments, cold chain, and other practical considerations. The efficacy of vaccines tested in clinical trials can vary widely in different settings and populations. Even if a vaccine has been shown in definitive clinical trials to be efficacious, the *effectiveness* of a vaccine in the field often is determined by practical considerations of cost-benefit, adverse-event profile, and the clinical relevance to the experience of the practitioner and of parents. Although pediatricians in the outpatient setting in the United States generally are strong advocates of proper vaccination, hospital physicians and staff who manage the peripartum period may be less acculturated to routine vaccination of neonates. Administration of multiple vaccines to all newborns before discharge after birth would require an infrastructure and culture that is still not currently present. Parents play a major role in decision making too, and appropriately so. Parents need assurance of the clinical benefit and the safety of any vaccines offered shortly after birth.

VACCINE STRATEGIES FOR PROTECTING NEONATES AGAINST INFECTION

There are four major vaccination strategies for protecting neonates: (1) maternal immunization during pregnancy, (2) passive immunization with antibodies or immune globulins, (3) active immunization of neonates, and (4) immunization of contacts to prevent transmission.

Maternal Immunization

Immunization of mothers during pregnancy is an attractive strategy for several reasons. Pregnant women typically are easy to identify, and in many areas of the world there is a high level of access to prenatal care. The principle of maternal immunization is to induce or boost the levels of antibodies against microorganisms in the mother's serum, causing a quantitative or qualitative enhancement of the IgG isotype antibodies that cross the placenta and circulate in the blood of the fetus. Maternal immunization has been shown to be safe and effective for several diseases, especially tetanus[16-18] and influenza,[18-22] has been tested for RSV,[23] and pertussis. Current recommendations for use of vaccines in women before, during, or after pregnancy are provided by the CDC (http://www.cdc.gov/vaccines/pubs/downloads/f_preg_chart.pdf) and are shown in Table 38-2.

Table 38-2 Vaccines That May Be Used in Mothers Before, During, or After Pregnancy

Vaccine (Type)	Before Pregnancy	During Pregnancy	After Pregnancy
Hepatitis A (inactivated)	Yes, if indicated	Yes, if indicated	Yes, if indicated
Hepatitis B (subunit)	Yes, if indicated	Yes, if indicated	Yes, if indicated
Human papillomavirus (HPV, subunit)	Yes, if indicated, through 26 years of age	Under study	Yes, if indicated, through 26 years of age
Influenza (inactivated)	Yes	Yes	Yes
Influenza (live attenuated)	Yes, if healthy and <50 years of age; avoid conception for 4 weeks	No	Yes, if healthy and <50 years of age; avoid conception for 4 weeks
MMR (live attenuated)	Yes, if indicated; avoid conception for 4 weeks	No	Yes, give immediately postpartum if rubella seronegative
Tdap (toxoid, inactivated)	Yes, if indicated	Yes, vaccinate in each pregnancy preferably between 27 and 36 weeks	Yes, immediately postpartum if not received previously
Td (toxoid)	Yes, if indicated	Yes, if indicated, Tdap preferred	Yes, if indicated
Varicella (live attenuated)	Yes, if indicated; avoid conception for 4 weeks	No	Yes, if indicated, give immediately postpartum if susceptible

Modified from http://www.cdc.gov/vaccines/pubs/downloads/f_preg_chart.pdf.
MMR, Measles-mumps-rubella; *Td,* tetanus-diphtheria; *Tdap,* tetanus–reduced diphtheria–acellular pertussis.

In 1979, the FDA introduced a classification of fetal risks resulting from pharmaceuticals given during pregnancy. Pregnancy category A is applied when adequate and well-controlled studies have failed to demonstrate a risk to the fetus in the first trimester of pregnancy and there is no evidence of risk in later trimesters. Pregnancy category B pertains when animal reproduction studies have failed to demonstrate a risk to the fetus and there are no adequate and well-controlled studies in pregnant women *or* animal studies have shown an adverse effect but adequate and well-controlled studies in pregnant women have failed to demonstrate a risk to the fetus in any trimester. Pregnancy category C is assigned when animal reproduction studies have shown an adverse effect on the fetus and there are no adequate and well-controlled studies in humans but potential benefits may warrant use of the drug in pregnant women despite potential risks. All vaccines that have been licensed by the FDA are categorized as pregnancy category C, except for the quadrivalent human papillomavirus vaccine, which is category B.

Maternal Immunization to Prevent Tetanus, Diphtheria, and Pertussis

In developed countries, tetanus and diphtheria are essentially controlled or eliminated. In the 1970s, there was a worldwide push to deliver tetanus-diphtheria (Td) vaccine to a broad segment of the population by targeting susceptible pregnant women. These campaigns were highly effective in markedly reducing or eliminating tetanus of the mother and infant in some areas. Still, in the 47 poorest countries in Africa and Asia, an estimated 128,250 babies and up to 30,000 mothers died of tetanus in 2004, according to the United Nations Children's Fund.[24] That agency set a goal to deliver 1 million doses of vaccine to mothers and infants in an effort to eliminate the disease in these groups by 2012. The World Health Organization (WHO) estimated that in 2010 (the latest year for which estimates are available), 58,000 newborns died from neonatal tetanus. As of November 2012, 31 countries still had not reached maternal and neonatal tetanus elimination status. There does not seem to be any problem with performance or safety of the vaccine in these groups; the shortfall stems simply from implementation.

Pertussis has been much more difficult to address. Major reductions in numbers of pertussis cases were accomplished by childhood pertussis vaccination through the middle of the 20th century; however, the disease has been rising in incidence for several decades. It is estimated that hundreds of thousands of cases occur in adults in the United States each year, which places infant contacts at risk. Many feel that the durability of solid vaccine-induced immunity may not extend beyond early adolescence, leaving a susceptible adult and older adolescent population.[25-29]

Pregnant mothers can be infected with *Bordetella pertussis* and suffer symptomatic respiratory tract disease, spanning from mild to severe. Surprisingly, there is little evidence in the literature that pregnant women are more susceptible to severe disease than other healthy adults. Also, there is little evidence that infection of pregnant mothers is associated with adverse outcomes for the fetus, such as fetal demise or altered development. Therefore the focus of maternal immunization against pertussis is on preventing severe disease in young infants *after* birth.

Most of the deaths caused by pertussis occur in infants younger than 2 months at a time before routine immunization is initiated. The optimal strategy to protect these young infants is not entirely clear. Immunization of women postpartum could maximize immunity in the mother to prevent the mother from acquiring a new infection and transmitting it to newborns. However, data suggest that mothers are the source of pertussis in less than a quarter of cases.[30] Therefore this strategy may have minimal effect on reducing risk in the first months of life. Immunization in the second or third trimester of pregnancy is of potential benefit to the mother by prevention of disease in her and induces higher levels of antibodies that can be transferred across the placenta. In the first half of the 20th century, pregnant mothers were commonly immunized with whole-cell pertussis vaccine, and it was clear that third trimester vaccination raised the level of antibodies in infants. Efficacy was not studied or proven in a rigorous way, however. There is the suggestion in clinical and epidemiology surveillance studies that maternal immunization reduces the incidence of disease in infants.[31-33] Tetanus–reduced diphtheria–acellular pertussis vaccine (Tdap) was licensed for use in adolescents and adults in the United States in 2005. This vaccine is commonly given to pregnant women without evidence of harm to mothers or fetuses. Recent changes in policies of the ACIP recommend that adolescents and adults should receive a single dose of Tdap (instead of a single dose of Td), if their last dose of Td was greater than 2 years ago (instead of >10 years ago). The American College of Obstetricians and Gynecologists (ACOG) and the AAP recommend that women should receive Tdap before pregnancy if possible. In 2012, the ACIP voted to recommend use of Tdap during every pregnancy. Vaccinating during the third trimester (optimally at weeks 30-32 of pregnancy) provides the highest concentration of maternal antibodies to be transferred to the newborn.[34] If not administered during pregnancy, Tdap should be given immediately postpartum. The issue of pertussis and pertussis immunization strategies for pregnant women and infants is discussed in detail in Chapter 21.

Maternal Immunization to Prevent Influenza

Immunization of pregnant women against influenza is important for the health of both the mother and the infant. The risk of influenza during pregnancy continues to be underappreciated. Seasonal influenza poses a significant risk to the health of pregnant women during annual winter seasonal epidemics.[35,36] Both pregnant women and their infants are at increased risk of morbidity from influenza, and both benefit from maternal immunization. During the 2009 H1N1 pandemic, rates of stillbirth and prematurity were greater in pregnant women with influenza infection.[37] Both infants and pregnant women were at greater risk of hospitalization and severe medical complications from the 2009 pandemic H1N1 infection, including death.[37-40] Both the ACIP and ACOG recommend that all pregnant women be immunized during the influenza season. Vaccination is recommended at any gestational age. The WHO also recommends that all pregnant women should receive the vaccine regardless of trimester. The indicated vaccine is conventional trivalent inactivated vaccine, given by the intramuscular route in the deltoid muscle. Although an intranasal live-attenuated trivalent vaccine is available, that vaccine is not recommended during pregnancy. Immunization during pregnancy has been shown to be safe for both the infant and the mother. Large numbers of pregnant women have been immunized with influenza vaccine; for example, during the 2009 to 2010 influenza season, according to the CDC, 51% of pregnant women in 10 states received the seasonal influenza vaccine.[41]

Pregnant mothers appear to respond well to inactivated influenza virus vaccination in a similar manner to nonpregnant women, achieving elevated antiviral antibody titers in both maternal serum and umbilical cord serum.[20] A careful prospective trial in 158 mother-infant pairs suggested that immunization of pregnant women could delay onset or reduce severity of disease in infants.[42] A 2004 to 2005 randomized study of 340 mothers receiving either inactivated influenza vaccine or the 23-valent pneumococcal polysaccharide vaccine showed that the influenza vaccine reduced proven influenza illness by 63% in infants up to 6 months of age and prevented about a third of all febrile respiratory illnesses in mothers and young infants.[43] This striking result reignited enthusiasm in the maternal immunization research community for testing this strategy more broadly for other respiratory virus infections, such as RSV. Influenza antibody titers in umbilical cord blood of immunized mothers do achieve protective levels; in fact, they can be higher than those of the mother. Higher levels of maternal antiinfluenza antibodies are associated with greater and longer protection of infants.

Maternal Immunization to Prevent Respiratory Syncytial Virus Infection

Respiratory syncytial virus causes hospitalization of infants for wheezing, pneumonia, or apnea, with a peak incidence at about 6 weeks of age. There appears to be some relative sparing of disease in the first weeks of life, possibly associated with maternal antibodies. It is difficult to contemplate inducing immunity in neonates before this age; therefore investigators have investigated maternal immunization against RSV to increase the titer of virus-neutralizing maternal antibodies that cross the placenta. The rationale is that, for every twofold rise in maternal antibodies that could be achieved, infants might be protected for an additional 3 weeks if a conventional IgG antibody half-life of 21 days is observed. A small experimental trial of an RSV subunit protein vaccine has been conducted in pregnant women. The vaccine, an immunoaffinity-purified protein isolated from infected cell culture–designated purified protein-2 (PFP-2), was safe but minimally immunogenic in a small trial.[23] New experimental vaccines for RSV based on the surface fusion (F) protein, which is the protective antigen, are being developed for maternal immunization using various technologies. Structure-based designs for RSV F subunit vaccines, including a stabilized prefusion form of F and a computationally designed epitope vaccine, have been described[44,45] and were enabled by the determination of the structure of prefusion and postfusion F protein at atomic resolution.[46,47] A method for reproducibly isolating aggregates of postfusion F protein expressed in insect cells, termed F nanoparticles, has been developed.[48] This vaccine candidate has been tested in human phase I trials,[49] and maternal immunization studies are planned.

Measles-Mumps-Rubella (MMR) Vaccine During Pregnancy

Women are advised not to receive the MMR vaccine during pregnancy because all components are live viruses. Rubella virus is of particular concern because there is the theoretical possibility of this live-virus vaccine causing congenital rubella syndrome. A number of women have inadvertently received this vaccine while pregnant or soon before conception. The CDC collected data about the outcomes of their births. From 1971 to 1989, 324 infants were born to 321 women who received rubella vaccine while pregnant and continued pregnancy to term, and no cases of congenital rubella syndrome were identified.[50] Given that the risk to the fetus appears to be negligible, a recommendation suggesting termination of pregnancy after inadvertent immunization is not warranted.

Maternal Vaccines in the Setting of Special Risk Factors

The ACIP recommends some other vaccines during pregnancy if particular risk factors are present— specifically, meningococcal and pneumococcal polysaccharide, and hepatitis A and B virus vaccines. If meningococcal conjugate vaccine (MCV4/MenACWY) is indicated, pregnancy should not preclude vaccination. There are two types of licensed pneumococcal vaccines: pneumococcal polysaccharide (PPSV23) and conjugate vaccine (PCV13). The safety of pneumococcal polysaccharide vaccine during the first trimester of pregnancy has not been evaluated formally; however, no adverse consequences have been reported among newborns whose mothers were inadvertently vaccinated during pregnancy. The use of PCV13 has been very limited among women of childbearing age, and the ACIP has not published pregnancy recommendations for PCV13. The ACIP recommends that all persons between the ages of 1 and 18 years should receive the hepatitis A virus (HAV) vaccine, as well as persons of any age who have risk-associated conditions.[51] Pregnancy is not a contraindication to HAV vaccination. Studies reveal no apparent risk for adverse events in the developing fetus when the current vaccine is administered to pregnant women.[51,52] The hepatitis A inactivated vaccine therefore is recommended if another high-risk condition or other indication is present. The ACIP recommends that the hepatitis B virus (HBV) vaccine should be administered to all patients before age 19 years, including unvaccinated pregnant women.[53] Hepatitis B vaccine also is not contraindicated in pregnancy. This inactivated vaccine should be given to pregnant women who are at elevated risk for acquiring HBV infection during pregnancy because they (1) have had more than one sex partner during the previous 6 months, (2) have been evaluated or treated for a sexually transmitted disease, (3) have recent or current injection drug use, or (4) have had a hepatitis B surface antigen (HBsAg)-positive sex partner.

Maternal Vaccines for Group B Streptococci Under Development

Group B streptococci (GBS) are desirable targets for maternal immunization because these bacteria mainly cause disease in infants younger than 3 months, especially early-onset disease in newborns. GBS are a significant cause of infant disease and mortality worldwide. There is no licensed GBS vaccine to date, but vaccine candidates are under development, and several clinical trials suggest that a capsular polysaccharide conjugate vaccine is well tolerated and immunogenic. There are 10 GBS serotypes, but the most likely candidate for a vaccine would be a multivalent conjugate vaccine incorporating capsular polysaccharides from the five most common serotypes. A capsular polysaccharide conjugate vaccine was given to pregnant women in a double-blind, randomized, controlled trial that showed that the vaccine was immunogenic in mothers and caused transplacental transfer of IgG to infants.[54] Additional vaccine studies are active and listed at http://Clinicaltrials.gov.[55]

PASSIVE IMMUNIZATION

Antibodies in the blood of otherwise healthy, previously infected adults can be collected in the form of plasma or serum, which can also be fractionated to isolate polyclonal immune globulins. If the collections are performed from large numbers of randomly selected healthy donors and pooled, then the resulting preparation of gamma globulin will contain an average titer of antibodies to microorganisms that is found in the donor population. Administration of antibodies to naïve recipients to confer temporary humoral immunity is termed passive immunization.

A large number of hyperimmune and conventional immune globulins and a monoclonal antibody have been licensed for use in humans (Table 38-3). Conventional immune globulin is used to treat a number of conditions, including congenital or acquired immunodeficiency, Kawasaki disease, and idiopathic thrombocytopenic purpura, and to provide postexposure prophylaxis for hepatitis A and measles. Donors can be screened by serology to identify subsets of individuals with high functional titers of specific antibodies, enabling polyclonal antibody preparations that are enriched in activity for a specific organism, termed hyperimmune globulin (e.g., immune globulin).[56] A large number of immune globulins have been produced, such as preparations for botulism, hepatitis B, tetanus, cytomegalovirus (CMV), varicella-zoster virus (VZV), rabies virus, and vaccinia virus. Most of these have been used in neonates.

Immunoglobulins are derived from human blood products, so there is the theoretical risk of transmission of adventitious infectious agents. These products are prepared from plasma by a process called Cohn fractionation, which removes most of the potential adventitious agents and purifies the product. Plasma is treated with ethanol in increasing concentrations up to 40%.

Table 38-3 FDA-Approved Products for Passive Immunization and Immunotherapy

Disease	Product	Indication
Infant botulism	Botulism immune globulin (BabyBIG)	Treatment of infant botulism
Cytomegalovirus	CMV immune globulin	Prevention or treatment in immunocompromised
Hepatitis B	Hepatitis B immune globulin	Postexposure prophylaxis
Tetanus	Tetanus immune globulin	Treatment of tetanus infection
Varicella (chickenpox)	Varicella-zoster virus immune globulin	Postexposure prophylaxis in high-risk individuals
Rabies	Rabies immune globulin	Postexposure prophylaxis (administered with rabies vaccine)
Vaccinia (smallpox vaccine)	Vaccinia immune globulin	Treatment of progressive infection
Hepatitis A	Pooled human immune globulin	Prevention of hepatitis A infection
Measles	Pooled human immune globulin	Prevention of measles infection
Congenital/acquired immunodeficiency	Pooled human immune globulin	Treatment of immunodeficiency
ITP/Kawasaki disease	Pooled human immune globulin	Treatment of inflammatory state
Respiratory syncytial virus	Palivizumab (humanized mouse monoclonal antibody)	Prevention of respiratory syncytial virus disease in high-risk infants

CMV, Cytomegalovirus; *FDA*, Food and Drug Administration; *ITP*, idiopathic thrombocytopenia purpura.

The pH is progressively reduced over the course of the fractionation, as is the temperature. Five major fractions are recovered, each containing a specific precipitate. In recent years, preparations have also been treated with a solvent-detergent viral inactivation process that is highly effective.[57]

Respiratory Syncytial Virus Immune Globulin and Monoclonal Antibodies

Respiratory syncytial virus immune globulin was partially effective in preventing hospitalization caused by severe RSV infection[58-60]; however, the intravenous (IV) route and large volumes needed brought challenges for administration. Subsequently, a neutralizing, humanized mouse monoclonal antibody to the RSV fusion protein (palivizumab) was developed and licensed and allowed intramuscular administration. The efficacy of palivizumab was assessed in a randomized, double-blind, placebo-controlled trial (designated the Impact-RSV Study) in high-risk infants, with a 55% reduction in hospitalizations.[61] This antibody is the only monoclonal antibody licensed to date to prevent virus infection. An affinity-matured, second-generation RSV monoclonal antibody (motavizumab) was tested in large clinical trials,[62] but skin events were increased in motavizumab recipients, raising safety concerns, and the development of this antibody has been halted.

Hepatitis B Immune Globulin

This immune globulin for intramuscular administration is used to treat babies born to mothers who test positive for HBsAg (or who have not been screened) with or without hepatitis B early antigen (HBeAg). Infants born to mothers known to be HBsAg positive should receive hepatitis B immune globulin (HBIG) after physiologic stabilization of the infant and preferably within 12 hours of birth. The hepatitis B vaccine series should be initiated simultaneously, if not contraindicated, with the first dose of the vaccine given concurrently with the HBIG but at a different site. Women admitted for delivery who were not screened for HBsAg during the prenatal period should be tested. Although test results are pending, the newborn infant should receive hepatitis B vaccine within 12 hours of birth. If the mother is later found to be HBsAg positive, the infant should receive HBIG as soon as possible and within seven days of birth; however, the efficacy of HBIG administered after 48 hours of age is not known.[63] Testing for HBsAg and anti-HBsAg antibodies is recommended at 12 to 15 months of age for infants who were born to HBsAg-positive mothers and who were immunized and given HBIG at birth. If HBsAg is not detectable and surface antigen–specific antibodies are present, the child is considered protected.[53]

Varicella-Zoster Immune Globulin (VZIG)

The varicella virus vaccine is a live virus, and because the effects of the varicella virus on the fetus are unknown, *pregnant women should not be vaccinated. Therefore passive immunization is an important consideration in exposed unimmunized subjects.* A hyperimmune globulin, VZIG, has been used to protect high-risk individuals after exposure. VZIG treatment is expected to be most effective when it is initiated as soon as possible after exposure, but it may be effective if administered as late as 96 hours after exposure. Treatment after 96 hours is of uncertain value. Small-particle aerosols transmit varicella, so assessing exposure is complex. The CDC has defined what constitutes a "substantial" varicella exposure, with the central concept that direct contact exposure is defined as greater than 1 hour of direct contact with an infectious person while indoors.[64] The onset of varicella in pregnant women from 5 days before to 2 days after delivery is estimated to result in severe varicella infection in about a quarter of those newborn infants, with a high risk of death.[65-67] Although the numbers of treated infants are not adequate to determine a rigorous efficacy, VZIG reduced disease. In the United Kingdom, surveillance studies suggested the proportion of deaths among neonates infected with varicella decreased from 7% to 0% after the onset of routine use of VZIG in this setting.[68] In October 2004, the Massachusetts Public Health Biologic Laboratories, the only U.S.-licensed manufacturer of VZIG, discontinued manufacturing this product. In December 2012, the FDA approved VariZIG, a VZIG preparation (Cangene Corporation, Winnipeg, Canada) for use in the United States for postexposure prophylaxis of varicella. Patient groups recommended by CDC to receive VariZIG[69] include the following:

- Newborn infants whose mothers have signs and symptoms of varicella around the time of delivery (i.e., 5 days before to 2 days after)

- Hospitalized premature infants born at greater than or equal to 28 weeks of gestation who have been exposed to varicella or herpes zoster and whose mothers do not have evidence of immunity to varicella
- Hospitalized premature infants born at less than 28 weeks of gestation or who weigh less than or equal to 1000 g at birth and who have been exposed to varicella or herpes zoster, regardless of their mothers' evidence of immunity to varicella
- Pregnant women without evidence of immunity who have been exposed to varicella or herpes zoster

Cytomegalovirus Immune Globulin (CMV-IVIG)

This preparation is a purified immunoglobulin for IV administration derived from pooled adult human plasma selected for high titers of antibody for CMV.[70] It is generally used for the prophylaxis of CMV disease associated with transplantation of a kidney, lung, liver, pancreas, or heart in older subjects. Only limited information is available about the use of CMV-IVIG in pregnancy or the neonatal period, and more study is needed to more fully evaluate the possible benefits and risks of passive immunization with CMV-IVIG in such situations. In a recent trial, 123 women in whom primary infection occurred at 5 to 26 weeks of gestation were randomized to receive CMV-IVIG or placebo every 4 weeks until 36 weeks of gestation.[71] Congenital infection was documented in 18 of 61 (30%) of the treated women and 27 of 62 (44%) of the controls. This 14% reduction in the infection rate (95% confidence interval [CI], −3% to 31%) was not statistically significant (P = .13), nor were there any significant differences in secondary outcome variables), although the number of adverse obstetric events was greater in the treatment group (13% vs. 2%, P = .06). Two additional randomized controlled trials addressing this question are underway. However, the use of CMV-IVIG to prevent congenital CMV infection is considered experimental at this time.

Botulinum Immune Globulin

Infant botulism is a form of human botulism caused by ingestion of *Clostridium botulinum* spores that colonize and grow in the infant's large intestine, resulting in the secretion of botulinum neurotoxin into the intestine. The toxin can cause flaccid paralysis with respiratory and feeding failure. Botulinum immune globulin is an orphan drug product with high titers of antibodies against botulinum toxin for IV administration that is indicated for the treatment of patients younger than 1 year with infant botulism caused by toxin type A or B. The approach, isolating immune globulin from the plasma of donors immunized with pentavalent (ABCDE) botulinum toxoid, was developed by the California Department of Health Services. Treatment within 3 days of admission to hospital shortened the mean hospital stay of all (type A and type B) infant botulism patients by several weeks, significantly shortened length of intensive care unit stay, duration of mechanical ventilation, and length of tube feedings.[72]

ACTIVE IMMUNIZATION

Immunization of individuals directly to stimulate adaptive immune responses characterized by memory is termed active immunization. This approach is preferred when feasible because long-lasting responses can be induced by brief medical encounters, without further intervention, or in some cases with periodic boosting.

The general approach to developing an effective vaccine starts with an understanding of pathogenesis and correlates of immunity. For instance, tetanus is caused by a toxin secreted by a bacterium, not by the organism itself, so the licensed vaccine was designed to induce antibodies to the toxin rather than the bacterium. Once the fundamentals of the disease are understood through epidemiology studies and animal model experiments, vaccine candidates are developed and tested in preclinical models, usually including small animals such as mice and then nonhuman primates. Human studies are conducted in phases, with increasing numbers of subjects. Phase I trials establish safety (typically in several dozen subjects), phase II trials investigate dose and expanded safety data collection (typically in hundreds of subjects), phase III trials establish efficacy (typically in many thousands of subjects), and phase IV surveillance is sometimes conducted after licensure. There are a large number of strategies for development of vaccines that have been successful to date (Box 38-2).

Box 38-2 Major Types of Vaccines

- Jennerian approach (use of inoculation with a naturally occurring animal pathogen to induce a cross-protective immune response to a human pathogen); e.g., vaccinia virus (the smallpox vaccine), rhesus rotavirus (withdrawn), human-bovine rotavirus reassortant viruses, bacillus Calmette-Guérin (BCG; a vaccine against tuberculosis)
- Live-attenuated viruses
- Naturally occurring avirulent isolates, e.g., the Jeryl Lynn strain of mumps virus
- Cell culture–passaged mutants (with in vitro marker, such as cold-adapted, temperature-sensitive, small plaque, or other phenotype), e.g., rubella virus Wistar Institute RA 27/3 strain, influenza, poliovirus, measles and mumps viruses, varicella virus, rotavirus
- Inactivated (killed or disrupted) virus, e.g., influenza, inactivated poliovirus, hepatitis A virus, rabies virus
- Toxoid, a bacterial toxin whose toxicity has been reduced; e.g., diphtheria and tetanus toxoids
  - Chemical treatment
  - Genetic manipulation of toxin sequence
- Subunit proteins
  - Purified from serum, cell, or egg culture; or recombinant expression systems, such as yeast, e.g., hepatitis B surface antigen, papillomavirus
  - Purified from bacterial culture, *Bordetella pertussis*
- Polysaccharides, e.g., *Haemophilus influenzae* type B, *Streptococcus pneumoniae*, *Neisseria meningitidis*; plain or conjugated to a protein
- Combined vaccines, e.g., MMRV, DTaP/Hib/IPV, HepA/B, and others
- Experimental approaches: vectored vaccines, DNA, peptides, mimotopes, nanoparticle RNA

DTaP, *Diphtheria-tetanus–acellular pertussis;* HepA/B, *hepatitis A/B;* Hib, Haemophilus influenzae *type b;* IPV, *inactivated poliovirus;* MMRV, *measles-mumps-rubella-varicella.*

Jennerian Vaccines

The simplest approach, pioneered by Jenner, uses an animal microorganism to infect humans to induce cross-protective immune responses. This approach was used to develop the smallpox vaccine vaccinia, which was also multiply passaged. BCG is a live mycobacterial strain that is used in many parts of the world as a tuberculosis vaccine during the neonatal period.

In recent years, a modified Jennerian approach has been used in which virus genes from animal viruses are combined with genes from the matching human virus to create chimeric viruses that retain the authentic human protective antigens but incorporate animal genes that perform suboptimally during virus replication, resulting in attenuation. Because these organisms often replicate in the recipients to some degree, they can often induce both T- and B-cell responses and can be very immunogenic. There are two principal ways that the chimeric vaccines are made. If the virus genome is segmented, then the animal virus and the human virus are used to coinfect cells in culture, and viruses with various combinations of gene origins arise, a process termed reassortment. If the genome is nonsegmented, then the viral genomes are cloned by molecular biology techniques to make a complementary DNA (cDNA) copy of each genome. By molecular means, these genomes can be manipulated to make chimeras, point mutations, gene deletions, or gene order shuffling. Once the altered cDNA is made, plasmid DNA is used to transfect mammalian cells and generate a live mutant virus, a process termed "virus rescue." The modified Jennerian approach has been successful using genes from nonhuman primate and bovine rotaviruses by reassortment. Bovine parainfluenza virus type 3 has been tested in infants as young as 2 months,[73] and chimeric experimental vaccines for RSV or human parainfluenza virus type 3 have been developed by rescue from cDNA by using the bovine virus backbone.[74,75]

Attenuation of Live Human Viruses

Live viruses have been attenuated in additional ways. Typically, viruses can be multiply passaged in cell culture, during which attenuated viral variants arise as a consequence of viral polymerase error. Mutation rate (or selection for survival of mutants in culture) can be accelerated by passaging and adapting in cells from a different species (resulting in "host range restriction" mutations), passaging in the presence of chemical mutagens that cause missense mutations in the virus genomes or selecting for an in vitro phenotype, such as cold adaptation, temperature sensitivity, or small plaque phenotype (e.g., the live-attenuated trivalent influenza vaccine). Vaccines for poliovirus, measles, rotavirus, rubella, and others have been derived in this way. In some cases, investigators have isolated naturally attenuated or avirulent virus strains from human subjects that can be used as vaccines with their native sequence. For example, Maurice Hilleman isolated a mumps virus isolate from his daughter, Jeryl Lynn, in the 1960s and developed this strain at Merck as the mumps vaccine. Six experimental live-attenuated vaccine candidates for RSV made by passage and phenotypic selection of plaques have been tested in clinical trials.[76-81] A live-attenuated vaccine candidate for parainfluenza type 3 (the main cause of croup in infants) was developed by multiple passaging in cell culture (designated *cp45*, because it had been cold passaged 45 times in culture) and has been studied in infants and found to be immunogenic.[82] A phase II trial has been conducted with combined experimental vaccines for RSV and for parainfluenza type 3.[83]

Inactivated Vaccines

Growing organisms in culture in the laboratory, followed by inactivation, is a simple approach that has been dramatically successful for some organisms. Organisms can be inactivated by β-propiolactone, formalin, ultraviolet irradiation, and other techniques. The Salk polio vaccine had a dramatic effect on polio epidemiology when implemented. Similar efforts with influenza led to the development of the inactivated trivalent influenza vaccine that is the mainstay of current prevention against influenza disease. Excellent inactivated vaccines also have been developed for hepatitis A and rabies virus. This approach is not without its potential problems, however. If a virulent strain is used to produce the virus stock, inadequate inactivation can lead to iatrogenic disease, such as occurred in the so-called Cutter incident. A number of children immunized with an inactivated poliovirus vaccine preparation containing inadequately inactivated Mahoney poliovirus developed paralytic poliomyelitis.[84] Also, unexpected adverse events have followed immunization with inactivated vaccines. In the 1960s, a formalin-inactivated RSV vaccine induced enhanced disease in children when they were later exposed to natural infection, resulting in several deaths.[85,86] Similarly, an inactivated measles vaccine induced a response known as "atypical" measles that was associated with giant cell pneumonia and an unusual rash on exposure to wild-type virus.

Toxoids

Diseases caused by bacterial toxins (generally exotoxins) have been successfully addressed by the development of toxoids. In some manner, the virulence of the toxin is reduced or removed, while preserving the immunogenicity of the resulting protein. Detoxification can be achieved by treating wild-type toxins with chemicals to alter them or by creating genetic mutant forms of toxin that can be expressed in the laboratory. These vaccines tend to be very immunogenic and effective. Tetanus toxoid and diphtheria toxoid are the prototypes for this approach. Toxoids are also used sometimes as the carrier protein to which polysaccharides are attached in conjugate vaccines.

Subunit Proteins

The success of inactivated virus vaccines led to the idea that nonreplicating materials could induce protective responses as long as the materials contained the protective antigens (usually the target of protective antibodies) in a conformationally intact presentation. Microbial proteins can be partially or highly purified from whole-organism cultures by extraction and purification, or individual proteins can be expressed in a recombinant fashion from DNA copies of the coding region of the protein. Using HBsAg, a highly effective vaccine was originally isolated from the plasma of naturally infected subjects, but now HBsAg is expressed in *Saccharomyces cerevisiae*. The use of nonreplicating proteins has the advantage that the antigen will not likely cause the disease produced by the microbe; however, inoculation with proteins usually does not induce major histocompatibility class I–restricted cytolytic T cells, and the response to subunit proteins is often weak in the absence of adjuvants.

Polysaccharide Vaccines

Encapsulated bacteria are some of the major pathogens of infancy. Immunity to most of these organisms is mediated by type-specific capsular polysaccharide antibodies. Therefore immunization with polysaccharides purified from the organism is immunogenic and protective in older individuals. For instance, there is a 23-valent polysaccharide vaccine for protection against invasive disease caused by *Pneumococcus*. Infants younger than 2 years, however, do not respond to polysaccharides. Investigators found, however, that conjugation of these polysaccharides to carrier proteins enabled young infants to respond to the immunizations with robust antibody responses to the polysaccharides. The intellectual concept was that the carrier protein would facilitate coupled helper T-cell induction by B cells specific for the polysaccharides that process and present peptides from the associated protein, thus inducing T-cell help for the response. Of interest, different carrier proteins exhibit differing performance levels. Now we know that some of these carrier proteins also work in part by stimulating pattern recognition receptors, such as Toll-like receptors (TLRs).

The first conjugate vaccines were aimed at *H. influenzae* type B (Hib), a former major cause of sepsis and meningitis in infancy. The polysaccharide Hib vaccine worked poorly in young children, whereas the conjugate vaccine has virtually eliminated the disease in the United States. Conjugated vaccines have been developed for *S. pneumoniae* that are effective, but a challenge is to incorporate as many type-specific polysaccharides as possible to cover circulating field strains. The frequency of strains varies in different geographic locations. The current pneumococcal conjugate vaccine, designated PCV13 or Prevnar 13 and containing antigens from 13 serotypes, was licensed in 2010 and can be used in children younger than 2 years. This conjugate vaccine has been incorporated into the childhood immunization schedule in the United States for infants aged 2 to 23 months. The European Medicines Agency approved a 10-valent pneumococcal conjugate vaccine (covering serotypes 1, 4, 5, 6B, 7F, 9V, 14, 18C, 19F, and 23F) for use in the European Union in 2009, a vaccine named Synflorix and marketed by GlaxoSmithKline (Philadelphia).

Subjects older than 2 years at high risk of disease can be given the 23-valent polysaccharide vaccines (designated PPV23 or PPSV). A conjugate strategy for a vaccine for older subjects has been developed for four meningococcus subtypes. A quadrivalent meningococcal polysaccharide vaccine (designated MPSV4, Menomune, Sanofi Pasteur, Swiftwater, Pa) was the only meningococcal vaccine available in the United States until a quadrivalent meningococcal conjugate vaccine (designated MCV4, Menactra, Sanofi Pasteur) was approved for young children in 2007. This vaccine is approved now in subjects aged 9 months to 55 years. MenACWY-CRM conjugate vaccine (Menveo, Novartis, New York) was licensed in 2010 and Hib-MenCY-TT conjugate vaccine (MenHibrix, GlaxoSmithKline) in 2012. A new meningococcal vaccine for serogroup B has been developed[87] to cover as many types as possible and was recently licensed in Europe.

Combination Vaccines

The relatively large number of successful childhood vaccines resulted in an inordinate number of needle injections to deliver all recommended vaccines. Therefore a push has been made over the years to combine vaccines to reduce injections, visits, and administration costs. Most childhood vaccines in use today are, in fact, combination vaccines. Various combinations are possible and depend in part on the intellectual property and the clinical experience of the manufacturer. Diphtheria and pertussis toxoids are routinely co-administered with pertussis antigens, but Hib conjugate vaccine and trivalent inactivated poliovirus can be added to this combination. Measles, mumps, rubella, and varicella live-attenuated viruses can be co-administered as a single inoculation. Even live or killed poliovirus and live or killed influenza virus vaccines can be considered to be combination vaccines because they each contain three different viruses representing antigenic variants.

When converting vaccines from a monovalent form to a combined form, manufacturers must demonstrate that the combination does not result in interference that reduces the efficacy of any of the components. For instance, the dose of each of the three live poliovirus vaccine strains was adjusted to achieve optimal immunogenicity for each without interference. Often serologic correlates of protection are followed for the purpose of analyzing whether interference occurs. Interpretation of these serologic tests is definitive only when a solid quantitative correlate of protection has been established, which is often lacking.

Experimental Approaches

A number of additional technologies are being explored for the development of new vaccines. Insertion of heterologous sequences into an attenuated organism is termed using a vectored approach. This approach is common in preclinical development today, using viral vectors such as poxviruses, adenoviruses, alphaviruses, and other organisms. Bacterial vectors such as *Salmonella* and BCG are also under investigation. DNA immunization using plasmid DNAs that encode microbial antigens that are expressed under the control of mammalian promoters is administered by needle injection or by "gene-gun" gold particle–mediated inoculation. Nonviral delivery of self-amplifying RNA encapsulated within nanoparticles to vaccinate against RNA viruses has been tested experimentally. These and other approaches are common in the preclinical arena and in phase I healthy adult trials, but they face significant regulatory hurdles before neonatal vaccine trials could be contemplated.

Adjuvants. Immunologic adjuvants are substances that enhance the magnitude, induction, or durability of antigen-specific immune responses when used in combination with specific vaccine antigens. Typically, adjuvants are not antigenic when administered in the absence of vaccine antigens. Historically, there has only been one type of adjuvant licensed for human use: aluminum salts (alum). These inorganic compounds, such as aluminum hydroxide and aluminum phosphate, mediate aggregation and physical deposition effects for the complexed antigens, but they also have additional effects. These and other adjuvants cause inflammatory responses, sometimes mediated by TLRs and other pattern recognition molecules. This mechanism is a two-edged sword because untoward effects of inflammation may occur, and alum may skew the cytokine responses to antigen toward a Th2-dominated profile.

Vaccines formulated with one of four additional adjuvants have now been licensed in Europe, including MF59 oil-in-water emulsion (Novartis; 1997); AS03 oil-in-water emulsion (GlaxoSmithKline; 2009); virosomes, which are a type of liposome (Berna Biotech, Allschwil/Basel, 2000); and the alum-absorbed TLR4 agonist AS04 (GlaxoSmithKline, 2005); only human papilloma virus (HPV) vaccine adjuvanted with AS04 has been approved for regular use in the United States. Many newer adjuvants are under development; a large number has been tested in adults in the context of experimental HIV vaccine trials. Various classes of new adjuvants include oil-based products, virosomes, and organic molecules, such as squalene. TLR agonists for TLR2, TLR3, TLR5, TLR7/8, and TLR9 are being investigated in an attempt to stimulate the innate immune system in a controlled fashion. Despite the explosion of knowledge of innate immune mechanisms in recent years, incorporation of adjuvants into vaccine development programs is still to some extent an empirical exercise.

Route of Inoculation. Various routes of inoculation are used for immunization, depending on the mechanism of action, convenience, and the technology used. Live-attenuated viruses intended to induce gastrointestinal tract mucosal immunity, such as rotavirus and poliovirus vaccines, are fed orally. Live-attenuated viruses intended to induce respiratory tract mucosal immunity, such as live-attenuated influenza vaccine, can be administered as intranasal drops or spray. Live viruses designed to induce high levels of systemic immunity marked by elevated serum levels of antibody, such as measles, mumps, rubella, and varicella, are given by a parenteral route, such as intramuscular or subcutaneous. This strategy makes sense because the pathogenesis of systemic diseases, such as measles, often involves a viremia during which the circulating viruses are susceptible to serum antibodies. Of interest, the site of intramuscular inoculation (deltoid, gluteus, quadriceps) can affect the immunogenicity of vaccination, so providers should follow the vaccine package insert to most closely replicate the conditions used in the successful efficacy trials.

Timing. The age of vaccine recipients and presence or absence of passively acquired maternal antibodies greatly affects response to vaccination. The antibody response to measles virus vaccine, for instance, is highly susceptible to inhibition by small amounts of maternal antibodies. Administration of vaccine before 12 months of age is associated with diminished responses in infants because of the presence of passively derived maternal antibodies, and administration before 6 months of age is associated with diminished responses, even in infants lacking passively acquired maternal antibodies.[88] Therefore vaccination is optimally initiated after 12 months of life.[88] This plan represents a major problem in developing world environments because the disease often occurs in infants younger than 1 year. It was reasoned that one effective approach might be to deliver an increased dose of attenuated virus in young infants in an attempt to overcome suppression mediated by maternal antibodies. In 1989, a high-titer measles vaccine using the Edmonston-Zagreb strain was recommended by the WHO for use in areas with a high incidence of measles in children younger than 9 months.[89] Three years later, that recommendation was withdrawn because reports from Haiti, Senegal, and Guinea-Bissau suggested an increased incidence of female mortality occurring after administration of the high-titer vaccine.[90,91] The pathogenesis of this process is not fully understood, and the association was not observed in all areas where high-titer vaccine was used. Nevertheless, the high-titer vaccine is no longer used.

Many childhood vaccines are initiated in the first weeks or months of life, including diphtheria-pertussis-tetanus (DPT) and diphtheria-tetanus–acellular pertussis (DTaP), polio, Hib, and hepatitis B vaccines. Multiple doses of these vaccines are often required to achieve sufficient immunogenicity and protection early in life. The interval between doses also may significantly affect the immunogenicity of particular vaccines. Often the optimal interval is not known or cannot be implemented because most countries develop a standard infant vaccine administration schedule. Having done so, the introduction of new vaccines early in life is typically designed to fit the established visit schedule, such as 2, 4, and 6 months of life in the United States.

Birth Dosing. Most infant vaccines are not actually administered during the neonatal period; however, there are a few notable exceptions. BCG is given in many countries of the world shortly after birth, and some also administer a birth dose of oral polio vaccine. A series of hepatitis B inoculations can begin shortly after birth as well. Universal immunization with hepatitis B vaccine is principally aimed at preventing sexually transmitted or bloodborne disease later in life; however, initiating the series near the time of birth can contribute to the interruption of mother-child transmission in the setting of maternal infection. If a mother is known to be infected, a combination of HBIG and hepatitis B vaccine is administered at the time of birth.

SPECIFIC VACCINES FOR INFANTS

Bacillus Calmette-Guérin

This organism is a live attenuated *Mycobacterium bovis* vaccine. It is given soon after birth in most countries in sub-Saharan Africa. It is estimated that approximately three quarters of the global birth cohort is immunized near the time of birth with this vaccine. It is not routinely used in the United States. Various substrains and preparations are used in different countries, and the efficacy of the vaccine against infection is questionable. However, there is a consensus that vaccination reduces the most severe forms of tuberculosis, disseminated processes marked by miliary disease or tuberculous meningitis, which among otherwise healthy individuals most commonly occur in children younger than 2 to 4 years. There are a large number of studies whose numbers conflict; however, meta-analysis suggests that vaccination prevents about 75% of miliary disease and tuberculous meningitis.[92,93] In contrast, it is not clear that BCG affects the rate of pulmonary tuberculosis disease.

The vaccine causes a significant local inflammatory reaction in many cases but is safe in immunocompetent children. It is estimated that fewer than 5 in 1 million healthy children develop disseminated disease with BCG,[94] and many of these children prove to have congenital immunodeficiencies. In contrast, a special concern with this live vaccine is that the geographic areas in which it is most used also are areas where HIV infection is especially common and often undiagnosed. As a consequence, universal vaccination of infants results in inoculation of a significant number of infants who will develop HIV infection and acquired immunodeficiency syndrome. The risk of disseminated BCG infection and disease is several–100-fold increased in infants with HIV infection (estimated incidence, 401-1300/100,000).[81] The WHO has now made HIV infection in infants a full contraindication to BCG vaccination.[95]

Diphtheria

Corynebacterium diphtheriae is an aerobic gram-positive bacterium that secretes a toxin that inactivates human elongation factor eEF-2, thus inhibiting translation during protein synthesis by human cells. The site of infection, generally the throat, becomes sore and swollen. The toxin can cause damage to the myelin sheaths in the central and peripheral nervous system leading to loss of motor control or sensation. Immunization with diphtheria toxoid has been in widespread use since the 1930s; the vaccine is one of the safest in use. The toxoid can be manufactured from diphtheria toxin treated with formalin to inactivate the toxicity but maintain immunogenicity, and it is administered as part of the DPT vaccine beginning at about 2 months. Pertussis toxin (PT) and diphtheria toxin (DT) also have been detoxified genetically by introduction of point mutations that cause a loss of enzymatic activity but retention of binding activity. One mutant DT protein, designated CRM_{197}, which is a toxoid with a single amino acid mutation at the enzymatic active site, is the protein carrier for a licensed *H. influenzae* type B vaccine.

Pertussis

B. pertussis is a gram-negative coccobacillus that causes an acute respiratory illness with multiple protracted phases. The organism secretes a number of toxins that affect respiratory tract epithelial cells and also some toxins that have systemic effects, such as the promotion of lymphocytosis. The disease is most severe in the youngest infants[96]; however, routine vaccination typically does not begin until age 6 to 8 weeks. The need for inducing herd immunity to reduce disease in the contacts of infants through immunizing healthy adults, adolescents, and pregnant mothers was discussed earlier. There are two principal types of pertussis vaccines: inactivated organisms ("whole-cell," often abbreviated P or wP) and a formulation that uses antigen fragments derived from the organism ("acellular," often abbreviated aP). Both vaccines are immunogenic and protective, but the acellular vaccine causes about a 10-fold lower rate of side effects such as fever or injection-site pain and erythema. Most developed countries use acellular pertussis vaccine, but many countries continue to use the whole-cell vaccine because it is cheaper and equally efficacious. The WHO Expanded Program on Immunization (EPI) uses the whole-cell vaccine in its vaccination efforts. More recently, the durability of immunity induced by aP vaccine has been called into question, and current research is focusing on mechanisms underlying better durability of response after whole-cell vaccine.[97,98]

It seems to be intuitive that if the most severe disease caused by pertussis occurs in the first months of life, then adding a dose of vaccine near the time of birth might be effective in reducing disease early in life, and indeed this approach has been investigated recently in three relatively small studies of neonatal acellular pertussis vaccination in the United States and Europe.[99-101] Although the protocols and vaccines differed somewhat, it is not clear that adding a birth dose of acellular pertussis vaccine increases immunity to pertussis without interfering with other vaccine responses or the long-term immunogenicity of pertussis vaccine. An Italian study showed that a birth dose of aP vaccine, followed by the standard Italian schedule for DTaP vaccination at 3, 5, and 11 months, resulted in earlier antibody responses but lower PT IgG levels at 7 to 8 months of age.[101] A U.S. trial studied DTaP administered at birth plus the conventional vaccination schedule at 2, 4, and 6 months. Pertussis antibody levels were similar at 6 months of age in the two groups, but 7-month levels were significantly lower in the group vaccinated at birth, an effect that was still noted at 18 months of age.[99] A German study of aP vaccine at birth revealed induction of a higher response to pertussis antigens at 3 months of age compared with control subjects and equivalent pertussis antibody titers at 8 months of age, with or without a birth dose.[100] Previous trials with whole-cell pertussis vaccine in this age group also generated data that raised the question of whether inhibition of response is caused by an early dose. More study is needed in this area. Pertussis immunization is reviewed in detail in Chapter 21.

Tetanus

Clostridium tetani, the bacterial cause of tetanus, enters through open wounds from environmental sources and produces a toxin that causes prolonged spasms and tetani. The tetanus toxoid vaccine was developed in 1926. The vaccine is a solution of formaldehyde-deactivated toxin isolated from the bacterium. It also is one of the safest vaccines in use and is perhaps the most immunogenic vaccine in use in children. Immunization of infants is routinely initiated at 2 months of age.

Tetanus neonatorum (neonatal tetanus) is caused by contamination of the stump of the umbilical cord. The symptoms of the disease often begin in the first 2 weeks of life, well before routine vaccination is initiated at 2 months, and the disease is often fatal. Maternal immunization and clean treatment of the umbilical cord stump are the best approaches to prevention of this disease.

Tetanus of mothers can occur during pregnancy after wound contamination. Most cases of obstetric tetanus occur in the puerperal or postpartum period; however, these cases often follow complicated deliveries or surgical or spontaneous abortions.[102]

Poliovirus

There are two types of poliovirus vaccines in use. The first is a trivalent live-attenuated vaccine developed by Albert Sabin in the 1950s and licensed in 1961, containing attenuated poliovirus, types I, II, and III, grown in monkey kidney cell tissue culture. This vaccine is administered orally, replicates in the intestine, but does not invade neurons; thus it induces long-lasting intestinal and humoral immunity. Shedding of vaccine viruses in the stool results in transmission of vaccine viruses to close contacts, which has both benefits and risks. The benefit is that many naïve contacts who were not vaccinated themselves become inoculated and immune, thus achieving a high level of herd immunity. For this reason, the live vaccine is preferred in most large-scale eradication efforts in areas where disease still occurs.

Attenuated polioviruses do mutate during replication, however, and lose aspects of attenuation. Rarely (about one case per million doses), these partial revertant viruses cause vaccine-associated paralytic poliomyelitis. The last case of wild-type poliovirus disease acquired in the United States occurred in 1979. For this reason, the United States discontinued use of the live vaccine in 2000. Live poliovirus vaccine is still used in many parts of the world, with many countries administering a dose to neonates at the same time BCG vaccine is given. The aim of the global polio eradication program is to cease use of this vaccine once wild-type poliovirus has been eradicated, with the goal of achieving this during the current decade (see http://www.polioeradication.org/Resourcelibrary/Strategyandwork.aspx). The live vaccine is contraindicated in pregnant women and subjects with primary immunodeficiency, especially common variable immunodeficiency and agammaglobulinemia. Oral poliovirus vaccine has been given to infants and children with HIV infection without adverse effects, although shedding of vaccine virus in stool may be prolonged in these subjects. The live vaccine is typically used in HIV-infected children in resource-limited settings. Children with symptomatic HIV infection should receive inactivated vaccine.

The inactivated polio vaccine (IPV) is a killed virus preparation, first developed by Salk and licensed in 1955. Killed vaccine induces principally humoral immunity but still exhibits excellent efficacy against disease. IPV does not have the benefit of causing herd immunity but also does not transmit virus to contacts and does not cause vaccine-associated paralysis. The enhanced-potency IPV vaccine that is in current use has been in use since 1998. It is a component of some combination vaccine formulations.

Varicella-Zoster Virus

Varicella-zoster virus is spread by the respiratory route by small-particle aerosol and is one of the most infectious agents that affect humans. Before implementation of vaccination, infection was universal in childhood, consisting of a febrile syndrome with vesicular rash. The disease, although often relatively mild, was sometimes complicated by pneumonia, central nervous system effects, including encephalitis; secondary infection, such as bacterial cellulitis or fasciitis; and hemorrhagic conditions. Varicella during pregnancy can have adverse consequences for the fetus and infant of a nonimmune mother, including congenital varicella syndrome. It has been estimated that several dozen cases of this syndrome occurred each year before universal immunization. There was close consideration for many years whether universal vaccination was warranted in the United States because there were only about 100 varicella-associated deaths per year, and it was expected that the vaccine strain would persist, dormant in the sensory-nerve ganglia, similar to what occurs with wild-type virus. Further, the durability of protection was not known. Because varicella disease is often more severe in older subjects, concern was raised about the possibility of waning immunity during adulthood leading to more severe disease. Nevertheless, based on an extended experience in Japan and excellent safety and efficacy data, the virus was licensed for universal immunization in the United States in 1995.[103]

This vaccine contains the Oka strain of live-attenuated VZV. The Oka strain was isolated in Japan in the early 1970s from vesicular fluid in a healthy child who had natural varicella and was attenuated through sequential propagation in cell monolayer cultures in the laboratory.[104] The virus in the Oka/Merck vaccine in use in the United States was further passaged in MRC-5 human diploid cell cultures for a total of 31 passages. The combination measles-mumps-rubella-varicella (MMRV) vaccine was licensed in 2005 on the basis of noninferiority of immunogenicity of MMRV compared with MMR and varicella vaccine given at different sites.[105] The ACIP recommends the use of either MMRV vaccine or the separate MMR and varicella vaccines for children at 12 to 15 months of age and expressed a preference for the MMRV vaccine for the second dose, given at 4 to 6 years of age.

Measles Virus Vaccines

The current measles vaccine is a live-attenuated strain given subcutaneously. There are numerous strains of attenuated virus that have been developed, and the strains used in the vaccine have varied between countries and over the years in the United States. The live-attenuated Edmonston B strain was licensed in 1963 and used until 1975. A further-attenuated vaccine, called the Schwarz strain, was introduced in 1965 and used for a number of years. Finally, a live, further-attenuated preparation of the Enders-Edmonston virus strain was developed and licensed in 1968 (designated the "Moraten" strain because it was more attenuated). This is the only measles virus vaccine currently used in the United States. The vaccine is highly immunogenic in seronegative subjects. Maternal antibodies inhibit vaccine immunogenicity in the first year of life. Therefore vaccination is delayed until 12 to 15 months of age in the United States and other countries of the developed world.

Mumps Virus Vaccine

Mumps virus causes a febrile illness most commonly associated with parotitis but also sometimes more severe conditions, including aseptic meningitis. Pregnant women who contract mumps infection during the first trimester of pregnancy suffer an increased risk for fetal death,[106] but pregnancies not resulting in fetal demise are not associated with congenital malformations.[107] In the early 1960s, an inactivated vaccine was used, but live-attenuated virus has been used exclusively since 1978. The current vaccine strain has an interesting history. The noted virologist Maurice Hilleman isolated the virus from the throat of his daughter, Jeryl Lynn, and developed it as the vaccine strain. Later studies revealed the vaccine strain is actually a mixture of two strains that have differing genetics and in vitro growth characteristics.[108] The vaccine is typically given as a component of MMR or MMRV vaccine at 12 to 15 months of age. The incidence of mumps in the United States has been remarkably reduced by universal vaccination since the 1960s, especially notable after the widespread use of a second dose of mumps vaccine among U.S. schoolchildren began in 1990. Recent outbreaks in the United States, however, raise the question of whether a new strain or strategy is needed.[109]

Rubella Virus Vaccine

Rubella virus is a member of the *Togaviridae* family that is spread by respiratory droplets, causing a mild infection with viremia. The rubella virus vaccine is a live-attenuated virus first licensed in 1969. It is given subcutaneously, now usually as a component of MMR or MMRV vaccine, beginning between 12 and 15 months of age. The live rubella virus vaccine currently distributed in the United States, prepared using the RA 27/3 strain grown in human diploid cell culture, was licensed in the United States in 1979. Several strains used previously, including the HPV-77 and Cendehill strains, induced more adverse events and less durable immunity.

The main goal of rubella immunization is prevention of congenital rubella syndrome. There are several approaches that have been used to achieve immunity in women of childbearing age. For many years in the United Kingdom, girls were inoculated against rubella in their early teens because the childhood disease in boys and girls is typically mild, and the focus was on prevention of congenital rubella syndrome. In the United States, an alternate strategy was used, that of immunizing all children in an effort to reduce circulation of the virus in the population and thus the risk of exposure of pregnant women to children with virus shedding. Both strategies showed some effectiveness, but universal immunization proved more effective. Rubella and congenital rubella syndrome have been eliminated in the United States because of high vaccine coverage and high rates of immunity in the population.[110]

Rubella vaccine has long been incorporated into the MMR or MMRV combination vaccines for universal immunization of both boys and girls starting at 12 to 15 months, followed by a booster dose at school entry. The WHO also recommends that countries undertaking measles elimination should also take the opportunity to eliminate rubella through the use of measles-rubella (MR) or MMR vaccine in their childhood immunization programs.

Hepatitis B Vaccines

Hepatitis B virus causes a potentially life-threatening liver disease that in many cases becomes chronic. HBV is transmitted between people by contact with blood or other body fluids. Children typically acquire hepatitis B infection in one of three ways: (1) perinatal transmission from an infected mother at birth, (2) early childhood infections through close interpersonal contact with infected household contacts, or (3) blood transfusion. Hepatitis B vaccines have been available since 1982. The strategy in the United States initially was to target vaccine to health care workers and patients at high risk; however, that strategy was not adequately effective because of poor compliance. Currently, the strategy is that all infants should receive the hepatitis B vaccine. This approach has several benefits. First, universal vaccination typically achieves higher coverage of those later at risk than targeted programs. Second, initiation of immunization near the time of birth interrupts vertical transmission from mother to child. In areas where mother-to-infant spread of hepatitis is common, the first dose of vaccine should be given within 24 hours of birth. When it is known that a mother is actively infected at the time of birth, the baby is treated with both HBIG and vaccine. The original vaccine was prepared from the plasma of patients infected with hepatitis B, but now the protective antigen, HBsAg, is produced in a recombinant form in yeast.

Apart from the direct metabolic effects of liver dysfunction, chronic infection with HBV also is associated with liver cancer. Therefore the hepatitis vaccine was the first licensed vaccine to prevent cancer.

Hepatitis A Vaccines

Hepatitis A virus is transmitted by the fecal-oral route and causes acute liver disease. Transmission is relatively common in daycare settings. This inactivated vaccine is recommended for all children, starting at 1 year of age. Two single-antigen vaccines are licensed in the United States, HAVRIX (GlaxoSmithKline) and VAQTA (Merck, Whitehouse Station, NJ,), and one hepatitis A vaccine combined with hepatitis B vaccine, Twinrix (GlaxoSmithKline). The vaccine is given as a two-dose series.

Influenza Virus Vaccine

Influenza virus is a respiratory virus spread by large-particle aerosol and fomites. This orthomyxovirus circulates in humans in two major types (A and B), with two distinct A subtypes currently causing disease in humans, designated H1N1 and H3N2. Therefore current seasonal influenza vaccines are trivalent or quadrivalent, including A/H1N1, A/H3N2, and one or two B antigens. The virus uses an RNA-dependent RNA polymerase to replicate that is error prone, and each year, point mutations occur in the major antigenic proteins hemagglutinin and neuraminidase, a process called antigenic drift. This constant variation in circulating strains requires that new antigens be considered for incorporation into influenza vaccines on an annual basis. Periodically, the segmented genome of this RNA virus reassorts (mixes segments genetically) with a heterologous influenza strain (typically of animal origin), causing a complete change in the hemagglutinin and/or neuraminidase, a process termed antigenic shift. When these shifts occur with a virus that replicates well and transmits well in humans, then pandemics occur. Pandemics are declared by the WHO when a new influenza virus subtype emerges that infects humans, causing serious illness, and the virus spreads easily among humans in more than one world region. Major worldwide pandemics occurred in 1918 (H1N1), 1957 (H2N2), 1968 (H3N2), and most recently in 2009 (novel H1N1).

Two types of influenza vaccines are currently licensed. The first is an inactivated preparation prepared by inactivating wild-type viruses prepared in eggs or cell culture. The effectiveness of inactivated trivalent vaccines is not entirely clear but, in general, is estimated by most experts to be about 70%.[111] The efficacy varies year-to-year based on the accuracy of the match of the prepared vaccine strain antigens (chosen based on prior-year data) and the eventual circulating antigens of the current year. The vaccine is most effective against severe disease and hospitalization but probably also reduces the absolute number of infections. The virus for production of vaccine antigens has been produced for decades in embryonated hen eggs, which limits production to a degree; however, in 2012, the FDA approved a mammalian cell culture–based vaccine for seasonal influenza (Flucelvax; Novartis).

Seasonal influenza vaccines are indicated for pregnant women of any gestational age and children as young as 6 months of age. Although the vaccine is not licensed for use in neonates, young infants and newborns can benefit greatly from a comprehensive influenza vaccination program if all of the intimate contacts of the infant, such as household contacts and caregivers, can be immunized, achieving a herd immunity effect. Some inactivated influenza vaccines still contain a preservative related to mercury, called thimerosal. Concern was raised in the past that thimerosal might be causally related to developmental disorders. In 2004, the Institute of Medicine published a comprehensive review of the question and concluded that there is no evidence of such a relationship.[112] Thimerosal-free inactivated influenza vaccine is available now, however.

The second type of influenza vaccine is a trivalent live-attenuated virus suspension that is delivered by nasal spray device. This approach was initially developed in 1960 but took several decades to bring to licensure. The attenuating genes and mutations have been defined, enabling scientists to coinfect new wild-type antigenic variants (drifted strains) with the attenuated strains, in the laboratory. Selection methods have been developed to isolate new strains that arise from reassortment of the segmented genomes, such that the new vaccine strains possess the new surface proteins for immunogenicity but also the established virus genes encoding the internal attenuating virus proteins. New vaccines need to be prepared each year to address antigenic drift. Live-attenuated vaccine has been shown to be highly efficacious, leading to its licensure in 2003.[113,114] Initially, the vaccine was licensed for persons 5 to 49 years of age. In 2007, the FDA approved an expanded label to include children 2 to 5 years of age. A comparative trial of inactivated vaccine and live-attenuated vaccine in children 6 to 59 months of age showed that 54.9% fewer cases of cultured-confirmed influenza occurred in the group that received live-attenuated vaccine than in the group that received inactivated vaccine.[115] Respiratory tract infection with wild-type influenza virus can cause wheezing. Current studies are investigating whether or not there will be a minor association of live-attenuated virus vaccination and wheezing. If safe, this vaccine would benefit younger infants who suffer a high burden of serious disease caused by influenza.

Streptococcus pneumoniae Vaccines

S. pneumoniae is a gram-positive encapsulated organism that causes invasive diseases in infants and young children, including meningitis, bacteremia and sepsis, and pneumonia. Disease is caused by dozens of different types, which are based on the capsular polysaccharide. Immunity is mediated by type-specific antibodies that bind the polysaccharides. Two types of vaccines are available to prevent pneumococcal disease (polysaccharide and conjugate vaccines), but only the conjugate vaccine is used in infants. The polysaccharide vaccine was developed first, with 14-valent vaccine in 1977 and 23-valent vaccine in 1983. Long chains of capsular polysaccharides are collected from inactivated bacteria. Polysaccharide vaccine is indicated for children and adults at high risk, but the vaccine is not effective in children younger than 2 years of age. The safety of the vaccine for pregnant women has not been studied carefully; however, adverse consequences have not been reported in newborns whose mothers were vaccinated with pneumococcal polysaccharide vaccine during pregnancy.

A conjugate vaccine (PCV7) was developed that showed a high level of safety and efficacy against invasive disease,[116] and it was licensed in 2000. The 7 serotypes of *S. pneumoniae* that were included in that first conjugate vaccine (designated types 4, 6B, 9V, 14, 18C, 19F, and 23F) were chosen because they were the strains that most commonly cause serious invasive disease in children in the United States. In February 2010, a new 13-valent product was licensed—PCV13 (Prevnar 13 or PCV13, Pfizer, New York), which added 6 new serotypes (1, 3, 5, 6A, 7F, and 19A [which causes the most common invasive pneumococcal disease in young children]). The combined 13 serotypes in PCV13 account for the majority of invasive disease in the United States. The ACIP recommended in 2010 that providers switch to using PCV13 for routine vaccination of children. All infants should be given a primary series of PCV13 at ages 2, 4, and 6 months, with a booster at age 12 to 15 months.

Rotavirus Vaccines

Rotavirus is the most common cause of dehydrating diarrhea in infants throughout the world. The infection, which is acute and can be treated by rehydration, causes a large number of hospitalizations in the United States and deaths in developing countries. Of interest, rotavirus infection in healthy full-term neonates often is asymptomatic or results in only mild disease, suggesting a possible short-lived protective effect from passively transferred maternal antibodies.[117]

Ongoing worldwide surveillance has revealed a wide diversity of strains causing disease, but it is clear that four or five types are the most common causes of severe disease. Scientists at the National Institutes of Health developed a tetravalent live-attenuated vaccine based on a modified Jennerian approach. One of the vaccine components was a rhesus monkey rotavirus (RRV), and the other strains were made by reassorting the genes that determine type with RRV to generate three additional strains. This vaccine showed efficacy against severe disease and was licensed in 1998.[118] The vaccine was recommended for universal childhood vaccination at ages 2, 4, and 6 months[119]; however, it was withdrawn within a year[120] because of a temporal association with intussusception.[121] There is a sense that the age of immunization may be critical for association with intussusception, with older infants being more susceptible. This rhesus rotavirus tetravalent vaccine has also been tested in neonates, with a 0-, 2-, 4-month three-dose schedule, where it did not cause fever or other serious adverse events.[122] It appeared to induce rotavirus antibodies adequately in this setting, although with lower magnitude and kinetics than in infants, starting at 2 months of age. This vaccine is not under further development, however.

Subsequently, two similar vaccines were developed that appear to be safe and immunogenic. The first, another modified Jennerian-approach vaccine, a pentavalent human-bovine reassortant rotavirus vaccine, RotaTeq, was licensed in the United States in 2006. It is a live, oral

vaccine that contains five reassortant rotaviruses developed from human and bovine parent rotavirus strains.[123] The parental bovine virus strain, Wistar Calf 3 (WC3), was isolated in 1981 from a calf with diarrhea in Pennsylvania, and then reassortants were made. The Rotavirus Efficacy and Safety Trial (REST) studied the vaccine in nearly 70,000 infants and found a high level of safety and efficacy against severe disease.[124] This vaccine is administered in a three-dose schedule at 2, 4, and 6 months of age.

A third live-attenuated rotavirus vaccine, Rotarix, was licensed in the United States in 2008 for oral administration and is based on a single attenuated human strain. Five phase III clinical trials were conducted worldwide to assess the safety and efficacy of the monovalent vaccine in support of United States licensure. The biologic license application included data from nearly 75,000 infants[125] and showed safety and efficacy against severe disease using a two-dose schedule, beginning at 2 months of age. The use of this vaccine was temporarily suspended by the FDA for several months during 2010 after it was found that the vaccine contained porcine circovirus type-1 (PCV-1). However, PCV-1 is commonly found in pigs and pork products and is not known to cause illness in humans or animals. Therefore use of Rotarix was resumed in May 2010.

Current recommendations are that rotavirus vaccines be used for universal immunization during infancy, with care to keep the initiation of the two- or three-dose series at a young age. The ACIP also recommends immunization of premature infants, unless they are still hospitalized (to avoid nosocomial transmission to other vulnerable patients in the hospital).

Haemophilus influenzae Type B (Hib) Vaccine

H. influenzae was a major cause of serious invasive bacterial disease before institution of vaccine programs, and there are still many areas of the world where disease occurs because vaccine is not available. The principal life-threatening diseases are meningitis; bacteremia with sepsis; buccal, preseptal, and orbital cellulitis; and epiglottitis. Immunity to the disease is conferred by antipolysaccharide polyribosylribitol phosphate (PRP) antibodies directed to the capsular polysaccharide. A purified polysaccharide vaccine was licensed in 1985; however, it was not effective in children younger than about 18 months because of their inability to mount robust antibody responses to polysaccharides. The vaccine was only marketed for 3 years. Subsequently, Hib polysaccharide-protein conjugate vaccines were developed that are effective in young infants.

The Hib polysaccharide has been successfully conjugated to several proteins: the meningococcal group B outer membrane protein complex (vaccine designated PRP-OMPC), tetanospasmin (toxoid of the *Clostridium tetani* neurotoxin, vaccine designated PRP-T), or the mutant diphtheria protein (CRM_{197}, vaccine designated HbOC). The vaccines all exhibit a high level of safety and immunogenicity. Hib conjugate vaccine is expensive to manufacture, limiting worldwide implementation, and occasional supply problems have limited full use in the developed world. Nevertheless, the vaccine has virtually eliminated the disease in countries where universal vaccination is used. Furthermore, it has been observed that widespread immunization reduces not only disease but also nasal carriage, resulting in extended benefits resulting from herd immunity and lack of transmission to even those not vaccinated.

Neisseria meningitidis Vaccines

N. meningitidis is also a significant cause of invasive bacterial disease in childhood, causing sepsis and meningitis. Again, antibodies to the capsular polysaccharide mediate protection against invasive disease. The first meningococcal vaccine was a monovalent polysaccharide vaccine first used in the early 1970s. A quadrivalent polysaccharide vaccine has been licensed since 1981, which protects against four subtypes of meningococcus: A, C, Y, and W-135. Children younger than 2 years of age do not mount an adequate response to the polysaccharide, so this vaccine is used only in older children. A tetravalent meningococcal conjugate vaccine, also containing the A, C, Y, and W-135 subtypes, was developed and was licensed in the United States in 2005. The conjugate induces more durable immunity in vaccinees. Currently, it is licensed for use in persons 9 months to 55 years of age. In 2013, the European Commission licensed a four-component protein-based meningococcal B vaccine (incorporating NHBA, NadA, fHbp, and PorA P1.4 proteins) to prevent meningitis and septicemia (Bexsero, Novartis).

PREMATURE INFANTS

Premature infants are at special risk for many infectious diseases for several reasons. First, if birth occurs before about 32 weeks of gestation, very little maternal antibody is transferred to the baby before birth. Second, the physiology of the airways, gastrointestinal tract, and other organ systems is not fully mature, and severe disease is more common on that basis. Third, premature infants are even more immature immunologically than term infants, who themselves mount immune responses to infection that are less robust than those of older children and adults. Therefore premature infants are an especially vulnerable population who should be the focus of high compliance with vaccination recommendations. Studies reveal, however, that immunizations are not being given in a timely manner to many of these infants.[126]

There are specific data on the use of a number of licensed vaccines in premature infants, especially for hepatitis B vaccine. The response of infants weighing less than 2000 g to this vaccine is lower than that of term infants[127]; however, there may be benefit to early vaccination. Current guidelines recommend that the initial vaccine dose be given as usual, but if the infant weighs less than 2000 g on initial immunization, this dose is not considered part of the routine three-dose vaccination series.

Rotavirus

Rotavirus vaccine should be given to premature infants if the recommended schedule can be accomplished in a timely manner. In the phase III trials of RotaTeq, vaccine or a placebo was administered to 2070 preterm infants (25-36 weeks of gestational age; median, 34 weeks).[123] The ACIP considers the benefits of rotavirus vaccine vaccination of premature infants to outweigh the theoretical risks of horizontal transmission by shedding. Given this recommendation, premature infants should be immunized with rotavirus vaccine upon discharge from the neonatal intensive care unit if between 6 and 12 weeks of chronologic age.

Influenza

Vaccinating all household contacts and caregivers of premature infants against seasonal influenza is indicated, as discussed previously. Neonates are not eligible for vaccination themselves.

Tetanus-Reduced–Diphtheria–Acellular Pertussis (Tdap) Vaccine

Again, all close contacts should be up to date on these immunizations, as discussed previously. In 2012, maternal Tdap vaccine was universally recommended in the United Kingdom and United States to protect infants against pertussis. Mothers should be offered postpartum immunization, if needed.

REGULATION OF VACCINES AND ADVISORY BODIES

Vaccines are regulated by national governments. The FDA's Vaccines and Related Biological Products Advisory Committee (VRBPAC) reviews and approves use of vaccines in the United States. Just because a vaccine is licensed by a regulatory agency, however, does not mean that it will automatically be used in practice. Various advisory boards review the feasibility and appropriateness of implementing vaccination, especially universal vaccination.

The ACIP of the CDC provides advice and guidance on effective control of vaccine-preventable diseases in the U.S. civilian population. The ACIP develops written recommendations for routine administration of vaccines to the pediatric and adult populations and suggests details of vaccination schedules in terms of dosage, frequency, and contraindications. ACIP statements are considered official U.S. federal recommendations for the use of vaccines and immune globulins.

The Committee on Infectious Diseases of the AAP publishes the *Red Book*, the official publication of the academy that contains guidelines pertaining to infectious diseases.[128] It is updated every 2 to 3 years; interim policy updates are issued in the academy's journal. The guidelines from these regulatory and advisory bodies occasionally vary from one another for a time, but in general, there is an effort to harmonize recommendations.

References

1. Mold JE, Michaëlsson J, Burt TD, et al: Maternal alloantigens promote the development of tolerogenic fetal regulatory T cells in utero, *Science* 322:1562-1565, 2008.
2. Gitlin D, Kumate J, Urrusti J, et al: The selectivity of the human placenta in the transfer of plasma proteins from mother to fetus, *J Clin Invest* 43:1938-1951, 1964.
3. Adams KM, Nelson JL: Microchimerism: an investigative frontier in autoimmunity and transplantation, *JAMA* 291:1127-1131, 2004.
4. Rayfield LS, Brent L, Rodeck CH: Development of cell-mediated lympholysis in human foetal blood lymphocytes, *Clin Exp Immunol* 42:561-570, 1980.
5. Granberg C, Hirvonen T: Cell-mediated lympholysis by fetal and neonatal lymphocytes in sheep and man, *Cell Immunol* 51:13-22, 1980.
6. Marchant A, Appay V, Van Der Sande M, et al: Mature CD8(+) T lymphocyte response to viral infection during fetal life, *J Clin Invest* 111:1747-1755, 2003.
7. Rastogi D, Wang C, Mao X, et al: Antigen-specific immune responses to influenza vaccine in utero, *J Clin Invest* 117:1637-1646, 2007.
8. Claas FH, Gijbels Y, van der Velden-de Munck J, et al: Induction of B cell unresponsiveness to noninherited maternal HLA antigens during fetal life, *Science* 241:1815-1817, 1988.
9. Tian C, Kron GK, Dischert KM, et al: Low expression of the interleukin (IL)-4 receptor alpha chain and reduced signalling via the IL-4 receptor complex in human neonatal B cells, *Immunology* 119: 54-62, 2006.
10. Weitkamp JH, Lafleur BJ, Greenberg HB, et al: Natural evolution of a human virus-specific antibody gene repertoire by somatic hypermutation requires both hotspot-directed and randomly-directed processes, *Hum Immunol* 66:666-676, 2005.
11. Kallewaard NL, McKinney BA, Gu Y, et al: Functional maturation of the human antibody response to rotavirus, *J Immunol* 180: 3980-3989, 2008.
12. Bowen AL, Tian C, LaFleur BJ, et al: Transcriptional control of activation-induced cytidine deaminase and error-prone DNA polymerases is functionally mature in the B cells of infants at birth, *Hum Immunol* 67:43-46, 2006.
13. Mold JE, Venkatasubrahmanyam S, Burt TD, et al: Fetal and adult hematopoietic stem cells give rise to distinct T cell lineages in humans, *Science* 330:1695-1699, 2010.
14. Shokrollah E, Ertelt JM, Kinder JM, et al: Immunosuppressive CD71+ erythroid cells compromise neonatal host defence against infection, *Nature* 504:158-162, 2013.
15. Siegrist CA: Blame vaccine interference, not neonatal immunization, for suboptimal responses after neonatal diphtheria, tetanus, and acellular pertussis immunization, *J Pediatr* 153:305-307, 2008.
16. Stanfield JP, Gall D, Bracken PM: Single-dose antenatal tetanus immunisation, *Lancet* 1:215-219, 1973.
17. Koenig MA, Roy NC, McElrath T, et al: Duration of protective immunity conferred by maternal tetanus toxoid immunization: further evidence from Matlab, Bangladesh, *AmJ Public Health* 88:903-907, 1998.
18. Englund JA, Mbawuike IN, Hammill H, et al: Maternal immunization with influenza or tetanus toxoid vaccine for passive antibody protection in young infants, *J Infect Dis* 168:647-656, 1993.
19. Murray DL, Imagawa DT, Okada DM, et al: Antibody response to monovalent A/New Jersey/8/76 influenza vaccine in pregnant women, *J Clin Microbiol* 10:184-187, 1979.
20. Sumaya CV, Gibbs RS: Immunization of pregnant women with influenza A/New Jersey/76 virus vaccine: reactogenicity and immunogenicity in mother and infant, *J Infect Dis* 140:141-146, 1979.
21. Deinard AS, Ogburn P Jr: A/NJ/8/76 influenza vaccination program: effects on maternal health and pregnancy outcome, *Am J Obstet Gynecol* 140:240-245, 1981.
22. Heinonen OP, Shapiro S, Monson RR, et al: Immunization during pregnancy against poliomyelitis and influenza in relation to childhood malignancy, *Int J Epidemiol* 2:229-235, 1973.
23. Munoz FM, Piedra PA, Glezen WP: Safety and immunogenicity of respiratory syncytial virus purified fusion protein-2 vaccine in pregnant women, *Vaccine* 21:3465-3467, 2003.
24. United Nations Children's Fund (UNICEF): *Participate, vaccinate, eliminate: together against maternal and newborn tetanus*, Geneva, 2008, UNICEF.
25. Güriş D, Strebel PM, Bardenheier B, et al: Changing epidemiology of pertussis in the United States: increasing reported incidence among adolescents and adults, 1990–1996, *Clin Infect Dis* 28:1230-1237, 1999.
26. Jenkinson D: Duration of effectiveness of pertussis vaccine: evidence from a 10 year community study, *Br Med J (Clin Res Ed)* 296: 612-614, 1988.
27. Wendelboe AM, Van Rie A, Salmaso S, et al: Duration of immunity against pertussis after natural infection or vaccination, *Pediatr Infect Dis J* 24(Suppl 5):S58-S61, 2005.
28. Wearing HJ, Rohani P: Estimating the duration of pertussis immunity using epidemiological signatures, *PLoS Pathog* 5:e1000647, 2009.
29. Zepp F, Heininger U, Mertsola J, et al: Rationale for pertussis booster vaccination throughout life in Europe, *Lancet Infect Dis* 11:557-570, 2011.
30. Bisgard KM, Pascual FB, Ehresmann KR, et al: Infant pertussis: who was the source? *Pediatr Infect Dis J* 23:985-989, 2004.
31. Cohen P, Scadron SJ: The effects of active immunization of the mother upon the offspring, *J Pediatrics* 29:609-619, 1946.

32. Cohen P, Schneck H, Dubow E: Prenatal multiple immunization, *J Pediatr* 38:696-704, 1951.
33. Cortese MM, Baughman AL, Zhang R, et al: Pertussis hospitalizations among infants in the United States, 1993 to 2004, *Pediatr* 121:484-492, 2008.
34. Centers for Disease Control and Prevention: Preventing tetanus, diphtheria, and pertussis among adults: use of tetanus toxoid, reduced diphtheria toxoid and acellular pertussis vaccine: recommendations of ACIP and recommendation of ADIP, supported by the Healthcare Infection Control Practices Advisory Committee (HICPAC), for use of Tdap among health-care personnel, *MMWR Morb Mortal Wkly Rep* 55:1-37, 2006.
35. Neuzil KM, Reed GW, Mitchel EF, et al: Impact of influenza on acute cardiopulmonary hospitalizations in pregnant women, *Am J Epidemiol* 148:1094-1102, 1998.
36. Irving WL, James DK, Stephenson T, et al: Influenza virus infection in the second and third trimesters of pregnancy: a clinical and seroepidemiological study, *BJOG* 107:1282-1289, 2000.
37. Pierce M, Kurinczuk JJ, Spark P, et al: Perinatal outcomes after maternal 2009/H1N1 infection: national cohort study, *BMJ* 342:3214, 2011.
38. Jamieson DJ, Honein MA, Rasmussen SA, et al: Novel Influenza A (H1N1) Pregnancy Working Group. H1N1 2009 influenza virus infection during pregnancy in the USA, *Lancet* 374:451-458, 2009.
39. Mosby LG, Rasmussen SA, Jamieson DJ: 2009 pandemic influenza A (H1N1) in pregnancy: a systematic review of the literature, *Am J Obstet Gynecol* 205:10-18, 2011.
40. Blanchard-Rohner G, Siegrist CA: Vaccination during pregnancy to protect infants against influenza: why and why not? *Vaccine* 29:7542-7550, 2011.
41. Centers for Disease Control and Prevention: Seasonal influenza and 2009 H1N1 influenza vaccination coverage among pregnant women—10 states, 2009-10 influenza season, *MMWR Morb Mortal Wkly Rep* 59:1541-1545, 2010.
42. Reuman PD, Ayoub EM, Small PA: Effect of passive maternal antibody on influenza illness in children: a prospective study of influenza A in mother-infant pairs, *Pediatr Infect Dis J* 6:398-403, 1987.
43. Zaman K, Roy E, Arifeen SE, et al: Effectiveness of maternal influenza immunization in mothers and infants, *N Engl J Med* 359: 1555-1564, 2008.
44. McLellan JS, Chen M, Joyce MG, et al: Structure-based design of a fusion glycoprotein vaccine for respiratory syncytial virus, *Science* 342:592-598, 2013.
45. Correia BE, Bates JT, Loomis RJ, et al: Proof of principle for epitope-focused vaccine design, *Nature* 507:201-206, 2014.
46. Swanson KA, Settembre EC, Shaw CA, et al: Structural basis for immunization with postfusion respiratory syncytial virus fusion F glycoprotein (RSV F) to elicit high neutralizing antibody titers, *Proc Natl Acad Sci U S A* 108:9619-9624, 2011.
47. McLellan JS, Chen M, Leung S, et al: Structure of RSV fusion glycoprotein trimer bound to a prefusion-specific neutralizing antibody, *Science* 340:1113-1117, 2013.
48. Smith G, Raghunandan R, Wu Y, et al: Respiratory syncytial virus fusion glycoprotein expressed in insect cells form protein nanoparticles that induce protective immunity in cotton rats, *PLoS One* 7:e50852, 2012.
49. Glenn GM, Smith G, Fries L, et al: Safety and immunogenicity of a Sf9 insect cell-derived respiratory syncytial virus fusion protein nanoparticle vaccine, *Vaccine* 31:524-532, 2013.
50. Centers for Disease Control and Prevention: Current trends rubella vaccination during pregnancy—United States, 1971-1988, *MMWR Morb Mortal Wkly Rep* 38:289-293, 1989.
51. Advisory Committee on Immunization Practices, Fiore AE, Wasley A, et al: Prevention of hepatitis A through active or passive immunization: recommendations of the Advisory Committee on Immunization Practices (ACIP), *MMWR Recomm Rep* 55(RR-7):1-23, 2006.
52. National Center for Immunization and Respiratory Diseases: General recommendations on immunization—recommendations of the Advisory Committee on Immunization Practices (ACIP), *MMWR Recomm Rep* 60:1-64, 2011.
53. Mast EE, Weinbaum CM, Fiore AE, et al: A comprehensive immunization strategy to eliminate transmission of hepatitis B virus infection in the United States: recommendations of the advisory committee on immunization practices (ACIP) part 1: immunization of infants, children, and adolescents, *MMWR Recomm Rep* 54(RR-16):1-31, 2005. Erratum in *MMWR Morb Mortal Wkly Rep* 55:158-159, 2006; *MMWR Morb Mortal Wkly Rep* 56:1267, 2007.
54. Baker CJ, Rench MA, McInnes P: Immunization of pregnant women with group B streptococcal type III capsular polysaccharide-tetanus toxoid conjugate vaccine, *Vaccine* 21:3468-3472, 2003.
55. U.S. National Institutes of Health: Clinicaltrials.gov. Available at https://clinicaltrials.gov/. 2013 Accessed October 1, 2013.
56. Siber GR, Leszcynski J, Pena-Cruz V, et al: Protective activity of a human respiratory syncytial virus immune globulin prepared from donors screened by microneutralization assay, *J Infect Dis* 165:456-463, 1992.
57. Horowitz B, Wiebe ME, Lippin A, et al: Inactivation of viruses in labile blood derivatives. I. Disruption of lipid-enveloped viruses by tri(*n*-butyl)phosphate detergent combinations, *Transfusion* 25:516-522, 1985.
58. Groothuis JR, Simoes EA, Levin MJ, et al: Prophylactic administration of respiratory syncytial virus immune globulin to high-risk infants and young children, The Respiratory Syncytial Virus Immune Globulin Study Group, *N Engl J Med* 329:1524-1530, 1993.
59. World Health Organization: The PREVENT Study Group: Reduction of respiratory syncytial virus hospitalization among premature infants and infants with bronchopulmonary dysplasia using respiratory syncytial virus immune globulin prophylaxis, *Pediatrics* 99: 93-99, 1997.
60. Groothuis JR: Role of antibody and use of respiratory syncytial virus (RSV) immune globulin to prevent severe RSV disease in high-risk children, *J Pediatr* 124:S28-S32, 1994.
61. Group TI-RS: Palivizumab, a humanized respiratory syncytial virus monoclonal antibody, reduces hospitalization from respiratory syncytial virus infection in high-risk infants, *Pediatrics* 102:531-537, 1998.
62. Abarca K, Jung E, Fernández P, et al: Safety, tolerability, pharmacokinetics, and immunogenicity of motavizumab, a humanized, enhanced-potency monoclonal antibody for the prevention of respiratory syncytial virus infection in at-risk children, *Pediatr Infect Dis J* 28:267-272, 2009.
63. Beasley RP, Hwang LY, Stevens CE, et al: Efficacy of hepatitis B immune globulin for prevention of perinatal transmission of the hepatitis B virus carrier state: final report of a randomized double-blind, placebo-controlled trial, *Hepatology* 3:135-141, 1983.
64. Centers for Disease Control and Prevention: Prevention of varicella: recommendations of the Advisory Committee on Immunization Practices (ACIP), *MMWR Morb Mortal Wkly Rep* 45:1-26, 1996.
65. Brunell PA: Fetal and neonatal varicella-zoster infections, *Semin Perinatol* 7:47-56, 1983.
66. Meyers JD: Congenital varicella in term infants: risk reconsidered, *J Infect Dis* 129:215-217, 1974.
67. Pastuszak AL, Levy M, Schick B, et al: Outcome after maternal varicella infection in the first 20 weeks of pregnancy, *N Engl J Med* 330:901-905, 1994.
68. Miller E, Cradock-Watson JE, Ridehalgh MK: Outcome in newborn babies given anti-varicella-zoster immunoglobulin after perinatal maternal infection with varicella-zoster virus, *Lancet* 2:371-373, 1989.
69. Advisory Committee on Immunization Practices: Updated Recommendations for use of VariZIG—United States, 2013, *MMWR Morb Mortal Wkly Rep* 62:574-576, 2013.
70. Snydman DR, McIver J, Leszczynski J, et al: A pilot trial of a novel cytomegalovirus immune globulin in renal transplant recipients, *Transplantation* 38:553-557, 1984.
71. Revello MG, McIver J, Leszczynski J, et al: A randomized trial of hyperimmune globulin to prevent congenital cytomegalovirus, *N Engl J Med* 370:1316-1326, 2014.
72. Arnon SS, Schechter R, Maslanka SE, et al: Human botulism immune globulin for the treatment of infant botulism, *N Engl J Med* 354:462-471, 2006.
73. Karron RA, Makhene M, Gay K, et al: Evaluation of a live attenuated bovine parainfluenza type 3 vaccine in two- to six-month-old infants, *Pediatr Infect Dis J* 15:650-654, 1996.
74. Haller AA, Miller T, Mitiku M, et al: Expression of the surface glycoproteins of human parainfluenza virus type 3 by bovine parainfluenza virus type 3, a novel attenuated virus vaccine vector, *J Virol* 74:11626-11635, 2000.
75. Schmidt AC, McAuliffe JM, Murphy BR, et al: Recombinant bovine/human parainfluenza virus type 3 (B/HPIV3) expressing the respiratory syncytial virus (RSV) G and F proteins can be used to achieve simultaneous mucosal immunization against RSV and HPIV3, *J Virol* 75:4594-4603, 2001.

76. Friedewald WT, Forsyth BR, Smith CB, et al: Low-temperature-grown RS virus in adult volunteers, *JAMA* 204:690-694, 1968.
77. Wright PF, Belshe RB, Kim HW, et al: Administration of a highly attenuated, live respiratory syncytial virus vaccine to adults and children, *Infect Immun* 37:397-400, 1982.
78. Karron RA, Wright PF, Belshe RB, et al: Identification of a recombinant live attenuated respiratory syncytial virus vaccine candidate that is highly attenuated in infants, *J Infect Dis* 191:1093-1104, 2005.
79. Karron RA, Buonagurio DA, Georgiu AF, et al: Respiratory syncytial virus (RSV) SH and G proteins are not essential for viral replication in vitro: clinical evaluation and molecular characterization of a cold-passaged, attenuated RSV subgroup B mutant, *Proc Natl Acad Sci U S A* 94:13961-13966, 1997.
80. Karron RA, Wright PF, Crowe JE Jr, et al: Evaluation of two live, cold-passaged, temperature-sensitive respiratory syncytial virus vaccines in chimpanzees and in human adults, infants, and children, *J Infect Dis* 176:1428-1436, 1997.
81. Wright PF, Karron RA, Belshe RB, et al: Evaluation of a live, cold-passaged, temperature-sensitive, respiratory syncytial virus vaccine candidate in infancy, *J Infect Dis* 182:1331-1342, 2000.
82. Karron RA, Belshe RB, Wright PF, et al: A live human parainfluenza type 3 virus vaccine is attenuated and immunogenic in young infants, *Pediatr Infect Dis J* 22:394-405, 2003.
83. Belshe RB, Newman FK, Anderson EL, et al: Evaluation of combined live, attenuated respiratory syncytial virus and parainfluenza 3 virus vaccines in infants and young children, *J Infect Dis* 190:2096-2103, 2004.
84. Nathanson N, Langmuir AD: The Cutter incident. Poliomyelitis following formaldehyde-inactivated poliovirus vaccination in the United States during the spring of 1955. II. Relationship of poliomyelitis to Cutter vaccine, *Am J Hyg* 78:29-60, 1963.
85. Kapikian AZ, Mitchell RH, Chanock RM, et al: An epidemiologic study of altered clinical reactivity to respiratory syncytial (RS) virus infection in children previously vaccinated with an inactivated RS virus vaccine, *Am J Epidemiol* 89:405-421, 1969.
86. Kim HW, Canchola JG, Brandt CD, et al: Respiratory syncytial virus disease in infants despite prior administration of antigenic inactivated vaccine, *Am J Epidemiol* 89:422-434, 1969.
87. Gossger N, Snape MD, Yu LM, et al: Immunogenicity and tolerability of recombinant serogroup B meningococcal vaccine administered with or without routine infant vaccinations according to different immunization schedules: a randomized controlled trial, *JAMA* 307:573-582, 2012.
88. Gans HA, Arvin AM, Galinus J, et al: Deficiency of the humoral immune response to measles vaccine in infants immunized at age 6 months, *JAMA* 280:527-532, 1998.
89. World Health Organization Global Advisory Group: Expanded programme on immunization, *Wkly Epidemiol Rec* 65:5-11, 1990.
90. Aaby P, Samb B, Simondon F, et al: Sex-specific differences in mortality after high-titre measles immunization in rural Senegal, *Bull World Health Organ* 72:761-770, 1994.
91. Aaby P, Samb B, Simondon F, et al: Five year follow-up of morbidity and mortality among recipients of high-titre measles vaccines in Senegal, *Vaccine* 14:226-229, 1996.
92. Trunz BB, Fine P, Dye C: Effect of BCG vaccination on childhood tuberculous meningitis and miliary tuberculosis worldwide: a meta-analysis and assessment of cost-effectiveness, *Lancet* 367: 1173-1180, 2006.
93. Rodrigues LC, Diwan VK, Wheeler JG: Protective effect of BCG against tuberculous meningitis and miliary tuberculosis: a meta-analysis, *Int J Epidemiol* 22:1154-1158, 1993.
94. Lotte A, Wasz-Hockert O, Poisson N, et al: Second IUATLD study on complications induced by intradermal BCG-vaccination, *Bull Int Union Tuberc Lung Dis* 63:47-59, 1988.
95. Hesseling AC, Cotton MF, Fordham von Reyn C, et al: Consensus statement on the revised World Health Organization recommendations for BCG vaccination in HIV-infected infants, *Int J Tuberc Lung Dis* 12:1376-1379, 2008.
96. Farizo KM, Cochi SL, Zell ER, et al: Epidemiological features of pertussis in the United States, 1980–1989, *Clin Infect Dis* 14:708-719, 1992.
97. Lavine J, King A, Bjørnstad O: Natural immune boosting in pertussis dynamics and the potential for long-term vaccine failure, *Proc Natl Acad Sci USA* 108:7259-7264, 2011.
98. Jackson DW, Rohani P: Perplexities of pertussis: recent global epidemiological trends and their potential causes, *Epidemiol Infect* 142:672-684, 2013.
99. Halasa NB, O'Shea A, Shi JR, et al: Poor immune responses to a birth dose of diphtheria, tetanus, and acellular pertussis vaccine, *J Pediatr* 153:327-332, 2008.
100. Knuf M, Schmitt HJ, Wolter J, et al: Neonatal vaccination with an acellular pertussis vaccine accelerates the acquisition of pertussis antibodies in infants, *J Pediatr* 152:655-660, 660.e1, 2008.
101. Belloni C, De Silvestri A, Tinelli C, et al: Immunogenicity of a three-component acellular pertussis vaccine administered at birth, *Pediatrics* 111:1042-1045, 2003.
102. Fauveau V, Mamdani M, Steinglass R, et al: Maternal tetanus: magnitude, epidemiology and potential control measures, *Int J Gynaecol Obstet* 40:3-12, 1993.
103. Weibel RE, Neff BJ, Kuter BJ, et al: Live attenuated varicella virus vaccine. Efficacy trial in healthy children, *N Engl J Med* 310:1409-1415, 1984.
104. Takahashi M, Otsuka T, Okuno Y, et al: Live vaccine used to prevent the spread of varicella in children in hospital, *Lancet* 2:1288-1290, 1974.
105. Merck: *I. ProQuad (measles, mumps, rubella, and varicella [Oka/Merck] virus vaccine live) (package insert)*, Whitehouse Station, NJ, 2005, Merck.
106. Siegel M, Fuerst HT, Peress NS: Comparative fetal mortality in maternal virus diseases. A prospective study on rubella, measles, mumps, chicken pox and hepatitis, *N Engl J Med* 274:768-771, 1966.
107. Siegel M: Congenital malformations following chickenpox, measles, mumps, and hepatitis. Results of a cohort study, *JAMA* 226: 1521-1524, 1973.
108. Amexis G, Rubin S, Chizhikov V, et al: Sequence diversity of Jeryl Lynn strain of mumps virus: quantitative mutant analysis for vaccine quality control, *Virology* 300:171-179, 2002.
109. Dayan GH, Quinlisk MP, Parker AA, et al: Recent resurgence of mumps in the United States, *N Engl J Med* 358:1580-1589, 2008.
110. Centers for Disease Control and Prevention: Elimination of rubella and congenital rubella syndrome—United States, 1969-2004, *MMWR Morb Mortal Wkly Rep* 54:279-282, 2005.
111. Wright PF: The use of inactivated influenza vaccine in children, *Semin Pediatr Infect Dis* 17:200-205, 2006.
112. Institute of Medicine: *Immunization safety review: vaccines and autism*, Washington, DC, 2004, National Academies Press.
113. Belshe RB, Mendelman PM, Treanor J, et al: The efficacy of live attenuated, cold-adapted, trivalent, intranasal influenzavirus vaccine in children, *N Engl J Med* 338:1405-1412, 1998.
114. Belshe RB, Gruber WC, Mendelman PM, et al: Efficacy of vaccination with live attenuated, cold-adapted, trivalent, intranasal influenza virus vaccine against a variant (A/Sydney) not contained in the vaccine, *J Pediatr* 136:168-175, 2000.
115. Belshe RB, Edwards KM, Vesikari T, et al: Live attenuated versus inactivated influenza vaccine in infants and young children, *N Engl J Med* 356:685-696, 2007.
116. Black S, Shinefield H, Fireman B, et al: Efficacy, safety and immunogenicity of heptavalent pneumococcal conjugate vaccine in children. Northern California Kaiser Permanente vaccine study center group, *Pediatr Infect Dis J* 19:187-195, 2000.
117. Bishop RF, Barnes GL, Cipriani E, et al: Clinical immunity after neonatal rotavirus infection. A prospective longitudinal study in young children, *N Engl J Med* 309:72-76, 1983.
118. Kapikian AZ, Hoshino Y, Chanock RM, et al: Efficacy of a quadrivalent rhesus rotavirus-based human rotavirus vaccine aimed at preventing severe rotavirus diarrhea in infants and young children, *J Infect Dis* 174(Suppl 1):S65-S72, 1996.
119. Centers for Disease Control and Prevention: Rotavirus vaccine for the prevention of rotavirus gastroenteritis among children. Recommendations of the Advisory Committee on Immunization Practices (ACIP), *MMWR Recomm Rep* 48(RR-2):1-20, 1999.
120. Centers for Disease Control and Prevention: Withdrawal of rotavirus vaccine recommendation, *MMWR Morb Mortal Wkly Rep* 48:1007, 1999.
121. Murphy TV, Gargiullo PM, Massoudi MS, et al: Intussusception among infants given an oral rotavirus vaccine, *N Engl J Med* 344:564-572, 2001.
122. Vesikari T, Karvonen A, Forrest BD, et al: Neonatal administration of rhesus rotavirus tetravalent vaccine, *Pediatr Infect Dis J* 25:118-122, 2006.

123. Heaton PM, Goveia MG, Miller JM, et al: Development of a pentavalent rotavirus vaccine against prevalent serotypes of rotavirus gastroenteritis, *J Infect Dis* 192(Suppl 1):S17-S21, 2005.
124. Vesikari T, Matson DO, Dennehy P, et al: Safety and efficacy of a pentavalent human-bovine (WC3) reassortant rotavirus vaccine, *N Engl J Med* 354:23-33, 2006.
125. Ruiz-Palacios GM, Pérez-Schael I, Velázquez FR, et al: Safety and efficacy of an attenuated vaccine against severe rotavirus gastroenteritis, *N Engl J Med* 354:11-22, 2006.
126. Langkamp DL, Hoshaw-Woodard S, Boye ME, et al: Delays in receipt of immunizations in low-birth-weight children: a nationally representative sample, *Arch Pediatr Adolesc Med* 155:167-172, 2001.
127. Linder N, Vishne TH, Levin E, et al: Hepatitis B vaccination: long-term follow-up of the immune response of preterm infants and comparison of two vaccination protocols, *Infection* 30:136-139, 2002.
128. Pickering LK, Baker CJ, Kimberlin DW, Long SS, editors: *Red book: 2012 report of the Committee on Infectious Diseases*, 29th ed, Elk Grove Village, Ill, 2012, American Academy of Pediatrics.

Index

Note: Page numbers followed by *f* indicate figures, *t* indicate tables, and *b* indicate boxes.

B

C

F

I

N

O

P

Q

R

S

T

U

V

W

Y

Z